Accession no.
36062440

WITHDRAWN

KU-508-381

Reference
Book
Only

WITHDRAWN

WIRRAL EDUCATION CENTRE
LIBRARY
0151 604 7291

CANCER NURSING

THE JONES AND BARTLETT SERIES IN ONCOLOGY

American Cancer Society's Consumer Guide to Cancer Drugs, Wilkes/Ades
American Cancer Society's Patient Education Guide to Oncology Drugs, Wilkes/Ades
Biotherapy: A Comprehensive Overview, Second Edition, Rieger
Blood and Marrow Stem Cell Transplantation, Third Edition, Ezzone
Cancer and HIV Clinical Nutrition Pocket Guide, Second Edition, Wilkes
Cancer Chemotherapy: A Nursing Process Approach, Third Edition, Barton-Burke/Wilkes/Ingwersen
Cancer Chemotherapy Care Plans Handbook, Third Edition, Barton-Burke, et al.
Cancer Nursing, Fourth Edition CD-ROM, Groenwald/Frogge/Goodman/Yarbro
Cancer Nursing: Principles and Practice, Fifth Edition, Yarbro/Frogge/Goodman
A Cancer Source Book for Nurses, Eighth Edition, American Cancer Society
Cancer Symptom Management, Third Edition, Yarbro/Frogge/Goodman
Cancer Symptom Management, Patient Self-Care Guides, Second Edition, Yarbro/Frogge/Goodman
Chemotherapy Care Plans Handbook, Second Edition, Barton-Burke/Wilkes/Ingwersen
A Clinical Guide to Cancer Nursing, Fifth Edition, Yarbro/Frogge/Goodman
A Clinical Guide to Stem Cell and Bone Marrow Transplantation, Shapiro, et al.
Clinical Handbook for Biotherapy, Rieger
Comprehensive Cancer Nursing Review, Fourth Edition, Groenwald/Frogge/Goodman/Yarbro
Contemporary Issues in Breast Cancer, Second Edition, Hassey Dow
Contemporary Issues in Colorectal Cancer, Berg
Contemporary Issues in Lung Cancer, Haas
Contemporary Issues in Lymphoma, Poniatowski, et al.
Contemporary Issues in Prostate Cancer, Second Edition, Held-Warmkessel
Fatigue in Cancer: A Multidimensional Approach, Winningham/Barton-Burke
Handbook of Breast Cancer Risk-Assessment, Vogel/Bevers
Handbook of Oncology Nursing, Third Edition, Johnson/Gross
HIV Homecare Handbook, Daigle
HIV Nursing and Symptom Management, Ropka/Williams
Homecare Management of the Bone Marrow Transplant Patient, Third Edition, Kelley, et al.
Human Embryonic Stem Cells, Kiessling/Anderson
Making the Decision: A Cancer Patient's Guide to Clinical Trials, Mulay
Medication Errors: Cause, Prevention, and Risk Management, Cohen
Memory Bank for Chemotherapy, Third Edition, Preston/Wilfinger
Nursing Care in the Genomic Era, Jenkins/Lea
Oncology Nursing in the Ambulatory Setting, Second Edition, Buchsel/Yarbro
Oncology Nursing Review, Third Edition, Yarbro/Frogge/Goodman
Instruments for Clinical Nursing Research, Third Edition, Frank-Stromborg/Olsen
OncoRN 2005(PDA), Wilkes, et al.
Outcomes in Radiation Therapy, Watkins-Bruner, et al.
Pocket Guide to Breast Cancer, Third Edition, Hassey Dow
Pocket Guide to Breast Cancer Drugs and Treatment, Wilkes
Pocket Guide to Colorectal Cancer, Berg
Pocket Guide to Colorectal Cancer Drugs and Treatment, Wilkes
Pocket Guide to Lung Cancer, Haas
Pocket Guide to Managing Cancer Fatigue, Schwartz
Pocket Guide to Prostate Cancer, Held-Warmkessel
Quality of Life: From Nursing and Patient Perspectives, King/Hinds
2005 Oncology Nursing Drug Handbook, Wilkes, et al.
Women and Cancer: A Gynecologic Oncology Nursing Perspective, Second Edition, Moore-Higgs, et al.

CANCER NURSING

PRINCIPLES AND PRACTICE

SIXTH EDITION

EDITED BY

Connie Henke Yarbro, RN, MS, FAAN
Adjunct Clinical Associate Professor
MU Sinclair School of Nursing
University of Missouri-Columbia
Columbia, MO
Editor, *Seminars in Oncology Nursing*

Margaret Hansen Frogge, RN, MS
Senior Vice President, Riverside Health Care
Kankakee, IL
Associate Faculty
Rush University College of Nursing
Rush University Medical Center
Chicago, IL

Michelle Goodman, RN, MS
Oncology Clinical Nurse Specialist
Rush Cancer Institute
Division of Oncology and Hematology
Assistant Professor of Nursing
Rush University College of Nursing
Rush University Medical Center
Chicago, IL

EDITORIAL CONSULTANTS

Barbara Holmes Gobel, RN, MS, AOCN®
Oncology Clinical Nurse Specialist
Northwestern Memorial Hospital
Adjunct Faculty
Rush University College of Nursing
Rush University Medical Center
Chicago, IL

Debra Wujcik, RN, MSN, AOCN®
Director, Clinical Trials Training and Outreach
Vanderbilt-Ingram Cancer Center
Associate Professor
Vanderbilt School of Nursing
Nashville, TN

0196442Z
LIBRARY
ACC. No. 36062440
DEPT.
CLASS No.
UNIVERSITY OF CHESTER

JONES AND BARTLETT PUBLISHERS
Sudbury, Massachusetts
BOSTON TORONTO LONDON SINGAPORE

World Headquarters
Jones and Bartlett Publishers
40 Tall Pine Drive
Sudbury, MA 01776
978-443-5000
info@jbpub.com
www.jbpub.com

Jones and Bartlett Publishers Canada
6339 Ormindale Way
Mississauga, ON L5V 1J2
CANADA

Jones and Bartlett Publishers International
Barb House, Barb Mews
London W6 7PA
UK

Copyright © 2005 by Jones and Bartlett Publishers, Inc.

Jones and Bartlett's books and products are available through most bookstores and online booksellers. To contact Jones and Bartlett Publishers directly, call 800-832-0034, fax 978-443-8000, or visit our website www.jbpub.com.

Substantial discounts on bulk quantities of Jones and Bartlett's publications are available to corporations, professional associations, and other qualified organizations. For details and specific discount information, contact the special sales department at Jones and Bartlett via the above contact information or send an email to specialsales@jbpub.com.

ISBN-13: 978-0-7637-4720-6
ISBN-10: 0-7637-4720-3

Production Credits
Chief Executive Officer: Clayton Jones
Chief Operating Officer: Don W. Jones, Jr.
President, Jones and Bartlett Higher Education: Robert Holland
V.P., Design and Production: Anne Spencer
V.P., Manufacturing and Inventory Control: Therese Bräuer
Manufacturing and Inventory Coordinator: Amy Bacus
Executive Publisher: Christopher Davis
Editorial Assistant: Kathy Richardson
Production Director: Amy Rose
Production Coordinator: Jenny Bagdigian
Marketing Manager: Emily Ekle
Cover Design: Anne Spencer
Composition: ATLIS Systems, Inc.
Technical Illustrations: Imagineering Art
Printing and Binding: Courier Westford
Cover Printing: Courier Westford

Library of Congress Cataloging-in-Publication Data

Cancer nursing: principles and practice / edited by Connie Henke Yarbro, Michelle Goodman, Margaret Hansen Frogge; editorial consultants, Barbara Holmes Gobel, Debra Wujcik.– 6th ed.
p. ; cm.
Includes bibliographical references and index.
ISBN 0-7637-4720-3 (case-bound)
1. Cancer—Nursing.
[DNLM: 1. Neoplasms—nursing. 2. Oncologic Nursing—methods. WY 156 C2197 2005] I. Yarbro, Connie Henke. II. Goodman, Michelle. III. Frogge, Margaret Hansen.
RC266.C356 2005
616.99′40231—dc22
6048

2005007372

LIBRARY
UNIVERSITY

All rights reserved. No part of the material protected by this copyright notice may be reproduced or utilized in any form, electronic or mechanical, including photocopying, recording, or any information storage or retrieval system, without written permission from the copyright owner.

Printed in the United States of America
10 09 08 07 06 10 9 8 7 6 5 4 3 2

Contents

Part IV Cancer Symptom Management 621

64 Stomach Cancer 1617

Katherine G. O'Connor, RN, MS, ANP, OCN®

65 Testicular Germ Cell Cancer 1630

Eric Zack, RN, APRN, ACNP, AOCN®

66 Vulvar and Vaginal Cancer 1647

Carol Guarnieri, RN, MSN

Part VII Dimensions of Cancer Survivorship 1663

Part VIII End-of-Life and Palliative Care 1727

Part IX Professional Issues for the Cancer Nurse 1757

Preface

We welcome our readers to the Sixth Edition of *Cancer Nursing: Principles and Practice.* The rapid changes and progress in the science of oncology and oncology nursing have necessitated the inclusion of new topics and the extensive revision of many chapters in this edition, which have been updated to include the latest developments in oncology nursing and cancer patient care. Over 42 new authors, all experts in their fields, contributed advanced knowledge and significant up-to-date information to our traditional chapter topics, as well as to the 11 newly designed chapters that we feel will be of profound interest to our readers.

The basic science chapters in Part I have been reorganized and updated to reflect the massive increase in scientific knowledge that has occurred in the past few years, especially as it relates to genes and cancer. The section on Prevention Detection and Diagnosis has new chapters devoted to the Dynamics of Cancer Prevention and the Screening and Detection of Asymptomatic Individuals. The Treatment section has two new additional chapters that cover the important developments of Hematopoietic Therapy and Complementary and Alternative Medicine. Cancer patients face numerous psychological symptoms, and in response to this we have added a chapter on Cancer-related Distress in the section on Cancer Symptom Management. In addition, because millions of patients are cancer survivors we felt it important to expand the section on Dimensions of Cancer Survivorship, to not only address late effects and the various rehabilitation problems, but to also address spiritual responses to cancer and why cancer survivorship is a critical aspect of our care. A new section on End-of-Life and Palliative Care, which includes new chapters on the Principles and Issues of Palliative Care and the Delivery of Comfort Care, has been added to this edition in response to requests from our readers. The section on Professional Issues for the Cancer Nurse includes new chapters on Evidence-Based Nursing Practice and Legal Issues.

Every chapter has been updated with the latest references and research studies, and many include website addresses and resources. As with previous editions, *Cancer Nursing: Principles and Practice* continues to present the most comprehensive information on oncology nursing from leading cancer nursing experts.

The editors would like to pay special tribute to our families, especially John, Jim, and Larry, and our colleagues who supported us through this lengthy, time-consuming process. We would like to thank the editorial staff at Jones and Bartlett Publishers, especially Jenny Bagdigian, whose efforts have made possible the production of the sixth edition. And, most importantly, we would like to extend our gratitude to those authors whose tireless review of the literature, and writing, revising, and updating of chapters have made this book possible. The dedication of these contributors and all involved with this sixth edition contributes to the quality of care provided to patients with cancer.

Connie Henke Yarbro
Margaret Hansen Frogge
Michelle Goodman

Contributors

Lois A. Almadrones, RN, MS, CFNP, MPA (51)
Clinical Nurse Specialist
Memorial Sloan Kettering Cancer Center
New York, NY

Lowell Anderson-Reitz, RN, MS, ANP, AOCN® (20)
BMT Nurse Practitioner
Baylor — Charles A. Sammons Cancer Center
Dallas, TX

Terri S. Armstrong, MS, APRN, BC (33)
Neuro-Oncology Nurse Practitioner
Department of Neuro-Oncology
M.D. Anderson Cancer Center
Assistant Professor School of Nursing
University of Texas — Houston
Houston, TX

Marie Bakitas, ARNP, MS, FAAN (18)
Oncology Nurse Practitioner
Norris Cotton Cancer Center
Dartmouth-Hitchcock Medical Center
Lebanon, NH

Tammy Baltic, RN, MS, AOCN® (18)
Oncology Clinical Nurse Specialist
Stanford University Medical Center
Stanford, CA

Linda A. Battiato, RN, MSN, OCN® (21)
Clinical Research Coordinator
Hoosier Oncology Group
Indianapolis, IN

Susan M. Bauer-Wu, DNSc, RN (2)
Director
Dana-Farber Cancer Institute
Harvard Medical School
Boston, MA

Susan Weiss Behrend, RN, MSN, AOCN® (13)
Clinical Nurse Specialist
Fox Chase Cancer Center
Philadelphia, PA

Karen Belford, RN, MS, AOCN® (47)
Clinical Nurse Specialist
Memorial Sloan Kettering Cancer Center
New York, NY

Catherine J. Bradley, PhD (69)
Associate Professor
Department of Medicine
Michigan State University
East Lansing, MI

Bridget A. Cahill, MS, APN/NP-C (27)
Nurse Practitioner, Gastrointestinal Oncology
Northwestern Medical Faculty Foundation
Chicago, IL

Dorothy A. Calabrese, MSN, RN, CNP (45)
Clinical Nurse Specialist/Nurse Practitioner
Cleveland Clinic Cancer Center
Cleveland, OH

Dawn Camp-Sorrell, RN, MSN, FNP, AOCN® (17)
Oncology Nurse Practitioner
Central Alabama Oncology
Alabaster, AL

Elizabeth D. Carlson, DSN, MPH, RN, NP-C (25)
Postdoctoral Fellow
The University of Texas
M.D. Anderson Cancer Center
Houston, TX

Ellen Carr, RN, MSN, AOCN® (54)
Case Manager, Surgical Oncology
The Rebecca and John Moores University of San Diego Cancer Center
San Diego, CA

Dianne D. Chapman, ND, RN, ANCP (46)
Nurse Coordinator, Comprehensive Breast Center and RISC Program
Rush Cancer Institute
Rush University Medical Center
Chicago, IL

Marlene Zichi Cohen, RN, PhD, FAAN (25)
John S. Dunn, Sr., Distinguished Professor in Oncology Nursing
The University of Texas Health Science Center at Houston School of Nursing
Houston, TX

JoAnn Coleman, RN, MS, ACNP, AOCN® (53, 61)
Acute Care Nurse Practitioner, Surgical Oncology
Johns Hopkins Hospital
Baltimore, MD

Diane G. Cope, PhD, ARNP, BC, AOCN® (34)
Nurse Practitioner
Florida Cancer Specialists
Fort Myers, FL

Patrick J. Coyne, MSN, APRN, FAAN (26)
Clinical Nurse Specialist
Virginia Commonwealth University
Richmond, VA

Regina S. Cunningham, PhD, RN, AOCN® (31)
Director Ambulatory Services
Chief Nursing Officer, The Cancer Institute of New Jersey
Assistant Professor Family Medicine
Research Division, Robert Wood Johnson Medical School
New Brunswick, NJ

Georgia M. Decker, MS, RN, CS-ANP, AOCN®, CN® (24)
Advanced Practice Nurse, Integrative Care
The Braverman-Panza Medical Group
Albany, NY

Karen Hassey Dow, PhD, RN, FAAN (67)
Professor
The University of Central Florida
Orlando, FL

Heidi E. Ehrenberger, PhD, RN, AOCN® (76)
Nurse Consultant
University of Maryland School of Nursing
Baltimore, MD

Peg Esper, MSN, RN, CS, AOCN® (71)
Nurse Practitioner
University of Michigan Comprehensive Cancer Center
Ann Arbor, MI

Carol Estwing Ferrans, PhD, RN, FAAN (9)
Professor
University of Illinois at Chicago
College of Nursing
Chicago, IL

Anne Marie Flaherty, MSN, RN, AOCN® (39)
Advanced Practice Nurse
Memorial Sloan-Kettering Cancer Center
New York, NY

Margaret Hansen Frogge, RN, MSN
Senior Vice President
Riverside Health Care
Kankakee, IL
Associate Faculty
Rush University College of Nursing
Rush University Medical Center
Chicago, IL

Mei R. Fu, PhD, RN, CNS (30)
Assistant Professor
New York University
Division of Nursing
New York, NY

Laura E. Gallagher, MSN, RN, CNS (43)
Clinical Nurse Specialist for Emergency Services
Division of Critical Care and Emergency Services
Medical University of South Carolina
Charleston, SC

Theresa W. Gillespie, PhD, RN (11)
Assistant Professor
Department of Surgery
Emory University School of Medicine
Atlanta, GA

Barbara A. Given, RN, PhD, FAAN (69)
University Distinguished Professor
College of Nursing
Michigan State University
East Lansing, MI

Charles W. Given, PhD (69)
Professor
Department of Family Practice
College of Human Medicine
Michigan State University
East Lansing, MI

Barbara Holmes Gobel, RN, MS, AOCN® (23, 29, 37)
Oncology Clinical Nurse Specialist
Northwestern Memorial Hospital
Adjunct Faculty
Rush University College of Nursing
Rush University Medical Center
Chicago, IL

Elizabeth G. Gomez, RN, MSN, AOCN® (76)
Director, Oncology Program
Putnam Hospital Center
Carmel, NY

Michelle Goodman, RN, MS (50)
Oncology Clinical Nurse Specialist
Rush Cancer Institute
Division of Oncology and Hematology
Assistant Professor of Nursing
Rush University College of Nursing
Rush University Medical Center
Chicago, IL

Tracy K. Gosselin-Acomb, RN, MSN, AOCN® (12)
Clinical Operations Director
Duke University Health System
Clinical Associate
Duke University School of Nursing
Durham, NC

Nina N. Grenon, MS, APRN-BC, CCRN, AOCN® (56)
Adult/Geriatric Nurse Practitioner
Dana Farber Cancer Institute
Center for Gastrointestinal Oncology
Boston, MA

Carol Guarnieri, RN, MSN (66)
Instructor
Assumption University
Bangkok, Thailand

Beth Kelly Hayden, RN, BSN, MBA (16)
Director of Nursing
Division of Hematology and Oncology
Rush University Medical Center
Chicago, IL

Pamela J. Haylock, RN, MA (77)
Doctoral Student
University of Texas School of Nursing
Galveston, TX

Jeanne Held-Warmkessel MSN, RN, AOCN®, APRN-BC (62)
Clinical Nurse Specialist
Fox Chase Cancer Center
Philadelphia, PA

Wendy Hobbie, MSN, CRNP (68)
Coordinator, Cancer Survivorship Program
Children's Hospital of Philadelphia
Associate Program Director
Pediatric Oncology Program
School of Nursing
University of Pennsylvania
Philadelphia, PA

Maureen B. Huhmann, MS, RD (31)
Nutritionist
University of Medicine and Dentistry of New Jersey
The Cancer Institute of New Jersey
Brunswick, NJ

Joanne K. Itano, RN, PhD, OCN® (4)
Associate Professor
Department of Nursing
University of Hawaii
Kailua, HI

Linda A. Jacobs, PhD, RN (68)
Program Coordinator
University of Pennsylvania
Abramson Cancer Center
Philadelphia, PA

Roberta Kaplow, RN, PhD, CCNS, CCRN (36)
Professor (Clinical)
Nell Hodgson Woodruff School of Nursing
Emory University
Atlanta, GA

Sharon Kozachik, RN, MSN (69)
Doctoral Candidate
Johns Hopkins University, School of Nursing
Baltimore, MD

AnnMarie K. McDonnell Keenan MS, RN/APN, AOCN® (32, 41)
Assistant Professor/Clinical Nurse Specialist, Adult Oncology
Rush University Medical Center
Chicago, IL

Carol S. Knop, RN, MS, AOCN® (57)
Clinical Educator
GlaxoSmithKline
Philadelphia, PA

Linda U. Krebs, RN, PhD, AOCN® (35)
Assistant Professor
University of Colorado School of Nursing
Denver, CO

Dale Halsey Lea, MPH, RN, APNG, CGC, FAAN (22)
Assistant Director, Genetics Program
Southern Maine Genetics Services
Foundation for Blood Research
Scarborough, ME

Colleen Lee, CDR, RN, MS, AOCN® (24)
Practice Assessment Program Manager
Office of Cancer Complementary and Alternative Medicine
National Cancer Institute
Rockville, MD

Victoria W. Loerzel, MSN, RN, OCN® (67)
Instructor, Project Director
Quality of Life Study
The University of Central Florida
Orlando, FL

Lois J. Loescher, PhD, RN, FAAN (1)
Assistant Professor
University of Arizona College of Nursing and Arizona Cancer Center
Tucson, AZ

Jean Lydon, RN, MS, AOCN® (42)
Program Manager of Oncology Services
Elmhurst Memorial Hospital
Elmhurst, IL

Karen E. Maher, RN, MS, ANP, AOCN® (14)
Nurse Practitioner, Radiation Oncology
Legacy Good Samaritan Hospital
Portland, OR

Suzanne M. Mahon, RN, DNSc, AOCN®, APNG (6)
Associate Clinical Professor
Division of Hematology/Oncology
Saint Louis University School of Nursing
St. Louis, MO

Alecia Malin, DrPH, CHES (3)
Assistant Professor
Meharry Medical College, Department of Surgery
Assistant Professor, secondary appointment
Vanderbilt University, Internal Medicine
Nashville, TN

Sharon D. Manson, RN, MS, ACNP (58)
Nurse Manager, Acute Care Nurse Practitioner
Rush University Medical Center
Chicago, IL

Virginia R. Martin, RN, MSN, AOCN® (60)
Ambulatory Care Clinical Director
Fox Chase Cancer Center
Philadelphia, PA

Mary S. McCabe, RN, MA (10)
Director, Survivorship Program
Memorial Sloan-Kettering Cancer Center
New York, NY

Roxanne W. McDaniel, PhD, RN (30)
Associate Dean of Undergraduate and Master's Programs
University of Missouri–Columbia
MU Sinclair School of Nursing
Columbia, MO

Deborah B. McGuire, PhD, RN, FAAN (26)
Professor and Coordinator, Oncology Specialty
Department of Organizational Systems and Adult Health
University of Maryland School of Nursing
Baltimore, MD

Carrie J. Merkle, PhD, RN, FAAN (1)
Associate Professor, Mursing
College of Nursing, The University of Arizona
Southern Arizona V.A. Health Care System
Tucson, AZ

Ida Marie (Ki) Moore, RN, DNS, FAAN (68)
Professor and Director
Division of Nursing Practice
College of Nursing
The University of Arizona
Tucson, AZ

Susan Moore, RN, MSN, ANP, AOCN® (38, 40, 46, 73)
Oncology Nurse Practitioner
Rush University Medical Center
Chicago, IL

Judith Kehs Much, CRNP, AOCN®, APRN-BC (7)
Oncology Nurse Practitioner
Integrated Oncology Care
Lehigh Valley Hospital and Health Network
Allentown, PA

Katherine G. O'Connor, RN, MS, ANP, OCN® (64)
Nurse Practitioner, Medical Oncology
Memorial Sloan-Kettering Cancer Center
New York, NY

Kathleen Farley Omerod, RN, MS, AOCN® (8)
Joint Practice Nurse Manager
Medical Oncology Outpatient Clinic
Division of Hematology Oncology
Rush University Medical Center
Chicago, IL

James C. Pace, DSN, RN, Mdiv, ANP-CS (43)
Professor of Nursing and Coordinator, Adult Nurse Practitioner Palliative Care Focus
Vanderbilt University Medical Center
Nashville, TN

Rose Mary Padberg, RN, MA (5)
Nurse Consultant
National Cancer Institute
Rockville, MD

Judith A. Paice, PhD, RN, FAAN (72)
Director Cancer Pain Program
Division of Hematology-Oncology
Northwestern University
Feinberg School of Medicine
Chicago, IL

Carlene Porter, RN, MS, ACNP (58)
Acute Care Nurse Practitioner
Rush University Medical Center
Chicago, IL

Janice Post-White, RN, PhD, FAAN (2)
Adjunct Associate Professor
University of Minnesota
Minneapolis, MN

Anita M. Reedy, RN, MSN, OCN® (52)
Nurse Manager, Hematologic Malignancies
Johns Hopkins Hospital
Baltimore, MD

Verna A. Rhodes, EdS, RN, FAAN (30)
Associate Professor Emeritus
Sinclair School of Nursing
University of Missouri–Columbia
Columbia, MO

Paula T. Rieger, RN, MSN, CS, AOCN®, FAAN (7)
Director, International Affairs
American Society of Clinical Oncology
Alexandria, VA

Dana N. Rutledge, PhD, RN (74)
Associate Professor
California State University
Fullerton, CA

Lisa Schulmeister, RN, MN, CS, OCN® (75)
Oncology Nursing Consultant
New Orleans, LA

Brenda K. Shelton, MS, RN, CCRN, AOCN® (28)
Clinical Nurse Specialist
The Sidney Kimmel Comprehensive Cancer Center at Johns Hopkins
Baltimore, MD

Judith J. Smith, MSN, RN, AOCN® (5)
Clinical Trials Nurse Specialist
U.S. Department of Health and Human Services
National Institute of Health, National Cancer Institute
Division of Cancer Prevention
Lung and Upper Aerodigestive Cancer Research Group
Bethesda, MD

M. Jayne Kennedy Sumner, RN, BA, PCRM (44)
Orthopaedic Oncology
University of Florida Shands Hospital
Gainesville, FL

Joseph D. Tariman, RN, MN, APRN-BC, OCN® (59)
Certified Nurse Practitioner
Multiple Myeloma Program
Northwestern University Faculty Foundation
Chicago, IL

Elizabeth Johnston Taylor, RN, PhD (70)
Associate Professor
School of Nursing
Loma Linda University
Loma Linda, CA

Susan Vogt Temple, RN, MSN, AOCN® (48)
Senior Clinical Educator
GlaxoSmithKline Oncology
Philadelphia, PA

Peter V. Tortorice, Pharm.D., B.C.O.P. (15)
Senior Manager, Pharmaceutical Services
U.S. Oncology
Schaumburg, IL

Nancy D. Tsottles, RN, BSN (52)
Research Nurse/Program Coordinator
Greater Baltimore Chapter of Oncology Nursing Society
Baltimore, MD

Ashby C. Watson, APRN, BC, OCN® (26)
Psychosocial Oncology Clinical Nurse Specialist
Massey Cancer Center
Virginia Commonwealth University Medical Center
Richmond, VA

Rita Wickham, PhD, RN, AOCN® (32, 50)
Associate Professor
Rush University College of Nursing
Rush University Medical Center
Chicago, IL

Gail M. Wilkes, RNC, MS, ANP, AOCN® (49)
Oncology Nurse Practitioner and Clinical Instructor
Boston Medical Center
Boston, MA

Laura S. Wood, RN, MSN, OCN® (45)
Renal Cancer Research Program Coordinator
Cleveland Clinic Cancer Center
Cleveland, OH

Debra Wujcik, RN, MSN, AOCN® (19)
Director, Clinical Trial Training and Outreach
Vanderbilt-Ingram Cancer Center
Vanderbilt School of Nursing
Nashville, TN

Susan Germann Yackzan, RN, MSN, AOCN® (63)
Oncology Clinical Nurse Specialist
Central Baptist Hospital
Lexington, KY

Connie Henke Yarbro, RN, MS, FAAN
Editor, *Seminars in Oncology Nursing*
Adjunct Clinical Associate Professor
MU Sinclair School of Nursing
University of Missouri–Columbia
Columbia, MO

Katherine A. Yeager, MS, RN (26)
Research Project Coordinator
Rollins School of Public Health
Emory University
Atlanta, GA

Eric Zack, RN, APRN, ACNP, AOCN® (65)
Charge Nurse
Bone Marrow Transplant Center
Rush University Medical Center
Chicago, IL

PART I

The Cancer Problem

CHAPTER 1

Biology of Cancer

Carrie J. Merkle, PhD, RN, FAAN
Lois J. Loescher, PhD, RN

Introduction

In his now classic writings on the origin of cancer, Sir Richard Doll[1] proposed three potential causative factors underlying tumor development: (1) environmental factors, particularly diet, industrial pollution, and viruses; (2) systemic factors, including breakdowns in immunosurveillance; and (3) genetic factors, such as the degree of susceptibility to cancer. Since Doll's publications in the late 1970s, the biology underlying these proposed causative factors — which were derived largely from epidemiologic studies — has been carefully scrutinized to determine the causes of cancer at the biochemical, cellular, and molecular levels. Because of the intensity of biological research and the rapidity with which findings have become available, we now know that cancer is a disease resulting from the interaction of multiple factors at the cellular, genetic, immunologic, and environmental levels.

A fundamental goal of cancer research is to discern mechanisms of cancer cell development, ways that cancers grow and spread, and, finally, the means to correct abnormal mechanisms and eradicate or control cancer cell populations. This chapter reviews theories and models of tumor development, properties of cancer and transformed cells, genetic influences on cancer, the cell cycle, apoptosis, and metastasis.

Theories and Research Models of Tumor Development

Several theories have been proposed that contain elements along the continuum from tumorigenesis to metastasis. Many of these theories share similar information. Nevertheless, complete explanation of how tumors develop remains an enigma. Table 1-1 lists some of the leading theories of tumorigenesis and their key points.[2–4] These theories, at the very least, should include explanations of (1) the lack of contact inhibition in cancer cells, (2) the inability of cancer cells to differentiate, (3) cancer cells appearing to derive from a single cell, and (4) tumor cells acquiring multiple genotypic and phenotypic changes during the process of carcinogenesis.[2]

Theory of Clonal Evolution

A prevailing paradigm in tumorigenesis is that the first major step consists of a normal cell becoming "immortalized" and subsequently transformed into a neoplastic cell.[2] Nowell's theory of clonal evolution specifies that all cells within a particular tumor must have the same genetic makeup; that homogeneity is necessary or any one gene could not be identified.[5] Even though a carcinogen may affect a large number of cells, the resultant tumor usually represents the progeny of only a single cell or very few cells (Figure 1-1).[6] Initiation of clonal evolution may involve a stem cell that is already dividing. In mitosis, however, the proportion of daughter cells increases, rather than proceeding to differentiation. Uncontrolled proliferation may be accompanied by morphological and biochemical changes or altered gene expression in early cancer cells. Eventually, proliferation may increase and show further evidence of escape from growth-control mechanisms.

Nowell suggests that biological events in tumor progression represent effects of acquired genetic instability.[5] Each new mutation bearing a causal role would be selected for expansion if it is associated with a growth advantage.[7] Similarly, clonal expansion of partially altered cells can substantially increase the population of cells that have acquired some of the mutations critical for tumor development. This situation increases the probability that one of these cells will acquire the remaining mutations needed for neoplastic transformation.[3]

Research Models of Tumor Development

Cell culture models

Cell culture models permit investigation of cancer development at the cellular level. These models consist of cells that were obtained as primary samples of normal and cancerous tissues from humans and other animals, then serially propagated in culture. Culturing cells requires very specific conditions, including defined growth media (usually with serum that contains growth factors), sterility, limited pH range, and optimal temperature. Compared with many animal models and human studies, cell culture models provide greater uniformity of the cell population, offer a higher degree of experimental control and manipulation, and are less costly.

Most normal cells proliferate for a particular number of mitotic divisions (the Hayflick limit), then attain replicative senescence.[8,9] Cancer cells, in contrast, typically acquire immortality and demonstrate an unlimited replicative life span. Normal cells growing in culture will sometimes spontaneously attain immortality. Furthermore, adding chemical or physical carcinogens, biological agents such as viruses, and genetic manipulation sometimes can transform normal cells into an immortal population, with or without other characteristics of tumor cells.

Table 1-1 Key Points of Major Theories of Tumorigenesis

Theory	Key Points
Multistep	Initiation: • Stem cell becomes initiated by acquiring one or more mutations, leading to partial escape from normal homeostatic control • Genetic mutations or epigenetic events responsible • Irreversible Promotion: • Initiated cell stimulated to proliferate but not terminally differentiate • Initiated cell acquires further genetic changes required for neoplasias • Interruptible and sometimes reversible Progression: • Malignant conversion of cell • Confers autonomous growth of initiated cell • Irreversible
Mutagenic versus epigenetic	Mutagenesis: • Results in qualitative or quantitative alteration of genetic information • Chronic insults produce two to three mutations in individual cells within particular tissues • These mutations initiate tumors Epigenetic process: • Chronic insults repeatedly injure and transiently excite many cells in particular tissues • These insults alter expression of genetic information at the transcriptional, translational, or posttranslational levels • Mutations are secondary events
Nature versus nurture	Mutagens found in the environment (nurture) must interact with DNA (germ or somatic cell) to induce mutations in genes affecting cancer processes directly (e.g., oncogenes/tumor suppressor genes) or indirectly (e.g., DNA repair genes, growth factors)
Oncogene and tumor suppressor gene	Oncogenes: Do not contact inhibit; do not terminally differentiate or undergo apoptosis Tumor suppressor genes: When mutated, do not stop unregulated cell growth, induce differentiation, or undergo apoptosis
Stem cell versus de-differentiation	Stem cell: • Pluripotent stem cells restricted to allow a finite number of cell divisions to only the specific lineage of cell types within the organs that arise from the stem cells • Daughter (progenitor) cells of these pluripotent stem cells would give rise to terminally differentiated cells of that lineage De-differentiation: Some progenitor cells could revert back to a pluripotent cell

Data from Trosko, Ruch[2], Moolgavkar, Luebeck[3], Jaffe[4]

Transformed cells may or not be tumorigenic, but they attain properties and characteristics that are typical of cancer cells (Table 1-2). One such property is loss of contact inhibition. When normal epithelial cells grow in culture, the cells often form a continuous single layer on a plastic surface, stopping at the boundaries of the chamber; at that point the population stabilizes and cell loss approximates cell growth. In contrast, tumor cells and some transformed cells will grow in multiple layers or clusters, reaching higher densities in culture, thus losing density-dependent contact inhibition. Another characteristic of tumor cells is anchorage independence. Normal epithelial cells will not remain viable if they become detached from the basement membrane or other substrate. Detached cancer cells, however, continue to thrive. Of course, the ultimate test for tumorigenicity is to inject the cells into compatible animals, immunosuppressed animals, to see whether tumors form.

Cancer, immortalized nontumor, and nonimmortal cell lines provide opportunities for investigation of many cellular processes and behavior. Nevertheless, extrapolation from cell culture to cells in vivo may be inaccurate or incomplete.

Animal models

Animal models have made immense contributions to both the understanding of the biology of cancer and the development of cancer treatment strategies. Conventional mouse models include inbred strains, transgenic mice, and conventional knockouts.[10] Inbred strains require multiple generations of sibling matings to develop mice that are suspectible to spontaneous or carcinogen-induced cancers. The *BALB/c* mouse, which develops plasmacytomas in response to the hydrocarbon pristane, is an example of an inbred strain.

Transgenic mice bear oncogenes, whereas and "knockout" mice are missing or carrying inactive specific tumor suppressor genes. For the past two decades, these mouse models have proved instrumental for developing many cancer-prone strains and elucidating the roles of certain genes and specific gene mutations in tumorigenesis.[10]

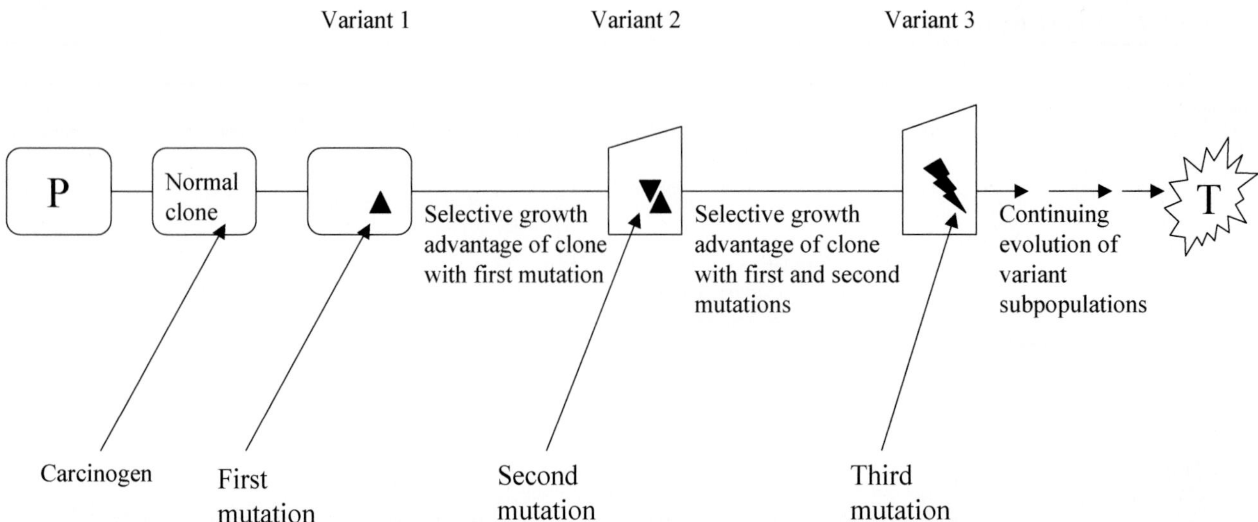

Figure 1-1. Clonal evolution in cancer. Specific generic alterations in evolving tumors may range from gene mutations to major chromosomal aberrations. This figure illustrates a carcinogen-induced genetic change in a progenitor normal cell (P), which produces a cell with selective growth advantage allowing clonal expansion to begin. In this case, gene mutations produce variant cells. Because they are at a disadvantage metabolically or immunologically, most variant cells are nonviable. If one variant has a selective advantage, its progeny become the predominant subpopulation until another variant appears. The sequential selection of variant subpopulations in each tumor (T) differs because of genetic instability, which positively or negatively affects cell proliferation. (Data from Nowell,[5] and Strachan, Read.[6])

Transgenic mice are derived from cells whoses genomes have been modified by the addition of exogenous, or foreign, DNA. This DNA can comprise a manipulated sequence from the same species or from another species that has some property desirable in a particular experiment. The operational gene in the exogenous DNA is called a transgene. In studies of cancer, transgenes are typically injected into cells. The foreign DNA becomes integrated into the cells randomly, without preference for a particular chromosomal location. Three weeks after birth, the offspring are tested for presence of the transgene.

Using transgenic adult mice offers many benefits in the study of cancer biology. Most important, this process allows the embryonic stem cells to be manipulated in vitro prior to injection into the embryo. Scientists then can produce mice with mutations in specific genes or replace a mutant gene with a wild-type (normal) gene.

Mouse models also can be problematic. Certain germ-line mutations can cause death during mouse embryonic stages, termed *embryonic lethality*. In addition, mutations are present in all mouse cells, not just the tissue of interest, thereby predisposing the animals to many different types of cancers that are not of interest to the particular study. These problems limit the study of sporadic cancers, which are believed to result from mutations in single cells.

Second-generation transgenic mouse models exhibit conditional gene-mutation strategies. In the commonly used *Cre/loxP* recombinase system, a tumor suppressor gene may be flanked by recombinase recognition *loxP* sites (the allele is said to be "floxed"), then the *Cre* recombinase is introduced by interbreeding with transgenic mice that have tissue-specific or drug-induced *Cre*. These models avoid embryonic lethality problems and can more closely mimic the time course and tissue specificity of sporadic cancers.[10] Second-generation transgenic mice permit scientists to address higher-order questions, such as "How does angiogenesis contribute to breast cancer development and progression?"[11] Conditional mouse models — along with improved fluorescence and bioluminescence imaging mechanisms that monitor tumor development, growth, and metastasis in living mice — help address complex questions in tumor biology.

Nevertheless, differences between mice and humans exist beyond the obvious phenotypic differences. For example, mouse cells have high levels of telomerase, which confer differences in the process of aging. Future models need to more closely mimic cancer development, progression, and drug actions in humans.

Properties of Cancer and Transformed Cells

Cancer cells are more autonomous than normal cells and are independent of growth-control pathways and

Table 1-2 Properties of Cancer and Transformed Cells

Property	Characteristics of Cancer and Transformed Cells	Explanation
Cytological changes	Increased size and number of nucleoli	• Reflects greater activity of tumor cells.
	Increased nuclear/cytoplasmic ratio	• Larger nucleus reflects more activity, more genetic information.
	Altered cytoskeleton	• Changes contribute to increased motility and variable sizes and shapes (pleomorphism).
Altered cell growth	Immortality	• Normal cells senesce (remain viable but do not divide). • During a crisis, cells mutate, proliferate indefinitely, become "immortal." • Telomeres (DNA segments at the ends of chromosomes) limit the number of cell doublings. Telomeres shorten with each chromosomal replication until reaching a threshold at which cells senesce. Telomere stability is critical for cancer progression. Many cancer cells contain telomerase, an enzyme that prevents telomere shortening and enables the cell to replicate indefinitely.[13]
	Decreased density-dependent growth inhibition (loss of contact inhibition)	• Normal cells stop growing when they contact other cells; crowding from contact compromises access to nutrients. • Transformed cells do not respond to physical contact with and chemical signals from neighboring cells, thereby continue to grow beyond normal limits. • Loss of contact inhibition may result from a faulty restriction point. (See text.)
	Decreased requirement for serum	• Serum normally provides growth factors necessary for cell development and survival. • Typically, the growth factor binds to a receptor on the cell surface, which in turn activates the intracytoplasmic portion of the receptor to send a message to the nucleus (signal transduction), where an effect on gene function occurs. Sometimes, an abnormal growth factor receptor on the surface of a cancer or transformed cell can activate the signal pathway spontaneously without exposure to a growth factor. • Cancer and transformed cell lines may grow in media without serum, suggesting that they can synthesize and secrete their own growth factors (autocrine stimulation).
	Loss of anchorage-dependent growth	• Cells require a substrate to grow. Transformed cells do not require a solid substrate. • Only tumor cells grow in soft agar (no anchorage); cell growth in soft agar is highly correlated with tumorigenicity.
	Loss of cell-cycle control	• Cell does not progress normally through cell-cycle pathways and checkpoints. (See text.)
	Reduced apoptosis	• Cancer cells are less susceptible to programmed death. (See text.)
Changes in cell membrane	New surface antigens	• Cancer and transformed cells exhibit new molecules on the surface. • Viruses can transform and alter multiple cell-surface antigens.
	New or altered glycoproteins (proteins complexed with polysaccharides)	• Transformed cells usually have profound changes in cell-surface glycoproteins. • Some changes may alter cell–cell and cell–matrix adhesion. • Mechanism by which polysaccharides are made and attached to proteins is deranged in transformed cells.
	New or altered glycolipids	• Content and complexity of glycolipids are reduced in transformed cell membranes. • Glycosphingolipid interacts with receptor proteins on the surface of normal cells to inhibit their responsiveness to growth factors.[14] • Transformed cells have less and/or altered glycosphingolipids on their cell surfaces, increasing their responsiveness to growth factors. Glycosphingolipids also serve as components of surface markers involved in cell–cell recognition.[15]

regulatory mechanisms. Cancer cells are also less differentiated than cells of the tissue of origin and behave more like embryonic cells, which also proliferate rapidly. Despite the importance of loss of differentiation in cancer, little is known about the genetic mechanisms and biochemical pathways involved in this phenomenon.[12]

Some cancer cells are so poorly differentiated (or anaplastic) that the tissue of origin cannot be determined. Normal cells may gradually become malignant, passing through the stages of metaplasia (the presence of a cell that appears mildly less differentiated), dysplasia (deranged cell growth with variable shape, size, and appearance), carcinoma in situ, and finally invasive cancer.[13] Cancer cells and other transformed cells may exhibit a variety of changes in cytology, cell growth patterns, and the cell membrane[14,15] (Table 1-2).

The microenvironment of cancer cells plays an important role in determining their properties.[16] The microenvironment consists of many cell types, the extracellular matrix (ECM), and the chemical milieu. The microenvironment includes tumor-associated macrophages, fibroblasts, vascular endothelial growth factor (VEGF), a mixture of cytokines,[17] the composition of the extracellular matrix, and various enzymes including specific matrix metalloproteinases (MMPs)[18–20] and urokinase plasminogen activator (uPA).

Genetic Influences Associated with Cancer

Mutations

A mutation is an alteration in a DNA nucleotide sequence — the order of the four bases adenine (A), cytosine (C), thymine (T), and guanine (G). Mutations can alter both the sequence of a gene and its regulatory sites.

Germ-line mutations in genes that predispose the organisim to cancers represent the strongest risk factors for these diseases.[21] Such mutations affect genes in the ova and sperm. During meiosis, each germ cell carries one of the two copies of mutated genes present in somatic cells, resulting in a 50% chance of a child inheriting a mutated gene copy from a parent. Such mutations are transmitted from generation to generation.

Mutation rate and cancer

Differing schools of thought exist regarding mutation rates and cancer. The historical view is that a raised mutation rate constitutes the most important factor in tumorigenesis.[22] For example, in humans, mutations occur at a rate of 1 in 1 million genes per cell generation. Because it takes as many as six independent mutations in specific genes to give rise to a tumor cell, the likelihood of a tumor developing is low, though everyone has cells with mutations in at least one gene.[6] The perplexing question is this: How can a normal cell accumulate all of these mutations? Increased mutation rates may be more critical in the rarer cancer predisposition syndromes and in cells with reduced DNA repair capability. These cells can have a mutation rate 1000-fold higher than that in cells with intact DNA repair mechanisms.[23,24]

A more recent view suggests that a higher mutation rate may accelerate tumorigenesis, but is not necessary for it to occur.[24] The presence of cancer-causing mutations accounted for by natural selection may be more important than the mutation rate.[24,25] Natural selection acts directly to increase the frequency of advantageous alleles (alternate forms of genes) in the population.[24] Proponents of this view argue that given clonal expansion and the fact that the rate of cell turnover probably exceeds the rate of tumor growth, raised mutation rates explain neither tumorigenesis nor the number of mutations observed in cancers.[24]

Causes of mutations

Mutations may arise spontaneously during DNA replication and recombination, or they may be caused by exogenous agents (environmental mutagens giving rise to mutations) or endogenous agents. DNA replication is a complex process resulting in the formation of DNA daughter strands with identical base pairing to the parent strand (i.e., replication of the genome). DNA replication errors are rare. More frequently, DNA rearranges itself by *recombination*, a process whereby DNA is either lost or inserted into the gene. Recombination may result in loss of control of gene expression or disrupt the coding sequence of the gene.

Exogenous agents may be environmental pollutants, pharmacological compounds, human-made chemicals (e.g., pesticides, organic chemicals, alkylating agents), or chemicals from lifestyle agents (e.g., tobacco smoke). These exposures damage DNA by directly binding to, or acting upon, the DNA molecules. Endogenous agents include reactive oxygen species and other free radicals resulting from normal cellular metabolism, exposure to ultraviolet radiation (UVR), and exposure to ionizing radiation. Exposure to these agents results in damaged DNA bases, thereby impairing transcription to RNA and replication.[26]

Types of mutations

Mutations commonly associated with cancer predisposition include point mutations, insertion and deletion mutations, and mutations affecting DNA repair mechanisms.

Point mutations. The substitution of a single base with another base is termed a point mutation. Point mutations are the most common types of mutations. Point mutations that occur in DNA sequences encoding proteins are further classified as silent, missense, or nonsense mutations.

A *silent point mutation* is a base substitution in the third position of a codon (a section of three DNA nucleotides that codes for an amino acid), in which the amino acid does not change. In other words, the protein product of the gene is not altered. In this regard, silent mutations may be considered "single nucleotide polymorphisms (SNPs)"; they are described in further detail later in this chapter.

Sometimes a base substitution results in generation of a codon that specifies a different amino acid, meaning that an amino acid is changed in the sequence of the gene product. This change is termed a *missense point mutation.* Such a mutation may or may not result in a deleterious gene product, depending on the amino acid that has been substituted. If the structure and properties of the normal and substituted amino acids are similar, no deleterious gene products will result. If the structure and properties of the two amino acids differ, however, a deleterious gene product may result.

A *nonsense point mutation* occurs when a base substitution results in the generation of a stop codon, meaning that the gene product will be truncated and probably nonfunctional. Nonsense point mutations are deleterious mutations.

Deletions and insertions. Deletions or insertions occur when one or more base pairs are removed from or added to the DNA. This process may result in a *frameshift* mutation. If one or two bases are deleted or added, the reading frame of the sequence is altered, usually resulting in a nonfunctional gene product. Deletions of three nucleotides or multiples of three nucleotides may be less serious because they preserve the reading frame.

Combinations of insertions and deletions are possible, and sometimes an insertion mutation will restore the reading frame of a gene with a deletion mutation (and vice versa). Such a gene product would then contain a garbled amino acid sequence between the insertion and deletion, but would otherwise be correct (Figure 1-2).[27]

Mechanisms to Repair DNA Damage

DNA repair is integral in protecting against mutations that could otherwise lead to cancer.[28] All humans have at least four mechanisms for repairing DNA damage in a cell: mismatch repair (MMR), base excision repair (BER), nucleotide excision repair (NER), and double-strand break repair. These repair mechanisms involve at least 80 different genes that play direct roles in DNA repair.[26] The MMR, BER, and NER mechanisms rely on DNA being a double-stranded structure with the same information contained in both strands. When damage affects just one strand, it can be accurately repaired by excision and replacement, with new DNA being synthesized using the complementary strand as a template.[26]

Mismatched base pairs, as well as single-base insertions and deletions, are generally repaired by MMR. This mechanism relies on a backup signal within the DNA to distinguish between the parental strand and the daughter strand containing the replication error. In humans, a protein called Msh recognizes and binds the mismatched base pair. A protein called Mih then binds to the protein Msh. Bound to the mismatch, the Msh/Mih complex likely activates a process that unwinds DNA in the direction of the mismatch, degrades the DNA strand, and repairs the error. An example of a disease resulting from MMR is colorectal cancer.

Base excision repair is a major repair mechanism that focuses specifically on repairing incorrect bases and filling base gaps. BER removes the incorrect base by a specific DNA glycosidase enzyme, which creates a baseless (AP) binding site on the DNA molecule. The enzyme AP endonuclease recognizes this site and cleaves the DNA to it. DNA repair synthesis occurs at the site, followed by sealing of the nicks by DNA ligase.[26]

The NER pathway involves genes that remove UVR-induced damage and DNA adducts associated with chemical exposures. NER is one of the most important repair mechanisms employed in response to a wide variety of DNA damages.[26] NER binds a protein at the damaged site, excises the damaged strand several nucleotides away from the damaged site on both sides, removes the damaged area, fills in the resulting gap with a DNA polymerase, and seals the gap with DNA ligase. A classic example of a disease caused by defective NER is xeroderma pigmentosum (XP), an inherited condition in which UVR-induced skin cancers result from defects in several genes in the NER pathway.[29]

The nonhomologous end-joining and homologous recombination repair pathways repair double-strand DNA breaks produced directly by exposure to ionizing radiation or indirectly by incomplete repair of other damages.[26] The primary activator of double-strand repair is the protein kinase ATM, the deficiency of which causes the inherited disorder ataxia-telangiectasia.

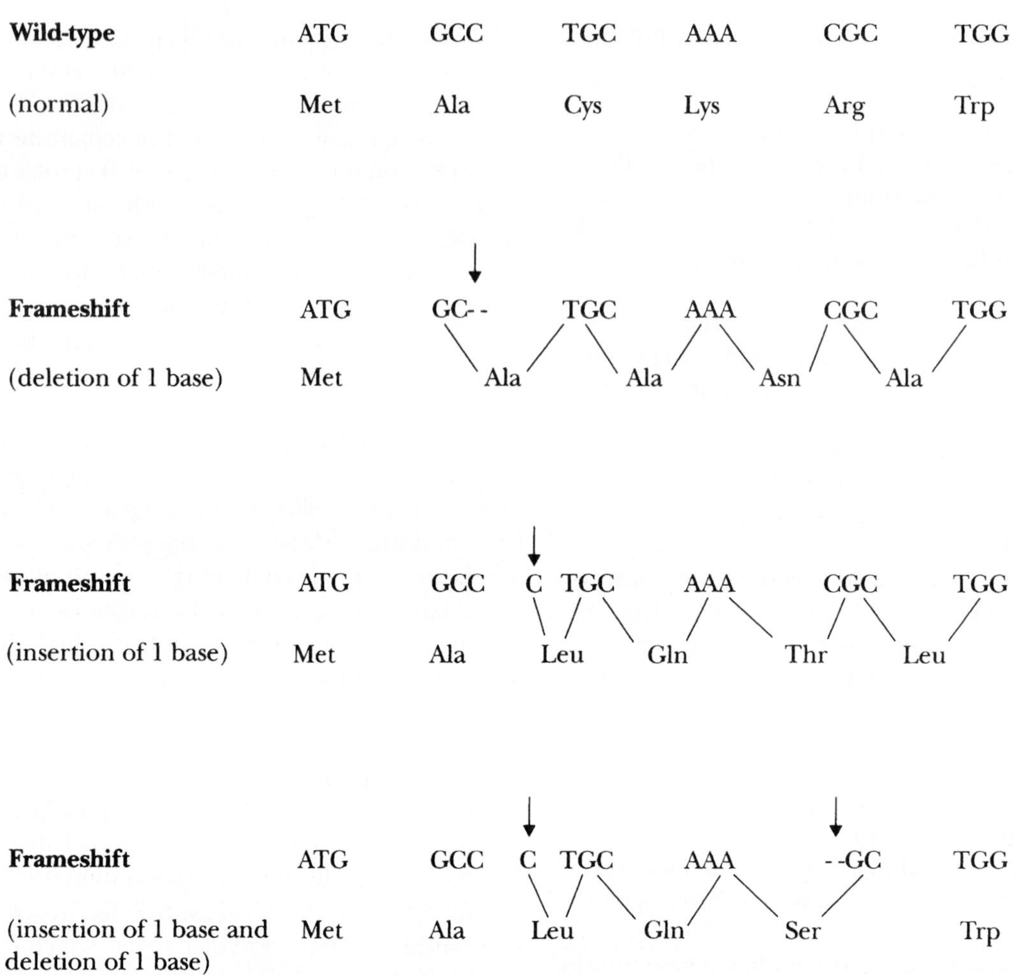

Figure 1-2. Frameshift mutations. Deletion and/or insertion of bases shifts the reading frame of the DNA sequence, thereby changing the expressed amino acids. Top rows in each set are DNA bases: A=adenine; T=thymine; C=cytosine; G=guanine. Bottom rows in each set are amino acids encoded by the bases: Ala=alanine; Arg=arginine; Asn=asparagine; Cys=cysteine; Gln=glutamine; Leu=leucine; Lys=lysine; Met=methionine; Ser=serine; Thr=threonine; Trp=tryptophan. (Reprinted with permission from Loescher LJ: DNA testing for cancer predisposition. *Oncol Nurs Forum* 25:1320, 1998.[27])

Polymorphisms

Polymorphisms, or genetic variants, represent another genetic influence on cancer. Polymorphisms comprise the occurrence together—in the same population—of more than one allele or genetic marker at the same locus, with the least frequent allele or marker occurring more often (i.e., occurrence of 1% or more) than can be accounted for by mutation alone.[30] Some polymorphisms result from the insertion or deletion of a section of DNA; these include microsatellite repeat sequences and gross genetic losses and rearrangement.[31] The simplest types of polymorphisms, however, are single-nucleotide polymorphisms (SNPs). SNPs, in which a single base substitutes for another, account for 90% of all DNA polymorphisms.[31]

Although SNPs are found in regulatory regions of the gene, most occur in noncoding regions and do not alter gene protein expression. In some instances, SNPs may cause subtle changes in a group of genes that under normal conditions are latent, meaning that the variations are not harmful on their own (i.e., they are switched "off"). With certain environmental exposures, however, they can be switched "on."[32] In other instances, the base substitutions are nonconservative, meaning that the wild-type (normal) genes and the variants have dissimilar structural or functional properties. In this situation, SNPs could influence protein function, DNA repair capacity, and cancer risk.[26,33]

Table 1-3 lists some of the polymorphisms in genes implicated in cancer susceptibility.[34] Well-studied SNPs include those found in genes encoding metabolizing enzymes, such as those in the p450 cytochrome system (*CYP* genes), glutathione-*S*-transferase (*GST*) genes, and the *N*-acetyl-transferase (*NAT*) genes.[32,35–39]

Table 1-3 Polymorphisms Implicated in Cancer Susceptibility

Gene	Chromosome Location	General Types of Cancer
ALDH2	12q24.2	Alcohol-related cancers
APC	5q21-q22	APC I1307K: colorectal cancer
CCND1	11q13	Head and neck cancers
COMT	22q11.2	Breast cancer
CYP 17	10q24.3	Prostate and breast cancers (female and male)
CYP1A1	15q22-q24	Lung, oral, and breast cancers; childhood leukemia
CYP1B1	2p22-p21	Breast cancer
CYP2A6	19q13.2	Lung cancer (and nicotine metabolism)
CYP2E	10q24.3-qter	Lung cancer
GSTM1	1p13.3	Bladder and breast cancers; lung cancer (tobacco smoke); childhood leukemia
GSTP1	11q13	Breast cancer
GSTT1	22q11.23	Head and neck and breast cancers
HRAS	11p15.5	Breast, ovarian, lung, and colorectal cancer risk
LTA	6p21.3	Myeloma
MC1R	16q24.3	Melanoma
MTHFR	1p36.3	Colon cancer; acute lymphoblastic leukemia
NAT1	8p23.1-p21.3	Bladder and lung cancers
NAT2	8p23.1	Bladder and colorectal cancers
SRD5A2	2023	Prostate and breast cancers
TNF	6p21.3	Myeloma

Modified from www.cancerindex.org/geneweb/gepidem.htm, 2003.[34]

Potentially, there could be millions of SNPs in the human genome. Some have a useful function. For example, if a SNP is frequently found close to a particular gene, it acts as a marker for that gene. Scientists can use SNPs as ways to catalog unique sets of changes involved in different cancers and as potential tools to improve cancer diagnosis and treatment planning. Additionally, SNPs may play a role in differing responses to treatments and individual cancer risk.[32]

Oncogenes

Oncogenes are genes that encode proteins (oncoproteins) whose action promotes cell proliferation. Oncogenes are the excessively or inappropriately active versions of normal cellular genes called *proto-oncogenes.* One mechanism for overexpression of oncogenes is amplification. In amplification, the number of copies of a gene increases, resulting in overexpression of the gene product. The gene itself remains unmodified. As tumor cells progress, they gain the ability to amplify genes as they lose cell cycle control (discussed later in this chapter). Oncogenes such as *MYC* and *HER2/NEU* often have amplified gene sequences, which may be related to tumor progression.[40]

Most proto-oncogenes participate in cellular signal transduction pathways, which can be visualized as molecular "bucket brigades" that relay growth-stimulating signals from the outside to the inside of the cell.[41] These complex signal transduction pathways control basic cell functions such as division, motility, and survival; consequently, they need to be highly regulated. Regulation occurs through alterations in the enzymatic activity of key components in the pathways and assembly of large multimolecular signaling complexes within the cell.

The pathways play an important role in tumor development. The large number of components constituting the pathways provide many potential targets for oncogene activation and explain the large number of proto-oncogenes that have been identified. Also, the intrinsic redundancy and interaction between the pathways explain why human cancers rarely, if ever, result from aberrant activation of a single oncogene.[42]

Classification of oncogenes

Broad classes of oncogenes can be distinguished according to their overall function. A number of these genes encode growth factors, growth factor receptors, nonreceptor tyrosine kinases, G-proteins, serine/threonine protein kinases, and transcription factors.[40–42]

Growth factors. Growth factors are polypeptides that influence cell growth, differentiation, and survival positively and negatively by binding to specific receptors in the cell membrane and, consequently, activating intracellular signal transduction. To do so, growth factors must interact with highly specific receptors. Growth factor activity results in transmission of a signal to the cell nucleus, where genes are turned off and on. The end result is change in expression (transcription into RNA) of certain genes.

Growth factors commonly regulate the cell through autocrine stimulation and paracrine stimulation. In autocrine stimulation, the growth factor stimulates the cell that produced it; in paracrine stimulation, the growth factor activates adjacent cells. Oncogenic growth factors can activate tumor cell proliferation by both forms of stimulation, but by themselves may not be sufficient to sustain the transformed cell.[41] For example, the oncogenes *FOS, JUN,* and *MYC* are early-response oncogenes that increase in activity soon after growth factor stimulation. These genes play key roles in cell proliferation. The overexpression of *MYC* coupled with the addition of fibroblast growth factor (FGF) will cause DNA synthesis, whereas each alone may not. Similarly, when platelet-derived growth factor (PDGF) is combined with another growth factor such as epidermal growth factor (EGF), PDGF can stimulate cell division in cultures; it cannot accomplish this effect alone.

Overproduction of several growth factors is implicated in cancer development. *Epidermal growth factor* stimulates a variety of cells such as epidermal cells, glial cells, vascular endothelial cells, and many cancer cells. Epidermal growth factors produce a mitogenic response in cells that have the EGF receptor (EGFR). High levels of EGFRs are noted in many epithelial carcinomas, and mutant EGF receptors have been found on high-grade glioblastomas.[43] Transforming growth factor alpha (TGF-α) is a member of the EGF family. It tends to stimulate endothelial cell proliferation. Transforming growth factor beta (TGF-β) tends to inhibit cell proliferation, largely through inhibition of cyclin 4 and cyclin-dependent kinase (CDK) 4 in the cell cycle. *Platelet-derived growth factor* receptors are normally located in fibroblasts and smooth muscle cells and appear to play a role in the development and support of brain tumors.[44] *Fibroblast growth factor* (FGF) stimulates the growth of fibroblasts and is released when cells are damaged or die, thereby stimulating surrounding tissue to proliferate. *Granulocyte-macrophage colony-stimulating growth factor* (GM-CSF) is involved in the proliferation and differentiation of granulocytes and monocytes/macrophages.

Growth factor receptors. A second type of oncogene encodes altered growth factor receptors (GFRs), which induce proliferative signals into the cell even in the absence of growth factors.[40] Most GFRs act through intrinsic tyrosine kinase activity, the ability to bond inorganic phosphate to the amino acid tyrosine. Increased tyrosine kinase activity leads to reactions that stimulate mitosis and can cause clonal expansion of cells. Point mutations may cause increased activity of tyrosine kinase. Nonmutation mechanisms for increasing tyrosine kinase activity include overexpression of GFR and autocrine stimulation.

When overproduced, EGFR is associated with poor prognosis for breast, bladder, colon, lung, and esophageal cancers.[45–47] HER2/NEU receptor (also known as ErbB2) overexpression is associated with poor prognosis for breast and ovarian cancers.[48,49] Together, EGFR and TGF-β serve as prognostic markers for tumor relapse and survival. HER2/NEU receptors in breast carcinoma also increase the risk of recurrence.[50]

Nonreceptor tyrosine kinases. The normal intracellular products of *src* proto-oncogenes have relatively low levels of tyrosine kinase activity. Although these proteins do not bind directly to growth factors, growth factors and other cellular activators may activate tyrosine kinases as part of the signal transduction process. For example, in platelets, thrombin activates tyrosine kinase. Platelet-derived growth factor activates *SRC* tyrosine kinase activity in fibroblasts. The *src* oncogene is activated in colorectal cancers and breast adenocarcinomas.

G-proteins. Guanine nucleotide-binding proteins (G-proteins) act as signal transducers for cell-surface growth factor receptors. An example of G-proteins is the RAS superfamily, which includes more than 50 members. The true RAS proteins (H RAS, K RAS, N RAS) act at the inner leaflet cell membrane to cause malignant transformation. Proteins encoded by unmutated *RAS* genes transmit stimulatory signals from other GFRs to other proteins. Mutated *RAS* genes cause activation of signaling pathways, even when unprompted by GFRs. Overall, *RAS* activation occurs in two ways: (1) loss of guanosine 5′-triphosphate activity (through point mutations that lead to transformation) and (2) increase in G-nucleotide exchange (point mutations with a lower affinity for G-nucleotide, leading to increased turnover). Mutant *RAS* genes are found in several tumors, including cancers of the colon and lung and 90% of pancreatic cancers.[51]

Serine-threonine kinases. Another category of oncogenes comprises the cytoplasmic oncoproteins with serine-threonine protein-kinase activity. Serine-threonine kinases are centrally involved in cell-cycle progression. The prototype for the serine-threonine kinase category is the Raf-1 protein, which is activated by tyrosine kinase–associated receptors.[41] The Raf-1 protein acts as an intermediary in the signal transduction pathway between *RAS* and the cell nucleus by activating other kinases, mitogen-activated protein (MAP) kinases. These MAP kinases phosphorylate critical substrates regulating cell division. To be active, raf-1 must move to the cell membrane. Recruitment to the membrane is accomplished by active *RAS*; however, this interaction alone is not sufficient to cause transformation. Other protein kinases (e.g., protein kinase C) are needed for transformation.[42]

Transcription factors. Transcription factor proteins bind to DNA and cause changes in gene expression. In many tumors, mutated transcription factors that regulate genes involved in cell growth and survival spur this transformation. Oncogenic transcription factors include proteins with activator protein-1 (AP-1) activity, such as Jun and Fos, which are part of signal-dependent processes that control cell growth.[52] The tumor suppressor gene *TP53* also acts as a transcription factor when it senses DNA damage and halts cell division by controlling the expression of other genes that directly regulate the cell cycle. Oncogenic transcription factors have been associated with many kinds of human leukemias and Ewing's sarcoma.[53]

Tumor Suppressor Genes

Tumor suppressor genes normally suppress or negatively regulate cell proliferation by encoding proteins that block the action of growth-promoting proteins. Thus, the hallmark characteristic of a mutated tumor suppressor gene is loss of function through loss of genetic material or information. Normally, tumor suppressor genes suppress oncogenes.[54] Tumor suppressor genes are recessive in that both alleles (forms of the gene) of a pair must mutate for the gene to be inactivated. In other words, loss or mutation of both copies of the gene is required for tumorigenesis.[21] Inactivation of tumor suppressor genes is a hallmark of cancers resulting from inherited predisposition.

Tumor suppressor genes have diverse functions. Some affect DNA transcription, such as *APC*, *MEN1*, *p53*, *RB*, and *WT1*. The tumor suppressor genes *BRCA1* and *BRCA2* play roles in DNA damage repair. The tumor suppressor genes *RB*, *p16*, and *TP53* are critical for operation of the cell cycle, suggesting that many tumor suppressor genes act as "gatekeeper" genes. Gatekeeper genes are responsible for maintaining a constant cell number by renewing cell populations or controlling proliferation in specific tissue types. A mutation in a gatekeeper gene may lead to more cell division than cell death, thereby permitting an increase in cell number.[55]

Loss of heterozygosity

Usually, the first (germ-line) mutation of a tumor suppressor gene affects the actual gene. The second mutation involves loss of a whole chromosome or loss of part of a chromosome. In each case, there is loss of one allele of any markers close to the tumor suppressor gene. Thus, if a patient with cancer was heterozygous for a genetic marker located close to the tumor suppressor gene, the tumor shows loss of heterozygosity (LOH). Most tumor specimens contain a mixture of tumor and nontumor tissue, indicating a decreased relative intensity of tumor, rather than total loss of genetic material from any one allele.[6,21]

DNA Repair Genes

DNA repair genes may be the best example of "caretaker" genes — genes involved in controlling or regulating genetic instability to ensure integrity of genetic information. Mutations in caretaker genes do not lead directly to cancer. Rather, mutations in these genes lead to inefficient replication or repair of DNA, which in turn allows subsequent mutations in tumor suppressor genes and proto-oncogenes to accumulate. As a result, the chance of a mutation in a gatekeeper gene is increased by the presence of a mutation in a caretaker gene. Once inactivation of a gatekeeper gene initiates a tumor, the tumor may progress more rapidly because of the increased rate of mutation in other genes.[55]

Many times DNA repair genes have microsatellite DNA — short stretches of DNA that include a simple repeating base sequence. The length of microsatellite DNA repeats varies in tumors and normal tissue. Microsatellite instability has been found in colorectal, gastric, breast, bladder, and non-small cell lung cancers. Microsatellites provide clues to gene stability. For example, LOH studies of hereditary nonpolyposis colon cancer (HNPCC) using microsatellite markers showed that rather than lacking alleles in DNA, some tumors appeared to contain extra, novel alleles.[56] Microsatellite instability also has a role in drug resistance in human tumors.[57]

Cytogenetic Abnormalities

The condition of ploidy indicates the number of repetitions of chromosomes in a cell. Normal somatic cells are diploid, in that they bear two sets of chromosomes (one from each parent). Normal germ cells are haploid, having only one chromosome. Many forms of cancer have incorrect ploidy numbers, owing to the accumulation of mutations that increase chromosome missegregation. As a result, cancer cells typically have bizarre, unstable chromosomal structures, with many gains, losses, deletions of segments, or rearrangements of chromosomes.

Translocations and deletions

Translocations are structural abnormalities in chromosomes that primarily affect oncogenes by causing overexpression and fusion at the points in the chromosome where abnormal breaks tend to occur (break points). In reciprocal translocations, exchange of genetic material occurs between two chromosomes or within the same chromosome. Leukemias and lymphomas typically involve translocations. For example, in chronic myelogenous leukemia, the reciprocal translocation between the q (long) arm of chromosome 9, band 34, and the q arm of chromosome 22, band 11 (9;22)(q34,q11), causes the *abl* proto-oncogene to be translocated to chromosome 22 (Philadelphia chromosome). This translocation produces a bcr-abl oncogenic protein with high tyrosine kinase activity. The translocation ultimately activates the *MYC* oncogene.[13,58]

Chromosomal deletions occur mostly in solid tumors, and commonly involve deletions of specific gene sequences (i.e., loss of a chromosomal band or LOH of a specific allele).[13] Deletions are the hallmark of tumor suppressor genes; for example, retinoblastoma shows the deletion del(13)(q14q14).

Aneuploidy

Aneuploidy entails an abnormal chromosome number reflecting gain or loss of chromosomes. It usually is seen with malignant transformation, in that gross changes in chromosome number usually occur as tumorigenesis progresses. Aneuploidy can be either random or nonrandom. In *random aneuploidy,* the change in chromosome number has no association with a tumor type; rather, it occurs late in tumorigenesis and reflects genetic instability of the tumor. *Nonrandom aneuploidy* involves a specific change in a given chromosome associated with a specific tumor. For example, trisomy 8 (three copies of chromosome 8) is associated with acute leukemia. Nonrandom aneuploidy tends to occur earlier in tumorigenesis than the nonrandom form.

Aneuploidy as a cause or a consequence of cancer has long been debated.[59] Recent research suggests that the function of telomeres — chromosomal structures that determine the domain of chromosomes within a nucleus and protect chromosomes from assault from internal and external environments — may have a greater role in cancer development than aneuploidy does.[60] However, the causes, involved mechanisms, and consequences of aneuploidy are currently under intense study and this thinking may change.

The Cell Cycle

Cell proliferation occurs as the result of coordinated events that include replication of DNA, mitosis, and cytokinesis. These events culminate with the division of a somatic cell into two daughter cells containing identical copies of the genome. The concept of a "cell cycle" to describe these events arose during the period when cell investigation relied mainly on light microscopy. Scientists could observe cycles of mitosis, a period of high activity in the cell, alternating with interphase, an inactive resting period.[61] After the discovery of DNA, further research into the biochemical events occurring in interphase elucidated several distinct phases.

Events of the Cell Cycle

The cell cycle is currently conceptualized as a four-phase process: (1) mitosis or (M) phase; (2) gap 1 (G1) phase; (3) synthesis (S) phase; and (4) gap 2 (G2) phase (Figure 1–3). In the M phase, the chromatids separate to form two sets of chromosomes and cytokinesis occurs. Two daughter cells form, containing identical sets of chromosomes and equal amounts of cellular constituents. Following the M phase, cells either reenter G1 to begin the cell cycle anew or exit the cell cycle by entering G0, a state of reproductive quiescence. In the G1 phase, the nucleus enlarges and transcription and translation activities occur in preparation for DNA replication. Late G1 is characterized by a restriction point (R), the point at which the cell becomes committed to replicate. Normal cells will often leave G1 and enter G0 at the restriction point if there is a shortage of nutrients or growth factors. In the S phase, the cell replicates the DNA and forms a complementary set of chromatids. Following replication, the cell proceeds to G2. Most of the cells in the adult body are in G0. Cells that are usually metabolically active, such as granulocytes and the epithelium of the gastrointestinal tract, are cycling cells.

The series of events that occur in the cell cycle is tightly controlled and regulated by proteins called *cyclins,* which combine with and activate enzymes called cyclin-dependent kinases (CDKs). Activation of cyclins and CDKs occurs at specific points in the cell cycle (see Figure 1-3).

Multiple factors in the microenvironment determine whether a particular cell will proliferate, become quiescent, or enter the postmitotic state.[62] The retinoblastoma protein (pRb) mediates most antiproliferative signals, thereby acting as a "master brake" on the cell cycle. Hypophosphorylated pRb blocks proliferation by altering E2F transcription factors[62] that control the gene expression needed for progression from G1 to the S phase. Transforming growth factor beta (TGF-β) acts to prevent phosphorylation of pRb by suppressing *c-myc* or blocking the formation of cyclin–CDK complexes. Hence, TGF-β blocks progression through G1. Phosphorylation of pRb liberates transcription factors called E2Fs, which in turn permit advancement through G1 to S phase.

Specific biochemical checkpoints within the cell cycle ensure that the cycle proceeds in the correct sequence and that one event has been completed before another begins. Checkpoints exist at the decisions to enter S phase, to enter mitosis (G2/M checkpoint), and to exit mitosis.[63] The checkpoint controlling entry into the S phase prevents replication of damaged DNA. The G2/M checkpoint detects damaged or unduplicated DNA and unduplicated centrosomes. A checkpoint in the M phase delays chromosome

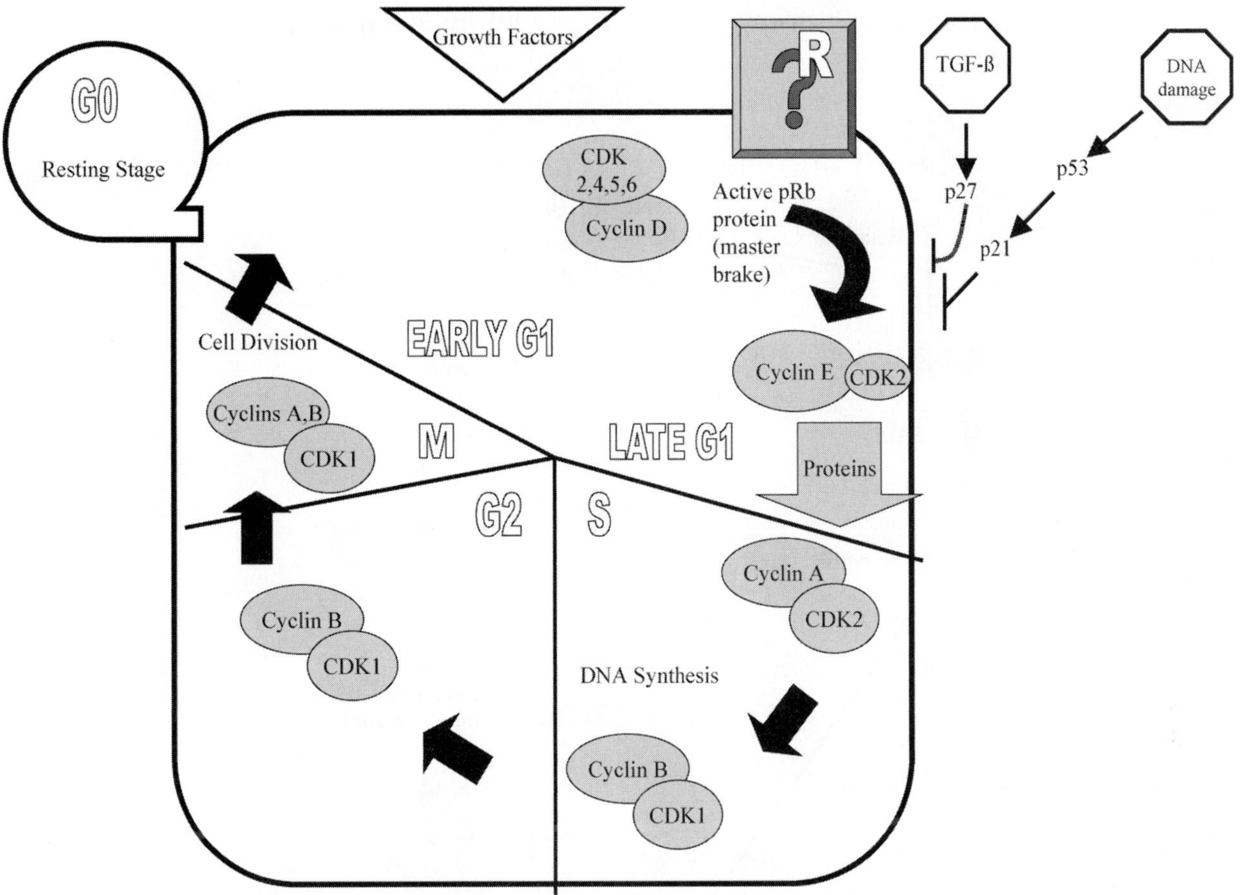

Figure 1-3. The cell cycle. The cell cycle consists of four stages (G1, S, G2, M) that are controlled by proteins called cyclins. The cyclins (D, E, A, B) are activated when complexed with enzymes called cyclin-dependent kinases (CDKs). Upon activation, the cyclin-CDK complex allows the cell to progress through each specific cell cycle stage. Present throughout the cell cycle, the cyclin-CDK complexes serve as checkpoints or monitors of the cell cycle. Inhibitory proteins prevent progression through the cell cycle if DNA damage is present or there is a lack of nutrients or oxygen to support cellular proliferation. Examples of inhibitory proteins include p21 p27, p53. The inhibitory proteins in turn are regulated by the presence of inhibitory growth factors and TGF-β. Once past R (the restriction point) the cell cycle is turned "on" and progression through the cell cycle is inevitable. Cyclin-CDK complexes and pRB (the "master brake") tightly regulate the R point. The stability of the inhibitory proteins and cyclin-CDK complexes are altered in cancer, thereby altering control of the cell cycle and uncontrolled cellular proliferation prevails.

segregation if all chromosomes have not become attached to the mitotic spindle fibers.[64]

The Cell Cycle and Cancer

Cancer cells often lack the ability to enter the G0 (quiescent) state, a condition attributed to having a deficient amount of the pRb protein. Functional pRb may be lost through mutation of the *RB* gene. Excessive cell proliferation may involve lack of signal transduction from TGF-β because of dysfunctional or insufficient numbers of receptors.[62]

Most likely, cancer cells have faulty cell-cycle checkpoints.[41,65] Genetic instability at the G1/S checkpoint in human cancers currently is best understood. Loss of the G1/S checkpoint leads to instability of the human genome, survival of genetically damaged cells, and clonal evolution. For example, the *TP53* gene is commonly mutated in several cancers, suggesting that abnormalities in the G1/S checkpoint are important in tumorigenesis.

Apoptosis

Apoptosis, often referred to as "programmed cell death" or "cell suicide," is a gene-directed method of cell destruction (see Figure 1-4). It can be triggered by environmental conditions, cellular receptor activation, and internal factors related to gene

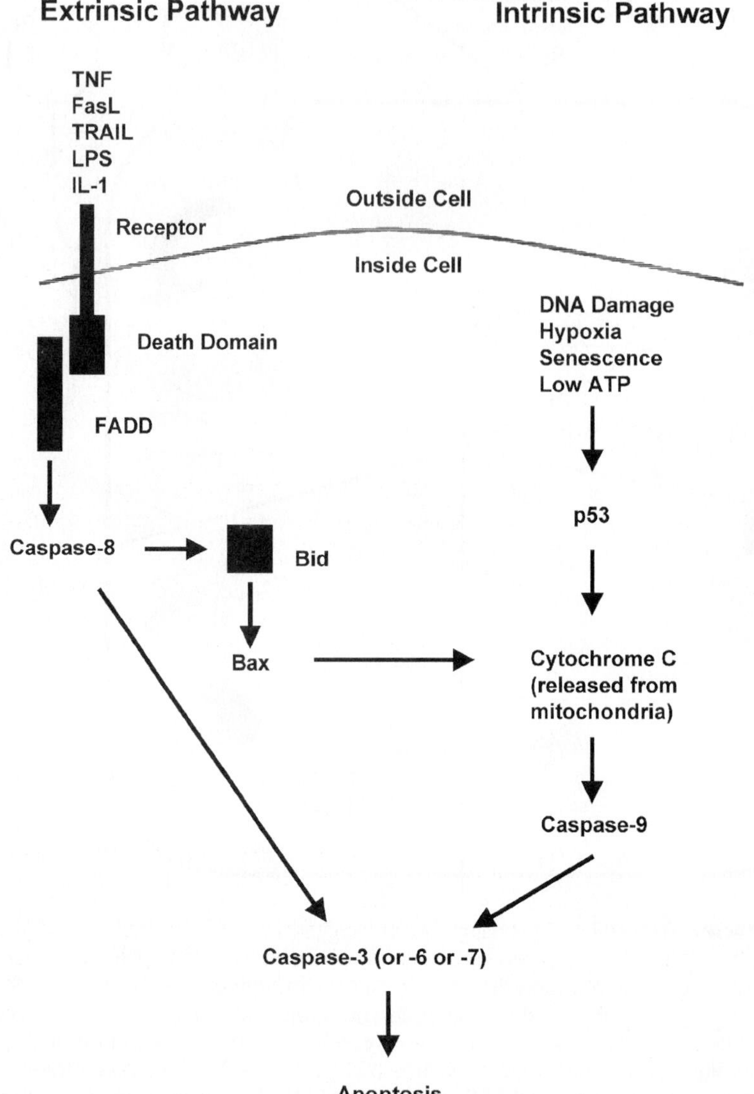

Figure 1-4. Apoptosis. The extrinsic and intrinsic pathways of apoptosis are normally activated by various cues occurring in the environment of the cell and/or within the cell. Activation of the pathways leads to activation of caspase-3 (and other executioner enzymes) which results in apoptosis. (See text for details)

expression.[66,67] Apoptosis is essential for normal development, orderly cell turnover, and tissue repair and remodeling. Two principal pathways mediate apoptosis: the extrinsic and intrinsic pathways. The extrinsic pathway involves activation of cell-surface receptors; the intrinsic pathway, or "mitochondrial pathway," is responsive to internal cues such as DNA damage, which increase p53 protein.[66,68] Because faulty apoptotic mechanisms are important factors in tumor development and survival, many forms of anticancer therapy focus on inducing apoptosis in tumor cells.[69] Furthermore, cancer therapy–induced apoptosis of healthy cells, especially those involved in inflammation and immunity, limits the dosage of chemotherapy.

Characteristics of Cells Undergoing Apoptosis

Structural changes

Structural changes during apoptosis include blebbing of the plasma membrane and breakage of the cell into apoptotic bodies. Apoptotic bodies help apoptotic cells to become phagocytized by cells that are not undergoing apoptosis. One way phagocytes and other healthy cells recognize apoptotic bodies is from specific changes in the composition of the phospholipids in the outer leaflet of the plasma membrane — that is, when phosphatidylserine translocates from the cytoplasmic leaflet to the extracellular leaflet of the membrane lipid bilayer.

The plasma membrane does not lose its integrity, so another cardinal feature of apoptotic cells is minimal leakage of cellular constituents into the extracellular space. This feature minimizes the inflammatory response and distinguishes apoptosis from necrosis, which usually results from trauma and causes injured cells to swell, lyse, and release cytoplasmic materials that activate inflammation.[70]

Apoptotic cells lose water, causing shrinking or condensation of the cytoplasm. Large vacuoles also form in the cytoplasm. In the nucleus, margins of chromatin become concentrated at the inside of the nuclear membrane. The nucleus condenses into multiple fragments characterized by an intact membrane.[70] The chromatin cleavage is associated with DNA degradation into small fragments.

Signaling pathways

The extrinsic signaling pathway is triggered by a number of primary signals that directly activate specific death receptors in the plasma membrane. These signals include the binding of proteins related to tumor necrosis factor (TNF), such as TNF-related apoptosis-inducing ligand (TRAIL);[71] Fas ligand, which is expressed on activated T cells and neutrophils;[66] increased oxidant production and hydrogen peroxide levels; high levels of glucocorticoids; and presence of endotoxins, such as lipopolysaccharide.[66] Receptor activation by these primary signals triggers secondary signaling pathways that induce death. Intermediate signaling proteins activate caspase-8, which acting in concert with other caspases, activates the main executioner enzyme, caspase-3.

The intrinsic (mitochondrial) pathway is activated by internal cues, such as DNA damage and hypoxia, through the p53 protein.[68] Changes in mitochondrial membrane potential release mitochondrial cytochrome c to the cytoplasm, which in turn leads to activation of caspase-9. Activated caspase-9 then activates caspase-3, allowing convergence of the intrinsic pathway with the extrinsic pathway. Furthermore, the extrinsic pathway can activate the intrinsic pathway by caspase-8–induced cleavage of the protein Bid to increase accumulation of Bax protein inside cells.[71] Bax, in turn, damages mitochondrial membrane and causes cytochrome c release and resultant caspase-3, -6, and -7 activation.

Genes and Proteins Involved in Apoptosis

Genetic alterations involving apoptosis are important factors in tumor development and biology. The *TP53* gene encodes the p53 protein, which is itself a transcription factor that helps regulate the cell cycle, DNA repair, and apoptosis. Half of all human cancers have *TP53* mutations,[68] and more than 50 tumor types demonstrate mutated *TP53*.[72] Studies using *TP53* cell lines transfected with a temperature-sensitive mutant of *TP53* have clearly shown that wild-type *TP53* function lowers the threshold for inducing apoptosis following genotoxic damage.[73]

Other genes and proteins important to apoptosis include members of the B-cell leukemia protein 2 (*Bcl-2*) gene family.[74] Certain members, including Bcl-2, Bcl-X_L, A1, and Mcl-1, are required for cell survival, whereas others, such as the Bax/Bak proteins, promote cell death. Overexpression of Bcl-2 on its own is weakly tumorigenic, but it is potently synergistic with other oncogenes that interfere with cell-cycle control. Bax can function as a tumor suppressor and may complement the actions of *TP53*.

Members of the TNF family of ligands and receptors,[71] such as TRAIL Apo 2L/TRAIL receptors and Fas/FasL systems, also influence apoptosis.[75,76] TRAIL causes death after activation of its receptors by the extrinsic pathway, but can also trigger the intrinsic pathway by stimulating Bax-induced release of cytochrome c into the cytoplasm. The activation of certain TRAIL receptors recruits a Fas-associated death domain (FADD) adapter protein to form a complex containing caspase-8 and -10. This complex activates caspase-3, -6, and -7 to execute apoptosis.[71]

When FasL is present, a death-inducing signaling complex is formed, similar to that described earlier for TRAIL. Responses of this system can be controlled by the *FasL* gene, which is usually inactive but is regulated by transcription factors such as nuclear factor kappa B (NF-κB).[77] The caspase-8 activity in the complex is regulated by a FADD-like interleukin 1B-interconverting enzyme (FLICE)–inhibitory protein (FLIP).[78] The FLIP protein can become incorporated into the death-inducing signaling complex, thereby thwarting the process.

Gene manipulation targeting apoptosis is being exploited for therapeutic purposes. For example, viral vectors are being examined to selectively destroy cells with *TP53* mutations and replace the mutated gene with nonmutated forms.[68] As a strategy to counteract drug resistance in multiple myeloma, genetic studies are focusing on perturbing NF-κB to induce apoptosis in cancer cells.[79] In studies targeting defective apoptosis signaling in cancer cells, strategies involving antisense-mediated down-regulation of Bcl-2 and Bcl-XL expression and small molecules that inhibit these proteins have shown promise.[80]

Metastasis

Metastasis is the major cause of death in individuals with solid tumors. The presence of metastatic sites is an important cancer prognostic factor; unfortunately, in many cases, metastases occur before initial diagnosis of cancer. The biology of the events involved in the process of metastasis represents a fundamental area of cancer research. Strategies are being developed to disrupt the metastatic process, thereby improving outcomes of cancer care.

Factors Contributing to Metastasis

Metastasis is the spread of tumor cells, usually via the bloodstream or lymphatic system, from the primary tumor site to a distant site in the body. Unlike tumorigenesis, in which the genetic basis may vary among cancer types, the cellular and molecular steps of metastasis are similar.[81] Mechanisms that contribute to the process of metastasis include angiogenesis, motility, alterations in cell adhesion, and secretion of proteolytic enzymes leading to barrier breakdown.[82–85] Furthermore, once in circulation, metastatic tumor cells must escape immune surveillance, and angiogenesis must occur for the cells to establish themselves in a new tissue site. Recently, the importance of the stromal microenvironment in cancer progression and metastasis has been recognized, and its role is under intense investigation.[81]

Angiogenesis

When a tumor is larger than 2 mm^3 in size, its growth will remain limited unless it receives an additional blood supply.[85] Formation of new blood vessels, a process termed *angiogenesis*, provides the nutrients and oxygen required by the growing tumor. Angiogenesis involves the migration and proliferation of endothelial cells from existing vasculature near the tumor. Additionally, circulating endothelial progenitor cells are now thought to play a role in tumor-associated angiogenesis.[86] Secreted MMPs promote endothelial cell proliferation by mediating degradation of the extracellular matrix (ECM) and releasing specific forms of vascular endothelial growth factor (VEGF). The newly formed blood vessels provide nutrition and oxygen to the growing tumor, as well as a potential route for metastatic tumor cells to leave the primary tumor site. These blood vessels tend to be "leaky," with loose cell–cell contacts, providing an easy route by which tumor cells can enter the bloodstream for potential transport to distant sites. Tumor-associated angiogenesis also involves the lymphatics; the events of lymphangiogenesis are currently being investigated.

Both positive and negative regulators of angiogenesis exist. Tumor cells produce positive angiogenic factors such as VEGF, basic fibroblast growth factor (bFGF), TNF, and angiopoietin-1, which serve as stimuli for the development of new capillaries. Angiogenic factors appear to promote locomotion and mitosis of vascular endothelium and to release endothelial growth factors, thus stimulating capillary proliferation. VEGF, which promotes growth and chemotaxis of endothelial cells in vitro, is found in high concentration in the microenvironment of many tumors. This growth factor has been proposed as the final pathway through which other angiogenic agents exert their influence.[87]

Negative regulators of angiogenesis are as important as the positive stimulatory agents and include TGF-β_1, alfa-interferon, angiostatin, and thrombospondin-1 and -2.[86,87] TGF-β_1 inhibits the proteolysis necessary for the formation of viable and effective endothelial sprouts emanating from parent vessels. Alfa-interferon, which was the first antiangiogenic substance to be used in a clinical trial, evolved following its use in the treatment of a life-threatening angioma.[86] Angiostatin, a fragment of the plasminogen molecule, generally prevents proliferation of endothelial cells.[87] Many tumors down-regulate the thrombospondins, a family of extracellular glycoproteins, during acquisition of an angiogenic phenotype.[86] Angiogenesis correlates with metastatic potential and is a prognostic factor for breast cancer.[88,89] Some researchers have reported that increased numbers of blood vessels associated with a tumor are the second most accurate prognostic factor, following lymph node status.[90]

Because many tumors remain indolent without increased vascularity, research now in progress is seeking to better understand the "angiogenic switch" that occurs in tumors. Some investigators have collected evidence for such a switch. This switch involves the production of low levels of thrombospondin-1 and -2, which interact with specific MMPs and VEGF to promote tumor-associated angiogenesis.[86] Furthermore, the use of antiangiogenic agents combined with conventional chemotherapy drugs may increase the effectiveness of the conventional agents.[91] The predicted improvement is related to a hypothesized "normalizing" process in tumor-associated vessels induced by antiangiogenic agents.[91] When the vessels become more normal, tumor pressure decreases, leading to improved uptake of chemotherapeutic agents by the tumor.

Similar to tumor development and progression, tumor angiogenesis is considered a complex process that involves contributions from other cells in the tumor microenvironment. Fibroblasts, inflammatory cells, and the ECM may all interact to control

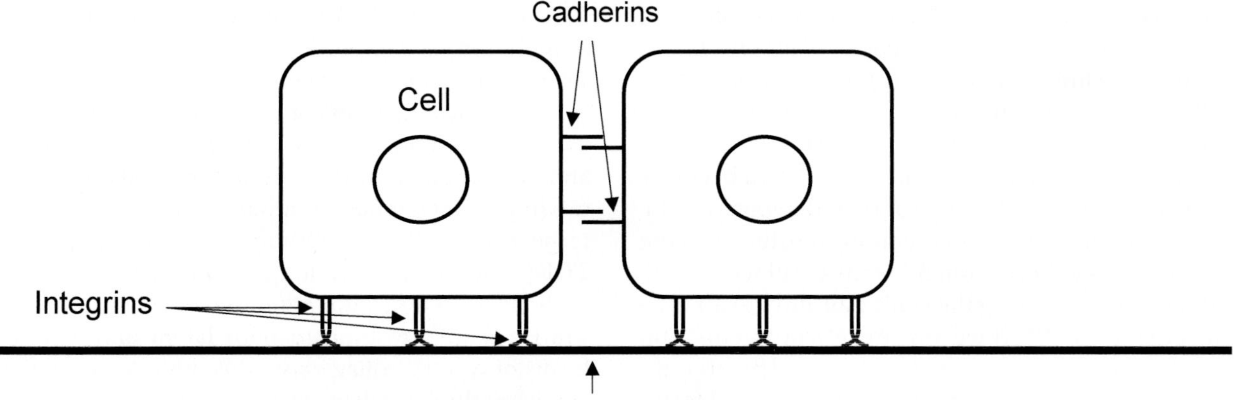

Figure 1-5. Cell adhesion. Cell adhesion molecules mediating cell–cell adhesion (cadherins) and cell–matrix adhesion (integrins) are important mediators of metastasis. Decreased cell–cell adhesion is required for detachment of metastatic cells from the primary tumor; and decreased cell–matrix adhesion is required with decreased anchorage dependence or cell–matrix adhesion.

angiogenesis. Some forms of VEGF have reduced activity and are sequestered by components of the ECM. High levels of particular MMPs in the vicinity may free active forms of VEGF. Thrombospondin-1 and -2 have antiangiogenic effects when they act directly on endothelial cells, but induce angiogenic effects on these cells when they are mediated by fibroblasts and immune cells.[86]

Motility and migration

A tumor cell must exhibit motile behavior to move from the primary tumor and enter the blood and lymph vasculature. Motogens, or motility factors, stimulate tumor cell motility.[83] Motility factors are produced by both tumor and normal cells and include EGF and interleukins-1, -3, and -6.

Changes in the cytoskeleton that affect cell shape are associated with increased motility of tumor cells.[92] The cytoskeleton, an internal supportive structure of a cell, consists of filamentous proteins including actin, keratin, vimentin, and tubulin. The distribution of these filaments and their coexpression are associated with metastatic disease in some cancers, such as melanoma and breast and cervical cancers.[92,93]

Antimotility factors that specifically target filamentous structures of the cytoskelton are currently in use or under investigation. Agents such as paclitaxel and colchicine work by altering microtubules. Cytochalasin D is associated with inhibition of cell motility following disruption of actin filaments.[83] Use of many of these agents is based on the premise that tumor cells migrate as single cells that become detached from the primary tumor, enter the blood and/or lymph vasculature, exit the circulation, and seed distant organs. These individual cells have amoeboid-like and mesenchymal-type movement patterns. It is now known that cancer cells can use collective migration strategies that include movement as cellular sheets, strands, and clusters.[94] These diverse migration strategies, which entail different morphological changes and varied reliance on integrins, proteases, cadherins, and gap junctions, may explain why therapies designed to target single-cell migration have not yet demonstrated effectiveness.[94]

Cell Adhesion

Cells express surface molecules, known collectively as cell adhesion molecules (CAMs), that mediate both attachments to the ECM and cell–cell adhesion (Figure 1-5). Changes in the adhesive properties of cells and CAMs are thought to have an important role in the tumor development and progression. Loss of attachments to the ECM and cell–cell adhesion contributes to a more invasive phenotype, by enabling tumor cells to (a) increase their motility and leave their sites of origin, (b) degrade the ECM, and (c) invade and metastasize.[95] Families of CAMs with known roles in tumor biology and metastasis include members of the immunoglobulin (Ig) superfamily, cadherins,[96] and integrins.[95,97]

Members of the Ig superfamily are calcium-independent adhesion molecules. Cell–cell adhesion molecule 1 (C-CAM1) may be a tumor suppressor of prostate cancer, as this disease shows reduced expression of the molecule.[95] Another member of the Ig superfamily, the product of the deletion in colon cancer (*DCC*) gene, is often absent in colon cancer cells and other cancers, including prostate and bladder cancer. Loss of the *DCC* gene is associated with increased muscle invasion and recurrence.[95] The cadherins are calcium-dependent cell–cell adhesion molecules that are important in adherens junctions. Cadherin family members include epithelial- (E-) and neuronal- (N-) cadherins. E-cadherin–mediated cell–cell adhesion is lost in many epithelial cancers. In cancer cells that have lost E-cadherin, many times N-cadherin becomes overexpressed and the cancer cells demonstrate increased motility. This phenomenon contributes to the idea that a "cadherin switch" from E-cadherin to N-cadherin occurs during the cell's transition to an invasive phenotype.[98,99] Integrins are glycoproteins that form heterodimers of alpha (α)and beta (β)subunits. Many combinations are possible, as 15 α and 9 β forms exist. Many of the integrins function as receptors for the components of the ECM. Expression of certain integrins may be lost or gained. The integrin $\alpha_v\beta_3$, for example, is not normally expressed in epithelial cells, yet can be expressed in breast and prostate cancer cells, where it mediates invasion to bone.[100]

Many investigations of CAMs and cancer are underway. These studies concern use of CAMs for diagnosing and staging cancers, assessing response to therapy and survival, and as potential targets for immune- and gene-based therapies.[95]

Proteolytic enzymes

To successfully metastasize, a tumor cell must cross a number of barriers, including the ECM, connective tissue, and the endothelial barrier.[82,101] The ECM serves as the first barrier that tumor cells encounter when migrating from the primary tumor site. The major components of the ECM include fibronectin, laminin, vitronectin, collagen type IV, and heparan sulfate proteoglycan. Prior to degrading the ECM, tumor cells bind components of the ECM. Integrins are a family of proteins that mediate cell–matrix interactions. Tumor cells interact with neighboring stromal cells to secrete a number of proteinases that assist with degradation of these barriers. Once secreted, the enzymes degrade components of the ECM, permitting passage of tumor cells through the interstitium or into the circulation. Increased levels of MMPs and uPA have been associated with highly metastatic tumors.[82,102]

Collectively, MMPs are able to degrade every component of the ECM.[103] In healthy tissues, the expression of potentially damaging MMPs is low and remains under tight regulation of cytokines and growth factors. By comparison, the quantity of MMPs is much higher in tumors. Historically, scientists thought that the tumor cells were responsible for producing MMPs. Current data support the hypothesis that cancer cells stimulate production and release of MMPs by the neighboring stromal cells.[103] For example, certain glycoproteins in the plasma membranes of cancer cells stimulate fibroblasts in the vicinity to secrete MMPs. Furthermore, the MMPS may release growth factors sequestered by components of the ECM. Hence, the stroma and tumor microenvironment play important roles in cancer progression.

Tissue inhibitors of metalloproteinases (TIMPs) and plasminogen activator inhibitors (PAIs) represent two important families of inhibitors of MMPs and uPA, respectively.[104] The TIMP members are regulated by TGF-β and other cytokines, and they are made in endothelial cells and some tumor cells.[105] Of the TIMPs, TIMP-2 is able to bind to both latent and activated forms of type IV collagenase; this inhibitor essentially abolishes the hydrolytic activity of all members of the metalloproteinase family.[106] Additionally, TIMP-2 has the capability to inhibit growth factor–stimulated proliferation of transformed cells in culture.[107]

The ratio of proteolytic enzymes to their inhibitors determines tumor invasiveness. For example, a small tumor may remain noninvasive until there are a sufficient amount of proteolytic enzymes to overcome the inhibitors. This enzyme–inhibitor ratio has been used as a marker of metastasis for patients with breast cancer.[108]

Because neoplastic cells will invade all primary site tissue barriers, including the local endothelial basement membranes and the basement membranes of the target organ, an inhibitor of proteinase activity would be a likely candidate to interrupt metastasis.[109] Unfortunately, many inhibitors of MMPs have failed to yield positive clinical effects in patients with advanced cancer.[103] Use of uPA-based naturally occurring inhibitors has been limited by their toxicity at therapeutic levels and nonspecific effects such as inhibition of tissue plasminogen activator, which is essential for clot lysis.[110] A better understanding of these proteases and their inhibitors will facilitate the development of effective drugs to inhibit this mechanism of metastasis.[111]

Immunogenicity

A tumor cell's ability to elicit an immune response will determine its ability to evade the immune system. The theory of immune surveillance suggests that malignant cells develop randomly and often, but immune cells destroy cancer cells before they proliferate. Cytotoxic T lymphocytes, activated macrophages, and natural killer (NK) cells are thought to be the predominant immune cells that protect the body from cancer.[82,112] For cytotoxic T-cell activation, the tumor antigen must be presented by an antigen-presenting cell (APC) to the T cell. The APC cell, in turn, depends on the presentation of tumor-associated antigens on the tumor cell surface.

Natural killer cells are large, granular lymphocytes that can naturally lyse a broad range of tumor cell targets, even if they have not had prior exposure to the tumor cells. The exact mechanism of how NKs recognize tumor cells is not clear. Natural killer cells do not require APC presentation of an antigen for spontaneous cytolytic activity, but NK activation is prevented when class I MHC (major histocompatibility complex) molecules are expressed on the tumor cell surface.[82,112] Macrophages are the tissue-based counterparts to blood monocytes; their natural antitumor activity is enhanced when they are "activated" by various substances. For example, interleukin-2 can heighten the antitumor actions of cytotoxic T cells and NK cells,[112] while gamma-interferon is a classic activator of macrophages.

Tumor cells evade or hide from the immune system in a multitude of ways. Many tumors down-regulate MHC expression, thereby escaping detection. Other tumors secrete immunosuppressive factors such as TGF-β, which decreases T-cell proliferation. Tumor cells can release soluble antigens or intracellular adhesion molecules that block T-cell interactions with APC. Alternatively, tumor cells may develop variants with no recognizable antigenic structures.[113] Chemotherapy and radiation treatments may depress the immune system in general.

Metastasis Suppressor Genes

The identification of tumor suppressor genes prompted the search for metastasis suppressor genes. To date, eight such genes have been identified: *NM23, MKK4, KAI1, BRMS1, KiSS1, RHOGDI2, CRSP3,* and *VDUP1.* These genes affect important signal-transduction pathways, including mitogen-activated protein kinases, RHO, RAC, and G-protein–coupled and tyrosine kinase receptors.[114]

The Metastatic Cascade

The process of metastasis is complex and involves multiple steps called a metastatic cascade.[82] In the metastatic cascade, cells first detach from the primary tumor, and then motile cancer cells invade and enter the bloodstream or lymphatic vessels. If cancer cells are successful at evading the immune system, blood and lymph transport them to distant sites such as the bones, lungs, and liver. To invade normal tissues and establish metastatic colonies, the tumor cells again must penetrate the endothelium, degrade the underlying basement membrane, and induce angiogenesis. Many of the molecular mechanisms that tumor cells use facilitate this cascade of events.

Steps of the metastatic cascade

Detachment. Detachment from the primary tumor begins as a tumor grows and begins to press on the surrounding tissue and blood supply. Detachment is further accomplished by down-regulation of E-cadherin and the hypothesized "cadherin switch" to N-cadherin at the tumor cell surface. This change decreases cell–cell contacts, facilitating complete detachment from neighboring tumor cells.

Invasion. Tumor cells can invade the surrounding tissue, a lymphatic vessel, or a blood vessel. Direct extension into an adjacent tissue or lymphatic vessels is mediated by pressure that the enlarged tumor exerts on the tissue as well as by motility factors. Invasion is accomplished by secretion of proteolytic enzymes that are not overcome by local inhibitors. The secreted enzymes cause barrier breakdown and subsequent tumor invasion. If a tumor enters a vessel, the cells may localize at the entry site or disseminate to other destinations.

Survival in transport. In the bloodstream, tumor cells are at risk for destruction due to mechanical factors and attack by the immune system. It is estimated that only one in every 5000 to 15,000 tumor cells that enter the vasculature survive to give rise to a metastatic colony of cancer cells.[115] Tumor cells rely in part on survival-enhancing mechanisms (see "Immunogenicity" in the previous section) to evade the immune system.

Arrest in distant organ capillary bed. Arrest of tumor cells in an organ capillary bed requires that they adhere to the endothelial layer or become lodged in the microcirculation as a result of the geometry of the capillary bed. To maximize their ability to adhere to a distant blood vessel, malignant cells may secrete substances that cause platelets to aggregate around them, resulting in a large, sticky mass. In turn, platelets secrete growth factors that favor continued survival of the adjoining tumor cells.[85]

Exactly where circulating tumor cells adhere depends on certain factors that are not entirely clear at this time. Selective patterns of tumor spread are known to exist for different cancers, however. Cell–cell adhesion molecules expressed on the surface of tumor cells may influence which organs or sites certain tumors will favor, because corresponding adhesion molecules might be present within the microvasculature of distant organs.[85] This phenomenon helps explain why prostate carcinoma cells so often go to bone and ocular melanomas arrive in the liver, while typically sparing other organs.

In addition to selective target tissue adhesion, specific chemotactic factors or growth factors may attract circulating malignant cells to a particular site.[85] Neoplastic cells with a higher affinity for laminin tend to metastasize to lung tissue, whereas other tumor cells with a higher affinity for fibronectin favor settlement in the liver.[85] Specific chemotactic substances have been isolated from various organ sources, including lung, brain, bone, and liver. For instance, melanoma cells that had metastasized to the brain were found to respond in culture preferentially to brain-derived chemotactic factors.[116]

Establishment of secondary tumor. The proteolytic process of degrading the endothelial basement membrane to enter the secondary site essentially mimics the process used by the tumor cell to gain initial entrance into the vascular system. Although the process must be repeated in the secondary organ, the conditions in the new microenvironment may be very different. The tumor cell may have to adapt to changes in nutrients or the presence of stimulatory growth factors. Additionally, the immune profiles of primary and secondary tumor sites may be quite different. For example, levels of interleukin-4 and TNF-α were found to be higher in the primary site of human colon carcinomas compared with metastatic sites.[117]

Models of Invasion and Metastasis

A number of in vitro and in vivo models of metastasis have been developed and used to gain insight into the process of metastasis and to assist in the testing of agents and strategies to treat metastasis. An example of a simple test of the ability of drugs, antibodies, and genetic manipulations to perturb cancer invasiveness is the fibrin plug invasion assay, in which the endpoint is the number of cancer cells in the plug. More complex cell culture models use porous filters coated with an artificial basement membrane and suspended in a dual-chamber system. The coated filter can be covered with endothelial cells, and the ability of cancer cells placed in the top chamber to cross the endothelial cells can be determined by counting the numbers of cancer cells that enter the bottom chamber.

Rodent models of metastasis also exist. Some involve injecting cultured cancer cells into the heart or tail vein of the animal, then monitoring metastasis. The injection of genetically engineered cells permits a high degree of experimental control and manipulation so as to gain greater insight into the mechanisms underlying the metastatic cascade. New fluorescence-labeling agents and sophisticated detection systems enable the evaluation and monitoring of metastases in living animals over time. Another method, the orthotopic model, involves transplantation of a tumor under the skin of a rodent.

Treatment of Metastasis

Tremendous progress in prolonging survival from metastatic cancer has been made in some tumor types, such as testicular cancer, whereas little progress has been made in other tumor types, such as breast cancer. Greater emphasis is now being placed on the development of treatment strategies that abrogate various steps of the metastatic cascade. Agents that inhibit tumor cell motility and invasiveness will have key roles as antimetastatic therapies.

Current technology and advances in genomics now enable profiling of gene expression in tumors. In some cancers — for example, breast cancer — genetic signatures or profiles of tumors highly likely to metastasize are emerging. Such gene expression profiles will enable the development of more targeted treatments to prevent metastasis and assist in more thoroughly delineating the molecular mechanisms involved in metastasis.

Conclusion

The biology of cancer is a complex, continually evolving phenomenon, and one that is difficult to keep abreast of unless immersed in cancer bioscience. Because cancer biology underlies every other aspect of cancer as a human disease, nurses need to have a basic understanding of cancer genetics, molecular and cell biology, immunology, and biochemistry. The relationships among these sciences will help us prevent and treat cancers based on knowledge of cancer development, growth, and metastasis.

References

1. Doll R: Introduction, in Hiatt H, Watson JR, Winsten JA (eds): *Origins of Human Cancer*. Cold Spring Harbor, NY, Cold Spring Harbor Laboratory, 1977, pp 1–12
2. Trosko JE, Ruch RJ: Cell–cell communication in carcinogenesis. *Front Biosci* 3:D208–236, 1998
3. Moolgavkar SH, Luebeck EG: Multistage carcinogenesis and the incidence of human cancer. *Genes Chromosomes Cancer* 38:302–306, 2003
4. Jaffe LF: Epigenetic theories of cancer initiation. *Adv Cancer Res* 90:209–230, 2003
5. Nowell P: The clonal evolution of tumor cell populations. *Science* 194:23–28, 1976
6. Strachan T, Read AD: *Human Molecular Genetics*. New York, Wiley-Liss, 1996

7. Bellacosa A: Genetic hits and mutation rate in colorectal tumorigenesis: versatility of Knudson's theory and implications for cancer prevention. *Genes Chromosomes Cancer* 38:382–388, 2003
8. Hayflick L, Moorhead PS: The serial cultivation of human diploid cell strains. *Exp Cell Res* 25:585–621, 1961
9. Houck J, Sharma VK, Hayflick L: Functional failures of cultured human diploid fibroblasts after continued population doublings. *Proc Soc Exp Biol Med* 137:331–333, 1961
10. Jonkers J, Berns A: Conditional mouse models of sporadic cancer. *Nat Rev Cancer* 2:251–265, 2002
11. Oshima RG, Lesperance J, Munoz V, et al: Angiogenic acceleration of Neu induced mammary tumor progression and metastasis. *Cancer Res* 64:169–179, 2004
12. Tenen DG: Disruption of differentiation in human cancer: AML shows the way. *Nat Rev Cancer* 3:89–101, 2003
13. Banks DA, Fossel M: Telomeres, cancer, and aging. Altering the human life span. *JAMA* 278:1345–1348, 1997
14. Hakomori S: Cancer-associated glycosphingolipid antigens: their structure, organization, and function. *Acta Anatomica* 161:79–90, 1998
15. Birkle S, Zeng G, Gao L, et al: Role of tumor-associated gangliosides in cancer progression. *Biochimie* 85:455–463, 2003
16. Bissell MJ, Radisky D: Putting tumours in context. *Nat Rev Cancer* 1:46–54, 2001
17. Dranoff G: Cytokines in cancer pathogenesis and cancer therapy. *Nat Rev Cancer* 4:11–22, 2004
18. Egeblad M, Werb Z: New functions for the matrix metalloproteinases in cancer progression. *Nat Rev Cancer* 2:161–174, 2002
19. Hojilla CV, Mohammed FF, Khokha R: Matrix metalloproteinases and their tissue inhibitors direct cell fate during cancer development. *Br J Cancer* 89:1817–1821, 2003
20. Stamenkovic I: Extracellular matrix remodelling: the role of matrix metalloproteinases. *J Pathol* 200:448–464, 2003
21. Knudson AG Jr: Mutation and cancer: statistical study of retinoblastoma. *Proc Natl Acad Sci USA* 68:820–823, 1971
22. Jackson AL, Loeb LA: The mutation rate and cancer. *Genetics* 148:1483–1490, 1998
23. Simpson AJ: The natural somatic mutation frequency and human carcinogenesis. *Adv Cancer Res* 71:209–240, 1997
24. Tomlinson I, Bodmer W: Selection, the mutation rate and cancer: ensuring that the tail does not wag the dog. *Nat Med* 5:11–12, 1999
25. Strauss BS: Hypermutability in carcinogenesis. *Genetics* 148:1619–1626, 1998
26. Hu JJ, Mohrenweiser HW, Bell DA, et al: Symposium overview: genetic polymorphisms in DNA repair and cancer risk. *Toxicol Appl Pharmacol* 185:64–73, 2002
27. Loescher LJ: DNA testing for cancer predisposition. *Oncol Nurs Forum* 25:1317–1327, 1998
28. Hoeijmakers J: Genome maintenance mechanisms for preventing cancer. *Nature* 411:366–374, 2001
29. Cleaver J, Karplus EK, Kashani-Sabet M, et al: Nucleotide excision repair: a legacy of creativity. *Mutat Res* 485:23–26, 2001
30. Griffiths A, Miller JH, Suzuki DT, et al: *Introduction to Genetic Analysis.* New York, WH Freeman, 1996
31. Chakravarthi A: Single nucleotide polymorphisms . . . to a future of genetic medicine. *Nature* 409:822–823, 2001
32. Bartsch H, Rojas M, Alexandrov K, et al: Impact of adduct determination on the assessment of cancer susceptibility. *Recent Results Cancer Res* 154:86–96, 1998
33. Miller RD, Kwok PY: The birth and death of human single-nucleotide polymorphisms: new experimental evidence and implications for human history and medicine. *Hum Mol Genet* 10:2195–2198, 2001
34. GeneticsWeb C: Polymorphisms implicated in cancer susceptibility. *http://www.cancerindex.org/geneweb/gepidem.htm*, 2003
35. Bartsch H, Nair U, Risch A, et al: Genetic polymorphism of CYP genes, alone or in combination, as a risk modifier of tobacco-related cancers. *Cancer Epidemiol Biomarkers Prev* 9:3–28, 2000
36. Risch A, Wikman H, Thiel S, et al: Glutathione-S-transferase M1, M3, T1 and P1 polymorphisms and susceptibility to non-small-cell lung cancer subtypes and hamartomas. *Pharmacogenetics* 11:757–764, 2001
37. Godschalk RW, Dallinga JW, Wikman H, et al: Modulation of DNA and protein adducts in smokers by genetic polymorphisms in GSTM1,GSTT1, NAT1 and NAT2. *Pharmacogenetics* 11:389–398, 2001
38. Vineis P, Marinelli D, Autrup H, et al: Current smoking, occupation, N-acetyltransferase-2 and bladder cancer: a pooled analysis of genotype-based studies. *Cancer Epidemiol Biomarkers Prev* 10:1249–1252, 2001
39. Wikman H, Thiel S, Jager B, et al: Relevance of N-acetyltransferase 1 and 2 (NAT1, NAT2) genetic polymorphisms in non-small cell lung cancer susceptibility. *Pharmacogenetics* 11:157–168, 2001
40. Cooper G: *Oncogenes.* Sudbury, MA, Jones and Bartlett, 1995
41. Weinberg RA: How cancer arises. *Sci Am* 275:62–70, 1996
42. Cantly L, Auger KR, Carpenter C, et al: Oncogenes and signal transduction. *Cell* 64:281–302, 1991
43. Wong A, Ruppert JM, Bigner SH, et al: Structural alterations of the epidermal growth factor receptor gene in human gliomas. *Proc Natl Acad Sci USA* 89:2965–2969, 1992
44. Chin LS, Murray SF, Zitnay KM, et al: K252a inhibits proliferation of glioma cells by blocking platelet-derived growth factor signal transduction. *Clin Cancer Res* 3:771–776, 1997
45. Kitagawa Y, Ueda M, Ando N, et al: Further evidence for prognostic significance of epidermal growth factor receptor gene amplification in patients with esophageal squamous cell carcinoma. *Clin Cancer Res* 2:909–914, 1996
46. Nicholson RI, Gee JM, Harper ME: EGFR and cancer prognosis. *Eur J Cancer* 37 (suppl 4):PS,9–15, 2001
47. Radinsky R, Risin F, et al: Level and function of epidermal growth factor receptor predict the metastatic potential of human colon carcinoma cells. *Clin Cancer Res* 1:19–31, 1995
48. Naidu R, Yadav M, Nair S, et al: Expression of c-erbB3 protein in primary breast carcinomas. *Br J Cancer* 78:1385–1390, 1998
49. Tsuda H, Sakamaki C, Tsugane S, et al: A prospective study of the significance of gene and chromosome alterations as prognostic indicators of breast cancer patients with lymph node metastases. *Breast Cancer Res Treat* 48:21–32, 1998
50. Ross JS, Fletcher JA, Linette GP, et al: The Her-2/neu gene and protein in breast cancer 2003: biomarker and target of therapy. *Oncologist* 8:307–325, 2003
51. Kita K, Saito S, Morioka CY, et al: Growth inhibition of human pancreatic cancer cell lines by anti-sense oligonucleotides specific to mutated K-ras genes. *Int J Cancer* 80:553–558, 1999
52. Papavassiliou AG: Molecular medicine. Transcription factors. *N Engl J Med* 332:45–47, 1995
53. Latchman DS: Transcription-factor mutations and disease. *N Engl J Med* 334:28–33, 1996
54. Weinberg RA: Oncogenes and tumor suppressor genes. *CA: Cancer J Clin* 44:160–170, 1994
55. Kinzler KW, Vogelstein B: Cancer-susceptibility genes. Gatekeepers and caretakers. *Nature* 386:761, 763, 1997
56. Cama A, Genuardi M, Guanti G, et al: Molecular genetics of hereditary non-polyposis colorectal cancer (HNPCC). *Tumori* 82:122–135, 1996

57. Picard SF, Franco N, Sergent C, et al: Analysis of microsatellite instability in acquired drug-resistance human tumor cell lines. *Oncol Rep* 9:971–976, 2002
58. Solomon E, Borrow J, Goddard AD: Chromosome aberrations and cancer. *Science* 254:1153–1160, 1991
59. Sen S: Aneuploidy and cancer. *Curr Opin Oncol* 12:82–88, 2000
60. Pathak S, Multani AS, Furlong CL, et al: Telomere dynamics, aneuploidy, stem cells, and cancer (review). *Int J Oncol* 20:637–641, 2002
61. Brown T: *Genomes.* New York, Bios Scientific, 2002
62. Hanahan D, Weinberg RA: The hallmarks of cancer. *Cell* 100:57–70, 2000
63. Hartwell LH, Kastan MB: Cell cycle control and cancer. *Science* 266:1821–1828, 1994
64. Pollard T, Earnshaw W: *Cell Biology.* New York, Saunders, 2002
65. Orr-Weaver TL, Weinberg RA: A checkpoint on the road to cancer. *Nature* 392:223–224, 1998
66. Lydon A, Martyn JA: Apoptosis in critical illness. *Int Anesthesiol Clin* 41:65–77, 2003
67. Martin TR, Nakamura M, Matute-Bello G: The role of apoptosis in acute lung injury. *Crit Care Med* 31:PS,184–188, 2003
68. Smith ND, Rubenstein JN, Eggener SE, et al: The p53 tumor suppressor gene and nuclear protein: basic science review and relevance in the management of bladder cancer. *J Urol* 169:1219–1228, 2003
69. Kim R, Tanabe K, Emi M, et al: Inducing cancer cell death by targeting transcription factors. *Anticancer Drugs* 14:3–11, 2003
70. Wyllie AH: Apoptosis and carcinogenesis. *Eur J Cell Biol* 73:189–197, 1997
71. Younes A, Kadin ME: Emerging applications of the tumor necrosis factor family of ligands and receptors in cancer therapy. *J Clin Oncol* 21:3526–3534, 2003
72. Hollstein M, Rice K, Greenblatt MS, et al: Database of p53 gene somatic mutations in human tumors and cell lines. *Nucleic Acids Res* 22:3551–3555, 1994
73. Lowe SW, Schmitt EM, Smith SW, et al: p53 is required for radiation-induced apoptosis in mouse thymocytes. *Nature* 362:847–849, 1993
74. Coultas L, Strasser A: The role of the Bcl-2 protein family in cancer. *Semin Cancer Biol* 13:115–123, 2003
75. Wajant H, Pfizenmaier K, Scheurich P: TNF-related apoptosis inducing ligand (TRAIL) and its receptors in tumor surveillance and cancer therapy. *Apoptosis* 7:449–459, 2002
76. Nagata S: Fas-induced apoptosis. *Intern Med* 37:179–181, 1998
77. Wajant H, Pfizenmaier K, Scheurich P: Non-apoptotic Fas signaling. *Cytokine Growth Factor Rev* 14:53–66, 2003
78. Wajant H: Targeting the FLICE Inhibitory Protein (FLIP) in cancer therapy. *Mol Interv* 3:124–127, 2003
79. Yang HH, Ma MH, Vescio RA, et al: Overcoming drug resistance in multiple myeloma: the emergence of therapeutic approaches to induce apoptosis. *J Clin Oncol* 21:4239–4247, 2003
80. Shangary S, Johnson DE: Recent advances in the development of anticancer agents targeting cell death inhibitors in the Bcl-2 protein family. *Leukemia* 17:1470–1481, 2003
81. Bogenrieder T, Herlyn M: Axis of evil: molecular mechanisms of cancer metastasis. *Oncogene* 22:6524–6536, 2003
82. Tannock I: Tumor progression and metastasis, in Tannock I, Hill R (eds): *The Basic Science of Oncology.* New York, McGraw-Hill, 1998, pp 219–262
83. Jiang WG, Puntis MC, Hallett MB: Molecular and cellular basis of cancer invasion and metastasis: implications for treatment. *Br J Surg* 81:1576–1590, 1994
84. Heppner GH, Miller FR: The cellular basis of tumor progression. *Int Rev Cytol* 177:1–56, 1998
85. Ruoslahti E: How cancer spreads. *Sci Am* 275:72–77, 1996
86. Lawler J, Detmar M: Tumor progression: the effects of thrombospondin-1 and -2. *Int J Biochem Cell Biol* 36:1038–1045, 2004
87. Folkman J, D'Amore PA: Blood vessel formation: what is its molecular basis? *Cell* 87:1153–1155, 1996
88. Morabito A, Magnani E, Gion M, et al: Prognostic and predictive indicators in operable breast cancer. *Clin Breast Cancer* 3:381–390, 2003
89. Sauer G, Deissler H: Angiogenesis: prognostic and therapeutic implications in gynecologic and breast malignancies. *Curr Opin Obstet Gynecol* 15:45–49, 2003
90. Weidner N, Semple JP, Welch WR, et al: Tumor angiogenesis and metastasis — correlation in invasive breast carcinoma. *N Engl J Med* 324:1–8, 1991
91. Jain RK: Molecular regulation of vessel maturation. *Nat Med* 9:685–693, 2003
92. Strauli P, Haemmerli G: The role of cancer cell motility in invasion. *Cancer Metastasis Rev* 3:127–141, 1984
93. Hendrix MJ, Seftor EA, Chu YW, et al: Role of intermediate filaments in migration, invasion and metastasis. *Cancer Metastasis Rev* 15:507–525, 1996
94. Friedl P, Wolf K: Tumour-cell invasion and migration: diversity and escape mechanisms. *Nat Rev Cancer* 3:362–374, 2003
95. Okegawa T, Li Y, Pong RC, et al: Cell adhesion proteins as tumor suppressors. *J Urol* 167:1836–1843, 2002
96. Mareel M, Leroy A: Clinical, cellular, and molecular aspects of cancer invasion. *Physiol Rev* 83:337–376, 2003
97. Mason M, Davies G, Jiang WG: Cell adhesion molecules and adhesion abnormalities in prostate cancer. *Oncol Hematol* 41:11–28, 2002
98. Cavallaro U, Schaffhauser B, Cristofori G: Cadherins and the tumour progression: is it all in a switch? *Cancer Letters* 176:123–128, 2002
99. Christofori G: Changing neighbours, changing behaviour: cell adhesion molecule–mediated signalling during tumour progression. *EMBO J* 22:2318–2323, 2003
100. Cooper CR, Chay CH, Pienta KJ: The role of alpha(v)beta(3) in prostate cancer progression. *Neoplasia* 4:191–194, 2002
101. Chambers AF, Matrisian LM: Changing views of the role of matrix metalloproteinases in metastasis. *J Natl Cancer Inst* 89:1260–1270, 1997
102. Choong PF, Nadesapillai AP: Urokinase plasminogen activator system: a multifunctional role in tumor progression and metastasis. *Clin Orthop* 415(suppl): S46–58, 2003
103. Pavlaki M, Zucker S: Matrix metalloproteinase inhibitors (MMPIs): the beginning of phase I or the termination of phase III clinical trials. *Cancer Metastasis Rev* 22:177–203, 2003
104. Gottesman M: The role of proteases in cancer. *Semin Cancer Biol* 1:97–160, 1990
105. Boone TC, Johnson MJ, De Clerck YA, et al: cDNA cloning and expression of a metalloproteinase inhibitor related to tissue inhibitor of metalloproteinases. *Proc Natl Acad Sci USA* 87:2800–2804, 1990
106. Goldberg GI, Marmer BL, Grant GA, et al: Human 72-kilodalton type IV collagenase forms a complex with a tissue inhibitor of metalloproteases designated TIMP-2. *Proc Natl Acad Sci USA* 86:8207–8211, 1989
107. Corcoran ML, Stetler-Stevenson WG: Tissue inhibitor of metalloproteinase-2 stimulates fibroblast proliferation via a cAMP-dependent mechanism. *J Biol Chem* 270:13453–13459, 1995
108. Alessandro R, Kohn EC: Molecular genetics of cancer. Tumor invasion and angiogenesis. *Cancer* 76:1874–1877, 1995
109. DeClerck YA, Imren S: Protease inhibitors: role and potential therapeutic use in human cancer. *Eur J Cancer* 30A:2170–2180, 1994

110. Chorostowska-Wynimko J, Swiercz R, Skrzypczak-Jankun E, et al: A novel form of the plasminogen activator inhibitor created by cysteine mutations extends its half-life: relevance to cancer and angiogenesis. *Mol Cancer Ther* 2:19–28, 2003
111. Yana I, Seiki M: MT-MMPs play pivotal roles in cancer dissemination. *Clin Exp Metastasis* 19:209–215, 2002
112. Brittenden J, Heys SD, Ross J, et al: Natural killer cells and cancer. *Cancer* 77:1226–1243, 1996
113. Nicholson G: Molecular mechanisms of cancer metastasis: tumor and host properties and the role of oncogenes and suppressor genes. *Curr Opin Oncol* 3:75–92, 1991
114. Steeg PS: Metastasis suppressors alter the signal transduction of cancer cells. *Nat Rev Cancer* 3:55–63, 2003
115. Alberts B, Johnson A, Lewis T, et al: *Molecular Biology of the Cell.* New York, Garland Science (Taylor-Francis Group), 2002
116. Hujanen ES, Terranova VP: Migration of tumor cells to organ-derived chemoattractants. *Cancer Res* 45:3517–3521, 1985
117. Barth RJ Jr., Camp BJ, Martuscello TA, et al: The cytokine microenvironment of human colon carcinoma. Lymphocyte expression of tumor necrosis factor-alpha and interleukin-4 predicts improved survival. *Cancer* 78:1168–1178, 1996

CHAPTER 2

Immunology

Susan M. Bauer-Wu, DNSc, RN
Janice Post-White, RN, PhD, FAAN

Introduction

Through understanding the immune system and factors that affect its function, oncology nurses can play an important role in promoting optimal immunologic responses and in preventing clinical complications in the patient with cancer. This chapter provides a basic review of immunology, including components of the immune system, key immunologic processes, and clinical implications. Cancer diagnosis and treatment are identified in conjunction with changes in immune function. For example, suppressed or inadequate immune processes are associated with the development of some cancers, while chemotherapeutic drugs and radiation therapy used to treat cancer can induce immunosuppression. Other cancer therapies, such as biotherapies, can selectively enhance the body's own immune system to fight off cancer. In addition, behavioral factors, such as nutrition, exercise, sleep, and stress, can affect immunologic functioning.

Overview

The immune system provides the body's defense against infectious and malignant disease. It is a complex arrangement of cells, tissues, and soluble mediators. Two overall functions of the immune system are to recognize foreign substances (nonself) and to eliminate the foreign substances with restoration of homeostasis.[1] Foreign organisms that invade the body are called *antigens* and initiate immune responses.

Immune responses may be either innate or adaptive.[1] *Innate immunity,* considered the body's first line of defense, provides nonspecific responses to foreign substances. Inflammation and phagocytosis are examples of such nonspecific responses. Phagocytosis involves general recognition and engulfment of foreign organisms.

Adaptive, or acquired, immunity differs from innate immunity in that it is highly specific for particular antigens. This type of immunity has memory, referred to as *anamnesis,* meaning that the responses improve with each successive encounter with the same antigen.[1] Humoral and cell-mediated immune responses are interdependent functional arms that fall within the domain of adaptive immunity. The specificity and memory associated with acquired immunity form the basis of vaccination to control certain diseases.

Immune responses can be characterized as appropriate, deficient, or overreactive. An *appropriate immune response* results in the elimination of antigen and the restoration of homeostasis with memory. *Immune deficiency* is an underreactivity of the immune processes, characterized by a pattern of repeated infections with a single organism. *Overreactive or inappropriate immune responses* are classified into three categories: (1) allergy, which involves inappropriate responses to innocuous foreign substances; (2) autoimmunity, which are responses to self-tissue antigens; and (3) graft rejection, as a result of transplanted organs.[1] The quality of immune responsiveness is quite variable and depends on myriad circumstances, such as genetics, age, medications, health behaviors, and environmental factors.

Components of the Immune System

Structures of the Immune System

Structures of the immune system are categorized as either primary or secondary lymphoid organs and tissues (Figure 2-1). The *primary lymphoid organs* are the anatomical locations in which lymphocytes develop immunocompetence: the bone marrow for B cells and the thymus for T cells.[1] *Secondary lymphoid organs* and tissues are where cellular and humoral responses take place. The spleen, lymph nodes, tonsils, Peyer's patches in the gastrointestinal tract, and the bone marrow are considered both primary and secondary lymphoid organs. The spleen responds to predominantly blood-borne antigens; lymph nodes mount immune responses to antigens circulating in the lymph system; and tonsils and Peyer's patches respond to antigens that have penetrated the mucosal barriers.

Cells of the Immune System

The cells of the immune system, *leukocytes,* arise from the pluripotent hematopoietic stem cells of the bone marrow, which give rise to two identified cell lines: myeloid and lymphoid (Figure 2-2). Immune cells are distinguished from one another through the expression of different surface molecules, or markers, referred to as clusters of differentiation (CD). Different markers may be characteristic of different lineages, of different stages of cell maturation, or of the presence of cell activation. An immune cell may have more than one marker, or CD number, associated with it.[1]

The myeloid lineage

The myeloid lineage produces monocytes, polymorphonuclear leukocytes (neutrophils, eosinophils, and basophils/mast cells), and platelets.[1] *Monocytes* are circulating leukocytes that give rise to the mononuclear phagocyte system, which includes the following: Kupffer cells in the liver, intraglomerular mesangium of the kidney, alveolar macrophages in the lung,

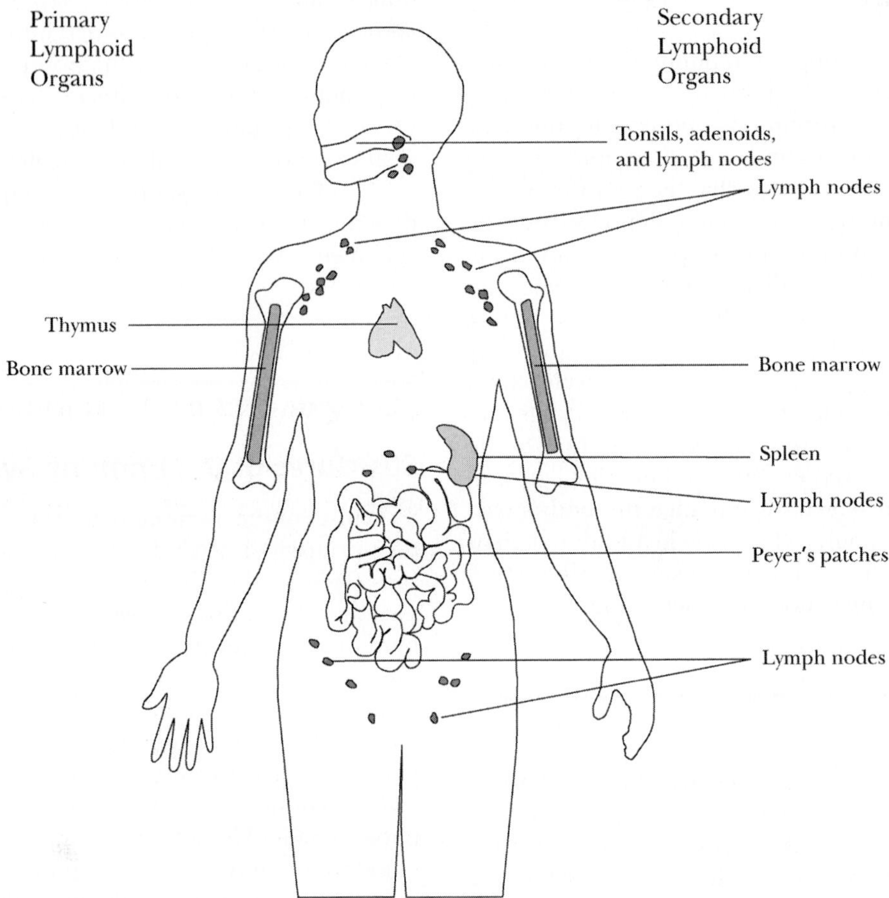

Figure 2-1 Primary and secondary lymphoid organs.

serosal macrophages, brain microglia, spleen sinus macrophages, and lymph node sinus macrophages. These cells play important roles in both innate and adaptive responses and have two main functions: (1) "professional" phagocytic macrophages remove particulate antigens; and (2) antigen-presenting cells (APCs) present antigen to lymphocytes.[1]

Polymorphonuclear granulocytes (polymorphs) make up 60%–70% of the total normal blood leukocytes but are also found in extravascular sites. They are rapidly produced in the bone marrow at a rate of about 80 million per minute and are relatively short-lived (two to three days) compared to monocytes/macrophages, which may live for months or years. *Neutrophils* constitute more than 90% of the circulating polymorphs. Their primary role is phagocytosis. Neutrophils are considered the cells providing the body's first line of defense. Significant loss of neutrophils, or neutropenia, can pose a serious threat to cancer patients receiving immunosuppressive therapies.

Eosinophils are polymorphs that constitute 2%–5% of blood leukocytes in healthy, nonallergic individuals. They play a role in dampening the inflammatory response but are also capable of phagocytosing and killing microorganisms. Eosinophils appear to play a specialized role in immunity to parasites and nematodes. Through a degranulating mechanism, eosinophils adhere to worm larva; granules then release a toxic protein substance.

Basophils constitute less than 0.2% of circulating leukocytes. *Mast cells* are indistinguishable from basophils, although the former are resident only in body tissues (i.e., mucosal epithelia and connective tissue). Basophils and mast cells play key roles in allergic responses through a degranulation process involving the release of histamine.

Although *platelets* are not leukocytes, they are derived from the myeloid lineage (megakaryocytes) and play important roles in various aspects of the immune response, in addition to their chief role in coagulation. Following damage to endothelial cells, platelets adhere to and aggregate at the surface of the damaged vascular tissue. They release mediators that increase

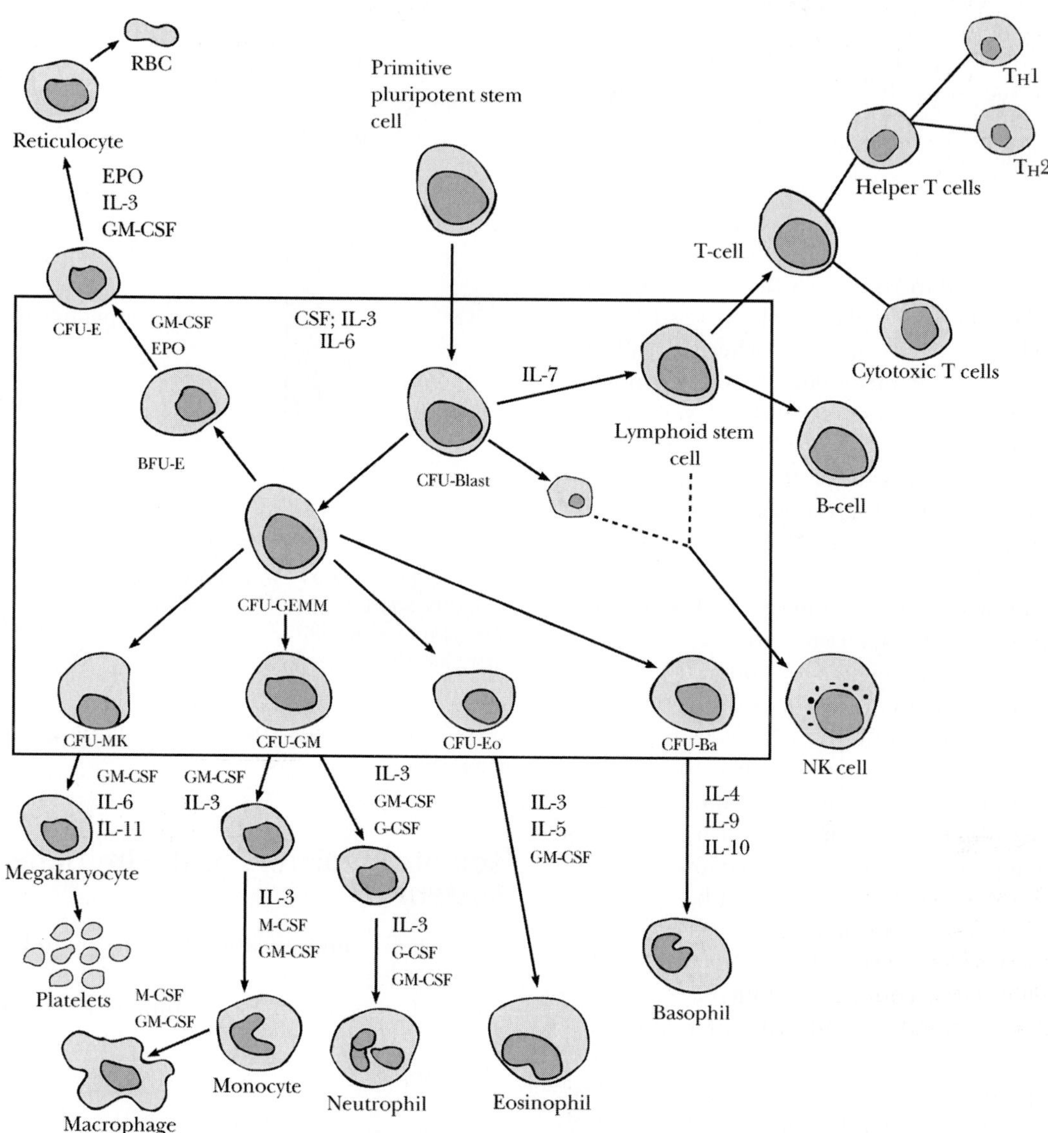

Figure 2-2 The hematologic cascade. Ba = basophil; BFU = burst-forming unit; CFU = colony-forming unit; CFU-GEMM = colony-forming unit-granulocyte/erythrocyte/monocyte/megakaryocyte; CSF = colony-stimulating factor; Eo = eosinophil; EPO = erythropoietin; G = granulocyte; GM = granulocyte/macrophage; M = macrophage; MK = megakaryocyte; NK = natural killer; RBC = red blood cells/erythrocytes; T_H = helper T cells.

permeability and activate complement, and therefore attract leukocytes.

The lymphoid lineage

The lymphoid lineage produces B lymphocytes (B cells), T lymphocytes (T cells), and large granular lymphocytes (LGL) called natural killer (NK) cells. *B cells,* so named because they were originally discovered in the bursa of birds, play a major role in the humoral arm of adaptive immunity through the production of antibodies, also called *immunoglobulins.*[1] On activation, B cells become antibody-secreting plasma cells. They have a less important role in the cell-mediated arm of adaptive immunity.

T cells, so named because they mature in the thymus, play the major role in cell-mediated immune responses and a less important role in humoral responses. Cell-mediated immunity provides the body's defense against intracellular viruses, transplanted tissue, tumor cells, fungi, and protozoa. T cells recognize antigen not in its intact form, as it is recognized by B cells, but rather as peptide fragments that are bound to cell-surface molecules, called *major histocompatibility complex* (MHC) molecules.[1] T cells have specialized receptors that recognize the antigenic fragments bound to a MHC molecule. Two classes of the MHC molecule exist: MHC class I and MHC class II.

T cells ($CD3^+$) are divided into three general subpopulations: helper T cells (T_H), suppressor T (T_S) cells, and cytotoxic T (T_C) cells. Helper T cells ($CD4^+$), which are restricted to MHC class II, are differentiated into two types: T_H1 cells play a role in the enhancement of cell-mediated responses, whereas T_H2 cells play a role in the enhancement of antibody production in humoral responses. Suppressor T cells, in general, act to shut off T_H2 when sufficient antibody has been produced. Cytotoxic T cells ($CD8^+$), which are restricted to MHC class I, are capable of recognizing and destroying specific target cells, usually virus infected cells, through cell–cell contact.

Natural killer cells are considered LGL because of their morphologic characteristics: distinct granules in the cytoplasm, a kidney-shaped indented nucleus, high nuclear–cytoplasmic ratio, and low density.[1] These characteristics distinguish NK cells from other lymphocytes. Natural killer cells appear to arise from stem cells other than the common lymphoid progenitors; however, this relationship is not clear. Maturation of NK cells depends on intact bone marrow but not on thymus. Although expression of a number of surface molecules has been identified on NK cells, the major marker characteristics are $CD16^+$, $CD56^+$, and $CD3^-$. Natural killer cells account for as much as 15% of peripheral blood lymphocytes. In addition to circulating in the blood, other locations of human NK cells include the spleen, tonsils, interstitial lung space, intestinal mucosa, and liver; mature NK cells are virtually absent in bone marrow. Natural killer cells, so named because of early identification of their activity of innate, non–MHC-restricted cytotoxicity of malignant and virally infected cells, play key roles in tumor surveillance and natural resistance against certain microbial infections.

Dendritic cells, also called interdigitating reticular cells, are not lymphocytes per se, yet their activity and locations connect them to the lymphoid system. Dendritic cells are found in T-cell areas of lymphoid tissue, are potent stimulators of T-cell responses,[1] and are considered the most powerful APCs. Because dendritic cells effectively deliver tumor-specific antigens and induce tumor-specific immune responses, they are useful for cancer immunotherapy. Genetically modified dendritic cell vaccination is a promising cancer treatment, with recent evidence of effectiveness for different solid tumors and hematologic malignancies.[2–4]

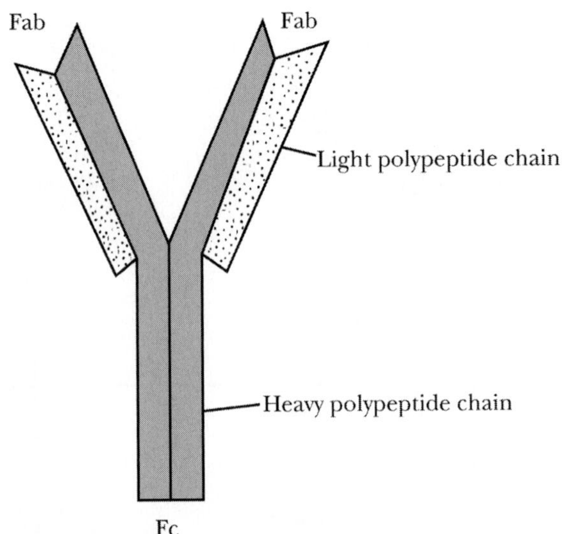

Figure 2-3 Basic antibody structure consists of a Y shape having two heavy and two light polypeptide chains, two antigen receptors (Fab), and one crystalline receptor (Fc) for binding to host cells or to soluble mediators.

Soluble Mediators of the Immune System

Cell-to-cell communication occurs due to the production and secretion of, and receptors for, various soluble mediators. Examples of soluble mediators include antibodies, cytokines, serum proteins, and prostaglandins.

Antibodies

Antibodies, also called immunoglobulins (Ig), are serum glycoproteins that have specificity to particular antigens. Each antibody is Y-shaped and consists of three fragments (Figure 2-3). Two identical fragments are for antigen-binding (Fab), and one crystalline fragment (Fc) is for nonspecific binding to other cells or soluble mediators of the immune system. The antibody molecule consists of four polypeptide chains: two identical light chains and two identical heavy chains. Both the light and the heavy chains are further divided into variable and constant regions. The sequencing of the amino acids, particularly with the heavy chains, determines the class of antibody, given here in decreasing order of abundance: IgG, IgA, IgM, IgE, IgD.[1]

IgG (γ) is the most abundant antibody, accounting for approximately 75% of serum antibodies. It is the only antibody able to cross the placenta. IgG is the major antibody produced in a secondary immune response. It consists of four subclasses. IgG is involved in the activation of complement as well as in binding of phagocytes.

IgA (α) is present in both serum and seromucous secretions, playing a key role in secretory immunity in response to upper respiratory infections. It represents about 15%–20% of the total serum antibody and consists of two subclasses.

IgM (μ) constitutes approximately 10% of serum antibodies. It is the major antibody expressed on B cells and the chief antibody in primary immune responses. IgM is also considered to be the most efficient activator of complement.

IgE (ϵ) accounts for less than 0.004% of serum antibodies. It binds to the Fc receptors on basophils and mast cells, playing the principle role in most hypersensitivity reactions.

IgD (δ) makes up less than 1% of serum antibodies. It is primarily expressed on B cells (along with IgM) and is a major B cell activator.

Cytokines

Cytokine is a general term for chemical (peptide) substances produced by a variety of immune cells, which serve to mediate the activity of other cells.[1,5] Examples of types of cytokines include interleukins (IL), interferons (IF), tumor necrosis factors (TNF), and colony-stimulating factors (CSF). Table 2-1 provides an overview of the more common cytokines. Pro-inflammatory cytokines (including IL-1α, IL-1β, TNF-α, IL-6) constitute a specific group of cytokines that cross the blood–brain barrier and cause "sickness behaviors" — symptoms of illness that include fever, hypersomnia, depressed activity, weakness, malaise, inability to concentrate, and memory loss. Interleukin-1 causes fever, pain and inflammation, slow wave sleep, and profound effects on learning, memory, and behavior.[5,6] Although intended to be restorative and adaptive, these cytokines create symptoms that can be prolonged in patients with cancer.

Serum proteins

Serum concentration levels of certain proteins increase during infection and are therefore called *acute-phase proteins.* Two key serum proteins are *C-reactive protein* (CRP) and *complement.*

C-reactive protein binds to and coats bacteria, while promoting the binding of complement and phagocytosis.[1] The complement system is a group of approximately 20 serum proteins whose overall function is to control inflammation and remove pathogens. Two mechanisms to activate the complement system exist: the alternate pathway and the classical pathway. The *alternate pathway,* which relies on CRP, is an innate, nonspecific reaction in response to antigen trigger, leading to complement coating a microorganism and subsequent uptake by phagocytes. The *classical pathway* is a specific, adaptive response activated by antibodies. The major mechanisms of the classical complement pathway include (1) opsonization (coating) of microorganisms for uptake by phagocytes; (2) chemotaxis, the attraction of phagocytes to sites of infection; (3) increased vascularity to the site of activation with increased permeability of capillaries to plasma molecules; and (4) damage to plasma membranes on cells or pathogens that have induced the activation, leading to lysis.[1]

Prostaglandins

Prostaglandins are important mediators involved in inflammation. They are major end products of arachidonic acid metabolism produced from inflammatory immune cells, such as monocytes/macrophages and basophils/mast cells, and triggering of IL-1. Prostaglandins are thought to be the central mediators triggering central nervous system responses to inflammatory processes, as they are small and lipophilic and are able to cross the blood–brain barrier. Further evidence comes from the inhibition of prostaglandins, and amelioration of the systemic sickness behaviors, produced by cyclooxygenase (COX) inhibitors.[7,8] Prostaglandins also increase platelet aggregation and inhibit the effects of heparin on smooth muscle cells and vascular endothelial cells.[9]

Mechanisms of Adaptive Immunity

Humoral and cell-mediated immune responses, involving both B cells and T cells, are interdependent functional arms that fall within the domain of adaptive immunity, as illustrated in Figure 2-4.

Humoral Immune Response

Humoral responses play important roles in the body's defense against extracellular pathogens (bacteria and some viruses) as well as in certain hypersensitivity reactions.[1] The main mechanism in humoral immune responses involves the binding of antibodies to antigens. B cells play a key role in these processes through the production of antibodies.

Two proliferative steps take place before antibody production can occur: clonal diversity and clonal selection.[1] *Clonal diversity* takes place in the bone marrow and is antigen independent and hormonally driven. It

Table 2-1 Cytokines: Sources and Main Functions

Type	Source	Major Functions
	INTERLEUKINS (IL)	
IL-1 (α and β)	Predominantly macrophages, T_H2	Activates T cells and B cells; inflammatory mediator (pro-inflammatory cytokine); crosses blood–brain barrier (BBB); ↑ glucocorticoids, ↓ dopamine, serotonin; fever and "sickness behaviors"
IL-2 (T-cell growth factor [TCGF])	T_H1 cells, NK cells	↑ T-cell proliferation and differentiation; ↑ cytolytic activity of NK cells and production of LAK cells; activates B cells to ↑ Ig
IL-3 (multi-CSF)	Predominantly T_H1 and T_H2 cells	↑ Production and differentiation of hematopoietic progenitor cells
IL-4 (B-cell growth factor)	T_H2 cells, T cells, macrophages, mast cells, B cells, basophils	Differentiation of $T_H0 \rightarrow T_H2$; induces proliferation and differentiation of B cells
IL-6	T_H2 cells, monocytes/macrophages, fibroblasts, hepatocytes, endothelial and neuronal cells	Activates hematopoietic progenitor cells; induces maturation and ↑ platelet number; ↑ growth and/or differentiation of various cells; ↑ acute-phase protein release
IL-7	Bone marrow stromal cells, fetal liver cells	↑ Proliferation and cytotoxic activity of T_C cells and LAK cells; support the growth of pre-B cells and proliferation of T cells
IL-8 (neutrophil chemotactic factor)	Monocytes, macrophages, endothelial cells	↑ Chemotactic activity of neutrophils, T cells, and basophils; ↑ phagocytic activity of neutrophils
IL-10 (cytokine synthesis inhibitory factor [CSIF])	T_H2 cells, macrophages, B cells	↓ Pro-inflammatory cytokine release of macrophages; inhibits T_H1; ↑ B-cell proliferation and Ig production
IL-12	Macrophages, B cells	Initiates cell-mediated immunity by inducing differentiation of $T_H0 \rightarrow T_H1$; ↑ growth and activity of NK and T_C cells
	INTERFERONS (IFN)	
IFN-α	T cells, B cells, macrophages	Antiviral activity; modulates MHC class I and II expression on various cells; ↓ B-cell proliferation, ↓ macrophage activity and production of IL-8
IFN-β	Fibroblasts, epithelial cells, macrophages	Antiviral activity; ↑ IL-6; ↓ IL-8
IFN-γ	T_H1 cells, T cells, NK cells	Activates NK cells; antiviral activity; ↑ MHC class I and II expression on macrophages; ↑ B-cell differentiation; ↑ macrophage activity
	TUMOR NECROSIS FACTOR (TNF)	
TNF-α (cachectin)	T_H1 cells neutrophils, activated lymphocytes, NK cells, fibroblasts, endothelial cells, malignant cells	↑ Macrophage activity; ↑ cytokines from NK cells; mediates expression of genes for growth factors and cytokines, inflammatory mediators, acute-phase proteins, and transcription factors
TNF-β (lymphotoxin)	T cells, malignant cells	Similar to TNF-α

(continued)

Table 2-1 Cytokines: Sources and Main Functions (continued)

Type	Source	Major Functions
	COLONY-STIMULATING FACTORS (CSF)	
Granulocyte CSF (G-CSF)	T cells, macrophages, neutrophils, endothelial cells, fibroblasts	↑ Differentiation and activation of neutrophils
Granulocyte-macrophage CSF (GM-CSF)	Macrophages, T cells, endothelial cells, polymorphs	↑ Growth and differentiation of multipotential progenitor cells; stimulates all cells in myeloid lineage
Macrophage CSF (M-CSF)	T cells, macrophages, neutrophils, fibroblasts, endothelial cells	↑ Growth and development of macrophage colonies; stimulates various functions of monocytes and macrophages
	OTHERS	
Transforming growth factors (TGF): α and β	Macrophages, malignant cells, other cells	Stimulates macrophages, ↑ fibroblasts, ↑ epithelial development and angiogenic activity, ↓ growth of various other cells
Stem cell factor (SCF)	Bone marrow stromal cells, epithelial cells, fibroblasts	Stimulates growth of myeloid, erythroid, and lymphoid progenitors; stimulates growth and proliferation of mast cells
Erythropoietin (EPO)	Liver, kidneys, macrophages	Stimulates growth and differentiation of erythroid progenitors; ↑ red blood cell production

↑, Increased; ↓, Decreased. See text for other abbreviations.

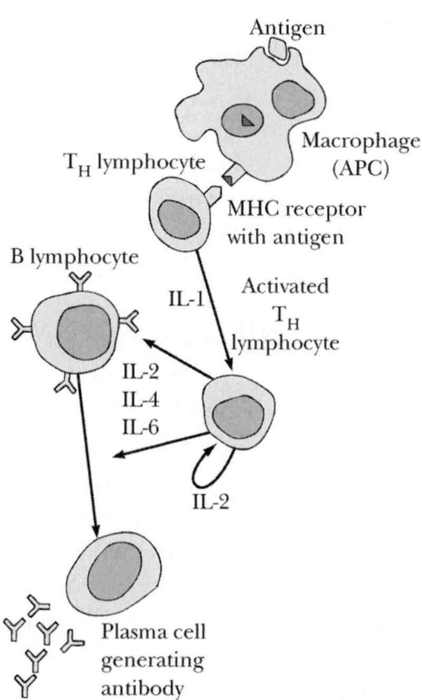

Figure 2-4 Major components of adaptive immune response. APC = antigen-presenting cell; T_H = helper T lymphocyte.

results in the generation of immature but immunocompetent B cells, with plasma-membrane receptors that can recognize any antigenic molecule. *Clonal selection,* the second step, occurs in secondary lymphoid organs such as the spleen and lymph nodes. Antigens can stimulate B cells to become antibody-producing plasma cells either with or without the help of T cells; the latter are called *T-independent antigens.*

When a B cell encounters a specific antigen, it matures and proliferates into plasma cells and a set of memory B cells. Plasma cells are active during the primary immune response; IgM is the main antibody produced during this phase. Memory B cells are active in secondary responses that occur on future exposure to the antigen and are responsible for long-term immunity. Gamma-immunoglobulin is the predominant antibody in secondary responses. Class switching of antibodies from IgG to other classes or subclasses occurs with the help of cytokines released by a type of helper T cells (T_H2).[1]

Antibody–antigen processes

An antibody circulates in the blood or in lymph fluid, or is suspended in body secretions until encountering and binding to its particular antigen. Binding of antigen (by antigenic-determinant sites) to the Fab portions of the antibody results in antigen–antibody complexes, also called *immune complexes.*[1] The class of the antibody and specific characteristics of the antigen determine subsequent processes. Most humoral immune responses are polyclonal; however, monoclonal antibodies generated in laboratories are single antibodies of known specificity that play important roles in clinical therapeutics and diagnostics with cancer patients.

In general, antibodies function to target extracellular pathogens and their products for disposal by phagocytes, particularly macrophages and neutrophils. Antibodies play three major roles: (1) they neutralize bacterial and viral toxins; (2) they opsonize (or coat) bacteria; and (3) they activate complement.[1] In *neutralization,* antibodies bind to and neutralize toxins, thereby preventing interactions with host cells that can cause pathology. Unbound toxin can react with receptors on host cells, whereas antigen–antibody complexes cannot. These immune complexes are then typically scavenged and degraded by macrophages. In *opsonization,* an antibody literally coats an antigen, rendering it recognizable as foreign by macrophages and polymorphonuclear leukocytes. These phagocytes then destroy and ingest the antibody-coated antigen complex. Finally, bound antibodies to antigens form a receptor to activate the first protein of the complement system, C3. This activation eventually forms a protein complex on the surface of the pathogen that favors its uptake and destruction by phagocytes.[1]

Cell-Mediated Immune Response

T cells are responsible for cell-mediated immunity, although interaction between both T cells and B cells oftentimes occurs. Maturation and initial proliferation of T cells take place in the thymus in processes similar to clonal diversity for B cells. While journeying through the thymus, lymphocytes destined to become T cells proliferate and develop the capacity to recognize a huge spectrum of antigens that the host will encounter throughout life. Antigen cluster differentiation on the plasma membrane of the T cells takes place in the thymus. On exiting the thymus through blood and lymph vessels, T cells mature and are antigenically committed. When these immunocompetent T cells encounter a recognizable antigen in the body, they proliferate.[1]

Naive CD8 cells leaving the thymus are predestined to become cytotoxic cells. In contrast, the differentiation of CD4 cells is much more complex. Depending on the first encounter with antigen, CD4 cells can either become type 1 helper (T_H1) or type 2 helper (T_H2) cells. Type 1 helper (T_H1) cells express interferon gamma (IFN-γ) and TNF-α and regulate cell-mediated immunity, whereas T_H2 cell subsets regulate humoral immunity and express cytokines IL-4, -6, and -10.[10,11] These T-cell subsets are modulated by hypothalamus-pituitary-adrenal (HPA) axis mediators, particularly by increased circulation of the stress hormones, glucocorticoids, and catecholamines, resulting in down-regulation of T_H1 cell activity and enhanced T_H2 humoral immune responses.[12]

Antigen processing, recognition, and presentation

After entering the host, an antigen flows through the bloodstream, is filtered through the spleen, and enters the lymphatics. Lymph nodes and other body tissues such as the skin and mucous membranes are lined with phagocytic cells, particularly macrophages, which ingest antigen. After its ingestion by a phagocyte, the antigen is degraded. A portion of the degraded antigen is reexposed, or expressed, on the plasma membrane of the phagocyte, which "presents" it to B and T cells. This antigen–phagocyte complex, referred to as Antigen Presenting Cell (APC), is necessary to induce most immune responses.[1] Three cell types that can serve as APCs are dendritic cells, macrophages, and B cells.

The only way a T cell can recognize antigen is when it is presented in the context of "self" material, such as MHC molecules. To activate naive T cells, APCs must be capable of processing antigen from intracellular and extracellular pathogens and presenting it on MHC class I and MHC class II molecules. The particular MHC class determines which cell will respond to the presentation of antigen. Inflammatory CD4 cells (T_H1) and helper cells (T_H2) both express the CD4 coreceptor and recognize antigen displayed at the cell surface by MHC class II molecules. Conversely, T_C (CD8) cells kill target cells (particularly viruses) bound to MHC class I molecules at the cell surface.

T-cell receptors (TCR) are the site on T cells where APC bind. These receptors are structurally similar to the Fab portion of an antibody and are antigen specific. The two known types, TCR1 and TCR2, express different gene chains and binding patterns.[1]

Intercellular communication is dynamic during the cell-mediated immune response. Various cytokines and adhesion molecules on the surface of each cell play important roles. For example, IL-1 is produced by the APC and helps the T cell respond, while IL-2 facilitates maturation of a functional T_H1 cell and binds to specific IL-2 receptors on the same cell that is producing it. This results in increased production of IL-2 and IL-2 receptor, further differentiation and proliferation of the T_H1 cell, and the production of other cytokines.

Delayed-Type Hypersensitivity

Delayed-type hypersensitivity (DTH) reactions, also called type IV responses, are mediated by T cells.[1] Specifically in response to a previously responded pathogen, inflammatory (T_H1) CD4 cells recognize receptors on MHC class II APCs. The T_H1 cells then release inflammatory cytokines, such as macrophage chemotactic factor (MCF), TNF-α, and IFN-γ, resulting in blood-vessel permeability and fluid and protein accumulation into the tissue. This process evolves over 24 to 72 hours. Delayed-type hypersensitivity is often used as an in vivo measure of cell-mediated immunity. The prototypic DTH reaction is the tuberculin skin test.

Cell-Mediated Cytotoxicity

Cell-mediated cytotoxicity entails the recognition and lysis of target cells (which may be tumor cells or viruses) by either T_C cells or NK cells.[1] It may or may not be antibody dependent (IgG). The mechanisms of action are quite similar regardless of the type of lymphocyte or involvement of IgG. The main difference lies in the different receptors and the binding of the cytotoxic cell to the target.

Cytotoxic T cells are antigen specific and have MHC-restricted T-cell receptors. In contrast, NK cells are not antigen specific; instead, they recognize determinants expressed on neoplastic cells. Lymphokine-activated killer (LAK) cells are NK cells with enhanced cytotoxic activity due to stimulation with IL-2. These cells are used in the treatment of certain types of cancer by stimulating a patient's own NK cells with IL-2 in vitro, then returning those cells to the patient.[13]

Antibody-mediated cytotoxicity involves the binding of an effector cell, referred to as a killer (K) cell, to antigen-bound IgG. Killer cells are usually T_C cells, but may also be NK cells. The K cell has Fc receptors that can bind to the Fc region of antibody that has coated a target cell. Through these receptors, the K cell can adhere indirectly to and kill an IgG-coated target.

The mechanisms involved in the killing are similar whether T_C cells, NK cells, or K cells are the effectors, and no matter what kind of receptor–target interaction is responsible (Figure 2-5). First, the effector cell recognizes and makes close contact with the target cell. Upon making contact with the target cell, changes occur within the effector cell cytoplasm; specifically, the granule-containing vesicles of the Golgi apparatus fuse with the cell membrane. Through a calcium-dependent process, a protein substance called *perforin* is discharged from the vesicles.[14] This release of perforin causes pores to form on the target cell membrane, leading to an influx of water, electrolytes, and enzymes. Within minutes, the target cell swells and bursts. The effector cell survives this process, possibly because of a protective protein in the cell membrane called *protectin,* and continues to recognize and cause lysis of other target cells. Cytokines, particularly TNF (α and β) and IFN-γ, appear to play important roles in and are products of cell-mediated cytotoxicity.

Tumor Surveillance

Natural killer cells lyse tumor cells without specific antigen recognition and, therefore, are important to tumor surveillance. Although it is unclear whether NK activity affects the development of cancer, some evidence supports the relationship between NK cytotoxicity and cancer recurrence and metastasis.[15–18] In addition, some studies suggest that lower NK levels at diagnosis influence prognosis and survival from cancer.[19]

In addition to NK cells, other mechanisms of cell-mediated immunity may be important for tumor surveillance. All stress hormones influence some aspect of immunity, and immune suppression and infection often accompany increased tumor risk, indicating that tumor surveillance depends on a healthy immune system.[20,21] Stress may contribute to tumorigenesis through neuroendocrine responses that alter T_H1 and T_H2 cells, resulting in lymphocyte apoptosis and lower NK cytotoxicity[21,22] and directly affecting genomic DNA.[23] Although not all tumors are directly responsive to immune control, innate and natural immune resistance is critical to malignant transformation of cells.[24] Some cancers may be more susceptible to stress-induced immune suppression, but all are nonspecifically responsive to NK lysis.

Tissue Destruction from Immune Responses

While attempting to rid the body of foreign organisms, products of certain immune processes have the potential to cause tissue damage. Specifically, neutrophils and macrophages produce toxins during inflammation and phagocytosis. For example, bacterial killing by neutrophils occurs through an oxidative process with lysosomal release of such mediators as superoxide, hydrogen peroxide, and hydroxyl radicals.[1] Fortunately, these free radicals are effective killers of pathogens. At the same time, release of these chemicals affects surrounding cells, leading to damage of healthy cells. This same mechanism supports the dietary intake of antioxidants.

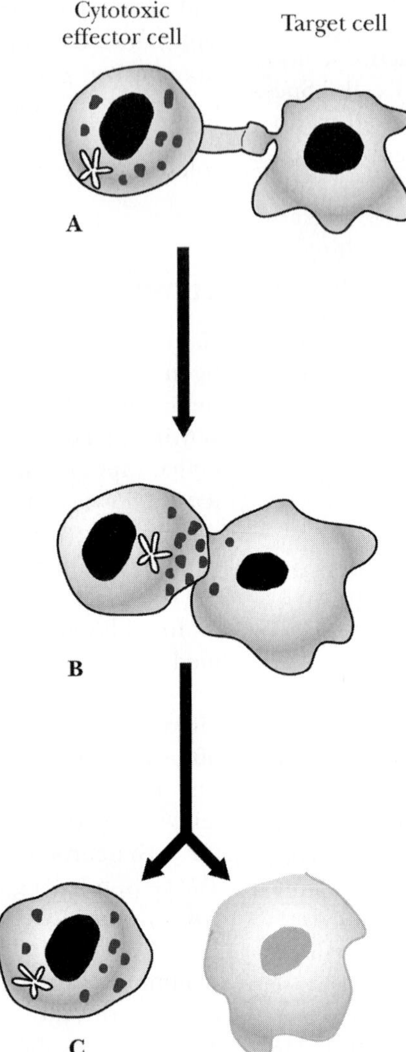

Figure 2-5 Cell-mediated cytotoxicity. **(A)** Target cell (e.g., tumor cell) binds to effector cell (e.g., NK cell). **(B)** Changes in the Golgi apparatus of the effector fuse with the cell membrane to release perforin, which forms pores on the target cell membrane. The target cell swells. **(C)** The target cell bursts, while the effector remains intact and ready to lyse other targets.

Factors Affecting Immune Responses

Stress

Stress generally refers to demands placed on the body that threaten *homeostasis* (internal stability).[25] Stressful stimuli may be either external or internal. External stress is considered to comprise cognitive sensory stimuli because of its initial processing through the peripheral and central nervous systems; death of a loved one is an example of a cognitive stressor. Internal sensory input, or noncognitive stress, is received by the immune system, which in turn relays this information to the neuroendocrine system; viral infection is an example of noncognitive stress. Regardless of the source, external or internal, stressful stimuli clearly have systemic effects. Chronic stress, in general, has immunosuppressive effects, while acute or short-term stress has stimulatory effects on immune function. The hypothalamus plays a key role mediating these processes.

The scientific field called psychoneuroimmunology (PNI) focuses on understanding the effects of stress on immune responses and related health outcomes through the dynamic interplay and bidirectional communication between the neuroendocrine and immune systems.[26] Substantial evidence implicates interaction of the cells of these systems in stress: (1) the immune system's interaction with the hypothalamic-pituitary-adrenal axis; (2) the innervation of lymphoid organs by the autonomic nervous system; and (3) the secretion of and receptors for identical soluble mediators such as cytokines, neuropeptides, and hormones.

The field of PNI first emerged in the late 1970s and now involves interdisciplinary collaboration among professionals of various basic science, social science, and clinical disciplines. Because of the substantial body of knowledge supporting the negative effects of psychological stress on immune function,[25–27] clinical studies are attempting to evaluate and identify the benefits of stress-reducing interventions. This area holds particular interest for nurses, due to its knowledge base rooted in both basic and social sciences, and is reinforced by a holistic perspective that is at the core of the profession.[28]

Stress-reducing interventions

A number of stress-reducing interventions have been shown to improve neuroendocrine, immune, and overall health outcomes — massage,[29–33] expressive or group therapies,[34–37] and mindfulness meditation.[38,39] Other interventions that are known to improve sense of well-being and to decrease symptoms of stress include acupuncture, music therapy, and energy therapies, although minimal research has been done to date on the effects of these therapies on immune function.

Aging

Advancing age is clearly associated with decline of immunologic functioning.[40–42] The thymus reaches its maximum size at about age 25, then begins involuting. Thymic size is only 15% of its maximum by age 50. Although numbers of T cells may not decrease with age, T-cell function does deteriorate. Older individuals (those more than 60 years of age) generally exhibit diminished responsiveness with various T-cell–mediated activities. In addition, antibody activities can decrease or become dysfunctional with increasing age, resulting in lowered resistance to infections and disease. Cytokine production also changes, with some cytokines showing no change (TNF), others increasing (IL-3, IL-4, IL-6) and others decreasing (IFN-α, IL-2, TGF-β).

Gonadal Hormones

Gonadal or sex hormones — specifically, estrogen, progesterone, and testosterone — are known to affect immune function. For example, superphysiological levels of 17-beta-estradiol that occur during pregnancy are immunosuppressive, whereas physiological levels of this hormone are immunostimulatory. Testosterone is also known to be immunosuppressive. While the exact mechanisms are not clear, it appears that IL-6 is central to these processes.[43,44]

Behavioral Factors

Behavioral factors known to suppress immune function include alcohol, caffeine, marijuana, morphine, nutrient deficiencies, smoking, and chronic stress. Other protective factors increase immune function — some nutritional and herbal therapies, physical exercise in moderation, adequate sleep, stress only during acute phases, and stress-reducing interventions. Because changes in these behaviors are often concurrent, it is difficult to fully comprehend the individual effects of these factors. For example, individuals who are distressed may be more likely to engage in self-destructive behaviors (e.g., increased smoking and alcohol/drug consumption) as well as experience changes in their appetite, energy level, and sleep pattern.

Nutrition

Nutritional status and dietary intake can influence immunocompetence and overall health function. Protein-calorie and zinc deficiencies are associated with alterations in both innate and cell-mediated immune mechanisms, for example, while essential amino acids, the essential fatty acid linoleic acid, and certain vitamins (A, B_6, B_{12}, C, and E) and minerals (e.g., selenium) play roles in the maintenance of healthy cells.[45,46] A controversial topic for patients with hormone-sensitive cancers is the use of soy foods. Soy proteins are considered weak estrogens and, therefore, are likely to exert effects on immunologic function and hormone-sensitive tumor growth; research in this area has produced mixed results, however, and final conclusions cannot be drawn.[47] Recent studies also have demonstrated immune-related benefits of other dietary products, such as maitake mushrooms[48] and green tea, which contains antioxidants and catechin, but requires extraordinary daily amounts to attain apoptotic effects on cancer cells.[49]

Alcohol and other CNS drugs

Consumption of alcohol (ethanol) and other CNS-acting drugs can affect immune function. Alcohol intake is associated with suppression of NK cytotoxicity in both animal models and humans.[50,51] The deleterious effects of marijuana on NK, antibody, and cytokine production have also been documented.[52]

Physical exercise

Changes in immune response to physical exercise have been recognized, with moderate and continued aerobic exercise having a general positive effect. With vigorous aerobic exercise, changes occur in cytokines (i.e., increases in CD8), hormones (i.e., β-endorphin), and NK cytotoxicity. The marked increase in NK function is followed by decline, which is thought to be due to skeletal stress, inflammatory responses, or the response to catecholamines.[53–56]

Sleep

Increasing evidence is clarifying the immunorestorative mechanisms involved in sleep.[57,58] Growth hormone and prolactin, known to be associated with enhanced immune function, are elevated during sleep; conversely, levels of immunosuppressive corticosteroids and catecholamines are depressed. Immune suppression, specifically NK cytotoxicity, has been associated with sleep disturbances.[59]

Implications for Nursing Practice

Nursing professionals strive to improve quality of life and clinical outcomes for their patients, with an emphasis toward self-care and changing behaviors. Independent nursing interventions can be educational or supportive. Educational programs and individual or group counseling sessions can be aimed at changing behaviors such as diet, exercise, sleep habits, and stress reduction. These interventions and topics are germane to nursing and ripe areas for refinement and research.

References

1. Janeway C, Travers P, Walport M, et al: *Immunobiology: The Immune System in Health and Disease.* Elsevier Science/Garland, London, 2001
2. Gabrilovich D: Dendritic cell vaccines for cancer treatment. *Curr Opin Molecular Therap* 4:452–458, 2002
3. Morse M, Lyerly H: DNA and RNA modified dendritic cell vaccines. *World Surg* 26:819–825, 2002
4. Vieweg J, Dannull J: Tumor vaccines: from gene therapy to dendritic cells — the emerging frontier. *Urol Clin North Am* 30:633–643, 2003
5. Besedovsky HO, Del Rey A, in Ader R, Fenton DL, Cohen N (eds): *Psychoneuroimmunology.* San Diego, Academic Press, 2001, pp 1–20
6. Kelley KW, Bluthe RM, Dantzer R, et al: Cytokine-induced sickness behavior. *Brain Behav Immun* 17:S112–S118, 2003
7. Hori T, Katafuchi T, Oka T, in Ader R, Felten DL, Cohen N (eds): *Psychoneuroimmunology.* San Diego, CA, Academic Press, 2001, pp 517–546
8. Maier SF, Watkins LR, Nance DM, in Ader R, Felten DL, Cohen N (eds): *Psychoneuroimmunology.* San Diego, CA, Academic Press, 2001, pp 563–583
9. Rabin BS: *Stress, Immune Function, and Health.* Wiley-Liss, New York, 1999
10. Curtsinger J, Schmidt C, Mondino A, et al: Inflammatory cytokines provide a third signal for activation of naïve CD4+ and CD8+ T cells. *J Immunol* 162:3256–3262, 1999
11. Elenkov I, Chrousos G: Stress hormones, proinflammatory and antiinflammatory cytokines, and autoimmunity. *Ann NY Acad Sci* 966:290–303, 2002
12. Eskandari F, Sternberg EM: Neural–immune interactions in health and disease. *Ann NY Acad Sci* 966:20–27, 2002
13. Dunbar P, Chen J, Chao D, et al: Cutting edge: rapid cloning of tumor specific CTL suitable for adaptive immunotherapy of melanoma. *J Immunol* 162:6959–6962, 1999
14. Smyth M, Thia K, Creteney E, et al: Perforin is a major contributor to NK cell control of metastasis. *J Immunol* 162:6658–6662, 1999
15. Antoni MH: Psychoneuroendocrinology and psychoneuroimmunology of cancer: plausible mechanisms worth pursuing? *Brain Behav Immunity* 17:S84–S91, 2003
16. Menon A, Janssen-Van Rhijn C, Morreau H, et al: Immune system and prognosis in colorectal cancer: a detailed immunohistochemical analysis. *Lab Invest* Feb 16, 2004
17. Lotze M, Rees R: Identifying biomarkers and surrogates of tumors (cancer biometrics): correlation with immunotherapies and immune cells. *Cancer Immunol Immunother* 53:256–261, 2004
18. Wu J, Lanier L: Natural killer cells and cancer. *Adv Cancer Res* 90:127–156, 2003
19. Fauriat C, Marcenaro E, Sivori S, et al: Natural killer cell-triggering receptors in patients with acute leukemia. *Leukemia Lymphoma* 44:1683–1689, 2003
20. Moynihan JA: Mechanisms of stress-induced modulation of immunity. *Brain Behav Immunity* 17:S11–S16, 2003
21. Shi Y, Devadas S, Greeneltech KM, et al: Stressed to death: implication of lymphocyte apoptosis for psychoneuroimmunology. *Brain Behav Immunity* 17:S18–S26, 2003
22. Stefanek M, McDonald PG: Biological mechanism of psychosocial effects on disease: implications for cancer control. *Brain Behav Immunity* 17:S2–S4, 2003
23. Yang EV, Glaser R: Stress-induced immunomodulation: implications for tumorigenesis. *Brain Behav Immunity* 17:S37–S40, 2003
24. Sheridan J: The HPA axis, SNS, and immunity: a commentary. *Brain Behav Immunity* 17:S17, 2003
25. Glaser R, Kiecolt-Glaser J: *Human Stress and Immunity.* Academic Press, San Diego, 1994
26. Ader R, Felten DL, Cohen N: *Psychoneuroimmunology.* Academic Press, San Diego, 2001
27. Buckingham J, Gillies G, Cowell A: *Stress, Stress Hormones and the Immune System.* John Wiley, West Suffix, UK, 1997
28. Bauer S: Psychoneuroimmunology and cancer: an integrated review. *J Adv Nurs* 19:1114–1120, 1994
29. Diego MA, Field T, Hernandez-Reif M, et al: HIV adolescents show improved immune function following massage therapy. *Int J Neurosci* 106:35–45, 2001
30. Goodfellow LM: The effects of therapeutic back massage on psychophysiologic variables and immune function in spouses of patients with cancer. *Nurs Res* 52:318–328, 2003
31. Ironson G, Field T, Scafidi F, et al: Massage therapy is associated with enhancement of the immune system's cytotoxic capacity. *Int J Neurosci.* 84:205–217, 1996
32. Post-White J, Kinney ME, Savik K, et al: Therapeutic massage and healing touch improve symptoms in cancer. *Integrative Cancer Therap* 2:332–334, 2004
33. Wikstrom S, Gunnarsson T, Nordin C: Tactile stimulus and neurohormonal response: a pilot study. *Int J Neurosci* 113:787–793, 2003

34. Fawzy F, Fawzy N, Hyun C, et al: Malignant melanoma. Effects of an early structured psychiatric intervention, coping, and affective state on recurrence and survival 6 years later. *Arch Gen Psych* 50:681–689, 1993
35. Fawzy F, Cousins N, Fawzy N, et al: A structured psychiatric intervention for cancer patients. II. Changes over time in methods of coping and affective disturbance. *Arch Gen Psych* 47:720–725, 1990
36. Rosenberg HJ, Rosenberg SD, Ernstoff MS, et al: Expressive disclosure and health outcomes in a prostate cancer population. *Int J Psych Med* 32:37–53, 2002
37. Stanton AL, Danoff-Burg S, Sworowski LA, et al: Randomized, controlled trial of written emotional expression and benefit finding in breast cancer patients. *J Clin Oncol* 20:4160–4168, 2002
38. Carlson L, Speca M, Patel K, et al: Mindfulness-based stress reduction in relation to quality of life, mood, symptoms, of stress, and immune parameters in breast and prostate outpatients. *Psvchosomatic Med* 65:571–581, 2003
39. Davidson RJ, Kabat-Zinn J, Schumacher J, et al: Alterations in brain and immune function produced by mindfulness meditation. *Psychosomatic Med* 65:564–570, 2003
40. Glaser R, MacCallum RC, Laskowski BF, et al: Evidence for a shift in the Th-1 to Th-2 cytokine response associated with chronic stress and aging. *J Gerontol Series A: Biol Sci Med Sci* 56:477–482, 2001
41. Kiecolt-Glaser JK, Preacher KJ, MacCallum RC, et al: Chronic stress and age-related increases in the proinflammatory cytokine IL-6. *Proc Natl Acad Sci* 100:9090–9095, 2003
42. Solomon GF, Morley JE, in Ader R, Felten DL, Cohen N (eds): *Psychoneuroimmunology*. San Diego, Academic Press, 2001, pp 701–717
43. Kovacs E, Messingham K, Gregory M: Estrogen regulation of immune responses after injury. *Molecul Cell Endocrinol* 193: 129–135, 2002
44. Verthelyi D: Sex hormones as immunomodulators in health and disease. *Intl Immunopharmacol* 1:983–993, 2001
45. Calder P, Kew S: The immune system: a target for functional foods? *Br J Nutrition* 88:S165–S177, 2002
46. Lopez-Varela S, Gonzalez-Gross M, Marcos A: Functional foods and the immune system: a review. *Euro J Clin Nutrition* 56(suppl 3):S29–S33, 2002
47. Tham D, Gardner C, Haskell W: Phytoestrogens and health: a review of the epidemiological, clinical and mechanistic evidence. *J Clin Endocrinol Metab* 83:2223–2235, 1998
48. Kodama N, Komuta K, Nanba H: Effect of maitake (*Grifola frondosa*) D-fraction on the activation of NK cells in cancer patients. *J Med Food* 6:371–377, 2003
49. Hall NS: Alternative medicine and the immune system, in Ader R, Felten DL, Cohen N (eds): *Psychoneuroimmunology*. San Diego, Academic Press, 2001, pp 161–171
50. Arbabi S, Garcia I, Baum G, et al: Alcohol (ethanol) inhibits IL-8 and TNF: role of the p38 pathway. *J Immunol* 162:7441–7445, 1999
51. Ochshorn-Adelson M, Bodner G, Toraker P, et al: Effects of ethanol on human natural killer activity: in vitro and acute, low-dose in vivo studies. *Alcohol Clin Exp Res* 18:1361–1367, 1994
52. Klein TW, Newton C, Snella E, et al, in Ader R, Felten DL, Cohen N (eds): *Psychoneuroimmunology*. San Diego, Academic Press, 2001, pp 415–432
53. Nieman D, Nehlsen-Cannarella S: The immune response to exercise. *Semin Hematol* 31:166–179, 1994
54. Shepard R, Rhind S, Shek P: Exercise and training: influence on cytotoxicity, interleukin-1, interleukin-2 and receptor structures. *Int J Sports Med* 15:154–166, 1994
55. Shephard RJ, Shek PN, in Ader R, Felten DL, Cohen N (eds): *Psychoneuroimmunology*. San Diego, Academic Press, 2001, pp 511–524
56. Hoffman-Goetz L, Pedersen BK, in Ader R, Felten DL, Cohen N (eds): *Psychoneuroimmunology*. San Diego, Academic Press, 2001, pp 123–132
57. Krueger JM, Majde JA, Obal F: Sleep in host defense. *Brain Behav Immunity* 17:S41–S47, 2003
58. Uthgenannt D, Schoolman D, Pietrowsky R, et al: Effects of sleep on the production of cytokines in humans. *Psychosomatic Med* 57:97–104, 1995
59. Cover H, Irwin M: Immunity and depression: insomnia, retardation, and reduction of natural killer cell activity. *J Behav Med* 17:217–223, 1994

CHAPTER 3

Epidemiology

Alecia Malin, DrPH, CHES

Introduction

Cancer epidemiology examines the frequency of cancer in populations, the role of certain risk factors that contribute to cancer rates, and the interrelationships or associations that exist between the host, the environment, and other conditions that may contribute to the development or inhibition of cancer.[1] The basic premise of epidemiology is that disease does not occur randomly, but rather in describable patterns that reflect the underlying etiology, or causes of cancer. Because disease does not occur randomly, individuals who have cancer must have been exposed to some factor, either voluntarily (through diet, medication, or smoking), or involuntarily (through factors such as cosmic radiation, air pollution, occupational hazards, or genetic constitution that contributed to the causation of disease).[2] The application of epidemiology to cancer research allows investigators to identify possible causes of disease by elucidating how those exposed and not exposed to risk factors toward cancer differ.

The first section of this chapter reviews basic epidemiological concepts. These concepts will help the reader better understand epidemiologic research, identify groups at higher risk for cancer development, and learn how to conduct research in the field of cancer epidemiology. After reading this chapter, the reader should understand the major issues involved in cancer research design, assessment, and estimation of cancer risks. A brief glossary of fundamental terms used in the field of epidemiology is given in Table 3-1. Table 3-2 includes rates and ratios frequently calculated in epidemiologic research.

Subsequent sections discuss causes of cancer, risk factors that influence cancer susceptibility, and the application of epidemiologic principles in nursing practice.

Basic Considerations in Epidemiological Research

Six primary components are considered when evaluating an epidemiological research project:

1. Definitions of the disease and exposures related to the research hypothesis
2. Study design
3. Eligibility and exclusionary criteria used to select study participants
4. Definition of the source and study populations to be used in the study
5. Statistical plan measuring the association between the exposures and the disease
6. Identification of potential sources of bias and confounding variables[3]

Study Designs

Several standard study designs are used in epidemiologic research. Although this section discusses the general features of these designs, the primary emphasis is on the three designs most commonly used in epidemiologic cancer research: the case-control, cohort, and clinical trial study designs. Other major study designs include experimental, ecological, and cross-sectional.[4]

In selecting the appropriate study design, several factors must be considered:

- The frequency of the disease or the exposure in the general population and the defined population to be studied
- The length of the latency period
- The anticipated size of the study sample
- The time allowed for subject recruitment
- The diagnostic characteristics of the disease and the measurability of the exposure[3]

Case-control studies

The case-control study design should be considered if at least one of the following criteria is met:

- The disease is rare in the general or source population (many forms of cancer meet this criterion).
- The investigation is preliminary.
- Time and funding limitations prohibit the use of larger, more expensive study designs.

The hallmark of the case-control study (as illustrated in Figure 3-1) is that it begins with people with the disease (cases) and compares them to people without the disease (controls).[5] Subjects in case-control studies are recruited on the basis of their disease status. Cases of the disease in question can be either preexisting or newly developed. Generally, a strict definition of the disease is used to identify eligible subjects. For example, pathology slides, cytology results, or medical records can be examined to identify the stage or histology of a cancer. The control subjects, or noncases, are defined as participants who do not have the disease at present but who, if the disease did develop, would have the same opportunity to be diagnosed as the case subjects.

The assumption that cases and controls originate from the same hypothetical source cohort is a critical issue affecting the validity of case-control data. Both cases and controls must originate from populations

Table 3-1 Glossary of Epidemiological Terms

Association	Statistical association refers to the strength of the relationship between two variables. In epidemiological terms, association indicates the degree to which the rate of disease in persons with specific exposure is either higher or lower than the rate of disease in persons without the exposure. The strength of this dependence is greater than what would be expected by chance.
Bias	Selection bias results from a systematic difference in the manner in which the case and comparison groups are selected for participation in the study. This bias may produce spurious associations due to the differential inclusion or exclusion of subjects from the disease or exposure groups.
Case-control study	A study where individuals are selected according to the disease status of interest — those who have the disease (cases) and those individuals who do not have the disease (controls). The cases and controls are examined to ascertain which proportions were exposed to the disease risk factors and which were not.
Cohort study	A study where individuals are classified according to their exposure and are observed to ascertain the frequency of disease occurrence or death among those in various exposure-defined categories.
Confounding	The systematic overestimation or underestimation of the effect of an exposure because the influence of a disease risk factor has not been taken into account. A confounding variable is a risk factor for the disease being studied that is associated with the exposure being studied and is not an intermediate step between the exposure and the disease.
Epidemiologic triangle	The traditional model of infectious disease causation. It consists of three components: an external agent, a susceptible host, and a environment that brings the host and the agent together. Also known as the epidemiologic triad.
Epidemiology	Nonexperimental investigation of disease causation through observational study of human population groups. Descriptive epidemiology is the study of the frequency of occurrence of (incidence) or death from (mortality) in a disease population stratified by time, place, and/or group characteristics. Analytical epidemiology is the ascertainment of whether a particular exposure, such as a physical, chemical, or biological agent, and a specific cancer or other disease are unrelated (independent) or associated.
Etiology	The study of the cause of disease.
False negative	In analyzing the validity of a screening test for disease, those people who truly have the disease who are erroneously called "negative" by the test.
False positive	In analyzing the validity of screening tests for disease, those people who do not have the disease who are erroneously called "positive" by the test.
Historical cohort	A study using a cohort defined in the past.
Incidence	The number of new events or cases of disease that occur in a defined population at risk within a specified period of time. Incidence rates can be used to evaluate the changing patterns of disease frequency within a population and to assess the effectiveness of screening programs and treatment modalities on disease development.
Intervention	A study employed to test the efficacy of a preventive or therapeutic measure to generate knowledge about the etiology and natural history of a disease so as to formulate strategies for its prevention. Clinical trials are intervention studies that focus on the individual. They compare the outcomes in a group of patients treated with the test treatment with those observed in a comparable group of patients receiving a control or placebo treatment, where patients in both groups are enrolled, treated, and followed over the same time period. Community interventions focus on the group or community and evaluate the benefits of new policies and programs, determining which have an effect on the health of those who receive the intervention and which do not.
Nested case-control	A study where a series of cases are identified using a case-control approach within the confines of a well-defined cohort study. The case group consists of a representative sample of individuals, with the disease of interest occurring in the defined cohort over a specified follow-up period.
Population	The number of persons in a defined group who are capable of developing the disease. Can also refer to the general population; a population specifically defined by geographic boundaries, physical or social characteristics, or risk; the sampling population; and the study population.

(continued)

having similar and relevant characteristics. In this instance, the control group can be regarded as a reasonably representative sample of the case reference population. The selection of an appropriate control group represents the major challenge with case-control studies and often serves as the source of selection bias introduced into the study.[6]

The information gained from case-control studies does not establish a causal relationship between the disease and the exposure, but it does explore the concurrent association between the two. If the strength of this association is significant and supported by other studies, it can be used to justify the use of larger cohort studies or clinical trials that can investigate causative relationships.

When conducting a case-control study, be aware that cases and controls may differ in characteristics and exposures aside from the ones that have been

Table 3-1 Glossary of Epidemiological Terms (continued)

Power	The probability that a study will have the statistical strength to detect relationships that exist between exposures and disease. The power of a study can be maximized by controlling for factors such as sample sizes, measurement error, and bias.
Prevalence	The number of new and existing cases of a given disease or condition in a defined population within a specified period of time. Point prevalence refers to prevalence at one point in time. Period prevalence refers to prevalence between two points in time. Prevalence rates can be used to compare disease frequencies across populations and to assess the magnitude of effect of certain diseases on the health status of a population.
Rates and ratios	Calculations used to compare the frequencies of diseases in a population. Commonly used rates and ratios are given in Table 3-2, which lists the rate names. The numerator and denominator values and the population factor are used to express the rate in a standard format.
Risk measures	Attributable risk is the arithmetic or absolute difference between the exposed group and the nonexposed group in terms of incidence rates or death rates. It estimates the number of disease cases that can be attributed to or explained by the exposure (e.g., the majority of lung cancer cases can be attributed to exposure to cigarette smoking). Relative risk (RR) is a ratio comparing the rates of a disease among the exposed group and the nonexposed group that serves as a measure of the association between the disease and the exposure. The RR is generally used in cohort studies. The formula for calculating it is $\frac{a(a+b)}{c\neq(c+d)}$ The odds ratio (OR) approximates the relative risk by comparing the rates of disease among the exposed and nonexposed groups. The OR is generally used in case-control studies with smaller sample sizes. The formula for calculating it is $\frac{ad}{cb}$ Both the RR and OR are expressed as ratios (e.g., an OR of 1.0 means the rate of disease among the exposed group equals the rate among the nonexposed group).
Sensitivity	Measures the probability that a screening test will correctly classify an individual as positive for a disease when he or she actually does have the disease.
Specificity	Measures the probability that a screening test will correctly classify an individual as negative for a disease when he or she actually does not have the disease.
Spurious	As applied to associations between exposures, a false relationship produced by methodological errors or confounding variables.
Validity	Internal validity is the extent to which the subjects in an epidemiological study are truly comparable with respect to general characteristics (e.g., if most of the cases are from an urban setting and the controls are mainly from a rural setting, the two groups are not comparable, and evaluation of the exposure–disease relationship may be affected by these differences). Internal validity is essential for the interpretability and reliability of a study. External validity, or generalizability, is the extent to which the study population can be compared with a larger population (e.g., the general population). External validity must be assessed before study results can be applied to a broader population (e.g., a study that uses as its population a specific profession, such as nurses, may yield results that are not relevant to all women in the general population; while the study may have strong internal validity, the participating nurses may not be representative of the women in the general population or in the nursing profession).

Adapted from Reid M: Cancer control and epidemiology, in Yarbro CH, Frogge MH, Goodman M, et al (eds): *Cancer Nursing Principles and Practice* (ed 5). Sudbury, MA, Jones and Bartlett, 2000, pp 60–82.[4]

targeted for the study. Suppose we were interested in conducting a case-control study to determine whether lung cancer was linked to cigarette smoking. With this study design, we would start with the disease outcome (e.g., lung cancer) and retrospectively examine the extent of smoking among cases and controls. Age, in this instance, is related to length of smoking history as well as to cancer of the lung. The confounding effect of age can be avoided by selecting cases and controls of the same age group or matching the two groups for age.[7]

Matching is the process of selecting controls for factors beyond the targeted factors for the study so that the controls are similar to the cases in certain characteristics, such as age, race, sex, social economic status (SES), menopausal status, and occupation.[5] Two matching techniques are used in epidemiologic research: frequency matching and individual matching. In frequency matching, the proportion of controls with a certain characteristic is identical to the proportion of cases with the same characteristic. In individual

Table 3-2 Rates and Ratios Commonly Used in Epidemiology

Rate Name	Rate Description	Population Factor
Crude birth rate	Number of live births / Average or midyear population	per 1000
Fertility rate	Number of live births / 15- to 41-year-old women at midyear	per 1000
Crude mortality rate	Total number of deaths / Total population at midyear	per 1000
Age-specific mortality rate	Deaths in specific age group / Midyear population in age group	per 100,000
Cause-specific mortality rate	Deaths from a specific cause / Total midyear population	per 100,000
Infant mortality rate	Deaths of children younger than 1 year of age / Number of live births	per 1000
Neonatal mortality rate	Deaths in infants younger than 28 days / Number of live births	per 1000
Case fatality rate	Number of deaths from a disease in a given period of follow-up / Number of diagnosed cases of disease at start of follow-up period	per 1000
Proportional mortality rate	Number of deaths from a given cause / Number of deaths from all causes	per 1000
Morbidity rate	Number of cases of the disease that develop in a given period / Total population at midperiod	per 100,000

Adapted from Reid M: Cancer control and epidemiology, in Yarbro CH, Frogge MH, Goodman M, et al (eds): *Cancer Nursing Principles and Practice* (ed 5). Sudbury, MA, Jones and Bartlett, 2000, pp 60–82.[4]

matching (also known as matched pairs), a control is selected for each case that is similar to the case in terms of the specific variable or variable of concern. If the first case enrolled in our study is a 50-year-old postmenopausal white woman, we would therefore seek a 50-year-old white postmenopausal control. The advantage of matching and analyzing the data for pairs of subjects is that fewer subjects are required in each group to discern a relationship between the exposure and the disease. Matching enhances the ability to substantiate a true association between exposure and disease outcome. It is useful when small numbers of case subjects with the disease are available for study and when efficiency is a major issue. Matching also provides a means for controlling potential confounding introduced by the selection of the control group.

The following example describes a case-control study that used matching to examine cervical cancer, a disease where little is known about the actual causes, though many suspected risk factors have been studied.

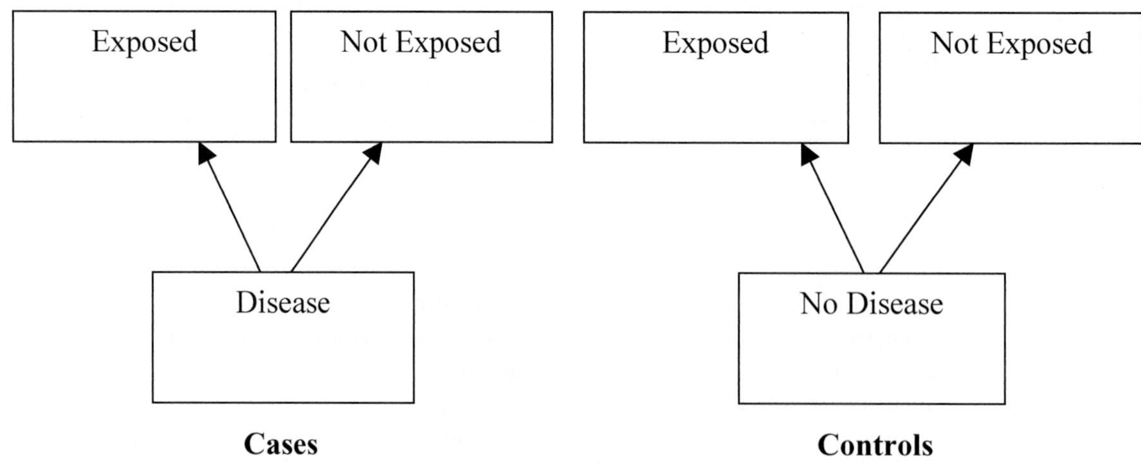

Figure 3-1 Design of a case-control study. Reprinted from *Epidemiology,* Gordis, L, pp. 118–119, Copyright 1996, with permission from Elsevier.[5]

SCHOOL OF HEALTH & SOCIAL CARE
Library
01 AUG 2008
Arrowe Park Site
UNIVERSITY OF CHESTER

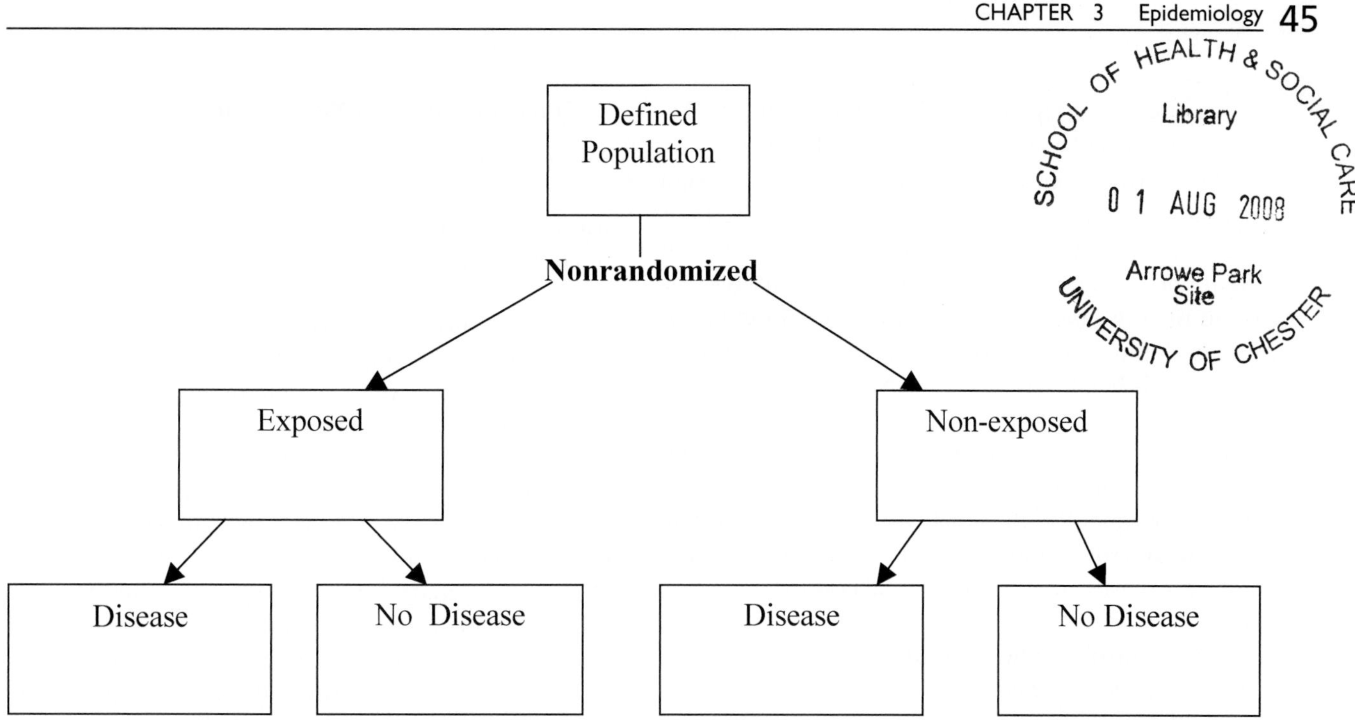

Figure 3-2 Design of a concurrent cohort study. Reprinted from *Epidemiology*, Gordis, L, pp. 118–119, Copyright 1996, with permission from Elsevier.[5]

The cases were 480 patients with invasive cervical cancer diagnosed at 24 different hospitals. Patients were between 20 and 74 years. A total of 797 controls were identified and matched by telephone exchange, race, and five-year age group. Data were collected through home interviews that included questions on hypothetical cervical cancer risk factors such as smoking, sexual behavior, pregnancy history, menstrual history, oral contraceptive use, medical history, diet, marital status, and family history. The results illustrated that compared to never-smokers, the women who smoked 30 or more cigarettes per day were 3.2 times more likely to have cervical cancer.[8]

Two immediate problems arise with matching. First, if an attempt is made to match too many characteristics, it may prove difficult or impossible to identify an appropriate control. Second, once cases and controls have been matched according to a given characteristic, that characteristic cannot be studied in relation to disease. Caution is advised on matching on any variable that may be of interest for exploring in a study.

Cohort studies

A cohort study seeks to investigate whether the incidence of an event is related to a suspected exposure. That is, a cohort study is an incidence study. It starts with a group of subjects who are at risk for developing a disease, yet are free of the disease at the beginning of the study, as shown in Figure 3-2.[5] Cohort studies can be envisioned as going from cause to effect. The exposure of interest is determined for each member of the cohort, and the group is followed to document incidence of disease in the exposed and nonexposed members.

Cohort studies can be prospective, retrospective, or ambidirectional. Cohort studies are considered *prospective* or *concurrent* when the cohort is assembled at the present time and the subjects are followed concurrently through calendar time until the point at which the disease does or does not develop. The disadvantages of prospective studies relate to the amount of time needed to conduct them to determine whether the outcome of interest has developed and their usually exorbitant costs.

The Nurses Health Study is one of the most prominent examples of a prospective cohort study.[9–11] Nurses between the ages of 25 and 42 years old, living in one of 14 selected states, were enrolled in the study when they responded to a questionnaire about their medical histories and lifestyles in 1976. Follow-up questionnaires were sent biennially to update information on risk factors and medical events. All eligible nurses were studied for weight gain, hypertension, dietary intake, reproductive behaviors, menopausal status, family history, hormone replacement therapy (HRT), physical activity, medical history, smoking status, and alcohol consumption. Blood samples have allowed researchers to explore biomarkers and genetic factors.[10] This study is now in its third wave of data collection and has addressed several hypotheses germane to women's health and female cancers, including the

LIBRARY, UNIVERSITY OF CHESTER

association of estrogens, tubal ligation, folate intake, menopausal status, and weight gain with cancer risk.

An alternative approach to the cohort study design is nonconcurrent cohorts, also known as *historical* or *retrospective cohort studies.* A previously defined cohort is identified and assembled in the past on the basis of existing records, and disease outcome (development or no development of disease) is ascertained at the time the study is begun (Figure 3-3). Nonconcurrent studies are notably less expensive and can be implemented more expeditiously than concurrent studies. Their main disadvantage is reliance on available information; consequently, the quality of exposure or outcome data is sometimes less than ideal for fulfilling the study objectives. Many occupational cohort studies are conducted retrospectively.

Case-control studies within a cohort study are known as *ambidirectional studies* or *nested case-control studies,*[11] because they combine some of the features and advantages of both cohort and case-control designs. The selection of participants is carried out using a case-control approach, as shown in Figure 3-4. A nested case-control design starts with a previously established cohort and continues subject follow-up into the future. Ambidirectional designs are being used increasingly for cost-efficiency reasons when analysis of all cohort members requires substantial resources.[11]

Clinical trials and intervention studies

A clinical trial or intervention study is a planned experiment testing medical treatments. This type of study is designed to assess the efficacy of a treatment by comparing outcomes in a group of patients who received the test treatment with outcomes observed in a comparable group of patients who receive a control treatment. Both groups of patients are enrolled, treated, and followed over the same time period.[12]

Once clinical trial patients have been screened for eligibility, they are randomly assigned to one of the study groups. There is an intervention or a treatment group and a control arm of the trial, which receives the placebo or the current therapy. A randomized clinical trial may, for example, randomly assign a group of cancer patients to a particular drug regimen and assign a similar group of cancer patients to a course of not receiving the drug. The two groups are monitored over the duration of the study, with researchers comparing the groups' survival or cure ratio of cancer.

To preserve the objectivity of the data gathered in clinical trials, the blinding approach is used. Participants are blinded as to which group assignment they will get, either the treatment or the control group. This technique prevents attrition when subjects who learn that they have been randomized to the placebo

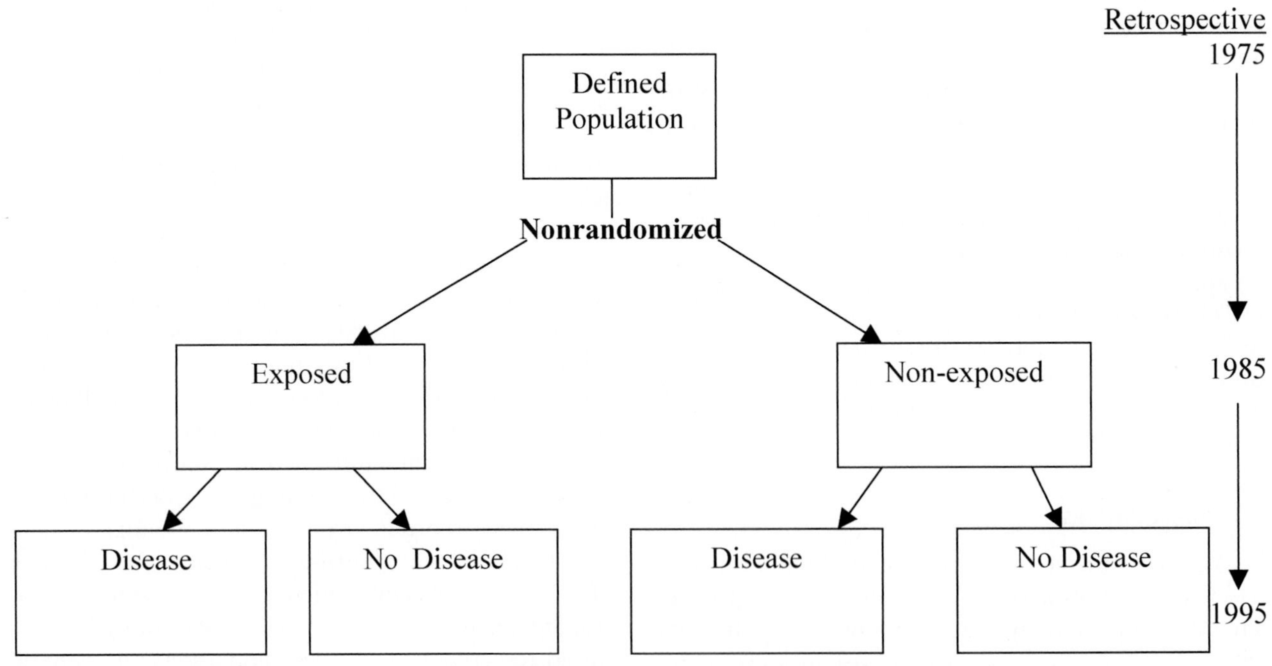

Figure 3-3 Design of a nonconcurrent cohort study. Reprinted from *Epidemiology*, Gordis, L, pp. 118–119, Copyright 1996, with permission from Elsevier.[5]

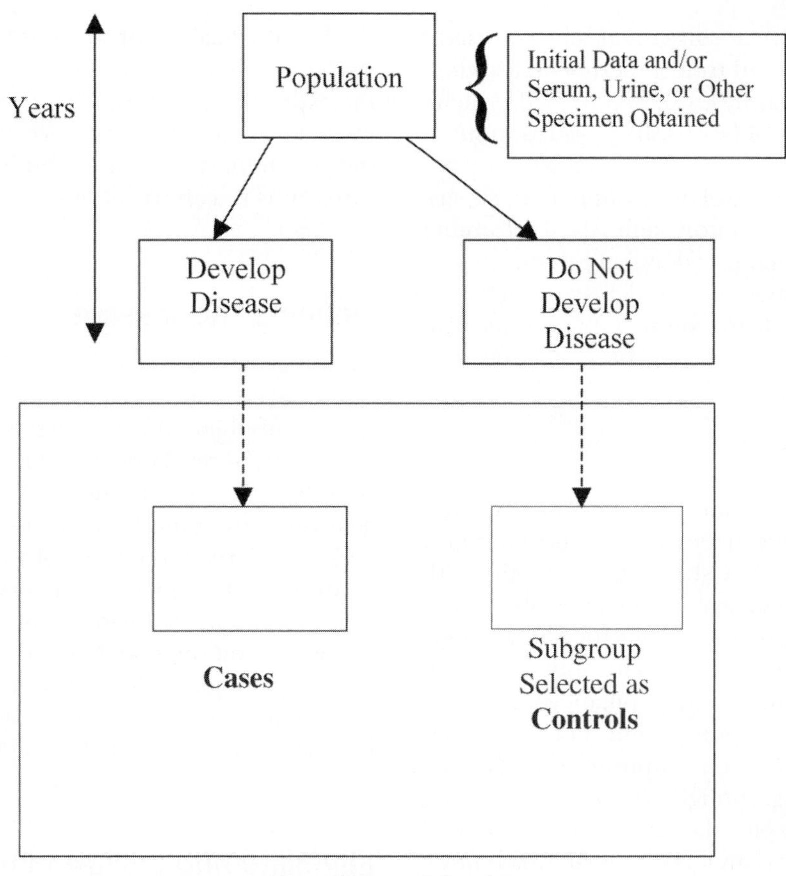

Figure 3-4 Design of a nested case-control study. Reprinted from *Epidemiology*, Gordis, L, pp. 118–119, Copyright 1996, with permission from Elsevier.[5]

arm of the trials subsequently drop out. Additionally, the investigator can be blinded as to the subject's group assignment, creating a double-blind design. A double-blind design protects against the investigator becoming biased as to the trial's outcome, particularly if a drug manufacturer is financing the trial.[2]

A major benefit of a double-blind, placebo-controlled clinical trial is that the random assignment of treatment groups helps to distribute potential confounding variables evenly between the two groups, thereby minimizing their effects on the measurement of the association between the exposure and the disease. If this control of confounding is successful and the primary difference between the two treatment groups is the intervention, then a clinical trial can definitively evaluate the efficacy of the intervention.

An example of a clinical trial is the Physicians' Health Study,[13] which randomized 22,071 licensed physicians into an expanded design to test the effectiveness of aspirin on decreasing the rates of heart attacks and the effect of beta-carotene on inhibiting the development of cancer. This study was defined as having a multifactorial design. After five years, the aspirin arm of the trial was stopped because a significantly lower risk of heart attack was observed among the subjects receiving aspirin. The beta-carotene arm of the trial was discontinued in December 1995; no effect of beta-carotene was observed on cancer incidence.[14]

A major limitation of the clinical trial design is that several years of subject follow-up may be required before significant changes in the rate of disease development are observed among treatment groups. The length of follow-up will depend on several factors, including the strength of the effect the treatment has on the risk of the disease. Long-term studies raise patient management issues, such as maintaining active participation of subjects, monitoring subject deaths and adverse events, and tracking subjects lost to follow-up. These factors, if unevenly distributed among the treatment groups, may confound the results of the project.

Experimental studies

Experimental studies maintain the greatest control over the research setting. Random allocation is used to assign subjects either to receive the treatment or to not receive it or to be assigned to either the exposed or the nonexposed group. Once substantial and consistent evidence has accumulated from experimental studies, other study designs may be employed to further demonstrate the feasibility of large-scale population interventions.

The randomized control trial dominates experimental research in laboratory animals. Performing such experiments on humans does have its drawbacks, however, the most important of which are ethical. It is obviously not acceptable to expose humans intentionally to a potential carcinogenic agent in an attempt to ascertain cancer causation.[11]

Ecological studies

Ecological studies in epidemiology occupy an intermediate position between descriptive and analytical investigations, in that they share characteristics with descriptive studies but serve etiologic objectives.[11] The exposure and disease under investigation in ecologic studies are not ascertained for specific individuals but rather across groups and whole populations. The unit of measure is the geographic region, not individuals within that region.[15] When an exposure is fairly common, such as smoking, sunlight, or fat consumption, ecological studies can elucidate the possible effects of these exposures. For example, skin melanoma is more common in geographic latitudes with more sunshine exposure, and countries with higher per capita intakes of dietary fat tend to be the same countries with high rates of breast cancer mortality.[16] The caveat of using ecological studies to prove disease causality is the phenomenon of ecological fallacy: "the bias that occurs because an association observed between variables on an aggregate level does not necessarily represent the association that exists at an individual level."[17]

Despite their limitations, ecological studies do have merit within epidemiologic research. They are quick, simple to conduct, and inexpensive. When little is known about the association between an exposure and disease, an ecologic study is a reasonable place to start generating hypotheses.[2]

Cross-sectional studies

Cross-sectional studies allow the investigator to study the relationship between an exposure (e.g., electromagnetic fields) and a disease outcome (e.g., leukemia) by surveying a population for each participant, and determining the exposure and disease outcome simultaneously.[7] The unit of analysis in cross-sectional studies is the individual. Cross-sectional studies are referred to as "snapshot" studies because they provide a one-time view of a population's rate of existing (prevalent) cases of the disease, the degree of exposure, and other demographic characteristics of interest at a single hypothetical point in time. While cross-sectional studies cannot establish a causal relationship between the exposure and the disease, they do provide descriptive statistics for the population and are often used as the preliminary step in establishing disease or exposure status in cohort studies.

Defining the Disease

Defining the disease in epidemiologic studies is the penultimate task in including and excluding the appropriate subjects in a study population. Disease may be defined by review of medical records, pathologic results, blood test results, physical exam, histologic characteristics, or results from a psychological battery of tests. To increase the rigor of this step, two different medical professionals, each unaware of the other's findings, should confirm disease status. Clearly stating disease definition guidelines at the outset can prevent enrolling subjects who are actually ineligible for the study. Once a disease status is confirmed for each subject, he or she is eligible for study enrollment.

Eligibility and Exclusionary Criteria

Study eligibility is determined by a set of criteria to gather a population of subjects with a sufficient prevalence of disease to test the hypothesis efficiently. Eligibility criteria in cancer research are typically age ranges, gender-specific factors, race, disease stage, life expectancy, absence of other cancers except nonbasal cell carcinoma, exposure to certain drugs, treatments, and current health status. A strict definition of exclusionary criteria should also be stated as part of the study subject screening process. Exclusionary criteria may involve previous medical history, inability to provide informed consent due to mental competency, a permanent address if the study design is conducted via the telephone or mail, and proficiency in a particular language if the study materials are written and administered in one language.

Interrelated with the definition of disease is how the disease was contracted, or exposure to which factors that lead to a disease state. An exposure in epidemiology comprises the subject's contact with the variable of interest, which may influence the development or improvement in disease status. Exposures run the gamut from microenvironmental exposures on an individual level, such as nutrients, medications, physical activity, and genes, to macroenvironmental exposures, such as air pollution and environmental conditions that affect an entire community.[11] In epidemiologic research, exposures are measured by their frequency and duration as well as their ability to synergistically react with one another.

Dose refers to a standardized, measured amount of exposure issued (e.g., standard milligrams, as in the case of drugs; gray [Gy] for radiation; number of packs of cigarettes per year; hours of exercise; drinks of alcohol per day). It is imperative to assess whether the dose has remained constant throughout the exposure or whether certain variables or conditions have affected the dose over time. The likelihood of an association between an exposure and disease being causal is stronger if a more intense "dose" of the exposure produces higher rates of disease.

Defining the Population

In addition to defining the type of study design appropriate for testing a research hypothesis and the disease/exposure, the source population for study subjects and the actual study population must be defined. This process clarifies to whom the research results can be generalized (external validity), whether the study population represents the total population and the source population, and what the overall characteristics of eligible subjects are.

The source population for the study is the larger group or population from which the study subjects are recruited. It might include, for instance, residents in a certain city or neighborhood, university students, or all patients attending a particular hospital. The source population is usually a subgroup of the total population.

The study population is the group of subjects actually recruited into the project from the source population. Recruitment into the study population, based on the defined eligibility and exclusionary criteria, is planned to access all potential subjects within the source population. It is important to review the types of subjects who were part of the source population but who were not eligible or not approached for recruitment. For example, if subjects were recruited from phone interviews, we could safely conclude that only subjects with telephones were eligible. Because the presence of a telephone in the household might be related to socioeconomic status (SES), it is possible that the study population might be biased toward subjects with a higher SES. The relationship of SES to the disease may be impossible to evaluate and may affect the results of the study.

Statistical Plan

Epidemiologic research measures disease outcomes in rates and ratios, frequencies, and distributions. Aside from these descriptive statistics, inferential statistics can be used to infer whether the exposure disease relationship that is observed in the study population is applicable to a larger population. This premise is called *external validity* or *generalizability*. Additional factors play a role in establishing causation between exposure to risk factors and disease outcome.

Potential Sources of Bias and Confounding Variables

To reasonably assert an uncompromised relationship between exposure and disease, we must account for any bias that exists in an epidemiologic study design. The most common forms of bias in a case-control study are (1) including noncases in the case series of subjects, (2) a systematic error in data collection, (3) an inordinate amount of random error in the collection of data, and (4) inappropriate analysis of data. These types of bias result in a mistaken estimate of an exposure's effect on the risk of disease.[18]

Two primary forms of bias are encountered in epidemiologic studies: selection bias and recall bias. *Selection bias* arises when the relationship between exposure and disease is different for those who participate in the study and those who would be theoretically eligible for the study but did not participate.[19] For instance, the healthy worker effect may occur in occupational cohort studies. Only employed individuals are eligible for such a study, but workers are relatively healthy people who are able to maintain employment.[2] The characteristics of these individuals are, therefore, not generalizable to the overall population. *Recall bias* results from inaccurate recall of past exposures. It is especially a concern in the context of case-control studies when cases and controls are queried for exposures in the past. Bias on the selection of subjects or the study results can lead to a spurious, or unrelated association as contributing to the exposure–disease relationship factor.

Another concern in epidemiologic studies is confounding variables. Confounding variables prevent study groups from being comparable. For instance, if a case-control study shows an association between alcohol intake and lung cancer, we must investigate whether a third factor might exist in the causal pathway of a lung cancer outcome, one that was not originally stated in the study hypothesis. Smoking is another complementary risk factor associated with drinking alcohol. Smoking in this case is a confounder. Although we were interested in the causal relationship between alcohol consumption and lung cancer, smoking is a known risk for lung cancer; it is associated with alcohol intake but is not a result of drinking alcohol.[5]

When planning an epidemiologic study, consult a biostatistician or epidemiologist to help design the research protocol. Sample a large enough study group to have the ability to draw causal inferences for the general population and to perform a rigorous statistical analysis. A variety of techniques can be used to control for bias and confounding variables in epidemiologic studies. Randomization, matching, and statistical analyses stratifying or controlling for confounding variables are commonly used methods. In summary, retain experienced researchers to minimize potential errors at the data-set phase of the study design. Various statistical[18,19] and epidemologic texts[2,5,7,11,20] are excellent resources for fundamentals of epidemiologic and statistical practice.

Data Sources

There are several types of data sources in epidemiology from which to glean information on cancer research and data sets, as shown in Table 3-3 — computerized bibliographic databases, repositories of vital statistics, disease registries, hospital clinic data, and survey research on the general population. When utilizing epidemiologic data from these sources, be cognizant of the availability and completeness of the data. Also, obtain the necessary permission to access the data. Legislation has been enacted to protect identifying information on medical patients. Additionally, a given data set for a target population may not be representative of the general population and lack generalizability.

Table 3-3 A Selection of Internet Addresses for Sites Dealing with Epidemiology and Cancer

American Cancer Society	www.cancer.org
American Lung Association	www.lungusa.org/
International Agency for Research on Cancer	www.iarc.fr
National Cancer Institute	cancer.gov/cancerinformation
National Center for Health Statistics	www.cdc.gov/nchs/
Office of Minority Health	www.omhrc.gov/OMH/sidebar/datastats.htm
Oncolink	www.oncolink.org/
SEER Cancer Statistics	seer.cancer.gov/
U.S. Census Bureau	www.census.gov
Virtual Library: Epidemiology (Biosciences and Medicine), University of California, San Francisco	www.epibiostat.ucsf.edu/epidem/epidem.html
World Health Organization	www.who.ch/whois/whois.htm

Causes of Cancer

Tobacco

The causal relationship between tobacco use and various forms of cancer has been primarily derived from epidemiologic research. Epidemiologic studies of tobacco have relied on mostly self-reported smoking histories. Unlike with dietary patterns, subjects participating in epidemiologic research are unlikely to seriously misreport their smoking habits owing to faulty recall.[21]

Active tobacco use has been linked to many cancer types: lung; lower urinary tract, including the renal pelvis and bladder; upper aero-digestive tract, including the oral cavity, pharynx, and esophagus; and pancreas. Smoking tobacco can also cause cancer of the nasal cavity, paranasal sinuses, and nasopharynx; stomach; liver; kidney; cervix uteri; adenocarcinoma of the esophagus; and myeloid leukemia. Cancer can be caused by smoking cigarettes, pipes, cigars, or bidis (a small amount of tobacco wrapped in the leaf of another plant, commonly used in South Asia).[22,23]

Passive Smoking

The carcinogenic effects of environmental tobacco smoke (ETS) or passive smoking on human lung tissues have been a hotly debated issue during the past decade. ETS can be defined as sidestream smoke and mainstream smoke exhaled by active smokers. Both forms of ETS contain about 40 different chemicals that are suspected or proven carcinogens.[21] In 1992, the U.S. Environmental Protection Agency (EPA) published a report that classified ETS as a group A carcinogen (known human carcinogen). Approximately 90% of the epidemiologic studies on ETS focused on nonsmoking women married to smokers. The annual number of cases attributable to spousal ETS is on the order of 50 in men and more than 500 in women. The corresponding estimates for ETS exposure at the workplace are about 200 cases among men and 270 cases among women.[24] Estimates from the EPA for the U.S. population, which considered spousal and background sources of ETS, predicted in 1930 cases among women and 1130 cases among men. The evidence for a causal association between ETS exposure and cancer in organs other than the lung is inconclusive.[8,25] The overall estimate of risk associated with ever being exposed to ETS and lung cancer is a 1.2 greater risk for lung cancer in married women based on spousal smoking.[26] Being exposed to ETS in the workplace also conveys a 1.2 greater risk of developing lung cancer. Although results from studies of passive smoking and breast cancer risk have been inconclusive, new findings on active smoking status and breast cancer reveal a 1.3-fold greater risk of breast cancer in smokers compared to women who have never smoked and were not exposed to passive smoking.[27]

Individuals who use smokeless tobacco, such as chewing tobacco and snuff, experience an increased risk of oral cancer. The evidence to date from epidemiologic studies indicates no relationship between smokeless tobacco and bladder cancer, but suggestive evidence links smokeless tobacco use to prostate cancer risk. Hemoglobin adducts to carcinogens present in smokeless tobacco products are found in measurable levels in the blood of smokeless tobacco users, indicating that smokeless-tobacco–related carcinogens circulate throughout the body. This prompts a concern that smokeless tobacco may increase risks of other cancers as well.[28,29]

Diet

Diet may be of great importance in cancer prevention. It has been proposed as a contributing factor in 20%–70% of cancer deaths[30,31] and is considered a modifiable risk factor. Interest and research in the role of diet in cancer have flourished in recent years, with many micronutrients (vitamins and minerals) and some macronutrients (proteins, fats, carbohydrates) being investigated for adverse or protective effects against cancer, in both human and animal studies.[32,33] The impetus for many of these studies came from the results of ecological studies. For example, a high correlation was found between national per capita daily meat consumption and country-specific colon cancer incidence rates.[34]

Cancer and macronutrients

Fat intake. Historically, results from case-control and cohort studies generally have supported high fat intake as a risk factor for colon cancer.[35–38] The role of fat in colon cancer is supported by both the rapid change in incidence with dietary change and the potential relationship of fat consumption to bile acids, which are known to be mutagenic.

Nevertheless, the relationship between fat and colon cancer has yet to be firmly established. Ecological studies that use data from many countries show a strong positive relationship between per capita fat intake and breast cancer mortality rates.[34] At the same time, case-control and cohort studies give conflicting results. In a combined analysis of 12 case-control studies of dietary factors and breast cancer, an association was found between high fat intake and breast cancer in postmenopausal women.[39] However, the analysis of data from seven cohort studies in four countries showed no evidence of a positive association between total dietary fat and the risk of breast cancer.[40] Two of the largest cohort studies, the Nurses Health Study[41] and the Iowa Women's Study,[42] showed no relationship between dietary fat intake and breast cancer risk, although some researchers suggest that this outcome may be because the range of fat intake in such studies was too small. Current dietary recommendations are for women to reduce fat intake to less than 30% of calories. In Willett's study, the range of fat intake was 32%–44% of calories.[41] The notion that fat intake may be related to breast cancer has persisted, but there has been an inability to provide individual — as opposed to national — statistics relating breast cancer to fat intake. This result has led to a wide acceptance that the relationship is not to fat but rather to total calories and especially to total calories consumed early in life.

Cancer, micronutrients, supplements, and intake of fruits and vegetables

One of the most consistent dietary findings in analytic epidemiological studies with regard to cancer is the protective effect of fruits and vegetables.[43] Which particular nutrient, non-nutrient, or combination in fruits and vegetables offers protection against cancer remains under investigation. The roles of several micronutrients in cancer prevention, including the carotenoid beta-carotene, vitamin A, vitamin E, and selenium, have been extensively investigated. Relatively high levels of these four micronutrients have been found to be associated with lower cancer risk in many studies, although again not all study results are in agreement.[31,33,44–47]

Some have speculated that the antioxidant effect of vitamin C might play a preventive role against cancer, but this relationship has not been well established.[48,49] Various studies strongly suggest that folate has effectiveness in cancer prevention.[50] Folate is critical for both DNA synthesis and DNA methylation, and various mechanisms have been hypothesized through which folate might influence carcinogenesis. Dietary and supplemental folate appear to be protective and reduce the risk of pancreatic,[51] breast,[52] and colorectal cancer.[53] The optimal dose of folate to minimize colorectal cancer has not been established. Preliminary evidence based on pooled results from nine cohort studies suggest that intakes of approximately 400–500 μg/d may be required to minimize risk.[53]

The antioxidant effects of lycopene may explain the reduction in gastrointestinal tract, breast, and cervical cancer incidence in some populations.[54] Various observational studies have explored the role of lycopene, a carotenoid derived from tomato products like pizza, spaghetti sauce, ketchup, and salsa, in conjuction with gastrointestinal, breast, prostate, lung, and cervical cancer incidence. The mechanisms for the cancer-preventing actions of carotenoids may involve antioxidant activity, induction of detoxifying enzymes, and inhibition of cellular proliferation.[54–56]

There has been a growing interest in the preventive and therapeutic effects of phytoestrogens on various hormone-responsive cancers, such as breast, endometrial, ovarian, and prostate cancer. The phytoestrogens are compounds found in plants such as soy. The isoflavones, which show structural similarity to mammalians estrogens,[57] are considered to be responsible for providing the anticancer benefit. Isoflavones are present in large amounts in soybeans and soy products such as miso and tofu, kudzu root, peanuts, and lentils.[58] Their chemopreventive properties result from soy isoflavones possessing estrogenic activity, competing with estradiol for the estrogen receptor complex, and inhibiting hormone response in cancer cells and tumor growth.[59]

Fiber intake. A majority of studies of differing epidemiological designs support the hypothesis that high fiber intake is protective for colon cancer.[60] The well-documented relationship between meat consumption and colon cancer likely reflects the role played by animal fat consumption. The role of fiber in colon cancer has repeatedly been postulated to relate to altered transit time, altered bacterial flora in the colon, and altered exposure of the colonic mucosa to potentially carcinogenic bacterially modified bile acids. Epidemiological studies have suggested an inverse relationship between dietary fiber and colon cancer, and animal studies suggest that the type of fiber may be important,[61] although not all results are supportive of this position. Vegetables as well as cereals are sources of fiber. In studies where the source of fiber has been examined, fiber from vegetables appears protective against colon cancer, whereas the data for cereal fiber are less supportive of a protective effect. According to the hypothesized mechanism, fiber affects the bile acid content of the aqueous portion of stool. These differing results may be due to the difference in composition of fiber in cereals and vegetables or to the lack of a large range in cereal fiber intake, or they may indicate that some other chemical or nutrient in vegetables is protective against colon cancer.[60,62]

Calcium intake. A protective role for high calcium intake against colon cancer has been reported in several studies[63–65] but not in all.[36,66,67] Data from supportive studies suggest that to reduce the risk of colon cancer, calcium intake should be 1500 mg for females and 1800 mg for males.[68] Calcium may inhibit colorectal carcinogenesis because of its ability to bind toxic bile acids, thereby rendering them inert, or by direct effects on the cell cycle.[69] The role of calcium in colon cancer etiology is linked to vitamin D, as this micronutrient mediates intestinal calcium absorption.[70]

Case-control and cohort studies of diet and cancer present some measurement problems:

1. The distribution of dietary components among individual foods varies greatly. The interactive roles of dietary components are not completely understood, particularly when several components are present in individual foods.[71]
2. Recall bias may be present if dietary assessment is conducted after the presentation of the disease, as in a case-control study. In essence, individuals' recall of their past diet may be affected by their knowledge that they have the disease.[72] To avoid the problems associated with self-reported dietary intake methods, direct assessment of some micronutrients has been developed, involving measuring serum micronutrient levels. Issues regarding measurement of micronutrients through biospecimens are discussed later in this chapter.

Alcohol

Alcoholic beverages consist primarily of ethanol, water, and volatile and nonvolatile compounds. Numerous additives are also used in the production of alcoholic beverages, such as hops, synthetic flavor enhancers, preservatives, and trace elements.[73] Certain contaminants with proven mutagenic and carcinogenic properties have been detected in alcoholic beverages, such as N-nitrosamines, asbestos, arsenic compounds, and pesticides. Moderate to heavy alcohol use has been linked to cancers of the oral cavity, esophagus, larynx, bladder, and liver.[73] The association of alcohol consumption with cancers of the stomach, colon, and pancreas is less well established. Rectal cancer is the exception, for it appears to be associated specifically with beer consumption.[74] Nitrosamines that are found in beer have been suggested as a possible cause of the association between rectal cancer and beer consumption.[75] A cohort study of men who were past drinkers or who reported drinking more than two drinks per day, were non-aspirin users, and had low levels of folate intake had more than a sevenfold greater risk of developing cancer of the distal colon.[76]

Studies focusing on the relationship between alcohol and breast cancer suggest a positive but weak association. Alcohol has been well documented as a risk factor in head and neck cancer and more recently has been implicated in breast cancer,[77–81] although this observation remains controversial. A majority of the findings from epidemiologic studies have shown a moderately increased breast cancer risk among women who consume moderate to high levels of alcohol.[80–82] Both the level of alcohol consumption required to significantly increase breast cancer risk[81] and the age at which exposure to alcohol becomes important[82] are unclear.

Physical Activity

Increased physical activity consistently has been found to be protective against prostate cancer,[83] colon cancer,[61,84-86] and precancerous colon polyps.[86–88] A mounting body of evidence suggests that increased physical activity is protective against breast cancer.[88–90] Intense physical activity at the age of usual menarche may be especially important, because it can cause a delay in onset of menarche. Lifetime physical activity has been proven protective against breast cancer in a large case-control study of women from Shanghai, China. Graded reductions in breast cancer risk were noted in premenopausal and postmenopausal women who exercised in both adolescence and adulthood. These women who engaged in exercise for 16 years or longer periods reduced their risk of breast cancer by 43% and 64%, respectively.[91] The close interrelationship of physical activity with obesity and diet — two factors associated with many cancers — also makes its role in relation to cancer risk important to assess.[92]

Occupational Exposures

At least 10% of cancer deaths in the United States are attributable to workplace exposures. The reasons to study occupational causes of cancer are numerous.

1. An immense number of individuals spend large amounts of time at their jobs, and a growing repertoire of chemicals and physical factors are found in diverse workplaces of today.
2. Workers are generally exposed to much higher levels of potentially hazardous chemical and physical factors than individuals who are exposed to similar hazards in nonoccupational settings. This phenomenon of increasing environmental cancer rates in the occupational group should be heeded by the community at large, which is itself potentially at risk.
3. Cancer stemming from occupational exposures should be considered preventable. Evidence from epidemiological research confirming causal cancer agents should prompt the removal of the agents or adequate prevention of potential exposed workers.[92]

Table 3-4 Cancers Associated with Various Occupations or Occupational Exposures

Cancer	Substances or Processes
Lung	Arsenic, asbestos, bis(chloromethyl) ether, chromium compounds, coal gasification, mustard gas, nickel refining, foundry substances, radon, soots, tars, oils, acrylonitrile, beryllium, silica
Bladder	Aluminum production, auramine and magenta manufacture, rubber industry, leather industry, 4-aminobiphenyl, benzidine, naphthylamine
Nasal cavity and sinuses	Formaldehyde, isopropyl alcohol manufacture, mustard gas, nickel refining, leather dust, wood dust
Larynx	Asbestos, isopropyl alcohol, mustard gas
Pharynx	Formaldehyde, mustard gas
Mesothelioma	Asbestos
Lymphatic and hematopoietic system	Benzene, ethylene oxide, chlorophenols, chlorophenoxy, herbicides, x-radiation
Skin	Arsenic, coal tars, mineral oil
Soft-tissue sarcoma	Cholorophenols, chlorophenoxy herbicides
Liver	Arsenic, vinyl chloride

Adapted from Reid M: Cancer control and epidemiology, in Yarbro CH, Frogge MH, Goodman M, et al (eds): *Cancer Nursing Principles and Practice* (ed 5). Sudbury, MA, Jones and Bartlett, 2000, pp 60–82.[4]

A summary of some occupational carcinogens that may cause cancer is found in Table 3-4.

Pollution

The relationship between drinking contaminated water and cancer has been established in Taiwan, where increased risk of lung cancer has been reported among people exposed to arsenic in drinking water. Trihalomethane, another more common pollutant of drinking water, may be linked to rectal and bladder cancer.[93] These compounds are produced by the action of chlorine on organic waste.

Assessing the association of air pollution with cancer in epidemiologic studies is more challenging. Specifically, it is complicated to measure past exposure to the relevant air pollution and the level of the exposure. Exposure to air pollution has been evaluated by counting the number of inhabitants in the community of residence near a major pollution source. These data mainly take into account suspended particulates, sulfur oxides, and nitrogen oxides, which are agents not responsible for the carcinogenic effect of air pollution.[11]

One type of pollution that may indirectly increase cancer risk involves chlorofluorocarbons (CFCs), which are destroying the ozone layer in the stratosphere.[94] It is predicted that this destruction will allow more ultraviolet light to reach the earth's surface, thereby increasing the risk for nonmelanoma and melanoma skin cancer. Exposure to ultraviolet-B (UV-B) radiation has been implicated by laboratory and epidemiologic studies as a cause of two types of nonmelanoma skin cancers: squamous cell cancer and basal cell cancer. Studies predict that for every 1% increase in UV-B radiation, nonmelanoma skin cancer cases would increase by about 1%–3% each year during which the condition of the deteriorating ozone exists. Recent epidemiologic studies suggest that UV-B radiation plays an important role in causing malignant melanoma skin cancer; for each 1% change in UV-B intensity, the incidence of melanoma could increase from 0.5% to 1%.[95]

Viruses and Other Biological Agents

Viruses may contribute to approximately 15%–20% of human cancers throughout the world.[96] Table 3-5 identifies viruses associated with certain cancer sites. Viruses produce cancer in the host only after a substantial incubation or latency period. This latency period usually extends for years, hindering studies in linking the particular viral exposure with a particular cancer. When the initial infection with the candidate virus is subclinical, verification after clinical features emerge to establish the exact time of infection is compromised.

Several epidemiologists and experimental studies have established a casual role of Hepatitis B virus (HBV) and Hepatitis C virus (HCV) in the occurrence of hepatocellular carcinoma (HCC) and liver cancer.[96] Viruses are etiologically linked to approximately 20% of all malignancies worldwide.

The Epstein-Barr virus (EBV) has been linked with Burkitt's lymphoma and other B-cell lymphomas and nasopharyngeal cancer. EBV has also been implicated in the development of Hodgkin's disease.

The human T-cell lymphotropic virus (HTLV-1), which contributes to the development of human T-cell leukemias, has the highest incidence rate in Japan. This virus is primarily spread from males to females, through transmission in semen, and from mother to child, with breast milk being the likely vector. After a long latent period, adult T-cell leukemia/lymphoma (ATL) occurs in 1 per 1000 carriers per year, resulting in 2500–3000 cases per year worldwide and over half of the adult lymphoid malignancies in endemic areas.

Human immunodeficiency virus 1 (HIV-1) accounts for a significant cancer burden. Kaposi's sarcoma (KS) is a very rare tumor except after HIV-1 infection, when its incidence is greatly amplified, being magnified 70,000-fold in HIV-infected homosexual men. Human herpesvirus 8 (HHV-8), which is also known as Kaposi's sarcoma–associated virus (KSHV), is a necessary but not sufficient etiological factor in KS. The dramatic decline of KS incidence in recent years is due to the introduction of highly active antiretroviral therapy (HAART). B-cell non-Hodgkin's lymphoma occurs as the first acquired immunodeficiency syndrome–defining diagnosis in 3%–4% of HIV-infected patients. Hodgkin's lymphoma is also associated with HIV infection, albeit at a lower risk.

Human papillomaviruses (HPVs) are linked to invasive cervical cancer and anogenital cancers among HIV-infected patients. HPVs are DNA viruses that have been causally linked to cancers of the uterine cervix. Subtypes HPV-16, -18, -31 and -45 have been linked to cervical, penile, and anal cancers of the aerodigestive tract. HPV DNA is found in 93% of all invasive cervical cancers, with 50% of cases being infected with subtype 16.

Human retroviruses cause malignancy via direct effects as well as through interactions with other oncogenic herpesviruses and other viruses. In no case in humans, in contrast to animal and cell culture systems, has a viral infection directly produced a malignancy; in humans, cancer is a multistep process.[97]

Radiation

Ionizing radiation

The greatest source of exposure to ionizing radiation is background radiation in the environment. For U.S. residents, ionizing radiation from natural sources

Table 3-5 Cancer Types Associated with a Virus or Other Biologic Agent

Virus or Biological Agent	Cancer
Hepatitis B virus	Hepatocellular carcinoma
Human papillomavirus (types 16 and 18)	Cervical cancer
Epstein-Barr virus	Burkitt's lymphoma
Human T-cell lymphotrophic virus type I	Adult T-cell leukemia/lymphoma (ATLL)
Human immunodeficiency virus	Kaposi's sarcoma; non-Hodgkin's lymphoma
Schistosoma	Bladder cancer
Heliobacter pylori	Gastric cancer

accounts for approximately 82% of the total exposure from all sources. Background radiation includes naturally occurring cosmic rays and radiation from ground sources, such as uranium, radon, potassium, and other substances. It is problematic to conduct epidemiologic studies of potential cancer risk from naturally occurring background radiation due to the difficulty of measuring an individual's lifetime or cumulative exposure.[98,99]

From the standpoint of prevention, little more can be done than is already being done: minimizing exposure to man-made radiation hazards. It is notable, however, that stopping smoking has the greatest potential for preventing radiation-induced cancer of the lung, as radon exposure acts synergistically with tobacco smoke. Smokers who were exposed to radon while working as miners had ten times the incidence of lung cancer as did nonsmokers.[100]

In 1987, the International Agency for Research on Cancer designated radon, a radionuclide existing normally as an inert gas, as a human carcinogen. Radon exposure increases the risk of lung cancer among underground miners, and indoor radon exposure is the second leading cause of lung cancer in the United States. Radon itself does not directly cause lung cancer; rather, alpha particles from radon progeny directly damage target lung cells to cause cancer. In 1999, the EPA released a report on the health effects of indoor radiation, integrating findings from epidemiologic studies with evidence from animal experiments and other lines of laboratory investigation. The agency's report also considered the limited evidence on the synergistic effect of smoking and radon. According to this study, an estimated 157,400 people died of lung cancer due to radon in homes (from all causes, including smoking and radon exposure) in the United States. Of the 95,400 men who died of lung cancer, approximately 95% were probably ever-smokers; of the 62,000 women, about 90% were probably ever-smokers. Approximately 11,000 radon-related lung cancer deaths are estimated to have occurred in never-smokers.[101]

Radiation exposure found in medical treatments and diagnosis largely centers on the use of x-rays or irradiation treatment for various illnesses. The therapeutic radiation dosages given to cancer patients are among the highest levels received by humans. A large body of evidence indicates that organs can develop secondary cancers caused by radiation used in the treatment of a primary cancer. Treatment with ionizing radiation for the prevention of breast cancer is a controversial issue for this reason. In a risk-versus-benefits issue, healthy women are subjected to radiation to diagnose breast cancer at an early stage through mammography, a procedure with known carcinogenic potential. Clearly, the benefits of mammography outweigh the risks, considering the reduced amount of ion radiation to which women are exposed from mammography versus the tremendous improvement in quality-control aspects of screening mammography.

Epidemiologic studies of occupational exposures to radiation have been targeting radiologists since the early twentieth century. These niche groups of physicians have higher incidences of lung, pancreas, thyroid, bone, and breast cancers than practitioners in other medical specialties. Occupational exposure to ionizing radiation is highest among underground uranium miners, commercial nuclear power plant workers, fuel fabricators, physicians, flight crews and attendants, industrial radiographers, and well loggers.[100] Other populations of interest include victims of the atomic bombings in Nagasaki and Hiroshima in World War II. The high doses of ionizing radiation contribute to cancers of the lung, breast, colon, ovary, stomach, and thyroid.

Non-ionizing radiation

Non-ionizing radiation includes microwaves, radio waves, and extremely low doses of electromagnetic fields (EMF). Early epidemiologic studies observed that residential exposure to the weak EMF surrounding power lines was associated with a small elevated risk of childhood cancers. When these studies have been evaluated for their validity and study design in two large case-control studies, no detectable effect of residential magnetic field exposure was found on the development of brain tumors in children.[101,102]

Cell phone usage has increased to include 65% of all U.S. households, up from 62% in 2002. As cellular telephones are a relatively new technology, no long-term follow-up on their biological effects is possible as yet. However, the lack of ionizing radiation and the low-power frequency EMF level emitted from cell phones and absorbed by human tissues make it unlikely that these devices can cause cancer.[103] Moreover, several well-designed epidemiologic studies have failed to find any consistent association between cell phone use and head and neck cancers.[104–106] It is impossible to prove that any product or exposure is absolutely safe, especially in the absence of very long-term follow-up. Nevertheless, the scientific data do not demonstrate that mobile phones are harmful. If individuals are concerned about the radiofrequency (RF) energy from these products, they might choose digital rather than analog telephones, because the former use lower RF levels.[107]

Ultraviolet radiation

Ultraviolet-A (UV-A) radiation from sunlight can suppress cellular immunity, and the suppression of immunity has been postulated as the factor for tumor growth. UV-A is the major cause of nonmelanoma skin cancer, with cumulative exposure and number of lifetime sunburns being predictive of risk. Incidence of melanoma, the most insidious form of skin cancer, is increasing worldwide more rapidly than incidence of any other cancer; mortality rates are also increasing by about 2% per year for this form of skin cancer.

Conversely, sunlight has been shown to protect against cancer development. Epidemiologic studies of prostate, breast, and colon cancer suggest an inverse relationship between sunlight exposure and the incidence and mortality rates for these diseases. Sunlight activation of vitamin D has been shown to retard the growth of colon and breast cancer cells. Unlike the zero tolerance given to tobacco products, it would be remiss to promulgate public health messages to completely avoid sunlight to people who have suffered little or no skin damage from UV-A.[108]

Drugs

Despite the vast array of chemicals discovered to cause cancer in animals, few chemicals (other than tobacco) exist for which there is strong evidence of causation of the common cancers in humans. Medications associated with malignancies include analgesics, cyclophosphamide, and barbiturates, which have been associated with an increased risk (or, in the case of barbiturates, decreased risk) of bladder cancer. Analgesics such as phenacetin have been linked to tumors of the renal pelvis, ureter, and urinary bladder.[109] Cyclophosphamide, an immunosuppressive drug used for the treatment of non-Hodgkin's lymphoma, is prescribed to 500,000 patients annually worldwide. The cumulative risk of bladder cancer in patients taking cyclophosphamide was found to be 10.7% at 12 years of follow-up.[110] Barbiturates, such as phenobarbital, have been shown to interact negatively with smoking in bladder cancer risk. This barbiturate deactivates bladder carcinogens found in tobacco smoke.[111]

Nonsteroidal anti-inflammatory drugs

Nonsteroidal anti-inflammatory drugs (NSAIDs) are among the most frequently used drugs in the United States. It is has been estimated that 75 million prescriptions for these agents are dispensed annually at a cost of about $2.5 billion.[112] NSAIDs were first introduced in 1949 for their anti-inflammatory properties in the treatment of arthritis. The term "NSAIDs" applies to all "aspirin-like" drugs that are used clinically as antipyretics, analgesics, and anti-inflammatory agents. The drugs inhibit enzymes of the cyclooxygenase (COX) family and, in doing so, prevent the production of certain eicosanoids (a large family of intracellular signaling molecules) in response to inflammatory or mitogenic stimuli.[113]

The antitumor effects of NSAIDs have been extensively studied in the last 25 years. Numerous observational and case-control studies reported since 1989 indicate that regular NSAID use is associated with a reduced risk of colorectal adenomas, cancer, and cancer mortality.[114] Antitumor effects have been associated with NSAID-mediated inhibition of COX activity. In particular, these drugs are linked to up-regulation of COX-2, an enzyme associated with tissue regulation of inflammation.[115] COX-2 is found wherever inflammation is present; it is markedly up-regulated in major epithelial cancers, including colon, esophagus, lung, breast, and prostate cancer. COX-2 may be a key component of epithelial tumorigenesis and its suppression of NSAIDs.

Observational evidence collected as part of epidemiologic studies indicates that regular use of nonspecific COX-inhibiting drugs, such as celecoxib, a commonly used COX-2 inhibitor, discourages polyp and tumor growth.[116] Patients taking aspirin or NSAIDs on a regular basis have roughly 50% less risk of developing colorectal polyps. Additionally, investigators have noted a 50% reduction in the incidence of carcinoma and in cancer-associated mortality with use of such drugs.[117]

Exogenous hormones

Combined oral contraceptives (OC) and postmenopausal hormones are the most vital source of exogenous estrogens for women today. In the past, synthetic hormones such as diethylstilbestrol (DES) were widely prescribed for the prevention of miscarriage and to suppress lactation. Epidemiologic studies of the risk of breast cancer in mothers exposed to DES during their reproductive and pregnancy years suggest a modest 20%–50% increased risk among the exposed women, with a latency period of about 15 to 20 years.

More than 50 epidemiologic studies have evaluated the relationship between OC use and breast cancer risk. Combined OCs contain ethyl estradiol and a progestin. The role of contraceptives in breast cancer risk is controversial and not clearly established, with most studies showing no relationship,[118,119] no significant increase in breast cancer risk with long duration of use, or a small increased risk of breast cancer based on the recency of OC use. The risk associated with OC use among current users was found to persist for ten years after discontinuation, yet no risk was associated with duration of use, age at first use, or dose and formulation. The study results suggest that the pattern of risk seems incompatible with a genotoxic effect, and that OC use may act as a late-stage promoter of preexisting tumors. Case-control studies have consistently demonstrated that the use of such contraceptives reduces the risk of endometrial cancer by 50% and the risk of ovarian cancer by 40%.

The association between hormone replacement therapy (HRT) and breast cancer is an issue of great public health importance, given the increasing size of the older female population. A large effect of HRT on breast cancer risk has not been detected. Some risk may be associated with current or long-term HRT among women who receive it for five to ten years or longer.[120] One factor to consider in these studies is detection bias. Current users of hormones must see a physician to review prescriptions and, therefore, are more likely to be screened for breast cancer.

Tamoxifen is a nonsteroidal antiestrogen medication that has been used successfully for 15 years in the treatment of breast cancer. Because tamoxifen acts by binding to estrogen receptor sites, it has been most effective in treating postmenopausal women, who are more likely to have cancers containing estrogen receptors. In contrast to its antiestrogenic tumor-suppressor action in the case of breast cancer, this drug has been associated with the development of endometrial carcinoma.[121] The trade-off between the effective use of tamoxifen in breast cancer prevention and the higher risk of endometrial cancer leads to a recommendation for routine screening for the latter cancer in tamoxifen users.

Table 3-6 Examples of Biomarkers of Internal Dose

Biomarker	Source of Exposure	Biologic Sample
Aflatoxin	Contaminated food	Urine
Bacterial mutations	Cigarette smoke	Cervical fluids
Benezene, toluene	Cigarette smoke	Urine, breath concentration
CFA	Occupational exposure	Urine
Cotine	Cigarette smoke	Serum, urine, saliva
DNA sequences	HPV	Cervicovaginal lavage
HDL Alkaline phosphatase	Alcohol	Serum
Lead-210	Cigarette smoke	Bone, soft tissues
Mutagens	Cigarette smoke, various occupational exposures	Urine
Nitrosamino acids	N-nitroso compounds in diet	Urine
Selenium	Diet	Hair, toenails
Vitamin levels	Diet	Serum

CFA: 3-chloro-4-fluoroaniline
HPV: human papillomavirus
HDL: high-density lipoprotein

Nasca PC: Biomarkers and epidemiological studies of cancer, in Nasca PC, Pastides H (eds): *Fundamentals of Cancer Epidemiology*. Sudbury, MA, Jones and Bartlett, 2001, pp 85–102; Perera FP: Molecular epidemiology in cancer prevention, in Schottenfeld D, Fraumeni JF (eds): *Cancer Epidemiology and Prevention*. New York, Oxford University Press, 1996, pp 101–115.

Biomarkers

As many as 80% of cancer cases are theoretically preventable because the controlling causative factors are exogenous rather than inborn or inherent. We can estimate that in the absence of external carcinogenic exposures resulting from lifestyle, occupation, and the ambient environment, 400,000 of the annual 500,000 cancer-related deaths in the United States could be averted. More effective methods are needed to identify groups and individuals at greatest risk of cancer at a stage where intervention is possible.

The field of molecular epidemiology offers a potentially powerful tool in cancer prevention by combining biomarkers, measurement of carcinogenic dose, biologic response, and susceptibility with epidemiologic methods. Biomarkers offer a strategy to assess precursors of disease and identify biologic markers of exposure. Traditional epidemiologic tools such as questionnaires and medical records are important for measuring the external dose of a particular environmental exposure. Because these epidemiological measures rely on human recall, however, a certain amount of misclassification can be expected to occur.

The term *biomarker* is used to describe the application of chemical, physical, radiologic, and immunobiologic tests to human biologic samples, such as blood, urine, and tissue. Table 3-6 provides examples of biomarkers that measure internal dose. In biomarkers of internal dose, the investigator examines the extent to which the biomarker correlates with the epidemiological measure. The accuracy of the epidemiological exposure data can be assessed by measuring body burden levels of the actual compound or one of its stable metabolites in human tissue.[122] Examples of biomarkers include plasma or salivary cotine from cigarette smoke, urinary aflatoxin indicative of dietary exposure, and N-nitroso compounds in urine from dietary sources and cigarette smoke.[123]

Table 3-7 Probability of Developing Invasive Cancers Over Selected Age Intervals, by Sex, US, 1998-2000*

		Birth to 39 (%)	40 to 59 (%)	60 to 79 (%)	Birth to Death (%)
All Sites†	Male	1.36 (1 in 73)	8.03 (1 in 12)	33.92 (1 in 3)	44.77 (1 in 2)
	Female	1.92 (1 in 52)	9.01 (1 in 11)	22.61 (1 in 4)	38.03 (1 in 3)
Bladder‡	Male	.02 (1 in 4603)	.40 (1 in 250)	2.36 (1 in 42)	3.46 (1 in 29)
	Female	.01 (1 in 9557)	.12 (1 in 831)	.64 (1 in 157)	1.10 (1 in 91)
Breast	Female	.44 (1 in 229)	4.14 (1 in 24)	7.53 (1 in 13)	13.36 (1 in 7)
Colon & rectum	Male	.06 (1 in 1678)	.806 (1 in 116)	3.94 (1 in 25)	5.88 (1 in 17)
	Female	.06 (1 in 1651)	.67 (1 in 150)	3.05 (1 in 33)	5.49 (1 in 18)
Leukemia	Male	.15 (1 in 649)	.20 (1 in 495)	.82 (1 in 122)	1.45 (1 in 70)
	Female	.13 (1 in 789)	.14 (1 in 706)	.46 (1 in 219)	1.00 (1 in 100)
Lung & bronchus	Male	.03 (1 in 3439)	1.02 (1 in 98)	5.80 (1 in 17)	7.69 (1 in 13)
	Female	.03 (1 in 3046)	.79 (1 in 126)	3.93 (1 in 25)	5.73 (1 in 17)
Melanoma of skin	Male	.12 (1 in 809)	.49 (1 in 205)	.97 (1 in 103)	1.81 (1 in 55)
	Female	.19 (1 in 532)	.39 (1 in 255)	.51 (1 in 197)	1.22 (1 in 82)
Non-Hodgkin's lymphoma	Male	.14 (1 in 739)	.45 (1 in 224)	1.27 (1 in 79)	2.10 (1 in 48)
	Female	.08 (1 in 1258)	.30 (1 in 332)	.98 (1 in 102)	1.76 (1 in 57)
Prostate	Male	.01 (1 in 12833)	2.28 (1 in 44)	14.20 (1 in 7)	17.15 (1 in 6)
Uterine cervix	Female	.16 (1 in 632)	.31 (1 in 322)	.27 (1 in 368)	.78 (1 in 128)
Uterine corpus	Female	.05 (1 in 1832)	.69 (1 in 144)	1.57 (1 in 64)	2.60 (1 in 38)

*For those free of cancer at beginning of age interval. Based on cancer cases diagnosed during 1998-2000. The "1 in" statistic and the inverse of the percentage may not be equivalent due to rounding.

†All sites exclude basal and squamous cell skin cancers and in situ carcinomas except urinary bladder. ‡Includes invasive and in situ cancer cases.

Data from DEVCAN: Probability of Developing or Dying of Cancer Software, Version 5.1. Statistical Research and Applications Branch, National Cancer Institute, 2003, http://srab. cancer.gov/devcan, and the American Cancer Society, Surveillance Research, 2004: http://www.cancer.org/downloads/STT/CAFF_final PWSecured.pdf. Accessed August 18, 2004.

Host Characteristics Influencing Cancer Susceptibility

Age

Age is a major risk factor for many health outcomes and is frequently associated with numerous exposures. Even if the effect of age is not among the primary objectives of the study, it is important to assess its relationship with exposures and outcomes, given its potentially confounding effects. The age distribution of new cancer cases by site reveals that leukemia is the leading cancer for individuals younger than age 20. New cervical cancers remain high in women aged 20–54, whereas the highest distribution of new testicular cancer cases occurs in the 20–34 age group.[124] An estimated one-third of deaths in children younger than age 14 involve leukemia.[125] As shown in Table 3-7, the greatest number of cancer deaths predicted for males in 2004 were expected from prostate cancers in the 60–79 age group. Women in the same age strata are predicted to primarily die of cancer of the uterine corpus to cancer of the breast.[124]

Because age is such an important determinant of cancer risk, it is critical in epidemiological studies to make adjustments for age in the statistical analysis, unless comparison groups have the same age distribution.

Sex

The distributions of new cancer cases in each sex are shown in Figure 3-5. The prostate is the leading site for cancer in men, followed by lung and bronchus and colorectal cancer. The leading site of new cancer cases in women is the breast, followed by lung and bronchus and colorectal cancer. Figure 3-6 shows the estimated number of cancer deaths by gender. The majority of cancer deaths for both genders derive from lung and bronchus cancers, followed by prostate cancers for men and breast cancers for women.[125]

Genetic Predisposition

Genetic epidemiology in cancer research is used to identify inherent susceptibility factors for primary, secondary, and tertiary prevention of cancer. The cumulative body of evidence indicates that genetic factors contribute to the development of most cancer cases,

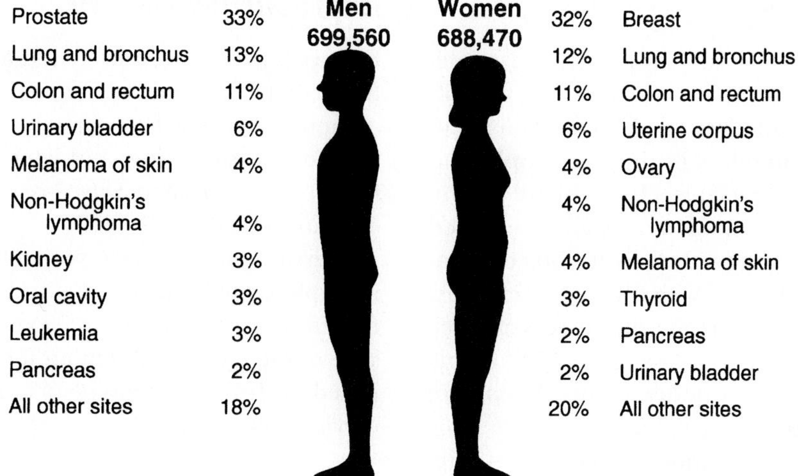

Excludes basal and squamous cell skin cancers and in situ carcinomas except urinary bladder.

Figure 3-5 Estimated U.S. cancer cases, 2004. Data from the American Cancer Society: *Cancer Statistics, 2004.* Atlanta, American Cancer Society, 2004.

including those without a clear familial aggregation. Epidemiologic studies of genetics in cancer etiology have been either family studies or genetic biomarker studies. Family studies can provide general information on the role and/or inheritance patterns of genetic factors in the etiology of cancer. Biomarker studies can target specific genetic factors suspected to be responsible for the pathology of cancer. Epidemiological investigation of genetic predisposition to cancer is increasing thanks to developments in molecular biology, which have made it possible to study genetic markers in large populations.[126] The ongoing Human Genome Project is almost certain to accelerate this work through the discovery of new genes or gene markers associated with increased genetic predisposition for cancer.[127]

Genes have been discovered that are associated with susceptibility to breast cancer and ovarian cancer (*BRCA1* and *BRCA2*), colon cancer (*APC*), and prostate cancer (*HPC1* and *HPC2*). Much work remains to be done to further investigate the effects of these genes, including elucidating how other known risk factors for these cancers modulate the risk conferred by each of these genes.

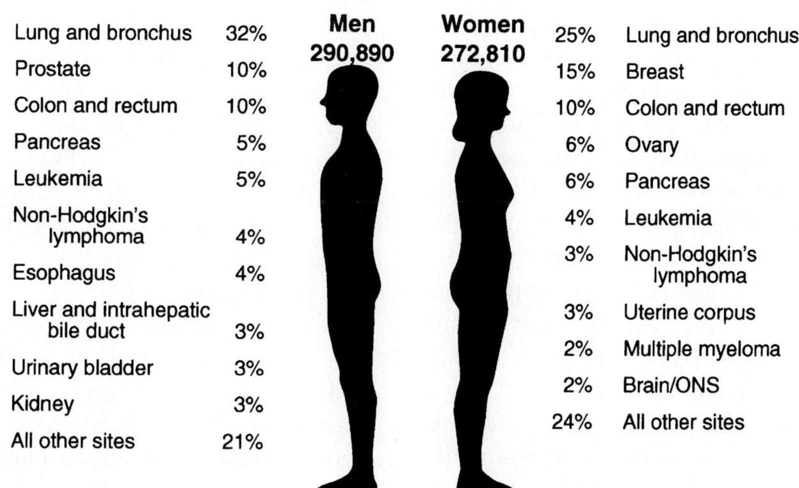

ONS = Other nervous system.

Figure 3-6 Estimated U.S. cancer deaths, 2004. Data from the American Cancer Society: *Cancer Statistics, 2004.* Atlanta, American Cancer Society, 2004.

Ethnicity and Race

The U.S. Bureau of the Census classifies race into categories such as white, African American, Asian or Pacific Islander, Mexican American, and Native American. Race is often similar to ethnicity, in that people who come from a particular racial stock may share a common ethnic identification. Caution should be used when trying to classify individuals with mixed racial parentage into a racial group with which they identify. Race does have implications for differences in incidence and prevalence of disease. Racial or ethnic groups may differ in their attitudes toward illness, care seeking, and prevention.

An illustration of the variation of race in cancer incidence and mortality from the Surveillance, Epidemiology, and End Results (SEER) data appears in Figure 3-7. The data on prostate cancer, which can be detected by physical exam and a prostate antigen test (PSA), reveal how cancer mortality adversely affects African Americans. Seventy-three prostate cancer deaths per 100,000 occurred in African American males compared to 30 prostate cancer deaths per 100,000 in white males.[128]

Socioeconomic Factors

Socioeconomic status (SES) is determined by income, education, occupation, or percentage below the poverty level. Lower SES is related to excess mortality, morbidity, and disability rates. Higher-poverty areas are characterized by later-stage diagnosis, poorer survival, and higher mortality rates. A substantial decline in mortality over time occurs in all socioeconomic groups, but a considerable gradient is still evident where the lower-SES group have worse outcomes. In 1999, for all cancers combined in men, the mortality rate was 13% higher in high-poverty areas. All-cancer mortality in women in 1999 was 3% higher in high-poverty areas. Lower-SES groups have a larger proportion of cancers with poorer prognosis in comparison with higher-SES groups. Poorer survival rates in the lower socioeconomic classes may be attributed to delay in seeking health care, health system barriers (e.g., lack of access to care and lack of insurance), and lack of information about cancer detection and treatment. For example, these high-poverty areas have substantially lower rates of mammography and colorectal cancer screening.[129] Residents of high-poverty areas are also less likely to receive optimal surgical treatment for breast, prostate, and lung cancers.

Reproductive History

Factors related to reproduction and sexual behaviors have been identified only for cancers in women. Earlier menarcheal age, later menopausal age, parity status, years of breast-feeding, and later age at first live birth have been associated with breast, endometrial, and ovarian cancers.[130–133]

Cervical cancer has a very different pattern, with multiple sexual partners being identified as a major risk factor. The number of sexual partners is a measure of the likelihood that an individual has been exposed to HPV, which has been implicated as a cause of cervical dysplasia.[8,134,135]

Other Applications of Epidemiology in Oncology

Cancer Pain

One facet of research that is entrenched in cancer nursing practice is determining the epidemiology of cancer pain. The undertreatment of cancer pain is a significant clinical problem. Unrelieved pain has serious negative consequences (e.g., depression, fatigue, and decreases in quality of life for both cancer patients and their family caregivers).[136] Epidemiological research in this area is deemed necessary to define the scope and magnitude of the problem. Epidemiological studies of cancer pain tend to focus on behavioral epidemiology, improving patient and family caregiver knowledge and attitudes, and changing their behaviors regarding cancer pain management. Randomized clinical trials (RCTs) have been undertaken to show that increasing patient or family caregiver knowledge and improving behaviors can significantly affect cancer pain management. RCTs comprise a target intervention in which all study participants in the intervention group receive an identical intervention, contrasted with a tailored intervention in which the study participants receive an intervention structured to meet their specific learning needs. These clinical trials evaluate the effectiveness of an intervention by randomly allocating subjects to groups that will undergo or not undergo a particular intervention.[11] Such studies evaluating the effectiveness of an intervention on attitudes and knowledge regarding the epidemiology of cancer pain were shown to be more successful if they employed a tailored intervention including teaching sessions, home visits, and follow-up phone calls.[137-139]

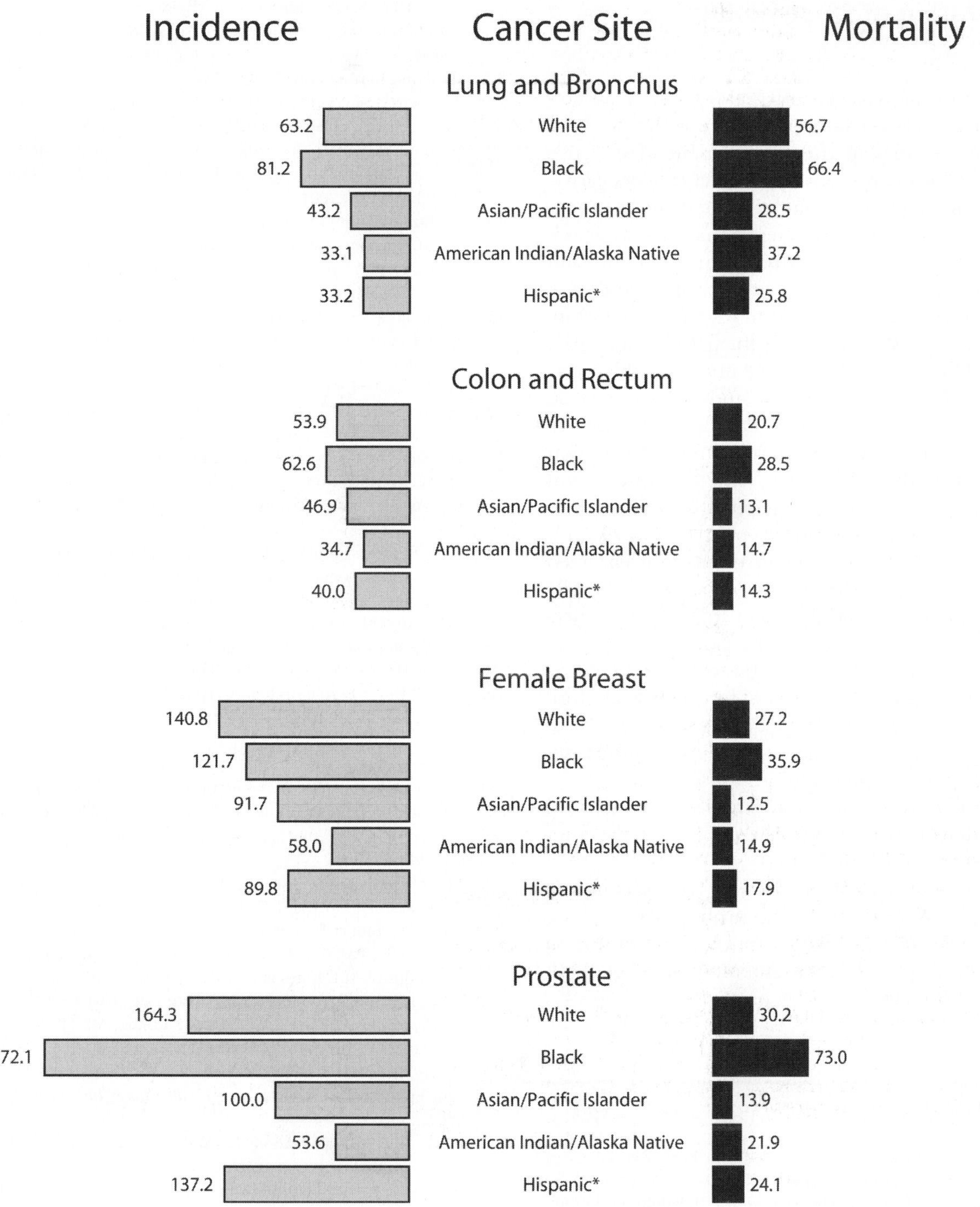

*Hispanic is not mutually exclusive from whites, blacks, Asian/Pacific Islanders, and American Indians/Alaska Natives. Incidence data for Hispanics exclude Detroit and Hawaii. Mortality data for Hispanics exclude cases from Connecticut, Oklahoma, New York, and New Hampshire.
Rates are per 100,000 and age-adjusted to the 2000 U.S. standard population by five-year age groups.

Figure 3-7 SEER cancer incidence and U.S. death rates, 1996–2000 (by cancer site and race). Data from SEER 12 areas and NCHS public use data file.

Application of Epidemiology to Nursing Practice

Nursing professionals play integral roles in all aspects of cancer prevention and cancer control. Nurses have played major roles in the development of effective means to educate, prevent, and detect cancers early.

Much of the progress that has been made in cancer control has stemmed from epidemiologic research that aims to understand environmental, genetic, and population risks for developing specific cancer(s). Nurses are constantly challenged to construct and interpret cancer risk assessments for patients and their families. This effort demands that nurses be able to accurately interpret epidemiologic studies of cancer risk.

Nurses have implemented the principles of primary, secondary, and tertiary cancer prevention through individualized cancer risk assessment and screening programs, cancer genetics counseling programs, government-sponsored programs, and programs that are offered at public events. A great need exists for nursing professionals to coordinate, implement, and help to provide cancer-control and education services.[140]

Nurses need to consider several common themes as they begin to design programs for cancer control. Some inherent cancer-control themes include consideration of the target population, resources of the institution or sponsor, opportunities for and value of collaboration, and resources for and approaches to public education, funding, marketing, and program evaluation.[141]

As cancer prevention and early detection continue to grow as a priority for oncology professionals and the institutions where they work, nurses will continue to play a critical role in the development, management, and success of cancer-control programs.

References

1. Trichopoulous D, Lipworth L, Petridou E: Epidemiology of cancer, in DeVita VT, Hellman S, Rosenberg SA (eds): *Cancer Principles and Practice of Oncology* (ed 6). Philadelphia, Lippincott-Raven, 2001, pp 231–257
2. Friis RH, Sellers TA: Study designs, in Friis RH, Sellers TA (eds): *Epidemiology for Public Health Practice.* Gaithersburg, Aspen, 1999, pp 187–229
3. Reid M: Cancer control and epidemiology, in Yarbro CH, Frogge MH, Goodman M, Groenwald SL (eds): *Cancer Nursing Principles and Practice* (ed 5). Sudbury, MA, Jones and Bartlett, 2000, pp 60–82
4. Rothman KJ: *Modern Epidemiology* (ed 2). Boston, Little Brown, 1998
5. Gordis L: *Epidemiology.* Phildelphia, Elsevier, 1996
6. Szklo M, Nieto FJ. *Epidemiology: Beyond the Basics.* Gaithersburg, Aspen, 2000
7. Page RM, Cole GE, Timmreck TC: Epidemiologic research, in Page RM, Cole GE, Timmreck TC (eds): *Basic Epidemiological Methods and Biostatistics: A Practical Guidebook.* Sudbury, MA, Jones and Bartlett, 1995, pp 81–143
8. Brinton LA, Schairer C, Haenszel W: Cigarette smoking and invasive cervical cancer. *JAMA* 255:3265–3269, 1986
9. Bertone ER, Willett WC, Rosner BA, et al: Prospective study of recreational physical activity and ovarian cancer. *J Natl Cancer Inst* 93:942–948, 2001
10. Colditz GA, Stampfer MJ, Willett WC, et al: Type of postmenopausal hormone use and risk of breast cancer: 12-year follow-up from the Nurses' Health Study. *Cancer Causes Control* 3:433–439, 1992
11. Adami H-O, Trichopoulos D: Concepts in cancer epidemiology and etiology, in Adami H-O, Hunter D, Trichopoulos D (eds). *Textbook of Cancer Epidemiology.* New York, Oxford University Press, 2004, pp 87–112
12. Piantadosi S: *Clinical Trials: A Methodologic Perspective.* John Wiley and Sons, New York, 1997
13. The Steering Committee of the Physicians' Health Study. Preliminary report: findings from the aspirin component of the ongoing Physicians' Health Study. *N Engl J Med* 318:262–263, 1988
14. Hennekens CH, Buring JE, Mason JE: Lack of effect of long-term supplementation with beta carotene on the incidence of malignant neoplasms and cardiovascular disease. *N Engl J Med* 334:1145–1149, 1996
15. Morgenstern H: Uses of ecologic analysis in epidemiologic research. *Am J Public Health* 72:1336–1344, 1982
16. Carroll KK: The role of dietary fat in breast cancer. *Curr Opin Lipidol* 8:53–56, 1997
17. Last JM: *A Dictionary of Epidemiology* (ed 3). New York, Oxford University Press, 1995
18. Breslow NE, Day NE: *Statistical Methods in Cancer Research: The Analysis of Case-Control Studies* (IARC Scientific Publications, no. 32) (ed 5). Lyon, International Agency for Research on Cancer, 1992
19. Greenland S: Response and follow-up bias in cohort studies. *Am J Epidemiol* 106:184–187, 1977
20. Nasca PC: Biomarkers and epidemiological studies of cancer, in Nasca PC, Pastides H (eds): *Fundamentals of Cancer Epidemiology.* Sudbury, MA, Jones and Bartlett, 2001, pp 85–102
21. Nasca PC: Tobacco and cancer, in Nasca PC, Pastides H (eds): *Fundamentals of Cancer Epidemiology.* Sudbury, MA, Jones and Bartlett, 2001, pp 139–174
22. Vineis M, Alavanja M, Buffler P, et al: Tobacco and cancer: recent epidemiological evidence. *J Natl Cancer Inst* 96:99–106, 2004
23. World Health Organization: *The World Health Report, 1999.* Geneva, World Health Organization, 1999
24. Boffetta P, Nyberg F: Contribution of environmental factors to cancer risk. *Br Med Bull* 68:71–94, 2003
25. International Agency for Research on Cancer: Tobacco smoking and involuntary tobacco smoke. *IARC Monographs on the Evaluation of the Carcinogenic Risk of Chemicals to Humans*, vol 83. Lyon, International Agency for Research on Cancer, 2002
26. Boffetta P, Agudo A, Ahrens W, et al: Multicenter case-control study of exposure to environmental tobacco smoke and lung cancer in Europe. *J Natl Cancer Inst* 90:1440–1450, 1998
27. Khuder SA, Simon VJ: Is there an association between passive smoking and breast cancer? *Eur J Epidemiol* 16:1117–1121, 2000
28. Reynolds P, Hurley S, Goldberg DE, et al: Active smoking, household passive smoking, and breast cancer: evidence from the California Teachers Study. *J Natl Cancer Inst* 96:29–37, 2004

29. Winn DM: Epidemiology of cancer and other systemic effects associated with the use of smokeless tobacco. *Adv Dent Res* 11:313–321, 1997
30. Gupta PC, Ray CS: Smokeless tobacco and health in India and South Asia. *Respirology* 8:419–431, 2003
31. Shatzkin A: Diet and cancer: future etiologic research. *Environ Health Perspect* 103:171–175, 1995
32. Bal DG, Foerster SB: Dietary strategies for cancer prevention. *Cancer* 72(suppl):1005–1010, 1993
33. Malin A, Dai Q, Shu X-O, et al: Intake of fruits, vegetables and selected micronutrients in relation to the risk of breast cancer. *Int J Cancer.* 105:413–418, 2003
34. Armstrong B, Doll R: Environmental factors and cancer incidence and mortality in two different countries, with special reference to dietary practices. *Int J Cancer* 15:617–631, 1975
35. Whittmore AS, Wu-Williams AH, Lee M, et al: Diet, physical activity and colorectal cancer among Chinese in North America and China. *J Natl Cancer Inst* 82:915–926, 1990
36. Jain M, Cook GM, Davis FG, et al: A case-control study of diet and colorectal cancer. *Int J Cancer* 26:757–768, 1980
37. Lyon JL, Mahoney AW, West DW, et al: Energy intake: its relationship to colon cancer risk. *J Natl Cancer Inst* 78:853–861, 1987
38. Potter JD: Diet and cancer of the colon and rectum: a case-control study. *J Natl Cancer Inst* 76:557–569, 1986
39. Howe GR, Jain M, Miller AB: Dietary factors and risk of pancreatic cancer: results of a Canadian population-based case-control study. *Int J Cancer* 45:604–608, 1990
40. Cho E, Spiegelman D, Hunter DJ: Premenopausal fat intake and risk of breast cancer. *J Natl Cancer Inst* 95:1079–1085, 2003
41. Willet WC, Hunter D, Stampfer MJ, et al: Dietary fat and fiber in relation to risk of breast cancer: a 8-year follow-up. *JAMA* 268:2037–2044, 1992
42. Kushi L, Potter J, Drinkard C, et al: Dietary factors and risk of breast cancer: combined analysis of 12 case-control studies. *Cancer Epidemiol Biomarkers Prev* 4:9–11, 1995
43. Steinmetz KA, Potter JD: Vegetables, fruits and cancer: I. epidemiology. *Cancer Causes Control* 2:325–327, 1991
44. Lampe JW: Health effects of vegetables and fruit: assessing mechanisms of action in human experimental studies. *Am J Clin Nutr* 70 (suppl):475S–490S, 1991
45. Zhang S, Hunter DJ, Forman MR, et al: Dietary carotenoids and vitamins A, C, and E and risk of breast cancer. *J Natl Cancer Inst* 91:547–556, 1999
46. Smith-Warner SA, Spiegelman D, Yaun SS, et al: Fruits, vegetables and lung cancer: a pooled analysis of cohort studies. *Int J Cancer* 107:1001–1011, 2003
47. Smith-Warner SA, Spiegelman D, Yaun SS, et al: Intake of fruits and vegetables and risk of breast cancer: a pooled analysis of cohort studies. *JAMA* 285:769–776, 2001
48. Johnson LJ, Meacham SL, Kruskall LJ: The antioxidants — vitamin C, vitamin E, selenium, and carotenoids. *J Agromedicine* 9:65–82, 2003
49. Seifried HE, McDonald SS, Anderson DE, et al: The antioxidant conundrum in cancer. *Cancer Res* 63:4295–4298, 2003
50. Stolzenberg-Solomon RZ, Albanes D, Nieto FJ, et al: Pancreatic cancer risk and nutrition-related methyl-group availability indicators in male smokers *J Natl Cancer Inst* 91:535–541, 1999
51. Li D, Jiao L: Molecular epidemiology of pancreatic cancer. *Int J Gastrointest Cancer* 33:3–14, 2003
52. Shrubsole MJ, Jin F, Dai Q, et al: Dietary folate intake and breast cancer risk: results from the Shanghai Breast Cancer Study. *Cancer Res* 61:7136–7141, 2001
53. Giovannucci E: Epidemiologic studies of folate and colorectal neoplasia: a review. *J Nutr* 132:2350S–2355S, 2002
54. Giovannucci E: A review of epidemiologic studies of tomatoes, lycopene, and prostate cancer. *Exp Biol Med (Maywood)* 227:852–859, 2002
55. Holick CN, Michaud DS, Stolzenberg-Solomon R, et al: Dietary carotenoids, serum beta-carotene, and retinol and risk of lung cancer in the alpha-tocopherol, beta-carotene cohort study. *Am J Epidemiol* 156:536–547, 2002
56. Cooper DA, Eldridge AL, Peters JC: Dietary carotenoids and lung cancer: a review of recent research. *Nutr Rev* 57(Pt 1):133–145, 1999
57. Peeters PHM, Keinan-Boker L, van der Schouw YT, Grobbee DE: Phytoestrogens and breast cancer risk. *Breast Cancer Res Treat* 77:171–183, 2003
58. Castle EP, Thrasher JB: The role of soy phytoestrogens in prostate cancer. *Urol Clin North Am* 29:71–81, 2002
59. Aldercreutz H: Epidemiology of phytoestrogens. *Baillieres Clin Endocrinol Metab* 12:605–623, 1998
60. Trock B, Lanza E, Greenwald P: Dietary fiber, vegetables, and colon cancer: critical review and meta-analyses of the epidemiologic evidence. *J Natl Cancer Inst* 82:650–651, 1990
61. Kiningham RB: Physical activity and the primary prevention of cancer. *Prim Care* 25:515–536, 1998
62. Negri E, Franceschi S, Parpinel M, La Vecchia C: Fiber intake and risk of colorectal cancer. *Cancer Epidemiol Biomarkers Prev* 7:667–671, 1998
63. Slattery ML, Sorenson AW, Ford MH: Dietary calcium intake as a mitigating factor in colon cancer. *Am J Med* 128:504–514, 1998
64. Garland C, Shekell RB, Barrett-Connor E, et al: Dietary vitamin D and calcium, and risk of colorectal cancer: a 19-year prospective study in men. *Lancet* 1:307–309, 1995
65. Sorenson AW, Slattery ML, Ford MH: Calcium and colon cancer: a review. *Nutr Cancer* 11:135–145, 1998
66. Alberts DS, Einspahr J, Ritenbaugh C, et al: The effect of wheat bran fiber and calcium supplementation on rectal mucosal proliferation rates in patients with resected adenomatous colorectal polyps. *Cancer Epidemiol Biomarkers Prev* 6:161–169, 1997
67. Kune S, Kune GA, Watson LF: Case-control study of dietary etiological factors: the Melbourne Colorectal Cancer Study. *Nutr Cancer* 9:21–42, 1987
68. Newmark HL, Lipkin M: Calcium, vitamin D and colon cancer. *Cancer Res* 52:2067s–2070s, 1992
69. Potter JD: Molecules and populations. *J Natl Cancer Inst* 91:916–932, 1999
70. Boyapati SM, Bostick RM, McGlynn KA, et al: Calcium, vitamin D, and risk for colorectal adenoma: dependency on vitamin D receptor B*sm*I polymorphism and nonsteroidal anti-inflammatory drug use? *Cancer Epidemiol Biomarkers Prev* 12:631–637, 2003
71. Nasca PC: Alcohol and cancer, in Nasca PC, Pastides H (eds): *Fundamentals of Cancer Epidemiology.* Sudbury, MA, Jones and Bartlett, 2001, pp 85–102
72. Bueno de Mesquita HB, Smeets FW, Ruina S, et al: The reproducibility of a food frequency questionnaire among control participants in a case-control study on cancer. *Nutr Cancer* 18:143–156, 1992
73. International Agency for Research on Cancer: *Alcohol Drinking,* no. 44. IARC Monographs on the Evaluation of Carcinogenic Risks to Humans. Lyon, France, World Health Organization, 1988
74. Simanowski UA, Homann N, Knuhl M, et al: Increased rectal cell proliferation following alcohol abuse. *Gut* 49:418–422, 2001
75. Spiegelhalder B, Eisenbrand G, Preussmann R: Contamination of beer with trace quantities of N-nitrosimethyl-amine. *Food Cosmet Toxicol* 17:29–31, 1979

76. Giovannucci E, Rimm EB, Ascherio A, et al: Alcohol, low-methionine–low-folate diets, and risk of colon cancer in men. *J Natl Cancer Inst* 87:265–273, 1995
77. Stampfer MJ, Colditz GA, Willett WC: Alcohol intake and risk of breast cancer. *Compr Ther* 14(5):8–15, 1988
78. Willett WC, Stampfer MJ, Colditz GA: Does alcohol consumption influence the risk of developing breast cancer? Two views. *Important Adv Oncol* 267–281, 1989
79. Willett WC, Stampfer MJ, Colditz GA, et al: Moderate alcohol consumption and the risk of breast cancer. *N Engl J Med* 316:1174–1180, 1987
80. Longnecker MP: Alcoholic beverage consumption in relation to the risk of breast cancer: meta-analysis and review. *Cancer Causes Control* 5:73–82, 1994
81. Longnecker MP, Newcomb PA, Mittendorf R, et al: Risk of breast cancer in relation to lifetime alcohol consumption. *J Natl Cancer Inst* 87:923–929, 1995
82. Smith-Warner SA, Spiegelman D, Yaun SS, et al: Alcohol and breast cancer in women: a pooled analysis of cohort studies. *JAMA* 279:535–540, 1998
83. Albanes D, Blair A, Taylor PR: Physical activity and risk of cancer in the NHANES I population. *Am J Public Health* 79:744–750, 1989
84. Slattery ML, Caan BJ, Benson J, Murtaugh M: Energy balance and rectal cancer: an evaluation of energy intake, energy expenditure, and body mass index. *Nutr Cancer* 46:166–171, 2003
85. Kono S, Shinchi K, Ikeda N, et al: Physical activity, diet habits and adenomatous polyps of the sigmoid colon: a study of self-defense officials in Japan. *J Clin Epidemiol* 44:1255–1261, 1991
86. Tavani A, Braga C, La Vecchia C, et al: Physical activity and risk of cancers of the colon and rectum: an Italian case-control study. *Br J Cancer* 79:1912–1916, 1999
87. John EM, Horn-Ross PL, Koo J: Lifetime physical activity and breast cancer risk in a multiethnic population: the San Francisco Bay area breast cancer study. *Cancer Epidemiol Biomarkers Prev* 12(Pt 1):1143–1152, 2003
88. Patel AV, Press MF, Meeske K, et al: Lifetime recreational exercise activity and risk of breast carcinoma in situ. *Cancer* 98:2161–2169, 2003
89. Lee IM: Physical activity and cancer prevention — data from epidemiologic studies. *Med Sci Sports Exerc* 35:1823–1827, 2003
90. Matthews C, Shu X-O, Jin F, et al: Lifetime physical activity and breast cancer risk in the Shanghai Breast Cancer Study. *Br J Cancer* 84:994–1001, 2001
91. Gerber M, Corpet D: Energy balance and cancers. *Eur J Cancer Prev* 8:77–89, 1999
92. Pastides H: Occupation and cancer, in Nasca PC, Pastides H (eds): *Fundamentals of Cancer Epidemiology*. Sudbury, MA, Jones and Bartlett, 2001, pp 123–137
93. Morris RD, Audet AM, Angelillo IF, et al: Chlorination, chlorination by-products, and cancer: a meta-analysis. *Am J Public Health* 82:955–963, 1992
94. McFarland M, Kaye J: Chlorofluorocarbons and ozone. *Photochem Photobiol* 55:911–929, 1992
95. World Health Organization: *Fluorides. Environmental Health Criteria 227.* Geneva, World Health Organization, 2002
96. Henderson BE: Establishment of an association between a virus and a human cancer. *J Natl Cancer Inst* 81:320–321, 1989
97. Blattner WA: Human retroviruses: their role in cancer. *Proc Assoc Am Physicians* 111:563–572, 1999
98. Nicholson WJ, Perkel G, Selikoff IJ: Occupational exposure to asbestos: population at risk and projected mortality — 1980–2030. *Am J Ind Med* 3:259–311, 1982
99. Lubin JH, Liang Z, Hrubec Z, et al: Radon exposure in residences and lung cancer among women: combined analysis of three studies. *Cancer Causes Control* 5:114–128, 1994
100. National Council on Radiation Protection and Measurements: *Exposure of the U.S. Population to Occupational Radiation.* National Council on Radiation Protection and Measurements. NCRP 101. Bethesda, NCRP, 1989
101. Environmental Protection Agency: *Health Risks of Exposure to Radon: BEIR VI.* Washington, DC, Commission of Life Sciences, National Academy Press, 1999
102. Gurney JG, van Wijngaarden E: Extremely low frequency electromagnetic fields (EMF) and brain cancer in adults and children: review and comment. *Neuro Oncol* 1:212–220, 1999
103. Frumkin H, Jacobson A, Gansler T, Thun MJ: Cellular phones and risk of brain tumors. *CA: Cancer J Clin* 51:137–141, 2001
104. Cook A, Woodward A, Pearce N, Marshall C: Cellular telephone use and time trends for brain, head and neck tumours. *N Z Med J* 116:U457, 2003
105. Warren HG, Prevatt AA, Daly KA, Antonelli PJ: Cellular telephone use and risk of intratemporal facial nerve tumor. *Laryngoscope* 113:663–667, 2003
106. Wrensch M, Minn Y, Chew T, et al: Epidemiology of primary brain tumors: current concepts and review of the literature. *Neuro Oncol* 4:278–299, 2002
107. Hardell L, Mild KH, Carlberg M: Further aspects on cellular and cordless telephones and brain tumours. *Int J Oncol* 22:399–407, 2002
108. Pastides H: Ionizing, nonionizing, and solar radiation and cancer, in Nasca PC, Pastides H (eds): *Fundamentals of Cancer Epidemiology*. Sudbury, MA, Jones and Bartlett, 2001, pp 207–222
109. McCredie M, Stewart JH, Day NE: Different roles for phenacetin and paracetamol in cancer of the kidney and renal pelvis. *Int J Cancer* 53:245–249, 1993
110. Pedersen-Bjergaard J, Ersboll J, Hansen VL, et al: Carcinoma of the urinary bladder after treatment with cyclophosphamide for non-Hodgkin's lymphoma. *N Engl J Med* 318:1028–1032, 1988
111. Olsen JH, Wallin H, Boice JD Jr, et al: Phenobarbital, drug metabolism, and human cancer. *Cancer Epidemiol Biomarkers Prev* 2:449–452, 1993
112. Conrad SA: Acute upper gastrointestinal bleeding in critically ill patients: causes and treatment modalities. *Crit Care Med* 30:365s–368s, 2004
113. Bertagnolli MM: The potential of nonsteroidal anti-inflammatory drugs (NSAIDs) for colorectal cancer prevention. *J Surg Oncol* 84:113–119, 2003
114. Thun MJ, Henley SJ, Patrono C: Nonsteroidal anti-inflammatory drugs as anticancer agents: mechanistic, pharmacologic, and clinical issues. *J Natl Cancer Inst* 94:252–266, 2002
115. O'Banion MK, Sadowski HB, Winn V, et al: A serum- and glucocorticoid-regulated 4-kilobase mRNA encodes a cyclooxygenase-related protein. *J Biol Chem* 266:23261–23267, 1991
116. Haller DG: COX-2 inhibitors in oncology. *Semin Oncol* 30(suppl 12):2–8, 2003
117. Giovannucci E, Rimm EB, Stampfer MJ, et al: Aspirin use and the risk for colorectal cancer and adenoma in male health professionals. *Ann Intern Med* 121:241–246, 1994
118. Barrett-Connor E: Postmenopausal estrogen replacement and breast cancer. *N Engl J Med* 321:319–320, 1989
119. Thomas DB: Do hormones cause breast cancer? *Cancer* 53(suppl):595–604, 1984
120. The Practice Committee of the American Society for Reproductive Medicine: Estrogen and progestogen therapy in postmenopausal women. *Fertil Steril* 81:231–241, 2004
121. Chasan-Taber L: Epidemiology of endogenous hormones and cancer, in Nasca PC, Pastides H (eds): *Fundamentals of Cancer Epidemiology*. Sudbury, MA, Jones and Bartlett, 2001, pp 275–295

122. Nasca PC: Biomarkers and epidemiological studies of cancer, in Nasca PC, Pastides H (eds): *Fundamentals of Cancer Epidemiology*. Sudbury, MA, Jones and Bartlett, 2001, pp 85–102
123. Perera FP: Molecular epidemiology in cancer prevention, in Schottenfeld D, Fraumeni JF (eds): *Cancer Epidemiology and Prevention*. New York, Oxford University Press, 1996, pp 101–115
124. American Cancer Society, Surveillance Research, 2004. *http://www.cancer.org/downloads/STT/CAFF_finalPWSecured.pdf*. Accessed August 12, 2004
125. American Cancer Society: Cancer Statistics, 2004, Atlanta, American Cancer Society, 2003
126. Zheng W: Epidemiological studies of genetic factors for cancer, in Nasca PC, Pastides H (eds): *Fundamentals of Cancer Epidemiology*. Sudbury, MA, Jones and Bartlett, 2001, pp 103–121
127. Human Genome Project: Implications for human genetics. *Am J Hum Gene* 49:687–691, 1991
128. Ries LAG, Eisner MP, Kosary CL, et al: SEER Cancer Statistics Review, 1975–2000, Bethesda, MD, National Cancer Institute, 2003
129. Reynolds T: Report examines association between cancer and socioeconomic status. *J Natl Cancer Inst* 95:1431–1433, 2003
130. Gao YT, Shu XO, Dai Q, et al: Association of menstrual and reproductive factors with breast cancer risk: results from the Shanghai Breast Cancer Study. *Int J Cancer* 87:295–300, 2000
131. Whiteman DC, Siskind V, Purdie DM, Green AC: Timing of pregnancy and the risk of epithelial ovarian cancer. *Cancer Epidemiol Biomarkers Prev* 12:42–46, 2003
132. Tung KH, Goodman MT, Wu AH, et al: Reproductive factors and epithelial ovarian cancer risk by histologic type: a multiethnic case-control study. *Am J Epidemiol* 158:629–638, 2003
133. Wise LA, Palmer JR, Harlow BL, et al: Reproductive factors, hormonal contraception, and risk of uterine leiomyomata in African-American women: a prospective study. *Am J Epidemiol* 159:113–123, 2004
134. Holly EA: Cervical intraepithelial neoplasia, cervical cancer, and HPV. *Annu Rev Public Health* 17:69–84, 1996
135. Munoz N, Bosch FX, de Sanjose S, et al: Risk factors for cervical intraepithelial neoplasia grade III/carcinoma in situ in Spain and Colombia. *Cancer Epidemiol Biomarkers Prev* 2:423–431, 1993
136. Miaskowski C: Pain management, in Given CW, Given B, Champion V, et al (eds). *Evidence-Based Cancer Care and Prevention*. New York, Springer, 2003, pp 274–291
137. Miaskowski C, Dodd M, West CM, et al: Randomized clinical trial of the effectiveness of the PRO-SELF pain control program in improving cancer pain management. *J Clin Oncol* 22:1713–1720, 2004
138. Rimer B, Levy MH, Keintz MK: Enhancing cancer pain control regimes through patient education. *Patient Ed Counsel* 10:267–277, 1987
139. deWit R, van Dam F, Zandbelt L: A pain education program for chronic cancer pain patients: follow-up results from a randomized clinical trial. *Pain* 73:55–69, 1997
140. Mahon SM: Overview: II. Cancer prevention, in Jennings-Dozier K, Mahon SM (eds): *Cancer Prevention, Detection and Control: A Nursing Perspective*. Pittsburgh, Oncology Nursing Press, 2002
141. Mahon SM: Overview: Section III. Cancer detection, in Jennings-Dozier K, Mahon SM (eds): *Cancer Prevention, Detection and Control: A Nursing Perspective*. Pittsburgh, Oncology Nursing Press, 2002

PART II

Prevention, Detection, and Diagnosis

CHAPTER 4

Cultural Diversity Among Individuals with Cancer

Joanne K. Itano, RN, PhD, OCN®

Special thanks to Karen Taoka for her contributions to the previous edition of this chapter.

Introduction

Culture is a fundamental element that uniquely shapes each individual. Cultural diversity encompasses more than just ethnic diversity, however. It is multifaceted and can include diversity in many forms, such as sexual orientation, nontraditional lifestyle, age, socioeconomic status, and religious beliefs. In this chapter, the focus of cultural diversity is on ethnic diversity.

Overview

Historically, the United States has taken pride in its "melting pot," or multicultural composition of peoples from many nations. Until recently, this cultural diversity was largely limited to white immigrants from Europe, who represented the majority of the population. In the twentieth century, immigration from areas such as Southeast Asia, China, Japan, Korea, the Philippines, Mexico, and the Caribbean began rapidly redefining the population composition of the United States. Projections by the U.S. Census Bureau predict that by the year 2050, the U.S. population will include the following distribution: white, 52.5%; Hispanic, 22.5%; black, 14.4%; Asian and Pacific Islander (API), 9.7%; and American Indian/Alaskan Native, 0.9%. These projections reflect a steady decrease in the white population, from 76% of the total population in 1990 to a projected 52.5% in 2050, as compared to steady growth in the minority populations.[1] In addition, ethnic minority populations will not be distributed uniformly across the United States. For example, it is projected that in 2020 nearly two-thirds (62%) of the API population will be concentrated in California, New York, Texas, Hawaii, and Washington.[2]

Unfortunately, this trend of increased ethnic diversity in the U.S. population is not matched in the composition of healthcare professionals. The representation of minority nurses increased from 7% in 1980 to 12% in 2000. Despite this increase, the diversity of the RN population is far lower than that of the U.S. population as a whole (30%).[3] The distribution of RNs by ethnicity is Hispanic, 2%; black, 4.9%; Asian, 3.5%; Native Hawaiian/Pacific Islander, 0.2%, and American Indian/Alaskan Native, 0.5%.

According to an Institute of Medicine (IOM) report,[4] evidence supports the importance of increasing racial and ethnic diversity among health professionals. Greater diversity is associated with improved access to care for ethnic minority patients, including higher patient satisfaction and improved patient–provider communication. Ethnic minority health providers are more likely to serve minority and medically underserved communities.

A fundamental challenge for healthcare providers is that the healthcare beliefs and practices of many ethnic groups may be incongruent with mainstream, Westernized medicine. The use of traditional healers and folk medicine, for example, often plays a major role in the provision of holistic care for blacks, APIs, Hispanics, and American Indians/Alaskan Natives.

This chapter provides an introduction to culture and cancer and describes the potential for oncology nurses to have a positive impact on the cancer experience of individuals and their families from different ethnic minority groups. Specific cultural information and nursing considerations for four ethnic minority groups (blacks, APIs, Hispanics, and American Indians/Alaskan Natives) are addressed. The discussion of these four ethnic minority groups is limited by several factors. Foremost is the diversity within each group. Blacks, APIs, Hispanics, and American Indians/Alaskan Natives are composed of several subgroups, each with its own subculture. For example, the subgroups under the term "Hispanic" include Mexican Americans, Puerto Ricans, Cuban Americans, and Central and South Americans. Added to the existence of subgroups and their unique cultures is the inherent heterogeneity due to intragroup differences, such as socioeconomic status, education attainment level, and degree of acculturation. Most important is the individual within the group. Although profiles of ethnic minority groups are provided in this chapter, each patient must be recognized as an individual with unique needs, regardless of his or her cultural background.

Epidemiology

Comparison data among the four major ethnic groups indicate differences in cancer incidence and morality. For example, blacks on the whole, have higher cancer incidence and mortality rates than do whites. Age-adjusted incidence and mortality rates by ethnicity are presented in Table 4-1.[5] There is also a difference in five-year survival rates, in that black men and women, American Indian/Alaskan Native men and women, and API men have lower five-year survival rates than non-hispanic Whites.[6]

Blacks

"Blacks" include immigrants from the African countries, the West Indies, the Dominican Republic, Haiti, and Jamaica and make up about 12% of the U.S. population.[7] Black men have the highest overall cancer incidence rates. Blacks have the highest cancer incidence for all sites compared to other major ethnic groups. This rate is about 10% higher than that for whites, 50–60% higher than that for Hispanics and

API, and more than twice as high as American Indians/Alaskan Natives. Death rates are higher than whites and more than twice as high as that for APIs, American Indians/Alaskan Natives, and Hispanics. Except for female breast cancer incidence and lung cancer death rates, where rates are higher in white females, ethnic and gender-specific incidence and death rates for the most common cancer types are higher for blacks than for any of the other ethnic minority groups.[8,9] In addition, blacks are more likely diagnosed with a later stage of cancer than whites and socioeconomic factors such as access to medical care and education play a role in this trend.

Asian and Pacific Islanders

Asian and Pacific Islanders were combined as one group until the 2000 census, which designated the Native Hawaiian and other Pacific Islanders as a separate group.[10] "Asian" refers to people having origins in any of the original peoples of the Far East, Southeast Asia, or the Indian subcontinent. The category includes Asian Indian, Chinese, Cambodian, Filipino, Korean, Japanese, Vietnamese, Hmong, Laotian, Thai, and other Asian (Bangladeshi, Burmese, Indonesian, Pakistani, or Sri Lankan) subcategories. This group makes up 3.6% of the U.S. population. More than half of all U.S. Asians live in three states: Hawaii, California, and Washington.[11]

"Native Hawaiians and other Pacific Islanders" refers to people having origins in any of the original peoples of Hawaii, Guam, Samoa, and other Pacific Islands (Tahitian, Northern Mariana Islander, Palauan, Fijian, or cultural groups such as Melanesian, Micronesian, or Polynesian). This group makes up 0.3% of the U.S. population.[12]

APIs are fourth in cancer incidence, behind blacks, whites, and Hispanics, and have the lowest mortality rate compared to blacks, whites, Hispanics, and American Indians/Alaskan Natives. However, given the diversity of the group, differences in incidence and mortality rates are noted among the various subgroups of the diverse API group. For example, there are variations in the age-adjusted incidence rate in the top five cancers for Asian groups compared to whites. Stomach cancer is included in this top five listing for Chinese, Japanese, Korean, and Vietnamese men, while liver cancer appears in the listing for Chinese, Filipino, Korean, and Vietnamese men. Thyroid and cervical cancer are among the top five cancers for Filipino women. Uterine cancer is first in incidence in Vietnamese women. There are also variations in the age-adjusted mortality rates in the top five cancers for Asian groups compared to whites. In Chinese men, esophageal cancer is in the top five. For Filipino men, liver cancer is in the top five. For Japanese men and women and Chinese women, stomach cancer is in the top five.[13]

Hispanics

Hispanics or Latinos constitute a heterogeneous group who trace their ancestry from Mexico, Puerto Rico, Cuba, and other countries in Central and South America or other Spanish cultures. They make up about 12.5% of the U.S. population and are the nation's fastest-growing minority group. Cancer occurrence and risk factors vary among Hispanics based on their status as U.S. or foreign born, their country of origin or heritage, their degree of acculturation, and their socioeconomic status. Hispanics have a lower incidence and mortality for all cancers combined and for the four most common cancers (breast, prostate, lung and bronchus, and colon and rectum) compared to non-Hispanic whites. Conversely, they demonstrate higher incidence and mortality rates from cancers of the stomach, liver, uterine, cervix, and gallbladder than non-Hispanic whites.[9,14,15]

American Indians/Alaskan Natives

The American Indian/Alaskan Native group includes people who have ancestors belonging to any of the original peoples of North and South America, including Central America, and who maintain tribal affiliation or community attachment. This group totals about 2.5 million individuals and represents 0.9% of the U.S. population.[10] As a group, they have the lowest cancer incidence rates and third lowest cancer mortality rates among blacks, whites, APIs, and Hispanics. In this group, the percentage of deaths from lung cancer increased 28.1% between 1990 and 1998, which reflects the higher percentage of American Indians/Alaskan Natives who smoke cigarettes. Of these men, 38.8% smoke, compared to 26.1% of men from all other ethnic groups; 31.7% of these women smoke, compared to 21.9% of women from all other ethnic groups.[16]

The poverty rate among the American Indians/Alaskan Native group was 24.5% in 2001, which is higher than comparable rates for non-Hispanic whites (7.8%), APIs (10.2%), Hispanics of any race (21.4%), and blacks (22.7%).[17] As a group, they are less likely to have health insurance than members of any other ethnic group. Based on a three-year average (1999–2001), 72.9% of the American Indian/Alaskan Native group have health insurance, compared to 66.8% of Hispanics, 80.8% of blacks, 81.5% of APIs, and 90.2% of non-Hispanic whites.[18]

Table 4-1 Age-Standardized Incidence and Mortality Rates* for Selected Cancer Sites by Ethnicity, United States, 1996 to 2000[5]

	White	Black	Asian/Pacific Islander	American Indian/Alaskan Native	Hispanic/ Latino†
			Incidence		
All Sites					
Males	555.9	696.8	392.0	259.0	419.3
Females	431.8	406.3	306.9	229.2	312.2
Breast (female)	140.8	121.7	97.2	58.0	89.8
Colon and Rectum					
Males	64.1	72.4	57.2	37.5	49.8
Females	46.2	56.2	38.8	32.6	32.9
Lung and Bronchus					
Males	79.4	120.4	62.1	45.6	46.1
Females	51.9	54.8	28.4	23.4	24.4
Prostate	164.3	272.1	100.0	53.6	137.2
Stomach					
Males	11.2	19.9	23.0	14.4	18.1
Females	5.1	9.9	12.8	8.3	10.0
Liver					
Males	7.3	11.0	21.1	6.1	13.8
Females	2.8	3.9	7.7	5.5	5.6
Uterine Cervix	9.2	12.4	10.2	6.9	16.8
			Mortality		
All Sites					
Males	249.5	356.2	154.8	172.3	176.7
Females	166.9	198.6	102.0	115.8	112.4
Breast (female)	27.2	35.9	12.5	14.9	17.9
Colon and Rectum					
Males	25.3	34.6	15.8	18.5	18.4
Females	17.5	24.6	11.0	12.1	11.4
Lung and Bronchus					
Males	78.1	107.0	40.9	52.9	40.7
Females	41.5	40.0	19.1	26.2	15.1
Prostate	30.2	73.0	13.9	21.9	24.1
Stomach					
Males	6.1	14.0	12.5	7.0	9.9
Females	2.9	6.5	7.4	4.2	5.3
Liver					
Males	6.0	9.3	16.1	7.6	10.5
Females	2.7	3.7	6.7	4.3	5.0
Uterine Cervix	2.7	5.9	2.9	2.9	3.7

*Rates are per 100,000 and age-adjusted to the 2000 U.S. standard population.

†Hispanics/Latinos are not mutually exclusive from whites, African Americans, Asian/Pacific Islanders, and American Indians/Alaskan Natives.

Data from Ries LAG, Eisner MP, Kosary CL, et al: *SEER Cancer Statistics Review, 1975–2000*. Bethesda, MD, National Cancer Institute, 2003, http://seer.cancer.gov/csr/1975–2000.

Ethnicity and Cancer

This section explores how ethnicity affects responses to the cancer experience. For each of the four major ethnic groups, information about health beliefs and practices, healing practices, social organization, communication, space and time, death and dying, and biologic variations is presented. Note that this information provides only a guideline for practice; each person is culturally unique. Nursing interventions that consider the patient and the family's cultural background must be based on a sound assessment and validation of the role culture plays in the life of both patient and family.

Many subgroups exist within the four major ethnic groups (black, API, Hispanic, and American Indian/Alaskan Native); however, it is beyond the scope of this chapter to provide an in-depth description of each subgroup's cultural beliefs and practices. Instead, relevant group characteristics regarding the cancer experience are presented. Various sources are available that further explore the individual subgroups.[19–24]

Blacks

Most blacks' ancestors were brought to the United States as slaves between 1619 and 1860 from the west coast of Africa. Blacks have also immigrated to the United States from other African countries, the West Indies, the Dominican Republic, Haiti, and Jamaica.[25] Blacks constitute about 12% of the total U.S. population but are disproportionately represented among the poor. They account for about 23% of the population below the poverty level, and 19% are medically uninsured compared to 10% of whites. Individuals in a lower socioeconomic group are generally at greater risk for illness, because seeking health care for early symptoms and preventive care generally are not priorities for those who struggle with day-to-day survival.[26]

Health beliefs and practices

The health beliefs of blacks include a tendency to categorize events as either desirable or undesirable. Illness is just another undesirable event, along with bad luck, poverty, and unemployment. Some believe illness results from their failure to live according to or to accept God's will. An individual may believe that cancer is an unnatural illness, caused by supernatural or sinful behavior, and that it cannot be treated by Western medicine.

For many blacks, a strong relationship exists between faith and healing. All blessings come from God, and only God can heal the sick. Illness may be perceived as a natural occurrence resulting from disharmony and conflict in some aspect of an individual's life, generally falling into one of three main areas: divine punishment, impaired social relationships, and environmental hazards. Divine punishment attributes illness to sin. An example of an impaired social relationship may be a spouse leaving or parents disowning a child. Environmental hazards include being struck by lightning or bitten by a snake.

Another belief among some blacks is that everything has an opposite. For every birth, there is a death; for every marriage, there is a divorce. Some may not distinguish between physical and mental illness and spiritual problems and may, therefore, present for treatment with a combination of somatic, psychological, and spiritual complaints. The nurse must acknowledge the patient's health belief system if he or she expects the patient to participate in Western practices. Some blacks may respond to pain stoically out of a desire to be a perfect patient; others may view pain as God's will.

Blacks tend to be less knowledgeable about cancer than whites. They are less likely to see a physician when experiencing warning signs or symptoms and are less aware of the benefits of specific cancer screening methods. Blacks are often more fatalistic about cancer and are less likely to believe that early detection or treatment can make a difference in the outcome of the disease. These factors lead to diagnosis at a later stage of illness, a poorer prognosis, and higher mortality rates for cancer.[27]

Blacks are more likely than whites to prefer to remain ignorant of their own cancer diagnosis. They are also less likely than whites to regard surgery, chemotherapy, and radiation as effective cancer treatment measures and are less optimistic about the chances of surviving cancer. In one study, 64% of blacks believed that cancer was a death sentence, and 65% believed that cancer treatment is worse than the disease. Eighty percent believed that cancer was spread by surgical treatment, and 20% indicated that they would rather not know that they had cancer.[28] Thus nurses may find black patients unwilling, uncooperative, or apparently noncompliant partners in their treatment.

Black attitudes about the U.S. healthcare system may be explained partially by history. During slavery, blacks received inconsistent and often barbaric healthcare treatment and developed a deep mistrust of their white masters and their harsh remedies and prescriptions. Even after slavery was abolished, blacks often received poor health care and inferior treatment in hospitals and clinics, which merely served to reinforce their negative view of Western medicine, and led to a high level of caution and mistrust.[29] Blacks may choose not to seek care if they perceive that their values will be compromised. To work effectively with black patients and families, the nurse will need to convey caring and understanding.

Healing practices

Different folk healers are used by some blacks. These healers are well-respected individuals and can be powerful resources for the healthcare team. They understand the beliefs and needs of the people they serve. Symptoms may be of minor importance. Cure may involve self-treatment or consultation with a neighbor knowledgeable in home remedies, a physician, or someone regarded to have unusual powers.

Often, religion is incorporated as part of therapy. A lay referral system typically services the health needs of the community and determines whether Western practitioners can be trusted and incorporated into the treatment. Openness, acceptance, and cooperation with this referral system by healthcare professionals may enhance acceptance and use of Western healthcare providers by blacks.

Help may be sought from an "old lady," a woman in the community who acts as a local consultant. She is knowledgeable about home remedies made from spices, herbs, and roots used to treat common illnesses. She also gives advice and makes appropriate referrals to another type of practitioner when an illness or a particular medical condition extends beyond her practice. The spiritualist is considered to have received the gift from God for healing incurable diseases or solving personal problems. This practitioner combines rituals, spiritual beliefs, and herbal medicines and is the most prevalent and diverse type of folk practitioner. A root doctor may also meet the needs for herbs, oils, candles, and ointments. The Voodoo priest/priestess may inherit this title only by birthright and is perceived to have a special gift. Voodoo, which combines African, Christian, and magical beliefs related to religion and health care, is practiced by some blacks. It is believed to cause, as well as prevent, the action of malevolent forces. Awareness of which home remedies have been used would help the nurse understand cultural practices and determine whether the remedies are helpful, harmful, or neutral.[30]

A treatment plan that is congruent with the patient's own beliefs has a better chance of being successful. Cultural health practices that are helpful should be encouraged. For example, use of herbal teas in place of water can serve both traditional and Western practices.

Social organization

The history of slavery likely contributes to the large number of female-headed households among blacks today. In 2000, female-headed households accounted for 44% of all black families. Thus, the wife or mother generally is charged with the responsibility for protecting the health of family members. Family members may enter the healthcare system at the advice of the matriarch of the family. The importance of the black woman in sharing information and helping the patient in decision making is important for the nurse to recognize.[30]

Some families have large social networks that can prove very supportive during times of illness. The added numbers may be helpful in provision of care and support but also may delay seeking help outside the network while consultation among the various members takes place. Including the members of the network in planning care may decrease the possibility of conflicting messages being given by the nurse and members of the network.[30]

The church plays an important role in the lives of many blacks by championing their interests and providing tangible assistance during periods of economic and social instability. The church is also a source of social identity and allows escape from the harsh realities of life. It promotes self-esteem among its membership and serves as a curator for maintaining the cultures of many blacks. Given the importance of the church in the lives of many blacks, inclusion of the clergy in the healthcare team may be very helpful.

Communication

The dialect that is spoken by many blacks is sufficiently different from Standard English in pronunciation, grammar, and syntax as to be classified as "Black English." The use of Standard English versus Black English varies among blacks and is sometimes related to educational level and socioeconomic status. Black English is a unifying factor for blacks in maintaining their cultural and ethnic identity. It is not uncommon for some blacks to speak Standard English when in a professional capacity or when socializing with whites and then revert to Black English when in black settings. Some blacks who have not mastered Standard English may become very quiet in settings in which they believe that Standard English is required. This may be incorrectly interpreted as hostility, submissiveness, or agreement.[30]

For more effective communication, the nurse who works with blacks must understand as much of the context of the dialect as possible. Viewing Black English as an unacceptable form of the English language may lead to labeling and stereotyping of the patient. Chiding and correcting the speech of blacks may result in the patient becoming quiet, passive, aggressive, or hostile. Conversely, attempting to use words common to the patient's vocabulary and mimicking the language may be interpreted as dehumanizing.

Slang also is used and may have different meanings among individuals and among cultural groups. Using words commonly understood by blacks in place of more sophisticated medical terms might make the patient more receptive to teaching and more cooperative. Examples of such words include "miseries" for pain, "tired or low blood" for anemia, "throw up" for vomit, and "pass water," "tinkle," or "peepee" for urinate.

When working with black patients, keep in mind that eye contact, nodding, and smiling do not necessarily mean that the black patient is paying attention. Validation of the message is very important in improving communication. Nurses may find it difficult to communicate with black patients who speak loudly and seem hostile and aggressive. However, it is the expressive quality of Black English that is often responsible for this behavior.[31]

Space and time

Many blacks have a "today" or "present" health orientation, and their approach to the prevention of cancer may be to work out problems as they occur, rather than trying to prevent them from occurring. This approach is based on the belief that planning for the future is hopeless and may reflect previous experiences with racism and discrimination.[32] In planning nursing care for individuals with such a time orientation, explain when flexibility of time is acceptable and when a delay might result in a serious problem. Acceptance of lateness in appointments is helpful when possible.

Many blacks are highly involved people who tend to have several activities going on at the same time. This may create conflict for the nurse, who, in an effort to complete nursing care, often may be interrupted by these activities. Negotiating with the patient and family to meet the needs of both the nurse and the patient may prove helpful.

Death and dying issues

In the African language, the primary time frames are past and present. No word exists for the distant future, as it has not yet happened. Consequently, the future and the past merge into the present. Life is viewed as cyclical in nature, and all events are given by God. Death is a natural part of the cycle of life and is unavoidable. It is familiar and near and evokes no great fear or awe.[33]

The strong family network of blacks may be called into action when a family member is seriously ill. Care of the terminally ill is a public rather than a private undertaking, with neighbors and friends sharing resources. The family develops plans for the care of the patient, identifies tasks, and assigns family members to assume them. The home is usually viewed as the place for the ill person to spend his or her final days. Frequent visitors are common. The patient generally remains an active and vital force within the family until he or she can no longer do so. The decision as to whether to inform the patient of terminal illness is made on an individual basis.[33]

It is not uncommon for blacks to plan their funerals and purchase grave plots long before their own deaths. Public and communal grief are openly expressed at traditional black funerals, which are termed "home-goings." People in the congregation often respond spontaneously and out loud to the sermon. A gradual increase in emotion occurs as the funeral progresses, and many of those attending express deep emotion. Music provides a means of sending the deceased joyfully on to the next leg of his or her journey.[33,34]

Biological variations

A major biological variation in blacks relates to skin color. That is, there is great variation in the darkness of skin color, and individuals who are fairer-skinned have a greater risk for developing skin cancers from sun exposure. A darker skin color makes the assessment of pallor, jaundice, ecchymosis, or erythema more difficult. Assessing areas of lighter melanin pigmentation such as the sclera, conjunctiva, soles of feet, and palms of the hands may be useful.

The diet of many blacks contains little fresh produce, is highly seasoned, and includes frequent use of smoked and fatty meats as seasoning for vegetables and soups. Pork is often a staple meat. As a consequence, saturated fat intake may be high. In comparison to white women, black women are more likely to be obese, while black men are more likely to be underweight. The eating habits and compromised nutritional status of blacks could be a factor in their generally higher incidence and mortality rates from cancer.[27]

Lactose intolerance affects 75% of blacks. Affected individuals lack the enzyme to convert lactose to glucose and galactose, resulting in gastrointestinal symptoms of bloating, cramping, and diarrhea after the ingestion of milk and other products containing lactose. The intolerance tends to occur primarily in infancy shortly after weaning and in the teen years or early twenties. Treatment is to avoid milk products. As milk products are often suggested to improve nutrition for patients with cancer, awareness of possible lactose intolerance in the black population is significant for the nurse in patient and family teaching.[30]

Alcoholism is a major health problem in the black community and a risk factor for cancers of the mouth, larynx, tongue, esophagus, lung, and liver. Factors associated with alcohol abuse include unemployment, the availability of the substance, peer pressure, a desire to escape from personal problems, and the prevalence of taverns as social centers in black communities. Thus the causes are complex social issues and difficult to treat.

Asian and Pacific Islanders

Asian and Pacific Islanders are very heterogeneous group, composed of individuals from 28 Asian countries and 25 identified Pacific Island cultures. This marked ethnic diversity is further compounded by inherent variations within each subgroup, such as degree of acculturation and socioeconomic status. It was estimated in 1990 that approximately 74% of the total API population were foreign born and were recent immigrants and refugees. Although many have good incomes, approximately one out of eight APIs lives in poverty. Similarly, many APIs have a college degree or postgraduate education, but a significant number are functionally illiterate.[11,12] Because the APIs are predominately Asian, this discussion primarily addresses Asian Americans.

Health beliefs and practices

Many Asians share traditional health beliefs and practices that are carried out in varying degrees within each group. Nevertheless, because of the common influence of Chinese culture, much similarity in beliefs and practices is noted among Asian groups. For example, one of the most common beliefs is that health is a state of harmony in body, mind, and spirit with nature and the universe.[25] Although Native Hawaiians are not of Asian descent, harmony with nature is also an important health belief in this culture.[35]

Many APIs believe that a balance between hot and cold elements is essential for good health. In the Chinese, Japanese, and Korean cultures, in particular, this balance is defined as *yin* (cold) and *yang* (hot).[36,37] *Yin* and *yang* are life forces in which *yin* (cold) is characterized as female, dark, negative energy, and *yang* (hot) is male, light, positive energy. Illness is believed to result from an imbalance of these two forces. The Chinese believe that the human body, illnesses, and foods possess *yin* or *yang* characteristics, and treatment is aimed at reestablishing the balance.[36–38] For example, cancer is a *yin* or cold illness and would be treated with foods, herbs, and healing ceremonies that possess "hot" properties. The Filipino, East Indian, and Southeast Asian cultures share similar beliefs about hot and cold balance and health. Other explanations for illness include an imbalance of humoral elements, an obstruction of *chi* (an essential life energy), a curse by a spirit, spiritual imbalance, punishment for immoral behavior, or an imbalance in the body caused by exposure to wind or air.[39]

There exists a widespread belief among some API groups that suffering is part of life, a philosophy that may result in postponement in seeking medical treatment, either traditional or Western. Fatalism is found in the Filipino culture where the attitude of *bahala na* — "It's in the hands of God" — exists, especially when illness and pain are seen as punishment.[39] In the Japanese culture, the term *shoganai* is used when misfortune strikes, such as an illness. Its translation, "It can't be helped," reflects an almost fatalistic view. Chinese Americans also have a fatalistic outlook on life, exemplified by their belief that they lack control over nature.[36]

Many APIs believe that blood is a life force that cannot be replaced or, if taken, will disrupt the body's balance, causing weakness and even death. Therefore, many APIs fear venipunctures. Hmong patients may be reluctant to receive blood transfusions because their perception is that the donor's spirit may enter the body via the transfusion. Chinese and Vietnamese patients may not agree to surgery when organs or body parts are to be removed because of their belief that the human body must be intact at the time of death to avoid potential adverse consequences in the afterlife. Vietnamese individuals may also avoid surgery because it is perceived as a last resort and associated with death. Hmong patients may refuse surgery because of their belief that cutting into the body releases spirits, causing an imbalance.[40,41]

Healing practices

As part of their traditional health beliefs, APIs use herbal medications, seek out traditional healers, and perform healing ceremonies. Because APIs often employ herbal preparations concurrently with Western medicine, it is important to ascertain if, and what, herbal preparations are being used to anticipate possible drug interactions. For example, *ma huang* is a Chinese herb that contains ephedrine. Complications can arise if, in addition to the *ma huang*, the patient takes ephedrine via a Western practitioner's prescription.[41] Ginseng, another popular herb, is considered a stimulant and has hypertensive effects. Undesirable side effects can result if the patient takes ginseng in conjunction with Western antihypertensive medication.[36]

Traditional healers among APIs include shamans (Laotian, Hmong), Chinese herbalists, *kahuna la'au lapa'au* (Native Hawaiian), and *Hilot* (Filipino). These healers are often consulted before Western medical practitioners. In some cases, the perceived cause of the illness determines who is consulted first. For example, if Southeast Asians believe that an illness is organic in origin, they may seek a Western physician. Conversely, if the cause of illness is thought to be supernatural, a traditional healer would be consulted. If the illness persists after consulting with traditional healers, then Western treatment might be sought. At this point, however, the disease may be at an advanced stage and untreatable. Because Western medicine cannot cure the illness, it is therefore seen as ineffective. This pattern may reinforce the use of traditional healers. For many APIs, the Western healthcare system is foreign. Greater comfort is found in consulting a healer who understands, with whom one can communicate, and whose practice is familiar to the patient. Additionally, healers are inexpensive and have a reputation for being effective for specific conditions.

Healing ceremonies or practices vary considerably across API groups. In the Native Hawaiian culture, healing includes special rituals, prayers, and chants as well as the use of special herbs and plants.[42] Other practices include moxibustion, cupping, acupuncture, massage, and skin scraping or coining.[36]

Moxibustion. This treatment, used to restore the *yin–yang* balance, involves a deeply penetrating heat. Small pellets or cones made of the herb *Artemesis vulgaris* (moxa) are placed at acupuncture points on the body and are then burned. The pellets or cones are removed when the patient feels the heat. This treatment leaves small, rounded or asymmetrical superficial burn marks. It is used in the treatment of ailments of the joints, muscles, bones, and back.[36,37]

Cupping. Like moxibustion, cupping uses heat but in a different fashion. A material, such as alcohol-soaked cotton, is placed in a special cup and set on fire to create a vacuum in the cup. When the flame is extinguished, the cup is then placed immediately on the treatment area of the body, where it creates suction. The cup is kept there for 15–20 minutes or until it is easily removed. Cupping is used to treat pain, body aches, and headaches. This painful procedure sometimes leaves circular burn marks approximately 2 inches in diameter. These burn marks have been misinterpreted as child abuse in Southeast Asian children who have been treated with cupping.[43]

Skin scraping or coining. This treatment involves the application of a special menthol oil or ointment to the symptomatic area. With the edge of a coin, the area is then rubbed in a firm, downward motion. This procedure is used to treat colds, heatstroke, headache, pain, vomiting, and indigestion.

Social organization

Asian and Pacific Islanders tend to have very strong, family-centered systems. The family exerts an extremely powerful force in an individual's life, and the needs of the individual are often secondary to those of the larger group. Healthcare decisions are often made by the family or social network.[36,44,45]

In many API groups, patrilineal authority, along with filial piety and respect for elders, often means that the eldest son or male head of the clan acts as the spokesperson for the patient. This individual is the designated family member with whom medical practitioners speak when information about the patient's condition is given or when treatment decisions need to be made.[45]

Because of the strong emphasis placed on the family, API family members are more likely to actively participate in the patient's daily care. Healthcare professionals need to be sensitive to these cultural needs and must support the family to prevent caregiver exhaustion, especially if one family member is the sole caregiver.

Communication

In many API groups, communication patterns are influenced by values that emphasize politeness, respect for authority, and avoidance of shame. These values prevent many API from asking health professionals questions or challenging a proposed diagnostic workup or treatment plan.[45] Instead, an individual may nod his or her head, in what is interpreted as agreement. In reality, the patient may not necessarily agree or understand what the practitioner has said.[34] Thus poor communication can occur between the API patient and the Western practitioner.

In communicating with members of some API groups, Western practitioners may need to avoid or limit engaging in direct eye contact, as such eye contact may be perceived as being rude, challenging, or just culturally unacceptable.[40,46] For example, in the Filipino culture, direct eye contact between an older man and a young woman usually implies seduction or anger.[44] In the East Indian culture, eye contact between a woman and a man other than her husband can have sexual significance.[47] Avoiding eye contact by the South Vietnamese is a sign of respect when talking with someone perceived to be of different rank in education, social status, age, or gender.[40]

Many APIs prefer limited or no physical contact.[36,40,45] In some API groups, the head is sacred and touching or patting the head is perceived as a rude gesture.[36] For some Southeast Asians, crossing the legs and pointing the foot at the individual is also considered to be insulting. Similarly, directing the sole of the shoe or foot toward Koreans is offensive to them.[46]

Many APIs do not speak English or have limited proficiency in English as their second language. Because of this language barrier, interpreters are often used. Such communication via a third party presents challenges in ensuring that the literal meaning of the conversation is translated correctly, along with the interpretation of nonverbal messages. When possible, use professional interpreters who can facilitate and ensure communication among the patient, family, and health professional.

In selecting an interpreter, first ascertain the specific dialect spoken by the patient and family. For example, several dialects are spoken by Filipinos, including Visayan, Tagalog, Ilocano, and Cebuano. Family interpreters are often used; however, the message relayed may not always be accurate. For example, if the message delivers a poor prognosis, the family member may modify it in an attempt to protect the patient. In addition, if interpreters are of the opposite sex, patients may not bring up symptoms or concerns that they perceive to be either embarrassing or culturally unacceptable to discuss in the presence of a member of the opposite sex. The traditional hierarchy in many API families where power and influence run from elders to youths represents another potential pitfall when using family interpreters. In some instances, especially with recent immigrants, children may be used as interpreters because they usually have a better command of English. This practice reverses the rank of the child in the family and may put undue stress on the family.[46]

Space and time

Asian/Pacific Islanders value privacy, and many are very modest. When physical examinations or procedures necessitate exposure of the body, it should be minimized by revealing only that part of the body that needs to be examined. Female API patients, such as East Indian and Chinese women, may feel more comfortable being examined by female practitioners.[22]

The concept of time varies among API groups. For example, Japanese patients, who are present and future oriented, are usually prompt and adhere to fixed schedules.[45] By contrast, Chinese are more present oriented, do not necessarily adhere to fixed schedules, and may be late for appointments.[36] Filipinos are past and present oriented and may disregard health-related matters. This time orientation is closely linked to their *bahala na* philosophy of leaving things in God's hands.[44]

Death and dying issues

Many issues arise regarding death and dying in API groups. Bioethics, truth telling, the patient's right to know, and advance directive decisions are based in the tenets espoused by Western culture. It is important to be aware that patient autonomy and self-determination in API groups may not be culturally acceptable or valued. As previously discussed, the family or family spokesperson frequently makes decisions about the patient's care, rather than the patient.

Conflict may arise between the value in Western medicine of open disclosure of a terminal illness and the value shared by many API groups that "to tell someone he or she is dying is not only rude but dangerous."[48] For example, East Indians prefer not to tell patients about the seriousness of their condition or to reveal the possibility of death. They believe that "speaking of possibilities may render them too real, and a traditional Indian does not speak lightly of death; . . . if a patient knows the gravity of the illness, he or she will give up hope and die."[49,p.269] This concept is also seen in the Hmong culture, where the disclosure of prognosis to a terminally ill patient "is the same as wishing death upon that person and may in fact bring about that person's death."[50] Muller and Desmond further note that in many Asian groups,

> People fear that openly acknowledging an impending death is like casting a death curse upon the person; it will make the person despair and die even sooner. Thus, to engage in discussions of code status or the possibility of hospice care, interventions that can be seen as explicit preparation for death, is courting bad luck.[48,p.325]

On the other hand, although hospice care discussions may not always be encouraged, some APIs prefer to die at home rather than in the hospital.[41,46] This preference is due, in large part, to the value placed on the family and

> The belief that the unfortunate who die among strangers and away from their familiar dwelling are forever condemned to wander in pain, so-called orphan souls, endlessly searching in vain for the family and home they missed when they died.[51,p.24]

Given the potential for conflict and frustration between the values of Western health care and the cultural values of various API groups, exploring life-support decisions with the patient and family is critical. Klessig suggests that information about the following be determined: sanctity of life, definition of death, religious background and extent of involvement, beliefs about causal agents in illness and how they relate to the dying process, social support system, and the family's decision maker.[52]

By facilitating communication about these issues between the patient, his or her family, and the health-care team, oncology nurses can assist in narrowing the gap between these two value systems and support the patient and family through this phase of the cancer experience.

Biological variations

The incidence rate for liver cancer is exceptionally high in API groups, particularly among the Southeast Asian groups. This increased rate is linked to the high incidence of hepatitis B infection, largely due to the fact that these groups originate from areas where hepatitis B is endemic.

Lactose intolerance is also common in APIs. Milk and cheese — common foods in the mainstream

American diet—may therefore be unacceptable to this group. When providing oral supplements that do not contain milk but have the appearance of a milk product, the patient and his or her family must be reassured that the supplement is not a milk product.

Many APIs also have a distinguishing yellow cast to their skin that ranges in tone. This yellow cast can make the recognition of jaundice more challenging. To assess for jaundice, the sclera and excreta need to be checked.

Although not a biological variation, the higher smoking rates among Southeast Asian men as compared to the general population deserve mention. This is a prime area for health promotion activities. Another area of concern is that APIs had the lowest self-reported rates for Pap tests within the past three years.[26] Possible reasons for this low participation rate include lack of health education programs targeted specifically at this group, fatalism belief, and decreased access to health care.

Hispanics

Hispanics, in general, identify themselves as members of the same ethnic group — not by demographic characteristics but by their cultural values and language. *Hispanic* is the term that has been used by the U.S. federal government to classify individuals who claim ties to Spain in their heritage. The term *Latino* includes all Latin American individuals and describes immigrants from those Spanish-speaking countries where the integration of Spanish, indigenous people, and Africans has occurred. Whether an individual prefers to be called Hispanic or Latino is generally a matter of choice. Some have strong opinions; others do not. It may be helpful to use the name of the country of origin when referring to individuals or to a specific ethnic group. *Chicano* is another term used when discussing Hispanics; it refers to all Americans of Mexican descent.

Generally, the cancer incidence and mortality rates among Hispanics rank at the median when compared to the rates among other ethnic groups.

Health beliefs and practices

For Hispanics, health often is believed to be the result of good luck or a reward from God for good behavior. The concept that a disease is God's will is widely accepted. Terminal illnesses especially are seen as the result of some indiscretion against God. Thus health and illness in Hispanic groups have a strong religious association.

In many cases, Hispanics espouse a fatalistic belief that one is at the mercy of the environment and has little control over what happens. Personal efforts are unlikely to influence the outcome of a situation. For this reason, Hispanics often do not believe that they are personally responsible for present or future successes or failures with regard to their health and otherwise.[53]

Several categories of disease exist in the Hispanic culture. The concept of hot and cold imbalance resembles *yin* and *yang* in the Chinese culture. To ensure good health, it is believed that individuals must ingest both hot and cold foods.[24] Internal factors such as a change in body temperature and external factors such as the foods eaten can affect the hot–cold balance. Many of the disorders caused by hot and cold imbalances are digestive in nature. A stomach ulcer is a "hot illness" caused by eating too much hot food. Excesses of heat developed from within the body and extending outward are believed to be related to cancer, rheumatism, tuberculosis, and paralysis.

Another group of illnesses is believed to be caused by magical interventions. *Mal ojo*, or "evil eye," occurs when someone with a powerful glance looks improperly at a child; it is believed to be a manifestation of witchcraft and, as a result, the child is said to be affected by evil spirits. Treatment entails a ceremonial ritual that includes passing an egg over the affected person's body while reciting prayers. *Susto*, or "sudden fright," occurs when an individual experiences a stressful event at some time prior to the onset of symptoms. The stressor may be the death of a significant person, a child's nightmare, or an inability to adequately fulfill social-role responsibilities. *Mal puesto* ("evil") is an illness caused by a hex bestowed by a *brujo* ("witch"), *curandero* ("folk healer"), or other person knowledgeable about witchcraft.[24]

In Hispanic culture, there are two types of emotional diseases: mental illness and moral illness. Mental illness is seen as inevitable, and the affected person is viewed as a victim of consequence. Moral illness, such as alcoholism, is said to be caused by the individual, and treatment is the responsibility of family members. The latter category includes scientific diseases that cannot be treated by traditional health practices and must be diagnosed and treated by the Western health-care system.

Hispanics commonly view cancer fatalistically as being God's will, and they believe it goes against principle to treat the disease aggressively. Family members with cancer, especially elders, often are not informed of their diagnosis, as it is believed such information will simply worsen the illness because it is considered deadly and engenders great fear. Patients often say, "I deserve to suffer." Cancer is viewed by Hispanics as contagious and difficult to prevent because it is caused by many things. Thus going to see the doctor early serves no useful purpose. Many Hispanic patients believe that chemotherapy does not work, that radiation may cause cancer, and that cancer will remain even after surgery to remove it. Some believe that certain cancer treatments may have side effects that can be passed on to family members (e.g., that family members may become radioactive if the patient receives radiation therapy).[54]

Hispanic individuals may believe that there is no need to see a physician unless a person is very ill. Hospitals are seen as places where people die. Therefore, medical attention may be sought only after symptoms develop or when the individual is too ill to be cared for by the family.

Approximately 21% of Hispanics live at or below the poverty level. The cost of being sick includes not only the amount of money needed for care, but also the loss of money in time missed from work. Many Hispanics fear that because of their economic status and ethnicity, they may receive inferior care in the U.S. medical system. Some Hispanics believe they should receive only health care that they can afford. As a consequence, if they cannot afford to pay, some Hispanic individuals may not seek care.[54]

In general, Hispanics are less likely than members of any other group to have medical insurance. Approximately 23% of Hispanics lack health insurance.[18] The outcome of this trend in relation to cancer is late diagnosis and higher mortality rates despite the lower overall incidence of cancer in the Hispanic population.[54] The high percentage of Hispanics who are migrant farm workers also contributes to the overall decreased access to health care for that group.[53]

Individuals of Hispanic origin often believe that it is inappropriate to question those giving care, as they fear retaliation. Because some Hispanics believe that physical touch can promote healing, if Western providers do not touch Hispanic patients during their visit, the patients may believe that they did not derive any benefit from the visit.

Martaus offers the following suggestions for assimilating Hispanic individuals to the U.S. health care system:[55]

- Healthcare providers must communicate their acceptance of the person's value system to establish trust.
- Providers should incorporate a culturally relevant interview in the admission process. This practice defines the individual's perception of illness and allows the healthcare provider to establish a workable treatment plan.
- The treatment plan must include a family focus, as illness intensifies the need for family involvement.
- Many Hispanics are very religious and may view treatment without prayer as ineffective.
- Healthcare workers must take responsibility for finding common ground that incorporates traditional beliefs and modern health care.
- Many Hispanics have a great fear of authority. They may believe that disease occurs because it is God's will and may place great emphasis on treating doctors with respect.

Healing practices

For Hispanics, home remedies represent the first line of treatment. To cure a hot or cold imbalance, the opposite quality of the causative agent is applied. For example, if the causative agent for a headache is thought to have a hot quality, cold herbs may be placed on the temples to absorb the heat. If the cause has a cold quality, hot herbs are applied. If the stool is green or yellow, the diarrhea is hot and the remedy is cold tea. If the stool is white, the diarrhea is cold and the remedy is hot tea.[53]

Usually a family folk healer, someone respected for her knowledge of folk medicine, plays a pivotal role. The healing practices are passed down in the family from mother to daughter. If home remedies do not work, Mexican Americans send for the *curandero* or *herbalista*, a traditional folk medicine healer. This person receives his or her skills through an apprenticeship or as a gift from God and is knowledgeable in the use of herbs, diet, massage, prayer, and ritual. Puerto Ricans seek out the *espiritismo*, a folk healer with the gift of contacting the spirit world and healing through the powers of spirits. Such healers analyze dreams, foretell the future, and use medals, prayers, and amulets as part of their treatment approach. The Cuban population may seek medical help from a *santero*, a medicine man who works with the spirits of good within a system to promote wellness. Animal sacrifices, rituals, chanting, and prayers are used to aid in healing.[56] A *yerbero* is a healer who uses herbs and spices to prevent illness and enhance healing. A *brujo* uses witchcraft for healing illnesses that may be related to jealousy or envy (*envidia*). If these remedies fail, then Western physicians may be sought out for help.[53,57]

It is essential that the nurse demonstrate acceptance of the spiritual and folk basis of Hispanic people's health beliefs. Once this acceptance is conveyed, there is the potential for influencing acceptance and understanding of the rationale for modern healthcare practices, thereby gaining the community's confidence.

Social organization

The nuclear family (parents and children) is the foundation of the Hispanic community. Men are the breadwinners, assume dominant roles in Hispanic families, and are considered to be big and strong (*macho*). The hesitancy of a woman or child to make a decision may be due to the need to inform and obtain approval of the husband and father.[57] In Hispanic culture, women have always been the primary caretakers. The extended family is valued, and the family's needs supersede those of the individual members. When a family member's illness becomes too serious for the wife and mother to handle alone, she may ask the extended family to help care for the sick individual. Family members may also speak for the patient. Because of its high value in the patient's treatment and recovery, the family should be used to help with the patient's care.

Roman Catholicism is the predominant religion aong Hispanics. Because religion is such an important factor in the health beliefs of many Hispanics, the patient may turn to religious practices, such as prayer, making special devotions, visiting shrines, or lighting a candle as an act of devotion and appeal to a patron saint, to help overcome the illness. Allowing time and providing privacy for the family to practice their religion during hospitalization will be helpful to many Hispanics.[53]

Communication

For Hispanics, Spanish is the primary language, though numerous dialectical differences exist. Many Hispanics are bilingual but have a strong preference for their native language; during times of illness, they often revert to it. There is some mistrust of whites and Western medicine, especially when the healthcare provider does not speak Spanish. Language may be a barrier, and Hispanics may not let the provider know that they do not understand. Translators may be necessary.

The traditional Hispanic approach to communication requires the use of much diplomacy and tactfulness. Concern and respect for another's feelings dictate that a screen always be provided to preserve the patient's dignity. The manner of expression is likely to be elaborate and indirect, so as to make a personal relationship at least appear harmonious, as respect of each person's individuality is important. Politeness and courtesy are highly regarded. Even if the Hispanic individual disagrees with another's point of view, direct argument or contradiction is considered rude and disrespectful. On the surface, he or she may seem agreeable, but only because manners dictate that his or her genuine opinions should not be expressed openly. This apparent agreement may lead to a false assumption on the part of the healthcare provider, who may believe that the patient understands and will follow through with whatever is proposed. In practice, this may not be true.

Body language may be dramatic when expressing pain or emotion. Hispanics in pain may moan and groan to let those around them know they are uncomfortable and suffering.[57]

Space and time

Adult Hispanics may be described as tactile in their relationships, yet display a high degree of modesty. This is one reason why Hispanics do not enter the U.S. healthcare system. They generally do not like being touched by others or having to touch themselves and are not comfortable being examined by healthcare professionals of the opposite sex. Embarrassment is a common reaction to invasive procedures or body exposure during an examination.[54]

Despite the fact that Hispanics like consistent, close relationships and physical touching, female nurses should always assist a male physician when examining a female patient; likewise, a male nurse should always assist a female physician when examining a male patient. Special care should be taken to guard against exposing body parts other than those that are the focus of the examination. Male patients may refuse a complete examination because of their modesty.

Hispanics generally have a relaxed concept of time —a present orientation—and may be late for appointments. The patient may be more concerned with a current activity than with the activity of planning ahead to be on time. Such a mindset suggests a belief that future-oriented activities can be recovered and that present-oriented activities cannot. The present time orientation helps explain why Hispanics often seek out the most accessible and affordable care first (folk healing and the folk practitioner). It is therefore useful for the nurse to focus on short-term problems. For example, if a medication is not taken in a timely manner, the immediate effects should be emphasized.[53]

Death and dying issues

The afterlife of heaven and hell exists in the Hispanic culture. As many Hispanics are Catholic, religious practices such as the sacrament of extreme unction, or anointing of the sick, are important. The family serves as a supportive network for helping the terminally ill and later their survivors. Often, the patient is not told directly by the family of his or her condition but still demonstrates some awareness of death's likelihood. Although Hispanics typically prefer to remain at home to die, dying in a hospital is an acceptable alternative. Public expression of grief is to be expected, especially among women.[58]

Biological variations

The traditional Hispanic diet is high in fiber and carbohydrates from staples such as rice, beans, and corn. It contains few leafy, green vegetables. Beans are a source of protein and daily intake tends to be small. The use of lard and the common practice of frying foods both contribute to the high fat content of the Hispanic diet.[54]

Among the high-risk behaviors in the Hispanic population are obesity, alcohol consumption, and sexual practices. Obesity is a common problem among Hispanics in the United States due to their diet and lack of physical activity. In general, the culture accepts obesity as part of the natural aging process and does not value low body weight. To older individuals, obesity may mean health and wealth. However, obesity is a risk factor in cancers of the breast, colon/rectum, uterus, and prostate. Hispanic men tend to drink at younger ages and to consume larger amounts of alcohol and more frequently than do whites. Alcohol contributes to cancers of the esophagus and pancreas. Cigarette smoking is on the rise in Hispanic adolescents, although adult Hispanics smoke less than whites or blacks. A high risk for cervical cancer is observed among Hispanic women because of sexual promiscuity and infrequent use of condoms by males, which predisposes females to sexually transmitted diseases. In addition, low socioeconomic status and low educational levels often result in infrequent Pap smears, infrequent use of barrier contraceptives, and lack of reporting of genital warts.[54]

Skin color in Hispanics can vary from a natural tan to dark brown. Those with lighter color have more Spanish ancestry, while darker-skinned individuals have more Indian ancestry.

American Indians/Alaskan Natives

American Indians and Alaskan Natives include natives of the continental United States, Aleuts, and Alaskan Eskimos. This very diverse group consists of many tribes and more than 560 federally recognized nations, each with its own traditions and cultural heritage. Until the 1800s, these native peoples lived in loosely formed, often nomadic bands and tribes and spoke more than 100 languages with countless dialects.[59] This section focuses on the natives of the continental United States.

The approximately 2.5 million descendants of native North American residents make up the smallest (0.9%) of the defined U.S. minority groups. The West has the largest Indian population as a result of forced westward migration. The largest American Indian nations reported in 2000 were Cherokee, Navajo, Latin American Indian, Choctaw, Sioux, and Chippewa. The largest Alaskan Native group reported was Eskimo.[59]

American Indians who live on reservations tend to lead a more isolated, rural type of existence. Reservations have a high percentage of very young members and a growing number of members older than 55 years of age. Because reservation land cannot support a growing and increasingly concentrated population, poverty and welfare dependency are common. American Indians who relocate from reservations tend to move to urban areas away from the secure network of their family, community, and tribal lifestyle. Although lured by greater opportunities and better jobs, many experience culture shock at the significant differences in the environment. In the past 25 years, there has been an ongoing migration to urban areas. Today, nearly two-thirds of all American Indians live in nonreservation communities.[24]

Cancer is ranked as the third leading cause of death among American Indians, preceded by accidents and heart disease. Because of the heterogeneity of the American Indian group, cancer rates likely vary among the tribes and the Alaskan natives.

The Indian Health Service, through the U.S. Public Health Service, provides inpatient facilities and outpatient clinics and serves American Indians residing on reservations in 25 states as well as the Aleut and Eskimo residents of Alaska. Although health care is available, barriers preventing American Indians from accessing it include poverty and lack of transportation. American Indians believe in living day-to-day rather than in planning for the future, so they may not have savings or insurance to pay for health care. Many live long distances from healthcare facilities and resist seeking out hospital treatment.[24]

Health beliefs and practices

Most tribes link health beliefs and religion. To the American Indian, religion is something that surrounds an individual at all times and has a profound influence on the entire being. Wellness encompasses harmony in body, mind, and spirit as well as resilience, the ability to survive under exceedingly difficult circumstances. It is the patient's response or attitude toward circumstances that creates harmony.[60]

American Indians believe that health reflects living in harmony with nature and that humans have an intimate relationship with nature. The earth is considered a living being, the body of a higher individual with a will and desire to be well. The earth is periodically healthy or ill, just as humans are. An American Indian is expected to treat both the physical body and the earth with respect. If an individual harms the earth, he or she harms himself or herself, and vice versa. Because of this relationship between humans and nature, American Indians believe that humans should respect their bodies and nature through proper treatment.[61]

In this culture, unwellness is seen as being caused by the disharmony of mind, body, and spirit. Natural unwellness is caused by the violation of a sacred or tribal taboo. Taboos can be moral, religious, or cultural. Violations affect not only the offender but also the family.[60]

American Indians believe that illness may be caused by witchcraft as well. Evil or negative energy comes from "one who is on the bad side" or "a person who walks at night." It can be premeditated or not, so American Indians must be careful how they think or talk because bad thoughts can cause illness. Hopi Indians associate illness with evil spirits.[24] Navajos believe that witches are able to interact with evil spirits and can bring sickness and other unhappiness to those who annoy them. Traditionally, illness, disharmony, and sadness are seen by Navajos as the result of "displeasing the holy people, annoying the elements, disturbing animal and plant life, neglecting the celestial bodies, misuse of a sacred Indian ceremony, or tampering with witches and witchcraft."[62,p.21]

The cause of disease, injury, damage to property, or continued misfortune of any kind can be traced back to an action that should not have been performed, such as breaking a taboo or contacting a ghost or witch. Thus the treatment of illness must focus on external causative factors and not on the illness or injury itself.[24]

All causes of illness or disease are believed to have supernatural aspects. Treatment depends on whether the origins of bodily ailments are internal or external. External causes of illness include fractures, dislocations, wounds, and snake or insect bites. If the cause is not apparent, then it is attributed to a supernatural agency. The beliefs that illnesses are caused by germs, a malfunctioning body part, or poor nutritional intake are foreign and unacceptable to American Indians.

Sickness indicates a discord with the laws of nature and, according to American Indians, is most often caused by sorcery or witchcraft, taboo violation, disease or object intrusion, spirit intrusion or being possessed by spirits, or loss of soul. Iroquois Indians also believe that unfulfilled dreams or desires can result in illness. Likewise, restriction violations are thought to cause sickness. Most tribes have prescriptions and prohibitions governing behavior and daily activities, many of which pertain to the prevention of illness. For example, a Navajo boy was diagnosed as having urinary retention caused by his urinating on an ant hill. The boy caused the ants to suffer, and the ants' revenge came in the form of an illness. The boy was out of harmony with living entities that share the universe. The cure entailed a healing ceremony involving chants, prayers, and herbs administered by a medicine man.[60]

Diseases of *object intrusion* refer to the invasion of the body by a worm, snake, insect, or small animal. This problem may be a result of witchcraft. Navajos may orally suck out the foreign object using a hollow tube or bone. *Spirit intrusion* involves being possessed by disease-causing spirits of humans and animals. The healing ceremony is an exorcism of the bad spirits. *Soul loss* usually occurs during a dream, when the soul leaves the body and travels about. Witches and evil spirits can steal a soul. It is believed that the individual is in danger of dying if the soul is not recovered.[24]

A cancer diagnosis is viewed by American Indians as a white man's disease, as punishment for their actions or a family member's actions, as a way to wear the pain to protect others in one's community, as a natural part of one's path and the lessons to learn, as the result of a curse or a personal violation of tribal mores (i.e., stepping on a frog or urinating on a spider), or as the result of the contagious cancer spirit.[63]

Frequently, American Indians use traditional medicine and Western medicine, either independently of each other or simultaneously. An American Indian patient may consult both a medicine person and a Western doctor at the same time. One helps heal the individual heal by restoring harmony, while the other treats the physical disease. To treat the spirit and mind, a healer must understand why the disease occurred and begin to resolve the conflict occurring in mind, body, and spirit. In most instances, the two systems are complementary and should be encouraged.[61]

Preventive measures are generally practiced to ward off the effects of witchcraft, to reestablish harmony, or to prevent possession by an evil spirit. The medicine person may prescribe wearing a talisman, a buckskin, or cloth herbal bag that has preventive or curative powers. Removal of such items by the nurse without permission could result in serious consequences for the patient.[61]

Some tribes are not receptive to invasive bodily procedures and may agree to surgery only reluctantly. Relatives may refuse to donate blood because they fear that if the recipient dies, they may die as well. American Indians should be asked whether they wish a body part back after surgery, as some tribes believe the body must be intact for burial or that body parts can be used as a means for spirits to enter the body and cause harm.[60]

Offering food to American Indian patients during appointments may be helpful. This practice is referred to as "the give away," a celebration that meets basic needs and shows welcome, concern, caring, friendship, and neighborliness. Offering food is a tangible expression of the link in a relationship and serves as something always to be remembered about that individual.

Because of their history of inconsistent care and disrespectful treatment, American Indians often are not comfortable with Western healthcare providers. Long waits in clinics, separation from their families, the unfamiliar routines of the hospital, and the often demanding and demeaning attitudes of nurses and physicians result in a variety of responses by the American Indian patient that may include silence or even leaving, never to return again.[24]

The pain threshold of American Indians is often thought to be high, as stoicism is greatly valued. This pattern stems from American Indians' tendency to look at things in totality, so that when sickness occurs it is viewed as an ailment of the whole body. Many will "grin and bear" fever and pain until the physical condition becomes disabling. Asking an American Indian, "Where does it hurt?" might commonly be responded to with "All over." It may be more useful to have the patient point to where it hurts most. When treatment is sought, medication generally is expected. If none is given, the American Indian may be disappointed, as his expectations for treatment were not met.[60]

Helpful interventions in working successfully with American Indian patients include conveying acceptance without judgment of physical appearance, beliefs, or practices; explicitly recognizing unique cultural beliefs and behaviors; and making staff and services available when the need arises rather than by scheduling appointments. An unwillingness to accept traditional healing practices may discourage many American Indians from using the Western healthcare system.

Healing practices

The traditional healer is the medicine person who is wise in the ways of the land and nature, and takes time to determine first the cause of the illness, then the proper treatment. He or she often performs special ceremonies that may take several days. These medicine men and women are "chosen" — that is, divinely inspired. They are gifted with extrasensory perception that allows them to make mythological associations, and they seek spiritual causes of illness.[24] Medicine men and women spend many years learning their skills and serving as apprentices to more experienced healers.[60]

Different types of medicine men and women play specific roles in American Indian culture. They range from those who assume a purely positive role and whose focus is to maintain cultural integration at a time of great stress, to the singer who is the medicine man and treats illnesses and disharmony.[61]

A cure often requires the involvement of several medicine men and women. Medicine people may use medicine bundles (*jists*) containing symbolic and sacred items or small jars of medicinal solutions; place red, gray, or black marks on the patient's skin; use tobacco; or burn cedar sage, grasses, or whatever is appropriate for that tribe. Bracelets of shells, seeds, beads, or arrowheads also may be used.

The goal of treatment is always to enhance total healing. If an herbalist treats a patient, prayers and songs are offered in conjunction for mental and spiritual renewal. An important component of the healing is the patient's motivation for recovery. American Indians believe an individual gets back in equal proportion what he or she gives in words and actions to another.[24]

Healing ceremonies differ from tribe to tribe, and are associated with varying degrees of complexity. Most of these ceremonies take place in the home with the participation of family members and other tribal members. Supporting the use of healing ceremonies in the hospital and providing adequate space and privacy for them is helpful for the American Indian patient and family. Objects may be left in the room that were used in the ceremony. Because these objects are associated with elements identified with the cause of illness, they should not be removed without the permission of the patient and his or her family.

Purification is often practiced to maintain harmony with nature and to cleanse the body and spirit. Many American Indians believe that for every natural disease, the earth provides a cure. Roots are often chewed to relieve pain, clear the mind, or treat a toothache. Herbs are viewed as being agents of nature.[24]

Traditional medicines include cedar incense (for purification) and corn pollen (for blessings). A "seat" in a sweat lodge is a type of purging that is useful for preventing and treating illness. Individuals may engage in monthly sweats because it is believed that the body periodically builds up bad or negative spirits that block energy. Note that Navajo women do not participate in sweats. Objects to guard against witchcraft may be carried by some tribes, especially at nonfamily gatherings.[61]

Western physicians are regarded by American Indians as herbalists who can cure symptoms but cannot restore the patient's harmonious relationship with nature because they lack knowledge of the important rituals. American Indians believe that a real medicine woman or man will know, without being told, what is wrong with a person. Western doctors ask many questions and often are unable to determine what is wrong. Some American Indians believe that healthcare providers from the Indian Health Service come to the reservations to "practice."[64]

Social organization

As members of a matrilineal society, American Indian patients may not give consent for any procedure or treatment until permission is obtained from the mother, grandmother, or aunt. Sometimes consent may be obtained only after a ceremony. If it cannot be performed in the hospital, the patient may leave and return after the ceremony.[61]

The extended family is very important, especially during periods of crisis. When a family member is hospitalized, an assortment of relatives will come expecting to visit the relative. Limiting visitors to only close relatives is not relevant for American Indians, as they do not distinguish between close and distant relatives. Family members may make great sacrifices by traveling long distances to visit their family member. The hospitalized patient expects the family to visit, and the family expects to visit the patient.[22]

Communication

Older American Indians may speak only their traditional language, and often there are no comparable medical terms in the tribal language. Although translators are needed, they must understand the nature of social, cultural, and familial lines of communication and respect. Some tribes believe that a discussion with one individual about another is a sign of disrespect and could break a cultural taboo, leaving the individual or family vulnerable to harm. For the Navajo, special emphasis is placed on individual rights. Each person speaks for himself or herself, and each individual's action should be self-initiated. In this case, trying to obtain information about another family member may be difficult. Limited ability to speak English may hamper the understanding of the patient. It is common for American Indians to be silent rather than to admit to not understanding.[60]

Making direct eye contact with an American Indian may be considered as looking into his or her soul, which could result in its loss. Consequently, American Indians who do not look directly at care providers should not be labeled as "inattentive" or "uninterested." Prolonged eye contact is considered a sign of disrespect and pointing is viewed as insulting.[61]

Interpersonal relationships are carefully spelled out among American Indian tribes. To whom one speaks, when the speaking occurs, how one speaks, and what sequence of speaking is followed are very important. For example, a mother-in-law cannot speak to her son-in-law or be in the same room with him.[60] Awareness of these relationships is helpful to the nurse who must communicate with American Indian patients and families.

The importance of observing periods of silence is a cultural trait. Silence helps formulate one's thoughts so that the spoken words will have significance. An individual who interrupts, interjects, or hurries toward abrupt conclusions is perceived to be immature. American Indians are very sensitive to body language. If a healthcare provider appears hurried, nervous, or impatient, American Indians are quick to sense these cues, and blocks to communication may occur. Because American Indians are comfortable with silence, they do not feel a need to talk constantly; as a result, continual talking by a healthcare provider trying to obtain an adequate history may not be well received.[60]

American Indians tend to be private people who do not readily volunteer information. Patients may not understand a question or may give responses they think the nurse wishes to hear, particularly if the question is regarded as inappropriate. Making a declarative statement about an obvious symptom and allowing time for the patient to respond may be a better approach.

It is common for American Indians to speak in a very soft voice. The listener is expected to be attentive so as to hear what is being said. Asking for a statement to be repeated is considered rude. Thus, it is helpful to speak with an American Indian patient in a quiet setting to improve communication.

Some American Indians consider a firm handshake to be a sign of aggression. Navajos extend their hand and lightly touch the hand of the person they are greeting. Knocking on the door before entering the room and introducing oneself in the native language are often appreciated.

Using body language that is open, without closing or crossing the arms, is suggested. Loud speech may be viewed as rude or angry, and speaking slowly may be perceived as condescending. Note-taking is considered taboo for some American Indians, as Indian history is passed on through verbal story telling.[24]

Initiating a visit with casual conversation about family, social functions, and the tribe may be helpful because American Indians are very private. This introductory period allows for a gradual easing into discussions about personal and family health. Never use second-person language when discussing risk factors (e.g., "If you don't stop smoking, you will get cancer"), as this may be perceived as putting a hex on the individual. For American Indians, a direct address with the second person involves one's spirit. Some American Indians may feel that talking with someone other than a family member about breasts, testicles, self-examination, and uterine bleeding is improper.

Space and time

Personal space is very important to some American Indians, who may have difficulty adapting to situations that place them in unfamiliar spaces such as clinics or hospitals. Hospitals may be considered a place to die, and American Indians are hesitant to be admitted or put into a room where another person has died. Some tribes would welcome having the room ritually purified before they enter it.

Modesty is very significant to the American Indian; limited exposure of body parts is suggested. Permission should be asked to perform a physical examination, and American Indian women may prefer a female practitioner.

American Indian time typically runs from one hour to a few days later than standard time. Homes often have no clocks. For American Indians, time is casual, present oriented, and relative to present needs that must be accomplished within a given time frame.[60] A present time orientation may cause a Navajo patient to eat two meals today, four meals tomorrow, no meals the next day, and three meals the following day. This would create difficulty if the patient were instructed to take a medication three times a day with meals.

Death and dying issues

Existence is circular and continuous for most traditional American Indians. They existed as spirit beings with the supreme creator before birth. At death, their spirit joins the creator and eventually returns to the physical world in another form. Death consists of joining one's ancestors, and good or bad deeds have nothing to do with this reunion.[61]

Attitudes and approaches to death and dying vary considerably among American Indian tribes. Some are very accepting of death, but others view dying people and death with fear. Some prefer that their family members die at home, while others prefer the hospital. Suffering is a major value in the American Indian culture, and dying and grief may be met with stoicism and silence. The opportunity to share feelings may be rejected by the patient or family. The family, including children, should be with the dying person, even though they often may avoid touching the dead person or articles associated with that person.[33]

Biological variations

There is a high incidence of obesity and alcohol abuse in American Indians. Some believe that the disruption and subsequent loss caused by the European settlement of North America left many American Indians feeling powerless and hopeless. These feelings may contribute to many of the social problems experienced today by American Indians.

The American Indian diet has changed over time. When these peoples were nomadic, their diet was high in fiber and low in fat. Today, the diet is likely to be high in refined carbohydrates, fat, and sodium and low in fiber, meat, eggs, cheese, and milk. Obesity is a major problem in this group. Many American Indians are also lactose intolerant.[60]

Nursing Issues

Cancer, Poverty, and Ethnicity

In the late 1970s, the question of poverty's role in the differences noted in cancer incidence, mortality, and survival in different ethnic groups was first raised. A landmark report by Freeman in 1989 concluded that poverty, not race, accounted for the 10%–15% lower survival rate from cancer in many ethnic groups.[65] In particular, the disproportionate number of blacks in the lower socioeconomic strata was found to account for the increased incidence.

The Institute of Medicine (IOM) released two reports, *The Unequal Burden of Cancer* (1999)[66] and *Unequal Treatment* (2003),[67] which documented the disproportionate cancer burden in blacks. According to these reports, even at the same socioeconomic and health insurance status, blacks are less likely to receive the most curative treatment for cancer.

According to the U.S. Census Bureau, in the United States 35 million people (12%) are poor and 44 million (15%) are uninsured. A disproportionate number of blacks (23%) and Hispanics/Latinos (21%) live below the poverty line compared to whites (8%).[16,18] Ward reports that residents who live in poorer counties have higher death rates due in part to the fact that the poor and uninsured people are more likely to be diagnosed with cancer at a later stage and are more likely to die from the disease.[26] Poverty is a significant factor in cancer disparities, being associated with a lack of resources, information, and knowledge; substandard living conditions; risk-promoting lifestyles, and diminished access to health care.[68]

The "culture of poverty" includes economic factors, such as unemployment, unskilled occupations, no savings, no health insurance, and frequent daily food purchases in small amounts; social factors, such as crowded living quarters, women as single parents, low educational attainment, and critical attitudes toward the dominant class; and psychological factors, such as feelings of helplessness, inferiority, fatalism, and dependency, and a present time orientation with an inability to defer gratification. These influences increase cancer incidence and mortality by increasing the risk factors of chronic malnutrition; occupational exposure through unskilled jobs; early initiation into sex and multiple partners; and smoking and alcoholism, contributing to cancers of the lung, oral cavity, prostate, cervix, or esophagus.[68]

Secondary prevention may be absent because of a present time orientation, where survival needs take precedence over screening and early detection. A critical attitude toward the middle class and a sense of fatalism may decrease participation in screening programs. Delayed tertiary prevention is often due to a lack of insurance, inability to pay for service, or limited care access. Emergency rooms are often used inappropriately, and referral to clinics may result in fragmented care, impersonal service, long waiting hours, and transportation and child care problems.[68]

The recommendations made by the American Cancer Society report, *Cancer in the Economically Disadvantaged,* as part of a plan to reduce cancer incidence and mortality in the poor would be effective in many ethnic groups.[69] These recommendations seek to improve access in three ways: (1) by establishing programs where the economically disadvantaged or ethnic minorities can gather in emergency rooms, neighborhood clinics, or churches; (2) by developing culturally relevant educational materials that may be translated into different languages; and (3) by recruiting and training healthcare providers and volunteers from the targeted groups to serve the special needs of the poor or of a particular ethnic group.

Strategies to Enhance Access to Health Care

A primary barrier to cancer care for many of the ethnic minority populations is access to health care, especially among the socioeconomically disadvantaged. Since 1989, when attention was directed to this particular need, several programs have been developed. Many of these programs focus on providing effective cancer screenings for ethnic minority populations by using culturally sensitive strategies, including (1) involvement of trusted and respected members of the community in the planning and delivery of healthcare services, (2) provision of social support by women in the social network, and (3) development of culturally sensitive patient education materials.[70]

One of these programs, The Witness Project, involves African American women volunteers who are cancer survivors. By "witnessing," or talking about their cancer experience at churches and community centers, these volunteers help to increase breast and cervical cancer awareness and stress the importance of early detection among minority women in rural central and eastern Arkansas.[71]

Another program is the American Cancer Society's Harlem Education and Detection Project in New York City. This program uses the Patient Navigator Model to assist individuals in overcoming healthcare access barriers. This model "attempts to guide the individual around and through the labyrinth of the healthcare system, through many of the social, community, health, and attitudinal barriers to ensure that patients receive timely diagnosis and treatment."[72,p.97] In addition, the navigator provides education and support to the individual.

The Wai'anae Coast Cancer Control Project in Hawaii also uses the navigator model. This project emphasizes community-driven cancer control as a means of improving breast and cervical cancer screening practices among Native Hawaiian women. The navigators in this project are community members who provide information on cancer and assist individuals in "navigating" the unfamiliar healthcare system by scheduling clinic appointments and patient follow-up services.[35]

Mujer a Mujer: Woman to Woman is an example of a successful, culturally sensitive patient education program targeting Hispanic women. It was developed to reduce the mortality from cervical cancer in this group.[73] Palos outlines some of the culturally appropriate strategies used in the development of this and other effective cancer-control programs:[73,p.112]

- Follow basic rules when initiating interpersonal communication, such as being courteous and respectful to establish trust or confidence.
- Use focus groups comprising grassroots (community) and professional individuals to validate promoters or barriers to attitudes, knowledge, and behavior related to cancer and its prevention.
- Use influential formal and informal leaders such as religious leaders, community gatekeepers, or opinion leaders.
- Integrate religious, cultural, and, when appropriate, traditional (folk) medicine and healing practices, beliefs, and taboos.
- Involve the family, friends, and members of other influential support systems.
- Determine a group's preferred communication process (verbal or nonverbal) as well as language preference.
- Determine an individual's degree of acculturation or assimilation, when appropriate.
- Involve paraprofessionals such as folk healers, when and if appropriate.

- Integrate cultural assessments into daily nursing practice.

The success of these culturally sensitive programs indicates that the targeted populations will use the services if they are available, accessible, and acceptable.[74]

Culturally Appropriate Public/Patient Education

Ethnic minority cancer patients are not much different from other cancer patients in their need for basic cancer information and in their experiences of learning barriers such as anxiety and feelings of being overwhelmed about the disease and treatment. Nevertheless, ethnic minorities present certain unique challenges, such as the need to communicate in a language other than English and cultural values, beliefs, and practices that can affect the teaching/learning process.

Strategies

Because of the challenges posed by ethnic minorities, several strategies have been identified to provide culturally sensitive patient education interventions:[72,73]

1. Developing culturally relevant and community-specific materials.
2. Keeping educational messages simple.
3. Determining the preferred language and learning process (e.g., video versus booklets; group versus one-on-one teaching).
4. Identifying the preferred communication style of the individual, such as the best way to address him or her and acceptable nonverbal communication. For example, as mentioned in the description of the different ethnic groups, the appropriateness and acceptance of direct eye contact varies among cultures.

In addition, determining decision-making patterns for the particular ethnic group is important. An example of this consideration is seen in many API groups, where the family, instead of the patient, makes treatment decisions. In these situations, teaching only the patient about a proposed chemotherapy treatment may not be appropriate if the educational effort needs to be directed to the family for subsequent decision making and consent to treatment.

Use of interpreters. Language frequently poses a barrier to effective patient education. The use of professional interpreters, if available, is the optimal choice. Family and friends may be used, but the correct or complete message may not be relayed. This distortion or omission of parts of the message may be due to the interpreter's own skill and fluency in the language, the interpreter's subjective censoring (e.g., to "protect" the patient), or the patient's comfort level in discussing personal issues in the presence of the family member or friend. Recommendations for using interpreters and steps to take if no interpreter is available are listed in Table 4-2.[75]

Translating written materials. Although translated cancer information materials are now available, additional resources are needed. Just as professional interpreters are desirable for clear, accurate communication, guidelines also exist for translating material. Translating material written in English into another language is not enough. To ensure that the content and tone are accurately captured and maintained throughout the translation, the newly translated material must be back-translated into English by independent translators. After making any needed text corrections, it is helpful to pilot-test the finished product with a sample of the target population for whom the translated material was created.[64]

Always assess the reading level of the original material before it is translated. Analyses of the reading levels of available cancer education materials have shown an average that is much higher than the reading level of the general population.[76] Thus the reading level of the material to be translated may need to be adjusted before it is translated. Just as literacy has been identified as a barrier to cancer patient education for the general population, it also represents a challenge faced by many ethnic minority groups. As mentioned earlier, a significant number of APIs are functionally illiterate. In addition, the literacy level of ethnic minority groups will be influenced by whether they are literate in their native language. For example, the Hmong culture is primarily an oral culture, and many of these people who immigrated to the United States are illiterate in the Hmong language.[22]

Preferred styles of learning. Determining an individual's preferred style of learning is important as well. The different styles include one-to-one versus group, oral tradition, story telling, peer educators, and receiving information from "powerful others." Some cultural groups may have preferences for one or more learning styles. For example, knowing the learning style of the targeted ethnic minority population helped in the development of a culturally sensitive cancer education video. Because story telling is used by many American Indians to relay information, one video, *Standing Strong Against the Cancer Enemy*, used the story format to

Table 4-2 Overcoming Language Barriers

Use of an Interpreter
• Before locating an interpreter, be sure that the language the client speaks at home is known, as it may differ from the language spoken publicly (e.g., French is sometimes spoken by well-educated and upper-class members of certain Asian or Middle Eastern cultures). • Avoid interpreters from a rival tribe, state, region, or nation (e.g., a Palestinian who knows Hebrew may not be the best interpreter for a Jewish client). • Be aware of gender differences between interpreter and client. In general, an interpreter of the same gender is preferred. • Be aware of age differences between interpreter and client. In general, an older, more mature interpreter is preferred to a younger, less experienced one. • Be aware of socioeconomic differences between interpreter and client. • Ask the interpreter to translate as closely to verbatim as possible. • An interpreter who is not a relative may seek compensation for services rendered.
Recommendations for Institutions
• Maintain a computerized list of interpreters who may be contacted as needed. • Network with area hospitals, colleges, universities, and other organizations that may serve as resources. • Utilize the translation services provided by telephone companies (e.g., American Telephone and Telegraph Company).
What to Do When There Is No Interpreter
• Be polite and formal. • Greet the person using the last or complete name. Gesture to yourself and say your name. Offer a handshake or nod. Smile. • Proceed in an unhurried manner. Pay attention to any effort by the patient or family to communicate. • Speak in a low, moderate voice. Avoid talking loudly. Remember that there is a tendency to raise the volume and pitch of your voice when the listener appears not to understand. The listener may perceive that the nurse is shouting and/or angry. • Use simple words, such as *pain* instead of *discomfort*. Avoid medical jargon, idioms, and slang. Avoid using contractions. Use nouns repeatedly instead of pronouns. Example: Do *not* say, "He has been taking his medicine, hasn't he?" *Do* say, "Does Juan take medicine?" • Pantomime words and simple actions while verbalizing them. • Give instructions in the proper sequence. Example: Do *not* say, "Before you rinse the bottle, sterilize it." *Do* say, "First, wash the bottle. Second, rinse the bottle." • Discuss one topic at a time. Avoid using conjunctions. Example: Do *not* say, "Are you cold and in pain?" *Do* say, "Are you cold [while pantomiming]? Are you in pain?" • Validate whether the client understands by having him or her repeat instructions, demonstrate the procedure, or act out the meaning. • Write out several short sentences in English, and determine the person's ability to read them. • Try a third language. Many Indo-Chinese speak French. Europeans often know three or four languages. Try Latin words or phrases, if the nurse is familiar with that language. • Ask who among the client's family and friends could serve as an interpreter. • Obtain phrase books from a library or bookstore, make or purchase flash cards, contact hospitals for a list of interpreters, and use both formal and informal networking to locate a suitable interpreter.

Adapted from M. Andrews: Transcultural considerations in assessment, in Jarvis C: *Physical Examination and Health Assessment* (ed. 4). Philadelphia, Elsevier, 2004.

convey its educational message on cancer prevention.[77]

Other successful educational strategies include the use of peer educators and "powerful others" to relay information. Enlisting fellow ethnic minorities to teach their peers is the basic principle behind the peer educator's strategy. The use of "powerful others" often involves the recruitment of respected community leaders who are recognized authorities or cancer survivors from the community.[64]

Providing effective public and patient education for ethnic minority groups presents many challenges and opportunities for oncology nurses. Using the strategies presented here as well as knowledge of the individual's cultural background can help oncology nurses develop and implement successful, culturally sensitive public and patient education interventions.

Clinical Trials and Cancer Research

Historically, minorities have been underrepresented in clinical trials. Barriers to their participation that have been identified include ethnic minorities' distrust of outsiders doing research in their communities (often referred to as "white-run research") and a lack of culturally sensitive and specific educational materials.

Brawley cites a number of additional barriers to recruitment of ethnic minorities in clinical trials, including difficulties in transportation, inconvenient clinic hours, lack of day care, differences in language, lack of understanding, fear of being denied care because of inadequate financial support, fear that researchers will take advantage, and not understanding the value of the research to the participant.[71] Other factors identified are a belief held by some healthcare providers that the medically underserved are less likely to comply with study protocols and treatment guidelines, and a lack of information about clinical trials participation and access.[70]

In response to this underrepresentation of minorities and in an effort to recruit more minorities to National Cancer Institute (NCI)–sponsored clinical trials, NCI developed the Minority-Based (MB) Community Clinical Oncology Program (CCOP). Since its inception, one of the fundamental factors that has facilitated the progress of this program is the healthcare providers' respect for, and increased understanding of, the unique cultures that they serve.[71]

Several factors facilitate participation in clinical trials by ethnic minorities who are socioeconomically disadvantaged:[78]

- Adequate information and education about the risks, benefits, costs, and time commitment required
- Endorsement of the goals of clinical trials by the gatekeepers of the community (i.e., church leaders, community leaders, or family physicians)
- Improved access to the healthcare system and the specific location where the trial is being conducted
- A perceived benefit to the individual from participation
- Minimal actual cost to the individual in terms of time lost from work, transportation, and child care
- Having recruiters of the same ethnicity as the potential subjects

Research studies

Conducting research involving ethnic minorities presents several unique challenges: selection of the research sample, appropriate instruments and research methodology, and translation of research instruments. Because of the heterogeneity of the major groups, study samples need to be selected carefully. For example, if the study sample were identified as American Indians, knowing which subgroups were studied would make a difference in interpretation of the research findings and in determining for whom the data are generalizable.

Also, knowing which particular ethnic group will be studied while the research study is being planned can make a difference in the development of appropriate instruments and the chosen research methodology. For example, several ethnic minority groups apparently have difficulty in using Likert scales.[79,80] Flaskerud further proposes that

> Problems in using Likert scales cross-culturally could be due to education, faulty translation, irrelevant content, lack of semantic equivalence, the differing character of social interactions in various groups, or the nature of the response required. It is also possible that the degree of variation Likert scales attempt to measure is meaningless in some cultural groups.[80,p.186]

Research instruments that are developed in English and translated into another language are also of particular concern. When such translation occurs, subtle cultural nuances and conceptual equivalency may be compromised, leading to difficulties in retaining the validity of the instrument. Strategies to overcome these potential problems include translating newly translated materials back into the original language, with the goal being to maintain the essence of the original meaning. Pilot-testing the instrument with the appropriate population is also recommended to establish reliability.[79]

As the U.S. population becomes more culturally diverse, there is an obvious need for more cancer research involving ethnic minorities. Expertise is needed to incorporate cultural considerations when cancer research studies are developed and conducted.

Resources

In response to the increasing awareness of the needs of the United States' culturally diverse population and the healthcare professionals who care for them, many resources are available. Table 4-3 lists programs and organizations at the national level whose focus is to eliminate the unequal burden of cancer among ethnic minorities. Other important resources include the American Cancer Society (www.cancer.org) and the NCI's Cancer Information Service (http://cis.nih.gov).

Several professional organizations aim to promote cultural awareness in nurses and to provide support to ethnic minority nurses, including the Oncology Nursing Society (ONS) (www.ons.org) and its Transcultural Nursing Issues Special Interest Group (TNI SIG). The National Coalition of Ethnic Minority Nurse Association (NCEMNA) advocates for equity and justice in nursing and health care for ethnic minority populations. It consists of five national ethnic nurse associations:

- Asian American/Pacific Islander Nurses Association (AAPINA) (www.aapina.org)
- National Alaska Native American Indian Nurses Association (NANAINA) (www.nanaina.com)

Table 4-3 Selected Programs and Resources Targeting Cancer Disparities

Name of Program and Web Address	Sponsors/Partners	Description
Intercultural Cancer Council (ICC) http://iccnetwork.org	Baylor College of Medicine	The ICC, established in 1995, promotes policies, programs, partnerships, and research to eliminate the unequal burden of cancer among racial and ethnic minorities and medically underserved populations in the United States and its associated territories. It prepares *Cancer Fact Sheets* that provide detailed information on cancer occurrence and risk factors among racial and ethnic minorities and the medically underserved.
National Center on Minority Health and Health Disparities (NCMHD)	National Institutes of Health (NIH)	The NCMHD was established in 2000. It leads and coordinates NIH efforts to improve the health of minority and medically underserved people.
Center to Reduce Cancer Health Disparities (CRCHD) http://crchd.nci.nih.gov	National Cancer Institute (NCI)	The CRCHD was created in 2001 to carry out NCI's Strategic Plan for Reducing Cancer Health Disparities. NCI's goal is to nearly triple the funding for cancer health disparities in four years. Research will investigate social, cultural, environmental, biological, and behavioral determinants of cancer disparities across the cancer-control continuum from prevention to end-of-life care.
Special Populations Networks for Cancer Awareness, Research and Training http://crchd.nci.nih.gov/spn	National Cancer Institute (NCI)	The Special Populations Networks is a program within the CRCHD. The first projects were funded in 2001. Its purpose is to build relationships between large research institutions and community-based programs and to find ways of addressing important questions about the burden of cancer in minority communities. The major goal is to build an infrastructure to promote cancer awareness within minority and medically underserved communities, and to launch from these communities more research and cancer-control activities aimed at specific population subgroups. Currently the Special Populations Networks consists of 18 projects in 15 states.
Racial and Ethnic Approaches to Community Health (REACH) http://www.cdc.gov/reach2010	Centers for Disease Control and Prevention (CDC)	The REACH program funds community coalitions to develop and implement activities to reduce the level of disparities in one or more of six priority areas, which include breast and cervical cancer screening. The first projects were funded in 1999. The program emphasizes the importance of working more closely with communities to identify culturally sensitive implementation.
National Breast and Cervical Cancer Early Detection Program (NBCCEDP) http://www.cdc.gov/cancer/nbccedp	Centers for Disease Control and Prevention (CDC)	The NBCCEDP was created by Congress in 1990 to help improve access to breast and cervical cancer screening among underserved women. This program, funded at $200.6 million for fiscal year 2003, provides both screening and diagnostic services and has been implemented in all 50 states, five U.S. territories, the District of Columbia, and 15 American Indian/Alaskan Native organizations.

Data from Ward, E., Jemal, A., Cukkinides, V. et al: Cancer Disparities by Race/Ethnicity and Socioeconomic Status. CA: A Cancer Journal for Clinicians 54: 78–93, 2004

- National Association of Hispanic Nurses (NAHN) (www.thehispanicnurses.org)
- National Black Nurses Association (NBNA) (www.nbna.org)
- Philippine Nurses Association of America (PNAA) (www.pnaa03.org)

NCEMNA's goals are support for the development of ethnic nurses who reflect the nation's diversity; advocacy for culturally competent, accessible, and affordable health care; promotion of the professional and educational advancement of ethnic nurses; education of consumers, healthcare professionals, and policy makers on health issues of ethnic minority populations; development of ethnic minority nurse leaders in areas of health policy, practice, education, and research; and endorsement of best practice models of nursing practice, education, and research for minority populations.[81]

Conclusion

Cultural diversity will remain a particular challenge in health care, as the composition of the population of the United States continues to change. The effects of cultural diversity on cancer care are multilayered. At one level, each ethnic group, with its unique values, health beliefs, and practices, responds to cancer somewhat differently. Additional factors such as degree of acculturation, socioeconomic status, and educational attainment add yet another layer to intergroup and intragroup diversity. A third level is an underlying, often negative perception among many ethnic minorities of the mainstream culture and Western medicine. This perspective primarily arises due to their history and experience with Western culture, which in turn influences their health behaviors, attitudes, and acceptance of mainstream health care.

In the midst of this diversity, one can still identify shared responses among the major cultural groups. Many of the ethnic minority groups believe in and practice folk healing, consult both traditional and Western practitioners, and use both traditional and Western medicine. Many groups also place a high value on the family. However, individual variations make it inappropriate to generalize certain group characteristics to all subgroups and to each member of each group. Regardless of ethnicity, the individual must come first.

The heterogeneity and marked cultural diversity of the U.S. population presents many challenges for oncology nurses. Because of the inherent differences between mainstream and ethnic minority cultures and the potential for misunderstanding and conflict, continued efforts at increasing knowledge, appreciation, and understanding of each culture are needed. Our challenge is to facilitate these efforts among health professionals and in the community at large.

References

1. Day JC: *Population Projections of the United States, by Age, Sex, Race, and Hispanic Origin: 1993 to 2050.* U.S. Bureau of the Census, Current Population Reports. Washington, DC, U.S. Government Printing Office, 1993, pp 25-1104
2. Campbell PR: *Population Projection for States, by Age, Race, Sex, and Hispanic Origin: 1993–2020.* U.S. Bureau of the Census, Current Population Reports, P25-111. Washington, DC, U.S. Government Printing Office, 1994
3. Spratley E, Johnson A, Sochalski J, et al: *The Registered Nurse Population,* Washington, DC, U.S. Department of Health Human Services, March 2000. *http://bhpr.hrsa.gov/healthworkforce/reports/rnsurvey/rnssl.htm#71.* Accessed May 25, 2004
4. Smedley BD, Butler AS, Bristol LR (eds): *In the Nation's Compelling Interest: Ensuring Diversity in the Healthcare Workforce.* Washington, DC, The National Academic Press, 2004
5. Ries LAG, Eisner MP, Kosary CL, et al (eds): *SEER Cancer Statistics Review, 1975–2000.* Bethesda, MD, National Cancer Institute, 2003, *http://seer.cancer.gov/csr/1975-2000*
6. Singh GK, Miller BA, Hankey BF, et al: *Socioeconomic Variations in US Cancer Incidence, Mortality, Stage, Treatment and Survival, 1975–1999.* NCI Cancer Surveillance Monograph Series, No. 4. NIH Publication No. 03-5417. Bethesda, MD, National Cancer Institute, 2003
7. American Cancer Society: *Cancer Facts and Figures for African Americans, 2003–2004.* Atlanta: American Cancer Society, 2003
8. American Cancer Society: *Cancer Facts and Figures — 2004.* Atlanta, American Cancer Society, 2004
9. Jemal A, Murray T, Samuels A, et al: Cancer statistics 2003. *CA: Cancer J Clin* 53:5–26, 2003
10. U.S. Department of Commerce: *Profiles of General Demographic Characteristics, 2000.* Washington, DC, U.S. Census Bureau, 2001
11. U.S. Department of Commerce: *The Asian Population, 2000.* Washington, DC, U.S. Census Bureau, 2002
12. U.S. Department of Commerce: *The Native Hawaiian and Other Pacific Islander Population, 2000.* Washington, DC, U.S. Census Bureau, 2002
13. Miller BA, Kolonel LN, Bernstein L, et al (eds): *Racial/Ethnic Patterns of Cancer in the United States 1988–1992.* NIH Publication No. 96-4104. Bethesda, MD, National Cancer Institute, 1996
14. American Cancer Society: *Cancer Facts and Figures for Hispanics/Latinos, 2003–2005.* Atlanta: American Cancer Society, 2003
15. O'Brien K, Cokkinides V, Jemal A, et al: Cancer statistics for Hispanics. *CA: Cancer J Clin* 53:208–226, 2003
16. Kepel KG, Peaercy JN, Wagener DK: Trends in racial and ethnic specific rates for the health status indicators: United States, 1990–1998. *Healthy People 2000,* 2002
17. U.S. Census Bureau: *Poverty in the United States: 2001.* 2001. *http://www.census.gov/prod/2002pubs/p60-219.pdf.* Accessed August 12, 2003
18. U.S. Census Bureau: *Health Insurance Coverage: 2001.* 2001. *http://www.census.gov/hhes/hlthins/hlthino01/hlth01asc.html.* Accessed August 12, 2003
19. Andrews MM, Boyle JS (eds): *Transcultural Concepts in Nursing Care* (ed 4). Philadelphia, Lippincott Williams & Wilkins, 2003
20. Frank-Stromborg M, Olsen SJ (eds): *Cancer Prevention in Diverse Populations: Cultural Implications for the Multidisciplinary Team.* Pittsburgh, PA, Oncology Nursing Society, 2001
21. Giger JN, Davidhizar RE (eds): *Transcultural Nursing: Assessment and Intervention* (ed 4). St. Louis, Mosby-Year Book, 2004
22. Lipson JG, Dibble SL, Minarik PA (eds): *Culture and Nursing Care: A Pocket Guide.* San Francisco, UCSF Nursing Press, 1996
23. Palafox N, Warren A (eds): *Cross-Cultural Caring: A Handbook for Health Care Professionals in Hawaii.* Honolulu, John A. Burns School of Medicine, 1980
24. Spector RE: *Cultural Diversity in Health and Illness* (ed 6). Upper Saddle River, NJ, Pearson Prentice Hall, 2004
25. Spector RE: Diversity in caring, in Potter PA, Perry AG (eds): *Fundamentals of Nursing: Concepts, Process, and Practice* (ed 5). St. Louis, Mosby-Year Book, 2001, pp 113–135
26. Ward E, Jemal A, Cokkinides V, et al: Cancer disparities by race/ethnicity and socioeconomic status. *CA: Cancer J Clin* 54:78–93.
27. Kosary CL, Ries LAG, Miller BA, et al: *SEER Cancer Statistics Review,* 1973–1992. NIH Publication No. 95-2789. Bethesda, MD, National Cancer Institute, 1995
28. Bloom JR, Hayes WA, Saunders F, et al: Physician induced and patient induced utilization of early cancer detection practices among black Americans. *Adv Cancer Control Innov Res* 293:279–296, 1989

29. Winbush GB: African-American health care: beliefs, practices and service issues, in Julia MC (ed.): *Multicultural Awareness in the Health Care Professions.* Boston, Allyn & Bacon, 1996, pp 8–22
30. Cherry B, Giger JN: African-Americans, in Giger JN, Davidhizar RE (eds): *Transcultural Nursing: Assessment and Intervention* (ed 4). St. Louis, Mosby-Year Book, 2004, pp 177–219
31. Glanville C: People of African American Heritage in Purnell LD, Paulanka BJ (eds): *Transcultural Health Care, a Culturally Competent Approach* (ed 2), Philadelphia, F.A. Davis Co. 2003, pp 40–53
32. Giger J, Davidhizar RE: Time, in Giger J, Davidhizar RE (eds): *Transcultural Nursing: Assessment and Intervention* (ed 4). St. Louis, Mosby-Year Book, 2004, pp 99–120
33. Kozier B, Erle G, Blais K, et al: Ethnicity and culture, in Kozier B, Erb G, Berman AJ, et al (eds): *Fundamentals of Nursing* (ed 6). Upper Saddle River, NJ, Prentice Hall Health, 2000, pp 201–218
34. Kemp C: Terminal Illness: *A Guide to Nursing Care.* Philadelphia, Lippincott, 1995
35. Itano JK, Clark F, Hussey LOL: Cancer prevention and early detection in Native Hawaiians, in Frank-Stromborg M, Olsen SJ (eds): *Cancer Prevention in Diverse Populations: Cultural Implications for the Multidisciplinary Team.* Pittsburgh, Oncology Nusing Society, 2001, pp 113–138
36. Xu Y, Chang K: Chinese Americans, in Giger JN, Davidhizar RE (eds): *Transcultural Nursing: Assessment and Intervention* (ed 4). St. Louis, Mosby-Year Book, 2004, pp 407–427
37. Lee P, Takamura J: The Japanese Americans in Hawaii, in Palafox N, Warren A (eds): *Cross-Cultural Caring: A Handbook for Health Care Professionals in Hawaii.* Honolulu, John A. Burns School of Medicine, 1980, pp 105–135
38. Chin P: Chinese Americans, in Lipson JG, Dibble SL, Minarik PA (eds): *Culture and Nursing Care: A Pocket Guide,* San Francisco, UCSF Nursing Press, 1996, pp 74–81
39. Baysa E, Cabrera E, Camilon F, et al: The Filipinos, in Palafox N, Warren A (eds): *Cross-Cultural Caring: A Handbook for Health Care Professionals in Hawaii.* Honolulu, John A. Burns School of Medicine, 1980, pp 197–212
40. Stauffer RY: Vietnamese Americans, in Giger JN, Davidhizar RE (eds): *Transcultural Nursing: Assessment and Intervention* (ed 4). St. Louis, Mosby-Year Book, 2004, pp 455–491
41. Kunz K, Lam C, Siu K, et al: The Chinese, in Palafox N, Warren A (eds): *Cross-Cultural Caring: A Handbook for Health Care Professionals in Hawaii.* Honolulu, John A. Burns School of Medicine, 1980, pp 26–50
42. Krauss BH: Medicine and medicinal herbs, in Krauss BH: *Plants in Hawaiian Culture.* Honolulu, University of Hawaii Press, 1993, pp 100–104
43. Andrews MM: Transcultural perspectives in the nursing care of children, in Andrews MM, Boyle JS (eds): *Transcultural Concepts in Nursing Care* (ed 4). Philadelphia, Lippincott Williams & Wilkins, 2003, pp 132–180
44. Vance AR: Filipino Americans, in Giger JN, Davidhizar RE (eds): *Transcultural Nursing: Assessment and Intervention* (ed 4). St. Louis, Mosby-Year Book, 2004, pp 429–453
45. Ishida D, Inouye J: Japanese Americans, in Giger JN, Davidhizar RE (eds): *Transcultural Nursing: Assessment and Intervention* (ed 4). St. Louis, Mosby-Year Book, 2004, pp 333–362
46. Earp JB: Korean Americans, in Giger JN, Davidhizar RE (eds): *Transcultural Nursing: Assessment and Intervention* (ed 4). St. Louis, Mosby-Year Book, 2004, pp 571–589
47. Miller SW, Lass KA: East Indian Hindu Americans, in Giger JN, Davidhizar RE (eds): *Transcultural Nursing: Assessment and Intervention* (ed 4). St. Louis, Mosby-Year Book, 2004, pp 493–515
48. Muller JH, Desmond B: Ethical dilemmas in a cross-cultural context — a Chinese example. *West J Med* 157:323–327, 1992
49. Ramakrishna J, Weiss MG: Health, illness, and immigration — East Indians in the United States. *West J Med* 157:265–270, 1992
50. Brotzman GL, Butler DJ: Cross-cultural issues in the disclosure of a terminal diagnosis: a case report. *J Fam Pract* 32:426–427, 1991
51. Tung TM: Death, dying, and hospice: an Asian-American view. *Am J Hosp Palliat Care* 7:23–25, 1990
52. Klessig J: The effects of values and culture on life-support decisions. *West J Med* 157:316–322, 1992
53. Gonzalez T, Kuipers J: Mexican-Americans, in Giger JN, Davidhizar RE (eds): *Transcultural Nursing: Assessment and Intervention* (ed 4). St. Louis, Mosby-Year Book, 2004, pp 221–253
54. Cohen RJ: Cancer prevention and screening among Hispanic populations, in Frank-Stromborg M, Olsen SJ (eds): *Cancer Prevention in Minority Populations: Cultural Implications for the Multidisciplinary Team.* Pittsburgh, PA, Oncology Nursing Society, 2004, pp 177–243
55. Martaus TM: The health seeking process of Mexican-American migrant farm workers. *Home Healthc Nurse* 4(5):32–36, 1986
56. Purnell LC: People of Cuban Heritage, in Purnell LD, Paulanka BJ (eds): *Transcultural Health Care: A Culturally Competent Approach* (ed 2). Philadelphia: FA Davis, 2003, pp 122–137
57. Zoucha R, Purnell LD: People of Mexican Heritage, in Purnell LD, Paulanka BJ (eds): *Transcultural Health Care: A Culturally Competent Approach* (ed 2). Philadelphia: FA Davis, 2003, pp 264–278
58. dePaula T, Lagana K, Gonzalez-Ramirez L: Mexican Americans, in Lipson JG, Dibble SL, Minarik PA (eds): *Culture and Nursing Care: A Pocket Guide.* San Francisco, UCSF Nursing Press, 1996, pp 203–221
59. Ogunwole SH: *The American Indian and Alaskan Native Population: 2000.* Washington, DC, U.S. Department of Commerce, 2000
60. Hanley CE: Navajo Indians, in Giger J, Davidhizar RE (eds): *Transcultural Nursing: Assessment and Intervention* (ed. 4). St. Louis, Mosby-Year Book, 2004, pp 255–277
61. Still O, Hodgins D: Navajo Indians, in Purnell LD, Paulanka BJ (eds): *Transcultural Health Care: A Culturally Competent Approach* (ed 2). Philadelphia: FA Davis, 2003, pp 279–293
62. Bilagody H: An American Indian looks at health care, in Feldman R, Buch D (eds): *Ninth Annual Training Institute for Psychiatrist-Teachers of Practicing Physicians.* Boulder, CO, WICHE, 1969
63. Burhansstipanou L, Lovato MP, Krebs LU: Native American cancer survivors. *Healthcare Women Int* 20:505–515, 1999
64. Burhansstipanou L, Olsen S: Cancer prevention and early detection in American Indian and Alaska Native populations, in Frank-Stromberg M, Olsen SJ (eds):, *Cancer Prevention in Diverse Populations: Cultural Implications for the Multidisciplinary Team.* Pittsburgh, PA: Oncology Nursing Society, 2001, pp 5–52.
65. Freeman HP: Cancer in the socioeconomically disadvantaged. *CA: Cancer J Clin* 39:266–288, 1989
66. Institute of Medicine: *The Unequal Burden of Cancer.* Washington, DC: National Academy Press, 1999
67. Institute of Medicine: *Unequal Treatment: Confronting Racial and Ethnic Disparities in Health Care.* Washington, DC, National Academy Press, 2003
68. Freeman HP: Poverty, culture and social injustice, determinants of cancer disparities. *CA: Cancer J Clin* 54:72–77, 2004
69. American Cancer Society: *Cancer in the Economically Disadvantaged: A Special Report.* Atlanta, American Cancer Society, 1989
70. Burhansstipanov L, Krebs LU, Bradley A, et al: Lessons learned while developing ''clinical trials education for Native Americans'' curriculum. *Cancer Control* 10(5):29–36, 2003
71. Brawley OW: Minority accrual and clinical trials. *Oncol Issues* 10:22–24, 1995

72. Black BL, Ades TB: American Cancer Society urban demonstration projects: models for successful intervention. *Semin Oncol Nurs* 10:96–103, 1994
73. Palos G: Cultural heritage: cancer screening and early detection. *Semin Oncol Nurs* 10:104–113, 1994
74. Black BL, Schweitzer R, Dezelsky T: Report on the American Cancer Society workshop on community cancer detection, education, and prevention demonstration projects for underserved populations. *CA: Cancer J Clin* 43:226–233, 1993
75. Andrews MM: Culturally competent nursing care, in Andrews MM, Boyle JS (eds): *Transcultural Concepts in Nursing Care* (ed 4). Philadelphia, Lippincott Williams & Wilkins, 2003, pp 15–35
76. Cooley ME, Moriarty H, Berger MS, et al: Patient literacy and the readability of written cancer educational materials. *Oncol Nurs Forum* 22:1345–1351, 1995
77. Brant J: Video review: Standing Strong Against the Cancer Enemy. *Transcultural Nursing Issues Special Interest Group Newsletter* 4:3, 1994
78. McCabe MS, Varricchio CG, Padberg RM: Efforts to recruit the economically disadvantaged to national clinical trials. *Semin Oncol Nurs* 10:123–129, 1994
79. Munet-Vilaro F: Methodologic issues in the implementation of a Latino population, in *Proceedings of the Third National Conference on Cancer Nursing Research.* Atlanta, American Cancer Society, 1994, pp 39–43
80. Flaskerud JH: Is the Likert scale format culturally biased? *Nurs Res* 37:185–186, 1988
81. National Coalition of Ethnic Minority Nurse Associations (NCEMNA): 2004. *http://www.ncemna.org/whatisncemna.html.* Accessed May 3, 2004

CHAPTER 5

Dynamics of Cancer Prevention

Judith J. Smith, RN, MSN, AOCN®
Rose Mary Padberg, RN, MA

Introduction

Cancer incidence and mortality have changed little in the United States over the past several decades despite major advances in biomedical science and technology. More than 1.3 million new cancer cases are diagnosed and more than 440,000 cancer deaths occur each year.[1] Given these staggering statistics, it is understandable that cancer prevention has evolved into one of the principal components of the National Cancer Program. Collaborative efforts among key federal programs, healthcare providers, researchers, policymakers, and legislators combine to shape cancer prevention policy and set prevention priorities for public health practice. This chapter presents an overview of the principles, practices, research, and nursing implications for cancer prevention as a dynamic and integral component of the national cancer control program.

Development of Cancer Prevention

The National Cancer Institute (NCI), under congressional mandate, directs the United States' national cancer prevention research effort. The ultimate goal of this effort is population-wide application of evidence-based interventions that are drawn from hypotheses and methods developed through basic biomedical research. The NCI, along with other federal, nonfederal, public, and private organizations and programs, has participated and contributed significantly to the development of cancer prevention science over the past several decades. Many examples of collaborative efforts and contributions exist; only a few are cited here.

The Surveillance, Epidemiology, and End Results (SEER) Program, a component of the NCI, is one such program.[2] SEER coordinates and manages a national network of cancer registries. Its primary goal is to accumulate accurate and complete cancer data to be used for cancer control and epidemiological research, public health planning, and healthcare development. SEER collects data for approximately 26% of the U.S. population, generated from 14 geographic areas, representing the diversity of the nation, including racial, ethnic, and medically underserved cohorts. Data include those dealing with demographic characteristics, primary tumor site, morphology, stage of disease at diagnosis, first course of treatment, and follow-up for vital status.

The Healthy People 2010 initiative, coordinated by the Office of Disease Prevention and Health Promotion within the U.S. Department of Health and Human Services, is another key component of the multidisciplinary approach to public health risk reduction.[3] Healthy People 2010 presents the national prevention agenda and provides a comprehensive statement of health-related objectives designed to achieve two overarching goals by the year 2010: to increase the quality and years of healthy life, and to eliminate health disparities. A key feature of this initiative is its list of ten leading health indicators (LHIs), reflecting major public health behavioral concerns. Three LHIs are directly related to cancer prevention: physical activity, overweight and obesity, and tobacco use.

The American Cancer Society (ACS) is internationally known for its dedication to eliminating cancer through research funding, professional and public education, advocacy programs, and cancer-related services to society.[4] Among ACS's many contributions to prevention science are two well-established prospective cohort studies: Cancer Prevention Study I (CPS I) and Cancer Prevention Study II (CPS II).[4] These studies have assessed and provided significant data on lifestyle and environmental factors related to cancer incidence since 1959. ACS also publishes cancer screening guidelines for breast, colorectal, cervical, endometrial, and prostate cancers, as well as annual national cancer statistics.

Professional organizations, such as the Oncology Nursing Society (ONS), support and promote cancer prevention and early detection through a variety of publications, professional education and training programs, special-interest groups, and research funding opportunities. Cancer prevention, risk reduction, and early detection consistently rank among the top ten research priority areas among oncology nurses, according to an ONS survey.[5] The ONS position statement, "Prevention and Early Detection of Cancer in the United States," informs and guides practicing oncology nurses in five core areas: professional education, public education, cancer prevention and detection services, research, and health policy.[6]

Framework of Cancer Prevention

Progressive development of innovative technologies based on scientifically sound principles has facilitated an increased understanding of cancer and the way it develops and progresses. Two fundamental concepts, multistep carcinogenesis and field carcinogenesis, provide the structural framework for a variety of innovative ideas and approaches in cancer prevention.

Multistep Carcinogenesis

The progression of epithelial tissue from premalignant to invasive disease follows a complex biological

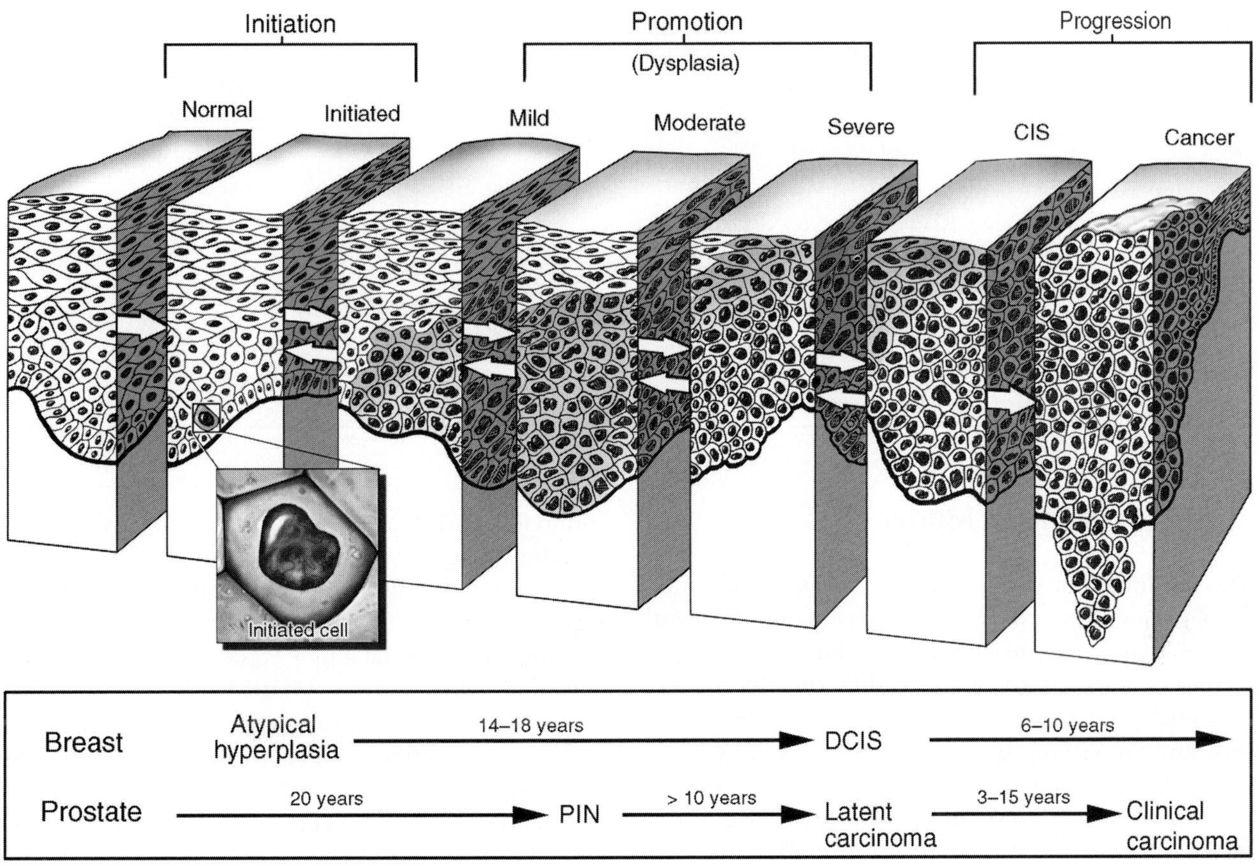

Figure 5-1 Carcinogenesis.

process called carcinogenesis.[7–11] Multiple successive stages of alterations to cellular DNA occur secondary to carcinogenic exposure. The steps in the process are identified as initiation, promotion, and progression (Figure 5-1). *Initiation* occurs rapidly upon exposure to an initiating agent (such as nitrosamines in tobacco smoke, ionizing radiation, or oncogenic viruses), resulting in an irreversible alteration in cellular DNA. *Promotion* is characterized by continued carcinogenic exposure causing cell proliferation, disorganization, and morphological changes.[12,13] Promotion may occur over a span of 20 to 40 years and is reversible, providing an opportunity to intervene to stop or reverse the process.[14,15] Further exposure or action by a promoting agent may lead to the final stage in the carcinogenic pathway, *progression*. Progression occurs over a period of one or more years, is irreversible, and is characterized by progression of genetically altered cells to malignancy.[16,17]

Field Carcinogenesis

The concept of field carcinogenesis suggests widespread tissue damage to an entire epithelial field from carcinogenic exposure, as when the entire respiratory and upper aerodigestive tracts are exposed to carcinogens during smoking.[12,13] Genetic alterations in premalignant and malignant lesions identified at one site of the exposed tissue field suggest an increased risk in other sites within the same field.[8,9,18-20] Field carcinogenesis explains the development of multiple primary tumors and locally recurrent disease in lung cancer and cancers of the upper aerodigestive tract in smokers and former smokers.[21]

Table 5-1 Chemoprevention versus Chemotherapy Trials

	Chemoprevention Trials	Chemotherapy Trials
Goal	Cancer prevention Decrease cancer incidence and mortality Prevent or reverse premalignant lesions Prevent second primaries	Cancer treatment Increase cure or remission Decrease mortality and morbidity
Target Population	Individuals without cancer General population High-risk population Persons with premalignant lesion(s) Persons previously treated, disease-free	Individuals with cancer
Endpoint	Cancer development Phenotype reversal	Cancer eradication Control/palliate cancer
Agent	None to minimal toxicity, acceptable Potentially long-term	Moderate toxicity, acceptable Relatively short-term

Cancer Prevention Model

The traditional model for cancer prevention is made up of primary, secondary, and tertiary levels. The most desirable approach to eliminating cancer is through *primary prevention.* Carcinogen avoidance, effective educational programs related to healthy lifestyle behaviors, and counseling by primary care providers offer the best hope for reducing cancer incidence in the context of primary prevention. Local and state governments, professional and volunteer organizations, employers, insurers, and primary care providers all share the responsibility for facilitating and supporting such approaches.[22] Optimal educational outreach strategies would ideally target young school children, emphasizing the importance of avoiding tobacco products, limiting exposure to ultraviolet sun light, and maintaining a healthy weight through proper diet and physical activity.[23] Another form of primary prevention is found in the evolving science of chemoprevention, the use of nutritional or pharmacologic agents to slow or reverse the development of cancer.

Secondary prevention refers to the early detection of subclinical malignancy through validated screening tests. Examples of effective evidence-based cancer screening procedures include the fecal occult blood test for colorectal screening, the mammogram for breast cancer screening, the digital rectal exam for prostate screening, and the Pap test for cervical cancer screening.[24] Evidence suggests the reduction of national mortality rates for these diseases secondary to screening. As yet, no effective guidelines for lung cancer screening have been developed. Based on evidence from three large, randomized, NCI-sponsored screening trials in the 1970s, no survival benefit was found for individuals screened with chest x-ray and/or sputum cytology. To evaluate new screening technology, the NCI, in collaboration with the American College of Radiology Imaging Network (ACRIN), is conducting the National Lung Screening Trial (NLST). This study will determine whether lung cancer screening using low-dose spiral computed tomography in high-risk populations reduces mortality from lung cancer compared with standard chest x-ray screening. It will evaluate 50,000 smokers and former smokers over eight years at 30 sites nationwide. Results from this study could potentially have major implications for public health policy.

Tertiary prevention involves appropriate supportive and rehabilitative services to minimize morbidity and maximize quality of life following cancer diagnosis and treatment. As the population of cancer survivors continues to grow, research aimed at identifying individuals at risk for post-treatment adverse outcomes, approaches to promoting optimal outcomes, and the nature and scope of problems experienced is under way. Monitoring individuals for early signs of recurrence or development of second malignancies through screening techniques is an example of tertiary prevention, as is investigational chemoprevention to prevent development of second primary tumors.[23]

While all three levels of prevention are necessary for a comprehensive cancer prevention program, primary prevention offers the best hope for reducing cancer incidence. Secondary and tertiary prevention can best be thought of as complementary strategies, as they attempt to minimize the effects of disease rather than to prevent its occurrence. The exploratory interventions and strategies discussed in this chapter are related to primary prevention efforts.

Table 5-2 Phases of Chemoprevention Clinical Trials

Phase	Design	Goal/Evaluation
Phase Ia	Small-scale (15–30), short-term (<12 months), single-arm	Safety and toxicity Dose-response on pharmacokinetics, pharmacology
Phase Ib	Small-scale (15–30), short-term (may be randomized or nonrandomized, dose-escalation, placebo-controlled, blinded)	Safety and toxicity Dose-response on pharmacokinetics, pharmacology Feasibility of intermediate endpoints
Phase IIa	Small-scale (50–100), short-term (>12 months), single or multiple dose	Safety, toxicity, and efficacy Feasibility of intermediate endpoints
Phase IIb	Small-scale (50–100), randomized, double-blind, placebo-controlled	Safety and toxicity Efficacy Evaluation of intermediate endpoints
Phase III	Large-scale, randomized, placebo-controlled design for specific indication	Long-term toxicity Evaluation of intermediate endpoints Cancer incidence and mortality
Phase IV	Postmarketing study	Assess agent's side effects in the general population

Cancer Prevention Research

The scope of cancer prevention research is broad and includes the reduction of underlying risk factors through chemical, immunological, and behavioral interventions. Current knowledge of the latency period between carcinogenic initiation and invasive progression, as described earlier, provides myriad opportunities for reducing cancer incidence through a variety of investigational strategies.

Chemoprevention

Chemoprevention, first described in 1976 by Michael Sporn, is the systemic use of natural or synthetic chemical compounds that inhibit the development of invasive cancer by blocking DNA damage or by arresting or reversing progression of preneoplastic cells that have already sustained such damage.[25] Once identified as potentially effective, based on epidemiological data and/or preclinical research, chemopreventive agents progress through the well-defined stepwise process of clinical trials research. Although similar to chemotherapeutic trials within the structure of the scientific framework, chemoprevention trials differ with regard to several key characteristics, as shown in Table 5-1.

Phases of clinical investigation

Following preclinical testing, promising agents must be investigated in the clinical setting. Table 5-2 summarizes the phases of chemoprevention clinical trials.

Agents are introduced to a limited number of cancer-free but high-risk human subjects (15 to 30) in phase I chemoprevention clinical trials. Phase I chemoprevention studies may be divided into phase Ia or Ib trials. A phase Ia trial is conducted as a small, single-dose study to determine the dose-response of a given chemopreventive agent in terms of pharmacokinetics, pharmacology, and toxicology before progressing to a longer and more comprehensive study. A phase 1b study is a sequential, short-term (3- to 12-months), dose-escalation trial (in some cases randomized, placebo-controlled, and blinded) involving a small number of subjects (15 to 30) in which the endpoints are pharmacokinetics, pharmacology, toxicology, and intermediate endpoint feasibility studies.[26] The maximum tolerated dose and the minimum effective dose are determined at this stage. Phase I trials may be omitted when a known safety profile exists for the agent in humans, allowing progression from preclinical study to phase II clinical trials. Unlike cancer treatment trials, which may accept or even expect moderate levels of toxicity, agents used in chemoprevention trials must have a low toxicity index. For the same reason, agent candidates with known toxicities are administered at doses well below the toxic level.

In addition to further safety and pharmacokinetic evaluations, the primary objective of phase II chemoprevention trials is the evaluation of intermediate endpoints. Intermediate endpoints consist of biochemical, genetic, molecular, cellular, and histological indicators that can be used to estimate possible neoplastic progression and predict future cancer incidence.[15,27,28] Prior to the establishment of a clearly defined and standardized intermediate biomarker, phase IIa chemoprevention clinical trials are conducted to evaluate the feasibility of candidate biomarkers, standardize assay conditions, establish quality control procedures, and define the pharmacodynamics of the biomarker responses.[29] Phase IIa trials typically

Table 5-3 Selected Completed Phase III Chemoprevention Trials

Trial	Target	Regimen	*N*	Outcome
Beta Carotene and Retinol Efficacy Trial (CARET)	Lung	Beta-carotene (30 mg) and retinol (25,000 IU) versus placebo	18,314	28% higher incidence of lung cancer and 17% increased mortality in beta-carotene group
Alpha-Tocopherol, Beta-Carotene Cancer Prevention Trial (ATBC)	Lung	Alpha-tocopherol (vitamin E) (50 mg) versus beta-carotene (20 mg)	29,133	No reduction in lung cancer incidence with alpha-tocopherol; 18% higher incidence of lung cancer and 8% higher mortality rate in beta-carotene group
Breast Cancer Prevention Trial (BCPT)	Breast	Tamoxifen (20 mg) versus placebo	13,388	49% reduction in breast cancer incidence in tamoxifen arm
Prostate Cancer Prevention Trial (PCPT)	Prostate	Finasteride (5 mg) versus placebo	18,822	25% reduction of prostate cancer in finasteride arm
Nutritional Prevention of Cancer	Second primary cancers in people with history of skin cancer	Selenium (200 μg) versus placebo	1312	Increase in both basal and squamous cell skin cancer in selenium arm 63% decrease in the incidence of prostate cancer
Nutritional Intervention Studies of Esophogeal Cancer (Linxian, China)	Esophageal cancer	Four arms: (1) oral vitamin C/molybednum; (2) beta-carotene, vitamin E, selenium; (3) retinol; (4) riboflavin, niacin	30,000	Beta-carotene, selenium, vitamin E group experienced lower incidence and mortality

comprise single-dose studies with a small number (50 to 100) of subjects. Once an intermediate biomarker is identified, phase IIb trials are conducted as randomized, blinded, placebo-controlled studies in high-risk subjects to further evaluate efficacy and safety, and to test the modulation of the biomarker by the chemopreventive agent. The placebo-controlled design allows for a description of the natural history of both groups.[26] The choice of a biomarker or precancerous lesion as an intermediate endpoint is based on the strength of its association with a specific cancer, the ability to evaluate it quantitatively, and the prevalence of the lesion in a study population.[30] Although investigation of intermediate endpoints is enthusiastic and vigorous, no biomarkers have as yet been validated as predictors of cancer incidence.

A celecoxib study provides an example of a phase IIb trial. Celecoxib, a nonsteroidal anti-inflammatory drug (NSAID) that selectively targets the cyclooxygenase (COX)-2 enzyme, has been used to reduce pain and inflammation associated with arthritis. COX-2 inhibition also appears to prevent the growth of tumor cells in the colon to some extent. A double-blind, placebo-controlled, randomized study evaluated the effect of celecoxib on colorectal polyps in individuals with familial adenomatous polyposis (FAP), a disease that has nearly 100% risk of developing colorectal cancer.[31] Seventy-seven subjects were randomized to receive 100 mg celecoxib, 400 mg celecoxib, or placebo twice daily for six months. Patients underwent endoscopy at the beginning and end of the study to evaluate the number and size of polyps before and after celecoxib. Results showed a significant reduction in the number of colorectal polyps in the group receiving 400 mg celecoxib. Based on evidence from this trial, the agent was approved by the Food and Drug Administration (FDA) in 1999 for cancer risk reduction in individuals with FAP.

Phase III chemoprevention trials are large (involving 1,000 to 50,000 or more subjects), randomized, placebo-controlled studies with cancer incidence as the primary endpoint. Such studies typically cost tens of millions of dollars and require thousands of participants, many years of follow-up, and years of analysis.[32] They also evaluate the long-term toxicity of the agent under investigation. Because of their size and expense, phase III trials must be based on strong evidence from early-phase trials or previous clinical experience. Findings from such studies are capable of dramatically influencing public health practice. Table 5-3 provides a list of current and completed phase III trials.

Two pioneering NCI-sponsored phase III chemoprevention trials, the Breast Cancer Prevention Trial (BCPT) and the Prostate Cancer Prevention Trial (PCPT), demonstrate the feasibility of successfully conducting such trials. BCPT is a clinical chemoprevention trial that involved more than 16,000 women deemed to be at increased risk for breast cancer. Subjects were randomized to receive either tamoxifen (Nolvadex) or placebo for five years. The women in the tamoxifen arm experienced a 49% lower incidence of invasive breast cancer. The trial also evaluated tamoxifen in terms of incidence of myocardial infarction (MI) and bone fractures. Results showed no difference between the groups in incidence of MI; however, the tamoxifen recipients had 20% fewer bone fractures. BCPT was the first trial of this size to identify an effective agent to reduce breast cancer incidence.

PCPT is a clinical trial designed to evaluate the efficacy of finasteride (Proscar) for the prevention of prostate cancer in men aged 55 and older. The study randomized more than 18,000 men with a PSA of 3.0 ng/mL or less to receive either finasteride or a placebo for seven years. The study was stopped when an interim data analysis revealed that finasteride reduced the risk of developing prostate cancer by 25%. Results also showed higher grade tumors in the finasteride arm.

The Study of Tamoxifen and Raloxifene (STAR) and the Selenium and Vitamin E Cancer Prevention Trial (SELECT) are two phase III, NCI-sponsored, chemoprevention clinical trials that build on information obtained from previous studies. STAR is being conducted in postmenopausal women at increased risk for breast cancer to determine whether raloxifene (Evista) is as effective as tamoxifen (Nolvadex) in reducing breast cancer incidence. Endometrial cancer and deep-vein thrombosis were identified as side effects of tamoxifen in an earlier study; STAR will evaluate raloxifene for these side effects as well. SELECT is a clinical trial to determine whether selenium and/or vitamin E can reduce prostate cancer incidence. Men 55 years and older have been randomized to one of four arms (selenium and vitamin E, selenium alone, vitamin E alone, or placebo) and will continue these courses daily for seven years. African American men, due to their increased risk of prostate cancer, may enter the trial at age 50. The study will also evaluate the molecular genetics of cancer risk and associations between diet and prostate cancer. At this time, no outcome data have been made available from either STAR or SELECT.

Agents

Agents used in chemoprevention clinical trials can be natural or synthetic compounds, dietary constituents such as micronutrients and vitamins, or pharmacologic agents such as NSAIDs, synthetic retinoids, and anti-estrogens. Although there is no widely accepted classification system for chemoprevention agents, two broad categories cover a spectrum of agents: antimutagenics and antiproliferatives. Based on multiple mechanisms of action, a number of agents cross over into both categories and exhibit an effect at different steps of the carcinogenic pathway.[9,33]

Table 5-4 Agent Categories and Selected Chemoprevention Agents

Agent Category	Potentional Chemoprevention Agents
Antimutagenic Agents	Calcium DHEA Oltiprax Polyphenols NAC NSAIDs Tea Protease inhibitors Soy isoflavones
Antiproliferative Agents	Retinoids Budesonide Finasteride NSAIDs Soy isoflavones Tamoxifen Polyphenols DFMO Calcium Vitamin D Selenium Vitamin E Folic acid Genistein Protease inhibitors

Antimutagenic agents are carcinogen-blocking compounds that prevent activation of carcinogens, enhance detoxification systems, or stop carcinogens before they reach their target sites.[33–35] Such agents appear to react directly with initiating and promoting carcinogens. For example, in animal models calcium has been shown to inhibit hyperproliferation and subsequent malignancy in the colon by binding to excess bile and free fatty acids.[29]

Antiproliferative agents typically act to block or retard the promotion and progression phases of the carcinogenic process.[33] Retinoids, the most well studied of the chemoprevention agents, belong to this class of agents. They act by inducing apoptosis and terminal maturation or differentiation. NSAIDs inhibit key enzymes in the arachidonic acid pathway, which can enhance the development and progression of cancers.[33] Other agents, such as tamoxifen, finasteride, and flutamide, act by modulating growth hormone activity.

Approximately 400 compounds are currently being evaluated as potential chemopreventive agents, mainly in laboratory research. More than 60 compounds have shown early potential and are under investigation in chemoprevention clinical trials.[36] Chemopreventive agents that have shown promise and are considered priorities for study are listed in Table 5-4.

Endpoints

While the traditional endpoint for establishing chemopreventive agent efficacy is cancer incidence, assessing this endpoint is feasible only in large phase III trials. Although cancer incidence is a major public health concern, the overall risk of any one individual developing malignant disease is relatively low. Thus cancer incidence as a study endpoint is a difficult standard to meet. The use of biomarkers as intermediate endpoints plays an important role in early-phase chemoprevention clinical trials, as they are intended to predict the development of disease and implement disease prevention practices.[37,38]

An intermediate endpoint is a marker representing a biological event that takes place between carcinogenic initiation and the development of cancer.[8,27,30,34,37,39] To be useful, a surrogate endpoint biomarker must be reliable, highly sensitive and specific, quantitative, readily obtained from study participants, part of the causal pathway for disease, and capable of being modulated by the agent, and have high predictive value for the disease.[36] Intermediate endpoints may take the form of premalignant lesions (e.g., oral leukoplakia, colon polyps, dysplastic nevi), histologic markers (e.g., hyperplasia, metaplasia, dysplasia), biochemical or molecular markers (e.g., ornithine decarboxylase prostaglandin synthetase), or cytogenetic abnormalities (e.g., DNA ploidy, oncogene activation/ suppression, micronuclei).[12,16,20]

Study populations

Potential participants in cancer prevention clinical trials include individuals who are at high risk of developing cancer due to genetic or environmental risk factors, individuals with a preneoplastic lesion such as oral leukoplakia, individuals previously cured of a malignancy and at risk for developing second primary tumors, or members of the general population.[9,29] In chemoprevention trials, in contrast to therapeutic trials, the target populations are frequently healthy, even though they may be at higher risk for developing cancer.[26] Factors that motivate individuals to enroll in an interventional study that requires agent ingestion, possible toxicity, and protracted follow-up differ from the motivational factors for diagnosed cancer patients considering trial participation. As a consequence, recruitment and retention approaches for chemoprevention clinical trials are particularly challenging and should be in place prior to the initiation of a study.

Eligibility criteria for participants in chemoprevention trials actively attempt to identify those individuals at highest risk for the disease. Enrolling high-risk individuals allows the trial to more rapidly reach its endpoint and offers a savings in time and resources. In addition, knowledgeable study participants concerned about their high-risk status tend to be more adherent to study requirements than average-risk participants.

Minority enrollment. The ultimate desired outcome of any clinical research is to have its findings be useful to those individuals in need of this information. According to recent SEER data, minority populations bear a large share of the cancer burden and would most benefit from research-derived interventions to reduce this risk (see Figure 5-2). However, minority populations historically have been underrepresented in chemoprevention clinical trials. Suggested barriers to their participation include attitudes, beliefs, perceptions, and knowledge regarding clinical research and cultural characteristics, all of which influence their willingness to enroll.[40] To reduce cancer incidence in minority populations, researchers must identify successful methods of addressing these potential barriers and enrolling minorities at risk. Experts on minority recruitment strategies have stressed the importance of having common goals between the research community and the minority community, exploiting local histories between the community and the academic research institution, and using key community people.[41,42] During the BCPT and PCPT, the first large phase III chemoprevention clinical trials, researchers realized that optimal minority enrollment was not occurring despite their targeted efforts. At the end of the studies, BCPT enrolled 3.5% minority women and PCPT enrolled 3.4% minority men. When the next large phase III chemoprevention clinical trials (STAR and SELECT) were launched, researchers had learned a great deal about the barriers and strategies for re-

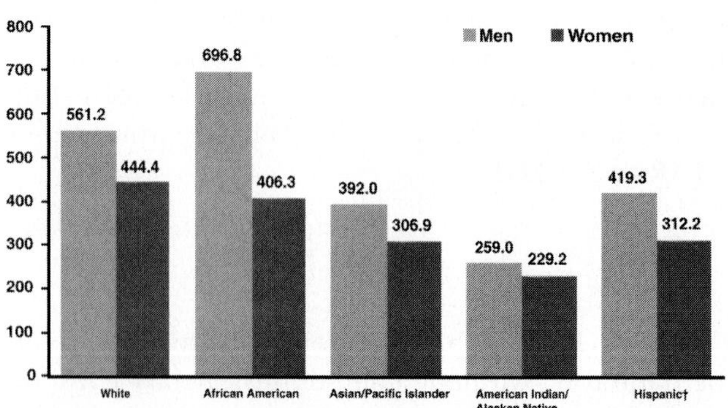

*Age-adjusted to the 2000 U.S. standard population.
†Hispanic is not mutually exclusive from whites, African Americans, Asian/Pacific Islanders, and American Indians.

Figure 5-2 Minority incidence. Cancer incidence rates* by race and ethnicity, 1996–2000 (Rate per 100,000). Data from Surveillance, Epidemiology, and End Results Program, 1975–2000, Division of Cancer Control and Population Sciences, National Cancer Institute, 2003.

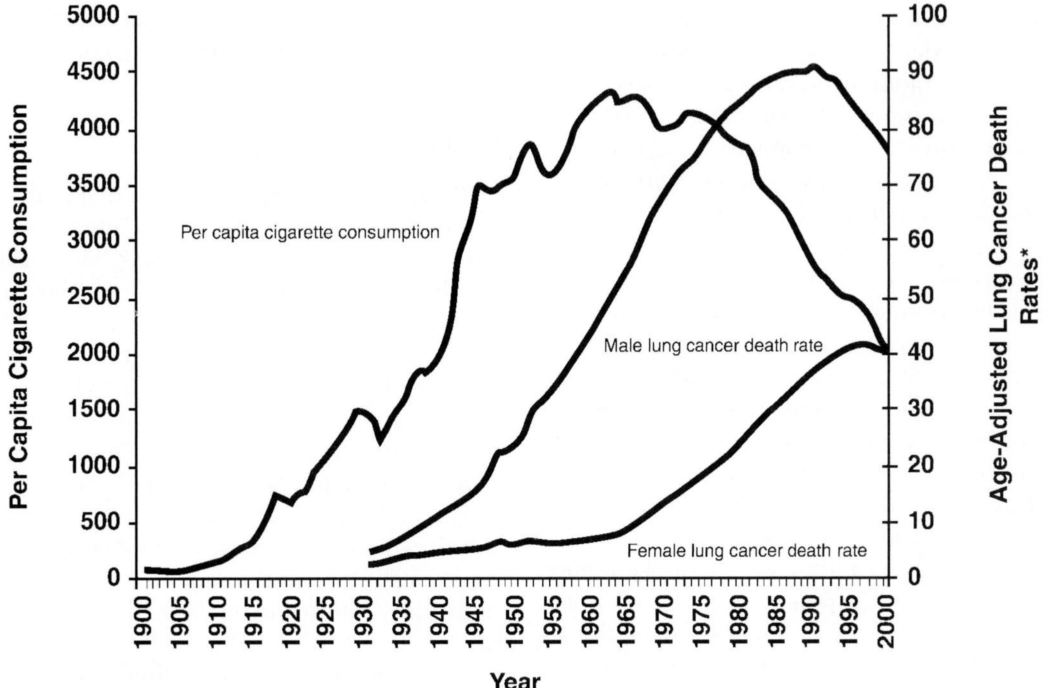

*Age-adjusted to the 2000 U.S. standard population.

Figure 5-3 Trends in tobacco use. Tobacco use in the United States, 1900–2000. Data from Death rates: U.S. Mortality Public Use Tapes, 1960–2000, U.S. Mortality Volumes, 1930–1959, National Center for Health Statistics, Centers for Disease Control and Prevention, 2002. Cigarette consumption: U.S. Department of Agriculture, 1900–2000.

cruiting minorities and had well-developed plans in place to address this challenge. At the time this chapter was written, SELECT minority enrollment was 14.5% and STAR minority enrollment was 6.5%.

Vaccines

Epidemiological and experimental evidence has established an association between several viruses — human papillomavirus (HPV), hepatitis B virus (HBV), and human immunodeficiency virus (HIV) — and the development of various malignancies. Vaccines that seek to prevent infections by oncogenic pathogens, thereby preventing progression to carcinoma, are under investigation. Currently, the only prophylactic cancer vaccine to receive FDA approval is the vaccine against HBV.

Tobacco Use

Despite an ever-increasing body of behavioral and scientific evidence linking smoking and cancer, tobacco use remains the leading cause of preventable death in the United States. Although a great deal of progress has been made toward cessation since the publication of the first Surgeon General's Report in 1964, more is needed. Figure 5-3 shows the downward trend in cigarette consumption since 1964.[43]

Tobacco use causes more than 440,000 deaths each year and results in more than $75 billion in direct medical costs and $82 billion in lost productivity annually.[44,45] An estimated 46.5 million, (23.5%) American adults are habitual tobacco users, while 44.3 million (22.2%) are former smokers.[4] Additionally, 4000 adolescents younger than age 18 begin using tobacco each day.[4] In fact, smoking rates are declining in all age groups except among 18- to 24-year-old individuals, where it is rising.[46] Smoking also has a substantial effect on nonsmokers. Environmental, or second-hand, smoke has been associated with increased risk for lung cancer and coronary heart disease.[47] Smoking during pregnancy has been associated with perinatal deaths, low-weight births, and preterm deliveries. The number of lives saved by smoking cessation among adults and prevention of smoking initiation among adolescents would be significant.

Among current smokers, 74% report a desire to quit and 70% have made previous attempts, yet the success rate remains low.[45] Behavioral and pharmaceutical approaches to tobacco cessation have demonstrated varied efficacy. Current cessation interventions include a myriad of self-help programs and resources: advice from primary care providers, group programs and classes, individual counseling sessions, pharmacologic interventions, and worksite and statewide cessation programs.[48] Clearly, innovative research initiatives exploring the causes of tobacco use and the nature of nicotine addiction are needed.

The NCI sponsors a broad spectrum of tobacco-related research initiatives seeking to evaluate educational and behavioral interventions to prevent the initiation of tobacco use, assessments of clinical treatment for nicotine addiction, and exploration of genetic and environmental factors leading to increased risk for cancer. As tobacco control programs are developed and enforced at the state level, new assessment tools are being developed to measure tobacco-use outcomes of taxation, clean indoor-air policies, marketing restrictions, youth access restrictions, and other strategies.

Chemoprevention may be an option for some of the apparent pulmonary pathology in smokers and former smokers. Two NCI-sponsored phase III trials designed to test the efficacy of beta-carotene, alpha-tocopherol, and retinol in lung cancer chemoprevention for smokers and former smokers have been reported: the Alpha-Tocopherol, Beta-Carotene Cancer Prevention Study (ATBC) and the Beta-Carotene and Retinol Efficacy Trial (CARET). ATBC was a randomized, double-blind, placebo-controlled lung cancer chemoprevention trial conducted from 1985 to 1993 involving 29,133 Finnish men between the ages of 50 and 69 with a history of heavy smoking. The study sought to determine the efficacy of 20 mg beta-carotene per day alone or in combination with 50 mg vitamin E in preventing lung cancer.[49] Results showed no evidence of a beneficial effect from supplemental vitamin E or beta-carotene in the prevention of lung cancer. In fact, men who received beta-carotene experienced an 18% increase in lung cancer incidence ($P = 0.01$) and an 8% increase in mortality. The findings were published in 1994 and later confirmed by the CARET results in 1996.[49]

CARET, a randomized, double-blind, placebo-controlled lung cancer chemoprevention trial was designed to compare the effects of 30 mg beta-carotene and 25,000 IU vitamin A (retinyl palmitate). Median follow-up was six years, and 18,314 men and women ages 45 to 74 who were smokers, were former smokers, and/or had been exposed to asbestos were enrolled.[50] The study intervention was stopped 18 months earlier than expected following an interim analysis that indicated no benefit from the agents and perhaps harm. Ultimately, 28% higher lung cancer incidence and 17% higher overall mortality occurred in the group taking the vitamin supplementation.

Despite the disappointing results, early-phase chemoprevention efforts to prevent lung cancer in smokers and former smokers continue, however. They include a variety of agents, such as zileuton, celecoxib, selenium, myo-inositol, green tea, and rofecoxib.

Diet and Nutrition

In 1981, Doll and Peto estimated that as many as 35% of all cancer cases in the United States may be attributed to poor diet and nutrition.[51] Since that time, a growing body of evidence from molecular biology, epidemiology, biochemistry, and clinical medicine continues to support an association between diet and increased risk of specific cancers.[52-54] Epidemiologic studies have associated diets rich in fruit and vegetable consumption with a decrease in risk for a variety of cancers (pharynx, larynx, lung, esophagus, stomach, cervix, uterus, colon, and rectum). Laboratory research efforts have focused on determining which dietary constituents and supplements are responsible for cancer protection and on defining their precise role in cancer development. Despite the progress made in this area, inconsistencies in clinical trial findings suggest that major biochemical complexities exist in the causal relationship. Clearly, further investigation is required.

Despite compelling epidemiological evidence, two NCI-sponsored studies of nutritional interventions in people at high risk for developing colorectal cancer reported no evidence that diet affects the growth of precancerous colorectal polyps in individuals with a history of polyps. The Polyp Prevention Trial and the Wheat Bran Fiber Study evaluated the effect of diet on the growth of new colorectal polyps in individuals with prior history of polyp removal.[55,56] The Polyp Prevention Trial randomized 2079 men and women either to receive intensive nutritional counseling about adopting a low-fat, high-fiber, fruit- and vegetable-enriched eating plan or to receive a standard brochure on healthy eating. Participants were enrolled for four years. The Wheat Bran Fiber Study randomized 1429 men and women to receive a daily cereal supplement with either a high level of wheat bran fiber (13.5 g of fiber in two-thirds cup of cereal) or a low level of wheat bran fiber (2 g of fiber in two-thirds cup cereal) over a three-year period. The negative results in the two studies may be due to several factors, including the short duration of the intervention (three and four years, respectively). Also, the influence of nutritional factors on critical molecular-, cellular-, or tissue-level events in colorectal cancer formation may take place well before polyps are formed. The study subjects will continue to be followed to evaluate the long-term effects of the dietary interventions.

The Women's Health Initiative (WHI), a 15-year national study focusing on strategies for preventing heart disease, breast and colorectal cancer, and osteoporosis in postmenopausal women, provides an example of a major nutritional research initiative sponsored by the National Institutes of Health.[57] WHI involves more than 161,000 women aged 50–79 and is one of the most definitive, far-reaching studies of women's health ever undertaken in the United States. It includes a clinical trial component to evaluate a number of women's health issues, among them dietary patterns and calcium/vitamin D supplements, and their effects on the prevention of cancer. More than 48,000 women are participating in this component of WHI. Participants are randomized either to follow their usual eating pattern and receive standard information on nutrition guidelines, or to follow a low-fat dietary program that limits their fat intake to 20% of their total daily calories, increases fruit and vegetable consumption to five or more servings per day, and increases grains to six or more servings per day. Participants are evaluated every six months for 8 to 12 years.

The effectiveness of calcium and vitamin D in decreasing risk for cancers of the colon and rectum will be evaluated in a supplemental study to WHI. Nearly 45,000 postmenopausal women aged 50–79 will be randomized into one of two study groups. One group will take calcium carbonate and vitamin D 400 IU daily; the other group will take a placebo. Participants will be followed for 7 to 11 years. Valuable information obtained from WHI and other ongoing nutritional clinical trials will help guide a new era of nutritional science in cancer prevention.

Cancer Prevention and Public Policy

Public policy influences cancer prevention at all levels of the cancer control continuum. A number of national organizations develop guidelines for cancer control. It then becomes the responsibility of local and state governments to implement those guidelines. Cancer prevention policy governs exposure to cancer risk and is operationalized primarily through public education programs and regulation of carcinogens.[58] Public education regarding cancer risk is promoted by several vehicles, such as school programs, product labeling (e.g., on tobacco, cosmetics, food), and mass media campaigns. The primary goal of public prevention education is to provide adequate information for an individual to make informed decisions about healthy lifestyle choices.

Regulation of carcinogenic exposure includes a number of policy interventions. Tobacco offers the best example of how regulatory provisions may be used to safeguard the public. Tobacco use has received unprecedented attention as a result of tobacco taxes, state lawsuits against tobacco companies, and sweeping legislative proposals to reduce smoking, especially among youth. Litigation has resulted in the release of many confidential documents from tobacco companies, including unpublished research on nicotine addiction and tobacco marketing practices. It has also produced changes in the way tobacco is advertised and sold nationwide.

Nursing Implications

As noted earlier, the ONS has developed a position statement titled "Prevention and Early Detection of Cancer in the United States."[6] This position statement provides a wide range of opportunities and responsibilities for nurses in cancer prevention and early detection. The statement identifies five specific areas where nurses, depending on their practice setting, may play a significant role:

1. Professional education
2. Public education
3. Cancer prevention and detection services
4. Research
5. Health policy

Nurses certainly have a presence in each of these areas. Nevertheless, the majority of ONS members—and perhaps all oncology nurses—work in clinical settings providing patient education and treatment. It is in this setting where the oncology nurse encounters a prime opportunity to inform a receptive patient, family, and friends about cancer screening guidelines. When a loved one is diagnosed with cancer, there is often an increased awareness of an individual's own vulnerability and desire to find out what can be done to avoid this disease. This time may be termed a "teachable moment." The oncology nurse in clinical practice frequently encounters these small but interested audiences who are open to hearing about healthy lifestyle choices and current cancer screening guidelines. The cancer patient is also part of this discussion, because having cancer once does not protect the individual from other cancers. Healthy lifestyle choices and vigilant screenings are also indicated.

The oncology nurse is also a member of a social community where healthy lifestyle choices, cancer prevention, and screening instruction can be provided to groups at churches, scout troops, sports teams, and local businesses. Educational materials can be found through ACS and NCI web sites.

Finally, the oncology nurse can be a role model. This can be accomplished by choosing not to smoke, maintaining a healthy weight with appropriate food choices, and following recommended sun safety practices.

Oncology nurses must expand their perspective beyond treatment. As stated earlier, the majority of oncology nurses treat patients with cancer and have excellent knowledge and skills regarding treatment and symptom management. However, the continuum of cancer care extends from prevention all the way to palliation. The oncology nurse is at the peak of practice when integrating the spectrum of cancer care into his or her clinical setting. Cancer nurses, due to their frontline experience with the ravages of the disease, are well suited to advocate powerfully for methods to intervene in halting or reversing the march of initiated cells toward metastatic cancer.

Conclusion

An impressive body of evidence in cancer prevention science has been accumulating over the past three decades. Pharmacologic and nutritional compounds continue to be identified as potential agents for testing in chemoprevention clinical trials. Currently, more than 60 agents have shown potential and are under investigation in NCI-sponsored chemoprevention clinical trials.

Refined epidemiological studies are providing more targeted information regarding lifestyle behaviors and cancer risk, thereby providing better direction for laboratory, clinical, and behavioral research efforts. As technology advances, exploration of intermediate biomarkers will become the focal point of prevention research. At the same time, prevention research must address effective ways to reach minorities and medically underserved populations, and explore social, cultural, and physical determinants of cancer incidence and outcomes, as well as behavioral and biologic factors that contribute to them.[48] The potential to reduce the nation's cancer burden is great, but it will require sustained and committed efforts by a cadre of federal agencies and programs, healthcare providers, researchers, legislators, policymakers, and support from the population at large.

References

1. American Cancer Society: Cancer prevention and early detection: facts and figures, 2004. *www.cancer.org/docroot/STT/stt_0.asp*. Accessed March 15, 2004
2. U.S. Department of Health and Human Services, National Institutes of Health, National Cancer Institute: *Surveillance, Epidemiology, and End Results Program: 30 Years of Measuring Our Nation's Progress Against Cancer.* NIH Publication No.03-5434. 2004
3. U.S. Department of Health and Human Services: Cancer, in *Healthy People 2010: With Understanding and Improving Health and Objectives for Improving Health* (ed 2). Washington, DC, U.S. Government Printing Office, 2002
4. American Cancer Society: Retrieved from the American Cancer Society home page at *www.cancer.org*. Accessed May 15, 2004
5. Ropka ME, Guterbock TM, Krebs LU, et al: Year 2000 Oncology Nursing Society research priorities survey. *Oncol Nurs Forum* 29:481–491, 2002
6. Oncology Nursing Society: Position statement: prevention and early detection of cancer in the United States. *www.ons.org/xp6/ONS/Information.xml/Journals_and_Positions.xml/ONS_Positions.xml*. Accessed March 15, 2004
7. Sporn M: Carcinogenesis and cancer: different perspectives on the same disease. *Cancer Res* 51:6215–6218, 1991
8. Schottenfeld D: Principles and applications of cancer prevention, in Schottenfeld D, Fraumeni JF (eds.): *Cancer Epidemiology and Prevention* (ed 2). New York, Oxford University Press, 1996, pp 1391–1409
9. Lippman S, Benner S, Hong WK: Cancer chemoprevention. *J Clin Oncol* 12:851–873, 1994
10. Greenwald P, McDonald S, Anderson D: An evidence-based approach to cancer prevention clinical trials. *Eur J Cancer Prev* 11:S43–S47, 2002
11. Wattenberg L: An overview of chemoprevention: current status and future prospects. *Proc Soc Experi Biol and Med* 216:133–141, 1997
12. Lippman S, Benner S, Hong WK: Chemoprevention. *Cancer* 72:984–990, 1993
13. Hong WK, Sporn M: Recent advances in chemoprevention of cancer. *Science* 278:1073–1077, 1997
14. Swan DK, Ford B: Chemoprevention of cancer: review of the literature. *Oncol Nurs Forum* 24:719–727, 1997
15. Kelloff G, Sigman C, Greenwald P: Cancer chemoprevention: progress and promise. *Eur J Cancer* 35:2031–2038, 1999
16. Shaw GL, Mulshine JL: Biomarkers and histology of premalignant and malignant lesion, in Greenwald P, Kramer B, Weed DL (eds.): *Cancer Prevention and Control.* New York, Marcel Dekker, 1995, pp 111–133
17. Volker D: Carcinogenesis: application to clinical practice. *Clin J Oncol Nurs* 5:225–229, 2001
18. Lippman SM, Spitz MR: Lung cancer chemoprevention: an integrated approach. *J Clin Oncol* 19: 74S–82S, 2001
19. Hong WK, Carbone P: Cancer chemoprevention: present status, future expectations. *Hosp Pract* 101–105, 1999
20. Lippman S, Lee JJ, Sabichi A: Cancer chemoprevention: progress and promise. *J Natl Cancer Inst* 90:1514–1528, 1998
21. Braakhuis BJ, Tabor MP, Kummer JA, et al: A genetic explanation of Slaughter's concept of field cancerization: evidence and clinical implications. *Cancer Res* 63:1727–1730, 2003
22. Loescher LJ, Reid M: Dynamics of cancer prevention, in Yarbro CH, Frogge MH, Goodman M, Groenwald S (eds.): *Cancer Nursing: Principles and Practices* (ed 5). Sudbury, MA, Jones and Bartlett, 2000, pp 135–149
23. Mahon SM: Principles of cancer prevention and early detection. *Clin J Oncol Nurs* 4:169–176, 2000
24. Champion VL, Rawl SM, Menon U: Population-based cancer screening. *Oncol Nurs Forum* 29:853–861, 2002
25. Sporn M: Approaches to prevention of epithelial cancer during the preneoplastic period. *Cancer Res* 36:2699–2702, 1976
26. Goodman GE: The clinical evaluation of cancer chemoprevention agents: defining and contrasting phase I, II, and III objectives. *Cancer Res* 52:2752S-2757S, 1992
27. Greenwald P: Cancer chemoprevention. *Brit Med J* 324: 714–718, 2002
28. Greenwald P: From carcinogenesis to clinical interventions for cancer prevention. *Toxicology* 166:37–45, 2001

29. Kelloff G, Boone CW, Steele VE, et al: Mechanistic considerations in the evaluation of chemoprevention data. *IARC Sci Pub* 139:203–219, 1996
30. Greenwald P, Dixon DW, Maline W, et al: Concepts in cancer chemoprevention research. *Cancer* 65:1483–1490, 1990
31. Steinbach G, Lynch PM, Phillips RKS, et al: The effect of celecoxib, a cyclooxygenase-2 inhibitor, in familial adenomatous polyposis. *New Engl J Med* 342:1946–1952, 2000
32. Ford LG, Minasian LM, McCaskill-Stevens W, et al: Prevention and early detection clinical trials: opportunities for primary care providers and their patients. *CA: Cancer J Clin* 53:82–101, 2003
33. Steele VE: Current mechanistic approaches to the chemoprevention of cancer. *J Biochem Molec Biol* 36:78–81, 2003
34. Lippman S, Benner S, Hong WK: in Greenwald P, Kramer B, Weed DL, (eds.): *Cancer Prevention and Control.* New York, Marcel Dekker, 1995, pp 329–335
35. Wattenberg L: Chemoprevention of cancer. *Cancer Res* 45:1–8, 1985
36. Greenwald P: Cancer prevention clinical trials. *J Clin Oncol* 20:14S–22S, 2002
37. Bonassi S, Neri M, Puntoni R: Validation of biomarkers as early predictors of disease. *Mutation Res* 480–481:349–358, 2001
38. Vourlekis JS, Szabo E: Predicting success in cancer prevention trials. *J Natl Cancer Inst* 95:178-179, 2003
39. Negm RS, Verma M, Srivastava S: The promise of biomarkers in cancer screening and detection. *Trends Molec Med* 8:288–293, 2002
40. Guiliano AR, Mokuau N, Hughes C, et al: Participation of minorities in cancer research: the influence of structural, cultural, and linguistic factors. *Ann Epidemiol* 10:S22–S34, 2000
41. Levkoff S, Sanchez H: Lessons learned about minority recruitment and retention from the Centers on Minority Aging and Health Promotion. *Gerontologist* 43:18–26, 2003
42. Moinpour CM, Atkinson JO, Thomas SM, et al: Minority recruitment in the prostate cancer prevention trial. *Ann Epidemiol* 10:S85–S91, 2000
43. U.S. Department of Health and Human Services, Centers for Disease Control and Prevention: Smoking and health: report of the Advisory Committee of the Surgeon General of the Public Health Service. Retrieved from *www.cdc.gov/tobacco/sgrlist1.htm#IRP* on March 15, 2004. 1964
44. U.S. Department of Health and Human Services, Centers for Disease Control and Prevention: Retrieved from Tobacco Information and Prevention Source at *www.cdc.gov/* on March 15, 2004
45. American Lung Association: State of tobacco control: 2003. Retrieved from *www.lungusa.org* on March 15, 2004
46. Schroeder SA: Tobacco control in the wake of the 1998 Master Settlement Agreement. *N Engl J Med* 350:293–301, 2004
47. National Cancer Institute: Cancer prevention overview www.nci.nih.gov/cancerinfo/pdq/ prevention/overview, 2002
48. Director of National Cancer Institute: The nation's investment in cancer research: a plan and budget proposal for fiscal year 2005. Rep. No. NIH Publication No. 03-5446, 2004
49. Albanes D, Heinonen OP, Huttunen JK, et al: Effects of alpha-tocopherol and beta-carotene supplements on cancer incidence in the Alpha-Tocopherol Beta-Carotene Cancer Prevention Study. *Am J Clin Nutr* 62:1427S–1430S, 1994
50. Omenn GS, Goodman G, Thornquist MD, et al: Risk factors for lung cancer and for intervention effects in CARET, the beta-carotene and retinol efficacy trial. *J Natl Cancer Inst* 88: 1550–1559, 1996
51. Doll R, Peto R: The causes of cancer: quantitative estimates of avoidable risks of cancer in the United States today. *J Natl Cancer Inst* 66: 1191–308, 1981
52. Greenwald P, Milner JA, Clifford CK: Creating a new paradigm in nutrition research within the National Cancer Institute. *J Nutrition* 130:3103–3105, 2000
53. Greenwald P, Clifford CK, McDonald S: The challenge of cancer prevention and control: diet, nutrition, and cancer prevention. Heber D, Blackburn GL, Go VL (eds.): *Nutritional Oncology*, San Diego Academic Press, 1999, pp. 325–341
54. Greenwald P, Clifford CK, Milner JA: Diet and cancer prevention. *Eur J Cancer* 37:948–965, 2001
55. Greenberg ER, Baron JA, Tosteson TD, et al: A clinical trial of antioxidant vitamins to prevent colorectal adenoma: Polyp Prevention Study Group. *N Engl J Med* 331:141–147, 1994
56. Alberts DS, Martinez ME, Roe DJ, et al: Lack of effect of a high-fiber cereal supplement on the recurrence of colorectal adenomas. *N Engl J Med* 342:1156–1162, 2000
57. Women's Health Initiative: Retrieved from *www.whi.org* on March 15, 2004
58. Warner KE: Public policy issues, in Greenwald P, Kramer B, Weed DL (eds.): *Cancer Prevention and Control.* New York, Marcel Dekker, 1995, pp 451–472

CHAPTER 6

Screening and Detection for Asymptomatic Individuals

Suzanne M. Mahon, RN, DNSc, AOCN®, APNG

Introduction

Improved survival from cancer has been a result of both improved treatment and the earlier detection of cancer. Oncology nurses are becoming increasingly involved in cancer prevention and detection services. This chapter provides an overview of the fundamental principles involved in the early detection of cancer, also referred to as cancer screening. Principles of cancer risk assessment will be addressed as well.

Conceptual Considerations in Cancer Screening

Intuitively, it makes sense to screen for and detect cancer in its earliest stages. Theoretically, treatment should be the least complicated and least toxic at this point, and there should be the greatest chance for long-term disease-free survival. Nurses are often confronted with questions about screening and the early detection of cancer. They need to be able to instruct patients and families on the principles of screening, the rationale for the recommendations put forth by national agencies, and controversies in screening.

Definitions

An understanding of commonly used terms for risk assessment and cancer screening is fundamental. Oncology nurses need to be able to explain each term to patients when educating about cancer screening. Once patients understand these terms, they find it easier to make appropriate choices regarding cancer screening. Table 6-1 lists some commonly used terms and their definitions.

Cancer screening is aimed at asymptomatic persons with the goal of finding disease when it is most easily treated. Screening tests seek to decrease both the morbidity and the mortality associated with cancer. This is the traditional definition of cancer screening. Some also consider screening for genetic or molecular markers that put an individual at high risk for developing cancer to be a form of cancer screening. Information on genetic testing is found in detail in Chapter 7 of this text. This chapter focuses on cancer screening in the more traditional sense.

Outcomes

Short-term outcomes may include measures of the number of persons who are screened or who undergo

Table 6-1 Definitions of Terms Used in Cancer Screening

Primary cancer prevention includes measures to avoid carcinogen exposure, improve health practices, and, in some cases, use chemoprevention agents. Primary prevention may also include the use of prophylactic surgery to prevent or significantly reduce the development of a malignancy.

Secondary cancer prevention includes the identification of persons at risk for developing malignancy and the implementation of appropriate screening recommendations. Terms often used interchangeably with secondary cancer prevention are *early detection* and *cancer screening*.

Tertiary cancer prevention is aimed at persons with a history of malignancy and includes monitoring for and preventing recurrence and screening for second primary cancers. In many cases, those who have had a diagnosis of cancer and who carry a mutation in a cancer susceptibility gene are at significantly higher risk for developing a second malignancy.

Cancer screening test is the method used to detect a specific target cancer. It may be a single modality, but often is a combination of tests. Laboratory tests of blood or body fluids, imaging tests, physical examination, and invasive procedures are all sometimes used for screening tests.

Asymptomatic means that the person being screened and the examiner are unaware of any signs or symptoms of cancer in the individual prior to initiating the screening test.

Diagnostic tests are used in those with symptoms of cancer or abnormal screening tests. The purpose of diagnostic testing is to determine the cause of symptoms or abnormal screening tests.

Target population is the number of persons in a defined group who are capable of developing the disease and would be appropriate candidates for screening. *Population* may refer to the general population, or a specific group of people defined by geographic, physical, or social characteristics. For example, nurses who provide cancer genetics counseling need to determine whether a person is of Ashkenazi Jewish background. This special population of Jewish people is at higher risk for three specific mutations for hereditary breast cancer.

Mortality is the number of persons who die of a particular cancer during a defined period of time such as one year.

Prevalence is the number of cancers that exist in a defined population at a given point in time.

Outcomes are the health and economic results that occur related to screening. Outcomes may include the benefits, harms, and costs of screening or genetic testing, and its incurred diagnostic evaluations. Outcomes may be short or long-term in nature.

Cost-effectiveness is achieved if the costs of the screening program are less than the costs in the unscreened group.

Table 6-2 Goals of Cancer Risk Assessment and Screening Programs

- Provide accurate information on the genetic, biologic, and environmental factors related to the individual's risk for developing a cancer
- Formulate appropriate recommendations for primary and secondary prevention
- Offer emotional and psychosocial support to facilitate adjustment to the information regarding risk and promote adherence to recommendations for prevention and early detection
- Increase the number of individuals who are offered screening
- Increase the number of individuals who complete screening
- Assure 100% follow-up of all abnormal screens
- Increase the number of premalignant lesions detected
- Long-term goals include an earlier stage distribution of detected cancer, decreased mortality, and decreased healthcare costs

Data from Clark, Reintgen[2]; Mahon.[3]

genetic testing, the number of persons with abnormal screens who have further diagnostic testing, the number of cancers detected, or the cost per cancer detected and risks associated with screening. Long-term outcomes may include site-specific cancers detected in the screened population, total costs, and the stage distribution of detected cancers.[1] Knowledge of outcome measures is important for nurses who provide risk assessments and cancer screening services. Goals of cancer screening are described in Table 6-2. Nurses need to be able to give detailed information about the risks and benefits that can arise during the screening process.

Cancer Risk Assessment: The First Step in the Cancer Screening Process

A *risk factor* is a trait or characteristic that is associated with a statistically significant and increased likelihood of developing a disease.[2,3] It is important to note, however, that having a risk factor does not mean that a person will inevitably develop a disease, such as malignancy, nor does the absence of a risk factor render one immune to developing a disease or malignancy.

Basic elements of a *cancer risk assessment* may include a review of medical history, a history of exposures to carcinogens in daily living, and a detailed family history. Once all information is gathered, it must be interpreted to the patient in understandable terms. Often this is accomplished by using various risk calculations such as absolute risk, relative risk, attributable risk, or specific risk models for various cancers.

Family History

A family history should focus on primary and secondary relatives. This includes an assessment of both paternal and maternal sides, as many autosomal dominant syndromes can be passed through either the father or the mother. First-degree relatives include parents, siblings, and children. Because first-degree relatives share 50% of their genes, these relatives will be the most likely to inherit similar genetic information. These families will often have multiple cases of cancer at an earlier age than expected in the general population. Information about second-degree relatives can also prove helpful. Second-degree relatives include grandparents, aunts, and uncles. Second-degree relatives have 25% of their genes in common. In particular, older second-degree relatives can provide important information about genetic risk, because they would have been expected to manifest an early-onset cancer if a hereditary trait is present in the family. The pedigree should also include nieces and nephews, because these younger family members can provide information about childhood cancers, which also has implications for the genetic risk assessment. Third-degree relatives (cousins, great-aunts and great-uncles, and great-grandparents) can be included as well, although the accuracy of reports on these relatives is not always high. These relatives share 12.5% of the same genes. Once all of this information is documented, it should be stored in a standard pedigree format. In families with multiple cases of malignancy, this pedigree can help to teach concepts of genetics, clarify relationships, and provide a quick reference. The recent availability of software to draw these pedigrees has greatly simplified the process of updating this information.

Reliability of patient information should be considered both when obtaining and when communicating the risk assessment. Reports suggest that personal recall of a family history of malignancy may be inaccurate. Family reports may be inaccurate as much as 17% of the time for first-degree relatives and even more frequently for second- and third-degree relatives.[4] It is important to order pathology reports or actual mammograms for review before determining risk and communicating risk information to the patient. For example, there is a big difference between the risk for development of breast cancer in a woman with a biopsy-proven fibroadenoma and in a woman with biopsy-proven ductal hyperplasia with atypia. Fibrocystic disease or change is a generic term and should not be equated with an increased risk for developing breast cancer. Obtaining accurate information is necessary to develop the most accurate risk assessment possible, correct misconceptions if indicated, and make the best possible recommendations for cancer screening.

The family history provides an organized way to document the risk factors related to family history, such as whether a relative is alive or dead, age at death if applicable, significant medical diagnoses, or a diagnosis of cancer. Space can be provided to describe in detail the specific type of cancer, age at diagnosis, and other characteristics such as whether a breast cancer was premenopausal or bilateral. Specific knowledge may influence recommendations for screening. Taking a detailed family history is not only useful for cancer risk assessment, but is also the first step in identifying families with a possible hereditary predisposition to malignancy and other illnesses. Healthcare providers should ask patients about specific relatives and their health individually rather than asking a more general question such as, "Have any of your relatives been diagnosed with cancer?" After gathering the family history, it is important to recheck whether any of the patient's relatives have been diagnosed with these cancers. It is amazing how often patients forget to provide this information, and reiterating this question may unearth valuable information.

Past Medical History/Lifestyle Factors

Assessment of past medical history and personal history factors that may increase the risk of developing cancer should be documented. Many of these risk factors are not within an individual's control and are not amenable to primary prevention efforts (e.g., age at menarche). In contrast, lifestyle factors complete the risk factor assessment and are often within the control of the individual. They provide a framework for providing education about primary prevention efforts, which is discussed in more detail in Chapter 5.

Structuring the interview in more of a traditional medical history format facilitates the information-gathering process. Trying to find risk factors by category or anatomical site can be confusing to the patient, resulting in a disjointed interview, and may not be as thorough as a comprehensive health history. Healthcare professionals need to realize that conducting an interview in this fashion demands that the clinician interpret the risk factors to the patient and document recommendations for cancer prevention and early detection somewhere on the chart. For that reason, specially designed forms to make documentation of risk factors comprehensive and the information easy to retrieve, update, and interpret to the patient are helpful.[3]

After all of the risk data are collected, the clinician must assimilate the risk factors mentally and provide information about them for each of the major cancers to the patient. For example, early menarche, nulliparity, and late menopause are risk factors for both breast and endometrial cancer. The communication of risk should therefore include a discussion of the risk for developing both of these cancers.

Risk can be communicated to patients in several different formats. Often, it is best to use several means, including absolute, relative, and attributable risk.

Absolute Risk

Absolute risk is a measure of the occurrence of cancer, either incidence (new cases) or mortality (deaths), in the general population. It can be expressed either as the number of cases for a specified denominator (e.g., 75 cases per 10,000 people annually) or as a cumulative risk up to a specified age (e.g., one in eight women will develop breast cancer if they live to age 85). Another way to express absolute risk is to discuss average risk of developing breast cancer at a certain age. For example, a woman's risk of developing breast cancer might be 2% at age 50 but 11% at age 85. Risk estimates will be much different for a 50-year-old woman than for a 85-year-old woman, as approximately 50% of the cases of breast cancer occur after the age of 65. These concepts are illustrated in Figure 6-1 and Table 6-3.

Patients who present for screening need to understand that certain assumptions are made to reach an absolute risk figure. For example, the "one in eight" figure describes the "average" risk of breast cancer in Caucasian American women and takes into consideration other causes of death over the life span. By necessity, this figure will overestimate breast cancer risk for some women with no risk factors and underestimate the risk for women with several risk factors.[5] This statistic actually means that the average woman's breast cancer risk is 2% to age 50; 6% from age 50 to 70; and 3% from age 70 to 85.[4] The 11% or "one in eight" risk is obtained by adding the risk in each age category (2% + 6% + 3% = 11%). When a woman who has an average risk reaches age 50 without a diagnosis of breast cancer, she has passed through 2% of her risk, so her risk to age 80 is 11% minus 2% which equals 9%. When she reaches age 70 without a diagnosis of breast cancer, her risk to age 80 is 11% – 2% – 6% = 3%. Time must always be considered for the risk figure to be meaningful. For example, the average 50 year old woman's risk is 6% to age 70 but 9% to age 80.[4] Absolute risk is helpful when a patient needs to understand the chances for all persons in a population of developing a particular disease. Screening tests often focus on cancers with higher absolute risk because they are more common in certain populations.

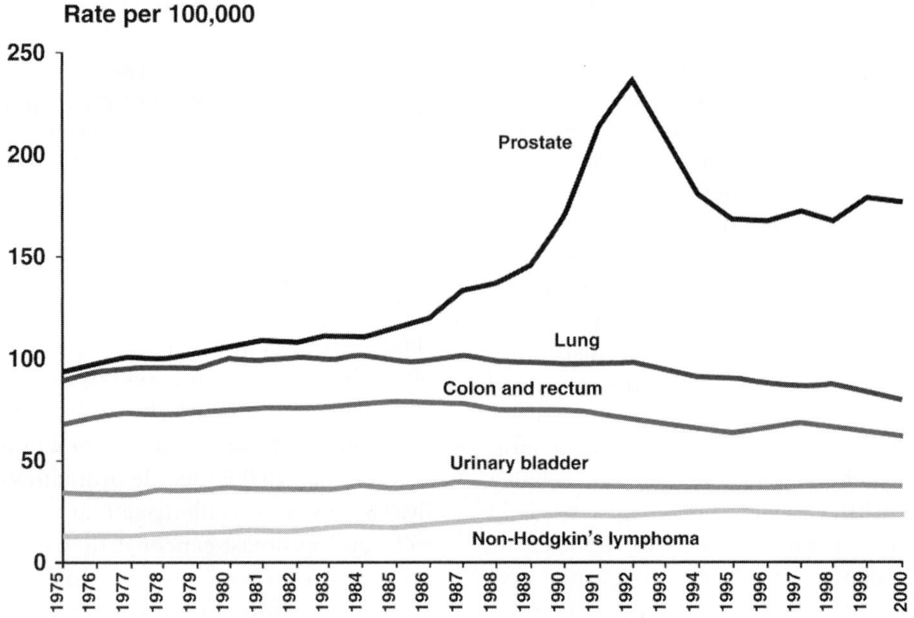

*Age-adjusted to the 2000 U.S. standard population.

Figure 6-1 Cancer incidence rates* for men, in the United States, 1975–2000. Data from Surveillance, Epidemiology, and End Results Program, 1975–2000, Division of Cancer Control and Population Sciences, National Cancer Institute, 2003.

Relative Risk

The term *relative risk* refers to a comparison of the incidence or deaths among those with a particular risk factor compared to those without the risk factor. By using relative risk factors, an individual can determine his or her risk factors and thus better understand personal chances of developing a specific cancer as compared to individuals without such risk factors. If the risk for a person with no known risk factors is 1.0, one can evaluate the risk of individuals with risk factors in relation to this figure. For example, for a woman whose mother had breast cancer in both breasts before age 40, the relative risk would be approximately 8.5 over her lifetime. That is, she has eight and a half times the chance of a woman with no known risk of developing breast cancer.

Table 6-3 Lifetime probability of developing cancer by site, for men, in the United States, 1998–2000

Site	Risk
All sites	1 in 2
Prostate	1 in 6
Lung and bronchus	1 in 13
Colon and rectum	1 in 17
Urinary bladder	1 in 29
Non-Hodgkin's lymphoma	1 in 48
Melanoma	1 in 55
Leukemia	1 in 70
Oral cavity	1 in 72
Kidney	1 in 69
Stomach	1 in 81

Data from DevCan: Probability of Developing or Dying of Cancer Software, Version 5.1 Statistical Research and Applications Branch, NCI, 2003. http://srab.cancer.gov/devcan.

Relative risk factors can confuse some patients. If one plans to give a patient information about his or her relative risk, it is important to specify exactly what comparison is being made. Often percentages are confusing when used with risk. If a news report states that there is a 30% to 50% increase in breast cancer risk in women who take a particular hormone therapy after menopause, it means, in absolute numerical terms, that there will be 0.6 more cases of breast cancer per 100 women from ages 50 to 70. The same concept applies if a person is informed that he or she has a 1% chance of developing cancer. This simply means that the risk has increased from 1 in 10,000 to 1.3 in 10,000.[6]

Nurses need to remember that the relative risk statistic is helpful only if it is clear what the baseline risk is. Unless the risk to the baseline group is clearly known, a comparison risk is not useful and can even prove misleading.

Relative risk can be very helpful when selecting screening recommendations. If a person's relative risk is significantly higher than most members of the general population, it will probably be necessary to modify a screening recommendation usually given in the general population.

Table 6-4 Models That Predict Risk of Developing a Particular Cancer or Having a Mutation for Developing a Particular Cancer

Model	Measurement	Reference
Gail	Provides a figure of absolute risk for developing breast cancer at the current age and in five years.	Constantino, Gail, Pee, et al, 1999.[7]
Claus	Provides useful age-specific risk estimates based on the number and age of first- and second-degree relatives with breast cancer.	Claus, Risch, Thompson, 1994[8]; Claus, Schildkrkaut, Thompson, et al, 1996[9]
Couch	Estimates the chance of carrying a *BRCA1* mutation.	Couch, DeShano, Blackwood, et al, 1997[10]
Shattuck-Eidens	Calculates the possibility of carrying a *BRCA1* mutation.	Shattuck-Eidens, Oliphant, McClure, 1997[11]
Berry	Uses principles of Mendelian inheritance and Bayes' theorem to calculate the probability that a woman with a family history of breast and/or ovarian cancer carries a mutation of *BRCA1/2*.	Berry, Parmigiani, Sanchez, et al, 1997[12]
Frank	Estimates the probability that a woman with breast cancer diagnosed before 50 years of age carries a mutation in *BRCA1/2*. Sometimes called the Myriad II model.	www.BRCAnalysis.com
Bethesda Criteria	Estimates the probability that an individual has a mutation for hereditary nonpolyposis colorectal cancer.	Lynch, Lynch, 2003[13]

Attributable Risk

Attributable risk is the amount of disease within the population that could be prevented by alteration of a risk factor. Although historically this component of risk assessment has not received much attention, assessment of attributable risk has important implications for public health policy. A risk factor could convey a very large relative risk yet be restricted to a few individuals; as a consequence, changing it would benefit only a small group. Conversely, some risk factors that can be altered (such as cigarette smoking) could potentially decrease the morbidity and mortality associated with malignancy in a large number of people.

One clinical example involves the use of attributable risk related to smoking and lung cancers. Attributable risk could be calculated to determine how many lung cancer cases could be prevented if everyone stopped or never started smoking. Another example is the number of cases of breast cancer that might develop in women taking a particular birth control pill. A package insert might report a relative risk for developing breast cancer of 2.35 in women younger than age 35 whose first exposure to the drug was within the previous four years. Because the annual incidence rate (absolute risk) for women age 30 to 34 is 26.7 cases per 100,000, a relative risk of 2.35 increases the possible risk from 26.7 to 62.75 cases per 100,000 women. The attributable risk of breast cancer is calculated to be 3.38 cases per 10,000 additional women per year. This slight increase in the number of cases may possibly be associated with the use of the contraceptive.

Explanation of Risk with Clinical Models

More recently, models have become available with which to calculate risk for developing a specific cancer. Most of the current models have been developed for use in women with a risk for developing breast cancer. A list of models, the measurements they provide, and appropriate references can be found in Table 6-4.[7–13] Note that some of these models are used to calculate risk for developing a disease, whereas others are used to calculate risk of having a cancer susceptibility mutation. Each model has its own strengths and weaknesses, which must be presented to the patient. The purpose of calculating these models is to guide or modify screening recommendations for each individual.

Principles of Cancer Risk Communication

Cancer risk communication has many goals. These goals are not limited to helping people understand the risks they face.[14] Other goals include building trust, influencing public policy, fulfilling legal obligations, denying responsibility for undesirable outcomes, and justifying past actions.

Risks can be communicated to patients in a numerous ways. Nurses need to be aware of the strengths and limitations of the various forms of risk communication and provide each patient with a balanced discussion of risks. Most risk discussions will include, at a minimum, a discussion of absolute risks and relative risks; in some cases, discussion of genetic risk assessment models may be warranted.

There is no perfect model that completely and accurately explains an individual's risk for developing a particular cancer.[15] Indeed, for most cancers, a portion of those cases diagnosed cannot be explained by recognized risk factors. For example, approximately 41% of breast cancer cases are attributable to later age at first birth, nulliparity, and family history of breast cancer.[4,15] Ideally, knowledge of risk factors should guide primary prevention efforts. In the case of breast cancer, however, the inability to readily alter these risk factors has limited their relevance for primary prevention. In some cancers, such as breast cancer, the central role of risk factor identification at this point is to identify women at higher risk, particularly those with a potential genetic susceptibility to breast cancer, and to screen them more aggressively. For example, women from these families may be advised to undergo mammographies at a younger age than usually recommended, or to have a clinical breast examination (CBE) twice a year instead of annually.[16]

Transmitting risk information is a central component of all screening and genetic counseling programs—a task that is much more difficult than it might appear. Risk assessment is a complex discipline that is often not fully understood by healthcare professionals and is even less clear to the lay public.[17,18] For professionals who practice risk assessment on a daily basis, continued debate exists over terminology and techniques.

Of course, decisions and behavior are not determined by knowledge of risk alone.[14] Being well-educated about risk and other issues offers no guarantee that good decisions will be made. Other factors may play even more powerful roles in determining how decisions about risk are made. These factors include emotions, personal values, social pressures, environmental barriers, and economic constraints

The transmission of information about risk is also often influenced by professional judgment.[19] Many professional groups have standards of practice or position statements that influence how risks are communicated to patients. In addition, professional opinions about emotionally charged issues such as genetic testing probably influence how risk information is communicated. These biases are probably communicated no matter how nonjudgmental a professional tries to be during a risk communication session.

Risk factor assessment is an ongoing part of oncology nursing practice. Risk factor profiles should be reviewed at least annually. Patients should be questioned about any change in their family history since the last assessment, development of any new health problems that may be associated with increased risk (e.g., abnormal Pap test, a change in breast examination), and initiation of any new medications that may change the risk profile (e.g., started estrogen replacement therapy or tamoxifen therapy). If significant changes have occurred, screening recommendations may need to be modified. If no significant changes have occurred, an annual review of the risk factor assessment offers an excellent opportunity to reinforce information on cancer prevention and early detection. It also communicates an ongoing concern for the patient as a dynamic individual and identifies the nurse as a resource for further information should a problem develop.

Oral Communication of Risk

Communication of cancer risk can be challenging because it includes both qualitative and quantitative components.[19] The quantitative component is usually relatively straightforward. It typically involves sharing risk figures such as absolute or relative risk, or the probability of having a mutation in a cancer susceptibility gene. Numerical data can be presented with the understanding that some individuals have a greater capacity than others to comprehend the meaning of such data. Qualitative information should follow the presentation of quantitative data. It includes a discussion of what the quantitative data specifically mean for the individual patient. Many experts in risk communication believe that all discussions of risk should include both qualitative and quantitative components.[6]

People often hold an inaccurate assessment of their personal risk for developing cancer.[20] That is, patients may perceive their risk to be lower or higher than it actually is. These biases may occur because persons have inaccurate information; are unable to comprehend complex, technical information; or have developed a psychologically protective coping mechanism.

An awareness of the individual's anxiety is important, because it can limit an individual's ability to actually understand his or her risk for developing cancer. The thought of cancer can be so anxiety provoking in some individuals that they fail to understand their actual risk for cancer.

Communication of risk information should reflect how much the patient or family wishes to know.[21] Timing may be important as well. Messages suggesting increased susceptibility to breast cancer may be less effective if delivered too soon after the breast cancer diagnosis of a close relative, but they might be appropriate several months after the diagnosis.[21]

Communication of a cancer risk assessment should be viewed as an information-sharing interview. Table 6-5 summarizes the steps involved. The manner in

Table 6-5 Steps in Cancer Risk Communication

1. Communication of the risk information should begin by reminding the patient of the strengths and limitations as well as the purpose of a cancer risk assessment. The patient should clearly understand that the assessment will be only as accurate as the information the patient provides.
2. Provide information on the risk factors for the cancer(s) for which the person desires screening.
3. Provide basic information on the cancer for which the person is at risk (e.g., number of people affected annually, average age at diagnosis, clinical presentation). Information about the general population can serve as a baseline against which individuals can measure the magnitude of their increased risk.
4. A review of basic anatomy and physiology using diagrams and models may be indicated to provide necessary background information.
5. Depending on the magnitude of the risk and the ability and desire of the patient to understand the content, the discussion can be expanded to include a more detailed discussion of absolute or relative risk. Care should be given to distinguish between absolute and relative risk and reinforce the fact that risk factors do not combine in a simple mathematical fashion.
6. Information about lifestyle factors amenable to changes should be discussed.
7. Patients should receive information about the strengths and limitations of screening tools.
8. Adequate opportunity for the patient to ask questions and express concerns must be provided to make the cancer risk assessment process effective and the interview truly information-sharing.

which the information is communicated (sometimes referred to as "framing") is also important.[22] If material is presented in a negative fashion, patients may assume that the risk is greater than it actually is. If the discussion is too positive, the magnitude of risk may be underestimated or minimized. Framing occurs with statistics, too. If an individual is told that he or she has a risk of a particular cancer of 1.4 in 10,000 compared to the general population's risk of 1 in 10,000 it will not be particularly impressive to most people. If the same risk is communicated using the format that the individual has a 40% greater risk than the general population, the situation is likely to be seen as "riskier" even though the two situations are equivalent.[17,23] Clearly, this is the most challenging aspect of cancer risk assessment communication. The goal is not to frighten a patient unnecessarily; conversely, if the risk is minimized too much, the patient may not see the value in recommended cancer prevention and screening activities.[24,25]

Achieving true informed consent may affect an individual's decision as to whether he or she truly desires to participate in cancer screening. Conveying a better understanding of one's risk for developing a particular cancer is part of this informed consent process. For example, informed consent can directly affect patient interest and desire to undergo prostate-specific antigen (PSA) screening.[26] Patients who receive more detailed information about the strengths and limitations of PSA screening are significantly less interested in undergoing PSA screening than control subjects. Conversely, giving more information about the benefits of a screening test when accompanied by information about personal risk may increase interest in participating in a specific screening.

Thus the importance of communicating risk individually should not be underestimated. A meta-analysis found that individualized risk communication generally leads to increased use of screening modalities.[27] Individualized counseling makes the risk more realistic to the individual.

Technological Communication of Risk

Today, technology is affecting the means of communication of cancer risk. The use of computers in educating people about cancer risk and the management of cancer risk is relatively new. A few programs are available for both the public and health professionals to utilize. Little is known about the effectiveness of these programs. An advantage of using some of the newer technologies and multimedia is that by accessing the medium, patients have active—rather than passive—involvement.[28] A multimedia approach also offers the advantage of being able to deliver a consistent message to a large number of persons at a relatively low cost. Disadvantages include the difficulty of ensuring that the individual understands the meaning and implications of the risk assessment.

Visual Aids in Risk Communication

Graphics can be a very effective means to communicate risk. They can be especially effective in communicating numerical risk.[29] Graphics can often reveal data patterns that might otherwise go undetected. Graphs also hold people's attention for longer periods of time, which might increase the understanding of data. To be useful, they must communicate the magnitude of risk, relative risk, cumulative risk, uncertainty, and interactions among risk factors. Despite the popularity of using graphics, little research has focused on the impact of graphics in communicating risk data. In many cases, a combination of formats is used to present risk information, including numerical, visual, and explanatory formats.[23]

Several considerations do enhance the usefulness of graphs. The graph should decrease the number of mathematical computations that the user must make. In some cases, it may be best to avoid communicating small-probability events with graphs.[29] Although most persons can understand a flip of the coin (0.5 chance), it is often very difficult for persons to understand the magnitude of a small-probability event such as a 0.0003 chance. A solution to this problem is to change the probabilities to frequencies (3 out of 10,000).

The risk ladder is often used to describe environmental hazards. It displays a range of risk magnitudes by showing increasing risks as being higher on the ladder. Perceptions of risk are, therefore, influenced by the location on the ladder. The ladder helps people to anchor risk to upper and lower reference points.

Pie charts are commonly and effectively used to communicate information about proportions. Most individuals are able to understand a pie chart. These graphics can sometimes be combined to explain subcategories of data.

Histograms are also commonly used. Most individuals have some understanding of how to read a simple histogram. These illustrations will often convey the magnitude of the risk more clearly than just using numbers.[29]

Psychological Concerns

Risk assessment and giving patients information about risk factors do not affect risk of developing cancer. Nevertheless, such information about risk may influence patients' choices regarding screening and may change the way in which some people think about their lives. A risk factor assessment can potentially improve patients' healthcare and ultimately their quality of life if it results in regular screenings and possibly the early detection of a malignancy. Conversely, if a person becomes distressed or upset by the information conveyed in a risk assessment, recommendations for screening may be ignored or the person may experience psychological harm and possibly increased morbidity if a malignancy is not detected early.

The psychosocial effects of risk factor communication have not received much attention.[4] Some degree of concern or anxiety about cancer might heighten an individual's vigilance and motivation to seek reassurance through repetitive screenings. Conversely, such notification may result in anxiety and cancer worries with a reduction in recommended screening. Of concern would be the potential for inappropriate decisions about the use of prophylactic surgery in persons who overestimate their risk for developing breast cancer or endometrial cancer. Clearly, the overall impact of risk assessment on quality of life is poorly understood. Similarly, it is not clear why two women with similar risk factors for developing breast cancer who receive risk factor information in a similar format can respond so differently to the information.

Table 6-6 Accuracy of Cancer Screening Tests

Results of Screening Test	Population Who Actually Have the Disease	Population Who Actually Do Not Have the Disease
Positive Test	75	225
Negative Test	25	775
Total	100	1000

True positives = 75
True negatives = 775
False positives = 225
False negatives = 25

Sensitivity = 75/(75 + 25) = 0.75

Specificity = 775/(775 + 225) = 0.78

Positive predictive value = 75/(75 + 225) = 0.25

Negative predictive value = 775/(775 + 25) = 0.97

Documentation of Risk Assessment

Documentation of a risk assessment is important and may enhance the risk communication process. The first time a patient is seen for risk assessment and screening services, information should be gathered about family history, pertinent medical background, and lifestyle factors. This information is necessary for the initial risk assessment and any subsequent reevaluation and update of the assessment. The choice of the format for documentation and risk factors to be included ultimately affect the risk assessment. For example, in a mammography center, a woman may be queried regarding risk factors for breast cancer. Some of the same risk factors may place the woman at higher risk for endometrial, ovarian, or colorectal cancer.

Few published reports describe documentation of a risk factor assessment.[3] A checklist form containing the major risk factors for the various cancers can be completed after an interview, with space being provided to encourage documentation specific to the risk factor, such as number of years of estrogen replacement therapy or number of years and packs of cigarettes a patient has smoked. Other items that should be documented are a pedigree and any numerical risk assessments that have been calculated. Components of patient education should be documented as well.

Measures of the Accuracy of Screening Tests

In addition to conveying information about cancer risk, nurses must communicate to patients about the accuracy of screening tests. It is not enough to simply recommend a screening test. Patients need to understand what the possibilities are regarding a truly positive or a truly negative test result.

Accuracy

The *accuracy* of screening tests is described using a number of terms. A *true-positive test* (TP) is a normal test for cancer in an individual who actually has cancer. In Table 6-6, the number of true-positive tests is 75. A *true-negative test* (TN) is a normal or negative screen for cancer in an individual who is subsequently found not to have cancer within a defined period after the last test. In Table 6-6, the number of true-negative tests is 775. A *false-negative test* (FN) is a normal test for cancer in an individual who actually has cancer. In Table 6-6, the number of false-negative tests is 25. A *false-positive test* (FP) is an abnormal test for cancer screening in an individual who actually does not have cancer. In Table 6-6, the number of false-positive tests is 225. An understanding of true and false test results is necessary to calculate information about sensitivity and specificity (Table 6-6). Other information about the accuracy of screening tests can be found in Table 6-7.[30]

Sensitivity

The *sensitivity* of a screening test is its ability to detect those individuals with cancer. It is calculated by taking the number of TPs and dividing it by the total number of cancer cases (TP + FN). For the data in Table 6-6, sensitivity would be calculated as 75/(75 + 25) = 0.75. Most people are unwilling to accept a test with a high false-negative rate because many cancers will be missed.

Specificity

The *specificity* of a test is its ability to identify those individuals who actually do not have cancer. It is calculated by dividing the TN by the sum of the TN and FP cases. For the data in Table 6-6, specificity is calculated as 775/(775 + 225) = 0.78. A high false-positive test rate can result in unnecessary follow-up testing and anxiety in persons who have a positive screen.

Positive Predictive Value

The *positive predictive value* is a measure of the validity of a positive test. It is the proportion of positive tests that are TP cases. The predictive value of a test depends on the disease prevalence. As the prevalence of a cancer increases in the population, the positive predictive value of the screening tests increases, even though its sensitivity and specificity remain unchanged.[2]

Negative Predictive Value

The *negative predictive value* is a measure of the validity of a negative test. It refers to the proportion of negative tests that are TNs.

Improving the Accuracy of Screening

Healthcare providers can take several steps to improve the accuracy of screening tests.[31,32] Attaining certification and following federal guidelines in the area of radiology and laboratory services represent one such

Table 6-7 Principles in Developing Cancer Screening Tests

- **The disease should be an important health problem.** There is little doubt that cancer is a significant health problem. Cancer is not just one disease. Some types of cancer are more significant health problems than other types. For example, the incidence of breast cancer is an estimated 217,440 new cases annually and that of lung cancer is an estimated 173,770 new cases, which make both of these cancers very significant.[30] The mortality associated with these cancers is also high, with an estimated 40,580 deaths annually from breast cancer and an estimated 160,440 deaths annually from lung cancer.[30] Clearly, both of these cancers are significant health problems.
- **The disease should have a preclinical stage before symptoms become obvious.** In breast cancer, mammography is able to detect breast cancers before the cancer is palpable. Although lung cancer has a high incidence, at present there is not an obvious preclinical stage.
- **The disease should be treatable.** There should be a recognized treatment for lesions identified following screening. Breast cancer is a disease that responds to surgery, chemotherapy, and radiation therapy, especially when the disease is detected early. Even more important, when breast cancer is detected early, it can often be treated with less radical surgery such as lumpectomy. The same is not true of cancers such as ovarian or lung cancer.
- **The test must be clinically relevant.** The test must be able to detect a condition for which intervention at a preclinical stage can improve outcome. The test must be accurate. The sensitivity and specificity must be acceptable.
- **The test must be acceptable to individuals being screened.** Highly invasive, painful, or risky procedures are generally unacceptable.
- **The test must be widely available and easily accessible.** Technology has made mammography readily available. Colonoscopy is becoming increasingly available. Medicare and insurance coverage of these screening tests makes them more financially accessible to a larger group of people.
- **The test must be cost-effective.** Measuring cost-effectiveness can be difficult. Different groups have different thresholds for what they consider to be cost-effective.

step. Guidelines are now in place for mammography centers and laboratories providing cancer screening services to ensure that a minimum acceptable standard is met. Certification from relevant agencies should be publicly displayed.

The person conducting the exam or interpreting the laboratory or radiological test results profoundly affects the effectiveness of a cancer screening test. For example, some healthcare professionals are clearly better at performing CBEs than others and are more likely to detect a subtle breast change. Monitoring the quality of clinical examinations is important. Monitoring and improving the quality of physical examinations in the clinical setting is far more challenging, but is nevertheless important to improve the sensitivity and specificity of the examination.[33]

Screening quality may also be improved by developing standardized instructions for patient preparation. This may not only improve patient compliance, but also help obtain the best possible screen. An example might be scheduling a breast screening a week after the menses begin, avoiding the use of deodorant prior to mammography, or instructing a patient to avoid douching for 24 hours prior to a Pap smear.

Providers need to be continually updated on the newest guidelines and techniques for cancer screening. Such training should include a staff competency evaluation. New equipment is constantly being developed to enhance screening and diagnostic procedures. Agencies that provide screening services need to not just review such equipment, but to develop policies on how they will test and possibly eventually adapt such equipment to their specific needs.

Implementing Cancer Screening

A screening protocol or recommendation defines how cancer screening tests should be used. Table 6-8 illustrates the American Cancer Society (ACS) recommendations for the early detection of cancer in asymptomatic individuals.[30] It is an example of a screening protocol. Such recommendations can vary among organizations and practitioners. A recommendation generally describes the target population to be served, the screening recommendation to be applied, and the interval at which the test should be undertaken.

Development of Screening Guidelines

Screening guidelines change over time. The ACS, for example, has been publishing guidelines for the early detection of cancer for more than 20 years.[34] In the past, the ACS has recommended screening for lung cancer using sputum cytology. Currently, the ACS does not have a recommendation for the early detection of lung cancer. All efforts are focused on prevention of and smoking cessation.[30] Although specific guidelines have changed over the years, the focus of the guidelines has changed very little. Healthcare providers are still expected to use the guidelines to select the best screening tests for an individual and to modify the guidelines in certain cases, such as if an individual has a particularly high risk for developing a specific malignancy.

Clinicians must remember that screening protocols are merely guidelines.[35] They are not practice standards to be used blindly with every individual. The goal of the ACS standards is the detection of malignancy. The U.S. Preventive Services Task Force (USPSTF) uses very strict criteria for assessing evidence of effectiveness. Cost-effectiveness of the screening recommendations is an important consideration for this group, for example. When providing information on cancer screening recommendations, nurses need to inform the individual why a certain recommendation is being made in his or her case.

Nurses will often make recommendations for various screening or detection measures, especially in persons who carry a higher risk for developing a particular cancer based on their family history and genetic background. Nurses need to be able to accurately explain the risks and benefits of these screening tools to their patients. This requires an understanding of the measures of validity of a screening test. Specific recommendations for a screening test often vary among organizations such as the ACS, the USPSTF, or the National Cancer Institute (NCI). The specific criteria that each organization uses to make recommendations may vary, which is why the recommendations are not universal and can prove very confusing to the general public. Tests are often combined to compensate for the limitations of any one test.[33]

There are, however, generally agreed-upon requirements and characteristics of acceptable screening tests. When presenting screening recommendations to individuals, it is important to include the rationale and strengths and limitations of each test and to present this information in light of the individual's own risk for developing cancer. The following issues are frequently considered before recommendations for screening for the general public are made. Often those individuals with a genetic susceptibility need recommendations that are more rigorous than those for persons with average risk.

First, nurses need to review the scientific basis for each guideline. Each agency that promulgates a guideline should make this information available. An

Table 6-8 American Cancer Society Recommendations for the Early Detection of Cancer

Breast Cancer

- ☐ Yearly mammograms are recommended starting at age 40 and continuing for as long as a woman is in good health.
- ☐ A clinical breast exam should be part of a periodic health exam, about every three years for women in their twenties and thirties, and every year for women 40 and older.
- ☐ Women should know how their breasts normally feel and report any breast changes promptly to their healthcare providers. Breast self-exam is an option for women, starting in their twenties.
- ☐ Women at increased risk (e.g., family history, genetic tendency, past breast cancer) should talk with their doctors about the benefits and limitations of starting mammography screening earlier, having additional tests (i.e., breast ultrasound and MRI), or having more frequent exams.

Cervical Cancer

- ☐ Screening should begin approximately three years after a woman begins having vaginal intercourse, but no later than 21 years of age.
- ☐ Screening should be done every year with regular Pap tests or every two years using liquid-based tests.
- ☐ At or after age 30, women who have had three normal test results in a row may get screened every 2–3 years. However, doctors may suggest a woman get screened more if she has certain risk factors, such as HIV infection or a weakened immune system.
- ☐ Women 70 and older who have had three or more consecutive Pap tests in the last ten years may choose to stop cervical cancer screening.
- ☐ Screening after a total hysterectomy (with removal of the cervix) is not necessary unless the surgery was done as a treatment for cervical cancer.

Endometrial Cancer

- ☐ All women should be told about the risks and symptoms of endometrial cancer and encouraged to report any unexpected bleeding or spotting to their doctors.
- ☐ Women at increased risk (e.g., family history, genetic tendency, past breast cancer) should talk with their doctors about the benefits and limitations of an endometrial biopsy starting at age 35.

Colorectal Cancer

Beginning at age 50, men and women should follow one of the following examination schedules:

- ☐ A fecal occult blood test (FOBT) every year
- ☐ A flexible sigmoidoscopy (FSIG) every five years
- ☐ Annual fecal occult blood test and flexible sigmoidoscopy every five years*
- ☐ A double-contrast barium enema every five years
- ☐ A colonoscopy every ten years

People who are at moderate or high risk for colorectal cancer should talk with a doctor about a different testing schedule.

Prostate Cancer

- ☐ The prostate-specific antigen (PSA) test and the digital rectal examination (DRE) should be offered annually, beginning at age 50, to men who have a life expectancy of at least ten years.
- ☐ Men at high risk (African American men and men with a strong family history of one or more first-degree relatives diagnosed with prostate cancer at an early age) should begin testing at age 45.
- ☐ For men at average risk and high risk, information should be provided about what is known and what is uncertain about the benefits and limitations of early detection and treatment of prostate cancer so that they can make an informed decision about testing.

Other Cancers

For people having periodic health examinations, a cancer-related checkup should include health counseling (such as information on quitting smoking) and, depending on a person's age, possible examinations for cancers of the thyroid, oral cavity, skin, lymph nodes, testes, and ovaries.

*Combined testing is preferred over either annual FOBT or FSIG every five years alone.
Data from American Cancer Society.[30]

excellent place to obtain information about the scientific basis and the review process for a guideline is from the individual agency that generates the guideline or at the National Guideline Clearinghouse (*www.guideline.gov*).

Second, nurses play a key role in interpreting these data to patients. Nurses need to explain why a particular set of guidelines is being used for an individual patient. They need to remind each patient that these recommendations are guidelines and that some modifications may be made based on personal risk factor assessment and findings on a clinical examination. With some persons in failing health, it is appropriate to discuss stopping cancer screening, although few of the guidelines provide specific direction in this area. Clearly, the benefits, risks, and potential limitations of each screening test need to be discussed individually and tailored to the risk factor assessment.

Many individuals will choose to undergo a screening examination, even if a test has a lower sensitivity and specificity, in hopes that it will prove effective for them. Screening for ovarian cancer is an excellent example. Highly specific and sensitive screening tests are currently unavailable for the early detection of ovarian cancer. Many women, however, still want an annual pelvic examination to assess for ovarian masses. This test is relatively inexpensive to perform and is usually tolerated fairly well by women. Some clinicians are better at detecting ovarian masses than others. Nevertheless, many ovarian cancers cannot be detected using this examination, even when performed by skilled clinicians. As long as a woman realizes that the test may fail to detect ovarian cancer and is willing to accept this limitation, utilizing the pelvic examination may be effective. Often women at higher risk for ovarian cancer will choose to have CA-125 antigen testing and a transvaginal ultrasound in hopes of finding early ovarian cancer. Neither of these tests has been proven to be effective in reducing the morbidity and mortality associated with ovarian cancer, yet women at higher risk continue to undergo these screening tests.

Informed Consent

After the risk assessment is completed and its information is interpreted to the patient, a consent form should be signed for the screening procedures that the patient intends to undergo. The consent form states who will provide the screening procedure, notes that not all cancers may be detected during a screening examination, and, if the patient declines recommended screening, specifies a waiver of which recommended procedures are being declined. This consent also helps to reinforce the recommendations for screening. Table 6-9 highlights the basic elements of an individual cancer screening.

Clearly, cancer risk communication influences decisions to undergo cancer screening examinations.[27] When a healthcare provider recommends a particular screening examination, there is an increased likelihood the individual will actually go on to have the recommended screening. Health providers can make good recommendations for screening based on the myriad of guidelines available only if they understand the biases of various guidelines and have completed an accurate assessment of risk.[31] In addition, decisions to undergo screening are influenced by how much benefit is perceived to result from undergoing the screening procedure. Such a decision must be balanced with a discussion of the risks associated with screening. Providing individuals with information about the sensitivity and specificity of a screening procedure is, indeed, challenging.

Table 6-9 Steps in a Basic Individual Cancer Screening Sessions

- Complete a comprehensive health history and risk assessment.
- Communicate the risk assessment to the patient.
- Complete a physical examination of all or selected at-risk sites. This may include skin, head and neck area, breasts, abdomen, prostate, rectum, gynecologic organs, and a survey of lymph nodes.
- Provide patient education that includes information about anatomy, physiology, risks, strengths and benefits of available screening tests, primary prevention strategies, sources for genetic counseling/testing when appropriate, early signs and symptoms of cancer, and self-examination techniques.
- Schedule and obtain appropriate laboratory and radiologic studies, including Pap test cytology and mammography. Schedule and obtain other screening tests, such as colonoscopy or endometrial biopsy.
- Ensure that the patient receives follow-up. All patients should receive the results of screening whether they are positive or negative. Patients with abnormalities should receive information about why follow-up is necessary. Those with normal screens should receive a reminder for follow-up screening in one year.

Follow-up

If the intended benefits of screening are to be realized, individuals need to have a clear understanding of the implications of tests both before they are screened and after they receive the results. The potential benefits of screening are lost if individuals are never informed of the test results or the meaning of those results. Providing patients with information about screening results generates another opportunity to reinforce the information included in the risk factor assessment. After screening tests are completed, risk may be more apparent and screening recommendations may need to be revised. For example, a 50-year-old woman may have a baseline flexible sigmoidoscopy examination that demonstrates a polyp that is subsequently biopsied and shows hyperplasia. Her risk for developing colon cancer is higher than initially perceived. She should be informed of this risk and be counseled about ACS's guidelines for a total colon examination.[30]

Nurses must also consider the various types of screening programs and which will best work in a particular environment. These options include mass screening and individual screening. To be successful, either mass screening or individual screening needs to include a strategy to follow up on both normal and abnormal test results. Procedures need to be in place to ensure that patients receive results in a timely fashion. In particular, recommendations for further follow-up or follow-up screening need to be clearly communicated to the patient.

Mass screening generally refers to screening programs in which large numbers of persons undergo screening, usually under fairly impersonal circumstances. An example would be screening 150 persons on two consecutive days for skin cancer.

Individual screening typically includes a more traditional approach. It might include risk assessment, education about primary and secondary cancer prevention strategies, screening tests, and results-based health recommendations.

Nursing Implications

Education of Healthcare Professionals

Risk assessment is the responsibility of many different healthcare professionals, including physicians, nurses, psychologists, and genetic counselors. Although formal and clinical education regarding risk assessment is limited in many professions,[32] historically assessment activities have received much attention in most healthcare professions. Risk factor assessment, by contrast, has received little attention in the formal educational setting. Education of healthcare professionals on techniques and tasks of risk assessment is important because healthcare professionals make initial recommendations for screening. Many oncology professionals have learned about genetics through self-study and clinical practice.[36] Although these professionals may understand oncology well, principles of risk communication may be less clear to them.

Statistics is one of the most challenging courses and a source of frustration for many nurses, both at the undergraduate level and especially at the graduate level. Many, however, do not recognize that this course has numerous ramifications for clinical practice. The challenge is for nurses to understand various statistical measures well enough to accurately critique and use existing literature and research and — more importantly — to interpret this information to patients and their families.

Educators need to consider adding information about risk factor assessment to both undergraduate and graduate curricula. In particular, these programs need to emphasize the fact that a cancer risk assessment is not merely collecting data but also communicating the meaning of those data to a patient, so that he or she can ultimately make informed decisions about cancer prevention and early detection behaviors. Specific content regarding cancer risk assessment that should be incorporated into a curriculum includes basic epidemiologic concepts, specific types of risk (absolute, relative), risk factors for specific cancers and etiologic factors (if known), basic statistics, information about cancer prevention and early detection measures, and counseling techniques.

Table 6-10 Barriers to Cancer Screening

Patient Factors
Patient does not understand the magnitude of risk
Patient does not understand benefits of screening
Inadequate social support
Patient distress or misconceptions related to screening
Lack of financial resources to pay for screening or follow-up care
Lack of transportation to get to screening
Screening considered too uncomfortable or embarrassing
Service System Factors
Lack of a wellness focus in healthcare system
Low awareness of the benefits of screening by some providers
Conflicting recommendations about screening
Lack of time to perform a comprehensive examination or risk assessment
Failure to recommend a screening procedure
Facilities may have access that is difficult or inconvenient

Data from Mahon[3]; Price[16]; Stoner, Mahon.[37]

Administrative Considerations

Administrators who want to introduce cancer risk assessments into a program of cancer screening or other oncology programs need to consider a number of issues. First, they must look at the rationale for implementing such a program. Increasing recruitment to health promotion programs is regarded as a major benefit of completing a health risk assessment. Screening programs that include risk assessments also can be incorporated into outreach programs to work site settings. Ultimately, the success of most screening programs depends on the effort taken at the beginning to completely assess the unique needs of the population or community being served.

Other important considerations include where services will be provided, marketing of services, and reimbursement issues. If the institution is unable to provide the screening that will be recommended following a risk factor assessment (e.g., genetic testing), what arrangements will be made for patients who desire such services? Administrators cannot overlook the need to hire nursing or other personnel who have the expertise and skills needed to provide this essential and comprehensive service. Barriers to consider are described in Table 6-10[3,37] Many innovative secondary cancer screening programs are described elsewhere.[37]

Economic Considerations

At the clinical level, the delivery of cancer risk information takes time, and how people who provide such information should be reimbursed for their risk assessment and counseling services is unclear. Such charges may be bundled with other service charges such as mammography. Without adequate reimbursement, however, risk assessment services are unlikely to be given adequate attention or provided by people with sufficient background and expertise. When providing genetic services, many providers report that a standard protocol states that individuals or families should be seen for two visits, with each session lasting about two hours. In the setting of genetic risk counseling, the use of multidisciplinary teams and multiple interactions is emphasized. The underlying concern is that individuals may be "overwhelmed" by all the information provided in a single one-hour visit.[4] Such attention usually is not given to people with an average risk for developing malignancy.

Much debate focuses on how much should be spent on cancer screening. Controversy continues regarding the threshold necessary to deem a screening or treatment as cost-effective. It is difficult to find a measure that allows comparisons between healthcare interventions that save lives and those that improve quality of life.[38]

Practice Considerations

The cancer risk assessment begins the educational process related to cancer prevention and early detection. Without an accurate and comprehensive risk assessment, it is impossible to provide the individual with appropriate and reasonable recommendations for primary and secondary cancer prevention. The risk factor assessment provides the oncology nurse with an opportunity to teach individuals about the epidemiology, risk factors, and signs and symptoms associated with the various cancers. It transmits the framework individuals need to understand the importance and rationale for primary and secondary cancer prevention strategies as well as information about signs and symptoms that merit further evaluation.

Empowering patients with enough information in understandable terms so that they can make an informed choice about cancer screening is the ultimate goal of cancer risk counseling. When a healthcare provider simply recommends a screening test or tries to scare a patient into undergoing a screening test or genetic test by telling a poignant or compelling story, the patient may select or fail to select a screening test for the wrong reasons. Thus it is important that providers offer balanced and accurate information. The downside of conveying a risk assessment such that the individual has enough information to make an informed decision is that it is extremely labor-intensive for the healthcare provider.[39]

Staff nurses can serve as case finders to identify individuals at increased risk for developing cancer who will benefit from a more detailed risk assessment, and possibly cancer genetic counseling.[40] Indeed, many staff nurses who work with patients and get to know their families are the best persons to initiate referrals and begin the cancer risk assessment process. To be an effective case finder, the nurse must understand basic cancer incidence, epidemiology, and the importance of an accurate family history.

Nurses with advance practice degrees can perform more in-depth risk assessments, recommend cancer screening procedures, explain the risks and benefits of a particular screening examination, and, in many cases, actually carry out the screening examination. They are well-suited to perform professional breast examinations, teach breast self-examination, do rectal examinations, complete a skin examination, or complete a pelvic exam and take a Pap smear. Some advanced practice nurses with additional subspecialty training are able to perform flexible sigmoidoscopy examinations.

Oncology nurses have a major responsibility to teach the public about cancer detection and screening. Individuals need to realize that cancer screening differs from diagnostic examinations for cancer. They also need to recognize that cancer screening is not perfect and, even when conducted properly, will still fail to detect some malignancies because of the strengths and limitations associated with different screening tests.

Research continues to suggest that the single most important factor in whether an individual has ever had a screening test, or has recently had a screening test, is a recommendation from the healthcare provider.[34] When nurses recommend screening to an individual, there is a far greater chance that the individual will actually go on to have appropriate screening. This recommendation can easily come in the form of patient education about cancer prevention and early detection.

Every cancer screening program should include a significant patient education component. Care needs to be taken in gathering appropriate and useful materials for this purpose.[5] These materials may include brochures that may come from cancer-related organizations or that are developed specifically for an agency's population. Posters can be obtained to provide additional education and be displayed in waiting and examination areas. Bulletin boards are a relatively simple means to provide brief public education specific to a population or topic. They have the advantage of being relatively easy to produce and change. Flip charts can be used for individual education; these can be either purchased or developed specifically for the group being served. Other educational aids might include anatomical charts and models, computer-assisted education, and professional samples (e.g., sunscreen or smoking cessation kits).

When providing patients with information on cancer prevention and early detection, it is important to use educational materials that focus on wellness. Ever more of these resources are becoming available. It is inappropriate to provide materials that focus on disease and treatment. In fact, some persons find them distressing. The message of education and materials should be that when detected early, cancer is associated with decreased morbidity and mortality and improved quality of life. Written materials with a prevention focus on nutrition; participation in chemoprevention trials; self-examination technique; Pap smears; and prostate, skin and colorectal cancer are available through the NCI and the ACS. Other examples of printed materials are readily available in the professional literature.[5]

How long a person can retain information after counseling about cancer risk factors is unclear. Information about risk and recommended screening can be reinforced by sending patients a post-visit letter that summarizes the discussion of risk and recommendations for screening or other follow-up. Consideration needs to be given to how individuals will be retained in cancer screening programs and genetic counseling programs so that risk assessments can be updated, recommendations for screening modified if needed, and regular routine screening completed.

Legal Considerations

Once cancer risks and screening recommendations are identified and communicated to the patient, the patient must make a decision as to which screening tests he or she desires. If a patient declines a recommended screening test, a waiver is signed on a consent form that acknowledges the patient was informed of the recommendation and is declining the recommended screening at that time. Information about cancer screening recommendations can be reinforced in a post-visit letter that summarizes the discussion of risk, informs the patient of the results of his or her screening tests, reiterates any recommended follow-up, and summarizes the recommendations for cancer prevention and early detection.

Interactions with the Media

New risk factors seem to emerge every day. An important educational role for nurses is to help patients understand which risks they should take seriously. Most people accept a wide variety of risks (e.g., driving at the posted speed limit, crossing a busy parking lot, riding a bike, flying across the country in an airplane) on a daily basis with little thought. For some reason, brief news segments about cancer risk seem to conjure up more fear. Nurses need to be aware of public news reports and go to the primary sources when new risk factors are presented so that they can interpret this information accurately to their patients. They also need to communicate concepts related to cancer risks carefully when providing information to the media. This effort may include providing the media with primary sources and reports and more integrated state-of-the-art information. Both the ACS and the other resources should be consulted prior to speaking with the media, to ensure that accurate statistics and figures are provided.

Each year the ACS publishes *Cancer Facts and Figures.*[30] Nurses can use this helpful reference to quickly gather incidence data about estimated cancer cases. The information is presented in several formats, including the estimated projected number of new cases of specific cancer (incidence) and estimated mortality rates. The incidence rates are also given by state. Oncology nurses can obtain this publication free of charge from the local unit of the ACS and may find it helpful to review so as to better understand the incidence of specific cancers in the geographical area in which they practice. The publication also offers detailed information about primary and secondary cancer prevention of the major tumors as well as projected survival data by stage. Once familiar with the format of the publication, oncology nurses will find it to be an invaluable resource.

Another source of commonly cited data is the Surveillance, Epidemiology, and End Results Program (SEER).[41] Currently, SEER data include incidence, mortality, and survival rates from 1973 through 1996. Data from the nine SEER geographic areas are used to represent an estimated 9.5% of the U.S. population. Currently, the database contains information on 2.3 million cases diagnosed since 1973. Approximately 125,000 new cases are added yearly. This information can be obtained easily at the NCI Web site (www.seer.ims.nci.nih.gov/) or by ordering *SEER Cancer Statistics Review 1973–1996* (publication number 99-2789) through the NCI (800-4CANCER).

Future Research

Future research should evaluate the process of risk notification and its effects on knowledge, attitudes, emotions and practices, and outcomes related to health and disease status. Most of the studies of perceived risk have been cross-sectional in nature, which makes it difficult to determine whether the perceived risk is a cause or an effect in relation to cancer screening.[18] This relationship could be better understood if longitudinal studies were conducted to measure perceived risk in defined populations with different cancer screening histories that include follow-up for screening and repeated measures of risk perception. Such investigations should include controlled clinical trials to evaluate different counseling protocols. This type of research will provide information on the impact and effectiveness of cancer risk assessment and counseling.

Clearly, more information is needed on the roles played by cognition, affective state of the individual, developmental differences, and personal values and the way in which these individual qualities influence cancer risk communication.[24] More research is also needed to determine the best persons (including an interdisciplinary approach) to communicate cancer and genetic risks.[32,41] Likewise, information is needed on how to facilitate decision making regarding the management of cancer risks.

Prospective studies are needed to determine the psychological and behavioral implications of risk information. Assessments should optimally be conducted at multiple time points and include outcome variables. More research is needed to understand why two individuals react differently to similar information regarding cancer risk. Little research has focused on how people cope with information related to their risk of disease. Models of coping with disease may not encompass the concept of coping with increased risk for developing a disease such as cancer. The effect of cancer risk assessment on cancer screening behaviors merits more attention.

There is also a lack of formal education for nurses and health professionals about communicating risk and genetic concepts. Future studies need to address effectiveness of this education.[18,41,42]

Conclusion

Oncology nurses need to view risk factor assessment as a wonderful opportunity for patient education on not only cancer risk factors, but also cancer prevention and early detection activities. Cancer risk assessment can be a technical process requiring expertise. Oncology nurses have an ethical responsibility to communicate risk information in understandable terms and as accurately as possible. Indeed, risk assessment is more than collecting assessment data from the patient. A critical component of the process is communicating the information to patients in a meaningful way.

Cancer risk communication is a continuous process. The risk assessment is a large component of this process. It demands effective communication with patients so that they are informed about the best possible choices regarding cancer prevention and early detection activities. Like other components of the cancer screening process, a cancer risk assessment is most effective if it is updated and reviewed annually.

Once risk is communicated, education about cancer screening options must be provided. This effort should include accurate information about the accuracy, benefits, and risks associated with the test(s). Each individual must decide what testing her or she is willing to accept.

Once testing is completed, the results must be interpreted to the patient. Individuals with normal screening results should understand when screening is again indicated. Patients with abnormal screens need to be directed through appropriate follow-up.

Nurses need to consider epidemiological terms and calculations when conducting risk assessments. They also need to teach patients and their families about the strengths and weaknesses of various screening or surveillance strategies. This education includes a discussion of the sensitivity and specificity of various screening tests, as well as a discussion of why screening is available for some cancers and not for others. Individuals at higher risk for developing cancer because of genetic susceptibility need to understand that the screening recommendations for people of average risk, which are issued by groups such as the ACS, may be inadequate for those with higher risk.

References

1. Lai D, Hardy RJ: Potential gains in life expectancy or years of potential life lost: impact of competing risks of death. *Int J Epidemiol* 28:894–898, 1999
2. Clark RA, Reintgen DS: Principles of cancer screening, in Reintgen DS, Clark RA (eds.): *Cancer Screening*. St. Louis, MO; Mosby Year-Book, 1996, pp 1–20
3. Mahon SM: Principles of cancer prevention and early detection. *Clin J Oncol Nurs* 4:169–176, 2000
4. Kelly PT: *Assess Your True Risk of Breast Cancer*. New York, Henry Holt, 2000
5. Mahon SM: Patient education regarding cancer screening guidelines. *Clin J Oncol Nurs* 7:581–584, 2003
6. Rothman AJ, Kiviniemi MT: Treating people with information: an analysis and review of approaches to communicating health risk information. *J Natl Cancer Inst Monogr* 25:44–51, 1999
7. Constantino JP, Gail MH, Pee D, et al: Validation studies for models projecting the risk of invasive and total breast cancer incidence. *J Natl Cancer Inst* 91:1541–1548, 1999
8. Claus EB, Risch N, Thompson WD: Autosomal dominant inheritance of early-onset breast cancer: Implications for risk prediction. *Cancer* 73:643–651, 1994
9. Claus EB, Schildkraut MM, Thompson WD, et al: The genetic attributable risk of breast and ovarian cancer. *Cancer* 77:2318–2324, 1996
10. Couch FJ, DeShano ML, Blackwood MA, et al: BRCA1 mutations in women attending clinics that evaluate the risk of breast cancer. *N Engl J Med* 336:4109–1415, 1997
11. Shattuck-Eidens D, Oliphant A, McClure M: BRCA1 sequence analysis in women at high risk for susceptibility mutations. Risk

factor analysis and implications for genetic testing. *JAMA* 278:1242–1250, 1997

12. Berry DA, Parmigiani G, Sanchez J, et al: Probability of carrying a mutation of breast-ovarian cancer gene BRCA1 based on family history. *J Natl Cancer Inst* 89:227–238, 1997
13. Lynch HT, Lynch JE: Hereditary nonpolyposis colorectal cancer. *Semin Surg Oncol* 18:305–313, 2003
14. Weinstein ND: What does it mean to understand a risk? Evaluating risk comprehension. *J Natl Cancer Inst Monogr* 25:15–20, 1999
15. Leventhal H, Kelly K, Leventhal EA: Population risk, actual risk, perceived risk, and cancer control: a discussion. *J Natl Cancer Inst Monogr* 25:81–85, 1999
16. Price AS: Primary and secondary prevention of colorectal cancer. *Gastroenterol Nurs* 26:73–81, 2003
17. Bottorff JL, Ratner PA, Johnson JL, et al: Communicating cancer risk information: the challenges of uncertainty. *Patient Educ Couns* 33:67–81, 1998
18. Vernon SW: Risk perception and risk communication for cancer screening behaviors: a review. *J Natl Cancer Inst Monogr* 25:101–119, 1999
19. Fischhoff B: Why (cancer) risk communication can be hard. *J Natl Cancer Inst Monogr* 25:7–13, 1999
20. Kreuter MW: Dealing with competing and conflicting risks in cancer communication. *J Natl Cancer Inst Monogr* 25:27–34, 1999
21. Hopwood P: Psychological issues in cancer genetics: current research and future priorities. *Patient Educ Couns* 32:19–31, 1997
22. Salovey P, Schneider TR, Apanovitch AM: Persuasion for the purpose of cancer risk reduction: a discussion. *J Natl Cancer Inst Monogr* 25:119–122, 1999
23. Kramer BS: Matching strength of message to strength of evidence: a discussion. *J Natl Cancer Inst Monogr* 25:85–87,1999
24. Maibach E: Cancer risk communication — what we need to learn. *J Natl Cancer Inst Monogr* 25:179–181, 1999
25. Meyerowitz BE, Chaiken S: The effect of message framing on breast self-examination attitudes, intentions, and behavior. *J Pers Soc Psychol* 3:500–510, 1987
26. Wolf AM, Nasser JF, Wolf AM, et al: The impact of informed consent on patient interest in prostate-specific antigen screening. *Arch Intern Med* 15:1333–1336, 1996
27. McCaul KD, Tulloch HE: Cancer screening decisions. *J Natl Cancer Inst Monogr* 25:52–58, 1999
28. Strecher VJ, Greenwood T, Wang C, et al: Interactive multimedia and risk communication. *J Natl Cancer Inst Monogr* 25:134–139, 1999
29. Lipkus IM, Hollands JG: The visual communication of risk. *J Natl Cancer Inst Monogr* 25:149–163, 1999
30. American Cancer Society: *Cancer Facts and Figures — 2004.* Atlanta, American Cancer Society, 2004
31. Foltz A: Issues in determining cancer screening recommendations: who, what and when. *Oncol Nurs Forum* 27(suppl 9):13–18, 2000
32. Arkin EB: Cancer risk communication — what we know. *J Natl Cancer Instl Monogr* 25:182–185, 1999
33. MacLean CD: Principles of cancer screening. *Med Clin North Am* 80:1–14, 1996
34. Smith RA, Mettlin CJ, Davis KJ , et al: American Cancer Society Guidelines for the Early Detection of Cancer. *CA Cancer J Clin* 50:34–49, 2000
35. Beck LH: Periodic health examination and screening tests in adults. *Hosp Pract* 34:117–119, 121–122, 124–126, 1999
36. Weitzel JN: Genetic cancer risk assessment. Putting it all together. *Cancer* 86(suppl):2483–2999, 1999
37. Stoner C, Mahon SM: Overview section IV: cancer control — local programs. Clinical application of cancer control: case examples, in Jennings-Dozier K, Mahon SM (eds.). *Cancer Prevention, Detection and Control: A Nursing Perspective.* Pittsburgh, Oncology Nursing Press, 2002, pp 769–866
38. Ubel P, Hirth RA, Chernew ME, et al: What is the price of life and why doesn't it increase at the rate of inflation? *Arch Intern Med* 163:1637–1641, 2003
39. Edwards A, Unigwe S, Elwyn G, et al: Effect of communicating individual risks in screening programmes: Cochrane systemic review. *BMJ* 327:703–709, 2003
40. Greco KE, Mahon S. Common hereditary cancer syndromes. *Semin Oncol Nurs* 20: 164–177, 2004
41. Ries LA, Kosary CL, Hankey BF, et al (eds): *SEER Cancer Statistics Review 1973–1996.* Bethesda, National Cancer Institute, 1999
42. Visser A, Bleiker E: Introduction: genetic education and counseling. *Patient Educ Couns* 32:1–7, 1997

CHAPTER 7

Genetic Risk for Cancer

Paula Trahan Rieger, RN, MSN, CS, AOCN®, FAAN
Judith Kehs Much, CRNP, APRN, BC, AOCN®

Introduction

An important component of cancer prevention is risk assessment. The ability to identify individuals who are at increased risk for developing cancer will allow intensive screening programs and prevention strategies to be targeted to those individuals most in need. Advances in the understanding of cancer biology and of the role of genetics in the development of cancer are dramatically changing the field of cancer care. This chapter focuses on how this new knowledge is being applied in the field of risk assessment.

The discovery of genes that, when altered, confer an increased risk for cancer development is having a profound effect on cancer care. It is currently estimated that 5%–10% of cancers arise in individuals who inherit one of these altered genes and are members of a family in which multiple individuals have an increased risk for developing certain types of cancer. The identification of affected members of these families is now possible. Predisposition genetic testing is having, and will continue to have, a significant impact on health care, even though many ethical, legal, financial, and psychosocial issues associated with testing remain unresolved.

In the coming years, it will be important for healthcare professionals to understand how advances in genetics can be integrated into cancer care. All nurses involved in cancer care will ultimately need to be knowledgeable about hereditary cancer syndromes, understand how to recognize characteristics that may indicate the presence of such a syndrome in a family, and know how to initiate appropriate referrals for risk management in members of such families.[1,2]

Human Genome Project

Errors in genes are known to be responsible for thousands of hereditary diseases, including cystic fibrosis, sickle cell anemia, and Huntington's disease. In addition, altered genes are known to influence the development of multifactorial diseases such as cancer, heart disease, and diabetes; these diseases result from the interaction of genes and environmental factors.[3,4] Advances in technology are making possible discoveries and achievements that were merely dreams a few years ago. We are on the verge of identifying the genetic changes responsible for a multitude of diseases.

A major reason for these achievements is the knowledge and technology generated from the landmark project known as the Human Genome Project (HGP). The HGP was an international collaborative research program established in 1990 through a partnership between the National Institutes of Health (NIH) and the U.S. Department of Energy. It was administered by the National Center for Human Genome Research, an institute within the NIH. Scientists from around the world sought to analyze the structure of human DNA and to determine the locations and sequences of an original estimate of 100,000 human genes. The initial major goals of the project included development of maps to assist in pinpointing the locations of genes and the decoding of the sequences of all nucleotide bases within the genome and thus the identification of specific genes. By identifying a gene's sequence, the protein product of that gene and its normal function in the body can be determined.[4] In 1998, a five-year plan was published in which human DNA sequencing was the major emphasis. The HGP was completed several years ahead of schedule in April 2003, with its finale coinciding with the 50-year celebration of the discovery of the structure of DNA by Francis Crick and James Watson. It is now estimated that the human genome comprises 30,000 to 35,000 genes. Understanding the complete set of genes within the human genome is expected to have profound effects on the management of disease.[4]

The pace of progress often surpasses society's ability to manage the changes that progress brings. To address these changes, the Ethical, Legal, and Social Implications (ELSI) program was established as part of the project to investigate four areas: (1) ethical issues of genetics research; (2) responsible clinical integration of new genetic technologies; (3) privacy issues and fair use of genetic information by employers, insurers, and others; and (4) professional and public education. To date, the ELSI office has sponsored conferences, courses, and research grants for studies evaluating the implications of this new knowledge.[5] Despite concerns, the HGP ultimately holds the promise of initiating a new chapter in medicine, involving molecular medicine, that will transform the diagnosis, treatment, and prevention of diseases.

Cancer Risk Assessment

The assessment of risk for developing cancer is an important component of oncology nursing practice and should include obtaining from the patient information about risk factors associated with the development of cancer (e.g., exposure to carcinogens), medical history, and a detailed family history. A *risk factor* is defined broadly as any event or characteristic associated with an increased probability of disease. A major requisite of fully using *primary prevention* (i.e., intervention before pathological changes have begun) as a means of cancer control is the ability to identify carcinogenic agents and host factors that make individuals susceptible to developing cancer. Cancer epidemiology is the field that studies the frequencies, patterns of distribution, and determinants of tumor occurrence in humans.[6] Both environmental and host factors (e.g., genetic predisposition) are examined in an effort to determine causal relationships. The identification of etiologic influences can facilitate prevention, especially in individuals at increased risk, and detection of cancer at an early stage when cure is a realistic expectation.

Advances in technology are also influencing the field of epidemiology. An emerging field is *molecular epidemiology*, which combines the standard tools of epidemiology (case histories, questionnaires, and monitoring of exposure) with sensitive molecular biology laboratory techniques. The goal is to uncover critical precancerous events taking place inside the body and to identify measurable biological flags or markers signaling their occurrence. These biological markers may ultimately be used to more precisely determine exposure to carcinogenic agents and resultant increased risk.[7]

An understanding of how individuals perceive their risk for developing cancer is crucial and will assist the healthcare professional when providing specific information about risks and prevention and screening recommendations. Research has demonstrated that many individuals tend to overestimate their risk for developing cancer,[8] and many worry about whether and when they may develop a cancer.[9] This perception can be influenced by many factors, including family history, life experiences (e.g., losing a parent to cancer at a young age), and understanding of information presented in the media. It is important that individuals recognize that the presence of a particular risk factor or trait does not mean that a person will inevitably develop a specific cancer and that the absence of a risk factor does not ensure that a person will not develop cancer. For example, many women who develop breast cancer do not have any of the known risk factors.[10]

The goals of risk assessment are to understand an individual's perceptions and concerns related to risk for developing cancer, to provide information regarding that risk, to outline recommendations for primary and secondary prevention (i.e., detect disease at its earliest stage and treat it promptly), and to offer psychosocial support so that an individual may better cope with information related to risk and adhere to the recommendations for prevention and screening.[11,12]

Medical History

A review of the individual's medical and lifestyle history will provide information related to risk for developing cancer. Specific information should be obtained about any previous diagnosis of cancer, the age at diagnosis, and the treatments for that cancer as well as about any preneoplastic lesions such as polyps or breast lesions. For women, information related to reproductive history should also be obtained (e.g., age at menarche, age at menopause, number of children and age at first live birth, hormone history, and sexual history). Information about exposure to carcinogens can be obtained by asking questions about occupation and lifestyle (e.g., smoking, alcohol use, sunlight exposure, dietary practices, and exposure to chemicals). The presence of physical findings associated with certain forms of inherited cancers, such as the mucocutaneous lesions seen in Cowden syndrome, should also be determined.

Family History

A review of family history is important to determine risk and identify whether characteristics indicative of a hereditary cancer syndrome are present. Visual representation of the family history in a pedigree is often helpful (Figure 7-1). While it is desirable to obtain complete information on three generations of the family, both affected (i.e., those with a cancer diagnosis) and unaffected individuals, this is often not realistic in clinical practice. At minimum, information related to parents, siblings, and both maternal and paternal grandparents and aunts and uncles should be obtained. Specific details related to cancers present, age at diagnosis, bilaterality of disease (e.g., bilateral breast cancer), presence of more than one primary tumor, preneoplastic lesions, and prophylactic surgeries will aid in the identification of individuals at an increased risk for cancer and those who should be referred for cancer genetic counseling because of the potential presence of a hereditary cancer syndrome.[13–16] Confirmation of the cancer diagnoses through pathology reports or death certificates is critical for accurate interpretation of risk in high-risk clinics, as recall of cancer diagnoses by family members may be inaccurate.

Models for Determining Risk

Models have been developed for determining risk in some cancers. In breast cancer, two tools are currently available for calculating risk. These tools, or models, use data derived from different epidemiological studies. Tabular data, compiled by Claus et al using information from the Cancer and Steroid Hormone Study, is especially useful for evaluating family history because it takes into account the age of affected relatives

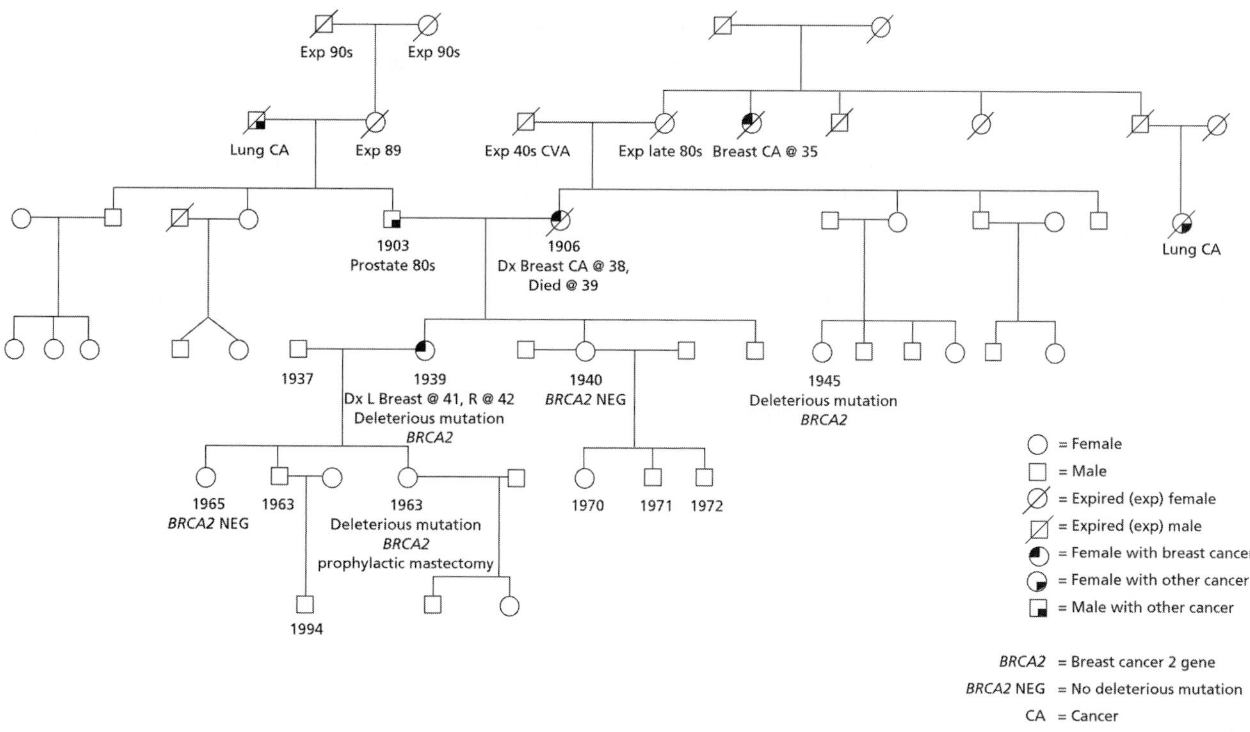

Figure 7-1 Example of a pedigree from a family with known mutation in *BRCA2*.

at cancer onset.[17] The second tool is the Gail Model, based on information gathered from the Breast Cancer Detection and Demonstration Project. The Gail Model uses five variables to calculate risk ratios: current age, age at first live birth, age at menarche, number of first-degree relatives with breast cancer, and number of breast biopsies. With respect to breast biopsies, high-risk indicators such as atypical ductal hyperplasia and lobular neoplasia are factored in.[10,18,19] Tables and computer programs are available to estimate individualized age-specific risk based on this model; a program disk is available from the National Cancer Institute (NCI). The Gail Model was used to determine eligibility for participation in the breast cancer prevention trial that led to the approval in 1998 of tamoxifen for chemoprevention in women at increased risk for breast cancer.

While these models are useful, both have limitations. Data were acquired primarily from white women, so the models may not apply to women of other races. In addition, both models were developed prior to the discovery of genes associated with hereditary cancer syndromes. As a consequence, they tend to underestimate the risk for individuals from families with hereditary breast cancer while overestimating the risk in others. The Gail Model also fails to factor in the powerful indicator of ovarian cancer in a close relative. To date, models are not yet available for use in estimating risk for the development of other types of cancers such as colorectal or prostate cancer, although data are available on the degree to which family history elevates risk.

Hereditary Cancer Syndromes

Many individuals voice the sentiment, "Everyone in my family has cancer." Cancer is a common disease affecting an estimated one in three individuals, contributing to a misconception of increased incidence within families. Aggregation of cancers in a family may occur because of shared cultural, lifestyle, and environmental factors, hereditary influences, chance, or a combination of these factors. Since the eighteenth century, it has been observed that certain types of cancers tend to cluster within some families at a higher rate than would be expected by chance alone. Although many believed that some cancers were hereditary, until recently no genetic basis had been elucidated. Today, as a result of advances in molecular biology and research efforts such as the HGP, genes associated with hereditary cancer syndromes are rapidly being identified (Table 7-1).[20–23] To date, more than 50 cancer-linked genes have been identified.[20,24] On the

American Society of Clinical Oncology (ASCO) Web site, an appendix of hereditary cancer syndromes and associated genes can be found under the continuing education section of the site.[22]

It is now accepted that all cancer is "genetic"—that is, that cancer occurs because of a series of stepwise mutations in genes that control important cellular processes such as cell growth, differentiation, DNA repair, and death. Most cancers are sporadic, resulting from a series of mutations in somatic, or body, cells. It is estimated that only 5%–10% of cancers are due to inheritance of a highly penetrant, rare cancer predisposition gene.[20,24] Mutated genes associated with hereditary cancer syndromes are carried in the germline cells, the cells responsible for reproduction; these genes have the potential to be passed from generation to generation and confer an inheritable predisposition for cancer development (Figure 7-2).[25] This means that a person who inherits a mutated gene known to cause cancer has an increased likelihood of

Table 7-1 Overview of Hereditary Cancer Syndromes

Hereditary Cancer Syndromes	Gene/Chromosome Locus	Type of Gene	Inherited Tumor(s)
Ataxia telangiectasia	*ATM*/11q22–23	DNA damage response	Lymphoid leukemias, lymphomas account for majority of tumors; breast cancer and possibly stomach and other cancers
Breast/ovarian cancer	*BRCA1*/17q21	Tumor suppressor Maintenance of genomic integrity	Early-onset breast, ovarian, prostate, pancreas, fallopian tube cancers
	BRCA2/13q12	Tumor suppressor Maintenance of genomic integrity	Early-onset breast, ovarian, male breast cancer, pancreatic cancer, and possibly other cancers such as stomach or bile duct
Cowden syndrome	*PTEN/MMAC1*/10q23	Tumor suppressor	Breast, thyroid, and endometrial cancer Associated with other clinical features such as hamartomatous polyps of the colon, breast, thyroid, skin, and mucous membranes; facial trichilemmomas, subcutaneous lipomas, and palmar pits
Colon cancer		DNA damage response genes; also termed mismatch repair genes	Colorectal carcinoma, gastric, endometrial, ovarian carcinoma
Hereditary nonpolyposis colorectal cancer (HNPCC)	*MSH2*/2p16 *MLH1*/3p21 *PMS1*/2q32 *PMS2*/7p22 *MSH6*/2p16		*MSH2* accounts for about 30% of HNPCC *MLH1* accounts for about 30% of HNPCC *PMS1* accounts for < 5% of HNPCC *PMS2* accounts for < 5% of HNPCC Variant: Muir-Torre syndrome (*MLH1, MSH2*)—colon, gastric, and sebaceous skin tumors, keratocanthomata of skin
Peutz-Jeghers	*STK11*/19p	Tumor suppressor	Breast, pancreas carcinomas, ovarian tumors, colon, testicular cancer, stomach; mucocutaneous pigmentation, polyps in the GI tract (especially jejunal polyps), bladder, and renal pelvis
Familial adenomatous polyposis (FAP)	*APC*/5q21	Tumor suppressor	Colorectal cancer: Characterized by multiple (hundreds) adenomatous polyps occurring in the colon and rectum; polyps may be found throughout the GI tract Nonmalignant features include epidermoid cysts, osteomas, desmoid tumors, and congenital hypertrophy of the retinal pigment epithelium (CHRPE) Variant: Turcot syndrome—polyps in association with brain tumor. In this syndrome, mutations have also been found in HNPCC-associated genes

(continued)

Table 7-1 Overview of Hereditary Cancer Syndromes (continued)

Hereditary Cancer Syndromes	Gene/Chromosome Locus	Type of Gene	Inherited Tumor(s)
Li-Fraumeni syndrome	*p53*/17p13	Tumor suppressor	Early-onset breast cancer, childhood bone and soft-tissue sarcomas, brain tumors, childhood leukemias, adrenocortical carcinoma
Malignant melanoma	*CDKN2A* (also termed *p16, MTS1*)/9p21	Tumor suppressor	Cutaneous melanomas; possibly pancreatic cancer and other GI cancers
	CDK4/12q14	Oncogene	*CDKN2:* About 20%–25% of melanoma-prone kindreds
Multiple endocrine neoplasia (MEN) type 1	*MEN1*/11q13	Function unknown	Characterized primarily by endocrine tumors, including parathyroid, pancreatic island cell, and pituitary. Hyperparathyroidism is a common presenting syndrome. Other features may include adrenocortical tumors, carcinoids, and thyroid abnormalities.
Multiple endocrine neoplasia type 2	*RET*/10q11.2	Oncogene	Pheochromocytoma and medullary thyroid carcinomas; parathyroid tumors and neurofibromas in some cases
			MEN2A: Characterized by mutations in exons 10 and 11 of *RET*
			MEN2B: Characterized by a single mutation in codon 918 (exon 16) in the majority of patients, mucosal neuromas, and marfanoid phenotype
			FMTC — characterized by later age of onset, indolent course, no pheochromocytoma or parathyroid disease
Nevoid basal cell carcinoma syndrome (Gorlin syndrome)	Patched/*PTCH*/9q22	Transmembrane receptor for human "sonic hedgehog protein" Tumor suppressor	Multiple basal cell carcinomas (one before age 30); medulloblastoma (5% affected individuals); ovarian carcinomas, fibrosarcomas Benign neoplasms include jaw cysts, palmar or plantar pits, cutaneous keratocysts and milia, ovarian fibromas, cardiac fibromas, and hamartomatous polyps of the stomach
Retinoblastoma	*RB*/13q14	Tumor suppressor Negative regulators of cell growth	Retinoblastoma; second primary sarcomas such as osteosarcoma of the leg and radiogenic sarcoma of the orbit; cutaneous melanoma
von Hippel-Lindau disease	*VHL*/3p25	Tumor suppressor	Renal cell carcinoma, pheochromocytoma (seen with or without renal cell cancer); additional features include hemangioblastoma; retinal angiomata; pancreatic, renal, and liver hemangiomas; subarachnoid hemorrhage

Data from American Society of Clinical Oncology[22]; Lindor, Greene[23]; Offit.[21]

developing cancer, although for a cancer to develop, other genetic mutations must also occur. In addition, the effects of environment, lifestyle, and other genetic factors on the development of cancer are currently not known. Thus, although cancer predisposition genes increase the likelihood of developing cancer, cancer is not an inevitable outcome. This concept is critically important for genetic counseling and as an underpinning for cancer prevention.

Patterns of Inheritance

The monk Gregor Mendel described the basic modes of inheritance in his pea garden in the 1850s. Different forms (alleles) of a gene may occupy a given genetic locus, or position on the chromosome. Each individual has two copies (alleles) of each gene. The two alleles may be identical or different; together they determine a disease or physical trait. The genetic

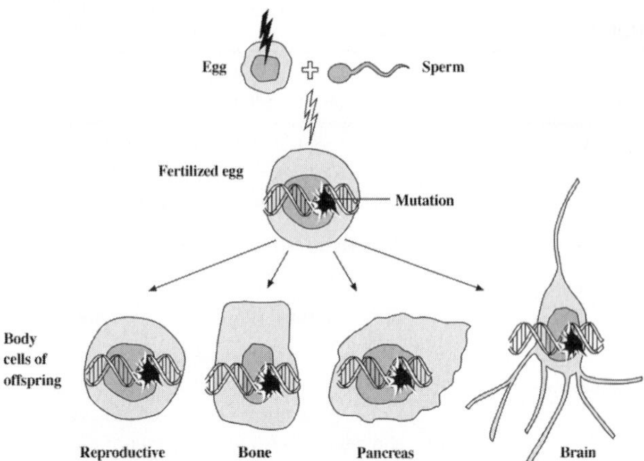

Figure 7-2 Hereditary mutations are carried in the DNA of the reproductive cells. When reproductive cells containing mutations combine to produce offspring, the mutation will be present in all of the offspring's body cells. Reprinted from the National Institutes of Health and National Cancer Institute: *Understanding Gene Testing* [NIH pub. no. 96–3905]. Washington, DC, U.S. Department of Health and Human Services, 1995.[25]

constitution of an individual is referred to as the *genotype*, whereas the physical, biochemical, or clinical characteristics of the trait are referred to as the *phenotype*.

For diseases produced by dominant genes, only one altered allele is required to produce the disease. Genes that predispose for the development of cancer are generally transmitted in an *autosomal dominant* fashion, meaning that individuals who harbor a mutated gene have a 50% chance of passing the mutated gene on to their children. Inheritance of the altered gene confers an increased risk for developing cancer. The pattern of transmission seen with cancer susceptibility genes is usually vertical (successive generations are affected), and depending on the disease, males and females are generally equally affected (Figure 7-3).[26] In classic autosomal dominant inheritance, every affected person in a pedigree has an affected parent. In reality, this may not be the case in hereditary cancer kindreds for several reasons. First, cancer is a multifactorial disease. The factors that influence the *penetrance*, or expression, of a gene that predisposes for the development of cancer have not been well elucidated. Thus, within a family, individuals may inherit a gene alteration that predisposes for the development of cancer yet never develop a cancer. Furthermore, the type of cancer usually caused by a specific gene alteration may not be equally expressed in males and females. For example, breast cancer 1 (*BRCA1*), the altered gene associated with hereditary breast and ovarian cancer, may be carried by a male yet not expressed. Males cannot develop ovarian cancer and generally do not develop breast cancer as a consequence of mutations in *BRCA1*. Thus skipped generations may be seen in families with a hereditary cancer syndrome.

Characteristics of Hereditary Cancer Syndromes

Table 7-1 reviews the most common hereditary cancer syndromes and the associated genes that, when altered, predispose for the development of cancers associated with that syndrome. Many other syndromes include an increased susceptibility to cancer in addition to other abnormalities or diseases. However, most of these syndromes, such as Cowden syndrome, are quite rare. (Table 7-1 lists some of these syndromes and their other associated clinical features.)

Several common characteristics are seen in families with a hereditary cancer syndrome:[11,27]

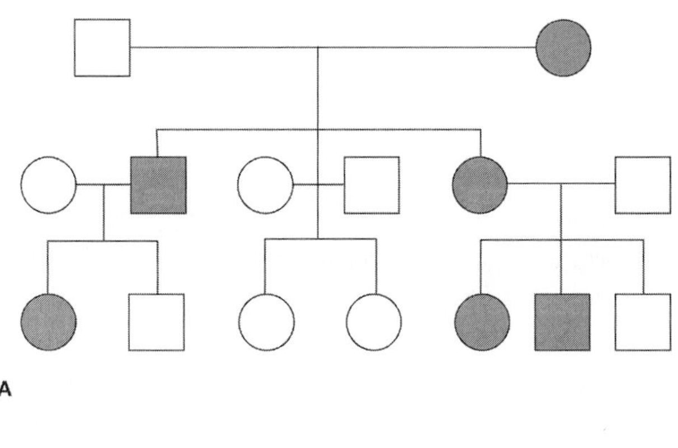

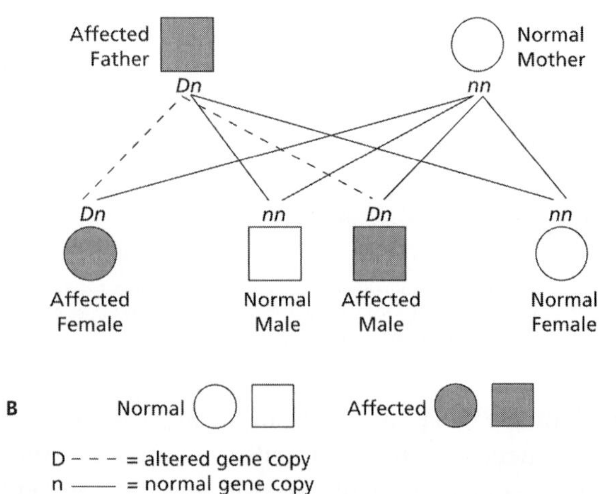

Figure 7-3 Autosomal dominant inheritance. **A.** A pedigree with affected family members. **B.** How an altered gene is passed. Reprinted with permission from Lea DH, Jenkins JL, Francoman O: *Genetics in Clinical Practice, New Directions for Nursing and Healthcare*. Sudbury, MA, Jones and Bartlett, 1998, p. 45.[26]

- The occurrence of multiple cases of cancer, especially cancers of the same type (e.g., melanomas or colorectal cancers) or types related to a specific syndrome (e.g., breast and ovary; bowel and endometrium; leukemia and sarcoma) within a single lineage (i.e., the maternal side or the paternal side)
- A diagnosis of cancer at an earlier age than is seen in the general population (e.g., breast cancer before age 50 years)
- The occurrence of multiple cancers in one person (e.g., a person with both colon and uterine cancer)
- The presence of rare tumors, such as retinoblastomas or brain tumors
- Cancer in paired organs (i.e., both breasts or both kidneys)
- Nonmalignant manifestations of a hereditary cancer syndrome (e.g., hamartomas of the skin and mucous membranes and palmar pits, as seen in Cowden syndrome)

When any of these conditions is present alone or in combination, the possibility of a hereditary cancer syndrome should be considered. During risk assessment, these criteria can serve as "flags" to identify individuals who should be referred for more intensive cancer genetic counseling. Following is a brief review of the hereditary cancer syndromes most commonly seen in clinical practice. The reader is referred to the *ASCO Curriculum Cancer Genetics and Cancer Predisposition Testing*, second edition,[11] for a comprehensive review of other hereditary cancer syndromes that may be seen in practice or for which cancer genetic testing may be available (e.g., hereditary gastric cancer, melanoma, and thyroid cancer).

Hereditary Breast and Ovarian Cancer Syndromes

Syndromes of breast cancer susceptibility have been linked to mutations in several genes, including *BRCA1* and breast cancer 2 (*BRCA2*). The *BRCA1* and *BRCA2* genes are both large tumor suppressor genes and the proteins they code for have roles in genomic stability.[28] The traditional approach to identifying genes that predispose to cancer has been to localize the gene to a particular chromosome by using a technique known as *linkage analysis*. In this approach, DNA from multiple family members is studied, and the gene is localized to a particular chromosome according to how it segregates with identified markers on the chromosome during the meiotic phase of cell division. This was accomplished for *BRCA1* in 1990,[29,30] and for *BRCA2* in 1994.[31]

The sequence of nucleotide bases in a gene codes for the production of a protein. Once a gene has been localized to a particular chromosome, the next step is to identify the gene and determine the precise sequence of nucleotide bases for that gene. This was accomplished for *BRCA1* in 1994[32] and for *BRCA2* in 1995.[33] *BRCA1* is located on chromosome 17q (long arm) and is thought to account for 30%–45% of breast cancer cases in families with a high incidence of early-onset breast and ovarian cancer. *BRCA2* is located on chromosome 13q and appears to account for about 35% of families with early-onset breast cancer. Thus, while *BRCA1* and *BRCA2* mutations account for a significant percentage of hereditary breast cancer, it is believed that other, as yet undiscovered genes, such as a proposed breast cancer 3 (*BRCA3*), may also increase susceptibility to breast and other cancers. In contrast, it is believed that *BRCA1* and *BRCA2* mutations account for the majority of familial ovarian cancers.

With respect to certain hereditary cancer syndromes, the concept of a *founder effect* is important. This effect is defined as an unusual prevalence of specific genotypes in a population and produces a greater-than-expected frequency of a specific mutation in common descendants of an ancestor. Founder effects frequently occur due to migration, a limited number of ancestors, and catastrophes. They have been seen in several hereditary cancer syndromes. For example, in *BRCA1* and *BRCA2* families, specific mutations are commonly seen in those of Ashkenazi Jewish, French Canadian, Dutch, and Icelandic heritage. Thus, it is always important to inquire about an individual's heritage.

The lifetime risk for developing breast cancer in *BRCA1*-linked families is relatively high. In the general population, the cumulative incidence for breast cancer by age 50 is 2%, with a lifetime risk of more than 10%. In families with multiple cancer cases, which were used to clone the *BRCA1* and *BRCA2* genes, the estimated lifetime risk of breast cancer is about 80%. In the general population, the lifetime risk for ovarian cancer is in the range of 1%–2%. In those women with an alteration in *BRCA1*, the lifetime risk may range from 20% to 60%. Deleterious mutations in *BRCA1* also lead to greater risks for cancer of the cervix, uterus, pancreas, fallopian tube, stomach, colon, and prostate cancer for male carriers.[34,35] Multiple studies have evaluated the current *BRCA1* and *BRCA2* mutation-associated breast cancer penetrance data, and these are thoroughly reviewed by Begg.[36] Depending on the population studied (e.g., families with multiple cases of breast cancer, heritage, or singly ascertained cases of breast cancer), the estimates will vary.[36-38]

A lifetime risk of breast cancer similar to that in families with *BRCA1* mutations is seen in families with *BRCA2* alterations, although some data indicate that the onset of breast cancer may occur at an older age. Ovarian cancer is also seen in women carrying mutations in *BRCA2,* albeit to a lesser extent than with *BRCA1.* Estimates for the lifetime risk of ovarian cancer range from 10% to 20% in women with *BRCA2* mutations. Other cancers that may be associated with *BRCA2* mutations include stomach, gallbladder, bile duct, and pancreatic cancers.[34] The estimated lifetime risk of breast cancer for male carriers of *BRCA2* mutations is roughly 6.9%, with carriers also having an increased risk of cancers of the prostate, pancreas, stomach, and melanoma.[39,40]

Some controversy has surrounded the risk estimates, with many suggesting that the estimates for lifetime risk may have been inflated by utilitzation in early studies of highly enriched patient populations, or multiple affected family members in any given sample. However, a recent study by King et al[35] confirmed risk estimates in a group of 1008 Ashkenazi Jewish women with as little as a single affected relative. Researchers found that of women with incident primary invasive breast cancer, approximately 10% carried a mutation of *BRCA1* or *BRCA2.* Lifetime risks to relatives were greater than 80%, with the risk conferred from *BRCA2* mutations being lower prior to the age of 65. Lifetime risks for ovarian cancer were confirmed as being greater than 50% for those with *BRCA1* mutations and greater than 20% for *BRCA2* mutation carriers. Interestingly, King et al also found that modifiable risk factors of health, weight at menarche and age 21, and exercise as a teen delayed onset of breast cancer in their sample.

Hereditary Colon Cancers

The lifetime risk of developing colorectal cancer in the United States is approximately 6%. Many studies have shown that the stronger one's family history of colorectal cancer, the greater one's risk of developing the disease. Highly penetrant cancer susceptibility syndromes account for about 5% of colorectal cancers. The most common syndrome is hereditary nonpolyposis colon cancer (HNPCC), with familial adenomatous polyposis (FAP) being much less frequent.

Hereditary nonpolyposis colon cancer

This cancer is evidenced by early-onset colorectal cancer (diagnosis before the age of 50 years), and extracolonic tumors such as uterine, ovarian, stomach, and small intestine tumors, and transitional cell tumors of the renal pelvis and ureter. Individuals who have HNPCC have inherited a germline mutation in one of the several genes responsible for repairing DNA mismatches. These genes have been termed *spell checker genes.* Normally functioning mismatch repair genes allow for accurate transmission of genetic information from a cell to its progeny by recognizing abnormal base pairs and correcting the sequence on one strand to restore normal base pairing. Mutations in the following genes have been found to cause HNPCC: *hMSH2* (found on chromosome 2p [short arm]), *hMLH1* (found on chromosome 3p), *hPMS1* (found on chromosome 2q), *hPMS2* (found on chromosome 7p), and *hMSH6* (found on chromosome 2p). *Microsatellites* are repetitive DNA sequences of one to four nucleotides found throughout the genome and usually do not encode for proteins. Most cancers in patients with HNPCC show a high degree of microsatellite instability (MSI). MSI is the abnormal situation in which tissues acquire variability in the number of nucleotides in their repeat sequences. It provided clues for the discovery of genes associated with this syndrome in the early 1990s.[41-43]

Individuals inheriting one of these genes can anticipate an approximately 80% lifetime risk of developing colorectal cancer. In some families, the penetrance may range as high as 90%. The median age at diagnosis is less than 45 years. In many families, *synchronous cancers* of the colon (several tumors presenting at the same time) and *metachronous tumors* (several tumors presenting at different times) have been documented. The lifetime risk for endometrial cancer is about 60% as compared to a populational risk of 3%.[21,43]

The International Collaborative Group on HNPCC defined criteria for identifying the syndrome at a meeting in Amsterdam in 1991. The *Amsterdam criteria* define the syndrome as histologically verified colorectal cancer in three or more relatives, one of whom is a first-degree relative of the other two; colorectal cancer involving at least two generations; and one or more colorectal cancer cases diagnosed before 50 years of age. A limitation of these criteria has been the omission of endometrial and other extracolonic tumors. A subsequent meeting developed the Bethesda criteria for HNPCC, which include the Amsterdam criteria, pedigrees with a colon cancer case before 40 years, and pedigrees with a high incidence of noncolonic tumors associated with HNPCC.[44] An NCI workshop was held in December 1997 to review and unify the field and develop recommendations on MSI and its use for cancer detection and identification of familial predisposition. At this meeting, the Bethesda guidelines were endorsed.[45] A subsequent meeting was held in 2002 to consider revision of the guidelines. Within the revised guidelines are recommendations for evaluation of MSI testing results. Depending on whether MSI testing results are high (MSI-H) or low (MSI-L), recommendations are given on those patients who should go on for molecular evaluation.[46]

Familial adenomatous polyposis

FAP is a rare syndrome (accounting for only about 1% of all colorectal cancers) characterized by hundreds to thousands of polyps carpeting the colon that inevitably progress to colon cancer. Although rare, because the lifetime risk for colon cancer approaches 100%, it is incumbent on the healthcare professional to be able to help identify this syndrome. Polyps usually begin to appear in an affected person's late teens and twenties. If left untreated (generally by prophylactic colectomy), death from colon cancer will occur in virtually all cases by age 50 years. Congenital hypertrophy of the retinal pigment epithelium (CHRPE) is a useful diagnostic marker for the syndrome and consists of pigmented lesions in the retina that can be detected by funduscopic examination. Individuals with a variant form of FAP known as Gardner's syndrome also exhibit sebaceous cysts, lipomas, desmoid tumors, fibromas, facial bone osteomas, and impacted or supernumerary teeth.[43] A subset of patients present with fewer colorectal polyps, later age in onset of both polyps and colorectal cancer, and more proximal location of tumors. These individuals are said to have attenuated familial adenomatous polyposis (AFAP).[47]

The *APC* gene is a tumor suppressor gene associated with FAP and AFAP. Like most of the genes associated with hereditary cancer syndromes, the *APC* gene is large, and a wide spectrum of mutations have been observed. However, genotype–phenotype correlations have begun to be identified in this gene. In the *APC* gene, most mutations in both the 5′ and 3′ ends are associated with AFAP, while the more central regions of the gene are associated with the FAP phenotype.[43]

Cancer Genetic Counseling

A variety of healthcare professionals with specialized training, such as oncologists, oncology nurses, genetic counselors, and clinical geneticists, now provide cancer risk and genetic counseling. It is helpful for the practicing oncology nurse to understand the process of cancer risk counseling and genetic testing so that when individuals are referred for these specialized services, the nurse will be knowledgeable regarding the type and scope of services that should be provided. Table 7-2 provides an overview of the cancer genetic counseling process.[12,26] A study evaluating oncology nurses' knowledge of cancer genetics found that patients often made inquiries regarding the subject but only about one-third of the nurses who responded were aware of referral resources for queries, counseling, or testing.[48]

Definition

Genetic counseling is a risk assessment, communication, and educational process by which individuals and family members receive information about the nature and limitations of genetic tests, benefits, risks, costs, and meaning of test results. Counseling and support concerning the implications of information gained from testing are a vital component of this process.[21,49] Regardless of the setting in which cancer predisposition genetic testing is offered (e.g., within the context of a clinical trial or as a commercially available test), individuals must receive adequate information to make an informed decision concerning their health and give informed consent to undergo testing. Genetic testing must be conducted only in conjunction with genetic counseling to ensure that this process occurs.

Although traditional genetic counseling assumes the wish/need for performing genetic testing, the motivation for testing in the setting of cancer risk assessment and counseling is less concrete. This difference is related to the fact that the etiology of cancers is multifactorial. Patients and family members may approach the nurse with concerns or worries about cancer risk that may be dispelled based on the family pedigree and individual history, thereby negating the need for genetic testing. Additionally, as the genetic "revolution" continues, genetic information will be used increasingly to understand the biology of cancer as a disease, select appropriate therapies, and identify specific somatic mutations that put individuals at risk. Increasingly, healthcare providers will need to have knowledge of human molecular genetics so as to "counsel" individuals regarding selection of therapeutic options, interpretation of pathology reports, and response to various drug therapies, as well as to provide the traditional interpretation of the family pedigree.[1]

Services Provided

Comprehensive services should include the following:

- Determinations of the individual's reasons for seeking cancer risk counseling
- Data collection that provides an in-depth review of the family history (a minimum of three complete

Table 7-2 The Cancer Genetic Counseling Process

Clinical Activity	Information to Be Discussed
Assessment and Information Gathering	
Reason for referral	Patient concerns and questions Physician recommendation
Information gathering	
Family history	Collect information on three generations when possible Minimum: parents, siblings, aunts, uncles, grandparents Cancers in the family: age at diagnosis, bilaterality in paired organs, more than one primary tumor Relevant genetic testing results Verification by pathology report or death certificates of cancers in the family is critical
Personal history	Past medical history and screening practices History relevant to cancer risk assessment (e.g., gynecologic history for breast/ovarian cancer) Lifestyle factors (e.g., smoking, alcohol, carcinogen exposure)
Patient perception of risk for cancer	Beliefs about cancer and its causation Patient perception of lifetime risk for developing cancer and probability of altered gene in the family that is "responsible" for cancer
Social, emotional, and cultural concerns	Cultural beliefs Support systems Economic factors
Evaluation and Analysis of Data	
Family history	Assess family for characteristics seen with hereditary cancer syndromes Estimate of probability that family would test positive for alteration in cancer predisposition gene
Focused physical examination	Dependent on syndrome present in the family (e.g., eye exam for FAP)
Laboratory testing	Dependent on syndrome present in the family
Communication of Genetic and Risk Information	
Natural history of condition	Discussion of types of cancer seen in the family Explanation of suspected hereditary cancer syndrome
Inheritance patterns	Review of autosomal dominant transmission of cancer predisposition genes
Discussion of risk for developing cancer	Populational risk and estimated risk for patient Review in terms of several types of risk (e.g., in terms of relative risk, lifetime risk)
Ramifications and appropriateness of cancer predisposition genetic testing	Benefits, risks, limitations, costs of testing Potential answers that may be obtained Who in the family is best to test
Strategies for managing risk	Lifestyle changes Options for screening and detection Signs and symptoms of cancer Chemoprevention Prophylactic surgery
Supportive Counseling	
Discussion of patient and family questions and concerns	Common concerns include potential risk for children, potential for discrimination due to cancer predisposition genetic testing
Providing emotional and social support	Determination of existing coping patterns and support systems Teaching new coping strategies as required Assisting patient in discussing genetic testing results with family Allow patient and family to voice fears and concerns Discussion of how to communicate results to relatives
Referral for additional counseling and support as needed	Available support systems for patients with extreme anxiety and distress

(continued)

Table 7-2 The Cancer Genetic Counseling Process (continued)

Clinical Activity	Information to Be Discussed
Follow-up Counseling	
Further discussion of genetic testing results (if performed) and risk for developing cancer	Review patient questions and concerns Review strategies for managing increased risk Discuss availability of clinical trials for long-term follow-up, chemoprevention, new screening technologies
Written summary and follow-up letter	Summary of discussion of family history, assessment of risk for developing cancer, probability of gene in the family, issues related to genetic testing, and strategies for managing risk
Coordination of care with other healthcare providers such as oncologist, primary care provider	Obtain permission from patient for release to other healthcare providers
Discussion with relatives about implications of results	Obtain permission from patients for release of information to relatives who may wish to come for cancer genetic counseling

Data from Lea, Jenkins, Francomano[26]; Mahon[12]; Rieger.[16]

generations) and patterns of transmission of cancers within the family

- Risk assessment as outlined earlier
- Determination of the client's level of knowledge regarding hereditary cancer syndromes and cancer genetics, self-perception of risk for developing cancer, determination of the wish to proceed with genetic testing (if appropriate), and motivation for seeking predisposition genetic testing
- Recommendations for management of risk (i.e., surveillance, chemoprevention, prophylactic surgery)
- Evaluation of the appropriateness of testing
- Education regarding the testing process and the benefits, risks, limitations, costs, and potential outcomes that may result from testing
- Disclosure of test results and their implications

All counseling should include an evaluation of the patient's psychosocial status, support systems, ability to receive and cope with test results, and referrals as appropriate for medical or surgical means of early detection or prevention of cancer.[16,21,50,51] It is considered mandatory—and is standard practice—that individuals receive a follow-up letter after counseling that documents clearly the information provided regarding family history, risk assessment, implications of testing and/or known results, and recommendations for management of risks. It is also critically important to attempt to obtain documentation of the cancers in the family by securing pathology records or death certificates.[11]

Healthcare Professionals Involved in Cancer Genetic Counseling

Cancer genetic counseling services are generally provided using a multidisciplinary approach. Most counseling is provided by advanced practice oncology nurses with specialized training in cancer genetics or by genetic counselors with specialized training in the field of oncology in collaboration with medical oncologists or clinical geneticists. In 2001, the International Society of Nurses in Genetics (ISONG) created a method by which nurses who are working in cancer risk assessment and counseling can become credentialed through completion of a portfolio for approval as a means of assuring competence. Credentialing can be completed on both the baccalaureate level as a Genetics Clinical Nurse (GCN) or on the master's level as an Advanced Practice Nurse in Genetics (APNG).

Traditionally, the nondirective provision of information was used as a guiding principle in genetic counseling to enable individuals to make their own decisions. This approach was applied to all components of the process, including discussion of the use of genetic testing to identify disease or predisposition for disease, and discussion of the specific features or management of the genetic condition. In essence, counselors did not make recommendations one way or the other as to which decision would be the "best."

With respect to cancer genetic counseling, this philosophy has been questioned because occasionally clear medical recommendations can be made about managing genetic risk. For example, effective surgical options exist for managing individuals at increased risk for developing colorectal cancer. The healthcare provider is obligated to recommend such options. Nevertheless, the ultimate goal is the provision of balanced and complete information so that an individual may make an informed decision concerning his or her health. Those providing counseling should be aware of their own biases and philosophy toward testing so that their opinions do not inadvertently influence an individual's decisions.

Patient Education

During the process of cancer genetic counseling, information that is often technically complex and emotionally laden must be presented to individuals. Oncology nurses are well versed in the provision of patient education, and the fundamentals for providing quality education can be applied to the counseling process. Assessment of an individual for any barriers to learning, such as hearing problems, decreased visual acuity, primary language other than English, low literacy level, or changes in emotional status (extreme anxiety, distress, or distrust), is important to guide both choice and adjustment of teaching and counseling methodologies. A variety of teaching methodologies, such as face-to-face communication and video, audio, and written materials, can be used to present information in a manner that best suits the person seeking consultation. The individual's understanding of the information given should be assessed periodically during the counseling session, and an opportunity for questions should be provided.[52–54]

Table 7-3 Factors Influencing Cancer Genetic Counseling

Individual Frame of Reference
- Personal philosophy about cancer
- Life experience with cancer
- Self-perception of risk
- Anxiety over cancer risk
- Opinions about obtaining genetic information

Family Considerations
- Differing opinions about obtaining genetic information
- Presence of family members during counseling

Cultural and Ethnic Considerations
- Views on cancer as a disease
- Views on genetics and genetic testing
- Decision-making process within the family

Structural Considerations
- Healthcare providers
  - Multidisciplinary team providing counseling and expertise in cancer care
- Setting
  - Wellness setting (e.g., prevention center)
  - Illness setting (e.g., within cancer treatment center)
- Payment for counseling services
- Payment for genetic testing
- Timing (e.g., near recent diagnosis of cancer, near recent death in the family from cancer)
- Record keeping
  - Documentation of services
  - Communication with other health care professionals

Data from Rieger, Pentz.[56]

Problems and Issues Related to Cancer Genetic Counseling and Genetic Testing

Predisposition genetic testing remains relatively new, and many issues surrounding its use persist. The major topics that must be addressed during the process of cancer genetic counseling include the setting for testing, informed consent, discussion of the accuracy of the test and interpretation of test results, psychosocial issues, and management of risk.

Setting for Testing

The American Society of Clinical Oncology (ASCO) has issued a statement on genetic testing for cancer susceptibility that speaks to indications for cancer predisposition testing.[55] When preparing the update on its position statement on cancer genetic testing, ASCO recognized that the majority of tests being performed at this time are carried out by commercial laboratories. As such, it recommended that these laboratories have strong oversite not only to regulate the materials utilized in performing the tests and reference samples, but also to assure access to all individuals who are in need of the tests.

Clinical trials continue to address issues regarding risk management, psychological responses, risk profiles, and so forth. Whenever possible, individuals should be enrolled in clinical trials to obtain answers to these questions in the most expeditious manner.

In its updated guidelines, ASCO recommends that genetic testing be offered when the individual has personal or family history features suggestive of a genetic cancer susceptibility condition; the test can be adequately interpreted; and the results will aid in diagnosis or influence the medical or surgical management of the patient or family members at hereditary risk of cancer. Testing should be done only in the setting of pre- and post-test counseling. The provision of cancer genetic counseling may be influenced by many factors. Table 7-3 outlines individual, family, cultural, ethnic, and structural factors that must be considered when providing services.[56]

Informed Consent

A principal concern about predisposition genetic testing is that individuals receive adequate information to

Table 7-4 Topics to Be Discussed During the Informed Consent Process

Purpose of the genetic test
Reason for offering testing
Type and nature of genetic condition being tested for
Accuracy of genetic test
Benefits of participating in testing
Risks associated with genetic testing, including unexpected results
Other available testing options
Available treatment and intervention options
Further decision making that may be needed on receipt of test results
Consent to use patient's DNA for further research purposes
Availability of additional counseling and support services
Acknowledgment of the right to refuse testing

Reprinted with permission from Lea DH, Jenkins JL, Francomano C: *Genetics in Clinical Practice: New Directions for Nursing and Health Care.* Sudbury, MA, Jones and Bartlett, 1988, p 85.[26]

give informed consent.[56–59] Numerous position statements have been published concerning the process of genetic testing and counseling,[55,60–64] and the majority of which speak to the necessity of informed consent. Table 7-4 reviews topics that should be discussed during the informed consent process.[26,56]

Accuracy of the Test and Interpretation of Results

Information about cancer predisposition genetic testing abounds in the lay media and on the Internet; as a consequence, individuals frequently seek predisposition genetic testing with unrealistic expectations of what testing can provide. During cancer genetic counseling, the counselor must assess the individual's risk for the syndrome in question, determine which tests are available for the syndrome, review how the test is performed, establish the type of test to be used (e.g., protein truncation versus full sequencing of the gene), investigate the sensitivity and specificity of the test, determine who in the family is the best person to test, identify the potential answers that may be obtained, and explain the meaning of each answer.

In the broadest sense, genetic tests are defined as the analysis of human DNA, RNA, chromosomes, proteins, and other gene products to detect disease-related genotypes, mutations, phenotypes, or karyotypes.[65] The tests may be helpful in identifying those at risk of getting the disease in question, identifying carriers of mutated genes, establishing diagnoses or prognoses, and establishing genetic identity (paternity). Commercially available genetic tests are based on a variety of techniques, including protein truncation assays, heteroduplex analysis, versions of single-strand conformational polymorphism (SSCP) analysis, and direct sequencing of the gene of interest. The first three techniques involve the use of gels to detect changes in mobility patterns of either proteins or single strands of DNA (SSCP) or double strands of DNA (heteroduplex analysis). The most sensitive technique to date, and the one considered to be the gold standard, is the test done to determine the DNA sequence of both copies of the gene. Although highly accurate, sequencing is both expensive and labor-intensive. It can be likened to trying to find a spelling error in one word in an article that is several thousand words long. The cost of commercial predisposition genetic testing may range from several hundred dollars (e.g., when confirming a known mutation that has been found in another family member or when using panels that assess for several mutations commonly seen in those of a specific heritage) to several thousand dollars for full sequencing of large genes such as *BRCA1* or *BRCA2*. Depending on the test being performed and the approach used, it often requires 4–6 weeks to obtain results.[66–68]

The meaning and likelihood of each genetic test result (positive, negative, or inconclusive) must be reviewed in detail. If a deleterious mutation is found (positive test result), the individual must clearly understand that it denotes a predisposition for the development of cancer — not a diagnosis or even inevitability of cancer development. Information related to the penetrance of the mutation must be reviewed. Because cancer susceptibility genes were discovered only recently, knowledge in this field continues to evolve. With some genes, such as the *APC* gene associated with FAP, penetrance is near 100%, and medical management is well defined; with others, such as the *BRCA1* gene, penetrance is less extensive, and recommendations for medical management continue to evolve as new data are generated through clinical trials.[21,55] When there is a known mutation in the family and an individual's test is negative for that mutation, it is important for the individual to realize that he or she still has the general population risk for the development of that type of cancer.

Some answers from testing may provide no additional information for an individual or the family. A negative test result is often difficult to interpret when no known mutation has yet been detected in a family. These tests are termed "uninformative." Negative test results may be obtained because the test missed something (i.e., a false-negative test may occur because of technical difficulties or the location of a mutation in a region of the gene not tested, such as promoter, enhancer, or intronic regions), because there is an as yet undiscovered gene responsible for the constellation of cancers seen in the family, or because the cancers may have resulted purely from chance. Other results are inconclusive and could include finding a "polymorphism," which is simply a harmless genetic variation within the population, or a variant of unknown significance (VUS), a sequence change found about which insufficient information currently exists to determine whether the change is deleterious. In such cases, it remains difficult to determine cancer risk. Depending on the family history, in many instances the individual would still be considered at high risk.[68–70] A study by Petrucelli and colleagues of registered members of the National Society of Genetic Counselors found significant diversity in the personal interpretation of a VUS result, which led to various clinical recommendations. This variation suggests a need for clinical management recommendations in how to approach such results.

To provide the most information for a family, it is best to test an affected individual (e.g., one who has already developed cancer). However, even this approach carries with it the risk of testing a person who developed a sporadic cancer within a family that has a specific genetic alteration. Many centers will test *only* affected individuals. In many families, this strategy may not be possible or practical. Therefore, when an unaffected individual is tested, it is important to reinforce the limitations of this approach and to emphasize how results will ultimately be interpreted within the context of the family. A positive test result for a known deleterious mutation in the family will provide the most information. Remember that a negative test result — one that finds no evidence of a mutation — may provide no information for the family as a whole. Rather, it provides information solely applicable to the individual being tested. Individuals must realize that testing for hereditary cancer syndromes is complex and may provide no additional information concerning risk for developing cancer.

Psychosocial Issues

Predisposition genetic testing for susceptibility to cancer carries with it unique psychosocial implications of which oncology nurses and those providing cancer risk counseling services must be aware and able to discuss openly with patients. Assessing the psychological impact of test results remains an important area of research. Early studies in women seeking medical advice who believed they were at high risk for breast cancer revealed that they frequently overestimated their risk; individuals undergoing counseling had a more accurate perception of their risk a year after counseling than those who did not undergo counseling.[71,72] Earlier fears that provision of accurate risk information would increase an individual's anxiety have not been found to pan out in women with family history of breast cancer.[73] Indeed, a study by Schwartz et al[74] suggests that true-negative test results lead to psychological benefit for individuals pursuing the testing, while positive or uninformative results do not increase psychological distress or risk perception.

While the majority of behavioral health research investigating psychological response to genetic testing has focused on the population with higher breast/ovarian cancer risk, Esplen et al[75] explored motivation for testing and psychological response to genetic testing for HNPCC. This motivation was not different than that of women seeking testing for breast/ovarian cancer risk, and psychological response and satisfaction with testing of the HNPCC population mirrored that of the breast/ovarian population.

Clearly, to prevent and manage a patient's potential adverse reactions to the disclosure of genetic status, healthcare professionals who provide cancer risk assessment and counseling services must be sure the patient understands the benefits, risks, and limitations of testing both prior to cancer susceptibility testing and before results are disclosed. The healthcare provider must evaluate family dynamics and the patient's cultural and healthcare beliefs, reinforce the patient's existing coping skills and teach new ones for handling the information provided, facilitate the patient's decision making through nondirective counseling, and identify patients who may need referral to a mental health professional.[76,77] Table 7-5 outlines some of the benefits and risks that are related to cancer predisposition genetic testing.

The confidentiality of results remains an area of question and concern. Many individuals harbor concerns over misuse of information or negative sequelae that may result from release of test results, such as discrimination with respect to employment opportunities, or health, life, disability, or mortgage insurance coverage.[76–82] To date, at least 41 states have enacted legislation prohibiting discrimination by health insurers and, in some cases, employers. Federal legislation passed in 1996, the Kennedy-Kassebaum bill,[81] includes safeguards against discrimination based on genetic information, but its effectiveness in protecting consumers has yet to be tested in the courts. Addressing genetic issues for federal employees, President Clinton provided Federal Executive Order 13145 (February 2000) to prohibit discrimination based on genetic information. Lastly, the Genetic Information Nondiscrimination Act of 2003 (S1053), supported by the Oncology Nursing Society and the majority of

Table 7-5 Benefits and Risks of Cancer Genetic Testing

Positive Results	Inconclusive Results	Negative Results*
	BENEFITS	
Ability to tailor more aggressive cancer screening and detection measures to those individuals carrying the highest risk	May provide feeling of empowerment (i.e., something was done to look for cause of multiple cancers within the family)	Extra surveillance unnecessary as cancer risk would be the same as for the general population
Reduction of uncertainty and anxiety		Relief that children cannot inherit the altered gene
Ability to test other family members for known mutation within the family		Financial savings from decreased surveillance
Reason as to "why" cancer developed		Decreased anxiety about ability to plan for the future
		Relief over not having greatly increased risk for developing cancer
	RISKS	
Anxiety and depression over increased cancer risk	Anxiety and depression over uncertain results	Delay in seeking recommended cancer screening measures
Fear that "nothing can be done" to minimize risk for developing cancer	Family continues to be monitored as high-risk family	Survivor guilt
Lowered life goals	"No news"	Depression because increased cancer risks can no longer serve as cause of problems
Strained relationships with family (e.g., guilt over passing mutation to children)	Current testing techniques and state of knowledge cannot classify all mutations as positive (deleterious) or negative	Strained relationships within the family
Potential for discrimination by employers, insurers, and state licensing agencies		
Financial costs of cancer screening and detection		
Positive tests predict risk of developing disease, not occurrence of cancer; age or time of developing cancer unknown		

*When there is a known mutation within the family.
Data from Lea, Jenkins, Francomano[26]; Loescher[67]; Rieger.[16]

other healthcare groups interested in genetic safeguards, was passed by the U.S. Senate in October 2003; as of August 2004, the House of Representatives had not taken action on it.[83,84]

Few, if any, cases of overt discrimination related to cancer genetic testing have been documented. Nevertheless, individuals' fears of discrimination have a direct impact on patients' willingness to seek genetic counseling and testing and on the practice of healthcare professionals.[77] Serious consideration must be given as to how results are documented, communicated, and managed to ensure confidentiality. Many institutions do not place results obtained from cancer predisposition genetic testing in the patient's medical record. In addition, they may require signed consent from the individual who has been tested to release or discuss results with family members, insurers, or other healthcare professionals. Table 7-6 lists questions patients should ask genetic testing providers.[67]

Management of Risk

The field of cancer prevention is changing rapidly, as information gleaned through better understanding of cancer at the molecular level and the ability to target those at the highest risk of developing cancer become integrated into new prevention and detection strategies. Because of the high lifetime risk for developing cancer associated with mutations in cancer predisposition genes, measures to manage risk for those carrying a mutation are a pressing issue. Options fall into three basic categories: (1) chemoprevention, (2) prophylactic surgery, and (3) screening and detection measures.

Chemoprevention

Preventive measures for those at high risk of developing cancer are just beginning to be evaluated. *Chemoprevention* is defined as the use of natural or synthetic chemical agents to reverse, suppress, or prevent carcinogenic progression to invasive cancer.[85] As more

Table 7-6 Questions for Patients to Ask During Cancer Genetic Counseling

Questions for Providers of Commercial Testing	Questions for Providers of Testing Performed as Research
• How much does the test cost?	• If the cost of testing is covered under the research protocol, what additional costs are borne by participants?
• Is payment for the test required at the time of testing?	• What is the turnaround time for receiving test results?
• What are the informed consent procedures for the test?	• Is the testing protocol approved by an IRB? Which IRB?
• Has the consent been approved by an institutional review board (IRB)?	• What are the informed consent procedures for the test? Have these been approved by an IRB?
• Is there established clinical/analytical validity of the test?	• Are protocols of tests in developmental phases being conducted in a laboratory certified under CLIA?
• Does the testing laboratory participate in internal or external (e.g., College of American Pathology molecular oncology program or American College of Medical Genetics medical genetics proficiency program) monitoring of procedures?	• Has a pilot phase been conducted verifying that all steps in the testing process are operating appropriately?
• Do laboratory personnel have formal training in human and medical genetics? Cancer genetics?	• Does the testing laboratory participate in internal or external monitoring of procedures?
• What types of follow-up data are/have been collected after marketing of the test?	• Do laboratory personnel have formal training in human and medical genetics? Cancer genetics?
• How is confidentiality maintained?	• How is confidentiality of results maintained?
• What are the qualifications of the personnel providing cancer genetic counseling?	• What are the qualifications of the personnel providing cancer genetic counseling?
• What type of support services are available?	• What type of support services are available?
• Are Clinical Laboratory Improvement Act (CLIA) regulations followed?	

Adapted with permission from Loescher LJ: DNA testing for cancer predisposition. *Oncol Nurs Forum* 25:1317–1327, 1998.[67]

is understood about the nature of carcinogenesis, the ability to intervene at the earliest stages is becoming a greater possibility. Recognition of dysplastic lesions as biologically significant at their preinvasive stage represents a paradigm shift that may lead to the design of effective prevention measures. In addition, study of the intrinsic biological mechanisms that may prevent these lesions from becoming invasive and metastatic can offer insight into the design of new, effective therapeutic strategies.[85–88]

Conceptually, chemoprevention agents may be classified into two categories: agents that prevent initiation of the carcinogenic process (blocking agents) and agents that prevent further promotion or progression of lesions that have already been established (suppressing agents). In reality, the distinction between these two categories is often artificial. Over the last 20 years, numerous trials have sought to evaluate the effectiveness of various agents in the chemoprevention of cancer.[86]

One example of how chemoprevention may potentially be applied to high-risk populations involves the use of nonsteroidal anti-inflammatory drugs (NSAIDs) for the prevention of colorectal cancer. Several large, observational, epidemiological studies for those who self-elect to take NSAIDs have demonstrated a lowering of the risk for colorectal cancer. Limitations of these studies are difficulty in controlling for confounding variables and lack of randomization. Nevertheless, based on these findings and those from basic research, the rationale for the use of NSAIDs in preventing colorectal cancer is supported.[89] The NCI has sponsored several chemoprevention trials using NSAIDs for the prevention of adenomas in those at high risk for developing colorectal cancer due to an inherited predisposition (FAP or HNPCC). Based on clinical research, celecoxib has received approval from the U.S. Food and Drug Administration (FDA)for use in decreasing the formation of colorectal polyps in patients with FAP.[90]

The finding of a decrease in contralateral breast cancer incidence following tamoxifen administration for adjuvant breast cancer therapy suggested that the drug might play a role in breast cancer prevention. To test this hypothesis, the National Surgical Adjuvant Breast and Bowel Project (NSABP) initiated the Breast Cancer Prevention Trial (BCPT) in 1992. Women at increased risk for breast cancer because they (1) were 60 years of age or older, (2) were 35–59 years of age with a five-year predicted risk for breast cancer of at least 1.67%, or (3) had a history of lobular carcinoma in situ were randomly assigned to receive placebo or tamoxifen 20 mg/day for five years. The Gail Model, based on a multivariate logistic regression model using combinations of risk factors, was used to estimate the probability (risk) of occurrence of breast cancer over time.

Results from the trial were publicly released in 1998. Tamoxifen reduced the risk of invasive breast cancer by 49%, with cumulative incidences through 69 months of follow-up of 43.4 and 22.0 per 1000 women in the placebo and tamoxifen groups, respectively. Risk was decreased 44% in women aged 49 years or younger, 51% in those aged 50–59 years, and 55% in those 60 years or older. Risk was also reduced 56% in women with a history of lobular carcinoma in situ and 86% in those with a history of atypical hyperplasia. In fact, risk was reduced in women in all risk categories. Tamoxifen reduced the risk of noninvasive breast cancer by 50% and the occurrence of estrogen receptor–positive tumors by 69%, though no difference in the occurrence of estrogen receptor–negative tumors was seen.[91] Although two small European trials failed to confirm the observations from the BCPT, tamoxifen received FDA approval for use in women at increased risk for developing breast cancer in 1998. Differences between these trials may result from reduced power in the smaller trials and different selection criteria.

The implications of these results for women who may be carriers of mutations in *BRCA1* or *BRCA2* were published in 2001, when King et al analyzed data from the NSABP prevention trial. Although the numbers were small, King et al suggested that tamoxifen would be less effective in *BRCA1* mutation carriers than in *BRCA2* mutation carriers. This seemed to make intuitive sense, as the vast majority of *BRCA1*-related cancers are found to be estrogen receptor–negative, while those found in *BRCA2* carriers are predominantly estrogen receptor–positive.[92] A study by Duffy and Nixon[93] confirmed this result in 2002 and suggested that individuals with *BRCA1* mutations should pursue an nonhormonal prevention strategy. Conversely, in 2002 Foulkes et al[94] disputed the use of tamoxifen only in *BRCA2* carriers when their study in Ashkenazi Jewish women showed a benefit of tamoxifen for *BRCA1* carriers. More research will likely be done on this subject to clarify the best chemoprevention strategies.

Oral contraceptives have been proven to protect against ovarian cancer in general, although further research is required to determine whether they also protect against hereditary forms of ovarian cancer. Narod et al enrolled 207 women with hereditary ovarian cancer and 161 of their sisters as controls in a case-control study.[95] Lifetime histories of oral contraceptive use were obtained by interview or by written questionnaire and were compared between patients and control women, after adjustment for year of birth and parity. Their results demonstrated that risk for developing ovarian cancer decreased with increasing duration of use of oral contraceptives. They concluded that oral contraceptive use may reduce the risk of ovarian cancer in women with pathogenic mutations in the *BRCA1* or *BRCA2* gene.[95] Modan and colleagues, in a subsequent study published in 2001, failed to confirm this result.[96] Although a risk reduction with oral contraceptive use was seen, the results were not statistically significant. Individualized management is important, and *BRCA1* and *BRCA2* mutation carriers considering using oral contraceptives must weigh the uncertain ovarian cancer risk-reducing potential against the possibility that breast cancer risk may be elevated.[97]

A number of early studies (animal and preclinical) are investigating the use of NSAIDs in prevention of ovarian cancer. In these studies, NSAIDS have been shown to inhibit ovulation, inhibit growth, and induce apoptosis.[98]

Prophylactic surgery

Many individuals faced with a high lifetime risk of developing cancer consider the option of prophylactic surgery as a means to manage their risk. This is particularly true in the cases of diseases for which surveillance/screening modalities do not pick up occult disease. For some conditions, such as FAP or hereditary medullary thyroid cancer, prophylactic surgery is accepted practice due to the high likelihood of developing cancer.[99] In other situations, such as hereditary breast and ovarian cancer, prophylactic surgery is more controversial. Although it is often assumed that prophylactic mastectomy will greatly decrease the risk of breast cancer, not all breast cells can realistically be removed. The precise degree of risk reduction associated with prophylactic mastectomy or oophorectomy has not yet been determined for individuals who carry a mutation that predisposes for breast or ovarian cancer. Individuals who choose the option of prophylactic mastectomy must realize that some risk remains.

Hartmann et al published results from a retrospective study of all women with a family history of breast cancer who underwent bilateral prophylactic mastectomy at the Mayo Clinic between 1960 and 1993.[100] The women were divided into two groups — high risk and moderate risk — on the basis of family history. A control study of the sisters of the high-risk probands and the Gail Model were used to predict the number of breast cancers expected in these two groups in the absence of prophylactic mastectomy. The study included 639 women with a family history of breast cancer who had undergone bilateral prophylactic mastectomy: 214 at high risk and 425 at moderate risk. Prophylactic mastectomy was associated with a reduction in the incidence of breast cancer of at least 90%. The authors concluded that in women with a high risk of breast cancer on the basis of family history, prophylactic mastectomy can significantly reduce the incidence of breast cancer. In 2001, Hartmann and colleagues published data that evaluated the risk-reduction benefit of surgery in women from this original group who tested positive for a mutation in the *BRCA1* or *BRCA2* gene; they concluded that prophylactic mastectomy provided a substantial reduction in risk.[101]

Prophylactic oophorectomy, with or without tubal ligation and hysterectomy, is becoming more common in women with *BRCA1/2* mutations as well as for individuals with HNPCC who carry a higher than normal risk of both ovarian and endometrial cancers. Because of the failure of CA-125 and ultrasound to diagnose early ovarian cancers when they may be curable, primary prevention through surgery is increasing. As in the case of prophylactic mastectomy, the risk reduction is not absolute (approximately 85%–95%). The benefit of oophorectomy appears to be greatest prior to the age of 60. Additionally, a reduction of risk of breast cancer of about 50% is found.[102,103] Early oophorectomy on the other hand, is complicated by an increased risk for osteoporosis and cardiovascular disease.

Two recent studies address the implications of proplylactic surgeries for women with *BRCA1/2* mutations. In the first study by Armstrong et al, a Markov decision analytic model used the most current epidemiologic data to assess the expected outcomes of prophylactic oophorectomy with or without HRT (to age 50 years or for life) in cohorts of women with *BRCA1/2* mutations. In this model, prophylactic oophorectomy lengthened life expectancy in women with *BRCA1/2* mutations, irrespective of whether HRT was used after oophorectomy. This gain ranged from 3.34 to 4.65 years, depending on the age at oophorectomy. On the basis of the results of this decision analysis, Armstrong and colleagues recommended that women with *BRCA1/2* mutations undergo prophylactic oophorectomy after completion of childbearing, decide about short-term HRT after oophorectomy based largely on quality-of-life issues rather than life expectancy, and, if using HRT, consider discontinuing treatment at the time of expected natural menopause, approximately age 50 years.[104]

A second study by Rebbeck and colleagues addressed the increased efficacy of prophylactic mastectomy when done at the same time as oophorectomy. In this case-control study, women who underwent a prophylactic mastectomy at the same time as oophorectomy or who had a previous oophorectomy had a 95% risk reduction as opposed to the 90% risk reduction observed in women with intact ovaries. In the control group, 48.7% of 378 matched controls who did not have the procedure developed breast cancer, with a mean follow-up of 6.4 years.[105]

Women who are carriers of a *BRCA1* or *BRCA2* mutation are at high risk for developing contralateral breast cancer; hence, bilateral mastectomy is increasingly considered a treatment option for newly diagnosed *BRCA1/2* carriers. A study by Schwartz and colleagues prospectively evaluated the impact on surgical decision making of pretreatment genetic counseling and *BRCA1* or *BRCA2* testing among breast cancer patients at high risk for carrying a mutation. Forty-eight percent of patients who were found to carry a *BRCA1/2* mutation chose bilateral mastectomy as their definitive breast cancer surgery. In contrast, 24% of patients in whom no mutation was detected and 4% of test decliners opted for bilateral mastectomy. Additional predictors of bilateral mastectomy included patients' self-reports of physician recommendations for *BRCA1/2* testing and bilateral mastectomy. This study highlights patient interest in, and the technical feasibility of, offering presurgery *BRCA1/2* testing to high-risk patients. Most importantly, these results demonstrate that *BRCA1/2* test results significantly affect patients' surgical decision making. The availability of genetic counseling and testing could serve as a valuable aid to decision making for newly diagnosed breast cancer patients at high risk for carrying a mutation.[106]

Prophylactic gastrectomy is also being employed for individuals with hereditary diffuse gastric cancer syndromes when mutations are identified in the *CDH1* gene. In a recent study, prevention of gastric cancer for young, asymptomatic carriers of *CDH1* involved gastrectomy. Results indicated that four of five individuals who had surgery had occult gastric cancer.[107]

Clearly, there is a need for studies of quality of life and evaluations by multidisciplinary teams for those contemplating prophylactic surgeries, as the risks of the surgeries and their sequelae are real and need to be assessed.

Screening and detection

Another option for risk management is more aggressive cancer screening beginning at an earlier age and at more frequent intervals for individuals who are at increased risk for cancer due to inheritance of a mutated cancer predisposition gene. Tables 7-7[21,97] and 7-8[21,43] review the recommended risk management strategies. Clinical trials to determine the most appropriate surveillance measures for those carrying mutated cancer susceptibility genes and the development of newer and more sensitive screening tests remain a high priority. Two methods for the early detection of breast cancer currently in clinical trials include ductal lavage and magnetic resonance imaging (MRI).

Ductal lavage involves introducing a small catheter into the milk ducts in the nipple and flushing the duct with saline solution. The cells are collected and cytologically examined. Although a series involving *BRCA1/2* mutation carriers has not been published, a body of literature exists showing that women with atypical ductal epithelial cells have an elevated risk of developing breast cancer and that ductal lavage is a safe

Table 7-7 Options for Cancer Prevention/Detection in Carriers of *BRCA1* and *BRCA2* Mutations

Chemoprevention
No known chemoprevention methods
Discuss option of entrance into chemoprevention trials
Data indicate that oral contraceptive pills may decrease the risk of ovarian cancer; the impact on breast cancer is unclear
Data on efficacy of tamoxifen in decreasing risk for developing breast cancer continue to emerge
Prophylactic Surgery
Discuss options and limitations of prophylactic mastectomy
Evidence suggests 90% reduction of risk
Discuss options and limitations of prophylactic oophorectomy
Evidence suggests 85%–95% reduction of risk for ovarian cancer, 50% for breast cancer
Screening
Instruction in breast self-exam
Perform monthly beginning at age 18 years
Clinical breast exam
Annual or semiannual beginning at age 25 years
Mammography
Annual beginning at age 25 years
MRI may be more sensitive, less specific
CA-125 blood level
Semiannual beginning at age 30–40 years*
Transvaginal ultrasound with color Doppler imaging
Semiannual beginning at age 30–40 years*

*May be considered at 25–35 years.
Data from Offit[21]; Offit, Garber, Greene, et al.[97]

and well-tolerated procedure and is a more sensitive method of detecting cellular atypia than nipple aspiration.[108] Hollingsworth and colleagues proposed that quantitative risk assessment is part of basic breast care and comprehensive management includes a discussion of the following: ductal lavage for improved risk stratification, multiple options for risk reduction, and high-risk surveillance strategies that might incorporate investigational imaging protocols.[109] More research is needed to determine the sensitivity and specificity of this technique for detection of malignancy or as a marker of risk.

It is well known that mammograms for young women are often not reliable because of the increased density of their breasts. Breast screening of young women who are at risk because of a *BRCA1/2* mutation has proved challenging. MRI has been studied for its utility in this setting.[110,111] In the largest study to date, results of the Dutch MRI Screening study (MRISC) were presented in the plenary session at the American Society of Clinical Oncology's annual meeting in 2003. More than 1900 women were screened, including al-

Table 7-8 Options for Cancer Prevention/Detection in Carriers of Mutations Causing HNPCC

Chemoprevention
No known chemoprevention methods
Discuss option of entrance into chemoprevention trials
Preliminary data indicate that use of nonsteroidal anti-inflammatory agents may decrease risk of cancer and formation of polyps
Prophylactic Surgery
Discuss options of prophylactic colectomy
Generally discussed following diagnosis of cancer or detection of adenomas
Discuss options of prophylactic hysterectomy/oophorectomy
Screening
Colonoscopy
Annually beginning at age 20–25 years (or 5 years before earliest onset in family)
Endometrial aspirate*
Annual beginning at age 25–35 years
Transvaginal ultrasound (endometrial cancer)*
Annual beginning at age 25–35 years

HNPCC = hereditary nonpolyposis colon cancer.
*Benefits unproven.
Data from Offit[21]; Offit, Garber, Greene, et al.[43]

most 300 proven *BRCA1/2* mutation carriers. MRI appears to be extraordinarily sensitive in detecting abnormalities (more so than mammography), although its lack of specificity may make additional procedures necessary. MRI is able to detect tumors less than 1 cm.[112] Larger prospective studies to examine the role of MRI in screening programs are justified.

Models for Cancer Risk Counseling Programs

As the integration of genetic information into the management of patients with cancer continues, there will be an increasing need for clinical services that provide cancer genetic counseling and address issues related to predisposition genetic testing for cancer susceptibility genes. There exists no standard model of a cancer risk evaluation program that specifically addresses the unique issues associated with genetic testing. An effective program would include clinical and psychosocial assessment, education, individualized cancer risk analysis, and genetic counseling, in addition to long-term screening and surveillance for cancer, preferably within the context of a strong prevention program. Large academic centers should provide a forum for ongoing genetic and clinical research. In many institutions, centers providing cancer genetic counseling services are housed within prevention centers, as opposed to disease site centers. As described earlier, cancer predisposition genes predispose to patterns of cancer that often do not respect current disease site boundaries. For example, women with HNPCC who are followed in a gastrointestinal clinic may not receive adequate surveillance for gynecologic cancers, such as endometrial and ovarian cancer, and vice versa. Utilizing a multidisciplinary mix of healthcare professionals is important so that patients will have full access to a range of professional services and skills.[21,113]

Implications for Oncology Nurses

As advances in technology continue to yield new methods of prevention, diagnosis, detection, and treatment of cancer, part of our professional responsibility as nurses is to expand our level of knowledge. Additionally, the abundance of information available to patients through the media and newer resources such as the Internet challenge us more than ever to keep up the pace of learning. All licensed registered nurses, regardless of their practice setting, will have a role in the delivery of genetic services and the management of genetic information. Nurses will require genetic knowledge to identify, refer, support, and care for persons affected by or at risk for manifesting or transmitting genetic conditions.[49]

As part of the nursing assessment, the family history should always be evaluated. Determination of the number of affected relatives and the age at diagnosis of cancer may provide clues to the possible existence of a hereditary cancer syndrome. How many first-degree relatives (e.g., mother, sibling, father) and second-degree relatives (e.g., aunt, grandmother) are affected with cancer or, more specifically, cancers that are part of a known syndrome? Are there characteristics of a hereditary cancer syndrome in the family? Not all oncology nurses will be experts in this new area. Nevertheless, knowledge and awareness of hereditary cancer syndromes will help in the identification of patients who should be referred to a specialized cancer risk assessment clinic for further evaluation and counseling. As a general rule, patients should be referred for further evaluation if they meet any of the following criteria:

- They have more than two first-degree relatives affected by similar cancers.
- They are members of families characterized by a high rate of cancer.
- They have features of hereditary cancers (e.g., young age at onset).
- They have relatives with rare cancers, such as retinoblastoma.
- They have relatives with a known mutation in a cancer susceptibility gene.

Knowing that tests are now available to identify some of the genes that predispose to the development of cancer can be useful in answering questions and referring individuals to appropriate resources for more specific information.

We are living in the age of information, in which knowledge multiplies exponentially. It is impossible to remain an expert in all areas of cancer care. One of an oncology nurse's greatest assets, therefore, is awareness of available resources. We may not have all the answers to questions raised by individuals who seek healthcare services, but we can direct them to the person, clinic, or source that will be able to answer their questions. In cancer genetics, we might begin by identifying experts in our institution, city, county, or state who provide cancer risk assessment and counseling. The NCI's Web site provides an online resource for the identification of professionals who provide cancer genetic counseling services across the United States. Nurses who specialize in the provision of cancer genetic counseling services can be identified through professional organizations such as the Oncology Nursing Society, which has a special-interest group in cancer genetics, or the International Society of Nurses in Genetics. These societies also serve as resources for information and continuing education,[16,21,114] Table 7-9 shows a partial list of current Web sites that address questions related to inherited cancers and genetic testing and that provide general information on genetics and cancer. Another excellent starting point is the NCI's information line (800-4CANCER).

Following evaluation at a specialized center, patients may return to a primary care provider or be referred to an oncologist for cancer screening and detection services. Nurse practitioners can provide physical assessments, coordinate and evaluate cancer screening examinations based on an individual's level of risk, and serve as a source of psychosocial support for those patients found to be carriers of a mutated cancer susceptibility gene. Both basic and advanced practice nurses can encourage and support patients in health-promoting behaviors and cancer screening and detection practices.

A new role for oncology nurses in the future will be to participate in the provision of cancer genetic counseling. Genetic counselors are healthcare professionals who provide information and support to families who may be at risk for a variety of inherited conditions.

Table 7-9 Genetic Resources for Healthcare Professionals

Societies

International Society of Nurses in Genetics (ISONG)
ISONG c/o Jean Anderson, Executive Director
2593 West 15th Street South
Newton, IA 50208-8500
janderson@isong.us
www.isong.org

Oncology Nursing Society
Cancer Genetics Special Interest Group
Position statements, educational materials
125 Enterprise Drive
Pittsburgh, PA 15275-1214
412-859-6100
www.ons.org

American Society of Clinical Oncology
Position statement, educational materials
1900 Duke Street, Ste 200
Alexandria, VA 22314
703-299-0150
www.asco.org

Web Sites

GeneTests: A national directory of DNA diagnostic laboratories; designed for healthcare providers; computerized directory of laboratories providing DNA diagnosis for clinical services and research. Requires registration.
www.genetests.org/

Genetics Education Center, University of Kansas Medical Center
www.kumc.edu/gec/

Blazing a Genetic Trail: online tutorial on human genetics
www.hhmi.org/genetictrail/start.htm

National Human Genome Research Institute
www.nhgri.nih.gov

National Cancer Institute
www.nci.nih.gov

Facing Our Risk Cancer Empowered (Force) Advocacy Group
www.facingourrisk.org

Search for genetic professionals
http://cancernet.nci.nih.gov/

Oncolink
www.oncolink.upenn.edu

Cancer Information Network
www.cancernetwork.com/

Stanford Human Genome Center
www-shgc.stanford.edu/

Understanding Gene Testing Book: online
www.cancer.gov/newscenterpublicationslocater

Secretary's Advisory Committee on Genetics, Health, and Society
www4.od.nih.gov/oba

Johns Hopkins University Genetics and Public Policy Center
www.dnapolicy.org

Hum-Molgen: International communication forum
www.hum-molgen.org

U.S. Department of Energy Genome Programs
www.doegenomes.org/

National Coalition for Health Professional Education in Genetics
www.nchpeg.org

Online Mendelian Inheritance in Man (OMIM): Catalogue of human genes and genetic disorders
www.ncbi.nlm.nih.gov/omim

Traditionally, genetic counselors have focused on prenatal counseling and, until recently, few have specialized in cancer risk assessment and counseling. The anticipated need for qualified healthcare professionals who can provide genetic counseling services, especially in cancer care, is expected to far exceed the number of genetic counselors who are qualified and trained to provide these services. Oncology nurses, because of their extensive background in cancer care and complement of professional skills, are well suited to assume these roles with appropriate specialized training and to participate fully as members of the multidisciplinary team providing cancer risk assessment and counseling services.[50] It is the position of both the Oncology Nursing Society and the International Society of Nurses in Genetics that counseling should be provided by advanced practice nurses with a master's degree or higher.[49,62] Oncology nurses with additional training in cancer genetics could also provide services at the basic level for individuals at increased risk for developing cancer and work closely with advanced practice nurses and physicians. The critical elements that distinguish advanced- from basic-level genetics nursing practice are the complexity of decision making, leadership, the ability to negotiate complex organizations, and expanded practice skills and knowledge in nursing and genetics.[48] Specialized practitioners at both the basic and the advanced levels would serve as professional resources and educators to both nursing colleagues and other healthcare professionals.

Future Directions

The rapid pace of the acquisition of knowledge related to cancer biology and causation and cancer genetics shows no signs of slowing. Global issues that relate to cancer risk assessment and counseling include improvement in testing technology, populational screening, management of information, timing of testing, and training of healthcare professionals to provide cancer genetic counseling services.

New Technology for Testing

New technologies are being developed that will provide more accurate results in a shorter period of time, test for multiple genes at once, and cost less. One exciting area of research is DNA chip technology. DNA chips are similar in construction and concept to the chips used in computers. The minute chips are filled with dense grids of DNA probes (i.e., short stretches of DNA). Extracts from cells are incubated with the chips so that gene fragments will bind to the DNA probes on the chips. The probes on the chips can be thought of as ''molecular tweezers,'' picking out gene fragments for which they are tailored or matched. For example, probes could be designed to pick out known alterations in genes associated with hereditary cancer syndromes or other diseases. Currently, a DNA chip is being marketed to detect *p53* mutations, the most common genetic mutation in human cancers; chips to detect *BRCA1* and *BRCA2* mutations are also being evaluated. In the future, DNA from a few cells might be placed in a DNA gene chip scanner and quickly analyzed to determine a person's risk for developing numerous diseases. Other areas of research include customizing cancer therapy for individuals by ''profiling'' them to identify all the genetic defects present and designing gene therapy to correct defects.[68,115,116]

Populational Screening

Genetic screening is the application of genetic testing to specific populations, independent of a family history of a disorder. Identification of individuals with a genetic condition, prior to the onset of symptoms, can allow for more effective treatment planning. This currently occurs for some diseases such as phenylketonuria. As the relationship between genes and disease continues to unfold, a determination must be made as to which diseases require genetic screening. Hence, discussions of genetics will become part of public policy debates. The ability of decision makers to balance such factors as benefits, costs, privacy, and other ethical considerations, as well as management of those found to be at risk for disease, will be paramount. Genetic screening may become possible for a multitude of single-gene diseases as well as multifactorial diseases such as cancer and heart disease. Nurses in a variety of settings may participate in discussions of relevant information that will allow individuals to make informed decisions and so should participate in the establishment of public policy.[3,26]

Information Management

How to manage the information obtained from genetic testing will remain a relevant issue in the near future. Who should have access to results will continue to be debated. Until individual fears related to potential discrimination when attempting to obtain health, life, mortgage, or disability insurance because of information obtained from genetic testing are addressed and conquered, appropriate handling of genetic information will remain a contentious issue. While no cases of genetic testing–related discrimination with respect to health insurance have yet been documented in the United States, in some countries genetic information is being used to guide decisions regarding life insurance. Cassells and colleagues published an ethical assessment framework for addressing global genetic issues in clinical practice in 2003.[117]

Timing of Testing

The question of when to test for genes that predispose for the development of cancer will continue to be posed. Should children be tested for adult-onset disease? Is it ethical to test for genes that predispose for cancer in the prenatal setting? Should prospective parents be allowed to request genetic testing on children they are considering adopting? Predictive genetic testing of apparently healthy children has been urged as a way to generate information about children's future health and to assist families in deciding whether to adopt. In January 2004, the Genetics and Public Policy Center convened a forum on preimplantation genetics and its evolving use in society.[118] In some diseases, such as multiple endocrine neoplasia types 2A and 2B and FAP, children are tested so that preventive measures such as prophylactic surgery can be taken at a young age.[82] However, the point at which testing should occur (e.g., upon diagnosis of a disease such as medullary thyroid cancer, at birth, or some other time prior to diagnosis of a disease) has yet to be determined. Genetic tests may offer medical or psychological benefits but may also create harm. Potential risks include stigmatization and alteration of the child's self-concept or of parent–child bonds.

Training of Healthcare Professionals

The need exists to train healthcare professionals concerning genetics and the integration of genetic information into practice. Today, few nurses receive education in basic genetic concepts during their training. A study funded by the HGP was one of the first to assess the ways in which nurses in the United States are currently managing genetic information. Fewer than 10% of nurses had a course in basic genetics during their basic nursing education, while almost 70% thought a course in human genetics should be required.[119] Future challenges will include integrating basic genetics into nursing programs as well as educating the millions of nurses currently practicing.

With respect to cancer genetics, debate continues as to the amount and type of education required to provide cancer genetic counseling services. Currently, no specially trained healthcare professional provides these services. While most oncology specialists (e.g., nurses and physicians) are knowledgeable in the field of oncology, few have received formal genetic education during their training. Conversely, few genetic counselors or clinical geneticists have received specialized training in oncology. The majority of professionals who currently practice in the field of cancer genetic counseling have acquired specific components of the required expertise through additional training, education, and clinical practice. Still undetermined are the amount of additional training required for each discipline and the best way to certify ''competence.'' Several initiatives are under way to address issues specific to cancer genetics and global genetic issues related to medical and nursing practice.

The National Coalition for Health Professional Education in Genetics (NCHPEG) is a consortium of leaders from approximately 120 diverse healthcare professional organizations, consumer and volunteer groups, government agencies, industry, managed care organizations, and genetics professional organizations. The idea for NCHPEG was catalyzed by the American Medical Association, the American Nurses Association, and the National Human Genome Research Institute in an effort to provide an organized, systematic, and national approach to the provision of genetics education to all healthcare professionals. The coalition's mission is to ensure that our U.S. healthcare providers have the knowledge, skills, and resources needed to effectively and responsibly integrate new genetic knowledge and technologies into the prevention, diagnosis, and management of disease.[120] Since its inception, NCHPEG has held annual meetings with a focus on topics ranging from religion in genetics to competencies in practice. Its Web site is an excellent resource for educational materials and a review of current and completed projects.

Both the Oncology Nursing Society and the American Society of Clinical Oncology have numerous initiatives targeted toward education of healthcare professionals in cancer genetics. The American Society of Clinical Oncology has published the second edition of its curriculum on genetics, has developed position statements, and continues to offer education targeted toward cancer genetics at its annual meeting. The Oncology Nursing Society held a ''think tank'' session on cancer genetics in 1996 to review the impact of advances in cancer genetics on oncology nursing and to develop strategies to address issues related to genetic testing in patients with cancer, ranging from basic education of Society members to ethics. Since that time, it has developed position statements, online courses, and published texts, and it offers continuing education in genetics at its annual meeting.

While not all oncology nurses will assume new specialized roles in genetic counseling, nurses must be aware of the changes and discoveries being made. The oncology nurse of the future will use this new knowledge to assess patients for a history of cancer within the family, to refer patients to appropriate resources and care centers, to support individuals who are found to be at increased risk for developing cancer, and to educate patients about the application of genetics to cancer care. Ultimately, the integration of genetics into cancer care will guide all aspects of the management of cancer: risk assessment, prevention, detection, prognostics, and treatment.[3,121] Today, we continue to prepare ourselves, and our profession, for a new era in cancer care.

References

1. Jenkins J, Masny A: Why should oncology nurses be interested in genetics?, in Straus Tranin A, Masny A, Jenkins J (eds.): *Genetics in Oncology Practice: Cancer Risk Assessment.* Pittsburgh, Oncology Nursing Society, 2003, pp 1–12
2. Greco KE: Cancer genetics nursing: impact of the double helix. *Oncol Nurs Forum* 27 (suppl):29–36, 2000
3. Collins FS, Green ED, Guttmacher AE: A vision for the future of genomic research. *Nature* 422:835–847, 2003
4. Collins FS, McKusick VA: Implications of the Human Genome Project for medical science. *JAMA* 285:540–544, 2001
5. A decade of ELSI research: a celebration of the first ten years of the Ethical, Legal, and Social Implications (ELSI) programs. *J Law Med Ethics* 29 (suppl):1–65, 2001
6. Thun MJ, Jemal A: Cancer epidemiology, in Kufe DW, Pollock RE, Weichselbaum RR, et al (eds.): *Cancer Medicine.* Hamilton, Ontario, BC Decker, 2003, pp 367–382
7. Perera FP: Molecular epidemiology: on the path to prevention? *J Natl Cancer Inst* 92:602–612, 2000
8. Iglehart JD, Miron A, Rimer BK, et al: Overestimation of hereditary breast cancer risk. *Ann Surg* 228:375–384, 1998
9. Loescher LJ: Cancer worry in women with hereditary risk factors for breast cancer. *Oncol Nurs Forum* 30:767–772, 2003

10. Vogel VG: Breast cancer risk factors and preventive approaches to breast cancer, in Kavanagh JJ, Singletary SE, Einhorn N, DePetrillo AD (eds.): *Cancer in Women.* Malden, MA, Blackwell Science, 1998, pp 58–91
11. Offitt K, Garber JE, Greene MH, et al: Cancer risk assessment and the genetic testing process, in Offitt K, Garber JE, Greene MH, et al (eds.): *ASCO Curriculum Cancer Genetics and Cancer Predisposition Testing* (ed 2). Alexandria, VA, ASCO Publishing, 2004, pp 3-1–3-50
12. Mahon SM: Cancer risk assessment: conceptual considerations for clinical practice. *Oncol Nurs Forum* 25:1535–1547, 1998
13. Loescher LJ: The family history component of cancer genetic risk counseling. *Cancer Nurs* 22:96–102, 1999
14. Rich EC, Burke W, Heaton CJ, et al: Reconsidering the family history in primary care. *J Gen Intern Med* 19:273–280, 2004
15. Ziogas A, Anton-Culver H: Validation of family history data in cancer family registries. *Am J Prev Med* 24:190–198, 2003
16. Rieger PT: Counseling about the genetics of breast cancer, in Vogel VG, Bevers T (eds.): *Handbook of Breast Cancer Risk-Assessment.* Sudbury, MA, Jones and Bartlett, 2003, pp 146–169
17. Claus EB, Risch N, Thompson WD: Autosomal dominant inheritance of early-onset breast cancer: implications for risk prediction. *Cancer* 73:643–651, 1994
18. Benichou J, Gail MH, Mulvihill JJ: Graphs to estimate an individualized risk of breast cancer. *J Clin Oncol* 14:103–110, 1996
19. Domchek SM, Eisen A, Calzone K, et al: Application of breast cancer risk prediction models in clinical practice. *J Clin Oncol* 21:593–601, 2003
20. Offitt K, Garber JE, Greene MH, et al: Overview of cancer genetics, in Offitt K, Garber JE, Greene MH, et al (eds.): *ASCO Curriculum Cancer Genetics and Cancer Predisposition Testing* (ed 2). Alexandria, VA, ASCO Publishing, 2004, pp 1-1–1-68
21. Offit K: *Clinical Cancer Genetics: Risk Counseling and Management.* New York, Wiley-Liss, 1998
22. American Society of Clinical Oncology: Appendix: genetic differential diagnoses by organ system neoplasms. *www.asco.org/ac/1,1003,_12-002519-00_18-0028816-00_19-0028817-00_20-001,00.asp,* Accessed August 30, 2004
23. Lindor NM, Greene MH: The concise handbook of family cancer syndromes. Mayo Familial Cancer Program. *J Natl Cancer Inst* 90:1039–1071, 1998
24. Knudson A: Hereditary cancer: Theme and variations. *J Clin Oncol* 15:3280–3287, 1997
25. National Institutes of Health and National Cancer Institute: *Understanding Gene Testing.* NIH Publication no. 96–3905. Washington, DC, U.S. Department of Health and Human Services, 1995
26. Lea DH, Jenkins JL, Francomano C: *Genetics in Clinical Practice: New Directions for Nursing and Healthcare.* Sudbury, MA, Jones and Bartlett, 1998
27. Knudson AG: Cancer genetics. *Am J Med Genet* 111:96–102, 2002
28. Venkitaraman AR: Cancer susceptibility and the functions of BRCA1 and BRCA2. *Cell* 31:55–59, 2002
29. Hall JM, Lee MK, Newman B, et al: Linkage of early-onset familial breast cancer to chromosome 17q21. *Science* 250:1684–1689, 1990
30. Narod SA, Feunteun J, Lynch HT, et al: Familial breast-ovarian cancer locus on chromosome 17q12–q23. *Lancet* 338:82–83, 1991
31. Wooster R, Neuhausen SL, Mangion J, et al: Localization of a breast cancer susceptibility gene, BRCA2, to chromosome 13q12–13. *Science* 265:2088–2090, 1994
32. Miki Y, Swensen J, Shattuck-Eidens D, et al: Isolation of BRCA1, the 17q-linked breast and ovarian cancer susceptibility gene. *Science* 266:66–71, 1994
33. Wooster R, Bignell G, Lancaster J, et al: Identification of the breast cancer susceptibility gene BRCA2. *Nature* 378:789–792, 1995
34. Thull DL, Vogel VG: Recognition and management of hereditary breast cancer syndromes. *The Oncologist* 9:13–24, 2004
35. King MC, Marks JH, Mandall JB, et al: Breast and ovarian cancer risks due to inherited mutations in BRCA1 and BRCA2. *Science* 302:643–645, 2003
36. Begg CB: On the use of familial aggregation in population-based case probands for calculating penetrance. *J Natl Cancer Inst* 94:1221–1226, 2002
37. Easton DF, Ford D, Bishop T, et al: Breast and ovarian cancer incidence in BRCA1-mutation carriers. *Am J Hum Genet* 56:2265–2271, 1995
38. Streuwing JP, Hartge P, Wacholder S, et al: The risk of cancer associated with specific mutations of BRCA1 and BRCA2 among Ashkenazi Jews. *N Engl J Med* 336:1401–1408, 1997
39. Liede A, Karlan BY, Narod SA: Cancer risks for male carriers of germline mutations in BRCA1 and BRCA2: a review of the literature. *J Clin Oncol* 22:735–742, 2004
40. Frank TS, Manley SA, Olopade OI, et al: Sequence analysis of BRCA1 and BRCA2: correlation of mutations with family history and ovarian cancer risk. *J Clin Oncol* 16:2417–2425, 1998
41. Bronner CE, Baker SM, Morrison PT, et al: Mutation in the DNA mismatch repair gene homologue hMLH1 is associated with hereditary nonpolyposis colon cancer. *Nature* 368:258–261, 1994
42. Liu B, Parson RE, Hamilton ST, et al: hMSH2 mutations in hereditary nonpolyposis colorectal cancer kindreds. *Cancer Res* 54:4590–4594, 1994
43. Offitt K, Garber JE, Greene MH, et al: Hereditary gastrointestinal cancer syndromes, in Offitt K, Garber JE, Greene MH, et al (eds.): *ASCO Curriculum Cancer Genetics and Cancer Predisposition Testing* (ed 2). Alexandria, VA, ASCO Publishing, 2004, pp 5-1–5-69
44. Rodriguez-Bigas MA, Boland CR, Hamilton SR, et al: A National Cancer Institute Workshop on Hereditary Nonpolyposis Colorectal Cancer Syndrome: meeting highlights and Bethesda guidelines. *J Natl Cancer Inst* 89:1758–1762, 1997
45. Boland CR, Thibodeau SN, Hamilton SR, et al: A National Cancer Institute Workshop on Microsatellite Instability for cancer detection and familial predisposition: development of international criteria for the determination of microsatellite instability in colorectal cancer. *Cancer Res* 58:5248–5257, 1998
46. Umar A, Boland R, Terdiman JP, et al: Commentary: revised Bethesda guidelines for hereditary nonpolyposis colorectal cancer (Lynch syndrome) and microsatellite instability. *J Natl Cancer Inst* 96:261–268, 2004
47. Hernegger GS, Moore HD, Guillem JG: Attenuated familial adenomatous polyposis: an evolving and poorly understood entity. *Dis Colon Rectum* 45:127–136, 2002
48. Peterson SK, Rieger PT, Marani SK, et al: Oncology nurse's knowledge, practice and educational needs regarding cancer genetics. *Am J Med Genet* 98:3–12, 2001
49. International Society of Nurses in Genetics, American Nurses Association: *Statement on the Scope and Standards of Genetics Clinical Nursing Practice.* Washington, DC, American Nurses Publishing, 1998
50. Greco K: How to provide genetic counseling and education, in Straus Tranin A, Masny A, Jenkins J (eds.): *Genetics in Oncology Practice: Cancer Risk Assessment.* Pittsburgh, Oncology Nursing Society, 2003, pp 189–224
51. Calzone KA, Masny A: Genetics and the oncology nurse. *Semin Oncol Nurs* 20:178–185, 2004
52. Doak CC, Doak LG, Friedell GH, et al: Improving comprehension for cancer patients with low literacy skills: strategies for clinicians. *CA Cancer J Clin* 48:151–162, 1998

53. Morra ME, Grant M: Cancer patient education. *Semin Oncol Nurs* 7:77–145, 1991
54. Baty BJ, Yeomans Kinney A, Ellis SM: Developing culturally sensitive cancer genetics communication aids for African Americans. *Am J Med Genet* 118A:146–155, 2003
55. American Society of Clinical Oncology: American Society of Clinical Oncology policy statement update: genetic testing for cancer susceptibility. *J Clin Oncol* 21:1–10, 2003
56. Rieger PT, Pentz RB: Genetic testing and informed consent. *Semin Oncol Nurs* 15:104–115, 1999
57. Calzone KA, Biesecker BB: Genetic testing for cancer predisposition. *Cancer Nurs* 25:15–25, 2002
58. Bove C, Fry ST, MacDonald DJ: Presymptomatic and predisposition genetic testing: ethical and social considerations. *Semin Oncol Nurs* 13:135–140, 1997
59. Geller G, Botkin JR, Green MJ, et al: Genetic testing for susceptibility to adult-onset cancer: The process and content of informed consent. *JAMA* 277:1471–1474, 1997
60. American Society of Human Genetics Social Issues Subcommittee on Familial Disclosure: ASHG statement on professional disclosure of familial genetic information. *Am J Hum Genet* 62:474–483, 1998
61. National Society of Genetic Counselors I: Predisposition genetic testing for late-onset disorders in adults. *JAMA* 278:1217–1220, 1997
62. Oncology Nursing Society: ONS position: the role of the oncology nurse in cancer genetic counseling. *Oncol Nurs Forum* 25:463, 1998
63. American Society of Clinical Oncology: Resource document for curriculum development in cancer genetics education. *J Clin Oncol* 15:2157–2169, 1997
64. Oncology Nursing Society: ONS position statement: cancer genetic testing and risk assessment counseling. *Oncol Nurs Forum* 25:464, 1998
65. Genetics and Public Policy Center: Berman Bioethics Institute Johns Hopkins University. *www.DNApolicy.org*. Accessed August 30, 2004
66. Jacobs LA: Hereditary nonpolyposis colon cancer: genetic basis, testing, and patient-care issues. *Oncol Nurs Forum* 25:719–725, 1998
67. Loescher LJ: DNA testing for cancer predisposition. *Oncol Nurs Forum* 25:1317–1327, 1998
68. Offitt K, Garber JE, Greene MH, et al: Clinical laboratory methods for cancer genetic susceptibility testing, in Offitt K, Garber JE, Greene MH, et al (eds.): *ASCO Curriculum Cancer Genetics and Cancer Predisposition Testing* (ed 2). Alexandria, VA, ASCO Publishing, 2004, pp 2-1–2-54
69. Wong N, Lasko D, Rabelo R, et al: Genetic counseling and interpretation of genetic tests in familial adenomatous polyposis and hereditary nonpolyposis colorectal cancer. *Dis Colon Rectum* 44:271–279, 2001
70. Petrucelli N, Lazebnik N, Huelsman KM, et al: Clinical interpretation and recommendations for patients with a variant of uncertain significance in BRCA1 or BRCA2: a survey of genetic counseling practice. *Genet Test* 6:107–113, 2002
71. Evans DG, Burnell LD, Hopwood P, et al: Perception of risk in women with a family history of breast cancer. *Br J Cancer.* 67:612–614, 1993
72. Evans DG, Blair V, Greenhalgh R, et al: The impact of genetic counselling on risk perception in women with a family history of breast cancer. *Br J Cancer* 70:934–938, 1994
73. Hopwood P, Shenton A, Lalloo F, et al: Risk perception and cancer worry: an exploratory study of the impact of genetic risk counselling in women with a family history of breast cancer. *J Med Genetics* 38:139–142, 2001
74. Schwartz MD, Peskin BN, Hughes C, et al: Impact of BRCA1/BRCA2 mutation testing on psychologic distress in a clinic-based sample. *J Clin Oncol* 20:514–520, 2002
75. Esplen MJ, Madlensky L, Butler K, et al: Motivations and psychosocial impact of genetic testing for HNPCC. *Am J Med Genet* 103:9–15, 2001
76. Hutson SP: Attitudes and psychological impact of genetic testing, genetic counseling, and breast cancer risk assessment among women at increased risk. *Oncol Nurs Forum* 30:241–246, 2003
77. Lerman C, Shields AE: Genetic testing for cancer susceptibility: the promise and the pitfalls. *Nat Rev Cancer* 4:235–241, 2004
78. Slaughter LM: Genetic information must remain private to prevent discrimination, spur research. *Gene Test* 2:17–35, 1998
79. Jacobs LA: At-risk for cancer: genetic discrimination in the workplace. *Oncol Nurs Forum* 25:475–480, 1998
80. Giarelli E, Jacobs LA: Issues related to the use of genetic material and information. *Oncol Nurs Forum* 27:459–476, 2000
81. Fleischer LD, Cole LJ: Health Insurance Portability and Accountability Act is here: what price privacy? *Genet Med* 3:286–289, 2001
82. Offitt K, Garber JE, Greene MH, et al: Ethical, legal, and social issues in cancer genetic testing, in Offitt K, Garber JE, Greene MH, et al (eds.): *ASCO Curriculum Cancer Genetics and Cancer Predisposition Testing* (ed 2). Alexandria, VA, ASCO Publishing, 2004, pp 4-1–4-39
83. National Human Genome Research Institute: Policy and ethics, health insurance and employment discrimination. *www.genome.gov*. Accessed August 30, 2004
84. Library of Congress. Thomas: legislative information on the Internet. *http://thomas.loc.gov*. Accessed August 30, 2004
85. Sporn MB, Dunlop NM, Newton DL, et al: Prevention of chemical carcinogenesis by vitamin A and its synthetic analogs (retinoids). *Fed Proc* 35:1332–1338, 1976
86. Sporn MB, Lippman SM: Chemoprevention of cancer, in Kufe DW, Pollock RE, Weichselbaum RR, et al: (eds.): *Cancer Medicine,* (ed 6). Hamilton, Ontario, BC Decker, 2003, pp 413–422
87. Hong WK, Spitz MR, Lippman SM: Cancer chemoprevention in the 21st century: genetics, risk modeling and molecular targets. *J Clin Oncol* 18 (suppl):9S–18S, 2000
88. Foltz AT, Mahon SM: Application of carcinogenesis theory to primary prevention. *Oncol Nurs Forum* 27 (suppl):5–11, 2000
89. Lee IM, Hennekens CH, Buring JE: Use of aspirin and other nonsteroidal antiinflammatory drugs and the risk of cancer development, in Devita VT, Hellman S, Rosenberg SA (eds.): *Cancer: Principles and Practice of Oncology* (ed 5). Philadelphia, Lippincott-Raven, 1997, pp 599–607
90. Steinbach G, Lynch PM, Phillips RK, et al: The effect of celecoxib, a cyclooxygenase-2 inhibitor, in familial adenomatous polyposis. *N Engl J Med* 342:1946–1952, 2000
91. Fisher B, Costantino JP, Wickerham DL, et al: Tamoxifen for prevention of breast cancer: report of the National Surgical Adjuvant Breast and Bowel Project P-1 Study. *J Natl Cancer Inst* 90:1371–1388, 1998
92. King MC, Wieant S, Hale K, et al: Tamoxifen and breast cancer incidence among women with inherited mutations in BRCA1 and BRCA2: National Surgical Adjuvant Breast and Bowel Progect (NSABP-1) Breast Cancer Prevention Trial. *JAMA* 286:2251–2256, 2001
93. Duffy SW, Nixon RM: Estimates of the likely prophylactic effect of tamoxifen in women with high risk BRCA1 and BRCA2 mutations. *Br J Cancer* 86:218–221, 2002
94. Foulkes WE, Goffin J, Brunet JS, et al: Tamoxifen may be an effective adjuvant treatment for BRCA1-related breast cancer irrespective of estrogen receptor status [correspondence]. *J Natl Cancer Inst* 94:1504–1506, 2002

95. Narod SA, Risch H, Moslehi R, et al: Oral contraceptives and the risk of hereditary ovarian cancer. Hereditary Ovarian Cancer Clinical Study Group. *N Engl J Med* 339:424–428, 1998
96. Modan B, Hartge P, Hirsh-Yechezkel G, et al: Parity, oral contraceptives, and the risk of ovarian cancer among carriers and noncarriers of a BRCA1 or BRCA2 mutation. *N Engl J Med* 345:235–240, 2001
97. Offitt K, Garber JE, Greene MH, et al: Hereditary breast and ovarian cancer syndromes, in Offitt K, Garber JE, Greene MH, et al (eds.): *ASCO Curriculum Cancer Genetics and Cancer Predisposition Testing* (ed 2). Alexandria, VA, ASCO Publishing, 2004, pp 6-1–6-65
98. Rodiguez-Burford C, Barnes MN, Oelschlager DK, et al: Effects of non-steroidal anti-inflammmatory drugs (NSAIDs) on ovarian carcinoma cell lines: Preclinical evaluation of NSAIDs as chemopreventive agents. *Clin Cancer Res* 8:202–209, 2002
99. Brose MS, Smyrk TC, Weber B, et al: Genetic predisposition to cancer, in Kufe DW, Pollock RE, Weichselbaum RR, et al (eds.): *Cancer Medicine* (ed 6). Hamilton, Ontario, BC Decker, 2003, pp 241–265,
100. Hartmann LC, Schaid DJ, Woods JE, et al: Efficacy of bilateral prophylactic mastectomy in women with a family history of breast cancer. *N Engl J Med* 340:77–84, 1999
101. Hartmann LC, Sellers TA, Schaid DJ, et al: Efficacy of bilateral prophylactic mastectomy in BRCA1 and BRCA2 gene mutation carriers. *J Natl Cancer Inst* 93:1633–1637, 2001
102. Rebbeck TR, Lynch HT, Neuhausen SL, et al: Prophylactic oophorectomy in carriers of BRCA1 or BRCA2 mutations. *N Engl J Med* 346:1616–1622, 2002
103. Kauff ND, Satogopan JM, Robson ME, et al: Risk-reducing salpingo-oophorectomy in women with a BRCA 1 or BRCA2 mutation. *N Engl J Med* 346:1609–1615, 2002
104. Armstrong K, Schwartz TS, Randall T, et al: Hormone replacement therapy and life expectancy after prophylactic oophorectomy in women with BRCA1/2 mutations: a decision analysis. *J Clin Oncol* 22:1045–1054, 2004
105. Rebbeck TR, Friebel T, Lynch HT, et al: Bilateral prophylactic mastectomy reduces breast cancer risk in BRCA1 and BRCA2 mutation carriers: the PROSE Study Group. *J Clin Oncol* 22:1055–1062, 2004
106. Schwartz MD, Lerman C, Brogan B, et al: Impact of *BRCA1/BRCA2* counseling and testing on newly diagnosed breast cancer patients. *J Clin Oncol, www.jco.org*. Accessed April 5, 2004
107. Weitzel JN, McCahill LE: The power of genetics to target surgical prevention. *N Engl J Med* 344:1942–1943, 2001
108. Dooley WC, Ljung B, Veronesi U, et al: Ductal lavage for detection of cellular atypia in women at high risk for breast cancer. *J Natl Cancer Inst* 93:1624–1632, 2001
109. Hollingsworth AB, Singletary SE, Morrow M, et al: Current comprehensive assessment and management of women at increased risk for breast cancer. *Am J Surg* 187:349–362, 2004
110. Stoutjesdijk MJ, Boetes C, Jager GJ, et al: Magnetic resonance imaging and mammography in women with a hereditary risk of breast cancer. *J Natl Cancer Inst* 93:1095–1102, 2001
111. Warner E, Plewes DB, Shumak RS, et al: Comparison of breast magnetic resonance imaging, mammography, and ultrasound for surveillance of women at high risk for hereditary breast cancer. *J Clin Oncol* 19:3524–3531, 2001
112. Kriege M, Brekelmans CT, Boetes C, et al: Efficacy of MRI and mammography for breast-cancer screening in women with a familial or genetic predisposition. *N Engl J Med* 351:427–437, 2004
113. Dimond E: Establishing a cancer genetics clinic, in Straus Tranin A, Masny A, Jenkins J (eds.): *Genetics in Oncology Practice: Cancer Risk Assessment*. Pittsburgh, Oncology Nursing Society, 2003, pp 225–241
114. Offitt K, Garber JE, Greene MH, et al: Appendix, in Offitt K, Garber JE, Greene MH, et al (eds.): *ASCO Curriculum Cancer Genetics and Cancer Predisposition Testing* (ed 2). Alexandria, VA, ASCO Publishing, 2004, pp A-1–A-4
115. Affymetrix. Products; gene chip arrays. *www.affymetrix.com/products/system.html*. Accessed August 30, 2004
116. The chipping forecast II. *Nature Genet* 32:461–552, 2002
117. Cassells JM, Jenkins J, Halsey Lea D, et al: An ethical assessment framework for addressing global genetic issues in clinical practice. *Oncol Nurs Forum* 30:383–390, 2003
118. Genetics and Public Policy Center: Custom kids? Genetic testing of embryos: thought leaders to examine policy options for preimplantation genetic diagnosis. *http://dnapolicy.stage.labvelocity.com/policy/pgdForum.jhtml*. Accessed August 30, 2004
119. Scanlon C, Fibison W: *Managing Genetic Information: Implications for Nursing Practice*. Washington, DC, American Nurses Association, 1995
120. National Coalition for Health Professional Education in Genetics. www.nchpeg.org/, accessed August 30, 2004
121. Collins FS: Shattuck lecture — medical and societal consequences of the Human Genome Project. *N Engl J Med* 341:28–37, 1999

CHAPTER 8

Diagnostic Evaluation, Classification, and Staging

Kathleen Farley Omerod, RN, MS, AOCN®

Diagnostic Evaluation

Factors Affecting the Diagnostic Approach

The etiology of most cancers remains unknown, and cancer prevention measures are complicated by multiple economic, behavioral, social, and cultural factors. Early detection efforts and comprehensive diagnostic evaluations hold the most promise for controlling the morbidity and costs associated with cancer. This chapter focuses on the process of diagnostic evaluation when cancer is suspected and classification, staging, and grading of the cancer once the diagnosis is confirmed.

The major goals of the diagnostic evaluation for a suspected cancer are to determine the tissue type, the primary site, and the cellular characteristics of the malignancy, which help to determine the potential for tumor recurrence. The approach to the diagnostic evaluation depends on several factors:

- Presenting signs and symptoms
- Clinical status and ability to tolerate invasive procedures
- Anticipated goal of treatment when diagnosis is made
- Biological characteristics of the suspected malignancy
- Diagnostic equipment available in the community
- Third-party payer approval of diagnostic procedures

Even with the most sophisticated technology and resources presently available for cancer diagnosis, the key to survival continues to be early detection of disease. The discovery of a precancerous lesion or a malignant neoplasm at its earliest stage affords the very best opportunity for cure, extended survival, and less extensive treatment. For example, the nonpalpable breast mass found on a screening mammogram or the isolated tumor found incidentally on a chest film is more likely to be diagnosed as localized disease amenable to treatment and cure. More typically, the tumor goes undetected until specific signs or symptoms become apparent, prompting the person to consult a health professional.

Most commonly, an individual with undiagnosed cancer will present with complaints of weight loss, persistent pain, unexplained fever, fatigue, or one of the seven warning signals that have brought the early detection of cancer into public awareness.[1] A patient's attitude, demographics, and behavior influence when medical attention is sought, as do geographic location, socioeconomic background, and insurance coverage. Changes in the framework of health care make it a priority to identify, address, and eliminate these potential barriers.

Healthcare providers can expect to see a steadily growing number of elderly patients with cancer as the U.S. population ages and cancer incidence and mortality continue to increase. Diagnosing cancer in the elderly is complicated by many issues. For example, these individuals often live alone and have limited resources. They often have a high prevalence of co-morbidities, decreasing hematopoietic reserves, cognitive impairment, functional decline, and depression. In addition, elderly patients' out-of-pocket expenses for diagnosis and treatment can be incurred at a time when their financial reserves are diminishing.

Those at highest risk for developing cancer are the poor, the uninsured, the elderly, minorities, and those with a low-level education. Unfortunately, many of the people at greatest risk for developing cancer have an inadequate understanding of the importance of early attention to symptoms and may lack access to available resources. A study of cancer knowledge among the elderly revealed that most respondents were uncertain about the seven warning signals of cancer and lacked awareness of their increased cancer risk.[2] Nurses need to make a concerted effort to gather information, analyze the data, and then identify ways to reduce the threat of cancer in these individuals. Table 8-1 identifies the most common warning signals of cancer, the significance of each signal or symptom, and the persons at greatest risk for developing an associated malignancy.[1,3,4]

The worst prognosis can be expected in those people who delay seeking medical evaluation at the onset of their symptoms, in those cancers for which technologic methods are unavailable to make an early diagnosis, and in people for whom the primary lesion cannot be found. For the person who presents with widespread extensive disease, the palliative goal of treatment may direct and abbreviate an otherwise exhaustive and expensive diagnostic workup.

An effective clinical evaluation of the person with a suspected malignancy includes a comprehensive history with the identification of risk factors, a thorough physical examination, laboratory and imaging tests, and, perhaps most importantly, a biopsy-proven histologic verification of the malignancy. Known biological characteristics of the suspected malignancy and the typical routes of regional and distant metastases will direct the choice of further diagnostic and staging procedures. In some situations, extensive laboratory and imaging examinations precede tissue biopsy in an attempt to locate the primary tumor or an accessible tumor. In other patients, results of a biopsy specimen

Table 8-1 Seven Warning Signals of Cancer and Their Significance

Warning Signals	Significance of Warning Signal	Persons at Greatest Risk
Change in bowel or bladder habits	Changes in stool caliber and regular bowel function are frequent signs of colorectal cancer; dependent on the area of intestine involved. A change in bladder function, frequency, dysuria, retention, or hematuria may indicate prostate or bladder cancer.	*Colorectal cancer:* Over age 40, personal or family history of polyps or colorectal cancer, family history of polyposis syndromes, inflammatory bowel disease *Prostate cancer:* Over age 65, black males, family history of prostate cancer *Bladder cancer:* Smokers, males, chemical exposure
Unusual bleeding or discharge	Any unusual bleeding or discharge can signify malignancy. Occult or bright red blood may be seen with colorectal cancer. Abnormal vaginal bleeding is the most frequent sign of endometrial or cervical cancer. A clear, milky, or bloody discharge from the nipple is the second-most common symptom of breast cancer. Hemoptysis is a sign of lung cancer. Hematuria is the most frequent sign of bladder cancer and is also seen in renal and prostate cancer.	*Endometrial cancer:* Postmenopausal women over age 50, family history of endometrial cancer, obesity, diabetes, hypertension, prolonged estrogen administration, nulliparity *Cervix cancer:* First vaginal intercourse at early age, multiple sexual partners, genital human papillomavirus, previous abnormal Pap smear, smokers, low socioeconomic status, HIV
A sore that does not heal	Delayed healing of a sore or a change in a skin lesion's size, color, or shape, particularly on a surface exposed to ultraviolet light, can represent basal cell or squamous cell cancer. Oral lesions and leukoplakia, particularly tobacco or alcohol users, need careful follow-up. Persistent sores or itching of the vulva can indicate a preinvasive or malignant lesion.	*Skin cancer (nonmelanoma):* Exposure to UV radiation, psoralens, and UV light, or chemical carcinogens; fair-skinned whites, family history *Oral cancer:* Males, over age 40, tobacco users (chewed or smoked), pipe smokers, combined tobacco and alcohol use, excessive sun exposure (lip lesions)
Obvious change in wart or mole	A change in a mole's color and pigmentation pattern, irregularities in border or surface topography, or increasing size causes suspicion of malignancy. Occurs in areas protected from or exposed to the sun.	*Melanoma:* Fair-skinned whites with history of sun exposure, family or personal history of melanoma or dysplastic nevi, large congenital moles
Thickening or lump in breast or elsewhere	A painless lump or mass is the most common presenting sign in cancer of the breast, testis, and soft tissue sarcoma. Persistent enlarged lymph nodes can signify lymphoma or metastatic nodal disease.	*Breast cancer:* All women, particularly over age 55, endogenous hormonal factors, personal history or family history of breast cancer (mutations of *BRCA1* and *BRCA2* genes), nulliparity or first child after age 30, history of early menses previous mantel field irradiation *Testis cancer:* Males aged 20–35, undescended testes
Nagging cough or hoarseness	Persistent, productive cough is the most frequently reported symptom of lung cancer. Hoarseness may indicate lung, laryngeal, or thyroid cancer.	*Lung cancer:* All smokers, black males, history of asbestos exposure *Larynx cancer:* Males over age 60, combined tobacco and alcohol use
Indigestion or difficulty in swallowing	Indigestion, gastroesophageal reflux, painful "spasms" after eating, or difficulty swallowing can be symptoms of cancer of the esophagus, stomach, or pharynx.	*Stomach cancer:* Males over age 50, Japanese emigrants, history of pernicious anemia, atrophic gastritis, tobacco use, and alcohol consumption *Esophagus cancer:* Males over age 60, history of Barrett's esophagus, achalasia, caustic injury to esophagus, tobacco use, and heavy alcohol consumption

that confirm the presence of malignancy direct further testing that will be done to accurately stage the extent of disease.

In the present era of cost containment in health care, the judicious selection and sequencing of diagnostic studies is stressed. The proper test is one that yields information on the suspicious site of malignancy and complements, rather than merely confirms, known information. Third-party payers, prospective payment systems, and managed care networks also play important roles as gatekeepers in the diagnostic evaluation. Blue Cross of California is an example of a health insurance provider with published practice guidelines for breast cancer screening, diagnosis, staging, and treatment.[5] Due to cost-containment and insurance directives, many diagnostic evaluations are now being completed in ambulatory or outpatient facilities, unless patients are acutely ill and require hospitalization.

Nursing Implications

Many opportunities exist for nurses to promote the early detection and diagnosis of cancer. As respected members of the healthcare profession, they are consulted formally and informally about perceived signs and symptoms of cancer. Through communication, education, and intervention, nurses can increase public awareness about cancer. For example, they have the necessary skills and opportunities to assess and teach patients about the importance of early detection. Nurses are well suited to provide education about prevention measures and general population screening guidelines for early detection and diagnosis of cancer. Relating principles of cancer risk assessment, discussing issues related to genetic testing, educating patients about performing self-examinations, reporting symptoms, and scheduling appropriate screening tests are some examples of their capabilities. Nurses also can facilitate entry into the healthcare system by encouraging appropriate follow-up without delay, providing accurate information on cancer detection and diagnostic procedures, clarifying misconceptions, and referring individuals to trusted healthcare providers or community programs. Nurses must explain risk assessment clearly to help patients understand which risk factors may be applicable and are of highest priority.[6,7]

Table 8-1 presents information on the significance of the early warning signals of cancer and can be used to design community education programs that target individuals who are at greatest risk for developing a malignancy and who are most likely to delay seeking medical attention. An immediate opportunity exists to implement this approach in men and women who are covered by Medicare and are already eligible for reimbursement of the respective screening tests for breast, cervical, colorectal, and prostate cancers. The program content should stress the importance of recognizing symptoms early to improve survival. In addition, the rationale for participating in screening or annual physical examinations that include rectal and pelvic examinations should be given. Nurses proficient in physical assessment and screening techniques can perform early detection examinations, including digital rectal examinations, pelvic examinations, Papanicolaou tests, and testicular and breast examinations.[8] Integrating instruction on breast self-examination, testicular self-examination, or skin self-examination in community education programs can be done by nurses in most practice settings. Displaying posters and making available pamphlets from the American Cancer Society that identify warning signals and recommendations for a cancer-related checkup are effective ways to reach many people.

Educational programs are most accessible and acceptable if they are based in the local church, work site, shopping center, health fair, senior center, or wherever participation can be maximized. Successful examples of community-based programs include breast cancer screening programs presented to women at their work sites and cancer awareness programs reaching the elderly in long-term care facilities and in home care. While these programs have been an effective strategy for reaching individuals, there is a need to establish more such programs and to monitor their effects on early detection.[9–12]

Nurses are integral members of the professional team, providing information and emotional support to individuals facing the potential threat of cancer. The time elapsed between the discovery of a suspicious symptom, such as a breast lump, the seeking of medical attention, and the completion of diagnostic evaluation varies for every person and for many reasons. However, the potential for stress, disruption, anxiety, and fear always exists for individuals suspected of having cancer and for their family members.

During the prediagnostic period, a delay in seeking attention can be attributed to the perceived threat or "importance" of the symptom, the severity of the symptom, personal beliefs about cancer and treatment, and personal and financial resources. Once the individual acts on his or her concerns and seeks medical attention, the diagnostic period begins and may take several weeks before a cancer diagnosis is confirmed. Anxiety about the results of examinations and fear and curiosity regarding the technology used in procedures are common.[13] Psychological responses after receiving a diagnosis of cancer are individualized and range from suspicion, shock, denial, grief, and helplessness to loss and fear of death. Guilt feelings may be apparent if the patient did not seek attention early or if lifestyle may have contributed to the cancer.[14] In such situations, professional nurses can intervene by taking time to listen to concerns, responding to questions, and providing support. Projecting optimism and hope helps to counter the worst-case scenarios often assumed by the patient and family.

Oncology nurses play a key role in providing information and support to reduce the stress of going through a diagnostic evaluation for a suspected malignancy. An accurate assessment of the individual's and family's desire to know, in addition to their ability to understand, coping abilities, and supportive resources, is the first step in providing this much-needed support. Education should be provided in a manner consistent with the cultural background and healthcare beliefs of the affected individual and his or her family. In addition, education materials provided should be language and literacy appropriate. Educational preparation for an examination should include the following elements:

1. An explanation of and necessary preparation for the procedure

2. A description of any physical sensations that might be expected, such as pain, discomfort, and facial flushing
3. The purpose of the examination, including what information can and cannot be gleaned from it
4. When and from whom the results can be expected

Reinforcing verbal information with written materials has proved helpful.[15] Scheduling of the procedure should be done in a timely manner to decrease the patient's stress level.

Nurses also must be cognizant of any potential for complications during or after a procedure, including reactions to contrast agents, bleeding, vasovagal response, and the need for intravenous analgesia or moderate sedation. Nurses may assist with a procedure, perform the procedure, or provide post-procedure care.

Including the family members in all aspects of the diagnostic evaluation benefits the individual, the family, and the healthcare team. Families can reinforce instructions and information, assist with preparation for an examination, observe for untoward effects from procedures, and provide emotional support to the patient. An assessment of the family's ability to cope with the cancer diagnosis may prompt referrals to a variety of support services, including social services, psycho-oncology support groups, and home care agencies.

Laboratory Techniques

Laboratory studies are performed to help formulate or confirm a clinical diagnosis and to monitor the patient's response to or relapse from a specific therapy. The data provide information on the functioning of specific organs and metabolic processes that may be altered by disease or a malignant process.

Biochemical analysis of blood, serum, urine, and other body fluids identifies chemical and hematologic values outside the narrow, homeostatic range. Specific malignancies characteristically alter chemical composition of the blood, but no single value is diagnostic for a malignancy. For example, elevated serum levels of bilirubin, alkaline phosphatase, and glutamic-oxaloacetic transaminase are seen in approximately 50% of individuals presenting with liver cancer, and these abnormalities are significant in their correlation with shorter survival. Nonspecific changes such as anemia, leukocytosis or leukopenia, and thrombocytosis or thrombocytopenia also may contribute to the diagnostic evaluation.

Tumor markers consist of proteins, antigens, genes, ectopically produced hormones, and enzymes that are *tumor derived* (expressed by the tumor) or *tumor associated* (produced by normal tissue in response to the tumor). Markers have been recognized in serum and body fluids, and in tissues at the cellular and genetic levels.

The accuracy of a particular laboratory study or imaging technique often is reported in terms of sensitivity or specificity. *Sensitivity* establishes the percentage of people with cancer who will have positive (abnormal) test results, known as *true-positive* results. Test results of people with cancer that are negative (normal) constitute *false-negative* findings. *Specificity* establishes the percentage of people without cancer who will have negative (normal) test results, known as *true-negative* results. People who are free of disease and show positive (abnormal) results are considered to have *false-positive* results. A clinically useful test will detect a malignant abnormality early in its development (sensitivity) and exclude nonmalignant sources for the abnormality (specificity). In reality, many tests are highly sensitive but not very specific. The *predictive value* of a test establishes the probability that a test result correctly predicts the actual disease status.

An increase or decrease in a tumor marker can indicate whether a patient is responding to a certain therapy, locate the tumor's origin, or determine recurrence. One of the best detectors for certain tumors is human chorionic gonadotropin (HCG).[16] Several other markers are clinically useful in monitoring tumor activity during treatment and in detecting recurrent cancer but lack the specificity required to be good screening tools. Carcinoembryonic antigen (CEA), although less specific, is a marker widely used as a prognostic factor in colon cancer, reflecting tumor burden, and is used to monitor other disease sites such as breast and lung.[16,17] CEA lacks specificity because the antigen is expressed by benign as well as many different malignant cells. Table 8-2 identifies several tumor markers and indicates their clinical significance in the diagnosis and monitoring of cancer.[17–22]

Recent technological advances in monoclonal antibody production, radioimmunoassay, and flow cytometry have provided diagnostic and prognostic information in a variety of cancers. Techniques to produce monoclonal antibodies that detect specific tumor antigens have been important to the diagnosis, classification, localization, and treatment of several solid tumors, T- and B-cell lymphomas, and leukemia. Identified tumor antigens include surface immunoglobulins (cytoplasmic membranes), surface epitopes (antigen sites), antigens in various stages of cell differentiation, and enzymes.[20]

Radioimmunoassay, an important technique in the measurement of tumor markers, determines the amount of tumor antigen in a serum sample. A known amount of radiolabeled antigen, combined with antibody, is added to a serum sample. The individual's

Table 8-2 Selected Markers in the Diagnosis and Monitoring of Malignant Disease

Laboratory Test	Associated Malignancy	Comments
	ENZYMES	
Lactic dehydrogenase (LDH)	Lymphoma, seminoma, acute leukemia, metastatic carcinoma	Elevated in 50% of patients with advanced disease; also in hepatitis and myocardial infarction
Prostatic acid phosphatase (PAP)	Metastatic cancer of prostate, myeloma, lung cancer, osteogenic sarcoma	Elevated in 80% of patients with bone metastases from prostate cancer; also in prostatitis, nodular prostatic hypertrophy
Placental alkaline phosphatase (PLAP)	Seminoma, lung, ovary, uterus	Elevated in pregnancy
Neuron-specific enolase (NSE)	Small cell lung cancer, neuroendocrine tumors, neuroblastoma, medullary thyroid cancer	
Creatine kinase-BB (CK-BB)	Breast, colon, ovary, prostate cancers, small cell lung cancer	Elevated in bowel infarction, renal failure, stroke
Terminal deoxynucleotidal transferase (TdT)	Lymphoblastic malignancy	Helpful in differentiating between AML and ALL
	HORMONES	
Parathyroid hormone (PTH)	Ectopic hyperparathyroidism from cancer of the kidney, lung (squamous cell), pancreas, ovary, myeloma	Elevated in primary hyperparathyroidism
Calcitonin	Medullary thyroid, small cell lung cancer, breast cancer, and carcinoid	
Antidiuretic hormone (ADH)	Small cell lung cancer, adenocarcinomas	Inappropriate secretion associated with pneumonia, porphyria, CNS disease, various drugs, and endocrinopathies
Adrenocorticotropic hormone (ACTH)	Lung, prostate, gastrointestinal cancers, neuroendocrine tumors	Elevated in Cushing's disease
Human chorionic gonadotropin, beta subunit (B-HCG)	Germ cell tumors of testicle and ovary; ectopic production in cancer of stomach, pancreas, lung, colon, liver	Elevated in almost all choriocarcinoma, 60% of testicular cancer; also in pregnancy
	METABOLIC PRODUCTS	
5-Hydroxyindoleacetic acid (5-HIAA)	Carcinoid, lung	Drugs and diet interfere with test
Vanillylmandelic acid (VMA)	Neuroblastoma	Drugs and diet interfere with test; detected in ganglioneuroma
	PROTEINS	
Protein electrophoresis (urine — Bence Jones) (serum — immunoglobulins)	Myeloma, lymphoma	Elevated in connective tissue disease, benign monoclonal gammopathy, chronic renal failure
IgG	IgG myeloma	
IgA	IgA myeloma	
IgM	Waldenström's macroglobulinemia	
IgD	IgD myeloma	
IgE	IgE myeloma	
	Advanced neoplasms	
Beta-2 microglobulin	Myeloma, lymphoma	Invalid if patient received radioactive dyes week prior to test
	ANTIGENS	
Alpha-fetoprotein (AFP)	Nonseminomatous germ cell testicular cancer, choriocarcinoma, gonadal teratoblastoma in children, cancer of the pancreas, colon, lung, stomach, biliary system, liver	Elevated in 80% of hepatocellular cancer, 60% of nonseminomatous germ cell cancer; also in cirrhosis, hepatitis, toxic liver injury

(continued)

Table 8-2 Selected Markers in the Diagnosis and Monitoring of Malignant Disease (continued)

Laboratory Test	Associated Malignancy	Comments
	ANTIGENS (cont.)	
Carcinoembryonic antigen (CEA)	Cancer of the colon-rectum, stomach, pancreas, prostate, lungs, breast	Elevated in smokers, chronic obstructive pulmonary disease, pancreatitis, hepatitis, inflammatory bowel disease
Prostate-specific antigen (PSA)	Prostate cancer	Elevated in prostatitis, nodular prostatic hyperplasia
Tissue polypeptide antigen (TPA)	Breast, colon, lung, pancreas cancer	Marker for cell proliferation in benign or malignant disease
CA-125	Ovary (epithelial), pancreas, breast, colon, lung, liver cancer	Elevated in >85% of ovarian cancer; also in endometriosis, pelvic inflammatory disease, peritonitis
CA-19-9	Pancreas, colon, gastric cancer	Differentiates benign from malignant pancreatobiliary disease
CA-15-3	Breast cancer	
CA-27.29	Breast cancer	
CA-72-4	Gastric cancer	
	OTHER	
Lipid-associated sialic acid (LSA)	Leukemia, lymphoma, melanoma, most solid tumors	
Chromosome rearrangements (deletion, translocation, inversion)	Melanoma, small cell lung, renal, testicular cancers, liposarcoma, neuroblastoma, lymphoma, leukemia, and others	
Amplified oncogenes		
MYC	Neuroblastoma, small cell lung cancer, lymphoma, breast cancer	
EP1B-B	Glioblastoma, squamous cell carcinomas, breast, gastric, esophagus cancers	
C-ERB-B2 (HER-2)	Breast and ovarian cancers, adenocarcinomas	

unlabeled antigen displaces the radiolabeled antigen, which permits quantification.

Flow cytometry rapidly measures and identifies DNA characteristics and cell-surface markers that correlate with patient prognosis and are useful in diagnosing a malignancy and monitoring response to therapy. A *cell sorter* measures fluorescence and light scatter as cells flow past an excitation source. In hematologic and lymphoid malignancies, fluorescent-marked antibodies directed against specific cell-surface antigens (T-cell antigens, common acute lymphocytic leukemia antigen) help to differentiate hematopoietic cell lines. The primary application of flow cytometry analysis in solid tumors has been to determine DNA content (ploidy) and the percentage of cells synthesizing DNA (the S-phase fraction). Normal DNA is characterized as diploid and contrasts with abnormal, disorganized DNA, which is aneuploid. The proliferative potential of a tumor is measured by the percentage of cells in the synthesis phase of the cell cycle. Both of these factors — aneuploidy and high S-phase fraction — correlate with the biological aggressiveness of several tumors.[23,24] Breast cancer is a tumor in which DNA aneuploidy and high S-phase levels appear to be predictors of poor prognosis for women, especially when correlated with other risk factors. Although no standard for treatment has been established, some physicians and research protocols are incorporating this information into adjuvant treatment decisions.[25]

Over the last decade, substantial progress has been made in cancer genetics. A great deal of this progress stems from the Human Genome Project (HGP) research, which was completed in 2003.[26] Researchers have unlocked the key to the genetic puzzle of many cancers. As a result of the rapid advances made in this area, patients and their families can benefit from cancer risk assessment, undergo effective genetic testing, and consider the options for preventive or definitive therapy. Unfortunately, along with this willingness and potential need for testing come heightened expectation and anxiety on the part of patients and families. Communicating risk information to patients in a way that facilitates patient understanding and addressing the psychological issues related to the communication of cancer risk information are essential components of the cancer risk assessment. Genetic testing can assist healthcare providers in determining the probability that an individual will be diagnosed with a certain cancer in the future. Correctly estimating the risk for certain cancers is a complex endeavor, as risk estimates associated with certain mutations are changing as more information becomes available. Equally important is the nurse's sensitivity to the emotional impact of genetic information and his or her ability to support patients and families through the process.

A significant number of ongoing clinical trials are studying gene therapy and its relationship to the treatment of cancer. One such study focuses on the suppression of the HER-2/NEU protein or receptor, which, when overexpressed, appears to make breast cancer more aggressive.[27,28] Practicing oncologists are now able to test patients diagnosed with breast cancer for HER-2/NEU, enabling them to determine appropriate therapies.

Genetic testing for breast, ovarian, and colon cancers, as well as melanoma, has only recently become available. Inheritance of the mutated form of the genes *BRCA1* and *BRCA2* place women at a 90% risk for developing breast cancer and a 60% risk for developing ovarian cancer at a relatively young age.[26,29] Mutation in the adenomatous polyposis coli gene leads to the colon cancer known as adenomatous familial polyposis, which affects patients early in life. Chromosome abnormalities have also been documented in hereditary nonpolyposis colorectal cancer (HNPCC).[26,29]

The American Society of Clinical Oncology recommends that physicians offering genetic testing be able to explain the risks, benefits, and limitations of the testing procedure.[30] Once the test results become available, the physician should discuss treatment options based on those results with the patient and family.

As genetic technology evolves and knowledge of cancer genetics expands, healthcare providers must respond by informing patients, families, and the public about developments in cancer prevention, early detection, and treatment. The challenge of problem solving and knowledge application in genetic risk assessment requires that members of the health profession seek continuing education in this area. Nurses providing comprehensive cancer genetic counseling must be advanced practice oncology nurses with specialized education in hereditary cancer genetics.[31,32]

Tumor Imaging

Many diagnostic procedures are available to ascertain the presence of a tumor mass, localize the mass for biopsy, provide tissue characterization, and further assess or stage the anatomical extent of disease. Although diagnostic imaging has benefited from the technology that produced computerized tomography and magnetic resonance imaging (MRI), an important role remains for the conventional diagnostic procedures. Examinations are selected that are efficient in detecting suspicious lesions and that also result in the least risk, discomfort, and expense for the patient. Table 8-3 identifies preferred imaging procedures for tumor definition and staging in several organ sites.[33–42] Table 8-4 elaborates on patient preparation and education for select examinations.[43]

Radiographic techniques

Radiographic studies, or x-ray films, allow for visualization of internal structures of the body. Distinction is made between normal and abnormal structure and function. X-rays, or gamma rays, are passed through the body and are absorbed variably by tissues of differing densities; they react on specially sensitized film or fluoroscopic screens. Radiographs may be site specific, such as the standard chest film or mammogram, or they may view the dynamic function of an entire organ system. For example, in a gastrointestinal series, a continuous flow of x-rays passes through the digestive tract to assess the action of peristalsis, to detect displacement of structures, and to visualize mucosal abnormalities.

Mammographic examination is performed primarily in radiology suites dedicated solely to this procedure. These units are distinguished by the incorporation of a tissue compression device or cone that improves the quality of the image and reduces the amount of primary and scatter radiation. Informing women that this examination offers a safe, low dose of radiation and a high-quality mammographic image that is sensitive to abnormalities has been necessary to promote participation in screening efforts. Since 1987, the American College of Radiology (ACR) has provided accreditation of mammography facilities, which has resulted in a standard of quality assurance.[44]

Diagnostic mammography is indicated when symptoms or clinical findings exist that suggest an abnormality. The examination requires that more views be taken than for the standard two-view screening mammogram, as well as spot compression and magnification views of suspicious spots. Ultrasound may also be used for clarification purposes as an adjunct to the mammogram. Frequently, mammography is used to guide the placement of a wire, needle, dye, or catheter near a suspicious lesion in preparation for biopsy or surgery. Figure 8-1 shows a mammographically guided needle localization of a nonpalpable breast lesion. The localizer penetrates and extends beyond the lesion for more reliable surgical excision.

Table 8-3 Preferred Imaging Procedures for Tumor Definition and Staging

Site	Imaging Techniques	Comments
Central nervous system	Positron emission tomography (PET)	Useful as a guidance tool in biopsy of lesions Ability to determine grade of tumor due to metabolic uptake
	Magnetic resonance imaging (MRI) with contrast	Superior to CT due to exquisite sensitivity of lesions <1 cm and lack of bone artifact in posterior fossa imaging
Head and neck	PET	Superior to CT in determining tumor necrosis versus tumor recurrence after radiotherapy
	Computerized axial tomography (CT)	Best for osseous change
	MRI	Superior for soft tissue lesions, tumor–tissue interface, parapharyngeal spaces
Lung	PET	Detects benign versus malignant in solitary pulmonary nodules Aids in staging of non–small cell lesions due to high sensitivity in depicting mediastinal involvement
	Chest x-ray (CXR)	Good for detection of peripheral lesions
	CT	Preferred for parenchyma and mediastinal nodes
	MRI	Advantage over CT in chest wall, hilum, and mediastinal vascular invasion
Esophagus	Esophagram with contrast	Preferred for measuring lesion length, necessary for staging
	Endoscopic ultrasound (EUS) CT	Superior to CT (except with severe stenosis) for depth of tumor invasion and lymph node assessment
Stomach	Barium studies with double contrast	Good for detection
	EUS	Preferred over CT for staging due to better detection of small nodes
Colon	PET	More sensitive than CT in diagnosing liver metastases and lymph node involvement with recurrent disease
	Barium enema with double contrast	Most tumors originate in mucosa, where barium studies will detect 90% of lesions >1 cm
Liver	Ultrasound (US)	Preferred for differentiating biliary obstruction from hepatic parenchymal disease
	CT or MRI with contrast	CT has been preferred for imaging, but MRI with contrast may be equivalent
Bladder	Intravenous pyelogram (IVP)	Detects lesions >1.5–2 cm
	MRI or CT	MRI preferred for bladder wall invasion, identifying large nodes, and separating them from vessels
Kidney	IVP	Preferred for detection
	CT	CT with contrast provides 90% accuracy for staging
Musculoskeletal	X-ray	For initial detection
	Bone scan	More sensitive than x-ray in identifying metastatic bone lesions (except multiple myeloma)
	CT or MRI	CT preferred for intraosseous lesion; MRI preferred for extraosseous lesion or intraosseous lesion extending into bone
Breast	Mammogram	Mammography provides the standard for breast imaging; sensitivity rate of >80% for screening purposes
Prostate	Transrectal ultrasound (TRUS)	Continues to be evaluated as a screening tool; detects extracapsular lesion extension Used as guidance tool for biopsy
	MRI or CT	MRI preferred for staging seminal vesicle invasion
Endometrium	MRI	Primary staging is by surgery; MRI assists with staging of local and nodal disease
Ovary	US (transvaginal and transabdominal) or CT	Tumor mass >1 cm can be defined by US or CT; primary staging is by surgery
Lymphoma and Hodgkin's disease	CXR CT of chest and abdomen	Required CT of abdomen images upper retroperitoneal and mesenteric nodes, liver, and spleen
	PET	PET replacing need for gallium scan or LAG in lymphoma and Hodgkin's disease

Table 8-4 Selected Tumor Imaging Techniques with Instructions for Preparing the Patient

Tumor Imaging Examination	Patient Instructions	Comments
Barium studies	• Restriction of diet, smoking, and most medication before examination • Laxatives and enemas to cleanse bowel before colon examination • Will lie on tilting x-ray table, secured • Barium will taste chalky, milkshake consistency • Barium enema (BE) will feel cool, may cause cramping • Laxatives to clear barium after UGI • *Time:* 30–60 min	Bowel cleansing and procedure are exhausting for elderly patients. BE must precede UGI and small bowel series. BE should follow other imaging examinations. Single contrast preferred for elderly. Double contrast requires full patient cooperation due to time frame.
Computerized tomography	• Diet restrictions before examination • Will lie still on adjustable table; x-ray tube rotates around patient to take many pictures • Machinery noisy • Test painless • May receive intravenous contrast dye; may feel burning sensation as injected • May report feelings of nausea, vomiting, flushing, itching, bitter taste • Drink fluids after examination to eliminate dye • *Time:* 30–90 min	Careful history required to determine prior adverse reaction to contrast. Cost depends on use of contrast and radiologist's interpretation. Discontinue Glucophage for 2 days prior to and 2 days past CT scan because it is incompatible with IV contrast dye. Careful history of prior kidney disease with evaluation of BUN and creatine. May need sedation if claustrophobic.
Angiogram	• Diet restriction before examination • May receive sedative just before examination • Will lie still on x-ray table • Skin over selected artery site cleansed and anesthetized • Cannula passed into artery or vein • Contrast die rapidly injected, may feel burning sensation as injected • Several x-ray films taken • May report feelings of nausea, vomiting, flushing, itching, bitter or salty taste • Cannula removed after examination, pressure applied, limb immobilized • *Time:* 1–3 h	Decreased use as diagnostic procedure. Being replaced by percutaneous procedures. Useful in preoperative planning and therapeutic embolization.
Positron emission tomography	• Diet restriction before exam to optimize sensitivity • Must lie still during exam • Receives injection of glucose-tagged radioisotopes with no adverse effect • Radiation exposure is minimal • Must refrain from excessive physical activity for minimum of 24 hours prior to test • A glucose level may be drawn prior to testing • *Time:* 4 h	Substances that alter metabolism, such as ETOH, caffeine, and nicotine, should be avoided. Use of sedatives may decrease test sensitivity.
Magnetic resonance imaging	• No diet restriction • Remove anything affected by a magnet • Lie still on table, secured with Velcro straps	Difficult to titrate medication for comfort and sedation during lengthy procedures. May need sedation if claustrophobic.

(continued)

Table 8-4 Selected Tumor Imaging Techniques with Instructions for Preparing the Patient (continued)

Tumor Imaging Examination	Patient Instructions	Comments
Magnetic resonance imaging (cont.)	• Table will move into narrow magnet opening • Knocking or beating sound in machinery is normal • Painless • May receive intravenous contrast dye • May report nausea, vomiting, itching if given contrast dye • *Time:* 45–60 min	•
Ultrasonogram	• Diet restriction before examination • Full bladder for pelvic ultrasound • Will lie on exam table • Ultrasound gel applied over skin of area to be examined • Transducer passes over skin • May feel pressure; no pain • No radiation involved • *Time:* 30 min	Increased use of probes introduced into the body (transrectal, transvaginal) for detection of cancer. Also has intraoperative use for intracranial and intraabdominal tumor localization.
Bone scan	• No diet restriction • Radioisotope injected before exam • Must void before scan to decrease tracer activity • Will lie on scanner table • Scanner moves back and forth, taking several pictures, emitting a clicking sound • Procedure painless • Radioisotope harmless • Patient instructed to drink water over 1–3 hours to aid renal clearance of radioisotope	Increased use of radioimmunoimaging using radiolabeled monoclonal antibodies. Highly sensitive over routine x-ray in detecting metastatic disease to bone.
Endoscopy	• Diet restriction before examination • Mild sedation before procedure, but patient remains conscious • Intravenous infusion for medications and hydration *Oral:* • Local anesthetic sprayed in mouth • Flexible tube passed through mouth to level to be examined • Tongue and throat feel swollen; difficult to swallow • May feel pressure and fullness if scope in stomach *Rectal:* • Prepared for exam with laxatives, enemas • Lubricated endoscope inserted anally • Feels cold, urge to defecate • May need to change positions during examination as scope is advanced • *Time:* 30–60 min	Screening sigmoidoscopy is recommended every 3–5 yr, beginning at age 50. Covered by Medicare. Colonoscopy requires more extensive preparation.

(continued)

Table 8-4 Selected Tumor Imaging Techniques with Instructions for Preparing the Patient (continued)

Tumor Imaging Examination	Patient Instructions	Comments
Mammogram	• Breast is compressed between two plates on x-ray cassette • Compression may feel tight, but not painful • Radiation exposure is minimal and safe *Screening:* • Two views are taken of each breast: one view from head to foot (craniocaudal), the other lateral • *Time:* 15 min *Diagnostic:* • Three views taken of breast; craniocaudal, lateral, oblique • Spot compression and magnification films • *Time:* 30 min	Clinical breast exam and instruction on breast self-examination should be included. Covered by Medicare.

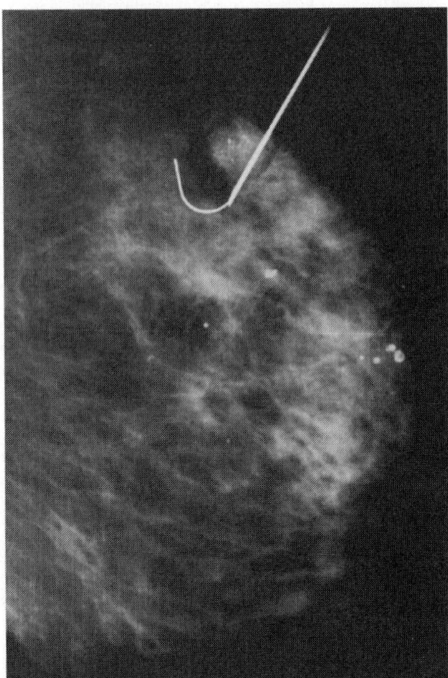

Figure 8-1 Mammographically guided hook-wire needle localization of nonpalpable breast lesion with multiple pathologic microcalcifications. (Courtesy of Scripps Memorial Hospital, Department of Radiology, La Jolla, CA.)

Digital mammography is similar to conventional film-screen mammography, but uses a dedicated electronic detector system that captures and changes the digital image into a fixed record. The transmitted image is converted into a number of images that are transmitted as electrical signals by telephone lines, dedicated telecommunication lines, or satellite in less than four minutes to display the x-ray information on a computer. Digital mammography is poised to eventually become the dominant medium for sending mammographic images. Although digital mammography promises to overcome the limitations of conventional film-screen mammography in dense fibroglandular breast tissue, it remains in the early stages of technical development and clinical trial.[45]

Computerized tomography (CT) also provides sectional (axial, coronal, or sagittal) views of structures in the body. After serial x-ray exposures are taken through different angles of the body, a computer analyzes the information and provides a three-dimensional, reconstructed picture of the area studied. Computerized tomography has become one of the most useful, informative, and available tests in the diagnosis and staging of malignancies. Due to its profound spatial resolution, it is the diagnostic tool of choice for evaluation of the thorax, as it is capable of visualizing small lung nodules much earlier than standard imaging tests.[46] A CT scan is able to detect minor differences between tissue densities in any area of the body. The major drawback is its production of artifact in areas of cortical bone content. MRI is the preferred imaging study, rather than CT, when evaluating musculoskeletal tumors.[47] The specificity of MRI is one reason it has become the superior examination for detection of spinal cord compression and for skeletal metastatic deposits.

Computerized tomography may be completed with or without radioiodinated contrast agents. Figure 8-2 demonstrates two different tumors imaged by CT with intravenous contrast. Computerized tomography frequently is used to direct a needle to a tumor site for percutaneous biopsy.

Several radiographic examinations rely on contrast materials to enhance or outline the structures to be visualized. Angiography, venography, cholangiography, and urography, in addition to CT, all rely on the intravascular administration of iodinated contrast agents for optimal visualization of body structure and function. An example is the excretory radiograph, also known as the intravenous pyelogram (IVP), which is used in the initial diagnostic evaluation of renal masses.

Patients who undergo studies requiring iodinated contrast material can experience minor, to intermediate, to life-threatening anaphylactoid reactions.[48] A metallic or bitter taste, becoming flushed, and a feeling of warmth all are common and transient sensations experienced during injection of contrast material. Vesicular reactions such as itching, angioedema, and mild urticaria may occur from a few minutes to several hours after contrast injection.[48] These symptoms do not require treatment and will not progress to life-threatening reactions. There is no good predictor for severe reactions; however, patients with a history of allergic response should be considered to be at high risk, closely monitored, and premedicated. Those considered to be at risk for adverse reactions can receive a test dose of the contrast agent and should be premedicated with diphenhydramine, steroids, or epinephrine. Delayed reactions in patients have been noted from 2 to 6 hours after testing.[49] On completion of an iodinated contrast examination, patients should be instructed to drink a minimum of eight glasses of fluid in 24 hours to prevent renal toxicity. Nonionic contrast agents are available, at considerable expense, for use with patients who have had serious reactions in the past.

Intrathecal contrast agents are used in myelography and in CT. Radiographs of the subarachnoid space are taken after the injection of either an oily or a water-soluble contrast agent. The contrast agent flows only to the point of obstruction, and more than one injection may be required.

Virtual colonoscopy (VC) is a promising new method for detecting colorectal polyps and cancers. Air is insufflated into a cleansed colon, and high-resolution, thinly collimated, spiral CT slices are acquired. The two-dimensional slices, as well as the postprocessed "fly-through" virtual colonoscopic images, are examined for polyps and tumors. These images can be saved, manipulated to achieve better viewing angles, and reviewed after the procedure. Preparing for a virtual colonoscopy requires administration of a laxative and insertion of a probe to push air into the colon. Moderate sedation is not required, so individuals can resume usual activities after completing a VC. In a clinical trial, 11,233 asymptomatic adults underwent both virtual and conventional colonoscopies. The sensitivity of virtual colonoscopy for adenomatous polyps was found to be 93.8% for polyps at least 10 mm in

A

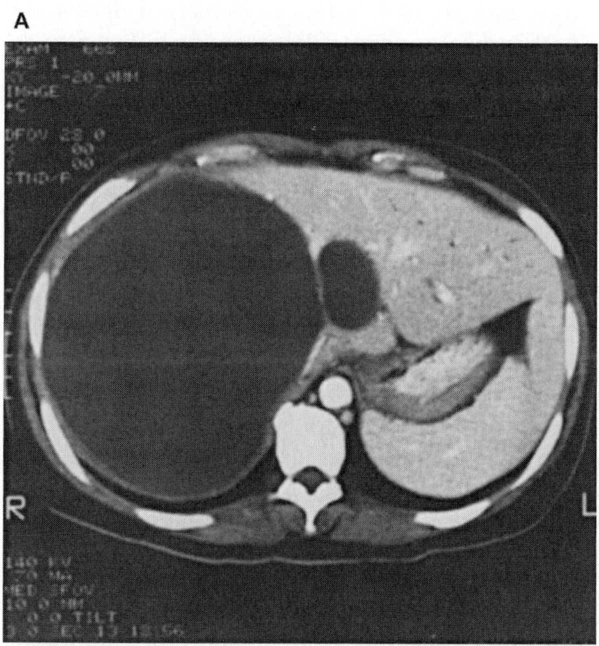

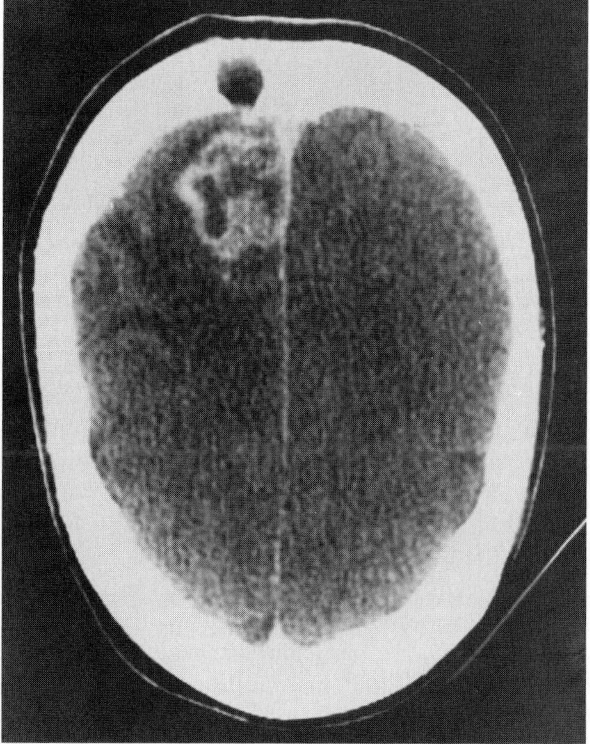

B

Figure 8-2 Examples of contrast-enhanced CT: CT abdominal scan revealing huge cystadenocarcinoma involving most of the liver (**A**), and CT head scan demonstrating lobular glioblastoma with peripheral rim enhancement (**B**). (Courtesy of Scripps Memorial Hospital, Department of Radiology, La Jolla, CA.)

diameter, 93.9% for polyps at least 8 mm in diameter, and 88.7% for polyps at least 6 mm in diameter. The sensitivity of optical colonoscopy for adenomatous polyps was 87.5%, 91.5%, and 92.3% for the three sizes of polyps, respectively. The specificity of VC for adenomatous polyps was 96.0% for polyps at least 10 mm in diameter, 92.2% for polyps at least 8 mm in diameter, and 79.6% for polyps at least 6 mm in diameter.[50] Indications for VC may include screening for polyps, incomplete or failed colonoscopy, and preoperative assessment of the colon proximal to an occlusive cancer.[51]

Barium sulfate is a nonabsorbable, radiopaque agent used to enhance the contrast between the lumen of the gastrointestinal tract and adjacent soft tissues. Studies that use barium include esophagography, upper gastrointestinal (UGI) series, small bowel series, barium enema, and hypotonic duodenography. Barium is ingested or introduced into the gastrointestinal tract and allowed to coat the intraluminal surfaces. Radiographs are taken that can detect primary malignancies of the gastrointestinal organs or extrinsic compression from other tumor sites. Figure 8-3 presents a classic annular lesion of the colon imaged with radiopaque contrast. By combining flexible sigmoidoscopy and double contrast (barium and air), sensitivity rates of 98% for cancer and 99% for adenomatous polyps are achieved.[52] Complications seldom result from this examination unless there is an obstruction or a perforation of the digestive tract. Retention of the barium may cause fecal impaction and discomfort in some patients. The administration of a laxative or an enema may be necessary to assist with bowel evacuation.

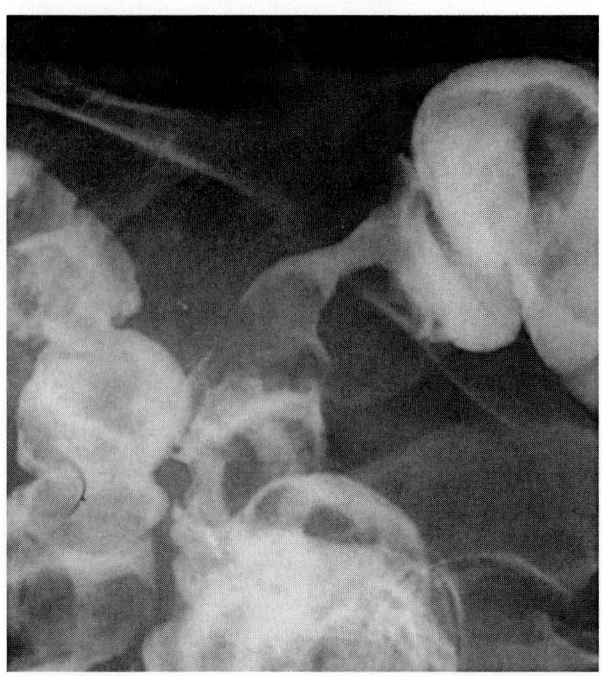

Figure 8-3 Barium enema visualizes annular, "apple core" lesion that is constricting the colon. (Courtesy of Scripps Memorial Hospital, Department of Radiology, La Jolla, CA.)

Nuclear medicine techniques

Nuclear medicine imaging involves the intravenous injection or the ingestion of radioisotope compounds, followed by camera imaging of those organs or tissues that have concentrated the radioisotopes. Nuclear medicine studies are extremely sensitive and often will detect sites of abnormal metabolism or early malignancy several months before changes are seen on a radiograph. Scans of the bones, liver and spleen, brain, thyroid, and kidneys are useful in the detection of malignancy. Figure 8-4 shows an abnormal bone scan suggestive of widespread metastasis from prostate cancer. Gallium scans are particularly sensitive in detecting bronchogenic carcinomas and lymphomas. Today, however, many radioisotope examinations are being replaced by CT because of the latter's greater sensitivity and ease of administration.

Positron emission tomography (PET) is an imaging modality that provides information based on the biochemical and metabolic activity of tissue. Infused biochemical compounds such as glucose are tagged with radioactive particles that emit positrons detectable by gamma camera tomography. F-18 fluorodeoxyglucose (FDG) is the most widely used radiopharmaceutical. Tumors have a higher rate of glycolysis, enabling FDG to trace glucose metabolism in cancerous tissues, unlike other diagnostic tests that examine only structural changes.[53] Figure 8-5 shows a PET image demonstrating a large lung tumor. To allow maximum accumulation of FDG in cancerous tissue, patients must fast for at least 8 hours prior to the examination.

Previously used for cardiac and neurologic disorders, PET has demonstrated accuracy in a variety of cancers, such as those of the head and neck, breast, and lung, as well as gastrointestinal malignancies, lymphomas, and melanoma.[53] The most extensive application of this technology in clinical oncology has been in brain imaging. PET can be used to define the most metabolically active targets for stereotactic biopsy, thereby improving diagnostic accuracy and reducing the number of biopsy samples required. It is also useful for evaluating residual or recurrent tumors following therapy, and can be used to survey patients with low-grade brain tumors for evidence of degeneration into high-grade malignancy.[54]

The PET scan is particularly useful in differentiating low-grade from high-grade tumors and in distinguishing treatment-induced tissue necrosis from recurrent tumor. It has proved highly effective when evaluating patients for metastatic disease. In a study

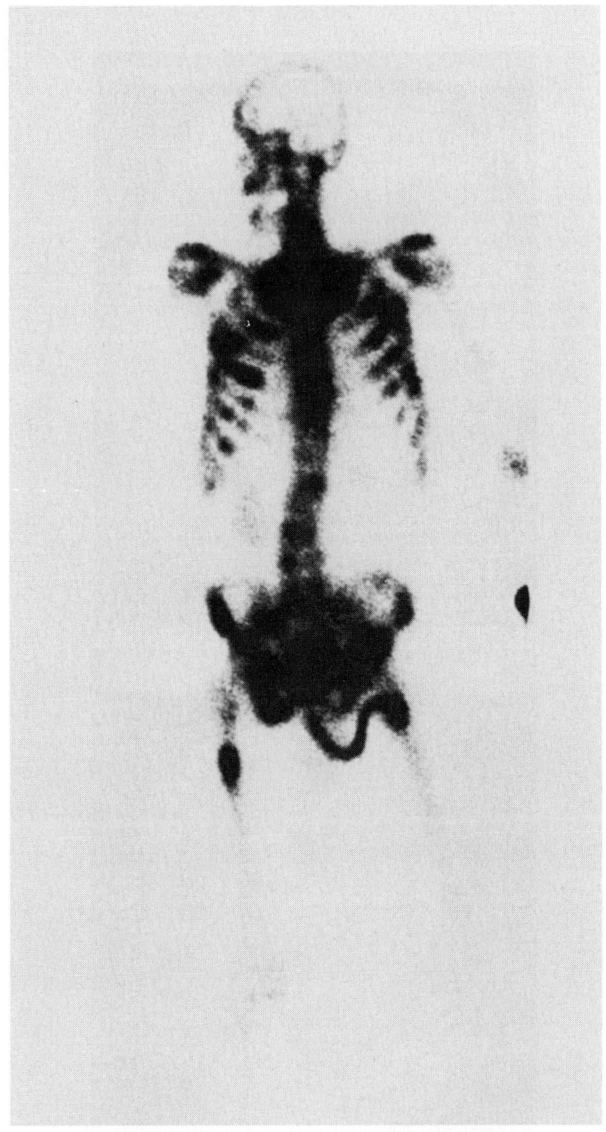

Figure 8-4 Abnormal bone scan suggesting widespread bony metastasis in central axial skeleton, pelvis, hips, and right proximal femur. (Courtesy of Scripps Memorial Hospital, Department of Radiology, La Jolla, CA.)

done by Zhuang et al,[55] 80 patients diagnosed with colon cancer were evaluated for recurrent disease in the liver using PET, CT scans, surgical pathology, and clinical outcome. PET proved more accurate than CT in diagnosing liver metastases and extrahepatic metastases.

Limitations of the PET scan include its expense, the need for a cyclotron to produce the isotopes, and the requirement that patients fast prior to the exam to allow for maximum tissue uptake of FDG. There is variable physiologic FDG uptake in the digestive tract, thyroid gland, skeletal muscle, myocardium, bone marrow, and genitourinary tract. Benign pathologic FDG uptake can occur in healing bone, lymph nodes,

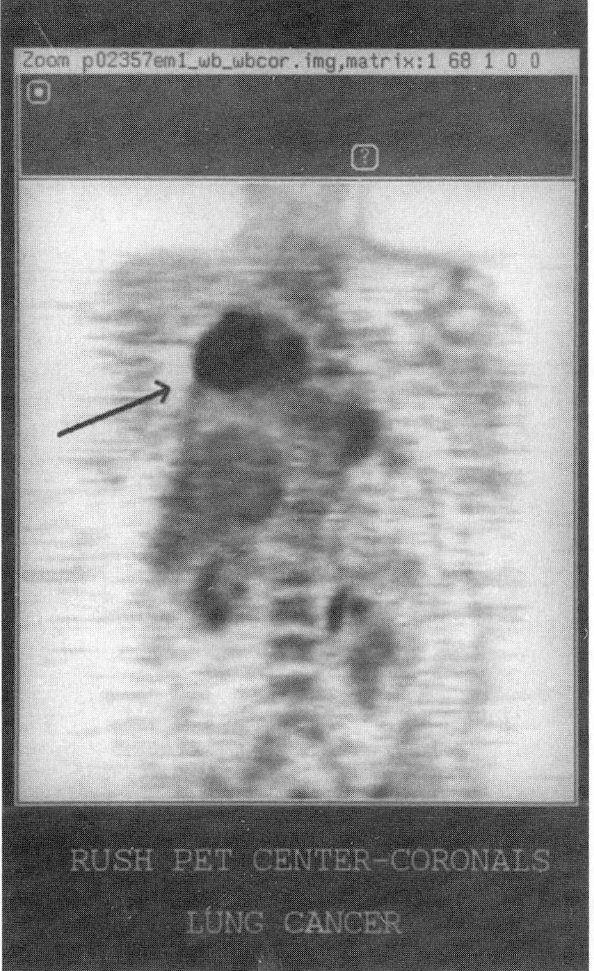

Figure 8-5 PET scan of lung. (Courtesy Rush PET Center.)

joints, sites of infection, and sites of aseptic inflammatory response.[54–57]

PET has emerged as a reliable method for evaluating and staging recurrent disease. Additionally, it plays an important role in differentiating benign and malignant primary tumors. Although FDG has emerged as the dominant radiopharmaceutical for PET imaging in oncology, numerous other compounds are being evaluated. The next decade will witness an explosive growth of PET technology in oncologic imaging.

Nuclear imaging with radiolabeled monoclonal antibodies visualizes microscopic sites of metastasis or suspected malignancy. This technique requires that a monoclonal antibody targeted against a specific tumor antigen be combined with trace amounts of radioactivity. After intravenous injection, the antibody binds to antigen on the tumor. Tumor sites then ''light up'' with imaging scanners. CYT-103 (OncoSCINT OV/CR) is the first FDA-approved radiolabeled monoclonal antibody for diagnostic use in cancer. The indium-111–labeled antibody targets the tumor-associated glycoprotein (TAG-72) found in mucin-producing adenocarcinomas.[58] Although data remain limited, this type of imaging is approved for colon and ovarian cancer and plays a role in assessing occult recurrent disease.[59]

After many years of rapid growth, diagnostic imaging technology is now being intensely scrutinized by healthcare providers. Hospitals and free-standing radiology centers are considered cost environments, and insurance carriers now require authorization or certification for all diagnostic studies. In the recent past, many studies were automatically added to clinical practice without considering whether it would be money well spent.[60]

Ultrasonography

Ultrasonography (US) is a nonradiographic and noninvasive technique for imaging deep soft-tissue structures within the body. The reflecting echoes of high-frequency sound waves directed into specific tissues are recorded on an imaging screen. The echoes are variable, depending on the tissue density, and can be used to discriminate masses. A limitation of the examination is its inability to visualize through bone or air. Ultrasonography is most applicable in detecting ascites, renal or biliary obstruction, or tumors within the pelvis of patients with cancer.[61] Masses greater than 2 cm in diameter can be detected and localized for possible percutaneous biopsy. Transrectal ultrasound is useful in guiding a needle biopsy of suspicious prostate lesions but has not proved to be an effective screening tool. In the diagnosis of breast cancer, ultrasound is an important adjunct to mammography for distinguishing cysts from solid lesions with 98%–100% accuracy.

A

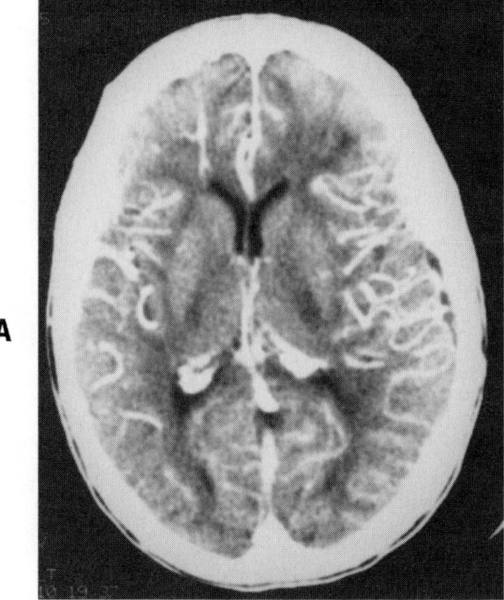

B

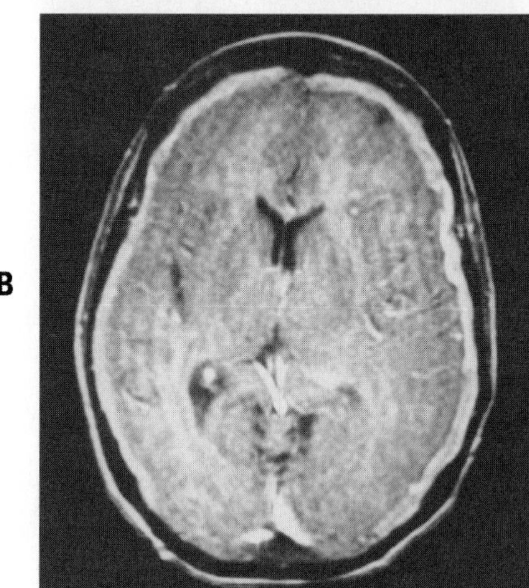

Figure 8-6 Contrast-enhanced CT **(A)** and contrast-enhanced MRI **(B)** of metastatic intracranial tumor. MRI shows "rind" of metastatic deposit around brain that was invisible on CT due to bone artifact. (Courtesy of Scripps Memorial Hospital, Department of Radiology, La Jolla, CA.)

Magnetic resonance imaging

Magnetic resonance imaging creates sectional images of the body, similar to CT, but does not expose the patient to ionizing radiation. Images are created by placing the individual within a powerful magnetic field that aligns the body's hydrogen nuclei in one direction. Radiofrequency pulses are used to excite the magnetized nuclei and change their alignment. Between radiofrequency pulses, the nuclei return to a state of relaxation, and variable signals are transmitted on the basis of tissue characteristics. These signals are analyzed by the computer, and multiplanar (sagittal, coronal, and axial) images are produced with exquisite clarity. Magnetic resonance imaging can be enhanced with use of two intravenous paramagnetic contrast agents, gadolinium diethylenetriamine pentaacetic acid (DTPA) and gadotetrate meglumine (DOTA).[62] These agents work by reducing tissue relaxation time, thereby increasing signal intensity and image production. Adverse reactions to gadolinium DTPA, which are rare, include nausea, pain localized to the injection site, and headache occurring several hours after the examination.

Magnetic resonance imaging is most applicable in the detection, localization, and staging of malignant disease in the central nervous system, spine, head and neck, and musculoskeletal system. At present, MRI enhanced with gadolinium and used for the detection of brain metastasis stands alone, continuing to be the best diagnostic tool for this diagnosis (Figure 8-6).[63]

MRI shows promise in staging cancers in women with dense breasts where mammography has been shown to provide less definitive results.[64] It may be appropriate for women at high risk for breast cancer or where a high degree of suspicion exists without evidence of disease on mammogram. In one study, the records of 367 women considered to be at high risk for breast cancer were reviewed. All had normal mammograms and underwent their first MRI of the breasts for screening due to high risk of breast cancer based on family history, previous breast cancer, or history of a precancerous lesion. Sixty-four of the MRIs showed an abnormality that warranted a biopsy. Fifty-nine of the patients underwent the recommended biopsy; of these cases, a cancer was found in 14 patients and a high-risk lesion was seen in 13 others. A high-risk lesion is one that can progress to cancer or is a marker for possible breast cancer in the future.[65] This study demonstrated that in these women MRI was more sensitive than mammogram in detecting early breast lesions. More research is needed before widespread use of MRI is indicated as a screening tool for early detection of breast cancer.

MRI does have some limitations to its utility. For example, persons with aneurysm or surgical clips, pacemakers, implanted pumps, tattooed eyeliner, or any ferromagnetic metallic implant cannot undergo this kind of examination. The magnetic pull of MRI is capable of dislodging an implant, interfering with its operation, or removing the object from the person's body. This limitation excludes use of this technology in acutely ill patients with life-support or monitoring devices. Nonferrous metallic implants may produce artifacts that distort the MRI image but are generally safe for the patient. Implanted ports, which are frequently used in cancer patients to provide vascular, peritoneal, and epidural access, are made from many different materials. Shellock and Kanl provide a list of ports that do not move or deflect during exposure to magnetic scanning.[66] Camp-Sorrell identifies ports causing the least artifact but concludes that attention must be paid to the manufacturer's recommendations, as materials tend to change and new ports may be developed.[67] High-grade titanium and nonmetal ports produce the least amount of or no artifact.

Claustrophobic individuals may require sedation if they are to undergo MRI, but also benefit from explanations prior to the procedure, a support person nearby, verbal contact, MRI-compatible headphones, prisms or mirrors to allow a view outside of the tube, and relaxation techniques.[66] Free-standing, open MRI facilities offer a welcome alternative for individuals who are claustrophobic. The cost of the MRI and length of the examination (1 to 2 hours for a total scan of the spine) are disadvantages.

Invasive Diagnostic Techniques

Endoscopy

Endoscopy is a method to directly visualize the interior of a hollow viscus by the insertion of an endoscope into a body cavity or opening. The endoscope contains fiber-optic glass bundles that transmit light and then return an image to the optical head of the endoscope. The instrument may be rigid or flexible. Visual inspection, tissue biopsy, cytologic aspiration, staging the extent of disease, and excision of pathologic processes are possible through the endoscope.

By passing a flexible scope through the mouth, endoscopic examinations can visualize directly the larynx, upper airway passages and bronchial tree, esophagus, stomach, and upper duodenum. Visualization of the distal sigmoid colon, rectum, and anal canal is performed by means of a rigid scope. The entire large intestine can be viewed with a flexible colonoscope that is inserted anally. Endoscopic retrograde cholangiopancreatography (ERCP) combines the diagnostic procedures of endoscopy and contrast-enhanced radiography to evaluate biliary tract obstruction and pancreatic masses.

The endoscopic ultrasound (EUS) may prove superior to other imaging modalities for assessing direct depth of tumor invasion and local lymph node status for esophageal, gastric, and colon malignancy. Where available, EUS is indicated to distinguish benign from malignant lesions, to stage neoplasms, to establish operability and surgical approach, and to determine response or recurrence.[68]

The cervix and vagina are directly visualized with the magnification lens of the colposcope. Peritoneoscopy or laparoscopy permits assessment of surfaces within the peritoneal cavity by the insertion of a peritoneoscope through a small incision below the umbilicus. Thoracoscopy allows visualization of the visceral and parietal pleura, mediastinum, and diaphragm by means of a thoracoscope passed through an incision in the midaxillary line of the sixth to the eighth intercostal space. The direct visualization of the tissues and organs of the mediastinum is performed by passing an endoscope into the mediastinum through a small incision above the manubrium.

Biopsy

A diagnosis of cancer requires tissue confirmation, usually as a result of a biopsy. The importance of obtaining accurate histologic or cytologic proof of malignancy cannot be overstated. Treatment decisions for cancers arising within the same organ differ on the basis of the histopathology report. An example is the very different treatment regimens for small cell cancer of the lung and adenocarcinoma of the lung. Exactly

Table 8-5 Instructions for Preparing the Patient for Image-Guided Fine-Needle Aspiration Biopsy

- Contrast agent may be required — intravenous or oral.
- Intravenous line established as a precaution or for sedation.
- Sedatives may be offered.
- Vital signs and oximetry will be monitored if intravenous sedation is used.
- Some pain may be experienced; local anesthetic is used.
- Skin at biopsy site is cleansed, and the needle inserted.
- Needle position is established by an imaging technique (e.g., CT, ultrasound, or chest fluoroscopy).
- Syringe is attached to the needle, and the fluid and tissue are aspirated.
- Patient is observed for infection, bleeding, or increase in pain.

what tissue should be biopsied depends on several factors: the clinical status of the person, his or her willingness to undergo invasive procedures, the size and location of the identified tumor, and the amount of tissue needed by the pathologist for analysis.[69]

The cytologic examination of aspirated fluid, secretions, scrapings, or washings of body cavities may reveal malignant cells that have exfoliated from a primary or metastatic tumor. Tissue will not be obtained by this method, however, and the pathologist's ability to establish the primary site of the malignancy may be limited. Cancer of the cervix is one example of a malignancy that is successfully detected by the cytologic examination of cells acquired from a Papanicolaou (Pap) smear.

The fine-needle aspiration biopsy, guided by palpation or an imaging technique, is used extensively and is available in the ambulatory setting. It provides not only cytologic information but also microhistologic information if adequate tissue fragments are obtained. Table 8-5 provides general instructions for preparing the patient for an image-guided fine-needle aspiration biopsy.[70]

Stereotactic localization is another diagnostic tool that utilizes CT or MRI to establish the coordinates of a lesion and accurately position a needle for the tissue biopsy. Stereotactic breast biopsy of nonpalpable lesions is comparable to conventional needle-localization surgical biopsy, with a sensitivity of 90%–95% for breast cancer detection.[71] Figure 8-7 demonstrates stereotactic images of a breast nodule and the accurate placement of a needle for biopsy. Stereotactic brain biopsy of suspicious lesions is a relatively safe and quick procedure. A stereotactic head frame is fixed to the skull under local anesthesia, the lesion is scanned for localizing landmarks (including the location of arteries and vessels), a small hole is made in the skull, and the biopsy is directed by an instrument attached to the frame.

Cooperation and skill are required of the surgeon, pathologist, and affiliated pathology lab to ensure that an accurate diagnosis is made. Local or topical anesthesia is commonly used. Table 8-6 lists specific details of each type of needle biopsy: (1) aspiration needles, (2) cutting or core needles, (3) large cutting needles, and (4) automated biopsy systems (biopsy guns). Some needles have carriers that shield and guide the actual biopsy needle, cup, or punch used to obtain the specimen. The carrier reduces the possibility that the needle tract will become contaminated with tumor cells from the specimen as the needle is withdrawn. An unfortunate limitation of both needle aspiration and core biopsy is the possibility that the tumor will be missed; for this reason, only a positive finding of malignancy is diagnostically significant.[72–74]

The biopsy needles are small bore, usually 20- to 23-gauge. Fine-needle biopsies are well tolerated by the patient, result in limited trauma to tissue, and cause minimal manipulation of the tumor. Hematoma and infection are potential complications.

Fluoroscopy, ultrasound, or CT are often used to guide the clinician during core biopsy procedures. Local anesthesia is used. Hematoma, infection, and pain are postbiopsy considerations.

Regional biopsy is performed using a variety of approaches and needles. It involves obtaining several samples of tissue from different locations within a tumor or within a diseased organ. Regional biopsies are used to diagnose metastatic disease in a defined, but not localized, region of the body. They also are used to sample diffuse disease within an organ or to sample multiple nodes within a region. Examples include transthoracic, pancreatic adrenal gland, liver, pelvic mass, prostate, renal, breast, thyroid, and bone regional biopsies.

For a definitive diagnosis of malignancy, it is imperative that the pathologist receive an adequate, representative, and well-preserved tissue specimen. A cytologic or histologic report that is negative for malignancy may suggest a specimen inadequate for diagnostic evaluation, necessitating repeat biopsy. Only a complete excisional biopsy can exclude malignancy with certainty. When the results of a biopsy are equivocal, the specimen should be sent to an outside source for a second evaluation. The Armed Forces Institute of Pathology in Washington, D.C., is used by pathologists worldwide as a reference and for review.

Not infrequently, the biopsied tissue will confirm malignancy, but the primary site or tissue of origin cannot be established by the pathologist or the clinician. An example is the individual who undergoes biopsy of a cervical node and is diagnosed with squamous cell carcinoma but for whom a thorough examination of the chest and head and neck area fails

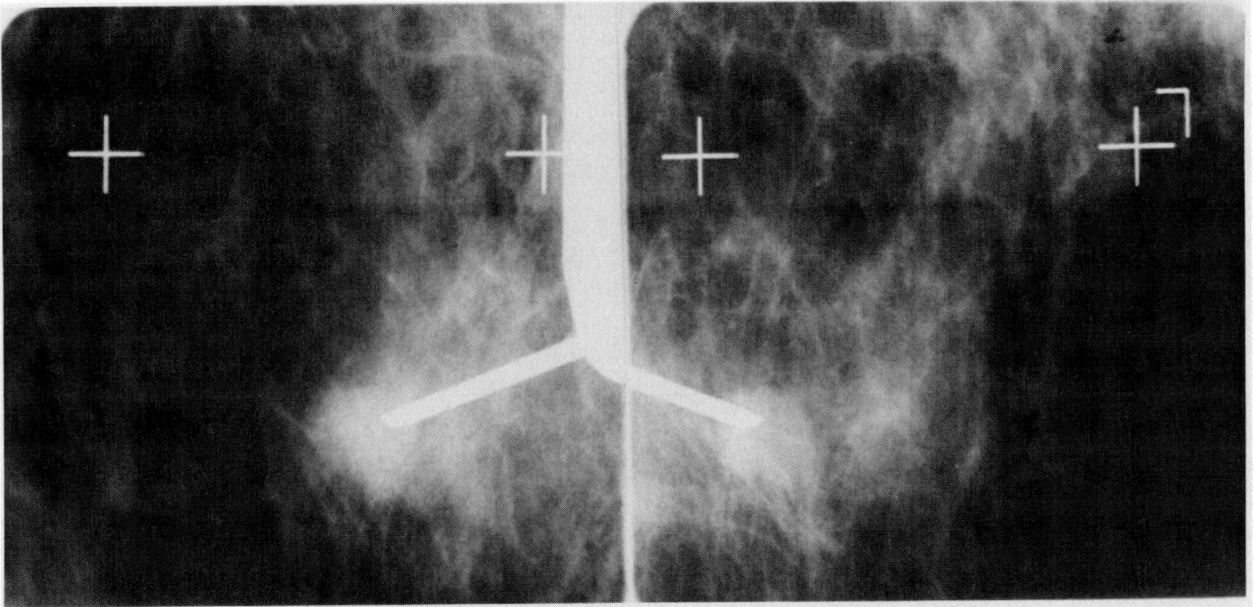

Figure 8-7 Pair of images confirming accurate placement of needle at the margin of a breast nodule for stereotactic core biopsy. (Courtesy of Scripps Memorial Hospital, Department of Radiology, La Jolla, CA.)

to yield the source of the malignancy. The goals for pursuing the primary site in this situation are discussed later in this chapter in "Tumors of Unknown Origin."

Surgical biopsy techniques

In some cases, such as tumors of the lip, nose, ear, or breast, excisional biopsy alone will be definitive therapy. The pathologist and the surgeon will determine whether the extent of the excisional biopsy is sufficient to eliminate the possibility of residual disease or whether more extensive surgery is indicated. The tissue is covered with ink, sliced, and then put on the slide for microscopic evaluation.

Incisional biopsies are generally selected for the diagnosis of large tumors that will require major surgery for complete removal. In this type of procedure, a portion of the mass is removed for pathologic examination. Incisional biopsy should be positioned in such a way that the biopsy site will be totally excised with subsequent definitive surgery.

Endoscopy is a surgical technique used to obtain biopsy specimens for diagnosis of tumors in accessible lumens.[75] Tumors of the gastrointestinal, genitourinary, or pulmonary system and, more recently, of the ductal system of the breast can be diagnosed by inserting an optical instrument into the lumen to examine the area and to secure a biopsy for analysis or secretions for cytologic examination. Flexible instruments have made endoscopy more tolerable for the patient and more functional for the clinician. Bleeding and infection are potential problems.

Laparoscopy

During the last decade, laparoscopy has been increasingly used for the detection, staging, and treatment of cancer, thereby legitimizing it as an acceptable surgical procedure. The development of high-resolution monitors and instrumentation as well as greater surgical experience have made this expansion possible.[76]

Laparoscopy has been used to diagnose and treat a wide variety of cancers, including lymphoma and gastrointestinal, urologic, and gynecologic malignancies.[77] It enjoys a distinct advantage over other diagnostic procedures in visualizing the abdominal cavity and lesions, and in evaluating adenopathy and liver abnormalities. Laparoscopy also offers the opportunity to visualize the diaphragm and peritoneal surfaces.

Patients facing a diagnosis of cancer of the pancreas, stomach, or esophagus have benefited from the use of laparoscopy rather than CT and US to determine resectability and nodal status. The surgical approach using this method decreases the need for, and may prevent putting the patient through, an unnecessary laparotomy. Accurate diagnosis and staging of Hodgkin's lymphoma can now be done thanks to current laparoscopic capabilities. Staging laparotomies have decreased by 70% in these patients due to the advent of laparoscopic liver and spleen biopsies.[78]

Table 8-6 Approaches for Biopsy

Type	What Used For	Where Done	Rationale
Needle Biopsy			
Fine-needle aspiration (21–22 g needle 5-cc syringe): Local anesthesia	Solid, palpable lesion (i.e., breast mass, thyroid nodule)	Outpatient setting Operating room	Involves only small amount of trauma to tissue, so if positive then surgical procedure is avoided. Used when there is a high level of suspicion of malignancy.
Sterotaxic fine-needle aspiration (21–22 g needle, sterotaxic equipment): Local anesthesia	Solid, nonpalpable lesion (i.e., mammographic abnormality)	Outpatient setting Radiology center	Same as for fine-needle aspiration, but able to sample small, *nonpalpable* lesions.
Core needle biopsy (special cutting needle): Local anesthesia; can use ultrasound to help guide	Solid, accessible tumor	Outpatient setting	Removes larger amount of tissue than fine-needle aspiration; may allow for more information (i.e., hormone receptor tests).
Surgical Biopsy			
Excisional biopsy: Usually local anesthesia	Solid, palpable mass (i.e., melanoma, breast mass)	Day surgery	Attempt is made to remove the whole mass only, without regard to clear margin. Result should be cosmetically acceptable.
Incisional biopsy: Usually local anesthesia	Solid, palpable large mass (i.e., large, ulcerating or bleeding mass)	Day surgery	Biopsy is for diagnosis; mass is too large to remove without major surgery. May bleed profusely.
Endoscopy (special endoscope): May use sedation	Solid mass in an accessible lumen (i.e., colon, esophagus)	Outpatient setting Day surgery	May be for diagnosis or treatment. Avoids surgical trauma.

Overall, for some patients who face the diagnosis of cancer, there may be an advantage to using laparoscopy as a diagnostic tool. A shorter hospital stay and recovery time, which lowers costs, along with decreased pain and a quicker return to activities of daily living, have a definite impact on the patient's quality of life. The future of laparoscopy holds promise, but emphasis must be placed on proper surgical training, gathering of scientific data, and evaluation of this procedure if patients are to benefit.

Classification and Nomenclature

Basic Terminology

The terms *cancer* and *tumor* often are used interchangeably and inappropriately and can be misleading for patients, families, and professionals. A *tumor* is a swelling or mass of tissue that may be benign or malignant. *Cancer,* synonymous with *malignant neoplasm,* is an uncontrolled "new growth" capable of metastasis and invasion that threatens host survival.

The term *primary tumor* is used to describe the original histologic site of tumorigenesis. A *secondary,* or metastatic, *tumor* resembles the primary tumor histologically but sometimes may be so anaplastic as to obscure the cell of origin. A *second primary lesion* refers to an additional, histologically separate malignant neoplasm in the same patient. Although this is a relatively unusual occurrence, it must be excluded at the time of an apparent recurrence. Tables of probability for recurrence exist to guide the clinician in making these determinations. A general rule is always to biopsy the first recurrence, because it may actually represent a new, curable or treatable malignancy — for example, a patient with a history of breast cancer who presents with suspicious lymph nodes and is found on biopsy to have lymphoma. Unfortunately, some recurrences present in sites where the morbidity from biopsy is so significant that the lesion is treated without tissue confirmation — for example, a woman with breast cancer who presents with a vertebral pedicle lesion.

Benign and Malignant Tumor Characteristics

Certain biological, histologic, and cytologic characteristics distinguish a benign tumor from a malignant tumor. However, with the exception of the properties of invasion and metastasis, which are found only in cancer, the differences between a benign process and a malignant process are relative. In some circumstances, a definitive diagnosis of benign tumor versus malignant tumor cannot be made. For example, a well-differentiated follicular carcinoma of the thyroid may be solitary and encapsulated and may mimic a benign adenoma of the thyroid. Occasionally, a benign tumor will transform into a malignant tumor over time. An adenomatous polyp of the colon is an example of a relatively benign process that can transform into cancer of the colon if left untreated.

In general, the following features distinguish benign tumors from those that are malignant. The *benign tumor* is relatively slow growing. Tumor stasis or regression may occur. Growth occurs as the tumor expands locally within a capsule of fibrous tissue. Benign tumors do not invade adjacent tissues, destroy normal tissue, or metastasize elsewhere in the body. Although death from a benign tumor is rare, distressing symptoms may result from a tumor's pressure on vital organs or from ectopic hormone production. Cytologic examination reveals uniform, well-differentiated cells that resemble those of the adult tissue of origin and demonstrate little or no anaplasia and rare mitoses.

In contrast, the *malignant tumor* is characterized by its generally high mitotic rate, rapid growth, and disregard for normal growth limitations. Malignant tumors are almost never encapsulated. The malignant cells invade surrounding tissue, lymphatic vessels, and blood vessels and metastasize to distant sites. They are anaplastic, vary in morphologic characteristics within the same tumor, are poorly differentiated, and have abnormal and inconstant numbers of chromosomes.

Tumor Classification System

The most relevant classification systems will universally communicate clinical and prognostic information. Tumors may be classified not only by their biological behavior (benign versus malignant), but also by their tissue of origin.

Virtually every cell type in the body is capable of transforming into a malignant cell. It is fairly well accepted that the malignant cell derives from a postembryonic cell that is arrested in the process of differentiation. Most tumors retain sufficient characteristics— such as function and structure of the normal, differentiated cell—to allow recognition of the type of tissue from which they were derived, which is the basis for the classification of human tumors by tissue type (Table 8-7).[79–81]

Tumors of Unknown Origin

Five to ten percent of patients diagnosed with cancer each year are found to have a malignancy from an unknown primary site.[82] Most frequently, the histologic classification will be adenocarcinoma, but the site of origin may never be determined, even on autopsy. The prognosis in such cases is poor, primarily because the disease is already metastatic. The overall median survival of persons with an unknown primary site ranges from 3 to 4 months.[83] The goal of proceeding with a diagnostic investigation in this situation is to identify those malignancies, even if they are disseminated, that are potentially curable or palliated with known, effective treatment. For example, lymphomas and germ cell tumors are potentially curable with systemic chemotherapy. Lesions in the nasopharynx may be cured with radiation. Local complications such as bowel obstruction, spinal cord compression, and pathologic fractures can be palliated with surgery or radiation treatment, even when the primary site of malignancy is unknown. Hormonal therapy may be recommended if the presumptive diagnosis, based on tumor markers or hormone receptor analysis, is breast, prostate, or endometrial malignancy.

Patients and their families who are facing cancer from an unknown source present unique challenges for the nurse. Not only do they need information and preparation for extensive imaging and laboratory testing, but they also need support when these tests fail to yield a definitive diagnosis. It is often hoped, though does not necessarily prove true, that a known primary source of malignancy will be more treatable or curable than an unknown primary source. Coping with any cancer diagnosis is difficult. Coping with an "unknown" cancer accentuates the feelings of loss of control, anxiety, and frustration. The involved nurse can offer the greatest assistance by identifying psychosocial concerns and available support systems early in the diagnostic period, clarifying and reinforcing known information and the rationale for extensive testing, and providing hope and reassurance that treatment is offered for the most probable and most treatable source of malignancy.[84]

Staging and Grading Classifications

Staging the Extent of the Disease

The staging process is a method of classifying a malignancy by the extent of its spread within the body. It is a clinical and histologic determination that depends on the natural course of each particular type of cancer. Staging is based on the premise that cancers with similar histologic features and sites of origin will extend and metastasize in a predictable manner. Although most staging classifications are based on the anatomical extent of disease, other criteria are included for specific malignancies. For thyroid cancer, the age of the patient and the histologic diagnosis (papillary,

Table 8-7 Selected Benign and Malignant Neoplasms Listed by Histogenetic Classification

Tissue of Origin	Benign Neoplasm	Malignant Neoplasm
Epithelial (Endodermal)		
Squamous	Squamous cell papilloma	Squamous cell or epidermoid carcinoma
Glandular	Adenoma	Adenocarcinoma
	Papilloma	Papillary carcinoma
	Cystadenoma	Cystadenocarcinoma
Respiratory tract		Bronchogenic carcinoma
Renal epithelium	Renal tubular adenoma	Renal cell carcinoma (hypernephroma)
Urinary tract	Transitional cell papilloma	Transitional cell carcinoma
Placental epithelium	Hydatidiform mole	Choriocarcinoma
Testicular epithelium		Seminoma
		Embryonal carcinoma
Liver	Liver cell adenoma	Hepatocellular carcinoma (hepatoma)
Biliary tree	Cholangioma	Cholangiocarcinoma
Stomach	Gastric polyp	Gastric carcinoma
Colon	Colonic polyp	Adenocarcinoma of the colon
Mesenchymal (Mesodermal)		
Connective		
Fibrous tissue	Fibroma	Fibrosarcoma
Adipose tissue	Lipoma	Liposarcoma
Cartilage	Chondroma	Chondrosarcoma
Bone	Osteoma	Osteosarcoma
Muscle		
Smooth muscle	Leiomyoma	Leiomyosarcoma
Striated muscle	Rhabdomyoma	Rhabdomyosarcoma
Endothelial		
Blood vessels	Hemangioma	Hemangiosarcoma
Lymphatic vessels	Lymphangioma	Lymphangiosarcoma
Hematopoietic and lymphoreticular		
Hematopoietic cells		Leukemias
Lymphoid tissue		Lymphomas
		Hodgkin's disease
Plasma cells		Plasmacytoma (multiple myeloma)
Neural (Ectodermal)		
Meninges	Meningioma	Meningeal sarcoma
Glia	Astrocytoma	Glioblastoma multiforme
Nerve cells	Ganglioneuroma	Neuroblastoma
		Medulloblastoma
Melanocytes	Nevus	Malignant melanoma
Mixed Tissues		
Kidney	Teratoma	Teratocarcinoma
Salivary gland		Wilms' tumor
	Mixed tumor of salivary gland (pleomorphic adenoma)	Malignant mixed tumor of salivary gland

follicular, medullary, or anaplastic) are included in the staging system. In the staging of prostate cancer, soft-tissue sarcomas, primary malignant tumors of the bone, and brain tumors, the histopathologic grade of the tumor is significant.

There are multiple objectives of solid tumor staging, but the most important is to provide the necessary information for individual treatment planning. In addition, uniform staging procedures reveal prognosis, evaluate various treatment modalities, facilitate the exchange of information, compare mortality and morbidity statistics among various treatment centers, promote exchange of information among treatment centers, and stratify individuals who may be eligible for clinical trials.[85]

With the goal of developing an internationally consistent system of staging solid tumor malignancy, the TNM committee of the International Union Against Cancer (UICC) and the American Joint Committee on Cancer (AJCC) have agreed on the TNM staging system. This system classifies solid tumors by the anatomical extent of disease, as determined clinically and histologically. Three categories are quantified, with gradations representing progressive tumor size or involvement. First, the extent of the primary tumor (T) is evaluated on the basis of depth of invasion, surface

Table 8-8 TNM Classification System for Describing the Anatomical Extent of Disease

TNM Definitions		
(T) Primary tumor		
	TX	Primary tumor cannot be assessed
	T0	No evidence of primary tumor
	Tis	Carcinoma in situ
	T1, T2, T3, T4	Increasing size and/or local extent of the primary tumor
(N) Regional lymph nodes		
	NX	Regional lymph nodes cannot be assessed
	N0	No regional lymph node metastasis
	N1, N2, N3	Increasing involvement of regional lymph nodes
(M) Distant metastasis		
	MX	Presence of distant metastasis cannot be assessed
	M0	No distant metastasis
	M1	Distant metastasis

TNM Classifications	
cTNM or TNM	*Clinical Classification:* Based on information obtained from the physical examination, laboratory and imaging studies, endoscopy, biopsy, and surgical exploration. Clinical staging uses all information available before the initiation of definitive treatment.
pTNM	*Pathologic Classification:* Based on information acquired before treatment, supplemented or modified by information from surgery and the pathologic examination of a resected specimen. This includes resected tumor (pT), lymph nodes (pN), and distant metastasis (pM).
rTNM	*Retreatment Classification:* Based on all information available after a disease-free interval or at the time of a second-look surgery. The extent or absence of disease recurrence is documented before retreatment planning is begun.
aTNM	*Autopsy Classification:* Based on all information available at the time of a postmortem examination. It is helpful in answering questions about the tumor's response to treatment, recurrence patterns, and the extent of disease at the time of death.

spread, and tumor size. Second, the absence or presence and extent of regional lymph node (N) metastasis are considered, with attention to the size and location of the nodes. Third, the absence or presence of distant metastasis (M) is assessed. A three-letter abbreviation may specify the site of metastasis. For example, M1 PUL denotes pulmonary metastasis. The TNM system is further classified by whether the assessment is obtained clinically (cTNM or TNM), after pathologic review (pTNM), at the time of retreatment (rTNM), or on autopsy (aTNM). For reporting purposes, the TNM stage classification remains constant throughout the disease process. Progression of disease does not change the initial stage of disease. Table 8-8 presents the nomenclature of the TNM system for classification.[85]

It is important to distinguish the cTNM, based on a clinical exam, from the pTNM, which is determined after surgery when the true extent of the disease is known and treatment decisions can be made. This is particularly true in breast cancer, where the lymph node status (pN) is the most precise prognostic indicator and directs adjuvant therapy decisions. Surgical nurses are well aware of the support needed by the woman with breast cancer in the first 24 to 48 hours after lymphadenectomy while she is awaiting the pathologist's review of lymph nodes. Another example occurs in the treatment of prostate cancer when the discovery of tumor in the pelvic lymph nodes (pN) at the time of surgery precludes the anticipated radical prostatectomy.

After numerical values are assigned to the T, N, and M categories, they are clustered into one of four stages (I through IV), or stage 0 for carcinoma in situ. Stage IV consistently includes distant metastases (M1) and predicts the worst prognosis. All tumor sites are grouped differently on the basis of characteristics of the disease.

Several established and accepted staging classifications other than TNM exist for particular malignancies. Melanomas have been staged not only by the level of invasion of the primary lesion but also by lesion thickness—both major determinants of prognosis. The Clark levels of invasion along with Breslow's measurement of vertical thickness are universal staging systems. The TNM system, which is now in use and highly valued in clinical practice, encompasses four stages utilizing both microstaging classifications for tumor assessment. For many years, the staging system of choice for colorectal cancer had been the Duke's system, which classifies tumors by their depth of invasion and presence of nodal metastasis. Only recently has the TNM system become widely accepted and incorporated into this medical arena. The issue of which staging system is preferred remains unresolved. The International Federation of Gynecology and Obstetrics has an accepted staging system for cervical and endometrial cancers. Hodgkin's disease and non-Hodgkin's lymphoma are routinely described by the Ann Arbor classification, which recognizes disease distribution and symptoms. Cancers of the brain are not entirely suited to the TNM system because there are no lymphatic structures with which to categorize nodal (N) involvement.

Nonsolid tumors do not conform to solid tumor staging principles because of their disseminated nature. Leukemias are best classified according to their predominant cell types (i.e., lymphocytic or nonlymphocytic), cell maturation, and acute or chronic nature. Clinical, morphologic, histochemical, and immunologic findings help to define favorable or unfavorable prognostic categories in acute lymphoblastic leukemia. The French-American-British classification has clinical and prognostic significance in acute myeloblastic leukemia but is not a staging system. In chronic lymphocytic leukemia, two staging systems exist: the Rai classification system and the Binet classification system. For patients with myeloma, a three-stage classification system correlates M proteins with myeloma cell mass to provide prognostic information.[86] The AJCC, with the UICC, continues to work on the development of staging systems for malignancies not yet classified by the TNM system. These include cancers of the small intestine, mesothelioma, spinal cord, carcinoid, and Kaposi's sarcoma. Additionally, they are likely to incorporate tumor markers into the present anatomical staging to produce a system with better prognostic indexes.[87] This development has important implications for patients with early-stage disease (based on anatomical staging) who are actually at risk for recurrence based on other measurements of malignant potential and who will need further treatment. The 30% of women with node-negative breast cancer who eventually experience a recurrence represent one subset of people with early-stage disease who have a less favorable prognosis. The staging system of the future will encompass an estimation of risk (of local extension and distant metastases) based on the sum of risks associated with anatomical stage, morphologic grade, biological grade, and genetic potential.[88] In breast cancer, it could include the TNM stage, degree of morphologic anaplasia, estrogen and progesterone receptor status, S-phase fraction and DNA ploidy, epidermal growth factor receptors, *HER-2* or *ERB-2,* and *MYC* oncogene expression.[88]

Patient Performance Classification

A multitude of factors affect treatment decisions at the time of diagnosis, with the patient's physical condition being a primary consideration. Patients who are bedridden are much less likely to respond to treatment than are those who are asymptomatic and able to maintain the activities of daily living. Performance scales that measure a person's functional status are used frequently in the eligibility criteria for cooperative group clinical trials and also periodically to evaluate the effects of treatment and disease. It is important to assess whether aggressive, toxic treatment protocols actually will permit people to feel better and to maintain their optimal functional status. The most prevalent performance scales are the Karnofsky Performance Status scale, the Eastern Cooperative Oncology Group (ECOG) scale, and the World Health Organization (WHO) scale.[89–91] The three scales are compared in Table 8-9. Nurses need to be familiar with the scoring systems, as they may be able to contribute the most accurate information to a primarily subjective rating.

Grading

Grading a malignant neoplasm is a method of classification based on histopathologic characteristics of the tissue. The pathologist assesses the aggressiveness or degree of malignancy of tumor cells by comparing the cellular anaplasia, differentiation, and mitotic activity with those of the cells' normal counterparts. Specific characteristics vary with each type of cancer.

The objective of grading a tumor is to quantify information so as to assist with treatment planning and prognostic determinations. For selected tumors, the grade is considered more significant than anatomical staging in terms of prognostic value and treatment. The histology of tumors that affect the brain and spinal cord is by far the most important variable with regard to prognosis, and in many cases it determines the treatment modalities that are employed. In soft tissue sarcomas, the grade is the primary determinant of stage of disease and of prognosis.

Two grading systems are commonly seen. One descriptively identifies the tumor as well-differentiated (i.e., retaining most of the morphologic features and behavior of the normal cell of the tissue of origin), moderately well-differentiated, poorly differentiated, or undifferentiated. The other system numerically grades from 1 to 3 or 4, with 1 being the most differentiated and 3 and 4 being the least well-differentiated; grade 4 applies to tumors with no specific differentiation. It is important to remember that the grade 1, well-differentiated tumor implies the best prognosis for the patient. The AJCC recommends the following grading classification:[85]

GX Grade cannot be assessed
G1 Well-differentiated
G2 Moderately well-differentiated
G3 Poorly differentiated
G4 Undifferentiated

Other grading systems under development offer more precise guidelines adding features of nuclear grade and mitotic activity to the evaluation of tissue differentiation. If there is evidence of more than one grade or of differentiation of the tumor, the least differentiated is recorded as the histopathologic grade, using only G2 through G4. For example, a colonic adenocarcinoma that is partially well-differentiated and partially moderately differentiated is coded as grade 2 (G2). The growing edge of the tumor is not generally assessed in grading because it may appear to be high grade—except in the breast, where that is the best reflection of prognosis.

For some anatomical sites, grades 3 and 4 are combined into a single grade—for example, poorly

Table 8-9 Comparison of Frequently Used Performance Status Scales

Karnofsky Scale		ECOG Scale		WHO Scale	
% Score	Status	Score	Status	Score	Status
100%	Normal; no complaints; no evidence of disease	0	Asymptomatic	0	Fully active, able to carry out all predisease activities without restriction
90	Able to carry on normal activity; minor signs or symptoms of disease	1	Symptomatic; fully ambulatory	1	Restricted in strenuous activity but ambulatory and able to carry out light work or pursue sedentary occupation
80	Normal activity with effort; some signs or symptoms of disease				
70	Cares for self; unable to carry on normal activity or to do active work	2	Symptomatic; in bed less than 50% of day	2	Ambulatory and capable of all self-care but unable to do any light work; up and about more than 50% of waking hours
60	Requires occasional assistance, but able to care for most needs				
50	Requires considerable assistance and frequent medical care	3	Symptomatic; in bed more than 50% of day but not bedridden	3	Capable of only limited self-care; confined to bed or chair more than 50% of waking hours
40	Disabled; requires special care and assistance				
30	Severely disabled; hospitalization indicated, although death not imminent	4	Bedridden	4	Completely disabled; unable to carry out any self-care and confined totally to bed or chair
20	Very sick; hospitalization necessary; active supportive treatment necessary				
10	Moribound; fatal processes progressing rapidly				
0	Dead				

differentiated to undifferentiated (G3–4). The combination is valid for carcinomas of the uterine corpus, ovary, prostate, urinary bladder, kidney, renal pelvis, ureter, urethra, and breast. Only three grades are used for melanoma of the conjunctiva and uvea. Grading does not apply to carcinomas of the thyroid, eyelids, and retinoblastoma or to malignant testicular tumors and melanoma of the skin.

Certain problems exist with grading classifications. Most notably, a tumor's level of differentiation may vary with time. Also, several grades of malignancy may exist within one tumor, in which case the tumor should be labeled as having the least favorable level of differentiation. It is essential that an adequate and representative biopsy specimen be obtained for a valid interpretation by the pathologist. Nurses who are aware of the significance of a malignant tumor's grade and stage, as well as new prognostic, molecular markers, will be able to respond realistically to the patient's questions about treatment and prognosis.

Future Trends

Biomarker research has benefited from advances in technology such as proteomics. The cellular proteome is a dynamic profile that is subject to changes in response to various signals as part of disease progression. This shifting occurs through interplay of post-translational modifications, translocation, protein–protein interactions, and protein–nucleic acid interactions. An important aspect of cancer proteomics is the ability to target and analyze subsets of proteins. Specific compartments under scrutiny include proteome analysis of mitochondria, lysosomes, peroxisomes, endoplasmic reticulum, Golgi apparatus, endocytic vesicles, and the nucleus.[92]

Proteomics complements genomic-based approaches in the study of cancer. Proteins represent the functional output of a cell and form an intrinsic part of its dynamic network. Their expression, activities, and location can be changed at any time through post-translational modifications. Studies indicate that as many as six different proteins form per gene in humans, and understanding their functional status in nondiseased individuals and in various stages of disease progression will provide insights into designing strategies for prevention, diagnosis, and therapeutics.[93] Proteomics is essential in detecting changes in protein profiles that can lead to more comprehensive understanding of the cancer process and the development and validation of new protein biomarkers.

Molecular imaging has become of the utmost importance in evaluating patients with cancer. Single-photon emission computed tomography (SPECT) and PET are accurate methods for detecting cancer and related metabolic abnormalities, but they often do not provide the anatomical landmarks needed to precisely localize lesions. MRI and CT scan offer excellent anatomical detail but are less sensitive because they do not provide functional detail.

Fusion imaging combines functional radiologic imaging with metabolic studies, overcoming the drawbacks associated with these modalities. Software-based fusion of independently performed scintigraphic and radiological images has proven time-consuming and impractical for routine use. Recently, dual-modality integrated imaging systems (SPECT/CT and PET/CT) have been developed: The acquired images are co-registered by means of the hardware in the same session. These new devices can be particularly useful, as the anatomical images provide precise localization of the tumor and allow for the exclusion of disease in sites of physiologic tracers' accumulation for SPECT and PET findings.[94]

Results of hybrid imaging in the diagnosis of cancer have proved very encouraging, indicating that these systems are well suited for routine use in clinical practice. Fused images provide additional information that improves diagnostic accuracy and can influence patient management. The efficacy of these modalities has been questioned due to their higher cost and limited availability, however.

The nurse's role is one of teacher, educating the patient about the testing procedure, and offering guidance and reassurance. Serving also as a liaison between physician and insurance carrier, the nurse will be called on to explain the procedure and purpose behind the diagnostic study.

Conclusion

The diagnostic phase of a cancer illness is a time of adjustment, learning, anxiety, and uncertainty for both patient and family. With adequate knowledge of the symptoms of disease and of the diagnostic process required for evaluation, nurses can help prepare patients, thereby easing the anxiety associated with the unknown. During this time, nurses will interact with the individual in several healthcare settings — primary clinics, inpatient and outpatient units, and extended care units — as well as in the community. Oncology nurses have used their expertise to do the following:

1. Facilitate early diagnosis of cancer by promoting awareness of "warning signals" of cancer and conducting screening programs
2. Educate and prepare individuals for a diagnostic evaluation of suspicious signs or symptoms
3. Perform or assist with diagnostic procedures and interpret or clarify results
4. Counsel and support the individual and family in a therapeutic relationship
5. Prepare the individual for the possible treatment options once a definitive diagnosis is made

Nurses have the power to promote the detection of cancer at the earliest possible stage and to assist the individual and family to regain hope, control, and quality of life once the diagnosis of cancer has been determined.

References

1. American Cancer Society: *Cancer Facts and Figures.* Atlanta, American Cancer Society, 2004
2. Fitch MI, Greenberg M, Levstein L, et al: Health promotion and early detection of cancer in older adults: assessing knowledge about cancer. *Oncol Nurs Forum* 24:1743–1748, 1997
3. Fink DJ, Mettlin CJ: Cancer detection: the cancer-related checkup guidelines, in Murphy GP, Lawrence W, Lenhard RE (eds.): *American Cancer Society Textbook of Clinical Oncology* (ed 2). Atlanta, American Cancer Society, 1995, pp 178–193
4. Carroll-Johnson, RM (ed.): Cancer prevention and early detection: oncology nursing's next frontier. *Oncol Nurs Forum* 27(suppl 9):1–61, 2000
5. Blue Cross of California Presents: *Breast Cancer Practice Guidelines.* Woodland Hills, Blue Cross of California, 1995
6. Mahon SM: Cancer risk assessment conceptual considerations for clinical practice. *Oncol Nurs Forum* 25:1535–1547, 1998
7. Rohan K, Frank-Stromborg M: The evolution of nursing's role in the prevention and detection of cancer, in Jennings-Dozier K, Mahon S (eds.): *Cancer Prevention, Detection, and Control: A Nursing Perspective.* Pittsburgh, PA, ONS Press, 2002, pp 7–32
8. ONS Board of Directors Position Paper: The role of the advanced practice nurse in oncology care. *Oncol Nurs Forum,* 30:549–550, 2003
9. Caplan LS, Couglin S: Worksite breast cancer screening programs: a review. *AAOHN J* 46:443–453, 1998
10. Gelfand DE, Parzuchowski J, Rivero-Perry M, et al: Work-site cancer screening: a Latino case study. *Oncol Nurs Forum* 27:659–666, 2000
11. Kenny J, Keenan P: A survey of breast cancer detection methods in long-term care facilities. *J Gerontol Nurs* 17:20–22, 1991
12. Williams R: Breast cancer detection in home health care of the older woman. *Home Healthcare Nurse* 8:25–29, 1989

13. Peteet JR, Stomper PC, Ross DM, et al: Emotional support for patients with cancer who are undergoing CT: semistructured interviews of patients at a cancer institute. *Radiology* 182:99–102, 1992
14. Shell J, Kirsch S: Psychosocial and quality of life issues, in Otto SE (ed.): *Oncology Nursing* (ed 4). St. Louis, Mosby, 2001, pp 948–972
15. Mahon SM, Casperson D: Teaching women about mammography through use of a brochure. *Oncol Nurs Forum* 18:1375–1378, 1991
16. McCance KL, Roberts LK: Biology of cancer, in McCance KL, Huether SE (eds.): *Pathophysiology: The Biologic Basis for Disease in Adults and Children* (ed 3). St. Louis, Mosby, 1998, pp 304–349
17. Schlom J, Abrams SI: Tumor immunology, in Kufe DW, Pollock RE, Weischelbaum R, et al (eds.): *Cancer Medicine* (ed 6). Hamilton, Ontario, BC Decker, 2003, pp 153–168
18. Wallach J: *Interpretation of Diagnostic Tests: A Synopsis of Laboratory Medicine* (ed 7). Boston, Little, Brown, 2000
19. Liotta LA, Liu Et: Essentials of molecular biology: basic principles, in DeVita VT, Hellman S, Rosenberg SA (eds.): *Cancer Principles and Practice of Oncology* (ed 6). Philadelphia, Lippincott, 2001, pp 3–15
20. Ravel R: *Clinical Laboratory Medicine: Clinical Application of Laboratory Data* (ed 6). St. Louis, Mosby, 1995
21. Stearns V, Yamauchi H, Hayes D: Circulating tumor markers in breast cancer: accepted utilities and novel prospects. *Breast Cancer Res Treat* 52:239–259, 1998
22. Chernecky C: *Laboratory Tests and Diagnostic Procedures.* Philadelphia, Saunders, 2004
23. Madeya ML, Pfab-Tokarsky JM: Flow cytometry: an overview. *Oncol Nurs Forum* 19:459–463, 1992
24. Mirza AV, Vlastos G, Singletary SE: Prognostic factors in node-negative breast cancer: a review of studies with sample size more than 200, follow up more than 5 years. *Ann Surg* 235:10–26, 2002
25. Herman C: Cytometric DNA analysis in the management of cancer: clinical laboratory considerations. *Cancer* 69(suppl 6):1553–1556, 1992
26. Loescher LJ: DNA testing for cancer predisposition. *Oncol Nurs Forum* 25:1317–1327, 1998
27. Liu K: Breakthroughs in cancer gene therapy. *Semin Oncol Nurs* 19:217–226, 2003
28. Mercic F, Hung M, Hortobagyi GN, et al: HER2/neu in the management of invasive breast cancer. *J Am Coll Surg* 194:488–501, 2001
29. Lerman C, Shields AE: Genetic testing for cancer susceptibility: the promise and the pitfalls. *Nat Rev Cancer* 4:235–241, 2004
30. Statement of the American Society of Clinical Oncology: Genetic testing for cancer susceptibility. *J Clin Oncol* 4:1730–1736, 1996
31. Calzone KA, Jenkins J, Masny A: Core competencies in cancer genetics for advanced practice oncology nurses. *Oncol Nurs Forum* 29:1327–1333, 2002
32. Oncology Nursing Society: Cancer predisposition genetic testing and risk assessment counseling. *Oncol Nurs Forum* 27:1349, 2000
33. Dillon WP: Head and neck imaging. *Am J Neuroradiol* 21:25–28, 2000
34. McLoud TC: Imaging techniques for diagnosis and staging of lung cancer. *Clinics Chest Med* 23:123–136, 2002
35. Hilton S: Imaging of renal cell carcinoma. *Semin Oncol* 27:150–159, 2000.
36. Soper JT: Radiographic imaging in gynecologic oncology. *Clin Obstet Gynecol* 44:485–494, 2001
37. Schiepers C, Filmont JE, Czermini J: PET staging of Hodgkin's disease and non-Hodgkin's lymphoma. *Eur J Nuclear Med Molec Imag* 30(suppl 1):82–83, 2003
38. Rubin P, Bragg DG: Principles of oncologic imaging and tumor imaging strategies, in Rubin P (ed.): *Clinical Oncology: A Multidisciplinary Approach for Physicians and Students* (ed 8). Philadelphia, Saunders, 2001, pp 241–251
39. Brenner RJ: Interventional procedures of the breast, in Bragg DG, Rubin P, Hricak H (eds.): *Oncologic Imaging* (ed 2). Philadelphia, WB Saunders, 2002, pp 295–310
40. Munden RE, Bragg DG: Primary malignancies of the thorax, in Bragg DG, Rubin P, Hricak H (eds.): *Oncologic Imaging* (ed 2). Philadelphia, WB Saunders, 2002, pp 313–341
42. Skarin AT: *Atlas of Diagnostic Oncology* (ed 3). London, Mosby-Wolfe, 2002
43. Miaskowski C: *Oncology Nursing: An Essential Guide for Patient Care.* Philadelphia, WB Saunders, 1997
44. 1998 MQSA (Mammographic Quality Standards Act) final rule released American College of Radiology: *Radiol Manage* 20:51–55, 1998
45. Roses DF: *Breast Cancer.* Philadelphia, Churchill-Livingstone, 1999
46. Clark RA: Imaging in lung cancer, in Berman CG, Brodsky NJ, Clark RA (eds.): *Oncologic Imaging* (ed 2). New York, McGraw-Hill, 1997, pp 119–132
47. Fishman EK, Urban BA: Cancer diagnosis: computed tomography, in DeVita VT, Hellman S, Rosenberg SA (eds.): *Cancer Principles and Practice of Oncology* (ed 6). Philadelphia, Lippincott, 2001, pp 659–668
48. Bittengle JR, Davis DC: Preventative care and emergency response to contrast media, in Tortorici M (ed.): *Administration of Imaging Pharmaceuticals.* Philadelphia, WB Saunders, 1996, pp 71–86
49. Pagana KD, Pagana TJ: *Mosby's Manual of Diagnostic and Laboratory Tests.* St. Louis, Mosby, 2003
50. Pickhart PJ, Pickhardt PJ, Choi JR, et al: Computed tomographic virtual colonoscopy to screen for colorectal neoplasia in asymptomatic adults. *N Engl J Med* 349:2191–2200, 2003
51. Ransohoff DF: Virtual colonoscopy: what it can do vs. what it will do. *JAMA* 291:1772–1774, 2004
52. Kewenter J, Brevinge H, Engaras B, et al: The yield of flexible sigmoidoscopy and double-contrast barium enema in the diagnosis of neoplasms in large bowel in patients with a postivie hemoccult test. *Endoscopy* 27:159–163, 1995
53. Metler FA, Guiberteau MJ: *Essentials of Nuclear Medicine Imaging* (ed 4). Philadelphia, WB Saunders, 1998
54. Berman CG, Brodsky NJ: New imaging modalities, in Berman CG, Brodsky NJ, Clark RA (eds.): *Oncologic Imaging* (ed 2). New York, McGraw-Hill, 1997, pp 367–381
55. Zhuang H, Purdehnad M, Duarte FS, et al: The role of positron emission tomography with fluorine-18-deoxyglucose in identifying colorectal cancer metastasis to the liver. *Nuclear Med* 219:793–798, 2000
56. Shafer K: Radiographic evaluation of cancer, in Skarin AT (ed.): *Diagnostic Imaging.* London, Mosby-Wolfe, 1996
57. Wahl RD, Hawkins RA, Larson SM, et al: Proceedings of a National Cancer Institute workshop: PET in oncology — a clinical research agenda. *Radiology* 193:604–606, 1994
58. Harrison KA, Tempero MA: Diagnostic use of radiolabeled antibodies for cancer. *Oncology* 9:625–631, 1995
59. Hendee WR: New imaging techniques, in Bragg DG, Rubin P, Hricak H (eds.): *Oncologic Imaging.* Philadelphia, WB Saunders, 2002, pp 39–54
60. Tengs TO: Radiological imaging: research on cost-effectiveness and the cost-effectiveness of research. *Acad Radiol* 6(suppl 1):20–27, 1999

61. Hamper UM: Cancer diagnosis: ultrasound, in DeVita VT, Hellman S, Rosenberg SA (eds.): *Cancer Principles and Practice of Oncology* (ed 6). Philadelphia, Lippincott, 2001, pp 708–714
62. Hohenschuln E, Watson AD: Constrast media: theory and mechanisms of contrast enhancing agnents, in Higgins CB, Hricak H, Helms CA (eds.): *Magnetic Resonance Imaging of the Body*. Philadelphia, Lippincott-Raven, 1997, pp 1439–1464
63. Li AE, Bluemke DA: Cancer diagnosis: magnetic resonance imaging, in DeVita VT, Hellman S, Rosenberg SA (eds.): *Cancer Principles and Practice of Oncology* (ed 6). Philadelphia, Lippincott, 2001, pp 669–672
64. Orell SD, Schnall MD: MR imaging of the breast for the detection, diagnosis, and staging of breast cancer. *Radiology* 220:13–30, 2001
65. Morris EA: Screening for breast cancer with MRI. *Semin Ultrasound CT MR* 24:45–54, 2003
66. Shellock FG, Kanl E: MRI biologic effects and safety considerations, in Higgins CB, Hricak H, Helms CA (eds.): *Magnetic Resonance Imaging of the Body*. Philadelphia, Lippincott-Raven, 1997, pp 175–204
67. Camp-Sorrell D: Magnetic resonance imaging and the implantable port. *Oncol Nurs Forum* 17:197–199, 1990
68. Levy MJ, Jondal ML, Clain J, et al: Preliminary experience with an EUS-guided trucut biopsy needle compared with EUS-guided FNA. *Gastrointest Endoscopy* 57:101–106, 2003
69. O'Hara CJ, Reed WP, Banner BF: Biopsy principles, pathologic evaluation of specimens and staging, in *Cancer Manual* (ed 9). Framingham, MA, American Cancer Society, Massachusetts Division, 1996, pp 55–74
70. Ell SR: Imaging techniques: fine-needle aspiration of various organs and body sites, in Bibbo M (ed.): *Comprehensive Cytopathology*. Philadelphia, WB Saunders, 1997, pp 615–620
71. Liberman L: Percutaneous image-guided core breast biopsy. *Radiol Clin North Am* 40:483–500, 2002
72. Daly JM, Bertagnoli M, De Cosse JJ, et al: Oncology, in Swartz SI, Shires GT, Spencer FC (eds.): *Principles of Surgery* (ed 7). New York, McGraw-Hill, 1998, pp 97–360
73. Moffat FL, Ketcham AS: Surgery for malignant neoplasia: the evolution of oncologic surgery and its role in the management of cancer patients, in McKenna RJ, Murphy GP (eds.): *Cancer Surgery*. Philadelphia, Lippincott, 1994, pp 1–20
74. Venta L: Image-guided biopsy of nonpalpable breast lesions, in Harris JR, Lippman ME, Morrow M, Osborne CK (eds.): *Diseases of the Breast*. Philadelphia, Lippincott, 1999, pp 149–164
75. Turner AF: Radiographically guided techniques of biopsy, in McKenna RJ, Murphy GP (eds.): *Cancer Surgery*. Philadelphia, Lippincott, 1994, pp 21–34
76. Ramshaw BK, Essartia D, Mason EM, et al: Lapraoscopy for diagnosis and staging of malignancy. *Semin Surg Oncol* 16:279–283, 1999
77. Pollock RE, Morton DL: Principles of surgical oncology, in Kufe DW, Pollock RE, Weischelbaum R, et al (eds.): *Cancer Medicine* (ed 6). Hamilton, Ontario, BC Decker, 2003, pp 448–458
78. Lefor AT: The role of laparoscopy in the treatment of intraabdominal malignancies. *Cancer J* 6(suppl 2):59–68, 2000
79. Ruddon RW: *Cancer Biology* (ed 3). New York, Oxford University Press, 1995, pp 3–18
80. Walter JB, Talbot C: *General Pathology* (ed 7). New York, Churchill-Livingstone, 1996, pp 471–487
81. Chandrasoma P, Taylor CL: *Concise Pathology* (ed 3). Stamford, CT, Appleton and Lange, 1998
82. Greco FA, Hainsworth JD: Cancer of unknown primary site, in DeVita VT, Hellman S, Rosenberg SA (eds.): *Cancer Principles and Practice in Oncology* (ed 6). Philadelphia, Lippincott, 2001, pp 2537–2560
83. Hainsworth JD, Greco FA: Neoplasms of unknown primary site, in Kufe DW, Pollock RE, Weischelbaum RE, et al (eds.): *Cancer Medicine* (ed 6). Hamilton, Ontario, BC Decker, 2003, pp 2115–2124
84. Hainsworth JD, Greco FA: Management of patients with cancer of unknown primary site. *Oncology* 12:563–567, 2000
85. Greene FL, Page DL, Fleming ID, et al: *American Joint Committee on Cancer: Cancer Staging Handbook* (ed 6). Philadelphia, Lippincott, 2002
86. Durie BGM, Salmon SE: A clinical staging system for multiple myeloma correlation of measured myeloma cell mass with presenting clinical features, response to treatment and survival. *Cancer* 36:842–854, 1975
87. Henson DE: Future directions for the American Joint Committee on Cancer. *Cancer* 69(suppl):1639–1644, 1992
88. Kates R, Schmitt M, Harbeck N: Advanced statistical methods for the definition of new staging models. *Rec Result Cancer Res* 162:101–113, 2003
89. Karnofsky DA, Abelmann WH, Craver LF, et al: The use of the nitrogen mustards in the palliative treatment of carcinoma. *Cancer* 1:634–656, 1948
90. Oken MM, Creech RH, Tormey DC, et al: Toxicity and response criteria of the Eastern Cooperative Oncology Group. *Am J Clin Oncol* 5:649–655, 1982
91. World Health Organization: *World Handbook for Reporting Results of Cancer Treatment*. Geneva, WHO, 1979
92. Srinivas PT, Srivastava S, Hanash S, et al: Proteomics in early detection of cancer. *Clin Chem* 47:1901–1911, 2001
93. Choi W, Song SW, Zhang W: Understanding cancer through proteomics. *Technol Cancer Res Treat* 1:221–230, 2002
94. Rollo FD: Molecular imaging: an overview and clinical applications. *Radiol Manage* 25:28–32, 2003

PART III

Treatment

CHAPTER 9

Quality of Life as an Outcome of Cancer Care

Carol Estwing Ferrans, PhD, RN, FAAN

Introduction

Over the past 30 years, quality of life has become an important gauge for evaluating healthcare outcomes. Providers of cancer care have been front-runners in the evaluation of quality of life, recognizing the need to assess outcomes more broadly than tumor response and length of survival. In 1985, the U.S. Food and Drug Administration (FDA) identified quality of life as a key parameter for approval of new anticancer drugs for advanced metastatic disease.[1] In 1988, improvement of quality of life was identified as one of the highest priorities of the Cancer Therapy Evaluation Program (CTEP) of the National Cancer Institute (NCI).[2] Increasingly, clinical trials have been designed with quality of life components in the cancer cooperative groups in the United States. In Canada, that country's National Cancer Institute now requires quality of life endpoints in all phase III clinical trials.[3] Quality of life issues are not limited to clinical trials, however. Such information is important for the entire spectrum of care for cancer patients, including palliative care, end-of-life care, and long-term survivorship.

The concept of quality of life is particularly salient for oncology nursing, because nurses traditionally have viewed patients from a holistic perspective, focusing on the quality of survival as well as the length of survival. The holistic perspective encompasses all aspects of life affected by cancer and treatment, such as physical symptoms, treatment toxicities, mental and physical functioning, body image, psychological state, work and role responsibilities, social and family life, and spiritual concerns. Because the concept of quality of life is a multidimensional construct that encompasses the whole of life, it provides a useful appraisal of outcomes important in oncology nursing.

Quality of Life as a Prognostic Indicator

It has generally been assumed that the "soft," subjective measures of quality of life are inferior to "hard," clinical indicators, such as histology and weight loss. In recent years, however, the field of measurement has grown in both methodological rigor and sophistication. A growing body of evidence suggests that patients' ratings of their quality of life before treatment are predictive of survival—in some cases even having more predictive power than traditional clinical factors. Studies reporting findings such as these primarily have been clinical trials of patients with advanced disease.[4–6] Because the studies used different instruments to measure quality of life, and the clinical trials focused on different treatment regimens, they provide greater confidence that a relationship between pretreatment quality of life and survival actually exists.

For example, Herndon et al explored this question in a study of 206 advanced non–small cell lung cancer patients treated on a clinical trial.[6] Survival was predicted by baseline scores of a quality of life instrument for pain, appetite loss, fatigue, lung cancer symptoms, physical functioning, and overall quality of life. However, when clinical factors such as histology, weight loss, dyspnea, and other factors were taken into account in the statistical analysis, one score from the quality of life instrument was still predictive. Self-rated pain was a predictor for survival, over and above the clinical factors. In another study of lung cancer patients, Montazeri et al found that patients' rating of global quality of life (prediagnosis) was the most significant predictor of length of survival even after adjusting for known prognostic factors.[7] Based on findings such as these, Ganz et al recommended that patient-rated quality of life assessment should be obtained as an integral part of cancer management to serve as a guide to patient needs, as an outcome measure, and as a prognostic variable for survival time.[5] Osoba has even suggested that pretreatment quality of life ratings could be used as an eligibility criterion and stratification variable in clinical trials.[8]

Using Quality of Life Information in Cancer Care

Information about quality of life is important for planning treatment, decision making, and the provision of supportive care. Table 9-1 lists examples of ways that quality of life information can prove valuable in clinical practice. Such information is useful for both clinicians and patients, as well as to promote communication between them. Oncology nurses play a critical role in providing this information to patients, so that they can evaluate the balance of risks and benefits associated with treatment. As early as 1984, Schipper and colleagues suggested that information about quality of life outcomes should be provided to patients, in addition to survival statistics, to enable them to make better-informed decisions about their treatment.[9] For patients to give informed consent, they must be able to decide whether the likelihood of longer life is worth the additional morbidity caused by treatment.[10] Examples of quality of life studies that have contributed to clinical decision making, the provision of supportive care, and improved communication are described in the following sections.

Table 9-1 Uses of Quality of Life Information in Cancer Care

- Determine whether a new therapy is preferable to standard therapy
- Compare two standard therapies having similar survival outcomes
- Identify the long-term negative effects of therapy, when survival time is long
- Discover whether a therapeutic regimen is better than supportive care only, when survival time is short
- Determine the negative effects of therapy given to prevent recurrence
- Identify the need for supportive care
- Target problems and facilitate communication in clinical practice

New Therapy Versus Standard Therapy

A classic use for quality of life data is to determine whether a new therapy is preferable to the standard therapy. The gold standard for these comparisons is the phase III clinical trial. An example of the importance of quality of life in a phase III study can be seen in the head-to-head comparison of imatinib (Gleevec) and interferon-alpha plus low-dose cytarabine in patients with newly diagnosed chronic myeloid leukemia.[11] After 12 months of treatment, the imatinib group had a significantly better quality of life than the interferon/cytarabine group. In particular, the imatinib group had better daily functioning, less fatigue, fewer cognitive problems, and better social functioning. In fact, the imatinib group actually had an increase in emotional well-being as compared to baseline, as patients felt better able to cope with illness, and were less worried and sad. In addition, patients who crossed over to imatinib experienced an improvement in quality of life, as compared with patients who continued with the interferon/cytarabine regimen.

Two Standard Therapies with Similar Survival Outcomes

When two treatments produce similar outcomes in survival, information about differences in quality of life outcomes can help determine the best choice. An example can be found in treatment for localized prostate cancer, which has equivalent survival rates for patients treated by radical prostatectomy or radiation therapy.[12] When Yarbro and Ferrans compared quality of life outcomes for men receiving radical prostatectomy or radiation therapy, they found that those treated by surgery had significantly worse urinary and sexual functioning.[13] Protective pads or adult diapers were worn daily by 32% of the men in the surgical group, as compared with only 6% of the radiation group. Ability to have an erection was reported to be very poor for 88% of the surgical group and for only 46% of the radiation group. In contrast, the radiation group had worse bowel functioning due to radiation damage to the rectal mucosa, although the differences between groups were smaller in this area. Diarrhea and cramping pain were problems for only a few men. Similar findings later were reported in a nationwide Prostate Cancer Outcomes Study[14,15] as well as in a prospective study.[16] These studies indicate that radiation therapy produces more favorable outcomes regarding long-term sequelae, which is an important consideration for men when deciding between these treatments.

Long-Term Negative Effects of Therapy

Quality of life information is critically important when it is not clear that treatment provides a survival advantage. For example, men with slow-growing, early prostate cancer face the prospect of watchful waiting, rather than prostatectomy or radiation, based on the assumption that comorbid conditions will cause death before the cancer will. A randomized trial of watchful waiting versus radical prostatectomy found that all-case mortality was not significantly different in the two groups, even though the rate of death from prostate cancer was slightly lower in the prostatectomy group.[17] In a companion study, quality of life outcomes were assessed an average of four years after randomization.[18] The prostatectomy group had significantly greater urinary leakage and compromised sexual function. These results are important for men to consider when newly diagnosed with prostate cancer, so that they can make an informed decision regarding treatment.

Treatment Versus Supportive Care Only

When survival time is expected to be short, quality of life information is critically important for clinical decision making. If chemotherapy cannot extend survival time significantly, the alternative is supportive care only, so that the last months of life can be enjoyed without the side effects of treatment. Before 1998, this was the situation faced by patients with metastatic colorectal cancer after fluorouracil failure. Because no treatment was known to be effective, supportive care was a reasonable alternative. Two studies then demonstrated that irinotecan was superior to second-line treatment with fluorouracil and, surprisingly, supportive care only.[19,20] The median survival time with irinotecan was two months longer than with fluorouracil, and three months longer than with supportive care only. However, for all three alternatives, the median survival time was still less than a year. Because survival time was so short, it was important to know whether irinotecan's side effects had a detrimental effect on quality of life, which might render the treatment undesirable. In comparison with patients receiving supportive care only, the irinotecan group had fewer tumor-related symptoms and a better quality of life, despite the side effects of treatment. They had better performance status, less weight loss, and less pain than the supportive care group. The only area in which the irinotecan group fared more poorly was diarrhea. These studies established irinotecan as the standard second-line therapy for metastatic colorectal cancer after fluorouracil failure.

Myelodysplastic syndrome is another example of a disease that at one time had no known effective treatment and a short survival time (6–12 months median survival). Quality of life data played a significant role in establishing azacytidine as a standard therapy. In a randomized clinical trial that compared azacytidine with supportive care only, the azacytidine group had better quality of life, greater treatment response, and longer time to death or transformation to acute myeloid leukemia. This group also had less fatigue and dyspnea, better physical functioning, more positive affect, and less psychological distress.[21,22]

Negative Effects of Therapy to Prevent Recurrence

When adjuvant therapy has been used to prevent cancer recurrence, quality of life concerns regarding toxicity and long-term disability have led to changes in practice. For example, cranial radiation has been used for central nervous system prophylaxis for acute lymphoblastic leukemia (ALL) in children. However, there was concern that cranial radiation contributed to deficits in attention and overall intellectual functioning. Hill and colleagues conducted a study that supported the conclusion that these problems were related to cranial radiation, rather than to some other aspect of ALL and treatment.[23] Two groups of survivors of childhood ALL were compared: One group had been treated with 24 Gy of cranial radiation and intrathecal methotrexate; the other had received systemic and intrathecal methotrexate but no cranial radiation. The group who had received cranial radiation had significantly worse academic achievement and greater psychological distress. As a result of these quality of life concerns, intensive efforts have been made to find effective alternatives to cranial radiotherapy to prevent relapse, such as high-dose systemic chemotherapy and intensive intrathecal therapy.[24]

Supportive Care

Quality of life information can play an important role in revealing needs for supportive care, both during treatment and afterward. For example, Ganz and colleagues examined the quality of life in 558 breast cancer patients during the period of time immediately after the completion of treatment, when women need to move beyond cancer to reestablish their normal life patterns.[25] They found that women experienced breast sensitivity, muscle stiffness, aches and pains, difficulty concentrating, and decreased energy, regardless of the type of treatment (mastectomy, lumpectomy, chemotherapy). These problems were all associated with poor physical functioning and emotional well-being. In addition, sexual functioning was worse for women who received chemotherapy, regardless of whether they underwent a lumpectomy or mastectomy. After chemotherapy, women experienced difficulties with sexual interest, lubrication, and pain with intercourse. These results target areas for more effective management to help women make a smoother transition to normal life.

Many of the problems caused by cancer and treatment can be anticipated intuitively, such as body image disruptions caused by mastectomy. Nevertheless, quality of life studies have identified some needs of patients that would not necessarily be expected. For example, although treatment for Hodgkin's disease does not commonly cause changes in appearance, one study reported that 26% of survivors believed that they were less physically attractive because of their cancer, and this belief was associated with depression and decreased sexual activity.[26] Another study found that 22% of Hodgkin's disease survivors were experiencing psychological distress severe enough to meet the criterion suggested for psychiatric diagnosis.[27] In addition, 39% still experienced conditioned nausea triggered by smells and sights that reminded them of chemotherapy. They reported problems with their sex life, employment, income, education, and denial of health and life insurance. Based on these findings, an intervention was implemented at the completion of treatment to facilitate adaptation by providing counseling via telephone.[28]

Other nurse-delivered interventions also have been instituted based on quality of life outcomes. For example, cancer outpatients diagnosed with major depressive disorder received a multicomponent intervention delivered by nurses.[29] The intervention was effective, in that 38.5% fewer patients in the treatment group were still depressed at the final six-month outcome, as compared with patients who received the usual care. In another study, breast cancer patients, who were three to four months postdiagnosis, received ten sessions of cognitive-behavioral therapy by telephone.[30]

The women who received the therapy had less anxiety and confusion at the final ten-month outcome, as compared to the control group.

Quality of life data can help to identify patients who may be at greater risk, over and above what would be expected based on their disease status. In a study of patients undergoing treatment for primary brain tumors, Weitzner et al found outcomes that would be expected, such as a poorer quality of life for patients who had bilateral tumor involvement, poorer functional status, or more aggressive treatment.[31] However, these researchers also found that patients who were female, divorced, or unable to work were at greatest risk for poorer quality of life while undergoing treatment. Similarly, based on an extensive review of studies of cancer survivors, Kornblith et al concluded that patients were at highest risk who had less social support to buffer stress, poorer prediagnosis psychological adjustment, fewer economic resources, and greater cancer-related physical problems and co-morbidities.[32] Length of time since completion of treatment played a role as well, in that adjustment tended to improve over time.

Still, not all problems disappear with the passage of time, even for long-term survivors who remain free of disease. For instance, some breast cancer survivors—particularly those with mastectomies or lymphedema—continue to experience significant problems with body image, sex life, depression, and symptoms of post-traumatic stress disorder years after treatment.[33–35] In addition, long-term survivors of various cancers have been found to experience many of the same problems—namely, chronic fatigue, fear of recurrence and death, infertility, issues of control and independence, altered meaning of health, and uncertainty about the future.[36] To help cancer patients cope with the array of cancer-related problems, Kornblith has recommended provision of both educational and counseling programs that are comprehensive in nature, provided either in groups or individually, to address these needs.[32]

As well as identifying problems, quality of life studies of long-term cancer survivors have revealed positive outcomes that can serve to encourage patients. For example, one large study found that the overall quality of life of breast cancer survivors was as good as or better than that of healthy aged-matched women, even though cancer survivors reported higher rates of physical symptoms.[37] In addition, many studies have identified positive changes in people's lives because of their experience with cancer.[32,33,36,37] Survivors have reported that they have become better people, understand life better, have reassessed their values and priorities, and are proud of their accomplishments. They characterize their lives as fuller and more meaningful, and have a greater appreciation for life and the other people in their lives. They also have reported a strengthening of spirituality and faith in God, as well as a more optimistic outlook and decreased fear of death.

Using Quality of Life Questionnaires in Clinical Practice

Quality of life questionnaires can be used in clinical practice to facilitate communication and identify problems that otherwise might go undetected, as shown in a study by Detmar and colleagues.[38] In this study, chemotherapy patients completed the questionnaires in the clinic before seeing their physicians, so that the physicians had the scores in hand at the time when they met with the patients. Quality of life issues were discussed more frequently by patients who completed the questionnaires, as compared to patients who did not. In addition, the physicians identified a larger proportion of patients with moderate or severe health problems when they had the questionnaires. All physicians and 87% of the patients thought the questionnaires facilitated communication and should continue to be used.

What Is Quality of Life?

The term *health-related quality of life* commonly is used to focus on the effects of illness and treatment. For example, because this chapter targets quality of life as an outcome of cancer care, it addresses health-related quality of life. The term "health-related quality of life" is used to draw a line between the facets of life that are primarily health related and those that are not. Cultural, political, or societal issues generally are categorized under non–health-related quality of life and fall within the purview of fields such as economics, demography, and sociology. Although social and economic problems can affect health adversely, some argue that these problems remain distant from the concerns of health-care providers.[39] At the same time, it has been pointed out that illness can make almost all aspects of life "health related."[39] It is interesting to note that the World Health Organization has chosen to define *quality of life* in a comprehensive manner:

> an individual's perception of their position in life in the context of the culture and value systems in which they live and in relation to their goals, expectations, standards, and concerns. It is a broad-ranging concept affected in a complex way by the person's physical health, psychological state, level of independence, social relationships, and their relationship to salient features of their environment.[40, p. 1570]

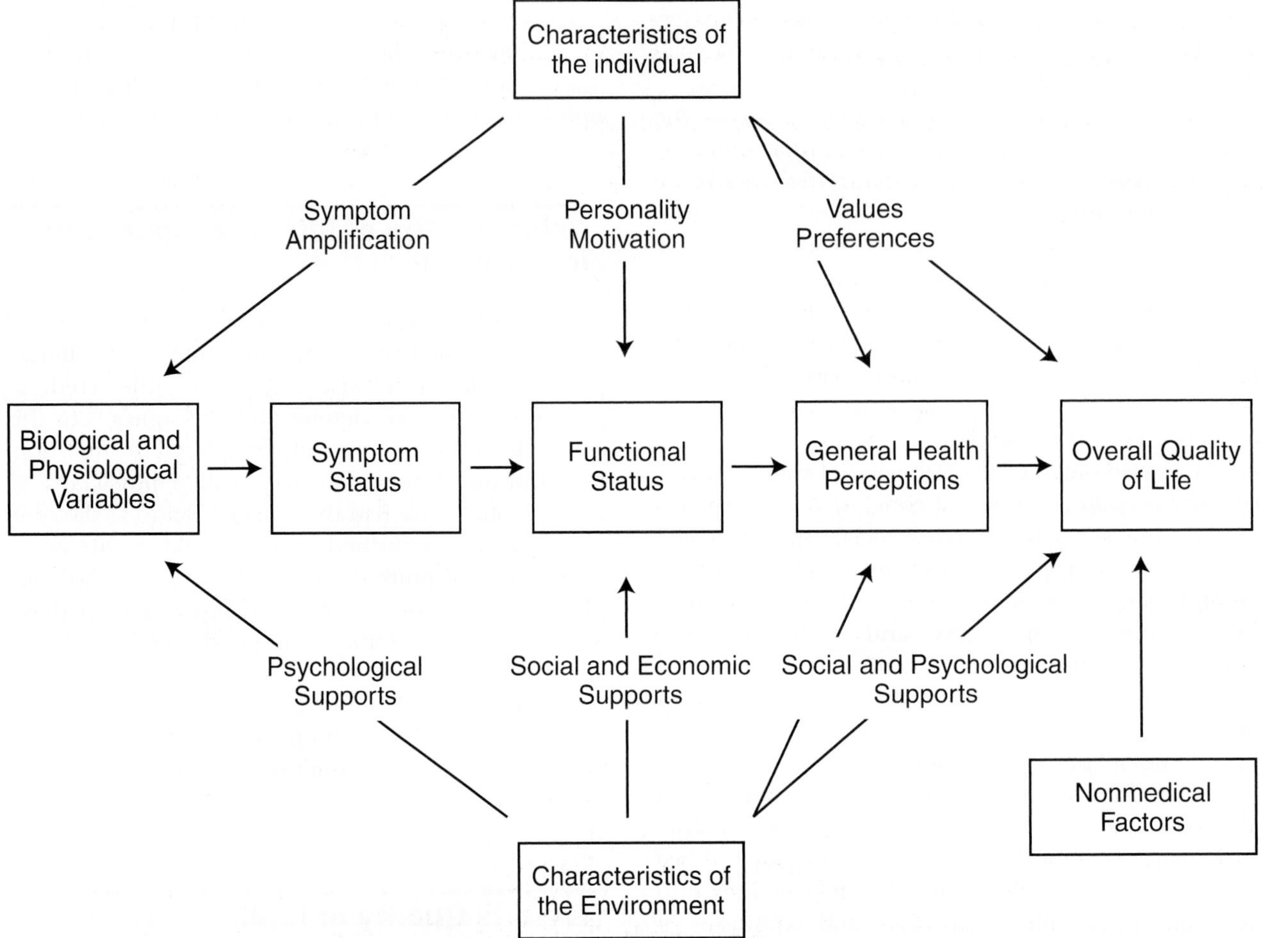

Figure 9-1 Wilson and Cleary's conceptual model for health-related quality of life. Reprinted with permission from Wilson IB, Cleary PD: Linking clinical variables with health-related quality of life. *JAMA* 273:59–65, 1995, American Medical Association. All rights reserved.[43]

Even when we consider only health-related quality of life, we find that this term has been used to mean many different things — health status, emotional adjustment, symptoms, physical functioning, well-being, life satisfaction, and happiness, for example. This ambiguity has led to a great deal of confusion, making it difficult to compare findings across studies and apply in clinical practice. Many differences stem from the fact that definitions and instruments were developed for a specific population and purpose, and the concept was tailored accordingly. Definitions and instruments should be selected based on their fit with the intended target population and purpose for use. This consideration is extremely important, because outcomes can differ depending on what is meant by "quality of life." For instance, 205 physicians were given a case description of an elderly man with chronic pulmonary disease and asked to make treatment decisions based on their own definitions of quality of life.[41] Their conclusions varied so widely that there was even disagreement regarding whether treatment should be given or withheld.

Conceptual Model of Quality of Life

A number of conceptual models have been developed to characterize health-related quality of life.[42] Wilson and Cleary developed a model that is particularly helpful for clarifying the concept.[43] Their model presents the relationships among the various types of patient outcomes that have been used to measure health-related quality of life (Figure 9-1). It focuses primarily on the five boxes in the center of the figure, which represent five levels of measurable patient outcomes. The first box, biological and physiological variables, focuses on the function of cells, organs, and organ systems. These are assessed through indicators such as physical assessment, laboratory tests, and histological findings. Symptom status, the second box, refers to physical, emotional, and cognitive symptoms, which are perceived by the patient. The third box, functional status, is composed of physical, psychological, social, and role functioning. General health perceptions, the fourth box, refers to a patient's subjective rating of health. This rating provides an integration of all of the boxes that precede it in the model. The fifth box is overall quality of life — that is, how happy or satisfied someone is with life as a whole. Values and preferences of patients are characterized as contributing to general health perceptions and overall quality of life.

Wilson and Cleary make clear that the model characterizes what they believe to be the dominant relationships, and acknowledge that some reciprocal relationships may not be pictured. Nevertheless, their model is helpful because it clearly displays the various concepts that have been used to measure quality of life outcomes. Use of this model should help researchers and clinicians to specify what exactly is meant by the term "quality of life," which will reduce some of the current confusion. Many of the definitions of quality of life that are most commonly used in health care today can be classified in relation to the components of the Wilson and Cleary model. For example, Ferrans provides a definition that characterizes overall quality of life in terms of life satisfaction (the fifth box): "a person's sense of well-being that stems from satisfaction or dissatisfaction with the areas of life that are important to him/her."[44, p. 15] Another example is provided by Gotay et al's definition, which focuses on the third and fifth boxes:

> Quality of life is a state of well-being that is a composite of two components: (1) the ability to *perform* everyday activities that reflect physical, psychological, and social well-being and (2) patient *satisfaction* with levels of functioning and the control of disease and/or treatment-related symptoms.[45, p. 576]

Domains of Quality of Life

As can be seen in the Wilson and Cleary model, quality of life is not limited to physical health status alone. There is general agreement among experts that quality of life is a multidimensional construct. As a consequence, each component of the Wilson and Cleary model should be thought of in terms of multiple domains. For example, symptom status refers to emotional and cognitive symptoms, as well as physical ones. In addition to physical functioning, functional status refers to psychological, social, and role functioning.

Leplege and Hunt have criticized many of the models developed to characterize the domains of quality of life, because they were not developed based on the viewpoints of patients themselves.[46] The two models of quality of life presented in this chapter were based on qualitative analysis of patients' perspectives and were validated with additional patient data. One model was developed by Ferrell et al (Figure 9-2) and the other by Ferrans et al (Figure 9-3 and Table 9-2). Both models are quite similar in terms of the domains identified. Both contain domains for physical health and functioning, as well as social, psychological, and spiritual domains. Additionally, the Ferrans model addresses economic elements and has a separate family domain. Because the two models were developed independently and simultaneously, the close match between them provides mutual validation. The Ferrell et al model was based on qualitative data from cancer patients with pain.[47,48] Subsequently, it was developed and validated further for patients with breast cancer, bone marrow transplantation, and cancer survivors.[49-52] The Ferrans model was based on descriptions of the components of a satisfying life given by dialysis patients.[53,54] It then was modified to include cancer patients[44] and later was validated with data from patients with breast cancer, sarcoma, bone marrow transplant, and other chronic illnesses, as well as cross-culturally.[55–60] By identifying the range of domains, both models guide the assessment of quality of life for research and clinical practice. One instrument or a battery of instruments may be needed to capture the broad nature of the concept.

Scope of Quality of Life for Research and Clinical Practice

It is clear that the idea of quality of life conveys an evaluation of the whole of life. This concept generally has been addressed by including the requisite domains. However, within each domain, a question remains as to whether the scope should be limited to those things appropriately addressed by healthcare professionals. This decision depends on the target population and the goals to be accomplished in the particular research study or clinical practice. For example, the definition of quality of life used for a chemotherapy clinical trial might focus primarily on toxicity and interference with functioning, so it might be narrow in scope. A study in end-of-life care would require a broader definition providing a balance between physical comfort and existential concerns, such as spirituality and personal meaning.

Ferrans recently developed a taxonomy for quality of life definitions based on their scope.[42] The first level is quality of life within the commonly recognized purview of health care. This level is the most narrow, in that the healthcare system is concerned primarily with the correction of problems. These definitions highlight the negative effects of illness and treatment, such as symptoms, sexual dysfunction, or disability. An example is Schipper et al's definition: "quality of life in clinical medicine represents the functional effect of an

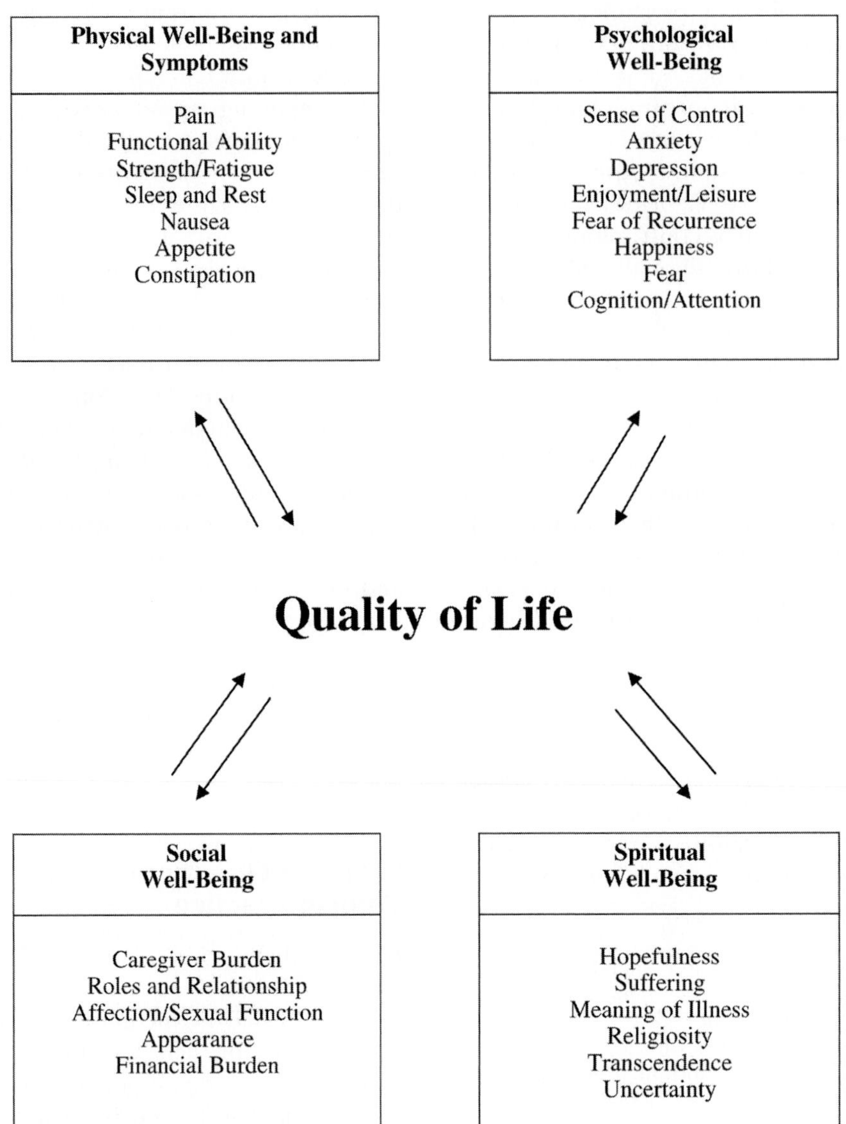

Figure 9-2 Ferrell and Grant conceptual model for quality of life. Reprinted with permission by BR Ferrell.

illness and its consequent therapy upon a patient, as perceived by the patient.''[61]

The second level in Ferrans' taxonomy is the impact of illness on quality of life. This level is broader, in that these definitions allow for consideration of the effects of illness on a wider range of aspects of life. For example, the impact of illness on a marital relationship is of interest, rather than just sexual dysfunction. Instead of focusing solely on the ability to work, the financial impact of an illness would be taken into consideration as well. An example is provided by Revicki et al, who define quality of life as ''the subjective assessment of the impact of disease and its treatment across the physical, psychological, social, and somatic, domains of functioning and well-being.''[62]

The third level in Ferrans' taxonomy is quality of life during illness. It is the most comprehensive in scope, in that these definitions address the quality of the whole of life for an individual who has an illness, including positive aspects. For example, this level includes positive changes reported to result from the experience of cancer and treatment, such as improved sense of purpose, changes in priorities, improved relationships, or increased faith in God.[33] An example is Padilla et al's definition of quality of life as ''the positivity or negativity of attributes that characterize one's psychological, physical, social, and spiritual well-being at a point in time when health, illness, and treatment conditions are relevant.''[63]

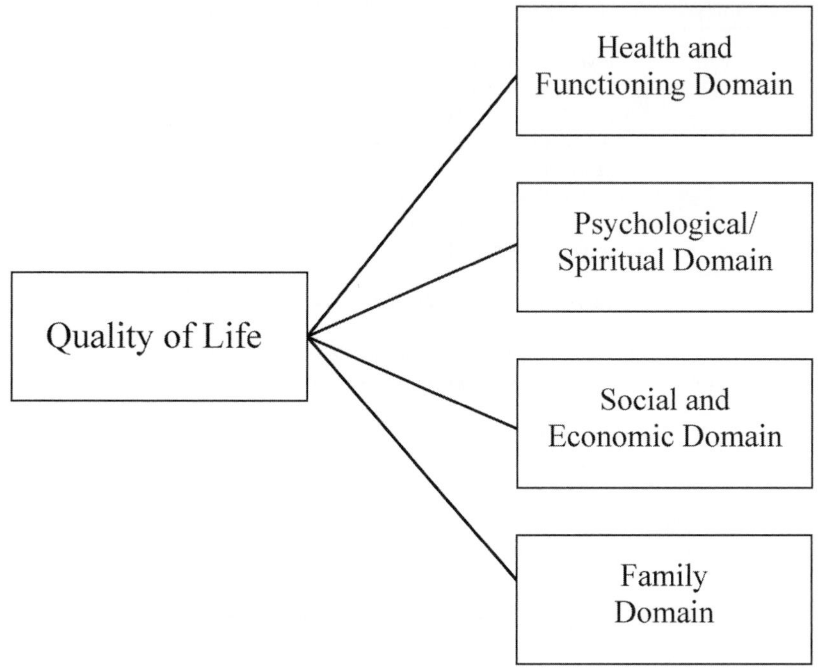

Figure 9-3 Ferrans conceptual model for quality of life.

Measuring Quality of Life

Choosing Instruments to Measure Quality of Life

There are many quality of life instruments from which to choose. To assist in narrowing the choice of instruments, Salek has produced a comprehensive compendium that contains both instruments and psychometric information.[64] In addition, the Quality of Life Instruments Database is an Internet resource that contains information on 430 instruments (*www.qolid.org*). Table 9-3 presents examples of multidimensional instruments that were developed for use with cancer patients, except for the SF-36, which was designed for use in the general population.[65] The domains of quality of life that each instrument measures are listed, as well as the availability of an overall quality of life score. Web sites for the instruments are identified; they are excellent sources for current and comprehensive information.

Evidence of reliability, validity, and responsiveness/sensitivity are prerequisites for the choice of an instrument, as they provide assurance that the instrument is reasonably free of random error, measures what it was intended to measure, and is sufficiently sensitive to detect change in quality of life. Of course, no one instrument is ideal for all situations in which quality of life outcomes can be assessed. When choosing instruments, clinicians and researchers need to consider the purpose of the evaluation, the nature of specific disease and treatment, and the characteristics of the patient population that will be assessed. In light of these considerations, instruments should be examined to determine which ones provide the best fit.

Generic Versus Disease-specific Instruments

Another distinction made among quality of life measures is whether the instrument is generic or disease specific. Generic instruments produce scores for all domains of quality of life, whereas disease-specific instruments focus on concerns that are most relevant to a specific illness and treatment.

There are advantages and disadvantages for both types of instruments. Generic instruments are useful for making comparisons with the general population, which is particularly helpful for the interpretation of results. They also can be used across treatment groups and illness populations, making it possible to evaluate the relative impact of therapies and healthcare programs.[39] In addition, they can put symptoms in the context of overall quality of life, which can help clarify the effectiveness of treatment.[75] They are particularly useful for documenting the range of treatment effects, which may help to identify unanticipated adverse effects.[39] The major disadvantage of generic instruments is that because they are so broad, they tend to cover

Table 9-2 Elements of the Ferrans Conceptual Model for Quality of Life

Health and Functioning Domain	Psychological/Spiritual Domain
Own health	Satisfaction with life
Pain	Happiness in general
Energy (fatigue)	Achievement of personal goals
Ability to take care of yourself without help	Peace of mind
Ability to take care of family responsibilities	Faith in God
Usefulness to others	Personal appearance
Worries	Satisfaction with self
Control over life	
Chances of living as long as you would like	**Social and Economic Domain**
Chances for a happy future	Friends
Sex life	Emotional support from friends
Leisure time activities	Home (house, apartment)
Health care	Neighborhood
	Job/unemployment
Family Domain	Ability to take care of financial needs
Family happiness	Education
Spouse, lover, or partner	
Children	
Emotional support from family	
Family health	

each area superficially and may not even address the primary symptoms.[75] Disease-specific instruments tend to be much more powerful in detecting treatment effects and are more responsive to changes in specific conditions.[39,75] However, these instruments are limited in scope, so they may miss critical aspects of quality of life. For these reasons, there is general agreement that both types of measures should be used, even in clinical trials.[76]

Many of the instruments used for cancer care are a blend of both generic and disease-specific measures. For example, the FACT/FACIT[69] and the EORTC QLQ-C30[68] are core instruments that are used for all cancer patients. In addition, modules have been developed for use with the core instruments, which are specific for different types of cancer, such as prostate, breast, and colon cancer.

Status and Evaluation Questions

Historically, a distinction between subjective and objective measures has been made in quality of life assessment. Objective indicators are directly measurable, such as blood pressure, hemoglobin levels, tumor size, income, or years of education. Quality of life instruments occasionally may assess things that are directly observable, such as the number of emeses. Normally, however, they assess things that are neither directly observable nor measurable, such as severity of nausea, so their results depend on subjective assessment. Subjective indicators rely on information from the patient.

Within this subjective realm, another important distinction has been recognized only recently. There are actually two types of subjective information produced by quality of life questionnaires.[42] One asks for information on the state (or status) of a particular aspect of life, such as "How much pain do you have?" The other asks for an evaluation of that state, such as "How satisfied are you with the amount of pain you have?" This distinction is important because the answers to these two types of questions (status and evaluation) provide different information. An evaluation requires additional steps in cognitive processing, because the person first must think of how much pain he or she has and then make a judgment about it—good or bad, satisfied or dissatisfied. This distinction is also important because some quality of life instruments are composed entirely of status questions, such as the EORTC QLQ C30 and SF-36, whereas others are composed entirely of evaluation questions, such as the Quality of Life Index (QLI) and the Quality-of-Life Scale for Cancer (QOL-CA). Others contain a mixture of both status and evaluation questions, such as the Functional Assessment of Cancer Therapy (FACT/FACIT).[42]

Different information (and different scores) is produced depending on whether status or evaluation questions are asked. This consideration is important both when selecting an instrument to use and when interpreting scores from it. Evidence can be seen in studies that have used two quality of life instruments with the same sample. For example, although the FACT/FACIT scale and the QLI—Cancer Version measure many of the same domains, the correlation between the two instruments was only .41 in a sample of patients with primary brain cancer.[31] Similarly, scores from the SF-36 and QLI were only moderately

Table 9-3 Multidimensional Instruments Used to Measure Quality of Life

Cancer Rehabilitation Evaluation System (CARES) — Short Form[66]
www.atsqol.org/cares.asp
Physical
Psychosocial
Marital
Sexual
Medical interaction
Overall quality of life

EORTC Quality of Life Questionnaire (EORTC QLQ-C30)[67,68]
www.eortc.be/home/qol/
Physical functioning
Pain
Fatigue
Nausea and vomiting
Overall symptoms
Role functioning
Cognitive ability
Psychological functioning
Social interaction
Finances

Functional Assessment of Cancer Therapy (FACT/FACIT)[69,70]
www.facit.org
Physical well-being
Social/family well-being
Emotional well-being
Functional well-being
Overall quality of life

Functional Living Index — Cancer (FLIC)[71,72]
www.qolid.org/public/FLIC.html
Overall quality of life
Physical well-being and ability
Nausea
Hardship due to cancer
Psychological well-being
Social well-being

McGill Quality of Life Questionnaire[73]
www.promotingexcellence.org/downloads/measures/mcgill_qol.pdf
Physical symptoms
Psychological symptoms
Outlook on life
Meaningful existence
Overall quality of life

Quality of Life Index — Cancer Version (QLI)[45,54,58]
www.uic.edu/orgs/qli
Health and functioning
Psychological/spiritual
Social and economic
Family
Overall quality of life

Quality of Life Scale for Cancer (QOL-A)[53]
www.qolid.org/public/QOL-CA.html
Physical well-being
Psychological well-being
Spiritual well-being
Social well-being
Overall quality of life

SF-36 Health Survey[65,74]
www. microfit.com/ l products/healthwizard/healthsurvey.html
Physical function
Physical role function
Vitality
Bodily pain
Mental health
Emotional role function
Social function
General health perceptions

Note: All the instruments listed were developed for use with cancer patients, except for the SF-36, which was designed for the general population.

correlated, even though they measured many of the same domains, in patients with angina or HIV.[77,78]

Most definitions of quality of life used in health care today focus on the evaluative aspect of quality of life.[42] The idea of quality of life, in its essence, requires a value judgment about a person's life. It is the incorporation of a patient's values that sets it apart from measures of health status. In this way it provides an understanding of the impact of illness from the viewpoint of the patient. However, both status and evaluation information are important for measuring outcomes in cancer care. Individuals may consider their quality of life to be good, even when faced with physical disabilities. Particularly in long-term illness, individuals make adaptations to compensate for physical limitations, which can preserve satisfaction with life.[47] Covinsky et al provided evidence of this adaptation in a study of 493 older patients, in which 43% of those with the worst physical functioning considered their quality of life to be good.[79] Conversely, 15% of those with the best physical functioning considered their quality of life to be fair or poor. Note that these findings also show that erroneous conclusions could be drawn if either the status or evaluation measures were used alone to determine the outcome for this study.

Importance and Preference Measures

The idea of quality of life conveys a judgment about a person's life, which requires the use of values. This concept is depicted in the Wilson and Cleary model, in that values and preferences are characterized as directly influencing general health perceptions and overall quality of life (Figure 9-1).[43] It raises the question of how values are captured in quality of life instruments. As discussed previously, evaluation-type questions, by their very nature, require an additional cognitive step in that they ask for a judgment to be made, which requires the use of personal values.[42] For example, values come into play when answering questions about how distressing something is, how much of a problem it is, how bothered you are by it, or how satisfied you are with it. Thus instruments that contain evaluation-type questions implicitly require the use of personal values for their questions to be answered.[42]

Some instruments incorporate values in a more structured manner. They use a variety of terms to elicit information regarding values, such asking patients to rate importance, distress, bother, or effect on quality of life. The answers are then incorporated into the quality of life scores by weighting. *Weighting* is based on the idea that highly valued areas of life have greater influence on quality of life than areas of less importance. Some instruments use ratings of importance of individual aspects of life as weights to produce scores, such as the Quality of Life Inventory (QOLI)[80] and the Quality of Life Index (QLI).[45] Other instruments ask respondents to rate the importance of an entire domain, but do not use the information in a weighting scheme. Examples include the FACT (original version),[70] the WHOQOL-100 instrument,[40] and the Prostate Cancer Index (PCI).[81] All of these instruments use the values of the respondents themselves in the quality of life assessment. Other instruments use weights based on the values of the general population or values gleaned from other groups of patients, rather than the individual completing the instrument. For these instruments, a person answers status-type questions that do not ask for an evaluation, and the score is computed using values previously obtained from groups of other people. Examples of this type of instrument that have been used with cancer patients include the EuroQol EQ-5D,[82] the Health Utilities Index,[83] and the Quality of Well-Being scale.[84] Feeny provides an excellent discussion of these and other preference measures.[85]

A different sort of preference measure that was developed specifically for cancer care is Q-TwiST (Quality-Adjusted Time Without Symptoms and Toxicity).[86] With this instrument, survival time is discounted to take into consideration the effect of treatment side effects and disease symptoms, using a utility weight ranging from 0 to 1. The utility weights, which reflect preferences, were determined by the investigators themselves, rather than patients with breast cancer. Q-TwiST has been used to demonstrate the additional burden of adjuvant chemotherapy in women receiving tamoxifen.[87] However, it has been pointed out that the summary scores of instruments such as Q-TwiST do not permit identification of specific problem areas. Guyatt et al have suggested that disease-specific instruments be used simultaneously with such measures to provide this information.[39]

The question about whose values to use for quality of life measurement can be addressed by considering the purpose of the assessment. The developmental work for the WHOQOL-100[40] demonstrated that some aspects of life are of universal relevance. However, individuals and cultural groups will differ from the general population in the values they attach to various aspects of life.[88] Changes in values also occur over time, as a result of adaptation in response to significant life events. These changes, which are referred to as ''response shift,'' can occur as a result of making accommodations to illness.[89] If the purpose is to determine the types of healthcare services that will be paid for by public resources, it has been argued that the general population's values should be used.[90] Conversely, if the purpose is to identify the needs of individual patients in clinical practice, there is no substitute for the values of the individual.

Populations Presenting Special Challenges

Proxy ratings

The term *quality of life* conveys the idea of a value judgment requiring some kind of rating, such as good/bad, high/low, or best/worst. It makes a difference who does the rating, because people use their own internal standards for what they consider a desirable or undesirable quality of life.[8] There is general agreement that quality of life is best evaluated by the patient, rather than by an outside observer. Nevertheless, in some situations the patient may not be able to provide the information needed, because of cognitive impairment, debilitating fatigue, severe nausea, pain, or other symptoms. These are often times when quality of life information is most needed, which makes the use of proxy raters appealing. A proxy rater is anyone other than the patient who evaluates the patient's quality of life.

Because patients' own perspectives differ from those of outside observers, ratings assigned by proxies may differ dramatically from the ratings patients would give themselves. These differences have been demonstrated in studies comparing patients' ratings with those of physicians, nurses, and significant others (spouse, family, friends). For example, one study reported that correlations between quality of life ratings by patients and physicians ranged only from .26 to .45, and that patient and nurse correlations were no better, ranging from .19 to .47.[91] A recent review of 23 of the most methodologically sound studies found that the agreement between patients and proxies was modest to good ($r = .42$ to .78), although there were a few studies whose correlations were very low.[92] Better agreement was found for physical functioning than for other domains. This is consistent with an earlier review of 49 studies,[93] which found that proxies provided more accurate information when they assessed things that are concrete and observable, such as functional status, cigarette smoking, and consumption of food, coffee, and alcohol. Proxies provided less accurate information when they assessed things that are subjective and unobservable, such as the patient's satisfaction, pain, cognitive functioning, depression, or psychosocial adjustment to cancer.

These findings demonstrate that proxies should be used for quality of life assessment only if absolutely necessary, and with the understanding that they are an imperfect substitute for the patient. In addition, whenever possible, the level of agreement between patients and the proxies should be determined when patients are still able to answer questions. Later, when patients are no longer able to provide information, the proxy ratings can be interpreted in light of the concordance found previously between proxy and patient. An example of this approach has been reported in a study of stroke survivors.[94]

Cognitive Impairment

Cognitive impairment may make it difficult or impossible for patients to complete the response scales of many quality of life instruments. Rather than relying on proxies, there are techniques to assist patients to provide valid responses to scales with multiple categories. Patients' understanding of response choices can be improved with the use of visual aids such as histograms with bars of increasing size, which depict the response categories.[60] In addition, it can be helpful to break the cognitive task into smaller parts. For example, the Quality of Life Index was administered in an interview format to patients with cognitive impairment (Mini-Mental State Examination scores ranging from 18 to 20).[95] Patients were able to provide valid responses to the six-point response scale when it was administered in a series of dichotomous questions. They were first asked whether they were satisfied or dissatisfied with an aspect of life. Next, they were given three options (slightly, moderately, or very satisfied/dissatisfied) from which to choose. To facilitate the decisions, a histogram characterizing the response choices also was shown to the patients.

Children

Work based on adults in the field of quality of life cannot be applied directly in pediatric oncology for several reasons. First, there is the complex interplay between the child's developmental stage and the experience of cancer.[96] Second, the sense of well-being in children can fluctuate in response to daily events and chronic problems, and is affected by their developing cognitive ability and personality.[97] Third, the child's quality of life has a complex interrelationship with that of the family as a unit and individual family members.[97]

For these reasons, it has been necessary to develop unique definitions, conceptual models, and instruments to address quality of life in children. Different conceptual approaches can be identified in the definitions and instruments developed. For example, the definition of quality of life of the Pediatric Oncology Group focuses primarily on functioning: "Quality of life is a multidimensional construct, incorporating both objective and subjective data, including (but not limited to) the social, physical, and emotional functioning of the child and, when indicated, his/her family. QOL measurement must be sensitive to changes that occur throughout development."[96, p. 89] An alternative definition, which focuses on the sense of well-being, is provided by Hinds: "Children's and adolescents' subjective and changeable sense of well-being which reflects how closely their desires and hopes match what is actually happening, and their orientation toward the future, both their own and that of others."[98, p. 285] Similarly, instruments have been developed that differ in their conceptual approach, as shown by a qualitative analysis of their content.[99] Some measure the individual's self-assessment of functioning in physical, psychological, and social domains, such as the KINDL[100] and the PEDsQL.[101] Others measure satisfaction of life in terms of the discrepancy between how life is and how one would expect it to be, such as the GCQ[102] and the TACQOL.[103] A third group of instruments measure health status, such as the CHQ[104] and the CHIP.[105]

It is common for quality of life evaluations to be provided by parents. Unfortunately, parents are imperfect proxies for children, as shown by well-designed studies measuring quality of life. For example, using the parent and child versions of the same instrument, correlations between scores of parents and children (ages 8–11) have been found to range from .44 to .61.[106] Children reported lower quality of life in the areas of positive emotions, physical complaints, motor functioning, cognitive functioning, and autonomy.

Because children generally are recognized as the preferred source of information, a number of instruments have been developed for children to complete themselves. Touch-screen computers that speak to children can be used to administer some instruments to young children who cannot read.[100] In addition, some instruments provide different versions for specific age groups. For example, the KINDL has versions for three age groups: 4–7, 8–12, and 13–16 years.[100] A few instruments have been developed specifically for children with cancer, such as the Pediatric Oncology Quality of Life Scale.[107] The majority of instruments were developed for use with a wide range of pediatric and adolescent populations, although some of these have cancer-specific modules, such as the PEDsQL[101] and the KINDL.[100]

End of Life

At the end of life, cancer care focuses on promoting comfort so as to provide the best possible quality of life. Rather than tumor response and survival time, success is achieved in terms of a "good death." Recognizing this shift in emphasis, symptom management and supportive care become of paramount importance. Cancer patients commonly experience pain, fatigue, constipation, dyspnea, and dry mouth at the end of life.[108,109] In addition to physical symptoms, Steinhauser et al[110] reported that the factors most important to patients at the end of life were mental awareness, peace with God, not being a burden to family, and feeling their life was complete. However, the SUPPORT study, which followed approximately 4000 patients at the end of life, found that more than half had inadequate pain control, and one-fourth suffered from emotional distress, social isolation, and feelings of abandonment.[111]

What are the implications for neglecting quality of life at the end of life? For dying patients, it can lead to loss of the will to live, which can result in premature death by active suicide or passive surrender.[112] Researchers have found that the will to live is highly correlated with the sense of well-being in cancer patients at end of life, along with depression, anxiety, and dyspnea.[113] There are also implications for caregivers, in terms of increased morbidity and mortality. A 63% higher mortality rate has been found for caregivers with mental and emotional strain, as compared with noncaregivers.[114]

Measuring quality of life at the end of life presents its own set of challenges. Although physical functioning and activities of daily living are still important, these eventually become less useful to measure, because physical status deteriorates until it eventually levels off. At some point, those scores become uniformly low and so no longer provide discrimination. Instead, measures of quality of life need to capture the elements that are important to patients at the end of life, such as meaning in life, spirituality, relationship issues, and positive aspects, in addition to symptoms. Instruments have been developed expressly for the purpose of measuring these concerns, such as the Hospice Quality of Life Index,[115] McGill Quality of Life Questionnaire,[73] and Missoula-VITAS Quality of Life Index.[116] In addition, palliative care modules have been developed for general quality of life measures, such as the FACT/FACIT.[117] These instruments all elicit information directly from the patient, rather than from a proxy. Information from the patient is preferred, because proxies are less able to provide accurate information about the subjective elements that are important to patients at the end of life.[118] Because patients become unable to answer questions as death approaches, inevitably family members need to provide information about the very end of life. The Quality of Dying and Death questionnaire was developed specifically for eliciting information from family members. It was designed for use after death and asks family members to rate 31 aspects of the patient's dying experience.[119] To help clinicians and researchers find measures for use at end of life, Teno and colleagues developed a Toolkit of instruments (*www.chcr.brown.edu/pcoc/toolkit.htm*).[120] The Toolkit Web site provides a review of 41 instruments that can be used to measure outcomes at the end of life, including the last month of life.

Culture and Language Differences

The major quality of life instruments are available in a number of languages and have been used throughout the world. When preparing the instruments for use with different cultural groups, the primary focus has been language issues. Linguistic equivalence does not necessarily ensure conceptual equivalence in terms of quality of life, an issue that often goes unaddressed.[121] Although many aspects of quality of life are universally shared, some are culturally unique.[60,122] In general, quality of life instruments have been developed based on nonminority, well-educated samples from one cultural group.[121] Continued work in this area is needed to provide assurance that quality of life is assessed validly for various cultural groups. Examples of instruments that have been developed expressly for cross-cultural international use include the EORTC QLQ-C30,[67] the Quality of Life Questionnaire of the EuroQol (EuroQol),[82] and the WHOQOL-100.[40]

Future Directions

Quality of life has become a respected outcome for cancer care. Increasingly, it is recognized as a valuable supplement to tumor response and survival data, providing information about the positive and negative effects of therapy from the patient's perspective. It is helpful in determining the trade-offs between toxicity and quality of life, and in evaluating whether small gains in life span come at too high a cost. Although interest in quality of life outcomes is expanding, fewer studies have included quality of life endpoints than might be hoped. Assessment of quality of life in research and clinical practice is relatively new, as compared to standard clinical indices, and significant work remains to be done. Much more information about quality of life outcomes is needed for clinical decision making, provision of supportive services, and health policy for cancer care.

References

1. Johnson JR, Temple R: Food and Drug Administration requirements for approval of new anticancer drugs. *Cancer Treat Rep* 69:1155–1157, 1985
2. Clinical Trials Cooperative Group Program: *Cancer Therapy Evaluation Program: Guidelines*. Bethesda, MD, Division of Cancer Treatment, National Cancer Institute, 1988
3. Osoba D: The quality of life committee of the clinical trials group of the National Cancer Institute of Canada: organization and functions. *Qual Life Res* 1:211–218, 1992
4. Cella D: Changes in quality of life predict survival in NSCLC. *Oncol News Int* 6:19, 1997
5. Ganz P, Lee J, Siau J: Quality of life assessment: an independent prognostic variable for survival in lung cancer. *Cancer* 67:3131–3135, 1991
6. Herndon J, Fleishman S, Kornblith A, et al: Is quality of life predictive of survival among patients with advanced non–small cell lung cancer? *Cancer* 85:333–340, 1999
7. Montazeri A, Milroy R, Hole D, et al: Quality of life in lung cancer patients as an important prognostic factor. *Lung Cancer* 31:233–240, 2001
8. Osoba D: Lessons learned from measuring health-related quality of life in oncology. *J Clin Oncol* 12:608–616, 1994
9. Schipper H, Clinch J, McMurray A, et al: Measuring the quality of life of cancer patients: the Functional Living Index — Cancer: development and validation. *J Clin Oncol* 2:472–483, 1984
10. Dean H: Multiple instruments for measuring quality of life. in Frank-Stromborg M, Olsen S (eds.): *Instruments for Clinical Health-Care Research* (ed 2). Sudbury, MA, Jones and Bartlett, 1997, pp 135–148
11. Hahn EA, Glendenning GA, Sorensen MV, et al: Quality of life in patients with newly diagnosed chronic phase chronic myeloid leukemia on imatinib versus interferon alpha plus low-dose cytarabine: results from the IRIS study. *J Clin Oncol* 21:2138–2146, 2003
12. Hanks GE: External beam radiation treatment for prostate cancer: still the gold standard. *Oncology* 10:17–20, 1992
13. Yarbro C, Ferrans C: Quality of life of patients with prostate cancer treated with surgery or radiation therapy. *Oncol Nurs Forum* 25:685–693, 1998
14. Potosky AL, Harlan LC, Stanford JL, et al: Prostate cancer practice patterns and quality of life: the Prostate Cancer Outcomes Study. *J Natl Cancer Inst* 91:1719–1724, 1999
15. Potosky AL, Legler J, Albertsen PC, et al: Health outcomes after prostatectomy or radiotherapy for prostate cancer: results from the Prostate Cancer Outcomes Study. *J Natl Cancer Inst* 92:1582–1592, 2000
16. van Andel G, Visser AP, Zwinderman AH, et al: A prospective longitudinal study comparing the impact of external radiation therapy with radical prostatectomy on health related quality of life (HRQOL) in prostate cancer patients. *Prostate* 58:354–365, 2004
17. Holmberg L, Bill-Axelson A, Helgesen F, et al: A randomized trial comparing radical prostatectomy with watchful waiting in early prostate cancer. *N Engl J Med* 347:781–789, 2002
18. Steineck G, Helgesen F, Adolfsson J, et al: Quality of life after radical prostatectomy or watchful waiting. *N Engl J Med* 347:790–796, 2002
19. Cunningham D, Pyrhönen S, James RD, et al: Randomised trial of irinotecan plus supportive care versus supportive care alone after fluorouracil failure for patients with metastatic colorectal cancer. *Lancet* 352:1413–1418, 1998
20. Rougier P, Van Cutsem E, Bajetta E, et al: Randomised trial of irinotecan versus fluorouracil by continuous infusion after fluorouracil failure in patients with metastatic colorectal cancer. *Lancet* 352:1407–1412, 1998
21. Kornblith AB, Herndon JE, Silverman LR, et al: Impact of azacytidine on the quality of life of patients with myelodysplastic syndrome treated in a randomized phase III trial: a Cancer and Leukemia Group B study. *J Clin Oncol* 20:2441–2452, 2002
22. Silverman LR, Demakos EP, Peterson BL, et al: A randomized controlled trial of azacitidine in patients with the myelodysplastic syndrome: a study of the Cancer and Leukemia Group B. *J Clin Oncol* 20:2429–2440, 2002
23. Hill J, Kornblith A, Jones D, et al: A comparative study of the long term psychosocial functioning of childhood acute lymphoblastic leukemia survivors treated by intrathecal methotrexate with or without cranial radiation. *Cancer* 82:208–218, 1998
24. MacLean W: Children's Cancer Group (CCG). *J Natl Cancer Inst Monogr* 20:87–88, 1996
25. Ganz PA, Kwan L, Stanton AL, et al: Quality of life at the end of primary treatment of breast cancer: first results from the moving beyond cancer randomized trial. *J Natl Cancer Inst* 96:376–387, 2004
26. Fobair P, Hoppe RT, Bloom J, et al: Psychosocial problems among survivors of Hodgkin's disease. *J Clin Oncol* 4:805–814, 1986
27. Kornblith AB, Anderson J, Cella DF, et al: Hodgkin's disease survivors at increased risk for problems in psychosocial adaptation. *Cancer* 70:2214–2224, 1992
28. Kornblith A: Cancer and Leukemia Group B (CALGB). *J Natl Cancer Inst Monogr* 20:67–71, 1996
29. Sharpe M, Strong V, Allen K, et al: Management of major depression in outpatients attending a cancer centre: a preliminary evaluation of a multicomponent cancer nurse-delivered intervention. *Br J Cancer* 90:310–313, 2004
30. Sandgren AK, McCaul KD, King B, et al: Telephone therapy for patients with breast cancer. *Nurs Forum* 27:683–688, 2000
31. Weitzner M, Meyers C, Byrne K: Psychosocial functioning and quality of life in patients with primary brain tumors. *J Neurosurgery* 84:29–34, 1996

32. Kornblith A: Psychosocial adaptation of cancer survivors, in Holland J (ed.): *Psycho-oncology*. New York, Oxford University Press, 1998, pp 223–254
33. Ferrans C: Quality of life through the eyes of survivors of breast cancer. *Oncol Nurs Forum* 21:1645–1651, 1994
34. Kornblith AB, Herndon JE, Weiss RB, et al: Long-term adjustment of survivors of early-stage breast carcinoma, 20 years after adjuvant chemotherapy. *Cancer* 98:679–689, 2003
35. Kornblith AB, Ligibel J: Psychosocial and sexual functioning of survivors of breast cancer. *Semin Oncol* 30:799–813, 2003
36. Dow K, Ferrell B, Haberman M, et al: The meaning of quality of life in cancer survivorship. *Oncol Nurs Forum* 26:519–528, 1999
37. Ganz PA, Rowland JH, Desmond K, et al: Life after breast cancer: understanding women's health related quality of life and sexual functioning. *J Clin Oncol* 16:501–514, 1998
38. Detmar S, Muller MJ, Schornagel JH, et al: Health-related quality of life assessments and patient–physician communication. *JAMA* 288:3027–3034, 2002
39. Guyatt GH, Jaeschke R, Feeny DH, et al: Measurements in clinical trials: choosing the right approach, in Spilker B (ed.): *Quality of Life and Pharmaeconomics in Clinical Trials* (ed 2). Philadelphia, Lippincott-Raven, 1996, pp 41–48
40. WHOQOL Group: The World Health Organization Quality of Life Assessment (WHOQOL): development and general psychometric properties. *Soc Sci Med* 46:1569–1585, 1998
41. Pearlman R, Jonsen A: The use of quality of life considerations in medical decision making. *J Am Geriatric Soc* 33:344–352, 1985
42. Ferrans CE: Definitions and conceptual models of quality of life, in Lipscomb J, Gotay CC, Snyder C (eds.): *Outcomes Assessment in Cancer*. Cambridge, UK, Cambridge University Press (In Press)
43. Wilson IB, Cleary PD: Linking clinical variables with health-related quality of life: a conceptual model of patient outcomes. *JAMA* 273:59–65, 1995
44. Ferrans CE: Development of a quality of life index for patients with cancer. *Oncol Nurs Forum* 17:15–19, 1990
45. Gotay C, Korn E, McCabe M, et al: Quality of life assessment in cancer treatment protocols: research issues in protocol development. *J Natl Cancer Inst* 84:575–579, 1992
46. Leplege A, Hunt S: The problem of quality of life in medicine. *JAMA* 278:47–50, 1997
47. Ferrell B, Wisdom C, Wenzl C: QOL as an outcome variable in the management of cancer pain. *Cancer* 63:2321–2327, 1989
48. Padilla G, Ferrell B, Grant M, et al: Defining the content domain of quality of life for cancer patients with pain. *Cancer Nurs* 13:108–115, 1990
49. Ferrell B, Grant M, Padilla G: Experience of pain and perceptions of quality of life: validation of a conceptual model. *Hospice J* 7:9–24, 1991
50. Ferrell B, Grant M, Schmidt G, et al: The meaning of quality of life for bone marrow transplant survivors. Part 1: the impact of bone marrow transplant on QOL. *Cancer Nurs* 15:153–160, 1992
51. Ferrell B, Dow K, Leigh S, et al: Quality of life in long term cancer survivors. *Oncol Nurs Forum* 22:915–922, 1995
52. Grant M, Ferrell B, Schmidt G, et al: Measurement of quality of life in bone marrow transplantation survivors. *Qual Life Res* 1:375–384, 1992
53. Ferrans CE, Powers M: Quality of Life Index: development and psychometric properties. *Adv Nurs Sci* 8:15–24, 1985
54. Ferrans CE: Development of a conceptual model of quality of life. *Schol Inq Nurs Pract Int J* 10:293–304, 1996
55. Anderson J, Ferrans CE: The quality of life of persons with chronic fatigue syndrome. *J Nervous Mental Dis* 106:359–367, 1997
56. Arzouman J, Dudas S, Ferrans C, et al: Quality of life of patients with sarcoma post-chemotherapy. *Oncol Nurs Forum* 18:889–894, 1991
57. Belec R: Quality of life: perceptions of long-term survivors of bone marrow transplantation. *Oncol Nurs Forum* 19:31–37, 1992
58. Ferrans C, Powers M: Psychometric assessment of the Quality of Life Index. *Res Nurs Health* 15:29–38, 1992
59. Ferrans C, Powers M: Quality of life of hemodialysis patients. *ANNA J* 20:575–581, 1993
60. Warnecke R, Ferrans C, Johnson T, et al: Measuring quality of life in culturally diverse populations. *J Natl Cancer Inst Monogr* 20:29–38, 1996
61. Schipper H, Clinch J, Olweny C: Quality of life studies: definitions and conceptual issues, in Spilker B (ed.): *Quality of Life and Pharmaeconomics in Clinical Trials* (ed 2). Philadelphia, Lippincott-Raven, 1996, pp 11–23
62. Revicki D, Osoba D, Fairclough D, et al: Recommendations on health-related quality of life research to support labeling and promotional claims in the United States. *Qual Life Res* 9:887–900, 2000
63. Padilla GV, Grant MM, Ferrell BR, et al: Quality of Life — Cancer, in Spilker B (ed.): *Quality of Life and Pharmaeconomics in Clinical Trials* (ed 2). Philadelphia, Lippincott-Raven, 1996, pp 301–308
64. Salek S: *Compendium of Quality of Life Instruments*. Chichester, John Wiley and Sons, 1999
65. Ware JE Jr, Sherbourne CD: The MOS 36-item short-form health survey (SF-36). *Med Care* 30:473–483, 1992
66. Shag C, Ganz PA, Heinrich R: Cancer Rehabilitation Evaluation System — Short Form (CARES-SF). *Cancer* 68:1406–1413, 1991
67. Aaronson N, Ahmedzai S, Bergman B, et al: The European Organization for Research and Treatment of Cancer QLQ-C30: a quality of life instrument for use in international clinical trials in oncology. *J Natl Cancer Inst* 85:365–376, 1993
68. Aaronson NK, Cull AM, Kaasa S, et al: The European Organization for Research and Treatment of Cancer (EORTC) modular approach for quality of life assessment in oncology: an update, in Spilker B (ed.): *Quality of Life and Pharmacoeconomics in Clinical Trials* (ed 2). Philadelphia, Lippincott-Raven, 1996, pp 179–189
69. Cella D, Bonomi A, Lloyd S, et al: Reliability and validity of the Functional Assessment of Cancer Therapy — Lung (FACT-L) quality of life instrument. *Lung Cancer* 12:199–220, 1995
70. Cella D, Tulsky D, Gray G, et al: The Functional Assessment of Cancer Therapy (FACT) scale: development and validation of the general version. *J Clin Oncol* 11:570–579, 1993
71. Morrow G, Lindke J, Black P, et al: Measurement of quality of life in patients: psychometric analysis of the Functional Living Index — Cancer (FLIC). *Qual Life Res* 1:287–296, 1992
72. Clinch J: The Functional Living Index — Cancer: ten years later, in Spilker B (ed.): *Quality of Life and Pharmacoeconomics in Clinical Trials* (ed 2). Philadelphia, Lippincott-Raven, 1996, pp 215–225
73. Cohen S, Mount B, Strobel M, et al: The McGill Quality of Life Questionnaire: a measure of quality of life appropriate for people with advanced disease. *Palliat Med* 9:207–219, 1995
74. Stewart AL, Hays RD, Ware JE: The MOS short-form general health survey. *Med Care* 26:724–735, 1988
75. Guyatt GH, Naylor CD, Juniper E, et al: Users' guide to the medical literature: XII. How to use articles about health-related quality of life. *JAMA* 277:1232–1237, 1997
76. Spilker B: Introduction, in Spilker B (ed.): *Quality of Life and Pharmaeconomics in Clinical Trials* (ed 2). Philadelphia, Lippincott-Raven, 1996, pp 1–10

77. Dougherty C, Dewhurst T, Nichol P, et al: Comparison of three quality of life instruments in stable angina pectoris: Seattle Angina Questionnaire, Short Form Health Survey (SF-36), and Quality of Life Index — Cardiac Version III. *J Clin Epidemiol* 51:569–575, 1998
78. Schlenk E, Erlen J, Dunbar-Jacob J, et al: Health-related quality of life in chronic disorders: a comparison across studies using the MOS SF-36. *Qual Life Res* 7:57–65, 1998
79. Covinsky KE, Wu AW, Landefeld S, et al: Health status versus quality of life in older patients: does the distinction matter? *Am J Med* 106:435–440, 1999
80. Frisch MB: The Quality of Life Inventory: a cognitive-behavioral tool for complete problem assessment, treatment planning, and outcome evaluation. *Behav Ther* 16:42–44, 1993
81. Litwin M: Measuring health related quality of life in men with prostate cancer. *J Urol* 152:1882–1887, 1994
82. EuroQol Group: EuroQol — a new facility for the measurement of health-related quality of life. *Health Policy* 16:199–208, 1990
83. Feeny DH, Torrance GW, Furlong WJ: Health Utilities Index, in Spilker B (ed.): *Quality of Life and Pharmacoeconomics in Clinical Trials* (ed 2). Philadelphia, Lippincott-Raven, 1996, pp 239–252
84. Patrick DL, Bush JW, Chen MM: Methods for measuring levels of well-being for a health status index. *Health Serv Res* 8:228–245, 1973
85. Feeny DH: The roles for preference-based measures in support of cancer research and policy, in Lipscomb J, Gotay CC, Snyder C (eds.): *Outcomes Assessment in Cancer.* Cambridge, UK, Cambridge University Press (In Press)
86. Gelber RP, Goldhirsch A, Cavelli F: Quality of life-adjusted evaluation of adjuvant therapies for operable breast cancer. *Ann Int Med* 114:621–628, 1991
87. Gelber RD, Cole BF, Goldhirsh A: Adjuvant chemotherapy plus tamoxifen compared with tamoxifen alone for postmenopausal breast cancer: meta-analysis of quality-adjusted survival. *Lancet* 347:1066–1071, 1996
88. Carr A, Higginson J: Measuring quality of life: are quality of life measures patient centered? *Br Med J* 322:1357–1360, 2001
89. Sprangers MAG, Schwartz CE: Integrating response shift into health-related quality of life research: a theoretical model. *Soc Sci Med* 48:1507–1515, 1999
90. Frost MH, Bonomi AE, Ferrans CE, et al: Patient, clinician, and population perspectives on determining the clinical signficance of quality of life scores. *Mayo Clin Proc* 77:488–494, 2002
91. Molzahn A, Northcott H, Dossetor J: Quality of life of individuals with end stage renal disease: perceptions of patients, nurses, and physicians. *ANNA J* 24:325–333, 1997
92. Sneeuw K, Sprangers M, Aaronson NK: The role of health care providers and significant others in evaluating the quality of life of patients with chronic disease. *J Clin Epidemiol* 55:1130–1143, 2002
93. Sprangers M, Aaronson N: The role of health care providers and significant others in evaluating the quality of life of patients with chronic disease: a review. *J Clin Epidemiol* 45: 743–760, 1992
94. Sneeuw KC, Aaronson NK, DeHaan RJ, et al: Assessing quality of life after stroke: the value and limitations of proxy rating. *Stroke* 28:1541–1549, 1997
95. Matano T: *Quality of Life of Persons with Alzheimer's Disease (dissertation).* Chicago, IL, University of Illinois at Chicago, 2000
96. Bradlyn AS, Pollock BH: Pediatric Oncology Group (POG). *J Natl Cancer Inst Monog* 20:89–90, 1996
97. Hinds PS, Hasse JE: Quality of life in children and adolescents with cancer, in King CR, Hinds PS (eds.): *Quality of Life from Nursing and Patient Perspectives.* Boston, Jones and Bartlett, 1998, pp 93–114
98. Hinds PS: Quality of life in children and adolescents with cancer. *Semin Oncol Nurs* 6:285–291, 1990
99. Rajmil L, Herdman M, Sanmamed MJF, et al: Generic health-related quality of life instruments in children and adolescents: a qualitative analysis of content. *J Adolescent Health* 34:37–45, 2004
100. Ravens-Sieberer U, Bullinger M: Assessing health-related quality of life in chronically ill children with the German KINDL: first psychometric and content analytical results. *Qual Life Res* 7:399–407, 1998
101. Varni JM, Seid M, Kurtin PS: Pediatric health-related quality of life measurement technology: A guide for health care decision makers. *J Clin Outcomes Manage* 6:33–40, 1999
102. Collier J, MacKinlay D, Phillips D: Norm values for the Generic Children's Quality of Life Measure (GCQ) from a large school-based sample. *Qual Life Res* 9:617–623, 2000
103. Vogels T, Verrips GHW, Verloove-Vanhorick SP, et al: Measuring health-related quality of life in children: the development of the TACQOL parent form. *Qual Life Res* 7:457–465, 1998
104. Landgraft JM, Abetz L, Ware J: *The Child Health Questionnaire User's Manual.* Boston, Health Institute, New England Medical Center, 1996
105. Starfield B, Riley A, Green B: The Child Health and Illness Profile: a population-based measure of health. *Med Care* 33:553–566, 1995
106. Theunissen NC, Vogels TGC, Koopman HM, et al: The proxy problem: child report versus parent report in health-related quality of life research. *Qual Life Res* 7:387–397, 1998
107. Goodwin DA, Boggs SR, Graham-Pole J: Development and validation of the pediatric oncology quality of life scale. *Psychol Assess* 6:321–328, 1994
108. McMillan SC, Weitzner M: How problematic are various aspects of quality of life in patients with cancer at the end of life? *Oncol Nurs Forum* 27:817–823, 2000
109. McMillan SC, Small BJ: Symptom distress and quality of life in patients with cancer newly admitted to hospice home care. *Oncol Nurs Forum* 29:1421–1428, 2002
110. Steinhauser KE, Christakis NA, Clipp EC, et al: Factors considered important at the end of life by patients, family, physicians, and other care providers. *JAMA* 284:2476–2482, 2000
111. SUPPORT Principal Investigators: A controlled study to improve care for seriously ill hospitalized patients: the Study to Understand Prognoses and Preferences for Outcomes and Risks of Treatments (SUPPORT). *JAMA* 274:1591–1598, 1995
112. Rummans TA, Bostwick JM, Clark MM: Maintaining quality of life at the end of life. *Mayo Clin Proc* 75:1305–1310, 2000
113. Chochinov HM, Tataryn D, Clinch JJ, et al: Will to live in the terminally ill. *Lancet* 354:816–819, 1999
114. Schultz R, Beach SR: Caregiving as a risk for mortality: the Caregiver Health Effects Study. *JAMA* 282:2215–2219, 1999
115. McMillan SC, Weitzner M: Quality of life in cancer patients: use of a revised hospice index. *Cancer Pract* 6:282–288, 1998
116. Byock IR, Merriman MP: Measuring quality of life for patients with terminal illness: the Missoula-VITAS quality of life index. *Palliat Med* 12:231–244, 1998
117. Cella D: Functional Assessment of Chronic Illness Therapy (FACIT) scales Web site. *www.facit.org.* Accessed March 14, 2004
118. McPherson CJ, Addington-Hall JM: Judging the quality of care at the end of life: can proxies provide reliable information? *Soc Sci Med* 56:95–109, 2003
119. Curtis JR, Patrick DL, Engleberg RA, et al: A measure of the quality of dying and death: initial validation using after-death

interviews with family members. *J Pain Symptom Manage* 24: 17–31, 2002

120. Teno JM, Byock I, Field MJ: Research agenda for developing measures to examine quality of care and quality of life of patients diagnosed with life-limiting illness. *J Pain Symptom Manage* 17:75–82, 1999
121. Stewart AL, Napoles-Springer A: Health-related quality of life assessments in diverse population groups in the United States. *Med Care* 38(suppl):II102–24, 2000
122. Meyerowitz B, Richardson J, Hudson S, et al: Ethnicity and cancer outcomes: behavioral and psychosocial considerations. *Psychol Bull* 123:47–70, 1998

CHAPTER 10

Principles of Clinical Research and Development

Mary S. McCabe, BA, RN, MA

Overview

Advances in molecular biology are rapidly adding to our knowledge of the cell and its function with a focus on understanding the basic mechanisms of disease.[1] Yet, scientific inquiry — and, in particular, clinical research — continues to be an incremental process, moving forward in a series of carefully planned steps. This process occurs through the conduct of clinical trials — experiments designed to evaluate the value of new therapies in people with disease or at risk of disease.

The Clinical Trials Process

Cancer clinical trials are the prospectively designed evaluations of new interventions for the prevention, diagnosis, treatment, and/or improvement of quality of life of individuals at risk of or diagnosed with cancer. Clinical trials require careful scientific planning and rigorous review, oversight, and conduct. Such scientific evaluation includes built-in safeguards for study participants who volunteer through a process called informed consent. The goal in conducting clinical trials is to provide "definitive answers to a well-defined question," and these studies usually proceed in a carefully planned series of steps, called phases. The process begins with small studies testing the safety of the intervention and moves to progressively larger studies testing the effectiveness of the new interventions compared to the current standard of care.

Types of Clinical Trials

The most common type of clinical trial is designed to evaluate new treatments. However, as cancer clinical research has evolved, studies are now being designed to develop new interventions across the entire cancer continuum, including evaluations for the prevention, detection, and improvement of quality of life of both patients and individuals at risk of developing cancer.

- *Prevention trials* are designed to evaluate interventions, such as lifestyle modifications, pharmalogical agents, and dietary supplements, for the prevention of cancer in individuals at risk for cancer. A breast cancer prevention study is an example of a prevention trial. One such trial compared the use of tamoxifen against placebo in women at high risk of developing breast cancer.[2]

- *Screening and early detection trials* are intended to find cancer as early as possible in individuals who do not yet have a diagnosis of cancer, but who may be at risk for developing the disease.

- *Diagnostic trials* are designed to evaluate new tests, interventions, or procedures that can identify a suspected cancer earlier and more accurately. Such studies include the evaluation of tumor markers based on the molecular signature of the malignant cell.

- *Treatment trials* are designed to evaluate the safety and effectiveness of new drugs, biologics, radiation therapy techniques, surgical procedures, or new behavioral interventions in individuals who have been diagnosed with cancer.

- *Quality of life and supportive care trials* are designed to improve the comfort and domains of life that can be adversely affected by cancer and its treatment, such as physical symptoms and psychosocial functioning.

Phases of Clinical Trials

Clinical trials usually proceed in four phases — 1, 2, 3, and 4 — and each phase is designed to answer a research question that builds on the information obtained in the previous phase of study (Table 10-1). In this section, the phases of clinical trials are explained in the context of drug treatment trials, but the same concepts generally apply to most types of clinical trials. Some basic questions are helpful in understanding the goals of the different phases of studies.

- *Phase 1 studies:* What dose is safe, how can the agent best be given, and how does the agent affect the body?

- *Phase 2 studies:* What effect does the agent have on the particular cancer, and what effect does the agent have on the body?

- *Phase 3 studies:* Is the new agent or combination better than the current standard of care?

- *Phase 4 studies:* What is the long-term safety and effectiveness of the intervention?

Phase 1 Trials

Current approaches. Most frequently, phase 1 trials are designed to determine the maximum tolerated dose (MTD) and the dose-limiting toxicities of a new agent. While the primary goal of a phase 1 trial is to determine toxic effects, pharmacological behavior, and recommended dosage for future studies, these studies are conducted with therapeutic intent. The dose and schedule established in these trials then

Table 10-1 Phases of Clinical Trials

	Phase 1	Phase 2	Phase 3	Phase 4
Number of Participants	15–30 people	Less than 100 people	Generally, from 100 to thousands of people	Several hundred to several thousand people
Purpose	• To find a safe dosage • To decide how the agent should be given • To observe how the agent affects the human body	• To determine if the agent or intervention has an effect on a particular cancer • To see how the agent or intervention affect the human body	• To compare the agent or intervention (or new use of a treatment) with the current standard	• To further evaluate the long-term safety and effectiveness of a new treatment

determines the dose and schedule that will be used in phase 2 studies of the agent. In addition to the evaluation of previously untested, new agents ("first in human" studies), phase 1 studies are conducted to evaluate a new dose and schedule of an already approved agent in an effort to improve the efficacy and broaden the application of the agent. Later phase 1 studies may be conducted to further evaluate the agent in populations not previously studied, and some are pilot trials designed to determine the interaction of a drug with another agent.

Patient selection. Eligibility requirements for phase 1 studies are broad. Almost all such trials include only patients who have proven malignancy for which no effective treatment currently exists or whose disease is refractory to known therapy. Because of this requirement, most patients in phase 1 studies have been extensively treated before entering the study. New agents are first tested in adults, followed by testing in pediatric studies.[3] Major organ function must be adequate so that the drug can be metabolized and excreted normally. This helps ensure that evaluation of major organ toxicity can be determined and that patients will not be placed at even greater risk of toxicity. Study participants must have a life expectancy of at least 1 to 2 months, as this time is considered to be the minimum period required to observe toxic effects.

Starting dose and dose escalation. In phase 1 studies that involve an agent that has never been administered to humans, the initial group of participants receives a dose that is based on preclinical testing. This dose is usually quite conservative, recognizing that animal models are not perfect predictors of toxicity in humans.[4] The study participants are usually divided into cohorts of three to six participants. Each cohort is treated with an increased dose of the new agent, and the results obtained with early participants greatly influence the doses that subsequent participants receive. If no serious side effects are seen in the initial group after a period of time, usually 3 to 4 weeks, the next group of participants receives a higher dose.

Until recently, the most common plan for dose escalation was the "modified Fibonacci" scheme.[5] This plan sets the second dose level at double the initial dose; the third level is 67% higher than the second; the fourth is 50% higher than the third; and each subsequent level is increased by 33%. The goal is to avoid the problems of escalating the dose too rapidly (potential exposure of patients to severe toxicity) or too slowly (depriving participants of potential benefit through administration of subtherapeutic doses). The dose that is found to cause moderate, reversible toxicity in the majority of patients is recommended for further evaluation in a phase 2 trial.

New approaches. As researchers continue to gain a fuller understanding of cancer's molecular basis, there will be ever more of a shift from using the MTD as the phase 1 endpoint to an approach of establishing an "optimal biological dose" as the relevant endpoint. This endpoint is established as the safe dose of the agent found to affect a specifically defined target (or targets) in the tumor. For example, an agent directed against epidermal growth factor receptor (EGFR), if found to suppress tumor growth in preclinical models, would next be evaluated in a phase 1 study with patients with EGFR-expressing tumors. In the future, the MTD will continue to be used when the mechanism of the drug is not known and when it is not possible to measure the activity of the drug.[6] A biologic endpoint will be used to define the dose for populations as the dose and schedule that inhibits the target(s) by at least x% in at least y% of patients treated for the desired period of inhibition.

Phase 2 Trials

Current approaches. Phase 2 trials are designed to evaluate the efficacy of the agent against specific tumors, using the dose and schedule determined to be safe in the phase 1 trials.[7] On the basis of the phase 1 study results, phase 2 studies focus on the evaluation of cancers for which no effective therapy exists and/or that are most likely to show a response to therapy.[8]

Patient selection. Phase 2 trials evaluate the response of the tumor to the new drug, so participants must have a specific diagnosis and measurable tumor. Participants in phase 2 studies should be individuals likely to benefit from the new treatment and for whom no effective therapy currently exists.[9] They should have good performance status and minimal prior exposure to chemotherapy. Usually, one or, at most, two prior regimens are acceptable since, in patients heavily pretreated with chemotherapy, a drug may not demonstrate its true activity. The inherent problem in phase 2 trials is that individuals who have failed standard treatment may be the least likely to provide a satisfactory evaluation of the new agent. Subjects must have adequate organ function and a life expectancy of at least 3 months to participate. Phase 2 studies usually enroll 15 to 30 (less than 100) patients in a cohort group.

Dose and schedule. In most phase 2 studies, all participants receive the same dose of the agent (or undergo the same intervention). The new treatment is assessed for efficacy, and additional safety information is obtained. Some phase 2 studies may compare different schedules of administering the agent; at the end of the study, the most promising regimen is chosen to move into phase 3 trials. Participants in this type of phase 2 study are randomly assigned to one group or the other.

Trial design. Drawing conclusions regarding treatment benefit from a phase 2 single-agent trial is complex. The usual measure of an agent's antitumor activity in such a trial is response rate.[10] While obtaining a response rate answers the basic question posed in the study, partial responses do not necessarily indicate patient benefit. A partial response (50% reduction in tumor mass) may be brief and complicated by toxicity. Even if the agent seems to demonstrate activity against the cancer, it usually requires further testing. Because the agent has not been compared to any other agent or intervention, its relative value is unclear, and it is impossible to rule out other factors that may have influenced its effectiveness. In addition, phase 2 studies are often too short to determine long-term benefits, such as survival.

Phase 2 studies are also used to evaluate the practicality and tolerability of combination regimens. Results of this type of study are difficult to interpret, however, because often the agents under study are known to be of some benefit alone. The combination of agents must demonstrate greater activity than its most active component or greater activity than another combination. A phase 2 trial in which participants are randomized to treatment groups avoids some of these difficulties. This type of design requires simultaneously testing two or more regimens and the availability of a large number of participants. For these reasons, randomized phase 2 trials are not common.

New approaches. For molecularly targeted therapies under development, finding antitumor activity in phase 2 studies will involve using either the MTD or the biologically active dose. Toxicities will be characterized in the same way, but there will be the additional need to understand the determinants of response. Patient selection for study will continue to include individuals with minimal prior therapy and good performance status, but selection criteria will focus on individuals with tumor types that possess the target of the new agent expressed. Endpoints for phase 2 studies will continue to include response rate, duration, and toxicities, but it will be important to include tumor analysis (using probes or assays) to determine on a molecular level the responders from nonresponders.

Phase 3 trials

In a phase 3 trial, a new therapy is compared to a standard therapy. A new agent enters this phase of testing if it has demonstrated significant efficacy in phase 2 trials. An agent may be tested as a single agent, as part of a drug combination, or by comparing a combined-modality treatment with a single modality. Phase 3 trials require hundreds to thousands of participants and are most often carried out by multiple institutions, including community settings. Because these study results guide healthcare professionals in making treatment decisions, they often include information about quality of life as well as survival.

Patient selection. The requirements for participation in phase 3 trials are similar to those in phase 2. Participants must have measurable disease, adequate organ function, good performance status, and little or no prior anticancer therapy. Debate has occurred regarding how narrow the eligibility criteria in phase 3 trials should be, given that narrow eligibility criteria limit the generalizability of the results.

Trial design. The standard design for phase 3 studies is a prospective, randomized trial. Randomization means that the participants are assigned randomly to one or the other of the agents and/or regimens being evaluated. The assignment is not biased by knowledge of specific individual characteristics. Rather, both known and unknown prognostic factors of participants are distributed randomly. This design allows results to be interpreted as being due to the therapy under evaluation, rather than due to nonrandom variations in the distribution of unknown prognostic factors.[11] Also, a randomized design is necessary to detect small, but significant differences between agents and/or regimens.

New approaches. Currently, phase 3 studies assess the average effects of an intervention or regimen on the study sample, and eligibility is determined in very broad terms, usually without reference to tumor biological features. This practice limits the extrapolation both to populations and to the individual. The future evaluation of agents in phase 3 studies will likely include several relevant tumor types in the same trial, as the eligibility will be determined by the molecular characteristics of the tumor. The effect on the molecular target would drive the trial process and be the main effect under evaluation; the findings would then be relevant to the entire population having the same molecular target, rather than just to a single tumor type.

Phase 4 Trials

Following approval by the Food and Drug Administration (FDA) of an agent or regimen, additional studies (usually considered postmarketing studies) can be and may be required to be conducted. Not all new agents will enter into phase 4 trials. The purpose of such trials is to accrue new information about any risks or side effects not previously identified. Phase 4 trials have proved extremely useful in identifying potential issues with agents that were not discovered during early-phase trials. The FDA may require such trials when approval of the new agent is based on limited data about long-term outcome, for example. For this reason, some refer to phase 4 trials as "long-term experiments."

Nonclinical Trial Access to Experimental Agents: Special Access Programs

Although only well-designed clinical trials can reliably determine whether promising agents actually help persons with cancer or at risk of developing cancer, individuals seeking access to agents being evaluated in clinical trials have specific programs available if they are not eligible for a clinical trial. These avenues include special access programs.

Group C Program

Since 1976, the National Cancer Institute (NCI) has offered a program that allows access to agents that have reproducible activity in one or more types of cancer and that are likely to alter the pattern of the treatment of the disease. These agents must be administered by properly trained physicians and cannot require specialized care facilities. Each Group C protocol specifies eligibility and reporting requirements. Group C drugs are provided free of charge, and the Centers for Medicare and Medicaid Services (CMS) provides coverage for beneficiaries for care associated with Group C therapy.

Treatment Referral Center (TRC)

TRC is another mechanism that the NCI offers to provide access to experimental agents when a patient population is identified for which an investigational agent should be available. The NCI develops and provides the TRC protocol to the requested Cancer Centers, which then may offer it to patients as a treatment option.

Expanded Access Program

Expanded access programs are available for a limited number of well-studied investigational agents when substantial evidence indicates that the agent has significant activity against a specific cancer and may provide benefit for persons with the particular type of cancer. These programs allow a wider group of individuals to be treated with the agent before the FDA approval process has been completed.

The investigational new drug (IND) sponsor must apply to the FDA to make the agent available through an expanded access protocol. It must provide adequate evidence from completed trials showing that the agent may be effective to treat a specific type of cancer and that the agent does not have unreasonable risks.

Special Exception (Compassionate Use/Compassionate Exception)

People who do not meet the eligibility criteria for a clinical trial of an investigational agent may be eligible to receive the agent. The person's physician must contact the study sponsor and provides the person's medical information and treatment history. Requests are then evaluated on a case-by-case basis, and the FDA must approve each request to provide the agent outside a clinical trial. To use an agent under this mechanism, there should be reasonable expectation that the agent will prolong survival or improve quality of life.

Clinical Trials Design and Implementation

Careful planning and organization are essential in the design and conduct of a clinical trial both to protect the participants and to assure scientifically sound results (Table 10-2). Due to the rapidly increasing ability to apply cancer biology to targeted drug development, the expansion of patient-centered endpoints, and the increased skills of multidisciplinary research teams, cancer clinical trials are being designed and implemented with an ever-increasing level of sophistication.

The Clinical Protocol

For each clinical trial, a formal document known as a *protocol* is developed to clearly describe the process of evaluation. The protocol includes a rationale for the study and provides clear, specific instructions for all individuals involved in its conduct. Each protocol includes essential elements that provide the framework for achieving the study goals (Table 10-3).[12]

Research Team Members

The conduct of a clinical trial requires the collaboration of a multidisciplinary research team, with each member being held responsible for specific functions. Typical team members include the following individuals:

- *Principal investigator.* This individual has responsibility for overseeing all aspects of the protocol, including development of the protocol, submission of the study to the Institutional Review Board (IRB), patient recruitment, informed consent, and data collection, analysis, interpretation, and publication.

Table 10-2 Essential Elements in the Design of a Clinical Trial

- Clearly stated testable hypothesis
- Well-defined primary endpoint
- Appropriate trial design
- Adequate resources to answer the study question
- Accrual of adequate number of patients to complete the study in a reasonable amount of time
- Appropriate statistical analysis of predetermined trial endpoints
- Conclusions drawn directly from the data

Table 10-3 Elements of a Protocol

1. Introduction and scientific background
2. Objectives
3. Selection of patients
4. Design of study (including schematic diagram)
5. Treatment plan
6. Drug information
7. Toxicities to be monitored and dosage modifications
8. Required clinical and laboratory data and study calendar
9. Criteria for evaluating the effect of treatment and endpoint definition
10. Statistical considerations
11. Informed consent and regulatory considerations
12. Data forms
13. References
14. Study chairperson, collaborating participants, addresses, and telephone numbers

- *Research nurse.* This individual educates staff, participants, and others involved in the clinical trial about all aspects of the study. The nurse serves as the communication link between the clinical setting and the principal investigator. The nurse often is responsible for monitoring toxicity and response, performs quality assurance reviews and participates in the data collection and analysis.
- *Data manager.* This individual collaborates with the principal investigator and research nurse in the management of the clinical trial data. The data manager also provides data to monitoring agencies and groups and prepares data summaries for interim reports and final analyses.
- *Staff physicians and nurses.* Members of the clinical team administer the intervention to the participants in the study as specified in the protocol; identify and record toxicities and adverse events; and provide overall clinical management.

Protection of Research Participants

The protection of the individuals who agree to participate in clinical research is paramount. This right has not always been respected and, in the past, there have been notorious abuses of human rights. In 1947, the post–World War II trial that led to the conviction of Nazi physicians and scientists in Nuremberg, Germany, brought international attention to the abuses of clinical research and highlighted the fact that the protection of human rights cannot be left solely to the integrity of researchers. This trial resulted in a formal

Table 10-4 Fundamental Principles of Biomedical Ethics

Respect for persons: autonomy, self-determination, the right to deliberate about personal goals and act accordingly without interference
Nonmaleficence: obligation to do no harm to others
Beneficence: obligation to do good or promote the good of others
Justice: fairness, equitable distribution of benefits and burdens

statement (called the Nuremberg Code) about the ethical conduct of research in humans, which continues to form the basis for international codes of research ethics today.[13]

In the United States, a number of unfortunate, infamous clinical trials also called attention to the need for increased protection for research participants. The most notable was the Tuskegee syphilis study, in which African American men with syphilis were followed. The observational study was conducted from 1932 to 1972 without the knowledge and consent of the men who participated.[14] Even in the 1940s, after penicillin was found to be effective in the treatment of syphilis, the researchers never informed the participants or treated them with the antibiotic.

In 1974, in response to the identified need for the government to assure the protection of human subjects in research, Congress passed the National Research Act. This act required research studies involving human subjects to be reviewed by an IRB before federal grants and contracts could be funded. This requirement was then codified in the Code of Federal Regulations Title 45, Part 46 (45CFR-46), and includes the specific functions and membership of the IRB. The National Research Act also created the National Commission for the Protection of Research Subjects. This commission was extremely important in developing seminal reports on various aspects of human subject protection.[15] Most influential was the *Belmont Report,* which first identified the set of ethical principles that continue to guide the ethics of clinical research today (Table 10-4).[16] Common to these national guidelines and regulations — and others used throughout the world — are a number of agreed-upon rules:[17]

- The research design must offer a high probability of generating useful knowledge.
- The probable benefits must outweigh the risks.
- The selection of subjects must be just.
- Subjects must give their informed consent.
- Subjects' rights to privacy and confidentiality must be protected.

Informed Consent

The Nuremberg Code established the positive requirement that the voluntary consent of the human subject is absolutely essential. This positive rule supports the principles of respect for autonomy and respect for persons in requiring that individuals be free to choose what will happen to them.[18] This requirement has been codified in the Common Rule, which requires the informed consent of the potential research participant, or his or her legally authorized representative, along with written documentation of the consent on a form approved by an IRB. Although specific requirements govern the content of the informed consent document, it is actually the informed consent process that is of greatest importance. Legal, regulatory, medical, and ethical groups have described the process as needing to contain four essential elements: understanding, comprehension, voluntariness, and competence.[19] Table 10-5 outlines the elements required under 45CFR-46 that must be included in the informed consent document to ensure that adequate information is presented to the potential participant for consideration.

Because clinical trials are often complicated and include tests and interventions that carry risks, the manner in which the information is presented is extremely important. The information should be written and presented using clear and understandable wording, taking into consideration the educational level, language requirements, and cultural needs of the individual. Presentation of the information is necessary but not sufficient for informed consent.[20] Although it can be a challenge, it is critical that the participant comprehend the information, especially in studies where the potential for significant risk exists. Recently, atten-

Table 10-5 Essential Elements of Informed Consent

- Statement that the trial involves research
- Explanation and description of the nature of the trial, purpose of the trial, duration of participation, procedures to be followed, and which procedures are experimental
- Description of foreseeable risks and discomforts
- Benefits to the participants and others
- Alternative procedures or treatments
- Description of the confidentiality of records
- Explanation of procedures if the project involves more than minimal risk (e.g., compensation, availability of medical treatment)
- Contact person for questions
- Statement that participation is voluntary, that there will be no loss of benefits on withdrawal, and that the participant may withdraw at any time
- Statement that the participant's signature indicates a decision to participate, having read and discussed the information presented

tion has targeted ways to improve the informed consent process. Numerous groups, including the NCI, have developed recommendations and templates to assist investigators in developing informed consent documents.[21]

Institutional Review Board

The IRB is a uniquely important, institutionally based component of the protection system for participants in research. It is responsible for assessing the balance of risks and benefits of the clinical trials it reviews, evaluating the ethical status of the study, and, once the study is approved, monitoring the overall conduct of the clinical trial. In recent years, the deaths of clinical trials participants have spurred major changes and improvements in the institutional support for IRBs and in the degree of independent oversight that must be in place to monitor clinical trials.

Federal regulations stipulate that the composition of the IRB must include at least five people, who must come from diverse occupations and backgrounds. In addition, one member must be from outside the institution. Typically, IRBs are composed of medical specialists, nurses, other healthcare specialists, ethicists, chaplains, and lay members of the community. Since greater attention has focused on the function of IRBs, national committees and commissions have recommended that IRB membership be revised to better represent the community of potential research participants. A number of proposals and pilot studies have also evaluated the use of central — rather than institutional — IRBs as a way to improve the quality of review, given the increasing complexity of clinical trials.

Federal Oversight Agencies

Two government organizations — the Office for Human Research Protections (OHRP) in the Department of Health and Human Services and the FDA — have regulations in place to protect clinical trials participants. Some studies fall under the jurisdiction of both groups and are subject to both sets of regulations, which are basically congruent in terms of their requirements for informed consent and rules for IRBs.

Office for Human Research Protections

Formerly known as the Office of Protection from Research Risks, the OHRP has responsibility for safeguarding the welfare of participants in the research conducted by the 17 federal agencies and departments that come under the Common Rule. This oversight spans standards for the development of informed consent documents, the formation and function of IRBs, and rules relating to especially vulnerable populations in research, such as children and prisoners.

Food and Drug Administration

The FDA is responsible for clinical trials of new drugs, biologics, or devices that come under its regulations, regardless of whether the studies are federally funded. The agency conducts audits of IRB operations and institutional safeguards for participants in clinical trials.

Barriers to Clinical Trials Participation

At a time when the number of new agents to be evaluated in clinical trials is increasing, there continue to be a limited number of people who participate in these studies. In 1999, for example, the American Society of Clinical Oncology released data showing that only 3% of adults with cancer participate in clinical trials. Several organizations have conducted surveys to understand the reason for this limited number of participants and found that the barriers to participation are multifactorial. These barriers include factors relevant to healthcare professionals, the public, and patients, especially the underserved. In surveys, physician groups state that participation is often limited by the physician's lack of awareness of appropriate trials for a particular patient population; the physician's unwillingness to "lose" control of the person's care; the common belief that standard therapy is best; the belief that participation in clinical trials adds cost and significant administrative burdens to the practice; and concerns about how the person or individual will react to the suggestion of participation in a clinical trial.

In a 2000 survey of 6000 adults, 85% of the respondents stated that they were unsure or unaware that participation in a clinical trial might have been an option. Interestingly, about 75% of respondents said that they would have enrolled in a clinical trial if they knew it was an option. Of the individuals who knew clinical trials were an option but declined to participate, they cited a variety of reasons: they thought that the care they would receive in a clinical trial was less effective than standard care; they might receive a placebo; they feared they would be treated like a "guinea pig"; or their insurance company would not cover the costs. Of those people in the survey who participated in a clinical trial, 97% said they were treated with dignity and respect and stated that the quality of care they received was "excellent" or "good."[22,23]

Unique, additional barriers exist for individuals who are members of certain ethnic groups and/or who are medically underserved. Due to past experiences, there is a long-standing fear and skepticism among some minority populations about medical research and distrust of the medical care system in general. Also, physicians may not discuss clinical trials with patients who belong to ethnic minorities out of concern of offending these individuals. Certainly, language and literacy barriers may make it difficult to communicate the needed information in a way that is understandable, especially the informed consent document. Costs may pose a significant barrier for the underserved, as it is most often assumed that the individual's health plan (either public or private) will cover the usual care costs. Health insurance plans vary on their coverage of clinical trials. The effort to precertify or assure this coverage can be difficult and untimely; thus it can serve as a disincentive for an individual needing immediate treatment for cancer.

Cancer Clinical Trials Programs

Currently, most clinical trials are conducted by the NCI, cancer centers, and the pharmaceutical industry, often in collaboration with one another. Although in past years the NCI was the primary developer of new cancer drugs, this role has now been increasingly assumed by the pharmaceutical industry. For phase 3 randomized studies, however, the cooperative groups remain the prime entities responsible for these evaluations, and the NCI cancer centers continue to be valuable resources for the conduct of studies funded by both NCI and industry.

NCI Cooperative Group System

The unique organization of the cooperative group system allows for the conduct of clinical trials in a multi-institutional setting. Established in 1955 by Congress, the cooperative groups primarily conduct large-scale studies, including combined-modality approaches and studies of cancer prevention, detection, quality of life, supportive care, and cost analysis. Currently, ten cooperative groups are conducting studies in the United States. They include thousands of physicians and nurses in academic medical centers, hospitals, and community physician offices (Table 10-6).

Table 10-6 NCI-Funded Clinical Cooperative Oncology Groups

- American College of Radiology Imaging Network
- American College of Surgeons Oncology Group
- Cancer and Acute Leukemia Group B
- Children's Oncology Group
- Eastern Cooperative Oncology Group
- Gynecologic Oncology Group
- National Surgical Adjuvant Breast and Bowel Project
- North Central Cancer Treatment Group
- Radiation Therapy Oncology Group
- Southwest Oncology Group

NCI Cancer Centers Program

The development of the NCI Cancer Centers Program began in the 1960s and was formally authorized under the National Cancer Act in 1971. This legislation, and the strong national support for it, promoted the formation of comprehensive cancer programs across the country that became national resources for research and led to the development of multidisciplinary approaches and national standards for oncology care. Cancer centers continue to be the research engines for oncology today; in addition, they are developing mechanisms to better integrate their work with community programs. This integration is essential to ensure better dissemination of research results and better design of applicable research so that it will benefit the majority of patients who are not treated in cancer centers.

Current Issues

Quality of Life Evaluations

In recent years, more clinical trials have included quality of life endpoints in addition to the traditional endpoints of response and survival as outcomes to be measured. These patient-reported evaluations of quality of life domains, which may include physical, psychosocial functioning, and symptom reduction, provide a much broader body of information about the intervention under study. The addition of such quality of life evaluations allows both clinicians and patients to weigh those items of most importance when making a decision about a particular treatment or a choice between treatments (Table 10-7). For example, one individual may choose the therapy (based on clinical trial results) that offers the opportunity for the maximum length of survival at the price of considerable toxicity, while another individual may choose less additional survival time to forgo the toxicity of treatment with the expectation of a better quality of life during this shorter survival period.

Table 10-7 Questions to Ask When Considering Participation in a Clinical Trial

The Study

1. What is the purpose of the study?
2. Why do researchers think the approach may be effective?
3. Who will sponsor the study?
4. Who has reviewed and approved the study?
5. How are study results and safety of participants being checked?
6. How long will the study last?
7. What will my responsibilities be if I participate?

Possible Risks and Benefits

1. What are my possible short-term benefits?
2. What are my possible long-term benefits?
3. What are my short-term risks, such as side effects?
4. What are my possible long-term risks?
5. What other options do people with my risk of cancer or type of cancer have?
6. How do the possible risks and benefits of these trials compare with those options?

Participation and Care

1. What kinds of therapies, procedures, and/or tests will I have during the trial?
2. Will they hurt, and, if so, for how long?
3. How do the tests in the study compare with those I would have outside the trial?
4. Will I be able to take my regular medications while in the clinical trial?
5. Where will I have my medical care?
6. Who will be in charge of care?

Personal Issues

1. How could being in this study affect my daily life?
2. Can I talk to other people in the study?

Cost Issues

1. Will I have to pay for any part of the trial, such as tests or the study drug?
2. If so, what will the charges likely be?
3. What is my health insurance likely to cover?
4. Who can help answer any questions from my insurance company or health plan?
5. Will there be any travel or child care costs that I need to consider while I am in the trial?

Tips for Asking Your Doctor About Clinical Trials

When you talk with your doctor or members of the research team:

1. Consider taking a family member or friend along, for support and for help in asking questions or recording answers.
2. Plan ahead what to ask — but don't hesitate to ask any new questions you think of while you're there.
3. Write down your questions in advance, to make sure you remember to ask them all.
4. Write down the answer, so that you can review them whenever you want.
5. Consider bringing a tape recorder to make a taped record of what is said (even if you write down answers).

Economic Evaluations

As a greater number of new agents and interventions undergo evaluation, there is increasing interest in including economic analyses in clinical trials. These economic evaluations form a relationship with the traditional study endpoints (i.e., response, survival, functional status, and symptom reduction) and require new theoretical and methodologic approaches to evaluate effects such as cost-effectiveness and cost-efficiency.[24] In an economic analysis, the cost of the therapy is compared to the effect of the therapy; the overall costs are presented in financial terms, while the effects of therapy are presented in terms of a clinical measure, such as disease-free years of survival, years of life saved, or quality-adjusted years of life saved (QALY).[25] The costs to be evaluated can be medical or nonmedical, depending on the focus of the proposed evaluation. When planning for an economic evaluation, it must be first determined what type of costs will be included in the analysis. This determination will depend on whose perspective is to be considered in the study — the healthcare provider, the patient, the health plan, or society.

The integration of economics into cancer clinical trials requires close communication between economists, policymakers, and clinical researchers so that the evaluations will provide useful information that benefits patients. Including cost analyses in research studies adds a serious element to the discussion of resource allocation and must be done carefully and with objective deliberation. As we begin to utilize the knowledge of the postgenomic era, it is important to be able to explore the new targeted approaches to therapeutic development, while at the same time acknowledging the need to develop a sound financial approach to providing the most effective agents.

Dissemination of Research Results

The completion of a clinical trial is not the end of the story in bringing new and better diagnostics, prevention strategies, and therapies to the public. A critical step remains — the actual introduction and use of these new interventions in the healthcare system. In the past, it often took more than a year for a scientific paper to be written and published despite the importance of the study results. Today's medical publishers have rapid-alert systems that enable them to publish immediately those studies of critical importance that have potential to affect the care being given to current patients or those at risk for cancer. These results can be made available immediately on the Internet and can then be picked up by the professional and lay press.

The next step — incorporating the study results into the healthcare system — can prove a difficult task, with multiple barriers to be overcome. Although the approval process for new agents and medical devices is clearly spelled out by FDA regulations, the coverage of their costs by health plans and their use by healthcare providers is not assured. Better systems for the evaluation of medical evidence that lead to insurance coverage are needed as well as the broader acceptance of standards of practice that outline the most effective method of treating or preventing a particular cancer-related problem.

Future Trends

Many challenges lie ahead in the development of new and more effective interventions for the prevention, diagnosis, and treatment of cancer. The postgenomic era offers tremendous opportunities for applying the understanding of preclinical drug pharmacology and molecular targeting to the design and development of clinical trials.[26] There is potential for new agents entering study to have well-defined theoretical mechanisms of action, and for investigators to design studies with biochemical and molecular endpoints.[27] At the same time, as the clinical inquiry becomes more specific to the particular molecular characteristics of the individual patient's disease, it will require new trial designs focused on these characteristics rather than the more broad-based traditional approaches. Communication and education will be needed to produce effective collaboration between investigators and to ensure participant understanding about the new clinical trials designs.

The opportunity also exists to more extensively utilize patient-centered endpoints, along with response and survival, in clinical trials. More patient groups and health professional organizations are working together to establish clinical outcomes of importance. The challenge to both the medical, nursing, and behavioral research communities is to design trials that focus on evaluating both the effects of the intervention on the disease and its effects on the overall quality of life of the individual.

References

1. Peltonen L, McKusick VA: Genomics and medicine: dissecting human disease in the postgenomic era. *Science* 291:1224–1229, 2001
2. Fisher B, Constantino JP, Wickerham DL, et al: Tamoxifen for prevention of breast cancer: report of the National Surgical Adjuvant Breast and Bowel Project P-1 study. *J Natl Cancer Inst* 90:1371–1388, 1998
3. Leventhal BG, Wittes RE: Phase I trials, in Leventhal BG, Wittes RE: *Research Methods in Clinical Oncology*. New York, Raven Press, 1988, pp 41–59
4. Leventhal BG, Wittes RE: *Research Methods in Clinical Oncology*. New York, Raven Press, 1998
5. Schneiderman MA: Mouse to man: statistical problems in bringing a drug to clinical trial, in *Proceedings of the Fifth Berkeley Symposium on Mathematical Statistical Probability*. Berkeley, University of California, 1967, p 855
6. Piantadosi S, Liu G: Improved designs for dose escalation studies using pharmacokinetic measurements. *Stat Med* 15: 1605–1618, 1996
7. Ratain MJ, Mick R, Schilsky RL, et al: Statistical and ethical issues in the design and conduct of phase I and II clinical trials of new anticancer agents. *J Natl Cancer Inst* 85:1637–1643, 1993
8. Simon R: Design and analysis of clinical trials, in De Vita VT, Hellman S, Rosenberg SA (eds.): *Cancer: Principles and Practice of Oncology* (ed 6). Philadelphia, Lippincott Williams & Wilkins, 2001, pp 521–538
9. Wittes RE, Marsoni S, Simon R, et al: The phase II trial. *Cancer Treat Rep* 69:1235–1239, 1985
10. Thiesse P, Ollivier L, Di Stefano-Louineau D, et al: Response rate accuracy in oncology trials: reasons for interobserver variability. *J Clin Oncol* 15:3507–3514, 1997
11. Pocock SJ: Randomized clinical trials. *Br Med J* 1:1161, 1977
12. Spriet A, Dupen-Spriet T: *Good Practice of Clinical Drug Trials*. Farmington, CT, Karger, 1997
13. Faden RR, Beauchamp TL: The development of consent requirements in research ethics, in Faden RR, Beauchamp TL: *A History and Theory of Informed Consent*. New York, Oxford University Press, 1986, pp 151–199
14. King P: The dangers of difference: the legacy of the Tuskegee Syphilis study, in Arras JD, Steinbock B (eds.): *Ethical Issues in Modern Medicine*. Mountain View, CA, Mayfield, 1995, pp 578–584
15. Ingelfinger FJ: Ethics of human experimentation defined by a national commission. *N Engl J Med* 296:44–45, 1977
16. The National Commission for the Protection of Human Subjects of Biomedical and Behavioral Research: *The Belmont Report: Ethical Principles and Guidelines for the Protection of Human Subjects of Research*. Washington, DC, U.S. Government Printing Office, April 1979, 1988-201-778/80319
17. Levine R, Lebacqz K: Ethical considerations in clinical trials. *Clin Pharmacol Ther* 25:728–749, 1979
18. Ramsey P: *The Patient as Person: Explorations on Medical Ethics*. New Haven, CT, Yale University Press, 1970
19. Faden RR, Beauchamp TL: The concepts of informed consent and competence, in Faden RR, Beauchamp TL: *A History and Theory of Informed Consent*. New York, Oxford University Press, 1986, pp 274–294
20. Daugherty CK: Impact of therapeutic research on informed consent and the ethics of clinical trials: a medical oncology perspective. *J Clin Oncol* 17:1601, 1999
21. National Cancer Institute. Simplification of Informed Consent Documents. (Available from *www.cancer.gov/clinicaltrials/understanding/simplification-of-informet-consent-docs*). Accessed August 24, 2004
22. Harris Interactive. *Health Care News* 1(3) [Poll]. Available from *www.harrisinteractive.com/news/newsletters/healthnews/HI_HealthCareNews2001Vol1_iss3.pdf*). Accessed August 24, 2004
23. Comis RL, Miller JD, Aldige CR, et al: Public attitudes toward participation in cancer clinical trials. *J Clin Oncol* 21:830–835, 2003
24. Integrating economic analysis into cancer clinical trials: the National Cancer Institute–American Society of Clinical Oncology economics workbook. *J Natl Cancer Inst* 24:1–3, 1998
25. Schulman KA, Glick HA, Yabroff RK, et al: Introduction to clinical economics: assessment of cancer therapies. *J Natl Cancer Inst* 19:1–10, 1995
26. Takimoto CH: Anticancer drug development at the US National Cancer Institute. *Cancer Chemother Pharmacol* 52(suppl 1): S29–S33, 2003
27. Szurmomi P, Vinson V, Marshall E: Rethinking drug discovery. *Science* 303:1795, 2004

CHAPTER 11

Surgical Therapy

Theresa Wicklin Gillespie, PhD, RN

Introduction

Surgery, whether utilized for diagnosis, staging, curative therapy, or palliation, remains the key component of oncology care. Surgery as the earliest form of cancer therapy dates back to the time of ancient Egypt. The first oncologic surgery of a more contemporary era occurred in 1809, when a large (22.5-pound) ovarian tumor was removed from a woman.[1] While rudimentary, the operation was successful in that the patient survived another 30 years. Critical dates in the history of surgery as cancer therapy are listed in Table 11-1.

Currently, more than 60% of all cancers are treated with surgery and this modality is used in diagnosis or staging of tumors in about 90% of all cases.[2] The advantages of surgery include a high potential for cure when the cancer is localized and the ability to obtain tissue for initial diagnosis as well as evidence for staging of disease. The unavoidable disadvantage of cancer surgery is the need to remove normal tissue as well as malignant tissue to assure an adequate margin of unaffected tissue when the cancer is resected. To undergo the anesthesia required for major surgery, an individual should have an acceptable performance status and organ function, especially cardiac and pulmonary.

The field of surgical oncology has progressed significantly since its inception, such that surgery is now considered part of a multidisciplinary approach to cancer therapy. The thoughtful combination and careful timing of surgery along with chemotherapy, radiation therapy, immunotherapy, and other novel therapeutic approaches are essential for optimal treatment planning. Because the initial consultation for most patients with a possible cancer diagnosis occurs with a surgeon, surgical oncology often functions as the gatekeeper for involvement of other oncologic specialties. Therefore, to guide the treatment approach properly, surgeons must be expert in not only the most current surgical techniques, but also the latest evidence related to other cancer therapy.[3] The initial treatment decisions by the surgical oncologist will often prove to be critical in terms of either allowing future treatment options or rendering certain therapies unfeasible.

Table 11-1 Critical Dates in History of Surgical Oncology

Date	Event	Significance in Surgical Oncology
1809	Resection of ovarian tumor	Patient survived long-term postsurgery
1884	Building of first U.S. operating room in Bellevue, New York	Promoted aseptic technique and allowed more invasive surgery
1889	Introduction of x-rays in surgical practice	Allowed visualization and localization of findings prior to surgery
1890	Radical mastectomy developed by William Halstead	Demonstrated long-term control of disease through radical surgery; emphasized anatomic precision and careful handling of tissue
1903	Initiation of neurosurgery by Harvey Cushing as independent specialty	Changed approaches to endocrine tumors
1975	Initiation of first adjuvant therapy trial for early-stage breast cancer	Demonstrated survival advantage for those randomized to chemotherapy postsurgery
1986	Publication of NSABP B-06 trial	Showed equivalency of segmental mastectomy (lumpectomy) plus radiation therapy compared to mastectomy

Roles of Surgery in Oncology Care

Prevention and Early Detection

As knowledge of cancer genetics and tumorigenesis has increased, understanding about interventions to prevent cancer progression and development from precancerous lesions has also advanced. The roles of hereditary and susceptibility genes have been investigated to elucidate important aspects of the process of carcinogenesis, with particular emphasis on how to prevent or interrupt this process.

Evidence has demonstrated that surgical resection of premalignant lesions can effectively prevent some types of tumors from developing further into invasive cancers. The removal of precancerous lesions of the cervix, vulva, and oropharynx are common examples of the role of surgery in cancer prevention.[4] Surgery also plays a key role in the prevention of colorectal cancer. Surgical removal of noncancerous polyps detected at time of screening or diagnostic colonoscopy effectively prevents further development of such polyps into malignancies.[5] Hereditary nonpolyposis colorectal cancer (HNPCC), familial adenomatous polyposis (FAP), and Peutz-Jeghers disease represent relatively rare causes of colorectal cancer. The development of colon cancer at a very early age, often before age 40, due to familial polyposis can be prevented through a prophylactic colectomy.[6]

Barrett's esophagus is a known premalignant condition for esophageal adenocarcinoma, and its incidence has increased over the past two decades. Esophageal adenocarcinoma develops in a stepwise progression from normal tissue to dysplasia to malignancy, with the diagnosis of high-grade dysplasia (HGD) in Barrett's esophagus, and an accompanying high risk of esophageal adenocarcinoma. The management of HGD in this case is controversial, with sur-

Table 11-2 Surgical Techniques for Tissue Diagnosis in Cancer

Surgical Technique	Description	Advantages and Disadvantages
Fine-needle aspiration	Fine needle (21–22 gauge) inserted into palpable mass; may remove fluid and/or cells in sample	Simple procedure; results available quickly; relies on cytology review of cells obtained for diagnosis
Core-needle biopsy	Core/cutting needle inserted into mass and core of tissue removed	More tissue trauma than with a fine needle; obtains larger sample and tissue for histology; may be used with interventional radiology for nonpalpable mass
Incisional biopsy	Used for larger tumors (usually >3 cm); piece of tumor removed from larger mass	Risk of bleeding; no information on margins of tumor; additional surgery or treatment needed for residual tumor; may be used when neoadjuvant therapy is expected
Excisional biopsy	Removal of entire tumor plus some additional tissue to obtain clear margins; accessible tumor usually <3 cm	May be definitive surgery; outcome should be aesthetically acceptable; limited use if tumor is too large or defect would be too obvious
Needle localization biopsy	Needle or wires placed by stereotactic procedure to mark site of tumor, then tumor excised based on marker location; used for nonpalpable or hard-to-visualize tumors	Radiographic documentation that specimen was removed is necessary; possible to miss mark and remove incorrect or inadequate sample of tissue
Endoscopy	Tumor visualized through lighted endoscope; piece of tumor or entire tumor removed; commonly used for GI, GU, and pulmonary tumors; may be incisional or excisional	Risk of perforation and hemorrhage; increases ability to access hard-to-reach tumors; avoids surgical trauma and postoperative complications associated with open surgery
Laparoscopy	Tumor visualized through lighted scope; specimen can be obtained through a variety of techniques (incisional, excisional, scraping, peritoneal washing)	Useful in staging disease; risk of perforation, hemorrhage, and other postoperative complications; avoids surgical trauma and postoperative complications associated with open surgery
Open biopsy	Exploratory or definitive surgery to obtain primary diagnosis, perform surgical resection of disease, and note visible or palpable metastases; used to help stage disease	Allows primary access to tumor and adjacent organs affected by cancer; typical surgical risks, including trauma, postoperative complications, perforation, hemorrhage, infection, and recurrence

gical resection considered by some to be the most appropriate therapy.[7] Likewise, the presence of the cancer susceptibility genes, *BRCA1* and *BRCA2*, confers a high risk for breast and/or ovarian cancer. In such cases, prophylactic mastectomy and/or oophorectomy may be one option recommended.[8] However, prophylactic surgery for individuals at high risk for developing breast and ovarian cancers, while offering some risk reduction, continues to be a source of controversy.[9]

Diagnosis

Surgery represents the primary method of obtaining tissue necessary for pathological or cytological diagnosis of malignancy. Common methods of biopsy for tissue diagnosis are described in Table 11-2. A tissue diagnosis is a requirement for new malignancies and generally for the first recurrence of a known primary tumor. Surgery is also utilized to diagnose second primary tumors and to differentiate the source of metastases if a second primary tumor is suspected. A tissue diagnosis obtained preoperatively is needed unless the surgery is planned for the purpose of diagnosis, staging, or treatment planning. A documented pathological diagnosis is imperative in cases of extensive surgery, such as mastectomy, limb amputation, or organ removal.

The location and extent of the tumor will determine which options might be pursued to obtain adequate tissue for diagnosis. Advances in interventional and guided imaging techniques have enabled clinicians to obtain necessary tissue using less invasive and often more precise procedures than open surgical approaches. CT-directed or stereotactic biopsies utilize computer imaging to pinpoint tumor locations and facilitate biopsy for diagnosis — for example, lung cancer and primary brain tumors. Colonoscopy provides a means to remove tissue (e.g., a polyp) for diagnosis, while also resecting a potentially premalignant lesion. Open biopsy may be reserved for lesions that are inaccessible by less invasive techniques, considered too risky (e.g., because of the risk of pneumothorax or other complications), or are best treated with debulking surgery.[10]

Cytology, using fine-needle aspiration (FNA), may be the optimal means for diagnosis in palpable tumors. Cytological examination can often confirm the presence of malignancy in a brief period of time. FNA may be used to obtain the initial tissue diagnosis, then additional surgical options can be explored. If complete removal of the tumor is possible, excisional biopsy with an adequate margin of tissue or more extensive surgery may be pursued following FNA diagnosis. FNA diagnosis is based on pathological examination of cells rather than tissue, and its accuracy often depends on the sample obtained, the preparation of the specimen, and the expertise of the cytopathologist interpreting the specimen. As with tissue biopsy in general, sampling error or nondiagnostic specimens may require additional interventions. Subsequent core-needle biopsy or open biopsy may be necessary to obtain adequate or precise specimens for definitive diagnosis.

Intraoperative diagnosis of tissue may be obtained using a pathological technique termed *frozen section*. With this procedure, a sample of the mass is taken from the operating room to be interpreted immediately by a pathologist. The precise histology may not be available from this initial intraoperative interpretation, but the presence of a malignancy can be confirmed. This information enables the surgeon to then pursue further surgical procedures or conclude the operation.

While ideally all lesions will have either preoperative or intraoperative confirmation of malignancy, in some cases this confirmation is not possible. A classic illustration of this dilemma is the patient with jaundice and an identified mass in the head of the pancreas. Removal of the mass requires extensive surgical resection (pancreatoduodenectomy; Whipple procedure) with known morbidity and mortality being associated with the intervention.[11] Unfortunately, the surgical procedure is necessary to both diagnose and treat a possible cancer in the head of the pancreas. Part of the preoperative work-up for any surgery must therefore include a clear discussion of possible outcomes and complications, including the risk of more extensive surgery for what may ultimately be shown to be a benign tumor.

Staging of Disease

Preoperative care for patients with a known or suspected diagnosis of cancer includes an adequate staging work-up. The size of the tumor, as determined by clinical and radiological evaluation, and the involvement of lymph nodes or distant sites are important factors for effective clinical decision making.[12] Preoperative staging is a critical element in deciding whether the patient would benefit from surgical approaches and what the goal of therapy might be — cure, control, or palliation. The use of CT scans, positron emission tomography (PET) scans, nuclear medicine scans, mammography, and other radiological techniques may aid in determining the extent of tumor involvement locally, regionally, and in distant organs. While pathological confirmation may be needed for some equivocal lesions seen on imaging exams, often these radiological methods are sufficient to establish stage of the cancer. For example, in non-small cell lung cancer (NSCLC), involvement of the mediastinum, as represented by positive lymph nodes, is a key prognostic indicator and a contraindication to surgical resection.

Pathological examination of the tumor, lymph nodes, and any other tissue removed is crucial for effective patient management. This examination will provide pathological staging criteria, prognostic factors, and rationale for any adjuvant therapy.[13] The stage, histological cell type and grade of tumor, status of margins of resection (whether involved with the tumor or not), and degree of vascular invasion contribute to the determination of risk of recurrence and assessment of whether the surgery is likely to represent a long-term control or cure of the malignancy. Accurate staging of disease continues to function as the principal prognostic factor for most cancers, because stage of disease is often directly correlated with long-term survival. Only a few cancers (e.g., testicular) remain curable even in advanced stages. Therefore, preoperative staging can assist in the decision making as to whether extensive surgical resection with the goal of cure is possible, or if a more palliative approach is justified.

Trends in surgical staging procedures have changed over time. Historically, the goals for staging via lymphadenectomy of regional nodes included prognosis, regional control of malignancy through removal of involved nodes, and improvement in other outcomes, including survival. However, removal of regional nodes was also associated with morbidity, reduced quality of life, loss of function, and surgical mortality.

Sentinel lymph nodes represent the initial set of nodes thought to receive drainage from the primary tumor. Thus, cancer cells are theorized to metastasize first to these draining nodes, and the removal and examination of one or more identified sentinel nodes is seen as an effective approach to staging regional nodes.[14] The use of blue dye, nuclear medicine technology, and other techniques has enabled surgeons to identify one or more sentinel nodes with a high level of accuracy. If no malignant cells are found in sentinel nodes, the remaining regional nodes are usually negative as well. The traditional methods for pathological examination of nodes have also undergone extensive revision as new laboratory methods to detect malignant involvement and micrometastases have become available. However, the prognostic significance of some newer pathological findings, such as micrometastases, remains to be determined.

Sentinel lymph node biopsy has replaced complete lymph node dissection as the standard of care in some tumors, and it is under investigation in other solid tumors. In certain tumor sites, such as melanoma, sentinel biopsy has been established over the past decade as the standard of care. For many centers, sentinel node mapping also represents the standard of care for breast cancer. The application of this technique remains under investigation in other solid tumors, including gastrointestinal malignancies.[15]

Resection for Cure

When a malignancy is diagnosed at an early or localized stage, surgical resection usually represents the best option for long-term survival and cure. The traditional surgical approach for cure remains en bloc resection of the primary tumor with negative margins, along with biopsy or removal of regional or draining lymph nodes where indicated.[16] Early-stage solid tumors, especially in situ or encapsulated tumors where margins are clearly defined and less radical surgery is indicated, are most amenable to surgical resection and offer the best clinical and functional outcomes. Knowledge of the biology of the tumor and natural history of the disease is imperative when planning surgical resection. This principle is demonstrated by a comparison of two types of skin cancer: malignant melanoma, where wide resection with adequate margins is required for long-term control of disease, versus basal cell carcinoma, where less aggressive resection is often adequate for cure.[17]

Surgical resection for cure can be problematic when the tumor is large or invades vital organs or tissues with critical functions. In these cases, decision making involves both clinician and patient input regarding the risk–benefit ratio. The need for an adequate surgical margin must be weighed against potential loss of function, change in body image, and the age and general health of the patient.[18] For example, surgical treatment for stage I and II NSCLC represents the standard of care.[19] With the goal of cure, the location, depth, size, and characteristics of the tumor may require different surgical approaches, including a wedge resection, a lobectomy, or pneumonectomy. In each case, the potential benefits of long-term survival resulting from removal of larger amounts of lung tissue must be judged in the context of anticipated loss of pulmonary function. Patients with head and neck cancers requiring extensive surgical resection to ensure adequate margins must be evaluated for, and informed of, both potential functional deficits and significant changes in self-image. In some cases, such as primary brain tumors, the location or extent of tumor involvement may be such that adequate resection is not possible without dramatic and unacceptable loss of function. In these cases, less radical surgery combined with chemotherapy or radiation may be the optimal approach to achieving the desired treatment goals.

Resection with Minimal Residual Disease

If the primary tumor is not amenable to complete resection with adequate margins, or if malignant cells are found in regional lymph nodes, then some form of adjuvant therapy may be considered following surgery. The presence of even minimal residual disease in surgical margins or draining nodes generally indicates a high risk of recurrence. The use of adjuvant chemotherapy or radiation therapy, or a combination of these modalities, is often recommended postoperatively. Novel therapies such as biological or targeted therapies may also prove effective in the setting of minimal residual disease. Aggressive tumor debulking may lend itself to the use of adjuvant treatment to eradicate remaining residual cancer cells. In the case of ovarian cancer, which is often diagnosed at a relatively advanced stage, cytoreduction in combination with chemotherapy can improve survival and prevent complications, such as bowel obstruction.[20]

Resection in Advanced Disease

Surgical resection of advanced disease is generally performed to achieve one of two goals: (1) resection of solitary or limited metastatic disease or (2) palliation of symptoms. Resection of a solitary metastatic lung or liver nodule is routinely performed in advanced disease to improve survival. Resectability of metastatic disease will depend on size, number, and anatomical location of the tumors, and it may require performance of more extensive surgery, such as removal of an entire lobe of the liver or lung. Five-year survival rates ranging from 20% to 45% have been noted with hepatectomy for metastatic liver lesions from colorectal cancer.[21] Unfortunately, fewer than 15% of patients with advanced colorectal cancer present with potentially resectable disease.[22] In patients whose disease is unresectable, neoadjuvant chemotherapy may be administered in an attempt to downstage the tumor to enable resection. Administration of preoperative chemotherapy has resulted in resectablity rates of 10%–40% for liver metastases from colorectal cancers that were previously considered unresectable. Postoperative five-year survival rates of 30%–60% were reported.[23]

Brain metastases occur in about 20%–40% of all cancer cases. For those patients with a good performance status and limited or controlled systemic disease, radiosurgery alone or surgical removal of a solitary brain metastasis often in combination with whole-brain radiation can yield favorable long-term results.[24]

Reconstruction

The goals of reconstruction in surgical oncology are fourfold: (1) restoration of function, (2) skin closure or wound covering for surgical defects, (3) restoration of cosmetic appearance (cosmesis) for improvement of body image changes, and (4) maintenance or enhancement of quality of life. Depending on the extent of reconstruction and the specialized expertise required, reconstructive surgery may be undertaken by the primary surgeon alone or in collaboration with various other specialists, such as plastic and reconstructive surgeons, urologic surgeons, and gynecologic surgeons.[25] Consultation with other specialists in advance of the scheduled surgery promotes interdisciplinary coordination of care, facilitates the patient's comprehension of anticipated postoperative results, and enhances the patient's understanding of reconstruction options and timing.

Considerable advances in the field of reconstruction have occurred for many types of cancer. Breast cancer may have experienced the greatest changes, from the time many decades ago when wound closure following radical mastectomy was the primary goal, to current approaches including immediate reconstructive techniques, such as implants placed behind the pectoralis muscle and gradually inflated over time (expanders) and transverse rectus abdominis mocutaneous (TRAM) flap, and the more recent technique of skin-sparing mastectomy.[26] The cosmetic appearance of the breast depends on the amount of skin that remains following mastectomy. If adequate skin is preserved, then the cosmetic appearance of the operative side is enhanced and the need to make surgical changes on the contralateral side to achieve symmetry is reduced.[27] Incidence rates for both local recurrence and wound complications are similar for skin-sparing mastectomy and non–skin-sparing mastectomy. The type of breast reconstruction technique, timing of reconstruction (immediate or delayed), and preference for any reconstruction at all are often difficult decisions needing to be made by the woman who has experienced a recent diagnosis of cancer. Such decision making demands careful patient education, presentation of options, and provision of adequate time to consider individual preferences. Therapeutic factors, such as timing of adjuvant chemotherapy or radiation therapy, must also be discussed. Complications related to the reconstruction, such as infection or necrosis that would warrant removal of the implant or flap repair, could lead to significant delays in the delivery of adjuvant therapy.[28]

Reconstruction for head and neck cancers, depending on size, location, and extent of tumor involvement, represents a significant challenge in reconstructive surgery. Radical neck dissection, laryngectomy, and other surgeries of the oropharynx require extensive efforts to provide skin and wound closure, reasonable cosmesis, and restoration of as much function as possible. Specialists in plastic surgery, otolaryngology, medical and radiation oncology, and rehabilitation medicine may all need to be involved in treatment planning. Limited surgical defects, such as occur with small tongue base, may undergo primary closure or be left to granulate and fill in the wound over time. Tissue flaps have their own adequate, reliable blood supply and are composed of segments of donor tissue that match the graft site in color, texture, and often sensitivity; they are used to close larger defects. Moderate-sized surgical defects may be closed by flaps such as those from the buccal mucosa.[29] Large surgical defects require flaps, termed *pedicle* flaps, from regional muscles, including the pectoralis major or latissimus dorsi, with adequate inherent vasculature. The pectoralis major myocutaneous pedicle flap (PMMPF) has been used extensively for reconstruction postsurgery for head and neck cancer. Flap procedures may be used for primary reconstruction, or for second-line or "salvage" procedures to repair defects arising from surgical or flap complications. Complications of head and neck reconstruction include infection, hematoma, partial or total flap failure, dehiscence, seroma, fistula, or similar problems at the donor site.[30] Risks of complications are greater in procedures done for salvage or reconstruction of the oral cavity, and they increase with the number of co-morbidities present and history of cigarette smoking. Flaps may also be utilized for repair of scars from previous surgery or reconstruction.[31] Examples of flaps are illustrated in Chapter 54.

Radical surgery for gastrointestinal, urinary, and gynecologic cancers can also require attention to needs for reconstruction and restoration of function. Tumors of the low to mid-rectum may require construction of a pouch to restore function, such as reconstruction with a colonic J-pouch–anal anastomosis.[32] Several randomized trials have evaluated different reconstructive pouches in terms of function and complications. Smaller pouches tend to be more effective, and reconstructive pouches may offer an advantage over traditional coloanal anastomosis (surgical connection between the colon and anus or anal canal) as the former are associated with less morbidity and anastomotic complications.[33]

Urinary diversion and reconstruction or replacement of the bladder following cystectomy have been pursued with multiple approaches, including the following: (1) creation of conduits to the skin using intestinal segments (conduit diversion); (2) creation of a rectal reservoir or diversion to the skin (continent diversion); (3) use of intestinal segments to replace bladder function; and (4) reconstruction of the removed bladder.[34] Outcomes are related to patient selection, based on assessment of co-morbidities, renal status, and ability to handle the care of the diversion or reservoir post surgery. Chronological age or locally advanced disease is not an automatic contraindication to urinary diversion.[35]

Gynecologic malignancies often require careful reconstruction techniques, as resection of these tumors may affect the function of the gastrointestinal, genitourinary, and reproductive systems. Invasive gynecologic cancer, such as cervical cancer, may call for extensive resection including pelvic exenteration. Use of diversion techniques for urinary continence, as well as fertility-sparing surgery, require decision making relating to the patient's age, prognosis, childbearing potential, and tumor characteristics and stage.[36]

Surgery as Ancillary Intervention

Surgery plays an important role in comprehensive cancer care outside the realm of diagnosis, tumor resection, staging, and reconstruction. The surgery team, along with interventional radiology specialists in some centers, is responsible for placement of central vascular access devices (VADs). Placement of VADs may be a routine part of patient work-up and staging when a diagnosis of cancer is known and the decision regarding systemic chemotherapy has been made. Placement of VADs may occur at the time of more definitive surgery to avoid the need for additional anesthesia. Other ancillary surgical procedures, including therapeutic bronchoscopy, thoracentesis for malignant pleural effusion, or repair of other complications (e.g., extravasation or removal of infected catheters), may be required throughout the course of the patient's care.

Clinical Decision Making in Surgical Therapy

Clinical decision making in the field of surgical oncology depends on the considerable data available at the time of consultation or diagnosis. These data might encompass specific characteristics of the primary tumor or stage of disease, characteristics or desires unique to the patient, and issues pertinent to the healthcare environment. During the entire preoperative work-up and treatment-planning phase, the nurse will guide and support the patient and family through an extensive and often confusing process of decisions, alternatives, and appointments. The extensive work-up process can be anxiety provoking and further complicated by overwhelming amounts of information and opinions from family and neighbors. The oncology nurse is in a pivotal position to help the patient and family assimilate the vast array of data and arrive at the decision of their choice.

Tumor Characteristics

Awareness of the differential diagnoses prior to definitive diagnosis, as well as knowledge of biological features and natural history of specific malignancies post-diagnosis, is critical in surgery for cancer. While general surgeons in some communities continue to perform the majority of cancer surgeries, in many settings specialized surgeons focus only on surgical oncology. In academic centers, surgeons may specialize even further and limit their practice to certain tumor types. This specialization enables surgeons to stay current in the latest research and findings related to optimal care of specific malignancies. For example, in breast cancer, the distinctive properties of lobular carcinoma, infiltrating adenocarcinoma, and inflammatory breast cancer all require different surgical approaches to treatment. Understanding the proclivity of high-grade or aggressive cell types of tumors to proliferate more rapidly or metastasize more quickly may alter decisions regarding care. Comprehension of the concept of residual disease after primary surgical resection would lead to a referral to medical or radiation oncology for adjuvant therapy.

Patient Characteristics

While complete resection of the primary tumor for cure may be the optimal overall goal in surgical approaches, knowledge of the specific patient's medical and surgical history, prior therapies, and demographics are all important factors in clinical decision making. Patients who have previously received radiation therapy to a tumor bed may not be candidates for surgical resection of a recurrence in the same area. Individuals with reduced pulmonary function may not be appropriate candidates for pneumonectomy, but may be able to tolerate a lobectomy or wedge resection of a primary lung cancer if more conservative surgery is an alternative. Performance status and the presence of significant co-morbidities, rather than chronological age alone, are more important indicators of the ability to tolerate surgery and anesthesia. Metastatic work-up and careful staging of the disease will help to determine appropriate therapeutic options.

The preoperative work-up should include the following elements: history and physical; concomitant medications; pathology of tumor (if available); staging of disease; evaluation of surgical and anesthesia tolerance; consultation by medical and/or radiation oncology as indicated; discussion of need for preoperative or neoadjuvant therapy; documentation and communication of the goals of therapy; plans for immediate or delayed reconstruction, with consultation by plastic or reconstructive surgery; consultation with any other specialists who may need to be involved in surgery depending on the extent of resection (e.g., urology in extensive colorectal or gynecologic surgeries); and plans for rehabilitation if needed. A checklist or careful documentation in the patient's record will facilitate the progression of the preoperative work-up, ensure that no items are missed, and promote interdisciplinary communication and coordination of care.

Environmental Factors

Several environmental factors may affect the outcomes associated with the surgery: any specialized physician and nursing expertise available at the patient's selected place of care; the technology and surgical techniques to be utilized; the volume of cases performed by the institution and by the attending surgeon with the patient's specific tumor type/stage; supportive care available, such as hematopoietic growth factor use, antibiotics, transfusions, nutritional supplementation, and related interventions; and availability of specialized nursing care or specialty units, such as critical care. Each of these environmental factors may have an effect on perioperative outcomes, from immediate postsurgical morbidity and mortality, to long-term rehabilitation and recovery of function.

Impact of Nursing Care on Surgical Outcomes

Outcomes in surgical oncology are often directly related to the quality of care provided by the entire team. Perioperative mortality may be due to wound infection; organ function, especially cardiac, pulmonary, and renal function; effects of anesthesia; anticipation and management of surgical complications; and effectiveness of patient self-care when discharged. Other outcomes may be related to postoperative changes in mobility, function, and quality of life. Nursing care plays a critical role in affecting outcomes through careful assessment, intervention, and evaluation. Patient teaching, both preoperatively and postoperatively, is key to ensuring that patients and families understand anticipated procedures and effects, and that desired outcomes are achieved.

Short-Term Outcomes

Short-term perioperative outcomes may be defined as those events occurring preoperatively and within 30 days of surgery.[37] Serious complications that can occur during this period include life-threatening cardiac or pulmonary events, renal failure, shock, hemorrhage, infection, and need for reoperation. All patients in the postoperative setting—and cancer patients in particular—are at increased risk for thromboembolic events, including pulmonary embolism. High-risk patients, such as those with brain tumors, lung cancer, or a preexisting coagulation dysfunction, may benefit from additional interventions beyond standard antithrombolic mechanical approaches of ambulation or passive exercise. A prospective study investigating low-molecular-weight heparin (LMWH) for prophylaxis of venous thrombosis in high-risk patients undergoing surgery for urologic cancer used subcutaneous LMWH administered daily beginning one or two hours prior to surgery and continuing three to seven days.[38] All 38 patients completed prophylaxis with LMWH, and none developed DVT or any other adverse hematologic events either intraoperatively or postoperatively.

Preoperative history, staging work-up, and documented co-morbidities are key factors in developing a model for risk factors predicting operative mortality. In a model for postoperative mortality developed in colorectal cancer, independent predictors of mortality were identified as patient age, American Society of Anesthesiology risk-assessment grade, stage of disease, extent of surgical resection, and the urgency with which the operation was undertaken.[39]

Surgical patients are subject to immune suppression, and cancer patients are generally already susceptible to immunosuppression as related to their disease. Nursing care in the perioperative period should be directed at assessing for causes of further depression of immune function, and at facilitating approaches to boost the immune system.[40] Potential factors that may affect immune function include surgery, anesthesia, pain, opioid medications, temperature changes, blood transfusion, and physiologic and psychological stress. The underlying mechanism of these immune changes is proposed to be a decrease in natural killer (NK) cell activity. Indeed, several of these factors are known to affect NK cell function. Interventions that may address immune changes encompass aggressive pain control, avoidance of unnecessary blood transfusions, selection of anesthetics and pain medications that may be less immunosuppressive, and delay in elective surgery until the patient has attained an improved immune status.[40]

Most often using colorectal cancer resection as the tumor type studied, recent data have indicated an inverse relationship between hospital volume for specific surgeries and certain outcomes and complications, including 30-day mortality.[41–44] Specialization by surgeons has also been shown to have an effect on outcomes (e.g., postoperative mortality rates). Specialists were found to have lower rates of complications, such as anastomotic leak rates [odds ratio 0.46 (95% confidence interval: 0.31 to 0.66)], higher local recurrence-free survival [hazard ratio 0.56 (0.44 to 0.71)], and increased overall long-term survival [hazard ratio 0.76 (0.71 to 0.83)].[45] Although volume of cases for individual surgeons and operative techniques were seen as being important for certain outcomes (e.g., ostomy rates), hospital volume was found to play a more critical role as a predictor of postoperative outcomes.[46] Thus, the hospital-based multidisciplinary care, including nursing care, was viewed as the primary factor affecting quality of cancer surgery and the area where education and quality improvement efforts should be focused.

Long-Term Outcomes

Long-term disease-free or recurrence-free survival was not predicted by hospital volume in those studies focused on colorectal cancer, although overall five-year survival rates were found to be related.[43] Besides survival, other long-term outcomes, such as incontinence, dysphagia, or loss of mobility, are important to note. Some surgically induced changes in function may recover after the immediate postoperative period, while other side effects may last for years or for the rest of the patient's life. Urinary incontinence and sexual impotence are two potential long-term outcomes associated with radical prostate cancer surgery, which even use of nerve-sparing surgical techniques may not prevent. A survey of 166 men who had prostate cancer surgery highlighted the extent of urinary incontinence as a problem, management strategies used to address the problem, and effective coping interventions.[47] Nearly 70% of the respondents reported dealing with incontinence postsurgery, with the majority experiencing stress incontinence, for periods up to five years or longer. Management techniques used by the respondents included absorbent pads, specialized undergarments, and pelvic muscle exercises. While most subjects (89 of 111) stated that they were informed prior to surgery that urinary incontinence could be a potential problem as a result of their surgery, few felt properly equipped to address or resolve this important issue in their lives.[47] This study demonstrates the pivotal role nurses can play in preoperative teaching and postoperative reinforcement of patient education and the need to help patients design effective strategies to address postoperative side effects.

Key long-term postsurgical changes commonly occur with tumors of other sites, such as breast cancer. Lymphedema secondary to axillary lymph node dissection or more extensive surgical resection can result in loss of mobility and function in the affected arm. While some improvement may be noted over time, often these postsurgical deficits are permanent. Other long-term outcomes associated with breast cancer surgery relate to reconstruction, either with implants and expanders or autologous tissue.[48] Even if the woman opts to undergo reconstruction immediately at the time of the surgical resection of the tumor, the reconstruction and adaptation process may take months before it is completed. One study pointed to mastectomy patients' needs to return to "normality" after surgery, highlighting decision making that might facilitate achieving that goal, including immediate reconstruction.[48]

Preoperative Teaching and Counseling

A variety of personnel may share responsibility for preoperative teaching, including surgeons, anesthesiologists, nurses, pain management teams, pharmacists, social workers, and house officers if the surgery will be performed in a teaching facility. The teaching may take place over several days or even weeks as the patient completes consultation with each specialist involved in the care. The volume of work-up–related activities required to be accomplished prior to the scheduled surgery may allow only limited time for comprehensive and coordinated teaching or verification of patient understanding of the information provided. Reinforcing teaching guides and educational materials can allow patients to absorb the material at their own pace.

Preoperative teaching generally encompasses informed consent for the planned surgery, optional procedures that may be done at the time of the expected surgery, and need for blood transfusion; the type of anesthesia to be given and anticipated side effects; physical preparation for the planned surgery (e.g., bowel prep); logistical information regarding the schedule of events; administration of regular medication during the perioperative period; laboratory or imaging studies required; insurance coverage; the plan for pain management; nutritional issues; and expected risks and benefits of the surgery. Patient teaching may be delivered verbally, through written pamphlets or forms, as a video, via interactive computer program, or through a combination of educational strategies.

The timing of teaching may also vary, although better comprehension and retention are reported when preoperative teaching takes place prior to admission for surgery.[49] Effective preoperative teaching may also serve to reduce postoperative pain and anxiety.[50]

When evaluating the effectiveness of preoperative patient teaching, the oncology nurse should be aware of the high level of anxiety commonly generated by impending hospital or day-surgery admission and surgical procedures. Individuals undergoing surgery for a known or suspected cancer diagnosis have the added burden of dealing with a potentially life-threatening disease. Consequently, comprehension and recall of teaching are often compromised. A study of 125 patients undergoing head and neck surgery who had received preoperative teaching about associated risks reported that the patients had an overall recall rate of 39% of the material presented.[51] Comprehension and recall may be affected by patient age, gender, educational level, stage of disease, and whether the cancer is newly diagnosed or recurrent. Patient preferences regarding the amount of information to be disclosed may vary from those desiring little or no information regarding risks, to those wanting to know of major risks, to individuals preferring to be told *all* possible risks.[52] While individual preferences and anxiety levels should be assessed, critical and relevant information, including the potential risk of death, must be given to ensure that informed consent has been achieved.

Postoperative Teaching and Counseling

Knowing the purpose of the surgical intervention will help the nurse determine the approach, content, and extent of postoperative teaching needed. It is important to know whether the surgery was performed to obtain a new diagnosis of cancer, resect with intent to cure, confirm recurrence of a previously diagnosed malignancy, or palliate the disease. The oncology nurse can tailor the information to provide education that supports the patient's and family's understanding of the goal of the surgery.

Helping patients and their families understand what to expect after an operation is critical as part of both preoperative and postoperative teaching. Often this information will need to be reinforced or modified if the extent of cancer or required surgical intervention was not known prior to surgery. Information related to pain management; wound care; restrictions on diet, exercise, or other activities; and signs and symptoms of complications in the immediate postoperative period must be explained in detail prior to discharge.

Cancer surgery, particularly for initial diagnosis, will usually be performed on an outpatient basis, so limited time may be available for extensive patient teaching. In these cases, coordination between the outpatient surgery center nurses and the patient's surgeon or oncologist is imperative to assure adequate dissemination of information. Even if the patient is admitted to the inpatient setting for more extensive surgery, the length of stay may be short and again will require careful coordination with outpatient services. A preoperative teaching checklist validating that information was given and offering some assessment of patient's level of understanding is helpful and may be shared among clinical sites where care is given. An example of a preoperative/postoperative patient teaching tool appears in Figure 11-1.

Teaching patients and their families about long-term outcomes following surgery for cancer may require considerable time, repeated sessions, and the involvement of a multidisciplinary care team. For example, the relatively high incidence of urinary incontinence and sexual dysfunction following radical prostatectomy may entail postoperative teaching and intervention over an extended period of time.[53] Patients whose surgery resulted in the formation of an ostomy will usually benefit from teaching by enterostomal therapists and other specialists to help patients learn to care for their ostomy, obtain and apply the needed medical devices and supplies, have nutritional counseling, and receive advice regarding potential effects of the surgery on sexuality and body image.[54]

Rehabilitation

The need for and degree of rehabilitation following cancer surgery will depend on multiple factors: (1) the extent of surgery performed and organ preservation achieved; (2) the age and performance status of individual; (3) co-morbid conditions; (4) the patient's physical activity/mobility level prior to surgery; (5) additional treatment (chemotherapy and/or radiation) given prior to or following surgery; and (6) the overall goals of therapy. Rehabilitation required for cancer surgery designed with curative intent may vary significantly from rehabilitation for surgery performed for palliation or symptom relief.

Individuals undergoing head and neck surgery may require consultation and services from specialists in fields including swallowing, audiology, speech pathology, nutrition, and plastic surgery. The amount and type of rehabilitative care required are determined by the functional abilities retained after surgery. It is important to note that more complete rehabilitation to an enhanced functional status usually translates into improved quality of life for the patient.[55] Complete discussion of tumor-specific surgeries and rehabilitation can be found in site-specific chapters throughout this book.

Preoperative Assessment of Patient Teaching

- ☐ Consultations completed
  - ☐ Primary surgeon
  - ☐ Anesthesia
  - ☐ Reconstruction
  - ☐ Other surgical subspecialty
- ☐ Lab work ordered and results checked
  - ☐ CBC
  - ☐ Chemistry
  - ☐ Anticoagulant studies
  - ☐ Preoperative tumor markers (CEA, CA-125, etc.)
  - ☐ Type and cross-match
  - ☐ Other ____________
- ☐ Imaging studies completed
  - ☐ CXR, CT scan, PET
  - ☐ Staging studies
  - ☐ Tumor localization
  - ☐ Other ____________
- ☐ Pathology report
  - ☐ Biopsy report available and reviewed
  - ☐ Outside consultation on slides reviewed
- ☐ Patient teaching
  - ☐ Schedule for OR, time for arrival, parking and transportation
  - ☐ Preoperative preparation
  - ☐ Medications day/night before
  - ☐ Medications day of surgery
  - ☐ Family location to wait
  - ☐ Contact numbers for waiting area, recovery room, ICU or patient floor
  - ☐ Instructions re: valuables, clothes
  - ☐ Review of surgery planned
  - ☐ Surgical consent signed and on chart
  - ☐ Transfusion consent signed and on chart
  - ☐ Other pertinent consent forms signed
  - ☐ Review of immediate postoperative period
  - ☐ Discussion of pain management
  - ☐ Discussion of postanesthesia management

Postoperative Assessment of Patient Teaching

- ☐ Review of findings from surgery
- ☐ Consultations ordered postsurgery
- ☐ Review of pathology
- ☐ Diagnosis and/or stage of disease
- ☐ Treatment planning
- ☐ Pulmonary exercises
- ☐ Discharge instructions:
  - ☐ Exercise
  - ☐ Nutrition
  - ☐ Sexual activity
  - ☐ Return for postoperative appointment set: ____________
  - ☐ Signs and symptoms to watch for and report

Figure 11-1 Preoperative and postoperative patient teaching tool

Trends in Surgical Oncology

Advances in oncology care and understanding of cancer biology and therapeutic implications have resulted in important developments in surgery as well as in such associated modalities as medical oncology, radiation, biotherapy, and targeted and small-molecule therapies. Recent advances in surgical oncology include a focus on organ preservation, use of neoadjuvant therapy, and expansion of the role of sentinel node mapping as a staging and prognostic tool.

Organ Preservation

In the case of extensive primary disease, the use of neoadjuvant chemotherapy or radiation prior to surgery may allow for surgical resection with adequate margins along with preservation of function or improved cosmesis. Organ preservation is important in most cancers, but particularly in cases where retention of the majority of the organ tissue is critical for either function or cosmetic appearance. Such cases include cancers of the anus, rectum, or bladder; sarcomas, especially of the extremities; breast cancer; and head and neck cancers. Both chemotherapy and radiation, either alone or in combination, have been utilized extensively, reflecting their important roles in organ preservation. Hyperfractionation, or the delivery of more than one fraction of radiation per day, allows higher radiation doses to be given to tumors while sparing normal tissues. The accelerated radiation fractionation regimen also addresses the heightened malignant cell proliferation that occurs during treatment.[56] Higher doses of radiation with little increase in associated toxicity can also be achieved using three-dimensional conformal and intensity-modulated radiation therapy.[57] Novel biologic and targeted therapies, such as monoclonal antibodies, antiangiogenesis, gene therapy, vaccines, signal transduction inhibitors, antisense technology, and small molecules, have sought to exploit advances in cancer biology. These new therapies could play a role in organ preservation because they have the potential to control or impede malignant growth.

The principles of organ preservation rely on multimodality therapy to achieve maximum shrinkage of the tumor prior to surgery (neoadjuvant), so as to render the tumor resectable while retaining organ function and possibly appearance. Response of the tumor to induction chemotherapy demonstrates its chemosensitivity and tends to correlate with clinical outcomes.[58] A less favorable response, or complete lack of response, indicates a poorer prognosis and the need for more radical surgery. Pathologic assessment of tumor response is also an important component in treatment planning for organ preservation. A pathologic response reflects sensitivity to the induction therapy and allows for more conservative surgery. Nevertheless, complete resection of the tumor while preserving as much organ as possible and potentially adjuvant therapy are indicated to promote long-term outcomes.

Neoadjuvant Therapy

Chemotherapy for solid tumors given preoperatively (termed "neoadjuvant") has been reported to produce significant improvements in clinical response rates as well as enhance the ability to perform organ-preserving therapy. Originally intended for large and/or locally advanced tumors, neoadjuvant therapy is increasingly being used to reduce the size of the primary tumor as part of an effort to achieve good cosmesis or improved function in organ conservation.

Adjuvant therapy in breast cancer has been used extensively for almost three decades and has demonstrated improved outcomes, including reduction in risk of recurrence and survival, in nearly all subsets of patients.[59] The use of neoadjuvant therapy has also shown the ability to increase clinical response rates as well as to achieve breast conservation.[60] Other advantages of neoadjuvant therapy include its use to demonstrate chemosensitivity in the presence of clinical, often measurable disease, as well as its role in allowing the analysis of biomarkers as potential predictors of response.[61] Although the exact biologic mechanisms underlying the prognostic significance of pathologically complete remission remain to be elucidated, the significance of reductions in proliferation of breast cancer cells, increases in apoptosis, and alterations in biomarkers such as *p53*, *bcl-2*, hormone receptors, and *HER2* remains under investigation.[62]

Sentinel Node Biopsy and Mapping

The use of sentinel lymph node (SLN) biopsy and mapping in breast cancer has gained considerable support, to the point where it is rapidly becoming adopted as the standard of care in many centers with practitioners experienced in these techniques.[63] The ability to assess lymph node involvement while avoiding potential additional co-morbidities associated with axillary lymph node dissection (ALND) is the major advantage of SLN mapping. This kind of biopsy and mapping was originally explored in melanoma. The primary indication for using SLN techniques involves palpable and nonpalpable T1 and T2 tumors, with limited data supporting SLN application for other stages of disease.

SLN mapping has been associated with less morbidity compared with complete axillary node dissection in patients with primary breast cancer.[64,65] Although the specifics of procedures for lymphatic mapping, case selection, surgical techniques, pathological analysis, definition and identification of micrometastatic disease, and related outcomes often vary by center or sometimes by practitioner, overall findings reported are similar. Experience is a prerequisite for accurate mapping, whether radioguided, blue dye, or other techniques are used. More recently, PET and SPECT/CT scanning have been explored to identify SLN. In one prospective trial of 154 patients with stage I and II breast cancer, using a combination of dye and radioisotope techniques, these lymph nodes were successfully identified in 147 of 154 (95.5%) patients, with agreement between SLN and axillary node status in 146 (99.3%) of cases. The false-negative rate was 1 in 42, or 2.4%.[66] Higher false-negative rates (11.3%) have been reported in patients with multifocal disease or for tumor size greater than 2 cm.[67] Although randomized trials evaluating SLN biopsy have not yet been published, some groups have developed clinical practice guidelines based on currently available evidence .[68–70]

Current clinical trials, being conducted through National Surgical Adjuvant Breast and Bowel Project (NSABP), British Association of Surgical Oncology (BASO), European Organization for Research and Treatment of Cancer (EORTC), and American College of Surgeons Oncology Group (ACOSOG), are investigating the outcomes, including survival of both sentinel node-negative and node-positive patients who do not undergo further axillary dissection. The prognostic importance of immunohistochemistry (IHC) detection of positive sentinel lymph nodes as well as IHC-positive bone marrow is not known.[71,72]

Special Considerations for Nursing Care

Older Patients and Surgical Therapy

More than half of all cancers and cancer deaths occur in elderly individuals (age ≥ 65 years old). The increased incidence of cancer with aging may be due to long-term accumulation of cellular and DNA mutations, heightened susceptibility of aging tissues to carcinogens, and the systemic effects of aging, including immune senescence and changes in cytokine production.[73]

Earlier studies reporting differences in therapeutic outcomes (e.g., survival), in older patients have focused on age and often ignored variations in care delivery.[74] Unfortunately, clinical decision making tends to be based on chronological age as a major criterion; however, no published data support the use of age alone as the primary means to determine contraindications for chemotherapy or optimal cancer care.[75]

Carbone reported that older patients are more likely to be given inadequate therapy or therapy without curative intent, and less likely to be referred to specialty cancer centers.[76] Currently, no evidence exists to withhold chemotherapy or standard treatment based solely on age.[77] Effective therapy can be given to elderly patients, and the outcomes and toxicities are the same as for younger patients for multiple tumor types.[78]

A stratified random sample of 1174 newly diagnosed, node-negative breast cancer cases, aged 50 years or older, were reviewed, with predictors of definitive loco-regional treatment identified through multiple logistic regression analysis. Results indicated that women 70 years or older were significantly less likely than younger women (aged 50–69 years) to receive definitive breast cancer therapy (48.7% versus 83.5%, $p < 0.0001$). Lower rates of breast-conserving surgery, radiation therapy, lymph node dissection, and chemotherapy were reported ($p < 0.0001$ for each modality) for older patients, while treatment with tamoxifen was equivalent (66.4% versus 64.7%, $p = 0.41$). Regression analysis, while controlling for co-morbidity and other disease characteristics, hospital site, and attending physician, revealed that age was a strong predictor of the probability of receiving definitive loco-regional therapy (odds ratio, 0.14; 95% confidence interval) for women 70 years or older compared to the younger cohort (50–69 years). Thus, less aggressive therapy was delivered to elderly breast cancer patients based primarily on chronological age, independent of co-morbidity status.[79]

More than half of all lung cancers are found in patients aged 65 years or older, yet surgical resection is performed less often in older patients than in younger individuals with NSCLC.[80] Clinical decisions to avoid surgery in such cases are often based on chronological age rather than documented risk factors. Progress in preoperative risk assessment and surgical approaches has greatly reduced morbidity and mortality associated with lung cancer surgery in older patients.

In contrast, prostate cancer diagnosed at an early stage in elderly men who are asymptomatic with slow-growing tumors may benefit from a "watch and wait" approach rather than radical prostatectomy.[81] Treatment options, including observation, should be reviewed in the context of the biologic characteristics of the tumor and associated risk–benefit ratio, co-morbidities, expected life span, and desired quality as well as quantity of life.[82]

Oncologic Emergencies

Most conditions that are classified as oncologic emergencies require immediate medical intervention. However, certain structural changes may call for emergency surgical intervention, such as spinal cord compression or increased intracranial pressure from brain tumors or brain metastases; spontaneous pneumothorax in chemosensitive tumors such as sarcoma;[83] malignant pleural effusion in lung cancer; intestinal obstruction in colon cancer; and obstructive uropathy in bladder cancer.[84] Careful assessment and rapid decision making with appropriate referral for surgical intervention or other modalities (e.g., radiation therapy) are needed to relieve these life-threatening conditions and maintain optimal quality of life.[85] Nurses and other members of the healthcare team need to remember that oncologic emergencies can occur in patients who have no prior diagnosis of cancer, and the index of suspicion may be low in an individual without a known malignancy.[86] Presenting symptoms may be vague and related to numerous other conditions besides cancer. Nevertheless, the differential diagnosis should include the possibility of malignancy even in the absence of a known tissue diagnosis if the medical history and risk factors support such a diagnosis.

Patients may also be at risk for oncologic emergencies as a result of recent surgery. Such risks include life-threatening infection, hemorrhage, postoperative complications, or multiple-organ failure. Surgical nursing care in the immediate postoperative period as well as postoperative follow-up and surveillance should focus on assessing wound healing and function of other organ systems, management of surgical deficits or physical changes, monitoring of laboratory results, and knowledge of clinical syndromes that might be associated with the specific tumor type under treatment.[87] If an emergency event does occur in the perioperative period or the patient's condition requires unexpected surgical intervention for resolution, nurses play a pivotal role in educating patients and family members about planned procedures and in reducing anxiety associated with urgent situations.

Perioperative Blood Transfusion

The need for allogeneic blood transfusion is a known risk associated with surgical procedures. The risk of requiring transfusion of red blood cells, platelets, or other blood products varies with the diagnosis, stage of disease, extent and type of surgical procedure planned, and decision to perform immediate reconstruction. Transfusion rates may be very low in some cases involving solid tumors (e.g., early-stage breast cancer undergoing breast conservation) or extremely high in other procedures and tumor sites. Radical neck dissection with flap reconstruction may be associated with a rate of transfusion as high as 80%.[88] Immunosuppression associated with allogeneic transfusion, in addition to the presumed immunosuppression due to the cancer itself, is thought to be the underlying etiology for poorer outcomes reported among patients who received blood transfusion along with surgery for their cancer diagnosis. Numerous studies, including randomized trials, have reported varying results over several decades. Allogeneic blood transfusion given perioperatively for multiple tumor types has been implicated as a factor leading to important outcomes such as increased rates of postoperative infection and reduced relapse-free survival and overall survival. In one prospective study of 281 patients with stage I lung cancer, the disease-free interval for those patients who received a blood transfusion in the perioperative period was significantly less than that for nontransfused patients, with median follow-up of 73 months (52% versus 71%; $p < 0.02$).[89] Similar findings have been reported for head and neck, gastrointestinal, and gynecologic cancers, although these results remain controversial due to issues related to the study designs and variations in blood products used.[90,91]

Considerable evidence has been gathered regarding the risk of postoperative infection associated with perioperative allogeneic blood transfusion. A meta-analysis involving more than 13,000 patients who underwent surgery found that the incidence of postoperative bacterial infection associated with allogeneic blood transfusion was 3.45 (odds ratio; range 1.43–15.15).[92] Risk of infection was also significantly increased in trauma patients (odds ratio 5.263; range 5.03–5.43). Thus, allogeneic blood transfusion represents a significant, yet often overlooked, risk factor associated with higher rates of bacterial infection postoperatively.

Nurses may play an important role in assessing risk factors prior to surgery, including anemia. Low preoperative hematocrit and low postoperative hematocrit, as well as increased blood transfusion rates, have been associated with increased mortality ($p < 0.01$), increased rates of postoperative pneumonia ($p \leq 0.05$), and increased hospital length of stay ($p < 0.05$), as shown by prospective data collected through the National Veterans Administration Surgical Quality Improvement Program (NSQIP).[93] Use of erythropoiesis-stimulating therapies, such as recombinant human erythropoietin (rHuEPO) or darbepoetin alfa, a longer-acting version of rHuEPO, should be considered if adequate time exists prior to scheduled surgery. A prospective, randomized double-blind study of rHuEPO ($N = 63$) administered at least seven days preoperatively and at least seven days postoperatively resulted in better outcomes for those patients who received erythropoietin. Patients in the rHuEPO group required significantly fewer transfusions perioperatively and demonstrated significantly higher hematocrit, hemoglobin, and reticulocyte counts postoperatively compared to the control group.[94] In addition, fewer postoperative complications and improved one-year survival were reported for the erythropoietin group.

Anxiety and Pain Control

As with any surgical procedure, patients should be carefully assessed for pain already present prior to surgery, approaches used to control pain, effectiveness of those pain control measures, and any adverse events associated with pain control currently in use or previously experienced. The anticipated surgical procedure, and any expected additional surgery or reconstruction, should be discussed in detail with the patient, including a plan for pain control postoperatively. For major surgical procedures, a pain management team, if part of the institutional program, should be consulted preoperatively. Plans for immediate postoperative as well as post-discharge pain control should be developed and discussed with the attending physician, patient, and other members of the healthcare team.

The reason for surgery (e.g., diagnosis, staging, curative resection, palliation) should be clear and documented. If the surgery is being planned for primary diagnosis or for staging of a newly diagnosed or recurrent cancer, all of these scenarios are associated with significant levels of anxiety. Fear of the unknown, which includes fear of possible cancer therapy associated with serious discomfort and well-publicized side effects, should be addressed and reduced by psychological, complementary, or pharmacologic interventions when possible.

Nutritional Support

Most types of surgery affect nutritional status to some degree, even if that impact consists of only dietary restrictions for a limited time prior to surgery. However, surgeries with known effects on patients' long-term nutrition require significant interventions before and after scheduled surgery to ensure adequate nutritional intake and to minimize negative influence on quality of life and overall postoperative recovery. Such surgeries include radical procedures performed for pancreatic, gastric, head and neck, and colorectal cancers. In addition, surgical complications, such as infection, may increase the nutritional needs of the patient. In all these cases, consultation with appropriate nutritional support services, if available, or generation of a thoughtful plan of care prior to surgery, is imperative to promote surgical healing and ensure a rapid return to presurgical quality of life.

Risk Assessment and Surveillance After Surgery

Individuals considered at high risk for malignancy due to a family history of the disease or other risk factors, including pathological evidence of precancerous lesions, may be followed by surgical oncologists or other specialists for risk assessment and surveillance. Individuals in a high-risk classification may benefit from genetic counseling, participation in regular screening programs, incorporating lifestyle changes, or taking chemopreventive agents to reduce known risks of cancer. They may also need to periodically undergo biopsy or invasive tests if high-risk lesions are identified. High-risk assessment and surveillance may focus on multiple types of cancers, including breast, colorectal, pancreatic, skin, melanoma, oropharyngeal, cervical, ovarian, and lung cancer.

At completion of cancer therapy—whether surgery, chemotherapy, radiation, or combined-modality treatment—patients who are considered to be cured or in long-term remission require oversight of their subsequent care. Often, surveillance after therapy is provided by the surgeon, who may obtain periodic screening tests, biomarkers, or imaging studies to evaluate for recurrence of disease or a new primary tumor. The nurse in this setting may be responsible for scheduling tests according to established protocols for follow-up care; assessing patients for signs of recurrence or need for further symptom management; teaching patients and families about rehabilitative needs or adaptation post-treatment; and addressing psychosocial issues related to quality of life, changes in role and functions due to the cancer or its treatment, and dealing with cancer as a chronic illness. The importance of complying with surveillance after therapy, and of reporting any new physical findings to the physician or nurse, should be stressed to both patients and their caregivers.

Conclusion

Surgery remains the cornerstone of oncology care, serving as an essential component for prevention, diagnosis, staging, therapy, and palliation of disease. Advances in surgical oncology have promoted significant improvements in organ preservation, multimodality care, rehabilitation, and treatment planning. Nursing care affects both short- and long-term surgical outcomes in oncology by playing a critical role in perioperative assessment, teaching, symptom management, and post-treatment surveillance.

References

1. Scott EA (ed.): *Surgery in America: From the Colonial Era to the Twentieth Century, Selected Writings*. Philadelphia, W. B. Saunders, 1965
2. American Cancer Society: *Cancer Facts and Figures — 2003*. Atlanta, American Cancer Society, 2003
3. Cady B: The changing role of the surgical oncologist. *Surg Clin North Am* 80:459–469, 2000
4. Morgan MA, Mikuta JJ: Surgical management of vulvar cancer. *Semin Surg Oncol* 17:168–172, 1999
5. Schulmann K, Reiser M, Schmiegel W: Colonic cancer and polyps. *Best Pract Res Clin Gastroenterol* 16:91–114, 2002
6. Blumberg D, Ramanathan RK: Treatment of colon and rectal cancer. *J Clin Gastroenterol* 34:15–26, 2002
7. Sharma P: Controversies in Barrett's esophagus: management of high grade dysplasia. *Semin Gastrointest Dis* 12:26–32, 2001
8. Shons AR, Cox CE: Breast cancer: advances in surgical management. *Plast Reconstr Surg* 107:541–549, 2001
9. Eerola H, Aittomaki K, Asko-Seljavaara S, et al: Hereditary breast cancer and handling of patients at risk. *Scan J Surg* 91:280–287, 2002
10. Wagman LD: Principles of surgical oncology, in Pazdur R, Coia LR, Hoskins WJ, Wagman LD (eds.): *Cancer Management: A Multidisciplinary Approach*. Melville, NY, PRR, 2000, pp 1–3
11. Schafer M, Mullhaupt B, Clavien PA: Evidence-based pancreatic head resection for pancreatic cancer and chronic pancreatitis. *Ann Surg* 236:137–148, 2002
12. Lloyd C, Silvestri GA: Mediastinal staging of non-small cell lung cancer. *Cancer Control* 8:311–317, 2001
13. Comptom CC: Colorectal carcinoma: diagnostic, prognostic, and molecular features. *Mod Pathol* 16:376–388, 2003
14. Krag DN, Weaver DL: Pathological and molecular assessment of sentinel lymph nodes in solid tumors. *Semin Oncol* 29:274–279, 2002
15. Kitagawa Y, Kitajima M: Gastrointestinal cancer and sentinel node navigation surgery. *J Clin Oncol* 79:188–193, 2002
16. Canter RJ, Williams NN: Surgical treatment of colon and rectal cancer. *Hematol Oncol Clin North Am* 16:907–926, 2002
17. Terando A, Sabel MS, Sondak VK: Melanoma: adjuvant therapy and other treatment options. *Curr Treat Options Oncol* 43:187–199, 2003
18. Sugarbaker DJ: Lung cancer: the case for limited surgical resection in non-small cell lung cancer. *Thorax* 58:639–641, 2003
19. Orlowski TM, Szczesny TJ: Surgical treatment of stage III non-small cell lung cancer. *Lung Cancer* 24 (suppl 2):S137–S143, 2001
20. Ozols RF: Update on the management of ovarian cancer. *Cancer J* 8 (suppl 1):S22–S30, 2002
21. Ong SY: Neoadjuvant chemotherapy in the management of colorectal metastases: a review of the literature. *Ann Acad Med Singapore* 32:205–211, 2003
22. Kadry Z, Clavien PA: New treatments with curative intent for metastatic colorectal liver cancer. *Expert Opin Pharmacother* 3:1191-1197, 2002
23. Adam R, Huquet E, Azoulay D, et al: Hepatic resection after down-staging of unresectable hepatic colorectal metastases. *Surg Oncol Clin North Am* 12:211–220, 2003
24. Soffietti R, Ruda R, Mutani R: Management of brain metastases. *J Neurol* 249:1357–1369, 2002

25. Hasen KV, Few JW, Fine NA: Plastic surgery: a component in the comprehensive care of cancer patients. *Oncology* 16:1685–1698, 2002
26. Harcourt D, Rumsey N: Psychological aspects of breast reconstruction: a review of the literature. *J Adv Nurs* 35:477–487, 2001
27. Simmons RM, Adamovich TL: Skin-sparing mastectomy. *Surg Clin North Am* 83:885–899, 2003
28. Petit J, Rietjens M, Garusi C: Breast reconstructive techniques in cancer patients: which ones, when to apply, which immediate and long term risks? *Crit Rev Oncol Hematol* 38:231–239, 2001
29. Sabri A: Oropharyngeal reconstruction: current state of the art. *Curr Opin Otolaryngol Head Neck Surg* 11:251–254, 2003
30. Liu R, Gullane P, Brown D, Irish J: Pectoralis major myocutaneous pedicled flap in head and neck reconstruction: retrospective review of indications and results in 244 consecutive cases at the Toronto General Hospital. *J Otolaryngol* 30:34–40, 2001
31. Clark JM, Wang TD: Local flaps in scar revision. *Facial Plast Surg* 17:295–308, 2001
32. Dehni N, Parc R, Church JM: Colonic J-pouch–anal anastomosis for rectal cancer. *Dis Colon Rectum* 46:667–675, 2003
33. Bruch HP, Schwandner O, Farke S, et al: Pouch reconstruction in the pelvis. *Lagenbecks Arch Surg* 388:60–75, 2003
34. Yog SM, Dublin N, Pickard R, et al: Urinary diversion and bladder reconstruction/replacement using intestinal segments for intractable incontinence or following cystectomy. *Cochrane Database Sys Rev* 1:CD003306, 2003
35. Clark PE: Urinary diversion after radical cystectomy. *Curr Treat Options Oncol* 3:389–402, 2002
36. Stehman FB, Rose PG, Greer BE, et al: Innovations in the treatment of invasive cervical cancer. *Cancer* 98(9 suppl): 2052–2063, 2003
37. Jimenez RE, Shoup M, Cohen AM, et al: Contemporary outcomes of total pelvic exenteration in the treatment of colorectal cancer. *Dis Colon Rectum* 46:1619–1625, 2003
38. Sawczuk IS, Williams D, Chang DT: Low molecular weight heparin for venous thromboembolism prophylaxis in urologic oncologic surgery. *Cancer Invest* 20:889–892, 2002
39. Tekkis PP, Poloniecki JD, Thompson MR, Stamatakis JD: Operative mortality in colorectal cancer: prospective national study. *BMJ* 327:1196–1201, 2003
40. Vallejo R, Hord ED, Barna SA, et al: Perioperative immunosuppression in cancer patients. *J Environ Pathol Toxicol Oncol* 22:139–146, 2003
41. Zingmond D, Maggard M, O'Connell J, et al: What predicts serious complications in colorectal cancer resection? *Am Surg* 69:969–974, 2003
42. Panageas KS, Schrag D, Riedel E, et al: The effect of clustering of outcomes on the association of procedure volume and surgical outcomes. *Ann Intern Med* 139:658–665, 2003
43. Meyerhardt JA, Catalano PJ, Schrag D, et al: Association of hospital procedure volume and outcomes in patients with colon cancer at high risk for recurrence. *Ann Intern Med* 139:649–657, 2003
44. Hodgson DC, Zhang W, Zaslavsky AM, et al: Relation of hospital volume to colostomy rates and survival for patients with rectal cancer. *J Natl Cancer Inst* 95:708–716, 2003
45. Smith JA, King PM, Lane RH, Thompson MR: Evidence of the effect of "specialization" on the management, surgical outcome and survival from colorectal cancer in Wessex. *Br J Surg* 90:583–592, 2003
46. Schrag D, Panageas KS, Riedel E, et al: Surgeon volume compared to hospital volume as predictor of outcome following primary colon cancer resection. *J Surg Oncol* 83:68–78, 2003
47. Palmer MH, Fogarty LA, Somerfield MR, et al: Incontinence after prostatectomy: coping with incontinence after prostate cancer surgery. *Oncol Nurs Forum Online* 30:229-238, 2003
48. Neill KM, Armstrong N, Burnett CB: Choosing reconstruction after mastectomy: a qualitative analysis. *Oncol Nurs Forum* 25:743–750, 1998
49. Hughes S: The effects of giving patients pre-operative information. *Nurs Stand* 16:33–37, 2002
50. Sjoling M, Nordahl G, Olofsson N, et al: The impact of preoperative information on state anxiety, postoperative pain and satisfaction with pain management. *Patient Educ Couns* 51:169–176, 2003
51. Chan Y, Irish JC, Wood SJ, et al: Patient education and informed consent in head and neck surgery. *Arch Otolaryngol Head Neck Surg* 128:1269–1274, 2002
52. Beresford N, Seymour L, Vincent C, et al: Risks of elective cardiac surgery: what do patients want to know? *Heart* 86:626–631, 2001
53. Fagermoen MS, Hamilton G: Preparing patients for urological surgery. *Int J Nurs Stud* 40:281–290, 2003
54. Shaaban AA, Mosbah A, El-Bahnasawy MS, et al: The urethral Kock pouch: long-term functional and oncological results in men. *BJU Int* 92:429–435, 2003
55. Maher KE: Organ preservation. *Semin Oncol Nurs* 15:270–281, 1999
56. Russell NS, Bartelink H: Radiotherapy: the last 25 years. *Cancer Treat Rev* 25:365–376, 1999
57. Joensuu H: Novel cancer therapies: more efficacy, less toxicity and improved organ preservation. *Ann Med* 32:31–33, 2000
58. Urban CE, Benesch M: Multimodal strategies as prerequisite for organ-salvaging tumor surgery. *Eur J Pediatr Surg* 6:144–147, 1996
59. Green M, Hortobagyi GN: Neoadjuvant chemotherapy for operable breast cancer. *Oncology* 16:871–884, 2002
60. Hutcheon AW, Heys SD, Sarkar TK, Aberdeen Breast Group: Neoadjuvant docetaxel in locally advanced breast cancer. *Breast Cancer Res Treat* 79 (suppl 1):S19–24, 2003
61. Goble S, Bear HD: Emerging role of taxanes in adjuvant and neoadjuvant therapy for breast cancer: the potential and the questions. *Surg Clin North Am* 83:943–971, 2003
62. Cleator S, Parton M, Dowsett M: The biology of neoadjuvant chemotherapy for breast cancer. *Endocr Relat Cancer* 9:183–195, 2002
63. Bonnema J, van de Velde CJ: Sentinel lymph node biopsy in breast cancer. *Ann Oncol* 13:1531–1537, 2002
64. Schijven MP, Vingerhoets AJ, Rutten HJ, et al: Comparison of morbidity between axillary lymph node dissection and sentinel node biopsy. *Eur J Surg Oncol* 29:341–350, 2003
65. Leidenius M, Leppanen E, Krogerus L, et al: Motion restriction and axillary web syndrome after sentinel node biopsy and axillary clearance in breast cancer. *Am J Surg* 185:127–130, 2003
66. Motomura K, Komoike Y, Inaji H, et al: Patient age affects identification rate of sentinel nodes in breast cancer. *Biomed Pharmacother* 56 (suppl 1):209S–S212S, 2002
67. Ozmen V, Muslumanoglu M, Cabioglu N, et al: Increased false negative rates in sentinel lymph node biopsies in patients with multi-focal breast cancer. *Breast Cancer Res Treat* 76:237–244, 2002
68. Cantin J, Scarth H, Levine M, et al: Clinical practice guidelines for the care and treatment of breast cancer: sentinel lymph node biopsy. *Can Med Assoc J* 165:166–173, 2001
69. McCready DR, Bodurtha AJ, Davis NL, et al: Sentinel lymph node biopsy in breast cancer. *Can J Surg* 42:406–407, 1999
70. Spillane AJ, Sacks NP: Role of axillary surgery in early breast cancer: review of the current evidence. *Aust NZ J Surg* 70:515–524, 2000

71. Wilke LG, Giuliano A: Sentinel lymph node biopsy in patients with early-stage breast cancer: status of the National Clinical Trials. *Surg Clin North Am* 83:901–910, 2003
72. Bonnema J, van de Velde CJ: Sentinel lymph node biopsy in breast cancer. *Ann Oncol* 13:1531–1537, 2002
73. Balducci L, Beghe C: Cancer and age in the USA. *Crit Rev Oncol Hematol* 37:137–145, 2001
74. Kimmick GG, Fleming R, Muss HB, et al: Cancer chemotherapy in older adults. A tolerability perspective. *Drugs Aging* 10:34–49, 1997
75. Bernabei R, Venturiero V, Tarsitani P, et al: The comprehensive geriatric assessment: when, where, how. *Crit Rev Oncol Hematol* 33:45–56, 2000
76. Carbone PP: Advances in the systemic treatment of cancers in the elderly. *Crit Rev Oncol Hematol* 35:201–218, 2000
77. van Rijswijk RE, Vermorken JB: Drug therapy for gynaecological cancer in older women. *Drugs Aging* 17:13–32, 2000
78. Berger DH, Roslyn JJ: Cancer surgery in the elderly. *Clin Geriatr Med* 13:119–141, 1997
79. Herbert-Croteau N, Brisson J, Latreille J, et al: Compliance with consensus recommendations for the treatment of early stage breast carcinoma in elderly women. *Cancer* 85:1104–1113, 1999
80. Jaklitsch MT, Mery CM, Audisio RA: The use of surgery to treat lung cancer in elderly patients. *Lancet Oncol* 4:463–471, 2003
81. Jani AB, Hellman S: Early prostate cancer: clinical decision-making. *Lancet* 361:1045–1053, 2003
82. Kakehi Y: Watchful waiting as a treatment option for localized prostate cancer in the PSA era. *Jpn J Clin Oncol* 33:1–5, 2003
83. Stein ME, Shklar Z, Drumea K, et al: Chemotherapy-induced spontaneous pneumothorax in a patient with bulky mediastinal lymphoma: a rare oncologic emergency. *Oncology* 54:15–18, 1997
84. Kemp C: Metastatic spread and common symptoms. Part one: introduction, bladder cancer, and brain cancer. *Am J Hosp Palliat Care* 15:355–360, 1998
85. Bridgen ML: Hematologic and oncologic emergencies. Doing the most good in the least time. *Postgrad Med* 109:143–146, 151–154, 157–158, 2001
86. Merrill P: Oncologic emergencies. *Lippincotts Prim Care Pract* 4:400–409, 2000
87. Woddard WL 3rd, Hogan DK: Oncologic emergencies: implications for nurses. *J Intraven Nurs* 19:256–263, 1996
88. Krupp NL, Weinstein G, Chalian A, et al: Validation of a transfusion prediction model in head and neck cancer surgery. *Arch Otolaryngol Head Neck Surg* 129:1297–1302, 2003
89. Nosotti M, Rebulla P, Riccardi D, et al: Correlation between perioperative blood transfusion and prognosis of patients subjected to surgery for stage I lung cancer. *Chest* 124:102–107, 2003
90. Blumberg N, Heal J: Immunomodulation by blood transfusion: an evolving scientific and clinical challenge. *Am J Med* 101:299–308, 1996
91. Hyung Wj, Noh SH, Shin DW, et al: Adverse effects of perioperative transfusion on patients with stage III and IV gastric cancer. *Ann Surg Oncol* 9:5–12, 2002
92. Hill GE, Frawley WH, Griffith KE, et al: Allogeneic blood transfusion increases the risk of postoperative bacterial infection: a meta-analysis. *J Trauma* 54:908–914, 2003
93. Dunne JR, Malone D, Tracy JK, et al: Preoperative anemia: an independent risk factor for infection, mortality, and resource utilization in surgery. *J Surg Res* 102:237–244, 2002
94. Kosmadakis N, Messaris E, Maris A, et al: Perioperative erythropoietin administration in patients with gastrointestinal tract cancer: prospective randomized double-blind study. *Ann Surg* 237:417–421, 2003

CHAPTER 12

Principles of Radiation Therapy

Tracy K. Gosselin-Acomb, RN, MSN, AOCN®

Introduction

The role of radiation therapy in the treatment of cancer and noncancerous conditions has expanded dramatically in recent decades. Since the introduction of radiation in the early 1900s, both the field of radiation oncology and the technology used for treatment have seen many advances. Based on a greater understanding of radiobiology and physics, patients can now receive radiation as a primary treatment modality. Radiation therapy may be used alone or in combination with chemotherapy, surgery, or biotherapy. Collaboration of the multidisciplinary team is critical to ensure optimal patient outcomes.

Radiation therapy involves the use of ionizing radiation in the treatment of patients with benign and malignant diseases. The aim of therapy is to deliver a precisely measured dose of irradiation to a defined tumor volume with as little damage as possible to surrounding healthy tissue, resulting in eradication of the tumor, high quality of life, and prolongation of survival at competitive costs.[1] Radiation therapy can be delivered to both outpatients and inpatients.

History of Radiation Therapy

Radiation occurs naturally in the environment. Although it is something we cannot see or feel, it is important to differentiate naturally occurring radiation from radiation produced by technologic means. In the course of everyday life, we are exposed to small amounts of radiation, but the amount of radiation needed to treat cancer is much larger.

The understanding and therapeutic use of radiation has evolved rapidly over the past century (Table 12-1). Wilhelm Conrad Roentgen, a German physicist, discovered the x-ray in 1895 while doing a laboratory experiment. Roentgen noticed that a cathode tube (developed by Sir William Crookers) shielded with black cardboard produced a fluorescent glow or ray after an electrical charge was passed through the tube. Roentgen eventually concluded that a new type of ray had been produced in the cathode ray tube that could be defined based on the distance it could travel. This new ray was given the designation X, the scientific symbol for the unknown. In 1901, Roentgen was awarded the first Nobel Prize in Physics for this discovery.

During the same historical time frame, Antoine Henri Becquerel was in France studying the chemical properties of naturally occurring elements. He is credited with discovering radioactivity in uranium. The Curies, Pierre and Marie, further advanced Becquerel's work because Marie Curie wanted to further understand the origin of this new energy source. The Curies would eventually discover polonium and radium. For the next 35 years, Madame Curie would concentrate her efforts on the investigation of radium and radioactivity, until her death from aplastic anemia in 1934.[2]

In the early 1900s, many radiobiological experiments were conducted in parallel with the development of radiation therapy. One of the most well-

Table 12-1 History of Radiation

460 B.C.	Democritus proposed that atoms were the building blocks of all materials
1600–1700s	Sir Isaac Newton and Benjamin Franklin produce developments that lead to the discovery of electricity
1800s	Sir William Crookes develops the vacuum tube and cathode ray
1895	Wilhelm Conrad Roentgen discovers the x-ray
1896	Antoine Henri Becquerel discovers that uranium is naturally radioactive
1897	Professor Freund uses x-rays to make a hairy mole disappear
1898	Marie and Pierre Curie discover polonium and radium
Early 1900s	Law of Bergonié and Tribondeau established X-rays are used therapeutically for benign and malignant diseases
1920–1940s	Deep-therapy x-ray machines are developed Atomic bomb developed during World War II Marie Curie dies of aplastic anemia in 1934
1950s	Cobalt therapy units become available and first-generation linear accelerators are developed Combined modality therapy is used
1970s	The term *radiation oncology* is employed to describe the scientific as well as the therapeutic discipline
1980s–early 1990s	Various treatment methods are studied in clinical trials (hyperthermia, intraoperative and radiolabeled antibodies) Research is conducted with radiosensitizers and radioprotectors Basic radiation metric terminology changes: gray (Gy) replaces rad
1990s	Development of multileaf collimation (MLC) and intensity-modulated radiation therapy (IMRT) FDA approves the first radioprotective agent — amifostine

known results of the experiments was the law of Bergonié and Triboneau, which states that radiosensitivity is highest in tissues with the highest mitotic index and lowest in well-differentiated tissues.[3]

Between 1920 and 1940, a series of experiments led to what we know today as fractionation. The development of x-ray mechanisms to treat deep tumors was under way, and brachytherapy was being performed with radium. With technological advances, the atomic bomb was developed during World War II and deployed on Hiroshima and Nagasaki, leading to radiobiological research for decades to follow.

In the 1950s, cobalt therapy machines became a standard for treatment and the first linear accelerators were developed. The role of combined modality treatment was pursued in clinical trials.

In the most recent decades, both technological and scientific advances related to radiation have occurred. The development of computers for treatment planning and optimizing dose permitted the emergence of three-dimensional (3-D) and 3-D conformal radiation therapy (3-DCRT) treatment planning. In the 1990s, intensity-modulated radiation therapy (IMRT) and multileaf collimation (MLC) were developed to assist in minimizing treatment-related toxicity. Hyperthermia, intraoperative radiation, brachytherapy, and stereotactic radiosurgery have undergone many refinements and are currently the focus of many clinical trials.

The radiation oncology team is a specialized group of healthcare providers who work collaboratively to meet patient care needs. A better understanding of radiobiology principles and the role of combined modality treatment have provided important information about both acute and late toxicities of treatment. Ongoing research continues to assess treatment techniques, combined modality treatment, the role of radiosensitizers and radioprotectors, and the effects of hypoxia on overall survival. The years ahead will support ongoing investigation into maximizing treatment dose without compromising quality of life.

Goals of Treatment Approaches

Radiation therapy plays a major role in the treatment of patients diagnosed with cancer. Approximately 60% of cancer patients will receive radiation at some point in their disease trajectory, either to cure, control, or palliate the disease.[1] If the tumor is diagnosed at an early stage, cure is possible. Patients undergoing a curative course of radiation therapy often face vigorous and lengthy treatment. In such cases, the total dose of radiation may be higher and the toxicities of treatment may be more severe. Chemotherapy may also be used to increase the therapeutic index. Patients with early-stage Hodgkin's disease, skin cancer, and carcinoma of the cervix are often treated with radiation alone.

For certain types of cancer and those in later stages, cure or eradication is not possible. In such cases, control of the cancer with radiation therapy for periods ranging from months to years may be the goal. Recurrent breast cancer, some soft-tissue sarcomas, and lung cancer are examples of cancers controlled by radiation therapy in combination with surgery or chemotherapy.

Palliation may be another goal of radiation therapy. Relief of pain, prevention of pathological fractures, and return of mobility can be achieved with radiation to metastatic bone lesions from primary sites such as breast, lung, and prostate. Pain relief often is dramatic, and it is not uncommon for one individual to receive multiple palliative courses to different bony structures over the course of several years. Radiation therapy contributes significantly to improved quality of life for the person with bone metastases. Palliative radiation therapy also is given for the relief of central nervous system (CNS) symptoms caused by brain metastasis or spinal cord compression. Hemorrhage, obstruction, ulceration, and fungating lesions can be effectively reduced — and in some instances eliminated — by palliative radiation therapy.

"Anticipatory" palliation is an application of radiation therapy that seeks to treat potentially symptomatic lesions before they become problematic. Examples of anticipatory palliation include treatment of a mediastinal mass that threatens to produce a superior vena cava syndrome and treatment of a vertebral lesion when spinal cord compression is impending. Prophylactic treatment may be used in patients with small cell lung cancer (SCLC) who receive whole-brain irradiation to minimize their risk of developing brain metastases.

Although treatment techniques and equipment may vary, the fundamental principles of radiobiology and radiation physics form the basis on which a course of treatment is selected and designed for each patient. Understanding these principles enables the oncology nurse to support and care for the patient receiving radiation therapy — attending to the emotional and physical needs that result from the disease and the therapy.

Applied Radiation Physics

The use of ionizing radiation in the treatment of cancer is based on the ability of radiation to interact with

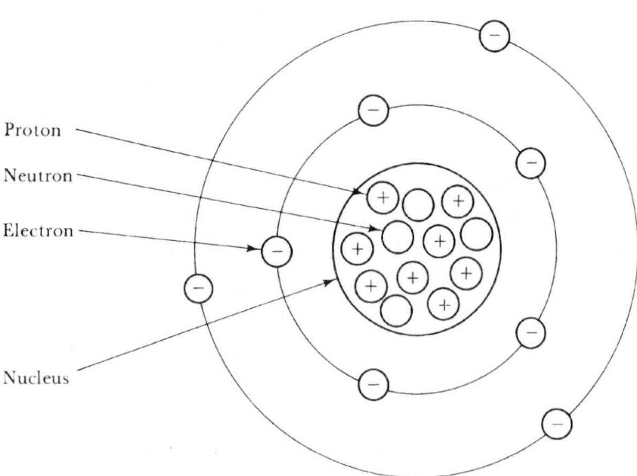

Figure 12-1 Basic structure of an atom. Protons, which are positively charged, and neutrons, which have no electrical charge, are the major components of the nucleus of an atom. The number of protons is equal to the number of negatively charged electrons orbiting the nucleus. Atoms of any given element may have different numbers of neutrons in the nucleus, thus giving atoms of the same element different atomic weights. An atom of a given element that differs only in its atomic weight is called an isotope.

the atoms and molecules of the tumor cells to produce specific harmful biological effects. Ionization affects either the molecules of the cell or the cell environment.

An understanding of atomic structure is essential to understanding the ionizing effects of radiation. The atom — the basic unit of molecular structure — has two parts: (1) the nucleus, containing positively charged protons and neutrons that have mass but no charge, and (2) the shells (orbits), containing negatively charged electrons (equivalent to the number of protons). Each shell can accommodate only a certain number of electrons; if this number is exceeded, a second or third shell is established more distant from the nucleus (Figure 12-1). The negatively charged electrons orbit the nucleus and are held in place by the attractive force of the positive protons in the nucleus; thus, a stable state is maintained. Certain atoms are known to be unstable, however; during the process of their decay or breakdown into a more stable state, alpha, beta, or gamma rays may be emitted. Radium, radon, and uranium are examples of unstable atoms that produce ionizing radiation.

Stable atoms also may be made to produce ionizing radiation through excitation, ionization, and nuclear disintegration. Radiation produced by these processes can be classified as electromagnetic radiation or particulate radiation. The electromagnetic spectrum can be further divided into five levels of decreasing wavelength: (1) radio waves, (2) infrared radiation, (3) visible light, (4) ultraviolet radiation, and (5) ionizing radiation.

Ionizing radiation has the shortest wavelength and the greatest energy of the electromagnetic spectrum and, therefore, is the form of energy used in radiation therapy. A classification system for ionizing radiation is shown in Figure 12-2. As seen in the figure, the terms *x-ray* and *gamma ray* both describe ionizing electromagnetic radiation. These forms differ only in their means of production. That is, x-rays are produced by specially designed equipment, and gamma rays are emitted by radioactive materials such as ^{60}Co undergoing nuclear transition. Both x-rays and gamma rays have no mass; rather, they are packets of available energy ready to be released on collision with a substance. Because they have no mass, x-rays and gamma rays can penetrate more deeply into tissue before releasing their energy. This process, which is commonly referred to as *photon* irradiation, is used to treat deep-seated tumors such as those located in the thoracic, abdominal, or pelvic areas. Photons are skin sparing, so skin toxicity is minimal.

Particulate radiation, by contrast, is composed of alpha and beta particles, as well as electrons and neutrons, which have mass. The relatively large size of alpha particles allows them to penetrate only a short distance into tissue before collision and energy release take place. Beta particles, which are smaller than alpha particles, penetrate more deeply but, because of their mass, do not have the ability to reach as deeply into tissues as do x-rays and gamma rays. The significance of these variations in ability to penetrate tissue will become obvious when treatment beams and equipment are discussed in Chapter 13.

X-rays are produced when a stream of fast-moving electrons, accelerated by the application of high voltage (between the filament and the target), strikes the target, and the electrons give up their energy. This radiation loss occurs because the electron is attracted to and slowed down by the nucleus of the tungsten (target) atom. Figure 12-3 illustrates the basic structure of an x-ray tube.

In addition to x-rays, some treatment machines (betatron, linear accelerator) are equipped to produce particle irradiation in the form of electrons. Electrons are small negatively charged particles produced in an x-ray tube by bypassing one of the steps used to produce x-rays. That is, electrons from the heated tungsten filament are injected into the vacuum tube and accelerated at a high velocity; they then emerge from a window in the vacuum tube, bypassing the tungsten target and emerging as electron particles. Electrons are used to treat surface lesions and sites located a few centimeters below the skin. They may also be used at the end of treatment in what is commonly

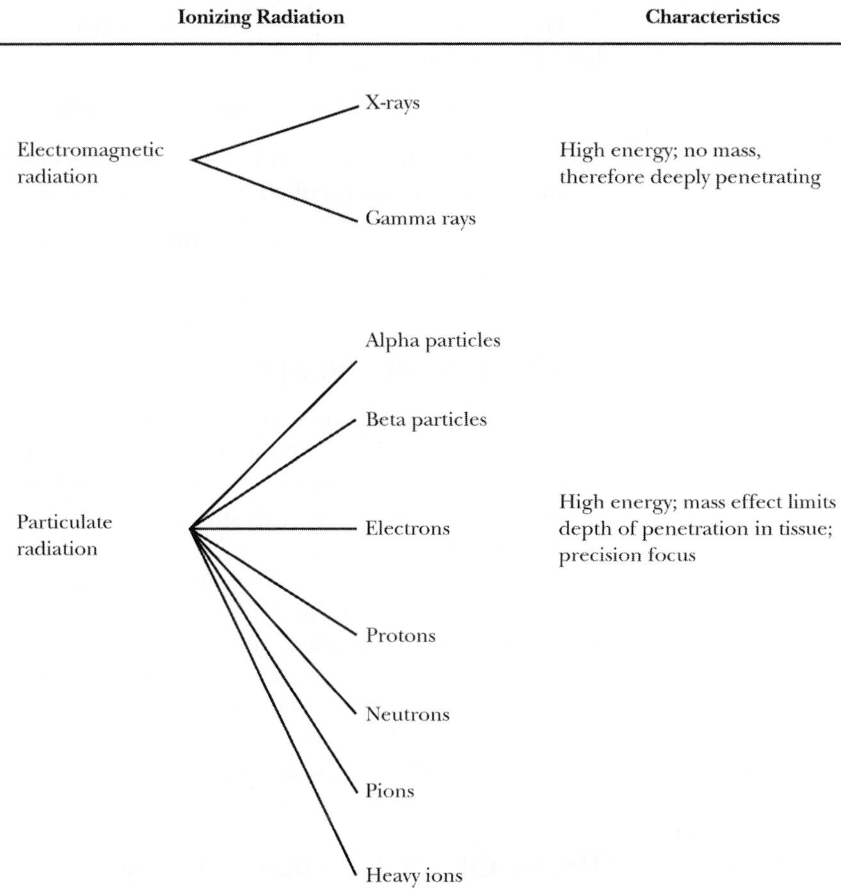

Figure 12-2 Characteristics of ionizing radiations.

referred to as a *boost*. A boost may be administered after a course of photons has been given to treat a surgical area where the tumor was excised in an effort to reduce the risk of local recurrence.

Electromagnetic and particulate radiations also are produced through the process of decay of radioactive elements and radioactive isotopes. This process, which produces radiation in the form of alpha, beta, or gamma rays, takes place as follows:

$$\text{atom} \xrightarrow{\text{radioactive decay}} \text{atom } y + \text{radiation}$$

The time required for half of the radioactive atoms present at any time to decay is known as the *half-life* of that radioactive element or isotope.

Because most radioisotopes are produced by neutron bombardment of stable elements (^{60}Co, ^{32}P, ^{182}Ta, ^{198}Au) or by nuclear fission of uranium in a nuclear reactor (^{90}Sr, ^{137}Cs), they are referred to as *artificial isotopes* to distinguish them from naturally occurring radioisotopes such as ^{226}Ra and ^{222}Rn. Radioactive isotopes are listed in Table 12-2.

High Linear Energy Transfer and Charged Particle Radiation Therapy

One important physical property of ionizing radiation is linear energy transfer (LET). *Linear energy transfer* describes the rate at which energy is deposited as radiation travels through matter on a given track. Electromagnetic radiation has no mass or charge and, therefore, is sparsely ionizing as it penetrates matter. X-rays, gamma rays, and electrons are electromagnetic and low-LET sources.

By contrast, the number of ionizing events produced by molecules of high-LET radiation is significant because of their considerable mass and charge. High-LET radiation, which includes neutron beams, heavy ions, and negative pi-mesons (pions), loses energy rapidly as it passes through matter. Multiple ionizing events occur in a relatively short distance with this type of radiation. Few high-LET radiation facilities exist, but two such centers operate at Loma Linda, California, and at the Massachusetts General Hospital in Boston. Years of research have shown that this form of therapy offers distinct advantages, yet the cost of the facilities and the technological sophistication needed for their operation have meant that they function pri-

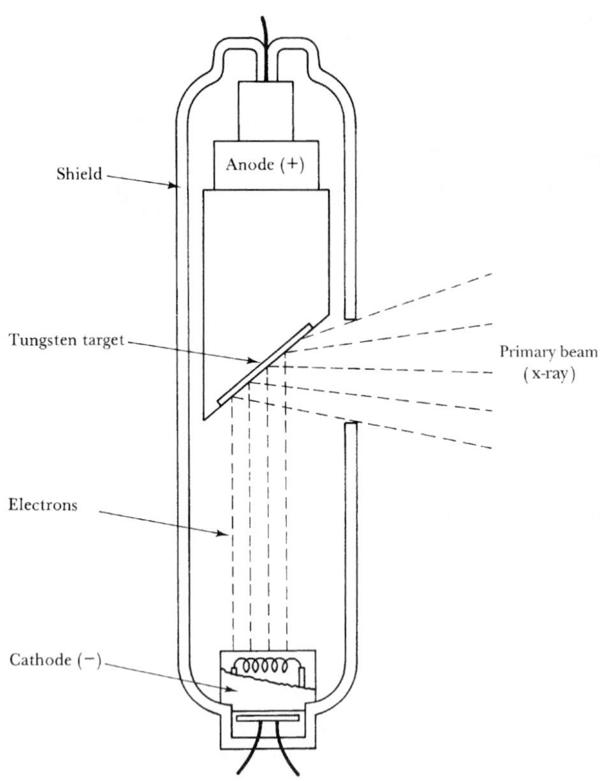

Figure 12-3 Basic structure of an x-ray tube. Electrons emitted from a heated tungsten filament are accelerated across a high-voltage source. These high-speed electrons strike a positively charged tungsten target, producing x-rays. The primary beam of radiation produced penetrates tissues. The greater the voltage, the greater the penetrating power of the beam.

marily as referral centers to treat salivary gland and prostate tumors.

High-LET radiation has several advantages over low-LET radiation:

- Greater relative biological effectiveness (RBE)
- Reduced relative radioresistance of hypoxic cells in tumors (low oxygen enhancement ratio [OER])
- Less intertreatment recovery of tumor cells in fractionated dosage

Neutron Beam Therapy

Fast neutrons are produced by a *cyclotron,* equipment in which high-energy neutrons bombard targets consisting of either beryllium or tritium. Neutrons have a lower OER, so the cancer cells do not need to be as well oxygenated to be damaged. Neutrons tend to be associated with less repair of both sublethal and potentially lethal damage to cells and with smaller variations in radiosensitivity according to the phase of the cell cycle.[3] Neutron therapy is less expensive than other high-LET energy producers; however, technological problems and the low dose rate (5–6 cGy/minute) are among the disadvantages of this form of therapy.

Heavy Charged Particle Therapy

Heavy ions, such as protons, helium ions, and nitrogen ions, are mainly useful for treating small tumors, because the dose distribution is best for treating a small volume. As the tumor size increases, treatment volume and OER also increase. Particle beams have an inverse dose profile compared to photons: The dose increases

Table 12-2 Radioactive Isotopes Used in Radiation Therapy

			Emissions		
Isotope	Symbol	Half-Life	Alpha	Beta	Gamma
Cesium	^{137}Cs	30 years			X
Cobalt	^{60}Co	5.3 years		X	X
Gold	^{198}Au	2.69 days		X	X
Iodine	^{125}I	60 days		X	X
Iodine	^{131}I	8.0 days		X	X
Iridium	^{192}Ir	74.5 days		X	X
Palladium	^{103}Pd	17 days			X
Phosphorus	^{32}P	14.3 days		X	
Radium	^{226}Ra	1622 days	X	X	X
Radon	^{222}Rn	3.83 days	X	X	X
Samarium	^{153}Sm	1.93 days		X	X
Strontium	^{89}S	50.5 days		X	
Strontium	^{90}S	28 years		X	
Tantalum	^{182}Ta	118 days		X	X
Yttrium	^{90}Y	64 hours		X	

with penetration depth, ranging from a low dose in the entrance to a sharp maximum dose at the end of the particle range.[4]

Negative Pi-meson Therapy

Negative pi-mesons (pions) are small, negatively charged particles found in the nuclei of atoms that "cement" protons and neutrons together. Pions are produced when protons are accelerated at approximately 131,000 miles/second before striking a carbon target. The pions are then collected by a system of magnets, and the beam of high-LET energy is directed at the target tissue. The first application of this form of treatment for humans took place at the Los Alamos Meson Physics Facility in Los Alamos, New Mexico, in 1974. The advantage of pion therapy, like other forms of high-LET radiation, is that the beam can be shaped to fit the tumor precisely, thereby minimizing the amount of radiation administered to surrounding normal structures. Pions can be aimed and stopped at a specific target site by adjusting the momentum of the particles.

At Los Alamos, a number of tumor sites and histologies were treated with good local cure rates and minimal morbidity, particularly in cancers of the head and neck, lung, bladder, cervix, and prostate gland. Tumors of the large bowel, pancreas, and brain did not respond equally well. The Los Alamos program was terminated in 1981, because overall results were not impressive and costs were prohibitive.

A second pion facility opened in 1979 in Vancouver, British Columbia, and a third opened in 1980 in Villigen, Switzerland. Approximately 500 patients were treated at Villigen, with a high incidence of long-term toxicities being noted. The severity of these late effects was attributed to the use of treatment volumes nearly three times those used by the Vancouver group. The program at Villigen was discontinued in 1993.

The Vancouver pion group completed two randomized trials in late 1995, comparing photon and pion irradiation as treatments for high-grade gliomas and advanced prostate cancers. The glioma study found no difference between the two treatment groups in terms of overall survival, time to recurrence, toxicity, and quality of life. Acute effects of pion therapy were increased over those seen with photon therapy; however, late toxicity was reduced in pion treatment.

Raju concludes that clinical results obtained with pions appear to be about equal to those achieved with photons for all sites investigated, except for the bladder.[5] Because of the cost and complexity of building and operating pion facilities, Raju also concludes that pion radiation will not likely be pursued in the future.

Radiobiology

The biological effects of radiation on humans are the result of a sequence of events that follows the absorption of energy from ionizing radiation and the organism's attempts to compensate for this assault. The effects of radiation take place at the cellular level, with consequences developing in the tissues, organs, and/or the entire body depending on the treatment site. Radiation's biological influences on these cells are mediated by a variety of biochemical, genetic, and kinetic factors. They are also affected by the dose, type, and rate at which radiation is given. The incidence and severity of these effects can be classified as acute and/or late depending on the tissue kinetics.

Cellular Response to Radiation

Target theory

Radiation effects at the cellular level may be either direct or indirect, according to the target theory. A direct hit occurs when any of the key molecules within the cell are damaged by energy that is directly deposited in the DNA or RNA. After high-dose radiation of DNA molecules in vitro, four types of damage are observed: (1) change or loss of a base (thymine, adenine, guanine, or cytosine); (2) breakage of the hydrogen bond between the two chains of the DNA molecule; (3) breaks in one or both chains of the DNA molecule; and (4) cross-linking of the chains after breakage. Such unrepaired breaks or alterations in a base lead to mutations that result in impaired cellular function or cell death.

An indirect hit, according to target theory, occurs when ionization takes place in the medium (mostly water) surrounding the molecular structures within the cell. Radiation absorbed by the water molecules results in the formation of a free radical when an electron is literally knocked out of orbit surrounding the ion. The free radicals produced in this way may trigger a variety of chemical reactions, producing new compounds that are toxic to the cell. Figure 12-4 illustrates the ionizing effect of radiation on the water contained within a cell.

It generally is agreed that a direct hit (i.e., DNA damage and chromosomal aberrations) accounts for the most effective and lethal injury produced by ionizing radiation.[3] However, because of the relative ratio of water to DNA in a single cell, the probability of indirect damage through ionization of intracellular water is much greater than the probability of damage from a direct hit. Loss of the cell's reproductive capacity is considered to be the most biologically significant endpoint of radiation damage.[6]

The final products of the ionization of water molecules (HOH) by radiation are an ion pair (H^+, OH-) and free radicals ($H^\cdot$, $OH^\cdot$), which are capable of damaging the cell. The ionization of water is shown in the following steps:

$$HOH \xrightarrow{\text{radiation}} HOH^+ e^-$$

The free electron (e^-) is captured by another available water molecule and, as shown in the next step, forms the second ion:

$$HOH + e^- \rightarrow HOH^-$$

Because the two ions (HOH^+, HOH^-) produced by these reactions are unstable, rapid breakdown occurs (in the presence of other, normal water molecules), forming yet another ion and a free radical:

$$HOH^+ \rightarrow H^\cdot + OH^\cdot$$
$$HOH^- \rightarrow OH^- + H^\cdot$$

Although the resulting pair of ions (H^+, OH^-) have some potential for cellular damage through chemical reactions, they are more likely to recombine and form water (HOH). The free radicals ($H^\cdot$, $OH^\cdot$) are extremely reactive, and they too may simply recombine to form water. However, free radicals appear to be more likely to undergo chemical interactions with other free radicals, forming cytotoxic agents, as shown in this reactions:

$$OH^\cdot + OH^\cdot \rightarrow H_2O_2 \text{ (hydrogen peroxide)}$$

Free radicals that result from the interaction of radiation with water are capable of triggering a variety of chemical reactions within the cell and are therefore believed to be a major factor in the production of damage in the cell.

Figure 12-4 The effect of ionizing radiation on water molecules.

In addition to the damage produced by a direct or indirect hit (Table 12-3),[7] experimental evidence shows that radiation can cause damage to proteins, carbohydrates, and enzymes within the cell. Damage to these additional molecules, as well as alterations in the permeability of the cell membrane, may contribute to the ultimate effect of radiation at the cellular level.

Cell cycle and radiosensitivity

According to Hall and Cox, radiosensitivity appears to be maximized during the M and G_2 phases of the cell cycle.[3] Thus, the maximum effect from radiation should occur just before and during actual cell division. In early research, Bergonie and Tribondeau suggested that the sensitivity of cells to irradiation is directly proportional to their reproductive activity and inversely proportional to their degree of differentiation.[8] A differentiated cell is one that is morphologically or functionally specialized (such as an erythrocyte) and does not undergo mitosis. An undifferentiated cell (such as a red blood cell, stem cell, or erythroblast) has few specialized morphological or functional characteristics, and its primary purpose is to divide and provide new cells to maintain its own population. Because the effect of radiation is known to be greatest during mitosis, undifferentiated cell populations generally are most sensitive to radiation. In contrast, well-differentiated cells are relatively radioresistant.

Changes in mitotic activity due to radiation can be classified as either delayed onset or complete inhibition. *Delayed onset of mitosis* indicates that although damage occurred at some point during prophase, repair was accomplished and division occurred. *Complete inhibition of mitosis,* or cell sterilization, renders the cell incapable of division, although it may continue to live in a nonreproducing state.

Cell death

According to McBride and Withers there are four types of cell death: (1) mitotic (or genetic), (2) interphase, (3) apoptotic, and (4) necrotic.[9] *Mitotic death* occurs after one or more cell divisions and usually with much smaller radiation doses than those required to produce interphase death. *Interphase death* occurs within four to six hours after irradiation, even with low doses of radiation. Affected cells can no longer contribute to the reproductive pool. *Apoptotic death* requires active metabolic processes and neighboring cells to phagocytose the cell remnants, with the entire process unfolding in just a few hours. *Necrotic death* involves the loss of membrane integrity, an increase in cell size, the release of lyposomal enzymes, and the generation of an inflammation response. This type of cell death may also represent a pathological response to vascular damage as well as a default pathway for cells that lack an effective apoptotic apparatus.

Contributing biological factors

A number of additional factors directly affect the biological response to radiation and, ultimately, the treatment outcome. Among these are the oxygen ef-

Table 12-3 Biologic Effects When Cells Are Exposed to Radiation

Single-strand DNA damage that can be accurately repaired
Single-strand DNA damage that is incorrectly repaired, leading to mutations
Double-strand DNA damage, which usually cannot be repaired
Delay in mitosis to allow repair of DNA, if possible
Apoptosis (programmed cell death) if the DNA damage is severe and not repaired
Cell division and repopulation with some of the cells containing mutations

Reproduced with permission from Dunne-Daly C: Principles of radiotherapy and radiobiology. *Semin Oncol Nurs,* 15:250–259, 1999.[7]

fect, LET, relative biological effectiveness, dose rate, radiosensitivity, and fractionation.

Oxygen effect. Well-oxygenated tumors show a much greater response to radiation; that is, they are more radiosensitive than poorly oxygenated tumors. Extensive laboratory and clinical research has shown that the existence of oxygen tension from 20 to 40 mm Hg at the time of radiation greatly enhances the radiosensitivity of the cells.[3,10] One theory suggests that the mechanism of the oxygen effect is related to the ability of oxygen to combine with the free radicals formed during ionization, thereby producing new and toxic combinations. A second theory holds that the presence of oxygen at the time of irradiation prevents the reversal (and thus the repair) of some of the chemical changes that occur as the result of ionization. The clinical significance of the *oxygen effect* is that oxygen modifies the dose of radiation needed to produce a given degree of biological damage. The magnitude of the oxygen effect is expressed as the oxygen enhancement ratio (OER). The OER is the ratio of radiation dose in the absence of oxygen (or hypoxia) to the radiation dose in the presence of oxygen required for the same biological effect. Cells that are hypoxic are considered to be radioresistant and therefore limit the effectiveness of radiation therapy. Studies in head and neck and cervical cancer have demonstrated poorer survival outcomes in patients with hypoxic tumors.[11,12] It has also been noted that patients with hypoxic tumors are more likely to be anemic.[13] The use of blood transfusions and erythropoietin continues to be evaluated.

Linear energy transfer. *Linear energy transfer* describes the rate at which energy is lost from different types of radiation while traveling through matter. Low-LET radiations (x-rays and gamma rays) are sparsely ionizing, having a random pathway that results in few direct hits within the cell nucleus. Radiation of higher LET (alpha particles, neutrons, and negative pions) has a greater probability of interacting with matter and producing more direct hits within the cell.

Relative biological effectiveness. Because different radiations have varying rates of energy loss, the biological responses of these treatments likewise will be different. Therefore, RBE is used to compare a dose of test radiation with a dose of standard radiation that produces the same biological response. The following formula is used to express RBE:

$$RBE = \frac{\text{Dose of reference radiation to produce a given biological effect}}{\text{Dose of test radiation to produce the same biological effect}}$$

Dose rate. *Dose rate* refers to the rate at which a given dose is delivered by a treatment machine or equipment. Dose rate becomes particularly significant when a course of therapy is fractionated over many days and weeks, as it is in standard external beam teletherapy. Studies have shown low dose rates to be much less effective in producing lethal cell damage than high dose rates, primarily because low dose rates permit cell repair to occur before the lethal dose has been reached in fractionated teletherapy.

Radiosensitivity. According to Bergonie and Tribondeau, ionizing radiation is most effective on cells that are undifferentiated and undergoing active mitosis.[8] Laboratory and clinical experience has shown this relationship to hold true in most tissues.

Fractionation. Fractionation is the treatment approach that takes the total dose of radiation and divides it into equal fractions, recognizing that the dose may need to be higher due to the plan of delivering multiple fractions. A single dose of radiation has more of a biological effect than the same dose divided or fractionated, but that single dose will not be able to spare normal tissues and also eradicate the tumor. Hyperfractionation uses smaller doses per fraction and treatment is given twice a day, separated by a minimum of six hours.

The four R's of radiobiology

The four R's of radiobiology (repair, redistribution, repopulation, and reoxygenation) explain the biological and chemical effects of fractionation on tumors and normal tissues.

Repair. Repair of intracellular sublethal damage by normal cells between daily-dose fractions is one benefit of fractionation. The goal of fractionation is to deliver a dose sufficient to prevent tumor cells from being repaired while allowing normal cells to recover before the next dose is given. Although some tumor cells may be repaired between daily doses, they also may reoxygenate, rendering them more radiosensitive when the next dose is administered. Thus, although some degree of repair of tumor cells may occur between fractionated doses, repeated daily doses ultimately would lead to tumor control.

Redistribution. Redistribution of cell age (within the cell cycle) as a result of daily radiation is advantageous because more tumor cells are made radiosensitive. Theoretically, with succeeding daily doses of radiation, increasingly more tumor cells would be delayed in the cycle and reach the mitotic phase as the next dose is given, thereby increasing the cell kill.

Repopulation. Repopulation of normal tissues takes place through cell division at some time during a multifraction treatment course. Fractionation of dose allows this repopulation to occur in normal tissues, sparing them from some of the late consequences that might arise if repopulation (new growth) was inhibited. Those tumor cells that succeed in dividing while undergoing a fractionated course of radiation therapy are usually incapable of surviving because of the radiation effect. Thus, fractionation favors normal tissue while eradicating tumor.

Reoxygenation. Reoxygenation is the fourth consideration favoring fractionation of the radiation dose. Whereas normal tissues usually are well oxygenated, tumors characteristically range from normal to hypoxic to anoxic. As discussed earlier, radiosensitivity is closely related to oxygen tension in the tumor cell; hypoxic or anoxic cells generally are radioresistant, whereas oxygenated cells are radiosensitive. Fractionating the dose allows the cells to become oxygenated as the tumor shrinks.

Tissue and organ response to radiation reflects the sensitivity of the affected cellular components. Both tissues and organs are composed of more than one cell type, with each category of cells having a different degree of radiosensitivity. Another factor that determines tissue response is related to the parenchymal versus stromal substances found in that tissue. The parenchyma is composed of cells characteristic of the tissue or organ. If those cells are radiosensitive (e.g., the testis), then ionizing radiation has its greatest effect on the parenchyma. Conversely, if parenchymal tissue is relatively radioresistant (e.g., the spinal cord), then radiation response in that organ is due to the indirect effects on the stromal components (especially the vasculature) that support the parenchyma. Table 12-4 lists various organs according to their degree of radiosensitivity as measured by parenchymal hypoplasia.

Table 12-4 Degree of Radiosensitivity of Various Organs Based on Parenchymal Hypoplasia

Organ	Radiosensitivity
Lymphoid organs, bone marrow, blood, testes, ovaries, intestines	High
Skin, cornea, oral cavity, esophagus, rectum, bladder, vagina, cervix, ureters	Fairly high
Optic lens, stomach, growing cartilage, fine vasculature, growing bone	Medium
Mature cartilage or bone, salivary glands, respiratory organs, kidneys, liver, pancreas, thyroid, adrenals, pituitary gland	Fairly low
Muscle, brain, spinal cord	Low

Apoptosis. A major focus of research in radiobiology is currently directed toward the study of various mechanisms regulating apoptosis. *Apoptosis,* or programmed cell death, occurs in both normal and malignant cells in a process that is distinct from cellular death due to hypoxia. Failure of the normal apoptotic process results in survival and uncontrolled proliferation of malignant cells.

As described earlier, repair of radiation injury (sublethal damage repair) takes place in healthy tissues but may also occur in the targeted malignancy, thereby reducing radioresponsiveness and diminishing the likelihood of cure. Ionization and direct damage to DNA account for the death during mitosis of most irradiated cells. It has been demonstrated that the process of apoptosis is also accelerated by radiation, particularly in lymphocytes, small bowel crypt cells, salivary gland cells, and germ cells.[14]

The role of certain genetic, molecular, and biochemical substances (*p53, pRb, BCL-2*), basic fibroblast growth factors (bFGF), and protein kinase C (PKC) inhibitors, among others, at the time of irradiation is thought to be significant in radiation-induced apoptosis.[14,15] The presence or absence of these substances and many others could enhance radioresponsiveness in various cell lines. Intensive research to identify the pathways that ultimately lead to apoptosis is under way. Manipulating these pathways may hold the key to increasing the therapeutic benefit ratio in radiation oncology.[16]

Radiobiology of Brachytherapy

The basic radiobiologic mechanism of cell kill in brachytherapy and teletherapy is the same, as the principles described previously as the four R's of radiobiology (i.e., repair, redistribution, repopulation, reoxygenation) apply to both forms of radiation delivery. However, the temporal and spatial principles of physics are what account for the effectiveness of both brachytherapy and teletherapy.[17] Standard brachytherapy delivers continuous radiation at a low dose rate over a period of several days. Standard teletherapy delivers low dose rate radiation in higher doses, given in daily fractions over a number of weeks.

Brachytherapy entails the use of implanted or injected radioactive sources, which capitalize on the effects of continuous rather than fractionated irradiation. These differences in effect occur when the dose rate is less than 5 cGy per minute.

Low dose rate brachytherapy

Low dose rate (LDR) brachytherapy, commonly used for gynecologic and head and neck cancers, delivers a continuous dose of radiation for as long as the source remains in place within the patient. This approach stands in contrast to the intermittent dosing that takes place when treating with fractionated external-beam teletherapy. Following doses of fractionated teletherapy, cellular sublethal damage repair (SLD-R) occurs within one to four hours following treatment, producing the initial portion of the cell-survival curve referred to as the *shoulder*. Recall that cells are most radiosensitive during the M and G_2 phases of the cell cycle. LDR brachytherapy increases the effectiveness of radiation by redistributing an even greater proportion of cells into the G_2 phase as compared with fractionated treatment. Irradiated cells that manage to divide are blocked in the G_2 phase by continuous LDR brachytherapy.

Hypoxia in a tumor being treated with LDR brachytherapy is a less significant negative factor than it is in teletherapy. Low dose rates reduce the OER, and SLD-R is inhibited under prolonged hypoxic conditions. Thus LDR brachytherapy enhances radiation effect by taking advantage of repair, redistribution, and repopulation principles even in poorly oxygenated tissue.

High dose rate brachytherapy

High dose rate (HDR) brachytherapy is the newest delivery method for brachytherapy. HDR sources deliver more than 1200 cGy of radiation per hour, administered as single, repeated fractions rather than continuously as in LDR treatments. The equipment used for this treatment modality is highly sophisticated, with computer optimization of dose distribution and sparing of normal tissues. In addition to the advantages of outpatient treatment and reduced staff exposure to radioactivity, HDR brachytherapy has shown a lower complication rate in treatment of cervix cancer than LDR therapy, without any decrease in local control.[18]

Capitalizing on Radionuclides and Radioimmunotherapy

The development of radiopharmaceuticals dates back to the early discoveries by Becquerel and the Curies. Interest and research efforts in this area have accelerated in recent decades. Radioimuunotherapy has been studied with a variety of solid tumor and hematologic malignancies. Among the numerous radioactive isotopes that have been administered therapeutically, ^{131}I and ^{90}Y in particular have been adopted for use in radiolabeled antibody therapy.

Radioimmunotherapy involves the fusion of a radioisotope and a monoclonal antibody through direct labeling or incorporation of an appropriate chelating agent.[19] These agents are typically administered via intravenous injection, but can be given via the intrathecal, intralesional, intraarterial, or intraperitoneal route. Because radionucleotides have short half-lives, radioimmunotherapy avoids prolonged radiation exposure to healthy cells while delivering lethal or sublethal doses to the tumor. Depending on the biologic properties of the given antibody, cell kill may be based on apoptosis, antibody-dependent cellular cytotoxicity (ADCC), complement dependent cytotoxicity (CDC), or a combination of the actions.[19] Among numerous phase 1, 2, and 3 clinical trials over the past three decades, some of the more significant results have been achieved in the treatment of thyroid cancer and hematologic malignancies, particularly B-cell malignancies.[19]

A major problem in delivering the intended dose of radiation to the target site is the fact that the radiolabeled antibody is rapidly cleared from the target organ by the normal blood flow, thus limiting the time of contact with the tumor target. A new delivery method has been developed and patented (U.S. Patent No. 5,424,288) that uses macroaggragated proteins injected directly into the organ site to block the rapid clearance of the radioactive substance.[20,21] This procedure, called *infusional brachytherapy,* is being employed to treat a number of advanced cancers, with the most extensive application in pancreatic adenocarcinoma.[21] Phase II multicenter trials have been initiated in the United States and in Europe, using macroaggragated albumin (MAA) as the blocking agent and P32 (chromic phosphate) as the radioactive source for treatment of pancreatic cancer.[20,21]

Iodine-131 has historically been used in the treatment of neuroendocrine tumors and is referred to as MIBG (meta-iodebenzylguanine). This isotope emits both beta and gamma rays, so patients who receive this agent are admitted to the hospital and placed on radiation precautions. Once their dose is 33 millicuries or less, they may be discharged. Iodine-131 tositumomab is a conjugated monoclonal antibody attached to the radioisotope ^{131}I. This unique compound targets a protein, the CD-20 antigen, found on the surface of malignant B cells in non-Hodgkin's lymphoma (NHL).[22] Clinical trials have demonstrated positive results in NHL patients.[23,24]

Yttrium ibritumomab tiuxetan is another radiolabeled monoclonal antibody. This beta-emitting source requires fewer precautions than ^{131}I, which emits both beta and gamma radiation. Trials of yttrium-90 have been conducted in patients with relapsed or refractory low-grade or follicular B-cell lymphoma and have shown positive results.[25,26]

Radioimmunotherapy continues to demonstrate efficacy in cancer treatment. Radioimmunotherapy agents may be administered in nuclear medicine or radiation oncology areas depending on the practice setting. In addition to the care provided by oncologists and oncology nurses, radioimmunotherapy administration requires the services of nuclear medicine physicians and technologists or radiation oncologists, radiopharmacists, and radiation safety officers.[26]

Chemical and Thermal Modifiers of Radiation

Radiosensitizers and Radioprotectors

The goal of radiation therapy is to achieve maximum tumor cell kill while minimizing injury to normal tissues (therapeutic ratio). Local tumor failure is the cause of 40% to 60% of cancer deaths and may occur in 60% to 80% of cancer patients at the time of death.[27] Efforts to improve the therapeutic ratio have resulted in the development of certain compounds that act to increase the radiosensitivity of tumor cells or to protect normal cells from the effects of radiation. Combined modality therapy, using both radiation and certain chemotherapeutic agents, also takes advantage of enhanced tumor cell kill. *Chemical modifiers* represent a broad class of agents that include radiosensitizers, radioprotectors, and chemotherapy agents. When used independently, radiosensitizers provide an oxygen substitute to poorly vascularized areas of the tumor that is needed at the time of radiation for the desired effect to occur.

Radiosensitizers are compounds that apparently promote fixation of the free radicals produced by radiation damage at the molecular level. The mechanism of this action is similar to the oxygen effect described previously, in which biochemical reactions in the damaged molecules prevent repair of the cellular radiation damage. Free radicals (such as OH^+) are captured by the electron affinity of the radiosensitizers, rendering the molecules incapable of repair.

The four most-studied sensitizers are metronidazole (Flagyl), misonidazole (RO-07-0582), etanidazole (SR-2508), and nimorazole. These agents are classified as hypoxic cell sensitizers because they replace oxygen in the chemical reaction that follows irradiation. The two most biologically active radiosensitizing compounds first tested in phase 2 and 3 studies were metronidazole and misonidazole. Major side effects of these agents were noted to relate to neurotoxicity, including peripheral neuropathies, somnolence, confusion, and transient coma. Nausea and vomiting are also frequent side effects that seem to be dose related.

Early clinical trials using misonidazole as a radiosensitizer indicated some degree of effectiveness in treatment of squamous carcinoma of the head and neck and of the uterine cervix. Overall results were disappointing, due to the severe toxicity and only marginal improvement in tumor control.[28] Misonidazole is the only such substance to have undergone extensive clinical trial evaluation. It has been shown to increase the cytotoxicity of alkylating agents, nitrosoureas, 5-fluorouracil (5-FU), cyclophosphamide, and melphalan. Unfortunately, the side effects commonly experienced with these agents are apparently enhanced by the addition of misonidazole. This nonselective enhancement significantly detracts from the potential benefits to be gained.

Etanidazole has been tested, with encouraging results, in early phase II and III trials. This member of the nimorazole group of compounds appears to be less toxic to the CNS tissue than misonidazole and crosses the blood–brain barrier in limited quantity. A phase 3 study of this agent showed an increase survival in the two-year local control in N_0 and N_1 disease with 55% in the etanidazole arm and 37% in the radiation-alone arm.[29]

Nimorazole is a member of the same structural class as metronidazole but is less toxic, allowing for higher doses. A phase 3 study of nimorazole versus placebo in subjects with squamous cell cancer of the supraglottic larynx and pharynx demonstrated a statistically significant difference (49% versus 33%) in improvement of locoregional control at five years post-treatment.[30] In a phase 2 study of nimorazole in patients with stage 3 or 4 squamous cell carcinoma of the head and neck who received continuous hyperfractionated accelerated radiation therapy (CHART), it was found that local control rates were higher than in other studies using CHART, suggesting a positive effect of nimorazole.[31]

Nonhypoxic cell sensitizers include the halogenated pyrimidines, bromodeoxyuridine (BUdR), and iododeoxyuridine (IUdR). These agents are taken up by the DNA of rapidly dividing cells, but their mechanism of action is not completely understood. In a study by Epstein et al,[32] subjects received hyperfractionated radiation with IUdR for locally advanced head and neck cancer. These researchers found a high complete response rate, but hematological and mucosal toxicities were severe.

Hypoxic cell cytoxic agents include mitomycin-C and tirapazamine. Mitomycin-C is a bioreductive alkylating agent that has been studied in pancreatic and head and neck cancer. Tirapazamine is another bioreductive agent that is preferentially cytotoxic to hypoxic cells in vitro. It differs from oxygen-mimetic sensitizers in that it requires metabolic activation, and enhancement is seen when this agent is given prior to or after radiotherapy.[33] Studies in lung and head and neck cancer have shown positive results. Side effects include nausea, muscle cramps, and hematologic toxicities.[33,34]

Motexafin gadolinium, which is currently being studied in clinical trials, is the first in a class of pharmaceuticals known as texaphyrins to reach human testing. Texaphyrins accumulate inside cancer cells due to their high rate of metabolism and induce programmed cell death. A phase 1 study of patients who are receiving hyperfractionated irradiation and concurrent 5-FU/cisplatin for head and neck cancer reported interim results recently.[35] Nine of the ten evaluable patients demonstrated a complete tumor response, and eight of these remained in complete remission with a median follow-up of one year. Side effects reported include mucositis and radiation dermatitis. A randomized phase 3 trial is currently investigating the use of motexafin in patients with brain metastases who receive whole-body radiation therapy.[35,36]

The utility of radiosensitizers in radiation oncology has yet to be definitively determined. Past clinical trials have demonstrated minimal to zero patient benefit and reported toxicities that adversely affected quality of life. The role of radiosensitizers in cancer care is being evaluated today both in clinical trials and in the laboratory setting. Studies are also looking at the roles of gene therapy, biologics (e.g., cytokines, hormones, growth factors), and oxygen therapy and considering how they may work in sensitizing cells.[37]

Radioprotectors are compounds that can protect oxygenated (nontumor) cells while having a limited effect on hypoxic (tumor) cells. This selective action serves to increase the therapeutic ratio by promoting the repair of irradiated normal tissues. Repair or return to a nondamaged state takes place through the chemical process of reduction. Free electrons are captured by the radioprotective substance, rendering them unavailable to participate in further chemical reactions that might lead to cellular damage. This process can be viewed as the opposite of what occurs when radiosensitizers are used.

The sulfhydryl groups contained in the nonprotein fraction of most cells aid in the reduction process following radiation damage. Thiophosphate compounds (such as cysteine and cysteamine) containing sulfhydryl and aminopropyl groups were among the earliest radioprotectors synthesized.

Amifostine (WR-2721) is one of today's most widely studied radioprotectors. The U.S. Army initially developed this agent during the Cold War at Walter Reed Army Institute of Research. The project, which began in 1959, sought to identify an agent that could be used to protect military personnel in the event of nuclear warfare.[38] Amifostine selectively protects a broad range of normal tissues, including the oral mucosa, salivary glands, lungs, bone marrow, heart, intestines, and kidney. A phase 3 study of patients who received radiation therapy for head and neck cancer demonstrated that those who received 200 mg/m^2 of amifostine, IVP 15–30 minutes prior to radiation daily, had a statistically significant decrease in acute (p = <0.001) and late (p = <0.0012) grade ≥ 2 xerostomia. Patients also experienced a statistically significant improvement (p = 0.0001) in the time to onset of grade II xerostomia (30 days versus 45 days).[39] Amifostine may be administered intravenously or subcutaneously and should be dosed daily before radiation therapy. Side effects of this agent include nausea, vomiting, and hypotension. When administered subcutaneously, the side effects may decrease, but the risk of a local injection site reaction increases. Daily patient assessment, prompt intervention, and symptom management are essential in caring for these patients.[40] Amifostine was the first FDA-approved radioprotector. Clinical trials with patients receiving head and neck, thoracic, and pelvic radiation therapy are ongoing.

Keratinocyte growth factor (KGF) is a glycoprotein member of the fibroblast growth factor family and a potent stimulant of the proliferation of normal epithelial cells. Clinical trials have investigated its use in patients being treated for metastatic colorectal cancer and in the bone marrow transplant setting to reduce the incidence and/or severity of mucositis from chemotherapy and/or radiation therapy.[41,42] A randomized, double-blind, placebo-controlled study of 212 patients undergoing bone marrow transplant showed a significant reduction in mucositis. The study also found that patients required less use of narcotics and total parenteral nutrition.

Combined Modality Therapy

The role of combined modality therapy (CMT) using chemotherapy, biotherapy, surgery, and radiation in combination with one another or at alternating intervals has shown not only clinical benefit, but also improvements in disease-free survival, local regional control, and overall survival. The goal of CMT is to improve quality of life whether it is for cure, control, or palliation by maximizing tumor cell kill.

In 1999, the NCI announced the results of studies showing that patients who received platinum-based chemotherapy concurrently with daily radiation for cervical cancer had a 30%–50% increase in survival. These clinical trials changed the standard of care for women receiving treatment for cervical cancer.[43–45]

Other studies with chemotherapy and radiation have shown a survival advantage in patients with rectal, head and neck, and lung cancer.[46–48] Vigorous CMT may also allow for organ preservation in some cases.[49]

Chemotherapeutic agents used for their radiosensitizing effect include carboplatin, cisplatin, mitomycin C, navelbine, paclitaxel, docetaxel, and 5-fluorouracil. Other potential agents include methotrexate, doxorubicin, vinblastine, VP-16, actinomycin D, and bleomycin. Cisplatin and 5-FU are two of the most commonly used radiosensitizing agents. In CMT, both radiation and certain chemotherapy agents are able to provide a greater cell kill than either therapy could achieve alone. However, CMT has the potential to increase both acute and late toxicities—possibilities that need to be assessed, documented, and managed promptly. It is important to know whether the chemotherapy agent selected has overlapping or differing toxicities than what may be expected from the radiation. Organ systems at greatest risk for acute toxicity include the gastrointestinal, integumentary, and myeloproliferative system. Late effects will typically be experienced at the site of radiation treatment; for example, lung cancer patients may experience fibrosis and/or pneumonitis and rectal patients may experience proctitis.

One of the most challenging aspects of effectively combining chemotherapy with radiation is determining the optimal timing, sequencing, and dose of each agent/modality.[50] Agents may need to be given immediately before or after treatment. Many times surgery may be performed before or after chemotherapy and radiation. Induction or neoadjuvant chemotherapy is given prior to radiation and/or surgery to reduce the size of the tumor before radiation (smaller treatment field) or surgery (reduced amount of tissues removed) takes place. It may decrease the patient's risk of metastasis. Concurrent chemotherapy is given while the patient is undergoing radiation. It may include daily, weekly, or continuous infusion depending on the drug, dose, and known toxicities. Chemotherapy is used during this time to increase the cell kill and maximize the tumor response to radiation. Sequential therapy, often referred to as the sandwich technique, also falls under the rubric of concurrent therapy and has been used in clinical trials with lung and head and neck cancers. This approach employs a split course of radiation in which the patient is treated with chemotherapy during a planned break in the total course of radiation. Lastly, adjuvant chemotherapy can be given once a course of radiation is completed to control micrometastases and subclinical disease.

Radiation therapy may also be given preoperatively or postoperatively depending on the site of disease. Preoperative radiation assists in shrinking the tumor prior to surgery, allowing for less extensive resection and increased potential for organ preservation. The issues with this approach are that surgical staging is often affected because the tumor has shrunk and the patient may be at risk for healing problems at the radiated site. Postoperative radiation therapy is delivered to patients to reduce their risk of a local recurrence.

Combined modality therapy is used in the treatment of numerous cancers, including squamous cell cancer of the cervix, anus, head and neck, and lung. Cancers of the bladder, esophagus, pancreas, and stomach frequently are treated with both chemotherapy and radiation therapy in varying schedules. Vigorous CMT has enabled organ preservation for some individuals with carcinoma of the larynx, bladder, or anus.[51,52] Symptom management is critical in caring for these patients, because each treatment approach has a unique side-effect profile that may prove to be synergistic or exacerbate the side effects of other treatments.

Hyperthermia

The use of hyperthermia in conjunction with other types of cancer treatment continues to be studied in clinical trials. The first references to hyperthermia occurred in an Egyptian papyrus scroll 5000 years ago.[3] Current interest focuses on the use of heat with radiation and chemotherapy and the ongoing development of treatment applicators. When hyperthermia is added to radiation, absolute complete response rates increase 20% to 30%.[53] Hyperthermia has an additive and synergistic effect when radiation is delivered prior to treatment. Its mechanisms of action appear to be complementary to the effects of radiation with regard to inhibition of potentially lethal damage and sublethal damage repair, cell cycle sensitivity, and effects of hypoxia and nutrient deprivation.[53] Tumor tissues appear to be preferentially sensitized compared to normal tissue. Several biological effects support the rationale for why heat is more damaging to malignant tumors:[3,54–59]

- Heat is directly cytotoxic.
- Cells in the S phase are considered to be radioresistant and more sensitive to heat.
- The combined effects of radiation and hyperthermia produce greater cell kill than either treatment alone.
- Hypoxic cells that are typically radioresistant have been found to be thermosensitive.
- Cells that have a low pH and are metabolically deprived are more sensitive to heat. Note, however,

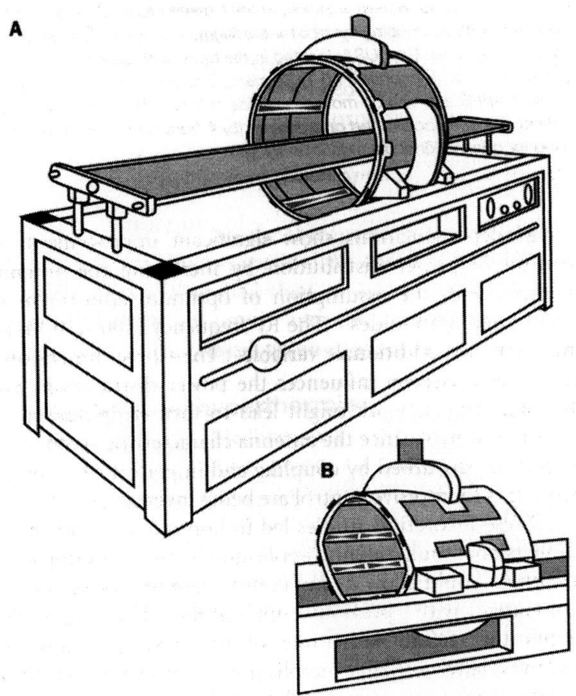

Figure 12-5 Two models of regional hyperthermia treatment devices used for large treatment areas and those tumors that are deep seated. **(A)** Using multiple antennae, widely spreads applicators distribute power-density and temperature. **(B)** Elliptical shape is more comfortable for the patient. Reprinted with permission from Wust P, Hildebrandt G, Sreenivasa G, et al: Hyperthermia in combined treatment of cancer. *Lancet Oncol* 3: 487–497, 2002.[59]

that cells can adapt to physical changes in 80–100 hours and lose their thermosensitivity.

- Heat inhibits the repair of radiation damage, thereby increasing the therapeutic ratio.

Heat preferentially damages tumor vasculature. After heating, blood flow decreases in tumors but increases in normal tissue.

Hyperthermia may be delivered locally, regionally, or systemically (whole body) depending on the malignancy. It has been used to treat cervix, head and neck, sarcoma, rectal, and breast cancers as well as melanoma. The type of treatment applicator will vary depending on the site of treatment (see Figures 12-5 and 12-6). Smaller applicators are used for superficial areas, such as skin cancer, whereas regional/deep applicators are used for deep-seated tumors, such as cervix and rectal cancers.

Treatment can last from 60 to 90 minutes, and the goal is to heat the tumor for 30 minutes or longer to a temperature of 40–43°C. Thermometry catheters are placed into the tumor itself, on the skin and/or in the body orifice. Heating may be achieved with ultrasound, low- or high-frequency microwaves, or radiofrequencies. As temperatures increase, the first tissue reaction that occurs is increased blood flow.[53] Thermotolerance is a transient adaptation to thermal stress that renders surviving heated cells more resistant to additional heat stress; it can develop during or after heat stress and can persist for several days.[53]

Treatments may be given twice weekly, once weekly, or monthly, depending on the combination with chemotherapy and radiation. Common side effects include first- or second-degree, superficial or subcutaneous tissue burns. For patients receiving regional deep hyperthermia, cardiovascular stress due to change in pulse and blood pressure will ensue.

Hyperthermia has been shown to have additive and synergistic effects with chemotherapy and radiation therapy. A recent resurgence of interest has inspired studies that have used radiation, chemotherapy, and hyperthermia as well as chemotherapy and hyperthermia.[56–58] Higher perfusion rates can increase drug delivery and reoxygenation, thereby increasing the efficacy of radiotherapy.[59] For most drugs (excluding 5-FU and perhaps other antimetabolites), the optimal sequence is to administer heat and the drug simultaneously or to give the drug immediately before the onset of heating.[53]

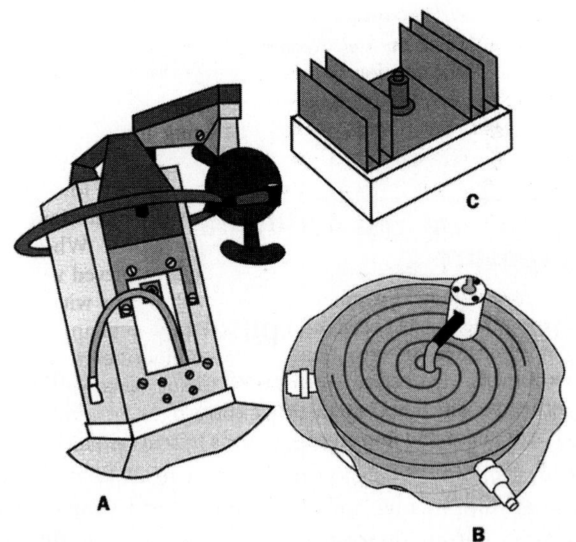

Figure 12-6 Different treatment devices are used to treat patients with small superficial lesions using local hyperthermia: **(A)** waveguide applicator; **(B)** spiral applicator; **(C)** sheet applicator. Although each device looks different, each holds a water bolus that is used to heat the respective area to be treated. Reprinted with permission from Wust P, Hildebrandt G, Sreenivasa G, et al: Hyperthermia in combined treatment of cancer. *Lancet Oncol* 3: 487–497, 2002.[59]

Table 12-5 Appropriate Mean Doses Relevant to Societal Low-Dose Radiation Risk Estimation

	Approximate Mean Individual Dose (mSv)
Some Societally Relevant Exposures	
Round-trip flight, New York–London	0.1
Single screening mammogram (breast dose)	3
Background dose due to natural radiation exposure	3/year
Dose (over a 70-year period) to 0.5 million individuals in rural Ukraine in the vicinity of the Chernobyl accident	14
Dose range over 20-block radius from hypothetical nuclear terrorism incident (FASEB scenario 1: medical gauge containing cesium)	3 to 30
Pediatric CT scan (stomach dose from abdominal scan)	25
Radiation worker exposure limit	20/year
Exposure on international space station	170/year
Some Low-Dose Epidemiological Studies	
A-bomb survivors (mean dose in LSS cohort)	200
Medical x-rays (breast dose in scoliosis study)	100
Nuclear workers (mean dose from major studies)	20
Individuals diagnostically exposed in utero	10

Notes: Absorbed doses in milligrays are numerically the same as equivalent organ doses in millisieverts. *Absorbed dose* is the physicial quantity describing energy deposited per unit mass. For radiation protection purposes, *equivalent dose* and *effective dose* are used, which include a radiation-dependent weighting factor. For x-rays or gamma rays, 1 mGy = 1 mSv.

All doses are effective whole-body doses with the exception of the medical exposures (mammography, CT scan, irradiation for scoliosis), which are to specific organs.

Reprinted with permission from Brenner DJ, Doll R, Goodhead DF: Cancer risks attributable to low doses of ionizing radiation: assessing what we really know. *PNAS* 100:13761–13766, 2003.[61]

Incidental and Accidental Radiation Exposure

Chronic Low-Dose Exposure

Chronic low-dose radiation exposure occurs to all individuals, due to background radiation from naturally occurring radioactive substances and cosmic rays. The dose of natural radiation received varies. Urban populations may receive more radiation on a yearly basis from human-made sources, including building materials.[60] It is estimated that the background dose an individual receives each year is approximately 3 mSv.[61] Table 12-5 reviews approximate societal doses of radiation. This exposure is largely unavoidable and is considered to be within safe limits as defined by federal regulations. Although radiation workers are exposed to additional ionizing radiation, the allowable limit is well below that which is known to produce ill effects.

Accidental exposure or low-dose exposure may occur in nuclear power plants or among people who handle isotopes. Accidental exposure of industrial radiation workers has been reported in the literature as case reports; in such instances, common injuries include skin changes, bone marrow changes, and chromosome translocations.[62–66]

Regulations require that institutions measure and monitor the radiation exposure to individuals and that they employ ALARA (As Low As Reasonably Achievable) guidelines. Staff caring for patients receiving radiation therapy as well as those working in radiology departments and on units caring for patients receiving therapy wear film badges, which monitor exposure to radiation. Personnel handling the loading and unloading of radioactive material may wear ring badges and, depending on the frequency of exposure, still others may use pocket ion chambers.

Most of the information concerning the effects of radiation comes from reactor accidents (e.g., Chernobyl) or from the atomic bombs dropped in Japan. The prodromal syndrome is immediate and follows whole-body exposure. Symptoms typically include nausea, vomiting, listlessness, headache, and hypotension. The length and severity of this syndrome depend on the amount of exposure. Treatment is primarily supportive and consists of antiemetics, intravenous fluids, and pain medications. The latent phase follows a variable course after the prodromal syndrome. With low-dose exposures the latent phase may last for several weeks, whereas with higher doses the prodromal and latent phases may be short and the patient may immediately experience one of the syndromes that may eventually prove fatal.

Total Body Radiation Syndrome

Total body radiation syndrome refers to the effects of acute exposure of an organism to doses of radiation received in a matter of minutes rather than hours or days. Acute exposure of humans has been studied through data obtained from industrial and laboratory accidents, individuals exposed at Hiroshima and Nagasaki, Pacific Testing Grounds fallout exposure, and medical treatment procedures.[67,68] More than 100,000 people in Japan were exposed to the effects of the atomic bombs in dose ranges of 0 to 600 rem, with an average of about 200 rem.[69] Among the epidemiologic findings to date is an increase in leukemia incidence among those who received radiation of 50 rem or more. This increase in incidence began two years following irradiation, peaked at seven to ten years, and returned to control levels after 20 years.[69,70] The April 1986 nuclear accident in Chernobyl, Ukraine, has yielded additional significant information about the somatic effects of exposure to high levels of radioactivity. Researchers generally agree that it takes longer for solid tumors to develop from exposure than leukemia. Total body radiation syndrome is manifested by the critical effects seen in the hematopoietic, gastrointestinal, and cerebrovascular systems.

Doses of 15–200 Gy delivered to the whole body in a short time produce life-shortening or lethal damage through effects on the hematopoietic, gastrointestinal, and central nervous systems. Three types of death from total body exposure have been delineated:

1. Doses on the order of 100 Gy or higher cause death in a matter of hours from effects on the central nervous system and cardiovascular collapse.
2. Intermediate doses of 10 to 20 Gy result in death within several days caused by elimination of the intestinal epithelium with intractable diarrhea.
3. Lower doses, from 1 to 5 Gy, result in depopulation of hematopoietic stem cells; death may occur several weeks after the exposure from infection or bleeding.[3]

Hematopoietic syndrome

Total body radiation exposure in a single dose ranging from 300 to 800 cGy leads to hematopoietic failure. Stem cells are most susceptible and are sterilized almost immediately on exposure. When the circulating cells begin to die off in a matter of a few weeks, and marrow replacement is insufficient, the crisis and symptoms appear. Generally, within three weeks after exposure, the patient experiences chills, fever, fatigue, petechiae, and mouth ulcerations — all symptoms of depressed blood components. Treatment typically includes transfusions, antibiotics, growth factors, and isolation. Death ensues unless marrow recovery or successful transplantation occurs. Ongoing research to treat this syndrome has focused on the use of growth factors, cytokines, and stem cell transplantation.[71]

Gastrointestinal syndrome

Following total body exposure of 10 Gy or more, death occurs within a few days to two weeks due to the severity of gastrointestinal damage. The highly radiosensitive intestinal epithelium is essentially denuded of villi, with total loss of the normal cell-renewal mechanism. The patient suffers nausea, anorexia, vomiting, lethargy, and severe, prolonged diarrhea leading to death. Sepsis is a critical issue in this population. Treatment is primarily supportive in nature and includes antiemetics, antimotility agents, IV fluids, TPN, narcotics, and antibiotics.

Cerebrovascular syndrome

No human has survived accidental total body exposure of more than 10 Gy. At this dosage level, death results from the cerebrovascular consequences. Although the exact mechanism of cerebrovascular death is not clear, symptoms include disorientation, lack of coordination, seizures, visual impairment, hypotension, respiratory distress, renal failure, and coma. This syndrome has short prodromal and latent phases. At this high-dose exposure level, gastrointestinal symptoms also occur almost immediately, and death due to neurovascular failure occurs in a matter of hours to a few days. Treatment is primarily supportive and consists of oxygen, anticonvulsants, sedatives, IV fluids, and narcotics. (For case descriptions of total body radiation syndrome, see Kato and Schull[67] and Schull.[68])

Radiation Effects on the Embryo and Fetus

Data regarding fetal and embryonic response to radiation have been obtained primarily from laboratory animals, for the obvious reason that human experimentation is unethical. Information that has become available on human fetal exposure has been acquired from studies of the surviving children who were in utero at the time of the atomic explosions in Nagasaki and Hiroshima.[72–74] Information has also come from medical radiation exposure in the early twentieth century before the fetal dangers were recognized. Radiation is considered a teratogen, and the developing embryo/fetus is more sensitive to the damaging effects of radiation due to its rapidly dividing cells.

Three critical periods in gestation have been identified: preimplantation, organogenesis, and the fetal period.[60] The classic triad of effects of radiation upon the embryo are (1) intrauterine growth retardation (IUGR); (2) embryonic, fetal or neonatal death; and (3) congenital malformation.[60] The frequency and severity of these effects in an irradiated population depends on a number of factors, including the stage of gestation at which irradiation occurs, the organ systems exposed, LET (linear energy transfer) of the radiation, the total dose (or absorbed dose equivalent), the dose rate, and fractionation.[60] During preimplantation or shortly afterward, radiation is almost always lethal. Surprisingly, a surviving embryo progresses to normal growth because, at this point in gestation, the only task of the cells is division, not differentiation.

During the next phase, organogenesis, the embryo is at greatest danger of developing malformations following exposure to radiation. Neonatal death is common, as multiple abnormalities that result from the radiation exposure are incompatible with life. When radiation exposure occurs during the growth or fetal period (after six weeks in humans), the most common effects are overall growth retardation, microcephaly, and mental retardation.[75] Other reported abnormalities in humans include spina bifida, hydrocephalus, blindness, clubfoot, and scalp alopecia.[76] Radioiodine administered to the mother after the embryo/fetus's thyroid has formed may destroy thyroid function, resulting in cretinism if untreated.[77] In the postpartum period, the infant has the ability to recover partially from the growth-retarding effects of high-dose irradiation.[78]

Radiation-Induced Malignancies

The carcinogenic effects of radiation, from both chronic low-dose exposure and therapeutic radiation, are of particular interest and concern to the nurse, especially when providing support to the individual who is hesitant about accepting treatment. The key to understanding lies in the fact that acute exposure occurring in radiation accidents is rare, and chronic low-dose occupational or environmental exposure is the exception. The therapeutic doses usually prescribed (in the range of 2500–6500 cGy) are believed to be less carcinogenic than lower doses given over a much longer time period. Theoretically, a cell that has survived in a damaged or altered state after low-dose irradiation may undergo carcinogenic mutation in the presence of other conditional factors. At the same time, a cell that has been sterilized or destroyed by therapeutic doses of radiation should be incapable of malignant changes.

Malignancies that have been associated with radiation exposure include skin carcinoma, leukemia, sarcoma, thyroid carcinoma, and lung cancer.[3,79] Other reports have suggested the possibility of inducing breast cancer in females by frequent radiographic exposure for screening for tuberculosis, lung disease, and breast cancer itself.[3,80,81] It is also important to consider the individual factors that contribute to carcinogenesis (e.g., lifestyle, geographic location, health history, and genetics). Both pediatric and adult cancer survivors are at greater risk for developing a secondary malignancy based on past treatment and genetics. Nurses caring for patients who have received radiation therapy need to encourage them to undergo routine physical exams, teach proper self-examination techniques, and assist patients in making lifestyle choices that decrease the development of a secondary malignancy.

Radiation carcinogenesis depends on a number of variables but is directly related to the exposure to radiation. These factors include a latent period of 1 to 30 years, radiation dose, concomitant factors in the radiated organism's environment, and the actual fate of the cell as it responds to radiation injury.[82]

Conclusion

The science of radiation oncology and medicine has achieved tremendous advances in the past century, from the early work of the Curies to the development of first-generation linear accelerators. The biologic effects of radiation therapy have long been observed, recognized, and acknowledged but not well understood. Today, researchers continue to investigate population-based exposure (Chernobyl), and the acute and late effects that patients experience while undergoing therapeutic irradiation. The recognition and pursuit of both basic and clinical radiobiologic research have led to the current emphasis on maximizing treatment outcomes while minimizing both early and late effects of treatment. This goal is being achieved with combined modality therapy, altered fractionation schedules, reduction in treatment volume and dose, and ever more sophisticated treatment planning and techniques of delivery. With the unraveling of the human genome now complete, the science behind therapy will develop at the molecular level by understanding patients' genetic make-up and tailoring treatments based on their unique profiles.

Knowledge of radiobiologic effects also has led to the expansion of radiation therapy for some nonmalignant conditions. Nonmalignant treatment indications being explored include cardiac and lung allograft rejection,[83,84] macular degeneration,[85,86] and endovascular brachytherapy for arterial restenosis following angioplasty.[87–89] Research in molecular and cellular biology will continue to be of primary importance in radiation oncology and improved cancer treatment.

References

1. Halperin EC, Schmidt-Ullrich RK, Perez CA, et al: Overview and basic science of radiation oncology, in Perez CA, Brady LW, Halperin EC, Schmidt-Ullrich RK (eds.): *Principles and Practice of Radiation Oncology* (ed 4). Philadelphia, Lippincott Williams & Wilkins, 2004, pp 1–95
2. Hilderley LJ: Radiation oncology: historical background, in Hassey-Dow K, Bucholtz J (eds.): *Nursing Care in Radiation Oncology* (ed 2). Philadelphia, W. B. Saunders, 1997, pp 3–5
3. Hall EJ, Cox JD: Physical and biological basis of radiation therapy, in Cox JD, Ang KK (eds.): *Radiation Oncology*. St. Louis, Mosby, 2003, pp 3–62
4. Weyrather WK, Debus J: Particle beams for cancer therapy. *Clin Oncol* 15:S23–S28, 2002
5. Raju MR: Particle radiotherapy: historical developments and current status. *Radiat Res* 145:391–407, 1996

6. Hilderley LJ: Principles of teletherapy, in Hassey-Dow K, Bucholtz J (eds.): *Nursing Care in Radiation Oncology* (ed 2). Philadelphia, W. B. Saunders, 1997, pp 6–20
7. Dunne-Daly C: Principles of radiotherapy and radiobiology. *Semin Oncol Nurs* 15:250–259, 1999
8. Bergonie J, Tribondeau L: Interpretation of some results of radiotherapy and an attempt at determining a logical technique of treatment. *Radiat Res* II:587, 1959
9. McBride WH, Withers HR: Biologic basis of radiation therapy, in Perez CA, Brady LW, Halperin EC, Schmidt-Ullrich RK (eds.): *Principles and Practice of Radiation Oncology* (ed 4). Philadelphia, Lippincott Williams & Wilkins, 2004, pp 96–136
10. Gray LH: Radiobiologic basis of oxygen as a modifying factor in radiation therapy. *Am J Roentgenol Radium Nucl Ther* 85: 803–815, 1961
11. Brizel DM, Scher RI, Dewhirst MW: Oxygenation of head and neck cancer: changes during radiotherapy and impact on treatment outcome. *Int J Radiat Oncol Biol Phys* 42:142, 1998 (abstr 46)
12. Dunst J, Kuhnt T, Strauss HG, et al: Anemia in cervical cancer: impact on survival, patterns of replase, and association with hypoxia and angiogenesis. *Int J Radiat Oncol Biol Phys* 56:778–787, 2003
13. Kumar P: Tumor hypoxia and anemia: impact on the efficacy of radiation therapy. *Semin Radiat Oncol* 37:4–8, 2000
14. Dewey WC, Ling CC, Meyn RE: Radiation-induced apoptosis: relevance to radiotherapy. *Int J Radiat Oncol Biol Phys* 33:781–796, 1995
15. Fuks Z, Haimovitz-Friedman A, Kolesnick RN: The role of the sphyngomyelin pathway and protein kinase C in radiation-induced cell kill, in DeVita VT, Hellman S, Rosenberg SA (eds.): *Important Advances in Oncology 1995*. Philadelphia, Lippincott, 1995, pp 19–31
16. Kim HE, Han JS, Kasza T, et al: Platelet-derived growth factor (PDGF) signaling mediates radiation-induced apoptosis in human prostate cancer cells with loss of p53 function. *Int J Radiat Oncol Biol Phys* 39:731–736, 1997
17. Orton C: Radiobiology in brachytherapy: biologic aspects and practical applications, in Nag S (ed.): *Principles and Practice of Brachytherapy*. Armonk, NY, Futura, 1997, pp 51–65
18. Patel FD, Sharma SC, Negi PS, et al: Low dose rate vs high dose rate brachytherapy in treatment of carcinoma of the uterine cervix: a clinical trial. *Int J Radiat Oncol Biol Phys* 28:335–341, 1994
19. Clapp KJ: Therapeutic aspects of radiopharmaceuticals. *Oncol Issues* 16(suppl):9–10, 2001
20. Order SE, Seigel JA, Lustig RA, et al: Infusional brachytherapy in the treatment of non-resectable pancreatic cancer: a new radiation modality (preliminary report of the phase I study). *Antib Immunoconj Radiopharm* 7:11–27, 1994
21. Westlin JE, Anderson-Forsman C, Garske U, et al: Objective responses after fractionated infusional brachytherapy of unresectable pancreatic adenocarcinomas. *Cancer* 80(suppl):2743–2748, 1997
22. Benkert TA: Bexxar (tositumomab and iodine I 131 tositumomab): an investigational drug for the treatment of low-grade and transformed low-grade non Hodgkin's lymphoma. *Oncol Issues* 16(suppl):18–19, 2001
23. Kaminski MS, Zelentz AD, Press OW, et al: Pivotal study of iodine I 131 tositumomab for chemotherapy-refractory low-grade or transformed low-grade B-cell non-Hodgkin's lymphoma. *J Clin Oncol* 19:3918–3928, 2001
24. Zelentz AD, Vose JM, Knox S, et al: Iodine I 131 tositumomab for patients with transformed low-grade non-Hodgkin's lymphoma: overall clinical trial experience. *Blood* 94:632a, 1999 (abstr)
25. Witzing TE, White CA, Gordon LI: Final results of a randomized controlled study of Zevalin radioimmunotherapy for B-cell NHL. *Blood* 96:831a, 2000 (abstr)
26. Hendrick CS, de Leon C, Dillman RO: Radioimmunotherapy for non-Hodgkin's lymphoma with yttrium 90 ibritumomab tiuxetan. *Clin J Oncol Nurs* 6:144–148, 2002
27. Wasserman TH, Chapman JD: Radiation response modulation. Part A: chemical sensitizers and protectors, in Perez CA, Brady LW, Halperin EC, Schmidt-Ullrich RK (eds.): *Principles and Practice of Radiation Oncology* (ed 4). Philadelphia, Lippincott Williams & Wilkins, 2004, pp 663–698
28. Brown JM: Hypoxic cell radiosensitizers: where next? *Int J Radiat Oncol Biol Phys* 16:987–993, 1989
29. Lee DJ, Cosmatos D, Marcial VA, et al: Results of an RTOG phase III trial (RTOG 85-27) comparing radiotherapy plus etanidazole with radiotherapy alone for locally advanced head and neck carcinomas. *Int J Radiat Onco Biol Phys* 32:567–576, 1995
30. Overgaard J, Hansen HS, Overgaard M, et al: A randomized double-blind phase III study of nimorazole as hypoxic radiosensitizer of primary radiotherapy in supraglottic larynx and pharynx carcinoma. Results of the Danish Head and Neck Cancer Study (DAHANCA) Protocol 5-85. *Radiother Oncol* 46:135–146, 1998
31. Henk JM, Bishop K, Shepherd SF: Treatment of head and neck cancer with CHART and nimorazole: phase II study. *Radiother Oncol* 66:65–70, 2003
32. Epstein AH, Lebovics RS, Van Waes C, et al: Intravenous delivery of 5′-iododeoxyuridine during hyperfractionated radiotherapy for locally advanced head and neck cancers: results of a pilot study. *Laryngoscope* 108:1090–1094, 1998
33. Von Pawel J, von Roemeling R, Gatzemeier U, et al: Tirapazamine plus cisplatin versus cisplatin in advanced non-small cell lung cancer: a report of the international CATAPULT I study group. Cisplatin and tirapazamine in subjects with previously untreated non-small cell lung tumors. *J Clin Oncol* 18:1351–1359, 2000
34. Lee DJ, Trotti A, Spencer S, et al: Concurrent tirapazamine and radiotherapy for advanced head and neck carcinomas: a phase II study. *Int J Radiat Oncol Biol Phys* 42:811–815, 1998
35. Pharmacyclics: *www.pharmacyclics.com/webpage_templates/tert.php3?page_name=pr_1078155733*. Accessed March 1, 2004.
36. Xu S, Zakian K, Thaler H, et al: Effects of motexafin gadolinium on tumor metabolism and radiation sensitivity. *Int J Radiat Oncol Biol Phys* 49:1381–1390, 2001
37. Coleman CN: Chemical sensitizers and protectors. *Int J Radiat Oncol Biol Phys* 42:781–783, 1998
38. Capizzi RL: The preclinical basis for broad-spectrum selective cytoprotection of normal tissues from cytotoxic therapies by amifostine. *Semin Oncol* 26:3–21, 1999
39. Brizel DM, Wasserman TH, Henke M, et al: Phase III randomized trial of amifostine as a radioprotector in head and neck cancer. *J Clin Oncol* 18:3339–3345, 2000
40. Gosselin TK, Pavilonis H: Head and neck cancer: managing xerostomia and other treatment induced side effects. *ORL Head Neck Nurs* 20:15–22, 2002
41. Spielberger R, Emmanoulides C, Stiff P, et al: Use of recombinant keratinocyte growth factor (rHuKGF) can reduce severe oral mucositis in patients with hematologic malignancies undergoing autologous peripheral blood progenitor cell transplantation (auto-PBSCT) after radiation-based conditioning: results of a phase 3 trial. *Proc Am Soc Clin Oncol* 22: 2003 (abstr 3642)
42. Meropol NJ, Somer RA, Gutheil J, et al: Randomized phase I trial of recombinant human keratinocyte growth factor plus

chemotherapy: potential role as mucosal protectant. *J Clin Oncol* 21:1452–1458, 2003
43. Morris M, Eifel PJ, Lu J, et al: Pelvic radiation with concurrent chemotherapy compared with pelvic and para-aortic radiation for high-risk cervical cancer. *N Engl J Med* 340:1137–1143, 1999
44. Rose PG, Bundy BN, Watkins EB, et al: Concurrent cisplatin-based radiotherapy and chemotherapy for locally advanced cervical cancer. *N Engl J Med* 340:1144–1153, 1999
45. Keys HM, Bundy BN, Stehman FB, et al: Cisplatin, radiation, and adjuvant hysterectomy compared with radiation and adjuvant hysterectomy for bulky stage IB cervical carcinoma. *N Engl J Med* 340:1154–1161, 1999
46. Wolmark N, Wieand HS, Hyams DM, et al: Randomized trial of postoperative adjuvant chemotherapy with or without radiotherapy for carcinoma of the rectum: National Surgical Adjuvant Breast and Bowel Project Protocol R-02. *J Natl Cancer Inst* 92:388–396, 2000
47. Brizel DM, Albers ME, Fisher SR, et al: Hyperfractionated irradiation with or without concurrent chemotherapy for locally advanced head and neck cancer. *N Engl J Med* 338:1798–1804, 1998
48. Lara PN, Goldberg Z, Davies A, et al: Concurrent chemoradiation strategies in the management of unresectable stage III non-small-cell lung cancer. *Clin Lung Cancer* 3(suppl):S42–48, 2002
49. Forastiere AA, Goepfert H, Maor M, et al: Concurrent chemotherapy and radiotherapy for organ preservation in advanced laryngeal cancer. *N Engl J Med* 349:2091–2098, 2003
50. Coleman CN: Clinical radiosensitization: why it does and does not work. *J Clin Oncol* 17:1–3, 1999
51. Marks L, Carroll P, Dugan T, et al: The response of the urinary bladder, urethra and ureter to radiation and chemotherapy. *Int J Radiat Oncol Biol Phys* 31:1257–1280, 1995
52. Komaki R: Combined chemotherapy and radiation therapy in surgically unresectable regionally advanced non-small cell lung cancer. *Semin Radiat Oncol* 6:86–91, 1996
53. Jones EL, Samulski TV, Vujaskovic Z, et al: Hyperthermia, in Perez CA, Brady LW, Halperin EC, Schmidt-Ullrich RK (eds.): *Principles and Practice of Radiation Oncology* (ed 4). Philadelphia, Lippincott Williams & Wilkins, 2004, pp 699–735
54. Martin CW, Whitehead T: Radiation modifiers chemical and thermal, in Watkins-Brumer D, Moore-Higgs G, Haas M (eds.): *Outcomes in Radiation Therapy.* Sudbury, MA, Jones and Bartlett, 2001, pp 102–120
55. Anscher NS, Lee C, Hurwitz H, et al: A pilot study of preoperative continuous infusion 5-fluorouracil, external microwave hyperthermia, and external beam radiotherapy for treatment of locally advanced, unresectable, or recurrent rectal cancer. *Int J Radiat Oncol Biol Phys* 47:719–724, 2000
56. Jones EL, Samulski TD, Dewhirst MW, et al: A pilot phase II trial of concurrent radiotherapy, chemotherapy, and hyperthermia for locally advanced cervical carcinoma. *Cancer* 98:277–282, 2003
57. Blackwell K, Vujaskovic Z, Rosen E, et al: A phase I dose escalation study of liposomal doxorubicin, paclitaxel, and hyperthermia in locally advanced breast carcinoma. *Proc Am Soc Clin Oncol* 21:200a, 2002 (abstr)
58. Kouloulias VE, Dardoufas CE, Kouvaris JR, et al: Liposomal doxorubicin in conjunction with reirradiation and local hyperthermia treatment in recurrent breast cancer: a phase I–II trial. *Clin Cancer Res* 8:373–382, 2002
59. Wust P, Hildebrandt G, Sreenivasa G, et al: Hyperthermia in combined treatment of cancer. *Lancet Oncol* 3:487–497, 2002
60. Ritenour ER: Health effects of low level radiation: carcinogenesis, teratogenesis, and mutagenesis. *Semin Nucl Med* 16: 106–117, 1986
61. Brenner DJ, Doll R, Goodhead DT, et al: Cancer risks attributable to low doses of ionizing radiation: assessing what we really know. *PSNA* 100:13761–13766, 2003
62. Jalil A, Rab Molla MA: Accidental exposure to ^{192}Ir source in industrial radiography: a follow-up study. *Health Phys* 62:74–76, 1992
63. Lucas JN, Poggensee M, Straume T: The persistence of chromosome translocations in a radiation worker accidentally exposed to tritium. *Cytogenet Cell Genet* 60:255–256, 1992
64. Ramalho AT, Nascimento ACH, Littlefield LG, et al: Frequency of chromosomal aberrations in a subject accidentially exposed to 137Cs in the Goiania (Brazil) radiation accident: intercomparison among four laboratories. *Mutat Res* 252:157–160, 1991
65. Raina S, Samuel AM: Isotope angiography and blood pool imaging as a procedure for assessing radiation-induced injuries to the hands. *Clin Nucl Med* 17:646–651, 1992
66. Scott BR, Lyzlov AF, Osovets SV: Evaluating the risk of death via the hematopoietic syndrome mode for prolonged exposure of nuclear workers to radiation delivered at very low rates. *Health Phys* 74:545–554, 1998
67. Kato H, Schull WJ: Studies of the mortality of A-bomb survivors. Mortality, 1950–78. I. Cancer mortality. *Radiat Res* 90:395–432, 1982
68. Schull WJ: *Effects of Atomic Radiation: A Half Century of Studies from Hiroshima and Nagasaki.* New York, Wiley-Liss, 1995
69. Beebe GW, Kato H, Land CE: Studies of the mortality of A-bomb survivors. Mortality experience of A-bomb survivors, 1950–74. *Radiation Effects of Research Foundation*, RERF Technical Report No. 1, 1977
70. Ishimaru T, Hoshina T, Ichimaru M, et al: Leukaemia in atomic bomb survivors. Hiroshima and Nagaski, 1 October 1950–30 September 1966. *Radiat Res* 45:216–233, 1971
71. MacVittie TJ: Therapy of radiation injury. *Stem Cells* 15(suppl 2):263–268, 1997
72. Wood JW, Johnson KG, Omori Y: In utero exposure to the Hiroshima atomic bomb: follow up at 20 years. *Pediatrics* 39:385–392, 1967
73. Otake M, Schull WJ: In utero exposure to A-bomb radiation and mental retardation: a reassessment. *Br J Radiol* 57:409–414, 1984
74. Izumi S, Koyama K, Soda M, et al: Cancer incidence in children and young adults did not increase relative to parental exposure to atomic bombs. *Br J Cancer* 89:1709–1713, 2003
75. Miller RW: Effects of prenatal exposure to ionizing radiation. *Health Phys* 59:57–61, 1990
76. Dekaban AS: Abnormalities in children exposed to x-radiation during various stages of gestation: tentative timetable of radiation to the human fetus. *Int J Nucl Med* 9:471–477, 1968
77. Glenn JE: What cancer centers should know about radioactive materials. *Oncol Issues* 16(suppl):13–15, 2001
78. Arnon J, Meirow D, Lewis-Roness H, et al: Genetic and teratogenic effects of cancer treatments on gametes and embryos. *Hum Reprod Update* 7:394–403, 2001
79. March HC: Leukemia in radiologists in a twenty-year period. *Am J Med Sci* 220:282, 1950
80. MacKenzie I: Breast cancer following multiple fluoroscopies. *Br J Cancer* 19:1–8, 1965
81. Myrden JA, Hiltz JE: Breast cancer following multiple fluoroscopies during artificial pneumothorax treatment of pulmonary tuberculosis. *Can Med Assoc J* 100:1032–1034, 1969
82. Bucholtz JD: Radiation carcinogenesis, in Hassey-Dow K, Bucholtz JD, Iwamoto R, et al (eds.): *Nursing Care in Radiation Oncology* (ed 2). Philadelphia, W.B. Saunders, 1997, pp 57-68
83. Wolden SL, Tate DJ, Hunt SA, et al: Long-term results of total lymphoid irradiation in the treatment of cardiac allograft rejection. *Int J Radiat Oncol Biol Phys* 39:953–960, 1997

84. Diamond DA, Michalski JM, Lynch JP, et al: Efficacy of total lymphoid irradiation for chronic allograft rejection following bilateral lung transplantation. *Int J Radiat Oncol Biol Phys* 41:795–800, 1998
85. Akmansu M, Dirican B, Ozturk B, et al: External radiotherapy in macular degeneration: our technique, dosimetric calculation, and preliminary results. *Int J Radiat Oncol Biol Phys* 40:923–927, 1998
86. Archambeau JO, Mao XW, Yonemoto LT, et al: What is the role of radiation in the treatment of subfoveal membranes: review of radiobiologic, pathologic and other considerations to initiate a multimodality discussion. *Int J Radiat Oncol Biol Phys* 40:1125–1136, 1998
87. Rubin P, Williams JP, Riggs PN, et al: Cellular and molecular mechanisms of radiation inhibition of restenosis. Part I: role of the macrophage and platelet-derived growth factor. *Int J Radiat Oncol Biol Phys* 40:929–941, 1998
88. Tripuraneni P: Coronary artery radiation therapy for the prevention of restenosis after percutaneous coronary angioplasty, II: outcomes of clinical trials. *Semin Radiat Oncol* 12:17–30, 2002
89. Crocker I, Robinson KA: Rationale for coronary artery radiation therapy. *Semin Radiat Oncol* 12:3–16, 2002

CHAPTER 13

Radiation Treatment Planning

Susan Weiss Behrend, RN, MSN, AOCN®

Introduction

Radiation oncology nurses are challenged to understand the scientific framework of treatment and the equipment used to plan and deliver radiation treatment. Radiation therapy centers include both technological and clinical components. Patient management issues are fundamental to the nursing process and evolve naturally during the course of treatment. This information needs to be supplemented and supported by the expertise of the multidisciplinary team, including radiation oncologists, nurses, medical physicists, dosimetrists, engineers, and radiation therapists.

Treatment Planning and Simulation Processes

Receiving radiation therapy is a multifaceted process. Initially, a thorough consultation must occur in which the patient and family are introduced to the radiation oncologist and the radiation oncology nurse. Later, the patient meets other members of the multidisciplinary team — dosimetrists, therapists, social workers, and administrative support staff. The initial consultation includes a thorough review of the patient's history, physical and psychosocial assessment, histologic reconfirmation of the cancer diagnosis, discussion of treatment options, and educational informed consent.

Treatment recommendations are based on potential for disease response and risk of acute and long-term toxicity. A variety of radiation treatment modalities may be offered, including external beam alone or a combined regimen with internal radiation. The type and length of treatment vary according to the diagnosis, radiation sensitivity of the tumor, and patient performance status. Once these parameters are considered, the patient is offered a therapeutic plan. The radiation oncologist, in conjunction with medical physicists, develops the radiation prescription. Treatment planning is a detailed and precise process that focuses on obtaining a series of radiographic studies to identify tumor type, size, and location. Simulation involves a series of fluoroscopic films that, combined with a computerized planning program, circumscribe the tumor and vital organs and tissues in the area. This information is used to determine the exact dose required for the target volume and surrounding normal tissues.

At the first appointment, the simulation procedure may require 1–2 hours. Thus, to allay anxiety, the patient should be prepared for an extended visit. At this time, the treatment field is identified and measured. Indelible small tattoos are injected on the patient's skin to mark the treatment area and enable daily replication of the target treatment field. Patients should be made aware that they will be partially disrobed during the simulation and daily treatments. The patient may be required to drink radio-opaque contrast or have intravenous contrast injected to enhance visualization of the tumor. Additionally, mold-room technicians will create customized blocks and immobilization devices to shield vital organs from scatter radiation and to safely secure the patient. At this time, the physician will obtain final informed consent. Depending on the facility policy, the patient may be required to return for a treatment setup prior to the initial dose so the plan can be checked methodically before actual administration. The aforementioned events can create tremendous anxiety for patients and families,[1] so it is incumbent on the professional radiation oncology nurse to provide an environment where patients feel physically comfortable and psychosocially supported.

During the initial consultation, the patient and family learn about the treatment process. The patient is required to maintain the same position throughout the treatment session. The machinery (typically a linear accelerator) rotates around the patient, and average treatment time varies between 10 and 15 minutes. The radiation beam is odorless, colorless, and painless. The patient is comfortably situated alone in the treatment room and is monitored at the therapist's control station with audiovisual cameras. Some patients may require pretreatment medication with antiemetics, steroids, or analgesics. Pediatric patients may need sedation or anesthesia to diminish the risk of movement during the treatment session.[2]

The typical treatment course is daily for 5 days and varies in the total number of weeks. Weekly planning films to monitor beam placement are checked by the radiation oncologist. In addition, weekly appointments are scheduled for all patients on treatment so that the radiation oncology nurse and the radiation oncologist can assess the patient for development of acute toxicities and overall status.

The planning and simulation processes depend on highly accurate measurements of patient characteristics to provide for differences in dose distribution. Dosimetric planning requires expert medical physicists, dosimetrists, and equipment. The data required by the physicists to plan treatment include body contour, outline and depth of internal structures, and location and size of the target.[3] Patient contours can be determined by mechanical, optical, ultrasonic, and computerized tomography (CT) equipment. The patient's contour must be assessed in the same position as the one proposed for actual treatment. Additionally, the tabletop should be included in the contour as a reference for beam angles, and bony landmarks and beam entry points should be indicated. Body contour should be

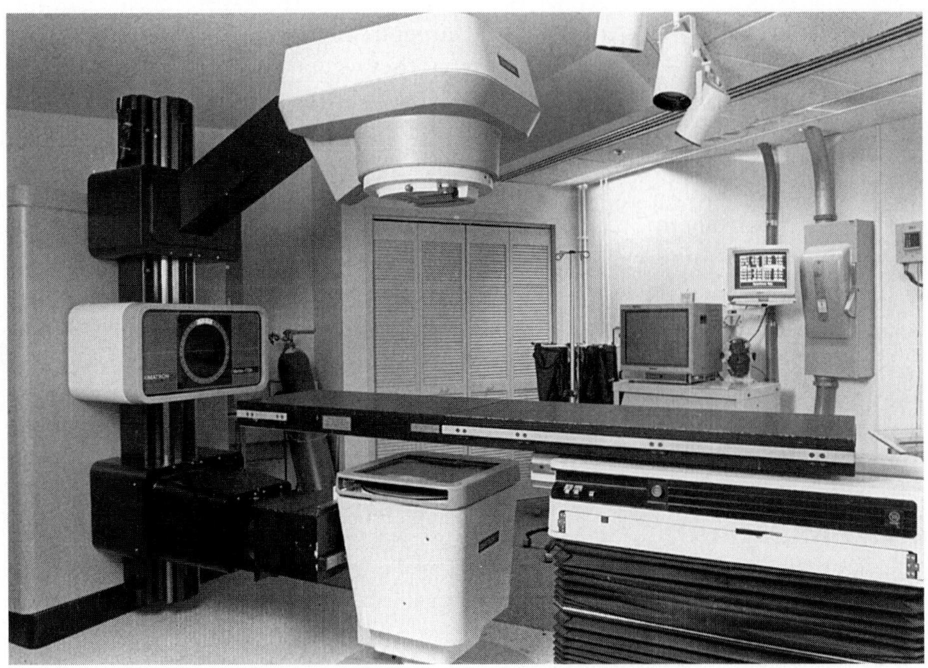

Figure 13-1 The treatment simulator is a conventional radiation treatment planning unit. It includes a fluoroscopy unit that geometrically duplicates an actual radiation treatment machine. (Photo courtesy of Fox Chase Cancer Center.)

continuously checked throughout treatment in anticipation of changes due to tumor response or weight change.

Internal structure identification provides vital information about the size and location of critical organs. These quantitative data complement the qualitative diagnostic radiographic findings that are essential for the identification of realistic contours. Several techniques and devices are used for localizing internal structures to facilitate treatment planning—transverse tomography, CT, ultrasound, treatment simulators, and port films, for example. The characteristics of treatment simulators and port films are explained next.

Treatment Simulators

A traditional treatment simulator is an x-ray machine that has the ability to duplicate the geometry and mechanics of radiation treatment machines (Figure 13-1). Pretreatment CT scans are often required to identify the target tumor and surrounding anatomical structures, and to guide the fluoroscopic simulation of the treatment position. The treatment simulator displays the treatment fields, ensuring the location of the target volume and identifying the surrounding normal tissues, thereby protecting them from excessive radiation. Radiographs are taken of the treatment field, and customized block templates are drawn on these films by the radiation oncologists. Next, mold-room technicians use these films to create customized lead blocks to protect normal tissues from the radiation beams.[4] Once the treatment field is confirmed, indelible marks on the skin surface serve as guides for treatment field placement and as permanent records if future radiation treatment should be required. As noted earlier, patients must assume and maintain the same exact position throughout the course of treatment. To facilitate this degree of precision, polystyrene plastic casts are created that conform to the body contours and help the patient to hold the same position. Additionally, laser lights are used to align patient position on the treatment machines.

Simulators have improved the precision of the delivery of radiation therapy. Their use evolved for three reasons:

1. The relationship between the radiation beam and external and internal anatomy cannot be assessed by diagnostic radiology.
2. The radiographic quality of the treatment machines is not sophisticated enough to be used for precise field localization.
3. The use of a treatment machine for field localization is impractical and creates time constraints.

Potential problems with patient treatment setup can be identified and solved during simulation. In addition, anatomical contours and thickness relating to tissue compensators or bolus designs can be obtained during simulation. The simulator can determine the adequacy of the fabrication of shielding blocks. Laser lights, contour makers, and shadow trays are equipment accessories to simulators that facilitate these functions.[3] More recently, traditional simulators are being replaced by CT simulators that combine traditional simulation and diagnostic CT scan to enable more complex radiation delivery techniques.

Port Films

Port films are radiographic images taken by linear accelerators to verify treatment fields. Although these high-beam energies do not produce images as detailed as standard diagnostic radiographs, they provide excellent information about treatment accuracy and quality.[4] Weekly port films should be considered mandatory for departmental quality assurance purposes. Patients frequently ask the radiation oncology nurse about the results of the "x-rays," or the port films. Nurses need to educate patients and families about the specific purpose of the port films, explaining that tumor filming for diagnostic and staging purposes usually occurs at the completion of treatment and beyond.

The Treatment Plan

Appropriate, effective radiation dose distribution is determined by the medical physicist and dosimetrists using the information from pretreatment diagnostic imaging (e.g., CT, MRI, PET scans) and the simulation. All of these calculations are computerized and include depth of beam dose and beam profile. The number of beams usually ranges from two to four and is determined by the medical physicist in conjunction with the radiation oncologist. The goal of treatment and appropriate dosing always remains constant: to maximize the tumor dose and minimize surrounding normal tissue exposure. The radiation oncologist is usually given a choice of several treatment plans, and the one that provides the optimal dose is selected. Specific planning computers are used to calculate the amount of time that each beam is on during treatment. The details of the treatment planning, including beam time, beam angles, compensators, casts, tattoos, lasers, and blocks, are documented in the patient's chart, which resides at the treatment machine. Therapists administering the treatment use the patient record to set up the patient each day.[4]

Delivery of Radiation Therapy: Machines and Complementary Equipment

Linear Accelerator

A linear accelerator (LINAC) delivers high-energy radiation to tumors (Figure 13-2). Such a device uses high-frequency electromagnetic waves to accelerate charged particles, such as electrons, to high energies through a linear tube. When a beam of electrons is generated and accelerated by the LINAC, the energy increases. The electron volt (eV) is the basic unit of energy used in radiation oncology, and the escalating energy levels are kilovolts (10^3 eV = 1 kV) and megavolts (10^6 eV = 1 MeV). The electrons produced by the LINAC strike a target and produce x-rays of varying energies in the 10- to 30-kV range; superficial units are between 30 and 125 kV, and orthovoltage units produce x-rays from 125 to 500 kV. The charged electrons of the LINAC can be used to treat surface lesions as well as deep tumor targets.[4]

In lower-energy LINAC machines (6 MeV), the electrons proceed straight down a short accelerator tube to strike a target and produce x-rays. In higher-energy LINAC machines (18 MeV), the accelerator structure is longer and therefore must be angled to bend the electrons before striking the target.[5] An elaborate beam transport system made of specific bending magnets and focusing coils is responsible for directing the highly charged angled electrons. The LINAC treatment head consists of a thick shell of shielding material to provide protection from the danger of radiation leakage.[3]

Collimation

Collimation refers to the treatment administration technique of shaping the radiation beam to the desired target. The collimator is located in the head of the LINAC. High-atomic-number collimators can vary the treatment field size from 4 × 4 cm to 40 × 40 cm.[4] Electrons disperse easily in air, so the beam collimator must be approximated to the patient; 80–100 cm is the most common distance. The collimation system basically consists of a primary fixed collimator situated beyond the target in the direction of the beam, and secondary movable collimators that shape the beam into square or rectangular fields. The two pairs of leaves in each secondary collimator can be moved in and out from the beam to increase or decrease the size of the treatment field. The leaves also can be closed or

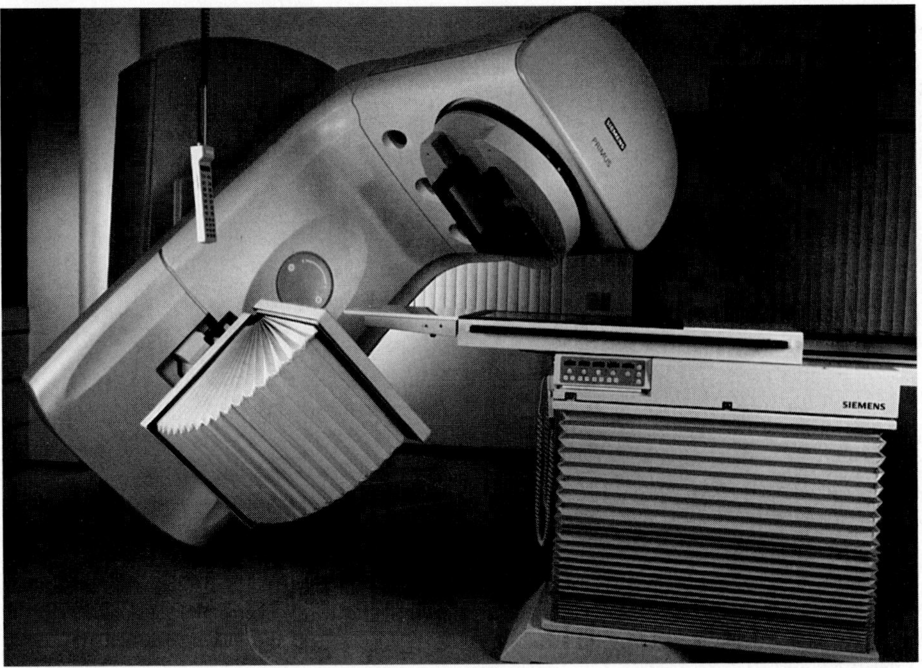

Figure 13-2 The linear accelerator (LINAC) is the most frequently used contemporary radiation therapy delivery unit. (Photo courtesy of Siemens Corporation.)

opened to provide the widest treatment field necessary.[5] Various sizes of cones are attached to the collimators and extend to the skin surface of the patient. Lead cutouts at the end of the electron cone can provide additional beam shaping.[5]

The introduction of multileaf collimators (Figure 13-3) installed in the gantry of the LINAC, directly in the path of the beam, has revolutionized treatment field shaping.[5] Multileaf collimators have proved useful in providing computerized customized blocking that does not require the physical creation of a new block for each field. This advance has lessened the workload of the mold-room technicians and minimized the amount of time required for treatment planning and administration. A multileaf collimator can be programmed to change the shape of the beam to match the target shape as the beam moves around the target. This technique, called *dynamic beam shaping*,[3] is considered to be clinically superior because it enhances tissue sparing.

The multifaceted role played by the radiation oncology nurse demands that the nurse develop an expanded knowledge base beyond clinical management issues. It is important for the radiation oncology nurse to understand the intricacies of treatment machine options, the associated costs, maintenance requirements, and pertinent information for patient education. This knowledge will provide a more comprehensive approach to patient care.

Orthovoltage Units

Orthovoltage units are x-ray machines that operate in the range of 150–500 peak kilovoltage (kV[p]). Filters are used to harden the x-ray beam and facilitate the limited penetration of these superficial x-rays. The maximum dose from this low-energy unit is found on the surface of the patient.[5]

Although orthovoltage machines continue to be used at some radiation oncology centers to treat superficial skin lesions, the advent of electron therapy to treat superficial cancers has made this equipment obsolete. Therefore, as these units begin to require repair and maintenance, they are being replaced.

Megavoltage Units

In recent decades, the megavoltage linear accelerator has been the machine of choice used to deliver radiation treatment. The production of x-rays with these devices is similar to that with the lower-voltage machines. The energy range of the megavoltage machines is broad: 4 to 20 MeV. The depth of the maximum dose ranges from 1.5 to 3.5 cm. The skin dose is 30%–40% of the delivered dose. The electron beam capabilities of the megavoltage machines range from 5 to 20 MeV. An electron beam is produced by the removal of the tungsten target from the path of the beam; this beam is used for treatment purposes. The electron skin dose is high from megavoltage machines, about 80%–95%

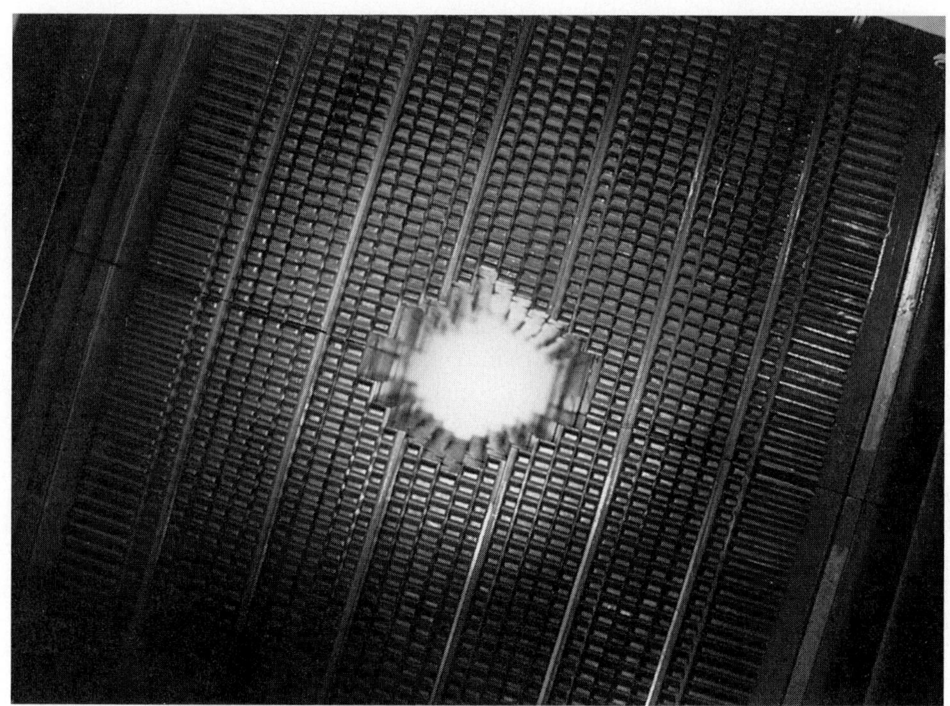

Figure 13-3 The multileaf collimator is used to define the treatment field configuration while shielding local and regional normal tissues. (Photo courtesy of Siemens Corporation.)

of the delivered dose. A standard formula relating to the depth of electron penetration states that 80% of the dose is delivered (in centimeters) at a depth corresponding to one-third of the electron energy in MeV. For example, a 12 MeV beam will deliver 80% of the dose at a depth of 4 cm.[4]

Machine Design

Radiation therapy devices are built to accommodate continual daily use for large cohorts of patients. The machines are compact and have a rotating feature that allows for 360-degree movement around the patient. This rotation offers a variety of options for beam angles to reach the target site. Distance must be provided between the patient and the beam-defining structures so as to allow for a safe rotation and to avoid collision with the patient and the treatment table or couch. The couch must be positioned to avoid potential interference of the beam by bars or rails. Treatment couches typically have removable sections that can be replaced either by thin polyester-film sheeting or a meshlike insert to support the patient. The removable sections provide two different options for patient treatment. First, removable side sections with a center spine for a continuous surface provide for treatment of posterior oblique fields without side rail interference. Second, a large removable center couch section allows for the treatment of a wide posterior field. Side rails are the link to support the segments of the couch, which are separated.[5]

Patient safety and comfort are priorities when treatment positioning occurs. The radiation therapists, together with the radiation nurses, must develop thorough preparatory information to ease patient fears and to ensure that a secure environment is provided throughout the treatment course. It may be appropriate to invite the patient and family to visit the treatment room to see the machines and associated equipment early in the process so that questions and concerns can be addressed prior to the actual planning and treatment sessions. Concerns about an unfamiliar environment, coupled with the multitude of anxieties associated with the entire cancer experience, can be alleviated by providing a personal introduction and tour.

Proton Therapy

Proton beams consist of energized particles that are accelerated using megavoltage energy. They conform the high-dose region to the targeted volume and minimize normal tissue injury, thereby reducing treatment-related side effects. This reduction in dose to normal tissue allows for an increase of radiation dose to the target, beyond that possible with conventional radiation. Protons can be delivered to an irregular three-dimensional volume in a variety of anatomical locations. Conforming the high-dose region of radiation beams to the tumor volume and avoiding unnecessary irradiation of normal tissue is the underlying premise of photons or electrons (standard x-ray) radiation treatment. Protons share radiobiological characteristics similar to those of standard radiation.

Protons were discovered in 1919 and were first accelerated to megavoltage energies in the 1930s. The clinical use of protons and the opening of treatment facilities began in the 1950s. Protons function by depositing a small portion of energy in the skin and superficial tissue, with the concentrated energy being delivered to the target volume. Protons are uniquely able to stop at the distal margin of the target, thereby sparing normal tissue.

Both conventional radiation therapy and proton beams work on the principle of selective cell destruction. A major advantage of proton treatment, however, is that the energy distribution of protons can be deposited more completely and more precisely in designated tissue than via standard (photon and electron) radiation. This capability provides superior targeting and enhanced tumor control.

Protons are energized to specific velocities. These energies determine the anatomical depth of penetration of the deposited protons. As these particles travel through the body, they slow down, allowing for increased interaction with orbiting electrons. Maximum interaction with electrons occurs as the protons approach their stopping point.

As noted earlier, protons release their maximum energy in the designated cancer volume. As a consequence, the surrounding healthy cells receive significantly less injury than cells in the designated target. The high-dose region of energy release occurs at a point called the Bragg peak. Protons' significant absorption characteristics result from their positive charge and heavy mass. Their energy upon entering the patient and the density of the tissue along their track determine the depth of penetration of the beam and the placement of the Bragg peak. The heavy mass results in minimal deviation and, therefore, minimal side scatter, which reduces unwanted side effects and maximizes treatment benefit.

Protons are administered through a proton accelerator. They pass through several components of the accelerator at boosted energies of 2 MeV. On their high-speed journey, they travel to the target about 10 million times per second. Each time they circulate, a boost of energy increases the protons' speed up to 250 MeV. These massively high energies can place the protons at any depth within the patient.

A series of steering and focusing magnets guide the particles through different chambers of the accelerator. The gantries of the proton accelerator are massive and include wheels that are 35 feet in diameter and weigh approximately 90 tons. These gantries revolve around the patient and direct the beam precisely where it is needed. For their part, patients simply see a revolving cone-shaped aiming device.

The computers that control the proton facility have safety measures to ensure that patients receive their prescribed treatments. These computers verify patient identification, set operational parameters for each patient's treatment plan, and direct the host computers to deliver a specified beam (*www.llu.edu/proton/physician/technical.html*).

Proton particle therapy is a superior treatment modality for treating a variety of solid tumors. Currently, the clinical delivery of this therapy remains extremely limited, being restricted to only a few U.S. sites and others worldwide. The installation of a proton facility poses tremendous financial and technical challenges and represents a significant limitation of this radiotherapy treatment technique.

Principles of External Beam Radiation Dosing/Dosimetry

Radiation dosing is a complex process that requires a strong background in physics. For purposes of this chapter, general definitions and key concepts are provided to serve as an adjunct to the radiation oncology nurse's clinical knowledge. Dose measurements of radiation are determined when the radiation beam hits the target (i.e., the patient). These measurements depend on the depth of the calculation point below the point of entry (depth), the penetrating power of the beam (energy), the tissue type that must be penetrated (density), the distance from the radiation source to the skin surface, the size of the field on the skin surface (field size), and the type and design of the collimator.

Measured data tables are created for each treatment machine and are planned using anthropomorphic phantoms, which are commercial systems that simulate various body tissues and are used to determine dose distribution. Frequently, water is used as the phantom material because it absorbs radiation similarly to human soft tissue. Sheets of varied tissue-equivalent plastics are also used for convenience. These measured data tables are referred to as *dosimeters* and are used by dosimetrists to quantify radiation dose distributions within phantom substances. These measurements are then used as patient controls for dose.[5]

The dose calculation must adhere to a strict check-and-balance system to ensure the utmost precision of the derived values. The components of dosing must include consistency of all aspects of the treatment machine and the data tables to avoid fatalities associated with either overdosing or underdosing. The radiation physics team is responsible for documenting the congruence of the machine settings with the treatment plans on a daily basis. Occasionally, dosimeters may be placed inside patient tissues to measure the actual dose delivered. This information can then be correlated with the treatment dose prescribed. Although dose calculations are often written to four significant figures, in practice the exact dose cannot be known with this degree of certainty. Although computers have enabled radiation treatment planners to carry dose calculations to large numbers, such large numbers do not ensure increased accuracy. Typically, medical physicists and dosimetrists round the numbers to the nearest whole number derived for dosing. This practice can be done with confidence, as it is not clinically possible to set treatment machines to fractions of dosing units.[5]

The *absorbed dose* of radiation is the energy deposited in a small fixed weight of the material (tissue) surrounding the point in question. The unit of dose measurement is the rad (radiation absorbed dose), which is considered equivalent to a dose or energy deposition of 100 erg per gram. In clinical practice, the rad is being replaced by the gray (Gy), which is 100 times larger (1 Gy = 100 rad). One rad is therefore the same as one-hundredth of a gray, or 1 centigray (cGy):

1 rad = 1/100 Gy = 1 cGy

Dose Delivery of Radiation

Dose delivery of radiation involves two major components. The first component identifies the output of the treatment machines from a specified point in the beam, to the specific distance from the target, and through a specific medium. The second component of dosing determines the actual absorbed dose within the medium. Both of these dose delivery concepts require precise calculations, thorough knowledge of the irradiated material, a geometric relationship with the proposed beam, and the size of the irradiated field.[3]

Secondary electrons are set in motion when high-energy photon beams strike a medium. These secondary electrons have the ability to penetrate to a depth that depends on the photon energy and the composition of the medium. When the electron equilibrium is reached at this depth, the maximum dose is achieved. The maximum depth is referred to and written as *Dmax*; the maximum dose is also referred to and written as *Dmax*. These abbreviations are used interchangeably. The Dmax is the point of build-up of peak radiation dose in tissue. As the x-ray energy increases, the Dmax extends more deeply in the tissue. It is a significant measurement due to the increased skin-sparing abilities of high-energy LINAC. The *build-up region* comprises the difference between the surface and this depth. The dose in the build-up region increases as the electrons add to the total dose administered. This premise underlies the technology's skin-sparing capabilities. The surface layer receives a smaller dose than layers between the surface and Dmax. If mechanical devices from the machines or if the patient's clothing intercepts the beam within a few centimeters of the skin surface, the skin-sparing effect is diminished or lost. More efficient skin sparing occurs with the use of higher energies, through which the Dmax increases. The beam dose falls gradually off at higher energies due to the combination of a smaller photon supply and increased distance from the target.

The *percent depth dose* (%DD) is the absorbed dose at a given depth expressed as a percentage of the absorbed dose at a reference depth. This value varies according to energy, field size, skin surface distance (SSD), and change in medium. The %DD falls less rapidly with higher energy.[3,5] It can be measured and plotted to form a %DD curve. As energy increases, the penetrative ability of the beam increases and the skin dose decreases (Table 13-1).

The *inverse square law of radiation* states that the intensity of a radiation beam is inversely proportional to the distance from the source squared. For example, the radiation dose at 2 cm will be one-fourth the dose at 1 cm. The inverse square law governs the theory of the intensity of an x-ray beam. Collimators and other scattering devices may cause deviations from the inverse square law. Consequently, the inverse square law must be checked for completion and accuracy to avoid serious errors in dosing.

Within the body, the radiation beam must pass through tissues of different densities. The variance in lung, bone, fat, muscle, and air affects both the beam penetration and the amount of scatter. The overall effect on the dose depends on the size of the treatment volume, the tissue density, and the beam energy. This variability of irradiated media requires complicated changes in dosimetry. The dose effect near the interface between layers of different densities is complex. Historically, outlining treatment borders was difficult and there were tremendous problems calculating a dose from beams that crossed nonhomogeneous volumes. In recent times, the use of CT to provide a detailed outline of irregularities and give information about the density of the target medium has improved dosing capabilities.

Radiation doses must be measured through different mediums to accurately determine patient dose.

Table 13-1 Dose Determination Measurements and Techniques for External Beam Radiation

Acronym	Term Defined
HVT	Half-value thickness: Penetration or quality or hardness of beam. The thickness of the material that reduces the intensity of the beam to half its original value. Low-energy beams and photon beams are described in terms of HVT.
SSD	Source surface distance: Measure of radiation dose in the absence of a scattering phantom. Sometimes referred to as "in air" measure.
SAD	Source axis distance: Measurements of radiation beam in air.
Dmax	The point of build-up of peak radiation dose in tissue.
%DD	The absorbed dose at a given depth expressed as a percentage of the absorbed dose at a reference depth.
TAR	Tissue–air ratio: Calculates radiation dose in rotation therapy; when source of radiation moves in a circle around the axis of the gantry rotation, TAR is the ratio of the dose at a given point in a medium to the dose at the same point in free space. $\text{TAR} = \frac{\text{Dose in tissue}}{\text{Dose in air}}$
TPR	Tissue–phantom ratio: Used in dosimetry of high-energy beams; eliminates unreliable in-air measurements. The ratio of dose at a specified point in tissue or in a phantom to the dose at the same distance in the beam at a reference depth of 5 cm. $\text{TPR} = \frac{\text{Dose in tissue}}{\text{Dose in phantom}}$
TMR	Tissue–maximum ratio: A special case of TPR; reference depth is at Dmax. TMR is the ratio of the dose at a specified point in tissue or in a phantom to the dose when it is at the depth of maximum dose. $\text{TMR} = \frac{\text{Dose in tissue}}{\text{Dose in phantom Dmax}}$
SAR	Scatter–air ratio: The ratio of the scattered dose at a given point in a medium to the dose in air at the same point. Used for calculating scattered dose in a medium.
Isocentric technique	Known as fixed source-axis technique to distance (SAD). Occurs when the axis of machine rotation (the isocenter) is placed in the target volume. Spares tissue around the target by limiting tissue exposure to the radiation beam.
Penumbra	Region near the edge of the field where dose rapidly falls.

Data from Bentel.[5]

Dosimetrists measure ionization of the radiation beam in air, identifing this quantity as the degree of exposure. The next steps in the process involve correcting for the presence of soft tissue in air and deriving the absorbed dose in units of grays.

Identification of dose variations within a field at prescribed depths is an essential component of radiation dosing techniques. The variety of clinical presentations requires that radiation treatment planning and dosing provide the capabilities to achieve a standard of safe, effective, and methodically planned treatment to targets while sparing surrounding anatomical structures. This treatment must also be reproducible on a daily basis to an exact standard, and concomitant accuracy checks and balances must be provided. Radiation oncology nurses benefit from understanding the conceptual framework that guides dosimetric treatment planning so that technical and clinical patient queries can be appropriately answered or referred.

Field-Modifying Instruments

Beam-modifying absorbers known as *filters* or *wedges* can be placed in the path of a beam. A typical beam-modifying filter is a wedge-shaped device made of dense material such as lead that progressively extends the beam across the field. The wedge has thick and thin sides, a shape that creates tilted isodose curves. The angle of the wedge is the angle through which an isodose curve is tilted at the central axis of the beam and at a specific depth. The degree of tilt changes with the depth; therefore, the predetermined depth is critical. Although the reference depth may vary, the wedge angle is commonly defined at the intersection of the central axis of the beam and the 50% isodose curve. The *wedge angle* refers to the tilt of the isodose curve, not the angle of the wedge filter. The wedge angle or tilt produced by a wedge has a different angle than the wedge material. Some wedge filters with standard isodose curves are prefabricated; others can be customized by technicians[5] (Table 13-2). In contemporary LINAC treatment units, physical wedges have largely been replaced by virtual wedges. The virtual wedge enhances efficiency and minimizes the physical workload of radiotherapists.

Tissue Compensation

When a radiation beam is projected along an irregular or sloping surface, it causes bending of the isodose curves. Such distortion may result in unacceptable nonuniformity of dose within the target and has the potential to cause excessive irradiation of sensitive structures such as the spinal cord. Several techniques are used to eliminate this problem, such as the use of wedges and the addition of bolus material or compensators. In addition, treatment fields with thinner tissue planes can be blocked for the last few treatments to reduce radiation dose.[3]

A *bolus* is a tissue-equivalent material that is put directly on the patient's skin to even the irregular contours and to create a flat surface that normalizes the

Table 13-2 Field-Modifying Instruments, Glossary

Instrument	Definition
Wedge transmission factor	Ratio of the dose rated on the central axis with and without the wedge. Must be included in the dose calculation to account for progressive attenuation of the beam by the wedge.
Universal wedge	A given angle, fixed in the beam and applied to all beam widths up to a specific limit; creates uniform attenuation across the field.
Individualized wedge system	Multiple wedges designed for a particular field width. Beam passes through minimal material and slightly reduces the dose.
Dynamic wedging	Wedge effect by driving a collimator leaf across the field to increase the field size. Starting position of moving leaf receives higher dose, then final position.

Data from Bentel.[5]

radiation z beam (Figure 13-4). The use of a bolus differs from the application of a bolus layer, which is sufficiently thick to provide adequate dose build-up over the skin surface. A bolus layer is often referred to as a *build-up bolus.* When higher-energy beams are used, bolus application on the skin surface eliminates the skin-sparing advantage.

Compensators are designed to provide the required beam arrangement that occurs in the "missing" tissue when the body surface is irregular. The compensator is positioned at a distance from the target (15–20 cm away from the skin) in an effort to preserve the skin-sparing effect of the megavoltage machines. It should have adjustable dimensions and shapes. The compensator must account for beam divergence, linear attenuation coefficients of the filter material and soft tissues, and the reduction in scatter at different depths. Compensators are constructed of a variety of materials so as to accomplish their multiple objectives. For example, compensating wedges (C-wedges) are used for oblique beam incidence or curved surfaces and are made from metals such as copper, brass, or lead. Their function is to compensate for a missing wedge of tissue in the treatment field.[3,5]

The difference between a wedge filter (Figure 13-5) and a C-wedge is as follows: Wedge filters can be used as compensators but are primarily used for tilting the standard isodose curves through a certain wedge angle in conjunction with the wedge-pair technique. In contrast, the C-wedge is used *only* as a compensator to facilitate the use of the standard isodose charts without modification. As such, C-wedges are more clinically practical than wedge filters as compensators because they can be used for partial-field compensation. The C-wedge is used to compensate for only a portion of the irregularly shaped contour. A wedge filter is designed to be placed in the field in a fixed position and, therefore, cannot partially compensate for the treatment field. Additional applications of compensating filters include compensators for tissue heterogeneity (for total body irradiation) and improvement of dose uniformity in fields where nonuniformity of the dose arises from sources other than contour irregularity, such as with large-mantle fields.[3,5]

Patient Positioning and Immobilization Techniques

Patient positioning and immobilization are critical components of radiation treatment delivery. To achieve the goals of tumor kill and preservation of normal organs and tissues, it is mandatory that daily treatment be reproducible and accurate. If patient positioning is not exact and if immobilization devices are inadequate, lethal consequences could occur. Accuracy of radiation treatment depends on both dosimetric and geometric exactness. This section focuses on the elements necessary to achieve *geometric accuracy,* which refers to issues of patient positioning and immobilization.

Patients must be positioned so that the target is at the isocenter.[6] The advantage of isocentric technique over SSD is that the patient is not moved between fields. If the patient lies supine on a horizontal treatment couch, a single skin mark (such as a tattoo or permanent ink) will locate the center of the target volume that imaging has shown to be at a certain depth (*d*) beneath the surface. Table 13-3 describes steps for treatment setup for isocentric radiation therapy plans.[6]

To achieve treatment setup accuracy, it is essential that continuous evaluation by the team of radiation oncology professionals occur. Patients must also be assessed for safety and comfort. Patients will move if they are uncomfortable, and initially tense muscles may relax during the treatment process. Using wedges, pillows, and head cups can avoid this unintentional patient movement. The laser crosshair system is useful for providing additional markings for treatment setup guides that can ensure the patient is in the same

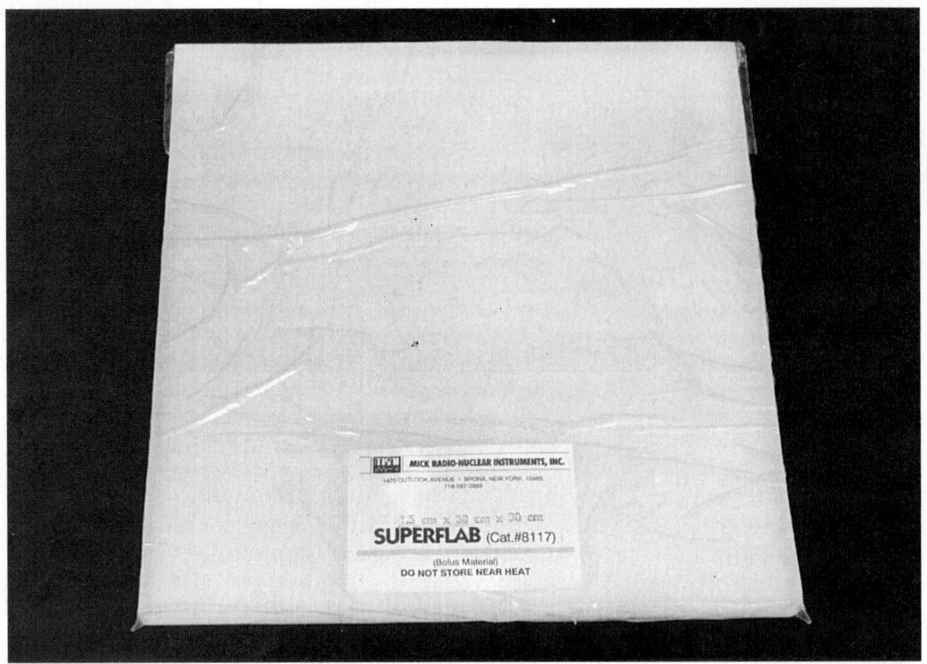

Figure 13-4 A bolus is a tissue-equivalent material placed in path of beam directly on the target surface. It modifies beam interaction with target surface. (Photo courtesy of Fox Chase Cancer Center.)

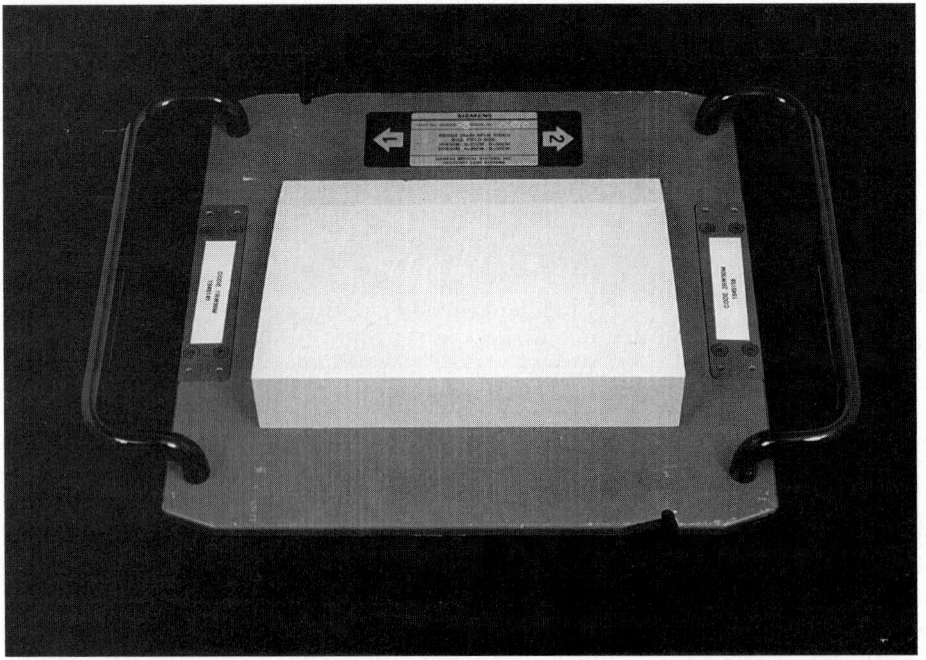

Figure 13-5 A wedge filter is placed in the path of radiation beam at a distance from the target and modifies radiation beam characteristics. (Photo courtesy of Fox Chase Cancer Center.)

position each day. Extending the skin markings as far superior and inferior to the central treatment plane will improve reproducibility of beams. External anatomical landmarks should always be referred to during daily treatment setup. The distance between several visible landmarks should be calculated to determine the accuracy of the positioning. In addition, immobilization devices should be used when appropriate. These

Table 13-3 Steps for Treatment Setup for Isocentric External Beam Radiation Therapy

1. Patient is positioned on the treatment couch in either a supine or prone position, with or without bolsters, wedges, or immobilization apparatus.
2. Treatment couch is raised to the required height to align patient coordinate system with the room coordinate system. Verification occurs by superpositioning of the orthogonal room lasers with the skin marks.
3. Gantry points straight down and secondary confirmation checks are made of the target-to-surface distance (TSD) using the optical distance indicator (ODI). This is identified as the proper treatment setup position.
4. Treatment plan is implemented for each field by proper rotation of the gantry and collimator as well as by choice of field and size beam modifiers. Before treatment, a secondary check of TSD should be made for each identified treatment field.
5. Complex treatment planning (multiple isocenters) may require further delineation of the patient coordinate system in relationship to the room and beam coordinate systems.

Data from Reinstein.[6]

devices begin as soft, flexible materials and then become rigid sanctuaries of comfort and security for patients during daily treatment.

Immobilization Devices

Immobilization devices help keep patients in a stationary position for daily treatment. These devices also help to minimize the potential for treatment setup errors, reduce the amount of radiation of normal tissues, and ensure appropriate treatment to the target volume. Patient immobilization equipment varies in terms of construction materials and style. Some are fabricated on site; others are available from commercial suppliers. Before implementing an immobilization system, it may be helpful to assess and evaluate the individual patient and treatment objectives. This inquiry can guide the radiation oncology team in creating a safe and comfortable physical environment for each patient.

The assessment begins by observing the patient's physical comfort and degree of relaxation. If the immobilization device touches the patient, it can serve as a reminder of how the position feels to the patient and therefore can be used to direct the therapists in replicating the setup. The patient must be secured in such a way as to preclude any movement. The immobilization equipment should be contoured to the patient's body surface. This equipment must fit the patient's anatomy properly and allow for variance in symmetry, body fat, and target location. The device should be able to position the patient in such a way as to minimize normal tissue complications. In addition, immobilization equipment should allow for unobstructed radiation beams and not interfere with the treatment plan. The material used to construct the devices should be radiotransparent, rigid, and able to be trimmed if necessary to remove sections. The devices must not cause mechanical obstruction by interfering with the LINAC gantry during beam rotation. Devices must be usable with all treatment planning systems to establish consistency for patient setup and treatment. If the radiation beam passes through the device, the effect on surface dose must be considered. Although the accumulation of surface build-up may be small, it must be documented.[6]

The immobilization device must allow sufficient space for reference marks to be seen so patient setup can be reproduced. The immobilization device defines the patient coordinate system, which must be aligned with the room coordinate system using reference marks. This alignment is achieved through the use of treatment tables and specialized adapters.[6]

The immobilization device must be rigid and maintain its shape over time. If the device loosens over time, the patient may move within it, which could potentially flaw the setup. Radiation therapists should assess the fit of the device daily, and determine normal wear and tear as well as changes in the patient's weight and environmental factors that may affect the required fit.

In recent times, every aspect of medical care has become subject to cost analysis. The costs of using complex immobilization systems must be evaluated in terms of the benefit to the clinical outcome. Factors affecting the cost of an immobilization system include materials, staff time for construction and setup, supplies, potential for recycling of materials, and available storage space.[6] Overall, immobilization devices have been identified as being beneficial and serve to enhance the administration of radiation treatments. Properly constructed immobilization devices can reduce daily setup times, increase efficiency, and reduce overall costs of treatment. Comfortable, well-fitting immobilization devices can reduce patients' fears and minimize misconceptions about treatment.

Immobilization devices have been identified by category. Following are the most common:

Hook-and-loop tape and straps

Many types of adhesive tape have been used in the past to secure patient position during treatment. Currently, straps with hook-and-loop backing are preferred to assist patient setup. Hook-and-loop tape can be affixed to the side rails of the treatment couch and then wrapped around the patient and attached to the

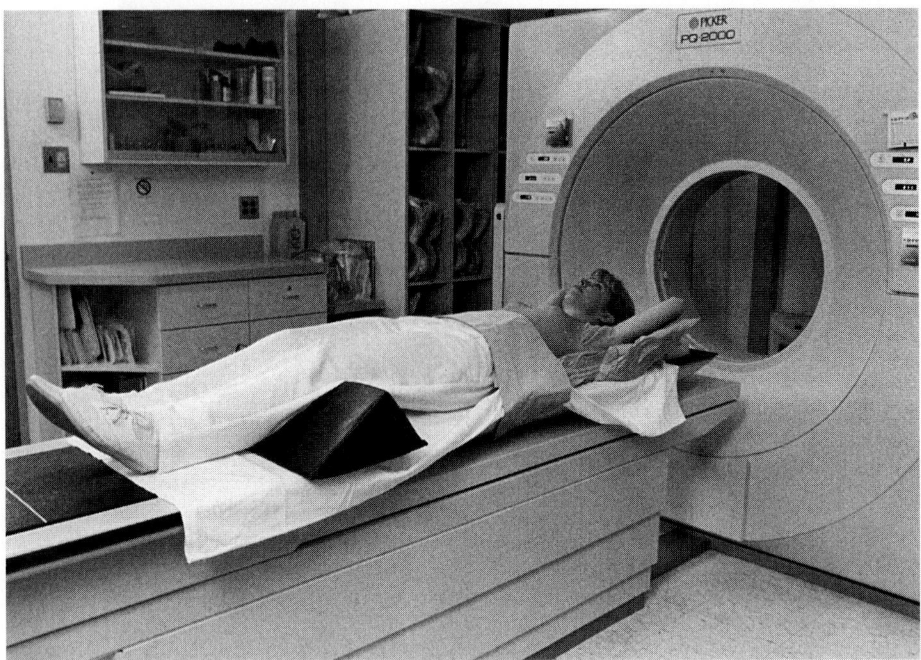

Figure 13-6 Various immobilization devices are used to maintain daily accurate reproducible patient positioning. Examples are the angle-wedged foam behind the knees and the custom-molded Alpha Cradle to support the head and torso. (Photo courtesy of Fox Chase Cancer Center.)

side rail hooks. These hook-and-loop straps are padded, reusable, and much more comfortable than adhesive tape. The hook-and-loop tapes can keep both of the extremities aligned and support the chin and head and neck region.

Generic body supports

Body supports include foam rubber wedges and supports, plastic head cups, neck rolls, knee and lumbar supports, thigh and heel stirrups, and prone face holders. This equipment provides comfort and stability during treatment. Indexed supports are a type of body support that are indexed by size, shape, and elevation above the treatment couch. These devices provide head and neck support as well as height and angle information for setup duplication.

Body casts

Methods and materials used to make effective body casts have evolved over the past two decades due to a need to reduce patient setup errors and to allow for three-dimensional (3D) conformal therapy treatment methods. Many of these materials originated in the specialties of orthopedics and dentistry and use modern packaging systems. For example, the Alpha Cradle (Smithers Medical Products, North Canton, Ohio) is a polyurethane foam cast that is created by placing the patient in the treatment position on a plastic bag held within a specialized form. The form is constructed of rigid polystyrene plastic blocks. When a combination of two chemicals known as Alpha Cradle Foaming agent is combined in the bag, the mixture reacts to form into a polyurethane foam. The foam rises and expands, supporting the patient's anatomical structures. When the foam hardens, the cast is ready to use. Alpha Cradles are effectively used for a variety of disease sites. They are rigid, are radiolucent, and fit snugly and comfortably to the patient's contours. Because, they are unable to prevent patient movement and rotation, they must be used in combination with other immobilization devices. Additional methods and materials used to create body casts are vacuum bags and thermoplastics (Figure 13-6).

Positioning Devices

Positioning devices secure patients in nontraditional positions for treatment (Figure 13-7). These devices are necessary to improve the therapeutic ratio and enhance patient comfort. Varied anatomical features coupled with nonrigid human body contours require the use of positioning devices to provide stability. Neck rolls, foam wedges, head holders, and Timo, a head and neck support (Bionix, Toledo, Ohio), are used to arrange body parts away from the path of the radiation beam and to improve positioning.

Arm boards, knee saddles, and thigh stirrups are other appliances used to position the extremities

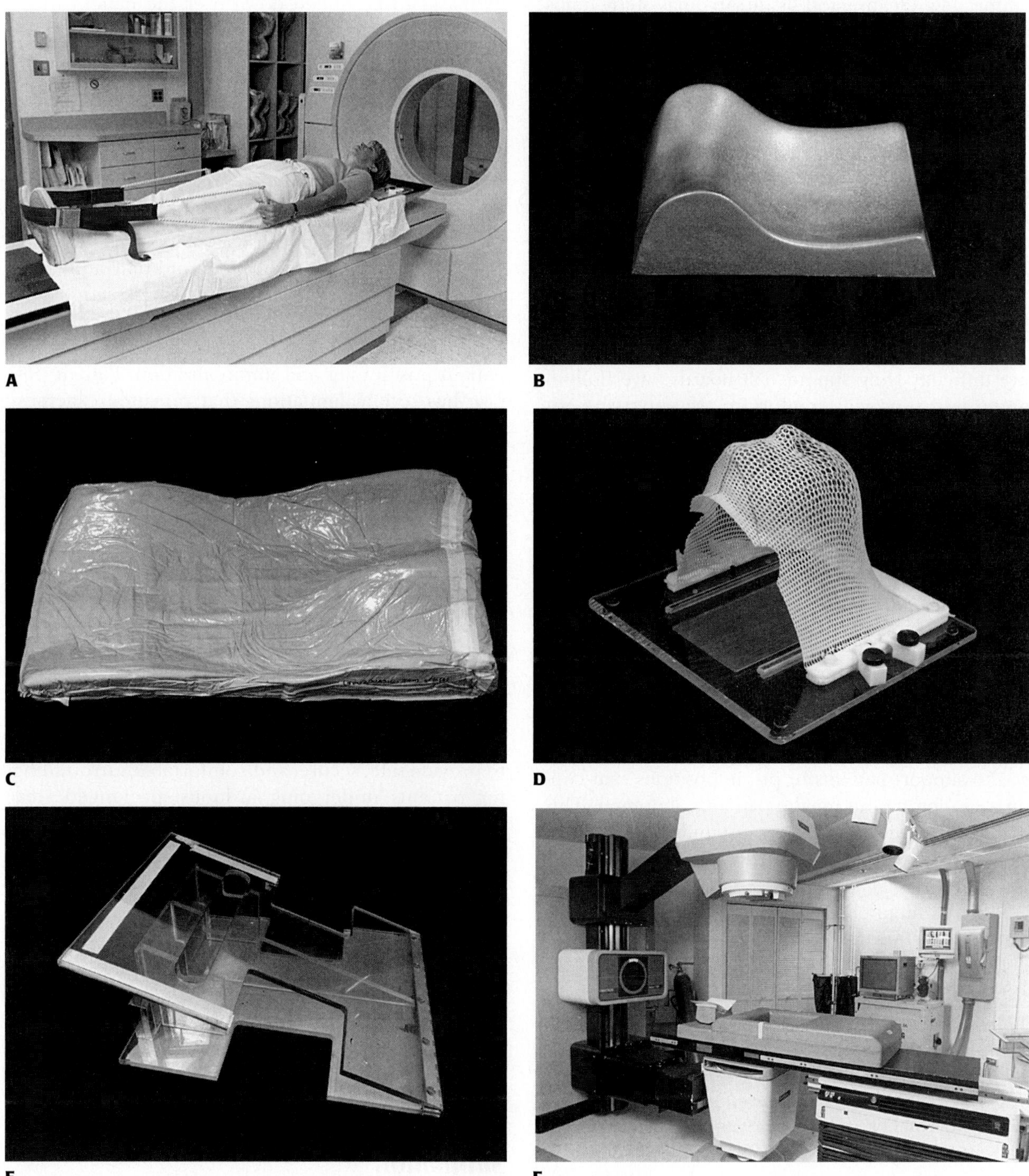

Figure 13-7 Positioning devices. **(A)** Hand and foot strap to pull shoulders down and out of the radiation path when treating the base of the neck. **(B)** Headrest for varying neck extension during treatment. **(C)** The Alpha Cradle is an anatomically molded custom positioning device. **(D)** Aquaplast is a head immobilization device of precut thermoplastic sheets that are attached to a rigid frame. **(E)** A breast board provides arms and breast support for improved treatment position. **(F)** A belly board is a prone position support with a window cutout for the abdomen that minimizes the amount of intestine in the treatment field. (Photos courtesy of Fox Chase Cancer Center.)

comfortably. Treating soft-tissue sarcomas of the limbs often requires careful positioning of the extremities, for example. Handgrips, overhead arm positioners, and shoulder retractors are also used to place extremities out of the path of critical treatment regions. Arms can be placed above the head or at the sides in reproducible locations with couch rail-mounted or tilt board-mounted handgrips and arm supports or with overhead arm positioners.

Patient elevation systems include tilt boards, slant boards, and breast boards. Patients who are required to maintain supine positions during treatment are often placed on tilting or slanting rigid plastic boards. These positioning devices can assist individuals who have difficulty lying supine. Tilt boards have built-in handgrips that provide comfort for arms-up treatment setups. The breast board is used most commonly for the treatment of breast cancer with parallel-opposed tangential fields. It allows for arm support above the shoulders and away from the lateral field. Additionally, it allows for unobstructed access to the breast by the lateral field, places the chest wall position horizontal to avoid angulation of the collimator, and by gravity pulls the large breast down for an improved treatment position. Several clinical circumstances must be considered when treating breast patients, such as stabilizing large pendulous breasts and minimizing skin reaction in the inframammary crease.

Belly boards are specialized positioning devices used to support patients in prone positions that contain a window cutout for the patient's abdomen. This equipment provides comfort and stability for obese patients and minimizes the amount of intestine in the field.

The treatment chair is a positioning device that is mounted on the treatment couch. It has head and neck supports and can accommodate a variety of arm positions. The treatment chair is used for patients with respiratory compromise and for mediastinal disease, as the position minimizes the amount of normal tissue that is irradiated during treatment.

Head fixation devices are used for immobilization during stereotactic radiosurgery and for treatment of head and neck cancer. Stereotactic radiosurgery requires the use of a frame that is bolted to the patient's skull before target localization. Metal stereotactic frames are not comfortable and are used for single fraction administration only. New noninvasive, relocatable frames are now available that enhance patient comfort and facilitate precise treatment planning. Nonstereotactic head immobilization is commonly used during treatment of head and neck regions. Such a device is commonly made of precut thermoplastic mesh sheets that are attached to a rigid frame. Warm water softens this system and enables the thermoplastic masks to be pulled down over the patient's face, molding to the facial contours; the masks are then attached to a base plate. Bite blocks use a dental impression mouthpiece supported by a solid base plate under the patient's head, which is fastened to the treatment couch. Adjustable bite blocks are often used in conjunction with a Timo support to steady the head and neck region.

Due to the enhancement of the specialty with 3D conformal therapy and dose escalation, it is essential that precise tumor control occur and that side effects be minimized. The ability to provide tight target margins, standardize dose, and maintain daily treatment reproducibility is directly related to the precision of patient positioning and immobilization. Patient position has several limitations that preclude exactness: variance among accelerators, simulators, and treatment planning coordinate systems; daily organ movement; organ movement during the treatment processes; patient movement during treatment; rotation of the skeleton; and treatment setup errors. Appropriate patient positioning and immobilization help to diminish errors and facilitate the delivery of precise radiation. Studies have concluded that immobilization systems assist in reducing the need for large target margins.[7–9] The combination of CT simulation with radiation therapy in the same treatment room and on the same machine has also become possible.

The multidisciplinary team must make it a priority to provide safe, secure, and comfortable surroundings for patients undergoing arduous, prolonged treatment. Nurses are in a key position to coordinate this effort by ensuring that patients are provided with comprehensive informed consent about these procedures and are encouraged to ask questions to demystify the fear of the unknown associated with radiation therapy and treatment protocols.

Treatment Techniques and Delivery: Advanced Topics

Computed Tomography–Based Simulation

In the past, computerized tomography and simulation were considered separate pretreatment procedures. Today, the two are considered a combined entity for radiation treatment planning. A CT simulator is a single diagnostic treatment planning machine that combines both procedures in one unit, minimizing the number of patient visits for pretreatment planning. In addition, CT simulation offers the advantages of increased speed, efficiency, and accuracy of treatment planning and delivery.

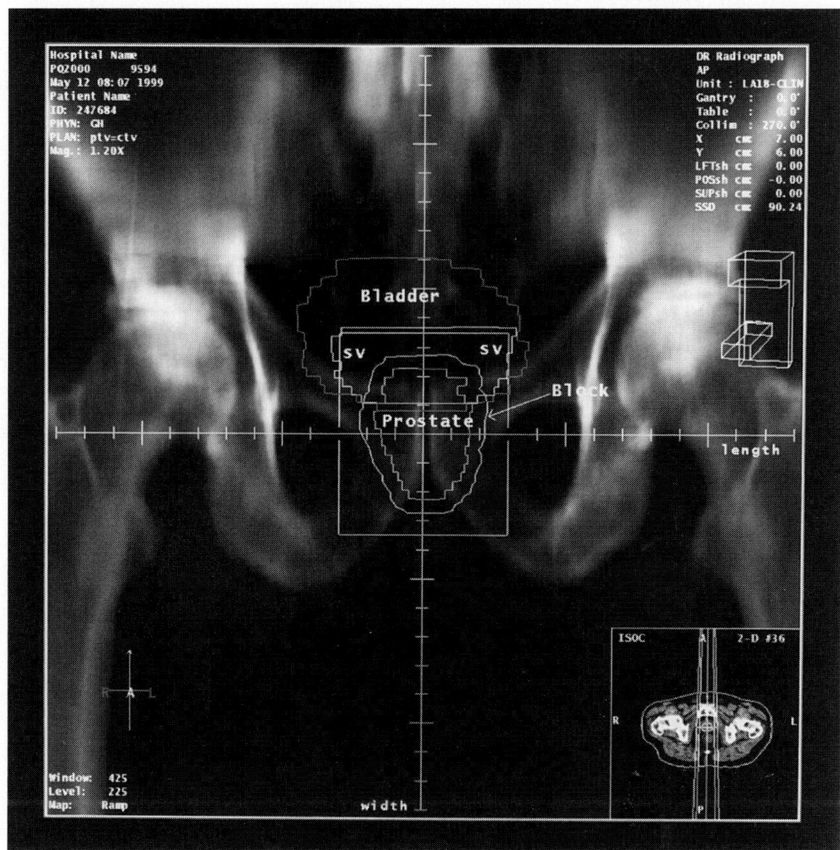

Figure 13-8 A digitally reconstructed radiograph of the pelvis is used for radiation therapy planning and documentation of radiation treatment fields. (Photo courtesy of Fox Chase Cancer Center.)

To accomplish this procedure, the patient is placed on the CT simulator table, and the tumor and normal structures are outlined on each CT slice. A computer performs a 3D transformation of the CT slices and creates a digitally reconstructed radiograph (DRR).[10] The DRR resembles a normal diagnostic film, but the images are digital and can be manipulated to improve contrast and detail (Figure 13-8). Radiation oncologists draw blocks directly on the DRR to accurately differentiate the tumor from normal surrounding tissue. The mold room uses the DRR to construct blocks. The DRR and all CT slices and outlines are then digitized into the treatment planning computer. One popular mode for retrieval and monitoring of DRRs entails use of a local area network (LAN), which enables physicians to obtain DRR and port film images on their desktop computers to ensure clinical quality assurance.[11]

Computer and other technological advances have also provided radiation oncology with the advantages of 3D conformal radiation therapy (3D CRT).[12] The virtual simulator is used to simulate the therapy machine and operates on a digital representation of the patient. Today, virtual simulation software is widely available for clinical treatment planning.[13] The process of virtual simulation differs from conventional simulation, yet still accomplishes the development of a fully documented beam arrangement. The steps to achieve virtual simulation are detailed in Figure 13-9.[14] Patients are immobilized in hemibody foam torso casts and custom foam head supports with thermal plastic face masks. Next, they are placed in the immobilization device and then registered electronically with the monitoring equipment on a CT scanner table. Head casts are secured to the CT table by use of a head holder. The body casts are also registered for daily alignment using lasers. A coordinate system is used to localize objects and is tailored to the individual patient.

Once the CT scans have been completed, the structures to be treated, target volumes, and critical structures to avoid are identified. Structures are outlined on a computer display of the scans. These outlines delineate the parameters for creating 3D graphical displays and for performing volume, dose volume, and other geometric calculations. Drawing and defining these parameters is a time-consuming endeavor. In the future, advances in computer algorithms for pattern

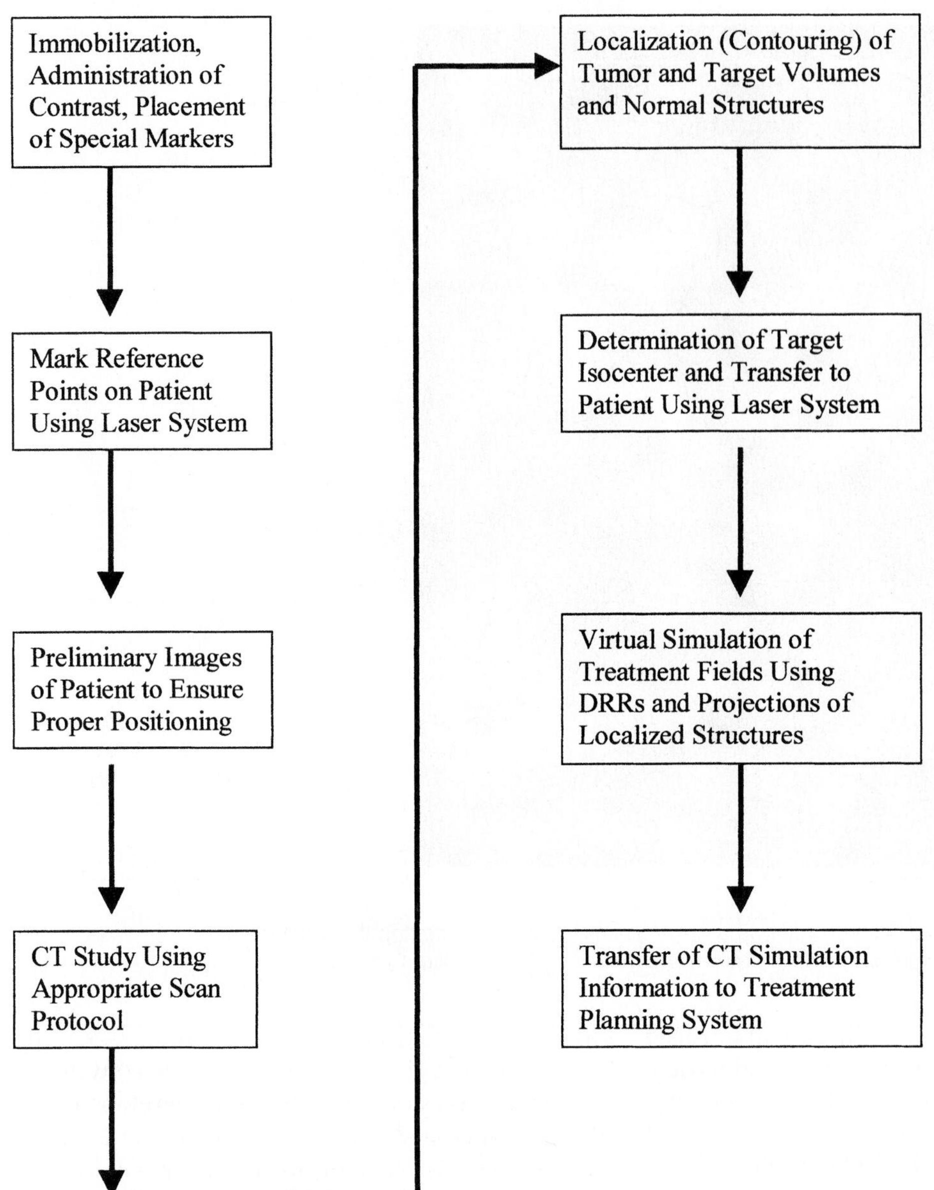

Figure 13-9 Computerized tomography simulation process. (Reprinted with permission from Hunt M: Localization and field design using a CT simulator, in Coia LR, Schultheiss TE, Hanks GE (eds.): *A Practical Guide to CT Simulation*. Madison, WI, Advanced Medical Publishing, 1995, p 37.[14])

recognition will likely eliminate the need for manual depictions.[13]

Virtual simulation is similar to physical simulation in that it requires a machine that can imitate the motions of the actual treatment machine. The virtual simulator display has seven panels that provide a superset of the functions of both a conventional simulator and a treatment machine. The unit control panel provides the same functions as the traditional simulator. The table can be oriented along three axes; the collimator or gantry can be rotated; and the jaws of the machine can be opened or closed by operating the corresponding control with a computer mouse. Documentation of conventional simulation consists of chart notes, simulation films, and skin marks. Virtual simulation documentation is related to these parameters and includes beam parameter settings and hard-copy block templates for the block fabrication room or multileaf collimator parameters. These are communicated over a computerized network that controls the multileaf collimator subsystem.[12]

Virtual simulation provides for the exact identification of structures that can be visualized on CT scans as well as conformation of beam outlines to target shapes

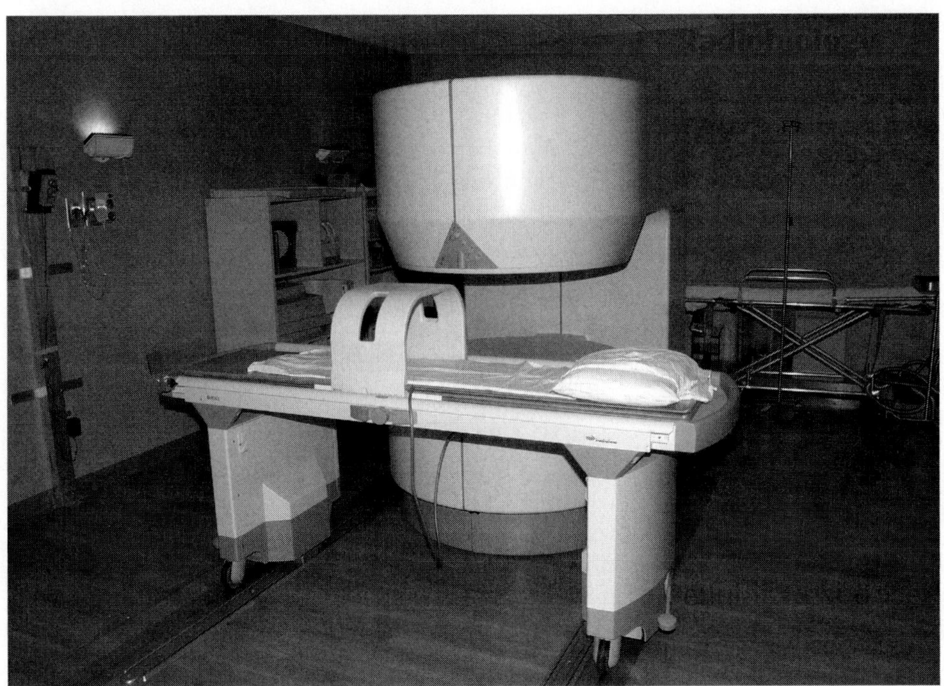

Figure 13-10 MRI Simulator The MRI simulator precisely identifies anatomic regions of tumor target and vital tissues and organs to be spared and provides information for accurate radiotherapy beam placement. Patients are positioned either prone or supine on the couch of the simulator and the MRI unit surrounds them. The MRI simulator is valuable for localization of deeply seated tumors such as pelvic malignancies. (Photo courtesy of Fox Chase Cancer Center.)

with small margins from any direction. Note that some precautions need to be considered when using this advanced practice technique. For instance, patient motion and internal organs are sometimes not visualized as clearly on virtual simulation as on fluoroscopic simulation. It is important to be aware of the potential for daily error due to the diminished visualization of structures. Virtual simulation often results in a CT study of greater than 100 scans, which is a large amount of data to review to form contours of structures. In addition, virtual simulation is sometimes unable to provide a well-defined clinical target volume (CTV) for some tumor sites. In this event, it becomes necessary for radiation oncologists and dosimetrists to rely on the natural history of the patient's disease to identify the appropriate CTV.

Virtual simulation is integral for conformal treatment planning and for achieving complicated configurations.[13] Magnetic resonance imaging (MRI) simulators are now being used to enable more accurate delineation of targets and critical normal structures where clinically indicated. (Figure 13-10)

Conformal Radiation Therapy: 3D Treatment Planning

Three-dimensional treatment planning and CRT delivers a radiation dose to a target with an improved margin for sparing normal tissue compared to standard two-dimensional treatment. Researchers working around the world have developed 3D and conformal treatment methods.[12,15] The overall goal driving the research and development of this treatment advance was to create a modality that would conform the radiation prescription to the target volumes and deliver lower doses to surrounding normal structures.[12] Today, the most common clinical application of 3D CRT is for prostate cancer.[12] Table 13-4 describes the process of 3D treatment planning and CRT.

The process of 3D CRT is complicated and requires radiographic verification of the simulation procedure in some patients to confirm the accuracy of 3D plans. Block checks and a comparison of portal films with the DRR using bony landmarks are performed. The dosimetrist provides dose calculations and treatment parameters, which are recorded on the treatment record. Common tumor sites treated with 3D CRT include the prostate, lung, head and neck, brain, and hepatobiliary tract. Clinical research in 3D CRT has focused on technical improvements with immobilization and dose delivery, reduction of dose to normal structures, and dose-escalation studies to increase dose to the target volume in an effort to improve local tumor control and survival.

Patient selection for 3D CRT must focus on individuals who will benefit from this treatment delivery system. Patients with tumors surrounded by complicated

Table 13-4 Process of 3D Treatment Planning and Conformal Radiation Therapy

- Clinical evaluation of patients, including tumor staging, functional status of uninvolved organs, and performance status
- CT simulation and placement of anatomical reference marks, and the creation of an immobilization device to assist with positioning
- Outline of target volumes (gross, clinical, and planning GTV, CTV, and PTV) and surrounding normal structures and transfer of these contour data to the 3D treatment planning system
- Virtual simulation with CT data for anatomical reconstruction and portal outline, dose planning, and beam selection for plan optimization, including the generation of DRRs
- Portals are designed using the beam-eye view (BEV) tool and beam arrangements using the room-eye view (REV), which is used to set the isocenter position and monitor beam arrangements
- Evaluations and rendering of the final plan once clinical precision is accomplished
- Review of final set of DRRs, and determination of cerrobend blocks or multileaf collimation settings

Data from Chao, Perez, Brady.[12]

anatomy, irregular-shaped tumors, or tumors near radiation-sensitive normal structures are considered good candidates for such therapy. In constrast, achieving dose escalation can be a challenge in patients with cancers affecting certain sites with serial architecture (spinal cord and brain) due to the potential for complications. Some identified benefits of 3D CRT include improved local tumor control due to better coverage of the target volume with a specific dose of radiation, less acute and late morbidity, the existence of dose-escalation studies, and improved survival. The efficiency of 3D CRT is improving, and more patients are being treated using this approach.

Three-dimensional treatment planning requires tremendous precision and accuracy. It is therefore essential that a quality assurance (QA) program include the entire multidisciplinary team, be thorough, and provide for monitoring and evaluation of all parameters of these advanced treatment modalities. The testing of hardware and software and the methodical review of individual patient treatment plans must be included as part of the program. Three-dimensional physics and treatment planning includes the use of multimodality imaging to define the gross tumor volume (GTV) and CTV more precisely. MRI and PET are used to supplement CT data. In the future, research will focus on the study of improved clinical outcomes as well as efficiency and cost-effectiveness in prospective clinical trials.[12]

Intensity-Modulated Radiation Therapy

Intensity-modulated radiation therapy (IMRT) is a novel technology that can deliver a precise dose of radiation to the target and spare normal surrounding tissues. The beam intensity in IMRT varies across the treatment field and irradiates the tumor using a series of small beams of different strengths. These small beams are created by the use of a multileaf collimator or a dynamic multileaf collimator.[12] The tumor receives the dose from these beams using a crossfire technique, which creates a uniform dose, sparing the surrounding tissues. The difference between IMRT and 3D CRT is that 3D CRT uses radiation beams of uniform strength. The treatment planning software used for IMRT is based on inverse planning. The inverse planning algorithms start with the ideal distribution and then find the beam characteristics or profiles necessary to produce the intended plan. This contrasts with conventional forward planning, in which a number of beams are directed from different directions. The conventional beams cannot treat a tumor surrounding a vital organ due to their inability to avoid dosing the normal tissue. Conversely, the IMRT technology provides for separation of the tumor from adjacent structures and tissues.[12] It is considered an advanced treatment planning system and may eventually replace 3D planning, although more clinical experience is needed before its application in the community becomes widespread.[16]

Stereotactic Radiosurgery

Stereotactic radiosurgery is a 3D technique that delivers the entire desired dose in one fraction. Stereotactic principles guide radiosurgery and target intracranial lesions through the use of multiple beams. The concept of radiosurgery evolved in 1951 from Lars Leksell, a Swedish neurosurgeon. His work focused on the use of a specially designed isotope unit known as the gamma knife, which was responsible for the evolution of many radiosurgical procedures. Limited availability of the gamma knife kept radiosurgery largely inaccessible until the mid-1980s,[16,17] when researchers began to adapt LINACs to administer radiosurgery. This made radiosurgery more widely available, as many radiation oncologists and neurosurgeons purchased hardware and software to upgrade their LINACs. Stereotactic techniques have since expanded beyond the scope of neurosurgical procedures. During this last decade, they have been applied to fractionated treatments, known as *stereotactic radiotherapy*, and applications outside of the brain.[17]

Radiosurgery techniques use a stereotactic frame fixed to the patient's skull to provide accurate land-

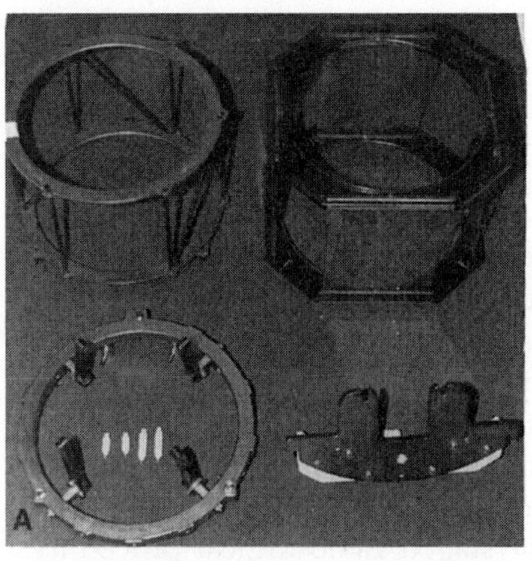

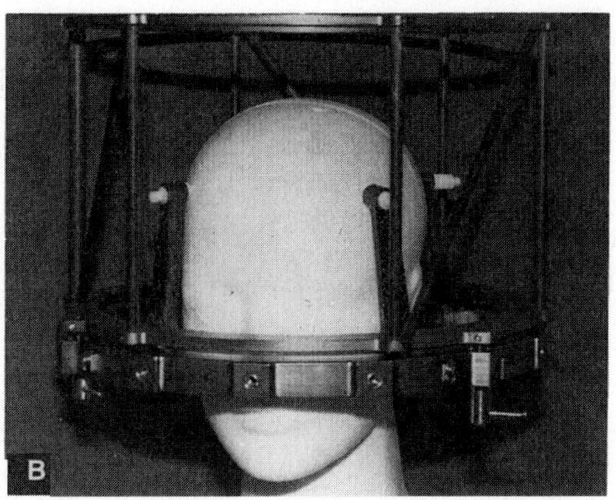

Figure 13-11 Stereotactic frame. **(A)** Basic stereotactic system with angiographic localizer *(upper right),* computerized tomographic localizer *(upper left),* head ring with post and pins *(lower left),* and a mount for positioning the patient onto the table *(lower right).* **(B)** Computerized tomographic localizer. (Reprinted with permission from Sherouse GW: Radiotherapy simulation, in Khan, FM, Potish RA (eds.): *Treatment Planning in Radiation Oncology.* Baltimore, Williams and Wilkins, 1998.[13])

Table 13-5 Unique Features of Stereotactic External Beam Irradiation to the Brain

- Small volumes of 1–30 cm^3 are treated.
- Single radiation fraction is commonly delivered.
- Target localization and treatment planning require expert and precise planning.
- High-dose gradients at field edges minimize dose deposition outside the target volume.
- Beams intersect at a common point within the skull; 3D distribution of beams minimizes the volume of normal tissue receiving moderate or high doses of radiation.

Data from Chao, Perez, Brady.[12]

marks for localization of intracranial targets (Figure 13-11). These targets are correlated with neuroimaging studies such as MRI, CT, and angiography. The purpose of the frame is to provide a basis for target identification within an *x*, *y*, and *z* coordinate system. This system is used to define the shape and extent of the target lesion.[12] Table 13-5 describes the unique features of stereotactic external beam irradiation.[12]

Radiosurgery is indicated for distinct lesions, less than or equal to 4 cm, with the potential to respond to a single fraction of radiation. Ideal targets for radiosurgery are almost entirely spherical and small ($\leq$ 3 cm in maximum dimension). Irregular volumes can present the challenge of treating many isocenters to achieve conformation to the target volume. Although primary and metastatic brain tumors are most commonly treated, the greatest clinical experience has involved treatment of arteriovenous malformations (AVMs).[12]

The two radiosurgery systems used are the gamma knife and the LINAC-based system. Both systems consist of a stereotactic frame, radiation delivery system, and computer hardware and treatment planning software. The radiosurgery system utilizes MRI or CT information to locate and determine target size and location, treatment planning needs, and type of radiation delivery. Although the systems vary, the clinical outcomes for treatment should be the same for similar patient groups.

The cost of the gamma knife system ranges from approximately $3.5 million to $4.2 million, including new facility construction. The cobalt sources decay after seven years and must be replaced at a significant cost. The unit contains cobalt distributed in 201 sources over a portion of a hemisphere so that circular beams from collimators may enter the skull through a large number of evenly distributed points. The gamma knife has a permanent 18,000-kg shield surrounding a hemispheric array of cobalt sources. Four interchangeable outer collimator helmets are used to vary the target volume. Individual collimators can be plugged in to conform the dose to the target shape. The target size is about 3–18 mm, with a 0.1-mm degree of accuracy.[12,18]

The LINAC can be adapted to administer stereotactic radiation and is available at a much lower cost ($50,000–$300,000) than the gamma knife. Target sizes of the LINAC range from 10 to 50 mm, with an accuracy of 0.1–1.0 mm. The LINAC administers radiosurgery in the following ways:

1. The gantry rotates through an arc for each of several stationary couch angles.

2. In dynamic stereotactic radiosurgery, the gantry and couch move simultaneously, and the beam of entry on the skull resembles a seam. This seam provides an advantage, in that beam entrance and exit doses do not overlap.
3. A rotating chair aligns and immobilizes the patient's head in a stationary radiation beam.

Approximately six months after radiosurgery, MRI is used to monitor the development of edema or potential radiation sequelae. The PET scan has emerged as a way to differentiate tumor from necrosis in previously irradiated patients.[12] Whole-body stereotactic treatment is now being implemented in some centers where appropriate.

Image-Guided Cyberknife Radiosurgery

The Cyberknife is an innovative frameless robotic radiosurgical system that is based on the original concept of frame-based radiosurgery. It includes three components: an advanced, lightweight LINAC; a robot; and x-ray cameras. The miniature LINAC produces high-energy (6 MeV) radiation. It is mounted on a robotic arm, which directs the LINAC to deliver radiation beams to the targeted tumor from multiple positions and angles. Image guidance cameras are used to locate the target, to take frequent pictures of the tumor during treatment, and to target the radiation beam emitted by the linear accelerator. The Cyberknife uses its robotic arm to deliver highly focused beams of radiation that converge at the tumor. Thus the tumor receives a cumulative dose of radiation to control or destroy the tumor cells while radiation exposure to surrounding tissue is minimized. The Cyberknife is able to compensate for patient movement to ensure highly accurate delivery of radiation during treatment. When patient movement occurs during treatment, the cameras detect the position change, and the robot is able to compensate for the movement by repositioning the LINAC before administering the radiation beam. This process of constantly correcting for beam placement ensures accurate tumor targeting.[19,20]

The first Cyberknife prototype was installed for clinical use at Stanford University in 1994. Cyberknife technology was finally approved by the FDA for general use in August 2001. Standard stereotactic techniques require that a rigid metal frame be affixed to a patient's skull for immobilization and target localization purposes. Although the frame-based systems have been effective clinically, they have many limitations, including restricting treatment fields to the brain, limiting the angles for radiation targeting, and patient discomfort. As an alternative to standard frame-based radiosurgical instruments, the Cyberknife uses noninvasive, image-guided localization and a robotic delivery system. This technological combination enables the Cyberknife to supercede the limitations of older frame-based radiosurgery such as the gamma knife and LINAC.

The unique mechanism of the Cyberknife provides a noninvasive, surgical-like outcome for lesions of the brain and spine. It is the first and only commercial application of robotic stereotactic radiosurgery for the spine and the spinal cord. Additionally, this technology has the benefit of enabling the Cyberknife system to be used for radiosurgical applications outside the brain as well as for staged radiosurgical procedures. Staged radiosurgery (i.e., fractionated radiosurgery) occurs when the total dose of stereotactic radiation is divided into several smaller doses with delivery spanning several days. The Cyberknife has provided radiosurgery (1–5) fractions on targets throughout the body.

Cyberknife radiosurgery has also been effectively used to treat selected lung malignancies.[21] The combination of investigational software and hardware with Cyberknife technology can deliver conformal radiation to moving primary and metastatic lung tumors if surgery is not an option. The Cyberknife accommodates lung and tumor motion, enabling modifications to be made so as to deliver a maximal therapeutic dose while minimizing surrounding tissue toxicity. Lung cancer patients have been treated on a dose-escalation study of 15–25 Gy and carefully monitored for toxicity.[21] This procedure involves a planning CT scan; foam mold construction for immobilization; and the placement of a radiographic fiducial, a gold seed that is implanted in the tumor and used for computer tracking. Once the radiation oncologist and the medical physicist design treatment plans, the patient receives the delivery of the prescribed radiation treatment using the Cyberknife. Its computer-controlled robotic device modifies radiation beam delivery as necessary to accommodate tumor movement. Patients are encouraged to breathe normally, as the rhythmic breathing enables the computer to track the process. The entire pretreatment evaluation and planning process spans several days. The actual treatment time takes approximately 1.5 hours.[21]

Treatment procedure

Once patients are assessed and evaluated by the multidisciplinary team, the treatment process commences. This process involves the following three steps: (1) treatment setup, (2) treatment planning, and (3) treatment delivery. Each of these procedures can occur either on the same day or on separate visits. Unlike with conventional stereotactic radiosurgery, the Cyberknife treatment planning procedure does not require that the patient be confined in an acute care setting while the plan is formulated. Patients are ambulatory and able to return home in between treatment planning appointments.

During treatment setup, the radiation oncology team plans the overall details of radiation delivery. If a cranial tumor is being treated, a custom-fit plastic mask is made for the patient. This mask serves the same purpose as the conventional metal head frame used during stereotactic radiosurgery, but is noninvasive and painless. The patient has a CT scan with iodinated dye contrast (and sometimes an MRI is obtained for full visualization) with the mask in place. The CT data are then integrated into the treatment planning software, and digitally reconstructed radiographs demonstrating various patient positions are correlated with images of the target so that the computer can identify in three-dimensional space exactly where the lesion is located.[22]

Cyberknife treatment planning utilizes the clinical experience of both the radiation oncologist and the physicist as well as the power of high-speed computers to determine the volume, dose, and pattern of radiation beam target. During this planning phase, the Cyberknife performs millions of calculations to determine the most effective radiation delivery plan.

Soon after treatment planning is complete, the patient returns for treatment delivery. During treatment, the patient lies supine on the treatment table and is fitted with the appropriate immobilization device. At the beginning of the actual treatment, the imaging system acquires digital x-rays of tumor localization and patient position. This information is transmitted to the robotic arm, which is used to move the LINAC to the appropriate position. As treatment proceeds, the robot moves and retargets the LINAC at multiple positions around the patient. At each position, a small radiation beam is delivered. This process is repeated at 50–300 different positions around the patient to complete treatment. At various intervals, the LINAC stops and takes additional pictures, allowing the Cyberknife to track and compensate for slight physical movement.

The total process takes 30–90 minutes to deliver radiation beams. One fraction or multiple treatments (fractionated) may be prescribed, which requires the patient to return for a repeat treatment session. The Cyberknife is able to treat larger lesions than conventional radiosurgery (up to 6 cm). Typically, patients are assessed and can be discharged immediately upon completion of treatment to resume their normal activities.

Patient education and preparation

Radiation oncology nurses assume the primary responsibility for educating patients who will undergo image-guided Cyberknife radiosurgery. For this reason, nurses must be involved in the initial assessment of patients. Educational goals should be formulated in conjunction with the entire multidisciplinary team. Patients and families require explicit verbal informed consent accompanied by comprehensive written information and visual materials, including the option of a tour of the equipment and treatment area. Each patient must be considered individually, and an accurate assessment made about the amount of information to be provided. Nurses must ensure that educational preparation commences prior to therapy, during therapy, upon discharge, and during follow-up encounters. It is vital that patients be given adequate time for understanding advanced concepts related to procedural details that will ensure safe and effective Cyberknife treatment outcomes.

Brachytherapy

Brachytherapy or implant therapy has been used clinically for more than 100 years. *Brachy* (from the Greek, meaning "short distance") describes radiation treatment where the radiation source comes in direct contact with the tumor. With brachytherapy, dose distribution is dependent on the inverse square law, because the source is usually directly located within the tumor volume. It is therefore crucial that the radiation sources be placed with high precision. Brachytherapy procedures can be done with either temporary or permanent implants. Temporary implants usually have long half-lives and higher energies than permanent implants. These radiation sources can be manufactured in several forms, such as needles, seeds, and ribbons (Figure 13-12). Temporary radiation sources are inserted into catheters that are surgically placed in the tumor. A few days postoperatively, the patient is brought to the radiation department for simulation. Wires with nonradioactive metal seeds are then threaded into these catheters. Films are taken, and the image of the seed placement is digitized into a brachytherapy treatment planning computer. Once the treatment plan is complete and the optimal dose rate is selected, the radioactive sources can be inserted. The implantation occurs in the patient's room. The duration is usually 1–3 days. Most temporary implants are loaded interstitially.[23]

Implantation techniques may be characterized in terms of the type of surgical approach within the target volume (interstitial, intracavitary, transluminal, or mold techniques), the means of controlling the dose delivered (temporary or permanent implants), and the dose rate (low, medium, or high). *Interstitial brachytherapy* is the surgical implantation of small radioactive sources directly into target tissues. Permanent

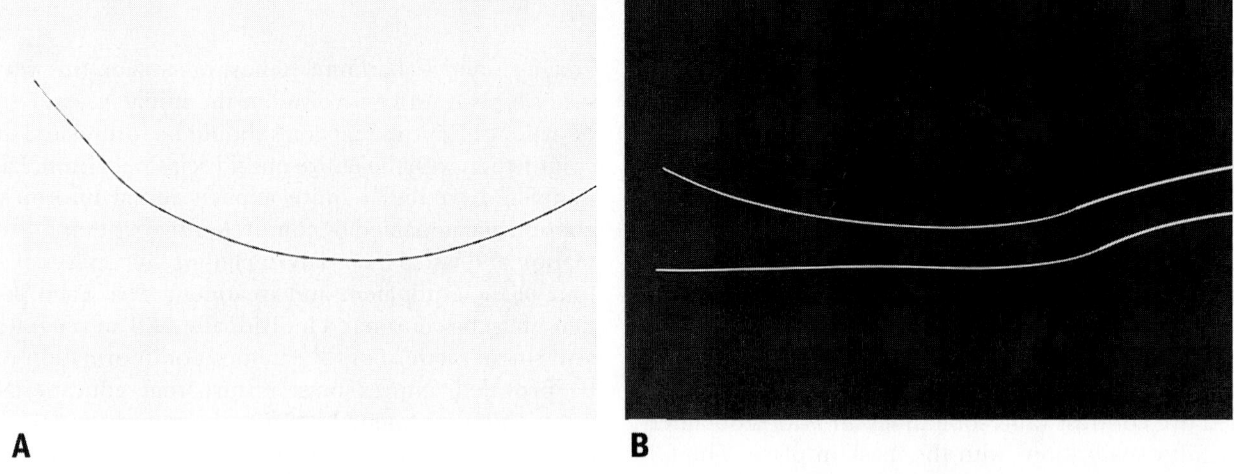

Figure 13-12 Brachytherapy sources. **A.** Iridium ribbon. **B.** Loading catheter for iridium seeds. (Photo courtesy of Fox Chase Cancer Center.)

interstitial implants remain in place forever. The initial source strength is chosen so that the prescribed dose is fully delivered when the implanted radioactivity has decayed to a negligible level. *Interstitial low-dose rate* (LDR) *brachytherapy* is commonly used to treat cancer of the oral cavity, oropharynx, prostate, and sarcoma. Intracavitary insertion consists of positioning applicators with radioactive sources into a body cavity close to the target tissue. The most commonly used intracavitary treatment technique entails insertion of a tandem and colpostat for cervical cancer. Intracavitary implants are temporary; they are inserted in the patient for a specified time (usually 24–168 hours after source insertion for LDR therapy). *Transluminal brachytherapy* is the insertion of a line source into a body lumen to treat its surface and adjacent tissues. *Plesiocurie* or mold therapy is a surface-dose application, which consists of an applicator containing a variety of radioactive sources designed to deliver a uniform dose distribution to the skin or mucosal surface.[12]

The International Commission on Radiation Units and Measurements (ICRU) determines dose rates of implants.[24] Low-dose rate (LDR) implants deliver doses at a rate of 40–200 cGy/hour (0.4–2.0 Gy/hour), requiring treatment times of 24–144 hours. High-dose rate (HDR) brachytherapy delivers dose rates in excess of 0.2 Gy/minute (12 Gy/hour). Modern HDR remote afterloaders contain sources capable of delivering dose rates of 0.12Gy/second (432 Gy/hour) at 1 cm distance, resulting in brief treatment times. A shielded vault and remote afterloading device are essential components of a HDR brachytherapy facility. LDR implant patients are confined to the hospital during treatment to manage the potential radiation safety hazard of the implant. HDR brachytherapy is performed as an outpatient procedure. Although the ultra-low-dose rate range is not recognized by the ICRU, it is important in the implementation of treatment with permanent iodine-125 (^{125}I) and palladium-103 (^{103}Pd) seed implants. The clinical application and usefulness of radionuclides depend on physical properties such as half-life, radiation output per unit activity, specific activity, and photon energy. In the past, radium was the primary isotope used in brachytherapy. Due to its long half-life and high energy output, radium has been replaced with cesium (Cs), gold (Au), and iridium (Ir). These isotopes have shorter half-lives than radium and can be shielded more easily due to their low energies.[12]

Traditional implant systems known as Manchester, Quimby, and Paris were developed before computer-assisted dosimetry for implant therapy became available. These classic systems continue to guide the radiation oncologist in arranging and positioning sources for target volumes identified intraoperatively by palpation and direct visualization. Additionally, they may serve as the basis for dose prescription independent of the use of computer-assisted planning. Classic systems are useful for preplanning of interstitial implants and for manually verifying postimplant computer plans.[12]

By using remote afterloading devices, radiation exposure can be diminished for hospital personnel and particularly for nursing staff who are primarily responsible for source loading and the care of implant patients. This delivery system consists of a pneumatically or motor-driven source transport system that robotically transfers radioactive material between a shielded safe and each treatment applicator. HDR and LDR are the two types of remote afterloading that can be used. The most common LDR source is ^{137}Cs, which has a dose rate of about 1 cGy/minute. The most common HDR source is ^{192}Ir, with a dose rate of 100 cGy/minute.[4,12]

Pretreatment brachytherapy procedures are similar to remote afterloading brachytherapy. The treatment plan is developed by the physicists and approved by the radiation oncologists, then the patient is escorted and set up in the treatment room. The LDR or HDR source is connected to the end of a cable inside the afterloading unit. This unit has data from the planning computer. The cable is directed out of the unit into one of the patient's catheters. Several catheters can be connected to the unit. Each catheter is irradiated, one at a time, until the designated dose is achieved. The motor that drives the source out of the treatment unit is connected electronically to the treatment room door. If the need arises for cessation of treatment, opening the door will cause the source to draw back into the unit by an interlocking system. This safety device lessens the danger of personnel exposure. This interlock is the safety advantage integral to the use of this delivery system compared to manual afterloading.[25]

LDR remote afterloading is commonly used for intracavitary treatment of uterine cancer. All LDR procedures are performed in the patient's room. The interlock is connected to the patient's door so nurses can give care and family members can visit without risk. The most common applications of HDR brachytherapy include treatment of sarcomas and tumors of the vaginal apex, esophagus, lung, and floor of the mouth. Most HDR treatments are performed on an outpatient basis, which constitutes a tremendous advantage for afterloading brachytherapy.[26,27]

Partial Breast Irradiation

Brachytherapy as a primary treatment modality for early-stage breast cancer is now being considered in selected patients following breast conservation surgery.[28–30] Historically, breast cancer treatment focused on the need to treat the entire breast to achieve local control. Over time, local recurrences have commonly occurred at the vicinity of the surgical incision and have arisen even if the entire breast was irradiated.[28] For this reason, the focus of treatment for individuals who qualify with early-stage breast cancer has changed to include the concept that partial breast irradiation (PBI) targeted at the lumpectomy cavity with a small surrounding margin will yield similar local control to whole-breast irradiation.

Two types of brachytherapy systems have been developed and are currently in clinical trials for targeting a specific population of early-stage breast cancer patients: the MammoSite Radiation Therapy System (Proxima Therapeutics, Georgia) and Intrabeam (Photoelectron Corporation, Massachusetts). Each system has a different administration technique for breast brachytherapy. The overall appeal of PBI is the avoidance of interstitial brachytherapy (with its requirements of insertion of multiple needles in the breast tissue, inpatient confinement, and concomitant infection risk) as well as a reduction of required treatment time for external beam therapy and concomitant side effects.[31]

MammoSite Radiation Therapy System

A targeted internal radiation therapy treatment modality referred to as MammoSite is indicated for patients with early-stage breast cancer who are candidates for lumpectomy. Approved by the FDA in 2002, the MammoSite system delivers high-dose radiation directly to the site of tumor excision, targeting the area where the cancer would most likely recur and sparing approximating healthy tissue.[32]

MammoSite can be used in conjunction with conventional external beam radiation as a boost or as primary treatment for a qualified patient. The new technology reduces the length of daily radiation treatment following surgery. Patients are able to receive a higher radiation dose due to targeted concentration to one specific area. MammoSite is considered the next generation of internal radiation therapy. It is minimally invasive, has a good safety profile, and can be performed as an outpatient procedure with high patient tolerance.

Treatment Procedure. The MammoSite balloon catheter is placed at the time of lumpectomy or within 10 weeks postsurgery. Catheter placement is performed either during the surgical procedure under general anesthesia or in an ambulatory procedure room under local anesthesia. The catheter is inserted into the surgical cavity either through a separate pathway created by a trocar or through the lumpectomy scar. Its balloon end is inflated with saline and a contrast agent to allow the surrounding tissue to conform to the balloon, the exit site is dressed, and the patient is discharged.

When surgical recovery is complete (usually within 24 hours), the patient is referred to radiation oncology for treatment planning. Radiation therapy is administered on an outpatient basis. During therapy, a ^{192}Ir seed (attached to a HDR remote afterloader) is inserted into the inflated balloon for a short duration (less than 10 minutes). When used as primary radiation therapy, two treatments are administered per day, for 5 days, to deliver the prescribed radiation dose (typically 34 Gy). When used as a boost with external beam radiation, a typical prescription requires treatment for 1–2 days. When the course of radiation therapy is complete, the balloon is deflated, the MammoSite catheter is removed, and no indwelling radioactive source remains.[33]

This technological advance is much more readily tolerated than conventional internal radiation therapy for breast cancer, in which radioactive seeds and multiple catheters are placed in the breast for each treatment. MammoSite is a simpler, more localized, and more effective treatment modality with a relatively low side-effect profile. Brachytherapy has been used successfully to treat many solid tumors but not commonly breast cancer. Now with the development of the MammoSite Radiation Therapy System, which allows the use of a single, flexible catheter and outpatient treatment, brachytherapy for early-stage breast cancer may eliminate the need to expose the entire breast to radiation. Currently, MammoSite is being prescribed alone and as a boost in conjunction with conventional external beam therapy. As more data are collected, the use of MammoSite without accompanying conventional external beam radiation therapy may become common practice in specific clinical situations.

Clinical data. Data are currently available from a number of studies indicating that PBI (restricted to the tumor bed after lumpectomy) can be used safely to reduce the time and toxicity associated with traditional radiation therapy, and to potentially make the option of breast conservation more widely available. A number of institutions over the past ten years have investigated the use of PBI as an alternative to whole-breast external beam radiation therapy (EBRT) with favorable results. Reported local recurrence rates are low and within the recurrence rates documented for patients treated with whole-breast EBRT.[28,34] These studies also demonstrated good or excellent cosmetic outcomes for patients treated with PBI. Patients enrolled in these studies were carefully selected to minimize the risk of significant residual tumor surrounding the lumpectomy cavity. Appropriate patient selection is essential to successfully treating patients with PBI as an alternative to whole-breast radiation therapy. Generally, patient criteria include a diagnosis of early-stage pathology of DCIS, breast cancer with tumors 3 cm or smaller in size, and age of 45 yeears or older.

Patient education and practice implications. The focus of patient care with the MammoSite system is percutaneous catheter and skin care. Nurses must assess catheters, provide routine care, and teach patients self-care. The skin at the insertion site should be assessed for erythema, edema, and exudate. Daily dressing of the entrance site includes cleansing with half-strength hydrogen peroxide and application of an antibiotic ointment and sterile dressing cover.[35] Patients are taught to keep catheters clean and dry (tub baths are permitted without submerging). Patients are taught the need for frequent temperature monitoring; an elevation of greater than 101°F, any redness or swelling of the breast, or increased tenderness or drainage from the catheter site must be reported immediately. Pain management can be assessed for and provided depending on the degree of incisional discomfort, which is usually mild.[31]

Upon completion of the final radiation therapy dose, the catheter is removed. The balloon is deflated, and then the radiation oncologist gently pulls the catheter from the breast cavity. Although it is not a painful procedure, the breast should be compressed gently over the lumpectomy site so that excess accumulated interstitial fluid is expressed. Additionally, the skin should be cleansed with half-strength peroxide solution and an antibiotic ointment applied to insertion site. This site should be covered with sterile gauze and redressed once daily until the skin is closed and scab formation occurs. Patients should be taught signs and symptoms of local and systemic infection and should avoid lifting the arm on the treatment side for a full 24 hours post-treatment. Side effects following MammoSite treatments have been reported as minimal and include pain, mild erythma, and dry desquamation.[35]

Intrabeam System

The Intrabeam brachytherapy system uses a single dose of intraoperative radiotherapy, in contrast to the fractionated dosing of MammoSite. Intrabeam is used both as primary treatment for specific breast cancer diagnoses and as a boost source to the tumor bed prior to external beam radiation. Candidates for Intrabeam therapy must meet the following criteria:

- Biopsy-proven breast cancer with lesions smaller than or equal to 2 cm
- Negative margin and infiltrating ductal pathology
- Negative node status
- Stage should be T1 (stage I)

If patients have bilateral, multifocal, or recurrent disease, they are excluded from treatment. Intrabeam has been used in stage II and stage III disease.[36]

The Intrabeam applicator is placed into the tumor bed in the operating room. The spherical applicator is between 1.5 and 5 cm in diameter, with 0.5-cm interval size increments available. The surgeon determines the appropriate applicator size and fit. Snug placement of the applicator in the lumpectomy cavity is recommended to ensure uniform treatment. Once breast placement is achieved, the applicator is attached to a small x-ray source and loaded with a probe approximately 3 mm in diameter. The radiation is then administered from the tip of the probe, which is inside the sphere from a 50 kV electronic generator, a device that resembles a small LINAC. Treatment energy emitted is low, and the radiation is absorbed quickly around the surface of the applicator. Thus skin and tissue sparing is provided. Radiation treatment time is about 30 minutes at a rate of 1 Gy/minute. Intrabeam intraoperative treatment is given once. When treatment is complete, the applicator is removed, and the surgical incision is closed.

Nursing care and practice implications. Patient education is paramount for this treatment approach. Preteaching and preparatory information, including candidacy criteria and procedures of applicator placement for Intrabeam therapy, will be invaluable to assist patients and to temper anxiety. Specific patient care needs with Intrabeam intraoperative treatment involves postsurgical wound care, minimizing risk of infection, and potential erythema at the insertion site, which may delay skin healing.[31]

Patient education, preparation, nursing, and interventions. It is challenging for patients experiencing a breast cancer diagnosis to comfortably navigate the nuances of the healthcare system. Individuals are required to make complicated choices regarding which treatment options to pursue, which healthcare professionals will prescribe and administer therapy, and which facility will offer the treatment. Patients experiencing a breast cancer diagnosis must be participative.[37] For their part, radiation oncology nurses must guide patients through the choices of technological treatment advances. Patients must understand the criteria for candidacy for breast-conserving surgical procedures as well as the options available postsurgery for brachytherapy treatment modalities. The prospective delivery of concise, detailed information is most effective for providing information, which describes new procedures, risks, benefits, and supportive research data.

Unsealed Radionuclide Therapy

Unsealed radionuclide therapy is used for the treatment of benign or malignant thyroid disease, hematological disease, malignant bone disease, and benign or malignant disease within a body cavity. Table 13-6 lists the currently approved nonsealed radionuclide sources. Strict guidelines exist for the use of these sources in women; hence verification of a nonpregnant and nonbreast-feeding condition must be established prior to the initiation of therapy. A negative B human chorionic gonadotropin test within 48 hours before therapy, documented hysterectomy or tubal ligation, a postmenopausal state with no menstrual bleeding for 2 years, or premenarche are sufficient clinical indicators to proceed with treatment. Breastfeeding must be stopped for 1 or 2 weeks prior to administration of an unsealed radioactive source.[12]

Specific Nuclear Regulatory Commission (NRC) guidelines must be followed for determining inpatient or outpatient dose, which is dependent on the total body burden of the radioisotope. Nurses must consistently but safely render care to patients receiving unsealed radioisotope therapy. It is essential that nurses reduce their exposure to emitted radiation by using the principles of time, distance, and shielding. Institutional policy and procedure must be in place to manage the total program and process as well as the possibility of emergency spills. Institutions administering both teletherapy and brachytherapy must have preestablished standards of nursing practice to ensure effective patient management as well as radiation safety. These nursing actions must focus on individual patient needs and provide detailed practice guidelines for both routine and emergency requirements. Table 13-7 provides an overview of nursing practice standards from a national comprehensive cancer center (Fox Chase Cancer Center, Philadelphia, Pennsylvania). These standards provide details of clinical actions for both routine and emergent situations.

Institutions administering unsealed radioactive sources must have strict quality assurance (QA) policies and procedures in place. These programs should be guided by the NRC recommendations and focus on the protection of patients, the public, and medical personnel from the potential hazards of unnecessary exposure. Table 13-8 lists the components of a QA program for administration of unsealed radioactive sources.[12]

Radioimmunotherapy

Radioimmunotherapy (RIT) is an FDA-approved treatment modality that combines the cytotoxicity of radiation with the specificity of monoclonal antibodies for tumor cell surface antigens.[38] RIT is a novel therapeutic modality that links radionuclides to monoclonal antibodies to form radioimmunoconjugates. Cell death occurs once the radioimmunoconjugate has become bound to the tumor cell antigen by either the antibody itself or the radiation from the radionuclide. RIT is a different approach from standard external beam radiation therapy in that RIT targets radiation directly to tumor sites, potentially giving lower doses of radiation to normal tissue. RIT is extremely specific and does not have a broad side effect profile associated with standard systemic or loco-regional treatment modalities.

Oncology nurses must develop a knowledge base regarding clinical trials, treatment protocols, and indications for RIT. Additionally, those nurses working in radiation, nuclear medicine, and medical oncology should participate in creating patient education plans for individuals receiving RIT. These educational programs must include information on background and rationale for RIT, administration information, and follow-up and safety guidelines. As RIT becomes used more frequently in the clinical setting, it is essential that nurses prioritize communication among the multidisciplinary professional team involved in RIT so that effective and safe patient administration is a reality.[39,40]

Multimodality Fusion

The ability to correlate 3D images from various common imaging modalities (CT, MRI, PET) has become a valuable tool in the practice of radiation oncology. Specialized computer software enables multimodality fusion and provides clinicians with the ability to identify structures in one imaging modality and then spatially register the structures in a different modality. The most frequently used 3D imaging modalities for treatment planning in radiation therapy are CT and MRI. Computerized tomography imaging is fast, is cost-effective, and provides high resolution between structures.

All of the 3D imaging techniques can be fused to any other technique. This is possible because 3D image data are stored in units known as voxels. A voxel is depicted on a computer screen by a gray-scale level that represents a level characteristic to its imaging modality. The volume and size of the voxels are not equal when comparing two different imaging modalities. To equate two image sets of different size, the fusion software must scale the lower-resolution study to the same size voxel as the other study. This is done by interpolating between the voxels of the lower-resolution study to create the same size voxel as the higher-resolution image set. The images are packaged into equal volumes, with the minimum data necessary to spatially register the studies consisting of three unique points. These points must represent the same point in space in each of the image sets. Having more points would increase the accuracy of the fusion. Scaling the images to the same resolution also allows them to be viewed together at any reference plane.[41,42]

Mathematical algorithms are often used in image fusion software. This registration technique works by trying to minimize the amount of error between selected points in each study that are supposed to represent the same point in space in each study. Other sources of error in image fusion can be attributed to the accuracy of the imaging technique itself. The spatial accuracy of imaging modalities varies. Computed tomography, for example, has a superior spatial accuracy with an error of only a few millimeters over 30 cm. Spatial accuracy in MRI is not as good and can have errors of as much as 3–4 mm over 20 cm. Variations in patient positioning and patient motion during each of the imaging sessions can also be a great source of error. These potential errors require that the image fusion concentrate on the area of interest.

The clinical application of multimodality image fusion will continue to be refined as imaging techniques and computer support evolve. This radiation planning technique has the potential to provide patients with the most exact treatment plan, which will enhance efficacy and minimize side effect profiles.

B-Mode Acquisition and Targeting System

The B-mode acquisition and targeting (BAT) system (NOMOS Corporation, Sewickley, Pennsylvania) is a patented ultrasound positioning system used for the

Table 13-6 Currently Approved Nonsealed Radionuclide Sources

Agent	Use
Sodium iodine (I-131)	Cure of hyperthyroidism; cure and palliation of thyroid carcinoma
Sodium phosphate (P-32)	Treatment of myeloproliferative disorders such as polycythemia vera and thrombocytosis
Colloidal chromic phosphate (P-32)	Intracavitary therapy for malignant ascites, malignant pleural effusion, and brain cysts
Strontium chloride (Sr-89)	Palliation of painful bony metastasis
Rhenium (Re-186)	Experimental. Investigated for use in treating radiation synovectomy, cystic craniopharyngioma, cystic astrocytoma, medullary thyroid carcinoma, bone metastasis. Intraperitoneal use for metastatic ovarian carcinoma.

Data from Chao, Perez, Brady.[12]

Table 13-7 Standards of Nursing Practice

Care of the Patient Receiving External Beam Radiation

1. Educate the patient with regard to the goal of therapy and treatment experience, including simulation, setup, tattoos, blocks, and casts.
2. Be aware of the patient's treatment field and teach the patient symptom management of the associated general and site-specific reactions to therapy. Site-specific reactions may include diarrhea, nausea and vomiting, dysuria, dysphagia, esophagitis, mucositis, xerostomia, hair loss, and skin reactions.
3. Encourage rest periods as needed during the course of therapy to combat the anticipated side effect of fatigue.
4. Provide nutrition counseling to minimize weight loss. Encourage the patient's consumption of an appropriate diet for side effect management (e.g., high protein, high calorie, low residue, or soft).
5. Use skin care products (i.e., soaps, creams, lotions, gels) only at the recommendation of the radiation oncology staff.
6. Initiate referral to home health services if the patient's symptoms require continued follow-up and assessment in the home.

Care of the Patient Receiving Brachytherapy

1. Provide preimplant teaching to patients and their families to promote basic knowledge and understanding of the goals of therapy and the treatment experience.
2. Observe principles of time, distance, and shielding while caring for the implant patient. Perform patient care from behind lead shields placed at the bedside.
3. Wear a radiation film badge or direct reading dosimeter to record radiation exposure when in proximity to the implant patient.
4. Pregnant nurses are not to care for implant patients while they are loaded with radioactive sources.
5. Body fluids are *not* radioactive and may be disposed of according to routine institutional policy.
   Exception: Patients receiving systemic radioactive iodine will have contaminated body secretions. Patients' linens must remain in the room in the linen bag. Patients should be served meals with disposable utensils and paper products. The trash bin will also remain in the room until a radiation safety officer verifies it is no longer contaminated. Everything should remain in the patient's room until cleared by a radiation safety officer.
6. Check radioactive sources at the beginning and end of each shift and document the status of the implant. Applicators should wear caps, and interstitial needles and catheters should be counted and observed for dislodgment.
7. If the implant becomes dislodged, the nurse will retrieve the radioactive source using the provided long forceps and place it in a source holder in the room. Notify the radiation oncologist immediately. There is 24-hour on-call coverage.
8. Know the correct course of action if the patient has a medical emergency.
9. Inform the patient and visitors of hospital policy regarding visitation while the patient has radioactive material in place. Children under 18 and pregnant women are prohibited from visiting. Any questions should be referred to the radiation safety officer.

Reproduced with permission of Fox Chase Cancer Center, Department of Nursing, Philadelphia, PA.

Table 13-8 Components of a QA Program for Administration of Unsealed Radioactive Sources

- Different foundations of the same isotope must be recognized when ordering them. For example, chromic P-32 is used for pleural or peritoneal instillation and sodium P-32 is used intravenously for polycythemia vera.
- The appropriate activity of isotope must be available on the date of administration, so the timing of the delivery and the availability must be considered.
- Safe handling is essential, and the packaging must appropriately protect the shipment on receipt.
- Radioisotope activity must be determined with a dose calibrator that has been tested for linearity, constancy, and accuracy.
- Administration of an activity of a radiopharmaceutical that differs from the prescribed activity by more than 20% (either smaller or larger) is a misadministration. If the difference is between 10% and 20%, it is a recordable event. Compliance with Nuclear Regulatory Commission policy is mandatory.
- Prior to radioisotope administration, the following must occur: signed and dated informed consent and advanced directive, prescribed activity correct within 10%, and patient identification using two methods.

Data from Chao, Perez, Brady.[12]

delivery of radiation treatment to the prostate gland (Figure 13-13). This system provides a noninvasive way to deliver more precise radiation therapy. The BAT technology combines an ultrasound probe and a 3D positioning tool to pinpoint target organs rapidly at the time of each radiation treatment session. It dramatically reduces the need to target an extra margin of tissue around the tumor site. These extra margins have traditionally been used to compensate for errors in localization of the radiation beam. As such, BAT results in a significant reduction in the amount of healthy tissue exposed to radiation. The BAT stereotactic localization device is essentially equivalent to CT scanning localization; it is accurate, is simple to use, and adds no significant time to overall treatment.

Preliminary feasibility trials first occurred in 1999 at the Fox Chase Cancer Center in Philadelphia and at the Cleveland Clinic. BAT is considered appropriate for any organ that can be visualized by ultrasound. Possible cancer sites for radiation treatment using this technology include the breast, liver, bladder, kidney, pancreas, and uterus. The ability of BAT to reduce treatment margins allows for more successful, higher-dose treatments while decreasing the risk of complications associated with either standard or escalated doses of radiation therapy.

Image-Guided Radiation Therapy: CT-on-Rails

Conventional methods of localizing cancers for delivery of radiation treatment are still widely utilized in a variety of settings. Today, however, their increased power and accuracy have enabled radiation oncologists to tailor radiation fields for three-dimensional conformal radiation therapy and for intensity-modu-

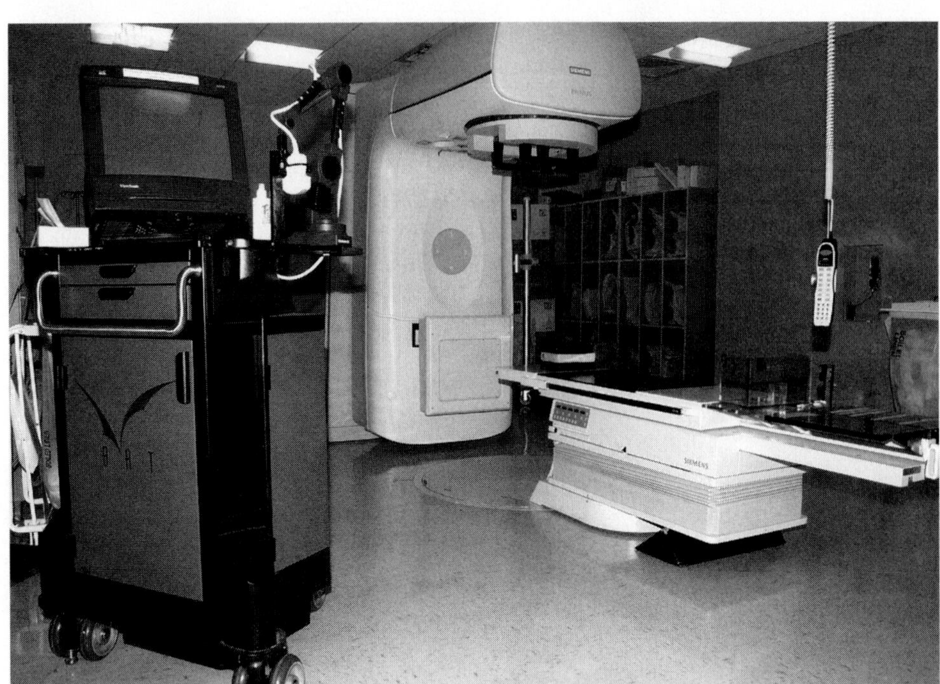

Figure 13-13 B-mode acquisition and targeting ultrasound localizing system. (Photo courtesy of Fox Chase Cancer Center.)

lated radiation therapy. Tumor localization occurs during a pretreatment planning session, during which the skin over the treatment field is tattooed and an immobilizing cast is constructed and marked to indicate the site above the tumor.[43] These methods assume that both the targeted tumor and the tattooed skin will remain still during treatment. In reality, neither of these assumptions is correct.[43] As individuals age, their skin loses elasticity and therefore can move before the radiation beam is aimed at the tattoo, which could cause the beam to miss part of the tumor. Casts can be ineffective immobilizers for patients with excess subcutaneous tissue, who may experience skin, muscle, and fatty tissue movement. These limitations demand that radiation treatment planners obtain images of the tumor before each treatment session. To do so, patients must physically move from the imaging system to the LINAC (which may cause tumor movement) or ultrasonography must be used (which provides inferior localization images).

Cutting-edge image-guided radiation therapy has been developed and is a multifunctional hybrid configuration consisting of a LINAC and a diagnostic CT scanner with a sliding gantry. This treatment planning advance brings image guidance to radiation treatment delivery, providing accurate, near-real-time target localization within the treatment room. The combination of a CT-on-rails/LINAC system provides a CT scan immediately before radiation treatment and gives information on the size, shape, and location of the target volume and nearby critical organs to ensure precise delivery of a prescribed course of radiation.

The Siemens CT-on-rails/LINAC was unveiled in the United States in 2000. It produces accurate, virtual, real-time, diagnostic-quality images of tumors within the treatment room. This system allows patients to remain on one table while the tumor is pinpointed and treatment is more accurately delivered.[44]

The gantry of the CT-on-rails/LINAC system moves along a series of high-precision rails that are embedded in the floor of the treatment room. The patient remains stationary on the treatment table while the CT scanner moves quickly and easily over the patient for imaging purposes. The gantry encircles the patient who is lying on the treatment table, making incremental movements during the scanning process. When image acquisition is complete, it retracts. Based on the updated tumor localization data, the system will then deliver the most optimal radiation therapy to the tumor while providing maximal sparing of normal tissue (Figure 13-14).

Precise treatment plans and targeting abilities are the most important features associated with high doses of radiation treatment delivery. Intensity-modulated radiation therapy (IMRT) provides clinicians with the techniques to customize the shape of the radiation beams to the tumor, though some organs, such as the prostate, may shift positions with body movement. CT-on-rails tracks organ movement just moments before treatment and adjusts the radiation treatment plan

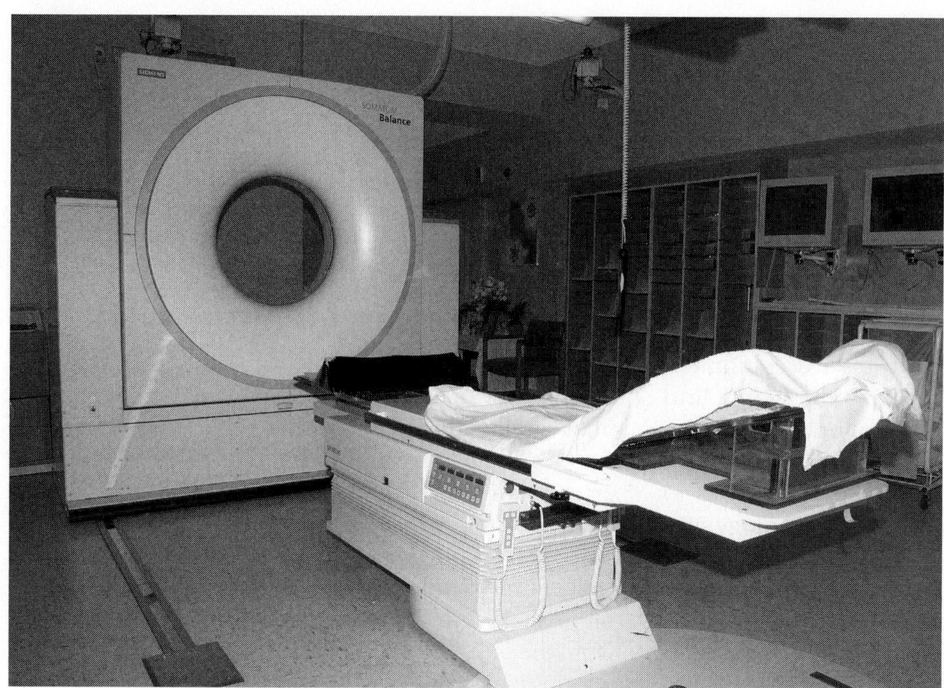

Figure 13-14 CT-on-Rails/LINAC System The CT-on-rails/LINAC system is a combination linear accelerator and CT scanner set on a sliding gantry. Patients lie stationary on the treatment couch while the CT scanner moves over them. Once CT target imaging is completed, treatment is then delivered immediately by the LINAC. The patient remains stationary for both tumor localization and treatment delivery, thus diminishing risk of organ movement, sparing normal tissue, and enabling delivery of precise treatment dose to the target. (Photo courtesy of Fox Chase Cancer Center.)

accordingly. It allows for the precise delivery of high-dose radiation therapy. Prostate cancer illustrates the challenges facing radiation treatment planners. The gland lies between the bladder and the rectum and is subject to frequent displacement due to intermittent distention. In an attempt to target the prostate gland, urinating on command and holding back urination are difficult requests of patients who are receiving radiation treatment. Prostate gland mobility has been documented, and studies have found significant differences in marker displacements on daily images obtained by electronic portal imaging during treatment sessions.[45] CT-on-rails permits accurate and noninvasive targeting of the prostate gland while avoiding the bladder and rectum.

Computerized tomography scans are used routinely in radiation treatment planning, but the pairing of the CT scan with daily radiation treatment is unique. CT-on-rails provides an additional technique for target localization, and in some settings is used in conjunction with ultrasound localization. The following are overall advantages offered by a CT-on-rails system:

- Fast, 3D tumor localization prior to any treatment fraction provides an opportunity to escalate dose, reduce complications, and evaluate the therapeutic effectiveness of treatment.
- CT functionality in the treatment room provides diagnostic-quality images with the patient in the actual treatment position, ensuring routine visualization of the tumor so as to check for anatomical movement.
- The CT scan operator in the radiation therapy department can perform the scheduling and acquisition of patients' CT image data for simulation, planning, and treatment purposes.

The addition of 3D localization and readily available diagnostic imaging to the clinical environment represents a major advancement in the support of oncology disease management. Future refinement of CT-on-rails is focusing on use of the LINAC for imaging. Theoretically, this could be accomplished by directing a series of narrow beams at regularly spaced sites on the gantry. The data would be captured using a large-area portal imaging device and reconstructed into a three-dimensional image. This technique, called cone-beam CT, remains in development phase but could eventually replace the hybrid CT scanner and LINAC.[46–48]

Patient preparation and nursing implications

Nurses are required to be flexible, dynamic, educated, and motivated to incorporate patient teaching materials when evolutionary equipment and treatment techniques are introduced into the radiation oncology setting. Patients must be prepared with detailed information and the rationale for the use of new equipment; description of the equipment (i.e., size, sound, increased amount of time for treatment setup); equipment location; personnel monitoring patient safety; and overall role of the equipment in the treatment plan and desired therapeutic outcome.

Radiation oncology nurses must embrace the evolving science of advanced treatment planning techniques by establishing a nursing presence in the multidisciplinary planning meetings to discuss equipment purchase, rationale for incorporating the system into the treatment setting, location of equipment, and ultimate effects on the treatment plan. Invoking evidence-based practice guidelines offers a way for nurses to understand the implications of new technology and provide appropriate educational plans for patients.

Respiratory Gating

Respiratory gating is a new technology that synchronizes radiation treatment regimens to the patient's respiratory cycle. It increases the accuracy of cancer radiotherapy by adjusting for tumor movements caused by respiration-induced movement. Varian Medical Systems' CT option for real-time position management (RPM) respiratory gating system turns off the radiation beam used in therapy when a tumor moves outside the treatment area. The CT option extends gating to the CT scanner so that diagnostic imaging can be correlated with the gating system that controls the LINAC. RPM respiratory gating technology provides treatment planning information that allows for the reduction of the radiation field to avoid hitting healthy, critical tissues while delivering high doses to tumors. The FDA approved the Varian RPM Respiratory Gating System in 2001.[49]

High-resolution conformal radiation therapy requires accurate tumor localization for identification of distinct tumor contours. This treatment planning process will maximize the dose delivered to the tumor while minimizing the dose administered to the surrounding healthy tissue. Physiological functions such as respiration can cause a change in the tumor position during treatment, which requires the use of a larger treatment volume to compensate for tumor movement.

A respiratory gating system allows for accurate monitoring and compensation for tumor motion during the course of treatment. The versatile system can be used anywhere that the effects of respiratory motion are encountered — for example, the lung, breast, liver, pancreas, kidney, and pelvis. Respiratory gating quickly and easily monitors respiration without compromising patient comfort. A video monitoring device is used to characterize the patient's breathing pattern. The pattern is obtained by tracking the motion of a lightweight, retro-reflective marker placed on the patient.[50] This respiration-related signal is derived from a transducer operated by the patient or from the CT scanner. The signal is fed into the CT system to be used as a gating mechanism for data acquisition.

Next, through video image analysis and signal processing, the system identifies both the full range of chest wall motion during respiration and the normal pattern of that motion. By correlating these data with the motion of the tumor in simulation, a treatment plan can be created that turns the treatment beam on only when the tumor falls within the planned beam aperture. Throughout this process, the RPM Respiratory Gating System allows the patient to breathe naturally and comfortably.[50]

Unanticipated patient movement during treatment such as sneezing and coughing, could interfere with the normal operation of the respiratory gating system. The system therefore features a predictive filter, which analyzes the patient's respiration, establishes a baseline respiratory pattern, and detects any deviations from the expected pattern. Deviations from this pattern result in an automatic hold of treatment delivery until the baseline respiratory pattern is re-established.[51]

Accurate treatment gating must be supported by a superior LINAC — one with a high-speed digital control system. These features provide less than 100-millisecond beam-on times with accurate gated dose rates and uncompromised beam flatness and symmetry.[51]

The respiratory gating system should be integrated with dynamic multileaf collimation (MLC). Treatment beam gating holds the MLC motion during ''beam-off'' times, even during dynamic conformal therapy treatments and IMRT. Leaf motion continues during the ''beam-on'' time, with precise registration to the MLC shape defined for treatment delivery. The objective of improved patient positioning accuracy is achieved using an integrative approach to treatment planning with the RPM Respiratory Gating System.[50]

Patient education and preparation

Patients need to know that respiratory gating during treatment planning is available in certain centers. They should be made aware that not all individuals are candidates for this treatment planning modality. The need to comply with specific breathing instructions may preclude some individuals with compromised respiratory status from participating. No risks or side effects are inherent in this treatment planning technique, but the time required for planning using respiratory gating is longer than that for conventional treatment planning. Patients should be assessed for candidacy and should be provided with succinct, yet complete written and verbal information regarding the details of how respiratory gating systems are used to enhance radiation treatment planning and to ultimately improve disease response.

Conclusion

The specialty of radiation oncology comprises a technological and clinical blend of skill and knowledge. This unique practice incorporates the talent and skills of a diverse team of professionals. Integral to the function of this complex environment is the professional oncology nurse. It is incumbent on these nurses to study, learn, and apply the scientific basis of radiation oncology practice to clinical situations. Patients treated with radiation are subject to rigorous procedures, prolonged treatment courses, and unfamiliar environments, all of which are compounded by the fear of a cancer diagnosis. Numerous questions and anxieties must be addressed. Nurses must creatively combine scientific and clinical knowledge into a pragmatic framework for patient management.

Radiation oncology continues to refine known treatment techniques and modalities and to investigate new technology. Research studies focus on the enhancement of treatment planning techniques in an effort to provide patients with the most refined modalities. Although advanced treatment planning has become popular, some institutions have not been able to implement it fully due to its expense, requirement for additional staffing, and need for sophisticated equipment. Economic constraints continue to plague institutions and hinder the installation of state-of-the-art equipment to deliver cutting-edge technology. By the time smaller, independent, less well-endowed radiation centers install a new technology, it has probably become dated. Thus it is not the pace of discovery and application of new treatment techniques that is problematic, but rather the struggle of institutions to keep pace economically. As such, radiation oncology professionals must advocate for the specialty so that scientific sophistication and clinical application are promoted and invoked in a timely, effective manner.

References

1. Rice AM: An introduction to radiotherapy. *Nurs Stand* 12:49–54, 1997
2. Bucholtz JD: Comforting children during radiotherapy. *Oncol Nurs Forum* 21:987–994, 1994
3. Khan FM: *The Physics of Radiation Therapy*. Baltimore, Williams & Wilkins, 1994
4. Gazda MJ, Coia LR: Radiation treatment planning and techniques in cancer management: a multidisciplinary approach, in Pazdur R, Coia LR, Hosians WJ, Wagman LD (eds.): *Medical, Surgical and Radiation Oncology* (ed 3). New York, PRR, 1999, pp 649–660
5. Bentel GC: *Radiation Therapy Planning*. New York, McGraw-Hill, 1996
6. Reinstein LE: Patient positioning and immobilization, in Khan FM, Potish RA (eds.): *Treatment Planning in Radiation Oncology*. Baltimore, Williams & Wilkins, 1998, pp 55–88
7. Rosenthal SA, Roche M, Goldsmith BJ, et al: Immobilization improves the reproducibility of patient positioning during 6 field conformal radiation therapy for prostate carcinoma. *Int J Radiat Oncol Biol Phys* 27:921–926, 1993
8. Soffen EM, Hanks GE, Hwang CC, et al: Conformal static field therapy for low volume, low grade prostate cancer with rigid immobilization. *Int J Radiat Oncol Biol Phys* 20:141–146, 1991
9. Verhey LJ: Immobilizing and positioning patients for radiotherapy. *Semin Radiat Oncol* 5:100–114, 1995
10. Hunt M: Localization and field design using a CT simulator, in Coia LR, Schultheiss TE, Hanks GE (eds.): *A Practical Guide to CT Simulation*. Madison, WI, Advanced Medical Publishing, 1995, pp 23–38
11. Das IJ, McGee KP, Desobry GE: The digitally reconstructed radiograph, in Coia LR, Schultheiss TE, Hanks GE (eds.): *A Practical Guide to CT Simulation*. Madison, WI, Advanced Medical Publishing, 1995, pp 39–50
12. Chao KSC, Perez CA, Brady LW: *Radiation Oncology: Management Decisions*. Philadelphia, Lippincott-Raven, 1999
13. Sherouse GW: Radiotherapy simulation, in Khan FM, Potish RA (eds.): *Treatment Planning in Radiation Oncology*. Baltimore, Williams & Wilkins, 1998, pp 39–53
14. Hunt M: Localization and field design using a CT simulator, in Coia LR, Schultheiss TE, Hanks GE (eds.): *A Practical Guide to CT Simulation*. Madison, WI, Advanced Medical Publishing, 1995, pp 25–38
15. Sterling TD, Knowlton KC, Weinkham JJ, et al: Dynamic display of radiotherapy plans using computer-produced films. *Radiology* 107:689–691, 1973
16. Khan FM, Potish RA: *Treatment Planning in Radiation Oncology*. Baltimore, Williams & Wilkins, 1998
17. Bova FJ, Meeks SL, Friedman WA: LINAC radiosurgery: system requirements, procedures and testing, in Khan FM, Potish RA (eds.): *Treatment Planning in Radiation Oncology*. Baltimore, Williams & Wilkins, 1998, pp 215–242
18. Schwartz M: Stereotactic radiosurgery: comparing different technologies. *CMAJ* 158:625–628, 1998
19. Fink L: Robot assisted surgery: futuristic trend enhances radiation therapy. *Adv Admin Radiol Radiat Oncol* 7:113–118, 1997
20. Adler JR, Chang SD, Murphy MJ, et al: The CyberKnife: a frameless robotic system for radiosurgery. *Stereotact Func Neurosurg* 69(pt 2):124–128, 1997
21. CyberKnife: *www/cksociety.org/PatientInfo/radiosurgery.asp*. Accessed May 24, 2004
22. Yamamoto M: Gamma knife radiosurgery: technology, applications, and future directions. *Neurosurg Clin North Am*, 10:181–202, 1999
23. Brenner DJ: Radiation biology in brachytherapy. *J Surg Oncol* 65:66–70, 1997
24. International Commission on Radiation Units and Measurements: *Dose and Volume Specification for Reporting Intracavitary Therapy in Gynecology*, Report No. 38. Bethesda, MD, ICRU, 1985
25. Orton CG, Ezell GA: Physics and dosimetry of high-dose-rate brachytherapy, in Perez CA, Brady LW (eds.): *Principles and*

Practice of Radiation Oncology (ed 3). Philadelphia, Lippincott-Raven, 1998, pp 469–485
26. Erickson B, Gillin MT: Interstitial implantation of gynecologic malignancies. *J Surg Oncol* 66:285–295, 1997
27. Gaspar LE: Brachytherapy in lung cancer. *J Surg Oncol* 67:60–70, 1998
28. Baglan K, Martinez A, Frazier R, et al: The use of high-dose rate brachytherapy alone after lumpectomy in patients with early-stage breast cancer treated with breast-conserving therapy. *Int J Radiat Oncol Biol Phys* 30:1003–1011, 2001
29. Polgar C, Fodor J, Major T, et al: Radiotherapy confined to the tumor bed following breast conserving surgery: current status, controversies, and future projects. *Strahlentherapie Onkologie* 178:597–606, 2002
30. Vicini F, Baglan K, Kestin L, et al: The emerging role of brachytherapy in the management of patients with breast cancer. *Semin Radiat Oncol* 12:31–39, 2002
31. Hogle WP, Quinne AE, Heron DE: Advances in brachytherapy: new approaches to target breast cancer. *Clin J Oncol Nurs* 7:324–330, 2003
32. Vicini F: Limited-field radiation therapy in the management of early-stage breast cancer. *J Natl Cancer Inst* 95:1205–1211, 2003
33. Keisch M, Vincini F, Kuske R, et al: Two-year outcome with the MammoSite breast brachytherapy applicator: factors associated with optimal cosmetic results when performing partial breast irradiation. Proceedings of the 45th Annual ASTRO meeting. *Int J Radiat Oncol Biol Phys* 57(suppl):S315, 2003
34. King TA, Bolton JS, Kuske RR, et al: Long-term results of wide-field brachytherapy as the sole method of radiation therapy after segmental mastectomy for T(is, 1,2) breast cancer. *Am J Surg* 180:299–304, 2000
35. Mitchell CK: *Patient Care Management: HDR Brachytherapy for Breast Cancer Utilizing MammoSite* [Patient care recommendations]. Alpharetta, GA, Proxima Therapeutics, 2002
36. Vaidya JS, Baum M, Tobias JS, et al: Targeted intra-operative radiotherapy (Targit): an innovative method of treatment for early breast cancer. *Ann Oncol* 12:1075–1080, 2001
37. Gordils-Perez J, Rawlins-Duell R, Kelvin JR: Advances in radiation treatment of patients with breast cancer. *Clin J Oncol Nurs* 7:629–636, 2003
38. Potamianos S, Varvarigou AD, Archimandritis SC: Radioimmunoscintigraphy and radioimmunotherapy in cancer: principles and application. *Anticancer Res* 20:925–948, 2000
39. Hendrix C: Radiation safety guidelines for radioimmunotherapy with yttrium 90 ibritumomab tiuxetan. *Clin J Oncol Nurs* 8:31–34, 2004
40. Riley MB, Byar K: The rationale for and background of radioimmunotherapy: an emerging therapy for B-cell non-Hodgkin's lymphoma. *Semin Oncol Nurs* 20:1–7, 2004
41. Quarantelli M, Alfano B, Larobina M, et al: Frequency and coding for simultaneous display of multi-modality images. *J Nucl Med* 40:442–447, 1999
42. McNeeley SW: Image fusion theory and demonstration, in *Proceedings Radiation Oncology Conference,* Philadelphia, Fox Chase Cancer Center, 1998, p 206
43. Bronson JG: *Imaging with a Linear Accelerator. www.imagingeconomics.com/library/200307-07.asp,* accessed May 22, 2004.
44. Wong JR, Cheng CW, Grim L, et al: Clinical implementation of the world's first PRIMATOM, a combination of CT scanner and linear accelerator, for precise tumor targeting and treatment. *Phys Med* 17:271–276, 2001
45. Vigneault E, Pouliot J, Laverdiere J, et al: Electronic portal imaging device detection of radioopaque markers for the evaluation of prostate position during megavoltage irradiation: a clinical study. *Int J Radiat Oncol Biol Phys* 37:205–212, 1997
46. Sidhu K, Ford EC, Spirou S, et al: Optimization of conformal thoracic radiotherapy using cone-beam CT imaging for treatment verification. *Int J Radiat Oncol Biol Phys* 55:757–767, 2003
47. Ford EC, Chang J, Mueller K, et al: Cone-beam CT with megavoltage beams and an amorphous silicon electronic portal imaging device: potential for verification of radiotherapy of lung cancer. *Med Phys* 29:2913–2924, 2002
48. Jaffray DA, Siewerdsen JH, Wong JW, et al: Flat-panel cone-beam computed tomography for image-guided radiation therapy. *Int J Radiat Oncol Biol Phys* 53:1337–1349, 2002
49. Varian Medical Systems: *www.varian.com,* 2004
50. Ramsey CR, Scaperoth D, Arwood D: Clinical experience with a commercial respiratory gating system. Proceedings of the 42nd Annual ASTRO Meeting. *Int J Radiat Oncol Biol Phys* 48:164–165, 2000 (abstr 106)
51. Ramsey CR, Scaperoth D, Arwood D, et al AL: Clinical efficacy of respiratory gated conformal radiation therapy. *Med Dosimetry* 24:115–119; 1999

CHAPTER 14

Radiation Therapy: Toxicities and Management

Karen E. Maher, RN, MS, ANP, AOCN®

Introduction

Approximately 60% of oncology patients will receive radiation therapy during the course of their treatment. Irradiation may be administered at multiple points in the treatment continuum — as neoadjuvant therapy, preoperative and postoperative therapy, and adjunctive treatment. Palliative irradiation may occur at multiple times depending on the disease course and patient response. Combined modality therapy with chemotherapy and/or surgery and/or radiation therapy is commonly used in the treatment of cancer. The additive effects of combining these treatments with radiation generally result in more acute and prolonged toxicities. Performance status and comorbid conditions contribute to patient tolerance of irradiation and may predispose the patient to a more difficult course of therapy. This chapter reviews the radiobiologic rationale for radiation toxicities, site-specific acute and late toxicities, and nursing assessment and management.

Radiobiology

Cellular response to radiation injury is directly related to the degree of mitotic activity. Actively replicating cells have four stages and one resting phase in their life cycle:

G_1	The gap between the end of mitosis and the start of DNA synthesis
S	DNA synthesis
G_2	The gap between DNA synthesis and mitosis
M	Mitosis
G_0	Resting phase

The cell is most sensitive to radiation during mitosis and the G_2 phase, with the greatest radioresistance occurring in the DNA synthesis phase.[1]

The term *radiosensitivity* refers to the response of tumor cells to radiation in terms of degree and speed of response. Poorly differentiated immature cells, rapidly proliferating cells, or cells with a high mitotic potential are more radiosensitive.

Another term frequently used is *radiocurability*. It refers to local or regional eradication of tumor cells by radiation, and means that the tumor-to-normal-tissue relations are such that curative doses of radiation can be applied without excessive damage to normal tissues. Examples of radiocurable tumors include carcinomas of the cervix, larynx, breast, and prostate.

The terms "radiosensitivity" and "radiocurability" are not interchangeable. For example, non-Hodgkin's lymphoma is very radiosensitive but may not be radiocurable. All tissues have a degree of radiosensitivity, but it is the effect on normal tissue surrounding the tumor that largely determines the maximum radiation dose and resulting toxicities.[2]

The goal of radiation therapy is to destroy cancer cells while maintaining the integrity of normal tissue. This range is defined as the *therapeutic ratio* (Figure 14-1).[2] Providing radiation doses within the therapeutic ratio allows for tumor eradication or reduction and minimal residual injury to surrounding normal tissues and structures. However, because ionizing radiation does not differentiate between normal cells and cancer cells, it damages both. Malignant and normal cells differ little in their overall response to ionizing radiation. Achieving the therapeutic ratio requires a delicate balance between desired treatment outcome and toxicities.

Normal cells and cancer cells undergo some degree of repair to sublethal damage between doses of radiation. A single dose of ionizing radiation will have a greater effect on cells than the same dose divided into several fractions. If the goal of radiation is maximizing tumor cell kill while sparing normal tissue, dividing the radiation into equal doses or fractions is crucial to achieving the therapeutic ratio. Radiation is most commonly administered in a daily fraction, although *hyperfractionation* (two or more fractions per day separated by 4–6 hours) can be used in some patients. Fractionation is designed to take advantage of the "four R's" of radiobiology:

1. *Repair:* The ability of cells to recover from sublethal radiation injury. Repair usually occurs within 24 hours but may occur in as little as 4 hours in some tissues. Normal cells are repeatedly repaired between daily doses. By contrast, tumor cells may be initially repaired, but as radiation continues their repair ability decreases, increasing the radiation damage to tumor cells.
2. *Redistribution:* Fractionated radiation doses disrupt the cellular life cycle, causing mitotic delays in the tumor cell cycle. This disruption theoretically enhances the effects of each succeeding radiation dose because more tumor cells are likely to be in mitosis at the same time, increasing the cell kill. Tumor cells may be more subject to redistribution, due in part to their erratic growth and development.
3. *Repopulation* (regeneration): Irradiated normal cells are able to complete their cell cycle and undergo successful mitosis between radiation doses. Tumor cells are more likely to die after radiation injury because of the abnormal features that result from growth and mitosis. Generally, tumor cell division stays ahead of cell death or loss, which contrasts with mature normal cell growth and division that matches cell loss.
4. *Reoxygenation:* It is believed that well-oxygenated cells do not allow reversal and repair of the chemical changes produced by radiation. The reoxygenation process involves radioresistant hypoxic tumor cells becoming radiosensitive aerated or oxygenated cells between radiation doses. In large tumors with necrotic central components, radiation continuously destroys the outer layers (like peeling an onion), allowing the central core to be exposed to capillary oxygenation and thus become more radiosensitive. This theory assumes there is adequate microcirculation of the tumor mass. It has been stated that reoxygenation may be the most important advantage of fractionation.[2]

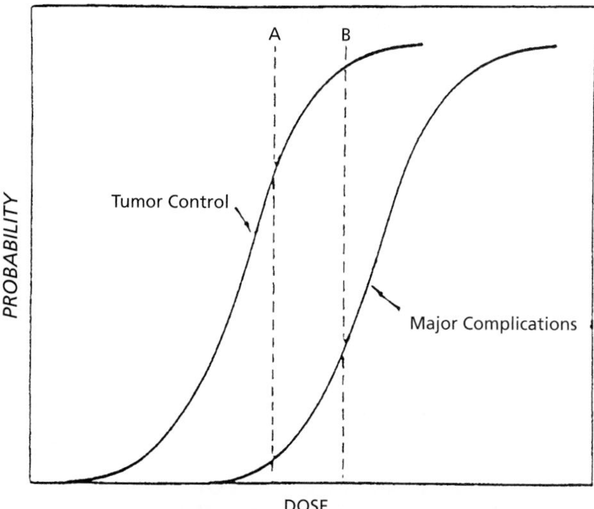

Figure 14-1 Therapeutic Ratio. Sigmoid curves of tumor control and complications. **(A)** Dose for tumor control with minimum complications. **(B)** *Maximum tumor dose with significant complications. (Reprinted with permission from Hellman S: Principles of cancer management: radiation therapy, in DeVita VT, Hellman S, Rosenberg SA (eds.): Cancer: Principles and Practice of Oncology* (ed 6). Philadelphia, Lippincott-Raven, 2001, pp 265–288.[2])

In summary, fractionation of the total radiation dose spares normal tissue because repair of sublethal damage allows repopulation between doses. The redistribution and reoxygenation that occur between the daily fractions increase the radiosensitivity of the tumor cells, thereby improving overall treatment outcome. The goal is to kill tumor cells and allow normal cells to regrow and repopulate surrounding tissue.[2]

Tissue and Organ Response to Radiation

Normal tissue response to ionizing radiation depends on the total dose, fractionation schedule (daily dose and overall length of treatment), and volume treated (Figure 14-2).[3] This concept, which will be repeated

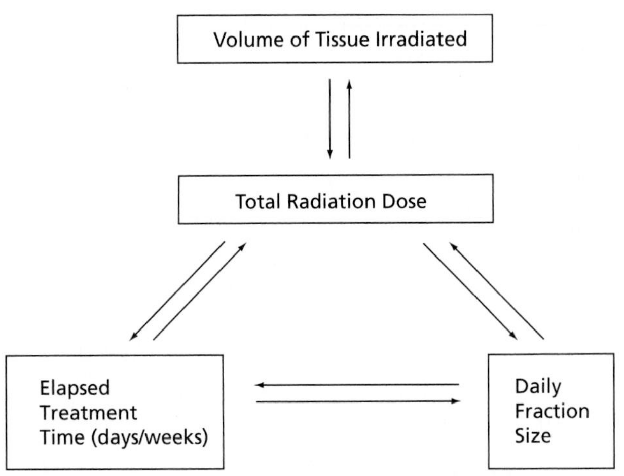

Figure 14-2 Basic Factors Affecting Normal Tissue Response to Radiation. (Adapted with permission from Chao KS, Perez CA, Brady LW: Fundamentals of patient management, in Chao DS, Perez CA, Brady LW (eds.): *Radiation Oncology Management Decisions.* Philadelphia, Lippincott-Raven, 2002, pp 1–13.[3])

throughout the chapter, is integral to understanding the pathophysiology and occurrence of both acute and late radiation-associated toxicities.[3] All cells and structures that lie within the path of the ionizing radiation beam are vulnerable to toxicities. Tissue and organ systems within the body are composed of multiple cellular components that have differing radiation-tolerance parameters. Normal tissue and organ tolerance determines the limit of radiation that can be safely administered to a specific target area in the body. A large body of literature has documented tolerance doses of tissues and structures within reasonably precise limits. Table 14-1 illustrates the cellular replacement times for certain body systems.[4,5]

Information on tolerance doses has been revised in recent years because of advances in combined modality therapy. When chemotherapy and radiation are used concurrently, acute and late reactions in various tissues generally occur at much lower doses than when radiation is used alone. In addition, combined modality therapy can produce acute and late radiation injuries that are not commonly seen with either modality alone. Patients treated with radiation alone and in combination with other modalities such as chemotherapy are at risk for multiple toxicities that can be classified as acute, subacute, and late effects (Table 14-2).[6]

Acute Effects

Acute effects of radiation occur primarily in rapidly renewing tissues.[2] Because the response of such tissues depends on the balance between cell birth and cell death, acute tissue reaction is affected by the time allowed for repopulation and is therefore dependent on field size, daily radiation dose, and overall length of treatment (number of treatments). The concept of fractionation of radiation therapy is *crucial* to allowing normal cell repopulation (recall the four R's of radiobiology). Uninterrupted treatment would quickly overwhelm the body's ability to repair normal tissues and therefore would cause unacceptable toxicities. As a result, treatment schedules are generally 5 days per week, with 2 consecutive days of break or rest. Occasionally, treatment breaks are necessary to allow healing of normal tissue. Acute toxicities vary with each patient, are site specific and generally short term, and resolve after completion of treatment. The time to complete resolution of acute toxicities depends on the specific tissues treated and the degree of reaction to the radiation.

Subacute Effects

Subacute effects are those toxicities that are clinically evident within weeks to a few months after completing radiation. Pneumonitis, for example, is a subacute

Table 14-1 Selected Cellular Systems in Normal Tissue and Approximate Turnover/Replacement Time

System	Turnover/Replacement Time*
Integumentary	
Epidermis	30 days
Basal cells	Nadir: 21 days Reepithelialization: 28–31 days
Endothelial cells	Unknown
Blood	
RBCs	120 days
Granulocytes	6–10 h in blood, 2–3 days in tissue
Lymphocytes	100–300 + days
Platelets	5–10 days
Respiratory tract	
Tracheal epithelium	50 days
Lung alveolar cells	10–30 days
GI tract	
Oral mucosa	10–14 days
Stomach	3–9 days
Small intestine	1.5 days
Colon	10 days
Skin	20 days
GU tract	
Urinary bladder	50 days
Testis	20 days
Eye	
Cornea	7 days

*Turnover/replacement time is the time required for replacement of number of cells equal to that in the whole population of the system.

Data from Coia, Moylan[4]; Archambieu, Pezner, et al.[5]

Table 14-2 Phases of Radiation Effect: Acute, Subacute, Late

Acute Effect Phase
- Evidence of radiation effect is seen in hours to days.
- Proliferating cells are more radiosensitive than quiescent cells.
- Brisk reactions heal completely, but some degree of residual damage may be present.
- Tissues most at risk:

Bladder	Ovary, testis
Bone marrow	Salivary gland
Colon	Skin
Esophagus	Small bowel
Lymph nodes	Stomach
Oral mucosa	Vagina

Subacute Effect Phase
- Evidence of damage of clinical significance is seen in weeks to a few months after completing radiation.
- Tissues most at risk:

Brain	Liver
Heart	Lung
Kidney	Spinal cord

Late Effect Phase
- If given sufficient doses of radiation, all tissues can manifest late effects.
- Late effects are the result of a perpetual cascade of cytokine expression causing progressive cellular and tissue destruction.
- Occurs in tissues with low cell turnover.
- Dependent on fractionation, treatment volume, and total radiation dose.
- Tissues most at risk:

Bile ducts	Lymph tissue
Bone	Pancreas (endocrine)
Brain	Pituitary
Breast	Thyroid
Cartilage	

Data from Williams, Chea, Rubin, et al.[6]

clinical syndrome that may occur after chest irradiation. (Pneumonitis is described in detail later in the chapter.)

Late Effects

The concern for development of late effects is the dose-limiting factor in radiation treatment delivery.[2] The extent and degree of late effects depend on the size of the daily fraction and the total radiation dose, total treatment time, size of the treatment field, type of radiation (photons versus electrons), and concurrent chemotherapy. The mechanism of late radiation injury is not definitively known. An older paradigm described gradual ablation of the fine microvasculature leading to permanent cell/tissue death due to hypoxia. A newer model suggests that a ''perpetual cascade'' of cytokine (primarily the TGF family) expression causes progressive cellular and tissue death.[6]

Assessment and Management of Skin Reactions, Fatigue, and Myelosuppression

Role of the Radiation Therapy Nurse

The role of the radiation therapy (RT) nurse has only recently been clearly defined, in contrast to the medical oncology nurse, who has had an established role in the administration of chemotherapy and management of symptoms.[7] With increasingly aggressive cancer treatment regimens being adopted, patients are at risk for multiple toxicities, and the RT nurse must be prepared to assess and intervene as indicated. New and innovative strategies for teaching about and managing toxicities necessitate a dialogue among all professionals involved in each patient's treatment to produce optimal outcomes. Radiation therapy nurses are responsible for teaching, assessing, and managing toxicities, and supporting patients through a course of irradiation. Radiation therapy can engender many fears for patients, their families, and friends. Misinformation is common, and a patient's friends and family may reinforce these concerns due to erroneous assumptions and lack of accurate information. It is essential that RT nurses and physicians educate both the patient and the family before beginning a course of treatment.

Hinds et al. evaluated the functions and methods preferred by patients for receiving information related to radiation therapy.[8] They concluded that information allowed patients to be active participants in their care, reduced anxiety, and helped patients feel better prepared for the treatments. Poroch demonstrated that RT patients who received structured teaching interventions, including sensory and procedural information, were significantly less anxious and more satisfied during the course of their treatment than members of a cohort control group who received standard information used in the radiation therapy department.[9] Bennenbroek et al. reported on their study that evaluated the effects of three different audiotapes on patients' subjective understanding of radiation therapy and validation of emotions related the cancer experience. The results indicated that the tapes had a positive effect, especially the procedural and coping tape.[10] These findings were similar to those in an earlier randomized study by Hagopian, who reported a benefit for patients using informational audiotapes. The conclusion was that patients who used the tapes were more knowledgeable about radiation therapy and side effects and practiced more helpful self-care measures.[11] Patient education should include an overview of the treatment plan, address any myths and misconceptions, information on the actual treatments (including sensory information), an explanation of the simulation process, expected outcome (cure, control, or palliation), specific side effects of treatment, and symptom management.[12]

The experience of cancer and its treatment generate high levels of distress and difficulty in coping. Even though cancer treatment is stressful, cessation of treatment may also be associated with emotional stress due to uncertainty about tumor recurrence.[13] The staff in radiation oncology departments form brief, intense relationships with patients and their families. Each individual staff member and radiation program deals with the ending of a course of therapy in a different way. While patients are always pleased to finish their treatment, it is important to acknowledge the ending of this portion of their cancer therapy. Often radiation therapy is the last treatment modality, after surgery and chemotherapy, and patients are indeed "finished" with treatment at the completion of the radiation course. This can be an uncertain time, with patients experiencing multiple concerns related to time to resolution of treatment-related toxicities, monitoring for cancer recurrence, and — perhaps most difficult — resuming a "normal" life. Cancer counseling or other supportive care can be extremely helpful at this point in the treatment continuum.

In general, the management of toxicities related to radiation therapy is similar to the management of chemotherapy-related side effects. It may not always be clear whether the chemotherapy or the radiation is causing the specific toxicity. It is important that medical and radiation oncology nurses collaborate in planning management of side effects. While the side effects of radiation are site specific, most patients are at risk for some degree of skin reaction, fatigue, and occasionally myelosuppression.

Skin Reaction (Radiodermatitis)

Early radiation machines used much lower and less penetrating energies, so most of the radiation dose was superficial. The degree of skin erythema was frequently used as an indication of overall radiation dose. Therefore, when the patient's skin became severely erythematous or desquamated, the radiation course ended. Modern megavoltage radiation equipment, such as the linear accelerator, have been called "skin-sparing" treatment machines. Despite advanced technology in the science and delivery of radiation, the radiation beam still must first pass through the skin to reach the targeted tissue or organ. Fortunately, the dreaded and frequently severe skin reactions previously associated with radiation therapy are rarely seen with the modern treatment techniques and equipment now in common use.

Typical skin response to radiation depends on numerous radiation- and patient-related factors. Radiation factors affecting skin reaction include the beam type and energy, daily treatment dose, tissue equivalent (bolus) material on the skin surface during treatment, accelerated dose fractionation, and location and size of the treatment fields. The field location and beam arrangement (single versus opposed versus multibeam) defines the skin surface(s) at risk. Patient factors affecting skin reaction include body habitus that creates significant skin folds in the treatment fields, nutritional status, individual radiosensitivity, and comorbid conditions such as ataxia-telangiectasias and autoimmune illness (Table 14-3).[14] Individual skin type is not predictive of a skin reaction; therefore it is not necessarily the case that fair-haired, light-skinned individuals are at greater risk for incurring severe skin reactions.

Skin response to radiation is dependent on dose and reflects changes in the cellular components of the epidermis, dermis, and vasculature. The epidermis and dermis are continuously renewing their cellular populations so that cell production equals cell loss. An acute skin effect is a reflection of the inability of cells in the epidermis and dermis to keep up with the accelerated loss caused by the radiation.[15]

Acute skin effects

Acute skin reactions vary in intensity and duration depending on the factors mentioned earlier. The single most important factor is the location of radiation field. For example, a woman undergoing breast irradiation is at greater risk for an acute skin reaction due to the curved, tangential radiation fields that result in a higher dose to the skin surface and skin folds. In contrast, a man receiving four-field radiation to the pelvis (small, relatively flat surfaces) for prostate cancer rarely experiences a skin reaction.

The degree of skin reaction can be visually assessed and may progress in a stepwise fashion from erythema to dry desquamation to moist desquamation. The stages of potential acute skin reactions are outlined in Table 14-4.[16] It is important to understand that not all patients experience each stage of skin reaction and that some patients have several stages occurring simultaneously. Most patients demonstrate some degree of skin dryness, itching, and erythema. Erythema can progress to dermal edema and discomfort. Dry desquamation of the skin can occur as erythema resolves. Moist desquamation of skin in the treatment field involves the epilation of the epidermis and exposure of the dermis. Patients with moist desquamation have pain and may need treatment suspended to allow for healing. *Burn* is not an appropriate term to describe a skin reaction to radiation, as it implies that too much radiation was administered or that an error was made in the treatment prescription.[17] Most radiation oncolo-

Table 14-3 Overview of Factors Influencing Skin Response to Radiation

Radiation Related	Patient Related
• Total dose and total time • Daily fraction size • Type of radiation beam (photons versus electrons) • Use of tissue-equivalent bolus material • Size of treatment field	• Anatomical location of treatment field(s) • Characteristics of skin in treatment field(s) • Proximity of tumor to skin surface • Concomitant chemotherapy • Co-morbid conditions • Nutritional status
Inflammatory Response • Histamine and serotonin released • Local microcirculation increases tissue perfusion • Infiltration by leukocytes	
Acute Changes • May occur within 2–3 weeks after start or completion of treatment • Usually repairable • Types: Erythema/epilation Dry desquamation Moist desquamation	**Chronic Changes** • May occur several months to years after completion of treatment • May be permanent • Types: Tissue necrosis or ulceration Fibrosis Edema Hyperpigmentation

Data from Strunk, Maher.[14]

gy nurses and staff avoid use of this word, although "burn" is how patients commonly describe their skin reactions. Generally, acute skin symptoms begin about 3 weeks (2700–3000 cGy) into a course of treatment and are confined to the treatment field. Acute skin reactions heal completely and are not always predictive of late skin manifestations.

Concurrent chemotherapy and irradiation can result in more severe and prolonged acute skin reactions. The degree of skin effect depends on the specific chemotherapeutic agents used and the site of radiation. For example, patients receiving concurrent chemotherapy and radiation for cancers of the oropharynx, hypopharynx, or nasopharynx (skin of the neck and face), or of the anus and vulva (perianal/perineal skin) are at higher risk due to body contours that result in skin folds where the skin dose is enhanced. An erythematous skin recall reaction may occur in patients who undergo irradiation and are then given anthracyclines (e.g., doxorubicin) in close proximity to completion of radiation. There are no systematic methods available to confirm skin recall, the doses of chemotherapy or radiation required, or the time interval involved.[5]

Late skin effects

The late changes to skin produced by radiation can be functionally limiting if neuropathy, arthropathy, contraction, and necrosis are produced. Management of late skin effects is directed at relieving symptoms, promoting healing, and surgical intervention as indicated. The late effects of radiation on the skin are dose dependent. The time interval to development of clinically evident skin changes results from the response of the cellular components in the epidermis, dermis, and microvasculature. The evolution of skin effects reflects a continuous remodeling of these cellular populations.[5]

A time period of varying length occurs in which the skin appears "normal" during radiation treatment. Then, within a period of time that may be measured in years, skin changes such as hyperpigmentation, scaling, atrophy, telangiectasias, subcutaneous fibrosis, and necrosis may develop and progress. Radiation dose schedules that produce late skin reactions are similar to those that produce acute skin reactions. Nevertheless, late effects on skin are more severe following schedules that include daily fractions of 250–300 cGy or higher. Most patients are treated using daily fractions of 180–200 cGy, thus markedly reducing the risk of late skin effects.[5] Potential late skin effects are outlined in Table 14-5.[16]

Skin care assessment and management

A major role carried out by RT nurses is assessing skin reactions, teaching skin care, and managing skin breakdown if it occurs.[17] Many preventive and interventional skin care regimens are currently in use, though limited scientific data support many practice interventions. It has long been believed that skin in the treatment field should have no product (such as topical emollients) applied prior to daily treatment. A common belief states that the product applied to the skin acts as a bolus and will enhance skin reaction. Burch et al. investigated what occurs on the skin surface when deodorants, powders, and creams are

Table 14-4 Acute Effects of Radiation on Skin

Tissue Response	Onset/Duration	Clinical Presentation	Physiological Rationale
Erythema			
Phase I (transient)	Within hours to days of first treatment Resolves after several days but will recur if treatment continues	Faint, often unnoticed redness	Thought to be a vascular response to extracapillary cell injury
Phase II (erythema proper)	Following 2–3 weeks of standard fractionated radiation therapy. Resolves 20–30 days following last treatment	Redness that outlines treatment field Intensifies as treatment continues	Intensity greater with higher radiation doses and larger treatment fields (greater amount of vasculature)
		Increased skin temperature	Increased blood flow through dermis from vasodilation.
		Edema	Capillary vasodilation with endothelial swelling and increased capillary permeability. Histamine and serotonin are released and microcirculation increases tissue perfusion allowing infiltration of the area by leukocytes.
Folliculitis	Occurs most commonly when exposure exceeds 20–28 Gy	Papular erythematous rash with itching	Inflammation of hair follicules
Hyperpigmentation	Following 2–3 weeks of standard fractionated radiation therapy. Usually resolves 3 months to 1 year following completion of treatment, but may be chronic	Tanned appearance	Cornified basal cells carry more melanin into superficial layers of the epidermis, and radiation stimulates tyrosinase to convert tyrosine to melanin. Increased melanocyte activity causes cells to become darker. Darker-skinned people may have more hyperpigmentation because they traditionally have more melanin.
Dry desquamation	Following 3–4 weeks of standard fractionated radiation therapy. Resolves 1–2 weeks after completion of treatment	Dryness, flaking, and peeling often accompanied by itching	Each dose of radiation destroys a fixed percentage of basal cells. Surviving basal cells become cornified and are shed at an increased rate. Noncycling basal cells are stimulated and cell cycle time is shortened.
Moist desquamation	Following 40 Gy or with trauma/excess friction. Recovery usually 2–3 weeks after completion of treatment	Brilliant erythema Sloughing skin Exposed dermis Serous exudate oozing from surface	Destruction of epithelium. All basal cells have been destroyed and no new cells are yet formed.
		Pain	Nerve endings in the dermis are exposed.
Skin regrowth following moist desquamation	Dependent on severity Usually complete 2–3 months following completion of treatment	Small areas of epithelium develop New skin is smooth, pink, thin, and dryer. Gradual thickening of skin over time, but skin does not regain former thickness	Epithelial cells migrate via proliferation from outside the treatment field and through peripheral migration. Migration occurs best over moist healthy tissue. Fewer sweat and sebaceous glands result in chronic dryness. Repopulation of the entire epidermis takes approximately 4 weeks.

Reprinted with permission from Goodman M, Hilderley LJ, Purl S: Integumentary and mucous membrane alterations, in Groenwald SL, Frogge MH, Goodman M, Yarbro CH (eds.): *Cancer Nursing: Principles and Practice* (ed 4). Sudbury, MA, Jones and Bartlett, 1997, pp 772–773.[16]

Table 14-5 Late Effects of Radiation on Skin and Connective Tissue

Tissue Response	Onset/Duration	Clinical Presentation	Physiological Rationale
Photosensitivity	Begins during treatment and is lifelong	Enhanced erythema over skin exposed to UV radiation from sun and tanning beds/booths	Destruction of melanocytes in the irradiated dermis and slower melanin production following irradiation reduce the skin's ability to protect itself from UV rays.
Pigmentation changes			
Hyperpigmentation	Refer to Table 14-4		
Hypopigmentation	May begin anytime following resolution of hyperpigmentation Permanent	Lack of skin color	Radiation doses necessary to eradicate cancer may permanently destroy melanocytes, which results in the skin's inability to form pigment.
Atrophy	Following epidermal regrowth Permanent	Thin and fragile epidermis	Newly formed epidermis is thinner. The epidermis thickens over time, but never attains its preirradiation thickness.
Fibrosis	Usually begins 4–6 months following completion of treatment May worsen over time	Dense, hard, uneven skin texture If extensive, may cause considerable induration and pain	Fibroblasts, responsible for producing collagen, proliferate due to a cytokine cascade that causes increased extracellular matrix that is unchecked by normal mechanisms. Fibrotic tissue results, giving the skin an uneven texture.
Telangiectasia	Occurs up to 8 years following radiation therapy Permanent	Purple-red, spiderlike appearance of blood vessels in skin	Dose and fraction size dependent. Basement membrane thickening results in a decreased permeability of material through capillary walls. With capillary occlusion, there are fewer functioning small vessels and a decreased capacity for capillary regeneration. This results in increased pressure of blood flow through remaining undamaged superficial structures.
Ulceration and necrosis	Rare May occur up to 20 years following treatment Usually occurs as a result of inflammation and trauma to previously irradiated tissue	Painful ulcers with red, raised edges and a shaggy, necrotic base. Usually shows little or no tendency to epithelialize or contract. Despite local treatment, ulcers tend to deepen and become more painful.	See fibrosis.

Reprinted with permission from Goodman M, Hilderley LJ, Purl S: Integumentary and mucous membrane alterations, in Groenwald SL, Frogge MH, Goodman M, Yarbro CH (eds.): *Cancer Nursing: Principles and Practice* (ed 4). Sudbury, MA, Jones and Bartlett, 1997, p 775.[16]

applied in the treatment area prior to radiation treatments. Their study was conducted using a phantom chamber to measure surface doses of radiation after various products were applied. Results showed essentially no difference in surface dose. One limitation of this study was that it was conducted using a phantom and not human subjects.[18]

Another study randomized 99 patients receiving radiation therapy to the breast or chest wall to one of three washing policies:

Group 1: No washing of skin in the treatment field
Group 2: Washing with water alone
Group 3: Washing with soap and water

This study concluded that there was little difference between washing with water alone and washing with soap and water. Overall, skin reactions were less frequent if the patients washed. Patients were also prescribed a topical cream for skin reactions, but whether the creams were beneficial was not tested; therefore no recommendations on their use can be made.[19]

At this time, the optimal skin care regimen remains unclear. The goals of skin care management are to

Table 14-6 Suggested Skin Care Guidelines for Patients During Radiation Therapy*

What to expect:

- When you are receiving radiation therapy, it is recommended that you pay special attention to your skin in the area being treated. Skin in the treated area will be more sensitive and can be more easily injured than usual.
- Skin in the treated area may become itchy, dry, red, and sore. Rarely, the skin blisters and peels. Your physician, nurse, and radiation therapist will be monitoring the skin. Ask questions if you have any symptoms or concerns.
- Most important: handle skin in the treated area gently.
- Do not remove temporary skin marks; tattoos are permanent and will not be affected.
- You will lose hair only in the immediate treated area.
- Wash skin in the treated area with warm — not hot — water.
- Wash — never scrub — the skin with care with a mild moisturizing soap (e.g., Dove) and pat dry.
- Avoid heating pads and ice packs on the treated area.
- Avoid using preshave lotions and hair removal products in the treated area.
- If possible, do not shave the treated area. If shaving is necessary, use an electric razor.
- Wear loose, soft clothing over the treated area.
- Do not expose the treated area to the direct sun. If sun exposure is unavoidable, use sunblock having SPF 30 or more.
- Avoid using tape on the treated area.
- Moisturizing the skin can be helpful. Talk with your nurse, radiation therapist, or physician; a list of recommended products may be available.

*Techniques for skin care management are institution specific and not necessarily based on established data as to the optimal regimen.

enhance patient comfort, promote healing, and prevent infection if skin breakdown occurs.[15] Some general guidelines have been suggested, including gentle care of the skin in the treatment field, sun protection with sun-block products (SPF ≥ 30), and moist wound-healing principles for management of moist desquamation.[15,17] Because of the lack of definitive data regarding the efficacy of skin care products and regimens, most skin care guidelines are institution specific and based on habit and anecdotal experience. However, there is a general agreement that hydration of the skin with an emollient, such as aloe vera, is helpful in promoting comfort and reducing pruritis. No products have been shown to definitively prevent or reliably reduce a skin reaction, with the exception of moist wound healing for moist desquamation. Most radiation oncology nurses and physicians have developed skin care protocols. Table 14-6 lists commonly suggested skin care guidelines.

Fatigue

Fatigue during radiation is subjective, almost universal, and affected by multiple factors such as the extent of disease, age, concurrent chemotherapy, weight loss, pain, anemia, and length of radiation treatment. The specific etiology of radiation-related fatigue is unclear. Frequently, patients have undergone a surgical procedure(s) and received chemotherapy prior to radiation therapy. Thus, many patients come to the radiation experience familiar with fatigue and its impact on their lives.

Although most cancer patients report that fatigue is a major obstacle to maintaining normal daily activities and quality of life, it is seldom assessed and treated in clinical practice.[20] Fatigue is best measured by patient self-report. Patients describe their fatigue in many ways, including tiredness, weakness, exhaustion, lack of energy, malaise, impaired ability to concentrate, and overall impaired ability to complete activities of daily living.[21] It follows that such a potentially dramatic influence on physical and mental functioning may adversely affect quality of life.

Patients and families should be taught that fatigue is an expected effect of treatment and may be increased when receiving combined modality therapy.[22] The degree of fatigue-related symptoms increases over the course of radiation treatment.[23,24] During a course of fractionated radiation therapy, fatigue is often cumulative and may peak after a period of weeks. Occasionally, fatigue persists for a prolonged period after the completion of radiation therapy.[20] An early study by King et al. examined 96 subjects weekly during radiation therapy, and then monthly for three months after completing treatment.[25] The patients were receiving radiation for cancers of the chest, head and neck, prostate, and bladder, and for gynecologic tumors. Overall, 65%–93% of patients reported fatigue that gradually increased, was continuous by the last two weeks of treatment, and persisted for several months postradiation. Fatigue symptoms tend to persist after other treatment-related side effects have resolved. It is important to watch for symptoms of clinical depression, especially in the patient experiencing prolonged fatigue.

Graydon et al. evaluated four strategies that patients use to manage fatigue while undergoing chemotherapy or radiation therapy: (1) reducing or stopping activity, (2) increasing activity (physical/social), (3) distraction, and (4) doing something different.[26] Another study of 76 women undergoing radiation therapy for breast cancer reported that the strategies of sitting and sleeping were consistently the most frequently reported and believed to be somewhat effective.[27] What may make the management of fatigue even more difficult is the fact that it is a subjective experience. Patients can generally cope with other side effects such as nausea, vomiting, diarrhea, and skin reactions, perhaps because concrete and effective

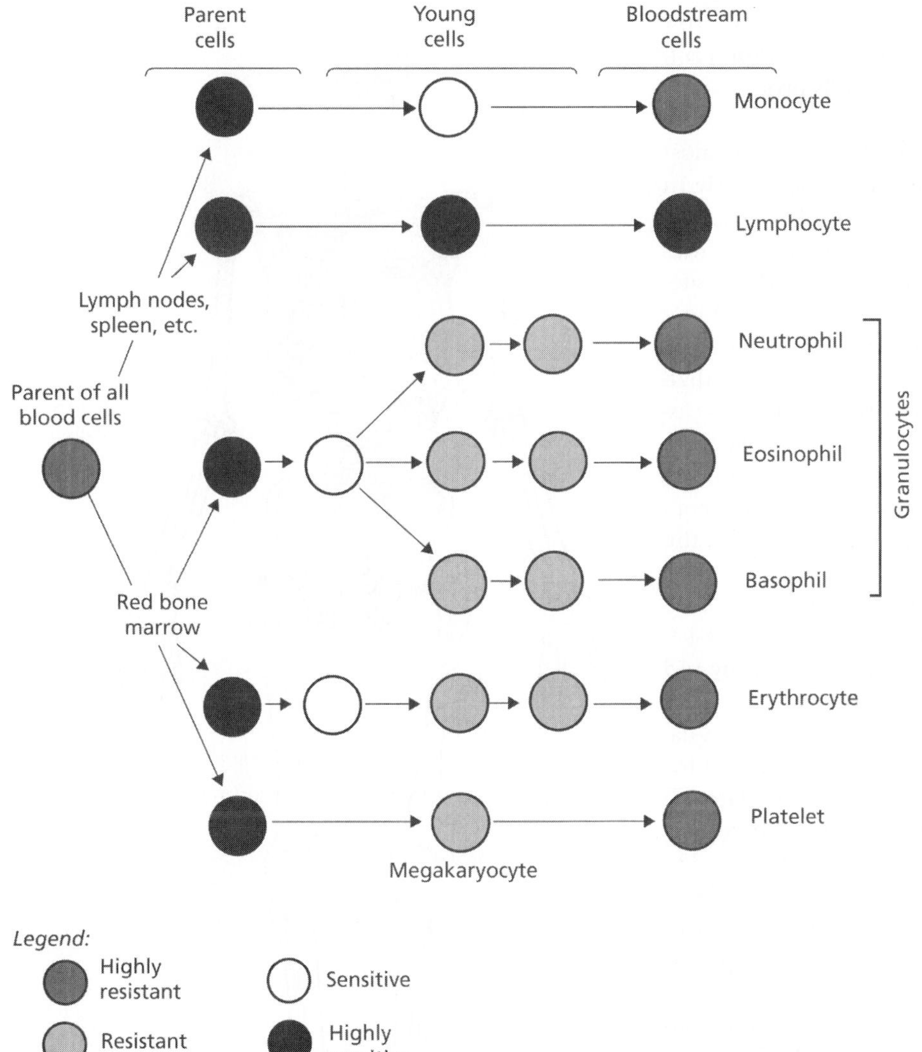

Figure 14-3 Radiosensitivity of Hematopoietic Blood Cells. Note that lymphocytes remain highly sensitive to radiation throughout their life cycle. (Reprinted with permission from Casarett GW: *Radiation Histopathology* (vol. 1). Boca Raton, CRC Press, 1980.[29])

interventions are available. Fatigue, by contrast, does not lend itself to such concrete management techniques.

Acknowledging fatigue as a "legitimate" toxicity of radiation therapy may be as important as making suggestions for its management. Educating patients and family members also includes helping them choose the most appropriate interventions to fight fatigue. Finding a balance of activity and energy conservation may be helpful for the chronic fatigue experienced with both chemotherapy and radiation therapy.[22] Physical activity must be tailored to each individual, but usually includes light exercise such as walking and gardening. Exercise has been shown to increase concentration and overall ability to think clearly, which allows patients to participate more fully in their care and daily activities. Other strategies to treat fatigue include modification of the patient's drug regimen, correction of metabolic abnormalities, and pharmacologic treatments for anemia (e.g., epoetin alfa), depression, or insomnia. Specific pharmacologic approaches include psychostimulant drugs and corticosteroids. Supportive therapies may also be helpful, including cognitive therapies, sleep hygiene strategies, and nutritional support.[20] Patients report acupuncture can be helpful for fatigue management. (See Chapter 30 for a detailed discussion of fatigue.)

Myelosuppression

Bone marrow is an important dose-limiting cell-renewal tissue for chemotherapy, wide-field irradiation, and autologous bone marrow transplantation.[28]

It is so highly radiosensitive that injury to bone marrow is produced by any dose of radiation. Following each dose of radiation, peripheral blood cells progressively decrease in number due to the destruction of both mature and precursor cells. Lymphocytes are the most sensitive cells; hence lymphopenia develops early in the course of radiation therapy. Figure 14-3 illustrates the relative radiosensitivity of hematopoietic cell lines throughout their life cycle.[29] The radiation dose, site, and tissue volume all affect the acute response of bone marrow to therapy. When small radiation fields comprising only 10%–15% of the bone marrow are radiated, the unexposed bone marrow responds by increasing its population of progenitor cells to meet the demands for hematopoiesis. Thus, treatment limiting myelosuppression is rarely seen unless large areas containing a substantial portion of marrow are within the radiation fields.[28] Approximately 40% of active bone marrow is in the pelvis, with the remaining 60% of active marrow distributed as illustrated in Figure 14-4.[30]

The acute effects of concurrent chemotherapy and radiation on bone marrow are complex. Any treatment regimen combining chemotherapy and radiation therapy must take into account the potential for increased dose-limiting marrow suppression.[28] Growth factors supporting development of all hematologic cell lines are seldom needed when radiation is used as a single modality. However, in combined modality therapy, growth factors are more commonly part of treatment regimens due to the increased risk of pancytopenia.

Patients at highest risk for developing cytopenias are those receiving concurrent chemoradiation, total body irradiation, extended-field (whole-abdomen) radiation, and splenic radiation. Most radiation fields are designed to limit the amount of bone marrow exposed to radiation. However, it may be necessary to irradiate marrow-producing areas in high-risk patients, such as those who have been heavily pretreated (chemotherapy and/or radiation) and those who have bony metastases that require radiation therapy for pain management. The frequency of monitoring blood counts varies by individual patient risk factors.

Chronic or late effects of radiation on bone marrow include increased hematopoietic activity in unexposed marrow segments, followed by extension of functioning marrow into previously quiescent areas such as the femora and humeri. Bone marrow regeneration is variable in each individual but generally lags behind the peripheral blood counts. Marrow recovery can occur over extended periods, with total recovery in 12–24 months, but this outcome depends on the volume of marrow irradiated.[28] Generally, patients are not at greater risk for infection during the chronic recovery phase.

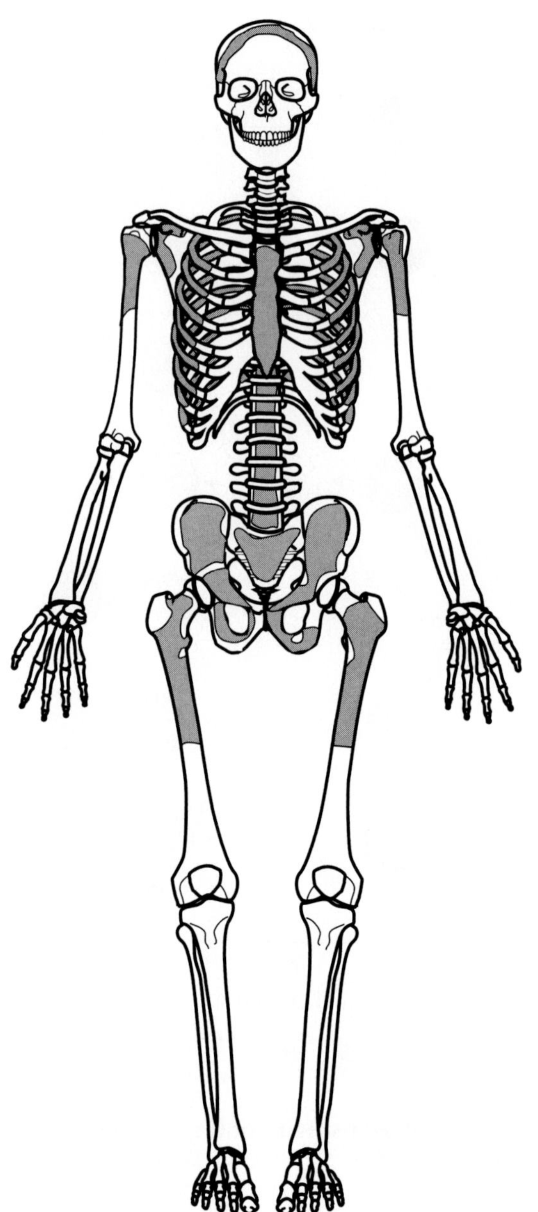

Figure 14-4 Bone Marrow Distribution. Bone marrow distribution in adult humans as determined by autopsy findings; active regions are shaded.

Acute Radiation Toxicities and Management: Site Specific

Acute toxicities or side effects are expected during a course of radiation therapy. Radiation toxicities directly correlate with the specific normal tissues and structures within the path of the radiation beam. Table 14-7 presents a representative list of site-specific acute toxicities. The goal of radiation is to maintain the therapeutic ratio so as to achieve maximum tumor cell kill with minimal toxicity to normal tissues and structures.

Because the radiation beam must pass through the skin, all patients are at some level of risk for an acute

Table 14-7 Selected Site-Specific Acute Toxicities of Radiation Therapy*

CNS (primary brain tumors, brain metastasis)
- Brain
  - Scalp, forehead erythema
  - Alopecia
  - External auditory canal irritation
  - Transient increased cerebral edema
  - Nausea/vomiting (rare)
- Spinal cord
  - Lhermitte's syndrome (subacute)

Head and Neck (nasopharynx, oro/hypopharynx, larynx)
- Skin erythema
- Oral mucositis
- Esophagitis → dysphagia → odynophagia
- Xerostomia
- Dysgeusia, ageusia → anorexia

Breast
- Skin erythema that may progress to moist desquamation

Chest/Lung (lung, esophageal, gastric cancers)
- Skin erythema (anterior and posterior fields)
- Esophagitis → dysphagia/odynophagia
- Dysgeusia → anorexia
- Gastric reflux symptoms
- Pneumonitis (subacute)

Abdomen/Pelvis (GI, GU, gynecologic cancers)
- Nausea/vomiting (radiation site dependent)
- Diarrhea
- Proctitis symptoms
- Cystitis symptoms
- Mucositis of perianal region
- Vaginal dryness

*Acute toxicities are dependent on the site treated (the normal structures in the field), daily dose, radiation energy used, and volume treated (size of the field).

skin reaction. Also, as previously described, fatigue is an almost universal reaction to radiation therapy. When assessing patients, the nurse should be aware of potential skin reactions, fatigue, and myelosuppression, in addition to site-specific effects. The following section addresses potential site-specific acute radiation-related toxicities and management. The list of toxicities is representative and reflects policies and practices currently advocated in the literature and at various institutions. It should be stressed that alternative methods for managing toxicities exist that are also appropriate. Acute toxicities are dependent on the site treated, daily dose, radiation energy used, and size of the treatment field (the radiation therapy mantra).

Brain

Used in treatment for primary brain tumors or metastases, head and brain irradiation can result in the following toxicities.

Alopecia and scalp erythema

Because of the high mitotic rate of hair follicles of the scalp, hair loss will occur when the head is irradiated. Alopecia starts approximately 2–3 weeks (2500–3000 cGy) into treatment. The extent of alopecia depends on the size of the field. If the whole brain is treated (i.e., diffuse or multiple metastases), total hair loss will result. Partial brain irradiation (i.e., primary brain tumor) results in alopecia that conforms to the edges of the treatment field(s). Hair almost always regrows with scalp doses of 5000–6000 cGy or less, and permanent hair loss usually occurs with doses of 6000 cGy or more.[31] Regrowth of hair may take from 3 to 6 months after completion of radiation, and the new hair may be a different color and/or texture. Alopecia secondary to irradiation of the head is inevitable, and there are no proven preventive strategies. Alopecia causes a major change in self-image and is a visible reminder of the cancer experience.

Management. Scalp irritation and erythema can be managed with gentle care to the scalp and hair. The hair should be washed with a mild shampoo. Irritants such as hair dyes, hot curlers and irons, and hair dryers that can further irritate the scalp should be avoided. Patients should be encouraged to consider hair coverings (e.g., wig, turban, scarf) prior to hair loss because it is much easier to match hair style and color before total alopecia occurs. The scalp tends to be sensitive after radiation-induced hair loss, especially with accompanying scalp erythema and irritation. Some patients cannot tolerate anything on the head.

Inform patients that significant body heat loss occurs from the head and that, without the insulation of hair, they might feel cold, especially during sleep. During the day, the head and scalp should be protected from the sun with hats and sun-block products. Psychological interventions, such as support groups or patient-to-patient assistance, may help the patient cope with the effects of alopecia on self-image.

Ear and external auditory canal

If the ear is in the treatment field, the pinna and external auditory canal may become irritated, sore, and pruritic. Symptoms generally resolve within 1–2 weeks after completion of therapy.

Management. Instruct the patient to protect the ear from sun and cold exposure. For discomfort in the external auditory canal, ear drops with hydrocortisone can be prescribed.

Cerebral edema

Increased intracranial pressure (ICP), secondary to cerebral edema, is often present at diagnosis. Radiation-induced ICP occurs, though the mechanism involved is not well understood.[32] The incidence of ICP increases with the size of the initial fraction(s); for example, fractions of 200 cGy or more per day commonly result in ICP. Symptoms include exacerbation of patients' presenting neurologic symptoms, such as headache, nausea and vomiting, muscle or extremity weakness, seizures, and mental status changes.

Management. Patients with known brain tumors or metastasis are usually taking corticosteroids, and titrating the dose will often alleviate symptoms of ICP. The patient who is not taking corticosteroids and who will begin brain radiation, especially whole-brain treatment, needs to be closely monitored. Cerebral edema can develop quickly. The steroid most commonly used to prevent cerebral edema is dexamethasone, which offers rapid onset of activity and a biologic half-life of 36–54 hours. The dose of dexamethasone varies, but a frequently used regimen is 12–16 mg per day (4 mg every 6–8 hours). Instruct patients not to abruptly discontinue the corticosteroid because of the risk of hypothalamic-pituitary axis (HPA) suppression, which can result in adrenal insufficiency. Symptoms of adrenal insufficiency include fatigue, nausea, vomiting, diarrhea, and weight loss.

Patients and families should be educated regarding the multiple side effects of steroids, such as gastrointestinal (GI) effects (reflux, nausea), candidiasis (especially in the oral cavity), hyperglycemia in diabetics, psychological changes such as mood swings, insomnia, and myopathy (especially proximal leg weakness). Antacid therapy (i.e., H_2 blocker or acid-pump inhibitor) is recommended for prophylaxis of GI symptoms. Other steroid-induced toxicities are managed with medications such as lorazepam and temazepam for relaxation or sleep, systemic antifungals for candidiasis, and titration of oral antidiabetic agents or insulin for hyperglycemia.

Although steroids relieve ICP symptoms relatively quickly, most patients do not feel well while taking them and want to stop steroid therapy as soon as possible. The timing of a steroid taper varies, but generally decreasing the dose by half every 4–7 days will not cause exacerbation of symptoms. If symptoms recur, instruct the patient to return to the previous steroid dose. Try not to begin a steroid taper on Friday (half-life of dexamethasone = 36–54 hours), because neurologic symptoms may recur on the weekend when radiation oncology staff are not as readily available.

Nausea and vomiting

Nausea and vomiting caused by brain irradiation are rare, short-lived effects and can be well controlled with antiemetics. Symptoms also may occur secondary to cerebral edema, and increasing the corticosteroid dose may relieve symptoms.

Management. Antiemetic regimens include the following:

Selective 5-HT_3 Receptor Antagonists

- Ondansetron 8 mg PO 1–2 hours prior to radiation and every 8 hours PRN
- Granisetron 2 mg PO 1 hour prior to daily radiation
- Dolasetron mesylate 100 mg PO 1 hour prior to radiation

Phenothiazines

- Prochlorperazine 5–10 mg PO 1 hour prior to radiation and every 4–6 hours PRN
- Prochlorperazine spansules 15 mg PO or suppositories 25 mg PR given approximately 1–2 hours prior to radiation
- Triethylperazine 10 mg PO 1 hour prior to radiation and every 8 hours PRN

Benzodiazepines

- Lorazepam 0.5–1.0 mg PO or sublingual three times a day PRN

Antidopaminergic (promotes gastric motility)

- Metaclopramide 10 mg PO four times a day PRN, or
- Metachlopromide (controlled release) 20–80 mg every 12 hours (maximum 12 weeks duration)

Corticosteroids (dosage varies with agent)

- Dexamethosone
- Prednisone
- Prednisolone

Somnolence syndrome (subacute)

Somnolence syndrome is a collection of symptoms consisting of excessive sleepiness and drowsiness, lethargy and fatigue, accompanied by anorexia and occasional mild headache. This syndrome is well recognized and occurs more frequently in children than in adults. The cause of the somnolence is unclear but is believed to be related to transient demyelination secondary to radiation's effect on oligodendrocytes. Symptoms occur 4–12 weeks after radiation is complete and can last for 2–8 weeks. In one study, adult patients who developed somnolence syndrome after cranial irradiation for primary brain tumors identified a cyclical pattern to the symptoms. Periods of drowsiness and fatigue occurred from day 11 to day 21 and from day 31 to day 35 after the completion of cranial radiation. Patients often attributed symptoms of somnolence to flu or other ailments. The unexplained and overwhelming nature of the symptoms caused anxiety.[33]

Management. Anticipatory guidance is a critical nursing intervention.[34] Management is directed at supportive care as the syndrome runs its course. Supportive measures include maintaining nutrition (especially in children who may sleep a greater portion of 24 hours) and prevention of problems related to prolonged immobilization, such as venous thrombosis and skin breakdown.

Head and Neck

Used in treatment for cancers of the nasopharynx, oropharynx, hypopharynx, and larynx, head and neck irradiation can result in multiple toxicities. Assessment and management of these toxicities present a major challenge for oncology nurses. There are numerous structures and systems in the head and neck region that result in multiple and often severe acute and late toxicities. Patients with head and neck cancer are more likely to have poor nutritional status, abuse tobacco and alcohol, and have functional deficits (i.e., speech, swallowing, chewing, airway compromise). Persons with head and neck cancer need advocacy and support from all members of the cancer care team to maintain compliance with the radiation schedule, as well as to manage the toxicities and needed self-care regimens. Suspension of radiation treatment may become necessary to allow for healing of affected tissues.

Oral mucositis (stomatitis)

The epithelial cells of the mucous membrane lining the oral cavity are highly radiosensitive.[31] The reaction of the oral mucosa can range from erythema to painful ulceration. A pseudomembrane can form and then slough off, leaving a painful, friable surface.[35] Areas of the buccal mucosa and buccal sulcus that are adjacent to metal tooth fillings are at greater risk for increased reaction due to radiation scatter from the metal filling. Mucositis will be enhanced and prolonged in patients who have preexisting poor oral or dental hygiene, continue to smoke, use chewing tobacco, consume alcohol, and have poorly fitting dentures. Combined modality therapy with chemotherapeutic agents such as 5-fluorouracil will enhance mucositis of the oropharynx. The onset of oral mucositis is seen approximately 2–3 weeks after the start of treatment. Symptoms generally begin as generalized oral discomfort and progress (depending on the radiation dose) to pain such that eating, swallowing, and speaking become extremely painful, if not impossible.

Assessment for oral mucositis involves frequent inspection of the oral cavity. Evaluation schedules are patient specific, though weekly inspection is adequate early in the course of treatment (first 2–3 weeks), and then as symptoms indicate. A mouth care regimen should focus on hygiene, dental prophylaxis, and comfort.

Management. Management strategies include avoiding products that will further dry the mucous membranes, such as mouthwashes with alcohol and any glycerin-based product. Instruct the patient to gently brush the teeth and tongue frequently with a soft toothbrush. Ideally, the patient should perform oral care four times daily and, if tolerated, continue flossing teeth. Mouth rinses with an isotonic saline solution (swish and spit) help loosen debris and cleanse the oral cavity. A common saline solution mixture is 1 teaspoon of salt and/or 1 teaspoon of baking soda in a quart of water. This solution is mild and rarely causes increased discomfort. Patients should be encouraged to swish and spit the solution as often as possible—ideally, every 1–2 waking hours. Topical anesthetics such as a 1:1:1 mixture of liquid antacid, diphenhydramine hydrochloride, and viscous lidocaine are helpful. Instruct patients to swish and swallow/spit 5–10 mL of the topical anesthetic 20 minutes prior to eating and drinking.

Many prepared topical anesthetics are commercially available. Systemic analgesics are often needed and are most convenient in liquid and transdermal forms if odynophagia is present. Other recommendations include using dentures only when eating and consuming a soft to liquid diet of bland foods at room temperature. Oral mucositis can dramatically decrease appetite and diminish caloric intake, which may necessitate nutritional supplements and intravenous hydration. (See the section on esophagitis later in this chapter for further discussion of nursing management.)

Oral candidiasis

Candidiasis is an infection of the oral mucosa with a yeast-like fungus, most commonly *Candida albicans*. In patients undergoing head and neck irradiation, candidiasis occurs frequently due to destruction of the protective oral mucosal barrier, resulting in an overgrowth of *Candida*. The infection is characterized by white patches and clusters in the mouth. Assessment of the entire oral cavity includes the tongue, roof of mouth, and buccal sulci. Although a culture can be sent for microbiologic confirmation, the diagnosis is usually made on the basis of clinical findings.

Management. Antifungal medication is prescribed. A variety of preparations of antifungal drugs are available, including swish-and-swallow, troches, and systemic oral agents. It is important to remember that most head and neck patients have concurrent xerostomia (see below), so troches will be generally ineffective because they will not dissolve well, if at all. A swish-and-swallow preparation demands a compliant patient, as it must be done four to five times daily and can further irritate already painful oral mucosa. Daily oral administration of an agent such as fluconazole, which is available in liquid form, may be more appropriate for these patients. Often, esophagitis and mucositis diminish somewhat when candidiasis is resolved. Head and neck patients endure multiple toxicities, and candidiasis is one of these many side effects. Reassure the patient that this infection is fairly easily treated with medication.

Oral herpes

Oral herpetic lesions may occur with or without candidiasis. Herpes lesions appear as vesicles on the oral mucosa. Diagnosis is made by clinical assessment, culture, and microbiologic confirmation.

Management. Treatment with oral antiviral medications such as acyclovir or famciclovir are generally effective.

Xerostomia

The major salivary glands (parotid, submandibular, and sublingual) are highly radiosensitive. Together, the salivary glands produce more than 1 liter of saliva per day. Typically, 60%–65% of the total salivary volume is produced by the parotid glands, 20%–30% by the submandibular glands, and 2%–5% by the sublingual glands. The parotid glands are composed of serous cells and produce watery and albuminous secretions. The submaxillary and sublingual glands, composed of mixed serous cells and mucous acini, have thicker secretions.

Saliva plays an important role in mastication, digestion, swallowing, and speech. The mean daily salivary output ranges from 500 to 1500 mL. The average volume of saliva present in the oral cavity is approximately 1 mL.[36] More than 99% of saliva is water. Saliva also contains inorganic ions, lipids, amino acids, proteins, and traces of hormone-like substances. The proteins, including the salivary enzymes, are derived from the serum or synthesized within the parotid glands. The secretory function of the salivary glands is controlled by the autonomic nervous system and may be stimulated by the sensation of taste, smell, or chewing, and by psychological factors and stimulation, such as esophageal and gastric irritations, from other organs.[36] Saliva provides lubrication for oral tissues and protection from bacterial infections. It also inhibits enamel decalcification and provides an important excretory route for blood-borne urea, uric acid, and ammonia.

The serous cells of the salivary glands are more radiosensitive and the mucous cells more radioresistant. A 50% or more reduction in salivary flow has been detected after the first week of fractionated radiation therapy to the head and neck area. This flow continues to decline and may become barely measurable by the end of a 6- to 8-week course of treatment. Because the parotid glands (serous, watery secretions) are more affected by the radiation, the remaining saliva becomes thick and ropy.[36] Generally, patients notice the onset of dry mouth within the first 2 weeks of radiation.

Management. Strategies for managing oral dryness include increasing oral fluids (most patients find water most helpful, but relief is of short duration), sugarless candy or gum, and sugarless lemon-flavored drinks.[35,37] Sugarless products sweetened with xylitol alone or in combination with sorbital are preferred. Some data suggest that xylitol has anticariogenic properties. Xylitol is associated with a decrease in *Streptococcus mutans* levels in saliva and dental plaque.[38] A dietary consult is helpful to assist patients with meal planning.

Saliva substitutes and chemical salivary gland stimulants are available. The so-called artificial saliva products are helpful for some patients but only afford short-term relief of dryness. These products are costly, and generally patients dislike their taste and consistency.

Pilocarpine hydrochloride is a cholinergic stimulant that acts on postganglionic cells innervating smooth muscles and exocrine glands (i.e., sweat and salivary glands).[36] Several studies have demonstrated that pilocarpine given orally can reduce the symptoms of postirradiation xerostomia in patients who have some residual salivary function.[39–42] The most common regimen consists of pilocarpine 5 mg qid but the dose can be increased to 10 mg qid as indicated. Side effects include sweating (usually within 30 minutes of administration) and other cholinergic effects that are relatively mild with the 5-mg dose regimen. Some data suggest that pilocarpine given concurrently and 3 months postirradiation may decrease overall postirradiation xerostomia.[43]

The radioprotectant potential of thiol-containing compounds has been established. Amifostine (WR-2721, Ethyol) is a free-radical scavenger and cyto/radioprotectant that has been tested extensively. Multiple studies have demonstrated its protective effects on the salivary glands during head and neck irradiation. In all studies, no tumor-protective effect by amifostine was detected.[44]

Acupuncture has also been shown to increase salivary flow. The mechanism of action is unknown, but this strategy is an option for xerostomic patients.[45–47]

Esophagitis and pharyngitis

The pharynx and esophagus are usually in the treatment fields for head and neck irradiation. The radiation causes inflammation and denudation of the surface epithelium of the pharynx and esophagus. The resulting mucositis leads to dysphagia and odynophagia that can be so severe that patients may be unable to take food and fluids or swallow oral secretions. Symptoms usually start approximately 2 weeks into a course of therapy. If the patient is receiving concurrent chemotherapy, symptoms may occur sooner and be more severe. As with oral mucositis, patients who continue to smoke and use alcohol are at greater risk for acute and prolonged symptoms.

Management. Nursing management and interventions are similar to those for oral mucositis. Esophagitis/pharyngitis is a potentially serious toxicity if patients are unable to maintain nutrition and hydration. Patients should be weighed once or twice weekly and carefully assessed as to oral intake. Enteral feeding and IV hydration are needed in many patients and should be discussed prior to initiating irradiation. When prescribing medication for the patient with odynophagia, liquids or crushable tablets should be considered. Patients quickly determine what they can swallow, and intake usually concentrates on soft to liquid foods. Consultation and collaboration with a dietitian may help the patient maintain the optimal protein and calorie intake.

Taste changes (dysgeusia, ageusia)

Taste buds (receptors) are primarily located on the tongue, soft palate, glossopalatine arch, and posterior wall of the pharynx. Taste sensations include sweet, sour, salty, and bitter. Because the taste buds are extremely radiosensitive, symptoms are noted early in the course of treatment, often during weeks 1 and 2.[35] Patients typically describe a decrease in taste (hypogeusia) and altered taste (dysgeusia). In some patients, this effect will progress to loss of all taste (ageusia).

Taste is integrally bound to appetite. When one cannot taste food, this problem may result in progressive anorexia and weight loss. Patients may describe a sensation of the food creating a "tasteless ball of goo" in their mouth. Add to this the symptoms of xerostomia and mucositis/esophagitis, and eating can become an ordeal.

Management. Encourage oral care prior to meals to help clear residual tastes and refresh the mouth for meals.[35] Strategies to enhance the palatability of foods are discussed in Chapter 33 and apply to patients undergoing radiation. The loss of "salt" perception can be particularly problematic for some patients if they add significant quantities of salt to their food. In such a case, a dietary consult can prove very helpful.

Laryngitis

If the larynx is in the radiation treatment field(s), patients will experience laryngitis due to edema of the vocal cords.[31] Symptoms include hoarseness that can be mild to so severe that speech becomes almost impossible.

Management. Patients should be instructed to avoid straining to speak; however, this is difficult to accomplish. Elderly patients or those who live alone may be anxious that they will not be able to communicate their needs should they be in an emergent situation. Speech therapists can be consulted regarding assistive devices such as those that amplify the voice.

Instruct patients to avoid tobacco and alcohol. It is important to remember that compliance with abstinence from tobacco and alcohol can be difficult, if not impossible, for this group of patients, as they often have many years of dependency and use. Management of laryngitis is similar to management of esophagitis and focuses on nutrition, hydration, lubrication, and pain relief.

Dental caries

Dental caries technically are not an acute toxicity of head and neck irradiation, but preventive management for them during treatment is mandatory. All teeth are at risk — not just those in the path of the radiation beam. Due to xerostomia, the pH of the mouth shifts toward a highly acid oral environment, and markedly cariogenic flora develop. The teeth rapidly demineralize and enamel defects appear, especially on the cervical and incisal/occlusal surfaces. The resulting dental demineralization almost always leads to radiation-induced caries, which constitute a risk factor for osteoradionecrosis of the mandible and maxilla.[48] Osteoradionecrosis is a potentially severe chronic complication that results in bony necrosis of the jaw (primarily the mandible) and requires intensive treatment that may include surgical resection and bone grafting.

Preventive management. Dentulous patients must have a dental evaluation prior to starting radiation. Questionable teeth should be extracted, ideally at least 14 days prior to the initiation of irradiation. Most often, dental prophylaxis consists of daily fluoride solution or gel applied to a mold (tray) and placed on upper and lower teeth, then held in place for several minutes. A home care fluoride regimen is essential but may not be possible to maintain if severe mucositis is present. This potential complication argues for even greater compliance with the oral care regimen until fluoride prophylaxis can be resumed.

Breast

Used in treatment for breast carcinoma, breast irradiation can result in several toxicities. This discussion focuses on the effects of breast irradiation after breast-preserving surgery.

Skin reactions

Skin reactions are the primary acute side effects of breast irradiation. Due to the tangential angle of the beam, the skin dose is enhanced. Skin in the treatment fields may demonstrate erythema and hyperpigmentation. Changes are usually clinically evident at approximately 3000 cGy with standard fractions of 180–200 cGy daily.[49] Skin reactions can progress to severe erythema and moist desquamation, especially in the inframammary crease and axilla. Women who are at most risk for developing moist desquamation are those with large pendulous breasts and those receiving concurrent chemotherapy.

Management. See the Assessment and Management of Skin Reactions section earlier in this chapter. The patient may also experience transient discomfort in the breast and axilla during radiation. The etiology of this effect is unclear, although surgical changes and possibly radiation-related edema may be the cause. Such symptoms usually respond to nonsteroidal anti-inflammatory drugs such as ibuprofen or naproxyn.

Esophagitis

Esophagitis may occur if the supraclavicular fossa is included in the treatment field. Symptoms are usually mild and limited in duration.

Management. See the discussion of management under esophagitis and pharyngitis in the Head and Neck section of this chapter.

Chest and Lung

Used in treatment for lung, esophageal, gastric cancers, Hodgkin's disease, and non-Hodgkin's chest lymphoma, chest and lung irradiation results in the following toxicities.

Esophagitis and pharyngitis

Most radiation treatment fields for treatment of lung, esophageal, and gastric cancers and some lymphomas include the mediastinum and thus affect the esophagus and hypopharynx. The resulting mucositis causes dysphagia and odynophagia that may become severe. Patients often describe the feeling of a "lump" in the throat and a feeling of obstruction when swallowing. Symptoms start 2–3 weeks after initiation of radiation, or sooner if the patient is receiving concurrent chemotherapy.[50] The treatment fields are usually angled (versus initial direct anterior-posterior fields) approximately two-thirds of the way into treatment, thereby minimizing some of the dose to the pharynx and esophagus. As a consequence, symptoms lessen. Depending on the length (top to bottom) of the field and the site of esophageal or gastric cancer (e.g., tumor at the gastroesophageal junction), patients may experience gastric reflux that can exacerbate esophagitis symptoms.

Management. Management is similar to that described under esophagitis and pharyngitis in the Head and Neck section of this chapter. Dietary modifications are helpful and include a soft to liquid diet and nutritional supplements. Antacid therapy can be started for patients who experience reflux symptoms. Close monitoring is essential, as oral intake can decrease with fluid imbalance and weight loss may occur rapidly. Patients presenting with upper gastrointestinal and lung cancers frequently have impaired nutritional status and a history of tobacco and alcohol abuse, which can present a challenge for optimal patient management.

Taste changes

It is unclear why patients receiving radiation to the chest experience taste changes. The cause is likely multifactorial, including prior or concurrent chemotherapy, fatigue, and medications such as opioids. Taste changes may lead to anorexia and, when combined with the previously described toxicities, can cause a cascade of effects including increased fatigue, weight loss, weakness, and delayed healing of acute side effects.

Management. Consultation with the oncology dietitian is helpful to define ways to maintain optimal nutritional status.

Pneumonitis (subacute)

Pneumonitis is not an infectious process; indeed, *pneumonopathy* might be a more appropriate term for this toxicity. Pneumonitis is caused by a decrease in surfactant produced by the alveolar type II pneumocytes in conjunction with endothelial cell and vessel permeability that negatively affects perfusion.[31] Symptoms occur 1–3 months after completion of radiation and can be seen within days after administration of certain chemotherapeutic agents, such as bleomycin, chlorambucil, the nitrosureas, cyclophosphamide, methotrexate, and procarbazine. Symptomatic pneumonitis occurs in approximately 5%–15% of patients irradiated for mediastinal lymphoma or lung cancer, and approximately 1% of women treated for breast cancer.[51]

The severity of the pneumonitis depends on the degree of pulmonary involvement, which is the amount of lung parenchyma in the treatment fields. Symptoms include low-grade fever and nonspecific respiratory symptoms such as congestion, nonproductive cough, and a feeling of fullness in the chest. If symptoms progress, the patient may experience dyspnea, pleuritic chest pain, and increasing cough that may result in small amounts of sputum with hemoptysis. On examination, altered breath sounds are usually absent. Pleural friction rub or pleural fluid may be detected. Generally, the symptomatic phase of pneumonitis is relatively short in duration, and symptoms resolve completely.

Diagnosis of pneumonitis is made clinically with radiologic studies and symptom review. A chest x-ray (CXR) may reveal a diffuse infiltrate and possibly functional lung volume loss corresponding to the radiation field. Computerized tomography (CT) scans are more sensitive in evaluating lung density. Ventilation/perfusion scans are also used for diagnosis. Pulmonary function tests (PFT) will not demonstrate an abnormality until 4–8 weeks after completion of irradiation. A decrease in diffusion capacity is generally the most outstanding parameter on PFTs.[51]

Management. Treatment of the acute symptoms of pneumonitis includes bed rest to conserve respiratory effort, bronchial dilators, oxygen therapy, and glucocorticoids. Treatment measures do not shorten the duration of pneumonitis; instead, they aim to palliate symptoms. In rare cases, radiation pneumonitis may be severe, with symptoms including fever and acute cor pulmonale that can lead to death. After the acute phase of pneumonitis, symptoms slowly improve, as inflammation resolves.[51]

Nursing assessment includes evaluation of symptoms and monitoring of the patient's oxygenation status and ability to complete activities of daily living. A physical/occupational therapy consultation can help patients adapt their daily activities to accommodate their respiratory disability.

Abdomen and Pelvis

Used in treatment for gastrointestinal, genitourinary, and gynecologic cancers, abdomen and pelvis irradiation can result in the following toxicities.

Nausea and vomiting

Radiation therapy is a localized treatment. As a consequence, nausea and vomiting will not occur unless radiation fields include the whole abdomen, extended pelvic fields, epigastric region, paraortic area, and, in rare cases, the chemoreceptor trigger zone (CTZ) in the cerebral cortex.[43] Symptoms of nausea and vomiting directly related to irradiation are fairly predictable and will occur 1–3 hours after the daily treatment. Nausea and vomiting are influenced by multiple other factors, including medications (e.g., opioids, antibiotics), chemotherapeutic agents, constipation, pain, and metabolic alterations such as hypercalcemia.[52]

Management. Patients who are at risk for nausea and vomiting should be premedicated with antiemetics approximately 1 hour prior to daily treatment, depending on medication and route of administration. The goal is to prevent an initial emetic episode. Around-the-clock administration of antiemetics may be necessary if symptoms warrant. It is difficult to definitively recommend whether patients should receive daily radiation treatment with an empty or full stomach. Generally, patients feel better and have less nausea if they eat small frequent meals or snacks, including prior to daily radiation. See the discussion of nausea and vomiting in the Brain section of this chapter for a brief discussion of antiemetics commonly used in radiation therapy.

Diarrhea and proctitis

The size of the abdominal/pelvic radiation field generally determines the risk for diarrhea and proctitis. Diarrhea is a result of denuding of the intestinal mucosa, leading to decreased absorptive capacity and increased motility and peristalsis.[53] The small bowel is much more radiosensitive than the colon or rectum, and the extent of the small bowel's involvement greatly influences the severity of the symptoms. A patient undergoing whole-abdomen radiation is at greatest risk to experience watery diarrhea and cramping, while the patient with a relatively small pelvic field (e.g., radiation for prostate cancer) will most likely have frequent soft bowel movements rather than pronounced diarrhea.

Proctitis can be accompanied by tenesmus. Proctitis occurs most frequently in patients receiving radiation for rectal, anal, and prostate cancers due to the location of the inferior border of the treatment fields. Symptoms are compounded if concurrent chemotherapy is administered.

Management. Patients should be instructed regarding a low-residue diet and the use of antidiarrheals. A low-residue diet guideline is helpful to assist in teaching and for patient reference. Ethnic and geographic food patterns should be considered to support compliance.[52] An oncology dietitian consult can be invaluable. The patient should ideally have antidiarrheal medication (e.g., loperamide or diphenoxylate/atropine) on hand in case diarrhea occurs unexpectedly. Severe or protracted diarrhea may require treatment with octreotide (Sandostatin). Octreotide, which is similar to the natural hormone sandostatin, suppresses secretions of serotonin and multiple GI peptides. It is effective in secretory-type diarrhea because it stimulates fluid and electrolyte absorption from the GI tract. This agent is administered by subcutaneous injection one to three times daily. A long-acting formulation is available as well. A clinical trial is currently recruiting patients receiving radiation therapy to the pelvis, with or without chemotherapy, to assess the efficacy of octreotide in controlling and preventing acute and chronic diarrhea.

Proctitis symptoms can be treated with conservative management, including sitz baths and anti-inflammatory agents such as pramoxine hydrochloride 1% and/or hydrocortisone acetate 1% (cream or foam). Gastrointestinal-specific antispasmodics may decrease tenesmus symptoms. Diarrhea and frequent stools can result in painful irritation of the perianal region secondary to frequent cleansing. Helpful interventions include gently cleansing the perianal region (after each bowel movement) with warm water using a squirt bottle, patting dry, and then applying a barrier cream and using pre-moistened towelettes.

Assessment should start with the patient's definition of diarrhea and specific stool characteristics and frequency. Of most concern are frequent, watery stools that have the potential for inducing electrolyte imbalance and dehydration. Patients most at risk for dehydration due to diarrhea or vomiting include children, the elderly, debilitated individuals, and those receiving concurrent chemotherapy (e.g., 5-fluorouracil, cisplatin). It is essential to monitor weight frequently (daily if necessary), check orthostatic blood pressure, and assess skin and mucosal turgor. Some patients may require intravenous hydration and a break from radiation treatment.

Cystitis

Acute cystitis symptoms include dysuria, nocturia, hesitancy, urgency, and urinary frequency. The intensity and duration of symptoms depend on the volume of bladder in the radiation treatment field. As the radiation dose escalates, patients may experience tenesmus and bladder spasms that potentiate existing symptoms. Hematuria is uncommon. Symptoms of acute bladder irritation frequently occur 3–5 weeks after the initiation of radiation therapy and usually subside 2–8 weeks after completion of treatment. Symptoms of cystitis subside with mucosal healing, pharmacologic intervention, and, if needed, a break from radiation treatment.[54]

Management. Pretreatment assessment of bladder function includes documentation of patterns of urinary elimination, such as symptoms of urgency, frequency, dysuria, nocturia, and past history of urinary tract infections and medications used for treatment.

Inflamed mucosa and ulceration of the bladder increase the potential for infection. Initial treatment consists of ruling out infection and administering antibiotic therapy if indicated. Infection often exacerbates bladder spasm and complicates delivery of radiation treatment. Antispasmodics help relieve dysuria and provide relief from bladder spasms. Optimal comfort is obtained if both infection and bladder spasm are treated simultaneously. Phenazopyridine hydrochloride is frequently used to treat dysuria symptoms. When taken orally, the majority of the drug enters the urine unchanged, where it acts as a topical analgesic within the bladder. When taking the drug, the patient's urine will be colored orange-red.

Symptoms such as mild urinary frequency occur due to a modest reduction in bladder capacity. To increase storage capacity, antispasmodic medications such as oxybutynin chloride and flavoxate hydrochloride may be prescribed to relax the bladder smooth muscle by inhibiting the muscarinic effects of acetylcholine. Side effects of antispasmodic therapy include hypertension, palpitation, arrhythmia, and stimulation of the central nervous system. Anticholinergic drugs should be used cautiously in patients with cardiovascular diseases and hyperthyroidism and avoided in patients with bladder outlet obstructive symptoms. Relaxation of bladder smooth muscle can also be produced by blocking the alpha-1 adenoreceptors in the bladder with medications such as terazosin and doxazocin, or alpha-IA blockers such as tamsulosin, and uroxatrol (extended release formulation) which can decrease bladder outlet obstruction without affecting contractility. Use alpha-1 blockers cautiously in patients on antihypertensive medication.[54]

Instruct patients to maintain an adequate intake of fluids to promote frequent voiding and to decrease the potential for infection by diluting the bacterial population. Recommended fluid intake is 1–2 L/day. If voided urine is clear to light yellow in color, hydration is probably adequate. In addition, teaching patients to avoid foods that irritate the bladder mucosa may help to delay the onset of cystitis and decrease symptoms; these foods include coffee, tea, alcohol, spices, and tobacco products.[54] Encourage patients to report any signs of bladder irritation, such as dysuria, frequency, urgency with decreased urine volume, and any signs of hematuria or excessive mucus shreds in the urine. The nurse should also be aware of the baseline hemoglobin and hematocrit values as well as any coagulation studies. Hematuria usually causes minimal blood loss and rarely anemia, but early documentation will assist in assessment of future problems. Acute cystitis symptoms cause discomfort and pain, and they may significantly disrupt the patient's life. Reassure the patient that symptoms subside gradually over 2–8 weeks after completion of radiation.

Vaginal dryness

The most immediate response to external beam radiation and/or brachytherapy of the vagina is loss of most or all of the vaginal epithelium. This acute reaction results in vaginitis, with thinning and inflammation of the mucosa causing dryness, pruritis, and possibly a mucoid discharge.[55] Dyspareunia is common.

Patients report itching and discomfort, especially at the vaginal introitus, that begin at variable points in the course of treatment. Onset of symptoms is usually early and more pronounced in women who have estrogen depletion.

Management. Vaginal lubricants (such as Astroglide), and vaginal moisturizers (either pectin based, such as Summer's Eve, or polycarbophil based, such as Replens) are advised to decrease discomfort and itching. Acute radiation reactions such as erythema, moist desquamation, and confluent mucositis will resolve within 2–3 months after completion of irradiation. (See Chapter 35 for more on sexuality issues.)

Extremity

Used in treatment of sarcoma and bony metastasis, radiation to the extremities, due to minimal surrounding structures, generally results in few acute toxicities. Some fields for radiation of an extremity, such as the hip or femur, include surrounding pelvic structures, so the patient will be at risk for diarrhea due to bowel sensitivity. (See management of diarrhea/proctitis in the Abdomen and Pelvis section in this chapter.)

Eye

Used in treatment of intraocular malignancies, lymphoma and leukemia, CNS cancers, head and neck cancers, and thyroid eye disease (benign pathology), eye irradiation can result in conjunctival edema and tearing.

Conjunctival edema and tearing

The eyelid, conjunctiva, cornea, sclera, and often the lacrimal gland are irradiated in treatment of ocular malignancies. Inflammatory response to radiation can occur within 24 hours following radiation, and the conjunctiva and other periocular tissues can develop edema secondary to diffuse infiltration by neutrophils. The conjunctiva will become erythematous, with periorbital edema occasionally developing within the first 24 hours after treatment. Other acute symptoms include transient eyelid erythema or edema, mild conjunctivitis, and loss of lashes. Patients may experience burning of the eye(s), sensation of a foreign body, diminished vision, and excessive tearing.[48] Depending on the size of the radiation field, alopecia of the eyebrow(s) may occur.

Management. Ocular lubrication with an artificial tears solution or ointment, patching, and antibiotic drops as indicated is helpful. Toxicity-related symptoms peak within 10–20 days, resolve within 2–4 weeks, and heal completely within 8 weeks.[56]

Late Effects of Radiation: Site Specific

Since the earliest application of radiation in treating cancer, providers have voiced concerns about the late effects of radiation therapy on normal tissues and organs. The inability to precisely predict manifestations of late normal-tissue injury emphasizes the importance of vigilant patient follow-up. Late effects are usually progressive and can become manifest months to years after completion of radiation therapy. Radiation-related second malignancies are a risk for some patients following successful radiation treatment.[57]

Radiation tissue tolerance, measured in degrees ranging from minimal to maximal, can be a valuable guide for estimating long-term effects. The clinical applicability of tolerance doses has changed as a result of the introduction of agents such as biologic response modifiers, chemotherapeutic drugs, new modalities (hyperthermia, high dose rate brachytherapy, and radiosurgery), and these modalities' concurrent and subsequent use with traditional irradiation, chemotherapy, and surgery.[57]

Tissue and organ tolerance is determined by the radiosensitivity of relevant stem cell subpopulations, which may not always be proliferating or dividing. Within the radiation field(s), the most radiosensitive vital cell population determines whether organ tolerance or organ failure will occur. Thus, the functional capacity of cells is often distinct from their regenerative capacity, permitting organ function to be preserved in the face of injury and allowing for recovery or repair from the radiation insult.[58] Complication probability rates have been calculated for each tissue/organ system. They define the 5% and 50% levels of a total radiation dose that are predicted to create late effects at 5 years — that is, the TD 5/5 (5% risk at 5 years) and TD 50/5 (50% risk at 5 years).[14]

All normal tissues do not follow the same behavior pattern in response to radiation. Late reactions occur in tissues that normally have low cell-cycle turnover or regeneration, such as the endothelium and connective tissues.[57] In such tissues, the radiation produces little change in the function of mature, differentiated cells, and therefore no evidence of tissue malfunction appears until those mature cells gradually die due to normal wear and tear or additional trauma. When the tissue attempts to replace the lost cells by cellular division, the radiation damage inflicted on the tissues months or years earlier becomes manifest, as the cells are unable to produce viable new cells. In contrast, tissues in which the cells are normally replaced every few hours or days (e.g., skin and mucosa) quickly recognize that cell replacement is impaired, even as treatment proceeds. These cells immediately activate compensatory mechanisms to speed up the rate of cell proliferation and thereby counteract the accelerated rate of cell loss. Molecular biology, gene expression, and cytokine cascade identification are key factors in the mechanisms responsible for late effects. Intercellular communication through autocrine, paracrine, and endocrine pathways via cytokine networks is the new pathophysiologic paradigm to explain the cellular process of late radiation effects.[59]

A model to aid understanding of the clinical outcome of late effects of radiation, as described by Marks, characterizes an organ as being composed of multiple functioning subunits (FSU) that operate in one of two ways: as a parallel system or as a series system.[60] In a *parallel system,* organ function is generally maintained if damage occurs because the remaining FSUs operate independently from the damaged region, assuming there is adequate function in the remainder of the organ. Hence, part of an organ can be sacrificed or damaged beyond repair, yet the organ will continue to function adequately. The lung, liver, and kidney are highly sensitive to relatively low doses of radiation, but damage to part of these organs does not render them incapable of function. In a *series system,* damage to one portion of an organ may render the entire organ or system dysfunctional because the system must work in sequence. Examples include the gastrointestinal tract and neural tissues. The series system concept can encompass organ-to-organ interactions as well. Damage produced in one organ can have serious consequences in another organ, such as renal failure leading to overall multisystem failure and death.[59]

Late radiation effects are now recognized as an important area of study, especially as they relate to quality of life. The dose-limiting organs in the treatment field define the amount of radiation prescribed. The risk of late effects related to radiation confirms the importance of accuracy in daily fraction dose, total radiation dose, volume treated, and patient co-morbidities. Optimal dose-response curves to avoid late effects remain difficult to define, despite extensive documentation of radiation injuries in the literature. The accuracy of commonly used scales for quantification of acute and especially late reactions is important.[58]

In 1992, one group developed a grading scale for late effects of normal tissues (LENT). The goal was to create a simple, widely applicable, reproducible, and accurate scale — in ascending order of severity — of the complications of radiation treatment. The descriptors were divided into four major categories: subjective, objective, management, and analytic (SOMA). Each SOMA scale is site specific so as to more precisely define outcomes.[57] The scales are reviewed and revised as needed when longer patient follow-up data become available. By monitoring different elements in the SOMA scales, it is hoped that the components of damage in individual organs may be differentiated, perhaps allowing for more appropriate medical intervention to manage and alleviate symptoms. By diligently measuring and reporting the outcomes of radiation treatment, one day toxicity-free survival may become possible, just like disease-free survival or local tumor control.[58]

The morbidity and burden of specific late effects and toxicities may be perceived quite differently by patients and healthcare providers. This is especially true if the late effects and toxicities are protracted, irreversible, uncontrollable, painful, or socially disabling.[57] It is important to remember that the overall risk of late effects is very small (but never zero) and that it varies by site treated. The risk of morbidity and mortality associated with no treatment for a primary or metastatic cancer is almost always greater than the risk of late effects. Ultimately, the patient and family must decide how to weigh the risks and benefits of treatment.

Selected late effects on organ systems are discussed next. Table 14-8 provides a more inclusive list of site-specific late effects.

Radiation-Induced Fibrosis: Subcutaneous and Soft Tissue

Radiation-induced fibrosis (RIF), commonly of subcutaneous and soft tissue, is defined as loss of pliability and flexibility of soft tissues down to the muscle layer. Deep tissue fibrosis involves muscle, fascia, and connective tissue down to bone. The most common regions affected are the breast, head and neck, and connective tissues. Onset is generally within 1–2 years after radiation. The severity of RIF can progress, and the time to onset may not plateau. Higher risk is associated with higher daily treatment doses and overall dose, combined modality therapy, and postoperative infection, seroma, wound drainage, and extensive hematoma.[61,62]

Initially there is a loss of tissue elasticity, which is followed by mild induration. This effect can progress to rigidity of the surface skin layers and retraction of surface contours. Fibrosis can lead to disuse atrophy, ulceration/necrosis, entrapment of neurologic structures (i.e., brachial or lumbar plexus), and stenosis or obliteration of vital anatomy in the head and neck, chest, abdomen, or pelvis.[61,62]

Management. Treatment options include pharmacologic agents such as pentoxifylline and vitamin E, which have been shown to increase tissue pliability and arrest neurologic deficits. A minimum of 3 months of treatment is needed to evaluate for response.[63] The efficacy of this regimen was examined in a randomized clinical trial of women who had undergone breast irradiation and developed clinically significant RIF. A significant surface reduction of RIF was seen in the treatment group.[64] Hyperbaric oxygenation has been shown to be helpful in decreasing pain and erythema. Physical therapy is important to help preserve function, especially in those patients with restricted movement or mobility. Impedance-controlled microcurrent therapy may significantly improve range of motion in the neck and decrease pain in patients with RIF.[65]

Central Nervous System

Brain necrosis

The onset of symptoms of brain necrosis can be as early as 6 months following radiation treatment, but the peak time of presentation of symptoms is 1–2 years after completion of radiation. Brain necrosis is typically not diffuse; instead, it is focal. Symptoms of brain necrosis include manifestations of increased intracranial pressure (ICP) such as headache, somnolence, intellectual and cognitive deficits, decrease in short- and long-term memory, seizures, and focal neurological deficits corresponding to the part of the brain irradiated. Magnetic resonance imaging (MRI) is the most sensitive tool available for diagnosing brain necrosis. Pathologic tissue confirmation may be necessary to differentiate necrosis from recurrent tumor.[58,66] Radiation-induced brain necrosis is usually progressive and most often fatal.

Management. If appropriate, surgical debulking of necrosis and use of corticosteroids can offer transient symptom relief.

Leukoencephalopathy

Leukoencephalopathy occurs almost exclusively after chemotherapy but can occur after brain irradiation, with or without chemotherapy.[58,66] It is characterized by multiple, noninflammatory necrotic foci in the white matter of brain tissue, with demyelination and reactive astrocytosis. Symptoms of leukoencephalopathy include lethargy, seizures, spasticity, paresis, and ataxia. Magnetic resonance imaging can be helpful in diagnosis. Leukoencephalopathy is generally irreversible.

Management. Treatment is limited to supportive measures, such as symptom management of seizures, and physical and occupational therapy consultations for assistance with motor dysfunction.

Table 14-8 Selected Site-Specific Late Effects of Radiation Therapy*

CNS
- Brain
  - Focal/diffuse necrosis
  - Leukoencephalopathy
  - Pituitary/hypothalamic dysfunction
  - Cognitive dysfunction
- Spinal cord
  - Myelopathy/necrosis

Head and Neck
- Mucosa
  - Paleness, thinning, telangiectasias
- Salivary gland
  - Xerostomia
- Teeth/mandible
  - Caries
  - Temporomandibular joint fibrosis
  - Osteoradionecrosis
- Thyroid
  - Hypothyroid/hyperthyroid
  - Thyroid cartilage necrosis
  - Laryngeal edema
- Eye
  - Cataracts
  - Skin changes, loss of lashes
  - Dry eye, corneal ulceration
  - Visual loss/blindness

Chest
- Lung
  - Pneumonitis (subacute)
  - Pulmonary fibrosis
- Heart
  - Cardiomyopathy
  - Pericarditis
  - Coronary artery disease
- Breast
  - Skin tanning, fibrosis, telangiectasias
  - Breast fibrosis, contraction, edema
  - Increased risk of pathologic rib fracture
  - Pneumonitis (subacute)
  - Pulmonary fibrosis
  - Pericarditis
  - Arm edema if axillary or supraclavicular lymph nodes treated

Bone
- Necrosis of femoral head

Gastrointestinal
- Esophagus
  - Dysmotility
  - Dysphagia/odynophagia
  - Esophageal stricture
- Stomach
  - Dyspepsia/gastritis
  - Contracture
- Small/large bowel
  - Mucosal injury
  - Decreased motility, malabsorption
  - Obstruction
- Rectum
  - Proctitis
  - Fistula
- Liver
  - Radiation hepatitis
  - Hepatic failure

Genitourinary
- Kidney
  - Anemia
  - Chronic radiation nephritis
  - Hypertension
- Bladder
  - Mucosal injury: hematuria
  - Fistula
  - Fibrosis
- Prostate
  - Impotence
- Penis
  - Mucosal changes
  - Urethral stricture
- Vagina
  - Thinning/atrophy/dry mucosa
  - Narrowing, shortening, fibrosis

Reproductive
- Ovaries/testis
  - Sterility

Hematopoietic
- Fibrosis
- Aplasia

Carcinogenesis
- Meningioma, nerve sheath glioma
- Sarcoma: bone/soft tissue
- Leukemias: acute myelogenous leukemia

*Because the tolerance levels of all tissues are known, the overall risk of radiation-related late effects is very low. The percentage of risk varies by tissue site.

Cognitive and emotional dysfunction

The incidence and extent of radiation-related cognitive and emotional dysfunction are difficult to determine due to multiple variables, including underlying disease (primary tumor, leukemia), specific brain site, increased ICP, and effects of therapies including surgery and chemotherapy. Cognitive and emotional deficits following brain radiation are well documented in children, but the contribution by radiation alone is unclear because patients often receive systemic and intrathecal chemotherapy.[58,66]

Management. Neuropsychiatric consultation can be valuable for behavioral and pharmacologic management of specific dysfunctions. A baseline neuropsychiatric evaluation can be helpful in assessing future mental status changes.

Pituitary and hypothalamic dysfunction

Radiation damage can affect the hypothalamic-pituitary axis and cause permanent dysfunctions. Clinical syndromes include hypothyroidism, Addison's disease, diabetes insipidus, and decreased sexual hormone levels.[66] Growth hormone is commonly affected in children and must be monitored and replaced as needed.

Management. Each specific syndrome is treated with replacement hormonal therapies and surveillance of hormone levels.

Spinal cord

Myelopathies are uncommon, but not rare, complications of cancer treatment. Because the multiple signs and symptoms of radiation myelopathy can occur in variable combinations at different rates of progression, it is not possible to make the diagnosis of radiation myelopathy based on symptoms alone. The initial signs are subtle and may not be noticed by patients. Symptoms include sensory deficits (unilateral or bilateral), which are often manifested as diminished temperature sensation, leg weakness, clumsiness, and diminished proprioception. Objective signs and symptoms include changes in gait (often foot drop), spasticity, weakness, hemiparesis, Brown-Séquard syndrome, and possibly incontinence. Hyperreflexia and Babinski signs are often found on neurological examination. Pain may accompany symptoms. The patient may be asymptomatic until some trauma initiates a progressive neurological deficit. No specific combination of signs or symptoms can distinguish radiation myelopathy from myelopathies of many other etiologies.[66]

Management. Management of radiation-induced spinal cord myelopathy has been primarily limited to administration of corticosteroids, with limited success. Response to corticosteroid therapy is transient with some improvement in symptoms and is likely due to a decrease in spinal cord edema. The prognosis in radiation myelopathy depends primarily on the degree to which the originally treated lesion transects the spinal cord and the anatomical level of the lesion. Complete transection of the cord is a sign of poor prognosis. Generally lesions at higher anatomical levels have a poorer prognosis than lesions at lower levels. The actuarial mortality from radiation-induced spinal cord myelopathy is 55% at 18 months for cervical lesions, and 25% at 18 months for thoracic lesions. Younger patients have a better prognosis than older patients.[65]

Head and Neck

There is the potential for multiple disabling late effects following head and neck irradiation. If the patient has also undergone surgical resection, structural dysfunction can occur in addition to the effects of irradiation. Persons with head and neck cancer usually require extensive rehabilitation to manage alterations related to speech, swallowing, eating, and respiratory function.

Xerostomia and dental caries

Xerostomia persists for months to years and almost always will be present to some degree. The extent of symptoms is dependent on the volume of salivary gland tissue irradiated, the total radiation dose, and individual patient response. As a consequence, patients may experience impaired ability to swallow, chew, talk, and wear dentures comfortably. Most patients permanently change the nature of their diet to some degree.

Radiation-induced dental effects are indirectly produced by salivary changes that occur when the parotid glands are included in the treatment portals, and less often by direct effect of radiation on the teeth. Alteration of the normal oral microfloral balance to a more cariogenic one occurs as a result of changes in the salivary contents and a lowered oral pH. (See the discussion of xerostomia in the Head and Neck section of this chapter for a more detailed outline of salivary composition.)

Dental decay and varying degrees of dental disintegration after irradiation typically develop along the gum line.[32] Thus, patients are at high risk for dental caries, periodontal disease, stomatitis, dysphagia, and altered taste.[31] Because of changes in the oral microflora secondary to xerostomia, candidiasis and other oral infections are more common. Long-term xerostomia and dental caries can be disabling and can significantly affect quality of life.[35–37]

Management. Management is as discussed under xerostomia in the Head and Neck section of this chapter. The most important aspect of xerostomia management is compliance with life-long dental surveillance and prophylaxis.

Osteoradionecrosis

Osteoradionecrosis is a serious complication secondary to the effects of xerostomia and radiation to the maxilla and mandible. Osteoradionecrosis is characterized as a hypocellular and hypovascular dissolution of bone. Osteocytes and the supporting vasculature may be irreversibly injured by radiation. Osteoradionecrosis is progressive, can lead to intolerable pain or fracture, and may necessitate surgical resection. Those patients at greatest risk are dentulous and require dental extractions after completing radiation therapy. It is not always necessary — nor advisable — to extract all teeth before treatment as a preventive measure;[36] however, teeth of questionable viability should be extracted prior to initiating radiation therapy (see the discussion of dental caries in the Head and Neck section of this chapter). Nonirritating, well-fitting dentures do not appear to increase the incidence of osteoradionecrosis. The overall risk of osteoradionecrosis is higher in patients with preexisting poor dentition, nutritional and/or immunologic compromise, and smoking during radiation. Patients remain at risk for development of osteoradionecrosis for years following radiation therapy.

Most cases of osteoradionecrosis develop in the mandible. This condition initially manifests as a nondescript erythematous change of the overlying mucosa, which then ulcerates to reveal the necrotic bone below. Necrotic bone has a dull appearance, unlike the pearly color of healthy periosteum.[37]

Management. Prevention of osteoradionecrosis includes meticulous oral and periodontal hygiene, with fluoride prophylaxis and frequent dental evaluation. Oral care must be maintained indefinitely because of the impaired potential for healing in response to physical irritation, chemical agents, and microbial organisms.[36,37] Attempts should be made to replace or increase salivary flow (see the Head and Neck section). Foods and beverages containing sucrose should be avoided. If caries develop, removal and restoration are advised immediately. Patients are at greater risk for developing oral *Candida albicans* infection due to xerostomia, and prompt treatment helps maintain oral integrity. Optimal nutritional status is important for bone maintenance and healing. Head and neck cancer patients are commonly at increased risk of nutritional compromise due to poor nutritional status at diagnosis and alterations in chewing and swallowing induced by surgery and radiation.

Treatment of osteoradionecrosis includes antibiotic therapy to help control acute pain, swelling, and suppuration. Surgical resection of osteoradionecrotic lesions is an option. In one study, 6 of 22 patients had lesions resected, with 3 patients demonstrating postsurgical recurrence. The preventive and therapeutic use of antibiotics and hyperbaric oxygenation (HBO) has been reported to be effective in some cases, but clear treatment guidelines are not defined. A series of HBO treatments are recommended for postradiation patients who must undergo dental extractions.[67]

Hypothyroidism

Hypothyroidism is the most common clinical consequence of irradiation to the thyroid in patients who have received therapeutic doses to the neck area.[68] Patients should be monitored with periodic serum thyroid-stimulating hormone (TSH) and free-thyroxin 4 (FT4) screening.

Management. Hypothyroidism can be effectively treated with thyroid replacement therapy.

Lung

Pulmonary fibrosis

Pulmonary fibrosis can develop insidiously in a previously irradiated lung field. Debate continues as to whether an acute phase of fibrosis, which may not be symptomatic but can be viewed radiographically, is always present. The degree of fibrosis stabilizes after 1–2 years. Radiation-induced lung injury is characterized by progressive fibrosis of the alveolar septa, which become thickened by bundles of elastic fibers. The alveoli subsequently collapse and are then obliterated by connective tissue. The hilum or mediastinum may become retracted with a densely contracted lung segment, resulting in compensatory hyperinflation of adjacent or contralateral lung tissue.[51] These changes can lead to the appearance (usually within 1–2 years after radiation) of lung scarring on CXR that corresponds to the shape of the radiation portal; CT scan may provide more definitive imaging for diagnosis.

Pulmonary function tests (PFTs) may suggest reduced tidal volume; however, PFTs do not demonstrate significant changes when small volumes of lung are irradiated, due to functional compensation by adjacent lung regions. Thus, PFTs are not the most accurate measurement of radiation-induced lung injury. Diffusion capacity may be the best measure of total lung function, because this test is least likely to be affected by compensatory changes in unirradiated portions of the lung.[51]

Not all areas of the lung are equally functionally important. The lung bases have a greater ventilation/perfusion ratio than at the apices. Should fibrosis develop, the location of the lung treatment field serves as an important predictor of degree of respiratory symptoms. It is important to understand that all patients will develop lung fibrosis if radiation encompasses any lung tissue. Whether that fibrosis becomes clinically apparent is the issue.[69] Most patients with radiation-induced pulmonary fibrosis are asymptomatic. Symptoms are directly related to the amount of lung parenchyma involved and the patients' preexisting pulmonary reserves. Symptoms generally remain minimal if fibrosis is limited to less than 50% of one lung. If the volume of one irradiated lung exceeds 50%, the patient will likely become symptomatic to some degree. Symptoms include dyspnea on exertion, reduced exercise tolerance, orthopnea, cyanosis, and finger clubbing. In some instances, chronic respiratory failure can occur and may result in cor pulmonale and subsequent right heart failure.[51]

Management. Management of radiation-induced pulmonary fibrosis consists of supportive care, such as steroids, oxygen therapy, and pulmonary rehabilitation exercises to manage respiratory symptoms. Clinical trials are looking at using amifostine (Ethyol) as a pneumoprotector.[69]

Heart

Cardiac complications are much less common in the "modern era" of radiotherapy. Most data related to heart disease after radiation have focused on childhood survivors of Hodgkin's disease. The risk of radiation-induced pericarditis, coronary artery disease, and cardiomyopathy is dramatically lower with current doses and treatment techniques. Long-term follow-up is required to confirm an actual decrease in cardiac toxicities resulting in symptomatic complications.

Pericarditis

Pericarditis is a result of fibrosis in the parietal pericardium that may progress to constriction of the heart. Patients may exhibit symptoms of acute pericarditis or have a chronic pericardial effusion.[70]

Management. If signs of heart failure occur, treatment focuses on increasing cardiac output to maintain system perfusion. Excessive pericardial fluid may accumulate rapidly to produce cardiac tamponade, which must be relieved by pericardiocentesis or pericardiectomy. Pericardial disease may develop several months to years after radiation therapy.[70]

Cardiomyopathy

The myocardium is involved less frequently than the pericardium. The myocardium can develop patches of diffuse fibrosis affecting the anterior wall of the left ventricle and, less frequently, the anterior wall of the right ventricle.[70]

Patients present with signs and symptoms of congestive heart failure. Left ventricular ejection function (LVEF) studies can be used for monitoring during chemotherapy and radiation.[69] The combination of radiation and doxorubicin affects left ventricular systolic function and mortality more significantly than either therapy used alone.[71]

Management. If signs of heart failure occur, treatment focuses on increasing cardiac output to maintain system perfusion.

Coronary artery disease

The main types of radiation damage to arteries are intimal disruption and luminal stenosis or occlusion. Vessel changes due to atherosclerosis and with the normal aging process are produced or accelerated by radiation. Pathological changes may be difficult to distinguish from typical atherosclerotic coronary disease.[72]

Management. Screening and treatment are the same as they are for patients with coronary artery disease who have not had radiation. It is recommended that all cancer survivors treated with chest radiotherapy be monitored for risk factors such as obesity, hypertension, dyslipidemias, and diabetes.[71]

Breast/Chest Wall

The total radiation dose to the whole breast for management of microscopic residual disease is 4500–5000 cGy. In this dose range, the incidence of late effects is very low. Higher doses to the whole breast (≥ 6000–6500 cGy) are associated with atrophy, fibrosis (see the earlier discussion of RIF), retraction, and telangiectasias that predispose the patient to a poor cosmetic outcome. Rarely, late effects occur that limit function, such as breast tissue contraction, necrosis, or neuropathy. Moist desquamation of the skin during radiation is not predictive of late skin effects.

Management. Management is directed at relieving symptoms; surgical intervention occurs as appropriate.[5] Surgical revision of a contracted painful breast can be difficult due to the risk of poor healing after definitive radiation doses to the breast and surrounding tissues. It must be emphasized that late effects, with a poor cosmetic outcome, are extremely rare today with the radiation doses used and modern high-energy equipment.

Abdomen and Pelvis

Small and large bowel injury

The radiation tolerance of the small and large bowel is a major dose-limiting factor in the treatment of many cancers of the abdomen and pelvis. Late radiation-related injury to the bowel is caused by intestinal wall fibrosis, vascular stenosis, and mucosal atrophy. The incidence of late effects to the bowel is 3%–5%. Some alteration of bowel function is likely the most dominant chronic postradiation toxicity. Interestingly, only a fraction of patients with postradiation bowel dysfunction seek medical treatment. Instead, they adjust their lifestyles to symptoms, and seem to have very little expectation for effective interventions.

Bowel late effects can be defined as symptoms altering the patient's lifestyle or hospitalization or surgical interventions.[73] Symptoms are related to malabsorption and dysmotility and include fecal frequency/urgency, tenesmus, bleeding, pain, fistula formation, and intractable diarrhea. Due to its anatomically smaller lumen size, obstruction is more common in the small bowel than in the large bowel or rectum. The most important factors contributing to the extent of bowel injury include radiation dose (the rectum is generally more tolerant than the remainder of the bowel), prior abdominal surgery, history of pelvic inflammatory disease, and concurrent chemotherapy. Some studies suggest that a history of hypertension or diabetes mellitus may be associated with a greater risk of late intestinal injury.[73,74]

Management. Chronic radiation injury to the small and large intestine can be managed by a low-residue diet, stool softeners, and use of loperamide or diphenoxylate with atropine. If reduced rectal sphincter compliance is a problem, fiber laxatives can be used to provide form, consistency, and softening of the stool. For diarrhea caused by small bowel injury, several studies have suggested the use of cholestyramine might be effective. This agent presumably helps by reducing the level of intraluminal bile salts. Octreotide, now available in a long-acting formulation, offers benefits in managing secretory diarrhea. Rectal bleeding is managed with products to help improve mucosal integrity, such as sucralfate or short-chain fatty acid enemas, topical formalin, and laser cauterization.[73,74] Partial small bowel obstruction may be managed by bowel rest and decompression followed by dietary modification. Surgery may be necessary to relieve more extensive bowel obstruction. Nevertheless, controversy persists as to the extent of surgical resection necessary—whether all adhesions within the bowel should be lysed versus limiting the resection to the area(s) acutely involved.

Late-occurring bowel toxicities (i.e., more than 10–20 years) generally have a poorer prognosis for optimal functional outcomes.[73]

Genitourinary System

Bladder

Most late radiation-induced complications of the bladder are related to contracture, bleeding, symptomatic cystitis, and (rarely) fistulas. Incontinence is not common, but if found is likely related to the additive effect of radiation and prior surgical manipulations of the bladder neck and urethra. The degree of late radiation-related symptoms depends on the amount of bladder included in the radiation treatment fields. Irradiation fields for prostate cancer include much less bladder volume than the treatment fields for bladder cancer.

Management. Treatment for late effects on the bladder is individualized, but may include drug therapy to reduce cystitis symptoms (e.g., pentosan polysulfate) or surgical intervention for bleeding or to manage fistulas (e.g., vesicovaginal fistula).

Vagina

Chronic effects to the vagina, occurring 12 months or more after completion of radiation, include thinning and atrophy of the vaginal epithelium and development of telangiectasias. Patients may experience a decrease in size of the vaginal vault due to narrowing, shortening (made more pronounced after radical hysterectomy), paravaginal fibrosis, loss of elasticity, adhesions, and marked decrease in vaginal lubrication. All of these manifestations may result in dyspareunia. Vaginal brachytherapy can contribute to late effects.[55]

Management. Management begins with preradiation teaching so patients know what to expect after radiation. If the patient is not sexually active, dilators can be used to maintain vaginal patency. Women should be instructed about the importance of keeping the vagina patent and minimizing fibrosis so as to facilitate future physical examinations essential for tumor surveillance. Problems with sexual adjustment after radiation therapy can be significant. Women may have depressive symptoms, fear of injury from intercourse, fear of recurrent cancer, poor communication with sex partner, feeling of being less feminine and desirable, and separation and loss of sex partner.[55] The nurse often is the most accessible and comfortable person with whom the patient can discuss this physically and emotionally complex topic.

Reproductive System

Ovary

The probability of sterility and endocrine insufficiency is related to radiation dose, fraction size, and patient age. Definitive external pelvic irradiation of doses exceeding 2400 cGy will produce permanent ovarian ablation in the adult female. If the woman is postmenopausal, few clinical consequences are likely. For the premenopausal woman, symptoms will be similar to those of menopause, including hot flashes, atrophic vulvitis, vaginitis with pruritis and dyspareunia, alterations in body fat distribution, changes in the breasts, accelerated bone demineralization, potential premature cardiovascular disease, and unpredictable effects on libido. The severity of these effects varies among individuals, based on body habitus and levels of estrogen production, both adrenal and peripheral.[55]

Management. Management of estrogen deficit produced by damage to the ovaries varies according to the specific cancer. Estrogen replacement in women with breast cancer is controversial and seldom advised. For women with gynecological cancers, estrogen replacement may have a role. Women are advised to discuss this issue with their oncologists. Nontraditional medicine — use of natural and herbal preparation — may be helpful in providing relief of menopausal symptoms. Women with breast cancer are generally advised to avoid all estrogens, including phytoestrogens, until more is known regarding the pathophysiology of these substances and the specific malignancy.

The premenopausal woman who requires radiation therapy that will include the ovaries may have concerns regarding conservation of potential reproductive capability. Preventing ovarian ablation is an achievable goal in patients treated with radiation. A thorough discussion of the available alternatives should occur prior to selection of a definitive plan for treatment. Strategies for conserving reproductive capability include utilization of reproductive technology such as in vitro fertilization and transplantation of one or both ovaries to sites remote from the radiation fields. If the patient is receiving high-dose chemotherapy, ovarian ablation may occur despite efforts to remove them from path of the radiation beam.[55]

Testis

The testis is highly radiosensitive, and a small dose of 200–1000 cGy or a fractionated dose of 100–200 cGy of radiation will cause permanent sterility. Young men who require radiation that may affect the testes should be referred for sperm analysis and sperm banking as appropriate. Although testicular shields can be used, they will not prevent internal radiation scatter; therefore, the testes will inevitably receive some radiation dose.[75]

The severity of the impairment in spermatogenesis and length of recovery depend on the radiation dose to the testis. In the typical patient receiving irradiation for a classic seminoma, the remaining testis receives a dose in the range of 30–180 cGy. An even greater dose is delivered to the contralateral testis if the hemiscrotum is irradiated. Radiation doses of this magnitude usually produce temporary oligospermia or azospermia followed by recovery 18–24 months later.[75]

Management. A patient may become fertile during the recovery phase, and should be counseled regarding this possibility. Mutations induced in germinal stem cells may produce abnormal spermatozoa. Fortunately, the potentially abnormal spermatozoa arising from these mutated stem cells tend to have poor fertilization potential. The occurrence of the mutations depends on the radiation dose delivered. No genetic abnormalities from ionizing radiation have been demonstrated in humans, which perhaps reflects the body's ability to repair such damage.[75] Patients are advised to practice birth control during and after irradiation. The length of time during which birth control should be continued is not entirely clear, but generally a duration of 24 months is recommended to allow for recovery of normal spermatogenesis.

Sexual dysfunction

A comprehensive discussion of sexuality and interventions is beyond the scope of this chapter; the reader is referred to Chapter 35 for more on this topic. However, it is important to recognize that sexual dysfunction in both men and women can occur after radiation therapy for various malignancies, especially gynecological and genitourinary cancers. Radiation therapy can cause significant sexual disruption. It is incumbent on oncology nurses to recognize that sexual dysfunction is a problem that may be of great concern to the patient and his or her partner and therefore affect quality of life. Patients and their partners rarely verbalize issues or concerns about sexual dysfunction. Obtaining a sexual history prior to initiating treatment may allow for implementation of preventive measures that can lessen dysfunction. The direct effects of irradiation on normal tissue may progress over a number of years; thus, sexual dysfunction may be progressive and require lifelong rehabilitation and interventions.[55]

Secondary Malignancies

In the retrospective evaluation of radiation-induced secondary malignancies, an important factor to remember is that many patients in the studies being reported were originally treated in the 1950s and 1960s, with some being treated as far back as 1925. Thus, patients were treated with techniques and doses different from the more refined radiation therapy currently in use.[76] Criteria for defining second cancer include the following:

- Secondary tumors must have a different histological appearance from primary tumors.
- Both the primary and secondary tumor must be malignant.
- Both must be anatomically separate, and the second tumor cannot be a metastasis from the primary tumor.
- Secondary tumors must produce their own metastases.[76]

With increasing longevity, many patients may develop second cancers anywhere from 6 months to 20 years or longer after completion of treatment for the primary cancer. Considering the difficulty of classifying and identifying secondary cancers induced by radiation, their incidence may be higher than current studies indicate. Vigilant follow-up and surveillance are essential for recent patients to determine whether changes in therapeutic technique and radiation doses have affected the incidence of second cancers.[76]

Most solid tumors (e.g., sarcoma) do not occur until 10 years or longer after radiation exposure, and for some cancer sites (e.g., breast and bladder) excess risks emerge only 15 years or longer after irradiation. Radiation-induced sarcomas of bone and soft tissue are the most frequent secondary malignant neoplasms in irradiated tissues. Sarcomas have a high tendency to recur locally, metastasize, and become a fatal complication of radiation therapy.[76]

Most of the knowledge about radiation effects in humans has come from epidemiological studies of atomic bomb survivors in Japan, occupationally irradiated workers, patients exposed to large amounts of diagnostic radiation, and patients treated with radiation for malignant and nonmalignant diseases. Studies in the atomic bomb survivors and in women treated for benign gynecological disorders have shown that the excess relative risk per gray tends to be fairly stable for at least 30 years following radiation. At present, it is not known whether the relative risk remains elevated throughout life or whether the risk for different solid tumors versus leukemia or lymphomatous cancers varies.

The risk of leukemia attributable to irradiation is observed within a few years from radiation exposure, with a peak after 5–9 years and a gradual decline thereafter. Continuous exposures, given at low-dose rates, are less leukomogenic than a single radiation dose. Age at exposure may be the greatest determinant of risk for radiation-induced cancer, especially in those patients who are irradiated as children or adolescents.[77]

Knowledge of the risk factors for second malignancy has made it possible to identify patient groups at high risk of developing second cancers due to treatments they received in the past. An example is the increased risk of breast cancer in women who were treated as youngsters with mantle irradiation for Hodgkin's disease. Previously irradiated patients should be closely monitored and screened as appropriate. Preventive strategies, such as smoking cessation, may substantially reduce the risk of developing a treatment-related cancer.

The issue of treatment-induced second cancers must always be viewed in relation to the dramatic improvement in survival rates for various malignancies. The carcinogenic effects of therapeutic irradiation deserve more investigation. Issues to be clarified include the shape of the radiation dose-response curve in the higher dose range, the duration of the radiation-induced cancer risk, the effects of dose fractionation, and age at radiation exposure. It is important to remember that not all second cancers are due to chemotherapy or irradiation. The occurrence of two primary malignancies in the same individual may reflect influences such as genetic predisposition, immunodeficiency, carcinogenic influences, clustering of risk factors, and a chance event or the interaction of multiple factors.[76] Because the mechanisms underlying the carcinogenic effects of radiation remain poorly understood, research should also focus on the identification of specific gene alterations associated with the development of radiation-induced cancer.[77]

The risk associated with cancer treatment should be weighed carefully against the consequences of not using such treatments. Changes in therapies to reduce the risk of late complications and second malignancies should be made only in the context of carefully designed clinical trials that evaluate whether the overall efficacy of treatment is maintained. In addition, for many new cancer treatments, the long-term risk of second malignancies is not known.[77]

Conclusion

Cancer treatment with radiation therapy can be rigorous, with multiple acute toxicities and the risk of late effects. The global radiation oncology community is hopeful that advances in technology (e.g., 3D conformal treatment planning, intensity-modulated radiation therapy, stereotactic radiosurgery, and high dose rate brachytherapy) will result in a decreased risk of long-term morbidities, while maintaining, or improving, optimal treatment outcomes. While a toxicity-free course of radiation probably is not realistic, oncology nurses are skilled at managing side effects and supporting patients through a course of therapy. Balancing treatment outcomes with quality of life, especially when palliation is the goal, remains a priority. Oncology nurses are integral in caring for cancer patients and their families at each point on the treatment continuum.

References

1. Hall E: *Radiobiology for the Radiologist.* New York, Lippincott-Raven, 1994
2. Hellman S: Principles of cancer management: radiation therapy, in DeVita VT, Hellman S, Rosenberg SA (eds.): *Cancer: Principles and Practice of Oncology* (ed 6). Philadelphia, Lippincott-Raven, 2001, pp 265–288
3. Chao KS, Perez CA, Brady LW: Fundamentals of patient management, in Chao DS, Perez CA, Brady LW (eds.): *Radiation Oncology Management Decisions.* Philadelphia, Lippincott-Raven, 2002, pp 1–13
4. Coia LR, Moylan DJ: *Introduction to Clinical Radiation Oncology* (ed 3). Madison, WI, Medical Physics Publishing, 1994
5. Archambieu JO, Pezner R: Pathophysiology of irradiated skin and breast. *Int J Radiat Oncol Biol Phys* 31:1171–1185, 1995
6. Williams J, Chen Y, Rubin P, et al: The biological basis of a comprehensive grading system for the adverse effects of cancer treatment. *Semin Radiat Oncol* 13:182–188, 2003
7. Wengstrom Y: Assessing nursing problems of importance for the development of nursing care in a radiation therapy department. *Cancer Nurs* 21:50–53, 1998
8. Hinds C, Streater A, Mood C: Functions and preferred methods of receiving information related to radiotherapy. *Cancer Nurs* 18:374–384, 1995
9. Poroch D: The effect of preparatory patient education on the anxiety and satisfaction of cancer patients receiving radiation therapy. *Cancer Nurs* 18:206–214, 1995
10. Bennenbroek FT, Buunk BP, Stiegelis HE, et al: Audiotaped social comparison information for cancer patients undergoing radiotherapy: differential effects of procedural, emotional and coping information. *Psychooncology* 12:567–579, 2003
11. Hagopian GA: The effects of informational audiotapes on knowledge and self-care behaviors of patients undergoing radiation therapy. *Oncol Nurs Forum* 23:697–700, 1996
12. Dunne-Daly CF: Nursing care and adverse reactions of external radiation therapy: a self-learning module. *Cancer Nurs* 17:236–256, 1994
13. Christman NJ: Uncertainty and adjustment during radiotherapy. *Nurs Res* 39:17–20, 1990
14. Strunk B, Maher KE: Collaborative nurse management of multifactorial moist desquamation in a patient undergoing radiotherapy. *J Enterost Ther Nurs* 20:152–157, 1993
15. Sitton E: Managing side effects of skin changes and fatigue, in Dow KH, Bucholtz JD, Iwamoto RR, et al (eds.): *Nursing Care in Radiation Oncology* (ed 2). Philadelphia, Saunders, 1997, pp 79–100
16. Goodman M, Hilderley LJ, Purl S: Integumentary and mucous membrane alterations, in Groenwald SL, Frogge MH, Goodman M, Yarbro CH (eds.): *Cancer Nursing: Principles and Practice* (ed 4). Sudbury, MA, Jones and Bartlett, 1997, pp 768–822
17. Dunne-Daly CF: Skin and wound care in radiation oncology. *Cancer Nurs* 18:144–162, 1995
18. Burch SE, Parker SA, Vann AM, et al: Measurement of 6-MV x-ray surface dose when topical agents are applied prior to external beam irradiation. *Int J Radiat Oncol Biol Phys* 38:447–451, 1997
19. Campbell IR, Illingworth MH: Can patients wash during radiotherapy to the breast or chest wall? A randomized controlled trial. *Clin Oncol* 4:78–82, 1992
20. Portenoy RK, Itri LM: Cancer-related fatigue: guidelines for evaluation and management. *Oncologist* 4:1–10, 1999
21. Piper BF: The Groopman article reviewed. *Oncology* 12:345–346, 1996
22. Clark PM, Lacasse C: Cancer-related fatigue: clinical practice issues. *Clin J Oncol Nurs* 2:45–54, 1998
23. Greenberg DB, Sawicka J, Eisenthal S, et al: Fatigue syndrome due to localized radiation. *J Pain Symptom Manage* 7:38–45, 1992
24. Munro AJ, Potter S: A quantitative approach to the distress caused by symptoms in patients treated with radical radiotherapy. *Br J Cancer* 74:640–647, 1996
25. King KB, Nail LM, Kraemer K, et al: Patients' descriptions of the experience of receiving radiation therapy. *Oncol Nurs Forum* 12:55–61, 1985
26. Graydon JE, Bubela N, Irvine D, et al: Fatigue-reducing strategies used by patients receiving treatment for cancer. *Cancer Nurs* 18:23–28, 1995
27. Irvine DM, Vincent L, Graydon JE, et al: Fatigue in women with breast cancer receiving radiation therapy. *Cancer Nurs* 21:127–135, 1998
28. Mauch P, Constine L, Greenberger J, et al: Hematopoietic stem cell compartment: acute and late effects of radiation therapy and chemotherapy. *Int J Radiat Oncol Biol Phys* 31:1319–1339, 1995
29. Casarett GW: *Radiation Histopathology* (vol. 1). Boca Raton, FL, CRC Press, 1980
30. Hashimoto M: The distribution of active marrow in the bones of the normal adult. *Kyushu J Med Sci* 11:103–111, 1960
31. Bruner DW, Bucholtz JD, Iwamoto R, Strohl R (eds.): *Manual for Radiation Oncology Nursing Practice and Education.* Pittsburgh, Oncology Nursing Press, 1998
32. Wara WM, Bauman GS, Sneed PK, et al: Brain, brain stem and cerebellum, in Perez CA, Brady LW (eds.): *Principles and Practice of Radiation Oncology* (ed 3). Philadelphia, Lippincott, 1997, pp 777–828
33. Faithfull S, Brada M: Somnolence syndrome in adults following cranial irradiation for primary brain tumors. *Clin Oncol (R Coll Radio)* 10:250–524, 1998
34. Ryan J: Radiation somnolence syndrome. *J Pediatr Oncol Nurs* 17:50–53, 2000
35. Iwamoto RR: Cancers of the head and neck, in Dow KH, Bucholtz JD, Iwamoto RR, et al (eds.): *Nursing Care in Radiation Oncology* (ed 2). Philadelphia, Saunders, 1997, pp 239–260
36. Diaz-Arnold AM, Marek CA: The impact of saliva on patient care: a literature review. *J Prosthet Dentist* 88:337–343, 2002

37. Davies AN: The management of xerostomia: a review. *Eur J Cancer Care* 6:209–214, 1997
38. Lynch H, Milgrom P: Xylitol and dental caries: an overview for clinicians. *J Calif Dent Assoc* 31:205–209, 2003
39. Mandel ID, Katz R, Zengo A, et al: The effects of pharmacologic agent on salivary secretion and composition in man. 1. Pilocarpine, atropine and anticholinesterases. *J Oral Ther Pharmacol* 4:192–199, 1968
40. Greenspan E, Daniels TE: Effectiveness of pilocarpine in postradiation xerostomia. *Cancer* 59:1123–1125, 1987
41. LeVeque FG, Montgomery F, Potter D, et al: A multi-center randomized, double-blind, placebo-controlled, dose-titration study of oral pilocarpine for treatment of radiation-induced xerostomia in head and neck cancer patients. *J Clin Oncol* 11:1124–1131, 1993
42. Johnson JT, Ferretti GA, Nethery WJ, et al: Oral pilocarpine for post irradiation xerostomia in patients with head and neck cancer. *N Engl J Med* 329:390–395, 1993
43. Zimmerman R, Mark R, Tran L, et al: Concomitant pilocarpine during head and neck irradiation is associated with decreased posttreatment xerostomia. *Int J Radiat Oncol Biol Phys* 37: 571–575, 1997
44. Maher K: Xerostomia, in Yarbro CH, Frogge MH, Goodman M (eds.): *Cancer Symptom Management* (ed 3). Sudbury, MA, Jones and Bartlett, 2004, pp 215–229
45. Blom M, Dawidson I, Fernberg JO, et al: Acupuncture treatment of patients with radiation-induced xerostomia. *Eur J Cancer B Oral Oncol* 32B:182–190, 1996
46. Blom M, Lundberg T: Long-term follow-up of patients treated with acupuncture for xerostomia and the influence of additional treatment. *Oral Dis* 6:15–24, 2000
47. Johnstone PA, Niemtzow RC, Riffenburgh RH: Acupuncture for xerostomia: clinical update *Cancer* 64:1151–1156, 2002
48. Rothstein JP: *Oral Care of Cancer Patients* (ed 7). Tampa, FL, American Cancer Society, 1998
49. Mazanec SR: Breast cancer, in Dow KH, Bucholtz JD, Iwamoto RR, et al (eds.): *Nursing Care in Radiation Oncology* (ed 2). Philadelphia, Saunders, 1997, pp 101–135
50. Knopp JM: Lung cancer, in Dow KH, Bucholtz JD, Iwamoto RR, et al (eds.): *Nursing Care in Radiation Oncology* (ed 2). Philadelphia, Saunders, 1997, pp 293–315
51. McDonald S, Rubin P, Phillips TL, et al: Injury to the lung from cancer therapy: clinical syndromes, measurable endpoints, and potential scoring systems. *Int J Radiat Oncol Biol Phys* 31:1187–1204, 1995
52. Hilderley LJ: Radiotherapy, in Groenwald S, Frogge MH, Goodman M, Yarbro CH (eds.): *Cancer Nursing: Principles and Practice* (ed 4). Sudbury, MA, Jones and Bartlett, 1997, pp 247–282
53. Stevens KR: Stomach and small intestine, in Cox JD (ed.): *Moss' Radiation Oncology: Rationale, Technique, Results* (ed 7). St. Louis, Mosby, 1994, pp 428–439
54. Maher KE: Male genitourinary cancers, in Dow KH, Bucholtz JD, Iwamoto RR, et al (eds.): *Nursing Care in Radiation Oncology* (ed 2). Philadelphia, Saunders, 1997, pp 184–221
55. Grigsby PW, Russell A, Bruner D, et al: Late injury of cancer therapy on the female reproductive tract. *Int J Radiat Oncol Biol Phys* 31:1281–1300, 1995
56. Gordon KB, Char DH: Late effects of radiation on the eye and ocular adnexa. *Int J Radiat Oncol Biol Phys* 31:1123–1140, 1995
57. Rubin R, Constine LS, Fajardo D, et al: RTOG late effects working group — overview: late effects of normal tissues (LENT) scoring system. *Int J Radiat Oncol Biol Phys* 31:1041–1042, 1995
58. Rubin P, Constine LS, Williams JP: Late effects of cancer treatment: radiation and drug toxicity, in Perez CA, Brady LW (eds.): *Principles and Practice of Radiation Oncology* (ed 3). Philadelphia, Lippincott, 1997, pp 155–211
59. Rubin P: The law and order of radiation sensitivity, absolute vs. relative, in Vaeth JM, Meyer JL (eds.): *Radiation Tolerance of Normal Tissues: Frontiers of Radiation Therapy and Oncology*. Basel, Switzerland, Karger, 1989, pp 7–40
60. Marks LB: The impact of organ structure on radiation response. *Int J Radiat Oncol Biol Phys* 34:1165–1171, 1996
61. Davis AM, Dische S, Gerber L, et al: Measuring postirradiation subcutaneous soft-tissue fibrosis: state-of-the-art and future directions. *Semin Radiat Oncol* 13:203–213, 2003
62. O'Sullivan B, Levin W: Late radiation-related fibrosis: pathogenesis, manifestations, and current management. *Semin Radiat Oncol* 13:274–289, 2003
63. Delanian S, Balla-Mekias S, Lefaix J-L: Striking regression of chronic radiotherapy damage in a clinical trial of combined pentoxifylline and tocopherol. *J Clin Oncol* 17:3283–3290, 1999
64. Delanian S, Porcher R, Balla-Mekias S, et al: Randomized, placebo-controlled trial of combined pentoxifylline and tocopherol for regression of superficial radiation-induced fibrosis. *J Clin Oncol* 21:2545–2555, 2003
65. Lennox AJ, Shafer, JP, Hatcher M, et al: Pilot study of impedance-controlled microcurrent therapy for managing radiation-induced fibrosis in head-and-neck cancer patients. *Int J Radiat Oncol Biol Phys* 54:23–34, 2002
66. Schultheiss TE, Kun LE, Ang KK, et al: Radiation response of the central nervous system. *Int J Radiat Oncol Biol Phys* 31:1093–1112, 1995
67. Andrews N: Dental implications and management of head and neck radiotherapy patients. *Ann Royal Austral Dent Surg* 15:90–97, 2000
68. Hancock SL, McDougall IR: Thyroid abnormalities after therapeutic external radiation. *Int J Radiat Oncol Biol Phys* 31:1165–1170, 1995
69. Marks LB, Yu X, Vujaskovic Z, et al: Radiation-induced lung injury. *Semin Radiat Oncol* 13:333–345, 2003
70. Stewart JR, Fajardo LF, Gillette LM, et al: Radiation injury to the heart. *Int J Radiat Oncol Biol Phys* 31:1205–1211, 1995
71. Adams MJ, Lipshultz SE, Schwartz C, et al: Radiation-associated cardiovascular disease: manifestations and management. *Semin Radiat Oncol* 13:346–356, 2003
72. Basavaraju SR, Easterly CE: Pathophysiologic effects of radiation on atherosclerosis development and progression, and the incidence of cardiovascular complications. *Med Phys* 29:2391–2403, 2002
73. Hauer-Jensen M, Wang J, Denham JW: Bowel injury: current and evolving management strategies. *Semin Radiat Oncol* 13:357–371, 2003
74. Coia LR, Myerson RJ: Late effects of radiation therapy on the gastrointestinal tract. *Int J Radiat Oncol Biol Phys* 31:1213–1236, 1995
75. Hussey DH: The testicle, in Cox JD (ed.): *Moss' Radiation Oncology: Rationale, Technique, Results* (ed 7). St. Louis, Mosby, 1994, pp 559–586
76. Haas R: Evaluating the risks of radiation-induced secondary cancers. *Radiat Ther* 4:104–112, 1996
77. van Leeuwen FE, Travers LB: Second cancers, in DeVita VT, Hellman S, Rosenberg SA (eds.): *Cancer: Principles and Practice of Oncology* (ed 6). Philadelphia, Lippincott-Raven, 2001, pp 2939–2963

CHAPTER 15

Chemotherapy: Principles of Therapy

Peter V. Tortorice, PharmD, BCOP

Historical Perspective

The term *chemotherapy* was first coined to describe the use of chemicals or drugs to treat microbial diseases and later neoplastic diseases.[1] In the 1940s, nitrogen mustard, the first cytotoxic drug, was introduced for cancer chemotherapy. Nitrogen mustard—a derivative of mustard gas, which was used as a chemical deterrent in the two world wars—was developed as an antineoplastic agent after it was learned that soldiers exposed to this drug developed reversible leukopenia. Soon after the introduction of nitrogen mustard, methotrexate, cyclophosphamide, and fluorouracil were made available for treatment of advanced cancers. Two significant developments occurred in the 1960s and late 1970s that opened the door for modern-day cancer chemotherapy: (1) the introduction of platinum-coordinated complexes as cytotoxic therapy, and (2) the introduction of combination chemotherapy to improve response rates and survival without significantly affecting toxicity.

The screening, synthesis, and clinical testing of new compounds or analogues of currently active agents continued through the 1970s and 1980s. Among the most useful agents discovered during this period were the semisynthetic podophyllotoxin etoposide and paclitaxel, a natural product isolated from the Western yew tree. The development of the anthracycline analog doxorubicin also had a significant impact on the treatment of breast cancer and sarcomas. The biologic response modifiers were first recognized as having antineoplastic activity in the 1980s. The search for new agents to treat cancer continues into the twenty-first century.

Current strategies being emphasized for drug development include drugs with novel mechanisms of action, monoclonal antibodies directed against specific cellular targets, drugs that modulate or reverse drug resistance, and drugs used for supportive care of the cancer patient. Supportive therapies that have made administering and managing chemotherapy easier and safer include simple and effective antiemetic therapy and hematopoietic growth factors.

Historically, the goals of early chemotherapy were primarily limited to palliation of symptoms. An increase in available agents and more experience with cytotoxic chemotherapy produced significant tumor regression and improved control of cancer. The development and acceptance of combination chemotherapy greatly improved the outcome for otherwise incurable neoplastic diseases. This approach to cancer treatment incorporated the theoretical point that targeting multiple biochemical processes would have a greater overall effect on tumor regression and remission. Eventually, the goals of chemotherapy shifted to a curative approach for those cancers in which complete responses to chemotherapy were seen. Cancers for which cures and increased survival have been accomplished using chemotherapy given alone or in combination with other modalities such as surgery and radiation therapy are listed in Table 15-1. Although chemotherapy has produced cures in a subset of patients with cancers such as acute leukemia, Hodgkin's disease, and testicular tumors, significant cure rates for the most common cancers such as breast cancer, lung cancer, and colon cancer have not been achieved.

The use of drugs to control or eradicate cancer has developed into the specialization of medical oncology. The treatment of individuals with cancer is one of the most rapidly expanding and dynamic fields in medicine and demands continuous reevaluation and reappraisal of both new and established therapies. To continue to develop and improve cancer treatments, more patients need to participate in controlled clinical trials. It is estimated that fewer than 10% of eligible pa-

Table 15-1 Chemotherapy-Sensitive Tumors

Relative Chemosensitivity and Expected Survival Outcome	Type of Cancer
Highly sensitive: Normal survival, possible cure	Acute leukemia in children Hodgkin's disease Diffuse large-cell lymphoma Burkitt's lymphoma Testicular carcinoma Embryonal carcinoma Ewing's sarcoma Wilms' tumor Skin cancer
Moderately sensitive: Increase in survival	Ovarian carcinoma Breast carcinoma Endometrial carcinoma Acute leukemia in adults Small cell lung cancer Prostate cancer Stomach cancer Cervical cancer Neuroblastoma
Minimally sensitive: Some increase in survival	Head and neck cancers Gastrointestinal cancers Endocrine gland tumors Malignant melanoma Osteogenic sarcoma Soft tissue sarcoma
Marginally sensitive: No documented increase in survival	Bladder cancer Esophageal cancer Non-small cell lung cancer Pancreatic carcinoma Hepatocellular carcinoma

tients actively being treated for cancer are enrolled in such trials. The clinician is a key figure in encouraging cooperation not only from the patient and his or her family but also from the healthcare community, including providers and sponsors (third-party payers). Increased survival and — more important — the maintenance or improvement of quality of life for patients with cancer can be achieved with the appropriate use of chemotherapy.

Cancer Chemotherapy Drug Development

Drug discovery and the eventual development of cancer treatment compounds involve numerous strategies. The most successful methods seek to combine current knowledge of the biology of cancer and the pharmacological properties of potentially therapeutic compounds. In particular, synthesis and testing of analogs of compounds with known antineoplastic activity is one approach that has had some success. Synthesis of chemically or mechanistically similar compounds having different pharmacokinetic or toxic properties has yielded clinically useful new agents. Recent advances in understanding the molecular and genetic operations that neoplastic cells possess have led to the development of targeted antitumor agents — for example, angiogenesis inhibitors and oncogene suppressors.

The oncology research community is composed of national and local study groups, university-based research programs, and pharmaceutical manufacturers. The National Cancer Institute (NCI) assists in coordinating the massive efforts of researchers and clinicians in screening and developing drugs for use in cancer treatment. In addition, a significant amount of research and development, primarily by pharmaceutical manufacturers, is conducted outside the auspices of the NCI.

The drug approval process in the United States is rigorous and comprehensive. New compounds undergo extensive testing in animals and then in humans before being submitted to the FDA for approval and becoming commercially available. Because of the unique and potentially life-threatening toxicities associated with antineoplastic drugs, this approval process may become both lengthy and expensive. The average time and cost to bring a drug to market may range from 10 to 12 years and from $40 to $80 million.

Preclinical Evaluation

The NCI coordinates the screening of more than 10,000 compounds each year in an effort to find new and potentially useful drugs for treating cancer. Less than 1% of these screened compounds proceed to clinical trials. Compounds with known or suspected antineoplastic activity are tested in animal tumor models and human tumor cell lines. Cell lines frequently used include lung, ovarian, and renal cell cancer; malignant melanoma; brain tumors; and leukemias. Because of the interest in how drug resistance may influence chemotherapy effectiveness, multidrug-resistant (MDR) variants of human breast cancer and murine leukemia cell lines are also available for testing.[2]

Compounds having demonstrated significant antineoplastic activity first undergo preclinical toxicology studies. The purpose of these studies is to determine a safe starting dose for use in humans. The lethal dose in 10% of animals tested (LD_{10}) is then used to calculate a starting dose for clinical trials. The LD_{10} is usually determined in mice and dogs to avoid excessive risk to humans. Body surface area (BSA) is the preferred reference point used for making interspecies dose comparisons.

Table 15-2 Different Phases of Clinical Trials Conducted in the United States

Phase	Purpose	Comment
I	Determines maximum tolerated dose and describes pharmacology and pharmacokinetics in humans	Dosing starts at 10% of the LD_{10} in mice Determine safe dose and schedule for phase II
II	Determines drug activity in specific tumors	Also determines administration schedule, toxicity, supportive care
III	New drug or drug combinations are compared against the standard therapy	Objective criteria: Response rate, duration of response, survival, toxicity, and quality of life
IV	Role of drug in adjuvant/ curative setting	Determines other uses, doses, schedules, and combination regimens

Clinical Trials

Following the initial development and pharmaceutical preparation in the preclinical phase, new compounds must be tested in humans to evaluate their activity and toxicity in treating cancers. Table 15-2 briefly describes the phases of clinical trials conducted in the United States and lists the purpose and goals of each phase of testing. Although healthy volunteers are usually recruited for phase I testing, because of the potential for significant toxicity with antineoplastic drugs, patients with advanced cancer are enrolled in trials of these agents. These patients may also benefit from the new therapies. The ideal patients for phase II testing are previously untreated; with antineoplastic agents, however, most tend to be patients who have shown little or no response to prior chemotherapy. Usually, response rates of higher than 20% indicate the agent may have therapeutic usefulness and warrants further clinical testing. Traditionally, response rates, duration of response, survival, and toxicity are measured, although quality of life has emerged as a focus of clinical trials in recent years. At the conclusion of phase III testing, it should be known whether the new treatment is better than the standard therapy in terms of response, survival, and toxicity, and how it affects the patient's quality of life. Phase IV studies generally involve the use of drugs in combination with other therapies where cure is the goal of treatment.

Scientific Basis of Chemotherapy

Only recently have researchers begun to identify what is thought to be the primary pharmacological activity of many antineoplastic agents. The actual mechanism or combination of mechanisms responsible for killing tumor cells remains elusive. This disparity is partly a function of the lack of a clear understanding of how cancer cells originate, grow, and regress. The next section addresses tumor cell biology and examines how chemotherapeutic drugs may selectively exert their cytotoxicity.

The Cell Cycle

Much of what is known regarding the effects of cytotoxic chemotherapy relies on understanding the cell cycle. The cycle consists of five phases: G_1, S, G_2, M, and G_0. The phases describe periods of time for different cellular processes that ultimately result in a cell's reproduction or death (Figure 15-1). In any population, only some cells are actively proliferating. The *growth fraction* is the portion of cells actively cycling compared to the entire population. Following mitosis, a cell can do any one of the following: leave the cycle, differentiate, and eventually die; enter a resting state (G_0) and reenter the cycle at some later time (stem cells); or enter the G_1 phase and continue to cycle.

Synthesis of RNA and proteins occurs predominantly in the *G_1 phase.* Synthesis, or *S phase,* is when DNA is being replicated and is a relatively short period compared with the overall time a cell is cycling. The *G_2 phase* is typically brief, occurring after DNA synthesis and just before cell division. Mitosis, or cell division, ensues during the *M phase,* resulting in two identical daughter cells. The time from mitosis to mitosis is described as the *cycling time.* Cells that have left the cycle to enter the *G_0 phase* are considered to be in a *resting* or *dormant phase.* These cells can actively synthesize RNA and proteins and differentiate; however, they are typically resistant to the cytotoxic effects of chemotherapy. Apoptosis, or programmed cell death, is an important cellular process that may be exploited for its antineoplastic effect by targeted chemotherapy.

Tumor Cell Kinetics

Tumor cells may be distinguished from cells of normal tissues by their loss of controlled cell division, lack of differentiation, and ability to invade surrounding tissues and establish new growth at distant sites in the body. Theoretically, most antineoplastic agents utilize the rapid proliferation rate of tumor cells as a target for their cytotoxic effects. The same mechanism explains many of the toxicities seen in cells of normal tissues, because these cells are also going through the cell cycle and dividing, albeit at a much slower rate. The selective effects of antineoplastic drugs on both normal and tumor cells may be explained by the following model: (1) tumor growth is often exponential,

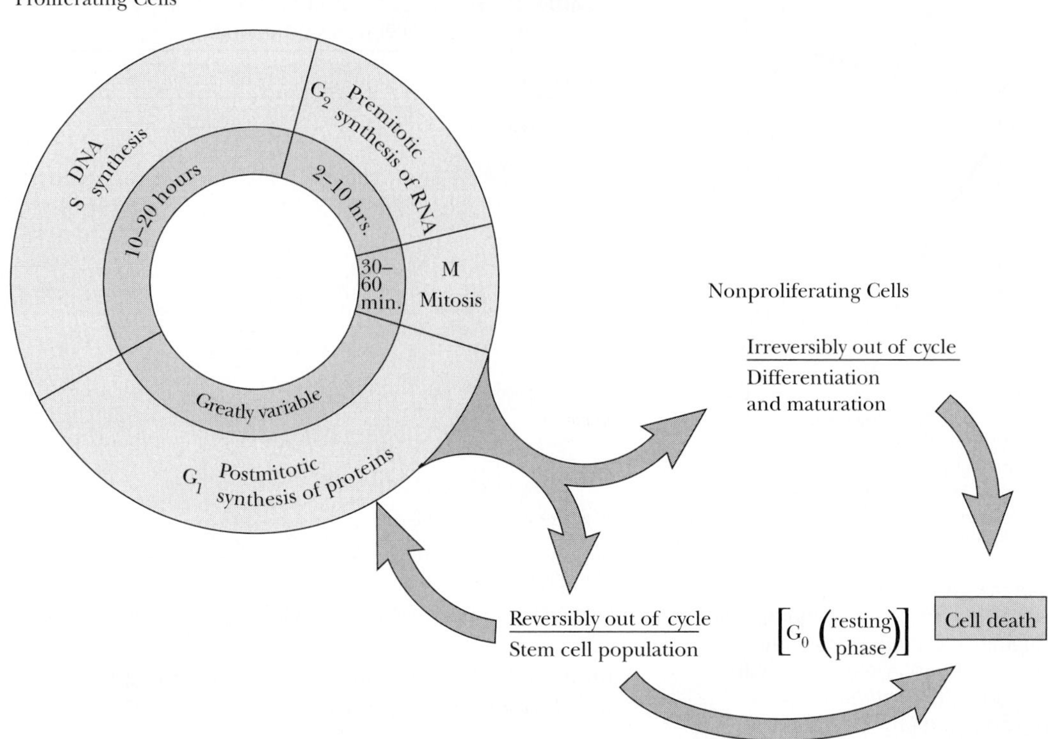

Figure 15-1 Diagrammatic representation of the life of a cell, emphasizing the relationships between the cell cycle and proliferating and nonproliferating cells.

(2) doubling times vary widely between tumors, and (3) chemotherapy-sensitive tumors tend to grow faster than slow-growing tumors that are less responsive to chemotherapy.

The doubling times of both malignant and normal tissues vary widely. Factors that affect doubling time include cell cycle time, growth fraction, and cell loss by either cell death (apoptosis) or differentiation or metastasis. Cells with a rapid cycling time and a tumor with a large growth fraction should be the most responsive to cytotoxic therapy. Although tumor cells may exhibit rapid cycling, the rate is not higher than what is seen with normal renewal tissues such as bone marrow and gastrointestinal mucosa. Therefore, uncontrolled proliferation is not the sole distinguishing trait of tumor cells. Loss of homeostatic mechanisms, such as contact inhibition, cell differentiation and maturation, leads to an increased proliferative rate, which exceeds cell death. Collectively, these processes lead to accumulation of tumor cells.

The Effects of Cytotoxic Chemotherapy on Tumor Cells

Cell kill hypothesis

The cell kill hypothesis is a basic principle often used to describe the effects of cancer chemotherapy on normal and tumor cells. The hypothesis describes a first-order kinetic process that predicts the number of cells killed based on the dose of chemotherapy given. It applies only to cells that are actively proliferating and assumes that treatment sensitivity does not change and that growth rate is constant. The model is based on a log-kill relationship for dose of chemotherapy and a constant proportion of cells killed per treatment. A treatment with a 3-log kill produces a tumor reduction of 99.9%. Essentially, no treatment can bring the number of tumor cells to zero; therefore, the net effect on viable tumor cells is calculated as surviving cells plus regrowth before the next treatment. Because of these limitations, the model is not applicable to most human tumors. Malignancies that do follow this model include Burkitt's lymphoma and germ cell tumors. The cell kill hypothesis is still used today in determining tumor cell growth inhibition of newly derived anticancer compounds.

Gompertzian curve

The effect of antineoplastic drugs on human tumors cannot be fully explained by the cell kill model because not all tumor cells are in a proliferative state. A Gompertzian growth curve (Figure 15-2) probably best describes the growth of human tumors and the responses observed with the administration of antineo-

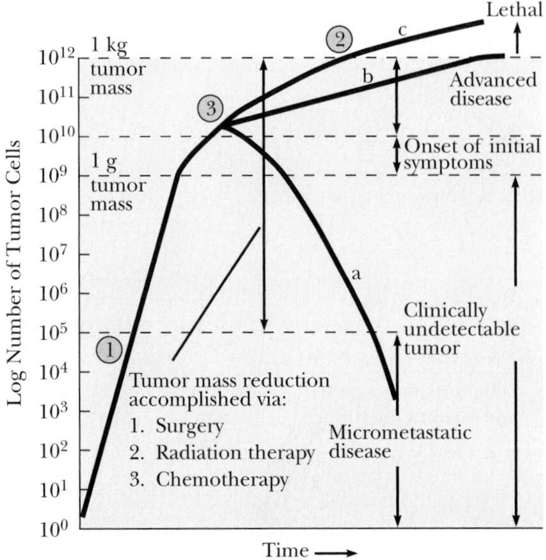

Figure 15-2 Gompertzian tumor growth curve: relationship of tumor mass, diagnosis, symptoms, and potential treatment regimens. Growth phases and chemotherapy response: (1) log phase (high growth fraction, short doubling time); (2) plateau phase (low growth fraction, longer doubling time); (3) initiation of chemotherapy treatments: (a) tumor cells responsive to drugs; (b) tumor exhibits initial response to treatment but develops resistance (secondary or somatic resistance); (c) tumor unresponsive to drug regimen (primary resistance). (Used with permission from Buick RN: Cellular basis of chemotherapy, in Dorr RT, Von Hoff DD (eds.): *Cancer Chemotherapy Handbook* (ed 2). Norwalk, CT, Appleton & Lange, 1994, pp 3-14.[3])

plastic drugs.[3] Tumor growth fraction and proliferative rate are not constant, but rather decrease with time as a tumor goes from a small, undetectable clump of cells to a large mass. The doubling time of a tumor increases as the mass grows in size. Eventually, the tumor reaches a growth plateau phase, where further increase in size becomes minimal because of the slower doubling time.

The Gompertzian curve also is useful in describing the observed tumor response to chemotherapy.[4] If cytotoxic chemotherapy is given in the growth phase of the tumor, the portion of cells actively proliferating (the growth fraction) is large; therefore, a high percentage of cells will be susceptible to the effects of the drugs. In contrast, in a more advanced stage of the disease, when growth has reached a plateau, fewer cells will be dividing and therefore will be less susceptible to chemotherapy.

When surgery or radiation therapy has been used to reduce the tumor mass, chemotherapy may prove beneficial in eradicating both residual and micrometastatic disease. However, because metastatic cells often result from numerous prior divisions, the possibility that either primary or secondary drug resistance has developed is significant.

Table 15-3 Targets for Anticancer Therapy and Associated Pharmaceutical Compounds

Therapeutic Target	Compounds
Signal transduction inhibition	Bryostatin* EGFR inhibitors (see Table 15-4) UCN-01 (staurosporine congener)* Thalidomide
Angiogenesis inhibition	Angiostatin* Bevacizumab (Avastin) Endostatin* Interferon alfa Thalidomide
Matrix metalloproteinase inhibitors	Marimastat* AG 3340* BAY 12-9566*
Cycline-dependent kinase inhibitors	Flavopiridol* UCN-01* PKC 412

*Drug in development.

Data from Dy, Adjei[5,6]; Nelson, Fingleton, Rothenberg, Matrisian.[7]

Mechanisms and sites of action of cytotoxic chemotherapy

Chemotherapeutic drugs induce their cytotoxicity on tumor cells and normal tissue by one or more mechanisms. Figure 15-3 illustrates the potential sites and proposed mechanisms of action for many of the drugs currently available for cancer chemotherapy. Central to the diagram is the genetic machinery, considered to be the focus for most effective cytotoxic drugs.

Targeted Therapies for Cancer

Until recently, the majority of cancer chemotherapy had been limited to drugs that are cytotoxic to the reproductive cycle and functions of tumor cells. A better understanding of the molecular biology of normal and tumor cells has allowed significant developments in targeting mechanisms of tumor growth, invasion, and metastasis. By targeting tumor cell growth, these types of therapies should be less toxic to normal tissues. Additionally, overall treatment of cancer may evolve from an acute tumor destruction approach to a more chronic management of malignant cells. Table 15-3 lists the proposed anticancer targets of selected compounds either currently available or under development.[5–7]

Inhibition of signal transduction

Epidermal growth factor receptor (EGFR; also known as HER-1) controls normal cell growth and

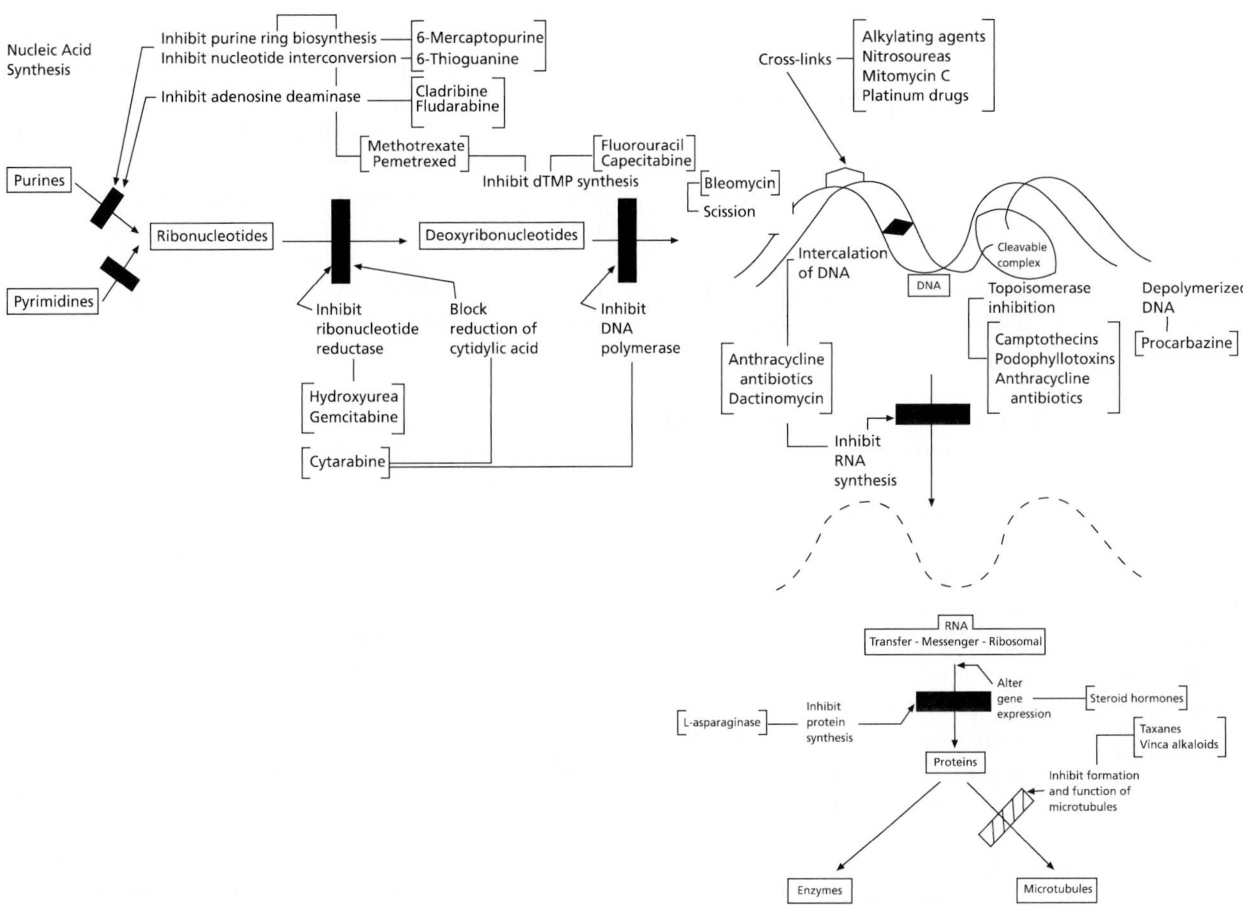

Figure 15-3 Proposed mechanisms of action of cytotoxic chemotherapeutic agents.

differentiation. Ligand binding to EGFR in tumor cells activates signaling pathways that regulate cell growth, DNA repair, adhesion, survival and development of metastases, and angiogenesis.[8,9] EGFR is overexpressed in many types of cancers, including non-small cell lung cancer (NSCLC), renal cell carcinoma, and cancers of the head and neck, pancreas, breast, ovary, and colon.[10] Interruption of signal transduction via inhibition of EGFR has been shown to inhibit cellular replication and tumor progression in tumors that overexpress this receptor.[11] Table 15-4 lists strategies that may be employed to inhibit the stimulation of EGFR and block signal transduction as well as compounds being investigated or currently available for targeted anticancer therapy.[5,6,12] The combination of EGFR tyrosine kinase inhibitors and cyclooxygenase 2 (COX-2) inhibitors such as sulindac is being investigated for its ability to reduce the number of adenomatous colon polyps.[13]

Table 15-4 Strategies to Block or Inhibit EGFR in Tumors and Drugs

Site of Activity	Pharmacodynamic Effect	Pharmaceutical Compounds
Block ligand binding to EGFR on cell surface	Interrupt signal transduction	*Monoclonal antibodies* • Cetuximab (Erbitux) • ABX-EGF* • H22-EGF*
Block EGFR tyrosine phosphorylation	Interrupt signal transduction	*Small-molecule tyrosine kinase inhibitors* • Gefitinib • Imatinib • Erlotinib*
Bind toxin to external domain of receptor	Cell death	No known compounds currently in development
Block translation of mRNA downstream	Block protein synthesis	*Antisense oligonucleotides* • ISIS 3521*

EGFR = epidermal growth factor receptor.

* Drug in development.

Data from Dy, Adjei[5,6]; Finley.[12]

Angiogenesis inhibition

Tumors need an adequate blood supply to provide individual cells with the nutrients and oxygen required for them to grow and develop. Angiogenesis, the formation of new blood vessels, occurs as a tumor mass expands and displaces cells farther away from the primary blood source. If angiogenesis does not occur, tumor growth remains limited to a small clump of nonproliferative cells that are usually incapable of metastasizing.[13] Disease progression and prognosis have been shown to depend on microvessel density of breast, lung, and prostate tumors.[14] In addition, metastasis can occur only if the primary tumor has nearby access to permeable vasculature, thereby allowing cells to travel to distant sites and invade other organs and tissues.

Several growth factors and oncogenes are known to stimulate angiogenesis. Among the most potent mitogens for normal and pathologic angiogenesis are vascular endothelial growth factor (VEGF) and beta fibroblast growth factor (β-FGF).[15] VEGF is responsible for endothelial cell mitogenesis and migration, extracellular matrix remodeling, increased vascular permeability, and maintenance of newly formed blood vessels. Increased levels of VEGF are found in tumors of the lung, breast, thyroid, GI tract, kidney, bladder, ovary, cervix, and glioblastomas of the brain.[16] Inhibition of these factors is being investigated as a potential therapeutic modality for controlling the growth of tumors and inhibiting the development of metastatic disease. Several strategies for targeting the vascular expansion necessary for tumor growth, reproduction, and metastasis are under investigation. Agents that block mitogenic signals or that bind to mitogen receptors such as vascular epithelial growth factor receptor (VEGFR) are currently available or being investigated in clinical trials. Among the most popular compounds that have demonstrated significant antiangiogenic activity are angiostatin, endostatin, interleukin-12, suramin, and thalidomide.[17,18] Colorectal cancer prognosis correlates negatively with VEGF expression.[16]

Matrix metalloproteinase inhibition

Matrix metalloproteinases (MMPs) represent a group of proteolytic enzymes associated with degradation of the extracellular membrane (ECM), including the basement membrane.[7] MMPs may aid tumor metastasis by disrupting the basement membrane integrity, thereby allowing tumor cells to spread both locally and distantly. MMPs may also play a key role in the creation and maintenance of a microenvironment that facilitates growth and angiogenesis of tumors at primary and metastatic sites. MMP expression is common in human tumors, including cancers of the breast, colon, rectum, lung, prostate, pancreas, and ovary. An imbalance in the amounts of MMPs and endogenous MMP inhibitors may contribute to the degradation of the ECM, permitting tumor cells to grow and metastasize.[19] As a consequence, inhibiting these enzymes might shift the balance away from activation of MMPs.

Matrix metalloproteinase inhibitors (MMPIs) are under investigation for their ability to inhibit not only invasion of tumor cells in target organs and tissues but also angiogenesis. Among the compounds being studied for oral use are marimastat, AG3340, and BAY 112-9566.[20] Three clinical strategies are being used to test the activity of MMPIs in anticancer therapy: (1) comparison of MMPIs against standard chemotherapy, (2) adding MMPIs to standard chemotherapy, and (3) long-term administration of MMPIs following successful chemotherapy (MMP1). Ultimately, the chronic administration of MMPIs may provide the optimal utilization of these agents in responsive tumors.

Cyclin-dependent kinase inhibitors

Cyclin-dependent kinases (CDK), along with complementary cyclins, are responsible for regulating key checkpoints on the cell cycle.[6] Inhibition of CDK activity appears to block the release of transcription factors, causing failure of activation of the transcription genes required for S-phase entry. This failure, in turn, induces cell cycle arrest in tumor cells and enhances cytotoxic chemotherapy-induced apoptosis. Currently, CDK inhibitors are being investigated in preclinical and phase I and II trials to determine their role in stalling or blocking progression of the reproductive cell cycle. Through inhibition of the phosphorylation or activation of CDKs, cells with unreplicated or damaged DNA will go on to replicate and produce nonviable cells or cell death.[21] Flavopiridol has been the most extensively studied CDK inhibitor. In a recently reported phase II trial in patients with metastatic NSCLC, flavopiridol administration was not associated with any clinical responses but did produce disease stabilization.[22]

Cytotoxic Drug Selection Criteria

There is wide variability in both therapeutic response and unacceptable toxicity observed in patients receiving chemotherapy. This variability may be explained by differences in factors involving the patient with cancer, the chemotherapy being given, and the type of tumor being treated.

Patient factors include response to toxicity, organ dysfunction, previous treatment, and age. The occurrence and severity of toxicity vary widely among patients and often necessitate chemotherapy dose reduction or treatment delay. Preexisting organ dysfunction, such as renal or hepatic insufficiency, may also require dose or schedule alteration. Patients who have previously received chemotherapy may not be candidates to receive the same drug again or, likewise, a drug with similar toxicity. In particular, the recommended maximum lifetime dose of anthracycline drugs (doxorubicin, daunorubicin, epirubicin, and idarubicin) should not be exceeded, as these agents greatly increase patients' risk for developing severe cardiomyopathy. Drugs that are neurotoxic should be avoided in patients with preexisting neurological defects, such as taxane use in patients with diabetic neuropathies. Previous bone marrow transplant or the use of severely marrow-toxic drugs may preclude the future use of full doses of myelosuppressive drugs. All of these factors may have adverse effects on a patient's antineoplastic response and the overall potential to cure or control the cancer.

Antineoplastic activity, pharmacokinetics, dose, and schedule are important drug factors that can influence chemotherapy response and toxicity. The relative cytotoxicity of any antineoplastic drug is dependent on the origin of the tumor and the presence of intrinsic drug resistance. Intrinsic resistance is probably a type of generic defense mechanism present in cells of certain histologic type. Pharmacokinetic factors determine the ability of chemotherapeutic drugs to reach their cellular targets. Changes in these factors, such as decreased metabolic activation or increased drug clearance from the body, may decrease antitumor response. Similarly, alterations in protein binding of certain drugs, such as etoposide or teniposide, may enhance clinical toxicity. Poorly lipophilic drugs administered systemically are ineffective for tumors found in lipophilic tissues such as the central nervous system. Administration of drugs such as methotrexate or cytarabine directly into the intrathecal space will circumvent this obstacle. The ability to deliver the optimal dose of chemotherapy for a specific cancer is often limited by the patient's individualized maximum tolerated dose. The clinical use of hematopoietic growth factors, such as granulocyte colony-stimulating factor (G-CSF) and granulocyte-macrophage colony-stimulating factor (GM-CSF), has allowed the doses of myelotoxic drugs to be escalated in an attempt to improve response.

Tumor factors such as growth and size significantly influence the response to chemotherapy. Larger tumors have small growth fractions and, therefore, are less responsive to the cytotoxic effects of antineoplastic drugs. In addition, the ability of chemotherapy to reach large solid tumors may be hindered by inadequate blood flow. Chemotherapy response is also influenced by tumor cell histology. Table 15-1 differentiates tumor types based on their sensitivity to chemotherapy and the outcomes that may be expected in patients successfully treated with chemotherapy.

Selectivity of certain types of malignancies for specific chemotherapeutic agents is also seen. Fluorouracil is most active in cancers of endodermal tissue, such as gastrointestinal and breast neoplasms. Epithelial tumors, such as squamous cell cancers, are especially sensitive to the cytotoxic effects of bleomycin.

Managing Chemotherapy Resistance

In addition to the patient and drug factors that play important roles in chemotherapy response, genetic instability of the tumor cell and emergence of drug resistance are currently considered the most significant determinants of response. Although much work has focused on changing the biology or genetic composition of tumor cells, strategies for overcoming resistance need to be developed and implemented.

Cytotoxic drug resistance may be expressed as a temporary or permanent insensitivity to one or more antineoplastic drugs. Temporary or relative resistance is usually a function of the drug's inability to reach the target cells. Reasons why this could happen include poor blood supply, existence of anatomical sanctuary sites such as the testes and central nervous system, or altered pharmacokinetic parameters. Likewise, as yet undefined host defense mechanisms may have a negative effect on treatment success. In some conditions, temporary resistance may be reversed by altering drug delivery, dose, or scheduling of drug administration.

Permanent or phenotypic drug resistance is an inheritable mechanism, which may result from a genetic mutation or preexisting trait.[23] This form of resistance may be present prior to treatment (*primary resistance*) or may develop after exposure to antineoplastic drugs (*secondary resistance*). *Point mutations* usually occur in a single cell and are independent of drug concentration. *Gene amplification* is influenced by drug concentration and occurs with repeated exposure over an extended period of time. For example, expression of the *MDR-1* gene is associated with the development of the MDR phenotype.[24]

Theoretical Basis for Cytotoxic Drug Resistance

The failure of chemotherapy to control tumor growth and induce remission from cancer is one of the most challenging problems facing the oncology clinician. Several theories and models have been developed to explain this phenomenon. The previously described cell kill model represented an early attempt to explain neoplastic cell growth and lack of response to cytotoxic chemotherapy. According to the model, increasing the dose of a cytotoxic drug or adding other drugs results in an increase in cell kill. Therefore, the theory suggests, failure of chemotherapy to eradicate a tumor is the result of inadequate dose intensity or the presence of biochemically resistant tumor cells. Although this theory is applicable to tumor regression, clinical data do not necessarily support it.[4]

Another possible explanation for treatment failure derives from the stem cell concept. Stem cells continually produce progeny that go on to become mature cells but do not differentiate themselves. These cells constitute a small portion of the total population of cells. Therefore, eradicating the stem cell population would, in theory, eliminate the source of malignant cells and induce tumor regression. However, this must be accomplished without greatly increasing the rate of genetic mutation and producing other biochemically resistant stem cell lines.

Chemotherapy treatment failures may be explained by the development of drug resistance to specific chemotherapeutic drugs. The Goldie-Coldman theory proposes that the genetic instability of tumor cells with high mitotic rates may be responsible for the emergence of resistant clones within a population of tumor cells. Treatment failure may then be explained by the development of drug-resistant cells arising from random genetic mutations occurring prior to or during cytotoxic chemotherapy. The optimal chance for curing cancer with chemotherapy would be to apply effective drugs early in treatment so as to reduce the total number of cancer cells while preventing resistant cells from developing, thus supporting the established concepts of combination chemotherapy.

Tumors that recur following effective initial treatment often present a treatment dilemma. Disease that recurs within 6 months usually is considered resistant to initial chemotherapy, and an alternative drug regimen is used. However, recurrence more than 6 months after treatment may be successfully treated with the same or a similar chemotherapy regimen. This phenomenon may be explained by either the reversion of resistant cells to drug-sensitive cells or the predominance of initially sensitive cells in the relapsed tumor.[4] Although the Goldie-Coldman model presents an important concept of quantitative drug resistance, the assumptions are not always applicable to human tumors. Continued diligence in exploring the mechanisms behind chemotherapy treatment failure is a goal of modern chemotherapy.

Types of Drug Resistance

Table 15-5 lists possible mechanisms of resistance and the drugs most often affected.[3,25]

Table 15-5 Possible Mechanisms of Cytotoxic Drug Resistance

Site or Type of Resistance	Mechanism of Resistance	Drugs Involved
Drug metabolism	Reduced drug activation	Cytarabine Fluorouracil 6-Mercaptopurine Methotrexate
	Increased drug deactivation	Alkylating agents Cytarabine Doxorubicin
Cytotoxic targets	Increased enzyme levels	Fluorouracil Methotrexate
	Alteration in enzyme–substrate binding	Doxorubicin Etoposide Fluorouracil 6-Mercaptopurine Methotrexate
Biochemical modification	Use of alternative (salvage) pathways	Cytarabine Fluorouracil 6-Mercaptopurine Methotrexate
	Decreased cofactor concentrations (reduced folate pool)	Fluorouracil
DNA repair systems	Increased DNA repair	Alkylating agents Cisplatin Mitomycin
Intracellular drug concentration	Decreased cellular uptake	Mechlorethamine Methotrexate
	Increased efflux (P-glycoprotein mediated)	Anthracycline antibiotics Etoposide Paclitaxel Vinca alkaloids
Cell cycle checkpoint (failure to induce apoptosis)	*p53* mutation	Cytotoxic chemotherapy

Data from Buick[3]; Yarbro.[25]

Phenotypic drug resistance

Phenotypic drug resistance is believed to arise from spontaneous genetic mutations that regularly occur in a population of tumor cells.[23] The model is based on early observations of the development of acquired resistance in bacteria. A mutational origin appears to explain the development of antibiotic resistance in bacterial cells, which is analogous to the cytotoxic drug resistance observed in tumor cells. Antibiotics and cytotoxic drugs selectively kill sensitive cells and leave behind phenotypically resistant ones that reproduce and expand the volume of resistant cells.

The development of drug resistance is dependent on the spontaneous mutation rate of tumor cells, the timing of a significant mutation relative to the tumor's growth, and the overall tumor burden. All biological systems have an inherent probability of undergoing genetic variation from random changes. These random changes may result in minor effects, no effect, or a mutation that alters the cell's characteristics and sensitivity to cytotoxic drugs. Neoplastic cells are genetically unstable and exhibit a high rate of mutation. If mutations occur early in the growth of a population of tumor cells, a high fraction of resistant cells would result. In contrast, a mutation occurring later would produce only a small fraction of resistant clones. If no resistant cells develop prior to treatment, then a cure would be probable with the appropriate chemotherapy. Cytotoxic therapy used to treat minimal tumor burden has a much greater likelihood of proving successful.

The Goldie-Coldman model provides a strong argument for the use of adjuvant and combination chemotherapy. Adjuvant chemotherapy is used in an attempt to eradicate undetectable or micrometastatic tumor cells. If the probability of cure decreases as the number of tumor cells or the mutation rate increases, then eliminating all possible tumor cells or clones should induce a cure or a complete response. The model also supports the use of combination chemotherapy with non-cross-resistant drugs to potentially eliminate subpopulations of resistant tumor cells. The likelihood of a cell being resistant to two or more antineoplastic drugs simultaneously is less than that of it being resistant to single agents when used alone.

Multidrug resistance

Tumor cells exposed to antineoplastic drugs sometimes develop mechanisms to protect themselves against the drug's cytotoxic effect. This resistance may result from alterations in cytotoxic drug metabolism, alterations in cytotoxic targets, biochemical cofactor presence or absence, ability of cells to repair DNA lesions, or decreased intracellular drug concentrations. Multidrug resistance (MDR) is observed in tumor cells that exhibit resistance to a group of drugs that are structurally dissimilar, have unrelated cytotoxic mechanisms, or both. Such resistance usually develops intrinsically or is acquired following exposure to a particular drug in the group.[24] It may occur as a result of overexpression of P-gp membrane efflux pump, enhancements of the glutathione detoxification pathway, or alterations in topoisomerase enzyme systems. The identification and further investigation of this type of resistance and strategies to prevent MDR will have broad clinical implications for the use of chemotherapy as a form of cancer treatment.

Table 15-6 Chemotherapeutic Drugs Exhibiting Cross-Resistance in P-Glycoprotein–Associated Multidrug Resistance

Dactinomycin
Daunorubicin
Doxorubicin
Etoposide
Mitomycin
Mitoxantrone
Paclitaxel
Trimetrexate
Vinblastine
Vincristine

Data from Dalton.[27]

P-glycoprotein (P-gp)-associated MDR. The classic form of MDR is associated with overexpression of the *MDR-1* gene, which encodes for an energy-dependent cell membrane efflux pump, P-gp. This phenomenon was first described in tumor cells selected for resistance to dactinomycin that also exhibited resistance to vinca alkaloids, daunorubicin, and mitomycin.[24] The pump naturally functions to transport toxic molecules from inside the cell to the external environment, and P-gp is found in low concentrations in normal tissues, including the renal tubules, colon, small intestine, bile canaliculi, and vascular epithelia of the brain and spinal cord.[26] Cytotoxic drugs that have entered the cell probably bind to a carrier protein before reaching their cellular targets and are transported out of the cell via the pump.[27] The actual process of drug binding and exit from the cell is unknown. The list of drugs exhibiting P-gp–associated cross-resistance includes several natural products and an antimetabolite (Table 15-6).

The detection of the *MDR-1* gene product from cells of tumors typically resistant to chemotherapy, such as colon, kidney, liver, and pancreas, further supports the importance of P-gp in chemotherapy failure.[28] The presence of the *MDR-1* phenotype and overexpression of P-gp have been found to be predictors of poor prognosis and shortened survival in patients with acute leukemias, multiple myeloma, and malignant lymphomas.[29,30] Much work has been done in an attempt to further elucidate the development of MDR and reverse it. As yet, only limited success in bringing these therapies to the bedside has been achieved.

Other mechanisms of MDR. Another type of MDR has been described in cells that are cross-resistant to topoisomerase poisons such as etoposide, doxorubicin, daunorubicin, and topotecan. Although most of the drugs associated with this type of MDR are also associated with P-gp–mediated MDR, the pattern of resistance is different and cells retain sensitivity to vinca alkaloids.[31] Resistance may be conferred by tumor cells' ability to decrease the activity of or change the binding properties of topoisomerase enzymes. Tumor cells that have developed resistance to one type of topoisomerase II poisons, such as intercalators (e.g., doxorubicin), may not be resistant to an alternative type, such as epipodophyllotoxins (e.g., etoposide). As a consequence, resistance may be overcome by utilizing different types of topoisomerase II poisons.

Multidrug resistance may also be demonstrated in cells with increased detoxifying systems, such as glutathione S-transferase (GST) enzymes, and elevated glutathione levels.[32] These enzymes catalyze conjugation of electrophilic hydrophobic compounds, such as alkylating agents and their metabolites, with glutathione, which facilitates elimination from the tumor cell. Alkylating agents, their metabolites, and platinum compounds are among the most frequent substrates of these enzymes. Strategies being investigated for reversing this type of resistance include administering inhibitors of GST and glutathione synthesis such as buthionine sulfoximine (BSO).[33] Further research is needed to determine the effects of BSO on chemotherapy response rates and duration before this modulator can be used in clinical practice.

Tumor Cell Death and Cytotoxic Drug Resistance

Although drugs can have numerous effects on tumor cells, the critical molecular mechanisms leading to cell death have never been clearly elucidated. For more than 30 years, the classic belief of anticancer drug action has held that cell death is a direct consequence of a specific interaction between a cytotoxic drug and its molecular target. In recent years, newer understanding of the molecular mechanisms controlling cell cycle and programmed cell death (apoptosis) has prompted the reexamination of the classic model of cytotoxic drug-induced cell death. Specific cytotoxic drug–target interactions are now believed to stimulate a pathway that eventually results in apoptosis. This pathway most likely involves processes or sensors that can detect an apoptotic signal, a signal transduction network, and cell machinery that brings about cell death.[34] This pathway is complex and highly dependent on the cell type, the anticancer agent, and the drug–target interaction environment.

p53 *and cell cycling*

Cells that are undergoing replication enter the cell cycle and progress through the four phases of the cycle, resulting in the formation of two identical daughter cells. Checkpoints along the cycle ensure that DNA is undamaged before the cell is allowed to enter into DNA synthesis (S phase). The regulator protein that provides a checkpoint for cells with undamaged DNA is known as p53.[35] When cells with damaged DNA enter the cell cycle, those with nonmutated *p53* genes will be prevented from entering S phase and instead undergo apoptosis. The ability of certain tumor cells to resist or overcome the cytotoxic effects of chemotherapy is believed to result from specific mechanisms possessed by the cell and unique to a drug. Resistance is now considered more directly linked to abnormalities in the cells' genetic machinery or to alterations in critical pathways of cell cycle control and apoptosis. In the clinical setting, support for this theory may be observed by examining the failure to overcome drug resistance when only the classic biochemical or molecular approaches to resistance are employed.

Sensitive cancer cells are initially killed in response to effective cytotoxic chemotherapy; if they survive, however, they develop resistance to further treatment. Mutations in their DNA result in disregulation of the genetic machinery and signaling pathways that control cell cycling and apoptosis. Mutations in the *p53* gene are among the most common genetic changes observed in tumor cells and may occur in at least 50% of all human tumors.[36] p53 is a tumor suppressor protein and critical transcriptional activator that causes both G_1 and G_2 arrest of the cell cycle and is a potent inducer of apoptosis in cells exposed to DNA-damaging drugs.[37,38] Resistance to both radiation therapy and a wide array of chemotherapy drugs have been demonstrated in in vivo models.[39,40] However, not all cells with *p53* mutations are resistant to various antitumor agents, thereby indicating that other factors play a role, such as the cytotoxic stimuli, differences in the overall genetic machinery, and intracellular signaling pathways.[41] An intact *p53* gene maintains the cell's genetic stability and, following exposure to DNA-damaging agents, will lead to apoptosis for the tumor cell, whereas the normal cell survives. When *p53* function is lost, the tumor cell's genomic stability decreases, the cell survives the apoptotic stimuli, and the disease progresses. The presence of a *p53* mutation usually indicates a poorer prognosis, though it does not always correlate with the ability to cure or not cure a cancer.[42]

Loss of mutations in *p53* have been found in a number of solid tumors and in chronic lymphocytic leukemia. Similarly, patients with advanced breast cancer who exhibited a poor response to doxorubicin chemotherapy and were more likely to relapse were more likely to have *p53* gene mutations.[43] Poor response to cisplatin chemotherapy and shorter disease-free survival were observed in 60% of patients with ovarian cancer who had inactivation of the *p53* gene. Other solid tumors with abnormal *p53* expression that show a reduced response to chemotherapy and radiation therapy include non-small cell lung cancer, gastric cancer, and colorectal cancers.[44,45] *p53* status was the strongest prognostic factor for survival in a multivariate analysis conducted in patients with B-cell chronic lymphocytic leukemia.[46]

Other cell cycle regulators

p53 influences the transcriptional activation of a number of genes that are known to regulate cell cycle checkpoint control. The cyclin-dependent kinases, when *p53* is fully active, act on other tumor suppressors to inhibit the cell from entering S phase of the cell cycle. The *MDR-1* gene has also been shown to be potentially influenced by *p53*. Wild-type (nonmutated) *p53* suppresses the promoter of the *MDR-1* gene, whereas the mutant protein can stimulate the promoter.[47,48]

Disregulation of the *p53* pathway leading to overproduction of gene products responsible for the cells entry into S phase and rapid cell growth may be a significant mechanism of cytotoxic drug resistance. Furthermore, resistance could be further suppressed through the stimulation of the *MDR-1* gene directly by mutant *p53*.[34] Therefore, the spontaneous development of resistance and the development of multidrug resistance appear to be related more to mutations in key genes in the cell cycle checkpoint control than to drug-specific mutations. Avoiding or reversing these genetic and molecular changes may provide an effective approach to preventing and reversing cytotoxic drug resistance.

BCL-2 and BAX are members of a large family of related proteins that control a cell's decision to enter apoptosis. The ratio of these proteins appears to be the critical determinant of whether a cell undergoes apoptosis. The BCL-2 protein blocks apoptosis, and elevated levels of it are associated with resistance to vincristine, methotrexate, fluorouracil, hydroxyurea, and cisplatin.[49] BCL-2 can also block apoptosis even in the presence of tumors with high levels of *p53* expression, which is known to promote apoptosis. Conversely, the BAX protein urges the cell to enter apoptosis and is associated with increased chemosensitivity to paclitaxel, vincristine, and doxorubicin.[50] Most of the research on ways to enhance chemosensitivity related to BCL-2 and BAX is being conducted in vitro. The sequencing of chemotherapy drugs to increase the phosphorylation of BCL-2 has been suggested as a way to optimize apoptosis in tumor cells.[51]

Chemotherapy as a Treatment for Cancer

Primary and Adjuvant Chemotherapy

Chemotherapy is considered primary treatment for cancers for which no effective alternative treatment is available or when the alternative treatment is less than optimal. *Induction* is a term commonly used to describe chemotherapy given to patients with leukemia or other advanced disease that is highly sensitive to drugs. *Neoadjuvant chemotherapy* describes chemotherapy given prior to the standard primary therapeutic approach — usually surgery — in patients who present with local disease. It has enjoyed significant success in preserving organ structure and function in cancers of the lung, larynx, and breast. Chemotherapy given concurrently, instead of sequentially, with radiation therapy is another popular approach for combining effective methods up-front to control and potentially eradicate disease. Cancers of the head and neck are often treated in this way.

Adjuvant chemotherapy is a routine part of treatment for cancers of the breast and bowel. Systemic therapy is usually given following surgical resection of the primary tumor with the intent of improving the potential for cure. Although effective chemotherapy would theoretically eradicate clinically undetected and micrometastatic disease, the overall effect on tumor recurrence has been less than dramatic for cancers of the colon and rectum. More success has been realized in patients with node-positive breast cancer.[52]

Therapeutic Strategies

Combination chemotherapy

Administering a combination of clinically effective anticancer drugs is the standard chemotherapeutic approach for most malignancies. Although individually the drugs are biochemically and clinically active, they are rarely used alone as single agents outside of metastatic disease. Combination chemotherapy was first applied with success in the treatment of leukemias and lymphomas and is now employed routinely for most other malignancies. The objectives of combination chemotherapy are to achieve maximal tumor cell kill without excessive toxicity, to provide cytotoxic drugs that are active against potentially resistant heterogeneous tumor populations, and to avoid selection of resistant cell lines. Table 15-7 delineates the principles by which antineoplastic drugs are usually chosen for combination regimens.

When overlapping toxicities are unavoidable, as is often the case with marrow-suppressive drugs, administration of less than full doses or longer intervals

Table 15-7 Principles for Selection of Antineoplastic Drugs for Combination Chemotherapy Regimens

1. Choose drugs with single-agent activity. Drugs producing complete responses are preferred.
2. Avoid drugs with overlapping toxicities.
3. Administer drugs at their optimal dose and schedule as previously determined by clinical trials.
4. Give chemotherapy at regular intervals (cycles) and minimize the time between cycles.

between treatments may be necessary. Recovery time for normal tissues is typically used to determine the retreatment or cycle time. The time for the bone marrow to reach its nadir (lowest counts) and recover differs depending on which drugs are administered. Nadir and recovery periods are critical for determining the length of a treatment cycle. Therefore, chemotherapy cycles for drugs with significant myelosuppression are approximately 3 to 4 weeks. The duration or cycles of treatment administered are usually based on the response rate or a predetermined number obtained from clinical trials.

Dose intensity. Delivering a sufficient amount of drug over a specified period of time is of great importance in curing drug-sensitive malignancies. However, many factors may prevent the proper dose from being delivered, such as the necessity for a dose reduction or a delay in treatment because of unacceptable toxicity. Although dose reductions as small as 20% do not affect clinical response rates for most drug-sensitive tumors, curative potential may be lost. Decreasing the dose or adjusting the schedule of treatment may explain the failure of chemotherapy to cure drug-sensitive tumors.

The concept of dose intensity has been developed to assist the researcher and clinician in evaluating the effects that these changes in doses have on treatment outcomes. Dose intensity is expressed as the amount of drug delivered per unit of time (mg/m^2/week). The effect of a new regimen on treatment outcome can be expressed as the relative dose intensity (RDI), which is calculated by dividing the dose intensity of a test regimen by that of a standard regimen. This calculation can be done for a single drug or an average can be calculated for all drugs in a combination regimen. The effects of dose reductions or treatment delays are best evaluated when dose intensity is based on actual or received doses instead of intended or protocol doses.

The dose intensity has been applied to a number of diseases to improve response rates. Increasing the dose has improved outcomes in lymphomas and advanced tumors of the ovary, breast, and colon.[53] Of particular interest is the recently demonstrated improvement in disease-free survival and overall survival with dose-dense adjuvant treatment of node-positive breast cancer.[52] Chemotherapy was given on an every 2-week schedule with hematopoietic support. High-dose chemotherapy with hematopoietic stem cell support also provides a way to administer larger doses for potentially sensitive cancers.

Chemoprotective and radioprotective agents

Antineoplastic drugs are among the most toxic compounds administered to humans. Some toxicities, such as nausea, vomiting, mucositis, alopecia, and fatigue, are not life-threatening. Although bone marrow suppression is both common and potentially life-threatening, it is dose dependent and can be managed by reducing doses, delaying therapy, or administering hematopoietic growth factors. Several drugs are known to induce life-threatening and permanent cellular injury.

Chemoprotective and rescue agents have been developed and are under investigation for use in preventing or reversing drug-induced toxicity for some anticancer agents, including cisplatin, cyclophosphamide, doxorubicin, ifosfamide, methotrexate, and paclitaxel. Availability of these compounds has permitted expanded clinical development and use of the anticancer drugs whose toxicity they ameliorate. Unfortunately, these agents may have significant toxicities of their own, possibly negatively affect the cytotoxicity of the anticancer agent, add significant cost to the patient's treatment, or lead to several of these scenarios. The American Society of Clinical Oncology (ASCO) has established guidelines for the appropriate use of chemoprotective and radioprotective drugs based on scientific evidence.[54] Table 15-8 lists currently available agents along with ASCO clinical guidelines for use, proposed mechanisms of action, and toxicities.

High-dose chemotherapy with peripheral blood stem cell support

High-dose chemotherapy with autologous rescue is being used more frequently in cancers that respond to increasing doses of marrow-ablative therapy, such as leukemias, lymphomas, breast cancer, and ovarian cancer. This form of therapy, once available only at select treatment centers, is now being offered at most major medical centers and many large community hospitals. Reasons for the expansion of this form of cancer treatment include its curative potential, more experience with administering and managing this type of therapy, and advancements in supportive care for patients. The introduction of hematopoietic growth factors (HGFs), such as G-CSF and GM-CSF, has been among the major advancements in supportive care

Table 15-8 Compounds Used as Chemoprotective and Radioprotective Agents and ASCO Guidelines for Use

Chemoprotective Agent	Protectant Mechanism	Adverse Effects	ASCO Clinical Practice Guidelines for Use [toxicity, drug, or disease based recommendation]
Amifostine (Ethyol)	Reduces DNA damage in renal and neurologic tissues	Hypotension, nausea and vomiting	1. Nephrotoxicity: *Consider in patients receiving cisplatin-based chemotherapy.* 2. Neutropenia (alkylating agents): *Alternative to dose reduction or growth factor use.* 3. Neurotoxicity: *Insufficient data to recommend routine use in cisplatin- or paclitaxel-induced effects.* 4. Thrombocytopenia: *Insufficient data to recommend use.* 5. Radiation-induced xerostomia: *Consider in patients undergoing fractionated radiation of the head and neck region. (Do not recommend for reduction of mucositis.)*
Dexrazoxane (Zinecard)	Inhibits free radical formation in cardiac tissue	Myelosuppression, nausea and vomiting	1. Metastatic breast cancer: a. *Routine use is not recommended in patients receiving initial anthracycline chemotherapy.* b. *Consider in patients who have received cumulative dose of ≥ 300 mg/m² of doxorubicin.* 2. Other tumors: *Consider in adults who have received > 300 mg/m² of doxorubicin. Caution should be used if chemotherapy is known to improve survival (dexrazoxane tumor-protective effects).* 3. Adjuvant chemotherapy: *Not recommended outside of clinical trials.* 4. Pediatric tumors: *Insufficient evidence to recommend use with epirubicin-based regimens.*
Mesna (Mesnex)	Binds toxic metabolites in bladder	Nausea and vomiting, hypersensitivity	1. Ifosfamide chemotherapy: Using standard doses, recommended for routine use to reduce urothelial toxicity. 2. High-dose ifosfamide: *Insufficient evidence to establish guidelines for use with ifosfamide > 2.5 g/m²/d.* 3. High-dose cyclophosphamide: Alternative to forced saline diuresis in stem cell transplant setting.

Data from Hensley, Schuchter, Lindley, et al.[54]

measures. Their availability has allowed for harvesting of hematopoietic stem cells from peripheral blood—in most situations, avoiding costly and painful bone marrow harvesting. Peripheral blood stem cells (PBSCs) are committed progenitor cells existing in peripheral blood that have the capacity to restore hematopoiesis.

Before receiving marrow-ablative chemotherapy, patients are given HGFs with or without chemotherapy—typically cyclophosphamide—to mobilize stem cells into the peripheral blood from the bone marrow.[55] Patients then undergo leukopheresis to remove mobilized stem cells from the peripheral blood.[56] Leukopheresis may be performed two to six times to collect an adequate number of cells. Following high-dose chemotherapy, radiation therapy, or both—a course intended to eradicate the cancer cells and hence the bone marrow stem cells—the patient's PBSCs are reinfused. As with other forms of hematopoietic cell transplantation, infused stem cells migrate to the bone marrow and engraft. Compared with patients receiving only autologous bone marrow, patients who receive PBSCs either alone or with bone marrow transplantation typically experience fewer days of neutropenia and thrombocytopenia. Major disadvantages of PBSC transplantation include nausea, vomiting, and hypertension associated with infusion of the large amounts of the cryopreservative dimethyl sulfoxide (DMSO) and the large volume of PBSCs. Another concern is the potential to reinfuse mobilized tumor cells as well as hematopoietic stem cells. The significance of this contamination for relapse rates is yet to be determined.[56] The use of monoclonal antibodies to manufacture a product devoid of tumor cells is currently under investigation.

Chemotherapy as a radiation sensitizer

The concomitant use of chemotherapy and radiation therapy has received significant attention in the literature.[57] The primary goal of this type of combined modality treatment is to increase the effectiveness of the radiation and improve local–regional control of disease. A number of theoretical considerations may explain the improved results seen when chemotherapy and radiation are given concomitantly for specific tumors. The modalities affect different tumor cell subpopulations; therefore, their combined use may better eradicate cells resistant to the other modality. Tumor cell regrowth following radiation therapy is slowed by the addition of chemotherapy, and cells undergoing growth are more vulnerable to the cytotoxic effects of chemotherapy. The cytoreductive effects of chemotherapy improve tumor oxygen supply, resulting in an increased susceptibility to radiation effects. In addition, direct interaction of the combined modalities, as yet undefined, may explain the improved response seen especially at a local–regional level. A *positive interaction* is defined as enhanced radiation effects in tumor cells and less observed toxicity. Significant improvement in quality of life may be achieved by using combined modality regimens to preserve organs affected by larynx, anal canal, bladder, and esophagus cancers.

Chemotherapy and radiation therapy with fluorouracil has demonstrated improved overall survival for individuals with cancers of the head and neck, rectum, pancreas, and lung.[57] Cisplatin has also been investigated as a radiation enhancer, with the greatest activity being seen in tumors sensitive to cisplatin. The combination of cisplatin with other antineoplastic drugs such as paclitaxel, fluorouracil, or etoposide for radiation enhancement has also been studied.[58,59] The results of clinical trials combining cisplatin and radiation, with or without fluorouracil, for head and neck cancer have shown improved disease-free survival over radiation alone.

Modulation of fluorouracil by leucovorin

Leucovorin, or folinic acid, has been developed primarily as an antidote for antifolate therapy. Another emerging role of leucovorin is found in the modulation of the cytotoxicity of fluorouracil. Although fluorouracil is the most active antineoplastic drug in cancers of the gastrointestinal tract, its ability to control progression of these cancers is modest. For this reason, investigators have sought to enhance fluorouracil's efficacy in an attempt to better control and potentially cure these cancers. In the presence of increased folate pools, the active form of fluorouracil binds more tightly to the target enzyme.[60]

The interaction of leucovorin and fluorouracil has been studied in more than 650 patients, with significantly improved response rates being seen with the combination compared with fluorouracil alone.[61] Although the optimal dose and schedule of leucovorin have not been determined, a prolonged or 5-day intermittent dosing schedule is preferred. Other drugs that have been tested as biochemical modulators of fluorouracil include methotrexate, N-(phosphonacetyl)-L-aspartate (PALA), and alfa-interferon.

Pharmacology of Chemotherapeutic Drugs

Most drugs used to treat cancer are unique from drugs used to treat other illnesses such as cardiac disease, gastrointestinal disease, or neurological problems. The primary pharmacological outcome is usually cell death. Tumor cells are the intended targets; however, similarities between normal cells and tumor cells often result in destruction of healthy tissues as well as malignant cells. Understanding the pharmacology of these agents can help the researcher and clinician in optimally designing the most effective and least toxic single and multiple drug regimens.

The basic pharmacological principles of drugs used to treat cancer will be reviewed in this portion of the chapter. An explanation of the principles of pharmacokinetics and how they are applied in chemotherapy is followed by a detailed description of probable and potential drug interactions. The final sections are an overview of the diverse pharmacological and mechanistic groups of anticancer drugs highlighting key features of individual drugs or drug classes.

Pharmacokinetics of Antineoplastic Drugs

Pharmacokinetics is the study of the movement of drugs in the body. The processes may differ individually and is most closely related to the physical and chemical properties of the compound. The physical and chemical individuality of the patient and the tumor type also play an important role in determining pharmacokinetics outcomes.

Principles of pharmacokinetics

Several parameters have been used to describe the pharmacokinetics of drugs.

The serum *half-life* of a drug is the time required for the serum concentration to decrease by one-half. Knowing the half-life of a chemotherapeutic drug is of greatest interest when trying to determine the amount of time required for a patient to eliminate most of a dose administered. This time period is equal to three to four half-lives of the drug.

Clearance is determined by blood flow to an organ, usually the kidney or liver, and the organ's efficacy in extracting the drug from the blood. If a drug is cleared from the body by more than one organ, then the total clearance is the sum of the individual clearances of the various extracting organs. This pharmacokinetic parameter determines the drug's steady-state concentration and is independent of half-life. Clearance may be altered by changes in blood flow to an organ, by enzyme function, and by protein binding. For example, cyclophosphamide is highly dependent on metabolizing enzymes for activation and inactivation. Therefore, induction or inhibition of enzymes may cause a more rapid or slower clearance of the drug.

The volume of distribution (V_D) relates the amount of drug in the body to the serum concentration. This parameter differs among individuals and is a function of the drug's protein-binding capabilities and its ability to distribute to extravascular compartments (tissue binding). Changes in protein binding caused by either hypoalbuminemia or interactions with other drugs may alter the removal of highly protein-bound drugs such as etoposide or teniposide.

Variability in a drug's pharmacokinetic parameters may help explain the differences in response and toxicity seen among patients treated with similar doses and schedules of chemotherapy. The basic principles of clinical pharmacokinetics may be divided into four major areas: absorption, distribution, metabolism, and elimination.

Absorption. Absorption from the gastrointestinal tract should be sufficient to ensure adequate bioavailability of the drug. Because the bioavailability of most anticancer drugs is poor and unpredictable, these agents are usually given parenterally to ensure accurate dosing and optimal systemic exposure. Drugs administered orally for cancer treatment include alkylating agents (cyclophosphamide, chlorambucil, and melphalan), etoposide, lomustine, methotrexate, and procarbazine. Although oral absorption is less than optimal for some of these drugs, the amount that reaches systemic circulation and—more important—the tumor is sufficient to produce a response.

Distribution. Distribution of drugs in the body is determined primarily by their ability to penetrate different tissues and their affinity for binding to plasma proteins. Drugs that are highly lipophilic tend to be more readily taken up by lipophilic tissues such as bone marrow, fat, and the central nervous system. Nitrosoureas such as carmustine and lomustine are useful for brain and hematopoietic malignancies because they readily penetrate these tissues. Decreased levels of plasma proteins, especially albumin, often occur in patients with cancer. This situation may be the result of nutritional deficiencies or decreased hepatic synthesis of albumin. The cytotoxic activity of highly protein-bound chemotherapy drugs such as etoposide and teniposide may be enhanced in these patients because a greater percentage of the drug is unbound. An increase in the unbound fraction can also occur if two highly bound drugs are administered concurrently. Methotrexate abnormally distributes in ascites and pleural effusions, delaying clearance and enhancing hematologic and mucosal toxicity.[62]

Table 15-9 Chemotherapy Drugs That Depend on Hepatic Metabolism for Activation and Clearance from the Body

Chemotherapy Drug	Activation	Clearance
Anthracycline antibiotics	X	X
Capecitabine	X	X
Cyclophosphamide	X	X
Dacarbazine	X	X
Hexamethylmelamine		X
Ifosfamide	X	
Nitrosoureas		X
Carmustine		
Lomustine		
Procarbazine	X	
Temozolomide	X	X

Metabolism. The metabolic activation and inactivation or catabolism of drugs is carried out primarily by the liver. Some of these enzymatic processes are also performed in normal and tumor cells. Several chemotherapy drugs require activation intracellularly or systemically before they can exert their cytotoxic effects (Table 15-9). Antimetabolites such as fluorouracil and cytarabine are phosphorylated to active nucleotides in tumor cells. Cisplatin undergoes a chemical aquation with water molecules intracellularly, which generates a positively charged species that, in turn, forms adducts with DNA molecules. Cyclophosphamide and ifosfamide are transformed by hepatic microsomal enzymes into active alkylating species. Some chemotherapeutic drugs are metabolized to inactive compounds, which are then excreted by the body. The rate of metabolic conversion may be affected by a number of factors, including hepatic dysfunction (either drug induced or tumor induced) or genetic differences in drug metabolism. Changes in liver function or metabolic enzymes may result in decreased cytotoxic activity, increased treatment-related toxicity, or both. Table 15-10 lists drugs known to alter microsomal enzymes and potentially affect antineoplastic drug disposition.

Elimination. The kidneys are responsible for the majority of the elimination of drugs and drug metabo-

Table 15-10 Drugs Known to Enhance or Inhibit Hepatic Microsomal Metabolism

Enhance	Inhibit
Cyclophosphamide	Cimetidine
Phenobarbital	Alfa-interferon
Phenytoin	Ketoconazole
Rifampin	Verapamil
	Aprepitant

Table 15-11 Chemotherapeutic Agents Cleared by Kidneys That Have Increased Toxicity in Renal Insufficiency

Drugs Requiring Dose Modification	
Bleomycin	Cyclophosphamide
Carboplatin	Etoposide
Cisplatin	Methotrexate
Oxaliplatin	Streptozocin

lites from the body. A number of anticancer drugs are highly dependent on renal function for their elimination. As a consequence, significant decreases in renal function can decrease their clearance from the body and cause excessive toxicity (Table 15-11). Cisplatin and methotrexate are both eliminated primarily by the kidney and are nephrotoxic themselves; therefore, decreased renal function may produce enhanced toxicity and a further decline in renal function. The biliary tract is the primary route of elimination for vinca alkaloids.

Pharmacokinetic principles applied to chemotherapeutic drugs

Chemotherapeutic drugs must reach their target site to exert their antineoplastic effects. Often their targets are intracellular structures and molecules such as DNA, enzymes, and microtubules. Adequate blood supply to tumor cells is necessary for optimal delivery of chemotherapy to the drug's site of action. Then, once in the tumor microenvironment, the drug must be transported intracellularly via passive, facilitated, or active transport mechanisms.[62] Transport mechanisms may either facilitate drug entry into the cell or hasten the drug's removal. As mentioned previously, efflux from the cell may be a major limitation of antineoplastic drug efficacy.

Systemic drug exposure is also an important parameter in ensuring the optimal cytotoxic response and minimal toxicity. The area under the serum concentration-time curve (AUC) is a measure of systemic drug exposure. Because the AUC depends on drug administration and elimination, changes in these parameters may greatly affect the therapeutic outcome. Patients with a more rapid drug clearance may need larger doses than those with a slower clearance. Currently, the dose for carboplatin is usually calculated using a target AUC and the patient's own renal function to predict the optimal individualized dose.

Pharmacokinetic parameters should be routinely applied in clinical practice to assist in delivering the optimal dose with the least risk of serious toxicity. Interpatient variability should always be considered when evaluating therapeutic or toxic response to therapy.

Drug Interactions in the Patient Receiving Chemotherapy

A drug interaction occurs when the effects of one drug—whether therapeutic or toxic—are modified by the presence of another drug. Interactions may result in a beneficial effect, such as improving therapeutic response or preventing or reducing toxicity. However, the majority produce undesirable outcomes, such as suboptimal therapeutic response or enhanced adverse effects. Chemotherapeutic and other drugs occasionally share similar toxicities, such as myelosuppression and gastrointestinal disturbances. Tables 15-12[63–71] and 15-13[63,72,73] list selected clinically significant drug interactions in patients undergoing cancer chemotherapy.

Not all drug interactions result in clinically significant therapeutic or toxic outcomes. Indeed, most interactions occur only under specific pharmacologic and physiologic situations; therefore, drug interactions should be judged by their overall effect on therapeutic response and patient care. The potential for serious interaction increases with the number of drugs a patient receives. Because most patients with cancer receive chemotherapy drugs, supportive-care drugs, and conceivably pain management drugs, the potential for drug interactions is relatively high. Many patients with advanced disease have significant organ dysfunction, are elderly, or have concomitant illness, all of which contribute to the potential for harmful drug interactions.

Antineoplastic Drugs

Cancer chemotherapeutic drugs have traditionally been classified by their mechanism of action, chemical structure, or biological source. Grouping antineoplastic drugs into categories is done primarily for convenience. Although drugs within a class share some characteristics, there are often major differences in their indications, toxicities, and pharmaceutical properties. (See Chapter 17 for detailed descriptions of chemotherapy-induced toxicities and management of side effects.)

Alkylating and alkylating-like agents

Classic alkylators. Alkylating agents were among the first drugs used to treat malignancies in humans, and they continue to play a major role in chemotherapy. This group includes a wide array of cytotoxic drugs

Table 15-12 Selected Clinically Significant Drug Interactions in Patients Receiving Cancer Chemotherapy

Chemotherapy Drug	Interacting Drug	Pharmacokinetic/Pharmacodynamic Effect[a]	Management of Interaction
Arsenic trioxide	Drugs that prolong QT interval (beta blockers, cisapride, dolasetron, terfenadine)	Additive toxicity	Avoid co-administration
Asparaginase	Methotrexate	↓ toxicity[b]	Give methotrexate 3–24 hours prior
Bleomycin	Cisplatin	↓ renal elimination, ↑ pulmonary toxicity	Monitor renal function in patients previously treated with cisplatin
	Oxygen	↑ risk of acute pulmonary inflammation	Avoid inspired oxygen above 25%
Busulfan	Phenytoin[c]	↑ metabolic clearance, ↓ bone marrow cytotoxicity	Begin phenytoin therapy briefly before busulfan
Carmustine	Phenytoin	↓ phenytoin blood level, ↓ antiseizure effect	Monitor phenytoin level and adjust dose
Cisplatin	Anticonvulsant drugs (carbamazepine, phenytoin, valproic acid)	↓ oral absorption of anticonvulsant drug, ↓ blood levels	Monitor levels and increase dose as needed
	Sodium thiosulfate, Mesna	Chemical incompatibility, ↓ cytotoxic and toxic effects Sodium thiosulfate may be used as an antidote for cisplatin toxicity	Do not administer in same infusion device
Corticosteroids (dexamethasone, hydrocortisone, methylprednisolone)	Aminoglutethimide Mitotane Aprepitant	↑ metabolic clearance, ↓ therapeutic effect ↑ bioavailability of corticosteroids	Adjust corticosteroid dose to avoid adrenal crisis Decrease corticosteroid dose by half
Cyclophosphamide	Allopurinol	↓ renal elimination of alkylating metabolite, ↑ toxicity	Monitor bone marrow and urologic toxicity
CYP3A4 metabolized drugs (docetaxel, paclitaxel, irinotecan, vinca alkaloids)	Aprepitant (Emend)	↓ metabolism, ↑ cytotoxic effect	Monitor myelosuppression and other toxicities
Etoposide	Highly protein-bound drugs	↓ protein binding, ↑ myelotoxicity	Avoid co-administration
Fluorouracil	Alfa interferon	↓ metabolic clearance, ↑ cytotoxicity	Monitor for severe gastrointestinal toxicity
	Metronidazole	↓ metabolic clearance, ↑ toxicity	Co-administer with caution
Ifosfamide	Antifungals (ketoconazole, itraconazole)	↓ clearance, ↑ toxicity	Avoid co-administration
	Phenobarbital	↑ metabolic activation, ↑ toxicity	Monitor bone marrow suppression and neurotoxicity
Interleukin-2	Corticosteroids	Block antitumor effect, ↓ tumor response rate	Use corticosteroids only for IL-2 toxicity management
Mercaptopurine	Allopurinol	↓ metabolic clearance, ↑ serum levels, prolonged bone marrow suppression	Decrease dose of mercaptopurine by 75%
	Cotrimoxazole (trimethoprim, sulfamethoxazole)	↑ oral absorption, ↓ metabolic activation	Monitor bone marrow suppression
Methotrexate	Cotrimoxazole	↓ renal clearance, additive antifolate activity, ↑ bone marrow toxicity	Monitor methotrexate levels and toxicity
	NSAIDs, salicylates	↓ renal clearance, ↓ protein binding, ↑ bone marrow and gastrointestinal toxicity	Monitor methotrexate levels and toxicity (*fatal* outcomes reported in cases of oral methotrexate and NSAID use)

(continued)

Table 15-12 Selected Clinically Significant Drug Interactions in Patients Receiving Cancer Chemotherapy (continued)

Chemotherapy Drug	Interacting Drug	Pharmacokinetic/Pharmacodynamic Effect[a]	Management of Interaction
Paclitaxel	Cisplatin	↓ total body clearance, ↑ myelotoxicity	Give paclitaxel before cisplatin
Procarbazine	Ethanol	Blocks metabolism of alcohol, disulfiram-like reaction	Avoid co-administration
	Sympathomimetic drugs (ephedrine, epinephrine) Tricyclic antidepressant drugs (amitriptyline, imipramine)	MAO inhibition,[d] hypertensive crisis, tremor, excitation	Most interactions are not clinically important
Vinblastine	Phenytoin	↓ phenytoin blood level	Monitor phenytoin level and adjust dose as needed
Vincristine	Asparaginase	↑ risk of peripheral neurotoxicity	Give vincristine first

a. Refers to chemotherapy drug unless otherwise specified.

b. Result of methotrexate-induced block of protein synthesis.

c. For seizure prophylaxis for patients receiving high-dose busulfan for bone marrow transplant therapy.

d. Monoamine oxidase inhibition decreases the metabolism of sympathomimetic drugs, neurotransmitters released by tricyclic antidepressants, and endogenous amines.

Data from Dorr, Von Hoff[63]; Hansten, Horn[64]; Balis[65]; Finley[66]; Loadman, Bibby[67]; Thyss, Milano, Kubar, et al.[68]; Ellison, Servi[69]; Fitzsimmons, Ghalie, Kaizer[70]; McCrea, Majumdar, Goldberg, et al.[71]

that possess single-agent tumoricidal activity as well as play significant roles in combination chemotherapy. Alkylating agents contribute electrophilic alkyl groups ($R\text{-}CH_2\text{-}CH_2$) to attack electron-rich nucleophilic sites on biological macromolecules such as DNA. The most common site of DNA alkylation is the N-7 position of guanine. These DNA adducts may produce a variety of lesions, including strand breaks, nucleotide base deletions, and ring openings. Cytotoxicity and mutagenicity of alkylating agents usually result from these DNA adducts as well as interference with replication and transcription.[74] Many of the DNA lesions may be restored by repair enzymes; however, if the repair is only partial, additional DNA damage may result. Alkylators are non-cell cycle phase specific and are most active in the resting phase (G_0). Most alkylating agents are considered mutagens and potentially carcinogenic; therefore, the healthcare professional should be especially careful to avoid exposure when working with these compounds.

Mechlorethamine (nitrogen mustard) was the first alkylating agent introduced for cancer therapy. The drug spontaneously undergoes molecular rearrangement in aqueous solution to form a reactive species with two chloroethyl groups available for formation of cross-links of DNA strands. Nitrogen mustard has a very short half-life and is usually undetectable in the blood within a few minutes of administration. This severe vesicant must be handled with caution to prevent exposure of the clinician and to prevent extravasation during administration. Dose-limiting toxicities are myelosuppression, which may be severe, and rapid-onset nausea and vomiting. The major therapeutic role of mechlorethamine is in the MOPP (mechlorethamine, vincristine, procarbazine, prednisone) chemotherapy regimen for Hodgkin's disease. Other uses include topical application for mycosis fungoides or skin cancer, and intracavitary instillation for malignant pleural or pericardial effusions.

Melphalan, busulfan, and chlorambucil are usually given orally. Melphalan and busulfan are currently available as injectable products for specific indications. Melphalan was developed as a targeted agent for selective uptake in tumors actively using phenylalanine and tyrosine, such as melanin-producing malignant cells. Absorption from the gastrointestinal tract is variable and is slowed when the drug is taken with food; as a consequence, this agent should be taken on an empty stomach. Melphalan may be given parenterally when the oral route is not appropriate. A 50% dose reduction should be considered in patients with significant decreased renal function. Chlorambucil is completely absorbed from the gastrointestinal tract. It has a predictable myelotoxicity profile and is a well-established agent in the treatment of chronic lymphocytic leukemia. Busulfan is a bifunctional alkylating agent with two reactive groups on opposite ends of the molecule, which form DNA adducts resulting in cross-linked strands. In addition to its use in chronic myelogenous leukemia (CML), this drug is used in high-dose chemotherapy conditioning regimens and allogeneic or autologous bone marrow transplantation.

Cyclophosphamide and ifosfamide undergo a multistep activation process in vivo involving both hepatic microsomal and cellular enzyme systems to generate reactive chemical species. The two active metabolites of cyclophosphamide responsible for the majority of

Table 15-13 Chemotherapy Drug Interactions with Warfarin

Chemotherapy Drug	Possible Mechanism of Interaction	Effect on Prothrombin Time
Mercaptopurine	Antagonize anticoagulant effect	Shortens
Mitotane	↑ metabolic clearance	Shortens
Tamoxifen	Unknown; enzyme inhibition and/or protein-binding displacement	Prolongs

Data from Dorr, Von Hoff[63]; Hall, Lind, Huang, et al.[72]; Tenni, Lalich, Byrne.[73]

the drug's cytotoxicity are phosphoramide mustard and acrolein.[75] Acrolein is also primarily responsible for inducing hemorrhagic cystitis in approximately 10% of patients. This complication may be avoided by keeping the patient adequately hydrated and encouraging frequent urination within 24 hours of cyclophosphamide administration. Ifosfamide administration is associated with a much higher incidence of urotoxicity than cyclophosphamide. This outcome is the result of an altered pharmacokinetic profile, which generates more urotoxic metabolite precursors than are found with cyclophosphamide. Cystitis can be prevented by the co-administration of mesna, a compound that inactivates urotoxic metabolites in the bladder. Because cyclophosphamide and ifosfamide rely on both the kidneys and the liver for elimination, their toxicity may be prolonged in patients with compromised renal or hepatic failure.

Thiotepa is a polyfunctional alkylating agent that induces multiple types of DNA damage, including interstrand cross-links. It may be administered by various routes: intravenous for breast cancer, intravesical for superficial bladder cancer, intrapleural for malignant pleural effusions, and intraperitoneal for refractory ovarian cancer. Thiotepa has some unique skin toxicities, including an acute erythroderma and dry desquamation of the palms and soles, and chronic darkening or bronzing of the skin when used in high-dose regimens.

Nitrosoureas decompose in aqueous solutions to form two reactive intermediates, a chloroethyldiazohydroxide and an isocyanate group. The chloroethyldiazohydroxide compound forms adducts with DNA and induces interstrand cross-links. Isocyanate groups deplete glutathione and inhibit DNA repair. Nitrosoureas are distinct from other alkylators in that they are highly lipid soluble and readily cross the blood–brain barrier, so that they are highly active in intracranial tumors. Other uses include Hodgkin's disease, non-Hodgkin's lymphoma, and malignant melanoma. Nitrosoureas may cause severe and prolonged myelosuppression because of their high lipophilicity.

Platinum-containing compounds. Cisplatin, carboplatin, and oxaliplatin make up a highly active category of antineoplastic agents widely used for cancer treatment. Platinum compounds undergo an aquation reaction that enables them to react with macromolecules with strong binding sites, such as DNA. Cisplatin-induced DNA adducts and formation of intrastrand DNA cross-links correlate well with the drug's cytotoxicity and antitumor activity.[76] Although cisplatin and other platinum analogs behave similarly to alkylators, their cytotoxicity is probably the result of a combination of mechanisms of action, including inhibition of DNA and protein synthesis, alteration in cell membrane transport, and suppression of mitochondrial function.

The currently available platinum analogs are highly dependent on renal elimination as their primary route of excretion. Cisplatin is removed from the blood in both its free and protein-bound forms following a triphasic elimination model. In the first two phases, primarily the unbound (free) form of cisplatin is eliminated. Because 90% of the drug is excreted by the kidneys, adequate renal function is important in preventing drug accumulation and excessive toxicity. Patients who previously received cisplatin may be at increased risk for toxicity with carboplatin and should be evaluated for decreased renal function. Cisplatin given intraperitoneally produces peak levels that are as much as 21 times higher than peak plasma levels using similar doses.[77] Concurrently intravenous-administered sodium thiosulfate may prevent severe systemic toxicities experienced with this route of cisplatin administration. Carboplatin and oxaliplatin elimination follows a triphasic pattern similar to that of cisplatin. A formula derived by Calvert et al. utilizing a patient's glomerular filtration rate and a desired systemic exposure (AUC) is widely used to calculate an individualized dose of carboplatin.[78] A measured or estimated creatinine clearance is commonly used for the glomerular filtration rate, and a target AUC is chosen based on prior and concurrent myelotoxic chemotherapy exposure. Cisplatin and carboplatin are effective in a number of similar tumors, but oxaliplatin given in combination with fluorouracil and leucovorin is the only platinum analog with significant activity in colorectal cancer.[79]

Although the platinum analogs all possess a similar antitumor mechanism of activity, significant differences are observed in their dosing, administration, and side effect profiles. The dose-limiting toxicity of cisplatin is nephrotoxicity. Acute renal failure may occur within 24 hours of drug administration. Patients at greatest risk for this complication are those who receive inadequate hydration. Nephrotoxicity may usually be avoided by adequately hydrating the patient and administering diuretics such as furosemide, mannitol, or both. Carboplatin and oxaliplatin, although dependent on good renal function for elimination, are not necessarily nephrotoxic and rarely require concomitant hydration and diuresis. Although nausea and vomiting are common in patients receiving any of the platinum compounds, emesis is often more severe and prolonged with cisplatin. Combination antiemetic regimens are usually necessary to prevent and treat this side effect, which is often the most feared by the patient. Dose-limiting myelosuppression is much more of an issue with carboplatin than with cisplatin. Neurotoxicity and ototoxicity are also common adverse events seen with cisplatin treatment. Oxaliplatin induced peripheral sensory neuropathy in more than 74% of patients in clinical trials. Acute neuropathies consisting primarily of peripheral sensory neuropathy and precipitated by exposure to cold temperatures were described. More persistent sensory neuropathies were also observed that lasted two weeks or longer and were characterized by paresthesia, dysesthesia, and numbness in the extremities and other anatomical locations.[80]

Other alkylating-like drugs. Other drugs with alkylating-like activity include dacarbazine, temozolomide, procarbazine, and altretamine (hexamethylmelamine). These drugs, like most other alkylating agents, depend on metabolic activation for the formation of reactive species.

Dacarbazine functions primarily as an alkylating agent but may also act as an antimetabolite by inhibiting purine nucleoside incorporation into DNA. Dacarbazine does not appear to be cell cycle–phase specific; it kills cells in all phases of the cycle. This drug is extremely sensitive to light and will undergo spontaneous decomposition to both active and inactive compounds. The most significant adverse events associated with its use are nausea and vomiting, which may decrease with repeated courses. Other toxicities include a flu-like syndrome, myelosuppression, and photosensitivity. Dacarbazine is also associated with hepatic venoocclusive disease characterized by fever and acute hepatic necrosis.

Temozolomide is a newer monofunctional alkylating agent that is similar to dacarbazine. It requires dealkylation to produce an unstable intermediate that rapidly decomposes to release methyldiazonium. Temozolomide is administered orally and has significant activity in patients with malignant brain tumors (glioblastoma multiforme, anaplastic astrocytoma) and in advanced metastatic malignant melanoma.[81,82]

Procarbazine is administered orally as a therapy for Hodgkin's disease and brain tumors. Two significant drug interactions are possible in patients taking procarbazine.[83] The first relates to the drug's ability to inhibit the enzyme monoamine oxidase, which is responsible for metabolism of amines. Inhibition of vasoactive amine metabolism may lead to hypertensive crisis, severe headache, sweating, and coma. Patients should avoid eating foods high in tyramine (e.g., wine, ripe cheese, chocolate, and liver) to prevent this drug interaction. The second interaction is seen when patients on procarbazine consume alcohol. They may experience a disulfiram reaction, which is characterized by nausea, vomiting, palpitations, and sweating.

Hexamethylmelamine is an orally administered agent whose mechanism of action is uncertain but is probably of an alkylating type.

Antitumor antibiotics

Anthracycline antibiotics. The antitumor antibiotics comprise a large and diverse group of antineoplastic drugs originally derived from natural sources. Anthracyclines are a family of highly colored compounds known as *rhodomycins,* which have both antineoplastic and antimicrobial activities. Anthracyclines (daunorubicin, doxorubicin, epirubicin, idarubicin) and the chemically related anthracenedione (mitoxantrone) have multiple mechanisms of cytotoxicity, including intercalation, covalent DNA binding, free radical formation, and topoisomerase II enzyme inhibition. The two mechanisms now thought responsible for the majority of the cytotoxicity are free radical formation and inhibition of topoisomerase II enzyme.

Anthracyclines interfere with the DNA unwinding process that is catalyzed by the nuclear enzyme topoisomerase II.[84,85] A "cleavable complex" is produced by inhibiting the enzyme's re-ligation function, thereby creating double-strand breaks in the DNA structure.

Anthracyclines generate oxygen radicals by donating an electron to an oxygen molecule, thereby generating a superoxide. The superoxide is converted first to hydrogen peroxide by superoxide dismutase and finally to a hydroxyl radical. Hydroxyl radicals are the most reactive compounds known and rapidly attack DNA and cell membrane lipids. An iron–anthracycline complex may also produce hydroxyl radical from hydrogen peroxide. Most normal tissues and tumor cells possess enzymes capable of detoxifying hydrogen peroxide; heart muscle cells, however, lack these enzymes. As a result, cardiac tissue is unable to detoxify hydrogen peroxide, which may then give rise to a reactive hydroxyl radical. A substantial body of evidence suggests that the drug–iron complex plays an important role in the cytotoxicity of anthracylines. Hydroxyl radical formation in cardiac tissue may be significantly decreased by the use of an edetate analog called dexrazoxane, which effectively chelates iron.

Anthracyclines are metabolized to both active and inactive compounds by the liver. The major metabolites of most anthracyclines are their alcohols, such as doxorubinicinol, which have antitumor activity—albeit not as significant as that of the parent compounds. The anthracycline dose should be reduced in patients with hepatic dysfunction, especially if the bilirubin level is elevated. Dose adjustment is not necessary in renal failure because renal clearance of anthracyclines is minimal.

Cardiac toxicity of anthracyclines may be manifested as acute changes in ECG and arrhythmias, which are more significant in patients with preexisting heart disease. However, the more common and often therapy-limiting cardiotoxicity is the development of cardiomyopathy leading to congestive heart failure. As many as 10% of patients receiving a cumulative dose of doxorubicin greater than 550 mg/m^2 will develop this toxicity. Cardiac function is usually monitored with serial measurements of left ventricular function and ECG. Potential strategies to prevent or lessen cardiotoxicity include prolonged infusions of doxorubicin and cardioprotectant drugs such as dexrazoxane (Zinecard).

Mitoxantrone may be associated with less nausea, vomiting, and alopecia. Cardiac toxicity in patients treated with this drug appears to be less than that seen with doxorubicin.[86] However, there may be no difference in the incidence of cardiomyopathy at doses equipotent to doxorubicin.

Daunorubicin, doxorubicin, epirubicin, and idarubicin are vesicants and can induce a severe extravasation injury characterized by pain, erythema, and tissue necrosis. Mitoxantrone is considered an irritant, and extravasation injury is much less common with this agent. Other toxicities of anthracyclines include mucositis, nausea, vomiting, and alopecia.

Liposomal encapsulation of doxorubicin and daunorubicin has provided two new anticancer agents with therapeutic and toxicity profiles different from those of the free forms of these drugs. The mechanism of action is believed to be unchanged; the liposomal formulation changes the pharmacokinetics, allowing for a longer half-life and increased uptake by tumor cells.[87] Liposomal daunorubicin and liposomal doxorubicin are currently established treatments for Kaposi's sarcoma in patients with acquired immunodeficiency syndrome (AIDS). Significant data also suggest that the liposomes may have activity in breast cancer and multiple myeloma. Liposomal doxorubicin is indicated for recurrent ovarian cancer. Less alopecia, nausea, vomiting, and neurotoxicity are seen with these agents compared with their nonliposomal or free drug formulations. In addition, cardiac toxicity appears to be less dose-limiting with the liposomal-encapsulated drugs. Doses greater than 1000 mg/m^2 have been given without significant changes in left ventricular function. An infusion reaction consisting of back pain, chest tightness, and flushing has been seen in approximately 7% of patients receiving their first dose of liposomal doxorubicin.[88] This problem rarely requires discontinuing treatment and may be managed with administration of diphenhydramine and restarting the infusion at a slower rate. Palmar-plantar skin eruptions with swelling, pain, erythema, and desquamation of skin are a fairly common problem complicating therapy with liposomal doxorubicin.

Other antitumor antibiotics. Bleomycin is a polypeptide composed of many low-molecular-weight proteins, isolated from the fungus *Streptomyces verticullus.* A drug–iron–oxygen complex binds to DNA by intercalation and generates oxygen radicals resulting in single- and double-strand DNA breaks. Tumor cells are most sensitive to bleomycin in the premitotic, or G_2, phase, or in the mitotic phase of the cell cycle. Bleomycin has been used to synchronize cells into the G_2 and S phases so that other antineoplastic agents that act in those phases may have an increased cell kill potential. This drug has also shown efficacy in combination chemotherapy regimens because of its lack of significant myelosuppressive effects. Bleomycin is highly dependent on renal clearance for its elimination from the body. Significant renal failure necessitates decreasing the dose by 50%–75% of full dose. Renal function of patients previously treated with renal toxic drugs or those who are currently receiving cisplatin should be monitored closely. Pulmonary toxicity of bleomycin may initially present as cough, dyspnea, and pleuritic chest pain. Patients at higher risk for developing bleomycin-related pulmonary fibrosis include older patients (70 years or older), those with preexisting pulmonary disease, and those who have received mediastinal radiation therapy. Although a cumulative dose greater than 450 units is associated with a higher incidence of fibrosis, clinically significant pulmonary toxicity has been documented at lower doses.

Dactinomycin (actinomycin D) binds to DNA by intercalation and induces single-strand breaks similar to those seen with doxorubicin. The drug is currently limited to use in pediatric tumors and gestational trophoblastic neoplasm. Dactinomycin is not metabolized to a significant extent, but instead is excreted unchanged in the urine and bile.

Mitomycin C is activated to an alkylating agent; its cytotoxicity results from formation of cross-links with DNA, leading to inhibition of DNA synthesis and cell death. The drug is preferentially activated in hypoxic tissues such as the environment common to solid tumors. Metabolism of mitomycin by the liver is poorly defined, and renal clearance plays only a minor role in total elimination. Mitomycin degrades at a pH lower than 6; therefore, when the drug is used intravesicularly for bladder cancer, a pH higher than 6 should be maintained in the bladder to ensure potency. A delayed and cumulative myelosuppression is seen with mitomycin. However, the development of a hemolytic-uremic syndrome resulting in renal failure, which is rarely reversible, prompts greater concern. Mitomycin is considered a vesicant, and it is not uncommon to observe bluish streaks tracking along veins distal to the administration site.

Antimetabolites

Antifolates. Antimetabolites used in cancer chemotherapy are structural analogs of nucleotide bases, which are the building blocks of DNA and RNA. The antineoplastic effect of this group of drugs is related to their ability to inhibit nucleic acid synthesis or to falsely be incorporated into the DNA double helix. The antifolate drugs methotrexate and trimetrexate inhibit the enzyme dihydrofolate reductase (DHFR), which catalyzes the reduction of dihydrofolate (folic acid) to tetrohydrofolate (folinic acid). Reduced folates act as 1-carbon donors necessary for the synthesis of purine and pyrimidine bases. Inhibition of DHFR by methotrexate depletes the intracellular reduced-folate pool, thereby blocking de novo synthesis of nucleotide bases. These compounds also inhibit other folate-dependent enzymes such as thymidylate synthase, which catalyzes uracil to thymidine. Cytotoxicity is the result of an arrest of folate-dependent enzymatic reactions, including DNA, RNA, and protein synthesis.[89]

Rapidly proliferating cells in the S phase are most susceptible to methotrexate-induced depletion of reduced folates. Therefore, longer exposure of tumor cells to methotrexate will allow more cells to enter the DNA synthesis phase of the cell cycle and result in enhanced cell kill. Most cells can function with relatively small amounts of DHFR to maintain sufficient reduced-folate pools. Therefore, a high intracellular concentration of antifolate drugs should be maintained to ensure complete enzyme inhibition. This may be accomplished by administering large amounts of methotrexate, such as those seen in treatment for malignant lymphomas and sarcomas. The ability to administer such high doses is possible only with the timely administration of leucovorin (folinic acid). Leucovorin circumvents methotrexate-induced enzyme blockade and "rescues" normal cells by providing them with the reduced folates they need for nucleic acid and protein synthesis.

Methotrexate is one of the most extensively studied antineoplastic drugs for its pharmacokinetics, in part because there is a simple and readily available assay to measure the blood concentration of methotrexate. This assay is frequently used to monitor for potential toxicity when administering moderate to high doses of methotrexate. The drug is well absorbed orally at moderate to low doses. Elimination occurs primarily through renal excretion via glomerular filtration and active secretion in the proximal tubule.[90] As previously mentioned, excretion is highly dependent on adequate renal function and may be inhibited by a number of compounds. Doses should be reduced in patients with decreased renal function, and blood levels should be monitored following each dose. Patients with blood levels greater than 0.5 μM at 48 hours postdose are at increased risk for severe myelosuppression and mucositis.[91] Leucovorin therapy should be continued in these patients until methotrexate blood levels are below 0.05 μM. Patients with a creatinine clearance of 10–50 mL/minute should receive 30%–50% of the original dose, and those with creatinine clearance less than 10 mL/minute should receive only 15% of the original dose.[90] A significant drug interaction exist between methotrexate and drugs that decrease glomerular filtration rate (see Table 15-12). The pharmacokinetics of methotrexate are altered by distribution into third-space fluid collections such as ascetic accumulation in the peritoneal cavity. Elimination is prolonged and toxicity is increased because of the slow redistribution of the drug from the peritoneum back into the blood.[62]

Methotrexate-associated toxicities, besides myelosuppression and mucositis, include nephrotoxicity, hepatotoxicity, and pulmonary fibrosis. Hepatotoxicity may result from high-dose therapy and result in acute and reversible elevations in liver function enzymes. Methotrexate is useful as a treatment or prophylaxis for meningeal leukemia; however, the drug is poorly distributed into the cerebrospinal fluid (CSF). For this reason, a preservative-free formulation of methotrexate must be injected directly into the CSF by lumbar puncture or intraventricular device (Ommaya reservoir). Toxicities seen with intrathecal administration include severe headache, nuchal rigidity, vomiting, and fever; in severe cases, a demyelinating encephalopathy may develop.

Pemetrexed (Alimta) is a multitargeted antifolate that is indicated in combination with cisplatin for the treatment of unresectable malignant pleural mesothelioma. The drug's primary mechanism is inhibition of thymidylate synthase, resulting in reduced levels of thymidine and slowing of DNA synthesis.[92] Pemetrexed also inhibits other folate-dependent enzymes, including DHFR. Severe hematologic toxicity was seen in clinical trials and correlated to poor nutritional status.[93] When patients were supplemented with folic acid and vitamin B_{12} during the study, significantly less toxicity was observed, therefore, all patients receiving premetrexed should receive these supplements. Other adverse events experienced with pemetrexed include nausea, vomiting, fatigue, diarrhea, and skin rash.

Pyrimidine analogs. The fluoropyrimidine 5-fluorouracil (5-FU) undergoes extensive metabolism intracellularly to evolve into an active metabolite, fluorodeoxyuridine monophosphate (FdUMP). FdUMP covalently binds with thymidylate synthase (TS) and inhibits the enzyme's ability to synthesize deoxythymidine triphosphate (dTTP), a precursor of DNA synthesis. Other metabolic pathways are conversion of 5-FU to fluorouradine triphosphate (FUTP), which may be incorporated into RNA, and conversion of FdUMP to the triphosphate form, which may be incorporated into DNA. The cytotoxicity of 5-FU in these metabolic pathways results in depletion of dTTP or false incorporation of other metabolites into DNA and RNA. The administration of 5-FU and leucovorin concurrently enhances this reaction and increases the cytotoxic effect of 5-FU (see Modulation of fluorouracil by leucovorin, in the Therapeutic Strategies section of this chapter).

Rapidly cleared by the liver, 5-FU has a plasma half-life of 6–20 minutes. There may be considerable variation in clearance among patients. The enzyme dihydropyrimidine dehydrogenase metabolizes 5-FU to dihydrofluorouracil in the liver and other tissues. Patients who are deficient in this enzyme experience greatly increased 5-FU levels and resultant toxicity.[94] When 5-FU or floxuridine is administered directly into the hepatic artery or portal vein, hepatic metastases are directly exposed to the drug with minimal systemic exposure because of the drug's significant first-pass clearance.

The major dose-limiting toxicity of 5-FU depends on the schedule of administration. Myelosuppression is more prominent when the drug is given by rapid bolus injection, whereas mucositis and gastrointestinal toxicity are more common with prolonged infusions over 2 to 5 days. Cholestatic jaundice and biliary sclerosis are complications of intrahepatic administration of fluoropyrimidines. Therapy with 5-FU has sometimes caused chest pain, elevation in cardiac enzymes, and ECG changes similar to those seen with myocardial ischemia. This syndrome may be associated with 5-FU–induced coronary vasospasm.[95]

Orally administered fluoropyrimidines have traditionally been avoided because of the erratic bioavailability observed. Recently, however, three new approaches to orally administering fluoropyrimidines have been developed. Capecitabine is now FDA approved for the treatment of patients with metastatic breast or colorectal cancer. This prodrug undergoes numerous metabolic steps in both the liver and tissues to ultimately become fluorouracil.[96] The cytotoxic metabolite is more concentrated in tumor cells than in normal cells because of the higher concentrations of thymidine phosphorylase, the enzyme responsible for the final conversion to fluorouracil. The major dose-limiting side effects include diarrhea, hand-and-foot syndrome, and stomatitis. Two other fluoropyrimidine compounds are under investigation for use in colorectal cancer. UFT is a combination of the fluorouracil prodrug ftorafur and uracil and is given orally. The pharmacokinetics of fluorouracil are significantly altered by the co-administration of 5-ethynyluracil, a potent inhibitor of dihydropyrimidine dehydrogenase that is responsible for the inactivation of fluorouracil.[97] The combination is being investigated for the orally administered treatment of colorectal cancer.

Cytarabine was originally isolated from the sponge *Cryptothethya crypta*. The parent drug is phosphorylated to ara-CTP, which competes with the normal substrate deoxycytidine triphosphate (dCTP) to inhibit DNA polymerase-alpha. DNA polymerases are critical enzymes in the synthesis and repair of DNA. The metabolite ara-CTP may also become incorporated into DNA and interfere with chain polymerization and repair of damaged DNA strands. As seen with other antimetabolites, tumor cells and normal tissues are most sensitive to cytarabine in the S phase of the cell cycle.

Cytarabine is rapidly converted to the inactive metabolite ara-U by the enzyme cytidine deaminase, which is present in many tissues, including the gastrointestinal epithelium and liver. Cytarabine is usually administered by continuous infusion following a bolus dose. This regimen is used to maintain cytotoxic levels despite the drug's rapid inactivation and to maximally expose all cycling cells to the cytotoxic effects during the S phase of the cell cycle. Cytarabine may be used alone or in addition to methotrexate for meningeal leukemia; however, direct intrathecal administration is necessary to obtain sufficient drug concentrations in the CSF. Only small amounts of cytarabine are needed intrathecally, because deamination is minimal in the CSF. Toxicities of cytarabine include myelosuppression and gastrointestinal epithelial injury. When high-dose cytarabine is used for refractory acute myelogenous leukemia (AML), 20% of patients may experience a cerebral and cerebellar dysfunction. This syndrome is more often seen in individuals older than age 50 and is characterized by slurred speech, ataxia, confusion, and coma.[98] High-dose cytarabine is also associated with conjunctivitis, which can usually be prevented by giving the patient steroid ophthalmic drops.

Gemcitabine is a pyrimidine analog of deoxycytidine that is converted intracellularly to its diphosphate and triphosphate metabolites. Gemcitabine diphosphate is an inhibitor of ribonucleotide reductase and thereby inhibits de novo nucleotide synthesis.[99] Gemcitabine triphosphate inhibits DNA synthesis by competing with the physiologic substrate, deoxycytidine triphosphate, for DNA polymerase and incorporation into DNA. The reduction of intracellular deoxycytidine triphosphate induced by gemcitabine diphosphate enhances the incorporation of gemcitabine triphosphate into DNA, a mechanism referred to as "self-potentiation." The half-life of gemcitabine is prolonged as a consequence of this phenomenon, so infusions should be limited to 30 minutes. Longer infusions are associated with a higher degree of myelotoxicity. Other important adverse effects include elevated liver transaminase enzymes, nausea and vomiting, and skin rash with or without pruritus.[100]

Purine analogs. The thiopurines 6-mercaptopurine (6-MP) and 6-thioguanine (6-TG) are converted to their respective monophosphates, which inhibit purine synthesis and cause an accumulation of nucleic acid precursors. These precursors, in turn, facilitate the conversion of 6-MP and 6-TG to their active nucleotide forms. The triphosphate nucleotides of these drugs are incorporated into DNA and induce strand breaks, which are correlated with cytotoxicity. Methotrexate, an inhibitor of de novo purine biosynthesis, acts synergistically with the 6-thiopurines by blocking purine synthesis and enhancing thiopurine activation.

Fludarabine is relatively resistant to deamination (deactivation) and possesses enhanced solubility over other adenine arabinoside analogs. Following intravenous administration, the drug is rapidly dephosphorylated to F-Ara-A, which enters cells via nucleotide-specific membrane transport.[101] The primary mechanism of action is inhibition of the DNA polymerases involved in DNA synthesis and repair. Fludarabine is most active in the treatment of chronic lymphocytic leukemia and indolent non-Hodgkin's lymphoma. In the initial trials of fludarabine, doses of 75 to 150 mg/m^2 four times a day for 5–7 days produced profound neurotoxicity characterized by cortical blindness, seizures, coma, and death. Subsequent trials demonstrated fludarabine could be given safely when administered at doses between 25 and 30 mg/m^2 daily for 5 days.[102] At these doses the most common toxicities are myelosuppression and immunosuppression. Patients on fludarabine should also be given prophylactic therapy for *Pneumocystis carinii*. A rare but sometimes life-threatening and potentially fatal autoimmune hemolytic anemia may occur in patients receiving fludarabine.[103] Patients rechallenged with fludarabine, whether pretreated or not with steroids, have experienced fatal outcomes.

2-Chlorodeoxyadenosine (2-CdA, Cladribine) is a deoxyadenosine purine nucleotide analog that, like fludarabine, is resistant to deamination. Cladribine enters lymphocytes via a nucleotide transporter system and accumulates until it reaches lymphotoxic levels. Following a series of phosphorylation steps, the drug is converted to cladribine triphosphate, which is falsely incorporated into DNA, eventually interrupting DNA synthesis and repair.[104] Cladribine can produce durable complete remissions in as many as 91% of patients with hairy cell leukemia.[105,106] Responses may be seen in patients with chronic lymphocytic leukemia (CLL) and non-Hodgkin's lymphoma; however, remissions tend to be brief.[107] Myelotoxicity is the dose-limiting toxicity, and recovery may take as long as three to five weeks after a single course of therapy. A severe autoimmune hemolytic anemia with fatal bone marrow aplasia has been described in CLL patients receiving repeated cycles.[108] Immunosuppression and opportunistic infections are seen less often than in patients who receive fludarabine.

Pentostatin (Nipent) or 2′-deoxycoformycin was developed as a potent inhibitor of adenosine diaminase. Blockage of this enzyme causes an accumulation of deoxyadenosine, which is mostly responsible for Cladribine's cytotoxicity.[109] Pentostatin is active in a number of lymphocytic diseases, including CLL, prolymphocytic leukemia, and T-cell lymphoma. A profound immunosuppression may persist for more than a year after the drug is discontinued.[110] Other adverse events seen with pentostatin therapy include ocular complications, dermatologic toxicity, and gastrointestinal toxicity.

Plant derivatives

Antineoplastic drugs derived from plant sources represent a large and diverse group of chemotherapeutic agents. Many of these drugs are naturally occurring compounds that were isolated from plant material (vinca alkaloids). Others are the result of synthetic and semisynthetic processes used to manufacture analogs of compounds originally extracted from plants. Examples include etoposide, docetaxel, paclitaxel, and topotecan. The discovery of new plant-derived compounds with antitumor activity is ongoing and will continue to provide important and novel agents for the treatment of cancer.

Vinca alkaloids. Natural alkaloids present in small quantities in the periwinkle plant play a major role in cancer chemotherapy. Although the drugs in this group are dramatically similar in chemical structure, their antitumor activity and toxicity differ greatly. Vincristine has a broad spectrum of activity, leading to its use in leukemia, lymphoma, breast cancer, lung cancer, and multiple myeloma, whereas vinblastine is used primarily in germ cell tumors and advanced Hodgkin's disease. Vinblastine is myelotoxic and neurotoxic; vincristine is also neurotoxic but has amazingly minimal myelotoxicity. Vinorelbine, the newest vinca alkaloid to become available in the United States, is active in breast cancer and non-small cell lung cancer and is both myelotoxic and neurotoxic. Vindesine is widely available in Europe but currently not available in the United States except in clinical trials.

Vinca alkaloids belong to a group of compounds known as the *tubulin interactive agents.* They exert their cytotoxic effects primarily by interfering with normal microtubule formation and function, which is critical for the mitosis phase of the cell cycle and ultimately cell division. Microtubules have other important cellular functions that are affected by the vinca alkaloids, including maintenance of cell shape and intracellular transport. Vinca alkaloids bind to specific sites on tubulin, preventing formation of tubulin dimers and inhibiting the formation of microtubule structures. Although mitotic arrest is the primary mechanism of cell death, vinca alkaloids may have a cytolytic effect on resting cells in the G_0 phase and other cells in the G_1 or S phase. Cells are sensitive to low concentrations of vincristine, and duration of exposure is critical in determining the cytotoxic effect.

Despite the wide range of clinical uses of the vinca alkaloids, surprisingly little information is available on their pharmacologic and pharmacokinetic profiles. This may be primarily the result of the lack of a sensitive drug assay for quantifying the low concentrations found in patients. Vincristine is highly bound to serum proteins, blood cells, and especially platelets. It is metabolized primarily by the liver and concentrates in the bile. Seventy percent of a dose is excreted in the feces, and approximately 10% is excreted in the urine.[111] Dose modification should be considered in patients with hepatic dysfunction, particularly patients with biliary obstructions. Vinblastine and vinorelbine have similar pharmacokinetic profiles, with excretion occurring primarily through the biliary tract. All of the vinca alkaloids have a prolonged terminal elimination phase half-life of 1–4 days.

Vinca alkaloids are known for their peripheral neurotoxicity, which is frequently a cumulative dose-limiting effect. Toxicity initially presents as sensory impairment (stocking-and-glove distribution) and paresthesias. Patients may later develop neuritic pain and motor dysfunction. Loss of deep tendon reflexes, foot and wrist drop, ataxia, and paralysis may occur with continued vinca alkaloid therapy. The only effective management is discontinuation of therapy. Accidental intrathecal administration of vincristine induces an ascending paralysis resulting in death. Constipation and abdominal pain are frequent complaints of older patients while on vincristine. Myelosuppression is also a dose-limiting toxicity of vinblastine and vinorelbine, but not vincristine. The vinca alkaloids are vesicants, and extravasation should be avoided.

Taxanes. The taxanes have emerged as an extremely important group of antitumor compounds that show activity in a wide range of cancers. These complex chemical structures are difficult to synthesize in the laboratory. Extraction and isolation from bark of the Pacific yew tree *Taxus brevifolia* was the only source for paclitaxel until the early 1990s, when a semisynthetic process using a taxane precursor was developed. Because of paclitaxel's poor water solubility, the injectable formulation must contain 50% polyoxyethylated castor oil (Cremophor EL) to maintain aqueous solubility. This vehicle creates problems with administration, as Cremophor EL can leach hepatotoxic plasticizer from PVC plastic infusion devices and is associated with severe hypersensitivity reactions.

Paclitaxel and docetaxel preferentially bind to microtubules over tubulin dimers, and they inhibit microtubule disassembly, which is necessary for normal functioning of microtubule structures.[112] Cells exposed to paclitaxel display many arrays of disorganized microtubules during all phases of the cell cycle. Although taxanes have distinct antimicrotubule effects on cells, the actual mechanism of cell death remains unclear. The mechanism of action and cytotoxic effect of docetaxel are similar to those of paclitaxel.

Hepatic metabolism and biliary excretion probably constitute the major routes of elimination for paclitaxel and docetaxel.[113,114] Urinary excretion accounts for less than 5% of total body clearance of the drugs. Paclitaxel clearance is reduced by as much as 30% when given following cisplatin.[115] This interaction results in increased peak plasma concentrations of paclitaxel and more severe myelotoxicity than is seen with the reverse administration schedule. For routine use with cisplatin or carboplatin, paclitaxel should be given first, followed by cisplatin or carboplatin. The taxanes also exhibit a high degree of protein binding (90%–95%). Among the most significant toxicities associated with taxanes are myelosuppression, neurotoxicity, hypersensitivity, total body alopecia, and transient myalgias and arthralgias. Nail separation may occur, especially when paclitaxel is given as a weekly

1–hour infusion. Hypersensitivity reactions were seen in 10% of patients receiving paclitaxel during early clinical trials.[116] These reactions usually occur within the first 10 minutes of the initial infusion and are characterized by hypotension, bronchospasm, dyspnea, abdominal and leg pain, and severe facial flushing. Major hypersensitivity reactions may be prevented in most patients by the preinfusion administration of a corticosteroid (dexamethasone), an antihistamine (diphenhydramine), and an H_2-blocking drug. Paclitaxel may be safely given parenterally with infusions lasting 24, 3, or 1 hours. The 3-hour infusion rate has been associated with less neutropenia than the 24-hour infusion.

The toxicity profile of docetaxel differs from that of paclitaxel.[117] The incidence of hypersensitivity reactions is lower with docetaxel, with severe reactions experienced in fewer than 1% of patients treated. Skin reactions, including pruritus, macular or papular lesions, erythema, and desquamation, are seen in 50%–70% of patients treated with docetaxel. Nail changes, consisting of an orange discoloration and thickening of the nails, were also observed in many patients in clinical trials. A more significant complication is fluid retention and weight gain, which can occur in 6% of patients. A 3-day regimen of corticosteroids is useful in preventing and lessening the fluid retention as well as for preventing of hypersensitivity reactions.

Two new formulations of paclitaxel are currently under development that avoid using a Cremophor EL base as a solubilizer. ABI-007 (Abraxane), also known as nab paclitaxel, is a nanoparticle albumin-bound formulation of paclitaxel that is free of Cremophor and other solvents. The drug actually uses red blood cells as a reservoir. Phase I studies of ABI-007 were conducted without steroid premedication and did not produce any acute hypersensitivity reactions.[118] The dose-limiting toxicity (DLT) in this trial was 375 mg/m^2, which is significantly higher than the DLT for conventional paclitaxel in Cremophor. In phase III clinical trials in patients with metastatic breast cancer, ABI-007 was administered as a 30-minute infusion at a dose of 260 mg/m^2 versus paclitaxel in Cremophor dosed at 175 mg/m^2 and given over 3 hours.[119] There was a superior response rate in the ABI-007 group as well as a longer time to progression. Less neutropenia and more manageable peripheral neuropathy were seen in the ABI-007-treated patients despite the higher dose of paclitaxel given.

Xyotax (CT-2103) is a polymer–drug conjugate of polyglutamate and paclitaxel. The polymer conjugates are taken up by tumor cells and the reticuloendothelial system, and free paclitaxel is released by esterolysis intracellularly.[120] CT-2103 allows for extended release of free paclitaxel; as a result, cells are exposed for a prolonged period compared to conventional paclitaxel. CT-2103 was well tolerated and highly active as a single-agent therapy in patients with recurrent ovarian cancer with platinum-sensitive or platinum-resistant tumors.[121]

Epipodophyllotoxins. Podophyllotoxin, an extract of the mandrake plant, is an antimitotic drug that binds to tubulin and inhibits microtubulin formation. This compound was not further developed as an antitumor agent because of its unacceptable toxicity in humans.

Etoposide and teniposide are glycosidic derivatives of podophyllotoxin that possess significant activity in many human tumors such as germ cell tumors and lung cancer, but offer a more predictable and mild toxicity profile. Initially, these drugs were thought to work as antimicrotubule agents similar to podophyllotoxin and vinca alkaloids. However, they produced no effect on microtubule assembly. Cell-cycle studies demonstrated epipodophyllotoxins induced arrest of cells in the late S or early G phase instead of the expected M-phase arrest commonly observed with antimitotic drugs. Along with the observation of drug-induced DNA strand breaks, scientists have suggested the primary cytotoxic mechanism of these compounds is inhibition of topoisomerase II.[122] Epipodophyllotoxins stabilize the enzyme–DNA complex, thereby inhibiting the reunion of the two DNA strands originally cleaved by the enzyme. Additionally, the synergy of the etoposide with antimetabolite drugs may result from inhibition of nucleoside transport into the cell.

Etoposide and teniposide are highly protein bound (94% and 99%, respectively) to the plasma protein albumin. Drugs that interfere with the protein binding of teniposide may induce greater toxicity in patients receiving both drugs (see the Drug Interactions in the Patient Receiving Chemotherapy section of this chapter). Renal clearance is the major route of elimination for etoposide, with approximately 40%–60% of the drug being excreted unchanged in the urine. Biliary excretion and hepatic metabolism are responsible for elimination to a lesser extent. Teniposide is more extensively metabolized, with only 5%–20% being excreted unchanged in the urine. Etoposide is available as an oral formulation, which has a bioavailability of approximately 50%.

The toxicities of both agents are similar, with myelosuppression, hypersensitivity, and infusion-related blood pressure changes being the most significant toxic effects. Both agents are also poorly water soluble, necessitating the addition of Tween 80 or Cremophor EL and other excipients to maintain the drugs in aqueous solution. The manufacturer of teniposide recommends avoiding the use of PVC plastic infusion devices to prevent exposing the patient to potentially hepatotoxic plasticizers leached from the plastic by the Cremophor vehicle.

Camptothecin derivatives. Camptothecin sodium was originally tested in the early 1970s as an antitumor compound. Despite the drug's significant activity in both preclinical and clinical trials, it was abandoned because of unpredictable and often severe hemorrhagic cystitis. Interest in related drugs was renewed with the introduction of two semisynthetic analogs of camptothecin, topotecan and irinotecan. Their proposed mechanism of action is inhibition of topoisomerase I, an enzyme responsible for maintaining the three-dimensional structure of DNA. Topoisomerase inhibitors bind with the DNA–enzyme complex, thereby inducing DNA strand breaks and cell death.[123]

Camptothecins appear to exist in two species in aqueous solutions: a closed lactone ring, which possesses cytotoxic activity, and an open carboxylate form, which does not. The conversion is pH dependent, with the open form predominating in an alkaline environment and the closed, or active, form predominating in an acidic solution. Much of the unpredictable urotoxicity seen in early trials of camptothecin sodium may be explained by the lack of knowledge of the pH-dependent conversion and the shift of the equilibrium toward the active species in the acidic environment of the bladder. Irinotecan is a prodrug and must be converted to its active form via carboxylesterase in the body.[124] Myelosuppression is the major dose-limiting toxicity of topotecan, while diarrhea is the primary dose-limiting toxicity for irinotecan when administered on a once-weekly schedule. To effectively manage the diarrhea associated with irinotecan, patients should be instructed to start a high-dose loperamide regimen (2 mg of loperamide every 2 hours) until they are diarrhea free for 12 hours.

Miscellaneous agents

L-asparaginase induces a rapid and complete depletion from the blood of the amino acid L-asparagine. This biochemical process is cytotoxic to tumor cells that are highly dependent on exogenous sources of the amino acid. The major cytotoxic effect is the inhibition of protein synthesis, with a secondary effect of inhibition of nucleic acid synthesis also observed in sensitive cells. L-asparaginase is considered cell cycle–phase nonspecific, despite the drug's ability to block cells in the G_1 and S phases of the cell cycle. Its only antineoplastic use is as part of the induction and consolidation therapy for acute lymphocytic leukemia in both children and adults. L-asparaginase is extracted from *Escherichia coli* bacteria and is associated with a high incidence of anaphylaxis. Patients who develop severe hypersensitivity reactions to the bacterial product may receive pegaspargase, which is chemically altered to be less immunogenic. Other toxicities seen with L-asparaginase include hyperglycemia, hypoprothrombinemia, and neurotoxicity.

Hydroxyurea is a DNA-selective antimetabolite that inhibits ribonucleotide reductase and has minimal inhibitory effects on RNA and protein synthesis. Its major indication is in rapidly controlling blood counts in acute leukemia and other myeloproliferative diseases such as polycythemia vera and essential thrombocytosis. Allopurinol should be used in conjunction with hydroxyurea to prevent tumor lysis syndrome.

Estramustine is a unique compound made up of a molecule of estradiol phosphate combined with nitrogen mustard. Originally believed to have alkylating properties, the drug's mechanism of action is now thought to be related to antimicrotubule activity.[125]

Thalidomide is thought to possess both antiangiogenic effects and immunosuppressant activity. This drug decreases vascular endothelial growth factor (VEGF) and beta fibroblast growth factor (β-FGF) levels in the plasma of patients with refractory multiple myeloma.[126] However, it is unclear if the antiangiogenic effects are the primary reason for the drug's anticancer effects. Somnolence, headache, dizziness, and rash were the most common adverse events seen in clinical trials with thalidomide.

Tyrosine Kinase Inhibitors

Several small-molecule tyrosine kinase inhibitors are in development that block epidermal growth factor receptor (EGRF) tyrosine phosphorylation by competing with ATP for the tyrosine kinase domain of the receptor.[127] Two drugs in this category currently available in the United States to treat malignancies are imatinib and gefitinib.

Imatinib (Gleevec) is approved for the treatment of Philadelphia chromosome-positive chronic myelogenous leukemia (CML) after failure of interferon therapy. In clinical trials involving interferon-refractory patients with CML treated with imatinib, 93% of patients with chronic-phase CML and 68% of those with accelerated-phase CML[128,129] had a complete hematologic response (normal WBC and platelet count). These patients also experienced a major cytogenetic response (disappearance of the Philadelphia chromosome): 61% of patients in the chronic phase and 25% of patients in the accelerated phase. Adverse events were moderate to mild and consisted primarily of nausea, vomiting, fluid retention, and diarrhea. Fluid retention may be managed by interruption of imatinib and supportive care. Imatinib offers the convenience of orally administered therapy and a manageable side effect profile at a significantly increased cost relative to interferon. This drug is also indicated in gastrointestinal stromal tumors (GIST) that express c-KIT and are unresectable, metastatic, or both. The drug offers effective management of a disease commonly unresponsive to chemotherapy in the advanced stage.[130]

Gefitinib (Iressa) is a tyrosine kinase inhibitor approved as monotherapy for patients with locally advanced or metastatic non-small cell lung cancer (NSCLC) who have failed both platinum- and docetaxel-based chemotherapy regimens. EGFR is present in almost all NSCLC specimens and overexpressed in most. Gefitinib reversibly binds to ATP sites on tyrosine kinase, blocking signal transduction and resulting in decreased angiogenesis, increased apoptosis, and less tendency for invasion and metastatic potential.[131] Two large multicenter trials of gefitinib in NSCLC demonstrated response rates of less than 20% for two different dose sizes.[132,133] However, those patients who did respond experienced a rapid and marked improvement in symptoms and quality of life. The primary adverse events observed in these trials were a skin toxicity manifested as an acneiform rash and diarrhea. The addition of gefitinib to first-line chemotherapy in NSCLC showed no benefit in two large randomized, placebo-controlled trials.[134]

Proteasome Inhibitors

The proteasome is a large, multiprotein complex found in the nucleus and cytoplasm of all cells that is responsible for the tagging and destroying of obsolete protein messages and short-lived proteins. The transcription factor NF-kappa B is associated with chemoresistance, apoptotic inhibition, and cell growth and proliferation; it is very active in multiple myeloma cells. When released from its inhibitor, NF-kappa B locates to the nucleus and promotes cell survival.[135] Bortezomib (Velcade) is a 26S proteasome inhibitor approved for relapsed and refractory multiple myeloma. By blocking the NK-kappa B downstream signal pathway, bortezomib stimulates apoptosis of myeloma cells.[136] In highly refractory disease, bortezomib produced a major response with a median duration of 12 months in approximately 28% of patients treated.[137] The majority of toxicities were mild to moderate and included peripheral neuropathy, thrombocytopenia, diarrhea, nausea, and neutropenia. Patients who develop sensorimotor neuropathy may need a change in their dose and schedule of bortezomib.

Hormonal Therapy

Hormonal manipulations were among the first treatments used to control cancer. Initially, they had limited potential to induce significant response in sensitive tumors. Currently, however, they are critical components in the treatment for many different neoplasms. Table 15-14 lists the commonly used hormonal agents and their primary indications. Steroids, steroid analogs and enzyme inhibitors constitute the majority of drugs used for hormonal therapy. Their mechanism of action is incompletely understood, but probably involves the inhibition of stimulation of steroid-specific receptors located on the surface of cells. Blocking these receptors prevents the cell from receiving normal hormonal growth stimulation, thereby decreasing the growth fraction of the tumor.

Antiestrogens

Tamoxifen is a frequently used drug in the adjuvant treatment of breast cancer and treatment of metastatic disease in estrogen receptor-positive tumors. Its primary mechanism of action is blocking estrogen stimulation of breast cancer cells.[138] This is achieved by inhibition of both the translocation and nuclear binding of the estrogen receptor. Tamoxifen is an estrogen antagonist (blocker) in breast tissue and an estrogen agonist (stimulator) in endometrium, bone, and lipids. The most prominent toxicity is hot flashes, which affect approximately half of the women who use it. Other side effects include a slightly increased incidence of thromboembolic events and endometrial cancer. In a large randomized trial comparing tamoxifen and placebo in the prevention of breast cancer in women, women at risk for developing a breast malignancy were 50% less likely to develop the disease if they took tamoxifen 20 mg daily.[139] Megestrol has also been used to treat metastatic breast cancer but more recently has been primarily used for the treatment of anorexia-cachexia related to cancer.[140]

A monthly administered, injectable antihormonal agent is now available for patients with estrogen receptor-positive metastatic breast cancer who have failed initial therapy with another antiestrogen (tamoxifen). Fulvestrant binds to the estrogen receptor, blocking both hormone-dependent and hormone-independent activation functions and preventing estrogen-induced cell growth.[141] Fulvestrant was found to be equivalent to anastrazole in terms of length of survival, time to progression, and tumor response in patients with locally advanced metastatic breast cancer following progression of disease while on tamoxifen or other endocrine therapies.[142] Both drugs were well tolerated, and few patients withdrew from the study due to adverse events.

Table 15-14 Commonly Used Hormonal Agents and Primary Indications

Pharmacologic Class	Drug Name(s)	Primary Indication(s)
Corticosteroids	Dexamethasone Hydrocortisone Methylprednisolone Prednisone	Leukemias Hodgkin's disease Malignant lymphomas Breast cancer Multiple myeloma
Androgens	Fluoxymesterone Testosterone	Breast cancer
Estrogens	Conjugated estrogens Diethylstilbesterol Estradiol	Prostate cancer Breast cancer
Antiestrogens		
Progestins	Medroxyprogesterone Megesterol	Endometrial cancer Breast cancer
Estrogen-receptor antagonists	Tamoxifen (Nolvadex) Toremifene (Fareston) Fulvestrant (Faslodex)	Breast cancer Breast cancer
Aromatase inhibitors	Mitotane Anastrozole (Arimidex) Letrozole (Femara)	Adrenal cancer Breast cancer Breast cancer
LH-RH analogs	Goserelin (Zoladex) Leuprolide (Lupron)	Prostate cancer Breast cancer
Antiandrogens	Flutamide (Eulexin) Nilutamide (Nilandron) Bicalutamide (Casodex)	Prostate cancer

Aromatase inhibitors

Aromatase inhibitors suppress postmenopausal estrogen synthesis by inhibiting the peripheral conversion of androgens to estrogens. These agents have been primarily developed for the treatment of hormonally sensitive breast cancer. Ovarian production of estrogen is unaffected; as a consequence, these agents are useful only in postmenopausal women or oophorectomized premenopausal women. Aminoglutethamide was the first such agent available but is now rarely used because of its poor tolerance and the need to replace corticosteroids. Newer agents include anastrozole and letrozole. Both drugs are potent aromatase inhibitors and equally effective to aminoglutethamide; however, they affect the synthesis of corticosteroids, aldosterone, or thyroid hormone only minimally and, therefore, are associated with fewer toxicities.

Gonadotropin-releasing hormone analogs

Luteinizing hormone-releasing hormone (LH-RH) agonists are synthetic analogs of the naturally occurring hormone. Initially, these drugs induce an increase in testosterone levels secondary to their stimulation of LH release. With continued use, the pituitary gland becomes desensitized, resulting in a dramatic decrease in the production of estrogens and androgens. Leuprolide and goserelin are both available as slow-release depot injections that are given at monthly or every 4-month intervals. Castration levels of testosterone are achieved within 3–4 weeks with leuprolide and within 1 month with goserelin.

Antiandrogens

Antiandrogens are used in men with hormone-responsive metastatic prostate cancer, either as initial therapy or in combination with a gonadotropin-releasing hormone analog. Their mechanism of action is binding to the androgen receptor and blocking the effects of dihydrotestosterone on prostate cancer cells.[143] Flutamide was the first antiandrogen available; the most frequent adverse events observed with its use include diarrhea, gynecomastia, and occasionally hepatotoxicity. Newer antiandrogens are nilutamide and bicalutamide, both of which have equivalent activity to flutamide. However, they are usually better tolerated because they produce less diarrhea and offer a simpler administration schedule.

Differentiation Agents

Retinoids

Retinoids, a class of compounds structurally related to vitamin A (retinol), have been found to influence proliferation and differentiation of both normal and tumor cells. The two compounds most studied for their effect on controlling or preventing tumor growth are 13-*cis* retinoic acid (isotretinoin) and all-*trans* retinoic acid (tretinoin). Isotretinoin is currently marketed as the antiacne product Accutane. However, it is under extensive investigation, often in combination with alfa-interferon, for the prevention of new and recurrent squamous cell tumors.[144] Isotretinoin reverses oral leukoplakia, a premalignant state of the oral cavity in heavy tobacco smokers.[145] Other potential uses for isotretinoin include myelodysplastic syndromes and acute and chronic leukemias. Tretinoin (Vesanoid) is approved for use in induction and maintenance regimens for acute promyelocytic leukemia.

Toxicity of these compounds is similar to the pharmacologic effects of hypervitaminosis A, which include dry lips and mucous membranes, skin fragility, brittle nails, photosensitivity, and conjunctivitis. Other side effects are headache, nausea and vomiting, transaminase and triglyceride elevations, arthralgia, and bone pain. Tretinoin is also associated with severe leukocytosis, which may induce fevers, respiratory distress, pulmonary and pericardial effusions, and hypotension.[146] All retinoids are teratogens, so they should never be given to female patients who are pregnant or are considering becoming pregnant.

Arsenic trioxide

Studies from China of arsenic stimulated interest in the West to further investigate this poison as a chemotherapeutic agent.[147] Arsenic trioxide induces a complete remission in a considerably higher proportion of patients with acute promyelocytic leukemia (APL) than that seen with all-*trans* retinoic acid (tretinoin).[148] Arsenic trioxide activity in APL is associated with a partial nonterminal differentiation, degradation of the PML-RAR alpha fusion protein, and activation of capsases leading to apoptosis.[149] The drug is generally well tolerated when administered in a low-dose daily schedule. Fatigue, lightheadedness during the infusion, and characteristic maculopapular skin eruptions are common adverse events. When administered for prolonged periods, arsenic trioxide can induce a peripheral neuropathy and severe neuropathic reactions including quadriparesis.[150] It is known to cause a prolongation of the QT interval on ECG. For this reason, patients should be monitored with weekly ECG, and administration of other drugs known to prolong the QT interval, such as amiodarone, beta blockers, cisapride, dolaestron, quinidine, terfenadine, and tricyclic antidepressants should be avoided. Patients on arsenic trioxide may also develop a leukocytosis and retinoic acid syndrome, as described previously for tretinoin.[151]

Conclusion

Drug therapy for the control and cure of cancer has come a long way from early experimentation with mustard gas derivatives. Currently, a multitude of drugs with a variety of treatment schedules are among the oncologist's armamentarium. Research efforts must continue to focus on improving the oncology patient's life by evaluating new drugs and therapies, as well as reevaluating old ones. Cytotoxic chemotherapy and biological agents account for the majority of pharmaceutical agents used in the treatment of patients with cancer. The further development of targeted therapies may change the overall treatment of cancer from a primarily acute approach to a more chronic one. In addition, the introduction of effective and safe gene therapy may hold great promise for the cure of many cancers for which there are currently limited therapeutic options available. Future directions for research in oncology should include combining chemotherapy and biological therapy, gene therapy, or all of these to achieve optimal patient outcomes.

References

1. Kennedy BJ: Evolution of chemotherapy. *CA Cancer J Clin* 41:261–263, 1991 (editorial)
2. Chu E, DeVita VT: Principles of cancer management: chemotherapy, in DeVita VT, Hellman S, Rosenberg SA (eds.): *Cancer: Principles and Practice of Oncology* (ed 6). Philadelphia, Lippincott, 2001, pp 289–306
3. Buick RN: Cellular basis of chemotherapy, in Dorr RT, Von Hoff DD (eds.): *Cancer Chemotherapy Handbook* (ed 2). Norwalk, CT, Appleton & Lange, 1994, pp 3–14
4. Norton L: The Norton-Simon hypothesis, in Perry MC (ed.): *Chemotherapy Source Book* (ed 2). Baltimore, Williams & Wilkins, 1996, pp 43–61
5. Dy GK, Adjei AA: Novel targets for lung cancer therapy: Part I. *J Clin Oncol* 20:2881–2894, 2002
6. Dy GK, Adjei AA: Novel targets for lung cancer therapy: Part II. *J Clin Oncol* 20:3016–3028, 2002
7. Nelson AR, Fingleton B, Rothenberg ML, et al: Matrix metalloproteinases: biologic activity and clinical implications. *J Clin Oncol* 18:1135–1149, 2000
8. Radinsky R, Risin B, Fan R, et al: Level and function of epidermal growth factor receptor predict the metastatic potential of human colon carcinoma cells. *Clin Cancer Res* 1:19031, 1995
9. Petit AM, Rak J, Hung MC, et al: Neutralizing antibodies against epidermal growth factor and ErbB-2/neu receptor tyrosine kinases down-regulate vascular endothelial growth factor production by tumor cells in vitro and in vivo: angiogenic implications for signal transduction therapy of solid tumors. *Am J Pathol* 151:1523–1530, 1997
10. Ritter CA, Arteaga CL: The epidermal growth factor receptor–tyrosine kinase: a promising therapeutic target in solid tumors. *Semin Oncol* 30(suppl 1):3–11, 2003
11. Mendelsohn J, Baselga J: Status of epidermal growth factor receptor antagonists in the biology and treatment of cancer. *J Clin Oncol* 21:2787–2799, 2003

12. Finley RS: Overview of targeted therapies for cancer. *Am J Health Syst Pharm* 60(suppl 9):4–10, 2003
13. Mendelsohn J: Targeting the epidermal growth factor receptor for cancer therapy. *J Clin Oncol* 20(suppl 15):1s–13s, 2002
14. Folkman J: What is the evidence that tumors are angiogenesis-dependent? *J Natl Cancer Inst* 82:4–6, 1990
15. Weidner N, Folkman J: Tumor vascularity as a prognostic factor in cancer. *Prin Pract Oncol Update* 11:1–5, 1997
16. Ferrara N: Role of vascular endothelial growth factor in regulation of angiogenesis, in Teicher BA (ed.): *Antiangiogenic Agents in Cancer Therapy.* Totowa, New Jersey, Humana Press, 1999, pp 119–142
17. Genentech: AVF2540g: An open-label, multicenter extension study of rhuMAB VEGF (bevacizumab) in subjects treated with rhuMAB VEGF in a previous Genentech-sponsored phase II cancer study. San Francisco, July 10, 2002
18. Masiero L, Figg WD, Kohn EC: Review of the clinical experience with CAI, thalidomide, TNP-470 and interleukin-12. *Angiogenesis* 1:23–28, 1997
19. Boehm T, Folkman J, Browder T, et al: Antiangiogenic therapy of experimental cancer does not induce acquired drug resistance. *Nature* 390:404–407, 1997
20. Brown PD: Matrix metalloproteinase inhibitors in the treatment of cancer. *Med Oncol* 14:1–10, 1997
21. Poon RYC, Jiang W, Toyoshima H, et al: Cyclin-dependent kinases are inactivated by a combination of p21 and Thr-14/Tyr-15 phosphorylation after UV-induced DNA damage. *J Biol Chem* 271:13283–13291, 1996
22. Shapiro G, Supko JG, Patterson A, et al: A phase II trial of cyclin-dependent kinase inhibitor flavopiridol in patients with previously untreated stage IV non-small cell lung cancer. *Clin Cancer Res* 7:1590–1599, 2001
23. Goldie JH, Coldman AJ: The genetic origin of drug resistance in neoplasms: implications for systemic therapy. *Cancer Res* 44:3643–3653, 1984
24. Shustik C, Dalton W, Gros P: P-glycoprotein-mediated multidrug resistance in tumor cells: biochemistry, clinical relevance, and modulation. *Mol Aspects Med* 16:1–78, 1995
25. Yarbro JW: The scientific basis of cancer chemotherapy, in Perry MC (ed.): *Chemotherapy Source Book* (ed 3). Baltimore, Williams & Wilkins, 2001, pp 3–18
26. Gill DR, Hyde SC, Higgins CF, et al: Separation of drug transport and chloride channel functions of the human multidrug resistance P-glycoprotein. *Cell* 71:23–32, 1992
27. Dalton WS: Overcoming the multidrug-resistant phenotype, in DeVita VT, Hellman S, Rosenberg SA (eds.): *Cancer: Principles and Practice of Oncology* (ed 4). Philadelphia, Lippincott, 1993, pp 2655–2666
28. Goldstein LJ, Galski H, Fojo A, et al: Expression of a multidrug resistance in human cancers. *J Natl Cancer Inst* 81:116–176, 1989
29. Dan S, Esumi M, Sawada U, et al: Expression of a multidrug-resistance gene in human malignant lymphoma and related disorders. *Leuk Res* 15:1139–1143, 1991
30. Epstein J, Xiao HQ, Oba BK: P-glycoprotein expression in plasma-cell myeloma is associated with resistance to VAD. *Blood* 74:913–917, 1989
31. Glisson BS: Multidrug resistance mediated through alterations in topoisomerase II. *Cancer Bull* 41:37–39, 1989
32. Mannervik B, Danielson UH: Glutathione transferases: structure and catalytic activity. *Crit Rev Biochem* 23:283–337, 1988
33. Davies SM, Robison LL, Buckley JD, et al: Glutathione S-transferase polymorphisms and outcome of chemotherapy in childhood acute myeloid leukemia. *J Clin Oncol* 19:1279–1287, 2001
34. Hickman JA: Apopotosis induced by anticancer drugs. *Cancer Metastasis Rev* 11:121, 1992
35. Symonds H, Krall L, Remington L, et al: p53 dependent apoptosis suppresses tumor growth and progression in vivo. *Cell* 73:703–711, 1994
36. Hollstein M, Sidransky DE, Vogelstein B, et al.: p53 mutations in human cancers. *Science* 253:49–53, 1991
37. Leonard CJ, Canman CE, Kastan MB: The role of p53 in cell-cycle control and apoptosis: implications for cancer, in DeVita VT, Hellman S, Rosenberg SA (eds.): *Important Advances in Oncology 1995.* Philadelphia: Lippincott-Raven, 1995, pp 33–42
38. Levine AJ: p53, the cellular gatekeeper for growth and division. *Cell* 88:323–333, 1997
39. Lowe SW, Schmitt EM, Smith SW, et al: p53 is required for radiation-induced apoptosis in mouse thymocytes. *Nature* 362: 847–849, 1993
40. Wu GS, El-Deiry WS: p53 and chemosensitivity. *Nature Med* 2:255–258, 1996
41. Wahl AF, Donaldson KL, Fairchild C, et al: Loss of normal p53 function confers sensitization to taxol by increasing G(2)/M arrest and apoptosis. *Nature Med* 2:72–88, 1996
42. Piris MA, Pezzella F, Martinez-Montero JC, et al: p53 and bcl-2 expression in high-grade B-cell lymphomas: correlation with survivial time. *Br J Cancer* 69:337–339, 1994
43. Aas T, Borresen AL, Geisler S, et al: Specific p53 mutations are associated with de novo resistance to doxorubicin in breast cancer patients. *Nature Med* 2:811–814, 1996
44. Rusch V, Klimstra V, Venkatramen E, et al: Aberrant p53 expression predicts clinical resistance to cisplatin based chemotherapy in locally advanced non-small cell lung cancer. *Cancer Res* 55:5038–5042, 1992
45. Hamada M, Fujiwara T, Hizuta A, et al: The p53 gene is a potent determinant of chemosensitivity and radiosensitivity in gastric and colorectal cancers. *J Cancer Res Clin Oncol* 122:360–365, 1996
46. Dohner H, Fischer K, Bentz M, et al: p53 gene deletion predicts for poor survival and non-response to therapy with purine analogs in chronic B-cell leukemia. *Blood* 85:1580–1589, 1995
47. Wang Q, Beck WT: Transcriptional suppression of multidrug resistance-associated protein (MRP) gene expression by wild-type p53. *Cancer Res* 58:5768–5771, 1998
48. Zhou G, Kuo MT: Wild-type p53-mediated induction of rat mdr 1b expression by the anticancer drug daunorubicin. *J Biol Chem* 273:15387–15394, 1998
49. Simonian PL, Grillot DA, Nunez G: bcl-2 and bcl-XL can differentially block chemotherapy associated cell death. *Blood* 90:1208–1216, 1997
50. Strobel T, Swanson L, Korsmeyer S, et al: BAX enhances paclitaxel-induced apoptosis through a p53 independent pathway. *Proc Natl Acad Sci USA* 93:14094, 1996 (abstr)
51. Lictra E, Todd MB, Dipaola RS: Vinblastine or paclitaxel enhance mitoxantrone antitumor activity in a sequence dependent manner in association with BCL-2 phosphorylation. *Proc Am Soc Clin Oncol* 17:247, 1998 (abstr)
52. Citron ML, Berry DA, Cirrincione C, et al: Randomized trial of dose-dense versus conventionally scheduled and sequential versus concurrent combination chemotherapy as postoperative adjuvant treatment of node positive primary breast cancer: first report of Intergroup trial C9741/Cancer and Leukemia Group B Trial 9741. *J Clin Oncol* 21:1431–1439, 2003
53. Bonadonna G, Valagussa R: Dose-response effect of adjuvant chemotherapy in breast cancer. *N Engl J Med* 304:10–15, 1981
54. Hensley ML, Schuchter LM, Lindley C, et al: American Society of Clinical Oncology clinical practice guidelines for the use of chemotherapy and radiotherapy protectants. *J Clin Oncol* 10:3333–3355, 1999
55. Bregni M, Sierna S, Magni M, et al: Circulating hemopoietic progenitors mobilized by cancer chemotherapy and by rhGM-

CSF in the treatment of high-grade non-Hodgkin's lymphoma. *Leukemia* 5(suppl 1):123–127, 1991

56. Cooper DL, Seropian S: Autologous stem cell transplantation, in DeVita VT, Hellman S, Rosenberg SA (eds.): *Cancer: Principles and Practice of Oncology* (ed 6). Philadelphia, Lippincott, 2001, pp 2767–2778
57. Vokes EE, Weichselbaum RR: Concomitant chemoradiotherapy: rationale and clinical experience in patients with solid tumors. *J Clin Oncol* 8:911–934, 1990
58. Kallman RF, Rapachhietta D, Zaghloul MS: Schedule dependent therapeutic gain from the combination of fractionated irradiation plus c-DDP and 5-FU or plus C-DDP and cyclophosphamide in C3H/Km mouse model systems. *Int J Radiat Oncol Biol Phys* 20:227–232, 1991
59. Pfeffer MR, Teicher BA, Holden SA, et al: The interaction of cisplatin plus etoposide with radiation with and without hyperthermia. *Int J Radiat Oncol Biol Phys* 19:1439–1447, 1990
60. Bleiberg H: Role of chemotherapy for advanced colorectal cancer: new opportunities. *Semin Oncol* 23:42–48, 1996
61. Piedbois P, Buyse M, Rustum Y, et al: Modulation of fluorouracil by leucovorin in advanced colorectal cancer: evidence in terms of response rate. *J Clin Oncol* 10:896–903, 1992
62. Ratain MJ: Pharmacokinetics and pharmacodynamics, in DeVita VT, Hellman S, Rosenberg SA (eds.): *Cancer: Principles and Practice of Oncology* (ed 6). Philadelphia, Lippincott-Raven, 2001, pp 335–344
63. Dorr RT, Von Hoff DD (eds.): *Cancer Chemotherapy Handbook* (ed 2). Norwalk, CT, Appleton & Lange, 1994
64. Hansten PD, Horn JR (eds.): *Drug Interactions and Updates.* Vancouver, WA, Applied Therapeutics, 1995
65. Balis FM: Pharmacokinetic drug interactions of commonly used anticancer drugs. *Clin Pharmacokinet* 11:223–235, 1986
66. Finley RS: Drug interactions in the oncology patient. *Semin Oncol Nurs* 8:95–101, 1992
67. Loadman PM, Bibby MC: Pharmacokinetic drug interactions with anticancer drugs. *Clin Pharmacokinet* 26:486–500, 1994
68. Thyss A, Milano G, Kubar J, et al: Clinical and pharmacokinetic evidence of a life-threatening interaction between methotrexate and ketoprofen. *Lancet* 1:256–258, 1986
69. Ellison NM, Servi RJ: Acute renal failure and death following sequential intermediate-dose methotrexate and 5-FU: a possible adverse effect due to concomitant indomethacin administration. *Cancer Treat Reports* 69:342–343, 1985
70. Fitzsimmons WE, Ghalie R, Kaizer H: The effect of hepatic enzyme inducers on busulfan neurotoxicity and myelotoxicity. *Cancer Chemother Pharmacol* 27:27–32, 1990
71. McCrea JB, Majumdar AK, Goldberg MR, et al: Effects of the neurokinin 1 receptor antagonist aprepitent on the pharmacokinetics of dexamethasone and methyprednisolone. *Clin Pharmacol Ther* 74:17–24, 2003
72. Hall G, Lind MJ, Huang M, et al: Intravenous infusions of ifosfamide/mesna and perturbation of warfarin anticoagulant control. *Postgrad Med J* 66:860–861, 1990
73. Tenni P, Lalich DL, Byrne MJ: Life-threatening interaction between tamoxifen and warfarin. *Br Med J* 298:93, 1989
74. Bohr VA, Phillips DH, Hanawalt PC: Heterogeneous DNA damage and repair in the mammalian genome. *Cancer Res* 47:6426–6436, 1987
75. Hilton J: Role of aldehyde dehydrogenase in cyclophosphamide-resistant L 1210 leukemia. *Cancer Res* 44:5156–5160, 1984
76. Bloommaert FA, van Kijk-Knijenburg HCM, Dijt FJ, et al: Formation of DNA adducts by the anticancer drug carboplatin: different nucleotide sequence preferences in vitro and in cells. *Biochemistry* 34:8474–8480, 1995
77. Markman M: Intraperitoneal therapy of ovarian cancer. *Semin Oncol* 25:356–360, 1998
78. Calvert AH, Newell DR, Gumbrell LA, et al: Carboplatin dosage prospect of evaluation of a simple formula based on renal function. *J Clin Oncol* 7:1748–1756, 1989
79. Culy CR, Clemett D, Wiseman LR: Oxaliplatin: a review of its pharmacological properties and clinical efficacy in metastatic colorectal cancer and its potential in other malignancies. *Drugs* 60:895–924, 2000
80. De Gramont A, Figer A, Seymour M, et al: Leucovorin and fluorouracil with or without oxaliplatin as firstline treatment in advanced colorectal cancer. *J Clin Oncol* 18:2938–2947, 2000
81. O'Reilly SM, Newlands ES, Glaser MG, et al: Temozolomide: a new oral cytotoxic chemotherapeutic agent with promising activitiy against primary brain tumors. *Eur J Cancer* 29A:940–942, 1993
82. Brock CS, Newlands ES, Wedge SR, et al: Phase I trial of temozolomide using an extended continuous oral schedule. *Cancer Res* 58:4367–4367, 1998
83. Holt GA (ed.): *Food and Drug Interactions: A Health Care Professional's Guide.* Chicago, Precept Press, 1992
84. Zhang H, D'Arpe P, Liu LF: A model for tumor cell killing by topoisomerase poisons. *Cancer Cells* 2:23–27, 1990
85. Zwelling LA: Topoisomerase II as a target of antileukemia drugs: a review of controversial areas. *Hematol Pathol* 3:101–112, 1989
86. Fisher GR, Patterson LH: Lack of involvement of reactive oxygen in the cytotoxicity of mitoxantrone, CI941 and ametantrone in MCF-7 cells: comparison with doxorubicin. *Cancer Chemother Pharmacol* 30:451–458, 1992
87. Forssen EA, Coulter DM, Proffitt RT: Selective in vivo localization of daunorubicin small unilamellar vesicles in solid tumors. *Cancer Res* 56:2066–2075, 1996
88. Product information: Doxil. Menlo Park, CA, Sequus Pharmaceuticals, 1995
89. Chu E, Mota AC, Fogarasi MC: Antimetabolites, in DeVita VT, Hellman S, Rosenberg SA (eds.): *Cancer: Principles and Practice of Oncology* (ed 6). Philadelphia, Lippincott, 2001, pp 388–415
90. Evans WE, Crom WR, Yalowich J: Methotrexate, in Evans WE, Schentag JJ, Juskow J (eds.): *Applied Pharmacokinetics: Principles of Therapeutic Drug Monitoring* (ed 2). Spokane, WA, Applied Therapeutics, 1986, pp 1009–1056
91. Stoller RG, Hande KR, Jacobs SA, et al: Use of plasma pharmacokinetics to predict and prevent methotrexate toxicity. *N Engl J Med* 297:630–634, 1977
92. Grindley GB, Shih C, Barnett CJ, et al: LY231514, a novel pyrrolopyrimidine antifolate that inhibits thymidylate synthase. *Proc Am Assoc Cancer Res* 33:411, 1993 (abstr 2451)
93. Niyikiza C: LY231514 (MTA) safety analysis, 3 December 1999. Submitted to the FDA as a Serial Number 95 to IND #40,061. On file
94. Diasio RB, Schuetz JD, Wallace HJ, et al: Dihydrofluorouracil, a fluorouracil catabolite with antitumor activity in murine and human cells. *Cancer Res* 45:4900–4903, 1985
95. Burger AJ, Mannino S: 5-fluorouracil-induced coronary vasospasm. *Am Heart J* 114:433–436, 1987
96. Budman DR, Meropol NJ, Reigner B, et al: Preliminary studies of a novel oral fluoropyrimidine carbamate: capecitabine. *J Clin Oncol* 16:1795–1802, 1998
97. Baccanari DP, Davis ST, Knick V, et al: 5-Ethynyluraci (766C85): a potent modulator of the pharmacokinetics and antitumor efficacy of 5-fluorouracil. *Proc Natl Acad Sci USA* 90:11064, 1993 (abstr)
98. Baker WJ, Royer GL, Weiss RB: Cytarabine and neurologic toxicity. *J Clin Oncol* 9:679–693, 1991
99. Baker CH, Banzon J, Bollinger JM, et al: 2′-deoxy-2′-methylenecytidine and 2′-dexoy-2′, 2′-difluorocytidine 5′-diphosphate:

potent mechansim-based inhibitors of ribonucleotide reductase. *J Med Chem* 34:1879–1884, 1991
100. Hue YF, Reitz J: Gemcitabine: a cytidine analogue active against solid tumors. *Am J Health-Syst Pharm* 54:162–170, 1997
101. Montgomery JA, Hewson K: Nucleosides of 2-fluoroadenine. *J Med Chem* 12:498, 1969
102. Cheson BD, Vena D, Foss F, et al: Neurotoxicity of purine analogs: a review. *J Clin Oncol* 12:2216–2228, 1994
103. Weiss RB, Freiman J, Kweder SL, et al: Hemolytic anemia after fludarabine therapy for chronic lymphocytic leukemia. *J Clin Oncol* 16:1885–1889, 1998
104. Kawasaki H, Carrera CJ, Piro LD, et al: Relationship of deoxycytidine kinase and cytoplasmic 5′-nucleotidase to the chemotherapeutic efficacy of 2-chlorodeoxyadenosine. *Blood* 81:597–602, 1994
105. Estey EH, Kurzrock R, Kantarjian HM, et al: Treatment of hairy cell leukemia with 2-chlorodeoxyadenosine (2-CdA). *Blood* 79:882–895, 1992
106. Juliusson G, Hedlal D, Hippe E, et al: Subcutaneous injections of 2-chlorodeoxyadenosine for symptomatic hairy cell leukemia. *J Clin Oncol* 13:989–999, 1995
107. Tallman MS, Hakimian D, Zonzig C, et al: Cladribine in the treatment of relapsed or refractory chronic lymphocytic leukemia. *J Clin Oncol* 13:983–995, 1995
108. Cheson B: Immunologic and immunosuppressive complications of purine analogue therapy. *J Clin Oncol* 13:2431, 1995
109. Plunkett W, Gandhi V: Cellular metabolism of nucleoside analogs in CLL: implications for drug development, in Cheson BD (ed): *Chronic Lymphocytic Leukemia: Scientific Advances and Clinical Developments.* New York, Marcel Dekker, 1993, pp 197–214
110. Kraut EH, Neff JC, Bouroncle BA, et al: Immunosuppressive effects of pentostatin. *J Clin Oncol* 8:848–865, 1990
111. Nelson RL: The comparative clinical pharmacology and pharmacokinetics of vindisine, vincristine, and vinblastine in human patients with cancer. *Med Pediatr Oncol* 10:115–127, 1982
112. Schiff PB, Fant J, Horowitz SB: Promotion of microtubule assembly in vitro by taxol. *Nature* 22:665–667, 1979
113. Rowisnky EK, Burke PJ, Karp JE, et al: Phase I clinical and pharmacokinetic study of taxol. *Cancer Res* 49:4640–4647, 1989
114. Extra JM, Rousseau F, Bruno R, et al: Phase I and pharmacokinetic study of taxotere (NSC 628503) given as a short intravenous infusion. *Cancer Res* 53:1037–1042, 1993
115. Citardi M, Rowinsky EK, Schaefer KL, et al: Sequence-dependent cytotoxicity between cisplatin and the antimicrotubule agents taxol and vincristine. *Proc Am Assoc Cancer Res* 31:2431, 1990 (abstr)
116. Weiss RB, Donehower RC, Wiernik PH, et al: Hypersensitivity reactions from taxol. *J Clin Oncol* 8:1263–1268, 1990
117. Chevallier B, Fumoleau P, Kerbrat P, et al: Docetaxel is a major cytotoxic drug for the treatment of advanced breast cancer. *J Clin Oncol* 13:314–322, 1995
118. Ibrahmin NK, Desai N, Legha S, et al: Phase I and pharmacokinetic study of ABI-007, a Cremophor-free, protein-stabilized, nanoparticle formulation of paclitaxel. *Clin Cancer Res* 8:1038–1044, 2002
119. O'Shaughnessy J, Tjulandin S, Davidson N, et al: ABI-007 (Abraxane), a nanoparticle-bound (nab) paclitaxel demonstrates superior efficacy vs. taxol in MBC: a phase III trial. 25th Annual San Antonio Breast Cancer Symposium, San Antonio, TX, December 3–6, 2003 (abstr)
120. Wolff AC, Donehower RC, Carducci MK, et al: Phase I study of docasahexaenoic acid–paclitaxel: a taxane fatty acid conjugate with a unique pharmacology and toxicity profile. *Clin Cancer Res* 9:3589–3597, 2003
121. Seidman AD: New advances in taxanes therapy. National Comprehensive Cancer Network 9th Annual Conference, Hollywood, FL, March 10–14, 2004 (presentation)
122. Yang L, Rowe RC, Liu LF: Identification of DNA topoisomerase II as an intracellular target of antitumor epipodophyllotoxins in simian virus 40–infected monkey cells. *Cancer Res* 45:5872–5876, 1985
123. Jones SF, Burris HA: Topoisomerase I inhibitors: topotecan and irinotecan. *Cancer Pract* 4:51–53, 1996
124. Rothenberg ML, Kuhn JG, Burris HA, et al: Phase I and pharmacokinetic trial of weekly CPT-11. *J Clin Oncol* 11:2194–2204, 1993
125. Stearns ME, Tew KD: Antimicrotubule effects of estramustine, an antiprostatic tumor drug. *Cancer Res* 45:3891–3897, 1985
126. Singhal S, Mehta J, Desikan R, et al: Antitumor activity of thalidomide in refractory multiple myeloma. *N Engl J Med* 341:1564–1571, 1999
127. Ciardiello F: Epidermal growth factor receptor tyrosine kinase inhibitors as anticancer agents. *Drugs* 60(suppl 1):25–32, 2000
128. Druker BJ, Talpaz M, Resta DJ, et al: Efficacy and safety of a specific inhibitor of bcr-abl tyrosine kinase in CML. *N Engl J Med* 344:1031–1037, 2001
129. Talpaz M, Silver RT, Druker B, et al: A phase II study of STI 571 in adult patients with Philadelphia chromosome positive chronic myeloid leukemia in accelerated phase. *Blood* 96:469a, 2000 (abstr)
130. Blanke CD, von Mehren M, Joensuu H, et al: Evaluation of the safety and efficacy of an oral molecularly-targeted therapy, STI571, in patients with unresectable or metastatic gastrointestinal stromal tumors (GISTS) expressing c-KIT (CD117). *Proc Am Soc Clin Oncol* 20:367, 2001 (abstr)
131. Culy CR, Faulds D: Gefininib. *Drugs* 62:2237–2248, 2002
132. Herbst RS, Maddox AM, Rothenberg ML, et al: Selective oral epidermal growth factor receptor tyrosine kinase inhibitor ZD1839 is generally well-tolerated and has activity in non-small cell lung cancer and other solid tumors: results of a phase I trial. *J Clin Oncol* 20:3815–3825, 2002
133. Baselga J, Rischin D, Ranson M, et al: Phase I safety, pharmacokinetic, and pharmacodynamic trial of ZD1839, a selective oral epidermal growth factor receptor tyrosine kinase inhibitor, in patients with five selected solid tumor types. *J Clin Oncol* 20:4292–4302, 2002
134. Miller VA, Johnson DH, Krug LM, et al: Pilot trial of the epidermal growth factor inhibitor gefitinib plus carboplatin and paclitaxel in patients with stage IIIB or IV non-small cell lung cancer. *J Clin Oncol* 21:2094–2100, 2003
135. Adams J: The proteasome: structure, function and role in the cell. *Cancer Treat Rev* 29(suppl 1):3–9, 2003
136. Yang HH, Ma MK, Vescio RA, Berenson J: Overcoming drug resistance in multiple myeloma: the emergence of therapeutic approaches to induce apoptosis. *J Clin Oncol* 21:4239–4247, 2003
137. Center for Drug Evaluation and Research. Application number 21–602 Medical Review. *www.fda.gov/cder/approval/index.htm.* Accessed March 21, 2004
138. Jaiyesimi IA, Buzdar AU, Decker DA, et al: Use of tamoxifen for breast cancer: twenty-eight years later. *J Clin Oncol* 13:513–529, 1995
139. Fisher B, Costantino JP, Wickerham DL, et al: Tamoxifen for prevention of breast cancer: report of the National Surgical Adjuvant Breast and Bowel Project P-1 study. *J Natl Cancer Inst* 90:1371–1388, 1998
140. Loprinzi CL, Ellison NM, Schaid DJ, et al: Controlled trial of megestrol acetate for treatment of cancer anorexia and cachexia. *J Natl Cancer Inst* 82:1127–1132, 1990

141. Howell A, Osborne CK, Morris C, Wakeling AE: ICI 182,780 (Faslodex): development of a novel, "pure" antiestrogen. *Cancer* 89:817–825, 2000
142. Robertson JFR, Osborne CK, Howell A, et al: Fulvestrant versus anastrozole for the treatment of advanced breast carcinoma in postmenopausal women. *Cancer* 98:229–238, 2003
143. Brogden RN, Chrisp P: Flutamide: a review of its pharmacodynamic, pharmacokinetic properties and therapeutic use in advanced prostatic cancer. *Drugs Aging* 1:104–118, 1991
144. Lippman S, Parkinson D, Itri L, et al: 13-*cis*-Retinoic acid and interferon alpha-2a: effective combination therapy for advanced squamous cell carcinoma of the skin. *J Natl Cancer Inst* 84:235–241, 1992
145. Hong WK, Endicott J, Itri LM, et al: 13-*cis*-Retinoic acid in the treatment of oral leukoplakia. *N Engl J Med* 315:1501–1505, 1986
146. Warrell RR: All-*trans*-retinoic acid, in *American Society of Clinical Oncology Educational Book*, 28th Annual Meeting, San Diego, May 17–19, 1992, pp 107–112
147. Zhang P, Wang SY, Hu XH: Arsenic trioxide treated 72 cases of acute promyelocytic leukemia. *Chin J Hematol* 17:58, 1996
148. Soignet S, Kantarjian H, Frankel S, et al. Arsenic trioxide in acute promyelocytic leukemia: results of initial U.S. pilot and multicenter trials. *Blood* 92(suppl):483a, 1998
149. Soignet SL, Maslak P, Wang Z-G, et al: Complete remission after induction of non-terminal differentiation and apoptosis in acute promyelocytic leukemia by arsenic trioxide. *N Engl J Med* 339:1341–1348, 1998
150. Westervelt P, Pollock J, Haug J, et al: Response and toxicity associated with dose escalation of arsenic trioxide in the treatment of resistant acute promyelocytic leukemia. *Blood* 90(suppl 1):249b, 1997
151. Warrel RP Jr, Chanel S, Ho R, Soignet S: Leukocytosis and retinoic syndrome in patients with acute promyelocytic leukemia treated with arsenic trioxide. *Proc Am Soc Clin Oncol* 18:21a, 1999 (abstr)

CHAPTER 16

Chemotherapy: Principles of Administration

Beth Kelly Hayden, RN, BSN, MBA
Michelle Goodman, RN, MS

Chemotherapy Administration

Chemotherapy is administered in a variety of care settings. The majority of cancer patients, however, receive systemic chemotherapy in a hospital-based outpatient center, physician office setting, or freestanding infusion clinic. Others may receive their chemotherapy at home. Few individuals actually require hospitalization for chemotherapy, despite the fact that treatment regimens are currently more aggressive and dose intensive in nature. Hospital admission is generally reserved for patients who require intensive monitoring or who are acutely ill. Even bone marrow transplant and peripheral blood stem cell transplant programs are moving to the outpatient setting. The shift to outpatient ambulatory care services has grown out of the need for more efficient and economical healthcare delivery systems as hospitals cope with a largely managed care environment. Indeed, managed care has virtually replaced indemnity insurance reimbursement. Over the past few years, Medicare reimbursement rules and regulation changes have presented a tremendous challenge, especially in the ambulatory setting.[1] Oncology nurses are challenged with the increased responsibility of coordinating quality patient care with limited resources and support. Through team building and working with other disciplines, the nurse must effectively assess and develop a plan of care that ensures continuity regardless of the care setting. The real challenge lies in finding ways to promote self-care in an aging population with limited personal, financial, and social resources. This chapter deals with both basic and advanced principles of chemotherapy administration. It focuses on clinical practice and methods of drug delivery, including vascular access devices (VADs).

Table 16-1 Institutional Policies and Procedures for Chemotherapy Administration

- Staff education for chemotherapy and other specialty procedures (i.e., vascular access devices [VADs], Ommaya reservoirs)
- Chemotherapy administration (all routes)
- Mechanisms for prevention and reporting of drug and dosing errors
- Vesicant management
- Allergic reactions
- Safe drug handling and disposal
- Patient and family education
- Management of VADs
- Documentation methods (extravasation record)
- Coordination of home care
- Outcome standards
- Oncology quality-improvement process

Professional Qualifications

Educational guidelines for nurses administering chemotherapy are almost universally implemented in a variety of practice settings. The Intravenous Nurses' Society, the Oncology Nursing Society, and the American Society of Clincal Oncology have all published position statements regarding the administration of antineoplastic agents.[2–5]

Basic qualifications for nurses administering antineoplastic agents include the following:

- Current licensure as a registered nurse
- Certification in CPR
- Intravenous therapy skills
- Educational preparation and demonstrated knowledge in all areas related to antineoplastic drugs, including pharmacology, drug preparation, drug disposition, metabolism, elimination, symptom management, various drug interactions, and side effects
- Demonstrated knowledge of prevention of medication errors and the skill of drug administration
- Ongoing education and competency assessment
- Knowledge of policies and procedures related to chemotherapy and biotherapy administration (Table 16-1)

Formal instruction in chemotherapy administration techniques and certification programs that have both a didactic and clinical component are essential to ensure quality patient care as well as to achieve and maintain high safety standards. Chemotherapy certification also provides proof of formalized training and skill demonstration, which is extremely important from a professional liability perspective. Antineoplastic agents have serious — even life-threatening — side effects, and it is in the best interests of the patient, nurse, and institution that educational preparation be obtained, maintained, and documented. Additionally, clinically oriented policies and procedures that are part of ongoing quality improvement help to provide a firm practical and legal foundation for this aspect of oncology nursing practice.

Handling Hazardous Drugs

Exposure to hazardous drugs is known to be potentially dangerous to one's health. Hazardous drugs may include cytotoxic, antiviral, biological, or immunosuppressive agents. Direct exposure to cytotoxic agents can occur during admixture, administration, or handling, and involves inhalation, ingestion, or absorption. The drugs are known to be mutagenic, teratogenic, and carcinogenic. Additionally, exposure has been reported to result in rashes, skin discolorations, scarring, blurred vision, and dizziness. Guidelines containing recommendations to prevent cytotoxic drug exposure of personnel and the environment have been established by the Occupational Safety and Health Administration (OSHA), Oncology Nursing Society, and American Society of Hospital Pharmacists. Detailed drug handling guidelines are outlined in Table 16-2.[6–9]

Table 16-2 Hazardous Drug Handling Guidelines

Preparation

- Don a disposable gown that is lint-free, low- or nonpermeable, long-sleeved, cuffed, and solid-fronted.
- Don a pair of powder-free, thick, surgical-quality latex gloves, ensuring that the cuffs of the gloves overlap the cuffs of the gown.
- Admix all cytotoxic drugs in a class II biological safety cabinet (vertical air flow) that meets national standards and is inspected appropriately.
- Use a disposable, plastic-backed liner for the preparation area and appropriate equipment such as Luer-Lock syringes.
- Clean the cabinet daily with 70% alcohol, and decontaminate it weekly or if spills occur.
- Use aseptic technique.
- Take care to avoid drug dispersement by venting vials, handling ampules carefully, avoiding overfilling of containers, and adding diluents slowly.
- Attach and prime IV tubing before adding the cytotoxic drug to the IV solution.
- Wipe all syringes and containers, and label them appropriately, including a warning label indicating that the contents are cytotoxic.
- Do not clip or recap needles; discard all sharps in an appropriately labeled, puncture-proof container.
- Discard protective clothing and used materials in a separate trash bag labeled "cytotoxic."
- Wash hands.

Administration

- Receive appropriately labeled cytotoxic drugs in clean, dry syringes or bags of IV fluids inside zipper-seal plastic bags. Inspect bags before opening to ensure no spillage in the bag.
- Wash hands. If dripping or splashing can occur, don a disposable gown that is lint-free, low- or nonpermeable, long-sleeved, cuffed, and solid-fronted.
- Don a pair of powder-free, thick, surgical-quality latex gloves, ensuring that the cuffs of the gloves overlap the cuffs of the gown, if a gown is being worn.
- Place a plastic-backed absorbent pad over the work area to absorb any drips.
- Use intravenous administration sets and syringes with Luer-Lock fittings.
- If the administration set is not attached to the intravenous fluids and primed by the pharmacist, it should be attached and primed with caution to prevent exposure of the drug to the environment. It may be primed into a gauze pad inside a zipper-seal bag, or it may be piggybacked to plain fluids and primed by retrograde flow ("back-primed").
- Secure all connections and Y-sites with tape.
- Keep a gauze pad at hand to wipe droplets off Y-sites or connecting points.
- Do not expel air from syringes. If air is in a syringe, hold it in such a way that the air is up near the plunger and simply stop pushing on the plunger when all of the drug is injected.
- Do not use intravenous bottles with venting tubes.
- Monitor administration sets and connection sites for leakage.
- Do not clip or recap needles. Discard the needle-syringe unit into a convenient and appropriately labeled, puncture-proof container.
- Discard all gauze, tubing, bags, bottles, etc., in appropriately labeled bags, and seal. Remove gown and gloves and discard in a similar manner.
- Wash hands.

General Handling and Disposal

- Dispose of all sharps, containers, and cytotoxic waste according to appropriate state and federal guidelines (usually, incineration or burial in a hazardous waste landfill).
- Contain all grossly contaminated linen of treated patients within 48 hours in labeled double bags, and wash twice (same procedure as for infectious wastes).
- Obtain spill kits, and place them in the admixture and administration areas.
- Clean up spills using available kits and disposable towels or sponges. For large spills, double gloving is recommended.
- If direct exposure occurs, immediately rinse the area with running water. For eye exposure, rinse with an eye wash solution or sterile saline.
- Report all episodes of exposure to employee health or the equivalent resource.

Personnel

- Identify all personnel who handle cytotoxic drugs.
- Educate and train personnel in proper drug handling.
- Establish a mechanism to monitor cytotoxic drug handling practices, from receipt through disposal.
- Provide ready access to information regarding hazardous drugs.
- Address pregnancy and medical surveillance issues.
- Monitor all spills and occurrences of direct exposure through a quality-improvement program.
- Develop patient education materials as needed, particularly for use in the home.

Data from Oncology Nursing Society[3]; American Society of Hospital Pharmacists[6]; Occupational Safety and Health Administration.[8]

Personnel policies regarding pregnancy are quite varied, despite OSHA's suggestion that appropriate protective practices should reduce any potential reproductive hazards.[8] While OSHA recommends that employees be informed of potential risks and, if necessary, reassigned to other duties, it is not uncommon to find institutional policies that prohibit pregnant or lactating women from working with hazardous drugs, particularly in drug preparation. These precautionary measures are undertaken to protect the mother and developing fetus from the potential effects of drug exposure and the institution from potential liability.

Another personnel issue is medical surveillance. Although the 1995 OSHA guidelines recommend that institutions have a medical surveillance program in place, a survey of 263 outpatient clinic nurses revealed that only 46% of the sites reported any type of medical monitoring. The most common method of surveillance identified was a preemployment physical.[10]

Patient education regarding hazardous drug handling is important so that patients and family members understand why gloves and gowns are being worn and do not feel alienated by the practice. Education is a crucial element if chemotherapy is being provided in the home setting, as family members need to be instructed in drug containment practices. The patient should be provided with written instructions specifying that gloves be worn when working with the medications, used materials be placed in the provided containers, care be taken to avoid direct exposure, spills be cleaned up with the spill kit provided, and direct external exposure be managed with copious flushing and washing. Despite proof that exposure to cytotoxic drugs can be harmful, a large percentage of health professionals continue to disregard personal protective measures.[7,10] There appears to be a perception that low-level exposure is not harmful, as no absolute scientific quantification of exposure has been defined. However, studies have consistently found evidence of surface contamination. One study found that cytotoxic drugs were detected in 65% of the administration area samples and 75% of the pharmacy samples.[11] It is also important to realize that the institution may incur stiff financial penalties if OSHA ascertains noncompliance with established guidelines. The minimum standards to be met include (1) knowledge of the latest scientific information, (2) established policies and procedures, and (3) ongoing monitoring to ensure compliance and continuous quality improvement.

Patient and Family Education

Educating patients and their family members about cancer is usually initiated by the physician, who explains the diagnosis of cancer, treatment options, their risks and benefits, alternatives, and prognosis. Nurses are responsible for giving the patient and family specific information about treatment side effects and measures to recognize and minimize their consequences. Teaching self-care measures is critically important given the often limited resources and support services available. Self-care guides such as those detailed by Yarbro et al. are ideal because they can be photocopied, individualized, and given to the patient to reinforce teaching.[12] Identifying problems or side effects that a patient might experience due to the chemotherapy as a whole rather than addressing potential problems for each drug separately is most efficient, due to the wide range of side effects encountered. Some basic steps to follow when planning and implementing patient education appear in Table 16-3.

Safe Practice Considerations

One of the primary responsibilities of the nurse in the delivery of chemotherapy is to ensure that the correct dose of the appropriate drug is given to the appropriate individual. Despite the fact that safeguards are in place, serious medication errors do occur. Such tragic events are regrettable but not so remarkable when one considers the number of chemotherapy doses given and the number of patients treated. The overall medication error rate is estimated to be 2%–10%.[13,14] However, one recent survey revealed that 63% of the respondents reported that errors had occurred at their workplace. In addition, only 3% of the errors were reported to drug manufacturers or national databases, though most were reported internally.[14]

As practitioners, it is important to consider the potential origins and the settings in which drug errors are likely to occur. Table 16-4 identifies common types of medication errors. Combinations of complicated regimens of potentially lethal drugs are currently being given in high doses in a variety of settings. Consequently, even though the caregiver may recognize a cumulative dose as being higher than the usual dose, he or she may still fail to question the order. In addition, institutions are being pressured to dramatically scale back costs. As resources diminish and individuals are required to do more with less, the risk of error increases. In some settings, in an effort to reduce expenditures, highly trained and experienced nurse practitioners are being replaced by individuals who are less qualified, which increases the possibility of error.

In an effort to reduce the risk for drug error, the following safeguards should be instituted wherever chemotherapy is admixed and administered.

Table 16-3 Chemotherapy Patient Education Guidelines

Preparation

- Accompany the physician when the treatment plan is explained to the patient and family to better reinforce what they have been told.
- Identify learning needs and specific written instructions for prevention and management of side effects.
- Emphasize the importance of self-care strategies and provide the patient and family with self-care guidelines that are clearly written at an eighth-grade level of understanding.
- Determine whether audiovisuals are appropriate teaching aids. Test equipment and establish a time for the patient and family to view them.
- Review policies, procedures, and documentation forms.

Planning

- Know the basics about the patient to be taught and the goal of the treatment plan. Review the chart. It is especially important to know if the patient speaks and reads English, if that is the language being used.
- If possible, separate the teaching session from the actual drug administration procedure.
- Encourage the patient to have a family member present during instruction sessions.
- Assemble all teaching materials, including the calendar, prescriptions, drug information sheets, and other teaching materials, before you begin, to avoid interruptions.

Presentation

- Introduce yourself and your purpose.
- Determine if the patient has any specific questions or concerns to address before proceeding.
- Discuss the treatment process (i.e., starting intravenous infusion, administering drugs, length of time, immediate events, expected follow-up, monitoring side effects, and home care). Describe any sensations the patient might have during the infusion/injection (e.g., coolness, perirectal burning, light-headedness, nasal stuffiness).
- Describe the potential side effects and interventions to minimize their consequences. Include specific information about what to look for, what is normal, how to take a temperature, where to buy a wig, which mouth care regimen to use, and other appropriate recommendations. Provide written information regarding when to call the physician or nurse.
- Avoid overloading the patient with information about rare or unusual risks of chemotherapy. Give written information regarding this aspect of his or her treatment and elaborate where appropriate.
- Ensure that informed consent (written or verbal) has been obtained.
- Maintain a responsive atmosphere that is open to questioning.
- Give written instructions regarding activity, diet, hygiene, medications, and other self-care behaviors for the patient to follow for the next few days or weeks.
- Recommend useful Internet sites for education reinforcement.

Follow-up

- Document the encounter and the patient's response. (See Chapter 17, Figure 17-1.)
- Question the patient to assess his or her understanding of the information imparted.
- When possible, observe the patient to determine if his or her actions indicate an understanding of the information (e.g., hydration, mouth care, medications).
- It is optimal to contact the patient within 24 hours of drug administration to determine if there are any questions or problems to be resolved, especially if the patient and nurse are no longer together in the same setting (i.e., hospital or home).

1. Only the most senior physician directly responsible for the care of the patient and most familiar with the drug regimen and dosing schedule should sign the chemotherapy orders.
2. The drug name should be written (typed) clearly and in full. Abbreviations are to be avoided, especially where drugs with similar-sounding names are concerned.
3. When the drug order is written (usually in triplicate), the drug name, dose in mg/m^2, dose to be given, total daily dose, and number of days that the dose is to be given are indicated on the order sheet.
4. The cumulative dose for the course of treatment is not written on the order sheet to avoid the possibility of that dose being given each day by mistake.

Table 16-4 Medication Errors

Type of Errors	Contributing Factors	Risk Management Strategies
• Underdosing and overdosing • Schedule and timing errors • Infusion rate errors • Improper preparation • Drugs given to the wrong patient	• Stress • Understaffing • Unclear orders • Lack of experience	• Comprehensive, ongoing training • Adherence to the "five rights" of medication administration • Adequate staffing • Two forms of patient identification

Data from Schulmeister.[14]

5. A copy of the original order written by the physician is sent to the pharmacy for drug preparation. It is most important that the drug order not be transcribed or rewritten before it reaches the pharmacy.
6. Once the order reaches the pharmacy, the order is checked by the pharmacist against previous orders. If the drug or dose varies from the previous order, the order should be verified. If the patient is on a research protocol, the pharmacy staff should have a copy of the protocol to verify the order.
7. When writing the order for the drug, eliminate the use of trailing zeros, because "100.0" may be misread as "1000." Spelling out the amount as "one hundred" is also preferred. Likewise, include a zero prior to the decimal point (0.25 mg) to avoid overdosing.
8. In most settings, computer-generated labels are used. Ideally, the computer should be programmed *not* to print the label if the dose/cumulative dose are out of the ordinary and customary range. To override the computer and print the label would then require verification and authorization.
9. Drugs should be dispensed in plastic zipper-lock bags large enough to hold all the drugs to be given to one patient. Drugs intended for one patient might be confused with another patient's order if they are not isolated in a bag.
10. Once the pharmacist signs off on the drug, verifying that it is the right dose of the right drug for the right patient, the complete order is given to the nurse. The nurse then checks the drugs against the original written order to again confirm the accuracy of the order prior to treating the patient.
11. If possible, the person preparing the drug should not be the same person double-checking the order. If a nurse is working alone in a clinic, the physician should be available to double-check the drugs prior to administration.
12. Everyone responsible for drug preparation and administration (pharmacist, pharmacy technicians, and nurses) needs to be properly trained in the specialty of chemotherapy drug preparation.
13. If the patient is receiving chemotherapy at home, the nurse must have proof of certification by an approved chemotherapy administration program.
14. Policies and procedures for preventing and reporting drug errors are reviewed regularly according to institutional policy and procedure.
15. Policies and procedures for drug preparation and administration should also be reviewed on an annual basis.
16. Everyone responsible for chemotherapy drug preparation and administration should be empowered with the ability to question the order. If any question arises related to the drug, dose, route, or schedule, the individual must clarify the order and be encouraged to do so.
17. Any protocol involving unusual dosing patterns or dose-intensive regimens should be reviewed carefully by all parties. No one should be expected to prepare or administer a drug with a dose-intensive schedule without the opportunity to review the protocol at least 24 hours in advance, especially if the study involves an investigational agent.
18. Establish and implement safe practice staffing guidelines.

It is not uncommon in a busy outpatient clinic for a nurse to have no prior knowledge that a patient is beginning a new chemotherapy protocol before the patient appears in the clinic ready to be treated. This situation is not optimal because the nurse has no time to review the protocol and to prepare the patient's learning packet. Errors can be made whenever drugs are given in a hurried and unprepared manner. Communication between the physician, pharmacist, and nurse is critical to providing a safe level of care.

Drug Administration

Dose Calculation

The dose of drug to be administered is generally based on the individual's body surface area, usually expressed in milligrams per square meter or milligrams per kilogram. The patient's body surface area is usually determined by a height and weight nomogram. There is controversy regarding the accuracy and safety of this method because some patients may have been heavily pretreated and therefore unable to tolerate higher doses of drugs or dose-intensive regimens. In addition, many patients are clinically obese, which is defined as weighing 30% or more over ideal body weight. Empiric decreases in the doses of anticancer agents given to obese patients based on ideal body weight are not supported by available data.[15] Georgiadis et al. found no significant association between obesity and toxicity measured primarily as white blood cell nadir.[16] Bear in mind that inappropriate dose reduction may compromise efficacy, which is particularly meaningful when the intent of treatment is cure. However, in situations where a dose reduction is necessary and the patient's weight is significantly greater than the ideal, a simple method of calculating the dose is to take the average of the ideal and actual weights. If an ideal weight table is not available, start with 100 pounds for 5 feet and add 5 pounds for each additional inch. Thus someone who is 5 feet 5 inches would ideally weigh 125 pounds. That weight, plus their actual weight divided by 2, would give the weight on which to calculate dose per square meter.

Attempts are often made to individualize the dose of a drug so that optimal therapeutic response is achieved without toxic effects. However, the outcome is generally less than ideal, and patients, especially the elderly, are frequently underdosed because of the potential for severe toxicity. It is often proposed that individual doses be calculated based on a person's physiological age rather than his or her chronological age. One example of this approach involves the application of the Calvert formula for carboplatin dosing.[17] The Calvert formula makes it possible to individualize the carboplatin dose so as to obtain a maximally effective dose with tolerable side effects.

Carboplatin is excreted by the kidneys — in particular, glomerular filtration with little excretion or reabsorption by the renal tubules. Therefore, pretreatment assessment of renal function or glomerular filtration rate (GFR) can be used to individualize carboplatin dose in adults. The GFR is essentially equivalent to the creatinine clearance, which can be estimated from the patient's age, serum creatinine, and weight by using the Cockroft-Gault method. Another factor in the Calvert formula involves the area under the curve (AUC), or target drug concentration for carboplatin. The AUC dosing correlates more closely with drug toxicity than do doses based on body surface area.[18] In the presence of impaired renal function, the delayed clearance of carboplatin would result in prolonged drug exposure (increased AUC); in patients with high renal clearance, decreased AUC could result in subtherapeutic dosing. Because AUC or carboplatin exposure, rather than toxicity, is the measurement, it is not influenced by concurrent myelosuppressive therapy or supportive treatment. The following formula is applicable in single-agent, combination therapy, or high-dose studies:

Carboplatin dose (mg) = Target AUC × (GFR + 25)

where

AUC = Area under the curve

GFR = Glomerular filtration rate (calculated according to the Cockroft-Gault formula)

The AUC ranges from 4 to 8 and is selected for appropriate clinical situations. For example, if the patient has had prior treatment or is receiving carboplatin in combination with another myelosuppressive agent, an AUC of 4 to 6 might be selected. If the patient is receiving carboplatin alone and has not been previously treated with ablative chemotherapy, an AUC of 6 to 8 might be selected. It is important to note that doses in the Calvert method are total mg, not mg/m^2 of carboplatin.

Pretreatment Considerations

Table 16-5 includes specific tasks involved in antineoplastic drug administration that are applicable in all practice settings. In addition, Appendices 16A and 16B describe the dosing, efficacy, metabolism, preparation, administration precautions, and special considerations regarding the administration of the more common oral and intravenous antineoplastic agents. An important pretreatment consideration is the potential for infusion-related reactions, including hypersensitivity reactions and anaphylaxis. All emergency medication and equipment should be available and in good working order. Standing orders for emergency care should be readily available as well as appropriate personnel in the event that an emergency situation should arise. In the current practice environment, it is not uncommon for one or two nurses to be the sole providers of care in an ambulatory care setting with a clinic full of patients who have seen the physician and are receiving their medicines or waiting to begin their treatment. The physicians often see their patients and leave the clinic to do rounds in the hospital or to go to another freestanding oncology facility. Standards of practice dictate that a physician be physically available when chemotherapy is administered. This recommendation applies to all settings where drugs of an experimental nature are given but, in fact, reactions and emergency situations can arise when more commonly used drugs such as etoposide are given. The first consideration is the safety of the patient, and the policies and procedures governing the setting in which chemotherapy is given should specifically indicate that a physician should be physically present, not just available by phone.

Another pretreatment consideration involves the sequencing of various drugs to either enhance cytotoxicity or minimize toxicity to normal tissues. For example, the administration of slightly higher doses of intravenous methotrexate 1 hour prior to 5–fluorouracil (5–FU), with leucovorin rescue 24 hours later, appears to enhance the cell kill effects of both methotrexate and 5–FU. Similarly, the sequence of cisplatin or carboplatin before paclitaxel induces more profound neutropenia than the alternate sequence. The incidence of neutropenia is believed to be due to the lower paclitaxel clearance rates when cisplatin or carboplatin precedes paclitaxel.[19] In addition, the cytotoxic effects of paclitaxel preceding platinol were found to be additive, whereas the reverse sequence resulted in

Table 16-5 Chemotherapy Administration Guidelines

Professional Preparation

- Maintain appropriate knowledge and skills regarding chemotherapy drug protocols and administration procedures.
- Review applicable policies and procedures.
- Review drug protocol and research guidelines.

Patient Preparation

- Verify patient identity (arm band, driver's license, verbalization of name) using two forms of patient identification (i.e., name and birth date).
- Ensure appropriate patient education.
- Confirm that appropriate laboratory tests have been completed and are within normal limits.
- Measure and record baseline vital signs.
- Verify patient's allergy history.
- Assess venous access status (i.e., need for VAD).
- Initiate pretreatment therapies, if ordered (e.g., hydration, test dosing).

Drug Preparation

- Verify drug order (including body surface area and dosage calculations).
- Obtain prepared drug, and double-check label for the correct drug, dose, route, and patient. If admixing, follow appropriate guidelines for cytotoxic drug admixture.
- Ensure rapid access to extravasation kit and medications necessary if allergic reaction occurs (parenteral diphenhydramine hydrochloride, epinephrine, and hydrocortisone should be immediately available).
- Obtain necessary supplies and equipment for safe drug administration.
- Wash hands, and don gloves and appropriate protective clothing.

Venipuncture Guidelines

- Establish work area with plastic-backed pad.
- Organize materials, needle box, syringes, flush, IV start materials, and IV fluids.
- Select needle size and type according to setting, patient's veins, and treatment to be administered.
- Determine appropriate site for venous access, avoiding:
  - Limbs with recent (i.e., 30 min) venipunctures
  - Limbs with axillary node dissections, extensive radiation therapy, or obstructive process
  - Antecubital fossa (for peripheral sticks)
  - Ecchymotic or sclerosed areas
  - Bony prominences and joints
- Ensure adequate lighting and visualization of area to be accessed.
- Remove jewelry near access site.
- Select a large vein if administering drugs known to be irritating.
- Administer vesicants only at sites designated by established policies and procedures, specifically in areas with underlying subcutaneous tissue. Areas to be avoided when administering vesicants include veins over joints, bony prominences, neurovascular bundles, tendons, and areas of existing soft tissue damage.
- For peripheral sites, begin at the most distal areas, and gradually proceed proximally.
- Utilize an appropriate sterile technique for access.
- Achieve a "clean" venipuncture and determine patency. The needle should not puncture through the back of the vein and then be resettled within the vein. There should be a brisk, immediate blood return and no swelling at the needle site.
- Secure needle with tape, but ensure visualization of the site.
- Flush needle with sterile NS or D5W to clear the line and establish patency. Observe the site at this time to ensure that swelling is not occurring at the needle site.
- Use Luer-Lok fittings for IV sets and syringes; use sterile gauze or alcohol pad for priming IV sets.

Drug Administration Guidelines

- Check patient's condition periodically during drug administration, and explain actions being taken, when appropriate.
- Monitor the status of the venous access site periodically during the process.
- If administering a vesicant, observe the site continuously throughout the injection.
- Administer antiemetics (if not already given).
- Ensure drug containment at all times. Wipe any droplets at the connector or Y-site with a gauze pad.
- Administer chemotherapy drugs as ordered, using slow, steady pressure.
- Check for a blood return every few milliliters and before and after each drug.
- Flush between each drug with sterile NS or D5W to avoid drug admixture and potential precipitation.
- When administering short-term drips or infusions, establish the infusion, taping all connections securely, and set the appropriate flow rate.
- Generally, place long-term infusions on an infusion pump.
- Flush after last drug with sterile NS or D5W.
- If appropriate, discontinue the IV needle. For peripheral sites, hold pressure manually over the site for a few minutes, then apply small, sterile dressing.
- Do not clip or recap needles.

Post Administration Guidelines

- Discard all materials (needles, syringes, bags, tubing, gown, gloves, etc.) appropriately.
- Assess patient's status and provide for follow-up:
  - *Inpatient:* Call button within reach; fluids available, etc.
  - *Outpatient:* Transportation ready; return appointment and prescriptions obtained; telephone number of physician or nurse available
  - *Home care:* Caregiver available; telephone number of nurse-on-call available
- Document all actions (flow sheets or specialized forms are recommended). (See Chapter 17.)

VAD = vascular access device; NS = normal saline; D5W = 5% dextrose in water.

pronounced antagonism.[20] A study by Clark et al. demonstrated that administering paclitaxel before carboplatin resulted in significantly greater cytotoxicity than administering the drugs in the reverse sequence.[21] The toxicity profile was *not* affected by sequence of drug administration. Therefore, to achieve the greatest efficacy with no increase in toxicity, the paclitaxel is routinely administered prior to carboplatin.

Another example of the importance of sequencing in chemotherapy administration involves the administration of doxorubicin and paclitaxel. A moderate to severe mucositis can occur when paclitaxel is given prior to doxorubicin but not when it is given in the reverse sequence. The paclitaxel-related mucosal damage concomitant with neutropenia has been thought to contribute to the development of typhlitis, which can be life-threatening. Pharmacokinetic data indicate that when paclitaxel is given immediately prior to doxorubicin, there is a 31.6% average decrease in the clearance of doxorubicin, which contributes greatly to profound neutropenia.[22] Based on this finding, the sequence of doxorubicin followed by paclitaxel is recommended.

Routes of Administration

Chemotherapy was designed as a systemic treatment for cancer, having the ability to travel throughout the body via the bloodstream and to damage or kill dividing cells. It is now possible to direct drugs systemically as well as to almost every anatomical region in the body. Intravenous chemotherapy remains the most common route of drug delivery, but other systemic routes include oral, intramuscular, and subcutaneous. Regional drug delivery routes include topical, intraarterial, intraperitoneal, intrapleural, intravesical, intrathecal, intraventricular, and intratumoral.

Topical

Cutaneous malignant lesions can be treated in a variety of ways, including the topical application of antineoplastic agents. This is most commonly done for cutaneous T-cell lymphoma, basal cell carcinoma, Kaposi's sarcoma, and squamous cell carcinoma. The agents used include nitrogen mustard for cutaneous T-cell lymphoma and fluorouracil for basal and squamous cell carcinomas.[23] The topical agent is usually applied once or twice daily until the lesions progress to the necrosis phase, which may take 1–3 weeks. The affected area is not washed vigorously during the treatment period. The expected result of topical antineoplastic administration is local sloughing of the affected area and eventual regranulation of normal tissue, so it is normal for the treated area to become red and tender, then to form a lesion that becomes necrotic, followed by superficial sloughing of the dead tissue and regrowth of healthy skin. It is unusual for the patient to experience any systemic side effects of the drugs unless the majority of the skin is being treated; incidences of mild, delayed side effects such as nausea have been reported.

Special nursing considerations for these patients include the following:

- Patient education, with special consideration of body image issues
- Application of the drug using cotton swabs or nonmetal applicators
- Close attention to application only in the prescribed (affected) area
- Careful avoidance of the eyes, nose, mouth, or other areas close to mucous membranes
- Utilization of safe drug-handling practices (e.g., gloves and strict attention to drug containment)
- When using nitrogen mustard, having sodium thiosulfate available (to neutralize the nitrogen mustard) and applying it to areas of the skin that may be inadvertently exposed (after removal of the drug)
- Application of dressings, if prescribed
- Observation for untoward sequelae (e.g., severe burning or rashes, which may require discontinuation of therapy or subsequent dose reduction)

Oral

A variety of antineoplastic agents are now administered orally to treat numerous types of cancer (Appendix 16A). It is estimated that 25% to 30% of all new drugs in development are oral agents.[24] While oral agents offer many advantages, they also present challenges, which are listed in Table 16-6.[25,26]

The nursing responsibilities for oral drug administration include safe handling (gloves are considered acceptable if physical contact with the tablet or capsule is required) and monitoring for drug absorption and compliance with the prescribed therapy. If the patient experiences emesis immediately after drug ingestion and the pills or capsules cannot be visualized, the drug is usually not repeated. Several oral antineoplastic agents are also available in parenteral forms, providing an option for patients who are intolerant of or noncompliant with oral regimens. Other recommendations include the following:

- Prescribe one "course" at a time, to avoid inadvertent overdosing that could be life-threatening.

Table 16-6 Pros and Cons of Oral Antineoplastic Agents

Advantages	Disadvantages
• Patient convenience	• Less professional monitoring
• Eliminates the need for intravenous access	• Potential for nonadherence to the treatment plan and schedule
• Few side effects	• Risk of overdosing or underdosing
• Ease of administration	• Inconsistency of absorption
• Ability to achieve sustained blood levels	• Limited Medicare coverage
• Fewer office visits	

Data from Bedell[25]; Hartigan.[26]

- Instruct the patient to take the medication on an empty stomach with water to enhance absorption, unless the drug is tolerated better with food, as is the case with prednisone, cyclophosphamide, and tamoxifen.
- Familiarize the patient with both generic and brand names of the drug, to avoid confusion or double dosing (many physicians prefer to prescribe brand-name antineoplastic agents to avoid the possibility of the generics not being bioequivalent).
- Instruct the patient to maintain a record of drugs being taken.
- Obtain a list of any drugs currently being taken by the patient to ensure compatibility.
- Advise the patient to avoid taking any over-the-counter drugs without first checking with the physician or nurse.
- Question the patient at each visit regarding the medication (i.e., how much was taken, whether any doses were omitted, and why).
- Provide information regarding medication assistance and medication discount programs as needed.

It is important that the patient comply with the treatment regimen to maximize the goal of therapy (i.e., remission or cure). Although oral agents give the patient control over drug administration, compliance can be a problem. Studies have reported noncompliance to range from 26% to 59%, especially among patients older than 60 years of age.[26] Due to the side effects, a patient might decide to omit a dose to feel better temporarily. The patient needs to understand how important dosing and scheduling are and how critical it is that the prescribed regimen be followed exactly. With therapy such as leucovorin following methotrexate, noncompliance could be fatal. It is common for patients receiving oral antineoplastic agents to be given a calendar with the doses indicated and space to record each dose. The nurse checks the previous treatment calendar and questions the patient about any omitted doses during each encounter. The regimen can often be modified to enhance the patient's tolerance of the side effects (e.g., administering an antiemetic to minimize nausea or changing the time of dose administration).

Intramuscular and subcutaneous

The development of the biological agents (e.g., interferon, colony-stimulating factors) has increased the number of drugs given intramuscularly or subcutaneously. Subcutaneous injections of small volumes are given in the usual sites and should be rotated if given daily. Many drug manufacturers have distributed videos, charts, or posters that clearly outline the steps to follow for patients self-administering subcutaneous medications. One drug that is administered subcutaneously in a rather unique way is goserelin acetate (Zoladex). This dry drug pellet is implanted in the soft tissue of the abdomen, where it gradually is absorbed over 1 to 3 months. A local anesthetic such as an anesthetic cream or ice is usually used to minimize discomfort, as the needle is large (16-gauge).

Intravenous

The intravenous route is the most common and most reliable method of drug delivery. Detailed nursing actions concerning intravenous drug administration are included in Table 16-5 and Appendix 16B. Selection of a vascular access device (VAD), an angiocath, or a butterfly needle will be determined by the type of therapy the patient is to receive and the condition of the patient's veins. For most patients, a 21-gauge needle is adequate for extended infusions for hydration and for 3- and 4-hour infusions of chemotherapy. If an IV needs to stay in for more than 1 hour, it is best to place an angiocath that will be less likely to infiltrate and will be less traumatic to the veins. If the patient is to receive only an injection of chemotherapy and intravenous antiemetics without hydration, a 23- or 21-gauge butterfly needle is preferred because it is easy to insert into small veins and is less traumatic. The problem with small butterfly needles (25-gauge) is that the blood return is often lost because the needle is so small. When giving a vesicant, it is always better to have blood return throughout the injection, so a smaller-gauge needle is not preferable in that situation. Unfortunately, patients often have such small veins that the smaller needles are needed. In this situation, choosing an angiocath that is thin walled, with an over-the-needle cannula, permits a large internal diameter once the stylet is removed without overly traumatizing the vein.

Choosing the appropriate device is important but taking the time to find the most appropriate vein is even more important. All too often the nurse fails to assess the veins properly, fails to distend the veins sufficiently prior to attempting venipuncture, and fails to apply adequate traction on the vein to prevent the vein from rolling. If a vein is not obvious, it is advisable to apply moist heat to the arms for 5–10 minutes and have the patient drink warm liquids prior to attempting venipuncture. If the patient is known to have small, hard-to-find veins, the patient should drink four to six glasses of fluid the morning of treatment, dress warmly, and squeeze a handball for 10 minutes prior to the nurse attempting venipuncture. If the nurse has difficulty accessing an appropriate vein after one or two attempts, she should seek the assistance of a colleague. If a patient repeatedly requires more than three sticks and the plan is to have chemotherapy for an extended period of time, a VAD is appropriate. Even if a person has adequate veins, if he or she has metastatic disease and will require an access device at some point, it is appropriate to propose it early on. The longer the patient has the VAD, the longer he or she can benefit from its use.

Another issue involves the order in which chemotherapeutic agents are given. Except where sequencing is important pharmacologically, the order of drug delivery is probably not critical. However, when administering a vesicant agent, it is wiser to administer the antiemetic and any antianxiolytic agent after the vesicant. No agent, except perhaps nitrogen mustard, causes emesis in the first hour, so giving the vesicant before the antiemetic is sound practice. It is important that patients be alert and able to communicate how they are feeling throughout the injection of the vesicant. There are several reasons to give the vesicant before any other agent: (1) the venous integrity is greatest earlier in the procedure; (2) the nurse's assessment skills and the patient's level of awareness and sensitivity are most acute at the initiation of the infusion; and (3) the possibility that the vein will be irritated by other drugs (e.g., decadron) or by movement is eliminated. The idea that if the vein takes the nonvesicants without any problem, then the vesicant will infuse without difficulty, is faulty reasoning. The risk of infiltration of any IV increases over time. Often, other drugs can cause venous irritation and even spasm that can result in a loss of blood return, a major assessment criteria for safe administration of chemotherapy.

Vesicant extravasation issues. A drug is categorized according to whether it is an irritant, nonirritant, or vesicant. The most benign, inconsequential local reaction to chemotherapy is venous flare (see Color Plate 1). This reaction occurs most commonly in patients receiving doxorubicin and is characterized by a localized erythema, venous streaking, and pruritus along the injected vein. This localized allergic reaction is distinguishable from an extravasation by the absence of pain or swelling and the presence of a blood return. Once this important distinction is made, it is safe to continue injecting the agent. Flushing the vein with saline and slowing the injection rate appear to ease the symptoms, which dissipate without treatment within 20–30 minutes of the injection.

Another local tissue reaction characterized by pain, venous irritation, and chemical phlebitis can occur with certain nonvesicant chemotherapy agents. These agents, which are called *irritants,* are identified in Appendix 16B. While any drug given in concentrated form in sufficient amount can cause tissue damage if infiltrated, these agents are not associated with ulceration if infiltrated. Irritants cause intravascular irritation often accompanied by pain (described as achiness or as tightness) only during the infusion and may, as is the case with carmustine, be a function of the diluent.

The most devastating skin reactions caused by chemotherapy occur when a vesicant agent is infiltrated, causing an extravasation injury. The degree of injury to local tissues is related to the vesicant properties of the drug infiltrated, the concentration of the drug, and the amount of the drug infiltrated. For example, in an animal model, 0.2 mL of doxorubicin at a concentration of 2 mg/mL produced a 1-cm diameter lesion taking 7–8 weeks to heal.[27] By definition, an *extravasation* is the infiltration of a vesicant chemotherapeutic agent. A *vesicant* is a drug that, if infiltrated, is capable of causing pain, ulceration, necrosis, and sloughing of damaged tissue. The damage can be severe enough to result in physical deformity or a functional deficit, such as loss of joint mobility, vascularity, or tendon function (see Color Plates 2 and 3).

While a few nonantineoplastic drugs are vesicants (e.g., levophed and dilantin), the number of antineoplastic vesicants is significant; they are identified in Appendix 16B. It is critical that the nurse administering chemotherapy be aware of the drugs that are vesicants and use safety measures to try to prevent extravasation.

Prevention of extravasation. The following guidelines are suggested to minimize the risk of extravasation:

1. Be aware of certain patients at increased risk for extravasation:
   a. Patients unable to communicate to the nurse about the pain of extravasation
   b. Elderly, debilitated, or confused patients with diabetes or general vascular disease
   c. Any patient with fragile veins
2. Generally, avoid infusing vesicants over joints, bony prominences, tendons, neurovascular bundles, or the antecubital fossa.
3. Never give vesicants intramuscularly or subcutaneously.
4. Avoid giving vesicant drugs in areas where venous or lymphatic circulation is poor (e.g., operative side for a mastectomy patient, patient with superior vena cava syndrome) or in sites that have been previously irradiated.
5. Make sure the peripheral IV site is adequate and less than 24 hours old. A brisk blood return and easy flow of fluids are to be determined before administering vesicants in any IV needle or catheter (peripheral or central).
6. Visualize the needle or catheter insertion site, and observe the site continuously. (Never leave the patient unattended when administering a vesicant peripherally.)
7. When giving more than one chemotherapy agent, give the vesicant agent first.
8. Give vesicants in a steady, even flow, checking frequently (every 1–2 mL) for a blood return. When checking for a blood return, do so gently to avoid excessive pressure in the vein.
9. If a vesicant is ordered as an *infusion,* it is given through a central line only and checked every 1–2 hours in healthcare facilities and every 2–4 hours when the patient is receiving vesicant infusions in the home.
10. An extravasation kit containing all materials necessary to manage an extravasation should be available wherever vesicant agents are administered. Include a copy of the extravasation policy and procedure in the kit.

Despite these precautions, vesicant extravasation does occur. Chemotherapy drug extravasation is a known complication of cancer treatment. The incidence of extravasation has been reported to range from 0.5% to 6% of all adverse effects associated with chemotherapy.[28] Ranges of 0.3% to 4.7% were reported for patients receiving chemotherapy via an implanted vascular access port.[29]

To infiltrate a vesicant agent is traumatic for patient and nurse, but it is not an act of negligence. Often the occurrence of an extravasation is more a function of venous integrity than the administration technique. Patients should be thoroughly informed regarding the vesicant potential of the drugs they are receiving and the importance of reporting any pain, burning, or stinging during the injection.

Assessment of extravasation. Detection of a vesicant extravasation in its earliest stage is most likely to result in the least possible soft tissue damage. The nurse should be aware of the following symptoms that could indicate extravasation; it is also important to note that an extravasation can occur without any symptoms:

- Swelling—bleb formation at the injection site (most common)
- Stinging, burning, or pain at the injection site (not *always* present)
- Redness (not often seen initially)
- Lack of blood return (if this is *only* symptom, the IV should be reevaluated; if there is still no blood return, consider other options); lack of a blood return alone is not always indicative of an extravasation, as extravasation can occur even if a blood return is present

While generally considered a reliable and safe means of drug delivery, implanted ports and, less commonly, tunneled catheters do sometimes result in extravasations of vesicant agents. In the case of implanted ports, the cause of drug extravasation is usually a misplaced or displaced needle. In this situation, the drug extravasates into the port pocket or area surrounding the port. Another mechanism for drug extravasation from ports involves retrograde subcutaneous leakage from percutaneously inserted catheters obstructed by a fibrin sheath.[30,31] Extravasation may also occur into the subcutaneous tunnel, either from thrombosis and backtracking or from a damaged or fractured central venous catheter. Extravasation may also occur into the intrathoracic cavity as a complication of catheter placement.[29]

Prior to injecting or infusing a vesicant into a tunneled central venous catheter or a nontunneled centrally or peripherally placed central venous catheter (e.g., peripherally inserted central catheter [PICC]), examine the exit site for leaks and the insertion site for evidence of swelling or venous thrombosis. Catheter displacement may be evidenced by the appearance of the cuff extruding from the exit site or of the obviously whiter segment of catheter at the exit site, indicating

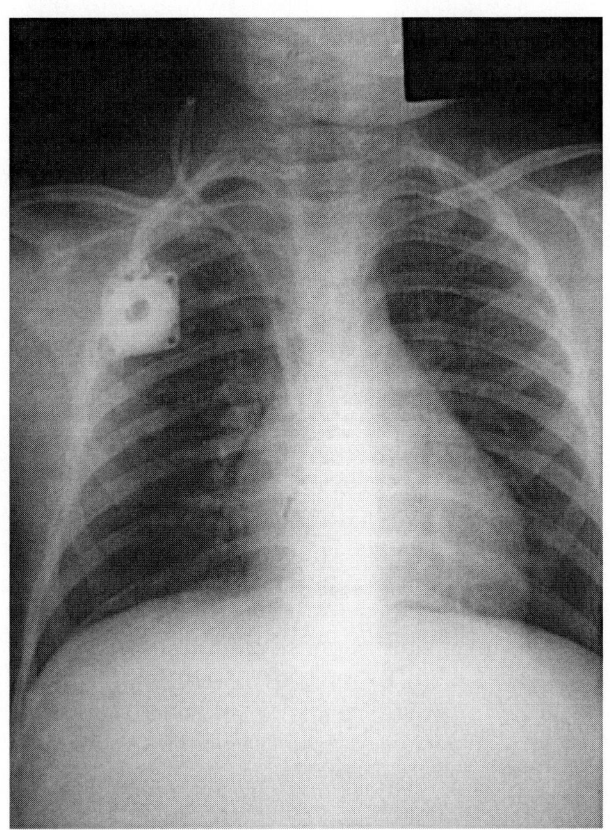

Figure 16-1 Catheter bent causing resistance during infusion and lack of blood return.

that the catheter has been pulled or slipped out of place. Observe the insertion site (usually the ipsilateral supraclavicular area) for evidence of swelling during fluid bolus. Any evidence of swelling or subjective complaints by the patient of pain or discomfort during fluid bolus warrants investigation.

The presence of a blood return from an implanted port or a tunneled catheter usually confirms catheter tip placement. However, it is not uncommon for a catheter to be properly placed without evidence of catheter damage and still have an absent or intermittent blood return. However, if the patient complains of discomfort with fluid injection or if the flow demonstrates resistance, becomes sluggish, or does not flow freely with gravity, it is possible that the catheter tip is somehow intermittently obstructed, the catheter has drifted or migrated into a smaller ancillary vein, or it has otherwise become bent or coiled, preventing back flow of blood (Figures 16–1 and 16–2). It is important in these situations to determine catheter placement by radiological means. The injection of fluid or chemotherapy should be withheld pending physician examination.

When giving vesicant agents through a port, whether by simple injection or by long-term infusion, it is important to use a 90-degree bent Huber-point needle

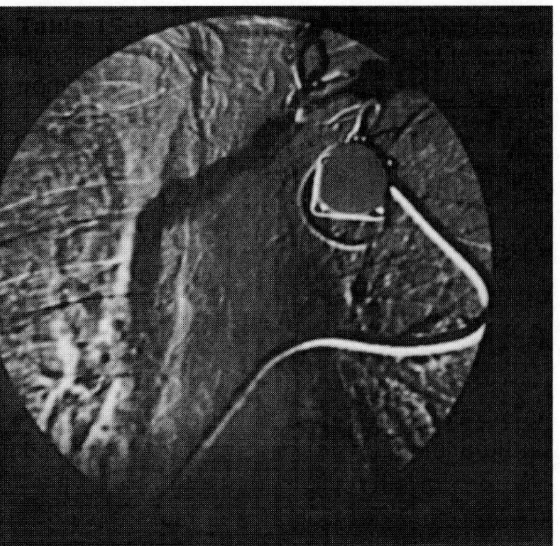

Figure 16-2 Catheter coiled around port as demonstrated by digital subtraction venogram.

rather than a straight needle. Straight needles can easily become dislodged because there is no way to stabilize them regardless of how brief the injection time. Patients are instructed to report any pain, burning, tightness, stinging, or discomfort over the chest area during the injection or infusion. When injecting a vesicant, the blood return is assessed before the injection and at the conclusion of the injection. During the short-term or long-term infusion of a vesicant, assessment of blood return is variable depending on the status of the patient. In some situations where the patient is confused or uncooperative, it is reasonable to question whether it is safe to use a port for long-term vesicant infusions because needle dislodgment can occur even under the best conditions.

It is difficult to determine how frequently a catheter should be aspirated during the infusion of a vesicant in the hospitalized individual to determine the presence or absence of a blood return. If the catheter or port never had a blood return prior to instituting the vesicant infusion, then assessment of the site every hour, as would be done with any intravenous infusion, seems appropriate. If a blood return is known to exist, then assessment of blood return will vary from institution to institution, but assessment at the beginning of each shift seems appropriate, with hourly visual examination of the infusion/insertion site. More frequent catheter aspiration, such as at the beginning and end of each shift or every 4 hours, would appear excessive and could significantly increase risk for infection.

The ideal catheter for infusion of vesicant agents in the outpatient/home environment is the tunneled externally based catheter or PICC line. In some situations where a port is already in place, this device can safely be employed for vesicant infusions provided the patient is capable of regularly assessing the site for proper needle placement.

Management of extravasation. If a frank extravasation has occurred, it will usually be obvious to patient and nurse at the time it occurs. In some situations, however, the actual symptoms are delayed for 24–48 hours. The patient may report redness over the injection site that is warm to the touch. Most often, these delayed symptoms indicate that only a small amount of drug actually infiltrated. Color Plate 4 depicts a doxorubicin extravasation 12 days after drug administration. There was no pain with movement of the area, which healed spontaneously without local treatment. Color Plate 5 demonstrates erythema and edema at the injection site one week after doxorubicin administration. At the time of administration, blood return was lost and the patient complained of slight pain at the site. The drug was stopped. After flushing with saline, slight swelling was noted over the area. Ice was applied. This area progressed to blister formation in three weeks, with clear demarcation of the damaged area (see Color Plate 6), which was surgically excised (see Color Plate 7).

When there is cause to believe that an extravasation of a vesicant agent has occurred during drug administration, prompt nursing action will, in general, minimize tissue damage. The nurse is responsible for ensuring that all antidotes and diluents are readily available and accessible. The following steps should be taken if an extravasation is suspected:

1. Stop the administration of the chemotherapeutic agent. If injecting through the side arm of a free-flowing IV, stop the fluid flow immediately; failure to do so further disperses the infiltrated drug into the tissues.
2. Disconnect the intravenous tubing or syringe and attach an empty 10-mL syringe. Attempt to aspirate any residual drug in the tubing and at the site. Stabilize the extremity and tape the syringe in place.
3. If unable to aspirate any blood or residual drug from the tubing, remove the needle. Gentle apply a sterile 2″ × 2″ gauze pad over the needle entrance site.
4. Prepare the antidote (if available) according to institutional policy and procedure.
5. Replace the syringe with an antidote-filled syringe and inject the antidote.
6. If the needle has been removed, inject the antidote subcutaneously into the extravasation site using a single injection of a 25-gauge needle.
7. Remove the needle.
8. Avoid applying direct manual pressure to the site.
9. Photograph the extravasation site prior to applying a loose sterile dressing.
10. Apply ice for 15 minutes or more every hour for 24–48 hours while awake.
11. Notify the attending physician that an extravasation has occurred or is suspected.
12. Instruct the patient on local care, systemic analgesics, and a plan for follow-up:
    a. Elevate the extremity for 48 hours.
    b. After the first 48 hours, the patient should be encouraged to use the extremity normally. Failure to do so may result in stiffness, neuropathy, and causalgia.[32]
    c. Arrange for a return appointment once or twice weekly depending on the amount of drug suspected to have extravasated and the patient's individual concerns.
    d. Photograph the site weekly as appropriate. Document degree of erythema, induration, pain, and any evidence of ulceration or necrosis.
    e. If pain persists beyond 7–10 days, confer with the physician regarding a plastic surgery consultation, especially if there is evidence of ulcer demarcation.
    f. Consider physical therapy consultation to encourage normal use of the extremity during healing.
13. Promptly complete an extravasation documentation record (see Figure 16–3), paying special attention to subjective complaints and objective observations of the details immediately surrounding the extravasation event.

Paclitaxel and docetaxel are similar antineoplastic agents that are considered to be moderate irritants with the potential to cause ulceration if large amounts of the drug infiltrate. These drugs are routinely infused via peripheral veins, some with the assistance of an infusion pump. In most healthcare settings, vesicants are not administered with the force of a peristaltic infusion pump into a peripheral vein. In the case of these drugs, it is important to use caution in the manner in which they are given. There is evidence clinically that both paclitaxel and docetaxel cause a moderate degree of tissue damage when infiltrated, and most clinicians consider them to be irritants. Once infiltrated, the amount of tissue damage appears to be related to the amount and concentration of the drug infiltrated.[33] Currently, the application of heat to the site of infiltration of either paclitaxel or docetaxel is not recommended. Color Plate 8 depicts a docetaxel infiltration. At four weeks, the area is peeling and somewhat tender. No ulceration occurred. The clear line of demarcation is the outline of the warm cloth that appeared to aggravate more than help the condition.[34]

Patient ______________________ DOB ____________ Date infiltration occurred ____________

Drug ______________________ Dilution mg/mL ____________ Vesicant ______ Irritant ______

Amount of Drug Infiltrated: < 1 mL ______ 1–3 mL ______ 3–5 mL ______ 5 mL ______ > 10 mL ______

Method of Drug Administration:

______ Two-syringe technique IV push

______ Side-arm with IV freely running

______ Continuous infusion: rate ______ mL/hour

Peristaltic pump: ______ yes ______ no

______ VAD: ______ Port ______ Tunneled catheter

Type of needle ________

______ Other ______________________

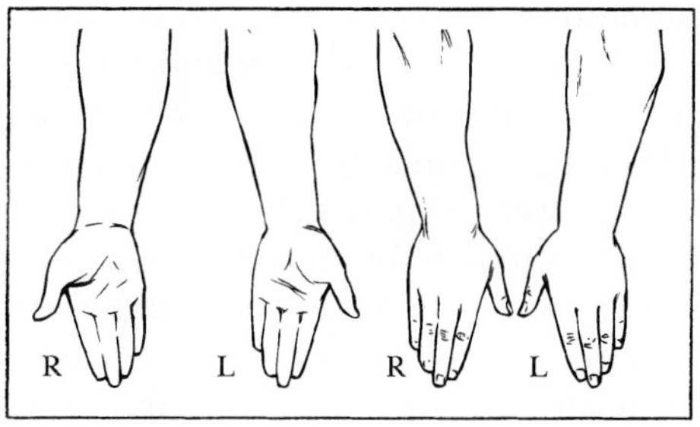

R L R L

Right arm Left arm

(attach photograph)

Description of Site:

Size ________ Color ________ Texture ________

(Indicate location on diagram)

Process Documentation: Describe the events that occurred during the drug administration

S: (Patient's Symptoms) ______________________

O: (Clinical Symptoms) ______________________

A: (Assessment) ______________________ Suspected extravasation ______ Definite extravasation ______

P: (Plan of care) Initial actions: ______________________

Physician notified: ____ Instructions: ______________________

Follow-up Instructions: ______________________

Additional Comments: ______________________

Consultations: ________ Plastic Surgery ______ Physical Therapy ______ Other ______________

Date of referral: ________ Follow-up ______________________

Return appointment: ________ Written instructions for site care reviewed with patient ______________

(RN Signature ______________________)

Follow-up visit #1 (date ______) Describe site and care instructions (attach photo): ______________

Follow-up visit #2 (date ______) Describe site and care instructions (attach photo): ______________

Follow-up visit #3 (date ______) Describe site and care instructions: (attach photo): ______________

Figure 16-3 Extravasation record. (Reprinted with permission from Goodman M, Rush University Medical Center, Chicago, IL.)

Ice should be applied to the site as with any infiltration of a vesicant or irritant.

Extravasation from a central venous catheter (tunneled, nontunneled, implanted port, or PICC line) may be substantial before it is detected because infusions are not monitored constantly and the vesicant may be more diluted than when given by intravenous injection. Therefore, pain at the site may not be noted early. Dressings over the port site may mask swelling. Because infusions tend to be given slowly, a considerable amount of drug can extravasate without obvious evidence of leakage. In the case of an implanted port, the cause is usually needle dislodgment from the port septum, where the needle is found lying in the subcutaneous tissue. The degree of tissue damage will depend on the concentration of the drug and the amount infiltrated. In some cases, there may be no tissue breakdown; in others, wide excision may be required for the wound to heal.

If an extravasation is suspected from a central venous catheter, the infusion is immediately stopped and the physician is notified. An attempt should be made to estimate the amount of drug extravasated. It may be possible to aspirate residual drug from the site. An antidote can be administered if available. Otherwise, the needle should be removed. Efforts to manually express fluid from the site should be avoided. Instead, a sterile dressing should be applied over the needle entrance site and changed frequently. Ice packs should be applied per institutional policy and procedure. Appropriate documentation (extravasation documentation record) should be completed, and plans for careful follow-up and additional consultation with a surgeon may be appropriate.

Intraarterial

Intraarterial drug administration, a drug delivery practice that gained popularity in the early 1980s, involves cannulation of the artery that provides a tumor's blood supply and subsequent administration of the drug directly through the arterial catheter to the tumor bed.[35] This practice increases the concentration of the drug to known areas of tumor and decreases the systemic drug concentration and thus the side effects. The primary use of this route is via the hepatic artery for the management of potential or actual metastasis of colon cancer to the liver. It has also been used for hepatocellular carcinoma. The antineoplastic drugs used include fluorouracil, floxuridine, and cisplatin, among others.

The most common method of intraarterial drug delivery involves placement of a silastic catheter into the main artery supplying the tumor. This catheter is then attached either to an implanted port or a pump (i.e., Arrow or Medtronics pump). The Arrow M-3000 (Arrow International, Walpole, Massachusetts) and the Synchromed Infusion System (Medtronics, Minneapolis, Minnesota) are examples of subcutaneously implanted pumps. The catheter is inserted into the appropriate artery and then attached to the pump located in a surgically created subcutaneous pocket, usually in the lower abdomen or upper chest. The pump chamber is accessed via a noncoring needle and filled with either chemotherapy or heparinized sterile saline. The flow rates are dependent on pump design and are either preset prior to implantation or adjustable via an external electronic wand that communicates with the internal pump. Obviously, care and maintenance of these devices by the nurse require a formalized educational program and ongoing monitoring of pump functioning.

The implantable pump offers the patient the greatest level of freedom when receiving intraarterial chemotherapy and has lower complication rates than external methods. One potential disadvantage is the cost. The pump plus the implantation can be extremely costly, and insurance coverage may be an issue. When compared to intermittent hospitalization, an ambulatory pump is usually deemed to be cost-effective if therapy is anticipated for a minimum of 3–6 months. In fact, long-term therapy with an external pump can eventually cost more due to the cost of disposable supplies.

Nursing care management includes monitoring for drug side effects and potential pump complications, such as infection, occlusion, extravasation, and malfunction.[36] Some unique nursing actions are necessary when dealing with implantable pumps, such as not aspirating the center septum, monitoring or establishing pump flow rate, and detecting malfunctions. The oncology nurse is referred to the manufacturers' instructions and guidelines regarding the management of these advanced nursing responsibilities.

Intraperitoneal

Regional delivery of chemotherapy into the peritoneal space has been found to be a safe and well-tolerated treatment for locally recurrent ovarian and colon cancers. The semipermeable nature of the peritoneal space allows high concentrations of the drugs to be delivered to tumor sites with lower concentrations entering the bloodstream. The procedure causes local side effects due to the large volume of fluid filling the space, and the drugs cause milder or delayed systemic side effects than traditional intravenous administration.

Three types of catheters are used to access the peritoneal space: (1) temporary indwelling catheters, (2) Tenckhoff external catheters, and (3) implantable peritoneal ports.[37–39] Intermittent placement might be used if the therapy is planned to last for a short time, such as for symptom relief or palliation. Tenckhoff catheters or ports are placed when several months of therapy are planned, especially when the treatment goal is cure of minimal or microscopic residual disease. Tenckhoff catheters have the advantage of rapid flow rate (10–15 minutes for 2 L) and allow for catheter manipulation to dislodge fibrin deposits, if necessary. Because they are external, these catheters require care and maintenance by the patient and may result in an increased incidence of infection or leakage around the catheter. In contrast, the implanted port is internal and requires no care when not accessed, so it has a potentially lower rate of infection. Disadvantages include a slower flow rate (30–45 minutes for 2 L), a needle stick required for access, a surgical procedure when removal becomes necessary, and the potential for drug extravasation. Nursing care management is outlined in Table 16-7.

Table 16-7 Nursing Care Management of Intraperitoneal Drug Administration

Patient Education

- Instruct the patient in the care of the catheter or port prior to its insertion.
- Immediately prior to initiating therapy, explain the drug administration process, side effects of the drugs, side effects of the route, and measures to manage/minimize the side effects.
- Teach the patient and/or family how to care for the catheter at home, if appropriate.

Pretreatment and Site Access

- Verify the drug order and normal serum electrolyte levels.
- Insert a urinary catheter to straight drainage, if ordered, and initiate intake and output measurements.
- Ensure that intravenous therapy is proceeding as ordered. (IP cisplatin infusions usually include prehydration for 12–24 hours with IV fluids containing potassium and magnesium supplements. A few moments before initiating the IP cisplatin, IV sodium thiosulfate is begun to neutralize the systemic cisplatin and to prevent renal toxicities and severe nausea and vomiting.)
- Gather appropriate supplies and materials, and wash hands.
- Assess the area around the catheter or port for redness, edema, warmth, or tenderness.
- Organize materials, don gloves (and gown if desired).
- Access external catheter directly after a thorough povidone-iodine scrub of the external hub using aseptic technique, *or*
- Access implanted port using aseptic technique and a large-gauge, noncoring, 90-degree needle of appropriate length (usually 1–1.5 in.); anesthetize the skin surface prior to access, if desired, with 2% xylocaine, Emla cream, or ice.
- Flush the catheter with 10–20 mL of nonbacteriostatic sterile saline; catheter should flush easily.
- Administer antiemetics, if ordered.

Drug Administration

- Initiate IV sodium thiosulfate, if ordered.
- Position patient comfortably in a semi-Fowler's position (elevate head of bed).
- Open the clamp on the tubing, and infuse the warmed IP chemotherapy at the prescribed rate (usually over 30 minutes to several hours).
- Stop infusion immediately if severe pain is experienced and check for catheter migration (usually with x-ray verification).
- Slow the rate of infusion if the patient experiences shortness of breath or discomfort.
- Administer analgesics as prescribed, if necessary.
- Apply blankets if patient feels chilled.
- Close the clamp on the tubing when the infusion is complete, and encourage repositioning from side to side every 15 minutes during the dwell time (usually 2–4 hours).
- Monitor patient's comfort levels and observe for shortness of breath, abdominal discomfort, or diarrhea.
- After the prescribed dwell time, open the clamp to the drainage bag and allow the solution to drain. If flow is sluggish, check tubing for kinks, help patient roll from side to side, have patient use the Valsalva maneuver, apply manual pressure to the abdomen, or irrigate the catheter with normal saline.
- Recognize that the volume of drained fluid may be less than that infused, and reassure patient that the fluid will be reabsorbed and metabolized.
- Clamp tubing on drainage bag after fluid has drained (usually 30 minutes to 2 hours), and send specimen, properly labeled as cytotoxic, to cytology or dispose of in proper hazardous waste container.

Post Administration Care

- Flush catheter or port with nonbacteriostatic sterile saline; if using a port, follow with heparinized saline.
- Secure site using standard technique (i.e., cap and secure catheter or remove needle from port, and cover site with a small dressing, if necessary).
- Establish IV fluids as prescribed, or discontinue IV needle.
- Assess patient's status; ensure ability to perform self-care, if appropriate.
- Document procedure in medical record.

IP = intraperitoneal; IV = intravenous.

Intrapleural

Care of the patient with a pleural effusion traditionally involves insertion of chest tubes, drainage of the fluid, and sclerosis of the pleural space to prevent recurrence of the effusion. Over the years, many different sclerosing chemicals have been used with varying degrees of effectiveness. Bleomycin, cisplatin, tetracycline derivatives, and sterilized talc are all agents that have been used for pleural installation.[40] This insertion is accomplished in the usual sterile manner by injecting the drug directly into the chest tube and clamping it for a specified time period. The procedure can be repeated daily for several days if necessary. Nursing management of intrapleural chemotherapy includes patient education, safe drug handling, and side effect management. In general, nursing care focuses on emesis control, pain control, respiratory status, chest tube security, and other comfort measures, depending on the drug used.

The process just described is a standard procedure that has been moderately successful for many years. The quest for newer and better forms of sclerosing therapy has uncovered a variety of alternatives to traditional therapy. One of the most noteworthy of these advances is small-bore catheter placement, which is easily accomplished with only mild discomfort and without the major trauma of regular chest tube insertion.[41,42] Also, for recurrent pleural effusion, thoracentesis can be performed repeatedly via an implantable port, with the catheter portion in the pleural space and the portal on the lower rib cage. Acceptance and clinical utilization of these techniques are variable, and the oncology nurse is encouraged to be aware of the specific procedures used and the established policies describing the nurse's role in administering intrapleural chemotherapy.

Intravesical

Direct instillation of chemotherapy into the bladder has proved to be an extremely effective and simple method of controlling superficial bladder cancer and carcinoma in situ. Agents such as thiotepa, doxorubicin, mitomycin C, and bacillus Calmette-Guérin (BCG) have all been shown to be effective, especially BCG. Instillation is usually weekly for 4–12 weeks and involves insertion of a urinary catheter, instillation of the drug (usually in 50–60 mL of sterile solution), and retention of the drug for 1–2 hours (with frequent movement to disperse the drug throughout the bladder) prior to unclamping the catheter or voiding. Some physicians prefer to have the urinary catheter remain clamped and in place for the dwell time. In this case, the fluid that drains from the catheter when it is unclamped should be contained and disposed of properly (i.e., sealed, then labeled as cytotoxic waste). If the physician prefers to withdraw the catheter after drug instillation and instructs the patient to void in 1–2 hours, the patient should flush the toilet twice after voiding. Local side effects such as bladder irritation or, with mitomycin C, dermatitis of the external genitalia can be experienced. A unique side effect of BCG is a "creepy-crawly" feeling, sometimes referred to as "BCG-osis."[43,44] Patients report feeling as if their skin is creeping or little things are crawling on them. Administration of a mild sedative can be considered if this side effect occurs.

While initial studies of intravesical chemotherapy demonstrated an apparent decreased incidence of recurrent bladder tumors, this finding has not been corroborated by long-term studies. Therefore, it appears that the role of intravesical chemotherapy will be as a single postoperative instillation rather than as long-term maintenance therapy.[45]

Nursing care management for patients receiving intravesical chemotherapy includes patient education (stressing hand washing and personal hygiene), drug administration, side effect monitoring, and safe drug handling. For most oncology nurses, it is unusual to have experience with this method of drug delivery, as it is commonly performed in urologists' offices as part of a postoperative office visit.

Intrathecal or intraventricular

Cancer cells can cross the blood–brain barrier and appear in the cerebrospinal fluid (CSF), resulting in central nervous system involvement of the malignancy. This phenomenon is seen most commonly in leukemia (meningeal leukemia) and to a lesser extent in other malignancies, such as breast cancer, lymphoma, and rhabdomyosarcoma (meningeal carcinomatosis). Unfortunately, available antineoplastic agents are unable to enter the CSF in sufficient concentrations to kill the cancer cells effectively, so chemotherapy is injected directly into the CSF as prophylaxis or to manage existing disease. The antineoplastic drugs used include methotrexate, cytarabine, thiotepa, and interferon. When prepared for use by this route, the preservative-free drug is always admixed under strictly sterile conditions with a preservative-free diluent such as sodium chloride USP (unpreserved) or Ringer's injection USP (unpreserved). Methotrexate is available in an unpreserved lyophilized form for intrathecal use. Cytarabine is supplied with a diluent that contains benzyl alcohol and should be replaced with an appropriate unpreserved diluent (sodium chloride or Ringer's solution).

The two primary methods of instillation are intrathecal and intraventricular. The intrathecal route is achieved by performing a standard lumbar puncture,

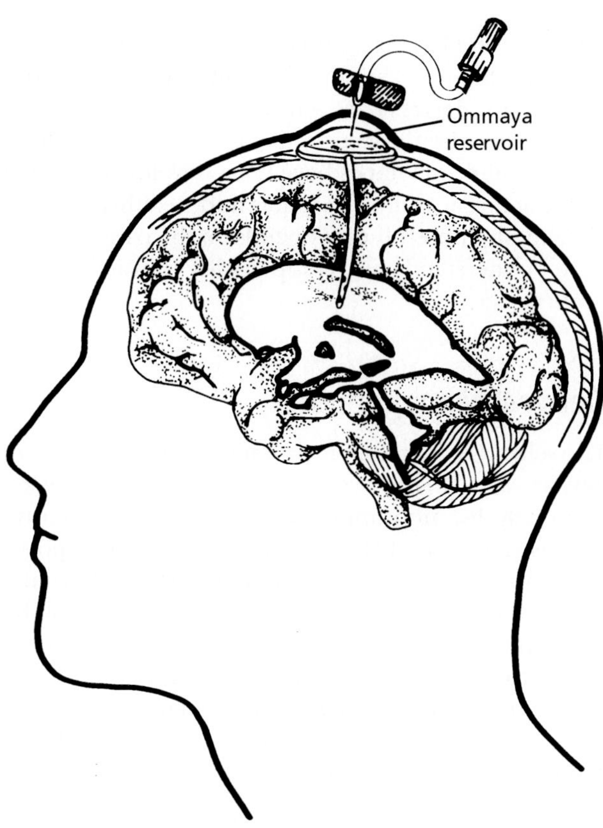

Figure 16-4 Ommaya reservoir placement.

using established techniques to ascertain placement, and injecting 10–12 mL of drug, followed by withdrawal of the needle. This procedure usually is performed by a physician or a nurse practitioner on a daily to weekly basis, depending on the protocol. This method is quick and easy to perform but has the disadvantage that the drug may reach only epidural or subdural spaces. Even when it reaches the subarachnoid space, therapeutic levels of the drug usually are not achieved in the ventricles. For this reason, many physicians prefer intraventricular drug administration.

Central instillation of the drug into the ventricle can be achieved via an Ommaya reservoir (Figure 16–4), which is surgically implanted through the cranium. A skin flap is created, and the Ommaya reservoir is placed underneath the skin, with the catheter extending from the reservoir to the ventricle. Once the surgical site has healed, the only visible evidence of the device is a small bump on the head. Placement of this reservoir obviously involves greater risk than performance of a lumbar puncture, but it provides permanent intraventricular access for those patients in whom repeated translumbar puncture is impractical. Ommaya reservoirs are usually accessed by specially trained nurses. Table 16–8 outlines the nursing procedure for administering chemotherapy via an Ommaya reservoir.

Table 16-8 Intraventricular Chemotherapy: Use of the Ommaya Reservoir

Description

The Ommaya reservoir has a catheter that rests in the lateral ventricle. The general uses of the reservoir include:

1. Sample CSF
2. Monitor CSF pressure
3. Administer analgesics into the CSF
4. Administer antibiotics into the CSF
5. Administer chemotherapy into the CSF

Equipment

Accessing the Ommaya reservoir is a sterile procedure. Assemble all equipment before you begin:

Sterile gloves
Antiseptic wash
Alcohol wipes #3
Shave/prep kit (optional)
Huber point needle — 22-gauge with attached tubing
Premixed drugs (preservative-free)
Equipment for specimen collection: 3-mL syringes, collection tubes, requisitions
Small dressing or adhesive strip

Procedure

NOTE: Shave area if needed prior to establishing a sterile field.

1. Assemble equipment; prepare a sterile field.
2. Position patient in a semirecumbent position. Support head with pillow.
3. Examine reservoir for any signs of infection. Palpate disc to locate center.
4. Cleanse area over disc in a circular motion with antiseptic swabs (x3).
5. Repeat using alcohol.
6. Using a sterile procedure puncture the disc perpendicularly with the needle. Normally, CSF is clear and colorless as it rises into the tubing. Aspirate slightly to collect 2–3 mL of CSF. Set aside to flush the reservoir after drug instillation. Aspirating the CSF from the reservoir is not contraindicated but should be done gently as it may cause the reservoir catheter to become obstructed. If this occurs, flush to clear and continue collection.
7. Obtain CSF specimens for cytology/microbiology with separate syringes and set aside.
8. Attach syringe of medicine and inject drug slowly over 5–10 minutes. The fluid being injected should be amply diluted to prevent irritation to the meninges (e.g., methotrexate is usually mixed in 12 mL of preservative-free solvent).
9. Follow medicine with 2–3 mL of CSF flush.
10. Remove needle, and apply a small dressing.

Regardless of the specific delivery method, nursing care management includes patient education, assessment of the access site, administration (or assistance with administration) of the drug, safe drug handling, and side effect management. Even though intravenous drugs do not cross the blood–brain barrier in sufficient concentration to treat meningeal disease, the intraventricular drugs are capable of entering the systemic bloodstream. Side effects of the drugs, such as nausea, stomatitis, and mild myelosuppression, are to be anticipated. Special care should be taken with methotrexate, particularly if it is given with another drug such as cytarabine or in conjunction with radiation therapy. Leucovorin may be given orally to prevent unnecessarily severe systemic toxicities. The expected side effects related to intraventricular drug administration include headache, nausea, vomiting, ataxia, blurred vision, and transient paresthesias. The most serious complication for which to observe is infection, which is manifested by tenderness, redness, drainage, warmth or fever, stiff neck, and headache (with or without vomiting). Acute chemical arachnoiditis characterized by headache, back pain, vomiting, fever, and nuchal rigidity has been reported. This reaction appears to be more common in the elderly and in the presence of reduced cerebral glucose and protein metabolism accompanied by altered blood–brain barrier permeability.[46]

Vascular Access Devices

The development of central venous catheters (CVCs) and other types of long-term VADs has enhanced the lives of oncology patients but added a new series of challenges for caregivers. Device selection, patient selection, use, maintenance, complication management, and product development continue to be refined by practice and research. Use of VADs is not restricted to the cancer population, and the oncology nurse often serves as an expert resource to other devise users.

Many different kinds of catheters, needles, and implantable ports are used for cancer chemotherapy delivery. Some of the major VAD types and features are outlined in Table 16-9. The nurse plays an important role in assessing the patient's vascular access needs and selecting or recommending placement of the proper device. Intermittent peripheral venous access is preferred for patients with good veins who are on limited intermittent therapies not involving vesicant infusions. Even multiday infusional therapy can easily be administered through peripheral veins when vascular integrity is good. A CVC should be considered in patients with poor veins, requiring multi-infusional therapy, requiring long-term therapy, or requiring continuous infusion of vesicants.

As with other aspects of chemotherapy administration, education of both the nurse and the patient and family is essential when dealing with VADs. The oncology nurse should be knowledgeable in all aspects of VAD care. There is no universal standard of care for these devices. Indeed, randomized prospective clinical trials are needed to help define the standards of care for VADs. The nurse is urged to be familiar with the particular brands of devices, the manufacturers' recommendations, existing clinical practice trends, and the established policies and procedures of the employing institution.[47,48] Patient and family education is critical, as many devices have self-care aspects that must be considered when selecting the VAD. Many excellent booklets and videotapes have been developed by VAD manufacturers and by hospitals and healthcare agencies, but their usefulness depends on the patient's ability to understand and comply with the actions described.

General Management

The selection, care, and maintenance of the long-term devices vary with the type of VAD and will be addressed separately for nontunneled CVCs, tunneled central venous catheters (TCVCs), and implantable ports. Many of the major complications are handled in similar ways, so the management of complications will be addressed together for all the devices. Most CVCs will be inserted such that the catheter tip ends in the superior vena cava, but for those patients in whom this positioning is not possible, a femoral approach with the catheter tip in the inferior vena cava may be an option.

Nontunneled central venous catheters

Short-term use of a nontunneled CVC, such as a standard subclavian line, is common practice in urgent situations. When an immediate need for a central line arises, it commonly is placed by a physician at the bedside, in the intensive care unit, or in the emergency room. For oncology patients, it is primarily intended to provide immediate access until the emergency can be resolved. In some practices, silastic catheters may be used for months with low infection rates.[49] These devices are also used when the need for multi-infusional therapy exceeds the capabilities of an existing tunneled CVC or implantable port. For example, a multilumen subclavian catheter might be placed in a patient with acute leukemia who is on chemotherapy, hydration, antibiotics, TPN, blood products, and other medications. The triple-lumen central catheter can augment the long-term device during the hospitalization and be removed prior to discharge or left in place for outpatient care. The oncology patient may also have a CVC in place for apheresis or dialysis. These catheters are usually dedicated to those procedures and care is directed by those departments.

For long-term use, the gap that exists between the trauma of subclavian lines and the investment in a long-term tunneled catheter or port has been narrowed with the use of PICCs.[50] From the patient's viewpoint, the PICC is the least expensive and most easily inserted long-term CVC, but it requires self-care capabilities and often a caregiver, because it is located at

Table 16-9 Overview of Available Vascular Access Devices

Type	Description	Longevity	Comments
Peripheral needle Scalp vein butterfly	• Stainless steel • Single lumen • 27- to 19-gauge	Minutes to days	• Excellent for short-term access, especially outpatient • Increased risk of infiltration with long-term use
Peripheral catheter Intima	• Catheter over needle • Teflon or polyurethane • Single and double lumen • 26- to 14-gauge	Hours to days	• Excellent for multiday infusional therapy • Provides greater patient mobility as less likely to infiltrate
Nontunneled central venous catheter	• Polyurethane or silicone catheter • Single, double, and triple lumen	Hours to months	• Excellent for emergency need for CVC • Can augment existing VAD for acute care needs or longer-term use • Inserted by physician at bedside or in procedure room
Peripherally inserted central catheter (PICC)	• Silicone elastomer or other polymers • Single and double lumen • 24- to 16-gauge	Weeks to months	• Excellent for continuous infusion over several weeks or months • Can be inserted at bedside by specially trained nurse • Quick, easy central access without surgical procedure • Requires external site care and routine flushing
Tunneled central venous catheter (TCVC)	• Silicone catheter with Dacron cuff • Single, double, and triple lumen • 4.2–19.2 Fr; 40- to 90-cm length • Groshong has slit valve, requiring less flushing	Months to years	• Excellent for long-term, continuous, or intermittent therapy • Preferred for long-term TPN administration • Preferred by many for vesicant infusional therapy • Requires external site care and routine flushing
Implantable port	• Titanium, stainless steel, silastic, or plastic portal attached to catheter • Single and double lumen • Access with noncoring needle • Low-profile ports available	Months to years	• Excellent for long-term, intermittent infusional therapy • No site care required when not in use so excellent for patients unable to perform site care • Surgical procedure required for removal
Peripheral port	• Titanium portal attached to silastic catheter • Single lumen • Access with noncoring 22-gauge needle	Months to years	• Ideal for intermittent access, particularly for those patients with active lifestyles or body image concerns • No external site care when not in use • Not ideal for blood draw due to small volume

CVC = central venous catheter; VAD = venous access device; TPN = total parenteral nutrition.

the antecubital fossa and self-care has to be one-handed. These small-gauge, thin-walled catheters are inserted at the antecubital fossa into the basilic or cephalic vein (Figure 16–5). The procedure is performed by a physician or a specially trained nurse at the patient's bedside. The catheter can be advanced into the superior vena cava, in which case x-ray verification of placement is required. A few state boards of nursing consider the placement of a CVC to be outside the role of a professional nurse, so it is important for the nurse to verify that placement of a PICC is within the scope of nursing practice as defined by the state. Some states allow PICC insertion by a nurse if it is considered a long-line catheter and is only advanced into the axillary or subclavian veins, in which case x-ray verification of placement is not necessarily required but is preferred, especially for vesicant administration. Formal training in the intricacies of PICC insertion is required, as the insertion techniques vary greatly among the specific devices and success is usually technique dependent and due to repeated practice.[49–51]

Peripherally inserted central catheters are ideal for short-term access in patients with adequate antecubital veins, self-care capabilities, and the need for a wide variety of intravenous therapies. However, the thin, flexible nature of the catheter does not lend itself well to

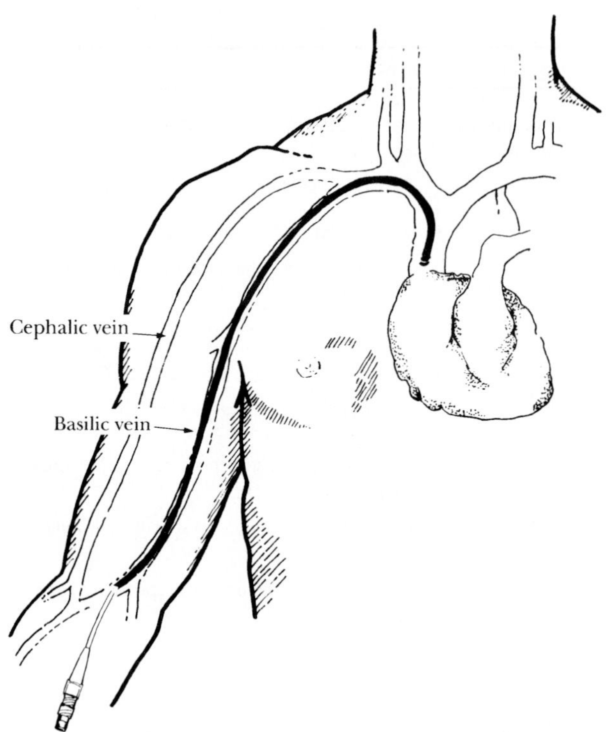

Figure 16-5 Placement of peripherally inserted center catheter (PICC).

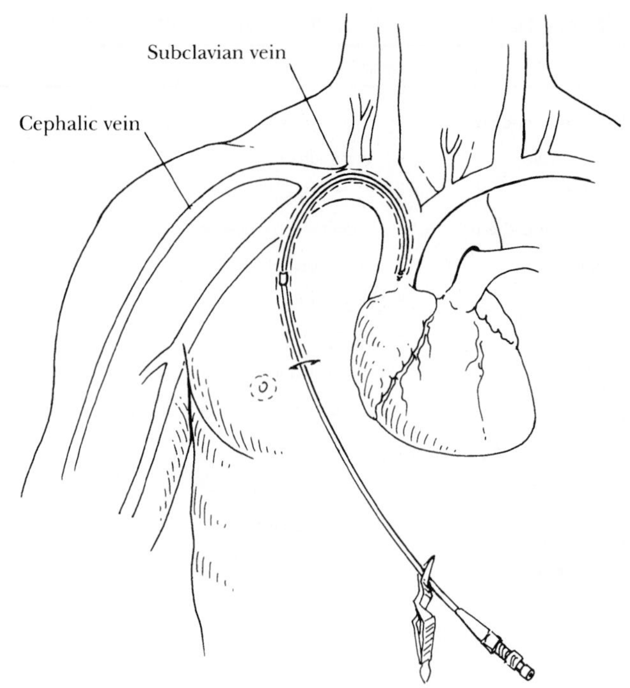

Figure 16-6 Tunneled central venous catheter placement.

blood withdrawal, but it is not contraindicated and may be successfully achieved with gentle application of pressure via the syringe used for blood withdrawal. The complication rate is similar to that for other VADs in terms of infection, clotting, and malfunction.[52] Some studies suggest a higher rate of phlebitis, which may be technique dependent or caused by powdered gloves. Meticulous attention to sterile technique during insertion and rinsing the powder off the gloves prior to handling the PICC seem to decrease these complications.[51]

Tunneled central venous catheters

The TCVC provides safe and reliable long-term access with a low incidence of infection, suitable for almost all hematology/oncology patients. Tunneled CVCs continue to be well accepted and have been modified by the various manufacturers that now market similar devices. The unique features of the TCVC (Figure 16–6) include a Dacron cuff around which granulation tissue forms, actually helping to hold the catheter in place. The 4- to 10-inch tunnel through which the catheter is channeled serves to prevent the easy passage of bacteria from the skin into the vein. Also, the cuff is thought to help stop bacteria from traveling along the subcutaneous portion of the catheter. A second cuff (VitaCuff; Vitaphore, San Carlos, California) impregnated with silver ions can be attached to any catheter to help decrease the infection rate. The catheter material is usually radiopaque silicone to aid insertion and subsequent placement verification. The external portion of the TCVC has a Luer-Lok hub (to allow direct access with an intravenous infusion set) or placement of an as-needed heparin-lock adapter (to allow access via a needle or needleless system). Single-, double-, and triple-lumen TCVCs are available in various gauges and lengths (Figure 16–7). Areas of development include newer materials and antibiotic-bonded catheters.[53]

One unique variation on the TCVC is the Groshong catheter (Figure 16–8), which features a closed-end radiopaque tip. Flow through the catheter is achieved via a patented slit valve, which opens out into the bloodstream when fluid is infusing into the catheter, opens inward into the catheter lumen when blood is being withdrawn from the catheter, and remains closed when no pressure is being applied. Groshong catheter technology has been applied to the other VADs, and Groshong ports and PICCs are available, as well as the tunneled and nontunneled Groshong CVCs. This design prevents the need for regular heparinization of the catheter, which usually is flushed with sterile normal saline (NS) once a week when not in use, making it advantageous in those patients for whom heparin is contraindicated.

Patient selection is a key issue with the TCVC because it requires regular care and maintenance. The patient or other caregiver must be willing and physically able to

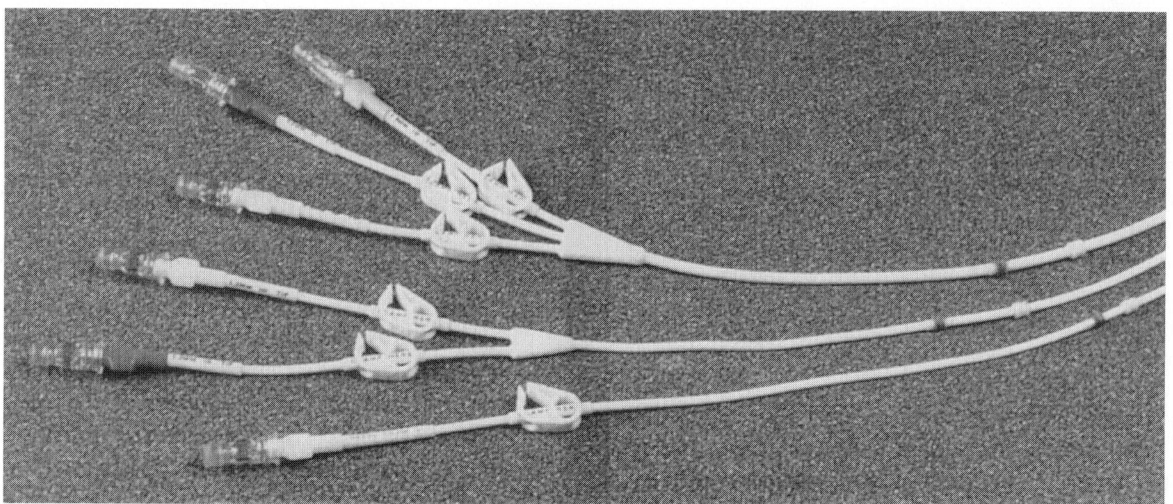

Figure 16-7 Hickman catheters – triple, double, and single lumen. (Courtesy of Bard Access Systems, Salt Lake City, UT.)

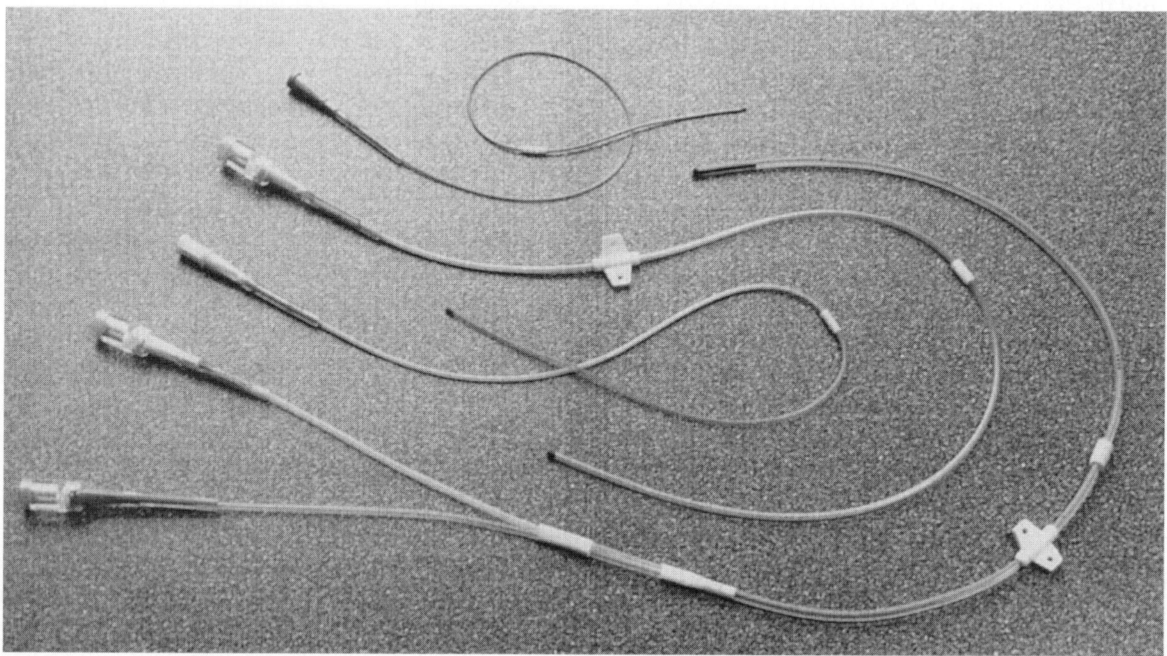

Figure 16-8 Various Groshong catheters. From top to bottom, pediatric, central venous catheter (CVC), tunneled central venous catheter (TCVC), dual-lumen TCVC. (Courtesy of Bard Access Systems, Salt Lake City, UT.)

clean the exit site, flush the catheter, change the cap, and assess and report complications. The patient must be able to afford the equipment (needles, syringes, heparin or saline, and dressing materials) and must have access to a clean area in the home in which to perform self-care. Body image and patient lifestyle can be issues because of the catheter exit through the chest wall, which can be distressing or embarrassing to some patients, particularly adolescents. Also, whereas swimming in chlorinated pools is allowed by some practitioners, swimming in ponds, rivers, or the ocean usually is not recommended.

The TCVC offers several major advantages, including its elimination of needle sticks for those people who have a needle phobia, and the ease with which it is removed when no longer needed for care. It also allows for a great deal of flexibility in terms of use, being a preferred device for long-term TPN, vesicant infusion therapy, and continuous infusions. It also is the only long-term device that offers a triple-access option. Finally, the TCVC is less expensive in terms of both the device and the insertion costs than an implantable port; however, there is some debate as to its long-term cost-effectiveness, because supplies are needed for care and their cost depends on the regimen of care and frequency and type of flushing.

Despite the common use of TCVCs for more than two decades, there is little standardization of their insertion and care. Insertion is not without risks, and complications include pneumothorax and arterial puncture.[54] Various techniques are used for placement, and experienced oncology nurses are beginning to work with physicians and patients prior to insertion to help select a site that is convenient when considering clothing and body contours. Adequate instruction of the patient and family both before and after placement is critical to a successful experience with a TCVC.

When developing policies and procedures governing the use of TCVCs, it is recommended that the following aspects of care be included:

- The TCVC requires sterile site care with dressings until the formation of granulation tissue and verification of normal absolute neutrophil counts, at which time site care involves bathing the chest wall and securing the catheter with tape to prevent dislodgment.
- When not in use, the catheter requires daily, every other day, or even weekly flushing with 3–5 mL of heparinized saline (10 U/mL).
- The TCVC allows blood withdrawal for all laboratory tests (except coagulation studies), which can be achieved via vacutainer technique, if desired. The vacutainer technique is preferred because it minimizes the risk of accidental needle sticks.
- Whenever blood has been aspirated into the catheter, it is flushed with 20 mL of saline prior to heparin-locking or resuming an infusion.
- One must avoid intraluminal mixing of potentially incompatible drugs, which can be achieved by flushing with plain fluid between each drug.
- The patient must avoid scissors, sharp objects, and needles longer than 1 inch.
- Access is either direct or via as-needed heparin-lock adapter cap; all connections must use Luer-Lok.
- Continuous infusions should be directly connected to the catheter hub.

One unique care issue related to TCVCs is the possibility of fracture, puncture, or cutting of the external portion of the catheter. Puncture can be prevented by not using scissors or sharp objects near the catheter and limiting needles used for access to 1 inch in length or by using needleless systems. It is also advisable to avoid clamping the catheter continuously or, if a clamp is used, padding and rotating the clamp site. As long as at least 2 inches of undamaged catheter exits the skin, it can be repaired using a repair kit available from the manufacturer. Most repair kits are designed only for a specific catheter, especially the double- and triple-lumen repair kits when the break occurs in the main portion of the catheter. Emergency repairs to a single-lumen can be conducted via the following steps:

1. Clamp the catheter close to the chest wall.
2. Clean the catheter with alcohol at the most distal undamaged point.
3. Using sterile scissors, cut the catheter.
4. Remove the inner metal stylus from a 14- or 16-gauge peripheral IV catheter, and insert the IV catheter into the TCVC until the cut edge touches the hub.
5. Secure with tape or suture.
6. Attach the heparin-lock adapter cap, and unclamp and gently flush catheter; heparinize or use it in the normal manner.
7. Obtain a repair kit as soon as possible for permanent repair.

One major advantage of the TCVC is the ease with which it is removed by the physician when no longer needed. by the patient. Prior to withdrawal of the catheter, some catheter manufacturers suggest a short surgical incision, under local anesthesia, to mechanically release the Dacron cuff from the subcutaneous tissue. If the cuff is not removed with the catheter, it may become infected later. Catheter removal is achieved by cleaning the exit site and manually pulling on the catheter until it loosens in the tunnel. Pressure is then applied manually over the entrance site into the vein and maintained for several minutes after catheter removal. Steady, slow pressure is applied while pulling on the catheter until the entire catheter is removed and inspected to ensure that it is intact, because breakage or splintering can occur. A small dressing is applied to the exit site, if necessary.

Implantable ports

The implantable port has proved to be a unique development in vascular access devices because when it is not in use, it requires almost no care or maintenance (Figures 16–9 and 16–10). A *port* is a hollow housing of stainless steel, titanium, or plastic that contains a compressed latex septum over a portal chamber connected via a small tube to a silicone or polyurethane catheter that is inserted into a blood vessel. It is placed subcutaneously and accessed percutaneously using a special noncoring needle. The needle has an offset bevel, which prevents coring the septum and allows 1000–3600 punctures per port, depending on the manufacturer and needle size. The plastic and

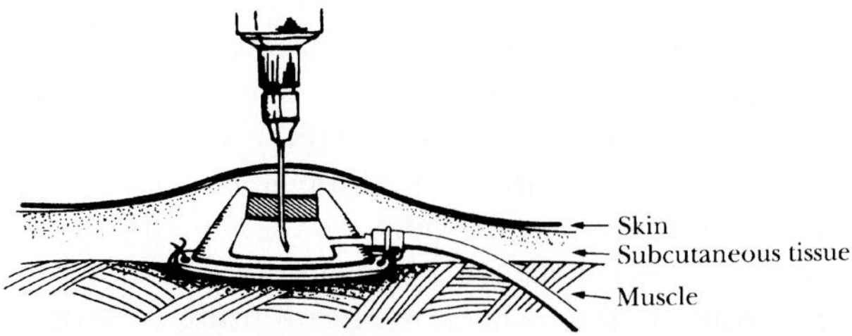

Figure 16-9 Schematic drawing of an implantable port.

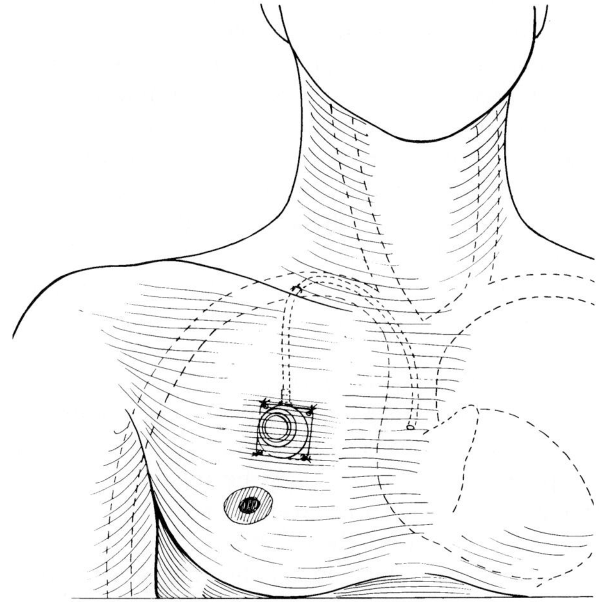

Figure 16-10 Venous port placement.

titanium ports are advantageous because they cause little, if any, disturbance on x-ray film during imaging procedures. Ports are available in two forms: (1) with the catheter permanently attached to the portal housing, in which case the surgeon adjusts the length by trimming the distal portion of the catheter prior to insertion, and (2) with the catheter separate from the portal housing, in which case the surgeon trims the proximal end prior to attaching and securing it to the portal during the implantation procedure. Ports are available in single and double designs, with the double port having two distinct portal chambers to allow simultaneous administration of separate solutions. Most ports are accessed through the top. A portal design that provides access via the side, allowing the needle to be positioned parallel to the skin, is available but is not commonly used by practitioners today.

Port routes. There are five major types of ports: venous, arterial, peritoneal, intrapleural, and epidural. The unique portal design allows access to more than just the vascular system. While the portal housings are all essentially the same, the catheters are designed, located, and cared for differently. Unfortunately, there is no standardized placement of the different types of ports, which creates major problems for the nurse unfamiliar with a new patient. It is imperative that the type of device and its purpose be determined prior to accessing the port. Though it is not common, ports can be located in other areas of the body. Most patients are given an identifying wallet card and information regarding their ports. If that information is unavailable and the patient is unsure of the device type, then the healthcare professional must seek the operative note in the hospital chart to confirm device type and catheter route.

Nursing issues related to arterial, peritoneal, epidural, and intrapleural ports are summarized in Table 16-10 and are discussed in some detail in the earlier section of this chapter dealing with routes of drug administration.

Port usage. The routine care of the venous port when not being used is to flush it once every 3–4 months with sterile heparinized saline (usually 5 mL of 100 U/mL solution). It is an ideal choice for patients who are unable or unwilling to care properly for an external device, receiving intermittent therapies, concerned about body image, or physically active (especially if swimming in unchlorinated bodies of water). Its major disadvantage is that it requires a needle to pass through the skin and into the port for usage. The procedure of accessing the port could introduce infective organisms, cause a hematoma in a thrombocytopenic patient, cause anxiety in a patient with a needle phobia, or result in extravasation of fluid around the port if performed incorrectly or if the needle subsequently becomes dislodged. There is also a remote possibility that the device could extrude through the skin.

Nursing management of ports involves assessing the site, accessing the device, infusing or withdrawing fluids, and flushing. The nurse should help select the portal site prior to implantation. With the patient erect and clothed, the nondominant side should be examined for a convenient location. Ideally, the port can be located over a rib in an area easy for the patient to visualize for care but not visible when clothed. Consideration should be given to clothing, brassiere straps, lifestyle (e.g., frequent holding of a telephone receiver between the head and shoulder), and physical activities (e.g., swimming). Thin patients may need low-profile ports; obese patients may need large ports. Also, in obese patients or large-breasted women, placement of the port near the sternum provides better needle stability and ease of access. Care should be taken to avoid placement of the port under the arm, under the breast, in the breast, or in the soft tissue of the abdo-

Table 16-10 Unique Types of Implantable Ports

Arterial

- Used to administer continuous or intermittent intraarterial chemotherapy.
- Catheter is placed into an artery, and port is usually placed on the lower rib cage.
- Accessed and managed in the usual manner, except heparinization procedure may be different, with increased frequency (i.e., weekly) or higher concentrations of heparin (100–1000 U/mL).
- Catheter has a small lumen and seems to form clots more easily than venous catheters; hence the need for at least weekly flushing.

Peritoneal

- Used to administer intermittent intraperitoneal chemotherapy for ovarian or colon cancer.
- Catheter is placed in the peritoneal space, and port is usually placed on the lower rib cage but can be in the lower abdominal area.
- Accessed and managed in the usual sterile manner, except 19-gauge noncoring needles are used to facilitate large-volume infusions; the portal is flushed after use with sterile saline, and heparinization usually is not required.
- Catheter has a very large lumen with several ridges or cuffs to secure placement and multiple exit holes in the distal portion for rapid fluid infusion.

Epidural

- Used to administer intrathecal or epidural medications, including chemotherapy and analgesics.
- Catheter is placed into the intrathecal or epidural space and tunneled through a long subcutaneous passage from the spinal area to the side of the abdomen, where the port is placed on the lower rib cage or the abdominal area. The portal is designed with a 60-μm screen filter to remove particulate matter.
- Accessed using special 24-gauge noncoring needles, *always* with meticulous sterile technique, including sterile gloves, prep drape, and procedure tray.
- **Never to be flushed with heparin.**
- Preservative-free chemotherapy or morphine is instilled or infused into the port.
- After usage, 1–2 mL of sterile, preservative-free saline may be used to flush the line.
- Catheter has a small lumen (0.5-mm inner diameter), which is suitable for this type of drug delivery.

Intrapleural

- Used to drain pleural effusions periodically in patients who are unresponsive to sclerosing.
- Accessed with noncoring needle only.
- Patient's position is changed frequently during "tap."
- Flushed with 3 mL of saline.

men (for nonvenous ports). The preferred site and an alternate should be marked on the skin as a reference for the surgeon. It is also helpful if the surgeon offsets the port pocket so that the suture line is 1–2 inches away from the top of the port.

Port access usually is achieved under sterile or aseptic technique after a betadine scrub using noncoring needles that can be either straight or bent at a 90-degree angle. The needle penetrates the septum and is advanced until it touches the bottom of the portal chamber. The most popular access needles are actually infusion sets consisting of needle, tubing, and Luer-Lok hub, and containing a Y-site and a clamp. These infusion sets allow great flexibility and multiple access sites and can be left in place for as long as 7 days. For long-term access, a sterile dressing (usually transparent) is placed over the site and assessed on a daily basis. Redness, rash, or blistering of the skin around the port could be indicative of an allergic reaction to the tape or dressing, and is resolved by using an alternative type of tape, dressing, or skin-disinfecting agent.

Several other aspects of port accessing are especially important to the patient. The area is tender and edematous for a week or so after implantation, causing manipulation of the device to be uncomfortable or even painful. Some practitioners prefer to wait until the site has healed and the edema is gone before using the port. When immediate use is indicated, the port should be accessed and dressed securely in the operating room. For routine use once the site is healed, the needle stick usually is not a concern to most patients and causes little discomfort. Occasionally, a patient will have a needle phobia or experience pain during insertion. An effective option is the application of an ice pack or a topical anesthetic cream prior to needle access.

Peripheral implantable port. A variation of the venous port that combines the properties of a PICC and a port is the peripherally inserted port.[55] The P.A.S.-Port (Peripheral Access System, SIMS Deltec, St. Paul, Minnesota) allows the peripheral insertion of a port near the antecubital fossa. Insertion and proper placement are achieved using an electronic device that enables insertion at the bedside or in the physician's office. The P.A.S.-Port is about half the size of a regular port and allows patients to experience the advantages of port placement (unobtrusive, long-term access, intermittent use) without having to expose the chest area to achieve access. Access is achieved through a short (½–¾ inch) noncoring needle or infusion set. In all other aspects except placement, it is managed like other implantable venous ports.

Complication Management

Occlusions, infections, and other complications can occur with all of the long-term VADs. Nurses must know and assess for signs and symptoms of complications with VADs. The incidence and type of complication depend on the device, insertion technique, care regimen, and, to a great extent, physiological factors inherent in the introduction of a long-term catheter into the venous system.[56–59]

Intraluminal catheter occlusion

The complete inability to withdraw blood or infuse fluid in a VAD is most commonly the result of a blood clot within the catheter. It can also be caused by incompatible drugs or lipids that have crystallized or precipitated and have obstructed the catheter. The nurse is instrumental in assessing the catheter and its most recent usage to determine which of these causes are most likely to have occurred. Blood clots can build up over time (i.e., sluggish catheter) but can also appear suddenly. Drug precipitates tend to be more directly related to a recent infusion and are seen more often with TPN and lipids.[60] Measures to prevent either occurrence include the following:[54,61–63]

- Maintain positive pressure within the catheter and vigorously flush the catheter provided no resistance is encountered. Intermittent resistance may mean that the catheter is being pinched off at the level of the clavicle and first rib. Vigorously flushing in this situation can cause an aneurysm in the catheter.
- Advise the patient to avoid excessive manipulation (i.e., pinching or bending) of external catheters.
- Vigorously flush with at least 20 mL of sterile NS after any blood has gotten into the catheter. This helps to prevent sludge build-up within the port.
- Document each patient's VAD experience, and adjust concentration, volume, and frequency of heparinized flush, as needed.
- Question the patient and family regarding actual catheter maintenance activities to assess compliance with recommended care and usage.
- Flush between each drug with at least 10 mL of plain IV fluid to avoid incompatible drug admixture.
- Vigorously flush the catheter every 8–12 hours when administering TPN or lipids.
- Do not administer IV fluid or TPN containing visible precipitates (which is more likely to occur if the solution is more than 24 hours old).

In the case of ports, the inability to infuse or aspirate is typically due to the needle being improperly placed in the septum rather than in the portal. Advancing the needle into the portal usually will solve the problem. Also, if the patient has a low-profile port, the septum is not very deep and a 1-inch Huber-point needle will result in a portion of the needle tip being occluded in the septum. When the patient has a low-profile port, a ¾-inch 22 Huber-point needle will clear the septum and function properly.

Management of an occluded catheter when a blood clot is suspected involves the instillation of alteplase, a tissue plasminogen activator (tPA). Alteplase is prepared as a 2 mg/2 mL syringe and is instilled into the occluded catheter and allowed to dwell for 2 hours. After 2 hours, the nurse attempts to withdraw blood from the catheter. Aspiration of several milliliters of blood ensures removal of the drug and residual clot. The catheter is then irrigated with several milliliters of 0.9% sodium chloride. Urokinase has been successful in clearing clotted catheters. The procedure for using it is as follows. A dose of urokinase 5000 units in 1–3 mL is instilled using a 3-mL or larger syringe and a gentle to-and-fro motion. The catheter is then clamped for 30 minutes or longer, after which an attempt is made to aspirate the catheter contents. If successful, the catheter is flushed and used; if unsuccessful, the procedure is repeated. Certain drug precipitates can be cleared using 0.1 N hydrochloric acid for some crystals or ethanol 70% for lipid deposits.[64,65] The process is similar to that used for urokinase, with the gentle instillation of 0.2–1.0 mL of drug. After a dwell time of 30–60 minutes, an attempt is made to aspirate the catheter contents. If TPN is not involved and a specific drug is known or suspected, a pharmacist should be consulted about possible agents that might dissolve the precipitate and enable it to be aspirated from the catheter. Figure 16-11 describes a possible decision-making matrix to consider when dealing with a completely occluded catheter.

Extraluminal catheter occlusion

Catheter sluggishness or partial occlusion can be due to two extraluminal phenomena: fibrin sheath formation and thrombosis. The catheter position can also affect flow, so a partial occlusion, in the absence of pain or discomfort, should first be managed by instructing the patient to change positions, raise the arms, breathe deeply, and/or cough (Figure 16–12). Each of these activities might release the open lumen of the catheter from the vein wall and allow easy flushing and blood withdrawal. If a withdrawal occlusion exists (flushes easily but back flow is sluggish or nonexistent), fibrin sheath formation or thrombosis should be considered. Fibrin sheaths can form at the

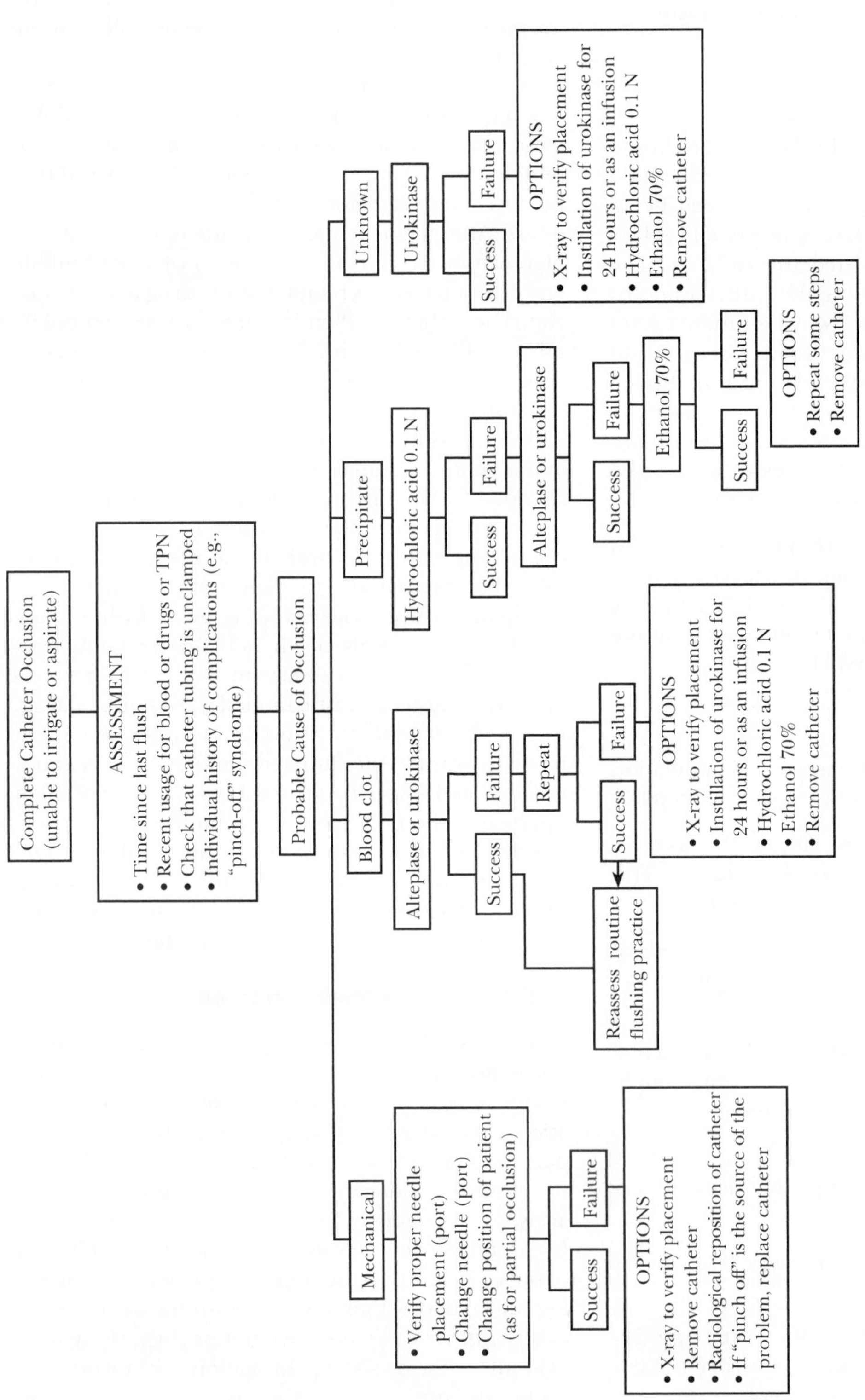

Figure 16-11 Managing complete catheter occlusion. (TPN = total parenteral nutrition.)

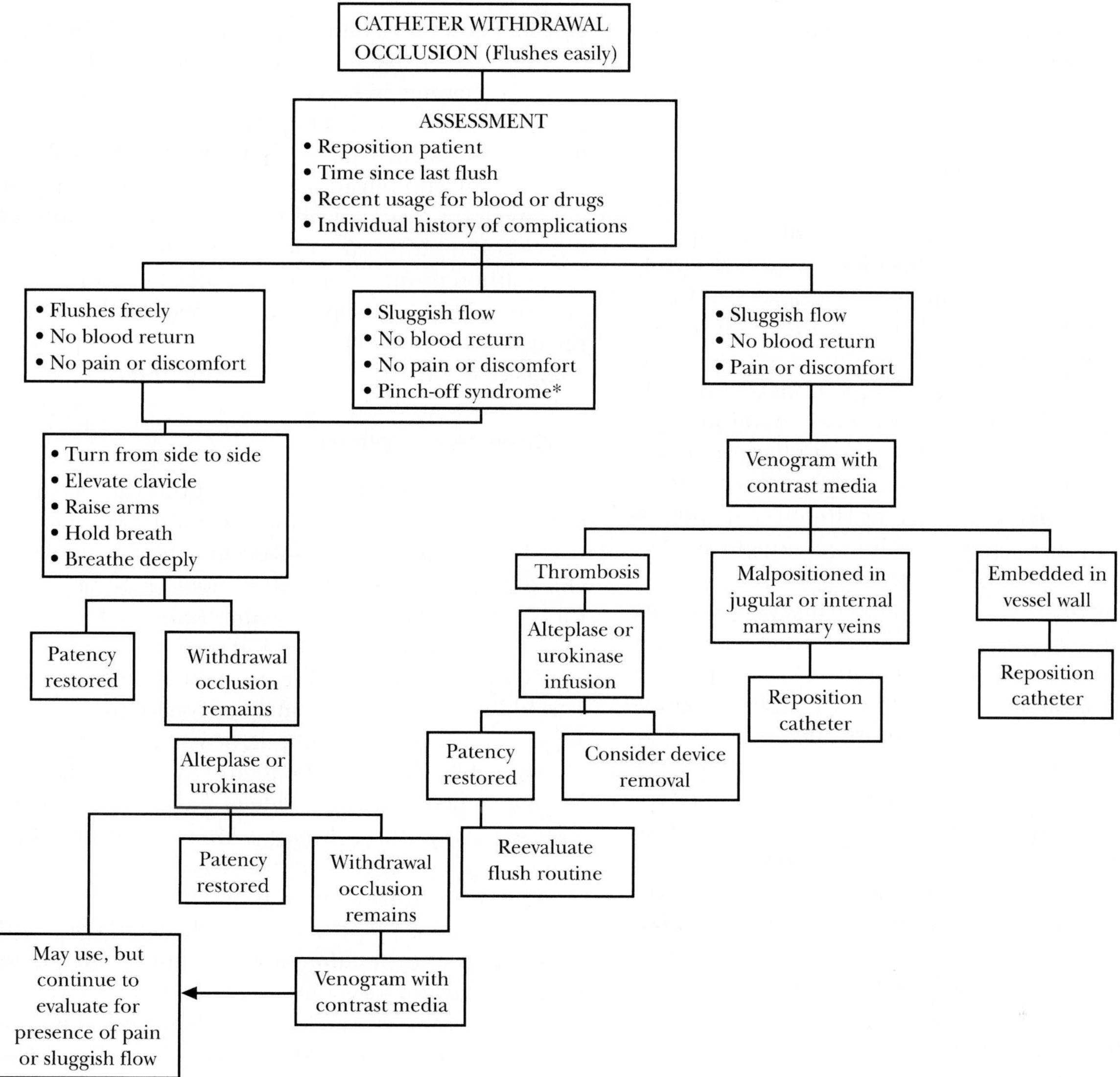

*Severe degree of pinch-off syndrome may require catheter removal.

Figure 16-12 Managing catheter withdrawal occlusion.

catheterinsertion site and float, like a sleeve, around the outside of the catheter. If the sheath extends beyond the lumen, it can cause withdrawal occlusions. Lysis of the sheath may be achieved by instilling alteplase 2 mg/2 mL prefilled syringe or (if available) urokinase 5000–10,000 units into the catheter with an extended dwell time of 1–24 hours.

Venous thrombosis can be caused by a variety of factors, including endothelial injury, hypercoagulability, multiple catheters, catheter stiffness (i.e., polyvinyl chloride), catheter size (i.e., larger bore), and catheter placement (i.e., left side or in a smaller vein). The incidence of catheter thrombosis with clinical symptoms appears to be as high as 10%. Actual incidence in the absence of clinical symptoms could be as high as 50%.[66] Signs and symptoms are related to impaired blood flow and include edema of the neck, face, shoulder, or arm; prominent superficial veins; neck pain; tingling of the neck, shoulder, or arm; and skin color or temperature changes. A variety of radiographic studies can be used to diagnose and define the extent of the thrombosis accurately.

Management of venous thrombosis usually involves anticoagulants or thrombolytic agents. Several authors report success with the continuous infusion, centrally and/or peripherally, of urokinase for 4–24 hours.[67] It is recommended that all lumens of a multilumenal device be treated. The serum fibrinogen level should be maintained at 80–100 mg/dL by titration of the urokinase.[67] The success of this treatment may be related to a short period of symptoms prior to the infusion. Prophylactic administration of low-dose warfarin (1 mg/day) appears to prevent or decrease the incidence of thrombus formation.[51,68]

Infection

Long-term central venous catheters are designed to minimize the risk of infection compared to regular venous catheters, but infection still occurs in 2.7%–60% of devices.[56,58] This wide range is probably dependent on the techniques used to insert and care for the VADs as well as the diagnoses and physical conditions of the patients involved. Infections can occur locally (on the skin), in the catheter tunnel/port pocket, or systemically. Infections are more common in patients with neutropenia (< 500 granulocytes/mm^3), those with multilumen catheters, and those receiving TPN or chemotherapy. A study by Howell et al. indicated that neutropenia was the only independent risk factor for catheter-related infections.[58]

Local infections at the catheter exit site or over the skin around the port needle insertion site usually are caused by organisms on the skin such as *Staphylococcus aureus* and *Staphylococcus epidermidis.* Symptoms can include redness, warmth, discomfort, and exudate. Management includes culture of the area, increased frequency of dressing changes with meticulous site care, and administration of appropriate oral or intravenous antibiotics. The needle should be removed from an implantable port if a skin infection occurs over the port, and it should not be reaccessed until the infection clears.

Infections in the catheter tunnel or port pocket usually involve a variety of organisms and are manifested by redness, edema, tenderness or discomfort, exudate, skin warmth, and/or fever. After cultures have been taken, including aspiration of any port pocket exudate, appropriate intravenous antibiotic therapy is initiated. If the causative organism is identified and appropriate antiinfective therapy fails to resolve the infection, consideration should be given to removal of the device.

Systemic infections can be thrombus related or caused by intraluminal catheter colonization with a wide variety of infective organisms. Signs and symptoms include fever and chills. Blood cultures are taken through each lumen of the device as well as peripherally and can be positive either in the device only or via both routes. Administration of appropriate antibacterial or antifungal therapy is initiated, and blood cultures are repeated. Failure to resolve the infection is cause to consider removal of the device.

Preventing infection is a primary concern when caring for all types of VADs. Attention should be focused on the techniques used in routine maintenance, and care should be taken to employ measures to minimize the risk of infection, such as decreasing the catheter manipulations and aseptic handling of the hubs. Another preventive measure that has proved successful in decreasing catheter infection rates is the "locking" of the device with a heparinized vancomycin solution (instead of only heparinized saline).[69] No toxicities or complications have been noted, and no patients have experienced bacteremia due to intraluminal colonization of vancomycin-susceptible organisms, although infection due to other organisms has occurred. Another approach has been to investigate the use of antibiotic-bonded catheters and the possible effects of these catheters on infection rates.[53]

Other complications

Occlusions and device malfunctions can occur for a variety of other reasons, and careful assessment of the device when occlusion occurs should always include consideration of malpositioning or breakage. Catheters can be kinked, compressed by tumor, compressed between the rib and clavicle ("pinch-off sign"), malpositioned due to patient manipulation ("twiddler's syndrome"), malpositioned for other reasons, severed, punctured, split, or separated. The port access needle can be embedded in the septum; be inaccurately placed into the side of the port or catheter, instead of the portal housing; or become dislodged from the port and remain under the skin.[29]

Thrombus formation can result in a retrograde flow of blood or fluid along the catheter tract, with subsequent extravasation into the subcutaneous tissues. Infusion of drugs into a severed, punctured, or separated catheter can also result in extravasation. Prevention of vesicant extravasation is discussed elsewhere in this chapter, but it is prudent to reiterate that all VADs should be patent and functioning appropriately before initiating vesicant therapy. Extravasation of vesicants into the chest wall or thorax can result in severe deformity, loss of function, or death.

All of the VADs are popular, and manufacturers are continually developing new designs with innovative features every year. Oncology nurses frequently review these new devices and are called on to evaluate their effectiveness. Cost-containment is a growing concern, and the best price usually can be achieved if all of the devices selected come from a limited number of vendors, thus consolidating buying power.

Reporting defects

The Safe Medical Devices Act of 1995 requires healthcare facilities and manufacturers to report device-related events that did cause or could have caused serious injury or death. The MEDWatch system enforced through the Food and Drug Administration (FDA) makes the reporting process simple and confidential. Forms can be obtained by calling 800–FDA-1088.[70]

Conclusion

Cancer chemotherapy administration is a rapidly evolving area of oncology nursing practice that offers exciting opportunities for both beginning and seasoned oncology nurses. The level of responsibility for monitoring patients receiving chemotherapy and managing many aspects of their care continues to increase. Expanded outpatient and home care settings, where the majority of chemotherapy is given, offer opportunities for triage assessment and nursing intervention at an increasingly autonomous level. The technical explosions in drug delivery systems pose a constant informational challenge, as does the process of maintaining the personal and rewarding relationships with patients for whom these advanced technologies are utilized.

Health care will continue to move toward more ambulatory and home care, with hospitals becoming virtually intensive care buildings. Reimbursement, lobbying, litigation, and legislation will continue to be issues of concern in the twenty-first century. The oncology nurse can play a vital role in establishing effective policies and procedures by serving on institutional practice or policy committees. An oncology clinical practice committee with responsibility for reviewing and recommending procedures can also serve to evaluate new technologies. Methods for assuring competency are being developed and documented as well. Patient care evaluation and quality improvement are key responsibilities recognized by the Joint Commission on the Accreditation of Healthcare Organizations, which initiated clinical indicators for oncology to more closely monitor quality in the healthcare setting.

References

1. Koceja V: Handle with care: nurses as pharmacists vs. nurses as nurses. *Oncol Issues* 19:22–25, 2004
2. Rutherford C: Position paper — administration of antineoplastic agents. *J Intraven Nurs* 15:8–9, 1992
3. Oncology Nursing Society: *Chemotherapy and Biotherapy. Guidelines and Recommendations for Practice.* Pittsburgh, Oncology Nursing Society Press, 2001
4. Oncology Nursing Society: *Position Statement — Preparations of the Professional Registered Nurse Who Administers and Cares for the Individual Receiving Chemotherapy.* Pittsburgh, Oncology Nursing Society Press, 1991
5. American Society of Clinical Oncology: *American Society of Clinical Oncology Statement Regarding the Use of Outside Services to Prepare or Administer Chemotherapy Drugs. www.asco.org/ac1, 1003–12–002477, 00. asp.* Accessed March 7, 2004
6. American Society of Hospital Pharmacists: *Safe Handling of Cytotoxic and Hazardous Drugs Study Guide.* Bethesda, MD, American Society of Hospital Pharmacists, 1990
7. Oncology Nursing Society: *Safe Handling of Hazardous Drugs.* Pittsburgh, Oncology Nursing Society Press, 2003
8. Occupational Safety and Health Administration: Controlling occupational exposure to hazardous drugs. *OSHA Technical Manual* (section VI, Chapter 2), 2003. *www.osha.gov/dts/osta/otm/otm_vi/otm_vi_2.html.* Accessed March 7, 2004
9. U.S. Department of Health and Human Services, Public Health Services, National Institutes of Health: *Recommendations for the Safe Handling of Cytotoxic Drugs.* NIH Publication No. 92–2621, 1996
10. Martin S, Larson E: Chemotherapy — handling practices of outpatient and office-based oncology nurses. *Oncol Nurs Forum* 30:575–581, 2003
11. Connor TH, Anderson RW, Broadfield L, Power LA: Surface contamination with antineoplastic agents in six cancer treatment centers in Canada and the United States. *Am J Health Syst Pharm* 56:1427–1432, 1999
12. Yarbro CH, Frogge MH, Goodman M (eds.): *Cancer Symptom Management* (ed 3). Sudbury, MA, Jones and Bartlett, 2003
13. Phillips D, Christenfeld N, Glynn I: Increase in U.S. medication error deaths between 1983 and 1993. *Lancet* 351:643–644, 1998
14. Schulmeister L: Chemotherapy medication errors: descriptions, severity, and contributing factors. *Oncol Nurs Forum* 26:1033–1042, 1999
15. Baker K, Grochow LB, Donehower R: Should anticancer drug doses be adjusted in the obese patient? *J Natl Cancer Inst* 87:333–335, 1995
16. Georgiadis MS, Steinberg SM, Hankins LA, et al: Obesity and therapy-related toxicity in patients treated for small cell lung cancer. *J Natl Cancer Inst* 87:361–366, 1995
17. Calvert AH, Newell DR, Gumbrell LA, et al: Carboplatin dosage: prospective evaluation of a simple formula based on renal function. *J Clin Oncol* 7:1748–1756, 1989
18. Riggs CE: Anti-tumor antibiotics and related compounds, in Perry MC (ed.): *The Chemotherapy Source Book.* Baltimore, MD, Williams & Wilkins, 1992, pp 318–358
19. Rowinsky EK, Gilbert MR, McGuire WP, et al: Serious hypersensitivity reactions related to its Cremophor EL formulation vehicle. *J Clin Oncol* 9:1692–1703, 1991
20. Van Hoefer U, Harstrick A, Wilke H, et al: Schedule dependent antagonism of paclitaxel and cisplatin in human gastric and ovarian carcinoma cell lines in vitro. *Eur J Cancer* 31A:92–97, 1995
21. Clark JW, Santos-Moore AS, Choy H: Sequencing of taxol and carboplatinum therapy. *Proc Am Assoc Cancer Res* 36:298, 1995 (abstr 1772)
22. Holmes FA, Newman RA, Madden T, et al: Schedule dependent pharmacokinetics (pk) in a phase I trial of taxol and doxorubicin as initial therapy for metastatic breast cancer. NCI Publication, A489, NCI-EORTC, 1–27 1994
23. Siegel RS, Pandolfino T, Guitart J, et al: Primary cutaneous T-cell lymphoma: a review and current concepts. *J Clin Oncol* 18:2908–2925, 2000
24. Akscin J: The future of oral chemotherapy drugs at ACCC's 27th annual national meeting. *http://222.accc-cancer.org/news/ornl.asp.* Assessed March 7, 2004
25. Bedell CH: A changing paradigm for cancer treatment: the advent of new chemotherapy agents. *Clin J Oncol Nurs* 7(suppl 6):5–9, 2003
26. Hartigan K: Patient education: the cornerstone of successful oral chemotherapy treatment. *Clin J Oncol Nurs* 7(suppl 6):21–24, 2003

27. Laughlin RA, Landeen JM, Habal MB: The management of inadvertent subcutaneous adriamycin infiltration. *Am J Surg* 137:408–412, 1979
28. Boyle DM, Engelking C: Vesicant extravasation: myths and realities. *Oncol Nurs Forum* 22:57–67, 1995
29. Schulmeister L, Camp-Sorrell D: Continuing education: chemotherapy extravasations from implanted ports. *Oncol Nurs Forum* 27:531–540, 2000
30. Viale PH, Yamamoto DS, Geyton JE: Extravasation of infusate via implanted port: two case studies. *Clin J Oncol Nurs* 3:145–151, 1999
31. Mayo DJ, Pearson DC: Chemotherapy extravasation: a consequence of fibrin sheath formation around venous access devices. *Oncol Nurs Forum* 22:675–680, 1995
32. Rudolph R, Larson DL: Etiology and treatment of chemotherapeutic agent extravasation injuries: a review. *J Clin Oncol* 5:1116–1126, 1987
33. Ajani J, Dodd LG, Daugherty K, el al: Taxol induced soft-tissue injury secondary to extravasation: characterized by histopathology and clinical course. *J Natl Cancer Inst* 86:51–53, 1994
34. Goodman M: Taxol and Taxotere infiltrations: special considerations in management. *Oncol Nurs Forum* 23:87, 1996
35. Martin R: Use of hepatic lines. *J Infus Nurs* 25:127–133, 2002
36. Barber FD, Fabugais-Nazario L: What's old is new again: patients receiving hepatic arterial infusion chemotherapy. *Clin J Oncol Nurs* 7:647–652, 2003
37. Winkelman LA: Ascities, in Yarbro CH, Frogge MH, Goodman M (eds.): *Cancer Symptom Management* (ed 3). Sudbury, MA, Jones and Bartlett, 2003, pp 401–412
38. Zook-Enck D: Intraperitoneal therapy via the Tenckhoff catheter. *J Intraven Nurs* 13:375–382, 1990
39. Malloy J: Administering intraperitoneal chemotherapy: a new approach. *Nursing* 21:58–62, 1991
40. Schrump DS, Nguyen DM: Malignant pleural and pericardial effusions, in DeVita VT, Hellman S, Rosenberg SA (eds.): *Cancer: Principles and Practice of Oncology* (ed 6). Philadelphia, Lippincott Williams & Wilkins, 2001, pp 2729–2744
41. Saffran L, Ost DE, Fein AM, et al: Outpatient pleurodesis of malignant pleural effusions using a small-bore pigtail catheter. *Chest* 118:417–421, 2000
42. Goldman DA: Effusions, in Yarbro CH, Frogge MH, Goodman M (eds.): *Cancer Symptom Management* (ed 3). Sudbury, MA, Jones and Bartlett, 2003, pp 420-436
43. Herr HW, Badalament RA, Amato DA, et al: Superficial bladder cancer treated with bacillus Calmette-Guérin: a multivariate analysis of factors affecting tumor progression. *J Urol* 141:22–29, 1989
44. Brosman SA, Lamm DL: The preparation, handling and use of intravesical bacillus Calmette-Guérin for the management of stage Ta, T1, carcinoma in situ and transitional cell cancer. *J Urol* 144:313–315, 1990
45. Lamm DL, Riggs DR, Traynelis CI: Apparent failure of current intravesical chemotherapy prophylaxis to influence the long-term course of superficial transitional cell carcinoma of the bladder. *J Urol* 153:1444–1450, 1995
46. Phillips PC: Methotrexate neurotoxicity, in Rottenberg DA (ed.): *Neurologic Complications of Cancer Treatment.* Boston, Butterworth-Heinemann, 1991, pp 123–155
47. Oncology Nursing Society: *Access Device Guidelines: Recommendations for Nursing Practice and Education* (ed 2). Pittsburgh, Oncology Nursing Society Press, 2004, pp 2–141
48. ACS Nursing Subcommittee: *Venous Access Devices Standards of Care.* Salt Lake City, American Cancer Society, 1990, p 8
49. Raad I, Davis S, Becker M, et al: Low infection rate and long durability of nontunneled silastic catheters. *Arch Intern Med* 153:1791–1796, 1993
50. Sansivero GE, Barton-Burke M: Chemotherapy administration: general principles for vascular access, in Barton-Burke M, Wilkes GM, Ingwerson K (eds.): *Cancer Chemotherapy: A Nursing Process Approach* (ed 3). Sudbury, MA, Jones and Bartlett, 2001, pp 645–670
51. Ryder M: Peripherally inserted central venous catheters. *Nurs Clin North Am* 28:937–971, 1994
52. Alexander HR: Infectious complications associated with long-term vascular access devices: etiology, diagnosis, treatment, and prophylaxis, in Alexander HR (ed.): *Vascular Access in the Cancer Patient: Devices, Insertion Techniques, Maintenance, and Prevention of Complications.* Philadelphia, Lippincott, 1995, pp 112–128
53. Centers for Disease Control and Prevention: Guidelines for prevention of intravascular and catheter-related infections. *MMWR* 51:1–29, 2002
54. Lucas A: Routine maintenance and care of long-term vascular access devices, in Alexander HR (ed.): *Vascular Access in the Cancer Patient: Devices, Insertion Techniques, Maintenance, and Prevention of Complications.* Philadelphia, Lippincott, 1995, pp 148–164
55. Winters V, Peters B, Coila S, et al: A trial with a new peripheral implanted vascular access device. *Oncol Nurs Forum* 17:891–896, 1990
56. Groeger S, Lucas A, Thaler H, et al: Infectious morbidity associated with long-term use of vascular access devices in patients with cancer. *Ann Intern Med* 153:1167–1174, 1993
57. Danzig L, Shat L, Collins K, et al: Bloodstream infections associated with a needleless system in patients receiving home infusion therapy. *JAMA* 23:1862–1864, 1995
58. Howell P, Walters P, Donowitz G, et al: Risk factors for infection of adult patients with cancer who have tunneled central venous access devices. *Cancer* 75:1367–1375, 1995
59. Keung Y, Watkins D, Chen S, et al: Comparative study of infectious complications of different types of chronic vascular access devices. *Cancer* 73:2832–2837, 1994
60. Kupensky D: Use of hydrochloric acid to restore patency in an occluded implantable port. *J Intraven Nurs* 18:198–201, 1995
61. Mayo DJ: Catheter related thrombosis. *J Intraven Nurs* 24(suppl 1):S13–S22, 2001
62. Wickham R, Purl S, Welker D: Long-term central venous catheters: issues for care. *Semin Oncol Nurs* 8:133–147, 1992
63. Wickham R, Purl S, McHale M: Long-term central venous catheters, in Kitt S, Selfridge-Thomas J, Proehl J, Kaiser J (eds.): *Emergency Nursing. A Physiologic and Clinical Perspective.* Philadelphia, Saunders, 1995, pp 640–664
64. Weinstein SM: Parenteral nutrition, in *Plumer's Principles and Practice of Intravenous Therapy* (ed 7). Philadelphia, Lippincott, 2001, pp 353–410
65. Thompson B, Veal D: Pharmacologic treatment of pediatric catheter occlusion. *Hosp Pharm* 27:137–141, 1992
66. Gray WJ, Bell WR: Fibrinolytic agents in the treatment of thrombotic disorders. *Semin Oncol* 17:228–237, 1990
67. Fraschini G, Jadeja J, Lawson M, et al: Local infusion of urokinase for the lysis of thrombosis associated with permanent central venous catheters in cancer patients. *J Clin Oncol* 5:672–678, 1990
68. Bern MM, Lokich JL, Wallach SR, et al: Very low doses of warfarin can prevent thrombosis in central venous catheters: a randomized perspective trial. *Ann Intern Med* 112:423–428, 1990
69. Schwartz C, Hendrickson KJ, Roghmann K, et al: Prevention of bacteremia attributed to luminal colonization of tunneled central venous catheters with vancomycin-susceptible organisms. *J Clin Oncol* 8:1591–1597, 1990
70. Dessler DA: Introducing MEDWatch, a new approach to reporting medication and device adverse effects and product problems. *JAMA* 269:2765–2768, 1995

Appendix 16A Oral Antineoplastic Agents

Drug and Disease Indications	Dose and Schedule	Side Effects: Acute or Delayed	Pharmacokinetics	Comments
Altretamine (Hexamethyl-melamine hexaline) Ovarian cancer	*Cap:* 50 mg and 100 mg clear *Dose:* 240–320 mg/m²/day	*Nadir:* 21–28 days Acute liver toxicity is dose limiting; nausea and vomiting are dose related Mild BMS (bone marrow suppression) Abdominal cramping Diarrhea Peripheral neuropathies Agitation, confusion	Variable absorption Rapid metabolism Urine excretion 90% in 72 hr	• Pyridoxine 50 mg/day may decrease neuropathy. • Take with food, prophylactic antiemetics. • May worsen vincristine-related peripheral neuropathy.
Bexarotene (Targretin) Cutaneous T-cell lymphoma	*Cap:* 75mg off white *Dose:* 300 mg/m²/day	*Nadir:* 4–8 weeks Lipid abnormalities that may be dose limiting Asthenia Headache Hypothyroidism Leukopenia Anemia Infection Sensitivity to the sun Allergic reactions GI disturbances Edema Teratogenicity	Hepatic metabolism Peak plasma concentration within 3 hr Short half-life Absorption enhanced with food	• Retinoid. • Avoid excessive sunlight. • Two reliable forms of contraception should be used for one month before, during, and after treatment. • Nighttime administration is recommended, at least 1 hr after the dinner. • Avoid vitamin A supplements and grapefruit juice. • Do not use with patients at risk for pancreatitis.
Busulfan (Myleran) Leukemia	*Tab:* 2 mg white *Dose:* 4–12 mg/day for several weeks	*Nadir:* 10–30 days delayed marrow recovery Potentially teratogenic Pulmonary fibrosis with long-term use Dermatologic hyperpigmentation Gynecomastia Amenorrhea	Well absorbed Extensive hepatic metabolism to inactive compounds Renal excretion	• Bone marrow recovery may be delayed; therefore caution is advised with long-term use. Hydration and allopurinol may be indicated to prevent hyperuricemia. Total cumulative dose: 600 mg. • Long-term daily administration is not recommended due to the risk of second malignancies with chronic alkylating agents.
Capecitabine (Xeloda) Metastatic breast cancer Metastatic colorectal cancer	*Tab:* 150 mg light peach, 500 mg peach 2500 mg/m²/day × 14 days q 21 days Swallow with water only; take with food	Mild BMS Dose-limiting toxicity is diarrhea Hand-foot syndrome, dermatitis, fatigue, anorexia, nausea, stomatitis	Metabolized to 5-FU; excreted in urine	• Administer in two oral doses, 12 hours apart, 30 minutes after a meal. • Monitor coagulation profile in patients also taking Coumadin.
Chlorambucil (Leukeran) Leukemia Hodgkin's disease	*Tab:* 2 mg white *Dose:* 4–8 mg/m²/day × 3–6 wk 16 mg/m²/wk q 4 wk	*Nadir:* 7–10 days Severe BMS Slight nausea and vomiting Occasional dermatitis Abnormal liver function Pulmonary fibrosis with prolonged use Second malignancy Sterility	Hepatic metabolism to active compound Renal excretion of 50% of unchanged drug	• Good oral absorption. • Concomitant barbiturate administration may enhance toxicity. Marrow suppression may be prolonged.
Cyclophosphamide (Cytoxan) Breast cancer Multiple myeloma Small cell lung cancer Malignant lymphomas Leukemias	*Tab:* 25–50 mg *Dose:* 1–5 mg/kg/day 60–120 mg/m² Adjust dose in presence of renal dysfunction	*Nadir:* 7–14 days Anorexia, nausea, and vomiting Alopecia Hemorrhagic cystitis with gross or microscopic hematuria Amenorrhea Sterility	Activated in the liver Oral absorption in 1 hr 30% of drug excreted unchanged in urine	• Vigorous hydration (3 L/day). • Encourage frequent voiding to prevent hemorrhagic cystitis (a sterile inflammation of the urinary bladder). If patient complains of burning on urination or bladder incontinence, urinalysis may reveal occult blood. Control by withdrawal of the drug and hydration. • May take pills in divided doses early in the day and with meals or all at one time. Better tolerated with cold foods. • Barbiturates and other inducers of hepatic microsomal enzymes may enhance toxicity (e.g., cimetidine). Allopurinol may enhance BMS.

(*continued*)

Appendix 16A Oral Antineoplastic Agents (continued)

Drug and Disease Indications	Dose and Schedule	Side Effects: Acute or Delayed	Pharmacokinetics	Comments
Gefitinib (Iressa) Advanced non-small cell lung cancer	*Tab:* 250 mg brown *Dose:* 250 mg daily	*Nadir:* No effects on the blood counts Diarrhea Rash Acne Dry skin Vomiting Nausea Pruritis Anorexia Eye irritation	Slowly absorbed after oral administration Extensive hepatic metabolism Elimination half-life is 48 hr	• Tyrosine kinase inhibitor. • May be taken with or without food. • If interstitial lung disease is confirmed, Iressa should be stopped immediately. • Monitor coagulation profile in patients on Coumadin. • Co-medication with rifampicin, phenytoin, and antacids may decrease efficacy. • Treat skin rash with topical clindamycin.
Hydroxyurea (Hydrea) Chronic myelocytic leukemia Melanoma Head and neck cancer	*Cap:* 500 mg *Dose:* 80 mg/kg/day every third day 750–1000 mg/m²/day × 5 Decrease dose in presence of renal dysfunction Store in tight container in a cool environment	*Nadir:* 13–17 days Acute nausea and vomiting Chronic and severe anemia Neurological seizures and hallucinations Dermatitis Dysuria Azotemia	Well absorbed Hepatic metabolism Renal excretion of 80% of compound in 12 hr Crosses into CSF	• Concomitant radiation and/or 5-fluorouracil (5-FU) may enhance neurotoxicity. • Dysuria and renal impairment may occur. • Consider pretreatment with allopurinol.
Imatinib (Gleevec) Chronic myelogenous leukemia Metastatic malignant gastrointestinal stromal tumors (GISTs)	*Tab:* 100 mg and 400 mg dark brown to brownish orange *Dose:* 400 mg daily chronic phase CML, 600 mg daily accelerated phase, 800 mg for blast crisis Laboratory abnormalities should be managed with dose reductions and/or interruption of treatment	BMS Nausea, vomiting Fluid retention and edema Muscle cramps Diarrhea Hemorrhage Muscle and joint pain Skin rash Headache Indigestion Hepatotoxicity	Major enzyme responsible for metabolism is CYP3A4 Absorbed well Eliminated predominately in the feces Elimination half-life is 18–22 hours	• Protein kinase inhibitor. • Take with a large glass of water to minimize nausea. Remain sitting or standing upright for 1 hour after drug ingestion. • Obtain complete blood counts weekly for the first month, biweekly for the second month, and every 2–3 months thereafter. • Dose reduction or interruption is effective in managing most cases of bone marrow suppression. • Do not take with grapefruit, grapefruit juice, or caffeine-containing products. • Calcium supplements may help relieve leg cramps. • Monitor liver function tests.
Lomustine (CCNU) Brain cancer Lymphomas	*Cap:* 100 mg/green/green, 40 mg green/white, 10 mg white *Dose:* 100–130 mg/m² q 6–8 week	*Nadir:* 28–42 days Severe cumulative BMS Nausea and vomiting 4–6 hr after dosing Anorexia Alopecia Stomatitis Hepatotoxicity	Absorbed rapidly (<60 min) Hepatic metabolism Renal excretion of 50% in 24 hr and 75% in 96 hr Crosses into CSF	• Dispense one dose at a time to prevent accidental overdose. • Take on an empty stomach just before bedtime. • Pretreat with aggressive antiemetics. • Protect pills from heat and humidity.
L-phenylanine mustard (melphalan, Alkeran) Multiple myeloma Ovarian cancer	*Tab:* 2 mg white *Dose:* 0.1–0.15 mg/kg/day × 2–3 wk Reduce dose with hepatic or renal impairment	*Nadir:* 10–18 days Nausea and vomiting usually mild Dermatitis Pulmonary fibrosis Long-term therapy can result in acute leukemia	Hepatic metabolism Renal excretion 20%–35% (10% unchanged) 20%–50% excreted in feces within 6 days	• Protect pills from sunlight. • Take on an empty stomach. • BMS may be cumulative in older patients. • Leukemogenic.
6-Mercaptopurine (6-MP) Leukemia	*Tab:* 50 mg off-white *Dose:* 80–100 mg/m²/day Titrate dose based on blood counts Reduce dose in presence of hepatic or renal dysfunction	*Nadir:* 10–14 days Nausea, vomiting Mucositis Diarrhea Drug fever Intrahepatic cholestasis Pulmonary toxicity with prolonged use	Incomplete oral absorption Hepatic inactivation Renal excretion 10% unchanged in 24 hr	• Protect pills from light. • Administer as single dose on an empty stomach. • Increased toxicity with allopurinal (reduce dose by one-third to one-fourth of the original dose). • Administer with caution to patients on sodium warfarin (Coumadin). • Monitor liver function tests.
Methotrexate Squamous cell carcinoma Lung cancer	*Tab:* 2.5 mg yellow *Dose:* 2.5–10 mg/day PO or 15–30 mg/day PO × 5 days q 1–3 wk	*Nadir:* 7–10 days Nausea and anorexia can occur; stomatitis and ulcerations can occur and are dose limiting.	Serum half-life lis 2–4 hr Excreted by the kidneys	• Dose is reduced with renal impairment; dosing on an empty stomach may enhance bioavailability. Excretion may be impaired in patients with simultaneous administration or weak acids such as salicylates or vitamin C; oral dosing is generally well tolerated. • Avoid administration of methotrexate with ketoprotein or probenecid because toxicity of methotrexate may be enhanced.

Appendix 16A Oral Antineoplastic Agents (continued)

Drug and Disease Indications	Dose and Schedule	Side Effects: Acute or Delayed	Pharmacokinetics	Comments
Procarbazine (Matulane) Hodgkin's disease	*Cap:* 50 mg *Dose:* 100 mg/m²/day × 14 days q 4 wk; reduce dose in presence of hepatic or renal dysfunction	*Nadir:* 4 wk BMS, nausea, vomiting, and diarrhea gradually subside; flulike syndrome, paresthesias, neuropathies, dizziness, and ataxia	Well absorbed from the gastrointestinal tract Metabolized in the liver with a biological half-life of about 1 hr 70% of the drug is eliminated by 24 hr in the urine; 5% appears as unchanged drug	• Drug and food interactions can occur. • Central nervous system (CNS) depression can occur with concomitant administration of procarbazine and CNS depressants. • Hypertensive crisis can occur when procarbazine is administered with certain antidepressants (tricyclics and monoamine oxidase inhibitors) and tyramine-rich foods. • Severe nausea and vomiting can occur if taken with ethanol, mixed drinks, and beer.
Temozolomide (Temodar) Astrocytoma	*Cap:* 5 mg green, 20 mg brown, 100 mg blue, 250 mg black *Dose:* 150 mg/m²/day × 5 days q month Dose escalation based on nadir counts	*Nadir:* Platelets by day 26, neutrophils by day 28 BMS is dose-limiting toxicity Nausea, vomiting, fatigue, and headache can be severe in 10% of cases	Rapidly absorbed with a mean elimination half-life of 1.8 hr Eliminated via the kidneys	• Take on an empty stomach at night with glass of water. • Capsules should not be opened or chewed.
Thalidomide (Thalomid) Erythema nodosum leprosum	*Cap:* 50 mg white, 100 mg tan, 200 mg blue *Dose:* 100–300 mg daily Higher dosages may be divided into a twice-a-day schedule. It is recommended to take one dose before dinner and the second dose after dinner or before bed.	Drowsiness, dizziness, weakness and fatigue Rash Orthostatic hypotension Neutropenia Bradycardia Constipation Peripheral neuropathy Sensitivity to sunlight Fluid retention HIV viral load increase	Slowly absorbed after oral administration Elimination half-life is 5–7 hours Exact metabolic route is not known in humans; appears to undergo a non-enzymatic hydrolysis in plasma to multiple metabolites	• Immunomodulating agent. • Can cause severe birth deffects or fetal death. • Two reliable forms of contraception must be used for one month before starting thalidomide. • Avoid co-administration with alcohol, reserpine, chlorpromazine, barbiturates, and other sedatives. • If drowsiness occurs, avoid hazardous activities, such as driving or operating heavy machinery. • Take 1 hr after the evening meal. • Consent form regarding safe birth control practices needs to be signed before treatment is initiated. • A pregnancy test must be completed 24 hours before starting and during treatment.
6-Thioguanine Leukemia	*Tab:* 40 mg green/yellow *Dose:* 80–100 mg/m² Reduce dose if stomatitis occurs	*Nadir:* 7–28 days Stomatitis Diarrhea Hepatotoxicity	Variable, incomplete absorption Hepatic metabolism Renal excretion	• Administer on an empty stomach. • Does not require dose reduction when used in conjunction with allopurinol.
VP-16 (etoposide, VePesid) Lung cancer Testicular cancer	*Cap:* 50 mg pink *Dose:* 2 × the IV dose or 100–200 mg/m²/day 3–5 × days q 3–4 wk	*Nadir:* 7–14 days (white blood cell count) Nausea and vomiting. 9–16 days (platelets) Alopecia BMS is dose limiting	Renal and hepatic metabolism Incomplete and variable absorption	• Nausea is mild though can be more severe with oral route than with IV route.

Adapted and revised from Goodman M: Delivery of cancer chemotherapy, in Baird S, McCorkle R, Grant M (eds.): *Cancer Nursing: A Comprehensive Textbook.* Philadelphia, W. B. Saunders, 1991, p 311.

Appendix 16B Intravenous Antineoplastic Agents

Dosage and Efficacy	Mechanism of Action and Metabolism	Administration Precautions	Side Effects
		ALEMTUZEMAB (Campath)	
Dosage: • Initial dose escalation: 3 mg daily until tolerated, advance to 10 mg daily until tolerated, advance to 30 mg daily. If tolerated begin maintenance dose of 30 mg 3 × a week on alternate days for 12 wk *Dose reductions:* • ANC < 250 or platelet count ≤ 25,000: First occurrence: Withhold Campath until ANC > 500 or platelet count ≥ 50,000. If delay > 7 days, restart at 3 mg and escalate to 10 mg and 30 mg. Second occurrence: Withhold until ANC > 500 and platelet count ≥ 50,000, and resume at 10 mg dose. Third occurrence: Discontinue permanently. • Decrease in ANC or platelet count to > 50% baseline in patients who start therapy with ANC < 500 or platelet count < 50,000: Withhold Campath until counts recover to baseline value. If delay > 7 days, restart at 3 mg, escalate to 10 mg and 30 mg. *Efficacy:* • Chronic lymphocytic leukemia	*Mechanism of action:* Humanized monoclonal antibody directed at CD52 antigen. *Metabolism:* • t½ = 12 days	*Administration precautions:* • Infuse over 2 hr. • Premedicate with diphenhydramine and acetaminophen 30 min prior to initiation of infusion. Corticosteroids may need to be added. • Anti-infective prophylaxis with Bactrim DS BID 3 × a week and antiviral prophylaxis with famciclivor 250 mg or equivalent BID upon initiation of treatment; continue for 2 months post-treatment. • Dilute in 100 mL of 0.9% sodium chloride or 5% dextrose in water solution. • Stable for 8 hr at room temperature. • Contraindicated in patients with active systemic infections and underlying immunodeficiencies.	*Side effects:* • Infusion reactions can be severe and present with rapid onset of hypotension, rigors, fever, bronchospasm, shortness of breath, and rash. Emergency medications should be readily available. Careful monitoring of blood pressure is necessary. • Severe pancytopenia including neutropenia, lymphopenia, thrombocytopenia, and anemia can occur. Weekly monitoring of CBC necessary. • Nausea, vomiting, diarrhea, stomatitis, and anorexia. • Headache and dysasthesia. • Asthenia and pain.
		ARSENIC TRIOXIDE (Trisenox)	
Dosage: • Induction: 0.15 mg/kg daily IV until bone marrow remission (not to exceed 60 doses) • Consolidation: 0.15 mg/kg daily × 25 doses over 5 wks, starting 3–6 wks after completion of induction therapy *Efficacy:* • Acute promyelocytic leukemia	*Mechanism of action:* • Causes morphological changes and DNA fragmentation. • Damages or degrades the fusion protein PML-RAR alpha. *Metabolism:* • Metabolized in the liver. • Excreted in the urine. • t½ = 4–17 hr	*Administration precautions:* • Dilute in 100–250 mL of D5W or 0.9% NS and infuse over 1–2 hr. May extend infusion time up to 4 hr if acute vasomotor reactions occur. • Stable at room temperature for 24 hr and 48 hrs under refrigeration.	*Side effects:* • Dizziness, lightheadedness, infusional hypotension, fatigue, skin reactions, musculoskeletal pain, mild hyperglycemia, nausea, vomiting, and diarrhea are the most common side effects. • Peripheral neuropathy can occur. • APL differentiation syndrome has been reported and can be fatal. Early signs include fever, weight gain, and dyspnea. High-dose steroids should be started immediately and continued until symptoms resolve. • Can cause prolongation of the QT interval, which can lead to complete atrioventricular block. Obtain baseline EKG and monitor weekly during treatment. Potassium, magnesium, calcium, and creatinine should be monitored twice weekly during induction and weekly during consolidation.

<table>
<tr><th colspan="4">BEVACIZUMAB (Avastin)</th></tr>
<tr>
<td>Dosage:
• 5 mg/kg IV infusion q 14 days
Efficacy:
• Metastatic carcinoma of the rectum or colon</td>
<td>Mechanism of action:
• Humanized monoclonal antibody
• Inhibits the action of vascular endothelial growth factor (VEGF) and angiogenesis
Metabolism:
• t½ = 20 days</td>
<td>Administration precautions:
• Dilute in 100 mL of 0.9% sodium chloride. Do not administer or mix with dextrose solutions.
• Infuse the initial dose over 90 mins; if tolerated well, infuse the second treatment over 60 mins. If the 60-min infusion is tolerated well, all subsequent infusions may be administered over 30 mins.
• Diluted Avastin solutions must be refrigerated. Stable for 8 hr under refrigeration.
• Avastin should not be started for at least 28 days following major surgery, and the surgical incision should be completely healed.
• Avastin should be discontinued for an appropriate interval prior to elective surgery.
• Protect from light.</td>
<td>Side effects:
• Gastrointestinal perforation and impaired wound healing.
• Hemorrhagic events such as epistaxis, embolism, hematemesis, and GI bleed can occur.
• Nephrotic syndrome and proteinuria may occur. Monitor urine protein closely.
• Hypersensitivity reactions can occur and often are characterized by fever, rigors, or chills. Emergency medications need to be available. Premedication and slowing the infusion rate substantially reduce the future occurrence.
• Asthenia, pain, hypertension, diarrhea, leucopenia, and hypertension were seen in clinical trails.
• Hypertension needs to be treated medically.</td>
</tr>
<tr><th colspan="4">BLEOMYCIN (Blenoxane)</th></tr>
<tr>
<td>Dosage:
• May be given IM, SQ, IV, intratumoral, intra-arterial.
• 10–20 U/m^2 once or twice a week
• Intrapleural/pericardial sclerosing dose: 50–60 U/m^2 in 50–100 mL NS or D5W; not to exceed 40 U/m^2 in geriatric population
Efficacy:
• Cervical cancer
• Head and neck cancer
• Penis, skin, and testicular cancer
• Hodgkin's and non-Hodgkin's lymphoma
• Kaposi's sarcoma</td>
<td>Mechanism of action:
• Cell-cycle phase specific for G_2 and M phase. Binds to DNA.
• Inhibits cell progression out of G_2, resulting in cellular synchronization for subsequent drug therapy.
Metabolism:
• t½ = 20 min
• Renal elimination.</td>
<td>Administration precautions:
• Administer with caution to patients with significant pulmonary or renal disease. Prior cisplatin therapy may reduce bleomycin clearance, increasing plasma half-life and toxicity.
• Test dose: Bleomycin is associated with HSR and a test dose of 2 U IV in 50 mL D5W over 15 min followed by observation. Observe for anaphylactic reaction for 1–2 hours post-test dose.
• Lymphoma patients are more at risk for HSR and should be tested for the first two doses.</td>
<td>Side effects:
• Lifetime cumulative dose is 400 U.
• 25% dose reduction for creatinine clearance of 30–50 mL/min.
• 50% dose reduction for creatinine clearance of 20–30 mL/min.
• Fever occurs in approximately 50% of patients. Premedicate with acetaminophen 1g and diphenhydramine 50 mg. (Repeat 6 hr later.)
• Dermatological reactions such as hyperpigmentation, hyperkeratosis, and erythema on palms and fingers; urticaria, rash, mucositis, and alopecia.
• Anorexia and mild nausea.
• Interstitial pneumonitis and pulmonary fibrosis occur more commonly in patients who also have mediastinal radiation, are elderly, and receive higher cumulative doses.</td>
</tr>
</table>

(continued)

Appendix 16B Intravenous Antineoplastic Agents (continued)

Dosage and Efficacy	Mechanism of Action and Metabolism	Administration Precautions	Side Effects
		BORTEZOMIB (Velcade)	
Dosage: • 1.3 mg^2 dose IV bolus twice weekly for 2 wk, followed by a 10-day rest period (21-day cycle) *Efficacy:* • Multiple myeloma	*Mechanism of action:* • Inhibits intracellular proteasome activity that induces cancer cell apoptosis, limits tumor growth and spread. *Metabolism:* • Hepatic and renal elimination. • Less than 10% eliminated unchanged in the urine. • $t½ < 10$ min.	*Administration precautions:* • Must maintain a strict 72-hour rest period between dosages to allow for restoration of normal proteasome function. • Reconstitute in 3.5 mL of 0.9% sodium chloride solution. • Stable for 8 hr at room temperature. • Growth factor administration is contraindicated within 24 hr of treatment. • Patients taking antidiabetic drugs may need dose adjustments during treatment. • Closely monitor patients concomitantly receiving CYP3A4 inhibitors or inducers for toxicities or decreased efficacy. • Administer with caution to patients receiving medications associated with neuropathy, such as antivirals, nitrofurantion, isoniazid, statins, and amiodarone. • Contraindicated for patients with allergies to mannitol and boron.	*Side effects:* • Asthenic conditions are commonly reported. • Nausea, vomiting, diarrhea, constipation, and anorexia. • Headache. • Peripheral neuropathy, predominantely sensory in nature, is common. • Thrombocytopenia may occur, but significant myleosuppression is uncommon. • Orthostatic hypotension, mostly moderate in nature, may occur and may be delayed. Seen most often in patients with diabetes and those on antihypertensive medications.
		CARBOPLATIN (Paraplatin)	
Dosage: • IV: 360 mg/m^2 q 4 wk • Higher doses are given in pretransplant protocols and intraperitoneally or intraarterially. • Dose calculations are most therapeutically based on the desired serum concentration (AUC), renal status, and whether or not the patient has been previously treated with chemotherapy (Calvert method). • Note that doses calculated according to the Calvert formula are total mg, not mg/m^2 (see text).	*Mechanism of action:* • Maximal cytotoxicity occurs when cells are in the S-phase although cell kill by intrastrand DNA cross-linkage occurs throughout G_1, S, and G_2 phases of the cell cycle. *Metabolism:* • 60% eliminated unchanged in the urine. • Major routes of elimination are glomerular filtration and tubular secretion. • $t½ = 2.5$ hr	*Administration precautions:* • Available as lyophilized (powdered) form to distinguish it from cisplatin, which is available only in aqueous solution. • Usually administered over 15–30 min in 500 mL of NS or D5W, without further hydration. • May also be administered as a continuous 24-hr or longer infusion. • Forms a precipitate when in contact with aluminum, causing loss of antitumor potency. • Injection site irritation and erythema can occur with infiltration but no ulceration or necrosis • Physically compatible with ondansetron.	*Side effects:* • DLT: myelosuppression, particularly thrombocytopenia. Nadir occurs at 2–3 wk. • Nausea and vomiting are mild and rarely last beyond 24 hr. • Ototoxicity and neurotoxicity (paresthesias) are uncommon. • Alopecia, mucositis, and abnormal liver functions have been reported. • Nephrotoxicity occurs but is less common than with cisplatin.

Efficacy:

- Ovarian carcinoma
- Testicular cancer
- Head and neck cancer
- Cervical cancer
- Lung cancer

CARMUSTINE (BiCNU)

Dosage:

- IV: 75–100 mg/m^2 iv/day × 2 days
- IV: 200–225 mg/m^2 q 6 wk
- IV: 40 mg/m^2/day on 5 successive days, repeating cycle q 6–8 wk
- Higher doses have been used in pretransplant protocols.

Efficacy:

- Brain tumors
- Multiple myeloma
- Hodgkin's disease
- Non-Hodgkin's lymphoma
- Melanoma

Mechanism of action:

- Inhibits enzymatic reactions involved in DNA synthesis.
- Inhibits DNA repair.
- Acts predominantly during late G and early S phase.
- Readily crosses the blood–brain barrier.

Metabolism:

- Metabolized by the liver.
- 80% eliminated via the kidneys.
- t½ = 15–20 min

Administration precautions:

- Soluble in water and absolute alcohol.
- Protect from light.
- Administer in 100–500 mL D5W or NS as a 1- to 2-hr infusion.
- Infusion may burn as it goes in and should be monitored closely.
- Heat provides symptomatic relief.
- Slowing the infusion rate eases vein discomfort.
- Hypotension can occur if the infusion is given rapidly.
- Facial flushing and dizziness occur infrequently.
- Compatible with ondansetron.
- Incompatible with polyvinylchloride infusion bags and with sodium bicarbonate.
- Avoid contact with skin; a brown stain may result.

Side effects:

- DLT: Leukopenia and thrombocytopenia occur 3–5 wk after treatment, recovery at 8 wk.
- Myelosuppression may be cumulative.
- Nausea and vomiting are common and require aggressive antiemetic therapy.
- Pulmonary fibrosis has been reported and generally presents as a dry cough and dyspnea.
- Alopecia is common.
- Elevation of LFTs and azotemia can occur with higher doses. Cimetidine has been shown to potentiate carmustine toxicity.

CETUXIMAB (Erbitux)

Dosage:

- Initial loading dosage: 400 mg/m^2 IV infusion
- Maintenance dose: 250 mg/m^2 IV infusion weekly

Dose reductions:

- Grades 1–2 infusion reaction: Reduce dose by 50%
- Grade 3–4 infusion reactions: Permanently discontinue the drug

Mechanism of action:

- Monoclonal antibody.
- Inhibits the binding of epidermal growth factor (EGF), resulting in the induction of apoptosis, inhibition of cell growth, and decreased growth factor production.

Metabolism:

- Exhibits nonlinear pharmacokinetics
- Mean elimination t½ = 97 hr

Administration precautions:

- Must be administered with a low protein binding 0.22 micron in-line filter.
- Infuse initial dose, over 120 min and subsequent infusions over 60 min.
- Maximum infusion rate is 5 mL/min.
- Must be administered via infusion pump or syringe pump.
- Premedication with an H_1 antagonist is recommended.

Side effects:

- Infusion reactions can be severe and usually occur during the initial infusion, presenting with rapid onset of airway obstruction, urticaria, and hypotention. Emergency medications should be readily available.
- Dermatological toxicities including acneform rash, dry skin, and fissuring are commonly reported. Sun exposure may exacerbate these effects, therefore protect skin from sunlight.

(continued)

Appendix 16B Intravenous Antineoplastic Agents (continued)

Dosage and Efficacy	Mechanism of Action and Metabolism	Administration Precautions	Side Effects
Efficacy: • Metastatic colorectal carcinoma		• Erbitux should be piggybacked to the main infusion line. • Observe the patient for a 1 hr period post-infusion for signs/symptoms of reaction. • Stable for 8 hr at room temperature and 12 hr under refrigeration.	• Asthenia conditions, diarrhea, nausea, vomiting, abdominal pain, constipation, and fever are commonly experienced. • Rare cases of interstitial lung disease are reported.
CISPLATIN (Platinol) AQUEOUS SOLUTION			
Dosage: • IV: 50–120 mg/m^2 q 3–4 wk • IV: 15–20 mg/m^2 × 5 q 3–4 wk, radio-sensitizing effect: • IV: 15–50 mg/m^2 1–3 times per week with concomitant RT • IP: 100–270 mg/m^2 in 2 L of warmed NS. Infuse via gravity over 10 min. Allow 4-hr dwell time. *Efficacy:* • Bladder cancer • Ovarian cancer • Testicular carcinoma • Non-small cell lung cancer • Head and neck cancer	*Mechanism of action:* • Binds to DNA affecting DNA replication. • Forms DNA protein cross-links. • Interacts with cellular glutathione. *Metabolism:* • 90% bound to plasma proteins. • 20%–45% eliminated unchanged via kidney. • 10% eliminated in bile. • t½ = 60–90 hr	*Administration precautions:* • Dose reductions: 25% dose reduction for patients with creatinine clearance of 30–50 mL/min and a 50% dose reduction for patients with creatinine clearance < 30 mL/min • Administer after appropriate hydration (1–2 L with mannitol). • Maintain urinary output (125 mL/hr). Mixing cisplatin in 0–9% NaCl maintains drug stability. • Cisplatin may react with aluminum, resulting in loss of cisplatin potency. • Physically compatible with ondansetron. • Sodium thiosulfate and mesna directly inactivate cisplatin. • Administer with caution in patients receiving other potentially nephrotoxic drugs (aminoglycosides).	*Side effects:* • Concomitant administration of probenecid enhances cisplatin renal toxicity. • Monitor patient for HSR: tachycardia, wheezing, hypotension, and facial edema. • Acute and delayed nausea and vomiting are preventable with aggressive antiemetics including receptor antagonists, dexamethasone, and metoclopramide. • High frequency hearing loss may occur in up to 30% of patients. • Tinnitis, vestibular dysfunction, and ototoxicity occur infrequently and are preventable with adequate hydration and mannitol diuresis. • Peripheral neuropathy including numbness, tingling, and sensory loss occurs in arms and legs with long-term administration. • Hypomagnesemia is seen with high dose (> 200 mg/m^2) and is preventable with oral and IV supplements. • Hemolytic anemia is seen with higher doses and responds to recombinant erythropoietin.
CYCLOPHOSPHAMIDE (Cytoxan)			
Dosage: • PO: 50–200 mg/m^2 PO each day × 14 days q 28 days • IV: 400 mg/m^2 IV × 5 days	*Mechanism of action:* • Activated by hepatic microsomal enzymes; prevents cell division by cross-linking DNA strands. • Non-cell cycle phase specific.	*Administration precautions:* • When doses > 1000 mg are given, patients should receive hydration of 500–1000 mL NS. • Administer IV dose slowly to prevent nasal congestion, headache, and dizziness.	*Side effects:* • Hemorrhagic cystitis occurs rarely with conventional doses. • Hydration and mesna are indicated with high-dose and pretransplant therapy.

• IV: 500 mg–1.5 g/m² IV q 3 wk or 60 mg/kg IV × 2 days prior to BMT *Efficacy:* • Breast cancer • Ovarian cancer • Leukemias • Lymphomas • Multiple myeloma • Lung cancer	*Metabolism:* • Metabolized in the liver. • Excreted in the kidney (15% unchanged). • 33% of drug is excreted unchanged in the stool. • t½ = 3–10 hr	• Encourage fluid intake of 3 L/day while taking cyclophosphamide. • When taking oral doses, encourage patient to take all pills before 5 P.M. to minimize bladder contact with toxic metabolites. • Phenytoin and chloral hydrate may enhance the conversion of cyclophosphamide to toxic metabolites, thereby increasing toxicity.	• SIADH can occur with high-dose cyclophosphamide. • Nausea and vomiting are preventable with aggressive antiemetic therapy. • Alopecia is common. Metallic taste occurs during injection and when taken orally. Encourage the patient to chew gum, peppermint, or lemon candy. • Myelosuppression (leukopenia) is dose limiting. • Amenorrhea and reversible oligospermia occur and are dose dependent. • Cyclophosphamide 1 mg/mL is compatible with doxorubicin, cisplatin, mesna, and other drugs. • Blurring of vision has been reported. • Cardiac toxicity can occur with high-dose therapy, especially if given with radiation to the chest area.

CYTARABINE (Cytosar: ARA-C Cytosine Arabinoside)

Dosage: • IV: 5–10 day CI (continuous infusion) of 100–200 mg/m² • Intrathecal: 5–70 mg/m² 1–3 × /week • Subcutaneous: 1 mg/kg 1–2 × /week or 100 mg bid × 5 days q 28 days *Efficacy:* • Acute leukemia • Myeloid leukemia • Acute nonlymphocytic leukemia • Meningeal leukemia	*Mechanism of action:* • Inhibits DNA polymerase causing DNA chain elongation and arrest. • Cell cycle phase specific for the S phase. • Antimetabolite. *Metabolism:* • Metabolized in the liver. • At 24 hr, 90% of the drug is eliminated in the urine. • t½ = 2–3 hr	*Administration precautions:* • Given IV push or IV infusion over 30 min. • 5- to 10-day continuous infusions may be optimal for antitumor cytotoxicity because of the S-phase specificity. • For intrathecal use, mix drug with lactated Ringer's solution or NS without preservatives. • Rotate sites for SQ injections.	*Side effects:* • Myelosuppression is the DLT. Nadir at 5–7 days, recovery in 2–3 wk. • Anemia is common. • Nausea, vomiting, anorexia, metallic taste, stomatitis, and diarrhea are reported. • Minimal alopecia. • Skin erythema can occur. Arthralgias and myalgias occur. • After intrathecal use, patients may experience nausea, vomiting, fever, and headache. • Ocular toxicity: excessive tearing, photophobia, and blurred vision. • High-dose therapy can lead to CNS toxicity: lethargy, confusion, ataxia. • Cytarabine may decrease the cellular uptake of methotrexate. • Compatible with vincristine, prednisolone, sodium phosphate, and ondansetron. • Physical changes are noted with methotrexate and 5-FU and heparin. • Compatible with vancomycin for 4–8 hr.

(continued)

Appendix 16B Intravenous Antineoplastic Agents (continued)

Dosage and Efficacy	Mechanism of Action and Metabolism	Administration Precautions	Side Effects
DACARBAZINE (DTIC)			
Dosage: • 375 mg/m^2 q 3–4 wk or • 150–250 mg/m^2/qd × 5 days q 3–4 wk or • 850 mg/m^2 on day 1 q 3–4 wk *Efficacy:* • Malignant melanoma • Soft tissue sarcomas • Hodgkin's disease	*Mechanism of action:* • Causes cross-linkage and breaks in DNA strands. • Inhibits RNA and DNA synthesis. • Cell cycle phase nonspecific, but has more activity in late G_2. *Metabolism:* • Activated by liver microsomes. • Excreted renally. • t½ = 35 mm	*Administration precautions:* • Reconstitute with D5W or saline. • Solution can be painful and should be administered slowly in 250–500 mL of solution over 30–60 min. Moist heat along the vein eases pain. • Stable for 8 hr at room temperature, 72 hr if refrigerated. • Drug should be protected from light. • May turn a pinkish color if exposed to light. • HSR can occur; hypotension occurs with high-dose therapy.	*Side effects:* • DLT: moderate degree of myelosuppression. • Nadir occurs at 21–25 days. • Anemia can occur. • Severe nausea and vomiting can occur. • Aggressive pretreatment with antiemetic therapy is needed. Nausea and vomiting lessen by days 3–4 of treatment. • Hepatotoxic; monitor liver functions. • Flulike syndrome may occur with fever, myalgia, and malaise at about 7 days, lasting 1–3 wk. • Photosensitivity can occur; protect skin from sunlight.
DACTINOMYCIN (Actinomycin D; ACT-D, Cosmegen)			
Dosage: • 10–15 μ/kg/day × 5 days q 3–4 wk or • 2–4 mg/m^2 in divided doses over 1 wk or • 2 mg/m^2 IV q 3–4 wk *Efficacy:* • Wilms' tumor • Embryonal rhabdomyosarcoma • Choriocarcinoma • Malignant melanoma • Hodgkin's and non-Hodgkin's lymphoma	*Mechanism of action:* • Binds between purine-pyrimidine base pairs in DNA. • Inhibits the synthesis of DNA-dependent RNA and messenger RNA. • Action is cell cycle nonspecific but is more active during G_1 and in cells that are cycling. *Metabolism:* • Excreted unchanged in bile and urine.	*Administration precautions:* • Reconstitute with preservative-free sterile water for injection. Preserved diluent may cause precipitation. Use drug as soon as possible. • Monitor liver functions; dose reductions may be necessary. • Use extreme caution during administration. • Dactinomycin is a severe vesicant. • Dactinomycin is compatible with ondansetron. • When calculating dose, double-check the order since the drug is ordered both as μg/kg and mg/m^2.	*Side effects:* • DLT: myelosuppression occurs within 7–10 days of dosing. • Nadir may be delayed, occurring at 3 wk. • Due to its immunosuppressive effects, avoid administering dactinomycin to patients who have an active viral infection. • Nausea and vomiting can be severe. Aggressive pretreatment with antiemetics is appropriate. • Mucositis and diarrhea can be severe; institute preventive oral hygiene regimen. • Alopecia occurs commonly. • Erythema, hyperpigmentation, and an acnelike rash occur commonly. • Dactinomycin can cause a radiation recall reaction. • Hepatic venoocclusive toxicity manifested as elevated SGOT and bilirubin can occur.

DAUNORUBICIN (Daunomycin, Cerubidine)			
Dosage: • 30–60 mg/m² daily × 3–5 days q 3–4 wk *Efficacy:* • ALL • AML • Acute monocytic leukemia • Acute nonlymphocytic leukemia	*Mechanism of action:* • Intercalates DNA, thereby blocking DNA, RNA, and protein synthesis. It is an anthracycline antitumor antibiotic. *Metabolism:* • Metabolized in the liver. • About 40% of the drug is eliminated via the bile. • 20%–25% is eliminated via the urine. • t½ = 20–25 hr	*Administration precautions:* • 20-mg vial is reconstituted with 4 mL of sterile water = 5 mg/mL. • QS to 15–20 mL of NS. • Stable for 24 hr at room temperature and 48 hr under refrigeration. • Incompatible with heparin, 5-FU, and dexamethasone. • Compatible with ondansetron. • Caution: Because the solution is red, as is doxorubicin and with a similar-sounding name, the vial should be double-checked against the order. • Urine will be pink to red for 12–24 hr after administration. • Daunorubicin is a severe vesicant. Extreme caution should be used in administration of this drug • Administer via the side arm of a freely running IV or by the two-syringe technique.	*Side effects:* • DLT: myelosuppression. • WBC nadir occurs at 7–14 days; recovery at 3 wk. Thrombocytopenia and anemia occur. • Stomatitis occurs, but is mild. • Diarrhea occurs infrequently. • Nausea and vomiting occur 1–5 hr after dosing but are prevented with aggressive antiemetic therapy. • Alopecia is abrupt and involves all body hair. • Hyperpigmentation of the nails occurs. Urticaria and a generalized rash have been reported. • Monitor liver functions. If elevated LFTs are noted, dose reduction is indicated. • Cardiac toxicity can occur. Dose is limited to 500–600 mg/m². • Manifestation of CHF is characterized by dyspnea on exertion, fatigue, and arrhythmias.

DENILEUKIN (Ontak)			
Dosage: • 9 or 18 μg/kg/day × 5 days q 21 days *Efficacy:* • Cutaneous T-cell lymphoma	*Mechanism of action:* • Recombinant DNA-derived cytotoxic protein • Interacts with high-affinity IL-2 receptors and inhibits cellular protein synthesis, resulting in cellular death. *Metabolism:* • Proteolytic degradation. • Terminal t½ = 70–80 min	*Administration precautions:* • Do not infuse through an inline filter. • Do not administer IVP. Must infuse over at least 15 mins. • Vials should be stored frozen at or below −10°C. • Bring up to room temperature before preparing dose. Never refreeze the drug. • Do not use with glass containers due to absorption issues. • Maintain the drug concentration at 15 mcg/mL or greater during all solution preparation. • Delay administration until serum albumin levels are at least 3.0 g/dL.	*Side effects:* • Hypoalbuminemia, elevated transaminases, fever, fatigue, and skin reactions are commonly seen. • Vascular leak syndrome (VLS) can occur and is characterized by two or more of the following symptoms: edema, hypotension, hypo-albuminemia. Closely monitor weight, edema, blood pressure, and serum albumin levels. • Acute HSRs have been reported, often within 24 hr of the first dose, regardless of the cycle. Emergency drugs and resuscitative equipment should be readily available. Premedication with 1 g of acetaminophen and diphenhydramine 25 mg PO is recommended. • Flulike syndrome is commonly reported. Symptoms are mild to moderate and are effectively managed with antipyretics and antiemetics.

(continued)

Appendix 16B Intravenous Antineoplastic Agents (continued)

Dosage and Efficacy	Mechanism of Action and Metabolism	Administration Precautions	Side Effects
		DOCETAXEL (Taxotere)	
Dosage: • 60–100 mg/m^2 q 3 wk as a 1 hr infusion *Efficacy:* • Ovarian cancer • Breast cancer • Non-small cell lung cancer	*Mechanism of action:* • Antimicrotubule agent — a mitotic spindle poison. Enhances microtubule assembly and inhibits the depolymerization of tubulin. This process leads to increased bundles of microtubules in the cell. The cell is then unable to divide. *Metabolism:* • Metabolized in the liver, excreted in the feces, and minimally excreted in the urine. • t½ = 11 hr	*Administration precautions:* • Docetaxel solution contains 2 mg (40 mg/mL) of docetaxel in polysorbate/tween 80. Refrigerated vial sits at room temperature for 5 min. Once mixed with solvent the solution contains 10 mg/mL. The appropriate amount of docetaxel is mixed with D5W in a concentration < 1 mg/mL. Once diluted, docetaxel is stable for 8 hr at room temperature. • Avoid infiltration: The drug is an irritant but can cause tissue damage depending on the concentration. • Hyaluronidase SQ injections (maximum volume of 3 mL) have been recommended for treatment of infiltration. Apply cold to the site, not heat. • Monitor liver functions carefully; dose adjustments are appropriate if LFTs are elevated 2.5 × normal.	*Side effects:* • The DLT for docetaxel is neutropenia and thrombocytopenia. • All patients receive dexamethasone 8 mg PO bid × 5 days starting 1 day prior to docetaxel to reduce the amount of fluid retention. • Diphenhydramine 50 mg is also given 30 min prior to prevent hypersensitivity reactions. • If mild HSR occurs with flushing, skin reactions, or pruritus, the infusion rate is slowed with observation. If the patient experiences rash, flushing, mild dyspnea, or chest discomfort, the infusion is stopped and the patient is treated with IV diphenhydramine and dexamethasone. The infusion may be resumed after symptoms abate. • If severe symptoms such as generalized urticaria, angioedema, or hypotension occur, the infusion is stopped and the patient is treated with antihistamine, steroid, and if necessary epinephrine or bronchodilators. The patient may still receive the docetaxel depending on the severity of the response. If the patient reacts a second time, the patient probably should not receive the drug again. • Nausea and vomiting are minimal. • Alopecia occurs within 3 wk of the first treatment. • Nail separation may occur. • Drug-associated fluid retention or edema including pleural effusions, ascites, and peripheral edema occur and may be managed with a diuretic, which may or may not be helpful.

DOXORUBICIN (Adriamycin, Rubex)

Dosage:

- IV: 30–75 mg/m^2 q 3–4 wk
- IV: 20-45 mg/m^2/IV × 3 days. Higher doses are used in dose-intensive regimens. Doxorubicin may also be given intraarterially, intrapleurally, and by bladder instillation.

Efficacy:

- Acute nonlymphocytic leukemia
- Acute lymphocytic leukemia
- Wilms' tumor
- Neuroblastoma
- Soft tissue sarcoma
- Breast cancer
- Hepatocellular carcinoma
- Ovarian carcinoma

Mechanism of action:

- Binds directly to DNA base pairs and inhibits DNA, RNA, and protein synthesis. Antitumor antibiotic. Cell cycle specific for the S phase.

Metabolism:

- Extensively metabolized by the liver.
- 40%-50% of the drug is eliminated in the bile.
- 5% is eliminated in the urine.
- t½ = 18–30 hr

Administration precautions:

- Available in liquid and lyophilized forms.
- Reconstitute with sterile water for injection, D5W, NS to form a solution of 2 mg/mL
- Stable for 35 days at room temperature.
- Incompatible with heparin, dexamethasone, 5-FU, furosemide, and aminophylline.
- Compatible with cyclophosphamide, cisplatin, dacarbazine, droperidol, vinblastine, vincristine, and ondansetron.
- Doxorubicin turns the urine a reddish orange for 8–10 hr after administration.
- Since doxorubicin is metabolized and eliminated by the liver, liver function tests are monitored frequently. Elevation in bilirubin to 1.2–3 mg/dL warrants a 50% dose reduction; bilirubin of 3 mg/dL calls for a 75% dose reduction.
- Administer with extreme caution. Doxorubicin is a severe vesicant. It will cause tissue damage, ulceration, and necrosis if infiltrated. Inject through the side arm of a freely running and well-established IV or by using the two-syringe technique.
- Caution: It has a similar name and color to daunorubicin. Check the drug order against the vial to ensure the right dose of the right drug.

Side effects:

- DLT: Myelosuppression, especially leukopenia. Nadir occurs at 10–14 days. Recovery is swift at 3 wk.
- Cardiac toxicity can occur. Dose is limited to 450–550 mg/m^2. Doxorubicin causes damage to the myocyte of the heart, causing various degrees of damage, but manifests as CHF as the heart begins to function less efficiently as a pump.
- MUGA scans are done periodically to monitor left ventricular function. Early symptoms of CHF include tachycardia, dyspnea on exertion, arrhythmias, and EKG changes.
- Alopecia occurs predictably and is dose dependent. Doses greater than 50 mg are associated with moderate to severe loss. Doses of 90–100 mg cause hair loss in 2–5 wk.
- Stomatitis is dose limiting and can be more severe with continuous infusions. Continuous infusions are only given through central lines, never through peripheral lines.
- Nail bed changes occur and include hyperpigmentation especially in blacks and in individuals of Mediterranean descent.

DOXORUBICIN HYDROCHLORIDE LIPOSOME INJECTION (Doxil)

Dosage:

- 20 mg/m^2 over 30 min q 3 wk
- 50 mg/m^2 q 4 wk × 4 cycles for metastic ovarian cancer

Mechanism of action:

- Antitumor antibiotic binds directly to DNA.
- Inhibits DNA and RNA synthesis.
- Drug is encapsulated in stealth liposomes to prolong circulation time.

Administration precautions:

- Dilute in 250 mL 5% dextrose USP.
- Drug is an irritant.

Side effects:

- Acute infusion reaction may occur with flushing, shortness of breath, facial swelling, headache, chills, back pain, chest and throat tightness, and/or hypotension. Stop infusion. Restart if symptoms abate.

(continued)

Appendix 16B Intravenous Antineoplastic Agents (continued)

Dosage and Efficacy	Mechanism of Action and Metabolism	Administration Precautions	Side Effects
Efficacy: • AIDS • Kaposi's sarcoma • Ovarian cancer	*Metabolism:* • Slower clearance from body than doxorubicin. • t½ = 55 hr		• Hand-foot syndrome may require dose reduction. • Stomatitis may occur. • BMS is dose limiting. • Cardiac toxicity may occur. • Less incidence of alopecia compared to doxorubicin.
EPIRUBICIN (Ellence)			
Dosage: • 100–120 mg/m^2 IV *Efficacy:* • Breast cancer	*Mechanism of action:* • Inhibits nucleic acid and protein synthesis. • Interferes with replication and transcription of DNA. • Semisynthetic derivative of daunorubicin and a 4′-epimer of doxorubicin. *Metabolism:* • Rapidly and extensively metabolized by the liver. • Excreted in the bile. • t½ = 30–35 hr	*Administration precautions;* • Administer with caution. Epirubicin is a vesicant. It can cause severe tissue damage, ulceration, and necrosis if infiltrated. • Refrigerate and protect from light. • Inject through the side arm of a free-flowing and well-established IV line or by using the two-syringe technique. • May cause the urine to turn a pink/red color for 2 days after administration.	*Side effects:* • Severe BMS may occur and is the dose-limiting toxicity. Monitor blood counts closely. May require colony-stimulating factors to avoid dose reduction and treatment delays. • Cardiotoxicity can occur. Do not exceed total cumulative dose of 0.9%–1 g/m^2. • Nausea, vomiting, stomatitis, and mucositis have been reported. Premedicate with $5HT_3$ antagonist and dexamethasone. • Amenorrhea and premature menopause may occur. • Concomitant use of calcium-channel blockers requires close monitoring of cardiac function. • Hypersensitivity reactions (HSRs) may occur, but are rare. • Discontinue cimetidine during treatment. • Alopecia is common, usually after the first or second treatment, and is transient. • Radiation recall may occur.
ETOPOSIDE (VePesid, VP-16)			
Dosage: • 50–100 mg/m^2 IV qd × 5 (testicular cancer) q 3–4 wk • 75–200 mg/m^2 IV qd × 3 (small cell lung cancer) q 3–4 wk. Oral dose is twice the intravenous dose. • 400 mg/m^2/day × 3 days prior to bone marrow transplant	*Mechanism of action:* • Inhibits DNA synthesis in S and G_2. Causes single-strand breaks in DNA. • Cell cycle phase specific for S and G_2 phases. *Metabolism:* • Extensively protein bound. Metabolized in the liver. Excreted in the bile and urine. • t½ = 8–14 hr	*Administration precautions:* • Following dilution in NS or 5% dextrose, the drug is stable for 72–96 hr at room temperature. At room temperature, stability is dependent on concentration: 0.6 mg/mL = 24 hr 1mg/mL = 4 hr 2mg/mL = 2 hr	*Side effects:* • DLT: Leukopenia, dose-related. Nadir occurs 7–14 days, recovery by day 21. • Nausea and vomiting are uncommon. Anorexia occurs, especially with oral dosing. • Alopecia occurs more commonly with IV dosing. Radiation recall and pruritus can occur. • HSR is rare.

Efficacy: • Small cell lung cancer • Testicular cancer		• Etoposide is administered slowly over at least 30–45 min. • Hypotension can occur if infused in less than 45 min. Monitor patients for drug sensitivity.	

5-FLUOROURACIL (5-FU, Adrucil)			
Dosage: • Doses vary: 300–600 mg/m^2 IV × 5 days q 3–4 wk • 450–600 mg/m^2 IV weekly • 800–1200 mg/m^2 continuous infusion × 14–21 days to toxicity *Efficacy:* • Breast cancer • Colon cancer • Rectal cancer • Pancreatic cancer • Stomach cancer • Head and neck cancer	*Mechanism of action:* • Inhibits the formation of thymidine, which is necessary for DNA synthesis. Causes abnormal RNA synthesis. Acts synergistically with methotrexate. • Cell cycle phase specific for the S phase. *Metabolism:* • Poorly absorbed by mouth. After IV administration, the drug is metabolized to active metabolites. • Approximately 45% of the drug is metabolized by the liver. • 15% is eliminated unchanged in the urine. • t½ = 10–20 min	*Administration precautions:* • May be given a variety of ways: IV as a continuous infusion, IV push, arterial infusion, intracavitary, or intraperitoneally. • Store at room temperature and protect from light. • Incompatible with daunorubicin, doxorubicin, idarubicin, cisplatin, cytarabine, and diazepam. • Compatible with vincristine, methotrexate, potassium chloride, and magnesium sulfate.	*Side effects:* • Myelosuppression may be dose limiting, but less common with continuous infusion. • Mucositis is most common dose-limiting toxicity with continuous infusions. Symptoms of erythema, soreness, and ulceration may begin within 5–8 days of therapy. Sucking on ice chips as tolerated may decrease oral stomatitis. Diarrhea can be severe, even life-threatening, especially when 5-FU is given in higher doses with leucovorin. • Nausea, vomiting, and anorexia occur less frequently, but are more common when 5-FU is given simultaneously with radiation to the abdomen. • Skin and nail bed changes occur, especially with continuous infusion. Partial nail loss can occur as well as banding. Palmar-plantar erythrodysesthesias can be severe, necessitating dose reduction and treatment delays. Hyperpigmentation and photosensitivity are common. Patients are cautioned to protect themselves from the sun. Excessive lacrimation due to tear duct stenosis and blurred vision occur in about 25% of patients. • Headache, cerebellar ataxia, nystagmus, and confusion occur with higher doses. • Administering 5-FU based on the patient's circadian rhythm may lessen toxicity in general. • Alopecia is dose dependent. • Ataxia occurs in elderly patients. Other CNS changes include headache, drowsiness, and blurred vision.

(continued)

Appendix 16B Intravenous Antineoplastic Agents (continued)

Dosage and Efficacy	Mechanism of Action and Metabolism	Administration Precautions	Side Effects
FLOXURIDINE (FUDR, 5-FUDR)			
Dosage: • 0.1–0.6 mg/kg/day by intrahepatic infusion. Therapy is continued to toxicity, usually 7–14 days. • Circadian infusion protocols have been used. • Intravenous doses range from 0.5–1.0 mg/kg/day for up to 2 weeks by continuous infusion. *Efficacy:* • Adenocarcinoma metastatic to the liver	*Mechanism of action:* • Antimetabolite, similar to 5-FU, interrupts DNA synthesis causing cell death. Cell cycle phase specific for the S phase. *Metabolism:* • Metabolized to 5-FU when given IV. • 70%–90% of the drug is metabolized by the liver, and metabolites are excreted by the kidneys and lungs. When given, intrahepatic FUDR has a much higher first-pass extraction rate compared to 5-FU and therefore the cytotoxic effect is more localized to the liver. • $t\frac{1}{2}$ = 0.3–3.6 hr	*Administration precautions:* • Caution should be exercised as both 5-FU and floxuridine (also called 5-FUDR) are supplied in 500-mg vials and the doses of each are dramatically different. With such similar names it is important to note that mistaking 500 mg of FUDR for 500 mg of 5-FU could be lethal. • FUDR 500-mg vial of lyophilized powder is reconstituted with sterile water. • Generally given via an intraarterial infusion pump. • Heparin is added to the FUDR to prevent clotting of the catheter due to the slow infusion rate.	*Side effects:* • When given as an intraarterial infusion an H_2 antihistamine such as ranitidine may be recommended (150 mg bid) to prevent peptic ulcer disease. • The intraarterial route is usually associated with less systemic toxicity. • BMS is more common with IV bolus injections. • Nausea, vomiting, and anorexia are common. Abdominal cramps with severe diarrhea are indications to interrupt therapy, • Mucositis does not occur often. If it does occur, it is an indication to interrupt the treatment and to reduce the dose. • Skin changes can occur and include edema, dermatitis, rashes, and pruritus as well as hyperpigmentation. • Alopecia can occur but is usually mild.
GEMCITABINE (Gemzar)			
Dosage: • 800–1000 mg/m^2 weekly × 3 weeks q 4 wk *Efficacy:* • Pancreas cancer • Non-small cell lung cancer • Breast cancer	*Mechanism of action:* • Antimetabolite. • Inhibits DNA synthesis. • Cell cycle specific for the S phase. *Metabolism:* • Eliminated by kidneys. • $t\frac{1}{2}$ = 20 min	*Administration precautions:* • Reconstitute with sodium chloride to a solution containing 10 mg/mL. • Dilute in 100–1000 mL of saline and infuse over 30 min to 3 hr. • Stable at room temperature for 24 hr.	*Side effects:* • Myelosuppression, especially thrombocytopenia, can be dose limiting. • Flulike syndrome with fever, mild nausea, and vomiting can occur. Fever generally occurs within 8 hr of dosing. Acetaminophen generally relieves symptoms. • Rash may occur within 2–3 days of the infusion. Topical steroids may be helpful. • Peripheral edema may occur.
GEMTUZUMAB OZOGAMICIN (Mylotarg)			
Dosage: • 9mg/m^2 IV of day 1and day 14 *Efficacy:* • CD33$^+$ acute myeloid leukemia	*Mechanism of action:* • Causes DNA strand breakage and apoptosis. • Necrotic mechanism of cytotoxicity is also suspected.	*Administration precautions:* • Protect from unshielded fluorescent light, direct and indirect sunlight during preparation and administration.	*Side effects:* • Pancytopenia is a common side effect and may be profound. Monitor blood counts very closely. Platelet and RBC transfusion are often necessary. Prophylactic antibiotics may also be helpful.

	• Consists of an antibody and a cytotoxic antitumor antibiotic. *Metabolism:* • Causes hydrolytic release of a calicheamicin derivative.	• Cover with a UV protectant bag and infuse over 2 hr. • Reconstitute with 5 mL of sterile water and dilute in 100 mL of 0.9% sodium chloride solution. • Must use a 1.2-micron terminal filter for administration. • Can be given in an ambulatory setting.	• Infusion reactions can be severe and usually resolve within 24 hrs. Fever, chills, hypotension, and hypoxia are often seen. Premedicate with diphenhydramine 50 mg and acetaminophen 650–1000 mg PO 1 hr before, followed by two additional doses of acetaminophen at hours 4 and 8. • Monitor vital signs before, during, and for the 6 hrs following infusion. • Observe for 4–6 hr after the completion of the infusion for side effects. • Emergency equipment and medications need to be readily available. • Venoocclusive disease (VOC) has been reported and can be fatal. A higher incidence has been seen with patients who have had a BMT.

IBRITUMOMAB TIUXETAN (Zevalin)

Dosage:	*Mechanism of action:*	*Administration precautions:*	*Side effects:*
• Step 1: Rituximab 250 mg/m^2 followed by Ibritimomab tiuxetan In-111 5 mCi • Biodistribution gamma scans within 2–24 hr post-step 1,48–72 hrs post-step 1, and an optional third image 90–120 hrs post-step 1 • Step 2: Rituximab 250 mg/m^2 followed by Ibritumomab tiuxetan Y-90 0.4 mCi/kg if platelet count > 50,000 or 0.3 mCi/kg if platelet count = 100,000–150,000. Dose not to exceed 32 mCi *Efficacy:* • Low-grade follicular or transformed CD20$^+$ non-Hodgkin's lymphoma	• Murine and chimeric monoclonal antibody conjugated with Y-90. Apoptosis due to complement-dependent cytotoxicity, antibody-dependent cellular cytotoxity, and ionizing radiation. *Metabolism:* • Mean effective half-life for Y-90 is 30 hr. 7% of activity excreted in urine.	• Rituximab infusion initiated at 50 mg/hr, increasing 50 mg/hr every 30 min to a maximum rate of 400 mg/hr through a 22-micron filter. • Zevalin In-111 and zevalin Y-90 infused over 10 min by licensed personnel. • Radiolabeled dose prepared by radiopharmacy and infused by licensed personnel.	• Infusion reaction: dyspnea, angioedema, bronchospasm, fever, chills, hypotension, rigors. Premedicate with diphenhydramine and acetaminophen. • Fever • Nausea, diarrhea, and vomiting. • Athralgias, myalgias. • Uticaria, pruritis. • Delayed BMS is common. Nadirs occur at 4–9 wk requiring weekly CBC for 10–12 wk post-treatment. Cytopenias may be prolonged. • Beta radiation precautions initiated after step 2 dose based on local or national regulatory agency guidelines.

(continued)

Appendix 16B Intravenous Antineoplastic Agents (continued)

Dosage and Efficacy	Mechanism of Action and Metabolism	Administration Precautions	Side Effects
IDARUBICIN (Idamycin)			
Dosage: • 12 mg/m²/day for 3 days • Doses vary • Generally given in combination with other drugs *Efficacy:* • Acute nonlymphocytic leukemia	*Mechanism of action:* • Cell cycle phase specific for the S phase. • Analog of daunorubicin. • Inhibits RNA synthesis. *Metabolism:* • Excreted primarily in the bile and urine. • 25% of the drug is eliminated over approximately 5 days. • Metabolized in the liver to the active form. • t½ = 13–26 hr	*Administration precautions:* • Reconstituted with NS. • Protect from light. • Caution is used during administration because drug is a vesicant. • Incompatible with 5-FU, etoposide, dexamethasone, heparin, hydrocortisone, methotrexate, and vincristine.	*Side effects:* • DLT: Leukopenia and thrombocytopenia are expected. • Urine can be pink to red for 48 hr after administration. • Nausea can be mild to moderate and preventable with standard antiemetic. • Diarrhea and mucositis can occur. • Alopecia occurs gradually. • Cumulative cardiomyopathy and CHF can occur with large cumulative doses.
IFOSFAMIDE (Ifex)			
Dosage: • IV: 1.0–1.2 g/m²/day over a 5-day period q 3–4 wk. Higher doses of 2.5–3.7 g/m²/day over a 2- to 3-day period. • Mesna at a dose of 20% of the ifosfamide dose is given just prior to the ifosfamide and q 4 h for 2 more doses. Mesna may be given IV or PO. *Efficacy:* • Testicular cancer • Soft tissue sarcoma • Hodgkin's and non-Hodgkin's lymphoma • Acute leukemias • Ewing's sarcoma • Osteosarcoma	*Mechanism of action:* • Ifosfamide is an alkylating agent. It is a prodrug and requires activation in the liver by microsomal enzymes. *Metabolism:* • Metabolized by the liver to inactive metabolites. • 15%–56% of the drug is excreted unchanged in the urine. • Drug elimination may be hindered by renal dysfunction. • t½ = 7–15 hr	*Administration precautions:* • Ifosfamide is administered over at least 30 min with aggressive hydration to reduce the incidence of hemorrhagic cystitis. • The uroprotectant mesna is also given either as a continuous infusion or in divided doses q 4 hr × 3 doses. • Ifosfamide and mesna are compatible and can be infused concurrently when high-dose ifosfamide is given.	*Side effects:* • Myelosuppression is dose limiting. • WBC nadir usually occurs 7–10 days post-treatment. • Urinary tract toxicity is a dose-limiting toxicity and is manifested as hemorrhagic cystitis. Patients may complain of dysuria and frequency 2–3 days after the infusion. Encourage oral intake of 2–3 L per day prior to and after dosing. Encourage patients to empty their bladders every 2–3 hr. • Nausea and vomiting are common with higher doses. Symptoms are preventable with serotonin antagonist therapy. • Avoid sedation with neurotoxic drugs that can exacerbate the lethargy and confusion that can occur due to the accumulation of chloracetylaldehyde, a metabolite with neurotoxic properties. • Alopecia is more common with higher doses and occurs usually within 3 wk of therapy.

<table>
<tr><th colspan="4">IRINOTECAN (Camptosar, CPT-11)</th></tr>
<tr><td>Dosage:
• 125–150 mg/m^2 IV over 90 min weekly × 4 wk q 6 wk
Efficacy:
• Adenocarcinoma
• Colon/rectal cancer</td><td>Mechanism of action:
• Topoisomerase I inhibitor.
• Blocks DNA and RNA synthesis in dividing cells.
Metabolism:
• Metabolized to its active form in liver.
• 20% drug excreted in the urine.
• 30% excreted in bile.
• t½ = 6–10 hr</td><td>Administration precautions:
• Dilute in 5% dextrose: stable for 24 hr at room temperature.
• Drug is an irritant.</td><td>Side effects:
• Dose-limiting toxicities are diarrhea and myelosuppression.
• Loperamide is administered for diarrhea.
• Flushing and diaphoresis may occur during infusion.
• Moderate to severe nausea and vomiting may occur.</td></tr>
<tr><th colspan="4">L-ASPARAGINASE (Elspar; Erwinia Asparaginase)</th></tr>
<tr><td>Dosage:
• Used in combination with other drugs, active in ALL 200 IU/day for 28 days, 1000 IU/kg × 10 days
or
• 20,000 IU/m^2/wk
Efficacy:
• ALL</td><td>Mechanism of action:
• Inhibits protein synthesis.
Metabolism:
• Biphasic elimination.
• Binds to vascular binding sites.
• May be eliminated by the liver.
• t½ = 4–9 hr and 1.4–1.8 days</td><td>Administration precautions:
• Dilute in NS or sterile water.
• Use within 8 hr.
• Refrigerate before and after reconstitution.
• Do not infuse through a filter.
• IV slow push over 30 min, or IM.
• Do not use if solution is cloudy.
• Skin test with 2 IU intradermal at least 1 hr prior to dosing.
• Administer subsequent doses with caution despite negative skin test.</td><td>Side effects:
• Anaphylactic reactions can occur in 20%-35% of patients.
• Monitor closely with appropriate support.
• IM use is associated with delayed allergic response.
• If HSR occurs, the Erwinia preparation may be used with prophylactic premedication.
• Urticarial eruptions are common.
• Incidence of reactions increases with each subsequent dosing.
• Slight anemia can occur; leukopenia is rare.
• Malaise, anorexia, nausea, and vomiting occur frequently.
• Hepatic toxicity is uncommon.
• Lethargy, somnolence, disorientation, and loss of recent memory occur with higher doses.</td></tr>
<tr><th colspan="4">MECHLORETHAMINE HYDROCHLORIDE (Nitrogen Mustard, Mustargen)</th></tr>
<tr><td>Dosage:
• IV: 6 mg/m^2 on days 1 and 8
• Topically 10 mg/60 mL ointment
Efficacy:
• Hodgkin's disease</td><td>Mechanism of action:
• Alkylating agent results in abnormal base pairing, causing DNA miscoding, cross-linking of DNA, and strand breakage.
• Cell cycle nonspecific.</td><td>Administration precautions:
• Once reconstituted with sterile water or NS the drug should be used within 60 min because of its instability.
• Nitrogen mustard should be administered by IV push via a freely running IV line.</td><td>Side effects:
• Myelosuppression is the DLT.
• Leukopenia occurs 8–14 days following treatment. Severe thrombocytopenia may occur.</td></tr>
</table>

(continued)

Appendix 16B Intravenous Antineoplastic Agents (continued)

Dosage and Efficacy	Mechanism of Action and Metabolism	Administration Precautions	Side Effects
• CML • Lymphosarcoma	*Metabolism:* • Rapidly deactivated in the blood. • t½ = 15 min	• Administering nitrogen mustard via direct IV push technique can cause venous thrombosis and pain. • Nitrogen mustard is a severe vesicant and must be given with extreme caution. • Assess for a blood return every 1 mL of injection. • If extravasation occurs, inject a solution of sodium thiosulfate (1/6 molar) into the area to neutralize the drug. • For 1 mg of nitrogen mustard infiltrated, inject 2 mL of the 10% thiosulfate solution. • Preparation: 4 mL sodium thiosulfate injection (10%) diluted with 6 mL of sterile water for injection.	• Severe nausea and vomiting within 1 hr of IV administration. Patients should be premedicated with aggressive antiemetic therapy. • Alopecia is common. A metallic taste is common during the injection and can be masked by encouraging the patient to chew gum or bite on a lemon rind. • Amenorrhea and impaired spermatogenesis occurs and is dose dependent.
MELPHALAN (Alkeran, L-PAM, L-Phenylalanine Mustard)			
Dosage: • IV: 16 mg/m² q 3 wk × 4 doses then q 4 wk • PO: 2 mg/kg/day × 5 days q 4–6 wk • BMT: 50–60 mg/m² IV *Efficacy:* • Multiple myeloma • Epithelial carcinoma of the ovary • BMT	*Mechanism of action:* • Alkylating agent; cycle specific. • Forms DNA cross-links. *Metabolism:* • 80%–90% of the drug is bound to plasma proteins. • 10%–15% of the drug is eliminated unchanged in the urine. • t½ = 1.5–4.0 hr	*Administration precautions:* • Reconstitute with 10 mL of supplied diluent for a concentration = 5 mg/mL. • Dilute in NS to a concentration of 0.45 mg/mL and use within 60 min. • Do not refrigerate reconstituted product. • When taken orally, peak plasma levels are reached within 2 hr. The drug is poorly absorbed when taken with food.	*Side effects:* • Myelosuppression is dose limiting. • GI: Mild anorexia, nausea, and vomiting when taken orally. Nausea and vomiting can be severe with higher IV doses. Mucositis, diarrhea, and oral ulceration occur infrequently. Leukopenia and thrombocytopenia peak at 2–3 wk and may be cumulative with a prolonged recovery period of 6 or more wk. • Pruritus, dermatitis, and rash may occur. Alopecia is not common with oral dosing. • Amenorrhea and oligospermia are common. • Second malignancies (leukemias) have been reported.
METHOTREXATE (MTX, Mexate, Amethopterin)			
Dosage: • IV Low: 10–50 mg/m² • IV Med: 100–500 mg/m² • IV High: 500 mg/m² and above with leucovorin rescue	*Mechanism of action:* • MTX tightly binds to dihydrofolate reductase, thereby blocking the reduction of dihydrofolate to tetrahydrofolic acid, the active form of folic acid. This process effectively arrests DNA, RNA, and protein synthesis.	*Administration precautions:* • Lower doses (< 100 mg) are usually given IVP without leucovorin rescue • When given with 5-FU for breast cancer, the MTX dose is followed in 1 hr by the 5-FU. The drugs are synergistic when given this way.	*Side effects:* • Myelosuppression is dose limiting. Leukopenia is dose dependent and is more likely to occur with prolonged exposure.

- IT: 10–15 mg/m² in 7–15 mL of preservative-free saline
- IM: 25 mg/m²

Efficacy:

- Trophoblastic neoplasms
- Acute leukemias
- Meningeal leukemias
- Carcinoma of the breast
- Osteogenic sarcoma
- Burkitt's lymphoma
- Hodgkin's disease
- Lung cancer
- CNS metastasis

- Antimetabolite.
- Cell cycle specific for the S phase.

Metabolism:

- MTX is distributed freely in water, which means that it will circulate in third-space fluid, increasing the toxicity of the drug since it is not being metabolized. Patients with effusions or ascites should be monitored carefully to avoid severe toxicity.
- MTX is highly protein bound and should not be given with acids that may compete for binding (elimination) sites, which would increase the AUC of the MTX, resulting in extreme toxicity.
- 90% of MTX is eliminated from the kidneys in the urine as unchanged drug.
- BUN and creatinine levels should be monitored regularly. If there is evidence of renal impairment, lower doses should be given with leucovorin rescue.

- Leucovorin rescue is needed because the dose of MTX is generally > 100 mg.
- Preservative-free MTX used for intrathecal injection should be prepared just prior to use.
- Protect infusions from light.

- Nausea and vomiting are common with higher doses. Diarrhea can be dose limiting. Stomatitis is more common with higher doses and more lengthy infusions.
- Skin erythema, hyperpigmentation, photosensitivity, rash, folliculitis, and pruritus may occur. MTX can cause enhanced radiation side effects if given simultaneously.
- Renal dysfunction is dose related and more common in patients who are dehydrated. When given in higher doses, the patient's urine pH must be > 7 to prevent precipitation of the MTX in the renal tubules, with subsequent renal damage. Administer bicarb as directed. The BUN and creatinine are monitored prior to high-dose therapy.
- Neurological dysfunction can occur with intrathecal administration, especially if cranial radiation has also been given.
- Photophobia, excessive lacrimation, and conjunctivitis have been noted.

MITOMYCIN (Mutamycin, Mitomycin C)

Dosage:

- 20 mg/m² as a single dose repeated q 6–8 wk
- IV: 2 mg/m² q day × 5 days
  or
  5–20 mg/m² q 6–8 wk
- Bladder instillation: 20–60 mg (1 mg/mL)

Efficacy:

- Adenocarcinoma of the stomach, pancreas
- Cancer of the bladder, breast

Mechanism of action:

- Antitumor antibiotic.
- Active during the G_1 and S phases of the cell cycle.
- Disrupts DNA synthesis secondary to alkylation.

Metabolism:

- Mitomycin is inactivated by microsomal enzymes in the liver and is metabolized in the spleen and kidneys.
- 10%–30% of the drug is eliminated unchanged in the urine.
- t½ = 0.5–1.0 hr

Administration precautions:

- Reconstitute in sterile water: 10 mL in 5 mg vial = 0.5 mg/mL. Use within 3 hr.
- Mitomycin is a severe vesicant. Administer with caution.
- Give IV push through the side arm of a freely running IV to minimize venous irritation. Assess for a blood return every 1 mL of drug. Discontinue the injection immediately if the patient complains of pain or burning.
- Mitomycin can cause tissue damage without evidence of drug infiltration.
- Skin ulceration may occur at sites distant from the site of drug administration

Side effects:

- Myelosuppression is dose limiting.
- Leukopenia and thrombocytopenia occur late at 4–5 wk with recovery at 7–8 wk. Both are cumulative.
- Anemia and hemolytic-uremic syndrome have been reported.
- Nausea and vomiting are mild.
- Alopecia is mild; photosensitivity, skin rash, and pruritus are uncommon.
- Venoocclusive disease of the liver with abdominal pain, hepatomegaly, and liver failure occur in patients receiving mitomycin and BMT.
- Pulmonary fibrosis has been reported.

(continued)

Appendix 16B Intravenous Antineoplastic Agents (continued)

Dosage and Efficacy	Mechanism of Action and Metabolism	Administration Precautions	Side Effects
MITOXANTRONE (Novantrone)			
Dosage: • 10–12 mg/m²/day × 5 days for induction of acute nonlymphocytic leukemia; 12 mg/m² q 3–4 wk *Efficacy:* • Acute monocytic leukemia • AML • Acute promyelocytic leukemia • Breast cancer • Primary hepatocellular carcinoma	*Mechanism of action:* • Antitumor antibiotic. • Intercalates into DNA; disrupts cell division. *Metabolism:* • Metabolized in the liver and excreted in the bile and urine. • $t_{1/2}$ = 24–37 hr	*Administration precautions:* • Dark blue solution in vials. • Dilute in at least 50 mL D5W or NS. • Stable for 7 days at room temperature. • Administer IV over at least 5 min as an infusion.	*Side effects:* • Leukopenia is dose limiting. • Nausea and vomiting are mild and preventable. Alopecia is common. Diarrhea and stomatitis may occur. • Cumulative cardiomyopathy can occur. Monitoring the left ventricular ejection fraction is indicated, especially in patients who are at risk for heart disease or who have received doxorubicin in the past. • Blue discoloration of the sclera may occur. The urine may remain blue-green for 48 hr following treatment.
OXALIPLATIN (Eloxatin)			
Dosage: • 85 mg/m² infusion q 2 wk. (Given in combination with 5-FU/leucovorin) *Dose Reductions:* • Persistent grade 2 neuropathies: 65 mg/m² • Grade 3 neuropathy: Discontinue oxaliplatin • Grades 3–4 gastrointestinal toxicity: 65 mg/m² • Grades 3–4 hematological toxicity: 65 mg/m² *Efficacy:* • Advanced colon or rectal cancer	*Mechanism of action:* • Cell cycle nonspecific. • Inhibits DNA replication and transcription. *Metabolism:* • Renal excretion is the major route of elimination. • Rapid and extensive nonenzymatic biotransformation.	*Administration precautions:* • Premedication with antiemetics, including 5HT, blockers with dexamethasone is recommended. • Prehydration is not required. • Eloxatin should not be given to patients with an allergy to platinum compounds. • Never reconstitute or dilute with sodium chloride-containing solutions. • Stable at room temperature for 6 hr at room temperature and 24 hr under refrigeration. • Administered over 2 hr in 250–500 mL of D5W. Dilute in 500 mL if infusion pain is experienced. This drug is a severe irritant. • Flush the infusion line with D5W before and after the administration of 5-FU due to incompatibility issues. • Do not use aluminum needles with this drug.	*Side effects:* • Neuropathy (acute and chronic persistent) are the dose-limiting toxicities. Baseline and ongoing neurological function assessment is critical. • Pharyngolaryngeal dysesthesia is seen in 1%–2% of patients. This side effect is usually worse with exposure to cold. • Pulmonary fibrosis has been reported and presents with unexplained respiratory symptoms. • Fatigue, nausea, vomiting, diarrhea, and bone marrow suppression are commonly seen. • Anaphylactic-like reactions have been reported and may occur within minutes of administration. Emergency medications including epinephrine, corticosteroids, and antihistamines should be readily available.

PACLITAXEL (Taxol)			
Dosage: • 200–250 mg/m² q 3 wk or in heavily pretreated patients • 135–175 mg/m² q 3 wk or weekly in divided doses *Efficacy:* • Ovarian carcinoma • Breast cancer • Non-small cell lung cancer • Head and neck cancer	*Mechanism of action:* • Promotes assembly of microtubules and stabilizes them, thereby blocking mitosis. • Paclitaxel also prevents transition of the cell from G_0 phase to S phase by blocking cellular response to growth factors. *Metabolism:* • The majority of paclitaxel is protein bound. • Elimination is primarily hepatic; minimal renal excretion. • t½ = 1.3–8.0 hr	*Administration precautions:* • Formulated in 50% polyoxyethylated castor oil (Cremophor EL) and 50% dehydrated alcohol. • Administer only in glass bottles or non-PVC containers (polyolefin containers using polyethylene-lined nitroglycerin tubing sets). • Cremophor-containing solutions will leach the plasticizer DEHP from PVC containers. DEHP can cause liver toxicity. • Inline filtration is needed (0.02 μm) due to the natural origins of the drug. • Administration rate varies from 1–3 hr to 24–96 hr. In general, the longer the infusion, the more likely the patient will experience myelosuppression that is dose limiting • Hypersensitivity reactions can occur with paclitaxel infusion and are thought to be related to the Cremophor EL. Patients are premedicated with dexamethasone 20 mg at 13 and 7 hr prior to treatment, with diphenhydramine 50 mg IV 30 min prior, and with an H² blocker (cimetidine 300 mg or Pepcid 20 mg) 30 min prior. • When administering paclitaxel with doxorubicin, the doxorubicin is given first; likewise, when paclitaxel is given with cisplatin or carboplatin, the paclitaxel is given first to avoid disruption in the elimination of the platinum compound and enhanced toxicity. • Synergistic with herceptin.	*Side effects:* • HSRs occur infrequently with proper premedication. Most HSRs occur within the first or second dosing. Symptoms include dyspnea, urticaria, flushing, and hypotension. • DLT: myelosuppression. • Leukopenic nadir occurs 7–10 days after dosing, with recovery at 15 days. Anemia and thrombocytopenia occur less frequently. • Peripheral neuropathy occurs more commonly in patients who are also receiving cisplatin. Hyperesthesias and burning pain in the feet may also occur. Myalgias and arthralgias occur usually 3–4 days after dosing. • Alopecia is complete at 3 wk • Mucositis occurs more commonly with prolonged infusions. Nausea and vomiting are mild. Diarrhea occurs infrequently. Paclitaxel is an irritant but can cause blistering and skin breakdown if large amounts of more concentrated drug are infiltrated.
PEMETREXED (Alimta)			
Dosage: • 500 mg/m² IV (21-day cycle) *Efficacy:* • Malignant pleural mesothelioma	*Mechanism of action:* • Disrupts the folate-dependent metabolic process essential for cell replication. *Metabolism:* • Eliminated by renal excretion.	*Administration precautions:* • To prevent skin rash, administer dexamethasone 4 mg po BID on the day before, day of, and day after treatment.	*Side effects:* • Contraindicated in patients whose creatinine clearance < 45 mL/min. • Nausea, vomiting, BMS, fatigue, stomatitis, pharyngitis, anorexia, and rash were commonly reported.

(continued)

Appendix 16B Intravenous Antineoplastic Agents (continued)

Dosage and Efficacy	Mechanism of Action and Metabolism	Administration Precautions	Side Effects
	• Elimination t½ = 3.5 hr	• Reconstitute in 20 mL of 0.9% NS (incompatible with diluents containing calcium). Then dilute in 100 mL of 0.9% NS and infuse over 10 mins, then wait 30 min before infusing cisplatin at the standard rate. • Administer folic acid daily of 350 ug to 1000-ug PO beginning 1 wk prior to treatment, and continuing throughout and after treatment to reduce toxicity. • One week prior to treatment, give 1000 ug IM injection of vitamin B_{12} and q 3 cycles thereafter. • Stable for up to 24 hr at room temperature.	• Conduct periodic blood tests to evaluate renal and hepatic function. • Exercise caution when administering concurrently with NSAIDs to patients with creatinine clearance < 80 mL/min.
RITUXIMAB (Rituxan)			
Dosage: • 375 mg/m² weekly for 4 or 8 more doses *Efficacy:* • Low-grade follicular $CD20^+$ B-cell non-Hodgkin's lymphoma	*Mechanism of action:* • Binds to the B-cell surface antigen CD20, causing cell death. *Metabolism:* • Unclear; possibly phagocytosis by the reticuloendothelial system. • Half-life varies with dose and sequence.	*Administration precautions:* • Do not administer by IV push or bolus. • Premedication with acetaminophen and diphenhydramine is recommended. • Administer the first infusion at 50 mg/m². If tolerated well, increase the rate by 50 mg/hr increments every 30 min to a maximum of 400 mg/hr. Subsequent infusions can be started at 100 mg/hr with a rate increase of 100 mg/hr every 30 min to a maximum of 400 mg/hr. • Due to potential of hypotension, consider holding antihypertensive medications for 12 hr before treatment. • Dilute in 0.9% NS or D5W to a final concentration 1-4 mg/mL into an infusion bag. Gently invert the bag to mix the solution. • Solutions are stable when refrigerated for 24 hr and for 12 additional hr at room temperature. • Protect from direct sunlight.	*Side effects:* • Severe infusion reactions can occur, usually within 30 min to 2 hr after starting the first infusion. Reactions are usually resolved by temporarily stopping the infusion or by giving additional diphenhydramine and steroids. If rigors occur, meperidine can also be given. Emergency equipment and medications should be readily available. • Severe mucocutaneous reactions can occur; some have been fatal. • Tumor lysis syndrome (rapid tumor lysis, hypocalcemia, hyperuricemia, hypokalemia, renal insufficiency) can occur, usually 12–24 hr after the initial infusion. • Mild, transient flulike symptoms have been reported.

TENIPOSIDE (Vumon, VM-26)			
Dosage: • 100 mg/m² 1-2 times weekly and 20–60 mg/m² × 5 days or 90 mg/m²/day × 5 days for lung cancer *Efficacy:* • Relapsed or refractory acute lymphoblastic leukemia • Small cell lung cancer	*Mechanism of action:* • Plant alkaloid, topoisomerase II inhibitor. • Phase specific, acts in late S phase and early G_2 phase. *Metabolism:* • Bound to plasma protein; metabolized in the liver with less than 10% of the unchanged drug in feces. • Eliminated in the urine. • t½ = 20 hr	*Administration precautions:* • Dosage is diluted in sodium chloride and is physically stable for approximately 24 hr at room temperature in glass containers. Drug may precipitate in plastic containers. • Administer over at least a 45-min period to avoid severe hypotension. • Avoid extravasation. • Local phlebitis may occur. • HSRs occur and include blood pressure changes, bronchospasm, tachycardia, urticaria, facial flushing, diaphoresis, periorbital edema, vomiting, and/or fever.	*Side effects:* • Leukopenia is the DLT occurring at 10–14 days. • Nausea and vomiting are rare. • Alopecia occurs gradually; skin rash is rare. • With high-dose therapy, severe skin rashes can occur. • Hemolytic anemia with renal failure has occurred. • HSR may be related to the Cremophor EL vehicle. • Secondary malignancies occur infrequently. • Hyperbilirubinemia, SGOT, and SGPT elevations can occur.

THIOTEPA (Thioplex)			
Dosage: • 12–16 mg/m² q 1–4 wk • 900 mg/m² (transplant dose) • 30–60 mg q wk × 4 wk for intravesicular use • 1.0–10 mg/m² 1–2 times per wk for intrathecal use *Efficacy:* • Breast cancer • Ovarian cancer • Superficial bladder cancer • Lymphoma • Hodgkin's disease	*Mechanism of action:* • An alkylating agent similar to nitrogen mustard. *Metabolism:* • Variably absorbed through the bladder mucosa following intravesical injection. • Metabolized in the liver. • t½ = 2–3 hr	*Administration precautions:* • 15-mg vial is reconstituted with 1.5 mL of sterile water and further diluted with saline for intrathecal use (preservative free). • Intravenous and intravesical solutions may be diluted with saline, D5W, or lactated Ringer's solution and are chemically stable for at least 5 days in the refrigerator and 24 hr at room temperature. • Intravesical instillation involves placement of a catheter in the bladder and instillation of the drug with retention of the liquid for up to 2 hr. The patient is repositioned q 15 min to maximize exposure to the tissues of the bladder. • Intrathecal doses are mixed in up to 20 mL of Ringer's lactate to maximize CNS distribution. • Intravenous administration may be given IVP or as an infusion. Thiotepa is not a vesicant.	*Side effects:* • Myelosuppression is the DLT and may be cumulative. • Leukopenia occurs 7–10 days postinjection. • Thrombocytopenia may be delayed. • Nausea and vomiting are not common in nontransplant doses. • Stomatitis may be severe in transplant doses. • Abdominal pain, hematuria, dysuria, frequency, and urgency occur with intravesical instillation. • Second malignancies have been reported.

(*continued*)

Appendix 16B Intravenous Antineoplastic Agents (continued)

Dosage and Efficacy	Mechanism of Action and Metabolism	Administration Precautions	Side Effects
TOPOTECAN (Hycamtin)			
Dosage: • 1.3–1.6 mg/m^2 IV infusion over 30 min, 2 hr, or 24 hr or • 1.5–2.0 mg/m^2/day as a 30-min infusion × 5 days *Efficacy:* • Small cell lung cancer • Ovarian cancer • Esophageal cancer	*Mechanism of action:* • Topoisomerase I inhibitor causes single-strand breaks in DNA, causing the cell to die during DNA replication. *Metabolism:* • Up to 48% of the drug is eliminated unchanged in the urine. • t½ = 3 hr	*Administration precautions:* • 5-mg vial is reconstituted with 2 mL of sterile water and diluted in D5W. • Stable for up to 48 hr at room temperature. • Given intravenously as an infusion.	*Side effects:* • Leukopenia is dose limiting, and the nadir occurs at days 10–12 with recovery at 3 wk. • Thrombocytopenia and anemia occur but are not usually dose limiting. • Mild to moderate nausea and vomiting may occur. Diarrhea has been reported to occur during or shortly after the infusion. • Fever and mild flulike symptoms are reported. • Alopecia and skin rash may occur. • Elevated LFTs are common. • Headache, dizziness, lightheadedness, and peripheral neuropathy have been reported.
TOSITUMOMAB (Bexxar)			
Dosage: • Dosimetry dose: tositumomab 450 mg followed by tositumomab 35 mg with I^{131} 5 mCi • Gamma scans to assess biologic clearance within 1hr of dosimetry, 2–4 days after dosimetry, and 6–7 days after dosimetry • Therapeutic dose: tositumomab 450 mg followed by tositumomab 35 mg with I^{131} based on biological clearance and platelet count • Platelet count > 150,000, deliver 75 cGy total body radiation, platelet count 100,000–150,000, deliver 65 cGy total body radiation *Efficacy:* • Follicular or transformed CD20$^+$ non-Hodgkin's lymphoma	*Mechanism of action:* • Murine monoclonal antibody conjugated with I^{131}. Apoptosis due to complement-dependent cytotoxicity, antibody-dependent cellular cytotoxity, and ionizing radiation. *Metabolism:* • Median clearance of tositumomab 68 hr. • 98% of free I^{131} eliminated in urine; 67% within 5 days of therapeutic dose.	*Administration precautions:* • Unlabeled tositumomab infused over 1 hr with a 22-micron filter. • Radiolabeled tositumomab infused over 20 min by licensed personnel. • Radiolabeled dose prepared by radiopharmacy and infused by licensed personnel. • Thyroid saturation with SSKI potassium iodide tablets, or Lugol's solution initiated day before treatment and continues for 14 days post-therapeutic dose. • Dilute unlabeled dose in 50 mL NS total volume. • Unlabeled tositumomab stable for 8 hr when refrigerated.	*Side effects:* • Infusion reaction: dyspnea, angioedema, bronchospasm, fever, hypotension, rigors. Premedicate with diphenhydramine and acetaminophen. • Fever. • Nausea, diarrhea, and vomiting. • Arthralgias, myalgias. • Uticaria, rash. • Delayed BMS common. Nadirs occur at 5–9 weeks requiring weekly CBC for 10–12 wk post-treatment. Cytopenias may be prolonged. • Thyroid dysfunction. Lifelong thyroid function assessment. • Gamma and beta radiation precautions initiated after therapeutic dose based on local or national regulatory agency guidelines.

TRASTUZUMAB (Herceptin)			
Dosage: • Loading: 4 mg/kg IV • Maintenance: 2 mg/kg IV weekly *Efficacy:* • Metastatic breast cancer with overexpression of HER2 protein	*Mechanism of action:* • Humanized monoclonal antibody. • Inhibits the proliferation of tumors that overexpress the HER2/neu protein. • Mediates antibody-dependent cellular cytotoxicity. *Metabolism:* • $t_{1/2}$ = 5.8 days	*Administration precautions:* • Do not administer by IVP or bolus. • Do not mix or administer with dextrose solutions. • Dilute in 250 mL of 0.9% NS and infuse the initial (loading) dose over 90 min; if tolerated well, infuse the weekly maintenance dose over 30 mins. • Reconstitute with 20 mL of bacteriostatic water for injections (BWFI) • When reconstituted with BWFI, the solution is stable for 24 hr at room temperature and 28 days under refrigeration.	*Side effects:* • Infusion-related reactions commonly consisting of chills and/or fever can occur that can be mild to moderate. Premedicate with pacetaminophen and/or diphenhydramine if reactions occur. • Cardiomyopathy can occur. Baseline cardiac assessment should be conducted. In addition, exercise caution when treating patients with preexisting cardiac dysfunction or prior cardiac therapy. • Nausea, vomiting, headache, and pain at the tumor site have been reported. • Increased incidence of anemia, leukcopenia, diarrhea, and infection is seen in patients receiving concurrent chemotherapy.

VINBLASTINE (Velban)			
Dosage: • 6–10 mg/m^2 q 2–4 wk; 1.7–2.0 mg/m^2/day weekly as a continuous infusion or over a period of 96 hr *Efficacy:* • Hodgkin's disease • Non-Hodgkin's lymphoma • Testicular cancer • Kaposi's sarcoma • Breast cancer • Melanoma • Cancers of the kidney, bladder, and cervix • Head and neck cancers • Lung cancer • Ovarian cancer	*Mechanism of action:* • Cell cycle phase specific for the M phase. • A plant alkaloid that binds to tubulin causing inhibition of the microtubule assembly, which inhibits mitotic spindle formation. *Metabolism:* • Metabolized by the liver. • Less than 1% is eliminated unchanged in the urine. • $t_{1/2}$ = 20 hr	*Administration precautions:* • Reconstituted with 10 mL of bacteriostatic NS to yield a concentration of 1 mg/mL. • Dose may be further diluted with D5W or NS for continuous infusion. • Continuous infusions may only be given through central lines because vinblastine is a severe vesicant if infiltrated. • Store in the refrigerator. Stable for 14 days at room temperature and for 30 days under refrigeration.	*Side effects:* • Leukopenia is dose limiting. • Thrombocytopenia and anemia are less common. • Nausea and vomiting, anorexia, diarrhea, and mucositis are rare. • Peripheral neuropathy, constipation, paralytic ileus, and urinary retention may occur. • Alopecia occurs with higher doses. • Rash and photosensitivity may occur. • Infiltration may cause ulceration depending on the amount of drug extravasated. • Treatment with hyaluronidase and heat may minimize ulceration. • Incompatible with heparin and furosemide. • Compatible in solution with doxorubicin, metoclopramide, dacarbazine, and bleomycin.

(continued)

Appendix 16B Intravenous Antineoplastic Agents (continued)

Dosage and Efficacy	Mechanism of Action and Metabolism	Administration Precautions	Side Effects
VINCRISTINE (Oncovin)			
Dosage: • 0.5–1.4 mg/m^2 q 1–4 wk • Continuous infusion regimens of 0.5 mg/day to 0.5 mg/m^2/day × 4 days may be used. *Efficacy:* • Acute leukemia • Hodgkin's disease • Non-Hodgkin's lymphoma • Rhabdomyosarcoma • Neuroblastoma • Wilms' tumor • Ewing's sarcoma • Melanoma • Multiple myeloma • Breast cancer • Lung cancer	*Mechanism of action:* • Plant alkaloid. • Binds to tubulin, causing inhibition of microtubule assembly, which inhibits mitotic spindle formation. • M phase specific. *Metabolism:* • Metabolized by the liver. • 40%–70% excreted in the bile. • t½ = 70–100 hr	*Administration precautions:* • Store in the refrigerator. • Stable for at least 30 days at room temperature. • Doses for continuous infusion are further diluted with NS or D5W. • Compatible with doxorubicin, bleomycin, cytarabine, fluorouracil, methotrexate, and metoclopramide. • Vincristine is a vesicant that should be given with caution and through a central line when given as a continuous infusion. • Hyaluronidase plus heat to disperse the antidote are indicated if the drug should infiltrate. • Greater than 2 mg total dose is usually contraindicated due to the toxicity of the drug. • Vincristine is lethal if given intrathecally and should be labeled as such when dispensed by the pharmacist. • Administer with caution in patients with obvious liver dysfunction.	*Side effects:* • Myelosuppression is mild. Nausea, vomiting, anorexia, and diarrhea are rare. • Constipation and abdominal pain may occur due to the neurological toxicity of the drug. • Prophylactic stool softeners and laxatives may be indicated in patients at high risk for constipation. • Alopecia is minimal. Paresthesias, ataxia, hoarseness, myalgias, headache, and seizures may occur. • Severe pain in the jaw may occur.
VINORELBINE TARTRATE (Navelbine)			
Dosage: • PO: 40-mg capsule for oral use • IV: 30–40 mg/m^2 weekly *Efficacy:* • Breast cancer • Ovarian cancer • Head and neck cancer • Esophageal cancer • Non-small cell lung cancer	*Mechanism of action:* • Cell cycle specific. • Produces cell blockade in G_2 and M phases. • Blocks polymerization of microtubules. • Impairs mitotic spindle. *Metabolism:* • Hepatic elimination. • Binds to plasma proteins. • Nonrenal elimination.	*Administration precautions:* • Venous irritation occurs in about 25% of patients. Symptoms include erythema and pain at the site, vein discoloration, and tenderness along the vein. • Administer drug over 6–10 min through the side arm of a freely running IV. Inject through the port farthest from the IV site. • Follow injection with 75–125 mL of IV fluid to flush the line (peripheral IV sites only).	*Side effects:* • DLT: Noncumulative neutropenia. • Alopecia/hair thinning after several treatments. • Anorexia. • Asthenia. • Peripheral neuropathy. • Constipation occurs in about one-third of patients and increases after several treatments. • Fatigue can be cumulative. • Arthralgias and myalgias. • Rash (rare).

• Lung cancer • Germ cell cancers		• Local tissue damage/necrosis, phlebitis may occur if the drug infiltrates. • Dose reduction may be appropriate for patients with impaired liver function. If bilirubin is > 2.1, the dose of vinorelbine is reduced 50%–75% (i.e., 15–7.5 mg/m^2). • Pain at the tumor site can occur during administration. • Vinorelbine is compatible with metoclopramide, ondansetron, chlorpromazine, promethazine, and dexamethasone. • Vinorelbine is incompatible with 5-FU, thiotepa, furosemide, amphotericin, ampicillin, piperacillin, aminophylline, and sodium bicarbonate.	• Typhlitis with abdominal pain and fever occur 3–4 days after treatment in heavily pretreated patients. • Jaw pain is rare.

ALL = acute lymphocytic leukemia; AML = acute myelogenous leukemia; AUC = area under the curve; BMT = bone marrow transplant; CHF = congestive heart failure; CI = continuous infusion; D5W = 5% dextrose in water; DLT = dose-limiting toxicity; 5-FU = 5-fluorouracil; 5HT^3 = serotonin receptor; GI = gastrointestinal; HSR = hypersensitivity reaction; IM = intramuscular; IP = intraperitoneal; IT = intrathecal; IV = intravenous; IVP = intravenous push; IU = International unit; LFT = liver function test; MUGA - ejection fraction; NS = normal saline; PO = oral; PVC = polyvinyl chloride; QS = quantity sufficient; SIADH = syndrome of inappropriate antidiuretic hormone; SGOT = serum glutamic oxaloacetic transaminase; SGPT = serum glutamic pyruvic transaminase; SQ = subcutaneous; t½ = half-life.

CHAPTER 17

Chemotherapy Toxicities and Management

Dawn Camp-Sorrell, RN, MSN, FNP, AOCN®

Introduction

Chemotherapy is administered based on a dose-response relationship (i.e., the more drug administered, the more cancer cells killed). Characteristically, chemotherapeutic agents have a narrow therapeutic index, with anticipated acute toxicities expressed in rapidly dividing normal tissues, such as bone marrow, the gastrointestinal tract, the gonads, and hair follicles. Acute and long-term toxicities from chemotherapy may also be a function of the drug's effect on specific cells of a given organ. The incidence and severity of toxicities are related to the drug's dosage, administration schedule, specific mechanism of action, as well as concomitant illness and specific measures used to prevent or minimize toxicities. Chemotherapeutic agents cause side effects that can appear immediately or after a few days (acute), within a few weeks (intermediate), or months to years after chemotherapy administration (long term).[1]

Because virtually every organ is affected by chemotherapy, the toxicities of the drug will commonly determine the maximum amount of drug that can be administered safely. Side effects such as stomatitis, alopecia, myelosuppression, nausea, vomiting, anorexia, and diarrhea are common, depending on the agent administered. These expected side effects can be managed effectively and generally do not warrant discontinuing the drug. *Toxic effects* refers to life-threatening, often dose-limiting effects that are characteristic of high dosages. Cumulative and irreversible damage to certain vital organs, such as the heart, limits the total dosage of chemotherapy.[1]

Pretreatment Evaluation: Risk Analysis

Individuals with an overall weak physical condition and poor nutritional status are not likely to tolerate a vigorous chemotherapy treatment regimine.[2] Patients previously treated with multiple chemotherapy agents, radiation, or biotherapy may lack marrow reserve, placing them at a higher risk for infection, bleeding, or anemia. The inability or unwillingness of an individual to perform self-care may increase the severity of a side effect and delay the seeking of appropriate care from healthcare professionals.

Preexisting disorders such as hepatic or renal dysfunction can alter the absorption, distribution, metabolism, and excretion of chemotherapy, causing abnormal accumulations of the drug and its metabolites.[3] Hypovolemia due to nausea and vomiting, diarrhea, inadequate dietary intake, third spacing (a shift of fluid from the vascular space to the interstitial space), or hypoalbuminemia may increase the risk of acute renal failure. Thus, the patient could be placed at a higher risk for organ toxicities.

Because the incidence of cancer increases with age, nurses must be aware of possible additional treatment risks for the elderly. Age-related changes in physical stature, body composition, kidneys, liver, and other organs influence the pharmacokinetic and pharmacodynamic properties of chemotherapy, possibly prolonging the drug's half-life.[4] Many elderly people, especially those older than age 85, are physically frail secondary to chronic and debilitating illness or poor nutrition or as a result of aging. Chronic illnesses such as arthritis, heart disease, diabetes, glaucoma, high blood pressure, cognitive deficits, and hearing and vision loss are common in the elderly.[3] These conditions may interfere with an individual's ability to perform basic activities of daily living. Consequently, elderly patients may be unable to perform preventive measures to minimize side effects from chemotherapy.

Gradual but substantial changes occur in body composition with age. The percentage of body fat increases with age, for example. Decreases occur in cardiac output, kidney function, hepatic blood flow, the ability to conjugate drugs, and the effectiveness of the immune system.[3] Cardiovascular changes may include thickening of blood vessel walls, atherosclerotic plaque formation, and loss of elastin fibers, which can lead to cardiac hypertrophy, diastolic dysfunction, and myocardial ischemia.[4] With advancing age, the kidneys atrophy, bringing subsequent decrease in renal function. Vasoconstriction of the renal vasculature decreases renal blood flow, glomerular filtration rate, and the ability to concentrate and dilute urine, resulting in a decreased creatinine clearance.[4] Bone marrow reserves decline, and the ability to replicate myeloid and erythroid progenitor cells decreases. In addition, the functional ability of peripheral mononuclear cells is impaired.[5,6]

Historically, elderly patients (over 60 years) with cancer have not been treated as aggressively as their younger counterparts because it was speculated that the elderly would not be able to tolerate the side effects of chemotherapy. This trend is changing, however, and many elderly patients now receive aggressive treatment for their cancer.[3–9] Numerous studies have looked at the consequences of treating older patients with chemotherapy.

In general, for many solid tumors, elderly patients tolerate chemotherapy, used for either adjuvant or palliative therapy, as well as young patients.[5] Cisplatin in moderate doses (60–100 mg/m^2) has been found to be safe in patients 80 years or older.[9] Geriatric patients with a systemic malignancy such as lymphoma or acute leukemia usually develop more treatment-related toxicity than younger patients. Nevertheless, geriatric patients can achieve complete response from chemotherapy if they survive the intensive initial therapy.[8]

While it is critical to be knowledgeable regarding the potential problems the elderly may encounter as a consequence of physiologic aging, age alone has not been shown to be a significant factor in the incidence and severity of toxicity to chemotherapy.[3–9] Chronic illness that often accompanies longevity is a better predictor for tolerance than age alone. The one exception has been hematologic toxicity, which is probably related to decreased marrow reserve or renal function. Healthcare professionals, therefore, should monitor hematologic values closely to minimize potential ill effects. Patients older than 70 years with normal renal and hepatic function and without serious medical conditions have been found to tolerate chemotherapy as well as individuals in younger populations.[7-9]

Quality of Life and Chemotherapy Toxicity

Treatment considerations include the patient's quality of life, the impact chemotherapy will have on the patient's quality of life, and the patient's physical and mental well-being.[10,11] Complications or side effects from chemotherapy are weighed against its potential antineoplastic benefits. In the past, cancer treatment was evaluated by tumor response and survival rates rather than by functional ability or quality of life.[12] Quality of life is based on the physical, psychological, social, and spiritual characteristics of what gives life value to the individual.[12] It is recognized as an acceptable endpoint in clinical trials, which have been influenced by viewing cancer as a chronic condition instead of as an acute event. Groups of cancer survivors have indicated to the healthcare community that quality of life is as important to the patient as the overall therapeutic effect.[13]

Physical symptoms (e.g., nausea, pain, rashes, stomatitis) can result in significant distress that has a marked impact on the patient's quality of life.[14] It is important to realize that the patient's perception of cancer and chemotherapy treatment will influence how the individual reacts and ultimately adapts.[14] Side effects can impair a person's abilities to function at work or at home, maintain sexual relationships, and engage in social activities. The degree of self-reported symptoms relates to the individual's perceived quality of life, such as when an increase in symptoms correlates with a decrease in quality of life.[10,11] Feelings of helplessness are heightened because patients are dependent on healthcare professionals to deliver their treatment. Anxiety can develop at key decision points, such as diagnosis, beginning of treatment, while awaiting test results, when the treatment plan is altered, or when the chemotherapy treatment plan has been successfully completed.[12] Chemotherapy-related changes in physical appearance are often described as a distressing aspect of cancer treatment. Weight changes and alopecia commonly occur and can be especially devastating because they are physical manifestations of having cancer.[12]

In an effort to minimize acute and chronic toxicities, chemoprotectant agents are being developed to improve the patient's quality of life.[15,16] Agents can be given prior to the chemotherapy to decrease the incidence of the expected toxicity, such as amifostine to minimize nephrotoxicity. Other agents, such as growth factors, are given concurrently with the chemotherapy and are directed at modulating the acute phase of the wound-healing response and decreasing inflammatory cascades. Rescue agents, such as leucovorin, are given after methotrexate to help minimize acute reactions.[15]

To help the patient cope with potential side effects, the nurse should foster a trusting relationship with the patient so that communication is open and sufficient information can be provided to help the patient retain control over his or her care. An important aspect of establishing a partnership with the patient and family in the pretreatment phase is knowing what concerns about the treatment need to be explored and what information needs to be provided. Such information helps patients formulate questions about available options when making difficult decisions about their care. When participating actively, the patient's feelings of control are enhanced, resulting in an improved functional status, sense of well-being, and performance of effective self-care.[17] Nurses must focus on developing practical interventions to reduce the psychological distress of treatment and to provide needed information, thereby increasing the patient's quality of life.

Self-Care

There is undeniable evidence that cost factors are dictating the administration of health care. Institutional, state, and federal regulatory bodies have assumed increasing jurisdiction over how and where patients will be treated. Diagnostic-related groups (DRGs) and prospective payment, cost-control measures by other insurers, and increased out-of-pocket medical expenses for consumers have all combined to create a shift from hospital-based care to outpatient and home care settings.[17] The change from inpatient to outpatient administration of chemotherapy shifts the responsibility for managing the treatment of side effects from healthcare providers to patients and their families. To facilitate self-care, nurses must understand the nature, incidence, and relative severity of each side effect, and be aware of effective self-care activities for reducing the severity of side effects.

With increasing severity of a side effect, patients become more immobilized and may delay initiating self-care behaviors for several days. Therefore, follow-up by the nurse must be initiated at least 1–3 days after chemotherapy to assess the patient and to determine whether side effects are being managed adequately. Patient education is essential to ensure that the patient and family understand what self-care measures need to be taken for the side effects experienced.[18]

A key goal of nursing care is to minimize toxicity, so the patient and caregiver must be instructed how to initiate self-care activities. *Self-care* is any activity initiated by patient, family, or friends to alleviate or minimize a side effect.[17] Self-care activities begin before treatment and continue throughout the treatment phase to manage or minimize side effects. In situations where patients are unable or unwilling to participate, efforts must be made to include family members or visiting nurses to ensure compliance. Without compliance, the side effects can be severe and may lead to further complications, which may result in hospitalization and death. Side effects that seem to be the most distressing to patients include fatigue, nausea, vomiting, alopecia, anorexia, and mouth sores.[12] Nurses must continue to develop effective strategies to assist patients in minimizing these side effects. Documenting strategies that have been successful, including those suggested by the patient, can serve as a useful resource for future patient instruction.

Patient Education and Follow-up

Although teaching may be initiated while the patient is still hospitalized, most teaching regarding chemotherapy takes place in the outpatient setting and is provided by the nurse who will administer the drugs. The intent of teaching is more than simply giving information: It provides support and knowledge to empower the patient to manage self-care effectively.[14,17] Teaching patients about their treatment reduces fear, increases self-confidence, improves compliance, and enhances their participation in self-care.[17]

One approach to identifying the informational needs of the patients and family members is to focus on the various phases of cancer care: diagnosis, treatment, rehabilitation, survivorship, and recurrent disease. Goals of chemotherapy teaching include the following:

1. Helping the patient adjust to the treatment
2. Explaining how the treatment will affect the cancer
3. Imparting the sequence of administration
4. Recognizing and controlling side effects
5. Encouraging self-care behaviors that minimize side effects
6. Listing side effects that should be reported to the healthcare professional

All information offered to the patient is documented in the patient's record (Figure 17-1) for future reference as well as to comply with professional regulations. It is important to reinforce teachings periodically, as retention without reinforcement may be short-lived.

In the outpatient setting, the nurse frequently screens phone calls and triages the patient to assist in evaluating symptomatology and initiating the appropriate treatment measures. The nurse must gather sufficient data to determine whether the patient needs medical intervention and, if so, whether the patient will be cared for most appropriately in the outpatient setting or in the hospital. Obviously, the nurse needs to be highly knowledgeable about what the patient's history is, when the last chemotherapy treatment took place, and whether this complaint is related to the treatment, is related to the disease, or is unrelated.

Objective and subjective data must be gathered methodically to formulate an opinion about the patient's account. After consulting with the physician or advance practice nurse, the nurse once again speaks to the patient, either to gather more information or to relay instructions to the patient or family regarding care. Examples of specific phone-triage flowcharts are included in the discussion of various chemotherapy side effects later in this chapter.

Chemotherapy Toxicities

Grading of Toxicities

Standardization of assessment and documentation of side effects are crucial in evaluating the therapeutic use of chemotherapy. Specific therapies can be assessed by comparing their benefits with toxicity occurrence. In the recognition and evaluation of toxicities, one must discriminate between an expected reaction and a toxic reaction to chemotherapy and distinguish these from complications related to the cancer. For example, if a patient with lymphoma presents to the clinic with a complaint of paresthesias, numbness, and tingling, he or she must be evaluated for possible spinal cord compression from tumor progression and for peripheral toxicity from vincristine administration.

CHEMOTHERAPY TEACHING CHECKLIST

Assessment Summary: ______________________________

Patient name: ______________________
Primary nurse: ______________________

Drugs: ______________________________

LEARNING NEED	TEACHING INITIATED (DATE & INITIALS)	KNOWLEDGE CONFIRMED (DATE & INITIALS)	COMMENTS
1. Patient education booklets/drug cards			
2. Viewed chemotherapy video/DVD/computer program Other:			
3. Common side effects and treatment			
a. Nausea and vomiting — antiemetics			
b. Stomatitis — mouth care			
c. Alopecia — wigs/scarves/hats			
d. Decreased white blood cells — infection precautions			
e. Decreased red blood cells — fatigue/SOB*			
f. Decreased platelets — bleeding precautions			
g. Skin and nail bed changes			
h. Loss of appetite — nutrition			
i. Diarrhea — medication/diet			
j. Constipation — diet/medication			
k. Flulike symptoms			
l. Urine discoloration			
m. Hemorrhagic cystitis — hydration			
n. Premedications (chemoprotectants, steroids, etc.)			
o. Other			
4. Specific teaching			
a. Subcutaneous injections			
b. Maintaining adequate nutrition			

*SOB = Shortness of breath.

Figure 17-1 Chemotherapy teaching checklist. (continued)

LEARNING NEED	TEACHING INITIATED (DATE & INITIALS)	KNOWLEDGE CONFIRMED (DATE & INITIALS)	COMMENTS
c. Precautions to report during drug administration:			
(1) Stinging, burning pain			
(2) Flushing of face			
(3) Metallic taste			
(4) Feeling of numbness			
(5) Itching at site (or generalized itching)			
(6) Allergic reactions			
d. Reproductive changes (1) Dyspareunia (2) Menopausal symptoms (3) Vaginal discomfort			
e. Activity			
f. Interaction with other drugs/food			
g. Vascular access device			
h. Perineal burning (Decadron)			
i. Peripheral edema			
5. Symptoms to report to physician:			
a. Bleeding			
b. Prolonged nausea or vomiting			
c. Fever/chills			
d. Stomatitis			
e. Diarrhea/constipation			
f. Numbness or tingling of extremities			
g. Difficulty breathing or shortness of breath			
h. Other			
6. Prescriptions given to patient with Instructions: □ Antiemetics ____ □ Wig □ Blood counts □ Other			
7. Schedule/calendar of drug treatment			
8. Instructions to obtain blood counts			
9. Follow-up or referral to community resources			

Comments: ____________________

____

____

____

Patient signature: ____________________

RN signature: ____________________

Figure 17-1 Chemotherapy teaching checklist (continued).

Using specific parameters and operational definitions to define the degree of a given toxicity ensures consistency in documenting observed reactions (Table 17-1). Toxicity grading scales have been developed by the World Health Organization and various cooperative study groups to provide consistency in reporting. Adequate assessment and documentation of the side effect experienced, the patient's overall response to the regimen, and subsequent quality of life can be essential for evaluating the impact of treatment. Decisions regarding the need for appropriate adjustments in the treatment plan can be determined on the basis of sound, objective data documented by the nurse.[12,19]

Specific guidelines need to be taught and given in written form to the patient and caregiver to ensure that they report any type of toxicity. Misinterpretation of a patient's report can negatively affect changes made in the treatment protocol. Nurses will continue to be challenged to design effective assessment and documentation systems that ensure accurate patient observation and reporting of toxicities, especially in the home setting.

Systemic Toxicities

Bone marrow suppression

Myelosuppression is the most common dose-limiting side effect of chemotherapy and can be the most lethal.[2,5,10] All hematopoietic cells divide rapidly, regardless of their developmental stage, and are therefore vulnerable to chemotherapy. Proliferating progenitor cells that produce the mature granulocytes, erythrocytes, and thrombocytes in the peripheral circulation are commonly destroyed by such treatment. As immature cells in the marrow and preexisting mature cells are destroyed, the nadir becomes apparent, usually 7–14 days after chemotherapy. At the same time, cells in the bone marrow are maturing and are ready to be released into the peripheral blood. Within a short period of time (3–4 weeks), the nadir will resolve.[20,21] However, when high doses of chemotherapy are administered, the stem cell population may fail to repopulate quickly enough, resulting in a prolonged nadir period.

The majority of chemotherapy drugs cause some degree of myelosuppression.[21] Agents most active against cells that are cycling or those active during a specific phase of the cell cycle can produce rapid cytopenia. Because alkylating agents and nitrosoureas affect both cycling cells and noncycling cells, these drugs are more likely to destroy the marrow stem cells. Antimetabolites, vinca alkaloids, and antitumor antibiotics are most damaging to cells that are in a specific phase of the cell cycle; thus, myelosuppression is less severe with these agents.[21] However, dose intensification and drug combinations can produce severe and prolonged neutropenia. For many drugs, myelosuppression can be the dose-limiting toxicity, especially for newer agents such as oxaliplatin, imatinib mesylate, bortezomib, pemetrexed, and gemcitabine.[21–25] Paclitaxel can cause neutropenia, with the severity depending on the administration schedule, dose, extent of previous treatment, and pharmacological exposure to the drug. Although preliminary data reveal that 3-hour infusion induces less neutropenia, the neutropenic effect is not cumulative, and permanent toxicity does not occur to the bone marrow. Gemcitabine can cause myelosuppression, especially thrombocytopenia. The hematologic toxicity has been found to be cumulative with the maximum tolerated dose of 1500 mg/m^2/week over a 30-minute infusion. Docetaxel results in an early, short-duration type of neutropenia at a dose of 100 mg/m^2 or greater when infused over 1 hour every 3 weeks. The nadir usually occurs at day 8 and resolves in 1 to 2 weeks, which has not been found to be a cumulative effect.

Oxaliplatin generally produces mild neutropenia and thrombocytopenia when given as a single agent. When oxaliplatin is administered in combination with 5-fluorouracil (5-FU) and leucovorin, myelosuppression can be a primary toxicity.[22] Imatinib mesylate produces neutropenia and thrombocytopenia with frequency of grade 3 to 4 when the patient is in an accelerated or blast phase of chronic leukemia. The duration is usually 2 to 3 weeks. Bortezomib causes mild neutropenia and thrombocytopenia, usually occurring on day 11 of a 4-day cycle.

Risk factors such as tumor cells in the bone marrow, prior treatment with chemotherapy or radiation, and a high negative nitrogen balance will compromise the marrow and increase the degree and duration of cytopenia.[21] It has been recognized that an increased risk of infection occurs among individuals suffering from protein-calorie malnutrition, which causes lymphopenia, diminished levels of the complement system, and decreased levels of certain immunoglobulins. In addition, myelotoxicity caused by chemotherapy and radiation therapy is enhanced by protein deprivation resulting from cancer cachexia. Younger patients are less likely to demonstrate severe cytopenia due to chemotherapy because their marrow is more cellular and has a decreased percentage of fat.

Differences in the lengths and kinetics of the life cycles of particular blood cells account for the frequency of neutropenia, thrombocytopenia, and anemia. Maturation of cells in the bone marrow takes 8 to 10 days, with variation in the life span for each cell type. Red blood cells (RBCs) have a life span of 120 days. Chemotherapy-induced anemia occurs less

Table 17-1 Grading Toxicities from Chemotherapeutic Agents

Toxicity	Grade ≥ 1	Grade 1	Grade 2	Grade 3	Grade 4
			HEMATOLOGIC		
WBC (1000/mm³)	≥4.0	3.0–3.9	2.0–2.9	1.0–1.9	<1.0
Granulocytes (1000/mm³)	≥2.0	1.5–1.9	1.0–1.4	0.5–0.9	<0.5
Platelets (1000/mm³)	≥100	75–99	50–74	25–49	<25
Hemoglobin (g/100 mL)	≥11	9.5–10.9	8.0–9.4	6.5–7.9	<6.5
Hemorrhage	None	Slight, no transfusion	Mild, 1–2 transfusions/episode	Gross, 3–4 transfusions/episode	Massive, >4 transfusions/episode
Infection/fever	None	Temp: <38°C No antibiotics	Temp: 38–40°C Broad-spectrum antibiotics	Temp: >40°C Antifungal coverage	Signs of sepsis: reevaluate medication
			GASTROINTESTINAL		
Nausea/vomiting	None	Slight nausea, 1 episode of vomiting Maintains intake	Occasional nausea, 2–5 episodes of vomiting Maintains intake	Frequent nausea, 6–10 episodes of vomiting Intake decreased	Constant nausea, >10 episodes of vomiting No intake
Diarrhea	None	2–3 stools	4–6 stools Moderate cramps	7–9 stools Severe cramps	>10 stools; needs rehydration
Constipation	None	Dry, hard passage of painful stool Stool softener	No stool >2 days Laxatives	No stool >4 days Rule out obstruction or cause	—
Stomatitis	None	Painless ulcers, erythema, or mild soreness	Painful erythema, edema, or ulcers, but can eat	Painful erythema, edema, ulcers, cannot eat	Requires parenteral or enteral support
Esophagitis/dysphagia	None	Painless ulcers, erythema, mild soreness, or dysphagia	Painful erythema, edema, ulcers, or moderate dysphagia, but can eat without narcotics	Cannot eat solids, or requires narcotics to eat	As above or complete obstruction or perforation
Taste	Normal	Slightly altered taste, metallic taste	Markedly altered taste	—	—
			DERMATOLOGIC		
Skin	None	Scattered macular or papular eruption or erythema; asymptomatic	Scattered macular or papular eruption, or erythema with pruritus or other associated symptoms	Generalized symptomatic macular, papular, or vesicular eruption	Exfoliative dermatitis or ulcerating dermatitis
Local	None	Pain	Pain and swelling with inflammation or phlebitis	Ulceration	Plastic surgery indicated
			OTHER		
Myalgia/arthralgia	None	Mild	Decrease in ability to move	Disabled	—

frequently because the bone marrow begins to recover before the number of circulating RBCs decreases significantly. Although low hemoglobin and hematocrit levels do not prevent administration of chemotherapy, low levels will affect how the patient feels and functions. Anemia is manifested by pallor, hypotension, headaches, irritability, and fatigue. Tachycardia and tachypnea may be present due to the hypoxic effects on the heart. Secondary problems include skin or mucous membrane breakdown arising from decreased tissue oxygenation as well as cardiopulmonary stress. The incapacitating symptoms of anemia have a profound impact on quality of life.[26,27] Anemia can usually be corrected with RBC transfusion.

Anemia of chronic disease is associated with erythroid hypoplasia of the bone marrow in underlying disease processes such as cancer, rheumatoid arthritis, and chronic infectious diseases.[11] Erythroid hypoplasia results in a slight decrease in reticulocytosis, hypoferremia, and a decrease in serum erythropoietin. Additionally, chronic inflammation and release of cytokines such as tumor necrosis factor, interferon, and interleukin-1 suppresses the production of erythropoietin, resulting in decreased red blood cell production. Actions of certain chemotherapeutic agents such as cisplatin may inhibit the maturation of the erythroid lineage cells in the bone marrow.[11]

Erythropoietin can be administered in an attempt to correct anemia induced by chemotherapy. This growth factor promotes erythroid progenitor cells' proliferation and maintains their survival.[26] Epoetin alfa has been available as a growth factor for red blood cells for more than a decade. Initially the usual dose is 150u/kg subcutaneously three times a week until the target hematocrit is reached. Weekly epoetin alfa administration at a dose of 40,000u to 60,000u is as effective compared to three weekly injections.[28] The target range, which is monitored weekly, is 36%–40%.[27] Once the patient reaches the target range, a maintenance dose is administered. Although a response from erythropoietin may take 2–8 weeks to occur, the maintenance dose is the dose the patient was receiving when the target hematocrit was reached. Only 50%–60% of anemic cancer patients respond to epoetin alfa, and it may require as long as 12 weeks of treatment to determine whether the patient is benefiting from the drug; monitoring assesses for increases in hemoglobin level and reticulocyte count.[28]

Another erythropoietin compound, darbepoietin alfa, has a prolonged half-life and increased biologic activity.[29] With the increase in serum half-life, dosing is less frequent, offering greater patient convenience, improved patient compliance, and decreased demands on healthcare professionals.[30] The initial dose for chemotherapy-induced anemia of darbopoietin alfa is 200μg every 2 weeks. If no response appears in 4–6 weeks, the dose can be increased to 300μg.[26,29] The most common side effects of both erythropoietin stimulators are hypertension and pain at the injection site; for this reason, the patient's blood pressure should be monitored frequently.[28] Patients with iron deficiency require iron supplementation because adequate iron stores are necessary to support erythropoiesis. Hemoglobin and hematocrit levels should be monitored prior to erythropoietin therapy to ensure the correct dose and the need for an injection.

The life span of platelets is 7–10 days. Thrombocytopenia usually occurs 8–14 days after chemotherapy — in most cases, concomitantly with neutropenia. Chemotherapy may be suspended if the count drops below 75,000–100,000 cells/mm^3. Thrombocytopenia is a potential or actual dose-limiting toxicity of gemcitabine, carboplatin, dacarbazine, 5-FU, lomustine, mitomycin-C, thiotepa, trimetrexate, imatinib mesylate, and bortezomib. A cumulative and delayed onset of thrombocytopenia has been observed with carmustine, fludarabine, lomustine, mitomycin-C, streptozocin, and thiotepa. When platelet levels are less than 50,000 cells/mm^3, a moderate risk of bleeding exists. As the platelet level continues to decrease below 10,000 cells/mm^3, a severe risk exists for fatal gastrointestinal, central nervous system, and respiratory tract hemorrhage.[31] Manifestations of thrombocytopenia are easy bruising; bleeding from gums, nose, or other orifices; and petechiae on the upper and lower extremities, pressure points, elbows, and palate (Figure 17-2). Transfusion of platelets is a common therapeutic intervention for a platelet count less than 10,000–20,000 cells/mm^3, although this step is often dependent on the patient's symptoms.[31]

In an attempt to minimize the occurrence of chemotherapy-induced thrombocytopenia, interleukin-11 (IL-11) has been approved as a growth factor for megakaryocytes in nonmyeloid malignancies and in non-myeloablative chemotherapy regimens. Interleukin-11 causes proliferation of hematopoietic stem cells and megakaryocyte progenitors and also induces megakaryocytic maturation.[32] Interestingly, IL-11 causes this effect independently of thrombopoietin. The dose is 50 μ/kg administered daily subcutaneously until the platelet count is greater than 50,000 cells/mm^3.[32,33] Interleukin-11 is discontinued 2 days prior to the next chemotherapy treatment. Side effects from IL-11 are thought to occur secondary to an increase in intravascular fluid from renal sodium retention and plasma volume expansion including dyspnea, edema, and an increase in pleural effusion formation.[32,33] As a consequence, patients with a history of congestive heart failure or coronary heart disease are usually not candidates for IL-11.

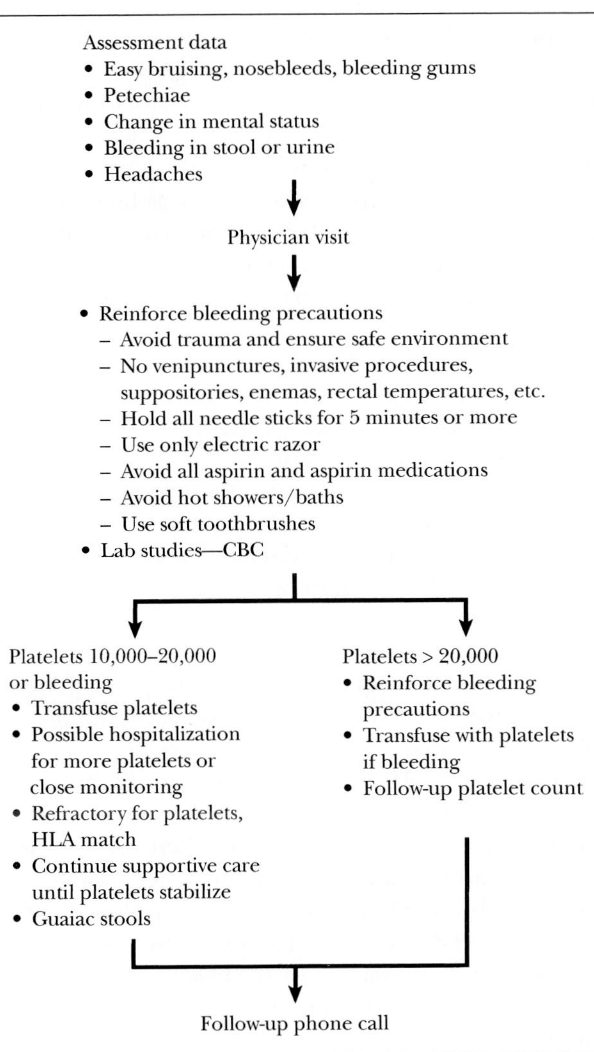

Figure 17-2 Thrombocytopenia telephone triage flowchart.

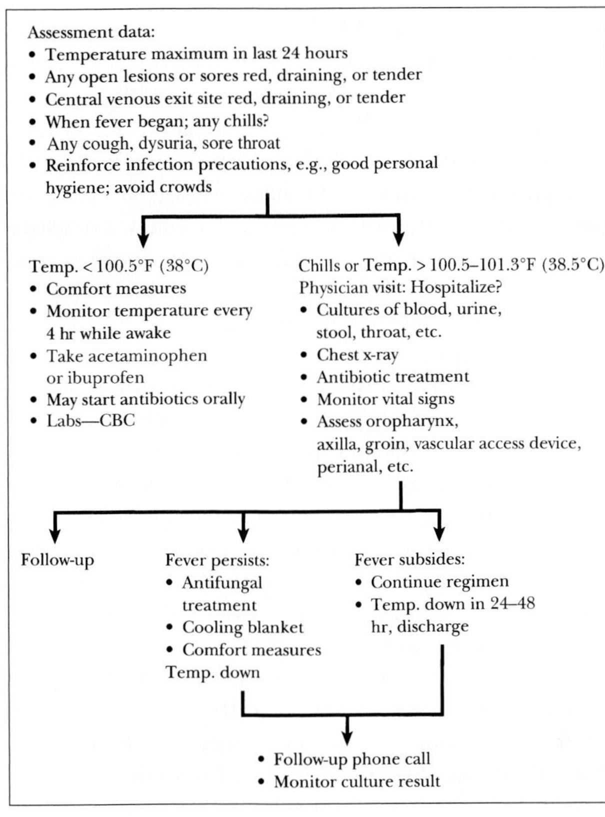

Figure 17-3 Fever telephone triage flowchart.

The life span of the granulocyte is 6–8 hours after release from the marrow. Neutropenia typically develops 8–12 days after chemotherapy, with recovery in 3–4 weeks. Chemotherapy is usually withheld if the patient's white blood cell (WBC) count is between 1000 and 3000 cells/mm^3 or if the absolute neutrophil count (ANC) is below 1500 cells/mm^3. Neutropenia generally is defined as an ANC less than 1500 cells/mm^3. In normal individuals, neutrophils, including both the segmented and slightly less mature band forms, are found in concentrations ranging from 1830 to 7250 cells/mm^3. Profound neutropenia (grade 4) usually is defined as an ANC less than 500 cells/mm^3.[10,34]

It is important to note that neutropenia can occur when the total WBC count is within a normal range (4000–10,000 cells/mm^3). Consequently, quantifying the ANC is essential to achieving a correct assessment of neutrophil status. The ANC is calculated by multiplying the total WBC count by the differential proportion of combined band and segmented neutrophils in a blood sample:

$$ANC = WBC\ (\text{segmented neutrophils} + \text{band neutrophils})$$

Thus, in a patient with a WBC count of 4000 cells/mm^3, a differential of 34% segmented neutrophils plus 3% band neutrophils yields

$$ANC = 4000\ \text{cells/mm}^3 \times 0.37 = 1480\ \text{cells/mm}^3$$

Monocyte count should also be monitored because an increase in monocytes precedes and predicts resolution of neutropenia.

Because the major function of neutrophils is phagocytosis, neutropenia eliminates one of the body's prime defenses against bacterial infection. Infections, due to invasion and overgrowth of pathogenic microbes, increase in frequency and severity as ANC decreases. In addition, risk for severe infections increases when the nadir persists for more than 7–10 days.[5]

Signs of an infection may not be apparent with the inhibition of phagocytic cells. The only response may be fever; at times, even it may not be present. It is estimated that 80% of the infections that occur arise from endogenous microbial flora of the gastrointestinal or respiratory tract.[20,34,35] When the neutrophil count is less than 500 cells/mm³, approximately 20% or more of febrile episodes will have an associated bacteremia caused principally by aerobic gram-negative bacilli (*Escherichia coli, Klebsiella pneumoniae, Pseudomonas aeruginosa*) and gram-positive cocci (coagulase-negative staphylococci, streptococci species, and *Staphylococcus aureus*).[35,36]

Chemotherapy-induced damage to the alimentary canal and respiratory tract mucosa facilitates the entry of infecting organisms; therefore, pneumonia and sinusitis are frequently seen. The nurse must assess for inflammation at the sites most commonly infected, including the periodontium, pharynx, lower esophagus, lung, perineum, anus, skin, and venous access exit sites. Prevention, early detection, good hand-washing technique, and prompt management of infections in patients with neutropenia are essential if sepsis and septic shock are to be avoided (Figure 17-3).[36]

Once appropriate cultures are obtained, broad-spectrum antibiotics are used to treat chemotherapy-induced infections (1) until cultures indicate eradication of the causative organism, (2) for a minimum of 7 days, or (3) until the neutrophil count is greater than 500/mm³.[37] Extended-spectrum cephalosporins (ceftazidime) and carbapenems (imipenem) are the agents most often used for empiric monotherapy. Combination therapy with antipseudomonal third-generation cephalosporins and aminoglycosides or penicillin is generally used.[37] Other combinations include a β-lactam (penicillin) with an aminoglycoside or another β-lactam.[35–38] With the increased predominance of gram-positive organisms in febrile neutropenic patients, the use of vancomycin with an antipseudomonal β-lactam agent has been beneficial. Although effective, such combinations should not be prescribed routinely because of the potential for emergence of vancomycin-resistant organisms. Empiric use of vancomycin is recommended in patients known to be colonized with methicillin-resistant organisms, in patients with a venous access device infection, and in patients on quinolone prophylaxis with severe mucositis who are at risk for a streptococcal infection or positive blood cultures prior to susceptibility information.[35]

Until recently, all febrile neutropenic patients were treated with hospital-based parenteral antibiotics. Risk assessment is now used to determine the need for hospitalization and the route of antibiotic therapy.[35,37,38] Neutropenia induced by solid tumor treatment usually lasts for less than 10 days, whereas neutropenia associated with hematologic malignancies often lasts for 15–20 days. High-risk patients include those with hematologic malignancies and bone marrow transplant recipients with prolonged neutropenia. These patients need to be hospitalized and given broad-spectrum parenteral therapy until resolution of their fever and neutropenia occurs and cultures indicate eradication of causative organisms. Moderate-risk patients include those with a co-morbidity such as hypertension or renal failure; these individuals need to be stabilized in the hospital and discharged early with parenteral or oral antibiotics. Low-risk patients can be given outpatient therapy with either oral ciprofloxacin or ciprofloxacin plus amoxicillin.[35,38]

Fever persisting for more than 3 days without identification of an infected site or organism suggests (1) a nonbacterial cause, (2) resistance to the antibiotic, (3) emergence of a second bacterial infection, (4) inadequate antibiotic serum and tissue levels, (5) drug fever, or (6) infection at avascular sites (abscess).[37] At this point, antifungal therapy is started. Antiviral drugs are usually not recommended unless mucosal lesions or viral disease is suspected. Risk for recurrent fever and infection are significant for neutropenic patients or those with poor marrow recovery such as in disease-related bone marrow dysfunction.[37]

Protective isolation has no effect on the host's endogenous flora or on organisms transmitted by water or food. It is not surprising that when careful hand washing and handling of food and other supplies are conducted, the addition of protective isolation offers no benefit in decreasing infections in neutropenic patients. Thus, hand washing is the best preventive method for minimizing infection in the neutropenic patient.[39]

Among all the problems identified with myelosuppression, infection is the most serious and is associated with significant morbidity and mortality.[35] For this reason, much attention has been focused on the therapeutic application of recombinant colony-stimulating factors (CSFs) to augment neutrophil counts. Hematopoietic growth factors constitute a family of glycoprotein hormones that act as natural regulators of hematopoiesis to promote the proliferation and differentiation of hematopoietic progenitor cells along multiple pathways.[40,41] While hematopoietic stimulants have not changed the decline rate of granulocytes, they have shortened the duration of neutropenia, thereby dramatically reducing the morbidity and mortality from infections. The discovery of CSFs offers hope that the myelosuppression associated with chemotherapy can be ameliorated and that full dosages of chemotherapy can be used in cancer therapy.

The American Society of Clinical Oncologists has developed clinical practice guidelines for appropriate use of CSFs.[40] After reviewing available literature, the following guidelines were developed to assist the practitioner in use of CSFs:

1. CSFs are appropriate if subsequent chemotherapy regimens are delayed from prolonged neutropenia and if dose reduction is not possible.
2. CSFs are appropriate in high-risk patients with febrile neutropenia in conjunction with antibiotics only in clinical deterioration such as multiorgan failure.
3. CSFs are appropriate when febrile neutropenia is expected in more than 40% of patients, such as results from high-dose or dose-dense chemotherapy.
4. CSFs are appropriate with autologous bone marrow transplants, to shorten neutropenia and infectious complications.
5. CSFs are effective in mobilizing peripheral blood progenitor cells for transplantation.
6. CSFs should be avoided in patients receiving combination chemotherapy and radiation, particularly involving the mediastinum.

Inconclusive data exist on the use of CSFs with other conditions, especially febrile neutropenia. Although growth factors have made tremendous inroads on decreasing duration of neutropenia, thereby decreasing the incidence of infections, reduced efficacy occurs with multiple courses and with bone marrow depletion. Another limitation is that specific lineage growth factors may affect only a segment of one tissue compartment.[41] Three CSFs are approved to stimulate the production and activation of neutrophils.[41–43] The granulocyte colony-stimulating factor (G-CSF) recommended dose is 5μg/kg/day for a maximum of 14 days. The granulocyte-macrophage colony-stimulating factor (GM-CSF) recommended dose is 250μg/m^2/day for a maximum of 21 days. In general, these CSFs are initiated 24 hours after chemotherapy administration and continued until the occurrence of an ANC greater than 10,000 cells/mm^3.[41] However, a shorter duration of CSF administration that is sufficient to achieve adequate neutrophil recovery is reasonable.[41]

Granulocyte colony-stimulating factor is available in a long-acting formulation for administration once per chemotherapy cycle.[42] Long-acting G-CSF (neulasta) is administered at a dose of 6 mg subcutaneously. This type of CSF appears to be self-regulated, remaining in the blood until the post-nadir ANC returns to normal. The serum concentration of the G-CSF begins to decline at the onset of neutrophil recovery.[42] The most common side effects of all CSFs are mild to moderate bone pain and injection site irritation.

Although clinical experience is limited, G-CSFs may have a potential role in treating fungal infections. Colony-stimulating factors have been shown to enhance activity of phagocytic cells against *Candida* species.[43]

Gastrointestinal tract

Chemotherapy-induced gastrointestinal toxicity can be the most devastating experience for the patient. Although numerous pharmacological interventions have been developed to minimize these toxicities, their occurrence can lead to delay of treatment, fluid and electrolyte imbalances, weight loss, and malnutrition. One agent, bevacizumab, has been found to cause gastrointestural perforation and wound dehiscence. Patients typically complain of abdominal pain with constipation and vomiting. To avoid disruption in wound healing, bevacizumab administration is delayed.

Diarrhea. Chemotherapy-induced diarrhea occurs due to a combination of factors, including an imbalance between absorption and secretion in the small bowel.[44,45] Diarrhea entails an increase in stool volume and liquidity, resulting in three or more bowel movements per day. Chemotherapy produces acute damage to the intestinal mucosa that is characterized by necrosis of the cells that line the intestinal crypt, resulting in extensive bowel wall inflammation. Without crypt cells, replacement of cells in the intestinal villi is hampered, resulting in a decreased absorptive surface. Because of the intestinal inflammation, factors such as prostaglandins and cytokines are secreted that further stimulate the secretion of intestinal fluids and electrolytes from crypt cells.[46]

The degree and duration of diarrhea depend on the agent, dose, nadir, and frequency of chemotherapy administration. Incidence and severity of diarrhea have increased with newer chemotherapy agents, adjunct therapies, and aggressive treatment approaches.[46] Alterations in mucosal integrity, coupled with the destruction of brush-border enzymes essential for carbohydrate and protein digestion, produce moderate to severe diarrhea immediately following chemotherapy and up to 14 days after chemotherapy. With 5-FU and leucovorin therapy, patients may experience abdominal cramps and rectal urgency, which can evolve into nocturnal diarrhea or fecal incontinence leading to lethargy, weakness, orthostatic hypotension, and fluid and electrolyte imbalance. Without adequate management, prolonged diarrhea will cause dehydration, nutritional malabsorption, and circulatory collapse.[46]

Although 5-FU is the chemotherapy drug that most commonly causes diarrhea, other agents potentially producing this effect include methotrexate, docetaxel, actinomycin D, doxorubicin, trimetrexate, irinotecan, bortezomib, arsenic trioxide, gefitnib, and capecitabine.[47] Combination chemotherapy and multimodal treatment can result in severe diarrhea. Antiemetics such as metoclopramide and prokinetic agents can cause diarrhea by increasing bowel transit time.[47]

Thorough evaluation to determine the cause of the diarrhea provides a firm foundation for planning interventions. Management may be limited to dietary measures, such as a low-residue, high-caloric, high-protein diet or pharmacological measures. Stool cultures need to be obtained initially to rule out an infectious process so that appropriate therapy can be implemented. *Clostridium difficile* has been reported in patients receiving chemotherapy who have had prior antibiotic exposure. Antidiarrheal agents should never be given to counteract diarrhea resulting from an infection, as these agents slow the passage of stool through the intestines, prolonging the mucosal exposure to the organism's toxins. When the diarrhea is a result of an infectious organism, it will typically resolve in a few days with the use of oral vancomycin or metronidazole.[48]

Pharmacological interventions for diarrhea vary. Anticholinergic drugs such as atropine sulfate and scopolamine reduce gastric secretions and decrease intestinal peristalsis. Opiate therapy binds to receptors on the smooth muscle of bowel, slowing down the intestinal motility and increasing fluid absorption. Loperamide is a long-acting opioid agonist without central opioid activity. Although the recommendation is a maximum of 16 mg in 24 hours, an increase of the loperamide dose must be used to control irinotecan-induced diarrhea. Current recommendations are 4 mg initially followed by 2 mg every 4 hours until the diarrhea stops.[48] Diphenoxylate is an opiate analog that inhibits intestinal peristalsis. Because diphenoxylate has codeine-like properties, atropine has been added to decrease abuse. Atropine can be used alone in a dose of 0.25 mg to 1 mg prior to irinotecan. It is thought that irinotecan-induced diarrhea may be cholinergic mediated, so atropine is beneficial in this setting in minimizing diarrhea.[48]

Octreotide acetate, a synthetic analog of the hormone octapeptide, inhibits the release of gut hormones, including serotonin and gastrin, from the gastrointestinal tract. It affects the gastrointestinal tract by prolonging intestinal transit time, increasing intestinal water and electrolyte transport, and decreasing mesenteric blood flow. Octreotide acetate is indicated for patients who have excessive diarrhea as a result of gastrointestinal resections or when other pharmacological treatments have proved ineffective in managing chemotherapy-induced diarrhea.[48]

Chemotherapy usually is administered despite the occurrence of diarrhea. However, diarrhea can be severe enough to be a dose-limiting toxicity of some chemotherapeutic agents such as irinotecan, oxaliplatin, capecitabine, gefitnib, or combination therapy — specifically, 5-FU and leucovorin. The nurse must carefully monitor the patient's status to provide appropriate therapy, such as antidiarrheal medications, fluid and electrolyte replacements, and perirectal care to prevent further complications (Figure 17-4).

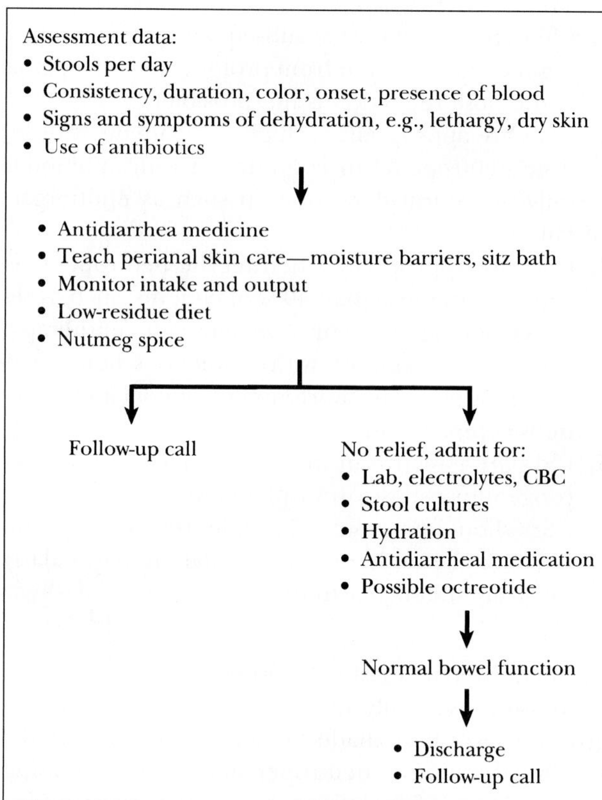

Figure 17-4 Diarrhea telephone triage flowchart.

Constipation. Constipation is defined as infrequent, excessively hard and dry bowel movements resulting from a decrease in rectal filling or emptying.[49] Risk factors that contribute to constipation include narcotic analgesics, a decrease in physical activity, a low-fiber diet, a decrease in fluid intake, and bed rest. Other medications such as anticholinergics, calcium-channel blockers, iron, calcium, and anticonvulsants decrease stool frequency. Vincristine, vinblastine, and vinorelbine are the most common chemotherapy agents to cause constipation, as a result of autonomic nerve dysfunction manifested as colicky abdominal pain and ileus. Rectal emptying is specifically diminished because nonfunctional afferent and efferent pathways from the sacral cord are interrupted. Symptoms occur 3–7 days after drug administration and may be accompanied by evidence of peripheral nerve dysfunction.[46]

Even though chemotherapy is usually administered despite constipation, patients are instructed to be aware of bowel movements. If a bowel movement does

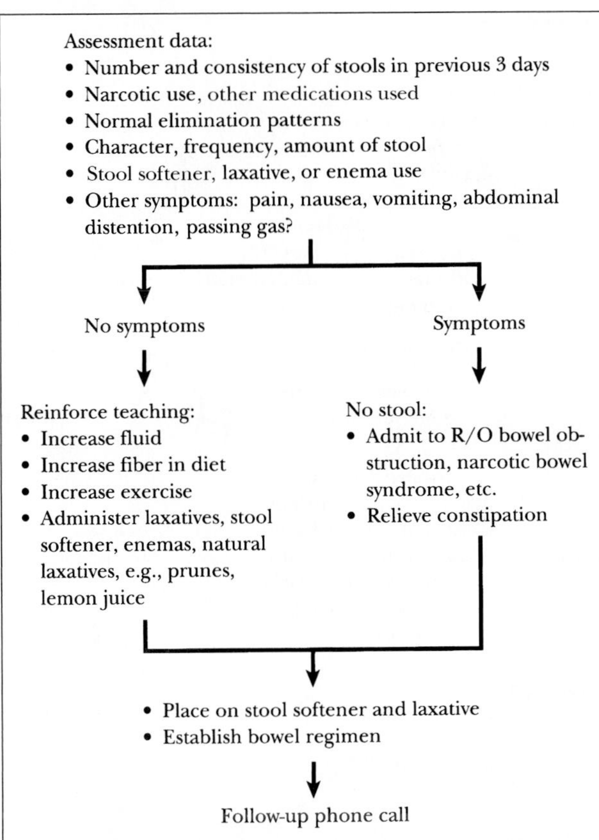

Figure 17-5 Constipation telephone triage flowchart.

not occur every other day, a laxative must be taken. If there are no results, the physician or advanced practice nurse should be consulted. Laxative therapy or prophylactic stool softener is recommended prior to the administration of drugs known to contribute to constipation, especially if the patient has a history of or is at risk for constipation. The patient should be encouraged to increase the amount of high-fiber foods in the daily diet as well as to increase fluid intake. He or she also should be encouraged to increase physical activity, if that is tolerated. It should be stressed to the patient never to wait more than 3 days for a bowel movement before calling the physician or nurse, as a complication such as impaction or ileus can arise (Figure 17-5).

Nausea and vomiting. During the past decade, the management of chemotherapy-related nausea and vomiting has vastly improved. Understanding the pathophysiology of the symptoms, the efficacy and limitations of pharmacological interventions, and the use of nonpharmacological techniques is essential in minimizing nausea and vomiting. Emesis is a complicated process that requires coordination by the vomiting center (VC) in the lateral reticular formation of the medulla (Figure 17-6). The VC lies close to the respiratory center on the floor of the fourth ventricle and is directly activated by the visceral and vagal afferent pathways from the gastrointestinal tract, chemoreceptor trigger zone (CTZ), vestibular apparatus, and cerebral cortex. When the VC is stimulated, emesis is induced via impulses to the salivation and respiratory centers and to the pharyngeal, gastrointestinal, and abdominal muscles.[50,51]

The VC is rich in neurotransmitter receptors that are sensitive to chemical toxins in the blood and cerebrospinal fluid.[52] The major receptors are dopamine, serotonin (5HT), neurokinin-1, and muscarinic cholinergic in the CTZ; muscarinic and dopamine in the VC, vestibular apparatus, and efferent vagal motor nuclei; and histamine in the VC and vestibular apparatus. Chemotherapy damages the enterochromaffin cells of the duodenal mucosa, causing serotonin release that binds to vagal afferent receptors. These afferent receptors, in turn, send impulses to the emetic center.[52]

Vestibular-cerebellar afferent pathway areas transmit impulses to the cerebellum and then to the VC, which are experienced as motion sickness. When rapid motion change occurs, the receptors of the labyrinth in the inner ear are stimulated, which is associated with nausea.[52] Obstruction, irritation, inflammation, or delayed gastric emptying may stimulate the gastrointestinal tract through vagal visceral afferent pathways.[51] Conditioned and anticipatory responses are controlled by the cerebral cortex and limbic system, which can be stimulated by sights, sounds, or odors that the patient associates with chemotherapy, thereby making the patient nauseated.[52]

Although nausea, retching, and vomiting commonly occur together, they are considered separate conditions.[52] *Nausea* is described as a subjective conscious recognition of the desire to vomit and is manifested by an unpleasant wavelike sensation in the epigastric area, at the back of the throat, or throughout the abdomen. It is mediated by the autonomic nervous system and accompanied by symptoms such as tachycardia, perspiration, light-headedness, dizziness, pallor, excess salivation, and weakness.

Retching is a rhythmic and spasmodic movement, involving the diaphragm and abdominal muscles, controlled by the respiratory center in the brain stem near the VC. Negative intrathoracic pressure and positive abdominal pressure result in unproductive retching. When the negative pressure becomes positive, vomiting occurs. *Vomiting* is a somatic process performed by the respiratory muscles causing the forceful oral expulsion of gastric, duodenal, or jejunal contents through the mouth.[53]

Nausea and vomiting can be classified as acute, delayed, and anticipatory. *Acute nausea and vomiting* occur from a few minutes to 1–2 hours after treatment,

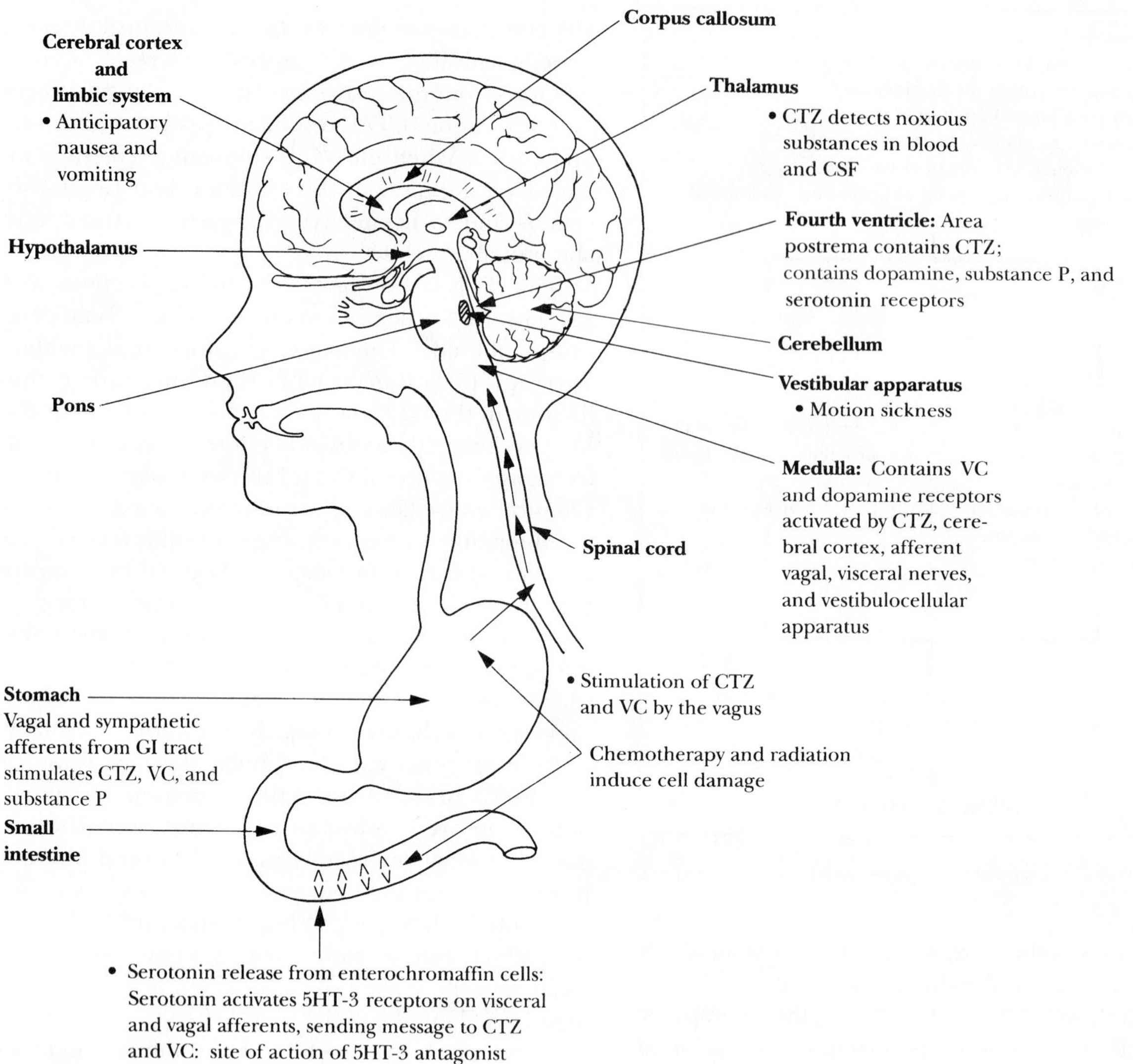

Figure 17-6 Pathways of nausea and vomiting.

resolving within 24 hours. The pattern is determined by the emetogenicity of the chemotherapy and pretreatment with an antiemetic agent. *Delayed nausea and vomiting* persist or develop 24 hours after chemotherapy, perhaps due to the ongoing effect that the metabolites of chemotherapy continue to exert on the CNS or gastrointestinal tract. Although cisplatin is thought to be the main culprit, cyclophosphamide, doxorubicin, carboplatin, and ifosfamide can cause delayed nausea as well. If nausea is controlled within the first 24 hours after therapy, delayed patterns are less likely to occur. However, despite effective antiemetic regimens, patients still experience a significant amount of delayed nausea and vomiting.[54,55] *Anticipatory nausea and vomiting* occur in 25% of patients as a result of classic operant conditioning from stimuli associated with chemotherapy, usually 12 hours prior to administration. Such conditioned responses are experienced after a few sessions of chemotherapy and occur most commonly when efforts to control emesis are unsuccessful. Lorazepam has been found to relieve anticipatory effects as well as delayed nausea.[56]

It is possible to predict the degree and severity of nausea and vomiting as well as the onset and duration (Table 17-2). Mechlorethamine, for example, induces emesis within 30 minutes of intravenous administration, whereas other highly emetic agents cause emesis at least 1 hour after infusion. With moderately to highly emetic drugs, emesis develops within 6 hours of administration. Drugs with low emetic potential usually cause emesis 12–48 hours after administration. The variability in their occurrence and onset suggests that each drug may cause emesis via a different mechanism or by stimulating a different pathway.[52,57] The rate and route of chemotherapy administration also affect emetic onset, intensity, and duration. For example, rapid infusion of cytarabine is more often associated with an earlier onset of severe emesis than is slower infusion.

Management begins with obtaining an in-depth emetic history and developing a preventive action plan with antiemetics (Table 17-3). Characteristics that affect the occurrence of nausea and vomiting include susceptibility to motion sickness, poor previous emetic control, fatigue, poor social functioning, and being young. Individuals with a heavy alcohol intake seem to have a decreased occurrence of nausea and vomiting.[52,54]

Successful antiemetic regimens interrupt the stimulation of the VC. Combination regimens must be individualized and developed according to the emetic potential of the chemotherapy regimen, expected duration of the nausea and vomiting, and current pattern of symptoms. Numerous combinations are being investigated extensively to eliminate the stimulation of the VC. These regimens use drugs with proven single-agent antiemetic activity, optimal doses, routes, and minimal overlapping toxicities (Figure 17-7).[58] For example, combinations of serotonin-receptor antagonists with steroids have been found to provide complete control of nausea and vomiting in as many as 100% of patients undergoing high-dose cisplatin-based regimens.

Experts generally agree that nausea and vomiting occur throughout the treatment phases and no one 5HT-3 receptor antagonist is superior to another, whether given intravenously or orally.[59,60]

Palonosetron is a newer 5HT-3 receptor antagonist and is unique because it has a 100-fold higher receptor-binding affinity compared to earlier serotonin antagonist.[61] Also, after intravenous administration, this agent has a half-life of 40 hours and a duration of 7 days. Studies reveal palonosetron to be superior to similar agents in controlling delayed nausea and vomiting.[61,62]

Aprepitant is the first substance P neurokinin-1 (NK_1) receptor antagonist. Chemotherapy-induced emesis is mediated by neurotransmitters such as serotonin, histamine, and substance P. Aprepitant prevents delayed nausea and vomiting because it effectively blocks substance P.[63] Following an oral dose, aprepitant has a half-life of 9–13 hours and a duration of 24 hours. This agent is given in a dose of 125 mg 1 hour prior to chemotherapy and 80 mg on days 2 and 3 after chemotherapy.[64] The agent is metabolized in the liver by CYP3A4. Subsequently, an increase in serum concentrations may occur with drugs metabolized by this enzyme, including docetaxel, paclitaxel, etoposide, irinotecan, ifosfamide, imatinib, vinorelbine, and vincristine.[63,64]

Another unique feature of this group of drugs is the fact that one, ondansetron, is available as an orally disintegrating tablet (ODT). The tablet dissolves quickly when placed under the tongue, where it is directly absorbed into the bloodstream. Ondansetron ODT is approved for delayed nausea following moderately emetogenic chemotherapy.

Further classification has been proposed to determine the emetogenicity of combination chemotherapy (see Table 17-2).[57] Initially, the most emetogenic agent in the combination is identified. Other agents are then assessed for emetogenic potential with these considerations: (1) Level 1 agents do not significantly contribute to the overall emetogenicity of the combination; (2) one or more level 2 agents increase the emetogenicity of the combination by one level greater than the most emetogenetic agents; and (3) the emetogenicity of the combination is increased by one level per agent when a level 3 or 4 agent is added to the regimen.[57]

Behavioral interventions such as progressive muscle relaxation, hypnosis, and systematic desensitization can be taught to the patient to help interrupt the association of nausea and vomiting with chemotherapy. The nurse can try to minimize any aversive sounds or smells in the environment that could stimulate the VC. Distraction with audiotapes, radio, or television programs should be provided in the treatment area to help minimize nausea. Each of these techniques has been found effective in decreasing the frequency and duration of vomiting as well as in decreasing anxiety.[53]

It is important to teach patients about the potential side effects of antiemetic therapy, such as drowsiness and diarrhea. If the patient is returning home after an emetogenic chemotherapy treatment, ensure that someone can provide transportation and care in the immediate hours following therapy. Phone follow-up 24–48 hours after treatment is essential to ensure that appropriate antiemetic management is being followed (Figure 17-8).

Mucositis. *Mucositis* is a general term that describes the inflammatory response of mucosal epithelial cells to the cytotoxic effects of chemotherapy. Painful ulceration, hemorrhage, and secondary infection may develop when mucositis is not detected early or continues untreated. Because all mucous membrane–covered surfaces exhibit similar patterns of growth, replacement, and function, any mucous membrane within the gastrointestinal tract, from the mouth to the rectum, can be adversely affected by chemotherapy.

The epithelial cells lining the gastrointestinal mucosa renew rapidly, which enables them to replace cells lost when food is chewed, swallowed, digested, and eliminated from the body. Mucositis results when these mucosal cells are damaged by chemotherapy

Table 17-2 Emetogenic Potential of Chemotherapeutic Agents

Incidence	Level	Agent	Onset (hours)	Duration (hours)
Very high (>90%)	5	Cisplatin (>50 mg/m^2)	1–6	24–48+
		Dacarbazine	1–3	1–12
		Mechlorethamine	0.5–2	8–24
		Melphalan — high dose	0.3–6	6–12
		Streptozocin	1–6	12–24
		Cytarabine — high dose (> 1 g/m^2)	1–4	12–48
High (60%–90%)	4	Carmustine (>100 mg/m^2)	2–4	4–24
		Cyclophosphamide (>600 mg/m^2)	4–12	12–24
		Procarbazine	24–27	variable
		Etoposide — high dose	4–6	24+
		Semustine	1–5	12–24
		Lomustine	4–6	12–24
		Dactinomycin	2–5	24
		Plicamycin	1–6	12–24
		Methotrexate — high dose	1–12	24–72
		Actinomycin-D	1–12	24–48
		Cytarabine (500 mg/m^2)	1–12	24–48
		Epirubicin	6–12	24+
		Idarubin	6–12	24+
		Oxaliplatin	1–6	24
Moderate (30%–60%)	3	Doxorubicin (>50–75 mg/m^2)	4–6	6+
		Mitoxantrone	4–6	6+
		5-fluorouracil	3–6	24+
		Mitomycin C	1–4	48–72
		Carboplatin	4–6	12–24
		Daunorubicin (<50 mg/m^2)	2–6	24
		L-asparaginase	1–4	2–12
		Topotecan	6–12	24–72
		Ifosfamide (<1.5 g/m^2)	3–6	24–72
		Irinotecan	6–12	24+
		Epirubicin	—	—
		Idarubicin	—	—
Low (10%–30%)	2	Bleomycin	3–6	—
		Cytarabine (<20 mg/m^2)	6–12	3–12
		Etoposide	3–8	—
		Melphalan	6–12	—
		6-Mercaptopurine	4–8	—
		Methotrexate (<100 mg/m^2)	4–12	3–12
		Vinblastine	4–8	—
		Hydroxyurea	—	—
		Teniposide	—	—
		Gemcitabine	—	—
		Vinorelbine	—	—
		Fludarabine	—	—
		Hydroxyurea	—	—
		Topotecan	—	—
		Capecitabine	—	—
		Trimetrexate	—	—
		Imatinib mesylate	—	—
			—	—
Very low (<10%)	1	Vincristine	4–8	—
		Chlorambucil	48–72	—
		Busulfan	—	—
		Thioguanine	—	—
		Hormones	—	—
		Paclitaxel	4–8	—
		Docetaxel	—	—
		Thiotepa	—	—
		Velcade	—	—
		Temozolomide	—	—
		Valrubicin	—	—
		Tretinoin	—	—
		Gefitnib	—	—

Table 17-3 Antiemetic Therapy

Classification	Drugs	Availability/Dose	Schedule	Duration	Half-Life	Comments
Benzodiazepines *Mechanism of action* CNS depressant; interferes with afferent nerves from cerebral cortex; sedative *Common side effects* Sedation, amnesia, confusion	Lorazepam	Tablet: 1–3 mg PO or sublingual IV: 0.5–2.5 mg	q3–4h	4–8 hr	10–15 hr	Reduces anticipatory nausea and vomiting. May aggravate CNS effects of ifosfamide. Use with caution in patients with hepatic and renal dysfunction.
	Diazepam	Tablet: 2–4 mg IV: 2–10 mg	q4–6h	4–8 hr	30–40 hr	
Butyrophenones *Mechanism of action* Dopamine antagonist in the CTZ, esophagus, and stomach *Common side effects* Sedation, hypotension, tachycardia, EPS	Droperidol	IM: 2.5–10 mg IV: 0.5–2.5 mg	q3–4h	2–4 hr	10 hr	Diphenhydramine 25–50 mg PO or IV will prevent EPS. EPS more common in young patients. May have additive effects. Use caution in patients with cardiac disorders.
	Haloperidol	Tablet: 3–5 mg IM: 1–5 mg IV: 1–3 mg	q4h q2–6h	2–6 hr	12–18 hr	
Cannabinoids *Mechanism of action* Suppresses pathways to VC (speculated) *Common side effects* Sedation, dizziness, dysphoria, dry mouth, disorientation, impaired concentration, orthostatic hypotension, tachycardia	Dronabinol	Tablet: 5–10 mg	q4h	4–6 hr		May be difficult to obtain in outpatient setting. Elderly patients generally do not tolerate side effects. Generally used for second-line antiemetic therapy.
Phenothiazines *Mechanism of action* Blocks dopamine receptor in the CTZ; inhibits VC by blocking autonomic afferent impulses via vagus nerve *Common side effects* Sedation, orthostatic hypotension, EPS, dizziness, drowsiness	Prochlorperazine	Tablet: 5–25 mg Sustained release: 10–30 mg PO IM/IV: 20–40 mg Rectal: 25 mg q4h	q4–6h q10–12h q3–4h q4–6h	3–4 hr 10–12 hr 3–4 hr 3–4 hr		Administer IV dose over 15–30 min. EPS more common in person < 30 years. Side effects can be cumulative in the elderly. Do not exceed 5 mg/min with IV dose. Dystonia can occur with chlorpromazine, especially with IV dosing. Chlorpromazine generally second-line antiemetic therapy. Diphenhydramine can prevent EPS and dystonia. Sustained-release form of prochlorperazine (currently not available) can prevent delayed nausea and vomiting.
	Promethazine	Tablet: 12.5–25 mg IM/IV: 10–25 mg Rectal: 25 mg	q4–6h	3–4 hr		
	Thiethylperazine	Tablet: 10 mg IM: 10 mg Rectal: 10 mg	q4–6h	3–4 hr 6–8 hr 6–8 hr		
	Chlorpromazine	Tablet: 25–50 mg IM/IV: 25–50 mg Rectal: 25–100 mg	q4–6h	3–4 hr		
	Perphenazine	Tablet: 4 mg IM/IV: 5 mg	q4–6h	3–4 hr		
	Trimethobenzamide	Capsule: 250 mg Rectal: 200 mg IM: 200 mg	q6–8h q6–8h q6–8h	3–4 hr 3–4 hr 3–4 hr		
Substituted Benzamide *Mechanism of action* Dopamine antagonist; accelerates gastric emptying and small-bowel transit; CTZ *Common side effects* Sedation, diarrhea, anxiety, EPS, fatigue, headache	Metoclopramide	Tablet: 5–10 mg IV: 1–3 mg/kg	q2–3h × 3–5 doses	2–3 hr	4–6 hr	EPS more common in young patients. Administer over 15 min to prevent intense anxiety. Use with caution in patients with renal dysfunction.

(continued)

Table 17-3 Antiemetic Therapy (continued)

Classification	Drugs	Availability/Dose	Schedule	Duration	Half-Life	Comments
5HT Agonists *Mechanism of action* Increases gastric emptying *Common side effects* Diarrhea, headache, abdominal pain, flatulence	Cisapride	Tablet: 10 mg	Before meals and at bedtime			Usually well tolerated.
Steroids *Mechanism of action* Antiprostaglandin synthesis activity? *Common side effects:* Insomnia, euphoria, anxiety, hypertension, edema, facial flushing	Dexamethasone	Tablet: 2–4 mg IV: 10–20 mg IV: 125–250 mg	q4–6 h q3h		2–3 hr	Rapid infusion causes perineal itching. Taper dose to prevent insomnia, anxiety, and euphoria. Acne may occur.
Antihistamines *Mechanism of action* Histamine H_1 receptor antagonist *Common side effects* Sedation, hypotension	Diphenhydramine	Tablet: 25–50 mg IM/IV: 12.5–50 mg	q3–4h		5–8 hr	Prevents acute dystonic reactions. Use with caution in patients with hepatic dysfunction.
Serotonin Inhibitors *Mechanism of action* Serotonin receptor; (5HT-3) antagonist *Common side effects* Hypotension, headache, constipation, sedation minimal	Ondansetron	IV: 16–32 mg/24 hr 0.15–0.18 mg/kg PO: 4-mg and 8-mg tablets Sublingual: ODT	 q12h q8h q8–12h	 8 hr	 3–4 hr	ODT approved for days 2 and 3 after moderate chemotherapy.
	Granisetron	IV: 10 mcg/kg	30 min prior to chemo	12 hr	8–10 hr	Single dose of granisetron may be sufficient for a 12-hr time period.
	Dolasetron	IV: 1.8 mg/kg PO: 100 mg		12 hr	8–10 hr	Classification not recommended for delayed or anticipatory nausea/vomiting.
	Palonosetron	IV: 0.25 mg	30 min prior to chemo	72 hr	40 hr	No redosing 7 days after treatment. Receptor binding affinity 30 × higher than that of other 5HT-3 antagonists.
Anticholinergics *Common side effects* Dry mouth, sedation, blurred vision, restlessness	Scopolamine	Patch: 0.5 mg/24 hr every 3 days		72 hr		May irritate skin. May be difficult to obtain.
Neurokinin I Receptor Antagonist *Common side effects* Constipation, diarrhea, headache, hiccups, anorexia	Aprepitant	PO: 125 mg 80 mg	1 hr prior to chemo days 2 and 3	24 hr	9–13 hr	Given as a part of 5HT-3 and steroid regimen.

VC = vomiting center; CTZ = chemoreceptor trigger zone; EPS = extrapyramidal symptoms; LFTs = liver function tests.

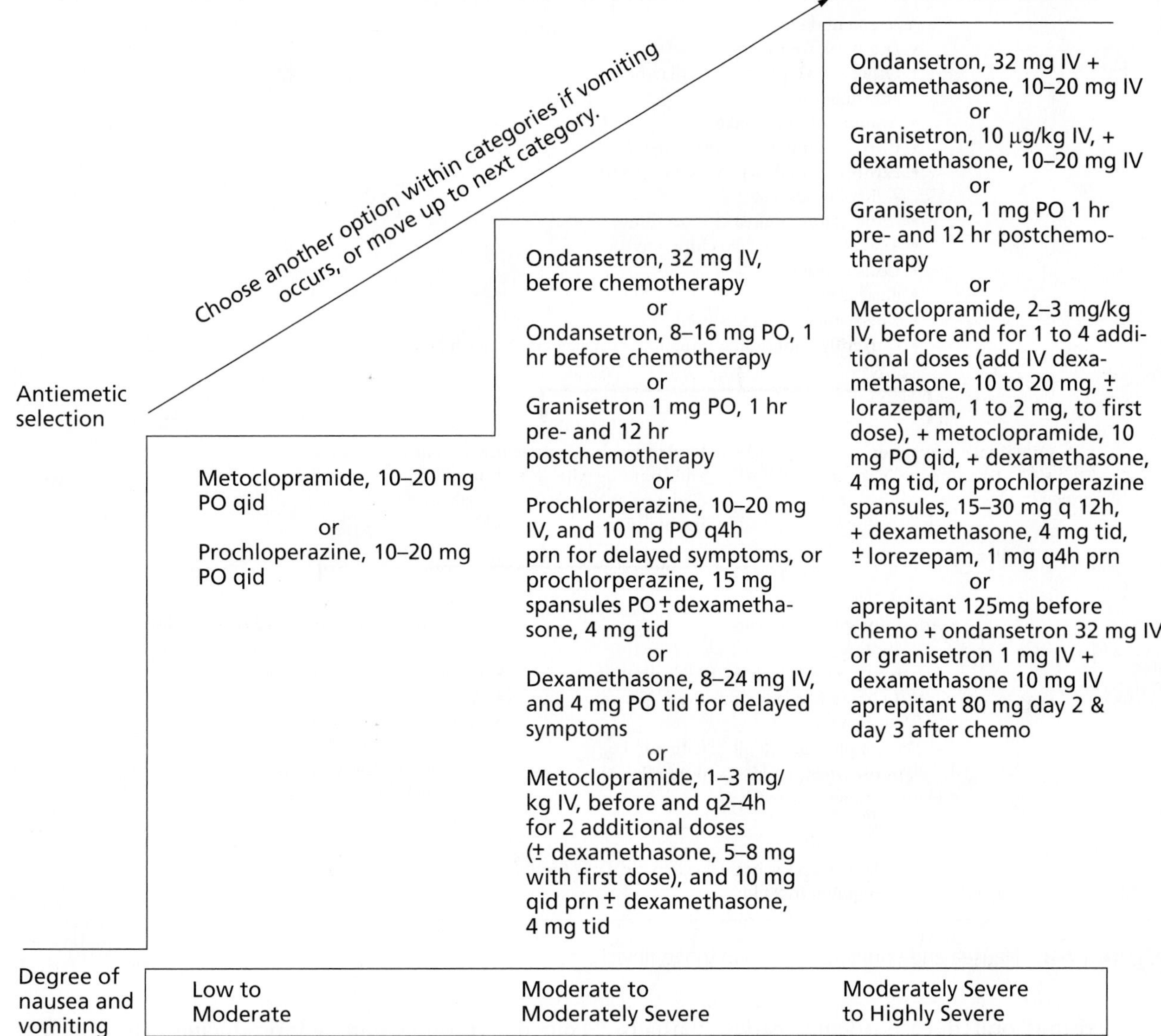

Figure 17-7 Antiemetic selection for chemotherapy. (Reprinted with permission from Wickham R: Nausea and vomiting, in Yarbro CH, Frogge MH, Goodman M (Eds.): *Cancer Symptom Management* (ed 3). Sudbury, MA, Jones and Bartlett, 2004.)[58]

and are unable to adequately repair and replace normal cell loss.[65,66] Manifestations of gastrointestinal toxicity include mucositis in the oral cavity (stomatitis), esophagus (esophagitis), and intestines (as diarrhea; enteritis).

Stomatitis. Chemotherapy-induced oral complications can be acute or chronic. Acute reactions include mucosal inflammation and ulceration, infection, and mucosal bleeding. Although chronic complications can occur from chemotherapy, these changes usually result from radiation-induced changes to healthy tissue and include xerostomia, taste alterations, trismus, and soft tissue and bone necrosis.

The risk of developing stomatitis is not the same for all patients, nor is it equal in similar drug regimens. Diagnosis and aggressiveness of the chemotherapy regimen are predictors of oral complications as well as prolonged or repetitive administration of lower doses of chemotherapy such as weekly 5-fluorouracil.[67] The frequency of oral problems is two to three times higher in patients with hematologic malignancies than with solid tumors. Stomatitis occurs more commonly in younger and elderly patients.[67]

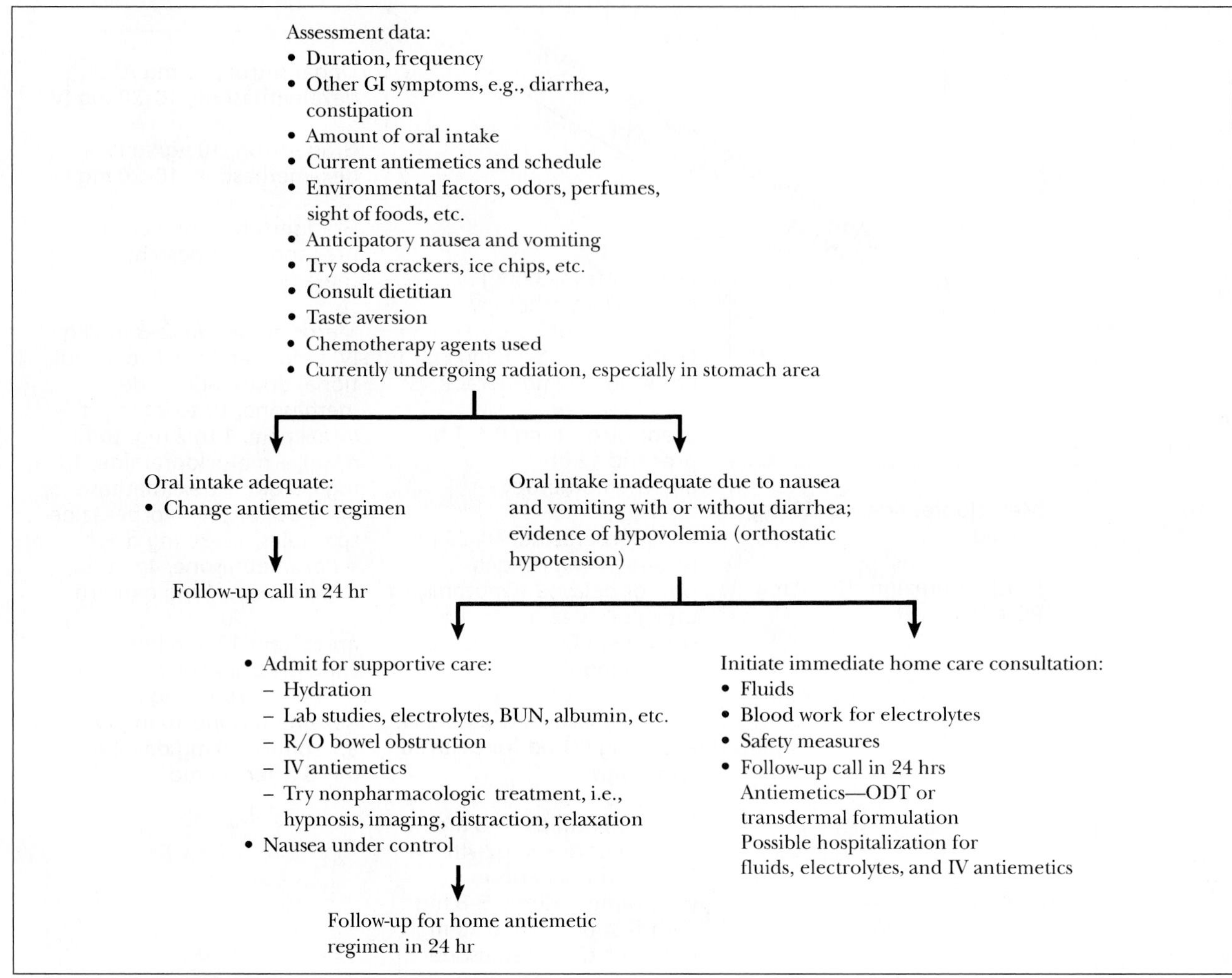

Figure 17-8 Nausea and vomiting telephone triage flowchart.

Preexisting oral disease (dental caries, partially erupted third molars) as well as poor oral hygiene and local irritants (ill-fitting dental prostheses, tobacco, alcohol) will predispose chemotherapy patients to an increased risk of oral complications. Periodontitis, a common oral disease, causes a tenfold increase in bacterial and fungal organisms in the oral cavity. Depletion of protein stores and malnutrition increase the risk of infection by altering the integrity of the epithelial barrier and depressing the immune system.[65,67]

The majority of chemotherapy agents can cause some degree of stomatitis. Those agents most associated with stomatitis are the antimetabolites and antitumor antibiotics — in particular, bleomycin, doxorubicin, daunorubicin, docetaxel, 5-FU, methotrexate, and high-dose therapy with busulfan, etoposide, melphalan, and thiotepa. Less commonly associated drugs include cytarabine, gefitnib, paclitaxel, vinblastine, gemcitabine, and vincristine. *Trans*-retinoic acid and arsenic trioxide can cause cracked and inflamed lips. Mucositis is observed more often with 5-FU when combined with other mucositis-producing drugs, such as methotrexate and doxorubicin, and when 5-FU is given concurrently with leucovorin.

Although stomatitis is dose related and is more common with higher doses, patients who develop stomatitis with one cycle of therapy will almost assuredly develop recurrence in subsequent courses unless the drugs or doses are changed.[67] This is especially the case when the body is unable to adequately eliminate a stomatotoxic drug. For example, in the presence of renal dysfunction or liver dysfunction, excretion of methotrexate and doxorubicin, respectively, may be compromised.

Direct stomatotoxicity results from the cytotoxic action of drugs on the cells of the oral basal epithelium, causing a decrease in the rate of cell renewal. The sequelae include a thinned atrophic mucosa and initiation of an inflammatory response (stomatitis). Most often affected are the nonkeratinized mucosal areas, including the buccal mucosa, tongue, soft palate, and floor of the mouth. Rarely are the gingiva or hard palate involved.[65–67]

Histologic changes can occur within 5–7 days of initial drug exposure. Dry mucosa, tongue, or lips; burning sensation in the oral cavity; and increased salivation result. Visible signs of inflammation and oral ulceration can be observed 7–10 days following therapy. Changes in the oral cavity correlate with the timing of myelosuppression, as leukocytes and the oral mucosal cells have similar cell renewal rates. Without complications and further insult from repeated drug administration, stomatitis is self-limiting and gradually reverses itself within 2–3 weeks as the granulocyte count returns to normal, often preceding bone marrow recovery by 2–3 days. Improvement in the status of the oral mucosa can therefore be predictive of a WBC count recovery.[65–67]

A baseline assessment of the oral cavity should be done prior to the initiation of treatment. Dental prophylaxis, restoration, and repair should be completed before treatment begins. Once treatment is initiated, an oral assessment should be repeated at regular intervals; outpatients should be instructed on self-assessment.[66] Nursing management of stomatitis will depend on its severity, which is often described as mild, moderate, or severe (see Table 17-1).

Oral complications can be reduced or eliminated by meticulous oral assessment with interventions before, during, and between courses of chemotherapy.[65–68] Table 17-4 describes various oral cleansing agents and devices, different means of lubricating and coating the oral cavity, and basic solutions and measures to manage oral discomfort. Developing a plan of care that the patient finds acceptable may be more beneficial than employing complicated regimens. Because reinforcement promotes compliance, nurses should continually review with the patient the individual plan for oral care and assess its continued acceptability. Generally, the recommendation is that routine oral care be performed at least after meals and at bedtime, and that the frequency increase as the severity of stomatitis increases.[66–68]

Mouth rinses enhance removal of loosened debris and should be nonirritating and nondehydrating. Several solutions for rinsing have been studied, including normal saline, chlorhexidine, benzydamine, sodium bicarbonate, and hydrogen peroxide, as well as several combinations of these options. Normal saline may be the least damaging. Sodium bicarbonate is effective as a cleansing agent, but some patients complain of the bad taste and a too concentrated solution can change the oral cavity pH. Hydrogen peroxide breaks down new tissues and should be avoided when fresh granulation surfaces are visible in the mouth. Chlorhexidine and benzydamine cleanse the oral cavity, yet poor taste yields poor compliance. To date, the optimal cleansing agent for stomatitis has not been determined.[65–68]

The oral cavity is indirectly susceptible to infection because of chemotherapy-induced neutropenia. Chemotherapy weakens host defenses by changing the oral flora to become primarily gram-negative and reducing salivary and mucous gland function.[66] An overgrowth of normal oral microorganisms results in invasion of both endogenous and exogenous pathological organisms capable of producing oral infections. Mucosal disruption becomes an important portal of entry and compromises the integrity of the oral mucosa as the first line of defense. Pathogenic organisms can further contaminate the lungs and gastrointestinal tract, disseminating infection systematically.

Bacterial, fungal, and viral infections are all common in the myelosuppressed patient. Organisms such as *Streptococcus* species, *Candida* species, and herpes simplex virus (HSV) are the major oral infectious pathogens. Each infection has certain clinical features, such as the white or "cottage cheese" appearance of *Candida albicans* and the painful vesicular lesions of herpes simplex, that assist in identifying the pathogen. The proper identification of the pathogen requires a culture, and management will depend on the identified pathogen.[65,67]

The most frequent cause of oral infection is fungal. *C. albicans* is the predominating organism and pseudomembranous candidiasis (oral thrush) is the most common clinical manifestation. Oral *Candida* infections are traditionally treated with topical antifungal agents such as nystatin oral rinses, clotrimazole troches, or fluconazole.[67] The nystatin liquid must be swished in the mouth for 5 minutes and then spit out or swallowed, four times daily. The troche, given five times daily, must be sucked in the mouth until dissolved, which takes approximately 30 minutes. Long-term use of oral troches should be avoided, however, as they contain large quantities of sugar that may result in dental caries. If xerostomia is present, the troche will take longer to dissolve. Patients should be instructed to cleanse the mouth before administering the agent and not to eat or drink for at least 30 minutes after application. This regimen will permit drug contact with the mucosal surfaces to exert an antifungal effect. Denture wearers should be instructed to soak their appliance overnight with 100 mL nystatin suspension. The plastic in dentures can act as a reservoir to reinfect the treated mucosa.

Alternatives for oropharyngeal candidiasis refractory to topical treatment include the systemic oral antifungal agents, ketoconazole 200 mg daily or fluconazole 100–200 mg daily. Absorption of ketoconazole is dependent on gastric acidity; therefore, patients are instructed to avoid the use of antacids and other

Table 17-4 Prevention and Management of Perioral Complications of Cancer Treatment

Plan/Agent	Schedule	Action	Comments
		BASIC ORAL CLEANSING	
Cleansing Mouth Rinses			
Normal saline	4×/day	Mechanical plaque control; removes and washes away loose debris Physical; moistens and soothes oral mucosa	Nonirritating; no unpleasant taste Mixture preparation: 1 teaspoon salt in 1 quart warm water; use sterile saline if granulocytopenic or mouth ulcers present
Sodium bicarbonate solution	4×/day	Mechanical plaque control; loosens hardened crusts and debris Mucosolvent Reduces acidity	Decreases odor; unpleasant taste reported Mixture preparation: 1 tsp baking soda in 8 oz water for thick paste of sodium bicarbonate; water applied to gingival sulcus for use in mechanical plaque debridement
Hydrogen peroxide	4×/day	Mechanical plaque control; loosens hardened crusts and debris	Mixture preparation: 1/2 water to 1/2 hydrogen peroxide
Antimicrobial Mouth Rinses			
Peridex	15 mL rinse 3×/day; do *not* swallow	Broad-spectrum antimicrobial agent used to suppress oral microflora and prevent dental plaque formation Decreases bacterial cloud in mouth Prevents oral candidal infections	Efficacy for the prophylaxis of therapy-induced mucositis is controversial Most common local side effect from long-term use is staining of teeth and tongue No systemic toxicity has been reported
Chlorhexidine	15-mL swish, gargle, and spit q8h	Antibacterial and antifungal action; used for high-risk patients	Augments protective effect of fluoride May cause brown discoloration of teeth Mixture preparation: dilute 3% hydrogen peroxide to 1/4 strength *Note:* Mix just prior to usage to maintain oxidizing effect; refrigerated solution may also provide local anesthetic effect
		MAINTENANCE OF ORAL MOISTURE	
Oral Care			
Orabalance	Use after rinsing mouth and after brushing	Relief of dry mouth	A nondrying moisturizing gel; may be applied around the teeth and along gum line
Saliva substitutes			
Moi-Stir	As needed	Mouth-moistening salivary supplement	Available in oral swabsticks and spray
Xerolube	As needed	Mouth moisturizer; caries inhibition	Includes fluoride as an added benefit
Sialogogues			
Salagen	5 mg 3×/day	Stimulates saliva production from functioning salivary glands	Contraindicated in patients with uncontrolled asthma or narrow-angle glaucoma; use caution with cardiovascular disease
Biotene	Use after rinsing mouth and after brushing	Relief of dry mouth	Available as mouthwash, gum, toothpaste, or oral gel

(continued)

Table 17-4 Prevention and Management of Perioral Complications of Cancer Treatment (continued)

Plan/Agent	Schedule	Action	Comments
	RELIEF OF PAIN AND INFLAMMATION		
Coating Agents			
Orabase	As needed	Topical anesthetic for localized areas of pain	Quick onset of action (30 sec), but short duration of action (5–15 min) Does not change consistency after application
Hurricane	As needed	Topical anesthetic	Available as spray, liquid, or gel Onset of action, 30 sec; duration, 15 min No systemic absorption
Oratect-gel	As needed, no more than 4×/day	Topical anesthetic	Gel dries in about 30–60 sec to form a protective film Maximum protection lasts about 2 hr Film dissipates gradually over 6 hr Do not try to mechanically remove Mild, transient stinging when applied
Zilactin	Dry lesions; apply 4×/day	Provides a protective coating and leads to pain relief	Forms protective film over oral ulcers that can last 5 hr Gel forms an opaque white film inside the mouth and a transparent film extraorally when dried Mild, transient burning sensation with application of gel
Gelclair	As needed	Moderate to severe pain	Adherent barrier forms over oral mucosa
Topical Anesthetic Rinses			
Xylocaine viscous 2% solution	15 mL swish and swallow q3h, as needed	Topical anesthetic for generalized areas of pain	Onset of action is 5 min Duration of action is approximately 20 min Systemically absorbed Watch for CNS and cardiac toxicity Swish and swallow for brief pain relief (e.g., before meals)
Dyclonine hydrochloride 0.5% or 1% solution	15 ml swish and spit, as needed	Topical anesthetic for generalized areas of pain	Minimally absorbed Decreasing potential for CNS and cardiac toxicity
Combination mixtures (e.g., viscous xylocaine 2%, Benadryl elixir 12.5 mg/mL, Maalox)	4×/day	Topical anesthetic for generalized areas of pain	Benadryl may exacerbate xerostomia
Ulcerease	15 mL swish	Anesthetic mouth rinse	Contains no alcohol Use full strength May apply directly to ulcers with cotton swab after rinsing
Sucralfate suspension	1 g/15 mL swish; 15 mL 4×/day	Binds to ulcerated tissue, protecting it from further insult, and may promote healing	No anesthetic action Suspension may aggravate nausea
Vitamin E	1 mL topically to oral lesions 2×/day	Promotes healing of mouth ulcers and controls pain	Anecdotal and research-based studies conclude vitamin E may help speed healing of chemotherapy-induced stomatitis
Systemic Analgesics			
Nonsteroidal anti-inflammatory agents (e.g., Trilisate)	Depends on agent used Doses vary	Mild to moderate pain	Longer duration of action than aspirin No effect on platelets Minimal GI side effects
Narcotic agents (e.g., morphine)	Depends on agent used Dose varies	Moderate to severe pain	
Capsaicin	4×/day	Moderate to severe pain	Active ingredient in chili peppers

medications that alter gastric pH within 2 hours of taking ketoconazole. Clotrimazole and fluconazole significantly reduce the incidence and duration of oropharnygeal candidiasis.[67] A course of low-dose intravenous amphotericin B is indicated for nonresponsive infection and in severe esophageal and disseminated candidal infections.[67]

Herpes simplex virus is the most common viral pathogen affecting the oral cavity. Vesicle fluid should be obtained for a culture to confirm the presence of HSV. When no vesicles are present, the base of the lesion should be swabbed using a viral culture swab. Swabs used for nasopharyngeal cultures (calcium alginate swabs) inactivate the virus and should not be used. Reactivation of latent HSV causes the majority of HSV infections.[67]

Immunocompromised patients who are seropositive are at risk for stomatitis. For patients with limited tissue involvement, acyclovir ointment can be applied topically every 3–6 hours while awake. Patients should be instructed to use gloves or cotton swabs when applying ointment, as autoinoculation with the virus can occur. Extensive tissue involvement for disseminated herpes requires systemic acyclovir therapy, either orally or parenterally. Acyclovir prophylaxis may be used to prevent infection in selected high-risk populations, such as individuals who have undergone bone marrow transplant.[67]

Bacterial infections may affect the gingiva, mucosa, or teeth. Bacterial culture isolate and positive blood cultures confirm the diagnosis, although clinical features (pain, fever, oral lesions) may be present without positive blood cultures. Parenteral antibiotic therapy based on the causative organisms is the treatment of choice.

Oral pain is the major clinical problem associated with stomatitis. Pain results due to sloughing of the superficial epithelium, inflammation of the oral mucosa, and ulceration, making it difficult for the patient to practice adequate oral hygiene, eat properly, and communicate. Minimizing the pain can be accomplished with topical anesthetics and systemic analgesics (see Table 17-4). The latest oral pain management option is Gelclair gel. This concentrated oral base gel contains the barrier-forming ingredient polyvinylpyrrolidone and sodium hyaluronate.[69] An adherent barrier forms over the oral mucosa after rinsing with the gel to decrease oral pain.

Oral bleeding and hemorrhage are indirect stomatotoxic sequelae from chemotherapy-induced thrombocytopenia. Bleeding results when the oral mucosa is traumatized or because of underlying periodontal disease; it may occur anywhere in the mouth. The lips, tongue, and gingiva are the most common sites. For patients with a platelet count less than 20,000 cells/mm^3, less vigorous oral hygiene regimens should be used to clean the oral cavity. Management of bleeding with topical coagulants (thrombin-soaked gauze) and pressure is often helpful.[70]

Although the treatment of stomatitis remains palliative and symptom-oriented, ongoing studies are evaluating prophylactic measures to alleviate this side effect. Clinical trials with CSFs administered to patients undergoing chemotherapy have incidentally reported a decrease in the occurrence and severity of stomatitis along with restoration of neutrophil counts and function.[65–68] Studies are under way examining the effectiveness of cytoprotective agents such as amifostine. Other agents, such as interleukin-11, keratinocyte growth factor, and epidermal growth factor, are also being studied. These agents stimulate growth, cellular differentiation, and cell migration of the oral epithelium.[67]

Taste alterations. Patients receiving chemotherapy may be susceptible to taste alterations. There can be actual or perceived changes in taste. The drugs cause direct injury to taste cells composing the taste buds, resulting in taste changes that vary widely and are highly individualized. Commonly induced changes include a lowered threshold for bitter taste, an increased threshold for sweet taste, and complaints of metallic taste. Chemotherapy drugs frequently associated with taste alterations include cyclophosphamide, dacarbazine, doxorubicin, 5-FU, methotrexate, nitrogen mustard, cisplatin, and vincristine.[71]

Some agents, such as doxorubicin and methotrexate may alter taste acuity; others, such as cyclophosphamide and vincristine, can be tasted while injected. Chemotherapy-induced taste alterations can further be influenced by poor oral hygiene, infection of the oral cavity, dentures, and unpleasant odors.[72]

Unless patients are specifically questioned, taste alterations are seldom reported spontaneously. When questioned, patients may report their taste changes as reasons for their loss of appetite or decreased weight. Nursing interventions are aimed at teaching patients self-care measures to maintain optimal nutrition. Eating hints should be customized in accordance with each patient's change in taste appreciation.

Esophagitis. Histologically, the mucosal lining of the esophagus is the same as the oral cavity. The esophagus is lined with stratified squamous epithelial cells. Destruction and inadequate replacement of these epithelial cells caused by chemotherapy agents will result in an inflammatory response called *esophagitis*. Similar to stomatitis, esophagitis can progress to ulceration, hemorrhage, and secondary infection and cause pain sufficient to make eating very difficult.[65]

Treatment may be discontinued temporarily to allow recovery of these cells, which parallels recovery of the WBC count.

The most common early symptoms of esophagitis include dysphagia (difficulty swallowing), odynophagia (painful swallowing), and epigastric pain. Esophageal pain that worsens and becomes continuous and substernal indicates progressive esophagitis. Any patient who develops oral mucositis following chemotherapy is at risk for spread to the esophageal mucosal tissue. Prior or concurrent radiation may augment the severity and extent of mucosal injury. Some drugs, such as dactinomycin and doxorubicin, potentiate radiation injury to the esophagus; others, including 5-FU, hydroxyurea, procarbazine, and vinblastine, produce an additive toxic effect with radiation.[65]

Although management of esophagitis varies greatly, all management is directed toward providing symptom relief and supportive care. Interventions are initiated to minimize irritation and promote comfort. This goal is best accomplished through dietary manipulation, topical anesthesia, and systemic analgesia when needed.

If nutritional status becomes compromised, patients may benefit from commercially prepared supplements. A nutritionist may be helpful in determining which products would best meet the individual needs of the patient. Some patients may require a feeding tube — usually a gastrostomy — if esophagitis is severe. Occasionally, a tube will be placed prior to initiating treatment if nutritional problems are anticipated.

Local anesthetics are often used every 3–4 hours as needed and prior to meals to help alleviate the pain associated with esophagitis (see Table 17-4). If topical anesthetic preparations do not relieve the discomfort, systemic narcotic analgesics may be needed. Tablets may need to be crushed and given in food, considering narcotic elixirs often contain alcohol, which can further irritate the mucosa.

Superimposed *Candida* infections may also present significant problems for patients with cancer.[67] Symptoms of *Candida* infection are often difficult to distinguish from treatment-induced esophagitis and may include dysphagia and pain. Prompt and appropriate medical treatment is necessary to prevent a systemic spread. Esophageal candidiasis is most commonly treated using ketoconazole, fluconazole, or nystatin oral suspension.[67]

Integument

Hyperpigmentation. Numerous chemotherapeutic agents are associated with hyperpigmentation (discoloration) of the skin, nails, and mucous membranes.

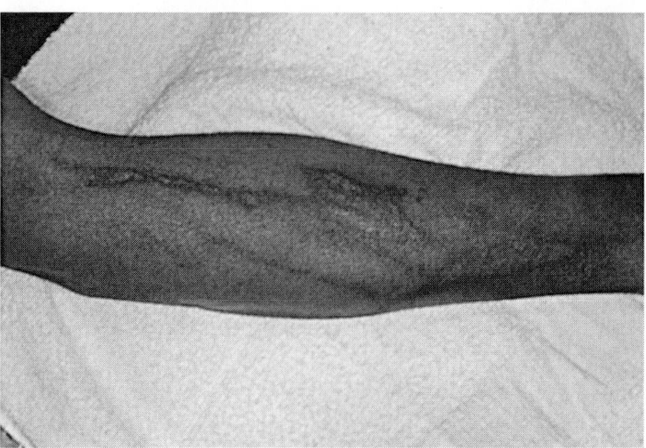

Figure 17-9 Serpiginous hyperpigmentation following 5-fluorouracil infusion.

While the etiology of hyperpigmentation is poorly understood, it is possible that the drug or a metabolic byproduct of the drug stimulates melanocytes to produce increased quantities of melanin.[73] It is unclear why some drugs are associated with widespread hyperpigmentation, whereas others cause darkening confined to a specific area such as the tongue, nails, or mucous membranes. Hyperpigmentation occurs more commonly in dark-skinned individuals.

Busulfan can cause hyperpigmentation involving the neck, upper trunk, nipples, and abdomen, which is frequently associated with busulfan-induced pulmonary fibrosis. Hyperpigmentation caused by cyclophosphamide may be diffuse or confined to the palms, soles, nails, or gums. Skin contact with carmustine or nitrogen mustard can result in a contact dermatitis followed by postinflammatory hyperpigmentation.[21] After several infusions, irinotecan can cause hyperpigmentation that fades after the drug regimen is stopped.[21] Arsenic trioxide commonly causes hyperpigmentation over the entire body surface.

5-fluorouracil can cause hyperpigmentation, especially in those patients who receive high-dose weekly infusions with or without leucovorin. Hyperpigmentation occurs most readily in sun-exposed areas.[73] Serpiginous hyperpigmented streaks overlying veins used repeatedly for 5-FU infusions occur without any clinical evidence of cutaneous inflammation, phlebitis, or sclerosis (Figure 17-9).

Bleomycin may cause hyperpigmentation over the veins into which the drug is administered. However, bleomycin is more commonly associated with hyperpigmentation over pressure points or with linear streaks occurring in areas of intense scratching, presumably due to localized vasodilation that results in an increased bleomycin concentration in the skin (Figure 17-10).[74]

Doxorubicin, busulfan, cyclophosphamide, 5-FU, and etoposide have all been associated with hyperpig-

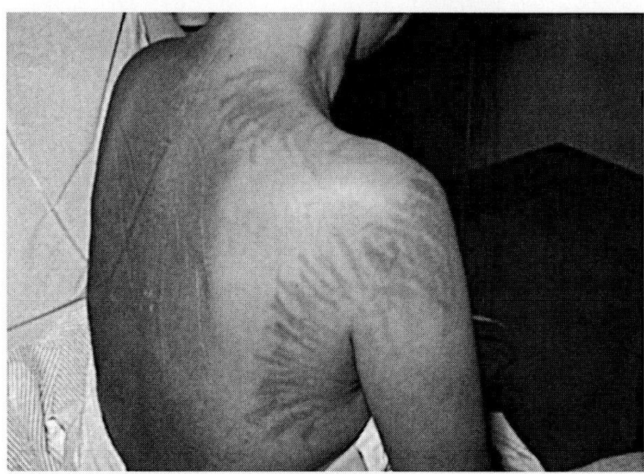

Figure 17-10 Flagellate streaks of hyperpigmentation in an Asian woman occurring in areas of intense scratching following intracavitary (intrapleural) bleomycin.

mentation of the oral mucosa and tongue, especially in African Americans. Doxorubicin and 5-FU also may cause skin darkening over the interphalangeal and metacarpophalangeal joints. The mechanism of this effect is not known, but phalangeal darkening decreases once therapy is terminated.[73]

Hypersensitivity. Cutaneous hypersensitivity reactions (HSRs) to chemotherapy occur infrequently and tend not to be dose related. Cutaneous manifestations of immediate HSRs (type I reactions) generally present as urticaria, angioedema, or anaphylaxis. L-asparaginase, for example, is a polypeptide of bacterial origin that causes HSR in 10%–20% of patients receiving the drug. Acute urticaria is the most frequent manifestation of L-asparaginase HSR, with 10% of these patients progressing to life-threatening anaphylaxis.[21]

Paclitaxel can cause hypotension, rash, dyspnea, and bronchospasm within 10 minutes of initiating the drug, suggesting a nonimmunologic anaphylactoid reaction.[21] The cause of this HSR is believed to be the drug vehicle, Cremophor EL (polyoxyethylated castor oil). Measures to minimize HSR with paclitaxel include prolonging drug infusion time (6–24 hours) and using a three-drug prophylactic regimen consisting of an antihistamine, corticosteroid, and H2 receptor antagonist. Despite these precautions, approximately 2% of patients will experience HSRs after receiving paclitaxel.[21]

Docetaxel is associated with HSR, most notably skin rash, anaphylaxis, and fluid retention. Pretreatment with 8 mg of dexamethasone twice daily starting 1 day prior to dosing and continuing for a total of 3 days has minimized these reactions.

Severe infusion reactions manifested as bronchospasm, stridor, hoarseness, urticaria, and/or hypotension have been noted with cetuximab infusions. Epenephrine, corticosteroids, intravenous antihistamines, and oxygen therapy may be necessary to stabilize vital signs.

Parenteral cisplatin, carboplatin, and nitrogen mustard have been found to cause a type I HSR in approximately 5% of patients.[21] Manifestations of this reaction include anxiety, pruritus, cough, dyspnea, angioedema, bronchospasm, rash, urticaria, and hypotension. These symptoms are usually relieved by prompt administration of antihistamines.

The incidence of HSR increases to 12% during retreatment of carboplatin in patients with recurrent ovarian cancer.[75] It is very high in patients receiving more than six cycles of carboplatin. Generally, the symptoms are moderate to severe, and include urticaria, tachycardia, chest tightness, wheezing, dyspnea, facial swelling, and hypotension.

Hypersensitivity reactions have been reported with oxaliplatin in 8% of patients.[76] Symptoms usually develop after the start of the infusion and include dyspnea, chills, wheezing, rigors, rash, and hypotension. The reaction has been described as a type I hypersensitivity IgE-mediated reaction similar to that seen with other platinum compounds.[76]

Teniposide and parenteral etoposide can cause HSR with the initial dosing, manifesting as dyspnea, wheezing, hypotension, urticaria, pruritus, angioedema, facial flushing, and rash. The incidence is higher with teniposide as it is admixed with Cremophor EL. Decreasing the infusion rate and premedicating with an antihistamine and a steroid generally permits further drug administration.[21]

Miscellaneous rash. Other drugs that can produce rash, urticaria, pruritus, or angioedema include procarbazine, cytarabine, levamisole, topotecan, trimetrexate, anthracycline antibiotics, melphalan, imatinib mesylate, pemetrexed, and methotrexate. *Trans*-retinoic acid causes dry skin with mild exfoliation similar to a rash associated with pruritus.[21] Arsenic trioxide can produce urticaria, dry skin, angioedema, rash, and exfoliation of the skin.

A common drug side effect is a morbilliform maculopapular rash sometimes associated with fever. The pruritic rash usually disappears and does not necessitate cessation of therapy. Rarely, it can progress and cause desquamation. Hydrocortisone may be given in higher than usual doses for the first 2 weeks of therapy in an attempt to decrease the severity of the skin rash.

Dactinomycin folliculitis presents as diffuse erythematous papules over the face and trunk, resembling acne, and appearing approximately 5 days after therapy. The rash resolves in 3–5 days. Folliculitis has also been reported following high-dose methotrexate.[21]

Erythema multiforme has been infrequently associated with chemotherapeutic agents. Patients receiving high-dose combination chemotherapy are at greater risk for this toxicity. The reaction is characterized by target lesions over the extremities, often involving the mucous membranes. Busulfan, etoposide, procarbazine, hydroxyurea, bleomycin, methotrexate, and cytarabine have been associated with such lesions, which occasionally develop into generalized blistering.[77] Gefitnib commonly causes an acneiform rash usually located on the face and upper torso. More than 80% of patients receiving this chemotherapy drug develop such as rash.[21]

Acral erythema. An intensely painful erythema, scaling and epidermal sloughing from the palms and soles, followed by desquamation and reepithelialization of the skin, has been reported with 5-FU, doxorubicin, paclitaxel, high-dose cytarabine, capecitabine, docetaxel, liposomal doxorubicin, and floxuridine. The condition, also called *palmar-plantar erythrodysesthesia,* may represent a direct toxic effect on the epidermis and dermal vasculature or an accumulation of the chemotherapeutic agent in eccrine structures, causing erythema of the palms and soles where there are a high concentration of eccrine glands.[21,74,78] Initially the patient may complain of tingling and pain of the feet and hands, which generally progress to edema, tenderness to touch, intense erythema, and desquamation. Strategies to prevent liposomal doxorubicin-induced reactions include avoiding pressure such as tight-fitting clothing over bony prominences, especially during drug infusion, and avoiding excessive heat beginning the day of infusion and for 5 days afterward. Management focuses on comfort measures. Chemotherapy is usually suspended until symptoms subside and then resumes at a lower dose. However, the symptoms may recur and may necessitate cessation of therapy.

Pruritus. An allergic dermatitis may result from chemotherapy causing localized and generalized pruritus. Pruritus can be overwhelming and distressing to the individual, as it commonly interferes with rest and sleep and can result in skin breakdown and infection.

Assessment requires a thorough evaluation of the possible cause of the itching and any factors that might aggravate the condition. If pruritus is chemotherapy induced, the condition generally resolves when the drug is stopped or gradually dissipates following antihistamine therapy.

Nursing management focuses on skin care and comfort. Medicated baths, anesthetic creams, and emollient creams may be soothing. Soaps made especially for sensitive skin should be used when skin cleansing is required. The patient is encouraged to use alternative cutaneous stimulation methods to relieve the urge to scratch, such as massage, pressure, or rubbing the area with a soft cloth. Distractions such as music, imagery, or relaxation may ease the itch sensation. Perfumes, cosmetics, starch-based powders, and deodorants should be avoided.[73]

Environmental factors include keeping the room humidity at 30%–40% and the room temperature cool. Cotton clothing and sheets should be washed in hypoallergenic soaps. Medications such as antihistamines or corticosteroids may be used to minimize itching.

Photosensitivity. Photosensitivity is an enhanced skin response to ultraviolet (UV) rays. This response may present much like a sunburn, with erythema, edema, blisters, hyperpigmentation, and desquamation or peeling.[21] Rarely, photoallergy, similar to contact dermatitis, with immediate wheal and flare reactions or delayed reactions may occur. Photosensitivity has been reported following skin exposure to UV light after administration of 5-FU, dacarbazine, *trans*-retinoic acid, vinblastine, and high-dose methotrexate. In general, the exposed area becomes erythematous within a few hours and gradually subsides. Dacarbazine, however, has been associated with pruritus and erythematous eruptions on the face, neck, and dorsal surfaces of both hands after sun exposure occurred within 1–2 hours following drug administration.[21]

Nurses must educate patients on the dangers of UV exposure. Verbal and written instructions concerning ways to reduce the risk of developing a photosensitivity reaction are given to the patient. Sun exposure, particularly between the hours of 10 A.M. and 3 P.M., and tanning booths should be avoided. Protective clothing and a hat should be worn even on cloudy days.

Most important, nurses should provide instructions regarding the proper use of sunscreen based on the individual's skin type. Sunscreens contain a sun protection factor (SPF) that defines the ratio of the time it takes to develop erythema with and without the sunscreen applied. For example, an individual who can be in direct sunlight for only 30 minutes without erythema may, by applying a sunscreen with an SPF of 8, remain outside for 240 minutes (30 × 8) without burning. The higher the SPF, the more complete the sun protection. Products with an SPF higher than 15 are recommended for protection following chemotherapy. Sunblocks with an SPF of 25 or higher are available and recommended for children and fair-skinned individuals. In general, the higher the SPF, the greater the chance of skin irritation. Some sunscreens are water resistant, but in general they should be applied frequently and directly to the skin. To maximize its effectiveness, the sunscreen should be applied at least 15–30 minutes before sun exposure and as often as indicated by activities in which the individual is engaged.

Alopecia. Alopecia is the most noticeable cutaneous side effect of chemotherapy and often one of the most distressing.[79] Although certainly not a life-threatening event, loss of hair has a profound social and psychological impact on individuals and their acceptance of treatment. Some may even refuse potentially curative therapy for fear of this effect.

Chemotherapy agents affect actively growing (anagen) hairs. Because anagen hair is the most rapidly proliferating cell population in the human body, alopecia is a common toxicity. Extent of hair loss can range from thinning of scalp hair to total body hair loss.[79] Chemotherapy causes the hair shaft to be fragile or defective and, therefore, subject to breakage with minimal trauma.

Higher doses of chemotherapy or more potent epilators cause complete mitotic arrest, resulting in atrophy of the root and loss of the hair root bulb. Hair falls out spontaneously or is lost easily when combed or washed. Drugs of less intensity temporarily inhibit or slow cellular activity, causing bulb deformity and narrowing of the hair shaft. When hair growth resumes, narrow, weakened hair shafts are prone to breakage at the point of constriction. The hair root however, remains intact and active, leaving a thinning pattern of hair loss.

With an average 85% of scalp hair follicles in the anagen phase at any given time, the most common location for hair loss is the scalp. The majority of other body hair follicles (eyebrows, axilla, pubic area) are in the less active catagen and telogen phases and therefore are not initially affected. However, with multiple exposures from long-term therapy, these hairs may also be lost as the hairs enter the anagen phase.[79]

Unlike natural hair loss, chemotherapy-induced alopecia occurs rapidly and usually starts 2–3 weeks following a dose of chemotherapy. Hair loss is usually asymptomatic; however, some patients have described intense scalp discomfort 1–2 days prior to and during hair shedding.

Chemotherapy-induced alopecia is temporary and reversible. After discontinuation of the drugs, regrowth is visible in 4–6 weeks, but complete regrowth may take 1–2 years. As hair grows back, alterations in hair pigmentation (lighter or darker), hair texture (finer or coarser), and hair type (straight or curly) may be evident.

The severity and duration of chemotherapy-induced alopecia are related to the type of drug, combination of drugs, dose of drug, method of administration, and pharmacokinetics. Hair loss can be described as minimal (less than 25%), moderate (25%–50%), or severe (more than 50%) loss of heat or body warmth from head as well as sun exposure, which indicates the need for head covering. Chemotherapy agents most frequently associated with moderate to severe hair loss include trimetrexate, cyclophosphamide, doxorubicin, dactinomycin, daunorubicin, etoposide, idarubicin, ifosfamide, irinotecan, mechlorethamine, paclitaxel, topotecan, and vincristine. Mild hair loss is associated with bleomycin, carmustine, epirubicin, 5-FU, methotrexate, melphalan, mitomycin, mitoxantrone, teniposide, temodar, and vinorelbine.

Bolus intravenous administration of chemotherapy results in immediate peak serum levels with subsequent exposure and damage of sensitive growing hairs, resulting in hair loss. Infusions over several hours or longer are associated with greater likelihood of alopecia. The risk of alopecia appears to be decreased with low-dose continuous infusion. This may be related to the fact that high peak serum levels are necessary to cause hair loss.[21]

A patient-related factor that may influence the degree of scalp hair loss is the variability of scalp hair growth among individuals. Individuals who have relatively few hairs in the anagen phase will be less sensitive to the effects of chemotherapy. Another factor to consider is the condition of the patient's hair before treatment. Damaged hair (tinted, permed) may potentiate the risk for alopecia.

Until the early 1990s, scalp hypothermia was the technique used to prevent or minimize hair loss. However, because there was risk of scalp micrometastasis, this technique is no longer recommended.[79] Therefore, more emphasis needs to be placed on the psychological support of the patient experiencing hair loss from chemotherapy and use of creative measures to preserve self-image.

It is essential that the patient and family be informed of the timing, extent, and duration of hair loss at the onset of therapy. While these factors are not always known, many times they are; for instance, when high-dose doxorubicin and cyclophosphamide are used, hair loss is nearly complete by 3 weeks. Patients should be encouraged to discuss their feelings regarding hair loss.[21] It is often helpful for patients to prepare for alopecia by procuring a scalp prosthesis (wig or hairpiece) before it becomes necessary. This strategy often reduces the anxiety associated with the uncertain timing of hair loss and makes it easier for a stylist to match color and style. Patients should be encouraged to question their insurance carriers regarding coverage for "cranial therapeutic prosthesis" for treatment-induced alopecia. Some insurance companies will reimburse with a physician's prescription or letter.

Certain measures can be used to minimize or delay hair loss and scalp irritation. Some clinicians advise patients to cut long hair short in anticipation of hair loss. Short hair may make hair loss less noticeable, make remaining hair appear thicker, and possibly decrease the weight on the hair shaft. Once hair loss is significant, the patient may be advised to shave the remaining scalp hairs. This practice allows the hair to grow in at the same length, often permitting the patient to go without a wig sooner. In addition, shaving the head rids the patient of the problem of continuous shedding of hair. Measures to minimize hair loss include use of mild protein-based shampoos with conditioners, avoidance of daily shampooing, allowing hair to dry naturally, and grooming hair with a wide-toothed comb. Hair care practices such as blow-drying, perming, or coloring hair are controversial and areas for further nursing research. Claims have been made that these practices cause the hair to become brittle and fall out earlier during chemotherapy.

Nails. Changes in the fingernails and toenails are commonly seen during chemotherapy.[74] Pigmentation is seen most commonly and occurs with more regularity and intensity in blacks than in whites. The pigment generally is deposited at the base of the nail, causing transverse dark bands that correlate with the times the drug was administered. This reaction occurs most commonly with paclitaxel, docetaxel, doxorubicin, and cyclophosphamide but has been reported with melphalan, 5-FU, daunomycin, idarubicin, and bleomycin. If continuous infusion therapy of these drugs is given, the nails darken evenly.[21]

Beau lines (transverse white lines or grooves in the nail) indicate a reduction or cessation of nail growth in response to chemotherapy. A partial separation of the nail plate (onycholysis) can be seen with 5-FU, doxorubicin, paclitaxel, docetaxel, and bleomycin.[21]

Organ Toxicities

Certain chemotherapy drugs may cause direct damage to specific cells of a given organ or cause indirect damage by the effects of cellular breakdown by-products. In general, organ toxicities are predictable based on the cumulative dose, the presence of concomitant organ dysfunction, the age of the patient, and the manner in which the drug is given. Of interest is the fact that the toxicity profile may be changing as a result of the more widespread use of dose-intensive regimens, multimodality treatment, chemoprotectants, and CSFs. These approaches to managing the disease are likely to result in more organ toxicities as myelosuppression becomes less prominent. Each of the major organ toxicities is discussed here. Tables 17-5 through 17-10 provide a review of major toxicities in terms of risk factors, signs of toxicity, preventive measures, grading, and management.

Cardiotoxicity

Cardiotoxicity is described as an acute or chronic process. The acute form consists of transient electrocardiogram (ECG) changes that occur in approximately 10% of patients receiving chemotherapy. Acute effects are immediate in onset and resolve quickly without serious complications. These effects are not dose related and are not an indication to stop the drug. Fewer than 5% of patients develop chronic cardiotoxicity from a cumulative drug effect that requires immediate discontinuation of the drug.[80] Chronic effects occur weeks or months after administration, involving nonreversible cardiomyopathy, presenting as a classic biventricular congestive heart failure (CHF) with a characteristic low-voltage QRS complex. Signs and symptoms are classical for CHF, including complaints of a nonproductive cough, dyspnea, and pedal edema. Generally, it is poorly responsive to diuretics or digitalis and becomes progressively worse, with a 60% mortality.

Anthracyclines are known to cause cardiotoxicity by directly damaging the cardiac myocyte cells. The incidence of cardiotoxicity is 2%–3% after cumulative doses are administered.[80] Total cumulative dosages have been established at 550 mg/m^2 for doxorubicin, 400 mg/m^2 for epirubicin, and 600 mg/m^2 for daunomycin, with a decrease in dose to 450 mg/m^2 if mediastinal radiation has been administered.[21,81]

The mechanism of action occurs in the presence of oxygen, where the anthracyclines form a bond or union with iron or copper. These complexes inhibit lipid peroxidation, allowing a free oxygen radical to damage the myocyte directly. The results are a loss of myocardial fibrils, mitochondrial changes, and cellular destruction. As a consequence, the myocyte has limited contractility, leading to hypertrophy of the cardiac muscle, which increases the demand for oxygen.[80]

In an attempt to decrease cardiotoxicity occurrence, altering the dose scheduling of doxorubicin to include frequent lower doses has resulted in reduction of cardiotoxicity without compromise of antitumor effects.[82] The use of liposome doxorubicin has demonstrated a reduction of cardiotoxicity.[21,81] Chemoprotectants are being evaluated for their ability to protect the cardiac tissue by blocking damage to the myocyte. In animal studies, calcium antagonists, catechin, and combination of selenium and amifostine have been found to reduce anthracycline-induced cardiotoxicity.[83,84]

Dexrazoxane (Zinecard) is currently approved for patients with metastatic breast cancer who have received cumulative doses of 300 mg/m^2 and are continuing treatment with doxorubicin (not for initial treatment). Patients have been able to tolerate greater cumulative doses of doxorubicin with a decreased risk of cardiac events. The agent is administered 30 minutes prior to doxorubicin, calculated on a 10:1 ratio. Thus, with a 50 mg dose of doxorubicin, 500 mg of dexrazoxane would be administered.[21] This compound has permitted doses of doxorubicin as high as 700 mg/m^2 to be administered without cardiotoxicity occurring. It appears to interfere with the intracellular process responsible for anthracycline-induced cardiomyopathy.[15] Dexrazoxane has been used in other types of malignancies in adult patients who received more than 300 mg/m^2 of doxorubicin.[15]

In an attempt to reduce further the cardiotoxicity from the anthracyclines, analogs that have greater antitumor activity and may have reduced cardiotoxicity have been developed. Epirubicin, idarubicin, esorubicin, and aclarubicin appear to be similar to doxorubicin, but their cardiotoxicity is significantly less. Although mitoxantrone has been associated with rare cardiac events, it is considered to be less cardiotoxic.[21] Congestive heart failure has been noted to occur in patients receiving bevacizumab therapy concurrent with anthracyclines or in those who received prior anthracyclines or left chest wall irradiation.

Acute pericarditis has been reported with high-dose cyclophosphamide therapy (90-270 mg/kg) used in the bone marrow transplant (BMT) population, with subsequent pericardial effusion and cardiac tamponade.[81] Cyclophosphamide damages the myocytes in a manner similar to that seen with anthracyclines, where swelling and decreased contractility lead to less effective pumping of the heart. Hemorrhagic myocardial necrosis has been reported, with leakage of blood through capillaries. Transient complete heart block requiring temporary pacemaker support has been reported as well. Toxicity ranges from minor, transient ECG changes and asymptomatic elevation of cardiac enzymes to fatal myopericarditis and myocardial necrosis.[81]

Myocardial ischemia has been reported with 5-FU infusion in patients with or without preexisting heart disease. Coronary vasospasm with resulting angina pectoris, myocardial infarction, S-T segment elevations, and ventricular ectopy have been described. The pathophysiology is unclear, although a direct cardiomyopathic effect from the release of vasoactive substances in the presence of 5-FU has been suggested.[85] It has been speculated that angina is a coronary artery spasm of the Prinzmetal type that responds to nitrates. Cessation of therapy does not appear to be absolutely necessary, as patients who have such a syndrome can be pretreated with calcium antagonists known to prevent coronary artery spasm.

Asymptomatic bradycardia has been reported in approximately 30% of patients with ovarian cancer who have received paclitaxel. Other cardiac disturbances, which have been reported in 5% of patients, include atrioventricular conduction blocks, left bundle branch blocks, ventricular tachycardia, and symptoms of cardiac ischemia. Most paclitaxel-related cardiac disturbances were not associated with clinical symptoms and were noted incidentally during continuous cardiac monitoring. Paclitaxel infusion is not discontinued unless it is associated with progressive atrioventricular conduction disturbances. Although the mechanism is unclear, it is speculated to be the result of the administration vehicle Cremophor EL, which causes activation of selected cardiac histamine receptors. Stimulation of these receptors in the cardiac tissue increases myocardial oxygen demand and produces coronary vasoconstriction.[21,81] Although cardiac disturbances are usually benign, a case report documents the occurrence of myocardial ischemia during paclitaxel administration that resulted in death.[86]

Cardiac function should be evaluated throughout therapy for patients who are at high risk for cardiotoxicity or who will be receiving high dosages of paclitaxel, an anthracycline, or cyclophosphamide. Methods to evaluate cardiac function include noninvasive monitoring with ECG, echocardiography, and radionuclide cardiography. An ejection fraction less than 45% or a decrease of 5% or more from the resting value is considered abnormal. Further doses of cardiotoxic chemotherapy are not recommended.[80] Although an endomyocardial biopsy can reveal damage to the myocyte prior to clinical detection, the procedure is costly and technically difficult and requires considerable expertise.

The lifelong cardiotoxic effects of conventional anthracycline therapy highlight the need for monitoring cardiac dysfunction. Radionuclide cardiography and echocardiograms are the noninvasive methods most commonly used, despite their insensitivity for detecting early signs of cardiotoxicity.[80] Considering the occurrence of late-onset cardiac dysfunction, long-term follow-up is recommended, with noninvasive testing based on the patient's risk factors and cardiac symptoms. Low-risk patients have been defined as those receiving less than 200 mg/m^2 of an anthracycline and no mediastinal radiation or exhibiting no cardiac abnormality. High-risk patients are considered to be those who received more than 400 mg/m^2 of an anthracycline, received mediastinal radiation, or have abnormal cardiac function. A follow-up evaluation 3 months after completing therapy with an echocardiogram or radionuclide angiograpy allows detection of late-developing toxicity. Long-term follow-up recommendations include a minimum of one echocardiogram yearly and a cardiac scan every 5 years if the patient remains asymptomatic.[80]

Accurate documentation and monitoring of total cumulative dosages of chemotherapy are essential. Cardiac assessment is imperative to evaluate for a third heart sound or gallop, which could indicate cardiac insufficiency. Cardiac monitoring may be necessary for administering high dosages of chemotherapy, such as with cyclophosphamide. Once the patient develops chronic cardiotoxicity, nursing interventions include teaching the patient about energy conservation, managing fluid retention, and minimizing sodium in the diet. Supportive care with digitalis, angiotensin-converting enzyme (ACE) inhibitors to enhance the cardiac output, and diuretics to manage fluid should also be instituted.[80] Eventually, the patient may need supplemental oxygen and vasodilator medications to relieve dyspnea. Heart transplantation has become an accepted procedure to treat end-stage heart disease from anthracycline cardiomyopathy.[87]

The degree of cardiac injury determines the limitations on activities of daily living that the individual will experience. Few patients are prepared for this debilitating effect, and nurses must initiate interventions that will assist patients and families in coping. Patients are also taught the importance of close cardiac follow-up, once the treatment is complete, to monitor for late cardiac effects (Table 17-5).

Neurotoxicity

Chemotherapy-induced neurotoxicity can arise in the form of direct or indirect damage to the CNS, peripheral nervous system, cranial nerves, or any combination of the three. Although the majority of patients experience temporary neurotoxicity, some will have permanent neurological deficits. Significant neurotoxicity usually requires suspending the treatment until the symptom resolves and reinstituting therapy with a 50% dose reduction or discontinuing the drug.[88]

The central and peripheral nervous systems are protected against potentially neurotoxic effects by the blood–brain barrier and blood–nerve barriers. If intact, these barriers exclude most water-soluble chemotherapeutic agents and relatively large molecules. Biopsies of nerves suffering damage from chemotherapy have demonstrated a mild decrease in the number of large-diameter myelinated nerve fibers, and ultrastructural studies have shown scattered degenerating nerve fibers both in axons and in myelin sheaths. The severity of neurotoxicity is usually dose related, with symptoms exhibited in a variable and unpredictable fashion.

The CNS consists of collections of neurons, and their connections are organized into the brain and spinal cord areas. Damage to the CNS primarily involves the cerebellum, which produces altered reflexes, unsteady gait, ataxia, and confusion. The peripheral nervous system is basically a set of communication channels located outside the CNS, consisting of the cranial and spinal nerves. Damage to the peripheral nervous system produces paralysis or loss of movement and sensation to those areas affected by the particular nerve. The autonomic nervous system (ANS) includes those peripheral nerves that regulate functions occurring automatically in the body, such as the cardiovascular, respiratory, and endocrine systems. Damage to the ANS causes ileus, impotence, or urinary retention.

Vincristine is well known for potential peripheral neuropathy characterized by myalgia and loss of the deep tendon reflex at the ankle, progressing to complete areflexia, distal symmetric sensory loss, motor weakness, foot drop, and muscle atrophy.[88] Autonomic neuropathy is characterized by ileus, constipation, impotence, urinary retention, or postural hypotension. The mechanism of damage is believed to involve disruption of the microtubule in the neural tissues, which inhibits the mitotic spindle movements necessary for the mitosis phase of cellular reproduction.[77] Vincristine doses greater than 2 mg increase the risk of neurotoxicity.

Neuropathy related to cisplatin is reversible, although cases of persistent progression after the discontinuation of the drug have been reported.[89] Cisplatin affects the large-diameter fibers of the neural tissues, resulting in sensory changes. The earliest sign of peripheral neuropathy is decreased vibratory sense, described as hand and feet paresthesia, with the classic stocking-glove distribution. Sensory loss occurs initially; without dose modification, loss of the Achilles reflex, muscle weakness, and loss of the deep tendon reflex occur. Symptoms of neuropathy are seen at cumulative doses of 300–500 mg/m^2. As the neuropathy progresses, position sense is impaired and a marked sensory ataxia develops. Peripheral neuropathy has been reported from combined therapy consisting of paclitaxel and cisplatin. Sensory-motor neuropathy occurs 1–21 weeks after initiation of therapy. Neuropathy appears to be progressive with additional courses, and more pronounced with higher doses of paclitaxel (cumulative dose ≥ 1500 mg/m^3).[90]

High-tone hearing loss is speculated to be related to the loss of hairs in the organ of Corti resulting from cisplatin administration. Rapid drug delivery,

Table 17-5 Organ Toxicity of Chemotherapy Agents: Cardiotoxicity

Toxicity/Symptoms	Grade	General Risk Factors	Chemotherapy Agent/Risk Factors	Mechanism of Damage	Protective/ Management Measures
• Tachycardia • Dyspnea • Nonproductive cough • Neck vein distention • Gallop rhythm • Rales • Pedal edema • Cardiomegaly • Dull or sharp precordial pain, may radiate to neck and shoulder • Cardiac friction rub • ST-T wave changes • Supraventricular tachyarrhythmias • T-wave flattening	Cardiac Dysrhythmias 0 = None 1 = Asymptomatic, transient, requires no therapy 2 = Recurrent or persistent, requires no therapy 3 = Requires treatment 4 = Requires monitoring; hypotension, ventricular tachycardia, or fibrillation Cardiac Function 0 = None 1 = Asymptomatic decline of resting ejection by less than 20% of baseline 2 = Asymptomatic decline of resting ejection fraction by more than 20% of baseline 3 = Mild CHF, responsive to therapy 4 = Severe or refractory CHF	• Age, geriatric and pediatric • Cumulative dose • Schedule of drug administration • History of cardiac disease (e.g., atherosclerosis, mitral valve prolapse, CHF, hypertension) • Use of combination drugs • Hepatic dysfunction • Prior mediastinum radiation • Prior anthracycline exposure	Anthracyclines • Doxorubicin (>550 mg/m²) • Daunorubicin (>600 mg/m²) • Dactinomycin • Doxorubicin-enhanced effect with actinomycin, mitomycin, vincristine, melphalan, bleomycin, cyclophosphamide • Mitoxantrone (>160 mg/m²)	Acute Changes • Hypereosinophilia of myocytes Chronic Changes • Loss of contractile elements • Mitochondrial changes • Myocyte damage	• Limit cumulative dose of doxorubicin to <550 mg/m² • Administer doxorubicin at lower doses more frequently • ECG before treatment • Radionuclide cardiac scan • Administer dexrazoxane before anthracycline dose • Administer calcium channel blockers before anthracycline dose
			• Cyclophosphamide, high-dose (>144 mg/kg × 4 days)	• Hemorrhagic myocardial necrosis	
			• 5-fluorouracil	• Fibrin deposition in interstitium • Coronary spasm of the Prinzmetal type	• Limit cumulative dose of daunorubicin to <600 mg/m²
			• Paclitaxel	• Speculated to be related to Cremaphor EL, the administration vehicle for paclitaxel that causes activation of selected cardiac histamine receptors	• Avoid alcohol, smoking, and cocaine use • Moderate exercise and low-fat, low-salt diet • Prevent thrombus with daily aspirin or warfarin • Herceptin is not given concurrent with doxorubicin
			• Arsenic trioxide	• Prolonged Q-T interval • Premature ventricular contractions • Potentially fatal • Torsades-de-pointes • Pericardial effusion	

CHF = congestive heart failure.

simultaneous administration of aminoglycosides, and dehydration seem to increase the potential for ototoxicity. Although the loss can be reversed with discontinuation of the drug, permanent damage has been reported, resulting in the need for a hearing aid.[89]

Neurotoxicity characterized by metabolic encephalopathy manifested as blurred vision, seizures, motor system dysfunction, urinary incontinence, cranial nerve dysfunction, subclinical electroencephalographic changes, or irreversible coma has been reported in 5%–30% of patients treated with ifosfamide.[88] Signs have occurred within 2 hours of bolus administration and as long as 28 days after therapy. Within 48–72 hours of cessation of ifosfamide, most abnormalities spontaneously resolve. Risk factors associated with neurotoxicity include duration of administration, hepatic insufficiency, previous cisplatin, presence of bulky disease, low serum albumin, and high serum creatinine.[88] Although the cause is not completely understood, the encephalopathy is thought to result from an accumulation of drug metabolites (chloracetaldehyde), which causes direct CNS damage. If the patient seems disoriented or demonstrates any neurological changes following ifosfamide infusion subsequent doses of ifosfamide should be withheld pending further investigation. Administration of additional doses of ifosfamide to an individual already demonstrating neurotoxicity from ifosfamide can result in worsening of symptoms and seizures. Methylene blue has been shown to be an effective treatment for ifosfamide-induced encephalopathy. Methylene blue (50 milligrams) in a 2% aqueous solution administered by slow intravenous injection has resulted in reversal of symptoms of encephalopathy. In patients with a history of ifosfamide-induced encephalopathy requiring additional doses of ifosfamide, the prophylactic use of methylene blue (50mg) 3 or 4 times daily, orally or intravenously, prevent, further episodes of encephalopathy.

After several courses, high-dose methotrexate (>1 g/m^2) occasionally causes encephalopathy that usually is transient and reversible.[89] Intrathecal methotrexate may cause a chemical meningitis, with fever, headache, muscle rigidity, and cerebrospinal fluid leukocytosis. This toxicity is rare, but it occurs within hours of the intrathecal injection and resolves spontaneously.

5-fluorouracil may cause an acute cerebellar dysfunction, which is usually more common in the elderly. It is characterized by rapid onset of gait ataxia, limb incoordination, dysarthria, nystagmus, and diplopia. Effects are reversible with drug withdrawal or dose reduction. Multifocal cerebral demyelination has been described to occur as the result of 5-FU and levamisole or leucovorin administration.[88] Symptoms that have been exhibited include acute confusion, ataxia, slurred speech, and restlessness. With steroid use and discontinuing chemotherapy, the patient's symptoms improve.

High-dose cytarabine can cause encephalopathy, leukoencephalopathy, and sometimes peripheral neuropathy with doses greater than 18 g/m^2. High doses increase the transport rate over the cell membranes, enhancing the intracellular drug concentrations and prolonging the cellular exposure to the drug's metabolites. CNS toxicity usually occurs 5–7 days after the start of therapy.[89] Ocular toxicity (conjunctivitis, photophobia, burning, and decreased acuity) and cerebellar and cerebral dysfunction can also occur. Once the drug is stopped, the neurological symptoms may resolve partially or completely.

Arthralgia and myalgia have been reported to occur infrequently with docetaxel administration. If symptoms occur, they are usually experienced a few days after administration and can last up to 4 days.[21] Severity of discomfort can be reduced by the use of prophylactic analgesics such as ibuprofen. Transient myalgia and arthralgia are common after paclitaxel therapy.[88] Symptoms usually occur 2–3 days after treatment and resolve in approximately 6 days. The shoulder and paraspinal muscles seem to be the most common area of occurrence, but other muscle groups can be affected. *Trans*-retinoic acid commonly causes myalgia, arthralgia, and muscle weakness.[21] Imatinib mesylate commonly causes arthralgia, myalgia, muscle cramps, and musculoskeletal pain.

One of the principal nonhematologic toxicities of paclitaxel is sensory neuropathy, which is experienced at doses of 250 mg/m^2 or greater. Symptoms consist of numbness, tingling, or burning pain of the lower extremities. Perioral numbness has been reported that may be asymmetrical at onset and progress in a symmetrical pattern. Neurotoxicity is typically cumulative; with large-fiber modalities (vibration, proprioception) being more frequently affected than small-fiber modalities (pain and temperature).[90] Mild symptoms improve or resolve within several months after the discontinuation of paclitaxel. Amitriptyline has been found to be beneficial in relieving the discomfort associated with the symptoms. Autonomic neuropathy has been reported with high doses of paclitaxel (250 mg/m^2 or greater) and is manifested as paralytic ileus and orthostatic hypotension. Patients with diabetes mellitus experience this neuropathy more frequently.[90] Transient encephalopathy has been reported after paclitaxel infusion and is exhibited as confusion, word-finding difficulty, and behavioral changes. Symptoms appear 1 week after paclitaxel infusion and resolve spontaneously.[91]

Docetaxel administration can produce mild sensory neuropathy. At a cumulative dose of 600 mg/m^2, severe and disabling neuropathy can develop. Symptoms include paresthesia, numbness, loss of sensory qualities, and a decrease in deep tendon reflexes.[88]

Oxaliplatin is a new platinum compound that can induce two types of neurotoxicity. An acute, reversible peripheral sensory neuropathy can occur within hours and as long as 2 days after infusion.[88] Symptoms may be precipitated by exposure to cold, such as cold air or cold drink. Although discontinuation of the drug is rarely necessary, this neuropathy frequently recurs with subsequent doses. Pharyngolaryngeal dysthesia characterized by subjective sensations of dysphagia, dyspnea, or tightness in the back of throat has occurred as well. During this sensation, no laryngospasm or bronchospasm has been observed. Motor neuropathy can also occur, characterized by paresthesia, dysesthesia, and hypoesthesia; it may be related to a cumulative dose of 780 mg/m^2.[22] Infusions of calcium gluconate and magnesium sulfate are being studied as ways to decrease the neuropathy. In addition, pretreatment with gluthathione may decrease the incidence of both neuropathies.[89] Patients are instructed to avoid cold drinks or exposure to cold immediately after infusion of oxaliplatin.[22]

Bortezomib is a proteasome inhibitor that can cause peripheral neuropathy. Symptoms include numbness, pain, or burning sensations in the feet or hands.[23] Doses greater than 1.3 mg/m^2 increase the incidence of neuropathy.

Cognitive function can be altered with the administration of standard-dose and high-dose chemotherapy. Problems are observed in the patient's short-term memory and ability to concentrate. Cognitive deficits can continue for as long as 10 years after treatment.[88]

Chemoprotectants have been evaluated in minimizing chemotherapy-induced neurotoxicity. Amifostine has been found to decrease cisplatin-induced neurotoxicity and may protect against ototoxicity.[15,88] Glutamine and vitamin B_{12} have been found to reduce chemotherapy-induced neuropathy.[88] Pyridoxine may be useful in docetaxel-induced paresthesias.

Astute neurological assessment is critical in patients receiving potentially neurotoxic agents. The baseline assessment should include sensory function, motor function, gait, range of motion, cranial nerves, and reflexes. Renal and hepatic functions should be monitored closely.[77] Chemotherapy agents such as ifosfamide and cytarabine will have increased neurotoxicity with renal dysfunction. Sedatives, antiemetics, and tranquilizers, which are CNS depressants, must be used with caution because their usage may increase toxicity. In addition, other causes of these symptoms — such as electrolyte imbalances, metastasis, or other medical conditions — can cause similar effects.

Neurotoxicity will affect patients by decreasing their mobility, ability for self-care, and ability to perform fine-motor skills such as writing and buttoning a shirt. An occupational therapist may need to be consulted to help the patient adapt to loss of motor skills. Patients must be taught the importance of reporting any change in status, such as numbness and tingling of the extremities. If neurological deficits become severe, safety measures must be initiated to protect the patient from harm (Table 17-6).

Pulmonary toxicity

Pulmonary toxicity that results from chemotherapy administration is usually irreversible and progressive. The initial site of damage seems to be the endothelial cells, with an inflammatory-type reaction resulting in drug-induced pneumonitis. Another type of damage occurs via an immunologic mechanism. Either the lung or the drug may act as the antigen in an allergic-type reaction.[92] Chronic exposure to chemotherapy causes an extensive alteration of the pulmonary parenchyma, with changes in the connective tissue, obliteration of alveoli, and dilatation of air spaces, known as *honeycombing*. Continuous injury and repair produce restrictive lung disease, increased work of breathing, and a functionally reduced lung volume, leading to impaired gas exchange. Hypoxemia results because oxygen does not diffuse in the damaged areas while perfusion continues.

Pulmonary toxicity usually presents clinically as dyspnea, unproductive cough, bilateral basilar rales, and tachypnea. The chest x-ray may be within normal limits, but can show a pattern of diffuse interstitial markings. Arterial blood gases reveal hypoxia, with hypocapnia and respiratory alkalosis. The most sensitive pulmonary function test is the carbon monoxide diffusion capacity, which becomes abnormal before clinical symptoms occur.[93] Other pulmonary function tests can show a restrictive pattern when pulmonary fibrosis has occurred. To establish a pathological diagnosis, the best method is to obtain involved tissues by an open-lung biopsy or a fiber-optic bronchoscopy. Bacterial or fungal infections and metastasis can then be ruled out.

Bleomycin is known to cause pulmonary toxicity. This effect's incidence is 5% for a total cumulative dose of 450 units and 15% for higher dosages. Bleomycin is concentrated preferentially in the lung and is inactivated by a hydrolase enzyme. This enzyme is relatively deficient in lung tissue as compared with other tissues, such as the liver. These findings may explain the relative sensitivity of bleomycin to lung tissue, causing (1) early endothelial cell damage, (2) decrease in type I pneumocytes, with subsequent proliferation, and (3) migration of type II pneumocytes into alveolar spaces, inducing interstitial changes.[94] Following destruction of type I cells, repair is characterized by hyperplasia and dysplasia of the type II pneumocytes. Fibroblast proliferation, with subsequent pulmonary fibrosis, is probably the basis for the irreversible changes induced by bleomycin.[94]

Cytarabine exerts a direct toxic effect on the pneumocytes and capillary endothelial cells by diminishing the integrity of cell membranes and increasing capillary permeability. A capillary leak syndrome, involving primarily the lung, occurs 2–21 days after the first dose, resulting in pulmonary edema and respiratory failure, with features of adult respiratory disease (ARD). It appears to be related to high doses and continuous administration.[77]

Mitomycin C damage to the lung presents as diffuse alveolar damage with capillary leak and pulmonary edema. Incidence ranges from 3% to 36%, occurring 6–12 months after therapy. In some patients, only a brief exposure suffices to produce damage. If dyspnea occurs with a normal chest radiograph, it may be necessary to discontinue mitomycin C from the treatment plan.[21]

Cyclophosphamide causes pulmonary toxicity in less than 1% of patients and is associated with high doses (120 mg/kg/day for 4 days). Histological

Table 17-6 Organ Toxicity of Chemotherapy Agents: Neurotoxicity

Toxicity/Symptoms	Grade	General Risk Factors	Chemotherapy Agent/Risk Factors/ Symptoms	Mechanism of Damage	Protective/ Management Measures
Cerebellar • Unsteady gait • Nystagmus • Ataxia • Dizziness • Seizures • Hemiparesis • Confusion • Coma Autonomic • Ileus • Constipation • Impotence • Urinary retention • Postural hypotension Peripheral/Cranial • Facial palsies • Diplopia • Paresthesia of hands and feet • Muscle atrophy • Foot drop • Loss of deep tendon reflexes • Areflexia • Sensory loss • Sensory perception loss • Hoarseness	Neurocerebellar 0 = None 1 = Slight incoordination dysdiadokinesis 2 = Intention tremor dysmetria, slurred speech 3 = Locomotor ataxia 4 = Cerebellar necrosis Neurocortical 0 = None 1 = Mild somnolence or agitation 2 = Moderate somnolence or agitation 3 = Severe somnolence or agitation, confusion, disorientation, hallucination, aphasia 4 = Coma, seizures, psychosis Neurosensory 0 = None 1 = Mild paresthesias, loss of deep tendon reflexes 2 = Mild or moderate objective sensory loss, moderate paresthesias 3 = Severe objective loss, or paresthesias that interfere with function Neuromotor 0 = None 1 = Subjective weakness 2 = Mild objective weakness 3 = Objective weakness with impairment of function 4 = Paralysis	• Dosage • Cranial radiation • Intrathecal administration • Age • CNS depressants (i.e., antiemetics, tranquilizers, and sedatives) • History of diabetes, chronic alcohol abuse	Ifosfamide • High doses • Cerebellar and cranial dysfunction Vincristine • Dose-related: >2 mg/m^2 of unit dose • Hepatic dysfunction • Autonomic, peripheral dysfunction Cisplatin • Dose-related • Renal dysfunction • Dehydration • Autonomic, peripheral dysfunction • Concurrent treatment with vincristine or etoposide Methotrexate • High dose (>1 g/m^2) • Cerebellar dysfunction • Concurrent cranial radiation therapy • Intrathecal dose • Increases effect with cytarabine, daunorubicin, salicylates, sulfonamides, vinblastine, vincristine Cytarabine • High doses (>2 g/m^2) • Cerebellar and peripheral effects 5-fluorouracil • Cerebellar dysfunction • Dose and schedule related Pemetrexed • Should not be adminstered to patients with impaired creatinine clearance Taxanes • Peripheral neuropathies • Myalgias/arthralgia Oxaliplatin • Peripheral neuropathy • Laryngopharyngeal dysesthia Bortezomib • Peripheral neuropathy	• Accumulation of drug metabolite (chloracetaldehyde) with direct CNS effect • Disrupts microtubules in the neural tissues • Damages large fibers, resulting in sensory change • Damage/loss of inner hair cells in the organ of Corti • Demyelination of nerve fibers	• Place on bowel regimen • Methylene Blue infusion • Oral diazepam 5 mg every 6 hr at the time of treatment, to manage muscle spasms • Eliminate furosemide • Avoid concurrent administration of aminoglycosides • Audiometric testing for high risk • Ethyol (amifostine) • Withhold therapy for severe toxicity, i.e., muscle weakness or pain • Neurologic recovery, start drug at 50% dose reduction • Monitor neurologic signs and symptoms • Monitor electrolytes • Institute safety measures • Administer amifostine with cisplatin • Glutamine and vitamin B_{12} may minimize symptoms • Folic acid and vitamin B_{12} supplements reduce toxicity of pemetrexed • Avoid cold drinks and cold in general

findings include endothelial swelling, pneumocyte dysplasia, edema, fibrosis, and fibroblast proliferation. The result of damage is alveolar hemorrhage and fibrin deposition.[77]

Carmustine inhibits lung glutathione disulfide reductase, which mediates the resultant cellular injury. Damage occurs after a long latency period, averaging 3 years, but may occur after only 6 weeks of therapy. High-dose carmustine has an incidence of 20%–30% when a cumulative dose of 1500 mg/m^2 is given. An insidious cough with dyspnea or sudden respiratory failure occurs. It has been suggested that this reaction may be more common when cyclophosphamide is given simultaneously.[21,77] Although glucocorticoid administration has improved symptoms, mortality still occurs in a small percentage of patients.

Methotrexate can also produce an acute or a chronic process related to endothelial injury.[95] Diffuse alveolar damage is characterized by the disappearance of type I pneumocytes, hyaline membrane formation, and the presence of inflammatory cells in the alveoli and interstitium. The incidence is less than 1%, with an acute onset of pulmonary edema producing ARD or more gradual systemic toxicity (such as fever or chills), and with malaise preceding the appearance of pulmonary symptoms. Radiographic features may be unique, with pleural effusion occurring either alone or in conjunction with pulmonary infiltrates, peripheral consolidations, or chronic eosinophilic pneumonia.

An uncommon side effect of docetaxel is fluid retention. Its incidence is related to the cumulative dose. This toxicity can be disabling, worsening with higher doses. Fluid retention is exhibited peripherally, as abdominal ascites, as a pleural effusion, or as a combination of the two. The fluid retention is reversible and can be controlled with diuretics.[21]

Trans-retinoic acid can cause a syndrome consisting of high fever, respiratory distress, pulmonary infiltrates, and pericardial or pleural effusion that occurs 2 days to 3 weeks after initiating treatment. This retinoic acid syndrome can be reversed with the administration of corticosteroids.[21] Irinotecan can cause dyspnea on exertion and pneumonitis with pulmonary infiltrates.[21] Busulfan can cause pulmonary fibrosis when a dose exceeding 500 mg is given.[21]

Gemcitabine can cause pulmonary symptoms ranging from mild, self-limiting dyspnea to fatal pulmonary toxicity. The symptoms exhibited include tachypnea, marked hypoxemia, and interstitial infiltrates on chest x-ray consistent with pulmonary edema. Administration of corticosteroids and diuretics seems to reverse the toxicity.[96]

Because lung damage is usually irreversible and progressive, it is imperative to detect pulmonary toxicity as early as possible. The causative agent may be discontinued or the dose reduced to prevent further damage to lung tissue. High concentrations of inspired oxygen are toxic to the lungs, and the simultaneous administration of various chemotherapy drugs may induce lung damage.[93] Nurses need to be aware of this phenomenon and must monitor the patient's oxygen saturation and breath sounds closely for early signs and symptoms of pulmonary toxicity.

When oxygen saturation is compromised due to restrictive lung damage, the patient experiences dyspnea on exertion or at rest. As a result, the patient must expend increased effort to perform simple activities of daily living. Nursing care centers on teaching the patient to prioritize daily activities and to use breathing techniques such as pursed lips to lessen the effects of dyspnea. Supplemental oxygen therapy may be necessary to relieve the dyspnea. The family and patient must be taught how to administer oxygen and what safety precautions are necessary with oxygen therapy. Steroids are usually administered to lessen the pulmonary symptoms. Single-lung transplantation may be an option for drug-induced pulmonary toxicity.[97] To prevent further complications, the nurse must also teach the patient how to mobilize secretions by maintaining an adequate fluid intake and performing effective cough and deep-breathing techniques (Table 17-7).

Hepatotoxicity

Chemotherapy agents can cause a variety of hepatotoxic reactions. The initial site of damage seems to be the parenchymal cells. Obstruction to hepatic blood flow results in fatty changes, hepatocellular necrosis, cholestasis, hepatitis, and venoocclusive disease (VOD). Hepatotoxicity usually is diagnosed initially by transient elevations of the hepatic enzymes during treatment, which can progress to hepatomegaly, jaundice, and abdominal pain. Unless extensive fibrosis or necrosis has occurred, hepatotoxicity is reversible.[21]

Liver toxicity induced by high-dose methotrexate is transient and usually does not result in chronic liver disease. Elevation of hepatic enzyme levels is common, rising with successive courses of therapy and tending to be higher in patients treated on a daily schedule than those treated on intermittent schedules. Chronic inflammatory infiltrates in the portal tracts, focal liver cell necrosis, fibrosis, and cirrhosis may occur. However, all abnormalities usually resolve within 1 month following cessation of methotrexate therapy.[98]

High-dose cytarabine may induce intrahepatic cholestasis, possibly as a result of injury to the hepatocyte transport system. Changes are reversible, so they do not appear to limit cytarabine use. 5-fluorouracil used in combination with levamisole has resulted in increases in alkaline phosphatase, transaminase, and bilirubin levels. These changes resolve with the

Table 17-7 Organ Toxicity of Chemotherapy Agents: Pulmonary Toxicity

Toxicity/Symptoms	Grade	General Risk Factors	Chemotherapy Agent/Risk Factors	Mechanism of Damage	Protective/ Management Measures
• Low-grade fever • Nonproductive cough • Dyspnea • Tachycardia • Diffuse basilar crackles • Wheezing • Pleural rub • Fatigue • Malaise • Chest pain • Night sweats • Tachypnea • Cyanosis • Edema	Dyspnea 0 = None 1 = Asymptomatic with abnormal PFTs 2 = Dyspnea on exertion 3 = Dyspnea at normal activity 4 = Dyspnea at rest Pulmonary Fibrosis 0 = Normal 1 = Radiographic changes, no symptoms 2 = N/A 3 = Changes with symptoms Pulmonary Edema 0–2 None 3 Radiographic changes and diuretics required 4 Requires intubation Pneumonitis (noninfectious) 0 = Normal 1 = Radiographic change, symptoms do not require steroids 2 = Steroids required 3 = Oxygen required 4 = Requires assisted ventilation Pleural Effusion 0 None 1–4 Present ARDs 0 = None 1 = Mild 2 = Moderate 3 = Severe 4 = Life-threatening	• Age • Preexisting lung disease, e.g., COPD, TB • History of smoking • Cumulative dose • Long-term therapy • Mediastinal radiation • High inspired concentration of oxygen • Renal insufficiency	Bleomycin • Synergistic with vincristine • Cumulative dose > 450 mg/m^2 • Oxygen exposure > 50%	• Initial injury to capillary endothelium cells • Necrosis of type I epithelial cells • Hypertrophy of type II alveolar pneumocytes • Pulmonary fibrosis	• Assess for risk factors • Obtain baseline pulmonary function tests • Monitor cumulative dose • Limit cumulative dose • Limit oxygen to keep arterial PO_2 > 60 mm Hg • Discontinue drug if dyspnea occurs • Assess for pulmonary symptoms • Administer steroids and oxygen • Monitor activities to minimize energy • Stop or reduce dose of drug • Fluid restriction • Administer diuretics • Follow-up with PFTs
			Mitomycin C • History of cyclophosphamide and/or methotrexate administration • Oxygen concentrations > 50%	• Hypersensitivity reaction or immune complex related • Damage similar to bleomycin • Increased effect with VM-26, vincristine	
			Carmustine • Dose-related (> 1500 mg/m^2) • Concurrent administration with cyclophosphamide	• Inhibition of glutathione reductase in alveolar macrophages	
			Busulfan	• Hyperplasia and dysplasia of the type II pneumocytes	
			Cyclophosphamide: • High dose > 120 mg/kg/day × 4 days	• Alveolar hemorrhage and fibrin deposition • Increased effect with cisplatin, VM-26, vincristine	
			Methotrexate	• Capillary leak syndrome, pulmonary edema • Interstitial pneumonitis	
			Cytarabine • High doses (5 g/m^2)	• Capillary leak syndrome • Capillary endothelial damage	
			Gemcitabine	• See cytarabine	

PFT = pulmonary function test; COPD = chronic obstructive pulmonary disorder; TB = tuberculosis.

discontinuation of therapy; no medical intervention is needed. Gemcitabine, irinotecan, trimetrexate, gefitnib, imatinib mesylate, oxaliplatin, and antitumor antibiotics can cause a transient increase of hepatic enzymes that resolves after discontinuing the drug.[21]

Fluorodeoxyuridine, usually administered as a continuous arterial dose, can cause chemical hepatitis, with increases in transaminases, alkaline phosphatase, and serum bilirubin levels. In addition, stricture of intrahepatic or extrahepatic bile ducts can occur. Toxicity appears to be both time and dose dependent. Although liver function usually normalizes when the drug is discontinued, the development of biliary sclerosis is irreversible.[21]

Hepatocellular disease occurs with the administration of 6-mercaptopurine in daily doses exceeding 2 mg/kg. The histological pattern includes features of intrahepatic cholestasis and parenchymal cell necrosis. Moderate elevations occur in transaminases, alkaline phosphatase, and serum bilirubin, with episodes of jaundice occurring 30 days after initiation of therapy.[21]

Few guidelines exist for the use of drugs when hepatic dysfunction is present. Known hepatotoxic drugs must be avoided when liver function test results are abnormal. Impaired liver function delays excretion and results in increased accumulation of the chemotherapy in the plasma and tissues, especially with drugs such as doxorubicin, daunorubicin, paclitaxel, docetaxel, vincristine, and vinblastine, all of which are excreted primarily by the liver into the bile. It has been recommended to reduce or to not administer these agents if the serum bilirubin is between 1.5 and 3 mg/dL. If the SGOT is between 60 and 180 international units, the dose should be reduced by 50%.[21]

Hepatic toxicity is uncommon, but it can be a serious consequence of chemotherapy administration, with effects ranging from transient enzyme elevations to permanent cirrhosis. Because many disease- and treatment-related factors can be hepatotoxic, it is difficult to attribute hepatic toxicity definitively to specific agents. During chemotherapy administration, the nurse should monitor liver function tests closely, as enzymatic changes may be the first clinical evidence of hepatotoxicity.

Third spacing (the shift of fluid from the vascular space to the interstitial space) can occur as a result of hepatotoxicity. Signs of fluid shift are decreased blood pressure, increased pulse rate, low central venous pressure, decreased urine output, increased specific gravity, low levels of serum albumin, and hemoconcentration. Albumin is administered to replace the plasma protein and assist with absorption of the fluid. Fluid restriction minimizes third spacing, so this measure enhances renal blood flow, decreases systemic congestion, and improves patient comfort. Other supportive care measures include diuretics, decreased protein intake, lactulose, and emotional support (Table 17-8).

Hemorrhagic cystitis

Hemorrhagic cystitis is a bladder toxicity resulting from cyclophosphamide and ifosfamide therapy. It ranges from microscopic hematuria to frank bleeding, necessitating invasive local intervention with instillation of sclerosing agents. Symptoms range from transient irritative urination, dysuria, and suprapubic pain to life-threatening hemorrhage. Transient cystitis has an early onset and short duration due to the direct effect of the deposition of acrolein, a by-product of metabolism, on the urothelium.[99]

After oral or intravenous administration, cyclophosphamide is metabolized by hepatic microsomal enzymes to hydroxycyclophosphamide and later by target cells to phosphamide mustard (active) and acrolein (urinary metabolite). The binding of acrolein to the bladder mucosa results in inflammation and ulceration. Approximately 10% of people receiving cyclophosphamide experience microscopic hematuria.[21] Early diagnosis is accomplished by urine dipstick or visual observation of red-tinged urine. If necessary, a confirmed diagnosis can be accomplished by cystoscopy, which shows discrete bleeding capillaries or diffuse mucosal ulceration, hemorrhage, and necrosis.[100]

When hemorrhagic cystitis develops, drug therapy probably should be discontinued. In many patients, discontinuation will lead to amelioration of the symptoms without sequelae; however, microhematuria may persist long after discontinuing cyclophosphamide. When therapy is not stopped, as many as 55% of patients will have persistent symptoms. Extensive chronic bleeding and mucosal inflammation can produce long-term cystitis, irreversible bladder fibrosis, bladder contraction, and an increased risk for bladder cancer.[100] In high doses, Mesna has been successful in protecting the bladder from the harmful effects of acrolein.[15]

Ifosfamide has a slower rate of metabolic activation into acrolein, allowing larger dosages to be administered as compared to cyclophosphamide. Mesna, a uroprotectant, contains a sulfhydryl group believed to bind acrolein within the urinary collecting system and detoxifies ifosfamide. It is administered before ifosfamide and then intermittently for as long as 24 hours afterward to protect the bladder. Mesna can be administered intravenously, orally, or subcutaneously.[99] Daily dose of mesna is 60% of the total daily dose of ifosfamide.

Gemcitabine can cause microscopic hematuria and proteinuria, especially with repeated cycles. In clinical trials, the occurrence was not found to be correlated

Table 17-8 Organ Toxicity of Chemotherapy Agents: Hepatotoxicity

Toxicity/Symptoms	Grade	General Risk Factors	Chemotherapy Agent	Mechanism of Damage	Protective/ Management Measures
• Elevated bilirubin, LDH, SGOT, alkaline phosphatase, SGPT • Chemical hepatitis • Jaundice • Ascites • Decreased albumin • Cirrhosis • Hepatomegaly • Right upper quadrant pain • Fatigue • Anorexia • Nausea • Decreased clotting factor synthesis • Hyperpigmentation of skin	Bilirubin 0–1 = Normal 2 = < 1.5 3 = 1.5–3.0 4 = > 3.0 SGOT/SGPT 0 = Normal 1 = < 2.5 2 = 2.6–5.0 3 = 5.1–20 4 = > 20 Alkaline Phosphatase 0 = Normal 1 = 2.5 2 = 2.6–5.0 3 = 5.1–20 4 = > 20 Liver Clinical 0–2 = No change 3 = Precoma 4 = Hepatic coma	• Prior liver damage, e.g., hepatitis • Dose • Diabetes mellitus • Tumor involvement • Irradiation of liver • Alcoholism • Liver infections • Concurrent administration of hepatotoxic drugs, e.g., phenothiazines • Age • Hepatic dysfunction • Total bilirubin > 2 mg/100 mL • Obesity	• Methotrexate • 6-Mercaptopurine • Cytarabine • Fluorodoxyuridine • Nitrosoureas • Etoposide, high dose • Cisplatin, high dose • L-asparaginase • Amsacrine • Cyclophosphamide, high dose • Doxorubicin • Vincristine • Vinblastine • Docetaxel • Irinotecan • Gemcitabine • Trimetrexate • Gefitnib • Imatinib mesylate • Oxaliplatin	Direct Toxic Effects • Parenchymal cell damage • Intrahepatic cholestasis • Hepatic fibrosis • Fatty changes	• Reduce dose in presence of liver dysfunction for drugs metabolized in liver, e.g., vinca alkaloids or doxorubicin • Avoid alcohol intake • Monitor liver function tests • If bilirubin > 1.5 mg, reduce dose by 50% • If bilirubin > 3.0 mg, reduce dose by 75% • Avoid hepatotoxic drugs

with a cumulative dose or with treatment duration.[21] In rare instances, irinotecan may cause hematuria.[21] In a case report, temozolamide was found to cause hemorrhagic cystitis.[101] Valrubicin is a recently approved anthracycline antitumor antibiotic that is administered intavesically. The agent is excreted almost completely with voiding and can cause urinary frequency, dysuria, hematuria, and bladder pain.[21]

Protection of the bladder from these drugs focuses on hyperhydration, frequent voiding, and diuresis. If cystitis occurs, the treatment includes bladder irrigation through a three-way Foley catheter to clear developing clots. The various solutions that cause a protein precipitate to form over the bleeding surfaces include saline, potassium aluminum sulfate, silver nitrate, and formalin. Vasopressins such as amino caproic acid may be administered intravenously or orally to decrease clotting. Cystoscopy may be necessary to cauterize bleeders, if the bladder irrigations were ineffective in controlling the bleeding. As a last resort, a cystectomy may be necessary.[100]

During administration of chemotherapy agents, the nurse should monitor the urine for blood, through dipsticking or observation. Strict intake and output measures are imperative to ensure minimal contact of acrolein with the bladder mucosa. The patient must be taught to maintain adequate hydration and to void frequently. If feasible, cyclophosphamide should be administered early in the day so that the patient can drink fluids and void frequently without interruption of sleep. Insertion of a Foley catheter may be necessary when high doses of cyclophosphamide are administered, to ensure that the agent is cleared from the bladder continuously (Table 17-9).

Nephrotoxicity

Nephrotoxicity is a dose-limiting side effect of some chemotherapeutic agents. Serious fluid and electrolyte imbalances that can progress to renal failure are the result of the direct and indirect effects of these agents on the kidney. Many chemotherapy agents are both metabolized and excreted by the kidneys; others are merely excreted as metabolites or as unchanged drugs including cisplatin, ifosfamide, high-dose methotrexate, mitomycin, mithramycin, and streptozocin. The manner in which chemotherapy damages the kidney varies from direct renal cell damage to an

Table 17-9 Organ Toxicity of Chemotherapy Agents: Hemorrhagic Cystitis

Toxicity/Symptoms	Grade	General Risk Factors	Chemotherapy Agent/ Risk Factors	Mechanism of Damage	Protective/ Management Measures
• Gross hematuria • Dysuria, urgency • Suprapubic pain	0 = None 1 = Micro only 2 = Gross, no clots 3 = Gross, with clots 4 = Requires transfusion	• Dose-related • Pelvic radiation	Cyclophosphamide • High dose (> 2.5 g) Ifosfamide • Single high dose versus multiple dose Gemcitabine Irinotecan	• Drug metabolite acrolein damages bladder mucosa Synergistic Effect • Cisplatin • VM-26 • Vincristine	• Vigorous hydration • Frequent emptying of bladder, especially at night • Monitor urine for blood • 3-way Foley irrigation with saline, alum, or formaldehyde
			Valrubicin	• Bladder wall affinity	• Administer amino caproic acid IV or PO • Mesna given in a dose of 60% total dose of ifosfamide q4h×3

obstructive nephropathy resulting from precipitate formation. Renal failure, acid–base disorders, or electrolyte abnormalities may also occur as a result of tumor lysis syndrome or uric acid nephropathy.[102] When the renal clearance rate for a specific drug with linear pharmacokinetics is 35%–40% and the patient has moderate to severe renal function, a significant increase in the drug's area under the plasma concentration curve (AUC) can occur.[103] For patients who have preexisting renal disease or who exhibit early signs of renal toxicity, the dosage may need to be reduced or the agent eliminated from the treatment plan.

Cisplatin can cause mild to severe nephrotoxicity, with specific damage occurring to the proximal and distal tubules. Platinum metal chelates in the renal tubules cause direct damage to the proximal tubular cells, injuring the tubular basement membranes, and can cause focal tubular necrosis.[103] Acute damage can occur within 3–21 hours after cisplatin administration, as evidenced by renal enzyme changes when precautions are not taken. Such renal dysfunction can persist for several years following cisplatin administration and may be irreversible.[102] Damage is characterized by degeneration of renal tubular epithelium, thickening of tubular basement membrane, and mild interstitial fibrosis. To avoid toxicity, patients should receive vigorous saline hydration of 1–2 L as well as diuresis during therapy, depending upon total cisplatin dose.

The use of mannitol in facilitating and inducing diuresis is a means of ensuring adequate urine flow. Mannitol may prevent immediate binding of cisplatin onto the renal tubules. Loop diuretics such as furosemide must be used with caution, however, as an increase in cisplatin toxicity has been reported following their administration. Frequent determinations of renal function should be obtained. If the creatinine clearance falls to less than 50 mg/mL, the drug should be withheld until renal function improves. If the serum creatinine level is elevated, cisplatin should be held. Daily magnesium supplementation may be indicated during cisplatin therapy, and electrolyte levels should be monitored frequently.[103]

Amifostine is an organic thiophosphate used to reduce the cumulative renal toxicity associated with repeated administration of cisplatin in patients with advanced ovarian or non-small cell lung cancer. This drug's ability to protect normal tissue without compromising tumor cell kill is attributed to its higher capillary alkaline phosphatase activity, higher pH, and better vascular bed of normal tissue as compared to cancer tissue. Other benefits seen with amifostine administration include (1) reduced occurrence of hypomagnesemia, (2) protection of the kidneys from nephrotoxic antibiotics, and (3) reduced cumulative nephrotoxicity associated with cisplatin.[104,105]

Amifostine is dephosphorylated at the tissue site by alkaline phosphatase to form free thiol. Within the cell, thiol neutralizes the reactive components of cisplatin before damage occurs to the DNA and RNA of the normal cell. Thiol acts as a potent scavenger of free radicals and superoxide anions. This phenomenon is important because free radicals can damage cell membranes, DNA, and other vital cell components.[104,105]

Amifostine 740 mg/m^2 or 910 mg/m^2 is administered to the patient over 5–15 minutes intravenously after the patient has been given antiemetics and adequately hydrated with a minimum of one liter of fluid intravenously. Fifteen minutes after the amifostine is given, cisplatin is administered. The most common side effect noted has been transient systolic hypotension; therefore, it is recommended that amifostine be administered with the patient in a supine position. Blood pressure should be monitored every 5 minutes throughout the infusion and 5 minutes after the infusion. If the blood pressure drops below the threshold level from the baseline, the infusion is interrupted. The infusion can be restarted if the blood pressure returns to threshold within 5 minutes and if the patient is asymptomatic. If the blood pressure does not return to threshold, the infusion is discontinued and the next dose is reduced to 740 mg/m^2.[104]

Transient systolic hypotension is short term and reversible. It is treated with fluid administration and by placing the patient in the Trendelenburg position. Increased nausea and vomiting have occurred with amifostine which may be a potentiating effect with cisplatin. Antiemetics must be given prior to amifostine administration and continued with cisplatin. Other side effects that have been observed include flushing, feeling of warmth or coldness, chills, syncope, somnolence, hiccups, and sneezing.[105]

Standard doses of methotrexate are not associated with renal toxicity unless the patient has preexisting renal dysfunction. High doses (>1 g/m^2) can cause an obstructive nephropathy from precipitation of methotrexate or its metabolites in the renal tubules. Risk factors associated with drug-induced nephrotoxicity include (1) low urine pH, (2) dehydration, (3) low methotrexate clearance, (4) decreased urine output, and (5) concurrent intrathecal treatment.[21] In general, urinary alkalization to maintain a urine pH greater than 7 with simultaneous administration of sodium bicarbonate or diamox prevents precipitate formation, permitting high-dose therapy to be administered. High doses of methotrexate should be accompanied by leucovorin rescue to counteract the effects of folic acid antagonists.

Streptozocin in doses exceeding 1.5 g/m^2 is associated with renal dysfunction in more than 65% of patients. Characteristically, streptozocin causes a tubulointerstitial nephritis and tubular atrophy due to direct damage of the tubules. This toxicity is manifested by hypokalemia, proteinuria, increased blood urea nitrogen (BUN), and increased creatinine levels.[102] Renal function tests and creatinine clearance tests should be obtained before beginning streptozocin therapy. Patients who develop an elevation of serum creatinine, even if the level subsequently returns to normal, are cautioned against receiving further streptozocin, as severe toxicity may occur.

Lomustine and carmustine can cause a delayed renal failure months or years following therapy. Azotemia and proteinuria are manifested, followed by progressive renal failure, often requiring dialysis. The incidence of renal failure appears to increase dramatically after a total dose of 1500 mg/m^2.[102]

Mitomycin C has been associated with a syndrome of renal failure and microangiopathic hemolytic anemia. This toxicity occurs in approximately 20% of patients who have received a cumulative dose of 100 mg or more after approximately 6 months of therapy and is characterized by an abrupt onset of microangiopathic hemolytic anemia, thrombocytopenia, azotemia, proteinuria, and hematuria.[102] Hemolytic uremic syndrome is associated with a high mortality rate, pegged at 50%.

Nurses play a vital role in preventing nephrotoxicity. Preventive management includes aggressive hydration with hypertonic saline, diuresis, urinary alkalinization, and careful monitoring of urine output. Renal function tests, especially creatinine clearance and serum creatinine, should be monitored before and after administering nephrotoxic drugs. Patients who must receive other nephrotoxic drugs, such as aminoglycosides or contrast dye, should be monitored closely for early signs and symptoms of toxicity. Assessment of renal function should continue throughout treatment and periodically after the completion of therapy (Table 17-10).

Conclusion

Advances in cancer therapy are made by continual investigations, evaluation of treatment results, and their incorporation into the practice of oncology. Successful prevention and management of toxicities of chemotherapy will occur because of grassroots research that has its origins in careful observation of patients' responses to cancer treatment. Because of the amount of time spent directly with the patient receiving chemotherapy, the nurse is often the healthcare provider best able to recognize subtle changes in the patient's status that could be indicative of pending complications from chemotherapy and therefore areas in need of research. Nursing responsibilities are expanding and multifaceted, and include patient education, ongoing physical assessments, identification of risk factors, and prompt therapeutic interventions, with continual evaluation for modification.

Occurrence of side effects does not necessarily preclude withholding of chemotherapy but instead alerts the nurse to the need for careful assessment, management, and follow-up evaluation. The nurse's

Table 17-10 Organ Toxicity of Chemotherapy Agents: Nephrotoxicity

Toxicity/ Symptoms	Grade	General Risk Factors	Chemotherapy Agent/Risk Factors	Mechanism of Damage	Protective/ Management Measures	General Management
• Increased BUN, creatinine • Oliguria • Azotemia • Proteinuria • Decreased creatinine clearance • Hyperuricemia • Hypomagnesemia • Hypocalcemia	Creatinine 0 = WNL 1 = < 1.5 2 = 1.5–3.0 3 = 3.1–6.0 4 = > 6.0 Proteinuria 0 = No change 1 = 1+ or < 3 g/L 2 = 2–3+ or 3–10 g/L 3 = 4+ or > 10 g/L 4 = Nephrotic syndrome Hematuria 0 = None 1 = Micro 2 = Gross, no clots 3 = Gross, with clots 4 = Requires transfusion BUN mg% 0 = WNL < 20 1 = 21–30 2 = 31–50 3 = > 50	• Age • Dose of agent • Preexisting disease of kidneys, renal insufficiency • Nutritional status • Duration of cancer therapy • Concurrent: — Aminoglycoside therapy — Amphotericin-B • Renal damage • Dehydration • Large tumor mass • Ileal conduits • Contrast dye • History of sodium-retaining states (e.g., cirrhosis, CHF, nephrosis) • K and Mg depletion	Nitrosoureas • Cumulative dose of 1200 mg/m^2 for carmustine and lomustine Mitomycin C • Increased effect with vincristine and VM-26 Anthracyclines • High dose (1.5 g/m^2/wk) Streptozocin • Dose (> 1.5 g/m^2/wk)	• Direct cell damage in glomerulus • Chronic interstitial nephritis • Tubular atrophy • Direct cell damage in glomerulus • Microangiopathic hemolytic anemia • Tubular atrophy • Diffuse tubulointerstitial nephritis	These four measures apply to all drugs: • Monitor renal function tests • Saline diuresis • Hydrate patient (3000 mL/day) • Decrease uric acid production with allopurinol	• Substitute analog drug • Reduce dose for creatinine clearance (normal 125 mL/min) 30–60 mL/min: Cisplatin, 50% Methotrexate, 50% Mitomycin, 75% Nitrosoureas, hold dose 10–30 mL/min Cisplatin, hold dose Mitomycin, 75% < 10 mL/min Cyclophosphamide, 50% Mitomycin, 50% Avoid nephrotoxic drugs and contrast dye
			Cisplatin • Multiple doses (> 50 mg/m^2) • High dose • Increased effect with cyclophosphamide	• Tubulointerstitial nephritis • Tubular atrophy • Direct cell damage in tubules • Necrosis of proximal and distal renal tubules	• Stop drug if creatinine does not return to baseline • Diuresis with mannitol • Administer amifostine 15 min before administration	
			Methotrexate • High dose (> 1 g/m^2) • Enhanced effect with cisplatin	• Precipitation of metabolites in the acid environment of the urine • Obstructive nephropathy	• Maintain alkalinization of urine pH > 7 • Administer leucovorin • Administer bicarbonate • Avoid vitamin C Acids (ASA, vitamin C) compete for drug elimination sites, which increases serum concentration of methotrexate	

Note: Pharmacokinetics of the following drugs suggest dose reduction when the patient has renal impairment:
Fludarabine
Carboplatin (increased thrombocytopenia with renal dysfunction)
Ifosfamide (increased CNS toxicity)
Melphalan IV
Pentostatin (increased serious toxicity)
Etoposide (increased bone marrow toxicity)
Topotecan (increased neutropenia)
Bleomycin (increased pulmonary toxicity)
Dacarbazine
Hydroxyurea (increased bone marrow toxicity)

assessment of a patient's response to treatment and assistance in preventing or managing side effects can make a difference in the patient's overall perceived quality of life. Once the treatment is complete, nurses can be instrumental in encouraging patients to have a yearly comprehensive physical examinations to detect cancer recurrence and long-term effects of chemotherapy.

References

1. Lowenthal RM, Eaton K: Toxicity of chemotherapy. *Hematol Oncol Clin North Am* 10:967–990, 1996
2. Hood LE: Chemotherapy in the elderly: supportive measures for chemotherapy-induced myelotoxicity. *Clin J Oncol Nurs* 7:185–190, 2003
3. Balducci L, Extermann M: Management of cancer in the older person: a practical approach. *Oncologist* 5:224–237, 2000
4. Balducci L, Yates J: General guidelines for the management of older patients with cancer. *Oncology* 14:2221–2227, 2000
5. Balducci L, Carreca I: The role of myelopoietic growth factors in managing cancer in the elderly. *Drugs* 62(supp 1):42–63, 2002
6. Ozer H: New directions in the management of chemotherapy induced neutropenia: risk models, special populations and quality of life. *Semin Oncol* 4(suppl 13):18–23, 2003
7. Gomez H, Mas L, Casanova L: Elderly patients with aggressive non-Hodgkin's lymphoma treated with CHOP chemotherapy plus granulocyte-macrophage colony stimulating factor: identification of two age subgroups with differing hematologic toxicity. *J Clin Oncol* 16:2352–2358, 1998
8. Cascinu S, Del Ferro E, Catalano G: Toxicity and therapeutic response to chemotherapy in patients aged 70 years or older with advanced cancer. *Am J Clin Oncol* 19:371–374, 1996
9. Thyss A, Saudes L, Otto J, et al: Renal tolerance of cisplatin in patients more than 80 years old. *J Clin Oncol* 12:2121–2125, 1994
10. Shelton B: Effects of neutropenia upon quality of life. *Oncol Supportive Care Quarterly* 1:6–17, 2003
11. Jakel P: The impact of cancer-related anemia on quality of life. *Oncol Supportive Care Quarterly* 1:18–30, 2003
12. Cella DR: Quality of life: concepts and definition. *J Pain Symptom Manage* 9:186–192, 1993
13. Youngblood M, Williams PD, Eyles H, et al: A comparison of two methods of assessing cancer therapy-related symptoms. *Cancer Nurs* 17:37–44, 1994
14. Chang VT, Ingham J: Symptom control. *Cancer Invest* 21:564–578, 2003
15. Schuchter LM, Hensley ML, Meropol NJ: 2002 update of recommendations for the use of chemotherapy and radiotherapy protectants: clinical practice guidelines of the American Society of Clinical Oncology. *J Clin Oncol* 20:3895–2903, 2002
16. Schuchter LM: Current role of protective agents in cancer treatment. *Oncology* 11:505–518, 1997
17. Dodd MJ, Miaskowski C: The PRO-SELF program: a self-care intervention program for patients receiving cancer treatment. *Semin Oncol Nurs* 16:300–308, 2000
18. Haley WE: Family caregivers of elderly patients with cancer: understanding and minimizing the burden of care. *J Supportive Oncol* 1(supp 2):25–29, 2003
19. Joshi TG, Ehrenberger HE: Cancer clinical trials in the new millennium: novel challenges and opportunities for oncology nursing. *Clin J Oncol Nurs* 5:147–152, 2001
20. Dale D: Current management of chemotherapy-induced neutropenia: the role of colony-stimulating factors. *Semin Oncol* 30(suppl 13):3–9, 2003
21. Fisher DS, Knobf MT, Durivage HT, et al: *The Cancer Chemotherapy Handbook* (ed 6). Philadelphia, Mosby, 2003
22. Berg D: Oxaliplatin: a novel platinum analog with activity in colorectal cancer. *Oncol Nurs Forum* 30:957–966, 2003
23. Adams J: Proteasome inhibition in cancer: development of PS–341. *Semin Oncol* 28:613–619, 2001
24. Deininger MW, O'Brien SG, Ford JM, et al: Practical management of patients with chronic myeloid leukemia receiving imatinib. *J Clin Oncol* 21:1637–1647, 2003
25. Michael M, Moore M: Clinical experience with gemcitabine in pancreatic carcinoma. *Oncology* 11:1615–1621, 1997
26. Bloomfield M, Jaresko G, Zarek J, et al: Guidelines for using darbepoietin alfa in patients with chemotherapy induced anemia. *Pharmacotherapy* 23(suppl 12 pt 2):110S–118S, 2003
27. Ross SD, Fahrbach K, Frame D, et al: The effect of anemia treatment on selected health-related quality-of-life domains: a systematic review. *Clin Ther* 25:1786–1805, 2003
28. Shasha D, George MJ, Harrison LB: Once weekly dosing of epoietin-alpha increases hemoglobin and improves quality of life in anemic cancer patients receiving radiation either concomitantly or sequentially with chemotherapy. *Cancer* 98:1072–1079, 2003
29. Glaspy J, Singh Jadeja J, Justice G, et al: A dose-finding and safety study of novel erythropoiesis stimulating protein (NESP) for the treatment of anaemia in patients receiving multiple chemotherapy. *Br J Cancer* 84(suppl 1):17–23, 2001
30. Beveridge RA, Rifkia RM, Moleski RJ, et al: Impact of long-acting growth factors on practice dynamics and patient satisfaction. *Pharmacotherapy* 23(suppl 12 pt 2):101S–109S, 2003
31. McCullough J: Current issues with platelet transfusion in patients with cancer. *Semin Hematol* 37(suppl 4):3–10, 2000
32. Demetri GD: Pharmacologic treatment options in patients with thrombocytopenia. *Semin Hematol* 37(suppl 4):11–18, 2000
33. Begley CG, Basser RL: Biologic and structural differences of thrombopoietic growth factors. *Semin Hematol* 37(suppl 4):19–27, 2000
34. Boxer L, Dale DC: Neutropenia: causes and complications *Semin Hematol* 39:75–81, 2002
35. Rolston KV: Expanding the options for risk-based therapy in febrile neutropenia. *Diagn Microbial Infect Dis* 31:411–416, 1998
36. Barber FD: Management of fever in neutropenic patients with cancer. *Nurs Clin North Am* 36:631–644, 2001
37. Hughes WT, Armstrong D, Bodey GP, et al: 1997 guidelines for the use of antimicrobial agents in neutropenic patients with unexplained fever. *Clin Infect Dis* 25:551–573, 1997
38. Innes HE, Smith DB, O'Reilly SM, et al: Oral antibiotics with early hospital discharge compared with in-patient intravenous antibiotics for low-risk febrile neutropenia in patients with cancer: a prospective randomized controlled single center study. *Br J Cancer* 89:43–49, 2003
39. Mank A, van der Lelie H: Is there still an indication for nursing patients with prolonged neutropenia in protective isolation? An evidence-based nursing and medical study of 4 years experience for nursing patients with neutropenia without isolation. *Eur J Oncol Nurs* 7:17–23, 2003
40. Ozer H, Armitage JO, Bennett CL, et al: 2000 update recommendations for the use of hematopoietic colony-stimulating factors: evidence-based clinical practice guidelines. *J Clin Oncol* 18: 3558–3585, 2000

41. Dale DC: Colony-stimulating factors for the management of neutropenia in cancer patients. *Drugs* 62(suppl 1):1–15, 2002
42. Crawford J: Safety and efficacy of pegfilgrastim in patients receiving myelosuppressive chemotherapy. *Pharmacotherapy* 23(suppl 8 pt 2):15S–19S, 2003
43. Rodriguez-Adrian LJ, Grazziutti ML, Rex JH, et al: The potential role of cytokine therapy for fungal infections in patients with cancer: is recovery from neutropenia all that is needed? *Clin Infect Dis* 26:1270–1278, 1998
44. Engelking C, Rutledge D, Ippoliti C, et al: Cancer related diarrhea: a neglected cause of cancer-related symptom distress. *Oncol Nurs Forum* 25:859–860, 1998
45. Hogan CM: The nurse's role in diarrhea management. *Oncol Nurs Forum* 25:879–886, 1998
46. Cope DG: Management of chemotherapy-induced diarrhea and constipation. *Nurs Clin North Am* 36:695–707, 2001
47. Viele CS: Overview of chemotherapy-induced diarrhea. *Semin Oncol Nurs* 19(suppl 3):2–5, 2003
48. Stern J, Ippoliti C: Management of acute cancer treatment-induced diarrhea. *Semin Oncol Nurs* 19(suppl 3):11–16, 2003
49. Vickery G: Basics of constipation. *Gastroenterol Nurs* 20:125–128, 1997
50. Campos D, Pereira JR, Reinhardt RR, et al: Prevention of cisplatin-induced emesis by the oral neurokinin-1 antagonist, MK 869, in combination with granisetron and dexamethasone or with dexamethasone alone. *J Clin Oncol* 19:1759–1767, 2001
51. Roscoe JA, Morrow GR, Hickok JT, et al: Nausea and vomiting remain a significant clinical problem: trends over time in controlling chemotherapy-induced nausea and vomiting in 1413 patients treated in community clinical practices. *J Pain Symptom Manage* 20:113–121, 2000
52. Osoba D, Zee B, Pater J, et al: Determinants of post chemotherapy nausea and vomiting in patients with cancer. *J Clin Oncol* 15:116–123, 1997
53. Eckert RM: Understanding anticipatory nausea. *Oncol Nurs Forum* 28:1553–1558, 2001
54. Marek C: Antiemetic therapy in patients receiving cancer chemotherapy. *Oncol Nurs Forum* 30:259–271, 2003
55. Dibble SL, Israel J, Nussey B, et al: Delayed chemotherapy-induced nausea in women treated for breast cancer. *Oncol Nurs Forum* 30: E40–E47, 2003
56. Malik IA, Khan WA, Qazilbash M: Clinical efficacy of lorazepam in prophylaxis of anticipatory, acute, and delayed nausea and vomiting induced by high doses of cisplatin. *Am J Clin Oncol* 18:170–175, 1995
57. Hesketh PJ, Kris MG, Grunberg SM, et al: Proposal for classifying the acute emetogenicity of cancer chemotherapy. *J Clin Oncol* 15:103–109, 1997
58. Wickham R: Nausea and vomiting, in Yarbro CH, Frogge MH, Goodman M (eds.): *Cancer Symptom Management* (ed 3). Sudbury, MA, Jones and Bartlett, 2004, pp 187–207
59. Koeller JM, Aapro MS, Gralla RJ, et al: Antiemetic guidelines: creating a more practical treatment approach. *Support Care Cancer* 10:519–522, 2002
60. Cope D: Oncology patient evidenced-based notes (OPEN): antiemetics for chemotherapy induced nausea and vomiting. *Clin J Oncol Nurs* 7:461–462, 2003
61. Gralla R, Lichinitser M, Vander Vegt S, et al: Palonosetron improves prevention of chemotherapy-induced nausea and vomiting following moderately emetogenic chemotherapy: results of a double-blind randomized phase III trial comparing single doses of palonosetron with ondansetron. *Ann Oncol* 14:1570–1577, 2003
62. Eisenbury P, Figueroa-Vadillo J, Zamora R, et al: Improved prevention of moderately emetogenic chemotherapy-induced nausea and vomiting with palonosetron, a pharmacologically novel 5–HT3 receptor antagonists. *Cancer* 98:2473–2482, 2003
63. Hesketh PJ, Grunberg SM, Gralla RJ, et al: The oral neurokinin-1 antagonist aprepitant for the prevention of chemotherapy-induced nausea and vomiting: a multinational, randomized, double-blind, placebo-controlled trial in patients receiving high-dose cisplatin — the aprepitant protocol 052 study group. *J Clin Oncol* 21:4112–4119, 2003
64. Patel L, Lindley C: Aprepitant — a novel NK1 receptor antagonist. *Expert Opin Pharmacother* 4:2279–2296, 2003
65. Hoffman HT: Oral mucositis: a challenging complication of radiotherapy, chemotherapy, and radiochemotherapy: part 1, pathogenesis and prophylaxis of mucositis. *Head Neck* 25:1057–1070, 2003
66. Rogers BB: Mucositis in the oncology patient. *Nurs Clin North Am* 36:745–760, 2001
67. Kostler WJ, Hejna M, Wenzel C, et al: Oral mucositis complicating chemotherapy and/or radiotherapy: options for prevention and treatment. *CA Cancer J Clin* 51:290–315, 2001
68. Wojtaszek C: Management of chemotherapy-induced stomatitis. *Clin J Oncol Nurs* 4:263–270, 2000
69. Innocenti M: Efficacy of gelclair in reducing pain in palliative care patients with oral lesions: preliminary findings from an open pilot study. *J Pain Symptom Manage* 24:456–457, 2000
70. Massler CF: Prevention and treating the oral complications of cancer therapy. *Dentistry General* 48:652–655, 2000
71. Sherry VW: Taste alterations among patients with cancer. *Clin J Oncol Nurs* 6:73–77, 2001
72. Wickham R, Rehwaldlt M, Kefer C, et al: Taste changes experienced by patients receiving chemotherapy. *Oncol Nurs Forum* 26:697–706, 1999
73. Gallagher J: Management of cutaneous symptoms. *Semin Oncol Nurs* 11:239–247, 1995
74. Remlinger KA: Cutaneous reactions to chemotherapy drugs. *Arch Dermatol* 139:77–81, 2003
75. Ottaiano S, Tambaro R, Greggi S, et al: Safety of cisplatin after severe hypersensitivity reactions to carboplatin in patients with recurrent ovarian carcinoma. *Anticancer Res* 23:3465–3478, 2003
76. Brandi G, Pantaleo MA, Galli C, et al: Hypersensitivity reactions related to oxaliplatin. *Br J Cancer* 89:477–481, 2003
77. Armstrong T, Rust D, Kohtz JR: Neurological, pulmonary, and cutaneous toxicities of high dose chemotherapy. *Oncol Nurs Forum* 24(suppl):23–33, 1997
78. Eich D, Scharffetter-Kochanck K, Eich HT, et al: Acral erythrodysesthesia syndrome caused by intravenous infusion of docetaxel in breast cancer. *Am J Clin Oncol* 25:599–602, 2002
79. Botchkarev VA: Molecular mechanisms of chemotherapy-induced hair loss. *J Investig Dermatol Symp Pro* 8:72–75, 2003
80. Keefe DL: Anthracycline-induced cardiomyopathy. *Semin Oncol* 28(suppl 12):2–7, 2001
81. Loerzel VW, Dow KH: Cardiac toxicity related to cancer treatment. *Clin J Oncol Nurs* 7:557–562, 2003
82. Pai VB, Nahata MC: Cardiotoxicity of chemotherapeutic agents: incidence, treatment, and prevention. *Drug Safety* 22:263–302, 2000
83. Kozluca O, Olcay E, Surucu S, et al: Prevention of doxorubicin induced cardiotoxicity by catechin. *Cancer Lett* 99:1–6, 1996
84. Dobric S, Dragojevic-Simic V, Bokonjic D, et al: The efficacy of selenium, WR–2721, and their combination in the prevention of adriamycin-induced cardiotoxicity in rats. *J Environ Pathol Toxicol Oncol* 17:291–299, 1998
85. Tsavaris N, Kosmas C, Vadiaka M, et al: Cardiotoxicity following different doses and schedules for 5-fluorouracil administration for malignancy — a survey of 427 patients. *Med Sci Monitoring* 8:151–157, 2002

86. Soe MS, Berkman A, Mardelli, J: Case report: paclitaxel-induced myocardial ischemia. *Med J* 45:41–43, 1996
87. Grande AM, Rinaldi M, Sinelli S, et al: Heart transplantation in chemotherapeutic dilated cardiomyopathy. *Transplant Proc* 35:1516–1518, 2003
88. Verstappen CC, Heimans JJ, Hoekman K, et al: Neurotoxic complications of chemotherapy in patients with cancer. *Drugs* 63:1549–1563, 2003
89. Plotkin SR, Wen PY: Neurologic complications of cancer therapy. *Neurol Clin North Am* 21:279–318, 2003
90. Berger T, Malayeri R, Doppelbauer A: Neurological monitoring of neurotoxicity induced by paclitaxel/cisplatin chemotherapy. *Eur J Cancer* 33:1393–1399, 1997
91. Perry JR, Warner E: Transient encephalopathy after paclitaxel (Taxol) infusion. *Neurology* 46:1596–1599, 1996
92. Abid SH, Malhotra V, Perry MC: Radiation-induced and chemotherapy-induced pulmonary injury. *Curr Opin Oncol* 13:242–248, 2001
93. Chap L, Shpiner R, Levine M, et al: Pulmonary toxicity of high-dose chemotherapy for breast cancer: a non-invasive approach to diagnosis and treatment. *Bone Marrow Transplant* 20:1063–1067, 1997
94. Sleijfer S: Bleomycin-induced pneumonitis. *Chest* 120:617–624, 2001
95. Cannon GW: Methotrexate pulmonary toxicity. *Rheum Dis Clin North Am* 23:917–937, 1997
96. Pavlakis N, Bell DR, Millward MJ, Levi JA: Fatal pulmonary toxicity resulting from treatment with gemcitabine. *Cancer* 80:286–291, 1997
97. Santamauro JT, Stover DE, Jules-Elysee K, et al: Lung transplantation for chemotherapy-induced pulmonary fibrosis. *Chest* 105:310–312, 1994
98. West SG: Methotrexate hepatotoxicity. *Rheum Dis Clin North Am* 23:883–915, 1997
99. Markman M, Kennedy A, Webster K, et al: Continuous subcutaneous administration of mesna to prevent ifosfamide-induced hemorrhagic cystitis. *Semin Oncol* 23(suppl 6):97–98, 1996
100. West NJ: Prevention and treatment of hemorrhagic cystitis. *Pharmacotherapy* 17:696–706, 1997
101. Islam R, Isaacson BJ, Zickerman PM, et al: Hemorrhagic cystitis as an unexpected adverse reaction to temozolomide: case report. *Am J Clin Oncol* 25:513–514, 2002
102. Kintzel PE: Anticancer drug-induced kidney disorders. *Drug Safety* 24:19–38, 2001
103. Choudhury D, Ahmed Z: Drug-induced nephrotoxicity. *Med Clin North Am* 81:705–717, 1997
104. Viele CS, Holmes BC: Amifostine: drug profile and nursing implications of the first pancytoprotectant. *Oncol Nurs Forum* 25:515–523, 1998
105. Alberts DS, Bleyer WA: Future development of amifostine in treatment. *Semin Oncol* 23(suppl 8):90–99, 1996

CHAPTER 18

Principles of Bone Marrow and Hematopoietic Cell Transplantation

Tammy Baltic, MS, RN, AOCN®
Marie Bakitas, MS, ARNP, AOCN, FAAN®

Introduction

Bone marrow transplantation (BMT) is now all but an historical term given the significant changes in conceptualization and terminology used to describe a treatment originally designed to cure disorders of the hematopoietic system. Rarely is "bone marrow" tissue actually transplanted to repair the diseased or dysfunctional hematopoietic system of persons with malignant and nonmalignant diseases. Rather, advances in technology have allowed an apheresis process, similar to donating a unit of blood, to become the major method of acquiring or "harvesting" hematopoietic "seeds" — the pluripotential stem cells. These cells, acquired from a healthy related or unrelated volunteer donor or the patient, are used in a variety of ways to aid in the cure or control of disease.

This chapter describes historical developments that have led to the current treatment traditionally known as BMT. Advances in science have led to broadened treatment indications and the development of practice and treatment standards for this therapeutic approach. The healthcare economic environment has also influenced current and likely future directions in transplantation. Recognizing this fact, the chapter concludes with a discussion of financial and reimbursement trends that have resulted in changes in care such as the movement of transplantation to the outpatient clinic and home. The transplant procedure is described in Chapter 19, and Chapter 20 discusses the acute and long-term effects of transplantation and nursing care.

The ABCs of Bone Marrow Transplantation

For clarity and consistency, a brief discussion of transplant terminology is important. Human bone marrow was the material previously used for transplantation — hence the acronym BMT. The term *autologous* resulted in the acronym ABMT and was used when an individual served as his or her own source of marrow. Discovery of the presence of hematopoietic stem cells in peripheral circulation, similar to those harvested from the bone marrow, led to the nomenclature *peripheral blood stem cell* (PBSC). However, due to the lack of worldwide scientific agreement on a single terminology, regional differences in language complicate the plethora of labels and acronyms referring to similar treatments formerly known as BMT. Common terms include peripheral blood stem cell transplantation (PBSCT), blood cell transplantation (BCT), blood and marrow transplant, and high-dose therapy with stem cell "rescue." More recently, the broad term hematopoietic cell transplantation (HCT) has gained acceptance.[1]

This confusing transplant terminology presents challenges to professionals as well as to patients and families who are trying to comprehend the type of treatment they are to receive and the goals of treatment. Use of the word *transplant* itself has led to confusion. For instance, in *traditional* BMT, healthy bone marrow was removed from a donor (allogeneic) and given to a patient with a bone marrow disease (e.g., leukemia) or a marrow defect (aplastic anemia) to replace the defective organ. This particular situation was truly a *transplant.*

When a tissue-compatible healthy donor was not available, control of the disease was sometimes possible by removal of the person's own bone marrow (autologous). Autologous marrow was purged of malignant cells with agents like chemotherapy or biological response modifiers and returned to the patient. In this case, the intent was also to replace the diseased hematopoietic organ with a presumably healthier one. Nevertheless, autologous marrow was not really *transplanted* but rather reinfused.

Concurrent with the development of autologous marrow removal and reinfusion technology was the advent of high-dose or dose-intensive chemotherapy regimens to cure previously incurable cancers like neuroblastoma.[2] The term *rescue* was used to indicate how this new procedure prevented treatment-related, lethal hematopoietic complications such as irreversible bone marrow destruction, immunosuppression, and fatal sepsis. The advent of autologous marrow rescue or support procedures signaled a new era in the field of transplantation for patients with both hematological and solid tumors. Today, patients with incurable cancers can safely receive potentially curative doses of chemotherapy and radiation therapy, while sparing their marrow from destruction.

Finally, the source of hematopoietic stem cells has evolved from being marrow derived (BMT) to being obtained primarily by pheresis from peripheral circulation (PBSCT). Most procedures known as BMTs involve neither bone marrow cells nor transplants. In fact, stem cells from healthy donors are obtained more frequently from peripheral blood than from the bone marrow.[3] For the remaining discussion in this chapter, the terms *transplantation* and HCT will be used regardless of whether stem cells are obtained from marrow or peripheral blood and administered for replacement. The terms *rescue* or *support* will be used rather than *transplant* when referring to the enhancement of a normal hematopoietic system following high-dose therapy.

Historical Developments

The notion of using bone marrow to treat patients with blood disorders dates back to the late nineteenth century, with the first reports describing bone marrow extract being given by mouth to patients with anemia. Over the next 50 years, sporadic attempts were made to use bone marrow orally, intramuscularly, and intravenously to treat anemia and leukemia. Figure 18-1 offers a timeline of developments in transplantation.

After World War II and detonation of the first nuclear bombs, interest in ameliorating the effects of radiation increased. In 1951, Jacobson et al. observed that lethally irradiated mice could survive if given an intraperitoneal injection of cells from the spleen.[4] Further studies that same year demonstrated the same result with an infusion of intravenous bone marrow from the animal's twin,[5] confirming that the recovery of marrow function was a result of the colonization of the transplanted marrow cells. Despite marrow recovery, death ensued due to severe diarrhea, weight loss, and skin lesions.[6] This so called *secondary disease* is now known to have been graft-versus-host disease (GVHD).

Based on this experience with animals, patients with leukemia were given high doses of radiation to treat their leukemia and infused with healthy donor marrow in an attempt to cure them. In 1957, Thomas et al. reported a successful human BMT and transient engraftment.[7] However, these early attempts at BMT were done without knowledge of tissue typing or GVHD and the results ultimately proved disappointing. After initial enthusiasm, attempts at human transplantation were largely abandoned.

Even so, animal—primarily canine—research continued and led to early understanding of the genetics of the histocompatibility system and development of immunosuppressive drugs to treat GVHD.[8] Understanding histocompatibility was crucial to success in transplantation. This knowledge led to human leukocyte antigen (HLA) typing, which allowed selection of appropriate donors and reduction in the incidence of GVHD resulting from poorly matched transplants. In 1963, the first BMT in a patient with leukemia with engraftment and survival for more than 1 year was reported.[9]

The modern era of transplantation is generally agreed to date from the late 1960s and early 1970s. Advances in supportive care including antibiotics, platelet collection and transfusion, and isolation techniques led to improved outcomes in transplant.[8] The Hickman catheter was developed to facilitate frequent and prolonged venous access.[10] Patients with aplastic anemia and leukemia were treated and cured with cyclophosphamide, with or without total body irradiation, and HCT.[8]

The last two decades have seen major changes in the field of transplantation. The use of peripheral blood, rather than bone marrow, as a source of stem cells has dramatically changed the way transplants are performed. The ability to cryopreserve peripherally derived stem cells and their ability to reconstitute the hematopoietic system more quickly than bone marrow have contributed to the increase in the use of autologous stem cell rescue.[2,11,12] In addition, peripheral blood stem cells are also being used in allogeneic transplants,[3] which allows for the collection of donor stem cells without the risks of an operative procedure. Peripheral blood stem cell collection contains a higher number of $CD34^+$ cells (stem cells) and T cells (immune cells responsible for GVHD) than bone marrow. Therefore, peripherally derived stem cells are expected to engraft sooner and hence lower the risk for life-threatening infections.

Umbilical cord blood is also used as a stem cell source.[13–15] However, use of cord blood in the adult population has been associated with slower engraftment and a higher rate of graft failure.[11] As a consequence, this treatment approach is primarily used in the pediatric transplant population.[12]

The use of colony-stimulating factors (CSF), such as granulocyte and granulocyte-macrophage colony-stimulating factors (G-CSF and GM-CSF), to facilitate collection of hematopoietic cells and to shorten the period of myelosuppression following transplant has had a significant effect on the safety, cost, and numbers of transplants performed.[16,17] Research has led to the investigation of many different CSFs (stem cell factor and interleukin-1, -3 and -6) that may improve mobilization and collection of stem cells. Ex vivo expansion to grow stem cell colonies may decrease the number of stem cell collections required, increase the number of mature post-progenitor cells (thereby reducing the duration of myelosuppression following high-dose chemotherapy), and generate populations of specific cells (dendritic cells) that may be used as adoptive immunotherapy after transplant.[18,19]

Major research issues concerning allogeneic transplant include improving conditioning regimens to reduce relapse rates from malignant disease, improving GVHD prevention and treatment, and improving prevention and treatment of infectious complications. With improvements in management of GVHD, which is a greater risk in unrelated donor transplant, the use of unrelated donors for allogeneic transplant has dramatically increased.[20] More recently, in an attempt to exploit the graft-versus-disease effect (described later) and explore the efficacy and feasibility of transplant for older patients or younger patients with co-morbid conditions, a nonmyeloablative transplantation approach has been used.[21]

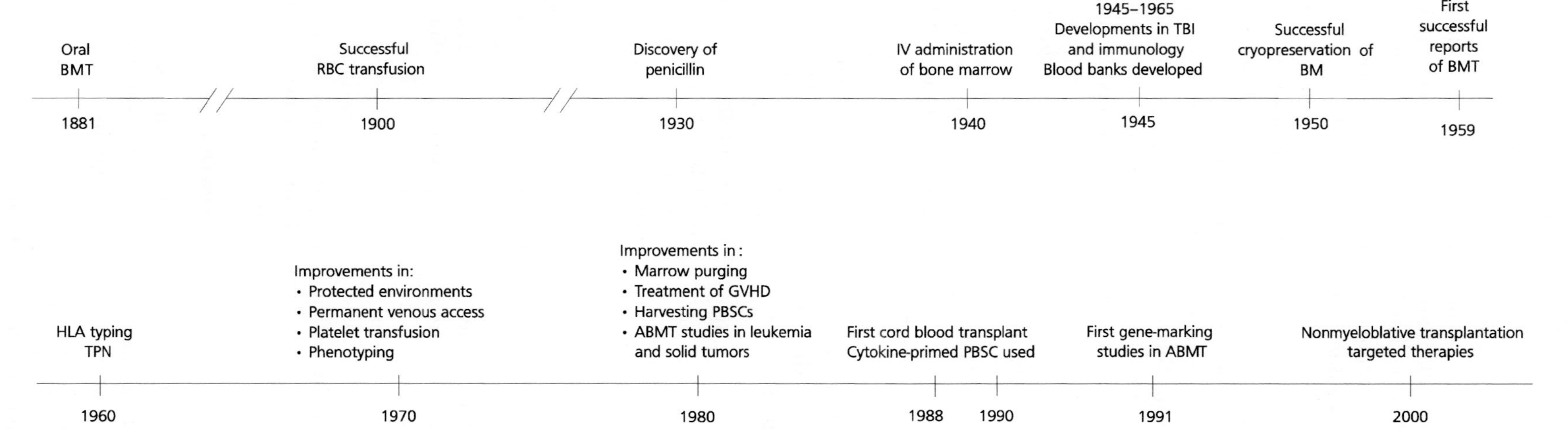

Figure 18-1 Time line to transplantation. (BMT = bone marrow transplant; RBC = red blood cell; IV = intravenous; TBI = total body irradiation; BM = bone marrow; HLA = human leukocyte antigen; TPN = total parenteral nutrition; GVHD = graft-versus-host disease; PBSC = peripheral blood stem cells; ABMT = autologous bone marrow transplantation)

In the ongoing attempt to reduce mortality associated with conditioning regimens and disease relapse, new targeted therapies have been incorporated into HCT research. Investigations of the efficacy of using monoclonal antibodies (e.g., rituximab), radioimmunotherapy (e.g., ibritumomab tiuxetan), and antiangiogenic agents (e.g., thalidomide) for transplant are under way. Rituximab is a CD20 targeted monoclonal antibody used in combination with chemotherapy as treatment for some non-Hodgkin's lymphomas (NHL). Clinical trials addressing the efficacy of rituximab as an in vivo purging agent pre-HCT and post-transplant to reduce the incidence of relapse have yielded promising results.[22–24] Radioimmunotherapy is a technique that attaches a radioisotope to a monoclonal antibody specific to a disease antigen. This approach allows the monoclonal antibody to deliver radiation directly to the tumor site and could potentially decrease the systemic toxicity associated with HCT preparative regiments.[25] Another targeted approach entails the use of thalidomide post-HCT to prevent disease relapse in multiple myeloma.[26]

Types of Transplantation

Different types of HCT are described in terms of the hematopoietic stem cell source: an identical twin (syngeneic), a donor (allogeneic), or the person's own (autologous). For each donor type, the stem cell source can be marrow or peripheral blood. Figure 18-2 compares relative numbers of allogeneic and autologous transplants worldwide since 1970.[27] Umbilical cord blood is another potential stem cell source primarily used in the pediatric setting.

Syngeneic

A syngeneic donor is an identical twin of the recipient. Both individuals share identical genes and thus are a perfect HLA match. Sharing identical tissue types may avoid the development and complications of GVHD. However, the risk of relapse is greater in patients who receive transplant for leukemia because of the lack of the graft-versus-disease effect.[28]

Allogeneic

Allogeneic transplant involves the removal of stem cells from a donor, which are then infused into the person with the disease. Allogeneic HCTs were originally done for bone marrow failure (e.g., aplastic anemia) or malignancy (e.g., leukemia). Allogeneic donors can be related or unrelated to the recipient. Because complications are reduced, the closer the HLA match between donor and recipient, the better. Indeed, an identical HLA match is the best scenario. The genes encoding the HLA are inherited, so the patient's family members (usually the siblings) are typed to determine how closely their HLA profile matches that of the patient. HLA typing involves taking a blood sample to test for these antigens on the surface of the blood lymphocytes.

A related donor is preferred because while the HLA system characterizes major histocompatibility antigens, minor antigens also exist that are not yet identifiable. A relative has a greater chance than an unrelated donor of sharing these minor antigens; thus the ideal donor is an HLA-identical relative.[29] However, given the small average family size in the United States, an individual has only a 35% chance of having an HLA-matched sibling.[30] A partially matched sibling or other family member can also serve as a donor, depending on the degree and character of the match.

If the patient does not have a suitable family donor, a search for an unrelated donor can be undertaken. The National Marrow Donor Program (NMDP), a donor registry developed in 1986, allows patients without a related donor to find an HLA-matched or partially matched unrelated donor. Approximately 8 million people have been registered as potential unrelated donors through 49 registries worldwide.[31] Although morbidity and mortality are generally greater in unrelated donor transplants (largely due to GVHD), the number of these transplants is increasing. Because HLA type is linked to ethnic origin and minorities are underrepresented in transplant registries, a major goal of the NMDP is to evaluate HLA type in more members of ethnic minorities. On a larger section, the NMDP collects HLA phenotypes of volunteer donors (stem cells and cord blood) and coordinates distribution of the products worldwide. Currently, there are 53 stem cell donor registries in 37 countries and 36 cord blood registries in 21 countries (*www.bmdw.org*).

The source of allogeneic stem cells, regardless of the donor, has historically been bone marrow. With the successful use of PBSCs in autologous transplant, these cells' use in allogeneic transplant has increased and continues to be investigated.[32] Advantages and disadvantages of using PBSCs in allogeneic transplants include:

Advantages

1. Shorter duration of myelosuppression, resulting in fewer transfusions; fewer bacterial, viral, and fungal infections; decreased use of antibiotic, antiviral, and antifungal agents; and potentially fewer deaths related to infection
2. Shorter length of hospitalization and lower costs

3. Decreased risk of developing acute GVHD compared to bone marrow as a stem cell source
4. Less donor morbidity, because an operative procedure is avoided

Disadvantages

1. Possible increased incidence of chronic GVHD related to the higher number of T cells in the PBSC product
2. Lack of data on the risk of using CSFs to mobilize stem cells in donors

The mid- to late 1990s brought research regarding the allogeneic nonmyeloablative transplant (Figure 18-3).[21,33] In nonmyeloablative transplant, low doses of total body irradiation and/or chemotherapy are administered to suppress the recipient's immune system. This conditioning regimen is followed by an infusion of PBSCs from a suitable donor. The infusion of the donor cells results in a mix of donor/recipient cells or a mixed chimerism. The nonmyeloablative approach is used to exploit a graft-versus-disease effect, a reaction that occurs when the donor graft recognizes residual recipient diseased cells (e.g., leukemia, multiple myeloma, etc.) as foreign and destroys them. This technique decreases the morbidity and mortality that occurs with myeloablative HCT. Complications of the nonmyeloablative preparative regimen are significantly reduced. As a consequence, older patients and younger patients with co-morbid conditions, who otherwise would not be candidates for HCT, can consider transplant as a treatment option. For diseases that do not respond well to high-dose chemotherapy, such as multiple myeloma and renal cell carcinoma, the nonmyeloablative approach with its graft (donor cells) versus disease effect, may prove beneficial[21,34]

Autologous

When the stem cell donor is the patient, the transplant is termed *autologous.* Autologous stem cells, collected and cryopreserved, are used as a rescue following dose-intensive chemotherapy, with or without radiation therapy that would otherwise be lethal to the hematopoietic system. Early autologous transplants used harvested bone marrow from the patient. In the early 1980s, however, it was found that stem cells also circulated in the peripheral blood, albeit in small numbers. The ability of PBSCs to restore hematopoiesis just as well and more quickly than bone marrow–derived stem cells caused this approach to become the major transplant technique used.[20]

Determining the number of stem cells needed to reliably reconstitute bone marrow function has been an active area of research. A number of techniques have been used. Cells with the CD34 antigen include committed hematopoietic progenitor cells as well as pluripotential stem cells.[35] Many transplant centers now use the number of $CD34^+$ cells present to determine whether adequate colonies are available to reconstitute hematopoiesis.[36] Studies have shown that infusion of 5×10^6 $CD34^+$ cells/kilogram (or more) reduces the time to platelet and neutrophil recovery.[17,35,37]

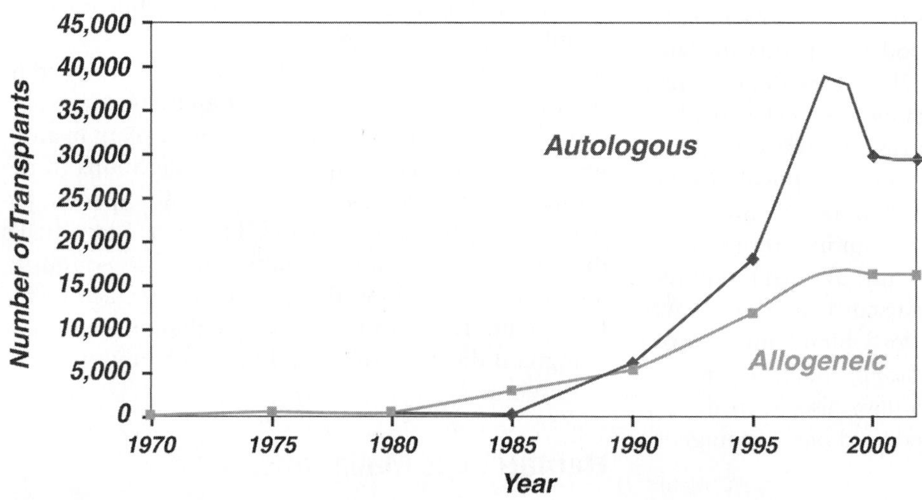

Figure 18-2 Annual numbers of blood and marrow transplants worldwide, 1970–2002. (Reprinted with permission from Loberiza F: Report on state of the art in blood and marrow transplantation – Part I of the IBMTR/ABMTR summary slides with guide. *Newsletter* 10:7, 2003.[27])

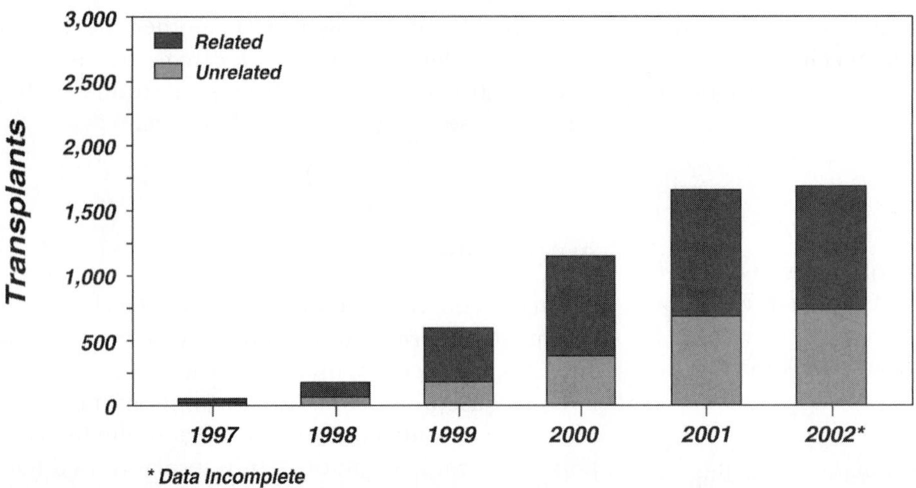

Figure 18-3 Nonmyeloablative allotransplants registered with the IBMTR, 1997–2002. (Reprinted with permission from Loberiza F: Report on state of the art in blood and marrow transplantation – part I of the IBMTR/ABMTR summary slides with guide. *Newsletter* 10:7, 2003.[27])

Umbilical Cord Blood

The presence of hematopoietic stem cells in umbilical cord blood was first reported in 1974.[38] Cord blood was first proposed as a possible stem cell source for transplant in the 1980s.[39] Currently, umbilical cord blood is used as a stem cell source for both related and unrelated donor transplants.

Cord blood represents a stem cell source that is abundant, correlated with lower infectious disease and tumor contamination risk, and associated with less GVHD.[40] Although the incidence of acute GVHD with cord blood appears no higher than with other stem cell sources, the incidence of chronic GVHD is unknown.[40,41] A disadvantage to the use of cord blood is the reality that the stem cell numbers may not be sufficient to restore hematopoiesis in adults (≥60–70 kg); for this reason, most cord blood transplants to date have been done in children. The ex vivo expansion and cryopreservation of cord blood stem cells are also being explored in view of their use in adults.[13]

Umbilical cord blood presents the possibility of greatly increasing the pool of donors for unrelated transplants as well as increasing minority representation in donor registries.[41] Currently, 37 cord blood registries from 21 countries provide cord blood units. As of 2002, more than 120,000 cord blood units were available worldwide (*www.bmdw.org*). Several private, commercial cord blood banks have also been developed for autologous and related cord blood storage.[15]

Transplantation Indications and Outcomes

Original indications for transplant comprised aplastic anemia or leukemias that were treated with syngeneic or allogeneic BMT. Although these diseases and acquired hematologic disorders are still treated with transplantation, the indications for transplant have expanded significantly over the last two decades. Figure 18-4 compares allogeneic and autologous transplants for different diseases performed in 2002.[27] Other indications for allogeneic transplantation include nonmalignant inherited diseases such as immunodeficiency disorders, sickle cell disease, storage diseases, thalassemia, and Fanconi's anemia. Currently investigation is treatment of some congenital disorders while the fetus is still in utero.

Most transplants are autologous and performed to treat a variety of solid tumors.[20] Researchers are also investigating the role of autologous transplant in autoimmune disorders.[20] Important considerations in determining the role of transplantation for specific patients are prognostic factors for that individual's disease, the timing of transplant in the disease course, and consideration of the patient's risk factors for transplant. Table 18-1 describes malignant and nonmalignant diseases treated with transplantation.

Hematologic Malignancies

Leukemias continue to be the most frequent diagnosis treated with allogeneic transplant.[20] HCT is the only potentially curative therapy for patients with acute myelogenous leukemia (AML) who fail induction

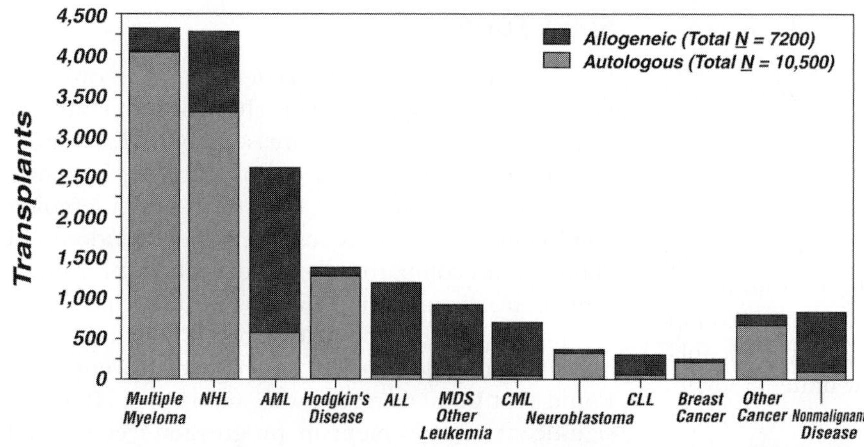

Figure 18-4 Indications for blood and marrow transplantation in North America, 2002. (AML = acute myelogenous leukemia; CML = chronic myelogenous leukemia; ALL = acute lymphocytic leukemia; MDS = myelodysplastic syndrome.) (Reprinted with permission from Loberiza F: Report on state of the art in blood and marrow transplantation – Part I of the IBMTR/ABMTR summary slides with guide. *Newsletter* 10:7, 2003.[27])

therapy. The best outcomes for allogeneic transplant are achieved in first complete remission; the five-year overall survival rate of 62% for patients in first complete remission is compared to a rate of 26% for patients experiencing a second complete remission or first relapse.[8] Compared to allogeneic transplant, autologous transplant results in a higher relapse rate but lower rate of treatment-associated mortality. Allogeneic transplant appears to have an advantage over autologous transplant when used in first remission for individuals with high-risk disease; results are comparable for allogeneic and autologous transplant in second remission.[30,31]

Acute lymphocytic leukemia (ALL) is the most common childhood leukemia. Allogeneic transplant is indicated in second remission and in first remission for children with poor prognostic features. In adults, the indications are similar to those in children: Allogeneic HCT remains the most effective therapy following initial relapse and is generally recommended for adults with high-risk disease (Philadelphia chromosome positive).[30] Autologous transplant is used in ALL for older patients and for those lacking a suitable donor, but relapse rates are much higher than with allogeneic transplant.

The introduction of imatinib mesylate (Gleevec), a targeted agent for treatment of chronic myelogenous leukemia (CML), marked a new era for the treatment of this disease.[42] While imatinib mesylate is not a cure for CML, it does provide sustained remissions for some patients. In first chronic phase CML, imatinib mesylate yields a complete hematological remission rate of 98%, although this rate drops to 8% for patients in blast crisis.[43] Despite these promising results, allogeneic HCT remains the only cure for CML. Patients who receive transplants in the early chronic phase within one year of diagnosis have the best outcomes. However, because the median age at diagnosis for CML is 60–65 years, patients may be ineligible for allogeneic HCT because of age and/or co-morbid conditions. Transplantation in later stages of CML

Table 18-1 Diseases Treated with Transplantation

Malignant Diseases	Nonmalignant Diseases
Hematologic malignancies	Hematologic disorders
Acute lymphocytic leukemia	Severe aplastic anemia
Acute myelogenous leukemia	Diamond-Blackfan anemia
Chronic lymphocytic leukemia	Fanconi's anemia
Chronic myelogenous leukemia	Sickle cell anemia
Myelodysplastic syndrome	Beta thalassemia major
Monosomy-7 syndrome	Chédiak-Hagashi syndrome
Non-Hodgkin's lymphoma	Chronic granulomatous disease
Hodgkin's lymphoma	Congenital neutropenia
Multiple myeloma	Reticular dysgenesis
Solid tumors	Congenital immunodeficiencies
Brain tumor	Severe combined immunodeficiency (SCID)
Testicular germ cell tumors	Wiskott-Aldrich syndrome
Breast cancer	Functional T-cell deficiency
Lung cancer	Mucopolysaccharidoses
Ovarian cancer	Hurler's disease
Melanoma	Hunter's disease
Sarcoma	Sanfilippo syndrome
Gastrointestinal tract cancer	Morquio syndrome
	Lipidoses
	Adrenoleukodystrophy
	Methachromatic leukodystrophy
	Gaucher disease
	Miscellaneous
	Osteopetrosis
	Langerhan cell histiocytosis
	Lesch-Nylan syndrome
	Glycogen storage diseases

(accelerated and blast phase) is associated with worse outcomes. Autologous transplant for CML, although not curative, may be associated with longer survival than conventional chemotherapy.[44]

The use of transplantation in chronic lymphocytic leukemia (CLL) is relatively new. Because it is largely a disease of older adults and often has an indolent course, conservative therapy has been the traditional approach. Given the decrease in the morbidity and mortality associated with transplant and the development of new drugs with activity in CLL, nonmyeloablative allogeneic transplantation is now under study for this indication.[45]

Patients with relapsed or resistant intermediate- and high-grade non-Hodgkin's lymphoma and relapsed/refractory Hodgkin's disease are candidates for transplantation. Patients whose tumors remain sensitive to chemotherapy and are treated with high-dose chemotherapy and stem cell rescue have a 40%–60% chance of 5-year disease-free survival.[31,46] Low-grade lymphoma, like CLL, is often a slowly progressive disease and has been managed conservatively in the past. Controversy persists over whether autologous transplant prolongs disease-free survival as compared with standard chemotherapy. Allogeneic transplant has been reserved for advanced low-grade lymphoma and shows promising disease-free survival rates.[45]

Myelodysplastic syndrome (MDS) and myeloproliferative disorders represent a variety of clonal hematopoietic diseases.[47] Allogeneic HCT is the only curative therapy available for myelodysplasia but is usually reserved for patients younger than age 55 with excess blasts or complex cytogenetic abnormalities.[47] Autologous HCT for MDS is also under investigation.[47] Allogeneic transplantation is an option for myeloproliferative disorders, primarily angiagenic myeloid metaplasia (myelofibrosis), and essential thrombocytopenia and polycythemia vera that does not respond to conventional therapy.

Transplantation is being increasingly used to treat multiple myeloma, a disease that cannot be cured with standard chemotherapy. Results of a randomized trial comparing high-dose chemotherapy and autologous HCT to conventional chemotherapy in multiple myeloma demonstrated that high-dose therapy with autologous HCT significantly improved disease-free and overall survival.[48–50] Allogeneic HCT is curative for some patients with advanced multiple myeloma.[51,52] This approach has high treatment-related mortality, however, and is generally reserved for patients who are younger than 50 years of age. Focus is now on the nonmyeloablative approach with the goal of decreasing toxicity and adding the advantage of the graft-versus-tumor effect.[26]

Solid Tumors

In the early 1990s, much excitement arose over the possibility of using autologous HCT for the treatment of solid tumors, specifically breast cancer.[53] Early, nonrandomized studies reported prolonged survival times for women with advanced breast cancer undergoing autologous HCT. Consequently, several randomized clinical trials comparing standard treatment for metastatic breast cancer versus autologous HCT have been performed.[54–60] Unfortunately, results of these trials were not as promising as anticipated. Recent trials found that women treated with autologous HCT had significant improvement in progression-free survival rates at one and two years, but no evidence of benefit in overall survival beyond the two-year period.[61] Follow up from these studies is incomplete because results extend just three to five years post-transplant.

Autologous HCT continues to be explored for use in solid tumors. Although the majority of patients with germ cell tumors are cured with conventional-dose chemotherapy, transplantation is an option for some patients who relapse following first-line chemotherapy.[62] Clinical trials are ongoing to establish the role of autologous HCT in germ cell tumors.[62] High-dose chemotherapy has also been used in brain tumors, neuroblastoma, and small cell lung cancer.[11] For cancers such as melanoma and renal cell that do not respond to high doses of chemotherapy, focus has shifted to the graft-versus-tumor effect with allogeneic HCT. In light of the significant morbidity and mortality associated with myeloablative allogeneic transplant, current clinical trials are investigating a nonmyeloablative approach.[63]

Nonmalignant Diseases

HCT is a novel approach employed in some incurable nonmalignant diseases, such as sickle cell anemia, inborn errors of metabolism, and autoimmune disorders. This treatment strategy arose after researchers realized that patients who underwent transplants for hematological malignancies and who had preexisting autoimmune diseases sometimes experienced a remission of their autoimmune disorders.[3] The mechanisms responsible for this response are not clear, but continue to be explored in animal models.[64] Clinical trials examining the feasibility and outcomes of allogeneic and autologous transplant for severe, life-threatening autoimmune diseases (e.g., rheumatoid arthritis) are being explored.[64] In adults, aplastic anemia is the most common nonmalignant disease treated with HCT.

Table 18-2 Estimated Five-Year Disease-Free Survival (DFS) Following Transplantation

Disease	Stage	Five-Year DFS Allogeneic	Five-Year DFS Autologous
AML	First CR	45%–65%	35%–70%
AML	Second CR	20%–45%	19%–56%
ALL	First CR	45%–60%	20%–50%
ALL	Second CR	20%–40%	0–20%
MDS	Combined	20%–45%	ND
CML	Chronic	60%–75%	50%
CML	Accelerated	30%–45%	25%
CML	Blast crisis	10%–20%	
NHL	First relapse, second CR	30%–50%	45%–60%
HD	First relapse, second CR	10%–30%	40%–60%
MM	Combined	30%–50%	16%–40%
CLL		20%–55%	ND
Germ cell	Recurrent	ND	15%–40%
Brain tumors		ND	13%

ALL = acute lymphocytic leukemia; AML = acute myelogenous leukemia; CLL = chronic lymphocytic leukemia; CML = chronic myelogenous leukemia; CR = complete remission; HD = Hodgkin's disease; MDS = myelodysplastic syndrome; MM = multiple myeloma; ND = no data; NHL = non-Hodgkin's lymphoma.

Outcomes

Cure

The goal for the transplant recipient is cure of the patient's disease. Transplantation is known to be curative in several malignant and nonmalignant disorders. Reductions in treatment-associated mortality have helped to make this outcome possible. Astute nursing care is one factor that can prevent deaths due to treatment complications. Other factors influencing the mortality rate include type and stage of disease at time of transplant, type of transplant (allogeneic versus autologous), degree of HLA match between donor and recipient in allogeneic transplant, age of patient, presence of co-morbid conditions, and experience of the transplant center. Overall, allogeneic transplant has a higher transplant-related mortality risk (20%–30%) than autologous transplant. The autologous transplant-related mortality is less than 5% at most centers.[20] Table 18-2 lists the estimated 5-year disease-free survival rates for various diseases following transplantation.

Even when cured of their original disease, survivors can have disabilities following transplant. (Acute and long-term complications are described in detail in Chapter 20.) Long-term complications that can have the greatest effect on the quality of life post-transplant include chronic GVHD (allogeneic), continued immune dysfunction resulting in infections (especially from chronic GVHD), pulmonary complications from conditioning therapy, reproductive effects, effects on sexual functioning, thyroid dysfunction, and the development of cataracts. Pediatric patients may experience adverse effects on growth and development and learning difficulties in school. The long-term sequelae of autologous transplant are generally less severe given the absence of GVHD and the avoidance, in most conditioning regimens, of the use of total body irradiation.

Nevertheless, allogeneic and autologous transplants share some potential long-term effects, including the risk of cognitive effects and second malignancies. Several studies have demonstrated cognitive deficits prior to transplant in some patients and impairment of cognitive functioning during transplant hospitalization.[65–68] Clinically, patients report difficulty with memory and concentration following transplant. Clearly, further study is needed in this area to delineate the effects of intensive therapy on cognitive functioning.

Secondary malignancies following treatment with chemotherapy and radiation are another potential consequence of transplantation.[65] Lymphoproliferative disorders, solid tumors, leukemia, and myelodysplastic syndrome have all been reported after transplantation. The incidence of solid tumors in one analysis was 6.7% at 15 years after transplantation.[65] For hematological malignancies, estimated incidence ranged from 4% to 18% in 1254 patients following autologous transplantation. Causes are thought to be multifactorial, including conditioning chemotherapy and radiation, immunosuppression, Epstein-Barr virus infection, and GVHD. Transplant patients should be evaluated for the development of secondary malignancies as an integral part of their preventive health care.

Relapse

Relapse of disease following transplant remains a major problem hindering the success of this procedure. Reasons for relapse depend on the stage of disease at transplant and differ between autologous and allogeneic transplants. In general, the later the transplant is performed in the course of a disease, the worse the outcome. Patients with leukemia who receive transplants during relapse have worse outcomes than those who receive transplants during remission. In solid tumors, patients with a minimal tumor burden at time of transplant fare better than those with more disease.

In allogeneic transplant, relapse results from inadequate conditioning therapy that fails to eradicate the cancer. The absence of a sufficient graft-versus-disease effect may also play a role in relapse. For example, syngeneic transplants for leukemia have higher relapse rates than allogeneic transplants, likely due to the former's lack of this effect.

Relapse following allogeneic transplant is very difficult for patients and families because this treatment is often the only hope for curing their disease. However, other possibilities are emerging. Second transplants have been performed for relapsed disease, though the risk of complications is high in such cases. Taking advantage of the graft-versus-disease effect in patients with CML, infusion of donor mononuclear cells can induce a complete remission in the majority of patients with less toxicity than a second transplant.[69] Withdrawal of immunosuppression in an attempt to trigger graft-versus-disease is another option in treating relapsed leukemias after allogeneic transplant.

In autologous transplant, the failure of high dose conditioning regimen to eradicate the tumor (inherent disease resistance) and acquired drug resistance are factors related to relapse. Further autologous transplant lacks the benefit of the graft-versus-disease effect. It is usually not possible to determine whether relapse resulted from insufficient tumor chemosensitivity or a developed drug resistance. Some transplant protocols are now incorporating strategies to overcome drug resistance. Promising post-transplant immunotherapy strategies to reduce disease relapse include the use of cytokines and interleukins (IL-2, IL-12, interferon), ex vivo activated cellular immunotherapy, immunomodulating agents such as cyclosporine and thalidomide, and monoclonal and bispecific antibodies.[22–24,26] Tumor contamination of autologous stem cell product is also a known contributor to relapse. Ways to purge stem cells of malignant cells continue to be investigated. After autologous HCT, second transplant is an option in selected patients, especially those who experience an extended disease-free interval after treatment.

Hematopoietic and Immunologic Concepts of Transplantation

The hematopoietic system and normal immunology are described in Chapters 2 and 29. Major concepts related to transplantation are reviewed here.

Normal Hematopoiesis and Peripheral Blood Stem Cells

The bone marrow contains a supply of all blood cells, from the earliest pluripotential stem cell to mature, fully functional red, white, and megakaryocytic blood cells (Figure 18-5). Although only about 5% of marrow cells are pluripotential stem cells, this amount is capable of dividing and differentiating (under the influence of various cytokines) into all lines of mature blood cells. Hence, an ongoing, lifetime supply of all blood cells necessary to support life is readily available. Exploitation of this principle has enabled stem cell transplantation and reconstitution of hematopoiesis into a recipient devoid of hematopoietic cells.[36] Similarly, removal of an adequate number of pluripotential stem cells from a patient that can then be reinfused following lethal doses of chemotherapy and radiation therapy allows the person to survive.[35,37]

Blood cells express certain antigens (referred to as cell differentiation or cluster designation antigens, or "CD" followed by a number) at different stages of maturation. These antigenic markers provide useful labels for identifying cells of interest. Hematopoietic cells that express (are positive for) the CD34 antigen are called $CD34^+$ (positive). These early cells are of greatest interest in transplantation. They are present at 10–100 times greater frequency in the bone marrow than in the peripheral blood. Moreover, the ability to identify this type of cell, increase its numbers, and separate it from other cells in the circulation allows $CD34^+$ cells to be obtained for transplantation using only minimally invasive harvesting techniques as compared to traditional bone marrow harvesting.[36]

In addition to containing hematopoietic stem cells, the marrow microenvironment must be intact for homing and reconstitution of hematopoiesis to occur. Both the "seed" and the "soil" are important aspects of normal recovery. It is truly remarkable that both marrow and peripherally derived stem cells, after infusion, can locate their appropriate places in the bone marrow. Destruction of marrow architecture by treatment (e.g., radiation) or disease can interfere with the resumption of normal hematopoiesis following stem cell infusion.

Hematopoietic Stem Cells

Mobilization

Hematopoietic stem cells have receptors on their cell walls for various cytokine growth factors. These growth factors, which are made endogenously, and their commercially available counterparts, which are made through recombinant DNA processes, stimulate pluripotential stem cells to differentiate and mature. The products are administered in transplantation and cause the body to overproduce pluripotential stem cells beyond the body's required needs and induce cell differentiation and maturation. Within 2 days of administration of hematopoietic growth factors (HGFs), the number of HSCs increases.[17] The administration of HGFs takes place right before pheresis so

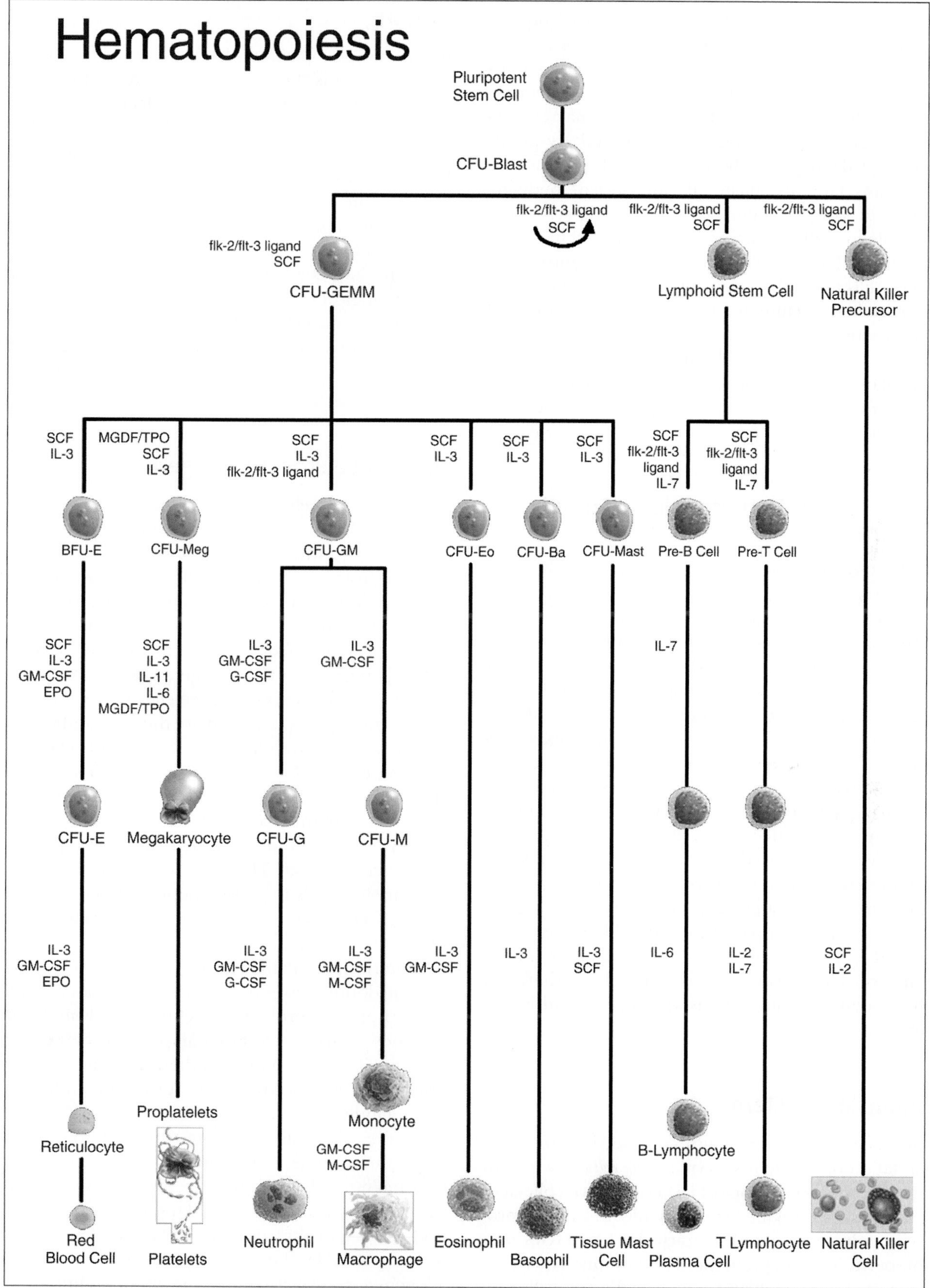

Figure 18-5 Hematopoietic tree. (Reprinted with permission from Amgen, Inc., Thousand Oaks, CA.)

that more cells are available to be collected from the circulation. This process is referred to as *mobilization*.[18]

Administration of chemotherapy (for autologous donors), usually cyclophosphamide, is another method to mobilize stem cells. Following the marrow-suppressive effects of chemotherapy, the body responds (within 2 days) with rebound stem cell production. Physicians take advantage of this normal body response to raise the number of circulating stem cells available for collection. Chemotherapy used in combination with HGFs yields higher numbers of autologous $CD34^+$ cells than administration of HGFs alone.[17] This mobilization technique reduces the number of phereses needed to collect adequate cells for reconstituting hematopoiesis. Mobilization has improved transplantation by making the collection procedure more efficient and the recovery period quicker and safer for the patient.[18]

Recombinant Hematopoietic Growth Factors

Hematopoietic growth factors used for mobilization include stem cell factor, IL-3, G-CSF, and GM-CSF alone or in combination. Collection of peripheral blood progenitor stem cells has been shown to have two effects: (1) It increases the yield of mononuclear cells expressing the CD34 antigen (e.g., $CD34^+$ cells) and other committed progenitor cells collected during pheresis, and (2) it hastens the hematopoietic recovery of the recipient.[17] Hastened recovery of neutrophils and platelets in mobilized cells versus steady-state peripheral stem cells or bone marrow is likely due to the maturational effect of the cytokines on the progenitors. Cytokine-induced maturational effects on some of the early progenitors decrease the normal lag time of cell maturation after infusion. The clinical significance of using cytokine-mobilized PBSCs is a decreased length of time for the patient's nadir (lowest point of blood counts following chemotherapy), which reduces complications of infection and bleeding.[17]

Expansion of Stem Cells

Another technique to obtain cells needed for transplantation or rescue is known as *stem cell expansion*. In this case, a select number of $CD34^+$ cells are collected, and in vitro a cytokine "soup" is added. In an appropriate culture medium, characterized by HGFs and slow perfusion of oxygen, the cells multiply. Thus it becomes possible to expand the few collected cells to a number of cells capable of replacing the adult hematopoietic system.

Purging

A concern of collection of HSCs from either marrow or circulation is the inability to assure that only nonmalignant normal cells will be collected.[31] This concern is especially troubling when harvesting cells from a person with a hematopoietic malignancy such as leukemia. It is also possible to harvest malignant cells metastatic to the bone in solid tumors, even if the patient has undetectable disease. A variety of techniques have been developed to attempt to eradicate these cells from the harvested product. Physical, chemical, and immunological methods are used to destroy or eliminate malignant cells, although it is unclear whether these methods are successful or reduce relapse of disease.[31,70]

Human Leukocyte Antigen

Blood-forming cells, like other human tissues, possess inherited characteristics (antigens) on their cell walls. Like a fingerprint, these antigens are unique to the individual from whom they are derived.[71] Also, just like the inherited characteristics of hair color or height, the HLA-6 antigen code on chromosome 6 (also known as the major histocompatibility complex [MHC]) is a result of a set of genes derived from each parent. Stem cells possess three classes of HLAs. Most important to transplantation are the A, B, and C genes on the class I region, and the D gene (broken down into the three subtypes of DR, DP, and DQ) on the class II region. Class I molecules are found on all nucleated cells of the body, and class II molecules are located primarily on immune cells such as lymphocytes and macrophages.[71] The most important function of these molecules is to present peptides to the immunological T cells so that body cells may be recognized as self.[71]

Determining compatibility between the patient and the donor is essential to the success of an allogeneic transplant. Serological, cellular, and molecular methods are used to test for compatibility between the HLA types of the donor and the recipient. Complications of HLA incompatibility can be life-threatening and include GVHD and rejection.

In the case of allogeneic transplantation, it is generally the immunocompetent donor graft that, after infusion into the immunoincompetent host, recognizes the host as "foreign." This response results in both acute and chronic forms of GVHD. The development of GVHD is the greatest predictor of outcome in allogeneic transplantation. (Prevention, clinical consequences, and treatment of GVHD are discussed in detail in Chapter 20.)

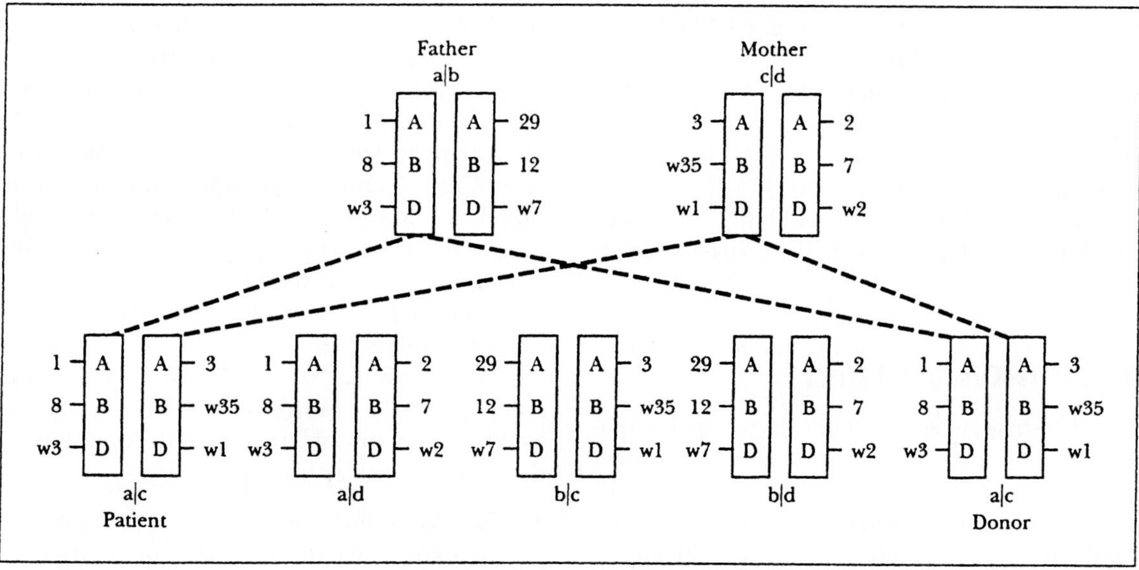

Figure 18-6 Diagram of possible combinations of human leukocyte antigen (HLA) region of chromosome 6 inherited by offspring from parents. The recipient and the donor have inherited the same two haplotypes and are genotypically HLA identical.

Identification of an HLA-compatible donor is a necessary first step in allogeneic transplantation. An identical twin is the most compatible donor for transplantation, as the HLA type is identical. Yet, as previously stated, a syngeneic transplant (twin as donor) poses a higher risk for relapse. The next step is to look within the recipient's immediate family for a donor. There is an approximately 25% chance of a person having an HLA match within his or her immediate family, as illustrated in Figure 18-6.[71] Lacking an acceptable match within the family, a search for a phenotypically compatible match from a volunteer donor registry (e.g., NMDP) is sought. A sample of the recipient's blood is HLA typed and matched by computer (NMDP search software; Translink) against the HLA types of volunteer donors from the registry. A BMT program can obtain the Translink software/training, which enables staff members to enter patient data and generate a report of potential donors in a matter of moments. If an acceptable match is found, the transplant may proceed. If a six-antigen match is not found, less compatible but acceptable matches may be identified. In such cases, the patient may be referred to a specialized center that performs mismatched unrelated transplants. Specialized centers are used because the physiologic consequences of transplanting mismatched stem cells can result in significant acute side effects that require the management of a team specialized in these complications.

Prophylaxis and Treatment of Graft-versus-Host Disease

The better the compatibility between donor and recipient, the lower the incidence and severity of GVHD.[71] Methods used to offset this serious complication include prophylaxis and treatment with immunosuppressive agents and T-cell depletion of the donor stem cell product.

Immunosuppression

Immunosuppressive medications such as cyclosporine, methotrexate, mycophenolate mofetil (MMF), FK506 (Tacrolimus), and steroids are used to prevent or treat GVHD. Immunosuppressive agents blunt the reaction of the newly developed donor immune system and keep it from identifying the host or patient as foreign. These drugs may need to be taken for months to years following an allogeneic transplant. Although this immunosuppression places the patient at prolonged risk for life-threatening bacterial, viral, and fungal infections, more harmful complications of GVHD are minimized or avoided.[72]

T-cell depletion

Under normal immunologic conditions, T cells play a major role in distinguishing self from nonself proteins. In the case of allogeneic transplantation, active donor T cells within the stem cell graft have this same capability. As a result, donor T cells may recognize the recipient tissues as foreign, initiating a GVHD reaction. To avoid or lessen this serious consequence, several methods have been attempted to deplete the donor product of T cells, including physical, immunological, and pharmacological techniques. Regardless of technique, the desired outcome is reduction or elimination of T cells capable of initiating life-threatening GVHD without losing the graft-versus-disease effect.

Graft-versus-Disease Effect

The donor marrow, in addition to causing the complication of GVHD, can exert a beneficial effect against the malignancy. The immunocompetent donor cells can recognize the patient's malignant cells as foreign and eliminate them. This effect was originally identified in leukemia patients. It was observed that relapses occurred less often in patients with GVHD than in patients who did not have this complication. Furthermore, syngeneic or autologous transplants lacking GVHD were noted to have higher relapse rates not only in leukemia but also in other disease types. "Graft-versus-disease effect" refers to this broader phenomenon.[28]

ABO Mismatch

Occasionally, a recipient may receive a HCT from a donor who possesses a different ABO blood type. Effective removal of red blood cells from the stem cell product has enabled successful transplantation in this case. After transplantation, the recipient will have the donor ABO blood type.

Standards for Transplantation

The unprecedented growth of transplant programs outside of established, academic centers in the late 1980s and 1990s raised many questions about the quality of care being provided. In response to this concern, the Foundation for the Accreditation of Cellular Therapy (FACT) was formed in 1996. FACT published *Standards for Hematopoietic Progenitor Cell Collection, Processing, and Transplantation* first in 1996 and then as an updated edition in 2002.[73] FACT standards were developed from and based on work of the International Society for Cellular Therapy (ISCT) and a subcommittee of the Clinical Affairs Committee of the American Society of Blood and Marrow Transplantation (ASBMT). To be considered for accreditation, a program must perform at least ten transplants of each type during the year prior to which accreditation is being requested. Therefore, a program seeking accreditation for both autologous and allogeneic transplantation must perform ten procedures of each type. This minimum requirement is consistent with earlier standards from the American Society of Hematology/American Society of Clinical Oncology and the American Society for Blood and Marrow Transplantation, following International Bone Marrow Transplant Registry (IBMTR) findings of higher treatment-related mortality and treatment failure in programs performing five or fewer transplants per year.

Although FACT standards deal primarily with the medical and laboratory practices of transplantation, standards for nurses are also addressed and include the following major points:

- Nurses and nurse supervisors need formal training and experience in the management of patients receiving hematopoietic progenitor cell transplants.
- Training should include hematology/oncology patient care, administration of high-dose therapy, growth factors, immunosuppressive medications, management of infectious complications associated with compromised host defense mechanisms, administration of blood components, and an appropriate degree of intensive medical/pediatric nursing care.[73]

Transplant nursing standards have come from a variety of sources. Within the Oncology Nursing Society (ONS), a special interest group (SIG) composed solely of nurses with an interest in caring for patients undergoing transplant and rescue procedures exists; this group has proposed educational and practice standards for the field.[74,75] The ONS/BMT SIG also publishes, on an annual basis, a directory of HCT programs that includes contact information and other program information to assist nurses in networking on clinical and administrative issues.[76] Similar organizations exist for transplant nurses in Canada and Europe (the European Bone Marrow Transplant [EBMT] group).

International and interdisciplinary collaboration and networking have assisted in defining standards for specialized education of nurses and quantifying appropriate nursing staff ratios to care for these patients.[77] Standards have been especially helpful in guiding programs under development to identify appropriate nursing care practice and educational requirements. Program standards for ratios or categories of personnel are less well described, especially for outpatient programs.

The complexity and specialization of transplant care within and across many different healthcare settings has given rise to multiple nursing roles within the field.[78–80] Transplant nursing coordinators and case managers are nurses who have specialized knowledge about patient evaluation, eligibility, and advocacy. Nurses fulfilling these roles assist patients in obtaining appropriate testing, education, and insurance eligibility prior to the procedure.[78] Following transplant, these same nurses maintain contact with patients to guide them through the postprocedure adaptation and continued medical follow-up phase. Changes in medical staffing and education have led to the incorporation of the nurse practitioner role as vital to the care of patients during the acute care phase of transplantation. A handbook of care practices has helped to define the scope of practice for nurse practitioners interested in the high-intensity care required by these patients.[80] Community and home care nurses also provide increasing amounts of specialized care, requiring in-depth HCT knowledge about issues formerly in the domain of the inpatient nurse.

National Marrow Donor Program

Prior to 1986, allogeneic transplant candidates lacking an HLA-matched relative either did not receive a transplant or were forced to independently canvas the world in search of a donor.[71] In July 1986, the U.S. Congress passed legislation creating a central registry of volunteers willing to donate marrow. The contract awarded to the NMDP created a registry that harnessed and regulated a national network of transplant, donor, and collection centers that work together to serve patients in need. As of July 2003, more than 8 million donors and 28,000 cord blood units were registered. The NMDP has facilitated more than 16,000 blood stem cell transplants throughout the world.[76]

International Bone Marrow Transplant Registry/Autologous Bone Marrow Transplant Registry

Since the development of BMT, thousands of procedures have been performed by hundreds of programs worldwide for many different diseases. Despite this, few programs treat a large enough volume of patients to determine overall procedure efficacy. The International Bone Marrow Transplant Registery (IBMTR) formed in 1970, the Autologous Bone Marrow Transplant Registry (ABMTR) formed in 1990, and the European Bone Marrow Transplant (EBMT) group are three international organizations studying and developing a scientific evidence base for the transplant procedure.[20,77,81] These groups maintain databases of procedures performed and their outcomes from a large percentage of transplant programs. For example, the IBMTR database includes information from 350 institutions performing allogeneic transplants worldwide and accounts for 40% of all allogeneic transplants done between 1998 and 2002.[27]

Table 18-3 Web Sites Containing Transplant Information

International Bone Marrow Transplant Registry (IBMTR) and Autologous Blood and Marrow Transplant Registry (ABMTR) *www.ibmtr.org* Provides scientific information to professionals on the state of the science of autologous and allogeneic HCT
National Marrow Donor Program (NMDP) *www.marrow.org* Provides information about becoming a marrow donor or searching for an unrelated marrow donor
Blood and Marrow Transplant Information Network *www.bmtinfonet.org* Provides access to the electronic newsletter and other publications in addition to HCT news items, a patient–survivor link service, and an attorney referral service regarding insurance reimbursement difficulties
American Society for Blood & Marrow Transplantation (ASBMT) *www.asbmt.org* Organization for physicians/investigators in the use of hematopoietic cell transplant. Developed national standards for laboratory and clinical handling of stem cells.
BMT Resource NetMarks *http://w3.duhsc.edu/hemaonc/bmtmark.htm* A directory of HCT-related information on the Internet
National BMT Link *www.nbmtlink.org* Connects HCT patients with survivors who can provide psychosocial support
Bone Marrow Donors Worldwide *www.bmdw.org* Collects HLA phenotypes of volunteer donors and assists with coordination in distribution of these products worldwide

Collaborating clinical treatment centers regularly and voluntarily report standardized information to these central agencies about the types of transplants performed, aspects of the process, and outcomes of the procedures. The growth of the database of autologous and hematopoietic procedures has been captured by the ABMTR, to which more than 200 centers contribute data; it summarizes about 50% of the autotransplants done between 1998 and 2002.[27] Updates of these data can be viewed on the IBMTR Web site (Table 18-3 gives examples of data available from IBMTR/ABMTR). The pooled data are regularly analyzed and shared through a variety of peer-reviewed mechanisms (journal articles, newsletters, Web sites, scientific slides, and presentations) to inform the scientific and lay communities about state-of-the-art care and promising trends related to the procedures.[27]

Future Directions

Financial/Reimbursement Issues

In the early 1990s, transplantation achieved distinction within and outside of the oncology community as much for its financial controversies as for its scientific discoveries. Reasons for this included:

- It was a costly, widely used procedure that lacked clear efficacy in some diseases.
- Insurance denials generated high-publicity court cases in which patients sued for insurance coverage.
- HCT programs were perceived to be high-profit centers, which led to exponential growth of programs.[82]
- Provision of an unprecedented level of high-intensity care in outpatient clinics and at home sought to decrease the economic burden.

Current financial issues in transplantation include transplantation program administrators' focus on balancing costs and charges, reducing actual treatment costs, and securing market share.[83–86] Costs for a transplant procedure range from $60,000 to $150,000, depending on the type (autologous versus allogeneic), complexity, hospital length of stay in a high-tech environment, use of high-cost pharmaceuticals, and stem cell procurement costs. Cost figures are generally more easily compared across institutions, in contrast to charges that are institution and insurance company specific. Even so, cost figures vary considerably from one program to the next, as there is no standardization regarding which costs are truly part of the transplant procedure. For instance, some programs do not include stem cell procurement in their cost estimates; instead, the institution and the insurance company may consider (and possibly reimburse) this phase of transplantation as a separate procedure from the actual transplant. In the case of allogeneic transplantation, typically the recipient (and rarely the donor's insurance company) is responsible for stem cell procurement costs. Reduced morbidity and mortality from procedural improvements and supportive care have increased the population of older patients who can be treated with this modality, thus stimulating the need for Medicare to develop reimbursement codes and standards for transplantation.[87] For instance, age and patient condition requirements may permit reimbursement for transplantation in patients older than age 65 for certain diseases, such as multiple myeloma.

Reducing costs of transplantation is a major focus for many programs that seek to achieve a positive (or at least balanced) margin between procedure costs, charges, and reimbursement. One of the most significant changes in HCT (clinically and financially) was the shift of care from the high-tech inpatient hospital environment to the outpatient environment. Some part of a program's financial viability could be secured by providing an increased volume of procedures outside the confines of the previously limited specialized inpatient isolation environments.[88] In addition to the financial benefit, lower costs per procedure could allow more eligible patients to receive this treatment. Of course, this trend does not account for the costs of care that have simply been shifted to unpaid at-home family caregivers and the out-of-pocket costs for services that were previously covered when procedures were performed exclusively on an inpatient basis (e.g., some medications, home care).

Finally, quality improvement initiatives to streamline and better coordinate care have likely benefited both the patient and program financial outcomes.

Outpatient and Home Care Issues

Several variations on traditional inpatient care have evolved for pediatric marrow transplantation,[89] patients receiving allogeneic PBSCTs, and adults undergoing HCT.[90] Patient evaluation and immunosuppressive therapies were the first interventions to be regularly performed outside of the inpatient setting. Later, chemotherapy administration and acute symptoms (such as neutropenia) were managed by a combination of outpatient nurses, home care nurses, and family or other caregivers. Positive patient outcomes from decreased isolation within confined environments include improved quality of life for patients without apparent increased morbidity or mortality.[88]

Targeted Therapy

Targeted therapies block a specific receptor site (e.g., epidermal growth factor receptor, CD20) thereby blocking the signal generated and causing cell death. With the emergence of these targeted therapies, HCT has changed yet again. Clinical trials addressing the efficacy of rituximab as a pre-HCT in vivo purging agent and a post-transplant adjuvant treatment to reduce the incidence of relapse are promising.[22–24] Other approaches to preventing relapse involve the use of thalidomide post-HCT for multiple myeloma[91] and the use of imatinib for CML.[43] Incorporating radioimmunotherapy (ibritumomab tiuxetan) into HCT is yet another exciting area of research. The ability to deliver radiation directly to the tumor site could significantly decrease systemic toxicity associated with HCT preparative regimens.[25] As new agents flow out of the research pipeline and into clinical practice, the future of cancer treatment and HCT continues to evolve.

Web Sites

The Internet contains a vast amount of information for patients and professionals regarding transplantation. Due to the lack of regulation on the Internet, nurses should explore patient online support groups or "chat rooms" before recommending them to patients. Nevertheless, a few online resources and support groups are well established and provide appreciated connections for patients who may feel isolated when separated from the treatment center. *Blood and Marrow Transplant Newsletter,* a quarterly paper version of an online site, is produced by BMT survivor Susan Stewart *Blood and Marrow Transplant Newsletter,* 2900 Skokie Valley Road, Suite B, Highland Park, IL 60035; phone: 847-433-3313; toll-free: 888-597-7674; fax: 847-433-4599; *www.bmtinfonet.org*). Originally created in 1994 under the name *BMT Newsletter,* with the cooperation of HCT medical and nursing professional volunteer writers and reviewers, it was one of the first comprehensive sources of information about the procedure for patients. This resource is a mainstay of HCT patient education. A listing of helpful Web sites is included in Table 18-3.

Conclusion

Since the earliest days of transplantation, nurses have been on the front lines, contributing to the art and science of patient care and research. Many scientific advances have led to a redesign of how care is provided. Nurses have lent the leadership and clinical expertise needed to ensure that patients and their families experience appropriate and safe levels of service. As the future brings new challenges in all aspects of health care, the lessons from areas ranging from transplant science (e.g., immunology, genetics) to economics (e.g., centers of excellence, high-tech outpatient care) will continue to guide the fields of oncology and oncology nursing.

References

1. Blume KG, Forman SJ, Appelbaum FR: *Thomas' Hematopoietic Cell Transplantation* (ed 3). Malden, MA, Blackwell Science, 2004
2. Wingard J: Bone marrow to blood stem cells: past, present, future, in Wujcik D (ed.): *Marrow and Blood Stem Transplantation: Principles, Practice and Nursing Insights* (ed 2). Sudbury, MA, Jones and Bartlett, 1997, pp 3–24
3. Wagner ND, Quinones VW: Allogeneic peripheral blood stem cell transplantation: clinical overview and nursing implications. *Oncol Nurs Forum* 25:1049–1055; quiz 1056-1047, 1998
4. Jacobson LO, Simmons EL, Marks EK, et al: Recovery from radiation injury. *Science* 113:510–511, 1951
5. Lorenz E, Uphoff D, Reid TR, et al: Modification of irradiation injury in mice and guinea pigs by bone marrow injections. *J Natl Cancer Inst* 12:197–201, 1951
6. Cohen J, Vos O, Van Bekkum D: The present status of radiation protection by chemical and biological agents in mammals, in Abbott J (ed.): *Advances in Radiology.* Edinburgh, Oliver and Boyd, 1957, pp 134–144
7. Thomas ED, Lochte HL Jr, Lu WC, et al: Intravenous infusion of bone marrow in patients receiving radiation and chemotherapy. *N Engl J Med* 257:491–496, 1957
8. Thomas E: A history of bone marrow transplantation, in Blume KG, Forman SJ, Appelbaum FR (eds.): *Thomas' Hematopoietic Cell Transplantation* (ed 3). Malden, MA, Blackwell Science, 2004, pp 3–8
9. Mathe G, Amiel JL, Schwarzenberg L, et al: Hematopoietic chimera in man after allogeneic (homologous) bone-marrow transplantation (Control of the secondary syndrome. Specific tolerance due to the chimerism). *Br Med J* 28:1633–1635, 1963
10. Hickman RO, Buckner CD, Clift RA, et al: A modified right atrial catheter for access to the venous system in marrow transplant recipients. *Surg Gynecol Obstet* 148:871–875, 1979
11. Appelbaum FR: The current status of hematopoietic cell transplantation. *Annu Rev Med* 54:491–512, 2003
12. Devine SM, Adkins DR, Khoury H, et al: Recent advances in allogeneic hematopoietic stem-cell transplantation. *J Lab Clin Med* 141:7–32, 2003
13. Almici C, Carlo-Stella C, Wagner JE, et al: Clonogenic capacity and ex vivo expansion potential of umbilical cord blood progenitor cells are not impaired by cryopreservation. *Bone Marrow Transplant* 19:1079–1084, 1997
14. Davison D: Bone marrow, peripheral blood stem cell, and umbilical cord blood procurement, in Rust D (ed.): *A Clinical Guide to Stem Cell and Bone Marrow Transplantation.* Sudbury, MA, Jones and Bartlett, 1997, pp 113–124
15. Fisher C, McGrath M, Cannon M: Related and autologous core blood banking, in Broxmeyer H (ed.): *Cellular Charateristics of Cord Blood and Cord Blood Transplantation.* Bethesda, MD, AABB Press, 1998, pp 199–216
16. Schmitz N, Linch DC, Dreger P, et al: Randomised trial of filgrastim-mobilised peripheral blood progenitor cell transplantation versus autologous bone-marrow transplantation in lymphoma patients [see comment] [erratum appears in *Lancet* 347:914, 1996]. *Lancet* 347:353–357, 1996
17. Kessinger A, Sharp JG: The whys and hows of hematopoietic progenitor and stem cell mobilization. *Bone Marrow Transplant* 31:319–329, 2003
18. Ng-Cashin J, Shea T: Mobilization of autologous peripheral blood hematopoietic cells for support of high-dose cancer therapy, in Blume KG, Forman SJ, Appelbaum FR (eds.): *Hematopoietic Cell Transplantation* (ed 3). Malden, MA, Blackwell Science, 2004, pp 576–587
19. Devine SM, Lazarus HM, Emerson SG: Clinical application of hematopoietic progenitor cell expansion: current status and future prospects. *Bone Marrow Transplant* 31:241–252, 2003
20. Horowitz M: Uses and growth of hematopoietic cell transplantation, in Blume KG, Forman SJ, Appelbaum FR (eds.): *Hematopoietic Cell Transplantation* (ed 3). Malden, MA, Blackwell Science, 2004, pp 9–15
21. Giralt S: Update on non-myeloablative stem cell transplantation for hematologic malignancies. *Int J Hematol* 76(suppl 1):176–183, 2002

22. Buckstein R, Imrie K, Spaner D, et al: Consolidative immunotherapy with Rituxan in autologous stem cell transplants for follicular lymphoma is associated wtih molecular remissions. *Proc Am Soc Clin Oncol* 2:26a, 2000 (abstr 94)
23. Flinn IW, O'Donnell PV, Goodrich A, et al: Immunotherapy with rituximab during peripheral blood stem cell transplantation for non-Hodgkin's lymphoma. *Biol Blood Marrow Transplant* 6:628–632, 2000
24. Magni M, Di Nicola M, Devizzi L, et al: Successful in vivo purging of CD34-containing peripheral blood harvests in mantle cell and indolent lymphoma, evidence for a role of both chemotherapy and rituximab infusion. *Blood* 96:864–869, 2000
25. Aksentijevich I, Flinn IW: Monoclonal antibody therapy with autologous peripheral blood stem cell transplantation for non-Hodgkin's lymphoma. *Cancer Control* 9:99–105, 2002
26. Kumar A, Loughran T, Alsina M, et al: Management of multiple myeloma, a systematic review and critical appraisal of published studies. *Lancet Oncol* 4:293–304, 2003
27. Loberiza F: Report on state of the art in blood and marrow transplantation — Part I of the IBMTR/ABMTR summary slides with guide. *Newsletter* 10:7, 2003
28. Fefer A: Graft-versus tumor responses, in Blume KG, Forman SJ, Appelbaum FR (eds.): *Hematopoietic Cell Transplantation* (ed 3). Malden, MA, Blackwell Science, 2004, pp 369–379
29. Goulmy F: Human minor histocompatibility antigens: new concepts for marrow transplantation and adoptive immunotherapy. *Immunol Rev* 157:125–140, 1997
30. Appelbaum FR: The use of bone marrow and peripheral blood stem transplantation in the treatment of cancer. *CA Cancer J Clin* 46:142–164, 1996
31. Oudshoorn M, Lie J, Bakker J, et al: Finding the most suitable allogenic hematopoietic stem cell donor, in Brenner M (ed.): *Clinical Bone Marrow and Blood Stem Cell Transplantation* (ed 2). Cambridge, UK, Cambridge University Press, 2004, pp 369–382
32. Korbling M: Mobilization regimens for harvesting autologous and allogenic peripheral blood stem cells, in Brenner M (ed.): *Clinical Bone Marrow and Blood Stem Cell Transplantation* (ed 3). Cambridge, UK, Cambridge University Press, 2004, pp 383–403
33. Giralt S, Khouri I, Champlin R: Non-myeloblative conditioning: induction of graft-versus-disease as a therapeutic modality, in Atkinson K (ed.): *Clinical Bone Marrow and Blood Stem Cell Transplantation* (ed 2). Cambridge, UK, Cambridge University Press, 2000, pp 1182-1188
34. Anagnostopoulos A, Giralt S: Critical review on non-myeloablative stem cell transplantation (NST). *Crit Rev Oncol Hematol* 44:175–190, 2002
35. Kiss JE, Rybka WB, Winkelstein A, et al: Relationship of CD34+ cell dose to early and late hematopoiesis following autologous peripheral blood stem cell transplantation. *Bone Marrow Transplant* 19:303–310, 1997
36. Wujcik D, Whedon M: *Blood and Marrow Stem Cell Transplantation: Principles, Practice, and Nursing Insights.* (ed 2). Sudbury, MA, Jones and Bartlett, 1997, pp 22–42
37. Sola C, Maroto P, Salazar R, et al: High dose chemotherapy (HDC) and peripheral blood stem cell (PBSC) autologous tranplantation: influence of the number of infused CD34+ cells in hematopoietic recovery and support measures required. *Proc Am Soc Clin Oncol* 15:538, 1996 (abstr)
38. Kundtzon S: In vitro growth of granulocytic colonies from circulating cells in human cord blood. *Blood* 43:357–361, 1997
39. Broxmeyer H, Kutzberg J, Gluckman E: Human umbilical cord blood as a potential source of transplantable hematopoietic stem/progenitor cells. *Proc Natl Acad Sci USA* 86:3828–3832, 1989
40. Weber-Nordt R, Schott E, Finke J, et al: Umbilical cord blood: an alternative to the transplantation of bone marrow stem cells. *Cancer Treat Rev* 22:381–391, 1996
41. Wagner JE: Allogeneic umbilical cord blood transplantation. *Cancer Treat Res* 77:187–216, 1997
42. Kantarjian H, Sawyers C, Hochhaus A, et al: Hematologic and cytogenetic responses to imatinib mesylate in chronic myelogenous leukemia [see comment] [erratum appears in *N Engl J Med* 346:1923, 2002]. *N Engl J Med* 346:645–652, 2002
43. Vandenberghe P, Boeckx N, Ronsyn E, et al: Imatinib mesylate induces durable complete remission of advanced CML persisting after allogeneic bone marrow transplant *Leukemia* 17:458–460, 2003
44. Bhatia R, McGlave P: Autologous hematopoietic cell transplant for chronic myelogenous leukemia, in Blume KG, Forman SJ, Appelbaum FR (eds.): *Thomas' Hematopoietic Cell Transplantation* (ed 3). Malden, MA, Blackwell Science, 2004, pp 1250–1261
45. Khouri I, Champlin R: Allogeneic transplantation for lymphoma and chronic lymphocytic leukemia, in Blume KG, Forman SJ, Appelbaum FR (eds.): *Thomas' Hematopoietic Cell Transplantation.* Malden, MA, Blackwell Science, 2004, pp 1105–1115
46. Anderlini P: Hematopoietic stem-cell transplantation for Hodgkin's disease (HD): current status. *Cytotherapy* 4:241–251, 2002
47. Delforge M, Boogaerts M: Autologous hematopoietic stem cell transplantation for myelodysplasia, in Brenner M (ed.): *Clinical Bone Marrow and Blood Stem Cell Transplantation* (ed 2) Cambridge, UK, Cambridge University Press, 2004, pp 613–619
48. Attal M, Harousseau JL: Standard therapy versus autologous transplantation in multiple myeloma. *Hematol Oncol Clin North Am* 11:133–146, 1997
49. Musto P, Arena G, Falcone A, et al: Intensive chemotherapy followed by single or multiple peripheral blood stem cell transplant (PBSCT) improves the prognosis of patients affected by multiple myeloma with proliferative activity. *Blood* 94:576, 1999 (abstr)
50. Lenhoff S, Hjorth M, Holmberg E, et al: Impact on survival of high-dose therapy with autologous stem cell support in patients younger than 60 years with newly diagnosed multiple myeloma, a population-based study. Nordic Myeloma Study Group. *Blood* 95:7–11, 2000
51. Bensinger WI, Buckner D, Gahrton G: Allogeneic stem cell transplantation for multiple myeloma. *Hematol Oncol Clin North Am* 11:147–157, 1997
52. Heffner LT Jr, Lonial S: Breakthroughs in the management of multiple myeloma. *Drugs* 63:1621–1636, 2003
53. Antman K: Hematopoietic cell transplantation for breast cancer, in Blume KG, Forman SJ, Appelbaum FR (eds.): *Thomas' Hematopoietic Cell Transplantation* (ed 3). Malden, MA, Blackwell Science, 2004, pp 1298–1307
54. Schmid P, Samonigg H, Nitsch T, et al: Randomised trial of upfront tandem high-dose chemotherapy compared to standard chemotherapy with doxorubicin and paclitaxel in metastatic breast cancer. *Proc Am Soc Clin Oncol* (abstr 171), *www.asco.org*, 2002. Accessed April 26, 2004
55. Cure H, Janvier M, Morvan F, et al: Intensive therapy and autograft of hematopoietic stem cells transplantation for metastatic breast cancer: results of the national program PEGASE 04. *Hematol Cell Ther* 41:71–74, 1999
56. Daly M, Goldstein L, Topolsky D, et al: Quality of life experience in women randomized to high-dose chemotherapy and stem cell support or standard dose chemotherapy for responding metastatic breast cancer in Philadelphia Intergroup Study (PBT-1). *Proc Am Soc Clin Oncol* (abstr 327), *www.asco.org*, 2000. Accessed April 26, 2004

57. Stadmauer E, O'Niell A, Goldstein LJ, et al: Conventional-dose chemotherapy compared with high dose chemotherapy plus autologous stem cell transplantation for metastatic breast cancer: 5-year update of the Philadelphia Trial (PBT-1). American Society of Clinical Oncology, *www.asco.org/cgi-bin/mem/abst.pl?absno=169&div-006&year-02abstracts*, 2002. Accessed April 26, 2004
58. Stadmauer E, O'Niell A, Goldstein L, et al: Conventional-dose chemotherapy compared with high dose chemotherapy plus autologous stem cell transplantation for metastatic breast cancer. *N Engl J Med* 345:1069–1076, 2000
59. Crump M, Gluck S, Stewart D, et al: A randomized trial of high dose chemotherapy with autologous preipheral blood stem cell support compared to standard therapy in women with metastatic breast cancer: a National Cancer Institure of Canada (NCIC) Clinical Trials Group Study. *www.asco.org*, 2001. Accessed April 26, 2004
60. Biron P, Durand M, Roche H, et al: High-dose thiotepa, cyclophosphamide and stem cell transplantation after 4 FEC 100 compared with 4 FEC alone allow better disease survival but the same overall survival in the first line chemotherapy for metastatic breast cancer: results of the PEGASE 03 French protocols (abstr) *www.asco.org*, 2002. Accessed April 26, 2004
61. Farquhar C, Basser R, Hetrick S, et al: High dose chemotherapy and autologous bone marrow or stem cell transplantation versus conventional chemotherapy for women with metastatic breast cancer. *Cochrane Database Syst Rev* 2003(1):CD003142.
62. Rosti G, Pico J, Wandt H, et al: High dose chemotherapy (HDC) in salvage treatment of patients failing first-line platinum chemotherapy for advanced germ cell tumors (GCT): first results of a prospective randomized trial of the European Group for Blood and Marrow Transplantation (EBMT): IT-94 study. *Proc Am Soc Clin Oncol* 21:180, 2002 (abstr)
63. Childs R, Sriniveson R: Transplantation for solid tumors, in Blume KG, Forman SJ, Appelbaum FR (eds.): *Thomas' Hematopoietic Cell Transplantation* (ed 3). Malden, MA, Blackwell Science, 2004, pp 1177–1187
64. Shizuru JA: The experimental basis for hematopoietic cell transplantation for autoimmune diseases, in Blume KG, Forman SJ, Appelbaum FR (eds.): *Thomas' Hematopoietic Cell Transplantation* (ed 3). Malden, MA, Blackwell Science, 2004, pp 324–343
65. Bhatia S, Bhatia R: Secondary malignancies after hematopoietic cell transplantation, in Blume KG, Forman SJ, Appelbaum FR (eds.): *Thomas' Hematopoietic Cell Transplantation* (ed 3). Malden, MA, Blackwell Science, 2004, pp 962–980
66. Harder H, Cornelissen JJ, Gool ARV, et al: Cognitive functioning and quality of life in long-term adult survivors of bone marrow transplantation. *Cancer* 95:183–192, 2002
67. Packer RJ, Mehta N: Neurocognitive sequelae of cancer treatment. *Neurology* 59:8–10, 2002
68. Ahles TA, Saykin AJ: Breast cancer chemotherapy-related cognitive dysfunction. *Clin Breast Cancer* 3(suppl 3):S84–S90, 2002
69. Porter DL, Antin JH: Infusion of donor peripheral blood mononuclear cells to treat relapse after transplantation for chronic myelogenous leukemia. *Hematol Oncol Clin North Am* 12:123–150, 1998
70. Colvin M: History of bone marrow transplant, in Blume KG, Forman SJ, Appelbaum FR (ed.): *Thomas' Hematopoietic Cell Transplantation.* Malden, MA, Blackwell Science, 2004, pp 254–257
71. Hegland J: HLA and issues of stem cell donation, in Wujcik D (ed.): *Marrow and Blood Stem Cell Transplantation: Principles, Practice and Nursing Insights* (ed 2). Sudbury, MA, Jones and Bartlett, 1997, pp 43–65
72. Sullivan KM: Graft-vs.-host disease, in Blume KG, Forman, SJ, Appelbaum FR (eds.): *Thomas' Hematopoietic Cell Transplantation* (ed 3). Malden, MA, Blackwell Science, 2004, pp 635–664
73. Foundation for the Accreditation of Cellular Therapy: *Standards for Hematopoietic Progenitor Cell Collection, Processing and Transplantation.* Omaha, NE, Foundation for the Accreditation of Cellular Therapy, 2002
74. Ezzone S: *Hematopoietic Stem Cell Transplantation: A Resource Book for Nurses.* Pittsburgh, ONS Press, 2004
75. Buchsel P, Kapustay P: *Stem Cell Transplantation: A Clinical Textbook.* Pittsburgh, PA, ONS Press, 2004
76. Oncology Nursing Society: *Bone Marrow Transplantation Nursing Resources Directory.* Pittsburgh, Oncology Nursing Press, 2004
77. Ezzone S, Fliedner M: Transplant networks and standards of care: international perspectives, in Wujcik D (ed.): *Marrow and Stem Cell Transplantation: Principles, Pratice and Nursing Insights* (ed 2). Sudbury, MA, Jones and Bartlett, 1997, pp 474–496
78. Ford R, Campbell J, Madison J: Nursing issues in hematopoietic cell transplantation, in Blume KG, Forman SJ, Appelbaum FR (eds.): *Thomas' Hematopoietic Cell Transplantation* (ed 3). Malden, MA, Blackwell Science, 2004: 469–482
79. Roach M, Whedon M: Bone marrow transplantation, in Gates R (ed.): *Oncology Nursing Secrets.* Boston, Henlay & Belfus, 1997, pp 62–72
80. Shapiro T, Davison D, Rust D: *A Clinical Guide to Stem Cell and Bone Marrow Transplant.* Sudbury, MA, Jones and Bartlett, 1997
81. Tyndall A, Gratwohl A: Blood and marrow stem cell transplants in auto-immune disease: a consensus report written on behalf of the European League Against Rheumatism (EULAR) and the European Group for Blood and Marrow Transplantation (EBMT). *Bone Marrow Transplant* 19:643–645, 1997
82. Engelking C: Peripheral blood stem cell therapy for breast cancer: arguing the case. *Innov Breast Cancer Care* 3:67, 1998
83. Vicent MG, Madero L, Chamorro L, et al: Comparative cost analysis of autologous peripheral blood progenitor cell and bone marrow transplantation in pediatric patients with malignancies. *Haematologica* 86:1087–1094, 2001
84. van Agthoven M, Groot MT, Verdonck LF, et al: Cost analysis of HLA-identical sibling and voluntary unrelated allogeneic bone marrow and peripheral blood stem cell transplantation in adults with acute myelocytic leukaemia or acute lymphoblastic leukaemia. *Bone Marrow Transplant* 30:243–251, 2002
85. Schweitzer SO, Scalzi CC: *The Cost Effectiveness of Bone Marrow Transplant Therapy and Its Policy Implications.* Washington, DC, Congress of the United States, Office of Technology Assessment, 1981
86. Meehan KR, Areman EM, Ericson SG, et al: Mobilization, collection, and processing of autologous peripheral blood stem cells: development of a clinical process with associated costs. *J Hematother Stem Cell Res* 9:767–771, 2000
87. Centers for Medicare and Medicaid (CMS): *Medicare Coverage Issues Manual, Transmittal 125. www.cms.hhs.gov/manuals/pm_trans/R125CIM.pdf,* August 29, 2000. Accessed February 2004
88. Meisenberg BR, Miller WE, McMillan R, et al: Outpatient high-dose chemotherapy with autologous stem-cell rescue for hematologic and nonhematologic malignancies. *J Clin Oncol* 15:11–17, 1997
89. Fidler PA, Hibbs CJ: Bone marrow transplant today — home tomorrow: ambulatory care issues in pediatric marrow transplantation. *J Pediatr Oncol Nurs* 14:228–238, 1997
90. Herrmann RP, Leather M, Leather HL, Leen K: Clinical care for patients receiving autologous hematopoietic stem cell transplantation in the home setting. *Oncol Nurs Forum* 25:1427–1432, 1998
91. Hahn T, Wingard JR, Anderson KC, et al: The role of cytotoxic therapy with hematopoietic stem cell transplantation in the therapy of multiple myeloma, an evidence-based review. *Biol Blood Marrow Transplant* 9:4–37, 2003

CHAPTER 19

Techniques of Hematopoietic Cell Transplantation

Debra Wujcik, RN, MSN, AOCN®

Introduction

Bone marrow transplantation (BMT) has been a treatment for patients with hematologic malignancies since the mid-1900s. The original procedure required harvesting pluripotent stem cells (PPSCs) from the bone marrow of a human leukocyte antigen (HLA)–matched donor. The patient received preparative therapy that included high-dose myeloablative chemotherapy and total body irradiation (TBI). The harvested cells were then reinfused into the patient. Intense supportive care was required for 4–6 weeks until the donor cells migrated to the bone marrow and began to produce new hematopoietic cells. This process was followed for allogeneic BMT.

High-dose chemotherapy for the treatment of solid tumors produced improved response rates, but the dose-limiting toxicity was myelosuppression. Patients needed a rescue of stem cells to recover hematopoietic function. Harvesting the patient's own stem cells, freezing them, and reinfusing them after conditioning therapy expanded the use of BMT to autologous BMT.

The discovery that PPSCs circulated in the peripheral blood led to new techniques to collect, preserve, and reinfuse cells. Collection of cells through apheresis was easier and less costly than bone marrow harvest. Controversy persists as to whether PPSCs and the peripheral blood progenitor cells (PBPCs) are equivalent in terms of durability of hematopoietic reconstitution. Nevertheless, transplantation with cells obtained from peripheral circulation is now the predominant type of transplant used in adults.[1–3]

The terminology for transplantation is confusing and ever changing. Despite attempts to achieve consensus, there is not universal acceptance of the nomenclature in this field. Key terms for understanding the literature are listed in Table 19-1. For the purposes of this chapter, the general term for transplantation is hematopoietic cell transplantation (HCT). Bone marrow transplantation designates transplant with hematopoietic cells obtained from the bone marrow. Blood cell transplantation (BCT) refers to transplant with cells from the peripheral circulation. Umbilical cord transplantation (UCBT) entails transplant with cells from the umbilical cord.

More than 40,000 HCTs are performed each year, with the number of procedures increasing at a rate of 10%–20% per year.[3,4] Several variables contribute to the growth: increased efficacy of HCT with increased use in more disease sites, better understanding of optimal timing for HCT, increased donor availability, improved conditioning strategies, and improved supportive care. Both allogeneic and autologous transplants are increasingly used in older patients. More than half of autologous transplants are in patients older than 50 years and 20% in patients older than 60 years.[3] Techniques for HCT differ according to the source of cells and type of transplant. The techniques for HCT must meet standards set by the Foundation for Accreditation of Cell Therapy (FACT; formerly FAHCT) (Table 19-2).[5]

This chapter reviews the various techniques employed in HCT. Procedures to obtain cells for transplant, cell processing and storage, preparative regimens, and reinfusion of cells are discussed. Nursing indications for patient education, assessment, and management of complications are presented.

Patient Evaluation

The first step in patient evaluation for HCT is determining whether the patient is a candidate for transplantation and which type of transplant is most appropriate. The disease, stage of disease, performance status of the patient, availability of an appropriate protocol, and donor availability are all considered. The type of transplant that the patient will receive is decided early in the process, because insurance preauthorization, timing, and scheduling are influenced by this information.[6,7]

Physical Evaluation

The clinical evaluation occurs simultaneously with the insurance preauthorization process. There is documented improved response to transplantation when the tumor burden is low and the disease is chemotherapy sensitive. Also, the earlier the stage of disease at the time of transplant, the better the survival rate. The clinical evaluation includes identification of any organ dysfunction secondary to disease or prior therapy. Specifically, the lungs and heart are evaluated. Other screening tests include viral studies to rule out HIV or hepatitis, among others (Table 19-3).[7]

Table 19-1 Terminology of Hematopoietic Cell Transplantation

Source of Hematopoietic Cells	Procedure
Bone marrow	Bone marrow harvest
Peripheral circulation	Apheresis
Umbilical cord blood	Delivery room collection
Type of Transplant	**Donor of Cells**
Allogeneic	HLA-matched related donor
	HLA-matched unrelated donor
Autologous	Patient
Syngeneic	HLA-identical twin

Table 19-2 Standards for Hematopoietic Cell Transplantation

	Personnel
Director	Licensed and board certified; 1 year of specific clinical training or 2 years as attending for patients undergoing transplantation
Other physicians	Trained under the director with demonstrated competency in the management of myelosuppressed patients
Surgeon	Skilled in catheter placement
Consultants	Consultants available who are board certified in pulmonary, gastroenterology, nephrology, infectious disease, cardiology, psychiatry, and radiation oncology
Nurses	Formally trained and experienced in care of transplantation patients; skills in administration of chemotherapy and blood components and management of infections
Technologist	Trained for handling of stem cells
	Cell Collection Facility Requirements
Facility medical director	Director shall have 1 year of experience in the collection procedure with 10 collection procedures of each type
Personnel	Adequate numbers of trained personnel
Laboratory	Accredited laboratory to perform all required tests
Facility	Transfusion facility or blood bank providing 24-hour blood component support, including irradiated blood components
Collection procedures	Standard operating manual describing all procedures
	Cell Processing
Laboratory director	Requires relevant doctoral degree with training and experience for the scope of activities
Processing procedures	Standard operating manual for all procedures; methods for processing shall be validated to result in acceptable hematopoietic progenitor cell viability and recovery
Records	Detailed worksheets maintained for all procedures; objectives and acceptable endpoints for each procedure are specified; director or designee reviews every record

Data from Foundation for the Accreditation of Hematopoietic Cell Therapy.[5]

Psychosocial Evaluation

The psychosocial evaluation begins with education of the patient and family about the rationale, risks, and benefits of HCT. This discussion should include both acute and long-term effects. The assessment of patient and family understanding of the informed consent provides the nurse with a basis for further counseling. The coping strategies of the patient and family are identified. Problems such as drug, alcohol, or tobacco addictions are addressed.[8] Sources of support and available resources are identified. A plan is developed for managing life activities during the transplant period, such as child care, transportation, employment, and who will stay with the patient during HCT.

Financial Evaluation

The insurance evaluation must occur early in the evaluation process due to the expense ($75,000–$150,000) and the frequent investigational nature of HCT.[9,10] An insurance counselor or transplant coordinator works closely with the transplant team to keep them advised of potential reimbursement obstacles. Preauthorization for insurance coverage purposes is usually required. Sometimes during this process, it is learned that the patient must go to a different transplant center where the insurance company has an existing contract. Successful preauthorization is dependent on the case manager's knowledge of the patient's history and the transplant process, as well as his or her experience in negotiations with the insurers.[7,11] It is common for institutions to negotiate with the insurer to provide all care for a set or capitated fee.

In general, insurers provide coverage of allogeneic and autologous BMT for patients with acute leukemia in remission, resistant non-Hodgkin's lymphoma, advanced Hodgkin's disease, recurrent neuroblastoma, and medulloblastoma. Often, patients without insurance coverage must raise their own funds and have a certain amount raised before the transplant.

Education

Beginning with the initial period of evaluation and continuing throughout the process of HCT, the

Table 19-3 Baseline Evaluation for Patients Undergoing Hematopoietic Cell Transplantation

Test	Comment
Complete blood count, including differential and reticulocyte	Establish baseline
Complete blood chemistry profile, urinalysis	Establish baseline; ensure renal and liver function
Prothrombin time, partial thromboplastin time	Establish baseline; ensure coagulation ability
Thyroid function tests	Establish baseline for comparison after total body irradiation
Chest x-ray (PA-Lat)	Establish baseline pulmonary status
Cardiac ejection fraction by (resting) MUGA scan, 12-lead ECG	Establish baseline cardiac function for comparison during and after conditioning therapy
Pulmonary function tests (including DLCO)	Establish baseline pulmonary function
Type and screen	Confirm patient blood typing
Herpes simplex virus serology, Epstein-Barr virus serology, *Varicella zoster* serology	Establish previous viral exposure and risk of reactivation of infection
Human immunodeficiency virus antibody, human T-cell leukemia virus I antibody	Rule out eligibility for transplantation
Toxoplasma serology (IgG)	Establish previous toxoplasma exposure and risk of reactivation of infection

PA-Lat = posterior, anterior, and lateral; MUGA = multigated angiogram; ECG = electrocardiogram; DLCO = diffusion of lung with carbon dioxide.

patient and family require extensive education (Table 19-4). It is useful to provide written and oral instructions and allow sufficient time for patients and family members to synthesize information and ask questions.[12,13] Use of critical pathways may allow the teaching to be presented in a consistent, sequential manner with reinforcement at appropriate points.[7,11,12]

Cells for Transplantation

The process of obtaining stem cells for HCT differs according to the type of transplant. With BMT, the cells are obtained through a bone marrow harvest. In BCT, the pluripotent stem cells and progenitor cells are collected from the peripheral blood. Each procedure has unique steps for donor preparation, the actual procedure, and management of complications.

Bone Marrow Harvest

The cells harvested from the bone marrow are PPSCs. These cells have the capacity for both myeloid and lymphoid (multilineage) differentiation, proliferation, and self-renewal.[2] The exact number of PPSCs needed to repopulate a marrow destroyed by chemotherapy and radiation has not been determined. However, 5% of the 1×10^6 or 1×10^7 nucleated cells found in adult human marrow contains sufficient PPSCs for transplant.[2,14] It is generally agreed that the minimum threshold below which acceptable hematopoietic reconstitution may not occur is $15–20 \times 10^4$ colony-forming units—granulocyte-macrophages (CFU-GM)/kg or 2.5×10^6 $CD34^+$ cells/kg of body weight.[14,15]

The cells needed for successful engraftment after high-dose chemotherapy and irradiation are difficult to isolate. The CD34 antigen is expressed on the surface of early progenitor cells; it does not appear on the PPSC but is present on the committed progenitors. Currently, the CD34 assay is the best technique available to identify the cells that have proved to be correlated with successful engraftment.[16]

Procedure

The bone marrow harvest is usually done in the operating room with the patient anesthetized. Multiple aspirations from each posterior iliac crest are required to obtain the necessary volume of PPSCs. Marrow may be aspirated from the anterior iliac crests and the sternum if the cell yield from the posterior iliac crests is not adequate. The marrow is placed in a heparinized tissue culture medium, filtered for removal of fat and bone particles, then sent to the laboratory for processing and cryopreservation. The procedure usually takes 1–2 hours.[6]

Postoperatively, pressure dressings are applied to the puncture sites. The nurse assesses the patient for bleeding, pain, and fluid balance. Because 400–600 mL of whole blood is aspirated during the harvest, the patient may receive an autologous unit of blood that was collected before the procedure. The complication rate for bone marrow harvest is low, and the patient is usually discharged following recovery on the same day

Table 19-4 Topics for Education of Hematopoietic Cell Transplantation Patients

Phase	Bone Marrow Transplant	Both	Blood Cell Transplant
Evaluation		Overview Tests Laboratory specimens Local housing	
Catheter		Placement Catheter care Complications	
Procurement of cells	Harvest procedure Complications		Mobilization Pheresis Complications
Conditioning	Specific drugs +/ – total body irradiation		Specific drugs Irradiation rare
Reinfusion		Preparation Procedure Complications	
Supportive care		Antibiotics Hematopoietic growth factors Blood products Total parenteral nutrition	
Discharge		Criteria for discharge Continued care at home	

or the next day.[6] The donor may experience pain at the collection sites, which is controlled by mild analgesics. The donor's body will replace the cells that were removed within a few weeks.

A double- or triple-lumen silicone catheter is placed centrally to use for reinfusion of bone marrow cells, administration of conditioning chemotherapy and hydration, and supportive therapies such as antibiotics and transfusions of blood products. The catheter is placed at the time of harvest or at the first day of conditioning therapy, unless the patient has a preexisting catheter from prior therapy. Catheter care includes insertion site care, dressing changes, and flushing procedures. The patient is instructed on the signs and symptoms of infection and management of complications such as occlusion or accidental puncture of the catheter.

Harvest for allogeneic bone marrow transplant

The replacement marrow for allogeneic BMT is obtained from a related or unrelated HLA-matched donor. Prior to harvest, several issues need to be addressed for the normal donor. Donor preparation includes education and medical evaluation. The standard physical evaluation of the donor includes a complete medical history and physical examination, psychosocial evaluation, ECG, chest x-ray, and laboratory evaluation. Laboratory evaluation includes CBC with differential, serum tests for major organ function (renal and hepatic), hepatitis screen (A, B, C), HIV, CMV, HSV, ABO and Rh, and histocompatible tissue typing.[6] The infectious disease screening should be performed within 30 days prior to the collection.[5]

To maintain maximum viability, cells harvested from a donor are transplanted as soon as possible. Thus the timing of allogeneic marrow harvest is carefully coordinated with the transplant team. Because cells are processed and delivered to the recipient within hours of collection, cryopreservation is unnecessary.

A thorough description of the harvesting procedure and the effects that the harvest may potentially have on the donor and the relationship with the recipient should be discussed with the donor. Unrelated donors should also receive counseling prior to donation. The donor should not feel pressured into donating. To preserve confidentiality and avoid contact between a potential donor and the patient or the patient's family, the identity of an unrelated donor remains unknown to both the patient and the transplanting center.[6]

There are many limitations to allogeneic BMT. The biggest drawback is the availability of an appropriate marrow donor. Despite the amount of attention paid to this need, only 30% of persons needing a BMT have related matches. The National Marrow Donor Program provides a pool of nearly 5 million potential donors and 28,000 cord blood units but the registry's efforts are constrained by the numbers of donors from different races. The best opportunity to find a match is within one's own race, and the largest race in the registry is white. The frequency of specific HLA types differs among racial and ethnic groups. Although most HLA pairs occur in all ethnic groups, a few are limited to a single ethnic group. The frequency of an HLA pair can also vary within the ethnic group, depending on the geographic location of the population.[17,18]

Histocompatibility is another limitation of allogeneic BMT. The greater the histoincompatibility between patient and donor, the greater the risk of graft failure, graft rejection, and graft-versus-host disease (GVHD).[17] If a major ABO incompatibility occurs between the donor and the recipient, the bone marrow will be depleted of red cells or plasma.[6]

Harvest for autologous bone marrow transplant

The process of obtaining bone marrow for autologous BMT is the same as for allogeneic BMT, but the volume harvested may be greater if purging or other manipulation is needed to remove tumor cells. The bone marrow is harvested when the patient is in remission and recovered from other treatment. The cells are then processed and frozen until needed.

Blood Cell Apheresis

Another option for transplant is to use stem cells obtained from the peripheral circulation. Some PPSCs circulate in the peripheral blood in small numbers, and committed progenitors circulate in greater numbers.[14] *Progenitors* are cells that have limited ability to divide and are irreversibly committed to one or more lines of differentiation.[19] The colony-forming unit—granulocyte, erythrocyte, macrophage, megakaryocyte (CFU-GEMM), and colony-forming unit—lymphocyte (CFU-L) are committed stem cells. Although they are irreversibly committed to the separate lineages, they remain capable of differentiating to form one of several cell lines. (Figure 18–5 in Chapter 18 illustrates the hematopoietic cascade.)

The PBPCs represent 1%–10% of the marrow progenitors. Once it was proved that these cells could be reinfused into animals (mice, dogs, and baboons) and restore hematopoiesis, the process was applied to humans.[20] The first transplant using cells obtained from peripheral blood was reported in 1985, with several more procedures taking place in the following year.[20,21]

This process has historically been referred to as peripheral blood stem cell transplant (PBSCT) or peripheral blood progenitor cell transplant (PBPCT). The process involves obtaining and infusing an unspecified number of true PPSCs with or without committed progenitor and precursor cells. The current terminology for this process is *blood cell transplant* (BCT). Blood cell transplant is considered to be more precise, so this term is preferred to differentiate the PPSC obtained from the bone marrow for allogeneic and autologous BMT from the combined PPSC and committed progenitors obtained from the peripheral blood for BCT.[2]

Using peripheral PPSCs and progenitor cells obtained from peripheral blood offers several advantages. Neutrophils and platelets recover more rapidly when progenitor cells are used,[19] because the committed progenitors collected for BCT are further along the differentiation pathway than are the PPSCs harvested from the bone marrow. Also, no anesthesia is required for BCT, so there is less risk of complications and fewer medical contraindications than with bone marrow harvest. Patients who cannot have bone marrow harvested due to contraindications to anesthesia, marrow involvement, or prior radiation therapy to large areas of bone marrow may be able to undergo BCT. Disadvantages to using PBSCs include the cost of multiple aphereses and purging procedures, the requirement for mobilization, and the necessity for vascular access.[22]

As with BMT, several types of BCT exist. A patient may use his or her own cells (autologous), cells obtained from an identical twin (syngeneic), or cells obtained from a matched related or unrelated donor (allogeneic).[23–25] The procedure for collection of the PBSCs and progenitors is the same for each type of BCT.

Blood cell transplant mobilization

Purpose. Mobilization for BCT seeks to release an increased number of PPSCs and progenitor cells into the peripheral blood. The number of progenitor cells in the bloodstream in the steady state is only 1%–10% of the marrow progenitors.[19] To collect enough stem cells from the blood, stem cells must be mobilized or moved from the bone marrow to the blood.[26,27] The number of PPSCs and progenitors can be increased 100- to 500-fold through the use of hematopoietic growth factors (HGFs), chemotherapy, or both.[28,29] The minimal number of cells required for BCT is 5–7 $\times 10^8$ mononuclear cells/kg or 1–5 $\times 10^6$ (or more) $CD34^+$ cells/kg.[4,15] Engraftment of both granulocytes and platelets is significantly influenced by the number of $CD34^+$ cells per kilogram infused, and some suggest that doses of 15×10^6 $CD34^+$ cells/kg shorten hematopoietic recovery and may improve quality of life.[30–32] With appropriate mobilization, this usually requires one to three apheresis procedures.

Chemotherapy mobilization. Chemotherapy is used for mobilization either alone or in combination with HGFs. Chemotherapy alone causes an increase in the number of circulating progenitor cells in the peripheral blood. However, the results of using chemotherapy are variable and less predictable than those found with HGFs. Rebound leukocytosis occurs after single-agent chemotherapy with high-dose cyclophosphamide or with multiple-drug regimens using etoposide, cyclophosphamide, and cisplatin.[33] Chemotherapy for mobilization is usually disease specific and follows standard dosing levels.[21,34] Blood counts are monitored daily or every other day to track the recovery of the absolute neutrophil count (ANC). Collection begins when the ANC is between 1000 cells/mm^3 and 5000 cells/mm^3.

The combination of chemotherapy and HGFs usually leads to the collection of more cells than either method alone.[25] The efficiency of the collection is influenced by both individual and technical factors. For example, the patient's pretreatment with chemotherapy or radiation therapy may cause bone marrow damage, making it difficult to mobilize a sufficient number of progenitors. Some data indicate that the patient's age and sex influence the yield of progenitors, with female patients and older patients (>55 years) having lower yields.[31]

Hematopoietic growth factor mobilization. The administration of HGFs alone can result in the collection of adequate numbers of stem cells. Hematopoietic growth factors stimulate enhanced proliferation and maturation of neutrophils and provide a much more controlled response for mobilization. Granulocyte-macrophage colony-stimulating factor (GM-CSF) and granulocyte colony-stimulating factor (G-CSF) are the agents most commonly used for mobilization.[25,35] Granulocyte colony-stimulating factor is indicated for mobilization at 10 μg/kg/day given subcutaneously for 4–6 days. Patients or a family member are taught self-administration. Collection of hematopoietic cells begins on day 4 or 5 of growth factor administration.[5] Daily injections continue until collection is completed. The type of growth factor employed results in different mobilization rates, with use of G-CSF producing a greater yield of stem cells than use of GM-CSF.[36]

Patient and caregiver education regarding administration and side effects of HGF/chemotherapy mobilization is important. Hematopoietic growth factors can produce adverse reactions including nausea, diarrhea, rash, fever, malaise, pleural effusion, increased clotting of the catheter, vomiting, bone pain, headache, chills, dyspnea, and edema.[37] Bone pain, the most predominant symptom, can be treated effectively with acetaminophen. Local irritation may occur at the injection site. Patients must be instructed to report this symptom immediately to prevent any skin breakdown and possible infection. Patients mobilized with chemotherapy need instruction regarding monitoring their temperature and reporting a temperature greater than 100.4°F (40.2°C), chills, or any change in their clinical condition.[26]

New agents. New strategies for mobilization of stem cells for BCT attempt to restimulate patients who show poor response, reduce the number of collection procedures, and/or decrease the amount of G-CSF required for adequate mobilization.[31,38] Pegfilgrastim, a long-acting G-CSF, was recently approved for reduction of neutropenia following myelosuppressive chemotherapy in patients with nonmyeloid leukemia. Studies are under way comparing the effectiveness of one injection of pegfilgrastim to standard G-CSF mobilization. The benefits of one injection versus 5–6 daily injections are obvious.[39] Other agents under investigation for mobilization include stem cell factor and G-CSF, erythropoietin (EPO), G-CSF and human growth hormone (hGH), and AMD-3100.[40–42]

Attempts are currently being made to amplify the number of stem cells ex vivo with stem cell factor and other investigational agents. This process allows for the collection of a small amount of cells, which are then grown and expanded in the laboratory until the desired number of cells is produced.[31]

Hematopoietic growth factor–mobilized PBSCs are being used more frequently as an alternative to marrow collection in the allogeneic transplantation setting.[23,24] Reports increasingly show that PBSCs alone are equal — or even superior — to bone marrow with regard to speed of engraftment and ability to provide long-term hematopoietic reconstitution.[31,40] The safety considerations for normal PBSC donors continue to be addressed. Short- and long-term effects of HGF mobilization and collection in normal donors are currently under investigation and are not yet well-defined. Further data are needed to answer the many questions regarding the safety of this practice.[23,24,40]

Blood cell transplant apheresis

A single apheresis can obtain the desired number of cells if there is no malignancy in the bone marrow, if the patient received minor pretreatment with chemotherapy, and if appropriate mobilization is used.[33] Although two or three procedures are usually needed, strategies are being investigated to decrease this number to one.[41] Two benefits of a single apheresis approach would be the decreased volume withdrawn from the patient and the decreased dimethylsulfate (DMSO) reinfused into the patient.[6]

Patient preparation

The preparation of the patient for apheresis includes extensive education, placement of a central venous catheter (CVC), and beginning specific medications. Teaching at this time focuses on catheter care, the apheresis process, mobilization, and potential complications.[12]

Catheter placement. The patient undergoing BCT requires a catheter that is stiffer than the traditional CVC used for BMT due to the need for high volume and pressure during apheresis (i.e., 60–70 mL/min versus 30 mL/min). Subclavian silicone catheters placed centrally and used in BMT are not stiff enough to withstand the rapid withdrawal of blood. A more rigid catheter used for dialysis was frequently used for BCT apheresis in the past. This catheter was replaced by another one after apheresis for extended use during BCT. The PermCath (Quinton, Bothell, Washington) is a double-lumen catheter suitable for use during apheresis, conditioning chemotherapy, and supportive care. A common choice is the Pheres-Flow (Horizan Medical Products, Inc., Manchester, Georgia), a triple-lumen catheter. This catheter is intended for long-term access, can withstand the pressures and flow rates required during apheresis, and offers the added benefit of a third port.

The catheter is inserted in an outpatient setting, usually at the beginning or during the period of mobilization; it is used throughout BCT. Normal donors for allogeneic transplantation may have large-gauge peripheral catheters placed in bilateral antecubital veins. If peripheral access is not achievable, a temporary CVC can be placed prior to collection and removed immediately following completion of the collection.

Medications. The mobilization process is initiated at the appropriate time. If an HGF is being used, the patient must learn subcutaneous administration. The growth factor is usually administered daily for 5–6 days, with the collection of cells beginning on day 4 or 5. If chemotherapy is used for mobilization, the drugs are given and the patient returns home. Blood counts are monitored daily or every other day, and apheresis begins when the desired WBC is achieved.[6] To prevent platelet clumping during apheresis, ibuprofen 200 mg is given daily, starting several days before apheresis begins. At the same time, calcium carbonate (Oscal-D) 500 mg orally, three times daily, is prescribed to minimize hypocalcemia during apheresis.

Procedure

Equipment. Blood cell separators have been used since the 1980s for various clinical indications such as plasma apheresis and leukapheresis. Cells can be harvested by automated continuous- or discontinuous-flow blood cell separators.[36] The Fenwal CS 3000 (Fenwal Laboratories, Deerfield, Illinois), Cobe Spectra (Cobe Laboratories, Lakewood, Colorado), and the Haemonetics V-50 or M30 (Haemonetics Corp., Braintree, Massachusetts) are the most commonly used machines.[6,36] Other collection equipment includes Amicus (Baxter Healthcare, Deerfield, Illinois), Spectra (Gambro BCT, software version 4.7), and CS 3000 Plus (Cobe Laboratories). These machines operate with cyclic phases of separation, spillover, concentration, and collection. Current research focuses on maximizing the number of $CD34^+$ cells while minimizing the platelets collected. The Amicus, when compared to the Spectra, was found to be superior due to the lower number of platelets collected.[43] Software programs such LP-MNC and LP-PBSC-LYM are also used to maximize cell collection. In one study, the LP-MNC program was more efficient in collecting $CD34^+$ cells, while the LP-MNC program resulted in less platelet loss.[44]

Collection. Collection of cells begins once the WBC count is adequate. When chemotherapy is used for mobilization, the WBC must be greater than 10,000 cells/mm^3 and clear evidence of rising counts must be present prior to collection of cells. If growth factor is used to stimulate neutrophil production, a count exceeding 20,000 cells/mm^3 indicates that the patient is ready to be apheresed. Baseline blood specimens — including RBC, platelet, and calcium samples — are drawn. Next, the patient is connected to the machine using the CVC. About 7–15 L of blood is processed through the machine in a 2- to 4-hour period. The mononuclear cell layer is drawn off of the blood, and the rest is returned to the patient. Chilling can occur due to the large volume of blood leaving the body, then cooling to room temperature before being returned to the patient. However, the patient is generally comfortable during the procedure and can watch television or use other diversional activities.

Large-volume leukapheresis. Cells are collected daily on an outpatient basis until the desired amount is obtained, which usually requires 2–4 days. Large-volume leukapheresis (LVL) is the standard procedure. The modernization of leukapheresis equipment makes possible the processing of large volumes of blood at one time.[42] Large-volume leukapheresis processes at least three blood volumes (15–35 L) during a single apheresis over approximately 3–5 hours.

Complications

Several potential procedure complications associated with apheresis can be avoided or minimized by early intervention.[13] A large volume of sodium citrate, an anticoagulant, is used to keep the blood from clotting.[41] The citrate binds to ionized serum calcium, producing hypocalcemia. As a result, the patient may experience tingling in the extremities and around the mouth. Nurses routinely give calcium carbonate (Tums, SmithKline Beecham) at the beginning of apheresis and as needed throughout the procedure. Intravenous calcium gluconate may be needed if the hypocalcemia becomes severe. Hypovolemia may also be problematic, especially for patients with a history of cardiac problems. Patients may complain of lightheadedness, chilling, dizziness, and shaking, and experience dysrhythmia. Thrombocytopenia is problematic with some types of equipment because platelets are destroyed by the process. Because platelet counts may drop by 50% during the apheresis procedure, the patient should have an adequate platelet count (>100,000/mm^3) before the procedure begins.[37] Occasionally, the blood flow rate through the CVC may be altered or decreased. In most cases, a position change by the patient will quickly remedy this problem.

Human Cord Blood

Another alternative for obtaining bone marrow stem cells is using placental or umbilical cord blood. Since 1998, an estimated 2500 related or unrelated donor umbilical cord blood transplants have occurred in the United States, and large-scale collection and storage of UCB stem cells is currently under way.[45,46] Unrelated donors have become the predominant source of UCB stem cells.[45] Cells are collected immediately after delivery of the placenta.

Advantages of using UCB include immediate availability, absence of donor risk, absence of donor attrition, and low risk of transmissible infectious disease such as cytomegalovirus and Epstein-Barr virus. A decreased risk of GVHD is considered an advantage because the fetal cells are not competent immunologically. Umbilical cord blood may allow expansion of available donor pools in targeted ethnic and racial minorities currently underrepresented in all marrow donor registries.[47,48] Disadvantages of using UCB include the lowered risk of GVHD in patients with hematologic malignancy. The lowered risk may potentially be associated with a higher risk of relapse, as there is no graft-versus-leukemia effect. Other disadvantages include an increased risk of genetic disorder transmission and insufficient numbers of cells for engraftment for larger recipients.

FACT standards require a personal and family history of the biological mother (and father, if available) to be obtained and documented prior to or within 48 hours of UCB collection. Infectious disease testing of the maternal donor is required no more than 30 days prior to or within 48 hours of UCB collection. Cord blood is not accepted for unrelated transplant if there is a history of a genetic disorder in the immediate family that could potentially affect the recipient.[5]

The outcomes from UCB transplants continue to be evaluated. There is one report of 143 UCB transplants from 45 centers. The 1-year survival rate of 78 recipients of UCB from related donors was 63%; in 65 patients receiving unrelated UCB transplants, 1-year survival was 29%.[49] Cohen and Nagler recently published a review of 10 unrelated-donor UCB studies in children and 6 related-donor UCB studies in adults. Although overall survival rates were not reported, improved survival was correlated with higher doses of UCB. The UCB transplants have been more successful in children than adults, a finding that is consistent with all types of transplants.[45] Many issues remain to be resolved, including optimal methods for harvesting, processing, and storing the cells; ethical and regulatory issues; minimum number of cells needed for engraftment in larger recipients; risk of chronic and acute GVHD with mismatched donors; malignancy relapse rate; potential for gene therapy; ex vivo expansion; and immunologic reconstitution following transplant.[48,50]

Cell Processing and Storage

Cell Identification

The cells obtained from the bone marrow, peripheral blood, or umbilical cord are processed and cryopreserved in the same way. The American Association of Blood Banking (AABB) and FACT have strict standards for processing and storage of the cells.[5,51] Processing begins with the identification of the cells needed for engraftment. The CD34$^+$ assay is an easy, standardized method that provides the real number of circulating progenitor cells, not a number predicted after growth in culture.[52] At present, CD34$^+$ selection is the most reproducible and consistent technique available. One new marker of more primitive hematopoietic progenitor cells is CD133.[53] However, further development of techniques to identify the number and type of cells essential for engraftment is needed.[51]

Processing

After collection, the stem cells are processed by weighing and calculating the concentration of cells per milliliter. For concentrations exceeding 2×10^8 nucleated cells/mL, additional plasma may be collected and added to adjust the volume to the optimal freezing concentration of 2×10^8 nucleated cells/mL. The product is tested for tumor or other outside contamination, total CD34+ count, mononuclear cell counts, and viability of the cells.[6] FACT describes this product as "minimally manipulated" cells because they have not been exposed to any ex vivo procedures that selectively remove, enrich, or expand the cell populations.[5]

Quality management of collected cells is strictly defined and monitored through the AABB and FACT (see Table 19-2). The laboratory must document the testing of the components, laboratory control procedures, and the sterility and accuracy of all supplies and reagents. Equipment must be kept clean and calibrated. Component identification and labeling should be done in a manner to prevent mislabeling of components.

Tumor Contamination

One of the main reasons for using blood rather than bone marrow–derived cells for autologous transplantation is to avoid tumor contamination from bone marrow.

Minimal residual disease is especially important for patients with hematologic malignancy. The outcome after either autologous BMT or BCT in patients with acute myelogenous leukemia is similar. Therefore, the shortened nadir period produced by BCT may be the only advantage of one procedure over the other. Gene-marking experiments have clearly indicated that relapses can originate from tumor cells contaminating the cryopreserved cells.[54] The development of sensitive methods for detecting tumor cells indicates that contamination of peripheral blood with malignant cells is common.[28,29]

Cell sorting

CD34 assays are useful for separating the malignant cells in a positive selection process. CD34 antigens are not present in breast tumors, neuroblastoma, lymphoma, and multiple myeloma cells.[29] Therefore, PPSCs and progenitor cell isolates should be free from tumor contamination. That is, in theory, selecting only CD34+ cells should give a product that is free from malignant cells for those diseases.[29,54]

Mobilized peripheral CD34+ progenitors can be highly purified with good recovery and can result in complete and sustained engraftment.[54] Methods currently in use include magnetic activated cell sorting of the product and continuous flow technology for cell enrichment. One method, Ceprate, a stem cell concentration kit (Cell Pro, Inc., Bothell, Washington) was recently approved by the Food and Drug Administration (FDA) for both bone marrow stem cell and PBPC processing.

Purging techniques

Purging of autologous bone marrow and peripheral blood cells is another strategy to decrease the risk of tumor contamination. Purging occurs after harvest or apheresis and before cryopreservation. A number of procedures are used to remove the malignant cells, all of which have the potential to harm the PPSCs and progenitor cells.[55,56] This manipulation often results in delayed or failed engraftment.

Several approaches are used for purging.[55] Pharmacologic methods use chemotherapeutic agents such as 4–hydroperoxycyclophosphamide (4HC), mafosfamide, etoposide, vincristine, or methylprednisolone. Immunologic methods use monoclonal antibodies (MoAbs) and toxins. A MoAb must specifically target the malignant cell and have no effect on hematologic stem cells to effectively purge the tissue. If the targeted antigen is present at high concentration on the cell surface, increased cell killing will occur. Because the MoAbs are not toxic themselves, they are combined with other agents or toxins. Physical methods are used to mark the malignant cells, then separate them from the isolate. Other techniques employ photosensitizing agents, membrane-active agents, and long-term bone marrow cultures.

Manipulation of hematopoietic progenitor cells includes ex vivo expansion, gene manipulation, and T-cell depletion. *Ex vivo expansion* involves the expansion in culture of one or more populations of cells. Reports indicate that selected CD34+ cells grown for 7–14 days in liquid culture systems with various combinations of HGFs, such as stem cell factor, IL-3 or IL-6 with G-CSF or GM-CSF, and EPO, produce an increase in numbers of CFU-GM. The long-term durability of these cells has not been determined.[1] Umbilical cord blood cells have also been expanded in culture using PIXY 321, flt-3 ligand, and EPO. To date, these expanded populations of cells have not shown improved recovery of bone marrow function.[48,50]

Gene manipulation involves the insertion of one or more genes into one or more populations of cells. An example is the insertion of the multidrug resistance gene (*MDR-1*) into PBPCs in an effort to confer resistance to drugs such as paclitaxel. Following engraftment of modified PBPCs, the patient can tolerate repeated exposures to high-dose paclitaxel.[57,58]

Although this strategy continues to be studied, results to date have not demonstrated improved outcomes.[58]

Marrow stem cells usually contain 10%–15% mature T lymphocytes. Patients who receive these T lymphocytes and have no post-transplant immunosuppression experience 80%–100% incidence of grade 2–4 acute GVHD.[59] Depletion of the T lymphocytes greatly decreases this risk and can be accomplished through a variety of laboratory techniques. Clinical trials continue to evaluate the most effective procedures.

Freezing of cells

Cells for autologous transplant or umbilical cord cells being harvested and stored for later use are frozen. Cryopreservation is necessary to prevent stem cell damage and assure viability of the stem cells. In this technique, cells are frozen and stored at temperatures below 0°C (32°F). Dimethylsulfate is added so that cells will not lyse when thawed. Freezing of the cells begins at −1°C (30°F)/minute down to −40°C (−40°F), and −2°C (28°F)/minute from −40°C (−40°F) to −80°C (−112°F). The cells are stored in liquid nitrogen between −100°C (−148°F) and −196°C (−321°F).[42] Freezers for component storage must have an alarm system that signals a change in temperature; this alarm system must be monitored 24 hours per day. Newer techniques for cryopreservation using a methanol bath and nonprogrammed freezer are being developed. Such a process would be simpler and less costly, enabling its use in almost any institution.[60,61]

Table 19-5 Toxicities of Total Body Irradiation

Toxicities	Onset	Duration
Acute		
Nausea	Immediate	48 hours
Severe vomiting	3–5 days	3–5 days
Diarrhea	3–5 days	3–5 days
Fever	Immediate	24 hours
Skin erythema	Immediate	3–4 days
Severe skin changes	4–10 days	Variable
Oral mucositis	4–10 days	Variable
Parotitis	24 hours	24–48 hours
Delayed		
Interstitial pulmonary pneumonitis	2 months	
Gonadal dysfunction	Variable	
Cataracts	10 years	
Second malignancy	10 years	

Conditioning Therapy

Conditioning therapy is the regimen used to prepare the patient to receive the transplanted stem cells. The goal of the preparative regimen varies depending on the type of transplant and the disease involved.[62–64] The goal for allogeneic transplantation is to eradicate remaining disease, ablate the marrow to make room for the donor marrow, and suppress the immune system to prevent GVHD. In autologous transplantation, immunosuppression is not needed, as the patient is the source of cells. Nevertheless, antitumor and ablative effects are still needed.

Total Body Irradiation

Total body irradiation (TBI) is used for immunosuppression and tumor eradication. Advantages of this systemic treatment include (1) no sanctuary sites of tumor, (2) even distribution of the dosage, (3) no detoxification or excretion needed after administration, and (4) ability to tailor the dose to the patient's specific needs (i.e., boosted or shielded).[65] Total body irradiation was originally given as a single fraction of 10 Gy. However, this dose produced idiopathic interstitial pneumonitis in more than 70% of patients. Today, the dose is fractionated and given at 1.5–2.0 Gy twice daily for 3 days for a total dose of up to 12 Gy.[66]

The procedure for TBI takes 20–30 minutes per fraction. The patient usually is placed in a side-lying position and changes to the opposite side midway through the procedure. Toxicities of TBI are both acute and delayed and can be more severe depending on the particular chemotherapeutic agents administered (Table 19-5).[67]

Chemotherapy

Total body irradiation and high-dose cyclophosphamide have been tested alone as preparative regimens for allogeneic BMT, but the results were not as good as hoped. The combination, however, provided an excellent response in hematologic malignancies and became the gold standard in the 1970s and 1980s.[4] Busulfan was tested to replace TBI and was found to be effective, although different toxicities result.[62] Cyclophosphamide and busulfan are most often used in allogeneic BMT centers that lack TBI capability. The regimens for preparation for autologous transplant vary according to the underlying disease. The agents are selected for maximum effect against specific malignancies (Table 19-6).[62–64,67] The dosages that constitute high-dose therapy increase systemic exposure threefold as compared to a standard dose.[62]

Reinfusion

Reinfusion of the bone marrow stem cells or PBPCs should occur 24 hours after high-dose chemotherapy so as to prevent damage to the reinfused stem cells by residual chemotherapy. The exception to this guideline is for thiotepa, which requires 48 hours for protection of the transplanted cells.

Blood cell transplant reinfusion

If PBPCs are collected in more than one apheresis procedure, the volume to be transplanted is contained in more than one bag. On the day of transplantation (day 0) the cells are transported in the frozen state to the patient's bedside. The primary container is sealed and aseptic. A secondary container is provided to prevent leakage. The outer shipping container is thermally insulated at whatever level is needed to maintain the frozen state until reaching the bedside. A basket of supplies needed during reinfusion should be available at the bedside. After patient identification is verified per patient armband, the cells are thawed quickly in a warm water bath 98.6–104°F (37–40°C). Rapid warming prevents small ice crystals from forming by recrystallization. Because the cells are fragile, they should not be manipulated prior to infusion. To preserve viability of cells, they are infused immediately, within 10–20 minutes of thawing the bag. A second bag of cells should not be thawed until the previous bag is completely infused.

A connector is inserted to break the vacuum and provide a needle puncture site. Using a 60–mL syringe, the cells are withdrawn from the collection bag. The cells are administered through a tunneled CVC by IV push via a separate line infusing preservative-free normal saline. The saline should help to minimize blood cell clumping. There should not be any filters on the IV line. The bag is emptied and rinsed with 10–20 mL of preservative-free saline. The process is repeated until each bag is infused.

Depending on the volume of the DMSO, the patient may receive 1–3 bags, wait several hours, then resume infusion. Dimethylsulfate makes up 10% of the volume of each bag. The maximum DMSO per day the patient should receive is 1 mL/kg; DMSO causes the patient to have an immediate garlic taste. Because DMSO is excreted by the lungs, the same odor is obvious in the immediate area of the patient's room.

Table 19-6 Common Chemotherapeutic Agents Used in Hematopoietic Cell Transplantation

Diseases	Conditioning Regimen	Acronym
Hematologic, general	Busulfan/cyclophosphamide	BU/CY
	Busulfan/cyclophosphamide/total body irradiation	BU/CY/TBI
	Busulfan/melphalan	BU/MEL
	Cyclophosphamide/total body irradiation	CY/TBI
	Cytarabine/total body irradiation	Ara-C/TBI
Hematologic, acute leukemia	Cyclophosphamide/etoposide/total body irradiation	CY/VP/TBI
	Cyclophosphamide/cytarabine/total body irradiation	TCC
	Etoposide/total body irradiation	VP/TBI
Non-Hodgkin's lymphoma	Carmustine/etoposide/cytarabine/cyclophosphamide	BEAC
Hodgkin's and non-Hodgkin's lymphoma	Carmustine/etoposide/cytarabine/melphalan	BEAM
	Cyclophosphamide/carmustine/etoposide	CBV, BCV
Hodgkin's, non-Hodgkin's lymphoma, multiple myeloma	Busulfan/cyclophosphamide/etoposide	BU/CY/VP
Multiple myeloma	Melphalan/total body irradiation	Mel/TBI
Breast	Mitoxantrone/etoposide/thiotepa	MVT
Breast, solid tumors	Cyclophosphamide/carmustine/cisplatin	CBP
	Cyclophosphamide/thiotepa/carboplatin	STAMP-5, CCT
	Cyclophosphamide/thiotepa/cisplatin	CTP
Breast, solid tumors, testicular	Cyclophosphamide/etoposide/cisplatin	CVP, CPE
Solid tumors	Ifosfamide/carboplatin/etoposide	ICE

Some patients report a lessened taste if they suck on hard candies during and after the infusion.

Nausea can be associated with reinfusion. Although it is temporary and usually not disturbing, patients are nevertheless premedicated with an antiemetic. Shortness of breath or complaints of chest tightness are associated with both the cells passing through the lungs and the temperature of the cells. Reducing the rate of infusion should alleviate these symptoms.

Bone marrow transplant reinfusion

Allogeneic hematopoietic cells are infused through the CVC much like any blood product would be given. The cells arrive at the bedside within hours of collection. Ideally, minimal manipulation of these life-giving cells will occur. Patient identity is verified using the patient armband. The patient is premedicated to lessen the side effects most commonly associated with the infusion. These premedications may include a prophylactic antiemetic such as lorazepam. Diphenhydramine chloride, meperidine hydrochloride, hydrocortisone, acetaminophen, and methylprednisolone may be given as prophylaxis for transfusion-related hemolytic reactions.

Furosemide and mannitol are given to prevent fluid overload. The patient is usually hydrated prior to, during, and following the infusion. Strict intake and output should be monitored to prevent fluid overload. Vital signs are monitored as per blood transfusion standards.

Cells are infused using an infusion pump. It is important to avoid any filters on the IV tubing. The infusion bags should be gently agitated periodically to prevent fat cells from clumping in the product.

Inpatient Issues

A number of factors have influenced the transition of transplant care from inpatient to outpatient settings: technological advances, improved symptom management, cost-containment initiatives, and patient advocacy.[12,68] Patients receiving allogeneic transplants generally receive the conditioning treatment and immediate post-transplant care in the hospital. Use of HGFs has decreased the length of the nadir, allowing for earlier discharge. In addition, many institutions have outpatient facilities (hotel accommodations) available 7 days per week to allow for daily assessments and treatments while providing for social/family needs.

Outpatient Issues

Blood cell transplant developments that support outpatient care have greatly influenced the move to outpatient care, including decreased number of aphereses, greater number and applications of HGFs, intravenous antibiotics and antiemetics,[7,12] increased numbers of BCT procedures, standardization of care, and increased numbers of community centers.[68] The cost-effectiveness of BCT is difficult to evaluate, however. A cost-effectiveness analysis that measures the value (years of life saved) over cost of medical interventions is frequently undertaken to support continued use of BCT.[9,10]

Advances in BMT include improved management of GVHD, increased long-term disease-free survival, increased availability of donors through the National Marrow Donor Program, and more diseases being treated with BMT. Also, more alternative care models and strategies are being utilized to provide safe, quality, cost-effective care that reduces or eliminates the need for hospitalization.[68] Ruiz-Arguelles et al. recently reported using noncryopreserved cells to successfully transplant patients in an outpatient setting using a 1–day conditioning regimen of high-dose melphalan in patients with hematologic malignancy.[69] Others have developed outpatient protocols as well.[7]

Successful outpatient models have modified chemotherapy regimens to decrease side effects such as mucositis and hemorrhagic cystitis. Drug combinations that have been used successfully for outpatient transplantation include melphalan, carmustine/triethylenethiophosphormide (thiotepa), cyclophosphamide/mesna/thiotepa, and busulfan. Duke's program has become the model for many outpatient centers. In the Duke program, women with breast cancer receiving autologous BMT are hospitalized for chemotherapy, then discharged to a nearby hotel. The women are seen daily in the outpatient clinic, and 67% are readmitted for a short period (< 5 days).[70] Other centers have also used a hotel to support outpatient care.[71] Patients in the Duke program receive empiric ceftazidime every 8 hours during the period of neutropenia. Two doses are administered in the outpatient clinic, and a night dose is administered at the hotel by a visiting nurse. This model adjusts the level of care provided in the clinic based on the length of time after transplant. During the first 2 weeks post-transplant, patients receive physician assessments one to two times per day. More stable patients are seen by the physician two to three times per week.

A program delivering autologous BCT in the home was reported by Hermann et al.[72] Twenty-five adults with multiple myeloma, non-Hodgkin's lymphoma, or Hodgkin's disease received all care at home except for the infusion of blood stem cells. Participation in the program required the availability of a caregiver. A clinical nurse specialist made visits to the home twice a day and reported to the physician and evening nursing staff on the BMT patient unit. Sixty percent of patients required admission to the hospital for a median of 5 days for management of complications, which is comparable to other outpatient models. Patients participating in the program expressed high satisfaction with the care received at home.

Outpatient TBI is also being evaluated. In one study, 68 pediatric patients received outpatient TBI in preparation for transplantation.[73] To control the nausea and vomiting usually associated with TBI, the patients received an oral 5HT-3 antagonist every 8 hours. Due to the efficacy of this classification of antiemetics, the nausea and vomiting were well controlled, with only one patient requiring intravenous hydration and one patient requiring hospitalization for intractable diarrhea and dehydration.

The clinic/home care option for transplant is not available for all patients. Patient selection requires assessment of the patient's medical condition, functional status, family support, and psychosocial history.[26] Geographical distance from the center is considered if no adequate housing is available nearby. Both the patient and the caregiver must be able to understand the treatment and demonstrate the ability to fully cooperate with all required treatments.

Studies comparing the cost and safety implications for patients receiving HCT in various settings are ongoing. Meisenberg and colleagues compared the cost and safety data for 94 patients receiving autologous BCT in three settings: inpatient, partial outpatient, and total outpatient.[74] The average lengths of stay were 17.3, 8.2, and 2.7 days, respectively. The mean procedure costs were $39,700, $36,200, and $29,400, respectively. No difference in toxicity or overall response was found. As efforts continue to reduce the cost of HCT, it will be interesting to see whether patients who have available caregivers providing a significant amount of care will receive direct benefits through premium discounts or reimbursement for care provided.

Conclusion

The applicability of hematopoietic transplant continues to increase as responses improve. As progress continues to be made in the isolation and expansion of stem cells, and as UCB use becomes more widespread, more patients will receive transplants. The nurse caring for patients undergoing HCT will continue to be challenged by the rapid progress and changes occurring in the field. The technical aspects of the mobilization, collection, processing, and reinfusion of hematopoietic cells require professionals who are committed to continual study. Participation in ongoing research will produce conditioning regimens modified for outpatient administration and more effective medications for symptom management. As HCT care continues to be delivered outside of the standard inpatient unit, the nurse must collaborate more closely with family caregivers and community health professionals.

References

1. Boiron JM, Reiffers J, Lowenthal RM: Blood cell transplantation: past, present and future. *Hematol Cell Ther* 38:399–407, 1996
2. Applebaum FR: The current status of hematopoietic cell transplantation. *Annu Rev Med* 54:491–512, 2003
3. *www.IBMTR.org*. Accessed May 28, 2004
4. Horowitz MM: Uses and growth of hematopoietic cell transplantation, in Thomas ED, Blume KG, Forman SJ (eds.): *Hematopoietic Cell Transplantation* (ed 2). Malden, MA, Blackwell Science, 1999, pp 12–18
5. *www.FACT.org*. Accessed May 28, 2004
6. O'Connell SA, Schmit-Pokorney K: Blood and marrow stem cell transplantation: indications, procedures, process, in Whedon MB, Wujcik D (eds.): *Blood and Marrow Stem Cell Transplantation: Principles, Practice, Nursing Insights* (ed 2). Sudbury, MA, Jones and Bartlett, 1997, pp 66–99
7. Flowers MED, Sullivan KM: Ambulatory care of patients undergoing marrow or blood stem cell transplantation, in Atkinson K (ed.): *Clinical Bone Marrow and Blood Stem Cell Transplantation*. New York, Cambridge University Press, 2000, pp 43–59
8. Blume KG, Amylon MD: The evaluation and counseling of candidates for hematopoietic cell transplantation, in Thomas ED, Blume KG, Forman SJ (eds.): *Hematopoietic Cell Transplantation* (ed 2). Malden, MA, Blackwell Science, 1999, pp 371–380
9. Yee GC: Peripheral blood progenitor cell transplantation: economic issues. *Pharmacotherapy* 18:9–16, 1998
10. Glaspy JA: Economic considerations in the use of peripheral blood progenitor cells to support high-dose chemotherapy. *Bone Marrow Transplant* 23(suppl 2):S21–S27, 1999
11. King CR: Peripheral stem cell transplantation: past, present, and future, in Buchsel PC, Whedon MB (eds.): *Bone Marrow Transplantation: Administrative and Clinical Issues*. Sudbury, MA, Jones and Bartlett, 1995, pp 187–211
12. Kelley CH, McBride LH, Randolph SR, et al: *Home Care Management of the Blood Cell Transplant Patient* (ed 3). Sudbury, MA, Jones and Bartlett, 1998
13. Walker FE, Roethke SK, Sandman V, et al: Guiding patients and their families through peripheral stem cell transplantation with the help of a teaching booklet. *Oncol Nurs Forum* 21:585–591, 1994
14. Anderson D, Weisdorf, D: Blood vs marrow allogeneic stem cell transplantation, in Laughlin MJ, Lazarus HM (eds.): *Allogeneic Stem Cell Transplantation*. Totowa, NJ, Humana Press, 2003, pp 103–115
15. To LB, Haylock DN, Simmons PJ, et al: The biology and clinical uses of blood stem cells. *Blood* 89:2233–2258, 1997
16. Shpall EJ, Warkentin PI, Jones RB: Guidelines for the procurement and manipulation of stem cells for transplantation, in Thomas ED, Blume KG, Forman SJ (eds.): *Hematopoietic Cell*

Transplantation (ed 2). Malden, MA, Blackwell Science, 1999, pp 417–430

17. Hegland J: Transplant immunology: HLA and issues of stem cell donation, in Whedon MB, Wujcik D (eds.): *Blood and Marrow Stem Cell Transplantion* (ed 2). Sudbury, MA, Jones and Bartlett, 1997, pp 43–65
18. *www.marrow.org.* Accessed May 28, 2004
19. Nandurkar HH, Begley CG: Molecular control of hematopoiesis, in Atkinson K (ed.): *Clinical Bone Marrow and Blood Stem Cell Transplantation.* New York, Cambridge University Press, 2000, pp 43–59
20. Thomas ED, Storb R: The development of the scientific foundation of hematopoietic cell transplantation based on animal and human studies, in Thomas ED, Blume KG, Forman SJ (eds.): *Hematopoietic Cell Transplantation* (ed 2). Malden, MA, Blackwell Science, 1999, pp 1–11
21. Cooper DL, Seropian S: Autologous stem cell transplantation, in DeVita VT, Hellman S, Rosenberg SA (eds.): *Cancer: Principles and Practices of Oncology* (ed. 6). Philadelphia, Lippincott, Williams & Wilkins, 2001, pp 2767–2778
22. Champlin RE: Peripheral blood progenitor cells: a replacement for marrow transplantation? *Semin Oncol* 2:15–21, 1996
23. Anderlini P, Korbling M, Dale D, et al: Allogeneic blood stem cell transplantation: considerations for donors. *Blood* 90:903–908, 1997
24. Arcese W, Aversa F, Bandini G, et al: Clinical use of allogeneic hematopoietic stem cells from sources other than bone marrow. *Haematologica* 83:159–182, 1998
25. Kapustay PM: Blood cell transplantation: concepts and concerns. *Semin Oncol Nurs* 13:151–163, 1997
26. D'Andrea B, Belliveau D, Birmingham J, et al: High-dose chemotherapy followed by stem cell transplant: the clinic/home care experience. *J Care Manage* 3:46–84, 1997
27. Poloquin CM: Overview of bone marrow and peripheral blood stem cell transplantation. *Clin J Oncol Nurs* 1:11–17, 1997
28. Kawabata Y, Hirokawa M, Komatsuda A, et al: Clinical applications of CD34+ cell-selected peripheral blood stem cells. *Therap Apher Dial* 7:298–304, 2003
29. Kondo M, Wagers AJ, Manz MG, et al: Biology of hematopoietic stem cells and progenitors: implications for clinical application. *Annu Rev Immunol* 21:759–806, 2003
30. Papayannopoulou T: Current mechanistic scenarios in hematopoietic stem/progenitor cell mobilization. *Blood* 103:1580–1585, 2004
31. Fruehauf S, Seggewiss R: It's moving day: factors affecting peripheral blood stem cell mobilization and strategies for improvement. *Br J Haematol* 122:360–375, 2003
32. Perez-Simon JA, Caballero M, Corral MJ, et al: Minimal number of circulating CD34+ cells to ensure successful leukapheresis and engraftment in autologous peripheral blood progenitor cell transplantation. *Transfusion* 38:385–391, 1998
33. Vriesendorp JM: Aims of conditioning. *Exper Hematol* 31:844–854, 2003
34. Childs R: Allogeneic stem cell transplantation, in DeVita VT, Hellman S, Rosenberg SA (eds.): *Cancer: Principles and Practices of Oncology* (ed 6). Philadelphia, Lippincott, Williams & Wilkins, 2001, pp 2779–2798
35. Pagliuca A, Carrington PA, Pettengell R, et al: Guidelines on the use of colony-stimulating factors in haematological malignancies. *Br J Haematol* 123:22–33, 2003
36. Moog R, Muller N: Technical aspects and performance in collecting peripheral blood progenitor cells. *Ann Hematol* 77:143–147, 1998
37. Wagner ND, Quinones VW: Allogeneic peripheral blood stem cell transplantation: clinical overview and nursing implications. *Oncol Nurs Forum* 25:1049–1055, 1998
38. Majado MJ, Gonzalez C, Marin L, et al: Second mobilization of peripheral blood progenitor cells in patients with poor first mobilization. *Transplant Proc* 35:2027–2028, 2003
39. Noga SJ, Oroszlan M, Zhang YL, et al: Single dose pegfilgrastim successfully mobilizes optimal numbers of autologous CD34+ cells for peripheral stem cell collection. *Blood* 100:826, 2002 (abstract)
40. Watanabe T, Takaue Y, Kawano Y: Peripheral blood stem cell transplantation: an update. *J Med Invest* 44:25–31, 1997
41. Szer J: Cryopreservation and functional assessment of harvested bone marrow and blood stem cells, in Atkinson K (ed.): *Clinical Bone Marrow and Blood Stem Cell Transplantation.* New York, Cambridge University Press, 2000, pp 201–207
42. Jeanne M, Bouzgarrou R, Lafarge X, et al: Comparison of CD34+ cell collection on the CS-3000+ and Amicus blood cell separators. *Transfusion* 43:1423–1427, 2003
43. Ikeda K, Ohto H, Nemoto K, et al: Collection of MNCs and progenitor cells by two separators for PBPC transplantation: a randomized crossover trial. *Transfusion* 43:814–819, 2003
44. Schwella N, Movassaghi K, Scheding S, et al: Comparison of two leukapheresis programs for computerized collection of blood progenitor cells on a new cell separator. *Transfusion* 43:58–64, 2003
45. Cohen Y, Nagler A: Hematopoietic stem-cell transplantation using umbilical-cord blood. *Leuk Lymphoma* 44:1287–1299, 2003
46. Cairo MS, Wagner JE: Placental and/or umbilical cord blood: an alternative source of hematopoietic stem cells for transplantation. *Blood* 90:4665–4678, 1997
47. Kline RM, Bertolone SJ: Umbilical cord blood transplantation: providing a donor for everyone needing a bone marrow transplant? *South Med J* 91:821–828, 1998
48. Koller MR, Manchel I, Maher RJ, et al: Clinical-scale human umbilical cord blood cell expansion in a novel automated perfusion culture system. *Bone Marrow Transplant* 21:653–663, 1998
49. Gluckman R, Rocha V, Boyer-Chammard A, et al: Outcome of cord-blood transplantation from related and unrelated donors. Eurocord Transplant Group and the European Blood and Marrow Transplantation Group. *N Engl J Med* 337:373–381, 1997
50. Barker JN, Wagner JE: Umbilical-cord blood transplantation for the treatment of cancer. *Nat Rev Cancer* 3:526–532, 2003
51. Apheresis, in American Association of Blood Banks, Standards Committee: *19th Edition Standards for Blood Banks and Transfusion Services* (ed 19). Bethesda, MD, American Association for Blood Banks, 1999, pp 47–55
52. Demirer T, Buckner CD, Bensinger WI: Optimization of peripheral blood stem cell mobilization. *Stem Cells* 14:106–116, 1996
53. Lang P, Bader P, Schumm M, et al: Transplantation of a combination of CD133+ and CD34+ selected progenitor cells from alternative donors. *Br J Haematol* 124:72–79, 2004
54. Handgretinger R, Lang P, Schumm M, et al: Isolation and transplantation: an update. *Bone Marrow Transplant* 21:987–993, 1998
55. Granena GA, Ferra CC: Autologous stem cell transplantation and purging in adult acute lymphoblastic leukemia. *Best Pract Res Clin Haematol* 15:675–693, 2002
56. Bradstock KF: The role of tumor cell purging in autologous hematopoietic stem cell transplantation for malignant disease: clinical results, in Atkinson K (ed.): *Clinical Bone Marrow and Blood Stem Cell Transplantation.* New York, Cambridge University Press, 2000, pp 414–422

57. Korbling M, Champlin R: Peripheral blood progenitor cell transplantation: a replacement for marrow auto- or allografts. *Stem Cells* 14:185–195, 1996
58. Keating A, Filshie RJA, Leslie KB: Gene therapy in blood and marrow transplantation, in Atkinson K (ed.): *Clinical Bone Marrow and Blood Stem Cell Transplantation.* New York, Cambridge University Press, 2000, pp 1302–1317
59. Kernan NA: T-cell depletion for the prevention of graft versus host disease, in Thomas ED, Blume KG, Forman SJ (eds.): *Hematopoietic Cell Transplantation* (ed 2). Malden, MA, Blackwell Science, 1999, pp 186–196
60. Hernandez-Navarro F, Ojeda E, Arrieta R, et al: Hematopoietic cell transplantation using plasma and DMSO without HES, with non-programmed freezing by immersion in a methanol bath: results in 213 cases. *Bone Marrow Transplant* 21:511–517, 1998
61. Straka C, Hebart H, Adler-Reichel S, et al: Blood stem cell collections after mobilization with combination chemotherapy containing ifosfamide followed by G-CSF in multiple myeloma. *Oncology* 65:94–98, 2003
62. Doroshow JH: Pharmacological basis for high-dose chemotherapy, in Thomas ED, Blume KG, Forman SJ (eds.): *Hematopoietic Cell Transplantation* (ed 2). Malden, MA, Blackwell Science, 1999, pp 103–122
63. Dix SP, Yee GC: Pharmacologic and biologic agents, in Whedon MB, Wujcik D (eds.): *Blood and Marrow Stem Cell Transplantation: Principles, Practice, and Nursing Insights* (ed 2). Sudbury, MA, Jones and Bartlett, 1997, pp 100–150
64. Conditioning regimens and management of common toxicities, in Shapiro TW, Davison DB, Rust DM (eds.): *Stem Cell and Bone Marrow Transplantation,* Sudbury, MA, Jones and Bartlett, 1997, pp 39–80
65. Shank B: Radiotherapeutic principles of hematopoietic cell transplantation, in Thomas ED, Blume KG, Forman SJ (eds.): *Hematopoietic Cell Transplantation* (ed 2). Malden, MA, Blackwell Science, 1999, pp 151–167
66. Lin H, Dryzmala RE: Total body and hemibody irradiation, in Perez CA, Bracy LW (eds.): *Principles and Practice of Radiation Oncology* (ed 3). Philadelphia, Lippincott-Raven, 1998, pp 333–342
67. Buckner CD, Bensinger WI: High-dose chemotherapy and chemoradiotherapy preparative treatment regimens, in Atkinson K (ed.): *Clinical Bone Marrow and Blood Stem Cell Transplantation.* New York, Cambridge University Press, 2000, pp 1147–1165
68. Buchsel PC, Kapustay PM: Models of ambulatory care for blood cell and bone marrow transplantation, in Wheden MB, Wujcik D (eds.): *Blood and Marrow Stem Cell Transplantation: Principles, Practice, and Nursing Insights* (ed 2). Sudbury, MA, Jones and Bartlett, 1997, pp 525–561
69. Ruiz-Arguelles GJ, Ruiz-Arguelles A, Perez-Romano B, et al: Non-cryopreserved peripheral blood stem cell autotransplants for hematological malignancies can be performed entirely on an outpatient basis. *Am J Hematol* 58:161–164, 1998
70. Peters WP, Ross M, Vredenburgh JJ, et al: The use of intensive clinic support to permit outpatient autologous bone marrow transplantation for breast cancer. *Semin Oncol* 21:25–31, 1994
71. McGuire TR, Tarantolo MD, Reed E: Peripheral blood progenitor cells: enabling outpatient transplantation. *Pharmacotherapy* 18:17S–23S, 1998
72. Herrmann RP, Leather M, Leather HL, et al: Clinical care for patients receiving autologous hematopoietic stem cell transplantation in the home setting. *Oncol Nurs Forum* 25:1427–1432, 1998
73. Applegate GL, Mittal BB, Kletzel M, et al: Outpatient total body irradiation prior to bone marrow transplantation in pediatric patients: a feasibility analysis. *Bone Marrow Transplant* 21:651–652, 1998
74. Meisenberg BR, Ferran K, Hollenbach K, et al: Reduced charges and costs associated with outpatient autologous stem cell transplantation. *Bone Marrow Transplant* 21:927–932, 1998

CHAPTER 20

Complications of Hematopoietic Cell Transplantation

Lowell Anderson-Reitz, RN, MS, ANP, AOCN®

Introduction

Hematopoietic cell transplantation (HCT) is a widely used therapy for malignant and nonmalignant diseases. *Transplantation* is defined as the transfer of living tissues or organs from one part of the body to another or from one individual to another. The three types of marrow and blood stem cell transplantation—autologous, allogeneic, and syngeneic—indicate the source of the marrow or blood stem cells that are transplanted into the recipient.

Numerous acute and chronic complications can occur with each type of transplant. The nature of some complications can be generalized to all transplant types, while others are specific to the transplant type or stem cell source. Complications are generally secondary to (1) the conditioning regimen (chemotherapy and radiation); (2) graft-versus-host disease (GVHD); (3) the presenting disease; and (4) the adverse effects of medications required during the transplant process. Acute complications are generally defined as those events occurring within the first 100 days after the transplant; chronic complications present after this time frame. The intricacies of both types of complications associated with stem cell transplantation present challenging management issues to the caregiver. This chapter reviews acute and chronic complications of stem cell transplantation as well as important supportive care issues that are faced by patients, families, and stem cell donors.

Acute Complications

Acute Graft-versus-Host Disease

Acute graft-versus-host disease (AGVHD) occurs within the first 100 days following allogeneic HCT. Despite advancements in prophylaxis and treatment of AGVHD, it remains one of the most challenging and debilitating complications of allogeneic HCT. Incidence can range from 30%–50% in matched sibling transplants to 50%–80% in mismatched sibling or unrelated donor transplants.[1,2] Graft-versus-host disease is an immunologic response that is mediated by the new immune system or graft against disparate human leukocyte antigen (HLA) host cell antigens. Cells known to be involved in this process include helper T cells, cytotoxic T cells, natural killer cells, lymphokine-activated killer (LAK) cells, and antigen-presenting cells.[3] Cytotoxic injury of host tissues is the result of this activated immune response.

Acute graft-versus-host disease usually occurs within 2–5 weeks following allogeneic transplant.[4] Risk factors that influence the incidence of AGVHD include the degree of HLA mismatch, related versus unrelated donor, gender match, patient and donor age, patient and donor parity, intensity of conditioning regimen, GVHD prophylaxis regimen, and viral seropositivity.[4] Table 20-1 describes how these factors may affect the incidence of GVHD.

Table 20-2 presents commonly used systems for staging and grading of AGVHD. Grade I AGVHD has a favorable outcome and does not require treatment. Moderate disease—grade II—is associated with multiorgan involvement and requires therapy to halt progression of the disease. Grade III AGVHD is severe and may lead to grade IV disease, which is life-threatening or fatal disease. Mortality rates rise significantly for patients developing moderate to severe disease due primarily to the increased risk of infection.

Acute graft-versus-host disease primarily presents in the skin, gastrointestinal tract, and liver. Skin GVHD is the most common clinical feature of AGVHD. Acute skin GVHD often presents as a pruritic or painful maculopapular erythematous rash that most commonly begins on the plantar or palmar surfaces. However, the rash can present anywhere and involve the entire body surface area. Staging of skin GVHD is based primarily on the extent of the body surface area involved (see Table 20-2).

Hepatic GVHD is the second most common manifestation of AGVHD. Isolated liver AGVHD is rare, but possible. Elevated alkaline phosphatase and hyperbilirubinemia are seen first, with eventual elevation of the transaminases. Hepatomegaly with associated tenderness are late symptoms of this disease. Although liver biopsy is helpful for a definitive diagnosis, it is rarely performed in the face of concomitant skin or gastrointestinal GVHD.[7,8] Staging of acute liver GVHD is based on the bilirubin level.

Gastrointestinal GVHD can present with voluminous diarrhea with bleeding and abdominal cramping. Staging for acute gastrointestinal GVHD is based on the volume of diarrhea and pain or ileus development. Upper gastrointestinal involvement is associated with nausea and vomiting, anorexia, dyspepsia, or early satiety. Endoscopy with biopsies must be completed to definitively diagnose gastrointestinal GVHD.[9] The triad of skin, hepatic, and gastrointestinal GVHD can occur independently or concomitantly.

Hyperacute GVHD also involves the previously mentioned organs, but is associated with fever, influenza-like symptoms, generalized erythroderma, and desquamation. This manifestation of AGVHD can present before signs of engraftment are clear. Biopsies of the involved organs are required for diagnosis.

The hematolymphoid system appears to be affected by AGHVD, and decreased hematopoietic precursors and low immunoglobulin production may result

Table 20-1 Influences on Incidence of Graft-versus-Host Disease (GVHD)

Risk Factor	Increased GVHD	Decreased GVHD
Donor relationship	Unrelated donor	Related donor
HLA match	Mismatched	Matched
Donor/recipient parity	Increased parity	Less parity
Donor/recipient age	Older	Younger
Donor/recipient viral seropositivity	Positive	Negative
Sex match	Mismatched: female to male	Sex matched
TBI dose	>12 Gy	<12 Gy
Immunosuppressive regimen	Less intensive	More intensive
T-cell depletion	No T-cell depletion	T-cell depletion

Data from Chao[3]; Przepiorka.[5]

from this complication. Thrombocytopenia has also been reported in AGVHD.[3] These factors compound the risks associated with AGVHD and resulting infection.

Prophylaxis

Discussion of prevention and prophylaxis of GVHD begins with a consideration of the donor selection process. Histocompatibility with molecular matching of class I and II antigens is the basis for decreasing incidence of GVHD. Matching viral-seronegative donors with viral-seronegative recipients also appears to decrease infection and GVHD incidence.[1] Although selective and nonselective T-cell depletion significantly decreases incidence of GVHD, it is associated with increased graft-rejection and disease relapse.[9] In addition, the intensity of chemoradiotherapy administered as part of the conditioning regimen is related to GVHD. The tissue damage associated with more intense regimens causes cytokine release, which allows for alloantigen presentation for donor T cells.[9] This effect, in turn, increases the incidence of AGVHD.

Combination immunosuppressive therapy is the mainstay of medical prophylaxis of GVHD. Cyclosporine or tacrolimus administered in combination with methotrexate has been shown to decrease GVHD and increase survival in numerous studies.[10–12] The benefit of adding corticosteroids remains unclear, with randomized studies providing conflicting results. Newer agents, such as mycophenolate mofetil, sirolimus, and pentostatin, are being studied to elucidate their roles in prophylaxis of GVHD. Studies are also ongoing with antithymocyte globulin, monoclonal antibodies such as Campath (anti-CD52), and extracorporeal photopheresis to determine these methods' effectiveness for AGHVD prophylaxis.

Treatment

Glucocorticoids remain the gold standard for treatment of confirmed AGVHD. Treatment is indicated for grades II–IV GVHD, consisting of the addition of glucocorticoids to the maintaining prophylactic regimen. Glucocorticoids are frequently administered in doses of 1–2 mg/kg/day IV or PO with a taper schedule based on patient response.[1,6] Antithymocyte globulin is also commonly used as a single agent or in combination with glucocorticoids for first-line therapy.[1,4] Many of the agents used for prophylaxis are also used in the treatment of GVHD.

Steroid-refractory AGHVD carries a poor prognosis. Continuing steroids in this population does not improve outcomes and is associated with increased infections. Recently, researchers have focused on the use of monoclonal antibodies to target specific T-cell populations (CD2, CD3, CD5, CD52) and agents that interfere or down-regulate interleukin receptors.[9]

Patients who develop AGVHD are at high risk for infection due to the impairment of their natural barriers against infection and in association with immunosuppressive agents used to treat GVHD. Supportive care should include prophylactic antibiotic, antiviral, and antifungal therapy. Patients who develop skin GVHD should meticulously care for their external central venous catheter sites. Skin integrity and cleanliness are also critical. Lower gastrointestinal GVHD may require gut rest with hyperalimentation and pain control for abdominal cramping. Upper gastrointestinal GVHD may require a regular antiemetic regimen.

Nursing management of patients who are at risk for, or who have developed, AGVHD is complex and requires an expert knowledge base. Nursing management issues include the following concerns:

- Careful assessment and physical examination to identify early clinical signs and symptoms of GVHD
- Identification of high-risk patients
- Meticulous skin care to prevent infection
- Monitoring fluid balance — intake/output, daily weights

Table 20-2 Staging and Grading of Graft-versus-Host Disease (GVHD)

Staging				
Skin	Grade I	Maculopapular rash < 25% body surface		
Skin	Grade II	Maculopapular rash 25–50% body surface		
Skin	Grade III	Generalized erythroderma > 50% body surface		
Skin	Grade IV	Generalized erythroderma with bullae formation		
Gut	Grade I	Diarrhea < 500 mL/day or persistent nausea		
Gut	Grade II	Diarrhea > 1000 mL/day		
Gut	Grade III	Diarhea > 1500 mL/day		
Gut	Grade IV	Severe abdominal cramping with or without ileus formation		
Liver	Grade I	Bilirubin 2.0–3.0 mg/dL		
Liver	Grade II	Bilirubin 3.1–6.0 mg/dL		
Liver	Grade III	Bilirubin 6.1–15 mg/dL		
Liver	Grade IV	Bilirubin > 15 mg/dL		
Overall Grade				
Grade	**Skin**	**Gut**		**Liver**
I	Stage I–II	None		None
II	Stage I–III	Stage I	or	Stage I
III	Stage II–III	Stage II–III	or	Stage II–III
IV	Stage II–IV	Stage II–IV	or	Stage II–IV

Data from Przepiorka, Cleary[6]; Chao.[7]

- Nutritional support, including monitoring of caloric intake and consulting with nutritional support team
- Monitoring serum electrolytes with appropriate supplementation
- Monitoring gastrointestinal output for signs of hemorrhage
- Pain management
- Monitoring for signs of infections, with knowledge that patients may not mount normal signs or symptoms while in an immunocompromised state
- Patient education regarding GVHD current therapies

Infection

Infections remain a significant cause of morbidity and mortality in HCT patients despite the significant strides made in terms of antimicrobial, antiviral, and antifungal therapies. Neutropenia following standard conditioning regimens lasts from 2 to 3 weeks. Data regarding neutropenia and infections following nonmyeloablative regimens are not well established. The number of patients developing neutropenia appears to range from 30% to 70%, and the duration of neutropenia ranges from 5 to 16 days.[13,14] Impairment of natural barriers — for example, mucositis development, central catheter placement, urinary catheter placement, and AGVHD — compounds the risk for infection. Likewise, humoral immunodeficiency with decreased IgG and antibody production increases the risk for infection long after transplant. Recovery of the humoral immune system occurs 3 to 6 months after autologous transplant and 6 to 12 months after allogeneic transplant. Recovery takes even longer in patients who develop GVHD and continue to require immunosuppressive agents.[1]

The use of prophylactic agents remains a topic of debate due to the emergence of resistant strains of microbes. Nevertheless, the Centers for Disease Control and Prevention (CDC) currently recommends prophylactic antimicrobial therapy for HCT patients. A wide range of prophylactic regimens exist, with most including a broad-spectrum antibiotic, an antiviral drug, and an antifungal agent. Post-transplant infections can generally be classified based on the time frame when they are most likely to occur (see Table 20-3). These time frames are associated with concurrent issues arising with regard to immune system status along the transplant continuum.

Bacterial infections are the most common infections, accounting for 90% of all infections occurring during the neutropenic phase. Most gram-negative and gram-positive pathogens are endogenous, and their portals of entry are tied to the physical barrier insults associated with the transplant process.[15] Viral infections also occur throughout the neutropenic phase, with herpes simplex virus (HSV) being the most common infectious agent. Antiviral prophylaxis significantly reduces the reactivation rate for HSV. Cytomegalovirus (CMV) tends to be a late infection, primarily

Table 20-3 Infection Time Frame after Hematopoietic Cell Transplant

Days 0–30	Days 31–100	Day > 100
Gram-positive bacteria	Gram-positive bacteria	Encapsulated organism
Gram-negative bacteria	Gram-negative bacteria	Pneumocystis
Herpes simplex	CMV	Varicella zoster
Candida	Varicella zoster	*Aspergillus*
Aspergillus	*Candida*	
	Aspergillus	

Data from Bashey[15]; Burt, Walsh[16]; Atkinson, Singhal.[17]

affecting allogeneic transplant recipients. Regular screening with polymerase chain reaction (PCR) has decreased CMV disease and allows for early treatment of CMV viremia. Fungal infections can occur at any time throughout the transplant process. Candidal infections are most common often arising from endogenous flora.[15] More serious fungal infections, such as that caused by *Aspergillus*, are associated with long-term immunosuppression and require extensive antifungal therapy.

Patients who develop febrile neutropenia or have strong suspicion of infection after neutrophil recovery require empiric antibiotic therapy. Broad-spectrum monotherapy or multidrug treatment is required until neutrophil recovery has occurred or until signs and symptoms of infection have resolved.

Early detection of infections is important in the nursing management of HCT patients. Frequent assessment of vital signs, catheter sites, impaired skin or mucosal barriers, pulmonary status, mental status, and laboratory values should be performed.

Gastrointestinal Complications

Chemoradiotherapy exhibits toxic effects upon rapidly proliferating cells such as those found in the gastrointestinal tract. Mucositis results from direct toxic effects on the oral mucosa from the conditioning regimen.[18] These effects lead to inflammation and ulceration of the mucosa, which is secondarily infected. One hypothesis suggests that this chain of events is accentuated by the release of interleukin-1 and TNF-alfa.[19,20] *Mucositis* is a general term referring to the inflammation and possible infection of mucous membranes, likely affecting the entire gastrointestinal tract. Resulting signs and symptoms include oral tissue erythema, denudation, bleeding, pain, esophageal spasms and dysphagia, nausea and vomiting, and abdominal cramping with diarrhea. Gastrointestinal complications occurring after HCT also include AGVHD, infection, and medication side effects.

Oral mucositis is reported to be one of the most distressing and toxic effects of HCT.[21] Its occurrence depends on the conditioning regimen, with overall incidence ranging from 75% to 99%.[19,22,23] Management of oral mucositis is simply supportive, with no proven means to prevent or treat the condition having emerged as yet. Traditionally, pain management with narcotic analgesics and routine oral care to help prevent superinfections have been the mainstays of therapy. Recent phase I and II studies suggest promising results with recombinant human keratinocyte growth factor (RHUKG). These studies report significant reductions in the severity and duration of mucositis in patients undergoing HCT.[24,25]

Candida albicans and HSV account for most oral infections. Incidence of these infections has been significantly reduced with the adoption of prophylactic antiviral and antifungal regimens. Close observation of the oral cavity should be performed to identify possible infections. Oral complications resulting from the conditioning regimen or AGVHD include altered taste and sicca syndrome. Treatment of GVHD and consultation with the nutritional support team will assist patients in combatting these difficult symptoms, which can significantly affect quality of life.[26]

Nausea and vomiting, whether associated with chemoradiotherapy, AGVHD, medications, or mucositis, remains a significant problem for HCT patients. Patients report them to be two of the most feared side effects of chemotherapy treatment.[27] The current standard of care for HCT patients calls for combination therapy with a 5HT-3 receptor antagonist and corticosteroids during chemotherapy administration.[28] Delayed nausea and vomiting is common and often more difficult to manage. Although current guidelines specify the use of corticosteroids in this situation, this approach is associated with significant immunosuppression, further increasing the risk for infection.[28] Combination therapy continues to be the standard of practice.

The etiology of abdominal cramping and diarrhea can be multifactorial. Gastrointestinal mucositis, AGVHD, infection, and medications are the most likely causative factors. Diarrhea is reported to affect 40% to 80% of HCT patients.[29–31] Management should focus on the most likely causative factor. Great care must be taken to maintain electrolyte replacements, fluid balance, and skin integrity. Antidiarrheal medications can be provided in appropriate situations.

Hepatic Complications

Numerous acute hepatic complications can arise following HCT. The most common complications include venoocclusive disease (VOD), AGVHD, infection, and drug-induced injury.

Venoocclusive disease is a clinical syndrome associated with high-dose chemotherapy and/or radiotherapy. Its reported incidence ranges from 0% to 70%, with mortality rates as high as 47%.[32] The diagnosis of VOD is based on clinical findings in the first 21 days following HCT. Diagnostic criteria include two or more of the following symptoms: hyperbilirubinemia, hepatomegaly, right upper quadrant pain, and fluid retention.[32] The pathophysiology of the syndrome begins with injury of the endothelial lining of hepatic venules and sinusoids. This endothelial injury leads to cytokine and tumor necrosis factor (TNF) activation, which stimulates coagulation and thrombosis.[33,34] The resulting impairment of blood flow produces the syndrome of hepatic VOD. Severe VOD often leads to renal insufficiency and, ultimately, multiorgan failure. Testing to support the diagnosis of VOD includes Doppler studies and liver biopsy. Biopsies obtained via a transjugular approach allow for measurement of hepatic venous pressure gradients, which are increased in VOD.[35]

Most patients who develop VOD recover spontaneously. Unfortunately, no proven therapies to prevent or treat VOD have been identified as yet. Treatment is primarily supportive in nature, and nurses play an integral role in this care for patients. Strict fluid restriction and fluid management are essential, especially when renal function is affected. Patients may be placed on dopamine to maximize renal function. Nurses need to be cognizant of medications that are renal toxic or are cleared via the kidney so that appropriate adjustments can be made. Patients may become encephalopathic, so safety measures need to be implemented. Severe disease can lead to coagulapathies, increasing patients' bleeding risk. With severe hepatomegaly, pain management becomes imperative. The intricacies of pain management are complicated by the encephalopathy that can arise in the syndrome.

Fungal and viral infections can arise in the liver in the post-transplant period. Patients often exhibit signs of infection with fever development in the absence of another site of infection. In addition, liver function tests are often elevated. Computerized tomography, ultrasound, and liver biopsy are most commonly performed to assist with diagnosis of an infectious process.

Drug-induced hepatitis can be a common side effect with the myriad of medications that are potentially hepatotoxic. Transaminitis, mimicking viral hepatitis, is the most frequently observed sign of a hepatic inflammation. Liver biopsy is diagnostic to determine the presence of drug-induced hepatitis. The insulting drug should be identified and removed or changed if possible.

Neurologic Complications

Neurologic complications in HCT patients generally arise from the underlying disease, initial treatment, conditioning regimen, immunosuppressive agents, or long-term immunosuppression.[36,37] The incidence of neurologic complications ranges from 0% to 50%.[36] The most common complications are metabolic encephalopathy associated with multiorgan failure or drug toxicity and cerebrovascular events.[36,38] Central nervous system infections are associated with extended immunosuppression and are more common in the allogeneic transplant population. Medications such as cyclosporine, tacrolimus, and corticosteroids that are required for the HCT patient can cause neurologic complications including leukoencephalopathy, peripheral tremor, and steroid-induced myopathy.

Nursing management of the HCT patient should include close observation for sometimes subtle neurologic changes. Rapid intervention in some situations may alleviate potentially deleterious outcomes.

Hematologic Complications

Pancytopenia following the conditioning regimen for HCT is an expected complication. Complications that arise as a result of this pancytopenia are associated with the specific roles of the particular blood components. Transplant patients are routinely treated with hematopoietic growth factors to hasten the recovery of neutrophils and red blood cells. Both granulocyte colony-stimulating factor (G-CSF) and granulocyte-macrophage colony-stimulating factor (GM-CSF) have been shown to speed recovery of neutrophils, thereby decreasing the neutropenic phase.[39,40] The specific start day for these particular factors remains under debate.

Red cell transfusion requirements have decreased with the advent of erythropoietin. However, patients undergoing fully ablative conditioning regimens still remain transfusion dependent. Transfusion requirements have been reported to range from 8 to 65 units of packed red cells throughout the transplant process.[41] The transfusion requirements for patients undergoing nonmyeloablative regimens appear to be less than those for their myeloablative counterparts. One report comparing transfusion requirements for myeloablative versus nonmyeloablative regimens found a significant decrease, from 96% of patients requiring transfusions to 63%, respectively.[42] Transfusion parameters vary according to the transplant center, with most maintaining hemoglobin levels above 8.0 g/dL. Erythropoietin therapy has not been shown to have benefits in the autologous transplant population.

However, due to the abnormal endogenous erythropoietin production in the allogeneic transplant population, it is an effective therapy for anemia following allogeneic HCT.[43]

Platelet transfusion requirements have been reported to range from 5 to 80 units throughout the transplant process.[42] Transfusion requirements following nonmyeloablative regimens appear to be significantly reduced, with one report indicating 23% of patients requiring platelet transfusions following a nonmyeloablative regimen compared to 100% of patients following a myeloablative regimen.[42] Research is ongoing to develop an effective growth factor for rapid platelet recovery.

Blood products for all HCT patients should be irradiated and leukopoor to decrease transfusion reactions, alloimmunization, and infectious risk.[44] Irradiated and leukopoor blood products lessen exposure to allogeneic white blood cells, which express antigens that lead to antibody production and worsening alloimmunization. Irradiated and leukopoor blood products also decrease possible exposure to CMV, because white blood cells harbor this virus.

Blood product administration should follow institutional policies. Transplant nurses need to remain vigilant to ensure that all HCT patients receive irradiated and leukopoor products. They should also carefully monitor ABO-incompatible allogeneic transplant patients as they convert their blood types to those of their donors to ensure appropriate typing and blood administration.

Primary graft failure occurs if no signs of engraftment appear within the first 3 to 4 weeks following HCT. Factors that increase the risk of graft failure include T-cell depletion, reduced-intensity immunosuppressive regimen, alloimmunization by multiple blood transfusions, low donor cell count, and HLA mismatch.[45,46] Patients experiencing primary graft failure must undergo a second transplant, which carries a high mortality rate — 70% to 80%.

Pulmonary Complications

Pulmonary complications following HCT are common and are a major cause of morbidity and mortality. Such complications account for nearly 40% of all deaths following HCT.[47] The complications that occur can be classified into three primary areas: parenchymal disease, pulmonary vascular disease, and infectious complications.

Three of the more common parenchymal diseases are idiopathic pneumonia syndrome, diffuse alveolar hemorrhage, and pulmonary edema. Idiopathic pneumonia syndrome occurs in approximately 15% of patients and is characterized by fever, dyspnea, hypoxemia, and nonproductive cough.[47] Diagnosis is made in the absence of an infectious process, with radiologic findings indicating diffuse alveolar infiltrates. Biopsy reveals fibrosis and inflammation most likely caused by high-dose chemotherapy and/or radiation. Although treatment has most often been corticosteroids, only anecdotal support for this therapy exists. Pulmonary edema in the post-transplant period is not well described in the literature, but has been reported in as many as 63% of patients.[47] Most patients develop pulmonary edema in the immediate post-transplant period, most likely as a result of volume overload. Patients present with classic signs of pulmonary edema, and treatment focuses on diuresis. Diffuse alveolar hemorrhage (DAH) has been reported in as many as 41% of patients.[47] This disease most often occurs within 2 weeks of HCT. Patients present with hypoxemia, dyspnea, cough, and fever, most often in the absence of hemoptysis. Radiography displays diffuse interstitial infiltrates, and histologic exam identifies alveolar injury with hemorrhage.[47,48] High-dose corticosteroids are the primary treatment for DAH.[49]

Pulmonary venoocclusive disease (PVOD) is the primary pulmonary vascular complication following HCT. This rare disease occurs 4 to 6 weeks after HCT.[47,48] Patients present with signs of pulmonary hypertension, cough, dyspnea and possible right heart failure. Diagnosis is made by biopsy with signs of pulmonary venular thrombosis. Corticosteroids are the treatment of choice, though few hard data exist to support this choice of therapy.

Infectious pulmonary complications remain the primary cause of pulmonary disease following HCT. Gram-negative bacteria are most commonly the infecting agents in the first 100 days post-HCT. Most of these infections are from endogenous sources. Bacterial infections after day 100 are more commonly attributable to community-acquired encapsulated organisms such as *Streptococcus pneumoniae* and *Haemophilus influenzae*.[47,48]

Viral pneumonitis is most often caused by CMV and herpes viruses. Herpes pneumonitis usually occurs in the early post-transplant period. Cytomegalovirus infections tend to occur after engraftment and account for approximately 40% of pneumonias in this population.[47] Patients present with a nonproductive cough, fever, hypoxemia, and dyspnea. Radiographs reveal diffuse reticulonodular or "ground glass" infiltrates. Early treatment with antiviral therapies such as gancyclovir or foscarnet and corticosteroids improves survival, although mortality rates for CMV pneumonitis remain high. Viral pneumonitis can also be caused by respiratory syncytial virus, adenovirus, influenza A and B, and parainfluenza. Effective treatments and outcomes of untreated disease with these viruses remain to be identified.

Fungal pneumonia caused by the *Aspergillus* fungi remains a serious problem for HCT patients. Invasive disease is difficult to treat, although extended therapy with new antifungal agents has greatly improved outcomes. Voriconazole is effective against *Aspergillus* and is in clinical trials as a potential prophylactic therapy.

Opportunistic infections such as *Pneumocystis carinii* pneumonia (PCP) present a risk for patients who are profoundly immunosuppressed for extended periods of time. Patients receiving immunosuppressive agents for GVHD should receive PCP prophylaxis until all immunosuppressive agents have been discontinued.

Cardiac Complications

High-dose cyclophosphamide is associated with a 5% to 10% incidence of detectable hemorrhagic cardiomyopathy in HCT patients. Clinical manifestations of this complication include congestive heart failure, pericardial effusion, loss of electrocardiogram (ECG) voltage, and cardiomegaly. Most patients experiencing cyclophosphamide-induced toxicity will experience minor ECG changes such as ST-T wave segment changes, supraventricular arrhythmias, or pericarditis without hemodynamically significant pericardial effusions. Cardiac toxicity due to cyclophosphamide is dose dependent and usually occurs within the first ten days following administration.[50] Factors that may contribute to the development of cardiac toxicity include prior anthracycline therapy, mediastinal radiation, and total body irradiation. Anthracycline therapy prior to HCT has been shown to decrease ventricular ejection fraction prior to transplant and appears to have predictive value for those developing cardiac complications.[51]

Patients generally undergo multiple gated aquisition (MUGA) scans or echocardiograms to determine left ventricular ejection fractions prior to HCT. Most centers will exclude patients with an ejection fraction less than 50% from receiving fully ablative regimens. Patients have been found to maintain ejection fractions following HCT despite possible cardiac toxic regimens.[52]

Treatment of cardiac complications consists of symptomatic support and fluid management. Significant cardiac effusions may require surgical intervention with pericardiocentesis or pericardial window placement. Nursing management begins with identification of high-risk patients. Routine fluid management and close assessment of cardiac status during the high-risk period should be the primary focus of care.

Table 20-4 Common Nephrotoxic Agents

Ifosfamide	Aminoglycosides
Foscarnet	Cyclosporine
Melphalan	Gancyclovir
Carboplatin	Acyclovir
Cisplatin	Amphotericin-B
Methotrexate	Tacrolimus

Data from Savdie[53]; Noel, Hazzan, Noel-Walter, et al.[54]

Renal Complications

Acute renal failure (ARF) and renal insufficiency (RI) occur in 30% to 80% of HCT patients in the first 3 months following transplant.[53–55] Nephrotoxic agents and VOD are the most likely causes of ARF/RI.[53] (See Table 20-4.) Patients who experience severe VOD often develop a hepatorenal syndrome. Decreased intravascular volume and low cardiac output lead to renal hypoperfusion and RI/ARF in severe VOD.[53] Patients who are receiving nephrotoxic agents or who are developing VOD need close observation of fluid balance. Nursing management includes the administration of diuretics and evaluating responses. Patients may require hemodialysis or continuous veno-venous hemodialysis for renal failure or fluid management.

Late Complications

Hematopoietic cell transplantation is becoming more common for treatment of a multitude of diseases. Advances in supportive care and development of less toxic conditioning regimens have improved the long-term survival rates for patients undergoing HCT. Hematopoietic cell transplantation carries with it the possibility of many long-term complications, ranging from chronic GVHD to infertility issues.

Chronic Graft-versus-Host Disease

Chronic graft-versus-host disease (CGVHD) is the most common long-term complication and the major cause of mortality following allogeneic HCT.[56] Incidence of CGVHD can range from 30% to 70%, and the disease is associated with several risk factors. The degree of HLA disparity, prior AGVHD, increasing age of donor and recipient, use of an unrelated donor, donor lymphocyte infusion (DLI), shortened cyclosporine courses and viral infections all appear to affect the incidence of CGVHD.[2,57] The effect of peripheral blood stem cells on CGVHD remains a topic of debate and is currently being studied in long-term clinical trials. Chronic GVHD can affect the skin, liver, gastrointestinal tract, oral mucosa, muscles, vagina, nerves, kidneys, lungs, and marrow function.[58,59] The grading of CGVHD is based on the extent of involvement of the affected organs and is generally of little use except to identify which patients require treatment. Patients with extensive CGVHD require treatment, whereas those with limited CGVHD may not require treatment.

Chronic GVHD occurs 100 or more days after HCT, with the highest incidence within the first 2 years post-transplant. Nevertheless, patients can develop CGVHD years after undergoing allogeneic HCT. Chronic GVHD that progresses directly from AGVHD is associated with the highest morbidity and mortality rates. Transplant recipients who develop CGVHD following a quiescent AGVHD period or who develop de novo CGVHD have lower morbidity and mortality rates.

Prevention of CGVHD is the same as for AGVHD. Numerous studies are investigating effective immunosuppressive regimens that could potentially lessen the incidence and severity of AGVHD and CGVHD. Currently, the treatment regimen of choice is alternating cyclosporine and prednisone every other day. Medications are then tapered based on response.[58] There are no universally accepted salvage regimens for refractory disease. Combination therapies include medications such as mycophenalate mofetil, sirolimus, thalidomide, azathioprine, and biological therapies such as infliximab and dacluzimab. Ultraviolet light therapy and extracorporeal photopheresis are also being studied in these patients.[60]

The most common cause of morbidity and mortality in CGVHD is infection. The combination of the immunodeficiency associated with CGVHD and the immunosuppressive agents used to treat CGVHD places these patients at high risk for incurring multiple infections. Prophylactic antibiotics, antivirals, and antifungals should be considered in profoundly immunosuppressed patients.

Nursing management of these patients is complex and requires frequent and in-depth holistic assessments. Signs and symptoms of infection may be masked by corticosteroid use and immunodeficient states. Psychosocial assessments and interventions may be required for patients who are often severely debilitated. A multidisciplinary approach to care of these patients is necessary to meet all of their complicated needs.

Infectious Complications

Late infectious complications following HCT are associated with several risk factors — namely, depressed T-cell and B-cell function, GVHD, anatomical barrier impairment, and immunosuppressive agents for treatment of GVHD. T-lymphocyte reconstitution may take months to years following HCT. There is often an inversion of the CD4/CD8 cell ratio, which may persist for a year and remain in the presence of CGVHD. B-cell/humoral immune system dysfunction usually lasts for 3 to 6 months following HCT. The recovery of immune globulin levels frequently occurs by 3 months following HCT. However, the immunosuppressive agents used to treat GVHD disrupt T-cell development, further delaying the recovery of T cells.[15,16,61] Graft-versus-host disease frequently damages natural anatomical barriers, leading to increased infection risk.

Bacterial infections seen in the late period are typically attributable to encapsulated organisms, due to the decreased humoral immune recovery. *Streptococcus pneumoniae* and *Haemophilus influenzae* are the most common pathogens. Although many centers have historically administered prophylaxis against these organisms, the development of resistant strains has called this practice into question. Vaccinations should be provided by one year post-transplant or when patients are no longer experiencing GVHD or receiving immunosuppression.[61]

The viral pathogen that most commonly causes infection late in the transplant course is CMV. Infections usually arise 30 to 80 days following HCT, although more CMV disease is being seen after day 100. Seropositive allogeneic HCT patients are at much higher risk for viral reactivation. Some centers prophylactically treat CMV with gancyclovir, decreasing the incidence of reactivation and CMV pneumonitis. Regular screening for CMV by polymerase chain reaction methods allows for early detection and therapy, decreasing the toxic effects of prophylactic gancyclovir.[61,62] Herpes viral infections occur in 70% to 80% of seropositive patients. Active infections can be painful but, when occurring alone, pose little danger to HCT patients. In contrast, profoundly immunosuppressed patients are at risk for disseminated disease and localized infections can become superinfected, leading to higher-risk infections.[61] Seropositive patients should receive viral prophylaxis until engraftment occurs, and consideration should be taken to continue prophylaxis for one year to help prevent varicella zoster activation.

Aspergillus infections pose the greatest risk of fungal disease late in the course of HCT. Patients who remain immunosuppressed due to GVHD and required treatment for that disease are at greatest risk for such infections. Some centers send routine fungal cultures from patients who are at high risk. Given the slow growth of fungal isolates, however, most patients will develop infection before the cultures grow.

Nonmyeloablative regimens are becoming more common for HCT. Although extensive data are not available, it appears that patients undergoing these regimens experience similar infections to those receiving myeloablative therapy, albeit with decreased incidence.[13,14]

Nursing management of late infectious complications focuses on close observation of signs and symptoms of infection. Patients may not exhibit classic signs or symptoms of infection due to the use of immunosuppressive agents and their altered immune function. Patient education regarding infections is imperative, as most patients are not being observed on a daily basis.

Ophthalmologic Complications

Cataract development and ocular GVHD are two of the most common late ophthalmologic complications seen in HCT patients. Cataract development is closely associated with radiation treatments. Patients who receive a single fraction of total body irradiation (TBI) have an 80% incidence of cataracts. Onset of cataracts usually occurs within a year following HCT. Fractionated TBI carries a 50% incidence of cataracts, and fractionated TBI with doses less than 1200 cGy causes cataracts in 30% to 35% of patients.[1,63] Long-term corticosteroids and prior cranial radiation also increase the risk of cataract development. Patients receiving high-dose chemotherapy alone have a 20% incidence of cataracts. Primary treatment is standard cataract removal.

Ocular GVHD affects approximately 40% of all long-term allogeneic HCT patients. Symptoms include eye dryness with associated gritty/sandy feelings. A sicca syndrome results from the damage to the lacrimal gland.[64] A Schirmer's test should be performed, with at least 10 mm of wetting being found in a negative test. Isolated ocular GVHD may be treated locally with lubricating eye drops and cyclosporine eye drops. Many patients also require obstruction of the nasolacrimal duct to decrease drainage of tears. Patients who do not respond to local therapy or who have concomitant GVHD involvement of other organs may require systemic therapy.[63] Patients should also be treated prophylactically to prevent any bacterial ocular infections.

Nursing management of ophthalmologic complications should include close observation of eye changes and patient education so that patients report any visual changes or eye symptoms.

Urologic Complications

Hemorrhagic cystitis is rare late in the transplant course. The cyclophosphamide metabolite acrolein can cause scarring of the bladder wall, which can in turn lead to protracted hematuria and urinary frequency. Bladder irrigation, cystoscopic fulguration, and — in severe cases — cystectomy are primary treatments for this diagnosis. Viral infections with CMV, BK virus, and adenovirus can also cause cystitis late in the allogeneic transplant course. No proven therapies for these infections exist, except decreasing immunosuppression. Supportive care with antispasmodics and hyperhydration help to reduce symptoms.

Renal insufficiency can develop late in the transplant course, due primarily to prior nephrotoxic agents and continued use of cyclosporine and tacrolimus. Renal insufficiency has been found in 20% to 25% of patients 2 years following HCT. Identification of renal insufficiency and possible causes is important to arrest further progression. Patients should be educated to report any urinary symptoms for prompt diagnosis and treatment. Renal damage can also diminish erythropoietin production, leading to anemia. Close observation of all laboratory data is required.

Oral/Dental Complications

Oral GVHD is the most common cause of late oral and dental complications following HCT. Patients may experience symptoms ranging from mild tenderness and food sensitivities to severe oral pain with marked dental decay. Chronic GVHD causes decreased saliva production, leading to a sicca syndrome and ensuing dental decay. Patients are often reluctant to perform good oral hygiene due to oral sensitivities, which contributes to poor dental health. Secondary fungal, bacterial, and viral infections can contribute to oral complications as well. Treatment of oral GVHD with steroid mouth washes is effective in most patients, but systemic therapy may also be required. Patients should perform meticulous oral hygiene and receive fluoride treatments to help prevent dental caries.[63,65]

Pulmonary Complications

Late-onset pulmonary complications affect approximately 15% of HCT patients. Sinopulmonary infections are the most common of these complications and have been discussed previously. Interstitial pneumonitis with resulting fibrosis and bronchiolitis obliterans (BO) or bronchiolitis obliterans organizing pneumonia (BOOP) and drug-induced fibrosis are the most common pulmonary complications. High-dose carmustine (BCNU), 450 mg/m^2 or greater, has been associated with pulmonary fibrosis with a peak onset approximately 6 weeks following HCT. High-dose corticosteroids are effective in halting the progression and alleviating any long-term damage.

Interstitial pneumonitis, BO, and BOOP all appear to have an association with CGVHD.[66–69] Interstitial pneumonitis is also associated with prior toxicities such as radiation therapy and infectious processes, most often viral in nature. It leads to interstitial fibrosis, resulting in symptomatology. Patients often complain of nonproductive cough with dyspnea and wheezing. High-dose corticosteroids are the treatment of choice in association with anti-infectives if secondary infections are suspected.

Bronchiolitis obliterans is a nonspecific inflammatory pulmonary injury thought to be initiated by GVHD. Histologic findings are consistent with GVHD found in other organs. Patients report progressive productive cough and shortness of breath. Concurrent infections are common and may be cofactors in the development of BO. Airway obstruction is found on pulmonary function tests, with these clinical findings sufficing for diagnosis for most patients. Reported incidence is between 5% and 20%.[67] Bronchiolitis obliterans has been reported to occur from 3 months to 2 years following HCT. Mortality rates are high in severe disease, which shows little response to standard GVHD treatment. Corticosteroids with anti-infective agents are first-line therapies.

Bronchiolitis obliterans organizing pneumonia is also associated with GVHD. This condition is rarely reported, with its incidence hovering between 1% and 2%. Patients present with nonproductive cough, fever, and dyspnea. Although definitive diagnosis requires biopsies, pulmonary function tests and radiography can be suggestive of disease.[67] Prognosis is favorable, as most patients respond to corticosteroids and anti-infectives.

Endocrine Complications

Hypothyroidism is common following HCT. Patients receiving TBI are at highest risk of developing thyroid dysfunction, with nearly 25% of these patients requiring thyroid supplementation.[2] High-risk patients should be evaluated every 6 months, with all patients receiving routine evaluation for this potential complication every year. Thyroid supplementation should be initiated when indicated.

Nursing management includes patient education regarding symptoms of hypothyroidism and close assessment to identify sometimes subtle presenting symptoms. Hypothyroidism is rarely life-threatening, but symptoms can significantly affect quality of life.

Avascular Necrosis

Avascular necrosis (AVN) is described as nontraumatic ischemic bone necrosis. It has been reported in up to 5% of HCT patients. Patients who have required corticosteroid therapy are at highest risk for the development of AVN.[70,71] Although the femoral head is most commonly affected by this complication, all joints are at risk of development of AVN. Patients will report progressive joint pain, especially with activity. Primary medical treatment is joint replacement. Nurses should be aware of patient complaints of progressive joint pain with clinical courses associated with this disease, including corticosteroid use.

Secondary Malignancies

The complication of secondary malignancies is increasing as patients enjoy increasingly longer lives following HCT. There appears to be a cumulative incidence effect: As survival increases, so does the risk of developing a secondary malignancy. Alkylating agents have long been associated with the development of secondary malignancies. Because most patients undergoing HCT have received alkylating agents prior to HCT, it is difficult to determine whether HCT is the greater causative effect. Secondary malignancies can be classified as one of three main types: myelodysplastic syndrome (MDS) with resulting acute myelogenous leukemia (AML), solid tumors, and post-transplant lymphoproliferative disorder (PTLD). Whereas secondary MDS and AML rarely develop following allogeneic HCT, MDS/AML occurs with some frequency following autologous HCT. The actuarial incidence of MDS has been reported to be as high as nearly 20% following autologous HCT.[72] Identification of MDS following HCT is difficult, as dysplastic changes occur following most types of chemotherapy. Treatment of secondary MDS/AML follows standard therapies, with allogeneic transplant providing the only possibility of cure.

Secondary solid malignancies more commonly develop in post-allogeneic HCT patients. There appears to be a close association between these complications and radiation therapy both prior to HCT and when used as a part of the conditioning regimen. Patients who develop GVHD and require immunosuppressive therapy are also at increased risk of developing solid malignancies. Chronic GVHD is associated with increased risk of squamous cell malignancies of the buccal mucosa and skin. Age-adjusted incidence has been reported to be as high as 4.2 times higher in transplant recipients than in the general population.[1,72,73]

Post-transplant lymphoproliferative disorder has been well described following solid organ transplant, with incidence reaching 10% in heart/lung transplant patients. This disorder is not well described in HCT patients. Reported incidence has ranged from 0.2% to 25%; the disease has been seen in both autologous and allogeneic HCT patients, albeit with higher incidence in the allogeneic transplant population.[72] Patients who receive T-cell–depleted grafts or who are treated with antithymocyte globulin or anti-CD3 monoclonal antibody are at greatest risk of developing PTLD. There is also association with Epstein-Barr viral infections. Treatment of PTLD includes combination chemotherapy and withdrawal of immunosuppression if possible.

Patients should receive ample education regarding the risk of secondary malignancies prior to undergoing HCT. Close observation for development of any secondary malignancy needs to be ongoing, as the incidence increases as survival lengthens.

Neurologic Complications

Late neurologic complications are rare to nonexistent following HCT; instead, most of the neurologic complications that can occur arise within the first 3 months following HCT. Magnetic resonance imaging of the brain has shown white matter lesions and brain atrophy, which were associated with CGVHD and immunosuppressive therapy. Neuropsychologic testing has indicated cognitive deficits that are also associated with long-term cyclosporine use and increased age.[74] Ongoing research is being conducted to determine the effects of HCT on cognitive ability in long-term survivors.

Graft Failure

Secondary graft failure (SGF) is a serious complication that occurs after initial engraftment. It has been reported in both autologous and allogeneic HCT patients. Note that improvements in HLA testing have significantly reduced SGF in the allogeneic transplant population. One recent report indicated that only 4 of 192 patients undergoing HLA-matched, unrelated-donor HCT developed SGF.[75] Historically, reported incidence has ranged from 2% to 25% depending on the donor type and HLA match.[76] Factors that affect SGF incidence include HLA disparity, T-cell depletion, related versus unrelated donor, GVHD, viral infections, inadequate donor cell counts, and stromal damage.

Treatment of SGF begins with a combination of growth factors, including G-CSF, GM-CSF, and erythropoietin. Immunosuppression should also be weaned if possible in allogeneic HCT patients. Patients who do not respond may require donor lymphocyte infusion or second transplant. Mortality rates are high if a second transplant is required.

Nursing management should focus on supportive care both physically and emotionally. Secondary graft failure is a traumatic event, and patients and families will require ample support and education to move through this time.

Gonadal Dysfunction

Gonadal dysfunction is common following HCT. Children — especially those close to puberty — experience the greatest long-term dysfunction or gonadal failure. High-dose chemotherapy can produce long-term dysfunction, and TBI has a high association with both gonadal dysfunction and failure. To date, large studies have not been completed following HCT to determine the incidence of gonadal dysfunction. Males have been reported to have fathered healthy children following HCT. Females have also been reported to have given birth to healthy children, although the number of these cases is minimal. Depending on their age, most womenn who undergo HCT will experience early chemical-induced menopause. Follicle-stimulating homone and luteinizing homone levels should be monitored to determine the need for hormone replacement therapy. Approximately 10% of males will recover spermatogenesis 2 to 5 years following HCT. Testosterone levels should be monitored in males reporting decreased libido and erectile dysfunction. Testosterone replacement therapy should be initiated in those with abnormally low levels.[63,77–79]

Nurses should have open discussions with patients and significant others regarding sexual function and fertility issues associated with HCT. Gonadal dysfunction can significantly affect quality of life, and the potential embarrassment of discussing sexual topics may keep patients from addressing these issues. Options for fertility should be discussed prior to HCT. Sperm banking may be possible if spermatogenesis remains following conventional therapies. Ovarian banking is also available, but the long-term success rate for this option is not known.

Osteoporosis

Osteoporosis can develop late after HCT. Prolonged corticosteroid use, ovarian failure, and decreased activity increase risk for osteoporosis.[77,80] Osteopenia occurs in 50% to 60% of HCT patients, while osteoporosis occurs in 20% of HCT patients.[2] Bone density testing should be completed for those patients deemed at high risk for these conditions. Osteoporotic patients need regular calcium supplementation, and those with severe osteoporosis should receive biophosphonate therapy.[81] Women in chemically induced menopause should consider hormone replacement therapy. Nursing management should seek to identify patients at high risk for osteoporosis development and initiate direct testing for the disease.

Supportive Management

Nutritional Support

Consultation with nutrition services is required for all HCT patients. Establishing baseline nutritional status will assist in identifying those patients at risk for malnutrition. The use of total parenteral nutrition (TPN) has decreased with the advent of growth factors, which decrease the neutropenic period and associated mucositis. In general, HCT patients have increased metabolic needs due to tissue damage, GVHD, and infection. These complicating factors may require nutritional support by TPN, enteral feedings, or simple dietary supplements. Maintaining nutritional status is often difficult but is imperative for overall recovery.

Pain Management

Individuals undergoing HCT may experience pain at various stages of the transplant process. Nurses need to assess for pain on an ongoing basis and identify the source and appropriate treatment options. Pain management may require both pharmacologic and nonpharmacologic therapies. Consultation with a dedicated pain team may be helpful for identifying alternative pain management options.

Vaccinations

Immunity to preventable diseases by vaccinations is lost over time following HCT, for both autologous and allogeneic transplant patients. Practices regarding vaccinations vary widely between transplant centers, and recommendations by the CDC can be followed. Vaccinations should be considered for the following diseases: diphtheria, *Haemophilus influenzae*, hepatitis B, measles, mumps, rubella, polio, tetanus, *Pneumococcus*, and seasonal influenza.[82,83] Nurses should maintain records detailing vaccination schedules to assure adequate immunization.

Psychosocial Issues

Quality of Life

Quality of life following HCT can be significantly affected by morbidity caused by the transplant process and subsequent long-term complications. Many studies evaluating quality of life post-transplant have already been conducted, and many more are currently enrolling patients. Quality of life has been reported to be affected for as long as 6 years following HCT.[84] Transplant centers face the challenge of developing plans of care that will improve quality of life and decrease the effects of complications on quality of life. Exercise during and following HCT has been shown to decrease the impact on quality of life and may be a simple, yet effective way to help patients recover from this life-altering therapy.[85]

Nursing management in this situation focuses on patient and family education. Providing patients with information regarding vocational counseling, financial counseling, rehabilitation programs, and support groups may help decrease the detrimental effects on quality of life.

Conclusion

Hematopoietic cell transplantation is a complex process that requires the care of expert nurses. The knowledge base required to care for these patients throughout the transplant process is extensive. Patients and families rely heavily on the expert and compassionate care of nurses to help guide them through very trying times. Consequently, transplant nurses need to be equipped with adequate knowledge regarding the multitude of complications that can occur to facilitate the smooth transition from patient to successful survivor.

References

1. Tabbara I, Zimmerman K, Morgan C, et al: Allogeneic hematopoietic stem cell transplantation. *Arch Intern Med* 162:1558–1566, 2002
2. Antin J: Long-term care after hematopoietic-cell transplantation in adults. *N Engl J Med* 347:36–42, 2002
3. Chao NJ: *Graft-Versus-Host Disease* (ed 2). Austin, TX, R. G. Landes, 1999
4. Deeg HJ, Yamaguchi M: Acute graft-versus-host disease, in Atkinson K (ed.): *Clinical Bone Marrow and Blood Stem Cell Transplantation* (ed 2). New York, Cambridge University Press, 2000, pp 681–699
5. Przepiorka D: Prevention of acute graft-versus-host disease, in Ball ED, Lister J, Law P (eds.): *Hematopoietic Stem Cell Therapy*. Philadelphia, Churchill Livingstone, 2000, pp 452–469

6. Przepiorka D, Cleary K: Therapy of acute graft-vs-host disease, in Ball ED, Lister J, Law P (eds.): *Hematopoietic Stem Cell Therapy*. Philadelphia, Churchill Livingstone, 2000, pp 531–540
7. Chao NJ: Graft-versus-host disease, in Burt RK, Deeg HJ, Lothian ST, Santos GW (eds.): *Bone Marrow Transplantation*. New York, Chapman & Hall, 1996, pp 478–497
8. Reddy P: Pathophysiology of acute graft-versus-host disease. *Hematol Oncol* 21:149–161, 2003
9. Davies JK, Lowdell MW: New advances in acute graft-versus-host disease prophylaxis. *Transfusion Med* 13:387–397, 2003
10. Gluckman E, Horowitz MM, Champlin RE, et al: Bone marrow transplantation for severe aplastic anemia: influence of conditioning and graft-versus-host disease prophylaxis regimens on outcome. *Blood* 79:269–275, 1992
11. Storb R, Deeg HJ, Farewell V, et al: Marrow transplantation for severe aplastic anemia: methotrexate alone compared with a combination of methotrexate and cyclosporine for prevention of acute graft-versus-host disease. *Blood* 68:119–125, 1986
12. Hiraoka A: Results of a phase III study on prophylactic use of FK506 for acute GVHD compared with cyclosporine in allogeneic bone marrow transplantation. *Blood* 90(suppl 1):2500, 1997
13. Mossad SB, Avery RK, Longworth DL, et al: Infectious complications within the first year after nonmyeloablative allogeneic peripheral blood stem cell transplantation. *Bone Marrow Transplant* 28:491–495, 2001
14. Busca A, Locatelli F, Barbui A, et al: Infectious complications following nonmyeloablative allogeneic hematopoietic stem cell transplantation. *Transplant Infect Dis* 5:132–139, 2003
15. Bashey A: Infection, in Ball ED, Lister J, Law P (eds.): *Hematopoietic Stem Cell Therapy*. Philadelphia, Churchill Livingstone, 2000, pp 510–520
16. Burt RK, Walsh T: Infection prophylaxis in bone marrow transplant recipients — myths, legends and microbes, in Burt RK, Deeg HJ, Lothian ST, Santos GW (eds.): *Bone Marrow Transplantation*. New York, Chapman & Hall, 1996, pp 438–451
17. Atkinson K, Singhal S: Bacterial infections, in Atkinson K (ed.): *Clinical Bone Marrow and Blood Stem Cell Transplantation*. New York, Cambridge University Press, 2000, pp 716–736
18. Filicko J, Lazarus H, Flomenberg N: Mucosal injury in patients undergoing hematopoietic progenitor cell transplantation: new approaches to prophylaxis and treatment. *Bone Marrow Transplant* 31:1–10, 2003
19. Stiff P: Mucositis associated with stem cell transplantation: current status and innovative approaches to management. *Bone Marrow Transplant* 27(suppl 2): S3–S11, 2001
20. Sonis S: Mucositis as a biological process: a new hypothesis for the development of chemotherapy-induced stomatotoxicity. *Oral Oncol* 34:39–43, 1998
21. Eilers J: When the mouth tells us more than it says — the impact of mucositis on quality of life. *Oncol Supportive Care* 1:31–43, 2003
22. National Cancer Institute: Oral complications of chemotherapy and head/neck radiation. PDQ, *www.cancer.gov/cancerinfo/pdq/supportivecare/oralcomplications/healthprofessonal*. Accessed March 10, 2004
23. Wardley A, Jayson G, Swindell R, et al: Prospective evaluation of oral mucositis in patients receiving myeloablative conditioning regimens and haemopoietic progenitor rescue. *Br J Haematol* 110:292–299, 2000
24. Durrant S, Pico JL, Schmitz N, et al: A phase I study of recombinant human keratinocyte growth factor (RKUGF) in lymphoma patients receiving high-dose chemotherapy (HDC) with autologous peripheral blood progenitor cell transplantation (AUTOPBCT). *Blood* 94(suppl 1):708a, 1999 (abstract)
25. Spielberger RT, Stiff P, Emmanouilides C, et al: Efficacy of recombinant human keratinocyte growth factor (rHuKGF) in reducing mucositis in patients with hematologic malignancies undergoing autologous peripheral blood progenitor cell transplantation (auto-PBPCT) after radiation-based conditioning — results of a phase 2 trial. *Proc Am Soc Clin Oncol* 20: 2001 (abstr 25)
26. Epstein JB, Phillips N, Parry J, et al: Quality of life, taste, olfactory and oral function following high-dose chemotherapy and allogeneic hematopoietic cell transplantation. *Bone Marrow Transplant* 30:785–792, 2002
27. Griffin A, Burtow P, Coates A, et al: On the receiving end: patient perceptions of the side effects of the cancer chemotherapy in 1993. *Ann Oncol* 7:189–195, 1996
28. Gralla R, Navari R, Hesketh P, et al: Recommendations for the use of antiemetics: evidence-based, clinical practice guidelines. *J Clin Oncol* 17:2971–2994, 1999
29. Van Kraaij M, Dekker A, Verdonck L, et al: Infectious gastroenteritis: an uncommon cause of diarrhea in adult allogeneic and autologous stem cell transplant recipients. *Bone Marrow Transplant* 26:299–303, 2000
30. Avery R, Pohlman B, Adal K, et al: High prevalence of diarrhea but infrequency of documented *Clostridium difficile* in autologous peripheral blood progenitor cell transplant recipients. *Bone Marrow Transplant* 25:67–69, 1999
31. Cox G, Matsui M, Lo R, et al: Etiology and outcome of diarrhea after marrow transplantation: a prospective study. *Gastroenterology* 107:1398–1407, 1994
32. Carreras E, Bertz H, Arcese W, et al: Incidence and outcome of hepatic venoocclusive disease after blood or marrow transplantation: a prospective cohort study of the European Group for Blood and Marrow Transplantation. *Blood* 92:3599–3604, 1998
33. Williams DB, Vickers CR: Hepatic complications, in Atkinson K (ed.): *Clinical Bone Marrow and Blood Stem Cell Transplantation*. New York, Cambridge University Press, 2000, pp 912–924
34. Khoury H, Adkins D, Brown R, et al: Does early treatment with high-dose methylprednisolone alter the course of hepatic regimen-related toxicity? *Bone Marrow Transplant* 25:737–743, 2000
35. Strausser SI, McDonald GB: Gastrointestinal and hepatic complications, in Thomas ED, Blume KG, Forman SJ (eds.): *Hematopoietic Cell Transplantation* (ed 2). Malden, MA, Blackwell Science, 1999, pp 627–658
36. Garrick R: Neurologic complications, in Atkinson K (ed.): *Clinical Bone Marrow and Blood Stem Cell Transplantation* (ed 2). New York, Cambridge University Press, 2000, pp 958–979
37. Magalhaes-Silverman M, Hammert L: Neurologic complications, in Ball ED, Lister J, Law P (eds.): *Hematopoietic Stem Cell Transplantation*. Philadelphia, Churchill Livingstone, 2000, pp 578–588
38. Colosimo M, McCarthy N, Jayasinghe R, et al: Diagnosis and management of subdural haematoma complicating bone marrow transplantation. *Bone Marrow Transplant* 25:549–552, 2000
39. Przepiorka D, Smith T, Folloder J, et al: Controlled trial of filgrastim for acceleration of neutrophil recovery after allogeneic blood stem cell transplantation from human leukocyte antigen-matched related donors. *Blood* 97:3405–3410, 2001
40. Wingard JR, Bartfield AA: Use of hematopoietic growth factors, in Ball ED, Lister J, Law P (eds.): *Hematopoietic Stem Cell Transplantation*. Philadelphia, Churchill Livingstone, 2000, pp 471–487
41. Lopez-Plaza I, Triulzi D: Transfusion support in hematopoietic stem cell transplantation, in Ball ED, Lister J, Law P (eds.): *Hematopoietic Stem Cell Transplantation*. Philadelphia, Churchill Livingstone, 2000, pp 589–597
42. Weissinger F, Sandman B, Maloney D, et al: Decreased transfusion requirements for patients receiving nonmyeloablative

compared with conventional peripheral blood stem cell transplants from HLA-identical siblings. *Blood* 98:3584–3588, 2001
43. Miller CB, Lazarus HM: Erythropoietin in stem cell transplantation. *Bone Marrow Transplant* 27:1011–1016, 2001
44. Dodds A: ABO incompatibility and blood product support, in Atkinson K (ed.): *Clinical Bone Marrow and Blood Stem Cell Transplantation.* New York, Cambridge University Press, 2000, pp 655–661
45. Georges G, Storb R: Failure of sustained engraftment: clinical manifestations and treatment, in Atkinson K (ed.): *Clinical Bone Marrow and Blood Stem Cell Transplantation.* New York, Cambridge University Press, 2000, pp 662–680
46. Chen J, Law P, Ball ED: Failure of engraftment, in Ball ED, Lister J, Law P (eds.): *Hematopoietic Stem Cell Transplantation.* Philadelphia, Churchill Livingstone, 2000, pp 521–530
47. Kreit JW: Respiratory complications, in Ball ED, Lister J, Law P (eds.): *Hematopoietic Stem Cell Transplantation.* Philadelphia, Churchill Livingstone, 2000, pp 563–577
48. Bryant D: Pulmonary complications, in Atkinson K (ed.): *Clinical Bone Marrow and Blood Stem Cell Transplantation.* New York, Cambridge University Press, 2000, pp 943–957
49. Bekele A, Tefferi A, Litzow MR: Outcome of diffuse alveolar hemorrhage in hematopoietic stem cell transplant recipients. *Am J Respir Crit Care Med* 166:1364–1368, 2002
50. Kupari M, Volin L, Suokas A, et al: Cardiac involvement in bone marrow transplantation: electrocardiographic changes, arrhythmias, heart failure and autopsy findings. *Bone Marrow Transplant* 5:91–98, 1990
51. Fujimaki K, Maruta A, Yoshida M, et al: Severe cardiac toxicity in hematological stem cell transplantation: predictive value of reduced left ventricular ejection fraction. *Bone Marrow Transplant* 27:307–310, 2001
52. Lehman S, Isberg B, Ljungman P, et al: Cardiac systolic function before and after hematopoietic stem cell transplantation. *Bone Marrow Transplant* 26:187–192, 2000
53. Savdie E: Renal complications, in Atkinson K (ed.): *Clinical Bone Marrow and Blood Stem Cell Transplantation.* New York, Cambridge University Press, 2000, pp 930–942
54. Noel C, Hazzan M, Noel-Walter MP, et al: Renal failure and bone marrow transplantation. *Nephrol Dialysis Transplant* 13:2464–2466, 1998
55. Gruss E, Bernis C, Tomas JF, et al: Acute renal failure in patients following bone marrow transplant: prevalence, risk factors and outcomes. *Am J Nephrol* 15:473–479, 1995
56. Wingard JR: The conundrum of chronic graft-versus-host disease. *Blood Marrow Transplant* 12:3–16, 2002
57. Bishop M: Emerging strategies in the treatment of chronic graft-versus-host disease. *Blood Marrow Transplant* 12:4–5, 2002
58. Volgelsang GB: How I treat chronic graft-versus-host disease. *Blood* 97:1196–1200, 2001
59. Spiryda LB, Laufer MR, Soiffer RF, et al: Graft-versus-host disease of the vulva and/or vagina: diagnosis and treatment. *Biol Blood Marrow Transplant* 9:760–765, 2003
60. Apisarnthanarax N, Donato M, Korbling M, et al: Extracorporeal photopheresis therapy in the management of steroid-refractory or steroid-dependent cutaneous chronic graft-versus-host disease after allogeneic stem cell transplantation: feasibility and results. *Bone Marrow Transplant* 31:459–465, 2003
61. Leather HL, Wingard JR: Infections following hematopoietic stem cell transplantation. *Infect Dis Clin North Am* 15:483–520, 2001
62. Boeckh M, Leisenring W, Riddell SR, et al: Late cytomegalovirus disease and mortality in recipients of allogeneic hematopoietic stem cell transplants: importance of viral load and T-cell immunity. *Blood* 101:407–414, 2003
63. Deeg HJ: Delayed complications, in Burt RK, Deeg HJ, Lothian ST, Santos GW (eds.): *Bone Marrow Transplant* New York, Chapman & Hall, 1996, pp 515–522
64. Cheok F: Eye complications, in Atkinson K (ed.): *Clinical Bone Marrow and Blood Stem Cell Transplantation* (ed 2). New York, Cambridge University Press, 2000, pp 1009–1016
65. Marcellus DC, Vogelsang GB: Chronic graft-versus-host disease, in Ball ED, Lister J, Law P (eds.): *Hematopoietic Stem Cell Therapy.* Philadelphia, Churchill Livingstone, 2000, pp 614–624
66. Wolff D, Reichenberger F, Steiner B, et al: Progressive interstitial fibrosis of the lung in sclerodermal chronic graft-versus-host disease. *Bone Marrow Transplant* 29:357–360, 2002
67. Afessa B, Litzow MR, Tefferi A: Bronchiolitis obliterans and other late onset non-infectious pulmonary complications in hematopoietic stem cell transplantation. *Bone Marrow Transplant* 28:425–434, 2001
68. Freudenberger TD, Madtes DK, Curtis JR, et al: Association between acute and chronic graft-versus-host disease and bronchiolitis obliterans organizing pneumonia in recipients of hematopoietic stem cell transplants. *Blood* 102:3822–3828, 2003
69. Sakaida E, Nakaseko C, Harima A, et al: Late-onset noninfectious pulmonary complications after allogeneic stem cell transplantation are significantly associated with chronic graft-versus-host disease and with the graft-versus-leukemia effect. *Blood* 102:4236–4242, 2003
70. Tauchmanova L, De Rosa G, Serio B, et al: Avascular necrosis in long-term survivors after allogeneic or autologous stem cell transplantation. *Cancer* 97:2453–2461, 2003
71. Wiesmann A, Pereira P, Bohm P, et al: Avascular necrosis of bone following allogeneic stem cell transplantation: MR screening and therapeutic options. *Bone Marrow Transplant* 22:565–569, 1998
72. Holman PR: Myelodysplasia and second malignancies, in Ball ED, Lister J, Law P (eds.): *Hematopoietic Stem Cell Therapy.* Philadelphia, Churchill Livingstone, 2000, pp 647–657
73. Lowsky R, Lipton J, Fyles G, et al: Secondary malignancies after bone marrow transplantation in adults. *J Clin Oncol* 12:2187–2192, 1994
74. Pavodan CS, Tarek AY, Schleuning M, et al: Neurological and neuroradiological findings in long-term survivors of allogeneic bone marrow transplantation. *Ann Neurol* 42:627–633, 1998
75. Hansen JA, Gooley TA, Martin PJ, et al: Bone marrow transplants from unrelated donors for patients with chronic myeloid leukemia. *N Engl J Med* 338:962–968, 1998
76. Chen J, Law P, Ball ED: Late graft failure, in Ball ED, Lister J, Law P (eds.): *Hematopoietic Stem Cell Therapy.* Philadelphia, Churchill Livingstone, 2000, pp 603–607
77. Winters SJ, Syed M: Endocrine and metabolic complications, in Ball ED, Lister J, Law P (eds.): *Hematopoietic Stem Cell Therapy.* Philadelphia, Churchill Livingstone, 2000, pp 625–636
78. Jacob A, Barker H, Goodman A, et al: Recovery of spermatogenesis following bone marrow transplantation. *Bone Marrow Transplant* 22:277–279, 1998
79. Chatterjee R, Kottaridis PD, McGarrigle HH, et al: Management of erectile dysfunction by combination therapy with testosterone and sildenafil in recipients of high-dose therapy for haematological malignancies. *Bone Marrow Transplant* 29:607–610, 2002
80. Cohen ML: Musculoskeletal complications, in Atkinson K (ed.): *Clinical Bone Marrow and Blood Stem Cell Transplantation* (ed 2). New York, Cambridge University Press, 2000, pp 988–992
81. Gandhi MK, Lekamwasam S, Inman I, et al: Significant and persistent loss of bone mineral density in the femoral neck

after haematopoietic stem cell transplantation: long-term follow-up of a prospective study. *Br J Haematol* 121:462–468, 2003

82. Guidelines for preventing opportunistic infections among hematopoietic stem cell transplant recipients. *MMWR* 49:1–128, 2000
83. Singhal S, Mehta J: Reimmunization after blood or marrow stem cell transplantation. *Bone Marrow Transplant* 23:637–646, 1999
84. Hensel M, Erger G, Schneeweiss A, et al: Quality of life and rehabilitation in social and professional life after autologous stem cell transplantation. *Ann Oncol* 13:209–217, 2002
85. Courneya KS, Keats MR, Turner AR, et al: Physical exercise and quality of life in cancer patients following high dose chemotherapy and autologous bone marrow transplantation. *Psychooncology* 9:127–136, 2000

CHAPTER 21

Biologic and Targeted Therapy

Linda A. Battiato, RN, MSN, OCN®
Vera S. Wheeler, RN, MN, OCN®

Introduction

Biological agents have gained acceptance as standard therapy in oncology care. They are used for primary or supportive care in solid tumors and hematological malignancies and in bone marrow transplants. Biological agents are used across the continuum of cancer care, including diagnosis, adjuvant therapy, treatment of metastatic disease, and even cancer prevention. Biologic therapy continues to mature with increased understanding of the human response and the identification of approaches to augment the function of immune effector cells to halt cancer cell growth. Recent advances in the science of molecular biology have led to the discovery of molecules involved in the initial development and progression of human cancers and to the development of targeted drugs that specifically inhibit these molecules. This chapter describes the major current applications of biologic and targeted therapy and those being investigated in clinical trials. Major toxicities commonly experienced by patients receiving these therapies are also addressed.

Foundation Concepts for Biotherapy

Immune Defense Against Malignancy: An Overview

Immune surveillance

Immune surveillance is a theory that was first proposed in the 1950s to explain the role of the immune system in defending against neoplastic cells. Tumor cells express abnormal tumor antigens on their surfaces that can be recognized and subsequently destroyed by immune cells. The immune system is believed to destroy many circulating malignant cells before they can become established sites of tumor. Although the response of immune defense cells to specific tumors has been demonstrated, the theory fails to explain why some cancers elude immune detection and response. Abbas et al. suggest that immunosurveillance may be most effective in a subset of virally caused cancers.[1]

Tumor escape mechanisms

Several mechanisms of immune evasion have been proposed to explain how tumors escape detection by the immune system. These mechanisms include downregulation of major histocompatibility class I expression, lack of costimulatory signals needed for antigen presentation, and tumor secretion of immunosuppressive products. Tumors may also escape immune system detection because they are weakly immunogenic. An *immunogenic tumor* is made of cells that express one or more antigens that could be recognized by the immune system. A tumor-bearing host may be immunologically tolerant to tumor antigens because of inappropriate antigen presentation to the immune system or because of neonatal exposure to such antigens. Induction of suppressor T cells may also inhibit the immune response to cancer.[2]

Effector mechanisms of immune function

Defense against foreign antigens, either exogenous microbes or endogenous altered or virally transformed cells, is accomplished through components of the immune response. Effector or cell-killing mechanisms are initiated through a complicated recognition system of self/nonself surface molecules known as the major histocompatibility complex (MHC). The primary defense against transformed cells is cell-mediated immunity carried out by T lymphocytes and aided by B cells and humoral immunity. Stimulated by the presence of an antigen, the macrophage activates a T-helper (TH) cell. The activated TH cell, along with cytokines, initiates a B-cell response and the generation of antibody, an increase in cytotoxic T8 cells, activation of natural killer (NK) cells, and the stimulation of hematopoietic stem cells.

Cytokines

Cytokines are glycoprotein products of immune cells, such as lymphocytes and macrophages, that coordinate and initiate effector defense functions. Cytokines include the interleukins, interferons, colony-stimulating factors, and tumor necrosis factor. Some of the interleukins have a primary role in hematopoiesis, others are more active in the immune system, and some have overlapping properties. Cytokines are not cytotoxic agents themselves, with the exception of tumor necrosis factor-alpha (TNF-α) and lymphotoxin (TNF-β). The primary host defense cytokines include interleukins 1, 2, 4, 6, and 12; interferons α, β, and γ; TNF-α; TNF-β; and transforming growth factor beta (TGF-β).

Cytokines generally share the following properties:

- They mediate and regulate the immune defense functions of the body by providing communication and coordination among a variety of diverse immune cells; they have been called the "hormones" of the immune system.
- They have brief half-lives and usually function over short distances.
- They are produced by many different cell types and act on diverse cell targets, both within the immune system and in other organs such as the liver.
- Their actions are overlapping, redundant, and sometimes contradictory. They can influence the stimulation of other cytokines to produce synergistic effects, as in a cytokine network, or to antagonize the actions of other cytokines.
- They bind to surface receptors of target cells and act as regulators of cell growth or as mediators of defense functions.[1,3]

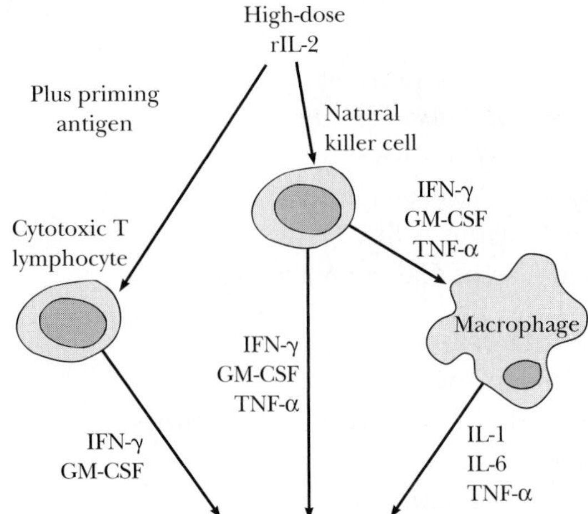

Figure 21-1 High-dose rIL-2 cytokine cascade: rIL-2 given parenterally can result in a massive release of cytokines and symptoms of inflammation from the activation of peripheral blood mononuclear cells and their pyrogenic cytokines.[3] (GM-CSF = granulocyte-macrophage colony stimulating factor; IFN = interferon; IL-1 = interleukin 1; IL-6 = interleukin 6; TNF-α = tumor necrosis factor-alpha)

The cytokine network is an overlapping, interactive communication pattern within the immune system. The secretion of one cytokine (or the administration of a recombinant form) can initiate a large release of secondary cytokines. Figure 21-1 illustrates one aspect of this network. When a bolus of high-dose interleukin 2 (IL-2) is administered, it potentially stimulates three cell types: NK, macrophage, and cytotoxic T-lymphocyte (CTL) cells. These cells secrete a variety of cytokines responsible for flulike symptoms and the potential killing of tumor cells. Other administered cytokines will engage in their own unique interactions within the cytokine network.

Origins of Biotherapy

Coley's toxins

William Coley, a New York surgeon, observed in 1893 that a patient with metastatic sarcoma had a complete remission of his cancer after two episodes of erysipelas, a streptococcal infection. Coley continued to explore the relationship between acute infection and tumor regression by injecting live and, later, killed bacterial extracts into patients' tumors. These extracts, known as Coley's toxins, were administered in a highly variable manner but are believed to have contained *Streptococcus pyogenes* with *Serratia marcescens* and *Bacillus prodigiosus*. Patients received these injections for weeks, months, or even up to a year. They reacted with

Table 21-1 Common Terms in Biotechnology

Biopharmaceuticals: Proteins, usually the product of recombinant DNA technology, that are used as drugs (e.g., interferon, human growth hormone).	*Polymerase chain reaction (PCR):* A method of gene amplication that does not require the use of bacterial vectors.
Gene: A unit of DNA that forms a discrete part of a chromosome of an organism.	*Recombinant DNA:* A genome containing genes from different sources that have been combined by genetic engineering methods.
Genetic engineering: The formation of new combinations of genes that are placed into an organism in which these genes do not occur naturally.	*Restriction enzymes:* Enzymes that act like "molecular scissors," cutting strands of DNA at specific cleavage sites to make specific DNA fragments.
Plasmid: An autonomously replicating, circular molecule of DNA. It is used as a vector for the introduction of a gene.	*Vector:* A carrier for the DNA in genetic engineering. Typical vectors are plasmids and viruses.

fever, chills, and other systemic effects that Coley believed were an essential part of the treatment. Although approximately one fourth of Coley's patients had a complete regression of their tumor, interest in these toxins waned with the onset of radiation therapy and chemotherapy.[3,4] It is now believed that the active ingredient in these toxins was endotoxin, a component in bacterial cell walls that generated TNF and other cytokines in the patient.

BCG and modern immunotherapy

In the 1960s and 1970s, nonspecific immunopotentiators such as bacillus Calmette-Guérin (BCG) were being tested in clinical trials. BCG was originally developed as a vaccine for tuberculosis. The use of BCG as adjuvant therapy after chemotherapy demonstrated increased survival of children with acute lymphoblastic leukemia and sparked interest in immunotherapy as a cancer treatment.[5] However, many subsequent clinical studies showed little difference in the cancer recurrence rates using BCG, *Corynebacterium parvum,* and other immunopotentiators. Interest in immunotherapy again faded.

Biological response modifiers

Advances in molecular biology and computerization, and the advent of genetic engineering in the early 1980s provided a large number of new substances from the mammalian genome that were capable of modulating immune functions. Oldham describes *biological response modifiers* (BRMs) as a "medicine cabinet" of new biologicals that may directly or indirectly have antitumor activity.[5] Unlike previous immunotherapeutic agents, these were homogenous, pure substances that were capable of more specific effects in the immune system. Biological response modifiers are defined as "agents or approaches that will modify the relationship between tumor and host by modifying the host's biological response to tumor cells, with resultant therapeutic benefit."[6,p3] These agents can be classified as (1) agents that restore, augment, or modulate host-antitumor immune mechanisms; (2) cells or cellular products, such as TNF, that have direct antitumor effects; and (3) biological agents that have other biological antitumor effects, for example, interfering with the metastatic ability of tumor or differentiating agents.[7] Today, BRMs are more broadly defined and encompass a greater number of substances than those used in the earlier field of immunotherapy, even though the terms are sometimes used interchangeably. *Biotherapy,* or *biologic therapy,* have become the more prevalent terms. *Biotherapy* is defined as the use of agents derived from biological sources or that affect biological responses.[8] It now describes agents that are biological in origin that may not have antitumor effects but have other biological effects such as affecting hematopoiesis.[9]

Recombinant DNA Technology

Recombinant DNA, or the combining of genes from different sources to produce an organism with new qualities, is an important basic principle in biotherapy. (Table 21-1 defines terms used in biotechnology.) This advance in molecular biology has enabled the current generation of biological agents to be made available for use in cancer therapy. When the process of recombinant DNA was discovered in the 1970s, there was much controversy over how this new technology might be used or misused. However, recombinant DNA technology produces proteins that have created a new class of drugs called *biopharmaceuticals.*

The process of creating recombinant DNA starts with the isolation of a specific segment of one strand of DNA (Figure 21-2). This segment, a sequence of base pairs responsible for the manufacture of a particular protein, is cut from the DNA strand, using a specific restriction enzyme. The remaining "sticky ends" enable the fragment to be joined to DNA in the plasmid by binding complementary base pairs, thymine to adenine and guanine to cytosine. The splice in the DNA strand is completed by another enzyme, and the plasmid is inserted into a bacterial cell and cultured to produce the desired protein.[10]

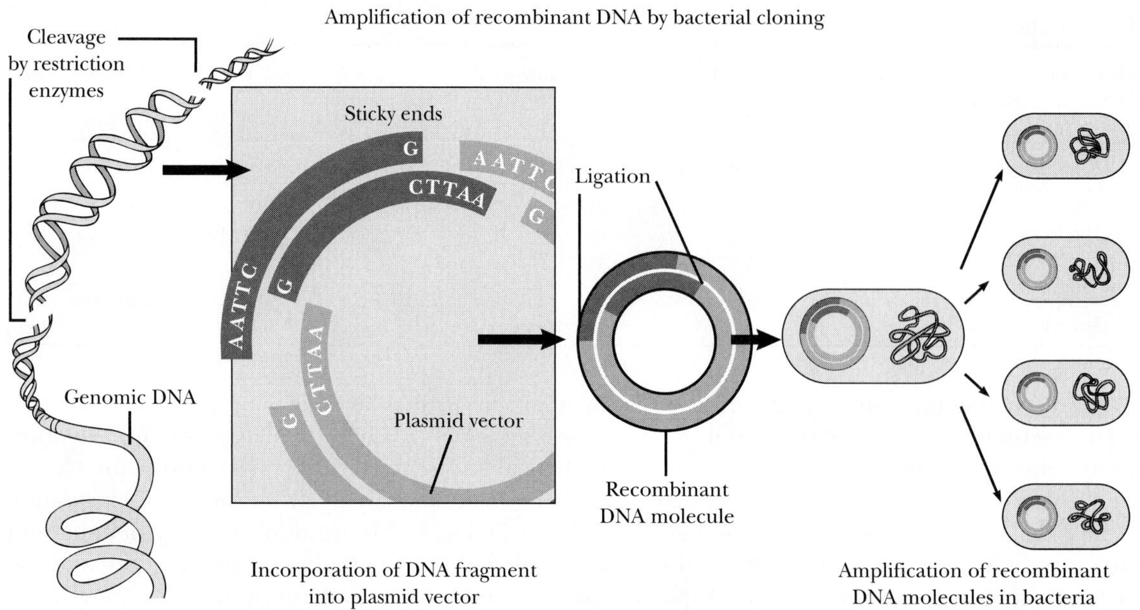

Figure 21-2 Amplification of recombinant DNA by bacterial cloning. In the example shown, the DNA segment to be amplified is separated by cleavage with a restriction enzyme that produces "sticky ends." The restriction enzyme cuts each strand as well as the plasmid DNA at a single site, generating "sticky ends" on the plasmid that are complementary to the ends of the DNA fragments. The cut ends of the DNA fragments and the plasmid form smooth joints with ligase enzyme. The new molecule is carried into bacteria that replicate the plasmid as they grow in culture. (Data from Rosenthal.[10])

This process, called a *polymerase chain reaction* (PCR), is used to create copies of a specific segment of DNA without vectors and bacteria. Short-stranded DNA fragments, known as *primers,* correspond to the short segment of DNA to be amplified. The DNA and primers are separated by heating and by the addition of DNA polymerase that generates new additions to the strands, doubling the number of DNA fragments. These cycles are repeated within minutes and can generate millions of copies of the DNA fragments.[10]

The future of biotherapy is influenced by new developments in biotechnology. The first generation of biotechnology produced recombinant versions of immune cell proteins such as alfa-interferon and interleukin 2. These were pure, homogenous, contaminant-free products used in clinical trials to modulate or initiate antitumor responses. A second generation of biotechnological products has now been evaluated. They are genes for the naturally occurring proteins that have been combined to make hybrid products.[11] The aim is to eliminate troublesome side effects and increase the effectiveness of the agents. These agents are called *fusion proteins.* An example of a fusion protein is DAB-IL-2, an immunotoxin. Consensus interferon is another example of such an agent, combining active portions of many separate subclasses of interferon into one molecule. Future generations of biological products will continue to develop with ongoing technological and theoretical advances.

Anticancer Cytokine Therapy

Interferon

Interferon (IFN) was the first cytokine to be explored as an anticancer biological agent. It has been extensively studied, both in natural and recombinant forms, in a variety of doses and schedules. The early enthusiasm for IFN as a "magic bullet" for cancer did not become a reality, but now IFNs are being used as part of biologic therapy in low- and high-dose regimens and in combination with other cytokines and chemotherapy regimens.[12]

Interferon was discovered in 1957 with the observation that cells infected with a virus produced a substance that prevented further viral infection to nearby cells.[13] In the 1970s and 1980s, the anticancer qualities of IFN led to clinical trials using a natural product extracted from leukocytes and later recombinant varieties when they became available. Table 21-2 describes the IFNs currently approved by the FDA for clinical use.

IFNs are classified into type I and type II. The type I IFNs include IFN-α, which has many subtypes (14 to 20 depending on the species); IFN-β; IFN-ω; and IFN-τ. All of the type I IFNs are structurally related and bind to a common receptor. Hematopoietic cells are the major producers of IFN-α and IFN-ω. Fibroblasts are a major cellular source of IFN-β, and IFN-β is also produced by macrophages. IFN-α is primarily made by

Table 21-2 Types of Interferons: A Comparison of Characteristics

Type/Subtype	Primary Function	Cell Source	Commercial Product	FDA-Approved Uses
Type I				
INF-α	Antiviral; antiproliferative	Leukocytes; host cells infected by virus	IFN alfa 2a Roferon (Roche)	• Chronic hepatitis C • Chronic myelogenous leukemia • Hairy cell leukemia • AIDS-related Kaposi's sarcoma
			IFN alfa 2b Intron A (Schering)	• Hairy cell leukemia; AIDS-related Kaposi's sarcoma • Chronic hepatitis B and C • Adjuvant therapy for follicular lymphoma with anthracycline-containing chemotherapy • Condyloma acuminata • Adjuvant melanoma
			Peginterferon alpha-2b PEG-Intron (Schering)	• Chronic hepatitis C, alone or in combination with Rebetol
			Infergen (Amgen)	• Chronic hepatitis C
IFN-β	Antiviral; antiproliferative	Fibroblast; endothelial cells	Interferon beta 1b Betaseron (Berlex/Chiron Labs)	• Relapsing, remitting multiple sclerosis
			Interferon beta 1a Avonex (Biogen/Idec)	
Type II				
IFN-γ	Immunomodulatory	Activated T cells; NK cells	IFN gamma 1b Actimmune (Genentech)	• Chronic granulomatous disease

virally stimulated leukocytes. IFN-γ is the only type II IFN. It is structurally unrelated to the type I IFNs and binds to a different receptor. It was initially thought that IFN-γ was exclusively produced by activated CD4-positive helper T cells, CD8-positive CTLs, and NK cells. There is also evidence that B cells and professional antigen-presenting cells (monocytes, macrophages, and dendritic cells) also secrete IFN-γ.[14]

A second-generation type of interferon is called consensus IFN (CIFN) (rIFN-con-1, Infergen). Consensus IFN, a type I interferon that does not occur in nature, was bioengineered by combining the amino acid sequences of the first eight known subtypes of IFN-α.[15] Toxicities are similar to those experienced with IFN-α. Consensus IFN is approved for use in chronic hepatitis C. A polyethylene-glycol-modified IFN-α2b (PEG-Intron) has shown reduced renal clearance and improved pharmacokinetic properties compared to its parent compound. Pegylated interferon has a 10-fold longer half-life than the naturally occurring protein and can be administered once weekly, with serum levels being sustained for nearly a week.[16] It is approved for chronic hepatitis C. Oncology trials of pegylated IFN-α2b are ongoing.

The IFNs have multiple activities that vary significantly among the interferon types. These activities include antiviral activity, direct antiproliferative activity, immunomodulation, inhibition of angiogenesis, regulation of differentiation, oncogene suppression, and enhancement of cell-surface antigen expression. Interferons α and β exert direct antitumor activity. They slow the growth and proliferation of tumor cells by prolonging the cell cycle, by reducing the availability of essential metabolites, and by increasing cell lysis. The antiviral activity of IFN occurs because of its ability to induce protein synthesis by binding to specific receptors and preventing viral replication. The chief function of IFN-γ is immunomodulation. It induces class II MHC receptor molecules, activates macrophages, and increases the cytotoxicity of T cells and NK cells. It also induces other cytokines such as IL-2 and TNF-α.[14,17–20] Because the IFNs have antiviral and antitumor properties, they are used to treat multiple medical conditions. Recombinant forms of IFNα, β, and γ have been developed and are approved for use in cancer and other diseases. IFN-α is the only type of IFN with approved indications in oncology.

IFN-α was first approved for use in hairy cell leukemia (HCL); however, other more active drugs have generally replaced its use in this malignancy. It is also approved for use in a high-dose regimen for AIDS-related Kaposi's sarcoma and chronic myelogenous leukemia (CML). IFN-α is approved for use in follicular lymphoma when used in combination with an anthracycline-containing regimen. The addition of IFN-α to a doxorubicin-containing regimen for patients with advanced-stage follicular lymphoma increased the progression-free survival and overall survival compared to chemotherapy alone.[21] IFN-α is also approved for use in various forms of hepatitis and for condyloma acuminata.

High-dose interferon-α (HDI) is used as an adjuvant for surgical patients with malignant melanoma who are at high risk for systemic recurrence because of the thickness of the primary lesion or local lymph node involvement. In the pivotal ECOG 1684 randomized clinical trial, HDI was associated with a 42% improvement in the five-year relapse-free survival (RFS) rate and an improvement in overall survival (OS) in the adjuvant setting in patients with resected Stage IIB and III melanoma.[22] The HDI adjuvant melanoma regimen involves a 4-week induction phase of IFN at 20 MIU/m^2 IV 5 days/week, followed by a 48-week maintenance phase of IFN at 10 MIU/m^2 SC 3 days/week. Side effects with this regimen may be substantial, but with appropriate monitoring, supportive care, and dose modifications, HDI can be given safely.[23]

The OS benefit initially seen with the ECOG 1684 trial showed a diminishing level of statistical significance with longer follow-up.[24] A subsequent follow-up large Intergroup trial, E1690, demonstrated an improvement in relapse-free survival but no statistically significant difference in overall survival.[25] In the ECOG 1694 trial, which enrolled a total of 880 patients, HDI demonstrated a significant RFS and OS benefit (with approximately two years median follow-up) compared with a ganglioside vaccine (GMK) that showed early promise in a randomized phase III trial.[26] ECOG trial 2696, a randomized phase II trial of GMK plus concurrent or sequential HDI versus GMK alone demonstrated that the combination of GMK and HDI reduced the risk of relapse compared with GMK alone.[27] A pooled analysis of 1916 patients on these four ECOG and Intergroup trials of adjuvant HDI for melanoma confirmed the durable RFS benefit of HDI compared with observation based on mature data from a large aggregate database. The multivariate analysis did not provide further evidence of an OS benefit associated with HDI.[24]

Although there seems to be consistent agreement that HDI prolongs RFS in patients with resected high-risk melanoma, the lack of a consistent overall survival benefit and the substantial toxicity of the regimen has caused an ongoing debate about the role of HDI as adjuvant therapy for malignant melanoma.[28] In an editorial on this subject, Schuchter noted, "While controversies are common in medicine, few aspects of the treatment of malignant melanoma have stimulated as much controversy as the interpretation of the adjuvant interferon alfa trials for patients with resected high-risk melanoma."[29,p7] Furthermore there is geographic variation in the interpretation of the data as well as ongoing debate regarding the optimal dose and schedule of IFN. The National Comprehensive Cancer Network (NCCN) recommends that decisions about the appropriateness of adjuvant interferon treatment be made on an individual basis after discussions with the patient that include an explanation of the trial results and side effects of HDI therapy.[30] Because of the toxicities associated with HDI, several trials have evaluated low-dose IFN in the adjuvant setting and have found no benefit in terms of OS.[28,29,31] It has been noted that progress beyond the initial trials of HDI will require more innovative and efficient trials and refinement of risk groups based on molecular genetic factors such as gene expression profiles.[29]

IFN-α has been widely studied in metastatic renal cell carcinoma and is associated with a 15% objective response rate and a modest survival benefit in this malignancy.[32] Two prospective randomized phase III trials have demonstrated that IFN-α prolongs survival in patients with metastatic renal cell cancer when combined with nephrectomy.[33,34] Trials evaluating IFN-α given as adjuvant therapy after complete resection by nephrectomy have not shown a delay in time to relapse or improvement in OS.[35] IFN-α has also demonstrated activity in multiple myeloma, cutaneous T-cell lymphoma, and squamous and basal cell cancer of the skin. It has been used in many clinical trials and continues to be evaluated in combination with other biological and targeted agents and chemotherapy in a wide variety of malignancies.

There is also ongoing interest in the antiangiogenic activity of IFN-α. Some of the activity of IFN-α in renal cell carcinoma is thought to result from its ability to inhibit angiogenesis by down-regulating an angiogenic factor, basic fibroblast growth factor (bFGF). Unlike the high doses used for melanoma, the best antiangiogenic effect may be obtained using low, frequent doses of IFN-α. Studies in mice have shown that the antiangiogenic activity of IFN-α is optimal at low doses and declines at higher doses. In addition to low, frequent doses, the antiangiogenic activity of IFN-α may be improved by combining it with other antiangiogenic agents. Ongoing phase III trials evaluating the antiangiogenic activity of IFN-α in metastatic renal cell cancer include a CALGB trial that randomizes patients to IFN-α alone versus IFN-α with bevacizumab (Avastin) and an ECOG trial comparing IFN-α with or without thalidomide.[36,37]

Toxicities associated with IFN-α treatment may include acute constitutional reactions to the initiation of therapy or more chronic effects. Many of the toxicities associated with IFN-α are related to the release of a

Table 21-3 IFN-Alfa: Common Toxicities and Management Considerations

Toxicity/Description	Pathophysiology	Management
Flulike symptoms Fever, chills/rigors, myalgia, headache, nausea, vomiting Worse with first dose — typically develop 2–4 hours after IFN and last approximately 8 hours Tachyphylaxis (the lessening of intensity and disappearance of symptoms) develops with continued administration. If the IFN is stopped and restarted, acute symptoms recur	Numerous cytokines — IL-1, IL-6, and TNF — acting together as part of inflammatory response. These cytokines are endogenous pyrogens. Nausea and vomiting are related to the effect of cytokines on serotonin	Prophylactic antipyretics Warm room with warm clothing and blankets for chills and rigors; severe cases may require meperidine Encourage adequate hydration (≥ 2L/day) Antiemetics for nausea and vomiting
Fatigue May be dose-limiting. Often worsens with continued therapy	Release of cytokines — IL-1, IL-2, IL-6, and TNF-α Cytokine-induced changes in neurotransmitter levels in areas of CNS that control alertness, attention, and energy may play a role Fatigue may be related to thyroid dysfunction, which can occur with IFN	Time management, priority setting Rest periods Pharmacologic intervention may be appropriate in selected patients
Anorexia/Weight loss Early satiety	Dry mouth and difficulty swallowing Nausea and GI dysmotility may contribute to early satiety Constipation and bloating Biochemical changes may result in food aversion or taste alterations Depression can contribute to anorexia — satiety-monitoring areas of brain affected by IFN-α, IL-1, and TNF-α	Assess weight Encourage small, frequent meals Food supplements Treat underlying disorders — nausea, GI dysmotility, pain, depression Consult with dietician
Impaired cognitive function May include decreased attention and short-term memory, psychomotor slowing, and poor coordination Incidence and severity increase with longer duration of therapy and in the elderly and patients with prior brain irradiation	Possibly related to decreased serotonin levels, changes in serum cortisol, and indirect effect of IFN on the hypothalamus followed by disturbance of neurotransmitters Possibly related to reduced central dopaminergic activity and reduced estradiol and progesterone levels	Assess for risk factors for neuropsychiatric side effects at baseline, i.e., history of mood/ psychiatric disorders Collaborate with mental health care providers
Depression Mild transient sadness to full clinical depression Sad, irritable mood, low energy and motivation Rare suicidal ideation	Indirect effect of IFN on the hypothalamus: Possibly related to increases in IL-6 and serum cortisol levels IFN effect on dopamine receptors Decreased serotonin levels	Assess for baseline history of depression For mild depression, encourage normal activities, social connections, and light to moderate exercise Pharmacologic intervention if necessary Collaborate with mental health care providers
Hematologic toxicities Acute, may occur early in the course of treatment. Neutropenia is the most common Neutropenia is rapidly reversible with dose interruption	Secondary cytokine release such as IP-10 inhibits bone marrow colony formation and hematopoiesis	Monitor CBC; dose modifications as appropriate for grade 3 and 4 neutropenia
Elevated liver enzymes AST, ALT, alkaline phosphatase, GGT	Poorly understood. Possible relationship to effects of IFN on hepatic CYP450 isoenzymes	Assess liver function tests, especially bilirubin. Dose modifications may be necessary
Thyroid dysfunction Transient hyperthyroidism followed by hypothyroidism	Related to autoimmune thyroiditis precipitated by the effects of IFN-α or secondary cytokines induced by IFN-α	Assess thyroid function tests at baseline and periodically

Data from Kirkwood et al,[23] Trask et al.[39]

cascade of cytokines initiated by the administration of exogenous IFN. Cytokines may be released directly or indirectly and include TNF-α, IL-1, IL-2, IL-6, IFN-γ, and IFN-inducible protein 10 (IP-10). The production of IFN-γ and IL-2 is increased indirectly through the activation of T cells by IL-1. The release of these cytokines initiates a complex cascade of processes that produce many of the toxicities associated with IFN therapy, including constitutional symptoms, fatigue, mood disorders, cognitive changes, and anorexia.[23,38,39]

Toxicities of IFN-α depend on the dose level and schedule. The severity of side effects can also be influenced by several patient variables, including age, performance status, and underlying disease. Younger

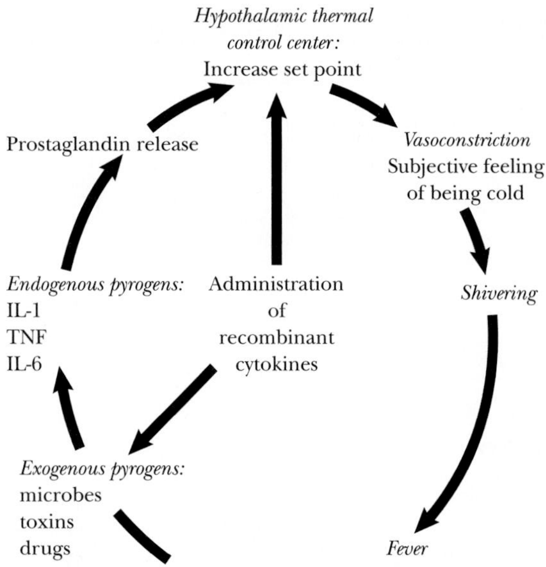

Figure 21-3 Pathogenesis of cytokine-related fever.

patients with a better performance status who require lower doses of IFN have reported fewer side effects with treatment. Table 21-3 lists typical toxicities associated with IFN-α, etiology, and management guidelines.[23,38,39]

Many of the cytokines released in response to IFN are mediators of the cellular and inflammatory immune response to viral infection, and they can cause similar constitutional symptoms. IL-1, IL-6, and TNF-α are the most important endogenous pyrogens. IL-1 and TNF-α also trigger production of prostaglandin E, which can reset the central thermostat and cause fever.[23] The pathophysiology of IFN-related fever is similar to the pathophysiology of fever related to the administration of certain other cytokines and provides a prototype for these reactions. See Figure 21-3.

Interleukins

Interleukins are cytokines that act primarily between lymphocytes. The word *interleukin* literally means "between white cells." However, since their discovery, interleukins have been found to have broader activity, interacting with other immune cells and body organs that have a role in the inflammatory immune response.

Interleukins are referred to by several names, as they were discovered by a variety of researchers and given functional names to describe their identified action. To minimize confusion, the International Congress of Immunology designates interleukins by number as soon as the interleukin gene is described. To date, 29 have been identified, and the search for new interleukins continues.[40] Unlike other forms of cancer therapy such as chemotherapy, interleukins are not directly cytotoxic to tumor cells. Rather, they act as messengers to initiate, coordinate, and sometimes amplify potent immune defense activities. As such, they require a functional, intact immune system to achieve their therapeutic effects.

Immunosuppressive agents such as corticosteroids can block the therapeutic actions of interleukins and other cytokines when they are used as anticancer therapy. This has implications for healthcare professionals when selecting medications for the management of symptoms commonly associated with cytokine therapy.

Many interleukins have been evaluated as anticancer agents. IL-2 is the only interleukin approved by the FDA as an anticancer agent. Several interleukins, such as IL-1, IL-6, and IL-4, have been evaluated as antitumor agents and have not shown significant antitumor effects. IL-12 is still being actively evaluated in clinical trials. The following section highlights IL-2 and its clinical use and briefly discusses IL-12.

Interleukin-2

First identified as a T-cell growth factor, IL-2 is a lymphokine that causes immune activation and release of other cytokines. IL-2 has no direct antitumor activity but stimulates the activation of immune cells capable of targeting and killing cancer cells. Produced by activated T lymphocytes, IL-2 increases and stimulates the following immune system cells: cytotoxic lymphoid cells, NK and lymphokine-activated killer (LAK) cells, B cells, complement factors, and monocytes and macrophages. It also stimulates the production of other cytokines such as IFN-γ, TNF, and granulocyte-macrophage colony-stimulating factor (GM-CSF) and facilitates the migration of immunologically active cells to the tumor site. Dose-dependent immunomodulatory and antitumor activity of IL-2 in animal models led to the development of high-dose IL-2 regimens for clinical investigation.[41,42]

Recombinant IL-2, also known as aldesleukin (Proleukin), was first approved for the treatment of metastatic renal cell cancer (RCC) and has subsequently been approved for metastatic melanoma. Initial approval for IL-2 in RCC was based on a multicenter study of 255 patients in which 14% of participants responded to the therapy. For those patients who responded, the remission was durable and averaged 20.3 months.[43] A 1996 update of the long-term response data from these patients indicated a 15% overall response rate and a median response duration for all objective responders of 54 months, with a range of 3 months to 8.9 years.[44] High-dose rIL-2 received approval for use in malignant melanoma based on a retrospective analysis of 266 patients treated in all trials of high-dose bolus IL-2 conducted between 1985 and

1993. The median response duration in this analysis was 6.5 months, with 60% of responders remaining progression-free at 5 years.[45] In selected patients with metastatic melanoma and clear-cell renal cancer, the *complete response* rate to high-dose bolus IL-2 is between 5% and 9%. According to follow-up data extending to 17 years, the majority of these completely responding patients will not relapse.[46,47]

In initial clinical studies, IL-2 was given by IV bolus infusion at doses of 600,000 to 720,000 IU/kg every 8 hours as tolerated. The regulatory approved dose of IL-2 for RCC and melanoma is 600,000 IU/kg every 8 hours by a 15-minute infusion for 5 days (maximum of 14 doses per cycle as tolerated). Following 9 days of rest, the schedule is repeated. Patients are retreated depending on the results of tumor evaluation 4 weeks after completion of a course of therapy and prior to starting another treatment course.

The toxicities associated with IL-2 are dose dependent. High-dose bolus IL-2 is associated with severe dose-limiting multisystem effects. Lower doses of IL-2 are associated with many of the same effects, but they are generally less severe. IL-2 induces proinflammatory cytokines such as IL-1, TNF-α, and IFN-γ. These and other substances such as nitric oxide play a major role in IL-2 toxicity.[48] Most side effects of IL-2 are reversible when therapy is stopped.[49]

Many toxicities associated with IL-2 are due to a dose-related capillary leak syndrome (CLS). Administration of IL-2 results in the release of cytokines, which contribute to an increased capillary permeability resulting in a fluid shift from the intravascular to the extravascular space. This fluid shift leads to decreased vascular resistance and hypovolemia and excessive fluid in the extravascular and interstitial spaces. Fluid accumulation from CLS may manifest as weight gain, generalized edema, pulmonary congestion, pleural effusion, and ascites. Hypovolemia associated with CLS may cause decreased blood flow to the kidneys, GI tract, heart, and brain and result in oligura, ischemia, and confusion. The earliest signs of CLS are hypotension and tachycardia, which can occur as early as two hours after the first dose of high-dose IL-2. Intravenous fluids are initial therapy for hypotension but are used judiciously because too much fluid can exacerbate generalized edema and pulmonary congestion. Persistent hypotension is treated with vasopressor support. Decreased urine output frequently occurs within the first eight hours of starting IL-2, and is due to hypotension and decreased intravascular volume. Renal dysfunction with IL-2 is prerenal in nature and transient, and there is no evidence of instrinsic renal damage. Patients may experience progressive shortness of breath from pulmonary congestion. When IL-2 therapy is stopped and BP stabilizes, diuresis is initiated, which results in weight loss and improvement in edema and pulmonary symptoms.[50]

During high-dose IL-2 therapy, toxicities are not managed with dose reductions. Rather, IL-2 doses are omitted and resumed according to recovery from the previous dose. Patients typically receive 8 to 12 doses of high-dose IL-2 in their first cycle of therapy and progressively less with subsequent treatments. Some toxicities require permanent discontinuation of therapy. Safe administration of high-dose IL-2 requires careful assessment of the many physiological changes that occur and expert clinical judgment on a dose-by-dose basis by the healthcare team. Treatment algorithms and clinical pathways are useful tools for managing patients receiving high-dose IL-2.[50,51]

Patients must be carefully screened prior to beginning IL-2 treatment to ensure adequate renal, hepatic, neurological, cardiac, and pulmonary function. Treatment-related mortality with high-dose bolus IL-2 has decreased significantly as clinicians have had more experience with this agent and have learned to select appropriate patients. Several groups with experience giving high-dose IL-2 have reported on a large series of patients with no treatment-related mortality.[52] The multiorgan toxicity of this regimen has limited its use to patients with excellent organ function and performance status who are being treated by experienced clinicians.[48,50] Toxicities associated with IL-2 and general management guidelines are described in Table 21-4.

In an attempt to minimize toxicity, clinical trials have examined various doses, routes, and schedules of rIL-2 in metastatic RCC. Numerous publications in the literature describe the use of IL-2 outside of the approved regimen. Lower-dose intravenous (bolus or continuous infusion) regimens have generally resulted in decreased toxicities. Subcutaneous (SC) IL-2 regimens have safely been given in the outpatient setting. These regimens are also associated with fewer side effects than high-dose bolus therapy. Transient inflammation and local induration at injection sites occurs in most patients receiving SC IL-2. Fever, chills, fatigue, and nausea are the most common side effects seen with SC IL-2.[53–56]

Alternate regimens of IL-2, alone or in combination with IFN, have successfully reduced acute toxicities and the expense associated with inpatient regimens. Patients with poorer functional status, such as the elderly and those with concomitant systemic disease, are more likely to tolerate the lower-dose regimens. Data suggest, however, that the duration of response may be less with low-dose regimens.[44,47,53,55,57] A three-arm randomized study compared response rates and overall survival of patients with metastatic renal cell carcinoma receiving high-dose bolus IL-2, low-dose bolus IV IL-2, or low-dose daily SC IL-2. The

Table 21-4 Interleukin-2: Toxicities and Management Considerations

System	Manifestation	Comment	Management Guidelines
General — flulike	Fever, malaise, chills/rigors Myalgias/arthralgias Headache Fatigue	Fever occurs within 2–8 hours of drug administration; most severe after initial doses Chills/rigors occur 2–8 hours after IV administration and within 30–60 minutes after SC administration	Premedicate with acetaminophen and/or NSAIDs Narcotics (i.e., meperidine or dilaudid) may be given to control chills Assess for potential sources of infection
Gastrointestinal	Nausea, vomiting, diarrhea, anorexia, taste changes, stomatitis	Mild to moderate and dose-dependent Resolve rapidly after treatment is discontinued	Antiemetics Avoid concomitant use of corticosteroids (may reduce effectiveness of therapy) Antidiarrheal agents Dietary modifications
Dermatologic	Pruritic, macular erythematous rash that can progress to dry desquamation Injection-site nodules and induration with SC administration Peeling skin on palms and soles	Dermatologic reactions can be mild to moderate or severe Skin nodules from SC injections usually disappear within a few months after treatment is discontinued	Antipruritics Water-based moisturizers Emollient lotions Avoid drying soaps, excessive heat Rotation of injection sites
Neurologic	Confusion, hallucination, agitation, cognitive changes, depression, sleep disturbances	Dose-related; may be dose-limiting with high-dose May be seen after a few doses; reversible	Establish safety measures; discontinuation of agent may be necessary Antidepressants as appropriate Sedative; antianxiety medication
Cardiovascular/ Pulmonary	Hypotension, tachycardia, arrhythmias, fluid retention, edema, weight gain, dyspnea	Partially related to capillary leak syndrome — increased capillary permeability causes fluid to leak from vascular bed into tissues	Assess heart/lung sounds, vital signs, weight Use of diuretics discouraged with high-dose IL-2 (may result in depletion of intravascular volume and hypotension) Vasopressors and judicious use of fluids for high-dose IL-2 Diuretics may be used at completion of high-dose therapy
Renal	Increased creatinine, BUN; oliguria, azotemia	Related to decreased renal perfusion associated with decrease in intravascular volume and peripheral vascular dilatation Concomitant use of NSAIDs may contribute further to renal toxicity	Monitor lab values, I & O Renal dose vasopressors may be needed to maintain kidney perfusion
Hepatic	Elevated SGOT, SGPT, LDH, alkaline phosphatase, bilirubin Jaundice	Dose-related Reversible	Monitor lab values Assess for jaundice, hepatomegaly
Hematologic	Thrombocytopenia, anemia leukopenia, eosinophilia Impaired neutrophil function with decreased chemotaxis	Generally mild	Monitor CBC Administer prophylactic antibiotics for patients with central lines receiving high-dose IL-2 Assess for infection, bleeding, fatigue, SOB Support with blood products

NSAIDs = nonsteroidal anti-inflammatories; I & O = intake and output; SOB = shortness of breath.

authors of this trial concluded that major tumor regression was more likely if patients received high-dose bolus IL-2, and that it appeared to produce greater biologic activity. Additionally, a quality of life assessment did not demonstrate major differences in patient perceptions of toxicity or quality of life between these high- and low-dose regimens. This study did not show an overall survival difference for high and low doses of IL-2.[47] The authors further concluded, as have several others, that low-dose IL-2 is a viable option for metastatic renal cell cancer patients with significant medical comorbidities or for physicians inexperienced in giving high-dose IL-2, but high dose IL-2 should be the therapy of choice for patients with metastatic renal cell cancer who are able to tolerate this therapy.[44,47,53,55,57] In metastatic melanoma, high-dose IL-2 has been associated with superior overall response rates that are more durable and of higher quality than those obtained with lower doses of IL-2 or alternative administration schedules or routes.[48]

IL-2 has been evaluated in the adjuvant setting for RCC. A prospective randomized phase III trial of high-dose bolus IL-2 given postoperatively as adjuvant therapy for patients with high-risk Stage III RCC failed to show significant clinical benefit.[58] Toxicity-reduction strategies such as administering IL-2 with agents that block the effects of IL-1 and TNF are being evaluated to ameliorate severe high-dose IL-2 toxicities.[48,59] Studies are also investigating the potential use of IL-2 in HIV infection[60] and as a vaccine adjuvant in cancer and infectious disease. Low-dose or ultra-low-dose long-term pulse therapy with IL-2 has been studied as a means of providing longer-lasting immune stimulation.[61]

IL-2 may have potential clinical applications in hematologic malignancies and in the transplant setting.[62] The combination of IL-2 and rituximab is being evaluated in phase II trials for the treatment of low-grade or follicular non-Hodgkin's lymphoma (NHL) in patients refractory to prior single-agent rituximab. The rationale for this combination is that the expansion of NK cells by IL-2 may enhance antibody-dependent cellular cytotoxicity (ADCC), which is the predominant mechanism of action of rituximab. Phase I trials showed that the combination was feasible, and that adding IL-2 to rituximab may be an effective strategy for enhancing monoclonal antibody efficacy mediated by ADCC.[63] IL-2 has been evaluated as consolidative immunotherapy using various schedules after autologous stem cell transplant (ASCT) at the time of minimal residual disease, with the intent of augmenting the graft versus tumor effect to reduce relapse rates, with mixed results.[64–66] Moderate-dose IL-2 given after ASCT has been associated with a low-regimen-related toxicity, and trial results have been suggestive of improved disease-free survival.

Interleukin-12

Interleukin-12 is a multifunctional cytokine that promotes cell-mediated immunity through its effects on T and NK cells. It facilitates type 1 helper T-lymphocyte responses, enhances the lytic activity of NK cells, augments the specific CTL responses, and induces the secretion of IFN-γ. Preclinical models of IL-12 have demonstrated significant antitumor activity. IL-12 inhibits angiogenesis by its induction of IFN-γ and IP-10. It has also been shown to play an important role in the promotion of the host resistance to infection by bacterial, fungal, and protozoan pathogens.[67–70]

Recombinant IL-12 has been studied in phase I and II clinical trials. Early studies of IV bolus IL-12 were complicated by severe toxicities and treatment-related deaths, and thus clinical development was temporarily halted.[71] Subsequent studies found that administering a test dose of IL-12 prior to initiating daily intravenous dosing is necessary to attenuate the severe toxicity. Recombinant IL-12 has been given safely as an IV bolus with the use of a test dose and in subcutaneous regimens. Prior exposure to IL-12 has been shown to protect against toxicity by attenuating the IFN-γ response following subsequent IL-12 administration. Common side effects seen with IL-12 include fever, chills, fatigue, stomatitis, liver function test abnormalities, and transient leukopenia.[48,71,72,73]

Clinical trials using rIL-12 in RCC and melanoma have shown limited responses, and trials in other malignancies are ongoing.[48,72] IL-12 has shown activity in Kaposi's sarcoma and cutaneous T-cell lymphoma.[74] The combination of IL-12 and rituximab has been shown to be safe and may be an active regimen in NHL.[70] Interleukin-12 has been evaluated after stem cell transplantation.[75] The fact that IFN-γ is down-regulated with repeated administration of IL-12 has raised concerns about its therapeutic potential, since IFN-γ is considered to be the key regulator of IL-12-mediated antitumor effects.[72] Studies have evaluated ways to reverse the down-regulation of IFN-γ induction and increase response rates. One potential strategy involves administering concurrent low-dose IL-2 with IL-12.[74] IL-12 has shown promise as a vaccine adjuvant and may be most clinically useful in this setting.[72]

Combination Therapy

In an attempt to improve and optimize response in certain malignancies, various combinations of cytokines and chemotherapeutic agents have been evaluated. The important variables of agent, dose, route, sequencing of agents, and duration of treatment are only a few that may significantly influence the therapeutic outcome for the patient. Many combinations of cytokines have been evaluated, such as IL-2 with IL-4 and IL-2 with TNF-α; the most widely studied combination is IL-2 with IFN-α. A clinical advantage from the addition of IFN-α to IL-2 has not been demonstrated in RCC and melanoma.[76,77]

Biochemotherapy is an example of combination therapy. This form of combination therapy involves combining a cytokine or group of cytokines with chemotherapy. This therapy attempts to preserve the immune function stimulated by the cytokines along with the tumoricidal effects of chemotherapy and improve response rates of either treatment modality alone. Synergy between chemotherapeutic and biological agents and the lack of cross-resistance provides a sound basis for the development of biochemotherapy regimens.[78] Numerous studies have evaluated IL-2 or IFN-α in combination with various chemotherapy agents in several malignancies.

Biochemotherapy has been most actively studied in metastatic melanoma. Encouraging results have been seen with studies that combine cisplatin-based chemotherapy with high-dose IL-2 alone or with lower doses of IL-2 and IFN. Combined results from a variety of regimens show a response rate of approximately 50%, with a median survival of 11–12 months. These regimens have been administered in either a sequential or concurrent fashion. Most biochemotherapy regimens require inpatient admission and are associated with significant side effects, including severe myelosuppression, nausea and vomiting, and moderately severe hypotension, as well as constitutional symptoms. Outpatient biochemotherapy regimens have also been developed. Although higher response rates have been seen with biochemotherapy regimens compared with chemotherapy or biotherapy alone, the long-term survival benefits to date have been marginal and may not justify the toxicity.[48,79]

Tumor Necrosis Factors

Tumor necrosis factors are a group of glycoproteins produced by immune cells in response to a pathogen. They are the active substances first seen in Coley's toxins. Cachectin, or TNF-α, is produced primarily by macrophages, NK cells, and T cells. These cells elicit a variety of immune response actions, including increased catabolism, enhanced phagocytosis, and tumor destruction.[18]

Lymphotoxin, or TNF-β, is also a cytokine produced by T cells in response to antigen. It is a cytotoxin that, when released, is capable of killing any nearby cells. The cell-killing ability of TNF-β is enhanced by IFN-γ.[18] Tumor necrosis factor is one of the few cytokines that has direct, tumoricidal capability. Although the exact method of cell killing is as yet unknown, TNF is capable of damaging tumor blood vessels, leading to necrosis and loss of nutrients and oxygen.[80]

The recombinant form of TNF-α was evaluated in phase I clinical trials in 1987. Toxicities included severe constitutional symptoms and hypotension, resembling symptoms of septic shock.[81] While TNF-α was shown to be effective in murine tumors in preclinical trials, the maximum tolerated dose (MTD) of TNF-α in clinical studies was substantially less than the effective dose in murine tumors.[82]

Subsequent clinical trials have focused on using TNF-α in a regional infusion as a way to limit systemic toxicity yet increase the dose to tumors to obtain local control and make limb-sparing surgery possible for melanoma or soft-tissue sarcoma.[83] Patients with melanoma and sarcoma whose tumors are confined to a limb have received TNF via isolated limb perfusions (ILP), most commonly with melphalan. TNF-α has been reported to improve the pharmacokinetics of concomitant chemotherapy by increasing drug concentration in tissues. Significant and sometimes dramatic necrosis of melanoma or sarcoma tumors has been seen with this treatment, which has produced response rates up to 90%.[84–87] A worldwide review of the experience with TNF-α-based hyperthermic ILP found that the majority of patients with limb-threatening soft-tissue sarcoma can be spared amputation with this treatment.[87] Hyperthermia is an important component of this therapy and acts by enhancing the tumoricidal effects of melphalan.[88] Side effects have included fever and chills, skin rash, limb swelling, and hypotension in the immediate postoperative period. Systemic toxicities are a result of the leak of TNF-α from the perfusate into the systemic circulation, resulting in a syndrome that resembles septic shock. This adverse event can be managed with generous fluid administration and short-term use of vasopressors and is largely preventable with the use of a leakage-free perfusion technique. Tumor necrosis factor is approved in Europe for isolated limb perfusion of locally advanced grade 2–3 soft-tissue sarcomas in extremities.[84–88]

Activated Cell Therapy (Adoptive Immunotherapy)

The discovery and development of recombinant cytokines such as IL-2 have facilitated the development of activated cell therapy. These activated cells are immune cells that are removed from the patient and placed in culture with rIL-2, which greatly increases their numbers and enhances their cytolytic capacity. The cells are then administered to the patient as adoptive immunotherapy. Activated cells are capable of targeting cancer cells without killing normal cells.

There are two types of activated cells: LAK cells and tumor-infiltrating lymphocytes (TILs). LAK cells are primarily made up of NK cells activated on exposure to high levels of IL-2. They are nonspecific killer cells that can lyse tumor cells without major histocompatibility complex (MHC) recognition and specificity.[89]

Lymphokine-activated killer cells

Therapy with LAK cells begins with the administration of high-dose IL-2 to stimulate cell production. These cells are then removed by a series of plasmaphereses and are cultured in IL-2 for several days. They are returned to the patient along with additional IL-2 doses as tolerated.

The side effects of the therapy are caused by the IL-2 administered with the cells and include fever, chills, hypotension, oliguria, weight gain, changes in mental status, and pruritus. Only pulmonary congestion and dyspnea are attributable to the LAK cells themselves.

One of the first patients with melanoma to be given IL-2/LAK therapy had a durable complete remission. However, long-term evaluation of IL-2/LAK therapy has shown that only 5% to 10% of patients with melanoma or RCC have responded to therapy. The addition of LAK cells has not demonstrated an advantage in response rates over patients receiving high-dose IL-2 alone.[90]

Tumor-infiltrating lymphocytes

TILs are a second type of activated cell used in cell transfer therapy. They are derived from tumor sites and are cytotoxic to autologous tumors (the patient's own tumors) but not to allogeneic tumors (tumors of the same type in other patients). They are also 50 to 100 times more potent than LAK cells. Although the TIL cell population may vary according to the type of cancer, in melanoma approximately 60% are CD4/CD8 cells, and NK cell numbers are low. They also differ from LAK cells in that they travel to tumor sites, recognizing MHC and tumor antigens.[91]

Therapy with TILs begins with isolation of these cells from a fresh resected tumor that is enzymatically digested into single-cell suspensions. Tumor cells and TILs are then cultured in a medium containing antibiotics and rIL-2. Within 2 weeks, tumor cells disappear; over 30 days, the number of TILs rapidly increases and is allowed to grow to a size predicted from preclinical studies to be therapeutically effective. The cells are then removed from the culture, washed, and prepared for reinfusion. They are administered intravenously in saline in divided doses depending on the total number of cells. High-dose rIL-2 is also administered as tolerated to keep the cells active.[92]

The toxicity of TIL therapy reflects the same side effects as high-dose rIL-2. Side effects directly related to TIL infusions are pulmonary symptoms such as dyspnea, pulmonary congestion, and hypoxia.

Rosenberg et al. reported the five-year National Institutes of Health (NIH) experience with TIL therapy in malignant melanoma: 86 patients were treated with TILs and rIL-2, with or without cyclophosphamide.[93] The objective response rate was 34%, with more patients responding to TILs derived from subcutaneous metastatic tumor deposits than to TILs derived from lymph nodes. No significant difference was reported for patients who also received cyclophosphamide. Some patients responded to TIL therapy who had previously failed to respond to high-dose rIL-2 alone; however, only one complete response and no durable responses occurred in this group. Considering that IL-2 plus TIL therapy is not sufficiently superior to IL-2 alone and that this regimen is costly and time- and labor-intensive, the clinical usefulness of this treatment modality appears limited.[48]

As cancer therapy moves to a molecular-based level, a new generation of more effective TILs may be created. Early gene therapy trials used TILs transduced with genes for cytokines such as TNF and IL-2 that were designed to deliver high concentrations of TNF to tumor sites with decreased systemic effects.[94] TILs have been instrumental in the identification of melanoma-associated antigens (MAAs), which have a role in cancer vaccine therapy. They also have shown an ability to recognize MAAs and have subsequently been used to clone the genes that encoded the MAA that they recognized. The availability of the gene sequences of MAAs has provided new opportunities for developing immunization strategies involving the delivery of the desired gene product to the patient in the form of a recombinant virus.[48]

Monoclonal Antibodies

Antibodies are proteins made by the immune system, each in response to a specific antigen. Monoclonal antibodies (MAbs) are artificially produced antibodies that are the product of a single clone of cells sensitized to a specific antigenic protein present on the surface of a target tumor. Monoclonal antibody therapy, also known as *serotherapy* or *passive immunotherapy*, was one of the first forms of modern biotherapy to use a highly specific agent directed against cancer cells while sparing normal tissue.

Manufacture of Antibodies and the Hybridoma Technique

In the 1970s, the hybridoma technique enabled researchers to create highly specific antibodies in large quantities, which made it possible to develop MAbs into a potential cancer therapy. However, it also introduced one of this therapy's biggest problems — the use of foreign immunogenic protein.

As shown in Figure 21-4, the hybridoma process begins by immunizing a mouse with a selected antigen. B cells within the spleen of the mouse soon produce immunoglobulin directed against the injected antigen. The mouse spleen cells are then fused in polyethylene glycol with immortal B cells — myeloma cells — that are capable of continued antibody production in cell culture. Thus, spleen B cells with the desired genetic antibody information are combined with cells having the potential to continue antibody production. These hybrid daughter cells are separated using a

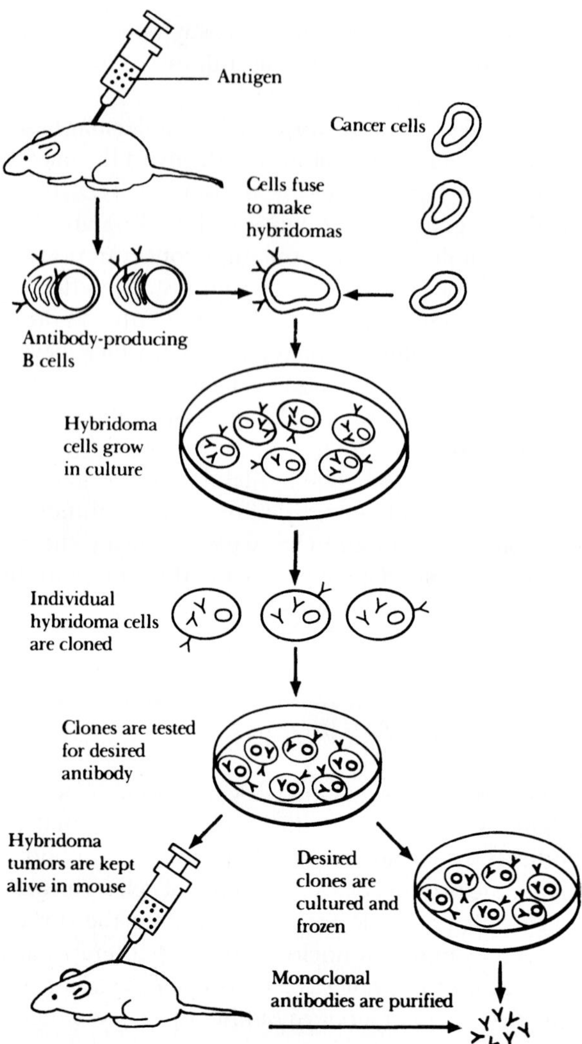

Figure 21-4 A diagram of the hybridoma technology for manufacturing monoclonal antibodies. (Reprinted from Schindler LW: *Understanding the Immune System.* NIH Publication No. 88-529. Bethesda, MD, US Department of Health and Human Services, 1988.[99])

medium that eliminates all nonhybrid cells; clones that produce the desired antibody against the immunizing antigen are then selected. Finally, the selected cell clones are stored or cultured for mass production.[95–99]

This classic method of MAb production has been modified through the use of genetic engineering techniques. Recombinant DNA allows the MAb structure to be reshaped to include portions made from human protein or allows undesired sections of the antibody structure to be deleted. Continued advances in genetic engineering have allowed the production of MAbs with more human and fewer murine components and have overall led to increased efficiency in MAb production.[98,100]

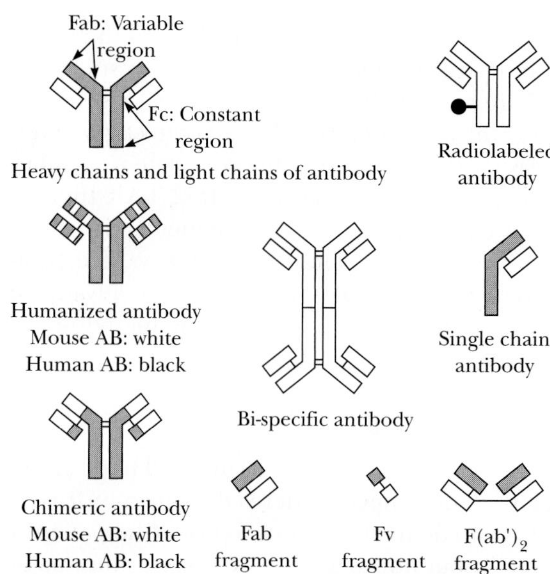

Figure 21-5 Antibody anatomy: variations on the structure of murine, human, and chimeric antibodies.

Structure of Monoclonal Antibodies

Monoclonal antibodies are made of two heavy and two light polypeptide chains that are linked by disulfide bonds to form a Y (Figure 21-5). The site where the antibody binds with the specific antigen is called the fragment antigen binding (Fab) or variable region because it varies greatly from one antibody to another. The stem of the Y links the antibody to other cells that participate in the immune response. This area is called the fragment crystallization or constant region (Fc) of the molecule because it is constant within all classes of antibodies.[95,98,101]

The first generation of MAbs was made from murine proteins. The repetitive use of antibodies containing foreign protein is strongly immunogenic in immunocompetent patients. It is estimated that 50% of patients develop human antimouse antibody (HAMA) on the first exposure, and up to 90% of patients who receive three or more MAb doses develop HAMA.[102] Human antimouse antibody can bind to the MAb, increasing its clearance from the body and potentially leading to increased toxicity.

In an attempt to decrease the incidence of HAMA, changes in the structure of MAbs have been made to include more human protein, which is less immunogenic. Figure 21-5 shows some of the major modifications of MAb. Chimeric antibodies combine the mouse variable region with a humanized constant region. These MAbs have a longer circulating half-life and an enhanced interaction with human effector cells, and they are less immunogenic than murine antibodies, allowing for repeated dosing.[103] The human Fc portion of a chimeric MAb improves its ability to mediate complement-dependent cytotoxicity (CDC) and ADCC, which makes it more potent than the parent murine MAb. Another MAb design is predominantly human protein and is called *humanized antibody*. Short segments of murine antibody have been inserted in the variable end on a human antibody structure.

Monoclonal antibodies are named according to their composition. The generic names of all monoclonal antibodies end with the suffix "mab" for monoclonal antibody. Usually the name for a murine antibody adds the letters *mo* to the suffix to become "momab." For a chimeric antibody, the letters *xi* are added to the suffix to become "ximab." The names for humanized antibodies add the letters *zu* to become "zumab", and for a fully humanized antibody the letters *mu* are added and the name ends in "mumab."[97]

Mechanism of action

Unconjugated monoclonal antibodies function like human immunoglobulin. The role of an antibody or immunoglobulin is to recognize an antigen and initiate an immunologic response to eliminate the antigen and/or destroy the cell associated with the antigen. This form of unaltered antibody is dependent on host immune mechanisms to kill cells because the antibody itself is not a cytotoxic agent. Some of these immune mechanisms include activation of ADCC or CDC. ADCC occurs when the Fc regions on the antibodies are recognized by receptors on natural killer cells, macrophages, granulocytes, and monocytes; these effector cells then enhance tumor cell destruction. The binding of antigen to antibody can activate the complement cascade, which can result in cell lysis through the release of enzymes and the augmentation of phagocytic cells that attach to and ingest tumor cells. Monoclonal antibodies can also cause cell destruction by the direct induction of apoptosis. Monoclonal antibodies can neutralize cell growth by interfering with the signal transduction of cell growth messages.[95,100,101,104]

Antigen identification

The specificity of MAbs is dependent on identifying antigenic proteins on the surface of tumors that are not present on normal tissues. MAbs have been developed and directed toward many tumor-associated antigens. Some of the categories of MAb antigen targets include oncofetal antigens (carcinoembryonic antigen, or CEA), differentiation antigens, tissue-specific antigens (prostate-specific antigen, or PSA), growth factors (epidermal growth factor), and oncogene products (c-erbB2). Anti-idiotypic antibodies can also be used as surrogate antigens. An *idiotype* is the specific binding region of an antibody. Anti-idiotype MAbs are directed to the antigen-binding sites of antitumor antibodies and mimic the original tumor antigen.[95,96,100]

The most widely studied target antigen in MAb therapy is the CD20 antigen, and several monoclonal antibodies have been developed against this antigen. The CD20 cell-surface antigen is expressed in more than 90% of B-cell lymphomas and to a lesser degree in chronic lymphocytic leukemias. It is suited for targeted therapy because it is not found on precursor B cells or stem cells. Furthermore, the CD20 antigen does not circulate in the bloodstream, nor does it impede tumor-cell targeting. Because CD20-anti-CD20 antigen-antibody complexes are not internalized by the cell, the cell-surface-bound antibody persists for a longer time, allowing optimal interaction between the antibody and host immune effector cells or complement.[104]

Monoclonal Antibodies in Cancer Therapy

MAbs may have a diagnostic or therapeutic role in cancer therapy. Radioisotope-labeled MAbs are capable of identifying sites of tumor in the patient that may not be detectable by other methods. In the investigational setting, MAbs are being evaluated to purge bone marrow after myeloablative cytotoxic conditioning regimens. Several conjugated and unconjugated monoclonal antibodies are approved for clinical use as a cancer therapy. The currently approved therapeutic monoclonal antibodies used in oncology, along with dosing guidelines, adverse events, and management considerations, are listed in Table 21-5 and are discussed in the following section. Cetuximab and bevacizumab are discussed in greater detail in the later sections on targeted therapy and angiogenesis inhibitors.

Unconjugated monoclonal antibodies

Unconjugated MAbs are the simplest of the MAb therapies. As noted earlier, these were the first generation of MAb to be studied. In this approach, the MAb itself mediates cell death through various immune mechanisms. Selecting the proper target antigen has been essential to the development of MAb therapy. Hematologic malignancies have been extensively studied as ideal tumor models for MAb therapy because they express a variety of well-defined cell-surface antigens.[105] The first MAb approved for therapeutic use in oncology, rituximab (Rituxan), is an unconjugated MAb directed against the CD20 antigen.

Rituximab

Rituximab is a chimeric murine/human MAb directed against the CD20 antigen found on the surface of B lymphocytes. It consists of variable regions from

Table 21-5 Therapeutic Monoclonal Antibodies Approved for Use in Oncology

Unconjugated Monoclonal Antibodies

Trade Name	Generic Name	Target/Type	Indication	Dose and Administration	Adverse Events	Management Considerations
Rituxan	Rituximab	CD20/ Chimeric	Relapsed or refractory, low grade or follicular NHL	375 mg/m^2 IV First infusion: Infuse at 50 mg/h for the first 30 minutes. Rate can be increased in 50 mg/h increments every 30 minutes to a maximum of 400 mg/h Subsequent infusions: Initial rate of 100 mg/h. Increase by 100 mg/h increments at 30-minute intervals to a maximum of 100 mg/h	*Most common* Infusion-related symptoms and lymphopenia *Less common* Tumor lysis syndrome Mucocutaneous reactions — Stevens-Johnson syndrome, lichenoid dermatitis, vesiculobullous dermatitis, and toxic epidermal necrolysis Arrhythmias, chest pain *Rare* Human antichimera antibodies	Increased risk of tumor lysis syndrome in patients with high number of circulating lymphocytes (> 25,000/mm^3) and/or high tumor burden
Herceptin	Trastuzumab	HER2/ Humanized	Metastatic breast cancer patients whose tumors overexpress HER2 As a single agent for second-line therapy in patients who have received one or more prior chemotherapy regimens With paclitaxel as first-line therapy for patients who have not received prior chemotherapy	Loading dose: 4 mg/kg IV over 90 minutes Maintenance doses: 2 mg/kg weekly. If loading dose is well tolerated, may infuse maintenance doses over 30 minutes	Infusion reactions Increased leukopenia and anemia in combination with chemotherapy *Other* Pain, asthenia, headache, diarrhea, nausea, vomiting Cardiotoxicity Rare severe pulmonary events leading to death	Assessment of HER2 overexpression should be performed Extreme caution in patients with preexisting cardiac dysfunction Assess baseline cardiac function and monitor while on treatment
Campath	Alemtuzumab	CD52/ Humanized	Patients with B-cell CLL who have been treated with alkylating agents and have not responded to fludarabine therapy	3 mg/day IV until tolerated, then 10 mg/ day IV until tolerated, then 30 mg 3 three times a week for up to 12 weeks	Infusion reactions Neutropenia, thrombocytopenia Increased risk of opportunistic infections	Contraindicated in patients with active systemic infection or underlying immunodeficiency Anti-infective prophylaxis to decrease opportunistic infections Monitor CBC/platelets
Erbitux	Cetuximab	EGFR/ Chimeric	In combination with irinotecan for the treatment of EGFR-expressing metastatic colorectal cancer in patients who are refractory to irinotecan-based chemotherapy As a single agent for the treatment of EGFR-expressing metastatic colorectal cancer in patients who are intolerant to irinotecan-based chemotherapy	In combination with irinotecan or as monotherapy: 400 mg/m^2 as an initial loading dose administered as an intravenous infusion Weekly maintenance dose: 250 mg/m^2	Acne-form rash, dry skin, fissuring, nail changes, hypersensitivity reaction, diarrhea, nausea, asthenia, malaise Human antichimera antibodies (rare)	Instruct patients to limit sun exposure — can exacerbate skin rash
Avastin	Bevacizumab	VEGF/ Humanized	In combination with intravenous 5-fluorouracil-based chemotherapy for first-line treatment of patients with metastatic carcinoma of the colon or rectum	5 mg/kg once every 14 days as an IV infusion until disease progression	*Most common severe adverse events* Asthenia, pain, hypertension, diarrhea, leukopenia *Other* Gastrointestinal perforations/wound-healing complications, thromboembolism hemorrhage (epistaxis most common bleeding event), proteinuria, CHF	Do not initiate therapy for at least 28 days following major surgery Surgical incision should be healed before starting therapy Monitor BP at baseline and every 2–3 weeks during treatment — more often for patients who develop hypertension during treatment Serial monitoring for proteinuria

(continued)

Table 21-5 Therapeutic Monoclonal Antibodies Approved for Use in Oncology (continued)

Conjugated Monoclonal Antibodies

Trade Name	Generic Name	Target/Type	Indication	Dose and Administration	Adverse Events	Management Considerations
Zevalin	(^{90}Y) ibritumomab tiuxetan	CD20/Murine	Relapsed or refractory low-grade or follicular or transformed B-cell NHL including rituximab refractory B-cell NHL	Day 1: Rituximab 250 mg/m^2 IV followed by ibritumomab labeled with ^{111}IN within 4 hours. If biodistribution is acceptable, rituximab 250 mg/m^2 IV is given between days 7 and 9 followed by ibritumomab labeled with ^{90}Y: 0.4 mCi/kg (or 0.3 mCi/kg for platelet count 100,000–149,000/mm^3). ^{90}Y ibritumomab tiuxetan is given as a slow IV over 10 minutes. Maximum total dose is 32 mCi	Severe delayed myelosuppression — median nadir 7–9 weeks after therapy with related infectious and hemorrhagic sequelae Most nonhematologic toxicities (i.e., infusion reactions, asthenia, nausea, chills, fever) are associated with the rituximab component	Should not be given to patients with > 25% lymphoma marrow involvement and/or impaired marrow reserves Should not be given to patients with ANC < 1500/mm^3 or platelets < 100,000/mm^3 Educate patient and family on radiation safety precautions Monitor CBC
Bexxar	tositumomab and Iodine ^{131}I tositumomab	CD20/Murine	Patients with CD20-positive follicular NHL with and without transformation whose disease is refractory to rituximab and has relapsed following chemotherapy	*Day 0:* "Cold" dose — 450 mg unlabeled tositumomab over 60 minutes followed by "hot dose" 5 mCi ^{131}I tositumomab (35 mg) over 20 minutes followed by whole-body gamma camera scans to determine whole-body ^{131}I counts *Days 2–4 and 6–7:* Whole-body gamma camera scans *Days 7–14:* 450 mg "cold" tositumomab over 60 minutes followed by ^{131}I tositumomab over 20 minutes (dose calculated to deliver 75 cGy total body irradiation (65 cGy for patients with mild thrombocytopenia) (based on clearance estimates from previous gamma scan counts)	*Myelosuppression* Severe and prolonged with nadir at week 5–6 with recovery of ANC and platelets by week 8–9 with related infectious and hemorrhagic sequelae *Nonhematologic short-term* Fatigue, nausea, fever, vomiting, infections, pruritus, rash *Long-term* Development of HAMA, secondary malignancies (MDS, AML) *Other* Hypothyroidism	Administer thyroid blocking agent (saturated solution of potassium iodide) to block uptake of ^{131}I by thyroid gland. Start 24 hours before dosimetric dose and continue for 2 weeks after therapeutic dose Monitor TSH at baseline and annually for life Educate patient and family on radiation safety precautions after release — provide written instructions Assess patient's ability for self-care and ability to follow radiation safety precautions Do not administer to patients with > 25% lymphoma bone marrow involvement and/or impaired marrow reserves Monitor CBC
Mylotarg	Gemtuzumab	CD33/ Humanized	Patients with CD33-positive AML in first relapse who are ≥ 60 and are not candidates for other cytotoxic chemotherapy	9 mg/m^2 IV infusion over 2 hours; repeat in 14 days	*Common* Severe myelosuppression — neutropenia/ thrombocytopenia Acute infusion-related symptoms Transient transaminase elevations *Rare* Hepatic venoocclusive disease	Reduction of WBC to < 30,000/mm^3 is recommended to decrease risk of tumor lysis syndrome and pulmonary complications, i.e., ARDS

Data from Cersosimo,[97] Plosker et al.,[106] Cersosimo,[135] Emmanouilides.[145]

the heavy and light chains of the murine anti-CD20 antibody (IDEC 2B8) grafted onto a human IgG1 constant backbone (Figure 21-6). Studies have shown that the human Fc regions enhanced the ability of the chimeric C2B8 antibody to initiate complement-mediated lysis and ADCC. The cytotoxic effects of rituximab on malignant B cells are not fully understood, but it is thought to cause cell lysis through the induction of ADCC and CDC (Figure 21-7). It also has been shown to trigger apoptosis (programmed cell death) through interaction with the CD20 antigen.[97,104] Since it is chimeric, rituximab stays in the circulation for long periods, effectively mobilizes immune effector mechanisms, and does not generate HAMA responses. The

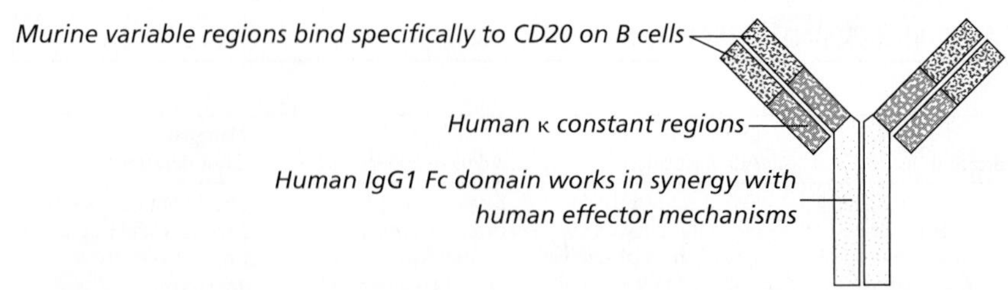

Figure 21-6 Chimeric rituximab-engineered antibody. The human Fc domain and kappa constant regions enhance the ability of rituxan to initiate complement-mediated lysis and ADCC. (Reprinted with permission from Genetech, Inc. San Francisco, CA, and IDEC.)

reduced immunogenicity of a chimeric antibody allows for repeated courses of rituximab.[104–107]

Treatment with rituximab resulted in an overall 48% response rate in a pivotal multicenter study in patients with relapsed or refractory low-grade or follicular CD20-positive B-cell non-Hodgkin's lymphoma. Side effects were mild to moderate and were mostly infusion related. The median time to progression for responders was 13.1 months, and the median duration of remission was 11.2 months.[108]

Rituximab is indicated for the treatment of patients with relapsed or refractory low-grade or follicular CD20-positive B-cell non-Hodgkin's lymphoma. It is administered by intravenous infusion once weekly for four or eight doses. Rituximab has been shown to be safe and effective for retreatment of relapsed low-grade or follicular NHL previously treated with rituximab. Grade 3–4 adverse events with retreatment were similar to those seen with initial treatment.[103] Rituximab has been shown to be effective for use in patients with bulky disease (> 10 cm), which is typically nonresponsive to treatment. Grade 3–4 adverse events were higher in patients with bulky disease and patients with a high number of circulating lymphocytes.[109]

The most common adverse events associated with rituximab are mild to moderate infusion-related symptoms, including fever, chills, rigors, nausea, headache, and asthenia. These common reactions are typical symptoms of an inflammatory process and are associated with an acute immune response resulting from antigen/antibody binding. Since most rituximab binds to CD20-positive B cells during the first infusion, causing rapid depletion of B cells, the incidence and severity of infusion-related events decrease with subsequent infusions. Additionally, rituximab has a long half-life, so it remains in the patient's bloodstream during subsequent infusions. Approximately 10% of patients develop more severe hypersensitivity reactions such as bronchospasm, hypotension, angioedema, or hypoxia.[97,106] Table 21-6 describes infusion-related reactions and management guidelines with rituximab and other monoclonal antibodies.

Grade 3–4 lymphopenia is seen in approximately 40% of patients receiving rituximab. Rituximab induces a rapid depletion of B lymphocytes that typically lasts about 6 months. Since CD20 is not expressed on stem cells, full recovery of B lymphocytes usually occurs 9 to 12 months after treatment. Aside from lymphopenia, other grade 3–4 hematologic adverse events occur infrequently with rituximab. The incidence of human antichimera antibodies (HACA) with rituximab is rare. Rare severe life-threatening events seen with rituximab include tumor lysis syndrome with associated renal toxicity, cardiac arrhythmias, and mucocutaneous reactions.[106]

A lack of overlapping toxicities, differing mechanisms of action, and evidence of in vitro synergy provide the rationale for combining rituximab with chemotherapy.[106] The activity of rituximab in combination with several chemotherapy regimens and bio-

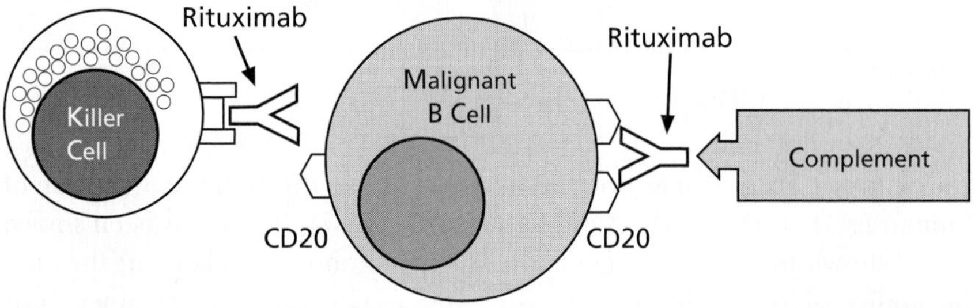

Figure 21-7 Rituximab mechanism of action. Rituximab binds CD20, which is present on normal and malignant pre-B mature B cells; may induce antibody-dependent cell-mediated cytotoxicity (ADCC) and complement-dependent cytotoxicity; and triggers apoptosis.

Table 21-6 Reactions to Monoclonal Antibody Infusion

Monoclonal Antibody	Frequency/Description	Premedication/Management
Rituximab (Rituxan)	*Mild to moderate* Most occur 30 minutes to 2 hours after start of infusion (77% frequency with first infusion). Decreased frequency with subsequent infusions. May include fever, chills, rigors, nausea, rash, pruritus, urticaria, rhinitis, myalgia, asthenia, headache, flushing, throat irritation, and pain at tumor sites *More severe hypersensitivity reactions* Hypotension, hypoxia, angioedema, and bronchospasm *Most severe* Pulmonary infiltrates, ARDS, MI, ventricular fibrillation, cardiogenic shock Severe reactions are more common among patients with pulmonary infiltration, CLL, mantle-cell lymphoma, and women Rare fatal reactions have occurred following an infusion reaction complex that included hypoxia, pulmonary infiltrates, acute respiratory distress syndrome, myocardial infarction, ventricular fibrillation, or cardiogenic shock	Premedication with acetaminophen, diphenhydramine *Mild to moderate reactions* Slow or stop infusion, administer diphenhydramine, acetaminophen, IV fluids, and vasopressors if necessary. Usually infusion can be restarted at reduced rate (50%) when symptoms resolve *Severe* Stop infusion/provide appropriate supportive therapy Medications for treatment of hypersensitivity reactions, i.e., epinephrine, antihistamines, and corticosteroids should be available Closely monitor patients with preexisting cardiac and pulmonary conditions, prior significant cardiopulmonary events, high number of circulating malignant cells (≥ 25,000) with or without high tumor burden
Herceptin (Trastuzumab)	*Mild to moderate — 40% frequency* Most common with first infusion. Fever, chills, nausea, vomiting, pain, headache, dizziness, dyspnea, hypotension, rash, asthenia *Infrequent — Severe hypersensitivity reactions* Anaphylaxis, bronchospasm, hypoxia, hypotension, urticaria, and angioedema *Rare* Pulmonary toxicity characterized by dyspnea, pulmonary edema, pulmonary infiltration, pleural effusion, noncardiogenic pulmonary edema, pulmonary insufficiency, hypoxia, and acute respiratory distress syndrome	Premeds not usually used with first infusion If infusion reaction occurs, stop or slow infusion and restart at a slower rate Acetaminophen, diphenhydramine, and meperidine may be used to treat infusion reaction. Premed with subsequent infusions if reactions occur Patients with lung disease or extensive tumor involvement of the lungs may be at greater risk of severe reactions Interrupt infusion for patients who have dyspnea or clinically significant hypotension Discontinue therapy for patients who develop anaphylaxis, angioedema, or acute respiratory distress
Alemtuzumab (Campath)	Rigors (90% frequency), fever (85% frequency), nausea, vomiting, rash Most common during first week of therapy; decline with continued administration Additional reactions may include dyspnea, hypotension, hypoxia	Diphenhydramine and acetaminophen 30 minutes before first dose and at each dose escalation. Patients who experience severe reactions should also be pretreated with hydrocortisone Monitor vital signs every 15 minutes during first infusion and with each dose escalation Antihypertensive meds
Cetuximab (Erbitux)	*Severe infusion reaction — (3% frequency)* Characterized by rapid onset of airway obstruction (bronchospasm, stridor, hoarseness), urticaria, and/or hypertension *Grade 1-2 infusion reactions (16%–23% frequency)* Chills, fever, dyspnea	Premedication with H_1 antagonist (i.e., diphenhydramine) recommended Severe reaction: immediately stop therapy and institute appropriate medical therapy Mild to moderate reaction: Slow infusion rate, use antihistamine, use with subsequent treatments
Bevacizumab (Avastin)	Infusion reactions with first dose uncommon (< 3%) — may include mild fever, chills, rigors, myalgia No grade 3–4 infusion reactions reported in trials	Interrupt infusion for severe reaction and administer appropriate treatment
Gemtuzumab (Mylotarg)	Acute infusion-related adverse events may include chills, rigors, fever, nausea and vomiting, urticaria, skin rash, fatigue, headache, diarrhea, and dyspnea. Usually occur within 4 hours of infusion in approximately 30% of patients Incidence decreases with second infusion Transient hypotension that responds to IV fluids can occur several hours after the end of the infusion	Acetaminophen and diphenhydramine prior to administration; can be repeated as needed A brief course of IV corticosteroids has been found to decrease infusion-related events Monitor vital signs during infusion and up to 4 hours after for delayed hypotension Administer IV fluids and supportive meds for hypotension
^{90}Y ibritumomab tiuxetan (Zevalin therapeutic regimen)	Most commonly associated with rituximab component of regimen Note: Prescribing information contains black box warning that deaths have occurred within 24 hours of rituximab infusion associated with infusion reaction symptom complex	Premedicate with acetaminophen and diphenhydramine prior to each dose of rituximab Manage infusion reactions per rituximab guidelines and prescribing information Discontinue therapeutic regimen for severe infusion reactions
Tositumomab and Iodine ^{131}I tositumomab (Bexxar therapeutic regimen)	Constellation of symptoms including fever, rigors, chills, sweating, hypotension, dyspnea, bronchospasm, and nausea have been reported during or within 48 hours of infusion of dosimetric dose Majority of infusion reactions grade 1 or 2	Premedicate prior to "cold" doses of tositumomab in dosimetric and therapeutic steps with acetaminophen and antihistamine For both tositumomab and ^{131}I tositumomab, reduce infusion rate by 50% for mild to moderate reaction; interrupt infusion for more severe toxicity. After severe infusion toxicity resolves, resume infusion at 50% rate reduction; symptomatic management for more severe reactions

Note: Emergency equipment and medications to manage acute hypersensitivity reactions and severe infusion reactions should always be available when administering monoclonal antibodies.

Data from Cersosimo,[97] Plosker,[106] Cersosimo.[135]

logic agents has been evaluated and continues to be studied. Several trials have been conducted of rituximab plus CHOP (cyclophosphamide, doxorubicin, vincristine, and prednisone) chemotherapy. The largest trial of rituximab plus CHOP is the Groupe d'Etude des Lymphomes de l'Adulte (GELA) study, which involved 399 newly diagnosed elderly patients with diffuse large B-cell lymphoma. Patients were randomized to receive rituximab plus CHOP or CHOP alone. Patients randomized to CHOP received one cycle every three weeks for eight cycles. Patients randomized to CHOP plus rituximab received CHOP every three weeks for eight cycles plus rituximab on day 1 of each cycle. The results showed a clear advantage for rituximab plus CHOP over CHOP alone in terms of event-free survival at two years (57% versus 38%, $p < 0.001$).[110] Many consider the combination of rituximab plus CHOP to be the gold standard for the treatment of aggressive NHL in elderly as well as younger patients. This combination has also become frequently used in the frontline therapy of patients with low-grade/follicular NHL.[111,112]

Several rituximab and chemotherapy combination regimens have been studied in aggressive NHL. Encouraging results have been seen in trials combining rituximab plus EPOCH (etoposide, prednisone, vincristine, cyclophosphamide, and doxorubicin), ICE (ifosfamide, carboplatin, and etoposide), or FCM (fludarabine, cyclophosphamide, and mitoxantrone) in patients with relapsed or refractory aggressive NHL.[97,106] The addition of rituximab to CVP (cyclophosphamide, vincristine, and prednisone) chemotherapy in patients with untreated follicular NHL resulted in improved response rates when compared to CVP alone.[113] Rituximab has been studied in combination with several other biotherapeutic agents, such as IFN-α, IL-2, IL-12, and alemtuzumab.

Rituximab has been evaluated in several clinical trials for the treatment of chronic lymphocytic leukemia (CLL)/small lymphocytic lymphoma (SLL). The CD20 antigen is expressed at lower levels in CLL than in other types of NHL. At standard doses, single-agent activity of rituximab has been disappointing in relapsed and refractory CLL/SLL patients; however, response rates have been higher in previously untreated patients. The most positive results have been seen with the use of rituximab in combination with fludarabine or fludarabine-containing regimens in untreated patients with CLL/SLL as well as in those with relapsed or refractory disease.[114,115] The role of rituximab in frontline or maintenance treatment of indolent and aggressive NHL is being actively investigated.[116] Rituximab is also being evaluated for other B-cell disorders such as Waldenstrom's macroglobulinemia and immune thrombocytopenic purpura and autoimmune disorders such as rheumatoid arthritis.[97,106]

Trastuzumab

Trastuzumab (Herceptin) is a MAb directed against the human epidermal growth factor receptor (HER2/neu) (also known as c-erbB2) proto-oncogene. HER2 is a member of the epidermal growth factor family of transmembrane proteins found on the surface of many epithelial cells. Stimulation of HER2 transmits signals to the cell nucleus regarding cell growth. Overexpression of HER2 may lead to increased cell division and cellular growth rates. Overexpression of HER2 is found in 25% to 30% of human breast cancers. Normally, a breast epithelial cell may have 20,000 to 50,000 HER2 receptors. With HER2 overexpression, there may be as many as 2 million receptors on the cell's surface. In clinical studies, HER2 protein overexpression and HER2 gene amplification have been associated with a higher frequency of tumor recurrence, a decreased overall survival time, and resistance to certain types of chemotherapy.[97,117–119]

Because of the role of the HER2 receptor protein in the pathogenesis of breast cancer, strategies to interfere with its function have been evaluated. Trastuzumab is a humanized MAb derived from recombinant DNA that binds to the extracellular domain of the HER2 protein. It has been shown to inhibit the proliferation of human tumor cells that overexpress HER2, both in vitro and in animals. Trastuzumab induces regression of tumors that are overexpressing HER2 by inhibiting signal transduction and cell proliferation and activating antibody cellular cytotoxicity. Additional activities of trastuzumab include suppressing angiogenesis by inducing antiangiogenic factors and repressing proangiogenic factors.[100,119]

In two pivotal clinical trials, trastuzumab demonstrated significant activity both as a single agent and in combination with traditional cytotoxic chemotherapy in the treatment of HER2/neu overexpressing metastatic breast cancer. A trial by Slamon et al. evaluated trastuzumab in combination with chemotherapy. In this trial, 118 (50%) of 235 patients who received chemotherapy plus trastuzumab responded, and 74 (32%) of 234 patients who received chemotherapy alone responded ($p < 0.001$). The addition of trastuzumab to chemotherapy significantly increased the median time to treat failure, the median survival time, and the one-year survival rate.[120] Another trial evaluated trastuzumab as a single agent in patients with disease that had progressed after prior chemotherapy and resulted in a overall response rate of 21.6%.[121] The beneficial treatment effects in these trials were limited to patients with the highest level (3+ by immunohistochemistry) of HER2 protein overexpression. Overall, trastuzumab was generally well tolerated in both studies. Mild infusion-associated symptoms such as chills and fever were reported by about 40% of patients and primarily occurred with the first infusion. An increased risk of cardiac dysfunction was observed in patients who received trastuzumab in combination with anthracyclines and cyclophosphamide. Anemia, leukopenia, diarrhea, and an increased incidence of infection were rarely seen with trastuzumab.[97,120,121]

Trastuzumab is indicated as a single agent for the treatment of patients with metastatic breast cancer whose tumors overexpress the HER2 protein and who have received one or more chemotherapy regimens for metastatic disease. Trastuzumab combined with paclitaxel is indicated for patients with metastatic breast cancer who have not received chemotherapy for metastatic disease and whose tumors overexpress the HER2 protein. Trastuzumab is approved for use as a weekly intravenous infusion. Several trials have confirmed the safety and efficacy of administering trastuzumab every three weeks as monotherapy or in combination with chemotherapy.[122–124] Trastuzumab is commonly continued beyond progression with an alternate chemotherapy regimen. In the pivotal trial, patients were allowed to continue trastuzumab alone or with an alternate chemotherapy regimen after progression as part of an extension trial that showed that prolonged use of trastuzumab is safe and well tolerated. Since safety was the primary objective of this extension trial, limited efficacy information is available. The limited efficacy results suggested that patients who received trastuzumab before disease progression may respond to a second trastuzumab-containing regimen.[125] Ongoing trials are evaluating the optimal duration of trastuzumab therapy and the use of trastuzumab beyond disease progression.

HER2 status is a critical determinant of response to trastuzumab and also provides important prognostic information. The American Society of Clinical Oncology (ASCO) recommends assessment of HER2 status in all primary breast tumors at the time of diagnosis or upon recurrence, and the NCCN recommends determination of HER2 expression as part of the initial workup and staging of a patient with invasive breast cancer. Several methods are available for assessing the HER2 status of tumors. Immunohistochemistry (IHC) and fluorescence in situ hybridization (FISH) are the two most common diagnostic methods used to measure HER2 levels in the clinical setting to identify appropriate candidates for trastuzumab therapy. IHC is an assay that measures overexpression of the HER2 protein, which is a result of gene amplification. When using commercially available IHC kits, the level of HER2 staining is graded on a scale from 0 (no detectable HER2) to 3+ (high HER2 expression). Tumors with a staining score of 3+ are the most responsive to trastuzumab. FISH detects actual HER2 gene amplification and allows for direct measurement of the number of gene copies. FISH is thought to be more sensitive and specific than IHC and less subject to variability in the reviewer's interpretation. With FISH, there are only two possible results, positive or negative. The superiority of FISH over IHC was suggested in a retrospective analysis of specimens from the phase III trial of trastuzumab and chemotherapy as frontline treatment of metastatic breast cancer. The NCCN guidelines recommend that an IHC result of 2+ be retested with FISH.[97,120,126]

The most serious toxicity observed with trastuzumab in clinical trials was cardiac dysfunction ranging from an asymptomatic reduced ejection fraction to congestive heart failure. Risk factors for cardiac dysfunction in patients receiving trastuzumab include age, preexisting cardiac disease, a history of cardiotoxic drug therapy, and radiation therapy involving the left side of the chest. The risk of cardiac dysfunction in clinical trials was highest in patients who received trastuzumab in combination with doxorubicin. The NCCN advises that the risk of cardiotoxicity with trastuzumab and doxorubicin-cyclophosphomide is too high to use outside of a clinical trial. Extreme caution should be used in treating patients with preexisting cardiac dysfunction. Patients should undergo a thorough cardiac assessment prior to treatment and be monitored frequenly for deteriorating cardiac function.[127,128]

The combination of trastuzumab with several chemotherapy, biological, and targeted agents has been studied in numerous clinical trials in metastatic breast cancer, and many combination trials are ongoing.[97,129] In phase II trials, the combination of vinorelbine and trastuzumab has been shown to be safe and effective as first-line therapy and in patients with previously treated HER2 positive advanced breast cancer.[130,131] The addition of carboplatin to trastuzumab and paclitaxel was evaluated in a randomized phase III clinical trial in women with HER2 positive metastatic breast cancer. The response rate was 52% for patients who received trastuzumab/paclitaxel/carboplatin (TPC) compared to 36% for trastuzumab/paclitaxel (TP) ($p = .04$), and time to progression was 11.2 months with TPC and 6.9 months with TP alone ($p = .007$).[132]

Given the survival benefit demonstrated with trastuzumab in advanced stage disease and poor outcomes in patients with HER2 positive breast cancer, the role of trastuzumab is being evaluated in the adjuvant setting. Four large-scale, multicenter, randomized adjuvant trials of trastuzumab are ongoing. These trials include the National Surgical Adjuvant Breast and Bowel Project (NSABP) trial B-31, North Central Cancer

Treatment Group (NCCTG) Intergroup trial N9831, Breast Cancer International Research Group trial (BCIRG) 006, and the Herceptin Adjuvant (HERA) trial. The different designs of these trials will attempt to determine the optimal schedule and duration of trastuzumab in relation to adjuvant therapy (concurrent, sequential, or both) and radiotherapy. The evaluation of cardiac dysfunction in the adjuvant setting is also a priority of these trials. Trastuzumab is also being evaluated in the neoadjuvant setting. Ongoing trials are also investigating ways to decrease cardiac dysfunction associated with trastuzumab.[133]

Alemtuzumab

Alemtuzumab (Campath) is a humanized monoclonal antibody directed against the CD52 antigen. The CD52 antigen is abundantly expressed on the surface of essentially all normal and malignant lymphocytes and a majority of monocytes, macrophages, and NK cells. It is also expressed by the tissues of the male reproductive system. CD52 is not expressed on hematopoietic stem cells, erythrocytes, and platelets. The proposed mechanism of action of alemtuzumab is lysis of leukemia cells after binding to the cell surface.[134,135]

The pivotal trial of alemtuzumab included 93 patients with relapsed or refractory B-cell CLL who had received prior alkylating agent therapy and had not responded to fludarabine. The overall response rate was 33%, including a 2% and 31% complete response (CR) and partial response (PR) rate, respectively. The median time to response was 1.5 months, the median duration of response was 8.7 months, and the median survival time for responders was 32 months.[136]

Alemtuzumab is indicated for the treatment of B-cell CLL in patients who have been treated with alkylating agents and who have failed fludarabine therapy. Alemtuzumab is associated with acute infusion-related events and delayed toxicities related to myelosuppression and immunosuppression. In the pivotal trial, the most frequent adverse events were infusion related and included rigors (90%), fever (85%), nausea, vomiting, and rash. Infusion-related events also included hypotension, rigors, shortness of breath, bronchospasm, chills, and/or rash. Rigors and fevers and other first-dose reactions were much less common in trials evaluating alemtuzumab as a subcutaneous injection. Local reactions at the injection site were experienced by 90% of patients, but were mostly grade 1 and 2.[134–138]

Because of the high density of the CD52 antigen on most lymphocytes of both T-cell and B-cell lineage, alemtuzumab induces profound lymphopenia, placing patients at an increased risk for infection. In the pivotal trial, 55% of patients experienced an infection. Antimicrobial prophylaxis, usually consisting of trimethoprim sulfamethoxazole and acyclovir, is suggested upon initiation of therapy and for a minimum of two months following the last dose of therapy.[134]

Conjugated monoclonal antibodies

Because of the limited efficacy seen with unconjugated MAbs in early trials, another strategy was developed to use the ability of MAbs to bind specifically to a target, spare normal tissues, and deliver a cell poison to the tumor cell. These carrier or conjugated MAbs are capable of killing cells and do not require the host's immune competence. The most common conjugated MAbs include immunotoxins, antibody drug conjugates, and radioimmunoconjugates. With conjugated antibody therapy, when the antibody attaches to the antigen, the radionuclide, toxin, or cytoxic drug is released, destroying the target cell and possibly surrounding cells as well.

An *immunotoxin* (IT) is a molecule formed when a MAb or fragment is conjugated to a plant or bacterial cell toxin. Ricin is the most commonly used plant toxin; however, some studies have tried saporin or gelonin. These are potent cell poisons, only minute amounts of which need to be incorporated into a cell to inhibit protein synthesis and cause cell death. Pseudomonas exotoxin (PE) and diphtheria toxin are the two most frequently used bacterial toxins. Most ITs have shown little activity in clinical trials and have been associated with significant toxicities such as dose-limiting vascular leak syndrome. Frequent development of HAMA or antitoxin responses have also occurred, which prohibited retreatment of patients. Of all MAb-based therapies, ITs may be farthest from clinical use as they are not as easy to use, as other MAb therapies and do not have the low side effect profile of the unconjugated MAbs.[105]

Antibody-drug conjugates are another type of conjugated monoclonal antibody. Monoclonal antibodies have been linked to chemotherapeutic agents with the goal of increasing drug concentration at the tumor site. However, difficulty getting sufficient concentrations of a drug at the site of bulky, often necrotic, and poorly vascularized tumors has been a limiting factor. Gemtuzumab is currently the only antibody-drug conjugate approved for therapeutic use in oncology.

Gemtuzumab

Gemtuzumab ozogamicin (GO) (Mylotarg) is composed of a humanized recombinant anti-CD33 monoclonal antibody, the antitumor antibiotic calicheamicin, and a linker that attaches the calicheamicin to the antibody. The antibody portion of this agent is specific for the CD33 antigen, which is expressed in over 90% of patients with acute myeloid leukemia (AML). The

CD33 antigen is expressed on most hematopoietic stem cells; on mature and immature myeloid cells, including colony-forming progenitor cells; and on erythroid, megakaryocytic, and multipotent progenitors. It is also found on leukemic blasts from the majority of patients with AML and myelodysplastic syndrome (MDS). CD33 has been identified as an attractive target for the treatment of AML because it has little expression outside of the hematopoietic system. With the administration of GO, antibody binding to the CD33 antigen on leukemic cells creates an antigen-antibody complex. After this complex is formed, the drug is internalized, the linker undergoes a hydrolysis reaction, and the calicheamicin is released into the lysosomes of the cell. The calicheamicin then exerts its cytotoxic activity by binding to DNA, resulting in double-strand DNA breaks and cell death by apoptosis.[135,138–140]

GO was evaluated in 142 patients in three single-arm open-label studies. All patients in these trials had CD33-positive AML in first relapse following a first CR of at least three months (for patients 60 and older) or six months (for patients younger than 60). After one dose of GO, 43% of patients had 5% or less blasts in the bone marrow. The overall response rate for the three pooled studies was 30%.[141] Based on data from these trials, GO was given approval from the FDA, conditional upon the completion of ongoing studies in patients with recurrent AML and the conduct of randomized clinical studies comparing the effects of GO in combination with induction chemotherapy with the effects of induction chemotherapy alone.[142]

GO is approved for the treatment of patients with CD33-positive AML in first relapse who are 60 years and older and are not considered candidates for conventional cytotoxic chemotherapy. In the phase II studies, GO resulted in fewer nonhematologic toxicities and appeared to be better tolerated than other cytotoxic regimens commonly used in the setting of relapsed AML. Importantly, GO induced responses in patients who would not be considered candidates for additional AML therapy.[135,138–140]

GO is administered as an IV infusion over two hours. It is recommended that the white blood cell count (WBC) be less than 30,000/mm^3 at the time of administration because higher WBC counts can result in severe acute respiratory distress. Severe myelosuppression, including thrombocytopenia, anemia, and neutropenia, is the major toxicity associated with GO. Myelosuppression occurs because the CD33 antigen is present on hematopoietic precursor cells, but it is reversible since the CD33 antigen is not present on the pluripotent stem cell. Patients may experience a rapid and profound thrombocytopenia and neutropenia, which may occur as early as within two days of the infusion. An acute infusion-related symptom complex occurs in approximately 30% of patients receiving this agent.[135,138–140] The administration of a brief course of intravenous corticosteroids has been shown to significantly reduce infusion-related events associated with GO administration.[143] Transient elevations of transaminases and bilirubin may occur with GO. Clinically serious, sometime fatal hepatic venoocclusive disease has been associated with GO, and ongoing trials are attempting to understand the pathophysiology of this syndrome.[135]

Radioimmunoconjugates

Radio-labeled monoclonal antibodies or *radioimmunoconjugates* are monoclonal antibodies with therapeutic radioisotopes chemically attached to them. Radioisotopes are atoms that emit energy in the form of radiation. When a radioimmunoconjugate is administered, the radioisotope is carried to the tumor by the monoclonal antibody, which then attaches to a specific antigen present on the surface of tumor cells, resulting in direct radiation to the targeted cells. Radioimmunotherapy uses systemically targeted continuous low-dose radiation to treat multiple tumor sites throughout the body while delivering minimal irradiation to normal cells. In addition to targeting tumor cells, radio-labeled monoclonal antibodies can indirectly target adjacent cells. This indirect targeting of adjacent cells is known as the crossfire or bystander effect. Radiation emitted from the radioisotopes may be deposited in an area covering several cell diameters. The crossfire effect is thought to increase tumor killing beyond that achieved with non-radio-labeled monoclonal antibodies because tumor cells in the emission path of the radionuclide that are not bound to the antibody or not physically accessible for antibody binding are killed by the energy released from nearby radiation decay. Radioimmunotherapy has been most widely studied in NHL and combines the targeting benefits of a monoclonal antibody with the efficacy of radiation in the treatment of this very radiosensitive malignancy.[144–148]

Monoclonal antibodies can be labeled with different radioisotopes or radionuclides, which can emit either gamma or beta radiation. Iodine 131 (^{131}I) and Yttrium 90 (^{90}Y) are two radionuclides that have been conjugated to monoclonal antibodies to CD20 as a form of radioimmunotherapy for NHL. ^{90}Y is a pure beta emitter, and ^{131}I emits both beta and gamma radiation. These radioiosotopes have a relatively short half-life and are capable of transmitting energy over a distance of several cell diameters. Two radioimmunotherapeutic agents are currently FDA approved for clinical use: yttrium ^{90}Y ibritumomab tiuxetan (Zevalin), and ^{131}I tositumomab (Bexxar). Table 21-7 com-

Table 21-7 Characteristics of ^{90}Y Ibritumomab Tiuxetan and ^{131}I Tositumomab

	^{90}Y Ibritumomab Tiuxetan	^{131}I Tositumomab
Radioisotope	Yttrium 90	Iodine 131
"Cold" Antibody for Preinfusion	Rituximab	Tositumomab
Type of Radiation	Beta	Beta and gamma
Half-life	64 hours	8 days
Imaging/Dosimetry	Imaging with ^{111}IN to assess biodistribution	Imaging/dosimetry to determine clearance and calculate dose
Elimination	Predictable	Intrapatient variability
Beta Path Length	5.3 mm	0.8 mm

Data from Emmanouilides[145;] Cheson[146]; Hendrix et al.[147]; Hernandez, Knox[148]; Gordon[151]; Zelentz.[157]

pares the key features of these two radioimmunoconjugates.[144–147]

^{90}Y Ibritumomab tiuxetan

Ibritumomab tiuxetan (Zevalin) is formed by the connection of ibritumomab (parent monoclonal antibody of rituximab) to ^{90}Y via the chelator tiuxetan, which stably links the ibritumomab and ^{90}Y together. Ibritumomab is a murine monoclonal antibody directed against the CD20 antigen. ^{90}Y ibritumomab tiuxetan releases high-energy beta particles with a long path length, which may be an advantage for bulkier or poorly vascularized tumors or those with poor antibody penetration or heterogeneous antigen expression. Since ^{90}Y ibritumomab tiuxetan does not have a gamma component, a surrogate isotope, indium 111 (^{111}In), is used for the imaging step of the treatment regimen. Tiuxetan binds ^{111}In to ibritumomab for imaging. The lack of a gamma component simplifies radiation precautions during the handing of ^{90}Y ibritumomab tiuxetan. Additionally, a short half-life of 64 hours results in rapid decay and a favorable radiation hazard profile.[144–147]

^{90}Y ibritumomab tiuxetan was compared with rituximab in a randomized phase III trial in patients with relapsed or refractory low-grade follicular or transformed CD20-positive B-cell NHL. The overall response rate in the ibritumomab tiuxetan group was 80% compared to 56% in the rituximab group ($p = .002$). A trial update reported a median duration of response of 23 months in complete responders in the ^{90}Y ibritumomab tiuxetan group.[149] In a single-arm phase II trial of ibritumomab tiuxetan in patients with rituximab refractory NHL, the overall response rate was 74%, and the complete response rate was 15%.[150]

^{90}Y ibritumomab tiuxetan, the first radioimmunotherapeutic agent approved by the FDA, is approved for the treatment of relapsed or refractory follicular/low-grade or transformed NHL, including rituximab-refractory follicular NHL. The ibritumomab tiuxetan therapeutic regimen is administered over eight days. On day 1, an initial unlabeled predose of rituximab 250 mg/m^2 (referred to as the "cold antibody" since there is no radioisotope) is delivered to clear the blood of normal B cells so that subsequent radio-labeled drug will be more likely to bind to tumor cells. The predose is followed within 4 hours by an imaging dose of indium 111 (^{111}In) ibritumomab. After the imaging dose, whole body scans are done at 2–24 hours (day 1) and 48–72 hours (days 3–4), with an optional third scan at 90–120 hours (days 4–5) to determine biodistribution. The images are assessed to ensure tumor targeting and to make sure that safe doses of radiation are delivered to normal organs. The therapeutic dose is delivered on day 8 following another predose of rituximab. Doses of ^{90}Y ibritumomab tiuxetan are adjusted for patients with mild thrombocytopenia.[147,151–153] In a phase II trial of 30 patients with relapsed or refractory low-grade follicular or transformed B-cell NHL and a baseline platelet count of 100×10^9 to 149×10^9, ^{90}Y ibritumomab tiuxetan at a reduced dose was safe and effective.[154]

The primary toxicity associated with ^{90}Y ibritumomab tiuxetan is a transient, delayed myelosuppression. Integrated safety data from 349 patients treated in five clinical trials showed that grade 3 or 4 thrombocytopenia occurred in 61% of patients and grade 3 or 4 neutropenia in 57%, with the median nadir occurring at approximately 7–9 weeks following therapy The duration of the nadir was approximately 2 weeks.[155] The likelihood of cytopenia correlates with higher bone marrow involvement with disease. Despite a high incidence of grade 3 to 4 neutropenia, a low incidence of infection seen with this regimen has been attributed to the maintenance of an intact GI mucosa and the preservation of IgM and T-cell counts and rapid recovery of NK cells. Most nonhematologic toxicities have been associated with the rituximab component of the therapy. The incidence of HAMA or HACA following ^{90}Y ibritumomab tiuxetan is less than 2%. The incidence of secondary malignancies, namely AML and MDS, after ^{90}Y ibritumomab tiuxetan therapy is 1.5%, with a median follow-up of less than 2 years.[135,145–147,153]

Tositumomab and ^{131}I Tositumomab

^{131}I tositumomab (Bexxar) is formed by the conjugation of radioactive iodine (^{131}I) to the murine monoclonal antibody tositumomab (B1), which affects cell kill by inducing apoptosis, CDC, and ADCC. Tositumomab was first approved as a diagnostic agent in 1982, and thus there is a long history of medical use with this agent. Iodine 131 decay produces a short-range beta particle and also a gamma component that allows total body gamma counts to be obtained over time, enabling calculation of patient-specific pharmacokinetics and determination of millicurie activity needed for delivery of an optimal therapeutic dose of total-body radiation. Variability in the excretion of ^{131}I tositumomab among patients has led to dosing according to a prediction of total body radiation exposure over time (total body dose [TBD]). The linkage between iodine and tositumomab is subject to a process called dehalogenation, which results in the release of ^{131}I into the bloodstream, where it may be taken up by thyroid tissue or excreted in the urine.[145–147,156,157]

A multicenter phase III trial evaluated this agent in patients with NHL who were rituxan-naïve and resistant to chemotherapy. This study compared the efficacy of ^{131}I tositumomab with the patient's last qualifying chemotherapy regimen (LQC). This trial resulted in an overall response rate of 65%, with 17% complete responders. The median duration of response was 6.5 months, which was significantly longer than that of the patient's most recent previous therapy.[156] ^{131}I tositumomab has shown activity in patients who failed to respond to or relapsed within 6 months of receiving rituximab.[145,146]

The tositumomab and ^{131}I tositumomab therapeutic regimen is approved for the treatment of patients with CD20-positive follicular NHL, with and without transformation, whose disease is refractory to rituximab and has relapsed following chemotherapy.

The ^{131}I tositumomab therapeutic regimen is given in two steps: the dosimetric and the therapeutic steps. On day 0, patients are given a predose of unlabeled or "cold" tositumomab to saturate accessible nontumor sites and increase tumor delivery of ^{131}I. Patients then receive a dosimetric dose of ^{131}I tositumomab. Because of the gamma component of ^{131}I tositumomab, dosimetry can be performed without a substitute radioisotope. The purpose of dosimetry is to determine the whole-body clearance and the therapeutic dose of ^{131}I tositumomab. Three whole-body gamma camera scans are performed — on day 0; on either day 2,3, or 4; and on day 6 or 7 — to help construct an elimination curve for each individual patient based on total body counts. Following dosimetry, the therapeutic dose is calculated and then adjusted based on the patient's platelet count. On day 7–14 the therapeutic dose is delivered. If biodistribution is found to be altered, the therapeutic step should not be administered. Patients must receive oral thyroprotection to prevent uptake of ^{131}I by the thyroid and subsequent thyroid irradiation. Premedication with diphenhydramine prior to the dosimetric and therapeutic steps is recommended. ^{131}I tositumomab can be safely given on an outpatient basis if it is determined by dose calculations that radiation doses to other individuals are at an acceptable level and that patients can be compliant with instructions regarding radiation safety precautions.[145,146,150]

The primary toxicities of ^{131}I tositumomab are mild to moderate: reversible neutropenia, thrombocytopenia, and anemia. The most common nonhematologic toxicities are asthenia, fever, nausea, and headache. Less commonly, chills, myalgias, anorexia, arthralgia, rash, and pruritus may occur. Even with thyroid protection, there is an 8.5% incidence of an elevated TSH level. The incidence of HAMA depends on the amount of prior treatment. In studies treating relapsed patients, the incidence of HAMA was generally less than 10%, but when used as a first-line treatment, the reported incidence was 65%. This increase incidence of HAMA is likely due to a more intact immune system in untreated patients. AML and MDS have been reported in up to 6.3% of patients; however, prior chemotherapy may contribute to this complication.[145–147,157] Longer follow-up and additional trials are needed to fully characterize the risk of secondary malignancies.

Radiation safety precautions with radio-labeled monoclonal antibodies

The type of radiation precautions required with radioimmunotherapy depend on the type and dosage of radiation emitted by the radio-labeled antibody. Because ^{90}Y is a pure beta emitter, it can be administered in an outpatient setting with minimal risk to healthcare workers or family members, and patients can be released immediately after treatment, with minimal restrictions. When administered intravenously, beta particles can penetrate soft tissue and into the epidermis but cannot penetrate beyond a patient's body. Beta emissions are absorbed by approximately 1-cm-thick materials with low atomic weights such as acrylic. Acrylic vial and syringe shields are necessary with the use of ^{90}Y ibritumomab tiuxetan. No additional precautions beyond standard universal precautions to avoid contact with body fluids are necessary for family members or healthcare workers. Clinical data have shown that the urinary excretion of ^{90}Y ibritumomab tiuxetan is minimal, with approximately 7.3% of the radiation excreted in the urine over seven days. Gamma radiation has a higher level of tissue penetration than beta radiation and can penetrate through a patient's body to the outside. Healthcare workers are required to use lead shielding when handling gamma-emitting radionuclides such as ^{131}I tositumomab, and radiation precautions for patients and family members are more stringent. Since ^{131}I can be cleaved from the monoclonal antibody and is rapidly excreted in the urine, patients are instructed to have sole use of the bathroom if possible. It is important to be familiar with institutional,

Table 21-8 Patient Release Instructions Following Radio-Labeled Monoclonal Antibody Therapy

^{90}Y Ibritumomab Tiuxetan therapeutic regimen[1]	Tositumomab and Iodine ^{131}I tositumomab therapeutic regimen[2]
Universal precautions	Avoid sleeping in common bed
Clean up spilled urine	Avoid traveling for more than 4 hours at close distance to others
Carefully dispose of material contaminated with body fluids	Keep distance of 6 feet from others
Wash hands after toilet use	Avoid contact with pregnant women and children
Use condoms for sexual relations	Have sole use of bathroom if possible
	Sit while urinating and flush toilet three times with lid down
	Wash hands frequently, shower daily
	Keep dishes and utensils separate from rest of household; wash separately
	Launder clothing and linen separately from rest of household
	Use separate toothbrush, towels, and washcloths
	Bag and throw out trash separately
	Avoid sexual relations for a short time

[1] Precautions are for approximately 3 days
[2] Precautions are for approximately 1–2 weeks

Data from Hendrix et al.[147]; Gordon[151]; Wagner et al.[152]; Tuninstra[153]; Hogenstein et al.[158]

state, and Nuclear Regulatory Commission (NRC) guidelines for radiation safety and patient release.[145–147,151–153,158] Table 21-8 describes common patient release instructions for patients receiving radiolabeled monoclonal antibodies.

Multidisciplinary management of the patient receiving radioimmunotherapy

The administration of radio-labeled monoclonal antibodies requires a multidisciplinary approach between hematologists/oncologists, nuclear medicine physicians and technicians, nurses, radiopharmacy, and the hospital radiation safety officer. Typically the oncologist administers the unlabeled or "cold" antibody and the imaging and therapeutic doses are given by a nuclear medicine physician or radiation oncologist. Good communication is essential regarding time and scheduling issues, since radioactive antibodies are ordered in an individualized manner only after the dose and treatment date are determined, and they have a very brief shelf life. It is useful to have a coordinator who acts as a liaison between team members, orders the drugs, and manages the treatment timeline.[147,151,158]

Monoclonal antibodies: Nursing management

The management of the patient receiving monoclonal antibodies is highly variable among the different agents. The adverse event profile and patient management strategies depend on the agent used, the amount of murine component of the antibody, and whether the MAb is conjugated and the nature of the conjugate. Because some or all of the MAb consists of foreign proteins, acute infusion-related reactions are common. Reactions can be mild to moderate and include fevers, chills, rigors, nausea and vomiting, fatigue, headache, rhinitis, and pruritus. More severe hypersensitivity reactions may include urticaria, pruritus, dyspnea, hypotension, bronchospasm, and rarely anaphylaxis. Type I hypersensitivity reactions (anaphylaxis) are rarely seen with the administration of biological agents; however, anaphylaxis is always a concern when administering agents that are designed to stimulate or potentiate immune function. Patients and families should be instructed about symptoms of hypersensitivity and to call their physician if symptoms occur or seek immediate medical assistance if symptoms develop rapidly. See Table 21-6 for a description of infusion reactions and management strategies for the FDA-approved monoclonal antibodies.

Fusion Proteins

As noted earlier, an immunotoxin is an MAb conjugated to a toxin. A fusion protein made of a growth factor or cytokine linked to a toxin is called a *recombinant toxin,* a *chimeric toxin,* or an oncotoxin. Sometimes, however, the term *immunotoxin* is loosely applied to all of these molecules.[96] Several fusion proteins have been evaluated as anticancer therapy, and DAB_{389}IL-2 is the first to be approved as a therapeutic cancer agent.

Denileukin Diftitox

Denileukin diftitox (DAB_{389}IL-2, Ontak) is a diphtheria toxin fused to IL-2. This fusion protein binds to cells containing IL-2 receptors and causes a series of reactions that inhibit protein synthesis, ultimately resulting in cell death. The human IL-2 receptor exists in three forms, and its expression has been reported to occur in patients with cutaneous T-cell lymphoma (CTCL), CLL, Hodgkin's, and non-Hodgkin's lymphoma. CD25 is one of the IL-2 receptor subunit components.[159–160]

In a phase III randomized trial of patients with CTCL, 30% of heavily pretreated refractory patients had objective responses to denileukin diftitox. In addition, treatment with denileukin diftitox improved quality of life in the responding patients.[161] It is approved for treatment of persistent or recurrent CTCL in patients whose malignant cells express the CD25 component of the IL-2 receptor. Side effects of denileukin diftitox include acute hypersensitivity-type reactions, vascular leak syndrome, flulike symptoms, nausea, vomiting, and diarrhea.[159–162] Steroid premedication has been found to significantly improve the tolerability of denileukin diftitox without compromising efficacy.[163] Subsequent to the pivotal phase III trial, it was found that CD25 expression is not necessary for activity of denileukin diftitox and that tumor expression of CD25 may not correlate with tumor response.[162] This agent has shown activity in CLL and NHL, and trials are ongoing in these malignancies.[164]

Other Immunomodulating Agents

An *immunomodulating agent* can be broadly defined as a substance that stimulates host defense mechanisms or indirectly augments aspects of immunity that are beneficial in cancer therapy. *Immunostimulants* are often nonspecific agents that target key immune cells such as the monocyte/macrophage, provoking secondary responses involving increased cytokines, cytotoxic cell activation, and increased immunoglobulins.

Nonspecific immunostimulation is based on the theory that the host's responsiveness to a tumor can be increased through overall stimulation of host defense mechanisms using nontumor-related antigenic agents such as microorganisms.[165] In localized therapy, the tumor may be an "innocent bystander" but may be killed in the reaction to the provoking agent. This concept has been pursued in numerous clinical studies since the 1970s, with occasional positive outcomes.[4] These results underscore the need to better understand the complexities of the host-tumor relationship in order to apply this theory to clinical practice.

Some immunomodulating agents, such as cancer vaccines, provide active specific immunotherapy directed to a specific tumor target. Immunomodulating agents also include those that target specific aspects of host defense to stimulate cell differentiation (e.g., thymic hormones acting on T-cell differentiation); chemical substances that act as nonspecific immunostimulants (e.g., levamisole); vitamin preparations such as retinoids; and even chemotherapeutic agents such as cyclophosphamide that may decrease suppressor T-cell function or stimulate immune cells after initial immunosuppression.[165]

Nonspecific immunomodulating agents require that the host be capable of developing an immune response. Permanent damage to the immune system or persistent immunosuppression will interfere with the agent's effectiveness. In addition, the patient's tumor burden should be low. Large, bulky tumors are believed to significantly suppress host defense mechanisms. Therefore, immunomodulators are frequently used as adjunctive therapy with surgery or chemotherapy to reduce the patient's tumor burden.[165,166]

The following sections briefly describe the immunomodulating agents that are approved for cancer therapy or for clinical trials.

BCG (Bacillus Calmette-Guérin)

This nonspecific immunostimulant was one of the earliest types of immunotherapy. The first human was vaccinated with BCG in 1921. BCG was originally derived from attenuated strains of the live virus *Mycobacterium bovis*. The immunostimulatory effect of BCG is thought to be initiated by a cascade of immunologic events involving humoral and cellular immunity and the activation of T cells, B cells, macrophages, dendritic cells, and natural killer cells, although the precise mechanism of action of BCG in cancer is unknown. BCG has been evaluated in several malignancies but has been used most successfully in the treatment of superficial bladder cancer. It has been most effective in decreasing bladder tumor recurrence after endoscopic resection and slowing its progression, especially in high-grade, superficial transitional cell carcinoma.

BCG (Thera Cys, Tice BCG) is FDA approved as a bladder instillation for intravesical treatment of carcinoma in situ of the bladder. Side effects of intravesical BCG instillation include symptoms of bladder irritability such as dysuria, frequency, and hematuria. BCG can cause a flulike syndrome consisting of fever, chills, malaise, and myalgias that can last for 1–3 days after bladder instillation. Hypersensitivity reactions have also been reported with BCG. Combination therapy with BCG and other cytokines such as IL-2 and IFN-α is being investigated to enhance the effectiveness of BCG treatment. BCG is also being evaluated as an adjuvant with antigen-specific vaccines in the treatment of urological tumors.[167,168]

Retinoids

Retinoids are a group of small-molecule hormones that are natural derivatives of retinol or vitamin A. They include all-*trans*-retinoic acid (ATRA, or tretinoin), 13-*cis*-retinoic acid (13-*cis*-RA, or isotretinoin), and 9-*cis*-retinoic acid (9-*cis*-RA, or alitretinoin).

Retinoids are essential in the physiologic processes of vision, fertility, and embryonal growth. In cancer, retinoids act as immunomodulators by inducing cellular differentiation and suppressing proliferation.[169,170] Cancers that may be responsive to retinoids include leukemias, melanoma, neuroblastoma, and various epithelial cancers.

Retinol is absorbed from the gastrointestinal tract and is bound in the circulation to retinol-binding plasma proteins in minute amounts. Intracellularly, retinol is oxidized to form 13-*cis*-RA, 9-*cis*-RA, and other compounds. They target receptors in the nucleus capable of binding retinol as well as steroids, estrogen, and thyroid. Here, they interact with DNA to affect cellular growth and functions. For example, retinol can suppress tumor cells' synthesis of stromelysin, a compound that allows tumors to metastasize by degrading stromal tissue.

Clinically, dramatic effects have been seen using retinoids in acute promyelocytic leukemia (APL). Tretinoin acts on APL cells to increase their differentiation into mature granulocyte cells and induce clinical remission.[170–171] Tretinoin (Vesanoid) is approved for the induction of remission in patients with APL. Trials have shown that in appropriate combinations with chemotherapy, incorporation of tretinoin into induction regimens doubles the disease event-free survival in APL. Used alone, tretinoin can induce a remission in the majority of newly diagnosed patients, but the remission often is not durable. Tretinoin may have a role as maintenance therapy in APL.[172] A serious side effect of retinol therapy in APL is retinoic acid syndrome.[169,173] Patients receiving retinoids can exhibit fever, respiratory distress, interstitial pulmonary infiltrates, pleural effusions, and weight gain. Retinoic acid syndrome can be fatal if not promptly recognized and treated, usually with high-dose corticosteroids. It occurs in approximately 25% of patients and can appear within 2–21 days of onset of therapy. Symptoms do not abate or reverse when the drug is discontinued.[174]

Isotretinoin (Accutane) is an actively studied retinoid in oncology. The combination of 13-*cis*-RA plus IFN-α improved response rates in RCC compared to IFN-α alone. Responses have also been achieved with this combination in advanced squamous cell carcinoma of the skin and cervix. Isotretinoin and other retinoids have shown activity in chemoprevention trials.[175–178]

Alitretinoin is a naturally occurring retinoid that activates all known retinoid receptor subtypes.[169] It is FDA approved as Panretin gel, which is indicated for the topical treatment of cutaneous lesions in patients with HIV-related Karposi's sarcoma.

Bexarotene (Targretin) is a retinoid approved for the treatment of cutaneous T-cell lymphoma in patients who are refractory to at least one prior systemic therapy. Common and often dose-limiting side effects of bexarotene include triglyceride and cholesterol elevations, which often require the administration of lipid-lowering agents. Other adverse effects of bexarotene include hypothyroidism, leukopenia, infection, headache, rash, dry skin, asthenia, edema, and mild gastrointestinal disturbances.[179]

Class effects of retinoids include photosensitivity and teratogenicity. Patients should be instructed to protect themselves from sunlight exposure. Retinoids are contraindicated in pregnancy, and pregnancy must be ruled out prior to starting therapy. Common retinoid side effects include headache, mucocutaneous dryness, alteration in liver enzymes, and elevation of triglycerides.[179]

Thalidomide

Thalidomide was originally marketed for use as a sedative, but was withdrawn from the market after it was found to be a potent teratogen that caused stunted limb growth. Subsequent identification of thalidomide's immune-modulating and antiangiogenic properties has led to the investigation of thalidomide in cancer therapy. Thalidomide has been classified as an immunomodulatory drug with antiangiogenic activity. The immunomodulatory effect of thalidomide was first reported in patients with erythema nodosum leprosum (ENL), an acute inflammatory presentation of lepromatous leprosy. Immunomodulatory effects of thalidomide include T-cell co-stimulatory activity and inhibition of TNF-α and other cytokines. The precise mechanism of the antiangiogenic effects of thalidomide is unknown, but it may exert some of its effects by blocking the action of potent angiogenic factors such as basic fibroblast growth factor and vascular endothelial growth factor. The antiangiogenic effects of thalidomide are thought to be responsible for the limb deformities seen in early use with this agent because it inhibited blood vessel formation in the developing limbs.[180–182]

Thalidomide (Thalomid) is FDA approved for the treatment of ENL. It is not FDA approved for the treatment of any cancer but has been widely studied in many malignancies as a single agent or in combination therapy. Thalidomide has been extensively studied in multiple myeloma (MM), a malignancy associated with increased levels of angiogenesis. In multiple myeloma, thalidomide has been investigated as a single agent, in combination with dexamethasone, and combined with cytotoxic chemotherapy. It has also shown activity in renal cell carcinoma. Side effects of thalidomide include sedation, dizziness, peripheral neuropathy, rash, orthostatic hypotension, neutropenia, bradycardia, and constipation. An increased risk of deep vein thrombosis has been seen in clinical trials using thalidomide for MM. Since thalidomide can cause severe birth defects or fetal death if taken by pregnant women, it is absolutely contraindicated in pregnancy, and detailed instructions for use in men and women of child-bearing potential are outlined in the drug's prescribing information.[180,183,184]

Structural analogues to thalidomide have been developed in an effort to find agents that have good activity in MM but fewer side effects than thalidomide. These agents are known as immunomodulatory drugs (IMiDs). IMiDs have multiple biological immunomodulatory effects, including stimulation of T-cell proliferation and production of IL-2 and IFN-γ and expansion of NK cells. CC-5013 (Revimid), an oral agent, is the IMiD farthest along in clinical development. CC-5013 is 50 to 20,000 times more potent than thalidomide in stimulating T-cell production. It triggers decreased secretion of TNF-α, IL-1β, and IL-6 and increases secretion of IL-10. CC-5013 specifically targets the bone marrow microenvironment by inhibiting the production of cytokines (IL-6, VEGF, TNF-α) in the bone marrow milieu that mediate the growth and survival of MM cells. It also decreases the binding of MM cells to bone marrow stromal cells, subsequently decreasing MM cell proliferation. CC-5013 also has antiangiogenic effects. Clinical trials have shown promising clinical activity with the use of CC-5013 in patients with relapsed refractory MM and an acceptable toxicity profile. CC-5013 has not been associated with somnolence, constipation, and neuropathy, but has been associated with myelosuppression.[183,185–187]

Cancer Vaccines

An improved understanding of immune recognition and antigen presentation has led to continued advancements of the science of cancer vaccines. Although no therapeutic cancer vaccines are approved for use in the United States, several phase III clinical trials of cancer vaccines are ongoing.

Cancer vaccine therapy is classified as a type of active specific immunotherapy. The term *vaccine* is commonly associated with the practice of administering microbes or derivatives of microbes to prevent infectious diseases.[188] A therapeutic cancer vaccine refers to the use of any antigen or antigen fragment or a collection of antigens used alone or together with an adjuvant to stimulate or modulate an immune response to destroy established cancer cells. For a cancer vaccine to be effective, the immune system must recognize that antigen as foreign, circulate, find the tumor expressing the same antigen, and "mediate" its destruction. The cellular arm of the immune response, in particular the CD8-positive cytotoxic T-cell (CTL) arm, has been identified as being best able to recognize tumor cells as foreign and lead to their destruction. Recent evidence indicates that CD4-positive T cells may be an equally important part of the antitumor immune response.[189,190]

Antigen presentation is required for the development of an effective antitumor CTL response. In the process of antigen presentation, the antigen is taken up by antigen-presenting cells (APCs), and then it is chopped into smaller fragments called peptides. These peptides combine with major histocompatibility complex (MHC) molecules and move to the cell surface for presentation to T cells and subsequent immune recognition. Antigens in combination with MHC class I molecules (antigen/peptide complex) are recognized by CD8-positive cytotoxic T cells, and antigens in combination with MHC class II molecules are recognized by CD4-positive helper T cells. Costimulatory molecules (such as molecules of the B7 family) are also required for complete T-cell activation to occur. Tumor vaccines may work to increase antigen presentation to immune cells or increase costimulatory signals to induce an immune response or a combination of both.[191,192]

Several features are necessary to generate an immune response with cancer vaccines. A target antigen must be present on the tumor cells to direct the immune response. A platform is required to present the vaccine-derived antigen to the immune system. Adjuvants are necessary to enhance the immune response and attract or activate various immune cells.[192]

Tumor Antigens

A prerequisite for the construction of tumor vaccines is the identification of tumor antigens recognized by T cells. In the past two decades, there has been a successful, focused effort in the field of tumor immunology to identify and characterize new tumor antigens. Several categories of antigens have been identified. *Unique tumor-* or *patient-specific antigens* are expressed only in the tumor from which they were identified and are unique to a certain patient. Unique tumor antigens represent the consequences of genetic alterations in tumors as they grow and progress. *Shared tumor-specific antigens* are expressed in many tumor types with a common histology but are not expressed in normal tissue or are expressed to a lesser extent or in a different form on normal tissues. *Tissue-specific differentiation antigens* are expressed by the normal tissue from which the tumor arose. Other antigen sources include mutated oncogenes (i.e., K-*ras*, HER2/neu), viral-transforming proteins, embryonic proteins, and mutated tumor suppressor proteins (i.e., p53).[155,163] Antibodies expressed by a patient's own tumor, called idiotype antibodies, can act as antigens and be incorporated into vaccines to trigger an immune response. A critical question in vaccine development is whether effective tumor immunity can be induced by immunization to a single antigen, or whether responses to multiple antigens on cancer cells are needed for cells to be destroyed.[188,189,191,193]

Vaccine Approaches

Intact tumor cells

The easiest way to make a cancer vaccine is to use intact, inactivated whole tumor cells as an antigen source. These vaccines may be either autologous or allogeneic.[194]

Among the earliest vaccines, *autologous vaccines* are derived by isolating proteins or peptides from a patient's tumor cells. These tumor cells are obtained from surgery or biopsy and then irradiated or somehow killed or attenuated before being reinfused to the patient. Autologous vaccines have many limitations, including the cost and time required to generate specific vaccines for each individual patient.[188,192,195] Heat-shock protein (HSP) vaccines are a type of autologous vaccine. Made by cells in response to heating or other stress, HSPs serve as carriers for peptides, some of which may have been derived from tumor proteins. They are autologous because they must be extracted from a given tumor and provide immunologic protection against only that tumor. HSPs play a role in the presentation of antigens to augment immune system recognition, and linking peptide antigens to certain HSPs enhances the immunogenicity of the antigen.[189,192]

Allogeneic tumor vaccines are developed by establishing tissue-culture lines from metastatic tumors of several patients, growing them in large batches, mixing the various cell lines, and inactivating them, usually by radiation. Allogeneic vaccines have more usefulness in a large population because they can be made from cell lines selected to provide multiple tumor-associated antigens and a broad range of human leukocyte antigen (HLA) expression. Allogeneic cells have been found to be more immunogenic than autologous cells. Canvaxin is an example of a whole-cell allogeneic vaccine composed of three melanoma cell lines expressing at least 38 tumor or melanoma-associated antigens. It is being administered after surgery in phase III clinical trials in patients with Stage III and IV melanoma. A related allogeneic strategy involves the preparation of crude extracts of tumor cells prepared from allogeneic cells. An example is the melanoma lysate vaccine, Melacine, which was developed from two melanoma cell lines and is administered to patients with the adjuvant, DETOX. Melacine was compared with a four-drug chemotherapy regimen in patients with advanced Stage III or IV melanoma in a multicenter phase III clinical trial. The response rates with chemotherapy and Melacine were similar, but Melacine was associated with less toxicity and a better quality of life compared with chemotherapy. Melacine is approved for clinical use in Canada.[194,196]

Purified extracts

Investigators have found chemical components on the surface of cancer cells and have been able to prepare vaccines consisting of purified or synthesized preparations of these components called *gangliosides.* Gangliosides are present on the surface of many melanoma cells and are important immunogenic antigens in melanoma patients. The ganglioside GM2 is found in the cell membrane of virtually all melanoma cells and is a normal component of other tissues. For use in a vaccine, GM2 is extracted from animal sources and then extensively purified. A polyvalent ganglioside vaccine that may be able to overcome the problem of antigenic heterogeneity and potentially induce a more potent immune response not possible with single ganglioside vaccines has been in development.[197] Another approach to ganglioside vaccination under investigation is the administration of anti-idiotype antibodies that mimic the ganglioside.[198]

Peptides

Intracellular proteins have been discovered that can be expressed on the cell surface in the form of small peptides. These proteins undergo intracellular processing and are broken down into units that are carried to the cell surface and bound to the MHC. These peptides can be characterized, synthesized, and used as vaccines. An example of peptide vaccines are those derived from a series of melanoma-associated proteins encoded by the melanoma antigen (MAGE) family of proteins. The MAGE proteins were first found in melanoma cells but have also been identified in some lung, gastrointestinal, and breast cancers. Another set of peptides found on the surface of most melanoma cells is made from proteins involved in the synthesis of melanin. These tissue-specific differentiation protein antigens are found on normal melanocytes in the skin and the choroid of the eye and include tyrosinase, gp100, and MART-1.[189,194]

Recombinant viral vaccines

Another immunization strategy involves the infection of allogeneic tumor cells with viruses such as the vaccinia virus to create oncolysates that are made of both viral and tumor antigens. The viral antigens act as an immunologic adjuvant that enhances immune responses to the tumor antigens. Two examples of this type of vaccine are the vaccinia melanoma oncolysate (VMO) vaccine and a vaccinia melanoma cell lysate (VMCL) vaccine.[188,199]

Gene-Modified Tumor Vaccines

The application of gene-transfer technologies has led to the development of cytokine gene-transduced tumor vaccines that have been shown to have enhanced immunologic activity. The use of GM-CSF-activated tumor peptide-pulsed dendritic cells (DCs) is supported by basic research on cytokine gene therapy applied to cancer immunotherapy.[200] Most current studies use retroviral vectors to add the desired cytokine gene to the tumor cell DNA. Innovations in gene therapy have also led to the development of recombinant and synthetic antigens. Scientists now have the ability to clone the genes encoding the tumor antigens recognized by tumor cells. Tumor-associated antigens can be made synthetically or by recombinant DNA technology.[188] Antigens made by synthetic or recombinant DNA technology can be altered to facilitate immune recognition. The inclusion of the costimulatory molecules, the B7 genes, into recombinant nucleic acid and viral vaccine vectors for antigen-specific vaccination is being evaluated.[201]

Viral and bacterial vaccine vectors have been identified as ways to deliver antigens. *Listeria monocytogenes* is a vaccine carrier that naturally infects APCs and may deliver immunogens to the antigen-processing and presentation pathways. Also, the bacterium itself acts as a danger signal for the immune system because it stimulates the innate immune response, producing cytokines and mediators that enhance antigen presentation.[202]

Dendritic cell vaccines

Many of the new cancer vaccine approaches are based on the understanding that the nature of the APC is a critical factor in the outcome of immune responsiveness. DCs are the most effective APCs. Approaches to effectively introduce antigen into activated DCs are an active area of clinical investigation. Dendritic cell-based vaccine therapy involves generating DCs from cancer patients, loading the DCs with antigen, and reinfusing them into the patient.[203] Vaccine development has also focused on the identification of molecules that induce DC proliferation and maturation and incorporating them into vaccines. Although the frequency of clinical responses with DC vaccines to date has not been superior to that using other vaccine approaches, the frequency of T-cell responses is increased when DCs are used. The approach of isolating DCs from individual patients is difficult and expensive, so alternative approaches are being investigated.[156,168,190,192,201]

Blockade of immunosuppression

A novel approach to vaccine therapy involves the combination of a vaccine together with a blockade of immunologic checkpoints. Normally, an immune response to an antigen is balanced by negative and positive signaling pathways. The negative signaling pathways "check" the immune response by dampening T-cell responses or costimulatory signaling pathways. Cytotoxic T-lymphocyte antigen 4 (CTLA 4) acts to down-regulate or turn off T-cell activity. Trials are investigating a blockade of CTLA 4 with a monoclonal antibody (anti-CTLA 4) administered at the time of vaccination in an effort to enhance vaccine potency.[192,201,204]

Tumor Vaccine Adjuvants

The development of adjuvants to boost the immune response to an antigen is critical to the development of effective vaccines. A vaccine adjuvant can be defined as an agent mixed with an antigen that enhances the immune response to that antigen. Adjuvants can activate APCs to more efficiently stimulate T cells and to activate natural killer cells or other immune system cells to produce cytokines or promote the survival of antigen-specific T cells.[193]

Multiple approaches to augment vaccine immunogenicity have been used, and several are under investigation. Bacterial products have been identified as being good stimulators of cytotoxic T lymphocytes. A bacterial preparation such as BCG is frequently used as a nonspecific immunostimulant. DETOX is an adjuvant composed of portions of *Salmonella minnesota* and *Mycobacterium phlei* combined with the tumor vaccine. In other studies, viral proteins, called *viral oncolysates,* are added to tumor cell preparations to stimulate the immune system. Other adjuvants include alum, or QS21, or slow-release vehicles such as liposomes. Other approaches include adding the antigen to strongly immunogenic molecules such as keyhole limpet hemocyanin (KLH).[188]

Several cytokines have been shown to augment antigen presentation during vaccine therapy and have been investigated as vaccine adjuvants. Cytokine gene-transduced cellular vaccines can avoid systemic toxicity associated with cytokines and have been shown to have enhanced immunologic activity. GM-CSF is the most potent cytokine gene used to modify tumor immunogenicity. Immunization has been enhanced by the incorporation of GM-CSF or its encoding gene into recombinant protein, DNA, or viral vaccines. Interferon-γ, IL-7, IL-2, IL-4, IL-12, and TNF-α gene-transduced tumor vaccines have also been evaluated and have been generally well tolerated. Administra-

Table 21-9 Selected Phase III Cancer Vaccine Trials

Trial Description	Population	Type of Vaccine
Polyvalent melanoma vaccine (Canvaxin) + BCG versus BCG + placebo after surgery	Stage IV melanoma	Allogeneic whole cell
BCG + polyvalent melanoma vaccine (Canvaxin) versus BCG + placebo	Surgically resected Stage III melanoma	Allogeneic whole cell
Keyhole limpet hemocyanin (KLH) + GM-CSF, with or without autologous lymphoma-derived idiotype-specific vaccination after standard CHOP	Stage III–IV follicular non-Hodgkin's lymphoma	Autologous idiotype
Cyclophosphamide, prednisone, and vincristine followed by KLH, with or without recombinant autologous tumor-derived immunoglobulin idiotype and adjuvant GM-CSF	Stage III–IV follicular non-Hodgkin's lymphoma	Autologous idiotype
Surgery + adjuvant autologous gp96 HSP-peptide complex after surgical resection	Locally advanced renal cell carcinoma at high risk for recurrence	Autologous heat shock protein
High dose IL-2, with or without gp100 antigens	Locally advanced or metastatic melanoma	Peptide
Provenge versus placebo	Metastatic prostate cancer after failure of hormonal therapy (androgen independent)	Dendritic cells + prostate acid phosphatase

Data from *www.cancer.gov/clinical trials*. Accessed May 22, 2004.

tion of liposomal cytokine preparations with vaccine has also improved immune response with less toxicity.[169] As previously noted, the presence of costimulatory molecules is essential to the immune response. Although the number of known costimulatory molecules is increasing, the most well-characterized costimulatory signals are members of the B7 or TNF family or various cytokines. Significant effort has been directed into engineering costimulatory molecules into vaccines to enhance their activity.[189,191,201]

Clinical Use of Cancer Vaccines

Because T-cell activation is critical to the development of an effective antitumor response, cancer vaccine trials usually involve some method of measuring T-cell responses to tumor antigens. Several techniques are available for monitoring immune response. Delayed type hypersensitivity (DTH) can be measured by the intradermal injection of antigenic material and measurement of the inflammatory response. The enzyme-linked immunospot (Elispot) assay is a more sensitive quantitative method and is considered the gold standard for measuring T-cell response. Intracellular cytokine measurement is another quantitative monitoring assay that may be less sensitive than Elispot. Immunologic results of vaccine trials are difficult to interpret and compare between trials due to the wide variety of methods used in evaluating the immunologic effects of vaccines.[191] In some patients, tumor regression has been associated with measurable immune responses; however, strong immune responses are often not associated with an objective measurable clinical benefit.[205] An ongoing challenge in vaccine therapy is to develop an immune monitoring system that has adequate sensitivity but also correlates with relevant clinical endpoints such as tumor shrinkage and improvements in time to progression and survival.[191,205]

Although many clinical trials have been carried out in patients with metastatic disease, cancer vaccine therapy may be most useful in the management of cancer patients after surgery, in patients with minimal residual disease, and in patients expected to have tumor recurrence. The amount of immune response needed to prevent tumor implantation is less than that required to slow the growth of an established tumor.[191,196] In contrast to chemotherapy, which exerts direct cytotoxic effects on tumor cells and causes prompt cell kill, vaccines act more indirectly, and immune response frequently takes 4–8 weeks to develop following initial immunization.[195] Studies of cancer vaccines are usually long-term and require years to demonstrate survival difference.[206]

Because they possess a degree of inherent immunogenicity, the most common targets for tumor vaccine strategies have been melanoma and, to a lesser degree, RCC. Melanomas are good candidates for vaccine therapy because they express well-characterized antigens, and since they often metastasize to superficial sites, tumors can be removed easily for cells to be extracted for vaccine preparation.[206] Other less immunogenic tumors have also been identified as targets for vaccine therapy.[189,193] With certain chemical manipulations and strategies to enhance immunogenicity, they also can be recognized by the immune system. In colorectal cancer, vaccines are being studied that immunize against carcinoembryonic antigen (CEA).[207] Several prostate cancer vaccines are also in development.[167] Breast cancer vaccine development has focused on induction of T-cell responses to HER2/neu. Several new breast cancer antigens, such as cyclin B1 or one of many cancer-germ-cell antigens unique to breast tumors, have recently been identified. Therapeutic vaccines against hematologic malignancies are in active clinical development. Two phase III trials of an idiotype vaccine are ongoing for patients with low-grade follicular non-Hodgkin's lymphoma. Some of the tumor vaccines that are in phase III clinical trials are shown in Table 21-9.

Vaccines have been administered by various routes, including intradermal (ID) subcutaneous, intravenous, intranodal, and intratumoral. Nursing management may vary depending on the route of administration. The ID route is more painful, and sometimes vaccines must be administered in several injections. Patients can develop fever and chills when some vaccines are given intravenously and may require pretreatment with antipyretics.[189,208]

Nursing assessment after vaccine administration involves measuring induration, erythema, or edema at vaccine sites and identifying systemic symptoms. Most vaccines studied in clinical trials thus far have been associated with little toxicity. Side effects with some vaccines have been related to the diluent. Local injection site reactions are the most common side effect. Local response to vaccines can include swelling, erythema and tenderness, or pruritus that can last from one to seven days. An acute reaction in the first 15 minutes suggests an antibody-mediated hypersensitivity allergic reaction that is different from the expected cellular immune response. Patients can become sensitized to proteins in the vaccine preparation and can develop a local hypersensitivity reaction. Part of the nursing role with vaccine therapy may include measuring and photographing vaccine sites and assisting with punch biopsies of vaccine sites as well as applying and interpreting of DTH skin tests.[108,208]

Targeted Therapy

Targeted therapy involves the administration of biotherapeutic agents with a specific molecular target in cancer cells. Targeted therapy has evolved as a result of translating basic principles of cancer biology into new clinical therapeutic strategies. It involves understanding, at a basic molecular level, differences between cancer cells and normal cells, such as how cells grow and divide. Tumor growth and progression depend on the activity of cell membrane receptors that control signaling pathways in the cell, which regulate proliferation, apoptosis, angiogenesis, adhesion, and motility. Targeted therapy involves blocking or interrupting the proteins associated with specific pathways involved in cancer transformation and progression. Traditional chemotherapy agents target all rapidly dividing cells and subsequently affect both healthy cells and cancer cells. Targeted therapies are based on tumor biology and selectively inhibit cancer cells with minimal harmful systemic effects on healthy cells. The best targets for therapy vary among cancers, since different genes and proteins are involved in the growth of different tumor types. Our improved understanding of the intracellular signaling process responsible for transformation and tumor progression has led to advances in the field of targeted therapy, including the approval of agents for clinical use as well as several agents undergoing clinical development.[209–211] Table 21-10 lists some of the terms commonly used in targeted therapy.

Table 21-10 Terms Used with Targeted Therapy

Ligand	A molecule that interacts with a protein by binding to the protein; binding occurs at a specific site in the protein molecule
Dimerization	The chemical union of two molecules
Dimer	A molecule made of 2 subunits linked together (in a homodimer, the two subunits are identical; in a heterodimer the two subunits are different)
Signal transduction	The movement of signals from outside the cell to the inside
Apoptosis	Programmed cell death
Tyrosine kinase	A class of enzymes that play an important role in regulating cell growth and division; enzymes that phosphorylate
Phosphorylate	Add a phosphate group
Downstream signaling	Growth-promoting events that occur after a ligand is bound to its receptor

Signal Transduction

Cell signaling, also known as *signal transduction*, is the communication/movement of growth signals from the outside of the cell to the nucleus inside the cell. Signal transduction is an extremely complex, intricate system of multiple cascades and chemical signals arranged in intersecting and overlapping networks. Signal transduction involves the binding of cell surface growth factor receptors with growth factors (often referred to as ligands) released from other cells. The binding of growth factor to receptor activates the receptor, triggering multiple events eventually resulting in cell growth and division. A subclass of growth factor receptors, known as tyrosine kinases (TKs), are enzymes, which are key regulators of the signal transduction process. TK growth factor receptors contain an extracellular ligand-binding domain, a transmembrane region, and a cytoplasmic TK region.[212–214]

Signal transduction is initiated when a ligand binds to receptor tyrosine kinases and promotes dimerization (pairing of receptor molecules). Receptors can dimerize with molecules identical to themselves (homodimerization) or with a different receptor (heterodimerization). Dimerization activates the TK enzyme on the intracellular portion of the receptor, which results in autophosphorylation of tyrosine residues in the cytoplasmic domain. Phosphorylation occurs when an adenine triphosphate (ATP) molecule binds to a pocket on the TK and a phosphate group is transferred from that ATP molecule to tyrosine residues on the intracellular domain of the receptor. Phosphorylated tyrosines serve as binding sites for a number of signal-transducing molecules. Phosphorylation essentially triggers the signaling cascade in most tyrosine receptors because once these transducing molecules have a binding site, two essential downstream signaling events can occur: (1) transcription factors near the cell's surface send a message via transduction proteins to the cell nucleus, and (2) the nucleus then produces transcription factors that induce the cell to enter the cell cycle, eventually resulting in mitosis and the production of two daughter cells. Critical downstream signaling events involve many additional complex intracellular processes and pathways. [212–215]

Because of their role in initiating the signal transduction process, the receptor TKs have a key role in cellular processes such as proliferation, migration, metabolism, differentiation, and survival. In normal resting cells, TK activity is tightly controlled, but when TKs become mutated or somehow altered, they become potent oncoproteins. The abnormal activation of receptor TKs is involved in the development and progression of many cancers. TK activity has been shown to promote invasion and metastasis and to be an important inducer of angiogenesis. TKs can facilitate the development of malignancy by inhibiting apoptosis.[212]

The characterization of the structure and function of receptor TK proteins and their ligands has substantially increased our understanding of the cell signaling process and paved the way for the development of targeted therapies for cancer. One of the first receptor TKs to be characterized was the epidermal growth factor receptor (EGFR). Preceding the discovery of EGFR was the discovery of one of its ligands, epidermal growth factor (EGF), which was identified in 1962. It wasn't until 1984 that advances in DNA cloning technologies allowed the characterization of the DNA sequence of human EGFR. This characterization was a milestone, as it provided the first complete amino acid sequence of a cell surface receptor that had the ability to generate signals essential for cell growth and division.[212]

EGFR was subsequently found to be part of a family of growth factor receptors known as the HER family. The HER family is made up of four closely related but distinct receptors: HER1/EGFR/ErbB-1, HER2/ErbB-2, HER3/ErbB-3, and HER4/ErbB-4. A great deal of overlap exists in the signaling pathways activated by all of the HER receptors. Ligands for HER1, HER3, and HER 4 have been identified, but the ligand of HER2 is not known. HER receptors are overexpressed and/or dysregulated in several solid tumor types. Members of the HER family are established therapeutic targets for the development of novel anticancer agents. The monoclonal antibody trastuzumab is the first example of a successful HER2 targeted therapy.[212,216,217]

Following the discovery of the EGFR, the sequences of several other TKs were discovered, including BCR-ABL, platelet-derived growth factor receptor (PDGFR), and KIT.[212] The presence or overexpression of HER2, BCR-ABL, C-KIT, and PDGFR is limited to specific cancer types. Other molecules pivotal to the progression of many tumor types have been identified that could be potentially more useful against a broader range of malignancies.[210] The names of receptor tyrosine kinases are usually derived from the tissue where they were first isolated, but the name does not imply that those tissues are the only ones that express that receptor.[218] Even though they have unique biological roles, TKs are highly related in structure and share many similarities to EGFR. The receptor TK class of cell surface receptors contains 58 known members and 20 subfamilies. More than half of these are overexpressed or mutated in hyperproliferative or hypoproliferative diseases and are considered to be targets for cancer therapy.[212]

TK inhibitors or antibodies to their receptors have been developed that inhibit activation of the intracellular pathways by growth factor receptors. Small-molecule TK inhibitors (TKIs) are orally available molecules that act intracellularly by blocking the ATP binding site of the TK enzyme. Oral TKIs have a relatively short half-life; thus daily oral dosing is common. Monoclonal antibodies are relatively large molecules that block the extracellular ligand-binding domain of the receptor. Monoclonal antibodies have a long half-life; thus weekly IV dosing is common. Imatinib was the first TK inhibitor to be approved for use with cancer.[218–220]

Non-EGFR Tyrosine Kinase Inhibitors

Imatinib mesylate

Imatinib mesylate (Gleevec) is a small-molecule antagonist that inhibits the protein TKs—BCR-ABL, PDGFR, and KIT. Imatinib targets the "molecular drivers" responsible for chronic myelogenous leukemia (CML) and gastrointestinal stromal tumors (GISTs), and it is FDA approved for these malignancies. An understanding of the activity of imatinib in these malignancies requires an understanding of the molecular pathogenesis of both diseases.[221,222]

Imatinib in CML

The hallmark of CML is the Philadelphia chromosome, which is a shortened chromosome 22 resulting from a genetic translocation between the long arms of chromosomes 9 and 22. This translocation creates a *BCR-ABL* gene, which results from the fusion of the *ABL* gene on chromosome 9 and the *BCR* gene on chromosome 22. The BCR-ABL protein is a tyrosine kinase that binds ATP and transfers phosphate from ATP to tyrosine residues on specific proteins. This phosphorylation stimulates other molecules to activate various signal transduction pathways in a nonregulated fashion, resulting in the uncontrolled cell division and overproduction of myeloid cells characteristic of CML. Imatinib acts by blocking the binding site of BCR-ABL for ATP, thus preventing the transmission of signals needed for BCR-ABL-driven cellular proliferation. The BCR-ABL protein has been recognized as an ideal target for imatinib since it is present in almost all patients with CML, it is expressed at high levels, and its tyrosine kinase activity is essential for its ability to induce leukemia.[221–224]

In a phase III multicenter trial that randomized a total of 1106 patients, imatinib was associated with a superior hematologic response, cytogenetic response, and time to progression to accelerated phase or blast crisis compared to IFN-α plus cytarabine in newly diagnosed patients.[225] In this same trial, imatinib also offered quality of life advantages compared to IFN and cytarabine.[226] Responses were rapid, with most patients achieving complete hematologic responses within the first 4–6 weeks of therapy. Imatinib has also shown activity in more advanced disease.

Imatinib in GISTs

Imatinib is not selective for BCR-ABL. It also blocks the kinase activity of KIT and PDGFR. KIT (CD117), a member of the receptor TK family, is the product of the C-KIT proto-oncogene. Binding of KIT to its receptor, stem cell factor (SCF), ultimately leads to activation of the signal transduction pathway and cellular proliferation and differentiation. Mutations of KIT occur in up to 90% of GISTs and result in ligand-independent activation of KIT signaling, uncontrolled cell proliferation, and resistance to apoptosis. In GISTs, imatinib inhibits the activity of the mutated tyrosine kinase, KIT, which plays a major role in the pathogenesis of this malignancy.[227]

An open-label multinational phase II study was conducted in patients with unresectable or metastatic KIT-positive GISTs. In this trial 147 patients were randomized to receive imatinib, 400 mg or 600 mg orally daily for up to 24 months. With a follow-up of more than 9 months, 120 patients remained in the study. Of these patients, 53.7% had a PR, and an additional 27.9% achieved disease stabilization. The clinical effect of imatinib on GISTs is often rapid, with improvements in well-being and cancer-related symptoms noted within a few days of starting therapy. Based on the results of the phase II trial, imatinib received FDA approval for use in GISTs. Phase III trials in the United States and Europe have been completed, and clinical trials of neoadjuvant and adjuvant therapy in GISTs are planned.[228]

Imatinib is indicated for the treatment of newly diagnosed adult patients with Philadelphia chromosome positive CML in chronic phase. It is also approved for the treatment of patients with CML in blast crisis, in accelerated phase, or in chronic phase after failing interferon-α therapy. Imatinib is indicated for the treatment of pediatric patients with Philadelphia chromosome positive chronic phase CML whose disease has recurred after stem cell transplant or who are resistant to interferon-α therapy. It is also indicated for the treatment of patients with KIT (CD117) positive unresectable and/or metastatic malignant GISTs.

Imatinib is administered orally at different doses depending on the indication. Since imatinib is a local irritant, it should be administered with food and a large glass of water. The most common nonhematologic adverse events seen in patients treated with imatinib include superficial edema (periorbital edema is most common), nausea, muscle cramps, musculoskeletal pain, rash, fatigue, diarrhea, headache, joint pain, abdominal pain, and myalgia. Myelosuppression is common with the use of imatinib in patients with CML, especially in patients with advanced disease. Inhibition of normal hematopoiesis with imatinib is minimal, and myelosuppression associated with imatinib is thought to be an expected therapeutic effect on the PH-positive leukemic clone. Imatinib is predominantly metabolized in the liver via the cytochrome p450 system, so patients need to be monitored for potential drug interactions.[229]

EGFR Inhibitors

The epidermal growth factor receptor (EGFR/HER1) TK is a cell membrane glycoprotein expressed in cells of epithelial origin (skin; respiratory, gastrointestinal and urinary tracts; and liver), but not on hematopoietic cells. EGFR function is essential for embryogenesis and organogenesis, and in adults the EGFR has a role in the repair of epithelial tissue.[210] The extracellular binding domain of the EGFR is the ligand-binding site for both the EGF and for transforming growth factor alpha (TGF-α). As described earlier, the binding of EGFR to EGF promotes receptor dimerization, activation of intracellular TK activity, and eventual initiation of signal transduction cascades leading to cell proliferation, differentiation, survival, angiogenesis, metastasis, and inhibition of apoptosis (see Figure 21-8). Normally, ligand binding is required to provide a stimulus for cell division, but mutations in the EGFR may allow cellular division to occur without ligand binding. This ligand-independent enzyme activation is known as constitutive activation.[212,213]

EGFR is overexpressed in a wide variety of tumors of epithelial origin, including non-small cell lung cancer (NSCLC), head and neck, pancreatic, colon, breast, kidney, ovarian, and bladder cancer, as well as gliomas. Of these, NSCLC has a very high level of expression, with 81%–93% EGFR overexpression.[210] Many studies have shown that EGFR overexpression correlates with poor prognosis, high proliferative index, increased recurrence rates, decreased survival, and increased resistance to chemotherapy. Because of its role in the malignant process, EGFR is an appealing target for cancer therapy. Different approaches to inhibiting EGFR have resulted in a number of EGFR-targeted agents in clinical development. The EGFR inhibitors farthest along in development include small-molecule TK inhibitors and monoclonal antibodies. Both approaches have the same objective, which is to stop the signal transduction that is initiated by activating the EGFR receptor.[210–215,230]

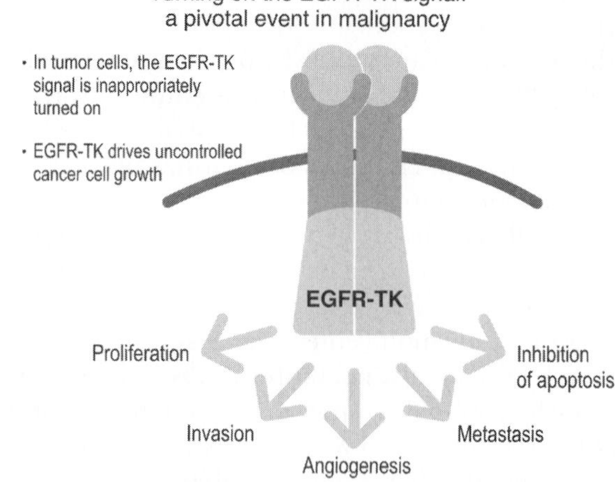

Figure 21-8 Mechanism of disease: Epidermal growth factor receptor is a cell surface receptor that dimerizes on ligand activation of the extracellular binding domain. Dimerization leads to activation of a tyrosine kinase in the receptor's cytoplasmic domain. Subsequent phosphorylation of the receptor's intracellular tyrosine residues initiates signal transduction. Aberrant activation of the EGFR-TK system in tumor cells derives from both extra- and intracellular events. The result is initiation of signal transduction programs associated with malignant progression. EGFR-TK, epidermal growth factor receptor–tyrosine kinase. Reprinted from *Seminars in Oncology*, 30(1):6, Ritter, CA, © 2003 Elsevier, Inc.[210]

Gefitinib

Gefitinib (Iressa), a quinazoline, is a potent and selective inhibitor of EGFR tyrosine kinase activity. Gefitinib inhibits EGF receptor signal transduction by interfering with the binding of ATP to the intracellular TK regions of the receptor.[218,219]

The antitumor activity of gefitinib has been confirmed in two large phase II randomized trials, where gefitinib was given to patients with pretreated NSCLC at doses of 250 or 500 mg/day. IDEAL 1 was a global trial and included patients who had received one or two prior chemotherapy regimens. IDEAL 2 was a U.S. trial that included patients who had been given two or more regimens including platinum and docetaxel. In IDEAL 1 the response rate was 18.4% and 19.0% and the disease control rate was 54.4% and 51.4% for the 250 and 500 mg/day doses, respectively. In IDEAL 2, the response rate was 11.8% and 8.8 % and the disease control rate (responding patients plus stable patients) was 42.2% and 36.0% for the 250 and 500 mg/day doses, respectively. Symptom improvement occurred in both trials at both doses. Quality of life improvement was seen in a significant number of patients and was consistent with disease-related toxicity. Overall, the 250 mg/day dose was determined to be as effective as and better tolerated than the 500 mg/day dose.[231,232] Two large, randomized phase III clinical trials (INTACT 1 and 2) conducted in chemotherapy-naïve patients with NSCLC failed to show any benefit to adding gefitinib to doublet platinum-based chemotherapy.[233,234]

Gefitinib is indicated as monotherapy for the treatment of patients with locally advanced or metastatic NSCLC after failure of both platinum-based and docetaxel chemotherapy. Gefitinib is administered orally. The most common adverse events reported with gefitinib at 250 mg/day were diarrhea, rash, acne, dry skin, nausea, and vomiting, all of which were mostly grade 1 or 2. In most patients, the skin disorders resolved either during treatment or with a temporary therapy interruption or following treatment cessation. In clinical trials, diarrhea was generally well controlled with antidiarrheal agents such as loperimide. Mild ophthalmic adverse events seen with gefitinib include conjunctivitis, blepharitis, keratitis, eye pain, dry eyes, and corneal erosion. Interstitial lung disease, which may be acute in onset, has been observed uncommonly (less than 1% worldwide incidence) in patients treated with gefitinib. These patients usually present with a fairly acute onset of dyspnea sometimes associated with cough or low-grade fever, which may become severe within a short period of time.[216,218,219]

Cetuximab

Cetuximab (Erbitux) is a chimeric monoclonal antibody derived from the murine monoclonal antibody C225. Cetuximab binds with high affinity to the EGFR and blocks the ability of EGF to initiate receptor activation and cell signaling. By interfering with the effects of EGFR activation, this blockade results in an inhibition of tumor growth.[216, 219] The antitumor activity of cetuximab occurs through several mechanisms. Cetuximab inhibits cell cycle progression and induces apoptosis. Cetuximab decreases the production of growth factors, including TGF-α, and angiogenic factors such as vascular endothelial growth factor (VEGF), bFGF, and interleukin-8. It may also inhibit tumor cell invasion and metastasis by inhibiting the expression of molecules that play a role in tumor cell adhesion. Preclinical data has demonstrated that combining cetuximab with marginally effective or ineffective chemotherapy resulted in marked synergy and dramatic improvement in antitumor activity for the combination therapy.[235]

A phase II trial evaluated cetuximab in 120 patients with advanced colon cancer after failure on irinotecan. The patients were treated with cetuximab plus continued irinotecan. Of the 120 patients who progressed on irinotecan, 22.5% achieved a partial response with the addition of cetuximab. These results were used to request FDA approval, but the FDA refused to file the submission due to concerns about the definition of progressive disease on irinotecan and the lack of single-agent data in colorectal cancer.[211] A confirmatory randomized phase II trial by Cunningham et al. evaluated cetuximab in combination with irinotecan or as a single agent in patients with EGFR plus metastatic, irinotecan-refractory colorectal cancer.[236] A total of 329 patients were randomized to receive irinotecan plus cetuximab (218 patients) or cetuximab alone (111 patients). Patients receiving single-agent cetuximab were allowed to switch to combination therapy if they experienced progressive disease. The overall response rate for the combination arm was 22.9% compared to 10.8% for cetuximab alone ($p = 0.0074$). Time to progression was 4.1 months for combination therapy and 1.5 months for cetuximab alone ($p < 0.0001$). The difference in median survival between the treatment groups was not statistically significant, which may have been due to crossover to the combination arm at progression.[236]

Cetuximab is approved for use in combination with irinotecan for the treatment of EGFR-expressing metastatic colorectal cancer in patients who are refractory to irinotecan-based chemotherapy. Cetuximab is also indicated as a single agent for the treatment of EGFR-expressing metastatic colorectal cancer in patients who are intolerant to irinotecan-based chemotherapy.

Cetuximab is associated with an acne-form skin rash and other dermatologic disorders that usually occur in the first three weeks of treatment (see Table 21-11). In the clinical trials, one or more dermatologic events were reported in 88% of patients receiving cetuximab plus irinotecan and in 90% of patients receiving cetuximab monotherapy. Studies have suggested a correlation between the presence and severity of rash and survival. It is hypothesized that rash is a surrogate indicator of an adequate degree of receptor saturation by cetuximab. Additionally, grade 3 or 4 allergic reactions characterized by symptoms of severe hypersensitivity that was rapidly responsive to standard management with epinephrine, antihistamines, and corticosteroids were seen in 3% of patients. This is

Table 21-11 EGFR Inhibitors: Dermatologic Toxicity

Gefitinib	Cetuximab
Rash 44%, acne 25% (at 250 mg/day dose), Grade 3–4 rash/acne 0% • Occurs between days 5 and 12 • Follicular pustules/papules, dry skin, pruritus • Some rashes spontaneously decrease even without therapy interruptions Management • No established effective treatment • A variety of topical agents have been used with varying success • Oral or topical antibiotics may be needed • For severe rash, therapy is usually interrupted until resolution or improvement and resumed at same dose • Obtain dermatologic consult if appropriate	Dermatologic toxicity overall 88% (n = 633), 12% grade 3–4 • Acne-form rash — described as acne, rash, maculopapular rash, pustular rash, dry skin, exfoliative dermatitis • Follicular/pustular rash, dryness, fissuring, inflammation, infection • Most common on face, upper chest, and back, can extend to extremities • Related nail disorder — paronychial inflammation with swelling of lateral nail folds of toes and fingers • Increased severity when combined with radiation therapy • Onset in first two weeks of therapy Management • Assess patients for infectious complications • Oral or topical antibiotics may be needed • Topical steroids not recommended • Instruct patients to wear sunscreen and hats and limit sun exposure — sunlight can exacerbate skin rash • Dose delays and modifications recommended for severe rash

Data from product prescribing information and Krozely[215]; Monti et al[237]; Doorn et al.[240]

likely due to an allergy to the mouse component of the protein in the antibody. Additional adverse reactions included diarrhea, nausea, asthenia, and malaise.[216,219,235,237]

Predicting response to EGFR inhibitors

Unlike trastuzumab and HER2 status, no predictive markers of sensitivity to EGFR inhibitors to select patients who might respond to therapy have been available during the initial clinical development of EGFR inhibitors. A retrospective analysis of tumor samples from the single-agent phase II trials of gefitinib in NSCLC confirmed a lack of correlation between EGFR expression levels in tumors and response. Likewise, analysis of the cetuximab trials did not demonstrate that the level of EGFR expression had any impact on response rates. In fact, a significant number of EGRF-positive colorectal tumors are resistant to cetuximab. A broad series of clinical as well as preclinical data confirm that there is no clear relationship between EGFR expression (as measured by currently available methods) and response to EGFR inhibition.[230,238]

Genomics and proteomics are being used to characterize response profiles at the cellular level to try to identify unique "molecular fingerprints" for responders versus nonresponders to EGFR inhibitors. The fact that most patients do not respond to gefitinib, while 10% of patients have a rapid and sometimes dramatic response, led to a search for the mechanisms underlying sensitivity to gefitinib, and a crucial first step has been made. Lynch et al. sequenced the entire coding region of EGFR in tumors from patients who responded to gefitinib and in tumors from those who did not respond to gefitinib. They determined that a subgroup of patients with NSCLC have mutations in the TK domain of the EGFR gene that correlate with clinical response to gefitinib. This finding could have immediate clinical implications with respect to the care of patients with NSCLC. If additional studies validate EGFR tyrosine kinase mutations as predictors of therapy, screening for such mutations may be done to identify patients who are likely to respond to gefitinib.[239]

Toxicity of EGFR inhibitors

Overall, the EGFR inhibitors have been well tolerated. Characteristics of the two major classes of EGFR inhibitors may be useful in predicting toxicity. The large size of MAbs may prevent penetration across the basement membrane of the alimentary tract, and thus minimal gastrointestinal toxicity is observed. The small size of TK inhibitors allows them to readily traverse basement membranes, thereby facilitating diarrhea, one of the primary dose-limiting toxicities of this class.[230] Diarrhea is usually well controlled with loperimide, although in rare cases IV hydration may be necessary.

Dermatologic toxicity is a unique and frequently reported adverse event with the use of EGFR inhibitors and is reported with gefitinib and cetuximab as well as with the investigational agent erlotinib. While the exact mechanism of the dermatologic toxicity is not fully understood, it is thought that they result from direct interference with the function of EGFR signaling in the skin. The EGFR is expressed in human skin by basal epidermal keratinocytes, outer root sheath cells, and sebocytes. In the skin the EGFR is activated by several karatinocyte-derived ligands, which stimulate proliferation and decrease the susceptibility to apoptosis. In the hair follicle, the EGFR-ligand system has an essential role in the regulation of the hair cycle. The cutaneous effects seen with these agents are thought to reflect the significance of the EGF signaling pathway in the skin and represent the results of inhibition of EGF receptor signal transduction in the epidermal and follicular epithelium.[240] Mild dermatologic effects can be treated with over-the-counter agents, but a dose

Table 21-12 Select Endogenous Angiogenesis Inducers and Inhibitors

Angiogenesis Inducers	Angiogenesis Inhibitors
Basic fibroblast growth factor (bFGF)	Angiostatin
TGF-α and β	Endostatin
Epidermal growth factor	Interferon-α, β, and γ
Hepatocyte growth factor	Interleukin 12 and 18
Insulin-like growth factor	Platelet factor 4
Platelet activating factor	Thrombospondin-1 (TSP-1)
Vascular endothelial growth factor (VEGF)	Tissue inhibitors of metalloproteinases (TIMPs)
Interleukin-8	

Data from Kerbel, Folkman[243]; Muehlbauer[244]; Hanahan, Folkman[246]; Bergers, Benjamin.[247]

interruption or dose reduction may be necessary for a severe rash.[215] See Table 21-11 for features of dermatologic toxicity associated with EGFR inhibitors and management guidelines.

Angiogenesis

Angiogenesis is the process of blood vessel formation. Physiologic angiogenesis is important for the formation of new blood vessels in the placenta, embryonic development, the menstrual cycle, and wound healing. In these normal processes, angiogenesis is brief and tightly controlled. Uncontrolled angiogenesis can lead to a variety of diseases, including psoriasis, arthritis, diabetic retinopathy, macular degeneration, gingivitis, hemangiomas, and malignant tumors. Tumor angiogenesis is the ability of a tumor to elicit growth of new capillaries from sprouts of preexisting vessels from the host tissue. Angiogenesis is dependent on endothelial cells, which line the lumen of all blood vessels. Tumor angiogenesis begins when the endothelial cells in a blood vessel adjacent to a tumor are stimulated and, through a series of complex steps, are formed into new blood vessels, which supply the tumor.[241–244]

In 1971, Dr. Judah Folkman was the first to propose that tumor growth depends on angiogenesis. Several in vitro and in vivo studies have demonstrated that tumors are angiogenesis-dependent for growth, progression, and metastasis. Tumors that are unable to elicit angiogenesis exist in a dormant state and are unable to grow beyond a few millimeters in size. Besides helping tumors grow in size, this blood vessel network provides an entry site into circulation for tumor cells to metastasize.[245]

Endogenous factors that both induce and inhibit angiogenesis have been identified (see Table 21-12). In normal tissues, inhibitors of angiogenesis are predominant, and the vessels are inactive. During tumor development an "angiogenic switch" occurs, resulting in an increase in the inducers or a decrease in the inhibitors of angiogenesis and allowing blood vessel growth to occur with resultant tumor growth and metastasis. Angiogenic factors are released in response to many different stimuli, including hypoxia, COX-2, and nitric oxide as well as multiple growth factors such as EGF, bFGF, IL-1, IL-6, transforming growth factor, and hepatocyte growth factor.[246,247] Many oncogenes can stimulate the production of molecules that are angiogenic factors.

Of the identified angiogenic factors, *vascular endothelial growth factor* (VEGF), also known as VEGF-A or vascular permeability factor, is the most potent and specific and has been identified as a crucial regulator of both normal and pathologic angiogenesis. VEGF is a cytokine that exerts a variety of effects on vascular endothelial cells that together promote the formation of new blood vessels. Increased expression of VEGF is identified in a majority of solid tumors as well as certain hematologic malignancies. VEGF is overexpressed by invasive cancer cells as well as by some premalignant lesions. The amount of VEGF expressed by cancer cells has been found to correlate with poor prognosis in several tumor types.[241,242,248]

VEGF acts by binding to and activating two structurally related membrane receptor TKs, VEGF receptor-1 (Flt-1) and VEGF receptor-2 (Flk-1 or KDR), that are selectively but not exclusively expressed by the vascular endothelium. As in the HER family of receptors, binding of VEGF to its receptors causes receptor dimerization to initiate multiple signaling pathways within endothelial cells to stimulate angiogenesis. VEGF stimulates the growth, survival, and proliferation of vascular endothelial cells and promotes the growth of tumors beyond the volume that can be supported by the existing vasculature. See Figure 21-9. One of the most important properties of VEGF is its ability to enhance microvascular permeability. Induction of vascular permeability is likely an essential first step in angiogenesis. VEGF acts as a vascular permeability factor and contributes to endothelial proliferation by promoting the extrasvascular leakage of plasma protein and the formation of a fibrin gel that functions as a substrate for endothelial and tumor cell growth.[248]

Angiogenesis Inhibitors

The discovery of tumor angiogenesis and an abundance of preclinical data supporting antiangiogenesis agents as a treatment for malignancy have led to the development of numerous agents in clinical trials. The angiogenesis inhibitors in clinical development target various steps in the angiogenic process, with the goal

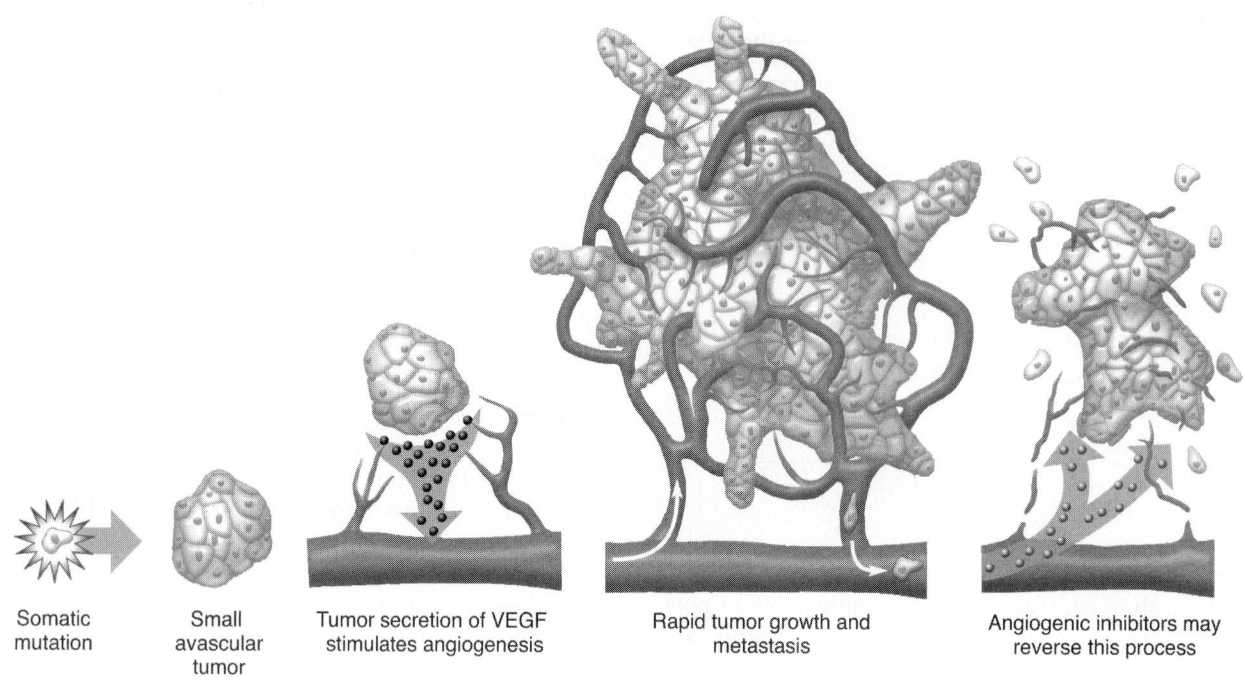

Figure 21-9 The effect of VEGF on tumor growth. Adapted with permission from Genetech, Inc. San Francisco, CA, and IDEC.

of halting the growth of malignant tumors and preventing tumor invasion and metastasis. Most antiangiogenic agents inhibit the growth of new microvessels in tumors, but they can also induce regression of newly developed microvessels.[243] Angiogenesis inhibitors can be classified as direct or indirect. Direct angiogenesis inhibitors prevent vascular endothelial cells from proliferating, migrating, or avoiding cell death in response to proangiogenic proteins. Direct angiogenesis inhibitors are not as likely to induce drug resistance, since they target endothelial cells, which are genetically stable. Indirect angiogenesis inhibitors prevent the expression of a tumor protein that activates angiogenesis or blocks the expression of its endothelial cell receptor. Endostatin and bevacizumab are examples of direct angiogenesis inhibitors, while the EGFR inhibitors cetuximab and gefitinib are considered indirect angiogenesis inhibitors.[243]

Certain chemotherapy agents and cytokines already in use for cancer therapy have been shown to be associated with antiangiogenic effects that are distinct from their cytotoxic or immunomodulatory effects. IFN-α for example, a cytokine with antiangiogenic properties, is know to have activity in diseases for which angiogenesis plays a critical pathophysiological role, such as hemangiomas, melanoma, renal cell carcinoma, and Kaposi's sarcoma. The taxanes have antiangiogenic activity when administered at lower doses and frequent intervals. Thalidomide, the COX-2 inhibitors, and IL-12 all have antiangiogenic activity.[249]

While the results of many clinical trials with antiangiogenesis agents have been disappointing, other results provide optimism regarding this therapeutic modality. Bevacizumab, the first FDA-approved angiogenesis inhibitor, was approved in February 2004. The encouraging results with bevacizumab have validated angiogenesis as a therapeutic target.

Bevacizumab

Bevacizumab (Avastin) is a recombinant humanized antibody against the VEGF molecule. It contains a human immunoglobulin G1 framework (93%) and murine binding sites (7%). Bevacizumab blocks the binding of VEGF to its receptors (Flt-1 and KDR) and inhibits VEGF-induced angiogenesis.

Bevacizumab was evaluated in a randomized double-blind phase III trial with irinotecan, 5-FU, and leucovorin (IFL) in patients with previously untreated metastatic colorectal cancer. Patients were initially randomized to receive bolus IFL plus placebo (arm 1), IFL plus bevacizumab (arm 2), or 5-FU/leucovorin plus bevacizumab (arm 3). Arm 3 was discontinued after therapy with IFL plus bevacizumab was determined to be safe. Overall survival was the primary end-

Table 21-13 Selected Angiogenesis Inhibitors and Agents with Antiangiogenic Activity in Clinical Trials

Cox-2 inhibitors	BMS-275291
Thalidomide	CC-4047
CC 5013 (Revimid)	TAC 101
PTK 787/2K222584	PI-88
Combretastatin A4 phosphate	MoAb Anti-alpha V beta 3 integrin (MEDI-552)
LY 317615	EMD 121974 (Cilengitide)
ZD 6474	SU-011,248
AE-941 (Neovastat)	S-3304
SU 6688	Interferon-α
VEG-F trap	2-methoxyestradiol
Angiostatin	AG-013736

point of this trial. Median survival with bevacizumab and IFL was 20.3 months, and 15.6 months with IFL alone. In addition to improving overall survival, the addition of bevacizumab to chemotherapy resulted in improvements in progression-free survival, duration of survival, and overall response rate.[250]

Bevacizumab is FDA approved for use in combination with intravenous 5-fluorouracil-based chemotherapy for first-line treatment of patients with metastatic colorectal cancer. It is administered as an IV infusion once every 14 days until disease progression. The most common adverse events of any severity in patients receiving bevacizumab were asthenia, pain, abdominal pain, headache, hypertension, diarrhea, nausea, vomiting, anorexia, stomatitis, constipation, upper respiratory infection, epistaxis, dyspnea, exfoliative dermatitis, and proteinuria. Other adverse events included gastrointestinal perforations/wound-healing complications, hemorrhage, thromboembolism, and congestive heart failure. Infusion reactions after the first dose of bevacizumab were uncommon (fewer than 3%).[251]

Bevacizumab is being evaluated in multiple ongoing trials in combination with various agents in multiple tumor types. It has shown activity in renal cell cancer. Inhibition of tumor angiogenesis is a rational approach for the treatment of renal cell cancer. Mutations in the von Hippel-Lindau tumor suppressor gene have been identified as the cause of most sporadic clear-cell kidney cancers. One consequence of mutation of the VHL gene is overproduction of VEGF by renal cell tumors. A randomized double-blind phase 2 trial was conducted that compared a placebo with bevacizumab in metastatic renal cell cancer and showed prolonged time to tumor progression in patients given bevacizumab 10 mg/kg every two weeks compared to placebo. Although survival was not a primary endpoint, there was no significant difference in survival of the bevacizumab-treated patients compared to those receiving the placebo.[252]

Numerous antiangiogenesis agents are in all phases of clinical trials. Table 21-13 is a partial listing of the agents currently being evaluated. Since the growth and regression of blood vessels is controlled by several pathways, a combination of antiangiogenic approaches that target more than one pathway may be most effective.[245] Antiangiogenic agents may find their place as a maintenance therapy to help prolong the dormancy of residual disease following chemotherapy or in the adjuvant setting. Ongoing trials are attempting to identify surrogate markers of the efficacy of angiogenesis inhibitors.

Targeted Therapy: Nursing Considerations

Oncology nurses play a key role in assessing and monitoring patients receiving targeted therapies and properly educating both patients and families. It is essential that patients understand how these agents work, what toxicities to expect, when and how to self-manage toxicities, and when to call a health professional. Understanding the complex, diverse, and unique mechanism of actions of these agents and then communicating this information effectively to patients and families provides an ongoing nursing challenge when patients are receiving targeted therapies. Some of the targeted agents are administered orally in the home setting, making them convenient and suitable for long-term chronic therapy. Orally administered agents present new challenges related to patient compliance and an increased need for patient self-assessment and management of side effects. The potential for dosing errors, missed doses, and self-initiated dose modifications are just of a few of the potential outcomes that may be avoided with effective education and communication. Although targeted therapies are generally well tolerated, serious and life-threatening events can occur with these agents. Knowledge of potential side effects and ongoing assessment are essential for managing patients on targeted therapies.[213,253]

Preparation, Administration, and Safe Handling of Biologic and Targeted Agents

Biologic agents such as recombinant growth factors are reconstituted predominantly by nurses and patients. Patients commonly self-inject these agents. Biopharmaceuticals must be handled differently than drugs. *Biopharmaceuticals* are protein-based agents that often require refrigerated storage. Patients who travel should be cautioned that these products cannot tolerate the extremes in temperature commonly found in car trunks and airplane baggage holds. When the lyophilized product is reconstituted, the vial should not be shaken or the diluent directed into the dried powder. Excessive foaming that can denature the protein may occur. Finally, some biopharmaceuticals are not compatible with all plastic syringes and intravenous tubing. The package insert can provide valuable information on storage and compatibility of a particular product. Many pharmaceutical companies offer toll-free numbers to answer questions and supply additional information regarding their products.

At present, there are no known safety hazards associated with exposure to cytokines, MAbs, or cell therapies. However, the use of simple barriers is recommended to prevent inadvertent exposure to immunogenic substances. The Oncology Nursing Society has published guidelines which provide specific instructions on preparation and handling of biotherapy.[254]

Guidelines have not yet been developed for handling oral targeted agents. It has not been documented whether or not to handle these targeted agents as oral chemotherapeutic agents. [213]

Table 21-14 Selected Targeted Agents in Clinical Trials

ABX-EGF (panitumumab)	Fully humanized monoclonal antibody against EGFR
OSI-774 (Tarceva)	Small-molecule EGFR tyrosine kinase inhibitor
Tipifarnib (Zarnestra/R115777)	Farnesyl transferase inhibitor — inhibits farnesyl transferase, an enzyme needed for activation of the RAS gene (a growth-promoting gene that acts like a cellular on-off switch)
GTI-2040	Antisense agent — targets R2 component of ribonucleotide reductase required for DNA synthesis
BAY 43-9006	RAF kinase inhibitor — targets the RAF/MEK/ERK signaling pathway at the level of RAF kinase Antiangiogenic effect by targeting the receptor tyrosine kinases VEGFR-2 and PDGFR and their associated signaling cascades
GW 572016	Small-molecule dual kinase inhibitor — inhibits tyrosine kinase activity of EGFR and HER2
EKB-569	Kinase inhibitor — inhibits activity of EGFR and HER2

Biologic and Targeted Therapy: Future Directions

The origins of biologic therapy date back to the 1800s with Dr. Coley and his toxins. In the many years since he treated his first patient, the field of biotherapy has grown considerably, and new agents and treatment approaches building on early experiences continue to be developed. The approval by the FDA of several biological agents began to establish biotherapy as a qualified cancer therapy. Numerous studies of cytokines, activated cells, and hematopoietic growth factors have been published, and vaccine therapy has experienced a rebirth. New indications have emerged for existing biological agents such as IL-2 and IFN. The approval of several new monoclonal antibodies has made biologic therapy a treatment option for several solid tumors and hematologic malignancies. Many monoclonal antibodies are also considered targeted therapies. The field of targeted therapy dates back only to the 1960s, and significant advances didn't occur until the 1980s, but rapid developments in the science of molecular biology and advances in drug development have brought these agents quickly into the clinic. Both of these classes of agents bring much-needed treatment options and clinical and quality of life benefits to oncology patients.

Many additional agents are in clinical trials that target the HER family and VEGF and some of the targets discussed here. Beyond these targets, many more pathways and targets have been identified in the pathogenesis of cancer, and multiple new anticancer agents are being investigated to disrupt one or more steps in the pathway. Some agents have dual TK activity and can affect more than one target; for example, agents targeting both EGFR and HER2 are in clinical development. Table 21-14 is a partial listing of additional targeted agents in clinical trials.

Cancer is a complex disease. It is likely that most advanced solid tumors gain their growth advantage from more than one abnormal molecular growth pathway. Because of crosstalk between key pathways that regulate cell growth, apoptosis, angiogenesis, and metastasis, combinations of agents that target one or more of these critical pathways will be necessary for optimal control and treatment of malignancy. An expanding number of combination molecular inhibitor approaches are underway in clinical trials, much like combination chemotherapy. It has been noted that the most significant advances in cancer therapy are likely to come from the identification of new targets rather than the identification of new drugs. Research will also continue to focus on the identification of predictors of response to targeted therapy and selection of patients most likely to respond to these therapies.

References

1. Abbas AK, Lichtman AH, Pober JS: *Cellular and Molecular Immunology*. Philadelphia, Saunders, 1991
2. Shu S, Plautz E, Krauss JC, et al: Tumor immunology. *JAMA* 278:1972–1981, 1997
3. Balkwill FR: *Cytokines in Cancer Therapy*. Oxford, Oxford University Press, 1989
4. Oettgen HF, Old LJ: The history of cancer, in DeVita VT, Hellman S, Rosenberg SA (eds.): *Biologic Therapy of Cancer*. Philadelphia, Saunders, 1991, pp 104–110
5. Oldham RK: Cancer biotherapy: General principles, in Oldham RK (ed.): *Principles of Cancer Biotherapy* (ed 2). New York, Marcel Dekker, 1991, pp 1–22
6. Mihich E, Fefer A (eds.): Biological Response Modifiers: Subcommittee Report. NIH publication no. 83–2606. Bethesda, MD, National Institutes of Health, 1983
7. Clark J, Longo D: Biological response modifiers. *Mediguide Oncol* 6:1–4, 1986
8. Rieger PT: *Biotherapy: a Comprehensive Overview* (ed 2). Sudbury, MA, Jones and Bartlett, 2001
9. Rieger PT: The use of biotherapy in patients with cancer, in *Anemia and Fatigue in Cancer Patients: Nursing Care Management. A Nursing Symposium*. Newtown, PA, Associates in Medical Marketing, 1997, pp 26–35
10. Rosenthal N: Tools of the trade — Recombinant DNA. *N Engl J Med* 331:315–317, 1994
11. Richards B: New ways for biotechnology to detect and treat old and new diseases. *Biotechnol Educ* 3:2–8, 1992
12. Jenks S: After the early hype, interferons spark interest. *J Natl Cancer Inst* 85:773–775, 1993
13. Johnson HM, Bazer FW, Fuller W, et al: How interferons fight disease. *Sci Am* 264:68–75, 1994
14. Schroder K, Hertzog P, Ravasi T, et al: Interferon-gamma: An overview of signals, mechanisms and functions. *J Leukocyte Biol* 75:163–189, 2004
15. Glaspy JA, Souza L, Scates S, et al: Treatment of hairy cell leukemia with granulocyte colony-stimulating factor and recombinant consensus interferon or recombinant interferon-alpha-2b. *J Immunother* 11:198–208, 1992
16. Bukowski RM, Tendler C, Cutler D, et al: Treating cancer with PEG intron. Pharmacokinetic profile and dosing guidelines for an improved interferon alpha-2b formulation. *Cancer* 95:389–396, 2002
17. Stadler R: Interferons in dermatology: Present day standard. *Dermatol Clin* 16:377–392, 1992
18. Tizard IR: *Immunology: An Introduction* (ed 3). Fort Worth, TX, Saunders, 1992
19. Rosenberg SA: Principles of cancer management: biologic therapy, in DeVita VT, Hellman S, Rosenberg SA (eds.): *Cancer: Principles and Practice of Oncology* (ed 6). Philadelphia, Lippincott-Raven, 2001, pp 307–333
20. Ballow M, Nelson R: Immunopharmacology: Immunomodulation and immunotherapy. *JAMA* 278:2008–2017, 1997
21. Sodal-Ceigny P, Lepage E, Brousse N: Doxorubicin containing regimens with or without interferon alfa-2b for advanced follicular lymphomas: final analysis of survival and toxicity in the Groupe d'Etude des Lymphomes Folliculaires 86 Trial. *J Clin Oncol* 16:2332–2338, 1998
22. Kirkwood JM, Strawderman MH, Ernstoff MS: Interferon-alfa-2b adjuvant therapy of high-risk resected cutaneous melanoma: The Eastern Cooperative Oncology Group Trial EST 1684. *J Clin Oncol* 14:7–17, 1996
23. Kirkwood JM, Bender C, Agarwala S, et al. Mechanisms and management of toxicities associated with high-dose interferon alfa-2b therapy. *J Clin Oncol* 20:3703–3718, 2002
24. Kirkwood JM, Manola J, Ibrahim J, et al. A pooled analysis of Eastern Cooperative Oncology Group and Intergroup trials of adjuvant high-dose interferon for melanoma. *Clin Cancer Res* 10:1670–1677, 2004
25. Kirkwood JM, Ibrahim JG, Sondak VK, et al: High and low-dose interferon alfa-2b in high-risk melanoma: first analysis of Intergroup trial E1690/S9111/C9190. *J Clin Oncol* 18:2444–2458, 2000
26. Kirkwood JM, Ibrahim JG, Sosman JA, et al: High-dose interferon alfa-2b significantly prolongs relapse-free and overall survival compared with the GM2–KLH/QS-21 vaccine in patients with resected stage IIB-III melanoma: Results of Intergroup trial E 1694/S9512/C509801. *J Clin Oncol* 19:2370–2380, 2001
27. Kirkwood JM, Ibrahim J, Lawson DH, et al: High-dose interferon α-2b does not diminish antibody response to GM2 vaccination in patients with resected melanoma: results of the Multicenter Eastern Cooperative Oncology Group Phase II Trial E2696. *J Clin Oncol* 19:1430–1436, 2001
28. Kefford RF: Adjuvant therapy of cutaneous melanoma: the interferon debate. *Ann Oncol* 14:358–365, 2003
29. Schuchter LM: Adjuvant interferon therapy for melanoma: High-dose, low-dose, no dose, which dose? *J Clin Oncol* 22:7–10, 2004 (editorial)
30. Houghton AN, Chu D, Coit DG, et al: *NCCN Clinical Practice Guidelines in Oncology: Melanoma*. V.I. 2004, nccn.org. Accessed 11/29/04.
31. Hancock, BW, Wheatley K, Harris S, et al: Adjuvant interferon in high-risk melanoma: The AIM HIGH Study — United Kingdom Coordinating Committee on cancer research randomized study of adjuvant low-dose extended-duration interferon alfa-2a in high risk resected malignant melanoma. *J Clin Oncol* 22:53–61, 2004
32. Glaspy, JA: Therapeutic options in the management of renal cell carcinoma *Semin Oncol* 29:41–46, 2002
33. Flanigan RC, Salmon SE, Blumenstein BA, et al: Nephrectomy followed by interferon alfa-2b compared with interferon alfa-2b alone for metastatic renal cell-cancer. *N Engl J Med* 345:1655–1659, 2001
34. Mickisch GH, Garin A, van Poppel H, et al: Radical nephrectomy plus interferon-alfa-based immunotherapy compared with interferon alfa alone in metastatic renal-cell carcinoma: a randomised trial. *Lancet* 358:966–970, 2001
35. Messong EM, Manola J, Wilding G, et al: Phase III study of interferon alfa as adjuvant treatment for resectable renal cell carcinoma: An Eastern Cooperative Oncology Group/Intergroup trial. *J Clin Oncol* 21:1214–1222, 2003
36. Hernberg M, Virkkunen P, Bono P, et al: Interferon alfa-2b three times daily and thalidomide in the treatment of metastatic renal cell carcinoma. *J Clin Oncol* 21:3770–3776, 2003
37. Rini BI, Halabi S, Taylor J, et al. Cancer and Leukemia Group B 90206: a randomized phase III trial of interferon-α or interferon plus anti-vascular endothelial growth factor antibody (bevacizumab) in metastatic renal cell carcinoma. *Clin Cancer Res* 10:2584–2586, 2004
38. Donnelly S: Patient management strategies for interferon alfa-2b as adjuvant therapy of high-risk melanoma. *Oncol Nurs Forum* 25:921–927, 1998
39. Trask PC, Esper P, Riba M, et al: Psychiatric side effects of interferon therapy: prevalence, proposed mechanisms, and future directions. *J Clin Oncol* 18:2316–2326, 2000
40. Gadina M, Ferguson PR, Johnston JA: New interleukins: are there any more? *Curr Opin Infect Dis* 16:211–217, 2003
41. Rubin JT: Interleukin-2: Its biology and clinical application in patients with cancer. *Cancer Invest* 11:460–472, 1993

42. Gale DM, Sorokin P. The interleukins, in Rieger PT (eds.): *Biotherapy: A Comprehensive Overview* (ed 2). Sudbury, MA, Jones and Bartlett, 2001, pp 195–227
43. Atkins MB: Interleukin-2: Clinical applications. *Semin Oncol* 29(suppl 7):12–17, 2002
44. Fisher RI, Rosenberg SA, Sznol M, et al: High-dose aldesleukin in renal cell carcinoma: long term survival update. *Cancer J Sci Am* 3(suppl):S70–S77, 1997
45. Atkins MB, Kunkel L, Sznol M, et al: High dose recombinant interleukin-2 therapy in patients with metastatic melanoma: long term survival update. *Cancer J Sci Am* 6(suppl 1):S11–S14, 2000
46. Rosenberg SA, Yang JC, Topalian SL, et al: Treatment of 283 consecutive patients with metastatic melanoma or renal cell cancer using high-dose bolus interleukin 2. *JAMA* 271: 907–913, 1994
47. Yang JC, Sherry RM, Steinberg SM, et al: Randomized study of high-dose and low-dose interleukin-2 in patients with metastatic renal cell cancer. *J Clin Oncol* 21:3127–3132, 2003
48. Atkins MB: Immunotherapy and experimental approaches for metastatic melanoma. *Hematol Oncol Clin North Am* 12:877–902, 1998
49. Parkinson DR, Sznol M: High-dose interleukin-2 in the therapy of metastatic renal cell carcinoma. *Semin Oncol* 22:61–66, 1995
50. Schwartzentruber DJ: Guidelines for the safe administration of high-dose interleukin-2. *J Immunother* 24:287–293, 2001
51. Mavroukakis SA, Muehlbauer PM, White RL, et al: Clinical pathways for managing patients receiving interleukin 2. *Clin J Oncol Nurs* 5:207–216, 2001
52. Kammula US, White DE, Rosenberg SA, et al: Trends in the safety of high dose bolus interleukin-2 administration in patients with metastatic cancer. *Cancer* 83:797–805, 1998
53. Rosenberg SA: Keynote address: Perspectives on the use of interleukin-2 in cancer treatment. *Cancer J Sci Am* 3(suppl 1):S2–S6, 1997
54. Gold PJ, Thompson JA, Markowitz DR, et al: Metastatic renal cell carcinoma: long term survival after therapy with high-dose continuous-infusion interleukin-2. *Cancer J Sci Am* 3(suppl 1):S85–S91, 1997
55. Yang JC, Rosenberg SA: An ongoing prospective randomized comparison of interleukin-2 regimens for the treatment of metastatic renal cell cancer. *Cancer J Sci Am* 3(suppl 1):S79–S84, 1997
56. Sleijfer DT, Janssen RAJ, Buter J, et al: Phase II study of subcutaneous interleukin-2 in unselected patients with advanced renal cell cancer on an outpatient basis. *J Clin Oncol* 10:1119–1123, 1992
57. Dutcher JP, Atkins M, Fisher R: Interleukin-2–based therapy for metastatic renal cell cancer: The Cytokine Working Group Experience, 1989–1997. *Cancer J Sci Am* 3(suppl 1):S73–S78, 1997
58. Clark JO, Atkins MB, Ura WJ, et al: Adjuvant high-dose bolus interleukin-2 for patients with high-risk renal cell carcinoma: a Cytokine Working Group randomized trial. *J Clin Oncol* 21:3133–3140, 2003
59. O'Day SJ, Agarwala SS, Naredi P, et al: Treatment with histamine dihydrocholoride and interleukin-2 in patients with advanced metastatic malignant melanoma: A detailed safety analysis. *Melanoma Res* 13:307–311, 2003
60. Levy Y, Capitant C, Houhou S, et al: Immunological efficacy of IL-2 therapy in HIV patients: results of a randomised trial comparing subcutaneous PEG, continuous IV IL-2 with antiretroviral therapy. *Blood* 92:169a, 1998 (abstr 681)
61. Lissoni P: Effects of low-dose recombinant interleukin-2 in human malignancies. *Cancer J Sci Am* 3(suppl):S115–S120, 1997
62. Fefer A: Interleukin-2 in the treatment of hematologic malignancies. *Cancer J Sci Am* 3(suppl 1):S35–S36, 1997 (editorial)
63. Gluck WL, Hurst D, Yuen A, et al: Phase I studies of interleukin-2 and rituximab in B-cell non-Hodgkin's lymphoma: IL-2 mediated natural killer cell expansion correlations with clinical response. *Clin Cancer Res* 10:2253–2264, 2004
64. Fefer A, Robinson N, Benyunes MC, et al: Interleukin-2 therapy after bone marrow or stem cell transplantation for hematologic malignancies. *Cancer J Sci Am* 3(suppl 1):S48–S53, 1997
65. Mazumder A: Experimental evidence of interleukin-2 activity in bone marrow transplantation. *Cancer J Sci Am* 3(suppl 1):S37–S42, 1997
66. Stein AS, O'Donnell MR, Slovak ML, et al: Interleukin-2 after autologous stem-cell transplantation for adult patients with acute myeloid leukemia in first complete remission. *J Clin Oncol* 21:615–623, 2003
67. Hiscox S, Jiang WG: Interleukin-12: An emerging antitumour cytokine. *In Vivo* 11:125–132, 1997
68. Fujiwara H, Hamaoka T: Antitumor and antimetastatic effects of interleukin 12. *Cancer Chemother Pharmacol* 38(suppl): S22–S26, 1996
69. Carreno V, Quiroga JA: Biological properties of interleukin-12 and its therapeutic use in persistent hepatitis B virus and hepatitis C virus infection. *J Viral Hep* 2(suppl 4):83–86, 1997
70. Ansell SM: Adding cytokines to monoclonal antibody therapy: Does the concurrent administration of interleukin-12 add to the efficacy of rituximab in B-cell non-Hodgkin's lymphoma? *Leuk Lymphoma* 44:1309–1315, 2003
71. Atkins MB, Robertson MJ, Gordon M, et al: Phase I evaluation of intravenous recombinant human interleukin-12 in patients with advanced malignancies. *Clin Cancer Res* 3:409–417, 1997
72. Portielje JEA, Gratama JW, van Ojik HH, et al: IL:12: a promising adjuvant for cancer vaccination. *Cancer Immunol Immunother* 52:133–144, 2003
73. Motzer RJ, Rakhit A, Schwartz LH, et al. Phase I trial of subcutaneous recombinant human interleukin-12 in patients with advanced renal cell carcinoma. *Clin Cancer Res* 4:1183–1191, 1998
74. Gollob JA, Veenstra KG, Parker RA, et al: Phase I trial of concurrent twice weekly recombinant human interleukin-12 plus low-dose IL-2 in patients with melanoma or renal cell carcinoma. *J Clin Oncol* 21:2564–2573, 2003
75. Pelloso D, Cyran K, Timmons L, et al: Immunological consequences of interleukin-12 administration after autologous stem cell transplantation. *Clin Cancer Res* 10:1935–1942, 2004
76. Mier J, Atkins MB: Pharmacology of cancer biotherapeutics, section 2 interleukin-2, in DeVita VT, Hellman S, Rosenberg SA (eds.): *Cancer: Principles and Practice of Oncology* (ed 6). Philadelphia, Lippincott, Williams and Wilkins, 2001, pp 471–478
77. Atkins MB, Sparano J, Fisher RI, et al: Randomized phase II trial of high-dose interleukin-2 either alone or in combination with interferon alpha-2b in advanced renal cell cancer. *J Clin Oncol* 11:661–670, 1993
78. Legha SS, Ring S, Eton O, et al: Development of a biochemotherapy regimen with concurrent administration of cisplatin, vinblastine, dacarbazine, interferon alfa, and interleukin-2 for patients with metastatic melanoma. *J Clin Oncol* 16:1752–1759, 1998
79. Mitchell MS: Combinations of anticancer drugs and immunotherapy. *Cancer Immunol Immunother* 52:686–692, 2003
80. Old LJ: Tumor necrosis factor. *Sci Am* 258:59–75, 1988
81. Feinberg B, Kurzrock M, Talpaz M, et al: A phase I trial of intravenously administered recombinant tumor necrosis factor-alpha in cancer patients. *J Clin Oncol* 6:1328–1334, 1988
82. Fraker DL, Alexander HR: The use of tumor necrosis factor in isolated limb perfusions for melanoma and sarcoma. *Princ Pract Oncol Upd* 7:1–10, 1993

83. Sleijfer S, Mulder NH: Tumour necrosis factor: the decline and fall of a biological agent and its resurrection. *Clin Oncol* 6:127–132, 1994
84. Gutman M, Inbar M, Lev-Shlush D, et al: High dose tumor necrosis factor-alpha and melphalan administered via isolated limb perfusion for advanced limb soft tissue sarcoma results in a >90% response rate and limb preservation. *Cancer* 79:1129–1136, 1997
85. Fraker DL, Alexander R, Andrich M, et al: Treatment of patients with melanoma of the extremity using hyperthermic isolated limb perfusion with melphalan, tumor necrosis factor, and interferon gamma: results of a tumor necrosis factor dose-escalation study. *J Clin Oncol* 14:479–489, 1996
86. Eggermont AMM, Schraffordt Koops H, Slausner JM, et al: Limb salvage by isolated limb perfusion with TNF and melphalan in patients with locally advanced soft tissue sarcomas: outcome of 270 ILPs in 246 patients. *Proc Am Soc Clin Oncol* 18:535a, 1999 (abstr 2067)
87. Rossi CR, Mocellin, S, Pilati P, et al: TNF-α- based isolated perfusion for limb-threatening soft tissue sarcomas: state of the art and future trends. *J Immunother* 26:291–300, 2003
88. Alexander HR: Specialized techniques in cancer management, section 3 isolation perfusion, in DeVita VT, Hellman S, Rosenberg SA (eds.): *Cancer: Principles and Practice of Oncology* (ed 6). Philadelphia, Lippincott, Williams and Wilkins, 2001, pp 769–776
89. Rosenberg SA: Adoptive immunotherapy for cancer, in Paul WE (ed.): *Immunology: Recognition and Response.* New York, Freeman, 1990, pp 109–121
90. Sznol M, Parkinson DR: Clinical applications of IL-2. *Oncology* 8:61–66, 1994
91. Platsoucas CD, Freedman RS: Tumor-infiltrating lymphocytes in gene therapy. *Cancer Bull* 45:118–124, 1993
92. Topalian SL, Solomon D, Avis FP, et al: Immunotherapy of patients with advanced cancer using tumor-infiltrating lymphocytes and recombinant interleukin-2: a pilot study. *J Clin Oncol* 6:839–853, 1988
93. Rosenberg SA, Yannelli JR, Yang JC, et al: Treatment of patients with autologous tumor-infiltrating lymphocytes and interleukin 2. *J Natl Cancer Inst* 86:1159–1164, 1994
94. Rosenberg SA: Gene therapy for cancer. *JAMA* 268:2416–2419, 1992
95. DiJulio JE: Monoclonal antibodies: overview and use in hematologic malignancies, in Rieger PT (ed.): *Biotherapy: A Comprehensive Overview.* Sudbury, MA, Jones and Bartlett, 2001, pp 283–316
96. Weiner LM, Adams GP, Von Mehren M: Therapeutic monoclonal antibodies: general principles, in DeVita VT, Hellman S, Rosenberg SA (eds.): *Cancer: Principles and Practice of Oncology* (ed 6). Philadelphia, Lippincott, Williams and Wilkins, 2001, pp 495–519
97. Cersosimo RJ: Monoclonal antibodies in the treatment of cancer, part 1. *Am J Health-Syst Pharm* 60:1531–1548, 2003
98. Berger M, Shankar V, Vafai A: Therapeutic applications of monoclonal antibodies. *Am J Med Sci* 324:14–30, 2002
99. Schindler LW: *Understanding the Immune System.* NIH publication no. 88-529. Bethesda, MD, US Department of Heath and Human Services, 1988
100. Schmidt KV, Wood BA: Trends in cancer therapy: role of monoclonal antibodies. *Semin Oncol Nurs* 19:169–179, 2003
101. Cheng JD, Rieger PT, von Mehren M, et al: Recent advances in immunotherapy and monoclonal antibody treatment of cancer. *Semin Oncol Nurs* 16(suppl 1):2–12, 2000
102. Gibbs WW: Try, try again. *Sci Am* 263:101–103, 1993
103. Davis TA, Maloney DG, Grillo-Lopez AJ, et al: Rituximab anti-CS20 monoclonal antibody therapy in non-Hodgkin's lymphoma: Safety and efficacy of re-treatment. *J Clin Oncol* 18:3135–3143, 2000
104. Johnson P, Glennie M: The mechanism of action of rituximab in the elimination of tumor cells. *Semin Oncol* 30(suppl 3):3–8, 2003
105. Multani PS, Grossbard ML: Monoclonal antibody-based therapies for hematologic malignancies. *J Clin Oncol* 16:3691–3710, 1998
106. Plosker GL, Figgett DP: Rituximab: A review of its use in non-Hodgkin's lymphoma and chronic lymphocytic leukemia. *Drugs* 63:803–843, 2003
107. Press O: Prospects for the management of non-Hodgkin's lymphomas with monoclonal antibodies and immunoconjugates. *Cancer J Sci Am* 4(suppl 2):S19–S26, 1998
108. McLaughlin P, Grillo-Lopez AJ, Link BK, et al: Rituximab chimeric anti-CD20 monoclonal antibody therapy for relapsed indolent lymphoma: half of patients respond to a four-dose treatment plan. *J Clin Oncol* 16:2825–2833, 1998
109. Davis TA, White CA, Grillo-Lopez AJ, et al: Single-agent monoclonal antibody efficacy in bulky non-Hodgkin's lymphoma: results of a phase II trial of rituximab. *J Clin Oncol* 17:1851–1857, 1999
110. Coiffier B, Lepage E, Briere J, et al: CHOP chemotherapy plus rituximab compared with CHOP alone in elderly patients with diffuse large B-cell lymphoma. *N Engl J Med* 364:235–242, 2002
111. Coiffier B: Immunochemotherapy: the new standard in aggressive non-Hodgkin's lymphoma in the elderly. *Semin Oncol* 30(suppl 2):21–27
112. Grillo-Lopez A: Rituximab (Rituxan/Mab Thera): the first decade (1993–2003). *Expert Rev Anticancer Ther* 3:767–779, 2003
113. Marcus R, Imrie K, Belch A, et al: An international multi-centre, randomized open-label, phase III trial comparing rituximab added to CVP chemotherapy alone in untreated Stage III/IV follicular non-Hodgkin's Lymphoma. *Blood,* 102: 2003 (abstr 87)
114. Byrd JC, Peterson B, Morrison VA, et al: Randomized phase 2 study of fludarabine with concurrent versus sequential treatment with rituximab in symptomatic, untreated patients with B-cell CLL: results from Cancer and Leukemia Group B 9712 (CALGB 9712). *Blood* 101:6–14, 2003
115. Montserrat E: Rituximab in chronic lymphocytic leukemia. *Semin Oncol* 30 (suppl 2):34–39, 2003
116. Hainsworth JD: First-line and maintenance treatment with rituximab for patients with indolent non-Hodgkin's lymphoma. *Semin Oncol* 30(suppl 2):9–15, 2003
117. Slamon DJ, Clark GM, Wong SG, et al: Human breast cancer: correlation of relapse and survival with amplification of the HER-2/neu oncogene. *Science* 235:177–182, 1987
118. Slamon DJ, Godolphin W, Jones LA, et al: Studies of the HER-2/neu proto-oncogene in human breast and ovarian cancer. *Science* 244:707–712, 1989
119. Nahta R, Esteva FJ: HER-2 targeted therapy: lessons learned and future directions. *Clin Cancer Res* 9:5078–5084, 2003
120. Slamon DJ, Leyland-Jones B, Shak, S, et al: Use of chemotherapy plus a monoclonal antibody against HER2 for metastatic breast cancer that overexpresses HER2. *N Engl J Med* 344:783–792, 2001
121. Vogel CL, Cobleigh MA, Tripathy D, et al: Efficacy and safety of trastuzumab as single agent in first-line treatment of HER-2 overexpressing metastatic breast cancer. *J Clin Oncol* 20:719–726, 2002
122. Castellon XC, Castandea-Soto NJ, Clemens M, et al: Efficacy and safety of 3–weekly Herceptin monotherapy in women with HER-2 positive metastatic breast cancer: preliminary data from a phase II study. *Proc Am Soc Clin Oncol* 21:2002, abstr 73

123. Leyland-Jones B, Gelmon K, Ayoub, et al: Pharmacokinetics, safety, and efficacy of trastuzumab administered every three weeks in combination with paclitaxel. *J Clin Oncol* 21:3965–3971, 2003
124. Gelmon K, Arnold A, Verma J, et al: Pharmacokinetics and safety of trastuzumab (Herceptin) when administered every three weeks to women with metastatic breast cancer *Proc Am Soc Clin Oncol* 20:2001, abstr 271
125. Tripathy D, Slamon DJ, Cobleigh M, et al: Safety of treatment of metastatic breast cancer with trastuzumab beyond disease progression. *J Clin Oncol* 22:1063–1070, 2004
126. Elkin EB, Weinstein MC, Winer EP, et al: HER-2 testing and trastuzumab therapy for metastatic breast cancer: a cost effectiveness analysis. *J Clin Oncol* 22:854–863, 2004
127. Seidman A, Hudis C, Pierri MK, et al: Cardiac dysfunction in the trastuzumab clinical trials experience. *J Clin Oncol* 20:1215–1221, 2002
128. Perez EA, Rodeheffer R: Clinical cardiac tolerability of trastuzumab. *J Clin Oncol* 22:322–329, 2004
129. Nahta R, Hortobagyi GN, Esteva FJ: Growth factor receptors in breast cancer: potential for therapeutic intervention. *Oncologist* 8:5–17, 2003
130. Burstein HJ, Harris LN, Marcom PK, et al: Trastuzumab and vinorelbine as first-line therapy for HER2–overexpressing metastatic breast cancer: multicenter phase II trial with clinical outcomes, analysis of serum tumor markers as predictive factors, and cardiac surveillance algorithm. *J Clin Oncol* 21:2889–2895, 2003
131. Burstein HJ, Kuter I, Campos SM, et al: Clinical activity of trastuzumab and vinorelbine in women with HER-2 overexpressing metastatic breast cancer. *J Clin Oncol* 19:2722–2730, 2001
132. Robert N, Leyland-Jones B, Asmar L, et al: Phase III comparative study of trastuzumab and paclitaxel with and without carboplatin in patients with HER-2/new positive advanced breast cancer. *San Antonio Breast Cancer Symposium,* 2002, (abstr 35)
133. Tan AR, Swain SM: Ongoing adjuvant trials with trastuzumab in breast cancer. *Semin Oncol Nurs* 30(suppl 5):54–64, 2003
134. Mavromatis B, Cheson BD: Monoclonal antibody therapy of chronic lymphocytic leukemia. *J Clin Oncol* 21:1874–1881, 2003
135. Cersosimo RJ: Monoclonal antibodies in the treatment of cancer, part 2. *Am J Health-Syst Pharm* 60:1631–1643, 2003
136. Keating MJ, Flinn I, Jain V, et al: Therapeutic role of alemtuzumab (CAMPATH-1H) in patients who have failed fludarabine: results of a large international study. *Blood* 99:3554–3561, 2002
137. Lynn A, Williams ML, Sickler JS, et al: Treatment of chronic lymphocytic leukemia with alemtuzumab: A review for nurses. *Oncol Nurs Forum* 30:689–696, 2003
138. Stull DM: Targeted therapies for the treatment of leukemia. *Semin Oncol Nurs* 19:90–97, 2003
139. Giles G, Estey E, O'Brian S: Gemtuzumab ozogamicin in the treatment of acute myeloid leukemia. *Cancer* 98:2095–2014, 2003
140. Shannon-Dorcy K: Nursing implication of Myelotarg: A novel antibody-targeted chemotherapy for CD 33+ acute myeloid leukemia in first relapse. *Oncol Nurs Forum* 29:52–59, 2002
141. Sievers EL, Larson RA, Stadmauer EA, et al: Efficacy and safety of gemtuzumab ozogamicin in patients with CD 33+ acute myeloid leukemia in first relapse. *J Clin Oncol* 19:3233–3254, 2001
142. Bross PF, Beitz J, Chen G, et al: Approval summary: Gemtuzumab ozogamicin in relapsed acute myeloid leukemia *Clin Cancer Res* 7:1490–1496, 2001
143. Giles FJ, Cortes JE, Halliburton TA, et al: Intravenous corticosteroids to reduce gemtuzumab ozogamicin infusion reactions. *Ann Pharmacother* 37:1182–1185, 2003
144. Chanan-Khan A, Czuczman, MS: Radioimmunotherapy in non-Hodgkin's lymphoma. *Curr Opinion Oncol* 14:484–489, 2002
145. Emmanouilides C: Radioimmunotherapy for non-Hodgkin's lymphoma. *Semin Oncol* 30:531–544, 2003
146. Cheson BD: Radioimmunotherapy of non-Hodgkin's lymphomas. *Blood* 101:391–398, 2003
147. Hendrix CS, de Leon C, Dillman RO: Radioimmunotherapy for non-Hodkgin's lymphoma with yttrium 90 ibritumomab tiuxetan. *Clin J Oncol Nurs* 6:144–148, 2002
148. Hernandez MC, Knox SJ: Radiobiology of radioimmunotherapy with 90Y ibritumomab tiuxetan (Zevalin) *Semin Oncol* 30(suppl 17):6–10, 2003
149. Witzig TE, Gordon LI, Cabanillas F, et al: Randomized controlled trial of yttrium-90-labeled ibritumomab tiuxetan radioimmunotherapy versus rituximab immunotherapy for patients with relapsed or refractory low-grade, follicular, or transformed B-cell non-Hodgkin's lymphoma. *J Clin Oncol* 20:2453–2463, 2002
150. Witzig TE, White CA, Flinn IW, et al: Zevalin radioimmunotherapy of rituximab-refractory follicular non-Hodgkin's lymphoma *Blood* 96:507a, 2000, (abstr 3149)
151. Gordon LI: Practical considerations and radiation safety in radioimmunotherapy with yttrium 90 tiuxetan (Zevalin). *Semin Oncol* 30(suppl 17):23–28, 2003
152. Wagner HN, Wiseman GA, Marcus CS, et al: Administration guidelines for radioimmunotherapy of non-Hodgkin's lymphoma with ^{90}Y labeled anti-CD20 monoclonal antibody. *J Nuc Med* 43:267–272, 2002
153. Tuninstra N: Outpatient administration of radiolabeled monoclonal antibodies. *Clin J Oncol Nurs* 7:106–108, 2003
154. Wiseman GA, Gordon LI, Multani PS, et al: Ibritumomab tiuxetan radioimmunotherapy for patients with relapsed or refractory non-Hodgkin's lymphoma and mild thrombocytopenia: a phase II multicenter trial. *Blood* 99:4336–4342, 2002
155. Witzig TE, White CA, Gordon KI, et al: Safety of yttrium-90 ibritumomab tiuxetan radioimmunotherapy for relapsed low-grade follicular, or transformed non-Hodgkin's lymphoma. *J Clin Oncol* 21:1263–1270, 2003
156. Kaminski MS, Zelenetz AD, Press OW, et al: Pivotal study of iodine I 131 tositumomab for chemotherapy-refractory low-grade or transformed low-grade B-cell non-Hodkgin's lymphomas. *J Clin Oncol* 19:3918–3928, 2001
157. Zelentz AD: A clinical and scientific overview of tositumomab and iodine I 131 tositumomab. *Semin Oncol* 30(suppl 4):22–30, 2003
158. Hogenstein MA, Augustine SC, Rutar F, et al: Establishing an institutional model for the administration of tositumomab and iodine I 131 tositumomab. *Semin Oncol* 30(suppl 4):39–49, 2003
159. Nichols J, Foss F, Kuzel RM, et al: Interleukin-2 fusion protein: an investigational therapy for interleukin-2 receptor expressing malignancies. *Eur J Cancer* 33(suppl):S34–36, 1997
160. Duvic M, Cather J, Maize J, et al: DAB389IL-2 fusion toxin produces clinical responses in tumor stage cutaneous T cell lymphoma. *Am J Hematol* 58:87–70, 1998
161. Olsen E, Dubic M, Frankel A, et al: Pivotal phase III trial of two dose levels of denileukin diftitox for the treatment of cutaneous T-cell lymphoma. *J Clin Oncol* 19:376–388, 2001
162. Walker PL, Dang NH: Denileukin diftitox as novel targeted therapy in non-Hodgkin's lymphoma. *Clin J Oncol Nurs* 8:169–174, 2004
163. Foss FM, Bacha P, Osann KE, et al: Biological correlates of acute hypersensitivity events with DAB 389 IL-2 (denileukin diftitox, Ontak) in cutaneous T-cell lymphoma: decreased frequency and severity with steroid premedication. *Clin Lymphoma* 1:298–302, 2001

164. Frankel AE, Fleming DR, Hall PD, et al: A phase II study of DT fusion protein denileukin diftitox in patients with fludarabine-refractory chronic lymphocytic leukemia. *Clin Cancer Res* 9:3555–3561, 2003
165. Hersh EM, Taylor CW: Immunotherapy by active immunization: use of nonspecific stimulants and immunomodulators, in DeVita VT, Hellman S, Rosenberg SA (eds.): *Biologic Therapy of Cancer.* Philadelphia, Lippincott, 1991, pp 613–626
166. Spreafico F: The use of levamisole in cancer patients. *Drugs* 19:105–116, 1980
167. Krejci KG, Markiewicz MA, Kwon ED: Immunotherapy for urological malignancies. *J Urol* 171:870–876, 2004
168. Rieger P: Biotherapy: an overview, in Rieger PT (ed.): *Biotherapy: A Comprehensive Overview* (ed 2). Sudbury, MA, Jones and Bartlett, 2001, pp 3–37
169. Parkinson DR, Smith MA, Cheson BD, et al: Trans-retinoic acid and related differentiation agents. *Semin Oncol* 19:734–741, 1992
170. Warrell RP: Applications for retinoids in cancer therapy. *Semin Hematol* 31(suppl 5):1–13, 1994
171. Miller WH, Dmitrovsky E: Retinoic acid and its rearranged receptor in the treatment of acute promyelocytic leukemia, in DeVita VT, Hellman S, Rosenberg SA (eds.): *Important Advances in Oncology 1993.* Philadelphia, Lippincott, 1993, pp 81–93
172. Slack JL: Recent advances in the biology and treatment of acute promyelocytic leukemia, in Perry MC (ed.): *American Society of Clinical Oncology Educational Book.* Alexandria, VA, ASCO, 1998, pp 54–65
173. Gillis JC, Goa KL: Tretinoin. *Drugs* 50:897–923, 1995
174. Moore DM, Kalvakolano DV, Lippman SM, et al: Retinoic acid and interferon in human cancer: mechanisms and clinical studies. *Semin Hematol* 31(suppl 5):31–37, 1994
175. Lippman SM, Lotan R, Schleuniger U: Retinoid-interferon therapy of solid tumors. *Int J Cancer* 70:481–483, 1997
176. Levine N: Role of retinoids in skin cancer treatment and prevention. *J Am Acad Dermatol* 39(suppl):S62–S66, 1998
177. Singh DK, Lipmann SM: Cancer chemoprevention, part 1: Retinoids and carotenoids and other classic antioxidants. *Oncology* 12:1643–1657, 1998
178. DiGiovanna JJ: Retinoid chemoprevention in the high-risk patient. *J Am Acad Dermatol* 39(suppl):S82–S85, 1998
179. Birner A: Pharmacology of oral chemotherapy agents. *Clin J Oncol Nurs* 7(suppl):11–19, 2003
180. Sparano JA, Gray R, Giantonio B, et al: Evaluating antiangiogenesis agents in the clinic: The Eastern Cooperative Oncology Group portfolio of clinical trials. *Clin Cancer Res* 10:1206–1211, 2004
181. Whang YE, Godley PA: Renal cell carcinoma. *Curr Opin Oncol* 15:213–216, 2003
182. Kerbel R, Folkman J: Clinical translation of angiogenesis inhibitors. *Nat Rev Cancer* 2:727–739, 2003
183. Barlogie B, Shaughnessy J, Tricot G, et al: Treatment of multiple myeloma. *Blood* 103:20–32, 2004
184. Wood LS, Perez C, Monroe D: The emergence of thalidomide in treating advanced renal cell carcinoma. *Oncol Nurs Forum* 30:501–509, 2003
185. Anderson K: The role of immunomodulatory drugs in multiple myeloma. *Semin Hematol* 40(suppl 4):23–32, 2003
186. Tariman JD: Understanding novel therapeutic agents for multiple myeloma. *Clin J Oncol Nurs* 7:521–528, 2003
187. Dredge K, Dalgeish AG, Marriott JB: Thalidomide analogs as emerging anti-cancer drugs. *Anti-cancer Drugs* 14:331–335, 2003
188. Restifio NP, Sznol M, Overwihk WW: Cancer vaccines, part 2, therapeutic cancer vaccines, in DeVita VT, Hellman S, Rosenberg SA (eds.): *Cancer: Principles and Practice of Oncology* (ed 6). Philadelphia, Lippincott-Raven, 2001, pp 3195–3217
189. Muehlbauer PM, Schwartzentruber DJ: Cancer vaccines. *Semin Oncol Nurs* 19:206–216, 2003
190. Engleman EG: Dendritic cell-based cancer immunotherapy. *Semin Oncol* 30(suppl 8):23–29, 2003
191. Berinstein N: Overview of therapeutic vaccination approaches for cancer. *Semin Oncol* 30(suppl 8):1–8, 2003
192. Ribas A, Butterfield LJ, Glaspy JA, et al: Current developments in cancer vaccines and cellular immunotherapy. *J Clin Oncol* 21:2415–2432, 2003
193. Flinn OJ: Cancer vaccines: between the idea and reality. *Nature Rev Immunol* 3:630–641, 2003
194. Berd D: Cancer vaccines: reborn or just recycled? *Semin Oncol* 25:605–610, 1998
195. Chan A, Morton D: Active immunotherapy with allogeneic tumor cell vaccines: present status. *Semin Oncol* 25:611–622, 1998
196. Parmiani G, Pill l, Castelli C, et al: Vaccination of patients with solid tumours. *Ann Oncol* 14:817–824, 2003
197. Livingston P: Ganglioside vaccines with emphasis on GM2. *Semin Oncol* 25:636–645, 1998
198. Foon K, Goutam S, Hutchins L, et al: Antibody responses in melanoma patients immunized with an anti-idiotype antibody mimicking disialoganglioside GD21. *Clin Cancer Res* 4:1117–1124, 1998
199. Mitchell M: Perspectives on allogeneic melanoma lysates in active specific immunotherapy. *Semin Oncol* 25:623–635, 1998
200. Simons JW, Mikhak B: Ex vivo gene therapy using cytokine-transduced tumor vaccines: molecular and clinical pharmacology. *Semin Oncol* 25:661–676, 1998
201. Pardoll DM: Spinning molecular immunology into successful immunotherapy. *Nature Rev Immunol* 2:227–238, 2002
202. Paglia P, Guzman CA: Keeping the immune system alerted against cancer. *Cancer Immunol Immunother* 46:88–92, 1998
203. Gilboa E, Nair SK, Lyerly KH: Immunotherapy of cancer with dendritic-cell-based vaccines. *Cancer Immunol Immunother* 46:82–87, 1998
204. Pardoll D: Does the immune system see tumors foreign or self? *Annu Rev Immunol* 21:807–839, 2003
205. Jager E, Jager D, Knuth A: Antigen-specific immunotherapy and cancer vaccines. *Int J Cancer* 106:817–820, 2003
206. Bystryn JC: Vaccines for melanoma: design strategies and clinical results. *Dermatol Clin* 16:269–275, 1998
207. Marshall J: Carcinogenic antigen-based vaccines *Semin Oncol* 30(suppl 8):30–36, 2003
208. Weber CE: Cytokine-modified tumor vaccines: an antitumor strategy revisited in the age of molecular medicine. *Cancer Nurs* 21:167–177, 1998
209. Gemmill R, Idell CS: Biological advances for new treatment approaches. *Semin Oncol Nurs* 19:162–168, 2003
210. Ritter CA, Arteaga CL: The epidermal growth factor receptor tyrosine kinase: a promising therapeutic target in solid tumors. *Semin Oncol* 30:3–11, 2003
211. Lage A, Crombet T, Gonzalez G: Targeting epidermal growth factor receptor signaling: early results and future trends in oncology. *Ann Med* 35:327–336, 2003
212. Gshwind A, Fischer OM, Ullrich A: The discovery of receptor tyrosine kinases: targets for cancer therapy. *Nature Rev Cancer* 4:361–370, 2004
213. Gale DM: Molecular targets in cancer therapy. *Semin Oncol Nurs* 19:193–205, 2003
214. Carpenter CL: Essentials of signal transduction, in DeVita VT, Hellman S, Rosenberg SA (eds.): *Cancer: Principles and Practice of Oncology* (ed 6). Philadelphia, Lippincott-Raven, 2001, pp 31–34

215. Krozely P: Epidermal growth factor receptor tyrosine kinase inhibitors: evolving role in the treatment of solid tumors. *Clin J Oncol Nurs* 8:163–168, 2004
216. Arteaga C: Targeting HER1/EGFR: A molecular approach to cancer therapy. *Semin Oncol* 30(suppl 7):3–14, 2003
217. Yarden Y: The EGFR family and its ligands in human cancer: signaling mechanisms and therapeutic options. *Eur J Cancer* 37:S3–S8, 2001
218. Cohen MH, Williams GA, Sridhara R, et al: United States Food and Drug Administration approval summary: Gefitinib (ZD 1839; Iressa) tablets. *Clin Cancer Res* 10:1212–1218, 2004
219. Mendelsohn J: Targeting the epidermal growth factor receptor for cancer therapy. *J Clin Oncol* 20:1S–13S, 2002
220. Herbst RS, Bunn PA: Targeting the epidermal growth factor receptor in non-small cell lung cancer. *Clin Cancer Res* 9:5813–5824, 2003
221. Savage DG, Antman KH: Imatinib mesylate: a new oral targeted therapy. *N Eng J Med* 346:683–693, 2002
222. Druker BJ: Imatinib as a paradigm of targeted therapies. *J Clin Oncol* 21:239S–245S, 2003
223. Goldman JM, Melo JV: Chronic myeloid leukemia: advances in biology and new approaches to treatment. *N Engl J Med* 349:1451–1464, 2003
224. Kurzrock R, Kantarjian JM, Druker BJ, et al: Philadelphia chromosome-positive leukemias: from basic mechanisms to molecular therapeutics. *Ann Intern Med* 138:819–830, 2003
225. O'Brian SG, Guillhot F, Larson RA, et al: Imatinib compared with interferon and low-dose cytarabine for newly diagnosed chronic-phase chronic myeloid leukemia. *N Engl J Med* 348:994–1004, 2003
226. Hahn EA, Glendenning GA, Sorensen MV, et al: Quality of life in patients with newly diagnosed chronic phase chronic myeloid leukemia on imatinib versus interferon alfa plus low-dose cytarabine: results from the IRIS study. *J Clin Oncol* 21:2138–2146, 2003
227. Connolly EM, Gaffney E, Reynolds JV: Gastrointestinal stromal tumours. *Br J Surg* 90:1178–1186, 2003
228. Demetri GD, von Mehren M, Blanke C, et al: Efficacy and safety of imatinib mesylate in advanced gastrointestinal stromal tumors. *N Engl J Med* 347:472–480, 2002
229. Deininger MWN, O'Brian SG, Ford JM, et al: Practical management of patients with chronic myeloid leukemia receiving imatinib. *J Clin Oncol* 21:1637–1647, 2003
230. Harari PM, Huang S: Searching for reliable epidermal growth factor receptor response predictors. *Clin Cancer Res* 10:428–432, 2004
231. Fukuoka M, Yano S, Giaccone G, et al: Multi-institutional randomized phase II trial of gefitinib for previously treated patients with advanced non-small cell lung cancer. *J Clin Oncol* 21:2237–2246, 2003
232. Kris MG, Natale RB, Herbst RS, et al: Efficacy of gefitinib, an inhibitor of the epidermal growth factor receptor tyrosine kinase, in symptomatic patients with non-small cell lung cancer: a randomized trial. *JAMA* 290:2149–2158, 2003
233. Giaccone G, Herbst RS, Manegold C, et al: Gefitinib in combination with gemcitabine and cisplatin in advanced non-small cell lung cancer: A phase III trial — INTACT 1. *J Clin Oncol* 22:777–784, 2004
234. Herbst RS, Giaccone G, Schiller JG, et al: Gefitinib in combination with paclitaxel and carboplatin in advanced non-small cell lung cancer: a phase III trial — INTACT 2. *J Clin Oncol* 22:785–794, 2004
235. Reynolds NA, Wagstaff AJ: Cetuximab in the treatment of metastatic colorectal cancer. *Drugs* 64:109–118, 2004
236. Cunningham D, Humblet Y, Siena S, et al: Cetuximab (C225) alone or incombination with irinotecan (CPT-11) in patients with epidermal growth factor receptor (EGFR)-positive, irinotecan-refractory metastatic colorectal cancer (MCRC). *Proc Am Soc Clin Oncol* 22:252, 2003 (abstr 1012)
237. Monti M, Mancini LL, Ferrari B, et al: Diagnosis in oncology: complications of therapy and a diagnostic dilemma case, case 2: cutaneous toxicity induced by cetuximab. *J Clin Oncol* 21:4650–4654, 2003
238. Ellis LM, Hoff PM: Targeting the epidermal growth factor receptor: an important incremental step in the battle against colorectal cancer. *J Clin Oncol* 22:1177–1179, 2004 (editorial)
239. Lynch TJ, Bell DW, Sordella R, et al: Activating mutations in the epidermal growth factor receptor underlying responsiveness of non-small cell lung cancer to gefitinib. *www.nejm.org*. Accessed April 29, 2004
240. Doorn RV, Kirtschig G, Scheffer E, et al: Follicular and epidermal alterations in patients treated with ZD 1839 (Iressa), an inhibitor of the epidermal growth factor receptor. *Br J Dermatol* 147:598–601, 2002
241. Ferrara N: Role of vascular endothelial growth factor in physiologic and pathologic angiogenesis: therapeutic implication. *Semin Oncol* 6(suppl 16):10–14, 2002
242. Ferrara N: Role of vascular endothelial growth factor in the regulation of physiological angiogenesis. *Am J Physiol* 280:C1358–1366, 2001
243. Kerbel R, Folkman J: Clinical translation of angiogenesis inhibitors. *Nat Rev Cancer* 2:727–739, 2003
244. Muehlbauer PM: Antiangiogenesis in cancer therapy. *Semin Oncol Nurs* 19:180–192, 2003
245. Ferrara N: VEGF and the quest for tumour angiogenesis factors. *Nat Rev Cancer* 2:795–803, 2002
246. Hanahan D, Folkman J: Patterns and emerging mechanisms of the angiogenic switch during tumorigenesis. *Cell* 86:353–364, 1996
247. Bergers G, Benjamin L: Tumorigenesis and the angiogenic switch. *Nat Rev* 3:401–410, 2003
248. Dvorak HF: Vascular permeability factor/vascular endothelial growth factor: a critical cytokine in tumor angiogenesis and a potential target for diagnosis and therapy. *J Clin Oncol* 20:4368–4380, 2002
249. Camp-Sorrell D: Antiangiogenesis: the fifth cancer treatment modality. *Oncol Nurs Forum* 30:934–944, 2003
250. Hurwitz H, Fehrenbacher L, Cartwright T, et al: Bevacizumab (Avastin, a monoclonal antibody to vascular endothelial growth factor) prolongs survival in first-line colorectal cancer (CRC): results of a phase III trial in combination with bolus IFL (irinotecan, 5-fluorouracil, leucovorin). *Proc Am Soc Clin Oncol* 20: 2003, (abstr 3646)
251. Avastin prescribing information, 2004, Genentech, Inc., San Francisco.
252. Yang JC, Haworth L, Sherry RM, et al: A randomized trial of bevacizumab, an anti-vascular endothelial growth factor antibody, for metastatic renal cancer. *N Engl J Med* 349:427–434, 2003
253. Bedell CH: A changing paradigm for cancer treatment: the advent of new oral chemotherapy agents. *Clin J Oncol Nurs* 7:5–9, 2003
254. Brown KA, Esper P, Kelleher L, et al: *i Chemotherapy and Biotherapy Guidelines and Recommendation for Practice*r. Pittsburgh, Oncology Nursing Society, 2001

CHAPTER 22

Gene Therapy

Dale Halsey Lea, RN, MPH, APNG, FAAN

Introduction

The diagnosis, management, and treatment of human disease are becoming individualized as a result of human genome discoveries. Gene therapy and pharmacogenetics are two major therapeutic interventions that take into account an individual's specific genetic makeup.[1] This chapter provides an overview of current clinical applications of gene therapy and the emerging field of pharmacogenetics, as well as social and ethical considerations. It presents new directions for oncology nursing practice, including assessing social, cultural, and family understanding of and responses to new genetic interventions, and assuring continuity and coordination of patient and family care across the various healthcare settings. Future issues for nurses in gene-based therapies are also discussed.

Genetic Disorders

Genes are made up of a chemical code (DNA) particular to each gene. Human genome discoveries have revealed that approximately 30,000 genes reside in each individual's human genome.[1] The code differs in sequence from gene to gene and directs the composition and production of proteins that in turn make up living tissue and regulate all of the body's functions. Genetic disorders arise when an error in the complex, multistep process of replication and cell division occurs. The error may be slight—perhaps just one unit of the code is misspelled, repeated, or deleted—but its corresponding protein will be similarly improperly put together. When the protein is essential enough, the error may lead to a sequence of events that can lead to disability or even death.[2,3]

Gene therapy interventions are being developed to treat three types of genetically caused conditions. These are single-gene, multifactorial, and acquired genetic conditions.[2] More than 10,000 genetic conditions are caused by a single altered gene. These are called *Mendelian genetic disorders* and include such conditions as cystic fibrosis, hemophilia, sickle cell anemia, and Huntington's disease.[4] Some forms of hereditary breast and colon cancer as well as other cancers are also caused by a single gene alteration. These and other single-gene disorders are inherited in families in either an autosomal dominant, recessive, or X-linked manner. Individually, these conditions are rare, but together they represent an important cause of disease and disability.[2] Conditions caused by a combination of genetic and environmental influences are called *multifactorial genetic disorders*. These conditions, which are more complex and less well-defined than the single-gene disorders, include heart disease, high blood pressure, cancer, and mental illness. Current research efforts are providing a better understanding of the genetic susceptibility to these and other multifactorial genetic conditions. *Acquired genetic conditions* are those that occur as a result of a viral infection such as hepatitis or acquired immunodeficiency syndrome. In these conditions, the disorder is caused by the new genetic information the virus carries into the host.[2]

Altogether, genetic disorders account for as much as 50% of pediatric and adult hospital admissions.[5] Gene therapy and other gene-based therapeutic interventions have the potential to offer alternative and possibly less invasive and less expensive ways of treating genetic-related health conditions. The current concept of gene therapy is based on the premise that definitive treatment for genetic disorders should be possible by directing the treatment to the site of the defect itself—the gene mutation—rather than to the secondary effects and symptoms of the mutant gene. Newer approaches to gene therapy unite pharmacotherapeutics with genetic principles and include the use of DNA to treat disease.[6] Gene therapy represents a comprehensive range of therapeutic interventions.

Principles and Goals of Gene Therapy

Gene Therapy Defined

Gene therapy seeks to provide therapeutic benefit to a patient by introducing normal genes into the patient's cell nuclei to repair, enhance, replace, or compensate for an altered gene. Gene therapy strategies under investigation include inserting a new functioning gene into the cells of a patient to correct a genetic abnormality or birth defect, thereby providing a new function for the cell. Gene therapy offers the potential for treating many genetic disorders as well as cancer, infectious diseases, and autoimmune disorders by genetically modifying cells in the human body.[7,8]

Current gene therapy initiatives are aimed at somatic cells, which are the nonreproductive cells of the body (e.g., skin, muscle, bone, and liver). This type of gene therapy, called *somatic gene therapy,* can correct inherited genetic disorders and is limited to only one generation. Gene therapy aimed at altering sperm and ova (reproductive cells) is called *germ-line gene therapy.* In the United States, only somatic gene therapy has been approved for use in clinical trials. Germ-line gene therapy has been limited to animal studies and is not currently considered to be ethically acceptable in the treatment of humans. The prospect of germ-line gene therapy raises several ethical issues. The introduction of an altered gene into a fertilized egg, for example, carries the potential risk of introducing a new gene mutation that would be present in an individual at birth and could then be passed on to future generations.[9]

Enhancement gene therapy and eugenics are two other possible uses of gene therapy. The principle behind *enhancement gene therapy* is the placement of genes in an embryo or offspring that would improve a societally desirable trait, such as decreased weight or increased height. Gene therapy used for *eugenic purposes* involves the introduction of specific genetic traits into a population to develop "desirable" human attributes such as intelligence. These two applications of gene therapy, like germ-line gene therapy, are not considered by most to be ethically acceptable.[9]

Gene Identification and Characterization

The normal function of the gene of interest and the characterization of the protein that it makes must be completely understood before a plan for gene correction can be made. Several mechanisms can cause an altered gene to produce a defective protein or result in abnormal regulation of gene expression. For example, an alteration may occur in a gene that is critical for cell survival. Depending on where in the gene the actual defect has occurred, the resulting defective protein is either nonfunctional or poorly expressed. An example of this type of gene defect is adenosine deaminase (ADA) deficiency, in which damage to the ADA gene results in T-lymphocyte death and severe combined immunodeficiency. An abnormality in a regulatory gene is another mechanism that can cause problems. Certain genes are responsible for controlling the production of a specific gene product. When these genes are defective, functional gene products are not produced in adequate quantities. The gene defect present in thalassemia is an example of this type of gene abnormality.[3]

Gene Transfer Methods

The most pressing technological hurdle facing gene therapy researchers is the lack of efficient methods for transferring genes into human cells.[10] Successful gene therapy requires efficient gene delivery and continuous corrective activity of the transferred gene in the patient.[11] Gene transfer methods currently under investigation include recombinant virus vectors; chemical, physical, and fusion methods; and liposomal and protein peptide transfer. Each of these techniques has demonstrated advantages and disadvantages, and each may someday find successful clinical application.[10]

Assuring that the transferred gene is integrated into the DNA of the target cell is as important as finding the proper transfer method. Stable integration of the corrected gene, for example, is critical when introducing modifications into cells that have not yet reached maturity or are rapidly dividing. These cells produce future cell populations; maintaining gene correction as the cells divide and reproduce helps to provide long-term benefit to patients. In contrast, gene insertion into nondividing and terminally differentiated tissues such as liver or skeletal muscle may not require integration as a feature of the gene transfer method.[10]

Gene transfer in vitro and in vivo

Two general approaches — in vitro and in vivo — have been used to transfer a corrected or altered gene to a patient.[8,10] The in vitro approach is used most widely in clinical trials because it has the advantage of eliminating the possibility of gene transfer into germ-line tissues. This technique is also often more efficient than in vivo transfer.

The *in vitro* approach requires that the defective cells or cells of interest be removed from the patient first. The corrected or marker gene is then inserted into the cells, and the altered cells are returned to the individual. The cells most commonly used for this approach include lymphocytes, skin fibroblasts, and tumor and bone marrow cells.[8] These cells are readily accessible, amenable to manipulation, and able to survive for long periods of time following reinfusion. The in vitro method has not been successful with nondividing cells such as kidney, liver, or brain cells because they cannot be grown in sufficient numbers for efficient stable gene transfer and are difficult to reimplant.

In vivo gene transfer involves the direct delivery of therapeutic genes to target body cells. This technique is more promising for its potential to directly affect disease sites with minimal risk to the individual. In vivo approaches to gene therapy have been used in clinical trials for cystic fibrosis (CF), muscular dystrophy, melanoma, and heart, lung, and metabolic conditions. With in vivo gene transfer, naked DNA can be delivered without the use of needles, using a gene gun or jet gun. Both methods use either high-pressure helium or liquid to deliver the DNA to interstitial places.[10]

Both in vitro and in vivo gene transfer methods require a carrier, or *vector*, to transfer the augmented or functional genes into the target cells. The two major vector systems currently used for gene transfer are viral and nonviral. These vectors are discussed in the next section.

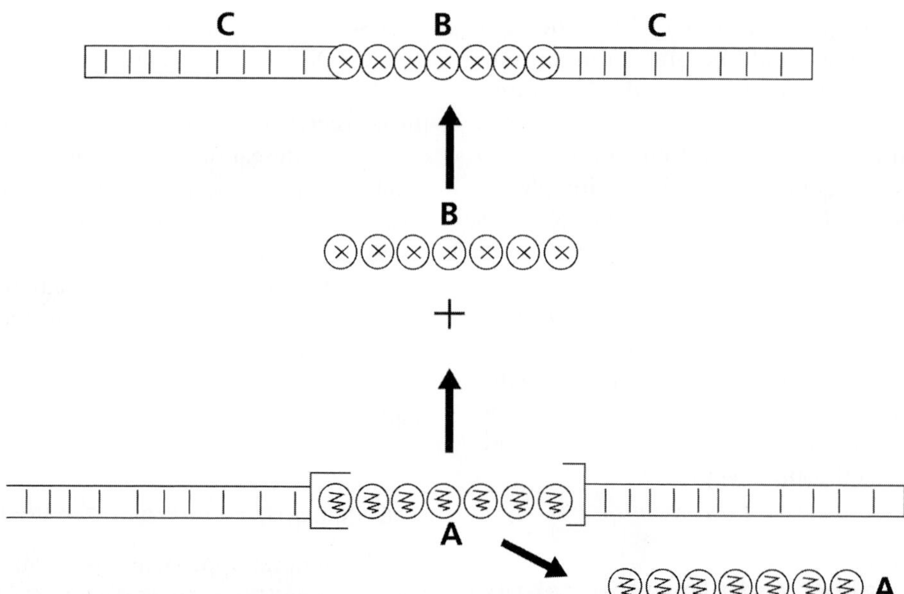

Figure 22-1 Viral vector with therapeutic gene. Viral vectors are prepared by removing the disease-producing viral gene **(A)** and replacing it with the therapeutic gene **(B)**. Viral genes necessary for invasion of the cell **(C)** are maintained.

Vectors for Gene Transfer

Effective use of gene therapy to treat inherited and acquired genetic disorders requires success in four main areas: (1) delivering the gene to the target tissue efficiently, (2) sustaining long-term gene expression, (3) ensuring that the gene transfer will not harm the patient in any way, and (4) transferring the corrected gene to nondividing cells. Another important goal is to develop a cost-effective means to manufacture the vector.[10,12] A variety of vector systems to deliver the genes have been developed and evaluated. These include viral vectors, such as retrovirus, adenovirus, adeno-associated virus, and herpes virus vectors. In addition, several nonviral vectors, including liposomes and protein peptides, have been created for gene transfer. Each vector has met with some success in delivering the therapeutic gene to the target tissue, and each has distinct problems and disadvantages. The ideal vector — one that is nontoxic, nonimmunogenic, easy to produce, and efficient in delivering DNA to cells with specificity for a particular cell type — has yet to be discovered.[10]

Viral Vectors

Most current gene therapy uses viral vectors to deliver the therapeutic gene to the target tissue. All viruses used have been disabled of any pathogenic effects by removing the genes required for replication of the virus and replacing them with therapeutic genes and selection markers (see Figure 22-1).[10] The use of viruses is a potentially powerful technique because many have evolved specific mechanisms for delivering DNA to cells. Humans, however, have an immune system designed to defend against viruses, and attempts to transfer genes by means of viral vectors have been complicated by host responses.[13]

Retroviral vectors

A retrovirus is composed of RNA that can insert itself readily into dividing cells. Retroviruses are considered the most promising gene transfer vehicle. Approximately 28% of the approved clinical gene therapy protocols use retroviral vectors.[14] These RNA viruses are able to carry out efficient gene transfer into many types of cells and can integrate into the host cell genes with stability. The therapeutic gene carried into the cell by the retrovirus will be inherited by all future generations of the cell and will provide the possibility of long-term gene expression (see Figure 22-2).[13] The murine leukemia virus (MuLV) in particular has traditionally been used as a vector of choice for gene therapy clinical protocols, and a variety of packaging methods to enclose the vector genome within the viral particles have been developed.[10]

Retroviruses, although advantageous in many ways, pose several challenges. One major concern is that the insertion of the retrovirus will disrupt normal genes essential for proper cell function, leading to harmful physiologic effects that favor cancer development. This is one of the most serious and current technical hurdles.[15]

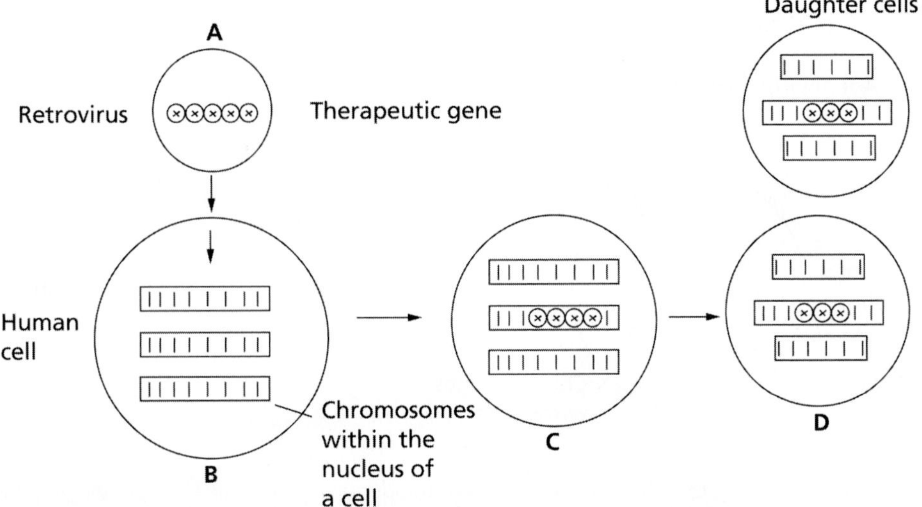

Figure 22-2 Retroviral delivery of a therapeutic gene. **(A)** A retrovirus with the therapeutic gene invades the cell. **(B)** Reverse transcriptase makes a DNA copy of the retroviral RNA. The viral DNA and the therapeutic gene are part of the nucleus and are incorporated into one of the 46 human chromosomes. **(C)** The therapeutic effect remains if the cell replicates, providing daughter cells with a copy of the therapeutic gene **(D)**.

Lentiviral vectors

Lentiviruses, which belong to the retrovirus family, are now being used in gene therapy because they can infect both dividing and nondividing cells. Human immunodeficiency virus (HIV) is the most well-known lentivirus used for gene transfer in vivo. When lentivirus vectors have been injected into rodent brain, liver, muscle, or eye cells, the viruses have produced sustained therapeutic gene expression over six months—the longest time tested thus far. To date, lentiviral vectors have not produced a cellular immune response at the site of the injection, nor have they generated any potent antibody response.[10,11,16]

Adenoviral Vectors

As of 2004, adenoviral gene therapy has been used in 26% of the clinical gene therapy trials worldwide.[14] Adenoviruses are a family of viruses that cause benign respiratory tract infections in humans. They also have the capacity to infect both dividing and nondividing cells, making them useful for gene therapy. Adenoviruses are large and can hold large segments of therapeutic DNA. They can also be produced in large amounts in culture. They have been the vectors of choice for many protocols designed to treat the pulmonary complications of cystic fibrosis as well as for a variety of clinical protocols to treat cancer. In contrast to retroviruses, which contain RNA, adenoviruses contain DNA and thus do not integrate into host DNA but instead replicate themselves outside of the nucleus of the host cell. Because of this limited integration, expression of the therapeutic gene is short-lived, and regular reapplication of gene therapy using adenovirus vectors is necessary (see Figure 22-3).[10]

The potential usefulness of adenoviral vectors stems from the fact that they do not require actively dividing cells to introduce their therapeutic gene. Adenoviruses, however, are a common cause of upper respiratory tract infections in humans. As a result, unfortunately, most of the human population may experience an active immune response to antibodies from a previous infection, which could reduce the effectiveness of gene therapy using this vector. Another potential concern with using adenoviral vectors is that the integrated gene may not lead to uniform correction of the gene defect, because it may not remain active in the host cell. Other viral vectors that may potentially enhance the delivery of therapeutic genes are therefore being explored.[10]

Newer adenoviral vectors

The adeno-associated virus (AAV) is one of the newer viral vectors under investigation; it is a simple, nonpathogenic virus composed of a single strand of DNA. In order to replicate, AAV needs additional genes. In the past, a helper virus, usually adenovirus or herpes simplex virus, served this purpose. Helper viruses are no longer required to produce AAV vectors. Plasmids are now used instead, essentially eliminating the practice of contaminating the wild type virus.

The AAV virus can infect a variety of types of cells, and although it appears to integrate in a nonspecific manner, it has been shown to integrate preferentially into chromosome 19. AAV gene therapy is being investigated for cystic fibrosis and for factor IX

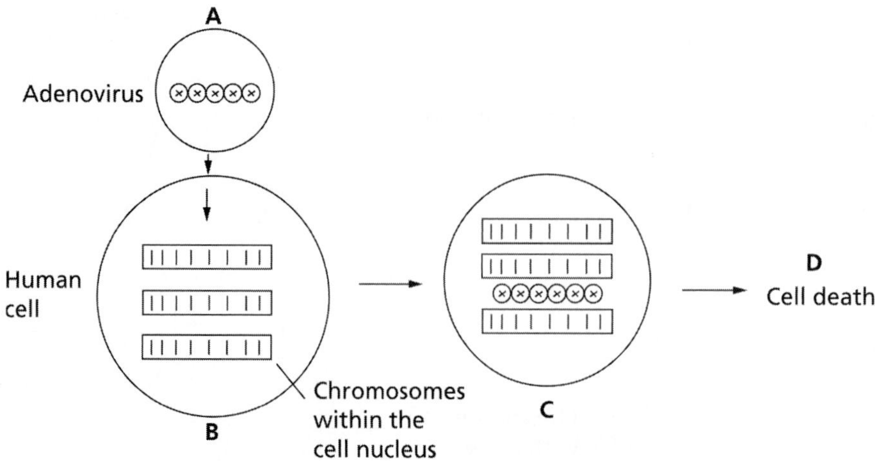

Figure 22-3 Adenoviral delivery of a therapeutic gene. **(A)** An adenovirus with the therapeutic gene invades the cell. **(B)** The viral DNA and the therapeutic gene are not incorporated into a chromosome. **(C)** The therapeutic effect is lost when the cell dies **(D)**.

hemophilia.[10] Other viruses that are being considered and developed for use as vectors for gene therapy are the herpes simplex virus, which infects cells of the nervous system, and the vaccinia virus. These viral vector systems produce a transient response, and many people have an immunity to components of the virus from being infected previously.[10]

Nonviral Vectors

Nonviral vector delivery systems for gene transfer may provide an alternative method of efficient gene delivery. To enhance integration into the human genome, nonviral methods transfer therapeutic genes into human cells by chemical methods such as precipitation with calcium phosphate and encapsulation of therapeutic genes into liposomes or molecular conjugates (complexes of lipids and DNA). Physical methods being explored and developed include direct microinjection of DNA into cells by particle acceleration. The efficiency of this process appears to be low, but intramuscular injection of "naked" DNA has been used successfully to establish cellular and humoral responses, suggesting that simple intramuscular administration of DNA could be used to create a gene vaccine.[17] During the past few years, researchers have become interested in the use of protein/peptide gene transfer. Limited information is available about the action, effectiveness, and safety of this method.[10]

Nonviral gene delivery systems may provide a means for achieving short-term expression of therapeutic gene products in certain tissues with a high degree of safety. Studies to date suggest that nonviral delivery systems have toxicities and safety profiles similar to those of conventional drugs and other biological products. There have been no reports of significant toxicity involving naked DNA in animal or human studies to date. Lung, liver, and endothelial tissue appear to be particularly acceptable targets for nonviral gene therapy. Other targets include tissues that are accessible to direct interstitial injection, such as muscle, skin, and tumor masses.[10]

One of the greatest challenges for gene therapy is the development of safe and cost-effective therapeutic gene delivery systems that can be used along with conventional pharmaceutical and biological products. Current viral and nonviral vectors do not yet provide a completely satisfactory means of propagating the therapeutic genes in proliferating cells. To increase the possibilities of success, the minichromosome, an artificial chromosome formed by reducing an existing chromosome, is under investigation. Using a method called telomere-mediated fragmentation, researchers reduce chromosomes to a size that can serve as a natural human vector for therapeutic genes. Nonviral gene therapy methods offer the potential for therapeutic interventions that may be acceptable to physicians and patients and offer safety and efficiency similar to those of conventional therapeutic modalities.[6,10]

Clinical Protocols for Gene Therapy

The Severe Combined Immunodeficiency Disease Protocol

The first approved clinical protocol for gene therapy was initiated in 1990. Two girls with ADA deficiency, a rare genetic condition that produces severe immunodeficiency in children, were injected with white blood cells carrying a therapeutic gene. The clinical protocol called for inserting the ADA gene into T lymphocytes.

ADA is an enzyme needed for normal immune system functioning. It prevents the buildup of deoxyadenosine, a metabolic product that becomes toxic to immune cells, especially lymphocytes, when present in high concentrations. ADA deficiency accounts for 25% of cases of severe combined immunodeficiency disease (SCID). The clinical protocol for treating ADA deficiency has served as a paradigm for both the benefits and the risks of gene therapy. It initially demonstrated the safety of retroviral gene transfer, and showed that patients could benefit from gene therapy.[10,18]

Treatment for ADA deficiency has also demonstrated the risks of gene therapy. In 2003, French researchers reported that two children with SCID who had been treated with retroviral gene therapy had developed a leukemia-like disorder 30 months after a single gene therapy treatment. In response to this discovery, the FDA put a hold on clinical trials that used retroviral vectors to insert the defective gene into hematopoetic cells. The American Society of Gene Therapy conducted its own investigation to determine why this occurred only in patients with SCID, and not in other trials with retroviruses.[18,19] Researchers have since discovered that the retrovirus used (Moloney murine leukemia virus, or MoMuLV) inserted the therapeutic genes next to a gene known to promote blood cancer. Insertional mutagenesis is a recognized complication of retroviral gene transfer attempts because gene integration occurs randomly. With MoMuLV, this appears to occur at the beginning of the gene, affecting how it works.[20]

Table 22-1 lists some examples of other single-gene disorders for which gene therapy is being investigated.

Gene Therapy Regulation

More than 700 clinical protocols have been approved throughout the world, and more than 4000 patients have been treated with therapeutic genes since the initiation of the SCID protocol.[14] Guidelines for clinical gene therapy protocols were established by the National Institutes of Health (NIH) in the document *Points to Consider in the Design and Submission of Human Somatic Cell Gene Therapy Protocols.* The guidelines require that proposals for human gene therapy go through several levels of review. Each proposed protocol must first be reviewed by local bioethics and biosafety committees and must be in accord with the standards of conventional research. The Human Gene Therapy Research Subcommittee and the Recombinant DNA Advisory Committee (RAC) then review the protocol. These two committees serve in an advisory capacity to the director of the NIH, who approves all gene transfer and gene therapy proposals.[21] The FDA addresses the scientific methodology and preclinical safety testing and has created a set of guidelines for the initiation of gene therapy. The FDA's guidelines are separate from the Human Genome Research Subcommittee and RAC guidelines and address the characteristics, production, and certification of the biological substances being used for gene transfer. The "Points to Consider" document is updated regularly and is found as an appendix of the NIH's guidelines on recombinant DNA research.[21–23]

As of early 2004, approximately 613 clinical protocols were approved in the United States. The majority of these (66%) are for the treatment of cancer. Genetic diseases such as cystic fibrosis and other single-gene disorders make up approximately 9.8% of clinical gene therapy protocols. Clinical gene therapy trials for the treatment of infectious disease (6.5%) and for conditions such as peripheral artery disease, rheumatoid arthritis, and coronary artery disease (10.9%) also are being carried out. The majority of these approved protocols are for phase I clinical trials.[14]

Cancer Gene Therapy

Treatment of cancer using gene therapy is aimed at inhibiting oncogene function and restoring tumor-suppressor function. *Proto-oncogenes* are normal cellular genes that are essential for cellular growth and development. Oncogenes stimulate neoplastic growth and are activated by proto-oncogenes that encode a growth factor or another protein and disturb normal cell development and regulation. *Antioncogenes* are those genes that block the action of growth-inducing proteins. These genes are also called tumor-suppressor genes to denote their ability to block the action of oncogenes. When functioning normally, tumor-suppressor genes and proto-oncogenes work together to enable the body to perform vital functions, such as replacing dead cells and repairing defective ones.[3]

Two types of gene transfer are used in clinical cancer gene therapy trials: gene marking and gene therapy. *Gene marking* involves labeling cells for future identification. A gene that has been genetically marked is introduced into cells, most commonly using a retrovirus as a vector for the desired gene. This approach is being used to determine the source of relapse in individuals undergoing autologous bone marrow transplantation. Gene marking studies have been used in the treatment of melanoma, leukemia, neuroblastoma, and stem cell transplantation.[24] *Gene therapy* studies involve modifying of the content or expression of altered genes in somatic cells by transferring the functional or enhanced genes.

Table 22-1 Examples of Approved Single-Gene Clinical Gene Therapy Trials

Inherited Genetic Condition	Target Tissue	Vector	Gene/Gene Product
Cystic fibrosis	Respiratory tract	Adenovirus, adeno-associated virus, liposomes	CFTR
Familial hypercholesterolemia	Hepatocytes	Retrovirus	LDL receptor
Severe immunodeficiency due to ADA deficiency	Lymphocytes	Retrovirus	ADA
Alpha-1 antitrypsin deficiency	Respiratory tract	Liposomes	Alpha-1 antitrypsin
Gaucher's disease	Lymphocytes	Retrovirus	Glulocerebrocidase
Hunter's syndrome	Lymphocytes	Retrovirus	Iduronate-sulfatase

CFTR = cystic fibrosis transmembrane conductance regulator; LDL = low density lipoprotein; ADA = adenosine deaminase.
Data from Balicki, Buetler.[10]

Cancer Gene Therapy Protocols

A number of protocols are investigating the transfer of genes to correct an error (gene alteration) or to add a new function (gene addition). These protocols use two general approaches. In one — a *tumor-directed* approach — the therapeutic gene is introduced into the tumor cells to destroy them. The other approach involves two forms of immunotherapy — active and adoptive. In the *active* immunotherapeutic approach, cytokines, tumor antigens, or tumor-associated antigens are introduced to stimulate the patient's immune system to mount an antitumor response. *Adoptive* immunotherapy involves the transfer of a genetically modified tumor lymphocyte to mediate tumor regression.[25,26] Such studies are founded on earlier gene marking studies that showed that a new gene could be safely inserted into patients and followed over time.

Tumor-directed gene therapy protocols

"Suicide gene" therapy protocols. These clinical trials involve the transfer of a gene that produces an enzyme whose activity converts a nontoxic prodrug to its toxic form — a "suicide gene." The gene transfer is targeted to tumor cells to make them susceptible to an agent that does not cause harm to normal cells but kills malignant cells. The suicide gene is toxic to dividing cells only, thus sparing the normal cells and nondividing tumor cells. The herpes simplex virus thymidine kinase gene (*HSV-TK*) is the one most commonly used. Any cell that incorporates the *HSV-TK* gene becomes sensitive to the antiviral drug ganciclovir and can be destroyed on exposure. Retroviral vectors transfer genes to actively dividing cells, making this type of gene therapy well suited for the treatment of brain tumors, as only the malignant cells are dividing and replicating. When a patient is treated with ganciclovir, the tumor cells are killed. Further modification of the promotor region of the vector creates tissue or organ specificity such that the suicide gene will be expressed only in cell types restricted by the specific promotor. For example, the insertion of a prostate-specific promotor directs the suicide gene to the prostate cells for expression and treatment of prostate cancer. Treatment with suicide gene vectors involves local injection into the tumor site. Anticipated complications are local and include bleeding, infection, and pain.[27]

Tumor-suppressor gene therapy. The tumor-suppressor gene, *TP53*, is found in approximately 50% of all cancers. In a number of clinical trials, a normal copy of the gene has been introduced to restore its function in patients with lung cancer, head and neck cancer, ovarian cancer, colorectal cancer, and bladder cancer. These treatments have met with some success. Clinical trials are now underway in which tumor-suppressor gene therapy is combined with chemotherapy to treat cancer.[28]

Antisense oligonucleotides. Genetic therapies for cancer treatment are being developed that specifically target DNA and RNA. The use of specific segments of DNA — antisense oligonucleotides — is one example of this new methodology. Antisense oligonucleotides are nucleic binding agents. They are short strands of nucleotides that predictably combine with other nucleotides. This property allows for the design of a treatment drug that can recognize a unique site on a specific gene. Oligonucleotides can be inserted into cells to interfere with the translation of RNA into an oncogene protein. When transferred into patients, they prevent the oncogene's RNA message from being translated into a functional oncogene protein. This approach is being used in clinical trials of anti-epidermal growth factor receptor in the treatment of head and neck squamous cell carcinoma.[29]

Oncolytic viral gene therapy. Oncolytic viruses reproduce in tumor cells, causing their lyses. These viruses can be used to treat cancers with a defective p53 pathway. In normal cells, p53 is destroyed by adenoviruses, producing a protein called E1B 55K. This protein binds with p53 and, in synchrony with another viral protein, directs p53 for destruction. Researchers have been able to modify a strain of adenovirus so that it does not encode E1B 55K and lose its ability to destroy p53. Normally, p53 activity causes a cascade of events that lead to the death of the affected cell, and viral replication cannot be established. In cancer cells that lack p53, however, the normal mechanism that leads to the death of the infected cells is abolished so that only the modified adenovirus can replicate and kill tumor cells. This approach is being used to treat head and neck cancer and, in some clinical trials, is being combined with chemotherapeutic agents.[30]

Active immunotherapy

Tumor-infiltrating lymphocytes. Host immunologic responses can be used to alter the natural course of some cancers, especially malignant melanoma. Tumor-infiltrating lymphocytes (TILs) that are able to mediate tumor regression in patients with melanoma have been identified. Using these TILs, researchers have mapped and cloned many genes encoding shared melanoma antigens and their antigenic epitopes. Administration of an epitope in conjunction with intravenous high dose IL-2 has been shown to mediate regression in patients with malignant melanoma. These findings have led to additional clinical trials using melanoma antigen genes to boost the immune system.[31]

Cytokine genes. Cytokines are molecules that enhance the body's immune response to tumor antigens. Cytokine genes are being used to augment the body's ability to mount an immune response to tumor cells. Two of the most commonly used cytokine genes are interleukein-2 (IL-2) and tumor necrosis factor. These cytokine genes are modified so that they will not proliferate but can still support expression of the introduced gene products. The modified cells are then injected into the patient via subcutaneous, intradermal, or intramuscular routes.[32]

DNA vaccines. Cancer vaccination is an example of an approach that is evolving into an effective and broadly applicable form of therapy. This approach circumvents the disadvantage of using common vectors such as adenovirus that cause the body to produce neutralizing antibodies or cellular immunity against the vector-derived gene products, rendering the vectors ineffective following administration. DNA vaccines that contain tumor-associated antigen genes or cytokine genes are now being used because the pure DNA encodes only the tumor-associated antigen gene. DNA vaccines are usually administered intramuscularly, alone or in combination with cytokine genes.[32]

Metastatic renal cell carcinoma is one cancer that has demonstrated responsiveness to immunotherapeutic intervention.[33] Therapeutic vaccine therapy is also being used in the treatment of prostate cancer. One phase III clinical trial is being conducted with a recombinant vaccine of prostatic acid antigen. This antigen is expressed in 95% of prostate cancers. When injected with the recombinant vaccine, the circulating immune cells recognize this antigen, and tumor response rates are boosted. Additional research is underway on tumor-specific vaccines using antigen-presenting cells such as dendritic cells to induce immune responses in T cells.[34]

Adoptive immunotherapy

Adoptive immunotherapy is a form of gene transfer therapy in which the patient's own lymphocytes (peripheral blood or from TILs) are modified outside of the body with genes that enhance their antitumor activity. The modified genes are then reinfused back into the same patient. Gene marking studies, although not therapeutic, use this approach to track, localize, and characterize the persistence of marked T cells.[32]

Chimeric receptors. Chimeric receptors are one example of adoptive immunotherapy. They consist of two different molecules brought together to form one functional molecule — an extracellular antibody molecule linked to intracellular signal domains of T-cell receptors. In this type of therapy, the patient's autologous T cells serve as the vehicle for inserted chimeric antibody molecules. The inserted antibody molecules have specificity for a tumor antigen. When transferred into patients, the modified T cells are redirected to recognize the tumor by virtue of the specific antibody on its surface. Once the tumor cells are engaged, the T-cells are activated via the signaling chain and mediate antitumor activity. This approach is being used in the treatment of patients with neuroblastoma, kidney cancer, and metastatic ovarian cancer.[32]

Tumor-specific T cells. Adoptive immunotherapy using transduction of the IL-2 gene into antitumor T lymphocytes is under investigation as a way of treating tumors and overcoming the limitation of toxicity following prolonged in vivo administration of IL-2. Transduction of an IL-2 gene into a TIL has been used with some success in the treatment of patients with melanoma and renal cell carcinoma.[10,32]

Pharmacogenetics: Gene-based treatment of cancer

Pharmacogenetics is an emerging field of individualized treatment that aims to identify the inherited basis for interindividual differences in drug response and to translate this to molecular diagnostics that can be used to indiviualize drug therapy. Many human genes involved in pharmacogenetic traits have now been identified, their molecular mechanisms elucidated, and their clinical use more clearly defined. Pharmacogenetics began with a focus on drug metabolism and has now been extended to include all aspects of drug disposition, absorption, distribution, and excretion.[35]

One of the most well-developed examples of clinical pharmacogenetics is the genetic polymorphism of thiopurine methyltransferase (TMPT). TMPT has been associated with altered drug metabolism and increased risk for severe toxicity from the anticancer agent 6-mercaptopurine. Testing for TMPT genotypes is now used to modify doses of 6-mercaptopurine and azothioprine that are used to treat acute lymphoblastic leukemia and inflammatory bowel disease. Individuals with deficient or intermediate TPMT activity are at risk for toxicity, including fatal myelosupression, at standard thiopurine doses. Testing for the presence of low-activity gene variants for TMPT has been done in clinical practice for more than 10 years in the United States. At present the testing applies to Caucasian populations in which the specific variant alleles are known. Further studies are needed to identify the variants that underlie the response in different populations.[36,37]

A similar example of pharmacogenetics has been observed with the antineoplastic agent 5-fluorouracil. Deficiency of the enzyme dihydropyrimidine dehydrogenase leads to severe toxicity from treatment with 5-fluorouracil using the usual doses. The dose of this drug therapy is now adjusted based on the DNA sequence of drug-metabolizing enzyme genes.[37]

Another example of individualized treatment is illustrated with trastuzumab (Herceptin). When overexpressed, HER2, a protein located in cell surfaces, causes cancers to become more aggressive. The HER2 oncogene is overexpressed in 20% to 30% of breast cancers, and these tumors seem to be more aggressive and somewhat more resistant to chemotherapy than those not overexpressing the oncogene. Clinical trials involving the use of gene therapy to deliver an antibody against the HER2 protein led to the creation of Herceptin, a humanized monoclonal antibody against the HER2 receptor that is linked to HER2 overexpression. It is now standard practice to test women with breast cancer for HER2 before initiation of treatment. Those with overexpression of HER2 benefit from treatment with Herceptin, either alone or in combination with chemotherapy, resulting in an improved response rate and overall survival advantage. Patients with breast cancer who do not have HER2 overexpression are prescribed alternate therapy.[38–40]

The discovery of the specific molecular defect BCR-ABL, which occurs as a result of the Philadelphia chromosome translocation, has created a new foundation for treating Philadelphia chromosome-positive leukemias. The Philadelphia chromosome translocation is present in more than 90% of patients with chronic myelogenous leukemia (CML). The translocation moves the *BCR* and *ABL* genes next to each other and causes the BCR-ABL tyrosine kinase to stay active. The activity of this kinase blocks apoptotic cell death and is the cause of chronic myeloid leukemia. The drug imitinib (Gleevac) was designed to target the molecular defect, and treatment with this specific medication has produced an 88% response in cases of Philadelphia chromosome-positive CML.[37]

Ethical, Social, and Legal Issues in Gene Therapy

As gene therapy has evolved over the past 30 years, professional and public scrutiny has focused on the ethical implications of the technology. Organized religions have taken an active part in discussions on the ethical implications of human gene therapy. The continuing dialogue among theologians, ethicists, and scientists has helped to shape and implement regulatory processes for gene therapy designed to safeguard against misuse.[9]

The NIH developed the guidelines "Points to Consider" in 1988 to solidify ethical concerns and to assist investigators and reviewers of human gene therapy proposals in addressing difficult issues.[9,21–23] The points, revised in 1990, provide a foundation for current and future clinical genome research. Information from the document was condensed to form six sets of ethical guidelines:

- Concern for the clinical benefit of all persons receiving gene therapy
- Assurance of informed consent
- Fair selection of persons for gene therapy research protocols
- Attention to the need for biosafety protocols
- Public involvement in genetic research policy
- Attention to long-term consequences of genetic research.

These considerations provide an ethical framework within which researchers and healthcare professionals can address the multitude of questions that are evolving as recombinant techniques and gene therapy become more common.[9,22,23]

Assessing Clinical Benefits

One guideline expressed in "Points to Consider" concerns the need to assess the clinical benefits of gene therapy. This refers to the researcher's responsibility to ensure that the risk to the participant for any gene therapy protocol is outweighed by the benefit of the treatment. To meet this responsibility, researchers must have adequate knowledge of the treatment to determine whether the participant will benefit more from the gene therapy trial than from any alternative treatment for the condition.

In 1995, the director of the NIH convened a panel to assess the NIH's investment in gene therapy research. The panel concluded that gene therapy had been oversold to the public and that the publicity surrounding gene therapy was already causing some patients to forgo conventional therapeutic interventions. Panel members emphasized the importance of research aimed at developing a better understanding of the underlying mechanisms that contribute to genetic disease. In October 1999, the first fatality related to gene therapy occurred and was reported. Subsequent investigations revealed the deaths of six additional gene therapy patients that had not received the usual public disclosure. In February 2000, the United States Senate held hearings on this topic, and the heightened scrutiny and awareness has resulted in an increase in the reporting of adverse effects and renewed oversight of gene therapy trials by both the NIH and the FDA.[9] This kind of research and public debate conducted to support ethical and scientifically sound development and application of gene therapy trials will better meet the needs of patients participating in the trials.[41]

Participant Selection and Informed Consent

The "Points to Consider" document also notes that potential research subjects should choose freely to participate in gene therapy. The choice of the participants must be equitable, and candidates for gene therapy research need to be chosen fairly from among multiple populations. Those populations considered to be vulnerable, such as prisoners, should not serve as subjects.[21,42] Participant selection also involves compassionate or "emergency" use of gene therapy. A request was made to the NIH RAC in 1993 for compassionate use of a gene therapy protocol, for example, for a patient with limited life expectancy. The request, although finally granted, generated many questions regarding emergency access to gene therapy and fairness to other participants. If one patient is granted permission, how can a researcher turn down other applicants? How does the researcher maintain the integrity of the research data if emergency-use patients, who do not meet the clinical trial research criteria, are accepted into the protocol? These and other concerns about subject selection presented to the RAC underscore some of the inherent issues in regulating of any new and as yet unproven therapy.[43]

Clinical research always involves an informed consent process to ensure that subjects participating in the research are doing so freely and voluntarily and with full information about the risks and benefits.[44–46] This precedent does not require that protocols be completely risk free or that the benefits be unequivocally established before clinical trials are proposed. Rather, the premise of informed consent is that the risks are honestly described, and the patient considering the research ultimately decides the value of the potential benefits, weighed against the possible risks. When minors are involved as participants in clinical gene therapy trials, the "Points to Consider" document emphasizes the need for informed consent by the minor in addition to obtaining parental permission.[21] The informed consent process for gene therapy protocols should also include a discussion of plans for follow-up with primary care providers, social workers, geneticists, and psychologists, in addition to the clinical investigators. Including these professionals in a follow-up plan ensures that participants will receive support in all areas of health care, including reproduction and psychological development, and normal processes that may be influenced by participation in gene therapy.

The issue of informed consent becomes more problematic when germ-line therapy is considered. Germ-line gene therapy would alter the genes of future generations and possibly create unknown long-term consequences. Germ-line gene therapy also raises the ethical concern that future unborn generations would not be able to give informed consent before gene therapy makes deliberate changes to their genetic code. For this and other ethical reasons, germ-line therapy is currently prohibited.[9,47]

Safety Issues

Short- and long-term side effects and toxicities associated with new gene therapy interventions also are of concern. Programs that implement human clinical gene therapy trials must emphasize staff expertise, training of professional support staff, and patient and family counseling. These factors are deemed essential to ensure the safety and successful implementation of gene therapy research.[8]

Patient safety

To date, a number of deaths due to gene therapy have been reported, and several children undergoing gene therapy for SCID have developed a leukemia-like

Table 22-2 Common Adverse Effects Reported in Worldwide Clinical Trials for Cancer Gene Therapy

Vector	Adverse Effect
Retrovirus	Erythema and induration, pruritus, pain, fever, elevation of LFTs, peritumor edema, abdominal pain, diarrhea, nausea, increased local edema, seizures abducens, paresis, confusion, intratumoral hemorrhage, mild exacerbation of graft-versus-host disease
Adenovirus	Fever, abnormal liver function, fatigue, pulmonary infiltrate, transient lung function abnormalities
Liposome	Injection pain, transient pneumothorax
Plasmid	Fever

LFTs = liver function tests.
Data from Cuaron, Gallucci[24]; Liu[32].

illness.[18–20] These toxicities have led to increased vigilance regarding patient safety. As with any research drug protocol, during administration, patients need to be observed and evaluated for an allergic reaction to the foreign protein. Common side effects reported thus far include fever, chills, headache, fatigue, myalgia, nausea, and vomiting. Less common side effects reported include anorexia, diarrhea, and central nervous system effects such as extremity weakness, anemia, and leukopenia. Table 22-2 summarizes side effects commonly reported with some of the more common vectors. Researchers cannot at this time predict the long-term risks to patients undergoing gene therapy or to their children. Some adverse effects may not become apparent for years. Vigilant follow-up care is needed to identify, diagnose, and prevent side effects. Long-term follow-up care may not be built into gene therapy protocols. Nurses caring for individuals who have undergone gene therapy must therefore be aware of this potential gap and develop a plan for following and monitoring patients.[8]

Public safety

The safety of those working with this new method of drug delivery is a second important concern. Safety involves protecting providers, families, and the public from the possibility of infectious transmission of recombinant genes with viral vectors. To date, infectious spread of recombinant viruses has not been observed, and the risk of this complication is considered to be remote. Not all gene therapy protocols use retroviral vectors, and those that do may not all use them in the same way. Implementing universal precautions in consultation with nursing and hospital infection control officers is one safety measure that has been put in place for clinical trials using viral vectors, as these precautions are considered sufficient to prevent transmission of known pathogens such as hepatitis and HIV.[42]

Equal Access to Gene Therapy and Confidentiality of Genetic Information

As more is learned about the safety and efficacy of gene therapies to treat cancer, additional ethical issues will arise concerning the cost, availability, and allocation of these therapies. Development of a new gene therapy trial costs over $1 million.[9] It is critical to consider the ethical implications of treatments developed for individuals with end-stage disease versus research directed toward prevention and cause of disease. As with any costly treatment, access to gene therapy may be provided to only a select few. Medical centers are the only institutions that can provide gene therapies, possibly meaning additional patient expense for travel and lodging, for which insurance companies do not pay. Patients could spend large amounts of their own money just to get to and stay near their treatment location unless this cost is covered by research money. The potential for an ever-widening disparity in health and quality of life among individuals thus becomes a greater possibility than before.[9]

The potential for gene therapy as a viable intervention raises several other ethical concerns. Genetic testing and gene therapies reveal information about individuals and family members. This information has the potential to label currently healthy individuals as being "at risk." As genetic testing and therapeutics become more common, personal and family genetic information may inadvertently become public. The Americans with Disabilities Act of 1990 offers protection against genetic discrimination in the workplace, but many questions remain about the possibilities for genetic discrimination by insurance companies and employers. Confidentiality, although viewed as the foundation of the patient–provider relationship, needs to be enforced in all areas of genetic testing and research. Ethical aspects of care, such as confidentiality, are core elements of professional nursing practice. The Code of Ethics for nurses created by the American Nurses Association provides an ethical foundation for nurses and a direction for practice.[8,48]

Emerging Ethical Issues in Gene Therapy

The RAC, which advises the NIH director on gene therapy, has engaged in discussions about fetal gene therapy. Two serious and life-threatening genetic disorders — ADA deficiency and alpha-thalassemia — are under consideration for fetal gene therapy. Current issues being debated include whether it is better to treat a disease for which backup therapies exist, as is the case for ADA deficiency, or to go forward with gene treatment for alpha-thalassemia, a blood disorder that is often fatal to fetuses. At this stage,

Table 22-3 Internet Sources for Gene Therapy

- *http://www.nci.nih.gov* — National Cancer Institute
- *http://www.nhgri.nih.gov* — National Human Genome Research Institute
- *http://www.nlm.nih.gov/medlineplus/genesandgenetherapy.html* — Medline Health Information
- *http://cis.nci.nih.gov/fact/7_18.htm* — National Cancer Institute: Cancer Facts. Questions and Answers about Gene Therapy
- *http://www.accessexcellence.org/AB/IWT/GENE_Therapy_Overview.html*— The National Health Museum. Gene Therapy: An Overview
- *http://www.georgetown.edu/research/nrcbl/scopenotes/sn24.html*— Background and historical information, religious and philosophical issues, public policy, and additional readings on gene therapy. From the Georgetown University National Reference Center for Bioethics Literature
- *http://www.fda.gov/cber/infosheets/genezn.htm* — Human Gene Therapy and the Role of the Food and Drug Administration

participants in the discussions agree that more data are needed about the safety and efficacy of fetal gene therapy as well as information on the possible alteration of fetuses' germ-line cells.[9,49] Information is available to educate the public about gene therapy and related social and ethical issues. Table 22-3 lists on-line resources for information regarding gene therapy and the Human Genome Project.

Practice Implications for Oncology Nurses

The evolution of genetics and its important role in health and disease are leading to continuous changes in nursing practice. To meet the changing clinical and educational needs of individuals, families, and communities, oncology nurses and the entire nursing community need to be knowledgeable and fluent in handling new genetic concepts and information.[8,50] Oncology nurses caring for individuals who are participating in gene therapy trials will be involved in providing direct care, educating individuals and the public, and advocating for fair and equitable use and for the confidentiality and privacy of genetic information. Table 22-4 outlines the roles for oncology nurses providing genetic-related health care in these areas.[51] Two emerging roles for oncology nurses are provider of genetic services and clinical investigator in nursing genetic research, as discussed in the next section.[8,50]

Provider of Genetic Services

The identification of genes that predispose certain individuals to cancer and developments in gene therapy are expanding the role for oncology nurses as genetic service providers. Oncology nurses now have the opportunity to participate in counseling individuals and families who are at increased risk of cancer by identifying risk factors and genes associated with cancer predisposition. Although these services are not uniformly available, many centers, clinics, and community practices are increasing their activities in this area.[50]

Genetic services include identifying individuals and families in need of further genetic evaluation and testing, referring these individuals to more specialized genetics professionals, and participating in the genetic counseling process. These services are a critical component of cancer risk assessment and treatment. Oncology nurses, by virtue of their specialized training in and knowledge of cancer and their sensitivity to the influence of family and cultural beliefs on healthcare decisions, can incorporate components of the genetic counseling process into the care of individuals receiving gene therapy and their families.[8,50] The Oncology Nursing Society has created a position statement titled "The Role of the Oncology Nurse in Cancer Genetic Counseling" that outlines the emerging roles for oncology nurses participating in the genetic counseling process.[52]

Nursing Research

Gene therapy as a clinical treatment for cancer is in its early stages. Many issues regarding response to gene therapy remain for patients undergoing gene therapy. The oncology nurse needs to consider the following issues:

- The long-term physical and psychosocial ramifications of gene therapy
- How individuals and families adapt to new genetic information and therapies
- How cultural and family backgrounds may influence individuals' decision making
- What educational materials and methods are best suited for providing information about gene therapy
- How to prepare primary care practitioners, especially nurses, to care for individuals and families throughout life following gene therapy

Oncology nurses as direct caregivers, educators, and advocates can have an instrumental role in initiating and participating in nursing research to help address these issues.[8] They can also play a leading role in developing longitudinal research efforts focusing on the continuum of identifying individual responses and adaptation to genetic cancer risk, testing, treatment, and

Table 22-4 Nursing Responsibilities in Caring for Patients and Families Undergoing Gene Therapy

Direct Caregiver
• Provides anticipatory guidance
• Assures informed decision-making/consent
• Develops treatment and management plans
• Administers gene therapy
• Observes patients for expected and unexpected side effects of treatment, including psychosocial and emotional response
• Participates in developing long-term follow-up plans
• Assures coordination and collaboration of care with all healthcare providers involved in patient/family care before, during, and after gene therapy
Educator
• Serves as an information source to patients, families, and the public
• Provides relevant, accurate, and understandable information to patients, in both written and verbal form
• Assures that all patient/family questions are answered
Advocate
• Assures privacy and confidentiality of genetic information
• Protects against discrimination
• Advocates for fair and equitable use of gene therapies for all populations
• Promotes public understanding of somatic gene therapy
Genetics Services Provider
• Gathers relevant family history information
• Identifies individuals and families in need of further genetic education and counseling
• Assesses psychosocial, ethnocultural, and educational background
• Provides psychosocial support in follow-up to genetic counseling
Research Investigator
• Participates in or conducts clinical research trials in gene therapy
• Serves as a preceptor to other nurses
• Develops research protocols that will address patient/family response and adaptation to genetic information, including gene therapy

Reprinted with permission from Lea DH: Gene therapy: Current and future implications for oncology nursing practice. *Semin Oncol Nurs* 13:115–122, 1997.[51]

post-treatment. Nurses can identify fluctuations in the coping process and recognize optimal times for psychosocial interventions and support. Other areas for oncology nursing research include determining effective means of tailoring information to individuals from differing educational and cultural backgrounds, and developing nursing management approaches to address family concerns with regard to gene therapy.[8]

Future Issues for Oncology Nurses

Human genome discoveries and the expanding roles of gene therapy, and pharmacogenetics, are leading to dramatic breakthroughs in cancer treatment. Gene therapy and pharmacogenetics hold the promise of increasing the ability to tailor treatments to certain populations or to individual patients, improving responsiveness to medications.[49,53] In the near future, nurses will increasingly care for patients participating in clinical trials and receiving targeted drug therapies, and will be called upon to assist families with decision making and to collaborate with other healthcare professionals to maintain continuity and coordination of care. In most acute and chronic healthcare settings, it is nurses who have the greatest contact with patients and who will administer the gene therapy or pharmacogenetic intervention. Nurses, as always, will have the obligation to detect changes in a patient's condition that may arise as a consequence of any of these therapies.[54]

Nurses will increasingly care for patients from diverse ethnic backgrounds and cultures. Culturally safe nursing care reflects the priorities and health needs of those receiving the care. Such care will be important with respect to gene therapy and pharmacogenetics. When ethnic differences are known to influence the choice of and responses to a particular gene-based intervention, the nurse needs to be observant and vigilant.[53] As technologies to create gene-based therapies advance, new and more individualized tools will become available that are more precise than ethnicity and will allow for culturally safe care for all populations.

Genomics research contributes to our knowledge and understanding of biology, health, and life. Although many aspects of this understanding will be of benefit to individuals, families, and communities, some applications will be controversial and will call for societal dialogues to define appropriate and inappropriate uses of genomics. Nurses need to contribute to those dialogues. As part of their responsibility to promote the health and welfare of individuals, families, and communities, oncology nurses must participate in the development of social policies regarding safety, financial, and ethical issues related to gene therapy and pharmacogenetics. One of the major ethical issues concerns equal access to and the affordability of health care, including reimbursement for gene-based technologies for targeted treatment. Oncology nurses are represented at the policy level on the Secretary's Advisory Committee on Genetic Health Care, which is addressing these issues. In this role, they are helping to shape new healthcare delivery options that include gene therapy and pharmacogenetics, to make these treatments available to all populations.[8]

Nurses are accustomed to viewing individuals in a holistic way that takes into account each person's physical, mental, spiritual, social, and cultural attributes. New genomic discoveries and technologies used to classify or categorize people by their race and ethnicity for the purpose of understanding human variation and to tailor diagnostics and therapeutics have the potential to redirect individual, family, and community identity from the social domain into the physical aspects of the body. The prominent focus on the genetic aspects may overshadow other factors, such as poverty and access to health services and the ways that each of these factors affects health and disease. Nurses and other healthcare providers will need to seek ways to utilize and interpret all aspects of health information in caring for individuals, families, and communities.

Oncology nurses practicing in all settings will be challenged as they care for individuals before, during, and after gene therapy interventions. They can meet these challenges by preparing to support and facilitate patients' decision making and their adaptation to genetic interventions, to face ethical and social issues, and to promote and advocate for the safe and fair use of this new technology. Oncology nurses can best prepare themselves for these tasks by becoming knowledgeable about all aspects of gene therapy and, as in any new clinical situation, by examining their views and values and their role in the effective delivery of genetic health care.

References

1. Collins FS, Green ED, Guttmacher AE: A vision for the future of genomics research: a blueprint for the genomics era. *Nature* 422:835–847, 2003
2. Rimoin DL, Connor JM, Pyeritz RE (eds.): *Emery and Rimoin's Principles and Practice of Medical Genetics* (ed 4). New York, Churchill Livingstone, 2002
3. Nussbaum RL, McInnes RR, Willard HF (eds.). *Thomson and Thomson: Genetics in Medicine* (ed 6). Philadelphia, Saunders, 2001
4. Omim: Online Mendelian Inheritance in Man. *www.ncbi.nlm.nih.gov/omim/*. Accessed September 3, 2004
5. McCandless SE, Brunger JW, Cassidy SB: The burden of genetic disease on inpatient care in a children's hospital. *Am J Hum Genetics* 74:121–127, 2003
6. Ulrich CM, Robien K, McLeod HL: Cancer pharmacogenetics: polymorphisms, pathways and beyond. *Nat Rev Cancer* 3:912–920, 2003
7. Hull, CD: Gene therapy trials: a patient pathway. *Nurs Standard* 17:39–42, 2002
8. Rieger, PT: The role of oncology nurses in gene therapy. *Lancet Oncol* 2:233–238, 2001
9. National Reference Center for Bioethics Literature: *Human Gene Therapy*. Scope Note 24. National Reference Center for Bioethics Literature, The Joseph and Rose Kennedy Institute of Ethics, Georgetown University, *www.georgetown.e3du/research/nrcbl/scopenotes/sn24.html*. Accessed February 2, 2004
10. Balicki D, Beutler E: Reviews in molecular medicine: Gene therapy of human disease. *Medicine* 81:69–86, 2002
11. Kafri T, Blomer U, Peterson DA, et al: Sustained expression of genes delivered directly into liver and muscle by lentiviral vectors. *Nat Genet* 17:314–317, 1997
12. Bilbao G, Feng M, Rancourt C, et al: Adenoviral/retroviral vector chimeras: a novel strategy to achieve high-efficiency stable transduction in vivo. *FASEB J* 11:624–634, 1997
13. Schneirle BS, Groner B: Retroviral targeted delivery. *Gene Ther* 3:1069–1073, 1996
14. *The Journal of Gene Medicine*, 2004, *www.wiley.co.uk/genmed/clinical*. Accessed September 3, 2004
15. NIH News — NHGRI Study. *www.nih.gov/news/*. Accessed September 3, 2004
16. Naldini L, Blomer P, Gallay D, et al: In vivo gene delivery and stable transduction of non-dividing cells by a lentiviral vector. *Science* 272:263–267, 1996
17. Kouraklis GP: Gene therapy for cancer: current status and prospects. *Dig Dis Sci* 48:854–855, 2003
18. Noguchi P: Risks and benefits of gene therapy. *N Engl J Med* 348:193–194, 2003
19. Marwick C: FDA halts gene therapy trials after leukaemia case in France. *BMJ* 326:181, 2003
20. Buckley R: Gene therapy for SCID: a complication after remarkable progress. *Lancet* 360:1185–1186, 2003
21. Jeungst E: The NIH "Points to Consider" and the limits of human gene therapy. *Hum Gene Ther* 1:425–433, 1990
22. U.S. Department of Health and Human Services: New initiative to protect participants in gene therapy trials. March 7, 2000. *www.fda.gov/fdac/features/2000/500_gene.html*. Accessed March 30, 2004
23. Points to consider in the design and submission of protocols for the transfer of recombinant DNA molecules into one or more research participants. *www4.od.nih.gov/oba/rac/guidelines_02/Appendix_M.htm*. Accessed March 30, 2004
24. Cuaron LJ, Gallucci B: Gene therapy and blood cell transplantation. *Semin Oncol Nurs* 13:200–207, 1997
25. McCormick F: Cancer gene therapy: fringe or cutting edge? *Nat Rev Cancer* 1:130–141, 2001
26. Rosenberg SA: Progress in human tumor immunology and immunotherapy. *Nature* 411:380–384, 2001
27. Hall SJ, Canfield SE, Yan Y, et al: A novel bystander effect involving tumor cell-derived Fas and FasL interactions following Ad. HSV-tk and Ad.mIL-12 gene therapies in experimental prostate cancer. *Gene Ther* 9:511–517, 2002
28. Nemunaitis J, Swisher SG, Timmons T, et al: Adenovirus mediated p53 gene transfer in sequence with cisplatin to tumors of patients with non-small-cell lung cancer. *J Clin Oncol* 18: 609–622, 2000
29. Ford AC, Grandix JR: Targeting epidermal growth factor receptor in head and neck cancer. *Head Neck* 25:67–73, 2003
30. Nemunaitis J, Khuri F, Ganly I, et al: Phase II trial of intratumoral administration of ONYX-015, a replication-selective adenovirus, in patients with refractory head and neck cancer. *J Clin Oncol* 19:289–298, 2001
31. Kawakami Y, Wang X, Shofuda T, et al: Isolation of a new melanoma antigen, MART-2, containing a mutated epitope recognized by autologous tumor-infiltrating lymphocytes. *J Immunol* 166:2871–2877, 2001
32. Liu K: Breakthroughs in cancer gene therapy. *Semin Oncol Nurs* 19:217–226, 2003
33. Vieweg J, Dunnull J: Tumor vaccines: from gene therapy to dendrite cells — the emerging frontier. *Urologic Clin North Am* 30:633–643, 2003

34. Gemmill R, Idell CS: Biological advances for new treatment approaches. *Semin Oncol Nurs* 19:162–168, 2003
35. Evans WE: Pharmacogenomisc: marshalling the human genome to individualize drug therapy. *Gut* 52 (suppl 11): ii10–ii18, 2003
36. Goldstein DB, Tate SK, Sisodiya SM: Pharmacogenetics goes genomic. *Nature Rev* 4: 837–947, 2003
37. Reidenberg MM: Evolving ways that drug therapy is individualized. *Clin Pharmacol Ther* 74:197–202, 2003
38. Hortobagyi GN: Treatment of breast cancer. *N Engl J Med* 339:974–984, 1998
39. Slamon D, Leyland-Jones B, Shak S, et al: Addition of herceptin (humanized anti-HER2 antibody) to first line chemotherapy for HER2 over-expressing metastatic breast cancer markedly increases anticancer activity: a randomized, multinational controlled phase III trial. *Proc Am Soc Clin Oncol* 17:98a, 1998, (abstr)
40. Tsai YJ, Hoyme HE: Pharmacogenomics: the future of drug therapy. *Clin Genet* 62:257–64, 2002
41. Orkin SH, Motulsky AG: *Report and Recommendations of the Panel to Assess the NIH Investment in Research on Gene Therapy. www.nih.gov/od/orda/panelrep.htm.* Accessed March 30, 2004
42. Subcommittee on Human Gene Therapy, Recombinant DNA Advisory Committee, National Institutes of Health. Points to consider in the design and submission of protocols for the transfer of recombinant DNA into the genome of human subjects. *Hum Gene Ther* 1:93–103, 1990
43. Capron A, Leventhal B, Post L: Requests for compassionate use of gene therapy: Memorandum from the subcommittee to the RAC, January 13, 1993. *Hum Gene Ther* 4:199–200, 1993
44. U.S. Surgeon General: *U.S. Public Health Service Investigation Involving Human Subjects, Including Clinical Research: Requirements for Review to Insure the Rights and Welfare of Individuals.* Public policy order no. 129, 1966
45. Code of Federal Regulations, Title 45, Part 46: *Protection of Human Subjects* (revised March 8, 1983), 1980
46. Faden R, Beauchamp T: *A History and Theory of Informed Consent.* New York, Oxford University Press, 1986
47. Fletcher JC, Richter G: Human fetal gene therapy: moral and ethical questions. *Hum Gene Ther* 7:1605–1614, 1996
48. American Nurses Association: *Code of Ethics for Nurses with Interpretive Statements.* Washington, DC, American Nurses Association, 2001
49. Jenks S: Researchers seek guidance on "preproposal" for *in utero* gene therapy. *J Natl Cancer Inst* 90:1507, 1998
50. Lea DH, Jenkins J, Francomano C: *Genetics in Clinical Practice: New Directions for Nursing and Health Care.* Sudbury, MA, Jones and Bartlett, 1998
51. Lea DH: Gene therapy: Current and future implications for oncology nursing practice. *Semin Oncol Nurs* 13:115–122, 1997
52. Oncology Nursing Society: The role of the oncology nurse in cancer genetic counseling. *Oncol Nurs Forum* 27:1348, 2000
53. Fibison, W: Gene therapy. *Clin Genetics* 35:757–772, 2000
54. Nicol MJ: The variation of response to pharmacotherapy: pharmacogenetics — a new perspective to "The right drug for the right person." *MEDSURG Nurs* 12:242–249, 2003

CHAPTER 23

Hematopoietic Therapy

Barbara Holmes Gobel, RN, MS, AOCN®

Introduction

Hematopoietic growth factors (HGFs), also called colony-stimulating factors, are glycoproteins that act on hematopoietic cells by binding to specific cell surface receptors and stimulating proliferation, differentiation, and commitment and some end-cell functional activation. The recombinant version of these HGFs is used as supportive therapy to prevent hematopoietic complications of myelosuppressive chemotherapy or hematopoietic stem cell transplantation (HSCT). Chemotherapy is associated with side effects including anemia, neutropenia, and thrombocytopenia. These side effects can affect outcomes related to therapy by interfering with dosing schedules, causing dose reductions, contributing to life-threatening complications (e.g., bleeding and infection), and contributing to an impaired quality of life.

Patients may need to be treated with blood component therapy at different times during the course of their disease or therapy. Unfortunately, even with the significant technological advances that have been made in blood transfusion therapy, there are still significant side effects related to this therapy. In addition, patients' blood counts may continue to be affected by cytotoxic therapy even when treated with the recombinant HGFs.

This chapter reviews the process of hematopoiesis and the role of the naturally occurring HGFs. It covers the recombinant HGFs, including both the single lineage and multilineage growth factors. The issues of anemia, neutropenia, and thrombocytopenia are considered in light of their treatment with the HGFs. The role of blood component therapy is also reviewed, including indications, treatment, and complications.

Hematopoietic Growth Factors

Hematopoiesis

Hematopoiesis is the process by which blood cells are formed. During fetal development, the blood-forming organs include the spleen, liver, and bone marrow. The bone marrow is the primary site of hematopoiesis at the time of birth. During childhood, hematopoiesis takes place in the ribs, skull, spleen, pelvis, liver, sternum, vertebrae, and the proximal epiphyses of the long bones; all these but the liver are involved in adult hematopoiesis. Bone marrow provides a specialized environment in which hematopoietic progenitor cells proliferate and become committed to differentiation. Within the marrow, various elements — including the structural or stromal elements (fibroblasts, endothelial cells, fat cells) and the accessory cells (macrophages and lymphocytes) — interact, either to enhance or inhibit hematopoiesis.

All of a person's blood cell lines derive from a pluripotent stem cell, or common progenitor cell, which is capable of extensive, possibly lifelong self-renewal and can differentiate to all cell lineages.[1] The stem cell is not normally in an active cycle, and only a small percentage of cells will reproduce. When the cell must undergo division, a daughter cell leaves the stem cell pool and passes through a series of divisions and maturational changes, culminating in the formation of mature blood cells that are found in the circulating blood. The processes of proliferation, differentiation, and commitment are mediated by various humoral factors, primarily by an expanding set of hematopoietic growth factors. See Figure 23-1 for an outline of blood cell development and the factors that mediate this process.

Early on in blood cell development, the progeny of the pluripotent stem cell form a population of multipotent progenitor cells that are uncommitted to any cell line and have a limited self-renewing capacity. The colony-forming unit CFU-GEMM is an example of the multipotent stem cell for granulocyte, erythroid, monocyte, and megakaryocyte lines and can develop into any one of these lines. The lymphoid cell line follows a separate course of development.

As cells continue to differentiate, they become committed to specific cell lines. At this level, progenitor cells are called *unipotent* or *bipotent*, describing their ability to follow one or two cell lines, respectively. These cells include colony-forming units for granulocytes, monocytes, and macrophages (CFU-GMM); colony-forming units for eosinophils (CFU-EO); burst-forming units for erythroid (BFU-E); colony-forming units for erythroid (CFU-E); and colony-forming units for megakaryocytes (CFU-MK) and are committed stem cells.[1] Committed stem cells become increasingly differentiated and morphologically recognizable as belonging to a specific cell line. Ultimately, the cell undergoes further division and becomes a mature component of the circulating blood.

Hematopoietic growth factors

HGFs are a set of hormonelike glycoproteins or cytokines that mediate hematopoiesis for all blood cell lines. They govern the production of blood at every level of cell development. Some HGFs appear to have an effect on more than one blood cell line. Interleukin-3 (IL-3), also called multi-colony-stimulating factor, is a growth factor for a variety of progenitor cells, as is granulocyte-macrophage colony-stimulating factor (GM-CSF). These HGFs stimulate the growth of multiple lines of the progenitor cells (*multilineage*) and cells already committed to myeloid, erythroid, or

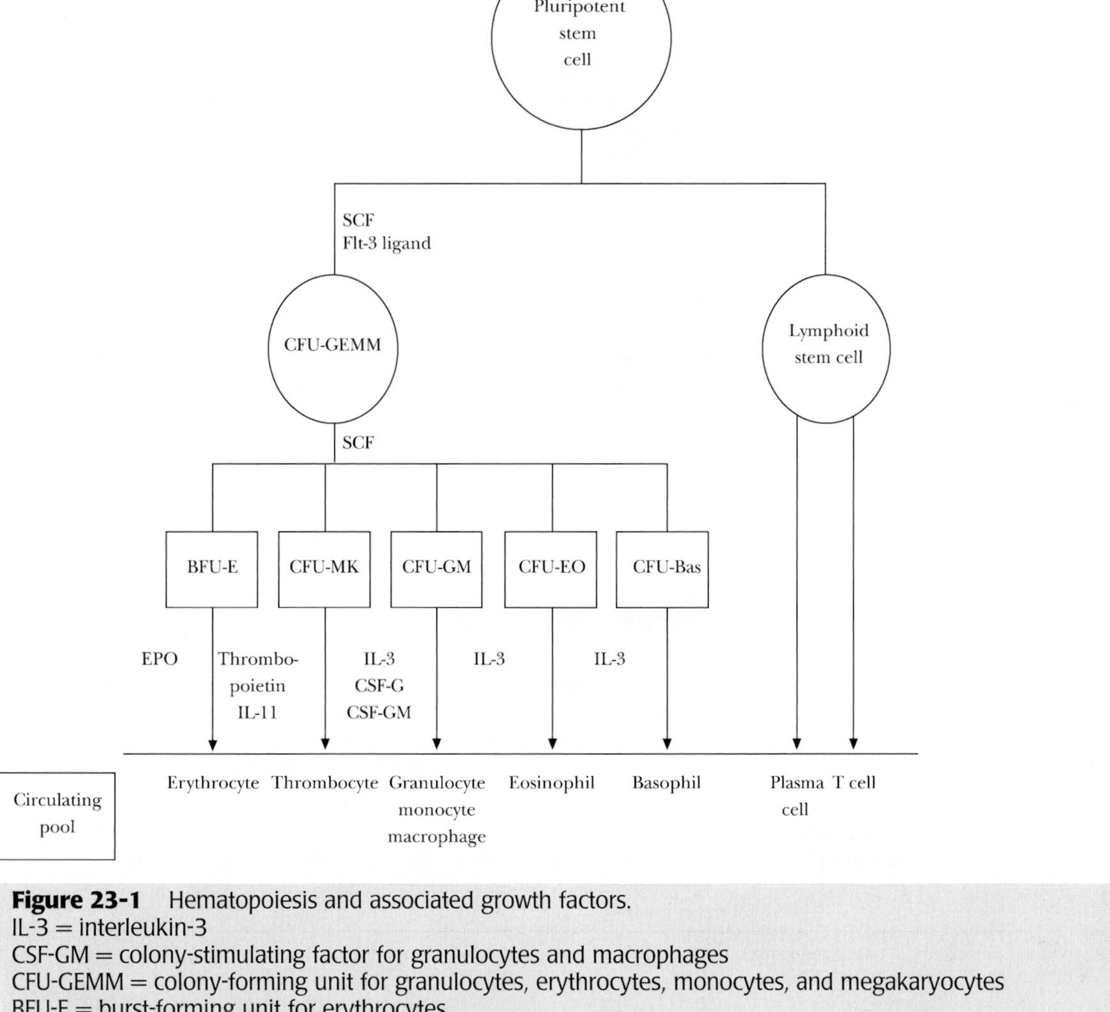

Figure 23-1 Hematopoiesis and associated growth factors.
IL-3 = interleukin-3
CSF-GM = colony-stimulating factor for granulocytes and macrophages
CFU-GEMM = colony-forming unit for granulocytes, erythrocytes, monocytes, and megakaryocytes
BFU-E = burst-forming unit for erythrocytes
CFU-MK = colony-forming unit for megakaryocytes
CFU-GM = colony-forming unit for granulocytes and macrophages
CFU-EO = colony-forming unit for eosinophils
CFU-Bas = colony-forming unit for basophils
EPO - erythropoietin
IL-11 = interleukin-11
CSF-G = colony-stimulating factor for granulocytes
SCF = stem cell factor
Flt-3 ligand = FMS-like tyrosine-3 ligand

megakaryocte lines.[2] Other HGFs stimulate production of cells along single blood cell lines (*lineage specific*). Granulocyte-CSF (G-CSF), macrophage-CSF, and erythropoietin (EPO) stimulate the growth predominantly of granulocytes, monocytes, and red blood cells, respectively. It is hypothesized that an overlap of the effects of one factor on another probably occurs and that the HGFs are not truly lineage specific.[3] HGFs appear to act on specific cells because of receptors that reside on the target cell membrane. The different distribution of these specific receptors may help to explain why they are responsive to some HGFs and not others.

Recombinant hematopoietic growth factors

Recombinant DNA technology has allowed for mass production of the naturally occurring hematopoietic growth factors for clinical use. Some of the recombinant HGFs are lineage specific, stimulating only a single blood cell line. Examples of lineage-specific growth factors include EPO, which stimulates the erythropoietin line of blood cells, and G-CSF, which stimulates the granulocyte blood cell line. Multilineage growth factors are developed to stimulate more than one line of blood cells. An example of a multilineage growth factor is GM-CSF, which stimulates the

Table 23-1 FDA-Approved Hematopoietic Growth Factors

Agent	Generic Name	Trade Name	Indications	Dose	Route
G-CSF	Filgrastim	Neupogen (Amgen, Inc., Thousand Oaks, CA)	Decrease neutropenia after chemotherapy in nonmyeloid malignancies; after induction/consolidation chemotherapy for AML, and in SCT PBPC mobilization	Chemotherapy: 5 μg/kg/day, administer 24 hr after chemotherapy, for up to 2 wk until ANC nadir >10,000/mm^3 BMT: 10 μg/kg/day, then titrate per counts	SC, IV
G-CSF	Pegfilgrastim	Neulasta (Amgen, Inc., Thousand Oaks, CA)	Decrease incidence of infection, as manifested by febrile neutropenia in patients with nonmyeloid malignancies receiving myelosuppressive chemotherapy	6 mg dose once per cycle of chemotherapy	SC
GM-CSF	Sargramostim	Leukine (Immunex Corp., Seattle, WA)	Accelerate bone marrow recovery after BMT; in allogeneic BMT with delayed or failed engraftment; after induction therapy in AML, and in PBPC mobilization	250 μg/m^2/day until ANC >1500/mm^3 × 3 days	SC, IV
Erythropoietin alfa	Epoietin alfa	Procrit (Ortho Biotech, Inc., Raritan, NJ); Epogen (Amgen, Inc., Thousand Oaks, CA)	Treatment of anemia in patients with chronic renal failure, cancer patients on chemotherapy, HIV+ patients receiving AZT, and surgical patients	For chemotherapy, recommended starting dose 150 units/kg, 3×/wk × 8–12 wk; adjust to maintain desired hematocrit	SC, IV
Erythropoietin alfa	Darbepoetin alfa	Aranesp (Amgen, Inc., Thousand Oaks, CA)	Treatment of anemia associated with nonmyeloid malignancies, chronic renal failure, including patients on dialysis and not on dialysis	For chronic renal failure, 0.45 μg/kg once a week, titrated to not exceed 12 g/dL	SC, IV
Interleukin-11	Oprelvekin	Neumega (Genetics Institute, Cambridge, MA)	Prevent thrombocytopenia and reduce need for patient transfusions following myelosuppressive chemotherapy	Adults: 50 μg/kg/day until post-nadir patient count is >50,000/mm^3 (max 21 days)	SC

AML = acute myelogenous leukemia; ANC = absolute neutrophil count; AZT = zidovudine; BMT = bone marrow transplantation; PBPC = peripheral blood progenitor cell; SCT = stem cell transplant.

granulocyte and the macrophage blood cell lines. Table 23-1 lists the HGFs that are FDA approved for clinical use.

Of the many HGFs that have been cloned over the years, only erythropoietin (EPO), G-CSF, and GM-CSF have widespread clinical use. Many clinical trials over the years have studied the role of recombinant thrombopoietin, but only a limited clinical role has been identified. Other HGFs that have been studied but have limited therapeutic value at the present time include stem cell factor and FMS-like tyrosine-3 ligand.

Erythropoietin growth factors

Mature red blood cells develop from the common multipotential progenitor cell, the CFU-GEMM, to a committed progenitor cell known as BFU-E. Under the influence of various growth factors, including erythropoietin, they proliferate and differentiate into erythroid colony-forming units (CFU-E) and then to reticulocytes and ultimately mature erythrocytes. Endogenous erythropoietin is the only hematopoietic growth factor that behaves as a hormone. Erythropoietin is produced primarily by the kidneys in response to hypoxia. It is secreted into the circulation and is delivered to the bone marrow via plasma. In general, plasma erythropoietin concentration levels reflect erythropoietin production and can be used as a measurement to determine deficient states that may be effectively treated with recombinant erythropoietin.[4]

Erythropoietin

Recombinant erythropoietin is marketed as two identical products of epoetin alfa or EPO: Epogen® (Amgen, Thousand Oaks, California) and Procrit® (Ortho Biotech, Raritan, New Jersey). Each company has unique marketing rights to their respective product. The recombinant forms of EPO are approved for the management of anemia associated with cancer chemotherapy, advanced renal disease when patients are on dialysis, anemia related to zidovudine (AZT) therapy in HIV-infected patients, and anemia in surgical patients to reduce the need for allogeneic transfusion.

Clinical practice guidelines of the American Society of Clinical Oncology and the American Society of Hematology found good evidence to recommend the use of erythropoietin as a treatment option for patients with chemotherapy-associated anemia with a hemoglobin level below 10 g/dL.[5] The recommendations also state that the use of erythropoietin for patients with less severe anemia (Hgb level below 12 g/dL but never below 10 g/dL) should be determined by clinical circumstances. The guidelines support the use of EPO given subcutaneously three times a week for a minimum of four weeks. Epoetin should be titrated once the hemoglobin concentration reaches 12 g/dL.[5] A newer, longer-acting version of epoetin is now available for clinical use. This agent, called darbepoetin alfa (Aranesp® Amgen, Thousand Oaks, California), can be administered less frequently than epoetin alfa. Darbepoetin alfa has been found to be as efficacious as epoetin alfa in a multicenter retrospective cohort study of outcomes of the use of darbepoetin alfa and epoetin alfa for chemotherapy-induced anemia.[6]

Multiple studies have demonstrated that epoetin alfa not only increases hemoglobin levels in patients with cancer being treated with chemotherapy, but it also significantly reduces transfusion requirements in these patients.[5,7-9] In recent years, many studies have focused on quality of life issues related to anemia and anemia-related fatigue. In a study by Cella,[10] fatigue was the most common complaint of 1171 patients with cancer and HIV, and reported more frequently than nausea, vomiting, and pain. The administration of epoetin alfa is correlated with a significant improvement in quality of life measures, as demonstrated in the literature and in large studies.[7,9,11] One of these studies involved 2030 patients with cancer in a community-based setting, and it was determined that treating anemia with epoetin alfa not only increased hemoglobin concentrations and reduced transfusion requirements but also improved patients' quality of life. The quality of life measures that were affected included an improvement in energy ($r = .30$, $p \leq .001$) and an improvement in activity ($r = .28$, $p \leq .001$).[9]

Myeloid growth factors

The monocyte/macrophage and neutrophil blood cell lineages develop from the common multipotential progenitor cell, the CFU-GEMM and, under the influence of a number of other growth factors, develop into the CFU-GM. The CFU-GM then differentiates into the neutrophils, monocytes, and macrophages in the circulation. G-CSF acts on the committed granulocytes to increase their progeny. Although G-CSF is considered to be a single lineage factor, it has been found to have some effect on multiple cell lines as well.

The myeloid growth factors have demonstrated enormous therapeutic value in patients with hematologic diseases over the years. The most common applications for these growth factors include myelodysplasia, stem cell transplantation, acute myeloid leukemia, acute lymphoblastic leukemia, and chemotherapy-induced neutroenia. The routine clinical use of these growth factors in the primary prevention of chemotherapy-induced neutropenia for solid tumors or lymphoma has not been significantly supported by research.[4]

Granulocyte colony-stimulating factor

The body's naturally occurring G-CSF regulates the production of neutrophils within the bone marrow and affects the proliferation, differentiation, and selected end-cell functional activation of the neutrophil progenitor. G-CSF is considered to be a single-lineage growth factor.

The recombinant version of G-CSF (filgrastim, Neupogen®, Amgen, Thousand Oaks, California) was approved by the FDA in the early 1990s as a safe and effective agent to accelerate the recovery of neutrophil counts following the administration of chemotherapy for nonmyeloid malignancies. The administration of filgrastim helps to facilitate the planned delivery of chemotherapy and dose-dense chemotherapy regimens by reducing the risk of infection.[12] Filgrastim has a short circulating time in the blood, and thus treatment with filgrastim may take up to two weeks of daily injections. A newer pegylated form of filgrastim, called Neulasta™ (Amgen, Thousand Oaks, California), has been approved by the FDA. The pegylation process extends the half-life of the agent and makes it a longer-acting version of Neupogen®. Neulasta™ is given once per cycle of chemotherapy, rather than daily for up to two weeks. A multi-institutional clinical trial was conducted to compare Neupogen® directly to Neulasta™ in patients being treated with chemotherapy.[13] These researchers concluded that Neulasta™ appeared to be as effective as Neupogen® in the treatment of neutropenia. The most frequent side effect of treatment with either version of G-CSF is bone pain. Other side effects include lethargy, myalgia, and injection site pain.

Treatment of myeloid malignancies with G-CSF has been a concern over the years due to the thought that this agent would stimulate leukemic blast proliferation. Over the past decade, 14 controlled trials of growth factors used after induction therapy in acute myeloid leukemia (AML) have been reported.[4] The vast majority of the data have demonstrated safety of use with the treatment of AML; the follow-up studies did not show any increase in the relapse rate or decreased survival among patients who went into a complete remission.[14]

The use of G-CSF is also recommended at any stage of therapy for acute lymphoblastic leukemia (ALL), either during induction or in subsequent intensification, as it reduces the period of neutropenia.[15] G-CSF is also indicated in the stem cell transplantation setting, for enhancement of neutrophil recovery and for mobilization of stem cells prior to the transplant.[16,17] The myeloid growth factors, including G-CSF, are reported to be occasionally beneficial in increasing the neutrophil count and function in patients with myelodysplasia. G-CSF is also approved for congenital, cyclic, or idiopathic neutropenia.[18]

Granulocyte-macrophage colony-stimulating factor

GM-CSF is a multilineage growth factor that regulates proliferation and differentiation of hematopoietic progenitors of neutrophils, monocytes, and eosinophils. It does not appear to have a role in the commitment of the neutrophil but does have an effect on maturing monocytes and macrophages.[19]

The recombinant version of GM-CSF (sargramostim, Leukine®) is FDA approved for use with HSCT and after induction therapy for AML. GM-CSF is used to enhance neutrophil recovery after HSCT, to prevent or provide therapy for graft failure, and to mobilize stem cells.[20] The incidence of graft failure is less common than in the past, due to the current technologies and measurement of precise numbers of CD34-positive cells in the donor pool. The administration of GM-CSF in the HSCT setting has been shown to reduce the rate of graft failure, accelerate hematopoiesis, and help in preventing lethal complications in patients after transplantation.[21,22] GM-CSF is also used during induction or subsequent intensification of ALL to help prevent life-threatening neutropenia. Like G-CSF, GM-CSF is reported to be occasionally beneficial in increasing the neutrophil count and function in patients with myelodysplasia.[4,23] The most prominent side effect of GM-CSF is bone pain. Other side effects include rash, fever, lethargy, myalgia, anorexia, and injection site redness.

Because of the effect that GM-CSF has on immune function, exciting studies are being done to determine new clinical applications. GM-CSF has been combined with a gene-transduced autologous tumor vaccine (GVAX). Preclinical trials demonstrated some benefit with this vaccine, and thus it has now been tested in early clinical trials of patients with non-small cell lung cancer. The study was small (34 patients), but the vaccine did show some survival benefit in patients who had previously failed chemotherapy.[24] GM-CSF may also prove to be useful as prophylaxis or as an adjunctive treatment of bacterial or fungal infections in patients with cancer who are receiving myelosuppressive chemotherapy.[20]

Multipotential growth factors

Stem cell factor

Stem cell factor is one of the HGFs that influence multipotential precursor cells to develop into myeloid or lymphoid blood cell lines. Stem cell factor, also known as steel factor or kit ligand, is a normal transmembrane glycoprotein produced by the *C-KIT* gene.[25] It stimulates undifferentiated multipotential progenitor cells and committed cell line precursors (e.g., CFU-GEMM) to further develop into mature blood cells.

Recombinant stem cell factor (r-metHuSCF) has demonstrated little colony-stimulating activity when administered alone. However, when administered along with other HGFs, particularly filgrastim, it increases the number and size of cell colonies, suggesting that it influences early progenitor activity.[26–28] Clinical trials suggest that r-metHuSCF may be clinically useful when combined with filgrastim for mobilization of peripheral blood progenitor cells (PBPCs) used in HSCT.[27,28] Treatment with r-metHuSCT and filgrastim was well tolerated, with mild to moderate skin rash being the most frequently reported adverse event.[28]

FMS-like tyrosine-3 ligand

FMS-like tyrosine-3 ligand (Flt-3 ligand) belongs to the same family of receptor tyrosine kinases as stem cell factor.[29] It is an early-acting growth factor that stimulates proliferation of stem cells and primitive progenitor cells in combination with other growth factors.[30] Flt-3 ligand has been shown to synergistically enhance G-CSF mobilization of hematopoietic stem and progenitor cells in preclinical studies.[31] Early clinical trials are underway to test its effectiveness in mobilizing PBPCs in humans.[32]

Platelet growth factors

The mature platelet cell in the circulation derives from the megakaryocyte in the bone marrow. The megakaryocyte develops from the multipotential myeloid progenitor cell. The first committed cell is the CFU-megakaryocyte (CFU-MK). It is stimulated by various growth factors, including thrombopoietin. The CFU-MK undergoes differentiation and proliferation under the influence of GM-CSF, IL-6, and IL-11, whereby it becomes committed to megarkaryocytes that will fragment into platelets.[18]

Interleukin-11

Interleukin-3, interleukin-6, and interleukin-11 all are potent stimulators of platelet production.

However, interleukin-3 and interleukin-6 have been found to be too toxic for clinical use. To date, only interleukin-11, known as oprelvekin (Neumega®, Genetics Institute, Cambridge, Massachusetts) has been FDA approved for the prevention of chemotherapy-induced thrombocytopenia. The use of IL-11 increases the likelihood of avoiding thrombocytopenia in patients undergoing chemotherapy and shortens the duration of the thrombocytopenia.[33,34] Two randomized controlled clinical trials of IL-11 have shown a reduction in the need for platelet transfusions in the setting of intensive chemotherapy.[35,36] However, when used in the setting of autologous transplantation, IL-11 did not reduce the need for platelet transfusion.[37] The most common adverse events associated with oprelvekin in clinical trials include dyspnea, tachycardia, peripheral edema, and conjunctival redness.

Thrombopoietin

Two recombinant forms of thrombopoietin have been studied extensively and demonstrate some clinical activity. The first is the full thrombopoietin molecule (TPO), and the other is the erythropoietin-like domain coupled with polyethylene glycol (PEG) to provide stability in vivo. This agent is known as polyethylene glycol-megakaryocyte and development factor (MGDF). Both of these agents have demonstrated some benefit in clinical studies for the prophylaxis of thrombocytopenia associated with chemotherapy, by reducing the duration of thrombocytopenia.[38] Clinical studies using MGDF have been stopped due to the development of neutralizing antibodies that were associated with thrombocytopenia.[39] Studies have continued with TPO to evaluate its clinical role in cancer care. It has been found that TPO acts synergistically with several growth factors to enhance megakaryocyte differentiation and proliferation.[40] Two randomized placebo controlled trials in patients with cancer have shown a benefit related to TPO administration in reducing thrombocytopenia related to chemotherapy.[41,42]

Transfusion Therapy

Despite the increasing use of hematopoietic growth factors, transfusion therapy continues to play a vital role in the care of the patient with cancer. A significant need exists for blood component therapy in the context of bleeding and/or hemorrhage, severe anemia, thrombocytopenia, and coagulation disorders caused by the disease, treatment, or both. The frequency of blood component therapy transfusions is driven by standards set in the industry regarding a safe "set point" for the need for transfusion and the individual patient's needs and tolerance of low blood counts.

Routine blood bank procedures identify most patients at risk for serious immune-mediated red cell transfusion reactions. These procedures include major ABO typing, antibody screening, and compatibility testing. Changes in the recruiting and screening of blood donors have dramatically reduced the risk of viral transmission in blood products in the United States and Europe. All units of blood in the United States are tested for hepatitis B, hepatitis C, human immunodeficiency virus 1 and 2 (HIV), human T-cell lymphotrophic virus I and II (HTLV-I/II), and syphilis. In Europe and the United States, nucleotide amplification testing is done for hepatitis C and HIV.[43]

In recent years, various professional societies and governmental organizations, including the American Society of Anesthesiologists, the American Society of Clinical Oncologists, and the College of American Pathologists, have developed guidelines and practice parameters for the use of blood component therapy. These guidelines are due in part to the fact that even though blood component therapies have clearly accepted benefits, significant risks remain. Risks of transfusion therapy that are common to all patients include acute and delayed hemolytic, febrile nonhemolytic, allergic, and septic reactions. Risks specific to patients with cancer, especially those patients who receive large amounts of allogeneic transfusions, include the development of human leukocyte antigen (HLA) alloimmunization and graft-versus-host disease (GVHD). The production of numerous recipient alloantibodies can severely limit the number of compatible units of blood that will be available for a patient. Also, a state of platelet refractoriness can develop when platelet alloantibodies develop.

Red Blood Cell Therapy

Red blood cell replacement therapy is no longer based on the patient's hemoglobin or hematocrit. The clinical concern for the adverse physiologic effects of anemia is now generally the basis for considering red blood cell replacement. The decision to transfuse is based on an overall clinical picture of the patient, including any underlying cardiac or pulmonary conditions that might impair the patient's tolerance of the anemia. Among the causes of anemia frequently seen in patients with cancer, the two most common are decreased red blood cell production secondary to myelosuppressive therapy and the primary disease. Patients with cancer often have more slowly developing chronic anemias that are tolerated better than rapid-onset anemias, due to the ability of the body's fluid compensatory mechanisms.

Most practice guidelines agree that red blood cell transfusions are rarely indicated when the hemoglobin concentration is greater than 10 g/dL, and they are not often considered until the hemoglobin drops below 8 g/dL.[44] To date, no controlled studies have been done to determine the hemoglobin concentration at which red blood cell transfusions improve clinical outcomes. Physiologic signs of anemia (pallor, fatigue, rapid pulse, hyperventilation, and shortness of breath) should be relieved when the hemoglobin level is raised to 10 or 11 g/dL. The transfusion of 1 unit of red blood cells increases the hematocrit by 3% or the hemoglobin concentration by 1 g/dL in a 70 kg patient who is not bleeding. Packed red blood cells are usually the therapy of choice. The advantage of red blood cells is that they provide approximately 70% of the hematocrit of whole blood with only one-third of the plasma load.

Red blood cells can be stored for up to five weeks at 1°–6° centigrade in solutions containing citrate, phosphate buffers, dextrose, and adenine (CPDA-1). Shelf life is further extended if an additive solution with higher concentrations of adenine is added to the red blood cells.[43] Red blood cells with rare antigen profiles can be frozen and stored for up to 10 years. Frozen red blood cells are indicated for patients with cancer who have an alloantibody to a high-incidence antigen or have multiple alloantibodies.[43]

Leukocytes in red blood cell transfusions can cause reactions if the recipient has antileukocyte antibodies, which can develop from previous transfusions or pregnancies. These antigenic reactions occur much more frequently in the oncology patient population compared with other patient groups.[45] Transfusion of packed red blood cells in these patients can cause fever and chills, and the patient can eventually become alloimmunized or refractory to transfusions. This condition is demonstrated when the transfusion of a unit of red blood cells fails to achieve the expected increase in the hemoglobin level. The use of leukocyte-reduced blood component therapy is indicated for these patients. Leukocyte-reduced of blood products may be obtained by the use of bedside leukocyte reduction filters or the use of prestorage leukocyte-reduced blood from the laboratory.

Platelet Therapy

Platelet therapy is used to control bleeding in the thrombocytopenic patient or to prevent bleeding in the severely thrombocytopenic patient. Most patients with cancer who receive platelets have malignancies associated with treatment-induced thrombocytopenia. Platelet transfusions are generally ineffective and unnecessary in patients with idiopathic thrombocytopenic purpura (ITP) and are contraindicated in patients with thrombotic thrombocytopenic purpura (TTP).

It is well established that spontaneous bleeding is rarely encountered when the platelet count is more than 20,000 μL. Recent studies have found that patients receiving chemotherapy can tolerate platelet counts as low as 5,000 to 10,000 μL.[46–48] Patients with bleeding or infection may benefit from prophylactic platelet transfusions when the platelet count drops below 20,000 μL. In addition, the coagulation status of the patient should also be considered, because patients with plasma coagulation factor disorders are more likely to bleed at marginal platelet counts.

Theoretically, one unit of platelets should increase the recipient's platelet count by 10,000 μL. However, the effectiveness of platelet transfusions is variable and depends on several factors. Failure to achieve adequate increases in the circulating platelet count may be due to fever, infection, disseminated intravascular coagulation (DIC), hypersplenism, prolonged storage of platelets, and HLA antibody grade.[49] Attempts should be made to lower a fever by administering acetaminophen if a patient has a fever when he or she is to receive a platelet transfusion. Fever and infection enhance the consumption of platelets and can increase the occurrence of hemorrhage. Acetaminophen, corticosteroids, and antihistamines may also be used to premedicate a patient prior to platelet therapy to minimize the chance of a febrile nonhemolytic reaction. Meperidine may be used if the patient experiences shaking chills.

Platelets can be obtained from differential centrifugation of donated whole blood or from platelet pheresis of single donors. A donor can be pheresed up to every other day if the donor's platelets provide the patient with good platelet count increases. One unit of platelets is routinely obtained from 500 mL of fresh whole blood (see Table 23-2). Platelets are stored at room temperature, and with gentle agitation, for up to five days. Contaminating organisms may reach unacceptable levels beyond five days.

Platelet refractory state

Platelet refractoriness is a major problem for patients with cancer who are dependent on platelet transfusions, occurring in about 10% to 15% of patients who require multiple platelet transfusions.[50] In many cases, platelet refractoriness is due to nonimmune cases such as sepsis, hypersplenism, and DIC.[51] The most common immune cause of platelet refractoriness is the development of antibodies directed against foreign (donor) leukocyte antigen (HLA) types, which may result in alloimmunization. Nonresponsiveness to platelet transfusions can be associated

Table 23-2 Platelet Transfusion Therapy

Specific Component	Content and Volume	General Indications	Complications	Nursing Considerations
Random donor (RD) • Fresh — best • Frozen and cryopreserved (limited application because of poor recovery)	• Multiple donors (4+) approximately 200 mL • Plasma, WBCs, few RBCs	• Bleeding and bleeding prophylaxis • Prophylactic for platelet count of 10,000–20,000/μL	• Exposure of patients to multiple tissue antigens, which initiates antigen-antibody formation, leading to refractoriness • Hepatitis (increased risk with pooled products) • Allergic reactions may be seen more often if leukocyte-reduced blood is not used	• Gently agitate bag occasionally to prevent platelet clumping • Rapid infusion (per patient tolerance) • Tubing should include a 170–220 μm in-line blood filter • A leukocyte reduction blood filter may be required or the use of prestorage leukocyte-reduced blood • Less expensive than single-donor or HLA-matched platelet concentrates • May require UVB irradiation if patient is severely immunosuppressed
Single donor (SD) • Fresh (maximum effectiveness up to 6 hr)	• One donor • 1 unit ∝ 300 mL • Plasma, WBCs, RBCs • Number of platelets in an SD unit equals approximately the number of platelets in 5 RD units	• Bleeding and bleeding prophylaxis • Severe febrile reactions associated with random donor platelets • Often used once a patient is refractory to random donor platelets • Patients who require long-term platelet therapy • Minimizes the transmission of viral disease	• Refractoriness to platelets may occur over time	• Rapid infusion (generally 30 min +) • Tubing as above • Leukocyte reduction of blood as above
Human-leukocyte antigen (HLA) matched concentrate	• One donor compatible at the HLA complex • 1 unit ∝ 300 mL • Plasma, WBCs, RBCs	• When patients become refractory to RD and SD platelets • Minimizes transmission of viral disease	• Minimal	• HLA-matched platelets minimize patient exposure to multiple tissue antigens (HLA complex found on all blood cells — acts as a genetic monogram) • Rapid infusion (30 min +) • Tubing as above. Generally see more effective increases in the platelet count than with RD or SD

∝ = approximately.

with hemorrhagic events secondary to thrombocytopenia.

Patients who are refractory to random-donor platelets may respond to either HLA-matched platelets or to single-donor platelet transfusions, as they significantly reduce the number of platelet and leukocyte antibodies to which the recipient is exposed. Antigen-presenting cells can be eliminated from platelet concentrates through the use of leukocyte-reduction blood filters or laboratory leukocyte-reduced blood, or by treating the platelets with ultraviolet light (UVB).[52] Platelet cross-matching has also been done at some blood centers to decrease the risk of alloimunization. Platelet cross-matches can detect antibodies in a patient's serum that will react with platelets in potential donor units. The cross-match may detect a variety of antibodies that can react with platelets. Thus, platelet products may be identified that provide good response for the patient.[50]

Plasma Therapy

Plasma is prepared by centrifuging whole blood and then freezing the plasma within eight hours of collection. This rapid freezing maintains the activity of the labile clotting factors.

Thawed plasma or fresh frozen plasma

Fresh frozen plasma (FFP) contains all of the coagulation factors, other plasma proteins, and complement. The most common indications for FFP in patients with cancer include deficiencies of multiple coagulation factors, as seen in liver disease, and for hypofibrinogenemia. It is often used for a quick reversal of warfarin therapy in bleeding patients and before procedures.[43] FFP is not recommended as a volume expander, because there is a risk of transfusion-transmitted disease. Also, FFP is not recommended to treat isolated factor deficiencies because of the large volumes that would be required to attain adequate levels. (A unit of FFP contains 180 to 270 mL of plasma.) Plasma is also used to treat thrombotic thrombocytopenic purpura by apheresis with plasma as a replacement fluid.

The amount and frequency of transfusions with plasma depend on several factors, including the severity of the deficiency, the specific factor deficiency, and the severity of bleeding. Generally, diffuse bleeding due to multiple coagulation factor deficiencies should be controlled when the clotting factor levels reach 20% to 50% of normal values. Appropriate concentrations of the levels can be obtained with infusions of 2 to 6 units of plasma in a 70 kg adult.[43] Plasma and plasma factors are infused rapidly, so the maximum plasma level is reached before metabolic changes or degradation of the product occur (due to a short half-life).

Cryoprecipitate

Cryoprecipitate contains fibrinogen, factor VIII, factor XIII, and some von Willebrand factor. Its use is generally limited to patients with severe hypofibrinogenemia (less than 100 mg/dL) and von Willebrand's disease. It is recommended that cryoprecipitate not be used in the management of DIC, as it contains no factor V. Each unit of cryoprecipitate contains approximately 250 mg of fibrinogen. The fibrinogen level should rise by approximately 8.5 mg/dL in a nonbleeding 70 kg adult per unit of cryoprecipitate.

Individual clotting factors

Purified factor preparations are usually preferred over FFP if the patient is deficient in only one coagulation protein, such as patients with hemophilia A (factor VIII), hemophilia B (factor IX), or acquired von Willebrand's syndrome.[53] In these cases, virally inactivated or recombinant proteins are available for use.

Transfusion Reactions and Complications

Many risks are associated with blood component therapy, including transfusion reactions and transmission of disease. While most reactions occur shortly after the transfusion, some reactions can occur several days to weeks afterward. Acute reactions include acute hemolytic transfusion reactions, febrile nonhemolytic transfusion reactions, allergic reactions, and bacterial contamination of blood resulting in sepsis. Delayed transfusion reactions include the development of GVHD and the transmission of diseases, particularly viral diseases. Table 23-3 lists transfusion reactions and complications, and Table 23-4 lists and explains the nursing management of transfusion reactions.

Immediate blood transfusion reactions

Acute hemolytic transfusion reactions

Immediate reactions to blood transfusions may be due to an immune response to the blood component, as occurs with acute hemolytic transfusion reactions (AHTRs). The most severe type of AHTR is caused by the transmission of ABO-incompatible blood. The most common cause of this reaction is clerical error involving a misidentification of the patient. A double check of all of the patient identifiers at every point, from dispensing the blood from the laboratory to hanging the unit of blood, is critical to avoid this type of error. Acute hemolytic reactions can present with

Table 23-3 Transfusion Reactions

Immediate
Acute hemolytic transfusion reaction (e.g., ABO incompatibility)
Bacterial contamination — shock, sepsis
Circulatory overload
Air embolism
Citrate toxicity
Hypocalcemia
Hyperkalemia
Hypothermia
Iron overload
Respiratory distress
Febrile reactions (temperature rise over 1.8°F), chills
Allergy — urticaria, anaphylaxis
Bacterial contamination
Delayed
Delayed hemolytic transfusion reaction
Graft-versus-host disease
Infection–hepatitis (A, B, or C), rotovirus, cytomegalovirus, HIV, HTLV-I parasites, malaria, babesiosis
Alloimmunization
Bacterial contamination

mild symptoms or as severe shock. Symptoms associated with this type of reaction include chills, fever, dyspnea, hematuria, flank pain, chest pain, and a "sense of impending doom." Laboratory testing for possible incompatibility of blood products usually reveals hemoglobinemia, a positive direct antibody test, and increased plasma levels of lactate dehydrogenase, hemoglobin, and bilirubin.[50]

Other immediate complications may be related to the method of administration (hypothermia, air embolism, citrate toxicity related to additives in the blood, and the age of the blood product). Bacterial contamination of blood, which results from bacteria entering blood bags during component preparation or from improperly cleansed skin at venipuncture sites, can cause fatal septic transfusion reactions. Treatment of acute reactions includes fluid infusion/resuscitation as well as blood product and respiratory support. Broad-spectrum antibiotics are used until the results of the blood cultures are available.

Acute nonhemolytic febrile transfusion reactions and allergic reactions

Cytokines released from damaged leukocytes can cause fever. The leukocytes may be damaged during storage of blood components or after entering the patient in patients who have antibodies that recognize antigens on foreign white blood cells. This usually occurs in patients who have had multiple blood transfusions and in multiparous women. A febrile reaction is generally diagnosed in an individual with a temperature increase of more than 1.8°F above the baseline temperature that occurs during or shortly after the transfusion without another identifiable cause. Shaking chills often accompany the fever. While these reactions are not dangerous, they may be a sign of a more serious reaction, such as a hemolytic transfusion reaction. Any febrile reaction in a patient receiving blood products should be investigated carefully. Treatment consists of acetaminophen for the fever, meperidine for severe rigors, and steroids for dyspnea. Patients who have a history of febrile reactions are premedicated with acetaminophen and steroids. Febrile reactions can generally be prevented by the use of leukocyte-reduced blood products. These products appear to be more effective than the post-storage use of leukocyte-reduction filters on blood products in preventing febrile nonhemolytic transfusion reactions.[54]

Allergic reactions account for about 1% of transfusion reactions. They may be mild, manifested by clinical signs and symptoms such as hives, urticaria, and cutaneous erythema, or they may be severe, manifested by bronchospasm, laryngeal edema, and anaphylaxis. A mild allergic reaction is treated with an antihistamine, and prevention also consists of premedication with an antihistamine. Washing the cells with saline helps to prevent allergic reactions by ridding the unit of plasma and suspending the cells in saline. If the patient has a severe allergic reaction, he or she will be treated like anyone with an anaphylactic reaction.

Delayed blood transfusion reactions

Graft-versus-host disease

A serious delayed transfusion reaction in patients who are severely immunocompromised is GVHD. Patients who are at risk of developing GVHD include bone marrow transplant recipients, peripheral blood stem cell recipients, patients undergoing combination treatment for Hodgkin's and non-Hodgkin's lymphoma, and patients with leukemia who are undergoing induction therapy. This complication can occur following the transfusion of blood products containing viable lymphocytes. The donor-competent T lymphocyte immunologically attacks the immunocompromised host tissue after transfusion.[55] GVHD generally manifests in the skin, liver, and gastrointestinal tract and can be fatal. Post-transfusion GVHD is fatal almost 90% of the time due to the development of bone marrow hypoplasia or aplasia.[43] To prevent GVHD, it is recommended that all blood products given to severely immunocompromised patients be irradiated before transfusion with 2500 cGy to inactivate donor lymphocytes. Leukocyte-reduction of blood components does not prevent GVHD.

Table 23-4 Nursing Management of Selected Transfusion Reactions

Type	Signs/Symptoms	Nursing Actions
Acute hemolytic transfusion reaction • ABO incompatibility	Fever, chills, hypotension, increased pulse rate, nausea/vomiting, flushing, low back pain, decreased urine output, hematuria, dyspnea, bleeding, anaphylaxis, shock	1. Stop transfusion. 2. Maintain patent IV line with normal saline. 3. Verify client and the blood unit with another nurse (the majority of reported fatalities with an acute hemolytic transfusion reaction involve human error). 4. Place in supine position. 5. Maintain open airway; provide CPR if necessary. 6. Obtain vital signs and record. 7. Notify physician. 8. Monitor intake and output. 9. Administer fluids and medications per physician order. 10. Monitor vital signs per institutional guidelines. 11. Obtain blood and urine specimens. 12. Notify blood bank and return remainder of blood to blood bank. 13. Document event. 14. Admit patient to hospital if outpatient.
Febrile nonhemolytic transfusion reaction (FNHTRS) • Antileukocyte antibodies in the recipient directed against the donor blood	Fever (>1.8°F) ± chills, headache, hypotension, increased pulse rate, dyspnea, chest pain, nausea/vomiting	1. Stop transfusion. 2. Maintain patent IV line with normal saline. 3. Obtain and monitor vital signs and record. 4. Notify physician. 5. Assist in ruling out infection. 6. Administer medications and fluids per physician order: acetaminophen for fever, meperidine for chills and rigors, antihistamine for dyspnea. 7. Continue transfusion if symptoms are not severe. 8. Notify blood bank. 9. Document event. 10. For clients who are known to have FNHTRS or for clients who are at high risk for FNHTRS (multiple transfused clients), acetaminophen and antihistamines/steroids may be given before the transfusion to minimize or eliminate the transfusion reaction. The use of a leukocyte-reduction filter or the use of prestorage leukocyte-reduced blood may be indicated.
Allergic (usually mild) reaction • Recipient antibodies against immunoglobulin components or other soluble proteins in the plasma	Hives, urticaria, cutaneous erythema; may develop severe allergic or even fatal anaphylaxis	1. Obtain and monitor vital signs and record. 2. Slow or stop transfusion rate, depending on symptoms. 3. Take measures to correct shock, maintain renal circulation, and correct the bleeding, depending on symptoms. 4. Notify physician. 5. Administer medications per physician order: antihistamines if reaction is mild. 6. Treat as anaphylactic reaction if severe. 7. Notify blood bank. 8. Document event.
Bacterial contamination • Cold-growing organisms	Fever, chills; may result in endotoxin shock	1. Stop transfusion. 2. Maintain patent IV line. 3. Take measures to correct shock and to maintain renal circulation. 4. Obtain vital signs and record. 5. Notify physician. 6. Notify blood bank and return remainder of blood to blood bank. 7. Obtain blood and urine cultures of the client and the unit of blood. 8. Administer antibiotics per physician order. 9. Document event. 10. Admit client to hospital if outpatient.
Delayed hemolytic reaction • Development of alloantibodies to transfused blood	Delayed (7–10 days to weeks) decreased hemoglobin, low-grade fever, jaundice (increase in bilirubin and LDH)	Notify blood bank.

Transfusion-transmitted disease

Transmission of disease, particularly viral disease, through blood products is a major concern of the public. Transmission of viral diseases has dramatically decreased over the years due to changes in the recruiting and screening of blood donors, as well as to advances in the testing of donor blood. Current estimates for the risk of transfusion-related HIV range from 1:500,000 to 1:750,000 units transfused.[56] Immunocompromised patients and splenectomized patients are most susceptible to severe infections caused by parvovirus B19, malaria, babesiosis, and cytomegalovirus.[57]

Approximately 40% to 60% of blood donors have been exposed to cytomegalovirus (CMV) infection at some point in their lifetime. These individuals then develop antibodies directed against CMV. Only about 2% of seropositive donors are actively infected, whereby they would transmit a potentially serious infection to an immunocompromised person.[43] The use of CMV-negative blood products is the standard of care for severely immunocompromised patients or for stem cell transplant patients who are seronegative for CMV.[58,59] The demand for CMV-seronegative blood products may exceed the supply at many blood centers and in geographical areas where CMV-seronegative blood cannot be found. Studies have shown that leukocyte-depleted blood products may significantly reduce the risk of CMV transmission.[60,61]

Conclusion

Patients with cancer, particularly patients with hematologic malignancies, are often treated with therapies that cause significant alterations in their blood counts. They may face alterations in their red blood cell counts, white blood cell counts, and platelet counts. Recombinant hematopoietic growth factors are biological agents that can help prevent negative outcomes related to low blood counts. While many of these agents have been available since the early 1990s, newer agents are now available that require less frequent dosing to maintain patients' blood counts. The hematopoietic growth factors have clearly established roles in the management of patients on cancer therapy. Exciting new work is being done to investigate new roles for these agents, such as their role in vaccine therapy.

Blood component therapy continues to be the cornerstone of treatment of the bleeding patient. Patients with cancer face bleeding from a number of causes, and the availability of red blood cells and platelets is crucial to the management of patients undergoing active cancer treatment. Significant advances have been made in recent years to make the role of blood component therapy safer in the United States.

References

1. Griffin JD: Hematopoietic growth factors, in DeVita VT, Hellman S, Rosenberg SA (eds): *Cancer: Principles and Practice of Oncology* (ed 6). Philadelphia, Lippincott Williams & Wilkins, 2001, pp 2798–2813
2. Quesenberry PJ: Hematopoietic stem cells, progenitor cells, and cytokines, in Beutler E, Lichtman MA, Coller BS, Kipps TJ (eds.): *Williams Hematology* (ed 5). New York, McGraw-Hill, 1995, pp 211–228
3. Zhan Y, Lieschke GJ, Grail D, et al: Essential roles for granulocyte-macrophage colony-stimulating factor (GM-CSF) and G-CSF in the sustained hematopoietic response of *Listeria monocytogenes*-infected mice. *Blood* 91:863–869, 1998
4. Rowe JM: Growth factors, in Furie B, Cassileth PA, Atkins MB, Mayer RJ (eds): *Clinical Hematology and Oncology: Presentation, Diagnosis, Treatment.* Philadelphia, Churchill Livingstone, 2003, pp 419–430
5. Rizzo JD, Lichtin AE, Woolf SH, et al: Use of epoetin in patients with cancer: evidence-based practice guidelines of the American Society of Clinical Oncology and the American Society of Hematology. *Blood* 100:2303–2320, 2002
6. Schwartzberg L, Shiffman R, Tomita D, et al: A multicenter retrospective cohort study of practice patterns about the outcomes of the use of darbepoetin alfa and epoetin alfa for chemotherapy-induced anemia. *Clin Ther* 25:2781–2796, 2003
7. Demetri GD, Kris M, Wade J, et al: Quality-of-life benefit in chemotherapy patients treated with epoetin alfa is independent of disease response or tumor type: results from a prospective community oncology study. Procrit Study Group. *J Clin Oncol* 16:3412–3425, 1998
8. Dunphy FR, Harrison BR, Dunleavy TL, et al: Erythropoietin reduces anemia and transfusions. A randomized trial with or without erythropoietin during chemotherapy. *Cancer* 86:1362–1367, 1999
9. Glaspy J, Bukowski R, Steinberg D, et al: Impact of therapy with epoetin alfa on clinical outcomes in patients with nonmyeloid malignancies during cancer chemotherapy in community oncology practice. Procrit Study Group. *J Clin Oncol* 15:1218–1234, 1997
10. Cella D: Factors influencing quality of life in cancer patients: anemia and fatigue. *Semin Oncol* 25:43–46, 1998
11. Mock V, Olsen M: Current management of fatigue and anemia in patients with cancer. *Semin Oncol Nurs* 19(4 suppl 2):36–41, 2003
12. Trillet-Lenoir V, Green J, Manegold C, et al: Recombinant granulocyte colony-stimulating factor reduces the infectious complications of cytotoxic chemotherapy. *Eur J Cancer* 29A:319–324, 1993
13. Green M, Koelbl H, Baselga JA: A randomized double-blind multicenter phase III study of fixed-dose single-administration pegfilgrastim versus daily filgrastim in patients receiving myelosuppressive chemotherapy. *Ann Oncol* 14:29–35, 2003
14. Johnson EM, Crawford J: Hematopoietic growth factors in the reduction of chemotherapeutic toxicity. *Semin Oncol* 25:552–561, 1998
15. Larson RA, Dodge RK, Linker CA, et al: A randomized controlled trial of filgrastim during remission, induction and consolidation chemotherapy for adults with acute lymphoblastic leukemia: CALGB study 9111. *Blood* 92:1556–1564, 1998

16. Linch DC, Milligan DW, Winfield DA, et al: G-CSF after peripheral blood stem cell transplantation in lymphoma patients significantly accelerated neutrophil recovery and shortened time in hospital: Results of a randomized BNLI trial. *Br J Haematol* 99:933–938, 1997
17. McQuaker IG, Hunter AE, Pacey S, et al: Low-dose filgrastim significantly enhances neutrophil recovery following autologous peripheral-blood stem cell transplantation in patients with lymphoproliferative disorders: evidence for clinical and economic benefit. *J Clin Oncol* 15:451–457, 1997
18. Battiato LA, Wheeler VS: Biotherapy, in Yarbro CH, Frogge MH, Goodman M, Groenwald SL (eds): *Cancer Nursing Principles and Practice* (ed 5). Sudbury, MA, Jones and Bartlett, 2000, pp 543–579
19. Glaspy JA: Hematopoietic management in oncology practice, part 2: erythropoietin factors. *Oncology* 17:1724–1730, 2003
20. Armitage JO: Emerging applications of recombinant human granulocyte-macrophage colony-stimulating factor. *Blood* 92:4491–4508, 1998
21. Greenberg P, Advani R, Keating A, et al: GM-CSF accelerates neutrophil recovery after autologous hematopoietic stem cell transplantation. *Bone Marrow Transplant* 18:1057–1064, 1996
22. Spitzer G, Adkins D, Mathews M, et al: Randomized comparison of G-CSF+GM-CSF vs G-CSF alone for mobilization of peripheral blood stem cells: effects on hematopoietic recovery after high-dose chemotherapy. *Bone Marrow Transplant* 20:921–930, 1997
23. Blinder VS, Roboz GJ: Hematopoietic growth factors in myelodysplastic syndromes. *Curr Hematol Rep* 2:453–458, 2003
24. Nemunaitis J, Nemunaitis J: Granulocyte-macrophage colony-stimulating gene-transfected autologous tumor cell vaccine: Focus on non-small-cell lung cancer. *Clin Lung Cancer* 5:148–157, 2003
25. Heinrich MC, Blanke CD, Druker BJ, et al: Inhibition of KIT tyrosine kinase activity: a novel molecular approach to the treatment of KIT-positive malignancies. *J Clin Oncol* 20:1692–1703, 2002
26. Berstein SH, Kufe DW: Future of basic/clinical hematopoiesis research in the era of hematopoietic growth factor availability. *Semin Oncol* 19:441–448, 1992
27. Wadhwa PD, Lazarus HM, Koc ON, et al: Hematopoietic recovery after unrelated-umbilical cord blood allogeneic transplantation in adults treated with in vivo stem cell factor (r-metHuSCF) and filgrastim administration. *Leuk Res* 27:215–220, 2003
28. Prosper F, Sola C, Hornedo J, et al: Mobilization of peripheral blood progenitor cells with a combination of cyclophosphamide, r-metHuSCF and filgrastim in patients with breast cancer previously treated with chemotherapy. *Leukemia* 17:437–441, 2003
29. Grundler R, Thiede C, Miething C, et al: Sensitivity towards tyrosine kinase inhibitors varies between different activating mutations of the FLT3 receptor. *Blood* 102:646–651, 2003
30. Pitler L: Hematopoietic growth factors in clinical practice. *Semin Oncol Nurs* 12:115–129, 1996
31. Yoshikazu S, Shimazaki C, Ashihara E, et al: Synergistic effect of Flt-3 ligand on the granulocyte colony-stimulating factor-induced mobilization of hematopoietic stem cells and progenitor cells into blood in mice. *Blood* 89:3186–3191, 1997
32. Lyman SD, Jacobsen SEW: C-KIT ligand and Flt-3 ligand: stem/progenitor cell factors with overlapping yet distinct activities. *Blood* 91: 1101–1134, 1997
33. Weich NS, Neben TY, Donaldson D, et al: Effects of interleukin 11 on megakaryocytes. *Blood* 88:(suppl 1)60a, 1996
34. Chu DT, Xu BH, Song ST, et al: Recombinant human interleukin 11 (Mega) promotes thrombopoiesis in cancer patients with chemotherapy-induced myelosupppressin. *Zhongguo Shi Yan Xue Ye Xue Za Zhi* 9:314–317, 2001
35. Isaacs C, Robert NJ, Bailey FA, et al: Randomized placebo controlled study of recombinant human interleukin 11 to prevent chemotherapy-induced thrombocytopenia in patients with breast cancer receiving dose-intensive cyclophosphamide and doxorubicin. *J Clin Oncol* 15:3369–3375, 1997
36. Tepler I, Elias L, Smith JW 2nd, et al: A randomized placebo-controlled trial of recombinant interleukin 11 in cancer patients with severe thrombocytopenia due to chemotherapy. *Blood* 87:3607–3621, 1996
37. Vredenburgh JJ, Hussein A, Fisher D, et al: A randomized trial of recombinant human interleukin 11 following autologous bone marrow transplantation with peripheral blood progenitor cell support in patients with breast cancer. *Biol Blood Marrow Transplant* 4:134–140, 1998
38. Kaushansky K: Use of thrombopoietic growth factors in acute leukemia. *Leukemia* 14:505–508, 2000
39. Vadhan-Raj S: Recombinant human thrombopoietin: clinical experience and in vivo biology. *Semin Hematol* 35:261–268, 1998
40. Broudy VC, Lin NL, Kaushansky K: Thrombopoietin (c-mpl ligand) acts synergistically with erythropoietin, stem cell factor, and interleukin 11 to enhance murine megakaryocyte colony growth and increases megakaryocyte ploidy in vitro. *Blood* 85:1719–1723, 1995
41. Basser RL, Rasko JE, Clarke K, et al: Randomized, blinded, placebo-controlled phase 1 trial of pegylated recombinant human megakaryocyte growth and development factor with filgrastim after dose-intensive chemotherapy in patients with advanced cancer. *Blood* 89:3118, 1997
42. Fanucchi M, Glaspy J, Crawford J, et al: Effects of polyethylene glycol-conjugated recombinant human megakaryocyte growth and development factor on platelet counts after chemotherapy for lung cancer. *N Engl J Med* 336:404–409, 1997
43. Perrotta PL, Snyder EL: Hematopoietic therapy, in DeVita VT, Hellman S, Rosenberg SA (eds): *Cancer Principles and Practice of Oncology* (ed 6). Philadelphia, Lippincott Williams & Wilkins, 2001, pp 2753–2767
44. Simon RL, Alverson DC, AuBuchon J, et al: Practice parameters for the use of red blood cell transfusions. *Arch Pathol Lab Med* 122:130–138, 1998
45. Mohandas K, Aledort L: Transfusion requirements, risks, and costs for patients with malignancy. *Transfusion* 35:427–430, 1995
46. Rebulla P, Finazzi G, Marangoni F, et al: The threshold for prophylactic platelet transfusions in adults with acute myeloid leukemia. Gruppo Italiano Malattie Ematologiche Maligne dell'Adulto. *N Engl J Med* 337:1870–1882, 1997
47. Navarro JT, Hernandez JA, Ribera JM, et al: Prophylactic platelet transfusion threshold during therapy for adult acute myeloid leukemia: 10,000/microL. versus 20,000/microL. *Haematologica* 83:998–1005, 1998
48. Wandt H, Frank M, Ehninger G, et al: Safety and cost effectiveness of a 10x10(9)/L trigger for prophylactic platelet transfusions compared with the traditional 20x10(9)/L trigger: a prospective comparative trial in 105 patients with acute myeloid leukemia. *Blood* 91:3601, 1998
49. Gobel BH: Bleeding, in Yarbro CH, Frogge MH, Goodman M, Groenwald SL (eds): *Cancer Nursing Principles and Practice* (ed 5). Sudbury, MA, Jones and Bartlett, 2000, pp 709–736
50. Sloan SR, Silberstein LE: Transfusion medicine, in Furie B, Cassileth PA, Atkins MB, Mayer RJ (eds): *Clinical Hematology and Oncology: Presentation, Diagnosis, and Treatment.* Philadelphia, Churchill Livingstone, 2003, pp 431–440

51. Contreras M: Diagnosis and treatment of patients refractory to platelet transfusions. *Blood Rev* 12:215–221, 1998
52. The Trial to Reduce Alloimmunization to Platelets Study Group: leukocyte reduction and ultraviolet B irradiation of platelets to prevent alloimmunization and refractoriness to platelet transfusions. *N Engl J Med* 337:1861–1869, 1997
53. Kumar S, Pruthi RK, Nichols WL: Acquired von Willebrand's syndrome: a single institution experience. *Am J Hematol* 72:243–247, 2003
54. Pruss A, Kalus U, Radtke H, et al: Universal leukodepletion of blood components results in a significant reduction of febrile non-hemolytic but not allergic transfusion reaction. *Transfus Apheresis Sci* 30:41–46, 2004
55. Vogelsang GB, Hess AD: Graft-versus-host disease: New directions for a persistent problem. *Blood* 84:2061–2068, 1994
56. Lackritz EM, Satten GA, Aberle-Grass J, et al: Estimated risk of the human immunodeficiency virus by screened blood in the United States. *N Engl J Med* 333:1721–1728, 1995
57. Moor AC, Dubbelman TM, VanSteveninck J, et al: Transfusion-transmitted diseases: risks, prevention, and perspectives. *Eur J Haematol* 62:1–8, 1999
58. Chang H, Haves J, Hall GA, et al: Prospective audit of cytomegalovirus-negative blood product utilization in hematology/oncology patients. *Trans Med* 9:195–198, 1999
59. Saavedra S, Sanz GF, Jarque I, et al: Early infections in adult patients undergoing unrelated donor cord blood transplantation. *Bone Marrow Transplant* 30:937–943, 2002
60. Bowden RA, Slichter SJ, Sayers MH, et al: A comparison of leukocyte-reduced and cytomegalovirus (CMV) seronegative blood products for the prevention of transfusion associated CMV infection after marrow transplantation. *Blood* 86:3598–3603, 1995
61. Fung MK, Rao N, Rice J, et al: Leukoreduction in the setting of open heart surgery: A prospective cohort-controlled study. *Transfusion* 44:30–35, 2004A

CHAPTER 24

Complementary and Alternative Medicine (CAM) Therapies

Georgia Decker, MS, RN, CS-ANP, AOCN®, CN®
Colleen Lee, RN, MS, OCN®

Introduction

Defining Complementary and Alternative Medicine (CAM) Therapies

Throughout this chapter, the reader will encounter many acronyms commonly used in discussing complementary and alternative medicine (CAM). These acronyms are summarized in Table 24-1. Professionals across multiple practice settings, including clinical practice, education, and research, contribute to the field of CAM (see Table 24-2). CAM is often termed "integrative," "integrated," or "complementary" when these therapies are combined with conventional approaches. It is often termed "alternative" or "unconventional" when its therapies are used instead of conventional approaches. Some therapies are considered both complementary and alternative. Table 24-3 provides several definitions of CAM found in the literature.[1–8] Conventional approaches, known as "standard" or "traditional" or "biomedical" approaches, are those that historically have broad application in Western medicine. To assist nurses in understanding CAM in cancer care, the Oncology Nursing Society (ONS) Position Statement entitled "The Use of Complementary and Alternative Therapies in Cancer Care" promotes standardizing terminology to enhance communication.[7] Throughout this chapter, the acronym CAM is used to refer to the broad range of complementary and alternative therapies, and the term "conventional biomedical" is used to refer to the traditional or standard approaches.

Two main approaches to categorizing CAM therapies exist. The National Center for Complementary and Alternative Medicine (NCCAM) classifies CAM therapies into five domains: (1) alternative medical systems, (2) mind-body interventions, (3) biologically based therapies, (4) manipulative and body-based methods, and (5) energy therapies.[5] The National Cancer Institute (NCI) Office of Cancer Complementary and Alternative Medicine (OCCAM)[9] expanded the NCCAM domains with three additional categories for clarification: movement therapy, pharmacological and biological treatments with a subcategory of complex natural products, and a miscellaneous domain.[10] *Alternative medical systems* are built upon complete systems of theory and practice. *Mind-body medicine* uses a variety of techniques designed to enhance the mind's capacity to affect bodily function and symptoms. *Biologically based therapies* in CAM use substances found in nature, such as herbs, foods, and vitamins. *Manipulative and body-based methods* in CAM are based on manipulation and/or movement of one or more parts of the body. *Energy therapies* involve the use of energy fields and are of two types: biofield therapies and bioelectromagnetic-based therapies. *Movement therapies* are modalities used to improve patterns of bodily movement. *Pharmacological and biological therapies* are drugs, vaccines, off-label use of prescription drugs, and other biological interventions not yet accepted in mainstream medicine. *Complex natural products,* a subcategory of the prior, consist of crude natural substances and unfractionated extracts from marine organisms used for

Table 24-1 Commonly Used Acronyms in Complementary and Alternative Medicine

Acronym	Full Name
ACS	American Cancer Society
ASCO	American Society of Clinical Oncology
CAM	Complementary and alternative medicine
DB	Double blind study
NB	Non-blinded study
EBP	Evidence-based practice
EBHC	Evidence-based health care
EBM	Evidence-based medicine
FDA	Food & Drug Administration
MA	Meta-analysis
NCCAM	National Center for Complementary and Alternative Medicine
NCI	National Cancer Institute
NLM	National Library of Medicine
NIH	National Institutes of Health
OCCAM	Office of Cancer Complementary and Alternative Medicine
ONS	Oncology Nursing Society
PDQ	Physicians Data Query®
RCT	Randomized controlled clinical trial
SR	Systematic review

Table 24-2 Professional Degrees and Certifications in CAM

Acronym	Degree or Certification
BA/BS	Bachelor of arts/Bachelor of science
MA/MS	Master of arts/Master of science
MPH	Master of public health
RN	Registered nurse
RD	Registered dietician
PhD	Doctor of philosophy
MBBS	British medical degree
ScD	Doctor of science
ND	Doctor of naturopathy
DO	Doctor of osteopathy
DNSc	Doctor of nursing science
DPH	Doctor of public health
PharmD	Doctor of pharmacy
MD	Medical doctor
OMD/DOM	Oriental medical doctor/doctor of oriental medicine
IMG	International medical graduate
LAc	Licensed acupuncturist
CNC	Certified nutritional consultant
CMT	Certified massage therapist
CHt/CMHt	Certified hypnotherapist/Medical hypnotherapist
CHTP	Certified healing touch practitioner
LMT	Licensed massage therapist

Table 24-3 Definitions of CAM

Source	Definition
Cassileth and Vickers[1,2]	CAM is an umbrella term used to describe diverse techniques. Unproven methods (alternative therapies for cancer treatment) should be distinguished from complementary methods applied to mainstream care for symptom management and to enhance quality of life.
Ernst[3]	CAM is any approach to improve a health problem that is not used or taught routinely to conventional Western practitioners. Alternative cancer treatments are CAM therapies that reduce tumor burden or replace mainstream therapy.
Micozzi[4]	CAM covers a broad range of health and medical systems often derived from ancient societies with the common theme that the body has energy along with material aspects, can heal itself, and healing comes from the inner resources of the body.
NCCAM[5,6]	CAM is a group of diverse medical and health care systems, practices, and products that are not currently considered to be a part of conventional medicine. Complementary medicine is used with conventional medicine. Alternative medicine is used in place of conventional medicine. Integrative medicine combines mainstream and CAM therapies for which scientific evidence of safety and efficacy exists.
Oncology Nursing Society[7]	CAM involves the interchangeable use of the terms "complementary," "alternative," and "integrative" therapies reflecting what may describe a therapy rather than how it is used. "Complementary" describes a therapy that is used with a conventional therapy, whereas "alternative" describes a therapy that is used "instead of" conventional therapy. "Integrative care" is defined as a combination of complementary and conventional approaches to care.
Segen[8]	Alternative health care systems constitute an array of treatments and ideologies that are based on no common or consistent philosophy. Three groups of philosophies are: (1) formal therapeutic systems such as traditional Chinese medicine, (2) informal therapeutic systems such as mind-body medicine, and (3) quackery involving potentially predatory practices in which the therapist or developer has been found guilty of fraud.

healing and treatment of disease. OCCAM classifications offer a usable framework for enhanced understanding of CAM as a whole and cancer CAM as a subcomponent. Table 24-4 further describes each domain as defined by the OCCAM and provides examples.

Historical Perspective

Therapeutic interventions relying on natural healing (nineteenth-century term), drugless healing (early twentieth-century term), or holistic healing (1970s to present term) are not new or original in the United States as the history of complementary and/or alternative medicine dates back to the 1700s. An awareness of the historical development of CAM as a distinctive field is essential for understanding the philosophical viewpoints between and among practice disciplines.[11]

Ancient traditions to the nineteenth century

In ancient traditions, healing methods were passed on in the form of hymns, prayers, incantations, and ritual formulas containing information on how to use plants for bodily healing. The stories remained oral for centuries before being written around 1200 BC into the first known versions called the Vedic texts. The word "*Ayurveda*" (meaning "life and knowledge") may have been coined around 400 BC to associate these plant remedies and recipes with basic Vedic texts. Like Ayurveda, Chinese medicine traces its history to unwritten legends that are thousands of years old. Chinese pharmacopoeias first appeared around 200 BC to AD 205. As early as 1000 BC, herbs from India, the Spice Islands, and the west coat of Africa were imported into China. Important roots of what is now considered modern medicine had developed by 500–400 BC in Greece.[12]

Hippocrates (460–370 BC) emphasized the art of clinical inspection, observation, and documentation of the science of medicine. Galen of Pergamum (AD 130–200) utilized animal studies to understand human disease and identified the four humors of blood, phlegm, black bile, and yellow bile. By the Middle Ages (AD 1100–1200), improvements in medicine had emerged, along with the simultaneous advent of nursing practice[13] as early research using herbs began in European hospitals. The Renaissance (1453–1600) represented the revival of learning and the casting aside of ancient Greek viewpoints such as the four humors. Through the understanding of blood circulation (Harvey, 1578–1657), the invention of the microscope (van Leeuwenhoek, 1632–1723), the use of vaccinations to prevent the spread of disease (Jenner, 1749–1823; Waterhouse in 1802), hand washing to prevent mortality (Semmelweiss, 1818–1865), the germ theory of disease (Pasteur, 1822–1895), bacteriology (Koch, 1843–1910), and the humoral components of host defense (Ehrlich, 1854–1915), advances in medicine unfolded in the United States.[14]

Unconventional methods of disease treatment with the intent to cure prior to the nineteenth century were considered folk medicine or quackery. Practitioners of the first generation of developing systems of alternative medicine in the early twentieth century (Thom-

Table 24-4 The OCCAM Domains of CAM and Their Modalities in Clinical Trials

Domain	Definition	Example(s)	Modality in Clinical Trials
Alternative medical systems	Systems built upon completed systems of theory and practice	Traditional Chinese medicine (acupuncture), Ayurveda, homeopathy, naturopathy, Tibetan medicine	Acupuncture Acupressure Electroacupuncture Traumeel S®
Manipulative and body-based methods	Methods based on manipulation and/or movement of one or more parts of the body	Chiropractic, therapeutic massage, osteopathy, reflexology	Distance healing Exercise-based counseling Group therapy Healing touch Music therapy Spirituality, religiosity Standard counseling Stress management training
Energy therapies	Therapies involving the use of energy fields	Reiki, therapeutic touch, pulsed fields, magnet therapy	Energy healing Energy therapy Reiki Touch
Mind-body interventions	Techniques designed to enhance the mind's capacity to affect bodily function and symptoms	Meditation, hypnosis, art therapy, biofeedback, mental healing, imagery, relaxation therapy, support groups, music therapy, cognitive-behavioral therapy, prayer, dance therapy, psychoneuroimmunology, aromatherapy, animal-assisted therapy	Distance healing, exercise-based counseling, group therapy, healing touch, music therapy, spirituality and religiosity
Movement therapy	Modalities used to improve patterns of bodily movement	T'ai chi, Feldenkrais, Hathayoga, Alexander technique, dance therapy, qi gong, Rolfing, Trager method, applied kinesiology,	none
Nutritional therapeutics	Assortment of nutrients and non-nutrient and bioactive food components that are used as chemopreventative agents, and the use of specific foods or diets as cancer prevention or treatment strategies	Dietary regimens such as macrobiotics, vegetarian, Gerson therapy, Kelley/Gonzalez regimen, vitamins, dietary macronutrients, supplements, antioxidants, melatonin, selenium, coenzyme Q10, ephedrine, orthomolecular medicine	Black cohosh Creatine Curcumin Flax seed Folid acid Fruit and vegetable extracts Garlic Ginger Herbal therapy Juven L-carnitine Low-fat diet Lycopene Macrobiotic diet Noni fruit extract Nutritional supplements Pomegranate juice Selenium Soy protein isolate *Valerian officinalis* Vitamins C and E Zinc sulfate
Pharmacological and biological treatments	Drugs, complex natural products, vaccines, and other biological interventions not yet accepted in mainstream medicine, off-label use of prescription drugs	Antineoplastons, products from honeybees, 714-X, low-dose naltrexone, met-enkephalin, immunoaugmentative therapy, laetrile, hydrazine sulfate, New Castle Virus, melatonin, ozone therapy, thymus therapy, enzyme therapy, high-dose vitamin C	Antineoplastons Pancreatic proteolytic enzymes

(continued)

Table 24-4 The OCCAM Domains of CAM and Their Modalities in Clinical Trials (continued)

Domain	Definition	Example(s)	Modality in Clinical Trials
Complex natural products	Subcategory of pharmacological and biological treatments consisting of an assortment of plant samples (botanicals), extracts of crude natural substances, and unfractionated extracts from marine organisms used for healing and treatment of disease	Herbs and herbal extracts, mixtures of tea polyphenols, shark cartilage, essiac tea, cordyceps, Sun soup, MGN-3	Chinese herbal extract Green tea extract (polyphenon E) Kanglaite injection Milk thistle Mistletoe Pycnogenol® Shark cartilage St. John's wort Virulizin®

Data reprinted from Lee.[9]

sonianism, Homeopathy, Hydropathy, Mesmerism, and Eclecticism) were held together by shared theoretical precepts and therapeutic regimens.[11] Established societies, journals, and schools gave credence to these systems, which captured about 10% of the practice.[15] Hahnemann, founder of the system of homeopathy that became popular in the United States in the 1830s, coined the word "allopathic," which is now a standard term for orthodox or conventional medicine. The second generation of developing systems (Osteopathy, Chiropractic, Naturopathy, and Hydropathy) took hold in the late twentieth century, capturing about 20% of all medical practice. During this time, contemporary holism emerged, focusing on treating the "whole" patient and promoting the self-care philosophy, leading to the current trend of lifestyle regulation and wellness promotion. Nursing curricula designed to distinguish between analyzing patient needs and problems from a medical diagnosis began in the 1950s in the United States.[13]

Cancer CAM in the United States today

Public education, legislative action, and medical advances in the mid-1970s to 1980s did not deter patients in the United States from seeking CAM. To address the mounting and significant issues, the Office of Alternative Medicine (OAM) was established in 1992, becoming the National Center for Complementary and Alternative Medicine in 1998. NCCAM is one of the 27 institutes and centers that make up the National Institutes of Health (NIH), which is one of eight agencies under the Public Health Service (PHS) in the U.S. Department of Health and Human Services (DHHS). NCCAM has four primary focus areas: research (clinical and basic science research), training and career development (predoctoral, postdoctoral, and career researchers), outreach (conferences, educational programs and exhibits, information clearinghouse), and integration (incorporating scientifically proven CAM practices into conventional medicine).[5]

To increase the amount of high-quality cancer research and information about CAM use, the National Cancer Institute (NCI) established the Office of Cancer Complementary and Alternative Medicine (OCCAM) within the Office of the Director in 1998. The OCCAM promotes and supports research within CAM disciplines and therapies as they relate to the prevention, diagnosis, and treatment of cancer, cancer-related symptoms, and side effects of conventional treatment. The OCCAM coordinates NCI's CAM research and informational activities and NCI's collaboration with other governmental and nongovernmental organizations on cancer CAM issues, and also provides an interface with health practitioners and researchers regarding cancer CAM issues.[9,16]

The White House Commission on Complementary and Alternative Medicine Policy (WHCCAMP) was established in March 2000 to address issues of access to and delivery of CAM, priorities for research, and the need to educate consumers and healthcare professionals (HCPs). WHCCAMP endorsed 10 principles, listed in Table 24-5.[17] A non-government agency established in 1970, the Institute of Medicine (IOM) of the National Academies, guarantees unbiased, evidence-based information and advice concerning health and science policy to policy-makers, HCPs, and the public. In 2003–2004, the IOM sponsored meetings to explore scientific, policy, and practice questions that arise from the increasing use of CAM by the American public. The final report of the IOM committee was released in January 2005.

Use of CAM Therapies in the United States

Consumer Issues

Issues relevant to understanding the use of CAM in the United States are as follows: the reasons for using CAM (motive), the frequency with which use occurs (preva-

Table 24-5 Guiding Principles Endorsed by the White House Commisison on CAM

- A wholeness orientation in healthcare delivery: delivery of high-quality health care must support care of the whole person
- Evidence of safety and efficacy: use science to generate evidence that protects and promotes public health
- Healing capacity of a person: support capacity for recovery and self-healing
- Respect for individuality: each person has the right to health care that is responsive, respects preferences, and preserves dignity
- Right to choose treatment: each person has the right to choose freely among safe and effective approaches and among qualified practitioners
- Emphasis on health promotion and self-care: good health care emphasizes self-care and early interventions for maintaining and promoting health
- Partnerships in integrated health care: good health care requires teamwork among patients, HCPs, and researchers committed to creating healing environments and respecting diversity of healthcare traditions
- Education as a fundamental healthcare service: education about prevention, healthy lifestyles, and self-healing should be part of the curriculum of all HCPs and made available to the public
- Dissemination of comprehensive, timely information: healthcare quality is enhanced by examination of the evidence on which CAM systems, practices, and products are based. This information should be widely, rapidly, and easily available
- Integral public involvement: input from informed consumers must be incorporated in proposing priorities for healthcare, research, and policy decisions

Data from White House Commission on Complementary and Alternative Medicine Policy.[17]

lence), and the people who use it (patient characteristics).[18] Among the reasons for the revival of complementary and alternative medicine in the twenty-first century in the United States are philosophical similarity (emphasis on holism, active patient role, natural treatments, spiritual dimension), personal control over treatment, positive relationship with therapist (time for discussion, including emotional aspects), accessibility, and increased well-being.[19] Factors that may contribute to the decreased use of conventional biomedical medicine in favor of CAM are dissatisfaction (ineffective therapies, adverse effects, poor communication with HCPs, insufficient time with HCPs, waiting lists), rejection (anti-science viewpoint), desperation, and cost of care. It is possible that the persuasive appeal of CAM is related to a perceived association of CAM with nature, a focus on energy forces promoting vitalism, intellectual traditions and sophisticated philosophies, extensive training involving complex systems and concepts, and a likely union of the physical (medical) and spiritual (truth, values, morals) realms.[18,20] Ultimately in the twenty-first century, patients have expressed a desire to take control of their own health, actively participate in decisions related to health and wellness, and choose treatment plans involving solely conventional biomedical medicine alone, CAM alone, or a combination of both.

The first U.S. national survey of the prevalence, cost of use, and pattern of use of CAM was published in 1993, at which time one in three respondents had used at least one "unconventional" therapy within the past year, and one third of these respondents had sought providers for "unconventional" therapy.[21] In the early to mid 1990s, CAM surveys were not disease specific. Trends over the past decade show a gradual increase in the prevalence of CAM use among patients in the United States.[22–25] Toward the end of the 1990s, more was known about CAM use among cancer patients, rural populations, and elderly patients, and similar trends in use were seen.[26–32] Studies conducted since 2000 (sample size $N \geq 100$) show CAM use in adults with cancer as being between 25% and 80%.[33–36]

Compared with non-CAM users, individuals who use CAM are more likely to be female, better educated, and have higher incomes.[22] Using a cross sectional design in females with gynecologic cancer, a recent study reported that characteristics associated with CAM use include annual incomes of more than $30,000, a cancer site of origin other than the cervix, and the use of CAM prior to the cancer diagnosis.[37] Respondents reported their reasons for using CAM as (1) hope of improved well-being and (2) possible anti-cancer effects of the particular CAM modalities used. In another study, 82% of the participants reported using CAM as a therapeutic intervention for medical conditions such as depression, anxiety, and insomnia.[28] Researchers conclude that the oncology community must improve patient–provider communication and initiate research to determine possible drug-herb-vitamin interactions.[36] Oncology nurses contribute a vital function in educating patients on the safe use of therapies[37] and in incorporating CAM modalities such as relaxation, imagery, or healing touch into cancer care.[28]

Consumers of CAM therapies are interested in choosing their providers, integrating CAM therapies into conventional care, limiting out-of-pocket expenses, and expanding insurance coverage. The amount patients are willing to pay for CAM may indicate the value they place on these therapies.[38] Reported mean out-of-pocket payments per visit for certain therapies were $9 for spiritual healing, $23 for herbal therapies, $33 for massage, $44 for acupuncture, and $49 for nutritional advice.[38] Consumers spent nearly $27 billion (out-of-pocket) dollars on alternative medicine professional services between 1990 and 1997, reflecting an increase of 45.2%. Given the financial investment in CAM therapies, an enduring question is

Table 24-6 Sample Clinical Trials Involving Conventional and CAM Modalities for Cancer Treatment

Type	Description	Example of Conventional Biomedical Trial	Example of Cancer CAM Trial
Prevention trials	Study ways to reduce risk of developing cancer	Phase IIB/III randomized chemoprevention study of celexicob in patients with superficial transitional cell carcinoma of the bladder at high risk for recurrence	Phase III randomized study of selenium and vitamin E for the prevention of prostate cancer (SELECT Trial)
Screening trials	Study ways to detect cancer in people who do not have any symptoms of cancer	Phase II pilot study of CA 125 screening in patients at high risk for ovarian cancer	None at this time
Diagnostic trials	Study tests or procedures that identify cancer earlier	Phase I/II diagnostic study of C11-methionine and FDG PET imaging in patients with progressive prostate cancer	None at this time
Treatment trials	Study new therapies or new indications of drugs, vaccines, or approaches to treatment	Phase II/III randomized study of paclitaxel and carboplatin with or without bevacizumab in patients with advanced, metastatic, or recurrent NSCLC	Phase II study of supplemental treatment with mistletoe in patients with stage IV NSCLC receiving palliative chemotherapy
Supportive care trials (Includes Quality of Life)	Study ways to improve cancer-related symptoms and quality of life	Phase III randomized study of octreotide versus standard care for chemotherapy-induced diarrhea in patients with colorectal cancer	Phase II/III randomized study of ginger for chemotherapy-related nausea in patients with cancer
Genetic studies	Study ways in which genetic makeup can affect detection, diagnosis, or treatment response.	Genetic study of familial factors in patients with colon cancer	None at this time

Data from Lee.[10]

whether CAM therapies can provide the beneficial health outcomes to justify the expense.[39]

Role of Evidence-Based Practice

Levels of evidence are guidelines used by researchers and clinicians to assess the degree to which interventions meet preestablished criteria. A frequent outcome of level of evidence data is clinical practice guidelines, which are used as a basis for recommendations for the care of patients with specific conditions. These guidelines are based on a systematic review of the available research, focusing on the strength of the evidence, and they involve value judgments as to how patients should be managed. In the past, guidelines focused on the effectiveness of interventions. Recently, however, more attention has been paid to the magnitude of the effect and the balance between the effect and the harm and costs to the patient.

The classification system used by the NCI Physician Data Query (PDQ) Adult Treatment Editorial Board ranks human cancer treatment studies according to the statistical strength of the study design and the specific scientific strength of the treatment outcomes. This classification system has been adopted for use in human studies involving CAM treatments. The strength of the study design is ranked in descending order from 1 to 4. Randomized controlled clinical trials (RCTs), doubled blinded or nonblinded, are a gold standard of study design. To achieve this, the study must be blinded to the physician before and after randomization and treatment assignment, thereby assuring protection from investigator bias and from bias in the outcomes caused by investigator and patient. Nonrandomized control clinical trials assign treatments by birth date, chart number, day of clinic appointment, bed availability, or any other strategy that would make the patient known to the researcher. Case series, ranking number 3 and 4, either population based or non-population based to a best-case series, are the weakest form of study design. For some CAM modalities, case series may be the only available or practical information known. Most CAM therapies have not undergone clinical trials. Table 24-6 provides examples of CAM therapies currently in clinical trials.

The scientific strength of study findings is determined by the endpoint. Two common endpoints are total mortality (the deceased proportion of the study population) and cause-specific mortality (the cause of death, such as cancer, a side effect of the treatment, or a co-morbidity). Quality of life endpoints are the most important endpoints to patients. The strength of quality of life findings, however, depends on the validity of the measurement instruments. Indirect surrogates such as disease-free survival, progression-free survival, and tumor response rate are additional endpoints.

Levels of evidence in CAM are generated in the same fashion as those in conventional medicine, beginning with clinical trials involving CAM modalities for the treatment of cancer and cancer-related side effects. The positive or negative clinical trial results form the foundation for systematic reviews and meta-analyses that in turn affect the development of evidence-based practice, research utilization, evidence-based health care, and practice guidelines. Levels of evidence are frequently used by organizations such as the NCI (clinical trials) and ONS (PRISM project), as well as in databases such as the Natural Medicines Comprehensive Database, the Natural Standard Database, and the Oxford Centre for Evidence-based Medicine.

Evidenced-base practice (EBP) is the care of patients using the best available evidence from the results of research to guide clinical decision making. Steps in EBP include defining the question, accessing the information, judging the credibility of the results, and applying these results to the care of patients. The process of defining EBP for certain CAM therapies is quite similar to that for conventional medicine, and it comes about as a result of integrating clinical expertise, epidemiological studies, and anecdotal evidence. Angell and Kassirer assert that there cannot be two kinds of medicine, conventional and alternative.[40] They state that there is only one type of medicine: one that has been adequately tested, reasoning that once a treatment has been tested rigorously, it no longer matters whether it was considered "alternative" at the outset. If the modality is found to be reasonably safe and effective, it can be accepted into clinical practice, but assertions, speculations, and testimonials do not substitute for evidence.[40]

Regulation of Dietary Supplements

Confidence in the contents of a single, active molecule of a substance, such as an herb, began to emerge in the late nineteenth century as a result of the need to have medicines tested, standardized, and patented. Two laws, the Biologic Control Act (1902) and the Food and Drugs Act (1906), formed the foundation of the present-day Food and Drug Administration.[41] After multiple fatalities involving an elixir, the federal Food, Drug, and Cosmetic Act of 1938 was passed, requiring that new drugs provide evidence of safety before being placed on the market. Following another fatality in 1962, legislation was passed requiring that drug manufacturers provide evidence of efficacy before marketing a drug. The U.S. Food and Drug Administration (FDA) governs all aspects of the development and manufacturing of drug products, product characterization, safety, efficacy, claims, and postmarket surveillance.

Prior to 1994, herbal products were not regulated; rather, they were marketed either as foods or as drugs, depending on their intended use and claims. Under the Dietary Supplement Health and Education Act (DSHEA) of 1994, a dietary supplement is now defined as a product intended to supplement the diet. A supplement may be a vitamin, mineral, herb, botanical, amino acid, or a combination of these ingredients, and may be in the form of a concentrate, metabolite, constituent, or extract, a supplement to increase total daily intake, or combinations of these ingredients.[42] The product must be intended for ingestion in pill, capsule, tablet, or liquid form, must not be a conventional food or the sole item of a meal or diet, and must be labeled as a "dietary supplement." The DSHEA provides for the use of various statements on a product label that do not need preapproval, although claims must not be made about the diagnosis, prevention, treatment, or cure of a specific disease. For example, a claim for an herb cannot read, "This product will cure cancer, heart disease, and obesity." Like foods, dietary supplements must bear ingredient labeling (including the name and quantity of each ingredient) and nutrition labeling (daily consumption recommendations). Botanical and herbal products must state the part of the plant from which the ingredient originated. The DHSEA grants the FDA the authority to develop good manufacturing practices governing the preparation, packing, and holding of products. The act also created the NIH Office of Dietary Supplements to promote, collect, and compile research and maintain a database on supplements and individual nutrients. From a consumer standpoint, the DHSEA provides for over-the-counter, ready access to a wide range of products without the requirement of standardization.

Efficacy and Safety of Common CAM Modalities

Despite the fact that CAM therapies are increasingly being used in the United States and abroad, limited data are available on the safety, efficacy, and mechanism of action of many individual therapies. One must be aware of this lack of complete data when making treatment decisions. Until recently, much information available was based on theoretical or personal opinion rather than on evidence. The concept of an evidence-based approach to CAM is still in its infancy. Recommending CAM therapies remains challenging for HCPs. Eisenberg[43] offered an algorithm for advising patients regarding CAM therapies. Ernst[44] strove to establish a base of evidence for CAM and offered a direction-of-evidence model. Increasingly, HCPs encounter patients who request information regarding CAM therapies for preventing or treating medical conditions. This interest may intensify when traditional therapies are not providing the desired result.[45] This desire for CAM therapies is complicated by the amount of information, much of it inaccurate, available from a variety of sources, including the Internet and well-meaning friends and family. Opinions differ, and methods for rating therapies vary even among experts. Ernst[44] uses "direction of evidence" (clearly positive, tentatively positive, uncertain, tentatively negative, clearly negative) and "weight of evidence" (low, moderate, and high). Eisenberg[45] uses "recommend," "tolerate," and "avoid."

Clinical Cancer CAM Research

In the investigation of medicine, there are six predominant types of research:[46] (1) a qualitative approach involving patient interviews, (2) laboratory and basic science involving in vitro and in vivo testing, (3) observational studies involving epidemiological and outcomes research, (4) RCTs involving the isolation or comparison of interventions, (5) meta-analyses and systematic reviews involving summaries of research, and (6) health technology assessment and health service research involving the utility and impact of interventions. While certain fields may seek out one or more types of research inquiry, comprehensive research involving all six types in the field of cancer CAM is forthcoming. Nonetheless, the key question for both conventional biomedical and cancer CAM research is whether the treatment under consideration is effective. Other considerations are also important: Is the treatment effective on average for patients with this condition? Is this feature of the treatment effective on average for patients with this condition? Is this treatment more effective on average than another treatment for patients with this condition? Does this treatment add anything to standard therapy? Is the effect of this treatment demonstrated biologically in laboratory experiments? CAM should be no different than conventional biomedical medicine in terms of the application of rigorous research methods.

A common criticism of CAM by conventional biomedical practitioners is the lack of scientifically conducted research. Evidence of effectiveness is critical to the widespread support of the use of conventional as well as CAM interventions. Since the RCT is the preferred method for evaluating the efficacy of interventions, significant support exists for evaluating CAM modalities using RCTs.[47] The goal is to ensure a methodologically rigorous trial without compromising the modality in a manner that is incomplete or inappropriate. The prevailing inquiry is no longer that RCTs be utilized, but rather, how best to apply the RCT results. The next step of integrating research and clinical evidence to create EBP in CAM requires a delicate and complex balance. Pelletier summarizes the views of many proponents and opponents of CAM:[48] Virtually any form of CAM is superior to any form of conventional biomedical practice, or any form of conventional biomedical practice is superior to any form of CAM. The balanced view is that both conventional biomedical medicine and CAM have benefits and limitations and that all therapeutic interventions can be held to the same rigorous standards of evidenced-based medicine. Not all CAM can be easily measured through clinical research, and thus three measurement areas should be included for consistency and accuracy: (1) philosophy and practice in healing in the CAM modality, (2) the relationship between the user and the practitioner, and (3) techniques used to enhance the healing process.[49]

Clinical Trials

Cancer clinical trials are research studies in humans designed to answer specific questions related to cancer. Clinical research may meet an individual's health needs in terms of quality care and treatment, although that is not the highest goal of research. Meticulously conducted cancer clinical trials are the fastest method to establishing safe and effective preventative, diagnostic, treatment, and/or supportive care interventions. Cancer CAM clinical trials are increasing in number and expanding in design. Three trial types are currently being conducted for cancer CAM: prevention, treatment, and supportive care trials (see Table 24-6).

Ethical Considerations in Cancer CAM

Ethics is a systematic method of answering questions about how and why individuals live and behave in daily life.[50] In regard to clinical research, the ethical questions are (1) *should* research be performed on human subjects? and (2) *how* should this research be performed? The primary ethical struggle in clinical research is that comparatively few individuals accept the risk of being research subjects in order to benefit others and society. Ethicists raise the point that asking subjects to bear the risk of harm for the good of others creates the potential for maltreatment or misuse.

Emanuel and colleagues[51] offers a framework for ethical clinical research composed of seven requirements: social value, scientific validity, fair subject selection, favorable risk-benefit ratio, independent review, informed consent, and respect for subjects. If the research inquiry has no social value, there is no justifiable reason to subject patients to risk in a clinical trial. Further, the research must be designed and conducted with rigorous methodology to ensure the validity of its findings. Studies without scientific validity are unethical because they expose patients to risk without the possibility of generalizable knowledge. HCPs often engage in conversations with patients regarding the role of nutrition, herbal medicine, and complementary approaches in cancer care. Conversations such as these are leading HCPs to reconsider their moral, ethical, and legal obligation to remain aware of the best available evidence in CAM, to present the evidence in patient-friendly terms, and to address choices from a comprehensive perspective.[52,53] Ethical struggles in cancer CAM research surrounding informed consent, malpractice, liability, and trial design are likely to be long-term considerations.

Methodological Challenges

The research methodology used pertains to how the study is conducted. It mainly involves the measurement of variables, aspects of control, and statistical analysis. Much is lacking in the amount of available information regarding the use of some CAM modalities: the number and type of patients who use various modalities, how the practices are delivered (method, dose, etc.), how well patients respond, and side effect profiles. A common criticism of CAM by conventional biomedical practitioners is the lack of scientifically conducted research. Since the RCT is the preferred method for evaluating the efficacy of conventional biomedical interventions, many scientists, researchers, and HCPs propose that CAM modalities be evaluated in the same manner. While agreeing that the RCT is a suitable design for some CAM modalities, others suggest the use of both explanatory ("gold standard") and pragmatic RCTs.[54] Pragmatic RCTs do not require that the patient or HCP be "blind" to the modality utilized, and they consider patient preference in the delivery of the modality. Design issues related to the use of a control and methods of assessing the effects of individual differences, minimizing therapist variability, determining acceptable inclusion-exclusion criteria, and assessing treatment outcomes are ongoing considerations in pragmatic trials. The overall goal of all research in cancer CAM is to ensure a methodologically rigorous trial that addresses the unique challenges without compromising the modality in a manner that is incomplete or inappropriate.[55]

In 2002, an NCI-sponsored expert panel on cancer symptom research identified the following challenges in CAM research methodology:[56] (1) the development of appropriate controls, shams, and placebo interventions, (2) the development of individualized versus standardized approaches, (3) the development of new drugs within the FDA regulations, (4) the current trend toward developing phase III trials versus I/II developmental trials, (5) ethical issues, (6) the implications for statistics, and (7) tools and measurement issues. The expert panel had the following major recommendations: (1) create truly inert controls that will not cause independent beneficial or harmful effects, (2) balance the need for replication in science with the desire to study interventions in a manner that is consistent with clinical practice, and (3) obtain an Investigational New Drug (IND) to ensure consistency in product quality and fulfillment of pharmacology and toxicology requirements. Richardson and Strauss[56], Carter,[57] and Hyland[58] comprehensively address the methodologic issues in CAM cancer clinical research. Ezzo[59] emphasizes the value in reporting all positive or negative cancer CAM trial results. Table 24-7 summarizes the pervasive methodologic challenges and offers practical solutions.

Pathways for Pursuing Cancer CAM Research

Pathways toward continued research in cancer CAM are multifold. Beginning with an idea alone, the researcher may conduct a literature search to identify cancer researchers who have published on topics related to the proposed mechanism of the CAM therapy. Researchers can then initiate contact, explain the theory, and suggest collaboration. Beginning with a study population but in need of funding, researchers can submit proposals to several grant programs that offer funding, such as the NIH (NCCAM and OCCAM) and the ONS Foundation. Numerous government sources for funding are available.

Preclinical and early drug development processes assist investigators who have a product (single chemical or biological entities) for potential commercial consideration. Two such programs are the NCI's Rapid Access to Preventative Intervention Development (RAPID) and Rapid Access to Intervention Development (RAID) programs. The RAPID program provides any or all of the in vitro preclinical and phase I clinical developmental requirements for phase II clinical efficacy trials with agents that have the potential to prevent, reverse, or delay carcinogenesis. This includes preclinical pharmacology and toxicology

Table 24-7 Methodologic Challenges and Proposed Solutions in Cancer CAM Research

Challenges	Solutions
Study accrual, adequate sample size, and randomization	Design both explanatory and pragmatic trials
Appropriate controls and placebo interventions	Create inert controls that do not cause independent effect
Individualized versus standard approaches	Combine the benefits of individualized and standardized approaches Design trials considering whole alternative systems instead of a core modality Design trials to study one intervention from a whole alternative system for a specific disease Propose alternate study designs involving detailed case histories and case series Seek a better understanding of the use of CAM by cancer patients
Herbs and nutritional supplements not characterized or standardized	Obtain an Investigational New Drug (IND) for herbs and supplements in clinical trials
New drug development requirements within FDA regulations	Clarify IND requirements
Applicability of RCTs to some CAM therapies	Use qualitative inquiry alongside quantitative measurement Combine the benefits of individualized and standardized approaches Seek collaboration among CAM researchers with varying approaches to design trials
Trial design	Conduct phase III trials versus I/II development trials
High-quality reporting of effectiveness	Systematically track ongoing studies Report negative trial results in indexed journals
Generalization of results	Conduct systematic reviews and meta-analysis
Lack of central location in listing cancer CAM clinical trials	Conduct periodic literature reviews of locations of primary clinical trial results
Funding to develop and implement meticulously designed clinical trials	Obtain sustained financial support from the government, industry, advocacy groups, and the public

studies, bulk supply, good manufacturing practices manufacturing and formulation, and regulatory and IND support. The RAID program assists in the translation of novel, therapeutic, and anticancer synthetic, natural product, or biologic interventions arising from the academic community to the clinic setting. This includes defining dose and schedules for in vitro and in vivo activity, assay and formulation development, IND-directed in vivo toxicology, and planning of clinical trials. Single chemical or biological entities or compounds are generally always evaluated in vitro before beginning in vivo testing. Since many CAM approaches are already in use with little or no preclinical or clinical research support, case reports or case series may be the only data available. The NCI Best Case Series program offers the opportunity to compile and submit case scenerios involving CAM for the treatment of cancer. A ''persuasive'' case is one that meets all of the following criteria: (1) a pathological diagnosis of cancer from a tissue specimen obtained prior to an alternative medicine intervention and after any conventional anticancer therapy, (2) documentation that a patient used the alternative medicine intervention under evaluation, (3) documentation of tumor regression appropriate for the disease type and location, and (4) absence of confounding and/or concurrent anticancer therapies. The medical records, radiographic imaging, and pathologic specimens are reviewed internally, and if potentially promising cases are identified (a CAM modality resulted in tumor regression without evidence of impact from confounders), the case undergoes advisory panel review. The main goal of the review is to make an overall assessment of whether further NCI-sponsored research is warranted.[60]

Integration of Evidence-Based Health Care and CAM Therapies

The Biomedical and Biopsychosocial Models

The dominant disease model is biomedical, with molecular biology as its basic scientific discipline. The biomedical model assumes disease to be a deviation from the norm of measurable variables, without accounting for the social, psychological, or behavioral dimensions of illness. Traditionally, cancer has been explained by the biomedical model, however, this model is limited in accounting for all of the facets of the cancer diagnosis.[61] A counterpart to the traditional biomedical model is the Engel biopsychosocial model that places the patient at center focus with inclusion of the affective states. This model has been widely endorsed in theory by contemporary medicine[62] and has been expanded in recent years to include more facets: culture,[63] health-related quality of life,[64] spirituality,[65] dignity and hope,[65] peer function,[66] environmental stimuli,[67] emotional function, role function, self-concept,[68] interdependence, and social support. Suggestive links between emotional distress and immune and neuroendocrine measures exist in patients with cancer.[68–70] The scientific and practice communities deliberate as to which model (biomedical versus biopsychosocial) better serves as the foundation for treating patients holistically.[65]

Locating Relevant and Reliable Research

Patients assume that healthcare decisions are firmly based on high-quality scientific research; however, in multiple clinical settings, unevaluated interventions are recommended and practiced. The publication of meta-analysis and systematic reviews is advantageous in reviewing the best available knowledge in CAM to facilitate public policy, practice decision-making, and integration into cancer care. Bringing together research findings, appraising their quality, and synthesizing the results broadens and publicizes knowledge on which to base healthcare decisions. Meta-analyses (MA) and systematic reviews (SR) are two methods of accomplishing this review and synthesis. An MA extracts relevant findings from research reports that are topic-specific and applies statistics to yield a combined analysis that may indicate greater overall strength than if reviewed individually. This is also known as quantitative pooling of results. An MA regards the findings from one study as singular data; therefore, combining singular data from multiple studies yields stronger positive or negative results. An SR is more comprehensive than an MA and uses explicit, rigorous methods in the identification and critical appraisal of relevant research studies. Intentions for SRs are clarity and accuracy in the aim of the review, selection and inclusion of studies, abstraction of data, validity of results, association between study variables, and review process. The processes and methods for conducting MAs and SRs have improved in the past decade. A premier source for SRs is the Cochrane Library, which represents the work of the Cochrane Collaboration. At the time of this printing, more than 150 Cochrane SRs have been completed in the field of CAM therapies, of which some include cancer CAM.

Since MAs and SRs are not available for all areas in cancer CAM, locating clinical trial results, unpublished data (dissertations), and case reports can be time-consuming due to various publication types and the increasing number of biomedical, social science, and nursing journals, some print based and some electronic. EMBASE (Excerpta Medica database) is a comprehensive biomedicine and pharmacology database that maintains a collection of more than 4500 domestic and international journals. Searchable databases include PDQ®, which offers two options: (1) PDQ® under the "closed trials" option in the advanced search mechanism and (2) PDQ® CAM Information Summaries. The American Society for Clinical Oncology (ASCO) sponsors the *Journal of Clinical Oncology* and the People Living with Cancer Web site, which contains abstracts and conference presentations that are viewable online. The NLM provides access to published results of clinical trials through (1) printed biomedical journals in the main library, (2) electronic full-text articles in publications available through Lonesome Doc, (3) PubMed or Medline searches with the "CAM" limitation for abstracts only in CAM journals (viewable under the "limits" option when searching for a topic), and (4) Medline Plus, which is a free online service of the NLM and the NIH presenting updated health information following clinical trials. Finally, a database sponsored by the University of Maryland Center for Integrated Medicine, known as the Complementary and Alternative Medicine and Pain Database (CAMPAIN), is continually expanding through a grant by the NCCAM. The best available evidence for several common CAM therapies is presented in the sections that follow.

Acupuncture

Description: Acupuncture has been used by many Americans and performed by many physicians, dentists, and acupuncturists for a variety of health conditions, particularly pain. It typically involves inserting a needle into the skin in specific sites (acupoints) for therapeutic purposes. Acupoint stimulation may also be via electrical current, laser, moxibustion, pressure, ultrasound, and vibration and of Japanese, Korean, or Chinese types. The underlying principle is that *qi* (pronounced "chee" and translated as meaning "energy") is present at birth and maintained throughout life. It circulates throughout the body, and 12 meridians provide a major path for the flow of *qi*. There are approximately 350 acupoints along the 12 meridians, with additional acupoints that lie outside the meridian pathways. Health is a balance of yin and yang (opposite forces present in everyone). Disease or any medical condition is a result of imbalance, usually a result of a blockage or deficiency of energy. Acupuncture theory embraces the belief that stimulating the appropriate acupoints helps the body correct any imbalance in the flow of energy, thus restoring balance. It is also held that changes in the balance of energy and flow of *qi* may be identified before disease has developed, and therefore, acupuncture has a role in the prevention of illness and maintenance of health. It has been and is routinely used in Eastern countries. It has also been integrated with allopathic and osteopathic medicine in the United States.[71] Acupuncture has been and continues to be used for pain and other disorders of the musculoskeletal system; headaches; stress; ENT conditions, including sinusitis, tinnitus, and vertigo; allergies; dental pain; addictions; and immune system support, among others.

Evidence: More than 30 MAs and SRs between 1996 and 2004 examined the use of acupuncture for symptom management, mostly related to pain. Nearly 400 RCT results are reported in Medline for the same time period. There is no evidence of the physical existence of *qi* or the meridians. The effects of acupuncture are reportedly better than placebo in most trials.[44] Opioid peptides, serotonin, and other neurotransmitters are released by acupuncture.[72,73] Conclusive evidence exists that acupuncture is effective in the treatment of dental pain[74] and post-operative nausea.[75] The efficacy of acupuncture in relief from asthma, back pain, drug dependency, fibromyalgia, migraine and tension headaches, neck pain, osteoarthritis, and stroke is considered inconclusive by some authors.[76] Others suggest that the evidence is equivocal and/or promising for some indications, including addiction, stroke rehabilitation, postoperative and chemotherapy-related nausea and vomiting, tennis elbow, carpal tunnel syndrome, and asthma.[71]

Contraindications: ''Needling'' technique is contraindicated in those patients with severe bleeding disorders or who are at increased risk for infection as in neutropenia, and during the first trimester of pregnancy, with the exception of treatment for nausea.[77] Patients with cardiac pacemakers should not be treated with electrical stimulation.[78] Caution is advised for the first treatment, and some authors recommend that treatment be administered with the patient in a supine position. Some patients become drowsy and should be cautioned against driving and operating machinery. Needles should not be re-used, and strict asepsis is mandatory.[78] Side effects include bleeding, bruising, pain with needling, and worsening of symptoms. Reported adverse events are rare but include pneumothorax and death.[78]

Opportunities: Since the diagnostic value of acupuncture has not been established it may constitute more risk than reward, however, it is worth consideration for a number of conditions. There is evidence that with accurate diagnosis it is safe, and for certain conditions it is more effective than placebo when administered by an appropriately trained practitioner.

Active Clinical Trials

- Phase III Randomized Study of Acupressure for Chemotherapy-Induced Nausea in Women with Breast Cancer Receiving One of Three Combination Therapy Regimens, MDA-NURO1–396
- Acupuncture to Prevent Postoperative Bowel Paralysis, AT 001065–2
- Randomized Study of Electroacupuncture for Treatment of Delayed Chemotherapy-Induced Nausea and Vomiting in Patients with Newly Diagnosed Pediatric Sarcomas, NCCAM-02–AT-0172
- Randomized Study of Acupuncture to Improve End-of-Life Symptom Distress in Patients With Metastatic Colorectal Cancer, UPITTS-010901
- Acupuncture to Improve Quality of Life in Patients with Advanced Cancer, 1 R21 AT01010–01
- Acupuncture for Shortness of Breath in Cancer Patients, 1 R21 AT010290–01

Practitioners: Nationally, acupuncturists can be certified in two ways. They can complete a formal, full-time educational program that includes both classroom and clinical hours, or they may participate in an apprenticeship program. Acupuncturists must also complete a Clean Needle Technique approved course. Medical doctors with training in acupuncture may also obtain board certification. The National Certification Commission of Acupuncture and Oriental Medicine (NCCAOM) established standards for certification that are accepted by some states for licensure. Medical doctors must possess a valid medical license and be certified through the American Academy of Medical Acupuncture. Some states require medical referral, while others allow nonmedical practitioners to see patients without a referral. A comparison of licensed versus certified acupuncturists is viewable at *www.asny.org*.

Qi gong

Description: Qi gong (chi kung) means ''energy cultivation'' and refers to movements that are believed to improve health, longevity, and harmony within oneself and the world.[79] There are thousands of such movements, and qi gong may include any done with the intention of enhancing energy. It is based on four common principles, sometimes referred to as the ''secrets'' of qi gong: mind (the presence of intention), eyes (the focus of intention), movement (the action of intention), and breath (the flow of intention). There are numerous styles, some of which include meditation, exercise, and self-massage. Mastery in qi gong is the achievement of the ultimate goal: harmonious existence and action in all situations. Elements that define this level of expertise include curiosity, ease in action, clarity of focus and intention, perseverance, nonattachment, resilience, openness, creativity, responsiveness, and fluid balance. Numerous books and teachers profess to teach the secrets of qi gong and the power of its applications. Authors agree that it is actually defined by a person's willingness to practice and experience — that is, the ability to learn.[80]

Evidence: Four MAs examined the use of qi gong from 1997 to 2004 for respiratory-related conditions. Nearly 100 RCTs are reported in Medline for the same time period for various conditions. Two trials involved patients with cancer (inspiratory muscle training and relief of breathlessness).[81,82]

Contraindications: Psychosis has been reported. It is not known if there was a latent condition.[44,83]

Opportunities: Ernst suggests that qi gong can be used for health promotion, functional disorders, and symptom control.[44] Yang predicts that it will be used in the treatment of arthritis.[80]

Practitioners: Because it is considered a form of Chinese medicine, consult acupuncturists and those appropriately credentialed in acupuncture and/or Oriental medicine.

Reiki

Description: Reiki means "universal life energy." It is an ancient form of healing. The practitioner is the conduit for the movement of energy. It is the energy — not the healer — that influences healing. In this respect Reiki differs from other healing systems. That is, energy travels through the healing, not from the healer. Reiki is said to alleviate physical, emotional, and spiritual blockages.[8] The five premises of Reiki are (1) there is an energy of unique properties applicable to physical and psychological conditions, (2) the energy has a source, (3) this source can be tapped, (4) a person can be taught to use this energy, and (5) the effects of this energy are palpable and subjective. The energy is considered pure because it is not influenced by the practitioner's faith or religion.[8] The practitioner gently places his or her hands on the client, in a particular series of positions. Typically, five minutes are spent on each of 12 positions, although this may vary based on the needs of the client. The client remains fully clothed at all times, and no pressure, massage, or manipulation is applied to the client. The environment is kept quiet and soothing, and the client should emerge feeling relaxed. Reiki is considered to be capable of healing anything because it works at very fundamental levels of reality. The limits to Reiki seem to be in the recipient's willingness to cast off old habits and patterns, to accept change, and to accept healing.[84] Ernst considers Reiki to be a form of spiritual healing.[44]

Evidence: Two MAs examining Reiki (with therapeutic touch) were reported between 1999 and 2004. More than 20 RCTs are reported in Medline for the same time period. Rexilius and colleagues[85] examined the effect of massage therapy and healing touch on anxiety, depression, subjective caregiver burden, and fatigue experienced by caregivers of patients undergoing stem cell transplant. The results showed declines in anxiety scores, depression, general fatigue, motivation fatigue, and emotional fatigue for individuals in the massage therapy group only. Anxiety and depression scores decreased in the healing touch group, and fatigue and subjective burden increased but without statistical significance.[85] Reiki may be helpful in the treatment of pain,[86] mood changes,[87] and fatigue.[88] Mansour and colleagues[89] tested a standardization procedure for placebo Reiki in an effort to provide a foundation for a subsequent randomized and placebo-controlled Reiki efficacy study. Based on the results, the authors plan a randomized three-arm Reiki efficacy clinical trial.

Contraindications: None are known.

Opportunities: Reiki appears to have no adverse effects and can eventually be self-administered. Clinical trials are sponsored by the National Center for Complementary and Alternative Medicine.

Active Clinical Trial

- Reiki/Energy Healing in Prostate Cancer, NCCAM, R21AT1120

Practitioners: Typically, Reiki is taught in three parts. Reiki Part I includes: history of Reiki, the Reiki hand positions, Reiki symbols and their names, and meditation manifestation. Part II involves intense training focusing on advanced techniques and includes a review of part I. The training for Reiki II brings knowledge of long-distance healing, scanning techniques, and the long-distance Reiki symbols and their names. Typically, there are two USUI-Reiki-Tibetan attunements at intervals throughout the course. Reiki III (Master) includes a review of previous training and practice and brings to the student knowledge for long-distance healing, scanning techniques, more meditation techniques, and an additional Reiki symbol. Typically, there is a Reiki attunement at the end of the course.

Reflexology

Description: Reflexology is a therapeutic method that uses a specific type of manual pressure applied to certain areas, or zones, of the feet (and sometimes the hands or ears) that are believed to correspond to areas of the body, in order to relieve stress and prevent and/or treat physical disorders. The organs, glands, and other components of the body are represented on the foot on the same side. Examining the feet to detect imbalances or obstructions to the flow of energy, which are expressed as tenderness or feelings of crepitus or gravel at the site, assesses body health. It is believed that stimulating these areas with pressure or massage can influence bodily function. Reflexology is purported to promote homeostasis and circulation, reduce stress and eliminate toxins. Skeptics believe that reflexology has an impact because it involves caring touch.[90] From a conventional biomedical framework, there is no known neurophysiological basis for connections between organs or glands and specific areas of the feet. Three investigations into the claimed correspondences are known: reflexologists' diagnoses were no better than chance in identifying medical conditions in one blinded study whereas in another their diagnostic success was better than chance but not clinically significant.[91] Reflexology foot massage may have general health benefits independent of any correspondence of the reflex with specific organs.

Evidence: Nearly twenty RCTs were conducted using reflexology for the relief of cancer symptoms between 1990 and 2004. One MA reviewing the evidence on efficacy and safety of massage was completed in 2002.[92] Reflexology may involve aromatherapy massage and therapeutic touch in some trials. Key findings were (1) aromatherapy and massage may reduce anxiety for short periods of time,[93] (2) therapeutic massage and healing touch induce relaxation,[89] (3) therapeutic back massage may enhance relaxation and reduce stress in caregivers,[94] and (4) reflexology may positively influence quality of life in patients in the palliative stage of cancer.[95] In noncancer populations, several key RCTs have been reported. Reflexology may be superior to placebo reflexology for the treatment of premenstrual symptoms.[96] It may also have beneficial effects on blood glucose in diabetics.[97] An RCT in patients with multiple sclerosis showed symptomatic improvements; however, the study experienced a high drop-out rate.[98] In a large observational study, 81% of patients with headaches reported themselves helped or cured at a three-month follow-up.[99]

Contraindications: Of concern would be conditions of the feet that might worsen or cause pain with applied pressure, such as gout and peripheral vascular disease. Ernst[44] suggests that reflexology may interfere with some drugs, including insulin.[46] The greatest risk would involve the use of reflexology as an alternative therapy. Reflexology should not be used alone for diagnostic purposes. When provided by an accountable practitioner, reflexology would probably do no harm and may possibly help.[44,90]

Practitioners: No regulatory system, licensure, or minimum training mandates exist for reflexology. Typically, healthcare professionals who may have licensure in another area, such as nursing, use it. Practitioners' backgrounds can range from self-taught to those who have attended training courses.[100]

Aromatherapy

Description: Aromatherapy is the controlled use of plant essences for therapeutic purposes.[101] *Essential oil* is the aromatic essence of a plant in the form of an oil or resin derived from plant leaf, stalk, bark, root, flower, fruit, or seed. The *carrier* is the diluent used with a concentrated essential oil for application. The *neat* is the direct application of the essential oil compound (essential oil plus carrier) to the skin. The *note* is the unique aromatic variable of an essential oil used when blending combinations of essential oil compounds. The *top note* is bright, the *middle note* is lingering, and the *base note* is grounding.[102] Essential oils can be applied directly to the skin through a compress or massage, inhaled via a diffuser or steaming water, or added directly to bath water. At the present time, there are about 150 essential oils.[103] The mechanism of action in the use of essential oils begins with the olfactory sense. After sensing the smell, the limbic system is activated in retrieving learned memories. Essential oils are also absorbed via the dermal route and subcutaneous fat into the bloodstream. Entry into the body via the oral route into the digestive system is not recommended. Often, aromatherapy is practiced with massage. Aromatherapy massage is used in palliative care settings to improve quality of life for patients with cancer. Published data on dosing, comparative methods of administration, and therapeutic outcomes in the use of essential oils in aromatherapy are limited.

Evidence: A 2003 Cochrane Database SR was performed involving aromatherapy for dementia. Nearly 20 RCTs are reported in Medline between 1998 and 2004 for the use of aromatherapy in various clinical settings, of which four involve patients with cancer. Cooke and Ernst[104] reviewed 12 trials in an SR. Six of these trials suggested that aromatherapy massage has a relaxing effect. Louis and Kowalski[105] measured the responses of 17 patients with cancer to humidified essential lavender oil, with a positive change noted in blood pressure, pulse, pain, anxiety, depression, and sense of well-being after both the humidified water treatment and lavender treatment. Olleveant and colleagues[106] compared drop size between six different essential oils and reported that the bottles differed in their method of delivery and recommended a universal standardization of measure to ensure equity and safety in administration. Massage and aromatherapy massage offer short-term benefits for psychological well-being, with the effect on anxiety supported by limited evidence.[107] Evidence is mixed as to whether aromatherapy enhances the effects of massage. Replication, longer follow-up, and larger trials are needed to accrue the necessary evidence.[107]

Contraindications: Contraindications to the use of essential oils are pregnancy, contagious disease, epilepsy, venous thrombosis, varicose veins, open wounds or skin sites, and recent surgeries of any type. Essential oils should not be administered orally or applied undiluted to the skin. Possible adverse events associated with the use of essential oils are photosensitivity, allergic reactions, nausea, and headache. Many essential oils have the potential to either enhance or reduce the effects of prescribed medications, including antibiotics, tranquilizers, antihistamines, anticonvulsants, barbiturates, morphine, and quinidine.[44] Cases of potentially serious reactions involving the use of essential oils have been reported in two individuals without known allergies or sensitivities prior to exposure.[108]

Opportunities: Campbell and colleagues[109] and Avis[110] offer the following guidelines for integrating aromatherapy safely into clinical practice:

- Identify certified staff to serve as resources and educators.
- Conduct a patient assessment.
- Select essential oils with low known risk potential.
- Choose one supplier with stringent product testing.
- Develop a range of oils and methods of application that can be used consistently.
- When blending oils, consider symptoms, patient allergies, and preference of aroma.
- Obtain a verbal consent.
- Place the oil on a tissue for patients in semiprivate rooms.
- Document the outcome of intervention.
- Avoid vaporizers in clinical settings.

Practitioners: Aromatherapy can be used in combination with massage therapy and holistic nursing care programs. Certification is available through the National Association for Holistic Aromatherapy (NAHA, *www.naha.org*). Schools must provide 200 hours of training and practice in the fields of aromatherapy, essential oil studies, anatomy, and physiology. In addition, students must submit a research paper and 10 case histories and must pass a written examination. Holistic nursing certification is available through the American Holistic Nurses' Certification Corporation (AHNCC, *ahna.org/edu/certification.html*). Requirements include a BSN, continuing education, one year of practice, and passing a written exam. Certification in aromatherapy or holistic nursing does not qualify a nurse to work independently, nor does it necessarily meet institutional requirements for practice.[111]

Antioxidants

Description: Antioxidant vitamins — E, C, and beta-carotene — are believed to have health-promoting properties. CoQ10 (Coenzyme Q 10, ubiquinone) is an antioxidant found in all living cells. It is involved in the production of energy within cells and is believed to have powerful antioxidant effects. Although the data are incomplete, up to 30% of Americans are taking some form of antioxidant supplement, and research has shown that patients with cancer take antioxidants, typically at doses higher than the recommended daily allowances (RDAs).[112] Antioxidants act by scavenging free radicals. The debate that surrounds antioxidants has focused on cancer therapies such as alkylating agents, antimetabolites, and radiation because of the purposeful creation of free radicals through cytotoxic mechanisms and, therefore, taking antioxidants could interfere in the action of these therapies. Limited research supports the belief that chemotherapy diminishes total antioxidant status,[113] but inconsistencies based on cancer site, cancer therapy, research methodologies, patient populations, variability in doses, duration of supplementation, and timing of interventions prevent the formulation of conclusions.[114]

Strength of Evidence: More than 45 MAs or SRs reviewing antioxidants (of which five involve patients with cancer) were reported between 1994 and 2004. More than 2000 RCTs involving antioxidants are reported in Medline during this same time period. The belief that antioxidants may interfere with the efficacy of cancer therapy is not new. The association between beta-carotene and increased risk of lung cancer in smokers is well known.[115,116] However, it has been suggested that selective inhibition of tumor cell growth is an action of antioxidants and that antioxidants may also promote cellular differentiation with enhanced cytotoxic effects.[117] Ray and colleagues[118] suggest that typically recommended doses may be insufficient to cover the higher production of reactive oxygen metabolites.[118] It has also been argued that inadequate coverage may actually contribute to malignant cell proliferation.[117] Researchers have been concerned that while antioxidants may decrease some kinds of toxicity associated with cancer chemotherapy, the therapeutic benefit of the cancer therapy may be compromised. Ladas and colleagues[114] reviewed more than 100 citations on antioxidant status and cancer outcomes and antioxidant use among patients receiving chemotherapy with or without radiation therapy. Of the 52 that met their research criteria, 31 were observational studies and 21 were intervention trials. Their findings showed a decline in the total antioxidant status of patients receiving cancer therapy but conflicting and inconsistent results regarding the effect of chemotherapy on the antioxidant status of patients receiving cancer therapy. Lenzhofer and colleagues[119] found that supplementation with vitamin E altered the metabolism of doxorubicin. Landas and colleagues[114] questioned whether this means decreased treatment efficacy, arguing that adjunctive agents such as mesna and amifostine are used to reduce free radicals and do not appear to interfere with therapeutic benefit. Among patients receiving chemotherapy and total-body irradiation for bone marrow transplantion, serum vitamin E levels decreased even among those receiving total parenteral nutrition.[120] Two randomized studies treating patients with gynecologic cancers with doxorubicin; cyclophosphamide; cisplatin with melphalan; and selenium and vitamin E, or placebo demonstrated increased serum selenium levels but not increased vitamin E levels after supplementation.[121] Studies among patients with breast cancer revealed a possible direct effect of selenium supplementation on serum and whole blood selenium.[114] The RDAs appear to be inadequate for maintaining plasma antioxidant levels in patients receiving high-dose chemotherapy before stem cell transplant. Antioxidants may have a role in cancer prevention. Holm and colleagues[122] and Ingram[123] suggest that high vitamin C intake prior to diagnosis of breast cancer has a positive effect on survival. Brawley and Parnes[124] reports that selenium and vitamin E supplementation may reduce the risk of prostate cancer. Variability in doses, duration of supplementation, and timing of interventions prevent the formulation of conclusions in this area of research as well. Except within the context of trials, conclusive recommendations as well as contraindications for the patient with cancer have not been established.

Contraindications: Contraindications exist for specific antioxidants. For example, beta-carotene increases lung cancer risk among smokers.

- *Vitamin C.* Potential interactions: aluminum antacids, cyclosporine, statins, calcium channel blockers and protease inhibitors, iron, vitamin E[125]
- *Vitamin E.* Potential interactions: cholestramine, colestipol, mineral oil, anticonvulsants, anticoagulants, verapamil[125]
- *Beta-carotene.* Potential interactions: cholestyramine, colestipol, mineral oil, orlistat[128]

Active Clinical Trial

- Phase III Randomized Study of Selenium and Vitamin E for the Prevention of Prostate Cancer (SELECT Trial), NCCAM, NCI, SWOG-S0000

Practitioners: Registered Dieticians have a minimum of a bachelors degree in dietetics. Certified nutritional consultants have education and training in clinical nutrition and may be nurses or other healthcare professionals. Caution should be taken when choosing a nutrition practitioner to be certain that he or she has expertise in cancer care as well as in supplements and nutrition.

Antineoplastons

Description: Antineoplastons are naturally occurring peptides and derivatives of amino acids that are hypothesized to control cancer cell growth with reportedly low toxicity.[126] Isolation of peptide fractions from urine have been achieved and named antineoplaston A1, A2, A3, A4, and A5.[126] The first active component was named A10. Two synthetic derivatives of A10 were named AS2-1 and AS2-5 prior to 1986.[126] The mechanism of action of A10 may be related to its structural and chemical resemblance to deoxythymidine and uridine, and it may act as a nucleoside antagonist (interfering with protein synthesis).[127,128]

Evidence: Antineoplastons demonstrated antitumor activity in early laboratory evaluations.[129–131] To date, no published SRs or MAs are available involving the treatment of cancer in humans with antineoplastons. One RCT involving antineoplastons has been reported. It evaluated the usefulness of the antineoplastons in combination therapy based on the imaging findings during the course of treatment. Disappearance or measurable shrinkage of the tumor lasting more than one month was visible diagnostically in 15 tumors. No increase in tumor size for more than three months was observed in 8 tumors. The authors asserted that antineoplastons A10 and AS2-1 were less toxic than chemotherapy and useful as maintenance therapy. Clinical trials performed between 1991 and 1995 involving A10 and AS2-1 were stopped prior to completion. Some reasons for early discontinuation involved quality assurance, delay in IND application approval, inclusion/exclusion of children and older adults in trials, length of treatment, and timing of evaluation. Patients are still being accrued to most of the open clinical trials. Conclusive evidence for the role of antineoplastons in the treatment of cancer has not been established.

Contraindications: Serious adverse reactions include anemia, hypernatremia, and fever in patients who received antineoplastons. Tsuda and colleagues administered A10 and AS2-1 formulations (oral and injectible) in an RCT.[132] The major adverse effects were general weakness, myelosuppression, and liver dysfunction, but effects were not seen when either A10 or AS2-1 was administered alone. The minor adverse effects were excess gas, maculopapular rash, finger rigidity, reduced cholesterol, reduced albumin, increased amylase, eosinophilia, increased alkaline phosphatase, headache, hypertension, palpitation, and peripheral edema, none of which limited use.[132]

Active Clinical Trials

- Multiple trials are underway in the United States at this time involving primary malignant brain tumors; colon, liver, esophageal, pancreatic, lung, and breast cancer; and non-Hodgkin's lymphoma.
- A listing of all clinical trials involving antineoplastons and cancer is available at *cancer.gov/cancerinfo/pdq/*. Two trials are underway in Japan.[160]

Practitioners: Insufficient evidence exists regarding the efficacy of antineoplastons for the treatment of cancer in humans.

St. John's wort

Description: Also known as amber touch-and-heal, devil's scourge, goatweed, hypericum, Klamath weed, millepertuis, rosin rose, Tipton weed, and witch's herb, St. John's wort (SJW) is a member of the *Hypericaceae* family and contains naphthodianthrones, flavinoids, bioflavinoids, phloroglucinols, tannins, volatile oils, and xanthones. The chemical composition is dependent upon the harvesting and drying processes and storage. The biologic activity of St. John's wort is believed to be due to several of its components.[133] It has been used topically and systemically for its medicinal properties for centuries. Uses include wound healing, burns, as a diuretic, and to treat melancholia, pain, gastritis, malaria, hemorrhoids and mental illness, among others.[134] Contemporary use is almost exclusively as an antidepressant.[135] The pharmacologic actions of this herb include antiretroviral and antidepressant action. The mechanism of action is not known. Possibilities include modulation of interleukin-6 and Gaba receptor binding, inhibition of serotonin reuptake, noradrenaline, and dopamine. There is some question regarding action as MAO inhibition. The active ingredients have not been identified, and therefore when considering safety the entire extract must be taken under consideration.[133] Some authors believe hypericin and hyperiform to be the active constituents.[135]

Evidence: Six MAs reviewed the efficacy of SJW in treating mild to moderate depression. More than 50 RCTs are reported in Medline between 1994 and 2004. A number of comparative RCTs have suggested this herb to be as effective as pharmaceutical antidepressants.[136–139] SJW has been shown to be as effective as light therapy in the treatment of seasonal affective disorder.[140] One study identified no antiretroviral effects in patients who were HIV positive.[141] Positive results have been reported with premenstrual syndrome,[18] menopausal symptoms,[140] and fatigue.[142] In an open-label crossover study design, six healthy men and six healthy women ages 22 to 38 years measured plasma pharmacokinetics of alprazolam as a probe for CYP3A4 activity before and after 14 days of SJW administration. A significant decrease in CYP3A4 activity as measured by alterations in alprazolam pharmacokinetics suggests that long-term therapy with SJW may cause diminished clinical impact or increased dose requirements for all CYP3A4 substrates. This represents approximately 50% of all available medications.[143] As monotherapy, SJW has a respectable safety profile considered superior to conventional antidepressants.[135,144]

Contraindications: SJW is contraindicated during pregnancy and lactation. It causes photosensitivity, gastrointestinal symptoms, fatigue, and anxiety. Cases of mania, subacute toxic neuropathy, and breakthrough bleeding (in patients taking oral contraceptives) have been reported. Concurrent use of SJW with serotonin reuptake inhibitors can result in serotonin syndrome. An episode of transplant rejection was reported in a patient receiving cyclosporine. Additional research suggests that the use of SJW reduced plasma levels of medications metabolized by hepatic cytochrome P450, including anticoagulants, anticonvulsants, digoxin, theophylline, and protease inhibitors. A single study indicated no interaction with alcohol.[135] There is inadequate evidence for use in severe depression.

Active Clinical Trial

- Phase III Randomized Study of Sertraline (Zoloft®) Versus *Hypericum Perforatum* (St. John's Wort) in Cancer Patients with Mild to Moderate Depression, CCCWFU-98101, CCCWFU-BGOI-152

Shark and bovine cartilage

Description: Also known as arthrelan, carticin, and haifischknorpel, shark cartilage is derived from the fin of the hammerhead and spiny dogfish sharks. It was thought that shark cartilage might have anticancer properties because sharks did not appear to get cancer.[145] Some believe that creative marketing, not science, promoted this hypothesis.[44] Chemical ingredients include glycoproteins sphyrnastatin 1 and sphyrnastatin 2. Cartilage accounts for 6% of a shark's total body weight.[146] Bovine (cow) cartilage and shark cartilage have been studied as cancer treatments for more than 30 years, and numerous products are sold as dietary supplements. Mechanisms of action have been proposed to explain the potential antitumor activity of cartilage: (1) direct cell kill, (2) immune system stimulation, and (3) angiogenesis. Three different angiogenesis inhibitors have been identified in bovine cartilage, and two have been purified from shark cartilage.[147]

Evidence: No MR or SA evaluating shark or bovine cartilage is reported. Seven RCTs (in vitro and in vivo) are reported in Medline for various conditions between 1995 and 2004. Few human studies of cartilage have been published, and the results are inconclusive. In animal studies, cartilage products have been administered orally, by injection, topically, and via surgical implant. The effects of cartilage on angiogenesis have been studied in chicken embryos, rabbit corneas, and mice conjunctiva. The antiangiogenic properties of oral shark cartilage in the rabbit cornea model appeared to produce systemic levels of angiogenesis inhibitors.[148] In human studies, cartilage products have been administered orally, topically, or via enema or subcutaneous injection. Oral administration presents a methodological challenge in trial design because human intestines do not allow the absorption of large molecules (sphyrnastatin) in quantities that are considered sufficient for therapeutic benefit.[149] The dosage and duration of cartilage treatment has varied due to the different products used in trials. To date, IND status has been granted to at least four groups of investigators to study cartilage as a cancer treatment.

Contraindications: There are significant differences in purity among commercially available cartilage products. Cases of hepatitis caused by shark cartilage[150] have been reported. Shark cartilage is contraindicated during pregnancy and lactation.

Active Clinical Trial

- Phase III Randomized Study of Induction Platinum-Based Chemotherapy and Radiotherapy with or Without Æ-941 (Neovastat) in Patients With Unresectable Stage IIIA or IIIB Non-Small-Cell Lung Cancer, MDA-ID-99303, NCCAM, NCI-T99–0046

Practitioners: Cartilage-containing products should not be recommended for the treatment of cancer because there is insufficient evidence of their safety or efficacy.

Mindfulness meditation

Description: Mindfulness meditation as practiced in mindfulness-based stress reduction (MBSR) is a self-regulatory approach to stress reduction and emotion management in widespread use for the past several decades. Mindfulness is a state in which an individual is highly aware of and focused on the reality of the present moment with acceptance and acknowledgement.[151] Growing interest in the use of MBSR reflects a desire for a more holistic approach to cancer treatment and a recognition of the links between social, psychological, and physiological health determinants. MBSR programs are usually six to eight weeks in length, involving daily individual activities and group activities up to several days per week. It is anticipated that individuals will continue to practice the activities for an extended period of time following completion of the structured program for full benefit of the intervention.

Evidence: There are currently no published MAs involving mindfulness meditation; however, eleven RCTs were reported in Medline between 1973 and 2004. Astin and colleagues tested the short- and long-term benefits of an eight-week MBSR intervention for individuals with fibromyalgia. The study results revealed no evidence that MBSR was superior to education and support as a treatment option.[152] Anxiety and emotional control improved in the treatment group as compared to the control in an RCT assessing the effectiveness of an MBSR program in patients with heart disease.[153] In two RCTs involving cancer, MBSR was effective in decreasing mood disturbance and stress symptoms in both male and female patients.[154]

Contraindications: None have been reported.

Practitioners: Trained individuals may administer MBSR interventions either separately or in a group situation. It is best practiced by those licensed in counseling, psychology, or social work.

Symptom Management

Patients use CAM for cancer treatment and/or symptom management. Symptom management in cancer care spans the prediagnosis to survivorship spectrum. Tremendous advances have been made in offering relief from symptoms ranging from those that are minor inconveniences to the major debilitating aspects of symptoms associated with the disease process, its treatment, and its possible physical, emotional, spiritual, and psychological long-term consequences. Oncology nurses are experts in managing cancer symptoms by reducing the overall impact of symptoms on health outcomes.[155] Quality cancer care, as identified by the Oncology Nursing Society[156], embraces appropriate symptom management as a supportive care component. The Priority Symptom Management (PRISM) project developed by the ONS Foundation Center for Leadership, Information, and Research (CLIR) in 2000 focused on six primary symptoms: anorexia, cognitive dysfunction, depression, fatigue, neutropenia, and pain. Conventional approaches to symptom management have been enhanced in the past several years by the popularity and availability of CAM therapies. Critical appraisal of the quality of CAM approaches in symptom management is available for a limited number of symptoms at this time, due to evolving approaches and impending clinical trials. Table 24-8 compares the traditional approaches and outcomes with the CAM approach and outcomes for several common symptoms.

Anorexia

Anorexia is defined as the loss of the compensatory increase in feeding.[203–204] Anorexia, involuntary weight loss, tissue wasting, poor performance, and ultimately death characterize the condition of advanced protein calorie malnutrition, also referred to as cachexia. The cancer anorexia-cachexia syndrome is a multidimensional maladaptation involving physiological and behavioral components correlated with compromised quality of life and poor outcomes. Aspects contributing to the anorexia-cachexia syndrome are abnormalities in the mouth and digestive tract (dysphagia, odynophagia, early satiety, erosive lesions), changes in taste and smell, learned aversion to specific foods, and cancer treatment (effects of chemotherapy). Traditional treatments for cachexia are: (1) curing the cancer, (2) increasing nutritional intake, (3) inhibiting muscle and fat wasting, and (4) identifying the causes of reduced food intake. First-line traditional interventions are glucocorticoids and progesterones. Second-line traditional interventions are cannabinoids, antiserotonergic drugs, and metoclopramide. CAM modalities either used or under review are branched-chained amino acids, eicosapentanoic acid, melatonin, and hydrazine sulfate.

Depression

Depression is a frequent, highly treatable, and yet often unrecognized source of distress among patients with cancer. Cancer or other medical illnesses, cancer therapy or side effects of other treatments, and adjunctive medications used in cancer care may cause symptoms of depression or psychological responses to the cancer experience. Changes in appetite, weight, and/or sleep patterns; fatigue; and loss of energy are indicators of depression in people who do not have a medical illness. Many of these same symptoms are not reliable indicators of depression in people with cancer. Surveys have identified depression as one of the most common reasons for using CAM.[205] The most popular therapies include exercise, herbal medicine, and relaxation.

Pain

Known as the fifth vital sign, pain is frequently referred to as a prevalent yet treatable and controllable aspect of the cancer experience. Patients may experience noncancer pain through comorbidities or injury predating a cancer diagnosis, further complicating management. Despite advances in frequent assessment and early pain management interventions, no failproof approach to pain management exists. Consultation frequency between HCPs and patients focusing on pain and pain-related concerns has been measured.[206] Regimens can be individually tailored for patients to meet preferences, life-style, and desired outcome. Traditional approaches with known effectiveness in pain management are antitumor therapy (surgery, chemotherapy, biologic or hormonal therapy),[207,208] nonsteroidal anti-inflammatory drugs,[209] opioids, adjuvant agents (bisphosphonates,[197] antidepressants[194]), and transcutaneous electrical nerve stimulation.[193] Potentially effective CAM approaches are acupuncture,[71] cognitive-behavioral therapy,[210] massage,[211] and relaxation with guided imagery.[198] CAM approaches with variable efficacy are topical capsaicin,[199] chiropractic manipulation,[211] music,[200] and distraction. Given the various types and causes of pain associated with cancer, multiple approaches to pain relief are under continual evaluation and remain a challenge for clinicians and patients.

Role of Oncology Nursing in Cancer CAM

Oncology nurses must become knowledgeable in understanding the role of CAM in cancer care, given the rapidly increasing use of CAM. The model for cancer CAM care begins with the nurse, the patient, and other healthcare team members and endorses three core actions: (1) distinguishing fact from fiction, (2) acknowledging misperceptions about CAM, and (3) mixing and unmixing therapies.[212] (See Figure 24-1.) A baseline knowledge of CAM, beginning with evaluating personal and professional beliefs, is mandatory. Oncology curriculums in the United States guide nurses to approach cancer care using the principles and practices of conventional biomedical, "Western" medicine. Lack of content, misperceptions, and biases surrounding CAM theory and practice within nursing academic programs can leave nurses essentially unprepared to evaluate CAM clinical care options. Nursing curricula without CAM content may inadvertently communicate the notion that CAM has no valid role in health care and convey a need to minimize a patient's choice to seek CAM. Knowledgeable nurses can begin to conduct peer education and establish standards of practice in CAM therapy delivery across practice settings. Nurses must ensure that staff with proper training deliver CAM therapies and that patients sign informed consent. The medical record must contain documentation of the consent procedures, tolerance

Table 24-8 Common Symptom Management Considerations in Cancer CAM

Traditional Approaches and Outcomes	CAM Approaches and Outcomes
Anorexia	
Hypercaloric feeding via total parenteral nutrition Ability to increase lean mass, improve quality of life, improve survival benefits, or decrease toxicity of chemotherapy has not been shown. Increase in infections and mechanical complications is reported[157]	Hydrazine sulfate No normalization of carbohydrate metabolism reported in cachectic cancer patients[158–160]
Glucocorticoids Limited effect of up to 4 weeks on appetite, food intake, sensation of well-being, and performance status[161]	Eicosapentanoic acid (EPA) Preclinical data shows Inhibition of lipolysis and muscle protein degradation. Inclusion of EPA increased weight gain, lean body mass, and performance status[162,163]
Progesterones Improvement of appetite, calorie intake, and nutritional status seen[164]	Melatonin Loss of more than 10% body weight was less common among those treated with melatonin compared to placebo[165]
Antiserotonergic agents (cyproheptadine) Possesses appetite-stimulant effect, decreases diarrhea but does not prevent progressive weight loss[166]	Soy NSD to end Dietary sources of protein (Grade A: strong scientific evidence)
5HT3 receptor antagonists Improves the ability to enjoy food but does not prevent weight loss[167]	Bromelian Nutritional supplementation (Grade C: unclear of conflicting scientific evidence)
Prokinetic agents (metaclopramide) Relief of anorexia and early satiety with minimal side effects is reported[168]	Omega-3 fatty acids, fish oil, alpha-linolenic acid Appetite/weight loss in cancer patients (Grade D: fair negative scientific evidence)
Cannabinoids (synthetic tetrahydrocannabinol) Improvement in mood and appetite with either no or some improvement in body weight reported[169]	Spirulina Malnutrition (Grade D: fair negative scientific evidence)[37]
Thalidomide Improvement in well-being, weight gain, insomnia, restlessness, and appetite is reported[170]	**Alfalfa, astragalus, betel nut, black cohosh, blessed thistle, camomille, cranberry, dandelion, devil's claw, essiac, eyebright, fenugreek, ginseng, hawthorn, hops, kava, lavendar, oleander, peppermint, sorrel, thyme, turmeric, valerian, white horehound** Appetite stimulant or anorexia (lack sufficient evidence)
Branch-chain amino acids (BCCA) Improvement in protein accretion and albumin synthesis is reported. Decrease in the severity of cancer-induced anorexia by oral BCCA is reported[171–173]	
Depression	
Antidepressants Tricyclic antidepressants and selective serotonin reuptake inhibitors (SSRIs) demonstrate efficacy in the treatment of depression.	**Acupuncture** seems to decrease symptoms of depression. Three RCTs demonstrated efficacy of electroacupuncture as similar to tricyclic antidepressants[174] RCTs using non-specific (sham) acupuncture show conflicting results Acupuncture improved the course of depression more than pharmacological treatment with mianserin alone in an RCT of 70 inpatients with a major depressive episode in three different treatment groups: verum acupuncture, placebo acupuncture, and a control group. All three groups were pharmacologically treated with the antidepressant mianserin[175]
Counseling/ psychotherapy Counseling and psychotherapy are common effective interventions for depression.	Surveys have identified depression as one of the most common reasons for using CAM. The most popular therapies are exercise, herbal medicine, relaxation and spiritual healing Herbal therapies St. John's wort (SJW) is effective in the treatment of mild to moderate depression. The value of SJW in severe depression is questionable Relaxation Three small RCTs have suggested that relaxation training is superior to no treatment and potentially similar to cognitive-behavioral therapy. While non-specific effects are difficult to control for with relaxation therapy the evidence is promising

(continued)

Table 24-8 Common Symptom Management Considerations in Cancer CAM (continued)

Traditional Approaches and Outcomes	CAM Approaches and Outcomes
	Autogenic training When utilized as a single therapy (2x/week x 10 weeks) resulted in reduction in symptoms similar to psychotherapy alone but not significantly more than with no intervention. Authors warned that autogenic training alone is not recommended as treatment for depression[176]
	Massage Massage (qd x 5 days) was more effective than viewing videos in children and adolescents. Improvements were measured symptoms of depression, anxiety, sleep and cortisol levels.[177] Massage should be used with caution when a patient has a hx of abuse, PTSD, and other psychiatric disorders[178,179]
	Exercise There is a large body of research, considered to be of questionable quality, that supports the antidepressant effects of exercise. There are RCTs that provide verification of the efficacy of exercise in the treatment of depression. Aerobic and nonaerobic forms of exercise have proven to be effective. In 3 RCTs data suggest that aerobic exercise may be as effective as psychological or drug treatment[180] The exact mechanisms are not known.
	Aromatherapy Aromatherapy is combined with massage for increased effectiveness in symptom relief for patients with cancer who are experiencing depression[181,182]
	Dance and movement therapy Dance and movement therapy are effective therapeutic interventions in reducing symptoms of depression and improving psychological well-being[183–186]
	Music therapy Patients with cancer are among those who can benefit from music as a therapy. Music provides unique opportunities and properties that promote well-being. Music has been effective in the treatment of the anxiety and fear associated with a cancer diagnosis and cancer therapy[187,188]. Music-driven psychoneuroimmunology identifies potential implications for cancer care[189-191]
Pain	
Surgery Curative excision or palliative debulking can relieve symptoms of obstruction or compression, improve prognosis, and may increase survival	Acupuncture National Institutes of Health Acupuncture Consensus Development Panel concluded that acupuncture may be useful for headache and low back pain
Antineoplastic therapy Antineoplastic therapy (chemotherapy, biological, or hormonal therapy) may provide palliation by reducing tumor burden. Chemotherapy is effective in prolonging time to disease progression and survival in patients with advanced colorectal cancer	Cognitive-behavioral treatment (CBT) Standard CBT (five 50 minute sessions) and profile-tailored CBT [based on results from Biobehavioral Pain Profile (measures factors related to pain experience)] showed greater improvement in pain relief than usual care
Radiation therapy Local or whole-body radiation enhances the effectiveness of analgesics and noninvasive therapies to relieve cancer pain. Single injections of beta particle-emitting agents can relieve pain secondary to bony metastases	Chiropractic SR of chiropractic manipulation for back, neck, headache disorders, non-spinal pain syndromes (excluding headache) failed to demonstrate efficacy
Nonsteroidal anti-inflammatory drugs (NSAIDS) NSAIDs appear to be more effective than placebo for cancer pain. Combinations of an NSAID with an opioid have none or slight significant difference compared with either single intervention	Massage RCTs using Swedish massage suggest efficacy for relieving back pain however the results were not uniform

(continued)

Table 24-8 Common Symptom Management Considerations in Cancer CAM (continued)

Traditional Approaches and Outcomes	CAM Approaches and Outcomes
Opioids Uncontrolled case series show that chronic pain (not associated with terminal disease) is relieved by a stable nonescalating dose of opioids with minimal risk of addiction. Opioids can induce abnormal pain sensitivity. Prolonged high-dose opioid therapy may have serious adverse sequellae (tolerance, sensitivity, hormonal effects, immunosuppression). Remaining questions are: are opioids beneficial over years (versus months) and does the dose of the opioid have an effect on the efficacy and safety of long-term therapy?[192]	**Relaxation with guided imagery** Relaxation with guided imagery can improve oral mucositis[198] Relaxation exercises are effective: slow rhythmic breathing; touch and massage; reflecting on peaceful past experiences; listening to music
Transcutaneous Electrical Nerve Stimulation (TENS) TENS may be effective for the treatment of neuropathic pain[193]	**Topical capsaicin** Moderate to poor efficacy in the treatment of chronic musculoskeletal or neuropathic pain. May be useful as an adjunct or sole therapy for pain that is unresponsive to other treatments[199]
Antidepressants SRs of antidepressants suggest efficacy in the treatment of neuropathic pain over placebo. First choice of drug class of antidepressants is uncertain[194]	**Physical modalities** Musculoskeletal pain may be treated with heat, cold, massage, and exercise therapy
Neurolytic blocks Effective in controlling cancer pain in select patients in addition to pharmacological therapy. Quality improves when placement is image-guided in collaboration with an interventional radiologist[195].	**Music versus distraction** Lack of definitive findings in RCT using music or distraction for controlling procedural pain versus standard approach (neither music nor distraction)[200]
Topical rubefacients containing salicylates Moderate to poor efficacy in the treatment of musculoskeletal and arthritic pain[196]	**Percutaneous electrical nerve stimulation (PENS)** PENS (acupuncture-like needle probes plus nerve stimulation) is a useful supplement to opioids for the management of bony metastases[201]
Bisphosphonates Bisphosphonates have a role in managing refractory pain from metastases where oncologic or orthopedic intervention is delayed or inappropriate[197]	**Distraction** Distraction via paced auditory serial addition task (mental math) was shown to inhibit pain perception[202]

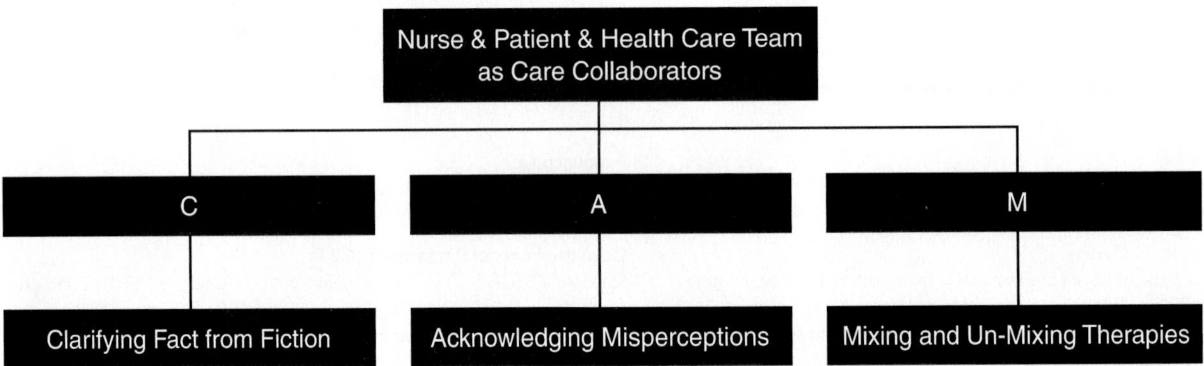

Figure 24-1 The CAM Model: approach cancer CAM from a nursing perspective.
Reprinted from Lee CO: CAM in the 21st Century in the US: role of nursing and evidence-based practice efforts, in *4th Annual Oncology Nursing Society Institutes of Learning*. Philadelphia, Oncology Nursing Society, 2003.[212]

of, and response to CAM therapy. Major endpoints for the role of nursing in cancer CAM are seen in Table 24-9.

Conducting an Integrative Assessment

The Hippocratic oath "do no harm" is apropos when CAM modalities are combined with conventional biomedical interventions.[213] Concurrent use of CAM and traditional approaches requires an examination of the safety and efficacy of the CAM modality and its potential interactions with surgery, chemotherapy, radiation, and/or biologic therapies. Mandatory pathways in clinical care are (1) incorporating evidence-based practice involving the use of CAM in oncology care, (2) assessing and documenting concurrent CAM use,

(3) verifying the safety and efficacy of CAM modalities under use, and (4) maintaining accountability in personal practice through proper licensure and continuing education.

Reliable Sources for Cancer CAM Information

Volumes of CAM information are presented online, in the media, and in lay literature. Distinguishing high-quality from poor-quality information is critical. Web sites volunteering medical resources should openly discuss who visits the site, who pays for the site, the purpose of the site, the sources of information, how information is selected for inclusion, how recent the information is, how links to other sites are selected, what information the site collects about visitors, and how the site manages interaction with visitors.[214] Selected sponsored Web sites, peer-reviewed journals indexed in Medline, and databases are listed in Table 24-10.

Future Trends

Given the widespread availability and affordability of many CAM therapies, integration of these therapies into cancer care is inevitable. To safely accomplish this integration, the clinical practice and scientific community must generate high-quality information in several ways: (1) collaborate with CAM practitioners to learn the theoretical basis for alternative systems and appropriate individualized regimens, (2) assist in the design of methodologically sound phase II and III trials, (3) perform periodic systematic reviews and meta-analyses, and (4) implement integrated curricula for students and continuing education for practitioners. Providing public education programs and forums that address the indications and contraindications creates an opportunity and arena for discussion between patients and practitioners. (See Figure 24-2.)

The law does not provide a definition of complementary and alternative medicine that is inclusive and official. A number of legislative codes and judicial decisions are emerging, however. Of concern is the issue of liability when a licensed practitioner refers a patient to a CAM provider who is not licensed. To complicate matters, some practitioners may be licensed in some states and not in others (for example, massage therapists). To date, we have seen a kind of *law of the majority* influencing decisions and law making. CAM has survived and emerged from an environment of rivalry and competition. Regulatory arenas that will need to be addressed include informed consent, licensure versus certification or registration, scopes of practice, malpractice, and professional discipline. In addition, serious consideration must be given to the possible regulation of CAM as a practice discipline. Issues of reimbursement have already emerged and may be connected to informed consent as well as insurance. Some patients might prefer acupuncture to narcotic analgesia if offered the choice. If a healthcare provider fails to offer CAM therapies as a treatment option, can that be interpreted as withholding treatment? Clarification of these issues is on the immediate horizon. Many HCPs are beginning to acknowledge that health and disease are as connected to nutritional, psychological, spiritual, mind-body, and environmental factors as to physical and chemical factors. Shared perspectives will create previously unimagined possibilities for evidenced-based research and practice.

Table 24-9 Endpoints for the Role of Nursing in Cancer CAM

Expand individual baseline knowledge regarding cancer CAM through oral and written modes and experiential learning	Establish institution-specific standards of practice for the use of CAM therapies within specific patient populations
Provide high-quality patient and peer education regarding the safety and efficacy of CAM therapies	Document patient consent procedures, tolerance, and response to CAM therapy
Facilitate partnerships between patients, conventional HCPs, CAM providers, and colleagues to discuss knowledge and perspectives about cancer CAM	Design a new integrative care program or assist in the quality maintenance of a preestablished program
Seek proper training, demonstrate competency, and obtain necessary credentials if practicing a CAM therapy	Develop and update a working knowledge of cost issues and reimbursement of CAM in the community
Request and require informed consent (with witness) of patients receiving a CAM therapy	Collaborate in the design of methodologically rigorous cancer CAM treatment and supportive care clinical trials
Ensure proper credentialing of a CAM provider prior to recommending the provider to patients	Contribute to the body of nursing knowledge in cancer CAM through publications and presentations in the United States and internationally

Data from Lee.[212]

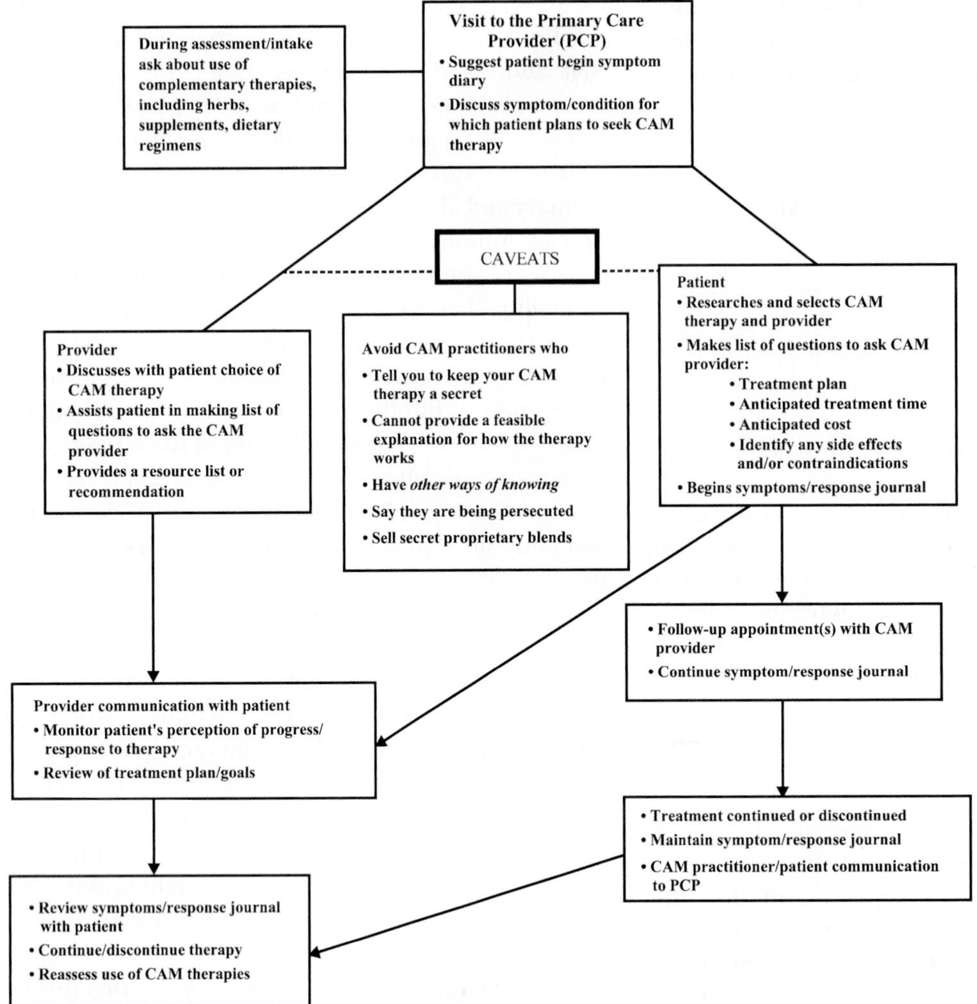

Figure 24-2 Discussing CAM therapies with patients. Reprinted from Decker.[215]

References

1. Vickers AJ, Cassileth BR: Unconventional therapies for cancer and cancer-related symptoms. *Lancet Oncol* 2:226–232, 2001
2. Cassileth BR, Vickers AJ: Complementary and alternative therapies. *Urol Clin North Am* 30:369–376, 2003
3. Ernst E: Complementary therapies for cancer, in *UpToDate Online.* Retrieved from *www.uptodateonline.com/application/topic/print.asp?file=gen1_cnc/8402.* Accessed April 12, 2004
4. Micozzi MS (ed.): *Fundamentals of Complementary and Alternative Medicine.* New York, Churchill Livingstone, 2001
5. NCCAM, *National Center for Complementary and Alternative Medicine,* 2004.
6. National Cancer Institute: *Levels of Evidence for Human Studies of Cancer Complementary and Alternative Medicine.* Retrieved from *www.nci.nih.gov/cancerinfo/pdq/levels=evidence=cam,* Bethesda, MD. Accessed May 10, 2004
7. Oncology Nursing Society: *The Use of Complementary and Alternative Therapies in Cancer Care.* Oncology Nursing Society, Pittsburgh, 2002
8. Segen JC: *Dictionary of Alternative Medicine.* Appleton & Lange, Stamford, 1998
9. OCCAM, *Office of Cancer Complementary and Alternative Medicine.* National Cancer Institute, Bethesda, MD, 2004
10. Lee CO: Clinical Trials in Cancer Part 1: Biomedical, Complementary, and Alternative Medicine: finding active trial and results of closed trials. *Clin J Oncol Nurs* 8:531–535, 2004
11. Whorton JC: *The history of complementary and alternative medicine,* in Jonas WB, Levin JS (eds.): *Essentials of Complementary and Alternative Medicine.* Philadelphia, Lippincott Williams and Wilkins, 1999, pp 16–30
12. Swerdlow JL: *Nature's Medicine: Plants That Heal.* Washington, DC: National Geographic Society, 2000
13. Black JM and Matassarin-Jacobs E: Nursing process, in Black JM, Matassarin-Jacobs E (eds.): *Luckman and Sorensen's Medical-Surgical Nursing: A Psychophysiologic Approach.* Philadelphia, W.B. Saunders, 1993
14. Gallin, JI: A historical perspective on clinical research, in Gallin JI (ed.): *Principles and Practice of Clinical Research.* San Diego, Academic Press, 2002, pp 1–11
15. Antman K, Benson MC, Chabot J et al: Complementary and alternative medicine: the role of the cancer center. *J Clin Oncol* 19(18 suppl):55S–60S, 2001

Table 24-10 Sources of Reliable Cancer CAM Information

	Sponsored Web Sites
Selected Sponsored Organizations	
Amerian Academy of Medical Acupuncture	http://www.medicalacupuncture.org
American Cancer Society	http://www.cancer.org
American Society for Clinical Oncology(ASCO, 2004a)	http://www.asco.org
National Institutes of Health(NIH, 2004)	http://www.nih.gov
• Cancer Information Service(CIS, 2004)	http://cis.nci.nih.gov
• Office of Cancer Complementary and Alternative Medicine(OCCAM, 2004)	http://www3.cancer.gov/occam
• National Center for Complementary and Alternative Medicine(NCCAM, 2004)	http://nccam.nih.gov
• Office Of Dietary Supplements(ODS, 2004)	http://ods.od.nih.gov
• Medline Plus(MedLine, 2004)	http://medlineplus.gov
• Cancer Patient Education Network	http://cpen.nci.nih.gov
People Living with Cancer(ASCO, 2004c)	http://www.plwc.org
The University of Texas MD Anderson Cancer Center(CIMER, 2004)	http://www.mdanderson.org/departments/cimer
The Dana-Farber Cancer Institute Zakim Center for Integrated Therapies(DFCI, 2004)	http://www.dana-farber.org/pat/support/zakim_default.asp
The Johns Hopkins Center for Complementary and Alternative Medicine(Hopkins, 2004)	http://www.hopkinsmedicine.org/CAM/links.html
The Rosenthal Center for Complementary and Alternative Medicine(Rosenthal, 2004)	http://rosenthal.hs.columbia.edu
Selected Peer-Reviewed Journals (Indexed in Medline)	
Alternative & Complementary Therapies(A&CT, 2004)	http://www.liebertpub.com/ACT/default1.asp
British Medical Journal(BMJ, 2004)	http://bmj.bmjjournals.com/
Clinical Journal of Oncology Nursing(CJON, 2004)	http://www.ons.org/publications/journals/CJON/index.shtml
Integrative Cancer Therapies(Therapies, 2004)	http://www.sagepub.com/journal.aspx?pid=286
Journal of Cancer Integrative Medicine(JCIM, 2004)	http://www.pnpco.com/index.html
Journal of Clinical Oncology(ASCO, 2004b)	http://www.jco.org/
Natural Pharmacy(Pharmacy, 2004)	http://www.liebertpub.com/NAP/default1.asp
Oncology Nursing Forum(ONF, 2004)	http://www.ons.org/publications/journals/ONF/
Seminars in Oncology Nursing(Nursing, 2004)	http://www.elsevier.com/wps/find/journaldescription.cws_home/623110/description#description
The Journal of Alternative and Complementary Medicine(JACM, 2004)	http://www.liebertpub.com/ACM/default1.asp
The Journal of the American Medical Association(JAMA, 2004)	http://jama.ama-assn.org/
Selected Sponsored Databases	
ClinicalTrials.gov(ClinicalTrials.gov, 2004)	http://clinicaltrials.gov/ct
Complementary and Alternative Medicine and Pain Database(University of Maryland School of Medicine, 2004)	http://www.campain.umm.edu/News.html
Directory of Information Resources Online (DIRLINE)	http://www.dirline.nlm.nih.gov
Food & Drug Administration (FDA, 2004)	http://www.fda.gov
Herbalgram.org(Herbalgram.org, 2004)	http://www.herbalgram.org/
HerbMed.com(HerbMed.com, 2004)	http://herbmed.com/
International Bibliographic Information on Dietary Supplements(IBIDS, 2004)	http://dietary-supplements.info.nih.gov/databases/ibids.html
Micromedex(Micromedex, 2004)	http://www.micromedex.com/products/hcs/
Natural Medicine	http://www.naturaldatabase.com/
Natural Standard(NaturalStandard, 2004)	http://www.naturalstandard.com/
PDQ(PDQ, 2004b)	http://cancer.gov/cancerinfo/pdq/
The Cochrane Collaboration(Cochrane, 2004)	http://www.cochrane.org/index0.htm

16. White JD: Complementary and alternative medicine research: A National Cancer Institute perspective. *Semin Oncol* 29:546–51, 2002, pp 546–551
17. WHCCAMP, *White House Commission on Complementary and Alternative Medicine Policy.* August 2003, United States Department of Health and Human Services: Washington, DC
18. Stevinson C: Why patients use complementary and alternative medicine, in Ernst E (ed.): *The Desktop Guide to Complementary and Alternative Medicine: An Evidence-Based Approach.* Edinburgh, Elsevier, 2001, pp 395–403
19. Furnham A: Why do people choose and use complementary therapies?, in Ernst E (ed.): *Complementary Medicine: An Objective Appraisal.* Oxford, Butterworth Heinemann, 1996, pp 71–88
20. Kaptchuk TJ, Eisenberg DM: The persuasive appeal of alternative medicine. *Ann Intern Med* 129:1061–1065, 1998
21. Eisenberg DM, Kessler RC, Foster C et al: Unconventional medicine in the United States. Prevalence, costs, and patterns of use. *N Engl J Med* 328:246–252, 1993

22. Eisenberg DM, Davis RB, Ettner SL et al: Trends in alternative medicine use in the United States, 1990–1997: results of a follow-up national survey. *JAMA* 280:1569–1575, 1998
23. Kessler RC, Davis RB, Foster DF, et al: Long-term trends in the use of complementary and alternative medical therapies in the United States. *Ann Intern Med* 135:262–268, 2001
24. Ni H, Simile C, Hardy AM: Utilization of complementary and alternative medicine by United States adults: results from the 1999 national health interview survey. *Med Care* 40:353–358, 2002
25. Basch E, Ulbricht C: Prevalence of CAM use among U.S. cancer patients: an update. *Cancer Integrative Med* 2:13–14, 2004
26. Ernst E, Cassileth BR: The prevalence of complementary/alternative medicine in cancer: a systematic review. *Cancer* 83:777–782, 1998
27. Bennett M, Lengacher C: Use of complementary therapies in a rural cancer population. *Oncol Nurs Forum* 26:1287–1294, 1999
28. Sparber A, Bauer L, Curt G et al: Use of complementary medicine by adult patients participating in cancer clinical trials. *Oncol Nurs Forum* 27:623–630, 2000
29. Bernstein BJ, Grasso T: Prevalence of complementary and alternative medicine use in cancer patients. *Oncology* 15:1267–1278, 1283, 2001
30. Vallerand AH, Fouladbakhsh JM, Templin T: The use of complementary/alternative medicine therapies for the self-treatment of pain among residents of urban, suburban, and rural communities. *Am J Pub Health* 93:923–925, 2003
31. Najm W, Reinsch S, Hoehler F et al: Use of complementary and alternative medicine among the ethnic elderly. *Altern Ther Health Med* 9:50–57, 2003
32. Herron M, Glasser M: Use of and attitudes toward complementary and alternative medicine among family practice patients in small rural Illinois communities. *J Rural Health* 19:279–284, 2003
33. Ashikaga T, Bosompra K, O'Brien P et al: Use of complementary and alternative medicine by breast cancer patients: Prevalence, patterns and communication with physicians. *Support Care Cancer* 10:542–548, 2002
34. Swisher EM, Cohn DE, Goff BA et al: Use of complementary and alternative medicine among women with gynecologic cancers. *Gynecol Oncol* 84:363–367, 2002
35. Maskarinec G, Shumay DM, Kakai H et al: Ethnic differences in complementary and alternative medicine use among cancer patients. *J Altern Complement Med* 6:531–538, 2000
36. Richardson MA, Sanders T, Palmer JL et al: Complementary/alternative medicine use in a comprehensive cancer center and the implications for oncology. *J Clin Oncol* 18:2505–2514, 2000
37. Lengacher CA, Bennett MP, Kipp KE et al: Design and testing of the use of a complementary and alternative therapies survey in women with breast cancer. *Oncol Nurs Forum* 30:811–821, 2003
38. Bridevaux IP: A survey of patients' out-of-pocket payments for complementary and alternative medicine therapies. *Complement Ther Med* 12:48–50, 2004
39. White A: Economic issues in complementary and alternative medicine, in Ernst E (ed.): *The Desktop Guide to Complementary and Alternative Medicine.* Edinburgh, Elsevier, 2001, pp 415–422
40. Angel M, Kassirer JP: Alternative medicine: The risks of untested and unregulated remedies. *N Engl J Med* 339:839–841, 1998
41. Zoon KC, Yetter RA: The regulation of drugs and biological products by the food and drug administration, in Gallin J (ed.): *Principles and Practice of Clinical Research.* San Diego, Academic Press, 2002, pp 123–132
42. *Dietary Supplement Health and Education Act of 1994,* in *Public Law 103–417.* 1994
43. Eisenberg DM: Advising patients who seek alternative medical therapies. *Ann Intern Med* 127:61–69, 1997
44. Ernst E (ed.): *The Desktop Guide to Complementary and Alternative Medicine: An Evidence-Based Approach.* Edinburgh, Elsevier, 2001
45. Eisenberg DM, Kaptchuk TJ, Laine C et al: Complementary and alternative medicine: an Annals series. *Ann Intern Med* 135:208, 2001
46. Jonas WB, Linde K: Conducting and evaluating clinical research on complementary and alternative medicine, in Gallin J (ed.): *Principles and Practice of Clinical Research,* San Diego, Academic Press, 2002, pp 401–420
47. Hilsden RJ, Verhoef MJ: Complementary therapies: evaluating their effectiveness in cancer. *Patient Educ Couns* 38:101–108, 1999
48. Pelletier K: *The Best Alternative Medicine.* New York, Simon & Schuster, 2000
49. Long AF: Outcome measurement in complementary and alternative medicine: unpicking the effects. *J Altern Complement Med* 8:777–786, 2002
50. Grady C: Ethical principles in clinical research, in Gallin JI (ed.): *Principles and Practice of Clinical Research,* San Diego, Academic Press, 2002, pp 15–25
51. Emanuel EJ, Wendler D, Grady C: What makes clinical research ethical? *JAMA,* 283:2701–2711, 2000
52. Miller FG, Emanuel EJ, Rosenstein DL et al: Ethical issues concerning research in complementary and alternative medicine. *JAMA* 291:599–604, 2004
53. Cohen MH: Legal and ethical issues in complementary and alternative medicine, in Ernst E (ed.): *The Desktop Guide to Complementary and Alternative Medicine: An Evidenced-Based Approach.,* Edinburgh, Elsevier, 2001, pp 404–411
54. Tunis SR, Stryer DB, Clancy CM: Practical clinical trials: increasing the value of clinical research for decision making in clinical and health policy. *JAMA* 290:1624–1632, 2003
55. Smith WB: Research methodology: implications for CAM pain research. *Clin J Pain* 20:3–7, 2004
56. Richardson MA, Straus SE: Complementary and alternative medicine: opportunities and challenges for cancer management and research. *Semin Oncol* 29:531–545, 2002
57. Carter B: Methodological issues and complementary therapies: Researching intangibles? *Complement Ther Nurs Midwifery* 9:133–139, 2003
58. Hyland ME: Methodology for the scientific evaluation of complementary and alternative medicine. *Complement Ther Med* 11:146–153, 2003
59. Ezzo J: Should journals devote space to trials with no results? *J Altern Complement Med* 9:611–612, 2003
60. Lee CO: Translational research in cancer complementary and alternative medicine: the National Cancer Institute's Best Case Series program. *Clin J Oncol Nurs* 8:212–214, 2004
61. Tacon AM: Attachment and cancer: a conceptual integration. *Integr Cancer Ther* 1:371–386, 2002
62. Munitz H, Rudnick A: The biopsychosocial model of medicine revisited: A meta-theoretical excursion. *Isr J Psychiatry Relat Sci* 37:266–277, 2000
63. Cooley ME, Jennings-Dozier K: Cultural assessment of black American men treated for prostate cancer: clinical case studies. *Oncol Nurs Forum* 25:1729–1736, 1998
64. Morales Lopez A, Grau Fibla G, Campoy Martinez P et al: Development of the ESCAP-CDV as measuring tool for the assessment of quality of life in prostatic cancer. *Actas Urol Esp* 26:242–249, 2002
65. Sulmasy DP: A biopsychosocial-spiritual model for the care of patients at the end of life. *Gerontologist* 42(suppl 3):24–33, 2002

66. Yeh CH: Health-related quality of life in pediatric patients with cancer: a structural equation approach with the Roy Adaptation Model. *Cancer Nurs* 25:74–80, 2002
67. White KL, Williams TF, Greenberg BG: The ecology of medical care. *Bull NY Acad Med* 73:187–212, 1996
68. Nuamah IF, Cooley ME, Fawcetet Jet al: Testing a theory for health-related quality of life in cancer patients: a structural equation approach. *Res Nurs Health* 22:231–242, 1999
69. Luecken LJ, Compas BE: Stress, coping, and immune function in breast cancer. *Ann Behav Med* 24:336–344, 2002
70. Syrjala KL, Chapko, ME: Evidence for a biopsychosocial model of cancer treatment-related pain. *Pain* 61:69–79, 1995
71. Mayer DJ: Acupuncture: an evidence-based review of the clinical literature. *Annu Rev Med* 51:49–63, 2000
72. Han JS, Terenius L: Neurochemical basis of acupuncture analgesia. *Ann Rev Pharmacol Toxicol* 22:193–220, 1982
73. Andersson S, Lundeberg T: Acupuncture — from empiricism to science: functional background to acupuncture effects in pain and disease. *Med Hypotheses* 45:271–281, 1995
74. Ernst E, Pittler MH: The effectiveness of acupuncture in treating acute dental pain: a systematic review. *Br Dent J* 184:443–447, 1998
75. Vickers AJ: Can acupuncture have specific effects on health? A systematic review of acupuncture antiemesis trials. *J R Soc Med* 89:303–311, 1976
76. Melchart D, Linde K, Fischer P et al: Acupuncture for recurrent headaches: a systematic review of randomized controlled trials. *Cephalalgia* 19:779–786, 1999
77. Aikins Murphy P: Alternative therapies for nausea and vomiting of pregnancy. *Obstet Gynecol* 91:149–155, 1998
78. Ernst E, White A: Life-threatening adverse reactions after acupuncture? A systematic review. *Pain* 71:123–126, 1997
79. Eichelberger B: *A qi gong primer.* Retrieved from *www.acupuncture.com.* Accessed May 19, 2004
80. Yang JM: A brief history of qi gong. Retrieved from *www.acupuncture.com.* Accessed May 10, 2004
81. Weiner P, Man A, Weiner M et al: The effect of incentive spirometry and inspiratory muscle training on pulmonary function after lung resection. *J Thorac Cardiovasc Surg* 113:552–557, 1997
82. Corner J, Plant H, A'Hearn R et al: Non-pharmacological intervention for breathlessness in lung cancer. *Palliat Med* 10:299–305, 1996
83. Wu CY: Spontaneous dynamic qigong and mental disorders. *Zhong Xi Yi Jie He Za Zhi* 10:497–498, 1990
84. Potter P: What are the distinctions between Reiki and therapeutic touch? *Clin J Oncol Nurs* 7:89–91, 2003
85. Rexilius SJ, Mundt C, Erickson Megel M et al: Therapeutic effects of massage therapy and handling touch on caregivers of patients undergoing autologous hematopoietic stem cell transplant. *Oncol Nurs Forum* 29:E35-E44, 2002
86. Olson K, Hanson J: Using Reiki to manage pain: a preliminary report. *Cancer Prev Control* 1:108–113, 1997
87. Lafreniere KD, Mutus B, Cameron S et al: Effects of therapeutic touch on biochemical and mood indicators in women. *J Altern Complement Med* 5:367–370, 1999
88. Post-White J, Kinney ME, Savik K et al: Therapeutic massage and healing touch improve symptoms in cancer. *Integr Cancer Ther* 2:332–344, 2003
89. Mansour AA, Beuche M, Laing G et al: A study to test the effectiveness of placebo Reiki standardization procedures developed for a planned Reiki efficacy study. *J Altern Complement Med* 5:153–164, 1999
90. Rosenfeld I: *Dr. Rosenfeld's Guide to Alternative Medicine.* New York, Knopf, 1996
91. White AR, Williamson J, Hart A et al: A blinded investigation into the accuracy of reflexology charts. *Complement Ther Med* 8:166–172, 2000
92. Weiger WA, Smith M, Boon H et al: Advising patients who seek complementary and alternative medical therapies for cancer. *Ann Intern Med* 137:889–903, 2002
93. Soden K, Vincent K, Craske S et al: A randomized controlled trial of aromatherapy massage in a hospice setting. *Palliat Med* 18:87–92, 2004
94. Goodfellow LM: The effects of therapeutic back massage on psychophysiologic variables and immune function in spouses of patients with cancer. *Nurs Res* 52:318–328, 2003
95. Hodgson H: Does reflexology impact on cancer patients' quality of life? *Nurs Stand* 14:33–38, 2000
96. Oleson T, Flocco W: Randomized controlled study of premenstrual symptoms treated with ear, hand, and foot reflexology. *Obstet Gynecol* 82:906–911, 1993
97. Wang XM: Treating type II diabetes mellitus with foot reflexotherapy. *Zhongguo Zhong Xi Yi Jie He Za Zhi* 13:536–588, 1993
98. Ernst E, Siev-Ner I, Gamus D: Complementary medicine — a critical review. *Isr J Med Sci* 33:808–815, 1997
99. Launso L, Brendstrup E, Arnberg S: An exploratory study of reflexological treatment for headache. *Altern Ther Health Med* 5:57–65, 1999
100. Decker G (ed.): *An Introduction to Complementary & Alternative Therapies.* Pittsburgh, Oncology Nursing Press, 1999
101. Ernst E: The current position of complementary/alternative medicine in cancer. *Eur J Cancer* 39:2273–2277, 2003
102. Perez C: Clinical aromatherapy, Part I: an introduction into nursing practice. *Clin J Oncol Nurs* 7:595–596, 2003
103. Thomas DV: Aromatherapy: mythical, magical, or medicinal? *Holist Nurs Pract* 16:8–16, 2002
104. Cooke B, Ernst E: Aromatherapy: a systematic review. *Br J Gen Pract* 50:493–496, 2000
105. Louis M, Kowalski SD: Use of aromatherapy with hospice patients to decrease pain, anxiety, and depression and to promote an increased sense of well-being. *Am J Hosp Palliat Care* 19:381–386, 2002
106. Olleveant NA, Humphris G, Roe B: How big is a drop? A volumetric assay of essential oils. *J Clin Nurs* 8:299–304, 1999
107. Fellowes D, Barnes K, Wilkinson S: Aromatherapy and massage for symptom relief in patients with cancer. *Cochrane Database Syst Rev* 2:CD002287, 2004
108. Maddocks-Jennings W: Critical incident: idiosyncratic allergic reactions to essential oils. *Complement Ther Nurs Midwifery* 10:58–60, 2004
109. Campbell L, Pollard A, Roeton C: The development of clinical practice guidelines for the use of aromatherapy in a cancer setting. *Aust J Holist Nurs* 8:14–22, 2001
110. Avis A: Aromatherapy in practice. *Nurs Stand* 13:14–15, 1999
111. Lee CO: Clinical aromatherapy, part II: Safe guidelines for integration into clinical practice. *Clin J Oncol Nurs* 7:597–598, 2003
112. VandeCreek L, Rogers E, Lester J: Use of alternative therapies among breast cancer outpatients compared with the general population. *Altern Ther Health Med* 5:71–76, 1999
113. Durken M, Herrnring C, Finckh B et al: Impaired plasma antioxidative defense and increased nontransferrin-bound iron during high-dose chemotherapy and radiochemotherapy preceding bone marrow transplantation. *Free Radic Biol Med* 28:887–894, 2000
114. Ladas EJ, Jacobson JS, Kennedy DD et al: Antioxidants and cancer therapy: a systematic review. *J Clin Oncol* 22:517–528, 2004
115. Omenn GS, Goodman GE, Thornquist MD et al: Effects of a combination of beta carotene and vitamin A on lung cancer and cardiovascular disease. *N Engl J Med* 334:1150–1155, 1996

116. Albanes D, Heinonen OP, Huttunen JK et al: Effects of alpha-tocopherol and beta-carotene supplements on cancer incidence in the Alpha-Tocopherol Beta-Carotene Cancer Prevention Study. *Am J Clin Nutr* 62(6 suppl):1427S-1430S, 1995
117. Conklin KA: Dietary antioxidants during cancer chemotherapy: impact on chemotherapeutic effectiveness and development of side effects. *Nutr Cancer* 37:1–18, 2000
118. Ray SD, Wong V, Bagchi D et al: In vivo protection of DNA damage associated apoptotic and necrotic cell deaths during acetaminophen-induced nephrotoxicity, amiodarone-induced lung toxicity and doxorubicin-induced cardiotoxicity by a novel IH636 grape seed proanthocyanidin extract. *Res Commun Mol Pathol Pharmacol* 107:137–166, 2000
119. Lenzhofer R, Ganzinger U, Rameis H et al: Acute cardiac toxicity in patients after doxorubicin treatment and the effect of combined tocopherol and nifedipine pretreatment. *J Cancer Res Clin Oncol* 106:143–147, 1983
120. Jonas CR, Puckett AB, Jones DP et al: Plasma antioxidant status after high-dose chemotherapy: a randomized trial of parenteral nutrition in bone marrow transplantation patients. *Am J Clin Nutr* 72:181–189, 2000
121. Sundstrom H, Korpela H, Sajanti E et al: Supplementation with selenium, vitamin E and their combination in gynaecological cancer during cytotoxic chemotherapy. *Carcinogenesis* 10:273–278, 1989
122. Holm LE, Nordevang E, Hjalmar ML et al: Treatment failure and dietary habits in women with breast cancer. *J Natl Cancer Inst* 85:32–36, 1993
123. Ingram D: Diet and subsequent survival in women with breast cancer. *Br J Cancer* 69:592–595, 1994
124. Brawley OW, Parnes H: Prostate cancer prevention trials in the USA. *Eur J Cancer* 36:1312–1315, 2000
125. Hendler SS, Rorvik D: *PDR for Nutritional Supplements.* Montvale, NJ, Thomson Healthcare, 2001
126. Burzynski SR: Antineoplastons: history of the research (I). *Drugs Exp Clin Res* 12(suppl 1):1–9, 1986
127. Michalska D: Theoretical investigations on the structure and potential binding sites of antineoplaston A10 and experimental findings. *Drugs Exp Clin Res* 16:343–349, 1990
128. Liau MC, Szopa M, Burzynski B et al: Quantitative assay of plasma and urinary peptides as an aid for the evaluation of cancer patients undergoing antineoplaston therapy. *Drugs Exp Clin Res* 13(suppl 1):61–70, 1987
129. Lee SS, Burzynski SR: Tissue culture and animal toxicity studies of antineoplaston A5. *Drugs Exp Clin Res* 13(suppl 1):31–35, 1987
130. Hendry LB, Muldoon TG, Burzynski SR et al: Stereochemical modelling studies of the interaction of antineoplaston A10 with DNA. *Drugs Exp Clin Res* 13(suppl 1):77–81, 1987
131. Burzynski SR. Mohabbat MO: Chronic animal toxicity studies on antineoplaston A2. *Drugs Exp Clin Res* 12(suppl 1):73–75, 1986
132. Tsuda H, Hara H, Eriguchi N et al: Toxicological study on antineoplastons A-10 and AS2-1 in cancer patients. *Kurume Med J* 42:241–249, 1995
133. Fetrow C, Avila A: *A Professional's Handbook of Complementary and Alternative Medicines.* Philadephia, Springhouse, 1999
134. Ernst E: Harmless herbs? A review of the recent literature. *Am J Med* 104:170–178, 1998
135. Ernst E: The risk-benefit profile of commonly used herbal therapies: Ginkgo, St. John's wort, ginseng, echinacea, saw palmetto, and kava. *Ann Intern Med* 136:42–53, 2002
136. Harrer G, Schmidt U, Kuhn U et al: Comparison of equivalence between the St. John's wort extract LoHyp-57 and fluoxetine. *Arzneimittelforschung* 49:289–296, 1999
137. Philipp M, Kohnen R, Hiller KO: Hypericum extract versus imipramine or placebo in patients with moderate depression: randomised multicentre study of treatment for eight weeks. *Br Med J* 319:1534–1538, 1999
138. Schrader E: Equivalence of St. John's wort extract (Ze 117) and fluoxetine: a randomized, controlled study in mild-moderate depression. *Int Clin Psychopharmacol* 15:61–68, 2000
139. Woelk H: Comparison of St. John's wort and imipramine for treating depression: randomised controlled trial. *Br Med J* 321:536–539, 2000
140. Wheatley D: Hypericum in seasonal affective disorder (SAD). *Curr Med Res Opin* 15:33–37, 1999
141. Gulick RM, McAuliffe V, Holden-Wiltse J et al: Phase I studies of hypericin, the active compound in St. John's wort, as an antiretroviral agent in HIV-infected adults. AIDS Clinical Trials Group Protocols 150 and 258. *Ann Intern Med* 130:510–514, 1999
142. Stevinson C, Ernst E: A pilot study of Hypericum perforatum for the treatment of premenstrual syndrome. *BJOG* 107:870–876, 2000
143. Markowitz JS, Donovan JL, DeVane CL et al: Effect of St. John's wort on drug metabolism by induction of cytochrome P450 3A4 enzyme. *JAMA* 290:1500–1504, 2003
144. Ernst E, Rand JI, Stevinson C: Complementary therapies for depression: an overview. *Arch Gen Psychiatry* 55:1026–1032, 1998
145. Lane IW, Comac L: *Sharks Don't Get Cancer.* Garden City Park, New York, Avery Publishing Group, 1992
146. Hunt TJ, Connelly JF: Shark cartilage for cancer treatment. *Am J Health Syst Pharm* 52:1756, 1760, 1995
147. PDQ, PDQ® Cancer Information Summaries: Complementary and alternative medicine, in *PDQ® Cancer Information Summaries: Complementary and Alternative Medicine.* Retrieved from *www.cancer.gov/cancerinfo/pdq/cam.* Accessed April 13, 2004
148. Gonzalez RP, Soares FS, Farias RF et al: Demonstration of inhibitory effect of oral shark cartilage on basic fibroblast growth factor-induced angiogenesis in the rabbit cornea. *Biol Pharm Bull* 24:151–154, 2001
149. Miller DR, Anderson GT, Stark JJ et al: Phase I/II trial of the safety and efficacy of shark cartilage in the treatment of advanced cancer. *J Clin Oncol* 16:3649–3655, 1998
150. Gotay CC, Dumitriu D: Health food store recommendations for breast cancer patients. *Arch Fam Med* 9:692–699, 2000
151. Bishop SR: What do we really know about mindfulness-based stress reduction? *Psychosom Med* 64:71–83, 2002
152. Astin JA, Berman BM, Bausell B et al: The efficacy of mindfulness meditation plus Qigong movement therapy in the treatment of fibromyalgia: a randomized controlled trial. *J Rheumatol* 30:2257–2262, 2003
153. Tacon AM, McComb J, Caldera Y et al: Mindfulness meditation, anxiety reduction, and heart disease: a pilot study. *Fam Community Health*, 26:25–33, 2003
154. Carlson LE, Ursuliak Z, Goodey E et al: The effects of a mindfulness meditation-based stress reduction program on mood and symptoms of stress in cancer outpatients: 6-month follow-up. *Support Care Cancer* 9:112–123, 2001
155. Ropka ME, Spencer-Cisek P: PRISM: Priority Symptom Management Project phase I: assessment. *Oncol Nurs Forum* 28:1585–1594, 2001
156. Oncology Nursing Society: *Quality Cancer Care (Oncology Nursing Society Position Statement).* Pittsburgh, Oncology Nursing Society, 2000
157. Body JJ: The syndrome of anorexia-cachexia. *Curr Opin Oncol* 11:255–260, 1999

158. Loprinzi CL, Goldberg RM, Su JQ et al: Placebo-controlled trial of hydrazine sulfate in patients with newly diagnosed non-small-cell lung cancer. *J Clin Oncol* 12:1126–1129, 1994
159. Loprinzi CL, Kuross SA, O'Fallon JR et al: Randomized placebo-controlled evaluation of hydrazine sulfate in patients with advanced colorectal cancer. *J Clin Oncol* 12:1121–1125, 1194
160. Kosty MP, Fleishman SB, Herndon JE et al: Cisplatin, vinblastine, and hydrazine sulfate in advanced, non-small-cell lung cancer: a randomized placebo-controlled, double-blind phase III study of the Cancer and Leukemia Group B. *J Clin Oncol* 12:1113–1120, 1194
161. Bruera E, Roca E, Cedaro L et al: Action of oral methylprednisolone in terminal cancer patients: a prospective randomized double-blind study. *Cancer Treat Rep* 69:751–754, 1985
162. Tanaka Y, Eda H, Fujimoto K et al: Anticachectic activity of 5'-deoxy-5–fluorouridine in a murine tumor cachexia model, colon 26 adenocarcinoma. *Cancer Res* 50:4528–4532, 1990
163. Wigmore SJ, Ross JA, Falconer JS et al: The effect of polyunsaturated fatty acids on the progress of cachexia in patients with pancreatic cancer. *Nutrition* 12(1 suppl):S27-S30, 1996
164. Mantovani G, Maccio A, Massa E et al: Managing cancer-related anorexia/ cachexia. *Drugs* 61:499–514, 2001
165. Lissoni P, Paolorossi F, Tancini G et al: Is there a role for melatonin in the treatment of neoplastic cachexia? *Eur J Cancer* 32A:1340–1343, 1996
166. Kardinal CG, Loprinzi CL, Schaid DJ et al: A controlled trial of cyproheptadine in cancer patients with anorexia and/or cachexia. *Cancer* 65:2657–2662, 1990
167. Tayek JA, Bistrian BR, Hehir DJ et al: Improved protein kinetics and albumin synthesis by branched chain amino acid-enriched total parenteral nutrition in cancer cachexia. A prospective randomized crossover trial. *Cancer* 58:147–157, 1986
168. Davis MP, Dickerson D: Cachexia and anorexia: cancer's covert killer. *Support Care Cancer* 8:180–187, 2000
169. Nelson K, Walsh D, Decter P et al: A phase II study of delta-9–tetrahydrocannabinol for appetite stimulation in cancer-associated anorexia. *J Palliat Care* 10:14–18, 1994
170. Klausner JD, Freedman VH, Kaplan G: Thalidomide as an anti-TNF-alpha inhibitor: Implications for clinical use. *Clin Immunol Immunopathol* 81:219–223, 1996
171. Argiles JM, Meijsing SH, Pallares-Trujillo J et al: Cancer cachexia: a therapeutic approach. *Med Res Rev* 21:83–101, 2001
172. Argiles JM, Lopez-Soriano FJ: Insulin and cancer (Review). *Int J Oncol* 18:683–687, 2001
173. Cangiano C, Laviano A, Meguid MM et al: Effects of administration of oral branched-chain amino acids on anorexia and caloric intake in cancer patients. *J Natl Cancer Inst* 88:550–552, 1996
174. Luo HC, Jia YK, Li Z: Electro-acupuncture vs. amitriptyline in the treatment of depressive states. *J Tradit Chin Med* 5:3–8, 1985
175. Roschke J, Wolf C, Muller MJ et al: The benefit from whole body acupuncture in major depression. *J Affect Disord* 57:73–81, 2000
176. Krampen G, Main C, Waelbroeck O: Optimizing the learning process in short-term autogenic training by practice protocols. *Z Klin Psychol Psychopathol Psychother* 39:33–45, 1971
177. Platania-Solazzo A, Field TM, Blank J et al: Relaxation therapy reduces anxiety in child and adolescent psychiatric patients. *Acta Paedopsychiatr* 55:115–120, 1992
178. Moyer CA, Rounds J, Hannum JW: A meta-analysis of massage therapy research. *Psychol Bull* 130:3–18, 2004
179. Jorm AF, Christensen H, Griffiths KM et al: Effectiveness of complementary and self-help treatments for depression. *Med J Aust* 176(suppl):S84–S96, 2002
180. Crevenna R, Zielinski C, Keilani MY et al: Aerobic endurance training for cancer patients. *Wien Med Wochenschr* 153:212–216, 2003
181. Hadfield N: The role of aromatherapy massage in reducing anxiety in patients with malignant brain tumours. *Int J Palliat Nurs* 7:279–285, 2001
182. Jones NA, Field T: Massage and music therapies attenuate frontal EEG asymmetry in depressed adolescents. *Adolescence* 34:529–534, 1999
183. Estivill M: Therapeutic aspects of aerobic dance participation. *Health Care Women Int* 16:341–350, 1995
184. Ostwald PF, Barron BC, Byl NM et al: Performing arts medicine. *West J Med* 160:48–52, 1994
185. Pappas GP, Golin S, Meyer DL: Reducing symptoms of depression with exercise. *Psychosomatics* 31:112–113, 1990
186. Gurley V, Neuringer A, Massee J: Dance and sports compared: effects on psychological well-being. *J Sports Med Phys Fitness* 24:58–68, 1984
187. Burns DS: The effect of the bonny method of guided imagery and music on the mood and life quality of cancer patients. *J Music Ther* 38:51–65, 2001
188. Cassileth BR, Vickers AJ, Magill LA: Music therapy for mood disturbance during hospitalization for autologous stem cell transplantation: a randomized controlled trial. *Cancer* 98:2723–2729, 2003
189. Zappa SB, Cassileth BR: Complementary approaches to palliative oncological care. *J Nurs Care Qual* 18:22–26, 2003
190. Hilliard RE: The effects of music therapy on the quality and length of life of people diagnosed with terminal cancer. *J Music Ther* 40:113–137, 2003
191. Yamashita A, Kato S: Music therapy used on a patient in the terminal stage of cancer who narrated a tale based on her fantasy. *Seishin Shinkeigaku Zasshi* 105:787–794, 2003
192. Ballantyne JC, Mao J: Opioid therapy for chronic pain. *N Engl J Med* 349:1943–1953, 2003
193. Martin LA, Hagen NA: Neuropathic pain in cancer patients: mechanisms, syndromes, and clinical controversies. *J Pain Symptom Manage* 14:99–117, 1997
194. McQuay HJ, Tramer M, Nye BA et al: A systematic review of antidepressants in neuropathic pain. *Pain* 68:217–227, 1996
195. Kongsgaard UE, Bjorgo S, Hauser M: Neurolytic blocks for cancer pain — still a useful therapeutic strategy. *Tidsskr Nor Laegeforen* 124:481–483, 2004
196. Mason L, Moore RA, Edwards JE et al: Systematic review of efficacy of topical rubefacients containing salicylates for the treatment of acute and chronic pain. *BMJ* 328:995, 2004
197. Mannix K, Ahmedzai SH, Anderson H et al: Using bisphosphonates to control the pain of bone metastases: Evidence-based guidelines for palliative care. *Palliat Med* 14:455–461, 2000
198. Pan CX, Morrison RS, Ness J et al: Complementary and alternative medicine in the management of pain, dyspnea, and nausea and vomiting near the end of life. A systematic review. *J Pain Symptom Manage* 20:374–387, 2000
199. Mason L, Moore RA, Derry S et al: Systematic review of topical capsaicin for the treatment of chronic pain. *BMJ* 328:991, 2004.
200. Kwekkeboom KL: Music versus distraction for procedural pain and anxiety in patients with cancer. *Oncol Nurs Forum* 30:433–440, 2003
201. Ahmed HE, Craig WF, White PF et al: Percutaneous electrical nerve stimulation (PENS): a complementary therapy for the management of pain secondary to bony metastasis. *Clin J Pain* 14:320–323, 1998
202. Terkelsen AJ, Anderson OK, Molgaard H et al: Mental stress inhibits pain perception and heart rate variability but not a nociceptive withdrawal reflex. *Acta Physiol Scand* 180:405–414, 2004

203. Inui A: Cancer anorexia-cachexia syndrome: are neuropeptides the key? *Cancer Res* 59:4493–4501, 1999
204. Inui A, Meguid MM: Cachexia and obesity: two sides of one coin? *Curr Opin Clin Nutr Metab Care* 6:395–399, 2003
205. Astin JA, Shapiro SL, Eisenberg DM et al: Mind-body medicine: state of the science, implications for practice. *J Am Board Fam Pract* 16:131–147, 2003
206. Rogers MS, Todd CJ: The 'right kind' of pain: talking about symptoms in outpatient oncology consultations. *Palliat Med* 14:299–307, 2000
207. Paice JA: Pain, in Yarbro CH, Frogge M, Goodman M (eds.): *Cancer Symptom Management,* (ed 3) Sudbury, MA, Jones and Bartlett, 2004, pp 77–96
208. Simmonds PC: Palliative chemotherapy for advanced colorectal cancer: systematic review and meta-analysis. Colorectal Cancer Collaborative Group. *Br Med J* 321:531–535, 2000
209. McNicol E, Strassels S, Goudas L et al: Nonsteroidal anti-inflammatory drugs, alone or combined with opioids, for cancer pain: a systematic review. *J Clin Oncol* 22:1975–1992, 2004
210. Dalton JA, Keefe FJ, Carlson J et al: Tailoring cognitive-behavioral treatment for cancer pain. *Pain Manag Nurs* 5:3–18, 2004
211. Ernst E: Manual therapies for pain control: chiropractic and massage. *Clin J Pain* 20:8–12, 2004
212. Lee CO: CAM in the 21st Century in the US: role of nursing and evidence-based practice efforts, in *4th Annual Oncology Nursing Society Institutes of Learning.* Philadelphia, Oncology Nursing Society, 2003
213. Markel H: "I Swear by Apollo": on taking the hippocratic oath. *N Engl J Med* 350:2026–2029, 2004
214. National Cancer Institute: *NCI Cancer Facts: How to Evaluate Health Information on the Internet.* NCI Cancer Information Service. Retrieved from *http://cis.nci.nih.gov/fact/2_10.html.* Accessed May 16, 2004
215. Decker GM: Discussing CAM therapies with patients, in Buchsel PC, Yarbro CH (eds.): *Oncology Nursing in the Ambulatory Setting: Issues and Models of Care* (ed 2). Sudbury, MA, Jones and Bartlett, 2004, pp 355–375

PART IV

Cancer Symptom Management

CHAPTER 25

Cancer-Related Distress

Marlene Zichi Cohen, RN, PhD, FAAN
Elizabeth D. Carlson, DSN, MPH, RN, NP-C

Introduction

Cancer remains a feared diagnosis that many individuals continue to link with death despite recent and continuing advances in early detection, treatment, and survival. Although psychological distress has long been identified as a significant issue for persons with cancer, a more thorough examination reveals a continuum of vulnerable periods along the cancer trajectory, from primary prevention to tertiary prevention periods, as well as variable levels of distress in any individual at any given time. Distress related to the cancer experience is a combination of multidimensional stressors that strain individual and family coping capabilities. Adaptation to these stressors can range from having normal feelings of fear, sadness, and anger to meeting diagnostic criteria for adjustment or mood disorders.

The ability to successfully adapt to the multitude of stressors that accompany the cancer experience often depends on intervention by the healthcare team. However, the evidence makes it clear that psychological distress is frequently undetected and, even more frequently, untreated by cancer professionals.[1,2] This chapter reviews the issues involved in the detection and treatment of distress for adult individuals with cancer. While quality of life, pain, and fatigue are inextricably linked to the experience of distress, these issues receive in-depth exploration in other chapters and are only briefly reviewed here.

Psychological adaptation to the experience of cancer requires a succession of ongoing coping responses by individuals and their supportive infrastructure of family and friends. While social and cultural norms value attending to the physical symptoms of cancer to some extent, both professionals and patients continue to diminish and stigmatize the psychological symptoms of the experience.[3] Indeed, labeling symptoms "psychological" suggests they differ from "physical" symptoms. In response to the stigmatization attached to words such as "psychiatric," "psychosocial," and "emotional," the National Comprehensive Cancer Network (NCCN) selected the word "distress" to denote the unpleasant emotional experience associated with the profusion of stressors that people encounter along the cancer continuum.[1] These stressors include cognitive, behavioral, emotional, social, and/or spiritual issues that may interfere with the ability to successfully adjust to the demands of the disease continuum. In line with the NCCN, this chapter explores the historical perspective, language issues, current incidence, etiology of risk factors, barriers to identification and treatment, clinical manifestations, assessment, and intervention strategies of distress precipitated by the numerous challenges associated with the cancer experience.

Historical Perspective

The notion that psychological features can cause cancer has a very long history. Hippocrates, in ancient Greece, believed that distorting the balance of humors caused disease, and that women with excess black bile in particular were melancholic and more likely to develop cancer. This connection between melancholic women and cancer was also made in 200 CE by the famous Roman doctor Galen.[4]

Early work on psychosocial factors and cancer linked anxiety and depression with cancer.[5] From the 1950s to 1970, psychosocial problems were discussed in relation to cancer and survival.[6,7] The review of this literature by De Boer and colleagues revealed that research support for this connection is mixed.[8] While some studies have found that social support and involvement are related to survival in patients with cancer, coping styles were not conclusively related to length of survival. They noted that important determinants of coping, such as uncertainty and information, have not been considered in the research.

While evidence is accumulating that distress can alter immune function, this is not the same as, or evidence that, emotions cause the disease. One recent study found that women with depressive symptoms had a lower risk of developing breast cancer.[9] We need to be cautious that our ideas do not blame those with cancer for their disease. As Sontag[10] pointed out in her classic work, a characteristic of diseases whose causation is not understood is the idea that a disease can have a variety of causes. Indeed, cancer is actually a label for many diseases that likely have different etiologies, different courses, varied symptoms, and different effective treatments. What is important for nurses is to remember, and tend to, patients' minds, bodies, and spirits. Nightingale[11] noted, "Volumes are now written and spoken upon the effect of the mind on the body. . . But I wish a little more was thought of the effect of the body on the mind." Care of the "whole" person is a central value in nursing.

Language

The language we use both reflects and shapes our views, and language for symptoms of distress is problematic. We chose to use the term "distress" in the title of this chapter after examining the origin of the word, which is from the Latin participial stem *distringere,* meaning "to draw asunder."[12] Distress is defined as "severe pressure of trouble, pain, sickness, or sorrow."[12] This seemed to us to reflect the experience of persons along the cancer continuum. In addition, as we discussed earlier, the NCCN panel developing

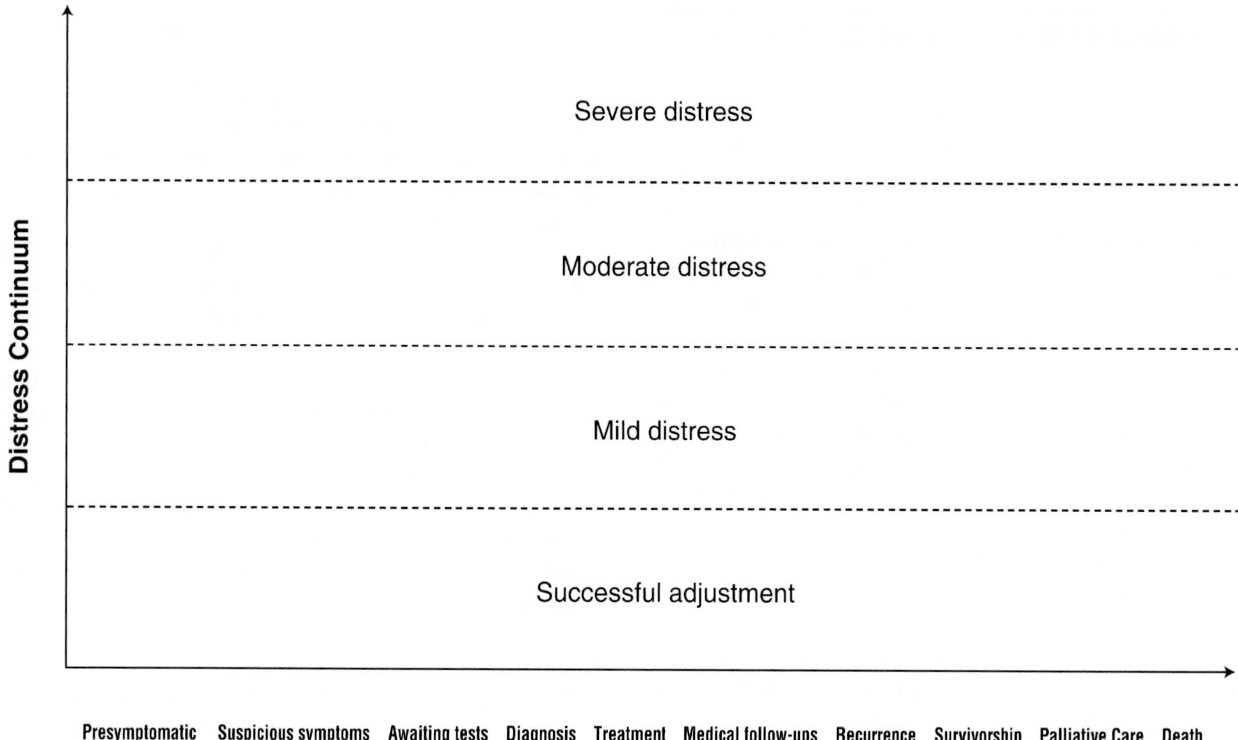

Figure 25-1 Psychological distress continuum of the cancer experience

standards for distress management selected the term "distress" because they viewed it as less stigmatizing and more acceptable than "psychiatric," "psychosocial," or "emotional."[1] They also noted that it sounds more "normal" and less embarrassing and can be defined and measured by self-report.

Incidence of Distress Associated with Cancer

As we noted earlier, the stressors experienced along the continuum of cancer begin even prior to diagnosis, continuing from primary prevention activities through tertiary care strategies related to treatment, survivorship, and palliative care (see Figure 25-1). As an example, adopting or continuing unhealthy lifestyle choices (such as smoking, alcohol intake, or excessive caloric intake) can be viewed as manifestations to external and internal stressors.[13] Decisions to engage in secondary prevention activities such as early detection screening can also be significant psychological stressors for some.[14,15] Other points along the cancer continuum that carry significant vulnerability to stressors include noticing suspicious symptoms, waiting for test results, and receiving a definitive diagnosis. These stressors may interfere with or impede optimal coping or adaptation.[16–18] In the past, health professionals have focused most of their attention on the active treatment period,[3,19] but susceptibility to the multiple demands of the cancer experience extends to issues of both survivorship and palliative care.[20–22]

Levels of perceived psychological distress are also significantly influenced by cancer type, stage of disease, and individual life circumstances. Although the overall rates of psychological distress were 35.1% in a large database of cancer patients (N = 9000), these rates varied significantly by cancer type.[23] Patients with lung cancer reported the highest rates of psychological distress (43.4%), while those with gynecological cancers reported the lowest rates of distress (29.6%). Distress is also significantly correlated with the stage of disease in both active treatment and palliative care patients, with the prevalence of distress increasing with the stage of disease.[24–26] Finally, both the life stage of the individuals and perceptions of their support significantly influenced the level of psychological distress experienced by cancer patients.[20,26]

Etiology of Risk Factors for Distress

Although the incidence of psychological distress varies by type of cancer and stage of disease, individual life circumstances play a significant role in the experience of distress. These factors include the effects of prior life experiences, perceptions of social support, and the burden of physical symptoms. The next section reviews these risk factors. Specific etiologies, risk factors, and the prevalence of specific symptoms are included in the sections on these symptoms.

Current work examining whether prior experience can exacerbate symptoms in persons with cancer has had mixed results. Several studies have found that the number of lifetime stressors (such as rape and abuse) and the perceived resolution of these stressors were related to symptoms such as anger, depression, and symptom-related distress in persons with cancer and their spouses.[27–29]

Baider and colleagues[30] examined the effects of interventions in persons with cancer who had had prior stressful experiences. Their early work[31] found that behavioral interventions, such as progressive muscle relaxation with guided imagery, resulted in a significant and sustained (for six months) decrease in psychological distress in cancer patients who were highly distressed. However, in a second study with Holocaust survivors who agreed to participate in the intervention, these interventions decreased distress over the short term, but the improvements were not seen three months later.[30] They concluded that the gravity of the Holocaust trauma had overburdened and outweighed the reservoir of positive images and prevented the participants from maintaining the benefits gained from the psychological intervention. They suggested that this finding may apply to other severely traumatized groups as well and that such groups may require long-term, ongoing psychological support.

Social support has been shown to mediate the effects of stress and coping on the level of distress in parents of children with cancer in Taiwan.[32] Hawkley and Cacioppo's[33] review of research linking loneliness (or social isolation, the reverse of social support) to disease suggested that loneliness can lead to altered health behaviors, excessive stress reactivity, and an inadequate or inefficient physiological repair and maintenance process. Even in situations thought to provide social support, such as support groups, emotional suppression (inhibiting the expression of negative emotions) has been found to be significantly associated with increased mood disturbance, in a study of a heterogeneous sample of cancer patients attending community cancer support groups, taking into account important demographic, medical, and group support variables.[34]

Evidence from autonomic, endocrine, and immune functioning suggests that these effects unfold over a long time. Therefore, providing instrumental support for the demands of coping with disease may be most clearly helpful. However, when patients and spouses were both highly distressed, they perceived little social support for either of them,[35] indicating the need to consider level of distress when providing social support. The complexity of these relationships is further indicated by the failure to find a relationship between job strain and cancer risks such as smoking, high alcohol consumption, low intake of fruits and vegetables, and lack of exercise in a study of 3309 persons in the Netherlands.[36]

The connections among physical symptoms, psychological symptoms, support, coping, and survival have been investigated. Symptom ratings among 218 patients who completed the Memorial Symptom Assessment Scale (MSAS) were correlated with survival, although when physical symptoms were entered into the model, it was found that other factors did not contribute to predicting survival.[37] The role of psychological symptoms independent of physical symptoms is therefore uncertain. These authors speculated that patients' self-reports captured aspects of disease severity that may not have been apparent to observers or by tumor burden alone.

Barriers to Identification and Treatment

Studies continue to show that between 20% and 50% of cancer patients routinely report significant levels of psychological distress, yet fewer than 10% of individuals with cancer are ever referred for psychosocial care.[18,23,26,38] Even among those identified as meeting clinical criteria for adjustment or mood disorders, few are prescribed pharmacological treatment regimens, and even fewer actually take the prescribed medication.[39] Several factors contribute to this lack of attention to psychological distress, including the reluctance of patients to report distress, clinical time constraints, and a tendency to focus on individual cancer symptoms (i.e., pain or fatigue) rather than the overall impact of the combined physical and emotional stressors as individuals experience them. In this section we review typical patient, provider, and system barriers to the recognition and treatment of psychological distress in cancer patients.

Patient Barriers

The reluctance of patients to report psychological distress to their healthcare providers is often influenced by an assumption that nothing can be done. Many individuals with cancer, and those in their support systems, assume that the stressors associated with the cancer experience are inevitable and are not amenable to intervention or alleviation.[3] In addition, the burden of psychological distress can impair the motivation and ability of patients to advocate for care that is not explicitly addressed by the healthcare team. Patients who are experiencing greater levels of anxiety and depression are the very individuals who are the least likely to report their psychological distress to professionals. In response, Cunningham[40] has argued that instead of waiting for patients or family to self-identify for treatment, professional advocacy is necessary for recognition and intervention.

In addition to erroneous assumptions that psychological distress is a natural by-product of the cancer experience, the inability to adapt to and cope with significant stressors continues to carry significant cultural and social stigmatization for cancer patients. As an example of the influence of this perceived stigmatization, McLachlan and colleagues[41] analyzed the response to intervention referrals in a group of 202 cancer patients. This intervention study assigned a triage nurse to offer appropriate referral services to meet patients' self-identified needs. The most frequently offered services were counseling (30% of referrals) and physical symptom management (20% of referrals). However, significantly more patients accepted referrals for physical symptoms than for psychological symptoms (57% versus 28%, respectively; $p = .0003$). Similarly, in a study of cancer patients in palliative care, none of the patients were in favor of obtaining psychological counseling, which they regarded as an indication of their inability to cope on their own.[21] This social stigmatization is often reinforced by the supportive infrastructure of family, friends, and providers. Cancer patients often experience considerable pressure to remain positive in the face of overwhelming physical and emotional symptoms, a perception that has been referred to by some as the "prison of positive thinking."[34,42]

Finally, many studies have reported that cancer patients feel a need to protect their families by minimizing or masking their own negative emotions. For instance, patients in a study of relaxation therapy versus cognitive-behavioral therapy noted that either form of therapy gave them a "space" to talk about their experiences with someone outside the family.[19] This safe context applied equally to both types of therapy and was an important aspect for patients. Patients described the therapy context as a time when they could discuss negative feelings without making their family members sad. In both forms of intervention, the therapist was identified as an objective listener whose feelings were not the patient's responsibility. Similarly, palliative care cancer patients involved in an aromatherapy massage study noted that these sessions provided an opportunity for them to talk about their concerns and fears without burdening their families.[21]

Clinician Barriers

Clinician barriers to the identification and treatment of psychological distress among cancer patients are also multidimensional. A recent study found that health professionals routinely elicited only 40% of patients' key concerns.[3] Impediments to the management of psychological distress in cancer patients include many of the same factors that impede adequate pain management.[43] Despite an increased recognition of distress, many healthcare professionals have inadequate knowledge concerning the manifestations of distress, conduct incomplete distress assessments, and hold misconceptions about their ability to deal with patient distress. In addition, cancer clinicians prioritize cancer cures over caring for the person with cancer. Subjective self-report of psychological distress symptoms are often minimized in comparison to objective data, such as lab values or physical findings. The clinical assessment of patient distress is often given a low priority and typically has not been a focus of ongoing assessment and monitoring efforts. In addition, clinicians are often uncertain about the clinical relevance of levels of distress and of the effectiveness of medications or psychotherapy to deal with distress, and they often have inadequate resources to address the problem.

Another common problem among cancer professionals is the use of distancing strategies designed to block patient disclosure of emotional issues. These distancing strategies typically take the form of normalization (e.g., "of course you are distressed"), but these normalizing tactics typically leave patients feeling that they have no right to talk about their distress. Researchers have identified three main reasons for the use of distancing strategies by health professionals: (1) the fear of unleashing strong emotions, (2) the lack of training in communication skills, and (3) the lack of support from professional colleagues.[3]

Finally, both clinicians and researchers have focused on one symptom at a time instead of the multidimensional experience of cancer. A cluster of symptoms, including pain, fatigue, sleep disturbances, depressed mood, and cognitive dysfunction, often accompanies the experience of cancer as a normal biological response to a life-threatening illness and its treatment. Indeed, this clustering of physiological and psychological symptoms has been referred to as sickness behaviors.[44] However, while these sickness behaviors may be a normal physiological response to illness, they represent additional stressors to an individual's coping capabilities.[45] At the same time, this is a dynamic process whereby sickness behaviors increase perceived levels of distress while higher levels of distress exacerbate the physiological tolerance threshold for sickness behaviors. Only recently has there been a deliberate attempt to focus on the clustering of distressing symptoms in cancer patients.[46]

System Barriers

A variety of system barriers noted for pain management apply equally well to distress management. These barriers include a lack of care coordination, which fragments care, and a lack of communication between specialists and primary care providers and among providers during transitions from settings, including from acute care or "cure" to hospice mode. In addition, reimbursement for symptom management is often lacking. Requiring standards for distress management may help initiate organizational changes to overcome system barriers to distress management. While pain standards, including those from the Joint Commission on Accreditation of Healthcare Organizations (JCAHO), are not sufficient to ensure adequate pain management, they have provided an important impetus for change in many organizations.[47]

Clinical Manifestations of Distress

Distress can be manifested in a number of ways, ranging from successful adjustment or adaptation to a continuum of severities of psychological distress. Our discussion of successful adaptation is followed by a range of symptoms of distress, from mild to moderate to severe.

Successful Adaptation

Successful adjustment to living with cancer is characterized by the ability to minimize disruptions to established social roles, regulate the experience of emotional distress, and maintain active engagement in meaningful life activities.[1] To maintain this successful adaptation to the multiple stressors associated with the cancer experience, coping efforts typically focus around three categories of strategies: those that are problem-focused, those that are emotion-focused, and those that are meaning-focused. Problem-focused strategies are directed at altering problem-specific stressors. These types of stressors might include aspects of the inevitable disruptions to work or school, financial issues, transportation problems, or family care concerns. Emotion-focused strategies are directed at minimizing the degree of emotional or psychological distress related to the cancer experience, the focus of this chapter. Finally, meaning-focused strategies help individuals integrate the spiritual significance of the disease process.

Mild Distress

Mild distress is defined by the NCCN guidelines as a score of less than 5 on the distress management assessment tool (see Figure 25-2).[1] However, successful intervention to alleviate more significant levels of distress requires consideration of the many physical and psychological stressors associated with the cancer experience. In this section we review the most significant physiological stressors that are typically reported by individuals with cancer. While these physiological symptoms may precipitate moderate or even severe levels of distress, we chose to address them here because they equally represent the perceptible manifestations of distress.

Fatigue

Fatigue is the most commonly occurring symptom among cancer patients, significantly affecting at least 70% of the population.[48–50] Expert cancer professionals have recently selected fatigue as one of the top symptom priorities for intervention.[51] Cross-sectional studies suggest that fatigue is a result of a combination of physical and psychological causes.[46,52] For instance, anemic cancer patients experienced statistically significant differences in fatigue compared to nonanemic cancer patients and controls.[53] Likewise, fatigue and depression typically occur together in cancer patients, suggesting a common etiology to stress. However, recent findings suggest that symptoms of fatigue are not ameliorated by antidepressant therapy.[50] Nevertheless, surveys consistently show that fatigue is associated with significant physical, emotional, psychological, and social consequences.

Sleep disturbances

Individuals with cancer report significantly poorer overall sleep quality than the general population, accompanied by more daytime dysfunction.[54] An estimated 30%–50% of cancer patients report significant distress related to sleep disturbances, typically insomnia or disruptions in the sleep-wake cycle.[55] Inadequate sleep is strongly correlated with both fatigue and mood disorders in people with cancer.[55,56] Cancer patients identified the most frequent causes of sleep disorders to be due to thoughts, concerns, and pain.[49]

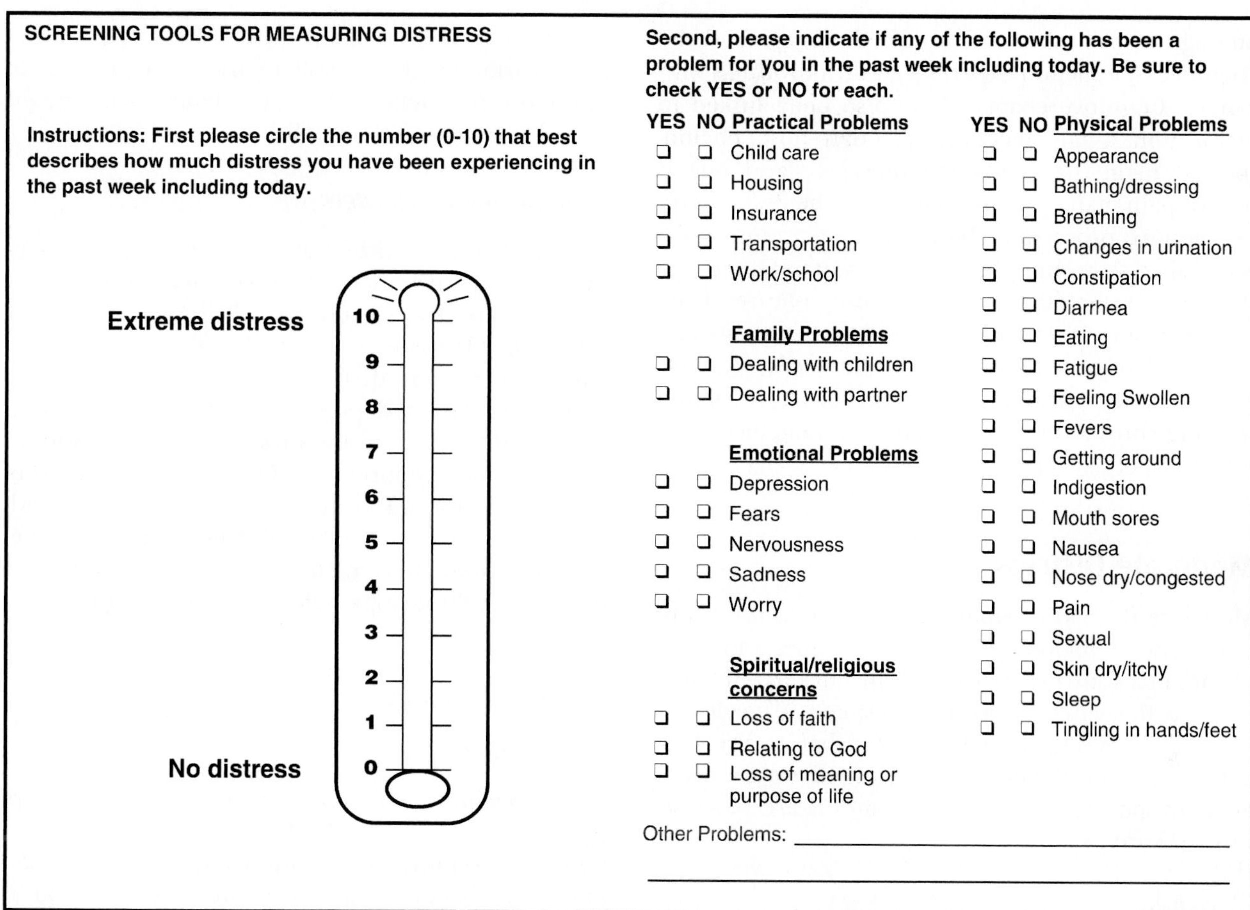

SCREENING TOOLS FOR MEASURING DISTRESS

Instructions: First please circle the number (0-10) that best describes how much distress you have been experiencing in the past week including today.

Second, please indicate if any of the following has been a problem for you in the past week including today. Be sure to check YES or NO for each.

YES	NO	Practical Problems
❑	❑	Child care
❑	❑	Housing
❑	❑	Insurance
❑	❑	Transportation
❑	❑	Work/school
		Family Problems
❑	❑	Dealing with children
❑	❑	Dealing with partner
		Emotional Problems
❑	❑	Depression
❑	❑	Fears
❑	❑	Nervousness
❑	❑	Sadness
❑	❑	Worry
		Spiritual/religious concerns
❑	❑	Loss of faith
❑	❑	Relating to God
❑	❑	Loss of meaning or purpose of life

YES	NO	Physical Problems
❑	❑	Appearance
❑	❑	Bathing/dressing
❑	❑	Breathing
❑	❑	Changes in urination
❑	❑	Constipation
❑	❑	Diarrhea
❑	❑	Eating
❑	❑	Fatigue
❑	❑	Feeling Swollen
❑	❑	Fevers
❑	❑	Getting around
❑	❑	Indigestion
❑	❑	Mouth sores
❑	❑	Nausea
❑	❑	Nose dry/congested
❑	❑	Pain
❑	❑	Sexual
❑	❑	Skin dry/itchy
❑	❑	Sleep
❑	❑	Tingling in hands/feet

Other Problems: ____________________

Data from National Comprehensive Cancer Network. These Guidelines are a work in progress that will be refined as often as new significant data becomes available.

The NCCN Guidelines are a statement of consensus of its authors regarding their views of currently accepted approaches to treatment. Any clinician seeking to apply or consult any NCCN guideline is expected to use independent medical judgment in the context of individual clinical circumstances to determine any patient's care or treatment. The National Comprehensive Cancer Network makes no warranties of any kind whatsoever regarding their content, use or application and disclaims any responsibility for their application or use in any way.

These Guidelines are copyrighted by the National Comprehensive Cancer Network. All rights reserved. These Guidelines and illustrations herein may not be reproduced in any form for any purpose without the express written permission of the NCCN.

Figure 25-2 Distress management assessment tool

Left unattended, sleep disorders may progress to a chronic state, lasting several years after the initial diagnosis and treatment period ends.[57] Family caregivers have also been found to have sleep problems, which were linked with depression and fluctuated over time.[58]

Cognitive dysfunction

Cognitive dysfunction is the inability to relate current to past events or to understand experiences. Evidence from several disciplines has shown that emotions and cognitive processing are intimately linked, and recent studies have linked cognitive performance with survival.[59,60] Cognitive changes occur from both cancer and its treatment and are significantly distressing to patients, to their family members, and to nurses.[61] Subtle cognitive changes are experienced quite frequently in cancer patients, with as many as 75% reporting mild to moderate cognitive impairment.[62] The distress patients experience from cognitive changes occurs regardless of the degree of the impairment, which can range from subtle memory changes noticeable only to the individual to more severe memory dysfunction, including acute delirium and dementia.[63]

Many factors influence cognitive function, and it is likely that several mechanisms may be operating simultaneously. Memory and concentration dysfunction often accompany fatigue, the most common complaint among cancer patients.[48] Anemia, depression, and age are all associated with both cancer and the cognitive dysfunction experienced by individuals with cancer. Cognitive changes have also been linked to medication usage, including standard-dose chemotherapy regimens,[62] radiation therapy,[59] and opioid use for pain management.[64] However, the dysfunction of cognitive processing abilities has been empirically established to occur even prior to active treatment, associated simply with the overwhelming nature of the cancer diagnosis.[16] Supporting evidence suggests that emotional distress systematically influences cognitive performance, including problem-solving abilities, working short-term memory, and the long-term consolidation of experiences.[65,66]

Moderate Distress

Moderate distress is experienced when symptoms of mild distress, including insomnia, fatigue, and sleep disturbances, are exacerbated. Delirium and dementia fall into this category, as do adjustment disorders, a category of anxiety-related disorders that involve difficulties coping with change. Generalized anxiety disorders and post-traumatic stress disorders are more severe and are discussed later.

Delirium

"Delirium," from the Latin *delirium*, meaning "deviate" or "deranged,"[12] is the diagnostic term used to describe an organic mental disorder that usually has an acute onset and an identifiable precipitating stressor. Also called acute confusion, delirium can have a short course and is reversible except when it occurs during the last 24 to 28 hours of life. Prolonged delirium may be a sign of infection or coagulopathy.[67] Delirium, in which both cognition and attention are disturbed, is experience by 15% to 40% of those with cancer and in more than 85% of those with terminal cancer.[67–70] In advanced disease, opioid dysfunction usually is in the form of delirium.[64] Standard-dose chemotherapy has also been linked with cognitive deficits in cancer patients.[62] Radiation therapy and combined radiation and chemotherapy are also neurotoxic.[59]

Dementia

"Dementia," from the Latin *dementare*, meaning "insane,"[12] is a chronic and irreversible cognitive disorder with more gradual onset than delirium. A simple definition of dementia is a deterioration of cognitive abilities that hinders people from performing their usual activities of daily living. Dementia is usually irreversible, may not have identified precipitating stressors, and includes impaired short- and long-term memory that causes significant social and occupational impairments. The result of the direct impact of tumors or treatment on the brain, dementia is thought to be less common than delirium.

Adjustment disorders

Adjustment disorders are "normal" reactions to stresses, generally related to a particular event. These reactions are also sometimes called "situational" or "reactive" depression. These disorders lack specific symptoms, making them difficult to diagnose and to differentiate from depression. Screening tools often fail to differentiate distress from major depression.[71] Unstructured supportive interactions with caring providers are helpful. Providers need to provide reminders to maintain hope, and need to listen and try to alleviate suffering.[72] Referral to mental health specialists is indicated if these approaches are not effective.

Severe Distress

Depression

Depression is a disabling syndrome that affects approximately 15% to 25% of cancer patients.[24,73–75] As we discussed in the section on barriers, patients often mistakenly believe both that depression is normal in those with cancer and that treatment is not helpful. Litofsky and colleagues[74] found poor concordance between physician and patient ratings of depression, and few received pharmacological therapy, even when depressive symptoms were recognized by physicians. Intervention is required when patients experience a depressive disorder, not for the normal sadness everyone experiences. The symptoms of major depression are summarized in Table 25-1. Depression is diagnosed in those without cancer when these symptoms last a minimum of two weeks. Of course, in those with cancer, it is important to distinguish between depression and the symptoms of cancer and cancer treatments. The most useful symptoms to examine in making this distinction are cognitive ones, such as feelings of worthlessness, guilt, and hopelessness; thoughts of suicide; and loss of pleasure in activities.

Anxiety

Anxiety in cancer is both common and poorly understood. This is indicated by the wide range in prevalence estimates, ranging in one literature review from 0.9% to 49%,[77] although when standardized psychiatric interviews and research diagnostic criteria are used, the range is more typically 10% to 30%.[78] Another source of variance for these estimates of prevalence is the differences in the samples studied, including

Table 25-1 Diagnostic Criteria for Major Depressive Disorder

At least one of the following three abnormal moods that significantly interfere with the person's life:	At least five of the following symptoms during the same two-week depressed period:

• Abnormal depressed mood most of the day, nearly every day, for at least two weeks
• Abnormal loss of all interest and pleasure most of the day, nearly every day, for at least two weeks
• If younger than 18, abnormal irritable mood most of the day, nearly every day, for at least two weeks
	• Abnormal depressed mood
	• Abnormal loss of all interest and pleasure
	• Appetite or weight disturbance;
	  ◦ Abnormal weight loss or decreased appetite
	  ◦ Abnormal weight gain or increased appetite
	• Sleep disturbance, either abnormal insomnia or abnormal hypersomnia
	• Activity disturbance, either abnormal agitation or abnormal slowing (observed by others)
	• Abnormal fatigue or loss of energy
	• Abnormal self-reproach or inappropriate guilt
	• Abnormal poor concentration or indecisiveness
	• Abnormal morbid thoughts of death (not just fear of dying) or suicide

Data compiled from the Diagnostic and Statistical Manual IV, 1994.[76]

differences in gender, age, type of cancer, and time since diagnosis. Patients with cancer can have one of several anxiety disorders, the most common being reactive anxiety/adjustment disorder, disease and treatment-related anxiety, substance-induced anxiety (from substances such as corticosteroids), and other anxiety disorders such as general anxiety disorders, panic, phobia, obsessive-compulsive disorder, and post-traumatic stress disorder.

Diagnosing anxiety in cancer patients is challenging, since the diagnosis in healthy persons is made based on somatic symptoms, including anorexia, fatigue, and weight loss, which in cancer are often symptoms of the disease itself and its treatment. The symptoms of worry, distractibility, restlessness, and fearfulness are more important for diagnosing anxiety among cancer patients.[79] Anxiety can be adaptive and can motivate actions to reduce the anxiety. Intervention is required when anxiety is severe or prolonged and interferes with activities of daily living and quality of life. Symptoms of anxiety result from autonomic overactivity and include intense fear out of proportion with the threat, the inability to absorb information, and the inability to cooperate with medical procedures. Somatic symptoms include shortness of breath, sweating, lightheadedness, and palpitations. Patients are generally distressed about their symptoms, and behavioral interventions and medications to treat anxiety are generally effective.

Post-Traumatic Stress Disorder

Post-traumatic stress disorder (PTSD) is a more severe anxiety-related disorder that is not acute and is the consequence of previous trauma. In 1994, the Diagnostic and Statistical Manual[76] added life-threatening illnesses, which had previously been explicitly excluded as stressors, to the list of factors that could precipitate PTSD. This change resulted in a great deal of attention to PTSD after a cancer diagnosis. PTSD develops in response to an unusually traumatic event that involved actual or threatened death or serious physical injury. Symptoms include feelings of intense fear combined with repeatedly reliving the event with intrusive, distressing recollections (thoughts, images); repeated, distressing dreams; and/or flashbacks, hallucinations, or illusions in which the individual acts or feels as if the event were recurring, accompanied by marked mental distress and physiological reactivity (such as rapid heartbeat and elevated blood pressure) (see Table 25-2).

Patients also repeatedly avoid stimuli related to the trauma and have a numbing of their general responsiveness, as shown by, for example, avoiding thoughts, feelings, or conversations concerning the event; avoiding activities, people, or places that recall the event; not being able to recall important features of the event; having a marked loss of interest or participation in activities important to the patient; feeling detached or isolated from other people; being restricted in the ability to love or feel other strong emotions; and having the feeling that life will be brief or unfulfilled (lack of marriage, job, children). In addition, symptoms of hyperarousal are present, as listed in Table 25-2. PTSD is diagnosed when the symptoms last longer than one month and cause clinically important distress or impair work, social, or personal functioning. It can occur even in very young children.[76]

Four recent reviews have examined studies of PTSD following cancer.[80–83] These studies found the incidence to range from 1.3% to 19%, with the range

Table 25-2 Diagnostic Criteria for Post-Traumatic Stress Disorder

The traumatic event is persistently reexperienced in one (or more) of the following ways:
• Recurrent and intrusive distressing recollections of the event, including images, thoughts, or perceptions
• Recurrent distressing dreams of the event
• Acting or feeling as if the traumatic event were recurring (includes a sense of reliving the experience, illusions, hallucinations, and dissociative flashback episodes, including those that occur on awakening or when intoxicated)
• Intense psychological distress upon exposure to internal or external cues that symbolize or resemble an aspect of the traumatic event and physiological reactivity upon exposure to internal or external cues that symbolize or resemble an aspect of the traumatic event
	Persistent avoidance of stimuli associated with the trauma and numbing of general responsiveness (not present before the trauma), as indicated by three (or more) of the following:
	• Efforts to avoid thoughts, feelings, or conversations associated with the trauma
	• Efforts to avoid activities, places, or people that arouse recollections of the trauma
	• Inability to recall an important aspect of the trauma
	• Markedly diminished interest or participation in significant activities
	• Feelings of detachment or estrangement from others
	• Restricted range of affect (e.g., unable to have loving feelings)
	• Sense of a foreshortened future
	• Persistent symptoms of increased arousal
	  ◦ Difficulty falling or staying asleep
	  ◦ Irritability or outbursts of anger
	  ◦ Difficulty concentrating
	  ◦ Hypervigilance
	  ◦ Exaggerated startle response
	• Duration of the disturbance is more than one month
	• The disturbance causes clinically significant distress or impairment in social, occupational, or other important areas of functioning

Data compiled from the Diagnostic and Statistical Manual IV, 1994[76]

related to the use of more or less stringent criteria. Several studies have also reported that between 10% and 40% of patients have intrusive and avoidance symptoms following cancer. The symptoms decline considerably for most patients within three months after diagnosis or after treatment is completed.

Several factors have been found to predict PTSD symptomatology. These include female gender, younger age at diagnosis, prior negative life stressors, history of psychological disturbance, increased distress subsequent to the diagnosis, lower education, poor social support, poor social functioning, reduced physical functioning, emotionally reactive temperament, and avoidant coping style. Mixed evidence supports the role of medical variables, including type, stage, severity, and prognosis of cancer in subsequent PTSD. Most studies have been small and cross-sectional, have relied on self-report measures, and have sampled mostly women with early to middle stage breast cancer, which is particularly an issue since most studies conclude that women are more likely to experience PTSD than men.

Assessment of Distress

As is true of all symptoms, effective interventions for distress require accurate assessment, which can be accomplished only with communication among health-care professionals, patients, and their families. While a great deal of cancer-related symptom assessment focuses on one symptom at a time, measures of multiple symptoms exist that include psychosocial symptoms.[23,84–86] However, attention to these symptoms has not always been a priority, as indicated by the fact that a stress management subscale has only recently been added to the Cancer Behavior Inventory, a measure of self-efficacy for coping with cancer.[87] The NCCN guidelines include a brief screening to assess the presence of problems and call for referral for further evaluation if the screening indicates symptoms such as delirium, dementia, mood disorders, adjustment disorders, anxiety disorder, substance abuse, and personality disorder.[1] The distress thermometer and problem list (see Figure 25-2) is a brief and useful screen for distress and related problems that patients can complete in only two or three minutes.

Self-report screening instruments must be scored, evaluated, and discussed with each patient. Triage, the process of communicating screening results, discussing each patient's needs, and determining the best course of further action, is vital to successful screening. The oncology team (oncologist, nurse, palliative care specialist, social worker, and counselor) is responsible for successful triage. In fact, screening without availability of appropriate treatment resources is considered unethical. Rapid methods of screening are needed to determine which patients need more in-depth clinical interviews for more precise diagnosis. These in-depth interviews require the skill of mental health specialists.[88] Ongoing evaluations and monitoring are also critically important.

Interventions

The NCCN standards of care suggest that distress rated as mild might result in a referral to a local self-help group or management by the primary oncology team only. Distress rated as moderate to severe warrants referral to other appropriate professionals (psychologists, psychiatrists, social workers, palliative care specialists, or pastoral counselors), depending on the nature of the distress. In some studies a significant percentage of patients who report moderate to high levels of distress do not get or want further assessment.[21,41] Thus, it is important to consider how the primary oncology team can introduce the need for further psychosocial assessment.

Interventions to minimize distress have focused on alleviating the physiological symptoms of cancer (i.e., fatigue, pain, and insomnia), improving coping strategies with cognitive-behavioral interventions, or providing a context of supportive therapy. Recently, complementary or alternative therapies have gained attention as interventions for distress in cancer patients. Ideally, cancer professionals should take a multifactorial approach to the alleviation of distress in cancer care. Factors associated with fatigue and pain management are found in the chapters specific to those symptoms. Here we review some of the more recent innovative initiatives aimed at managing the cluster of distress symptoms.

Symptom Management Strategies

Addressing the cluster of symptoms that accompany the cancer experience is an obvious focus, and an important approach, to alleviating distress. For instance, activity management—whether exercise or energy conservation — has consistently been shown to benefit the burden of fatigue.[89,90] In a similar vein, researchers have used cognitive-behavioral interventions to improve insomnia in women with metastatic breast cancer.[91] Both of these approaches significantly improved mood, fatigue, and quality of life.

Likewise, sensory stimulation approaches have been successful in alleviating or minimizing physiological symptoms. Cimprich and Ronis[16] have tested an environmental intervention in women newly diagnosed with breast cancer aimed at alleviating cognitive dysfunction. The intervention entailed 120 minutes of weekly exposure to an aesthetically pleasing environmental stimulus such as observing a sunset, walking through a park, or gardening. The intervention group significantly recovered their capacity to direct attention (CDA) compared to the control group, suggesting the beneficial effects of early intervention aimed at restoring cognitive functioning.

Japanese researchers have also used sensory stimulation interventions to alleviate the distress associated with chemotherapy.[92] The intervention, the Bedside Wellness System, integrates visual, auditory, and olfactory sensory stimuli and is targeted to individual preferences. Patients experienced a visual selection of a lake, a forest, or a country town. Auditory stimulation was selected and delivered by either headphones or speakers, and the system delivered a gentle, scented breeze. Each aspect (visual, auditory, and olfactory) of the sensory stimulation session was selected by the patient and lasted approximately 20 minutes. The sessions could be repeated as many times during the chemotherapy as the patient desired. The intervention had a positive effect on improving physical symptoms and decreasing negative mood states in the intervention group compared to the control group.

Cognitive-Behavioral Strategies

Most interventions aimed at alleviating psychological distress in cancer patients have typically focused on cognitive-behavioral interventions targeting either problem-focused or emotion-focused coping strategies. Problem-focused coping strategies are designed to help patients manage specific problems by directly trying to alter the problem situation. Emotion-focused coping strategies are aimed at helping to regulate the experience of psychological distress.[93] The most optimal outcomes are obtained when there is a good match between the appraisal of the situation and the coping strategy selected.[94] For instance, when there is a perception of high control over the situation, problem-focused coping strategies result in less psychological distress. In contrast, when the perception is that there is little control over the situation, emotion-focused coping strategies provided the best approach to alleviating distress.

As an example of a problem-focused strategy, Given and colleagues[95] randomized individuals with cancer (N = 237) to either a nursing intervention or the conventional care group. Individuals in the intervention group identified their unique problems with the nurse and selected specific interventions proposed by the nurse. The patient and nurse then together evaluated the outcomes of the selected interventions. Patients in the intervention group who entered the study with severe symptoms reported significantly lower severity scores at 10 and 20 weeks. Controlling for demographic and disease-specific variables did not attenuate the findings.

In contrast, emotion-focused interventions are aimed at alleviating psychological distress through stress reduction strategies. As an example, mindfulness-based stress reduction programs have reported significant decreases in mood disturbance and stress symptoms for up to six months in both male and female cancer patients as a result of a seven-week intervention.[96] Similarly, Jacobsen and colleagues[97] compared self-administered stress management training, professionally administered stress management training, and conventional care among patients about to start chemotherapy (N = 411). Patients receiving professionally administered stress management training did no better than those who administered it themselves. However, both training groups did significantly better on a variety of distress measures compared to persons receiving conventional care only.

Someone Who Cares

Several decades of research have associated levels of social support with individual coping capabilities.[94] Interventions aimed at providing a supportive environment focus on the provision of a safe, neutral context for the expression of emotions as a distress-alleviating strategy. Support groups for cancer patients are a common intervention strategy and have shown significant results. For example, Goodwin and colleagues[22] randomized patients with metastatic breast cancer to either supportive-expressive group therapy or conventional care. The intervention consisted of weekly 90-minute sessions of 8 to 12 women and professional group leaders (psychiatrists, psychologists, social workers, or nurse clinicians). Women in the intervention arm of the study reported significantly improved mood states and decreases in perceived pain compared to the control group.

The provision of a supportive environment as a safe, neutral context takes many forms. Interestingly, MacCormack and colleagues[19] found little difference in patient perception of benefit between cognitive-emotional therapy and relaxation therapy, as long as there was nonspecific time for the patient to talk to the therapist. Likewise, relaxation and counseling were both shown to relieve psychological distress symptoms in a group of newly diagnosed cancer patients.[98] Similarly, individuals receiving aromatherapy from a registered nurse reported significant stress-relieving benefits. Indeed, patients conveyed that the sessions provided a safe space where they could discuss their concerns and feelings without burdening their families or bothering their physicians.[21] Central to the beneficial findings in all of these studies was the opportunity to safely discuss thoughts and feelings with an attentive, empathetic, professional listener.

Complementary Strategies

As shown by the examples just cited, the division between professional and complementary or alternative therapies is increasingly blurred. Indeed, the importance of emotional expression has been highlighted in interventions aimed at alleviating the psychological distress of the cancer experience.[42] Supportive listening and massage therapy play a significant role in both aromatherapy[21] and reflexology.[99] Gilbar and colleagues[100] found that individuals with cancer who sought out complementary therapies in addition to conventional therapy reported significantly lower levels of distress than those individuals who did not seek outside treatment modalities, irrespective of the type of alternative treatment chosen. In contrast, Risberg and Jacobsen[101] found that among 158 cancer patients in Norway, those with higher levels of mental distress used more alternative medicine. Further research is needed to understand the intricacies of these approaches to alleviate distress.

Pharmacological Management

Persons with the clinically significant distress symptoms described in this chapter may benefit from medications. The most common medications used to treat both anxiety and depression are benzodiazepines. In persons with physical illness, the short-acting agents (alprazolam, lorazepam, and oxazepam) are best tolerated. In addition, nonbenzodiazepines, neuroleptics, antihistamines, and tricyclic antidepressants (TCAs) are useful in treating anxiety.[79] Antidepressant medications, used to treat both anxiety and depression, include TCAs, selective serotonin reuptake inhibitors (SSRIs), selective serotonin-norepinephrine reuptake inhibitors (SSNRIs), beta-blockers, antihistamines, lithium, sympathomimetic stimulants, monoamine oxide inhibitors (MAOIs), and central nervous system stimulants. See both Gobel[102] and Barsevick and Much[103] for a more comprehensive review of these medications, their doses, and side effects.

Conclusion

The importance of alleviating physical and psychological symptoms is underscored by the finding that the burden of physical symptoms experienced by individuals with cancer is significantly correlated with the desire for a hastened death in both patients in active treatment and those receiving palliative care.[24,25] Effective interventions are most available when multidisciplinary teams work together and involve patients and their families. Nurses play key roles in symptom control, since they have more time and closer relationships with patients than other professionals. The roles of psychiatrists, oncologists, clergy, and the rest of the interdisciplinary team, including social workers, psychologists, and nurses, are important, as they have unique disciplinary expertise with counseling, psychotherapy, education, pastoral care, and, when indicated, medications. The need for centralized sources of information about treatment, care, and support has been recognized. An example of a program to centralize resources, described by Nemetz and Mercardante,[104] was developed by a coalition of patients with cancer, volunteers, and hospital staff.

Learning from efforts to manage pain may help guide the development of effective support for symptoms of distress. The Joint Commission on Accreditation of Health Care Organizations (JCAHO)[15] instituted pain standards in 1999, although cancer pain has long been recognized as a serious problem for persons with cancer. While relief of cancer pain remains a problem, no JCAHO standards exist for the management of distress, and many barriers exist to both effective pain and distress management. The need for systematic examination to overcome these barriers, such as staff and patient education and examination and elimination of system barriers, is important. The added burden of societal stigma of psychological problems needs to be addressed.

Further work is needed to establish brief but effective ways to assess distress with reliable, valid, and clinically useful measures of distress. The NCCN distress thermometer may be useful for initial screening, although research is still needed to confirm its clinical utility.[1,105] Akizuki and colleagues[106] found that one question (asking patients to rate their mood on a 0 to 100 scale) and the distress thermometer were comparable in screening for depression in individuals with cancer, but both detected less depression than the Hospital Anxiety and Depression Scale when results were compared with diagnoses made by psychiatrists using DSM IV criteria.

Interesting links between pain, disease severity, and survival are beginning to be established in both animal and clinical research. Data about these links are now conflicting, so the underlying mechanisms need to be explicated. This important beginning evidence indicates that symptom management is vital. The role of immune mediation is being explored.[107–109] Extending this research beyond pain to symptoms of distress and clarifying the "mind-body" connection will also be important in future research.

We are coming to appreciate the complexity of the experience of cancer for everyone involved. This includes those who do not have cancer but whose lifestyles make them more or less prone to the disease, patients everywhere along the trajectory of disease, their family and loved ones, and professional caregivers. Thorne and Paterson,[110] in their review of research on the elements of chronic illness experiences, noted that researchers shifted their focus in the early 1980s when the insider perspective was first obtained. Early research (1980 to 1985) focused on loss and burden (e.g., suffering, sick role), and later a more optimistic perspective predominated (e.g., being courageous, maintaining hope, finding meaning, and transformation). This shift was accompanied by the view of ill persons as being the experts in their own health. Thorne and Patterson appropriately caution us to remember the complexity of illness, nowhere more appropriate than with cancer, where persons experience joys and sorrows, problems and possibilities. While patients are the experts, especially in describing their symptoms, they also need and seek the expertise of professionals. Providing a full range of resources to match needs as they change over the health and illness continuum will serve to best enable patients to live their lives as fully and productively as possible.

References

1. National Comprehensive Cancer Network: Distress management. Available from *www.nccn.org/physians_gls*. Accessed November 18, 2004
2. Rodin GM: Suffering and adaptation to cancer: What to measure and when to intervene. *J Psychosom Res* 55:399–401, 2003
3. Maguire P, Pitceathly C: Improving the psychological care of cancer patients and their relatives: the role of specialist nurses. *J Psychosom Res* 55:469–474, 2003
4. Olson J: *Bathsheba's Breast: Women, Cancer, and History*. Baltimore, MD: John Hopkins University Press, 2002
5. Gendron D: *Enquiries into the Nature, Knowledge and Cure of Cancer*. London, J. Taylor, 1701
6. Bard M: The sequence of emotional reactions in radical mastectomy patients. *Pub Health Rep* 76:1144–1148, 1952
7. Renneker R, Cutler M: Psychosocial problems to adjustment to cancer of the breast. *JAMA* 148:633–638, 1952
8. De Boer MF, Ryckman RM, Pruyn JF, et al: Psychosocial correlates of cancer relapse and survival: a literature review. *Patient Educ Counsel* 37:215–230, 1999
9. Nyklicek I, Louwman WJ, Van Nierop PW, et al: Depression and the lower risk for breast cancer development in middle-aged women: a prospective study. *Psychol Med* 33:1111–1117, 2003
10. Sontag S: *Illness as Metaphor*. New York, Farrar, Straus, and Giroux, 1978
11. Nightingale F: *Notes on Nursing: What It Is and What It Is Not*. New York, Dover, 1969

12. Brown L: *The New Shorter Oxford English Dictionary*. Oxford, Clarendon Press, 1993
13. McEwen BS: From molecules to mind: stress, individual differences, and the social environment. *Ann NY Acad Sci* 935:42–49, 2001
14. Klassen AC, Smith AL, Meissner HI, et al: If we gave away mammograms, who would get them? A neighborhood evaluation of a no-cost breast cancer screening program. *Prev Med* 34:13–21, 2002
15. Philips DM: JCAHO pain management standards are unveiled. *JAMA* 284:428–429, 2000
16. Cimprich B, Ronis DL: An environmental intervention to restore attention in women with newly diagnosed breast cancer. *Cancer Nurs* 26:284–292, 2003
17. Gates MF, Lackey NR, Brown G: Caring demands and delay in seeking care in African American women newly diagnosed with breast cancer: an ethnographic, photographic study. *Oncol Nurs Forum* 28:529–537, 2001
18. Lebel S, Jakubovits G, Rosberger Z, et al: Waiting for a breast biopsy. *J Psychosom Res* 55:437–443, 2003
19. MacCormack T, Simonian J, Lim J, et al: 'Someone who cares': a qualitative investigation of cancer patients' experiences of psychotherapy. *Psychooncology* 10:52–65, 2001
20. Cimprich B, Ronis DL, Martinex-Ramos G: Age at diagnosis and quality of life in breast cancer survivors. *Cancer Pract* 10:85–93, 2002
21. Dunwoody L, Smyth A, Davidson R: Cancer patients' experiences and evalutaions of aromatherapy massage in palliative care. *Int J Palliat Nurs* 8:497–504, 2002
22. Goodwin P, Leszcz M, Ennis M, et al: The effect of group psychosocial support on survival in metastatic breast cancer. *N Engl J Med* 345:1719–1726, 2001
23. Zabora J, Brintzenhofeszoc JK, Curbow B, et al: The prevalence of psychological distress by cancer site. *Psychooncology* 10:19–28, 2001
24. Jones JM, Huggins MA, Rydall AC, et al: Symptomatic distress, hopelessness, and the desire for hastened death in hospitalized cancer patients. *J Psychosom Res* 55:411–418, 2003
25. Kelly B, Burnett P, Pelusi D, et al: Factors associated with the wish to hasten death: A study of patients with terminal illness. *Psychol Med* 33:75–81, 2003
26. Norton TR, Manne SL, Rubin S, et al: Prevalence and predicors of psychological distress among women with ovarian cancer. *J Clin Oncol* 22:919–926, 2004
27. Andrykowski MA, Cordova M: Factors associated with PTSD symptoms following treatment for breast cancer: test of the Anderson model. *J Trauma Stress* 11:189–203, 1998
28. Green B, Krupnick J, Rowland J, et al: Trauma history as a predictor of psychological symptoms in women with breast cancer. *J Clin Oncol* 18:1084–1094, 2000
29. Silver-Aylaian M, Cohen LH: Role of major lifetime stressors in patients' and spouses' reactions to cancer. *J Trauma Stress* 14:405–412, 2001
30. Baider L, Peretz T, Kaplan De-Nour A: The effect of behavioral intervention on the psychological distress of Holocaust survivors with cancer. *Psychother Psychosom* 66:44–49, 1997
31. Baider L, Uziely B, Kaplan De-Nour A: Progressive muscle relaxation and guided imagery in cancer patients. *Gen Hosp Psych* 16:340–347, 1994
32. Yeh CH: Psychological distress: testing hypotheses based on Roy's adaptation model. *Nurs Sci Q* 16:255–263, 2003
33. Hawkley LC, Cacioppo JT: Loneliness and pathways to disease. *Brain Behav Immun* 17(suppl 1):S98–S105, 2003
34. Cordova MJ, Giese-Davis J, Golant M, et al: Mood disturbance in community cancer support groups: the role of emotional suppression and fighting spirit. *J Psychosom Res* 55:461–467, 2003
35. Baider L, Ever-Hadani P, Goldzweig G, et al: Is perceived family support a relevant variable in psychological distress? A sample of prostate and breast cancer couples. *J Psychosom Res* 55:453–460, 2003
36. van Loon AJ, Tijhuis M, Surtees PG, et al: Lifestyle risk factors for cancer: the relationship with psychosocial work environment. *Int J Epidemiol* 29:785–792, 2000
37. Chang V, Thaler H, Polyak T, et al: Quality of life and survival: The role of multidimensional symptoms assessment. *Cancer* 83:173–179, 1998
38. Carlson LE, Bultz BD: Cancer distress screening: needs, models, and methods. *J Psychosom Res* 55:403–409, 2003
39. Sharpe M, et al: Major depression in outpatients attending a regional cancer centre: Screening and unmet treatment needs. *Br J Cancer* 90:314–320, 2004
40. Cunningham AJ: Adjuvant psychological therapy for cancer patients: putting it on the same footing as adjunctive medical therapies. *Psychooncology* 9:367–371, 2000
41. McLachlan SA, Allenby A, Matthews J, et al: Randomized trial of coordinated psychosocial interventions based on patient self-assessments versus standard care to improve the psychosocial functioning of patients with cancer. *J Clin Oncol* 19:4117–4125, 2001
42. Zakowski SG, Harris C, Krueger N, et al: Social barriers to emotional expression and their relations to distress in male and female cancer patients. *Br J Health Psychol* 8:271–286, 2003
43. Jacox AK, Carr D, Payne R, et al: *Management of Cancer Pain. Clinical Practice Guideline No. 9.* AHCPR Publication No. 94–0592. Rockville, MD, Agency for Health Care Policy and Research, U.S. Department of Health and Human Services, Public Health Service, 1994
44. Kelley KW, Bluthe RM, Dantzer R, et al: Cytokine-induced sickness behavior. *Brain Behav Immun* 17:S112–S118, 2003
45. Miller AH: Cytokines and sickness behavior: Implications for cancer care and control. *Brain Behav Immun* 17:S132–S134, 2003
46. Patrick DL, Ferketich SL, Frame PS, et al: National Institutes of Health State-of-the-Science Conference statement: symptom management in cancer: Pain, depression, and fatigue, July 15–17, 2002. *J Natl Cancer Inst* 95:1110–1117, 2003
47. Cohen MZ, Easley M, Ellis C, et al: Cancer pain management and the JCAHO's pain standards: an institutional challenge. *J Pain Symptom Manage* 25:519–527, 2003
48. Curt GA: Impact of fatigue on quality of life in oncology patients. *Semin Hematol* 37(suppl 6):14–17, 2000
49. Davidson JR, MacLean AW, Brundage MD, et al: Sleep disturbance in cancer patients. *Soc Sci Med* 54:1309–1321, 2002
50. Morrow GR, Hickok J, Roscoe JA, et al: Differential effects of paroxetine on fatigue and depression: a randomized, double-blind trial from the University of Rochester Cancer Center Community Clinical Oncology Program. *J Clin Oncol* 21:4635–4641, 2003
51. Cella D, Paul D, Yount S, et al: What are the most important symptom targets when treating advanced cancer? A survey of providers in the National Comprehensive Cancer Network (NCCN). *Cancer Invest* 21:526–535. 2003
52. Stone P, Richards M, Hardy J: Fatigue in patients with cancer. *Eur J Cancer* 34:1670–1676, 1998
53. Cella D, Lai J, Chang CH, et al: Fatigue in cancer patients compared with fatigue in the general United States population. *Cancer* 94:528–538, 2002
54. Owen DC, Parker KP, McGuire DB: Comparison of subjective sleep quality in patients with cancer and healthy subjects. *Oncol Nurs Forum* 26:1649–1651, 1999
55. Savard J, Morin CM, Akechi T: Insomnia in the context of cancer: A review of a neglected problem. *J Clin Oncol* 19:895–908, 2001

56. Ancoli-Israel S, Moore PJ, Jones V: The relationship between fatigue and sleep in cancer patients: a review. *Eur J Cancer Care* 10:245–255, 2001
57. Morin CM, Rodrigue S, Ivers H: Role of stress, arousal, and coping skills in primary insomnia. *Psychosom Med* 65:259–267, 2003
58. Carter P: Family caregivers' sleep loss and depression over time. *Cancer Nurs* 26:253–259, 2003
59. Meyers C, Hess K, Yung WKA, et al: Cognitive function as a predictor of survival in patients with recurrent malignant glioma. *J Clin Oncol* 18:646–650, 2000
60. Sherman A, Jaeckle K, Meyers C: Pretreatment cognitive performance predicts survival in patients with leptomeningeal disease. *Cancer* 95:1311–1316, 2002
61. Breitbart W, Gibson C, Tremblay A: The delirium experience: delirium recall and delirium-related distress in hospitalized patients with cancer, their spouses/caregivers, and their nurses. *Psychosom* 43:183–194, 2002
62. Ahles TA, Saykin A: Cognitive effects of standard-dose chemotherapy in patients with cancer. *Cancer Invest* 19:812–820, 2001
63. Cohen MZ, Armstrong T: Cognitive dysfunction, in Yarbro CH, Frogge MH, Goodman M (eds.): *Cancer Symptom Management* (ed 3). Sudbury, MA, Jones and Bartlett, 2004, pp 635–650
64. Lawlor P: The panorama of opioid-related cognitive dysfunction in patients with cancer: a critical literature appraisal. *Cancer* 94:1836–1853, 2002
65. Ashby FG, Isen AM, Turken AU: A neuropsychological theory of positive affect and its influence on cognition. *Psychol Rev* 106:529–550, 1999
66. Bremner JD: *Does Stress Damage the Brain? Understanding Trauma-Related Disorders from a Neurological Perspective.* New York, Norton, 2002
67. Tuma R, DeAngelis LM: Altered mental status in patients with cancer. *Arch Neurol* 57:1727–1731, 2000
68. Breitbart W, Strout D: Delirium in the terminally ill. *Clini Geriatric Med* 16:357–372, 2000
69. Casarett DJ, Inouye SK: Diagnosis and management of delirium near the end of life. *Ann Intern Med* 135:32–40, 2001
70. Lawlor PG, Fainsinger RL, Bruera ED: Delirium at the end of life: critical issues in clinical practice and research. *JAMA* 284:2427–2429, 2000
71. Passik S, Lundberg J, Rosenfeld B, et al: Factor analysis of the Zung self-rating depression scale in a large ambulatory oncology sample. *Psychosom* 41:121–127, 2000
72. Angelino AF, Treisman GJ: Major depression and demoralization in cancer patients: diagnostic and treatment considerations. *Support Cancer Care* 9:344–349, 2001
73. Bodurka-Bevers D, Basen-Engquist K, Carmack CL, et al: Depression, anxiety, and quality of life in patients with epithelial ovarian cancer. *Gyn Oncol* 78:302–308, 2000
74. Litofsky NS, Farace E, Anderson F, et al: Depression in patients with high-grade glioma: results of the Glioma Outcomes project. *Neurosurg* 54:358–366, 2004
75. Lloyd-Williams M, Friedman T: Depression in palliative care patients: a prospective study. *Eur J Cancer Care* 10:270–274, 2001
76. American Psychiatric Association: *Diagnostic and Statistical Manual of Mental Disorders* (ed 4). Washington, DC, American Psychiatric Association, 1994
77. van't Spijker A, Trijsburg RW, Duivenvoorden HJ: Psychologic sequelae of cancer diagnosis: A meta-analytical review of 58 studies after 1980. *Psychosom Med* 59:280–293, 1997
78. Stark D, Kiely M, Smith A, et al: Anxiety disorders in cancer patients: their nature, associations, and relation to quality of life. *J Clin Oncol* 20:3137–3148, 2002
79. Kerrihard T, Breibart W, Dent R, et al: Anxiety in patients with cancer and human immunodeficiency virus. *Semin Clin Neuropsych* 4:114–132, 1999
80. Gurevick M, Devins GM, Rodin GM: Stress response syndromes and cancer: conceptual and assessment issues. *Psychosom* 43:259–281, 2002
81. Kangas M, Henry JL, Bryant RA: Posttraumatic stress disorder following cancer: a conceptual and empirical review. *Clin Psych Rev* 22:499–524, 2002
82. Neel ML: Posttraumatic stress symptomatology and cancer. *Int J Emerg Ment Health* 2:85–94, 2000
83. Smith MY, Redd WH, Peyser C, et al: Post-traumatic stress disorder in cancer: a review. *Psycho-Oncol* 8:521–537, 1999
84. Dugan W, McDonald MV, Passik SD, et al: Use of the Zung self-rating depression scale in cancer patients: feasibility as a screening tool. *Psychooncology* 7:483–493, 1998
85. Kirsh KL, Passik S, Holtsclaw E, et al: I get tired for no reason: a single item screening for cancer-related fatigue. *J Pain Symptom Manage* 22:931–937, 2001
86. Love AW, Kissane DW, Bloch S, et al: Diagnostic efficiency of the Hospital Anxiety and Depression Scale in women with early stage breast cancer. *Austr N Zeal J Psych* 36:246–250, 2002
87. Merluzzi TV, Nairn RC, Hedge K, et al: Self-efficacy for coping with cancer: revision of the Cancer Behavior Inventory (version 2.0). *Psychooncology* 10:206–217, 2001
88. Nicholas D, Veach T: The psychosocial assessment of the adult cancer patient. *Prof Psychol* 31:206–215, 2000
89. Barsevick AM, Dudley W, Beck S, et al: A randomized clinical trial of energy conservation for patients with cancer-related fatigue. *Cancer* 100:1302–1310, 2004
90. Nail L: Fatigue in patients with cancer. *Oncol Nurs Forum* 29:537–544, 2002
91. Quesnel C, Savard J, Simard S, et al: Efficacy of cognitive-behavioral therapy for insomnia in women treated for nonmetastatic breast cancer. *J Consult Clin Psychol* 71:189–200, 2003
92. Oyama H, Kaneda M, Katsumata N, et al: Using the bedside wellness system during chemotherapy decreases fatigue and emesis in cancer patients. *J Med Systems* 24:173–182, 2000
93. National Cancer Institute: Normal adjustment, psychosocial distress, and the adjustment disorders. (2004) Available from *www.cancer.gov/cancertopics/pdq/supportivecare/adjustment/healthprofessional.* Accessed November 18, 2004
94. Zakowski SG, Hall MH, Klein LC, et al: Appraised control, coping, and stress in a community sample: a test of the goodness-of-fit hypothesis. *Ann Behav Med* 23:158–165, 2001
95. Given C, Given B, Rahbar M, et al: Effect of a cognitive behavioral intervention on reducing symptom severity during chemotherapy. *J Clin Oncol* 22:507–516, 2004
96. Carlson LE, Ursuliak Z, Goodey E, et al: The effects of a mindfulness meditation-based stress reduction program on mood and symptoms of stress in cancer outpatients: 6-month follow-up. *Support Care Cancer* 9:112–123, 2001
97. Jacobsen PB, Meede CD, Stein KD, et al: Efficacy and costs of two forms of stress management training for cancer patients undergoing chemotherapy. *J Clin Oncol* 20:2851–2862, 2002
98. Petersen RW, Quinlivan JA: Preventing anxiety and depression in gynaecological cancer: a randomised controlled trial. *Br J Obstet Gynaecol* 109:386–394, 2002
99. Milligan M, Fanning M, Hunter S, et al: Reflexology audit: patient satisfaction, impact on quality of life and availability in Scottish hospices. *Complementary Ther* 8:489–496, 2002
100. Gilbar O, Iron G, Goren A: Adjustment to illness of cancer patients treated by complementary therapy along with conventional therapy. *Patient Educ Couns* 44:243–249, 2001
101. Risberg T, Jacobsen BK: The association between mental distress and the use of alternative medicine among cancer patients in north Norway. *Qual Life Res* 12:539–544, 2003
102. Gobel B: Anxiety, in Yarbro CH, Frogge MH, Goodman M (eds.): *Cancer Symptom Management* (ed 3). Sudbury, MA, Jones and Bartlett, 2003, pp 651–664

103. Barsevick A, Much J: Depression, in Yarbro CH, Frogge MH, Goodman M (eds.): *Cancer Symptom Management* (ed 3). Sudbury, MA, Jones and Bartlett, 2003, pp 668–684
104. Nemetz S, Mercardante M: The evolution of a cancer support center: a work in progress. *Oncol Nurs Forum* 29:1397–1399, 2002
105. Holland JC, Jacobsen P, Riba M: NCCN distress management. *Cancer Control* 8(suppl):88–93, 2001
106. Akizuki N, Akechi T, Nakanishi T, et al: Development of a brief screening interview for adjustment disorders and major depression in patients with cancer. *Cancer* 97:2605–2613, 2003
107. Kawashima I, Yoshida Y, Taya C, et al: Expansion of natural killer cells in mice transgenic for IgM antibody to ganglioside GD2: demonstration of prolonged survival after challenge with syngeneic tumor cells. *Int J Oncol* 21:381–388, 2003
108. Kiecolt-Glaser J, Page G, Marucha P, et al: Psychological influences on surgical recovery. *Amer Psychol* 53:1209–1218, 1998
109. Page GG, Ben-Eliyahu S: The immune-suppressive nature of pain. *Semin Oncol Nurs* 13:10–15, 1997
110. Thorne S, Paterson B: Shifting images of chronic illness. *Image* 30:173–178, 1998

CHAPTER 26

Assessment of Cancer Pain

Patrick J. Coyne, MSN, APRN, BC-PCM
Ashby C. Watson, APRN, BC, OCN®
Deborah B. McGuire, PhD, RN, FAAN
Katherine A. Yeager, MS, RN

Introduction

Pain is one of the most prevalent symptoms faced by patients with cancer. Fear of unrelieved pain is rightly a concern for both patients and their families, because despite the availability of information and technology that can relieve most cancer pain, it often remains undertreated.[1] This chapter describes the causes and manifestations of cancer pain, the scope of the cancer pain problem, key components of assessment, and the evaluation of populations at special risk for experiencing pain. Chapter 27, discusses the management of cancer pain.

Scope of the Cancer Pain Problem

Pain in the patient with cancer has long been recognized as a challenging clinical problem. The Oncology Nursing Society's (ONS) position paper on cancer pain management[1] emphasized the fact that cancer pain often is managed inadequately, despite nearly a decade of work attempting to alleviate this problem. A comprehensive understanding of the scope of the cancer pain problem, and the reasons why it is still not adequately managed, requires knowledge of its significance, its prevalence, and the professional issues involved in its management.

Significance

Although cancer pain clearly is a multidimensional phenomenon, its effects on patients who have it, or on their families and friends, are just beginning to be understood. Cancer pain is a significant problem for a variety of reasons. It is well known that individuals with cancer-related pain exhibit a variety of pain-related behaviors[2] and experience many physical and psychosocial problems.[3] Additionally, recent years have witnessed an explosion of clinical research, sociocultural, political, regulatory/legal, health policy, and professional activities that have increased knowledge about pain and have influenced in both positive and negative ways how pain is managed. These developments encompass issues such as quality of life, family and home care issues, ethical concerns related to use of advanced technologies, financial costs associated with cancer pain, managed care, regulatory influences on use of controlled substances, legal impediments to adequate management of pain, health policy initiatives in pain, increased emphasis on cancer pain by national and international agencies, and increased federal and private research funding opportunities. The brief discussion that follows provides a cursory overview of these developments and demonstrates the far-reaching significance of the cancer pain problem.

Quality of life is a construct that has been examined in people with cancer pain as a domain of concern[4,5] as well as a potential outcome variable in treatment. Research has included a quality of life tool in the clinical arena to evaluate pharmacological interventions with respect to their effects on pain intensity as well as on the total person.[6] Additional research has documented the scope and extent of pain's influence on quality of life. For example, in a study of 84 patients with cancer-related pain, Strang and Qvarner demonstrated that there was not only significant physical suffering but also negative influences on daily functional activities and concentration.[7] McMillan and Small found that physical correlates of symptom distress or intensity, including symptom distress and pain, were significantly correlated to quality of life in a sample of 178 adult hospice home care patients with advanced cancer. Higher ratings of distress or intensity were related to lower quality of life scores. While pain scores ranged from 0 to 10 (i.e., from none to the worst pain imaginable), the mean score of 3 indicated that pain was not severe in these patients. However, among all symptoms, pain caused one of the highest levels of distress.[8] Pain, anxiety, and depression were associated with impairment in emotional and physical aspects of quality of life in a study of patients with advanced cancer.[9] Anxiety and depression continued to be significantly associated with impairment of physical, psychological, and social aspects of quality of life even after controlling for the effects of pain and symptom severity. Pain was found to be a more important predictor of quality of life than limitations of physical performance, and it had a greater impact across the dimensions of quality of life.

Ferrell and colleagues validated a conceptual model of quality of life in patients with cancer pain that included four domains: physical well-being and symptoms, social concerns, psychological well-being, and spiritual well-being.[10] Research utilizing this model has demonstrated quite clearly that quality of life is significantly affected by cancer pain, and that its assessment is important in evaluating both patients' responses to pain interventions and their overall status.[11]

The impact of pain on family caregivers, particularly in the home environment, is an area that has been studied in some depth. A study of 85 family caregivers of patients with cancer pain[12] revealed that pain caused a significant burden for families. Descriptions of pain centered on four themes: anatomical descriptions of pain, hidden pain (i.e., patient hides it), family fear and suffering, and overwhelming or unendurable pain. Families' experiences of pain highlighted three themes: helplessness, coping by denial of their own feelings (i.e., pretending to "be strong"), and a wish for the patient's death (a "welcome relief" from the suffering).

A second part of this same study[13] documented that family members played a major caregiving role in managing their loved one's pain. With respect to pharmacological interventions, they decided which medications to give and when, monitored the patient around the clock, kept records, dealt with fears of addiction, and assumed total responsibility for pain medications.[14] In the realm of nonpharmacological interventions, they provided a number of physical interventions (e.g., positioning and/or mobility, massage, application of cold and heat) as well as cognitive interventions (e.g., being there, touch, talk). The same research also revealed the questions and concerns family caregivers had about pain and its management, including their advice to professional caregivers (i.e., be there, offer hope, explain, be honest, listen, educate, give enough medicine) and their own personal perspectives (the future, understanding why, death, and fears about medications and handling pain at home).

Data from this same study, which was conducted in a community hospital, a national cancer center, and a home-based community hospice, were examined in relation to caregiver burden and family factors influencing pain management.[15] Areas of burden included physical dimensions, psychological responses, and interference with normal activities. Families of patients cared for in all three sites rated patients' pain and distress as severe, but caregivers in the home hospice setting reported having a lower burden, better mood, less distress, and more feelings of being supported in their attempts to care for their loved one.

Research suggests that patients and their family caregivers do not always agree on the presence and severity of pain and other symptoms.[16] A study of 170 caregivers of cancer patients who died in 1994 found that caregivers reported effective pain relief in only 46% of the patients.[17] No differences were observed in the degree of pain or effectiveness of pain interventions when comparing rural, urban, or suburban locations or different care settings. Another study of 78 patient–caregiver dyads found that when dyads were noncongruent in assessment of patients' pain, caregivers experienced higher caregiver strain.[18] These issues document the significant impact that pain has on the family system of cancer patients.

Self-efficacy may play an important role in predicting cancer patients' adjustment over time as well as their response to intervention.[19] In one investigation, 30 dyads of newly diagnosed lung cancer patients and their primary caregivers were studied. Results revealed that noncongruence between patients and their caregivers regarding patient self-efficacy was associated with higher levels of psychological distress on the part of both the patient and the caregiver. Variables associated with caregiver overestimation of patient self-efficacy were higher levels of caregiver strain, lower levels of patient satisfaction with the relationship, and higher levels of patient-rated symptoms, including pain. The authors found that patients who had high levels of self-efficacy had lower levels of symptoms; when caregivers perceived patients to be high in self-efficacy, both caregivers and patients reported lower levels of symptoms.

In another study of 63 family caregivers of hospice-eligible cancer patients, caregivers who rated their self-efficacy as high reported much lower levels of caregiver strain, decreased negative mood, and increased positive mood.[20] High caregiver self-efficacy in pain management was correlated with the patient's physical well-being, but not with the patient's pain ratings. The authors suggested that highly self-efficacious caregivers were able to help patients control the impact of pain, which in turn positively reflected on quality of life. In those dyads where the caregiver reported high self-efficacy, the patient also reported having more energy, feeling less ill, and spending less time in bed.

Ethical concerns related to the use of high technology in medicine[21] are important issues, particularly with respect to costs, access, social justice, informed consent, and autonomy. In the management of cancer pain, the potential for violations of accepted principles of biomedical ethics (autonomy, beneficence, nonmaleficence, and justice) has been clearly explicated.[22] Examples include decision making by health caregivers who as experts feel they can make decisions for patients, lack of respect for patients' values, inadequate concern for the vulnerability of people in pain, conflicts of interest when caregivers have ownership in companies that manufacture or distribute high-technology equipment, selection of therapies that may not provide the best benefits for patients, implementation of therapies that increase risk of harm, denial of access to needed therapy because of reimbursement issues, and use of inappropriate interventions to increase reimbursement. Whedon and Ferrell provide an excellent discussion of considerations in using high-technology management in cancer patients with pain.[23] They emphasize the appropriate use of such technology, delineating the need for specific guidelines in clinical practice and for use of pain management principles in deciding on, selecting, and implementing various advanced technologies.

The costs associated with caring for patients with cancer-related pain have been explored empirically. Data from admissions records over a 12-month period in a national cancer center revealed that 26% of 5772 patients studied had at least one hospital admission for inadequately controlled pain, and that 54% of admissions for uncontrolled pain occurred within 2 weeks of the patient's most recent discharge.[24] The 255 readmissions for uncontrolled pain observed in this study cost approximately $5 million over a 1-year period. The investigators suggested that predischarge education related to pain management and potential barriers to effective pain management in the home and/or community need careful exploration. Because reimbursement for unplanned readmissions for pain control may be limited, tremendous costs to both patients and healthcare facilities may result from such hospital stays. Because nurses influence both the cost and the effectiveness of care for patients with cancer-related pain, assessing the cost-effectiveness of different approaches of pain management is an important part of the nurse's role in the changing healthcare environment.[25]

A different perspective on costs is provided by a landmark legal case that involved the inadequate management of pain in a terminally ill cancer patient admitted to a nursing home in North Carolina.[26] In this case, opioid analgesics were withheld from the patient by the nurse because of concerns about addiction, and other medications were substituted in their stead. The family of the patient proved that failure of the nurse and her employer to fulfill their obligations and responsibilities resulted in increased pain and suffering and in "emotional and mental anguish." This "inhuman treatment" resulted initially in a $15 million jury award for compensatory and punitive damages. Although the award was later set aside and a confidential settlement figure agreed on,[27] the case underscored the importance of ethical and professional obligations to relieve pain and suffering and of individualized plans of care for patients with pain.

Problems of inadequate medical coverage and uneven reimbursement policies for health care, including prescription drugs, medical equipment, and professional services, affect pain management for cancer patients — particularly, the elderly, poor, and minorities. Access to opioid analgesics is limited by some states' controlled substance regulations and by some mail-order pharmacy policies.[28–30] Ferrell and Griffith presented an in-depth analysis of cost issues related to pain management — specifically, costs associated with oral medications, parenteral and spinal analgesics, personnel, surgical and anesthetic procedures, radiation therapy, unrelieved pain at home, nondrug interventions, and morbidity.[31] They also discussed cost savings by various care settings, costs to justify services, reimbursement biases, conflict of interest, and indirect costs to patients and families.[31] In the world of managed care, many blame changing healthcare delivery systems (including managed care organizations) for creating roadblocks to effective pain treatments. Some argue that a broad range of social and political issues create roadblocks, including organized medicine's failure to meet the needs of people in pain.[32,33] The Oncology Nursing Society recognizes that the cost-reduction emphasis in healthcare restructuring threatens the delivery of quality cancer care and calls on nurses to make decisions guided by quality rather than costs alone when caring for patients in pain.[34] Opportunities have been identified for improving the response to managed care, including curbing the practice of providing excess care, placing greater emphasis on palliation and supportive care, allowing for flexible provider roles, reallocating research dollars to reward innovations and reduce duplication, and providing more community education.[34]

Regulatory and legal developments also have come to the forefront in the cancer pain issue. Because fear of regulatory scrutiny has been identified as a barrier in cancer pain management, state and national laws and regulations can be problematic.[35–38] Pain management advocates, especially state-based cancer pain initiatives[39] throughout the United States, have helped to defeat legislation that might potentially limit patient access to opioids. For example, state-run multiple-prescription programs and prescription monitoring programs, which are intended to decrease substance abuse fraud and drug abuse, have resulted in rapid decreases in the number of appropriate prescriptions written for controlled substances. Several states have considered repealing their triplicate prescription laws.[40] At the same time, positive efforts in the legislative arena include the passage of intractable pain treatment laws, pain summit meetings, and the establishment of state pain commissions.[41]

This brief review has highlighted several areas that demonstrate the far-reaching significance of the cancer pain problem. In addition, health policy initiatives and professional organizational efforts to reduce pain and improve its management are important developments.[41,42] Such initiatives have occurred both within the United States and internationally. Increased funding opportunities for basic and applied research on pain are available, with some agencies specifically targeting pain.[43]

Finally, another area of enormous significance to the cancer pain problem is the extensive body of evidence suggesting that cancer pain is poorly managed worldwide by health professionals from a number of disciplines. Nurses, in particular, suffer from a lack of research-based knowledge about the prevalence of pain, the impact it has on patients and others, and effective ways of managing it. The next section explores a number of professional issues that influence management of pain. Research indicates that patients may live longer when their pain and symptoms are managed aggressively.[44–47]

Prevalence

The incidence of cancer pain for all cancer diagnoses during all stages of the disease has proved difficult to quantify. Most studies report prevalence data rather than incidence data. Problems affecting the accuracy of prevalence data include (1) lack of systematic data collection and pain measurement techniques, (2) lack of documentation regarding the extent of patients' disease, (3) lack of identification of pain's etiology, and (4) inclusion of multiple cancer diagnoses as a single group.[48] Despite these problems, however, researchers have examined the prevalence of cancer pain in a number of studies. Prevalence of pain by clinical setting, regardless of cancer diagnosis, indicates that patients in hospice and specialty units report a higher prevalence of pain than patients in other settings. This observation can be understood by recognizing that patients with advanced, metastatic disease are often referred to these settings for terminal care. Likewise, patients with advanced disease report more severe pain than those who are in the early stages of their illness.[49,50]

The severity of cancer pain, as opposed to the presence of pain, has been used as a means of reporting not only prevalence of pain but also its characteristics. Cancer-related pain is described as ranging from mild or moderate to severe to excruciating. Most patients, however, report pain in the mild to moderate rather than in the severe range.[51] Examination of pain prevalence data by cancer diagnosis shows that pain is more likely to become a significant problem with the progression of disease, particularly in common solid tumors such as lung and breast cancer. Several cancers — most notably pancreatic and primary bone — exhibit relatively high prevalence rates for pain across all stages of disease.[52,53] Literature related to pain from cancer treatment (i.e., peripheral blood stem cell and bone marrow transplantation, postmastectomy) has identified unique concerns and treatment challenges.[54]

Estimates of pain rates for those afflicted with cancer range from 28% to 80%, depending on the stage of the disease.[54] Data from published studies should be examined carefully, taking several factors into consideration. First, knowledge of cancer pain comes primarily from prevalence studies, as few published reports have examined the incidence of cancer pain. Second, pain is more prevalent in those patients with advanced-stage disease and those being treated in hospice or specialty units. Third, certain common malignancies are more often associated with cancer pain, and it is these malignancies in which pain is better studied and understood. Finally, much of the available data is derived from patients with tumor- and/or treatment-related pain, rendering accurate rates for any specific type of pain difficult to ascertain.

Because of the complicated nature of cancer pain, with its different etiologies,[55] varied presentations,[56–58] multiple dimensions,[58,59] and variety of treatments, and the previously mentioned difficulties encountered when studying the incidence and prevalence of the problem, we can speculate that the true prevalence of pain is much greater than existing reports indicate.

Definitions of Pain

Historically, pain has not been easy to define. During the seventeenth century, pain was viewed as a signal of bodily injury, with scant attention being paid to its nonphysical aspects. In the twentieth century, researchers formulated concepts of pain that recognized and included not only the physical "alarm" aspect but also other neurological activities, cultural factors, individual personality, and experiential variables.

The International Association for the Study of Pain (IASP) developed a definition of pain acceptable to both clinicians and researchers: "Pain is an unpleasant sensory and emotional experience associated with actual or potential tissue damage, or described in terms of such damage."[60,p.250] This definition accounted for both sensory and emotional aspects of pain as well as for pain of pathophysiological and psychological origin. It incorporated the essential elements of subjectivity and individual uniqueness in the pain experience.

It is commonly accepted that chronic pain and acute pain are distinctly different phenomena. Bonica defined acute pain as "a complex constellation of unpleasant sensory, perceptual, and emotional experiences and certain associated autonomic, psychologic, emotional, and behavioral responses."[61,p.19] IASP further defined it as "pain of recent onset and probably limited duration," which usually has "an identifiable temporal and causal relationship to injury or disease."[62,p.2] McCaffery and Pasero's definition of pain remains the standard for pain assessment: "Pain is whatever the experiencing person says it is, existing whenever he says it does."[63,p.5] This definition points out the importance of relying on the patient's self-report. Nurses must be even more vigilant when individuals cannot report pain. Chronic pain generally continues past the time of injury and may not have an identifiable etiology or be associated with any overt behavioral signs or physiological changes. Bonica noted that acute pain may recur periodically when an individual has recurrent acute pathophysiological processes, such as those commonly seen in persons with cancer.[61] Thus, cancer pain can simultaneously be chronic (in the case of progressive disease) or acute, depending on the status of the disease.

Cancer Pain as a Multidimensional Phenomenon

The notion of sensory and reactive aspects of pain — developed and nurtured through the gate control theory of pain — has been used by researchers to develop a multidimensional conceptual framework for cancer pain. Ahles et al. hypothesized five dimensions: (1) *physiologic* (organic etiology of pain); (2) *sensory* (intensity, location, quality); (3) *affective* (depression, anxiety); (4) *cognitive* (manner in which pain influences an individual's thought processes, how the individual views herself or himself, or the meaning of pain); and (5) *behavioral* (pain-related behaviors such as medication intake and activity level).[64] Ahles and colleagues confirmed this framework in a study of 40 patients with cancer who had tumor-related pain. One conclusion reached by these researchers was that treatment for cancer pain could consist of specific therapeutic modalities targeted to each of the five dimensions.[64]

McGuire adapted Ahles et al.'s conceptual framework to conduct a descriptive study of 40 cancer patients with pain and 40 cancer patients without pain and found support for the five dimensions of the model.[65] Individuals with cancer pain used a number of cognitive and behavioral coping strategies that they reported as moderately effective at reducing and controlling their pain.[66] McGuire's results suggested, however, that there was a sixth important area — the *sociocultural dimension,*[66] which includes demographic, social, and cultural characteristics that are related to the experience of pain. The six dimensions are complex, are interrelated, and contribute to the individual's perception of and response to pain.[66] Reviews of research literature indicate substantial support for this conceptualization of pain, both for cancer pain and other types of pain.[66,67] Further discussion of each dimension follows.

Physiological Dimension

Ahles et al. originally described the physiological dimension as consisting of the organic etiology of pain.[64] This definition was based on earlier work by researchers at Memorial Sloan-Kettering Cancer Center in New York, who described three types of pain observed in patients with cancer, each with a different etiology: (1) pain associated with direct tumor involvement, (2) pain associated with cancer therapy, and (3) pain unrelated to either the tumor or its treatment.[68] Sources of pain associated with cancer treatment are many, ranging from initial diagnostic procedures causing acute, short-term pain, to standard therapeutic modalities (surgery, radiation therapy, chemotherapy) causing acute, short-term and/or chronic, long-term pain. An example of acute, short-term pain is that associated with mucositis in patients receiving bone marrow transplantation.[69,70] Additional work aims to describe more fully treatment-related pain syndromes in specific populations, such as marrow transplant patients.[71] The third type of pain described by Foley was pain unrelated to either cancer or its treatment.[68] She estimated that it accounted for 3%–10% of the pain seen in cancer patients. Individuals with cancer pain are just as likely as the average individual to have pain from migraine headache, osteoarthritis, or degenerative disk disease. The presence of such pain, however, is important, and should be carefully assessed to confirm that it is *not* cancer related.

The work of these researchers has led to a greater understanding of the epidemiology and pathophysiology of cancer pain, including three specific pain syndromes that occur in patients with cancer and are usually caused by tumor.[72,73] These syndromes of somatic, visceral, and neuropathic pain are characterized by pain of different qualities, located in different anatomical parts of the body, and caused by different mechanisms. Distinctions between somatic and visceral pain, and neuropathic pain, reflect not only the mechanisms causing the pain but also responses to treatment. Characteristics of these pain syndromes are described in Table 26-1. Although these three syndromes are usually associated with tumor-related pain, they may apply to treatment-related pain as well.[73,74] Note that many cancer patients with pain will have one or more of these three syndromes simultaneously, and that each syndrome responds differently to therapeutic modalities. These three syndromes are described in detail by Caraceni,[75] who also discusses pain due to treatment and draws clinical correlations to the various types of cancer pain.

Breakthrough or *incident pain* is defined as episodes of pain that "interrupt a tolerable background pain," which is usually chronic cancer-related pain. Breakthrough pain can be somatic, visceral, and/or neuropathic in origin.[76,77] Related to etiology of pain are two other characteristics. *Duration* of pain refers to whether pain is acute or chronic. The second characteristic related to etiology of pain is the *pattern* that pain displays. Cancer pain is often described as continuous or

Table 26-1 Cancer Pain Syndromes

Type of Pain	Physiological Structures	Mechanism of Pain	Characteristics of Pain	Examples of Acute Pain	Sources of Chronic Pain
Somatic pain	Cutaneous: Skin and subcutaneous tissues Deep somatic: Bone, muscle, blood vessels, connective tissues	Activation of nociceptors	Localization of cutaneous pain: Well localized Localization of deep somatic pain: Less well defined Common descriptions: Constant, achy	Postoperative incisional pain Pain at the insertion sites of tubes and drains Bone of hip fractures Skeletal muscle	Bony metastases Degenerative or osteoarthritis Rheumatoid arthritis Compression fractures from osteoporosis Back pain Peripheral vascular disease Chronic stasis ulcers
Visceral pain	Organs and linings of body cavities	Activation of nociceptors	Localization: Poorly localized, diffuse, deep Common descriptions: Cramping, splitting	Chest and abdominal tubes and drains Bladder distention or spasms Intestinal distention Pericarditis Constipation	Organ metastases Spastic bowel Inflammatory bowel disease Hiatal hernia Chronic hepatitis
Neuropathic pain	Nerve fibers Spinal cord Central nervous system	Nonnociceptive Injury to the nervous system structures	Localization: Poorly localized Common descriptions: Shooting, hot-burning, fiery, electric shocklike, sharp, painfully numb	Phantom limb pain Postmastectomy pain Nerve compression	Diabetic neuropathy Herpes zoster–related pain Cancer-related nerve injury Chronic phantom limb pain Trigeminal neuralgia Central poststroke pain Postmastectomy syndrome

constant, but it is also intermittent, brief, or transient, as evidenced by breakthrough pain, pain on movement, and other clinical manifestations of pain. Additionally, patients with cancer may have pain that lasts 1 hour or more through the entire day,[78] and many experience two or more patterns of pain simultaneously.

Sensory Dimension

The sensory dimension of cancer-related pain relates to where the pain is located and what it feels like. Three specific components of this dimension are location, intensity, and quality.

Location. This component of pain is important. Many patients with cancer have pain at two or more locations. The number of separate locations of pain has clear implications for the sensory dimension, for the entire pain experience, and for assessment and management.

Intensity. Intensity of pain — that is, how strong it feels — is the second important component of the sensory dimension. Intensity is a perceived, and therefore subjective, phenomenon that varies based on the individual's sensation threshold (defined by Twycross[79] as the least stimulus at which a person perceives a sensation). The individual's threshold may be affected by a variety of factors, such as physical comfort, mood, medications, and social environment, thus causing perceived intensity of pain to increase or decrease. Intensity is the most commonly assessed aspect of pain and is characterized by words such as *none, mild, moderate, severe, intolerable, excruciating, bad,* and *intense.* Recent data suggest, however, that intensity of cancer pain may be less for many patients than the intensity of common pains such as headache, stomachache, or toothache.[80] Patients did report that when their cancer pain was at its worst, it was severe and often inadequately controlled.

Quality. The third component of the sensory dimension is the quality of pain — that is, how it actually feels. Melzack and Torgerson were among the first to systematically study words that people used to describe pain.[81] They composed a list of 102 words from the clinical literature on pain and organized them into classes that described sensory, affective, and evaluative properties of pain. Words in the sensory category referred to temporal, spatial, pressure, and thermal aspects. Examples of these sensory words are *pulsing, radiating, penetrating,* and *burning,* respectively. Some studies have revealed that patients with cancer pain use certain words more commonly than others to describe sensory aspects of their pain.[82–84] Words commonly used by patients in these studies included *sharp, tender, aching, throbbing, sore, stabbing, heavy, shooting,* and *gnawing.*

Affective Dimension

The affective dimension consists of depression, anxiety, or other psychological factors or personality traits associated with pain. Research and review articles support the importance of the affective dimension in cancer pain, especially as related to mood changes and other transient affective states. Parameters relevant to the affective dimension of pain range from specific personality traits (e.g., neuroticism) to affective disorders (e.g., depression and anxiety) to general concepts such as psychological distress.[3,9,85]

Pain, anxiety, and depression were associated with impairment in emotional and physical aspects of quality of life in a study of patients with advanced cancer.[9] Anxiety and depression continued to be significantly associated with impairment of physical, psychological, and social aspects of quality of life even after controlling for the effects of pain and symptom severity. Pain was found to be a more important predictor of quality of life than limitations of physical performance, and it had a greater impact across the dimensions of quality of life.

In a small study by Kai-hoi et al.,[86] the researchers failed to find any difference in the nature or severity of pain and in the level of disability between depressed and nondepressed cancer patients. The study also suggested that depression does not correlate with severity of pain in patients with advanced cancer, leading the authors to speculate that this lack of correlation between depression and pain could best be explained by the effect of the cancer process. Also, disability in cancer patients was thought to be largely determined by disease stage and complications of malignancy. Treatment of depression was determined to be important but should not be expected to bring about less pain or disability.

Taking into account the strong and weak points of studies in this area, it is possible to conclude the following:

1. Specific personality factors probably are not related to the experience of cancer pain.
2. There is little evidence that affective disorders such as depression and anxiety are *strongly* related to pain.
3. There is a complicated association among symptoms of psychological distress and pain.
4. Much more research is needed on relationships among these psychological parameters and the experience of cancer pain.

Cognitive Dimension

The cognitive dimension of cancer pain, as conceived by Ahles et al.,[64] encompassed the manner in which the pain influences a person's thought processes or the manner in which the person views herself or himself. In their study, Ahles and colleagues found support for this dimension by assessing the meaning of each patient's pain. Almost two-thirds believed their pain was an indicator of progressive disease, and these individuals had significantly elevated anxiety and depression scores.

Spiegel and Bloom found that in patients with metastatic breast cancer, the belief that pain indicated worsening disease was significantly correlated with reports of more pain, more anxiety, and more depression.[87] Barkwell reported that cancer patients with pain used words like *challenge, punishment,* and *enemy* to describe their pain. She found that patients who viewed pain as a challenge reported less pain and had lower depression and higher coping scores than those who viewed pain as punishment or as an enemy.[88] Ferrell and Dean emphasized the importance of helping cancer patients determine the meaning of their pain so that they could better cope with it.[89]

In another aspect of the cognitive dimension, researchers have examined the effects of opioid analgesics on the cognitive function of patients with pain. They found that cognitive deficits occurred as opioids were first prescribed or when doses were adjusted upward, but that these deficits were transient, with functioning returning to baseline when drug doses were stabilized for approximately 2 weeks.[90,91] Thus, level and quality of cognition in relation to pharmacologic therapy appear to be part of the cognitive dimension of pain, as these factors may influence the ability of individuals to report pain.

Finally, several researchers have examined cognitive strategies used by patients with cancer to cope with pain. Such strategies clearly fall within the cognitive dimension of pain because they result from cognitive processes. Specific strategies include various forms of distraction (e.g., reading, watching television), use of coping self-statements, reinterpretation of painful sensations, selective inattention, withdrawal, suppression of pain, and trying to accept pain.[92,93]

Behavioral Dimension

The behavioral dimension of pain includes a variety of observable behaviors related to pain. Until recently, little research supported this dimension of the cancer pain experience. Ahles et al. focused on level of activity and intake of analgesics as manifestations of this dimension in their study.[64] They found that cancer patients with pain spent significantly less time walking or standing than those who did not have pain. Furthermore, 77% of the patients with pain reported that people in their immediate environment could tell when they were in pain because of their facial expressions, changes in mood or activity, or verbal complaints.

Communication of pain to others, however, remains problematic in some patient populations. For example, Francke and Theeuwen learned that patients who had undergone breast cancer surgery did not readily report their pain and expressed concern about "annoying" the staff.[94] A variety of behaviors have been described that indicate the presence — and possibly even the severity — of cancer pain. Keefe et al. conducted a study of the behavioral manifestations of pain in patients with head and neck cancer who were undergoing treatment for their disease.[95] Guarded movements and grimacing were the major behavioral indicators of pain, with grimacing correlating significantly with patients' reports of pain intensity. In addition, the amount of time patients spent walking or standing tended to decrease over the treatment period, whereas time spent reclining increased. As treatment progressed, the number of simple daily activities that caused pain increased significantly.

Another component of the behavioral dimension of pain consists of simple strategies or activities in which patients engage to control pain. In a survey of 351 hospitalized patients, some of whom had cancer, researchers noted that the most commonly cited (≥33%) pain reduction methods involved medications, rest or lying down, heat, and distraction.[96] Cancer patients use an array of nonanalgesic, behaviorally oriented pain control methods, including heat, distraction, position change, massage, non-narcotic drugs, exercise, pressure/manipulation, immobilization, guarding, and analgesics.

Activity restriction was found to mediate the impact of pain, public self-consciousness, and social support on depressed affect in 95 women with breast cancer. The effects of illness severity (i.e., general bodily pain) on symptoms of depression depended on the extent to which illness severity influenced the ability to conduct routine activities.[97] Also, older cancer patients were examined prior to their cancer diagnosis and were found to exhibit higher levels of physical functioning than their counterparts with previously diagnosed cancer in the U.S. population. At 6 to 8 weeks after diagnosis, the symptoms of pain, fatigue, and insomnia were significant and independent predictors of loss of patient functioning. These symptoms were found to be unrelated to cancer treatment or co-morbid conditions.[98]

It has been suggested that a complex relationship exists among the symptoms of pain, psychological distress, and performance status in patients with unresectable non-small cell lung carcinoma.[85] Psychological factors, such as anxiety and depression, had a greater negative impact on distress than the physical symptom of pain.[85]

Sociocultural Dimension

The sociocultural dimension of cancer pain encompasses a variety of demographic, economic, ethnic, cultural, spiritual, and related factors that influence a person's perception of and response to pain. Historically, few researchers have examined relationships among these factors and cancer pain, but research activity in these areas is increasing as healthcare providers recognize the important influences of demographic and cultural characteristics on responses to pain and its treatment.

Sociocultural variables studied in patients with cancer pain have included sex, race, age, and cultural background. In a study of cancer inpatients, McGuire noted that females and nonwhites had significantly lower scores on the McGill Pain Questionnaire than males or whites.[99] In a subsequent study of inpatients and outpatients, blacks and older patients had less pain and depression.[100] A study by Greenwald indicated that despite few differences between ethnic identity and pain report, the ways in which people described affective aspects of pain using the McGill Pain Questionnaire varied across ethnic groups.[101] He concluded that specific ethnic identities conditioned the individual expression of pain, even though assimilation into the U.S. population had occurred. Anderson et al.[102] reported that both African Americans' and Hispanics' pain were underestimated by healthcare professionals and that these patients received insufficient analgesia for pain.

McMillan found that cancer patients with pain who were older than 55 years reported less pain intensity than their younger counterparts.[103] By contrast, another study found that the pain intensity of patients who were older than 65 years of age was similar to that of patients younger than 65.[104] More recently, age has been related to doses of opioids in patients with cancer. Vigano et al. reported that while elderly patients reported similar pain intensity to younger patients, they required significantly lower doses of opioids.[105]

Cleeland et al., using the Brief Pain Inventory (BPI), reported in their landmark study that female patients with metastatic cancer were significantly more likely to experience inadequate management of their pain, manifested by less and shorter pain relief, and more pain-related functional impairment.[106] These results suggest that gender may be linked, in as yet unclear ways, to efficacy of pain management in patients with cancer.

As noted earlier, the research literature supporting the sociocultural dimension of cancer is just beginning to emerge. When Fink and Gates reviewed relationships among culture, pain, and cancer, they clearly demonstrated that, in both noncancer and cancer populations, demographic and cultural factors are important in patients' perceptions of and responses to pain.[107] For example, Taiwanese patients who ascribe more positive meaning to their pain, such as viewing pain as a challenge rather than as a threat or a profound loss, tended to have a higher degree of hope. Patients' cognitions or interpretations of events or crises determine their level of hope rather than relatively objective measures of stressful events such as pain intensity or disease stage.[108]

One additional component in this dimension that influences cancer pain assessment and management is the patient's family. A significant amount of literature has accumulated that addresses areas such as differences in perceptions of pain between patient and family caregivers,[109] influences of the family on pain management[109] including drug prescriptions,[18] and relationships between knowledge of pain and pain reporting.[17] Clearly, family caregivers, particularly in the home setting, play a major role in assessing and managing pain.[110,111] This role is being explored by clinicians and researchers.

Implications of the Multidimensional Model

The multidimensional conceptualization of cancer pain has been described as consisting of six interrelated dimensions,[59] a proposition that is confirmed by research findings. Glajchen and colleagues studied 191 outpatients with cancer and found that pain disrupted their mood, activities, and enjoyment of life.[112] They demonstrated relationships among pain intensity, family communication related to pain, and patients' educational level. These investigators concluded that psychological factors (affective and behavioral dimensions), demographics (sociocultural dimension), and medical factors (physiological, sensory, and behavioral dimensions) could interfere with assessment and management of cancer pain. In another study, Lancee et al. tested a model for determinants of distress in cancer patients in 1309 individuals with cancer.[113] Among their most striking findings was that pain (and other symptoms) had a direct effect on distress (affective dimension), and that pain was the single most significant factor related to distress. Additionally, pain exerted an indirect effect on distress through its effects on functional impairment (behavioral dimension) and cancer-related fears (cognitive dimension). Williamson and Schulz demonstrated in 268 younger (30–64 years) and older (65–90 years) patients with cancer that the effects of pain on depression (affective dimension) are mediated by functional disability (behavioral dimension).[114] This impairment was more distressing to the younger patients than to the older ones. These investigators also noted that patients' overall levels of depression were below those considered at risk for clinical depression.

The multidimensional conceptualization of cancer pain, as initially defined by Ahles et al.,[64] expanded by McGuire,[59] and supported by the research of many investigators, provides a relevant conceptual approach to pain assessment and management. Various parameters within the dimensions of pain (e.g., duration and pattern in the physiological dimension; intensity and quality in the sensory dimension; mood changes in the affective dimension; effects of pain on functioning in the behavioral dimension) are important for nurses to assess. Similarly, various parameters within the dimensions of pain can be targeted for specific interventions that affect the organic etiology causing pain, transmission of pain, or patients' responses to pain (see Chapter 27). As examples, a painful bony metastatic lesion (physiological dimension) can be treated with radiation therapy; pain intensity (sensory dimension) can be ameliorated using analgesics; and responses to pain (cognitive dimension) can be altered using distraction strategies.

Professional Issues

Organizational Efforts

Organizations and agencies involved with cancer treatment and pain management have directed their efforts toward improving pain management. The most recent ONS position paper[1] highlighted the fact that control of cancer pain is largely inadequate. Further, the paper pointed out that individuals with cancer pain have the right to have their pain recognized as a problem and dealt with expediently. Similarly, the World Health Organization (WHO) has designated the relief of cancer pain as one of the goals of its cancer control program.[115] The National Institutes of Health (NIH) consensus statement[116] recommended using multiple treatment modalities to help control cancer pain. At a national level, the American Pain Society (APS) published revised performance improvement standards on pain management[117] as well as the fourth edition of its principles for using analgesics to treat acute and cancer pain.[118] The American Society of Clinical Oncology (ASCO) issued a formal statement on the rights of patients to receive adequate pain management and published an educational curriculum for oncologists and oncologists in training.[119] The Agency for Health Care Policy and Research (AHCPR) has developed clinical practice guidelines for the management of cancer-related pain, which are currently being updated by the American Pain Society.[120] The National Comprehensive Cancer Network has also published guidelines.[121] Finally, the International Association for the Study of Pain (IASP) published a pain curriculum for use in basic nursing education,[122] predicated on the notion that because nurses have frequent contact with patients receiving care in many settings, they need comprehensive knowledge about pain. The position papers, guidelines, recommendations, and curricula from these various groups have been developed in part in response to the compelling evidence documented over at least two decades that unrelieved cancer pain is a significant clinical problem.

Obstacles to Successful Management

A number of obstacles to pain management can be attributed to healthcare professionals, patients and family, and the healthcare system (Table 26-2). Inaccurate knowledge about pharmacological principles represents a major problem area, as documented by many studies. Questionnaires administered to nurses, physicians, and students, as well as reviews of patients' records, indicate that in those individuals with cancer pain, problems arise such as prolonged dosing intervals (i.e., not commensurate with the duration of action of the drug), lack of knowledge about equal analgesic doses, misconceptions about morphine's effectiveness as an oral analgesic, and use of doses too low to provide relief of pain.[123–128] In a landmark case, the Oregon Board of Medical Examiners took action against a physician for undertreatment of pain. The physician was required to go through an educational program and work with another physician in his field to assess his practice and make improvements.[129]

Issues surrounding addiction and potential toxicities of potent opioids also have been cited as reasons for suboptimal pain control. Although some evidence strongly suggests that addiction is not a problem for individuals who require opioids,[130] nurses, physicians, and medical students fear iatrogenically induced addiction and certainly overestimate its risk when opioids are prescribed.[131–133]

Table 26-2 Obstacles to Successful Pain Management

- Lack of understanding about pain
- Expectation that pain should be present
- Relief of pain not viewed as a goal of treatment
- Inadequate or nonexistent assessment
- Undertreatment with analgesics
- Inadequate knowledge of analgesics and other drugs
- Fears of addiction, sedation, and respiratory depression
- Inadequate knowledge of other interventions for pain
- Perceptual differences between patients and healthcare providers
- Legal impediments

Ferrell et al. reviewed 14 pharmacology or medical-surgical nursing textbooks and found that only one defined opioid addiction correctly and described accurately the likelihood of addiction developing with legitimate opioid use.[134] This finding underscores the principal reason why so much confusion persists about addiction. A more fundamental problem that nurses have demonstrated is a deficiency in the assessment of pain.[135] A lack of basic assessment skills, failure to acknowledge and document the existence of pain, and inaccurate or nonexistent documentation when the problem is known to exist prevent patients from receiving reasonable pain control. Although strong evidence supports the notion that systematic pain assessment and documentation can improve pain management,[136] these very basic nursing actions are not performed consistently.

Several other problems have been identified as obstacles to successful management of pain.[33] Patients' reluctance to report pain to their healthcare providers and concerns about analgesics is a major problem.[137] In addition, perceptual differences between patients and professionals about the severity of existing pain have been documented.[138] Physician fear of regulatory scrutiny of prescriptive practices by governmental agencies, such as the Drug Enforcement Agency, coupled with the existence of vaguely worded state regulations and statutes, have contributed to inadequate prescribing of FDA-approved medications for pain.[37,139,140]

Improvements in Management

Nurses and physicians have acknowledged their educational deficiencies related to cancer pain and its management.[77,141] The development of structured educational content in basic health professions' educational programs has been encouraged.[116,122,142–147] Spross and colleagues delineated positions involving not only basic and graduate nursing school education but also continuing education.[148] ASCO recommends education about cancer pain management for all fellowship training programs,[119] and, as noted earlier, the IASP has recommendations on pain curriculum in basic nursing education.[122]

Initial efforts at improving pain management focused on integrating both patients and caregivers into quality assurance efforts[149] and using a multidisciplinary team to get current pain knowledge into practice.[150] More recently, clinicians have implemented a variety of creative programs in clinical and institutional settings that have improved pain management outcomes.[151–154] A structure common to several of these programs is teams or clinical partners who participate jointly in the educational activities, thereby supporting the interdisciplinary nature of cancer pain practice.

In addition to such institutional programs, improvement of pain management can be accomplished through formal performance improvement programs.[155–157] The APS quality improvement guidelines for acute and cancer pain are applicable to both inpatient and outpatient settings.[155] Major programmatic efforts, such as the state-based cancer pain initiatives and the WHO's Cancer Control Program, have made the cancer pain problem much more visible, leading to heightened efforts to improve the care of patients with cancer pain.

Delivery of Pain Management Services

The delivery of pain management services remains a controversial issue.[158] Individual practitioners who take care of oncology patients should possess basic skills in assessment and management. Recognizing the significant educational needs mentioned earlier, some practitioners may feel more comfortable in referring a patient to a "specialist" for pain management, if one is available. A specialist may be an anesthesiologist, a medical or radiation oncologist, a neurologist, a neurosurgeon, a nurse, a palliative care specialist, a pharmacist, a psychologist, a psychiatrist, or a social worker. Instead of an individual specialist, a multidisciplinary pain team may provide services.[159] Often, poor communication across different settings (i.e., hospital and community care settings) compounds this problem.[160]

Principles of Assessment and Management

Effective clinical assessment and management of cancer pain rest on recognition and use of a number of critical principles. First is the importance of the nursing role in assessment and management.[161,162] The ONS position paper[148] delineated the nurse's role as (1) describing pain, (2) identifying aggravating and relieving factors, (3) determining the meaning of pain, (4) determining its cause, (5) determining individuals' definitions of optimal pain relief, (6) deriving nursing diagnoses, (7) assisting in selecting interventions, and (8) evaluating efficacy of interventions. Although nurses certainly contribute to the goals of the physician (i.e., establishing and treating the cause of pain), nurses' emphasis is on the individual as a whole person, and on his or her response to pain. Thus, nurses' focus is on individual definitions of optimal pain relief, psychosocial and physical problems amenable to nursing interventions, and evaluation of the overall response to treatment. Nurses must evaluate how the analgesic regimen affects the patient's and family's quality of life. This endeavor includes constant assessment of the effectiveness of medication and the amount of relief obtained, the impact on the patient's ability to function, the presence of side effects and the ability of the patient and family to manage them, and the accessibility, affordability, and practicality of obtaining and taking the medication.

In addition to the critical importance of the nurse's role, other principles of assessment and management are implicit in successful nursing management of cancer pain. These principles consist of a well-conceived scope of practice for nurses, thorough assessment and documentation, incorporation of guidelines and standards into clinical practice and evaluation of outcomes, and approaches to managing pain in special populations of individuals. These areas are explored in the remainder of the chapter.

Nursing's Scope of Practice and Responsibilities

Nurses are an integral part of the interdisciplinary team approach to managing cancer pain. Because of their prolonged contact with cancer patients in a variety of settings, and their relationships with these individuals and their families, oncology nurses are best prepared to assume a leadership role in the assessment and management of cancer pain. Assumption of such a role is consistent with the ONS's mission of improving the care of persons with cancer.[1] The ONS position paper[148] delineated a scope of practice for nurses with different levels of expertise (e.g., nurses and oncology clinical nurse specialists). These levels of expertise were made operational, with specific knowledge and skills being associated with each level.

With the publication of the scope and standards of oncology nursing practice,[163] the idea of levels of expertise can be easily translated into general oncology nursing practice and advanced oncology nursing practice described in this publication. At the generalist level, the nurse needs a cancer pain-specific knowledge base that enables appropriate assessment, development of a care plan based on the nursing process, evaluation of the plan, and consultation with others when needed. At the advanced level, the nurse (an individual with a master's degree) should have substantially more theoretical knowledge and clinical expertise in cancer pain that allows assessment, diagnosis, analysis of complex problems, and the use of relevant research and theory to problem-solve.[164] It is clear that assumption of a leadership role in effective management of cancer patients' pain is a nursing responsibility. The scope of nursing practice delineated in the original ONS position paper on pain[148] as well as the newer paper on cancer pain management[1] provide the foundation for all positions relevant to nurses' roles and responsibilities in caring for persons with cancer-related pain.

Assessment and Documentation

The body of literature documenting nurses' problems with assessing cancer pain has been discussed previously, including the relationship between pain assessment and barriers to adequate pain management. This section presents the rationale for and basic principles of assessment, assessment parameters, tools for assessing pain, documentation of pain assessment, and strategies for incorporating assessment into institutional practice, including evaluation of outcomes.

Rationale and basic principles

Systematic nursing assessment of pain is important for several reasons. First, it establishes a baseline from which to plan and begin interventions. Second, it assists in the selection of interventions. Third, it makes evaluation of the interventions possible. Assessment of pain is a critical process that aids in the clinical management of pain and, indeed, goes hand-in-hand with successful management. Current clinical guidelines and other sources identify assessment as key to managing pain.[117–120]

The timing of assessments is critical as well. Any cancer patient with pain who enters any healthcare setting should have an initial or baseline assessment. After the initiation of interventions, continuous or ongoing assessment is necessary for evaluation and revision of treatment plans. This approach to assessment is modeled on the nursing process. Collection of pain assessment data should be systematic and organized, as is the collection of general nursing data.

Assessment parameters

The multidimensional conceptualization of pain described previously provides guidance in assessing pain.[59] The range of assessment parameters is quite wide and represents each of the multiple dimensions of cancer pain. Key clinical parameters that require assessment in each dimension are highlighted in Table 26-3. Basic techniques for assessing pain, including the extremely important pain history, are discussed in other sources.[63,164,165]

Assessment tools

An extensive body of literature describes instruments to measure clinical pain, but a lengthy discussion is impossible here. The reader is referred to several publications in which such tools are reviewed and discussed, both in relation to pain in general and cancer pain in particular.[63,161,165] This section presents a general discussion of the various types of tools, their appropriate uses, and considerations in selecting tools.

Pain assessment tools can be classified by the number of dimensions of pain they assess.[165] Unidimensional tools focus on one dimension of the pain experience, such as the sensory dimension, and within that dimension may focus on a specific parameter, such as pain intensity. Ten-centimeter visual analog scales (VAS; anchors of no pain and worst possible pain) or verbal descriptor scales (VDS; words such as *none, mild, moderate,* and *severe*) measuring pain intensity are examples of commonly used unidimensional tools. Although these scales have documented reliability and validity in measuring cancer-related pain,[100,165] they measure only one parameter of one dimension of pain and thus are limited in their representation of the total pain experience. However, because pain intensity is such a salient aspect of pain, these scales are an excellent means by which to evaluate the success of specific interventions for pain.[166] Note, however, that patients' reports of cancer pain intensity may vary in relation to their reported intensity of other types of pain,[82] which has implications for interpretation as well as patient teaching. Indeed, the APS quality improvement guidelines[117] recommend regular use of pain intensity and relief scales, as do the AHCPR guidelines for both cancer pain and acute pain management.[120,167] Other unidimensional tools include body diagrams to assess location of pain and rating

Table 26-3 Assessment Parameters Using the Multidimensional Conceptualization of Cancer Pain

Physiological	Sensory	Affective
• Onset • Associated factors • Duration • Type of pain (acute or chronic) • Syndrome • Anatomy • Physiology	• Location • Intensity • Quality • Pattern	• Distress • Anxiety • Depression • Mental state • Perception of suffering • Irritability/agitation • Pain relief
Cognitive	**Behavioral**	**Sociocultural**
• Meaning of pain • Thought processes • Coping strategies • Knowledge • Attitudes/beliefs • Previous treatments • Influencing factors (positive and negative) • Level of cognition and/or impairment	• Activities of daily living • Behaviors (pain-related, preventive, or controlling) • Use of medications • Sleep/rest patterns • Fatigue and other symptoms	• Ethnocultural/background • Family/social life • Work/home responsibilities • Environment • Familial attitudes/beliefs/behaviors • Personal attitudes/beliefs • Communication with others • Interpersonal relationships

scales to assess behavioral indicators of pain[161] (see Table 26-3).

Multidimensional tools focus on two or more dimensions of the pain experience (see Table 28–4). The McGill Pain Questionnaire (MPQ)[168] is perhaps the most well-known example. The MPQ was originally developed to measure multidimensional aspects of pain in many diseases but has since been shown to be reliable and valid in a number of different populations of patients with cancer.[161] Another comprehensive multidimensional (sensory, affective, cognitive, behavioral, sociocultural) tool is the Brief Pain Inventory (BPI), which was developed initially for assessing pain in general but is now used fairly extensively for cancer pain.[161] Recent research suggests that the BPI is a good tool for use in different populations.[100,169,170] Several other multidimensional tools are short and easy to administer. For example, Melzack developed the short-form version of the MPQ[171] to assess sensory (including intensity and quality) and affective dimensions of pain; the BPI also exists in a short version. Clinicians and researchers have recently begun to recognize the importance of interactions between pain and other symptoms such as fatigue, sleep, and psychological distress.[172,173] Studies indicate that patients with cancer often suffer from not only pain but also numerous other symptoms.[174,175]

The choice of tool for assessing pain depends on several considerations. Of foremost concern are the dimensions of pain that are most relevant in a given situation. For example, the behavioral dimension assumes primary importance in an adult patient with cancer experiencing acute confusion or cognitive failure,[176,177] whereas the sensory and affective dimensions may predominate in an alert and oriented postoperative patient. The tool selected should be able to assess the relevant parameters of the dimension(s) of interest. The purpose of the assessment (i.e., baseline versus ongoing) is a second major consideration. In general, baseline assessments will require a more detailed and comprehensive tool, while ongoing assessments can use brief, simple tools.

Finally, issues related to time, feasibility, and relevance to the clinical setting are a major consideration. Important aspects include the amount of time required to complete tools, format and amount of writing, overlap with existing documentation, relevance of parameters to setting and to clinicians, personal comfort and preference, and lines of responsibility and accountability.

Problem identification and documentation

The outcome of a thorough baseline assessment of the patient with cancer-related pain should be identification of problems that structure the design and implementation of the management plan. McCaffery and Pasero cited 18 nursing diagnoses that the nurse should consider as part of the assessment process: anxiety, constipation, ineffective individual coping, diversional activity deficit, fatigue, fear, knowledge deficit (specify), impaired physical mobility, powerlessness, feeding self-care deficit, bathing/hygiene self-care deficit, dressing/grooming self-care deficit, toileting self-care deficit, sexual dysfunction, sleep pattern disturbance, social isolation, spiritual distress (distress of the human spirit), and altered thought processes.[63] Other nursing diagnoses include activity intolerance, anxiety, constipation, family coping, fatigue, and fear, among many others.[178] The inclusion of *all* relevant clinical problems and nursing diagnoses will emphasize the need for multiple disciplines being involved in using multiple interventions for pain.

Of critical importance is the need for nurses to document their assessment in a manner appropriate for their clinical settings. The APS quality improvement standards[117] recommend the documentation of pain intensity and pain relief on standard patient records, such as the vital signs sheet or patient flow sheet. Similarly, the AHCPR guidelines on cancer pain management[120] suggest incorporation of assessment data into routine institutional records. The use of standardized pain assessment and documentation appears to have a positive impact on pain intensity and to facilitate management of pain.[136,179,180]

Special At-Risk Populations

Because cancer is a group of diseases that affects individuals across the life span, the pain associated with it likewise occurs in groups of varying age, background, and clinical characteristics. Several populations — the elderly, individuals with a history of substance abuse, individuals with diverse sociocultural backgrounds, and the terminally ill — require special consideration in the areas of pain assessment and management.

The elderly and cognitively impaired

The elderly population in the United States (individuals aged 65 and older) more than doubled between 1950 and 1980 (from 12.3 million to 25.5 million), and one projection for the year 2030 is that the elderly population will increase to 70.3 million people.[181] As this population increases in number, one would expect to see a corresponding increase in the incidence of cancer and cancer-related deaths. Current American Cancer Society statistics indicate that 76% of all cancers are diagnosed at age 55 and older.[182]

The problem of cancer pain in elderly patients with cancer has long been neglected,[183] and prevalence surveys of pain are lacking. Ferrell reviewed 11 geriatric medicine textbooks and found only two with chapters on pain in the elderly, with negligible content focusing on cancer-related pain.[184]

A misconception that lay individuals have about pain among the elderly is that pain is a normal sequela of aging. As a result of this belief, elderly patients may not report pain as a problem because it is considered "normal." In one study of "younger" elderly versus "older" elderly, there was a trend for the older elderly to report pain less often.[185]

Another unique problem is that the elderly may experience significant sensory and cognitive impairment.[186,187] Parmalee, Smith, and Katz studied 758 elders in skilled and intermediate nursing facilities. Residents with cognitive impairment slightly underreported their pain, but their pain reports were as valid as those patients who were cognitively intact. The authors emphasized the importance of attending to nonverbal pain indicators among the cognitively impaired.[188]

Caregivers of individuals with dementia of the Alzheimer's type (DAT), who belonged to a DAT society, were asked to identify patient behaviors indicating pain. No nonverbal behaviors were identified by the caregivers. Prior to their dementia diagnosis, these patients had experienced a number of painful conditions, including osteoporosis, arthritis, migraine, and Raynaud's disease. However, these symptoms were no longer reported and analgesic medication had been discontinued in all of those cases.[189]

Horgas and Tsai determined that nursing home residents are prescribed and administered significantly less analgesic medication, in terms of both number of drugs and dosage of those drugs than patients who are more cognitively intact, even after controlling for the presence of painful conditions.[190] In another study, analgesia administration largely eliminated behaviors associated with discomfort. When behaviors persisted, a change in analgesia brought about the desired effect.[191] Marzinski[192] and Herr[193] have also concluded that identification of pain behavior in the nonverbal cognitively impaired elderly is important. The American Geriatric Society[194] has published guidelines for assessment and treatment of pain in the cognitively impaired (see Table 26-4). The reader is referred to an excellent overview of pain assessment and assessment tools that can be used in cognitively impaired older adults who have cancer.[195]

When healthcare professionals are told about pain by elderly patients, they may dismiss the complaint as insignificant, assuming that pain is a manifestation of the aging process. While it may be true that people develop more chronic diseases as they age,[196] the experience of pain does not need to be an expectation.

The normal process of aging creates unique problems in the management of cancer pain, especially as related to assessment. Ferrell and colleagues found that 71% of patients in a long-term care facility had

Table 26-4 Nonverbal Behavioral Indicators of Pain In Cognitively Impaired Older Persons

Facial expression	Sad, frightened, rapid eye blinking, slight frowning
Vocalizations	Noisy breathing, moaning or groaning, calling out, chanting, increase in profanity and abusive language
Body movements	Increase in restlessness, agitation, guarding, rocking and/or pacing, changes in gait
Interpersonal interaction	Withdrawn, resists care, increase in disruptiveness or combativeness
Activity pattern	Refuses food, increase in wandering, increase in length and frequency of rest periods, sleep difficulties, ceases normal routines
Mental status	Increase in confusion, irritability, crying

Note: Some patients will not exhibit any specific behaviors when experiencing pain.

Data from American Geriatric Society: The management of persistent pain in older persons. *J Am Geriatr Soc* 50(suppl):205–224, 2002.[194]

pain and an average of five chronic medical conditions.[197] With the prevalence of more chronic diseases, there potentially will exist multiple causes of the same complaint. The elderly experience greater alterations in the musculoskeletal system and are more vulnerable to acute and soft tissue pain.[186] Chronic problems such as arthritis, degenerative disk disease, osteoporosis, and peripheral neuropathy may confuse the picture for individuals who also have cancer-related pain. The symptoms associated with these potential impairments should alert the healthcare professional to be especially astute in obtaining a careful, detailed pain history.

The risk of historical inadequacies through the underreporting of symptoms, memory deficits, and concomitant depression-related symptomatology may lead to an inaccurate pain diagnosis and inappropriate treatment. A very important piece of assessment data to obtain in the elderly is any change from baseline behaviors, usual routines, and social interactions. A gradual loss of physical health, changes in family structure, limited economic resources, and a loss of social status can greatly influence a patient's quality of life and, therefore, the problem of pain.[198]

The most important aspects of pain assessment in elderly adults are regular assessment of the patient, using a standardized tool, and consistent documentation of findings. Use of a pain scale that is short, concise, and clear and that meets the needs of the individual patient is important as well. Unmet comfort needs should be addressed, such as hunger, thirst, and toileting. Possible causes of pain should be explored (e.g., infection, undetected fracture, and skin ulceration). The use of intuitive perception — an internal feeling that something is not right with a patient — is a skill that should not be underestimated and that should be used to start the pain management process for a cognitively impaired adult.[195] An empiric trial of analgesia should be initiated, especially during and after potentially painful procedures. When pain is suspected, give Tylenol three or four times daily. If behaviors decrease or appear to respond to the analgesic, institute around-the-clock analgesia.[195]

Yet another major unique problem is the issue of elderly patients' sensitivity to both perception of pain and pharmacological interventions. The literature about perceptual sensitivity reveals contradictions. Bayer et al. reviewed symptoms of acute myocardial infarction in elderly patients and found that chest pain was reported less frequently than other symptoms, especially by patients more than 85 years old.[199] They proposed several explanations to account for this finding: higher pain threshold, autonomic dysfunction, or cortical failure from neurological disease.

The final issue relevant to pain in the elderly follows naturally from the issues already discussed. If assessment of cancer pain in the elderly is complicated by the possibility of multiple causative factors, sensory and cognitive impairment, differences in sensitivity, and pain relief because of normal physiological aging, does this population of patients receive adequate analgesic management? A study of 13,625 patients in nursing homes found that 4003 of these patients reported daily pain.[196] Only 26% of the patients received morphine, and 26% of the patients who reported daily pain received no analgesia. Independent predictors of failing to receive analgesic agents were minority race, low cognitive performance, and the number of other medications being administered. Several reports indicate that the elderly have fewer opioids prescribed for them than younger patients.[187,200] Portenoy and colleagues raised a very important issue in this regard: If the elderly perceive pain less often, indicating a lower prevalence of pain, then less frequent prescribing of analgesics is appropriate.[200] If, however, the elderly experience pain in a manner similar to the younger population of patients and choose not to report the pain, or respond more slowly to painful stimuli, indicating a higher prevalence of pain, then underprescribing creates needless suffering. As in other areas related to cancer pain, more well-controlled, epidemiological studies of the prevalence of pain in the elderly are needed to help delineate the scope of the problem in this vulnerable population and to assist in answering questions about appropriate management.

In summary, the problem of cancer pain in the elderly population is an important one. As individuals enter the later stages of life, the risk of developing cancer increases, and thus the risk of cancer pain increases. Specific attention to the unique physiological, pharmacological, psychological, and sociological issues for these individuals, especially those who are cognitively impaired, is crucial for appropriate, successful management of cancer pain. Like all other patients, older patients require aggressive pain assessment and management.

Substance abuse history

The national problem of drug abuse creates challenges for healthcare professionals when pain and substance abuse occur simultaneously. Compton identified specific management strategies in dealing with patients with active addiction.[201] The first step in treating a patient with a current or past history of addiction is for the clinician to acknowledge his or her personal biases and make a conscious effort to put those biases aside. General guidelines for treating these patients include openly discussing the patient's addiction and encouraging the patient to express fears of how this condition may affect treatment; accepting and acting on the patient's report of pain with appropriate assessment and treatment; developing a treatment plan and, if feasible, giving the patient a written copy; consulting an addiction specialist and a pain specialist if available; beginning with nondrug or non-opioid analgesia but if pain relief is inadequate, using opioids; and assessing the patient's motivation for drug treatment and having referral references available. For patients in the inpatient setting, consider using intravenous patient-controlled analgesia to give the patient more control and to reduce potential confrontations with the staff. For patients in the outpatient setting, if opioid analgesics are required, select long-acting formulations such as transdermal fentanyl or controlled-release morphine.

With all patients having any previous or current substance abuse history, it is important that an adversarial relationship should not begin or escalate between patient and staff. As with any other patient, the substance abuse patient's report of pain should not be questioned or doubted.[202] Appropriate medications should not be withheld as a form of punishment,[202] and pain relief should not become a bargaining tool.[203] Communication among all members of the healthcare team, including the patient, about how pain will be managed should be begun early in the course of contact with the patient. Sometimes a contract may be useful for establishing realistic goals between the healthcare provider and the patient. Regularly scheduled meetings to review the goals of care may avoid unnecessary conflict. To provide a consistent approach to management, several authors recommend having only one physician assume responsibility for writing all opioid orders and, likewise, having one nurse assume responsibility for coordinating nursing care.[204,205] The assistance of professionals experienced in substance abuse, analgesic management, and cognitive-behavioral approaches to pain may prove helpful in developing a successful plan of care.

Individuals with a history of substance abuse may require much higher doses of opioids for pain because of tolerance.[205] When a patient reports increasing pain that requires higher doses of opioids, the clinician should focus on the changing pain pattern as the reason for the need for more opioids and *not* on "drug-seeking behavior." Twycross recommends changing a patient from parenteral analgesics to oral or rectal routes so that the association between street drugs and pain relief is not present.[79] Regardless of any history of substance abuse, the patient is entitled to receive reasonable, adequate care for a concomitant cancer pain problem. Obstacles to achieving this goal need to be discussed, examined, and resolved to ensure pain relief.

Special Populations

Nurses' assessment and management of individuals with cancer pain can be influenced by a number of factors, ranging from attitudes, beliefs, and personal history of pain to stereotypical notions about how people of specific ethnocultural backgrounds respond to pain.[206] As the racial and cultural diversity of the United States increases, more nurses will find themselves caring for patients with ethnocultural backgrounds different from their own. The notion of "cultural competence" has come to the forefront of clinical practice and is exceedingly important in relation to pain assessment and management. Different ethnic groups express pain and suffering differently. The nurse's interpretation of individuals' behaviors and verbalizations related to pain should be based on knowledge of how each patient's culture views responses to pain. Respect for cultures other than one's own and for the fact that people have specific beliefs and behaviors that emanate from their cultural background is known as *cultural sensitivity*. Approaches for dealing with culturally diverse patient populations are discussed next.

Children

Pain management in children is often dismal. Reports of fewer than 40% of dying children having adequate pain management before death validate this reality.[207] Approximately 90% of children with cancer have been reported to suffer "a lot" as described by their parents. Children with pain often feel helpless, and parents describe having similar feelings.

Pain in children often is related to the treatment or procedures rather than to the disease process itself, and is affected by numerous factors including age, developmental level, disease process, previous pain experience, and parental style.[208] Children's ability to understand and quantify their pain may be limited by their cognitive development. Appropriate scales for assessing pain in each child need to be established upon initiation of care. Observation, parental assessment, and use of intuitive feelings may often prove to be the only means of assessment. While many scales can be used, trials of different instruments may be necessary to determine the best and most appropriate tool for assessing a specific child's pain. Essential issues in the treatment of this population include carrying out adequate assessment and giving appropriate preemptive analgesic interventions before procedures. It is important to remember that when a child hurts, the entire family suffers from the pain.

Palliative care

In 1987, Twycross wrote that "the aim of terminal care is to help the patient, despite the cancer and increasing physical limitations, to go on having a good quality of life until he dies."[209,p.173] Wanzer et al. describe the physician's responsibility toward dying individuals, emphasizing the "art of deliberately creating a medical environment that allows a peaceful death."[210,p.846] The parallel for nursing is obvious—the nurse must practice the art of creating a nursing environment that allows a peaceful death.

In recent years, this approach has evolved into the multidisciplinary specialty of palliative care. Philosophical, organizational, and practical aspects of providing palliative care to terminally ill individuals with cancer pain have been described for home hospice settings,[211–215] the home care setting,[214] extended care facilities,[216] and general inpatient and cancer settings.[217–220] Several key aspects of caring for these individuals cut across all settings and need to be considered by nurses who are involved in palliative care.

The focus of palliative care is on relief of pain and other symptoms and on psychological support of both the patient and the family. Teamwork is requisite to the success of these efforts. Death often is accompanied by great fear—a normal human response that is part of the survival instinct. Not only are the dying afraid of death, but the living are as well. Withdrawal from those who are dying is a common reaction, yet remaining with the individual is one of the most important aspects of terminal care. For individuals dying with pain, the knowledge that healthcare providers and others are not only present but continually focusing on relieving the pain and associated symptoms serves as a great comfort.

Many nurses do not know how to manage patient pain when pain worsens or when new pain appears. A flexible and adjustable care plan to meet the patient's changing needs as the disease progresses is essential.[221] Research indicates that pain and other symptoms during the last 4 weeks of life assume tremendous variability.[222] Tailoring of palliative care to meet these diverse needs involves the use of multiple interventions, including pharmacological therapies, and the expertise to use these interventions properly. Often there is inadequate knowledge of pharmacokinetics, neurology, and medical oncology.[221] Similarly, underutilization of opioids and adjuvant drugs can erode patients' confidence in the medical system and bring their dying into sharper focus.

Research has indicated the importance of addressing family factors that influence pain management, as well as the burdens shouldered by home caregivers.[12,13,15] As with all areas of health care, the cost aspects of palliative cancer care are being closely scrutinized.[223] Hospice care is often perceived as being less expensive, but data do not support this view. The analysis of this issue is difficult because some of the savings may be derived from home care where cost shifting occurs. Family members may be paying out-of-pocket costs and providing labor and losing wages due to time out of work.[223] These activities, the ongoing need for assessment of pain, coordination of pain management, and support of the family members are well within the scope of practice for oncology nurses engaged in palliative care.

The issue of suicidal ideation or actual suicide in persons with progressive cancer accompanied by severe pain has been followed closely by those working in palliative care.[224–226] Foley reviewed the issues surrounding patients' requests for physician-assisted suicide as an option in the face of uncontrolled pain and multiple other adverse symptoms.[227] She commented that physicians are not adequately trained to care for dying patients and, furthermore, are deterred from appropriate terminal care by economic considerations. She urged improved physician–patient communication, patient-centered care, better judgments about when to withhold or withdraw care, and familiarity with concepts of palliative care as ways to reduce physician-assisted suicide and euthanasia. Breitbart described specific factors that may make patients more likely to engage in suicidal ideation: pain and suffering, advanced disease with poor prognosis, depression and hopelessness, delirium, loss of control, preexisting psychopathology, prior family or personal history of suicide, and exhaustion or fatigue.[228]

Conclusion

Nurses should base their assessment and management of cancer pain on basic principles. Foremost is the need for an interdisciplinary approach. Nurses should also have a thorough understanding of the scope of nursing practice in pain management, possess accurate assessment and diagnosis skills, and pay attention to developmental, clinical, cultural, and palliative care issues. Awareness and use of the information just presented will help nurses to identify and assess cancer pain and to plan, implement, coordinate, and evaluate its interdisciplinary management. Specific approaches to the management of cancer pain are presented in Chapter 27.

References

1. Oncology Nursing Society: Cancer pain management. *Oncol Nurs Forum* 25:817–818, 1998
2. Wilkie D, Lovejoy N, Dodd M, et al.: Cancer pain control behaviors: description and correlation with pain intensity. *Oncol Nurs Forum* 15:723–731, 1988
3. Butler LD, Koopman C, Cordova M, et al.: Psychological distress and pain significantly increase before death in metastatic breast cancer patients. *Psychosom Med* 65:416–426, 2003
4. Padilla GV, Ferrell B, Grant MM, et al.: Defining the content domain of quality of life for cancer patients with pain. *Cancer Nurs* 13:108–115, 1990
5. Ferrell BR, Wisdom C, Wenzl C: Quality of life as an outcome variable in the management of cancer pain. *Cancer* 63:2321–2327, 1989
6. Ferrell B, Wisdom C, Wenzl C: Effects of controlled release morphine on QOL for cancer pain. *Oncol Nurs Forum* 16:521–526, 1989
7. Strang P, Qvarner H: Cancer-related pain and its influence on quality of life. *Anticancer Res* 10:109–112, 1990
8. McMillan SC, Small BJ: Symptom distress and quality of life in patients with cancer newly admitted to hospice home care. *Oncol Nurs Forum* 29:1421–1428, 2002
9. Smith EM, Gomm SA, Dickens CM: Assessing the independent contribution to quality of life from anxiety and depression in patients with advanced cancer. *Palliat Med* 17:509–513, 2003
10. Ferrell BR, Grant M, Padilla G, et al.: The experience of pain and perceptions of quality of life: validation of a conceptual model. *Hospice J* 17:9–24, 1991
11. Ferrell BR: The quality of lives: 1,525 voices of cancer. *Oncol Nurs Forum* 23:907–916, 1996
12. Ferrell BR, Rhiner M, Cohen MZ, et al.: Pain as a metaphor for illness: part I. Impact of cancer pain on family caregivers. *Oncol Nurs Forum* 18:1303–1309, 1991
13. Ferrell BR, Cohen MZ, Rhiner M, et al.: Pain as a metaphor for illness: part II. Family caregivers' management of pain. *Oncol Nurs Forum* 18:1315–1321, 1991
14. Mazanec P, Bartel J: Family caregiver perspective of pain management. *Cancer Pract* 10(suppl):66–69, 2002
15. Ferrell BR, Ferrell BA, Rhiner M, et al.: Family factors influencing cancer pain management. *Postgrad Med J* 67:S64–S69, 1991
16. Kurtz ME, Kurtz JC, Given CC, et al.: Concordance of cancer patient and caregiver symptom reports. *Cancer Pract* 4:185–190, 1996
17. Bucher JA, Trostle GB, Moore M: Family reports of cancer pain, pain relief, and prescription access. *Cancer Pract* 7:71–77, 1999
18. Miaskowski C, Zimmer EF, Barrett KM, et al.: Differences in patients' and family caregivers' perceptions of the pain experience influence patient and caregiver outcomes. *Pain* 72:217–226, 1997
19. Porter LS, Keefe FJ, McBride CM, et al: Perceptions of patients' self-efficacy for managing pain and lung cancer symptoms: correspondence between patients and family caregivers. *Pain* 98:169–178, 2002
20. Keefe FJ, Ahles TA, Porter LS, et al.: The self-efficacy of family caregivers for helping cancer patients manage pain at end-of-life. *Pain* 103:157–162, 2003
21. Ishay R: High technology in medicine: ethical aspects. *Isr J Med Sci* 25:274–278, 1989
22. Ferrell BR, Rhiner M: High-tech comfort: ethical issues in cancer pain management for the 1990s. *J Clin Ethics* 2:108–112, 1991
23. Whedon M, Ferrell BR: Professional and ethical considerations in the use of high-tech pain management. *Oncol Nurs Forum* 18:1135–1143, 1991
24. Ropchan R, Ferrell BR, Grant M, et al.: Pain management as a nursing administration concern. *Oncol Nurs Forum* 19:317, 1992 (abstract)
25. Bruner DW: Cost-effectiveness and palliative care. *Semin Oncol Nurs* 14:164–167, 1998
26. Angarola RT, Donato BJ: Inappropriate pain management results in high jury award. *J Pain Symptom Manage* 6:407, 1991
27. Cushing M: The legal side: pain management on trial. *Am J Nurs* 92:21–22, 1992
28. Angarola RT, Joranson DE: Healthcare reimbursement policies: do they block acute and cancer pain management? *APS Bull* 4:7–9, 1994
29. Joranson DE: Are health-care reimbursement policies a barrier to acute and cancer pain management? *J Pain Symptom Manage* 9:244–253, 1994
30. Coyne P, Watson A: Taking the lead in managing your cancer pain: breaking barriers to obtain relief. *Coping.* 15(2):3, 2001
31. Ferrell BR, Griffith H: Cost issues related to pain management: reports from the cancer pain panel of the Agency for Health Care Policy and Research. *J Pain Symptom Manage* 9:221–234, 1994
32. Coyne P, Lyckholm L, Smith T: Clinical interventions, economic outcomes, and palliative care, in Ferrell B, Coyle N (eds.): *Textbook of Palliative Nursing.* Oxford, Oxford University Press, 2001, pp 317–327
33. Steig RL, Lippe P, Shepard TA: Roadblocks to effective pain treatment. *Med Clin North Am* 83:809–821, 1999
34. Oncology Nursing Society: Position paper on quality cancer care. *Oncol Nurs Forum* 24:951–953, 1997
35. Simmons WJ, Goforth L: The impact of managed care on cancer care: review and recommendations. *Cancer Pract* 5:111–118, 1997
36. Angarola RT, Wray SD: Legal impediments to cancer pain treatment, in Hill CS, Fields WS (eds.): *Advances in Pain Research and Therapy,* vol 11. New York, Raven Press, 1989, pp 213–231
37. Portenoy RK: The effect of drug regulation on the management of cancer pain. *NY State Med J* 91:13–18, 1991

38. Joranson DE, Gilson AM: Regulatory barriers to pain management. *Semin Oncol Nurs* 14:158–163, 1998
39. Joranson DE, Gilson AM, Ryan KM: *Achieving Balance in Federal and State Pain Policy: A Guide to Evaluation* (ed. 2). Madison, WI, Pain and Policy Studies Group, University of Wisconsin Comprehensive Cancer Center, 2003
40. American Alliance of Cancer Pain Initiatives. *www.aacpi.org*, accessed May 7, 2004
41. Angarola RT, Bormel FG: Proposed legislative changes and access to pain medications. *APS Bull* 6:8–9, 1996
42. Joranson DE: State pain commissions: new vehicle for progress? *APS Bull* 6:7–9, 1996
43. Spross JA: Cancer pain relief: an international perspective. *Oncol Nurs Forum* 19(suppl):5–11, 1992
44. National Institute of Nursing Research: Symptom management: acute pain RFA: NR-94–003. *NIH Guide* 23. Washington, DC, 1994
45. Smith T, Staats T, Deer T, et al.: Randomized trial of an implantable drug delivery system compared with comprehensive medical management for refractory cancer pain: impact on pain, drug-related toxicity, and survival. *J Clin Oncol* 20:4040–4049, 2002
46. Staats P, Hekmat H, Sauter P: The effects of alcohol celiac plexus block, pain, and mood on longevity in patients with unresectable pancreatic cancer: a double-blind, randomized, placebo-controlled study. *Pain Med* 2:28–34, 2001
47. McBeth J, Silman A, Macfarlane GJ: Association of widespread body pain with an increased risk of cancer and reduced cancer survival: a prospective population based study. *Arthr Rheum* 48:1686–1692, 2003
48. Coyle N, Foley K: Prevalence and profile of pain syndromes in cancer patients, in McGuire DB, Yarbro CH (eds.): *Cancer Pain Management.* Philadelphia, W. B. Saunders, 1987, pp 21–46
49. McGuire DB: Occurrence of cancer pain. *J Natl Cancer Inst*, (in press)
50. Grond S, Zech D, Diefenbach C, et al.: Assessment of pain: a prospective evaluation in 2266 cancer patients referred to a pain service. *Pain* 64:107–114, 1996
51. Twycross R, Harcourt J, Bergl S: A survey of pain in patients with advanced cancer. *J Pain Symptom Manage* 12:273–282, 1996
52. Berry DL, Wilkie DJ, Huang H, et al.: Cancer pain and common pain: a comparison of patient-reported intensities. *Oncol Nurs Forum* 26:721–726, 1999
53. Miaskowski C, Dibble SL: The problem of pain in outpatients with breast cancer. *Oncol Nurs Forum* 22:791–797, 1995
54. Stevens PE, Dibble SL, Miaskowski C: Prevalence, characteristics, and impact of postmastectomy pain syndrome: an investigation of women's experiences. *Pain* 61:61–68, 1995
55. Kelly JB, Payne R: Pain syndromes in the cancer patient. *Neurol Clin* 9:937–953, 1991
56. Banning A, Sjogren P, Henriksen H: Pain causes in 200 patients referred to a multidisciplinary cancer pain clinic. *Pain* 45:45–48, 1991
57. Lyne M, Coyne P, Watson A: Pain management issues for cancer survivors. *Cancer Pract* 10(suppl):28–33, 2002
58. Cherney N: Cancer pain: principles of assessment and syndromes, in Berger A, Portenoy R, Weissman D (eds.): *Principles and Practice of Palliative Care and Supportive Oncology* (ed 2) Philadelphia, Lippincott, Williams and Wilkins, 2002, pp 3–52
59. McGuire DB: The multiple dimensions of cancer pain: a framework for assessment and management, in McGuire DB, Yarbro CH, Ferrell BR (eds.): *Cancer Pain Management* (ed 2): Sudbury, MA, Jones and Bartlett, 1995, pp 1–17
60. International Association for the Study of Pain Subcommittee on Taxonomy: pain terms: a list with definitions and usage. *Pain* 6:249–252, 1979
61. Turk D, Okifuji A: Definitions and taxonomy of pain, in *Bonica's Management of Pain* (ed 3). Philadelphia, Lippincott, Williams and Wilkins, 2001, pp 17–25
62. International Association for the Study of Pain Task Force on Acute Pain: *Management of Acute Pain: A Practical Guide.* Seattle, International Association for the Study of Pain Press, 1992
63. McCaffery M, Pasero C (eds.): *Pain: Clinical Manual* (ed 2). St. Louis, Mosby, 1999
64. Ahles TA, Blanchard EB, Ruckdeschel JC: The multidimensional nature of cancer-related pain. *Pain* 17:277–288, 1983
65. McGuire DB: Cancer-related pain: a multidimensional approach. *Dissert Abstr Int* 48(03), Sec B:705, 1987
66. McGuire DB: Coping strategies used by cancer patients with pain. *Oncol Nurs Forum* 14:123, 1987 (abstract)
67. NINR Priority Expert Panel on Symptom Management: Acute Pain: *Symptom Management: Acute Pain,* vol 6. NIH publication No. 94–2421. Bethesda, MD, National Institute of Nursing Research, U.S. Department of Health and Human Services, U.S. Public Health Service, National Institutes of Health, 1994
68. Foley KN: Pain syndromes in patients with cancer, in Bonica JJ, Ventafridda V (eds.): *Advances in Pain Research and Therapy,* vol 2. New York, Raven Press, 1979, pp 59–75
69. Gaston-Johansson F, Franco T, Zimmerman L: Pain and psychological distress in patients undergoing autologous bone marrow transplantation. *Oncol Nurs Forum* 19:41–48, 1992
70. McGuire DB, Altomonte V, Peterson DE, et al.: Patterns of mucositis and pain in patients receiving preparative chemotherapy and bone marrow transplantation. *Oncol Nurs Forum* 20:1493–1502, 1993
71. Yeager KA, McGuire DB, De Loney V: Profiles of pain in bone marrow/stem cell transplant and leukemia patients. *Oncol Nurs Forum* 26:358, 1999 (abstract)
72. Portenoy RK: Cancer pain: epidemiology and syndromes. *Cancer* 63:2298–2307, 1989
73. Payne R: Cancer pain: anatomy, physiology, and pharmacology. *Cancer* 63:2266–2274, 1989
74. Kelly JB, Payne R: Pain syndromes in the cancer patient. *Neurol Clin* 9:937–953, 1991
75. Caraceni A: Clinicopathologic correlates of common cancer pain syndromes. *Hematol Oncol Clin North Am* 10:57–78, 1996
76. Hwang S, Chang V, Kasimio B: Cancer breakthrough pain characteristics and responses to treatment at a VA medical center. *Pain* 101:55–64, 2003
77. Ferrell B, Juarez G, Borneman T: Use of routine and breakthrough analgesia in home care. *Oncol Nurs Forum* 26:1655–1661, 1999
78. Arathuzik D: Pain experience for metastatic breast cancer patients. *Cancer Nurs* 14:41–48, 1991
79. Twycross R: *Pain Relief in Advanced Cancer.* Edinburgh, Churchill Livingstone, 1994
80. Berry DL, Wilkie DJ, Huang H, et al.: Cancer pain and common pain: a comparison of patient-reported intensities. *Oncol Nurs Forum* 26:721–726, 1999
81. Melzack R, Torgerson WS: On the language of pain. *Anesthesiology* 34:50–59, 1971
82. Bressler LR, Hange PA, McGuire DB: Characterization of the pain experience in a sample of cancer outpatients. *Oncol Nurs Forum* 13:51–55, 1986
83. Zimmerman L, Duncan K, Pozehl B, et al.: Pain descriptors used by patients with cancer. *Oncol Nurs Forum* 14:67–71, 1987
84. Padilla GV, Ferrell B, Grant MM, et al.: Defining the content domain of quality of life for cancer patients with pain. *Cancer Nurs* 13:108–115, 1990
85. Akechi T, Okamura H, Nishiwaki Y, et al: Psychiatric disorders and associated and predictive factors in patients with unresectable nonsmall cell lung carcinoma. *Cancer* 92:2609–2622, 2001

86. Kai-hoi Sze F, Wong E, Lo R, et al: Do pain and disability differ in depressed cancer patients? *Palliat Med* 14:11–17, 2000
87. Spiegel D, Bloom J: Pain in metastatic breast cancer. *Cancer* 52:341–345, 1983
88. Barkwell DP: Ascribed meaning: a critical factor in coping and pain attenuation in patients with cancer-related pain. *J Palliat Care* 7:5–14, 1991
89. Ferrell BR, Dean G: The meaning of cancer pain. *Semin Oncol Nurs* 11:17–22, 1995
90. Bruera E, Macmillan K, Hanson J, et al.: The cognitive effects of the administration of narcotic analgesics in patients with cancer pain. *Pain* 39:13–16, 1989
91. Sjogren P, Banning A: Pain, sedation and reaction time during long-term treatment of cancer patients with oral and epidural opioids. *Pain* 39:5–11, 1989
92. Wilkie DJ, Keefe FJ: Coping strategies of patients with lung cancer-related pain. *Clin J Pain* 7:292–299, 1991
93. Arathuzik D: The appraisal of pain and coping in cancer patients. *West J Nurs Res* 13:714–731, 1991
94. Francke AL, Theeuwen I: Inhibition in expressing pain: a qualitative study among Dutch breast cancer patients. *Cancer Nurs* 17:193–199, 1994
95. Keefe FJ, Brantley A, Manuel G, et al.: Behavioral assessment of head and neck cancer pain. *Pain* 23:327–336, 1985
96. Barbour LA, McGuire DB, Kirchhoff KT: Non-analgesic methods of pain control used by cancer outpatients. *Oncol Nurs Forum* 13:56–60, 1986
97. Williamson G: Extending the activity restriction model of depressed affect: evidence from a sample of breast cancer patients. *Health Psychol* 19:339–347, 2000
98. Given B, Given C, Azzouz F, et al: Physical functioning of elderly cancer patients prior to diagnosis and following initial treatment. *Nurs Res* 50:222–232, 2001
99. McGuire DB: Assessment of pain in cancer inpatients using the McGill Pain Questionnaire. *Oncol Nurs Forum* 11:32–37, 1984
100. McGuire DB, Strickland OL: Assessment of cancer-related pain in low-income African Americans: reliability, validity, and clinical utility of the Brief Pain Inventory and three pain intensity scales, in *Proceedings of the 8th World Congress on Pain*. Seattle, WA, International Association for the Study of Pain, 1996, p 174
101. Greenwald HP: Interethnic differences in pain perception. *Pain* 44:157–163, 1991
102. Anderson KO, Mendoza TR, Valero V, et al: Minority cancer patients and their providers: pain management attitudes and practice. *Cancer* 88:1929–1938, 2000
103. McMillan S: The relationship between age and intensity of cancer-related symptoms. *Oncol Nurs Forum* 16:237–241, 1989
104. Ferrell BA, Ferrell BR: The experience of pain and quality of life in elderly patients. *Gerontology* 28(suppl):76A, 1988
105. Vigano A, Bruera E, Suarez-Almazor ME: Age, pain intensity, and opioid dose in patients with advanced cancer. *Cancer* 83:1244–1250, 1998
106. Cleeland CS, Gonin R, Hatfield AK, et al.: Pain and its treatment in outpatients with metastatic cancer. *N Engl J Med* 330:592–596, 1994
107. Fink RS, Gates R: Cultural diversity and cancer pain, in McGuire DB, Yarbro CH, Ferrell BR (eds.): *Cancer Pain Management* (ed 2). Sudbury, MA, Jones and Bartlett, 1995, pp 19–39
108. Chen ML: Pain and hope in patients with cancer: a role for cognition. *Cancer Nurs* 26:61–67, 2003
109. Yeager KA, Miaskowski C, Dibble SL, et al.: Differences in pain knowledge and perception of the pain experience between outpatients with cancer and their family caregivers. *Oncol Nurs Forum* 22:1235–1241, 1995
110. Elliott VA, Elliott TE, Murray DM, et al.: Patients and family members: the role of knowledge and attitudes in cancer pain. *J Pain Symptom Manage* 12:209–220, 1996
111. Ferrell BR: Patient and family caregiver perspectives. *Oncology* 13(suppl):15–19, 1999
112. Glajchen M, Fitzmartin RD, Blum D, et al: Psychosocial barriers to cancer pain relief. *Cancer Pract* 3:76–82, 1995
113. Lancee WJ, Vachon MLS, Ghadirian P, et al.: The impact of pain and impaired role performance on distress in persons with cancer. *Can J Psychiatry* 39:617–622, 1994
114. Williamson GM, Schulz R: Activity restriction mediates the association between pain and depressed affect: a study of younger and older adult cancer patients. *Psychol Aging* 10:369–378, 1995
115. World Health Organization: *Cancer Pain Relief* (ed 2). Geneva, World Health Organization, 1996
116. National Institutes of Health: The integrated approach to the management of pain. *NIH Consensus Development Conference, Statement* 6, 1986
117. American Pain Society Quality of Care Committee: quality improvement guidelines for the treatment of acute pain and cancer pain. *JAMA* 274:1874–1880, 1995
118. American Pain Society: *Principles of Analgesic Use in the Treatment of Acute Pain and Cancer Pain*. Skokie, IL, American Pain Society, 2004
119. Ad Hoc Committee on Cancer Pain of the American Society of Clinical Oncology: Cancer pain assessment and treatment curriculum guidelines. *J Clin Oncol* 10:1976–1982, 1992
120. Jacox A, Carr DB, Payne R, et al.: *Management of Cancer Pain: Clinical Practice Guideline No. 9*. AHCPR publication No. 94–0592. Rockville, MD, Agency for Healthcare Policy and Research, U.S. Department of Health and Human Services, Public Health Service, 1994
121. National Comprehensive Cancer Network. *www.nccn.org*, accessed March 3, 2004
122. Ad Hoc Committee: Pain curriculum for basic nursing education. *IASP Newsletter* Sept/Oct:4–6, 1993
123. Sheidler VR, McGuire DB, Grossman SA, et al.: Analgesic decision-making skills of nurses. *Oncol Nurs Forum* 19:1531–1534, 1992
124. Schauer PK, Wetterman TL, Schauer AR: Physicians' attitudes and knowledge about the management of cancer-related pain. *Conn Med* 52:705–707, 1988
125. McCaffery M, Ferrell BR: Nurses' knowledge about cancer pain: a survey of five countries. *J Pain Symptom Manage* 10:356–369, 1995
126. Hill CS: The barriers to adequate pain management with opioid analgesics. *Semin Oncol* 20:1–5, 1993
127. Wallace KG, Reed BA, Pasero C, et al.: Staff nurses perceptions of barriers to effective pain management. *J Pain Symptom Manage* 10:204–213, 1995
128. Ferrell BR, McCaffery M: Nurses' knowledge about equianalgesia and opioid dosing. *Cancer Nurs* 20:201–212, 1997
129. Barnett EH: Case marks big shift in pain policy. *The Oregonian* September 2, 1999
130. Porter J, Jick H: Addiction rare in patients treated with narcotics. *N Engl J Med* 302:123, 1980
131. Weissman DE, Dahl JL: Attitudes about cancer pain: a survey of Wisconsin's first-year medical students. *J Pain Symptom Manage* 5:345–349, 1990
132. Edgar L, Hamilton J: A survey examining nurses' knowledge of pain control. *J Pain Symptom Manage* 7:18–26, 1992
133. McCaffery M, Ferrell BR, O'Neil-Page E, et al.: Nurses' knowledge of opioid analgesic drugs and psychological dependence. *Cancer Nurs* 13:21–27, 1990

134. Ferrell BR, McCaffery M, Rhiner M: Pain addiction: an urgent need for change in nursing education. *J Pain Symptom Manage* 7:117–124, 1992
135. Coyne PJ: When the World Health Organization analgesic ladder fails: the role of invasive analgesic therapies. *Oncol Nurs Forum* 30:777–783, 2003
136. Faries JE, Mills DS, Goldsmith KW, et al.: Systematic pain records and their impact on pain control: a pilot study. *Cancer Nurs* 14:306–313, 1991
137. Ward SE, Goldberg N, Miller-McCauley V, et al.: Patient-related barriers to management of cancer pain. *Pain* 52:319–324, 1993
138. Grossman SA, Sheidler VR, Swedeen K, et al.: Correlation of patient and caregiver ratings of cancer pain. *J Pain Symptom Manage* 6:53–57, 1991
139. Weissman DE, Joranson DE, Hopwood MB: Wisconsin physicians' knowledge and attitudes about opioid analgesic regulations. *Wis Med J* 90:671–675, 1991
140. Von Roenn JH, Cleeland CS, Gonin R, et al.: Physician attitudes and practice in cancer pain management: a survey from the Eastern Cooperative Oncology Group. *Ann Intern Med* 119:121–126, 1993
141. Pilowsky I: An outline curriculum on pain for medical school. *Pain* 33:1–2, 1988
142. Ferrell BR, McGuire DB, Donovan MI: Knowledge and beliefs regarding pain in a sample of nursing faculty. *J Prof Nurs* 9:79–88, 1993
143. Wisconsin Cancer Pain Initiative Nursing Education Committee: *Competency Guidelines for Cancer Pain Management in Nursing Education and Practice.* Madison, WI, Wisconsin Cancer Pain Initiative, 1995
144. Zahn ML: Pain management instruction in nursing curricula. *J Nurs Educ* 34:262–267, 1995
145. Weissman DE: Cancer pain education for physicians in practice: establishing a new paradigm. *J Pain Symptom Manage* 12:1–8, 1996
146. Dalton JA, Blau W: Changing the practice of pain management. *Pain Forum* 5:266–272, 1996
147. Breitbart W: The practice of pain management — change from within or from without. *Pain Forum* 5:275–278, 1996
148. Spross JA, McGuire DB, Schmitt R: Oncology Nursing Society position paper on cancer pain. *Oncol Nurs Forum* 17:595–614, 751–760, 825, 944–955, 1990
149. Miaskowski C, Donovan M: Implementation of the American Pain Society Quality Assurance Standards for Relief of Acute Pain and Cancer Pain in oncology nursing practice. *Oncol Nurs Forum* 19:411–415, 1992
150. Weissman DE, Abram SE, Haddox AD, et al.: Educational role of cancer pain rounds. *J Cancer Educ* 4:113–116, 1989
151. Weissman DE, Dahl JL: Update on the cancer pain role model education program. *J Pain Symptom Manage* 10:292–297, 1995
152. Ferrell BR, Dean GE, Grant M, et al.: An institutional commitment to pain management. *J Clin Oncol* 13:2158–2165, 1995
153. Ferrell BR, Grant M, Ritchey KL, et al.: The pain resource nurse training program: a unique approach to pain management. *J Pain Symptom Manage* 8:545–556, 1993
154. McMenamin E, McCorkle E, Barg F, et al.: Implementing a multidisciplinary cancer pain education program. *Cancer Pract* 3:303–309, 1995
155. Ward SE, Gordon D: Application of the American Pain Society quality assurance standards. *Pain* 56:299–306, 1994
156. Bookbinder M, Kiss M, Coyle N, et al.: Improving pain management practices, in McGuire DB, Yarbro CH, Ferrell BR (eds.): *Cancer Pain Management* (ed 2). Sudbury, MA, Jones and Bartlett, 1995, pp 321–361
157. Ferrell B, Whedon M, Rollins B: Pain and quality assessment/improvement. *J Nurs Care Qual* 9:69–85, 1995
158. Portenoy RK, Coyle N: Controversies in the long-term management of analgesic therapy in patients with advanced cancer. *J Pain Symptom Manage* 5:307–319, 1991
159. Williams A, Kedziera P, Osterlund H, et al.: Models of healthcare delivery in cancer pain management. *Oncol Nurs Forum* 19(suppl):20–26, 1992
160. Redmond K: Organizational barriers in opioid use. *Support Care Cancer* 5:451–456, 1997
161. McGuire DB, Kim HJ, Lang X: Measuring pain, in Frank-Stromborg M, Olsen SJ (eds.): *Instruments for Clinical Health-Care Research* (ed 3). Sudbury, MA, Jones and Bartlett, 2004, pp 603–644
162. Watson AC, Coyne PJ: Recognizing the faces of cancer pain: learn how to distinguish the types and causes to help your patient manage his pain. *Nursing* 33:32 HN1–8, 2003
163. American Nurses Association and Oncology Nursing Society: *Statement on the Scope and Standards of Oncology Nursing Practice.* Washington, DC, 1996
164. Coyne PJ: The evolution of the advanced practice nurse within palliative care. *J Palliat Med* 6:769–770, 2003
165. Vallerand AH: Measurement issues in the comprehensive assessment of cancer pain. *Semin Oncol Nurs* 13:16–24, 1997
166. Collins SL, Moore RA, McQuay HJ: The visual analogue pain intensity scale: what is moderate pain in millimetres? *Pain* 72:95–97, 1997
167. Acute Pain Management Guideline Panel: *Acute Pain Management: Operative or Medical Procedures and Trauma. Clinical Practice Guideline.* AHCPR publication No. 92–0032. Rockville, MD, Agency for Healthcare Policy and Research, Public Health Service, U.S. Department of Health and Human Services, 1992
168. Melzack R: The McGill Pain Questionnaire: major properties and scoring methods. *Pain* 1:277–299, 1975
169. Uki J, Mendoza T, Cleeland CS, et al: A brief cancer pain assessment tool in Japanese: the utility of the Japanese Brief Pain Inventory — BPI-J. *J Pain Symptom Manage* 16:364–373, 1998
170. Saxena A, Mendoza T, Cleeland CS: The assessment of cancer pain in north India: the validation of the Hindi Brief Pain Inventory — BPI-H. *J Pain Symptom Manage* 17:27–41, 1999
171. Melzack R: The short-form McGill Pain Questionnaire. *Pain* 30:191–197, 1987
172. McGuire DB, Grimm PM, Baxendale-Cox L, et al: Pain, fatigue, and sleep alterations in cancer: a multidimensional perspective, in *Proceedings of the 12th Annual Meeting of the American Pain Society.* Glenview, IL, American Pain Society, 1994, p A-12 (abstract)
173. Portenoy RK, Thaler HT, Kornblith AB, et al.: Symptom prevalence, characteristics and distress in a cancer population. *Qual Life Res* 3:183–189, 1994
174. Donnelly S, Walsh D: The symptoms of advanced cancer. *Semin Oncol* 22:67–72, 1995
175. Miaskowski C, Lee K: Pain, fatigue, and sleep disturbance in oncology outpatients receiving radiation therapy for bone metastases: a pilot study. *J Pain Symptom Manage* 17:320–322, 1999
176. Stiefel F, Fainsinger R, Bruera E: Acute confusional states in patients with advanced cancer. *J Pain Symptom Manage* 7:94–98, 1992
177. Bruera E, Fainsinger RL, Miller MJ, et al.: The assessment of pain intensity in patients with cognitive failure: a preliminary report. *J Pain Symptom Manage* 7:267–270, 1992
178. North American Nursing Diagnosis Association: *Nursing Diagnoses: Definitions and Classification.* Philadelphia, North American Nursing Diagnosis Association, 2000
179. Jadlos MA, Kelman GB, Marra K, et al.: A pain management documentation tool. *Oncol Nurs Forum* 23:1451–1454, 1996

180. Kravitz RL, Delafield JP, Hays RD, et al.: Bedside charting of pain levels in hospitalized patients with cancer: a randomized controlled trial. *J Pain Symptom Manage* 11:81–87, 1996
181. Administration on Aging: Older populations by age: 1900 to 2050. *www.aoa.dhhs.gov./aoa/stats/AgePop2050chart-numbers.htlm.* Accessed May 7, 2004
182. American Cancer Society: *Cancer Facts and Figures.* Atlanta, GA, American Cancer Society, 2004
183. Harkins SW: Geriatric pain: pain perceptions in the old. *Clin Geriatr Med* 12:434–459, 1996
184. Ferrell BA: Pain in the elderly, in Watt-Watson JH, Donovan MI (eds.): *Pain Management: Nursing Perspective.* St. Louis, Mosby, 1992, pp 349–369
185. Thomas MR, Roy R: Age and pain: a comparative study of the "younger and older" elderly. *Pain Manage* 1:174–179, 1988
186. Newton PA: Chronic pain, in Cassel KY, Walsh JR (eds.): *Geriatric Medicine, vol. 2. Fundamentals of Geriatric Care.* New York, Springer-Verlag, 1984, pp 236–274
187. Ferrell BA, Ferrell BR, Rivera L: Pain in cognitively impaired nursing home patients. *J Pain Symptom Manage* 10:591–598, 1995
188. Parmalee PA, Smith G, Katz IR: Pain complaints and cognitive status among elderly institution residents. *J Am Geriatr* Soc 41:517–522, 1993
189. Fisher-Morris M, Gellatly A: The experience and expression of pain in Alzheimer patients. *Age Aging* 26:497–500, 1997
190. Horgas AL, Tsai P: Analgesic drug prescription and use in cognitively impaired nursing home residents. *Nursing* 47:235–242, 1998
191. Simons W, Malabar R: Assessing pain in elderly patients who cannot respond verbally. *J Adv Nurs* 22:663–669, 1995
192. Marzinski LR: The tragedy of dementia: clinically assessing pain in the confused nonverbal elderly. *J Geront Nurs* 17:25–28, 1991
193. Herr K: Pain assessment in cognitively impaired older adults: new strategies and careful observation help pinpoint unspoken pain. *Am J Nurs* 102:65–67, 2002
194. American Geriatric Society: The management of persistent pain in older persons. *J Am Geriatr Soc* 50(suppl):205–224, 2002
195. Soscia J: Assessing pain in cognitively impaired older adults with cancer. *Clin J Oncol Nurs* 7:174–177, 2003
196. Bernabei R, Gambassi G, Lapane K, et al.: Management of pain in elderly patients with cancer. *JAMA* 279:1877–1882, 1998
197. Ferrell BA, Ferrell BR, Osterweil D: Pain in the nursing home. *J Am Geriatr Soc* 38:409–414, 1990
198. Ferrell BR, Grant MM, Riner M, et al.: Home care: maintaining quality of life for patient and family. *Oncology* 6(suppl):136–140, 1992
199. Bayer AJ, Chadha JS, Farag RR, et al.: Changing presentations of myocardial infarction with increasing old age. *J Am Geriatr Soc* 34:263–266, 1986
200. Portenoy RK, Kanner RM: Patterns of analgesic prescription and consumption in a university-affiliated community hospital. *Arch Intern Med* 145:439–441, 1985
201. Compton P: Chronic pain, substance abuse and addiction. *Nurs Clin North Am* 38:525–537, 2003
202. Coyne P, Ropka M: Pain, in Ropka M, Williams A (eds.): *HIV: Nursing and Symptom Management.* Sudbury, MA, Jones and Bartlett, 1998, pp 493–527
203. McCaffery M, Vourakis C: Assessment and relief of pain in chemically dependent patients. *Orthoped Nurs* 11:13–27, 1992
204. Hoffman M, Provatas A, Lyver A, et al.: Pain management in the opioid-addicted patient with cancer. *Cancer* 68:121–122, 1991
205. McGuire DB, Sheidler VR: Pain, in Groenwald SL, Frogge MH, Goodman M, Yarbro CH (eds.): *Cancer Nursing: Principles and Practice* (ed 4). Sudbury, MA, Jones and Bartlett, 1997, pp 529–584
206. Lavizzo-Mourey R, Macknzie E: Cultural competence: essential measurements of quality for managed care organizations. *Ann Intern Med* 124:919–921, 1996
207. Wolfe J, Grier HE, Klar N, et al: Symptoms and suffering at the end of life in children with cancer. *N Engl J Med* 342:326–333, 2000
208. Hockenberry M, Wilson P, Winkelstein M: *Wong's Nursing Care of Infants and Children* (ed 7). St. Louis, Mosby, 2003
209. Twycross RD: Terminal care: organization and technical aspects, in Swerdlow M, Ventafridda V (eds.): *Cancer Pain.* Lancaster, UK, MTP Press, 1987, pp 173–184
210. Wanzer SH, Federman DD, Adelstein SJ et al.: The physician's responsibility toward hopelessly ill patients. A second look. *N Engl J Med* 320:844–849, 1989
211. Ferrell B, Virani R, Grant M: Beyond the Supreme Court decision: nursing perspectives on end of life care. *Oncol Nurs Forum* 27:445–455, 2000
212. Johnston Taylor E, Ersek M: Ethical and spiritual dimensions of cancer pain management, in McGuire DB, Yarbro CH, Ferrell BR (eds.): *Cancer Pain Management* (ed 2). Sudbury, MA, Jones and Bartlett, 1995, pp 41–231
213. Burchman SL: Hospice care of the cancer pain patient, in Abram SE (ed.): *Cancer Pain.* Boston, Kluwer, 1989, pp 153–169
214. Austin C, Cody OP, Eyres PJ, et al.: Hospice home care pain management: four critical variables. *Cancer Nurs* 9:38–65, 1986
215. Pickett M, Cooley ME, Gordon DB: Pallative care: past, present and future. *Semin Oncol Nurs* 14:86–94, 1998
216. Degner LF, Fujii SH, Levitt M: Implementing a program to control chronic pain of malignant disease for patients in an extended care facility. *Cancer Nurs* 5:263–268, 1982
217. Walsh TD: Continuing care in a medical center: the Cleveland Clinic Foundation Palliative Care Service. *J Pain Symptom Manage* 5:273–278, 1990
218. Bruera E, MacMillan K, Hanson J, et al.: Palliative care in a cancer center: results in 1984 versus 1987. *J Pain Symptom Manage* 5:1–5, 1990
219. Miller RD, Walsh TD: Psychosocial aspects of palliative care in advanced cancer. *J Pain Symptom Manage* 6:24–29, 1991
220. Chan H, Woodruff RK: Palliative care in a general teaching hospital: Assessment of needs. *Med J Aust* 155:597–599, 1991
221. White K, Coyne PJ, Patel U: Are nurses adequately prepared for end of life care? *J Nurs Schol* 33:147–151, 2001
222. Coyle N, Adelhardt J, Foley KM, et al.: Character of terminal illness in the advanced cancer patient: pain and other symptoms during the last four weeks of life. *J Pain Symptom Manage* 5:83–93, 1990
223. Bailes JS: Cost aspects of palliative cancer care. *Semin Oncol* 22:64–66, 1995
224. Foley K: Competent care for the dying instead of physician-assisted suicide. *N Engl J Med* 336:54–58, 1997
225. Emanuel E: Pain and symptom control: patients' rights and physicians' responsibilities. *Hematol Oncol Clin North Am* 10:41–56, 1996
226. Goldstein F: Inadequate pain management: a suicidogen. *J Clin Pharmacol* 37:1–3, 1997
227. Foley KM: Pain, physician-assisted suicide, and euthanasia. *Pain Forum* 4:163–178, 1995
228. Breitbart W: Cancer pain and suicide, in Foley KM, Bonica JJ, Ventafridda V (eds.): *Advances in Pain Research and Therapy.* New York, Raven Press, 1990, pp 399–412

CHAPTER 27

Management of Cancer Pain

Bridget A. Cahill, MS, APN/NP-C

Introduction

New developments in the understanding of pain and its effects on human responses have led to advances in the utilization of pharmacotherapy, nonpharmacological approaches, and invasive interventional techniques that target the physiological and psychosocial aspects of the pain experience. The multidimensional aspects of pain associated with cancer often require a combination of these modalities to achieve maximum pain-relieving benefits. Pain management, while still evolving as a specialty in health care, is now based on proven scientific principles and evidenced-based information. Research into the basis for pain and its specific mechanisms has guided the implementation of a wide variety of therapies that now offer patients with cancer-related pain better pain control and improved physical and emotional well-being. The content presented in this chapter will enable nurses to identify effective pharmacotherapy and nonpharmacologic interventions so that these may be implemented to prevent the worsening of pain and to alleviate suffering. Figure 27–1 demonstrates the hierarchy of pain management.[1]

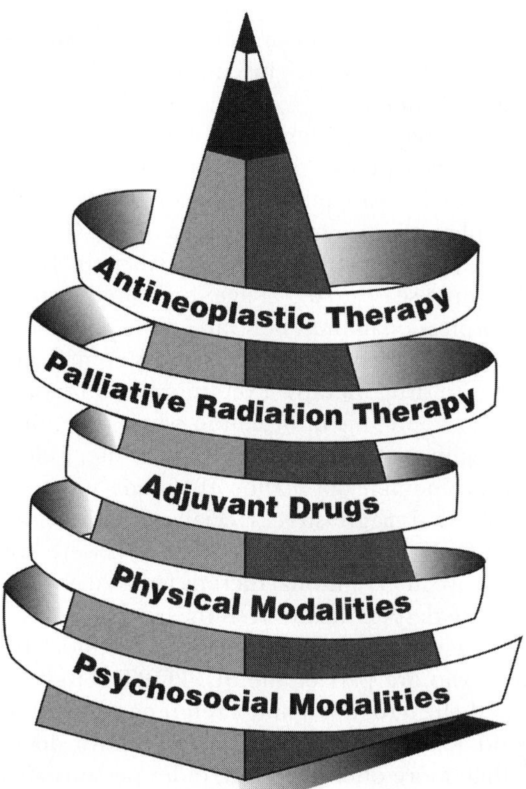

Note: The pyramid depicts a hierarchy of pain management strategies from least invasive (at the base) to most invasive (at the apex). Therapies depicted on the ribbon may benefit many patients who are receiving concurrent treatments at any level of invasiveness.

Data from Jacox, Carr, Payne, et al.[1]

Figure 27-1 Pain management strategies: a hierarchy.

Specialized Pain Care

Growing numbers of healthcare professionals (e.g., advanced practice nurses, medical oncologists, internal medicine physicians, anesthesiologists, clinical pharmacists) have sought specialization in pain care. The integration of interdisciplinary services (pain management teams, hospice, palliative care and supportive care teams, and pain clinics and centers) into the healthcare system has significantly affected the education of health professionals and the delivery of pain care. Such multidisciplinary groups have generated databases that have proved useful in understanding the incidence of pain syndromes and referral patterns for the treatment of complex pain problems requiring more attention.[2,3]

Nurses and other healthcare professionals need to be aware of inpatient, outpatient, and home care resources that are available to them and their patients, both through their institutions and health systems and referral agencies.[4] In addition, many health systems,[5] professional organizations,[6–10] government agencies,[1,11,12] and international organizations[13] have published evidence- and consensus-based guidelines to define "best practices" for the management of acute and chronic cancer pain. These documents offer a compilation of assessment and treatment clinical care guidelines in the form of protocols, algorithms, and outcome-based criteria; information on pharmacotherapy and other interventions; citations from the literature; and educational resources that are available to both clinicians and patients to promote optimal pain practices.

End-of-Life Issues

End-of-life issues are now being addressed by professionals who provide palliative and supportive care services in hospitals, at home, in long-term care facilities, and in freestanding institutions. However, many believe that these services should be rendered much sooner, and that patients should be able to make informed decisions about their care before they become too sick to determine what level of care is needed.[14] Changes in patterns for healthcare reimbursement, active cancer treatment at the end of life, and the reluctance of health professionals to refer patients for end-of-life care clearly emphasize the importance of implementing more aggressive pain care earlier in the course of the disease. Constraints imposed by managed care organizations on end-of-life services reinforce the need for clinicians who care for patients in all phases of their illness to be educated and trained in pain management.[15]

A growing body of evidence-based information addresses palliative care for specific populations such as the elderly. Older patients with cancer present with more complex clinical problems and pain. Cancer pain is often accompanied by long-term pain from nonmalignant diseases. To manage this pain effectively, health professionals must be aware of the physiological changes associated with aging that may complicate treatment with drug therapy. Even more important is the ability to apply this information when designing analgesic regimens for elders at the end of life. Elders represent a vulnerable population of patients who may not be afforded aggressive, specialized pain care. Cleary and Carbone documented that elders were less likely to receive interventional therapy for pain and expert pain care despite the fact that they experienced a higher incidence of symptoms at the end of life.[16] Investigators who are part of the SUPPORT (Study to Understand the Prognosis and Preferences for Outcomes and Risks of Treatment) project have documented that, more often than not, older persons who are seriously ill die in the hospital with significant pain and distressing symptoms.[17]

Interventions

Interventions and techniques for managing cancer pain can be categorized into three major approaches (Figure 27-2). The first approach, *treat the underlying pathology*, uses treatments targeting the underlying pathophysiological mechanisms for pain with antineoplastic therapies or surgical interventions. The primary goal of these treatments is to control, reduce, or eradicate the tumor. The second category, *change perception or sensation of pain*, utilizes pharmacological and interventional techniques to either diminish or interrupt painful sensory input from the periphery or alter pain perception and sensations at the level of the sensory cortex in the brain. The third category, *diminish emotional or reactive component*, implements cognitive or behavioral strategies as a means to alter the central processing of pain. The goal of this last approach is to positively affect the contextual aspects of pain by alleviating or reducing emotional distress or negative reactions to pain. A wide variety of nonpharmacological techniques can be used to achieve this outcome. More often than not, any combination of these three major approaches will be applied simultaneously to achieve the greatest level of pain relief.

Because pain management has evolved as a specialty among multiple groups of healthcare professionals, interdisciplinary efforts typically afford the greatest benefits in treating cancer-related pain. Multitreatment modalities have become the mainstay in managing chronic cancer pain; therefore, the following sections address specific interventions within each of the three major treatment categories. Successful plans of care for managing pain demand advanced knowledge of the physiology and pathophysiology of pain, underlying principles of pain control, and indications and mechanisms of action for pharmacotherapy, nonpharmacological strategies, and interventional techniques. Moreover, nurses must collaborate with physicians and other health professionals to assess pain, design optimal analgesic therapy, and evaluate responses to pain treatments.

Treatment of Underlying Pathology

Typically, the three major cancer treatment modalities — chemotherapy, radiation therapy, and surgery — are employed as curative and adjunctive therapies; however, they can also be effective in the control and palliation of cancer pain. The primary intent of palliation is to reduce symptoms and improve quality of life. Hormonal therapy, another treatment modality, is similar to chemotherapy in that hormonal agents can be administered for the purpose of arresting cancers and relieving symptoms. Whether treatments are given to control or palliate advanced cancer, the assessment of pain and pain relief are paramount in monitoring the success of therapy (see Chapter 26 for more on pain assessment). A new complaint of discomfort should warrant investigation of tumor progression, not just of intolerance to medication treatment. A multitude of pain interventions can now be used across the continuum of care.

Chemotherapy

Only recently has pain relief been measured as an outcome criterion for evaluating responses to chemotherapy. Because concerns with quality of life are now emphasized with palliative chemotherapy,[18] clinicians are encouraged to incorporate assessments of pain and its relief into clinical care practices. Pain intensity, perceptions of pain relief, quality and character of the pain, analgesic requirements, and functional level are all critical endpoints that can be used to evaluate responses to palliative therapy. The toxicities of any therapeutic modality must be weighed against the benefits of relieving pain and distressing symptoms from advanced cancer. Comprehensive staging systems for evaluating cancer pain provide a systematic way to

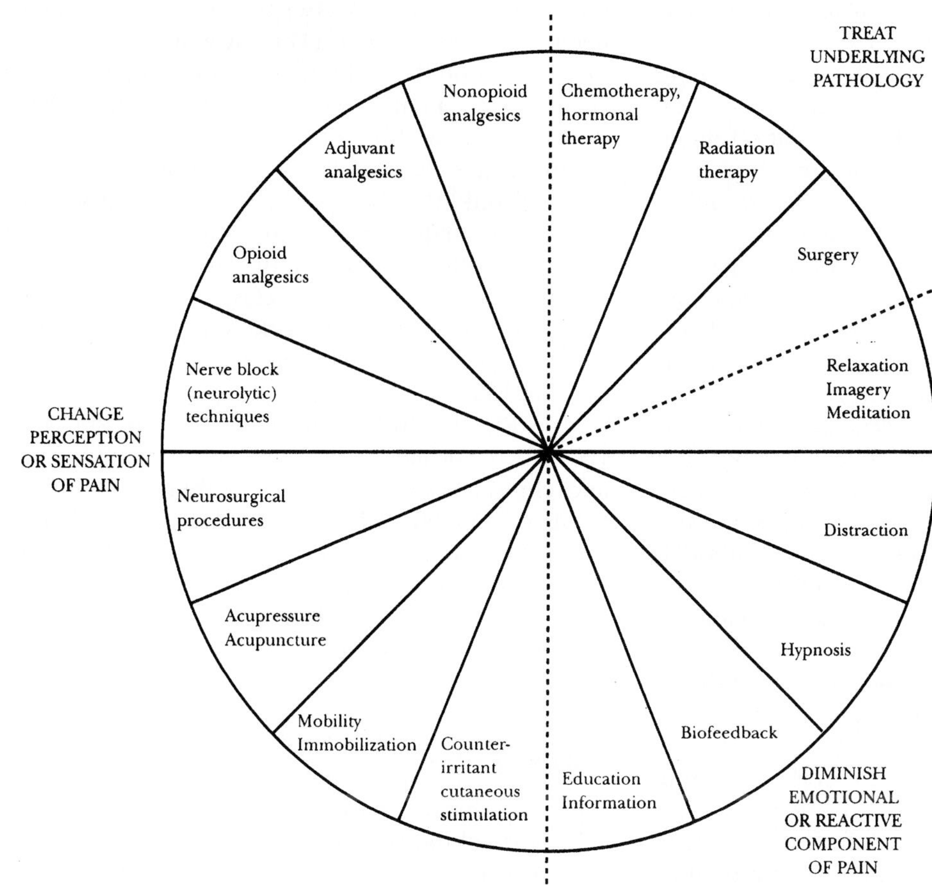

Figure 27-2 Three major approaches to interventions for cancer pain. Data from Polomano, McGuire, Sheidler.[4]

measure pain as an indicator of the efficacy of cancer treatment protocols with chemotherapy and other treatments.

Hormonal therapy plays an important role in the palliation of painful symptoms. While this form of therapy has relatively few side effects, hormonal manipulation is only an option for patients with certain types of cancer, such as cancers of the breast and prostate. Specific hormones can reduce the size of the tumor or slow its growth, typically in painful locations such as the bone and soft tissues. The time course for improvement is more gradual with hormonal therapy than with other treatments, sometimes taking 3–6 weeks before improvements in pain can be observed.[19] Hormonal therapy provides palliation with fewer side effects and may afford significant relief of pain, sometimes even for prolonged periods of time. Investigators have reported favorable responses in painful bony metastases from breast and prostate cancers using a variety of therapies, including estrogen, androgen, progestin, aminoglutethimide, and corticosteroids. The benefits of chemotherapy and steroids have also been investigated for the palliation of hormone-resistant prostate cancer. In a randomized, controlled trial with endpoints of pain control and quality of life, the addition of mitoxantrone to prednisone therapy prolonged the duration of palliation compared to prednisone therapy alone.[20]

Radiation Therapy

Alleviation of pain and improvements in symptoms and quality of life have been the major objectives for palliative radiation therapy. Radiotherapy is a valuable adjuvant to analgesic therapy in alleviating bone pain and an effective tool in the prevention of pathologic fractures, spinal cord compression, and treatment of spinal nerve damage. The presence of pain does not correlate to the type of tumor, location, size, or number of metastatic sites. Unfortunately, there is no way of knowing who will benefit from radiation for palliation of symptoms; however, characteristics of pain prior to treatment may be important predictors. Rutten et al. found that the presence of radiating pain and the pain intensity before therapy are predictors of responses to treatment.[21] Scott stresses the importance of assessing quality of life during palliative radiation therapy and provides a variety of measurement tools that incorporate measures for pain.[22]

External beam radiation therapy (EBRT) has long been an important component of the treatment regimen to relieve localized pain.[23] Local radiation therapy using a variety of dose-fractioning methods and dose schedules has been shown to be effective in relieving pain, especially when pain is limited to one site or region, producing improvements in 60%–90% of patients in several studies.[24,25] Indications for radiotherapy for bone metastases include pain, risk for pathologic fracture, and neurological complications arising from spinal cord compression, nerve root pain, or cranial nerve involvement.[26] Palliative EBRT for bone pain is well tolerated. Side effects are related to total dose or fraction size, and may arise from adjacent healthy tissue.[27] These effects may include nausea, vomiting, diarrhea, and myelosuppression. Although spinal cord compression can be treated with either surgery or radiotherapy, radiotherapy is the treatment of choice because of its convenience and lower cost.[27] The recommended maximum dose for the spinal cord is 40–45 Gy delivered in two Gy fractions five days a week.[27]

The onset and duration of pain relief are influenced by several factors, including the radiation energy source, dose per fraction, total dose, length of treatment, and type and location of cancer. The optimal dose and fractionation of palliative radiation for bony metastases remains controversial. When Gaze et al. studied the effects of two fractionation schedules, they found that a single treatment with 10 Gy was just as effective as 22.5 Gy in five fractionated doses.[28]

The cost of palliative radiation therapy for metastatic bone disease remains a concern. A preliminary evaluation of radiation therapy and chronic opioid therapy showed that brief courses of radiation therapy were significantly better in reducing pain and more cost-effective.[29]

Bone-seeking radioisotopes are commonly used to alleviate pain caused by bone metastases. These radioisotopes are administered parenterally, and all bony metastatic sites are targeted at once, unlike with EBRT.[30] Generally, radioisotopes can be considered in patients with multifocal pain caused by metastatic disease. Available data document the efficacy of radiopharmaceutical agents in relieving pain caused by bone metastases. Strontium-89 and samarium-153 are the most commonly used radioisotopes for relieving pain caused by bony metastases.[31,32] Both are available in the United States. A substantial body of evidence indicates that samarium-153 offers a greater therapeutic benefit than strontium-89.[32] Toxicities include myelosuppression and a temporary painful flare in the location of the pain within a few days following administration. For the first week after administration, patients need to be advised about (1) using a toilet instead of a urinal, (2) double flushing of the toilet after use, (3) cleaning excreta off of the toilet and flushing it down the toilet, (4) washing hands after using or cleaning the toilet, and (5) immediately laundering clothes separately should they be soiled with blood or urine.[33]

There is no difference in the degree or duration of pain relief offered by EBRT or radioisotope therapy. The average onset of pain relief is, however, somewhat slower following the administration of radioisotopes: 2–4 weeks for strontium-89 and 2 days to 2 weeks for samarium-153.[31,32]

186–Re 1,1–hydroxyethylidene disphosphonate (HDEP) is not licensed for use in the United States, and clinical experience with this therapy is limited. Sciuto et al. published a study of 60 patients looking at the short-term effects of HDEP. A total of 80% of patients had prompt relief of pain, 31% experienced complete relief, 34% achieved partial relief, and 14% had only minimal relief of pain.[34]

Surgery

Surgical intervention as a palliative measure is generally performed to prevent or treat complications or oncological emergencies such as obstruction or compression of vital organs or the spinal cord. Palliative surgery can help resolve these serious and often life-threatening complications. In addition, surgical intervention can alleviate tumor burden so as to maximize responses to other modalities such as radiation therapy or chemotherapy. Studies have shown that surgical palliation for pancreatic cancer, gastric and esophageal cancers, and pleural mesothelioma has improved quality of life, disease symptoms, and morbidity.[35–37] Few data, however, demonstrate the long-term outcomes for pain control with these procedures.

Surgical ablation of endocrine glands may indirectly affect tumor growth that depends on the production of certain hormones (e.g., hypophysectomy or bilateral oophorectomy for advanced breast cancer, and orchiectomy for advanced prostate cancer), thereby alleviating pain. Orthopedic procedures are performed to prevent or stabilize fractures of the long bones, spine, and pelvis.

Data are available that document the success of palliative surgical procedures in relieving pain. Harrington described the various innovations in surgical interventions for bony structures invaded by tumors and summarized the favorable outcomes, including pain relief by location and type of procedure.[38] For example, 82% of patients with compromised neurological function from vertebral metastases improved by at

Table 27-1 Examples of Palliative Surgical Procedures

Site and Clinical Condition	Type of Tumor	Palliative Surgical Procedures
Soft tissue/skin metastasis	Breast carcinoma	Surgical excision
	Ulcerating or fungating lesions	Simple mastectomy
	Melanoma	Local excision
Abdominal		
Intestinal obstruction	Colorectal and ovarian carcinoma, peritoneal carcinomatosis	Colectomy (resection and anastomosis)
		Colostomy
		Gastrointestinal bypass
		Placement of gastric or intestinal tube for decompression
	Pancreatic carcinoma	Choledochojejunostomy
Serious ascites	Colon, breast, and ovarian carcinomas	Peritoneovenous shunt
		Paracentesis, Thoracentesis
Acute urinary tract obstruction	Upper tract: Flank and retroperitoneal tumor	Nephrostomy
	Pelvic tract: Cancer of cervix, prostrate, rectum	Cutaneous ureterostomy, cystotomy
Rectovessical fistula	Rectal and cervical carcinoma	Colostomy
Rectovaginal fistula		Colostomy
Malignant lesions of the skeleton	Sarcomas, epithelial tumors, metastatic visceral tumors	Reductive surgery (amputation)
Lesions of the extremities		Disarticulation
Pathological fractures		
Extremities	Metastases from lung, breast, prostate, renal, thyroid carcinomas	Intramedullary fixation
		Prosthetic or replacement reconstruction
	Primary advanced bone and soft tissue tumors	Amputation
Vertebra	Same as above	Spine stabilization
Neuraxial nervous system involvement		
Spinal cord compression	Metastases from lung, breast, prostate, renal, thyroid carcinomas	Decompression laminectomy
	Lymphomas, sarcomas	

Data from Lillemoe[35]; Harrington.[38]

least one functional grade following decompression and stabilization.

Other surgical palliative techniques for pain include the procedures outlined in Table 27-1.[35,38] Therapeutic paracentesis is often indicated for symptomatic relief in the patient with malignant ascites. Abdominal pressure, nausea and vomiting, and dyspnea or orthopnea result in part from a taut abdominal wall and from restricted diaphragmatic excursion.[39] Large-volume paracentesis is considered a safe therapeutic option in such cases. Accumulation of peritoneal fluid can be disastrous for a patient's quality of life — restricting breathing, limiting movement, and requiring frequent visits to the office. Although no treatment is entirely satisfactory, abdominal paracentesis remains the most practical effective measure for most patients with ascites.[40] The main concern post-procedure is hypotension. No more than 4 liters should be drained at any one time. Instead of repeating the paracentesis, an interventional radiologist can place a subcutaneous venous access port. Studies are needed to determine this procedure's long-term effectiveness and safety.

Another palliative procedure is therapeutic thoracentesis. The amount of fluid removed from the lung should be limited to 1–1.5 liters.[41] Dyspnea is the most common presenting symptom, but patients may also report a cough or chest discomfort. Chest discomfort is related to involvement of the pleura, ribs, and other intercostal structures. Repeat thoracentesis is recommended for palliation of breathlessness in patients with a very short life expectancy.[41]

Technological advancements allow for less invasive techniques for tumor ablation and relief of pain. Interventional radiologists may, for example, insert percutaneous transhepatic biliary drains to relieve hepatic congestion and pain associated with biliary obstruction. Embolization and chemoembolization may alleviate pain from organ enlargement or tumor encroachment. Gastroenterologists may perform endoscopic placement of stents to relieve pressure, and drains to alleviate congestion. Photodynamic therapy can be used to reduce tumors in certain areas. (For specific information on these techniques for pain control, consult these sources.[42,43]) A variety of neurosurgical procedures can be performed to interrupt the transmission of pain by disrupting pain pathways; these are discussed in the next section.

The treatment modalities previously described offer one approach to relieving cancer pain — treatment of the underlying pathology. Nursing responsibilities in caring for patients are fairly standard and

Table 27-2 Common Terminology Associated with Analgesics

Efficacy	Degree of analgesic provided by a given dose of an analgesic administered under a particular set of conditions
Dose response	Increase in dose accompanied by increase in effectiveness
Relative analgesic potency	Ratio of doses of two drugs
Relative analgesic potential	Relationship between efficacy and adverse effects
Half-life	Time it takes a drug to fall to half its original concentration in the blood
Opiate receptors	Specific recognition sites on which opioids produce their actions
Tolerance	A state of adaptation in which exposure to a drug induces changes that result in a diminution of one or more of the drug's effects over time
Physical dependence	A state of adaptation that is manifested by a drug class–specific withdrawal syndrome that can be produced by abrupt cessation, rapid dose reduction, decreasing blood level of the drug, and/or administration of an antagonist
Addiction	A primary, chronic, neurobiologic disease, with genetic, psychosocial, and environmental factors, influencing its development and manifestations. It is characterized by behaviors that include one or more of the following: impaired control over drug use, compulsive use, continued use despite harm, and craving.

Data from Bruera, Sweeny[30]; Fitzgibbon[47]; Reisinc, Pasternak[48]; McCaffery, Pasero[49]; American Academy of Pain Medicine.[50]

quite similar to those when the same methods are used as first-line, curative therapies.

Change in Perception/Sensation of Pain

The second major approach to treating cancer pain, changing the perception and sensation of pain, requires knowledge and skills regarding pharmacotherapy and invasive and noninvasive interventional techniques. Figure 27–2 represents a number of interventions that can be used to modify noxious sensory input in the periphery and at the level of the spinal cord and brain.

Pharmacologic Therapy

Pharmacologic therapy with several classes of drugs (e.g., nonopioids, opioids, and adjuvant agents) is generally considered the mainstay for treating cancer pain and is employed for a wide variety of painful conditions. Nurses have a major responsibility to be familiar with all of the pharmacological options for pain, including indications for their use, drug classifications, mechanisms of action, routes of administration, usual starting doses, adverse effects and interventions to manage them, and important outcome measures for monitoring their effectiveness.

Drug therapy with opioid and nonopioid adjuvant medications remains the primary method used to control cancer-related pain. Regardless of the point at which a patient with cancer experiences pain, pharmacological interventions should be considered. (For a comprehensive overview of pharmacological agents used in the management of cancer pain, consult these references.[44–46])

It is critical to understand the classifications of analgesics, pharmacological properties, mechanisms of action, adverse effects, and associated terminology for analgesic medications that are outlined in Table 27-2.[30,47–50] These terms are especially important as they relate to the administration of opioid analgesics. Dosing of opioids has been guided by a simple principle: Provided the source of pain cannot be treated, higher pain levels require opioid doses, with the chief limitation on dose being unacceptable side effects.[51] Confusion exists among health professionals regarding the meanings of *tolerance, physical dependence,* and *addiction.* The American Academy of Pain Medicine, the American Pain Society, and the American Society of Addiction Medicine recognize the definitions of addiction, physical dependence, and tolerance as outlined in Table 27-2. As generally understood, addiction is a state of dependence caused by habitual use of drugs, alcohol, or other substances. The terminology used in pain practice deliberately separates dependence from addiction. Physical dependence is an inevitable consequence of continuous opioid use that is rarely associated with aberrant behavior when opioids are used for the treatment of pain.[50] Unfortunately, widespread misconceptions about these conditions have negatively influenced prescribing patterns for opioid analgesics.

Nonopioids

Nonopioid analgesics are important to the successful use of oral pharmacotherapy in cancer patients with pain.[47] These drugs control pain independently or help reduce the dose of opioid needed for pain control. Three groups of nonopioid analgesics exist:

acetylsalicylic acid (ASA), acetaminophen, and nonsteroidal anti-inflammatory drugs (NSAIDs). All of these drugs possess antipyretic and analgesic properties and exert their analgesic effects in the periphery. Para-aminophenol derivatives such as acetaminophen have no anti-inflammatory properties. In addition, nonopioid drugs have a maximum ceiling effect for their analgesic potential. Acetaminophen and choline magnesium trisalicylate have no antiplatelet properties, while the NSAIDs and aspirin do affect platelet function and coagulation. Antipyretic analgesics are the first line of pain relief therapy, according to the sequence scheme for cancer pain developed by the World Health Organization (WHO).

Acetylsalicylic acid (ASA). A salicylate, ASA is one of the oldest nonopioid analgesics. After oral administration, ASA has an onset of action in 5–30 minutes, peaking after 0.5–2.0 hours, and lasting approximately 3–7 hours.[47] The standard dose is 500–600 mg every 4–6 hours. The administration of greater than 4 g per day can lead to toxic side effects. D'Agati reviewed ASA effects on renal function and found that chronic administration can cause analgesic-associated neuropathy.[52] Gastric problems and bleeding are common adverse effects of therapeutic doses of ASA.[53] This drug should not be given to children younger than age 12 years who have viral illness due to a possible association with Reye's syndrome.

ASA hypersentivity can present in one of two clinical scenarios. Some patients can develop a respiratory reaction with rhinitis, asthma, or nasal polyps.[53] Other patients develop more serious symptoms including urticaria, wheals, hypotension, shock, and syncope within minutes of ingestion. Patients with ASA sensitivity can develop sensitivity to other NSAIDs.

Acetaminophen. Acetaminophen is a nonsalicylate indicated for noninflammatory pain and for fever control. It has no anti-inflammatory action and no antiplatelet activity.[47] A proposed mechanism of action for acetaminophen is inhibition of the third isoform of cyclooxygenase (COX-3), which occurs within the CNS; it may account for the analgesic and antipyretic effects but not the anti-inflammatory action of acetaminophen.[54] Hepatic toxicity increases with dosage of greater than 4 g per day but can occur at lower doses with coexisting liver disease or regular alcohol consumption.[55] The maximum dose for long-term use is 4–6 g per day.[47,53] Acetaminophen is preferred to NSAIDs in the elderly because of its low gastrointestinal and renal toxicity.[56] It is an underrecognized cause of excessive anticoagulation in patients taking warfarin.[57]

Acetaminophen overdose is common because this drug is found in many prescriptions and over-the-counter medications. It is important to discuss the overuse of acetaminophen with patients and their families. The opportunity for providers to educate patients about over-the-counter medications and acetaminophen is tremendous yet is often missed.[58] The maximum daily dosage of acetaminophen is 4 g for adults and 3 g for the elderly.[59] Liver damage has been reported in adults taking daily dosages as low as 6 g. Doses of 5–8 g every day can lead to liver failure.[59] Acetaminophen is hidden in many medications, including over-the-counter cold and cough medicines and opioid/acetaminophen combinations (Vicodin). Certain drug interactions increase the dangers of acetaminophen, such as excessive consumption of alcohol, anticonvulsants, isoniazid, and oral anticoagulants. Patients and their families should be advised that over-the-counter medications should be treated with the same care as prescribed medicines and that advice on recommended doses, contraindications, and interactions should be heeded.[60]

Nonsteroidal anti-inflammatory drugs. Traditional *nonselective NSAIDs*, such as ibuprofen, naproxen, and related agents, are nonselective inhibitors of both COX-1 and COX-2, which catalyze prostaglandin synthesis.[61] This inhibition accounts not only for the analgesic, anti-inflammatory, and antipyretic effects of these agents, but also for side effects such as gastric mucosal damage and renal toxicity. Although NSAIDs are widely believed to be helpful in the management of malignant bone pain, specific clinical data about pain-reducing responses to NSAIDs in cancer patients are sparse.

COX-1, the first isoform identified, is found in platelets, the gastrointestinal tract, the kidneys, and most other tissues. COX-2 is found only in the kidneys and central nervous system and is induced in the peripheral tissue by noxious stimuli that cause inflammation and pain.[53] The therapeutic effects of NSAIDs are due to COX-2 (not COX-1) inhibition. In the 1990s, COX-2 selective NSAIDs became available in the United States. Today, two COX-2 selective NSAIDs are available: celecoxib (Celebrex) and valdecoxib (Bextra).

Nonselective NSAIDs can produce multiple adverse effects on all organs. Common side effects include gastrointestinal upset, dizziness, and drowsiness.[47] NSAIDs may also cause bleeding, alter platelet function, or produce gastric irritation. Nonselective NSAIDs can interfere with oral anticoagulation, prolong prothrombin times, and cause bleeding.

COX-2 *selective NSAIDs* provide the efficacy of the nonselective NSAIDs with significantly less risk of gastrointestinal ulcers and bleeding problems.[62,63]

Much debate has focused on the increased risk of thrombotic cardiovascular events with NSAIDs because of their potential to decrease production of vascular prostaglandin, a vasodilator and inhibitor of platelet aggregation.[26] To date, few clinical trials have been published on the incidence of cardiovascular events of valdecoxib. One study compared the efficacy and safety of valdecoxib and naproxen, and one thrombolytic event was reported in each arm. At this time, no conclusive evidence shows that COX-2 inhibitors cause ischemic vascular events, and no specific randomized trials have been done as yet.[64] Hypertension is also a concern with NSAIDs. Fox et al. completed a clinical trial with a selective COX-2 inhibitor, lumiracoxib, in rats and found that it may offer a potential benefit in treatment of bone pain.[65]

NSAID-associated pain relief is typically characterized both by a ceiling dose, beyond which adding more drug fails to yield further pain relief or produces more severe side effects, and by a lack of demonstrated physical tolerance. One cannot predict the minimal effective analgesic dose, the ceiling dose, or the toxic dose in advance for patients with cancer pain. In general, the following guidelines for nonopioid dosing may be used:

- An increase in dose generally results in increased side effects.

- There is a questionable ceiling effect in cancer pain. To correctly titrate NSAIDs or nonopioids in cancer patients, limit dosing to 1.5 to 2 times the standard recommended dose. At this higher level, check patients' stools for occult blood, monitor protein, and check plasma creatinine levels bimonthly.

- Titrate doses at weekly intervals. If there is no response at the higher levels, then decrease the dose.[47]

Both nonselective and COX-2 selective NSAIDs can induce renal insufficiency.[53] Mechanisms by which NSAIDs affect renal function include decreased synthesis of the renal vasodilator prostaglandin, interstitial nephritis, impaired renin secretion, and enhanced tubular water and sodium reabsorption. COX-2 inhibitors do not seem to have renal-sparing effects and should be considered equally as nephrotoxic as the traditional NSAIDs. These drugs should be used cautiously in patients with underlying risk for NSAID-related nephrotoxicity.[66] Affected patients may develop an abrupt onset of oliguria with sodium and water retention. This condition is usually reversible after discontinuation of the NSAIDs.[53]

Guidelines for dosing in the elderly are available at *www.geriatricsatyourfingertips.org/ebook*. Therapy with either nonselective or selective medication should start at the lowest dose and be titrated slowly in the elderly.[56] Both cancer and nonmalignant pain may respond to selective COX-2 inhibitors, but their uses in cancer pain are not well studied.

The selection of a nonopioid drug for an individual patient is often based on the prescriber's preference and experience with particular agents. To date, little evidence indicates any advantages for one agent over another. Table 27-3 lists the commonly used nonopioid agents and usual dosages. Table 27-4 lists drugs and routes of administration that are *not* recommended.[53–55] Drugs that are available in tablet, suspension, and suppository formulations and that can be administered less frequently may simplify drug-dosing schedules. Table 27-5 highlights important considerations for the use of nonopioids.

The benefits of nonopioids for patients with severe pain who require higher than usual doses of opioids have not been established. Nonopioids can be considered either alone or in conjunction with an opioid when pain is mild. In summary, nonopioids are useful in the management of cancer-related pain. Optimal use of this group of drugs requires a careful medical and analgesic history, especially for patients with complex health problems.[67]

Opioids

Opioid analgesics constitute a class of analgesics that act centrally by interfering with pain perception in the brain. They are classified into three major categories:

1. *Morphine-like opioid agonists.* Opioid agonists are the subclass of opioids that are most useful for managing cancer pain. These agents bind with mu and kappa opioid receptors. The mu opioid receptor is responsible for supraspinal analgesia, respiratory depression, euphoria, and physical dependence. In contrast, the kappa receptor affects spinal analgesia, miosis, and sedation. Commonly used opioids classified as morphine agonists include codeine, fentanyl, hydrocodone, hydromorphone, levorphanol, meperidine, morphine, methadone, and oxycodone.
2. *Opioid antagonists.* These agents exert no agonistic effects on opioid receptor activity; therefore, they possess no analgesic properties. Naloxone (Narcan) is a pure opioid antagonist.
3. *Opioid agonist-antagonists.* Drugs in this category include partial agonists and mixed agonist-antago-

Table 27-3 Nonopioids Commonly Used in Analgesic Treatments of Cancer Pain

Name	Half-Life	Dosing Interval	Starting Dose (mg/day)	Maximum Dose (mg/day)
Acetaminophen	2–3 h	q4h–6h	2000	4000
Acetylsalicylic acid	2–3 h	q4h	2000	6000
Celecoxib (Celebrex)	11 h	q12–24h	200	400
Choline magnesium trisalicylate	9–17 h	q12h	2000	4000
Diclofenac	1–2 h	q8–12h	75–100	200
Diflunisal	8–12 h	q8–12h after loading dose	500–1000	1500
Ibuprofen	3–4 h	q4–6h	1600	3200
Ketorolac (IV, po)	4–9 h	q6h after loading dose	60–120	150
Naproxen	10–20 h	q6–8h	750	1250
Valdecoxib (Bextra)	8–11 h	q12–24h	10	40

Data from American Pain Society.[53]

Table 27-4 Drugs and Routes of Administration *Not* Recommended for the Treatment of Cancer Pain

Drugs	Rationale for Not Recommending
Meperidine	Short duration of analgesia (2-3 hours) Repeated administration may lead to CNS toxicity (tremors, confusion)
Pentazocine butorphanol (Nalbuphine)	Analgesic ceiling effect Risk of withdrawal in opioid-dependent patients Possible psychotomimetic effects (hallucinations, delusions)
Buprenorphine	Analgesic ceiling effect May precipitate withdrawal
Naloxone naltreoxe	May precipitate withdrawal Use limited to treatment of life-threatening respiratory depression
Brompton's cocktail	No evidence of analgesic benefit
DPT (meperidine, promethazine, and chlorpromazine)	Poor efficacy Increased adverse effects
Benzodiazepines (example: alprazolam)	Added sedation Analgesic properties not demonstrated to be effective in neuropathic pain
Barbiturates (benzodiazepines)	No analgesic properties demonstrated Added sedation
Routes	
Intramuscular	Absorption unreliable Should not be used in children May cause abscesses and fibrosis of muscle tissue Causes pain with injection
Transnasal	Only FDA drug approved is butorphanol, which is not recommended

Data from American Pain Society[53]; Chandraseharan et al[54]; Gloth.[55]

nists. Mixed agonist-antagonists block or are neutral at one type of opioid receptor while activating a different opioid receptor. Mixed-agonist analogs include pentazocine, butorphanol titrate, dexzocine, and nalbuphine hydrochloride.[53] It is generally accepted by cancer pain experts that opioid agonist-antagonist drugs have very limited usefulness in cancer pain management because of their propensity to induce opioid withdrawal and cause severe CNS side effects. As a result, these drugs are not discussed in this chapter.

There is certain critical information that nurses, physicians, and pharmacists must know before opioids are prescribed, dispensed, or administered to patients with cancer-related pain. Mechanism of action, purpose and category, common starting dose, equivalence to other analgesics, duration of effect, half-life of the drug, available routes, and adverse effects that are common and unique to certain agents must be known. Table 27-6[53,68,69] contains information about the relative potencies of commonly used analgesics for moderate to severe pain.

All opioid analgesics share common effects as a result of their action. Central nervous system, respiratory, cardiovascular, gastrointestinal, genitourinary, and dermatological effects of these drugs are outlined in Table 27-7. The most common adverse reactions are nausea, somnolence, and constipation. Sedation, a common problem, is addressed in the section that follows on psychostimulants.

Respiratory depression rarely occurs if opioids are given based on rational use and commonly accepted principles. If it does occur, it can be treated easily and successfully with naloxone or with nalmefene, which has a longer duration of action than naloxone. The amount of naloxone a patient receives should be

Table 27-5 Considerations in the Use of Nonopioid Analgesics

Problem	Suggested Nonopioids
Need for strong anti-inflammatory activity	All drugs except acetaminophen
Need for parenteral route	Ketorolac
Risk of thrombocytopenia or other hematological disorder	Acetaminophen, choline magnesium trisalicylate
Impaired renal function	Acetaminophen, diflunisal, sulindac
Altered gastrointestinal function	Acetaminophen, choline magnesium trisalicylate, salsalate, cox-2
Compliance	Diflunisal, naproxen, piroxicam, choline magnesium trisalicylate
Risk of significant adverse side effects	Avoid phenylbutazone, oxyphenbutazone
Need for chronic use	Avoid mefanamic acid, maclofenamate
Cost	Aspirin, acetaminophen

Data from Polomano, McGuire, Sheidler.[4]

titrated to reflect changes in respiratory rate. Rapid bolus injections of naloxone should be avoided in opioid- tolerant patients to avoid precipitating acute physiological withdrawal that can cause nausea, vomiting, agitation, diaphoresis, and intense pain, and lead to life-threatening seizures. Respiratory depression is a concern when patients who have been maintained on opioid agonist drugs receive an interventional anesthetic procedure that may totally eliminate their pain. The stimulus of pain on respiratory function is eliminated, which places the patient at risk for respiratory depression.

Table 27-6 Opioid Analgesics for Severe Pain

Drug	Brand	Oral (mg)	Parenteral (mg)	Half-life (hours)	Duration of analgesia (hours)
Morphine					
Immediate-release	Generic MSIR, Roxanol	30	10	2–4	4–5
Controlled-release	MS Contin, Oramorph SR, Avinza,				8–12
	Kadian				24
Hydromorphone	Dilaudid	8	2	2–3	3–4
Levophanol	Levo-Dromoran	4	2	12–18	4–6
Methadone	Dolophine	10*	5	30–60	5–6
Oxycodone					
Immediate-release	Roxicodone, Tylox, Percocet, Percodan	20	—	3–6	3–6
Controlled-release	Oxycontin				12
Oxymorphone	Numorphan	5 (rectal)	5	2–3	3–6
Tramadol	Ultram	50		7	4–6
Codeine/ acetaminophen	Generic	200	130	3–4	2–4
Hydrocodone/ acetaminophen	Vicodin, Lorcet, Lortab	30	—	3–4	3–4
Fentanyl	Duragesic patch	—	0.1	30–60 min	

*Depends on previous dose; not recommended.

Data from American Pain Society[53]; Portenoy, Rowe[68]; Lynch.[69]

Table 27-7 Common Side Effects of Opioid Analgesics

System	Side Effect
Central nervous	Sedation, drowsiness, mental clouding, euphoria, analgesia, nausea, vomiting, ↓ physical activity, lethargy, mood changes
Respiratory	↓ Respiratory rate, ↓ ventilatory minute volume, ↓ tidal exchange, ↓ PO_2, ↑ PCO_2
Cardiovascular	Hypotension from peripheral vasodilation or histamine release
Gastrointestinal	*Stomach:* ↓ motility; *small intestine:* ↓ propulsive contractions, delayed digestion from ↓ biliary and pancreatic secretions; *large intestine:* ↓ or absent propulsive peristaltic waves, causing delay in passage of contents; *biliary tract:* ↑ pressure from morphinelike drugs, causing epigastric distress to biliary colic
Genitourinary	↑ Tone and amplitude of ureter contractions, ↑ tone of bladder muscles→urgency, ↑ tone of vesical sphincter
Dermatological	Vasodilation of cutaneous blood vessels→ ↑ warmth and flushing of skin on face, neck, and upper thorax, sweating, pruritus

↑ = increased; ↓ = decreased; → = leading to

Data from Bruera, Sweeney[30]; McCaffery, Pasero.[49]

The chemoreceptor trigger zone (CTZ) in the brain is sensitive to chemical stimuli such as opioids. Similar to the effect of chemotherapy-related nausea and vomiting, the CTZ and the vomiting center can be stimulated to produce nausea and vomiting. If a patient experiences opioid-related nausea and vomiting, many options are available.

1. Treat aggressively on initial presentation.
2. Use antiemetics that act at the CTZ, such as prochlorperazine and thiethylperazine.
3. Use metoclopramide if gastroparesis is a possible etiology of the nausea and vomiting.
4. Use an antivertigo drug such as cyclizine or scopolamine if symptoms worsen with movement.
5. Consider drug combinations.
6. Maximize dose response, especially if symptoms partially improve.
7. Prescribe antiemetics on an around-the-clock basis for 1–2 weeks.
8. Switch opioids if other therapies are ineffective.

All patients should begin a bowel regimen with a stool softener when opioid therapy is started.[70] To prevent constipation, patients taking opioid analgesics should take stimulating laxatives such as senna or bisacodyl to increase bowel motility, with or without stool softeners as indicated by stool consistency.[53] Constipation is a significant clinical problem for patients taking chronic opioid therapy. The gut rarely accommodates or becomes tolerant to the effects of opioid analgesics; therefore, measures to prevent constipation must always accompany opioid administration. If measures to prevent and aggressively treat constipation are not instituted, patients can experience serious problems such as a bowel obstruction. The problem may be compounded by change in eating patterns, decreased fluid intake, inactivity, intraabdominal metastases, or concurrent administration of other drugs that cause constipation (e.g., vinca alkaloid antineoplastic agents, tricyclic antidepressants). Dietary measures include encouraging patients to increase their fluid intake, although dietary fiber consumption is rarely sufficient by itself. The patients or a family member should keep a record of when the patient has had a bowel movement.

Use of laxative preparations and stool softeners generally is necessary when patients must take opioids. Table 27-8 lists laxatives that are and are not recommended for treatment of opiate-induced constipation.[69,71,72] Patients frequently require laxatives from more than one category, such as a stimulant laxative and a detergent laxative. It is also important to keep in mind that stool softeners alone have little effect on opioid-induced constipation. Additionally, little evidence supports a strong correlation between opioid dose and the need for a laxative. In the clinical setting, however, an increase in the dose of opioids often necessitates an increased need for laxatives.

Oral naloxone has been investigated as an agent to reverse opioid-induced constipation. Latasch et al. studied 15 patients with opioid-induced constipation.[73] For 12 patients, bowel evacuation occurred within 1–4 hours. Because of the drug's poor bioavailability, higher doses of naloxone administered by the parenteral route are necessary. For managing constipation due to opioid use, some recommend dosages starting as low as 0.8 mg twice daily, with a maximum of 5 mg per day, titrated up to 12 mg per day, monitoring for toxicity and loss of analgesic effect.[74,75]

Alvimopam, a new opioid antagonist, is currently being investigated for cancer pain. Taguchi et al.[75] performed a clinical trial with this agent in postoperative patients. Their results suggest that gastrointestinal opioid receptors play an important role in the recovery of postoperative ileus and decreased length of hospitalization. Alvimopam is not yet approved by the FDA, and further clinical trials are ongoing.

Responsiveness to opioids may be a function of the mechanism producing the pain. Although opioids are commonly used to treat chronic neuropathic pain, limited data are available to guide this practice and few controlled trials have been performed. Considerable controversy has arisen over the last few years regarding

Table 27-8 Laxatives and Opiate Use

A. Laxatives Used for Opiate-Induced Constipation

Category	Common Preparations	Mechanism of Action	Precautions
Saline	Milk of magnesia Magnesium citrate Sodium phosphate	Draw water into the intestinal lumen. The accumulation alters the stool consistency, distends the bowel, and induces peristaltic movements.	Repeated use can alter fluid and electrolyte balance. May cause abdominal cramping.
Osmotic	Lactulose, sorbitol, glycerin, polyethylene glycol	Increase volume in colon and promote water retention.	May cause flatulence. Sweet taste may cause nausea. Excessive amounts can cause diarrhea. Polyethylene glycol: better tolerated; for short-term use only; no studies performed for long-term use.
Stimulant	Bisacodyl, Senna, Ex Lax, Dantrhon	Increase motor activity of bowels by direct action on the intestines.	Bisacodyl: avoid taking within one hour of taking antacids, and avoid with ulcerative lesion in the colon. May cause severe cramping. Prolonged use can cause laxative dependency and loss of normal bowel function.
Detergent	Docusate	Reduce surface tension.	May increase the systemic absorption of mineral oil when administered together.

B. Laxatives ***Not*** Recommended for Opiate-Induced Constipation

Category	Common Preparations	Action	Reasons for Not Recommending
Bulk	Metamucil, Maltsupex Psyllium	Increase size, weight, and frequency of stool, which requires increased fluid intake.	Effectiveness and feasibility in patients is doubtful.
Lubricant	Mineral oil	Reduce friction and coat the stool.	Causes decreased absorption of fat vitamins. May cause incontinence. Long-term use can cause perianal irritation.

Data from Lynch[69]; Mercadante[71]; DiPalma, DeRidder, Orlando, et al.[72]

the use of opioids for neuropathic pain. Historically, neuropathic pain was thought to be less responsive to opioid analgesics. Recently, Rowbotham et al.[76] conducted a double-blind dose-response study,[76] which revealed a greater reduction in the intensity of neuropathic pain during treatment with high doses of opioids than with lower doses. Higher doses did produce more side effects.[76] Patients with a definite or possible/probable component of neuropathic pain experienced significantly less pain relief compared to subjects with nociceptive pain. Patients with head and neck cancer who were experiencing neuropathic pain required greater escalations in their opioid doses compared to patients with other pain syndromes.[77]

In addition to pain mechanisms, factors such as age influence requirements for opioid analgesics. While older patients have been noted to have the same pain intensity levels as younger adults, elderly patients may require smaller amounts of opioid analgesics to achieve a comparable pain relief effect.[78]

Specific drug selection. In some circumstances, the selection of an opioid or other analgesic may be arbitrary or based on the prescriber's experience. The World Health Organization's Analgesic Ladder and Guidelines for cancer pain relief have been utilized widely, both in the United States and internationally. When this stepwise model based on pain severity is used appropriately, there are major benefits and substantial evidence to support guidelines for analgesic prescribing.[79]

Some investigators have attempted to describe physician-prescribing patterns for the treatment of cancer pain. Cherny et al. conducted a survey to determine strategies used by physicians in selecting opioid analgesics and routes of administration for inpatients with cancer pain.[80] There were 182 changes in opioid regimens or doses for 80 of the 100 patients evaluated. The frequency of changes before discharge or death were attributed to the following causes: 31.4% for convenience and adequate pain relief, 25% to diminish side effects, 19.3% to reduce invasiveness of the therapy, and 17.7% to improve pain control and decrease opioid toxicity.

Various patient-related factors influence the selection of a specific opioid, including pain intensity,

Table 27-9 Guidelines for the Use of Opioids in Chronic Cancer Pain

1. Consider the role of this treatment in a multimodal approach.
2. Drug selection
   a. Consider pain intensity, age, whether major organ failure is present (especially renal, hepatic, or respiratory), and presence of coexisting disease.
   b. Consider pharmacological issues (e.g., accumulation of metabolites and effects of concurrent drugs and possible interactions).
   c. Consider individual differences (note prior treatment outcomes) and patient preference.
   d. Be aware of available routes of administration (e.g., oral, intravenous, subcutaneous, transdermal) and formulation (e.g., controlled release or immediate release).
   e. Be aware of cost differences.
3. Route selection
   a. Use least invasive route possible.
   b. Consider patient compliance and convenience.
4. Dosing and dose tritration
   a. Consider previous dosing requirement and relative analgesic potencies when initiating therapy.
   b. Start with low dose and increase until adequate analgesia is achieved or dose-limiting side effects are encountered.
   c. Consider dosing schedule (e.g., around-the-clock or as needed).
   d. Consider "rescue" doses for breakthrough pain.
   e. Recognize that tolerance is rarely the "driving force" for dose escalation; consider disease progression or psychological factors when increasing dose requirements occur.
5. Trials of alternative opioids: Given individual differences in the response to various opioids, consider a trial of another opioid following treatment failure; be aware of incomplete cross tolerance.
6. Treatment of side effects
   a. Be aware of the prevalence and impact of opioid side effects.
   b. Consider a preventive approach in the management of constipation.
7. Monitoring
   a. Monitor pain intensity and pain relief on an ongoing basis.
   b. Make necessary modifications to treatment plan.
   c. Be aware of potential for withdrawal if considering cessation of opioid therapy and need for tapering schedule.

Reprinted with permission from Coyle N, Cherny N, Portenoy RK: Pharmacologic management of cancer pain, in McGuire DB, Yarbro CH, Ferrell BR (eds.): *Cancer Pain Management* (ed 2). Sudbury, MA, Jones and Bartlett, 1995, pp 131–158.[44]

patient age, concomitant medical illnesses, and specific drug characteristics. Opioid administration guidelines are described in Table 27-9.[44] The sections that follow outline specific analgesic drugs and considerations for the clinical management of cancer pain.

Morphine. Morphine remains the standard by which equianalgesic comparisons are established. It is available for oral, parenteral, rectal, and neuraxial (intraspinal, epidural, or subarachnoid) administration. Controlled-release or long-acting morphine permits 8- to 12-hour (MS Contin, Oramorph) or 24-hour (Kadian, Avinza) dosing schedules as opposed to 3- to 4-hour dosing. Klepstad et al.[81] found that sustained-release morphine taken once a day was as effective as immediate-release morphine taken every 4 hours.[81] Depending on the manufacturer, controlled- or sustained-released preparations come in multiple dosing strengths (15, 30, 60, 100, and 200 mg) to allow flexibility in dosing schedules.

Even though morphine is considered an effective oral analgesic agent, it is much less potent when taken orally than when administered parenterally. Parenteral (IV) morphine at 10 mg is equal to 30 mg of oral morphine.[53] A possible explanation for this discrepancy from single to chronic oral dosing might be related to the by-products of morphine metabolism—morphine-3-glucuronide and morphine-6-glucuronide. The accumulation of these metabolites with repeated dosing not only is responsible for analgesia, but also contributes to the development of adverse side effects, especially in patients with altered renal function.[82]

Fentanyl. Fentanyl is available as a parenteral agent and in transdermal and transmucosal delivery systems. Further information regarding fentanyl's use in the management of cancer pain is provided in later sections.

Hydromorphone. Hydromorphone (Dilaudid) can be administered orally, rectally, and parenterally and is a useful alternative to morphine, particularly for the elderly, as there are no known toxic metabolites that may accumulate with repeated dosing.[48]

Methadone and levorphanol. Methadone is an opioid agonist with a number of unique properties—a lack of known active metabolites; a long and unpredictable half-life; high lipid solubility; excellent absorption following rectal and oral routes of administration; longer administration intervals; and extremely low cost.[83–85] Because of methadone's long half-life, dose escalation must be implemented with caution, especially for elderly patients, to reduce the occurrence and severity of side effects.[86] This drug has been used in patients with renal disease who were unable to tolerate morphine because of the accumulation of morphine-6-glucuconide.[35] Methadone is available in a powder that can be used in the preparation of oral, rectal, and parenteral solutions. Its unique pharmocodynamic properties include activity at both the opioid and *N*-methyl-D-aspartate (NMDA) receptors and inhibition of the uptake of catecholamine.[87] The NMDA antagonistic activity results in increased efficacy against hyperalgesia and may explain methadone's greater effectiveness against neuropathic pain.

Recent data reveal that when oral or parenteral methadone is administered at proper doses and intervals, it is a very safe drug for all patients, both in and out of the hospital.[88–90] According to the guidelines for conversion of oral morphine to oral methadone, for patients on lower doses of morphine (30–90 mg), the ratio should be 4:1 morphine to methadone. For patients taking 91–300 mg of morphine, the ratio is 8:1. For example, 300 mg of morphine is approximately 35 mg of methadone. For patients on higher doses of morphine (greater than 300 mg), the ratio should be 12:1.[84] Methadone is generally given three times a day when used for analgesia.[85]

Methadone has a very high oral bioavailability. Thus, when converting from IV to oral methadone, the prudent approach is to perform 1:1 conversion, keeping in mind that some patients will require upward titration close to or equal to a 1:2 ratio. Conversely, when converting oral to IV methadone, the approach is a 2:1 conversion, keeping in mind that some patients switched to the lower IV dose may require upward titration.[84] When IV methadone is administered at a constant infusion rate, the analgesic and sedative effects will increase over the first 12 hours. As a consequence, the rate should not be increased during the initial 12-hour period; instead, as-needed dosing should be used.

In general, methadone should be reserved as a second-line option in the treatment of moderate to severe cancer pain. Bruera et al. published a randomized, double-blind study in which methadone did not produce superior analgesic efficiency or overall tolerability at 4 weeks compared with morphine when used as a first-line strong opioid for the treatment of cancer.[91]

Because dosing schedules for methadone can vary, it is generally recommended that initial therapy begin with longer dosing intervals of 6–8 hours, until responses to analgesia and the effects of the drug's long plasma half-life can be evaluated. Methadone is one of the preferred opioids for patients who are allergic to morphine because its chemical structure is so different.[45]

Levorphanol, a morphine congener with a long half-life (12–16 hours) is available in both oral and parenteral formulations.[83] It is approximately five times more potent than morphine. The normal starting dose is 2 mg every 6 hours. As with methadone, drug accumulation may follow initiation of therapy or dose escalation. Guidelines similar to those suggested for methadone may be helpful for managing patients taking high doses of levorphanol. Because levorphanol may be infrequently prescribed, it may be difficult to obtain from retail pharmacy chains. Similar to methadone, its extended serum half-life makes it less desirable for the elderly.

Oxycodone. Oxycodone, a semisynthetic μ-agonist opioid, has been prescribed for decades. Oxycodone is the only opioid beside morphine currently available in the United States. Levy described this drug as the ideal opioid because of its short half-life, long duration, and rapid onset of action.[92] Historically, oxycodone has been used in relatively low doses (e.g., 10 mg q4h), either alone or in combination with aspirin or acetaminophen. It is available in both immediate- and controlled-release formulations. Research and extensive clinical use of controlled-release oxycodone have shown it to be comparable to controlled-release morphine and more convenient than immediate-release opioids for treatment of cancer pain.[92] Current equianalgesic tables suggest that oxycodone 20 mg given orally provides the same dose as morphine 30 mg given orally. Oxycodone is now available as a controlled-release preparation (OxyContin) in 10-, 20-, 40-, and 80-mg tablets for every-12-hour dosing.

Opioids not recommended for cancer pain. Meperidine (Demerol) is not recommended for the treatment of chronic cancer pain.[12] Even though its use has declined considerably, some clinicians are not aware of its risk for producing serious toxic side effects such as agitation, tremors, myoclonus, and seizures. Additionally, it has poor oral efficacy.[48]

Proproxyphene, the active opioid in Darvocet, is structurally similar to methadone, but is a very weak opioid with few advantages in the treatment of chronic pain. Its short analgesic duration and longer plasma half-life with accumulation of a toxic metabolite present several risks when the drug is administered to elders.[8]

Other agents

Tramadol has dual action. It is an opioid agonist and blocks the reuptake of serotonin and norepinephrine. This drug can be considered a weak opioid similar to codeine. The normal dose range is 50–100 mg every 4–6 hours, and side effects include dizziness, nausea, sedation, dry mouth, and diaphoresis. To minimize side effects, the dose should be gradually titrated over a few weeks to a month and should not exceed 400 mg per day in any situation.[53] Caution should be taken when tramadol is used in patients also receiving tricyclic antidepressants because of the increased risk of CNS depression, seizure, and psychomotor impairment. Tramadol is not a controlled substance in the United States.[53]

Adjuvant analgesics

Adjuvant analgesics were originally indicated primarily for uses other than pain management. ''Adjuvant analgesic'' can be used to describe any drug that has a primary indication other than pain but that is analgesic in some painful conditions.[68] In cancer patients, this type of agent is given to enhance pain relief when there is a poor response to the opioids or it becomes necessary to reduce the dose of opioids because of intolerable side effects. According to Breitbart, psychotropic drugs such as antidepressants, anticonvulsants, and psychostimulants play an important role at each step of the WHO Analgesic Ladder, especially in the treatment of neuropathic pain.[93] Breitbart provides an excellent overview of the considerations that apply when selecting these agents for pain control and offers guidelines for their use in clinical practice. Although several classes of adjuvant analgesics exist, only the most common agents are discussed here.

Tricyclic antidepressants. Tricyclic antidepressants (TCAs) have demonstrated significant benefits for the management of neuropathic pain. The analgesic effects of TCA may be seen at lower doses (25–100 mg/day) than commonly recommended antidepressant doses (150–300 mg/day). Amitriptyline is the most common adjuvant analgesic used in cancer patients with neuropathic pain.[94] This antidepressant has demonstrated efficacy in the treatment of many chronic nonmalignant neuropathic pain syndromes, headache, and somatic pain.[53,95] For the treatment of cancer pain, TCAs have been effective in relieving pain caused by infiltration of nerves or by treatment-related injury such as postmastectomy pain syndrome.[96] Tricyclic antidepressants help to reduce continuous dysesthetic and burning sensations and the cutaneous hypersensitivity associated with nerve injury. Mercadante et al. conducted a clinical trial on 16 cancer patients with neuropathic pain, and concluded that amitriptyline does not provide a substantial decrease in the amount of pain experienced.[94] In light of their results, the use of amitriptyline should be questioned. More clinical trials are needed to determine definitively the usefulness of TCAs in cancer patients.

Although selective serotinin reuptake inhibitors (SSRIs; e.g., fluoxetine, paroxetine, sertraline) have not been proven to exert analgesic effects, treatment with any of these agents can substantially improve the depression that accompanies chronic pain. Interactions do occur with concomitant administration of TCAs and SSRIs, so nurses should consult the literature for recommended dosing modifications and approaches for monitoring adverse effects. The drug-to-drug interaction with citalopram (Celexa) and escitalopram (Lexapro) makes these two agents the SSRIs of choice for concurrent treatment with a TCA.[53]

Payne recommends that a low starting dose of 10 mg be administered at bedtime, especially for elderly patients.[45] The dose can be increased to 25 mg in 3 days, then escalated by 25 mg every 3–7 days as tolerated. Analgesic effects usually occur within 4–7 days after achieving an effective daily dose, which consists of 50–150 mg of amitriptyline.[68] It is often necessary to administer daily doses of 75–150 mg before significant pain-relieving effects are observed. Tricyclic antidepressants are contraindicated in patients with cardiac conduction abnormalities. Slower and lower incremental increases may be necessary for elderly patients.

The major adverse effects from TCAs are anticholinergic effects such as dry mouth, constipation, postural hypotension, urinary retention, and sedation. These effects can be troublesome, especially if a patient is already receiving opioid analgesics that cause similar problems. If treatment is unsuccessful, the dose should be tapered, which will decrease the risk of withdrawal.

Anticonvulsants. The site and mechanism of action for anticonvulsants given for cancer-related pain are not well understood. Although anticonvulsants are used widely in chronic pain, surprisingly few trials show analgesic effectiveness.[97] The actual improvement of pain scores in those who received gabapentin in clinical trials was not dramatic.[98] Likewise, the magnitude of response to other anticonvulsants has been limited. Nevertheless, very few effective treatments for neuropathic pain exist, so even a modest benefit is meaningful.[55] Similar to TCAs, anticonvulsants are used to treat neuropathic pain. Agents such as carbamazepine (Tegretol), gabapentin (Neurontin), phenytoin (Dilantin), valproate, and clonazepam (Klonopin) are particularly effective for neuropathic pain syndromes. Anticonvulsant drugs may offer benefits in the treatment of direct peripheral nerve injuries such as herpes zoster–related pain or centrally mediated pain from nerve damage. Studies have documented the efficacy of gabapentin for the treatment of neuropathic pain.[99,100] McCaffery provides anecdotal evidence that gabapentin is effective for lancinating pain.[101]

Gabapentin is the best-tolerated anticonvulsant for neuropathic pain.[53] It has significant advantages over the other agents because of its relatively low toxicity.

Table 27-10 Anticonvulsants for Pain Management

Drug	Dose	Indications	Adverse Effects
Carbamazepine	100–200 mg PO bid Increase every other day to 800 mg/day in divided doses.	Useful for paroxysmal and lancinating, shooting, electric shock–like pains	Sedation, drowsiness, diplopia, ataxia, hematological toxicity
Clonazepam	0.5–1.5 mg/day PO Maximum 3–4 mg/day in divided doses.	Same as above Useful for preexisting anxiety	Sedation, ataxia, behavioral disturbances, mood or mental changes
Gabapentin	300–900 mg tid (900–2400 mg) PO Initial dose 100 mg tid, then increase by 100 mg/day as tolerated. May titrate up to 3600 mg/day. For elders, increase slowly: 100 mg/day q3–5 days.	Same as above	Sedation, ataxia, dizziness, difficulty concentrating, visual abnormalities
Phenytoin	300–500 mg/day PO	Same as above	Sedation, drowsiness, ataxia, diplopia, nausea, skin rash, or hypertrichosis
Valproic acid	15–60 mg/kg/day PO in divided doses	Same as above	Behavioral, mood, or mental changes; hepatotoxicity, visual disturbances, coagulopathy or thrombocytopenia, bleeding

Data from Payne[45]; Rowbotham, Harden, Stacey, et al.[102]

Unlike carbamazepine and clonazepam, gabapentin is less sedating. In addition, gabapentin does not produce the hematological effects that are often a concern with carbamazepine and phenytoin. While somnolence, dizziness, ataxia, fatigue, and cognitive dysfunction have been linked to gabapentin, many of these adverse effects can be prevented with slow dose escalations. An initial dose of 100 mg twice daily can be administered, with dose increases of 100 mg/day every 3–5 days, as tolerated, to achieve a thrice-daily dosing schedule. Typically, patients will require at least 900–1200 mg per day; however, higher daily doses of 3600 mg have been suggested to maximize pain control.[102] Gabapentin dosing must be reduced for patients with renal insuffiency. Table 27-10 lists common doses and toxicities of five common anticonvulsants.

Many new anticonvulsants have been developed but not yet studied in cancer patients. These anticonvulsants include topiramate (Topamax), tiagabine, oxcarbazepine, and levetiracetam (Keppa). In the United States, zonisamide and levtiracetam are available and may be considered in refractory cases.[68]

Antispasmodic agents. Baclofen is generally used for spasticity but may also be administered to treat neuropathic pain. Long clinical experience with this drug suggests that it may be useful in all types of neuropathic pain. The dose ranges from 30 mg/day to greater than 200 mg/day.[68] Baclofen can be administrated orally or intrathecally. Side effects include drowsiness, confusion, nausea, vomiting, and ataxia. The drug has been reported to produce analgesic effects in the absence of muscle spasms in patients with neuropathic pain who did not respond to opioids.[103] Of note, patients with neuromuscular disease who are given antispasmodic agents may become immobile due to the drugs' effects if their spasticity is needed for movement. Gradual escalation from a low initial dose optimizes the benefit of baclofen.

Local anesthetics. Local anesthetics may be used in the treatment of pain. To date, limited data have been published to show the effectiveness in neuropathic pain in cancer patients. See the section on topical medication to learn more about EMLA cream and Lidoderm. Oral local anesthetic congeners available as systemic antiarrhythmic agents have proved disappointing for neuropathic pain due to their low efficacy and extensive side effects.[53] Both mexiletine and tocainide have provided disappointing results.

NMDA receptor antagonists. Data from animal models suggest that NMDA (*N*-methyl-D-aspartate) receptor activity plays an important role in many chronic pain states. Small human clinical trials showed a response to NMDA receptor antagonists and relief of some types of neuropathic pain.[104] However, these agents' use is restricted by their tendency to cause unpleasant adverse reactions such as hallucinations, vivid dreams, and delirium. The NMDA receptors may also be responsible, in part, for tolerance that develops to opiate analgesics.[58]

Both dextromethorphan (DM) and ketamine are NMDA antagonists. The effectiveness of dextromethorphan in humans has not been well studied either as monotherapy for in combination with other analgesics. Mercadante et al. added DM to therapy with NSAIDs and morphine and found that no significant benefits were provided by the inclusion of DM.[105]

Ketamine, a parenteral anesthetic, has potent analgesic properties at lower doses. It has been used as an analgesic in palliative care for approximately 10 years.[106] It also seems to exert its greatest effect on neuropathic pain syndromes. Bell et al. reviewed the results of clinical trials utilizing ketamine over the past few years.[107] The evidence base for ketamine as an adjuvant to opioid for cancer pain is weak. The available literature allows for only a cautious conclusion that ketamine may have potential efficacy as an adjuvant to opioids for cancer pain.[107]

Psychostimulants. Psychostimulants are useful in counteracting the sedation that accompanies opioid analgesics. If the sedation is present without any other CNS problems, such as delirium or confusion, and if pain occurs when the opioid dose is lowered, a psychostimulant may be indicated. In addition, these agents can potentiate opioid analgesia and allow for more rapid escalations of opioid doses to treat complex pain syndromes.

Typically, amphetamines (e.g., dextroamphetamine) or the drug methylphenidate is used to counteract opioid-induced sedation. Amphetamines are more powerful CNS stimulants than methylphenidate; however, both decrease the central depression caused by sedating drugs. The recommended starting dose for methylphenidate is 5–10 mg; the recommended starting dose for dextroamphetamine is 2.5 mg. The initial dose is given in the morning. If the morning dose is well tolerated, an early-afternoon dose may be administered to counteract midday sedation. Modafanil has been used but no studies have proved its effectiveness.

Psychostimulants' more desirable side effects include increased alertness, increased ability to concentrate, mood elevation, euphoria, and an increase in motor and speech activity. Unpleasant side effects include confusion, agitation, dysphoria, and apprehension.

The use of psychostimulants has become an acceptable practice based on data from earlier studies of patients with cancer. Bruera et al. conducted a study to assess the effectiveness of patients receiving methylphenidate for cancer-related fatigue.[108] The preliminary data suggest that methylphenidate rapidly improves fatigue and other symptoms, although more clinical trials are needed to elucidate its effects more fully. Methylphenidate has the advantage of a short half-life, which may enable it to provide clinical improvement in fatigue during the second half of the day without causing signs of anxiety or residual insomnia.[108]

Phenothiazines/antihistamines. According to Dundee and Moore, the myth that promethazine potentiates analgesia originated from "observations after its promethazine's use with large doses of pethidine [meperidine] or other analgesics, and erroneously attributing reductions in barbiturate dosage and side effects during anesthesia to the promethazine."[109,p.96] Even though promethazine was purported to have antianalgesic properties almost 30 years ago, the potentiation myth is still widely believed today. Keats and colleagues found that promethazine did not increase analgesic efficacy, increase meperidine-induced respiratory depression, or prevent meperidine-induced nausea and vomiting, but that it did increase the sedative effects of meperidine.[110] Methotrimeprazine (Levoprome) is the only phenothiazine that has demonstrated analgesic properties, but it is not available in the United States.

Haloperidol (Haldol) has not been found to possess any opioid-sparing effects. However, this agent can be prescribed to treat opioid-induced acute confusional states, including hallucinations and agitation from delirium.

Hydroxyzine (Vistaril) does have mild analgesic, antiemetic, sedating, and antihistamine effects, but its analgesic benefits have been demonstrated only with intramuscular injection. Oral hydroxyzine is a useful adjunct for nausea and anxiety.

Steroids. Steroids are essential for reducing swelling, inflammation, and compression that result from the direct or indirect effects of tumor growth and that may lead to permanent nerve damage. Emergent steroid therapy is warranted for impending spinal cord compression and the severe pain that accompanies tumor encroachment on spinal nerves.[111] The pain-relieving qualities of steroids when used as adjuvant analgesics with opioids have been observed clinically and have been reported in the literature. Dexamethasone has been shown to reduce pain and fatigue and to increase activity levels for patients with advanced lung cancer.[112] Clinical practice encourages once-daily dosing to decrease glucocorticoids' side effects, such as sleep disturbances. Corticosteroids such as dexamethasone can increase the appetite and assist in providing some patients with an improved sense of well-being.[113]

Glucocorticoid treatment (dexamethasone 16 mg/day or its equivalent) may be useful in managing pain caused by malignant lesions. Effects of dexamethasone may diminish after 4–6 weeks.[114] Rapid withdrawal of glucocorticoids may exacerbate pain.[53]

Some adverse effects caused by steroids — in particular, increased appetite and elevation of mood — may be desirable for some patients, especially those with advanced disease. Other toxicities, such as proximal myopathy, steroid-induced hyperglycemia, and cushinoid side effects, need to be considered seriously if steroids are used early in the disease course to treat pain. It is generally recommended that steroids be reserved for those patients with advanced disease or for short-term use.[45]

Bisphosphonates

Bisphosphonates clearly have palliative effects on bone pain and may improve quality of life or delay its decline for patients with bone metastases. Intravenous bisphosphonates, such as pamidronate and zoledronic acid, have clinically relevant analgesic effects in patients with metastatic bone pain.[115] Baseline serum creatinine level should be measured before every dose of IV bisphosphonates, and the rate of infusion should be monitored closely.[116] Berenson reported mild to moderate elevation of serum creatinine in approximately 10% of patients receiving IV bisphosphonates.[117] Bisphosphonate administration has become the mainstay of treatment for malignancy-induced hypercalcemia because this class of drugs is well tolerated and effective.[118] Data support the usefulness of these agents for relieving bone pain and improving outcomes for patients with metastatic bone involvement.

Pamidronate has significant benefits in relieving pain from bony metastases that do not respond to NSAIDs and steroids. Small et al. conducted a multicenter, randomized, placebo-controlled study of pamidronate in patients with metastatic prostate cancer.[119] Pamidronate disodium failed to demonstrate a significant benefit compared with placebo in palliation of bone pain or reduction of adverse side effects.[119] However, when Theriault et al. conducted a trial on 372 females with breast cancer, they found patients who received pamidronate had less skeletal complications and longer times to the first skeletal-related events.[120] While the cost of therapy and the time necessary to administer the infusion are important to consider with pamidronate's use, economic considerations must be weighed against more costly alternatives such as surgery or radiation.[121]

Zoledronic acid, a newer-generation bisphosphonate, has been approved for patients with bone metastases secondary to prostate, lung, renal cell, and other solid tumor cancers[116] Its indication is broader than that of pamidronate, and it is a highly potent bisphosphonate.[117] Three large, double-blind, randomized, phase III trials were conducted to investigate the efficacy of zoledronic acid.[122,123] In these trials, zoledronic acid was shown to be highly active in the treatment of bone metastatic. Saad et al. conducted a study of 643 patients randomized to receive either zoledronic acid or placebo.[124] Pain scores in all patient groups increased throughout the study but were lower in the zoledronic acid group. Zoledronic acid has also been compared with pamidronate and shown to have superior efficacy.[125] The recommended dose is 4 mg intravenously over more than 15 minutes every 3–4 weeks.[126]

Table 27-11 Routes of Opioid Administration

Route	Comments
Oral	Preferred in cancer pain management; effective, convenient, and safe
Sublingual	Used for short-term management; may yield flucuating serum concentration with erratic pain control
Transmucosal	Optimal dose found via titration; available in fentanyl
Transdermal	Available in fentanyl; application every 3 days, 12–16 hours to achieve therapeutic effect and 18 hours to achieve a steady state
Rectal	Available in hydromorphone, oxymorphone, and morphine; absorption is variable
Topical	First few application often associated with increase in pain but over time (days) a decrease in pain; Lidocaine patch 12 hours on and 12 hours off; may use up to 3 patches to cover the affected area
Parenteral	IM administration is not recommended; clearest indication is use subsequent to an inability to tolerate oral medication
Intraspinal	Morphine is the gold standard; usually administrated via implantable infusion pump; may be cost-effective

Data from Polomano, McGuire, Sheidler[4]; American Pain Society.[53]

Routes of opioid administration

A variety of routes of opioid administration are available. Individualized plans of care should be developed in collaboration with the patient and the physician. Table 27-11 briefly describes the routes of opioid administration. Six routes of opioid administration are briefly described here: (1) oral (which may also include sublingual and transmucosal routes, although they are infrequently used), (2) transdermal, (3) rectal, (4) topical, (5) parenteral (which includes subcutaneous and intravenous routes) delivered by intermittent bolus or infusion, and (6) intraspinal or neuraxial (which includes epidural, subarachnoid, and intraventricular routes) by intermittent bolus or continuous infusion via external or implanted pumps.

Oral. The oral route is preferred over all other routes because it is an effective, comparatively inexpensive, convenient, and safe way to administer opioids. Oral dosing schedules should be used for as long as possible. If patients have a functional gastrointestinal system and can swallow the required number of tablets or amount of oral solution to achieve adequate pain control, then the oral route is the most appropriate route of administration.

Switching patients from the oral route to an alternate route should be considered if high doses of oral opioids are ineffective or if toxicities occur that cannot be successfully managed. For example, severe nausea and vomiting that cannot be controlled with aggressive antiemetic therapy may be one reason to convert patients to another route of administration. Difficulty swallowing, mechanical obstruction of the gastrointestinal tract, and inability to ingest large amounts of oral medication may necessitate the use of other dosing formulations. Some tablets can be crushed and put into concentrated suspensions. Oral controlled-release opioids must never be crushed because doing so renders them in an immediate-release form and can cause severe toxicity.[53] Oral morphine controlled-release capsules containing beads (Kadian, Avinza) can be opened and sprinkled on food to assist patients who have difficulty swallowing pills. High doses of oral opioids are often necessary, but as long as effective pain relief can be achieved, high doses are not a reason to switch patients to alternate routes of administration. In general, assessing the patient's response to several different oral opioids is advisable before changing the oral route to a more invasive route of delivery.

Onset of action occurs within 45 minutes and peak drug effects in 1–2 hours after administration for most immediate-release and some controlled-release medications. Patients may, therefore, take a second opioid safely if they have not achieved pain control with the first dose.

The scheduling of oral medications should be on a fixed-interval basis, except in a few circumstances when it may be necessary to use a variable dosing schedule. These situations include (1) initial dose titration with methadone and levorphanol; (2) use of concomitant therapies, such as radiation and chemotherapy, that may relieve pain, thereby reducing the need for scheduled opioid analgesics; (3) simultaneous scheduling with around-the-clock administration to provide for incident or breakthrough pain (this also applies to continuous infusions); and (4) pain that is intermittent.

Sublingual. The sublingual route using concentrated oral solution preparations can administer opioids such as morphine or oxycodone. For patients who are unable to take oral medication, this route can be used intermittently for short-term management of breakthrough pain or on a regular schedule in the last few days or weeks of life. It is important, however, to recognize that sublingual administration may yield fluctuating serum concentrations with erratic pain control; thus, vigilant assessment is necessary.

Transmucosal. Oral transmucosal fentanyl citrate (OTFC) has been shown to be an effective delivery method for breakthrough pain.[127] Farrar et al. conducted a randomized, double-blind, placebo-controlled trial to evaluate the safety and efficacy of transmucosal fentanyl citrate in the treatment of breakthrough pain in cancer patients.[128] The OTFC consisted of fentanyl incorporated in a lozenge. The preparation proved effective in relieving pain within 15 minutes, and patients receiving the transmucosal fentanyl required fewer "rescue" doses with other opioids. Approximately half of the dose dissolves in the saliva and is absorbed rapidly through the oral mucosa; the rest is swallowed and absorbed in the GI tract. Plasma concentrations peak 5–10 minutes after lozenge consumption, which typically takes 15 minutes.[129] This direct entry of fentanyl into the circulation avoids first-pass metabolism, allowing the patient to attain effective opioid levels more rapidly than with oral administration. The optimal dose is found through titration and not predicated by around-the-clock dosing of opioids. OTFC is available in six dosage strengths—200, 400, 600, 800, 1200, and 1600 μg—to allow for individualization of therapy.[130] Consult the manufacturer's documentation for information about dosing guidelines and equinanalgesic conversions to other opioids.

Transdermal. The transdermal fentanyl system (Duragesic) is currently the only commercially available opioid preparation in the form of a patch, with dosing strengths of 25, 50, 75, and 100 μg. Fentanyl, which is 75–100 times more potent than morphine, is delivered through the skin in a constant-release delivery system. Approximately 92% of the drug is absorbed into the systemic circulation by 72 hours,[33] requiring applications of the patch every 3 days. While the preparation has been shown to produce effects on pain relief, sleep, and symptoms comparable to controlled-released oral morphine, greater patient satisfaction has been reported with the transdermal system.[131] Its use, however, is reserved for patients with steady-state pain. Significant delays in achieving analgesia can be encountered if this system is used for patients with rapidly escalating pain. A total of 12–16 hours is needed after application of the patch to achieve a therapeutic effect and 18 hours to achieve a steady state in the blood. Rescue or supplemental opioid medication is generally required to control incident or breakthrough pain. Patterns of supplemental medication usage must be assessed as well. The patch dose should be raised if additional supplemental medication is needed 48 hours following the application. Some patients may require patch changes every 48 hours, but this step should be considered only when an increase in the dose has been tried.

The potency of the transdermal fentanyl patch relative to other opioids has not been well established. The package insert suggests fentanyl 25 μg every hour is equivalent to oral morphine 30 mg every 8 hours.[53] Donner et al. suggest that 25 μg per hour may be replaced by approximately 45 mg per day oral morphine in cancer patients.[132] It has been proposed that conversion from the transdermal form to the intravenous form is a 1:1 ratio.[54]

Multiple studies of transdermal fentanyl have been performed in both cancer and noncancer patients. Ahmedzai and Brooks confirmed the efficacy of transdermal fentanyl patch in cancer patients.[133] Recently, van Seventer et al. found transdermal fentanyl to be equal to oral morphine as a treatment for the pain of cancer patients.[134]

Several unique features of the transdermal delivery system have important clinical implications. First, after removing the patch, release of the drug from the skin depot will continue for several hours. This issue is important if patients experience significant sedation or respiratory depression, because simply removing the patch does not eliminate the risk of further problems from drug toxicity. Therefore, continued monitoring for side effects is necessary. Second, variability in body temperature of 3°C can increase the serum concentration by 25%. Finally, variability in skin thickness can significantly affect serum concentrations. Thin skin can produce 1.5 times and broken skin 5 times the normal serum value. Death has resulted from extraneous uncontrolled heating of the fentanyl patch.[53] Using a research-based approach, Wakefield et al. identified the need for nursing education to ensure the appropriate use of more expensive drug delivery systems.[135] It is critical that nurses understand the pharmacodynamics of the transdermal fentanyl system, proper placement of the patch on the upper torso of the body, and—more important—practice implications should side effects occur.

Rectal. With the advent of the transdermal fentanyl system and innovations in infusional delivery devices, there is no longer as much need for rectal administration of opioids. In some circumstances, however, the rectal route is an acceptable alternative. When administered rectally, opioids appear to undergo prompt systemic absorption.[136] Patients who are unable to take oral medication in the last few days of life may benefit from rectal opioids. Rectal preparations are commercially available for nonopioids (e.g., acetaminophen, aspirin, indomethacin) and opioids (e.g., morphine, hydromorphone, oxymorphone). In the United States, rectal suppositories are available in hydromorphone (3 mg), oxymorphone (5 mg) and morphine (5, 10, 20, and 30 mg).[53] Oral to rectal conversion is 1:1 ratio. The rectal route of administration is not recommended for patients who have diarrhea, anal or rectal lesions, mucositis, neutropenia, or thrombocytopenia.

Moolenaar et al. conducted a study and found controlled-release morphine sulfate suppositories to be safe and effective in cancer pain relief.[137] In the clinical trial, the media plasma concentration of the suppository form was found to be 30% higher than that of the oral form. Although not yet approved by the FDA, rectal administration of the controlled-release form is a widely used method of opioid delivery in the palliative care setting.[138] Table 27-12 summarizes the advantages and disadvantages of rectal opioid administration.

Topical. Topical agents are generally effective in reducing inflammation and the cutaneous hypersensitivity that accompanies neuralgias and neuropathic pain. Capsaicin, manufactured from hot peppers, is a safe and effective analgesic agent that is used for the treatment of arthritis pain, herpes zoster–related pain, diabetic neuropathy, and postmastectomy pain.[139] When applied regularly to the skin of painful areas, capsaicin depletes the nerve terminals of substance P, a peptide responsible for the transmission of pain. The first few applications are often associated with increased pain, but over time (typically a few days), some patients will experience a decrease in pain and hypersensitivity of the skin. In Paice et al.'s study of the efficacy of capsaicin in treating HIV-associated peripheral neuropathy, the researchers found no improvement in measures of pain, pain relief, sensory perception, quality of life, mood, or function when patients received capsaicin compared to placebo.[140] The dropout rate was high. Adding a topical anesthetic when using capsaicin and initiating therapy with the lower concentration of the cream or lotion may improve compliance with initial therapy. Capsaicin is available in nonprescription strengths of 0.025% (Zostrix Cream, Capzacin-P Cream, Capsin Lotion) and 0.075% (Zostrix-HP Cream, Capsin Lotion). Patients are advised to wash their hands thoroughly after use and to avoid touching the affected area after applying the preparation.

EMLA cream (eutectic mixture of local anesthetics—specifically, prilocaine and lidocaine) is another topical agent that reduces the cutaneous hypersensitivity associated with neuropathic pain. Once applied, it is necessary to cover the area with an occlusive

Table 27-12 Advantages and Disadvantages of Rectal Opioid Administration

Advantages	Disadvantages
• Absorption is not delayed by alterations in GI tract, such as vomiting	• Wide variation in systemic availability
• Useful if patients have difficulty swallowing, are unconscious, or NPO	• Delayed or limited absorption due to small surface area
• Drug can be removed if an adverse drug reaction develops	• Defecation or constipation may impair absorption
• Digestive enzymes do not affect drug breakdown	• Rectal-wall enzymes or microorganisms may degrade drug
• No unpleasant taste	• Invasive
• Significant first-pass effect from the liver may be avoided	• Self-medication may be difficult or impossible
• Easier to learn than sophisticated pump technology	
• Low cost	

GI = gastrointestinal; NPO = nothing by mouth.

Data from American Pain Society.[53]

dressing such as a transparent (TegaDerm, or plastic wrap) or nonabsorbable covering. While the efficacy of topical NSAIDs has not been established, a variety of preparations (e.g., ketoprofen gel) are compounded for individual client use. Maximal anesthesia is reached in 2–3 hours after application and lasts approximately 1–2 hours after removal.

Topical lidocaine 5% patches (Lidoderm) are approved for postherpetic neuralgia and have been successful in treating a variety of neuropathic pain syndromes.[53] The patches are worn for 12 consecutive hours per day (12 hours on/12 hours off). A potential handicap is that some patients do not find pain relief lasting 24 hours.[141] Clinical evidence suggests that when the lidocaine patch is removed for 12 hours, one-third of patients will continue to report pain relief, one-third will report a gradual increase in pain, and one-third will have a rapid return of pain within 1 hour.[142] Overall, skin reactions at patch applications are minimal and resolve without clinical intervention. Recent studies have shown that the application of a topical drug onto painful skin areas appears to be a safe therapy.[143] The patches can be cut to fit the affected area, and as many as three patches can be used simultaneously. The patches are an alternative for neuropathic pain, especially in small, localized areas.

Parenteral. Although intramuscular (IM) injections are commonly used, this route of analgesic administration should be abandoned.[53] The mere act of giving IM injections can add to patients' emotional and physical trauma. Giving IM injections is not a benign procedure, and numerous accounts in the literature describe complications related to improper administration of injections.[144] Complications include nerve damage, abscesses at injection sites and muscle fibrosis. This route is not recommended for children or older adults.[53,145] Slowed IM absorption can result in delayed or prolonged effects, altered serum levels, and toxicity at the injection site. Large IM opioid doses often produce a peak serum concentration that overshoots the serum concentration needed for effective analgesia.[146] Absorption is variable, depending on the site of injection. Alternative drug routes of delivery—most commonly subcutaneous—are more reliable and less painful. Intermittent subcutaneous injections can be administered to control both acute and chronic cancer-related pain, if peripheral or central venous access is not possible. If prolonged analgesic administration is required, intermittent injections should not be used and other routes that do not produce pain on administration should be considered.

Intravenous bolus is a common alternative to intramuscular or subcutaneous injections; however, scheduled bolus injections produce significant peak-and-trough effects with fluctuating levels of pain relief. If doses need to be given every 2 hours or less, then continuous parenteral infusion may be more appropriate Time to peak effect varies, ranging from 1–5 minutes for fentanyl to 15–30 minutes for morphine.[53] For patients who cannot absorb adequate amounts of oral medication because of nausea, vomiting, or gastrointestinal disturbances, the parenteral route can be used.

Continuous infusions provide the patient with steady blood levels of the opioid and can avoid the potential side effects and return of pain associated with intermittent dosing. Guidelines are useful for initiating infusions and determining parameters for titrating doses. A summary of the management of continuous infusional therapy appears in Table 27-13.

Continuous subcutaneous. Continuous subcutaneous opioid infusions provide an acceptable alternative to intravenous administration in circumstances when long-term intravenous access is not available or is limited. Ambulatory, computerized infusion devices have facilitated the use of subcutaneous infusions at home. Because subcutaneous infusions are relatively easy to

Table 27-13 Suggestions for the Management of Continuous Intravenous or Subcutaneous Infusion of Opioid Analgesics

1. All infusions should be administered with a flow-calibrated infusion pump.
2. Convert the patient's current opioid drugs to an equal analgesic parenteral dose of the drug that will be used for the infusion.
3. If the drug to be used for the infusion is the same one the patient is currently receiving, divide the parenteral dose by 24 to determine the hourly infusion rate.
4. If the drug to be used for the infusion is a different drug, use half of the parenteral dose, and then divide by 24 to determine the hourly infusion rate.
5. Administer a loading dose at the beginning of the infusion and with each increase in the infusion rate. The amount of the loading dose depends on the patient's current opioid requirements.
6. Titrate the infusion until the patient reports pain relief or unacceptable side effects. Titration may occur the following ways:
   a. Increase the infusion rate by 10%–20% every few hours if the patient is receiving close monitoring.
   b. Administer additional doses of a short-acting opioid (preferably the same drug as the infusion) q1–2h PRN. Give 25%–50% of the hourly dose for PRN dosing. Increase the infusion rate q12–24h by the amount equal to the total number of milligrams during the preceding period divided by the number of hours in that period. Use this method if the patient is not receiving dose monitoring.
   c. If using IV/SQ for breakthrough pain, use 50%–100% of hourly rate every 15 min.
7. Opioids with a longer half-life (methodone, levophanol) should not be used for rapid titration.
8. Change site every 72 hours or if signs/symptoms of erythema occur at the site.
9. Limit the amount of volume to less than 5–10 mL/hr.

Data from American Pain Society.[53]

initiate, patients can be switched over to a subcutaneous infusion in the home providing that necessary resources (drug delivery system, skilled home care professionals) are in place. The subcutaneous route avoids problems associated with intramuscular or subcutaneous injections.

Continuous subcutaneous infusions of opioids are indicated for patients who (1) are unable to take oral medication due to nausea, vomiting, or a mechanical obstruction in the gastrointestinal tract; (2) are unable to use alternative routes because doses may be too high; (3) have limited or no venous access; and (4) are unable to maintain control with oral administration. Problems associated with subcutaneous continuous infusions include local skin irritation, leakage, swelling, and discomfort at the needle site.

An important clinical issue for subcutaneous infusions is the volume and concentration of the drug infused. Differences in volume and concentration and their implications for pain relief have been studied. Morphine and hydromorphone can be reconstituted to make concentrations as high as 60 mg/mL and 100 mg/mL, respectively.[42]

Limited data are currently available regarding continuous subcutaneous infusions of opioids. Watanabe et al. found that continuous subcutaneous fentanyl is a useful alternative for cancer patients.[147] No local toxicities were noted in their study.

Patient-controlled analgesia. The choice of opioid for patient-controlled analgesia (PCA) is guided by the same principles as the choice of any other opioid. Advances in computerized software for infusion devices have made PCA a common and acceptable method for delivering opioid analgesia through parenteral (IV and SQ) routes. Intravenous PCA for postoperative pain has become the mainstay for intravenous administration of opioids. Use of PCA for chronic cancer-related pain has also evolved into an effective approach for parenteral drug delivery. Patient-controlled analgesia allows patients to self-administer analgesics within a preset interval that is programmed into the infusion device. Regimens for acute pain such as postoperative pain include a self-administered or demand dose, but a continuous background infusion or basal rate of an opioid analgesic (e.g., morphine, fentanyl, hydromorphone, and less often meperidine) may be added. Demand-dosing schedules usually include doses of the opioid with *lock-out intervals* (15 minutes), the time allowed between doses. Patients can access self-administered doses frequently to control short-term pain. This approach avoids the peaks and troughs in serum levels that are often associated with conventional as needed (PRN) parenteral administration. In contrast, PCA regimens for the management of chronic cancer pain almost always include a basal rate that is supposed to deliver the bulk of the analgesic therapy. Higher demand doses at less frequent intervals are used to supplement the basal rate. This practice is intended to prevent the patient from working too hard to maintain adequate analgesia. In general, the benefits of PCA include better overall pain control, more prompt administration of opioids to control predictable or unpredictable bouts of pain, increased onset of analgesic action, and greater patient satisfaction.

Patient-controlled analgesia has also been used successfully in adolescents and adults to treat severe mucositis pain from the preparative regimen for bone marrow transplantation. In a multicenter study, Radbruch et al. found that PCA is appropriate for a small group of patients.[148] Higher treatment costs and risk of complications are drawbacks to using the PCA method of delivery when compared with conventional oral titration. While morphine and hydromorphone remain the opioids most frequently administered opioids via PCA, methadone and fentanyl can also be safely administered by this route.[149]

Table 27-14 Advantages and Disadvantages of Intraspinal Drug Administration

System	Advantages	Disadvantages
Percutaneous temporary catheter	Low cost; ease of insertion; limited life expectancy of 1–2 weeks	Mechanical problems include catheter dislodgement, kinking, or migration
Epidural catheter	Local anesthetic can be used; minor procedure; can deliver bolus injections, continuous infusions, or PCA	Catheter dislodgement; may develop fibrosis at epidural site that limits drug delivery into the epidural space
Subcutaneous injection port	Increased stability; less risk of dislodgement; can deliver bolus or continuous infusions	More invasive; approved only for epidural catheter in the United States; potential for infection increases with frequent injections
Implantable pumps	Continuous infusion of analgesics is possible; reservoir requires intermittent accessing and filling; patient is not hampered by external pump	Greater expertise is required for insertion; need more costly equipment

Data from Jacox, Carr, Payne, et al.[1]; American Pain Society.[53]

Sophisticated computer software technology for infusion devices as well as demonstrated efficacy and safety have contributed to more frequent use of PCA infusion devices by both inpatients and outpatients. While its use with inpatients is rarely disputed, the appropriateness of PCA for control of chronic cancer-related pain at home has been debated. Ferrell et al. caution that PCA is *not* appropriate with increased sedation or confusion; if oral therapy is not maximized; in case of potential conflict of interest when the prescribers and owners of the equipment or supplier are the same; when convenience is assumed; and if home healthcare nurses are inadequately trained.[150]

Intermittent subcutaneous. When it is not possible to administer continuous subcutaneous infusions due to outside restraints, short-term, intermittent subcutaneous injections are possible.[53] A subcutaneous needle system can be placed in a fashion similar to that for continuous infusions. The same needle and administration set are used for multiple scheduled injections throughout the day. This approach can also be used on an intermittent, as-needed basis for breakthrough pain in patients who are using transdermal fentanyl and are unable to take medications orally.

Intraspinal (neuraxial). The identification of opiate receptors in the brain and spinal cord and the results of early animal work involving spinal opioids have provided the bases for use of intraspinal or neuraxial (epidural and intrathecal [subarachnoid]) opioid administration for cancer pain. Epidural therapy is delivered into the epidural space, an area outside the dura over the subarachnoid space. The epidural space consists of fat, veins, and some arteries. The subarachnoid space, below the dura, is where cerebral spinal fluid circulates. The route of delivery into the subarachnoid space is termed *intrathecal administration.* The potency of opioids is approximately 10 times greater when injected into the subarachnoid space by intrathecal administration compared to the epidural route.

Although morphine currently represents the gold standard for intrathecal analgesia by infusion of a single drug, other opioids (e.g., fentanyl, hydromorphone, sufentanil and meperidine) are now being used successfully in patients who cannot tolerate morphine.[151,152] Clonidine and bupivacaine are drugs that are frequently used in clinical practice. Published reports endorse their effectiveness and lack of adverse effects when given intrathecally in a well-defined dose range. Hildebrand et al. found that the addition of clonidine appears to be more effective than opioid monotherapy in treating neuropathic pain and may help with other pain syndromes.[153]

Administration of intraspinal analgesics can be accomplished through a percutaneous externalized catheter, tunneled implantable externalized catheter (DuPen, Davol Inc., Cranston, Rhode Island), implantable reservoir or port for injection (either as a bolus injection or as a continuous infusion [Port-a-Cath, SIMS Delta, Inc., St. Paul, Minnesota]) and totally implantable drug delivery systems (SynchroMed Infusion System, Medtronic, Inc., Minneapolis, Minnesota). Factors that determine which type of system should be used include life expectancy, route of administration (epidural versus intrathecal), clinician expertise, opioid and anesthetic requirements, home care support, and economic considerations. Externalized catheters and implantable ports are generally used for epidural therapy and require an infusion device for drug delivery. Totally implantable drug delivery systems are more costly and are typically used when life expectancy is believed to be greater than 3 months. Table 27-14 describes the advantages and disadvantages of intraspinal delivery.

Smith et al. conducted a prospective, multicenter, randomized study of 200 patients with advanced cancer and refractory pain.[154] They found that the implantable delivery system improved pain control, reduced pain, significantly reduced common drug toxicity, and improved survival in patients with refractory cancer pain better than comprehensive medical management. A significant reduction in fatigue and depressed level of consciousness was observed in patients randomized to the pump. For 60% of patients who received the implantable pump, pain scores at 4 weeks fell below 4–10. Recently, Rauck et al. confirmed the greater efficacy of intrathecal opioid therapy in patients with cancer pain as compared to use of the implantable pump.[155]

Paice et al. conducted a multicenter survey of physicians to examine use of intraspinal opioids for both cancer- and non-cancer-related pain.[156] They concluded that there was little agreement as to the critical outcomes that should be measured to evaluate the success of therapy. Numerous reports have documented the outcomes of intraspinal therapy. Complications and rates of their occurrence have been attributed to the type of technology or catheter, placement of the catheter (epidural versus intrathecal), and duration of therapy. Complications include catheter-related problems, such as dislodgement, obstruction or occlusion, breakage, or leakage. Externalized epidural catheters are more vulnerable to kinking and tearing. Overall, the incidence of intraspinal catheter–related problems (10%–40%) was similar to the rates reported for other catheters. Of interest, patients with neuropathic pain tended to require higher doses at 6 months of therapy.

Drug-induced toxicities such as urinary retention, pruritus, nausea, vomiting, and respiratory depression can occur with intraspinal therapy. Respiratory depression, although potentially life-threatening, is rare. Epidural hematoma is a rare complication that requires immediate diagnosis and treatment to avoid a catastrophic event. Motor impairment is more pronounced with the use of a local anesthetic such as bupivacaine that acts on both sensory and motor nerves. Ropivacaine, which is selective for just sensory nerves, tends to produce fewer motor problems.[157] This agent may be a better option for patients who are elderly or who are already weak and debilitated. Another major concern is the risk of infection, which is possible with all types of delivery systems but is greater with externalized infusion systems. Catheters are removed only if a patient has a positive culture or if an infection is present in the epidural space.

Recently, intraspinal clonidine has been administered for the treatment of neuropathic pain. This alpha$_2$-agonist is believed to interfere with norepinephrine and epinephrine at the level of the spinal cord. Both neurotransmitters have been implicated in the transmission of pain from nerve injury.

The care of patients who are receiving intraspinal therapy at home requires coordination between the physician and team responsible for maintaining therapy and the home health agency professionals. Nurses must possess an understanding of the anatomy and physiology of the spinal cord, pharmacological properties of drugs used in neuraxial therapy, potential complications of therapy, and care of external catheters and the exit site. Nurses must also be familiar with the operational features of external infusion devices and implantable infusion systems. Guidelines for patient monitoring, drug administration, and protocols involving potential complications and emergency situations must be defined in the plan of care.

Prior to initiating intraspinal therapy, the patient and family should be informed about the expectations for the therapy, possible complications, the need for diagnostic tests, the costs involved, possible expected outcomes, alternative forms of therapy, signs and symptoms of infection, and options for home care. Next, the patient and family must be prepared for the placement procedure. Nursing diagnoses include (1) potential alteration in respiratory function; (2) potential alteration in comfort related to pruritus, nausea, vomiting, pain on injection, and inadequate pain relief; (3) potential alteration in elimination (urinary); (4) knowledge deficit regarding epidural analgesia; and (5) potential infection at the catheter site. After careful assessment, a decision about inserting a permanent catheter or an implantable infusion system is made.

Externalized catheters (e.g., Dupen catheter, Arrow International Inc., Reading, Pennsylvania) and implantable ports (e.g., Arrow Port-a-Cath) that are accessed require local skin care at the exit site. Admittedly, no universally accepted protocols for cleansing and dressing the site exist; nevertheless, many agree that caustic agents such as iodine and acetone might potentially migrate into the epidural space. Paice et al. recently conducted a study to evaluate potential hazards of using providine-iodine to cleanse the catheter exit site.[158] Cleansing with commercially available pledgets rather than with iodine swabs or gauze pads was associated with the least amount of contamination into the catheter.

Plans for home care focus on optimizing the patient's regimen before discharge. Because hospital length of stay may be limited, dose titration often must resume at home. Plans for follow-up, outpatient management, and coordination of home care activities are essential. It is critical to ensure that any home health or home infusion agency to which the patient is referred is familiar with prescribed protocols for catheter care and patient monitoring. The agency should have experience in the home management of intraspinal therapy and should be able to identify problems and promptly respond to them. The availability of agency resources must be determined, especially to safeguard against a disruption in therapy should problems with the catheter or infusion device occur. Implantable SynchroMed Infusion Systems require a portable computer for programming and interrogating the internal device. Should a patient experience side effects, it is critical that the agency be able to immediately access and use the computer or be able to promptly transport the patient to a facility where a computer is available.

When oral and parental analgesics fail, intraspinal medication may offer patients enhanced relief with lower doses of opioids and minimize adverse effects associated with conventional measures of opioid administration.[159]

Technology-Supported Pain Care

Concerns about the appropriateness of some of the routes of administration described previously, such as PCA and home use of neuraxial opioids, reflect the broader dilemma facing technology-supported pain care. The Oncology Nursing Society developed a resolution to address the appropriateness of technology in pain management, including use of neuraxial (intraspinal, epidural, and subarachnoid) routes, intravenous administration, and subcutaneous infusions.[160] This document delineated the appropriate applications for technology-supported pain care and stressed the significant financial, physical, and psychological burdens that are placed on the patient and family when such therapy is used. While no one would argue that all patients are unequivocally entitled to receive pain relief, the process of selecting the methods to provide such relief and allocating resources remains an issue for debate. Ferrell and Rhiner used a biomedical ethical perspective in approaching this problem.[161] Ethical principles and decision making are relevant to the determinations of who should receive technology-supported pain therapies. Whedon and Ferrell provided a case-study analysis of patient situations to illustrate the importance of appropriate patient selection, the need for a thorough assessment to determine the efficacy of the treatment, informed consent issues, financial implications, burden placed on the family, conflict of interest, and complications or morbidity.[162] Indiscriminate use of these therapies without clear indications can lead to undue emotional stress for the patient and family, disruptions in the home environment, financial worries, and inappropriate use of healthcare resources.

Nurses are seldom able to make the final decision about whether a patient should receive technology-supported pain care, but they are in a position to identify appropriate indications and weigh the benefits against the risks and costs of therapy. Nurses can also assume a lead role in establishing standards for the use of pain technology, as evidence suggests that clinicians are generally inconsistent in how they implement such therapies.[162]

Drug Therapy for the Elderly

Treatment of pain in the elderly requires knowledge of their specialized needs due to the physiological and lifestyle changes that occur with aging. The application of information regarding the pharmacodynamics of analgesics is critical in selecting agents that have more benign side effect profiles. Of the aging-related pharmacokinetic changes, two of the most important are the decline in the glomerular filtration rates and the reduction in the activity of the cytochrome P450 system, which is responsible for the activation and metabolism of many opioids.[163] Opioids are the mainstay for treatment of cancer pain even in the elderly. Morphine is probably the most often used opioid in the elderly. Because morphine is excreted in the kidneys and there is a decline in the glomerular filtration rate with age, neurotoxicity may develop in older patients. Hydromorphone undergoes the same metabolic changes. Unlike morphine and hydromorphone, fentanyl is lipophilic and suitable for transdermal administration. With chronic administration or hepatic failure, fentanyl may accumulate in the circulation due to saturation of storage sites.[163] Oxycodone is another popular opioid that is eliminated by hepatic metabolism. The fact that oxycodone's pharmacokinetics is largely independent of age, renal function, and serum albumin concentration makes this compound a favorable choice in the elderly. Meperidine is best avoided in the elderly because its metabolite normeperidine is excreted in the kidneys, accumulates in the circulation in the presence of renal insufficiency, and may cause seizures.[55,56] Table 27-15 outlines the important considerations for use of analgesics in the elderly.[8,56,164–168]

Acetaminophen is the analgesic of choice for most elderly patients. This medication works in the central nervous system but has no anti-inflammatory properties. For this reason, it may be less effective than NSAIDs. NSAIDs are beneficial in the presence of bone metastases, but gastrointestinal bleeding, renal toxicity, and drug-to-drug interactions need to be considered when prescribing them.

For the treatment of neuropathic pain, gabapentin is probably the agent of choice due to its safety profile.[169] It should be noted that this drug's pharmacokinetics is unpredictable and that gabapentin may have a prolonged half-life.[56] For peripheral painful

Table 27-15 Special Considerations for Pain Assessment in the Elderly

Age-Related Changes	Specific Interventions for the Elderly
Mental status ↓ Mental acuity Short-term memory problems ↓ Information processing ↑ Susceptibility to sedation of analgesics	• Initiate therapy with one-half of the usual starting dose for adults. • Start low and go slow. • Select adjuvant agents with ↓ sedating effects. • Initiate safety precautions.
Vision and hearing ↓ Visual acuity and hearing	• Use pain assessment measures and teaching materials that are easy to read. • Speak clearly and maintain eye contact. • Avoid drugs that are contraindicated with glaucoma (agents with anticholinergic effects).
Musculoskeletal Osteoporosis Joint stiffness ↓ Mobility	• Begin with nonopioid agents. • Do not exceed the daily recommended dose of acetaminophen (> 4 g/day). • Use NSAIDs for inflammatory pain. • Stop treatment with NSAIDs if not effective. • May consider corticosteroids rather than NSAIDs for short-term use with bone pain. • Encourage exercise or physical therapy.
Pulmonary COPD Emphysema ↓ Pulmonary reserves	• Use caution with opioid and other analgesic agents that cause sedation. • Initiate opioid therapy at one-half the starting dose for adults. • Remember risk of respiratory depression is minimal if dosed correctly.
Cardiovascular Reduced blood volume Conduction abnormalities ↓ Cardiac output Cardiac reserve and circulation	• Drug absorption, distribution, and excretion may be altered due to aging. • Adminster NSAIDs cautiously to patients with congestive heart failure because a reduction in renal profusion may cause fluid retention. • Avoid TCA if patients have cardiac conduction problems.
Gastrointestinal Dehydration ↓ Fluid intake ↓ Gastric emptying	• Avoid NSAIDs in patients with peptic ulcers or in patients taking anticoagulants. • Use caution in patients who are dehydrated, as they may be more susceptible to opioid-related side effects. • Use caution with TCA with ↑ anticholinergic effects (amitriptyline).
Renal ↓ Renal filtration and clearance Renal insufficiency	• Obtain baseline renal function tests (BUN, creatinine, and creatinine clearance) prior to starting therapy. • Consider lower doses of NSAIDs to reduce the risk of renal toxicity. • Consider risk of metabolite accumulation in patients with severe renal dysfunction. • Administer short-acting NSAIDs on a PRN basis rather than around the clock.
Genitourinary Urinary incontinences Males: benign prostatic hypertrophy Females: stress incontinence	• Patients who are opioid naïve are at greatest risk for urinary retention. • Anticholinergic agents may cause urinary retention, so use caution. • Instruct patients to monitor for signs of urinary tract infections.

↓ = decreased; ↑ = increased; BUN = blood urea nitrogen; COPD = chronic obstructive pulmonary disease; NSAID = nonsteroidal anti-inflammatory drug; TCA = tricyclic antidepressant

Data from American Pain Society[53]; Davis, Srivastava[56]; Gibson, Helme[164]; Fine[165]; Freedman[166]; American Geriatric Society[167]; Dellasega, Keiser.[168]

neuropathy, transdermal lidocaine should be the first-line treatment.[56]

Effective treatment of pain in older patients is compelling, because pain may compromise the general health and even shorten the survival of the elderly. The assessment of pain in older patients may require a more comprehensive assessment than that in younger patients. In general, one should initiate treatment with lower doses and longer dose intervals than would be used in younger patients.[163] Individual pain relief should guide dose escalation. Combination products — those that have both an opioid and a nonopioid — should be avoided because of the limited dosing available due to the ceiling dose for the nonopioid, which may lead to severe effects if excess medication is taken.[55]

Nerve Blocks and Neuroablative Procedures

Temporary nerve blocks and permanent neurolytic blocks or neuroablation are procedures used to modulate neural responses to noxious stimuli in cancer-related pain. The injection of a local anesthetic into a nerve, nerve root, or epidural space prevents the generation and conduction of nerve impulses. Temporary or nondestructive nerve blocks serve two functions: (1) They are used for the treatment of intractable pain such as neuropathic pain caused by invasion or compression of intraspinal nerve roots; and (2) they are helpful as a prognostic/diagnostic technique to differentiate visceral pain from somatic pain, demonstrate neural pathways for selected pain conditions, and determine who might benefit from a more permanent block or neuroablative procedures.[170] While adequate relief of pain may be achieved, it is only temporary, with the effects of the local anesthetic generally wearing off in 6–8 hours.

Neurolytic or destructive nerve blocks provide more prolonged pain relief than nondestructive nerve blocks and can minimize the need for systemic medication, thereby reducing drug-related toxicities. Procedural management of cancer pain should be pursued after a thorough neurological examination has been performed, a normalized coagulation profile is obtained, the patient is in an optimized immunologic state, and the procedure has been extensively discussed with the patient. Because neurolysis of nerves may not be permanent and some regeneration can be expected within weeks to months, neurolytic procedures are generally reserved for patients with a limited life expectancy. The short-term success rate of the blocks is very high (approximately 90%) regardless of the underlying type of cancer.[171]

Unfortunately, neurolytic agents cannot discriminate between pain fibers, A-delta and C-fibers, and other fibers (e.g., motor). Therefore, both sensory and motor impairment can result from neurolytic procedures. Two neurolytic blocks commonly used to provide analgesia and assist with pain control are the celiac plexus block (CPB) and the superior hypogastric plexus block (HPB).[172] Although these interventions may provide complete analgesia in some cases, they are especially used as adjuvants to opioid therapy to optimize treatment of cancer pain.

Celiac plexus block is useful in the treatment of pain associated with pancreatic cancer and intraabdominal cancer. Mercadante et al. conducted a prospective, multicenter study of 22 patients with pancreatic cancer.[173] In this study, CPB produced immediate analgesia and allowed for the reduction in the opioid dose.[173] A reduction in the amount of opioids needed may have a positive impact on the patient's quality of life. In the study, CPB had therapeutic effects for 4–5 weeks, after which symptoms' intensity worsened. CPB can be performed by a pain specialist or during an intraoperative procedure. The most common side effects are diarrhea and hypotension. Diarrhea occurs in approximately 50% of patients and lasts for a few days.[174] Significant hypotension occurs in approximately 38% of patients. These side effects are more likely to occur in dehydrated and debilitated patients.[175] Rare complications include pneumothorax, renal puncture, paraplegia, groin pain, and neurolytic drug spread.

HPB is used to alleviate visceral pain associated with pelvic pain. The aortic plexus bifurcates to form the superior and inferior hypogastric plexus.[176] The superior hypogastric plexus contains both sympathetic and parasympathetic fibers, which descend and pass through the colon, splenic flexure, and descending and sigmoid colon.[176] The inferior hypogastric plexus supplies pelvic organs and viscera along the internal iliac artery such as the rectum, bladder, prostate, uterus, and vagina.[176] Although the evidence for use of HPB is less strong than that for CPB, in patients with intractable pelvic pain the benefit/risk ratio is favorable.

Alcohol and phenol are the two agents most commonly used for chemical neurolysis. Alcohol is administered directly into the nerve, nerve root, or plexus. Injections can be painful, but this discomfort is transient and the pain can be effectively managed with additional pain medication. The alcohol can be absorbed, and depending on the concentration and volume, patients may experience short-term systemic effects of alcohol intoxication. It may be necessary to implement patient safety measures and close observation should this occur. Regardless of the agent used, patients may experience heightened pain 12–24 hours following the procedure. A flexible schedule with short-acting analgesics should be used to treat transient exacerbations of pain. Twenty-four to 48 hours following the procedure and regularly thereafter for 1–2 weeks, the patient should be assessed for a decrease in pain and a reduction in analgesics.

The nursing responsibilities for patients undergoing anesthetic and neurodestructive procedures include being knowledgeable about the (1) purpose of the procedure and how it is performed; (2) potential complications based on type of block, agent, and location; and (3) potential benefit of the procedure. An efficient way of obtaining some of this information is to participate in the explanation of the procedure to the patient and to talk with the anesthesiologist or neurosurgeon. Because this requisite information is based on the patient's individual pain problem, standard reference materials may provide incomplete information.

Complementary and Alternative Medicine

Complementary therapies are defined as those that patients use along with conventional medicine. Studies indicate that between 7% and 72% of adult cancer patients have used some form of complementary therapy in addition to conventional medicine.[177] The reasons for using complementary and alternative medicine (CAM) fall into three categories: physical (providing symptom relief), psychological (coping with the disease), and social (distrust of conventional medicine).[178] Alimi et al. found that acupuncture did show a benefit in cancer patients who were in pain despite stable analgesic treatment.[179] Their study was the first properly randomized trial to demonstrate the efficacy of acupuncture for neuropathic chronic pain, a pain that has been resistant to effective intervention.

As cancer patients continue to use CAM, the need for further reliable scientific data will grow. The National Cancer Institute (NCI) is devoted to rigorous investigation of any potential treatments and modalities in the prevention and treatment of cancer. In 1998, the National Institutes of Health (NIH) established the National Center for Complementary and Alternative Medicine to support the study of CAM modalities.[180] Oncology professionals, both nurses and physicians, need to take steps to become more familiar and comfortable with the topic of complementary medicine.

Diminishing the Emotional and Reactive Components of Pain

This approach to managing pain is an area in which nurses can discuss cognitive, behavioral, informational, and other strategies; prepare patients for these therapies; and mobilize the necessary resources to implement them. Interventions included in this approach do not generally affect the underlying pathology or alter the perception or sensation of pain, but rather help in a variety of ways to decrease patients' emotional responses to pain, enabling them to deal with it more positively and proactively. Distraction, relaxation, guided imagery, and symptom monitoring are interventions that can be taught to provide patients and caregivers with tools to help control the perception and experience of pain. Evidence from multiple studies suggests that a variety of mind-body medicine treatments can improve mood, quality of life, and symptoms such as pain, nausea, and vomiting.[181]

These techniques clearly serve as adjuvants to standard pharmacological therapy.[182] Drugs are used to treat the somatic (physiological and sensory) dimensions of pain, while nondrug methods are aimed at treating the affective, cognitive, behavioral, and sociocultural dimensions of pain. The benefits of many of the techniques are that they may increase the patient's sense of personal control, reduce feelings of helplessness, provide opportunities to become actively involved in care, reduce stress and anxiety, elevate mood, raise pain threshold, and thereby reduce pain.

McCaffery and Pasero address nonpharmacologic pain interventions.[49] They note that although sufficient research still does not exist to document the efficacy of these techniques, a number of them are easily and quickly implemented—specifically, cutaneous stimulation, distraction, and relaxation. They recommend that these techniques be incorporated into the care plan where appropriate and when patients are willing.

Many of the treatment strategies aimed at diminishing the emotional and reactive components of pain are classified as cognitive, behavioral, or cognitive *and* behavioral techniques. *Cognitive methods* attempt directly to modify thought processes in an effort to attenuate or relieve pain; they can be applied to thoughts, images, and attitudes. Examples include information, distraction, imagery, calming self-statements, identification of detrimental responses to pain, and informational or educational programs about pain and its management. *Behavioral methods* modify physiological reactions to pain or behavioral manifestations of pain. Examples include relaxation, meditation, music therapy, and various desensitization strategies. Sometimes cognitive and behavioral techniques are used together, such as relaxation and guided imagery.

Another category of nonpharmacologic interventions comprises those that diminish the emotional and reactive components of pain by providing cutaneous stimulation; examples include applications of heat, cold, massage, and vibration. Although these methods technically fall within the major treatment approach of changing perception or sensation of pain, they are included here because they are traditional nursing interventions that also involve use of specific behaviors to ameliorate pain.

Finally, a separate category of behavioral interventions that change perception or sensation of pain and also diminish affective reactions is based on mobility/mobilization and immobilization in an attempt to improve functional status. Most of these interventions are simple and can be initiated when ongoing assessment of pain suggests a need for them.

In each of the following sections, selected interventions are discussed briefly. The discussion here is limited to those techniques that are clearly within the scope of nursing practice and can be used without significant additional training. Table 27-16 provides additional information about these techniques.

Cutaneous Stimulation

Cutaneous stimulation is thought to help relieve pain by physiologically altering the transmission of nociceptive stimuli; these methods are based on the gate-control theory of pain and additional basic and clinical research findings related to mechanisms of pain.[183] Heat can be applied with hot packs, a heating pad, a hot water bottle, or a shower or bath. Cold can be applied with cold packs, cold cloths, ice, gel packs, or cold

Table 27-16 Selected Nonpharmacological Interventions for Pain

Technique	Examples	Advantages	Disadvantages
Cutaneous stimulation	Superficial heating or cooling, vibration, massage	Many methods; makes pain tolerable; reduces pain, patients are receptive; can apply stimulation at site of pain or other sites; can provide distraction	Not for therapeutic or curative purposes; can damage tissue if applied incorrectly
Immobilization/mobilization	Splinting, bracing, walking, exercise, rest	Decreases pain, improves range of motion, conserves energy, improves functional status, promotes relaxation	Discomfort on physical exertion; decrease in functional status
Distraction	*Internal:* Mental images, counting, singing silently; *external:* music, reading, television, conversation	Decreased pain intensity, increased pain tolerance; more acceptable pain sensation; greater sense of control; improved mood	Not helpful for vigilant patients; may have no effect on pain intensity; may be hard to enact; may not "look like" they are in pain, resulting in doubt about pain and/or failure to medicate after distraction; awareness of pain and fatigue may increase; irritability
Relaxation	Slow breathing, progressive muscle relaxation, relaxing mental imagery, repetitive activity or thought	Reduces anxiety, may reduce pain; promotes sleep; decreases fatigue and skeletal muscle tension; increases confidence in ability to handle pain	Can be time-consuming; difficult to teach, practice, and use effectively; is an adjunct method that does not directly relieve pain; often difficult to distinguish between relaxation and imagery
Comprehensive models	Cognitive/behavioral interventions, psychoeducational approaches	Address multiple dimensions of pain; individualized; include patient and family; problem-focused; requires interdisciplinary team	May be difficult to assemble an appropriate interdisciplinary team depending on setting and resources; can be complex and time-consuming

Data from McCaffery, Pasero.[49]

water. Cold treatments reduce swelling and may provide longer-lasting relief than heat applications. Massage is administered via fingers or hands and can be accompanied by a variety of topical local anesthetic agents such as capsaicin, EMLA, or lidocaine.[49] Tumor masses should not be aggressively manipulated. Note that massage is not a substitute for active exercise. Vibration can be administered with a variety of stimulators, including transcutaneous electrical nerve stimulators in some cases. Some of these methods are used frequently at home by patients with pain, and combinations are common. The research evaluating these methods remains somewhat sparse.

Transcutaneous electrical nerve stimulation (TENS) delivers controlled, low-voltage electrical stimulation via cutaneous electrodes to inhibit pain transmission. Patients with mild to moderate pain may benefit from a trial of TENS.[54]

Immobilization/Mobilization and Functional Status

Even when effective pharmacological therapy has been instituted, some individuals may still experience pain on movement. Immobilization can be helpful in the management of acute pain. A prolonged period of immobilization may cause more problems. Repositioning can maintain correct body alignment, decrease pain, and prevent painful pressure ulcers. In other circumstances, mild exercise such as joint range of motion and stretching may help decrease pain. Finally, rest or lying down may help in some instances, perhaps partly because of the relaxation that occurs. Pain assessment tools that address patients' functional status, such as the Brief Pain Inventory,[184] can be helpful in determining the impact of pain on daily activities or sleeping and provide a rationale for implementing some of these interventions in an effort to improve functional status.

Distraction

Distraction is usually defined as a method of diverting one's attention away from sensations or feelings related to pain. Distraction can be significantly helpful in reducing pain. A classic example is the focusing exercises (accompanied by relaxation techniques) taught in childbirth education classes. Many individual distraction techniques and strategies exist; examples include conversation, verbalization to self or others, deep thinking, visualization and imagery, mind-body separation, routines/rituals, breathing exercises, counting, reading, and watching television.

Many professional caregivers do not realize the broad scope and variety of distraction strategies, nor do they recognize that some strategies may work for one individual and not for another. A careful appraisal of patients' preferences and willingness to try such techniques is an important part of the care plan. Although the scientific evidence is not strong, it is sufficient for caregivers to consider incorporation of such distraction strategies into the pain management plan.

Relaxation and Guided Imagery

Relaxation training helps produce physiological and mental relaxation. Broadly defined, relaxation techniques include those practices whose goal is the elicitation of a pyschophysiological state of relaxation or hypoarousal.[181] In certain cases, the goal may be decreased muscle tension. Ultimately, the primary goal is to achieve a hypometabolic state of reduced sympathetic arousal. The two most commonly employed methods are *progressive muscle relaxation,* which is the systematic tensing/relaxing of 16 muscle groups, and *self-relaxation,* which is the passive, quiet, and still use of autogenic phrases such as "my arms are warm and heavy." Training usually occurs in six to ten sessions with a therapist. Audiotapes can be used at home afterward, and individuals are encouraged to practice and use their new skills. *Guided imagery,* in which an individual visualizes pleasant places or things, is frequently used in conjunction with relaxation. These images are typically visualized with the goal of a psychophysiological state of relaxation or with some specific outcome in mind.

Although the literature on these techniques in the patient population with cancer remains scanty, it was recently reviewed and discussed in depth by Wallace.[185] Effects of relaxation and imagery on the affective dimension of pain, or other components such as perceptions of control over pain or functional status, appear to be equivocal. Overall, however, the effectiveness of this group of interventions stills needs careful investigation, particularly when used with opioid analgesics.

Comprehensive Cognitive/Behavioral/ Educational Methods

Several individuals have proposed comprehensive cognitive, behavioral, and educational approaches for cancer pain. These approaches are based on cognitive and social learning models in which pain can be described in terms of objective qualities (e.g., location and intensity) and psychological significance. Indeed, a mounting body of evidence indicates that nurses have developed effective cognitive/behavioral/educational approaches to symptom management and, more important, that collaborative interdisciplinary teams of healthcare providers have developed management approaches that improve patient outcomes.[186–188]

In summary, the evidence available suggests that many of the nonpharmacological techniques described may be useful in alleviating cancer pain, but clearly much more systematic research is needed to document their efficacy, whether they are used alone in selected pain situations or as part of a comprehensive treatment plan. Most of these techniques are familiar to nurses and can be employed in a variety of settings. Specific references can assist nurses with the information needed to apply the techniques effectively.[49] Many of these techniques require patient and family education and a willingness to try them as adjuncts to pharmacological therapy. Integrated with the use of such techniques, however, should be the nurse as coach — a professional education counseling model that complements patient teaching.[189] The nurse as coach focuses on facilitating the cognitive emotional processing of the patient and enhances self-care skills and cognitive control, areas particularly important in pain management.

Education and Information

Accurate and appropriate education and information for patients with cancer-related pain and their caregivers represent an essential aspect of comprehensive pain management. Patients' knowledge about and attitudes toward cancer pain can positively or negatively affect its management. For example, Oliver et al. found that patients who were randomized to an intervention that provided individual coaching had better pain control.[190]

Barriers, challenges, and solutions to the problem of pain education for patients, families, and nurses have been discussed in depth by Ersek and Wilson,[191] Cohen et al.[192] and McCaffery and Pasero.[49] When Redinbaugh et al. conducted a study on the accuracy of caregivers' perceptions of pain, they found healthcare providers needed to consider the family members' interpretation of patients' pain when providing pain management educational information.[193] A comprehensive list of resources for pain would include professional and volunteer organizations, publications, and information on patient service programs, as well as Web sites with useful information for patients, their families, and professional healthcare providers.[49] With the explosion of Internet technology and patients' use of it, nurses and other healthcare providers need to be aware of these many resources.

Although an in-depth discussion of patient and family education is beyond the scope of this chapter, two key areas must be emphasized. First is the need to select appropriate content for pain education. Much of this content is based on the AHRQ guidelines,[1] the Alliance of State Cancer Pain Initiatives, and work by individual investigators.[194] Recent research testing pain education programs for cancer pain indicates that patients, families, and healthcare providers can all benefit from systematically implemented comprehensive programs.[195] Pain education is clearly an essential role for nurses caring for patients with cancer-related pain, as it helps patients and families cope with pain and improves quality of life.

Conclusion

Future changes in the healthcare system will make it necessary for nurses to use research-based data and published clinical care guidelines to define "best practices" that yield maximum benefits for pain relief. Nurses will need to closely examine their practices as they are asked to do more with fewer healthcare resources. Employers, managed care, and third-party healthcare payers will hold nurses accountable for their practice; therefore, it will be imperative to monitor nursing care through patient-oriented outcomes. As advances in pain therapy expand, greater demands will be placed on nurses to acquire the higher levels of knowledge necessary to care for patients with cancer-related pain. The greatest challenge will be to integrate this knowledge to its fullest, to continue to investigate innovative ways to treat pain, and to impart this knowledge to patients and other health professionals.

References

1. Jacox A, Carr DB, Payne R, et al: *Management of Cancer Pain: Adults' Quick Reference Guide No. 9.* AHCPR publication No. 94–0593. Rockville, MD, Agency for Health Care Policy and Research, U.S. Department of Health and Human Services, Public Health Service, 1994
2. Kiar M: The therapy of cancer pain and its integration into a comprehensive supportive care strategy. *Ann Oncol* 8(suppl 3):S15–S19, 1997
3. Janjan NA, Payne R, Gillis T, et al: Presenting symptoms in patients referred to a multidisciplinary clinic for bone metastases. *J Pain Symptom Manage* 16:171–178, 1998
4. Polomano RC, McGuire DB, Sheidler VR: Management of cancer pain, in Yarbro CH, Frogge MH, Goodman M, et al. (eds.) *Cancer Nursing Principles and Practice* (ed 5). Sudbury, MA, Jones and Bartlett, 2000, pp 657-690
5. Wisconsin Cancer Pain Initiative Nursing Education Committee: *Competency Guidelines for Cancer Pain Management in Nursing Education and Practice.* Madison, WI, Wisconsin Cancer Pain Initiative, 1995
6. Spross JA, McGuire DB, Schmitt R: Oncology Nursing Society position paper on cancer pain. *Oncol Nurs Forum* 17:595–614, 751–760, 825, 944–955, 1990
7. Ad Hoc Committee on Cancer Pain of the American Society of Clinical Oncology: Cancer pain assessment and treatment curriculum guidelines. *J Clin Oncol* 10:1976–1982, 1992
8. American Pain Society: *Principles of Analgesic Use in the Treatment of Acute Pain and Cancer Pain* (ed 4). Skokie, IL, APS Press, 1999
9. American Geriatrics Society Panel on Chronic Pain in Older Persons: The management of chronic pain in older persons. *J Am Geriatr Soc* 46:635–651, 1998
10. Practice guidelines for cancer pain management. A report by the American Society for Anesthesiologists Task Force on Pain Management, Cancer Pain Section. *Anesthesiology* 84:1243–1257, 1996
11. Acute Pain Management Guideline Panel: *Acute Pain Management: Operative or Medical Procedures and Trauma: Clinical Practice Guidelines.* AHCPR publication No. 92–0032. Rockville, MD, Agency for Health Care Policy and Research, Public Health Service, U.S. Department of Health and Human Services, 1992
12. World Health Organization: *Cancer Pain Relief* (ed 2). Geneva, WHO, 1996
13. Portenoy RK: Report from the International Association for the Study of Pain Task Force on cancer pain. *J Pain Symptom Manage* 12:93–96, 1996
14. Pickett M, Cooley ME, Gordon DB: Palliative care: past, present, and the future. *Semin Oncol Nurs* 14:86–94, 1998
15. Randal J: Hospice services feel the pinch of managed care. *J Natl Cancer Inst* 88:860–862, 1996
16. Cleary JF, Carbone PP: Palliative medicine in the elderly. *Cancer* 80:1335–1347, 1997
17. Lynn J, Teno JM, Phillipps RS, et al: Perceptions by family members of the dying experience of older and seriously ill patients. SUPPORT Investigators. Study to understand prognosis and preference for outcomes and risks of treatment. *Ann Intern Med* 126:97–106, 1997
18. Ellison NM: Palliative chemotherapy. *Am J Hosp Palliat Care* 15:93–103, 1998
19. Janjan NA, Weissman DA: Primary cancer treatment: antineoplastic, in Berger AM, Portenoy RK, Weissman DE (eds.): *Supportive Oncology Care.* Philadelphia, Lippincott-Raven, 1998, pp 43–59
20. Tannock IF, Osoba D, Stocker MR, et al: Chemotherapy with mitoxantrone plus prednisone or prednisone alone for symptomatic hormone-resistant prostate cancer: a Canadian randomized trial with palliative endpoints. *J Clin Oncol* 14:1756–1764, 1996
21. Rutten EH, Crul BJ, van der Toorn PP, et al: Pain characteristics help predict the analgesic efficacy of radiotherapy for the treatment of cancer pain. *Pain* 69:131–135, 1997
22. Scott CB: Issues in quality of life assessment during cancer therapy. *Semin Radiat Oncol* 8(suppl 4):5–9, 1998
23. Di Lorenzo G, Autorino R, Ciardiello F, et al: External beam radiotherapy in bone metastatic prostate cancer: impact on patients' pain relief and quality of life. *Oncol Rep* 10:399–404, 2003
24. Gaze MN, Kelly CG, Kerr GR, et al: Pain relief and quality of life following radiotherapy for bone metastases: a randomised trial of two fractionation schedules. *Radiother Oncol* 45:109–116, 1997

25. Niewald M, Tkocz HJ, Abel U, et al: Rapid course radiation therapy vs. more standard treatment: a randomized trial for bone metastases. *Int J Radiat Oncol Biol Phys* 36:1085–1089, 1996
26. Jeremic B: Single fraction external beam radiation therapy in the treatment of localized metastatic bone pain. A review. *J Pain Symptom Manage* 22:1048–1058, 2001
27. Saarto T, Janes R, Tenhunen M, et al: Palliative radiotherapy in the treatment of skeletal metastases. *Eur J Pain* 6:323–330, 2002
28. Gaze MN, Kelly CG, Kerr GR, et al: Pain relief and quality of life for bone metastases: a randomized trial of two fractionation schedules. *Radiat Oncol* 45:109–116, 1997
29. Macklis RM, Cornelli H, Lasher J: Brief courses of palliative radiotherapy for metastatic bone pain: a pilot cost-minimization comparison with narcotic analgesics. *Am J Clin Oncol* 21:617–622, 1998
30. Bruera ED, Sweeney C: Bone pain, in Bruera ED, Portenoy RK (eds.): *Cancer Pain Assessment and Management*. Cambridge, UK, Cambridge University Press, 2003, pp 413–428
31. Ben-Josef E, Porter AT: Radioisotopes in the treatment of bone metastases. *Ann Med* 29:31–35, 1997
32. Serafini AN: Samarium Sm-153 lexidronam for the palliation of bone pain associated with metastases. *Cancer* 88(suppl 12):2934–2939, 2000
33. United States Pharmacopeial Convention, Inc.: *USP DI Drug Information for the Health Care Professional* (ed 19). Englewood, CO, Micromedex, 1999
34. Sciuto R, Tofani A, Festa A, et al: Short- and long-term effects of 186Re-1,1-hydroxyethylidene diphosphonate in the treatment of painful bone metastases. *J Nucl Med* 41:647–654, 2000
35. Lillemoe KD: Palliative surgery for pancreatic cancer. *Surg Clin North Am* 7:199–216, 1998
36. Branicki J, Law SY, Fok M, et al: Quality of life in patients with cancer of the esophagus and gastric cardia: a case for palliative resection. *Arch Surg* 133:316–322, 1998
37. Soysal O, Karaoglanoglu N, Demiracan S, et al: Pleurectomy/decortication for palliation in malignant pleural mesothelioma: results of surgery. *Eur J Cardiothoracic Sur* 11:210–213, 1997
38. Harrington KD: Orthopaedic surgical management of skeletal complications of malignancy. *Cancer* 80(suppl 8):1614–1627, 1997
39. Gotlieb WH, Feldman B, Feldman-Moran O, et al: Intraperitoneal pressures and clinical parameters of total paracentesis for palliation of symptomatic ascites in ovarian cancer. *Gynecol Oncol* 71:381–385, 1998
40. Stephenson J, Gilbert J: The development of clinical guidelines on paracentesis for ascites related to malignancy. *Palliat Med* 16:213–218, 2002
41. Antunes G, Neville E, Duffy J, et al: BTS guidelines for the management of malignant pleural effusions. *Thorax* 58(suppl 2):29–38, 2003
42. Polomano RC, Soulen M, McDaniel C: Sedation and analgesia with interventional radiology for oncology patients. *Crit Care Nurs Clin North Am* 9:335–353, 1997
43. Kochman ML, Soulen M, Polomano RC: Palliative endoscopy and interventional radiology, in Berger A, Portenoy RK, Weissman DE (eds.): *Principles and Practice of Supportive Oncology*. Philadelphia, Lippincott-Raven, 1998, pp 651–666
44. Coyle N, Cherny N, Portenoy RK: Pharmacologic management of cancer pain, in McGuire DB, Yarbro CH, Ferrell BR (eds.): *Cancer Pain Management* (ed 2). Sudbury, MA, Jones and Bartlett, 1995, pp 131–158
45. Payne R: Pharmacological management of pain, in Berger A, Portenoy RK, Weissman DE (eds.): *Principles and Practice of Supportive Oncology*. Philadelphia, Lippincott-Raven, 1998, pp 61–75
46. Levy MH: Pharmacological treatment of cancer pain. *N Engl J Med* 335:1124–1132, 1996
47. Fitzgibbon DR: Cancer pain: management, in Loeser JD (ed.): *Bonica's Management of Pain*. Philadelphia, Lippincott, Williams and Wilkins, 2001, pp 659–703
48. Reisine T, Pasternak G: Opioid analgesics and antagonists, in Hardman JG, Gilman AG, Limbard LE, et al. (eds.): *Goodman and Gilman's The Pharmacological Basis of Therapeutics* (ed 9). New York, McGraw-Hill, 1996, pp 521–556
49. McCaffery M, Pasero C: *Pain: Clinical Manual* (ed 2). St. Louis, Mosby, 1999
50. American Academy of Pain Medicine, American Society of Pain, American Society of Addiction Medicine: Definitions Related to the Use of Opioids for the Treatment of Pain. *www.ampainsoc.org/advocacy/opioids2.htm*, 2004. Accessed May 25, 2004
51. Ballantyne JC: Chronic pain following treatment for cancer: the role of opioids. *Oncologist* 8:567–575, 2003
52. D'Agati V: Does asprin cause acute or chronic renal failue in experimental animals and in humans? *Am J Kidney Dis* 28:s24–29, 1996
53. American Pain Society: *Principles of Analgesic Use in the Treatment of Acute Pain and Cancer Pain* (ed 5). Glenview, IL, American Pain Society, 2003
54. Chandrasekharan NV, Dai H, Roos KL, et al: COX-3, a cyclooxygenase-1 variant inhibited by acetaminophen and other analgesic/antipyretic drugs: cloning, structure, and expression. *Proc Natl Acad Sci USA* 99:13926–13931, 2002
55. Gloth FM: Pain management in older adults: prevention and treatment. *J Am Geriatr Soc* 49:188–199, 2001
56. Davis MP, Srivastava M: Demographics, assessment and management of pain in the elderly. *Drugs Aging* 20:23–57, 2003
57. Hylek EM, Heiman H, Skates SJ, et al: Acetaminophen and other risk factors for excessive warfarin anticoagulation. *JAMA* 279:657–662, 1998
58. Gunn VL, Taha SH, Liebelt EL, et al: Toxicity of over-the-counter cough and cold medications. *Pediatrics* 108:E52–57, 2001
59. Acello B: Administering acetaminophen safely. *Nursing* 33:18, 2003
60. Bond C, Hannaford P: Issues related to monitoring the safety of over-the-counter (OTC) medicines. *Drug Saf* 26:1065–1074, 2003
61. Chavez ML, DeKorte CJ: Valdecoxib: a review. *Clin Ther* 25:817–851, 2003
62. Bombardier C, Laine L, Reicin A, et al: Comparison of upper gastrointestinal toxicity of rofecoxib and naproxen in patients with rheumatoid arthritis. VIGOR Study Group. *N Engl J Med* 343:1520–1528, 2000
63. Silverstein FE, Faich G, Goldstein JL, et al: Gastrointestinal toxicity with celecoxib vs nonsteroidal anti-inflammatory drugs for osteoarthritis and rheumatoid arthritis: the CLASS study: a randomized controlled trial. Celecoxib Long-term Arthritis Safety Study. *JAMA* 284:1247–1255, 2000
64. Fowles RE: Potential cardiovascular effects of COX-2 selective nonsteroidal antiinflammatory drugs. *J Pain Palliat Care Pharmacother* 17:27–50, 2003
65. Fox A, Medhurst S, Courade JP, et al: Anti-hyperalgesic activity of the COX-2 inhibitor lumiracoxib in a model of bone cancer pain in the rat. *Pain* 107:33–40, 2004
66. Perazella MA: Drug-induced renal failure: update on new medications and unique mechanisms of nephrotoxicity. *Am J Med Sci* 325:349–362, 2003
67. Ruoff G: Management of pain in patients with multiple health problems: a guide for practicing physicians. *Am J Med* 105:53S–60S, 1998

68. Portenoy RK, Rowe G: Adjuvant analgesics drugs, in Bruera ED, Portenoy RK (eds.): *Cancer Pain Assessment and Management.* Cambridge, UK, Cambridge University Press, 2003, pp 188–198
69. Lynch MP: *Oncology Nursing Essentials.* New York, Professesional Publishing Group, 2002, pp 111–120
70. Perron V, Schonwetter RS: Assessment and management of pain in palliative care patients. *Cancer Control* 8:15–24, 2001
71. Mercadante S: Diarrhea, malabsorption and constipation, in Berger AM, Portenoy RK, Weissman DE (eds.): *Principles and Practice of Supportive Oncology.* Philadelphia, Lippincott, Williams and Wilkins, 2002, pp 191–205
72. DiPalma JA, DeRidder PH, Orlando R, et al: A randomized, placebo-controlled, multicenter study of the safety and efficacy of a new polyethylene glycol laxative. *Am J Gastroenterol* 95:446–450, 2000
73. Latasch L, Zimmermann M, Eberhardt B, et al: Treament of morphine-induced constipation with oral naloxone. *Anaesthesist* 46:191–194, 1997
74. Scholz M: Managing constipation that's opioid-induced. *RN* 63:103, 2000
75. Taguchi A, Sharma N, Saleem RM, et al: Selective postoperative inhibition of gastrointestinal opioid receptors. *N Engl J Med* 345:935–940, 2001
76. Rowbotham MC, Twilling L, Davies PS, et al: Oral opioid therapy for chronic peripheral and central neuropathic pain. *N Engl J Med* 348:1223–1232, 2003
77. Mercadante S: Opioid responsiveness in patients with advanced head and neck cancer. *Support Care Cancer* 6:482–485, 1998
78. Vigano A, Bruera E, Suarez-Almazor ME: Age, pain intensity, and opioid dose in patients with advanced cancer. *Cancer* 83:1244–1250, 1998
79. Zech DF, Grond S, Lynch J, et al: Validation of World Health Organization guidelines for cancer pain relief: a 10-year prospective study. *Pain* 63:65–76, 1995
80. Cherny NJ, Chang V, Frager G, et al: Opioid pharmacotherapy in the management of cancer pain: a survey of strategies used by pain physicians for the selection of analgesic drugs and routes of administration. *Cancer* 76:1283–1293, 1995
81. Klepstad P, Kaasa S, Jystad A, et al: Immediate- or sustained-release morphine for dose finding during start of morphine to cancer patients: a randomized, double-blind trial. *Pain* 101:193–198, 2003
82. Faura CC, Moore RA, Horga JF, et al: Morphine and morphine-6–glucuronide plasma concentrations and effect in cancer pain. *J Pain Symptom Manage* 11:95–102, 1996
83. Miyoshi, RH, Leckband SG: Systemic opioid analgesics, in Loeser JD (ed.): *Bonica's Managment of Pain* (ed 2). Philadelphia, Lippincott, Williams and Wilkins, 2001, pp 1682–1709
84. Manfredi RL, Houde RW: Prescribing methadone, a unique analgesic. *J Support Oncol* 1:216–220, 2003
85. Bruera E, Neumann CM: Role of methadone in the management of pain in cancer patients. *Oncology* 13:1275–1282; discussion 1285–1288, 1291, 1999
86. Cleary JF: Cancer pain management. *Cancer Control* 7:120–131, 2000
87. Gutstein HB, Akil H: Opioid analgesics, in Hardman J, Limbard LE (eds.): *Goodman and Gilman's The Pharmacological Basis of Therapeutics* (ed 10). New York, McGraw-Hill, 2001, pp 569–619
88. Mercadante S, Casuccio A, Agnello A, et al: Morphine versus methadone in the pain treatment of advanced-cancer patients followed up at home. *J Clin Oncol* 16:3656–3661, 1998
89. Santiago-Palma J, Khojainova N, Kormick C, et al: Intravenous methadone in the management of chronic cancer pain: safe and effective starting doses when substituting methadone for fentanyl. *Cancer* 92:1919–1925, 2001
90. Rosen SH, Zeldin G, Davidson EM: Methadone is safe for treating hospitalized patients with severe pain. *Cancer J Anaesthol* 48:1109–1113, 2001
91. Bruera E, Palmer JL, Bosnjak S, et al: Methadone versus morphine as a first-line strong opioid for cancer pain: a randomized, double-blind study. *J Clin Oncol* 22:185–192, 2004
92. Levy MH: Advancement of opioid analgesia with controlled-release oxycodone. *Eur J Pain* 5(suppl A):113–116, 2001
93. Breitbart W: Psychotropic adjuvant analgesics for pain in cancer and AIDS. *Psychol Oncol* 7:333–345, 1998
94. Mercadante, S, Arcuri E, Tirelli W, et al: Amitriptyline in neuropathic cancer pain in patients on morphine therapy: a randomized placebo-controlled, double-blind crossover study. *Tumori* 88:239–242, 2002
95. Hammack JE, Michalak JC, Loprinzi CL, et al: Phase III evaluation of nortriptyline for alleviation of symptoms of *cis*-platinum-induced peripheral neuropathy. *Pain* 98:195–203, 2002
96. Martin LA, Hagan NA: Neuropathic pain in cancer patients: mechanisms, syndromes, and clinical controversies. *J Pain Symptom Manage* 14:99–117, 1997
97. Wiffen P, Collins S, McQuay H, et al: Anticonvulsant drugs for acute and chronic pain. *Cochrane Database Syst Rev,* 2000(3):CD001133
98. Pappagallo M: Newer antiepileptic drugs: possible uses in the treatment of neuropathic pain and migraine. *Clin Ther* 25:2506–2538, 2003
99. Beydoun A, Uthman BM, Sackellares JC: Gabapentin: pharmacokinetics, efficacy, and safety. *Clin Neuropharmacol* 18:469–481, 1995
100. Rosner H, Rubin L, Kestenbaum A: Gabapentin adjunctive therapy in neuropathic states. *Clin J Pain* 12:56–58, 1996
101. McCaffery M: Gabapentin for lancinating pain. *Am J Nurs* 98:12, 1998
102. Rowbotham M, Harden N, Stacey B, et al: Gabapentin for the treatment of postherpetic neuralgia: a randomized controlled trial. *JAMA* 280:1837–1842, 1998
103. Harmer JP, Larson BS: Pain relief from baclofen analgesia in a neuropathic pain patient who failed opioid and pharmacotherapy: case report. *J Pain Palliat Care Pharmacother* 16:61–64, 2002
104. Fisher K, Coderre TJ, Hagen NA: Targeting the *N*-methyl-D-aspartate receptor for chronic pain management. Preclinical animal studies, recent clinical experience and future research directions. *J Pain Symptom Manage* 20:358–373, 2000
105. Mercadante S, Casuccio A, Genovese G: Ineffectiveness of dextromethorphan in cancer pain. *J Pain Symptom Manage* 16:317–322, 1998
106. Prommer E: Ketamine to control pain. *J Palliat Med* 6:443–446, 2003
107. Bell RF, Eccleston C, Kalso E: Ketamine as adjuvant to opioids for cancer pain. A qualitative systematic review. *J Pain Symptom Manage* 26:867–875, 2003
108. Bruera E, Driver L, Barnes EA, et al: Patient-controlled methylphenidate for the management of fatigue in patients with advanced cancer: a preliminary report. *J Clin Oncol* 21:4439–4443, 2003
109. Dundee JW, Moore J: The myth of phenothiazine potentiation. *Anaesthesiol* 16:95–96, 1961
110. Keats AS, Telford J, Kurosu Y: "Potentiation" of meperidine by promethazine. *Anesthesiology* 22:34–41, 1961
111. Loblaw DA, Laperriere NJ: Emergency treatment of malignant extradural spinal cord compression: an evidenced-based guideline. *J Clin Oncol* 16:1613–1624, 1998
112. Robertson CL, Marques CB, Gralla RJ, et al: Documenting the rapidity of pain relief and palliation of other lung cancer symp-

toms with the use of dexamethasone. *Proc Am Soc Clin Oncol* 16:A280, 1997 (abstr)
113. Cordes ME, Brueggen C: Diffuse malignant pleural mesothelioma: part II. Symptom management. *Clin J Oncol Nurs* 7:545–552, 2003
114. Ross DD, Alexander CS: Management of common symptoms in terminally ill patients: part II. Constipation, delirium and dyspnea. *Am Fam Physician* 64:1019–1026, 2001
115. Van Poznak CH: The use of bisphosphonates in patients with breast cancer. *Cancer Control* 9:480–489, 2002
116. Maxwell C, Swift R, Goode M, et al: Advances in supportive care of patients with cancer and bone metastases: nursing implications of zoledronic acid. *Clin J Oncol Nurs* 7:403–408, 2003
117. Berenson JR: Zoledronic acid in cancer patients with bone metastases: results of Phase I and II trials. *Semin Oncol* 28:(suppl 6):25–34, 2001
118. Viale PH, Sanchez Yamamoto D: Bisphosphonates: expanded roles in the treatment of patients with cancer. *Clin J Oncol Nurs* 7:393–401, 2003
119. Small EJ, Smith MR, Seaman JJ, et al: Combined analysis of two multicenter, randomized, placebo-controlled studies of pamidronate disodium for the palliation of bone pain in men with metastatic prostate cancer. *J Clin Oncol* 21:4277–4284, 2003
120. Theriault RL, Lipton A, Hortobagyi GN, et al: Pamidronate reduces skeletal morbidity in women with advanced breast cancer and lytic bone lesions: a randomized, placebo-controlled trial. Protocol 18 Aredia Breast Cancer Study Group. *J Clin Oncol* 17:846–854, 1999
121. Strong KM, McPherson ML: Pamidronate. *Am J Hos Palliat Care* 15:54–55, 1998
122. Rosen LS, Gordon L, Davidson EM: Zoledronic acid versus pamidronate in the treatment of skeletal metastases in patients with breast cancer or osteolytic lesions of multiple myeloma: a phase III, double-blind, comparative trial. *Cancer J* 7:377–387, 2001
123. Lipton A, Small E, Saad F, et al: The new bisphosphonate, Zometa (zoledronic acid), decreases skeletal complications in both osteolytic and osteoblastic lesions: a comparison to pamidronate. *Cancer Invest* 20(suppl 2):45–54, 2002
124. Saad F, Gleason DM, Murray R, et al: A randomized, placebo-controlled trial of zoledronic acid in patients with hormone-refractory metastatic prostate carcinoma. *J Natl Cancer Inst* 94:1458–1468, 2002
125. Major P, Lortholary A, Hon J, et al: Zoledronic acid is superior to pamidronate in the treatment of hypercalcemia of malignancy: a pooled analysis of two randomized, controlled clinical trials. *J Clin Oncol* 19:558–567, 2001
126. Li EC, Davis LE: Zoledronic acid: a new parenteral bisphosphonate. *Clin Ther* 25:2669–2708, 2003
127. Portenoy RK, Payne R, Coluzzi P, et al: Oral transmucosal fentanyl citrate (OTFC) for the treatment of breakthrough pain in cancer patients: a controlled dose titration study. *Pain* 79:303–312, 1999
128. Farrar JT, Cleary J, Rauck R, et al: Oral transmucosal fentanyl citrate: randomized, double-blind, placebo-controlled trial for treatment of breakthrough pain in cancer patients. *J Natl Cancer Inst* 90:611–616, 1998
129. Egan TD, Sharma A, Ashburn MA, et al: Multiple dose pharmacokinetics of oral transmucosal fentanyl citrate in healthy volunteers. *Anesthesiology* 92:665–673, 2000
130. Lee M, Kern SE, Kisicki JC, et al: A pharmacokinetic study to compare two simultaneous 400 microg doses with a single 800 microg dose of oral transmucosal fentanyl citrate. *J Pain Symptom Manage* 26:743–747, 2003
131. Payne R, Mathias SD, Pasta DJ, et al: Quality of life and cancer pain: satisfaction and side effects with transdermal fentanyl versus oral morphine. *J Clin Oncol* 16:1588–1593, 1998
132. Donner B, Zenz M, Tryba M, et al: Direct conversion from oral morphine to transdermal fentanyl: a multicenter study in patients with cancer pain. *Pain* 64:527–534, 1996
133. Ahmedzai S, Brooks D: Transdermal fentanyl versus sustained-release oral morphine in cancer pain: preference, efficacy, and quality of life. The TTS-Fentanyl Comparative Trial Group. *J Pain Symptom Manage* 13:254–261, 1997
134. van Seventer R, Smit JM, Schipper RM, et al: Comparison of TTS-fentanyl with sustained-release oral morphine in the treatment of patients not using opioids for mild-to-moderate pain. *Curr Med Res Opin* 19:457–469, 2003
135. Wakefield B, Johnson JA, Kron-Chalupa J, et al: A research-based guideline for appropriate use of transdermal fentanyl. *Oncol Nurs Forum* 29:1505–1513, 1998
136. Davis MP, Walsh D, LeGrand SB, et al: Symptom control in cancer patients: the clinical pharmacology and therapeutic role of suppositories and rectal suspensions. *Support Care Cancer* 10:117–138, 2002
137. Moolenaar F, Meijler WJ, Frijlink HW, et al: Clinical efficacy, safety and pharmacokinetics of a newly developed controlled release morphine sulphate suppository in patients with cancer pain. *Eur J Clin Pharmacol* 56:219–223, 2000
138. Walsh D, Tropiano PS: Long-term rectal administration of high-dose sustained-release morphine tablets. *Support Care Cancer* 10:653–655, 2002
139. Hautkappe M, Roizen MF, Toledano A, et al: Review of the effectiveness of capsaicin for painful cutaneous disorder and neural dysfunction. *Clin J Pain* 14:97–106, 1998
140. Paice JA, Ferrans CE, Lashley FR, et al: Topical capsaicin in the management of HIV-associated peripheral neuropathy. *J Pain Symptom Manage* 19:45–52, 2000
141. Gammaitoni AR, Alvarez NA, Galer BS: Safety and tolerability of the lidocaine patch 5%, a targeted peripheral analgesic: a review of the literature. *J Clin Pharmacol* 43:111–117, 2003
142. Endo Parmaceuticals: *Lidoderm*. Chadds Ford, PA, 2002
143. Meier T, Wasner G, Faust M, et al: Efficacy of lidocaine patch 5% in the treatment of focal peripheral neuropathic pain syndromes: a randomized, double-blind, placebo-controlled study. *Pain* 106:151–158, 2003
144. Nicoll LH, Hesby A: Intramuscular injection: an integrative research review and guideline for evidence-based practice. *Appl Nurs Res* 15:149–162, 2002
145. Titler MG, Herr K, Schilling ML, et al: Acute pain treatment for older adults hospitalized with hip fracture: current nursing practices and perceived barriers. *Appl Nurs Res* 16:211–227, 2003
146. Golembiewski JA: Morphine and hydromorphone for postoperative analgesia: focus on safety. *J Perianesth Nurs* 18:120–122, 2003
147. Watanabe S, Pereira J, Hanson J, et al: Fentanyl by continuous subcutaneous infusion for the management of cancer pain: a retrospective study. *J Pain Symptom Manage* 16:323–326, 1998
148. Radbruch L, Loick G, Schulzeck S, et al: Intravenous titration with morphine for severe cancer pain: report of 28 cases. *Clin J Pain* 15:173–178, 1999
149. Fitzgibbon DR, Ready LB: Intravenous high-dose methadone administered by patient controlled analgesia and continuous infusion for the treatment of cancer pain refractory to high-dose morphine. *Pain* 72:259–261, 1997
150. Ferrell BR, Nash CC, Warfield C: The role of patient-controlled analgesia in the management of cancer pain. *J Pain Symptom Manage* 7:149–154, 1992

151. Krames ES: Practical issues when using neuraxial infusion. *Oncology* 13(suppl 2):37–44, 1999
152. Anderson VC, Burchiel KJ: A prospective study of long-term intrathecal morphine in the management of chronic nonmalignant pain. *Neurosurgery* 44:289–301, 1999
153. Hildebrand KR, Elsberry DD, Hassenbusch SJ: Stability and compatibility of morphine–clonidine admixtures in an implantable infusion system. *J Pain Symptom Manage* 25:464–471, 2003
154. Smith TJ, Staats PS, Deer T, et al: Randomized clinical trial of an implantable drug delivery system compared with comprehensive medical management for refractory cancer pain: impact on pain, drug-related toxicity, and survival. *J Clin Oncol* 20:4040–4049, 2002
155. Rauck RL, Cherry D, Boyer MF, et al: Long-term intrathecal opioid therapy with a patient-activated, implanted delivery system for the treatment of refractory cancer pain. *J Pain* 4:441–447, 2003
156. Paice JA, Penn RD, Shott S: Intraspinal morphine for chronic pain: a retrospective, multicenter study. *J Pain Symptom Manage* 11:71–80, 1996
157. Scott DA, Emanuelsson BM, Mooney PH, et al: Pharmacokinetics and efficacy of long-term epidural ropivacaine infusion for postoperative analgesia. *Anesth Analg* 85:1322–1330, 1997
158. Paice JA, DuPen A, Schwertz D: Catheter port cleansing techniques and entry of povidone-iodine into the epidural space. *Oncol Nurs Forum* 26:603–605, 1999
159. Rosenthal K: Implantable pumps deliver innovative pain management. *Nurs Manage* 34:46–49, 2003
160. Oncology Nursing Society: *Resolution: Use of Technology in Pain Management.* Pittsburgh, Oncology Nursing Society, 1991
161. Ferrell BR, Rhiner M: High-tech comfort: ethical issues in cancer pain management for the 1990s. *J Clin Ethics* 2:108–112, 1991
162. Ferrell BR, Rhiner M: Use of technology in the management of cancer pain. *J Pharm Care Pain Symptom Control* 2:17–35, 1994
163. Balducci L: Management of cancer pain in geriatric patients. *J Support Oncol* 1:175–191, 2003
164. Gibson SJ, Helme RD: Age-related differences in pain perception and report. *Clin Geriatr Med* 17:433–456, 2001
165. Fine PG: Opioid analgesic drugs in older people. *Clin Geriatr Med* 17:479–487, 2001
166. Freedman GM: Chronic pain. Clinical management of common causes of geriatric pain. *Geriatrics* 57:36–42, 2002
167. American Geriatric Society: The management of persistent pain in older persons. *J Am Geriatric Soc* 50PS,2–5, 2002
168. Dellasega C, Keiser CL: Pharmacologic approaches to chronic pain in the older adult. *Nurse Pract* 22:20–24, 1997
169. McQuay H, Carroll D, Jadad AR, et al: Anticonvulsant drugs for management of pain: a systematic review. *BMJ* 311:1047–1052, 1995
170. Hogan OH, Abram SE: Neural blockade for diagnosis and prognosis. *Anesthesiology* 86:216–241, 1997
171. Chambers PC: Coeliac plexus block for upper abdominal cancer pain. *Br J Nurs* 12:838–844, 2003
172. de Leon-Casasola OA: Critical evaluation of chemical neurolysis of the sympathetic axis for cancer pain. *Cancer Control* 7:142–148, 2000
173. Mercadante S, Fulfaro F, Casuccio A: Pain mechanisms involved and outcome in advanced cancer patients with possible indications for celiac plexus block and superior hypogastric plexus block. *Tumori* 88:243–245, 2002
174. Waldman SD: *Atlas of Interventional Pain Management.* Philadelphia, W.B. Saunders, 1998
175. Ischia S, Polati E, Finco G, et al: Celiac block for the treatment of pancreatic pain. *Curr Rev Pain* 4:127–133, 2002
176. Rigor BM: Pelvic cancer pain. *J Surg Oncol* 75:280–300, 2000
177. Hann DM, Baker F, Denniston MM: Oncology professionals' communication with cancer patients about complementary therapy: a survey. *Complement Ther Med* 11:184–190, 2003
178. Correa-Velez I, Clavarino A, Barnett AG, et al: Use of complementary and alternative medicine and quality of life: changes at the end of life. *Palliat Med* 17:695–703, 2003
179. Alimi D, Rubino C, Pichard-Leandri E, et al: Analgesic effect of auricular acupuncture for cancer pain: a randomized, blinded, controlled trial. *J Clin Oncol* 21:4120–4126, 2003
180. Smith WB: Research methodology: implications for CAM pain research. *Clin J Pain* 20:3–7, 2004
181. Astin JA, Shapiro SL, Eisenberg DM, et al: Mind-body medicine: state of the science, implications for practice. *J Am Board Fam Pract* 16:131–147, 2003
182. Spross JA, Burke MW: Nonpharmacological management of cancer pain, in McGuire DB, Yarbro CH, Ferrell BR (eds.): *Cancer Pain Management* (ed 2). Sudbury, MA, Jones and Bartlett, 1995, pp 159–205
183. Wilkie DJ: Neural mechanisms of pain: a foundation for cancer pain assessment and management, in McGuire DB, Yarbro CH, Ferrell BR (eds.): *Cancer Pain Management* (ed 2). Sudbury, MA, Jones and Bartlett, 1995, pp 61–87
184. McGuire DB: Measuring pain, in Frank-Stromborg M, Olsen S (eds.): *Instruments for Clinical Health-Care Research* (ed 2). Philadelphia, W.B. Saunders, 1997, pp 528–564
185. Wallace KG: Analysis of recent literature concerning relaxation and imagery interventions for cancer pain. *Cancer Nurs* 20:79–87, 1997
186. Dalton JA, Blau W, Lindley C, et al: Changing acute pain management to improve patient outcomes: an educational approach. *J Pain Symptom Manage* 17:277–287, 1999
187. Donovan MI, Evers K, Jacobs P, et al: When there is no benchmark: designing a primary care-based chronic pain management program from the scientific basis up. *J Pain Symptom Manage* 18:38–48, 1999
188. Miaskowski C, Crews J, Ready LB, et al: Anesthesia-based pain services improve the quality of postoperative pain management. *Pain* 80:23–29, 1999
189. Lewis FM, Zahlis EH: The nurse as coach: a conceptual framework for clinical practice. *Oncol Nurs Forum* 24:1695–1702, 1997
190. Oliver JW, Kravitz RL, Kaplan SH, et al: Individualized patient education and coaching to improve pain control among cancer outpatients. *J Clin Oncol* 19:2206–2212, 2001
191. Ersek M, Wilson SA: The challenges and opportunities in providing end-of-life care in nursing homes. *J Palliat Med* 6:45–57, 2003
192. Cohen MZ, Easley MD, Ellis C, et al: Cancer pain management and the JCAHO's pain standards: an institutional challenge. *J Pain Symptom Manage* 25:519–527, 2003
193. Redinbaugh EM, Baum A, DeMoss C, et al: Factors associated with the accuracy of family caregiver estimates of patient pain. *J Pain Symptom Manage* 23:31–38, 2002
194. Rhiner M, Coluzzi PH: Family issues influencing management of cancer pain, in McGuire DB, Yarbro CH, Ferrell BR (eds.): *Cancer Pain Management* (ed 2). Sudbury, MA, Jones and Bartlett, 1995, pp 207–230
195. De Wit R, van Dam F, Sandbelt L, et al: A pain education program for chronic pain patients: follow-up results from a randomized clinical trial. *Pain* 73:55–69, 1997

CHAPTER 28

Infection

Brenda K. Shelton, MS, RN, CCRN, AOCN®

Scope of the Problem

Despite tremendous progress in the management of infections in patients with cancer during this last decade, infection remains one of the most significant etiologies of morbidity and mortality for these patients. It is estimated that more than 25%–40% of patients with cancer[1] will experience infection during the course of their treatment, and some sources suggest that the management of infectious complications accounts for 45% of inpatient care for certain patient groups.[2] Localized infection can result in progression to systemic dissemination of the microbes in 10%–20% of patients[3,4] and a shock response in 15%–20%, which is today associated with a mortality rate of only 6%–10%.[5,6] Although much is known about the distribution, etiology, and clinical complications associated with infection, no predictive models exist to identify which patients will develop the most life-threatening of the associated complications.[7,8]

Definitions

Infectious complications are commonly described in terms of the type of infectious microorganism, the physiologic location of the infection, and the degree of tissue invasion. Types of infecting microbial organisms include bacteria, fungi, viruses, and opportunistic organisms. Each of these categories includes multiple microbial species, with unique propensities to infect specific locations, and production of specific signs and symptoms. The most common microbial sources of infection and their key clinical features are described in Table 28-1.[9–11] Two decades ago, the most common infections among immunocompromised patients involved gram-negative bacteria, which were thought to be primarily translocated from the gastrointestinal tract.[12–14] Today, with the use of more invasive vascular access lines and prolonged exposure to antimicrobials, gram-positive organisms are more prevalent.[8,13,15]

Infections are also described by the specific body location that is infected. For instance, infection involving the airway is termed pneumonia, whereas the same infection affecting the meninges is termed meningitis. The specific terms and clinical manifestations of infections of different body locations are detailed in Table 28-1.[10,11]

The presence of microbes in and on body tissues may indicate anything from the presence of normal resident flora to the invasion of body tissues by virulent and toxic foreign microbes. Bacteria that normally reside within the body include examples such as *Escherichia coli* that are commonly found within the gastrointestinal tract. These same organisms can cause infection if they are accidently ''tracked'' to another part of the body. Typical normal flora and their resident human tissues are listed in Table 28-2.[16–18] It can be assumed that these normal flora are pathogenic if discovered in a different part of the body.

Infections are graded and defined according to severity based on the level of tissue penetration. When organisms are present on body tissues, but are not viable, multiplying, or invading the epithelial layer, the situation is termed *colonization*, a form of microbial invasion that is not usually pathogenic.[19] Colonization may

Table 28-1 Signs and Symptoms of Infection

Body System	Complication	Signs and Symptoms*	Infectious Organisms
Neurologic	Encephalitis	Confusion, lethargy, difficulty arousing, headache, visual difficulty/photosensitivity, nausea, hypertension	*Neisseria meningitidis*, *Toxoplasma*, herpes simplex, cytomegalovirus
	Meningitis	Lethargy and somnolence, confusion, nuccal rigidity	*N. meningitidis*, streptococcus, *Listeria*, *Cryptococcus*, herpes simplex
Head/neck	Conjunctivitis	Reddened conjunctiva, excess tearing of eye, pus-like exudate from eye, blurred vision, swelling of eyelid, eye itching	Pneumococcus, streptococcus, staphylococcus, *N. meningitidis*, adenovirus, rotovirus
	Otitis media	Earache, difficulty hearing, itching inner ear, ear drainage	Streptococcus, aspergillus
	Sinusitis	Discolored nasal mucous, nasal congestion, face pain, eye pain, blurred vision	Staphylococcus, *Haemophilus influenzae*, aspergillus, *Histoplasma*
	Oropharyngeal infection	Oral ulcerations or plaques, halitosis, reddened gums, abnormal papillae of the tongue, sore throat, difficulty swallowing	Streptococcus, *Candida*, herpes simplex
	Lymphadenitis	Swollen neck lymph glands, tender lymph glands, a lump felt when swallowing	*Mycobacterium avium-intracellulare*
Pulmonary	Bronchitis	Persistent cough, sputum production, gurgles in upper airways, wheezes in upper airways, hypoxemia and/or hypercapnea	Streptococcus, staphylococcus

(continued)

Table 28-1 Signs and Symptoms of Infection (continued)

Body System	Complication	Signs and Symptoms*	Infectious Organisms
	Pneumonia	Chest discomfort pronounced with inspiration, persistent cough, sputum production, diminished breath sounds, crackles or gurgles, asymmetrical chest wall movement, labored breathing, nasal flaring with breathing, hypoxemia	Staphylococcus, pneumococcus, streptococcus, *N. meningitidis, Corynebacterium diphtheriae, Klebsiella,* proteus, *Pseudomonas,* actinomyces, *Nocardia,* aspergillus, *Cryptococcus, Blastomyces, Histoplasma,* cytomegalovirus, *Pneumocystis carinii,* legionella, Mycobacterium (*Mycobacterium tuberculosis, M. avium-intracellulare*), *Toxoplasma*
	Pleurisy	Chest discomfort pronounced with inspiration, sides of chest more painful, usually unilateral discomfort, splinting with deep breaths	*Listeria, Histoplasma*
Cardiovascular	Myocarditis	Dysrhythmias, murmurs or gallops, elevated jugular venous pulsations, weak thready pulses, hypotension, point of maximal impulse shifted laterally	*Toxoplasma*
	Pericarditis	Aching constant chest discomfort unrelieved by rest or nitrates, pericardial rub, muffled heart sounds	Staphylococcus, pneumococcus, streptococcus, *N. meningitidis, Histoplasma*
Gastrointestinal	Gastritis	Nausea, vomiting within 30 min of eating, heme-positive emesis, aching stomach that initially improves by eating	Salmonella
	Infectious diarrhea	Greater than six loose stools per day, clay-colored stools, foul-smelling stools, abdominal cramping, abdominal distention	Staphylococcus, *Corynebacterium diphtheriae,* actinomyces, *Klebsiella,* proteus, shigella, *Pseudomonas,* legionella, cytomegalovirus
	Cholelithiasis/pancreatitis	Epigastric discomfort, intolerance to high-fat meal, clay-colored stools, nausea and vomiting, hyperglycemia, hypocalcemia, hypoalbuminemia, increased lipase and amylase	*Nocardia, Candida,* cytomegalovirus, *Cryptosporidium*
	Hepatitis	Jaundice, right upper quadrant discomfort, hepatomegaly, elevated transaminases and bilirubin, fatty food intolerances, nausea and vomiting, diarrhea	Cytomegalovirus, mycobacterium (*M. tuberculosis, M. avium-intracellulare*), *Toxoplasma*
Genitourinary	Urethritis	Painful urination, difficulty urinating, itching of genitourinary orifice	*Escherichia coli, Candida*
	Cystitis	Small frequent urination (urinary urgency) feeling of fullness of the bladder	Streptococcus, *Pseudomonas, E. coli, Candida*
	Nephritis	Flank discomfort, oliguria, protein in urine	Streptococcus, *E. coli, Candida*
	Vaginitis	Itching of vaginal area, vaginal discharge	*N. meningitidis,* herpes simplex
Musculoskeletal	Arthritis	Joint discomfort, swollen and warm joints	Streptococcus, *Nocardia*
	Myositis	Aching muscles, weakness	
Dermatologic	Superficial skin infection	Rashes, itching, raised and/or discolored skin lesions, open draining skin lesions, patterns are unique to specific microorganism	Any organism
	Cellulitis	Redness, warmth and swelling of subcutaneous tissue area, radiating pain from area toward middle of body	*Staphylococcus aureus,* streptococcus, actinomyces
Hematologic/ Immunologic	Bacteremia	Low diastolic blood pressure, headache, confusion, oliguria, decreased bowel sounds, warmth, flushing, positive blood cultures	Any organism, although most common are those bacteria that infect the mucous membranes, lung, and gastrointestinal tract, and select fungi (eg, *Candida*), viruses (eg, cytomegalovirus), and opportunistic organisms (eg, mycobacterium).

*The signs and symptoms presented in this table are unique features of each process and do not include the common constitutional signs and symptoms seen with all infections, such as fever, chills, malaise, leukocytosis, positive tissue culture for microorganisms or increased erythrocyte sedimentation rate.

Reprinted with permission from Shelton BK: Sepsis. *Seminars in Oncology Nursing* 15:214–215, 1999.[10]

Table 28-2 Normal Flora within the Body

Body Tissue	Normal Flora at This Location
Eyes (cornea)	*Neisseria* Staphylococcus Streptococcus
Gastrointestinal tract, large intestine, rectum	*Bacteroides* *E. coli* *Enterobacter* *Klebsiella* *Proteus*
Gastrointestinal tract, small intestine	*Bacteroides* *E. coli* *Enterococcus* *Lactobacillus*
Oral mucosa	*Actinomyces israeli* *Candida albicans* *Entamoeba gingivalis* *Diptheroids* Streptococcus *Trichomonas tenax*
Reproductive system	*Candida* *E. coli* *Neisseria* Staphylococcus Streptococcus
Skin surface	*Candida* *Diptheroids* *Proprionibacteria* Staphylococcus epidermis
Stomach	*Candida* *Lactobacillus*
Upper respiratory tract	*Bronhamella* *Haemophilus* *Neisseria* Staphylococcus Streptococcus

Data from Mims, Nash, Stephen[16]; Todar[17]; Virginia Academy of Science.[18]

cause infection in severely immunocompromised patients, so it is considered an aspect of the patient's clinical data that is important to follow.[20] Definitions of levels of infection have been defined by the American College of Chest Physicians and Society of Critical Care Medicine;[19] these definitions are summarized in Table 28-3.

Infections are also defined in the context of the *chain of infection,* which relates to the spread of infection from one person to another. Not all infections are transmissable, but this theoretical model is useful for addressing all aspects of infection control for those microbial infections that can spread.[21,22] The six-step model describes the process from microbe to clinical disease. Infectious agents (e.g., bacteria, fungi, viruses, rickettsiae, parasites) are harbored in a sanctuary site called a *reservoir.* Reservoirs may comprise people, water, food, medications, equipment, or the environment. Microbes exit reservoirs by excretions, secretions, or droplets and are acquired by a host via one or more of the four modes of transmission: contact, airborne, vehicle, or vector. Microbes enter the host's body through breaks in the barrier defense or via one of the natural orifices. The susceptibility of the host is the primary variable determining whether infection will occur, and the link of transmission is the easiest to break and thereby halt the chain of infection spread.[21] Infections are described by where or how they are acquired (community acquired versus hospital acquired or nosocomial), as well as whether they are confined to the host (noncommunicable) or can spread from one person to another (communicable). Some clinical situations warrant differentiation of whether an infection is a primary (first to occur) or secondary (related to the presence or treatment of another infection).

Incidence

The prevalence of specific risk factors for infection, such as neutropenia and T-cell suppression, has been a focus of research, but less information is available regarding the incidence of actual infection resulting from these risks. This may be in part due to the limitations of diagnostic procedures to validate and reveal the source of infection, or in the varied approaches to care that make data collection a difficult task.[8] In patients with fever, only 48%–60% will have a documented infection.[8] Infection may be treated with intravenous antimicrobials on an inpatient basis, treated with oral antimicrobials on an outpatient basis, or not treated, allowing the body's normal immune mechanisms to overcome the microbe.

Systemic or bloodstream infection, which is termed sepsis, is estimated to occur in 10%–20% of patients who have a febrile neutropenic event.[23] Sepsis is better defined and tracked than most infections. Its incidence approaches 750,000 cases annually. In the United States, sepsis is the leading cause of death in noncardiac intensive care units and the eleventh leading cause of death overall.[24] Mortality associated with sepsis ranges from 28% to 50%.[24–26] In a recent study of more than 190,000 patients with severe sepsis, the additional cost of care for this complication amounted to an estimated $22,100 per case, and its annual costs exceeded $16.7 billion.[24] Although less well documented than in the critical care literature, sepsis has an estimated 45% incidence in patients with cancer, and the associated patient mortality exceeds 30%.[5]

Table 28-3 American College of Chest Physicians/Society of Critical Care Medicine Definitions of Infections and Sepsis

Infection: Microbial phenomenon characterized by an inflammatory response to the presence of microorganisms or the invasion of normally sterile host tissue by those organisms.

Bacteremia: The presence of viable bacteria in the blood.

Systemic inflammatory response syndrome: The systemic inflammatory response to a variety of severe clinical insults; the response is manifested by two or more of the following conditions:
Temperature > 38°C or < 36°C
Heart rate > 90 beats/min
Respiratory rate > 20 breaths/min or PaCO2 < 32 mm Hg (< 4.3 kPa)
WBC > 12,000 cells/mm^3, < 4000 cells/mm^3, or > the 10% immature (band) forms

Sepsis: The systemic response to infection; the response is manifested by two or more of the following conditions as a result of infection:
Temperature > 38°C or < 36°C
Heart rate > 90 beats/min
Respiratory rate > 20 breaths/min or PaCO2 < 32 mm Hg (< 4.3 kPa)
WBC > 12,000 cells/mm^3, < 4000 cells/mm^3, or > 10% immature (band) forms

Severe sepsis: Sepsis associated with organ dysfunction, hypoperfusion, or hypotension; hypoperfusion and perfusion abnormalities may include, but are not limited to, lactic acidosis, oliguria, or an acute alteration in mental status.

Septic shock: Sepsis with hypotension, despite adequate fluid resuscitation, along with the presence of perfusion abnormalities that may include, but are not limited to, lactic acidosis, oliguria, or an acute alteration in mental status; patients who are on inotropic or vasopressor agents may not be hypotensive at the time that perfusion abnormalities are measured.

Hypotension: A systolic blood pressure < 90 mm Hg or a reduction > 40 mm Hg from baseline in the absence of other causes for hypotension.

Multiple organ dysfunction syndrome: Presence of altered organ function in an acutely ill patient such that homeostasis cannot be maintained without intervention.

Reprinted with permission from Members of the American College of Chest Physicians/Society of Critical Care Medicine Consensus Conference Committee. Definitions for sepsis and organ failure and guidelines for the use of innovative therapies in sepsis. *Crit Care Med* 20:864–874, 1992.[19]

Etiology and Risk Factors

The causes of infection in the patient with cancer are varied, involving both host and environmental factors. To some degree, the type of invading microbe or site of infection may also be associated with specific risk factors. Examples of defective protective mechanisms and factors contributing to infection in people with cancer are listed in Table 28-4.[27–45] In some cases, specific microbial characteristics, such as extent of exposure or organism virulence, influence the incidence and severity of infection. However, it is clear that neither the presence of a potentially pathogenic microbe nor a defined risk factor conclusively leads to infection, so other, as-yet-undefined mediating factors may exist.

Physiologic Alterations

Normal Anatomy, Physiology, and Scientific Principles

The body's defensive systems are divided into nonspecific and specific defenses. The nonspecific defensive system of the body functions to rapidly recognize foreign antigens and mount an aggressive destruction of these proteins. It includes the skin and mucosal barriers, granulocytes, and the complement protein pathway. The specific immune system seeks to find specific antigenic material and to create targeted biologic agents that selectively destroy this unique substance.

The two systems work in an integrated fashion to produce both an immediate and a delayed response to pathogens entering the body. The specific response is a more delayed response, but is more selective in its pattern of destruction. The specific immune response is led by lymphocytes and their cytokines or immunoglobulins. It is divided into the primary (initial) response and the secondary response. The primary response recognizes foreign proteins and causes the release of cell killer substances termed cytokines (e.g., interferon, interleukin-2), a process termed *cellular immunity*. The secondary immune response relies on the immune memory of antigens that have been previously recognized by the lymphocytes, and involves the recall of immunoglobulins that were created upon initial exposure to the antigen. This activity is also termed the *humoral immune response*.

Inadequate nonspecific immune responses (e.g., breaks in the integumentary system, neutropenia, complement deficiency) usually result in bacterial infection. In contrast, inadequate specific immune responses may result in viral or opportunistic infection. Inappropriate specific immune responses constitute a

Table 28-4 Characteristics and Risks for Immunocompromised Patient Populations

Patient Characteristics	Physiologic Mechanism of Risk	Possible Consequences of Risk Factor
Abuse of intravenous drugs	• Chronic altered barrier defense leads to reduced white blood cells and slowed phagocytic responses. • Constant viral exposure may alter T-cell function.	Topical antimicrobial agents are used to prevent local infections induced by needles. Recognition of the T-cell defects and propensity for viral infections caused by IV drug abuse may allow for closer monitoring strategies and early treatment for viral infection.
Alcoholism	• Decreased neutrophil activity: increased bacterial infections, more rapid dissemination of infection. • Hepatic/splenic congestion also slows phagocytic response.	The risk of aspiration is more common in patients who use alcohol excessively, so oral and upper gastrointestinal infectious organisms are the usual suspects in patients with symptoms of pneumonia. Altered liver and spleen function may diminish immune memory and make patients prone to encapsulated organisms.
Antibiotics	• Destruction of normal flora, enhanced growth of resistant organism, fungal superinfection.	When normal bacterial flora are destroyed by the antimicrobial therapy, resistant organisms may emerge, and fungal organisms may flourish. Antifungal prophylaxis may be prescribed.
Autoimmune disease	• Diseases manifested by self-rejection that implies inappropriate sensitization of foreign substances.	General immunocompromised precautions are implemented in patients with poor immune recognition.These disorders are treated with immune-suppressing agents and corticosteroids, so the effects and management strategies are the same as those risk variables.
Blood transfusions	• Some viral illnesses are difficult to detect in blood screening, particularly in the incubation phase. Blood products infected with viruses can transmit viral disease to the recipient. • Blood products that are aged, left in room air, or not handled aseptically can become contaminated with bacteria (both gram positive and gram negative) and be transmitted as a bacteremia.	Increased awareness of possible pathogen transmission via blood products has led more patients to donate autologous blood prior to procedures where blood transfusion is anticipated. Careful evaluation of the hematologic malignancy and transplant patient's viral status (e.g., cytomegalovirus) allows for planned prophylaxis during the immunocompromised period when the patient is at greatest risk for infections.
Burns	• Altered barrier defenses allow pathogen entry. • Physiologic stressor thought to decrease phagocytic responses.	Loss of integument predisposes the patient to invasion by many different microbes. The additional immunologic response of neutrophil depression adds to this risk. Specific species of microbial infection may depend on the site of injury, host colonization, or environmental factors (e.g., exposure to soil).
Cancer	• Structural disruption may lead to bone marrow or lymphatic abnormalities. • Barrier defenses are affected when tumors erode into soft tissue and mucous membranes. • Certain cancers have specific immune defects (e.g., diminished phagocytic activity or T-cell defects). • Antineoplastic therapy can cause infection from several different mechanisms: (1) it destroys reserve of all white blood cells when the bone marrow is affected; (2) it destroys the lymphatic continuum when the lymph system is affected; (3) macrophages in specific organs may be damaged by therapy; and (4) immune memory may be lost when cancer involves the B lymphocytes or when lymphocyte suppression is intended (e.g., blood and marrow transplant).	Cancer is a reflection of inadequate immune surveillance and abnormalities of the lymphatic system. Biological anticancer therapies are based on the premise that we can support the body's normal immune processes. Certain cancers will predispose patients to infection with normal flora from nearby tissues or organisms most likely to invade that area (e.g., airborne organisms via respiratory tract). Antineoplastic therapy also compromises barrier defenses and inhibits cell growth within the bone marrow, predisposing to infection.
Diabetes mellitus	• Decreased numbers of neutrophils and slowed phagocytic activity: more frequent infections, more disseminated infections, increased risk of infections with antimicrobial-resistant organisms. • Hyperglycemia causes decreased phagocytic activity and immunoglobulin defects. • Neuropathy and glycosuria predispose to decreased bladder emptying and urinary tract infections.	The extremely high risk for serious and rapidly disseminating infections prompts prophylaxis against infection for some patients, a low threshold for treatment of presumed infection, more thorough diagnostic work-ups for sources, and pathologic diagnosis of infections. Patient education to help prevent infection may include foot safety, drinking plenty of fluids, and recognition of subtle symptoms.

(continued)

Table 28-4 Characteristics and Risks for Immunocompromised Patient Populations (continued)

Patient Characteristics	Physiologic Mechanism of Risk	Possible Consequences of Risk Factor
Frequent hospitalizations	• Frequent exposure to environmental organisms other than one's own normal environment. • Exposure to other people's organisms via staff, equipment, or supplies. • Potential exposure to resistant organisms	Hospitalizations are avoided whenever possible to reduce the patient's exposure to foreign microbes that are more pathogenic than the ones in their normal living environment. When hospitalization cannot be avoided, careful separation of patient care items, single-patient-use items, or thorough cleaning between use reduces the transference of microbes and development of resistance microbes.
Gastrointestinal disease	• Decreased bowel motility allows normal flora to translocate across the GI wall to the bloodstream. • Breaks in the mucosal integrity of the GI tract predispose patients to microbial transference into the bloodstream. • Poor circulation to the GI tract causes decreased peristalsis and mucosal atrophy. Normal flora and intestinal gram-negative organisms can become pathogenic.	Maintaining minimal normal GI motility and mucosal integrity reduces the amount of infection via the GI tract. Using the gut consistently for food and fluid consumption helps maintain normal function. Enteral feeding is always attempted, if at all possible, to enhance GI integrity and function.
HIV disease	• Viral incorporation into the RNA, then the DNA of immune cells having the $CD8^+$ molecule, disrupts normal WBC function and replication, leading to lymphopenia, lymphocyte dysfunction, and macrophage dysfunction. • Disruption of these cells leads to many different infections (e.g., unusual bacteria, fungi, opportunistic bacteria, viruses) and lymphoproliferative disorders/malignancies (e.g., Kaposi's sarcoma, lymphoma).	HIV disease is directly treated with antiretrovirals and immune-reconstituting agents such as interleukin-2. Stabilization of lymphocyte counts reduces the risk and incidence of opportunistic infections. When the lymphocyte count does drop, prophylactic antimicrobial agents specific to the organisms likely to infect these patients are prescribed in a well-defined and protocol-determined manner. Avoidance of activities likely to expose patients to infection and attempts to maintain care in the ambulatory environment may also reduce the risk of serious or resistant infections.
Immunosuppressive agents and corticosteroids	• Decreased phagocytic activity. • Altered T-cell recognition of pathogens, especially viral. • Lack of immune memory to recall antibodies to previously encountered pathogens.	Immune-suppressing agents have multiple immune-depressing functions, putting patients at risk for all kinds of infections. Special precautions are implemented, and prophylactic antimicrobial agents against common opportunistic organisms may be indicated. These patients also lose immune memory and are candidates for vaccinations, provided that the vaccine does not contain live agents. Patients are taught that they will have blunted inflammatory responses and that subtle symptoms may indicate infection.
Indwelling intravenous catheters	• Indwelling venous or arterial access devices break the barrier defenses, with subsequent risk of microbial invasion. • The presence of an intravenous device may irritate the venous wall and induce inflammatory damage, resulting in a higher risk for microbial invasion.	Intravenous catheters breach the barrier defenses and increase the risk of microbial invasion into the body. Some companies have developed catheters that have been coated or treated with active antimicrobial agents such as silver ions, chlorhexidine, or heparin. Catheters have also been designed with structural variations in an attempt to reduce the irritation of veins, thereby minimizing phlebitis and infection (e.g., angled catheter tips, modified catheter anchoring devices). Clinicians must choose the smallest lumen size, least number of lumens, and most appropriate permanence of a device to reduce infection rates. Heightened sterile technique when accessing these devices may also reduce the rate of associated infection.
Infants/elderly	• Immature thymus in infants: increased viral and opportunistic infection. • Atrophy of thymus in the elderly: increased viral infection. • Decreased antigen-specific immunoglobulins in elderly: diminished immune memory, delayed hypersensitivity reactions.	Immature and atrophied immune systems can lead to infection with a variety of organisms from any additional breach in the body's defenses. Frequent complex or polymicrobial infections are expected and are guarded against by careful infection prevention techniques and strategies. Recognition of the variety of infectious complications and the potential for their rapid

(continued)

Table 28-4 Characteristics and Risks for Immunocompromised Patient Populations (continued)

Patient Characteristics	Physiologic Mechanism of Risk	Possible Consequences of Risk Factor
	• Slowed macrophage activity: more fungal infection, diminished immune memory. • Appearance of autoimmune antibodies: increased incidence of autoimmune disease.	dissemination causes increased vigilance in monitoring and early aggressive interventions for infection. Prophylactic strategies are not usually recommended in these populations, but a low threshold for treatment is implemented.
Invasive devices (e.g., Foley catheter, nasogastric tube)	• Altered barrier defenses allow pathogen entry, especially skin organisms.	Invasive devices breach the barrier defenses and increase the risk of microbial invasion into the body. Catheters and invasive devices have been coated or treated with active antimicrobial agents such as silver ions, chlorhexidine, or heparin, in an attempt to reduce related infection. Some devices also have structural variations in an attempt to reduce the irritation or mucosal injury produced, with the hope of reducing the rate of related infection (e.g., altered bluntness of the tip of a tracheal suction catheter). Infection monitoring for microbial colonization may also help detect early presence of potential pathogens in high-risk patients.
Malnutrition	• Inadequate white blood cell count. • Reduced neutrophil activity.	Altered nutrition increases the risk of all infections. Efforts to boost immune-related nutrition deficits may focus on inclusion of glutamine, arginine, and other essential amino acids in nutrient supplements as well as other measures aimed at enhancing nutrition well-being.
Hepatic disease	• Decreased neutrophil count. • Decreased phagocytic activity. • Lost immunoglobulin production.	Hepatic disease increases the risk of bacterial infection and rapid dissemination of that infection. Loss of immunoglobulins leads to failed immune memory. Special infection precautions for immunocompromised patients are implemented.
Neutropenia	• Inadequate neutrophils to combat infection.	The lack of neutrophils places the patient at high risk for bacterial infections that will rapidly disseminate and potentially cause septic shock. Hematopoietic growth factors may be administered as primary or secondary prophylaxis to abrogate the severity (depth of nadir) or longevity of the period of neutropenia.
Pulmonary disease	• Inadequate oxygenation decreases neutrophil activity.	Infection risk is increased and can be abrogated by implementing immunocompromise precautions.
Radiation therapy	• Radiation to the long bones will interfere with WBC production. • Radiation in the area of certain endocrine organs can lead to endocrine failure (hypoadrenalism, hypothyroidism, pituitary dysfunction) and infection risk. • Radiation damage to the barrier defenses will predispose the patient to invasion by microbes.	Destruction of stem cells and existing bone marrow reserve of hematopoietic cells is a common dose-limiting toxicity of radiation therapy involving the long bones where cells are produced. Destruction of the normal skin and soft tissue barriers is treated with specialized skin care to reduce the incidence of infection.
Renal disease	• Decreased neutrophil activity. • Decreased immunoglobulin activity.	Patients with renal dysfunction are provided extra precautions against bacterial infection, recognizing that they may also show blunted or reduced symptoms of infection. These patients are appropriate candidates for vaccinations against many microorganisms.
Splenectomy	• Inability to recognize and remove encapsulated bacteria (e.g., streptococci, mycobacteria).	Postsplenectomy, either functional or anatomical, the patient is at risk for specific infections. Vaccination against pneumococci is recommended for these patients. A low threshold of suspicion for streptococci with oropharyngeal or urinary tract symptoms may allow for early antimicrobial therapy.
Surgical procedures/ wounds	• Normal flora may be translocated by surgical procedure. • Altered barrier defenses due to surgical entry. • The stress of surgery or anesthetic agents may reduce neutrophil activity.	Careful surgical preparation of the planned surgical site with chlorhexidine scrubs is recommended prior to many surgical procedures. Shaving the involved area remains a debatable practice, with some believing that hair removal reduces risk, and others believing that skin nicks from the

(continued)

Table 28-4 Characteristics and Risks for Immunocompromised Patient Populations (continued)

Patient Characteristics	Physiologic Mechanism of Risk	Possible Consequences of Risk Factor
		razor may increase the risk of infection. Operating room staff may also perform a surgical scrub of the site followed by placement of a clear sterile barrier film, which is subsequently cut through for the actual procedure. Conscientious postoperative care with fluids, coughing and deep breathing, and early mobility may decrease the risk of infection. Being aware of previous colonization or infection prior to surgery may assist in defining the source of fever postoperatively.
Traumatic injuries	• Altered barrier defenses allowing pathogen entry. • Type of infection dependent upon source and severity of injury (e.g., soil contamination, water contamination, skin flora).	Altered barrier defenses are treated with frequent cleansing, antimicrobial cleansing, covering with sterile dressings to prevent infectious organisms from entering the bloodstream via the open wound. Antimicrobial ointments have not been proven effective. If a wound is thought to be clean and sterile, a clear protective barrier dressing may provide better occlusiveness and guard against microorganism entry.

Data from Wade, Rubenstein, Brown, et al[3]; Shelton[10]; Allen, Shelton[27]; Balducci, Carreca[28]; Bartlett, Gallant[29]; Buchsel, Forgey, Grape, et al[30]; Camp-Sorrell[31]; Crnich, Maki[32]; Eggimann, Pittet[33]; Ellerhorst-Ryan[34]; Gilliam[35]; Hanna, Raad, Hackett, et al[36]; Masur, Kaplan, Holmes, et al[37]; Moran, Camp-Sorrell[38]; O'Grady, Alexander, Dellinger, et al[39]; Raber-Durlacher, Epstein, Raber, et al[40]; Rubin[41]; Shelton[42]; Yadegarynia, Tarrand, Raad, et al[43]; Regazzoni, Khoury, Irrazabal, et al[44]; Roback.[45]

reaction that involves reaction against self or foreign substances not normally considered antigenic. This reaction may be manifested as an allergic response or autoimmune disease.

Integumentary, mucosal, and chemical barriers

Intact skin constitutes the most important barrier against invasion by both exogenous and endogenous organisms. The skin is made up of cornified layers of epithelial cells that cover the body and protect tissues against dehydration and invasion by harmful bacteria. When a break in the skin occurs, environmental microbes and those organisms that normally inhabit hair follicles and sebaceous glands may enter the body and cause infection.

A second major defense against infection is the mucocilliary activity found in the mucous membranes. The cilia of the epithelial cells that line the respiratory tract beat rhythmically to propel mucous and entrapped foreign particles toward the nose and throat. In the gastrointestinal tract, the cilia propel bacteria and waste products to be removed in the feces. Microorganisms account for as much as 60% of the weight of the stool; therefore, an intact gastrointestinal mucous membrane is essential to prevent infection.

A variety of other mechanisms serve to protect the body from microbial invasion. Resident microbial flora prevent pathogenic colonization by competing for surface-binding sites and nutrients and by producing metabolic products that are toxic to other organisms.[17] Acidic pH inhibits or prevents bacterial growth on the skin and in the stomach, bladder, and vagina. Microbicidal elements found in prostatic fluid and tears also provide a protective effect.

Leukocytes

Granulocytes. Leukocytes, particularly polymorphonuclear neutrophils (PMNs), represent a significant defense against infection. Polymorphonuclear neutrophils, which are also referred to as polys or segmented neutrophils (segs), are short-lived white blood cells (WBCs) that respond quickly to bacterial invasion. They are the most numerous of the leukocytes, constituting 35%–76% of circulating WBCs. The primary function of PMNs is the destruction and elimination of microorganisms through phagocytosis, the process of engulfing and ingesting foreign matter. In addition, PMNs secrete chemotactants, chemical substances that alert the body to the presence of an invader. Chemotactants, or monokines, stimulate increased production of PMNs, macrophages, and complement proteins and direct them to the site of invasion. Without sufficient PMNs, the body's ability to mount an inflammatory response is compromised.

Monocytes and macrophages. Monocytes and macrophages constitute what was previously referred to as the reticuloendothelial system. Monocytes are released from the bone marrow before they complete the maturation process; thus they are initially capable of only limited phagocytosis. After migrating into the tissues, full maturation occurs; the cells are then referred to as macrophages. Under normal conditions, more than 95% of these cells are mature tissue macrophages, while less than 2% are circulating monocytes. Monocytes represent only 1%–10% of the circulating WBCs.

Macrophages can survive from several months to several years. They are highly phagocytic and play an important role in the inflammatory, cellular, and humoral responses. Following initial contact with a foreign protein, macrophages process and present antigens to lymphocytes, which in turn stimulate the immune response and cytokine production. Monocytes also produce specific components required for the complement cascade.[42]

Lymphocytes. Lymphocytes, the cells responsible for cellular and humoral immunity, provide long-term protection against a variety of microorganisms. They usually constitute 17%–44% of the total WBC count. B lymphocytes, which are responsible for humoral immunity, produce antibodies that neutralize, destroy, or facilitate phagocytosis of foreign proteins. T lymphocytes, which provide cellular immunity, initiate a variety of activities that directly or indirectly result in elimination of microorganisms or other foreign substances. Cytokines released from T lymphocytes have direct cytotoxic activity and enhance the activity of other differentiated T lymphocytes. T helper cells are the most numerous of the T-lymphocyte subsets, normally constituting more than 75% of total lymphocyte counts. T helper cells serve as the principal regulators of immune function through secretion of protein mediators (cytokines) that act on other cells involved in the immune and inflammatory responses. Cytokines produced by T helper cells include interleukin-2, -3, -4, -5, and -6; gamma interferon; and granulocyte-macrophage colony-stimulating factor (GM-CSF). See Chapter 2 for more detailed discussion of the immune response.

Pathophysiology

Once microbes invade the body's tissues, a multifaceted immune reaction occurs that involves changes in normal neurologic, cardiovascular, and coagulation pathways. Even nonpathogenic endogenous microbes cause infection when translocated from one area of the body to another. A large percentage of infections in immunocompromised hosts derive from endogenous organisms.[8,13,44] Microbial tissue invasion precipitates a well-documented immunologic pathway involving cytokines and coagulation proteins. This process is a continuum that is replicated in both inflammation and infection leading to sepsis (see Chapter 38 for detailed information).

Infections occur in a defined pattern according to the immune deficit and length of immune compromise. Bacterial infections are the usual results with granulocyte defects, although fungal infections are common after seven to ten days of granulocyte defects. T-cell dysfunction can result in bacterial or fungal infection, but opportunistic and viral infections are more prevalent in cellular immune defects. Infections occurring early in immune compromise are usually bacterial, with common bacteria being the infecting organisms that develop in the first 3 days, and atypical bacteria developing between days 4 and 7. The risk of fungal infection begins between day 7 and 10, and viral or opportunistic infections occur after the tenth day of immune compromise.[16,20]

Infection involving specific sites demonstrates characteristic pathophysiologic manifestations and consequences. The most common types of infection in patients with cancer are alimentary tract (oropharynx, stomach, bowel), blood (bacteremia), indwelling venous catheter–associated infection, pneumonia, skin, and urinary tract infections.[3,8,13,20,23]

Clinical Manifestations

The patient with cancer who is infected may not display the usual signs and symptoms of infection due to the degree of immune compromise and blunting of normal phagocytic and inflammatory responses.[46] Infection is clinically recognizable by organ-specific signs and symptoms, as well as constitutional symptoms. Multiple systemic symptoms indicate a more severe or extensive infection, with some symptoms being highly characteristic of sepsis or septic shock.

The patient with localized infection will demonstrate evidence of the inflammatory response on an isolated, local level. Pain, erythema, and swelling at the site of infection are usually the first symptoms of an infection. As leukocytes respond to the infection, an exudate may form. The nature of these exudates will depend on the location of infection and on the infecting microbe. Some of these characteristics are defined in Table 28-1.[3,10,11] If the infection remains confined to the site of origin, symptoms are limited to the local level.

When infection becomes systemic, or if a strong inflammatory response is required by the body to counteract the microbes, constitutional symptoms occur. Fever is one of the most well-recognized symptoms of infection.[3,47] Patients will experience rigors or shivering as the temperature begins to rise in response to a sudden presence or increase in microbes. This reaction is particularly prevalent in infections where there is periodic "showering" of microorganisms into the bloodstream, such as occurs with catheter-related infection after flushing the catheter, with administration of contaminated blood products, or with subacute bacterial endocarditis.[47] Other systemic symptoms may include influenza-like complaints such as myalgias, arthralgias, headache, fatigue, anorexia, or nausea. These symptoms are thought to be related to the cytokine response of the body to the presence of foreign microbes.[47]

Assessment and Grading

Patient and Family History for Risk Factors

Assessment for potential infection begins with evaluation of the patient's personal and family history of infections or risk factors for development of infection (see Table 28-4).[3,10,27–45] Familial risks may include inherited disorders involving any organ where immune cells are produced or stored. Family history of infections in common organs often connotes an anatomical abnormality that leads to infection of that part of the body. Certain clinical diseases also place patients at risk for infection due to their interruption of various immune functions. Other variables increasing the risk of infection involve intrinsic host-related changes in health such as malnutrition or disrupted barrier defenses (e.g., venous access devices). Additional factors to be considered in assessing the risk for, or type of, infection would be recent travel, pets, and children.[3] Certain characteristics of some of the risk factors defined in Table 28-4 can be further delineated to more precisely define the degree of risk for infection.[3,10,24,27,29–43] For instance, when neutropenia lasts longer than 7 days, the risk of infection increases exponentially. Additionally, the risk of infection due to venous access devices can be reduced by inserting cuffed permanent/semipermanent lines, using single-lumen lines, inserting catheters prior to the onset of immune suppression, or having catheters inserted and cared for by a limited number of skilled operators.

Patient interview will also reveal any previous history of infections. Patients will often present repeatedly with infections in the same site or with the same microorganisms. A history of microbial colonization at a site that now presents with symptoms of infection will often be treated with the presumption that colonization has become infection.

Physical Examination

Physical examination for the signs and symptoms of infection requires a complete head-to-toe assessment for signs or symptoms of inflammation. Erythema, local pain, swelling, and induration may be present at the site of infection. If the infection is systemic, the signs of compensatory hyperdynamic cardiovascular effects will be apparent, including tachycardia; warm, flushed, and dry skin; and full bounding pulses. The blood shunting to major organs such as the heart, lungs, and brain may result in decreased bowel sounds or oliguria.[10] Prolonged oliguria is considered a signal of infection that has progressed to sepsis.[10] When perfusion becomes more severely compromised, even the heart, lungs, and brain are less than optimally perfused. Altered mental status is considered an ominous sign of impending severe sepsis.[27] Breaks in the skin integrity or dark, moist, skin folds are particularly at risk for invasion by microbes. Examination of these sites for unusual skin color, texture, exudate, or lesions may yield evidence of infection.

Vital signs, particularly the temperature, are monitored frequently. Oral temperature monitoring is considered the most accurate for routine patient assessment.[47] Rectal probes are contraindicated due to potential injury to the rectal mucosa. Other methods of obtaining core body temperature include tympanic thermometers and bladder thermometers. The accuracy of tympanic thermometers is notoriously operator dependent, and bladder thermometers require insertion of a Foley catheter. The temperature threshold usually defined as significant for potential infection is 38.3°C (100.5°F) orally once or 38.0°C for 1 hour.[3] This degree of fever is thought to demonstrate a systemic reaction to injury or microbial invasion. Not all patients will display fever, so an increase in baseline temperature of 1°C may be considered a symptom of infection in the presence of risk factors and other clinical findings.[3] Low temperatures may also occur with infections and are thought to be associated with gram-negative organisms.

Fever patterns may also vary with different infecting organisms. Some have suggested that bacterial infections produce high, spiking fevers with periods of return to normal. Disseminated fungal infections usually produce high, spiking fevers without any such return to a baseline. Viral infections may be characterized by low continuous fevers.

Most patients who have infection are tachycardic and tachypneic, except when the infection is so severe as to cause acidosis. When patients are febrile, their diastolic blood pressure also drops, causing lower mean (average) pressures. This vasodilation will first present as orthostasis, followed by systolic hypotension.

Diagnostic Studies

The gold standard for diagnosis of infection is quantitative cultures obtained from the involved body organ. These results are not usually available for 24–72 hours, so screening tests may be used to evaluate the probability of infection.[48] While the most common and useful test is the complete blood count, other laboratory tests that will assist in the differential diagnosis include serum chemistry (inclusive of electrolytes, creatinine, and blood urea nitrogen), bilirubin levels, hepatic transaminases, and lactate.[3]

The complete blood count with the total white blood cell count and differential is the first diagnostic test used to screen for infection. White blood cells are elevated in the presence of infection. The normal white blood cell count is 5000–10,000/mm^3. In patients with normal immune reactions, infection causes mild to moderate elevations of 10,000–20,000/mm^3.[42] The extent of white blood cell elevation can vary depending on the specific microbe involved, severity of infection, organs involved, and host's immune competence. Extremely high white blood cell counts are associated with meningitis, associated with necrotizing organisms, or are found in children. White blood cell counts higher than 25,000/mm^3 are unlikely to be related to infection; instead, lymphoproliferative disorders are considered the more likely etiology.[42]

The white blood cell differential is interpreted by assessing the specific percentage of each of the major categories of white blood cells: granulocytes (neutrophils, eosinophils, and basophils), monocytes, and lymphocytes. Granulocytes (inclusive of all neutrophils, eosinophils, and basophils) normally account for 35%–76% of the total white blood count, monocytes are 1%–9%, and lymphocytes represent 17%–44%. The only cell that will be released from the bone marrow in an immature form is the granulocyte. Granulocytes are elevated with bacterial infection or with inflammatory conditions, but immature cells are noted in the circulating serum only if infection is present. This situation is dubbed a ''left shift'' in the differential because there are increased numbers of immature cells.[42] The term ''left shift'' is derived from the tradition of diagramming cells on a horizontal line with immature cells on the far left and completely mature cells on the far right. Monocytes normally differentiate into tissue macrophages and are seldom present in the serum. If an excessive number are present, then an unusual viral or opportunistic infection is most likely to blame. Lymphocytes are elevated when the body reacts to foreign antigenic agents or tissue. Elevated lymphocytes usually indicate viral infection, allergy, or rejection of transplanted tissue. Used in conjunction with risk assessment and clinical findings, the white blood count and differential can be a valuable tool in evaluating the probability of a serious infection requiring interventions such as hospitalization or intravenous antimicrobials.

Other laboratory tests that predict the risk for infection include the absolute neutrophil count (ANC), absolute lymphocyte count (ALC), and immunoglobulin levels. Recognition of low levels of these essential immune components can allow for proactive prevention of infection. An ANC of less than 2000/mm^3 is defined as a grade 1 neutropenia according to the Cancer Therapy Evaluation Program. Grade 2 neutropenia is an ANC of 1000–1500/mm^3. Grade 3 neutropenia is an ANC of 500–1000/mm^3, and grade 4 toxicity is less than 500/mm^3.[49] The lower the neutrophil count, the greater the risk for bacterial infection. When neutrophil levels are suppressed for more than 7 days, the risk for infection increases and the scope of possible infecting organisms broadens to include fungi, viruses, and opportunistic organisms. Patients are also at greater risk for infection with resistant microbes. A low ALC is common with HIV infection, although it may also occur in transplant patients or those on long-term corticosteroids. When the ALC is less than 200/mm^3, the patient is at risk for opportunistic organisms such as *Pneumocystis carinii*; when the ALC is less than 100/mm^3, infection with organisms such as toxoplasmosis may also occur.[29] Immunoglobulin levels less than 300 mg/dL predispose the patient to sinus and pulmonary infections. Immunoglobulin infusions are administered daily for three days to compensate for this condition.

Radiologic tests may also be performed to screen for pockets of infection such as pneumonia or abscesses.[3] The computed tomography (CT) scan often provides useful information to aid in diagnosis of infection in most areas of the body. Some locations that are prone to motion or dense with close organs are the abdomen and pelvis; ultrasound may be used for diagnosis of infections in these areas. Changes in neurologic tissue and joints are sensitive to magnetic resonance imaging (MRI), so MRI may be used to diagnose infections in these organs.

Definitive diagnosis of infection is determined by culture for microbes. The organisms for culture will always include aerobic and anaerobic bacteria, but when infection risk has extended beyond 3–5 days, cultures may also include assessment for fungi, viruses, or opportunistic organisms. The technique used when obtaining culture specimens is important for attaining valid and reliable results. Inadequate specimens can result in false-positive cultures. Contaminants in the culture media from lack of sterile technique can lead to false-positive cultures, although contamination is often suspected because the bacteria cultured may not be multiplying as usually seen with actual infection, and contaminants are slower to become positive.[48] Techniques for obtaining culture specimens are outlined in Table 28–5.[21,22,50–52] Special culture media are suggested to replace aerobic media when the patient is already receiving antimicrobial therapy.[10,50] The prevalence of infection with gram-positive organisms (approximately 75% of all infections) has led many clinicians to simultaneously obtain culture specimens for Gram stain testing.[53,54] Gram-positive organisms stain darkly when covered with Gram stain. Gram stain evaluation may be performed by the physician near the patient care area or the specimen may be sent to the laboratory for analysis.[53]

After cultures are determined to be positive for the presence of a microbe, they are evaluated for sensitivity to various antimicrobial agents, a process known as "sensitivity testing." The selection of agents tested for sensitivity is based on the usual ability of those agents to destroy the microbe. Sensitivity testing reveals resistant microbial strains and permits clinicians to continually monitor the ability of common antimicrobial agents to destroy various microorganisms in their clinical region. The agent with the narrowest spectrum of activity, but with effective destruction of the infecting microbe, is chosen for treatment of the infection. This strategy limits development of antimicrobial resistance.[55]

Therapeutic Approaches and Nursing Care

Prevention

The most important objective in management of inevitable risk factors for infection is proactive prevention. Infection can be prevented by control of environmental exposures to microorganisms, modification of patient care routines, and primary prophylactic measures such as growth factor or antimicrobial administration.

Environmental control

The Centers for Disease Control and Prevention (CDC) offers guidelines for construction, air handling, and water sanitation in the management of immunocompromised patients.[56–58] Construction barriers and alternative transportation routes must be provided to protect immunocompromised patients from microbes such as *Aspergillus* or *Coccidioides* that become airborne when the ground is disturbed or walls and ceilings are removed.[56] High-efficiency particulate air handling (HEPA) systems are required in care of blood and marrow transplant patients and have proved useful in preventing fungal and opportunistic airborne infections.[58] All immunocompromised patients are advised to use only sterile water for drinking or rinsing feeding tubes. Hospitals following the CDC guidelines for prevention of infection in immunocompromised patients have water sanitation and intermittent monitoring plans in place to assess and treat *Legionella* and *Pseudomonas* in their water systems.[58]

Although CDC guidelines do not recommend any kind of "protective" or "strict" isolation for prevention of infection, many institutions require additional protective barriers when caring for immunocompromised patients.[59,60] The CDC has carefully reviewed the scientific evidence and does not recommend barrier protection, but does emphasize that hand washing remains the single most significant measure for preventing infection.[61] Institutional practices vary from no special precautions, to masks only during influenza season, to full isolation barrier protection for all patient contact. At a minimum, whenever possible, immunocompromised patients should be placed in private rooms when hospitalized. If this is not feasible, cohorting of immunocompromised patients is recommended.[61] Screening visitors for infection exposure or limiting children visitation may be other strategies for controlling environmental risks for infection.[58,61]

Fastidious cleaning routines for all aspects of the environment are important for prevention of infection. Regular floor cleaning, curtain cleaning, and bathroom sanitation support prevention of infection in these patients. Environmental precautions may also prohibit fresh flowers and plants.[58]

Patient care routines

Patients who are immunocompromised should have their specific routines altered to limit the possibility of developing infection. Whether the granulocytes or the lymphocytes are affected, risk for infection is increased in case of immune compromise. Most measures are appropriate to implement regardless of which cell line is suppressed.[54] Patients are advised to maintain vigilant personal hygiene and to avoid exposure to people or places where communicable diseases are a prevalent issue. If they have pets, patients should maintain the animals' vaccinations, cleanse them frequently, and wash after handling the animals. When possible, patients should refrain from cleaning their excrement. If patients like to garden, they should wear gloves, cover their body, and wash thoroughly after each session.

Particularly in the hospital, single-use and throwaway items will reduce the risk of transferring infection from patient to patient. Staff must be careful to follow up these hospital measures with additional precautions such as making sure their stethoscopes are cleaned between patients, and wearing cover gowns if carrying soiled linens to a hamper far away from the

Table 28-5 Types of Cultures and Recommended Techniques

Type of Culture	Technique for Obtaining	Special Considerations/Comments
Blood culture, invasive line	• Assemble supplies for sterile blood drawing procedure: mask, sterile gloves, drape, hub and culture bottle disinfectant, and culture media (one aerobic, one anaerobic, possibly one viral medium). • Prepare tops of culture media bottles by thoroughly cleansing with alcohol and leaving alcohol swab on top of bottle until ready to access. • Don mask, lay barrier, and don sterile gloves • Using sterile gloves, cleanse catheter connection site thoroughly with alcohol and allow to dry. • Using sterile gloves, disconnect the line and cover with a sterile cap. • Connect blood drawing equipment (follow institutional policy for drawing a discard or not). • Draw at least 5 mL for each culture bottle.	• Some institutions recommend no blood withdrawal prior to the blood for culture; others require a waste withdrawal equivalent to at least 1.5 times the catheter volume. • Some institutions suggest obtaining cultures from each line or lumen during the first fever work-up, especially if the line has been in place 7 day or longer.
Blood culture, peripheral	• Assemble supplies for sterile blood drawing procedure: mask, sterile gloves, drape, skin disinfectant (chlorhexidine), culture bottle disinfectant (alcohol), and culture media (one aerobic, one anaerobic, possibly one viral medium). • Prepare tops of culture media bottles by thoroughly cleansing with alcohol and leaving alcohol swab on top of bottle until ready to access. • Don mask, lay barrier, and don sterile gloves. • Using sterile gloves, cleanse skin site thoroughly with chlorhexidine and allow to dry. • Using sterile gloves, prepare the needle with adapter for culture bottles. • Connect blood drawing equipment. • Draw at least 5 mL for each culture bottle.	• Cultures should be drawn no closer than 10 minutes, and no further apart than 20–30 minutes.
Drainage from a tube/drain (e.g., biliary stent, chest tube)	• Assemble supplies for sterile blood drawing procedure: mask, sterile gloves, drape, connection hub or access port, culture bottle disinfectant, and culture media (one aerobic, one anaerobic, possibly one viral medium). • Prepare tops of culture media bottles by thoroughly cleansing with alcohol and leaving alcohol swab on top of bottle until ready to access. • Don mask, lay barrier, and don sterile gloves. Using sterile gloves, cleanse connection/hub site thoroughly with alcohol and allow to dry. • Using sterile gloves, disconnect the tubing and cover with a sterile cap.	• Drainage should be removed from the cleanest tubing possible. At times, it may be advisable to change to new sterile drainage tubing prior to obtaining the culture specimen.
Nasopharyngeal cultures	• For bacteria: Use a dry swab for each nostril and insert gently until resistance is met. Turn the swab in a complete circle and remove. • For virus: With the patient leaning his or her head back slightly, instill 3–5 mL of preservative-free sterile water into first one nostril, then have the patient lean forward and blow the nose into a sterile specimen cup without having the secretions touch the face. Repeat the procedure on the other side if the patient can tolerate it.	• Cultures for bacteria have a greater yield with simple swabbing. Upper respiratory viruses are notoriously difficult to obtain valid positive cultures. False-negative results are common.
Sputum culture	• Common bacterial sputum cultures require patients to attempt to cough into a sterile specimen cup, attempting not to let the sputum touch their tongue. Some institutions suggest tooth and tongue brushing prior to obtaining a specimen. • Suctioned sputum culture: Using a new sterile suction catheter, the catheter is passed into the nasopharynx and can be used to obtain a specimen for culture.	• Culture for specific organisms may require an early-morning specimen to ensure a specimen from deep in the lungs and with best organism yield (e.g., *pneumocystis carinii*). • Bronchodilator therapy prior to obtaining the specimen may enhance the sputum yield. • A light water-soluable lubricant may be used if absolutely necessary.

(continued)

Table 28-5 Types of Cultures and Recommended Techniques (continued)

Type of Culture	Technique for Obtaining	Special Considerations/Comments
		• If there is limited sputum and it is stuck inside the suction catheter, a small amount of preservative-free sterile water can be drawn up from a sterile cup to wash the sputum from the tubing.
Stool culture	• Assemble sterile specimen cup, sterile gloves, and cleansing wipes. • Have the patient defecate into a clean bedpan or bedside commode/toilet receptacle. • Wearing clean gloves, use a wooden spatula (e.g., tongue blade) to remove specimen, attempting to not touch the receptacle or to use stool that was directly touching the receptacle. • Place specimen in a sterile specimen cup.	• Minimum volume is 1 ounce or approximately 1 inch.
Throat culture	• For bacteria: Using a dry culture swab, swipe one side across the distal pharynx on side; turn the swab over and swab the other side of the distal pharynx.	• Best yield is for bacterial infections.
Urine culture	• Assemble sterile specimen cup, sterile gloves, and cleansing wipes. • Cleanse the perineal area and allow to dry. • Ask patient to urinate into the sterile cup (approximately 5–15 mL is sufficient volume). • Cover quickly with the sterile cap. • Obtaining a culture from a Foley catheter: Don sterile gloves, and lay a sterile barrier while draining old urine down tubing. Cleanse the access area with alcohol and allow to dry, with catheter access site in a level position to allow pooling of fresh urine in tubing loop. Obtain needle access to the specimen port and remove 5–15 mL of urine. Transfer urine to sterile specimen cup.	• Clean-catch midstream urine specimens for culture have not been determined to be more "sterile" than a normal urine specimen.
Wound culture	• If the wound is obviously dirty or contaminated, rinse it with sterile saline and pat dry prior to performing a culture. • Assemble gloves, sterile drape, culture swabs, and culture media. • Don sterile gloves and uncap appropriate culture swab (calcium alginate or rayon swab — *not* cotton swab). • Swab with the sterile applicator in a rotary and clockwise fashion. • For ulcer: Scrape into the deepest section of the wound, but do *not* culture pus, exudates, or hard eschar.	• Ensure that the wound is clean of dirt or debris that may produce false-positive culture results. • Cotton swabs may leave fine fibers in the wound and worsen infection. • Wide wounds may alternatively be brushed side-to-side in a Z pattern • Minimum specimen is 0.25 mL.

Normal infection control guidelines (e.g., hand washing before and after each procedure) are assumed and not defined in this table.

Data from Schaffer, Garzon, Heroux, Korniewicz[21]; Mayhill[22]; Bell, Leckie, McKendrick[50]; Elsayed, Gregson, Lloyd, et al.[51]; Lifshitz, Kramer.[52]

patient's room. Supplies should be carefully covered to prevent dust and environmental contaminants. Universal precautions are conscientiously maintained for all care delivery.

Requiring that patients eat a "low-microbial diet" has been a long-time theoretical protection to guard against infection. This diet does not permit fresh fruits, vegetables, or contaminated food items such as nuts or bleu cheese. Cooked foods are permitted and assumed to protect the patient against food-borne organisms. This diet has inspired much controversy and little evidence supports its use.[54,58,62–64] In addition, these diets are inconsistent in their directions regarding more realistic risks such as consumption of mayonnaise that may be contaminated with *Salmonella*. General healthy eating instructions for patients should be discussed. Patients should be instructed to cook all meats thoroughly, avoid serving meat on platters where raw meat was prepared, avoid any products with eggs unless known prompt refrigeration was employed, and avoid eating any foods stored for more than 48–72 hours.

Table 28-6 Models for Assessing Risk for Infection and Recommended Actions for Specific Populations

Patient Population	Increased Risks for Infection	Clinical Applications
Breast cancer, adjuvant therapy, traditional	• First-cycle ANC after treatment without prophylaxis is grade IV toxicity level • First-cycle Hgb after treatment without prophylaxis is grade IV toxicity level • Concurrent chemotherapy and radiation • Previous radiation	• Growth factor prophylaxis after first-cycle assessment in patients receiving traditional adjuvant chemotherapy
Elderly patients	• Age > 70 years • Chemotherapy regimen with toxicity similar to CHOP chemotherapy	• Primary prophylaxis with growth factors and/or prophylactic antimicrobials in treatments regimens equivalent to CHOP chemotherapy
Indwelling intravenous catheters	• Large lumen • Multilumen • Percutaneous (not cuffed) line • Line placed after the onset of immune compromise • Previously infected catheter	• Choice of catheter • Timing of catheter placement • Catheter maintenance routine
Non-Hodgkin's lymphoma	• Bone marrow involvement with lymphoma • Low albumin prior to chemotherapy • LDH > 600 units prior to chemotherapy • Poor performance status • Late stage of disease	• Evaluate complete chemistry panel at the onset of chemotherapy • Primary prophylaxis for selected patients

Abbreviations: ANC = absolute neutrophil count; Hgb = hemoglobin; CHOP = cyclophosphamide, doxorubicin (Adriamycin), vincristine (Oncovin), prednisone; LDH = lactate dehydrogenase

Data from Balducci, Yates[65]; Balducci, Hardy, Lyman[66]; Blay, Gomez, Sebban, et al[67]; Chang[68]; Garcia-Suarez, Krsnik, Reyes, et al[69]; Intraguntornchai, Sutheesophon, Sutcharitchan, et al[70]; Lyman[71]; Lyman, Balducci, Agboola[72]; Silber, Fridman, Shpilsky, et al[73]; Silber, Fridman, DiPaolo, et al[74]; Paesmans.[75]

Primary prophylaxis against infection

Primary prophylaxis involves the administration of agents in an attempt to prevent a complication prior to the onset of risk. Recognition of patients at high risk for infection prior to immune suppression permits implementation of strategies to alter the course of immune suppression so as to prevent infection. Some researchers have retrospectively and prospectively studied factors that increase the risk of infection during periods of neutropenia. Three primary populations have been studied based on the perceived high risk–benefit relationship, and risk models have been defined. The variables that increase the risk of infection during periods of neutropenia or T-cell suppressions are summarized in Table 28-6.[65–74]

Administration of prophylactic antimicrobial agents or growth factors prior to the onset of immune suppression are common strategies used to prevent infections in patients perceived as being at high risk for infection, particularly antineoplastic therapy–induced neutropenia.[3,6,8,23,75]

Antimicrobial prophylaxis is viewed as appropriate in patients with HIV infection,[76] with neutropenia,[3] after organ or blood cell transplant,[58] with rheumatic heart disease, or as a surgical adjunct in specific procedures. The process of prescribing antimicrobial agents prior to chemotherapy, prior to blood cell transplant, and after severe lymphocyte depletion with HIV disease has evolved as the natural history of infections with these disorders has become better defined. Prophylactic antimicrobial therapy is reserved for situations in which there is a high risk for infections and their associated morbidity or mortality. Agents chosen as prophylactic medications should provide adequate microbial coverage with limited resistance. An overview of common antimicrobial prophylaxis regimens appears in Table 28-7.[3,11,20,29,58,77–81]

Hematopoietic growth factors promote the differentiation, maturation, and proliferation of hematopoietic cells within the bone marrow. These agents are used to shorten and reduce the severity of neutropenia after chemotherapy and after blood and marrow stem cell transplants. They may also be used as priming agents prior to pheresis of hematopoietic stem cells. Specific growth factors are used to enhance growth of specific cell lines: erythropoietin for erythrocytes, and granulocyte colony-stimulating factor for granulocytes. Initially, growth factors were primarily used reactively after chemotherapy when a patient demonstrated a post-therapy febrile neutropenic event, but no clear benefit was realized in this situation. This practice has evolved over time, and the most recent clinical guidelines suggest that it is cost-effective and clinically prudent to administer growth factors prior to therapy when the planned antineoplastic therapy is likely to produce significant neutropenia in at least 40% of patients receiving that regimen.[2,82] More recent studies applying cost-benefit analysis suggest that growth factor administration is cost-effective when the regimen is likely to reduce significant

Table 28-7 Antimicrobial Prophylaxis Management for Immunocompromised Patients

Patient Population	Specific Criteria	Organisms Likely to Lead to Infection	Suggested Antimicrobial Agents
HIV infection	All patients	1. Pneumococcus 2. Influenza 3. Hepatitis B	1. Pneumovax 2. Influenza vaccine — must be attenuated or dead organisms, or Amantadine 3. Recombivax HB or Energix B
	CD4 count < 200/mm³	*Pneumocystis carinii*	1. TMP-SMX or dapsone preferred, pyrimethamine
	CD4 count < 100/mm³	1. *Toxoplasma gondi* 2. *Histoplasma**	1. TMP-SMX or dapsone, pyrimethamine 2. Itraconazole
	CD4 count < 50/mm³	1. *Mycobacteria avium* complex 2. *Candida** 3. *Cryptococcus** 4. *Coccidiomycosis** 5. Cytomegalovirus* 6. *Varicella**	1. Clarithromycin or azithromycin 2. Fluconazole 3. Fluconazole or itraconazole 4. Fluconazole or itraconazole 5. Ganciclovir 6. Varicella IVIG or acyclovir
	Positive PPD or prior positive PPD	*M. tuberculosis*	INH and pyridoxine or pyridoxine alone
Neutropenia	Absolute neutrophil count (ANC) < 500/mm³, expected to last > 7 days	1. *Candida* 2. Gram-negative bacteria 3. *C. difficile**	1. Fluconazole, although some alternate with itraconazole 2. Norfloxacin or other fluoroquinolone 3. Oral metronidazole (Flagyl) or vancomycin
	ANC < 500/mm³ for shorter period of time but with other risk factors for infection (e.g., older age, chronic lung disease)	1. Gram-negative and gram-positive bacteria	Norfloxacin or other fluoroquinolone
	Neutropenia as above and a central venous access device	Staphylococcus†	Broad-spectrum cephalosporin or penicillin
Blood and marrow transplant	All patients	1. Pneumococcus 2. Influenza 3. Hepatitis B	1. Pneumovax 2. Influenza vaccine — must be attenuated or dead organisms, or Amantadine 3. Recombivax HB or Energix B
	Allogeneic transplant	1. *Candida*† 2. Gram-negative organisms†	1. Fluconazole or itraconazole 2. Norfloxacin or other fluoroquinolone
	Allogeneic transplant with prior herpes simplex and (HSV+)	Herpes simplex	Acyclovir
	Recipients of CMV-positive graft with CMV-negative status	Cytomegalovirus	Acyclovir or ganciclovir with CMV immunoglobulin

*Prophylaxis against these microbes is implemented only in the setting of significant risk and exposure; it is not implemented at all for individuals with normal immune systems.

† Depends on the depth and anticipated length of aplasia.

Data from Wade, Rubenstein, Brown, et al[3]; Shelton, Friese[11]; Hughes, Armstrong, Bodey, et al[20]; Bartlett, Gallant[29]; Sullivan, Dykewicz, Longworth, et al[58]; Kaplan, Masur, Holmes, et al[76]; Finberg, Talcott[77]; Fishman[78]; Furrer, Fux.[79]

neutropenia with fever about 22% of the time.[83] Specific guidelines for administration of these agents are provided in Chapter 23.

Management

The mainstay of infection management is administration of antimicrobial agents. Neutropenia or T-lymphocytic suppression increase the risk for more frequent and severe infections, so these conditions are treated aggressively. At the onset of fever in high-risk patients, aggressive treatment is implemented immediately to prevent sepsis and shock, but lower-risk patients may be closely observed rather than treated immediately. Prior to starting antimicrobial therapy, a focused physical examination for potential sites of infection is performed along with a complete culture work-up. Cultures of all excrement, wounds, lines, and drains are standard. Chest x-rays are usually ordered, but the yield is relatively low if the patient does not have accompanying respiratory symptoms; hence, this step is considered a lower priority than starting antimicrobial therapy.[3] In the setting of neutropenia, the general standard of care is a time frame of two hours from fever to administration of the first antimicrobial agent. This is obviously modified when patients are coming from outside the hospital. Antimicrobial agents selected for treatment may also be more potent and comprehensive in coverage when treating immunocompromised patients.

The National Comprehensive Cancer Network (NCCN) has defined specific thresholds and choice of agents for management of fever in neutropenic patients.[3] It recommends antimicrobial changes every 72 hours if the patient remains consistently febrile, unless there is a clear decline in the patient's stability warranting an earlier change.[3,20] This schema incorporates the conceptual belief that most initial infections are bacterial in nature, but as immune compromise and antibiotic exposure are prolonged, the spectrum of potentially infecting microbes can be broader. Common antimicrobial agents and key nursing implications are described in Table 28-8.[3,11,27,84,85]

Serious, refractory infections occur in a small number of patients with cancer. Risk factors for development of refractory infection and sepsis include complex polymicrobial infections, infections lasting more than 21 days, infectious lesions larger than 5 cm, hematologic malignancy, shock associated with infection, and low albumin at the onset of symptoms of sepsis.[3,9,86]

Although many neutropenic patients who are febrile are at risk for serious infection and require hospitalization with intravenous antimicrobial therapy, approximately 2%–15% of patients have a low risk of serious or disseminated infection, and can safely receive oral antimicrobial therapy on an outpatient basis.[87,88] Several studies have considered variables that favor successful outpatient therapy or early conversion to oral therapy with discharge from the hospital after 3–4 days of intravenous antibiotics. In general, although not considered mandatory or exclusive, contraindications to ambulatory oral antimicrobial therapy for treatment of fever in neutropenia include hematologic malignancy, blood and marrow transplantation, suspected pneumonia, history of invasive fungal infection, active malignant disease, serious comorbid health conditions, and hospital-acquired infections.[20,87–90]

In cases where antimicrobial therapy has failed to manage the infection, additional immune reconstitution therapies may be implemented. Studies to date have not shown proven benefit in using growth factors after the onset of infectious symptoms.[3,23] Immune globulin levels are usually normal at the beginning of the cancer illness continuum; however, in chronic disease, in children with cancer, or after blood and marrow transplant, the levels may become depleted and thus increase the risk of sinus or pulmonary infections.[90–92] Infusion of IgG may replenish immune globulins needed by the body to recognize foreign antigens.

When all other supportive measures fail, infusion of granulocytes may be considered a reasonable strategy, but it is associated with significant morbidity.[3,93] A meta-analysis of articles describing the administration of granulocyte transfusions demonstrated reasonable benefit against bacterial infections in prolonged neutropenia, and refractory fungal infections.[94,95] Granulocytes are harvested from normal, healthy individuals and pooled in plasma for reinfusion. The patient is usually premedicated with acetaminophen, diphenhydramine, and, occasionally, corticosteroids. After baseline vital signs are taken, the infusion is started slowly, and the rate is gradually increased to a set dose per minute. The bag of granulocytes is agitated frequently to prevent rapid infusion of the cells that settle in the bottom of the bag. The patient is closely observed, as granulocytes usually go to the site of infection and can cause severe symptoms of "white-out" within that organ.[96]

Conclusion

The clinical management of infections in the patient with cancer involves integration of a complex and dynamic body of evidence. Even as we find ourselves being able to define risk factors for severe infection and limiting exposure to antimicrobial therapy, we are challenged with new variations in microbial resistance. Currently, the most effective method of managing infection is prevention. As we look to the future, we hope to find increasing evidence-based risk models to define risk for neutropenia, risk for infection, risk for microbial resistance organisms, risk for sepsis, or risk for death. Scientists must also continue to press for more studies assessing the specific impact of infection-prevention interventions, such as low-microbial diets and specialized intravenous catheters. During the last two decades the risk of death from infection has decreased approximately 50% to less than 10%. Eventually, the hope is to eradicate this complication of cancer and antineoplastic therapy.

Table 28-8 Commonly Used Antibiotics

Antibiotic	Coverage	Nursing Implications
Aminoglycosides Gentamycin Amikacin Tobramycin Kanamycin	Most gram-negative enterobacteria (*Serratia, Proteus, Klebsiella, E. coli*), *Pseudomonas, Erwinia*	• Dose reduced in renal failure: excess serum levels are renal toxic. • Long-term use causes partially reversible vestibular and auditory damage. Administering the dose more slowly may reduce incidence. Assist in hearing evaluation after course of therapy. • Administered once to twice daily to decrease renal toxicity. Slower administration may reduce toxicity and does not alter antimicrobial effects, as the aminoglycoside destroys bacteria by entering the cell and killing from inside. • Apply antihistamine or steroid creams if needed for rash. • Alters platelet function and may enhance bleeding tendency. Avoid other anticoagulant or antiplatelet medications, such as aspirin or nonsteroidal anti-inflammatory agents. • Serum blood levels are monitored for the presence of medication prior to and after a dose. These medications' toxicity is determined by persistent and high blood levels. Based on the presence of medication just before a dose is due, the dosage or frequency may be decreased.
Penicillins Penicillin G Penicillin V Ampicillin Amoxicillin Ticarcillin Pipercillin Carbenicillin	*Actinomyces, Clostridium,* meningococcemia, *Proteus* (ampicillin), *Salmonella, Streptococcus, Staphylococcus* (second line)	• Frequent dosing to achieve steady-state blood level. • Peak-and-trough levels measured to assess whether the minimum inhibitory concentration (MIC) is achieved. The MIC is the serum blood level at which specific microbes are sensitive to death for the circulating drug. • Administer as rapidly as ordered to achieve a good peak blood level. • Idiosyncratic glomerulonephritis may occur due to glomerular basement membrane damage. • Administer antihistamine or steroid creams for itchy rash as needed (especially with ampicillin and amoxicillin). • Persistent, unexplained fever may be a manifestation of hypersensitivity. Antipyretics are only partially helpful in abrogating this effect. • Some hypersensitivity reactions are anaphylactoid and require emergency respiratory support, including epinephrine. The reaction does not involve the IgE antibody and, therefore, is not predictable in incidence or severity. • Administer antidiarrheals as needed (especially with ampicillin). • Administer with food and avoid concomitant caffeine to reduce drug-induced nausea. • Alters platelet function and may enhance bleeding tendency (especially with carbenicillin and ticarcillin). Avoid other anticoagulant or antiplatelet medications such as aspirin or nonsteroidal anti-inflammatory agents. • Adminster potassium supplements, because most agents enhance renal excretion of potassium and cause hypokalemia. • Neuromuscular twitching may occur (especially with imipenam), and the seizure threshold may be lowered in patients with preexisting seizures. Assess for resting tremors and seizure activity. Place on seizure precautions.
Carbapenams Imipenem cilastin Meropenam	Respiratory, skin/structure, gynecologic infections that are gram positive and gram negative	• Do not give carbenicillin or probenecid, as they interfere with absorption. • May increase hepatic transaminase levels. • May lower blood counts. • Avoid mixing with aminoglycosides, which may be physically imcompatible. • The drugs are dialyzable, so administer them after dialysis treatment. • The most common CNS toxicities are a lowered seizure threshold, dizziness, and confusion. • Irritating to veins — give low doses over approximately 30 minutes, higher doses over 1 hour.
Quinolones Norfloxacin Ciprofloxicin	Resistant enterobacteria	• Administer with food and avoid concomitant caffeine to reduce drug-induced tendency to cause gastric upset. • Administer acetaminophen as needed for headache. • Avoid concomitant nonsteroidal anti-inflammatory agents that enhance the potential bleeding tendency. • Implement safety precautions for potential dizziness or visual disturbances (blurred, diplopia).

(continued)

Table 28-8 Commonly Used Antibiotics (Continued)

Antibiotic	Coverage	Nursing Implications
		• Provide an environment conducive to sleep. • Perform care in increments, providing frequent rest periods due to drug-induced fatigue and malaise. • Assess for depressive tendency that may be worsened by drug-related fatigue and malaise. • Monitor hepatic transaminases for elevations indicating drug toxicity, or an increased risk of worsening of transaminase elevations while receiving this agent.
Other Gram-Positive Coverage Nafcillin Oxacillin Vancomycin	Staphylococcus, *Clostridium difficile*, *Corynebacterium diphtheriae*	• Persistent, unexplained fever may occur (especially with vancomycin). Antipyretics are only partially helpful in abrogating this effect. • Administer vancomycin over at least 2 hours, as too-rapid infusion may cause warmth, flushing, tachycardia, hypertension ("red man syndrome," "Antabuse-like reaction"), or hypotension. • Apply antihistamine or steroid creams if a macular, itchy rash occurs. • Periodically monitor complete blood count for leukopenia (vancomycin). Drug may be discontinued if it occurs. • Monitor blood levels of vancomycin for the necessary minimal inhibitory concentration (MIC) of the drug against the patient's specific organism. If the organism is resistant at lower MICs, the dose may be increased as tolerated.
Cephalosporins Cefamandole Cefazolin Cephalothin Cefuroxime Ceftazidime Cefuraxime Ceftriaxone Cefepime	General enterobacter coverage (*E. coli, Klebsiella, Proteus, Serratia*), *Staphylococcus aureus, Haemophilus influenzae*	• Administer via central venous access whenever possible. Administer slowly through large peripheral vessel to reduce incidence of phlebitis. • Administer antidiarrheals as needed. • Hypersensitivity reactions including macular, itchy rash may occur. Apply antihistamine or steroid creams if needed. • Persistent, unexplained fever may be a manifestation of hypersensitivity. Antipyretics are only partially helpful in abrogating this effect. • Some hypersensitivity reactions are anaphylactoid and require emergency respiratory support, including epinephrine. • Alters platelet function and may enhance bleeding tendency. Avoid other anticoagulant or antiplatelet medications such as aspirin or nonsteroidal anti-inflammatory agents (rarely occurs).
Tetracyclines Tetracycline Democycline Monocycline	Tick fever, *Chlamydiae, Klebsiella* urinary tract infections, *Mycoplasma pneumoniae* (second)	• Take with food to reduce drug-related nausea. • Avoid concomitant caffeine that will enhance GI upset. • Implement safety precautions for potential vertigo. • Administer steroid vaginal creams for itching due to vaginitis, and antifungal cream if secondary fungal vaginitis occurs. • Monitor hepatic transaminases for elevations indicating contraindication for treatment or drug toxicity. • Administer oral preparations with a straw to avoid teeth staining. • Avoid bright lights that will hurt the eyes due to drug-related photosensitivity.
Other Antibacterials Clindamycin	Gastrointestinal bacilli	• Take with food to reduce drug-related nausea. • Avoid concomitant caffeine that will enhance GI upset. • Administer antidiarrheals as needed. • Monitor stools for quantity, fluid loss, and blood, as colitis may occur. • Apply antihistamine or steroid creams if a macular, itchy rash occurs.
Erythromycin	*Campylobacter, Chlamydia* conjunctivitis, *Corynebacterium diphtheriae, Legionella, Mycoplasma pneumoniae*	• Administer via central venous access whenever possible. Administer slowly through a large peripheral vein to reduce incidence of phlebitis. • Administer antidiarrheals as needed. • Maintain good oral hygiene to reduce discomfort. • If stomatitis occurs, perform oral rinsing with saline or bicarbonate rinses four times a day, and use oral anesthetic agents (e.g., viscous xylocaine, Ulcerease) to reduce discomfort. • Monitor hepatic transaminases for elevations indicating contraindication for treatment or drug toxicity. • Apply antihistamine or steroid creams if a macular, itchy rash occurs. • Long-term use leads to partially reversible vestibular and auditory damage. Administering the dose more slowly may reduce incidence. Assist in hearing evaluation after course of therapy.

(continued)

Table 28-8 Commonly Used Antibiotics (Continued)

Antibiotic	Coverage	Nursing Implications
Metronidazole	*Bacteroides*, various normal flora, *Clostridium difficile*	• Administer with food. Sweet hard candies may best abrogate the metallic taste. • Administer acetaminophen as needed for headache. • Administer via central venous access whenever possible. Administer slowly through a large peripheral vein to reduce incidence of phlebitis. • Monitor peripheral sensation (soles of feet and fingertips) where peripheral neuropathies are first noted. Implement safety precautions for hands and feet, as the patient will be less aware of injury to these areas. When neuropathies occur, consider changing antimicrobial therapy. • Never administer with alcohol or alcohol based preparations (e.g. many oral elixirs) due to antabuse-like reaction (warmth, flushing, tachycardia, hypertension).
Sulfa-trimethoprim	*E. coli* UTI, *Haemophilus influenzae, Shigella, Pneumocystis carinii*, some strains *Pseudomonas, Salmonella, Yersinia*	• Hypersensitivity reactions including macular, itchy rash may occur. Apply antihistamine or steroid creams if needed. • Persistent, unexplained fever may be a manifestation of hypersensitivity. Antipyretics are only partially helpful in abrogating this effect. • Some hypersensitivity reactions are anaphylactoid and require emergency respiratory support, including epinephrine. • Take with food to reduce drug-related nausea. • Avoid concomitant caffeine that will enhance GI upset. • Periodically monitor complete blood count of leukopenia and thrombocytopenia. The drug may be discontinued if it occurs.
Sulfonamides (Gantricin)	Nocardia	• Hypersensitivity reactions including macular, itchy rash may occur. Apply antihistamine or steroid creams if needed. • Persistent, unexplained fever may occur. Antipyretics are only partially helpful in abrogating this effect. • Enhance fluid intake while on the drug to reduce the risk of crystalluria. • Take with food to reduce drug-related nausea. • Avoid concomitant caffeine that will enhance GI upset. • Avoid bright lights that will hurt the eyes due to drug-related photosensitivity.
Antifungals Ketoconozole Itraconazome Voriconazole	Widely spread localized fungal infections, oral/mucotaneous *candida*; itraconazole and vorizonazole are also approved for treatment of visceral or systemic *Candida* infection	• Take with food to reduce drug-related nausea. • Avoid concomitant caffeine that will enhance GI upset. • Monitor hepatic transaminases for elevations indicating contraindication for treatment or drug toxicity. • Prepare patient and family for altered body image (gynecomastia), secondary sex characteristics (dysmenorrhea, testes size), and decreased libido due to decreased testosterone levels. • Drugs interfering with stomach acidity may alter absorption. • Agents may potentiate action of benzodiazepines. • Agents may cause potassium depletion; monitor and replace potassium as needed.
Amphotericin-B	Topical-mucotaneous fungal infections, IV-disseminated fungal infections (*Candida, Aspergillus, Cryptococcus*)	• Severe, high, spiking fever may occur 30–45 minutes into the infusion. Premedication with antipyretics is only partially helpful in abrogating this effect. Some patients require steroids to abrogate fever and chills. • Rigors accompanying fever may be abrogated by covering with warm blankets or administering of intravenous morphine, Demerol, or a benzodiazepine. • Administer acetaminophen as needed for fever or headache. • Administer potassium supplements, as renal excretion of potassium is enhanced with this agent, which causes hypokalemia. • Prehydration with high-sodium fluid is thought to reduce renal toxicity. • Dose should be reduced in case of renal failure. • Periodically monitor complete blood count for anemia. The drug may be discontinued if it occurs. • Administer via central venous access whenever possible, or give slowly through a large peripheral vein to reduce phlebitis. • Tachycardia with hypertension or hypotension may occur. Monitor vital signs frequently during administration. • Consider lipid formulations of the drug if renal insufficiency or severe infusional toxicity occurs.

(continued)

Table 28-8 Commonly Used Antibiotics (Continued)

Antibiotic	Coverage	Nursing Implications
Flucytosine	Disseminated or septicemic *Candida, Coccidioides, Cryptococcus*	• Administer concomitant antiemetics to abrogate nausea and vomiting. • Administer with food and avoid concomitant caffeine to reduce drug-induced nausea. • Apply antihistamine or steroid creams if a macular, itchy rash occurs. • Monitor hepatic transminases for elevations indicating contraindication for treatment or drug toxicity. • Periodically monitor complete blood count for anemia, leukopenia, and thrombocytopenia. The drug may be discontinued if they occur. • Implement safety precautions and frequently check orientation, as confusion may occur with this drug.
Caspofungin	Disseminated *Candida* or *Aspergillus* refractory to oral therapy or amphotericin-B	• Not compatible with glucose-containing solutions; administer only with normal saline. • The drug is a venous irritant, so administer cautiously through peripheral IV, slowing the 1-hour infusion if necessary. • Transient mild transaminase elevations may occur, but severe or prolonged changes warrant drug discontinuation. • Hypersensitivity reactions may occur. Monitoring for itching, rash, erythema, or respiratory difficulty should be performed, being particularly vigilant during the first few doses. • Assess for baseline nausea and vomiting, and manage supportively if these effects increase during therapy. • Assess for baseline history of headache and advise the patient of this possible adverse effect. Discuss with the physician use of analgesic medications for management of this adverse effect.
Antivirals Acyclovir	Herpes simplex I and II, varicella zoster	• Administer through central venous access, if possible, to prevent irritation at the infusion site. • Dose should be reduced in case of renal failure. • Slower infusion rate decreases renal toxicity. Usually given intravenously over 1 hour. • Monitor hepatic transaminases for elevations indicating contraindication for treatment or drug toxicity. • Apply antihistamine or steroid creams if a macular, itchy rash occurs. • Periodically monitor complete blood count for leukopenia and thrombocytopenia. The drug may be discontinued if either occurs. • Monitor ammonia level, serum chemistry values, and glucose levels if mental status changes occur. Drug-related metabolic encephalopathy must be differentiated from clinical causes. The drug may be discontinued if it causes encephalopathy.
Ganciclovir	Cytomegalovirus	• Periodically monitor complete blood count for leukopenia and thrombocytopenia. The drug may be discontinued if either occurs. • Apply antihistamine or steroid creams if a macular, itchy rash occurs. • Monitor hepatic transaminases for elevations indicating contraindiction for treatment or drug toxicity. • Administer acetaminophen as needed for headache. • Persistent, unexplained fevers may be partially abrogated by antipyretics. • Perform frequent mental status assessment. Monitor ammonia level, serum chemistry values, and glucose levels if mental status changes occur. Drug-related metabolic encephalopathy must be differentiated from clinical causes. • Assess muscle strength and motor activity. Implement physical therapy to maintain muscle tone. Myopathy occurs idiosyncratically or with long-term use.

Data from Rubenstein, Brown, Elting, et al[3]; Shelton, Friese[11]; Allen, Shelton[27]; Khare, Sharland[84]; Shelton.[85]

References

1. Dale DC: Colony-stimulating factors for the management of neutropenia in cancer patients. *Drugs* 62(suppl 1):1–15, 2002
2. Lyman GH, Kuderer N, Greene J, et al: The economics of febrile neutropenia: implications for the use of colony-stimulating factors. *Eur J Cancer* 34:1857–1864, 1998
3. Wade JC, Rubenstein EB, Brown AE, et al: National Comprehensive Cancer Network practice guidelines for fever and neutropenia. *Cancer Control* 8(suppl 2):16, 21, 2001
4. Safdar A, Armstrong D: Infectious morbidity in critically ill patients with cancer. *Crit Care Clin* 17:531–570, 2001
5. Toney JF, Parker MM: New perspectives on the management of septic shock in the cancer patient. *Infect Dis Clin North Am* 10:239–253, 1996
6. Viscoli C, Castagnola E: Treatment of febrile neutropenia: what is new? *Curr Opin Infect Dis* 15:377–382, 2002
7. Blot F, Cordonnier C, Buzin A, et al: Severity of illness scores: are they useful in febrile neutropenic adult patients in hematology wards? A prospective multicenter study. *Crit Care Med* 29:2125–2131, 2001
8. Viscoli C, on behalf of the EORTC International Antimicrobial Therapy Group: Management of infection in cancer patients: studies of the EORTC International Antimicrobial Group (IATG). *Eur J Cancer* 38:S82–S87, 2002
9. Dellinger RP, Carlet JM, Masur H, et al: Surviving Sepsis Campaign Management Guidelines Committee: Surviving Sepsis Campaign guidelines for management of severe sepsis and septic shock. *Crit Care Med* 32:858–873, 2004
10. Shelton BK: Sepsis. *Semin Oncol Nurs* 15:209–221, 1999
11. Shelton BK, Friese CR: Anti-infectives, in Gay BG, Chernecky C (eds.): *Manual of Medical-Surgical Nursing*. Philadelphia, W.B. Saunders, 2002, pp 348–357
12. Carter LW: Bacterial translocation: nursing implications in the care of patients with neutropenia. *Oncol Nurs Forum* 21:857–867, 1994
13. Garcia-Carbonero R, Paz-Ares L: Antbiotics and growth factors in the management of fever and neutropenia in cancer patients. *Curr Opin Hematol* 9:215–221, 2002
14. Guinan JL, McGuckin M, Nowell PC: Management of healthcare–associated infections in the oncology patient. *Oncology* 17:415–420, discussion 423–426, 2003
15. Wisplinghoff H, Seifert H, Wenzel RP, et al: Current trends in the epidemiology of nosocomial bloodstream infections in patients with hematological malignancies and solid neoplasms in hospitals in the United States. *Clin Infect Dis* 36:1103–1110, 2003
16. Mims CA, Nash A, Stephen J: *Mim's Pathogenesis of Infectious Disease* (ed 5). San Diego, Academic Press, 2001
17. Todar K: *Bacteriology 303, Updated 2002.* University of Wisconsin–Madison Department of Bacteriology, *www.bact.wisc.edu/Bact303/Bact303normalflora.* Accessed May 30, 2004
18. Virginia Academy of Science: *Microbiology Course — Chapter 17: Normal Flora of the Human Body, Updated 2001. www.vacadsci.org/PUB/micro17.pdf.* Accessed May 30, 2004
19. Members of the American College of Chest Physicians/Society of Critical Care Medicine Consensus Conference Committee: American College of Chest Physicians/Society of Critical Care Medicine Consensus Conference. Definitions for sepsis and organ failure and guidelines for the use of innovative therapies in sepsis. *Crit Care Med* 20:864–874, 1992
20. Hughes WT, Armstrong D, Bodey GP, et al: 2002 guidelines for the use of antimicrobial agents in neutropenic patients with cancer. *Clin Infect Dis* 34:730–751, 2002
21. Schaffer SD, Garzon LS, Heroux DI, et al: *Pocket Guide to Infection Prevention and Safe Practice.* St Louis, CV Mosby, 1996
22. Mayhill CG: *Hospital Epidemiology and Infection Control.* Philadelphia, Lippincott, Williams and Wilkins, 2004
23. Pizzo PA: Current concepts: fever in immunocompromised patients. *N Engl J Med* 341:893–900, 1999
24. Angus DC, Linde-Zwirble WT, Lidlicker J, et al: Epidemioligy of severe sepsis in the United States: analysis of incidence, outcomes and associated costs of care. *Crit Care Med* 29:1303–1310, 2001
25. Sands KE, Bates DW, Lanken PN, et al: Epidemiology of sepsis syndrome in 8 academic medical centers. *JAMA* 278:117–123, 1997
26. Zeni F, Freeman B, Natanson C: Anti-inflammatory therapies to treat sepsis and septic shock: a reassessment. *Crit Care Med* 25:1095–1100, 1997
27. Allen MA, Shelton BK: Sepsis and septic shock, in Wright JE, Shelton BK (eds.): *Desk Reference for Critical Care Nursing.* Sudbury, MA, Jones and Bartlett, 1993, p 1252
28. Balducci L, Carreca I: The role of myelopoietic growth factors in managing cancer in the elderly. *Drugs* 62(suppl 1):47–63, 2002
29. Bartlett JG, Gallant JE: *Medical Management of HIV Infection.* Baltimore, MD, Johns Hopkins University, Department of Infectious Diseases, 2003
30. Buchsel PC, Forgey A, Grape FB, et al: Granulocyte macrophage colony-stimulating factor: current practice and novel approaches. *Clin J Oncol Nurs* 6:198–205, 2002
31. Camp-Sorrell D: Chemotherapy: toxicity management, in Yarbro CH, Frogge MH, Goodman M, Groenwald SL (eds.): *Cancer Nursing: Principles and Practice* (ed 5). Sudbury, MA, Jones and Bartlett, 2000, pp 444–486
32. Crnich CJ, Maki DG: The promise of novel technology for the prevention of intravascular device-related bloodstream infection. II. Long-term devices. *Clin Infect Dis* 34:1362–1368, 2002
33. Eggimann P, Pittet D: Overview of catheter-related infections with special emphasis on prevention based on educational programs. *Clin Microbiol Infect* 8:295–309, 2002
34. Ellerhorst-Ryan J: Infection, in Yarbro CH, Frogge MH, Goodman M, Groenwald SG (eds.): *Cancer Nursing Principles and Practice* (ed 5). Sudbury, MA, Jones and Bartlett, 2000, pp 691–708
35. Gilliam K: Oral care for patients undergoing cancer therapy. *Dentistry Today* 21:50–55, 2002
36. Hanna HA, Raad II, Hackett B, et al: Antibiotic-impregnated catheters associated with significant decrease in nosocomial and multidrug-resistant bacteremias in critically ill patients. *Chest* 124:1030–1038, 2003
37. Masur H, Kaplan JE, Holmes KK, et al: Guidelines for preventing opportunistic infections among HIV-infected persons. Recommendations of the U.S. Public Health Service and the Infectious Diseases Society of America. *Ann Int Med* 137(pt 2):435–478, 2002
38. Moran AB, Camp-Sorrell D: Maintenance of venous access devices in patients with neutropenia. *Clin J Oncol Nurs* 6:126–130, 2002
39. O'Grady NP, Alexander M, Dellinger EP, et al: Centers for Disease Control and Prevention: Guidelines for the prevention of intravascular catheter-related infections. *MMWR Recomm Rep* 51(RR-10):1–26, 2002
40. Raber-Durlacher JE, Epstein JB, Raber J, et al: Periodontal infection in cancer patients treated with high-dose chemotherapy. *Support Care Cancer* 10:466–473, 2002
41. Rubin RH: Importance of CMV in the transplant population. *Transpl Infect Dis* 1(suppl):3–7, 1999
42. Shelton BK: Hematological and immune disorders, in Sole ML, Lamborn ML, Hartshorn JC (eds.): *Introduction to Critical*

Care Nursing (ed 3). Philadelphia, W.B. Saunders, 2001, pp 431–432
43. Yadegarynia D, Tarrand J, Raad I, et al: Current spectrum of bacterial infections in patients with cancer. *Clin Infect Dis* 37:1144–1145, 2003
44. Regazzoni CJ, Khoury M, Irrazabal C, et al: Neutropenia and the development of the systemic inflammatory response syndrome. *Intensive Care Med* 29:135–138, 2002
45. Roback JD: CMV and blood transfusions. *Rev Med Virol* 12:211–219, 2002
46. Rolston KVI, Rubenstein EB: *Textbook of Febrile Neutropenia*, London, Martin Dunitz, 2001
47. Henker R: Evidence-based practice: fever-related interventions. *Am J Crit Care* 8:481–487, quiz 488–489, 1999
48. Raad I, Hanna HA, Alakech B, et al: Differential time to positivity: a useful method for diagnosing catheter-related bloodstream infections. *Ann Intern Med* 140:18–25, 2004
49. Cancer Therapy Evaluation Program, 1999. *http://ctep.cancer.gov/forms/ctcv2nom-4/30/99/final3.pdf*. Accessed May 29, 2004
50. Bell D, Leckie V, McKendrick M: The role of induced sputum in the diagnosis of pulmonary tuberculosis. *J Infect* 47:317–321, 2003
51. Elsayed S, Gregson DB, Lloyd T, et al: Utility of Gram stain for the microbiological analysis of burn wound surfaces. *Arch Pathol Lab Med* 127:1485–1488, 2003
52. Lifshitz E, Kramer L: Outpatient urine culture: does collection technique matter? *Arch Intern Med* 160:2537–2540, 2000
53. Murdoch DR, Greenlees RL: Rapid identification of *Staphylococcus aureus* from BacT/ALERT blood culture bottles by direct Gram stain characteristics. *Clin Pathol* 57:199–201, 2004
54. Shelton BK: Evidence-based care for the neutropenic patient with leukemia. *Semin Oncol Nurs* 19:133–141, 2003
55. Mutnick AH, Kirby JT, Jones RN: CANCER Study Group. CANCER resistance surveillance program: initial results from hematology-oncology centers in North America. Chemotherapy Alliance for Neutropenics and the Control of Emerging Resistance. *Ann Pharmacother* 37:47–56, 2003
56. Bartley JM, 1997, 1998, and 1999 APIC Guidelines Committee: APIC state-of-the-art report: the role of infection control during construction in health care facilities. *Am J Infect Control* 28:156–169, 2000
57. Sehulster L, Chinn RY: Guidelines for environmental infection control in health-care facilities. Recommendations of CDC and the Healthcare Infection Control Practices Advisory Committee (HICPAC). *MMWR Recomm Rep* 52(RR-10):1–42, 2003
58. Sullivan KM, Dykewicz CA, Longworth DL, et al: Preventing opportunistic infections after hematopoietic stem cell transplantation: the Centers for Disease Control and Prevention, Infectious Diseases Society of America, and American Society for Blood and Marrow Transplantation Practice guidelines and beyond. *Hematology* (Am Soc Hematol Educ Program): 392–421, 2001
59. Garner JS, Hospital Infection Control Practices Advisory Committee: guideline for isolation precautions in hospitals. *Infect Control Hosp Epidemiol* 17:5–80, 1997
60. Mank A, van der Lelie H: Is there still an indication for nursing patients with prolonged neutropenia in protective isolation? An evidence-based nursing and medical study of 4 years experience for nursing patients with neutropenia without isolation. *Eur J Oncol Nurs* 7:17–23, 2003
61. Boyce JM, Didier P: Centers for Disease Control and Prevention: Guideline for hand hygiene in health-care settings: recommendations of the Healthcare Infection Control Practices Advisory Committee and the HICPAC/SHEA/APIC/IDSA Hand Hygiene Task Force. *MMWR Recomm Rep* 51(RR-16):1–44, 2002
62. Smith LH, Besser SG: Dietary restrictions for patients with neutropenia: a survey of institutional practices. *Oncol Nurs Forum* 27:515–520, 2000
63. Wilson BJ: Dietary recommendations for neutropenic patients. *Semin Oncol Nurs* 18:44–49, 2002
64. Moody K, Charlson ME, Finlay J: The neutropenic diet: what's the evidence? *J Pediatr Hematol Oncol* 24:717–721, 2002
65. Balducci L, Yates J, Senior Adult Task Force Members of the National Comprehensive Cancer Networks: General guidelines for the management of older patients with cancer. *Oncology* 14:221–227, 2000
66. Balducci L, Hardy CL, Lyman GH: Hematopoietic growth factors in the older cancer patient. *Curr Opin Hematol* 8:170–187, 2001
67. Blay JY, Gomez F, Sebban C, et al: The international prognostic index correlates to survival in patients with aggressive lymphoma in relapse: analysis of the PARMA trial. *Blood* 82:3562–3568, 1998
68. Chang J: Chemotherapy dose reduction and delay in clinical practice. Evaluating the risk to patient outcome in adjuvant chemotherapy for breast cancer. *Eur J Cancer* 36(suppl 1):S11–14, 2000
69. Garcia-Suarez J, Krsnik I, Reyes E, et al: Elderly haematological patients with chemotherapy-induced febrile neutropenia have similar rates of infection and outcome to younger adults: a prospective study of risk-adapted therapy. *Br J Haematol* 120:209–216, 2003
70. Intraguntornchai T, Sutheesophon J, Sutcharitchan P, et al: A predictive model for life-threatening neutropenia after the first course of CHOP chemotherapy in patients with aggressive non-Hodgkin's lymphoma. *Leuk Lymph* 37:351–360, 2000
71. Lyman GH: A predictive model for neutropenia associated with cancer chemotherapy. *Pharmacotherapy* 20(pt 2):104S–111S, 2000
72. Lyman GH, Balducci L, Agboola Y: Use of colony-stimulating factors in the elderly cancer patient. *Oncol Spectrums* 2:414–421, 2001
73. Silber JM, Fridman M, Shpilsky A, et al: Modeling the cost-effectiveness of granulocyte colony-stimulating factor use in early-stage breast cancer. *J Clin Oncol* 16:2435–2444, 1998
74. Silber JH, Fridman M, DiPaolo RS, et al: First-cycle blood counts and subsequent neutropenia, dose reduction, or delay in early-stage breast cancer therapy. *J Clin Oncol* 16:2392–2400, 1998
75. Paesmans M: Risk factors assessment in febrile neutropenia. *Int J Antimicrob Agents* 16:107–111, 2000
76. Kaplan JE, Masur H, Holmes KK, et al: Guidelines for preventing opportunistic infections among HIV-infected persons. Recommendations of the U.S. Public Health Service and the Infectious Diseases Society of America. *MMWR Recomm Rep* 51(RR-8):1–52, 2002
77. Finberg RW, Talcott JA: Fever and neutropenia — how to use a new treatment strategy. *N Engl J Med* 341:362–363, 1999
78. Fishman JA: Prevention of infection caused by *Pneumocystis carinii* in transplant recipients. *Clin Infect Dis* 33:1397–1405, 2001
79. Furrer H, Fux C: Opportunistic infections: an update. *J HIV Ther* 7:2–7, 2002
80. Sepkowitz KA: Opportunistic infections in patients with and patients without acquired immunodeficiency syndrome. *Clin Infect Dis* 34:1098–1107, 2002
81. Wingard JR: Opportunistic infections after blood and marrow transplantation. *Transpl Infect Dis* 1:3–20, 1999
82. Ozer H, Armitage J, Bennett C, et al: Update of recommendations for the use of hemtopoietic colony-stimulating factors: evidence-based, clinical practice guidelines. *J Clin Oncol* 18:3558–3585, 2000

83. Lyman GH, Kuderer NM, Balducci L: Cost-benefit analysis of granulocyte colony-stimulating factor in the management of elderly cancer patients. *Curr Opin Hematol* 9:207–214, 2002
84. Khare MD, Sharland M: Cytomegalovirus treatment options in immunocompromised patients. *Expert Opin Pharmacother* 2:1247–1257, 2001
85. Shelton BK: Neutropenia, in Hebra J, Kuhn MA (eds.): *Manual of Critical Care Nursing.* Boston, Little, Brown, 1996, pp 223–225
86. Elting LS, Rubenstein EB, Rolstin KV, et al: Outcomes of bacteremia in neutropenic cancer patients: observations from two decades of epidemiologic and clinical trials. *Clin Infect Dis* 25:247–259, 1997
87. Freifield A, Marchigiani D, Walsh T, et al: A double-blind comparison of empirical oral and intravenous antibiotic therapy for low-risk febrile patients with neutropenia during cancer chemotherapy. *N Engl J Med* 341:305–311, 1999
88. Kern WV, Cometta A, deBock R, et al: Oral versus intravenous empirical antimicrobial therapy for fever in patients with granulocytopenia who are receiving cancer chemotherapy. *N Engl J Med* 341:312–318, 1999
89. Klatersky J, Paesmans M, Rubenstein EB, et al: The Multinational Association for Supportive Care in Cancer risk index: a multinational scoring system for identifying low-risk febrile neutropenic cancer patients. *J Clin Oncol* 18:3038–3051, 2000
90. Koh A, Pizo PA: Empirical antibiotic therapy for low risk febrile cancer patients with neutropenia. *Cancer Invest* 20:420–433, 2002
91. Takahashi T, Chiba S, Matsumura T, et al: A case of severe B cell deficiency after allogeneic stem cell transplantation. *Bone Marrow Transplant* 30:397–400, 2002
92. Maury S, Mary JY, Rabian C, et al: Prolonged immune deficiency following allogeneic stem cell transplantation: risk factors and complications in adults patients. *Br J Haematol* 115:630–641, 2001
93. Hubel K, Carter RA, Liles WC, et al: Granulocyte transfusion therapy for infections in candidates and recipients of HPC transplantation: a comparative analysis of feasibility and outcome for community donors versus related donors. *Transfusion* 42:1414–1421, 2002
94. Strauss RG: Granulocyte transfusion therapy. *Hematol Oncol Clin North Am* 8:1159–1164, 1994

CHAPTER 29

Bleeding

Barbara Holmes Gobel, RN, MS, AOCN®

Scope of the Problem

Bleeding represents one of the most complex clinical challenges in the supportive care of the patient with cancer. The numerous and unique complications of each cancer, combined with the often toxic effects of various cancer treatments, create a difficult problem in the diagnosis and management of bleeding. Multiple hemostatic abnormalities may be involved in cancer-associated bleeding. Considerable differences exist in the presentation, proper management, and implications of these clinical problems. Minor bleeding may be the initial symptom that leads to the diagnosis of cancer. More severe bleeding may indicate the onset of a progressive or terminal phase of the cancer. Because the morbidity and mortality of many bleeding problems are significant, prevention of the problem is clearly the best management plan. Rapid recognition, assessment, and knowledgeable treatment of the bleeding complications of cancer will significantly improve the patient's quality of life and potential for survival.

No specific incidence rates have been identified for this complication, as bleeding can occur with any cancer. Tumors themselves increase the risk for bleeding. Bleeding does occur more frequently in individuals with hematologic cancers compared with solid tumors. Hematologic cancers affect the bone marrow, usually resulting in thrombocytopenia or platelets with altered function. The bone marrow also becomes the target of antineoplastic therapy in these cancers, in an attempt to eradicate tumor cells. The incidence and severity of bleeding in a patient with an acute leukemia are greater than for a patient with a solid tumor. A much higher percentage of patients dying from acute leukemia (52%) will have a fatal hemorrhage, compared to the incidence of hemorrhage in patients dying with solid tumors (1.5%).[1]

The platelet count is considered to be the single most significant factor for predicting bleeding in the patient with cancer. Gaydos et al. first reported an association between a low platelet count and an increased risk of bleeding in 1962.[2] It was demonstrated that for a patient with leukemia, hemorrhage rarely occurred when the platelet count remained higher than 20,000 cells/mm^3.

Increased bleeding may also be due to other factors, including leukostasis, leukoencephalitis, and the presence of liver metastases in patients with solid tumors.[3] Solid tumors more prone to having hemostatic abnormalities include the mucin-producing adenocarcinomas, including those of the lung, breast, stomach, pancreas, and prostate.[4,5] These solid tumors are more commonly associated with disseminated intravascular coagulation (DIC).

This chapter reviews the processes of hemostasis and coagulation, then discusses fibrinolysis. Pathophysiology of bleeding covers platelet abnormalities and the problems associated with hypocoagulation, as well as a variety of other causes of bleeding. Care of the individual with cancer who is experiencing bleeding, including both nursing and medical support, is reviewed.

Physiology of Bleeding

Hemostasis

Hemostasis is the process by which the fluid component of blood becomes a solid clot. This process is initiated by vascular or tissue injury and culminates in the formation of a firm mechanical barrier, or a clot (made up of platelets and fibrin). The sequence of events after injury includes local constriction, platelet adherence to structures in the vessel wall, aggregation of platelets to form a hemostatic plug, and coagulation or solid-clot formation.

When blood vessel injury occurs, vasoconstriction initially provides minimal control of bleeding. Within seconds, platelets are attracted to and adhere to the underlying layer of collagen of the exposed subendothelial tissue. Platelets then release a number of components, including calcium, serotonin, proteolytic enzymes, cationic proteins, thromboxane A, and nucleotide adenosine diphosphate (ADP)[6]; ADP causes platelets to swell and become "sticky," thereby increasing their adherence to one another. Increasing levels of ADP lead to clot contraction, degranulation, and ultimately fusion of the platelets. The end result of ADP-mediated platelet accumulation is the formation of a large platelet aggregate, or a hemostatic plug. Activated platelets also provide an anionic phospholipid surface for the clotting reactions that lead to thrombin generation, an essential precursor to fibrin. The resulting mass of platelets fills the gap in the vessel wall and arrests bleeding, usually within 5 minutes. This primary hemostatic mechanism produces only a temporary cessation of bleeding, however.

Coagulation

Coagulation may be considered a mechanism for rapid replacement of an unstable platelet plug with a stable fibrin clot. A series of interdependent, enzyme-mediated reactions activate fibrin; the fibrin clot is the final product of hemostasis. When these enzymes or coagulation factors are stimulated, they become active in a sequential manner, not in numerical order (Table 29-1). This process is often referred to as the *coagula-*

Table 29-1 Normal Coagulation Factors

Factor	Factor Name	Normal Range
I	Fibrinogen	142–366 mg/dL
II	Prothrombin	80%–120%
III	Tissue factor, tissue thromboplastin (extrinsic prothrombin activator)	80%–120%
IV	Calcium	8.5–10.5 mg/dL
V	Proaccelerin, accelerator globulin	50%–150%
VI	Not assigned	
VII	Proconvertin, serum prothrombin conversion accelerator (SPCA)	60%–140%
VIII	Antihemophilic globulin (AHG), antihemophilic factor (AHF)	60%–150%
IX	Plasma thromboplastin component (PTC), Christmas factor	60%–150%
X	Stuart-Prower factor	60%–150%
XI	Plasma thromboplastin antecedent (PTA)	60%–135%
XII	Hageman factor	50%–150%
XIII	Fibrin-stabilizing factor (FSF)	Present

tion cascade. Multiple inhibitors and control mechanisms keep these reactions localized to the site of the injury. Figure 29-1 shows the mechanism of normal blood coagulation.

The coagulation cascade is initiated when procoagulant substances — most significantly, tissue factor (TF) — are released during blood vessel injury. *Tissue factor* is a transmembrane glycoprotein present on the surface of many cell types that is not normally in contact with the circulation but is exposed to blood after vascular damage; it also plays a significant role in inflammation.[7] Upon activation, TF binds with coagulation factors that, in turn, trigger both the intrinsic and the extrinsic pathways of coagulation. The intrinsic pathway of coagulation, known as the *contact activation pathway,* is activated by trauma or infection that causes inflammatory proteins to be released into the circulation. The extrinsic pathway of coagulation is activated by tissue injury. These two pathways collaborate at various stages and collectively make up the *common pathway of coagulation.*

The activation of prothrombin is an intermediary step in the activation of thrombin. Prothrombin is converted to thrombin, the most powerful of the coagulation enzymes. Thrombin then acts on fibrinogen to form fibrin.[8] The fibrin clot is soluble until it becomes polymerized by factor XIIIa (fibrin-stabilizing factor), which converts it into a stable (i.e., insoluble) clot. Hemostasis is complete when the fibrin network alone is able to resist the hydrostatic pressure in the vessel.

Figure 29-2 depicts the mechanisms of fibrinolysis. Fibrin formation is an essential component of hemostasis, inflammation, and tissue repair, but it is a temporary reaction. The fibrin clot must be remodeled and removed to restore normal tissue structure and function, as well as to restore normal blood flow. This is accomplished by the fibrinolytic system, which controls the enzymatic degradation of fibrin.

Fibrinolysis

Fibrinolysis, or clot breakdown, is initiated by enzymes known as *plasminogen activators,* which are present in most body fluids and both normal and neoplastic tissues (Figure 29-2). Plasminogen, an inactive precursor of plasmin, is activated to plasmin in the presence of thrombin. Plasmin is responsible for the lysis of fibrin clots. The breakdown of fibrinogen and fibrin results in polypeptides called *fibrin degradation products* (FDPs) or *fibrin split products* (FSPs). The FDPs are powerful anticoagulant substances that have a destructive effect on fibrin in the platelet plug. When these products are increased in the circulation, there is a predisposition to bleeding.

Pathophysiology of Bleeding

Bleeding or hemorrhage may occur when the processes of hemostasis or coagulation are overwhelmed, such as when blood vessel injury occurs and blood escapes. Multiple mechanisms exist in a patient with cancer that may cause bleeding, including altered platelet count and function, altered coagulation mechanisms, altered vascular integrity, and cancer treatment–related effects. Patients with cancer may have one or multiple causes of altered hemostasis.

Platelet Abnormalities

Thrombocytopenia

Thrombocytopenia, a reduction in the number of circulating platelets, is the platelet abnormality most frequently associated with cancer. It may be caused by a decrease in platelet production, a change in platelet distribution (e.g., sequestration of platelets in the spleen), platelet destruction, vascular dilution, drug therapies, or disseminated intravascular coagulation (DIC; see Chapter 37).

Platelet production. The most common cause of thrombocytopenia in patients with cancer is a disorder

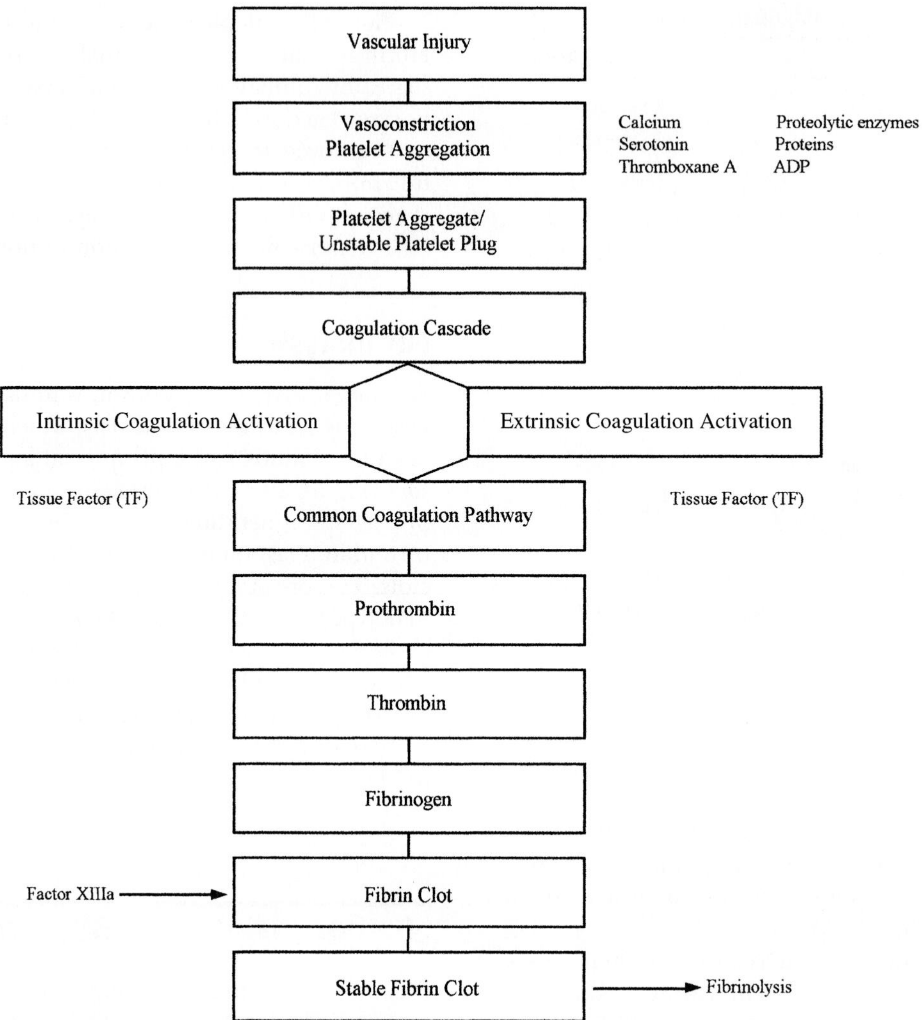

Figure 29-1 Mechanism of normal blood coagulation.

involving decreased megakaryocytopoiesis (i.e., platelet production in the bone marrow). This decreased production of platelets may be due to tumor invasion of the bone marrow or to acute or delayed effects of chemotherapy or radiation therapy. A low platelet count is directly proportional to the degree of bone marrow infiltration by tumor cells. When tumor invasion is the cause of the decrease in platelet production, the resulting thrombocytopenia is generally a part of the total picture of pancytopenia. The degree of thrombocytopenia due to chemotherapy depends on the type of chemotherapy, dose of chemotherapy, and intervals between treatments. The extent of thrombocytopenia associated with radiation depends on the amount of bone marrow in the radiation field.

Platelet distribution. Thrombocytopenia due to an abnormal distribution of platelets can occur in cancer patients with hypersplenism. An enlarged spleen may sequester as much as 90% of the platelet population, making these cells unavailable to the circulation. The bone marrow attempts to respond to the thrombocytopenia by increasing platelet production; platelets, however, continue to be sequestered by the spleen, thereby increasing the splenomegaly.[9] Tumor metastasis to the spleen, particularly due to lung, breast, colon, prostate, and stomach cancers and lymphomas, is known to cause hypersplenism and subsequent platelet sequestration. Thrombocytopenia can also be due to congestive splenomegaly related to splenic vein obstruction in pancreatic cancer.[10,11] The thrombocytopenia related to hypersplenism is generally mild (platelet count of 40,000–100,000 cells/mm^3). The absence of a palpable spleen rules out this type of thrombocytopenic disorder.

Platelet destruction. Thrombocytopenia can also be due to an immune-mediated thrombocytopenia, or idiopathic thrombocytopenia purpura (ITP). The rapid destruction of platelets in ITP is caused by an

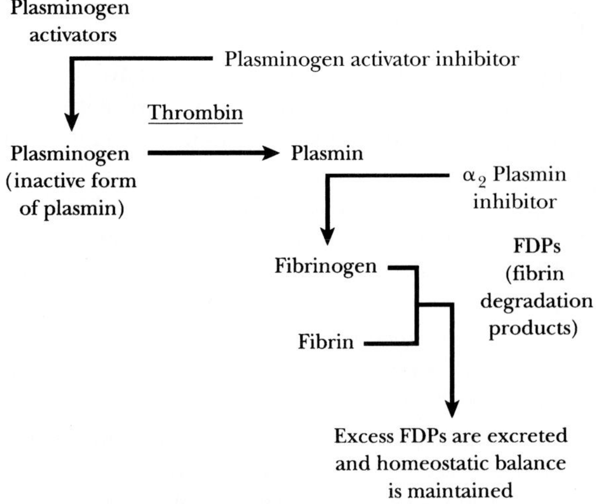

Figure 29-2 Fibrinolysis.

autoimmune process in which antibodies are formed against the individual's own platelets. This condition results in normal or increased numbers of megakaryocytes (immature platelets) in the bone marrow and decreased numbers of circulating platelets in the general circulation. Signs and symptoms of ITP include petechiae, purpura, ecchymosis, menorrhagia, epistaxis, thrombocytopenia, and bleeding (gingival, urinary, gastrointestinal, and occasionally cerebral).[12] ITP occurs most frequently in individuals with lymphoproliferative disorders such as chronic lymphocytic leukemia (CLL), acute lymphocytic leukemia (ALL), and Hodgkin's and non-Hodgkin's lymphoma.[13] It is rarely associated with solid tumors.

Platelet alloimmunization. Patients who have received multiple blood transfusions may develop antibodies to human leukocyte antigens (HLA) due to exposure to transfusion-related antigens. A significant percentage of patients who receive multiple platelet transfusions develop antibodies against these foreign antigens and become alloimmunized. This process impairs the patient's response to platelets. The use of leukoreduced platelets or HLA-matched platelets may decrease the incidence of this problem.[14]

Thrombocythemia/thrombocytosis

Thrombocythemia and thrombocytosis are a result of overproduction of platelets. Thrombocythemia, also known as *essential* or *primary thrombocythemia,* is characterized by an abnormal expansion of the megakaryocytic progenitor cell portion of the marrow. It occurs in a group of related chronic myeloproliferative disorders that includes polycythemia vera, chronic myelogenous leukemia (CML), agnogenic myeloid metaplasia, and idiopathic myelofibrosis.[3] Thrombocytosis, also known as *secondary* or *reactive thrombocytosis,* occurs in approximately 30%–40% of patients with cancer. It is associated with hemorrhage, inflammatory disorders, iron deficiency, hemolytic anemia, and splenectomized patients, and frequently occurs in individuals with widespread cancer.[15]

The major complications related to an increased platelet count are bleeding and thrombosis, albeit rarely in association with thrombocytosis. The most common sites of bleeding and potential hemorrhage associated with these conditions are the mucosa and the gastrointestinal tract. Bleeding can also occur in other sites, such as the skin and the genitourinary tract. Thrombosis may result in symptoms associated with venous thrombosis, pulmonary embolism, transient cerebral ischemia, myocardial infarction, and angina, or in portal mesenteric vein occlusion.

Altered platelet function

At times, patients with cancer may bleed despite normal platelet counts and coagulation factors. Alterations in platelet function may be responsible for this type of bleeding. A variety of hematologic diseases are associated with abnormal platelet function. Hemostatic abnormalities associated with abnormal platelet function include multiple myeloma, Waldenström's macroglobulinemia, acute myelogenous leukemia, and CML.[16] The major abnormality noted in these diseases is a decrease in the procoagulant activity of the platelets, which is a measure of platelet factor III. Also noted in these diseases are platelets that are larger or smaller than normal, abnormally shaped platelets, and a variation in the number of storage pool granules. In addition, abnormal platelet function has been described in patients with thrombocytosis associated with the myeloproliferative disorders; this phenomenon may help to explain the increased incidence of hemorrhage in patients with an increased platelet concentration.

Hypocoagulation

Conditions related to hypocoagulation are less common than the other types of hemostatic alterations discussed in this chapter. Although any type of coagulation abnormality can lead to bleeding, hypocoagulation disorders cause serious bleeding less frequently when they do occur. Hemorrhages tend to develop in the deeper areas of the body, such as the subcutaneous or intramuscular tissues. Bleeding into the joints, especially of the distal extremities, may occur in hypocoagulation disorders.

The most significant factor leading to a state of hypocoagulation is liver disease. Liver disease may result from infection, chemotherapy, tumor invasion, or surgical resection. Regardless of its etiology, liver disease has been reported to cause prolonged bleeding time, reduced platelet aggregation, and increased procoagulant activity.[17] Liver disease interferes with the synthesis of plasma coagulation factors I, II, V, VII, IX, and X. In addition to decreasing the production of these factors, liver disease may interfere with their functioning. Decreased liver function contributes to diminished liver clearance of FDPs and activated clotting factors, which further inhibits the coagulation mechanism.

A deficiency of vitamin K may also cause a hypocoagulation syndrome. This effect may be seen in patients with cancer who lack vitamin K in their diet, with resulting biliary obstruction, malabsorptive states, intestinal sterilization due to antibiotic administration, and impaired clotting factor synthesis due to liver disease.[18] A deficiency of vitamin K produces a greatly reduced chemical activation of vitamin K–dependent proteins, resulting in a state of decreased hemostasis.

Individuals who undergo extensive surgical procedures and receive large amounts of frozen plasma may demonstrate a prolonged prothrombin time and a prolonged partial thromboplastin time. These individuals are prone to postsurgical bleeding. Frozen plasma has deficient levels of factors V and VIII, which can also lead to a state of decreased hemostasis.

Isolated factor deficiencies are also related to cancer. Acquired von Willebrand's disease has been demonstrated to occur in solid tumors, hematologic cancers, myeloproliferative disorders, macroglobulinemia, and lymphoproliferative disorders. A small number of patients with malignant B-cell disease and Wilms' tumor have been reported to develop acquired von Willebrand's disease.[19] Patients with this syndrome demonstrate bruising, mucosal bleeding, and gastrointestinal hemorrhage. Coagulation studies show a prolonged bleeding time and diminished or absent factor VIII procoagulant activity (VIII:c), von Willebrand's factor antigen (vWF:Ag), and ristocetin cofactor activity.

Tumor Effects

Tumor-related bleeding in cancer can occur through a variety of mechanisms. Tumor invasion in the bone marrow, due either to solid tumors or hematologic malignancies, can cause bleeding. Tumor-related bleeding may also be due to tumor extension into surrounding structures or blood vessels. Tumor-related bleeding may be manifested as DIC as well.

Tumor invasion

Tumor invasion into the bone marrow can be caused by primary tumors in hematologic diseases that are intrinsic to the marrow or by metastatic spread of tumor to the marrow from cancers of various organs. This type of tumor invasion is called *myelophthisis*. Tumor invasion that causes bleeding is common in Hodgkin's and non-Hodgkin's lymphoma, leukemia, malignant melanoma, and neuroblastoma. Bleeding related to tumor invasion is also common in carcinoma of the lung, breast, prostate, thyroid, kidney, and adrenal glands.[20] Tumor invasion can result in anemia, thrombocytopenia, granulocytopenia, and neutropenia. The decrease in production of normal marrow elements is thought to comprise a response to the physiologic "crowding out" of normal cells, competition for cell nutrients, and the invading cells' metabolic end products, which are toxic to normal cells.

Tumor extension

Tumor extension may occur in surrounding structures or blood vessels. Bleeding is a common presenting symptom of cancer, generally occurring as a result of tumor and local invasion. Blood loss and the resulting iron-deficiency anemia are frequently the initial signs of lung, gynecologic, genitourinary, or colorectal carcinomas.[21,22] Clinically, the individual may present with symptoms ranging from minor incidents of bleeding to gross blood loss.

Frequently, the most dramatic cause of bleeding in the patient with cancer is the invasion, erosion, and sudden massive hemorrhage of the blood vessel. Any tumor involvement of vascular tissue or any tumor lying in close proximity to major vessels is seen as a risk for bleeding. Cancers of the large bronchi or lung may erode into the bronchial artery or branches of the pulmonary artery. Hemoptysis from tumor erosion into pulmonary blood vessels may appear as streaks of blood or gross blood loss. Head and neck tumors may also be associated with serious bleeding. Invasive cancers, particularly at the base of the tongue, can erode branches of the external carotid artery.

More gradual bleeding involving smaller circulatory structures is usually less obvious and therefore more difficult to diagnose. Melena due to colorectal carcinoma or the microscopic bleeding of macroglobulinemia can persist undetected until manifested by iron-deficiency anemia. A continual loss of 6–8 mL of blood per day will eventually precipitate classic iron deficiency, because the compensatory need for cell production exceeds the iron-producing capacity of the normal adult diet.

The homeostatic mechanisms in the body provide such remarkable compensatory adaptation that iron-deficiency anemia may be quite serious before the person actually develops significant symptoms. For this reason, it is important to remember that the onset of symptoms may reflect the rate of the progression of the anemia better than the severity does. Fatigue, weakness, irritability, dyspnea, and tachycardia are typical clinical symptoms experienced by individuals with anemia.

Treatment Effects

Bleeding in cancer may be related to chemotherapy, biotherapy, radiation therapy, surgery, or medication effects.

Chemotherapy/biotherapy effects

Chemotherapy is the cancer treatment most often associated with hematologic toxicity, including thrombocytopenia. The effects of chemotherapy are due in large part to the particular drugs used, dosages, schedules, routes of administration, previous cancer treatments, and any concomitant therapies. Chemotherapy-induced thrombocytopenia is usually caused by the destruction of the proliferating cells of the platelet line. As these cells are destroyed, the circulatory platelets are cleared at the end of their life span, and the nadir of a patient's blood cell count occurs. Considering that the average life span of a platelet is only 7 days, this phenomenon accounts in part for the high incidence of thrombocytopenia related to chemotherapy.

The chemotherapy agents mithramycin, carmustine, and daunorubicin are associated with abnormal platelet aggregation and other coagulapathies. Vincristine and vinblastine are associated with platelet dysfunction.[23]

Thrombocytopenia related to the biotherapy agents is not as common as that seen with chemotherapy. Table 29-2 lists chemotherapy, biotherapy, and radiotherapy agents associated with moderate to severe thrombocytopenia. Chemotherapy and biotherapy doses may be decreased or eliminated depending on the degree of toxicity manifested as thrombocytopenia. Altering doses of these agents has important implications for treatment outcomes.

Radiation therapy effects

Radiation therapy can cause hematologic toxicity, particularly when large areas of bone marrow are treated. The most significant factor that determines the risk of bone marrow suppression related to radiation therapy is the volume of productive bone marrow in the radiation field. Megakaryocytes are affected 1–2 weeks after exposure to the radiation, and they take about 2–6 weeks to recover from such damage. Radiation therapy is local treatment, except for total nodal or total body irradiation, and rarely causes the nadirs in blood counts seen with chemotherapy. The localized nature of this treatment generally allows the untreated marrow to compensate for the damage to the treated marrow.

Radiolabeled monoclonal antibodies have a therapeutic radioisotope that is chemically bound to the antibody. The advantage of using radiolabeled monoclonal antibodies is that the antibodies deliver the radiation primarily to the tumor cells with less radiation to the normal cells.[24] Side effects associated with radiolabeled monoclonal antibodies include reversible decreases in blood counts, including anemia, leukopenia, and thrombocytopenia.[25] Table 29-2 lists the radiolabeled monoclonal antibodies associated with moderate to severe thrombocytopenia.

Surgical effects

Bleeding may result from surgery performed in an attempt to manage the cancer itself. For example, carotid artery rupture could potentially occur after a radical neck dissection for the treatment of head and neck cancer. Carotid artery rupture occurs more frequently when the patient has received prior radiation therapy. Prophylactic arterial ligation may be performed to minimize the risk of a carotid hemorrhage. The patient who undergoes a ligation of the external carotid arteries runs the risk of a stroke. Small transient bleeding usually occurs before any vessel rupture. Careful observation can assist in predicting and controlling such a complication.

Medication effects

Numerous drugs are known to affect platelet number and function. Thrombocytopenia is the most common of the drug-induced blood dyscrasias, as any drug can cause unexpected thrombocytopenia.[26] Drug-induced thrombocytopenia may be caused by immune-mediated suppression or destruction of platelets, decreased production of platelets, or a nonimmune direct effect on circulating platelets (such as occurs with the use of heparin). Quinine and quinidine are drugs known to produce drug-induced immune thrombocytopenia.[27] When patients have been sensitized to the use of these drugs, their platelet count may drop rapidly, with bleeding occurring within hours or days of ingestion. Many drugs can cause a decreased production of platelets, including thiazide diuretics as well as furosemide, phenothiazines, antimetabolites, antimitotic agents, antitumor antibiotics, benzene and benzene derivatives, ionizing radiation, nitrogen mustard, estrogens, tricyclic antidepressants, and alcohol. If bleeding or prolonged thrombocytopenia becomes

Table 29-2 Chemotherapeutic Agents Associated with Significant Thrombocytopenia

Chemotherapeutic Agent	Degree of Suppression	Nadir (days)	Recovery (days)
Busulfan	Moderate	21–28	42–56
Carmustine	Severe	28–42	35–42
Chlorambucil	Moderate	21–28	42–56
Cladribine	Moderate	14	60
Cyclophosphamide	Moderate (dose-related — 100 mg/m^2)	7–14	21
Cytarabine	Severe	10	21
Dacarbazine	Marked (dose-related — 200 mg/m^2 IV daily × 5 days)	10–14	21–28
Dactinomycin	Severe	14	21–28
Daunorubicin hydrochloride	Severe	10	21–28
Docetaxel	Moderate to severe	8	14
Doxorubicin	Moderate to severe (dose-related)	10–14	21
Epirubicin hydrochloride	Moderate	10–14	21
5-Fluorouracil	Moderate (dose-related — 12–15 mg/kg)	9–21	21
Gemcitabine	Moderate		
Gemtuzumab ozogamicin	Moderate to severe		Prolonged
Hycamptin	Moderate	10–12	15–21
Hydroxyurea	Moderate	7	14
Ibritumomab tiuxetan	Moderate to severe	7–14	14–21
Idarubicin	Moderate	10–15	25
Irinotecan	Severe (rare)		
Lomustine	Severe	21–28	42
Mechlorethamine	Moderate	10–14	21–28
Methotrexate	Moderate (dose-related — 100 mg/m^2)	10	14
Mitomycin C	Severe	21–28	42–56
Oxaliplatin	Moderate		
Paclitaxel	Severe	8–15	21
L-phenylalanine	Moderate	14–21	21–28
Plicamycin	Moderate	14	21
Procarbazine	Moderate	14	21–28
Rituximab	Moderate to severe (rare)		
Streptozocin	Moderate		
6-Thioguanine	Moderate to severe	14–28	28–35
Tositumomab	Moderate to severe	7–14	14–42
Triethylenephosphoramide	Moderate	14–21	40–50
Vinblastine	Moderate to severe	10	21
Vinorelbine	Mild to moderate	14	21

a problem, these medications should be stopped or altered.

Heparin is the most common cause of drug-induced thrombocytopenia; this problem may arise either due to a direct aggregating effect of heparin, leading to reversible platelet clumping in which complications are unlikely, or due to heparin-induced thrombocytopenia (HIT). The latter condition is more serious and can lead to bleeding. In HIT, heparin binds to platelet membranes, which results in platelet clumping and a lower peripheral platelet count. Low-molecular-weight heparins are associated less often with HIT.[28]

Many drugs are known to affect platelet aggregation, as demonstrated by a prolonged bleeding time. Nevertheless, only aspirin has been shown to cause a significant increased risk of bleeding. Aspirin works primarily by inactivating platelet cyclooxygenase. Inactivation of cyclooxygenase decreases platelet aggregation, prevents release of vasoactive substances, and prolongs the bleeding time.[29] This platelet aggregation abnormality is so characteristic that abnormal platelet aggregation patterns of any etiology are often termed *aspirin-like.* The bleeding time can be prolonged for as long as 4 days after a single dose of aspirin, until normal platelet turnover results in a significant number of new platelets with normal function. The mechanism of action of nonsteroidal anti-inflammatory drugs (NSAIDs) appears to be similar to that of aspirin inhibition of platelet cyclooxygenase; these drugs have only a temporary effect, causing inhibition only as long as the active drug remains in the circulation. The newer class of NSAIDs (COX-2 inhibitors) have minimal platelet effects and are an important option for patients with cancer.[30]

Antibiotics are frequently associated with causing bleeding. High-dose β-lactam antibiotics (e.g., carbenicillin, ticarcillin, penicillin) inhibit platelet function and prolong the bleeding time. Maximal platelet dysfunction occurs 3–5 days after initiation of therapy and resolves within 3–4 days after therapy is stopped.[31] The cephalosporins and maxalactam may cause a similar pattern of platelet dysfunction. Vitamin K may be given parenterally to counter this effect.

Infection-Related Effects

Localized infections, including viral and bacterial infections that occur at sites of blood vessels, may cause cavitational or local ulcerations that lead to bleeding. Systemic infections — particularly gram-negative bacteremias — can stimulate DIC, which can result in life-threatening bleeding and thrombosis.

Miscellaneous Effects

The production of high-viscosity proteins in multiple myeloma and Waldenström's macroglobulinemia can cause bleeding. Although rare, this overproduction of abnormal proteins has been identified in 4% of individuals with immunoglobulin G (IgG) myeloma and in 5%–10% of individuals with immunoglobulin A (IgA) myeloma.[32] In multiple myeloma, this overproduction of proteins (immunoglobulins) increases the viscosity of the blood, resulting in poor circulatory movement with increased risk for clotting and bleeding.[33] A clinical triad of symptoms is associated with this hyperviscosity syndrome — namely, bleeding, visual changes, and neurologic deficits.

Thrombocytopenia associated with multiple myeloma usually occurs following chemotherapy or radiation therapy. Thrombocytopenia may also be seen when the myeloma expands within the marrow, further contributing to the risk of bleeding. Moreover, a qualitative defect in platelet function can occur, as the M protein (myeloma protein or malignant protein of myeloma) coating the platelet interferes with its function.[16]

Assessment for Bleeding

Assessment for bleeding in the patient with cancer begins with a thorough history and physical examination. The assessment may be comprehensive, as when interviewing a person suspected of having cancer, or cursory, as when caring for an individual with acute blood loss due to cancer. A number of laboratory screening tests provide information about the risk of bleeding, measure actual blood loss, and help to determine the pathophysiology of the bleeding. Diagnostic tests may also be ordered to evaluate internal hemorrhage, including magnetic resonance imaging and angiography (MRI/MRA) scans, computerized tomography (CT) scans, plain film radiographs, and ultrasound. The information gathered in the assessment of bleeding is critical in preparing an appropriate plan of care.

Patient/Family History

The patient/family history is a vital component of a complete assessment. Because bleeding is a common problem in many malignancies, it is important to remain alert to findings that suggest bleeding disorders. Key aspects of a comprehensive history for the individual at risk for bleeding include the following:

- Bleeding tendencies, including easy bruising, excessive nosebleeds, gingival bleeding, presence of petechiae, change in color of stools or urine, stomach discomfort, vision problems, and painful joints
- Signs or symptoms of anemia, which may signify undetected long-term bleeding
- Medications, including chemotherapy or any over-the-counter medications (including herbal medications) that might interfere with the coagulation

mechanism or that might uncover an important symptom for which the person is taking medication

- Acute bacterial or viral infections that may increase the risk of disseminated intravascular coagulation
- General performance status that helps to identify the effects of the disease or the presence of complications
- Transfusion history, including blood components required and the response to therapy (may provide information regarding potential risk of alloimmunization to prior blood products)
- Nutritional status, to identify vitamin K or vitamin C deficiency or generalized malnutrition that will affect the person's hematologic system
- Immunologic disorders, such as ITP, that increase the risk of bleeding
- Family history of any bleeding abnormalities

Physical Examination

Physical examination of the patient with actual or potential bleeding requires a thorough head-to-toe approach. Diagnostic signs can be subtle, including skin petechiae noticed while bathing the patient, traces of blood as the patient brushes his or her teeth, and oozing from venipuncture sites or sites of injections. Such observations can lead to early diagnosis of bleeding problems and might prevent an incident of spontaneous hemorrhage.

The major problem associated with active bleeding is hemorrhage. Although bleeding can occur from any part of the body, common sites of hemorrhage include the gums, nose, brain, bladder, and the gastrointestinal tract. An examination of all body systems is done on a routine basis for any patient known to have a bleeding disorder (Table 29-3).

Table 29-3 Physical Examination of the Patient with Actual or Potential Bleeding

System	Findings
Central Nervous System	Mental status changes including confusion, lethargy, restlessness, changes in cognition, alteration in level of consciousness, obtundation, seizures or coma; changes in neurologic signs including widening pulse pressure, pupil size and reactivity, motor strength and coordination, speech and paralysis, and complaints of headache (all may indicate intracranial hemorrhage or impaired tissue perfusion)
Eyes[a] and Ears	Visual disturbances including diplopia, blurred vision, and partial field loss; increased injection on the sclera, periorbital edema, subconjunctival hemorrhage (homogeneous red color that is sharply outlined on the sclera); eye or ear pain
Nose, Mouth, and Throat	Petechiae on nasal/oral mucosa, ulcerations, gingival or mucous membrane bleeding, epistaxis
Cardiovascular	Changes in vital signs, color and temperature of all extremities, peripheral pulses (all may demonstrate changes in peripheral perfusion); tachycardia, hypotension; observe for angina
Pulmonary	Respiratory rate and depth; dyspnea, tachypnea, and shortness of breath (may indicate an inability to compensate for blood loss); crackles, wheezes, stridor, dyspnea, tachypnea, orthopnea, hemoptysis (usually bright red in color and frothier than hematemesis); and cyanosis (all possible signs of bleeding in the lungs)
Abdominal	Pain (close attention to location); right upper quadrant pain and abdominal distention may be indicative of hepatomegaly; left flank or shoulder pain may be indicative of splenomegaly; vague abdominal pain may be indicative of retroperitoneal bleeding; palpable spleen, blood around rectum, tarry stools, frank or occult blood in stools, hematemesis; observe for bleeding hemorrhoids (may respond to local measures)
Genitourinary System	Blood in the urine (measure for frequency and size of clots); dysuria, burning, frequency and pain on urination (all are associated with hematuria); character and amount of menses; decreased urine output (if urine drops below 30 mL/hr it may be due to acute tubular necrosis secondary to thrombi, bleeding, or hypovolemia and associated shock)
Musculoskeletal System	Warm, tender, swollen joints with diminished mobility for active and passive range of motion (may indicate bleeding into the joints)
Integumentary System[b]	Bruising, petechiae, purpura, ecchymoses, hematomas, acrocyanosis (irregularly shaped cyanotic patches on the periphery of the arms and legs associated with bleeding due to DIC); pallor and jaundice (indicative of anemia and liver dysfunction); oozing from venipuncture sites or injections, biopsy sites, central lines, catheters, or nasogastric tubes

DIC = disseminated intravascular coagulation.

[a] Bleeding in the optic fundus could lead to permanent visual impairment.

[b] Assess entire skin surface, including intertriginous areas.

Screening Tests

Several screening tests provide information about hemostatic function, more specifically about the phases of hemostasis and fibrinolysis. The hematologic alterations leading to bleeding are complex, and test results vary depending on the degree of the original coagulation dysfunction and the cascading effect of related hemostatic mechanisms. Some of the most common screening tests of hemostatic functions are discussed next. A listing of tests of hemostasis is found in Table 29-4.

Platelet count

The platelet count is the best indicator of potential risk of bleeding in a patient with cancer. Normal platelet counts are considered to be 150,000–400,000 cells/mm^3; platelet counts below 100,000 cells/mm^3 are considered indicative of thrombocytopenia. Spontaneous hemorrhage generally is not a concern until

Table 29-4 Tests of Hemostasis

Test	Measures	Normal Value
	PLATELET FUNCTION	
Platelet count	Number of circulating platelets	150,000–400,000 cells/mm^3
Bleeding time	Platelet plug formation; response of small vessels	1–9 min
Bone marrow biopsy	Etiology of thrombocytopenia	Megakaryocytes present
	COAGULATION	
Partial thromboplastin time (aPTT)	Intrinsic and common pathways of coagulation cascade	Varies; compare with normal control (usually 30–40 sec)
Prothrombin time (PT)	Diminished or absent coagulation factors	Varies; compare with normal control (approximately 70%–130%)
International normalized ratio (INR)	Coagulation state	<2; >2 shows anticoagulation
Thrombin time	Fibrinogen concentration; structure of fibrinogen; presence of inhibitors	Varies: compare with normal value (approximately 200–400 mg/dL)
Specific factor assays	Concentration of functional factors in plasma	50%–150% activity in pooled normal plasma
	FIBRINOLYSIS	
Fibrin degradation product (FDP) assay	Presence of FDPs in serum	<10 μg/mL
D-dimer assay	Presence of FDPs in serum	30–400 ng/mL

the platelet count drops below 15,000 cells/mm^3. Thrombocytosis occurs when the count rises above 400,000 cells/mm^3.

Bleeding time

This test measures the time it takes for a small skin incision to stop bleeding. The results depend on the platelet number and function and the ability of the capillary wall to vasoconstrict. A normal bleeding time varies from 1–9 minutes. The bleeding time is prolonged when platelets are lacking or with a severe factor deficiency. Examples of disease states in which a prolonged bleeding time may be found include thrombocytopenia, von Willebrand's disease, infiltration of the marrow by tumor, and consumption of platelets in DIC. A prolonged bleeding time is also found with drugs that affect platelet function, such as aspirin.

Bone marrow aspirate

In most cases, the definitive test to determine the etiology of thrombocytopenia is the bone marrow aspirate. If the platelet count is low, the bone marrow aspirate will demonstrate few megakaryocytes because of underproduction of cells. This may occur when there is crowding of the marrow by disease. The bone marrow aspirate will demonstrate adequate to increased levels of megakaryocytes if the platelets are being destroyed in the peripheral blood by the immune system. This may occur with diseases such as ITP or as a result of marrow toxic therapy.

Partial thromboplastin time (activated)

A normal activated partial thromboplastin time (aPTT) is approximately 30–40 seconds. The aPTT screens for coagulation deficiencies in the intrinsic and common pathways of coagulation. A prolonged aPTT is evidenced when any clotting factor, except for factors VII or XIII, exists in inadequate quantities. A prolonged aPTT may be seen with DIC, liver disease, biliary obstruction, and with circulating anticoagulants such as heparin. There is a risk of spontaneous hemorrhage if the aPTT is greater than 100.

Prothrombin time

The prothrombin time (PT) screens for coagulation deficiencies along the extrinsic or common pathways of coagulation. The PT is prolonged when clotting factor I, II, V, VII, or X is deficient. Prolonged PT values are seen in liver disease (hepatitis and tumor involvement), in obstructive biliary disease (e.g., bile duct obstruction secondary to tumor), and with coumarin, heparin, streptokinase, and urokinase ingestion.[34]

Taken together, the aPTT and the PT can give a fair indication of the nature of the clotting defect. If both the aPTT and the PT are normal and the patient is bleeding, the vessels or platelets are probably defective. Likewise, if either the aPTT or the PTT is prolonged and the patient is bleeding, the defect is likely in the clotting mechanism.

International normalized ratio

The effects of anticoagulation therapy are often measured by the international normalized ratio (INR). The normal INR is less than 2.0. An INR greater than 2.0 is considered anticoagulated (e.g., for the treatment of deep-vein thrombosis or pulmonary embolus).

Factor assays

Measurement of specific factors identifies specific factor deficiencies, which may help in the diagnosis of bleeding.

Fibrin degradation products test and the D-dimer assay

The measurement of FDPs provides an indication of the activity of the fibrinolytic system. Agglutination is demonstrated if the patient's blood contains degradation fragments or products. Levels of FDP greater than 10 g/mL indicate increased fibrinolysis, as seen in DIC and primary fibrinolytic disorders. The D-dimer is a neoantigen formed as a result of plasmin digestion of fibrin. This test also measures the amount of FDPs in the blood.[35]

Therapeutic Approaches and Nursing Care

Prevention of Bleeding

General measures

Bleeding precautions are instituted for any patients at risk for bleeding to maintain their physical safety. These measures are taught to both the patient and the family so that they are aware of the potential risks of bleeding. Table 29-5 presents a care plan for a patient experiencing thrombocytopenia or bleeding. Environmental safety is critical in patients at risk for bleeding; bumps or falls can be dangerous and even fatal.

Diligent measures to maintain skin integrity are instituted. Personal hygiene is essential for maintaining skin integrity. The use of a good emollient lotion helps to minimize dryness and potential breaks of the skin. In addition, paper tape or similar tapes should be used rather than adhesive tape to avoid trauma to the skin.

All unnecessary procedures are avoided in the patient at risk for bleeding, including intramuscular or subcutaneous injections, rectal temperatures or suppositories, and indwelling catheters. If the patient requires parenteral administration of medications, the intravenous route is used whenever possible. Intramuscular and subcutaneous injections place the patient at risk for the development of hematomas, which can become sites of infection when granulocytopenia is present. If injections are unavoidable, the smallest-gauge needle possible is used. Pressure to the injection site is applied for several minutes, followed by the application of a pressure bandage to avoid a hematoma. Cold compresses may be used to assist in vasoconstriction. Similar care is taken at venipuncture sites.

The mouth and gums are easily damaged when the platelet count is low, and they become an excellent potential source of bleeding and infection. A systematic mouth care regimen should be instituted to minimize this problem. A lubricant to the lips, gums, and tongue will help avoid dryness and cracking. Soft-bristled toothbrushes help avoid trauma to sensitive gums. If the platelet count drops below 20,000–30,000 cells/mm^3 or if the gums and mouth are bleeding, bristled toothbrushes should be avoided and mouth swabs or Toothettes used. Most commercial mouthwashes should be avoided, as they contain a high alcohol content that is irritating and drying to the gums and mouth. When the gums and mouth are irritated, dentures should not be replaced, particularly if they fit poorly. Patients requiring oxygen via nasal cannula or endotracheal tube are assessed for irritation to the mucosa. A lubricant may need to be applied to the nares to minimize drying and cracking.

Prevention of forceful coughing, sneezing, nose blowing, or vomiting can be critical in a patient at risk for bleeding. Reducing the risk of bleeding helps to avoid increased intracranial pressure, which is critical in preventing intracranial hemorrhage in patients with low platelet counts.[36] Cough medications, especially those containing codeine or hydrocodone, may help to minimize bleeding related to coughing. For significant hemoptysis, in addition to cough suppressants the patient may need anxiolytics to promote decreased anxiety during this frightening event. Teaching the patient to gently clean the nares with tissue or a cotton swab dipped in saline may minimize bleeding related to nose blowing. Antiemetics minimize the potential of nausea and vomiting as well as keeping gastric juices from irritating the esophagus. The risk of upper gastrointestinal bleeding is minimized by treating patients who are on corticosteroids with H_2 blockers or proton pump inhibitors.

Bowel strain caused by constipation can initiate rectal bleeding. Laxatives and stool softeners may be necessary to avoid constipation. Instruction regarding proper diet and exercise to avoid constipation is also appropriate. The valsalva movement that may be used

Table 29-5 Care Plan for the Patient at Risk for Bleeding Related to Thrombocytopenia

Patient Problem	Expected Outcomes	Nursing Interventions
Potential for bleeding related to thrombocytopenia	The patient will have minimal or no bleeding. The patient/significant other will be able to state signs/symptoms indicative of bleeding. The patient/significant other will be able to demonstrate knowledge of their understanding of bleeding precautions.	1. Monitor platelet count and other coagulation tests and report abnormal values. 2. Assess vital signs q4h or as indicated. 3. Hold myelosuppressive agents as indicated. 4. Test all excreta for occult blood and report positive results. 5. Assess patient for any signs/symptoms of bleeding (see Table 29-3). 6. Teach patient/significant other about the signs/symptoms of bleeding. 7. Maintain and reinforce bleeding precautions when the patient's platelet count is ≤ 20,000 cells/mm^3 or the patient is bleeding. a. Use an emollient lotion on patient's skin. b. Use only electric razor. c. Use soft bristled toothbrush or moistened cloth to clean teeth. d. Use only alcohol-free mouthwash. e. Avoid use of dental floss and toothpicks. f. Avoid venipuncture, invasive procedures, rectal thermometers or suppositories, and indwelling catheters. g. Apply pressure to puncture sites for at least 5 min. h. Avoid forceful coughing, sneezing, nose blowing, or nausea/vomiting. i. Avoid constipation; may require laxatives and/or stool softeners. j. Avoid cutting toenails and fingernails. k. During menses, monitor pad count. l. Avoid aspirin or any medications that may cause/aggravate thrombocytopenia. m. Avoid tight-fitting or constrictive clothing. n. Use only humidified oxygen. 8. Administer recombinant thrombopoietin (rhIL-11) as indicated. 9. Administer platelet transfusion if ordered. a. Premedicate patient as indicated. b. Use leukocyte reduction filter on platelet transfusion as indicated. c. Use HLA-matched platelets, if refractory to platelets. d. Monitor, document, and notify physician if any allergic reaction (fever, chills, rash, hives, skin flushing) occurs. e. Obtain post-transfusion platelet count.

by patients with hard stool may increase intracranial pressure, which may in turn lead to intracranial hemorrhage.

Prophylactic blood component therapy transfusions

Transfusions of red blood cells (RBCs), platelets, and plasma may be administered to prevent bleeding in the thrombocytopenic patient. Red blood cell transfusions are generally given prophylactically when the hemoglobin level drops below 8 gm/dL. To date, no controlled studies have been done to determine the hemoglobin concentration at which RBC transfusions improve clinical outcomes.

A recent ASCO Platelet Transfusion Expert Panel recommendation regarding prophylactic platelet transfusions identified a platelet threshold of 10,000 cells/mm^3 in adult patients receiving therapy for acute leukemia. Transfusions at higher threshold levels may be needed in patients with signs of hemorrhage, high fever, hyperleukocytosis, or rapid fall of the platelet count in cases of coagulation abnormalities, and in patients undergoing invasive procedures or in circumstances in which platelet transfusions may not be readily available.[14,37,38] Plasma transfusions are generally given in patients with coagulation abnormalities who require surgical procedures.

Colony-stimulating factors

The use of recombinant colony-stimulating growth factors to accelerate hematologic recovery following intensive chemotherapy or radiation therapy continues to be an area of intensive investigation. Studies in both animals and humans have clearly shown that the administration of growth factors can reduce the hematopoietic toxicities that follow exposure to chemotherapy and radiation therapy. For a more thorough discussion of these factors, see Chapter 23.

Recombinant human interleukin-11 (rhIL-11). Several different cytokines or growth factors have been evaluated for their ability to stimulate megakaryocyte proliferation and maturation in patients undergoing chemotherapy,[39–41] but to date only rhIL-11 has demonstrated significant clinical efficacy in a randomized, placebo-controlled trial.[42] The use of rhIL-11 increases the likelihood of avoiding thrombocytopenia in patients undergoing chemotherapy and shortens the duration of the thrombocytopenia.[43] Another, more recent study involving rhIL-11 demonstrated effective reduction of chemotherapy-associated thrombocytopenia in patients with breast cancer who were receiving dose-intensive chemotherapy.[44] This study is of particular interest because it showed that the reduction of treatment-associated thrombocytopenia and the need for platelet transfusions in patients who receive dose-intensive chemotherapy may allow for chemotherapy to be administered at the intended doses as planned.[44]

Erythropoietin. The hematopoietic growth factor that regulates the proliferation, differentiation, and viability of erythrocyte progenitor cells and mature erythrocytes is erythropoietin (EPO). Erythropoietin (also known as epoietin alfa) has been shown to be an effective treatment for anemia associated with cancer and chemotherapy-associated anemia in some patients. Cloning of the erythropoietin gene was accomplished in 1985,[45,46] which allowed for large-scale production of this growth factor using recombinant DNA technology. Darbepoietin alfa is a novel erythropoiesis-stimulating protein developed for the treatment of anemia. Because of its longer half-life, compared to erythropoietin, it is given less frequently than erythropoietin (once weekly versus three times weekly).[47]

Erythropoietin administration is well tolerated and effective in the management of anemia associated with cancer and cancer chemotherapy. The administration of EPO increases the hemoglobin concentration and reduces red cell transfusion requirements (thereby decreasing exposure to donor blood products) in patients with cancer who receive chemotherapy and are anemic.

Chemotherapy protectors

Another approach to preferentially protecting normal tissues from the toxicities of chemotherapy entails the administration of cytoprotectant agents before the cancer treatment. Some of these agents have been used for many years, including leucovorin (prevents myelosuppression and mucositis associated with high-dose methotrexate) and mesna (prevents hemorrhagic cystitis associated with cyclophosphamide and ifosfamide). Saline diuresis or forced saline diuresis is also recommended to decrease the incidence of hemorrhagic cystitis associated with high-dose cyclophosphamide in the setting of stem cell transplantation.[48]

Management of Bleeding

General measures

If acute bleeding occurs, direct measures to stop the bleeding are instituted immediately. Direct, steady pressure is applied at the site of bleeding. Mechanical pressure, such as is produced by the insertion of an occlusion balloon catheter into the bronchus or the use of nasal packing during epistaxis, can be applied if the site of bleeding is not directly exposed. For epistaxis, the patient is placed in high Fowler's position. Gentle, steady pressure on the nares and a cold compress to constrict the bleeding vessels generally helps to stop the bleeding. Other measures implemented to stop the bleeding may include topical thromin or topical epinephrine to the affected nares. Iced saline gastric lavages or enemas may help to control gastrointestinal bleeding. Hypovolemic shock is to be avoided in situations of acute hemorrhage. Control of life-threatening hemorrhage is generally achieved with a combination of packed red cells with crystalloids or albumin as opposed to whole blood.

Intracranial bleeding in the thrombocytopenic patient may occur due to increased intracranial pressure from coughing, sneezing, or vomiting, or related to a valsalva maneuver. The immediate action with an intracranial bleed is to transfuse platelets. Corticosteroids are also given to decrease the concomitant intracranial edema and resultant increase in intracranial pressure.[36] Close monitoring of the patient with increased intracranial pressure is imperative, along with frequent vital sign and neurological monitoring.

Minor vascular bleeding due to capillary destruction is best controlled by treating the underlying malignancy. If iron-deficiency anemia arises, oral or parenteral iron supplements are indicated. Oral iron supplements are often recommended because they are safe and usually correct the anemia within 6 weeks, but therapy generally continues for 4–6 months to adequately replace the iron stores.[49] Parenteral iron supplements may be given if the patient cannot tolerate oral therapy or has a malabsorption problem. Iron dextran, generally given intravenously, requires a test dose because it is associated with a small risk of anaphylaxis.[49]

Physical and emotional rest are essential when the patient is bleeding. Rest helps to decrease pulse rate and blood pressure, allowing for clot formation. A state of active bleeding is frightening and anxiety-producing for the patient and family. A calm approach and reassurance are essential when managing an individual who is actively bleeding. Sedation can also be used to decrease anxiety and the metabolic rate.

Thrombocytopenia

Although thrombocytopenia may be the immediate cause of bleeding in individuals with platelet disorders, therapy must address the underlying cause of the decreased platelet level. When decreased platelet production results from tumor infiltration of marrow, the best therapy is treatment of the tumor itself. The hematologic complications will remain or worsen as long as marrow involvement persists. Platelet transfusions are often given to maintain a safe level of circulating thrombocytes until tumor regression occurs and marrow function returns. If platelet production has been depressed by chemotherapy or radiation therapy, in addition to platelet support the dosage or administration schedule of the treatment can be altered to maintain safe levels of platelet production.[50]

Platelet distribution. Thrombocytopenia related to platelet sequestration due to an enlarged spleen is treated most effectively by aggressive tumor therapy. Chemotherapy and radiation therapy are usually most effective for this condition. Sequestration of platelets is sometimes reversible with epinephrine, which causes a release of trapped platelets from an enlarged spleen. Transient control of platelet sequestration has also been achieved with corticosteroid therapy. Steroids have a capillary-stabilizing effect that is important in minimizing the bleeding potential of thrombocytopenia. Splenectomy may be considered if other methods fail to control the sequestration of platelets.

Platelet destruction. Individuals with asymptomatic ITP may be followed closely with no treatment. Patients who experience severe thrombocytopenia, however, are generally treated with glucocorticoid therapy.[13] Platelet transfusions are seldom indicated for patients with ITP because the survival time of transfused platelets is shortened. Intravenous immunoglobulin therapy plays an important role in managing acute bleeding. The efficacy of platelets has been found to be improved immediately after an infusion of intravenous immunoglobulin. Patients who are refractory to steroids and high-dose intravenous imunoglobulins may also benefit from anti-D immunoglobulin.[51]

Splenectomy was used for the management of ITP for many years before the advent of glucocorticoids. The decision to perform splenectomy for the treatment of ITP is determined by the course and severity of the disease. Splenectomy may be done early on in the course of severe thrombocytopenia that is unresponsive to prednisone, or it may be undertaken after several months if disease remission cannot be attained.[52] If patients fail prednisone therapy or show no response to splenectomy, other treatments include splenic radiation or partial splenic embolization, vincristine, vinblastine, bleomycin, danazol, colchicine, anti-D antibody, and alfa-interferon.[53,54]

Altered platelet function. Drug-induced platelet abnormalities must be assessed carefully in the context of the patient's total clinical profile. Aspirin has been demonstrated to increase the risk of bleeding. For this reason, the patient with cancer should avoid taking aspirin or any compounds containing aspirin. The clinical risk for bleeding associated with NSAIDs is much less than the risk associated with aspirin ingestion. However, the former drugs should be used cautiously in patients with preexisting thrombocytopenia. The potential for β-lactam–induced bleeding generally does not prohibit patients from being treated with appropriate antibiotic coverage; these patients need to be monitored closely for any signs or symptoms of bleeding. Platelet transfusions may be used during periods of thrombocytopenia to avoid hemorrhage as well as during periods of acute bleeding.

Hypocoagulation

Effective tumor therapy is the best means to control abnormalities related to hypocoagulation. Plasma and plasma derivative therapy may be used discriminately in specific clinical situations. Replacement of specific diminished factors is difficult because of the complex nature of these abnormalities. Generally, the treatment of specific inhibitors of coagulation factors depends on the severity of the abnormality.

Liver disease associated with bleeding and clotting can be treated with infusion of fresh-frozen plasma or prothrombin complex concentrate (which contains prothrombin and factors VII, IX, and X) when rapid correction of abnormalities is required. Prothrombin complex may also be given when attempting to shorten a prolonged prothrombin time, such as before a needle biopsy of the liver. Albumin can be used as a volume expander in cases of active bleeding. Albumin is safer than plasma because it carries no risk of hepatitis transmission. It may, however, precipitate congestive heart failure in patients with compromised cardiovascular function. When albumin is used as a volume expander, the patient's cardiac and renal status must be monitored closely. Desmopressin may be infused when the patient with liver disease has a prolonged bleeding time, with mild to moderate amounts of bleeding.[55,56]

Generally, subcutaneous vitamin K (menaphthone, AquaMEPHYTON) is administered to correct the protein defects when this vitamin is deficient, as demonstrated by prolonged prothrombin and bleeding times. The patient is also instructed about consuming dietary sources of vitamin K if absorption of the vitamin is not a problem. The major sources of dietary vitamin K are liver, broccoli, and spinach.[57,58] Prothrombin complex concentrates or fresh-frozen plasma can be used in situations of vitamin K deficiency with concomitant severe bleeding.

Isolated factor deficiencies are best treated with specific plasma components if they can be identified. Patients with acquired von Willebrand's disease are generally treated when they experience bleeding or when they require an invasive procedure. The severity of the bleeding dictates the type and amount of therapy used. Treatment for bleeding due to this syndrome includes fresh-frozen plasma, cryoprecipitate, packed RBCs and platelet concentrates, along with high-dose corticosteroids, factor VIII concentrates, desmopression infusions, epsilon-aminocaproic acid (amicar), intravenous gammaglobulin, and extracorporeal immunoabsorption.[59,60]

Blood Component Therapy

In recent years, several professional societies and governmental organizations, including the American Society of Anesthesiologists, ASCO, and the College of American Pathologists, have developed "guidelines" and "practice parameters" for the use of blood component therapy. These guidelines have been prompted by the recognition that even though blood component administration has clearly accepted benefits, it still has significant complications, including transfusion reactions, transmittal of bacterial or parasitic diseases, immunosuppression, and high cost.

Platelet therapy

Platelet transfusions have proved to provide tremendous therapeutic value in controlling and preventing hemorrhage in patients undergoing chemotherapy for leukemia and other cancers.[14] Theoretically, one unit of platelets should increase the recipient's platelet count by 10,000 cells/mm^3. In reality, the effectiveness of platelet transfusions is variable and depends on several factors. Failure to achieve adequate increases in the circulating platelet count may be due to fever, infection, hypersplenism, DIC, previous administration of amphotericin B, prolonged storage, and HLA antibody grade.[61]

Fever and infection enhance the consumption of platelets and can increase the occurrence of hemorrhage. Patients with fever or sepsis may require more frequent platelet transfusions to maintain adequate platelet counts. Patients with fever can be premedicated with antipyretics prior to platelet transfusion in an attempt to minimize platelet destruction; premedication may also consist of corticosteroids and antihistamines. Demerol may be given if the patient is having shaking chills.

Patients with hypersplenism who are receiving platelet transfusions will have a reduced recovery of circulating platelets that is generally proportionate to the size of the spleen. If platelets are transfused while the patient is actively bleeding, increased increments will not be detectable in blood counts. Instead, the effectiveness of platelet transfusions is determined by clinical improvement and control of the bleeding.

The preparation and storage of platelets are also important factors in determining the quality of the platelet transfusion. To be most effective, platelets must be fresh and metabolically active. Maximum effectiveness remains for as long as six hours after platelets are obtained. When platelets are properly collected and preserved, however, they can be stored for as long as five days.[14]

Red blood cell therapy

In any patient, the clinical concern for the adverse physiologic effects of anemia is usually the basis for considering RBC replacement. Generally, the decision to transfuse is based on the overall clinical picture, including any underlying cardiac or pulmonary conditions or any concurrent conditions that might impair the patient's tolerance of anemia. Among the causes of anemia frequently seen in patients with cancer, the two most common are decreased RBC production secondary to myelosuppressive therapy and the primary disease process.

The transfusion of one unit of red blood cells increases the hematocrit by 3% or the hemoglobin concentration by 1 g/dL in a 70-kg nonbleeding patient. Packed erythrocytes are typically the therapy of choice. The advantage of packed red blood cells is that they provide more than 70% of the hematocrit of whole blood with only one-third of the plasma. Their use prevents unnecessary volume, electrolyte load, and anticoagulants that might otherwise be transfused.

Plasma therapy

Fresh-frozen plasma, the most frequently used of the plasma products, contains all of the labile clotting factors and the plasma proteins. Plasma proteins such as albumin and cryoprecipitate can be isolated and removed from plasma. The most common use of plasma and plasma components in cancer occurs with coagulation disorders. Plasma component therapy is also administered for shock, severe bleeding, bleeding associated with infections, and management of acute DIC. Fresh-frozen plasma is generally not the treatment of choice for replacing most individual clotting factors, because large volumes would be required to obtain adequate factor levels. The patient's cardiovascular and pulmonary status may preclude the use of large amounts of plasma.[61]

The amount and frequency of transfusions depend on several factors, including the severity of the deficiency, the specific factor deficiency, and the severity of bleeding. Another important dosing consideration in plasma therapy is the metabolic half-life of the plasma and plasma derivatives. Replacement therapy is given in doses high enough to compensate for the decrease in plasma level as it is metabolized. The metabolic half-life varies for each of the factors. Typically, plasma and plasma factors are infused rapidly so that the maximum plasma level is reached before metabolic changes or degradation occurs.

Conclusion

Bleeding associated with cancer presents a complex clinical challenge to the nurse. It can occur as a result of the cancer itself or as a complication of the treatment of the cancer. Bleeding can be occult and chronic, or acute and life-threatening. Nurses who work with cancer patients must be prepared to meet the complex needs of these patients. Early detection of the signs and symptoms of bleeding allows for prompt diagnosis and treatment of the bleeding, thereby preventing further complications. Management of bleeding is often as complex as the bleeding process itself. A variety of medications may be used to prevent and treat bleeding disorders. The cornerstone therapy in the prevention and management of bleeding is blood transfusion therapy. An important adjunct to blood transfusion therapy in preventing and treating a bleeding problem is recombinant colony-stimulating factors. Exciting research continues in this area to identify as yet unknown CSFs that may benefit the patient with bleeding.

References

1. Belt R, Leite C, Haas CD, et al: Incidence of hemorrhagic complications in patients with cancer. *JAMA* 239:2571–2574, 1978
2. Gaydos LA, Frierich EJ, Mantel N: The quantitative relation between platelet count and hemorrhage in patients with acute leukemia. *N Engl J Med* 266:905–909, 1962
3. Arnold SM, Patchell R, Lowry AM, et al: Paraneoplastic syndromes, in DeVita VT, Hellman S, Rosenberg SA (eds.): *Cancer Principles and Practice of Oncology* (ed 6). Philadelphia, Lippincott, Williams and Wilkins, 2001, pp 2511–2536
4. Avances C, Oumaya C, Granger V, et al: Prostate cancer and acute disseminated intravascular coagulation. Therapeutic management based on three cases. *Prog Urolo* 2:303–312, 2003
5. Gobel BH: Disseminated intravascular coagulation, in Yarbro CH, Frogge MH, Goodman M (eds.): *Cancer Nursing Principles and Practice* (ed 5). Sudbury, MA, Jones and Bartlett, 2000, pp 869–875
6. Packham MA: Role of platelets in thrombosis and hemostasis. *Can J Physiol Pharmacol* 72:278–284, 1994
7. Versteeg HH, Peppelenbosch MP, Spek CA: The pleiotropic effects of tissue factor: a possible role for factor VIIa-intracellular signaling? *Thromb Haemost* 89:592–593, 2001
8. Howell DC, Laurent GJ, Chambers RC: Role of thrombin and its major cellular receptor, protease-activated receptor-1, in pulmonary fibrosis. *Biochem Soc* 30(part 2):211–216, 2002
9. CancerSourceRN.com: Bleeding in cancer. Updated August 24, 2000. *www.cancersourcern.com/Nursing/CE/CECourse.cfm?courseid=62&contentid=20166.* Accessed March 15, 2004
10. Yamakado K, Nakatsuka A, Tanaka N, et al: Malignant portal venous obstructions treated by stent placement: significant factors affecting patency. *JVIR* 12:1407–1415, 2001
11. Yamakado K, Nakatsuka A, Tanaka N, et al: Portal venous stent placement in patients with pancreatic and biliary neoplasms invading portal veins and causing portal hypertension: initial experience. *Radiology* 220:150-156, 2001
12. Lynch MP: Idiopathic thrombocytopenic purpura, in *Clinical Manual for the Oncology Advanced Practice Nurse.* Pittsburgh, Oncology Nursing Press, 2001, pp 689–691
13. Silverman MA: Idiopathic thrombocytopenic purpura. Updated August 27, 2003. *www.emedicine.com/emerg/topic282.htm.* Accessed April 1, 2004
14. Schiffer CA, Anderson KC, Bennett CL, et al: Platelet transfusion for patients with cancer: clinical practice guidelines of the American Society of Clinical Oncology. *J Clin Oncol* 19:1519–1538, 2001
15. Eichinger S, Bauer KA: Coagulopathic complications, in Holland JF, Bast RC, Morton DL, et al (eds.): *Cancer Medicine* (ed 4). Baltimore, Williams and Wilkins, 1997, pp 3179–3190
16. Munshi NC, Tricot G, Barlogie B: Plasma cell neoplasms, in DeVita VT, Hellman S, Rosenberg SA (eds.): *Cancer Principles and Practice of Oncology* (ed 6). Philadelphia, Lippincott, Williams and Wilkins, 2001, pp 2465–2499
17. Gralnick A, Ginsberg D: Von Willebrand's disease, in Beutler E, Lichtman MA, Coller BS, Kipps TJ (eds.): *Williams Hematology* (ed 5). New York, McGraw-Hill, 1995, pp 1458–1480
18. Patel P: Vitamin K deficiency. Updated January 5, 2004. *www.emedicine.com/emerg/topic2385.htm.* Accessed April 19, 2004
19. Murakawa M, Okamura T, Tsutsumi K, et al: Acquired von Willebrand's disease in association with essential thrombocythemia: regression following treatment. *Acta Haematol* 87:83–90, 1992
20. Elting LS, Rubenstein EB, Martin CG, et al: Incidence, cost, and outcomes of bleeding and chemotherapy dose modification among solid tumor patients with chemotherapy-induced thrombocytopenia. *J Clin Oncol* 19:1137–1146, 2001

21. Garcia AA: Ovarian cancer. Updated December 2, 2002. *www.emedicine.com/emerg/topic1698.htm.* Accessed April 19, 2004
22. Wauters H, VanCasteren V, Buntix F: Rectal bleeding and colorectal cancer in general practice: diagnostic study. *BMJ* 321:998–999, 2000
23. Smith MR, Khan N: Transfusion therapy, bleeding, and clotting, in Skeel RT (ed.): *Handbook of Cancer Chemotherapy* (ed 5). Philadelphia, Lippincott, Williams and Wilkins, 1999, pp 63–143
24. Idec Pharmaceuticals Corporation: *A Practical Guide for the Healthcare Professional.* San Diego, CA, Idec Pharmaceuticals Corporation, 2002
25. Tuinstra N: Outpatient administration of radiolabeled monoclonal antibodies. *Clin J Oncol Nurs* 7:106–108, 2003
26. Drews RE: Critical issues in hematology: anemia, thrombocytopenia, coagulation, and blood product transfusion in critically ill patients. *Clin Chest Med* 24:607–622, 2003
27. Reddy JC, Shuman MA, Aster RH: Quinine and quinidine-induced thrombocytopenia: a great imitator. *Arch Intern Med* 164:218–220, 2004
28. Hirsh J, Heddle N, Kelton JG: Treatment of heparin-induced thrombocytopenia: a critical review. *Arch Intern Med* 164:361–369, 2004
29. PDR Nurses Drug Handbook. Clifton Park, Delmar Learning, a division of Thomson Learning, 2003
30. Verburg KM, Maziasz TJ, Weiner, et al: COX-2-specific inhibitors: definition of a new therapeutic concept. *Am J Ther* 8:49–64, 2001
31. Cotran RS, Kumar V, Collins T: Red cells and bleeding disorders, in Cotran RS, Kumar V, Collins T (eds.): *Pathological Basis of Disease* (ed 6). Philadelphia, W.B. Saunders, 1999, pp 601–643
32. Kupas DF: Hyperviscosity syndrome. Updated June 29, 2001. *www.emedicine.com/emerg/topic756.htm.* Accessed April 11, 2004
33. Kwaan HC, Bongu A: The hyperviscosity syndromes. *Semin Thromb Haemost* 25:199–208, 1999
34. Furie B: Presentation of bleeding disorders, in Furie B, Cassileth PA, Atkins MB, Mayer RJ (eds.): *Clinical Hematology and Oncology.* Philadelphia, Churchill Livingstone, 2003, pp 265–271
35. Bick RL: Disseminated intravascular coagulation: pathophysiological mechanisms and manifestations. *Semin Thromb Haemost* 24:3–18, 1998
36. Friend PH, Pruett J: Bleeding and thrombotic complications, in Yarbro CH, Frogge MH, Goodman M (eds.): *Cancer Symptom Management* (ed 3). Sudbury, MA, Jones and Bartlett, 2004, pp 233–251
37. Pisciotto PT, Benson K, Hume H, et al: Prophylactic versus therapeutic platelet transfusion practices in hematology and/or oncology patients. *Transfusion* 35:498–502, 1995
38. Norfolk DR, Ancliff PJ, Contreras M, et al: Consensus conference on platelet transfusion. Royal College of Physicians of Edinburgh, 27–28 November, 1997. *Br J Haematol* 101:609–617, 1998
39. Demetri GD: Pharmacologic treatment options in patients with thrombocytopenia. *Semin Hematol* 37(suppl 4):11–18, 2000
40. Reid TJ, Rentas FJ, Ketchum LH: Platelet substitutes in the management of thrombocytopenia. *Curr Hematol Rep* 2:165–170, 2003
41. Vadhan-Raj S: Clinical experience with recombinant human thrombopoietin in chemotherapy-induced thrombocytopenia. *Semin Hematol* 37(suppl 4):28–34, 2000
42. Weich NS, Neben TY, Donaldson D, et al: Effects of interleukin-11 on megakaryocytes. *Blood* 88 (suppl 1):60a, 1996 (abstr)
43. Chu DT, Xu BH, Song ST, et al: Recombinant human interleukin 11 (Mega) promotes thrombopoiesis in cancer patients with chemotherapy-induced myelosuppression. *Zhongguo Shi Yan Xue Ye Xue Za Zhi* 9:314–317, 2001
44. Isaacs C, Robert NJ, Bailey FA, et al: Randomized placebo-controlled study of recombinant human interleukin-11 to prevent chemotherapy-induced thrombocytopenia in patients with breast cancer receiving dose-intensive cyclophosphamide and doxorubicin. *J Clin Oncol* 15:3368–3377, 1997
45. Erslev AJ: Erythropoietin. *N Engl J Med* 324:1339–1344, 1991
46. Erickson N, Quesenberry PJ: Regulation of erythropoiesis. *Med Clin North Am* 76:745–755, 1992
47. Cases A: Darbepoietin alfa: a novel erythropoiesis-stimulating protein. *Drugs Today* 39:477–496, 2003
48. Schuchter LM, Hensley ML, Meropol NJ, et al: 2002 update of recommendations for the use of chemotherapy and radiotherapy protectants: clinical practice guidelines of the American Society of Clinical Oncology. *J Clin Oncol* 20:2895–2903, 2002
49. Jayakumar S, Jayakumar S: Iron–dextran anaphylactic-like reaction with a negative test dose and subsequent successful administration of 3 doses. *Dialysis Transpl* 29:198, 200, 2000
50. Camp-Sorrell D: Chemotherapy: toxicity management, in Yarbro CH, Frogge MH, Goodman M (eds.): *Cancer Nursing Principles and Practice* (ed 5). Sudbury, MA, Jones and Bartlett, 2000, pp 444–486
51. Longhurst HJ, O'Grady C, Evans G, et al: Anti-D immunoglobulin treatment for thrombocytopenia associated with primary antibody defiency. *J Clin Pathol* 55:64–66, 2002
52. Zimmer J, Andres E, Noel E, et al: Current management of adult idiopathic thrombocytopenia purpura in practice: a cohort study of 201 patients from a single center. *Clin Lab Haematol* 26:137–142, 2004
53. Maloisel F, Andres E, Zimmer J, et al: Danazol therapy in patients with idiopathic thrombocytopenia purpura: long-term results. *Am J Med* 116:590–594, 2004
54. Stasi R, Provan D: Management of idiopathic thrombocytopenia purpura in adults. *Mayo Clin Pro* 79:504–522, 2004
55. Carpenter CL: Platelet disorders: acquired and congenital, in Furie B, Cassileth PA, Atkins MB, Mayer RJ (eds.): *Clinical Hematology and Oncology Presentation, Diagnosis, and Treatment.* Philadelphia, Churchill Livingstone, 2003, pp 485–497
56. Kessler CM, Tfayli A: Coagulation disorders: acquired and congenital, in Furie B, Cassileth PA, Atkins MB, Mayer RJ (eds.): *Clinical Hematology and Oncology Presentation, Diagnosis, and Treatment.* Philadelphia, Churchill Livingstone, 2003, pp 498–510
57. Johnson SR, Ernst ME, Graber MA: Commonly overlooked sources of Vitamin K. *Ann Pharmacother* 37:302, 2003
58. Booth SL, Centurelli MA: Vitamin K: a practical guide to the dietary management of patients on warfarin. *Nutr Rev* 57 (part 1):288–296, 1999
59. Jakaway JL: Acquired von Willebrand's disease. *Hematol Oncol Clin North Am* 6:1409–1417, 1992
60. Eikenboom JCJ, VanderMeer FJM, Briet E: Acquired von Willebrand's disease due to excessive fibrinolysis. *Br J Hematol* 81:618–624, 1992
61. Perrotta PL, Synder EL: Transfusion therapy, in DeVita VT, Hellman S, Rosenberg SA (eds.): *Cancer Principles and Practice of Oncology* (ed 6). Philadelphia, Lippincott, Williams and Wilkins, 2001, pp 2753–2766

CHAPTER 30

Fatigue

Mei R. Fu, PhD, RN, CNS
Roxanne W. McDaniel, PhD, RN
Verna A. Rhodes, EdS, RN, FAAN

Scope of the Problem

Fatigue is a symptom we all experience at some point in our lives. For healthy individuals, it occurs as a result of physical exertion, stress, or lack of sleep. Fatigue in healthy people serves a protective function by signaling people to restore energy by taking a rest. Generally, a good night's sleep or a few hours of rest will rejuvenate a healthy individual to a normal level of functioning. Unfortunately, fatigue experienced by individuals with cancer is not limited to the period of active disease and treatment; indeed, it may linger for months or years after treatment is completed.[1–4] Individuals with cancer typically describe their fatigue as being intense, severe, chronic, debilitating, distressing, and less likely to be relieved by rest.[5–9] For individuals with cancer, fatigue is one of the most common and distressing symptoms and has multifactorial etiologies, including cancer disease, treatment modalities, psychological factors, or decreased functional capacity.[6,8,10–17]

Definitions

Several definitions have been proposed to define fatigue.[18–20] The North American Nursing Diagnosis Association (NANDA) defined fatigue as "an overwhelming sustained sense of exhaustion and decreased capacity for physical and mental work at usual level."[18,p.89] Ream and Richardson define fatigue as "a subjective, unpleasant symptom which incorporates total body feelings ranging from tiredness to exhaustion creating an unrelenting overall condition which interferes with individuals' ability to function to their normal capacity."[19,p.527] Piper defines fatigue as "a universal feeling of tiredness that is expected to occur normally at certain times of the day (because of circadian rhythmicity) or after certain types of activity or exertion."[20,p.279] However, no single succinct definition has been formulated that applies to every situation of fatigue. Sufficient research has led scholars and researchers to reach the consensus that fatigue is a subjective and multidimensional phenomenon characterized by tiredness, weakness, exhaustion, lethargy, lassitude, listless, malaise, or lack of energy.[6,21–24]

In the last decade, fatigue has been defined by its cause. For example, cancer-related fatigue (CRF) refers to the fatigue caused by cancer or its treatment. Researchers have recognized that CRF occurs with a rapid onset and produces a persistent, relapsing, severe, intense, unpleasant, distressing, and debilitating sensation in individuals with cancer.[6,7,13,17] For many cancer patients, CRF is a common and significant contributor to decreased quality of life that exerts a great impact on the individual's sense of well-being and usual functioning, including daily performance, activities of daily living, relationships with family and friends, and compliance with treatment.[6,8,25] In a study of 379 cancer patients with a prior history of chemotherapy, 91% of the patients who experienced fatigue reported that fatigue prevented a "normal"[(p. 353)] life, and 88% reported that fatigue caused an alteration in their daily routine and made it more difficult to participate in social activities and perform typical cognitive tasks.[26]

Cimprich identified attentional fatigue as occurring in cancer patients.[27–29] *Attentional fatigue* is a decrease in mental acuity and physical discomfort that an individual experiences when trying to focus attention or concentrate on an activity. For example, when concentrating on listening, a person may try to block out distractions such as unwanted noise or thoughts. Directing attention also helps in planning and organizing daily or weekly activities. Cimprich believes that prolonged demands on attention can lead to attentional fatigue and related impairments in key areas of functioning.[27–29] Systemic fatigue may influence attentional fatigue, and individuals with cancer are at particular risk for developing attentional fatigue due in part to the systemic nature of the disease, metabolic changes in their bodies, treatment effects, and the overwhelming amounts of information given to them regarding their disease.

Incidence

Fatigue is one of the most common and distressing symptoms associated with the diagnosis and treatment of cancer.[30,31] Individuals with cancer were the first to identify fatigue as a cancer-related symptom. It is estimated that 60%–100% of individuals with cancer report fatigue during the course of their disease and treatment.[6,8,11,17,26,29,32–35] In individuals who are receiving chemotherapy, the incidence of fatigue has ranged from 65%–100%.[31,35] In a population-based study, Curt and colleagues found that 76% of cancer patients reported experiencing fatigue at least a few days each month during their most recent chemotherapy, compared with 54% reporting nausea, 23% reporting depression, and 20% reporting pain.[26] Thirty percent of patients reported experiencing fatigue on a daily basis; women tended to be more likely than men to report experiencing daily fatigue. Fatigue has been associated with surgery;[29] the use of interleukin-2, tumor necrosis factor, and colony-stimulating factor;[6,36] radiation therapy;[37,38] and chemotherapy;[25,39] and concurrent illness.[40]

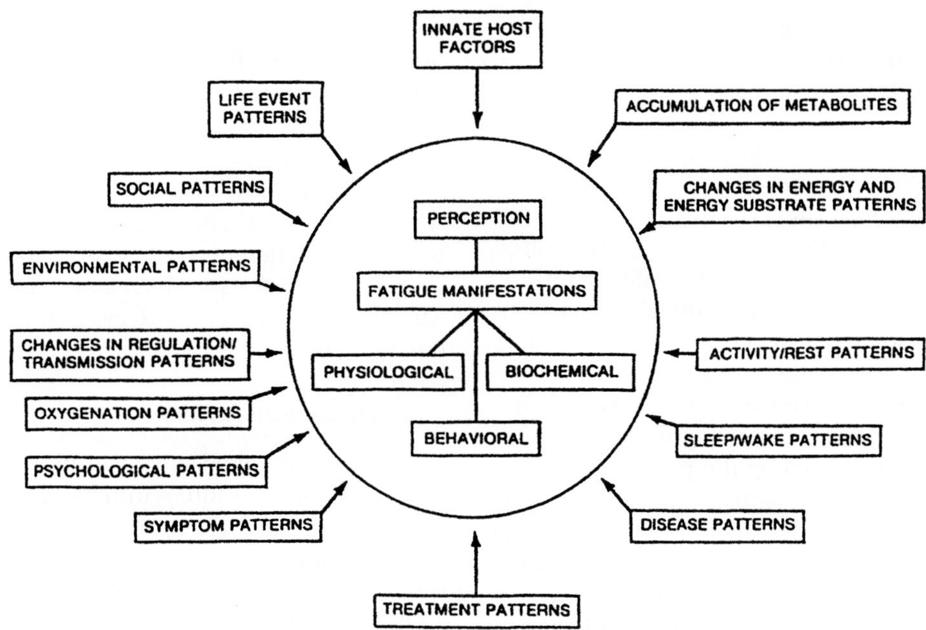

Figure 30-1 Piper's Integrated Fatigue Model. (Reprinted with permission from Winningham ML, Nail LM, Burke MB, et al: Fatigue and the cancer experience: the state of the knowledge. *Oncol Nurs Forum* 21:23–36, 1994.)[41]

Etiology and Risk Factors

Although the exact mechanism that causes fatigue in patients with cancer is not well understood, it is considered to involve a complex feedback system of regulated physiologic, psychological, and situational factors.[40] Various models and frameworks have been proposed to explain the mechanisms underlying fatigue. Two models that are frequently cited in relation to fatigue in cancer patients are Piper's Integrated Fatigue Model (IFM) (Figure 30-1)[41] and Winningham's Psychobiologic-Entropy Model.[42] Piper's IFM considers fatigue in relation to physical, psychological, and treatment factors, as well as symptom patterns. Winningham's model considers fatigue as an energy deficit that leads to decreased activity and secondary fatigue, causing decreased functional status.

Several physiologic factors have been associated with fatigue in individuals with cancer. They include anemia,[30,43,44] chronic pain,[45] infection, fever, surgery,[46] and inadequate nutrition related to gastrointestinal disturbances such as nausea, vomiting, and retching. Dehydration and electrolyte imbalances, acid–base imbalances, pain, hypoxia, neurologic toxicities, effects of drug therapies, cardiac abnormalities, dizziness, fever, constipation, and hormonal changes are other physiologic factors associated with cancer fatigue. Cancer fatigue is also related to radiation therapy, chemotherapy, biologic response modifiers, and multimodal therapy.

Anemia

Anemia is one of the most frequently encountered disease-related or treatment-related causes of fatigue. This common complication of cancer has been associated with nutritional deficiencies (iron or vitamin deficiency), hemorrhage, myelosuppression caused by cancer treatments, hemolysis or tumor involvement of the marrow, hemodilution, infection, and paraneoplastic syndromes. Severe myelosuppression can occur as the result of chemotherapy and radiation therapy to the bone marrow, particularly in the pelvis or spine. The use of higher doses of chemotherapy and more intense courses of chemotherapy and radiation has made stem cell depletion more common in recent years. Iron-deficiency anemia occurs most often in individuals with cancer when chronic blood loss is common, such as those with genitourinary and gastrointestinal cancers and cancers of the head and neck. In a retrospective review of 202 patients with cancer who underwent radiation therapy, Harrison and colleagues found that 57% of the patients had hemoglobin levels lower than 12 g/dL by the end of their radiotherapy.[47] Although chronic anemia associated with cancer is seldom life-threatening, it causes quality of life problems for individuals with cancer and is often exacerbated by intensive chemotherapy or combined modalities such as chemotherapy plus radiation therapy.[48] The relationship between anemia and fatigue was demonstrated in a study by Cella, who found that patients with hemoglobin levels greater than 12 g/dL reported significantly less fatigue and fewer nonfatigue anemia symptoms than patients with hemoglobin levels less than 12 g/dL.[30] Anemia has also been associated with decreased survival.[49]

Pain

Pain associated with cancer can interfere with the activities of daily living. Many studies report decreased functional capacity, diminished strength, and decreased endurance in cancer patients. Pain has been associated with psychological effects that contribute to fatigue, such as personal distress, depression, and increased anxiety, fear, and somatic preoccupation. One study found that pain and fatigue, mobility, and difficulties in sleeping were among the problems that patients with colorectal and gastric cancer were most concerned about following surgery.[50] In a retrospective study of 50 patients receiving radiation therapy for histologically diagnosed lung cancer, Hickok and colleagues found that 40 had pain.[51] Fatigue ultimately developed in 39 of the patients but closely followed development of pain in only 11 patients. Pain was independently associated with lack of energy in a study of 187 patients with metastatic and locally advanced cancer.[45] Fatigue and pain were found to be frequent and problematic side effects for women who were receiving treatment for breast cancer.[52]

Surgery

Fatigue is a frequent sequela of surgery. It is thought to be caused by injury to tissue and the surgical stress response, with subsequent increased demands on organ function, and by the effects of anesthesia and analgesics given before and after surgery. Changes in organ function may result from endocrine and metabolic changes due to the trauma of surgery.[53] Salmon and Hall have proposed that postoperative fatigue is the result of physiologic, psychological, and cultural factors that serve to maintain homeostasis while retaining the capacity to respond to new stressors.[54] This response is supported by cultural belief in the necessity of convalescence.[54] Fatigue following surgery has been found to last 6 months or longer. In a study of 60 patients with colorectal cancer, those who had conventional surgery experienced greater fatigue than those who underwent laparoscopic surgery.[50] A time-series study of women who had surgery for breast cancer found that fatigue and pain were the most frequently reported symptoms at 6 weeks, 3 months, and 6 months following surgery.[55] Advances in surgical techniques, such as laparoscopic surgery, may decrease the fatigue experienced by individuals with cancer. In a study of 60 patients with colorectal cancer, postoperative fatigue and analgesic requirements were lower after laparoscopic colorectal surgery than after conventional surgery.[46] Attentional fatigue has also been identified following surgery. In a study of women with breast cancer, Cimprich found that being older and having more extensive surgery increased the likelihood of attentional fatigue.[27]

Inadequate nutrition related to gastrointestinal disturbances such as nausea, vomiting, and retching has been well documented in the literature. Fatigue can also be the cause of decreased nutritional intake, which leads to a cycle of decreased nutrition and increased fatigue.

Psychological factors

Several psychological factors have been associated with fatigue in individuals with cancer, including anxiety, depression,[37,56–58] anticipatory nausea and vomiting, and pain. Anxiety and depression in individuals with cancer are frequently related to the stress associated with the diagnosis and treatment of cancer. Those patients with cancer at greatest risk for depression have inadequate pain control, preexisting mood disorders, or advanced disease, or are in poor physical condition.[59] Depression is often associated with fatigue, and this condition is quite common in the cancer population, with an estimated 15%–25% of cancer patients being affected.[60] A survey of 1957 breast cancer survivors revealed that those individuals who experienced fatigue had higher levels of clinical depressive symptoms.[61] Depression may be a co-morbid and disabling syndrome in cancer patients and survivors that elicits anxiety, sadness, and fatigue. Nearly 90% of patients with co-morbid depression had longer lengths of stay, higher hospital readmission rates, and higher medical costs than cancer patients experiencing no depression.[62] A higher incidence of anxiety and depression in individuals with cancer has been correlated with treatment-related fatigue. However, Hickok and colleagues found fatigue in 39 of 50 patients (78%) with lung cancer, but only 12% had depression.[51] It is difficult to differentiate whether the fatigue causes the depression or the depression causes the fatigue. Anecdotally, cancer patients are less sad when treated with antidepressants, but such therapy rarely appears to ease the problem of fatigue.

Situational factors associated with fatigue include sleep disturbances, decreased activity, immobility, and polypharmacy for concomitant health problems. Frequently, individuals who are experiencing fatigue are encouraged to get more rest, but this decreased activity leads to muscle wasting and lowers functional capacity and endurance. In their study, Foltz and colleagues found that more than 50% of patients who had received at least one cycle of chemotherapy as inpatients reported having fatigue and sleeping difficulties following their hospitalization.[63] Another study compared 61 women who had received chemotherapy for breast cancer to 59 women with no history of cancer. Those who had received chemotherapy had more severe fatigue that was correlated with poorer quality of sleep.[64]

Radiation therapy

Fatigue associated with radiation therapy may be caused by anemia, an accumulation of cell-destruction end products, or increased energy requirements to repair damaged epithelial tissue. Radiation therapy has known and predictable side effects depending on the site of radiation treatment. For example, individuals who receive radiation to the bronchus experience cough and difficulty swallowing, while those who receive radiation for gynecologic cancer experience diarrhea, urinary frequency, and urinary burning.[65] The incidence of fatigue in individuals receiving radiation therapy has been well documented.[37,38]

Fatigue is the most commonly reported systemic side effect of radiation therapy. It has been reported to affect 65%–80% of individuals receiving radiation therapy[51,66] and has been related to length of treatment, pain, depression, and weight loss. Radiation therapy has a cumulative effect, and many individuals report worsening symptoms later in their treatment. A study of cancer patients receiving radiation therapy found that just after radiation therapy, fatigue either increased or remained stable, whereas depression decreased.[58] At 9 months, fatigue had decreased, whereas levels of depression remained stable. Vogelzang and colleagues conducted a survey of 419 cancer patients who had received chemotherapy, radiation therapy, or both, and found that 78% experienced fatigue during the course of their disease and treatment.[31] Thirty-two percent of these patients experienced daily fatigue; in addition, 32% reported that fatigue significantly affected their daily routine. Most of these patients considered fatigue to be a symptom that had to be endured; half of these patients did not discuss treatment options for fatigue with their oncologists.

The cumulative effect of radiation therapy was demonstrated in a study of 76 patients with breast cancer who received external radiation therapy and were followed from the start of treatment to 6 months posttreatment.[37] Fatigue significantly increased over the course of treatment, peaking at the last week of treatment. Three months after treatment, fatigue returned to pretreatment levels. In this study, fatigue was not found to be influenced by age, stage of disease, time since surgery, weight, or length of time since diagnosis. It was significantly related to symptom distress, psychologic distress, and self-reported fatigue-relief strategies. Chronic fatigue was found in prostate cancer patients with radiation therapy.[4] In a study of patients who had completed radiation treatment for prostate or breast cancer, Walker and colleagues found that fatigue was the most frequently reported continuing side effect.[67]

Chemotherapy

Fatigue is frequently reported by individuals during the course of their chemotherapy. Chemotherapy-related fatigue may be associated with anemia or with an accumulation of cell-destruction end products. The side effects associated with chemotherapy vary according to the type and dose of chemotherapy, but fatigue is the side effect most frequently reported.[1,36,41,52] Chemotherapy agents that are more likely to cause anemia include thiotepa, mechlorethamine hydrochloride, dactinomycin, cytarabine, cyclophosphamide, cladribine, cisplatin, carboplatin, busulfan, and aldesleukin.[68] Persistent fatigue has often been reported as a long-term side effect of adjuvant chemotherapy.

The impact of fatigue associated with chemotherapy has been demonstrated in numerous studies. Patterns of fatigue, activity, and rest were examined in a study of 72 women receiving adjuvant chemotherapy for breast cancer.[69] The Piper Fatigue Scale was used to measure fatigue at 48 hours after treatment and at treatment cycle midpoints. Wrist actigraphs, which provide continuous monitoring of activity and motion, were used to measure activity and rest cycles for 96 hours during each treatment and for 72 hours at each treatment-cycle midpoint. Fatigue scores varied significantly over time and were higher at treatment and lower at cycle midpoints. Activity levels also varied significantly over time and reflected the fatigue pattern. In a study of 307 women receiving treatment for breast cancer, fatigue was the most common and problematic side effect.[52]

A qualitative study of 127 adult patients was conducted to explore the experience of fatigue from the perspective of patients undergoing chemotherapy. Eight major categories of fatigue were identified, along with the dimensions and properties of fatigue. The descriptions provided by these patients demonstrate the subjective nature of the phenomenon as well as the impact of fatigue on their lives.[12] Another qualitative study of cancer patients receiving chemotherapy examined patients' perceptions of fatigue and tiredness and the nature, pattern, and causes of fatigue in relation to cancer and its treatment. Data were collected during two interviews at the beginning and the end of a cycle of chemotherapy and with a diary. Fatigue at some point during the chemotherapy cycle was reported by almost 90% of the patients. It was most frequently associated with type of cancer, chemotherapy regimen, and changes in sleep patterns.[70]

Several studies have reported fatigue as a long-term side effect of chemotherapy. In a study of 21 women with breast cancer, fatigue was among the most frequently described problems immediately after completing chemotherapy and 6 months later. Most patients had not expected to experience chemotherapy-related problems 6 months after treatment. Fatigue interfered with the daily lives of these women.[1] The long-term effects of chemotherapy were examined in a study of 86 women who had completed adjuvant cytotoxic and/or hormonal therapy for early-stage breast cancer between 2 and 5 years prior to the study.[71] The Functional Living Index — Cancer, the Symptom Distress Scale, and the Medical Outcomes Study Short Form 36 were used to collect data. Overall, the women reported a high level of quality of life. Fatigue was the most frequently reported symptom (31.4%), followed by insomnia (23.3%), and local numbness at the surgical site (22.1%).

The characteristics of fatigue were examined in a comparison study of 61 women who had completed chemotherapy for breast cancer an average of more than 15 months prior to the study and 59 women with no history of cancer.[64] The women who had received chemotherapy reported more severe fatigue and worse quality of life because of fatigue. Their fatigue was significantly related to other symptoms, including poorer sleep quality and more menopausal symptoms. A study of 109 women who had completed treatment for stage I to stage III breast cancer within the previous 1 to 6 years produced similar findings. Low to moderate fatigue was found to persist in these women. When other variables were taken into account, fatigue was found to be significantly related to treatment with chemotherapy.[72]

These studies demonstrate the prevalence and severity of fatigue in individuals receiving chemotherapy for cancer. Fatigue is not just the most prevalent side effect — it interferes with activities of daily living and has a negative impact on quality of life. The persistent fatigue that has been demonstrated following chemotherapy needs to be investigated further.

Biologic response modifiers

Biologic response modifiers have the potential to improve both quality and quantity of life for many individuals. Unfortunately, their effectiveness is often limited by their side effects. One of the most common side effects associated with biologic response modifiers is fatigue.[73–76] The fatigue caused by biologic response modifiers may be due to neuromuscular fatigue,[74] changes in sleep patterns,[77] or immune-mediated endocrine disease that occurs during alfa-interferon therapy.[75]

The prevalence of fatigue in individuals receiving this therapy has been demonstrated in several studies. In a study of 92 patients with multiple myeloma who were receiving alfa-interferon, neutropenia and fatigue were the most common adverse effects.[78] A study by Johnston and colleagues evaluated the efficacy and toxicity of combination biochemotherapy compared to chemotherapy alone in 65 patients with metastatic melanoma.[79] Patients treated with combination chemotherapy had significantly higher fatigue rates than those treated with chemotherapy alone (26% versus 13%), and response rates were not improved with combination therapy. The dose-limiting effects of interferon were shown in a study of 13 patients with metastatic melanoma; in this study, 7 patients required a 50% dose reduction because of fatigue and other side effects.[80]

The fatigue and other side effects associated with biologic response modifiers have led to decreased dosages of these therapies and termination of treatment in some cases. Because fatigue is one of the dose-limiting side effects associated with biologic response modifiers, the positive results found by Karp with low-dose interleukin-2 are particularly encouraging.[81] This study also highlights the need for more research into low-dose biotherapy.

Physiologic Alterations

Pathophysiology

The mechanisms underlying the onset and persistence of fatigue are not well understood.[82] Several hypotheses have been proposed to explain the possible physiologic causes of fatigue in cancer patients. The causes of fatigue may be related to the primary tumor and metastasis to one or more systems. For example, cardiac or pulmonary function may be compromised as a result of a tumor, or severe anemia may lead to decreased oxygenation. In addition, the malignant process is thought to cause changes in protein turnover and abnormalities in glucose and lipid metabolism that causes physiologic changes in tumor-free muscle tissue in individuals with cancer, which can result in fatigue.[83] Another possible mechanism for cancer-related fatigue is the activation of the immune system through the central and peripheral release of pro-inflammatory cytokines in response to the tumor itself or to treatments.[74] The release of pro-inflammatory cytokines, such as interleukin-1 beta (IL-1 beta), interleukin-6 (IL-6), and tumor necrosis factor-alpha (TNF-alpha), is the result of the body's response to tumor, tissue damage, depletion of immune cells, or cytokine therapy.[74,84] Interleukin-1 (IL-1) and other cytokines are associated with muscle loss, decreased activity, slower recovery time following activity, increased somnolence, anorexia, and social withdrawal.[74] Increased levels of cytokines have been found in individuals with chronic fatigue syndrome,[85] and evidence indicates that some cytokines are involved in sleep regulation.[86] Elevated serum markers associated with pro-inflammatory cytokine activities (IL-1 receptor antagonist and soluble tumor necrosis factor receptor type II) were also found in breast cancer survivors who reported fatigue.[84]

The neurophysiological model proposes that impairment of the central component causes lack of motivation, impaired spinal cord transmission, exhaustion, or malfunction in the hypothalamic region.[87] *Central fatigue* originates in the central nervous system and refers to impairments or efforts in the central processing of stimuli that originate in working muscles. Causes of central fatigue may include impaired spinal cord transmission, inhibition of voluntary effort, or nerve cell malfunction. Another cause of central fatigue may be increased levels of 5-hydroxytryptamine (5-HT). According to Davis, a growing body of evidence suggests that increased brain serotonin (5-HT) can lead to central fatigue, thereby causing a deterioration in performance.[88] The processes of the central component and problems with sleep and loss of motivation are further compounded by the concomitant use of analgesics, hypnotics, antidepressants, antiemetics, or anticonvulsants, all of which depress the central nervous system. Disruption of sleep patterns and the feeling that sleep is not refreshing or restorative indicate that the normal function of the central nervous system is affected, supporting the neurophysiologic model of fatigue.[87] *Peripheral fatigue* refers to muscle exhaustion during exertion; it occurs because of impairments in the peripheral nerves and contracting muscles.[89] Concomitant health problems such as chronic obstructive pulmonary disease may contribute to or exacerbate cancer fatigue. Clearly, cancer fatigue is a complex problem that is influenced by myriad factors, including the malignancy, tumor metastasis, psychological factors, and treatment effects.

Clinical Manifestations

The manifestations of fatigue can be either subjective or objective. Subjective signs are those that only the individual can evaluate; objective signs can be assessed by another person. Subjective manifestations are the individual's perception of the occurrence and distress caused by the fatigue.[41] This perspective may include the emotional or psychological and physical feelings of fatigue, the perception of interference with daily living activities, and the amount of distress caused by the fatigue. Objective manifestations may include weight loss, decreased energy, apathy, anemia, weakness, lack of motivation, decreased attention, excessive sleepiness, or changes in sleep patterns.

Assessment of Fatigue

Fatigue is a subjective and multidimensional phenomenon. Its assessment should, therefore, reflect its multidimensionality and subjectivity. Fatigue should be assessed in relation to the individual's expectations, daily patterns of living, physical functioning, state of health, environmental conditions, and prescribed diagnostic, therapeutic, and rehabilitative measures. The occurrence and distress of tiredness, weakness, lack of energy, and decreased concentration must be assessed as different entities.

Researchers from a variety of disciplines have attempted to measure fatigue by assessing observable biological manifestations, such as changes in adenosine triphosphate (ATP) levels, serum lactate, pH levels, and physical ability/strength.[24,84,90] Other researchers consider such objective measurements to be inappropriate because of the subjective nature of fatigue and its multidimensionality. Using objective measurements may not accurately capture an individual's perception of fatigue because the objective and subjective indicators of fatigue might not be highly correlated.[84] Thus, self-report instruments that measure an individual's subjective perception of fatigue are essential in assessing fatigue. In a study of 2252 patients with cancer of the prostate, significant differences in patient and physician assessments of several domains, including fatigue, were noted.[91] Physicians underestimated all patient symptoms. The differences in patient and nurse assessments of symptoms were also demonstrated in a study of hospice patients' perceptions of their symptom experiences and the perceptions of the hospice nurses assessing them.[92] Patients and nurses both completed the Adapted Symptom Distress Scale (ASDS-2) Form 2 upon patient admission, at 2 weeks after admission, and at 4 weeks after admission. In this study, hospice nurses overestimated their patients' symptom experiences, including fatigue. Another study investigated the agreement between family caregivers' reports and cancer patients' reports of symptoms. Although the rate of agreement between patient and caregiver was highest for fatigue, the overall accuracy of caregiver reports was approximately 71%.[93] These studies highlight the importance of having patients assess their own fatigue.

Several instruments have been developed to assess an individual's level of fatigue in clinical practice and research studies. They include single-item self-report scales, comprehensive instruments that include measures of fatigue or fatigue subscales, and multiple-item fatigue instruments. The most commonly used single-item scales are visual analog scales and Likert-type scales that ask individuals to rate the presence or severity of fatigue. The Rhoten Fatigue Scale, an example of a visual analog type of scale, rates fatigue from 0 ("not tired, peppy") to 10 ("total exhaustion").[94] It can be completed in a minimal amount of time and can be used by either the patient or the healthcare provider. Comprehensive instruments include the Brief Fatigue Inventory,[95] the Functional Assessment of Cancer Therapy—Fatigue,[30] the Revised Piper Fatigue Self-Report Scale,[96] the Schwartz Cancer Fatigue Scale,[97] and the Fatigue Symptom Inventory.[98] The Revised Piper Fatigue Scale (PFS) is a concise and user-friendly instrument utilizing a 22–item Likert-type scale, with four subscales and four short-answer questions.[96] The Revised PFS measures the subjective multidimensionality of fatigue and has been employed in several studies on fatigue in cancer patients and healthy women.[6,21,69]

The choice of which instrument to use for assessing fatigue depends on the individual population and the purpose of the assessment. Single-item scales are easy to administer and time-efficient in clinical practice. Multiple-item fatigue instruments generally have demonstrated greater reliability and validity, but may be too time-consuming and taxing to use in daily clinical practice. The comprehensive instruments generally have similar advantages and disadvantages to the multiple-item fatigue instruments but are able to assess multiple symptoms. The subscales of the comprehensive instruments have demonstrated reliability and validity and can be used separately to assess individual symptoms, thereby decreasing the number of items to assess a symptom such as fatigue.

Cognitive, mental, affective, and temporal effects have also been identified as components of fatigue. Cimprich examined loss of concentration and decrease in memory or alertness. Assessment tools used in the past to evaluate attention and concentration focused on global impairments such as psychiatric disturbances, but were not always able to detect subtle impairments.[27–29] Clinical assessment for loss of concentration should begin with the initial contact and continue over time. Areas to be assessed include level of alertness, attention span, ability to focus and concentrate on an intended activity, and subjective perception of loss of concentration in daily life.

The temporal component of fatigue is linked to an individual's 24–hour circadian pattern. This component considers what time of day individuals might have more energy and looks for patterns of fatigue. Assessment of the temporal component examination is important in differentiating between acute and chronic fatigue and in determining appropriate interventions. The affective dimension of fatigue includes distress, irritability, impatience, and lack of motivation. These factors represent the emotional meanings that fatigue may have, and they raise the question of depression and how it relates to fatigue.

Patient and Family History

Assessment of fatigue should include a careful history describing the pattern of fatigue and identifying the factors that contribute to its development. The initial assessment should include the pattern, onset, duration, and intensity of fatigue. Factors that increase or alleviate fatigue should be explored as well. The history should include concurrent health problems, current medications, treatment history, and associated side effects. Patterns of sleep and rest and the effects of fatigue on activities of daily living and lifestyle are important history issues to assess. Likewise, fatigue assessment should include nutritional intake, change in appetite and weight, and psychological factors. A complete history obtained from the patient and family is essential to determine the best approaches for the individualized management of fatigue.

Physical Examination

A comprehensive assessment is necessary to provide information about both the physical and the psychological factors producing fatigue in the individual with cancer. A complete physical examination helps differentiate between physical weakness and fatigue; it should include complete physical examination encompassing the assessment of gait, posture, and range of motion; diagnostic and laboratory tests for anemia and weight change; and other physiologic causes of fatigue.

Daily or ongoing assessment and evaluation of fatigue is also an important part of a comprehensive assessment. Initial and ongoing assessments reveal information essential for effective education. Goals for education based on the assessment and deficits should be established with the individual and family. Ongoing assessments must be sensitive to comments from the individual or family that may indicate fatigue or decreased energy; remarks revealing any other limiting factors must also be considered. The Rhoten Fatigue Scale is a good starting point for assessing and documenting the severity of fatigue and providing an opportunity to open up discussion with the patient and family.[94]

Personal and Sociocultural	Rationale
Age: 36 Gender: Female Family: Married (2nd marriage); 2 daughters, 15 and 8 years, and an 8–month-old son (older daughter from first marriage); mother and father deceased, 1 sister, 2 brothers; husband is self-employed carpenter	Assessment of factors affecting patient's perspective of health situations
Educational Level: College graduate Occupation: Teacher (elementary) Religion: Church of God (attends regularly) Sociocultural Orientation: White, middle class, raised in a rural Midwest community Relevant Life Experiences: Both parents died with cancer at an early age (before patient turned 28) Social Roles: Wife, mother, sister, breadwinner	Experiences influencing the seeking and securing of appropriate medical assistance and management of health state
Patterns of Living Living Environmental and Family System: Lives with husband and children 100 miles from treatment center Health Habits (Self-Care Practices): Considers herself to have good personal hygiene: teeth in good repair; sees dentist regularly; overweight; doesn't exercise; inconsistent with BSE: has not enrolled in cancer-screening program; sees doctor for yearly Pap smear; obtains a suntan every summer — occasionally sunburns; Tylenol for headaches; daily multiple vitamins; birth control pills for 13 years, and again after birth of 8–month-old son	Factors to be considered when assisting this patient: Modifying self-concept, self-image, and learning to live with the effects of pathologic conditions (e.g., fatigue and medical care measures).
• Activity Patterns Usual/Routine: Household, church/community/school (children and employment) Preferred/Selected: Maintain employment; selected church and family activities • Sleep/Rest Patterns Usual: 6–7 hours/weeknight Preferred: 8 hours/night	Considerations for maintaining a balance of activity and rest: Regularly evaluate the severity of fatigue, and the individual's perception of what limitations are acceptable.
Nutritional Patterns Number of Meals/Snacks per Day: 3 meals (light breakfast, large evening meal) and 2 snacks, A.M. and P.M. Food Likes and Dislikes: Prefers starches, desserts; limited meat, dairy products (except ice cream), fresh fruits or vegetables	Data helpful to develop a nutritional dietary plan for potential energy requirements of health
Preferred Learning Style: Is an avid reader; feels comfortable in groups but prefers reading and one-to-one demonstrations	A guide regarding the type of patient education
Health State and Healthcare Systems Present Health State: Recently diagnosed with breast cancer; sought medical help after she discovered a breast lump while taking a shower; had (L) mastectomy with reconstruction; preparing to take adjuvant chemotherapy. Regular menstrual cycle since age 12 years. Questions the amount of time treatment will take from her many activities.	Provide information on coping strategies
Previous Health Concerns and Self-Care Actions: 3 normal pregnancies — only hospitalizations were for childbirth Perception of Health Care: Views system as helpful — patient wants to be an informed customer and involved in decision making	An index of patient's life experiences and possible effects on perceptions of present health state
Developmental State: Early adult transitions Self-Management System for Care — Physical, Emotional, Spiritual: Acknowledges some fear of cancer due to experience with parents. Lack of preventive healthcare due to fear of cancer experience with parents; looks to close friends for emotional support; feels she has strong spiritual faith; considers minister a close friend.	

Figure 30-2 Patient assessment form

A comprehensive assessment of the patient's healthcare situation must include the perspectives of both physician and patient. For an example of an initial assessment form that includes data based on the patient's perspective, see Figure 30-2. These data — the pathophysiology of the present and past medical diagnoses, clinical manifestations, usual treatment, and nursing management — are essential for the development of an appropriate patient-centered plan of care.

The importance of comprehensive assessment of fatigue was demonstrated in a qualitative study by Glaus and colleagues that explored themes of fatigue in individuals with cancer and compared fatigue/tiredness in 20 patients with cancer and 20 healthy individuals.[7] In unstructured interviews undertaken to discover the experiences and descriptions of fatigue, three categories emerged in both groups. Fifty-nine percent of patients with cancer and 55% of healthy individuals provided themes that were classi-

Table 30-1 ICD-10 Criteria for Cancer-Related Fatigue

The following symptoms have been present every day or nearly every day during the same two-week period.

Significant fatigue, diminished energy, or increased need to rest, disproportionate to any recent change in activity level, plus five or more of the following:

1. Complaints of generalized weakness, limb heaviness
2. Diminished concentration or attention
3. Decreased motivation or interest to engage in unusual activities
4. Insomnia or hypersomnia
5. Experience of sleep as unrefreshing or nonrestorative
6. Perceived need to struggle to overcome inactivity
7. Marked emotional reactivity (e.g., sadness, frustration, or irritability) to feeling fatigued
8. Difficulty completing daily tasks attributed to feeling fatigued
9. Perceived problems with short-term memory
10. Post-exertional fatigue lasting several hours

The symptoms cause clinically significant distress or impairment in social, occupational, or other important areas of functioning.

There is evidence from the history, physical examination, or laboratory findings that the symptoms are a consequence of cancer or cancer therapy.

The symptoms are not primarily a consequence of co-morbid psychiatric disorders such as major depression, somatization disorder, somatoform disorder, or delirium.

fied as physical, including decreased physical performance, weakness, and unusual need for rest or sleep. Themes classified as affective, including decreased motivation, no energy, anxiety, and sadness, were identified by 29% of patients with cancer and 21% of healthy individuals. More healthy individuals (24%) identified themes in the cognitive category than did patients with cancer (12%). Both groups identified physical themes as being most frequent, but patients with cancer described the fatigue as unusual tiredness while healthy individuals described it as normal tiredness.

Diagnostic Studies

There is no definitive physiological diagnostic test for the diagnosis of fatigue. Generally, a diagnosis of fatigue depends on a patient's subjective validation of fatigue by using various self-report instruments or diagnostic tests of hemoglobin and iron level to verify fatigue caused by anemia. The tenth revision of the *International Classification of Disease—Clinical Modification* (ICD-CM) defines cancer-related fatigue as a diagnostic syndrome with diagnostic criteria (see Table 30-1).[87] Ideally, this definition will lead to increased awareness of the fatigue diagnosis and more attention paid to possible management strategies. It may also be helpful in establishing a realistic and ongoing clinical documentation regarding fatigue and promote a more proactive attitude to the management of fatigue. At the same time, defining CRF as a cluster of symptoms may prevent some patients from receiving prescribed fatigue management if they suffer from fatigue but do not have all the symptoms listed in the ICD-10 diagnostic criteria.

Therapeutic Approaches and Nursing Care

A variety of therapeutic approaches are required to assist the patient who is experiencing fatigue. Assisting the patient with cancer-related fatigue to maintain his or her quality of life is the desired outcome of nursing care. Nursing interventions must satisfy both the psychological and the physical needs of the patient and consider the causes of fatigue. Interventions related to fatigue that are discussed in this section include prevention and management of fatigue.

Prevention

Prevention is the optimal intervention for cancer-related fatigue. It should aim at minimizing or eliminating the potential underlying causes of fatigue and providing preparatory sensory information. Fatigue related to anemia caused by cancer or treatment, for example, can be prevented by treating the underlying causes. Nutritional deficiencies, such as iron, folic acid, or vitamin B_{12}, should be assessed and identified in patients with cancer prior to the beginning of cancer treatment. If a nutritional deficiency is identified, the appropriate supplemental therapy should be prescribed.[99] In many patients with mild anemia, supplemental therapy can help to establish an acceptable hemoglobin level and relieve anemia symptoms, such as fatigue.[99,100] Recently, researchers have begun investigating serum erythropoietin (EPO) levels and soluble transferring receptor (sTfR) levels in patients with cancer prior to the initiation of cancer treatment. In one study, 35 lung cancer patients receiving no antineoplastic therapy were found with lower serum EPO and sTfR, suggesting that anemia may have existed in these patients due to the impairment of erythropoietin production.[101] Some researchers have hypothesized that anemia in cancer patients might increase energy expenditure, resulting in fatigue, wasting, and cachexia. They suggest that prophylactic administration of exogenous recombinant human erythropoietin (rHuEPO) might prevent the development of anemia, decrease patients' feelings of fatigue, and enable them to maintain higher levels of physical function.[102] Mercadante and colleagues[103] suggest that administration of prophylactic rHuEPO early in cancer therapy may serve as a means of preventing adverse effects from anemia, thereby improving quality of life in patients with cancer.[103] More studies are needed to investigate the role of erythropoiesis-stimulating therapy in preventing fatigue caused by cancer-related anemia.

Preparatory sensory information incorporates sensory, procedural, and temporal information that reflects the experience of an event from the patient's point of view. Information that clearly describes what patients can expect before, during, and after treatment is crucial for effective patient education.[22,104] This information should be conveyed in a positive, nonthreatening manner and given before the treatment, thereby allowing the patient to formulate a more effective mental image about the pending experience. An accurate mental image also decreases ambiguity about the event, activates innate coping strategies, and permits effective cognitive management of the fatigue experience. The goals and behaviors of patients with cancer are largely determined by their perceptions of the illness. For this reason, it is important to understand an individual's perception and its potential influence on actual experience and self-care and coping behaviors. For example, symptoms such as fatigue and weakness require that individuals modify their behavior to maintain normal self-care functions and continue with valued activities. In addition, the individual's expectations about an experience and the actual experience have been shown to be related.[23] Studies have demonstrated that preparation for stressful happenings can reduce symptom experience (occurrence and distress) and facilitate adaptation.[22,105–107] Rhodes and colleagues found a statistically significant relationship (p = .015) between patients' expectations of symptom experience and the symptom distress they actually experienced.[23] Often, fatigue is referred to as a side effect, a description that may convey a sense of secondary importance to the disease process and treatment.[12] In reality, fatigue is often a chief concern of individuals receiving chemotherapy.[12,25] The preparation individuals receive may yield unrealistic expectations about their experience, as the dimensions of cancer-related fatigue are unlike anything they have previously experienced.[12]

Information about fatigue, including neutral descriptions of specific sensations to be experienced and realistic expectations, helps the patient cope and develop self-care behaviors more easily. For example, if an individual is starting a treatment regimen in which participants have generally experienced little or no fatigue, then it is appropriate to give this factual information to prepare the patient. The amount of factual information provided will depend on what individuals want to know and what they need to know to safely live with their treatment and its side effects. For example, if a treatment regimen consists of combination antineoplastic agents, it is not important for the individual to know which drugs are most likely to cause neutropenia (and hence fatigue), but it is important for the patient to know when this potential side effect might occur and how to manage it. Kim and colleagues conducted a randomized clinical trial with 152 patients to examine the effects of an informational intervention on the severity of side effects resulting from radiation therapy for prostate cancer.[104] Specific, objective information about what to expect during their radiation treatments was given to patients in the informational intervention arm at the first and fifth treatments, whereas patients in the comparison group received general information at the same point in time. Patients in the informational intervention group reported significantly fewer problems with sleep and less fatigue than those in the comparison group. Individualized educational strategies are considered to be the most effective preventive interventions; however, definitive research is needed to confirm this belief.

Management

As noted earlier, cancer-related fatigue is a multidimensional phenomenon with multiple potential causative factors that may work alone or together to produce overwhelming fatigue affecting all aspects of cancer patients' lives. A single intervention (e.g., treatment of anemia) is unlikely to be the sole solution to managing fatigue given this problem's complex nature. A variety of management interventions have been identified and recommended, including self-care strategies, conservation of energy, exercise, rest and sleep, treatment of anemia, and motivational strategies.

Self-care activities

Individuals with cancer have attempted to alleviate their fatigue by adopting various self-care behaviors.[6,25] In a study evaluating the strategies that patients use to cope with fatigue during chemotherapy, patients identified 31 different self-care actions to relieve their fatigue.[41] These actions provided partial relief 53.7% of the time, nearly complete relief 25.5% of the time, and complete relief only 11.5% of the time. Most self-care activities (e.g., resting, napping, and modifying activity) were chosen because they seemed sensible; less than 7% of self-care was based on the advice of others. Self-care activities attempted for fatigue are only partially effective against this severe treatment side effect.[25,41]

Orem defines self-care as the activities that individuals initiate and perform on their own behalf to maintain life, health, and well-being.[108] Self-care includes not only self-responsibility, independence, interdependence, and attendance to mind, body, and spirit, but also prophylactic measures, self-determination regarding therapy, and the decision to seek and secure appropriate healthcare assistance. Individuals learning to live with the effects of their pathologic conditions and medical care measures frequently have to develop a new repertoire of skills and knowledge.

As the patient encounters health-related limitations in self-care, the goal of nursing is to teach strategies that will allow the individual to continue self-care. The nursing management of fatigue may best be addressed by instruction for self-care activities. This effort includes teaching about energy conservation, relaxation techniques, diversional activities, medication information, dietary modifications, and emotional support. A general teaching guide about fatigue for patients has been developed to assist nurses in designing and implementing individualized teaching (Table 30-2).

Conservation of energy

The conservation of energy in the patient experiencing CRF can be accomplished by rescheduling activities so as to allow for rest periods or to decrease the amount of time that energy is needed.[109] An individual may develop an activity plan that enlists others to perform activities that are deemed less important, allowing the patient to conserve energy for activities that are deemed more important.[40] Other activities may need to be abandoned or completed in a different manner. The environment may also need modification to decrease energy demands.

Employers, family, and friends must be made aware of the likelihood of this unseen symptom and be willing to develop flexible strategies to help the patient manage fatigue, such as decreasing nonessential activities, enlisting the aid of others, and allowing a flexible work schedule. Table 30-3 provides a patient guide with strategies to manage fatigue.

Exercise

Exercise as an intervention to manage fatigue has been investigated by researchers. To date, most exercise intervention studies have been conducted with breast cancer patients undergoing cancer treatment.[15,110] All of these intervention studies used aerobic exercise of varied types: a walking program,[15,109] bicycling,[111] patients' own choices of type and time of exercise.[110] The studies demonstrated that exercise significantly reduces fatigue in patients undergoing cancer treatment. For example, a study of 46 women receiving radiation therapy for breast cancer found that a self-paced walking exercise decreased fatigue during treatment.[15] Suh and Lee cited similar findings when they investigated the effects of a walking exercise on fatigue in 34 women receiving adjuvant chemotherapy for breast cancer.[112] In their study, fatigue scores were considerably lower for women in the walking group.

Exercise interventions for reducing fatigue in cancer survivors usually include a variety of physical activities undertaken throughout the day. In one study, a range of physical activities was prescribed to patients with advanced-stage cancer.[8] For example, a patient might walk for five minutes, perform arm exercise with a resisted rubber band in a chair, march on the spot in the kitchen, or dance to his or her favorite music. As studies reveal, an inverse relationship exists between level of physical activity and level of fatigue in cancer survivors.

Graydon and colleagues conducted two interviews with women receiving either chemotherapy or radiation therapy for cancer to determine their level of fatigue and the effectiveness of the strategies used to relieve fatigue.[113] Patients were significantly more fatigued at the time of the second interview, the midpoint of any chemotherapy cycle, or the end of a 5- or 6-week course of radiation therapy. Those with more effective fatigue-relieving strategies were less fatigued, relatively speaking, at that time. Sleep and exercise were the most effective strategies used to relieve fatigue. Another study reported that exercise and rest were the most commonly used strategies to manage fatigue in 219 cancer survivors.[114] Of interest, patients with breast cancer reported greater benefits from exercise than did patients with non-Hodgkin's lymphoma. The findings from these studies indicate that exercise is an effective intervention for fatigue.

Table 30-2 Teaching Guide About Fatigue

Self-Care Behaviors/Interventions	Expected Patient Outcome
Nursing Diagnosis: lack of understanding of fatigue and possible causes and effects.	
• Assess and differentiate potential causes of patient's feelings of fatigue, tiredness, or weakness. • Fatigue (related to cancer): subjective experience; intensity, duration and distress vary; not completely relieved with rest or sleep; multidimensional and multicausal. • Tiredness: subjective experience; relieved with rest or sleep. • Weakness: subjective and objective; lack of physical strength of a given anatomical part or a generalized feeling of insufficient strength.	Patient and significant others understand the causes of fatigue and the difference between fatigue, tiredness, and weakness. The patient and participants also understand the purpose of antineoplastic therapies and are better prepared.
• Explain that fatigue is multicausal: Therapeutic interventions of physiologic/biochemical changes Psychosocial, economic stress factors Imbalance of rest and activity (decreased activity) Insufficient sleep Inadequate nutrition	Patient will verbalize descriptions of fatigue and its sensations.
• Explain the purpose of antineoplastic therapy (e.g., chemotherapy, radiation therapy, biological response therapy [to destroy cancer cells]). • Discuss possible patterns of fatigue occurrence; provide possible patterns (e.g., nadir 10–14 days postchemotherapy). • Provide preparatory information (procedural, temporal, and sensory for specific therapy and diagnosis, if known).	An understanding of fatigue patterns based on kind of therapy.
• Appraise the existence of fatigue; measure fatigue occurrence and fatigue distress separately on a scale from 1 to 10. • Suggest recording level of fatigue at multiple points in time. • Encourage patients to discuss fatigue with family and healthcare providers; cumulative effect of radiation therapy and energy changes may be gradual. • Assess usual activity level and threshold. • Check laboratory reports and appraise effects.	Uses a numerical visual analog scale to measure the occurrence and distress of fatigue.
Nursing Diagnosis: insufficient knowledge to institute appropriate self-care actions to manage fatigue.	
• Decrease nonessential activities; increase dependence on others for home management (meal preparation, cleaning, grocery shopping), transportation; avoid unscheduled extra demands; plan, prioritize, pace, and modify activities.	Patient and participants develop helpful strategies to manage fatigue by utilizing family and friends for essential activities.
• Suggest a journal, log, or diary of activities, feelings, and an evaluation of self-care actions.	Patient will use a journal of self-care actions.
• Teach diversional techniques, relaxation procedures, and distraction/diversion. • Provide information concerning counseling or support groups. • Maintain a list of names and phone numbers of individuals volunteering assistance. • Limit energy expenditure.	Diversional activity and relaxation techniques will be incorporated in daily life.

Friendenreich and Courneya conducted a comprehensive review of the literature on exercise and rehabilitation of patients with cancer.[115] The nine studies available all involved patients with breast cancer. Based on a qualitative review, Friendenreich and Courneya concluded that exercise improves physiologic and psychological well-being; however, their findings should be considered preliminary because of methodological problems in the original studies. Nevertheless, the findings from this meta-analysis support the need for more research to identify the optimal level of exercise for managing fatigue, and the need for studies to determine which individuals will benefit most from exercise to reduce fatigue.

Assessment and prescriptions for managing fatigue should be a vital aspect of care for cancer patients and survivors during treatment and follow-up care. Exercise and physical activity should be considered as one important fatigue management strategy. Prescription of exercise or physical activities should consider individual health status, exercise type, intensity, duration, frequency, and progression. In addition, exercise programs must be tailored to the individual based on age, gender, condition, and concurrent major health problems. For example, if a patient has other health prob-

Table 30-3 Strategies to Manage Fatigue: A Patient Guide

Energy Conservation

- Limit energy expenditure.
- Determine the amount of activity you can do comfortably; preserve normality (e.g., going to work, maintaining a routine).
- Plan/schedule and rearrange activities and work (e.g., schedule therapy at most convenient hour or prior to weekend or days off work).
- Plan a variety of new/enjoyable activities to avoid the performance of a routine. Reserve energy for fun activities.
- Develop some meaningful goals, both short-term and long-term.
- Decrease nonessential activities.
- Increase dependence on others for home management (e.g., cleaning, shopping, meal preparation), transportation, and care.
- Avoid energy-consuming activities.
- Consider energy-saving techniques of daily living (e.g., avoid toweling — use a terry cloth robe; sit rather than stand for chores and other pertinent activities; use assistive devices).
- Invite family members' energy-saving ideas and aids:
  Wear school clothes 2 days to reduce laundry.
  Eliminate homemade desserts and eat prepared desserts.

Rest, Sleep, and Exercise

- Space periodic rest periods with activity/exercise during the day. Rest before becoming too tired! Try to keep ahead of the game!
- Avoid the use of stimulants, including caffeine.
- Avoid alcohol.
- Use relaxation techniques (e.g., progressive muscle relaxation, guided imagery).
- Follow an individualized plan of exercise with intermittent rest periods during the day.
- Participate in nonstrenuous exercise (e.g., walking may help to relieve fatigue).
- Participate in yoga, stretching exercises.
- Establish a regular bedtime.
- Take a warm bath.
- Sip warm milk or herbal teas.
- Listen to soothing music.
- Have a back massage.
- Read a relaxing book.
- Establish a quiet environment.

Motivation

- Encourage verbalization of thoughts and feelings regarding what makes life meaningful.
- Emphasize the positive aspects of life (e.g., the quality of our days, not the number of days makes life worthwhile). Uncertainty exists except for the present moment.
- Encourage participation and control in the treatment plan.
- Provide reminders that although illness is not desired, *everyone* can choose the way they wish to respond.
- Utilize appropriate humor (e.g., cartoons, videos, enjoyable people).
- Encourage communication with friends and loved ones.
- Encourage environmental change (e.g., indoor/outdoor).
- Encourage storytelling (e.g., life's accomplishments/events).

lems such as cardiovascular disease or gross obesity (50% over ideal body weight), rhythmic walking activity should be modified. It is important to assess what the patient has previously been doing and what he or she currently is able to do comfortably. Patients who have been accustomed to an active exercise program may need to be cautioned about the intensity, frequency, and type of activity that may be appropriate. Clearly, additional studies on the effectiveness of specific exercise interventions for fatigue are needed.

INSTRUCTIONS

Please keep daily records in this journal, beginning on the day of your outpatient visit. Carry the journal and a pencil with you at all times so that you can record activities and results as they occur. The more detailed your journal is, the more valuable it will be in assessing your progress. In addition, your careful records will assist us in planning your care and in serving other patients. Your help is greatly appreciated.

The directions below will help you determine what information to put in each column of the journal. In addition, please refer to the sample entries on the next page.

Date, time	Record the date and time of each entry.
How I felt before self-care activity	Record entries as often as desired and on awakening; at noon, midafternoon, or early evening; and before going to bed at night.
Self-care activity	Record the names of the medications taken and describe any action you took to improve how you were feeling.
Result	Describe how you felt an hour after completing the self-care activity; you may use the following code: 1 = I felt better 2 = no change 3 = I felt worse

Self-Care Journal Sample

Sample journal entries are shown below. Remember that details are important; if in doubt, include it.

Date/Time	How I Felt Before Self-Care Activity	Self-Care Activity	Result
6/18/99 7 A.M.	Awakened by alarm, tired, no energy. Hungry	Showered. Dried with terry cloth robe. Ate wheat toast & jam, boiled egg, orange juice, & coffee	2
8:15	Need to rest after dressing	Sat in recliner on patio listening to birds	1
8:50	Lack of stamina	Husband drove to work	2
10:30	Weary from decision making	Walked in courtyard for 10 minutes	1
12:00	Looking forward to seeing friends	Enjoyed lunch with two friends	1
3:00	Less able to concentrate	Called neighbor for ride home from work	2
5:30	Frustrated with children's lack of understanding about tiredness	Explained tiredness using marbles to represent mother's energy; removed ½ marbles to show energy needed to fight disease	1
7:30	Tired, but more able to cope	Reading, while husband takes children to mall	1

Figure 30-3 Self-care journal for fatigue. (Copyright 2000 by Verna A. Rhodes and Roxanne W. McDaniel. All rights reserved. Used with consent of the authors.)

Rest and sleep

Rest and sleep are often the most recommended interventions for individuals with cancer who are experiencing fatigue. Rest may include napping, taking it easy, or removing oneself from areas of high activity and noise. Rest and napping were among the most frequently cited self-care strategies in the study by Richardson and colleagues[116] but were less effective in relieving fatigue than going to bed early. Fatigue, the second most common symptom in a study of individuals who had received chemotherapy, was most often managed by increasing time spent resting and sleeping. For some individuals, rest and sleep can relieve or reduce fatigue.

In caring for the individual with fatigue, it is important to schedule medications, treatments, and other activities around periods of rest and sleep. Corticosteroids are frequently used in antineoplastic drug regimens and in antiemetic drug protocols. While several adverse neurologic effects may arise with use of glucocorticoids, sleep disruption, insomnia, restlessness, and increased motor activity are the most offensive to the patient combating fatigue. An inability to concentrate or to maintain attention is extremely distressful and may lead to increased uncertainty, anxiety, and depression.[53] Other symptoms that may increase fatigue or interfere with rest and sleep must be assessed. A balance of activity and rest—neither too little nor too much—is essential to avoid increased perceptions of fatigue.

A journal or diary of self-care activities and outcomes can be an extremely useful aid for reassessment, planning, and instruction.[63,116] In fact, this tool often fosters patient introspection that may direct a change in the individual's self-care activities. The nurse may detect patterns of cause and effect that will help in guiding the patient's care. Figure 30-3 is an example of a self-care journal for fatigue.

Treatment of anemia

Anemia is one of the major causes of cancer-related fatigue. Cancer-related fatigue (CFR) caused by anemia may be due to myelosuppression resulting from treatment, hemolysis, blood loss, tumor involvement, nutritional abnormalities, or iron or vitamin deficiency.[6,43,100,117,118] Treatment of CRF caused by anemia improves the quality of life in cancer patients.[119,120] Interventions to prevent and manage anemia in cancer patients have traditionally focused on minimizing and eliminating the etiologies of anemia. Interventions for managing anemia include supplemental therapy for nutritional deficiency (iron, folic acid, or vitamin B_{12}), red blood cell (RBC) transfusion, and erythropoiesis-stimulating therapies.

For mild anemia in cancer patients, oral or intravenous supplemental therapy of iron, folic acid, or vitamin B_{12} is generally effective in relieving symptoms of anemia (such as fatigue) and increase or maintain hemoglobin level.[100] Functional iron deficiency can result in an inadequate response to rHuEPO. Iron supplements have been used in combination with erythropoiesis-stimulating therapies. For example, iron supplements have been combined with rHuEPO to achieve effective anemia management and to reduce the total amount of rHuEPO needed to attain adequate hemoglobin level.[121] In a pilot study on 20 patients with rectal cancer undergoing preoperative chemotherapy and radiation therapy, Levine and colleagues found that oral iron supplement with rHuEPO use decreased transfusion requirement and maintained higher hemoglobin levels in the patients.[122]

With the advent of erythropoiesis-stimulating therapies, RBC transfusions have been reserved for acute anemia characterized by severe symptoms and symptomatic chronic anemia that does not respond to iron supplemental therapy.[100] Although strict screening of blood donors has made the blood supply in the United States safe, several potential risks are still associated with RBC transfusions, such as transmission of infectious agents, transfusion reactions, or immunosuppression. Nevertheless, in cases of severe anemia with severe symptoms, RBC transfusion may be administered immediately if an inadequate time frame does not allow for the use of erythropoiesis-stimulating therapies.

Erythropoiesis-stimulating therapies represent a new approach to the management of anemia in cancer patients. More than a decade ago, advances in the recombinant DNA technology used to manufacture hematopoietic growth factors, such as rHuEPO (epoetin-alfa), opened up the possibility of using erythropoiesis-stimulating therapies. The use of rHuEPO has been effective in increasing hemoglobin concentration and hematocrit, and in significantly reducing transfusion requirements in cancer patients with anemia brought on by chemotherapy and surgery.[123–125] In a randomized, placebo-controlled study of 375 cancer patients undergoing chemotherapy, 251 patients who received rHuEPO demonstrated significantly improved hemoglobin levels in comparison with 124 other patients who received placebo.[126] Erythropoietin has been effective in preventing and managing anemia in approximately 50%–60% of the patients who received rHuEPO.[127,128] Studies have shown that treatment with erythropoietin is associated with a significant increase in energy and activity level, functional status, and overall enhanced quality of life.[119,127,129–131] Two large-scale, multicenter studies[119,131] demonstrated that thrice-weekly dosing of rHuEPO (epoetin-alfa) was effective in increasing hemoglobin levels and improving quality of life. Concerns about the financial cost of the thrice-weekly dosing schedule for epoetin-alfa and patient compliance have led researchers to investigate a once-weekly dosing schedule for epoetin-alfa. Gabrilove and colleagues found that this once-weekly dosing schedule was similarly effective in increasing hemoglobin levels, improving quality of life, and decreasing blood transfusion requirements as darbepoetin or thrice-weekly dosing.[119,131,132]

Darbepoetin-alfa, a erythropoiesis-stimulating protein, has the potential to treat cancer-related anemia; it offers a longer serum half-life than epoetin-alfa and requires less frequent administration.[132–134] More studies are needed to investigate its effectiveness in treating cancer-related anemia.

The treatment of cancer-related anemia with blood transfusion or erythropoietin is costly. Meadowcroft and colleagues found that blood transfusions were less expensive than erythropoietin for managing anemia in breast cancer patients, but no standard guidelines for transfusion exist.[135] Other studies have examined the financial costs of transfusions and the costs to the patient in terms of risk.[136,137] Their findings highlight the need for careful assessment and monitoring of patients receiving transfusions or erythropoietin. More studies that examine the cost-benefit trade-offs of these treatments for anemia are needed.

Motivational strategies

Limited information is available regarding the use of a cognitive approach to motivate individuals with cancer to participate in fatigue management. Cognitive interventions focusing on increasing individuals' self-efficacy belief hold promise in motivating individuals to engage in activities that alleviate fatigue symptoms. Self-efficacy, a component of social cognitive theory, has been found to be the strongest predictor of exercise behavior among diverse populations.[138,139] Self-efficacy belief is a personal assessment of one's ability to successfully perform a given behavior.[138] Research related to self-efficacy in the cancer population has focused on disease prevention and early-detection behaviors.[140] In addition, addressing self-efficacy may promote smoking cessation, encourage consumption of a healthy diet, and increase use of relaxation techniques that may improve fatigue management.[141]

Motivational strategies to foster and enhance fatigue management should aim at initiating and sustaining individuals' motivation to actively participate in fatigue management. The theory of self-determination (SD) can be a fundamental framework for developing effective strategies for fatigue management.[142,143] According to the SD theory, individuals are motivated to initiate and continue specific behaviors when they feel that their behaviors are self-determined or autonomous, when they feel competent to accomplish the behaviors, and when they feel that they are understood or supported by others.[142,143] Thus, it is essential to inspire a patient's own pursuit of health and self-care for fatigue management. Motivational strategies to initiate and enhance fatigue management can be designed to mobilize the human spirit and empower the individual to take self-improving actions. Some of these strategies are outlined in Table 30-3.

Using a cognitive approach in motivating individuals with cancer to participate in activities for fatigue management is an important direction for future research. Cognitive interventions focusing on increasing individuals' self-efficacy beliefs and fostering individuals' perceived autonomy, competency, and sense of relatedness hold promise in motivating individuals to actively engage in fatigue management.

Future Trends

Fatigue is a complex, subjective symptom that is prevalent at all stages of the cancer trajectory. It is also a major debilitating symptom for individuals with cancer, affecting activities of daily living, influencing treatment choices, and decreasing quality of life. Recent research efforts have provided a scientific basis for understanding fatigue, its impact, and its management.

Fatigue is a multidimensional phenomenon, so its management correspondingly requires an integrative approach. A systematic and integrative program for fatigue management remains lacking. Future practice and research on fatigue management, therefore, should focus on providing systematic and integrative management programs based on strategies of prevention, relief of other related symptoms (pain or nausea), exercise, effective energy conservation, managing anemia through supplemental nutrition or erythropoiesis-stimulating therapies, and cognitive-oriented motivational strategies to encourage self-management of fatigue. Such systematic and integrative programs should encompass a variety of interventions — for example, systematic assessment of risk factors for fatigue, educational programs on fatigue and management, prescribed or scheduled aerobic exercise and progressive muscle relaxation, planned rest and nap periods during the day, modification of dietary needs, and assessment and meeting of emotional and spiritual needs. Such an integrative approach to fatigue management will improve cancer patients' and survivors' coping ability to meet their needs to manage fatigue. As future research documents the effectiveness of such integrative intervention programs in managing fatigue, the quality of life in patients with cancer will be improved.

References

1. Beisecker A, Cook MR, Ashworth J, et al: Side effects of adjuvant chemotherapy: perceptions of node-negative breast cancer patients. *Psychol Oncol* 6:85–93, 1997
2. Dow KH, Ferrell BR, Leigh S, et al: An evaluation of the quality of life among long-term survivors of breast cancer. *Breast Cancer Res Treat* 39:261–273, 1996
3. Loge JH, Abrahamsen AF, Ekeberg O, et al: Fatigue and psychiatric morbidity among Hodgkin's disease survivors. *J Pain Symptom Manage* 19:91–99, 2000
4. Vordermark D, Schwab M, Flentje M, et al: Chronic fatigue after radiotherapy for carcinoma of the prostate: correlation with anorectal and genitourinary function. *Radiother Oncol* 62:293–297, 2002
5. Andrykowski MA, Curran SL, Lightner R: Off-treatment fatigue in breast cancer survivors: a controlled comparison. *J Behavior Med* 21:1–18, 1998
6. Fu MR, Anderson CM, McDaniel R, et al: Patients' perception of fatigue in response to biochemotherapy as a treatment for metastatic melanoma. *Oncol Nurs Forum* 29:961–966, 2002
7. Glaus A, Crow R, Hammond S: A qualitative study to explore the concept of fatigue/tiredness in cancer patients and in healthy individuals. *Support Care Cancer* 4:82–96, 1996
8. Porock D, Kristjanson L, Tinnelly K, et al: An exercise intervention for advanced cancer patients experiencing fatigue: a pilot study. *J Palliat Care* 16:30–36, 2000
9. Schwartz A, Nail L, Chen S, et al: Fatigue patterns observed in patients receiving chemotherapy and radiotherapy. *Cancer Invest* 18:11–19, 2000
10. Nail LM: Fatigue in patients with cancer. *Oncol Nurs Forum* 29:537–546, 2002
11. Irvine DM, Vincent L, Graydon JE, et al: Fatigue in women with breast cancer receiving radiation therapy. *Cancer Nurs* 21:127–135, 1998
12. Messias DKH, Yeager KA, Dibble SL, et al: Patients' perspectives of fatigue while undergoing chemotherapy. *Oncol Nurs Forum* 24:43–48, 1997
13. Schwartz A: Patterns of exercise and fatigue in physically active cancer survivors. *Oncol Nurs Forum* 25:485–491, 1998
14. Aaronson LS, Teel CS, Cassmeyer V, et al: Defining and measuring fatigue. *Image J Nurs Schol* 31:45–50, 1999
15. Mock V, Hassey Dow K, Meares C, et al: Effects of exercise on fatigue, physical functioning, and emotional distress during radiation therapy for breast cancer. *Oncol Nurs Forum* 24:991–1000, 1997

16. Buckingham R, Fitt J, Sitzia J: Patients' experiences of chemotherapy: side-effects of carboplatin in the treatment of carcinoma of the ovary. *Eur J Cancer Care* 6:59–71, 1997
17. Ferrell BR, Grant M, Dean GE, et al: "Bone tired": the experience of fatigue and its impact on quality of life. *Oncol Nurs Forum* 23:1539–1547, 1996
18. North American Nursing Diagnosis Association (NANDA): *Nursing Diagnosis: Definitions and Classification 2001–2002.* Philadelphia, NANDA, 2001, p 89
19. Ream E, Richardson A: Fatigue: a concept analysis. *Int J Nurs Stud* 33:519–529, 1996
20. Piper B: Fatigue, in Carrieri-Kohlman V, Lindsey AM, West CM (eds.): *Pathophysiological Phenomena in Nursing: Human Responses to Illness* (ed 3). St. Louis, Saunders, 2003, pp 279–302
21. Fu M, LeMone P, McDaniel R, et al: A multivariate validation of the defining characteristics of fatigue. *Nurs Diagnosis: Int J Nurs Language Classification* 12:15–27, 2001
22. McDaniel RW, Rhodes VA: Development of a preparatory sensory information videotape for women receiving chemotherapy for breast cancer. *Cancer Nurs* 21:143–148, 1998
23. Rhodes VA, Watson PM, McDaniel RW, et al: Expectation and occurrence of postchemotherapy side effects. *Cancer Pract* 3:247–253, 1995
24. Tiesinga L, Dassen TWN, Halfens RJG: Fatigue: a summary of the definitions, dimensions, and indicators. *Nurs Diagnosis* 7:51–62, 1996
25. Richardson A, Ream E: Self-care behaviors initiated by chemotherapy patients in response to fatigue. *Int Nurs Stud* 34:35–43, 1997
26. Curt GA, Breitbart W, Cella D, et al: Impact of cancer-related fatigue on the lives of patients: new findings from the Fatigue Coalition. *Oncologist* 5:353–360, 2000
27. Cimprich B: Age and extent of surgery affect attention in women treated for breast cancer. *Res Nurs Health* 21:229–238, 1998
28. Cimprich B: Pre-treatment symptom distress in women newly diagnosed with breast cancer. *Cancer Nurs* 22:185–194, 1999
29. Cimprich B, Ronis DL: Attention and symptom distress in women with and without breast cancer. *Nurs Res* 50:86–94, 2001
30. Cella D: The Functional Assessment of Cancer Therapy—Anemia (FACT-AN) Scale: a new tool for the assessment of outcomes in cancer anemia and fatigue. *Semin Hematol* 34(suppl 2):13–19, 1997
31. Vogelzang NJ, Breitbart W, Cella D, et al: Patient, caregiver, and oncologist perceptions of cancer-related fatigue: results of a tripart assessment survey. The Fatigue Coalition. *Semin Hematol* 34(suppl 2):4–12, 1997
32. So WKW, Dodgson J, Tai JWM: Fatigue and quality of life among Chinese patients with hematologic malignancy after bone marrow transplantation. *Cancer Nurs* 26:211–219, 2003
33. Jacobsen PB, Hann DM, Azzarello LM, et al: Fatigue in women receiving adjuvant chemotherapy for breast cancer: characteristics, course and correlates. *J Pain Symptom Manage* 18:233–242, 1999
34. Furst CJ, Ahsberg E: Dimensions of fatigue during radiotherapy: an application of multidimensional fatigue inventory. *Support Care Cancer* 9:355–360, 2001
35. Sitzia J, Dikken C: Survey of the incidence and severity of side effects reported by patients receiving six cycles of FEC chemotherapy. *Cancer Nurs* 1:61–73, 1997
36. Dean GE, Spears L, Ferrell BR, et al: Fatigue in patients with cancer receiving interferon alpha. *Cancer Pract* 3:164–172, 1995
37. Irvine DM, Vincent L, Graydon JE, et al: Fatigue in women with breast cancer receiving radiation therapy. *Cancer Nurs* 21:127–135, 1998
38. Munro AJ, Potter S: A quantitative approach to the distress caused by symptoms in patients treated with radical radiotherapy. *Br J Cancer* 74:640–647, 1996
39. Mast ME: Correlates of fatigue in survivors of breast cancer. *Cancer Nurs* 21:136–142, 1998
40. Nail L, Winningham M: Fatigue and weakness in cancer patients: the symptom experience. *Semin Oncol Nurs* 11:272–278, 1995
41. Winningham ML, Nail LM, Burke MB, et al: Fatigue and the cancer experience: the state of the knowledge. *Oncol Nurs Forum* 21:23–36, 1994
42. Winningham ML: The role of exercise in cancer therapy, in Eisinger M, Watson RW (eds.): *Exercise and Disease.* Boca Raton, FL, CRC Press, 1992, pp 63–70
43. Cella D: Factors influencing quality of life in cancer patients: anemia and fatigue. *Semin Oncol* 25(suppl 7):43–46, 1998
44. Koeller JM: Clinical guidelines for the treatment of cancer-related anemia. *Pharmacotherapy* 18:156–169, 1998
45. Hwang SS, Chang VT, Corpion C, et al: A preliminary study of clinical predictors for lack of energy in patients (pts) with advanced cancer. *Proc Am Soc Clin Oncol* 16:A241, 1997 (abstr)
46. Schwenk W, Bohm B, Muller JM: Postoperative fatigue after laparoscopic or conventional colorectal resections: a prospective randomized trial. *Surg Endosc* 12:1131–1136, 1998
47. Harrison LB, Shasha D, White C, et al: Radiotherapy-associated anemia: the scope of the problem. *Oncologist* 5(suppl 2):1–7, 2000
48. Cella D: Factors influencing quality of life in cancer patients: anemia and fatigue. *Semin Oncol* 25:43–46, 1998
49. Grogan M, Thomas GM, Melamed I, et al: The importance of hemoglobin levels during radiotherapy for carcinoma of the cervix. *Cancer* 86:1528–1536, 1999
50. Forsberg C, Bjorvell H, Cedermark B: Well-being and its relation to coping ability in patients with colo-rectal and gastric cancer before and after surgery. *Scand J Caring Sci* 10:35–44, 1996
51. Hickok JT, Morrow GR, McDonald S, et al: Frequency and correlates of fatigue in lung cancer patients receiving radiation therapy: implications for management. *J Pain Symptom Manage* 11:370–377, 1996
52. Longman AJ, Braden CJ, Mishel MH: Pattern of association over time of side-effects burden, self-help, and self-care in women with breast cancer *Oncol Nurs Forum* 24:1555–1560, 1997
53. Kehlet H: Multimodal approach to control postoperative pathophysiology and rehabilitation. *Br J Anaesth* 78:606–617, 1997
54. Salmon P, Hall GM: A theory of postoperative fatigue. *J R Soc Med* 90:661–664, 1997
55. Wyatt GK, Friedman LL: Physical and psychosocial outcomes of midlife and older women following surgery and adjuvant therapy for breast cancer. *Oncol Nurs Forum* 25:761–768, 1998
56. Dimeo F, Stieglitz RD, Novelli-Fischer U, et al: Correlation between physical performance and fatigue in cancer patients. *Ann Oncol* 8:1251–1255, 1997
57. Longman AJ, Braden CJ, Mishel MH: Side effects burden in women with breast cancer. *Cancer Pract* 4:274–280, 1996
58. Visser MR, Smets EM: Fatigue, depression and quality of life in cancer patients: how are they related? *Support Care Cancer* 6:101–108, 1998
59. Breitbart W: Identifying patients at risk for, and treatment of, major psychiatric complications of cancer. *Support Care Cancer* 3:45–60, 1995
60. Henriksson MM, Isometsa ET, Hietanen PS: Mental disorders in cancer suicides. *J Affective Disorders* 36:11–20, 1995

61. Bower JE, Ganz PA, Desmond KA, et al: Fatigue in breast cancer survivors: occurrence, correlates, and impact on quality of life. *J Clin Oncol* 18:743–753, 2000
62. Stoudemire A, Bronheim H, Wise TN: Why guidelines for consultation-liaison psychiatry patients? *Psychosomatics* 39:S3–S7, 1998
63. Foltz AT, Gaines G, Gullatte M: Recalled side effects and self-care actions of patients receiving inpatient chemotherapy. *Oncol Nurs Forum* 23:679–683, 1996
64. Broeckel JA, Jacobsen PB, Horton J, et al: Characteristics and correlates of fatigue after adjuvant chemotherapy for breast cancer. *J Clin Oncol* 16:1689–1696, 1998
65. Fieler VK: Side effects and quality of life in patients receiving high-dose rate brachytherapy. *Oncol Nurs Forum* 24:545–553, 1997
66. Jereczek-Fossa BA, Marsiglia HR, Orecchia R: Radiotherapy-related fatigue. *Crit Rev Oncol Hematol* 41:317–325, 2002
67. Walker BL, Nail LM, Larsen L, et al: Concerns, affect, and cognitive disruption following completion of radiation treatment for localized breast or prostate cancer. *Oncol Nurs Forum* 23:1181–1187, 1996
68. McEvoy GK (ed.): *American Hospital Formulary Service Drug Information.* Bethesda, MD, American Society of Health-System Pharmacists, 1998
69. Berger AM: Patterns of fatigue and activity and rest during adjuvant breast cancer chemotherapy. *Oncol Nurs Forum* 25:51–62, 1998
70. Richardson A, Ream E: The experience of fatigue and other symptoms in patients receiving chemotherapy. *Eur J Cancer Care* 5(suppl):24–30, 1996
71. Lindley C, Vasa S, Sawyer WT, et al: Quality of life and preferences for treatment following systemic adjuvant therapy for early-stage breast cancer. *J Clin Oncol* 16:1380–1387, 1998
72. Mast ME: Survivors of breast cancer: illness uncertainty, positive reappraisal, and emotional distress. *Oncol Nurs Forum* 25:555–562, 1998
73. Borden EC, Parkinson D: A perspective on the clinical effectiveness and tolerance of interferon-alpha. *Semin Oncol* 25(suppl 1):3–8, 1998
74. Dalakas MC, Mock V, Hawkins MJ: Fatigue: definitions, mechanisms, and paradigms for study. *Semin Oncol* 25(suppl 1):48–53, 1998
75. Jones TH, Wadler S, Hupart KH: Endocrine-mediated mechanisms of fatigue during treatment with interferon-alpha. *Semin Oncol* 25(suppl 1):54–63, 1998
76. Weiss K: Safety profile of interferon-alpha therapy. *Semin Oncol* 25(suppl 1):9–13, 1998
77. Spath-Schwalbe E, Hansen K, Schmidt F, et al: Acute effects of recombinant human interleukin-6 on endocrine and central nervous sleep functions in healthy men. *J Clin Endocrinol Metab* 83:1573–1579, 1998
78. Blade J, San Miguel JF, Escudero ML, et al: Maintenance treatment with interferon alpha-2b in multiple myeloma: a prospective randomized study from PETHEMA (Program for the Study and Treatment of Hematological Malignancies, Spanish Society of Hematology). *Leukemia* 12:1144–1148, 1998
79. Johnston SR, Constenla DO, Moore J, et al: Randomized phase II trial of BCDT [carmustine (BCNU), cisplatin, dacarbazine (DTIC) and tamoxifen] with or without interferon alpha (IFN-alpha) and interleukin (IL-2) in patients with metastatic melanoma. *Br J Cancer* 77:1280–1286, 1998
80. Rosenthal MA, Oratz R: Phase II clinical trial of recombinant alpha 2b interferon and 13 *cis* retinoic acid in patients with metastatic melanoma. *Am J Clin Oncol* 21:352–354, 1998
81. Karp SE: Low-dose intravenous bolus interleukin-2 with interferon-alpha therapy for metastatic melanoma and renal cell carcinoma. *J Immunother* 21:56–61, 1998
82. Miaskowski C, Portenoy RK: Update on the assessment and management of cancer-related fatigue. *Prin Pract Support Oncol Updates* 1:1–10, 1998
83. Mulligan K, Bloch AS: Energy expenditure and protein metabolism in human immunodeficiency virus infection and cancer cachexia. *Semin Oncol* 25(suppl 6):82–91, 1998
84. Bower JE, Ganz PA, Aziz N, Fahey J: Fatigue and proinflammatory cytokine activity in breast cancer survivors. *Psycho Med* 64:604–611, 2002
85. Gupta S, Aggarwal S, See D, et al: Cytokine production by adherent and non-adherent mononuclear cells in chronic fatigue syndrome. *J Psychiatr Res* 31:149–156, 1997
86. Vgontzas AN, Papanicolaou DA, Bixler EO, et al: Elevation of plasma cytokines in disorders of excessive daytime sleepiness: role of sleep disturbance and obesity. *J Clin Endocrinol Metab* 82:1313–1316, 1997
87. Portenoy RK, Itri LM: Cancer-related fatigue: guidelines for evaluation and management. *Oncologist* 4:1–10, 1999
88. Davis JM: Central and peripheral factors in fatigue. *J Sports Sci* 13:549, 1995
89. Porth CM: *Pathophysiology: Concepts of Altered States.* Philadelphia, Lippincott, 1998
90. Piper BF: Measuring fatigue, in Frank-Stromborg M, Olsen SJ (eds.): *Instruments for Clinical Health-Care Research* (ed 2). Sudbury, MA, Jones and Bartlett, 2004, pp 538–569
91. Litwin MS, Lubeck DP, Henning JM, et al: Differences in urologist and patient assessments of health related quality of life in men with prostate cancer: results of the CaPSURE database. *J Urol* 159:1988–1992, 1998
92. Rhodes VA, McDaniel RW, Matthews C: Comparison of hospice nurses and patients perceptions of symptom experience. *Cancer Nurs* 21:312–319, 1998
93. Kurtz ME, Kurtz JC, Given CC, et al: Concordance of cancer patient and caregiver symptom reports. *Cancer Pract* 4:185–190, 1996
94. Rhoten D: Fatigue and the postsurgical patient, in Norris CM (ed.): *Concept Clarification in Nursing.* Rockville, MD, Aspen Systems, 1982, pp 277–300
95. Okuyama T, Akechi T, Kugaya A, et al: Development and validation of the Cancer Fatigue Scale: a brief, three-dimensional, self-rating scale for assessment of fatigue in cancer patients. *J Pain Symptom Manage* 19:5–14, 2000
96. Piper BF, Dibble SL, Dodd MJ, et al: The revised Piper Fatigue Scale: psychometric evaluation in women with breast cancer. *Oncol Nurs Forum* 25:677–684, 1998
97. Schwartz AL: The Schwartz Cancer Fatigue Scale: testing reliability and validity. *Oncol Nurs Forum* 25:711–717, 1998
98. Armitage JO: Management of anemia in patients with cancer. *Clin Oncol Updates* 1:1–12, 1998
99. Groopman JE, Itri LM: Chemotherapy-induced anemia in adults: incidence and treatment. *J Natl Cancer Inst* 91:1616–1634, 1999
100. Gillespie TW: Anemia in cancer: therapeutic implications and interventions. *Cancer Nurs* 26:119–130, 2003
101. Dowlati A, R'Zik S, Fillet G, Beguin Y: Anaemia of lung cancer is due to impaired erythroid marrow response to erythropoietin stimulation as well as relative inadequacy of erythropoietin production. *Br J Haematol* 97:297–299, 1997
102. Daneryd P, Svanberg E, Korner U, et al: Protection of metabolic and exercise capacity in unselected weight-losing cancer patients following treatment with recombinant erythropoietin: a randomized prospective study. *Cancer Res* 58:5374–5379, 1998

103. Mercadante S, Gebbia V, Marrazzo A, et al: Anaemia in cancer: pathophysiology and treatment. *Cancer Treat Rev* 26:303–311, 2000
104. Kim Y, Roscoe JA, Morrow GR: The effects of information and negative affect on severity of side effects from radiation therapy for prostate cancer. *Support Care Cancer* 10:416–421, 2002
105. Moore SM: Effects of interventions to promote recovery in coronary artery bypass surgical patients. *J Cardiol Nurs* 12:59–70, 1997
106. Gammon J, Mulholland CW: Effect of preparatory information prior to elective total hip replacement on psychological coping outcomes. *J Adv Nurs* 24:303–308, 1996
107. Johnson JE: Coping with radiation therapy: optimism and the effect of preparatory interventions. *Res Nurs Health* 19:3–12, 1996
108. Orem DE: *Nursing Concepts of Practice* (ed 6). St. Louis, Mosby, 2001
109. Mock V: Breast cancer and fatigue: issues for the workplace. *AAOHN J* 46:425–431, 1998
110. Schwartz A: Exercise and weight gain in breast cancer patients receiving chemotherapy. *Cancer Pract* 8:231–237, 2000
111. Dimeo F, Fetscher S, Lange W, et al: Effects of aerobic exercise on the physical performance and incidence of treatment-related complications after high-dose chemotherapy. *Blood* 90:3390–3394, 1997
112. Suh E, Lee EO: The effects of rhythmic walking exercise on physical strength, fatigue, and functional status of breast cancer patients in adjuvant chemotherapy. *Oncol Nurs Forum* 25:331, 1998
113. Graydon JE, Bubela N, Irvine D, et al: Fatigue-reducing strategies used by patients receiving treatment for cancer. *Cancer Nurs* 18:23–28, 1995
114. Schwartz AL: Patterns of exercise and fatigue in physically active cancer survivors. *Oncol Nurs Forum* 25:485–491, 1998
115. Friendenreich CM, Courneya KS: Exercise as rehabilitation for cancer patients. *Clin J Sport Med* 6:237–244, 1996
116. Richardson A, Ream E, Wilson-Barnett J: Fatigue in patients receiving chemotherapy: patterns of change. *Cancer Nurs* 21:17–30, 1998
117. Barrett-Lee PJ, Bailey NP, O'Brien MER, et al: Large-scale UK audit of blood transfusion requirements and anaemia in patients receiving cytotoxic chemotherapy. *Br J Cancer* 82:93–97, 2000
118. Coiffier B: The impact and management of anaemia in hematological malignancies. *Med Oncol* 17(suppl 1):S2–S10, 2000
119. Demetri GD, Kris M, Wade J, et al: Quality-of-life benefit in chemotherapy patients treated with epoetin alfa is independent of disease response or tumor type: results from a prospective community oncology study. *J Clin Oncol* 16:3412–3425, 1998
120. Gabrilove JL: Cancer therapy. New strategies and treatment modalities for optimizing patient outcomes. *Semin Hematol* 38(suppl 7):1–7, 2001
121. Adamson JW: Epoetin alfa: into the new millennium. *Semin Oncol* 25(3 suppl 7):76–79, 1998
122. Levine EA, Laborde C, Hambrick E, et al: Influence of erythropoietin on transfusion requirements in patients receiving preoperative chemoradiotherapy for rectal cancer. *Dis Colon Rectum* 42:1065–1069, discussion 1069–1071, 1999
123. Scott SN, Boeve TJ, McCulloch TM, et al: The effects of epoetin alfa on transfusion requirements in head and neck cancer patients: a prospective, randomized, placebo-controlled study. *Laryngoscope* 112(pt 1):1221–1229, 2002
124. Sturgis EM, Gianoli GJ, Miller RH, et al: Avoiding transfusion in head and neck surgery: feasibility study of erythropoietin. *Laryngoscope* 110:51–57, 2000
125. Adamson JW, Ludwig H: Predicting the hematopoietic response to recombinant human erythropoietin (epoetin alfa) in the treatment of the anemia of cancer. *Oncology* 56:46–53, 1999
126. Littlewood TJ, Bajetta E, Nortier J, et al: Effects of epoetin alfa on hematologic parameters and quality of life in cancer patients receiving nonplatinum chemotherapy: results of a randomized, double-blind placebo-controlled trial. *J Clin Oncol* 19:2865–2874, 2001
127. Ludwig H, Fritz E: Anemia of cancer patients: patient selection and patient stratification for epoetin treatment. *Semin Oncol* 25(suppl 7):35–38, 1998
128. Beguin Y: Prediction of response to optimize outcome of treatment with erythropoietin. *Semin Oncol* 25(suppl 7):27–34, 1998
129. Glaspy J: The impact of epoetin alfa on quality of life during cancer chemotherapy: a fresh look at an old problem. *Semin Hematol* 34(suppl 2):20–26, 1997
130. Henry D: Haematological toxicities associated with dose-intensive chemotherapy, the role for and use of recombinant growth factors. *Ann Oncol* 8(suppl 3):S7–S10, 1997
131. Gabrilove JL, Cleeland CS, Livingston RB, et al: Clinical evaluation of once-weekly dosing of epoetin alfa in chemotherapy patients: improvements in hemoglobin and quality of life similar to three-times-weekly dosing. *J Clin Oncol* 19:2875–2882, 2001
132. Glaspy J, Jadeja J, Justice G, et al: Randomized, active-controlled, phase I/II, dose-escalation study of darbepoetin alfa every 2 weeks in patients with solid tumors. *Eur J Cancer* 37(suppl 6):353, 2001
133. Pirker R, Smith R: Darbepoietin alfa: potential role in managing anemia in cancer patients. *Expert Rev Anticancer Ther* 2:377–384, 2002
134. Smith R, Meza L, Tchekmedyian S, et al: An open-label, dose-finding study of novel erythropoiesis stimulating protein (NESP; darbepoetin alfa; Aranesp) administered by subcutaneous (sc) injection for the treatment of anemia in patients with chronic anemia of cancer. *Eur J Cancer* 37(suppl 6):355, 2001
135. Meadowcroft AM, Gilbert CJ, Maravich-May D, et al: Cost of managing anemia with and without prophylactic epoetin alfa therapy in breast cancer patients receiving combination chemotherapy. *Am J Health System Pharm* 55:1898–1902, 1998
136. Mohandas K, Aledort L: Transfusion requirements, risks, and costs for patients with malignancy. *Transfusion* 35:427–430, 1995
137. Ortega A, Dranitsaris G, Puodziunas A: A clinical and economic evaluation of red blood cell transfusions in patients receiving cancer chemotherapy. *Int J Tech Assess Health Care* 14:788–798, 1998
138. Bandura A: *Self-Efficacy: The Exercise Control.* New York, Freeman, 1997
139. Conn V: Older women: social cognitive theory correlates of health behavior. *Women Health* 26:71–85, 1997
140. Lev EL: Bandura's theory of self-efficacy: applications to oncology. *Schol Inquiry Nurs Pract* 11:21–37, 1997
141. Haas BK: Focus on health promotion: self-efficacy in oncology nursing research and practice. *Oncol Nurs Forum* 27:89–97, 2000
142. Deci EL, Ryan RM: The "what" and "why" of goal pursuits: human needs and the self-determination of behavior. *Psychol Inquiry* 11:227–268, 2000
143. Sheldon KM, Ryan R, Reis HT: What makes for a good day? Competence and autonomy in the day and in the person. *Society Personality Social Psycho* 22:1270–1279, 1996

CHAPTER 31

Nutritional Disturbances

Regina S. Cunningham, PhD, RN, AOCN®
Maureen B. Huhmann, MS, RD

Scope of the Problem

In the United States, recognition of the relationship between cancer and nutrition began in the 1930s[1] and became the subject of systematic research in the 1970s.[2] The research studies could be classified into two main categories: (1) the relationship of nutrient intake to the development of cancer, and (2) cancer-induced nutritional problems and their management, which is the primary subject of this chapter.

Undernutrition is the most common nutritional problem in both pediatric and adult populations with cancer.[3,4] However, the evidence that both undernutrition and overnutrition negatively affect morbidity, survival, and quality of life[4–6] emphasizes the need for oncology nurses to evaluate the nutritional status of all individuals under their care.

Definitions

The two opposite endpoints of malnutrition in individuals with cancer are obesity and cancer cachexia. *Obesity* is frequently defined as a body mass index (BMI) of greater than 30 kg/m^2, but this definition can be misleading. While obesity is identified with surplus fat, weight above the normal range can occur secondary to increased muscle mass or fluid retention. As such, evaluation of body composition should be made when weight tables are used to diagnose obesity.

Terms used to describe nonmalignant nutritional deficiencies, and occasionally malignant starvation, are *kwashiorkor* (protein malnutrition with an adequate caloric intake) and *marasmus* (simple starvation with protein-calorie malnutrition). *Cachexia,* a general term meaning ill health, can occur in non-neoplastic diseases, such as sepsis, cardiac failure, and starvation. The term *anorexia-cachexia cancer syndrome* (ACCS) is often used to refer to the nutritional disorder in individuals with cancer. Cancer cachexia is characterized by anorexia, weight loss, skeletal muscle atrophy, and asthenia (loss of strength). Other symptoms of cancer cachexia include early satiety, edema, anemia, reduced attention span, organ dysfunction, metabolic abnormalities, and susceptibility to other diseases.

Cancer-associated cachexia can be differentiated into primary and secondary types.[6] *Primary cachexia* results from tumor-produced metabolic abnormalities or host responses. Successful treatment of primary cachexia relies on effective cancer treatment. When cure or significant control is not possible, palliation of cachexia may be possible for some interval of time. *Secondary cachexia* results from mechanical effects of the tumor or treatment. Secondary cachexia can be treated with a variety of approaches and is often more amenable to intervention than the primary form. *Repletion* describes the reestablishment of adequate nutritional status and normal body composition.

Other terms are commonly used to describe conditions that result from cancer or its treatment. These include *hypogeusia* (decreased taste sensitivity), *dysgeusia* (perverted taste perception), *odynophagia* or *dysphagia* (painful swallowing), *hyposmia* (diminished ability to smell), and *inanition* (progressive deterioration with muscle wasting and energy loss).

Incidence

Neither the incidence nor the prevalence of malnutrition is accurately documented in patients with cancer. Most individuals with cancer develop some degree of malnutrition during their illness. The exact incidence of malnutrition in specific cancer types is difficult to quantify for several reasons. First, nutritional status is rarely assessed when cancer is diagnosed, especially in the obese. Because assessment of nutritional status frequently is delayed, the opportunity to find more easily treated, minimal nutrient deficiencies in early stages is often lost. Second, no consensus exists regarding which indicators of nutritional status should be routinely assessed in cancer patients. Although weight is universally accepted as part of nutritional assessment, there is little agreement on which other parameters must be included. Recommendations vary from a careful clinical examination to the use of an array of laboratory tests.[7] There is also no agreement on how malnutrition should be graded. In clinical trials, study groups have developed toxicity scales for weight change and anorexia; however, these scales are better suited to determining side effect profiles rather than malnutrition levels. The American Dietetic Association is in the process of developing nutrition diagnosis categories and labels to be used in classifying alterations in nutrition status.[8]

Overnutrition is most commonly documented in breast cancer. The incidence of obesity among women recently diagnosed with breast cancer ranges from 24%–36%.[9,10] In addition, 40%–100% of women with breast cancer receiving adjuvant chemotherapy gain weight, and some become obese.[11,12] Concern about weight changes arises not only because of cardiac or quality of life issues, but also because of findings that women with breast cancer who are obese have poorer survival rates than women who are not obese.[13,14] However, specific characteristics that predispose cancer patients to weight gain are still being sorted out. Borugian et al. found that obesity as evidenced by an elevated waist-to-hip ratio was linked to increased mortality in postmenopausal patients with estrogen receptor–positive breast cancer, but there was no such effect in premenopausal women.[14] Overnutrition can exist in other cancers as well. Whether increased weight has negative consequences in types of cancer other than breast cancer is not clear.

Risk Factors

Individuals who are nourished adequately at the time of the cancer diagnosis have fewer problems with both the cancer and its treatment. The body's response to the tumor and the tumor-initiated metabolic changes are primary sources for malnutrition.[15] In addition, treatment imposes a burden by requiring repair of treatment-induced damage and by reducing the ability of the body to absorb nutrients.

External and internal factors

External factors include the environmental and political climate surrounding an individual. This climate encompasses the overall health of the country's economy, which has an impact on transportation, access to food shopping, availability of different nutrients, adequacy of housing and food preparation facilities, and availability of programs that offer food assistance. These environmental factors influence the individual, who possesses cultural and attitudinal concepts about nutrition and eating behaviors. Internal factors that influence a person's tendency to develop nutritional deficiencies include age, body image, past history of food fads or eating disorders, social support, educational level, alcohol or tobacco intake, and presence of comorbid diseases. Much more research in this area is needed before individuals at risk can be reliably identified.

Cancer-related factors

The type of cancer affects the probability of malnutrition. Individuals with breast cancer or leukemia are at low risk, whereas 31%–48% of patients with non-Hodgkin's lymphoma have significant weight loss; unfavorable histologies are correlated with higher weight loss.[16] Individuals with cancers of the aerodigestive (upper respiratory and digestive) and gastrointestinal tracts are at special risk for undernutrition from mechanical obstruction and physiological dysfunction due to local tumor compression.[17] Host responses to the cancer and the cancer itself cause changes in metabolism and energy needs and may explain why those individuals with advanced disease are more likely to have nutritional problems.[6]

Treatment-related factors

All cancer therapies can cause nutritional deficiency. The magnitude of the treatment-related risk depends on the area of treatment, type of treatment, number of therapeutic modalities used, dosages of therapy used, and length of treatment.

Surgery. The effects of surgery on an individual's nutritional status depend on the extent of the procedure as well as the site of operation. Complications associated with surgery also are related to the nutritional status of the individual prior to the operation. Malnourished individuals have higher incidences of morbidity and mortality than do those patients who are adequately nourished.[18] This fact has particular relevance for individuals with cancers of the aerodigestive or gastrointestinal tract. These patients may come to surgery with nutritional deficits because of cancer-related disruption of intake or absorption. In addition, they often have undergone multiple tests requiring restricted diets.

Surgery itself alters function. Major aerodigestive resections may produce hyposmia, dysgeusia, or impaired swallowing, resulting in reduced intake. Rearranged anatomy, which is common with gastric and esophageal resections, can create multiple lesions affecting nutrition. Patients with abdominal and pelvic incisions may experience an ileus after surgery, complicating the ability to take adequate nutrition postoperatively.[19] Resections of large segments of the bowel can lead to malabsorption of fat, inadequate caloric intake, vitamin B_{12} deficiency, anemia, and fluid–electrolyte imbalance.[17] These problems can become chronic, resulting in reliance on enteral or parenteral feedings.

For individuals with cancers affecting other sites, nutritional problems resulting from surgery are often limited to the immediate perioperative period. Interruption of oral intake is usually minimal. Use of antibiotics in the perioperative period, although disruptive to digestive processes that utilize intestinal bacteria, can be offset by intake of acidophilus-containing products such as yogurt. Surgical procedures create the same response to injury as does surgery for nonmalignant diseases. This stress is added to the psychological stress of dealing with a cancer diagnosis. Catecholamine, glucocorticoid, and glucagon outputs increase, resulting in increased energy needs, loss of nitrogen, and water and sodium retention. Surgery can increase energy requirements by 1.5–1.82 times basal energy needs or more.[20] For this reason, surgical candidates must be assessed carefully prior to treatment so that any nutritional deficiencies can be addressed proactively.

Radiation. Radiation therapy can alter nutritional status by exerting both systemic and local effects. The extent of the alteration varies with the area of the body being treated, the size of the area being treated, and the duration of treatment.[21] Radiation alters function in the treatment area and poses particular problems for patients with aerodigestive or gastrointestinal cancers. Acute effects are transient and include anorexia, diarrhea, bleeding, nausea, vomiting, weight loss, mucositis, esophagitis, gastritis, xerostomia, and changes in taste. Local desquamation reactions can temporarily increase energy needs. Some of these changes—especially xerostomia, taste changes, and diarrhea—can become chronic.[21]

Indirect effects of radiation can also influence nutritional status. Fatigue and appetite changes commonly occur among individuals receiving radiation therapy. These symptoms can alter the person's desire and ability to procure, prepare, and ingest food. Delayed effects of radiation, such as intestinal strictures, fibrosis or obstruction, fistulas, and hepatic or pulmonary fibrosis, may cause mechanical problems in gut function and oxygenation. These, in turn, interrupt the person's ability to absorb, process, and ingest food and may necessitate long-term management.

Chemotherapy. Chemotherapy has a number of direct and indirect effects on nutrition. Direct effects include alteration of the intestinal absorptive surface, excitation of the chemoreceptor trigger zone and true vomiting center, and interference with specific metabolic and enzymatic reactions. The majority of chemotherapeutic agents, because of the damage they cause to frequently reproducing cells, alter the length and surface area of intestinal villi. The reduced ability of the gut to absorb nutrients and water that results can induce diarrhea and malabsorption.

Direct excitation of the centers for nausea and vomiting occurs to varying degrees with the majority of chemotherapy drugs.[22] This variability is dependent on the drug, dosage, and individual response. In addition to these nonspecific changes in nutritional intake, some drugs cause specific nutritional problems. For example, cisplatin can cause magnesium wasting, which may require replacement therapy.

Indirect effects of chemotherapy on nutrition status may occur as a result of symptoms that interfere with intake. Common symptoms in patients receiving chemotherapy include anorexia, fatigue, constipation, taste changes, food aversions, anxiety, and depression. The number and magnitude of these effects depend on the drugs chosen, their dosages, and the frequency and duration of drug administration. Although these side effects clearly alter nutrient intake during treatment, their significance to overall nutritional status has not been adequately studied.

Biotherapy/immunotherapy. The effects of biotherapy on nutritional status are both direct and indirect. Agents such as the interferons and interleukins cause anorexia, malaise, mucositis, nausea, and vomiting. Biotherapy-induced fevers directly increase energy and fluid needs. Indirect influences, such as fatigue and flulike symptoms, can make food procurement and preparation difficult. The magnitude and duration of these side effects are variable and may decrease over time. Their clinical effect on nutritional status is not well documented.

Targeted therapies. Targeted therapies represent a relatively new approach to the treatment of cancer. These pharmaceutical and biological agents work by interfering with key tumor molecules or signaling pathways that drive tumor biology. Early agents have demonstrated improved tolerability when compared to chemotherapy. Several therapies that target key molecular pathways are under study. Growth factors and their receptors have been extensively investigated, including epidermal growth factor receptor (EGFR), vascular endothelial growth factor (VEGF), vascular endothelial growth factor receptor (VEGFR), and human epidermal receptor 2 (HER2). Drugs that inhibit EGFR cause mechanism-based side effects, which include gastrointestinal alterations such as diarrhea and, to a lesser extent, nausea and vomiting.

The effects of targeted therapies on nutritional status have not been investigated. As therapeutic interventions evolve, it is essential to consider how they will influence the patient's ability to consume adequate nutrition.[23,24]

Multimodality therapy. Cancer patients often receive therapeutic modalities in combination. Patients with early-stage breast cancer, for example, typically have care that includes surgical intervention followed by chemotherapy and radiation. Patients with lung cancer or gastrointestinal malignancies are often treated with multimodality therapy. When such combinations are part of the therapeutic regimen, the patient's risk for nutritional disturbance is increased.

Normal Nutritional Physiology

Several models depict the complex relationships influencing nutrition; those used in much of the cancer literature are specific to the disease state.[13] An alternative approach, relying on a model of normal nutrient intake, demonstrates the effect of a variety of diseases on nutrition. This model can be especially helpful for persons with co-morbid diseases, which are common in the older cancer population. One such universal and historically classic model suggests that nutritional status is a function of an energy exchange system made up of four compartments: the reference compartment, set point, controller, and body storage.[25]

The *reference compartment* is the repository of the standards governing nutrient intake. The standards have physiological (e.g., growth factors, insulin, glucose, thyroxine, smell/taste transmitters), psychological (e.g., body image, self-esteem, meaning/sight/smell of food), and cultural (e.g., acceptable foods, eating patterns, social importance of food) determinants. These standards are monitored by the *set point.* The standards are maintained by the *controller,* largely through balancing energy intake and expenditure. Energy is obtained through the ingestion, digestion, and metabolism of macronutrients (carbohydrates, protein, lipids, and water) and micronutrients (minerals and vitamins). The controller requires an intact gastrointestinal tract, including proper secretory and motility function, to work properly.

The result of the controller activity is the *body storage,* or body composition. The components of the body compartment include fat, protein (skeletal muscle, viscera, plasma, bone, cartilage, collagen), glycogen, minerals, and water (intracellular and extracellular). The percentage of each of these components varies with genetics, gender, and age. The body storage provides feedback to the set point regarding its status via physiological, psychological, and cultural perceptions (e.g., serum glucose, conditioned responses, perceived images). Under stress, feedback may be directed to the reference compartment, with the possibility that standard levels will be changed. The interplay among the compartments, in the setting of an adequate nutrient intake, results in sufficient body storage for energy needs and protection from illness.

Pathophysiology

Cancer, host response, and cancer treatment all alter normal physiology. The alterations that affect nutritional status occur in the reference compartment, set point, and controller. These changes result in modified body storage, with the potential for development of obesity or cachexia.

Cancer-Induced Changes in the Reference Compartment

Changes in appetite

Much evidence indicates that loss of appetite is related to circulating factors produced by the cancer and the host.[15,26,27] These factors may be produced peripherally but have a central effect on the reference standards for appetite. Cytokines, including tumor necrosis factor (TNF), gamma interferon, leukemia inhibitory factor, and interleukin-1 and -6, have been proposed as one class of circulating anorectic agents.[15] Additionally, wasting can be induced by tumor products such as lipid-mobilizing factor and proteolysis-inducing factor (PIF), which can directly affect tissue metabolism.[15,28] Some evidence also supports an effect of neurotransmitters such as serotonin and dopamine on appetite suppression, although this effect is believed to be interrelated with the effects of hormones and cytokines.[27,29] Animal studies support the importance of serotonin and ammonia as anorectics in cancer; to date, studies in humans have been limited.[27]

Loss of appetite may be precipitated by cancer-induced psychological distress as well. Depression, anxiety, pain or pain medications, or situational factors (isolation, hospital food) may negatively influence food intake. Cancer-related fatigue, the most commonly reported symptom in cancer patients, has also been associated with diminished intake. Fatigue often interferes with activities of daily living and may limit the patient's ability to procure and prepare food. This problem may linger long after cancer treatment has been completed.

Increased appetite has been reported among women with breast cancer. Investigators suggest that increased as well as decreased appetite may occur as a function of psychological distress.[30–32] Many healthy women regularly limit their food intake. Following a breast cancer diagnosis, these women may lose their restraint, eat more, and gain weight. It has been suggested that extremes in diet, sometimes seen in the breast cancer population, may be associated with poor survival.[33] Additional studies in this area are needed.

Changes in taste and smell

Altered taste and smell sensors, with loss of taste and olfactory cues, change the normal references that are part of appetite and intake. Changes may be caused by direct tumor invasion; cancer-induced deficiencies of zinc, copper, nickel, vitamin A, and niacin; or cancer-associated circulating factors. Circulating factors are hypothesized to be the sources of taste changes occurring early in the disease process.

Physiological increases in the recognition thresholds for sweet, sour, and salty and decreases in the recognition levels for bitter are common. These threshold changes can lead to meat and other food aversions. Psychological factors may also contribute to food aversions. The hedonistic component of eating can be negatively influenced by alterations in taste or smell, leading to a reduced interest in eating and loss of appetite.

Changes in electrolyte balance

Alterations in micronutrient availability occur in paraneoplastic syndromes. Cancer can cause hypercalcemia and hypocalcemia, hyponatremia, or hyperphosphatemia and hypophosphatemia. At least some of these abnormalities are caused by tumor-produced hormones and can be life-threatening. They also cause altered mental status as well as taste changes, with associated problems in intake and adherence to treatment regimens.

Cancer-Induced Changes in the Controller

Changes in energy expenditure

Patients with cancer can have increased energy needs initiated by cancer-induced sepsis, fistulas, or lesions. These energy demands can produce malnutrition in some patients, but they are not responsible for cachexia. Although early research suggested that cachexia results from tumor-driven increases in energy expenditure, data in this area are inconsistent and a definitive etiology for cancer cachexia has not been explicated. In studies, cancer patients have exhibited increased, decreased, and normal resting energy rates. Proposed mechanisms for those patients who do have increased energy expenditure include heightened cytokine activity, especially TNF and interleukin-6, increased use of futile metabolic cycles, and inappropriate energy production in response to decreased intake.[15,26,27,34] Although some support exists for each of the mechanisms in some patients, none is universally found in cachexic patients. Regardless, increased energy expenditure may be a problem for a subset of patients with cancer, although it does not explain cancer cachexia in all cases.

Changes in nutrient metabolism

Cancer is associated with abnormalities in carbohydrate, protein, and lipid metabolism. Changes in carbohydrate metabolism include increased Cori cycle activity, altered peripheral utilization of glucose, increased glucose turnover, and glucose intolerance.[35,36] Glucose intolerance has been linked to insulin resistance, delayed glucose clearance, reduced glucose uptake in skeletal muscles, and an inability to produce glycogen in muscle. Unlike diabetics, individuals with cancer have normal plasma insulin levels. It is not known whether cancer patients also have normal insulin secretion. Although the origin of the glucose intolerance remains unknown, researchers have suggested that some cases may result from the cytokines produced by the host in response to the tumor.[35] Indirect effects of cancer that alter glucose metabolism include reduced activity and infection.

Increased hepatic glucose production has been reported in both undernourished and normal-weight patients with cancer.[35,36] The elevated glucose level is one of the features that differentiates cancer starvation/cachexia from normal starvation responses. In normal starvation, hepatic glucose production falls; this effect does not occur in cancer cachexia. The lack of a normal response to decreased intake may be related to the reliance of cancer on glucose or it may be the product of a cancer-associated abnormal growth hormone.

Individuals with cancer may develop altered protein metabolism. Some studies indicate that tumors preferentially take up nitrogen-containing materials.[26,35] Glutamine, an abundant amino acid required for DNA synthesis, may be one substance taken up by cancers to the detriment of the host. In addition to the shunting of needed proteins to the cancer, increased muscle breakdown and hepatic protein activity may occur.[15] Despite the increased hepatic activity, protein synthesis does not match protein catabolism. The net result is increased whole-body protein turnover. However, not all researchers have observed increased protein turnover, especially among cancer patients who are maintaining their weight.[37]

Abnormal lipid metabolism noted in cancer includes increased lipid mobilization and turnover, elevated triglyceride levels, decreased lipogenesis, altered glycerol transport, and decreased lipoprotein lipase activity.[26,35] To some degree, the alteration in fat metabolism may be related to insulin resistance, with preferential oxidation of fat rather than carbohydrates.

Changes in the gastrointestinal tract

Controller function is heavily dependent on an intact gastrointestinal system. Cancer can produce direct negative effects on the digestive system. Cancers of the aerodigestive structures can cause primary reduction in food and nutrient intake associated with the following problems:

- Difficulty chewing or swallowing
- Partial or complete obstruction
- Dysmotility
- Inactivation of bile salts or pancreatic enzymes
- Blind loop syndrome
- Fistulas
- Interference associated with pain (e.g., ulceration, nerve compression)

- Bowel wall and mesenteric infiltration
- Protein-losing enteropathy

The type and magnitude of the nutritional deficit depend on the tumor site and size. Nongastrointestinal cancers can cause alterations in nutritional status by interfering with food intake or increasing energy demand. Examples of these types of direct and indirect interference with intake include pain, dyspnea, blockages of mesenteric or peritoneal lymphatics, paraneoplastic syndromes that alter fluid or mineral balance, and altered cognitive function. Ulcerated lesions, both external and internal, increase nutrient need.

Changes in body storage

The degree of body storage alteration varies along the continuum of malnutrition. With small changes in nutrient intake or absorption, there may be no obvious change in body composition. In patients with weight gain, the compartment in which the change occurred should be determined. The most commonly affected compartments are the extracellular fluid and adipose tissue compartments. The most striking change in body composition is seen in cachexia. The total body fat and skeletal muscle components can decrease by as much as 85% and 75%, respectively.[15] Reduction in intracellular water and mineral supplies also occurs, albeit not to the same degree. Feedback signals from the body storage compartment are deranged, reflecting the effect of cytokine activity and metabolic dysfunction. The altered feedback perpetuates the nutritional deficiencies, making this condition extremely difficult to treat.

Treatment-Induced Changes in the Reference Compartment

Changes in appetite

Just as cancer causes changes in appetite, so can therapy. Depressed appetite can be caused by biotherapeutic agents — notably, TNF, interferon, and the interleukins.[22–24] Psychological responses to having and being treated for cancer with any modality may alter mood and change appetite. Medications prescribed for treatment may also affect mood and appetite. Some drugs produce increased — rather than decreased — appetite or nutrient intake. For example, corticosteroids, which are prescribed in both pediatric and adult populations, can increase appetite.

Surgical anesthesia, chemotherapy, and radiation produce indirect effects on appetite through the induction of treatment-related side effects such as nausea, vomiting, and food aversions. Anticipatory nausea and vomiting may develop if emetic control is poor during early cycles of chemotherapy. This conditioned response may have a substantial effect on appetite. The clinical significance of these changes is unclear, because some patients alter their choice of foods and eating patterns but not their total intake when faced with these symptoms.[38]

Taste changes can follow head and neck surgery, radiation, and chemotherapy. In addition, such changes may result from oral infections, use of antibiotics, or administration of other medications. These changes may be temporary and are sometimes related to zinc deficiency. In contrast, radiation and surgical alterations in gustatory and olfactory structures can be permanent. This change may result in an alteration of the normal references for food acceptability or in a general reduction in intake over time.

Treatment-Induced Changes in the Controller

Changes in energy expenditure

Treatment can affect energy needs both directly and indirectly. Some biotherapeutic agents elicit shaking chills and fever, which increase energy demands. Increased energy needs from fever and infection can also accompany bone marrow suppression. Moreover, antifungal agents administered to immunocompromised patients may produce fever and chill responses. Nutritional needs increase as the body responds to repair damage induced by surgery, radiation, or chemotherapy. Energy requirements are related to the type and magnitude of the treatment.

Changes in the gastrointestinal tract

Surgical resection removes or bypasses areas of the aerodigestive or gastrointestinal tract, causing a number of nutritional lesions. Chemotherapy and radiation cause direct injury to the intestinal villi, reducing the absorptive surface. Secondary candidiasis throughout the gastrointestinal tract can occur following antibiotic therapy associated with any treatment. These problems represent major threats to the proper absorption of both macronutrients and micronutrients. Side effects of treatment include anorexia, nausea, vomiting, lactose intolerance, diarrhea, and constipation, all of which can create obstacles to normal gut function and intake. In addition, chronic changes can occur. Total bowel resection, bone marrow transplant–induced graft-versus-host disease, and radiation enteritis can lead to long-term patient dependence on parenteral nutritional support.

Clinical Manifestations

The most common clinical manifestation identified with cancer is cancer cachexia, which is characterized by skeletal muscle wasting, weight loss, and reduced function. The patient may complain of loss of appetite, inability to eat, or early satiety. Because the nutrient deficiencies occur along a continuum, however, nutritional deficits can exist without these cardinal or extreme signs and symptoms. This is especially true of obese individuals, in whom weight loss can be overlooked. Fluid changes, such as edema or effusions, can mask protein and fat loss. The fact that nutritional disturbances can be subtle and are frequently nonspecific renders the need for assessment that much more important.

It is clear that cancer patients experience changes in body weight. Patients with lung, GI, and head and neck tumors experience not only weight loss exceeding 10% of total body weight, but also loss of both muscle and fat. Individuals with GI malignancies experience the largest decreases (>50%) in muscle mass and protein content, as well as 30%–40% loss of body fat. However, even patients who experience severe wasting retain some body fat. Visceral muscle is also preserved to some extent, whereas skeletal muscle loss is the primary form of lean body mass loss.[39] A recent study revealed that patients with solid tumors could lose as much as 1.34 kg of fat-free mass (FFM) in as little as 4 weeks.[40]

Screening, Assessment, and Grading

The goal of screening in nutrition is to identify those persons who are at risk of developing nutritional problems associated with their cancer. Nutritional screening is a far newer entity than nutritional assessment, and standardized approaches remain to be developed. Nutritional assessment, a more precise and diagnostic procedure, consists of four elements: anthropometrics, laboratory findings, clinical examination, and dietary evaluation. Although nurses play an integral part in accurate nutritional assessment, registered dietitians and nutritionists are more frequently responsible for the nutritional assessment. Nurses should enlist the aid of trained dietary specialists to assist with this aspect of nutritional care. Nurses often conduct screening for, and early detection tests of, nutritional deficits or excesses. For this reason, the discussion here concentrates on screening and anthropometrics. For more detailed information on assessment, the reader is referred to other sources.[41–43]

Nutritional Screening

The Joint Commission on Accreditation of Healthcare Organizations' (JCAHO) standards require the identification of clients who are nutritionally at risk by means of an initial screening mechanism. This screening must be completed within 24 hours of admission to a hospital, within 14 days of admission to a long-term care facility, or within a facility-defined period of time in ambulatory care and home care settings.[44] The American Society for Parenteral and Enteral Nutrition (ASPEN) published guidelines for nutritional screening in 2002. These guidelines state that a nutritional screen should include the following items: height, weight, weight change, primary diagnosis, and presence of co-morbid conditions.[45] In 2003, the American Dietetic Association implemented its Nutrition Care Process model, which is intended to direct the nutritional care of individuals with and without complex disease states. Nutritional screening is an essential preliminary step on which the success of an effective nutritional care plan depends.[8]

The need to assess nutritional status quickly and efficiently has inspired the development of a number of screening instruments. The Patient-Generated Subjective Global Assessment (PG-SGA) is currently endorsed by the American Dietetic Association for oncology patients and has been used by oncology nurses in a variety of settings. The PG-SGA was modified by Ottery from the Subjective Global Assessment of Nutritional Status (SGA), an instrument with proven sensitivity and specificity.[46–49] Both the SGA and PG-SGA evaluate weight change, dietary intake changes, gastrointestinal symptoms lasting more than 2 weeks, and activity levels. The PG-SGA includes cancer-specific symptoms and a refinement of the activity-level estimation. The patient is able to complete a portion of the assessment, thereby decreasing the amount of clinician time required for data collection. The clinician, taking into consideration the diagnosis, stage of cancer, estimated treatment- and tumor-associated metabolic demand, and findings from a focused physical examination, determines a rating of well-nourished, moderately (or suspected) malnourished, or severely malnourished. The PG-SGA takes only a few minutes to complete, making it a practical screening tool in a busy clinical setting. PG-SGA forms and additional information about scoring can be found on the Society for Nutritional Oncology and Adjuvant Therapy's (NOAT) web site, *www.ctrf.org/history.cfm.*

A number of formulas integrate several objective measures into assessment of prognosis (Table 31–1), including the Nutritional Index (NI), the Prognostic Nutritional Index (PNI), the Hospital Prognostic Index (HPI), and the Nutrition Risk Index (NRI). These indices are especially helpful in identifying

Table 31-1 Prognostic Nutrition Assessment Formulas

Nutritional Formula	Formula	Key to Formula
Nutritional index (NI)	1.9579 − 0.0017 × (IgM × prealbumin) − (0.0075 × complement factor C3) − (0.0066 × fibrinogen) + (0.033 × cholesterol) − (0.1858 × vitamin A–binding protein) + (0.6636 × thyroxine-binding globulin)	IgM, complement, fibrinogen, cholesterol, vitamin A–binding protein, and thyroxine are measured in mg/dL
Prognostic nutritional index (PNI)	158 − (16.6 × albumin) − (0.78 × triceps skin fold) − (0.2 × transferrin) − (5.8 × delayed hypersensitivity reaction)	Albumin is measured in g; triceps skin fold in mL; transferrin in mg/dL; delayed hypersensitivity as 0 (nonreactive), 1 (<5 mm reactivity), or 2 (≥5 mm reactivity)
Hospital prognostic index (HPI)	(0.91 × albumin) − (1.00 × delayed hypersensitivity) − (1.44 × sepsis rating) + (0.98 × diagnosis rating) − 1.09	Albumin is measured in g; delayed hypersensitivity as 1 (positive to 1 or more antigen) or 2 (nonreactive); sepsis as 1 (present) or 2 (absent); diagnosis as 1 (cancer present) or 2 (cancer not present)
Nutrition risk index (NRI)	(15.19 × albumin) + (0.417 × % usual body weight)	Albumin is measured in g; % usual body weight is actual weight/usual weight × 100

which individuals undergoing head and neck or gastrointestinal surgery might benefit from nutritional intervention prior to and following surgery.[50] The HPI and NRI utilize measures that are commonly used and readily available.

Nutritional Assessment

Nutritional assessment has historically been performed by a registered dietitian (RD). The nutritional care provided by an RD is often termed medical nutrition therapy (MNT). MNT is defined by the 2001 Medicare MNT benefit legislation as "nutritional diagnostic, therapy, and counseling services for the purpose of disease management which are furnished by a registered dietitian or nutrition professional."[8]

In 2003, the American Dietetic Association published the Nutrition Care Process (NCP) model. The NCP provides a structure for the provision of nutrition care to all patients and provides a framework by which the RD can think critically and make decisions regarding medical nutrition therapy. There are four steps to the process: nutritional assessment, nutritional diagnosis, nutritional intervention, and nutritional monitoring and evaluation.[8] The *nutritional assessment* is a comprehensive evaluation of a client's nutrition status, performed by an RD. Components of the assessment include medical, social, nutritional, and medication history; physical examination; anthropometric measurements; and laboratory data. The nutritional assessment builds on the information collected as part of the nutritional screening.[51] Its goal is to develop an effective nutrition plan of care that can address issues identified as part of the assessment and screening.[7] Based on the assessment, a decision about the individual's nutritional diagnosis is made. A *nutritional diagnosis* describes "an actual occurrence, risk of, or potential for developing a nutritional problem that dietetics professionals are responsible for treating independently."[8] *Nutritional intervention* is the activity intended to address that problem. The effects of this intervention are then monitored and evaluated, with changes being made as necessary.

Anthropometrics

Anthropometrics, the measurement of the weight, size, and proportions of the body, commonly includes height, weight, and skin-fold thickness. Serial weight measurement is perhaps the single most important indicator of nutritional status for the clinician, although its importance is often underemphasized. Weights need to be measured from a reliable baseline using instruments that are periodically calibrated to maintain their accuracy and precision. Serial weight measurement is also the anthropometric measure most often provided by nursing staff. Standard weight measurement is inexpensive, quick, and practical.

Weight should not be considered the sole determinant of nutritional status, however, as weight alone does not reveal body composition. Weight among individuals with cancer may reflect tumor mass or fluid retention while masking loss of lean body mass. For example, children with abdominal masses are at risk for being considered at normal weight for height, despite loss of lean body mass. Adults with ascites are at similar risk. Attempts have been made to improve body composition determination through a variety of measures: ultrasound, computerized tomography, magnetic resonance imaging, dual-photon and dual-energy radiographic absorptiometry, neutron activation, total body potassium, total body water, and bioelectrical impedance. These techniques vary in their invasiveness, availability, and expense. Currently, the primary use of these measures is in research, not routine assessment.

For the most part, clinical body composition estimates utilized in daily patient care rely on weight measures coupled with additional anthropometrics, such as height or skin folds.

Bioelectrical impedance analysis (BIA) provides an estimate of total body water (TBW) via a measure of electrical impedance within the body. Using values of TBW derived from BIA, one can then estimate FFM and body fat. BIA is based in the principle that the body is a biological circuit, such that a fixed, low-voltage, high-frequency current introduced into the human body is conducted almost completely through the greater electrolyte content of the fluid compartment of FFM. It is assumed that the total conductive volume of the body is equivalent to TBW. The opposition to the flow of this current, called resistance, is measured.[52,53] The measured resistance is approximately equivalent to that of muscle tissue. Impedance measures vary with the frequency of current used. The current typically used with single-frequency BIA (SFBIA) is 50 kHz, the characteristic frequency for skeletal muscle tissue.[53] BIA has the potential to provide valuable information about changes in oncology patients' body composition. This technology is inexpensive, does not require specific operator skills, and provides no burden to the subject.[54] Studies of ambulatory normal-weight and underweight cancer patients have concluded that the SFBIA parameter ht^2 R is highly correlated with TBW in this population. Note that BIA systematically overestimates TBW in underweight patients (BMI < 19.6) by 5.0% when a prediction model that was developed for normal-weight healthy subjects is used.

Weight combined with height measurement, or ideal body weight (IBW), is an indirect indicator of body composition. It can be used to screen for both undernutrition and overnutrition. The Metropolitan Life Insurance Company Height–Weight Table was used at one time as such a screening device.[55] Because of its possible inaccuracy, stemming from (1) its use of clinician estimation rather than calculation of frame size and (2) its reliance on data from white, insured persons aged 25–59 as the basis of the table, concerns have arisen about using the Metropolitan table. Although Metropolitan standards have been shown to be applicable to nonwhite U.S. populations, few comparisons have been made with black women and the majority of Asian Pacific populations. Moreover, considerable controversy continues over what should be considered the normal range of age-related weight increases. Thus, the Metropolitan tables should be used in conjunction with other measures to determine nutritional status and with an understanding of their limitations.

Table 31-2 Classification of BMI in Adults

	Degree of Adiposity
Underweight	< 18.5 kg/m^2
Normal weight	18.5–24.9 kg/m^2
Overweight	25–29.9 kg/m^2
Obesity (class 1)	30–34.9 kg/m^2
Obesity (class 2)	35–39.9 kg/m^2
Extreme obesity (class 3)	≥40 kg/m^2

Data from National Institutes of Health.[58]

Another method of calculation of ideal body weight more commonly utilized is the Hamwi method. This method estimates weight for height based on frame size.[56] It provides only a rough estimate of ideal body weight, however, and it does not take into account age, race, and the differences in body composition that occur in athletes.[57]

Males

- Medium frame: 106 pounds for the 1st five feet, plus 6 pounds for every inch over.
- Small frame: Subtract 10% from the medium-frame number.
- Large frame: Add 10% to the medium-frame number.

Females

- Medium frame: 100 pounds for the first 5 feet, plus 5 pounds for every inch over.
- Small frame: Subtract 10% from the medium-frame number.
- Large frame: Add 10% to the medium-frame number.

Weight and height can also be used to calculate the BMI. The BMI (Table 31-2) is considered a more accurate estimation of total body fat than the Metropolitan weight tables. The BMI has limited utility in individuals with increased lean muscle mass or with large frames. It is also more relevant for determining obesity than for assessing undernutrition. The formula for BMI calculation is

Weight in kilograms/height in meters squared

OR

Weight in pounds/height in inches squared × 704.5

In an oncology population a weight measure that is more important than ideal body weight is the percent of usual body weight (UBW). This calculation determines the change in an individual's weight over time, using that individual as a standard to which measure-

Table 31-3 Categories of Weight Loss and Malnutrition

Degree of Malnutrition	
Mild	85%–90% UBW
Moderate	75%–84% UBW
Severe	<74% UBW
Significant Weight Loss	
5% loss in 1–3 months	
7.5% loss in 3–6 months	
10% loss in 6 or more months	
Severe Weight Loss	
>5% loss in 1 month	
>7.5% loss in 3 months	
>10% loss in 6 months	

UBW = usual body weight.
Data from Blackburn, Bistrian.[59]

ments are compared. The degree of change in body weight is used to assess the degree of malnutrition. Table 31-3 provides a description of how change in usual body weight is classified.

Despite the overall importance, practicality, and clinical relevance of weight and height measurements in nutritional assessment, the reliability of both measures is questionable when calibration checks of scales and uniform measuring methods are not practiced. Scales should be calibrated regularly. Self-calibrating scales also should be tested periodically. Using patient-reported weight and height should be discouraged. Training in accurate measurement and monitoring for quality assurance could improve the assessment process.

Additional anthropometrics used in nutritional assessment include skin-fold thickness and body-part circumferences to assess fat and muscle compartments. The assumptions underlying the use of skin-fold measures in this way remain the subject of debate, as do the number and specific skin-fold measures that should be included in assessment. In addition, reliability of measurement is dependent on training and quality control. For these reasons, skin-fold measures are rarely used; when cause for their use presents itself, the procedure is best performed by a registered dietitian or nutritionist.

Calculating Energy Needs

Another important function of the anthropometric measures of height and weight relates to their use in calculating an individual's energy needs. Currently, a very accurate assessment of energy needs can be obtained via indirect measurement of energy expenditure. Indirect calorimetry is one example of such an assessment. Indirect calorimetry requires the measurement of an individual's oxygen and carbon dioxide content of expired and inspired breath. It can be expensive and is not always practical in ambulatory settings. Much research has been devoted to creating equations that generate estimates of energy needs similar to those obtained through indirect calorimetry. To date, more than 200 equations have been designed for estimating the nutritional needs of various patient groups. A small representation of these equations is presented in Table 31-4. Caloric prescriptions for individuals with cancer are frequently based on the Harris-Benedict (HB) equation. Another equation used in critically ill oncology patients is the Ireton-Jones equation.

These equations indicate the number of calories expended while the individual is at rest, or the *resting energy expenditure* (REE). This number is corrected for the level of required energy and varies according to activity, treatment, and co-morbid condition (Table 31-5). Kondrup et al. advise factoring for activity level, stress, and desired weight gain.[63] However, few estimates have focused on the energy required by individuals with cancer; those that are available suggest that determining the appropriate caloric need is difficult. Ulander et al. found that although 66% of patients with colon cancer expended less than their estimated basal energy postoperatively, they also lost weight, indicating that providing adequate nutrition based on HB estimates did not translate into weight maintenance.[19] Ringwald-Smith et al. reported that the HB equation overestimated energy requirements before bone marrow transplant and underestimated energy needs after transplant. Thus, careful choice of correction factors is needed.[64]

Laboratory Tests

Laboratory tests are commonly used to evaluate nutritional status.[46,50] It is important to remember that most laboratory tests are nonspecific for malnutrition. Example test results include low blood count, decreased lymphocyte count, and delayed hypersensitivity testing, all of which can be affected by both cancer and cancer treatment. In addition, the tests are often not sensitive to nutritional deficiencies. For example, severe nutritional deficiencies may exist before albumin levels fall. Serum albumin is a poor marker for screening or early detection purposes but an excellent indicator of prognosis.[65] Because laboratory parameters can be influenced by a number of other factors, it is essential that all values be considered within the patient's specific clinical context.[66]

Table 31-4 Selected Adult Nutritional Assessment Equations

Nutritional Assessment Method	Formula	History
Calorie per kilogram	25–35 Calories/kg	Extrapolated from the WHO calculations. Estimated based on nonobese population. ASPEN recommends that predictive energy requirements should fall within the range of 20–35 Calories/kg.
World Health Organization (WHO)	Women: 18–30 years = 15.3(weight in kg) + 679 30–60 years = 11.6(weight in kg) + 879 >60 years = 8.8(weight in kg) + 1128(height in m) − 1071 Men: 18–30 years = 14.7(weight in kg) + 496 30–60 years = 8.7(weight in kg) + 829 >60 years = 9.2(weight in kg) + 637(height in m) − 302	Developed by FAO/WHO in 1974 for a healthy population.[60]
Harris-Benedict	Women: REE = [655 + 9.6(weight in kg) + 1.7(height in cm)] ÷ 4.7(age in years) Men: REE = [66 + 1.37(weight in kg) + 5(height in cm)] ÷ 6.8(age in years)	Developed in 1919 from studies of indirect calorimetry of 239 men and women. Random error calculations female equation ($r^2 = 0.53$), male calculation ($r^2 = 0.75$).[57,61]
Ireton-Jones	Ventilator dependent: EEE = 1784 − 11(a) + 5(w) + 244(s) + 239(t) + 804(b) Spontaneous breathing: EEE = 629 − 11(a) + 25(w) − 609(o) a = age (years) w = body weight (kg) s = sex (male = 1, female = 0) t = trauma (present = 1, absent = 0) b = burn (present = 1, absent = 0) o = obesity [BMI > 27] (present = 1, absent = 0)	Developed for critically ill and hospitalized patients using indirect calorimetry.[61]
Mifflin-St. Jeor	Women: REE = −161 + 10(weight in kg) + 6.25(height in cm) − 5(age) Men: REE = 5 + 10(weight in kg) + 6.25(height in cm) − 5(age)	Developed in 1990 from studies of 247 women and 251 men. ($r^2 = 0.71$)
Dietary reference intake for energy	Women: EEE = 354 − 6.91(age) + PA[9.36(weight in kg) + 726(height in m)] Men: EEE = 662 − 9.53(age) + PA[9.36(weight in kg) + 539.6(height in m)] PA (physical activity coefficient): Sedentary = 1.00 Low active = 1.11 Active = 1.25 Very active = 1.48	Developed in 2002 by the Institute of Medicine from studies of doubly labeled water for use in a healthy population.[62]

REE = resting energy expenditure.
EEE = estimated energy expenditure.

Physical Examination

Physical examination is limited in its ability to distinguish between the effects of cancer and the effects of nutritional deficiency. The fact that physical changes such as glossitis, muscle wasting, or diarrhea exist in many patients with cancer secondary to their disease or treatment does not minimize these changes' usefulness as indicators of problems in energy intake, absorption, or need. The patient's general appearance is important. The level of mobility may provide informa-

Table 31-5 Correction Factors for Use with Measures of Resting Energy Expenditure

	Energy Correction Factor
Activity Factors	
Confined to bed	1.2 × REE
Sedentary	1.4–1.9 × REE
Active	2.0–2.4 × REE
Stress Factors	
Fever	1.0 + 0.13 per 1°C > 37°C × REE
Elective surgery	1.0–1.1 × REE
Sepsis	1.2–1.4 × REE
Multiple trauma	1.4 × REE
Cancer	1.1–1.45 × REE
Burns	1.5–2.1 × REE
Infection with trauma	1.3–1.55 × REE
Severe infection	1.2–1.6 × REE

Data from Edel, Murray, Schurer, et al.[57]

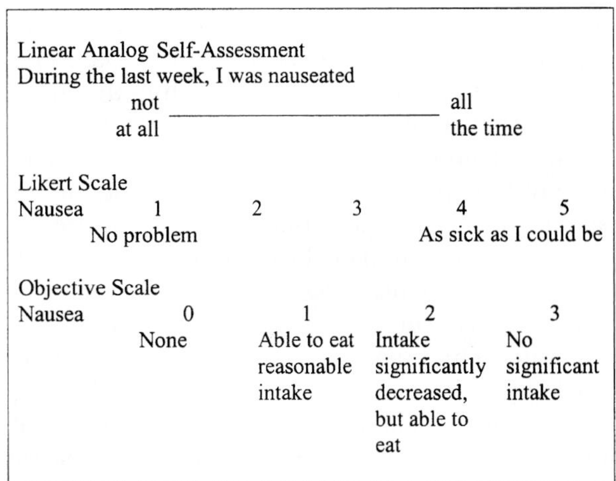

Figure 31–1 Examples of nutritionally linked symptom measurement

tion about functional status; fat and muscle status can be assessed by visualizing the posterior ribs, scapula, or spine. Skin tone and turgor should be noted. Scaling skin may indicate vitamin (niacin) or trace element (zinc) deficiencies. An assessment of fluid status should also be conducted.[66] In addition, physical examination may identify other cancer-related changes, such as fevers, fistulas, or external lesions that influence the intake or expenditure of energy.

Dietary Information

Dietary intake information is used to identify existing and potential nutritional excesses and deficits. In a full diet history, information that reflects both diet and general health is included. General questions alert the nurse to the need for more in-depth study of dietary intakes. Dietary information is obtained by using a number of approaches: 24-hour recall surveys, food frequency measures, diet diaries, calorie counts, or monthly purchase records. The last method is rarely used in clinical practice. Any of the types of food-intake recordings provide information about energy, nutrient, vitamin, and mineral intakes. Obtaining this information requires variable amounts of time to input the data into nutrient analysis programs. The need for this depth of assessment will depend on the setting. Full dietary assessments are usually conducted by registered dietitians or nutritionists. However, the nurse should be alert to nursing assessment items of weight change, recent changes in intake, symptoms that influence eating or food preparation, and indications that alternative or complementary nutritional products are being used.

Functional Assessment

Assessment of the ability to perform the activities of daily living, especially in the areas of food procurement and preparation, are part of a thorough nutritional assessment. For the past two decades, performance level assessments have also been used to determine the relationship of nutrition to function.[67,68] The use of more specific measures, such as muscle strength, have likewise been suggested as sensitive indicators of both positive and negative changes in food intake.[69,70] However, the use of such measures remains uncommon except in research situations.

Nutrition-Related Symptom Assessment

Assessment of symptoms that interfere with intake is part of an oncological nutritional assessment. These symptoms may include anorexia, nausea, vomiting, diarrhea, constipation, mouth sores, dry mouth, pain when eating or swallowing, other pain, taste change, fatigue, difficulty in swallowing, indigestion, early satiety, cramping, and bloating. Linear analog self-assessment, Likert scales, or narrative grading scales are useful in identifying the severity of the problem and the effectiveness of intervention[71] (Figure 31–1). A proactive approach with anticipatory interventions is the most effective means of minimizing the negative effects of symptoms on nutritional status.[72]

Therapeutic Approaches and Nursing Care

Because malnutrition is associated with poor outcomes, including increased morbidity and mortality and decreased quality of life,[73,74] interventions that might prevent or minimize nutritional problems represent a worthy goal. Ongoing research in this area is exploring nutritional manipulation in cancer prevention, as an adjunct to standard cancer therapy and as a mode of therapy. In addition, continuing studies are examining interventions that could minimize the threats of treatment to the host's nutritional status.[75,76] Optimal nutrition planning utilizes a nutritional team with expertise in cancer-associated malnutrition. When such a program is not available, a general nutritional support team may be of assistance. Development of a nutritional care plan may require the collaboration of nurses, physicians, dietitians, pharmacists, speech therapists, and social workers. The patient and family or significant others are an integral part of this effort. Without their participation in goal setting and method choice, it is unlikely that any intervention will succeed.

Interventions must also be based on realistic goals and ethical considerations. Goals may target specific or general dietary components to influence morbidity, mortality, appetite, function, or well-being. For patients in whom response to treatment is expected or for whom morbidity will be reduced, intervention is a sound practice. Goal setting within an ethical context can be more difficult for individuals with progressing disease, anorexia, and weight loss. Often, family members concentrate on reversing the patient's lack of appetite and weight loss, which can put undue stress on the patient and the family relationship. Since eating is often a major source of comfort and enhances quality of life, the use of interventions that improve appetite and alter the metabolic abnormalities should be considered where appropriate. In situations where the patient is in the terminal stages of illness and unable to eat or drink fluids, then allowing dehydration to proceed is ethically and legally acceptable.[77,78]

Oncology nurses play a key role in assessing nutritional issues across the continuum of cancer care. Nurses should be knowledgeable about nutritional issues commonly encountered in the cancer population and anticipate those issues in patients for whom they provide care.

Nutritional Interventions

The nutritional assessment, described previously and performed by members of the nutritional team, provides the basis for the nutritional prescription and development of intervention strategies. Possible prescriptions range from oral supplementation or deletion of specific nutrients to institution of total parenteral nutrition. Strategies include verbal counseling to alter intake or manage symptoms, prescription of medications to minimize side effects, and identification of resources to facilitate treatment with oral supplements, tube-administered enteral nutrition, or total parenteral nutrition. The level of intervention and accompanying strategy are dictated by the patient's baseline nutritional state, disease status, risks for malnutrition from treatment, anticipated response to therapy, and resources. Algorithms for individuals at normal weight and those who are undernourished are provided in Figures 31–2 and 31–3.

Nutritional Prescription

Alteration in specific dietary components

The development of some nutrient deficiencies is common across diseases. For example, low serum iron and potassium are not unusual in a number of chronic diseases. In patients with cancer, these deficits arise from a combination of chemotherapy-related effects on bone marrow, anemia of chronic disease, medications for co-morbid conditions, and antibiotic use. Other deficiencies that are more specific to cancer include hypomagnesemia related to platinum chemotherapy; hyponatremia and hypercalcemia, resulting from paraneoplastic syndromes; and zinc deficiency accompanying head and neck cancers. Intervention with parenteral fluids or supplements may be required for some patients; in others, oral mineral supplementation is used to control these problems. Educating the patient about foods that are good sources of the deficient mineral may also be helpful.

In addition to reversing known deficiencies, supplemental nutrients are given to minimize the side effects and maximize the therapeutic effect of standard treatment. The role of immunonutrition, or specific nutrients, such as arginine, omega-3 fatty acids, and glutamine, in the diet remains controversial. Consensus recommendations, published in 2001, concluded that immune-enhancing diets containing arginine, glutamine, omega-3 fatty acids, and RNA nucleotides are beneficial to severely malnourished patients undergoing major surgery. Subsequent analysis indicated a possible benefit in critically ill patients and no benefit in the postoperative period.[79,80] Glutamine supplementation may provide the benefits of protection from chemotherapy-induced mucositis, diarrhea, neuropathy, hepatic venoocclusive disease, and cardiotoxicity. Oral glutamine supplementation may also protect normal tissues from, and sensitize tumor cells to, radiation therapy.[81] The increased use of these approaches depends on additional study to verify their

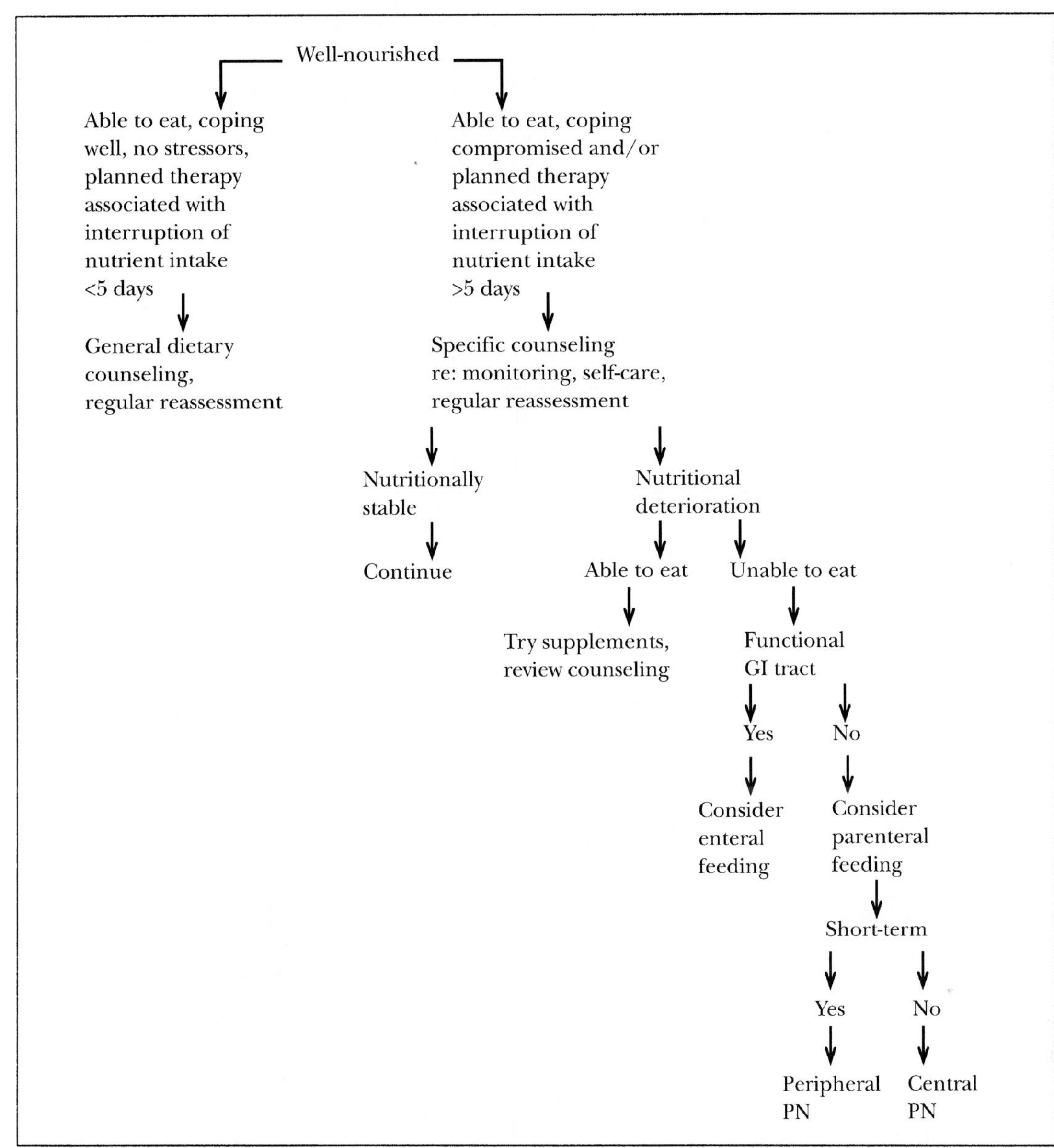

Figure 31–2 Nutritional support algorithm for individuals well-nourished at baseline. (GI = gastrointestinal tract; PN = parenteral nutrition)

effectiveness, target population, dosages, and scheduling.

Similarly, reduction of specific macronutrients has been the target of nutritional intervention. Dietary fat intake has become a target for specific treatment, especially among patients with breast cancer.[13,82] Clinical trials indicate that verbal counseling results in significantly decreased fat intake within 3 months among patients with breast cancer.[83] The altered intake pattern is sustained past the period of counseling. Several of the trials have found documented increased survival among participants.[84] Reduction of fat in combination with other diet manipulations are also being tested.[85]

Alteration in general intake

A more traditional nutritional goal has been the improvement of the patient's overall intake to aid general nutritional status, minimize treatment side effects, and maximize treatment delivery. Increases in nutrient intake can significantly reduce the morbidity and mortality among severely malnourished patients in certain settings. However, the complex interaction of nutrition, cancer, and host can alter the usual response to increased intake. Investigators report that increased caloric intake may neither reverse weight loss nor improve survival.[86] Because of this complexity, specialized nutritional augmentation is not recom-

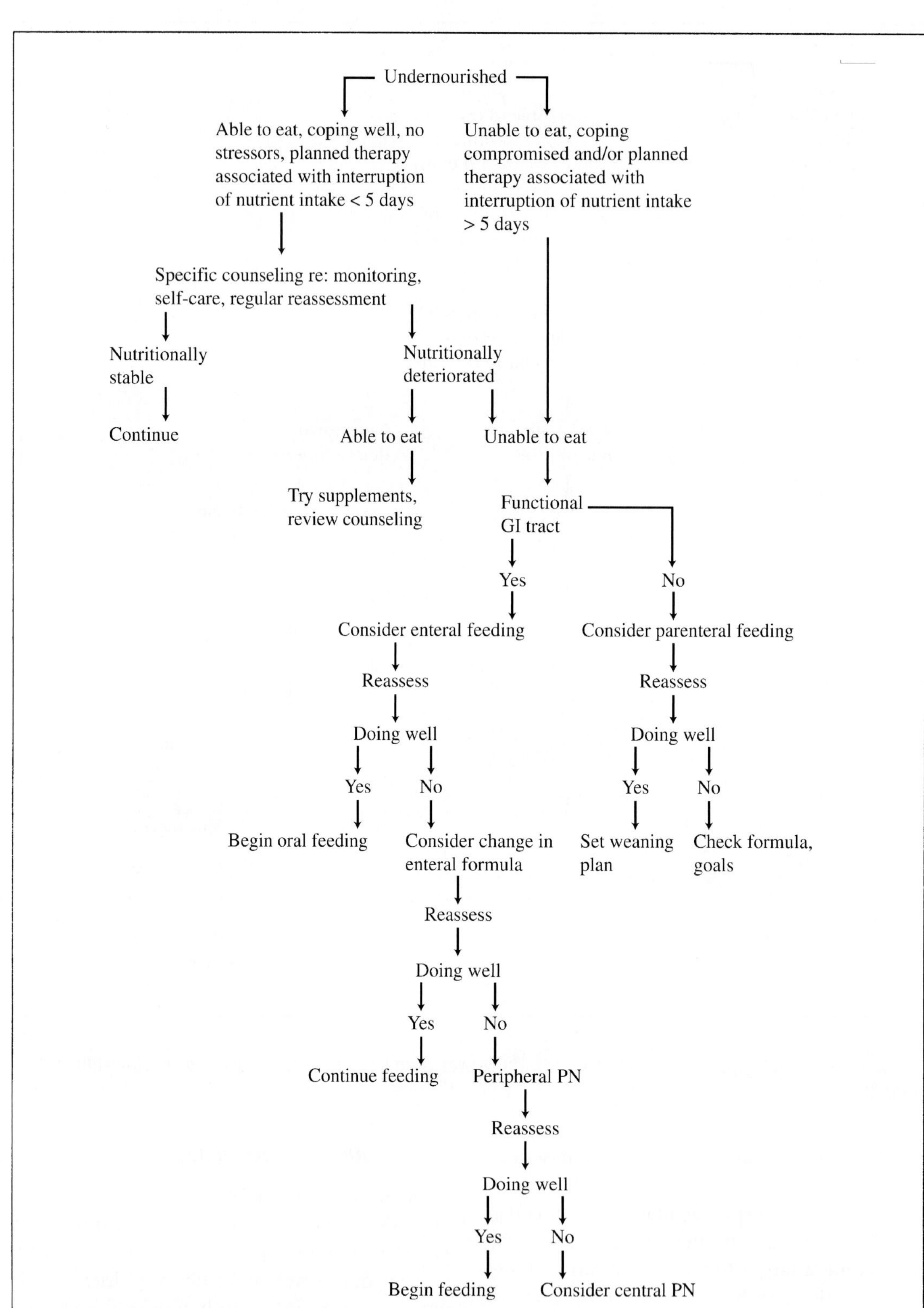

Figure 31–3 Nutritional support algorithm for individuals undernourished at baseline. (GI = gastrointestinal tract; PN = parenteral nutrition)

Table 31-6 Suggested Interventions for Nutrition-Related Side Effects

Side Effect	Suggested Interventions*
Appetite change	Alter food choice, increase oral hygiene; avoid sight, smell of food; eat sour foods; eat cold foods; use straw; increase seasoning; use plastic utensils; small amount of alcohol.
Constipation	Increase liquid intake; eat more fiber; eat more fruit; exercise; take laxative; drink hot beverages; add bran to foods.
Diarrhea	Take medicine; increase fluids; drink rehydration fluids; low-residue diet; avoid spices and caffeine, avoid milk products; take soluble-fiber supplement; eat low-fat diet.
Dry mouth	Take medicine (pilocarpine, saliva substitutes in xerostomia); increase fluids; chew gum; suck on sugarless candy; blend foods; avoid acid, salty, or spicy foods; moisten food, humidify air; apply oil to oral cavity.
Early satiety	Eat frequently, eat small meals; drink between meals; limit liquids at meals.
Mucositis	Take medicine (sucralfate, capsaicin, GSF, antibiotic pastilles, interleukin-1); apply cold (ice) to oral cavity during chemotherapy administration; increase oral hygiene; drink liquids; use soft toothbrush; avoid spicy food; humidify air; avoid use of gravy; use baking-soda mouthwash; apply mucosa-adhesive film, avoid alcohol and tobacco; use straws; use supplements; use glutamine.
Nausea	Take medicine; alter diet; practice relaxation; listen to music; rest after meals; avoid sight, smell of food; eat cold foods; increase oral hygiene; eat small frequent meals; eat slowly; get fresh air; drink clear liquids; keep busy/distracted; chew food well; drink between meals; eat crackers; breathe through the mouth; eat sour foods; eat low-fat foods; avoid spicy foods; eat sweet foods.
Conditioned nausea	Practice relaxation or deconditioning imagery, self-hypnosis; take medication.
Taste change	Alter food choice; increase oral hygiene; avoid sight, smell of food; eat sour foods; eat cold foods; increase seasoning; use straw; avoid tart foods; chew sugarless gum; eat less fat; use plastic utensils.
Vomiting	Take medicine; practice relaxation; rest after meals; drink clear liquids; avoid sight, smell of food; eat slowly; eat crackers; eat cold foods; get fresh air; chew mint candy; eat room-temperature foods; alter diet; increase oral hygiene; eat small frequent meals; eat low-fat diet; avoid spicy foods.

GSF = granulocyte-stimulating factor.
*Boldface type indicates that research support exists for the intervention.

mended for individuals who are adequately nourished, who are not anticipated to be unable to eat for 10–14 days, or who have uncontrolled disease.[45] These criteria may provide direction for healthcare providers who are considering the ethics of either supplying or withholding nutritional supplementation.

Nutritional Strategies

Verbal counseling and education

Verbal counseling can be extremely effective in assisting patients to choose calorie-dense foods and treat symptoms that interfere with oral intake.[86] A number of self-care actions have been proposed for treatment of cancer-induced nutritional problems. Patient education material commonly includes interventions related to decreased appetite, nausea, vomiting, constipation, taste changes, and mucositis. To date, little research has explored the effectiveness of most of these actions. Of those studies that employed an experimental approach, the majority have included nonpharmacological interventions. Much of what is suggested to patients regarding treatment of side effects is not based on scientific evidence or systematic review of patient experience. Moreover, some of the interventions are global in nature. For example, counseling and psychoeducational approaches have benefited patients having nausea. However, the actual content of the counseling and psychoeducational interventions has not been standardized, so research application is difficult. Table 31-6 lists common nutritional interventions; those that have been supported by research are highlighted. Much more research is needed before nurses can accurately predict which intervention will prove effective for a specific patient in a given situation.

Patients and their families may identify self-care activities that differ from those commonly suggested in the cancer patient education literature. The oncology nurse must be aware of these actions and the beliefs underlying them. If the nurse determines there is no potential harm, then ways to integrate the beliefs can be devised. Discovery of such beliefs and folkways takes some perception and skill, but is basic to a full assessment of the patient.

Pharmacological interventions

Medications are used by patients to prevent or treat a number of nutrition-related problems. Taking medicine is the most effective self-care technique reported in controlling constipation, diarrhea, nausea, vomiting, and mucosal irritation.[74,87] Psychotropic drugs also may assist those patients for whom depression is a factor in diminished appetite. Medications have been prescribed to improve appetite and increase nutrient intake, offset cancer-induced metabolic disturbances, and limit or reverse losses of lean body mass.

The medications most often prescribed counter loss of appetite. They include alcohol, corticosteroids, megestrol acetate, metoclopramide, and dronabinol.[26,75,88] Trials of cyproheptadine hydrochloride, a drug used in nonmalignant disease for appetite stimulation, have not prevented weight loss among individuals with cancer.[88]

No formal trials have examined the effectiveness of alcohol as an appetite stimulant, although anecdotal evidence supports its benefit. Alcohol has the advantage of being readily available and inexpensive, although cultural, religious, and physical conditions may restrict its use. There are also relatively few trials of corticosteroids, although they have been used for more than 20 years to treat anorexia.[89–91] The studies that are available report temporary, symptomatic improvement in appetite and function, especially in individuals with asthenia and tumor-induced fever.

Megestrol acetate has been found to improve appetite, cause weight gain, control nausea, and improve quality of life among individuals with cancer.[91–94] However, this weight gain appears to be fat gain, not the desired increase in lean body mass.[91] Megestrol acetate's mechanism of action may be related to its effect on cytokine activity and adipocytes. Dosages range from 160 to 800 mg/day. Factors to be considered in evaluating the use of this drug include the number of pills, cost, and potential side effects. Megestrol acetate now comes in a liquid form, reducing the mechanical problem of swallowing numerous tablets. Its side effects include edema and hyperglycemia, with some increase in risk of an embolism. For this reason, megestrol acetate should be avoided in individuals with congestive heart failure, pericardial effusions, or history of thrombotic problems. More recently, reports have described severe symptomatic adrenal suppression in pediatric oncology patients at doses of 10 mg/kg per day.[95] Diabetics should monitor themselves closely, especially during initiation of treatment.

Metoclopramide has been used to improve oral intake based on its effect on nausea, gastric motility, early satiety, and reflux.[88,91] The usual dose is 10 mg taken orally before meals and at bedtime. Very few trials have been performed to study the drug's effect on intake and weight, and more studies are needed.

Dronabinol, like metoclopramide, has been explored largely in terms of its effect on chemotherapy-induced nausea and vomiting. Few randomized trials have investigated the effect of the drug on appetite. Increases in weight have been reported at doses ranging from 2.5 mg twice per day to 15 mg per day.[91] Changes in weight may be related to fluid retention or fat rather than increased lean body mass. Dronabinol's effectiveness may be greater in individuals who have used the drug before. Side effects are more common in older persons, especially at higher doses, but may be reduced with timing administration of the drug after a meal. Cost and concerns about the abuse of cannabinoids may limit its acceptance, even though abuse of dronabinol is not common.[96]

Eicosapentaenoic acid (EPA) is an essential fatty acid, most abundantly found in fish oils and plant sources such as algae, flaxseed, and walnuts, and a new addition to the fight against cancer-induced weight loss. Multiple studies have utilized liquid nutritional supplements as a vehicle for administration of 1–2 g of EPA to patients with weight loss or cachexia. To date, the majority of the research with EPA has involved patients with pancreatic cancer. Results indicate slowing or reversing of weight loss in these patients. Noncompliance with the regimen is a commonly cited problem.[97–100]

Several drugs have been tested for their normalizing effect on metabolism, including insulin, hydrazine sulfate, and pentoxifylline.[91] Unfortunately, clinical trials suggest that these drugs are not useful. Insulin use is complicated by the difficulties of side effect management. Hydrazine sulfate and pentoxifylline showed promise in early trials, but placebo-controlled studies have indicated that neither offers a significant benefit. Additional drugs being tested in the cachectic AIDS population include thalidomide and melatonin, both of which have been associated with weight stabilization or reduced weight loss. Preliminary studies in cancer patients indicate reduced weight loss and some gain in lean body mass. [91,101]

Drugs that have been investigated for their ability to maintain lean body mass include the anabolic steroids fluoxymesterone, nandrolone, and oxandrolone and the growth hormone rhGH. Available research indicates that nandrolone is associated with significant improvements in weight, lean body mass, and quality of life in patients with AIDS but not in patients with lung cancer. Oxandrolone induces weight gain or maintenance in 81% of patients with cancer cachexia.[102] Growth hormone use results in short-term conservation of protein in patients with AIDS. Studies in more diverse cancer populations and with rigorous designs are needed before the use of these drugs can be supported as routine care.

Table 31-7 Guidelines for the Use of Nutrition Support in Cancer Patients

ADA Goals of Medical Nutrition Therapy[103]

- Maintain adequate intake of calories and protein.
- Select foods to limit the side effects of treatments.
- Maintain stable weight.
- After treatments, adopt healthy eating plans.

2002 ASPEN Guidelines[45]

- Specialized nutrition support is appropriate in patients receiving active anticancer treatment who are malnourished and are anticipated to be unable to ingest and or absorb adequate nutrients for a prolonged period of time.
- Preoperative specialized nutrition support may be beneficial in moderately or severely malnourished patients if administered for 7–14 days preoperatively, but the potential benefits of nutrition support must be weighed against the potential risks of the nutrition support itself.
- Specialized nutrition support should not be used routinely in patients undergoing major cancer operations. Use of nutrition support in patients undergoing major cancer operations does not improve surgical outcome.
- Specialized nutrition support should not be used routinely as an adjunct to chemotherapy.
- Specialized nutrition support should not be used routinely in patients undergoing head and neck, abdominal, or pelvic irradiation.
- The palliative use of specialized nutrition support in terminally ill patients with cancer is rarely indicated.

NCI Contraindications to Enteral Nutrition Support[104]

- Malfunctioning gastrointestinal tract.
- Malabsorptive conditions.
- Mechanical obstructions.
- Severe bleeding.
- Severe diarrhea.
- Intractable vomiting.
- Gastrointestinal fistulas in locations difficult to bypass with an enteral tube.
- Inflammatory bowel processes:
    - Prolonged ileus.
    - Severe enterocolitis.
- Overall health prognosis not consistent with aggressive nutrition therapy.

NCI Contraindications to Parenteral Nutrition Support[104]

- Functional gut.
- Limited life expectancy (<40 days).
- Lack of adequate vascular access.
- Lack of severe nutritional deficit such as temporary inability to eat (e.g., postsurgery).

ADA = American Dietetic Association.
ASPEN = American Society for Parenteral and Enteral Nutrition.
NCI = National Cancer Institute.

Enteral and Parenteral Nutrition

When severe malnutrition exists or oral intake is threatened for longer than a week, alternative methods of intake should be explored. Table 31-7 provides guidelines for the use of nutritional support in cancer patients.

If the gastrointestinal tract is functioning, enteral feeding is the intervention of choice. It is crucial for individuals with aerodigestive or upper gastrointestinal surgery. Enteral feeding protects suture lines postoperatively and is also effective for individuals with gastrointestinal obstructions that can be bypassed by tube placement. This feeding option, especially in the upper gastrointestinal tract, maintains the normal stimulation of enzymatic and mucosal activity in the gut, an important attribute when oral feeding is to be resumed.[43,45,105]

For individuals without a functioning gastrointestinal tract, total parenteral nutrition (TPN) may be the nutritional treatment of choice. A number of studies have reported the effect of TPN on the morbidity and mortality in malnourished patients undergoing surgery and have been critically reviewed.[45,105] Total parenteral nutrition has been associated with reduced morbidity in bone marrow transplant treatment when administered either before cytoreduction or when gastrointestinal reaction denudes the gut mucosa.[45] Patients with significant gastrointestinal malfunction, but otherwise with cured, controlled, or indolent disease, may also benefit from parenteral feeding. The largest group of cancer patients receiving home parenteral nutrition are those with chronic obstruction.[106]

Other uses of aggressive nutritional support remain controversial, in part because of problems of de-

Table 31-8 Common Enteral Feeding Problems and Solutions

Problem	Solution
Diarrhea	Give formula at room temperature; use lactose-free formula; add fiber; add antidiarrheal medicine; reduce rate of feeding; reduce volume or use continuous feeding schedule; reduce strength of formula; review other potential sources (medications, treatment)
Regurgitation	Check tube placement; check residuals and withhold feedings if more than 100–200 mL; keep in Fowler's position; use small bore tube; place tube distally (jejunum, duodenum); consider drugs to increase motility
Nausea	Check tube placement; reduce rate; reduce anxiety; change formula; review other potential sources (infection, medications, treatment)
Distention	Use low-fat or hydrolyzed formula; encourage activity; review other potential sources (obstruction, constipation, organomegaly)
Dehydration	Increase water intake to ensure adequate amounts (usually 1 mL/kcal); control (diarrhea, nausea); watch for glucosuria
Fluid overload	Reduce water intake; use concentrated formula
Constipation	Increase water; increase fiber; increase activity
Local irritation	Clean area around tube; apply skin-protecting agents; monitor for otitis media if using nasal tubes
Mouth dryness	Frequent mouth rinsing; use xerostomia products; sugarless gum or mints if medically allowed
Tube obstruction	Use room-temperature feedings; irrigate with water; use pump with high-density formulas (>1.5 kcal/mL) or small-bore tubes; use liquid medicines rather than crushing pills whenever possible
Metabolic imbalance	Monitor carbon dioxide levels; reduce carbohydrate in formula; monitor glucose; monitor potassium and supplement if needed

sign or methodology in the extant research. Many of the relevant studies have small sample sizes. Studies also frequently have different nutritional outcomes, differing patient populations, and different feeding formulas. They reveal that, although subsets of patients benefit from nutritional repletion, aggressive nutritional intervention does not alter morbidity or mortality for the majority of individuals with cancer. In addition, the risks associated with the various treatments must be considered. The problems and common solutions associated with enteral and parenteral nutritional interventions are listed in Tables 31-8 and 31-9. The role of aggressive nutritional intervention in cancer treatment clearly requires more study. As the nutritional abnormalities created by cancer are better understood, more appropriate interventions will be developed.

Physical Activity

Physical inactivity can lead to muscle atrophy, contributing to loss of cardiorespiratory fitness and fatigue. Weight loss that occurs secondary to catabolic activity or cytokine-mediated changes in metabolism or corticosteroid use can also contribute significantly to decreased muscle mass. The structure and function of muscle and bone depend on physical activity combined with appropriate nutritional intake and a hormonal milieu that supports anabolism.[107] An evolving body of knowledge supports the role of physical activity in enhancing a number of clinical outcomes. Improvements have been documented in functional capacity, fatigue, medication requirements, self-esteem, mood, sense of control and well-being, and immunological parameters.[108–111] Physical activities might include walking programs, stretching, use of resistance bands, swimming, cycling, or dancing, as tolerated.

Complementary and Alternative Nutritional Interventions

Selected traditional cancer centers are engaging in rigorous study of complementary and alternative medicine (CAM). This recent interest arises from at least two factors. First, research has shown that 20%–66% of

Table 31-9 Parenteral Feeding Considerations

General Indications: Nonfunctioning gastrointestinal tract; unable to begin enteral feedings for 7 or more days; high-output fistulas; in combination with enteral feedings for some bowel resections; severe radiation enteritis with or without malignant disease; temporary malabsorption secondary to aggressive therapy (e.g., bone marrow transplant); obstructed bowel but otherwise acceptable quality of life; pancreatitis

COMMON PARENTERAL FEEDING PROBLEMS AND SOLUTIONS

Problem	Solutions
Pneumo-hemothorax	Put patient in Trendelenburg position for line placement; check x-ray postprocedure
Embolism	Follow flushing regimen; avoid use of small-diameter syringes when flushing; avoid exposure to free air
Obstruction	Flush per protocol; check for flow per protocol; treat with antiembolics per institutional protocol
Dislodgment	Assess for patency; be alert to patient complaints of pain or swelling in area of catheter insertion
Metabolic abnormalities	Monitor levels of glucose, ammonia, phosphate, liver enzymes, magnesium, potassium, hemoglobin/hematocrit
Infection	Perform careful site care and evaluation; monitor temperature, glucose levels, glucosuria
Trace element deficiency	Monitor vitamin and trace element
Bleeding	Monitor vitamin K administration

Table 31-10 Questionable Dietary Treatments for Cancer

Diet/Additive	Proposed Activity	Comments/Side Effects
Antineoplastin/Burzynski therapy (peptide preparation originally derived from blood and urine)	Peptides are cytotoxic to cancer cells	FDA clinical trial showed no efficacy.
Cancell (nitric acid, sodium sulfate, sulfuric acid, potassium hydroxide)	Combination of ingredients alters electrical charges, creating lower voltage in cells. Cancer cells are susceptible to change and are converted to waste material.	Clinical trials showed no efficacy.
Gerson diet (daily coffee enemas, vegetarian diet, no sugar or salt, organic food purchased from Gerson Clinic)	Cleanses body of cancer toxins; reverses liver damage caused by toxins	Food requires extensive processing; expensive; enemas may cause perforated colon, enzyme imbalances
Macrobiotic diet (50%–60% calories from whole grains, 25%–30% from vegetables, 10%–25% from beans, seaweed, soy products); some rely heavily on rice with mineral and vitamins, including Laetrile; lifestyle changes (clothing choice, family involvement)	Cleanses body; "starves" cancer cells	Although properly constructed macrobiotic diets are adequate, many practitioners do not provide sufficient balanced nutrients. Protein, calorie, iron, vitamin B_{12}, and vitamin D deficiencies can occur.
Nieper diet (restricted flour, red meat, sugar, coffee, tea; emphasizes eggs, whole-grain products, B_{17} [Laetrile], carrot juice, high doses of vitamins A, E, C, D, zinc, magnesium, calcium)	Cleanses body; "starves" cancer cells	Oral Laetrile associated with cyanide poisoning; high-dose vitamins associated with decreased immune function, liver damage, and renal toxicity

individuals with cancer combine conventional and alternative or complementary therapies.[112–116] Nutritional approaches are the most commonly used complementary treatments. Second, a growing body of evidence has demonstrated the effectiveness of some of the products used in CAM. These elements make it essential for nurses to understand both the benefits and the disadvantages of CAM.

A number of therapeutic approaches rely heavily on nutritional components and have questionable or potentially harmful effects; these are listed in Table 31-10. A number of readily available herbs and chemical supplements of unknown efficacy are also advertised as helpful in improving health (Table 31-11).[117–120] (See Chapter 24 for more detailed information on CAM.) Knowledge about these products is constantly changing. It is essential for the nurse to remember several important details in general counseling about the use of herbs or chemical supplements:

- Preparations that may be useful in prevention of disease do not always have a salutary effect when the disease already exists (e.g., saw palmetto reduces prostate size, possibly through phytoestrogenic action, and may alter the effectiveness of hormonal drug treatment in prostate cancer).
- Preparations may be adulterated or contaminated with dangerous materials (e.g., lead and plant fillers containing digitalis or phytoestrogens have been found in some products).
- The complex interaction of nutrients, host, cancer, and cancer treatment, herbs, and supplements can alter the metabolism of drugs, cancer, and the host in unknown ways (e.g., antioxidant supplements may alter the effectiveness of radiation or antimetabolite chemotherapy).
- There are positive effects from some supplements, and identifying accurate information can be difficult (e.g., Internet sites abound; information from those selling products should be questioned).

Conclusion

Nutrition influences carcinogenesis itself as well as the quantity and quality of life once the disease exists. The nurse's ability to take full advantage of nutritional interventions is hampered by insufficient understanding of the pathophysiology of the tumor–host relationship. Without this knowledge, it is difficult to match a specific intervention with a specific nutritional problem.

This lack of knowledge emphasizes the importance of nursing care. Nurses are in the best position to detect undernutrition and overnutrition among individuals with cancer throughout the disease course. The nurse attends to basic nutritional information during the diagnostic process: height, weight, recent weight change, eating problems, unhealthy and healthful

Table 31-11 Herbal, Vitamin, and Mineral Supplementation Associated with Complementary and Alternative Treatments for Cancer

Herb/Vitamin/Mineral	Claims/Proposed Activity	Clinical Trial Results	Comments/Side Effects
Angelica root	Diuretic; diaphoretic	None available.	GRAS in medicinal tea and steam-distilled oil, may be unsafe if root, herb, or seed is eaten; contains coumarin constituents that may promote anticoagulation; may increase stomach acid; may cause photosensitivity and photodermatitis
Astragalus	↑ Immune system; ↑ red blood cells; antibacterial; antiviral; liver protectant; anti-inflammatory; antioxidant; diuretic; vasodilator; antihypertensive; ↑ interferon, T-cell count, stem cells; reduces side effects	Used in China and Korea; no clinical trial data available for the United States.	Possible immune suppression with high doses; may interfere with immunosuppressants
Black cohosh	↓ Menopausal symptoms; estrogen-like effects without binding to estrogen receptors, up-regulating estrogen-dependent genes, or stimulating the growth of estrogen-dependent tumors; anti-inflammatory	Animal studies indicate no benefit in breast cancer. Preliminary research suggests that black cohosh should not be used by women with breast cancer or women with a high risk of developing breast cancer. May increase metastatic cancer in animals.	GI upset; rash; headache; dizziness; weight gain; feeling of heaviness in the legs; cramping; may increase toxicity of doxorubicin and docetaxel; endometrial hyperplasia and vaginal bleeding with tamoxifen use; may increase risk of metastasis in patients with history of breast cancer; may produce estrogenic effects in patients with hormone-sensitive cancers
Buckthorn (sea buckthorn)	↑ Immune system; antioxidant; antihypertensive; reduction of chemotherapy toxicity; anticoagulant; cytotoxic action	Used in China and Asia; no clinical trial data available for the United States.	Likely safe when consumed in the amounts found in foods; may promote anticoagulation and interact with anticoagulant and antiplatelet drugs
Burdock, turkey rhubarb, sorrel, slippery elm (essiac)	↑ Immune system; improving appetite; analgesic; cytotoxic combination	NCI-led animal studies negative; case studies describe minimal, possibly psychological, positive effects.[118]	Contamination of burdock with belladonna in the past; may cause diarrhea
Cartilage (bovine or shark)	Antiangiogeneic; anti-inflammatory; antimutagenic; antioxidant; analgesic activity	May be of some benefit to survival in renal cell carcinoma; no benefit with advanced cancer of any type. AE-941 (Neovastat), a component of shark cartilage, is well studied in the United States.	Can cause taste disturbances, dyspepsia, constipation, osmotic diarrhea, nausea, hypotension, dizziness, hyperglycemia, hypoglycemia, hypercalcemia, altered consciousness, decreased motor strength, decreased sensation, erythema, peripheral edema, generalized weakness, fatigue, and decreased performance; acute hepatitis; local allergic reaction if used subcutaneously or intramuscularly
Cascara sagrada	Laxative; cytotoxic activity	A component of cascara (emodin) is currently being investigated for antitumor properties in vitro. No clinical trial information is currently available for the United States.	Increases intestinal musculature; diarrhea; may lead to cholestatic hepatitis; long-term use can lead to dependence, hypokalemia, albuminuria, hematuria, disturbed heart function, muscle weakness, finger clubbing, cachexia

(continued)

Table 31-11 Herbal, Vitamin, and Mineral Supplementation Associated with Complementary and Alternative Treatments for Cancer (continued)

Herb/Vitamin/Mineral	Claims/Proposed Activity	Clinical Trial Results	Comments/Side Effects
Cat's claw	Toxic to herpes simplex; analgesic; anti-inflammatory; ↓ production of proinflammatory cytokines; antioxidant; antiviral; antimutagenic; ↑ immune function; scavenges free radicals; alkaloid component treats leukemia	Several components: quinovic acid alkaloids, pteropodine, and isopteropodine — under investigation for possible roles in cancer prevention. There is preliminary evidence that cat's claw extracts can induce apoptosis and inhibit proliferation of leukemia and lymphoma cells.	Headache, dizziness, vomiting; hypotension; may inhibit cytochrome P450 3A4 (CYP3A4) enzymes and interfere with drugs that utilize this pathway; may interfere with immunosuppressants; may adversely affect patients with autoimmune disorders
Echinacea	Stimulates TNF-α, interferon, and IL-1; ↑ immune system function; ↑ wound healing; antibacterial action; antifungal; antiviral; ↑ phagocytosis; anti-inflammatory	Results are conflicting as to the benefit of echinacea in the treatment of the common cold/upper respiratory infections. Does not seem to improve herpes outbreaks. An isolated polysaccharide fraction of *Echinacea purpurea* given intravenously might reduce leukopenia caused by chemotherapy.	Overall well tolerated; rarely allergic reactions, fever, nausea, vomiting, unpleasant taste, abdominal pain, diarrhea, sore throat, dizziness, and disorientation; not recommended for long-term use in HIV; long-term use may decrease effectiveness; may inhibit cytochrome P450 3A4 (CYP3A4) enzymes and interfere with drugs that utilize this pathway; may interfere with immunosuppressants
Garlic	Anti-hyperlipidemic; antihypertensive; anti-inflammatory; ↑ immune system; antifungal; antibacterial; anthelmintic; antiviral; antispasmodic; diaphoretic; expectorant; ↑ immune system; antithrombotic	Some evidence from population studies that increased dietary consumption of garlic leads to decreased risk of gastric and colorectal cancer, but garlic supplements may not provide the same benefit. Dietary and supplemental garlic intakes may decrease the risk of prostate cancer. Dietary garlic does not seem to decrease the risk of breast or lung cancer. May protect intestinal mucosa from methotrexate and 5-FU-induced toxicity.	GI irritation; supplements containing allicin may inhibit cytochrome P450 3A4 (CYP3A4) enzymes and interfere with drugs that utilize this pathway; may promote anticoagulation; may decrease the effectiveness of cyclosporine, non-nucleoside reverse transcriptase inhibitors (NNRTIs), oral contraceptives, and saquinavir
Ginseng	American: antidiabetic; antihypertensive; ↓ luteinizing hormone; phytoestrogen Panax: ↑ immune function; CNS stimulant; analgesic; anti-inflammatory; cytotoxic activity; phytoestrogen; antiviral; antifungal Siberian: diuretic; appetite stimulant; ↓ severity of herpes simplex outbreaks; antioxidant; phytoestrogen	American ginseng extract may reduce breast cancer cell growth, but estrogenic effects may negate this activity. Components of Panax ginseng may inhibit tumor cell invasion in lymphocytes. Siberian ginseng may exert an antiproliferative effect on leukemia cells.	American: without reported side effects; hypoglycemia; may interact with antipsychotic drugs, MAOIs, stimulant drugs; may promote anticoagulation; may cause arrhythmias when taken in combination with ephedra; may produce estrogenic effects in patients with hormone-sensitive cancers Panax: (above listed plus) may cause insomnia; may contribute to diuretic resistance; may interfere with immunosuppressants; may inhibit cytochrome P450 2D6 (CYP2D6) enzymes and interfere with drugs that utilize this pathway Siberian: drowsiness; anxiety; irritability; melancholy; hypoglycemia; may promote anticoagulation; may inhibit cytochrome P450 1A2, 2C9, 2D69, and 3A4 enzymes and interfere with drugs that utilize these pathways; may promote digoxin toxicity

(continued)

Table 31-11 Herbal, Vitamin, and Mineral Supplementation Associated with Complementary and Alternative Treatments for Cancer (continued)

Herb/Vitamin/Mineral	Claims/Proposed Activity	Clinical Trial Results	Comments/Side Effects
Gotu kola	Contains flavinoids; ↑ wound healing; ↓ venous pressure; anti-inflammatory; antioxidant; neuroprotectant; cytotoxic agent	Dried powder extract seems to promote selective toxicity toward tumor cells.	May cause GI upset; nausea; pruritus; photosensitivity; sedation; may increase serum cholesterol; may cause hyperglycemia
Kombucha mushroom (Manchurian kargasok) tea	Fermentation product of yeasts and bacteria thought to be cytotoxic	None available.	Stomach problems; yeast infections; allergic reactions; jaundice; nausea; vomiting; head and neck pain; anthrax; possibly death; high risk of contamination; risk of transmission of opportunistic infections; fermentation in lead-glazed ceramic pot for 6 months led to lead poisoning in 2 people; high acid content of tea can interfere with acid-sensitive drugs
Milk thistle (silymarin)	Protects liver cells from damage; antioxidant; inhibitor of tumor necrosis factor; anti-inflammatory; ↑ immune system; phytoestrogen	May protect kidney cells from the nephrotoxic effects of cisplatin and vincristine. Components of milk thistle (silymarin, silibinin) may exert antiproliferative effects on prostate tumor cells.	Laxative effect; pollen allergy reaction; may inhibit cytochrome P450 2C9 and 3A4 enzymes and interfere with drugs that utilize these pathways; may produce estrogenic effects in patients with hormone-sensitive cancers; may interfere with estrogen, glucuronidated drugs, indinavir
Mistletoe (iscador)	American: smooth muscle stimulant; antihypotensive European: ↓ chemotherapy side effects; ↑ immune system; ↑ secretion of IL-1, IL-6, TNF-α; induces apoptosis; contains cytotoxic plant products; used in Europe	Subcutaneous European mistletoe administration does not improve survival in pancreatic, kidney, or head and neck cancer, glioma, or melanoma. European mistletoe extract may improve survival in breast, colon, and gastric cancer. May induce cytotoxicity via the inhibition of cellular protein synthesis or the induction of apoptosis. Lectin standardized mistletoe extract used adjuvantly in postoperative breast cancer patients improved side effect symptom scores.[119]	American: considered unsafe; abortifacient; nausea; bradycardia; hypertension; delirium; hallucinations; vasoconstriction; cardiac arrest European: considered safe at low doses; may have cardiotoxic and negative inotropic effects; vomiting; diarrhea; intestinal cramps; hepatitis; hypotension; seizures; coma; death; may interfere with immunosuppressants
Omega-3 fatty acid (fish oil)	Antihyperlipidemic; anti-inflammatory; antithrombotic; ↓ pro-inflammatory cytokines; ↓ red blood cell hemolysis; ↓ heart rate; ↓ T-cell and B-cell proliferation; ↓ secretion of IL-1, IL-6, TNF-α; ↓ cachexia-related cytokines; cytotoxic activity	Decreased risk of prostate cancer in individuals with high EPA and DHA levels in erythrocytes. May prevent prostaglandin and cyclooxygenase promotion of tumor growth via competition with precursors. May prolong cancer remission via a decrease in lactic acid in tumor cells. May cause tumor cell membrane perforation and cell death. May protect against cyclosporine-induced nephrotoxicity.	GRAS in fish oil form; may promote anticoagulation (doses > 3g/day); may ↓ immune function; risk of vitamin A and D toxicity with some preparations; may reduce vitamin E levels; may interfere with etretinate oral contraceptives; hypotension; hypomania; hyperglycemia (doses > 3g/day)
PC-SPES (da qing ye, licorice, panax pseudo-ginseng, reishi mushroom, baikal skullcap, chrysanthemum, rabdosia rubescens, saw palmetto)[120]	Phytoestrogen; ↓ PSA; analgesic; ↓ testosterone; induction of apoptosis; reduction of tumor cell proliferation; antimutagenic; anti-inflammatory;	Clinical trial stopped due to contaminated product. Transcriptional-effects in androgen sensitive prostate cancer cells. May inhibit tumor growth in all types of prostate cancer. Significantly decreases PSA levels. May improve QOL and reduce pain in patients with metastatic prostate cancer.	Recalled in February 2002 due to contamination with warfarin, indomethacin, diethylstilbestrol, and alprazolam. May promote anticoagulation; breast tenderness or enlargement (occurs in 90% of individuals); sexual dysfunction; hot flashes; leg cramps; GI symptoms; rapid rise in PSA with discontinuation of treatment; may interfere with conventional hormone therapies

(continued)

Table 31-11 Herbal, Vitamin, and Mineral Supplementation Associated with Complementary and Alternative Treatments for Cancer (continued)

Herb/Vitamin/Mineral	Claims/Proposed Activity	Clinical Trial Results	Comments/Side Effects
Pycnogenol	Antioxidant; ↑ natural killer cell cytotoxicity; anti-inflammatory; analgesic; antihypertensive; ↑ immune system; neuroprotectant	Pycnogenol has no effect on levels of pro-inflammatory cytokines. May increase resistance to UVA and UVB light damage. Improves natural killer cell, T-cell, and B-cell activity in animal models.	May interfere with immunosuppressants; may adversely affect patients with autoimmune disorders
Rosemary	Antioxidant; antibacterial; antifungal; ↓ gastric upset	None found.	GRAS in amounts found in foods; may be unsafe if the essential oil is ingested; large amounts of oil might cause deep coma, spasm, vomiting, gastroenteritis, uterine bleeding, kidney irritation, pulmonary edema, and death
Saw palmetto	↓ Benign prostatic hyperplasia; diuretic; sedative; anti-inflammatory; antiandrogenic; antiproliferative; anti-estrogenic	Improvement in urinary symptoms resulting from BPH, with no reduction in prostate size or PSA. May reduce the proliferation of prostate cells, possibly by inhibiting COX-2 expression.	Side effects generally mild; may promote anticoagulation; may interfere with oral contraceptives and hormone therapy
Tea (green or black)	Antioxidant; antimutagenic; anticarcinogenic; ↑ cognitive performance; antidiarrheal; weak phytoestrogen; diuretic; CNS stimulant; antiangiogenic (green tea only)	Several flavanols in green tea under investigation as angiogenesis inhibitors as well as cytotoxic agents. Green tea may enhance the effects and activity of doxorubicin. May increase resistance to UVA and UVB light damage.	Inhibitory effect on platelets with tea flavinoid supplements; tannins in tea reduce nonheme iron absorption; caffeine in tea can interfere with multiple medications; may produce estrogenic effects in patients with hormone-sensitive cancers; may promote anticoagulation
Tumeric (curcumin)	Antioxidant; anti-inflammatory; antiangiogenic; induction of apoptosis; antithrombotic; ↑ immune system	Chemopreventive and growth inhibitory activity in several tumor cell lines. May stabilize treatment refractory colorectal cancer. Numerous studies ongoing.	May promote anticoagulation; can cause gallbladder contractions; use with caution in individuals with gallbladder disease
White willow	Anti-inflammatory; antipyretic; antithrombotic; contains salicylate (salicin); may mimic aspirin-like effects in prevention of esophageal, gastric, and colorectal cancers	None available.	GI upset; may promote anticoagulation; may interact with other salicylate-containing drugs; tannin content may cause precipitation of some drugs; may exacerbate kidney or liver problems
DHEA (dehydroepiandrosterone)	Changes circulating androgen/estrogen ratio; androgenic effects; estrogenic effects; ↑ immune function; ↓ viral load (HIV)	Stimulates growth of estrogen receptor–positive breast cancer cells.	Will interfere with antiestrogen and estrogen receptor–blocking medications such as tamoxifen; may inhibit cytochrome P450 3A4 (CYP3A4) enzymes and interfere with drugs that utilize this pathway; ↑ insulin resistance; may exacerbate liver problems; may increase risk of psychiatric events in individuals with mood disorders

(continued)

Table 31-11 Herbal, Vitamin, and Mineral Supplementation Associated with Complementary and Alternative Treatments for Cancer (continued)

Herb/Vitamin/Mineral	Claims/Proposed Activity	Clinical Trial Results	Comments/Side Effects
Niacin	Antihyperlipidemic; ↑ histamine secretion; antithrombotic; ↑ immune function; ↑ healing; free radical scavenger	Numerous studies exploring antihyperlipidemic properties. Suboptimal niacin status may promote carcinogenesis. Topical nicotinamide (active form of niacin) prevented immunosuppression-induced skin tumors in animal studies.	Low doses: flushing High doses (>3 g): hepatotoxicity, hyperglycemia, cardiac dysrhythmias, cardiac arrest, nausea, vomiting, diarrhea, hypotension, myopathy; may promote carbamazepine toxicity; may exacerbate gallbladder, kidney, or liver problems
Vitamin A, retinoids	↑ immune function; ↑ wound healing; ↓ chemotherapy induced GI events; multiple medical uses	Preliminary evidence suggests that retinoic acid might increase the production of cytokines, such as IL-1. In vitro studies suggest retinoids may induce tumor suppressor genes known as retinoic acid receptors. Topical administration may increase resistance to ultraviolet light damage. Oral administration does not seem to decrease incidence of chemotherapy-induced GI side effects.	Acute toxicity following doses of 15,000 μg (50,000 units), nausea, vomiting, headache, increased cerebrospinal fluid pressure, vertigo, blurred vision, muscular incoordination; hepatotoxicity; hypervitaminosis A; benign intracranial hypertension (with concomitant tetracycline); may promote anticoagulation; may exacerbate liver problems; may promote osteoporosis
Vitamin B_6 (pyridoxine)	Reverses 5-FU-induced erythrodysesthesia; ↓ risk of lung cancer; antioxidant	Oral pyridoxine may be effective in partially reversing fluorouracil-induced erythrodysesthesia in metastatic colon cancer patients. Epidemiological research suggests that male smokers with higher serum levels of pyridoxine have a lower risk of lung cancer.	Nausea, vomiting, abdominal pain, loss of appetite, headache, paresthesia, somnolence, increased serum AST (SGOT), decreased serum folic acid concentrations, skin and other allergic reactions, breast soreness or enlargement, and photosensitivity; doses of 1000 g or more produce neuropathy; may interfere with amiodarone, levodopa, phenytoin, and phenobarbital
Vitamin C	Antioxidant; ↑ differentiation; repair; ↑ immune function; antihistamine; ↑ iron absorption; ↓ risk of mouth, esophageal, and stomach cancers	Epidemiological research suggests dietary vitamin C may decrease the risk of developing mouth, esophageal, and gastric cancer; there is no evidence of benefit in breast, ovarian, or bladder cancers. High-dose oral vitamin C (10 g) has no effect on survival in patients with advanced cancer. Preliminary clinical evidence suggests high doses of vitamin C given intravenously might have a beneficial effect on survival rate in patients with terminal cancer, but this has not been proven. Topical administration with vitamin E or A may increase resistance to ultraviolet light damage.	Doses > 2000 mg/day increase the risk of nausea, vomiting, esophagitis, heartburn, abdominal cramps, gastrointestinal obstruction, fatigue, flushing, headache, insomnia, sleepiness, diarrhea, DVT; increases risk of urate, oxalate, and cysteine kidney stones; may interfere with acetaminophen, aluminum-containing antacids, aspirin, HMG-CoA reductase inhibitors, dobutamine, ethinyl estradiol, protease inhibitors, heparin, and warfarin; may decrease the effectiveness of radiation and some chemotherapeutic drugs
Vitamin D	Prevents corticosteroid-induced osteoporosis; antiproliferative effects	Preliminary epidemiological evidence indicates that people with vitamin D deficiency may be at an increased risk of colon, breast, and prostate cancer.	Vitamin D intoxication (azotemia, hypercalcemia, and anemia); may increase the risk of arrhythmias in people taking cardiac glycosides

(continued)

Table 31-11 Herbal, Vitamin, and Mineral Supplementation Associated with Complementary and Alternative Treatments for Cancer (continued)

Herb/Vitamin/Mineral	Claims/Proposed Activity	Clinical Trial Results	Comments/Side Effects
Zinc	Adequate zinc levels promote healing; ↑ immune function; ↓ diarrhea in malnutrition; ↓ duration of colds; ↓ severity of herpes simplex outbreaks; improves hypogeusia; ↓ incidence of sickle cell crises; anti-inflammatory	Results are conflicting as to the benefits of zinc in treatment of the common cold. Decreases incidence of sickle cell crisis and infection in individuals who are zinc deficient.	Nausea, vomiting, metallic taste, irritation and corrosion of the gastrointestinal (GI) tract, acute renal tubular necrosis, interstitial nephritis; high-dose supplementation (300 mg) may ↓ immune function; risk of copper deficiency (450–1600 mg); ↑ risk BPH; ↑ risk prostate cancer; ↑ cytotoxicity of cisplatin in the presence of EDTA; may interfere with fluoroquinolones and tetracyclines; ↓ survival in individuals with HIV and high intakes of zinc

GRAS = generally recognized as safe.
TNF-α = Tumor necrosis factor alpha.
IL-1 = interleukin-1.
IL-6 = interleukin- 6.
CNS = central nervous system.
PSA = prostate-specific antigen.
QOL = quality of life.
AST = aspartate transaminase.
DVT = deep-vein thrombosis.
HMG-CoA = beta-hydroxy-beta-methylglutaryl-CoA.
EDTA = ethylenediaminetetraacetic acid.

Data from Natural Medicines Comprehensive Database.[117]

food choices, social situations that interfere with food procurement, and psychological responses that alter intake. Given this base, the nurse can work with other care providers to prioritize and define nutritional care. The nurse continues the assessment function throughout the patient's treatment and follow-up. Nutritional intervention can be devised in the overall context of the clinical situation and in accordance with the patient's beliefs and desires.

Although the scientific information is still far from complete, early nutritional intervention—when the tumor burden is relatively small—has the best chance to alter patient outcomes. This is particularly true for those undergoing surgery. Appropriate nutritional intervention reduces morbidity, length of hospital stay, and possibly mortality in these patients. For some patients, the need for nutritional support will continue for a period following hospitalization. Understanding the limitations of nutritional interventions is important for both nurses and patients. Assisting patients to make the best decisions for themselves may reduce frustration and minimize use of questionable methods.

Nurses also should be attuned to newer approaches in the use of nutrition as therapy. Determining what role nutritional interventions will play in the cancer armamentarium needs additional study. Further, nurses have an obligation to continue research into the self-care actions routinely prescribed in dealing with nutritional disturbances. Many of the actions commonly suggested are based solely on anecdotal evidence. Much more study is needed before a nurse can accurately predict which self-care actions will be effective for a given patient. With the base of nursing research added to that of other disciplines, oncology nurses can positively influence the incidence and prevalence of nutritional deficiencies in cancer.

References

1. Warren S: The immediate causes of death in cancer. *Am J Med Sci* 184:610–615, 1932
2. Shils ME: Nutrition and diet in cancer management, in Shils ME Olson JA Shike M. (eds.): *Modern Nutrition in Health and Disease* (ed 8). Philadelphia, Lea and Febiger, 1994, pp 1319–1342
3. McCarter MD, Gentilini OD, Gomez ME, et al: Preoperative oral supplement with immunonutrients in cancer patients. *J Parenter Enteral Nutr* 22:206–211, 1998
4. Andrassy RJ, Chwals WJ: Nutritional support of the pediatric oncology patient. *Nutrition* 14:124–129, 1998
5. de Lorgeril M, Salen P, Martin JL, et al: Mediterranean dietary pattern in a randomized trial: prolonged survival and possible reduced cancer rate. *Arch Intern Med* 158:1181–1187, 1998

6. Cunningham RS, Bell R: Nutrition in cancer: an overview. *Semin Oncol Nurs* 16:90–98, 2000
7. Shopbell J, Hopkins B, Shronts E: Nutrition screening and assessment, in Gottschlich M (ed.): *The Science and Practice of Nutrition Support.* Dubuque, American Society for Parenteral and Enteral Nutrition, 2001, pp 107–140
8. Lacey K, Pritchett E: Nutrition Care Process and Model: ADA adopts road map to quality care and outcomes management. *J Am Diet Assoc* 103:1061–1072, 2003
9. McTiernan A, Rajan KB, Tworoger SS, et al: Adiposity and sex hormones in postmenopausal breast cancer survivors. *J Clin Oncol* 21:1961–1966, 2003
10. Harvie M, Hooper L, Howell AH: Central obesity and breast cancer risk: a systematic review. *Obes Rev* 4:157–173, 2003
11. Del Rio G, Zironi S, Valeriani L, et al: Weight gain in women with breast cancer treated with adjuvant cyclophosphamide, methotrexate and 5–fluorouracil. Analysis of resting energy expenditure and body composition. *Breast Cancer Res Treat* 73:267–273, 2002
12. Costa LJ, Varella PC, del Giglio A: Weight changes during chemotherapy for breast cancer. *Sao Paulo Med J* 120:113–117, 2002
13. Cheblowski R, Aiello E, McTiernan A: Weight loss in breast cancer patient management. *J Clin Oncol* 20:1128–1143, 2002
14. Borugian M, Sheps S, Kim-Sing C, et al: Waist to hip ratio and breast cancer mortality. *Am J Epidemiol* 158:963–968, 2003
15. Tisdale M: Pathogenesis of cancer cachexia. *Support Oncol* 1:159–168, 2003
16. Bozzetti F: Rationale and indications for preoperative feeding of malnourished surgical cancer patients. *Nutrition* 18:953–959, 2002
17. Bloch A, Charuhas P: Cancer and cancer therapy, in Gottschlich M (ed.): *The Science and Practice of Nutrition Support.* Dubuque, Kendall/Hunt, 2001, pp 643–661
18. Nguyen T, Yueh B: Weight loss predicts mortality after recurrent oral cavity and oropharyngeal carcinomas. *Cancer* 95:553–562, 2002
19. Ulander K, Jeppsson B, Grahn G: Postoperative energy intake in patients after colorectal cancer surgery. *Scand J Caring Sci* 12:131–138, 1998
20. Martin C: Calorie, protein, fluid, and micronutrient requirements, in McCallum P, Polisena C (eds.): *The Clinical Guide to Oncology Nutrition.* Chicago, American Dietetic Association, 2000, pp 45–60
21. Polisena C: Nutritional concerns with the radiation therapy patient, in McCallum P, Polisena C (eds.): *The Clinical Guide to Oncology Nutrition.* Chicago, American Dietetic Association, 2000, pp 70–78
22. Wickham R: Nausea and vomiting, in Yarbro CH, Frogge MH, Goodman M (eds.): *Cancer Symptom Management* (ed 3). Sudbury, MA, Jones and Bartlett, 2004, pp 187–214
23. Herbst RS, Giaccone G: Novel molecular strategies in lung cancer: EGFR inhibition and anti-angiogenesis. *Lung Cancer Principl Pract* 2:1–19, 2002
24. Kim ES: Targeted therapies in non-small-cell lung cancer. *Lung Cancer Principl Pract* 3:1–19, 2003
25. Cioffi L: General theory of critical periods and the development of obesity, in Smogyi J (ed.): *Nutritional, Psychological and Social Aspects of Obesity.* Basel, Karger, 1968, pp 17–28
26. MacDonald N, Easson AM, Mazurak VC, et al: Understanding and managing cancer cachexia. *J Am Coll Surg* 197:143–161, 2003
27. Laviano A, Russo M, Freda F, Rossi-Fanelli F: Neurochemical mechanisms for cancer anorexia. *Nutrition* 18:100–105, 2002
28. Tisdale MJ: The "cancer cachectic factor" *Support Care Cancer* 11:73–78, 2003
29. Laviano A, Rossi-Fanelli F: Pathogenesis of cancer anorexia: still doubts after all these years? *Nutrition* 19:67–68, 2003
30. McInnes JA, Knobf MT: Weight gain and quality of life in women treated with adjuvant chemotherapy for early-stage breast cancer. *Oncol Nurs Forum* 28:675–684, 2001
31. Demark-Wahnefried W, Peterson BL, Winer EP, et al: Changes in weight, body composition, and factors influencing energy balance among premenopausal breast cancer patients receiving adjuvant chemotherapy. *J Clin Oncol* 19:2381–2389, 2001
32. Goodwin PJ: Weight gain in early-stage breast cancer: where do we go from here? *J Clin Oncol* 19:2367–2369, 2001
33. Goodwin PJ, Ennis M, Pritchard KI, et al: Diet and breast cancer: evidence that extremes in diet are associated with poor survival. *J Clin Oncol* 21:2500–2507, 2003
34. Palesty JA, Dudrick SJ: What we have learned about cachexia in gastrointestinal cancer. *Dig Dis* 21:198–213, 2003
35. Nebeling LC: Changes in carbohydrate, protein, and fat metabolism in cancer, in McCallum P, Polisena C (eds.) *The Clinical Guide to Oncology Nutrition.* Chicago, American Dietetic Association, 2000, pp 53–60
36. Tisdale MJ: Metabolic abnormalities in cachexia and anorexia. *Nutrition* 16:1013–1014, 2000
37. Mulligan K, Bloch AS: Energy expenditure and protein metabolism in human immunodeficiency virus infection and cancer cachexia. *Semin Oncol* 25(suppl 6):82–91, 1998
38. Cooley ME, Short TH, Moriarty HJ: Symptom prevalence, distress, and change over time in adults receiving treatment for lung cancer. *Psychooncology* 12:694–708, 2003
39. Marian M: Cancer cachexia: prevalence, mechanisms, and interventions. *Support Line* 20:3–12, 1998
40. May P, Barber A, D'Olimpio J, et al: Reversal of cancer related wasting using oral supplementation with a combination of B-hydroxy-B-methylbutyrate, arginine, and glutamine. *Am J Surg* 183:471–479, 2002
41. Ottery F, Bender F, Kasenic S: The design and implementation of a model nutritional oncology clinic. *Oncol Issues: Integrating Nutrition into Your Cancer Program* 17:2–6, 2002
42. Gabbard D, Luthringer S, Eldridge B: Oncology nutrition standards of care. *Oncol Issues: Integrating Nutrition into Your Cancer Program* 17:8–10, 2002
43. McCallum P, Polisena C: *The Clinical Guide to Oncology Nutrition.* Chicago, American Dietetic Association, 2000
44. Joint Commission on Accreditation of Healthcare Organizations (JCAHO): Crosswalk of 2003 standards for hospitals to 2004 provision of care, treatment, and service standards for hospitals. Joint Commission on Accreditation of Healthcare Organizations. *www.jcaho.org/accredited+organizations/hospitals/standards/new+standards/pc_xwalk_hap.pdf.* Accessed December 31, 2003
45. American Society for Parenteral & Enteral Nutrition (ASPEN): Guidelines for the use of parenteral and enteral nutriton in adult and pediatric patients. *J Parenteral Enteral Nutr* 26:1SA–138SA, 2002
46. Wojtaszek C, Kochis LM, Cunningham RS: Nutritional screening and assessment: an overview. *Oncol Issues: Integrating Nutrition into Your Cancer Program* 17:11–12, 2002
47. Bauer J, Capra S, Ferguson M: Use of the scored Patient-Generated Subjective Global Assessment (PG-SGA) as a nutrition assessment tool in patients with cancer. *Eur J Clin Nutr* 56:779–785, 2002
48. Barbosa-Silva MC, de Barros AJ: [Subjective global assessment: part 2. Review of its adaptations and utilization in different clinical specialties]. *Arq Gastroenterol* 39:248–252, 2002
49. Barbosa-Silva MC, de Barros AJ: [Subjective nutrition assessment: part 1. A review of its validity after two decades of use]. *Arq Gastroenterol* 39:181–187, 2002

50. Schneider SM, Hebuterne X: Use of nutritional scores to predict clinical outcomes in chronic diseases. *Nutr Rev* 58(pt 1):31–38, 2000
51. Hammond K: Dietary and clinical asssessment, in Mahan L, Escott-Stump S (eds.): *Krause's Food Nutrition and Diet Therapy* (ed 11). Philadelphia, W.B. Saunders, 2003, pp 407–435
52. Wagner DR, Heyward VH: Techniques of body composition assessment: a review of laboratory and field methods. *Res Q Exerc Sport* 70:135–149, 1999
53. Hills A, Byrne N: Bioelectrical impedance and body composition assessment. *Malaysian J Nutr* 4:107–112, 1998
54. Toso S, Piccoli A, Gusella M, et al: Bioimpedance vector pattern in cancer patients without disease versus locally advanced or dissmeinated disease. *Nutr Cancer* 19:510–514, 2003
55. Robinett-Weiss N, Hixson ML, Keir B, Sieberg J: The Metropolitan Height-Weight Tables: perspectives for use. *J Am Diet Assoc* 84:1480–1481, 1984
56. Hamwi G: Changing dietary concepts, in Danowski T (ed.): *Diabetes Mellitus: Diagnosis and Treatment,* Vol 1. New York, American Diabetes Association, 1964, pp 73–78
57. Edel J, Murray M, Schurer W, et al: Nutrition assessment of adults, in Rychlec G (ed.): *Manual of Clinical Dietetics* (ed 6). Chicago, American Dietetic Association, 2000, pp 3–38
58. National Institutes of Health: *The Practical Guide: Identification, Evaluation, and Treatment of Overweight and Obesity in Adults.* Bethesda, MD, National Institutes of Health, 2000
59. Blackburn G, Bistrian B: Nutritional and metabolic assessment of the hospitalized patient. *J Parenteral Enteral Nutr* 1:11–22, 1977
60. World Health Organization: *Energy and Protein Requirements. Report of a Joint FAO/WHO/UN Expert Consultation.* Geneva, World Health Organization, 1985
61. Frankenfield D: Energy and macrosubstrate requirements, in Gottschlich M (ed.): *The Science and Practice of Nutrition Support.* Dubuque, Kendall/Hunt, 2001, pp 31–52
62. Food and Nutrition Board Institute of Medicine: Energy, in Institute of Medicine (ed.): *Dietary Reference Intakes for Energy, Carbohydrates, Fiber, Fat, Protein, and Amino Acids.* Washington, DC, National Academy Press, 2002, pp 1–79
63. Kondrup J, Bak L, Hansen BS, et al: Outcome from nutritional support using hospital food. *Nutrition* 14:319–321, 1998
64. Ringwald-Smith K, Williams R, Horwitz E, et al: Determination of energy expenditure in the bone marrow transplant patient. *Nutr Clin Pract* 13:215–218, 1998
65. Vanek V: The use of serum albumin as a prognostic or nutritional marker. *Nutri Clin Pract* 13:110–112, 1998
66. Cunningham RS: The anorexia-cachexia syndrome, in Yarbro CH, Frogge MH, Goodman M (eds.): *Cancer Symptom Management* (ed 3). Sudbury, MA, Jones and Bartlett, 2003, pp 137–167
67. Luk JK, Or KH, Woo J: Using the comprehensive geriatric assessment technique to assess elderly patients. *Hong Kong Med J* 6:93–98, 2000
68. Extermann M: Studies of comprehensive geriatric assessment in patients with cancer. *Cancer Control* 10:463–468, 2003
69. Schmid A, Weiss M, Heseker H: Recording the nutrient intake of nursing home residents by food weighing method and measuring the physical activity. *J Nutr Health Aging* 7:294–295, 2003
70. Bales CW, Ritchie CS: Sarcopenia, weight loss, and nutritional frailty in the elderly. *Annu Rev Nutr* 22:309–323, 2002
71. Naliboff BD: Choosing outcome variables: global assessment and diaries. *Gastroenterology* 126(suppl 1):S129–S134, 2004
72. Wojtaszek CA, Kochis LM, Cunningham RS: Nutrition impact symptoms in the oncology patient. *Oncol Issues: Integrating Nutrition into Your Cancer Program* 17:15–17, 2002
73. Laviano A, Meguid MM, Rossi-Fanelli F: Cancer anorexia: clinical implications, pathogenesis, and therapeutic strategies. *Lancet Oncol* 4:686–694, 2003
74. Wigmore SJ, Todorov PT, Barber MD, et al: Characteristics of patients with pancreatic cancer expressing a novel cancer cachectic factor. *Br J Surg* 87:53–58, 2000
75. Miller M, Kearney N: Chemotherapy-related nausea and vomiting — past reflections, present practice and future management. *Eur J Cancer Care* 13:71–81, 2004
76. MacDonald N: Is there evidence for earlier intervention in cancer-associated weight loss? *Support Oncol* 1:279–285, 2003
77. Quill TE, Byock IR: Responding to intractable terminal suffering: the role of terminal sedation and voluntary refusal of food and fluids. ACP-ASIM End-of-Life Care Consensus Panel. American College of Physicians — American Society of Internal Medicine. *Ann Intern Med* 132:408–414, 2000
78. Maillet JO, Potter RL, Heller L: Position of the American Dietetic Association: ethical and legal issues in nutrition, hydration, and feeding. *J Am Diet Assoc* 102:716–726, 2002
79. Sacks GS, Genton L, Kudsk KA: Controversy of immunonutrition for surgical critical-illness patients. *Curr Opin Crit Care* 9:300–305, 2003
80. McCowen KC, Bistrian BR: Immunonutrition: problematic or problem solving? *Am J Clin Nutr* 77:764–770, 2003
81. Savarese DM, Savy G, Vahdat L, et al: Prevention of chemotherapy and radiation toxicity with glutamine. *Cancer Treat Rev* 29:501–513, 2003
82. Hebert JR, Ebbeling CB, Olendzki BC, et al: Change in women's diet and body mass following intensive intervention for early-stage breast cancer. *J Am Diet Assoc* 101:421–431, 2001
83. Djuric Z, DiLaura NM, Jenkins I, et al: Combining weight-loss counseling with the weight watchers plan for obese breast cancer survivors. *Obes Res* 10:657–665, 2002
84. Rock CL: Diet and breast cancer: can dietary factors influence survival? *J Mammary Gland Biol Neoplasia* 8:119–132, 2003
85. Seyfried TN, Sanderson TM, El-Abbadi MM, et al: Role of glucose and ketone bodies in the metabolic control of experimental brain cancer. *Br J Cancer* 89:1375–1382, 2003
86. Nitenberg G, Raynard B: Nutritional support of the cancer patient: issues and dilemmas. *Crit Rev Oncol Hematol* 34:137–168, 2000
87. Epstein JB, Schubert MM: Managing pain in mucositis. *Semin Oncol Nurs* 20:30–37, 2004
88. Von Roenn J: Pharmacologic interventions for cancer related weight loss. *Oncol Issues: Integrating Nutrition into Your Cancer Program* 17:18–21, 2002
89. Wooldridge JE, Anderson CM, Perry MC: Corticosteroids in advanced cancer. *Oncology (Huntingt)* 15:225–234, discussion 234–226, 2001
90. Lelli G, Montanari M, Gilli G, et al: Treatment of the cancer anorexia-cachexia syndrome: a critical reappraisal. *J Chemother* 15:220–225, 2003
91. Inui A: Cancer anorexia-cachexia syndrome: current issues in research and management. *CA Cancer J Clin* 52:72–91, 2002
92. Tomiska M, Tomiskova M, Salajka F, et al: Palliative treatment of cancer anorexia with oral suspension of megestrol acetate. *Neoplasma* 50:227–233, 2003
93. Ulutin HC, Arpaci F, Pak Y: Megestrol acetate for cachexia and anorexia in advanced non-small cell lung cancer: a randomized study comparing two different doses. *Tumori* 88:277–280, 2002
94. Jatoi A, Windschitl HE, Loprinzi CL, et al: Dronabinol versus megestrol acetate versus combination therapy for cancer-associated anorexia: a North Central Cancer Treatment Group study. *J Clin Oncol* 20:567–573, 2002
95. Orme LM, Bond JD, Humphrey MS, et al: Megestrol acetate in pediatric oncology patients may lead to severe, symptomatic adrenal suppression. *Cancer* 98:397–405, 2003
96. Calhoun SR, Galloway GP, Smith DE: Abuse potential of dronabinol (Marinol). *J Psychoactive Drugs* 30:187–196, 1998

97. Barber MD, Ross JA, Voss AC, et al: The effect of an oral nutritional supplement enriched with fish oil on weight-loss in patients with pancreatic cancer. *Br J Cancer* 81:80–86, 1999
98. Barber MD, Fearon KC, Tisdale MJ, et al: Effect of a fish oil–enriched nutritional supplement on metabolic mediators in patients with pancreatic cancer cachexia. *Nutr Cancer* 40:118–124, 2001
99. Wigmore SJ, Barber MD, Ross JA, et al: Effect of oral eicosapentaenoic acid on weight loss in patients with pancreatic cancer. *Nutr Cancer* 36:177–184, 2000
100. Hardman WE: Omega-3 fatty acids to augment cancer therapy. *J Nutr* 132(suppl):3508S–3512S, 2002
101. Khan ZH, Simpson EJ, Cole AT, et al: Oesophageal cancer and cachexia: the effect of short-term treatment with thalidomide on weight loss and lean body mass. *Aliment Pharmacol Ther* 17:677–682, 2003
102. Von Roenn J, Tchekmedyian S, Hoffman R, et al: Safety of oxandrolone in cancer-related weight loss. *Proc Am Soc Clin Oncol* 22:749, 2003 (abstract)
103. Luthringer S: Cancer (medical) medical nutrition therapy protocol, in Gilbreath J, Inman-Felton AE, Johnson EQ, Robinson G, Smith KG (eds.): *Medical Nutrition Therapy Across the Continuum of Care* (ed 2). Chicago, American Dietetic Association, 1998, pp. 1–15
104. National Cancer Institute: Nutrition in cancer care. National Cancer Institute. *www.cancer.gov/templates/page_print.aspx?viewid=56fc02ab-59c1-4860-8c90-5fea5040366a&version=1#Section_96.* Accessed March 1, 2004.
105. Charney P: Enteral nutrition: indications, options, and formulations, in Gottschlich M (ed.): *The Science and Practice of Nutrition Support.* Dubuque, Kendall/Hunt, 2001, pp 141–166
106. Finocchiaro C, Gervasio S, Fadda M, et al: Home parenteral nutrition (HPN): survival in advanced cancer patients. *Clin Nutr* 22(suppl 1):S65, 2003
107. Ottery F, Kasenic SR, Cunningham RS: Multimodality approaches to optimize survivorship outcomes: body composition, exercise, and nutrition. *Issues in Nutrition and Cancer: Update 2004* 19:11–14, 2004
108. Schwartz AL, Mori M, Gao R, et al: Exercise reduces daily fatigue in women with breast cancer receiving chemotherapy. *Med Sci Sports Exerc* 33:718–723, 2001
109. Kolden GG, Strauman TJ, Ward A, et al: A pilot study of group exercise training (GET) for women with primary breast cancer: feasibility and health benefits. *Psychooncology* 11:447–456, 2002
110. Fairey AS, Courneya KS, Field CJ, et al: Effects of exercise training on fasting insulin, insulin resistance, insulin-like growth factors, and insulin-like growth factor binding proteins in postmenopausal breast cancer survivors: a randomized controlled trial. *Cancer Epidemiol Biomarkers Prev* 12:721–727, 2003
111. Na YM, Kim MY, Kim YK, et al: Exercise therapy effect on natural killer cell cytotoxic activity in stomach cancer patients after curative surgery. *Arch Phys Med Rehabil* 81:777–779, 2000
112. Eng J, Ramsum D, Verhoef M, et al: A population-based survey of complementary and alternative medicine use in men recently diagnosed with prostate cancer. *Integr Cancer Ther* 2:212–216, 2003
113. Navo MA, Phan J, Vaughan C, et al: An assessment of the utilization of complementary and alternative medication in women with gynecologic or breast malignancies. *J Clin Oncol* 22:671–677, 2004
114. Henderson JW, Donatelle RJ: Complementary and alternative medicine use by women after completion of allopathic treatment for breast cancer. *Altern Ther Health Med* 10:52–57, 2004
115. Spiegel W, Zidek T, Vutuc C, et al: Complementary therapies in cancer patients: prevalence and patients' motives. *Wien Klin Wochenschr* 115:705–709, 2003
116. Gray RE, Fitch M, Goel V, et al: Utilization of complementary/alternative services by women with breast cancer. *J Health Soc Policy* 16:75–84, 2003
117. Therapeutic Research Faculty: Natural Medicines Comprehensive Database. *www.naturaldatabase.com/(aosor1vlexfide45u3pSqte1)/nd/Search.aspx?li=1&st=2&cs=&sND.* Accessed March 2, 2004
118. U.S. Congress Office of Technology Assessment: Office of Technology Assessment reports: unconventional cancer treatments. U.S. Government Printing Office. *www.quackwatch.org/01QuackeryRelatedTopics/OTA/ota04.html.* Accessed March 1, 2004
119. Schumacher K, Schneider B, Reich G, et al: Influence of postoperative complementary treatment with lectin-standardized mistletoe extract on breast cancer patients. A controlled epidemiological multicentric retrolective cohort study. *Anticancer Res* 23:5081–5087, 2003
120. Weiger W, Smith M, Boon H, et al: Advising patients who seek complementary and alternative medical therapies for cancer. *Ann Intern Med* 137:889–913, 2002

CHAPTER 32

Hypercalcemia

AnnMarie K. McDonnell Keenan, RN/APN, MS, AOCN®
Rita S. Wickham, RN, PhD, AOCN®

Scope of the Problem

Definition

Hypercalcemia is the most common metabolic complication of malignancy and can be life-threatening for some patients. Hypercalcemia is diagnosed when the serum calcium exceeds 11.0 mg/dL (or is greater than 5.5 mEq/L, or 2.74 mmol/L; or is greater than 1.35 mmol/L of *ionized* calcium). However, this definition is simplistic and does not capture the severity of hypercalcemia, which can be symptomatic with relatively small increases in serum calcium levels. Other factors, such as the rapidity of development, renal function, age, performance status, concomitant medications, and previous episodes of hypercalcemia, are also important.[1] Hypercalcemia occurs because of a breakdown of normal calcium homeostasis and almost always develops in patients whose cancer is advanced. Without effective antitumor therapy, survival beyond weeks to months is unlikely. Nevertheless, prompt recognition and treatment usually enhance quality of life, and antiresorptive therapies may increase duration of survival for some individuals.

Incidence

It is estimated that 10%–40% of cancer patients experience hypercalcemia as a relatively late complication of malignancy, but incidence varies widely by tumor type. The distribution of tumor types associated with hypercalcemia remains relatively unchanged, with squamous cell carcinomas of the lung, head, and neck; breast neoplasms; and multiple myeloma accounting for the majority of cases[1,2] (Table 32-1).[3–12] Hypercalcemia is rare in some common malignancies, such as colorectal and prostate cancer, and it virtually never occurs in patients who have primary bone tumors. An iatrogenic cause of transient hypercalcemia in some women with breast cancer is tumor flare, which occurs with the initiation of hormone therapy.[3] It has been proposed that the incidence of hypercalcemia may actually be decreasing because of the widespread use of bisphosphonates.[13]

Etiology and Risk Factors

More than 90% of patients who develop hypercalcemia have primary hyperparathyroidism or malignant disease. Other causes of hypercalcemia are infrequent and include drug effects, congenital problems, thyroid or renal dysfunction, and immobilization (Table 32-2).[4,14–16]

Hyperparathyroidism is the most frequent etiology of hypercalcemia, but patients with this condition usually are not acutely symptomatic because hypercalcemia develops over a long period of time, and homeostatic mechanisms can come into play. Thus, patients with primary hyperparathyroidism are commonly ambulatory, and hypercalcemia is typically diagnosed by routine laboratory tests.[4] In contrast, hypercalcemia due to cancer is usually steadily and rapidly progressive, so homeostatic mechanisms are overwhelmed. Cancer-induced hypercalcemia most often rapidly leads to symptoms, even with relatively low serum calci-

Table 32-1 Incidence of Hypercalcemia in Particular Malignancies

Malignancy	Reported Incidence	References
Lung		3,7,12
Squamous cell	35%	
Other	11%	
Breast	17%–40%	4,12
Hematologic		6,11,12
Multiple myeloma	20%–40%	
Lymphoma	<10%	
Genitourinary	12%	12
Head and neck (squamous)	2.5%–25% (varies by site)	5,12
Renal cell	6%	3
Unknown primary	7%	3
Liver (primary)	3%	3,12
Other: cholangiocarcinoma, clear cell carcinoma of the ovary, pancreatic islet cell, vipoma	1%	4,8
Prostate, uterine, colorectal, primary bone, parathyroid, chronic lymphocytic leukemia, chronic myelogenous leukemia, acute leukemia, small cell lung cancer	<1%	4,9–12

Table 32-2 Etiologies of Hypercalcemia

Relative Frequency	Comments
	FREQUENT
Primary hyperparathyroidism	• Develops over a long period, usually asymptomatic • Parathyroid adenomas cause >80% of cases
Malignancy	• More likely to occur rapidly, leading to neurological, cardiovascular, gastrointestinal, and fluid volume deficit symptoms • May be accompanied by other symptoms of advanced cancer
	RARE
Dietary (or drug)	
Vitamin D intoxication	• Chronic ingestion of >50,000 IU/day or excessive ingestion of foods high in vitamin D
Vitamin A intoxication	• Chronic ingestion of >50,000 units/day
Milk-alkali syndrome	• Associated with chronic use of milk and antacids; leads to mild metabolic alkalosis and renal calcium reabsorption
Drugs	
Lithium	• Alters "set point" for PTH secretion, causing mild hypercalcemia
Thiazide diuretics	
Tamoxifen, estrogens, antiestrogens	• Increases bone resorption
Endocrine disorders	• No specific information available regarding mechanisms
Hyperthyroidism	
Pheocromocytoma	
Adrenal insufficiency (Addison's disease)	
Thyrotoxicosis	
Granulomatous diseases	
Sarcoidosis	• Increased 1-alpha-hydroxylase activity leading to elevated serum 1,25-dihydroxyvitamin D
Histoplasmosis	
Tuberculosis	
Coccidioidomycosis	
Other	
Familial hypocalciuric hypercalcemia	• Autosomal dominant inherited condition
Diuretic phase of acute renal failure	• Increased renal calcium reabsorption
Acute and chronic renal failure	• Increased resorption of calcium from bone
Paget's disease	• Increased renal calcium reabsorption
Immobilization	• Increased resorption of calcium from bone

PTH = parathyroid hormone.

um levels, which necessitates hospitalization, prompt diagnosis, and treatment. Most patients have obvious widespread metastases when hypercalcemia is diagnosed but may or may not have bone metastases, depending on the primary pathogenic mechanisms involved.

Hypercalcemia of Malignancy: Physiologic Alterations

The fundamental cause of hypercalcemia is excessive bone resorption with impaired renal clearance of the increased circulating calcium.[17] Tumors, or normal tissues surrounding them, produce and secrete one or several hormone-like polypeptides (cytokines) or other regulatory factors, which subsequently act systemically or locally to impair normal calcium homeostasis. The pathophysiology of hypercalcemia differs somewhat depending on the underlying malignancy, but these mechanisms result in only subtle differences in organ effects that do not generally require different treatments. Therefore, it is probably most useful to bear in mind that there are no absolute divisions in types of malignancy-induced hypercalcemia, and pathogenic processes most likely occur along a continuum rather than being discrete etiologic groups.[2]

One of two mechanisms is usually the primary cause of hypercalcemia: humoral hypercalcemia of malignancy (HHM) or local osteolytic hypercalcemia (LOH). Humoral hypercalcemia occurs most frequently and is estimated to cause nearly 80% of hypercalcemia cases, whereas LOH causes 20%–30% of cases.[12,17] The broad classifications of HHM and LOH are not totally inclusive for all malignancies, and particular tumors may express other cytokines or hormones that have effects on organ systems involved in calcium homeostasis. For instance, hematologic malignancies may produce 1,25-dihydroxyvitamin D, which causes increased calcium resorption from bone, increased absorption of dietary calcium from the gut, and possibly impaired glomerular filtration of calcium.[11] In addition, immobilization because of poorly controlled pain or other symptoms, or renal failure may worsen hypercalcemia.

Humoral Hypercalcemia of Malignancy

Patients with HHM, who may or may not have bone metastases, have tumors that elaborate and secrete humoral factors (hormones and cytokines) that act systemically or locally to induce excessive calcium resorption from bone and resultant hypercalcemia.[7] The most important hormone is parathyroid hormone–related protein (PTHrP), which is elevated in the serum of about 80% of hypercalcemic patients who have solid tumors.[17] Parathyroid hormone–related protein has a structure closely resembling native parathyroid hormone (PTH) which accounts for its ability to mimic the biologic function of PTH.[2] That is, the release of either is associated with increased osteoclast bone resorption, reduced bone formation, and increased renal tubular reabsorption of calcium. Parathyroid hormone and PTHrP are both normally expressed in fetal and adult tissues, but serum PTHrP levels are undetectable in healthy adults. Parathyroid hormone–related protein has multiple roles in the differentiation and physiologic functioning of normal tissues, including cartilage and bone, skin, breast, pancreatic islets, kidney, mammary epithelium, placenta, and smooth muscle function, and in immune functions.[18,19]

Parathyroid hormone–related protein has some distinct roles, such as in the stimulation of growth factors that are capable of creating a microenvironment within bone that supports tumor growth.[20] It is also expressed by some malignant tumors that are not accompanied by extensive bone metastases, including squamous cell carcinomas of the lung, head, and neck; breast malignancies; and adenocarcinomas of the kidney, lung, pancreas, or ovary.[21] Ectopic PTHrP does not respond to normal negative feedback loops, and serum calcium levels rise to dangerous levels.[22]

Tumor-produced PTHrP probably does not account for all of the clinical features of HHM, and effects on the bone, kidney, and intestine of patients with cancer may be influenced by other tumor-produced factors, such as interleukins, tumor growth factor (TGF), tumor necrosis factor (TNF), and epidermal growth factor (EGF).[22,23] Recently, squamous carcinoma cell lines have been shown to secrete an osteoclast differentiation factor (ODF), also known as tumor necrosis factor–related activation-induced cytokine (TRANCE), which increases the number of osteoclasts.[2] High production of any of these factors can directly increase osteoclastic bone resorption, and these cytokines can also potentiate the effects of PTHrP on osteoclast activity and calcium homeostasis.[21] Furthermore, PTHrP-induced renal tubular calcium resorption occurs in many patients with solid tumors as well as in some patients with multiple myeloma and breast cancer, in whom circulating PTHrP is usually not an important factor. In these patients, volume depletion impairs glomerular filtration and leads to increased sodium and calcium resorption in the proximal convoluted tubules. However, increased renal tubular calcium reabsorption persists even after dehydration is corrected.[21]

Local Osteolytic Hypercalcemia

In patients who have breast cancer or multiple myeloma, hypercalcemia usually occurs late in the disease and almost never develops unless the patient has extensive osteolytic bone metastases.[2] Tumor cells typically do not resorb bone, but rather produce local cytokines or other regulatory factors that induce local bone resorption, osteolysis, and hypercalcemia.[21] Increased levels of osteoclast-regulating factors are found adjacent to and within skeletal metastases, and they induce osteoclasts to migrate to the tumor site and become active. This activity leads to uncoupling of bone formation and destruction of bone.[24–26] Local production of PTHrP by tumor cells is probably the most important mechanism of LOH. Breast cancer patients with LOH, for example, have been shown to have increased PTHrP near tumor cells in bone. This finding is consistent with the "seed and soil" theory. That is, bone provides a fertile environment for tumor cell growth, which is enhanced by PTHrP production in this micorenvironment. Similarly, multiple myeloma almost always causes destructive osteolytic bone lesions throughout the skeleton, leading to diffuse osteopenia. Bone destruction is the consequence of myeloma-produced mediators, such as IL-6, IL-1β, and TNF-α, and lymphotoxin.[11] Along with bone destruction, patients with multiple myeloma frequently have reduced glomerlar filtration rates caused by light-chain nephropathy, further hampering the kidney's ability to excrete excess calcium.

Normal Anatomy and Physiology: Scientific Principles

Normal Calcium Homeostasis

The body's total calcium content is approximately 1 kg, of which 99% is bound in bones and teeth. Only the remaining 1% of calcium, which is found in the serum, is of interest. Forty-five to 50% of serum calcium is ionized (Ca^{2+}), which is the biologically active form. Forty percent is bound to protein, primarily albumin, and a small amount is bound to globulin.[2] The remaining 10%–15% is complexed with bicarbonate, citrate, or phosphate. Normal serum calcium levels reflect both ionized and bound forms (unless ionized calcium is specifically measured) and are maintained in a constant narrow range. The ranges vary slightly by gender. For men, they are 9.0–10.3 mg/dL (or 4.5–5.2 mEq/L, or 2.25–2.57 mmol/L); for women, they are 8.9–10.2 mg/dL (or 4.4–5.1 mEq/L, or 2.22–2.54 mmol/L).[27]

Only ionized Ca^{2+} is physiologically active and filtered in the kidney. Among its most important activities, Ca^{2+} regulates many intracellular and extracellular functions, particularly the electrical potential of cells and thus neuromuscular conductivity and transmission.

Despite the fact that calcium levels fluctuate each day with dietary calcium consumption and bone remodeling, serum calcium remains within a remarkably narrow range because of the actions of several calciotropic hormones (parathyroid hormone, 1,25-dihydroxyvitamin D, and calcitonin) on target organ systems (bone, gastrointestinal tract, and kidney). For instance, 200–400 mg of calcium is released and is taken up by bone each day during bone remodeling. Under normal circumstances, calcium fluxes across bone surfaces not involved in remodeling are greater than those involved in remodeling.[6] Bone surface cells not actively involved in bone remodeling communicate with deeper osteocytes, which can rapidly interact to regulate calcium transport from the extraosseous extracellular fluid to the serum. This system has the potential capacity to move large volumes of calcium from bone to serum, which occurs under the influence of parathyroid hormone.

Each day, approximately 900 mg of calcium is consumed in the diet, and the influence of 1,25-dihydroxyvitamin D causes about 350 mg to be absorbed from the gastrointestinal tract. Of this amount, 150 mg is released into intestinal secretions, so the net absorption of dietary calcium is 200 mg. The excess is excreted by the kidney and maintains serum calcium balance.[14]

Calciotropic Hormones

Normally, calcium and bone metabolism are regulated by the action of three main hormones: PTH, 1,25-dihydroxyvitamin D, and calcitonin. The first two hormones serve to increase the serum calcium level, while calcitonin will decrease it over the short term. Other hormones (e.g., thyroxin, glucocorticoids, estrogens) also influence bone cell function.

Parathyroid hormone. Parathyroid hormone is a single-chain polypeptide secreted by the chief cells of the parathyroid gland in response to low serum calcium levels. The secretion of PTH may also be influenced by other factors, such as prostaglandins, adrenergic agonists, magnesium, and vitamin D metabolites, which can recruit and attract osteoclasts to bone surfaces and lead to subsequent bone resorption. Parathyroid hormone acts predominantly on bone and kidney. In bone, it increases the size and volume of the ruffled border of osteoclasts, which leads to increased bone resorption, and inhibits osteoblasts. The net effect is an increase in calcium release from bone.[6,28] Parathyroid hormone also has a powerful action on the kidney's ability to reabsorb calcium in the distal convoluted tubule, and it promotes the synthesis of 1,25-dihydroxyvitamin D in the proximal tubules of the kidney. This, in turn, increases calcium absorption in the gut.

1,25-Dihydroxyvitamin D. 1,25-dihydroxyvitamin D is synthesized by the body via conversion of precursors in the skin by ultraviolet light (sunlight), which are further acted on by the liver and ultimately by the kidney.[6,28] Final hydroxylation occurs in the kidney and may be stimulated by PTH or low extracellular phosphate levels; other hormones (e.g., calcitonin, estrogen, growth hormone, prolactin) may also have some influence. Conversely, when serum calcium or phosphate is high, synthesis is inhibited. The major effect of 1,25-dihydroxyvitamin D is to provide sufficient amounts of calcium and phosphate for bone mineralization. In the face of low serum calcium levels or during periods of increased physiologic need, 1,25-dihydroxyvitamin D acts primarily on the gut to promote absorption of dietary calcium.

1,25-dihydroxyvitamin D has powerful stimulatory effects on bone resorption and enhances the differentiation of osteoclast precursors into osteoclasts; it also influences both the resorption of bone and the mineralization of the matrix, along with calcium and phosphate resorption from bone.[6,28] In addition, it stimulates calcium and phosphate absorption in the gut.

Calcitonin. Calcitonin is synthesized by the parafollicular (C) cells of the thyroid. It acts primarily to lower serum calcium levels and secondarily to control the movements of other ions (e.g., phosphate, magnesium, sodium). The synthesis of calcitonin is regulated by extracellular calcium, food intake, and some gastric hormones (gastrin, glucagon, secretin, and cholecystokininpancreozymin).[6,28] The prime target organs are calcitonin receptors in the bone (osteoclasts) and the kidney.

Although calcitonin does not play a major role in day-to-day serum calcium homeostasis, it does enhance the body's ability to deal with rapid changes in serum calcium load or depletion. Thus, calcitonin is released in response to a rapid increase in serum calcium, such as would occur after the ingestion of a high-calcium-containing meal. As extracellular calcium levels decline, calcitonin release is inhibited.[6] Calcitonin also acts to decrease serum calcium by exerting a direct effect on osteoclast differentiation, maturation, number, mobility, and cellular function.[28] Under the influence of calcitonin, osteoclasts rapidly lose their ruffled border and move away from the resorptive surface, so calcium is not transported from bone to the extracellular fluid. In the kidney, calcitonin receptors are found in the ascending limb of the loop of Henle, the proximal end of the distal convoluted tubule, and the cortical segment of the collection tubule. When calcitonin binds to these receptors, tubular resorption is reduced and, consequently, calcium, sodium, potassium, chloride, phosphate, and water are excreted.

Other factors. Other factors, including other hormones and cytokines, are known to play some role in calcium balance. For instance, thyroid hormone stimulates osteoclasts and thus bone resorption; glucocorticoids exert complex effects on bone metabolism, and their prolonged use may inhibit bone matrix synthesis; and estrogens have complex and interactive effects with calcitonin, PTH, and vitamin D. Estrogen receptors have been identified on the osteoblasts and osteoclasts of humans and animals.[29] When estrogen is administered over a long period, the net effects are a decreased rate of bone turnover, osteoclast inhibition, and bone stabilization.[28]

Several cytokines interact synergistically and antagonistically with one another or with other hormones to exert important effects on bone cell function, metabolism, and bone turnover.[28] Cytokines involved mainly in bone formation include insulin-like growth factors 1 and 2 and bone morphogenetic proteins. Those that primarily cause bone resorption include IL-6 and colony-stimulating factors. Those that both form and resorb bone include TGF-β, platelet-derived growth factors, and IL-1. Prostaglandins may also influence local bone cell activity.

Bone

Living bone is specialized connective tissue consisting of bone cells and hydroxyapatite, an organic matrix composed mainly of calcium and phosphate and strengthened by crystalline salts.[30] Bone cells include osteoclasts and osteoblasts, as well as bone-lining cells and osteocytes, which arise from osteoblasts. The functions of osteoblasts and osteoclasts are controlled by hormones and local factors, including weight bearing. Both types of bone cells are intimately involved in remodeling bone (each elaborates and secretes substances that induce the formation and activity of the other) and in releasing and depositing calcium into bone.[6,30]

Osteoclasts arise from pluripotent hematopoietic bone marrow stem cells — specifically, the monocyte cell line. As such, osteoclasts share a common initial differentiation pathway with macrophages, but their differentiation is influenced by the sequential expression of different sets of genes, cytokines, and growth factors. Osteoclasts are morphologically, cytochemically, and immunophenotypically similar to other cells in the mononuclear-phagocytic system. They are rich in enzymes that degrade bone matrix, and can release local factors that contribute to resorption of bone. Osteoclasts play a major role in bone remodeling and are the *only* cells that can resorb bone; they can increase bone resorption to fulfill calcium requirements of body homeostasis when necessary.[25]

Osteoblasts arise from local mesenchymal osteoprogenitors (preosteoblasts) found near bone-forming surfaces. The primary role of these cells is to synthesize the mineralized bony matrix; they also can mature to become flattened bone-lining cells that cover bone surfaces or migrate into bone to become osteocytes maintaining the bone matrix. Osteoblasts and preosteoblasts, but not osteoclasts, have receptors for PTH, PTHrP, and 1,25-dihydroxyvitamin D.[24] Osteoblasts produce several factors (e.g., granulocyte-macrophage colony-stimulating factor [GM-CSF], granulocyte colony-stimulating factor [G-CSF], and macrophage colony-stimulating factor [M-CSF], IL-1, IL-6, TNF) that have subsequent effects on osteoclast differentiation and function.[29,30]

After skeletal maturation, remodeling occurs in which a fraction of bone is removed and replaced each

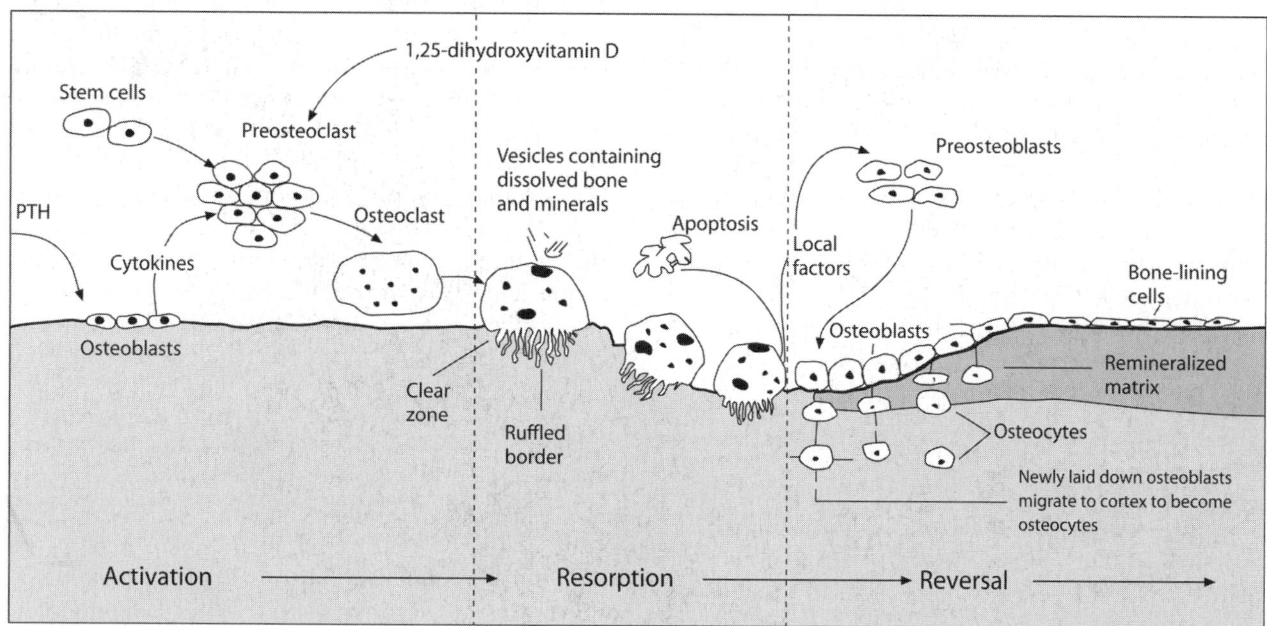

Figure 32-1 Bone remodeling involves coordinated processes of osteoblasts and osteoclasts that maintain bone mass. Activation commences as the parathyroid gland secretes parathyroid hormone (PTH), signaling osteoblasts to secrete cytokines. These cytokines, along with calcitriol, cause preosteoclasts to fuse into multinucleated osteoclasts. During resorption, osteoclasts are firmly attached to bone surfaces by the clear zone. The clear zone encloses an acidic environment, in which the ruffled border dissolves the bone matrix. The dissolved bone and minerals are resorbed via endocytosis into vesicles, transported through the cell cytoplasm, and released from the opposite cell membrane into the serum. At the end of resorption, osteoclasts release local factors to induce preosteoblast formation and then undergo apoptosis. During reversal, osteoblasts secrete new bone matrix, and some osteoblasts migrate to the cortex to become osteocytes. The remaining osteoblasts become bone-lining cells.

year without changing the size or shape of the bone. Bone remodeling, which takes place on the bone surfaces and within bone, is integral to maintaining the structural integrity and tensile strength of bone and to serum calcium regulation.[6,30] At any one time, only about 10% of the skeleton is undergoing active remodeling.[26] Bone remodeling continues throughout life and is *coupled;* that is, resorption at a particular site exactly equals bone formation at that site. Sometime after the fifth decade of life, bone remodeling becomes uncoupled, and bone formation does not keep pace with resorption. Thus, skeletal mass decreases, skeletal strength is reduced, and the risk for fractures increases.[30]

The functions of remodeling are to replace bone matrix that has developed defects from normal use, to prevent the propagation of fatigue cracks that can progress to fractures, and to play a role in mineral homeostasis.[28] It is not known how the body determines and controls the sites of remodeling, but weight bearing is an important factor and osteocytes may act as mechanosensors with bone.[25] The minimal intensity and type of mechanical forces (load) necessary to maintain normal bone density have not been identified, but empirical and clinical evidence suggest that markedly decreased loading has negative effects on bone strength and mass. For instance, prolonged immobilization of a limb or skeletal traction causes bone resorption to exceed bone formation. Even vigorous activity after such restriction can delay regained bone density for many months in children, and bone density may never reach previous levels in older people.[28]

Normal Bone Remodeling

The cycle of bone remodeling lasts approximately 3 months in adult bone. It comprises three phases: activation, resorption, and reversal.[26] This process maintains bone mass and equilibrates the balance between resorption and formation (Figure 32–1).

Activation

The activation phase initiates remodeling and corresponds to osteoclast differentiation in response to soluble factors released by osteoblasts.[29] Activation is not random but rather occurs at sites where remodeling and restructuring are necessary; osteoclasts are also found at active bone resorption sites in pathologic conditions characterized by extensive osteolysis.[6] Mononuclear preosteoclasts that have proliferated in the bone marrow are attracted to bone sites where resorption of bone will occur.[25] Resident bone cells, genes, and growth factors induce mononuclear precursors to fuse into multinucleated osteoclasts. Local osteoblasts and bone marrow stromal cells affect PTH, PTHrP, and prostaglandins to stimulate the formation of osteoclasts and resorptive activity. Genes that may be important for osteoclast formation and activity include the proto-oncogenes *FOS, MYC,* and *SRC.*[29] Growth factors that have been identified near bone and are known to play some role in the formation of osteoclasts include M-CSF, cytokines (IL-1, IL-6, IL-11), leukemia inhibitory factor, and TNF.[6] Calcitriol is also essential for the formation of osteoclasts and the differentiation of osteoclast precursors.

Resorption

The second phase of bone remodeling, resorption, lasts 15–30 days.[6,29] During this time, osteoclasts resting directly on the bone surface have two specialized plasma membranes: a ruffled border and a clear zone. The ruffled border is the bone-resorbing organ, and the clear zone surrounding it attaches the osteoclast to the underlying bone by means of integrins.[24,25,29] The highly infolded ruffled border is a specialized lysosomal membrane that forms by rapid fusion of acidic intracellular vesicles and secretes proteolytic enzymes, such as lysosomal cysteine proteinases and matrix metalloproteinases, which can dissolve hydroxyapatite crystals. In vitro studies using rat cells showed that osteoclasts are tightly sealed to the bone surface during resorption, which isolates the resorption area from the extracellular fluid. Dissolved bone mineral is endocytosed in vesicles through the ruffled border membrane, transported through the osteoclast, and emptied from a secretory area in the opposite cell membrane into the serum.[31–33] Osteoclasts are probably removed by apoptosis (programmed cell death) after they fulfill their resorptive task.[25]

Reversal

In the reversal phase of bone remodeling, osteoclasts from the old matrix release local factors that stimulate undifferentiated mesenchymal cells, or *preosteoblasts,* to start filling the resorption cavity. These precursor cells assume the appearance of osteoblasts and secrete a specialized extracellular matrix, which subsequently mineralizes.[28] Approximately 10%–20% of the osteoblasts become embedded in the mineralized matrix and evolve into osteocytes; the remainder become flattened and elongated to cover the bone surface.[26,34]

The Role of the Kidney

The kidney is the major regulator of serum calcium levels. As mentioned previously, under normal circumstances it excretes the excess dietary calcium that has been absorbed in the gut (approximately 200 mg/day). Renal excretion can increase to approximately 600 mg per day when necessary to maintain a normal serum calcium.[35] Severe hypercalcemia, however, overwhelms the kidney's ability to concentrate urine and excrete high amounts of calcium liberated from the bone. This effect is exacerbated in HHM, in which a tumor elaborates and secretes PTHrP into the serum. The PTHrP causes the kidney to reabsorb calcium despite the presence of hypercalcemia. Furthermore, high concentrations of calcium in the urine impede sodium and water reabsorption, which results in excessive urine formation (polyuria).[27] If uncorrected, fluid volume is lost and dehydration results. This sets up a vicious circle, because renal blood flow decreases in the face of dehydration and fluid volume deficit; glomerular filtration decreases; and sodium and calcium are reabsorbed in the proximal tubules, which worsens hypercalcemia.

The Role of the Gastrointestinal Tract

With the exception of rare tumors that produce 1,25-dihydroxyvitamin D, the gastrointestinal tract does not play a role in HHM. This is because 1,25-dihydroxyvitamin D is produced only when serum calcium is low and is inhibited by high serum calcium levels.

Clinical Manifestations

Individuals who develop hypercalcemia exhibit a constellation of unpleasant, nonspecific signs and symptoms that may be misinterpreted as manifestations of terminal cancer or as side effects of chemotherapy, radiation therapy, or other medications (e.g., opioids). There is great variability in how patients present: some are asymptomatic, and few have all of the symptoms associated with hypercalcemia. The predominant signs and symptoms reflect calcium's roles in neuromuscular (CNS and peripheral), gastrointestinal, renal, and cardiovascular functioning (Table 32–3).[1,6,14,27] In general, elevated calcium levels exert a depressive effect on neuromuscular excitability.

Little relationship exists between symptoms and serum calcium levels. Nevertheless, patients with serum calcium levels greater than 14 mg/dL usually have symptoms; those who rapidly develop hypercalcemia are likely to have severe symptoms; and older or debilitated individuals are more likely than young people to experience neuromuscular signs and symptoms.[1,2,27]

Table 32-3 Manifestations of Hypercalcemia Associated with Cancer

Organ System	Signs and Symptoms
Neurological	
Central nervous system	Altered cognition Confusion Apathy Drowsiness or lethargy Pain **Late:** Obtundation, coma
Peripheral neuromuscular	Muscle weakness Hypotonia Decreased respiratory muscle capacity Decreased or absent deep-tendon reflexes
Renal	Polyuria Polydipsia Dehydration (dry mucous membranes, orthostatic hypotension, etc.) Occasional nephrocalcinosis
Cardiovascular	Prolonged P-R interval Widened QRS Shortened QT, ST intervals Bradycardia (with rapid increases) **Late:** Widened T-waves, broadened T-wave, heart block, ventricular arrhythmias, asystole Enhanced sensitivity to digitalis Hypertension (if intravascular volume is maintained)
Gastrointestinal	Increased gastric acid secretion Anorexia Nausea and vomiting Constipation Acute pancreatitis (rare) **Late:** Obstipation

Neuromuscular

Neurologic effects of hypercalcemia occur in the central nervous system and in the periphery. The CNS effects are more obvious, whereas the peripheral effects are more likely to be attributed to advanced cancer. Effects in the CNS begin with impaired concentration and perhaps mild confusion or disturbing nightmares.[6] Bone pain may occur not only due to the presence of bony metastases but also because calcium may act as a neurosensitizer, decreasing the pain threshold.[2] Progressive confusion, lethargy, other CNS symptoms, and ultimately coma occur if hypercalcemia is uncorrected and serum calcium rises to greater than 15 mg/dL. Conversely, when hypercalcemia is adequately treated, severe CNS effects may resolve more slowly than serum calcium normalizes. (The clinical picture of hypercalcemia varies in patients with hyperparathyroidism, who are more likely to experience anxiety, memory difficulties, and restlessness.[14]) Peripheral effects occur because elevated serum calcium depresses neuromuscular excitability in smooth and striated muscle, and results in weakness, hypotonic muscles, and absent deep-tendon reflexes.[27]

Gastrointestinal

The dampening effect of increased serum calcium on neuromuscular excitability also occurs in the autonomic nervous system. Gastrointestinal signs and symptoms occur in most symptomatic patients. Gastrointestinal motility slows and gastric acid secretion increases, which may intensify nausea, vomiting, and anorexia.[27] Constipation is aggravated by dehydration and may progress to obstipation, which in turn worsens nausea and anorexia.

Renal

Hypercalcemia reduces the kidney's ability to concentrate urine. Polyuria results in dehydration and reduced extracellular volume, which in turn leads to decreased renal perfusion and decreased glomerular filtration rate (GFR). In the face of decreased GFR and dehydration, more sodium and calcium are reabsorbed in the proximal tubules.[2] Signs of dehydration are evident and may include thirst, dry mucosa, decreased or absent perspiration, poor skin turgor, and concentrated urine (late).

Cardiovascular

High levels of serum calcium increase cardiac contractility and irritability, and slow cardiac conduction.[27] Electrocardiogram changes may include a prolonged P-R interval, a widened QRS, or a shortened Q-T interval. T-waves appear wide secondary to the increased Q-T interval. As in other organ systems, symptoms worsen as serum calcium increases. Bradycardia is unusual but may occur when calcium levels increase rapidly. Bradyarrhythmias can progress to bundle branch block; at a serum concentration of 18 mg/dL, atrioventricular block may occur and can progress to complete heart block or asystole.[27] For the most part, cardiac manifestations have minimal clinical significance unless the patient is taking cardiac glycosides.[2]

Assessment and Grading

While no standard grading toxicity criteria for hypercalcemia have been established, several authors concur on the levels of severity based on a range of normal serum calcium values of 8.5–10.5 mg/dL.[27] Hypercalcemia may be graded as mild (<12 mg/dL), moderate

(12–14 mg/dL), severe (14–16 mg/dL), or life-threatening (>16 mg/dL). These values assume a normal serum albumin and must be adjusted if this is not the case (see Diagnostic studies later in this chapter). Grading, in conjunction with clinical symptoms, is useful in diagnostic and treatment decisions.

Diagnostic Work-up for Hypercalcemia

The diagnostic work-up for hypercalcemia includes a history, physical examination, and laboratory tests. It is an important step because 20%–25% of patients with cancer may experience hypercalcemia from other causes. These alternative etiologies include primary hyperparathyroidism (4%); hormone manipulation with tamoxifen, estrogens, androgens, or progestins for breast cancer (2%); vitamin D intoxication (2%); or other idiopathic causes (16%).[4] Confirming hypercalcemia therefore depends on confirming a syndrome, and single symptoms are insufficient to diagnose the problem.

Patient and family history

The patient or family history is important in identifying hypercalcemia and confirming a cancer-related cause. The patient — or family members if the patient is confused or obtunded — provides important information that guides further diagnostic tests as well as medical treatment and nursing care. Most patients who present with hypercalcemia have a known diagnosis of malignant disease and exhibit obvious signs of advancing disease. If the primary diagnosis is not immediately known, the patient's gender, general appearance, and duration and pattern of symptoms may provide some clues regarding the underlying cause. For example, the incidence of primary hyperparathyroidism is greatest in elderly women who have symptoms of mild hypercalcemia for longer than 6 months, whereas hypercalcemia related to malignancy has a rapid onset of symptoms.[21] The nurse should gather information regarding the patient's chief complaints, the presenting symptoms over time, the cancer diagnosis (if confirmed), known metastases, current antineoplastic therapy (especially estrogen or antiestrogen therapy), medication and dietary supplement history, and concomitant health problems (Table 32–4).[3,21,27,36] It is also important to do a pain assessment, particularly when the patient has known bone metastases, because poorly relieved pain can interfere with physical activity and mobility.

Physical examination

The physical examination is not specific for hypercalcemia per se, because of the previously discussed nonspecificity of signs and symptoms in multiple systems. Instead, when hypercalcemia is suspected, a broad-based assessment focuses on the patient's neurological assessment (level of consciousness, presence of confusion), muscular assessment (muscle weakness, flaccidity, absent deep-tendon reflexes), gastrointestinal assessment (nausea, abdominal distention, diminished bowel sounds, palpable feces in the colon), fluid volume status (obvious signs of dehydration), and cardiovascular assessment (irregular or slow heart rate). In addition, the nurse assesses the patient's performance status and physical appearance. Patients who have advanced disease may appear to be weak or fatigued and demonstrate muscle wasting and obvious weight loss.

Diagnostic studies

In most instances, the history and physical examination support a clear diagnosis of cancer-related hypercalcemia. In these individuals, the serum calcium confirms the diagnosis. However, it is not unusual for patients with advanced cancer to experience anorexia and cachexia, which result in low serum protein levels. Under normal circumstances, ionized calcium and calcium bound to albumin are at approximately equilibrium. When a patient has less serum albumin to bind with calcium, however, a greater portion of the total serum calcium portion *must* be ionized. One formula used to adjust serum calcium measurements is based on a normal serum albumin value of less than 4.0 g/dL and can be adjusted for serum calcium values expressed as mg/dL, mEq/L, or mmol/L calcium (Table 32–5).[3,15,21] The results are considered to be rough estimates of total serum calcium but are easily calculated and clinically useful.

In rare instances, patients with cancer will have primary hyperparathyroidism. If this condition is suspected, the immunoradiometric assay (IRMA) for PTH may be done. This test can confirm a malignant cause of hypercalcemia if PTH is suppressed; PTH levels will be elevated in primary hyperparathyroidism.[21]

Therapeutic Approaches and Nursing Care

Treatment decisions are based on the severity of hypercalcemia, the necessity of hospitalization for treatment, and whether a decision not to treat hypercalcemia is appropriate if all definitive treatment options have been exhausted.[2] Most patients will be treated, and those who have moderate or severe hypercalcemia will be hospitalized for treatment and close monitor-

Table 32-4 Focused History for Suspected Hypercalcemia

Focus	Comments
Chief complaint/reason for seeking care	Most commonly neurological/mental status symptoms, but may be other symptom(s) of advanced cancer, GI symptom, pain, polyuria, etc.
Symptom(s)	
Onset/duration	Recent onset or long-standing symptoms?
Progression	Rapid or slow worsening of symptoms?
Severity	Patient's rating.
Associated symptoms	If patient does not volunteer, ask about frequent urination, thirst, constipation (ask if patient is taking an opioid analgesic), weakness, fatigue.
Effects on important ADLs, QOL	Altered ambulation, nightmares.
Diagnosis of cancer confirmed?	Is this a malignancy in which hypercalcemia occurs?
Known bone metastases?	Breast cancer and multiple myeloma are frequently associated with hypercalcemia.
Previous episodes of hypercalcemia	Associated with increased risk for occurrence.
Current therapy for cancer	
Chemotherapy	Can therapy be the cause of some of the symptoms?
New estrogen or antiestrogen	Has bone pain increased with new hormone (may indicate tumor flare)?
Medications	Ask about over-the-counter medications and alternative/complementary supplements in addition to prescription drugs.
Megavitamins	
Nutritional supplements	Do CV assessment; report bradycardia or irregular HR to MD; hold digoxin until after consulting with MD.
Calcium	
Vitamin A, D	
Shark cartilage	
Thiazide diuretic	
Lithium	
Digoxin	
Other	Ask about: Activity level, especially bed rest Whether pain, nausea/vomiting, or other unrelieved symptoms interfere with activity Current/usual appetite and diet Weight loss in last 6 months; calculate percent weight loss (>10% may indicate protein/calorie malnutrition).

GI = gastrointestinal; ADL = activities of daily living; QOL = quality of life; CV = cardiovascular; HR = heart rate; MD = physician.

ing. A summary of treatment options is included in Table 32-6.[1,2,27,37,38]

No consensus exists regarding the treatment of patients with mild hypercalcemia whose symptoms may go unnoticed or are thought to be caused by other problems.[27] These individuals may be managed with oral fluids and antiresorptive therapy in ambulatory settings. In cases of moderate hypercalcemia, severity of symptoms guides the choice and speed of therapy. Thus, moderately hypercalcemic patients who have serious manifestations (e.g., altered mental status, ECG changes, nausea and vomiting, polyuria) are treated in the same manner as those with more severe hypercalcemia. Severe and life-threatening hypercalcemia (>15 mg/dL) are always considered medical emergencies, and patients require immediate antiresorptive therapy in addition to saline. Initial treatment may include the use of the most rapid osteoclast inhibitor, calcitonin, in conjunction with the bisphosphonate pamidronate or zoledronic acid.

Goals of Therapy

The medical goals of hypercalcemia management are fourfold: (1) to correct dehydration; (2) to increase renal excretion of calcium with vigorous saline diuresis; (3) to inhibit calcium resorption from bone with antiresorptive agents; and (4) to treat the underlying malignancy, if possible. No matter how mild or severe hypercalcemia is, dehydration with oral or intravenous saline-containing fluids is always the essential first step to restore fluid balance and subsequently increase urinary calcium excretion.

Saline Diuresis

Rehydration with intravenous 0.9% normal saline is critical to restore intracellular, extracellular, and vascular volumes, thereby increasing GFR, calcium filtration, and excretion. The rate of normal saline administration is based on patient parameters, such as severity

Table 32-5 Formulas for Adjusting Serum Calcium for Low Serum Albumin

Calcium in mg/dL =
(base albumin concentration [4.0 mg/dL] – measured serum albumin concentration [g/dL]) × 0.8 mg/dL + reported serum calcium

Example: The patient's reported serum calcium is 11.8 mg/dL, and serum albumin is 2.5 g/dL.

(4.0 g/dL – 2.5 g/dL) = 1.5 g/dL × 0.8 = 1.2
11.8 + 1.2 = 13 mg/dL (corrected serum calcium)

Calcium in mEq/L =
(base albumin concentration [4.0 mg/dL] – measured serum albumin concentration [g/dL]) × 0.4 mg/dL + reported serum calcium

Example: The patient's reported serum calcium is 5.9 mEq/L, and serum albumin is 2.5 g/dL.

(4.0 g/dL – 2.5 g/dL) = 1.5 g/dL × 0.4 = 0.6
5.9 + 0.6 = 6.5 mEq/L (corrected serum calcium)

Calcium in mmol/L =
(base albumin concentration [4.0 mg/dL] – measured serum albumin concentration [g/dL]) × 0.2 mg/dL + reported serum calcium

Example: The patient's reported serum calcium is 2.95 mmol/L, and serum albumin is 2.5 g/dL.

(4.0 g/dL – 2.5 g/dL) = 1.5 g/dL × 0.2 = 0.3
2.95 + 0.3 = 3.25 mmol/L (corrected serum calcium)

of hypercalcemia, severity of dehydration, and cardiovascular tolerance for volume expansion. If tolerated, the patient may receive 300–400 mL (or more) of normal saline for several hours to correct dehydration. Saline diuresis may be contraindicated in patients experiencing renal failure or congestive heart failure. Such patients must be treated cautiously, and a loop diuretic (most commonly furosemide) must be added *only* after fluid balance has been restored. Because furosemide can increase dehydration and electrolyte imbalance (particularly potassium), it is not generally recommended unless fluid overload is a major concern.

Pharmacologic interventions

The effect of normal saline diuresis is temporary, so definitive therapy including an antiresorptive drug to correct hypercalcemia is necessary (Table 32-7). According to recent reviews, the agent of choice to treat cancer-related hypercalcemia is a bisphosphonate, particularly for all patients whose corrected serum calcium is greater than 13 mg/dL (or 3.0 mmol/L).[1,2,27,37–40] Other therapeutic options for hypercalcemia include corticosteroids in hematologic malignancies and calcitonin combined with a bisphosphonate for the acute management of severe hypercalcemia. Other antiresorptive agents include gallium nitrate and plicamycin. In rare instances, dialysis may be indicated for severely hypercalcemic patients.

Bisphosphonates

Bisphosphonates are specific inhibitors of osteoclasts that act via multiple mechanisms: inhibit tumor cell binding to bone matrix; prevent differentiation of osteoclast precursors; inhibit secretion of protons that dissolve bone mineral matrix; and induce proapototic effects on tumor cells.[41] Three generations of bisphosphonates have been developed, with each subsequent class exhibiting greater potencies. Etidronate, a first-generation bisphosphonate, demonstrates little clinical utility in the treatment of hypercalcemia. Second- and third-generation bisphosphonates are potent antiresorptive agents that normalize calcium levels, reduce skeletal complications from bone metastases, and most recently have been found to inhibit bone metastases.[40,41] These agents are associated with few adverse effects when compared to other antiresorptive agents. Bisphosphonates are administered intravenously because oral formulations are poorly absorbed with limited bioavailability. Following intravenous administration, the drugs are rapidly taken up by the skeleton, remaining there for a prolonged period.[41] Approximately 20%–40% of these drugs are excreted unchanged in the urine within 24 hours.[41]

Pamidronate. Pamidronate (Aredia) has been the most effective and least toxic agent used to treat hypercalemia and thus has been the standard of care for LOH of breast cancer and multiple myeloma.[42] There is a dose-related response to pamidronate. In one study, 30% of patients who received 30 mg experienced normocalcemia, while response rates of patients who received 60 mg and 90 mg were 61% and 100%, respectively.[43] Pamidronate can be safely administered to patients with impaired renal function. The drug is given as an intravenous infusion over a relatively short period (2, 4, or up to 24 hours). The onset of action is 24–48 hours, the calcium nadir is reached at 5–6 days, and normal calcium is maintained for an average of 21–28 days.[44] Calcitonin, in addition to pamidronate, may be administered to patients experiencing severe or life-threatening hypercalcemia to achieve a more rapid reduction of serum calcium.

The adverse effects of pamidronate are few and mild. They include fever, flulike syndrome with malaise, infusion site reaction, gastrointestinal distress, hypophosphatemia, hypokalemia, and hypomagnesemia.[44]

Table 32-6 Therapy Options Based on Severity of Hypercalcemia

Grade/Level	Serum Calcium	Treatment Options
Normal	8.5–10.5 mg/dL 4.25–5.25 mEq/L 2.2–2.65 mmol/L	
Mild	<12 mg/dL <6 mEq/L >2.65–3.0 mmol/L	• Rehydrate with oral fluids or IV 300–400 mL/hr of normal saline × 3–4 hr in severely dehydrated patients and observe. • Manage associated symptoms. • Antineoplastic therapy for primary cancer. • If symptomatic, treat as for moderate to severe hypercalcemia.
Moderate	12–14 mg/dL 6–7 mEq/L 3.0–3.5 mmol/L	• Rehydrate with IV normal saline (3–4 L in first 24 hr) to induce diuresis. • Add furosemide 20–40 mg q12h, *only* after dehydration corrected, if indicated (e.g., CHF, peripheral edema related to low albumin). • Pamidronate 60–90 mg IV over 2–24 hr or zoledronic acid 4 mg IV over 15 min. • Antineoplastic therapy for underlying cancer.
Severe	14–16 mg/dL 7–8 mEq/L 3.5–4.0 mmol/L	• Rehydrate with IV normal saline (4–6 L in first 24 hr) to induce diuresis. • Add furosemide 20–40 mg q12h, after dehydration corrected, if indicated (as above). • Pamidronate 90 mg IV over 2–24 hr or zoledronic acid 4 mg IV over 15 min. • Antineoplastic therapy for underlying cancer.
Life-threatening	>16 mg/dL >8 mEq/L >4.0 mmol/L	• Rehydrate with IV normal saline (4–6 L in first 24 hr) to induce diuresis. • Add furosemide 20–40 mg q12h, after dehydration corrected, if indicated (as above). • Calcitonin 4 IU/kg SQ q12h; increase dose to 8 IU/kg SQ q6h if no response within 6 hr. • Pamidronate 90 mg IV over 2–24 hr (or plicamycin 25 μg/kg IV over 15–30 min) or zoledronic acid 4 mg IV over 15 min. • Antineoplastic therapy for underlying cancer.

Zoledronic acid. Unlike other third-generation bisphosphonates, zoledronic acid (Zometa) contains an imidazole ring structure with two nitrogen atoms, making it the most potent inhibitor of bone resorption currently available. Recently, zoledronic acid has demonstrated superiority over pamidronate in clinical trials.[39] A total of 275 patients with moderate to severe hypercalcemia were treated with a single dose of zoledronic acid (4 or 8 mg) via 5-minute infusion or pamidronate (90 mg) via a 2-hour infusion. The complete response rates at day 10 were 88.4%, 86.7%, and 69.7% for zoledronic acid 4 mg and 8 mg and pamidronate 90 mg, respectively. At day four, 50% of patients treated with zoledronic acid had normal calcium levels, compared to 33.3% of pamidronate-treated patients. The median durations of complete response were 32, 43, and 18 days for zoledronic acid 4 mg and 8 mg and pamidronate 90 mg, respectively.[39] Further studies, designed to evaluate prolonged skeletal effects of bisphosphonates, have shown safety and efficacy of both pamidronate and zoledronic acid when used for greater than 24 months in patients with breast cancer and multiple myeloma.[45]

Zoledronic acid 4 mg is initially administered as an intravenous infusion over a minimum of 15 minutes. The onset of action is 24–48 hours, with normal calcium levels being maintained for 4 to 6 weeks. Adverse effects are similar to those noted with pamidronate. Renal effects have been noted infrequently.[2,39] Refractory or relapsed hypercalcemia may be treated with 8 mg zoledronic acid. Advantages of this drug include superior efficacy, short infusion time, efficacy in both LOH and HHM, and a safe side effect profile.[38,39,45]

Calcitonin

Calcitonin has the most rapid onset of action. It lowers serum calcium primarily by decreasing renal tubular reabsorption of calcium and secondarily by blocking osteoclast resorption.[2] Calcium reductions of 2–3 mg/dL may occur in 4–6 hours. Calcitonin is useful for initial treatment but rapidly loses its effectiveness. Tachyphylaxis develops in 2–3 days. Occasionally, a corticosteroid is administered with calcitonin to enhance and prolong its effect.[44] Calcitonin may be

Table 32-7 Antiresorptive and Other Agents to Treat Hypercalcemia

Agent	Mechanism of Action	Administration Considerations	Adverse Reactions	Comments
Bisphosphonates Pamidronate (Aredia)	Bind to hydroxyapatite; inhibit number and action of osteoclasts	60–90 mg IV over 2–24 hr	Transient fever Flulike syndrome Site reaction	• Aredia is highly effective, low toxicity
Zoledronic acid (Zometa)	As above	4 mg IV over 15 min 8 mg IV over 15 min for relapsed or refractory cases	As above	• Agent of choice to treat hypercalcemia because it is the most potent bisphosphonate available • Superior efficacy • Short infusion time
Calcitonin	Inhibits osteoclast action; decreases renal reabsorption of calcium	4 IU/kg SQ q12h Increase to 8 IU/kg q6h prn	Allergic reactions Nausea and vomiting	• Most rapid onset of action • Administer intradermal test dose • Wheal or mild erythema contraindicate further use • Tachyphylaxis occurs in 2–3 days
Plicamycin (Mithracin)	Causes death of osteoclasts by DNA intercalation Inhibits renal tubular reabsorption of calcium	25 μg/kg IV over 4–6 hr	Nephrotoxicity Hepatotoxicity Increased prothrombin time Nausea and vomiting Thrombocytopenia	• Rapid onset of action • Dose may be repeated in 24–48 hr if no decrease in calcium • More toxic than bisphosphonates • Contraindications: renal insufficiency, thrombocytopenia, hepatic failure • Not recommended
Gallium nitrate (Ganite)	Stabilizes bone crystals Inhibits osteoclasts	100–200 mg/m^2 over 24 hr for up to 5 days	Nephrotoxicity (noncumulative) Nausea and vomiting	• Patient must be hospitalized for treatment • Not recommended
Corticosteroids Hydrocortisone	Inhibit lymphoid tissue growth	100–300 mg IV or PO over 3–5 days	Hyperglycemia Fluid retention	• Not used except for steroid-sensitive tumors (multiple myeloma, lymphoma) • May enhance effect of calcitonin
Prednisone	Inhibit down-regulation of steroid receptors Increase urinary excretion of calcium	40–100 mg/day		• Slow acting, not specific; never used routinely or alone • Adverse effects preclude long-term use

combined with pamidronate if the patient's serum calcium is greater than 13 mg/dL (3.3 mmol/L).[2]

Calcitonin can cause allergic reactions, so an intradermal test dose should be given. If a wheal forms or mild erythema occurs at the site, further treatment with calcitonin is contraindicated. Other toxicities include nausea, flushing of face and hands, and abdominal cramps.[2,44]

The usual initial dose of calcitonin is 4 IU/kg given subcutaneously every 12 hours. Most patients will start to respond within 2–4 hours, so the serum calcium should be rechecked 5–6 hours after the first dose. If there has been no response, intravenous hydration with normal saline (plus furosemide, as indicated) will continue, and the dose of calcitonin may be increased to 8 IU/kg every 6 hours.

Other agents

Plicamycin. Plicamycin (Mithracin) was developed as an antineoplastic agent that was noted to cause hypocalcemia; it was recognized as a useful agent to treat hypercalcemia before bisphosphonates were available. Plicamycin is a potent inhibitor of RNA synthesis in osteoclasts.[44] It has a rapid onset of action and begins to lower calcium within 12 hours. However, only 30%–50% of patients achieve normocalcemia, which typically persists for only 2–14 days, when rebound hypercalcemia may occur.[44]

Plicamycin is an irritant, and its infiltration may lead to local tissue reactions. The usual dose is 25 μg/kg administered as an intravenous infusion over 4–6 hours. The dose may be repeated in 24–48 hours if serum calcium does not decrease, and it is not unusual for patients to require multiple doses to control hypercalcemia.[44] Plicamycin is more toxic than bisphosphonates, which poses a problem in patients who may already have received a great deal of chemotherapy. This drug can cause cumulative nephrotoxicity, hepatotoxicity, nausea and vomiting, thrombocytopenia, and an increased prothrombin time. As a consequence, it is reserved for patients who do not respond to other treatments.[44]

Gallium nitrate. In 1991, gallium nitrate (Ganite) became available to treat cancer-related hypercalcemia unresponsive to hydration. It was withdrawn from the market in 1995 because of its adverse effect profile; at that time, pamidronate was available. Recently, gallium nitrate was reintroduced for the treatment of symptomatic hypercalcemia unresponsive to adequate hydration. It is a highly effective agent that normalizes calcium in almost all hypercalcemic patients. Gallium nitrate localizes to sites of bone resorption, binds to hydroxyapatite (which stabilizes bone crystals and produces hydroxyapatite more resistant to osteoclast-mediated absorption), and inhibits osteoclasts.[1] Serum calcium levels start to decrease within 24–48 hours; normocalcemia occurs in 4–7 days and lasts for approximately 1 week.

Gallium nitrate is not generally used because of its expense, inconvenience, and toxicities. Patients must be hospitalized for several days to receive this agent, which is administered by continuous intravenous infusion with adequate intravenous hydration. The recommended dose is 100–200 mg/m^2 over 24 hours for up to 5 days.[1] Gallium nitrate can exacerbate renal insufficiency or lead to reversible, noncumulative nephrotoxicity in some patients. This outcome can be prevented by maintaining the patient's urine output at 2 liters per day. Concurrent use of nephrotoxic drugs should be avoided. Other minor adverse effects include nausea and vomiting and constipation (may be related to hypercalcemia).

Corticosteroids

Corticosteroids do not play a major role in managing hypercalcemia but are occasionally useful in treating hypercalcemia associated with steroid-sensitive malignancies, such as multiple myeloma and lymphomas. In the past, these agents were used as adjuncts to calcitonin to prevent attenuation of the latter's effect.[44] Corticosteroids may be administered orally or parentally and act to inhibit 1,25-dihydroxyvitamin D–mediated absorption of calcium from the gut.[44] Corticosteroids induce a slow response over 1–2 weeks.

Dialysis

Peritoneal dialysis and hemodialysis are rarely used to treat hypercalcemia. An indication for dialysis is the severely hypercalcemic patient who has a treatable malignancy but is experiencing renal insufficiency.[27] Dialysis can reduce serum calcium by 3–12 mg/dL in 24–48 hours. Unfortunately, large amounts of phosphate are lost in the process, which aggravates hypercalcemia. Thus, phosphate is typically added to the next dialysate or to the diet.

Prevention

Until recently, there were no preventive measures for hypercalcemia. Pamidronate and zoledronic acid have now been approved by the U.S. Food and Drug Administration for patients who have osteolytic bone metastases and who are not hypercalcemic; these agents are recommended postdischarge to maintain normal serum calcium levels.[21,42] This recommendation is based on data that confirm the ability of pamidronate and zoledronic acid to decrease skeletal complications, including hypercalcemia, pathologic fractures, bone pain, and the need for radiation therapy or surgery.[42] In addition, patients experience recalcification of lytic metastases and fewer new lytic metastases to bone, which enhances their quality of life. Such benefits occur in patients with breast cancer, multiple myeloma, and bony metastases from other diseases. Pamidronate 60–90 mg administered intravenously over 2 hours every 3–4 weeks and zoledronic acid 4 mg administered over 15 minutes every 3 weeks are both effective to preventively treat hypercalcemia and bone metastases.[42] Preventive management is advantageous and less costly because patients are treated in outpatient settings and avoid complications that require hospitalization.

Other General Measures and Nursing Care

When caring for patients at risk for or actually experiencing hypercalcemia, nurses focus not only on administering medically ordered therapies but also on managing associated symptoms, maintaining patient safety, and minimizing risk for recurrence, which includes patient/family education. In addition, when patients no longer respond to anticancer or hypercalcemic therapies, nurses focus on the emotional and physical care of these individuals at the end stage of disease.

During the initial treatment phase of moderate to life-threatening hypercalcemia, patients are receiving large volumes of intravenous normal saline to induce rehydration and urinary calcium excretion. It is important to assess and manage fluid balance and potential electrolyte imbalance that may occur during vigorous diuresis, including marked decreases in sodium, potassium, phosphate, and magnesium. Laboratory results of these electrolytes should be assessed daily or more often if necessary. Vital signs and symptoms of fluid overload should also be monitored at least every 4 hours during hydration and drug treatment. Cardiovascular status should be assessed, and the patient may require cardiac monitoring. If any question arises regarding the patient's cardiac status, the nurse should hold a dose of digoxin until after consultation with the patient's physician. Likewise, if the patient has been taking tamoxifen or another hormone for breast cancer, the nurse should discuss administration procedures with the physician.

Safety is another major concern for patients who have altered thinking, confusion, sleepiness, and muscle weakness. A major goal is to protect patients from falls and injury, particularly if they are voiding frequently and get up to use the bathroom or commode. In addition, the family or care providers may misconstrue lethargy as depression, which might be assumed to be a normal emotional response to the diagnosis.[27] Performing a Mini-Mental Status examination can help to differentiate confusion and lethargy from depression.

The nurse also focuses on increasing patient activity and ambulation, particularly in patients who are bedridden, because exercise and weight bearing are critical to maintaining bone mass; inactivity leads to lost bone mass. This may mean controlling other symptoms that are interfering with the patient's ability or willingness to be active. For instance, it is not unusual for hypercalcemic patients to have painful bone metastases or nausea and vomiting, either of which may limit activity.

Continuity of Care

Unless prophylactic treatment for hypercalcemia or treatment for the underlying malignancy is planned, the patient is likely to become hypercalcemic again. It is therefore useful not only to teach the patient and family the most common signs and symptoms of hypercalcemia, but also to explore with them the pattern of symptoms experienced by the patient. Helping them to strategize about actions to decrease the risk for hypercalcemia and advice on when to seek medical attention can then be personalized. Teaching should include instructions to maintain fluid intake at 3–4 liters per day (and telephoning the nurse or physician if they are unable to do so), along with liberal salt intake (unless there is a medical contraindication). Pain control and management of nausea and vomiting and other symptoms are important. The goal to maintain or increase mobility must be addressed within the context of performance status, pain and other symptom control, and nutritional status. Most patients can be encouraged to eat whatever tastes good, and calcium does not need to be withheld from the diet; it is not an important contributor to hypercalcemia in most patients with cancer.[1,2]

Conclusion

Hypercalcemia occurs as a relatively late complication of advanced cancer in a significant number of individuals. It negatively affects patients' quality of life and may ultimately lead to their death. It is important that nurses recognize risk factors for, and signs and symptoms of, hypercalcemia. While the currently recommended "best" therapy for hypercalcemia—zoledronic acid—may not prolong survival, it represents a major advance because it can be used prophylactically and can be administered over a minimum of 15 minutes in an outpatient setting. Many patients therefore may not experience common unpleasant and distressing signs and symptoms of hypercalcemia. Managing hypercalcemia is a reasonable palliative care goal that enhances most patients' quality of life.

References

1. Warrell RP: Metabolic emergencies, in DeVita VT, Hellman S, Rosenberg SA (eds.): *Cancer: Principles and Practice of Oncology* (ed 6). Philadelphia, Lippincott, Williams & Wilkins, 2001, pp 2633–2645
2. Morton AR, Ritch PS: Metabolic disorders: hypercalcemia, in Berger AM, Portenoy RK, Weissman DE (eds.): *Principles and Practice of Palliative Care and Supportive Oncology* (ed 2). Philadelphia, Lippincott, Williams & Wilkins, 2002, pp 493–507
3. Harvey HA: The management of hypercalcemia of malignancy. *Support Care Cancer* 3:123–129, 1995
4. Raue F: Epidemiological aspects of hypercalcemia of malignancy, in Raue W (ed.): *Recent Results in Cancer Research.* Berlin, Springer-Verlag, 1994, pp 99–106
5. Muggia FM: Overview of cancer-related hypercalcemia: epidemiology and etiology. *Semin Oncol* 17(suppl 5):3–9, 1990

6. Mosekilde L, Eriksen EF, Charles P: Hypercalcemia of malignancy: pathophysiology, diagnosis and treatment. *Crit Rev Oncol Hematol* 11:1–27, 1991
7. Warrell RP: Etiology and current management of cancer-related hypercalcemia. *Oncology* 6:37–43, 1992
8. Orloff JJ, Stewart AF: Disorders of serum minerals caused by cancer, in Coe FL, Favus MJ (eds.): *Disorders of Bone and Mineral Metabolism.* New York, Raven, 1992, pp 539–561
9. Mao C, Carter P, Schaefer P, et al: Malignant islet cell tumor associated with hypercalcemia. *Surgery* 117:37–40, 1995
10. Brown EM, Harris HW, Vassilev PM, et al: The biology of the extracellular Ca^{2+}-sensing receptor, in Bilezikian JP, Raisz LG, Rodan GA (eds.): *Principles of Bone Biology.* New York, Academic, 1996, pp 243–262
11. Roodman GD: Mechanisms of bone lesions in multiple myeloma and lymphoma. *Cancer* 80:1557–1563, 1997
12. Heys SD, Smith IC, Eremin O: Hypercalcemia in patients with cancer: aetiology and treatment. *Eur J Surg Oncol* 24:139–142, 1998
13. Mundy GR: Mechanisms of bone metastasis. *Cancer* 80:1546–1556, 1997
14. Bleyer A, Goldfarb S: Calcium metabolism, in Szerlip HM, Goldfarb S (eds.): *Workshops in Fluid and Electrolyte Disorders.* New York, Churchill Livingstone, 1993, pp 165–191
15. Kaye TB: Hypercalcemia: how to pinpoint the cause and customize treatment. *Postgrad Med* 97:153–155, 159–160, 1993
16. Kovacs CS, MacDonald SM, Chik CL, et al: Hypercalcemia of malignancy in the palliative care patient: a treatment strategy. *J Pain Symptom Manage* 10:224–232, 1995
17. Solimando DA: Overview of hypercalcemia of malignancy. *Am J Health-Syst Pharm* 58(suppl 3):S4–S7, 2001
18. Rankin W, Grill V, Martin TJ: Parathyroid hormone–related protein and hypercalcemia. *Cancer* 80:1564–1571, 1997
19. Philbrick WM, Wysolmerski JJ, Galbraith S, et al: Defining the roles of parathyroid hormone–related protein in normal physiology. *Physiol Rev* 71:127–173, 1996
20. Davidson TG: Advanced prospectives on the clinical usefulness of bisphosphonates: introduction. *Am J Health-Syst Pharm* 58(suppl 3):S3–S4, 2001
21. Mundy GR, Guise TA: Hypercalcemia of malignancy. *Am J Med* 103:134–145, 1997
22. Molina PE: Parathyroid gland and CA++/PO4 regulation, in Molina PE (ed.): *Endocrine Physiology.* New York, Lange Medical Books/McGraw-Hill, 2004, pp 99–122
23. De La Mata J, Uy HL, Guise TA, et al: Interleukin-6 enhances hypercalcemia and bone resorption mediated by parathyroid hormone–related in vivo. *J Clin Invest* 95:2846–2852, 1995
24. Athanasou NA: Cellular biology of bone-resorbing cells. *J Bone Joint Surg* 78–A:1096–1113, 1996
25. Vaananen K: Osteoblast function: biology and mechanisms, in Bilezikian JP, Raisz LG, Rodan GA (eds.): *Principles of Bone Biology.* New York, Academic, 1996, pp 103–113
26. Kanis JA, McCloskey EV: Bone turnover and biochemical markers in malignancy. *Cancer* 80:1538–1545, 1997
27. National Cancer Institute: *PDQ Health Professional: Hypercalcemia.* Updated May 2003, *www.cancer.gov/cancerinfo/pdq/supportivecare/hypercalcemia/HealthProfessional.* Accessed April 9, 2004
28. Buckwalter JA, Glimcher MJ, Cooper RR, et al: Bone biology. Part II: formation, form, modeling, and regulation of cell function. *J Bone Joint Surg* 77–A:1276–1289, 1995
29. de Vernejoul MC: Dynamics of bone remodelling: biochemical and pathophysiological basis. *Eur J Clin Chem Biochem* 34:729–734, 1996
30. Marks SC, Hermey DC: The structure and development of bone, in Bilezikian JP, Raisz LG, Rodan GA (eds.): *Principles of Bone Biology.* New York, Academic, 1996, pp 3–14
31. Nesbitt SA, Horton MA: Trafficking of matrix collagens through bone-resorbing osteoclasts. *Science* 276:266–269, 1997
32. Mostov K, Werb Z: Journey across the osteoclast. *Science* 276:219–220, 1997
33. Salo J, Lehenkari P, Mulari M, et al: Removal of osteoclast bone resorption products by transcytosis. *Science* 276:270–273, 1997
34. Aubin JE, Liu F: The osteoblast lineage, in Bilezikian JP, Raisz LG, Rodan GA (eds.): *Principles of Bone Biology.* New York, Academic, 1996, pp 51–67
35. Mundy GR: General concepts of calcium homeostasis, in Mundy GR (ed.): *Calcium Homeostasis: Hypercalcemia and Hypocalcemia.* New York, Oxford University Press, 1990, pp 1–16
36. Lagman R, Walsh D: Dangerous nutrition? Calcium, vitamin D, and shark cartilage nutritional supplements and cancer-related hypercalcemia. *Support Care Cancer* 11:232–235, 2003
37. Hurtado J, Esbrit P: Treatment of malignant hypercalcaemia. *Expert Opin Pharmacother* 3:521–527, 2002
38. Major P: The use of zoledronic acid, a novel, highly potent bisphosphonate, for the treatment of hypercalcemia of malignancy. *Oncologist* 7:481–491, 2002
39. Major P, Lortholary J, Hon E, et al: Zoledronic acid is superior to pamidronate in the treatment of hypercalcemia of malignancy: a pooled analysis of two randomized, controlled clinical trial. *J Clin Oncol* 19:558–567, 2001
40. Body JJ, Mancini I: Bisphosphonates for cancer patients: why, how, and when? *Support Care Cancer* 10:399–407, 2002
41. Ramaswamy B, Shapiro CL: Bisphosphonates in the prevention and treatment of bone metastases. *Oncology* 17:1261–1270, 2003
42. Maxwell C, Swift R, Goode M, et al: Advances in supportive care of patients with cancer and bone metastases: nursing implications of zoledronic acid. *Clin J Oncol Nurs* 7:403–408, 2003
43. Nussbaum SR, Younger J, VandePol CJ, et al: Single-dose intravenous therapy with pamidronate for the treatment of hypercalcemia of malignancy: comparison of 30–, 60–, and 90–mg dosages. *Am J Med* 95:297–304, 1993
44. Davidson TG: Conventional treatment of hypercalcemia of malignancy. *Am J Health-Sys Pharm* 58(suppl 3):S8–S15, 2001
45. Ali SM, Esteva FJ, Hortobagyi G, et al: Safety and efficacy of bisphosphonates beyond 24 months in cancer patients. *J Clin Oncol* 19:3434–3437, 2001

CHAPTER 33

Paraneoplastic Syndromes

Terri S. Armstrong, MS, APRN, BC

Introduction

Symptoms often occur as a direct effect of a neoplasm. Paraneoplastic syndromes (PNSs) are those symptoms or signs that result from damage to organs or tissues that are remote from the site of a malignant neoplasm or its metastases.[1] As paraneoplastic syndromes may occur in several body systems, including endocrine, hematologic, neurologic, and dermatologic, they often must be distinguished from those symptoms caused directly by the tumor, metastases, toxicities of therapy, or concomitant medical problems. This distinction is important, as recognition of a PNS may lead to earlier diagnosis of a cancer, allow for treatment of associated symptoms, or serve as a surrogate marker of response to therapy.

Paraneoplastic syndromes arise from multiple etiologies, including the secretion of substances such as growth hormones, growth factors, cytokines, antibodies, and other immune products by the primary tumor or its metastases (see Figure 33-1). Although the true incidence of PNSs is not known, it is estimated that they occur in 10%–15% of all cancer patients at the time of diagnosis and in as many as 50% over the course of their disease. Some authors have classified the more generalized conditions associated with cancer — anorexia-cachexia, tumor fever, and anemia of chronic disease — as PNSs. If these conditions are included, then almost all patients with cancer will experience at least one paraneoplastic manifestation.

The most common cancer diagnosis associated with PNS is small cell lung carcinoma, but PNS can be associated with any malignancy.[2] This syndrome occurs uncommonly in childhood malignancies, with the exception of Wilms' tumor and neuroblastoma. It may precede the diagnosis of cancer or occur at any point in the illness trajectory. Its severity may not be correlated with the extent of malignancy, but frequently its existence predicts a poor prognosis. In general, the primary treatment of PNS entails treatment of the underlying malignancy.[3] However, symptoms associated with the PNS may be permanent despite adequate treatment of the cancer.

In general, PNSs are extremely rare, with only a few case reports in the literature. Despite their rarity, PNSs are now being viewed as mechanisms for providing a greater understanding of tumor immunity.[4] Tumor cells rely on normal tissue or produce naturally occurring hormones or other proteins to cause PNS. Normal cells are either mistaken for tumor cells by the patient's autoimmune response, as occurs in neurologic PNSs, or the normal systems are recruited through tumor secretion of hormone, cytokine, or endocrine mediators to produce the endocrine, hematologic, and cutaneous PNSs.

Endocrine Paraneoplastic Syndromes

Scope of the Problem

Endocrine PNSs occur frequently and result from ectopic (tumor) production of naturally occurring peptide proteins (hormones) or hormone precursors.[5] The endocrine PNSs are the most well defined in terms of their etiology, clinical presentation, and disease course. Diagnosis depends on the following conditions being present: coexistence of a hormone-excess syndrome and malignancy; increased hormone levels in the blood or urine; and improvement in the syndrome with successful treatment of the malignancy. The most common and well-known endocrine PNSs are hypercalcemia, paraneoplastic adrenocorticotropic hormone (pACTH) syndrome, and syndrome of inappropriate antidiuretic hormone (SIADH). However, tumor cells produce almost every known hormone and hormone-releasing factor, resulting in the potential existence of multiple endocrine PNSs (Table 33-1).

Definitions

Paraneoplastic or *humoral hypercalcemia* occurs when the patient has a calcium level exceeding 11.0 mg/dL in the absence of bony metastases. The elevation is caused by tumor secretion of parathyroid hormone–related protein (PTHrP). *Paraneoplastic ACTH syndrome* is the development of Cushing's disease caused by the secretion of ACTH by malignant cells in the absence of a pituitary neoplasm or hyperplasia.[6] *Syndrome of inappropriate antidiuretic hormone secretion (SIADH)* is defined as the presence of hyponatremia with plasma hyperosmolality and inappropriately concentrated urine.[5] It is characterized by failure of the normal regulatory influences to suppress arginine-vasopressin (AVP) release, which results in the inability to excrete free water.

Incidence

Hypercalcemia is a common metabolic complication of malignancy, occurring in approximately 10% of patients with cancer. An estimated 15% of malignancies are associated with endocrine paraneoplastic syndromes, with hypercalcemia most commonly being associated with squamous cell carcinomas of the lung (15%), head and neck, and esophagus, followed by breast, uterine, cervical, lymphoma, multiple myeloma, and renal cell carcinomas.[7] It is estimated that 10%–15% of cancer patients with hypercalcemia do not have metastatic bone disease.

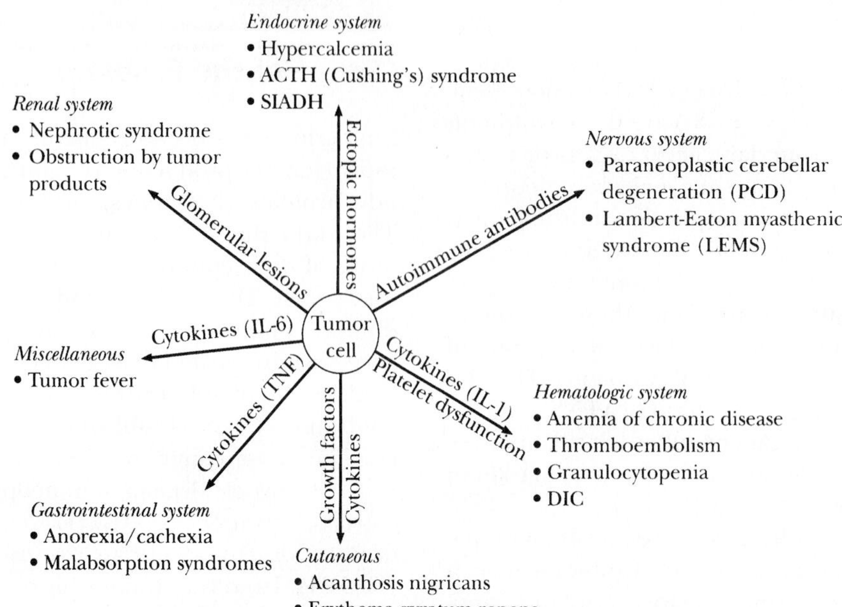

Figure 33-1 Paraneoplastic syndromes: Ectopic tumor effects. (ACTH = adrenocorticotropic hormone; SIADH = syndrome of antidiuretic hormone secretion; DIC = disseminated intravascular coagulation.)

Although pACTH syndrome occurs rarely, it is encountered more often than the benign form of Cushing's disease and is considered the second most frequent PNS. It occurs most often in patients with small cell lung cancer; approximately 5% of these patients will experience it at some time during the course of their disease. Bronchogenic carcinoma accounts for 60%–70% of the total cases of pACTH syndrome. Other malignancies associated with pACTH syndrome include pancreatic carcinoma, carcinoid tumors, hepatocellular carcinoma, pheochromocytoma, colon carcinoma, and medullary thyroid cancer.

Syndrome of inappropriate antidiuretic hormone secretion is associated with many types of malignancies, and has been reported to occur in 3% of patients with head and neck cancer, in 0.7% of patients with non-small cell lung cancer, and in 15% of patients with small cell lung cancer.[8] Most of these patients may have some aspects of SIADH without clinical evidence of the syndrome. Although their incidence is extremely limited, other cancers associated with SIADH include primary brain tumors; pancreatic, prostate, lymphoma, thymoma, and duodenal cancers; and Ewing's sarcoma.[8]

Etiology and Risk Factors

The etiology of paraneoplastic hypercalcemia involves tumor secretion of bone-resorbing cytokines. Although prostaglandins, transforming growth factors, and 1,25–dihydroxyvitamin D have all been reported to be associated with the development of the condition, PTHrP is considered the primary factor in the development of paraneoplastic hypercalcemia. These cytokines may also be important in the development of hypercalcemia in the setting of bone metastases, as some patients never develop hypercalcemia and no relationship has been found between the incidence of hypercalcemia and the extent of bony disease.[9] A recent study found that elevated PHTrP levels were associated with male gender, squamous cell histology, tumor located in the chest and mediastinum, decreased performance status, increased creatinine levels, and later stage of disease.[10]

Ectopic secretion of ACTH by neoplastic cells leads to bilateral adrenal hyperplasia and the symptoms of Cushing's disease in pACTH syndrome. The prognosis for patients with this condition is poor because ACTH may function as a growth factor for neoplastic cells and excessive cortisol levels suppress immune function, leading to an increased risk of infection, especially fungal infections.[6] The median survival time for small cell lung cancer patients with pACTH is 3–7 months.[11] In addition, patients are at risk for developing gastrointestinal ulceration and bleeding due to their high cortisol levels.[12]

The etiology of SIADH as a PNS is theorized to occur as a result of the ectopic production of vasopressin. Small cell carcinoma of the lung accounts for 80% of the malignancies associated with SIADH. Clinical

Table 33-1 Endocrine Paraneoplastic Syndromes

Syndrome	Hormone	Associated Malignancy	Clinical Presentation	Comments
Hypercalcemia	Parathyroid hormone–related protein (PTHrP)	*Solid Tumors:* Squamous cell • Lung cancer • Head and neck • Esophagus • Cervix • Breast • Ovarian • Bladder	• Confusion • Weakness • Lethargy	
	Osteoclast-activating factors 1,25-hydroxyvitamin D	*Hematologic:* Multiple myeloma Acute leukemia Lymphoma		
Paraneoplastic ACTH (Cushing's) syndrome	Adrenocorticotropic hormone (ACTH)	Small cell lung carcinoma (6%) Carcinoid Pancreatic Medullary thyroid Pheochromocytoma	• Hypokalemia • Muscle weakness/ atrophy • Weight loss • Hypertension	
Syndrome of inappropriate antidiuretic hormone secretion	Arginine vasopressin (AVP) Atrial natriuretic hormone (ANP)	Small cell lung carcinoma (80%) Pancreatic Thymus Breast	• Water intoxication • Hyponatremia	
Paraneoplastic growth hormone–releasing hormone syndrome (acromegaly)	Growth hormone–releasing hormone (GHRH)	Bronchial carcinoid Pancreatic carcinoma	• Acromegaly	Rapid onset
Paraneoplastic osteomalacia	1,25-hydroxyvitamin D	Soft tissue, bone tumors • Hemangioma • Angiosarcoma • Osteoblastoma	• Skeletal pain • Muscle weakness	Occurs in young adults
Paraneoplastic secretion of human chorionic gonadotropin	Human chorionic gonadotropin (HCG)	Ovarian Testicular Large cell lung cancer Gastric Breast Melanoma	Usually asymptomatic • Dysfunctional bleeding • Gynecomastia	
Hypoglycemia	Insulin-like growth factors	Mesothelioma Fibrosarcoma Neurofibrosarcoma Hepatoma	• Diaphoresis • Confusion — may progress to stupor/coma	Many patients asymptomatic unless fasting
Paraneoplastic erythrocytosis	Erythropoietin	Uterine fibroma Cerebellar hemangioblastoma Hepatocellular carcinoma	• ↑ RBCs • ↑ Hgb/Hct • ↑ Red blood cell mass	Remission achieved by surgical resection of tumor

RBC = red blood cell; Hgb = hemoglobin; Hct = hematocrit.

SIADH has been reported to occur in 30%–70% of these patients.[5] Other factors contributing to the multifactorial etiology of SIADH in the patient with small cell lung cancer include smoking (nicotine), stress, pain, nausea, and the use of morphine, all of which can increase AVP production.[12] No correlation has been shown between the extent of disease and the occurrence of SIADH or the stage of disease or survival.[13]

Pathophysiology

The underlying pathophysiology with endocrine PNSs focuses on the effects of ectopic hormone production, which then influences various physiologic pathways and release of other hormones. Paraneoplastic hypercalcemia is often associated with tumor secretion of PTHrP; this protein is similar to parathyroid hormone

(PTH), which is associated with bone resorption and osteolysis. PTHrP binds to PTH receptors, thereby inducing bone resorption and phosphaturia, and resulting in hypercalcemia.[14] In addition to inducing hypercalcemia, PTHrP may act as a growth factor for malignant cells. In patients with multiple myeloma and lymphoma, local bone destruction — not secretion of PTHrP — is associated with hypercalcemia. These tumors secrete osteoclast-activating factors, made from one or several cytokines, such as interleukin-1–β, which stimulate osteoclasts to resorb bone.[15] In patients with multiple myeloma, another cytokine, tumor necrosis factor beta (TNF-β), is secreted by multiple myeloma cells, which stimulates bone resorption. Finally, in patients with lymphoma, small cell lung cancer, and malignant melanoma, production of active metabolites of vitamin D is thought to stimulate calcium absorption from the gut.[16]

In patients with paraneoplastic ACTH syndrome, the tumor produces a precursor molecule, which contains ACTH, immunologic forms of beta-endorphin, and melanocyte-stimulating hormone (MSH). The secretion of ACTH stimulates the adrenal cortex to produce excessive amounts of glucocorticoids, which in turn leads to the development of Cushing's disease. Although as many as one-third of small cell lung cancer patients exhibit increased serum ACTH levels, only 1%–2% actually develop Cushing's syndrome, as a result of the inactivity of many of the products of the precursor molecule.[15]

Paraneoplastic SIADH is caused by excess stimulation of the neurohypophyseal peptide AVP. Normally, the body's fluid and sodium balance are maintained by the effect of AVP on the kidney. Excess stimulation of AVP leads to increased permeability of the collecting duct to water, resulting in water reabsorption. The excess AVP stimulation creates a scenario of water intoxication from an expanded extracellular volume, serum hypoosmolality, hyponatremia, and hypertonic urine.[15]

Clinical Manifestations

It is not uncommon for patients with hypercalcemia to be asymptomatic as a result of the gradual onset of this condition. However, a rapid increase in calcium can occur with highly proliferative tumors, when excessive bone reabsorption overwhelms the kidney's ability to excrete calcium. Symptoms of hypercalcemia may include polyuria, polydipsia, nausea, vomiting, anorexia, constipation, lethargy, weakness, and dehydration. Dehydration may then decrease the glomerular filtration rate and perhaps worsen the hypercalcemia. Excess calcium ions adversely affect cardiac muscle contractility, cell membrane permeability, and the conduction of electrical impulses through the heart. The resulting cardiovascular effects include heart block, bradycardia, ventricular arrhythmias, and asystole.[17] Late signs may include headaches, irritability, anxiety, insomnia, confusion, disorientation, hallucinations, and coma.

The symptoms associated with pACTH depend on the condition's underlying cause. Patients with small cell carcinomas rarely have all of the classic signs of Cushing's syndrome. In these patients, the most common symptoms include proximal myopathy, moon faces, hypokalemia, and hyperglycemia.[18] As a result of the increased levels of MSH, patients with pACTH also have hyperpigmentation. Symptoms associated with Cushing's disease unrelated to cancer, including plethora and cutaneous hyperpigmentation, may be absent because these patients do not survive long enough to develop these characteristics.

As with other endocrine PNSs, patients with SIADH may be asymptomatic. Water intoxication accounts for the signs and symptoms seen with SIADH, and most occur when the serum sodium level has fallen to 115–120 mEq/L (normal range = 137–145 mEq/L). These signs and symptoms include nausea, weakness, anorexia, fatigue, and muscle cramps. Neurologic symptoms are the most frequent manifestation of SIADH. They can include altered mental status, psychotic or combative behavior, lethargy, and weakness; if the hyponatremia is extremely severe, seizures, coma, and death may occur.[3] The symptomatology that a patient exhibits depends on both the severity of the hyponatremia and the rate at which it developed.[12]

Assessment

Diagnostic Studies

Diagnosis of hypercalcemia involves evaluation of serum calcium and findings on clinical exam. Hypercalcemia is defined as a serum calcium level greater than 11.0 mg/dL. Measurement of ionized calcium levels is preferred to total serum calcium because the former measure does not include protein-bound calcium and, as a result, is considered more accurate.

Paraneoplastic ACTH syndrome is made by evaluation of plasma cortisol and 24-hour urinary free-cortisol levels. The diagnosis is confirmed as a paraneoplastic condition and not a primary adrenal disorder when the 24-hour urinary-free cortisol level is elevated in the setting of a elevated serum ACTH level. More standard tests, such as dexamethasone suppression and metyrapone tests, may be misleading and are often not clinically useful. If the diagnosis remains in doubt, further imaging, including MRI of the pituitary gland,

^{111}In-octreotide scanning, and positron emission tomography have been used to localize somatastatin-receptive tumors.[19,20]

In some cases, SIADH may be diagnosed inadvertently when asymptomatic hyponatremia is found through routine laboratory studies. The diagnostic features of SIADH include serum hyponatremia and hypoosmolarity; less than maximally dilute urine with a urine sodium concentration greater than 20 mEq/L; euvolemia; and otherwise normal renal, adrenal, and thyroid function. Measurement of serum AVP levels is possible by radioimmunoassay but is rarely done. The levels may be normal or elevated.[21] Other conditions that cause hyponatremia must be ruled out, such as dehydration, fluid retention, or renal, adrenal, or thyroid dysfunction.

Therapeutic Approaches and Nursing Care

Humoral hypercalcemia is associated with a poor prognosis, with a median survival of 1 month.[22] Treatment of hypercalcemia includes correcting dehydration, enhancing the renal excretion of calcium, inhibiting the accelerated bone resorption, and treating the underlying cancer. A variety of agents, including mithramycin, gallium nitrate, and calcitonin, have been used with some efficacy, albeit often with serious side effects. Biphosphonates, such as pamidronate, tend to be the agents used most often, both for their tolerance and long-lasting effect. Recognition of subtle early signs of hypercalcemia and management of the toxicities ensuing from its treatment are important components of oncology nursing care. Chapter 32 includes a more detailed discussion of nursing assessment and interventions related to the occurrence of hypercalcemia.

The prognosis for patients with Cushing's syndrome related to tumor production of ACTH is poor, with a median survival of approximately 5 months.[18] It is common for patients to have extensive disease and have a poor response to chemotherapy. Treatment may consist of surgical removal of the tumor (with carcinoid tumors) or use of medication to inhibit steroid biosynthesis. Medications may include metryrapone, ketoconazole, and somatostatin analogs (octreotide).[5] Achieving control of Cushing's syndrome through normalization of cortisol levels prior to initiating chemotherapy may reduce the potential for infection.

The most effective long-term therapy for paraneoplastic SIADH is treatment of the underlying tumor.[5] In patients with small cell lung cancer, administration of chemotherapy leads to resolution of the SIADH in 80% of cases.[13] Correction of the hyponatremia and stabilization of the patient are essential while directing treatment at the underlying tumor. Management includes fluid restriction and administration of medications to increase the serum sodium level; other agents to control neurologic symptoms, such as anticonvulsants, are also used. Demeclocycline, which decreases the renal response to ADH, thereby decreasing the kidney's ability to concentrate the urine, has been shown to be effective in SIADH. Nursing management of patients experiencing SIADH focuses on thorough neurologic assessment and monitoring fluid balance. (See Chapter 41 for more on SIADH.)

Neurologic Paraneoplastic Syndromes

Scope of the Problem

Any part of the nervous system can be affected by paraneoplastic neurologic disorders. In general, only a single area or single cell type is affected, but neurologic PNS that affects multiple levels of the nervous system can also occur. Although most symptomatic paraneoplastic neurologic syndromes are rare, affecting approximately 1% of all cancer patients, certain neurologic PNSs are more common. Examples include conditions such as Lambert-Eaton myasthenic syndrome (LEMS), which affects about 3% of patients with small cell lung cancer; demyelinating peripheral neuropathy, which affects 50% of patients with a rare osteosclerotic form of plasmacytoma; and myasthenia gravis, which affects about 15% of patients with thymoma.[1] Although the symptoms can be quite diverse, certain features are common across conditions. In general, the neurologic disorder appears before the cancer is identified, and often the cancer is not diagnosed for several months or years after the appearance of the neurologic condition. In addition, although the cancer itself maybe indolent, the PNS often appears rapidly and may be severe and disabling and, in some instances, lethal.[23]

Unlike non-neurologic PNSs, which often occur as a result of the tumor secreting substances that mimic normal hormones or interfere with circulating proteins, most neurologic PNSs are immune-mediated. The tumor's ectopic expression of an antigen that is normally produced exclusively in the nervous system is recognized as foreign by the body and generates an immune response. It is thought that this response may control the growth of the cancer. The presence of autoimmune antibodies, indicating a significant antitumor immune response by the patient, has been associated with the spontaneous regression of small cell lung carcinoma and improved response to treatment and survival.[24,25] However, the attack on the identical

Table 33-2 Two Neurologic Paraneoplastic Syndromes and Their Associated Antibodies and Cancer Type

Syndrome	Antibody	Cancer Type[a]
Lambert-Eaton myasthenic syndrome	Anti-VGCC	SCLC
Subacute cerebellar degeneration	Anti-Hu	SCLC
	Anti-PCA-2	SCLC
	Anti-CRMP5/CV2	SCLC, thymoma
	ANNA-3	SCLC
	Anti-Yo	Breast, ovary
	Anti-Ta/Ma2	Testis
	Anti-Ma	Miscellaneous
	Anti-Ri	Breast
	Anti-Tr	Hodgkin's lymphoma
	Anti-Hu	Neuroblastoma

SCLC = small cell lung cancer.
[a]Most frequent.
Data from Voltz.[27]

neuronal-based antigen is what leads to the neurologic syndrome. Identification of these antibodies and their target neural antigens offers the most important diagnostic clue. Often levels of these antibodies will be elevated in the serum as well as the cerebrospinal fluid. Unfortunately, not all patients with neurologic PNSs will have identifiable antibodies in their serum.

The neurologic PNSs can be categorized according to whether they affect the central nervous system (CNS) or the peripheral nervous system (PNS). Two of the major neurologic PNSs, paraneoplastic cerebellar degeneration (PCD) and LEMS, are discussed in greater detail. Table 33-2 outlines antibodies and cancer types associated with these two neurologic PNSs.

Definitions

Subacute cerebellar degeneration is characterized by progressive cerebellar dysfunction, manifested as loss of coordination and ataxia.[3] Malignancies associated with this condition include small cell lung cancer, breast cancer, ovarian cancer, and Hodgkin's disease. A number of antibodies have been identified in relation to PCD, including anti-Yo, anti-Hu, anti-Ri, and PCD/LEMS. In more than 50% of patients, the onset of PCD predates diagnosis of the cancer by several months; in some cases, the malignancy is not detected for years or only at autopsy.[26]

Lambert-Eaton myasthenic syndrome (LEMS) is a paraneoplastic antibody-mediated autoimmune disorder, characterized by weakness and easy fatigability of muscles, often in the lower extremities. Ocular muscles may also be affected, and respiratory failure can occur. LEMS primarily affects patients with small cell lung carcinoma and occurs in 3% of patients with this diagnosis. It has also been reported in patients with lymphoid malignancies and other solid tumors.[27]

Incidence

Paraneoplastic cerebellar degeneration is extremely rare, with fewer than 300 cases reported in the literature. The malignancy most often associated with PCD is ovarian cancer. Other cancers in which PCD may occur include small cell lung cancer, Hodgkin's lymphoma, and, to a lesser extent, breast cancer. The autoantibody involved may differ depending on the malignancy (see Table 33-2).

Lambert-Eaton myasthenic syndrome occurs most commonly in patients with small cell lung cancer, affecting approximately 3% of these patients. It has also been incidentally reported in patients with breast, gastric, prostate, bladder, ovarian, and rectal cancers. This syndrome is more common in patients with autoimmune diseases, with 40% of cases occurring in patients with rheumatoid arthritis, scleroderma, and multiple sclerosis.[28]

Etiology and Risk Factors

Paraneoplastic neurologic syndromes are believed to be autoimmune diseases, but the exact immunopathogenetic mechanisms remain unclear.[29] The PCD disorders arise from the presence of antineuronal antibodies associated with specific neoplasms, which mistakenly attack Purkinje cells in the cerebellum with devastating neurologic consequences.[30] LEMS occurs as a result of abnormal release of acetylcholine into the neuromuscular junction, which subsequently causes autoantibodies to attack the neuromuscular structures involved in muscle nerve contraction. Small cell lung carcinoma is thought to originate from neuroectodermal tissue; as a consequence, these tumor cells may express neural antigens containing voltage-gated calcium channels (VGCCs) on their cell surface.

The immune response generated by the body to the presence of malignant cells produces immunoglobulin G (IgG) antibodies against these neural antigens. These IgG antibodies also mistakenly attack VGCCs in normal nerve tissue, leading to the development of LEMS.[27,28]

Pathophysiology

The pathophysiology of neurologic PNSs is related to tumor cell expression of one or more "onconeural" antigens that are identical to molecules normally expressed by neurons. An autoimmune response initially arising against the tumor "spills over" to attack neurons expressing the related "normal" antigens.[29] For some neurologic PNSs, antineuronal autoantibodies are thought to be directly involved in causing the clinical disease. In other syndromes, the autoantibodies are thought to be epiphenomena for autoimmunity but not directly involved in causing injury to the neurons.

Several antibodies, including anti-Yo, anti-MA, and anti-Ri, have been associated with PCD. Each antibody is associated with different malignancies, and PCD has since been categorized according to the autoantibody involved. The presence of antibodies appears to have a positive prognostic significance, as it is associated with a more indolent tumor course. These antibodies may be indirectly related to the syndrome, with recent studies indicating that cell-mediated immunity may cause the damage to Purkinje cells in the cerebellum. Not all patients with PCD exhibit antibodies in their serum and CSF, but the syndrome in such individuals appears to be clinically identical to that in patients with antibodies. The cerebellum is involved in coordination of movement, balance, eye movements, and muscle tone by processing sensory information and regulating the activity of the descending motor pathways. When the Purkinje cells are injured or destroyed, dizziness, visual problems (diplopia, blurry vision, or oscillopsia), nausea, vomiting, and dysarthria may occur.[26,31]

Lambert-Eaton myasthenic syndrome occurs as a result of the abnormal release of the neurotransmitter acetylcholine (ACh) into the neuromuscular junction from the presynaptic membrane. In normal neural function, a nerve impulse is communicated from one neuron to a target by transmission of neurotransmitters. These transmitters then open calcium channels on the target, allowing depolarization of the postsynaptic cell. In LEMS, the presence of tumor cells stimulates an autoimmune response that produces IgG antibodies against calcium channels expressed by both the cancer and the neuromuscular junction. The IgG autoantibodies block the VGCCs in the presynaptic nerve terminal, resulting in insufficient ACh release into the synaptic cleft and very-low-amplitude muscle action potentials.[32]

Clinical Manifestations

Paraneoplastic cerebellar degeneration may occur prior to the diagnosis of cancer, and it is not uncommon for the tumor to be found only after repeated searches.[29] Cerebellar dysfunction is usually bilateral, symmetric, and progressive. The deterioration in coordination of movement may occur over days or weeks, with the movements of the arms, legs, and trunk becoming progressively uncoordinated. The patient may experience dysarthria, nystagmus, vertigo, and oscillopsia (i.e., a sense that objects in the visual field are oscillating). Nearly all activities of daily living, including the ability to sit, walk, and communicate, may be affected. Other mild neurologic symptoms, such as sensorineural hearing loss, dysphagia, diplopia, and peripheral neuropathy, may occur. The symptoms of PCD usually progress, then peak in their severity, and finally stabilize. The degree of severity of PCD varies widely. Despite treatment, the neurologic symptoms are often permanent, with functional outcomes generally being better for patients who have anti-Ri antibodies as compared to those with anti-Yo or anti-Hu antibodies.[30]

Proximal muscle fatigue and weakness characterize LEMS. As noted earlier, the lower extremities tend to be primarily affected, with the arms and shoulders affected to a lesser extent. This weakness affects the muscles of the pelvis and thighs, resulting in difficulty in getting up from a chair or toilet and climbing stairs. If the ocular muscles are affected, double vision, ptosis, and blurred vision may occur. Additional symptoms may include dysarthria, dysphagia, and muscle pain, as well as symptoms of autonomic nervous system dysfunction, such as constipation, urinary retention, abnormal sweating, postural hypotension, and dry mouth.[33]

Assessment

Diagnostic Studies

In general, the onset of new neurologic symptoms in a patient with cancer warrants neuroimaging. These studies may include magnetic resonance imaging (MRI), computerized tomography (CT) scan of the brain, and/or lumbar puncture. Neurologic PNSs are often a diagnosis of exclusion, as tumor metastases, neurotoxicity of treatment, and metabolic derangements are more often the cause of neurologic symptoms in the patient with cancer. The initial MRI or CT of the brain may be normal in patients with PCD, but eventually these scans may exhibit diffuse cerebellar atrophy and a dilated fourth ventricle. CSF obtained via lumbar puncture may be normal or show elevated protein levels, increased IgG levels, and increased lymphocytes.[34] Antineuronal antibodies can also be a useful tool in identifying the neurologic condition as paraneoplastic and in searching for the underlying malignancy.

Lambert-Eaton myasthenic syndrome must be distinguished from another neurologic disorder — myasthenia gravis (MG). These two conditions are similar, but demonstrate some differences: In LEMS, muscle strength improves with exercise; edrophonium (Tensilon) has little effect in LEMS; and unlike some patients with MG, patients with LEMS do not have the presence of ACh receptor antibodies in their serum. Electromyography is usually the diagnostic test performed to evaluate patients suspected of having LEMS. Repeated nerve stimulation will cause an increase in muscle action potential, resulting in a temporary increase in muscle strength in LEMS. In contrast, patients with MG will experience a progressive decrease in muscle response.

Therapeutic Approaches and Nursing Care

Unfortunately, deficits associated with PCD are often permanent. A variety of immunomodulating treatments, including corticosteroids and plasmapheresis, have been attempted. Clonazepam may be prescribed to reduce the ataxia associated with PCD; doses range from 0.5 to 1.5 mg daily. Fewer than 10% of patients with PCD show significant neurologic improvement despite aggressive treatment of the underlying malignancy and the use of a variety of immunosuppressive therapies.[29]

The primary goal in caring for patients with PCD is providing emotional support and supporting maximal neurologic function. Deficits may have occurred rapidly and are often permanent, even if cure or improvement of the patient's cancer is possible.[12] An interdisciplinary approach to management, including rehabilitative service and psychological support, is needed to assist the patient and family to adjust to these deficits and to changing roles.

Unlike with PCD, symptoms associated with LEMS often improve with tumor response. If the neurologic symptoms do not improve, medications and plasmapheresis may be used. Pharmacologic agents that promote ACh release from the nerve terminal, such as 3,4-diaminopyridine and guanidine, are often used to treat LEMS. 3,4-Diaminopyridine affects K^+ channels, thereby increasing the amount of ACh released into the synaptic cleft. In addition, gamma globulin, steroids, and plasmapheresis have been used with mixed success. Weekly plasmapheresis, in combination with prednisone and azathioprine, has produced the most sustained clinical benefit, whereas plasmapheresis alone is associated with short-term clinical improvement.[33]

Like their counterparts with PCD, patients with LEMS require a multidisciplinary management approach, including rehabilitative and psychological services. These patients require emotional support, ongoing assessment of neurologic status, rehabilitative therapies, and comprehensive patient education regarding measures to cope with the chronic muscle weakness and fatigue.[35]

Hematologic Paraneoplastic Syndromes

Scope of the Problem

Hematologic and blood coagulation abnormalities occur commonly in cancer patients.[36] Tumor infiltration of bone marrow and the effects of antineoplastic therapy are typical etiologies. Hematologic disorders can also occur as a paraneoplastic condition, as a result of tumor secretion of cytokines, colony-stimulating factors, and factors that affect coagulation. In particular, anemia, granulocytopenia, eosinophilia, thrombocytosis, thromboembolism, nonbacterial thrombotic endocarditis, thrombocytopenia, and coagulopathies such as disseminated intravascular coagulation (DIC) can occur as a result of paraneoplastic involvement. Anemia of malignancy and thromboembolism will be discussed in more detail here.

Definitions

Anemia commonly occurs in the patient with cancer due to the effects of the cancer therapy or bone marrow invasion by tumor. Anemia as a remote effect is less common and can be due to an autoimmune hemolytic anemia (AIHA), pure red cell aplasia (PRCA), or anemia of chronic disease (ACD).[3] The most common of the three, ACD is characterized by a normocytic/normochromic anemia, usually with reduced serum iron and total iron-binding capacity and low erythropoietin levels.

As a result of the hypercoagulable state induced by malignancy, patients with cancer have a higher risk of thromboembolism (TE) or clot formation.

Paraneoplastic TE, also termed *Trousseau's syndrome,* was initially defined as the occurrence of migratory thrombophlebitis in the person with cancer. Its definition has been expanded over the years to reflect a better understanding of the effect of cancer cells on vasculature and the coagulation pathways. Trousseau's syndrome now describes a variety of thromboembolic disorders affecting both veins and arteries, including specific types of peripheral vascular disease and ischemic heart disease.[36] Paraneoplastic TE is characterized by venous or arterial thrombosis that may be recurrent and migratory, frequently occurring in veins in which deep-vein thrombosis (DVT) is uncommon.

Incidence

The incidence of anemia of malignancy is not known, as many patients will experience some degree of anemia during the course of the disease, primarily related to treatment effects. The diagnosis of ACD is most commonly applied to patients with advanced disease. Although PRCA is most commonly associated with thymoma, it can be seen in patients with adenocarcinoma of the stomach, breast, squamous cell carcinoma of the lung, and cancers of unknown primary. In contrast, AIHA is usually associated with leukemia and lymphomas and is less commonly seen with solid malignancies such as lung, renal cell, ovarian, breast, stomach, colon, cervical carcinoma, and seminoma.[3]

The incidence of TE in patients with cancer has been estimated to range between 1% and 11%, and this condition may not be identified until autopsy. Thromboembolism is reported to occur commonly in patients with mucin-secreting adenocarcinoma of the gastrointestinal tract. It is also commonly associated with small cell and non-small cell lung cancer, colon cancer, and pancreatic cancers, and has been reported to occur in patients with cancers of the breast, prostate, ovary, bladder, and brain. The incidence of TE appears to increase during chemotherapy and hormonal therapy, possibly related to the thrombogenic effect of antineoplastic agents and hormones. Although the exact mechanism remains unknown, it may involve a reduction in antithrombin fibrin and fibrinolytic activity.[37]

Etiology and Risk Factors

The etiology of anemia of malignancy is multifactorial. It includes tumor secretion of cytokines, such as interleukin-1 (IL-1), affecting red cell metabolism; protein-calorie malnutrition; bone marrow failure; and chronic hemorrhage. Patients with protein-calorie malnutrition often have insufficient iron and folic acid stores, leading to anemia. Bone marrow failure can occur in heavily treated patients who have received multiple courses of chemotherapy and radiation. Finally, chronic microscopic bleeding in patients with primary or metastatic disease of the gastrointestinal tract, genitourinary system, or upper and lower respiratory tract can result in anemia as a result of chronic hemorrhage.[38]

Thromboembolism occurs when tumor cells affect systemic activation of coagulation and cause platelet dysfunction. Thromboembolic disease that is refractory to anticoagulation therapy is often indicative of underlying cancer, with several prospective studies confirming a relationship between recurrent, episodic idiopathic DVT and the subsequent development of malignancy.[39,40] Idiopathic DVT (no identifiable risk factors) is associated with an estimated 10%–20% risk of malignancy. A significant proportion of these tumors are very small, present at an early stage, and are therefore potentially curable.[40]

Pathophysiology

Tumor secretion of cytokines, such as interleukin-1 (IL-1), affects red cell metabolism and function and is one factor associated with anemia of malignancy. Interleukin-1 has the ability to interfere in the process in which iron molecules are transferred from the reticuloendothelial system to red cell precursors in the bone marrow, resulting in an iron-rich bone marrow but iron-deficient erythrocytes.[37] Another function of IL-1 is stimulation of macrophages in the spleen, causing a decrease in red cell life span. Tumors are also known to secrete an anemia-inducing factor that shortens the life span of erythrocytes, reduces erythropoiesis, and results in severe anemia.[41]

Cancer may cause disturbances in the hemostatic system by numerous mechanisms, including activation of the coagulation pathway, damage to the endothelial lining of blood vessels, or platelet activation.[42] Cancer cells are known to play a role in activation of the extrinsic clotting pathway. They may induce the cleavage of fibrinogen to fibrin and activate clotting factors such as factor VII or factor X, thereby initiating the clotting cascade. This activity may reflect the combined direct and indirect effects of cancer cells. Stimulation of the patient's immune system by tumor cell antigens may activate monocyte-macrophages. These monocyte-macrophages, in turn, activate the clotting pathway through the expression of tissue factors. Patients with cancer experience a variety of platelet disorders, such as thrombocytopenia and platelet dysfunction. The exact mechanisms by which tumor cells influence these disorders are unclear. One theory focuses on the production of thrombin. Malignant cells may indirectly inflict damage on vascular endothelium via their activation of platelets. Platelets facilitate tumor cell adhesion to blood vessel walls through two mechanisms: the secretion of substances that promote further endothelial damage and the stimulation of increased platelet aggregation. This ability to affect platelet function is integral to the tumor's ability to invade, implant, and promote angiogenesis.[39]

Clinical Manifestations

Hemoglobin levels less than 10 g/dL are associated with anemia of malignancy. Commonly encountered symptoms include fatigue, dyspnea on exertion, headache, cognitive dysfunction, anorexia, and reduced overall quality of life.[41,43] On clinical exam, pallor, postural hypotension, edema, and splenomegaly can be seen. Patients with paraneoplastic TE may experience pain and edema of the extremity, or more generalized symptoms of dyspnea, hypotension, and anxiety.

Assessment

Diagnostic Studies

Anemia as a remote effect of cancer is a diagnosis of exclusion. More often, anemia occurs as a direct result of tumor infiltration of bone marrow or as an effect of therapy. On laboratory analysis, the hemoglobin, serum iron, and iron-binding capacity will be low. Treatment-related anemia can be excluded by the clinical history. Bone marrow biopsy and aspirate may be performed if marrow infiltration by tumor is a concern. Trousseau's syndrome is diagnosed on the basis of the clinical presentation in a patient with malignancy, combined with ultrasound or radiographic confirmation of a thrombosis. Doppler ultrasound is most commonly performed.

Therapeutic Approaches and Nursing Care

Management of anemia involves treating the underlying cause of the anemia and providing supportive measures such as improved iron consumption, blood transfusions, energy conservation techniques, and erythropoiesis-stimulating factors.[41] Trousseau's syndrome is treated with anticoagulation, but can recur despite continued therapy. Acute episodes may require hospitalization. Supportive care measures may include management of dependent edema with compression stockings and elevation, and maintenance of adequate oxygenation.

Renal Paraneoplastic Syndromes

Scope of the Problem

Renal complications of cancer are common and include tumor infiltration of the kidney, renal vein thrombosis, amyloidosis, urethral obstruction, and complications of antineoplastic therapy. Renal complications as a paraneoplastic syndrome are rare, however, and include nephrotic syndrome, intrarenal obstruction by mucoprotein secreted by pancreatic tumors, and lysozyme secretion in patients with acute leukemia, which results in wasting of potassium and calcium. Nephrotic syndrome will be discussed in more detail here.

Definitions

Nephrotic syndrome results when renal glomerular lesions or obstruction of the glomerulus by tumor products occurs.[44] Impaired renal function ensues, leading to massive proteinuria. Like other PNSs, nephrotic syndrome often occurs prior to the cancer being diagnosed and may herald tumor recurrence.

Incidence

The incidence of nephrotic syndrome as a PNS is not certain, but is considered rare.[45] Lung cancer is the diagnosis most commonly associated with nephrotic syndrome, but this condition has also been reported in Hodgkin's lymphoma and, to a lesser degree, non-Hodgkin's lymphoma.[44,46] Case reports also exist for patients with lung, breast, colon, and prostate carcinomas as well as carcinoid tumors. Nephrotic syndrome may appear at any point in the disease trajectory. It is reported to precede the cancer diagnosis by months to years in approximately 45% of cases, is found concurrently in 30%–40% of cases, and follows the diagnosis of cancer in 15%–20% of cases.[47]

Etiology and Risk Factors

Nephrotic syndrome is commonly associated with primary glomerular disease or occurs secondary to infection, drugs, or systemic diseases such as diabetes mellitus, systemic lupus erythematosus, or rheumatoid arthritis.[48] The etiology of paraneoplastic nephrotic syndrome depends on the type of malignancy involved. For example, with carcinoma, products of the immune system, specifically antigen–antibody complexes, may become trapped within the glomerulus and impair glomerular function. No association between the site, size, or nature of malignancy and any particular glomerular appearance has been identified.[45] Nephrotic syndrome may regress if the malignancy is treated successfully. Nevertheless, the occurrence of nephrotic syndrome is associated with a poor prognosis, with median survival averaging 12 months following the diagnosis of nephrotic syndrome, and approximately 3 months following a malignant diagnosis.[49]

Pathophysiology

The pathogenesis of nephrotic syndrome is immunological, associated with involvement of tumor-associated antigen, reexpression of fetal antigens, and/or viral antigens. In rare cases, nephrotic syndrome may occur as a result of intravascular coagulation or amyloidosis.[45] Typically, the glomerulus, (i.e., the functional unit of the kidney responsible for the ultrafiltration of plasma and urine formation) is affected. The basement membrane of the glomerular capillaries serves as the main filtration barrier to plasma proteins and is the location of most glomerular lesions.[44] The glomerular lesions associated with the presence of a malignancy vary with the type of malignancy involved. The most common nephropathy identified is membranous glomerulonephritis, which occurs in 70% of patients reported to have a malignancy-associated nephrotic syndrome.[45] Carcinomas are most often associated (80%–90%) with membranous glomerulonephritis, which is thought to result from antigen–antibody complexes that become trapped in the glomerulus, resulting in lesions that adversely affect renal function. These types of complexes have been isolated from the kidneys of patients with lung and colon carcinomas and nephrotic syndrome.

Clinical Manifestations

Clinical symptoms may include brown, foamy urine and mild to moderate hypertension. In addition, facial and peripheral edema may result from leakage of plasma proteins into the urine, with resultant hypoalbuminemia and reduced plasma oncotic pressure. The low plasma oncotic pressure triggers a series of homeostatic mechanisms, such as increased vasopressin secretion, that attempt to restore the plasma volume. This activity results in retention of sodium and water, which further aggravates the peripheral edema, leading to anasarca. Another effect of insufficient plasma oncotic pressure is increased hepatic lipoprotein synthesis, resulting in hyperlipidemia — specifically, elevated cholesterol and low-density lipoprotein levels. These clinical manifestations may precede the diagnosis of cancer by 2–18 months.

Assessment and Grading

Diagnostic Studies

In patients with cancer who are experiencing renal symptoms, laboratory studies include urinalysis, 24-hour urine collection, and a serum chemistry profile. Paraneoplastic nephrotic syndrome is associated with moderate heme, 2^{+}-4^{+} protein, and 2^{+} granular casts on urinalysis. A 24-hour urine examination may contain protein levels of 3800–7000 mg. The chemistry profile may reveal elevated creatinine, BUN, and cholesterol levels, with a decreased albumin level.

As with many PNSs, diagnosis of paraneoplastic nephrotic syndrome is made by exclusion. Other processes, such as renal-vein thrombosis, amyloidosis, and drug-related etiologies, must be ruled out. Renal ultrasound may be used to eliminate hydronephrosis or renal-vein thrombosis as a cause of symptoms. Percutaneous renal biopsy is then performed. Findings on biopsy may include hyalinization of the glomeruli and narrowing or obliteration of the capillary walls, but completely normal capillary basement membranes without evidence of immune deposits. A gallium scan will show uptake by the kidneys; this type of imaging can be utilized as a screening tool for patients with idiopathic nephrotic syndrome to screen for occult lymphoma.[50]

Therapeutic Approaches and Nursing Care

Treatment of paraneoplastic nephrotic syndrome is aimed at treating the underlying malignancy. Resolution can occur rapidly if the tumor responds to therapy. Management centers on symptomatic treatment by appropriate diuretic therapy, treatment of any electrolyte abnormalities, removal or treatment of the underlying tumor, and avoidance of other nephrotoxic agents.[45] Both diuretics and steroids may be prescribed to manage the syndrome. Standard therapy includes the use of high-dose glucocorticoids, which are eventually tapered off. Additional symptomatic treatment may include the use of loop diuretics to relieve edema and consumption of a high-protein diet. Cytotoxic drugs such as cyclophosphamide and chlorambucil may be used but are typically reserved for patients who cannot tolerate steroids.[51]

Miscellaneous Paraneoplastic Syndromes

Cutaneous Paraneoplastic Syndromes

Cutaneous PNSs occur most frequently in patients with pulmonary, gastrointestinal, and breast cancer, but can arise with nearly any type of malignant disease. These PNSs are extremely rare, with most existing as case reports in the literature (Figure 33-2).[52] Dermatoses range from those that occur rarely but are almost always associated with malignancy to those that are equally associated with benign and malignant disease. The pathophysiologic mechanism by which cutaneous PNSs occur remains unknown. These phenomena are thought to result from a triadic interaction among the tumor, some mediating fact, and the target tissue involved.[53] Mediators may include polypeptide hormones, cytokines, antibodies, and growth factors, which act by disrupting communication between cells, thereby producing either abnormal or increased cellular activity.[12]

Physical exam and skin biopsy are used for diagnosis. Paraneoplastic dermatoses may be the first sign of an occult malignancy, and prompt recognition may assist in cancer detection.[54] According to McLean and Haynes, for a cutaneous paraneoplastic syndrome to occur, it must follow a parallel course to the malignancy.[55] Often the recognition of the skin condition and the malignancy take place at the same time. The dermatoses considered to be true PNSs are described in Table 33-3.

Treatment of cutaneous PNSs targets the underlying malignancy. Supportive measures include analgesics for pain relief, antihistamines to treat pruritus, and both systemic and topical corticosteroids to reduce inflammation and block tumor production of prostaglandins thought to sensitize peripheral nerve endings to pruritogenic substances.[56] Nursing care is supportive, including wound dressings as well as education and emotional support.[53]

Cancer Anorexia-Cachexia Syndrome

Cancer anorexia-cachexia syndrome (CACS) is the most well-known PNS affecting the gastrointestinal system. It is estimated to occur in as many as 80% of patients with cancer and to be associated with 20% of cancer deaths.[57] Cachexia is a complex metabolic condition associated with progressive weight loss and depletion of host reserves of adipose tissue and skeletal muscle.[58] If a patient losses more than 5% of his or her premorbid weight in a six-month period, CACS should be considered.[58] Patients often experience anorexia, lose body fat and lean body mass, and may experience early satiety, profound weakness, anemia, fatigue, impaired immune function, and poor performance status.[58] Note that CACS does not result from the nutritional demands of the malignancy or reduced food intake, but rather from multiple metabolic and physiologic abnormalities. It occurs as a consequence of a chronic, systemic inflammatory response that results in depletion of essential amino acids by high hepatic synthesis of acute-phase proteins.[58] Symptoms associated with cancer cachexia result from macrophage production of TNF and IL-1, whereas metabolic effects result from release of IL-6 from tumor cells.[59] This syndrome differs from other PNSs in that CACS is not associated with a specific malignancy but can occur with any cancer. Although it is more commonly associated with end-stage disease, it may appear at any time during the disease process and is usually related to the amount of tumor burden. The timing of the syndrome differs with the type of histology. It can severely affect a patient's physical condition, quality of life, and prognosis.[60]

Treatment of CACS focuses on weight increase and appetite stimulation and may include progestational agents such as medroxyprogesterone acetate or megestrol acetate for long-term treatment. Prokinetic agents (i.e., metoclopramide) should be used if patients need concomitant opioid treatment. Corticosteroids may provide short-term benefits.[59] Nursing assessment of the cancer patient's nutritional status, including appetite, weight, and weight loss, is critical in allowing early diagnosis and intervention. (See Chapter 31 for more information on nutritional and pharmacologic interventions.)

Tumor Fever

Fever occurs in two-thirds of cancer patients during the course of their disease, and paraneoplastic fever is the second most common cause.[61] Tumor fever as a paraneoplastic syndrome occurs primarily in patients with lymphoma, but has also been associated with leukemias, myelodysplastic syndromes, renal cell carcinoma, hepatoma, osteogenic sarcoma, and metastatic liver disease. Tumor secretion of one or more pyrogenic cytokines (specifically, IL-1α, IL-1β, interferon-α, TNF-α, TNF-β, and IL-6), that act directly on the

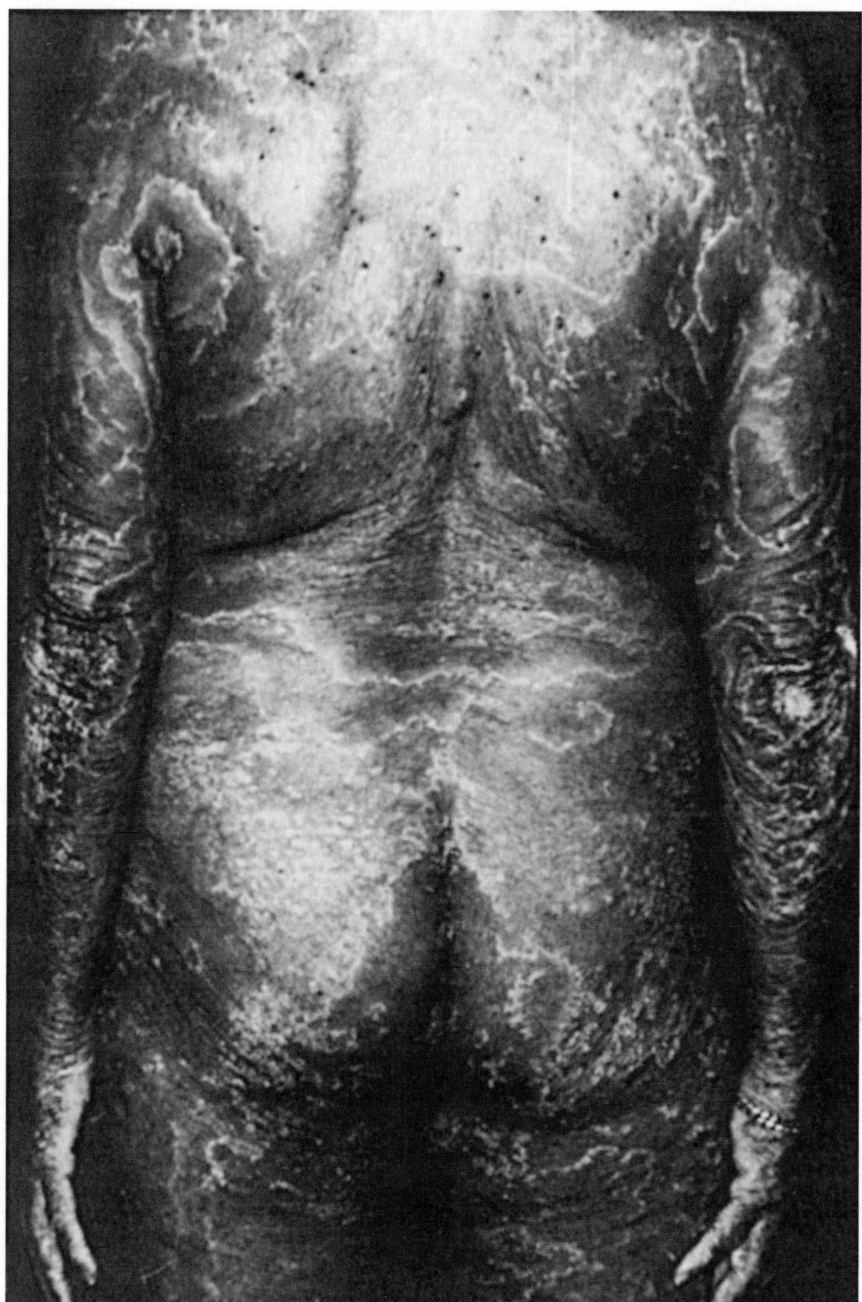

Figure 33-2 Patient with erythema gyratum repens showing classic "wood grain" pattern most pronounced in the intertriginous areas. (Photo reproduced with permission from Appell ML, Ward WQ, Tyring SK: Erythema gyratum repens – A cutaneous marker of malignancy. *Cancer* 62:548–550. Copyright © 1988 American Cancer Society. Reprinted by permission of Wiley-Liss, Inc., a subsidiary of John Wiley and Sons, Inc.)

hypothalamus causes the release of prostaglandin E2, which increases the body's temperature set-point, resulting in fever. Both lymphoma and leukemia cell lines produce these cytokines, whereas solid tumors may promote cytokine release from "bystander" endothelial cells or monocytes.[62]

Rarely, a specific fever pattern occurs, such as can be seen with Pel Epstein fever in Hodgkin's lymphoma. Affected patients have a 3- to 10-day febrile period followed by an afebrile period. Paraneoplastic fever has a poor prognostic value.[61] As with other PNSs, the primary therapy for tumor fever is treatment of the

Table 33-3 Paraneoplastic Cutaneous Syndromes

Disorder	Clinical Presentation	Associated Malignancy	Comments
Pigmented lesions			
• Acanthosis nigricans	• Velvety, brown, symmetrical lesions with hyperkeratosis that occur primarily in flexural areas — axilla, posterior neck, perineum, umbilicus	• 90% of cases associated with malignancy • 60% gastric carcinoma • 5% lung carcinoma	• Usually associated with advanced disease
• Sign of Leser-Trelat	• Multiple seborrheic (wart-like) lesions	• Adenocarcinomas • Non-Hodgkin's lymphoma • GI malignancies — 43%	• Rapid development signals malignancy • Pruritic
• Sweet's syndrome (acute, febrile neutrophilic dermatosis)	• Painful erythematous plaques covering arms, head, and neck	• 10%–15% of cases associated with a malignancy, usually hematologic, leukemias (AML), myeloma • GU, GI, breast — less common	
• Bazex's syndrome	• Scaly, pruritic psoriasiform rash affecting nails, nose, ears, elbows, knees, fingers, and toes	• Squamous cell carcinomas of head and neck, esophagus, lung • Vulvar, esophageal, and uterine carcinomas	• Males primarily affected • Females less common • 100% association with malignancy
Erythemas			
• Erythema gyratum repens (*repens* is Latin for "to crawl or creep")	• Expanding, scaly, concentric bands (gyri) with a "wood grain" pattern	• 32% lung carcinoma • Breast • Esophagus • Uterine	• Pruritic • Moves rapidly across skin surface — about 1 cm per day • 2:1 male to female ratio • 100% association with malignancy • Tumor resection results in complete resolution within 6 weeks
• Glucagonoma syndrome (necrolytic migratory erythema)	• Erythematous patches • Stomatitis	• Islet cell tumors of pancreas	• Tumor resection results in clearance of the eruption within 48 hours
• Flushing	• Intermittent episodes of facial flushing	• Carcinoid • Medullary thyroid carcinoma	
Endocrine/metabolic lesions			
• Porphyria cutanea tarda	• *Early:* Photosensitive subepidermal vesicles, fragile skin, hyperpigmentation • *Late:* Alopecia, scarring, sclerodermoid changes	• Liver carcinoma	• Often painful, pruritic
• Systemic nodular panniculitis	• Fever, erythematous SQ nodules, fat necrosis of bone marrow, lungs, and other organs; abdominal pain	• Pancreatic adenocarcinoma	• Occurs rarely; also associated with benign pancreatic disease
Miscellaneous			
• Pruritus	• Generalized itching with areas of excoriation from scratching • Chronic, intensive itching of nostrils associated with advanced brain tumors	• Hodgkin's and T-cell lymphomas • Polycythemia vera • CNS malignancies	• 25% of Hodgkin's lymphoma patients experience generalized itching • May be presenting symptom of malignancies
• Hypertrichosis lanuginosa (malignant down)	• Fine, silky hair occurring primarily on forehead and ears	• Lung, colon carcinomas, also bladder, uterine	• Rapid onset • 90% association with malignancy
• Hypertrophic pulmonary osteoarthropathy (HPO)	• Painful, symmetric arthropathy involving fingers, wrists, elbows, and knees caused by periostitis	• Intrathoracic malignancies, primarily lung carcinomas (88%) • Most common histologies are large cell and adenocarcinoma of the lung	• Associated with clubbing of fingers and toes • May resemble rheumatoid arthritis • Usually precedes diagnosis of malignancy

GI = gastrointestinal; AML = acute myelogenous leukemia; GU = genitourinary; SQ = subcutaneous; CNS = central nervous system.

underlying malignancy. Temporary relief of symptoms can occur with the use of nonsteroidal anti-inflammatory drugs (NSAIDs) — specifically, naproxen, indomethacin, or diclofenac, which are all equally efficacious. These drugs have also been used as a diagnostic tool in patients with cancer who have fever of unknown origin (FUO), based on the response to the agents. The mechanism by which NSAIDs affect tumor fever is unknown but may involve their ability to block prostaglandin E_2 synthesis.[62]

Ocular Paraneoplastic Syndromes

Extremely rare PNSs reported to occur in both adults and children are those involving the eyes. The two syndromes that have been most clearly defined are opsoclonus and cancer-associated retinopathy.

Opsoclonus is when the eyes move primarily horizontally, with frequent vertical and rotating jerks, regardless whether the eyes are closed or the person is sleeping.[63] Associated with neuroblastoma in children, opsoclonus often leads to the diagnosis of the malignancy. In adults, opsoclonus occurs most frequently in patients with small cell lung cancer or breast cancer. It usually affects patients older than age 40, and is often associated with tremors and gait disturbances.[29] Patients may also show evidence of cerebellar degeneration, and both anti-Hu and anti-Purkinje cell antibodies have been found in the serum of patients with opsoclonus.[64] Treatment focuses on resolving the underlying malignancy. In addition, oral steroids and intravenous immunoglobulin have been used with variable success.[23]

Cancer-associated retinopathy (CAR) is a paraneoplastic syndrome in which patients experience retinal degeneration (including abnormal vasculature and a reduced number of retinal ganglion cells), which results in unilateral or bilateral visual loss. This condition has primarily been reported in patients with small cell lung cancer but also has been documented in patients with non-small cell lung cancer and cervical, breast, and endometrial carcinomas. Antiretinal antibodies, known as anti-CAR antibodies, have recently been identified and are the basis for the theorized pathophysiology of an abnormal autoimmune response. Initially, patients may report blurred vision, abnormal color perception, and visual disturbances such as sparkles, shimmering, or distortions. Symptoms may either progress rapidly or occur over several years. The use of oral steroids may result in stabilization or improvement in vision.[23]

Conclusion

The PNSs are a complex group of disorders associated with malignancy that may affect most body systems, including the endocrine, neurologic, hematologic, renal, gastrointestinal, and cutaneous systems. Most syndromes are extremely rare, and outcome can be quite variable. Nursing management of these syndromes is complex, depending on the system affected as well as concomitant symptoms of the cancer itself or associated treatment. Often a multidisplinary approach, including nursing, medicine, and rehabilitative services, is required. The implications of PNSs for understanding the etiology of the cancer itself and available therapies have only just begun to be explored. As we gain a more thorough understanding of the substances secreted by tumor cells, the mechanisms involved, and their effect on normal tissue, we may be able to provide better treatments for PNSs, prevent their occurrence, and enhance the diagnosis and management of cancer itself.

References

1. Darnell RB, Posner JB: Paraneoplastic syndromes involving the nervous system. *N Engl J Med* 349:1543–1554, 2003
2. Thomas L, Kwok Y, Edelman MJ: Management of paraneoplastic syndromes in lung cancer. *Curr Treat Options Oncol* 5:51–62, 2004
3. Wallach PM, Flannery MT, Stewart JM: Paraneoplastic syndromes for the primary care physician. *Prim Care* 19:727–746, 1992
4. Albert ML, Darnell RB: Paraneoplastic neurological degenerations: keys to tumour immunity. *Nat Rev Cancer* 4:36-44, 2004
5. Mazzone PJ, Arroliga AC: Endocrine paraneoplastic syndromes in lung cancer. *Curr Opin Pulm Med* 9:313–320, 2003
6. Beuschlein F, Hammer GD: Ectopic pro-opiomelanocortin syndrome. *Endocrinol Metab Clin North Am* 31:191–234, 2002
7. Bollanti L, Riondino G, Strollo F: Endocrine paraneoplastic syndromes with special reference to the elderly. *Endocrine* 14:151–157, 2001
8. Sorensen JB, Andersen MK, Hansen HH: Syndrome of inappropriate secretion of antidiuretic hormone (SIADH) in malignant disease. *J Intern Med* 238:97–110, 1995
9. Ralston SH: Pathogenesis and management of cancer associated hypercalcaemia. *Cancer Surv* 21:179–196, 1994
10. Furihata M, Sonobe H, Iwata J, et al: Lung squamous cell carcinoma producing both parathyroid hormone–related peptide and granulocyte colony stimulating factor. *Pathol Int* 46:376–379, 1996
11. Marchioli CC, Graziano SL: Paraneoplastic syndromes associated with small cell lung cancer. *Chest Surg Clin North Am* 7:65–80, 1997
12. Zumsteg MM, Casperson DS: Paraneoplastic syndromes in metastatic disease. *Semin Oncol Nurs* 14:220–229, 1998
13. List AF, Hainsworth JD, Davis BW, et al: The syndrome of inappropriate secretion of antidiuretic hormone (SIADH) in small-cell lung cancer. *J Clin Oncol* 4:1191–1198, 1986
14. Odell WD: Endocrine/metabolic syndromes of cancer. *Semin Oncol* 24:299–317, 1997
15. Becker KL, Silva OL: Paraneoplastic endocrine syndromes, in Becker KL (ed.): *Principles and Practice of Endocrinology and Metabolism.* Philadelphia, Lippincott, 1995, pp 1842–1852
16. John WJ, Foon KA, Patchell RA: Paraneoplastic syndromes, in Devita VT, Hellman S, Rosenberg SA (eds.): *Cancer: Principles and Practice of Oncology.* Philadelphia, Lippincott-Raven, 1997, pp 2397–2422

17. Midthun DE, Jett JR: Clinical presentation of lung cancer, in Pass HI, Mitchell JB, Johnson DH, et al (eds.): *Lung Cancer: Principles and Practice.* Philadelphia, Lippincott-Raven, 1996, pp 421–435
18. Delisle L, Boyer MJ, Warr D, et al: Ectopic corticotropin syndrome and small-cell carcinoma of the lung. Clinical features, outcome, and complications. *Arch Intern Med* 153:746–752, 1993
19. Matte J, Roufosse F, Rocmans P, et al: Ectopic Cushing's syndrome and pulmonary carcinoid tumour identified by ^{111}In-DTPA-D-Phe1 octreotide. *Postgrad Med J* 74:108–110, 1998
20. Dewey TM, Yeung H, Downey RJ: Localization of adrenocorticotropic hormone-producing pulmonary carcinoid by somatostatin receptor scintigraphy. *J Thorac Cardiovasc Surg* 112:832–833, 1996
21. Shepherd FA, Laskey J, Evans WK, et al: Cushing's syndrome associated with ectopic corticotropin production and small-cell lung cancer. *J Clin Oncol* 10:21–27, 1992
22. Takai E, Yano T, Iguchi H, et al: Tumor-induced hypercalcemia and parathyroid hormone–related protein in lung carcinoma. *Cancer* 78:1384–1387, 1996
23. Bataller L, Dalmau J: Paraneoplastic neurologic syndromes: approaches to diagnosis and treatment. *Semin Neurol* 23:215–224, 2003
24. Darnell RB, DeAngelis LM: Regression of small-cell lung carcinoma in patients with paraneoplastic neuronal antibodies. *Lancet* 341:21–22, 1993
25. Douglas CA, Ellershaw J: Anti-Hu antibodies may indicate a positive response to chemotherapy in paraneoplastic syndrome secondary to small cell lung cancer. *Palliat Med* 17:638–639, 2003
26. Gatti G, Simsek S, Kurne A, et al: Paraneoplastic neurological disorders in breast cancer. *Breast* 12:203–207, 2003
27. Voltz R: Paraneoplastic neurological syndromes: an update on diagnosis, pathogenesis, and therapy. *Lancet Neurol* 1:294–305, 2002
28. Lang B, Newsom-Davis J: Immunopathology of the Lambert-Eaton myasthenic syndrome. *Springer Semin Immunopathol* 17:3–15, 1995
29. Dropcho EJ: Neurologic paraneoplastic syndromes. *Curr Oncol Rep* 6:26–31, 2004
30. Shams'ili S, Grefkeins J, de Leeuw B, et al: Paraneoplastic cerebellar degeneration associated with antineuronal antibodies: analysis of 50 patients. *Brain* 126(pt 6):1409–1418, 2003
31. Dalmau J, Gultekin HS, Posner JB: Paraneoplastic neurologic syndromes: pathogenesis and physiopathology. *Brain Pathol* 9:275–284, 1999
32. Lennon VA, Kryzer TJ, Griesmann GE: Calcium-channel antibodies in the Lambert-Eaton syndrome and other paraneoplastic syndromes. *N Engl J Med* 332:1467–1474, 1995
33. Newsom-Davis J: Lambert-Eaton myasthenic syndrome. *Rev Neurol (Paris)* 160:177–180, 2004
34. Cao Y, Abbas J, Wu X, et al: Anti-Yo positive paraneoplastic cerebellar degeneration associated with ovarian carcinoma: case report and review of the literature. *Gynecol Oncol* 75:178–183, 1999
35. Struthers CS: Lambert-Eaton myasthenic syndrome in small cell lung cancer: nursing implications. *Oncol Nurs Forum* 21:677–683, quiz 684–685, 1994
36. Lin JT: Thromboembolic events in the cancer patient. *J Womens Health (Larchmt)* 12:541–551, 2003
37. Bick RL, Strauss JF, Frenkel EP: Thrombosis and hemorrhage in oncology patients. *Hematol Oncol Clin North Am* 10:875–907, 1996
38. Wenzel L, Vergote I, Cella D: Quality of life in patients receiving treatment for gynecologic malignancies: special considerations for patient care. *Int J Gynaecol Obstet* 83(supp 1):211–229, 2003
39. Silverstein RL, Nachman RL: Cancer and clotting–Trousseau's warning. *N Engl J Med* 327:1163–1164, 1992
40. Prandoni P, Lensing AW, Buller HR, et al: Deep-vein thrombosis and the incidence of subsequent symptomatic cancer. *N Engl J Med* 327:1128–1133, 1992
41. Cunningham RS: Anemia in the oncology patient: cognitive function and cancer. *Cancer Nurs* 26(suppl):38S–42S, 2003
42. Sorensen HT, Johnsen SP, Norgard B, et al: Cancer and venous thromboembolism: a multidisciplinary approach. *Clin Lab* 49:615–623, 2003
43. Ludwig H, Strasser K: Symptomatology of anemia. *Semin Oncol* 28(suppl 8):7–14, 2001
44. Ebert B, Shaffer K, Rennke H: Some unusual paraneoplastic syndromes. Case 4. Paraneoplastic nephrotic syndrome in a patient with lung cancer. *J Clin Oncol* 21:2624–2625, 2003
45. Davison AM: Renal diseases associated with malignancies. *Nephrol Dial Transplant* 16(suppl 6):13–14, 2001
46. Shikata Y, Hayashi Y, Yamazaki H, et al: Effectiveness of radiation therapy in nephrotic syndrome associated with advanced lung cancer. *Nephron* 83:160–164, 1999
47. Burstein DM, Korbet SM, Schwartz MM: Membranous glomerulonephritis and malignancy. *Am J Kidney Dis* 22:5–10, 1993
48. Glassock RJ, Brenner BM: The major glomerulopathies, in Isselbacher KJ, Braunwald E, Wilson JD (eds.): *Harrison's Principles of Internal Medicine.* New York, McGraw-Hill, 1994, pp 1295–1306
49. Eagen JW, Lewis EJ: Glomerulopathies of neoplasia. *Kidney International* 11:297–306, 1977
50. Robinson WL, Malleson P, Lirenman D, et al: Remission and exacerbation of tumor-related nephrotic syndrome with treatment of the neoplasm. *Cancer* 54:1082–1084, 1984
51. Juweid M, Kim CK, Heyman S: Nephrotic syndrome as an unusual paraneoplastic syndrome of Hodgkin's disease demonstrated on gallium-67 scan. *Clin Nucl Med* 19:224–227, 1994
52. Appell ML, Ward WQ, Tyring SK: Erythema gyratum repens. A cutaneous marker of malignancy. *Cancer* 62:548–550, 1988
53. Weiss P, O'Rourke ME: Cutaneous paraneoplastic syndromes. *Clin J Oncol Nurs* 4:257–262, 2000
54. Boyce S, Harper J: Paraneoplastic dermatoses. *Dermatol Clin* 20:523–532, 2002
55. McLean D, Haynes H: Cutaneous manifestations of internal malignant disease, in Freedberg IM (eds.): *Dermatology in General Medicine.* New York, McGraw-Hill, 1999, pp 2106–2120
56. Twycross R: *Symptom Management in Advanced Cancer.* Abingdon, Radcliffe Medical Press, 1997
57. Albrecht JT, Canada TW: Cachexia and anorexia in malignancy. *Hematol Oncol Clin North Am* 10:791–800, 1996
58. Martignoni ME, Kunze P, Friess H: Cancer cachexia. *Mol Cancer* 2:36, 2003
59. Lelli G, Montanari M, Gilli G, et al: Treatment of the cancer anorexia-cachexia syndrome: a critical reappraisal. *J Chemother* 15:220–225, 2003
60. van Halteren HK, Bongaerts GP, Wagener DJ: Cancer cachexia: what is known about its etiology and what should be the current treatment approach? *Anticancer Res* 23:5111–5115, 2003
61. Penel N, Fournier C, Clisant S, et al: Fever and solid tumor: diagnostic value of procalcitonin and C-reactive protein. *Rev Med Interne* 22:706–714, 2001
62. Dinarello CA, Bunn PA Jr.: Fever. *Semin Oncol* 24:288–298, 1997
63. Amin AR, Jakobiec FA, Dreyer EB: Ocular syndromes associated with systemic malignancy. *Int Ophthalmol Clin* 37:281–302, 1997
64. Hersh B, Dalmau J, Dangond F, et al: Paraneoplastic opsoclonus-myoclonus associated with anti-Hu antibody. *Neurology* 44:1754–1755, 1994

CHAPTER 34

Malignant Effusions and Edema

Diane G. Cope, PhD, ARNP, AOCN®

Introduction

An effusion is an accumulation of fluid in body tissue or cavities. Malignant effusions are the accumulation of fluid caused by a neoplastic process and are associated with morbidity and mortality in the patient with cancer. Malignant effusions can be a presenting sign and symptom at the time of diagnosis but are more often seen in patients with advanced metastatic disease.[1] Overall, the prognosis of patients with malignant effusions is poor. The types of malignant effusions most frequently encountered are pleural, pericardial, and peritoneal.

Pleural Effusions

Scope of the Problem

Malignant pleural effusions are the accumulation of excess fluid in the pleural space. They can occur as the result of a neoplastic process due to direct pleural invasion or secondary to impaired pleural lymphatic drainage from a mediastinal tumor.

Approximately 40%–50% of pleural effusions are due to malignancy and, in patients older than 50 years of age, cancer is the second leading cause of pleural effusion.[2,3] As a result of the increasing incidence of breast and lung cancer, an estimated 200,000 to 250,000 new cases of malignant pleural effusions are identified annually.[4] The most common carcinomas associated with malignant pleural effusion are lung cancer, breast cancer, and lymphoma, with lung and breast cancer accounting for approximately 75% of all malignant pleural effusions.[5] In male patients, approximately 50% of malignant effusions are caused by lung cancer, 20% by lymphoma or leukemia, 7% by gastrointestinal primaries, 6% by genitourinary primaries, and 11% by tumors of unknown primary sites. In female patients, about 40% of malignant effusions are caused by breast cancer, 20% by gynecological tumors, 15% by lung primaries, 8% by lymphoma or leukemia, 4% by gastrointestinal primaries, and 9% by tumors of unknown primary sites.[6]

Physiologic Alterations

The pleurae are composed of mesothelial cells that envelop the lungs. They encompass the visceral pleura, the outer lining of the lung, and the parietal pleura, the inner lining of the thoracic cavity (Figure 34-1).[7] The pleural space is between the visceral and parietal pleura and normally contains 5–15 mL hypoproteinemic plasma at one time, although 100–200 mL of fluid moves through the pleural space in a 24-hour period.[5]

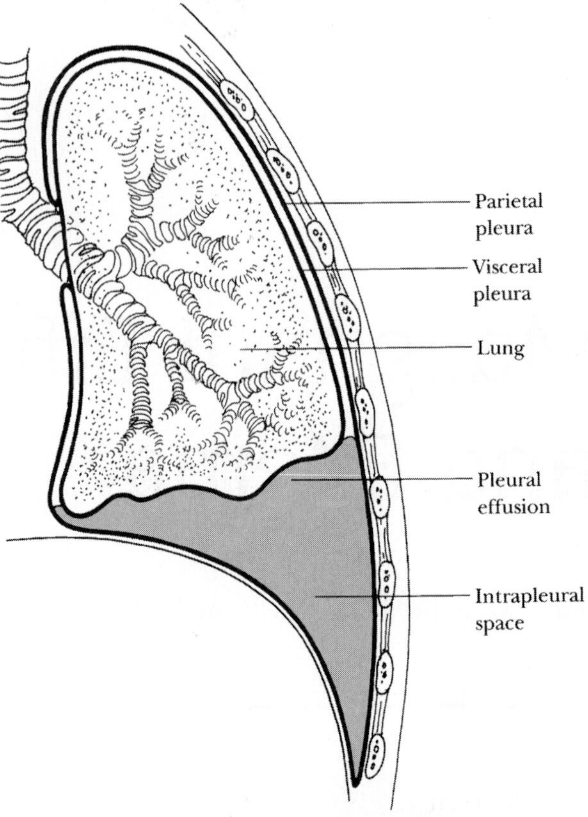

Figure 34-1 In the lung, fluid is constantly being filtered across the intrapleural space from the parietal pleural surface and reabsorbed through the visceral pleura. When obstruction by malignant processes prevents reabsorption, fluid accumulates in the intrapleural space and pleural effusion results.

Normally, a dynamic balance between the osmotic and hydrostatic pressures controls the secretion and reabsorption of pleural fluid. Alterations in fluid movement and changes in capillary permeability, hydrostatic and colloidal osmotic pressures, and lymphatic drainage can be caused by several neoplastic processes—for example, pleural implantation, lymphatic obstruction, venous obstruction, and tumor cell shedding.[1] Pleural implantation occurs when cancer cells seed or become implanted on the pleural surface, causing increased capillary permeability and inflammation of the pleural surface with leakage of fluid into the pleural space. This phenomenon is most commonly seen in patients with lung cancer. Lymphatic obstruction occurs when pulmonary lymphatic drainage becomes obstructed, causing alterations in fluid and protein reabsorption. This problem may occur with bulky tumor obstruction or lymph node involvement and is most commonly seen with lymphomas and metastatic breast and lung cancer. Pulmonary venous obstruction causes alterations in hydrostatic pressure, resulting in decreased fluid reabsorption. It may be seen with lung cancer. Tumor cell shedding into the pleural space decreases osmotic pressure, resulting in decreased fluid reabsorption; it may be seen with lung and breast cancers.[1,6]

Clinical Manifestations

Decreased respiratory function depends on the amount and rate of pleural fluid accumulation and the patient's baseline pulmonary status. Fluid accumulation restricts lung expansion, reduces lung volume, alters the ventilation and perfusion capacity, and results in abnormal gas exchange and hypoxia. Malignant pleural effusions usually develop slowly, in contrast to other etiologies that cause rapid onset with sudden dyspnea. Presenting symptoms typically include severe dyspnea, especially with exertion, cough, and chest discomfort. The dyspnea progresses to orthopnea as the effusion increases.

Assessment

A thorough history and physical examination with diagnostic studies are critical in guiding the evaluation and diagnosis of a malignant pleural effusion, because several other conditions can produce pleural effusion and must be included in a differential diagnosis list. These alternative etiologies may include benign pleural effusion, congestive heart failure, coronary artery bypass graft surgery, acute bacterial pneumonia, pulmonary embolism, trauma, and chemotherapy-induced effusions. The definitive diagnosis of malignant pleural effusion is based on a positive cytological analysis of pleural fluid, although fluid analysis is diagnostic in only 70%–80% of individuals with malignant pleural effusion.[2]

A patient's history should focus on pulmonary complaints. Further questioning of the patient and family member or caregiver about the pulmonary complaints will facilitate the diagnostic process (Table 34-1). Cough associated with pleural effusions is described as a dry, nonproductive cough that increases with activity, conversation, or deep inspiration. Chest discomfort is usually present near the involved lung. The patient may also report decreased appetite and oral intake as well as excessive fatigue.

A patient's physical examination should include baseline vital signs, patient appearance, mental status, and lung assessment (Table 34-2). Alterations suggestive of pleural effusion may include hypertension, tachycardia, tachypnea, low-grade fever, weight gain, cyanosis, shortness of breath with conversation or exertion, decreased level of consciousness, intercostal prominence, dullness on percussion, decreased tactile fremitus, and decreased breath sounds.[3,4]

Table 34-1 Patient History and Assessment: Pleural Effusion

1. When did the shortness of breath begin?
2. Are you able to carry on your normal activities?
3. Are you able to lay flat or supine to sleep?
4. Do you need several pillows to sleep?
5. Is your cough dry or productive?
6. Have you seen any blood in your sputum?
7. Do you have any chest discomfort or pain and, if so, where is it located?

Initial diagnostic studies should include a posterior-anterior chest film, a lateral decubitus film, and arterial blood gases or oxygen saturation evaluation. Posterior-anterior chest x-rays with effusion will reveal costophrenic angle blunting and an opaque shadow in the involved lung (Figure 34–2). A lateral decubitus will identify small effusions less than 200 mL. Oxygen saturation may be compromised with pleural effusions.

Table 34-2 Physical Examination for Pleural Effusion

Baseline vital signs: blood pressure, pulse, respiratory rate, temperature, weight

Patient appearance: color, respiratory patterns, pain

Mental status: level of consciousness, orientation

Lung assessment: diaphramatic alterations, percussion, auscultation

Further diagnostic testing includes a thoracentesis with pleural fluid analysis. Pleural fluid analysis requires a sample of at least 25–50 mL for adequate analysis and evaluates for transudate versus exudate, color, glucose, protein, lactate dehydrogenase (LDH), and lymphocyte content and cytology.[1] Fluids termed *transudate* are low in protein and are clear, watery, or lightly straw colored. By contrast, fluids termed *exudates* are high in protein and are dark yellowish, cloudy, or bloody in appearance. Positive pleural fluid cytologic analysis is found in approximately 50% of patients with pleural effusions, with an additional 20% being diagnosed as positive with repeat thoracentesis.[5] A therapeutic thoracentesis is usually performed at the same time as the diagnostic thoracentesis to provide immediate relief of symptoms.

The majority of malignant pleural effusions are classified as exudates. Pleural fluid consistent with malignancy characteristically is blood-tinged or grossly hemorrhagic, secondary to disruption of capillaries or venules by direct tumor invasion; is hypercellular with

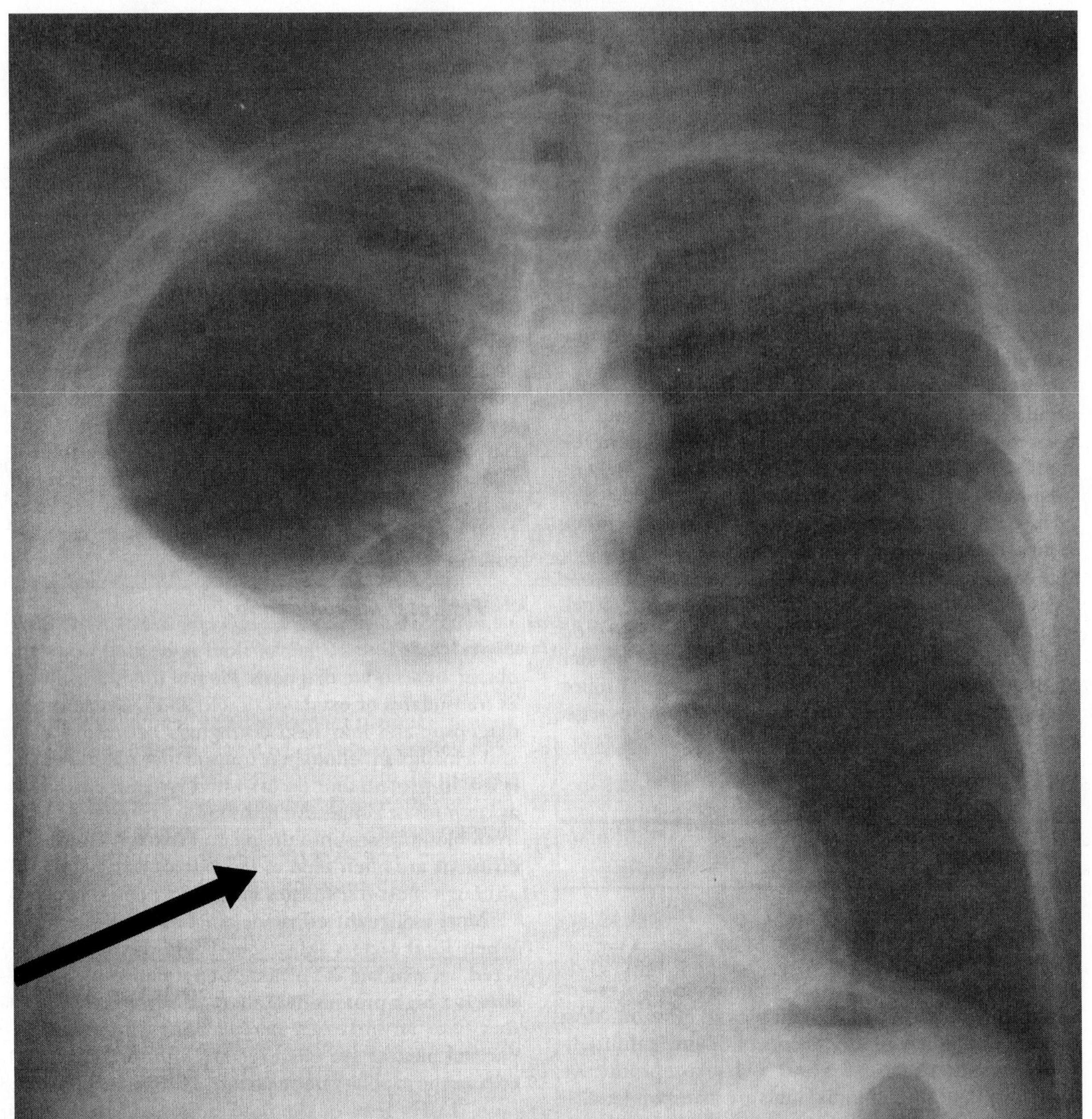

Figure 34-2 Chest x-ray film showing right pleural effusion. (Courtesy of Rush University Medical Center, Chicago, IL.)

leukocytes (predominantly lymphocytes and monocytes), and possesses an elevated LDH level, low pH, and a low glucose level (Table 34-3). Tumor marker concentrations in pleural fluid have been evaluated for their significance in determining benign versus malignant pleural effusion. At present, no tumor markers have been proved useful as a diagnostic study.[3]

Therapeutic Approaches and Nursing Care

The approach to treatment of a malignant pleural effusion depends on the type of tumor and previous therapy (Figure 34-3). Patients with chemosensitive tumors, such as small cell lung cancer and high-grade non-Hodgkin's lymphomas, and small, asymptomatic

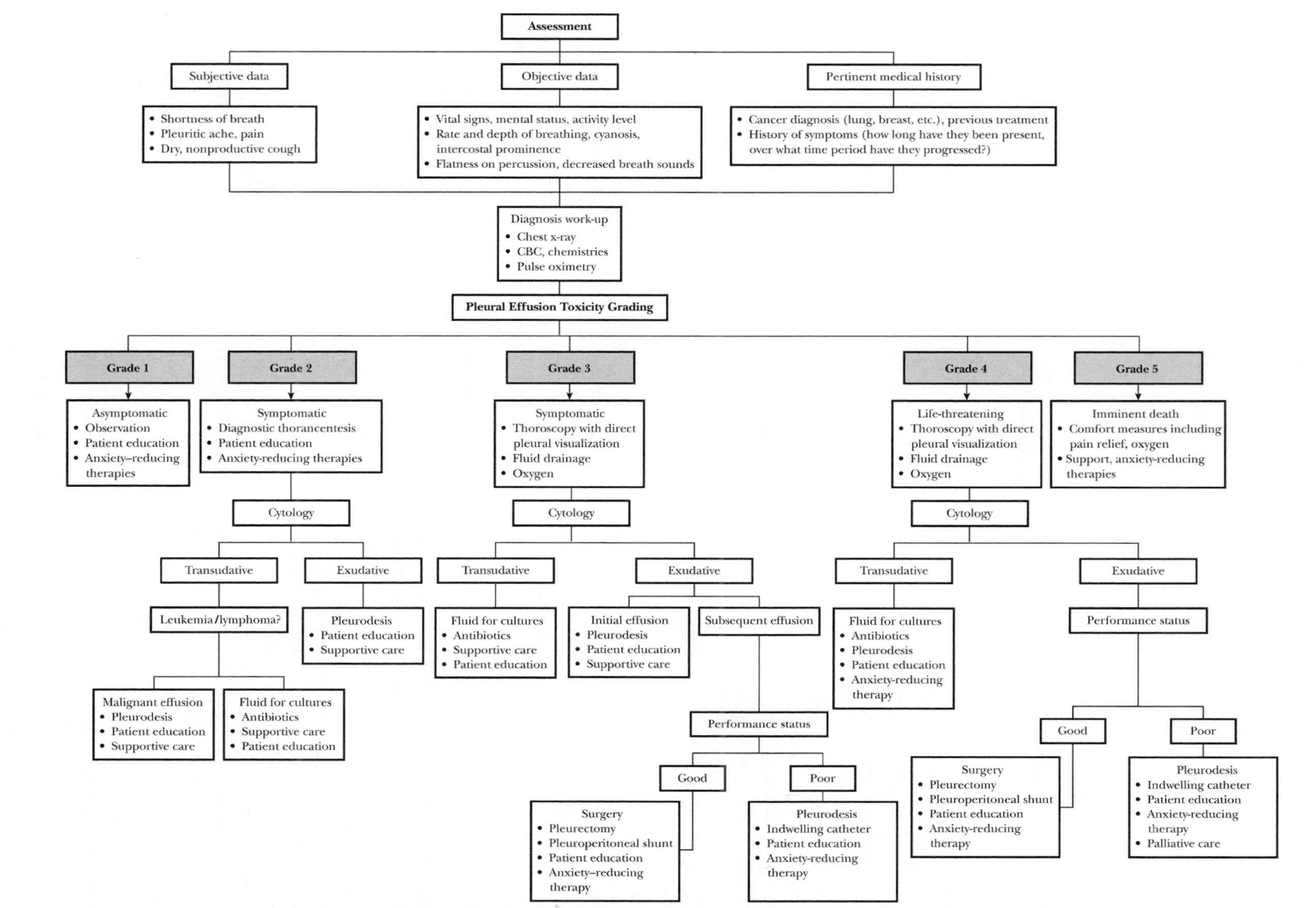

Figure 34-3 Algorithm for the management of pleural effusion.

Table 34-3 Characteristics of Malignant Pleural Fluid

Color	Cloudy, straw-colored, bloody or purulent
pH level	<7.3
LDH level	>200 U/mL
Fluid-serum LDH ratio	>0.6
Fluid-serum protein ratio	>0.5
Glucose-serum ratio	<0.5
Leukocytes	1000–10,000 cells/mm^3

Data from: Schrump DS, Nguyen DM: Malignant pleural and pericardial effusions, in DeVita VT, Hellman S, Rosenberg SA (eds.): *Cancer: Principles and Practice of Oncology* (ed 6). Philadelphia, Williams & Wilkins, 2001, p 2731.

effusions will usually respond to systemic chemotherapy or hormonal therapy. Patients who have been treated aggressively in the past or who possess a chemoresistant tumor will require other treatment approaches, which should take into account the patient's performance status and prognosis. With malignant pleural effusion, survival is related to the histology of the underlying disease. Patients with breast cancer may live more than 1 year; by comparison, patients with ovarian cancer have an average survival of 9 months and patients with lung or gastric cancer typically survive less than 3 months.[8]

The major goal of other treatment strategies is the relief of symptoms, which can be achieved when the pleural fluid is removed. Fluid, however, will reaccumulate if the underlying disease is not controlled. In this situation, obliteration of the pleural space is required to prevent pleural fluid reaccumulation.

Thoracentesis

In thoracentesis, the pleural fluid is removed by needle aspiration through the chest wall. The patient is placed in an upright sitting position, with arms and shoulders raised. This position elevates and separates the ribs to make needle insertion easier. Fluid should be relieved slowly to avoid reexpansion pulmonary edema. Prior to thoracentesis, patients should be educated about the procedure and provided with supportive care. After the thoracentesis has been completed, they should be assessed for complications. Complications of thoracentesis may include bleeding, vasovagal reaction, pain from reexpansion of the lung and apposition of pleural surfaces, and, in approximately 5% of cases, pneumothorax requiring tube thoracostomy.[2]

Recurrent effusions occur within 30 days after thoracentesis in 97% of individuals. Because repeated thoracentesis can increase risk of pneumothorax, empyema, electrolyte imbalances, infection, and pleural fluid loculations, it is not recommended.[1,2] Pleurodesis — infusion of a sclerosing agent into the pleura — immediately after thoracentesis is not effective, because residual pleural fluid may dilute the sclerosing agent.[2]

Thoracentesis via an implanted port and intrapleural catheter is an alternative approach that can be advantageous for the patient whose cancer is refractory to treatment and thus is likely to experience repeated pleural fluid reaccumulation. Pleural fluid removal via an implanted port and interpleural catheter can be completed by the nurse in the ambulatory or home setting (Figure 34-4). Use of the implanted port reduces the risk of pneumothorax and infection that can occur with repeated traditional percutaneous aspiration approaches. In addition, there can be significant reduction of healthcare resources consumed with this approach, because nurses can evacuate the fluid accumulation before the symptoms of effusion become disabling. There is also a reduced need for repeat radiological examinations. Because a Huber-point needle is used to access the implanted port, the patient experiences less pain than occurs with the large-gauge thoracentesis needle or thoracostomy tube. The greater ease of performing the thoracentesis procedure, along with reduced pain and anxiety, significantly improves the patient's experience.

Indwelling catheter

Another option for the management of recurrent pleural effusion is placement of a silicone Pleurx (Denver Biomaterials, Inc., Golden, Colorado) catheter. This catheter is ideal for patients with recurrent effusions unresponsive to therapy and is intended for long-term use. An externally draining catheter is surgically placed in the pleural space under local anesthesia. The patient, family caregiver, or home health nurse may empty the fluid accumulation as needed and provide for relief of the patient's symptoms without repeated hospital visits.[9]

Tube thoracostomy

A thoracostomy tube may be inserted via video-guided thoracoscopy to facilitate fluid drainage and then left in place to assess the degree of fluid reaccumulation. In reality, the chest tube drainage alone is only partially effective. Measures to prevent fluid reaccumulation are needed as well. Nursing assessments while a thoracostomy tube is in place include observing for pneumothorax, pain, hypotension, and pulmonary edema as well as care of the closed-chest drainage system.[10] Care must be taken to ensure that the chest tube remains patent, as exudative fluid tends to clot. Thoracostomy tubes can also be used to instill sclerosing agents into the pleural space.

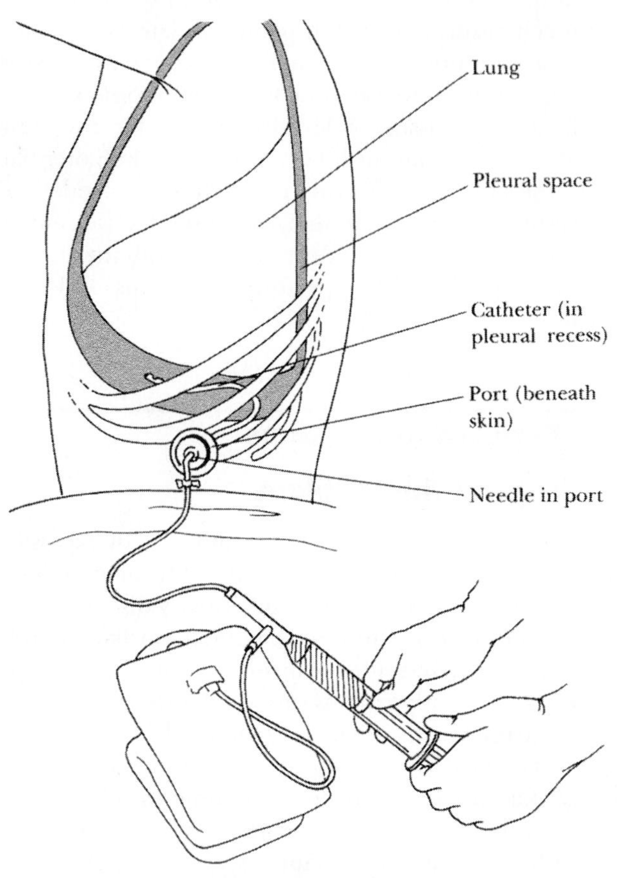

Assemble equipment:

1. Thoracentesis tray
2. Size 19-guage 90° Huber-point needle with tubing and clamps
3. Heparin-saline solution (100 μ/mL/3 mL)
4. Betadine swabs
5. Sterile gloves (2 pairs)

Procedures:

1. Place patient in a comfortable position on side.
2. Open thoracentesis tray.
3. Place sterile Huber needle on sterile tray.
4. Don sterile gloves.
5. Connect 60-mL syringe to 2-way connector.
6. Connect one end of 2-way connector to the drainage bag and one end to sterile Huber needle (see illustration).
7. Prep site over port using sterile technique
8. Change gloves.
9. Clamp Huber needle tubing.
10. Access port.
11. Tape needle securely.
12. Unclamp Huber needle tubing.
13. Draw back on plunger (fluid should yellowish).
14. Fill syringe. Push on plunger to empty syringe into drainage bag. Repeat procedure until desired amount is obtained
15. If the tube seems plugged, clamp the catheter, disconnect at 2-way valve, and clear mucous plug.
16. If drainage seems to slow down or stop, have patient change position.
17. When tap is complete (1500 mL or so), clamp catheter, Disconnect drainage tube and flush with 3-5 mL of heparinized saline.
18. Withdraw needle from port.
19. Apply bandage.

Do not attempt to access port with thoracentesis needle. Must use Huber-point needle. Procedure can be repeated as necessary.

Figure 34-4 Thoracentesis via an implanted port. (Procedure compliments of Michelle Goodman, RN, MS, Rush University Medical Center.)

Tube thoracostomy with pleurodesis

A tube thoracostomy is placed to completely evacuate pleural fluid and to allow apposition of the visceral and parietal pleura after a thoracentesis and reexpansion of the lung. A chest tube is inserted at the level of the sixth or seventh intercostal space laterally and directed posteriorly to the most dependent portion of the pleural cavity.[2] A sclerosing agent is instilled into the pleural space via the chest tube when complete drainage is confirmed by chest radiograph and daily drainage is less than 150 mL. The sclerosing agent is dissolved in 100–150 mL of normal saline. Once it is administered, the chest tube is clamped for 1–2 hours. During this time period, the patient changes positions to distribute the agent. The tube is then unclamped and attached to suction. The tube is removed when the daily drainage is less than 150 mL. Nursing management during chest tube insertion and pleural sclerosing includes patient education and reassurance, pain control, positioning, and the management of the chest tube drainage as well as maintaining the drainage system.[11,12]

Over the past 50 years, numerous agents have been used to achieve pleurodesis (Table 34-4). Nitrogen mustard was initially used and produced a response rate of 52%. Its complications included bone marrow suppression, pain, fever, nausea, and vomiting.[2] Tetracycline eventually became the sclerosing agent of choice because of its low cost, efficacy and relatively benign side effect profile. Since 1991, however, tetracycline has not been available in the United States.

Bleomycin and sterilized talc are the two agents now commonly used for pleurodesis.[2,13] Bleomycin is the only agent known to possess antitumor activity and is well tolerated. It is expensive, however, and can be associated with pain, fever, and nausea.[1,2] Talc was first utilized in 1950 and has been shown to be superior to other sclerosing agents, including tetracycline, doxycycline, and bleomycin.[2,13,14] Talc possesses a high response rate with minimal side effects, which include fever and pain, and is cost effective.

Table 34-4 Sclerosing Agents Commonly Used to Treat Pleural Effusion

Talc
Bleomycin
Tetracycline
Doxycycline
Quianacrine
Nitrogen mustard
Minocycline
Mitomycin

Biologic response modifiers have been used to treat malignant pleural effusions because of their antitumor activity, which stands opposed to that of chemical agents, which cause inflammation and adhesion of the pleurae and prevent reaccumulation of pleural fluid. Biological response modifiers — interferons and interleukin-2 — must be given in high systemic doses and are associated with severe side effects, such as flu-like syndromes, fever, transient increase in pleural effusion, skin rashes, and pruritus.[2,13] None of these agents are routinely administered for malignant pleural effusions.

Surgical approaches

If a pleural effusion persists after other treatment methods have been performed, surgery is another option for patients with good performance status and good life expectancy. Pleurectomy — stripping of the parietal pleura — is highly effective for some patients. More recently, pleurectomy via video-assisted thoracoscopic surgery has been performed, although further research into this option is needed.

Radiation therapy

Radiation is indicated for treatment of the underlying disease, although it is not recommended for first-line management of malignant pleural effusions. Radiation used to treat the mediastinal tumors seen with lymphoma and lung cancer has been effective in decreasing obstruction due to bulky tumor, thereby improving pleural fluid reabsorption. Side effects of radiation therapy to the lung field include radiation pneumonitis, cough, and increased sputum production.

Future Trends

Overall, the prognosis for patients with malignant pleural effusion is poor, with 65% dying within 3 months and 80% dying within 6 months.[2] Treatment for malignant pleural effusion at present focuses on treatment of underlying malignant disease and palliation. Recently gained knowledge into the molecular mechanisms involved in pleural inflammation has focused attention on new substances, such as transforming growth factor beta and vascular endothelial growth factor, as possible sclerosing agents for the future. More studies are needed to elucidate the potential of these substances. Further research is also needed to investigate procedures that are cost-effective and produce minimal side effects with consideration of patients' quality of life, performance status, and activity levels.

Pericardial Effusions

Scope of the Problem

Pericardial effusion is an accumulation of excess fluid in the pericardial sac that can result from infection, inflammation, or metastatic or primary disease. Pericardial effusion is the most common cardiac complication associated with cancer and indicates a poor prognosis, with patients surviving 1–13 months after its occurrence regardless of treatment.[15]

Pericardial effusions are present in as many as 20% of patients with cancer at the time of autopsy.[16] Approximately 50% of pericardial effusions in patients with cancer are malignant.

Malignant pericardial effusion is most often associated with lung (36.5%) and breast (22.3%) cancer. However, other malignancies are also associated with increased risk of pericardial effusion, such as leukemia and lymphoma (17.2%), sarcoma (3.5%), and melanoma (2.7%) (Figure 34-5).[17] Patients with cancer may develop pericardial effusion as a result of direct tumor extension with lung or esophageal cancers or as a result of chemotherapy-induced pericarditis or anthracycline therapy. Radiation therapy greater than 4000 cGy to the mediastinal area can lead to radiation-induced pericarditis. In addition, pericardial effusions can be related to hypothyroidism, hypoalbuminemia, renal failure, collagen vascular disease, chest trauma, aneurysm, improper insertion or placement of central venous catheters, or viral or bacterial pericarditis.[1,18]

Physiologic Alterations

The heart is surrounded by the pericardium, a thin, fibrous sac composed of two membranous layers, the visceral pericardium and the parietal pericardium (Figure 34-6). The visceral pericardium is the inner membrane that is connected to the surface of the heart. The parietal pericardium is the outer fibrous membrane that is in direct contact with the chest wall

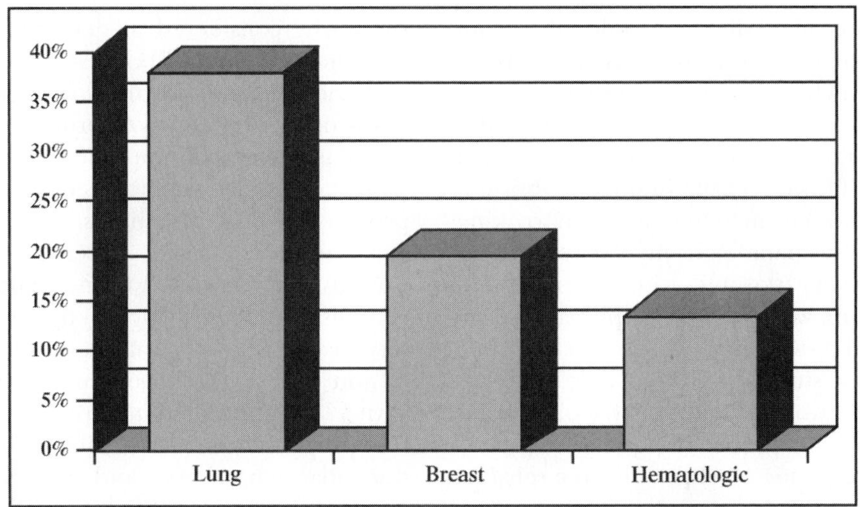

Figure 34-5 Tumor types associated with pericardial effusions. Incidence is illustrated as a percent of all pericardial effusions. Data from Taubert J.[17]

and provides structure and protection for the heart. The pericardial sac between the two membranes normally contains 15–50 mL of clear, serous, lubricating fluid that decreases friction during cardiac contraction. This pericardial fluid is produced by the lymphatic channels surrounding the heart and is reabsorbed by the lymphatic system into the mediastinum and right heart cavities.

Malignant pericardial effusions occur as a result of excess fluid accumulation from obstruction of the venous and lymphatic drainage by direct tumor invasion or from lymphatic or hematogenous spread. The majority of malignant pericardial effusions result from

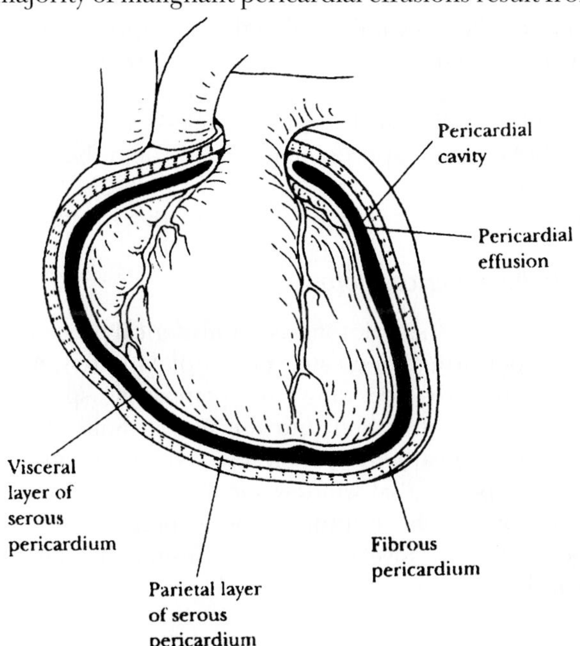

Figure 34-6 Structure of the pericardium with effusion present.

blockage of the lymphatic drainage of the heart. The effects of pericardial effusion accumulation depend on the rate of fluid accumulation, the physical compliance capacity of the pericardial cavity, ventricular function, myocardial size, and blood volume. If the fluid accumulation is gradual, the pericardium is able to stretch and accommodate as much as 2 liters of fluid without symptoms.[10] However, normal compensatory mechanisms are unable to adapt, with rapid fluid development of only 150–200 mL resulting in severe cardiac compromise and symptoms.[18]

Clinical Manifestations

Symptoms associated with pericardial effusion are related to the rate of effusion accumulation. The most common symptoms include dyspnea, cough, orthopnea, and chest pain, although patients may also report weakness, dysphagia, syncope, and palpitations. The most common signs of pericardial effusion are paradoxical pulse, tachypnea, tachycardia, hypotension, peripheral edema, distant heart sounds, rales, and pericardial rub.

Assessment

In most patients with cancer, malignant pericardial effusions may be asymptomatic and go undiagnosed until the late stages of the disease.[1,2] Although the symptoms of pericardial effusion — dyspnea, cough, orthopnea, and chest pain — can be related to numerous other etiologies, the clinician should have a high index of suspicion for pericardial involvement whenever patients with cancer present with cardiovascular symptoms.

The physical assessment should include a thorough examination focusing on the cardiac system. This examination should include blood pressure, pulse, respiratory rate, color, breath sounds, jugular venous distention, peripheral pulses, heart sounds, and abdominal girth. Physical exam findings consistent with pericardial effusion include cyanosis, narrowing pulse pressure, pulsus paradoxus, jugular venous distention, weak distant heart sounds with arrythmias and possible friction rub, weak peripheral pulses, and increased abdominal distention.

Initial diagnostic studies should include an echocardiogram, an electrocardiogram, and an anterior-posterior chest film. The echocardiogram is the most commonly used diagnostic tool because it is a reliable, noninvasive test that can evaluate the effect of a pericardial effusion on ventricular function.[16,19] Changes on the electrocardiogram associated with pericardial effusion include tachycardia, atrial and ventricular arrhythmia, low QRS voltage, and nonspecific ST- and T-wave changes. Chest radiographic changes associated with pericardial effusion include cardiomegaly, bilateral pleural effusions, mediastinal widening, and hilar lymphadenopathy. The heart may have a "water-bottle" appearance. Computerized tomography (CT) scan of the chest can identify fluid as well as pericardial thickening and masses.[19,20]

Pericardiocentesis is another diagnostic tool, albeit one that requires an invasive procedure. For this reason, its use is reserved for individuals who are symptomatic from a large effusion. While the patient is supine, a local anesthetic is administered. The pericardial sac is entered by passing an 18- or 19-gauge needle attached to a large syringe cephalad at an angle of approximately 45 degrees and directed at the patient's scapula. The fluid is analyzed to determine whether it is a transudate or an exudate, and is sent for bacterial, fungal, and mycobacterial cultures and cytology. Malignant pericardial fluid is exudative or bloody in appearance. Positive cytologic examination is confirmed in only 50%–60% of pericardial effusions in patients with cancer.[2]

Therapeutic Approaches and Nursing Care

The goals of treatment for pericardial effusion are relief of symptoms, identification of positive cytology and prevention of fluid reaccumulation. The patient's diagnosis, stage of disease, and performance status should be considered in determining treatment approaches (Figure 34-7).

Pericardiocentesis can be used as a diagnostic tool but is most frequently performed in symptomatic patients as a therapeutic procedure. Although it has a high success rate, fluid reaccumulation occurs in approximately 50% of patients; therefore, other definitive medical or surgical treatment is necessary to prevent recurrence.[19,20] Complications of pericardiocentesis include laceration of the heart or coronary artery, laceration of the internal mammary artery, penetration and possible contamination of the pleural cavity, laceration or puncture of the lung with resultant pneumothorax, aspiration of blood from the intracardiac chambers, and ventricular fibrillation. Nursing care during the pericardiocentesis includes explanation of the procedure to the patient; positioning the patient in a semi-Fowler's position; maintaining asepsis; and having available a defibrillator, oxygen, and emergency medications. The nurse must continuously monitor the patient and the ECG during the pericardiocentesis and after the procedure to detect any cardiac or pulmonary abnormalities.

Subxiphoid pericardiostomy

Subxiphoid pericardiostomy (pericardial window) is the most commonly performed procedure for pericardial effusions and can be performed under local anesthesia. A small, vertical skin incision is made in the subxiphoid region. The anterior pericardium is incised, and fluid is drained. Next, the pericardium is explored and a sample is obtained for pathologic studies. A pericardial tube is then placed in the upper abdominal wall into the pericardial space to allow for postoperative drainage. For subxiphoid pericardiostomy, the overall mortality rate is approximately 46%, the overall morbidity rate is approximately 1.53%, and the recurrence rate for effusion is approximately 3.5%.[2] Nursing care is the same as for the pericardiocentesis.

Balloon pericardiotomy

Balloon pericardiotomy is a nonsurgical procedure that is performed to create a pericardial window. After percutaneously accessing the pericardial space, a guide wire is threaded into the pericardium. A balloon-dilating catheter is then inserted and inflated to create a pericardial window for fluid drainage. This procedure has been found to be helpful in the management of massive pericardial effusions in patients with poor performance statuses.[21]

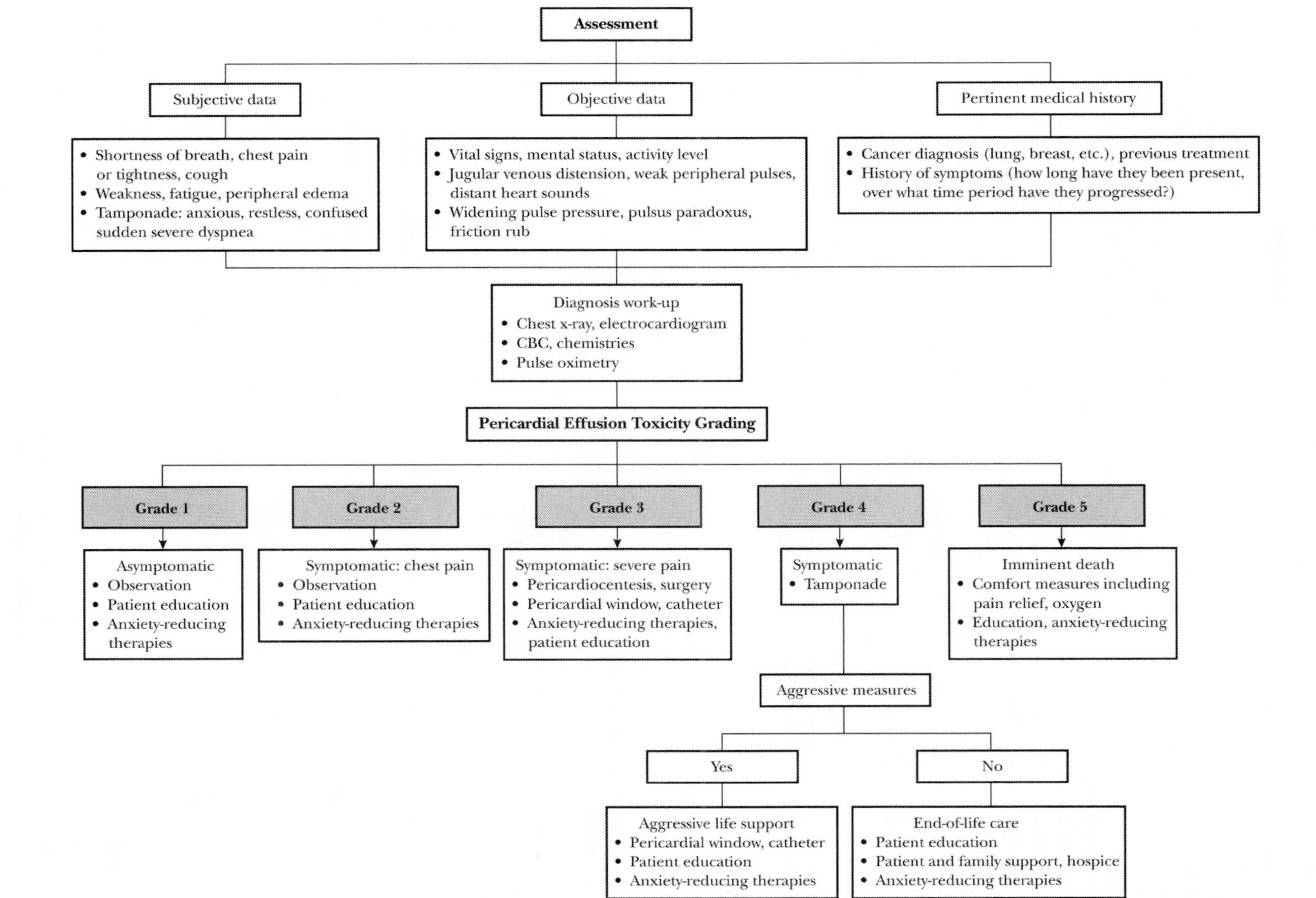

Figure 34-7 Algorithm for management of pericardial effusion.

Pericardiocentesis with sclerosing agent instillation

Pericardiocentesis with the instillation of sclerosing agents has been used to obliterate the pericardial space by inducing an inflammatory response with resultant fibrosis and sclerosis in the pericardium. Sclerosing agents used in pericardial effusions include tetracycline, doxycycline, thiotepa, bleomycin, minocycline, 5–fluorouracil, cisplatin, and nitrogen mustard; of these options, tetracycline and doxycycline have been the most extensively evaluated sclerosing agents.[2] This treatment approach controls the pericardial effusion for longer than 30 days in more than 90% of patients. In a small prospective study,[22] doxycycline and bleomycin were compared as sclerosing agents in the treatment of pericardial effusions. The findings suggested that the agents had similar efficacy but patients treated with bleomycin had shorter hospitalizations and less retrosternal pain. Other sclerosing agents found to be associated with minimal side effects and successful in controlling malignant pericardial effusions include carboplatin[23] and cisplatin.[24,25]

Surgery

Surgical intervention, including transthoracic pericardial window via thoracotomy and pericardiectomy, is generally reserved for individuals who require repeated pericardiocentesis and are able, medically appropriate patients because general anesthesia and thoracotomy are required. Patients undergoing transthoracic drainage versus subxiphoid pericardiostomy are at increased risk for complications including pneumonia, pleural effusion, respiratory failure, cardiac arrhythmia, deep-vein thrombosis, and pulmonary embolism. In comparison to thoracotomy, a preferred option is video-assisted thoracoscopy, which is less invasive.[26,27]

Radiation therapy

Radiotherapy is generally indicated for patients with lymphoma or breast carcinoma.[2] Radiation therapy is associated with several weeks of daily treatments or prolonged hospitalization, and can potentially cause acute pericarditis or myocarditis.

Future Trends

At the present time, subxiphoid pericardial window is the preferred surgical treatment for pericardial effusion. Further research is needed to investigate sclerosing agents, patient characteristics, and low-invasive, cost-effective procedures that may enhance patients' quality of life.

Malignant Peritoneal Effusions

Scope of the Problem

Malignant peritoneal effusion, commonly termed ascites, is fluid accumulation in the peritoneal cavity, a sac located between the parietal and visceral peritoneum. The most likely cause of ascites in a patient with known intraabdominal cancer is spread of disease. This condition is associated with a poor prognosis. Treatment is usually aimed at palliative care, with survival typically lasting only a few months.

Although ascites may occur with many types of carcinomas, its exact incidence is not well documented. Ascites is most often associated with ovarian cancer, with approximately 33% of patients having ascites at presentation and more than 60% having ascites at the time of death.[28]

Malignant ascites occurs commonly in patients with lymphoma, mesothelioma, ovarian, breast, gastric, hepatic, pancreatic, and colon carcinomas.[28] It is associated with advanced or progressive disease.

Physiologic Alterations

The peritoneal cavity is covered by a serous lining composed of the visceral peritoneum, which lines and supports the abdominal organs, and the parietal peritoneum. The parietal peritoneum covers the abdominal and pelvic walls and the undersurface of the diaphragm (Figure 34-8). Normally, a small amount of fluid is present to lubricate the cavity. Malignant ascites occurs when the fluid production exceeds the ability of the lymphatic channels to drain the cavity, because of increased peritoneal fluid production or lymphatic obstruction with decreased fluid reabsorption. The most common cause of ascitic fluid collection is tumor seeding of the peritoneum, resulting in obstruction of the diaphragmatic and abdominal lymphatics. This phenomenon occurs primarily with gynecological cancers.[7]

Widespread peritoneal carcinomatosis or tumor seeding results in damaged capillary endothelium and increased capillary permeability with increased peritoneal fluid formation. Tumors may also elaborate humoral factors that cause increased capillary leakage of proteins and fluids into the peritoneum. Tumor obstruction of the main thoracic duct or of the hepatic venous system will result in blockage of the lymphatic channels and impair normal lymphatic drainage. Patients with diffuse hepatic metastases and venous obstruction may develop a transudative ascites, as this condition is caused by hypoalbuminemia and increased portal vein pressure.

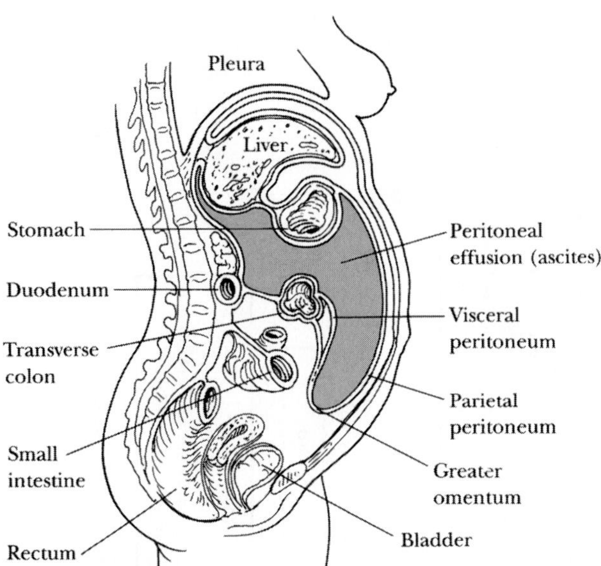

Figure 34-8 The peritoneal cavity is covered by the visceral peritoneum that lines and supports the abdominal organs, and the parietal peritoneum that covers the abdominal and pelvic walls and the undersurface of the diaphragm. If, due to malignant processes, the volume of fluid accumulating in the peritoneal space exceeds the capacity of lymphatic channels to drain the cavity, ascites develops.

Clinical Manifestations

Symptoms of ascites vary depending on the amount of peritoneal fluid present. As the amount of ascitic fluid increases, its pressure on abdominal organs and visceral structures becomes restrictive. The abdomen is distensible and able to accommodate large volumes of ascitic fluid. Patients may become symptomatic when the fluid amount present is 500 mL or greater.[7]

Assessment

Patient and family history

A detailed history should include the patient's recent dietary intake, urinary and bowel patterns, and abdominal complaints. Symptoms associated with ascites include abdominal distention, weight gain, indigestion, dyspnea, orthopnea, early satiety, anorexia, fatigue, abdominal or back pain, constipation, and urinary urgency, frequency, and decreased output. In severe cases, massive ascites can cause intestinal obstruction, resulting in nausea and vomiting, and lower extremity lymphatic obstruction with the development of peripheral edema.

Physical examination

The physical examination should focus on a detailed abdominal and respiratory assessment. The abdomen is usually distended with tightly stretched, shiny skin and bulging flanks. The abdominal girth should be obtained as a baseline. Abdominal percussion reveals tympany in the upper and mid-abdominal regions and dullness over the flanks.[7] A fluid wave may also be present and may be elicited by placing the ulnar surface of the hand on the midline of the patient's abdomen and applying pressure. Bowel sounds may be high-pitched, diminished, or absent, depending on the amount of ascitic fluid. Ascites may also involve the respiratory system, with physical findings revealing diaphragm elevation and pleural effusions. The presence of pleural effusions will produce dullness upon percussion over the involved lung fields, with diminished breath sounds upon auscultation.

Diagnostic studies

The presence of malignant ascites is assessed by several diagnostic studies, including abdominal x-ray, ultrasound, and CT scan, and paracentesis with fluid evaluation. An abdominal x-ray may reveal a generalized ground-glass appearance, with central positioning of the small bowel loops and separation of the bowel loops by ascitic fluid. Abdominal ultrasound and CT scan are very sensitive examinations to detect small amounts of fluid. A paracentesis should be performed to confirm the diagnosis and provide relief of symptoms.

The fluid appearance can provide important information regarding the etiology of the fluid accumulation. Bloody ascites, likely characterized as exudate, is often seen in ovarian or hepatocellular carcinoma but may also be associated with peritoneal carcinomatosis. Chylous ascites or a milky appearance may result from obstruction of the thoracic duct by lymphoma. Serous fluid may be suggestive of congestive heart failure or nephrotic syndrome. A cloudy appearance may be due to an infectious process. The fluid should be cultured for bacterial, fungal, and mycobacterial organisms and analyzed for protein, glucose, LDH, and amylase levels. Malignant ascites usually reveals elevated total protein and LDH levels.[7,29]

Therapeutic Approaches and Nursing Care

Malignant ascites is usually difficult to control in those individuals who develop fluid accumulation rapidly and are refractory to treatment. The majority of therapeutic approaches for malignant ascites focus

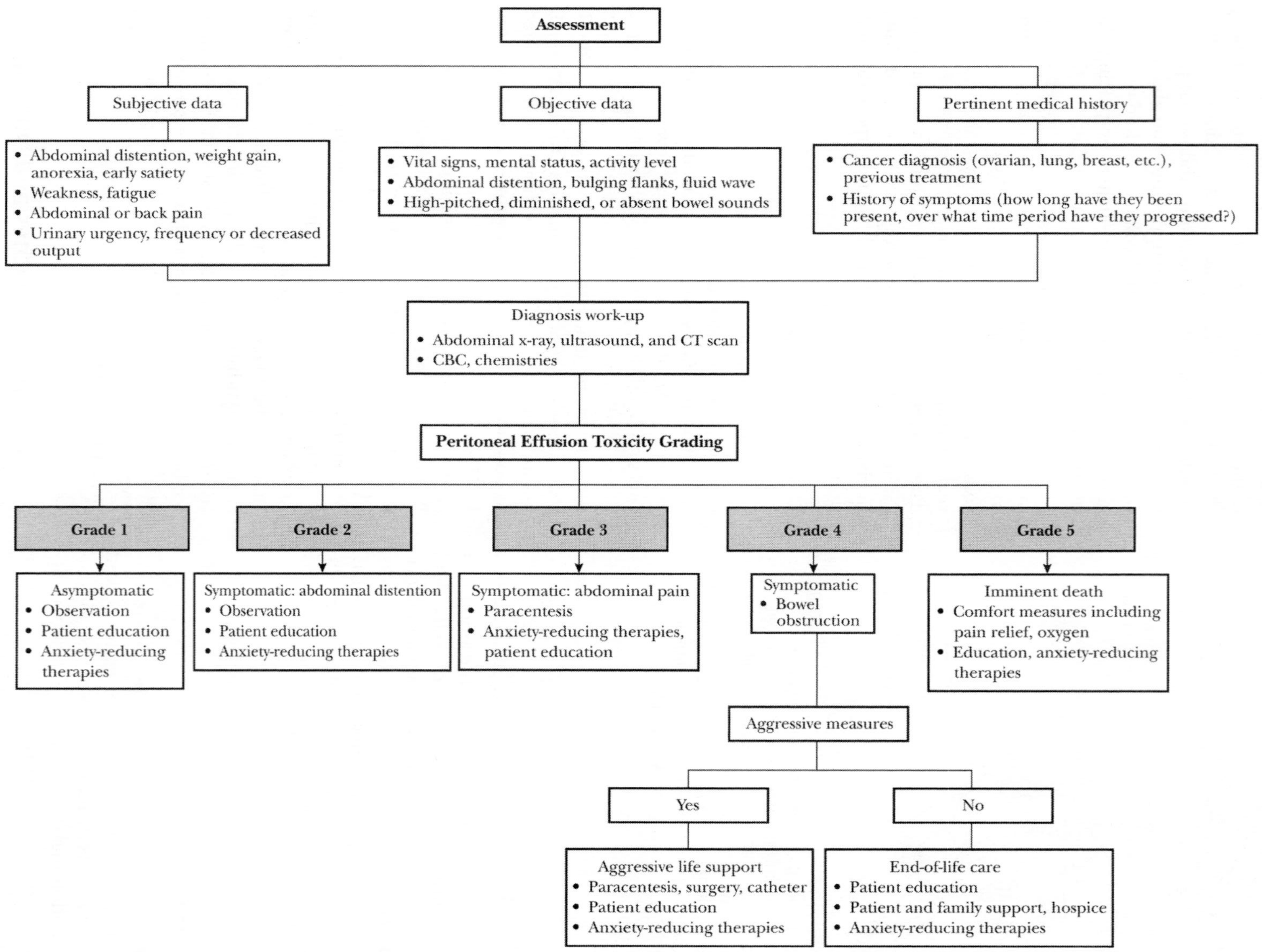

Assessment

Subjective data
- Abdominal distention, weight gain, anorexia, early satiety
- Weakness, fatigue
- Abdominal or back pain
- Urinary urgency, frequency or decreased output

Objective data
- Vital signs, mental status, activity level
- Abdominal distention, bulging flanks, fluid wave
- High-pitched, diminished, or absent bowel sounds

Pertinent medical history
- Cancer diagnosis (ovarian, lung, breast, etc.), previous treatment
- History of symptoms (how long have they been present, over what time period have they progressed?)

Diagnosis work-up
- Abdominal x-ray, ultrasound, and CT scan
- CBC, chemistries

Peritoneal Effusion Toxicity Grading

Grade 1
Asymptomatic
- Observation
- Patient education
- Anxiety-reducing therapies

Grade 2
Symptomatic: abdominal distention
- Observation
- Patient education
- Anxiety-reducing therapies

Grade 3
Symptomatic: abdominal pain
- Paracentesis
- Anxiety-reducing therapies, patient education

Grade 4
Symptomatic
- Bowel obstruction

Aggressive measures

Yes
Aggressive life support
- Paracentesis, surgery, catheter
- Patient education
- Anxiety-reducing therapies

No
End-of-life care
- Patient education
- Patient and family support, hospice
- Anxiety-reducing therapies

Grade 5
Imminent death
- Comfort measures including pain relief, oxygen
- Education, anxiety-reducing therapies

Figure 34-9 Algorithm for the management of malignant peritoneal effusion. (Data from U.S. Department of Health and Human Services: Common terminology criteria for adverse events (CTCAE) (v 3.0), 2003, p 19.)

on palliative care and symptom management (Figure 34-9). Goals of nursing care are the maintenance of fluid and electrolyte balance, comfort measures, and early recognition of complications.

Diet and diuresis

Loop and aldosterone-inhibiting diuretics and sodium-restricted diets have not been found to be beneficial in the control of malignant ascites, because sodium retention is not the cause of malignant ascites.[29] In addition, the administration of albumin has not been shown to delay fluid reaccumulation.

Fluid removal – paracentesis

Removal of peritoneal fluid by paracentesis is useful as a diagnostic tool but has little therapeutic benefit because the fluid reaccumulates rapidly without other interventions. Removal of 2–3 liters of fluid and repeated paracentesis procedures can lead to severe protein depletion, postural hypotension, intraperitoneal visceral injury, infection, and electrolyte abnormalities. Unlike ascites secondary to other etiologies, malignant ascites may be removed in large volumes without altering hemodynamic equilibrium.

Obliteration of the intraperitoneal space

In the past, intracavity therapy consisted of instillation of a radioactive colloid suspension (no longer in favor) or a chemotherapeutic agent. The chemotherapy instillation is designed to provoke an inflammatory response, leading to sclerosis of the peritoneal space membranes. Modest responses to bleomycin instillation for palliation have been reported with no significant side effects. Doxorubicin, cisplatin, carboplatin, etoposide, nitrogen mustard, and tetracycline have also been used as intraperitoneal sclerosing agents. Biologic response modifiers have been used as an alternative to chemotherapeutic agents, although further research is needed to elucidate their effectiveness.[25]

Obtaining access to the peritoneal cavity for drug administration is an important technical problem. The peritoneum can be entered on a temporary basis with various catheters, but repeated puncture of the abdominal wall and peritoneum can lead to increased risk of adhesions, bowel perforation, and peritonitis. Placement of a long-term catheter, such as a Tenckhoff or Groshong catheter, is often used to provide access for repeated paracentesis. The catheter can remain in place indefinitely and allows for peritoneal fluid sampling in addition to drug instillation. The catheter needs to be monitored to evaluate for patency and signs of infection. In general, however, indwelling catheters enhance patient comfort by alleviating symptoms and reducing the need for repeated percutaneous paracentesis.[28,30,31]

Peritoneovenous shunting

Shunt devices (LeVeen and Denver) can be used to recirculate ascitic fluid continuously to the intravascular space. One end of a catheter is implanted in the peritoneal cavity, and a tube is channeled through the subcutaneous tissue to the superior vena cava, where the other end of the catheter is implanted. A pressure differential between the abdominal cavity and the thoracic vein enables fluid to ascend from the peritoneal cavity into the superior vena cava. Peritoneovenous shunting is usually reserved for patients who have failed all other medical management options. Median survival time after shunt placement is usually 2–4 months, although when the shunt is functioning well, palliation is optimal. Complications can include clotting, disseminated intravascular coagulation, and pulmonary embolism.[32] Nursing care of the patient with a peritoneovenous shunt includes teaching the patient and family about the purpose and care of the shunt, signs and symptoms of problems with the shunt, and recognition and prevention of infection.

Future Trends

At present, no definitive management guidelines for malignant ascites exist, although the mainstays of treatment include diuretics and recurrent large-volume paracentesis. Recent evidence suggests that immune modulators, vascular permeability factors, and metalloproteinases may be significant contributing factors in the pathophysiologic process of malignant ascites.[32,33] Based on this rationale, new, more targeted therapies, such as matrix metalloproteinase inhibitors and VEGF antagonists, may offer better management of malignant ascites. Further research is needed to investigate these novel therapies.

References

1. Goldman D: Effusions, in Yarbro CH, Frogge MH, Goodman M (eds.): *Cancer Symptom Management* (ed 3). Sudbury, MA, Jones and Bartlett, 2003, pp 420–439
2. Schrump DS, Nguyen DM: Malignant pleural and pericardial effusions, in DeVita VT, Hellman S, Rosenberg SA (eds.): *Cancer: Principles and Practice of Oncology* (ed 6). Philadelphia, Lippincott, Williams & Wilkins, 2001, pp 2729–2744
3. Walker DL, Casciato DA: Malignant effusions, in Haskell CM (ed.): *Cancer Treatment* (ed 5). Philadelphia, W.B. Saunders, 2001, pp 1578–1590
4. Light RW: Pleural effusion. *N Engl J Med* 346:1971–1977, 2002
5. Camp-Sorrell D: Malignant pleural effusion. *Clin J Oncol Nurs* 3:36–37, 39, 1999

6. Pass HI: Malignant pleural and pericardial effusions, in DeVita VT, Hellman S, Rosenberg SA (eds.): *Cancer: Principles and Practice of Oncology* (ed 5). Philadelphia, Lippincott-Raven, 1997, pp 2586–2598
7. Works C, Maxwell MB: Malignant effusions and edema, in Yarbro CH, Frogge MH, Goodman M, et al (eds.): *Cancer Nursing: Principles and Practice* (ed 5). Sudbury, MA, Jones and Bartlett, 2000, pp 813-830
8. Fenton KN, Richardson JD: Diagnosis and management of malignant pleural effusion. *Am J Surg* 170:69–74, 1995
9. Brubacher S, Gobel BH: Use of the Pleurx pleural catheter for the management of malignant pleural effusions. *Clin J Oncol Nurs* 7:35–38, 2003
10. Robinson LA, Ruckdeschel JC: Management of pleural and pericardial effusions, in Berger A, Portenoy RK, Weissman DE (eds.): *Principles and Practice of Supportive Oncology*. Philadelphia, Lippincott-Raven, 1998, pp 327–3552
11. Luketich JD, Kiss M, Hershey J, et al: Chest tube insertion: a prospective evaluation of pain management. *Clin J Pain* 14:152–154, 1998
12. Spiea AI, Brahmer JR: Effusions, in Abeloff MD, Armitage JO, Niederhuber JE, et al (eds.): *Clinical Oncology*. New York; Churchill Livingstone, 2004, pp 1179–1212
13. Marchi E, Teoxeora R, Vargas FS: Management of malignancy associated pleural effusion: current and future treatment strategies. *Am J Respir Med* 3:261–273, 2003
14. Shaw P, Agarwal R: Pleurodesis for malignant pleural effusions. *Cochrane Database System Rev* 1:CD002916, 2004
15. Dragonette P: Malignant pericardial effusion and cardiac tamponade, in Chernecky C, Berger B (eds.): *Advanced and Critical Care Oncology Nursing*. Philadelphia, W.B. Saunders, 1998, pp 425–443
16. DeMichele A, Glick J: Cancer related emergencies, in Lenhard R, Osteen R, Gansler T (eds.): *Clinical Oncology*. Atlanta, American Cancer Society, 2001, pp 733–764
17. Taubert J: Management of malignant pleural effusion. *Nurs Clin North Am* 36:665–683, 2001
18. Bullock B: Altered cardiac function, in Bullock B, Henze R (eds.): *Focus on Pathophysiology*. Philadelphia, Lippincott, 2000, pp 455–502
19. Retter A: Pericardial disease in the oncology patient. *Heart Dis* 4:387–391, 2002
20. Palacios IF: Pericardial effusion and tamponade. *Curr Treat Options Cardiovasc Med* 1:79–89, 1999
21. Wang HJ, Hsu KL, Chiang FT, et al: Technical and prognostic outcomes of double-balloon pericardiotomy for large malignancy-related pericardial effusions. *Chest* 122:893–899, 2002
22. Liu G, Crump M, Goss PE, et al: Prospective comparison of the sclerosing agents doxycycline and bleomycin for the primary management of malignant pericardial effusion and cardiac tamponade. *J Clin Oncol* 12:3141–3147, 1996
23. Moriya T, Takiguchi Y, Tabeta H, et al: Controlling malignant pericardial effusion by intrapericardial carboplatin administration in patients with primary non-small cell lung cancer. *Br J Cancer* 83:858–862, 2000
24. Maisch B, Ristic AD, Pankuweit S, et al: Neoplastic pericardial effusion. Efficacy and safety of intrapericardial treatment with cisplatin. *Eur Heart J* 20:1625–1631, 2002
25. Tomkowski WZ, Wisniewska J, Szturmowicz M, et al: Evaluation of intrapericardial cisplatin administration in cases with recurrent malignant pericardial effusion and cardiac tamponade. *Support Care Cancer* 1:53–57, 2004
26. Liu HP, Chang CH, Lin PJ, et al: Thoracoscopic management of effusive pericardial disease: indications and technique. *Ann Thorac Surg* 58:1695–1704, 1994
27. Lin JC, Hazelrigg SR, Landreneau RJ: Video-assisted thoracic surgery for diseases within the mediastinum. *Surg Clin North Am* 80:1511–1533, 2000
28. Iyengar TD, Herzog TJ: Management of symptomatic ascites in recurrent ovarian cancer patients using an intra-abdominal semi-permanent catheter. *Am J Hosp Palliat Care* 1:35–38, 2002
29. Marincola FM, Schwartzentruber DJ: Malignant ascites, in DeVita VT, Hellman S, Rosenberg SA (eds.): *Cancer: Principles and Practice of Oncology* (ed 6). Philadelphia, Lippincott, Williams & Wilkins, 2001, pp 2745–2752
30. Lee A, Lau TN, Yeong KY: Indwelling catheters for the management of malignant ascites. *Support Care Cancer* 6:493–499, 2000
31. Richard HM, Coldwell DM, Boyd-Kranis RL, et al: Pleurx tunneled catheter in the management of malignant ascites. *J Vascul Intervent Radiol* 3:373–375, 2001
32. Smith EM, Jayson GC: The current and future management of malignant ascites. *Clin Oncol*, 15:59–72, 2003
33. Aslam N, Marino CR: Malignant ascites: new concepts in pathophysiology, diagnosis, and management. *Arch Intern Med* 22:2733–2737, 2001

CHAPTER 35

Sexual and Reproductive Dysfunction

Linda U. Krebs, RN, PhD, AOCN®

Scope of the Problem

Although increasingly recognized as consequences of cancer or cancer therapy, sexual and reproductive dysfunctions often have been dismissed as normal side effects about which the caregiver can do little or nothing. Indeed, these dysfunctions frequently have gone underdiagnosed, underrated, or both, because of lack of concern, information, or knowledge on the part of the caregiver, or because of fear, lack of knowledge, or embarrassment on the part of the patient or family. Often, problems related to sexuality and reproduction are not addressed unless the patient is extremely assertive or presents to the healthcare provider in a crisis situation. However, linking sexuality with health, initiating discussion of potential sexuality-related issues and concerns, and conducting a brief sexual assessment may prevent or minimize future complications.[1]

Of all the complications associated with cancer, difficulties in the ability to feel comfortable with one's own sexuality and body image, to be sexually intimate, and to bear children have remained major concerns that affect all aspects of the patient's and his or her family's lives. For some patients, sexual or reproductive dysfunctions may be temporary, with full recovery expected when therapy is completed. For many others, alterations in sexual or reproductive function are permanent, requiring adaptations in management of intimate relationships and lifelong plans to bear and raise children. Even short-term, temporary alterations can have long-term effects on the patient and family, influencing lifestyles and life choices.

Sexuality and reproductive ability are intrinsic components of every individual, involving all aspects of our being.[2] The sexuality and reproductive capacity of the individual with cancer may be affected by a variety of factors, including the biological process of cancer, the effects of treatment, additional health problems and medications, and the psychological and social issues, such as religious and cultural norms, surrounding the patient and family.[3] Physiological problems of infertility and sterility, changes in body appearance, and the inability to have intercourse are exacerbated by the psychological and psychosexual issues of alteration in body image, fear of abandonment, loss of self-esteem, alteration in sexual identity, and concerns about self. Without appropriate education, counseling, and support, it may be difficult for the patient and family to adapt to the alterations that cancer can produce.

Physiological Alterations

The pituitary and the hypothalamus regulate gonadal function. The pituitary is divided into two distinct parts — the anterior and posterior portions — and is attached to the hypothalamus by the pituitary or hypophysial stalk, through which runs a minute blood vessel system, the hypothalamic-hypophysial portal vessels.[4,5]

Hypothalamic-releasing or hypothalamic-inhibiting hormones are secreted within the hypothalamus and then spread via the portal vessel system to the anterior pituitary, where they act to influence glandular secretion. When produced in appropriate amounts, these hormones institute a feedback mechanism that shuts off hormonal secretion at the hypothalamus and pituitary level.[4,5]

In gonadal function, luteinizing hormone–releasing hormone (LHRH) or gonadotropin-releasing hormone (GnRH) is secreted by the hypothalamus and stimulates the anterior pituitary to produce luteinizing hormone (LH) and follicle-stimulating hormone (FSH). Luteinizing hormone and FSH stimulate the testis and ovary to produce the appropriate hormones. When blood levels of these hormones are adequate, the hormones exert a negative feedback on the pituitary, thereby decreasing glandular secretion.[4,5]

Follicle-stimulating hormone and LH play major roles in the control of male sexual function. Luteinizing hormone acts on the interstitial Leydig cells to produce testosterone; FSH, in conjunction with testosterone, is responsible for the conversion of spermatogonia into spermatocytes. A reciprocal inhibition of hypothalamic/anterior pituitary secretion of gonadotropic hormones by testicular hormones keeps the level of hormones stable. In this system, the hypothalamus secretes GnRH, which causes the anterior pituitary to secrete LH. In turn, LH stimulates the Leydig cells to produce testosterone. The testosterone then negatively feeds back to the hypothalamus, inhibiting production of GnRH. Spermatogenesis is controlled in much the same manner, with FSH stimulating the Sertoli cells to convert spermatids into sperm. The Sertoli cells then secrete a hormone called *inhibin* that, through negative feedback, causes a decrease in FSH production, thus keeping spermatogenesis at a constant rate (Figure 35–1).[4,5]

The female hormonal system, like its male counterpart, consists of three levels of hormones: GnRH from the hypothalamus, LH and FSH from the anterior pituitary, and estrogen and progesterone from the ovary. In the nonpregnant female, monthly rhythmic

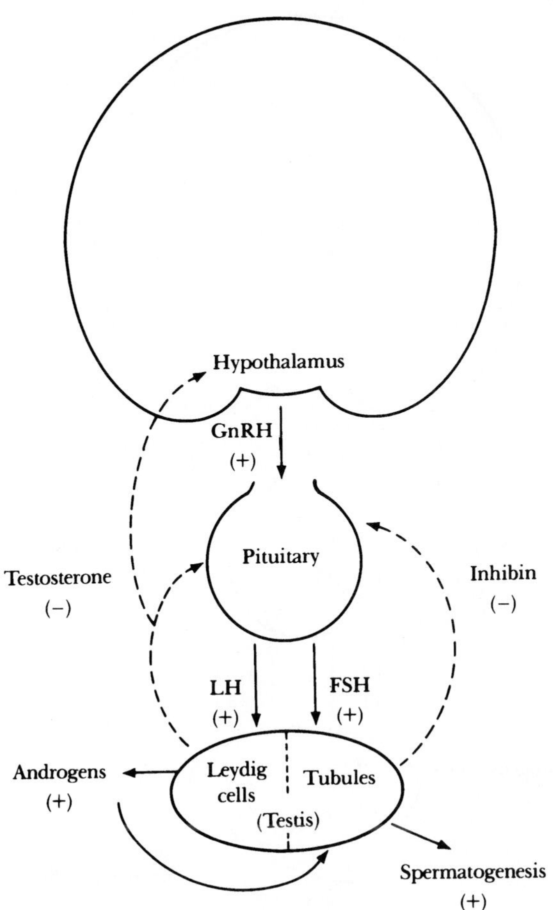

Figure 35–1 Normal testicular function. FSH = follicle-stimulating hormone; GnRH = gonadotropin-releasing hormone; LH = luteinizing hormone. (Data from Marieb.[5])

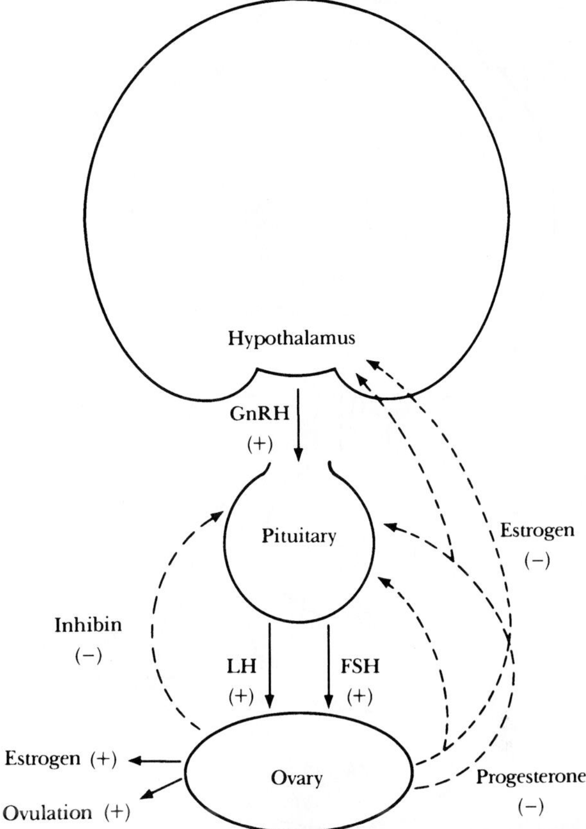

Figure 35-2 Normal ovarian function. FSH = follicle-stimulating hormone; GnRH = gonadotropin-releasing hormone; LH = luteinizing hormone. (Data from Marieb.[5])

changes in the rates of secretion of female hormones and responding changes in the sexual organs result in the female sexual (menstrual) cycle. As a result, a single mature ovum is released from an ovary, and the endometrium of the uterus is prepared for implantation. Follicle-stimulating hormone is responsible for growth of the ovarian follicle, which eventually will become the mature ovum. At the beginning of menstruation, FSH and LH increase, causing rapid cellular growth in about 20 follicles. Eventually, one follicle begins to outgrow the others, causing atresia of the remaining follicles. During follicle growth, estrogen is secreted, probably causing a positive feedback mechanism that results in a surge of LH. This surge of LH, which occurs two days before ovulation, is necessary for follicular growth and ovulation. Around the time of ovulation, the ruptured follicle, under the stimulation of LH, becomes the corpus luteum, which secretes both estrogen and progesterone. After several days, the estrogen and progesterone create negative feedback, decreasing secretion of FSH and LH. The corpus luteum, which also secretes inhibin, slowly degenerates, leading to a loss of the feedback mechanism and an associated rise in secretion of FSH and LH, beginning a new ovarian cycle, and leading to menstruation (Figure 35–2).[4,5]

Ovarian failure and germinal aplasia can occur as a result of disease, therapy, nutritional status, psychological factors, or any combination of these. Ovarian failure also is related to age; as women near menopause, ovarian failure is more likely. In ovarian failure, damage to ovarian follicles causes decreased levels of estrogens and progesterones, which results in increased levels of LH and FSH with no compensating feedback mechanism. In addition, inhibin may be produced and may react further to alter FSH production. Ovulation ceases, menstruation becomes erratic or ceases, and early menopause often results (Figure 35–3).[4,5] In the male, damage to the Leydig cells results in decreased testosterone production; LH and FSH levels will be elevated. Initially, Leydig cell activity may be sufficiently compensated to produce adequate amounts of testosterone, but continued damage results in temporary, but more often permanent, sterility (Figure 35–4).[4,5]

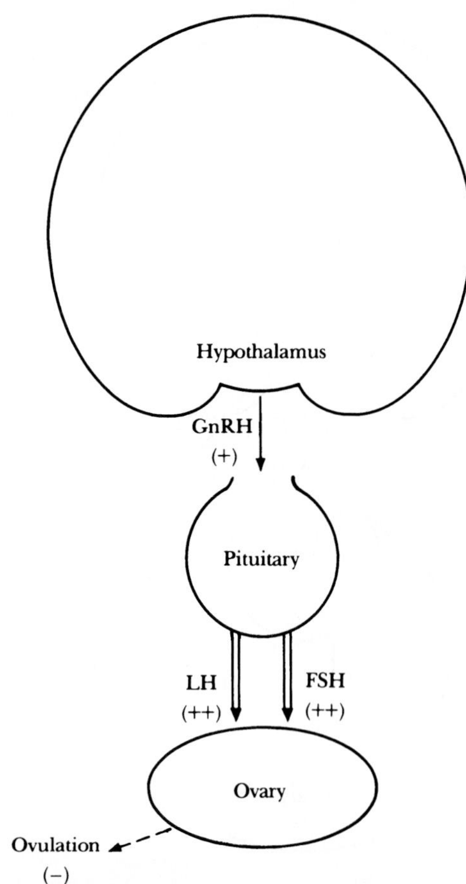

Figure 35-3 Ovarian failure. (FSH = follicle-stimulating hormone; GnRH = gonadotropin-releasing hormone; LH = luteinizing hormone.) (Data from Deneris, Huether and Robinson[4]; Marieb.[5])

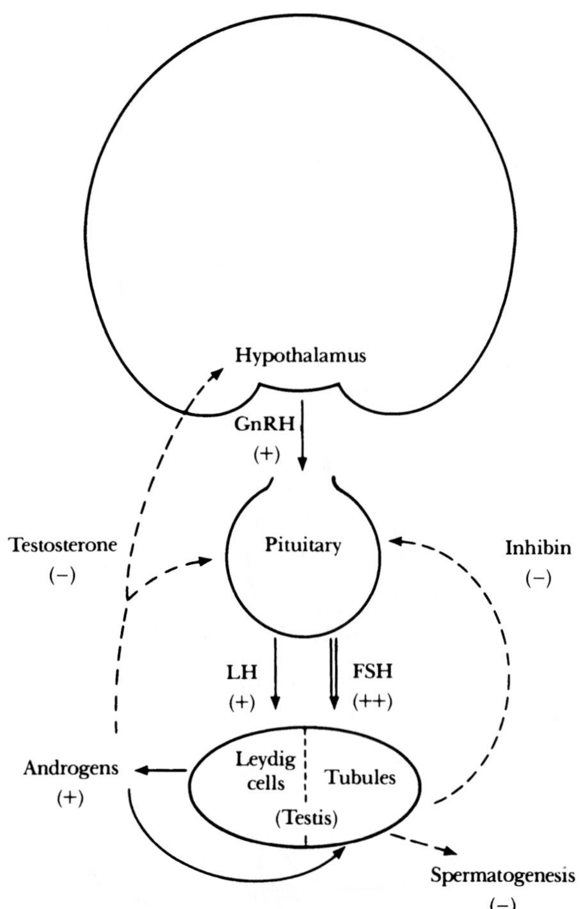

Figure 35-4 Germinal aplasia. (FSH = follicle-stimulating hormone; GnRH = gonadotropin-releasing hormone; LH = luteinizing hormone.) (Data from Deneris, Huether and Robinson[4]; Marieb.[5])

Clinical Manifestations: Effect of Cancer Therapy on Gonadal Function

Surgery

Some surgical procedures for cancer of the gastrointestinal and genitourinary tracts cause sexual dysfunction through the removal of sexual organs, damage to nerves that enervate sexual organs, or alteration of normal function. In addition, surgery for cancers of the head and neck and the breast, and amputation alter body image and may affect sexual identity. Organ dysfunction, either through loss of or alteration in normal function, is most common in cancers of the colon, rectum, bladder and associated urinary structures, and male and female genital tracts. Even when organs are not removed, normal function may be disrupted through removal of tumor tissue surrounding an organ, lymph node dissection, or associated physiological and psychological abnormalities related to the type of surgery required.

Cancer of the colon and rectum

Surgery for cancer of the colon and rectum may cause sexual dysfunction in both men and women. In general, sexual dysfunctions in women are more commonly related to psychosocial issues, whereas dysfunctions in men may be both physical and psychosocial. The most common surgery for colon cancer is some degree of colectomy, with or without a colostomy. While previously cancer of the rectum and anus often required an anterior or an abdominoperineal resection (APR), sphincter-preserving surgery without need for an ostomy is now the most common surgical procedure for rectal cancer.[6,7] Although this technique saves the sphincter, the surgery is associated with increased bowel frequency, a sense of urgency, fecal leakage, rectovaginal fistula and bladder, and erectile dysfunction in many patients.[8,9]

For those patients in whom an APR is necessary, sexual dysfunction may be related to the placement of the colostomy, removal of or interference with sexual organ function, or some combination of the two. A colostomy can be associated with sexual dysfunction because of negative changes in the patient's body image and self-esteem as well as the responses of family and friends. In an extensive review of quality of life literature focusing on patients with and without a stoma, the majority of patients with a stoma had some type of sexual dysfunction. The most common complaints were erectile dysfunction and ejaculatory erectile dysfunction in men and dyspareunia and orgasmic dysfunction in women. As a group, individuals with a stoma were less sexually active and experienced more generalized distress than those without a stoma. Of additional importance was the finding that all patients with colorectal cancer experienced some degree of sexual dysfunction and decreased quality of life, regardless of the type of therapy.[7,8]

For the woman with an APR, the ovaries or uterus may be removed at the time of surgery in addition to the colostomy being performed, causing dysfunction from primary inability to bear children or from alterations in normal hormonal patterns. In addition, women may have part of the vagina removed, or healing of the perineal wound may result in vaginal scarring that causes painful or incomplete vaginal intercourse. A decreased incidence of orgasm and vaginal lubrication, reduced libido, and dyspareunia has also been noted, but these outcomes are much less common.[7,10,11]

For the man who has an APR, sexual dysfunction is more severe, with 30%–60% of men experiencing decreased desire, 30%–75% having erectile dysfunction, and 65%–85% experiencing ejaculatory dysfunction.[11] Age appears to be a factor, with the older patient being more likely to suffer complete or incomplete erectile dysfunction.[12] This effect is most likely due to damage to the parasympathetic and sympathetic nerves that control both erection and ejaculation. In addition to erectile dysfunction, decreased amount and force of ejaculation or retrograde ejaculation may occur. This result, which may be temporary or permanent, adds to the trauma of surgery for the patient because the outcome is unpredictable. Sexual dysfunction defined by cessation of sexual relationship, absence of erection, absence of ejaculation, or inability to penetrate occurs in 15% of men who have a high anterior resection, whereas 54% of men with an APR experience some type of dysfunction.[13] For all patients, damage to nerves enervating the pelvic plexus appears to be the most common denominator in organic sexual dysfunction. If a complete nerve-sparing procedure is undertaken successfully, erectile and ejaculatory functions are maintained and the majority of men are able to have sexual intercourse and achieve orgasm.[10,14] Recently, the use of sildenafil (Viagra) has been shown to be effective in reversing or improving erectile dysfunction in 79% of patients who underwent rectal excision for either cancer or inflammatory bowel disease.[15]

Cancers of the genitourinary tract

Bladder cancer. The treatment of bladder cancer may alter sexual function in both men and women. Repeated cystoscopy for local treatment of transitional cell cancer has been noted to cause pain with coitus for women, transient pain during erection and ejaculation in men, and temporary decrease in desire for both. Transurethral resection or partial cystectomy may result in mild pain or dyspareunia; however, normal sexual function should not be altered. For some patients, urinary incontinence may cause cessation of normal activities for fear of having an accident. In addition, body image and self-esteem may be altered due to the need to use incontinence pads or other protective materials.

Radical cystectomy results in sexual dysfunction for both men and women because of organ removal and damage to nerves. Erectile dysfunction has been noted to occur in more than 90% of men undergoing radical cystectomy.[16] Orgasm may be experienced but is usually less intense and without ejaculate.[11] Sexual interest and penile sensation are not altered.[17] For the woman who undergoes a radical cystectomy, the surgery usually includes removal of the bladder and urethra, uterus, ovaries, fallopian tubes, and anterior portion of the vagina. Although vaginal reconstruction typically is performed, the resulting vagina may be more narrow and shallow and provide less lubrication than before surgery, leading to difficulty with penetration. In addition, the removal of the ovaries, with associated estrogen loss, leads to dryness, inelasticity of the vagina, dyspareunia, and menopausal symptoms. Vaginal dilation and the liberal use of lubrication may provide relief.[2,11,12]

For both sexes, urinary diversion is a necessity with radical cystectomy; this may result in alterations in self-esteem and body image and lead to a decrease or cessation of all sexual activities, with women reporting decreased desire and feelings of decreased attractiveness.[16,18,19] In the past, the ileal conduit, which necessitated the continuous use of an ostomy appliance, was the most common method for urinary diversion. Today, the surgical development of a Koch pouch, or continent reservoir, has become more widely employed, resulting in overall improved sexual adjustment due to decreased odor and leakage.[16,19] Most recently, the construction of a neobladder, made from the ileum and the large intestine, has allowed patients to maintain bladder function and normal voiding patterns.[18,20] While most commonly used in men, women also may benefit from this technique; however, women have a 70% chance of being hypercontinent, requiring self-catheterization.[21] In studies comparing the neobladder to the ileal conduit, improved quality of life and decreased alterations in sexual functioning were noted in both men and women who had bladder substitution.[18,19]

Penile cancer/cancer of the male urethra. Cancer of the penis and male urethra are rare. Primary treatment is total or partial penectomy. The degree of limitation primarily relates to the amount of tissue removed.[17] Partial penectomy does not result in loss of erectile, ejaculative, or orgasmic abilities, whereas erectile ability obviously is absent with total penectomy.[11,22] Desire remains, and stimulation of the remaining genital tissue can produce orgasm.[15,23] Ejaculation, through the perineal urethrostomy, should continue. New techniques to create a penis have been used after a total penectomy. A semirigid or inflatable prosthesis restores the ability to have intercourse and has been reported to increase erectile ability, libido, and frequency of intercourse.[23,24] Successful placement rates of 83% for malleable and mechanical prostheses and 67% for inflatable prostheses have been reported, with an overall mechanical failure rate of 7%.[25] Those patients treated with radiation therapy had significantly fewer concerns related to sexual dysfunction than those undergoing partial or total penectomy, who noted decreased interest, enjoyment, frequency, and ability.[26]

Testicular cancer. The treatment of testicular cancer includes an orchiectomy and typically retroperitoneal lymph node dissection and removal of a pelvic mass, usually followed by chemotherapy or radiation therapy. Unilateral orchiectomy will not result in infertility or sexual dysfunction, providing that the contralateral testis is normal and the individual is fertile at diagnosis. Infertility before any definitive therapy begins is well documented and may be related to hormonal imbalance or result from subacute chronic illness.[27–29] If bilateral orchiectomy is performed, sterility and decreased libido, related to loss of testosterone, will result. Retroperitoneal lymph node dissection (RPLND) done for staging or as treatment may result in temporary or permanent loss of ejaculation, whereas potency and the ability to have an orgasm remain.[29–31] Whenever possible, nerve-sparing RPLND should be done, as this procedure is associated with preservation of ejaculatory function and fertility.[16,29,32] In some individuals, retrograde ejaculation has been noted. Additionally, decreased libido and arousal, decreased pleasure and intensity of orgasm, and erectile dysfunction have been described.[16,33] Between 10% and 25% of those patients undergoing retroperitoneal surgery experience complete absence of ejaculation.[33] For most patients, discussions about sexuality before, during, and following treatment are crucial.[34] Prior to therapy, an important aspect of discussion should involve providing information about sperm banking.

Prostate cancer. Therapy for prostate cancer consists of various combinations of surgery, chemotherapy, radiation therapy, and hormonal manipulation, all of which have a potential to alter sexual function. Surgical treatment of prostate cancer includes prostatectomy or bilateral orchiectomy. Transurethral resection of the prostate generally does not cause erectile dysfunction; however, retrograde ejaculation occurs in approximately 90% of all patients. Transabdominal resection of the prostate results in retrograde ejaculation in 75%–80% of patients and may cause erectile dysfunction.[16,35]

The perineal approach, or radical prostatectomy, may result in permanent damage to erectile function with concomitant loss of emission and ejaculation.[15,16,35] Alterations in desire, penile sensation, and the ability to reach orgasm should not occur.[32] Radical prostatectomy is associated with a statistically significant decrease in sexual function, including the ability to achieve and frequency of erections, when patients are compared to those treated solely with radiation therapy.[36]

Nerve-sparing or potency-sparing surgery was developed by Walsh in the 1980s and, according to Church,[37] probably has been the most significant surgical development in the treatment of prostate cancer. Prior to the development of this procedure, 2%–15% of patients experienced urinary incontinence, and 80%–90% experienced erectile dysfunction. With current techniques, 60%–70% of men will maintain potency,[38] although the exact percentage varies among individual reports and by whether the patient had a non–nerve-sparing, unilateral nerve-sparing, or bilateral nerve-sparing procedure.[39,40] Because radical prostatectomy still results in a significant level of erectile dysfunction, a number of new procedures are being tested to maintain potency. Among them are intraoperative cavernous nerve stimulation and nerve grafting. The CaverMap surgical probe allows identification of the cavernous nerves, whose preservation relates to maintenance of potency. Results of studies to date have been conflicting, but some evidence indicates that potency can be maintained in as many as 70% of patients for at least one year following radical prostatectomy.[35] Additionally, cavernous nerve reconstruction has been undertaken to preserve spontaneous erectile function, with potency and the ability to have intercourse being maintained in 33%–43% of patients.[40,41]

Bilateral orchiectomy causes sexual dysfunction through gradual diminution of libido, erectile dysfunction, gynecomastia, penile atrophy, and body image changes.[17,35] Testicular implants filled with saline may be of benefit in managing body image changes. Various methods, including the use of penile prostheses, suction or vacuum devices, intracorporeal injections of papaverine hydrochloride or prostaglandin E_1, and medications such as yohimbine hydrochloride, have been used to restore erectile potential. Indeed, those who used erectile aids after surgery had the best sexual outcomes when compared to those who did or did not have nerve-sparing surgery and did not use them.[42] Sildenafil citrate (Viagra) has been tried to manage erectile dysfunction in men who have had radical prostatectomy, with 80% of patients who had undergone a bilateral nerve-sparing procedure being able to achieve erection and maintain vaginal intercourse for a mean of 6.92 minutes. All reported spousal satisfaction. None of the patients with unilateral or non–nerve-sparing procedures was able to attain an erection.[43] Most recently, two additional PDE5 (phosphodiesterase type 5) inhibitors, vardenafil (Levitra) and tadalafil (Cialis), have received FDA approval. Vardenafil half-life is similar to sildenafil half-life (4–6.5 hours); tadalafil has a half-life of 16–18 hours, allowing for longer potential for erection and intercourse.[44]

Fear of failure may also play a role in erectile dysfunction. Because return of full erection potential may take as long as 2 years, it is suggested that the patient wait a minimum of 6 months after surgery to see whether function will return.[35]

With new techniques, sterility in individuals with retrograde ejaculation is not as frequent. Because of the ability to separate sperm from urine, artificial insemination of the mate may be possible.[32]

Gynecologic malignancies

Surgical management of gynecologic malignancies includes surgery of the vulva, vagina, uterus and uterine cervix, ovary, and fallopian tube, and pelvic exenteration. Although the majority of gynecologic surgeries are invisible assaults to femininity, sexual identity and sexual functioning are often permanently affected. It is imperative that sexual and reproductive counseling be provided to the patient and family before surgical intervention, because most surgeries permanently alter fertility and may alter sexuality. Studies have shown that women treated for gynecologic malignancy are likely to experience alterations in sexuality and sexual functioning, including decreased desire, dyspareunia, recurrent vaginal infections, vaginal atrophy and dryness, decreased sense of feeling feminine, cessation of all sexual activities, and difficulties related to menopausal symptoms and infertility.[45–49]

Vulvar cancer. Treatment for vulvar cancer will not alter fertility but may affect sexuality, with 21%–90% of women reporting cessation of all sexual activities following radical vulvectomy.[45] In general, good cosmetic results occur with treatment of early disease except for the simple vulvectomy, which removes the labia and subcutaneous tissue, with retention of the clitoris. Introital stenosis may result but may be easily managed through the use of lubrication and vaginal dilators. Whenever possible, conservative therapy should be employed to minimize cosmetic alterations, maintain body image, and minimize sexual dysfunction.

Radical vulvectomy frequently results in delayed wound healing, altered body image, abnormalities in sensory perception of the genital area, leg edema, decreased range of motion in lower extremities, altered orgasmic potential, and introital stenosis.[47,49,50] Evaluation of lymph nodes prior to radical surgery may allow for more limited surgeries with less compromise to sexuality.[51] In those women who undergo radical pelvic surgery, generalized sexual dysfunction, including pain, anxiety, and decreased desire, is common, occurs earlier, and persists unless appropriately treated. In general, if cure is a possibility, women have been willing to live with sexual dysfunction and body image changes, provided adequate information and discussion about causes of dysfunction and alternative methods of sexual satisfaction are given.[52] All women need education on the effects of removal of tissue and on body image prior to surgery to promote self-esteem, function, and compliance with care.

Vaginal cancer. Vaginal cancer is rare. Surgery for the majority of gynecological cancers results in some abnormality and need for reconstruction of the vagina. Potential sexual side effects include alterations in body image and loss of femininity and body image.[49] A shortened vagina can cause considerable sexual dysfunction because of decreased vaginal length and width, lack of lubrication, and pain on intercourse. Total vaginectomy without reconstruction precludes vaginal intercourse; however, multiple techniques for vaginal reconstruction exist. Reconstruction can be accomplished using the large or small bowel, the umbilicus, gracilis or rectus musculocutaneous flaps, or a pedicle graft from the greater omentum.[53–55] In 30%–70% of patients who do have reconstruction, there is a return of orgasmic sensations if they existed before surgery. Despite this finding, reconstruction should not be considered a panacea for sexual dysfunction, as some women complain that the new vagina is too large, is too small, or has a persistent, annoying discharge.[55,56]

Cervical cancer and endometrial cancer. Surgical treatment for cervical intraepithelial neoplasia and carcinoma in situ includes conization, laser therapy, cryosurgery, loop electrosurgical excision (LEEP), or simple hysterectomy.[52,57] All but the last usually have no effect on fertility (conization may result in cervical stenosis or incompetence), nor should they cause any physiological sexual dysfunction. Simple hysterectomy precludes further childbearing but should not affect sexual functioning. Early-stage disease may be treated with radical trachelectomy and pelvic lymphadenectomy to preserve fertility.[57] Treatment for invasive disease is usually radical hysterectomy, with or without bilateral salpingo-oophorectomy. If oophorectomy is included, menopausal symptoms, with hot flashes and decreases in vaginal lubrication and elasticity, may severely alter sexual functioning.[49,51,56] Approximately 50% of patients treated for early-stage cervical cancer have a marked decrease in their sexual relationships and experience extreme fatigue, lack of energy, depressed mood, weight gain, and anxiety.[58,59]

In women with endometrial cancer, effects of treatment and uncertainty about the future increase sexual difficulties.[60] However, in a review of studies, consensus has shown that the majority of women experience no lasting sexual side effects, although grieving for lost fertility and inability to bear children is of concern.[61] Of those satisfied with their current sexual functioning, the majority noted that return to normalcy occurred gradually over a prolonged period.

Although sexual feeling should not be altered after a radical hysterectomy, delayed bowel and bladder function may occur and necessitate discharge from the hospital with a urinary catheter. Long-term catheter placement may alter body image and affect sexuality. Intercourse can be accomplished by securing the catheter to the abdomen and making changes in coital position.[51,60] It also should be remembered that many women measure femininity by the ability to bear children. If this ability is removed, sexual dysfunctions may occur even in the absence of organic cause.

Ovarian cancer. Initial treatment for ovarian cancer is surgery, usually consisting of a radical hysterectomy with bilateral salpingo-oophorectomy and omentectomy. Fertility is lost and the associated menopausal symptoms occur. Additionally, alterations in body image, decreased sense of desirability, and vaginal dryness may occur, resulting in decreased sexual interest.[62] In the young woman with ovarian teratoma or borderline malignant epithelial neoplasia, it is possible to maintain fertility if disease is confined to one ovary and is of low grade. Adequate staging is essential, and the patient must be willing to comply with all follow-up recommendations.[62–65] Treatment usually continues with combination chemotherapy, further compounding sexual and reproductive dysfunctions, including alterations in libido, frequency of intercourse, and desire for close physical contact.[45,62,65]

Pelvic exenteration

Although pelvic exenteration may be performed in the man or woman with advanced colorectal or bladder cancer, the most common indication for this procedure is a locally advanced gynecologic malignancy. An anterior pelvic exenteration preserves the rectum, whereas a posterior exenteration preserves the bladder. A total pelvic exenteration involves removing the vagina, uterus, ovaries, fallopian tubes, bladder, and rectum; in the man, the prostate, seminal vesicles, and vas deferens are removed.[52,57] In patients with total pelvic exenteration, a urinary conduit and colostomy are created and a neovagina may be constructed.[52,55] In the woman, reproductive and sexual dysfunctions are profound. Dysfunction related to removal of all pelvic organs with resulting ostomies is obvious. An Indiana pouch, a continent urinary pouch made from a piece of bowel and placed behind the umbilicus, requires catheterization, but may decrease some body image alterations.[66] In addition, body image, sexual identity, and self-esteem are disturbed, and appropriate interventions and education need to be provided. In the woman with vaginal reconstruction, intercourse may be possible; however, the physiological and psychological ramifications of this surgery may result in inability and lack of desire to participate in sexual activities.[56,64,65]

Breast cancer

Although some surgeries may not be strictly related to sexual functioning, they may cause dysfunction as a result of the psychological issues related to the particular body part. The most likely assault to body image and sexual identity with resultant sexual dysfunction is surgical removal of all or part of the breast. Although fertility is not altered by mastectomy or lumpectomy, the inability or difficulty in breast-feeding should pregnancy be accomplished may be a major assault to the woman's femininity. In addition, removal or partial removal of a breast may result in sexual dysfunction because of fear of rejection, physical discomfort, anxiety about initiating sexual activities, feelings of being defective or different, or any combination of these factors.[45,67] In particular, Lewis and colleagues noted that single women with children were more likely to be burdened by a breast cancer diagnosis than their married counterparts.[68]

Although it had been previously reported that the use of breast-preserving surgery (lumpectomy) caused significantly less alteration in body image, sexual desire, and frequency of intercourse, studies have shown no difference between women receiving lumpectomy and radiation therapy and women undergoing mastectomy.[67,69,70] Having the ability to choose the type of therapy also does not appear to play a role in overall sexual adjustment.[69] In general, breast reconstruction does not appear to influence overall sexual adjustment following mastectomy.[70] Neill, Armstrong, and Burnett reported decreased consequences of breast cancer in 11 women who did undergo reconstruction.[71] Yurek, Farrar, and Andersen noted that women with modified radical mastectomy and breast reconstruction had significantly more sexual dysfunction, including fewer sexual encounters and responsiveness than women receiving breast-conserving surgery or a modified radical mastectomy without reconstruction.[72] The research of Al-Ghazal and Blamey did not support this finding, however.[73] Whenever possible, surgical options, including breast reconstruction, should be made available to the woman with breast cancer.

Head and neck cancer

Although not generally considered an area responsible for sexual dysfunction, surgical treatment for cancers of the head and neck region is responsible for varying degrees of alteration in body image, leading to changes in sexuality and intimacy. Results of disease and treatment are readily apparent. Even with reconstructive surgery or the use of prostheses to ameliorate deformities, sexuality may be affected by the alterations in sensation, breathing, and voice; by the ability to use the mouth and tongue; or similar abnormalities. Difficulty with arousal and orgasm and cessation of sexual activities also have been reported.[60,74,75] Presurgical counseling and long-term follow-up may be necessary for sexual rehabilitation.[3,60]

Radiation Therapy

Radiation therapy can cause sexual and reproductive dysfunction through primary organ failure (e.g., ovarian failure and testicular aplasia), alterations in organ function (e.g., decreased lubrication and erectile dysfunction), and the temporary or permanent effects of therapy not associated with reproduction (e.g., diarrhea and fatigue). Permanent effects most commonly are related to total dose, location, length of treatment, age, and prior fertility status.[76,77] In women, fertility depends on follicular maturation and ovum release. Radiation therapy to the ovaries has its most direct effect on the intermediate follicles. If these follicles are damaged by radiation and insufficient small follicles remain, permanent sterility results. In men, although the Leydig cell and mature sperm are relatively radioresistant, immature sperm and spermatogonia are extremely radiosensitive. Small doses of radiation will begin the process of infertility, which, depending on total dose, may be permanent.[78]

In women, temporary or permanent sterility is related to the dose of radiation, the volume of tissues radiated, the time period during which the ovaries are exposed to radiation, and age.[76,78] Because a woman has fewer oocytes as she nears menopause, radiation injury at that point in the life span is more likely to be permanent. A radiation dose of 600–1200 cGy is capable of inducing menopause. Younger women appear to be more resistant to this effect and may not experience permanent sterility until a dose of greater than 2000 cGy. In women older than 40, a dose of 600 cGy often is associated with subsequent menopause and the associated menopausal symptoms of hot flashes, amenorrhea, dyspareunia, loss of libido, and vaginal atrophy.[76,79] For some women, the use of exogenous estrogens may alleviate these side effects.

Movement of the ovaries out of the radiation field (oophoropexy), with appropriate shielding, has helped maintain fertility even when relatively high doses of radiation have been given. Ovaries can be moved to the midline of the uterus or to the iliac crests. In young women or those desiring to maintain both reproductive capacity and hormonal function, ovarian transposition, with the ovaries moved to the upper abdomen, can be undertaken.[76] Successful pregnancies, without evidence of fetal congenital anomalies, have been reported following oophoropexy.[76,79–81]

In addition to sterility or transient infertility, radiation therapy can produce other sexual dysfunctions, which may be temporary or permanent. Decreases in sexual enjoyment, ability to attain orgasm, libido, and frequency of intercourse and sexual dreams, as well as vaginal stenosis or shortening, vaginal irritation, increased risk of infection, and decreased lubrication and sensation have been reported in women treated with radiation therapy. Painful intercourse and menstrual changes have also been reported.[3,82–84] Recently, a small, handheld device called Eros Therapy has been tested with woman experiencing severe sexual dysfunction following radiotherapy for Stage I and II cervical cancer. The Eros Therapy device increases blood flow to the clitoris and surrounding tissues. After three months of use, all participants noted a significant improvement in sexual desire, arousal, lubrication, and satisfaction as well as a decrease in dyspareunia.[85]

In men, temporary or permanent azoospermia is a function of age, dose, tissue volume, and exposure time. When the testis is exposed to radiation, a reduction in sperm count begins within 6–8 weeks and continues for up to 1 year after completion of therapy. Doses less than 500 cGy usually are associated with temporary sterility, whereas doses greater than 500 cGy typically result in permanent sterility.[78,79] The return of normal spermatogenesis is related to total testicular dose, with a dose of less than 100 cGy taking 9–12 months for recovery, whereas recovery from 200–300 cGy may take 2–3 years and 400–600 cGy 5 years or more.[86]

Below-diaphragm irradiation for Hodgkin's disease has been associated with long-term elevation of FSH, with the majority of patients remaining azoospermic more than a decade following treatment.[87] In a follow-up of 60 long-term survivors of childhood acute lymphoblastic leukemia, Sklar and colleagues found that 50% of men exposed to craniospinal and extended abdominal field radiation experienced decreased testicular volume, abnormal germ cell function, and elevated FSH levels.[88] Generally, shielding the testicle results in a mean dose of less than 44 cGy to the testicle. Thus, for those patients not requiring primary testicular irradiation, adequate testicular shielding may alleviate the sequelae of infertility.[89]

The majority of men treated by external beam for prostate cancer experience temporary or permanent erectile dysfunction. Erectile dysfunction is believed to be caused by fibrosis of pelvic vasculature or radiation damage of pelvic nerves. In addition to erectile dysfunction, patients experience decreased frequency of ejaculation and libido. Those who receive irradiation to the whole pelvis are likely to experience more severe side effects.[90] Interstitial therapy appears to decrease the incidence of erectile dysfunction even in those individuals who have undergone prior prostate surgery, provided the patient received a bilateral nerve-sparing procedure.[91] A more recent review, however, suggests that erectile dysfunction ranges between 6% and 90%.[92] Increased doses to the proximal penis appear to be associated with a higher incidence of erectile dysfunction.[93] Newer radiation delivery methods, such as three-dimensional conformal radiation therapy, and use of smaller radiation therapy ports have decreased the incidence of erectile dysfunction in patients with prostate cancer, although the addition of hormone therapy may negate this decrease.[94–97] In addition to difficulty in gaining or maintaining an erection, a decreased libido, inability to ejaculate, inability to lubricate, inability to achieve orgasm or reduced intensity of orgasm, and decreased sexual pleasure are common findings in men who receive radiation to the pelvis. The addition of phosphodiesterase 5 inhibitors, such as sildenafil, may help to preserve potency.[98,99]

Along with direct assaults to sexual and reproductive function, the general side effects and accompanying psychological effects of radiation therapy frequently can alter sexual function. Mild to severe fatigue is reported to occur in as many as 80% of those receiving radiation therapy.[100] Severe fatigue can limit all activity. Nausea, vomiting, and diarrhea can decrease energy, sexual desire, and feelings of desirability and can interfere with a sense of general well-being. Inflammation, pain, and limited range of motion may make sexual activities difficult or impossible. In addition to physical limitations, fear, depression, anxiety, stress, body image alterations, and lowered self-esteem may be burdens. The appropriate use of energy-conserving strategies, medications, lubricants, dilators, prostheses, time, and counseling may alleviate side effects, promote a sense of well-being, and improve sexual function.[76–78,98]

Chemotherapy

Chemotherapy-induced reproductive and sexual dysfunction is related to the type of drug, dose, length of treatment, age and sex of the individual receiving treatment, and length of time after therapy. In addition, the use of combination therapy, with multiple agents and drugs given to combat side effects of chemotherapy, plays a role in infertility or sexual dysfunction.

Infertility and sterility after chemotherapy have been noted since the early 1970s, with reports of amenorrhea and azoospermia after single-agent or combination therapy.[101] Adult men are more likely to experience long-term side effects regardless of age, whereas women are more apt to have permanent cessation of menses as they near age 40.[102,103] The principal drugs that induce infertility are the alkylating agents, but others have been implicated — in particular, cytosine arabinoside, 5-fluorouracil, vinblastine, vincristine, cisplatin, and procarbazine. Combinations of these drugs appear to prolong infertility[104–108] (Table 35-1).

Men

Infertility occurs in men primarily through depletion of the germinal epithelium that lines the seminiferous tubules. On testicular biopsy, the interstitial Leydig cells appear normal, whereas the tubules are abnormal, contain Sertoli cells, and have depleted or absent germinal epithelium. Clinically, testicular volume decreases, oligospermia or azoospermia occurs, and infertility results.[109] Leydig cell dysfunction, mani-

Table 35-1 Chemotherapeutic Agents Affecting Sexual or Reproductive Function

Agent	Complication
	Alkylating
Altretamine	Amenorrhea, oligospermia, azoospermia, decreased libido, ovarian dysfunction, erectile dysfunction, testicular atrophy, gynecomastia
Busulfan	
Chlorambucil	
Cisplatin	
Cyclophosphamide	
Ifosfamide	
Melphalan	
Nitrogen mustard	
Estramustane	
	Antimetabolites
Cytosine arabinoside	As for alkylating agents
5-Fluorouracil	
Methotrexate	
Fludarabine phosphate	
	Antitumor Antibiotics
Daunorubicin	As for alkylating agents
Doxorubicin	
Dactinomycin	
Plicamycin	
Epirubicin	
Idarubicin	
	Plant Products
Vincristine	Retrograde ejaculation, erectile dysfunction
Vinblastine	Decreased libido, ovarian dysfunction, erectile dysfuncton
	Miscellaneous Agents
Aminoglutethimide	Masculinization (women)
Androgens	Masculinization (women)
Antiandrogens	Decreased libido, erectile dysfunction, gynecomastia, breast tenderness, hot flashes
Antiestrogens	Gynecomastia, erectile dysfunction, menstrual irregularities, hot flashes
Corticosteroids	Irregular menses, acne
Estrogens	Gynecomastia, acne, decreased libido, erectile dysfunction
Goserelin acetate	Erectile dysfunction
Interferons	Transient erectile dysfunction, amenorrhea, pelvic pain
Leuprolide	Decreased libido, amenorrhea, gynecomastia, erectile dysfunction
Nonsteroidal aromatase inhibitors	Hot flashes, vaginal dryness
Procarbazine	As for alkylating agents
Progestins	Menstrual abnormalities, change in libido

Data from: Schilsky and Erlichman[102]; Wilkes, Ingwersen, Burke[104]; Otto[105]; Cleri, Haywood[106]; Gullatte[107]; Chu, DeVita.[108]

fested by a raised LH level and low or normal testosterone level, is usually seen.[110] Following drug-induced azoospermia, the process of spermatogenesis must start all over, as if the patient were going through puberty. Initially, the germ stem cell must repopulate the testicle, then spermatogenesis should occur. This process may take several years.[111]

Both single-agent and combination chemotherapy have been reported to cause germinal aplasia, with alkylating agents being the most extensively studied in terms of this effect. Cumulative doses of greater than 400 mg/m^2 of cisplatin have been associated with irreversible damage to gonadal function.[112] Stoter and colleagues evaluated 48 men with testicular cancer who had been treated with platinum, vinblastine, and bleomycin (PVB) plus maintenance chemotherapy.[113] With a minimum follow-up of 7 years, 40% of participants reported a negative alteration in sexual life, with 21% experiencing decreased sexual desire, 8% experiencing erectile dysfunction, and 15% experiencing ejaculatory dysfunction. In an additional 59 patients treated with the same chemotherapy, but only for two cycles, Bohlen and colleagues did not see an adverse effect in either future fertility or in sexual activity.[114] Fertility may improve with time, however, and some reports describe slow recovery of spermatogenesis, culminating with the ability to father children, in patients who had initially been rendered azoospermic or oligospermic following combination chemotherapy for testicular cancer.[115–117]

Hormonal manipulation and treatment with estrogens are well known as a cause of sexual dysfunction. The majority of patients who receive androgen-ablative therapy experience a major reduction in interest in sexual intercourse and are unable to attain or maintain an erection.[118] The incidence of hot flashes in men with prostate cancer treated with GnRH analogs, antiandrogens, or estrogens ranges from 10% to 45%. Hot flashes may be managed with drugs such as transdermal estradiol, diethylstilbesterol, oral progesterones, or venlafaxine.[119] In some instances, the addition of finasteride has been shown to maintain potency while maintaining the androgen-abalative effect.[108] Gynecomastia and decreases in libido, sexual excitement, and the ability to achieve sexual fulfillment are significant problems.[104,106,108]

Other potential side effects of chemotherapy include partial or total erectile dysfunction, ejaculatory difficulties, and decreased desire, arousal, and orgasmic ability. Sexual dysfunction may be related to chemotherapy-induced angiopathy, particularly with drug regimens that contain cisplatin, vinblastine, and bleomycin sulfate.[120] Semen cryopreservation prior to initial therapy should be considered for all men interested in fathering a child.[121]

Women

Women experience sexual and reproductive dysfunction from chemotherapy as a result of hormonal alterations or direct effects that cause ovarian fibrosis and follicle destruction. Previous sexual health may also play a role. Follicle-stimulating hormone and LH levels are elevated and the estradiol level is decreased, leading to amenorrhea, menopausal symptoms, dyspareunia, and vaginal atrophy and dryness.[104,109,122]

Like men, women experience reproductive dysfunction from both single-agent and combination chemotherapy. However, age appears to play a more significant role in infertility in women than in men, with women younger than 30 years able to tolerate much higher doses of chemotherapy without resultant permanent amenorrhea and premature menopause.[123,124] Amenorrhea has been noted in women with breast cancer who were treated with daily doses of cyclophosphamide and in women with Hodgkin's disease or breast cancer who were treated with combination chemotherapy, particularly when the regimen contained an alkylating agent.[104,123,125,126] In those patients experiencing temporary amenorrhea, menstruation returns in approximately 50% of those younger than 40 years of age within 15 months.[126] Permanent amenorrhea may be evident by cessation of therapy but often occurs gradually over time.[127] In younger women, permanent amenorrhea may appear in 6–16 months, in women closer to normal menopause, amenorrhea may occur in only 2–4 months. In an analysis of nine studies, Chapman and colleagues concluded that amenorrhea occurred more commonly in women older than 40 and that the ovarian failure rate was correlated most closely to that seen in women treated solely with cyclophosphamide.[123] Additionally, these researchers postulated that ovarian dysfunction occurs at all ages but is more frequently reported and diagnosed in women closer to menopause.

It appears that any combination of drugs containing an alkylating agent is apt to cause infertility, and as women near menopause, permanent cessation of menses becomes more likely. When hormonal manipulation includes androgens, not only sexual and reproductive function but also body image and feelings of sexual identity are affected. Chemotherapy contributes significantly to sexual dysfunction through menopausal symptoms as well as through increased risk of urinary tract infections and candidal infections, vaginal irritation, exacerbations of genital herpes and human papillomavirus, and alterations in desire and arousal due to decreases in circulating androgens. In addition, the use of hormonal therapies, such as tamoxifen, aminoglutethimide, and letrazole, has been associated with menopausal symptoms and decreased sexual desire.[104,122,127–129] Appropriate support and counseling should be provided to affected individuals. More research into the best methods to decrease menopausal side effects in the cancer patient needs to be undertaken. Additionally, long-term survivors have noted lack of sexual interest, difficulty reaching orgasm, and inability to relax and enjoy a sexual encounter.[130]

Children

The effect of chemotherapy on gonadal function in children has been extensively studied.[131,132] Primary effects include delayed sexual maturation and alterations in reproductive potential. While chemotherapy affects girls and boys differently, the primary effects appear to be age-related. Prepubescent boys seem to be minimally affected by chemotherapy and progress into and through puberty without major difficulty.[132] Young men treated during puberty appear to be more likely to have gonadal dysfunction, with profound effects on both germ cell production and Leydig cell function, resulting in increases in FSH and LH and a decrease in testosterone levels.[84,111] In a study of 77 men who had been treated for childhood cancer more than 13 years previously, 63% were found to be normozoospermic, while 20% had oligospermia and 17% had azoospermia.[133] Because the reserve supply of spermatogonia in young men is much smaller than in adults, however, chemotherapy has the potential to significantly alter spermatogenesis. This effect cannot be easily assessed until puberty.[111] The majority of girls treated with combination therapy appear to have normal ovarian function, although long-term follow-up is needed to assess whether these individuals will experience premature menopause.[111,132]

In reviews of female and male participants of the Childhood Cancer Survivor Study, no adverse pregnancy outcomes were found for either the women or the partners of men who had received chemotherapy when children.[134,135] Of importance, many children who receive therapy for childhood cancer experience decreased quality of life, including lower rates of marriage and parenthood and fears about their reproductive capacity.[136]

Other issues

Drugs used to manage chemotherapy side effects can alter sexual function. Erectile dysfunction, decreased sexual desire, decreased sense of sexual fulfillment, and decreased ability to achieve orgasm all have been associated with these agents (Table 35-2).[104,106,108,137]

Table 35-2 Cancer-Associated Drugs That Affect Sexual and Reproductive Function

Agent	Complication
	Antidepressants
Amitriptyline	Erectile dysfunction, altered libido
Bupropian hydrochloride	Irregular menses, anorgasmia
Clonazepam	Altered libido
Imipramine	Altered libido
Selective serotonin reuptake inhibitors (SSRIs)	Altered libido, painful erection
Venlafaxine hydrochloride	Altered libido
	Antiemetics/Sedatives/Tranquilizers
Prochlorperazine Chlorpromazine Diazepam Lorazepam Metochlopramide Scopolamine	Sedation, orgasm without ejaculation, erectile dysfunction, decreased sexual interest, decreased intensity of orgasm, gynecomastia
	Antihistamines
Diphenhydramine	Sedation, decreased sexual interest
	Steroids
(See Table 35-1)	
	Narcotics
Morphine Hydromorphone Codeine Fentanyl	Decreased libido, sedation, impaired potency
	Miscellaneous
Cimetadine	Erectile dysfunction
Dronabinol	Altered libido, sedation
Gabapentin	Amenorrhea, erectile dysfunction
Ketoconazole	Decreased libido, gynecomastia, oligospermia, erectile dysfunction

Data from: Wilkes, Ingwersen, Burke[104]; Otto[105]; Cleri, Haywood[106]; Gullatte[107]; Chu, DeVita[108]; Wilson.[137]

Biological Response Modifiers

Although frequently used in the adjuvant setting and for treatment of early-stage disease, biological response modifiers (BRMs) have not yet been studied sufficiently with regard to their sexual side effects. Rieger noted that most changes in sexuality are related to known BRM side effects, including fatigue, mucous membrane dryness, flulike symptoms, and body image changes.[138] Some information is available on the use of the interferons — in particular, alfa-interferon — alone or in combination with other agents. Decreased libido, amenorrhea, pelvic pain, uterine bleeding, and erectile dysfunction have been reported with alfa-interferon, and animals exposed to all interferons have demonstrated an increased rate of spontaneous abortion.[104–107,138] Likewise, the retinoids have been associated with spontaneous abortion and fetal malformation.[138] In addition to drug-induced dysfunction, the usual side effects of fatigue and flulike symptoms affect interest in and comfort with sexual activities. No studies have examined the effects of BRMs on human pregnancy and lactation; information often is extrapolated from animal data. Currently, use of these agents during pregnancy and while lactating is contraindicated. Future research on the subject of gonadal dysfunction related to BRMs is extremely important.

Targeted Therapies

Use of the novel anticancer therapies that inhibit cancer cell growth is increasing. These agents affect specific molecular targets that are responsible for the growth of tumors. Among these are epidermal growth factor tyrosine kinase inhibitors (i.e., gefitinib, imatinib), fusion proteins (e.g., denileukin diftitox), and antiangiogenic agents (i.e., bevacizumab, thalidomide). The sexual side effects related to these agents are unclear. The use of thalidomide requires two types of contraception and pregnancy tests prior to each cycle due to the potential for fetal malformations. Currently, all of these agents are contraindicated during pregnancy and breast-feeding.[139–142]

Stem Cell and Marrow Transplantation

As long-term survival from transplantation increases, issues related to sexuality and sexual dysfunction have become more evident. The late effects of bone marrow transplantation (BMT) include chronic fatigue, body image alterations, gonadal dysfunction, and infertility. Women experience decreased sexual desire and satisfaction, vaginal atrophy and decreased vaginal lubrication, premature menopause, failure to achieve orgasm, and painful intercourse, as well as feelings of loss of femininity.[143–145] Men frequently experience ejaculatory difficulties, while long-term consequences may include decreased desire, body image alterations, and erectile dysfunction most often related to arteriogenic insufficiency.[144,146,147] Other side effects may include gynaecomastia, Leydig cell insufficiency, and decreased libido.[148] The hospitalization often required in conjunction with transplantation can affect sexuality and intimacy due to lack of privacy and limited physical contact. The combination of high-dose chemother-

Table 35-3 Sexual and Reproductive Dysfunction: High-Risk Characteristics

Characteristic	Women	Men
Age	Older than age 30	Postpuberty
Surgery	Gynecologic surgeries Abdominal perineal resection Pelvic exenteration	Prostate, orchiectomy Abdominal perineal resection Pelvic exenteration
Radiation therapy	Pelvic	Pelvic
Medications	Antidepressants, antihistamines, antihypertensives, antiemetics, antiestrogens, narcotics, sedatives, tranquilizers, alcohol	Antidepressants, antihistamines, antihypertensives, antiemetics, estrogens, narcotics, sedatives, tranquilizers, alcohol
Psychosocial issues	Alterations in body image and self-esteem, decreased sense of femininity	Alterations in body image and self-esteem, decreased sense of masculinity

Data from Krebs.[158]

apy and total body irradiation (TBI) exacerbates sexually-related side effects.[143–146]

Primary gonadal dysfunction has been described in all transplant patients, whether or not the patients received TBI. Recovery of gonadal function is rare in both men and women (<10%) and is related to age as well as the use of TBI and combination versus single-agent chemotherapy.[143–145] Nevertheless, successful pregnancy has been reported following transplantation. Increasing age and the use of TBI seemed most integral to the inability to conceive or father a child.[149] Assisted reproduction techniques have been shown to benefit those individuals desiring a child following transplant.[150] Additionally, the use of testosterone and/or sildenafil has been shown to be of benefit in decreasing or preventing erectile dysfunction.[147]

Numerous authors have investigated quality of life in survivors of BMT.[151–154] Decreased energy and moderate to severe fatigue were experienced by more than 50% of BMT survivors as long as ten years after transplant.[151,152] Other major concerns included infertility, inability to perform sexually, and alterations in sexual intimacy, pleasure, and ability to achieve orgasm and an erection.[143–145,151,152] Other potential side effects include anxiety, depression, and current life stressors.[143] Sexual and reproductive implications of treatment should be discussed and counseling provided prior to, throughout, and following treatment.

Therapeutic Approaches and Nursing Care

Sexual Counseling

All patients should receive information about the possible side effects of disease and treatment on sexuality and reproduction. Potential side effects include alterations in physical function and libido, menopausal symptoms, problems with erection and ejaculation, and infertility. Patients deserve the opportunity to have their sexual problems thoughtfully identified, and good communication among all parties is essential. Potential side effects and possible methods for management should be discussed with the patient (and partner if available) at diagnosis, throughout treatment, and during follow-up visits.[155]

To effectively assess a patient for alterations in sexuality, the nurse must understand the patient's medical, psychiatric, and psychosexual status; evaluate present relationships; and provide recommendations and encouragement.[156] Nurses should include sexuality in their assessment of all patients and should provide hope, reassurance, and basic information.[157] While all patients should be assessed, it is important to recognize those who may be at high risk for sexual dysfunction. Characteristics include advancing age; surgery or radiation therapy to the pelvis; higher doses of chemotherapy; the use of medications for pain, hypertension, and nausea; and alterations in body image and self-esteem (see Table 35-3).[158] Potential methods for assessment of sexual dysfunction include the use of the ALARM model and the model proposed by Auchincloss (Table 35-4).[156,158]

Once sexual functioning has been assessed, interventions are necessary to maintain optimal sexual functioning and to promote adaptation to the sexual and reproductive side effects of disease and treatment. Interventions should include the patient's partner

Table 35-4 Evaluation of Sexual Dysfunction

ALARM Model	Auchincloss Model
A: Activity (sexual) L: Libido/desire A: Arousal and orgasm R: Resolution/release M: Medical data	Evaluate sexual status: Present sexual function Past experiences Relationships Evaluate medical, psychological, and cancer status

Data from: Andersen, Lamb[156]; Auchincloss.[157]

Table 35-5 PLISSIT Model for Intervention

P: Permission
LI: Limited information
SS: Specific suggestions
IT: Intensive therapy

Data from Annon.[159]

whenever possible. The PLISSIT model, another method of intervention (Table 35–5), can help the majority of patients without the need for intensive therapy.[159] To maintain integrity and to improve quality of life, it is essential that all patients receive counseling about sexual dysfunction, that open communication be encouraged, and that interventions be individualized and valued by the participants.

Nursing Assessment and Management

Although not every nurse can be a sexual counselor, listening to the concerns of the patient and family, presenting factual information in a nonthreatening manner, managing noncomplex disease- and treatment-related symptoms, and providing appropriate referrals can be easily incorporated into routine care. Many healthcare providers rarely discuss issues related to sexual and reproductive concerns for a variety of personal and professional reasons. Primary reasons cited include personal discomfort, lack of training or knowledge, and fears of embarrassing themselves or their patients. Additional reasons include lack of time, concerns about the appropriateness of such discussions when dealing with a life-threatening illness, and the belief that these subjects are not part of the nurse's job description.[3,160,161]

Although not always accurately portrayed, sexuality is more than the act of intercourse. It includes intimacy, touching, a multitude of activities to show affection, and a variety of methods to communicate with others. Cancer and treatment may disrupt or permanently alter one's ability to maintain previous sexual patterns or may cause infertility; at the same time, cancer cannot alter the fact that one is a sexual being. This information needs to be reiterated and reinforced to the patient and family.[3,160]

Assisting patients and families with sexual alterations is congruent with and integral to the nurse's role in providing holistic care. Many simple, easy-to-follow methods exist, but for nurses to provide assistance, they must first understand their own sexual identity, what constitutes acceptable sexual patterns and practices, as well as the sociocultural, environmental, and other beliefs that may influence how the nurse interacts with others as sexual beings. Being comfortable with one's own sexuality as well as having basic knowledge about sexual issues and concerns facilitates providing assistance.[3,83,160–166]

Asking about the patient's sexual practices early in the clinical assessment legitimizes and normalizes the subject and gives patients permission to discuss sexual issues. Current practices, cultural and religious beliefs, and general intimacy issues should be incorporated in the discussion. Whenever possible and appropriate, the patient's partner should be included. Medical jargon and value-oriented terminology should be avoided, and questions and responses should acknowledge the subject and related concerns as being normal and important.[3,160–166]

Nurses must provide factual information about disease, treatment, and potential side effects. Discussing potential alterations in sexual functioning, including fertility issues, prior to or early in treatment and continuing these discussions well into the follow-up phase is essential. Information is needed to dispel myths, decrease anxiety, minimize embarrassment, provide a basis for alternative strategies, and open lines of communication between the patient and others.[3,160,161,163,165–167]

Managing the side effects of cancer and treatment is also integral to the nurse's role. Offering simple suggestions and appropriately managing side effects may be sufficient for most patients to continue or reinstitute sexual activities and enhance intimacy. In addition to management of such traditional symptoms as pain, nausea, vomiting, and bone marrow depression, nurses should provide information and strategies about less commonly recognized symptoms that affect sexual function, such as peripheral neuropathies, malnutrition, stomatitis, fatigue, hand-foot syndrome, and incontinence.[104,155] They also should stress the importance of communication and openness; potential alterations in body image and self-esteem; the need for exercise, rest, and adequate nutrition; the use of contraception; setting the stage for sexual activities (candles, music, sexy clothing); experimentation with alternative methods of intimacy; and the liberal and adequate use of lubricants, foreplay, and more comfortable positions. Energy conservation techniques and information on the timing of medications and methods to maintain cleanliness and personal hygiene are important as well.[3,83,155,159–165]

Knowing when to make referrals and recognizing appropriate community resources are essential. Areas of referral include hormonal therapies, vacuum devices or medications to manage erectile dysfunction, sperm banking and other fertility-preserving options, and reconstructive surgery and prostheses. Some patients will require psychosexual counseling; others will not. Individualization of education and counseling is important for each patient. It is crucial that the nurse (or others) not invent sexual concerns for those who do not have them; rather, the nurse anticipates, recognizes, advocates, and assists those who do.

Finally, integrating the topic of alterations in sexual and reproductive function into practice requires many skills that most nurses do not obtain in basic nursing education. Participating in continuing education programs and in journal clubs focused on sexually related issues and the use of role models can provide the novice nurse with initial skills for sexual assessment. Additional skills can be gained through continual incorporation of sexuality assessment and counseling into daily nursing practice, role playing, attending advanced seminars, taking part in values clarification exercises, and participating in interdisciplinary rounds and educational offerings.[166]

Fertility Considerations and Procreative Alternatives

Fertility and pregnancy following cancer diagnosis are fraught with a multitude of concerns, particularly the ability to conceive, carry to term, and deliver a healthy newborn with no congenital abnormalities and no increased risk for future malignancies because of either parent's previous diagnosis and treatment for cancer. Radiation therapy and chemotherapy, alone or in combination, have the potential to induce infertility. Proved fertility is measured by pregnancy rates. Even when fertility is preserved, conception may be delayed. Information about procreative alternatives, the potential for infertility, and issues related to genetic inheritance, mutagenicity, and timing of pregnancy must be thoroughly discussed with potential parents prior to their attempting conception.[168,169]

Mutagenicity

Mutagenicity is the ability to cause an abnormality in the genetic content of cells, resulting in cell death, alteration(s) in growth and replication, or no noticeable alteration in cell function. Possible germ cell mutations may not be evident for generations of offspring.[170]

Numerous researchers have investigated the offspring of individuals exposed to chemotherapy or radiation therapy as children, adolescents, or young adults as a method to adequately assess mutagenicity following therapy.[111,171–174] While several specific instances of fetal wasting or congenital malformations, such as an increase in first pregnancy miscarriages[171] and congenital cardiac abnormalities,[172,173] were identified, no statistical difference in congenital malformations, stillbirths, or low birth weights was seen.[171–174] Additionally, chromosome analyses of offspring of parents treated for Hodgkin's disease were normal,[171–175] and no increased risk of genetic disease was identified in more than 4500 children of adult survivors of childhood cancer.[176] In all studies, it has been difficult to specifically implicate germ cell mutations as the cause of adverse outcomes of pregnancy. Follow-up over several generations of patients and their offspring will be needed before definitive answers are obtained.

Teratogenicity

Teratogenicity is the ability of a toxic compound to produce alterations in an exposed fetus. Both chemotherapy and radiation therapy are known to have teratogenic effects on the fetus, causing spontaneous abortion, fetal malformation, or fetal death, especially during the first trimester. Low-dose radiation has also been implicated in fetal malignancy.[177–179]

Radiation exposure during the first trimester represents the greatest risk to the fetus, with an exposure of 100 cGy or more resulting in fetal death, microcephaly, eye anomalies, and intrauterine growth retardation. In the second or third trimester, fetal death is unlikely, but growth retardation, sterility, and cataracts are common findings.[179]

Chemotherapy, particularly when received during the first trimester, has been related to congenital abnormalities, with approximately 10% of fetuses experiencing some type of anomaly. In general, the alkylating agents and antimetabolites have been most often associated with fetal malformations. Chemotherapy during the second or third trimester may cause premature birth or low birth weight, but congenital abnormalities are not increased over the incidence with normal pregnancy.[177,180–182] The timing of chemotherapy is critical. Therapy given prior to the fifth week of gestation is most likely to result in spontaneous abortion if severe damage to the blastocyst occurs. Between the fifth and twelfth weeks, structural damage is most common and congenital malformations tend to occur. After the twelfth week, fetal growth restriction is most common. Effects may be related to drug dose, length of exposure, frequency of administration, and type and number of drugs administered as well[181] (Table 35-6).

Reproductive Counseling

Discussions concerning fertility and reproduction issues need to be held prior to the onset of therapy and should continue well into post-treatment and follow-up. Current fertility status, desire for future childbearing, and contraception practices should be investigated during the initial assessment. Potential

Table 35-6 Teratogenetic Effects of Chemotherapy

Agent	Complication
	Alkylating
Altretamine	Spontaneous abortions
Busulfan	Skeletal malformations
Chlorambucil	
Cyclophosphamide	
Dacarbazine	
Ifosfamide	
Nitrogen mustard	
Nitrosoureas	
	Antimetabolites
Capecitabine	
Cytosine arabinoside	Spontaneous abortions
5-Fluorouracil	Skeletal malformations
Gemcitabine	
6-Mercaptopurine	
Methotrexate	
Trimetrexate	
	Miscellaneous Agents
Antitumor antibiotics	Spontaneous abortions
Arsenic trioxide	Skeletal malformations
Asparaginase	Skeletal malformations
Glucocorticoids	Spontaneous abortions
Hydroxyurea	Spontaneous abortions
Imatinib mesylate	Malformations
Irinotecan	Spontaneous abortions
Procarbazine	Atrial/septal defects
Retinoids	Spontaneous abortions, skeletal malformations
Thalidomide	Skeletal malformations
Vinblastine	Spontaneous abortions, malformations
Vinorelbine tartrate	Malformations

Data from: Wilkes, Ingwersen, Burke[104]; Otto[105]; Cleri, Haywood[106]; Chu, DeVita[108]; Rieger[138]; Green, Zevon, Lowrie, et al.[173]; Robinson, Krebs[177]; Barnicle.[180]

alterations should be openly discussed and referrals made as appropriate. Counseling for possible risks of mutagenicity, increased cancer risk, and unknown sequelae of treatment for progeny should be included.[169,183,184] Birth control methods need to be implemented to minimize the possibility of an unplanned pregnancy during therapy. In addition, methods to maintain fertility during therapy should be investigated.

For those patients receiving radiation therapy, appropriate shielding of the testes or ovaries or oophoropexy to position the ovaries outside the radiation field may be of benefit.[83,184,185] Birth control pills in women and GnRH analogs in men and women have been postulated to protect the germ cells from damage by chemotherapeutic agents. To date, no study has shown benefit in treating men with GnRH analogs, although some benefit has been found in animal studies.[186] The use of a GnRH analog before and during polychemotherapy was evaluated in 19 postmenarchal young women aged 14.7 to 20 years. Menstruation resumed from 45 to 120 days after the last dose of the analog, and ovulation resumed one to six cycles after resuming menstruation.[187]

Because it is often difficult to predict when an individual receiving chemotherapy is infertile, it is extremely important that methods to prevent pregnancy be discussed and appropriate contraceptive drugs or devices be provided. It has been suggested that following cancer therapy an individual should wait a minimum of two years before attempting conception. This suggestion is made both to prevent pregnancy during the time when recurrence is most likely and to allow for the recovery of spermatogenesis or ovarian function if it has been temporarily altered by therapy.[177,188] It should be noted, however, that this time frame may be too long for some women at risk for early menopause and that no benefit is known to be derived from a prolonged waiting time.[168,178]

Newer methods to preserve fertility remain under investigation. These measures include ovarian tissue transplantation,[189] which has been successful in a monkey and other animals; oocytes harvesting and cryopreservation;[155] the use of progestins in young women with endometrial cancer;[190] the use of goserelin as an ovarian protectant for women receiving adjuvant chemotherapy for breast cancer;[191] and ovarian and testicular tissue cryopreservation.[155]

Semen Cryopreservation and Sperm Recovery

Semen storage for use in artificial insemination has been available for many years, with the first pregnancy from frozen sperm reported in 1953.[192] Although initially used to establish pregnancy in infertile couples, sperm banking has more recently been used to preserve procreation abilities in men undergoing cancer therapy. Unfortunately, the option to bank sperm will not be available to every man undergoing cancer therapy. Many men will be subfertile or infertile at the time of diagnosis, particularly those with testis cancer or Hodgkin's disease.[193,194] Although techniques such as mapping and fine-needle aspiration of the testis to recover sperm after treatment[185] are being investigated, sperm banking is most effective when completed prior to initiation of therapy. Thus, anyone with rapidly progressing disease frequently cannot delay the start of therapy to complete the cryopreservation process. Even so, cryopreservation of sperm has provided a viable option for improving fertility prospects in men with various forms of cancer,[124,192,193,195,196] and any semen sample that contains even one motile or viable sperm can be preserved.[185,192]

Cryopreserved samples can be used in a variety of ways. The initial technique is usually intrauterine insemination (IUI), in which the thawed and washed semen samples are introduced into the partner's uterus around the time of ovulation. More technical procedures, such as in vitro fertilization (IVF) or intracytoplasmic sperm injection (ICSI), in which a single sperm is injected into a single egg, will be tried if this procedure is unsuccessful or if the number of cryopreserved semen samples is inadequate or the samples do not contain sufficient numbers of viable sperm.[197,198] In a study of 28 young men who had cryopreserved semen prior to chemotherapy, Agarwal and colleagues noted that a total of 87 assisted reproduction technique cycles (using IUI, IVF, or ICSI) were performed. In 18% of the cycles, pregnancy resulted, with 75% of the pregnancies resulting in a live birth.[199] Additionally, sperm may be obtained through testicular sperm extraction (TESE) and testicular sperm aspiration (TESA).[200]

Even if artificial insemination is never completed, the knowledge that semen has been banked and is available when needed can provide a significant psychological boost for the man undergoing cancer therapy.[195,200] All aspects of the sperm-banking process, from the initial visit through the completion of insemination, should be fully discussed with the patient so that informed decisions can be made.

For those men who have maintained some degree of fertility but experience retrograde ejaculation, a trial of a sympathomimetic agent may prove beneficial. If this procedure is not helpful, sperm can be harvested from urine, washed, and used for insemination. For true ejaculation, a rectal probe that electrically stimulates the vas deferens, seminal vesicle, and prostate to initiate the ejaculatory reflex may be of benefit. In addition, some men will benefit from sperm aspiration from the vas deferens or epididymis, followed by ICSI.[185,192] Finally, scientists are investigating the potential for restoration of spermatogenesis through transplantation of the male germ cell.[185,192]

In Vitro Fertilization/Embryo Transfer

In vitro fertilization, used for male infertility due to low sperm counts or for female infertility due to severe endometriosis, immunological infertility, or absent or damaged fallopian tubes, has experienced remarkable technological advances, with more than 30,000 fertilization cycles now being undertaken each year.[201] This technique requires ovarian stimulation followed by ova retrieval via ultrasound-guided needle aspiration of the preovulatory follicles. Laparoscopy also may be used. The retrieved oocytes are then incubated with sperm for 5–26 hours. Following incubation, the embryos are transferred to the uterus and released. The rate of successful pregnancy with IVF is approximately 20%. The process for ICSI is the same except that a single sperm is injected directly into the oocytes.[197] The use of ICSI has increased the rate of successful fertilization, thereby increasing the potential for a successful pregnancy.[185,192,194,196] Human embryo cryopreservation has been used for more than 15 years and is now considered to be a routine procedure. The process of retrieval is the same as with IVF and ICSI. For those who used both fresh and cryopreserved embryos, the rate of successful pregnancy increases by 8%.[202]

Researchers are investigating new techniques to cryopreserve oocytes that could later be autotransplanted into the infertile woman or isolated and allowed to mature in vitro. Concerns about the best method for implantation and the potential for reintroduction of malignant cells have affected the use of these approaches although the thawed oocytes appear to be viable and the procedure promising. Currently, it appears that in vitro maturation followed by ICSI and IVF will be most beneficial for patients desiring to have a child.[203–205]

Pregnancy and Cancer

Although pregnancy complicated by a diagnosis of cancer is a rare event, it creates multiple problems for all concerned. Uncertainty about the prognosis of mother and fetus, the rigors of treatment, and the long-term sequelae of cancer for patient, infant, and family compound events that normally are surrounded by a myriad of conflicting emotions. Only with comprehensive care by many healthcare and ancillary individuals can a positive outcome for mother, fetus, and family be anticipated.

Cancer is the second-leading cause of death during the reproductive years. It is estimated that cancer complicates about 1 in 1000 pregnancies and that approximately 1 in 118 women with cancer has a concomitant pregnancy. The most commonly associated cancers are lymphoma, leukemia, malignant melanoma, and cancers of the breast, cervix, ovary, and colorectum — the cancers with the highest incidence during the reproductive years.[206–208]

In general, most cancers do not adversely affect a pregnancy, nor does pregnancy adversely affect the cancer outcome, although the treatment necessary to manage the cancer may potentially have an adverse effect on the pregnancy. Therapeutic abortion has not been shown to be of benefit in altering disease progression and should not be considered unless continued pregnancy will compromise treatment and thus prognosis. The wishes of the patient and family must be considered, with therapeutic options, including prognosis for mother and fetus, being fully explained.

In the past, it was believed that cancer associated with pregnancy was more aggressive and that the outcome for all patients was dismal. Today, it is recognized that delay in diagnosis may be a more likely cause of advanced disease at the time of diagnosis. Diagnosing cancer during a pregnancy is difficult, and signs and symptoms of the disease may be misconstrued or underestimated. Treatment options should be evaluated as though the patient were not pregnant and therapy instituted when appropriate.[177,188,206,209]

Medical Management of Commonly Associated Cancers

Breast cancer

Breast cancer is the cancer most commonly associated with pregnancy, occurring in 1 of every 3000 pregnancies or in approximately 10%–20% of women of childbearing age.[177,210–212] Among all women with breast cancer who are still in their childbearing years, 1 in 3 will be pregnant at the time of diagnosis;[177,206] of those younger than age 40, about 1 in 200 is at risk of developing breast cancer.[126]

Breast examination should be part of the initial prenatal visit, and any woman 40 or older who is planning a pregnancy should consider having a screening mammography prior to attempting conception.[213] Although breast enlargement during pregnancy makes examination difficult, it is essential that all women have a thorough examination. If a mass is felt, prompt evaluation is necessary. Although a mammogram is difficult to interpret because of the density of the breast, it may be safely undertaken if appropriate fetal shielding is used.[214] Even if a mammogram shows negative results, a breast mass must be investigated until a definitive diagnosis is made.[210,215–219]

Treatment of breast cancer in the pregnant woman should be the same as in the nonpregnant woman. Initial diagnosis should be attempted by fine-needle aspiration, followed by open biopsy if a definitive diagnosis cannot be made.[210] Biopsy with the patient under local anesthesia has not been shown to cause fetal harm and should be performed without delay.[215,216,220] Once a definitive diagnosis is made, further therapy can be tailored to time of gestation, physician recommendations, and patient wishes. In general, modified mastectomy with lymph node sampling is the standard treatment for early disease. Depending on gestational age, adjuvant chemotherapy can often be delayed until after delivery. For the woman desiring breast-conserving surgery, lumpectomy with lymph node sampling may be done if she is close to term, with radiation therapy and chemotherapy being delayed until after delivery. For advanced disease, surgery and chemotherapy should be undertaken without delay. Therapeutic abortion may be suggested during the first trimester to prevent chemotherapy exposure to the fetus.[210,214–217,220–222] Chances for survival have been considered poor, with reports of 30%–57% survival rates.[218] When patients are matched stage for stage with nonpregnant control subjects, however, there appear to be no differences in survival rates.[219,223] Delay in diagnosis, often for more than 3 months, may be the most important factor leading to decreased survival.

Pregnancy safety following cancer treatment has been extensively evaluated, particularly for women treated for breast cancer.[224] There appears to be no decrease in survival for women who become pregnant following breast cancer treatment.[225–231] It is even possible that a further pregnancy may actually protect against recurrence. In reality, there may be inherent differences between those able to conceive and those unable to conceive, which may alter the survival statistics for this population.[232,233] While increasing, the number of reported pregnancies remains small and thus most likely represents a select and nongeneralizable subset of women with breast cancer. For those desiring future pregnancies, a wait of from 1–5 years following cessation of all treatment, including adjuvant tamoxifen, is recommended.[210,214,225,230,233] Women who are known to be *BRCA1* positive should consider seeking genetic counseling prior to attempting conception.[234]

Breast-feeding after breast cancer diagnosis has been the subject of much debate. For the woman who has received primary breast radiation, it has been suggested that breast-feeding occur only on the nonirradiated side, primarily because of the possible increase in mastitis associated with breast-feeding in the irradiated breast but also because of diminished or absent lactation.[211,214,225,229] Pregnancy subsequent to breast irradiation often results in breast asymmetry, with little enlargement of the irradiated breast and minimal to no lactation from the radiated side.[225]

Cancer of the cervix

The second most common cancer during pregnancy is cancer of the cervix, which occurs in 1 in 400 pregnancies. Approximately 1 in every 100 women diagnosed with cervical cancer will be pregnant at the time of diagnosis. Carcinoma in situ is most commonly found, with invasive disease seen in only 2%–5% of all patients. Signs and symptoms of cervical cancer are similar to those found in the nonpregnant patient, with the majority of pregnant patients experiencing vaginal bleeding or discharge.[235] Diagnosis is most commonly made by Papanicolaou smear. If the smear is abnormal, colposcopy with appropriate biopsies should be undertaken. Cone biopsy is rarely indicated but may be used to confirm a diagnosis of microinvasion. However, it is not without risks and is associated with a 30% complication rate, including hemorrhage, premature delivery, and infection.[177,211,236] More recently, loop electrode excision has been proposed to minimize the potential complications of conization; this type of excision does not appear to improve disease-free surgical margins; it is associated with an increased incidence of cervical hemorrhage;[201] and women who have a loop excision are more likely to have preterm births and low-birth-weight infants.[237] Laser vaporization may be of benefit but has not been tested in pregnancy. Importantly, it does not affect subsequent pregnancies, as is common with conization.[238]

In patients with cervical intraepithelial neoplasia (CIN 2–3), the pregnancy may be allowed to continue. Cytology and colposcopy should be repeated every 6–10 weeks and, unless progression occurs, definitive therapy should be delayed until after delivery.[239] If frank invasion is found, treatment consistent with standard practice for nonpregnant women should not be delayed. During the first two trimesters, surgery or radiation therapy without therapeutic abortion is usually undertaken. Early-stage disease (IA and IB) may be treated with radical hysterectomy and pelvic lymph node dissection; in advanced disease, radiation therapy is the most common treatment. During the third trimester, fetal viability usually can be awaited and the baby can be delivered by cesarean section, after which the appropriate cancer therapy is given.[211,235,240–244] For some patients with invasive disease, treatment with radical trachelectomy, rather than radical hysterectomy, has resulted in the ability to conceive and carry the pregnancy to a viable birth, with one study reporting 22 pregnancies in 18 patients, 12 full-term births, and 6 preterm births, most commonly due to premature rupture of membranes.[245]

Controversy exists over the safety of vaginal delivery. In reviewing the current literature, Nevin and colleagues found that many believed vaginal delivery would disseminate the cancer or cause hemorrhage or infection;[242] as a result, cesarean section was recommended. Others have suggested that vaginal delivery may be associated with an improved overall survival and should be allowed if possible. Recurrence in the episiotomy has been reported following vaginal delivery.[246,247] Careful follow-up for recurrence is essential. The definitive approach remains unclear.

Ovarian cancer

Ovarian masses are common during pregnancy, occurring once in every 81 pregnancies. In general, only 2%–5% of these masses are malignant, for an estimated 1:9000 to 1:25,000 case ratio. Most patients are asymptomatic, with an adnexal mass being noted at the first prenatal visit.[177,248] There are a variety of ways to approach a pelvic mass during pregnancy, including the use of ultrasonography and magnetic resonance imaging.[248,249] In general, any mass that is unilateral, greater than 6 cm, and solid, and that lasts into the second trimester must be evaluated.[248,250]

If malignancy is diagnosed, treatment should proceed as in the nonpregnant woman. Early-stage disease (IA) with low-grade histological findings can be managed by unilateral oophorectomy and biopsy of the other ovary. The pregnancy may be allowed to continue.[251] For all other stages, standard therapy of radical hysterectomy, omentectomy, node biopsy, and peritoneal washings should be carried out. If the woman is near term, a cesarean section, followed by the appropriate therapy, may be performed. Unfortunately, 30%–50% of all women will be diagnosed with stage III or IV disease. Although recent management approaches for stage III disease have resulted in improved survival, in general the prognosis for long-term survival is poor.[248,252] As in the treatment of all cancers, the wishes of the patient must be considered. It is not uncommon for a pregnant woman with advanced disease to delay treatment until the fetus is viable. Palliative treatment should be instituted at the earliest possible time.

Malignant melanoma

Malignant melanoma is one of the most rapidly increasing cancers. It occurs most often in a preexisting mole in fair-haired individuals with blue or green eyes and an inability to tan when exposed to the sun; the peak incidence is during the third and fourth decades. At least 35% of women diagnosed with melanoma will be in their childbearing years.[253,254]

Melanoma arising during pregnancy has been postulated to be associated with poor prognosis because it is hormonally influenced and thus exacerbated by pregnancy. At present, this hypothesis does not appear to be true.[255] What is known is that melanoma that occurs during pregnancy more often is found on the trunk, a site associated with a poor prognosis.[253] Also, these melanomas tend to be thicker, which is also synonymous with a poor prognosis.[256] In addition, all pigmented areas darken during pregnancy, making diagnosis of early changes more difficult. Biopsy and removal of questionable lesions are indicated. There appears to be no difference in survival between the pregnant and nonpregnant woman with melanoma.[253,255,257,258]

Treatment consists of wide excision with skin graft if necessary. While lymph node dissection remains controversial, sentinel node biopsy is recommended.[255] Adjuvant therapy, including the use of melanoma vaccines, remains under investigation, but no definitive answers are available for the pregnant patient. The benefits of chemotherapy and BRMs remain unclear.[255,259] While chemotherapy regimens can be safely administered during the second and third trimesters,[259] the adjuvant use of alfa-interferon should be delayed until postpartum due to the increased rates of fetal and maternal complications associated with high-dose regimens.[253] For individuals with advanced disease, therapeutic abortion followed by palliative chemotherapy is advised. For the individual with brain metastasis, surgery or radiation therapy with appropriate fetal shielding may be undertaken. The use of MRI for metastatic work-up is known to be safe, while the use of the PET scan during pregnancy is not indicated.[260]

Malignant melanoma is known to metastasize to the placenta and fetus. The placenta should be carefully evaluated at delivery and the infant monitored for development of melanoma.[261–263] Further pregnancies should not be undertaken until at least two years after diagnosis and treatment, due to the increased risk of recurrence during this time for all patients with malignant melanoma.[264]

Lymphomas

Both non-Hodgkin's lymphoma (NHL) and Hodgkin's disease (HD) may occur during pregnancy, although the incidence is rare, with HD occurring in 1 in 6000 pregnancies and NHL rarely associated.[265,266] Hodgkin's disease usually occurs as asymptomatic lymphadenopathy of the cervical, supraclavicular, or mediastinal regions. Disease confined to the neck or axilla usually can be treated with radiation therapy combined with fetal shielding. Because more extensive disease requires combination chemotherapy, a therapeutic abortion is suggested during the first half of pregnancy. During the last half of pregnancy, therapy will be defined by the stage of the pregnancy. If fetal viability is imminent, therapy may be delayed or single-drug treatment instituted and delivery awaited. For rapidly progressing disease, combination chemotherapy should be instituted immediately.[265–267] Pregnancy does not appear to negatively affect the clinical course of HD.[268]

Fewer than 100 cases of NHL and pregnancy have been reported in the literature. In general, pregnant patients tend to be diagnosed later and have a poor prognosis with increased risk of relapse after remission.[269] Although NHL is known to metastasize to the placenta and fetus and thus requires careful observation at delivery, NHL has not developed in these infants so affected .[270]

Leukemia

Leukemia occurs in 1 in 75,000 pregnancies. Diagnosis is often made on routine complete blood count. Treatment should be instituted immediately unless the fetus is viable or near viability. If the fetus is viable, delivery should not be delayed. If the fetus is near viability, leukapheresis may be utilized until delivery is possible. Combination chemotherapy has been administered safely in the second and third trimesters, with no increased incidence of neonatal birth defects.[271] Improved treatment and supportive care regimens have decreased the incidence of life-threatening complications and increased remission induction rates; as a consequence, initial survival of the pregnant woman and her fetus is common.[267] Therapeutic abortion is suggested in the first trimester to avoid fetal exposure to chemotherapy.[272,273]

Effects of Treatment and Malignancy on the Fetus

Surgery

Maternal surgery can be safely accomplished with minimal risk to the fetus.[211,248] Pelvic surgery is more easily accomplished during the second trimester and is associated with a lower rate of preterm birth.[274] There is little risk to the fetus from short exposure to anesthetic agents after the first trimester; however, longer exposure may lead to decreased birth weight.[274] Adequate ventilation and prevention of hypotension are of prime importance. As long as competent surgeons and anesthesiologists with appropriate fetal monitoring equipment are available, no harm to the fetus should occur.[215,248] MRI and ultrasound can safely be used to evaluate presurgical conditions.[275]

Radiation

Radiation doses of greater than 250 cGy during pregnancy have been associated with fetal damage—for example, mental retardation, skin changes, and spontaneous abortions (depending on stage of gestation). Low doses of radiation associated with diagnostic x-ray studies (<0.5 cGy) are probably not harmful if adequate fetal shielding is provided.[214,276] Radiation to the pelvis should be avoided.[179,214,277] Lethal effects are greatest during preimplantation (conception to day 9 or 10), while during organogenesis (weeks 3–12) retarded growth, microcephaly, and ocular problems can occur. Weeks 20–25, the fetal period, are associated with functional abnormalities of the liver, kidney, and bone marrow and sterility.[278] Because fetal death, malformation, and mental retardation are associated with doses of 100–200 cGy and higher, as long as fetal doses remain less than 100 cGy, therapeutic abortion need not be considered.[279] Long-term effects of low-dose radiation remain unknown, but the concerns about chromosomal aberrations and increased rates of childhood cancer in children exposed in utero remain. Follow-up over many generations may be necessary to determine the exact effects.[210,280]

Chemotherapy

Chemotherapy has been administered prior to and concurrent with pregnancy. As previously noted, chemotherapy during the first trimester has been associated with fetal wastage, malformations, and low birth weights. Many studies indicate that the incidence of fetal malformation is low (<10%) and may be minimized or avoided with careful selection of agents. Latent effects are still unknown, and offspring need continuous evaluation. Note that the pharmacokinetics of chemotherapeutic agents may be altered by the normal physiological changes of pregnancy. As a result, monitoring for unexpected toxicities or altered response patterns is of extreme importance. Additionally, evaluation of the fetus for toxicities from administration of drugs immediately prior to delivery is paramount. Both neonatal metabolism and drug excretion may be suboptimal, and the placenta, which is the normal mechanism for excretion, has been eliminated.[158,181,211,281,282]

Maternal–fetal spread

Only a few cancers spread from the mother to the fetus, with melanoma, NHL, and leukemia being the most common.[283] Because few studies have been compiled, the exact incidence is unknown. Dildy and colleagues reviewed literature related to maternal malignancy metastatic to the fetus and reported on 53 cases.[284] The most common cancer was malignant melanoma; metastasis to the placenta occurred in 12 patients and spread to the fetus in 7 cases. The second most common cancers were hematological malignancies (leukemia and lymphoma), involving 8 instances of placental spread and 4 cases of fetal spread. Breast and lung cancers were the next most common, although no cases of spread to the fetus have been reported. In most instances, the cancer spreads to the placenta but no fetal involvement ensues. There is no evidence that fetal malignancy spreads to the mother.[282]

Because of the rare incidence of metastatic involvement affecting the infant, evaluation of the placenta and fetus is essential in women with disseminated cancers, in additional to a full physical exam of the newborn.[252,282] If there is no incidence of spread to the newborn, prophylactic treatment should not be undertaken, but close follow-up is needed.[282]

Nursing Management of the Pregnant Patient

Nursing management of the pregnant patient with a concomitant diagnosis of cancer can be extremely complicated. Interventions including psychosocial, educational, and ethical considerations must be developed and implemented. It has been suggested that pregnancy and cancer be treated as a high-risk event with all the associated needs.[206,211,255] Careful explanations of all aspects of care, with special emphasis on support of the patient and her family, need to be provided. Normal activities of pregnancy may be delayed or prevented by disease or treatment, and fears of fetal demise, cancer therapy, and death may prevent resolution of ambivalence toward pregnancy and establishment of emotional affiliation to the growing child. Ethical considerations become apparent as plans for pregnancy are contrasted with needs for therapy. In some instances, therapeutic abortion may be necessary for optimal treatment; in other instances, therapy delays may be requested to provide for the safety of the fetus. Nonjudgmental care by healthcare personnel is essential during these difficult times.

Nursing care of the woman with cancer and her baby is extremely complex and of utmost importance. With a focus on educational interventions, psychological support, and coordination of care, the nurse has an important role in the final outcome. Treatment plans; coordination of follow-up; education about cancer, pregnancy, and treatment; and emotional support of the patient and significant others are integral components of the comprehensive care needed by the pregnant woman with cancer. Without these essential elements, it may not be possible to provide the necessary care that will ensure a positive or improved maternal and fetal outcome.

Conclusion

Sexual and reproductive dysfunction in patients with cancer occurs much more frequently than previously recognized. Almost every patient exposed to cancer or cancer treatment may experience some form of sexual dysfunction at some point during his or her illness. With cancer survival rates improving, and with the understanding that sexual and reproductive function are important to all individuals, it is essential that sexuality and sexual function be assessed and evaluated prior to therapy and that appropriate interventions be implemented throughout treatment and the follow-up period.

References

1. McKee AL Jr, Schover LR: Sexuality rehabilitation. *Cancer* 92:1008–1212S, 2001
2. Anastasia PJ: Altered sexuality, in Carroll-Johnson RM, Gorman LM, Bush NJ (eds.): *Psychosocial Nursing Care Along the Cancer Continuum*. Pittsburgh, Oncology Nursing Press, 1998, pp 227–240
3. Nishimoto PW: Sexuality, in Gates RA, Fink RM (eds.): *Oncology Nursing Secrets*. Philadelphia, Hanley & Belfus, 2001, pp 426–440
4. Deneris A, Huether SE, Robinson KM: Structure and function of the reproductive system, in Huether SE, McCance KL (eds.): *Understanding Pathophysiology* (ed 3). St. Louis, Mosby, 2004, pp 861–887
5. Marieb EN: *Human Anatomy and Physiology* (ed 6). Menlo Park, CA, Benjamin/Cummings, 2004, pp 1030–1077
6. Enker WE: Total mesorectal excision — the new golden standard of surgery for rectal cancer. *Ann Med* 29:127–133, 1997
7. Berg DT: *Pocket Guide to Colorectal Cancer*. Sudbury, MA, Jones and Bartlett, 2003
8. Sprangers MAG, Taal BG, Aaronson NK, et al: Quality of life in colorectal cancer: stoma vs. nonstoma patients. *Dis Colon Rectum* 38:361–369, 1995
9. Chatwin NA, Ribordy M, Givel JC: Clinical outcomes and quality of life after low anterior resection for rectal cancer. *Eur J Surg* 168:297–301, 2002
10. Chorost MI, Weber TK, Lee RJ, et al: Sexual dysfunction, informed consent and multimodality therapy for rectal cancer. *Am J Surg* 179:271–274, 2000
11. Andersen BL: How cancer affects sexual functioning. *Oncology* 4:81–88, 1990
12. Kim NK, Aahn TW, Park JK, et al: Assessment of sexual and voiding function after total mesorectal excision with pelvic autonomic nerve preservation in males with rectal cancer. *Dis Colon Rectum* 45:1178–1185, 2002
13. Koukouras D, Spiliotis J, Scopa CD, et al: Radical consequence in the sexuality of male patients operated for colorectal carcinoma. *Eur J Surg Oncol* 17:285–288, 1991
14. Masui H, Ike H, Yamaguchi S, et al: Male sexual functioning after autonomic nerve-sparing operation for rectal cancer. *Dis Colon Rectum* 39:1140–1145, 1996
15. Lindsey I, George B, Kettlewell M, et al: Randomized, double-blind, placebo-controlled trial of sildenafil (Viagra) for erectile dysfunction after rectal surgery for cancer and inflammatory bowel disease. *Dis Colon Rectum* 45:727–732, 2002
16. Ofman US: Preservation of function in genitourinary cancers: psychosexual and psychosocial issues. *Cancer Invest* 13:125–131, 1995
17. Smith DB, Babaian RJ: The effects of treatment for cancer on male fertility and sexuality. *Cancer Nurs* 15:271–275, 1992
18. Horenblas S, Meinhardt W, Ijzerman W, et al: Sexuality preserving cystectomy and neobladder: initial results. *J Urol* 166:837–840, 2001.
19. Bjerre BD, Johansen C, Steven K: A questionnaire study of sexological problems following urinary diversion in the female patient. *Scan J Urol Nephrol* 31:155–160, 1997
20. Kelly LP, Miaskowski C: An overview of bladder cancer: treatment and nursing interventions. *Oncol Nurs Forum* 23:459–468, 1996
21. Hautmann RE, Paiss T, de Petriconi R: The ileal neobladder in women: 9 years experience with 18 patients. *J Urol* 155:76–81, 1996
22. D'Ancona CA, Botega NJ, DeMoraes C, et al: Quality of life after partial penectomy for penile carcinoma. *Urology* 50:593–596, 1997
23. Dobkin PL, Bradley I: Assessment of sexual dysfunction in oncology patients: review, critique, and suggestions. *J Psychosoc Oncol* 9:43–74, 1991
24. Tefilli MV, Dubocq F, Rajpurkar A, et al: Assessment of psychosexual adjustment after insertion of inflatable penile prosthesis. *Urology* 52:1106–1112, 1998
25. Nukui F, Okamoto S, Nagata M, et al: Complications and reimplantation of penile implants. *Int J Urol* 4:52–54, 1997
26. Opjordsmoen S, Waehre H, Aass N, et al: Sexuality in patients treated for penile cancer: patients' experience and doctors' judgement. *Br J Urol* 73:554–560, 1994
27. Foster RS, McNulty A, Rubin LR, et al: The fertility of patients with clinical stage I testis cancer managed by nerve-sparing retroperitoneal lymph node dissection. *J Urol* 152:1139–1143, 1994
28. Nonomura N, Nishimura K, Takaha N, et al: Nerve-sparing retroperitoneal lymph node dissection for advanced testicular cancer after chemotherapy. *Internat J Urol* 9:539–544, 2002
29. Brock D, Fox S, Gosling G, et al: Testicular cancer. *Semin Oncol Nurs* 9:224–236, 1993
30. Joly F, Heron JF, Kalusinski L, et al: Quality of life in long-term survivors of testicular cancer: a population-based case-control study. *J Clin Oncol* 20:73–80, 2002
31. Arai Y, Kawakita M, Okada Y, et al: Sexuality and fertility in long-term survivors of testicular cancer. *J Clin Oncol* 15:1444–1448, 1997
32. Ohl DA, Sonksen J: What are the chances of infertility and should sperm be banked? *Semin Urol Oncol* 14:36–44, 1996
33. Kuczyk M, Machtens S, Bokemeyer C, et al: Sexual function and fertility after treatment of testicular cancer. *Curr Opin Urol* 10:473–477, 2000
34. Aass N, Grunfeld B, Kaalhus O, et al: Pre- and posttreatment sexual life in testicular cancer patients: a descriptive investigation. *Br J Cancer* 67:1113–1117, 1993
35. Montorsi F, Salonia A, Zanoni M, et al: Counselling the patient with prostate cancer about treatment-related erectile dysfunction. *Curr Opin Urol* 11:611–617, 2001
36. Yarbro CH, Ferrans CE: Quality of life of patients with prostate cancer treated with surgery or radiation therapy. *Oncol Nurs Forum* 25:685–693, 1998
37. Church PA: Prostate cancer, in Steele G, Cady B (eds.): *General Surgical Oncology*. Philadelphia, Saunders, 1992, pp 275–285
38. Richie JP: Localized prostate cancer: overview of surgical management. *Urology* 49(suppl 3A):335–337, 1997

39. Talcott JA, Rieker P, Clark JA, et al: Patient-reported symptoms after primary therapy for early prostate cancer: results of a prospective cohort study. *J Clin Oncol* 16:275–283, 1998
40. Kim RD, Nath R, Kadmon D, et al: Bilateral nerve graft during radical retropubic prostatectomy: 1-year followup. *J Urol* 165:1950–1956, 2001
41. Chang DW, Wood CG, Kroll SS, et al: Cavernous nerve reconstruction to preserve erectile function following non–nerve-sparing radical retropubic prostatectomy: a prospective study. *Plast Reconstr Surg* 111:1174–1181, 2003
42. Perez MA, Meyerowitz BE, Lieskovsky G, et al: Quality of life and sexuality following radical prostatectomy in patients with prostate cancer who do or do not use erectile aids. *Urology* 50:740–746, 1997
43. Zippe CD, Kedia AW, Kedia K, et al: Treatment of erectile dysfunction after radical prostatectomy with sildenafil citrate (Viagra). *Urology* 52:963–966, 1998
44. Kunthe A: Phosphodiesterase 5 inhibitors in male sexual dysfunction. *Curr Opin Urol* 13:405–410, 2003
45. Thranov I, Klee M: Sexuality among gynecologic cancer patients: a cross-sectional study. *Gynecol Oncol* 52:14–19, 1994
46. Auchincloss SS: After treatment: psychological issues in gynecologic cancer survivorship. *Cancer* 76(suppl 10):2117–2124, 1995
47. Steginga SK, Dunn J: Women's experiences following treatment for gynecologic cancer. *Oncol Nurs Forum* 24:1403–1408, 1997
48. Anderson BL: Stress and quality of life following cervical cancer. *Monogr J Natl Cancer Inst* 21:65–70, 1996
49. Gossfield LM, Cullen ML: Sexuality and fertility, in Moore-Higgs GJ (ed.), *Women and Cancer: A Gynecologic Oncology Nursing Perspective* (ed 2), Sudbury, MA, Jones and Bartlett, 2000, pp 466–500
50. Door A: Less common gynecologic malignancies. *Semin Oncol Nurs* 18:207–222, 2002
51. DiSaia PJ, Creasman WT: *Clinical Gynecologic Oncology* (ed 5). St. Louis, Mosby, 1997
52. Corney RH, Crowther ME, Howells A: Psychosexual dysfunction in women with gynaecological cancer following radical pelvic surgery. *Br J Obstet Gynaecol* 100:73–78, 1993
53. Chun JK, Behnam AB, Dottino P, et al: Use of the umbilicus in reconstruction of the vulva and vagina with a rectus abdominus musculocutaneous flap. *Ann Plastic Surg* 40:659–663, 1998
54. Esrig D, Freeman JA, Stein JP, et al: New technique of reconstruction following anterior exenteration. *Urology* 49:768–771, 1997
55. Louis-Sylvestre C, Haddad B, Paniel BJ: Creation of a sigmoid neovagina: technique and results in 16 cases. *Eur J Obstet Gynecol Reprod Biol* 75:225–229, 1997
56. Andersen BL, Lamb M: Sexuality and cancer, in Murphy GP, Lawrence W, Lenhard RE (eds.): *American Cancer Society Textbook of Clinical Oncology* (ed 2). Atlanta, American Cancer Society, 1995, pp 699–713
57. Schlaerth JB, Spirtos NM, Schlaerth AC: Radical trachelectomy and pelvic lymphadenectomy with uterine preservation in the treatment of cervical cancer. *Am J Obstet Gynecol* 188:29–34, 2003
58. Wilmoth MC, Spinelli A: Sexual implications of gynecologic treatments. *J Obst Gynecol Neonatal Nurs* 29:413–421, 2000
59. Bergmark K, Avall-Lundqvist E, Dickman PW, et al: Patient rating of distressful symptoms after treatment for early cervical cancer. *Acta Obstet Gynecol Oncol* 81:443–450, 2002
60. Shell JA: Impact of cancer on sexuality, in Otto S (ed.): *Oncology Nursing* (ed 4). St. Louis, Mosby Year Book, 2001, pp 973–999
61. Porter S: Endometrial cancer. *Semin Oncol Nurs* 18:200–206, 2002
62. DeGaetano C: Ovarian cancer — it whispers . . . so listen. *Nurs Spectrum* January: 28–32, 2001
63. Tserkezoglou AJ: Malignant ovarian neoplasms: the place of conservative therapy. *Ann NY Acad Sci* 816:362–368, 1997
64. Zanetta G, Chiari S, Rota S, et al: Conservative surgery for stage I ovarian carcinoma in women of childbearing age. *Br J Obstet Gynaecol* 104:1030–1035, 1997
65. Fitch MI: Psychosocial management of patients with recurrent ovarian cancer: treating the whole patient to improve quality of life. *Semin Oncol Nurs* 19(suppl 1):40–53, 2003
66. Fischer M: Cancer of the cervix. *Semin Oncol Nurs* 18:193–199, 2002
67. Amichetti M, Caffo O: Quality of life in patients with early stage carcinoma treated with conservation surgery and radiotherapy: an Italian monoinstitutional study. *Tumori* 2:78–84, 2001
68. Lewis FM, Zahlis EH, Sjands ME, et al: The functioning of single women with breast cancer and their school-aged children. *Cancer Pract* 4:15–24, 1996
69. Wilmoth MC, Townsend J: A comparison of the effects of lumpectomy versus mastectomy on sexual behaviors. *Cancer Pract* 3:279–285, 1995
70. Fallowfield L: Offering choice of surgical treatment to women with breast cancer. *Patient Educ Couns* 30:209–214, 1997
71. Neill KM, Armstrong N, Burnett CB: Choosing reconstruction after mastectomy: a qualitative analysis. *Oncol Nurs Forum* 25:743–750, 1998
72. Yurek D, Farrar W, Andersen BL: Breast conserving surgery: comparing surgical groups and determining individual differences in postoperative sexuality and body change stress. *J Consulting Clin Psychol* 68:697–709, 2000
73. Al-Ghazal SK, Blamey RW: Subcutaneous mastectomy with implant reconstruction: cosmetic outcome and patient satisfaction. *Eur J Surg Oncol* 26:137–141, 2000
74. Monga U, Tan G, Ostermann HJ, et al: Sexuality in head and neck cancer patients. *Arch Phys Med Rehab* 78:298–304, 1997
75. Bjordal K, Ahlner-Elmqvist M, Hammerlid E, et al: A prospective study of quality of life in head and neck cancer patients. *Laryngoscope* 111:1440–1452, 2001
76. Granai CO, Amado PM, Goldstein AS, et al: The effects of cancer therapy on fertility. *Clin Adv Oncol Nurs* 3:1, 3, 7–9, 1992
77. Kelly LD: Nursing assessment and patient management. *Semin Oncol Nurs* 15:282–291, 1999
78. Iwamoto RR, Maher KE: Radiation therapy for prostate cancer. *Semin Oncol Nurs* 17:90–100, 2001
79. Rubin A, Williams JP: Principles of radiation oncology and cancer radiotherapy, in Rubin A (ed.): *Clinical Oncology: A Multidisciplinary Approach for Physicians and Students* (ed 8). Philadelphia, Saunders, 2001, pp 99–125
80. Haie-Meder C, Milka-Cabanne N, Michel G, et al: Radiotherapy after ovarian transposition: ovarian function and fertility preservation. *Int J Radiat Oncol Biol Phys* 25:419–424, 1993
81. Morice P, Thiam-Ba R, Castaigne D, et al: Fertility results after ovarian transposition for pelvic malignancies treated by external irradiation or brachytherapy. *Hum Reprod* 13:660–663, 1998
82. Jensen T, Groenvald M, Klee MC, et al: Longitudinal study of sexual function and vaginal changes after radiotherapy for cervical cancer. *Int J Radiat Oncol Biol Phys* 56:937–949, 2003
83. Cartwright-Alcarese F: Addressing sexual dysfunction following radiation therapy for a gynecologic malignancy. *Oncol Nurs Forum* 22:1227–1232, 1995
84. Fieler VK: Side effects and quality of life in patients receiving high-dose rate brachytherapy. *Oncol Nurs Forum* 24:545–553, 1997

85. Goodman A: In small study, hand-held device offers hope for women alleviating radiation-induced sexual dysfunction in women. *Oncol Times* December: 44–46, 2002
86. Rowly MJ, Leach DR, Warner GA, et al: Effects of graded doses of ionizing radiation on human testes. *Radiat Res* 59:665–678, 1974
87. Shafford EA, Kingston JE, Malpas JS, et al: Testicular function following the treatment of Hodgkin's disease in childhood. *Br J Cancer* 68:1199–1204, 1993
88. Sklar CA, Robison LL, Nesbit ME, et al: Effects of radiation on testicular function in long-term survivors of childhood acute lymphoblastic leukemia: a report from the Children's Cancer Study Group. *J Clin Oncol* 8:1981–1987, 1990
89. Centola GM, Keller JW, Henzler M, et al: Effect of low-dose testicular irradiation on sperm count and fertility in patients with testicular seminoma. *J Androl* 15:608–613, 1994
90. Beard CJ, Lamb C, Buswell L, et al: Radiation-associated morbidity in patients undergoing small-field external beam irradiation for prostate cancer. *Int J Radiat Oncol Biol Phys* 41:257–262, 1998
91. Formenti SC, Lieskovsky G, Simoneau AR, et al: Impact of moderate dose of postoperative radiation on urinary continence and potency in men with prostate cancer treated with nerve sparing prostatectomy. *J Urol* 155:616–619, 1996
92. Merrick GS, Wallner KE, Butler WM: Permanent interstitial brachytherapy for the management of carcinoma of the prostate gland. *J Urol* 169:1643–1652, 2003
93. Merrick GS, Butler WM, Wallner KE, et al: The importance of radiation dose to the penile bulb vs. crura in the development of postbrachytherapy erectile dysfunction. *Int J Radiat Oncol Biol Phys* 54:1055–1062, 2002
94. Valicenti RK, Bissonette EA, Chen C, et al: Longitudinal comparison of sexual function after 3–dimensional conformal radiation therapy or post brachytherapy. *J Urol* 168:2499–2504, 2002
95. Sharkey J, Chovnick SD, Behar RJ, et al: Outpatient ultrasound-guided palladium 103 brachytherapy for localized adenocarcinoma of the prostate: a preliminary report of 434 patients. *Urology* 51:796–803, 1998
96. Zeitlin SI, Sherman J, Raboy A, et al: High dose combination radiotherapy for the treatment of localized prostate cancer. *J Urol* 160:91–95, 1998
97. Zelefsky MJ, Wallner KE, Ling CC, et al: Comparison of the 5-year outcome and morbidity of the three-dimensional conformal radiotherapy versus transperineal permanent iodine-125 implantation for early-stage prostate cancer. *J Clin Oncol* 17:517–522, 1999
98. Stipetich RL, Abel LJ, Blatt HJ, et al: Nursing assessment of sexual function following permanent prostate brachytherapy for patient with early-stage prostate cancer. *Clin J Oncol Nurs* 6:271–274, 2002
99. Valicenti RK, Choi E, Chen CT, et al: Sildenafil citrate effectively reverses sexual dysfunction induced by three-dimensional conformal radiation therapy. *Urol* 57:769–773, 2001
100. Jereczek-Fossa BA, Marsiglia HR, Orecchia R: Radiotherapy-related fatigue. *Crit Rev Oncol Hematol* 41:317–325, 2002
101. Longo DL, Fisher RI: Medical problems in long-term survivors of Hodgkin's disease. *Intern Med Spec* 4:165–171, 1983
102. Schilsky RL, Erlichman C: Late complications of chemotherapy: infertility and carcinogenesis, in Chabner B (ed.): *Pharmacologic Principles of Cancer Treatment.* Philadelphia, Saunders, 1982, pp 109–128
103. Chapman RM: Effect of cytotoxic therapy on sexuality and gonadal function. *Semin Oncol* 9:84–94, 1982
104. Wilkes GM, Ingwersen K, Burke MB: *2003 Oncology Nursing Drug Handbook.* Sudbury, MA, Jones and Bartlett, 2003
105. Otto S: Chemotherapy, in Otto S (ed.): *Oncology Nursing* (ed 4). St. Louis, Mosby Year Book, 2001, pp 638–683
106. Cleri LB, Haywood R: *Oncology Pocket Guide to Chemotherapy* (ed 5). Philadelphia, Mosby, 2002
107. Gullatte MM (ed.): *Clinical Guide to Antineoplastic Therapy: A Chemotherapy Handbook.* Pittsburgh, Oncology Nursing Society, 2001
108. Chu E, DeVita VT: *Physicians' Cancer Chemotherapy Drug Manual 2001.* Sudbury, MA, Jones and Bartlett, 2001
109. Schilsky RL, Lewis BJ, Sherins RJ, et al: Gonadal dysfunction in patients receiving chemotherapy for cancer. *Ann Intern Med* 93:109–114, 1980
110. Howell SJ, Radford JA, Smets EM, et al: Fatigue, sexual function and mood following treatment for haematological malignancy: the impact of mild Leydig cell dysfunction. *Br J Cancer* 82:789–793, 2000
111. Chapman RM: Gonadal toxicity and teratogenicity, in Perry MC (ed.): *The Chemotherapy Sourcebook.* Baltimore, Williams & Wilkins, 1992, pp 710–753
112. Pont J, Albrecht W: Fertility after chemotherapy for testicular germ cell cancer. *Fertil Steril* 68:1–5, 1997
113. Stoter G, Koopman A, Vendrik CP, et al: Ten-year survival and late sequelae in testicular cancer patients treated with cisplatin, vinblastine and bleomycin. *J Clin Oncol* 7:1099–1104, 1989
114. Bohlen D, Burkhard FC, Mills R, et al: Fertility and sexual function following orchiectomy and 2 cycles of chemotherapy for stage 1 high risk nonseminomatous germ cell cancer. *J Urol* 165:441–444, 2001
115. Lampe H, Horwich A, Norman A, et al: Fertility after chemotherapy for testicular germ cell cancers. *J Clin Oncol* 15:239–245, 1997
116. Peterson PM, Giwercman A, Skakkebaek NE, et al: Gonadal function in men with testicular cancer. *Semin Oncol* 25:224–233, 1998
117. Stephenson WT, Poirier SM, Rubin L, et al: Evaluation of reproductive capacity in germ cell tumor patients following treatment with cisplatin, etoposide, and bleomycin. *J Clin Oncol* 13:2278–2280, 1995
118. Shrover L: Sexual rehabilitation after treatment for prostate cancer. *Cancer* 71 (suppl 3):1024–1030, 1993
119. Spetz A-C, Zetterlund E-L, Varenhorst E, et al: Incidence and management of hot flashes in prostate cancer. *J Supportive Oncol* 1:263–273, 2003
120. Brufsky A, Fontaine-Rothe P, Berlane K, et al: Finasteride and flutamide as potency-sparing androgen-ablative therapy for advanced adenocarcinoma of the prostate. *Urology* 49:913–920, 1997
121. Van Basten JP, Hoekstra HJ, van driel MF, et al: Sexual dysfunction in nonseminoma testicular cancer patients is related to chemotherapy-induced angiopathy. *J Clin Oncol* 15:2442–2448, 1997
122. Knopf MT: Natural menopause and ovarian toxicity associated with breast cancer therapy. *Oncol Nurs Forum* 25:1519–1530, 1998
123. Chapman RM, Sutcliffe SB, Malpas JS: Cytotoxic-induced ovarian failure in women with Hodgkin's disease: II. Effects on sexual function. *JAMA* 242:1171–1181, 1979
124. Averette HE, Boike GM, Jarrell MA: Effects of chemotherapy on gonadal function and reproductive capacity. *CA Cancer J Clin* 40:199–209, 1990
125. Young-McCaughan S: Sexual functioning in women with breast cancer after treatment with adjuvant therapy. *Cancer Nurs* 19:308–319, 1996
126. Minton SE, Munster PN: Chemotherapy-induced amenorrhea and fertility in women undergoing adjuvant treatment for breast cancer. *Cancer Control* 9:466–472, 2002

127. Schover LR: Sexuality and body image in younger women with breast cancer. *Monogr Natl Cancer Inst* 16:177–182, 1994
128. Pansacreta JV, McCorkle R: Providing accurate information to women about tamoxifen therapy for breast cancer: current indications, effects, and controversies. *Oncol Nurs Forum* 25:1577–1583, 1998
129. Sitzia J, Huggins L: Side effects of cyclophosphamide, methotrexate and 5FU (CMF) chemotherapy for breast cancer. *Cancer Pract* 6:13–21, 1998
130. Broeckel JA, Thors CL, Jacobsen PB, et al: Sexual functioning in long-term breast cancer survivors treated with adjuvant chemotherapy. *Breast Cancer Res Control* 75:241–248, 2002
131. Meadows AT: Follow-up and care of childhood cancer survivors. *Hosp Pract* 15:99–108, 1991
132. Levy MJ, Stillman RJ: Reproductive potential in survivors of childhood malignancy. *Pediatrician* 18:61–70, 1991
133. Relander T, Cavallin-Stahl E, Garwicz S, et al: Gonadal and sexual function in men treated for childhood cancer. *Med Ped Oncol* 35:52–63, 2000
134. Green DM, Whitton JA, Stovall M, et al: Pregnancy outcome of female survivors of childhood cancer: a report from the childhood cancer survivor study. *Am J Obstet Gynecol* 187:1070–1080, 2002
135. Green DM, Whitton JA, Stovall M, et al: Pregnancy outcome of partners of male survivors of childhood cancer: a report from the childhood cancer survivor study. *J Clin Oncol* 21:716–721, 2003
136. Langeveld NE, Stam H, Grootenhuis MA, et al: Quality of life in young adult survivors of childhood cancer. *Support Care Cancer* 10:579–600, 2002
137. Wilson B: The effects of drugs on male sexual function and fertility. *Nurse Pract* 16:12–24, 1991
138. Rieger PT: Patient management, in Rieger PT (ed.): *Biotherapy: A Comprehensive Overview* (ed 2). Sudbury, MA, Jones and Bartlett, 2001, pp 461–503
139. Krozely P: Epidermal growth factor receptor tyrosine kinase inhibitors: evolving role in the treatment of solid tumors. *Clin J Oncol Nurs* 8:163–168, 2004
140. Walker PL, Dang NH: Denileukine diftitox as novel targeted therapy in non-Hodgkin's lymphoma. *Clin J Oncol Nurs* 8:169–174, 2004
141. Schmidt KV (ed.): Emerging therapies. *Semin Oncol Nurs* 1:153–229, 2003
142. Birner A: Pharmacology of oral chemotherapy agents. *Clin J Oncol Nurs* 7:11–19, 2003
143. Tierney DK: Sexuality following hematopoietic cell transplantation. *Clin J Oncol* Nurs 8:43–47, 2004
144. Lee HG, Park EY, Kim HM, et al: Sexuality and quality of life after hematopoietic stem cell transplantation. *Korean J Int Med* 17:19–23, 2002
145. Watson M, Wheatley K, Harrison GA, et al: Severe adverse impact on sexual functioning and fertility of bone marrow transplantation, either allogeneic or autologous, compared with consolidation chemotherapy alone: analysis of the MRC AML 10 trial. *Cancer* 86:1231–1239, 1999
146. Chatterjee R, Andrews HO, McGarrigle HH, et al: Cavernosal arterial insufficiency is a major component of erectile dysfunction in some recipients of high-dose chemotherapy/chemo-radiotherapy for haematological malignancies. *Bone Marrow Transplant* 25:1185–1189, 2000
147. Chatterjee R, Kottaridis PD, McGarrigle HH, et al: Management of erectile dysfunction by combination therapy with testosterone and sildenafil in recipients of high-dose therapy for haematological malignancies. *Bone Marrow Transplant* 29:607–610, 2002
148. Harris E, Mahendra P, McGarrigle HH, et al: Gynaecomastia with hypergonadotrophic hypogonadism of high dose chemotherapy or chemo-radiotherapy. *Bone Marrow Transplant* 28:1141–1114, 2001
149. Milliken S, Powles R, Parikh P: Successful pregnancy following bone marrow transplantation for leukaemia. *Bone Marrow Transplant* 5:135–137, 1990
150. Rio B, Letur-Konirsch H, Ajchenbaum-Cymbalista F, et al: Full-term pregnancy with embryos from donated oocytes in a 36-year-old woman allografted for chronic myeloid leukemia. *Bone Marrow Transplant* 13:487–488, 1994
151. Whedon M, Stearns D, Mills LE: Quality of life of long-term adult survivors of autologous bone marrow transplantation. *Oncol Nurs Forum* 22:1527–1537, 1995
152. Haberman M, Bush N, Young K, et al: Quality of life of adult long-term survivors of bone marrow transplantation: a qualitative analysis of narrative data. *Oncol Nurs Forum* 20:1545–1553, 1993
153. Ferrell B, Grant M, Schmidt GM, et al: The meaning of quality of life for bone marrow transplant survivors: part 1. The impact of bone marrow transplant on quality of life. *Cancer Nurs* 15:153–160, 1992
154. Ferrell B, Grant M, Schmidt GM, et al: The meaning of quality of life for bone marrow transplant survivors: part 2. Improving quality of life for bone marrow transplant survivors. *Cancer Nurs* 15:247–253, 1992
155. Thaler-DeMers D: Intimacy issues: sexuality, fertility and relationships. *Semin Oncol Nurs* 17:255–262, 2001
156. Andersen BL, Lamb M: Sexuality and cancer, in Murphy GP, Lawrence W, Lenhard RE (eds.): *American Cancer Society Textbook of Clinical Oncology* (ed 2). Atlanta, American Cancer Society, 1995, pp 699–713
157. Auchincloss S: Sexual dysfunction after cancer treatment. *J Psychosoc Oncol* 9:23–42, 1991
158. Krebs LU: Sexual and reproductive issues, in Yasko JM (ed.) *Nursing Management of Symptoms Associated with Chemotherapy* (ed 5). West Conshohocken, PA, Meniscus, 2001, pp 205–214
159. Annon JS: *The Behavioral Treatment of Sexual Problems.* Honolulu, Mercantile Printing, 1974, pp 43–47
160. Smith DB: Sexuality and the patient with cancer: what nurses need to know. *Oncol Patient Care* 4:1–3, 15, 1994
161. Shell JA: The psychosocial impact of ostomy surgery. *Progressions* 4:3–6, 8–11, 14, 15, 1992
162. Ofman US: Psychosexual aspects of sexuality in the patient with cancer. *Oncol Patient Care* 4:7, 8, 14, 15, 1994
163. Shell JA, Smith CK: Sexuality and the older person with cancer. *Oncol Nurs Forum* 21:553–558, 1994
164. Small EC: Psycho-sexual issues. *Obstet Gynecol Clin North Am* 21:773–780, 1994
165. Baron RH: Dispelling the myths of pregnancy-associated breast cancer. *Oncol Nurs Forum* 21:507–512, 1994
166. Wilmouth M, Bruner DW: Integrating sexuality into cancer nursing practice. *Oncol Nurs Patient Treatment Support* 8:1–14, 2002
167. Hughes MK: Sexuality issues: keeping your cool. *Oncol Nurs Forum* 23:1597–1600, 1996
168. Nicholson HS, Byrne J: Fertility and pregnancy after treatment for cancer during childhood or adolescence. *Cancer* 71(suppl):3392–3399, 1993
169. Klein CE: Fertility and the cancer survivor. *Coping* 9:48–49, 1995
170. Byrne J: Fertility and pregnancy after malignancy. *Semin Perinatol* 14:423–429, 1990
171. Hawkins MM: Is there evidence of therapy-related increases in germ cell mutation among childhood cancer survivors? *J Natl Cancer Inst* 83:1643–1650, 1991

172. Senturia YD, Peckham CS: Children fathered by men treated with chemotherapy for testicular cancer. *Eur J Cancer* 26:429–432, 1990
173. Green DM, Zevon MA, Lowrie G, et al: Congenital anomalies in children of patients who received chemotherapy for cancer in childhood and adolescence. *N Engl J Med* 325:141–146, 1991
174. Swerdlow AJ, Jacobs PA, Marks A, et al: Fertility, reproductive outcomes, and health of offspring of patients treated for Hodgkin's disease: an investigation including chromosome examinations. *Br J Cancer* 74:291–296, 1996
175. Hansen PV, Glavind K, Panduro J, et al: Paternity in patients with testicular germ cell cancer: pretreatment and posttreatment findings. *Eur J Cancer* 27:1385–1389, 1991
176. Byrne J, Rasmussen SA, Steinhorn SC, et al: Genetic disease in offspring of long-term survivors of childhood and adolescent cancer. *Am J Hum Genet* 62:45–52, 1998
177. Robinson WA, Krebs LU: Oncologic disease, in Abrams R, Wexler P (eds.): *Medical Care of the Pregnant Patient: Concepts and Management.* Boston, Little, Brown, 1983, pp 307–319
178. Reichman BS, Green KB: Breast cancer in young women: effect of chemotherapy on ovarian function, fertility, and birth defects. *Monogr Natl Cancer Inst* 16:125–129, 1994
179. Mayr NA, Wen B, Saw CB: Radiation therapy during pregnancy. *Obstet Gynecol Clin North Am* 25:301–321, 1998
180. Barnicle MM: Chemotherapy and pregnancy. *Semin Oncol Nurs* 8:124–132, 1992
181. Buekers TE, Lallas TA: Chemotherapy in pregnancy. *Obstet Gynecol Clin North Am* 25:323–329, 1998
182. Zemlickis D, Lishner M, Degendorfer P, et al: Fetal outcome after in utero exposure to cancer chemotherapy. *Arch Intern Med* 152:573–576, 1992
183. Shahin MS, Puscheck E: Reproductive sequelae of cancer treatment. *Obstet Gynecol Clin North Am* 25:423–433, 1998
184. Rieker PP: How should a man with testicular cancer be counseled and what information is available to him? *Semin Urol Oncol* 14:17–23, 1996
185. Turek PJ, Lowther DN, Carroll PR: Fertility issues and their management in men with testis cancer. *Urol Clin North Am* 25:517–531, 1998
186. Kreuser ED, Klingmuller D, Thiel E: The role of LHRH-analogues in protecting gonadal functions during chemotherapy and irradiation. *Eur Urol* 23:157–164, 1993
187. Pereyra Pacheco B, Mendez Ribaz JM, Milone G, et al: Use of GnRH analogs for functional protection of the ovary and preservation of fertility during cancer treatment in adolescents: a preliminary report. *Women's Oncol Rev* 1:371–372, 2001
188. Mott-Smith ME, Stolberg L: Sexual function and pregnancy, in Casciato DA, Lowitz BB (eds.): *Manual of Clinical Oncology* (ed 3). Boston, Little, Brown, 1995, pp 575–582
189. Lee DM, Yeomann RR, Battaglia DE, et al: Live birth after ovarian tissue transplant. *Nature* 428:137–138, 2004
190. Gotlieb WH, Beiner ME, Shalmon B, et al: Outcome of fertility-sparing treatment with progestins in young patients with endometrial cancer. *Obstet Gynecol* 102:718–725, 2003
191. Recchia F, Sica G, DeFilippis S, et al: Goserelin as ovarian protection in the adjuvant treatment of premenopausal breast cancer: a phase II pilot study. *Anti-cancer Drugs* 13:417–424, 2002
192. Anger JT, Gilbert BR, Goldstein M: Cryopreservation of sperm: indications, methods and results. *J Urol* 170:1079–1084, 2003
193. Lass A, Akagbosu F, Abusheikha N, et al: A programme of semen cryopreservation for patients with malignant disease in a tertiary infertility centre: lessons from 8 years' experience. *Human Reprod* 13:3256–3261, 1998
194. Petersen PM, Skakkebaek NE, Vistisen K, et al: Semen quality and reproductive hormones before orchiectomy in men with testicular cancer. *J Clin Oncol* 17:941–947, 1999
195. Sweet V, Servy EJ, Karow AM: Reproductive issues for men with cancer: technology and nursing management. *Oncol Nurs Forum* 23:51–58, 1996
196. Naysmith TE, Blake DA, Harvey VJ, et al: Do men undergoing sterilizing cancer treatments have a fertile future? *Hum Reprod* 13:3250–3255, 1998
197. Leonard M, Hammelef K, Smith GD: Fertility considerations, counseling, and semen cryopreservation for males prior to the initiation of cancer therapy. *Clin J Oncol Nurs* 8:127–131, 2004
198. Koeppel KM: Sperm banking and patients with cancer: issues concerning patients and healthcare professionals. *Cancer Nurs* 18:306–312, 1995
199. Agarwal A, Ranganathan P, Kattal N, et al: Fertility after cancer: a prospective review of assisted reproductive outcome with banked semen specimens. *Fertil Steril* 81:342–348, 2004
200. Salihu HM, Aliyu MH: Sperm retrieval in infertile males: comparison between testicular sperm extraction and testicular sperm aspiration techniques. *Wiener Klinisch Wochenschrift* 115:370–379, 2003
201. Meacham RB, Lipshultz LI: Assisted reproductive technologies for male factor infertility. *Curr Opin Obstet Gynecol* 3:656–661, 1991
202. Mandelbaum J, Belaisch-Allart J, Junca AM, et al: Cryopreservation in human assisted reproduction is now routine for embryos but remains a research procedure for oocytes. *Hum Reprod* 3(suppl 13):161–177, 1998
203. Abir R, Fisch B, Raz A, et al: Preservation of fertility in women undergoing chemotherapy: current approach and future prospects. *J Assist Reprod Genet* 15:477–496, 1998
204. Donnez J, Bassil S: Indications for cryopreservation of ovarian tissue. *Hum Reprod Update* 4:248–259, 1998
205. Newton H: The cryopreservation of ovarian tissue as a strategy for preserving the fertility of cancer patients. *Hum Reprod Update* 4:237–247, 1998
206. Krebs LU: Pregnancy and cancer. *Semin Oncol Nurs* 1:35–41, 1985
207. Waalen J: Pregnancy poses tough questions for cancer treatment. *J Natl Cancer Inst* 83:900, 1991
208. Ward RM, Bristow RE: Cancer and pregnancy: recent developments. *Curr Opin Obstet Gynecol* 14:613–617, 2002
209. Zemlickis D, Lishner M, Degendorfer P, et al: Maternal and fetal outcome after invasive cervical cancer in pregnancy. *J Clin Oncol* 9:1956–1961, 1991
210. Sorosky JI, Scott-Connor CEH: Breast disease complicating pregnancy. *Obstet Gynecol Clin North Am* 25:253–263, 1998
211. Krebs LU: Cancer and pregnancy, in Gates RA, Fink RM (eds.): *Oncology Nursing Secrets* (ed 2). Philadelphia, Hanley & Belfus, 2001, pp 502–514
212. Petrek J, Seltzer V: Breast cancer in pregnant and postpartum women. *J Obstet Gynaecol Canada* 25:944–950, 2003
213. Hindle WH, Gonzalez S: Diagnosis and treatment of invasive breast cancer during pregnancy and lactation. *Clin Obstet Gynecol* 45:770–773, 2002
214. Pelsang RE: Diagnostic imaging modalities during pregnancy. *Obstet Gynecol Clin North Am* 25:287–300, 1998
215. Fiorica JV: Special problems: breast cancer and pregnancy. *Obstet Gynecol Clin North Am* 21:721–732, 1994
216. Petrek JA: Breast cancer during pregnancy. *Cancer* 74(suppl):518–527, 1994
217. Zemlickis D, Lishner M, Degendorfer P, et al: Maternal and fetal outcome after breast cancer in pregnancy. *Am J Obstet Gynecol* 166:781–787, 1992
218. Shapiro CL, Mayer RJ: Breast cancer in pregnancy. *Adv Oncol* 8:25–29, 1992
219. Samuels TH, Liu FF, Yaffe M, et al: Gestational breast cancer. *Can Assoc Radiol J* 49:172–180, 1998

220. Hoover HC: Breast cancer during pregnancy and lactation. *Surg Clin North Am* 70:1151–1163, 1990
221. Barnavon Y, Wallack K: Management of the pregnant patient with carcinoma of the breast. *Surg Gynecol Obstet* 171:347–352, 1990
222. Van der Vange N, van Dongen JA: Breast cancer and pregnancy. *Eur J Surg Oncol* 17:1–8, 1991
223. Petrek JA, Dukoff R, Rogato A: Prognosis of pregnancy-associated breast cancer. *Cancer* 67:869–872, 1990
224. Dow KH (ed.): *Pocket Guide to Breast Cancer* (ed. 2). Sudbury, MA, Jones and Bartlett, 2002, pp 231–255
225. Higgins S, Haffty BG: Pregnancy and lactation after breast-conserving therapy for early stage breast cancer. *Cancer* 73:2175–2180, 1994
226. von Schoultz E, Johansson H, Wilking N, et al: Influence of prior and subsequent pregnancy on breast cancer prognosis. *J Clin Oncol* 13:430–434, 1995
227. Dow KH, Harris JR, Roy C: Pregnancy after breast conserving surgery and radiation therapy for breast cancer. *Monogr Natl Cancer Inst* 16:131–137, 1994
228. Shivvers SA, Miller DS: Preinvasive and invasive breast and cervical cancer prior to or during pregnancy. *Clin Perinatol* 24:369–389, 1997
229. Surbone A, Petrek JA: Childbearing issues in breast carcinoma survivors. *Cancer* 79:1271–1278, 1997
230. Danforth DN: How subsequent pregnancy affects outcome in women with a prior breast cancer. *Oncology* 5:23–35, 1991
231. Collichio FA, Agnello R, Staltzer J: Pregnancy after breast cancer: from psychosocial issues through conception. *Oncology* 12:759–769, 1998
232. Sankila R, Heinavaara S, Hakulinen T: Survival of breast cancer patients after subsequent term pregnancy: ''healthy mother effect.'' *Am J Obstet Gynecol* 170:818–823, 1994
233. Petrek JA: Pregnancy safety after breast cancer. *Cancer* 74:528–531, 1994
234. Johannsson O, Loman N, Borg A, et al: Pregnancy associated breast cancer in BRCA1 and BRCA2 germline mutation carriers. *Lancet* 352:1359–1360, 1998
235. Roberts JA: Management of gynecologic tumors during pregnancy. *Clin Perinatol* 10:369–382, 1983
236. Connor JP: Noninvasive cervical cancer complicating pregnancy. *Obstet Gynecol Clin North Am* 25:331–342, 1998
237. Crane JM: Pregnancy outcome after loop electrosurgical excision: a systematic review. *Obstet Gynecol* 103:1058–1062, 2003
238. Van Rooijen M, Persson E: Pregnancy outcome after laser vaporization of the cervix. *Acta Obstet Gynecol Scand* 78:346–348, 1999
239. Vlahos G, Rodolakis A, Diakomanolis E, et al: Conservative management of cervical intraepithelial neoplasia (CIN (2–3)) in pregnant women. *Gynecol Obstet Invest* 54:78–81, 2002
240. Sood AK, Sorosky JI: Invasive cervical cancer complicating pregnancy. *Obstet Gynecol Clin North Am* 25:343–352, 1998
241. Duggan B, Muderspach LI, Roman LD, et al: Cervical cancer in pregnancy: reporting on planned delay in therapy. *Obstet Gynecol* 82:598–602, 1993
242. Nevin J, Soeters R, Dehaeek K, et al: Cervical carcinoma associated with pregnancy. *Obstet Gynecol Surv* 50:228–239, 1995
243. Sivanesaratnam V, Jayalakshmi P, Loo C: Surgical management of early invasive cancer of the cervix associated with pregnancy. *Gynecol Oncol* 48:68–75, 1993
244. Charkviani L, Charkviani T, Natenadze N, et al: Cervical carcinoma and pregnancy. *Clin Exper Obstet Gynecol* 30:19–22, 2003
245. Bernardini M, Barrett J, Seaward G, et al: Pregnancy outcomes in patients after trachelectomy. *Am J Obstet Gynecol* 189:1378–1382, 2003
246. Cliby WA, Dodson MK, Podratz KC: Cervical cancer complicated by pregnancy: episiotomy site recurrences following vaginal delivery. *Obstet Gynecol* 84:179–183, 1994
247. Goldman NA, Goldberg GL: Late recurrence of squamous cell cervical cancer in an episiotomy site after vaginal delivery. *Obstet Gynecol* 101:1127–1129, 2003
248. Boulay R, Podczaski E: Ovarian cancer complicating pregnancy. *Obstet Gynecol Clin North Am* 25:385–399, 1998
249. Bromley B, Benacerraf B: Adnexal masses during pregnancy: accuracy of sonographic diagnosis and outcome. *J Ultrasound Med* 16:447–452, 1997
250. Grendys EC Jr, Barnes WA: Ovarian cancer in pregnancy. *Surg Clin North Am* 75:1–14, 1995
251. Schilder JM, Thompson AM, DePriest PD, et al: Outcome of reproductive age women with stage IA or IC invasive epithelial ovarian cancer treated with fertility-sparing therapy. *Gynecol Oncol* 87:1–7, 2002
252. King LA, Nevin PC, Williams PP, et al: Treatment of advanced epithelial ovarian cancer in pregnancy with cisplatin-based chemotherapy. *Gynecol Oncol* 41:78–80, 1991
253. Squatrito RC, Harlow SP: Melanoma complicating pregnancy. *Obstet Gynecol Clin North Am* 25:407–416, 1998
254. Teplitzky S, Sabates B, Yu K, et al: Melanoma during pregnancy: a case report and review of the literature. *J LA State Med Soc* 150:539–543, 1998
255. Katz VL, Farmer RM, Dotters D: Focus on primary care: from Nevus to neoplasm: myths of melanoma in pregnancy. *Obstet Gynecol Surv* 57:112–119, 2002
256. Travers RL, Sober AJ, Berwick M, et al: Increased thickness of pregnancy-associated melanoma. *Br J Dermatol* 132:876–883, 1995
257. Slingluff CL, Reintgen DS, Vollmer RT, et al: Malignant melanoma arising during pregnancy: a study of 100 patients. *Ann Surg* 211:552–559, 1990
258. Wong JH, Sterns EE, Kopald KH, et al: Prognostic significance of pregnancy in stage I melanoma. *Arch Surg* 124:1227–1231, 1989
259. Dipaola RS, Goodin S, Ratzell M, et al: Chemotherapy for metastatic melanoma during pregnancy. *Gynecol Oncol* 66:526–530, 1997
260. Nicklas AH, Baker ME: Imaging strategies in the pregnant cancer patient. *Semin Oncol* 27:623–632, 2000
261. Anderson JF, Kent S, Machin GA: Maternal malignant melanoma with placental metastasis: a case report with literature review. *Pediatr Pathol* 9:35–42, 1989
262. Brossard J, Abish S, Bernstein ML, et al: Maternal malignancy involving the products of conception: a report of malignant melanoma and medulloblastoma. *Am J Pediatr Hematol Oncol* 16:380–383, 1994
263. Ferreira CM, Maceira JM, Coelho JM: Melanoma and pregnancy with placental metastases. Report of a case. *Am J Dermatol* 20:403–407, 1998
264. Mackie RM, Bufalino R, Morabito A, et al: Lack of effect of pregnancy on outcome of melanoma. *Lancet* 337:653–655, 1991
265. Ward FT, Weiss RB: Lymphoma in pregnancy. *Adv Oncol* 8:18–22, 1992
266. Kennedy BJ: Hodgkin's disease. *CA Cancer J Clin* 43:325–346, 1993
267. Peleg D, Ben-Ami M: Lymphoma and leukemia complicating pregnancy. *Obstet Gynecol Clin North Am* 25:365–383, 1998
268. Anselmo AP, Cavalieri E, Enrici RM, et al: Hodgkin's disease during pregnancy: diagnostic and therapeutic management. *Fetal Diagn Test* 14:102–195, 1999

269. Gelb AB, van de Rijn M, Wamke RA, et al: Pregnancy-associated lymphomas: a clinicopathologic study. *Cancer* 78:304–310, 1996
270. Meguerian-Bedoyan Z, Lamant L, Hopfner C, et al: Anaplastic large cell lymphoma of maternal origin involving the placenta: case report and literature survey. *Am J Surg Pathol* 21:1236–1241, 1997
271. Ramirez-Smiley M, Ingle B: Leukemia during pregnancy. *Oncol Nurs Forum* 22:1363–1368, 1995
272. Henderson ES: A selected overview, in Gunz FW, Henderson ES (eds.): *Leukemia* (ed 4). Orlando, FL, Grune & Stratton, 1983, pp 785–798
273. Caligiuri MA: Leukemia in pregnancy. *Adv Oncol* 8:10–17, 1992
274. Jenkins TM, Mackey SF, Benzoni EM, et al: Non-obstetric surgery during gestation: risk factors for lower birthweight. *Austral N Zealand J Obstet Gynaecol* 43:27–31, 2003
275. Kawabata I, Takahashi Y, Iwagaki S, et al: MRI during pregnancy. *J Perinatal Med* 31:449–458, 2003
276. Damilakis J, Perisinakis K, Prassopoulos P, et al: Conceptus radiation dose and risk from chest screen-film radiography. *Euro Rad* 13:406–412, 2003
277. Cygler J, Ding GX, Kendal W, et al: Fetal dose for a patient undergoing mantle field irradiation for Hodgkin's disease. *Med Dosim* 22:135–137, 1997
278. Dow KH: Pregnancy and breast cancer. *J Obstet Gynecol Neonatal Nurs* 29:634–640, 2000
279. Kusama TOK: Radiological protection for diagnostic examination of pregnant women. *Congen Anomalies* 42:10–14, 2002
280. Jankowski CB: Radiation and pregnancy: putting the risks in proportion. *Am J Nurs* 86:260–265, 1986
281. Doll DC: Chemotherapy in pregnancy, in Perry MC (ed.): *The Chemotherapy Sourcebook.* Baltimore, Williams & Wilkins, 1992, pp 703–709
282. Leslie KK: Chemotherapy and pregnancy. *Clin Obstet Gynecol* 45:153–164, 2002
283. Tolar J, Neglia JP: Transplacental and other routes of cancer transmission between individuals. *J Pedtr Hematol Oncol* 25:430–434, 2003
284. Dildy GA, Moise KJ, Carpenter RJ, et al: Maternal malignancy metastatic to the products of conception: a review. *Obstet Gynecol Surv* 44:535–540, 1989

PART V

Oncologic Emergencies

CHAPTER 36

Cardiac Tamponade

Roberta Kaplow, RN, PhD, CCNS, CCRN

Scope of the Problem

Definitions

Cardiac tamponade results from an excess accumulation of fluid in the pericardial sac, which presents as a pericardial effusion. This fluid collection increases the hemodynamic pressure around the heart, gradually causing compression of the heart and a diminished flow of blood to the ventricles.[1–3] The net effect is a decrease in cardiac output and impaired cardiac function. The body tries to compensate for the heart's inability to pump by stimulating the sympathetic nervous system, resulting in an increase in myocardial workload. Eventually, compensatory mechanisms fail, which leads to cardiovascular collapse, shock, cardiac arrest, and death.[3] Hence, cardiac tamponade is a life-threatening complication of cancer. It is present when the pericardial effusion evolves into the aforementioned hemodynamic instability and compensatory mechanisms are no longer effective.[1,4]

Incidence

The diagnosis of cardiac tamponade is often missed because many patients with pericardial effusions are asymptomatic.[1] Patients with pericardial effusions are at risk for developing cardiac tamponade if those complications are left untreated due to the increase in pressure in the pericardial space.[1] Malignancies are the most common cause of cardiac tamponade, occurring in as many as 21% of individuals with cancer.[1,3,5,6]

Etiology and Risk Factors

Pericardial effusions develop secondary to malignant involvement of the pericardium by metastatic disease, metastatic disease to the heart, or primary heart malignancies. Malignant involvement of the pericardium by metastatic disease has been reported as a sequela to mesotheliomas, sarcomas, and teratomas. Metastatic disease to the heart occurs with breast and lung cancers, leukemia, and lymphoma. It is seen less often in melanoma, liver, gastric, esophageal, and pancreatic malignancies.[1,3] Lung and breast cancers are the malignancies most commonly associated with the development of cardiac tamponade.[5] When tumors metastasize to the pericardium or myocardium, obstruction of venous and lymphatic drainage occurs and an excess amount of pericardial fluid accumulates, resulting in a pericardial effusion. Cardiac tamponade (hemodynamically significant compression of the heart by pericardial fluid)[2] can also result from constriction of the pericardium by tumor or postradiation pericarditis.[6]

Cardiac tamponade often occurs when a tumor metastasizes to the pericardium or when tumor invades the pericardium from adjoining tissue.[3] Individuals who have received more than 4000 cGy of radiation therapy to the pericardium may also develop cardiac tamponade due to postradiation pericarditis.[3] The incidence of this complication depends on the dose, duration/fractionation of radiation therapy, amount of heart tissue in the radiation field, and radiation sources used.[7] Certain chemotherapeutic agents, such as doxorubicin, daunorubicin, paclitaxel, and docetaxel, may also cause pericardial effusions due to their effects on cardiac tissues.[1,6]

Small effusions usually do not cause signs and symptoms, so patients with cardiac tamponade may be challenging to identify in the early stages of this condition.[3,7,8] Often, clinical manifestations are vague or attributed to other causes. In particular, many of the symptoms associated with the presence of cardiac tamponade are not specific to that disorder and may be related to other unrelated conditions. This uncertainty poses a challenge for the nurse and other members of the healthcare team. Knowing that cardiac tamponade is a potential complication of both the malignant process and cancer treatment enables the nurse to identify the early and subtle changes in a patient's vital signs and clinical status, signaling the need for prompt and aggressive treatment so that the life-threatening complications of cardiac tamponade may be averted.[3]

Physiologic Alterations

Normal Anatomy and Physiology

The pericardium is a thin, double-layered sac surrounding the heart. It protects the heart from friction, infection, and inflammation.[1,3,5] Approximately 50 mL of low-protein fluid in the pericardium helps attain these goals.[1–3,7] This fluid is drained by the lymphatic system into the mediastinum.[3]

Normally, intrapericardial pressure is lower than ventricular diastolic pressure and is equal to pleural pressure. This normal pressure gradient between the heart chambers and the pericardium allows the heart chambers to fill.

Pathophysiology

The amount of fluid surrounding the heart in an individual with pericardial effusion can range from 50 mL to greater than 1 L.[2] As the fluid accumulates, the ventricle's ability to fill during diastole becomes impaired. The degree of pathophysiologic changes that occur depends on how quickly the excess fluid builds up.[7]

When it accumulates gradually, the pericardium has time to compensate for the increased volume before a tamponade (decreased cardiac output) will occur. When fluid accumulates acutely, intrapericardial pressure rises. This increase in pressure accounts for the hemodynamic instability and impaired cardiac function associated with cardiac tamponade.[1,4]

When an excess amount of fluid fills the pericardial sac, the heart is unable to fill during diastole and pump adequately. Right ventricular filling is contingent upon the existence of a gradient between central venous pressure and right ventricular diastolic pressure. The increase in intrapericardial pressure that results from the excess fluid accumulation affects this gradient, such that right ventricular filling cannot be adequately sustained. Decreased right ventricular filling and compression of the right ventricle results in a decrease in blood leaving that chamber. Thus, a smaller amount of blood enters, and leaves, the left side of the heart.[9] The compression also causes an increase in intracardiac diastolic pressures on the right and left sides of the heart as well as equalization of filling pressures in each of the heart chambers.[4,7,10]

Hence, the development of cardiac tamponade from a pericardial effusion is based on the compliance of the pericardium, the rate of accumulation of fluid, and the amount of fluid that accumulates.[4,10] If the fluid accumulates slowly, the pericardium will expand to accommodate the excess fluid[4] as the body attempts to compensate for this change.

Compensatory mechanisms include an increased production of endogenous catecholamines from the sympathetic nervous system.[10] Catecholamine production results in tachycardia, increased contractility, and increased peripheral vasoconstriction of the arterial and venous beds. If the tamponade is severe, compensatory mechanisms include an increase in systemic vascular resistance — the amount of work the heart has to do to eject blood.[10,11] If rapid fluid accumulation occurs, the pericardium will not stretch,[4] compensatory mechanisms cannot be activated, and hemodynamic instability ensues.

Clinical Manifestations

The signs and symptoms of cardiac tamponade are variable and depend on the rate and amount of pericardial fluid accumulation and the individual's underlying cardiovascular function.[1–3,6,8] A summary of the signs and symptoms appears in Tables 36–1a and 36–1b. If fluid accumulation occurs slowly, signs and symptoms may include fatigue, shortness of breath, nausea, vomiting, diarrhea, hepatomegaly, and abdominal distention.[6] As the amount of fluid increases, cardiovascular signs and symptoms become more prominent. One of the earliest noted is an elevation in central venous pressure, which results from the increase in intrapericardial pressure caused by the fluid accumulation.[6] Elevation in central venous pressure may be indicated by neck vein distention. Ordinarily, when a person inspires, there is a decrease in intrathoracic pressure with a resultant increase in blood return to the heart and collapse of neck veins. When an individual has cardiac tamponade, blood cannot return to the heart and neck vein distention occurs.[12]

Other signs and symptoms of increased fluid accumulation in the pericardial space include the presence of distant or muffled heart sounds, decreased or absent apical pulse, and decreased cardiac output.[2,6] Distant or muffled heart sounds are the result of fluid surrounding and compressing the heart.

If fluid accumulation is rapid, the body does not have time to develop compensatory mechanisms. The resultant clinical signs include an increase in ventricular diastolic and pulmonary venous pressures, and a decrease in stroke volume (the amount of blood ejected by the heart with each beat), cardiac output, and arterial blood pressure. These signs of hemodynamic compromise are accompanied by tachypnea, dyspnea, and orthopnea. Other signs with which the individual will present include hypotension and tachycardia.[6]

Tachypnea and dyspnea on exertion can progress to air hunger at rest. This evolution is, in part, due to an increase in lung stiffness.[10] Tachypnea may also follow from the decrease in cardiac output and resultant hypoxia. Cyanosis results from the decrease in venous return and venous hypertension. No adventitious sounds are audible with the disorder, as no pulmonary congestion is present. However, a patient may present with a pericardial friction rub if a tumor is present or if the patient has an inflammatory effusion.[1,4,6]

Individuals with cardiac tamponade often have a pulsus paradoxus — that is, a decrease in systolic arterial blood pressure of greater than 10 mm Hg during inspiration.[1,4,6] The etiology of pulsus paradoxus is believed to be due to impaired cardiac filling, and this condition should be suspected when a palpated pulse decreases in intensity or disappears upon inspiration.[10] It is important to remember that pulsus paradoxus, like other signs and symptoms of cardiac tamponade, is not specific to tamponade. It can also be found in patients with chronic obstructive pulmonary disease, pulmonary embolism, right ventricular infarction, extreme obesity, constrictive pericarditis, and restrictive cardiomyopathy.[2,11]

To measure the extent of a pulsus paradoxus, the blood pressure cuff should be inflated above the level of the individual's systolic pressure and deflated at a rate of 3 mm Hg/second. The first systolic pressure

Table 36-1a Cardiac Tamponade: Clinical Presentation and Pathologic Response

Pathology	Clinical Presentation: Signs and Symptoms	Pathophysiology and Compensatory Mechanism
Decrease in cardiac output	Tachycardia	Increased heart rate is associated with a decrease in cardiac output (sympathetic nervous system stimulation as a compensatory mechanism).
	Peripheral vasoconstriction causing cyanosis	Blood is shunted from the peripheral circulation to supply vital organs (due to decreased venous return).
	Decreased urinary output (oliguria or anuria)	Decreased renal perfusion.
	Narrowing pulse pressure, hypotension, increased systemic vascular resistance	Systolic pressure falls as cardiac output decreases; arteries constrict to maintain perfusion.
	Pulsus paradoxus	With inspiration, the diaphragm compresses the pericardial sac. The left ventricle receives less blood and cardiac output is reduced, causing a decrease in systolic blood pressure on inspiration (impaired cardiac filling).
	Anxiety, restlessness, confusion, mental status changes, dizziness, lightheadedness, agitation, fatigue	Cerebral anoxia due to inadequate perfusion.
	Symptoms of shock	Cardiac decompensation. Compensatory mechanisms have been exhausted/failed.
	Dyspnea, tachypnea, orthopnea, shortness of breath, air hunger	Hemodynamic changes/instability and decreased cardiac output result in hypoxia.
	Weakness, fatigue, cool extremities	Decreased cardiac output causes decreased peripheral perfusion, visceral congestion, venous stasis, and hepatic and visceral congestion.
Compression of heart and structures in chest	Dysphagia, cough, retrosternal chest pain and heaviness, hoarseness, hiccups	Fluid collection around heart compresses the trachea, esophagus, and adjacent nerves and bronchi.
Venous congestion	Peripheral edema, jugular venous distention	With decrease in ventricular filling, venous return is reduced, causing vascular congestion.
Distention and filling of pericardial sac	Dullness to percussion, weak heart sounds, chest fullness/discomfort	With decrease in ventricular filling, venous return is reduced, causing vascular congestion.
Increase in central venous pressure	Nausea, vomiting, diarrhea, hepatojugular reflux, hepatomegaly, abdominal distention	Increase in pericardial pressure causes increase in central venous pressure.

reading heard only during exhalation should be noted. This sound disappears upon inspiration. The systolic pressure reading that is audible during both inspiration and exhalation is then noted. If the difference between the two systolic pressure sounds is greater than 10 mm Hg, the individual has a pulsus paradoxus.[7,13]

As the cardiac tamponade increases, stroke volume continues to decrease, systemic vascular resistance increases, systolic blood pressure falls, diastolic blood pressure increases, and pulse pressure (the difference between the systolic and diastolic blood pressures) narrows. The "classic" signs of cardiac tamponade — distant heart sounds, hypotension, and increased jugular venous distention — constitute "Beck's triad."[2,11] It has been reported, however, that most patients with cardiac tamponade do not manifest this combination of symptoms.[11]

Individuals with cardiac tamponade may also present with mental status changes, anxiety, dizziness, lightheadedness, and agitation. These signs and symptoms result from the hemodynamic instability and decreased cardiac output and hypoxia.[3] Individuals may also exhibit hepatojugular reflux, an increase in jugular venous pressure of 1 cm Hg or more.[7] To determine whether hepatojugular reflux is present, the individual is placed in a supine position with the head of the bed elevated so that jugular venous palpations are discernible. Pressure is exerted for 30–60 seconds over the right upper quadrant of the abdomen. The test is positive if an elevation in the jugular venous pressure occurs. Such a result is due to the elevation of central venous pressure. Gastrointestinal side effects may include nausea and vomiting due to visceral congestion and venous stasis.[3]

Prolonged periods of hypotension cause hypoperfusion to the kidneys, which can result in oliguria or anuria.[6] Prolonged hypotension and decreased cardiac output may also result in decreased peripheral perfusion, which may be manifested as weakness, fatigue, dyspnea, and cool, clammy extremities.[3,5,6] Other findings may include apprehension, cough, hiccups, hoarseness, and dysphagia.[1,3,6] The latter four symptoms are thought to be related to compression of the

Table 36-1b Cardiac Tamponade: Symptoms Based on Rate of Fluid Accumulation

Gradual Accumulation of Fluid	Acute Accumulation of Fluid
Tachycardia	Hemodynamic instability
Increased cardiac contractility	Impaired cardiac function
Increased peripheral vasoconstriction of arterial and venous beds	Chest pain or heaviness
Fatigue	Increased ventricular diastolic and pulmonary venous pressures
Shortness of breath	Decreased stroke volume
Nausea	Decreased cardiac output
Vomiting	Hypotension
Diarrhea	Tachypnea
Hepatomegaly	Dyspnea
Abdominal distention	Orthopnea
	Tachycardia
	Cyanosis
As Fluid Increases	**As Fluid Increases**
Increased central venous pressure	Increased systemic vascular resistance
Neck vein distention	Narrowing pulse pressure
Distant, muffled heart sounds	
Diminished or absent apical pulse	
Decreased cardiac output	
	If Hypotension Is Prolonged
	Oliguria or anuria
	Weakness
	Fatigue
	Increased dyspnea
	Cool and clammy extremities
	Hepatojugular reflux
	Mental status changes
	Apprehension
	Cough
	Hiccups
	Hoarseness
	Dysphagia

esophageal and tracheal nerves and bronchi.[2,3,6] Individuals may also develop chest pain or heaviness if fluid accumulation is large or rapid.[1,3] Chest pain is enhanced when the patient is supine but decreases when the patient leans forward because of compression of the heart.[3]

Less common signs and symptoms include peripheral edema, low-grade fever, pallor, increased jugular venous pressure, hepatomegaly, abdominal distention, abdominal pain, and nausea.[1,6,14] The latter two symptoms are believed to be due to hepatic and intestinal congestion.[1,6]

Assessment and Grading

Physical Exam

Any of the aforementioned clinical manifestations may be noted on physical exam, depending on the rate of accumulation of the fluid, the amount of fluid accumulated, and the baseline cardiac function of the individual. (See Figure 36–1, Clinical Pathway for Cardiac Tamponade). Conversely, assessment for physical findings alone is not adequate, as patients may be asymptomatic.[11]

Diagnostic Tests

Several tests and procedures aid in the diagnosis of cardiac tamponade. These include echocardiography, chest radiograph, computerized tomography (CT) scan, magnetic resonance imaging (MRI), pulmonary artery catheterization, electrocardiogram, and pericardiocentesis with pericardial fluid evaluation.

Echocardiography. Echocardiography is the most sensitive and precise method for the diagnosis of cardiac tamponade. It is considered the "gold standard" for diagnosis.[8] During an echocardiogram, ultrasonic waves are produced via a probe.[3] These waves create a picture of the heart and can depict heart functioning. An echocardiogram will reveal fluid in the pericardial sac, compression of the right ventricular free wall during early diastole, inspiratory changes in ventricular size, and collapse of the right atrial and ventricular

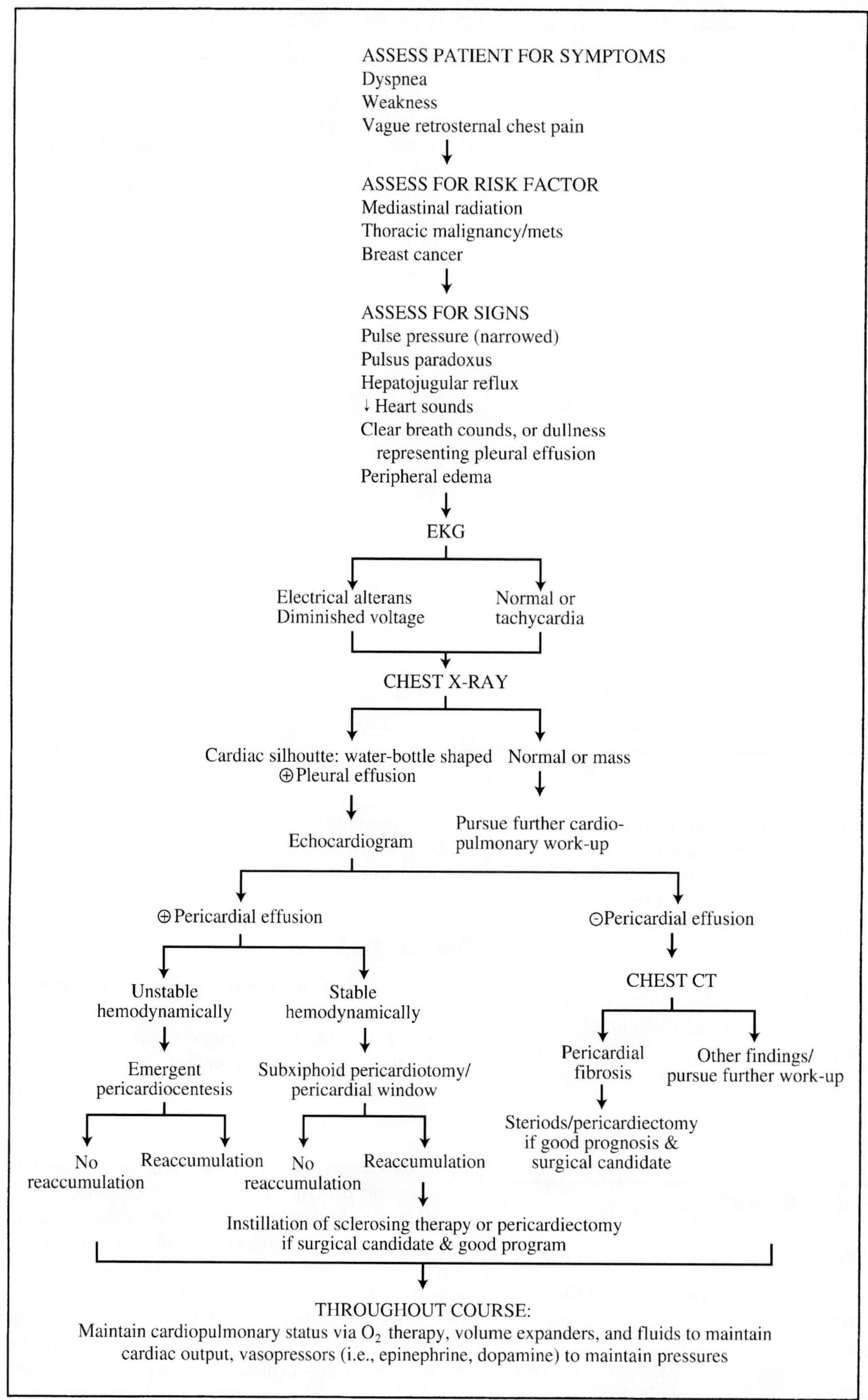

Figure 36-1 Clinical pathway for cardiac tamponade.

free walls during diastole in individuals with cardiac tamponade.[7] Because the right side of the heart contains less myocardium than the left side, the pressure being exerted by the pericardial fluid can cause the right side to collapse.

In addition to pericardial fluid, an echocardiogram will reveal a low ejection fraction and, possibly, a pericardial mass. Quantification of the pericardial fluid is also possible.[7] Similarly, echocardiography may prove helpful in the assessment of hemodynamic effects of the tamponade.[13] A two-dimensional echocardiography is useful for the detection of fluid as well as for selecting the appropriate site at which to perform a pericardiocentesis.

Radiograph. Chest radiograph is not a definitive diagnostic method for cardiac tamponade, because fluid may not appear radiographically if the effusion is small. Nevertheless, cardiac tamponade may be suspected if the chest radiograph reveals an enlarged heart, increased mediastinal width, and dilated cardiac silhouette. The cardiac silhouette will appear enlarged only after at least 200–250 mL of pericardial fluid has accumulated.[2,5,7] In affected patients, it may have the appearance of a "water bottle heart." Lung fields are usually clear in individuals with cardiac tamponade unless pulmonary disease is present.[10] A confirmation of the diagnosis must be made with either echocardiography, ultrasound, MRI, or CT scan. Each of these imaging techniques can show fluid in the pericardium better than an ordinary radiographic study.

Computerized tomography. A CT scan may indicate the presence of a cardiac tamponade, and it is useful for determining the pericardial thickness and presence of a pleural effusion or masses.[7] It will reveal large effusions and provide an estimate of the volume of the effusion.[1] As a diagnostic test, however, a CT scan has limited usefulness.[6,8,15] For example, a CT scan will provide no data regarding cardiac functioning in the presence of a tamponade[6] and is not as readily available as echocardiography.[4]

Magnetic resonance imaging. Magnetic resonance imaging also has limited usefulness in the diagnosis of cardiac tamponade. While MRI does afford the clinician a more defined view of the myocardium compared to CT, it offers no benefit over echocardiography.[4,8,15] It will reveal large effusions and provide an estimate of the volume of the effusion[1] and detect small and large effusions, masses, and pericardial thickening.[1,3,7] Results may have limited value in patients with dysrhythmias.[5]

Pulmonary artery catheterization. Insertion of a pulmonary artery catheter will reveal equalization of right- and left-sided heart pressures and a decrease in cardiac output.[6] Right atrial mean, right ventricular diastolic, and pulmonary artery wedge pressures equalize in individuals with cardiac tamponade. Hemodynamic changes include decreased pulse pressure, tachycardia, increased systemic vascular resistance, increased central venous pressure, increased left atrial pressure, increased pulmonary artery pressures, increased pulmonary artery occlusive pressure (wedge pressure), decreased blood pressure, and decreased cardiac output. As insertion of a pulmonary artery catheter is invasive and not without associated complications, this step is rarely indicated given that echocardiography is a reliable, noninvasive diagnostic method.[6]

Electrocardiography. Findings on electrocardiogram are nonspecific. Those findings consistent with the diagnosis of cardiac tamponade include presence of sinus tachycardia, premature contractions, changes in shape and amplitude of the P wave, low-voltage QRS complexes, T waves, and electrical alternans. The decrease in voltage of the complexes may be the result of the fluid in the pericardium compressing the heart. ST-segment elevation or depression may be present and will depend on the cardiac lead being viewed. The ST-segment elevation and T-wave changes may be due to inflammation.[1,6,8,10] Electrical alternans — a change in the direction and amplitude of the QRS complex and T wave — is usually seen with every other beat. It may result from changes in cardiac position during depolarization or the heart "swinging" or moving within the pericardial sac.[1,2]

Another sequela to cardiac tamponade is pulseless electrical activity. It will be manifested as the presence of electrical activity on electrocardiogram in the absence of a detectable pulse.

Pericardial fluid evaluation. To determine whether a pericardial effusion is malignant in nature, a pericardiocentesis may be performed in individuals with a large effusion. Pericardial fluid that is aspirated via this procedure is sent to the lab for analysis to determine whether the fluid is a transudate or an exudate. Malignant effusions are usually exudates and contain debris from sloughed cancer cells.[3] The procedure is usually done under echocardiography guidance so as to minimize the risk of complications such as cardiac puncture, ventricular tachycardia, or tension pneumothorax. The fluid is sent to the lab for cytology, lactic dehydrogenase (LDH), glucose, cell count, and protein levels. In addition, the specific gravity of the fluid will be measured, and the fluid will be cultured for the presence of bacteria or fungi.[1] Malignant effusions may appear bloody, serosanguinous, or serous as opposed to straw-colored, normal pericardial fluid.[1,3]

Grading

The World Health Organization has developed a grading system for acute and chronic toxicities of different body systems. The grading system has five levels (Grades 0–4):

- Grade 0: No change
- Grade 1: Asymptomatic, but have an abnormal cardiac sign
- Grade 2: Transient asymptomatic dysfunction, but no therapy is required
- Grade 3: Symptomatic dysfunction responsive to therapy
- Grade 4: Symptomatic dysfunction non-responsive to therapy

Therapeutic Approaches and Nursing Care

Prevention

A preventive measure for cardiac tamponade is successful treatment of the underlying malignancy. Treatment of the underlying cause may prevent reaccumulation of fluid. Long-term therapeutic interventions include instillation of a sclerosing agent, insertion of a pericardial window, and pericardiectomy.[12]

Management

Several therapeutic approaches are available to treat pericardial effusions and subsequent cardiac tamponade. Factors that are considered in selecting an intervention include the individual's presenting symptoms, the etiology of the tamponade, and the patient's level of stability.[2]

Individuals may require stabilization of their hemodynamic status prior to initiation of any other therapeutic intervention.[2] Regardless of the therapeutic approach selected, the goals of therapy include enhancing cardiac function, removing pericardial fluid, preventing its reaccumulation, and minimizing complications.[7] Ongoing monitoring by the nurse should include assessment for and recognition of subtle changes in the patient's clinical status, monitoring of vital signs, monitoring for the presence of a pulsus paradoxus, assessment of intake and output, and electrocardiographic monitoring.[3] These indicators are essential, as a patient's level of stability is a primary factor in determining which and when treatment procedures are performed. In reference to age differences and management strategies, there is no reported difference in etiology, clinical course, and prognosis between elderly and younger patients with moderate to large pericardial effusions. It is, therefore, suggested that management be similar in different age groups.[16]

Supportive care

Prior to treatment for cardiac tamponade, individuals can be stabilized with oxygen to reduce cardiac workload, anxiety, and respiratory distress; with aggressive fluid volume resuscitation; and with administration of inotropic agents to enhance cardiac output and prevent cardiovascular collapse.[6,7,9,10] Administration of intravenous fluids such as crystalloids (e.g., normal saline), blood, or plasma will increase ventricular filling (preload) and cardiac output.[3,6,7,9] Attainment of a systolic blood pressure of 90 mm Hg or higher will improve ventricular filling pressure. Titration of inotropic agents such as dopamine, norepinephrine, or dobutamine, all of which stimulate $beta_1$ receptors, may be employed to enhance contractility and cardiac output.[10] Logically, then, use of beta blockers should be avoided.

Agents that stimulate alpha-receptors, thereby causing vasoconstriction, will increase the amount of work the heart must do to eject blood and decrease cardiac output. Conversely, use of arterial vasodilators such as nitroprusside will decrease the amount of work the heart must do to eject blood and may help increase blood pressure.[10] Administration of diuretics will decrease circulating volume, thereby decreasing ventricular filling; for this reason, these agents should not be given.[6] Use of positive-pressure ventilation should, ideally, be avoided, as it is associated with an increase in intrathoracic pressure and subsequent decrease in cardiac output.[4,10] Maintaining the individual on bed rest in semi-Fowler's position may be helpful, as it further decreases cardiac workload.

Pericardiocentesis

Echocardiogram-guided paracentesis is considered the best initial treatment for cardiac tamponade.[4,10] Pericardiocentesis — removal of fluid from the pericardial sac — is also the approach most commonly used for management of cardiac tamponade.[7] It relieves the increased end diastolic pressure and decreased ventricular filling. Improvement in clinical status is usually seen after as little as 25–50 mL of fluid is removed.

200–400 Gy can be delivered to the heart, pericardial structures, and lower mediastinum.[1] For this reason, radiotherapy may be recommended for the individual with lymphoma or leukemia who has not received radiotherapy in the past[1] and who is hemodynamically stable.

Nursing care of individuals receiving systemic chemotherapy and radiotherapy for cardiac tamponade includes providing patient education materials to facilitate the decision-making process regarding treatment options and specific information related to antineoplastic toxicities.

Continuity of Care

Management of an individual with cardiac tamponade poses several challenges for the nurse. Such care encompasses assessment and management of physiologic alterations, psychosocial support, and individual and family education. Patients may need referral for home nursing services or hospice, depending on their symptomatology and disease status.[3]

Assessment

Ongoing assessments must be performed to detect pericardial fluid accumulation.[1] According to some reports, as many as 12% of patients experience reaccumulation of fluid after treatment.[1] Any signs and symptoms suggestive of reaccumulation should be investigated immediately.[3] This effort may include assessment for presence of hepatojugular reflux and measurement of abdominal girth to detect ascites.[3] Monitoring for the presence of edema, intake and output status, amount of catheter drainage, and presence of oliguria or anuria are important.[3,6] Identification of patients at risk for initial and subsequent development of cardiac tamponade as well as the performance of a complete review of systems can help assure prompt identification of patients and prevent lift-threatening sequelae.[3] Postprocedure wound assessments must also be performed, whether in the home, the ambulatory setting, or the hospital.[12]

Physiologic management

Nursing care associated with cardiac tamponade therapy includes ongoing assessment: monitoring of vital signs, respiratory, hemodynamic, and cardiovascular status; positioning; administration of supportive therapies; premedications; and ECG monitoring.[3] In addition, following any therapeutic intervention, nursing management encompasses monitoring for signs and symptoms of any specific complications related to the procedure. Pain management and catheter care will be indicated.[3] Physiologic management also entails administration of oxygen, intravenous therapy, and inotropic agents, as clinically indicated.[1]

Psychosocial support

Cardiac tamponade is a life-threatening oncologic emergency that can cause anxiety for both the patient and his or her family. This distress may be related to the significance of the presence of the tamponade with respect to disease progression or complications of treatment. In such cases, emotional support is pivotal.[7] Once fluid has accumulated and interventions are required, this kind of support must be provided to combat the fear and anxiety associated with experiencing a life-threatening emergency.[6] The acute onset of the signs and symptoms as well as the need for possible admission to a critical care unit are other sources of anxiety.

Providing an explanation of anticipated interventions and allowing the individual to verbalize concerns are essential. In addition to the reduction in psychosocial distress, emotional support may result in a concomitant decrease in cardiac workload. As part of their patient care management, nurses should assess for signs of ineffective coping and depression.[3]

Patient and family education

Patients should be prepared for the procedures they will be undergoing as treatment for the cardiac tamponade. An explanation of the sensations they will be feeling during and after the procedure may help allay some of the anxiety associated with this complication. Both patients and families must be educated about signs and symptoms of recurrence and actions to take in the event of recurrence.[6] Early intervention is crucial in trying to decrease complications and improving individual outcomes. Educational endeavors should also include information about the diagnostic and therapeutic interventions that the individual will be experiencing.[7] Other educational efforts should focus on signs and symptoms and complications to observe for and report once the patient has been discharged from the hospital.[3]

Nursing care

In addition to the nursing care delineated for the specific therapeutic interventions, several nursing diagnoses can be derived for the individual with a cardiac tamponade. A plan of care addressing the diagnoses appears in Table 36–3.

Table 36-3 Cardiac Tamponade: Nursing Care

Decreased cardiac output r/t decreased ventricular filling

Expected outcome:	Individual's cardiac output will return to within normal limits.
Interventions:	Assess for signs and symptoms of decreased cardiac output: Decreased blood pressure Increased heart rate Decreased level of consciousness Cool, pale, and clammy skin Decreased urine output (less than 0.5 mL/kg/hr) Faint or absent peripheral pulses Distant or muffled heart sounds Weakness Dizziness Shortness of breath
	Assess for signs and symptoms of cardiac tamponade.
	Monitor vital signs and hemodynamic parameters (blood pressure, heart rate, respiratory rate, central venous pressure, pulmonary artery pressures) and O_2 saturation hourly and PRN.
	Auscultate breath sounds q4h and PRN.
	Hourly I/O.
	Assess cardiac rhythm and ECG tracings for electrical alternans, dysrhythmias, and changes.
	Administer aggressive fluid therapy and vasoactive agents, as prescribed.
	Administer supplemental oxygen as prescribed.
	Assist individual to assume a position of comfort.

Alteration in tissue perfusion r/t decreased cardiac output

Expected outcome:	Individual will attain and maintain normal tissue perfusion.
Interventions:	Assess for signs and symptoms of altered tissue perfusion: Cool skin Altered mental status Increased capillary refill time
	Monitor ABG results for acid–base imbalance.
	Administer supplemental oxygen as prescribed.

Impaired gas exchange r/t pericardial effusions (compensation by respiratory system for change in cardiac output could lead to impaired gas exchange)

Expected outcome:	Individual will maintain adequate gas exchange.
Interventions:	Assess for signs and symptoms of impaired gas exchange: Mental status changes Tachypnea Tachycardia or bradycardia Dyspnea Orthopnea Use of accessory muscles Presence of adventitious breath sounds Activity tolerance SPO_2 levels
	Monitor ABG results.
	Administer supplemental oxygen, as prescribed.
	Monitor vital signs hourly and PRN.
	Auscultate breath sounds q4h and PRN.
	Provide measures to minimize anxiety (e.g., anxiolytics, calm environment, relaxation techniques).
	Assist to assume a position of comfort (e.g., semi-Fowler's).
	Plan activities to allow for frequent rest periods.

(continued)

Table 36-3 Cardiac Tamponade: Nursing Care (continued)

Potential for infection r/t procedure and antineoplastic therapy	
Expected outcome:	Individual will not develop infection related to invasive procedures or antineoplastic therapy.
Interventions:	Assess for signs and symptoms of infection: Fever Tachycardia Tachypnea Increased WBCs Redness or discharge from catheter sites Positive blood culture results
	Maintain aseptic or sterile technique with all indwelling catheters according to institutional policy and procedure.
	Administer antibiotic therapy as prescribed.
	Perform sterile dressing changes to catheter sites according to institutional policy and procedure.
Anxiety r/t procedure, symptoms, and onset of critical illness compounding a cancer diagnosis and lack of information	
Expected outcome:	Individual will verbalize a decrease in anxiety related to presence of symptoms and potential treatment modalities.
Interventions:	Assess patient's degree of anxiety by observing behavioral manifestations and listening for verbal cues.
	Encourage patient to verbalize feelings.
	Explain all procedures and rationale for symptoms to individual, and clarify misconceptions.
	Allow time for individual and significant other to ask questions.
	Anticipate that information may need to be reinforced.
	Administer anxiolytics for treatment modalities, as prescribed.
Lack of knowledge r/t procedures and possible symptoms	
Expected outcomes:	Individual will verbalize an increase in knowledge of symptoms and treatment modalities.
	Individual will verbalize the signs and symptoms to report.
Interventions:	Explain all procedures and rationale for symptoms to individual.
	Allow time for individual and significant other to ask questions.
	Assess individual understanding of information; reinforce as needed.
	Provide written education information when preparing for discharge (e.g., signs and symptoms of reaccumulation of fluid and actions to take).

$SPO_2 = PO_2$ saturation.

Conclusion

No one therapeutic intervention is preferred in the management of cardiac tamponade. The decision is based on numerous factors, including the individual's disease type and clinical status. Prompt and accurate nursing recognition and knowledge of the etiology, signs and symptoms, pathophysiology, and management of the problem are essential to decrease the morbidity and mortality associated with this oncologic emergency.[3]

References

1. Camp-Sorrell D: Cardiac tamponade, in Gates RA, Fink RM (eds.): *Oncology Nursing Secrets*. Philadelphia, Hanley & Belfus, 2001, pp 446–448
2. Hawley J, Dreher H, Vasso M: Under pressure: treating cardiac tamponade. *Nurs Manage* 34:44D, 44F, 44H, 2003
3. Flounders JA: Cardiovascular emergencies: pericardial effusion and cardiac tamponade. *Oncol Nurs Forum* 30:E48–E55, 2003
4. Spodick DH: Current concepts: acute cardiac tamponade. *N Engl J Med* 349:684–690, 2003
5. Valley VT, Fly CA: Pericarditis and cardiac tamponade. *EMedicine Journal* 2, *www.emedicine.com*. Accessed December 8, 2003
6. Reid-Finlay M, Kaplow R: Oncologic emergencies, in Schell H, Puntillo K (eds.): *Critical Care Nursing Secrets*. Philadelphia, Hanley & Belfus, 2001, pp 216–225
7. Knoop T, Willenberg K: Cardiac tamponade. *Semin Oncol Nurs* 15:244–255, 1999
8. van Steijn JH, Sleijfer DT, van der Graaf WT, et al: How to diagnose cardiac tamponade. *Neth J Med* 60:334–338, 2002
9. Bullock BL: Altered cardiac function, in Bullock BL, Henze RL (eds.): *Focus on Pathophysiology*. Philadelphia, Lippincott, Williams and Wilkins, 2000, pp 455–502
10. Spodick DH: Pericardial diseases, in Braunwald E, Zipes DP, Libby P (eds.): *Heart Disease. A Textbook of Cardiovascular Medicine*. Philadelphia, W.B. Saunders, 2001, pp 1823–1876

11. Tsang TSM, Oh JK, Seward JB: Diagnosis and management of cardiac tamponade in the era of echocardiography. *Clin Cardiol.* 22:446–452, 1999
12. Kaplow R: Cardiac tamponade, in Yarbro CH, Frogge MH, Goodman M, Groenwald SL (eds.): *Cancer Nursing Principles and Practice.* Sudbury, MA, Jones and Bartlett, 2000, pp 857–868
13. Keefe DL: Cardiovascular emergencies in the cancer patient. *Semin Oncol* 27:244–255, 2000
14. Au J: Role of surgical intervention, in McConachie I, Roberts DH (eds.): *Handbook of Cardiac Emergencies.* London, Greenwich Medical Media, 2000, pp 221–234
15. Sagrista SJ: Clinical decision making based on cardiac diagnostic imaging techniques. Diagnosis and therapeutic management of patients with cardiac tamponade. *Revista Espanola de Cardiologia* 56:195–205, 2003
16. Sagrista MJ, Permanyer MG, Carballo J, et al: Pericardial effusion in the elderly: a different disease? *Revista Espanola de Cardiologia* 53:1432–1436, 2000

CHAPTER 37

Disseminated Intravascular Coagulation

Barbara Holmes Gobel, RN, MS, AOCN®

Scope of the Problem

Definitions

Disseminated intravascular coagulation (DIC) is the most common serious thrombotic state that occurs in individuals with cancer. DIC represents an inappropriate and exaggerated overstimulation of normal coagulation, in which thrombosis and then hemorrhage occurs. This seemingly paradoxical situation results in hypercoagulation, in which multiple small clots are formed in the microcirculation of many organs, and fibrinolysis, in which there is consumption of clots and clotting factors. Ultimately the body becomes unable to respond to vascular or tissue injury through stable clot formation, and hemorrhage occurs. The hemorrhage associated with DIC may be profound, but it is the intravascular coagulation that leads to irreversible morbidity and mortality in this population of patients.[1] The resulting thrombosis of DIC leads to ischemia, impairment of blood flow, and end-organ damage.[1]

DIC can be chronic or acute in nature. If only a minor imbalance is present related to the intravascular coagulation, the syndrome may be chronic. Chronic DIC generally presents as localized thrombotic events, for example, deep-vein thrombosis. Acute DIC, which can be life-threatening, occurs when the intravascular coagulation becomes overwhelming to the body. Acute DIC is seen in certain defined clinical situations such as sepsis, acute leukemia, and tumor lysis. This chapter will deal with the acute form of DIC.

Incidence

Although DIC is considered to be a problem commonly associated with malignancy, its incidence is difficult to estimate as it varies depending on the type of associated neoplasm and concomittant disorders (e.g., sepsis). Abnormal blood coagulation studies that demonstrate laboratory evidence of DIC are frequently reported in patients with disseminated solid malignancies (particularly the adenocarcinomas) and leukemia (particularly acute promyelocytic leukemia [APL]).[2–5] DIC is estimated to occur in 10% of all patients with solid tumor malignancies,[5] and in as many as 85% of patients with APL.[2] Although clinical bleeding is the predominant finding in APL, disseminated thrombosis is found at autopsy in some patients.[6]

Etiology and Risk Factors

DIC in the cancer population is always secondary to either the malignancy itself or to an underlying condition such as infection. Table 37-1 lists common causes of DIC in cancer. The most common cancers associated with acute DIC include acute leukemia and the mucin-producing adenocarcinomas.

Table 37-1 Common Causes of DIC in Cancer

Neoplasms
- Solid tumors — lung, breast, ovary, renal, stomach, pancreas, prostate, melanoma, gallbladder
- Leukemia — acute promyelocytic, acute myelogenous, chronic myelogenous, acute lymphoblastic

Infections
- Gram-negative bacteria — meningococcus, pseudomonas, salmonella, hemophilus, enterobacteriaceae
- Gram-positive bacteria — pneumococcus, staphylococcus, hemolytic streptococci
- Viremias — hepatitis, varicella, cytomegalovirus, human immunodeficiency virus
- Septic shock

Liver Disease
- Obstructive jaundice
- Fulminant hepatic failure

Intravascular Hemorrhage
- Acute hemolytic transfusion reaction
- Multiple transfusions of whole blood
- Minor hemolysis

Prosthetic Devices
- Peritoneovenous shunts

APL is the malignancy most commonly associated with DIC. DIC associated with APL can occur before and in conjunction with chemotherapy administration. A procoagulant substance has been identified on the promyelocytic blast cells that is similar to thromboplastin. This substance is believed to initiate the clotting response.[7] APL cells also contain an abnormally high level of annexin II. This phospholipid-binding protein is found on the surface of endothilial cells and serves to bind plasminogen and its activator, tPA.[8] Increased levels of annexin II lead to increased production of plasmin, with resultant bleeding from unopposed fibrinolysis.[9] It is important to note that with the use of new antileukemic drugs and the use of antifibrinolytic medications (to prevent bleeding), the mortality rate associated with APL has decreased significantly. One of the antifibrinolytic agents that has shown great promise in the reduction of bleeding during treatment of APL is tretinoin (Vesanoid® all-*trans*-retinoic acid).[4]

The solid tumors that are most commonly associated with DIC are the adenocarcinomas, including those of the lung, breast, stomach, pancreas, and prostate. Of these solid tumors, breast and prostate cancers are probably the most commonly seen DIC-related cancers.[10] (The incidence of these cancers is significantly higher than the incidence of APL.) In addition to an unidentified procoagulant substance thought to be released from these cancers directly stimulating the coagulation system, tumors may release necrotic tissue or tissue enzymes into the circulation, thereby activating the coagulation mechanism.[11]

Infection and sepsis associated with cancer are the most common causes of acute DIC, and can be associated with a variety of bacterial, fungal, and viral infections. Sepsis, especially from meningococcemia and other gram-negative bacteria, is the most frequent cause of DIC. In fact, DIC may occur in 30%–50% of patients with sepsis.[12] It is believed that bacterial endotoxins released from gram-negative bacteremia activate one of the clotting factors (factor XII) of the clotting cascade; this factor can initiate coagulation as well as stimulate fibrinolysis (the breakdown of clots), thus setting up DIC. Gram-positive organisms are thought to initiate coagulation by the same mechanism as endotoxins.[1] The triggering mechanism associated with viruses, including varicella, hepatitis, cytomegalovirus (CMV), or human immunodeficiency virus (HIV) is unclear. Antibiotic therapy can also initiate DIC. Antibiotic therapy may alter intestinal flora, which is a source of vitamin K, thereby altering the coagulation process.[13]

Primary liver disease, liver metastasis, or liver damage due to chemotherapy or radiation therapy can increase the risk of DIC. The liver replaces clotting factors and inhibitors as they are consumed. The liver also clears activated coagulation factors and fibrinolytic degradation products from the systemic circulation. Hepatic failure then disrupts the normal balance of coagulation, which can lead to DIC.[1]

Hemolytic transfusion reactions may be complicated by shock, renal failure, and DIC with severe bleeding. These reactions are probably due to generalized endothelial injury caused by activated complement, cytokines, and neutrophil products occuring during acute hemolytic transfusion reactions.[1] DIC may also occur after massive transfusions, but its etiology is unknown.

Prosthetic devices, such as a peritoneovenous shunt, are used to shunt ascitic fluid into the systemic circulation. Ascitic fluid contains collagen and other procoagulant substances. When these substances are shunted into the general circulation, DIC can be triggered.[14]

Physiologic Alterations

Pathophysiology

Although DIC is triggered by a number of defined clinical events such as infection or the malignancy itself, once initiated the pathophysiology is similar in all disorders. When one of these events occurs, the coagulation system is activated, thus activating thrombin and eventually activating the fibrinolytic system with the production of plasmin.[12] As discussed in Chapter 29 on Bleeding Disorders, in which there is a thorough discussion of the physiology of coagulation, thrombin is the central proteolytic enzyme of blood coagulation. The presence of thrombin is also necessary for the breakdown of clots, or fibrinolysis.

The systemic formation of fibrin (the end result of coagulation is a stable fibrin clot) that occurs in patients with DIC results from excess circulating thrombin, suppression of the anticoagulation mechanisms, and impaired removal of fibrin.[6] The alterations in these processes are mediated by several pro-inflammatory cytokines, including interleukin-6 (IL-6) and tumor necrosis factor-alpha (TN-α).[6]

The excess formation of thrombin in DIC is driven by a transmembrane glycoprotein, called tissue factor (TF), and activated factor VII of the extrinsic coagulation pathway.[15] Tissue factor is present on the surface of many cell types (including endothilial cells, macrophages, and monocytes) and is exposed to the general circulation after vascular damage. It is released in response to exposure to cytokines, endotoxin, and tumor necrosis factor, which plays a major role in the development of DIC in septic conditions.[16]

Excess circulating thrombin yields fibrinogen, which leaves behind fibrin monomers that polymerize into fibrin clots in the circulation.[1] These excess clots trap platelets that lead to primarily microvascular thrombosis with subsequent ischemic impaired organ perfusion and end-organ damage.[1,4,12] This entrapment of platelets also leads to a worsening of the thrombocytopenia, which is generally seen with acute DIC. As this process continues, clotting factors are consumed, overwhelming their potential for production. At the time of maximal coagulation during DIC, the fibrinolytic system is largely suppressed.[4] This inhibition is caused by high levels of plasminogen activator inhibitor type 1, which is the main inhibitor of fibrinolysis. This impairment of fibrin removal creates increased fibrin levels in the microvascular leading to further damage.[6]

Eventually, the excess circulating thrombin also assists in the conversion of plasminogen to plasmin, causing fibrinolysis, which in turn results in increased amounts of fibrin degradation products (FDPs) that have strong anticoagulant properties, leading to hemorrhage.[17] Excess plasmin can inactivate clotting factors, but it can also activate the complement and kinin systems. Activation of these systems can lead to increased vascular permeability, hypotension, and shock. The clinical picture of acute DIC is a hemodynamically unstable patient who is experiencing a

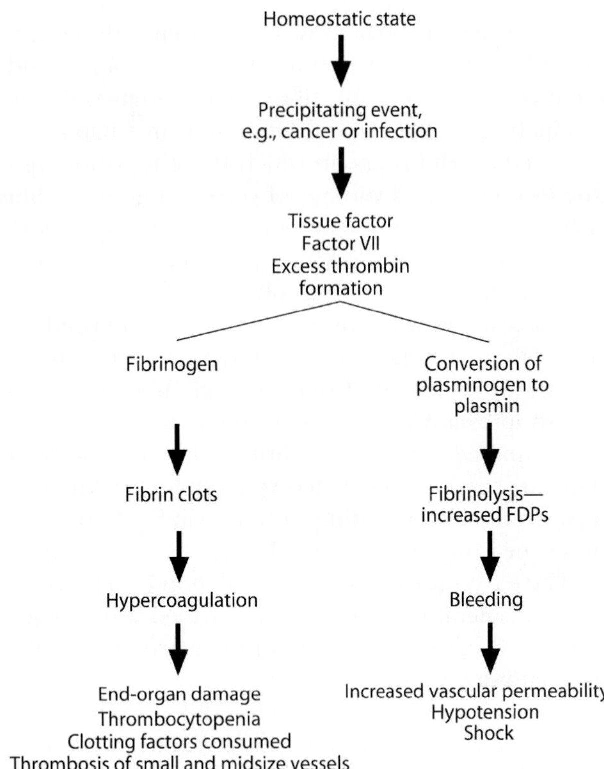

Figure 37-1 The process of DIC.

combination of extreme thrombosis and bleeding. Figure 37-1 depicts the process of DIC.

Clinical Manifestations

Signs and symptoms of acute DIC are variable and complex. Recognizing this syndrome in its early phase and treating it promptly are crucial to the prognosis of the affected patient. Unfortunately, DIC is often a fatal process as it frequently goes unrecognized until severe hemorrhage occurs.

Thrombus formation often occurs early and simultaneously with bleeding in DIC. Thrombi generally form in the superficial and smaller veins, and may be clinically undetectable. Subtle signs and symptoms of thrombi include red indurated tender areas indicating ischemia found over organ sites. When thrombosis occurs, the signs and symptoms may include focal ischemia, acrocyanosis, superficial gangrene, frank gangrene, altered sensorium, ulceration of the gastrointestinal tract (including stress ulcers with frank gastrointestinal bleeding), jaundice due to the release of excess bilirubin during hemorrhage, decreased urinary output if the renal system is affected by thrombosis,[18] and dyspnea (which can lead to acute respiratory distress syndrome). Widespread thrombosis (purpura fulminans — irregular hemorrhagic skin lesions) and significant bleeding can occur simultaneously.[19]

Bleeding is the most obvious sign of a hemorrhagic disorder and can occur from any orifice or opening on the surface of the skin. Patients may ooze blood from surgical, venipuncture, or wound sites. Skin hemorrhages in the form of purpura, petechiae, ecchymoses, and hematomas can be readily apparent.[13] Overt hemorrhage involving multiple unrelated sites is not uncommon in the patient with acute DIC. See Table 37-2 for the physical examination of the patient with actual or potential bleeding. Hemoptysis, intraperitoneal hemorrhage, and intracranial bleeding all pose life-threatening events for the patient with DIC.

Systemic signs and symptoms of DIC are based on the underlying pathophysiology of this process. The signs and symptoms can include fever, hypoxia, acidosis, hypotension, and proteinuria. If severe, the patient may demonstrate a clinical picture of shock.[20]

Assessment

There is no specific laboratory finding that is absolutely diagnostic of DIC. A battery of lab tests in conjunction with clinical evidence must be used to confirm the diagnosis, as well as to monitor response to treatment. A number of clinical conditions will affect these tests, which makes their interpretation difficult. For example, multiple blood product transfusions will dilute clotting factors or platelets, and liver disease with portal hypertension can lead to thrombocytopenia and the activation of the fibrinolytic system.

The platelet count and the plasma fibrinogen level (long used to help determine the diagnosis of DIC) are almost always decreased in the presence of DIC. Neither of these tests is sensitive nor specific for DIC, but normal levels exclude the possibility of DIC.[21] The presence of shistocytes, or red cell fragments, in the blood smear is a frequent but nonspecific finding for acute DIC. The presence of shistocytes supports the diagnosis of chronic DIC more significantly, as they are found in almost all such cases. Other coagulation studies often done to support the diagnosis of DIC are the prothrombin time (PT), activated partial thromboplastin time (aPTT), and the international normalization ratio (INR).[2,6,22] All of these global clotting times are expected to be prolonged in DIC; they are nonspecific as they can be shortened or normal in the presence of DIC. Table 37-3 describes laboratory studies for DIC.

Two of the newer and more sophisticated tests that are done to help determine a diagnosis of DIC include

Table 37-2 Physical Examination of the Patient with Actual or Potential Bleeding

Integumentary System
- Bruising, petechiae, purpura, ecchymoses, acrocyanosis (irregularly shaped cyanotic patches on the periphery of arms and legs associated with bleeding due to DIC)
- Oozing from venipuncture sites or injections, biopsy sites, central lines, catheters, or nasogastric tubes
- Color and condition of gingival tissues
- Cool and clammy skin

Eyes[a] and Ears
- Visual disturbances, increased injection on the sclera, periorbital edema, subconjunctival hemorrhage (homogeneous red color that is sharply outlined on the sclera), headache, eye or ear pain

Nose, Mouth, and Throat
- Petechiae on nasal/oral mucosa, epistaxis, tenderness or bleeding from gums or oral mucosa

Cardiopulmonary System
- Crackles, wheezes, stridor, dyspnea, tachypnea, orthopnea, hypoxia, cyanosis, and hemoptysis (all possible signs of bleeding in the lungs), vital sign changes, decrease in color and temperature of all extremities, decreased peripheral pulses, tachycardia, peripheral edema
- Assess for angina

Gastrointestinal System[b]
- Pain, bleeding, blood around rectum, tarry stools, frank or occult blood in stools, hematemesis
- Observe for bleeding hemorrhoids (may respond to local measures)

Genitourinary System
- Bleeding, character, and amount of menses
- Monitor intake and output (if urine drops below 30 mL/hr, it may be due to acute tubular necrosis secondary to thrombi, bleeding, or hypovolemia)

Musculoskeletal System
- Check for complaint of painful joints while performing active or passive range of motion, which may indicate bleeding into the joints

Central Nervous System
- Mental status changes, including restlessness, confusion, lethargy, dizziness, obtundation, seizures, or coma (may indicate intracranial hemorrhage or impaired tissue perfusion)

[a] Bleeding in the optic fundus could lead to permanent visual impairment.

[b] Guaiac all excreta for blood.

the D-dimer and the FDP assay. These tests can be performed alone or in combination. The D-dimer is a neoantigen formed as a result of plasmin digestion of fibrin. This test is specific for FDPs, which are found in increased levels in acute DIC.[1] Likewise, the FDP assay tests for increased levels of FDPs; FDP assays are also elevated in acute DIC. These tests reflect the microangiopathy of DIC and have been found to be sensitive, specific, and efficient in the diagnosis of DIC.[22]

Other tests may be done to document accelerated coagulation and accelerated fibrinolysis, which may also help to support a diagnosis of DIC. However, many of these tests are not currently clinically available as they are in clinical trials.[6,23] A decreased level of antithrombin III (AT III) demonstrates accelerated coagulation, which is suggestive for DIC. Measuring the products of coagulation factor activation provides more information about the dynamics of DIC. Other tests that are done to determine accelerated coagulation include the plasma level of fibrinopeptide A, levels of prothrombin activation peptide (F1 and F2), and thrombin–antithrombin complexes (TAT).[23]

In addition to FDP titers and the D-dimer assay tests to detect accelerated fibrinolysis in DIC, plasminogen and α2–antiplasmin levels may be drawn. The presence of lower or falling levels of plasminogen and α2–antiplasmin levels suggests hyperfibrinolysis.[14] These tests also help to support the diagnosis of DIC.

Therapeutic Approaches and Nursing Care

Prevention of Complications

DIC related to cancer cannot necessarily be prevented, as it often occurs as a result of the malignancy itself or treatment of the malignancy (e.g., administration of chemotherapy or blood products). The potential for preventing DIC related to infection may result from aggressive management of the neutropenic patient. Early detection of the signs and symptoms of DIC allows for the best chance for prompt diagnosis and treatment, resulting in a better prognosis for the patient with DIC.

Prevention of further complications of DIC includes removal of any tight or restrictive clothing. If edema is present, it should be measured daily. Elastic support stockings may help minimize stasis and promote venous return. Other measures to decrease stasis and promote venous return include assisting the patient with leg lifts or elevating the legs to 15–20 degrees at intervals, and teaching the patient to wiggle his or her toes and perform ankle circles frequently while in bed. Compression to the knee vessels is minimized by avoiding placing anything under the knees while in bed (pillows, knee gatches), by avoiding crossing of the knees or legs, and by avoiding dangling the legs over the side of the bed.[17]

Management

Treatment of the underlying etiology is critical in the management of DIC. Until the underlying stimulus of DIC is managed successfully, all other therapy will merely provide an interval of symptomatic relief. The patient with DIC can become unstable very quickly because of the complications of bleeding and thrombus

Table 37-3 Laboratory Studies for DIC

Test	Result	Comments
D-dimer assay	Elevated	Neoantigen formed when plasmin digests fibrin Specific for increased FDPs
FDP titer	Elevated	Increased consumption of clots Specific for increased FDPs
Platelet count	Decreased	Frequent, but nonspecific finding in DIC
Fibrinogen	Decreased	Nonspecific in DIC
Prothrombin time	Prolonged	Nonspecific in DIC; can be prolonged, shortened, or normal
Activated partial thromboplastin time	Prolonged	Nonspecific in DIC; can be prolonged, shortened, or normal
International normalization ratio	Prolonged	Nonspecific in DIC; can be prolonged, shortened, or normal
Peripheral smear	Schistocytes	Frequent, but nonspecific finding in DIC
Antithrombin III level	Decreased	Demonstrates accelerated coagulation
Fibrinopeptide A level	Elevated	Reflects the rate of fibrin formation, demonstrates accelerated coagulation
Prothrombin fragments (F1 and F2)	Elevated	Reflects the rate of thrombin formation, demonstrates accelerated coagulation
Thrombin–antithrombin (TAT) complexes	Elevated	Reflects the rate of thrombin formation, demonstrates accelerated coagulation
Plasminogen levels	Decreased	Suggests hyperfibrinolysis
α2-antiplasmin levels	Decreased	Suggests hyperfibrinolysis

formation, and must be supported hemodynamically to alleviate shock. The patient with DIC must be monitored closely for signs and symptoms of bleeding. A thorough review of organ systems must be done to minimize blood loss.

Oxygen therapy is initiated immediately for the hypoxia and associated acidosis. Fluid replacement therapy must also be initiated promptly, as the patient can quickly become hypovolemic with significant bleeding. Fluid replacement therapy will help manage the associated proteinuria (from thrombosis occuring in the kidneys) and hypotension. Fluid replacement may include simple crystalloids such as Ringer's lactate, artificial colloids such as dextran and hydroxyethyl starch, or human albumin.[24] The administration of plasma substitutes (dextran, hydroxyethyl starch, or plasma proteins) may result in adverse reactions ranging from allergic urticarial reactions to life-threatening anaphylaxis.[24] The administration of blood components such as red blood cells, platelets, and fresh frozen plasma may also double for use as replacement fluids. Caution must by used in treating the bleeding patient to avoid fluid overload and complications such as congestive heart failure.

Education is a necessary component of care when a patient is at risk for or is experiencing DIC. Patients and families are taught to report any bleeding or unusual symptoms. They are taught to save all excreta for the nurse to examine for blood. The patient and family will also need excellent psychosocial support should the patient develop this paradoxical situation of hemorrhage and thrombus formation.

Managing intravascular clotting

Although the bleeding associated with DIC is obvious and may be dramatic, it is the thrombotic process that has the greatest impact on morbidity and mortality in patients with DIC. Thus, an anticoagulant such as heparin may be initiated to stop the intravascular clotting process. Adequate prophylaxis is also needed to eliminate the risk of venous thromboembolism. Patients with DIC are usually given relatively low doses of heparin (300–500 U per hour) as a continuous infusion.[4] Effectiveness of low-dose heparin is generally seen within about 3 to 4 hours after initiation of therapy, first by correction of lab values and then by a cessation of clinically significant bleeding and thrombosis. Low-molecular-weight heparin (LMWH) may be an alternative to unfractionated heparin. LMWH has higher bioavailability, a longer half-life, and a more predictable antithrombotic effect.[25] Heparin use is contraindicated in patients with any signs of intracranial bleeding (e.g., cerebral vascular accident or headache), open wounds, or recent surgery. Antithrombin III is another anticoagulant that may be used for acute DIC.[16] Antithrombin III may be used for moderately severe to severe DIC when levels of antithrombin III are markedly depressed.[12]

Blood component therapy

After attempts have been made at treating the underlying stimulus of DIC and managing the thrombotic state of the patient, blood component replacement therapy may be initiated. Most reports regarding blood component replacement therapy stress the importance of identifying the missing or lacking component and administering that specific component.

Washed, packed red blood cells may be given if the patient continues to bleed or the hemoglobin level drops below 8 g/dL. When red blood cells are stored in the blood bank, they become deficient in the labile clotting factors V and VIII. Thus, it is recommended that for every 4–6 units of banked red blood cells given to the patient, 2 units of fresh-frozen plasma (FFP) also be administered to the patient to replete these factors.[24] The use of FFP in the management of DIC is somewhat controversial because FFP contains fibrinogen, which can potentially create higher levels of FDPs that will further impair hemostasis.[1]

Cryoprecipitate (a concentrated source of fibrin and factor VIII) may be used to treat the severely bleeding patient who is hypofibrinogenemic, yet it too may create increased levels of FDPs. Platelets may be given if the platelet count drops below 20,000 cells/mm^3 or if the patient is actively bleeding.

Fibrinolytic inhibitors

In rare instances, fibrinolytic medications may be used in managing ongoing DIC. These medications may be administered when the patient continues to bleed after being treated by the other three measures mentioned earlier: treating the underlying stimulus of DIC, treating the thrombotic process, and administering missing blood components. Two of these medications are epsilon-amino-caproic acid (EACA, Amicar) and tranexamic acid (tretinoin). These medications are given only after the intravascular coagulation process and fibrin deposition have been alleviated, as they can lead to widespread fibrin deposition in the microcirculation and result in ischemic organ dysfunction.[26] Amicar is generally given by slow IV push every hour for 24 hours, or until bleeding stops. In addition to the problem of increased fibrin deposition, Amicar can cause ventricular arrhythmias, severe hypotension, and severe hypokalemia.[1] Tretinoin is a newer agent with fewer undesirable effects. It is being used more frequently in the management of APL, where there is a high risk of DIC. The addition of retinoic acid to the treatment plan of APL may result in less hemorrhage and transfusion requirements.[4]

Continuity of Care

The care of patients with acute DIC is complex and challenging. Most patients experiencing this syndrome will be managed primarily in the intensive care setting. The patient who is bleeding and intravascularly clotting at the same time will require aggressive hemodynamic support. The treatments used for the bleeding and clotting—anticoagulants, blood components, and possibly fibrinolytic inhibitors—have serious potential side effects that require intensive assessment and monitoring. However, because the process of DIC may occur over hours to days, patients at risk for DIC may be cared for in any setting. Nurses need to be aware of risk factors for the development of acute DIC related to cancer. With prompt recognition of a bleeding or clotting problem, there is the potential for prompt treatment of this potentially fatal syndrome.

Conclusion

Acute DIC related to cancer can be due to a number of causative factors, including the cancer itself or a process such as infection. The primary management of patients with acute DIC is to treat the underlying pathology creating the DIC condition. Patients may also be treated aggressively to maintain their hemodynamic status, as well as with a variety of medications and blood components.

Because DIC contributes greatly to morbidity and mortality in patients with cancer, nurses play a valuable role in the prompt recognition of its signs and symptoms. Early recognition of the signs and symptoms of bleeding or clotting can lead to prompt treatment of this challenging problem. It is hoped that future research will identify more clearly the most appropriate treatment for acute DIC.

References

1. Bick RL: Disseminated intravascular coagulation: pathophysiological mechanisms and manifestations. *Semin Thromb Hemost* 24:3–18, 1998
2. Ezzone S: Disseminated intravascular coagulation, in Camp-Sorrell D, Hawkins RA (eds.): *Clinical Manual for the Oncology Advanced Practice Nurse.* Pittsburgh, Oncology Nursing Society, 2000, pp 683–688
3. Messmore HL, Wehrmacher WH: Disseminated intravascular coagulation: a primer for primary care physicians. *Postgrad Med* 111, 2002. *www.postgradmed.com/issues/2002/03_02/messmore.htm.* Accessed February 22, 2004
4. Levi M, Ten Cate H: Disseminated intravascular coagulation. *New Engl J Med* 341:586–592, 1999
5. Gouin-Thibault I, Achkar A, Samama MM: The thrombophilic state in cancer patients. *Acta Haematol* 106:33–42, 2001
6. Levi M, de Jonge E: Current management of disseminated intravascular coagulation. *Hosp. Pract* 8, 2000. *www.hosppract.com/issues/2000/08/celevi.htm.* Accessed February 22, 2004
7. Schmaier AH: Disseminated intravascular coagulation. *EMedicine* 577, updated December 10, 2003. *www.emedicine.com/med/topic577.htm.* Accessed February 22, 2004

8. Hajjar KA, Menell JS: Annexin II: a novel mediator of cell surface plasmin generation. *Ann NY Acad Sci* 811:337–349, 1997
9. Menell JS, Cesarman GM, Jacovina AT, et al: Annexin II and bleeding in acute promyelocytic leukemia [see comments]. *N Engl J Med* 340:994, 1999
10. Avances C, Oumaya C, Granger V, et al: Prostate cancer and acute disseminated intravascular coagulation. Therapeutic management based on three cases. *Prog Urol* 13:308–312, 2003
11. Gobel BH: Disseminated intravascular coagulation, in Yarbro CH, Frogge MH, Goodman M, et al (eds.): *Cancer Nursing Principles and Practice* (ed 5). Sudbury, MA, Jones and Bartlett, 2000, pp 869–875
12. Furlong MA, Furlong BR: Disseminated intravascular coagulation. *EMedicine* 150, updated September 11, 2001. *www.emedicine.com/EMERG/topic150.htm.* Accessed February 22, 2004
13. Gobel BH: Disseminated intravascular coagulation in cancer: providing quality care. *Topics in Adv Pract Nurse J* 2, 2002. *www.medscape.com/viewarticle/442737.* Accessed February 1, 2004
14. Staudinger T, Locker GJ, Frass M: Management of acquired coagulation disorders in emergency and intensive-care medicine. *Semin Thromb Hemost* 22:93–104, 1996
15. Carey MH, Rogers GM: Disseminated intravascular coagulation: clinical and laboratory aspects. *Am J Hematol* 59:65–73, 1998
16. Gando S, Nanzaki S, Sasaki S, et al: Significant correlations between tissue factor and thrombin markers in trauma and septic patients with disseminated intravascular coagulation. *Thromb Haemost* 79:111–115, 1998
17. Gobel BH: Disseminated intravascular coagulation. *Semin Oncol Nurs* 15:174–182, 1999
18. Linker CA: Blood, in Tierney LM, McPhee SJ, Papdakis MA (eds.): *Current Medical Diagnosis and Treatment* (ed 40). New York, Lange Medical Books, 2001, pp 505–558
19. Marder JV, Martin SE, Coleman RW: Clinical aspects of consumptive thrombohemorrhagic disorders, in Coleman RW, Hirsh J, Marder JV, et al (eds.): *Hemostasis and Thrombosis* (ed 3). Philadelphia, Lippincott, 1993, pp 665–693
20. Lin EM: Oncologic emergency: case 3, in Lin EM (ed.): *Advanced Practice in Oncology Nursing Case Studies and Review.* Philadelphia, W.B. Saunders, 2001, pp 312–319
21. Mammen EF: Disseminated intravascular coagulation (DIC). *Clin Lab Sci* 13:239–245, 2000
22. Yu M, Nardella BS, Pechet L: Screening tests of disseminated intravascular coagulation: guidelines for rapid and specific laboratory diagnosis. *Crit Care Med* 28:1777–1780, 2000
23. Wada H, Sakuragawa N, Nori Y, et al: Hemostatic molecular markers before the onset of disseminated intravascular coagulation: *Am J Hematol* 60:273–278, 1999
24. Letsky EA: Disseminated intravascular coagulation. *Best Pract Res Clin Obstet Gynaecol* 4:623–644, 2001
25. Dolovich LR, Ginsberg JS, Douketis JD, et al: A meta-analysis comparing low-molecular-weight heparins with unfractionated heparin in the treatment of venous thromboembolism. *Arch Intern Med* 1603:181–188, 2000
26. Wilkes GM, Ingwersen K, Barton-Burke M (eds.): Molecularly targeted therapies, in *Oncology Nursing Drug Handbook.* Sudbury, MA, Jones and Bartlett, 2003, pp 394–483

CHAPTER 38

Septic Shock

Susan Moore, RN, MSN, ANP, AOCN®

Scope of the Problem

Septic shock is one stage in a continuum of infection and inflammation. It is characterized by multiple hemodynamic changes and alterations in organ function that can result in death. In this disorder, bacterial, viral, or fungal infection triggers immune and inflammatory responses in the body. Early recognition and intervention often decrease the odds of mortality in this oncologic emergency. Oncology nurses are in a pivotal position to optimize patient outcomes by understanding the risk factors, pathophysiology, clinical presentation, and therapeutic interventions of septic shock.

Definitions

In a classic paper by Bone and colleagues,[1] definitions of the spectrum of sepsis syndromes (see Table 38–1) were standardized in 1991 by the American College of Chest Physicians/Society of Critical Care Medicine (ACCP/SCCM). In increasing order of severity, the phases were categorized as infection, bacteremia, systemic inflammatory response syndrome (SIRS), sepsis, severe sepsis, and septic shock. Definitions were also standardized for acute respiratory distress syndrome (ARDS), acute lung injury (ALI), and multiple organ dysfunction syndrome (MODS), all of which can be manifestations of sepsis or other conditions.[1,2]

Sepsis is a systemic inflammatory response in the presence of infection as evidenced by elevation of temperature, heart rate, and respiratory rate. The white blood count may be greater or less than normal. When sepsis progresses to a state of organ dysfunction, hypoperfusion, or hypotension, severe sepsis is present. Septic shock is marked by sepsis-induced hypotension despite reasonable fluid resuscitation or sepsis that requires vasopressors or inotropic agents to maintain normal blood pressure.[1] MODS, which is defined as the presence of altered organ function in an acutely ill patient such that homeostasis cannot be maintained with intervention,[1] is the final common pathway for the critically ill patient. Although MODS is potentially reversible, the pathophysiologic abnormalities in this syndrome are so severe that homeostasis cannot be maintained without prompt and exact intervention. The presence of MODS is an important prognostic indicator for septic shock; in fact, severe prolonged dysfunction of three or more organs correlates with a mortality rate of 70% or greater.[3]

Table 38-1 Definitions of Sepsis

Term	Definition
Bacteremia/fungemia	Presence of viable bacteria (or fungi) in the blood, as evidenced by positive blood cultures
Systemic inflammatory response syndrome (SIRS)	At least two of the following conditions in response to a variety of clinical insults: • Oral temperature > 38°C or < 36°C • Respiratory rate > 20 breaths/min or $PaCO_2$ < 32 mm Hg • Heart rate > 90 beats/min • Leukocyte count > 12,000 cells/μL or > 10% immature (band) forms
Sepsis	The presence of two or more SIRS criteria in the presence of infection
Severe sepsis	Sepsis with one or more signs of organ dysfunction, hypoperfusion, or hypotension, such as metabolic acidosis, acute alteration in mental status, oliguria, or adult respiratory distress syndrome (ARDS)
Septic shock	Sepsis with hypotension that is unresponsive to fluid resuscitation plus organ dysfunction or perfusion abnormalities as listed above for severe sepsis
Multiple organ dysfunction syndrome (MODS)	Dysfunction of more than one organ, requiring intervention to maintain homeostasis

Data from Bone, Balk, Cerra, et al.[1]

Incidence

Novel methods of treatment and supportive care in the presence of sepsis have increased survival rates among both previously healthy and immunocompromised patients. An estimated 750,000 cases of sepsis, resulting in 210,000 deaths, occur annually in the United States.[3,4] Angus and colleagues project an increase in the rate of sepsis of 1.5% per year on the basis of the growth and aging of the U.S. population.[4] Septicemia is the tenth leading cause of death overall in the United States.[5] Septic shock is the second leading cause of death among patients in noncoronary intensive care units[6] with mortality rates approaching 20%–50%.[7] Severe sepsis results in annual total costs of $126.7 billion nationally.[4]

Although fungal, viral, and protozoal infections can cause septic shock, the most common source continues to be bacterial infection, which is responsible for 40%–60% of cases. Gram-negative organisms were the predominant organisms causing sepsis from 1979 through 1987, whereas gram-positive bacteria were reported most commonly in each subsequent year. In cases where a causative organism was identified, gram-positive bacteria accounted for 52.1% of cases; gram-negative bacteria for 37.6%; polymicrobial infections for 4.7%; anaerobes for 1%; and fungi for 4.6%. In an estimated 20% of cases of septic shock, an initiating organism is never identified.[3]

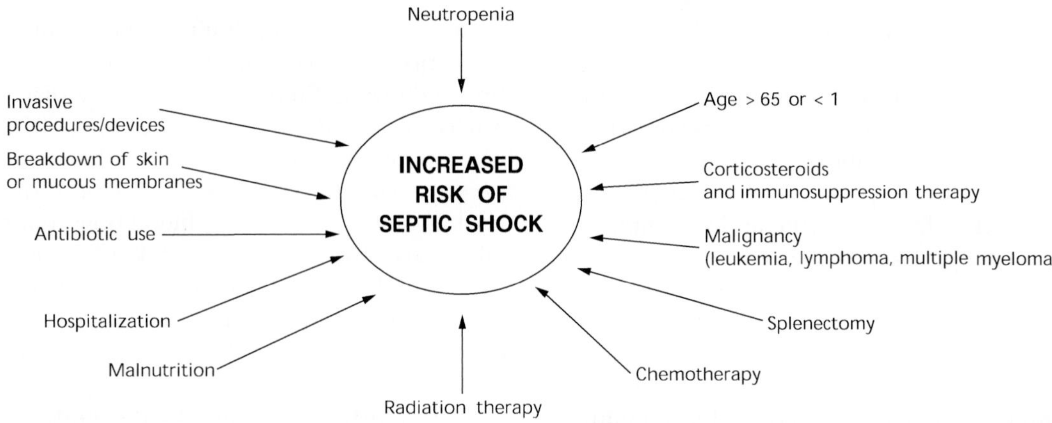

Figure 38-1 Risk factors for septic shock

Etiology and Risk Factors

The risk of septic shock in the oncology patient is related to the type, degree, and duration of immune deficiency. The immune function of individuals with cancer is threatened by numerous factors, including the nature of their malignancy, antineoplastic therapy, and any co-morbid conditions (see Figure 38-1). Understanding the normal immune function is key to recognizing the risk factors for sepsis and septic shock in the oncology population. In general, the individual is armed with nonspecific host defenses such as intact skin and mucous membranes, stomach acidity, flow of secretions, and proper nutrition. These protective mechanisms may be threatened by cytotoxic drugs, radiation, surgery, invasive procedures, or the tumor itself.

Safdar and Armstrong[8] classify the immune-specific host defenses into three categories: (1) granulocytes, (2) cell-mediated immunity, and (3) humoral immunity. In the first category of host defense, granulocytes phagocytize and kill microbes. A decrease in the number of functional granulocytes is termed *granulocytopenia.* It is the single most important risk factor for sepsis in individuals with cancer.[8] Granulocytopenia can occur as a result of leukemia, bone marrow infiltration by tumor cells in solid tumors, total body irradiation, and cytotoxic chemotherapy. The potential for infection is proportional to the degree and duration of granulocytopenia.[8,9]

The second category of host defense is cell-mediated immunity, which serves to eliminate pathogens, malignant cells, and viruses by employing monocytes, macrophages, and T lymphocytes. Patients with relapsed or refractory hematologic cancers have markedly impaired T lymphocytes.[8] The third type of host defense involves humoral immunity, consisting of B lymphocytes that produce antibodies to foreign antigens. Antibodies tag microorganisms to be phagocytized. A humoral immunity defect can occur in patients with multiple myeloma, Waldenstrom's macroglobulinemia, chronic lymphocytic leukemia, asplenism, and cytotoxic chemotherapy.

An important component of humoral immunity is antibody-dependent cellular cytotoxicity (ADCC). It involves the activation of lymphocytes by the interaction of immunoglobulin and leukocyte surface receptors, leading to the elimination of bacteria and parasites by cytolytic perforins.[8] Patients with humoral immune deficiencies are susceptible to fulminant infections caused by *S. pneumoniae* and other encapsulated organisms that require complement for elimination. The complement cascade induces inflammation and activation of phagocytic cells. Chapter 2 provides a detailed review of the immune system.

Physiologic Alterations

Normal Physiology

If a microbial intruder such as a bacterium, fungus, or virus invades the body, it is recognized as foreign by white blood cells (WBCs). An adequate, intact immune system promptly recruits neutrophils, macrophages, lymphocytes, and antibodies to the site of infection to prevent host colonization. At this point, microbes and their toxins are neutralized and eliminated via phagocytosis. If the virulence of the pathogen exceeds the capabilities of the host's defense, however, sepsis and possibly septic shock may follow. As previously noted, an individual with cancer is particularly at risk for this outcome due to the presence of multiple immune defects.

Pathophysiology

According to the prevailing theory, septic shock represents an uncontrolled inflammatory response.[10]

Initially, septic shock may be characterized by a pro-inflammatory response to ensure short-term survival. As infection persists, a shift toward an anti-inflammatory immunosuppressive state occurs.[11,12] Widespread systemic inflammation and shock may occur if the pro- and anti-inflammatory responses are imbalanced. The immunosuppressive features of the anti-inflammatory state may worsen preexisting immunosuppression in many cancer patients. As a result, these individuals have a loss of delayed hypersensitivity, an inability to clear infection, and a predisposition to nosocomial infections.[10–12]

If the invading organism overcomes local immune efforts, translocation into the bloodstream by the organism itself or by its cellular components occurs. Endotoxin, a structural component in the cell membrane of gram-negative bacteria, is a potent trigger that ultimately causes the cellular and hemodynamic alterations seen in septic shock. According to Parrillo and colleagues, human and animal research have demonstrated that small doses of endotoxin injected into subjects produce fever, tachycardia, hypotension, decreased systemic vascular resistance, and myocardial depression.[6] In addition, higher levels of endotoxemia generally correlate with an increased severity of septic shock.[6] Similarly, gram-positive organisms trigger septic shock via liberation of exotoxins, enterotoxins, peptidoglycans, and lipoteichoic acid.

The presence of bacterial toxins in the bloodstream initiates an immune reaction by the host against the invading pathogen. This counterattack by the host's immune system consists of the stimulation of macrophages, monocytes, neutrophils, and plasma cells, which in turn activates an outpouring of endogenous cytokines and mediators (see Figure 38-2).[1,6,7] Cytokines interact extensively with neutrophils and endothelial cells. When triggered by endotoxin or exotoxin, tumor necrosis factor (TNF) and interleukin-1 (IL-1) act synergistically to promote endothelial cell–leukocyte adhesion, release proteases and arachidonate metabolites, and activate clotting mechanisms. Interleukin-8 is a granulocyte chemotaxin that may promote tissue inflammation. Interleukin-4, IL-10, IL-13, and transforming growth factor-beta (TGF-β) have anti-inflammatory functions by suppressing gene expression and synthesis of IL-1 and TNF.[13,14] Both TNF and IL-1 are potent vasodilators and pyrogens.[14]

Septic shock is the most common cause of circulatory collapse in patients with malignancies.[13] The predominant hemodynamic feature of this condition is arterial vasodilation. Diminished peripheral arterial vascular tone may produce dependency of blood pressure on cardiac output, causing vasodilation to result in hypotension and shock if insufficiently compensated by a rise in cardiac output. Early in septic shock, the rise in cardiac output is limited by hypovolemia and a fall in preload secondary to low cardiac filling pressures. Following fluid resuscitation, cardiac output is usually elevated during a phase known as the hyperdynamic phase of septic shock. Cardiac performance, however, is depressed. Myocardial depression in septic shock is caused by coronary blood flow abnormalities, pulmonary hypertension, cytokine activity, nitric oxide, and down-regulation of beta receptors.[15] As septic shock progresses, fibrinolysis, coagulopathies, and disseminated intravascular coagulation (DIC) may occur.[16]

In response to endotoxin, the endothelium releases endothelium-derived relaxing factor, or nitric oxide, which causes vasodilation and decreased arterial and venous tone. The primary compensatory role of nitric oxide is to sustain visceral blood flow.[17] Nitric oxide production is increased in septic shock as a result of increased expression of the inducible form of nitric oxide synthase.[17,18] The increased synthesis of nitric oxide contributes to hypotension and resistance to vasopressor drugs that occur in vasodilatory shock. In all forms of vasodilatory shock, plasma catecholamine concentrations increase and the renin–angiotensin system becomes activated.[18] Venous pooling due to decreased venous return and maldistribution of blood volume are also present. In addition, increased microvascular permeability renders vessels porous to fluids and solutes, resulting in hypovolemia via capillary leak and third spacing.[13,19] Migration and adhesion of neutrophils, platelets, red blood cells (RBCs), and fibrin form sludging in the microvasculature, leading to obstruction of blood flow and inadequate nutrient exchange, and resulting in tissue hypoxia and metabolic abnormalities.[16,20]

Clinical Manifestations

The initial presentation of septic shock is generally manifested as fever, shaking chills, hypotension, tachycardia, tachypnea, and mental status changes. Such manifestations vary according to the stage of septic shock as well as the immunologic integrity of the individual with cancer. Frequently, signs and symptoms are subtle or absent. Fever is defined as a single oral temperature of 38.3°C or higher or a temperature of 38.0°C or higher for 1 hour or longer.[21] Fever may be absent, especially in elders.[2,22] Attention to all clinical changes, therefore, is crucial for early recognition and treatment of the sepsis syndrome. The clinical picture of septic shock illustrates the effects of coagulopathy, hypotension, hypoperfusion, and ultimately tissue ischemia on virtually every organ system in the body (see Table 38-2).

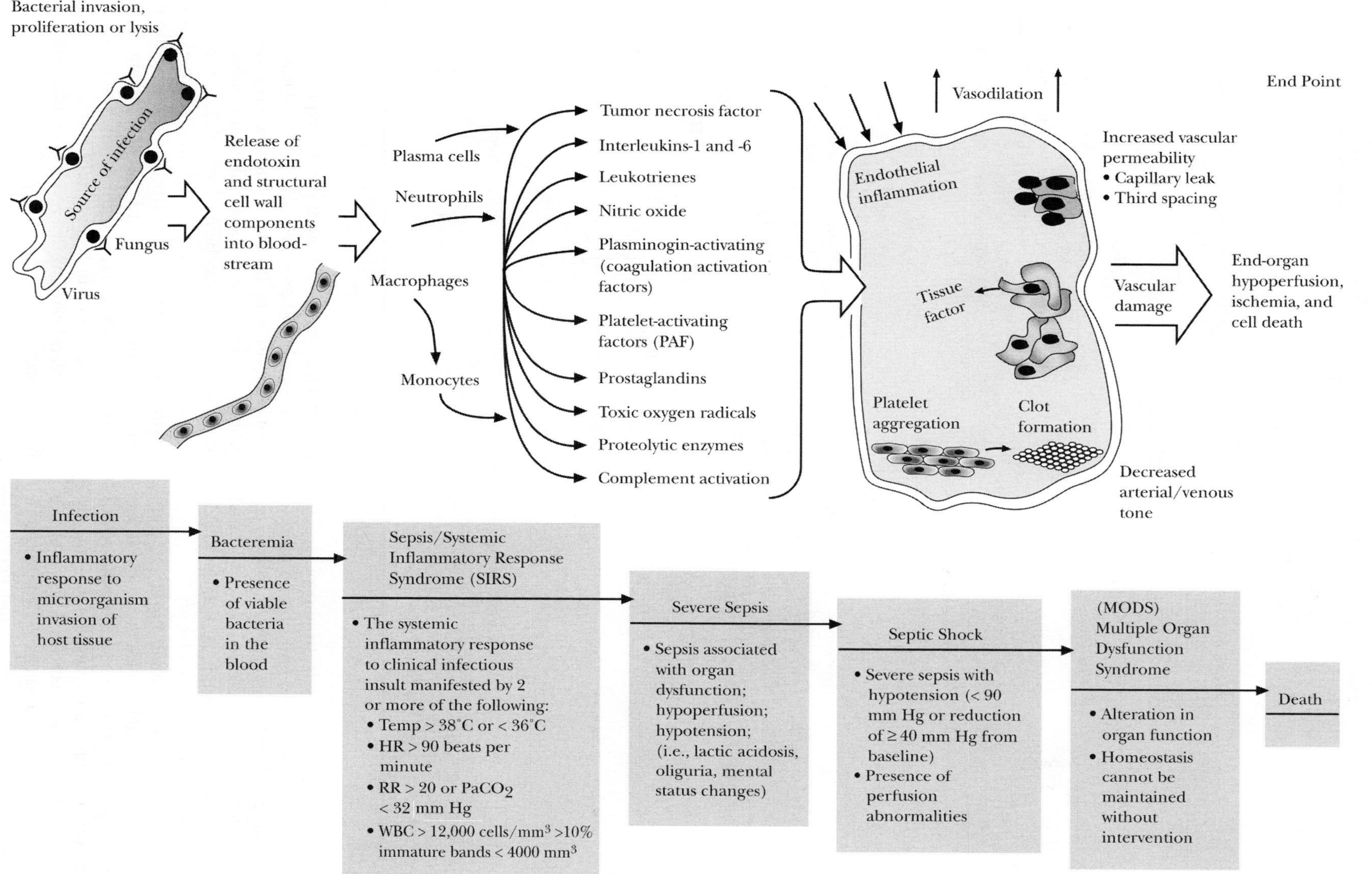

Figure 38-2 Pathophysiology of the septic shock cascade. (Data from Bone, Balk, Cerra, et al.[1]; Parillo, Parker, Natanson, et al.[6]; Wheeler, Bernard.[7])

Table 38-2 Clinical Manifestations of Organ Dysfunction in Septic Shock

Organ System	Severe Sepsis	Septic Shock
Central nervous system	- Apprehension - Confusion - Disorientation - Agitation	- Obtundation - Coma
Cardiovascular	- Sinus tachycardia - Cardiac output normal to increased - BP < 90 mm Hg, or 40 mm Hg ↓ baseline - Systemic vascular resistance ↓	- Acrocyanosis - Tachycardia - Dysrhythmias - Hypotension - Cardiac output normal or high - Systemic vascular resistance ↑ or ↓
Pulmonary	- Tachypnea - Shallow breaths - Hypoxic on room air - Respiratory and metabolic acidosis - ↓ Breath sounds and crackles	- Shortness of breath (if not ventilated) - Refractory hypoxemia - Respiratory and metabolic acidosis - ↓ Breath sounds, crackles, and wheezes - Pulmonary edema - Acute respiratory distress syndrome
Renal	- ↓ Urine output - Increased osmolality	- Oliguria - Anuria - BUN ↑ - Creatinine ↑ - Acute renal failure
Hematology	- Leukopenia or leukocytosis - Thrombocytopenia - PT/PTT prolonged - Fibrinogen ↓ - Fibrin degradation products ↑	- Leukopenia or leukocytosis - Thrombocytopenia - Anemia - PT/PTT prolonged - Fibrinogen ↓ - Fibrin degradation products ↑
Metabolic and electrolyte	- Temp > 38°C or < 36°C - Lactic acidosis - Hyperglycemia	- Temp > 38°C or < 36°C - Lactic acidosis - Hyperglycemia or hypoglycemia - ↓ Albumin - ↓ Potassium - ↓ Sodium - ↓ Calcium - ↓ Magnesium - ↓ Phosphate
Integument	- Dry, warm, and flushed skin	- Cold, pale, and clammy skin
Gastrointestinal	- Nausea and vomiting - ↓ GI motility	- ↓ GI motility - GI bleeding - ↑ Liver function tests - Jaundice

Mental status changes range from apprehension, agitation, withdrawal, confusion, and obtundation to coma. These changes arise from cerebral hypoxia, cerebral edema, and metabolic abnormalities. Mental changes may precede hypotension and temperature abnormalities in septic shock presentation.[19]

Shock is caused by an inadequate supply or inappropriate use of oxygen, which results in lactic acidosis and tissue damage. Cardiovascular manifestations of septic shock include increased heart rate and increased cardiac output (CO), decreased systemic vascular resistance (SVR), hypovolemia, hypotension, widened pulse pressure, arrhythmias, and decreased ejection fraction.[23] Although shock is typically defined as a systolic blood pressure of less than 90 mm Hg that is unresponsive to fluids or that requires vasoactive drugs,[1] use of blood pressure alone to assess for the presence of shock may be misleading. The administration of vasoactive drugs and fluid resuscitation can normalize blood pressure without correcting the fundamental underlying defect.[7] The skin and extremities are initially warm, dry, and flushed due to massive vasodilatation. Later in septic shock, the skin becomes cold, pale, and clammy as a result of maldistribution of blood flow.[24]

Pulmonary symptoms may herald the onset of septic shock. Dyspnea and tachypnea are almost universally observed; respiratory alkalosis is the result of hyperventilation.[25] Hypoxemia, pulmonary edema, adult respiratory distress syndrome (ARDS), respiratory acidosis, and ultimately respiratory failure will follow if the septic shock cascade is not averted.[7] Transient oliguria is a common finding and may be related to hypotension; in contrast, anuria is rare. Correcting volume deficits and hypotension usually reverses oliguria but may not prevent moderate elevation in serum creatinine.[7]

Blood dyscrasias may be present throughout the spectrum of septic events. Elevation of WBC count—that is, leukocytosis—results from increased neutrophil production and demargination of WBCs from the vessel wall into circulation. Leukopenia occurs due to consumption, sequestration, or decrease in the number of WBCs from underlying malignancy. Thrombocytopenia may result from decreased production, increased destruction, pooling, and sludging of platelets in the microvasculature. Granulocytopenia in septic shock generally correlates with a poor prognosis.[8] Subclinical coagulopathy, as evidenced by mild elevation of PT/PTT, is quite common. Although overt DIC is rare, development of DIC in septic patients roughly doubles the risk of death.[26] Clinical indicators of DIC include thrombosis, ischemia, and bleeding. Anemia is commonly seen as a result of hemodilution, hemorrhage, and shortened RBC survival.

Hyperglycemia may be present in both sepsis and severe sepsis. Blood glucose levels rise sharply in response to the sympathetic nervous system's release of endogenous catecholamines, epinephrine, norepinephrine, and glucocorticoids, as well as simultaneous gluconeogenesis. Hypoglycemia may be seen in prolonged septic shock, where it indicates hepatic failure and loss of compensatory mechanisms. Elevated serum lactate levels reflect anaerobic metabolism in response to tissue hypoxia that can occur early in the process. Also observed are lowered levels of albumin, sodium, potassium, calcium, and magnesium.[10]

The gastrointestinal (GI) tract is highly vascular and thus sensitive to ischemic conditions during septic shock. Septic shock usually causes ileus that typically persists for one to two days.[7] As a result of coagulopathies and tissue injury, GI bleeding and stress ulcers occur later in septic shock. Although hyperbilirubinemia and transaminase elevation are common, frank liver failure is rare.[7]

Assessment and Grading

Patient History

Septic shock risk factors generally relate to past and present medical history. The suspected source of infection may be identified by judiciously reviewing recent treatment, degree of myelosuppression, and lifestyle. Information regarding current cancer treatment (chemotherapy, radiation, steroids or other immunosuppressive drugs, dosages, and schedule) is important in determining the type, degree, and duration of immunosuppression. Most patients who show evidence of septic shock are transferred to an intensive care unit. The oncology nurse may be called upon to furnish essential information on the patient's cancer history and treatment. History of prior infections and antibiotic use may provide clues to the development of secondary infections or resistant organisms. Individuals who are older than 65, who have indwelling catheters, or who have poor nutritional status are at a significant risk for sepsis and possibly septic shock.[2,22]

Physical Exam

The patient with known or suspected sepsis requires a complete physical examination with focus on high-risk sites of infection. Common sites of infection include the oropharynx, skin, respiratory tract, perianal region, urinary tract, skin, and catheter site. Evaluation of the patient's hemodynamic and respiratory stability through monitoring vital signs should be ongoing. If the patient is not being transferred to an intensive care unit, his or her vital signs should be recorded using an electronic monitoring device. The blood pressure trend is particularly important, as is monitoring of subtle changes in other body systems that may indicate low organ perfusion. Oliguria, decreased bowel sounds, and mild lethargy or confusion may be indicators of organ compromise.[24] A thorough assessment should be performed, given that almost every organ system is affected during septic shock (see Table 38-2).

Most cancer patients are treated in the ambulatory setting and care for themselves at home despite immune dysfunction secondary to chemotherapy. In most situations, the initial assessment of sepsis and early septic shock occurs over the telephone by a practitioner in the outpatient setting. Figure 38-3 includes guidelines for a verbal assessment to examine risk factors, determine the severity of the patient's condition,

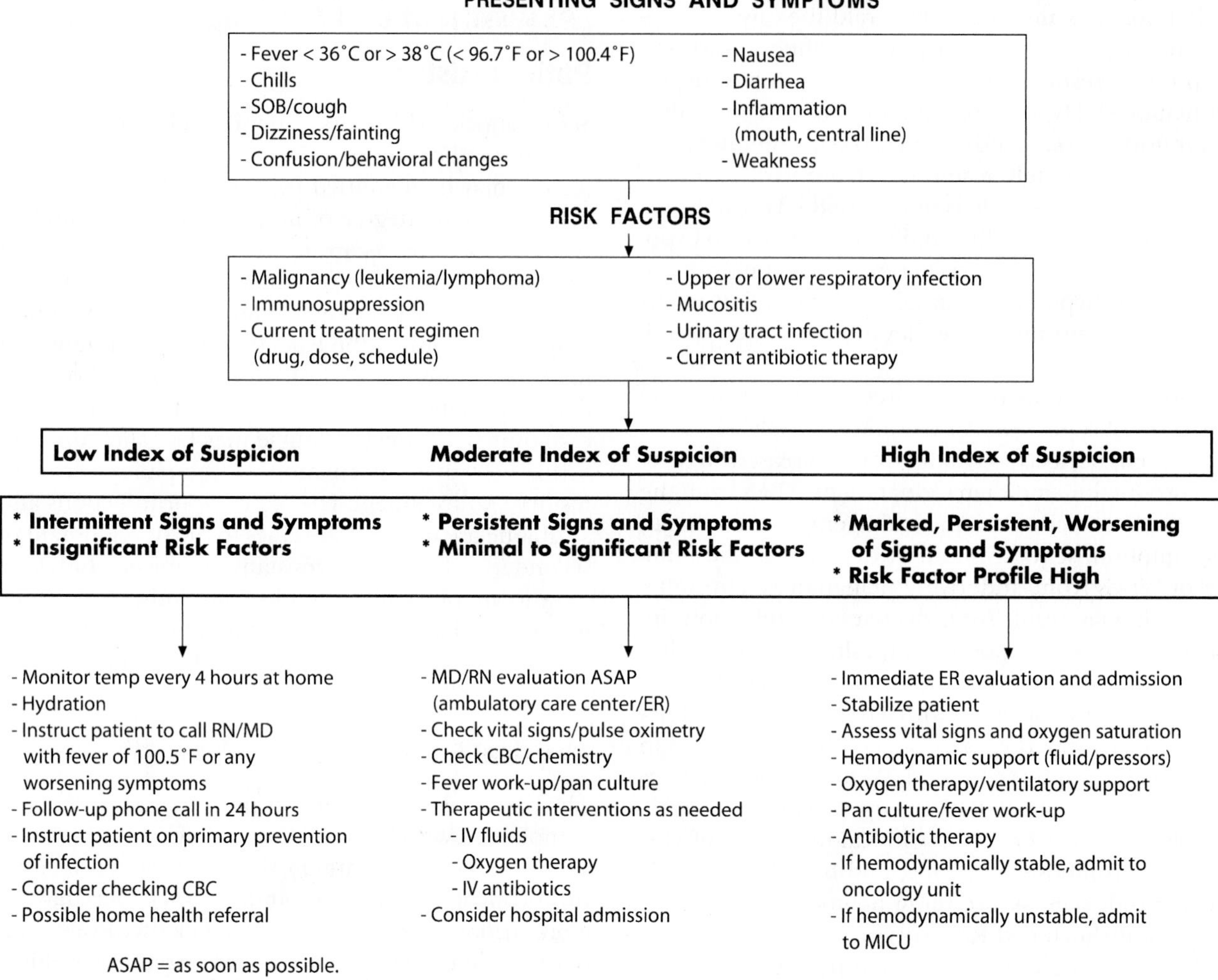

Figure 38-3 Telephone triage evaluation for suspected septic shock for patients in the home setting.

and identify the urgent need to seek medical evaluation.

Diagnostic Studies

Many diagnostic tests are available to evaluate severity of septic shock and to determine the source of infection. Blood cultures are drawn expeditiously from two separate sources (two venipuncture sites, or one venipuncture site and one central line) using 70% isopropyl alcohol, allowed to dry, as a skin preparation. Central line access and the culture bottles are cleansed with 70% isopropyl alcohol.[27,28] Chlorhexidine may also be used for skin preparation. Studies of chlorhexidine v 10% povidone-iodine indicated that chlorhexidine is superior to iodophors and should be the antiseptic of first choice for vascular access, particularly when accessing a venous access device.[29] Raad and colleagues found that a differential time to positivity of 120 minutes or more is highly sensitive and specific in diagnosing catheter-related bloodstream infections.[28] The only way to establish a definitive diagnosis of a central venous catheter (CVC) infection is removal of the catheter for culture. Thus, if the CVC is suspected as the source in a patient with negative blood cultures, the catheter should be removed and sent for culture.[27]

Cultures of body fluids such as urine, stool, sputum, or other exudate are collected as clinically relevant. Cultures should be repeated every 24 hours if septic shock persists. Frequent monitoring of the complete blood count (CBC), electrolytes, lactic acid, arterial blood gases (ABGs), coagulation profiles, and liver functions provides information about the severity of septic shock, organ dysfunction, and response to therapeutic interventions.[27] To further evaluate organ function and to determine the infectious source, other tests such as echocardiograms, computerized tomography (CT) scans, ventilation/perfusion scan, and angiography may be performed (see Table 38-3). Pleural, peritoneal, and paranasal sinus infections can

Table 38-3 Common Diagnostic Studies in Septic Shock Evaluation

Diagnostic Studies	Implications/Comments
Cultures of blood and body fluids (urine, sputum, drainage, stool)	Should be obtained expeditiously before starting antibiotics to properly identify pathogen Should be repeated every 24 hours if sepsis persists Results will show presence of a specific organism or no growth
Complete blood count	↑ WBCs in presence of infection or inflammation ↓ hemoglobin/hematocrit may reflect hemorrhage, hemodilution, or RBC destruction. ↓ platelet count may reflect decreased production, ↑ destruction, pooling or sludging; a ↓ platelet count may also signal early coagulopathies (DIC)
Chemistry (electrolytes and liver function tests)	↑ BUN, ↓ creatinine may reflect dehydration and/or renal hypoxia Initial ↑ in glucose due to the body's compensatory anti-inflammatory response and gluconeogenesis ↓ in glucose in prolonged shock as liver failure occurs Initially liver function test may remain normal but ↑ transaminase and bilirubin occur in prolonged septic shock
Serum lactate	↑ Levels are indicative of tissue hypoxia and anaerobic metabolism; helpful in evaluating metabolic acidosis
Prothrombin time/ partial thrombo-plastin time (PT/PTT)	Prolonged PT/PTT commonly occur during septic shock and may or may not indicate DIC ↓ PT may indicate hepatic failure
Pulse oximetry	↓ levels indicate decreased tissue perfusion and oxygenation; pulse oximetry should be monitored frequently Evaluates oxygenation efforts and respiratory status; if septic shock persists, more invasive monitoring of oxygenation is done via an arterial line in intensive care
Arterial blood gases (ABGs)	↓ percentage oxygen saturation indicates oxygenation of blood and decrease tissue perfusion ABGs indicate presence and degree of severity of respiratory and metabolic acidosis
Chest x-ray	Evaluates presence or progression of pulmonary edema, pneumonia, adult respiratory distress syndrome Posterior/anterior/lateral views are preferred but if only a portable x-ray is possible, films should be obtained with the patient in an upright position
Electrocardiogram	↑ heart rate in presence of fever, hypoxia, hypotension, hypermetabolism Dysrhythmias
Urinalysis	↑ in WBCs and bacteria may indicate infectious source ↑ RBCs/occult blood may be suggestive of bleeding due to coagulopathy
Antibiotic levels	The timing of blood level will depend on the chosen antibiotic These levels provide valuable information regarding appropriate posing based in renal function and drug clearance
Fibrinogen degradation products (FDPs)	↑ levels seen during fibrinolysis and DIC

BUN = blood urea nitrogen.
DIC = disseminated intravascular coagulation.

easily be overlooked, even with the use of CT scans. No imaging study can definitively rule out infection.[7]

The protein C pathway represents one of the major regulatory systems of hemostasis and exhibits anthrombotic, profibrinolytic, and anti-inflammatory properties. Acquired protein C deficiency is prevalent in the majority of septic patients (>85%) and is associated with increased morbidity and mortality in patients with severe sepsis and septic shock.[26] Serial protein C measurement may be a helpful biomarker in differentiating sepsis from other causes of shock. Activation of coagulation is significantly more pronounced in sepsis patients. Boldt, Papsdorf, and Rothe showed that levels of protein C were the lowest in sepsis patients at baseline (mean, 47.8%) and remained significantly lower than in other critically ill patients throughout the study period.[30] Protein C deficiency has been shown to occur in the presence of a wide range of infectious organisms.[26]

Therapeutic Approaches and Nursing Care

Prevention

The key to preventing progression from infection to septic shock is early recognition and intervention. Physicians and nurses must have the knowledge, experience, and advanced clinical judgment to anticipate and manage the complications associated with septic shock. Also, patients should be informed of the importance of reporting signs and symptoms of infection promptly. The sophisticated technology and advanced skills inherent in supportive ancillary disciplines such as pharmacy, respiratory care, and laboratory services as well as the consultative services of specialists in infectious disease, pulmonology, and intensive care are essential. Early administration of antibiotic and supportive therapy remains the cornerstone in preventing progression from sepsis to septic shock.

Management

Management of patients with severe sepsis and septic shock involves hemodynamic support, treatment of infection, treatment of inflammation, and oxygenation support.

Hemodynamic support

Major fluid volume depletion occurs in patients with septic shock due to decreased venous tone, vascular pooling, capillary leak, and third spacing of fluid. The hallmark of septic shock is profound hypotension. Reinstating adequate circulating volume raises blood pressure and enhances cardiac performance, systemic perfusion, and normalization of oxidative metabolism. Early goal-directed therapy is now routinely used in intensive care units for management of severe sepsis and septic shock. This approach involves adjustments of cardiac preload, afterload, and contractility to balance oxygen delivery with oxygen demand, thereby preventing further deterioration of cardiovascular function.[31] Endpoints include normalized values for mixed venous oxygen saturation, arterial lactate concentration, base deficit, and pH. Mixed venous oxygen saturation can be used as a surrogate for the cardiac index as a target for hemodynamic therapy.[31] Early goal-directed therapy requires placement of a central venous catheter for accurate measurement of hemodynamics.[23]

Fluid resuscitation

Fluid administration should be guided by the response to therapy as measured by blood pressure, urine output, and skin characteristics. Colloids offer no proven advantages over crystalloid fluids.[7] When colloids and crystalloids are titrated to the same level of filling pressure, they restore tissue perfusion to the same degree; however, four times more crystalloid is required than colloid, along with slightly longer infusion periods.[32] The goals of fluid resuscitation in septic shock are restoration of tissue perfusion and normalization of cellular metabolism. Therefore, fluid infusion should be the initial step in cardiovascular support and should be titrated to clinical endpoints of blood pressure, heart rate, and urine output.[32] If fluid resuscitation is given in the absence of central hemodynamic monitoring, bolus fluid therapy (250–1000 mL crystalloid over 5–15 minutes), repeated as long as the patient remains hypotensive or until early clinical manifestation of fluid overload (crackles on auscultation or drop in oxygen saturation) occurs, is appropriate.[23] If administration of 2–3 liters fails to show rapid clinical benefit as evidenced by increased blood pressure and urine output, then intravascular monitoring (pulmonary artery catheter or central venous catheter) is indicated, if not already in place.

Complications of fluid resuscitation include peripheral and pulmonary edema as well as hemodilution. The clinical benefits of restoring hemoglobin levels via packed RBC transfusion vary on an individual basis. Transfusion will increase the volume and oxygen-carrying capacity of blood, which can be beneficial for underlying cardiac disease. Raising the hemoglobin and hematocrit increases viscosity levels in the circulating volume, however, which reduces cardiac output, blood flow, and perfusion, most notably in the microvasculature. The optimal hemoglobin and hematocrit levels for patients with septic shock remain unclear, although a hemoglobin level of 9–10 g/dL is generally recommended. Most patients can tolerate this level of anemia. The minimum hemoglobin concentration should be 7–8 g/dL.[32] In a large randomized study by Hebert and colleagues,[33] ICU patients showed no benefit of transfusion to a hemoglobin level of 10 versus 7g/dL; in fact, use of the lower hemoglobin level for transfusion resulted in improved survival.

Vasopressors and inotropic support

Maximum volume restoration should be given before adding vasoactive drugs. Aggressive fluid resuscitation compensates for capillary leak, increased venous capacity, and increased pulmonary resistance by reestablishing adequate left ventricular blood return.[23] When fluid resuscitation fails, vasopressor and inotropic drugs are added to support cardiovascular function. In most cases, patients requiring vasoactive drugs will be cared for in intensive care units. Detailed information regarding the administration of vasopressor and inotropic drugs for septic shock is beyond the scope of this chapter.

Dopamine, epinephrine, norepinephrine, phenylephrine, and vasopressin have been demonstrated to be effective in raising blood pressure in patients with septic shock (see Table 38-4).[7,23,34] Dopamine is employed as first-line therapy for its vasopressor and inotropic effects. It also stimulates dopaminergic receptors, potentially increasing renal blood flow.[7] Norepinephrine is a more potent agent than dopamine in refractory septic shock. If dopamine alone

Table 38-4 Vasopressor Agents for Use in Septic Shock

Agent	Pharmacologic Role	Clinical Effect	Usual IV Dose Range
Dopamine	Dopamine and beta-adrenergic agonist; progressive alpha-adrenergic effect with increasing doses	Chronotropism Inotropism Vasoconstriction	2–25 μg/kg/min
Norepinephrine	Alpha- and beta-adrenergic agonist	Chronotropism Inotropism Vasoconstriction	1–30 μg/min
Phenylephrine	Alpha-adrenergic agonist	Vasoconstriction	40–180 μg/min
Epinephrine	Alpha- and beta-adrenergic agonist	Chronotropism Inotropism Vasoconstriction	1–20 μg/min
Dobutamine	Beta-adrenergic agonist	Chronotropism Inotropism Vasoconstriction	5–15 μg/kg/min
Vasopressin	Antidiuretic hormone (ADH)	Vasoconstriction	0.01–0.04 unit/min

Data from Wheeler, Bernard[7]; Dellinger[23]; Chen.[34]

proves inadequate, norepinephrine may be added for increased vasopressor support, or dobutamine for increased inotropic support. If these measures fail to restore hemodynamic stability, epinephrine is given, which generally heralds a very poor prognosis. Recent literature supports the use of vasopressin as an option to raise blood pressure in septic shock; this agent can also be used when trying to wean patients off traditional vasopressors. When vasopressin is given, it is most often used in patients already requiring high-dose vasopressors when blood pressure remains inadequate.[23]

Treatment of inflammation

While their use remains controversial, the rationale for administering corticosteroids stems from the understanding of septic shock as a profound inflammatory response to infection. Corticosteroids prevent complement activation, inhibit the inducible form of nitric oxide synthase, and prevent neutrophil aggregation and adherence induced by endotoxin. In a series of complex interactions between the inflammation and coagulation systems, pro-inflammatory cytokines activate the coagulation cascade.[35] A state of relative adrenal insufficiency is believed to exist during critical illness.[36] Numerous clinical trials have been conducted to evaluate the efficacy of corticosteroids on severe sepsis and septic shock. Although there may be some benefit to corticosteroid administration in physiologic doses (200–300 mg/day of hydrocortisone) in the patient with vasopressor-dependent septic shock,[37] the data appear to suggest that high-dose corticosteroids are not beneficial.[36] Administration of high doses (e.g., 30 mg/kg of methylprednisolone) does not improve survival among patients with sepsis[35] and may increase the frequency of secondary infections.[10] Administration of physiologic doses in placebo-controlled trials resulted in decreased duration of vasopressor support and a trend toward improved survival.[38,39] Adrenal function should be tested prior to hydrocortisone administration, as there may be no benefit for septic shock patients with a normal (>9 μg/dL) increase in plasma cortisol in response to corticotropin testing, making such testing important.[40]

Activated protein C Recombinant human activated protein C, an anticoagulant, is the first anti-inflammatory agent that has proved effective in the treatment of sepsis. Activated protein C inactivates various coagulation factors, thereby preventing the generation of thrombin, and decreases inflammation by inhibiting platelet activation, neutrophil recruitment, and mast-cell degranulation. It also has direct anti-inflammatory properties, including blocking the production of cytokines by monocytes and blocking cell adhesion.[10] Administration of activated protein C has been demonstrated to reverse hemostatic alterations and organ dysfunction in septic patients.[26,41] The primary risk associated with its use is hemorrhage. In both placebo-controlled and open-label trials, intracranial hemorrhage or bleeding requiring three or more units of blood were reported.[10] Due to the risk of hemorrhage, a platelet count and international normalized ratio (INR) should be obtained for any patient for whom activated protein C is considered as therapy. Administration of this anticoagulant to patients with an INR greater than 3.0 or a platelet count less than 30,000 cells/mm^3 is not recommended.[10]

Treatment of infection

The most important management strategy of septic shock is immediate treatment with intravenous antimicrobial therapy.[24] Blood cultures can provide critical information regarding offending pathogens and antibiotic sensitivity and therefore must be collected before any antimicrobial therapy begins. In 20%–30% of patients, a definitive site of infection is not determined.[7] Gram-positive bacteria now account for 60%–70% of microbiologically documented infections.[21] Until a definitive source of infection can be identified, empiric treatment with broad-spectrum antibiotics is initiated. Antibiotic coverage is subsequently narrowed as microbiologic data become available.[7] Immunocompromised individuals require broad-spectrum antibiotic coverage against common gram-negative organisms (*Pseudomonas aeruginosa, Escherichia coli, Klebsiella*) and gram-positive organisms (coagulase-negative staphylococci, *S. aureus,* streptococci, *S. pneumoniae, Corynebacterium*).[7,21,42] Monotherapy with a third- or fourth-generation cephalosporin (ceftazidime or cefepime) or carbapenem (imipenem-cilastatin or meropenem) may provide sufficient initial coverage while awaiting microbiologic data.[21,43] The National Comprehensive Cancer Network (NCCN) advisory panel on fever and neutropenia recommends therapy with a carbapenem, an aminoglycoside, and vancomycin as initial empiric therapy for all neutropenic patients with fever who present with SIRS.[42] Additionally, the NCCN panel recommends dual therapy with an antipseudomonal beta-lactam (cephalosporin or penicillin) plus an aminoglycoside or ciprofloxacin if the patient also has hypotension when he or she presents with fever and neutropenia or has a prior history of *P. aeruginosa* colonization.[42]

Patients on monotherapy must be closely monitored for nonresponse, secondary infections, adverse effects, or development of drug-resistant organisms. Addition of other antibiotics may be necessary during the clinical course. The most commonly used two-drug antimicrobial regimens combine an aminoglycoside (gentamicin, tobramycin, or amikacin) with an antipseudomonal carboxypenicillin or ureidopenicillin (ticarcillin–clavulanic acid or piperacillin–tazobactam); an aminoglycoside with an antipseudomonal cephalosporin; and an aminoglycoside with a carbapenem.[21,42,43]

Routine use of vancomycin in the initial antimicrobial regimen for granulocytic patients is not recommended unless (1) line sepsis is strongly suspected; (2) there is a high rate of nosocomial infection in the hospital with methecillin-resistant *Staphylococcus aureus* (MRSA) or the patient has a known MRSA colonization; (3) the patient is in shock with respiratory distress and there are strong reasons to suspect hemolytic viridans streptococcal bacteremia; or (4) the patient is at risk for endocarditis (e.g., has a prosthetic heart valve). Vancomycin should be reserved for microbiologically confirmed infections with coagulase-negative staphylococci or other resistant gram-positive organisms.[43] Treatment with aminoglycosides alone is suboptimal, even if the offending bacteria may be susceptible in vitro.[21] If aminoglycosides are used, serum levels of the drug should be monitored as needed in patients with impaired renal function and dosages adjusted accordingly to achieve optimal therapeutic concentrations. When considering combinations of antimicrobials, drugs such as amphotericin B, vancomycin, and aminoglycosides should be avoided in combination, if possible, due to their renal toxicity. Other drugs associated with a high incidence of renal toxicity, such as cisplatin and cyclosporine, should also be avoided when using antibiotics with potential for renal toxicity.[21] The primary advantages of combination therapy are potential synergistic effects against some gram-negative bacilli and decreased risk of development of drug-resistant strains during treatment.[21]

A phenomenon known as the *Jarisch-Herxheimer reaction* (J-HR) may occur following antimicrobial therapy against certain microbes—specifically, those caused by spirochetes such as Lyme disease and syphilis.[44] Relapsing fever, chills, petechiae, purpura, jaundice, and associated symptoms may occur. Originally thought to be due to the release of an endotoxin, the current hypothesis is that J-HR is a physiologic manifestation of a pro-inflammatory cytokine cascade that takes place after the destruction of spirochetes.[44,45] Attempts to treat J-HR by blunting the cytokine cascade have been largely unsuccessful.[45] Instead, appropriate antimicrobial therapies for relapsing fever, such as penicillin, tetracyclines, erythromycin, or chloramphenicol, are given along with supportive care.

The incidence of systemic fungal infections has increased during the past two decades, with the rise most likely being attributable to the existence of prolonged, profound neutropenia and the extensive use of broad-spectrum antibiotics.[42] The most common fungal infections in neutropenic patients include superficial and systemic infections due to *Candida* and invasive aspergillosis. Fluconazole is effective therapy for uncomplicated candidemia in patients with intact immune systems. Its role in neutropenic patients is unclear, however.[42] Amphotericin B and its liposomal formulations are approved for treatment of aspergillosis. The liposomal formulations have less renal toxicity than the conventional formulations.[42,43] New antifungal agents, including echinocandins and late-generation azoles, show promise for treating and/or preventing invasive fungal infections with greater efficacy and less toxicity.[42] Amphotericin B has been the standard empiric antifungal for patients with prolonged fever during neutropenia (e.g., after 5–7 days of broad-spectrum antibiotics). Itraconazole has recently been demonstrated to have efficacy in this setting as well.[46] Caution should be observed in the use of itraconazole as empiric therapy due to the possibility of liver failure.[47]

Oxygen therapy and supportive care

Oxygen therapy should be initiated by nasal cannula and increased as needed based on oxygen saturation, ABGs, and lactate levels. Targeting a specific threshold of high oxygen delivery is not recommended as therapy for septic shock.[23] As interstitial and alveolar edema continue to worsen, ventilation/perfusion mismatch occurs, taxing the respiratory effort and increasing oxygen demands. Respiratory complications of septic shock include ARDS, which is a severe form of acute lung injury (ALI) in the cascade of respiratory dysfunction.[25] The mortality associated with ALI and ARDS is in excess of 40%.[25] As part of goal-directed therapy, early endotracheal intubation and mechanical ventilation are encouraged to increase oxygen delivery and decrease oxygen demand until septic shock can be reversed. One of the chief benefits of mechanical ventilatory support in ARDS is to reduce the patient's work of breathing so that blood flow may be directed to other vital organs.[25]

Basic supportive care of patients with severe sepsis and septic shock is essential. Enteral nutrition, prevention of nosocomial infections, stress ulcers, skin breakdown, and deep-vein thrombosis (DVT) may play more important roles in the outcome of septic shock than was once appreciated. Histamine antagonists, proton-pump inhibitors, or sucralfate is indicated in mechanically ventilated patients who cannot be fed enterally. Unless contraindicated, low-molecular-weight heparin (LMWH) or fixed-dose unfractionated heparin should be used to prevent DVT.[7,48]

Protein and caloric requirements are high and underlying malnutrition is prevalent in patients with sepsis. Although prolonged starvation is likely to be harmful, short periods of several days without nutrition are not likely to have adverse effects. Therefore, feeding may be withheld until hemodynamic stability has been achieved.[7] Enteral nutrition is the preferred method of nutritional support in the critically ill patient. Parenteral nutrition should be reserved for those patients who cannot tolerate enteral feeding or in the presence of co-morbidities such as mesenteric ischemia or bowel obstruction.[48] Continuous-infusion insulin to achieve tight glucose control significantly reduces mortality and is an important element of effective management.[41]

Conclusion

Current predictions suggest that by the year 2030, more than 17% of the U.S. population will be older than 65 years of age.[49] Elders may have preexisting conditions such as diabetes or pulmonary dysfunction and may also manifest unexplained or unusual organ dysfunction as early signs of the septic process. Older patients with sepsis have decreased physiologic reserves compared with younger patients and are at increased risk for incidence of septic shock and MODS. In general, elders have increased mortality from sepsis and septic shock.[2,15,22]

Genetic factors that may predispose individual patients to increased mortality from sepsis remain under investigation. It is clinically recognized that not all patients who become infected will develop septic sequelae. The study of the genetic basis of disease is a rapidly emerging field of medicine. Among the few known genetic polymorphisms (a stable gene mutation that is sustained within a population)[50] that appear to affect the risk and progress of infection is the tumor necrosis factor 2 (TNF2) allele, which is responsible for the generation of TNF-α. This cytokine plays a central role in the initiation of septic shock.[50] The possibility TNF or other gene polymorphisms could either protect against septic shock or increase sensitivity to bacterial infection is a current topic of clinical investigation.[51] Functional genomic approaches may lead to a broader understanding of the complex pathophysiology involved in the septic shock cascade and yield individualized care based on genotype considerations and targeted therapies. Today, cloned proteins and monoclonal antibodies are among the new therapeutic agents being developed to regulate specific steps of the inflammatory response.

The use of growth factors and interferon-gamma (IFN-γ) during sepsis for modulation of neutrophil function to prevent progression to septic shock remains controversial. Colony-stimulating factors (CSFs) have been used to stimulate the proliferation of leukocytes during myelosuppressive chemotherapy. American Society of Clinical Oncology guidelines recommend the use of granulocyte CSF (G-CSF) or granulocyte-macrophage CSF (GM-CSF) to reduce the likelihood of febrile neutropenia under certain conditions. The benefit of a CSF for cancer patients with fever and neutropenia has not been proven, however.[52] The use of G-CSF or GM-CSF during septic shock continues to be studied due to the presence of both immunostimulatory and immunosuppressive effects.[9] Ongoing research into the pathophysiology of sepsis indicates the presence of a hypo-inflammatory phase during which immune stimulation with cytokines such as IFN-γ may prove beneficial. For this indication, IFN-γ has been studied only in small, pilot studies.[9] Further research may lead to new uses for cytokines in sepsis.

Sepsis, severe sepsis, and septic shock represent increasingly severe levels of systemic response to infection. With each level comes a higher toll in organ damage, life-support requirements, and mortality. Although significant advances have been made in our understanding of the septic cascade and our ability to manage patients with septic shock, this condition remains an oncologic emergency of great significance. Oncology nurses can play a major role in preventing septic shock and advocating for research into new and more effective therapies. An understanding of the population at risk for developing a life-threatening infection along with early recognition and treatment are the best resources to ensure improved patient outcomes. Future clinical studies of new therapies must be conducted to further characterize the disease process relative to targeted biological mediators causing organ dysfunction or death.

References

1. Bone RC, Balk RA, Cerra FB, et al: The American College of Chest Physicians/Society of Critical Care Medicine consensus conference: definitions for sepsis and organ failure and guidelines for the use of innovative therapies in sepsis. *Chest* 101:1644–1655, 1992
2. Balk RA: Severe sepsis and septic shock. Definitions, epidemiology, and clinical manifestations. *Crit Care Clin* 16:179–192, 2000
3. Martin GS, Mannino DM, Eaton S, et al: The epidemiology of sepsis in the United States from 1979 through 2000. *N Engl J Med* 348:1546–1554, 2003
4. Angus DC, Linde-Zwirble WT, Lidicker J, et al: Epidemiology of severe sepsis in the United States: analysis of incidence, outcome, and associated costs of care. *Crit Care Med* 29:1303–1310, 2001
5. Hoyert DL, Arias E, Smith BL, et al: Deaths: Final Data for 1999. National Vital Statistics Reports. Hyattsville, MD, National Center for Health Statistics, 2001
6. Parrillo JE, Parker MM, Natanson C, et al: Septic shock in humans. Advances in the understanding of pathogenesis, cardiovascular dysfunction, and therapy. *Ann Intern Med* 113:227–242, 1990
7. Wheeler AP, Bernard GR: Treating patients with severe sepsis. *N Engl J Med* 340:207–214, 1999
8. Safdar A, Armstrong D: Infectious morbidity in critically ill patients with cancer. *Crit Care Clin* 17:531–570, vii–viii, 2001
9. Glauser MP: Neutropenia: clinical implications and modulation. *Intensive Care Med* 26:S103–S110, 2000
10. Hotchkiss RS, Karl IE: The pathophysiology and treatment of sepsis. *N Engl J Med* 348:138–150, 2003
11. Lederer JA, Rodrick ML, Mannick JA: The effects of injury on the adaptive immune response. *Shock* 11:153–159, 1999
12. Oberholzer A, Oberholzer C, Moldawer LL: Sepsis syndromes: understanding the role of innate and acquired immunity. *Shock* 16:83–96, 2001
13. Bogolioubov A, Keefe DL, Groeger JS: Circulatory shock. *Crit Care Clin* 17:697–719, 2001
14. Nasraway SA: The problems and challenges of immunotherapy in sepsis. *Chest* 123:451S–459S, 2003
15. Sharma S, Mink S: Septic shock, July 21, 2003. *www.medicine.com/MED/topic2101.htm*. Accessed October 30, 2003
16. Nimah M, Brilli RJ: Coagulation dysfunction in sepsis and multiple organ system failure. *Crit Care Clin* 19:441–458, 2003
17. Vincent JL, Zhang H, Szabo C, et al: Effects of nitric oxide in septic shock. *Am J Respir Crit Care Med* 161:1781–1785, 2000
18. Landry DW, Oliver JA: The pathogenesis of vasodilatory shock. *N Engl J Med* 345:588–595, 2001
19. Stoll EH: Sepsis and septic shock. *Clin J Oncol Nurs* 5:71–72, 2001
20. Vincent JL, de Carvalho FB, De Backer D: Management of septic shock. *Ann Med* 34:606–613, 2002
21. Hughes WT, Armstrong D, Bodey GP, et al: 2002 guidelines for the use of antimicrobial agents in neutropenic patients with cancer. *Clin Infect Dis* 34:730–751, 2002
22. Krieger BP: Sepsis in the geriatric age group, in Fein AM, Abraham EM, Balk RA, et al (eds.): *Sepsis and Multiorgan Failure.* Baltimore, Williams & Wilkins, 1997, pp 373–380
23. Dellinger RP: Cardiovascular management of septic shock. *Crit Care Med* 31:946–955, 2003
24. Shelton BK: Sepsis. *Semin Oncol Nurs* 15:209–221, 1999
25. Martin GS, Bernard GR: Airway and lung in sepsis. *Intensive Care Med* 27:S63–S79, 2001
26. Fisher CJ Jr, Yan SB: Protein c levels as a prognostic indicator of outcome in sepsis and related diseases. *Crit Care Med* 28:S49–S56, 2000
27. Llewelyn M, Cohen J: Diagnosis of infection in sepsis. *Intensive Care Med* 27:S10–S32, 2001
28. Raad I, Hanna HA, Alakech B, et al: Differential time to positivity: a useful method for diagnosing catheter-related bloodstream infections. *Ann Intern Med* 140:18–25, 2004
29. O'Grady NP, Alexander M, Dellinger RP, et al: Guidelines for the prevention of intravascular catheter-related infections. Centers for Disease Control and Prevention. *MMWR* 51:1–29, 2002
30. Boldt J, Papsdorf M, Rothe A: Changes of the hemostatic network in critically ill patients — is there a difference between sepsis, trauma and neurosurgery patients? *Crit Care Med* 28:445–450, 2000
31. Rivers E, Nguyen B, Havstad S, et al: Early goal-directed therapy in the treatment of severe sepsis and septic shock. *N Engl J Med* 345:1368–1377, 2001
32. Vincent JL: International Sepsis Forum: Hemodynamic support in septic shock. *Intensive Care Med* 27:S80–S92, 2001
33. Hebert PC, Wells G, Blajchman MA, et al: A multicenter, randomized, controlled clinical trial of transfusion requirements in critical care. *N Engl J Med* 340:409–417, 1999
34. Chen P: Vasopressin: new uses in critical care. *Am J Med Sci* 324:146–154, 2002
35. Carlet J: Immunological therapy in sepsis: currently available. *Intensive Care Med* 27:S93–S103, 2001
36. Balk RA: Steroids for septic shock: back from the dead? (pro). *Chest* 123:490S–499S, 2003
37. Annane D: Corticosteroids for septic shock. *Crit Care Med* 29:S117–S120, 2001
38. Annane D, Sebille V, Charpentier C, et al: Effect of treatment with low doses of hydrocortisone and fludrocortisone on mortality in patients with septic shock. *JAMA* 288:862–871, 2002
39. Briegel J, Forst H, Haller M, et al: Stress doses of hydrocortisone reverse hyperdynamic septic shock: a prospective, randomized, double-blind, single-center study. *Crit Care Med* 27:723–732, 1999

40. Sessler CN: Steroids for septic shock: back from the dead? (con). *Chest* 123:482S–489S, 2003
41. Patel GP, Gurka DP, Balk RA: New treatment strategies for severe sepsis and septic shock. *Curr Opin Crit Care* 9:390–396, 2003
42. NCCN Fever and Neutropenia Panel Members. Fever and neutropenia, in Rubenstein EB (ed.): *NCCN Practice Guidelines.* National Comprehensive Cancer Network, Jenkintown, PA, April 9, 2003. www.nccn.org/physician_gls/f-guideline.html. Accessed December 10, 2003
43. Donowitz GR, Maki DG, Crnich CJ, et al: Infections in the neutropenic patient — new views of an old problem. *Hematology* 1:113–139, 2001
44. Griffin GE: Cytokines involved in human septic shock: the model of the Jarisch-Herxheimer reaction. *J Antimicrobiol Chemother* 41:25–29, 1998
45. Cooper PJ, Fekade D, Remick DG, et al: Recombinant human interleukin-10 fails to alter proinflammatory cytokine production or physiologic changes associated with the Jarisch-Herxheimer reaction. *J Infect Dis* 181:203–209, 2000
46. Boogaerts M, Winston DJ, Bow EJ: Intravenous and oral itraconazole versus intravenous amphotericin B deoxycholate as empirical antifungal therapy for persistent fever in neutropenic patients with cancer who are receiving broad-spectrum antibacterial therapy. *Ann Intern Med* 135:412–422, 2001
47. Anonymous: Itraconazole, terbinafine possibly linked to liver failure. *Am J Health Sys Pharm* 58:1076, 2001
48. Perez J, Dellinger RP: Other supportive therapies in sepsis. *Intens Care Med* 27:S116–S127, 2001
49. Rordriguez MJ, Fein AM: Diagnostic approach and clinical manifestations of severe sepsis, in Fein AM, Abraham EM, Balk RA, et al (eds.): *Sepsis and Multiorgan Failure.* Baltimore, Williams & Wilkins, 1997, pp 269–276
50. Kumar A, Short J, Parrillo JE: Genetic factors in septic shock. *JAMA* 282:579–581, 1999
51. Casey LC: Immunologic response to infection and its role in septic shock. *Crit Care Clin* 16:193–213, 2000
52. Ozer H, Armitage JO, Bennett CL, et al: 2000 update of recommendations for the use of hematopoietic colony-stimulating factors: evidence-based, clinical practice guidelines. *J Clin Oncol* 18:3558–3585, 2000

CHAPTER 39

Spinal Cord Compression

Anne Marie Flaherty, RN, MSN, AOCN®, APNc

Scope of the Problem

Definition

Although rare, spinal cord compression is a devastating complication of cancer. It is a malignant process that causes disruption in neurological function when a tumor and its destructive effects on the spinal cord compress neural tissue or interfere with its blood supply.[1]

Incidence

Spinal cord compression occurs in 5%–10% of patients with cancer and is the second most common neurological complication of cancer.[2] More than 25,000 cases are diagnosed annually, about twice the number of traumatic spinal cord injuries.[3] The incidence of spinal cord compression may actually be increasing due to improved treatments and prolonged survival currently seen in various cancers such as breast and prostate cancers, improved quality and availability of diagnostic tests, and earlier screening.[1,3] Spinal cord compression is now referred to as a skeletal-related event or a consequence of bone metastases, reflecting the fact that almost 90% of cases are due to involvement of the vertebral column with metastatic disease. The majority of spinal cord compressions in these cases are due to cancers of the lung, breast, and prostate. Approximately 10% of patients present with spinal cord compression as their initial symptom of cancer, and half of those patients will ultimately be diagnosed with lung cancer.[3]

In this chapter, the discussion is primarily related to metastatic epidural spinal cord compression and not primary spinal cord tumors, as less than 5% of cases are related to primary spinal cord tumors. Oncology nurses are in the best position to identify those individuals at risk to develop spinal cord compression and those with early-stage spinal cord compression so that treatment is instituted prior to neurological deterioration. The primary goal is to preserve and maintain the neurological status of the individual, thereby maintaining the patient's quality of life. The most important prognostic factor is the neurological function prior to the initiation of treatment. In the classic study by Gilbert and colleagues, the majority of those patients who were ambulatory prior to treatment remained so after its completion.[4]

Pathophysiology

Anatomy of the Spinal Cord

The spinal cord consists of ascending and descending nerve tracts that carry impulses to and from the brain and peripheral nerves. These impulses result in sensory information and motor ability.[5] The spinal cord is protected by three connective tissue membranes known as the leptomeninges: (1) pia mater, the innermost layer; (2) arachnoid, the middle layer; and (3) dura mater, the outermost layer. See Figure 39-1(A). The spinal cord is surrounded by the vertebral column — a bony structure that consists of stacked vertebrae and provides flexibility and support.[6] Each vertebra consists of a vertebral body, two laminae, two pedicles, and a spinous process. See Figure 39-1(B). The spinal cord starts at the base of the brain and ends in the space between the first two lumbar vertebrae. The cauda equina refers to a group of lumbar and sacral nerve roots emerging from the end of the spinal

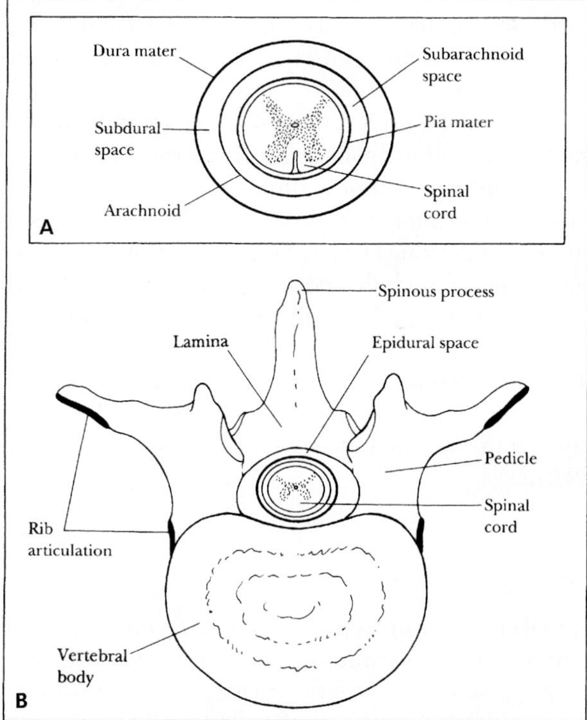

Figure 39-1 **(A)** The cross section illustrates the leptomeninges or membranes surrounding the spinal cord and spaces between the membranes. **(B)** Cross-section of vertebra and spinal cord. The vertebra consists of the vertebral body, pedicles, laminae, and spinous process. The spinal cord spans the length of the vertebral column in the canal formed by the vertebrae.

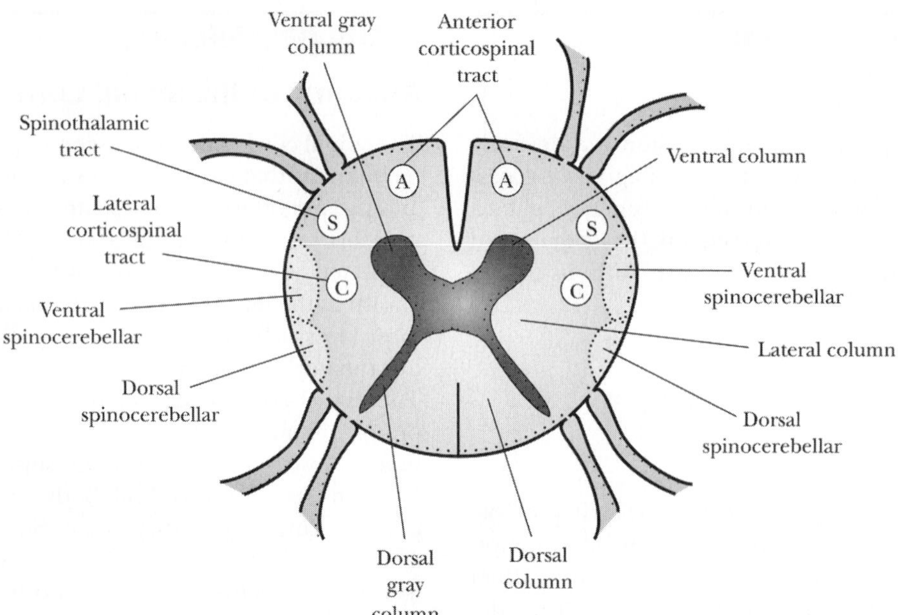

Figure 39-2 Cross section of spinal cord and spinal tracts.

cord. The spinal cord is larger in the cervical and lumbar regions and consequently these vertebrae are also larger to accommodate the cord.

The spinal cord is arranged into several distinct regions. The butterfly-shaped gray matter has anterior horns controlling motor function, lateral horns controlling autonomic functions, and posterior horns related to sensation. The lateral and anterior spinal cord white matter includes corticospinal tracts and additional nerve tracts that control fine motor control and tone. The spinocerebellar tracts are associated with muscle stretch and tone sensation. The lateral spinothalamic tract carries pain fibers, and the dorsal columns transmit fine touch and positional sense (Figure 39-2).[7]

Etiology

Spinal cord compression can arise from either primary tumors within the spinal cord and its protective layers or as a result of metastatic disease. Primary tumors of the spine that arise within the cord itself are called *intramedullary;* those that develop within the dural layers are called *extramedullary-intradural.* These tumors include malignancies such as ependymoma, astrocytoma, oligodendroglioma, and meningioma.[5]

Metastasis to the spine can be classified as intramedullary (within the spine itself), leptomeningeal (within the lining of the spinal cord), and epidural (outside the lining of the spinal cord). Intramedullary and leptomeningeal metastases are rare and arise from hematogenous spread via paravertebral and extradural plexi as well as growth along nerve roots from paravertebral tumors. Intramedullary metastases are most often associated with breast and lung cancer, whereas leukemia and lymphoma are more likely to result in leptomeningeal carcinomatosis.[8,9] Epidural metastasis — the most common type of metastasis to the spine — occurs because of the extension of a tumor or bone from the vertebral column, extension of a tumor through the intervertebral foramina, or direct tumor deposits in the epidural space (Figure 39-3). Eighty-five percent of cases of epidural metastasis involve the vertebral column, whereas 10%–15% of cases develop compression from paravertebral tumors that extend through the foramina. Direct epidural metastasis is rather uncommon and accounts for less than 5% of cases.[9]

The skeleton is the third most frequent site of metastasis after the lung and liver, and the vertebral column is the most common site for skeletal metastasis.[10] The vertebral body — rather than the pedicles or laminae — is most often involved. The vertebral column is rich with growth factors, which are present in the bone marrow and help support malignant growth. Another factor encouraging metastatic growth in the vertebral column is its blood supply. The Batson plexus is a low-pressure, valveless venous system that drains thoracic, abdominal, and pelvic organs when thoracic and abdominal pressure is raised during coughing or straining. Tumor cells travel from the primary site to the spinal canal through these paravertebral and extradural venous plexus. The proximity of the plexus may also explain why most spinal cord compression occurs anteriorly or anteriolaterally closest to the posterior portion of the vertebral body.[11] Epidural

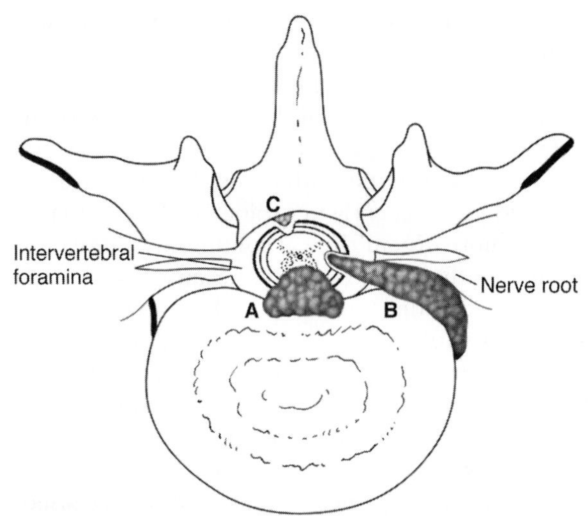

Figure 39-3 Primary types of epidural metastases: **(A)** tumor extension from vertebral body **(B)** tumor traveling along nerve root into intervertebral foramina, and **(C)** direct epidural metastasis.

compression occurs when bony disease in the vertebra causes either extraosseous extension of tumor or destruction and collapse of bony structures into the epidural space.[9] While extraosseous extension of a tumor most often causes compression, if vertebral collapse and angulation of the spine are present, the prognosis is not as favorable.[2] Cancers associated with epidural compression via vertebral metastasis include cancers of the breast, lung, prostate, and kidney, and multiple myeloma and melanoma.

While vertebral metastasis is the most common mechanism for spinal cord compression, tumors can compress the cord by direct extension through the intervertebral foramina.[9] Lymphomas and neuroblastoma travel through this space and compress the spine without invasion of the bony structures. Some tumors (e.g., colon, kidney, prostate, and head and neck) can extend directly into the vertebral structures or epidural space without metastases.[12]

Pathogenesis

Early in spinal cord compression, compression of the epidural venous plexus or direct mechanical injury causes vasogenic cord edema and decreased capillary blood flow.[2,13] This results in ischemia, conduction block, and demyelination of mostly white matter. New evidence indicates that compressed neural tissue leads to a series of neurochemical changes caused by the release of serotonin, prostaglandin, and vascular endothelial growth factor (VEGF). These neurotoxic chemicals cause further tissue damage and neurological changes.[2,13] Later in the course of spinal cord compression, the parenchymal blood supply is disrupted, which causes additional white matter injury.

Site of Compression

The site of epidural metastasis and cord compression is related to the origin of the primary cancer and depends on the anatomical location of the tumor, vascular supply, and venous drainage. The thoracic spine is the most frequent site of epidural compression accounting for about 70% of cases.[13] Its predominance can be explained by the fact that the cancers most frequently associated with bone metastases—breast, lung, and prostate—most often cause thoracic compression. In addition, there are more thoracic vertebrae than lumbosacral or cervical vertebrae. Although lumbosacral metastases on autopsy are more common, they are asymptomatic and often go undetected.[14] About one-third of all patients with spinal cord compression will have multiple noncontiguous sites of metastases.[15]

Clinical Manifestations and Physical Assessment

It is not clear which specific pathophysiologic changes cause each of the clinical manifestations associated with spinal cord compression. These manifestations of cord compression depend on the level of the lesion and compression but not necessarily on which part of the cord—anterior, posterior, or lateral—is actually compressed.[13]

The symptoms of cord compression usually start as mild and noncontributory, but eventually become more pronounced. These symptoms most often follow a progressive pattern that the clinician must recognize to diagnose cord compression early and preserve neurological function. The initial symptom is back pain that is accompanied or followed by motor weakness and decreased sensation. This weakness then progresses to motor and sensory loss, and loss of proprioception, vibratory sense, and bowel and bladder function.[16]

Back Pain

Back pain is the presenting symptom in more than 95% of individuals with spinal cord compression. Approximately one-third of individuals who present with back pain have significant spinal cord compression despite a normal neurological exam.[17] Central back pain is caused by vertebral collapse or stretching of the periosteum of the involved bony structure. The pain is localized within one or two vertebrae of the compression in about half of the cases of epidural compression that involve one vertebra.[7] The pain, however, can occur in multiple areas in cases that involve multiple noncontiguous areas of vertebral metastases. Back pain can also be radicular in nature, meaning that the pain moves or radiates from one location to another. Such a pattern is caused by the tumor irritating the nerve roots such that the pain follows the distribution of the nerve. Radicular pain with cervical and lumbosacral compression is usually unilateral, whereas thoracic compression is usually associated with bilateral pain.[16] Radicular pain with thoracic compression is described as a constrictive-band-like pain; in contrast, cervical and lumbosacral compression may cause pain that radiates to a limb. Radicular pain is more common in lumbar and cervical spinal cord compression.[15]

Back pain often heralds an impending cord compression and can be present a few days to months. The pain is similar to that associated with degenerative disease or herniated disc in that it can be elicited with movement, valsalva maneuver, cough, and straight leg raising or neck flexion. Back pain from cord compression differs from degenerative disease in that lying supine does not alleviate the pain. Lying down increases venous congestion and edema, both of which exacerbate pain. Individuals complain of being unable to sleep at night and feel more comfortable in a recliner or chair. Epidural compression can occur at any level in the spine, whereas degenerative changes are most often seen in the cervical and lumbar spine.[10] Sometimes it may be difficult to distinguish pain related to spinal cord compression, but suspicion should be raised when the nature, intensity, or location of back pain changes.

On physical exam, the clinician tries to elicit the back pain by percussing the vertebrae and having the patient perform leg rising or neck flexion. This exercise will help identify the level of compression. The assessment also includes a description of the nature and character of the pain, its intensity, and alleviating as well as aggravating factors.

Motor Weakness and Motor Loss

In general, muscle weakness follows pain as cord compression progresses. Rarely is weakness, which is a prelude to loss of motor function, the only presenting symptom of cord compression. Approximately three-fourths of affected individuals are obviously paraparetic at the time of diagnosis, and even more cases are identified during a neurological exam. The weakness is usually described as a heaviness or stiffness and involves proximal muscles that are used to climb stairs or get out of a chair.[2]

Roughly 95% of patients who have weakness have a significant compression of the spinal cord.[4] On physical exam, the strength of the extremities and gait are assessed to determine motor loss. This step is important in identifying early neurological deficits that represent a more urgent clinical condition. Ambulation at the time of diagnosis is critical because less than 25% of paralyzed patients will regain their ability to ambulate after treatment of spinal cord compression.[18]

On physical exam, weakness is evaluated by having the patient get out of a chair, walk, and push an extremity against a resisting force. The clinician carefully observes for any gait disturbances. Sometimes back pain will be accompanied by ataxia, which is caused by compression of the spinocerebellar tracts.[1,18] This ataxia is unrelated to other neurological findings and may be confused with central nervous system pathology. In addition to muscle strength and gait, muscle tone is assessed for spasticity and flaccidity.

Reflexes are also evaluated: tendon reflexes in elbow, knee, and ankle; Babinski sign; and abdominal reflexes. In cervical compression, tendon reflexes may be hyperactive; in thoracic and lumbosacral compression, they are decreased or absent.[19]

Sensory Disturbances and Sensory Loss

Sensory changes are less common than motor weakness, but early complaints include numbness or paresthesia. The sensory loss ascends from the toes to the level of the compression as it progresses and can correspond to within two vertebral bodies of the site of the lesion. Clinicians should be aware that this finding is not always reliable because multiple lesions may be present and multiple dermatomes may be affected. In addition, many sensory and motor pathways cross and overlap, making identification of the level of the lesion extremely difficult. In cauda equine compression, sensory loss involves the perianal region, or lateral or posterior thighs, and is dermatome specific and usually bilateral.[1]

As the compression progresses, sensory loss is accompanied by loss of proprioception, position sense, vibration, temperature sense, and deep pressure.[19] Loss of pain and temperature sensation below a specific dermatome indicates disruption of the spinal thalamic pathway in the lateral column of the spinal cord's white matter. Loss of vibration accompanies sensory loss and is associated with disruption in the posterior spinocerebellar pathways or posterior columns.[13,20] Deep-tendon reflexes may be decreased at the level of the lesion and hyperactive below that level.[20]

Table 39-1 Relationship of Pretreatment Neurologic Status to Ambulation after Treatment

Pretreatment Neurologic Status	Treatment	Post-treatment Neurologic Status
52% of patients ambulatory with minimal impairment	Dexamethasone 10 mg IV followed by 4 mg q6h	94% of patients ambulatory
39% of patients paraparetic and nonambulatory	Radiation 200–300 cGy every day for a total of 2000–3000 cGy	60% of patients ambulatory
9% of patients paraplegic		1% of patients ambulatory

Data from Maranzano, Latini.[31]

On physical exam, the clinician assesses for any numbness or parasthesia by testing for light touch with a cotton-tipped applicator, pain with a pin-prick technique, and proprioception by moving the big toe and fingers in various positions. For an accurate assessment of spinal cord disease, the clinician begins at the feet and works upward to determine the highest level of intact sensory function.[19]

Autonomic Dysfunction

Autonomic dysfunction includes an array of bowel and bladder disturbances that are due to disruption in lower motor neuron function.[16] This late sign of spinal cord compression includes sphincter problems that result in bowel and bladder incontinence or retention. The individual may experience difficulty initiating urinary flow, sometimes in conjunction with retention, frequency, or incontinence. Urinary retention is defined as a postvoid residual of greater than 150 mL when one is catheterized after micturition.

Early bowel problems may be present when the individual complains of difficulty expelling stool and experiences loss of feeling. This problem may eventually lead to constipation or incontinence. Poor sphincter tone is a late sign of autonomic dysfunction and is a poor prognostic sign.[13] Usually, those individuals who have autonomic dysfunction are also nonambulatory and rarely regain the ability to ambulate (Table 39–1).

Diagnostic Evaluation

Plain Films and Bone Scans

The type of evaluation is dictated by the clinical condition of the patient. If the patient presents with vague complaints that do not help direct the evaluation, a bone scan and plain films will assist the practioner in ordering the appropriate diagnostic studies. Plain radiological films of the painful area of the vertebral column will demonstrate vertebral body collapse, pedicle erosion, and osteolytic or osteoblastic lesions in more than 80% of cases of epidural metastasis.[20] The degree of vertebral destruction caused by metastatic disease as seen on plain films may be directly related to the incidence of spinal cord compression. For plain films to demonstrate osteolytic osseous destruction, more than 50% of bone must be affected.[21] While bone scan is more sensitive than x-rays, it is often not as helpful as plain films in diagnosing areas of potential cord compression. Bone scans pinpoint the area of disease but do not identify the degree of bone destruction or epidural cord compression. Also, if widespread disease is present, many vertebral bodies may be positive and the level or degree of actual compression not identified.

Magnetic Resonance Imaging

Magnetic resonance imaging (MRI) has emerged as the safest and preferred tool for the diagnosis of spinal cord compression.[22] This noninvasive technique provides a variety of images to help visualize different abnormalities in the spinal cord and surrounding structures. While it is equivalent to a myelogram with computerized tomography (CT) scan in diagnosing cord compression due to extradural masses, MRI is far superior in diagnosing paravertebral masses, intramedullary disease, and bone metastases.[23] An MRI is performed with and without gadolinium, as paravertebral masses, leptomeningeal disease, and intramedullary tumors are better visualized with gadolinium.

Based on the bone scan, spine films, and clinical presentation, the site of compression can be generally identified. If only a specific area of the spine is examined by MRI, additional sites of compression may not be identified and go untreated. Given that 10%–30% of patients with clinical symptoms of spinal cord compression have multiple lesions, the entire spine should be imaged to identify additional areas that are not near the symptomatic lesion. A sagittal MRI survey of the entire spine can be obtained to identify sites of compression, and then more detailed images at that level can aid in further visualizing the type and degree of compression.[2]

Individuals who suffer from claustrophobia may not be able to tolerate the MRI exam. In such a case, patients may be referred to an "open" MRI facility or a sedative such as lorazepam may also be given. Persons who have a pacemaker or metal implantation near the area to be imaged cannot undergo an MRI, nor can patients with a very large body habitus.

Myelogram with Computerized Tomography

If an MRI cannot be performed, myelography with CT scan is comparable in adequately diagnosing spinal cord compression. With CT guidance, contrast is injected via a lumbar puncture into the subarachnoid space, and flow is observed to identify any defects. If a complete block is found, a cervical or cisternal puncture is required to determine the upper level of the block. If multiple complete blocks are suspected, then additional punctures are required. Cerebrospinal fluid (CSF) withdrawn prior to the instillation of contrast is analyzed for malignant cells, cell count, glucose, and protein. Presence of malignant cells in the CSF confirms leptomeningeal carcinomatosis or tumor in the lining or meninges. This disease may be present along with spinal cord compression.

Myelography is not without risks. An invasive procedure, it requires proper coagulation as well as adequate renal function for the use of contrast. The MRI technique is preferred if available to the patient because of its lower cost, greater convenience, and better anatomical detail. The positron emission tomography (PET) scan is currently being evaluated in the diagnosis and management of spinal cord compression. Although its role is still evolving, it has been used to evaluate cervical spine changes following cord compression and intramedullary metastasis in renal cell cancer.[24,25]

Several algorithms have been developed to aid clinicians in promptly diagnosing spinal cord compression (Figure 39-4).[10,13] There are also differing opinions about how to treat symptomatic individuals regardless of the presence of actual spinal cord compression. In any case, it is important to identify all areas of disease, distinguish which areas may cause neurological sequelae, and identify adequate treatment ports for radiation. The goal is to accomplish this in the most efficient and cost effective manner. If the clinical condition demonstrates obvious signs of epidural compression, however, then MRI with gadolinium is warranted. In addition, if other areas of early cord compression are not identified, they may go untreated and become symptomatic with neurological deterioration.[10]

Therapeutic Approaches and Nursing Care

Medical Management

Epidural spinal cord compression is a life-threatening condition requiring immediate intervention so that the patient's neurological condition is at least preserved, if not improved. Disease progression can cause rapid deterioration and paraplegia, quadriplegia, and even respiratory arrest if the cervical spine is involved. The major therapeutic approaches include steroids, radiation therapy, and surgery, including either laminectomy or vertebral body resection with stabilization and chemotherapy. While controversy exists over which treatment or combination of treatments is the best approach, post-treatment neurological status is most directly related to pretreatment neurological status.[17,26] The goals of treatment include decompression of neural tissue, eradication of tumor, relief of pain, preservation of neurological function and stability of spine, and prevention of recurrence and progression.[2,13,27]

Steroids

The usual treatment for spinal cord compression, regardless of the type of cancer, comprises steroids combined with radiotherapy. Steroids are instituted when there is a high level of suspicion of spinal cord compression and prior to definitive treatment because they relieve pain and improve neurological function by reducing spinal cord edema. The one exception occurs when spinal cord compression is the presenting symptom of cancer and lymphoma is suspected. Due to the oncolytic effect, tissue diagnosis may be difficult.[10,23] The mechanism that mediates this phenomenon is related to prostaglandin synthesis, VEGF down-regulation, and prevention of certain effects of vascular permeability.[2]

The dosing of steroids is not standardized, and experts differ on the proper dose. The traditional dosing for steroids is either moderate dose, consisting of a bolus of dexamethasone 10 mg intravenously (IV) followed by 4 mg every 6 hours, or high dose, consisting of a bolus of 100 mg followed by 24 mg every 6 hours. One nonrandomized study compared high-dose dexamethasone to a lower dose and found no difference in overall neurological recovery.[28] Higher doses of steroid (100 mg) should be reserved for those patients with significant neurological symptoms or rapidly progressing symptoms, as higher doses are associated with more significant side effects.[9]

The steroid therapy continues during the early phase of definitive treatment and may begin to be tapered if the individual's neurological status is improving or stabilized. The taper continues unless symptoms worsen, in which case doses should be increased until improvement and tapered again after restabilization.[9] Tapering is a priority to avoid the long-term side effects of steroid therapy, such as hyperglycemia, gastric ulceration, immunosuppression and opportunistic infections, psychosis, and proximal muscle weakness, in an already compromised individual. One steroid

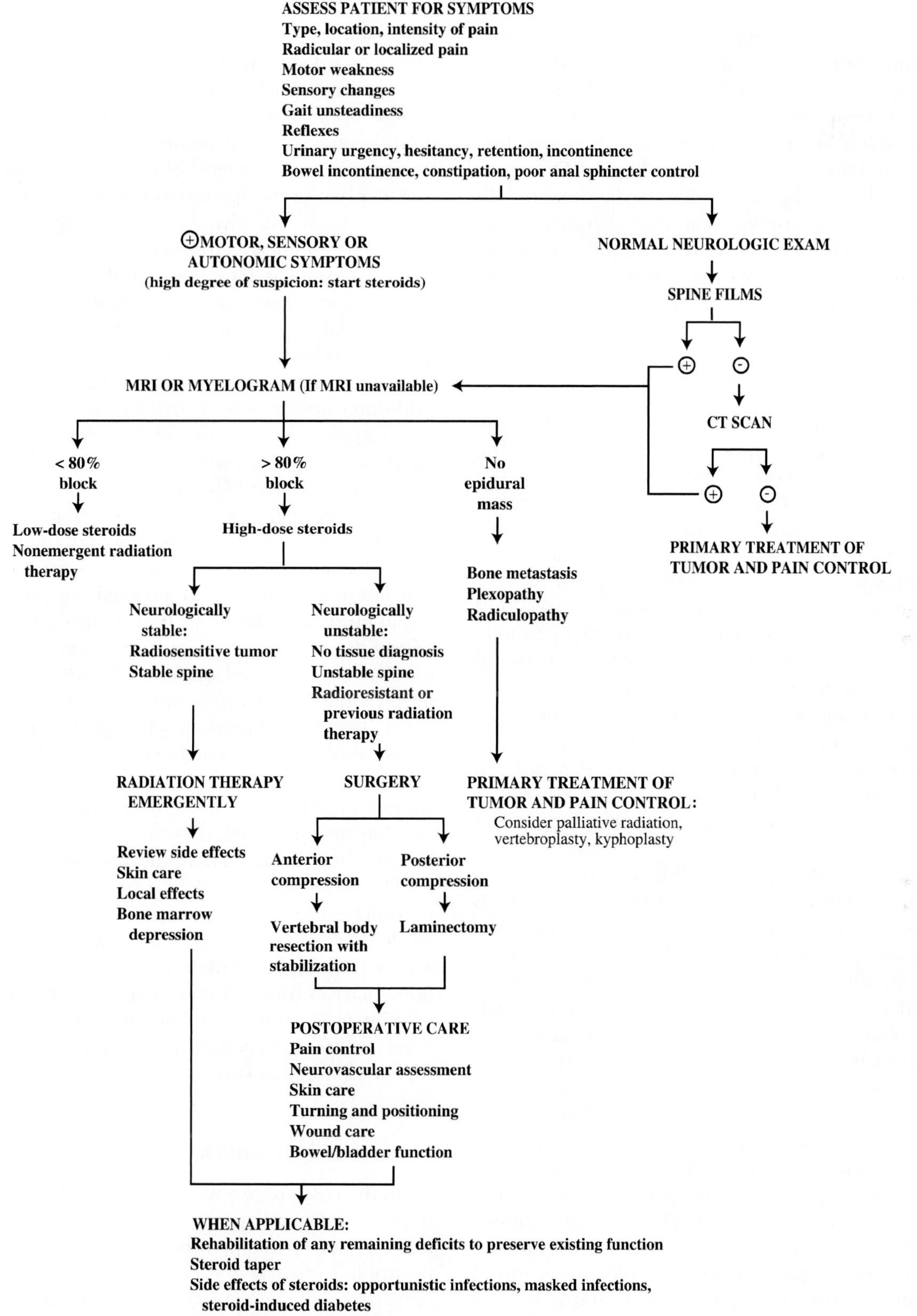

Figure 39-4 Clinical pathway for spinal cord compression.

complication that is unique to patients with spinal cord compression is gastrointestinal perforation from straining with constipation.[12] Complications associated with steroid use are more common when serum albumin is low, length of administration is longer than 3 weeks, and the cumulative dose is high.[2,10] One study looked at eliminating the use of steroids completely in patients who had normal neurological function and minor compression of the cord at the time of diagnosis. In this group of patients, steroids were not required during the course of treatment.[29]

Radiation

Radiation therapy is the standard treatment for spinal cord compression from epidural metastasis. The radiation port is identified by MRI and extends two vertebrae above and below the level of the compression. This field ensures that the metastatic disease is fully treated and prevents nearby recurrences. The usual dosage range is 2000–4000 cGy given in 5–20 fractions over 2–4 weeks. The dose of radiation and length of treatment are determined partly by histology, as most solid tumors respond at 3000 cGy delivered in 10 fractions. Neuroblastoma and lymphoma have favorable histologies and respond to 2000–3000 cGy, whereas more radiation-resistant tumors such as melanoma require more than 3000 cGy. Overall, breast and prostate cancer, myeloma, and lymphoma respond to radiation better than melanoma, sarcoma, lung, colon and renal cancer.[30]

As demonstrated in Table 39-1, the degree of neurological impairment prior to initiating treatment is predictive of recovery of ambulation post-treatment. In a classic study, Maranzano and Latini evaluated the effect of radiation and steroids on neurological status in cord compression.[31] The majority of individuals were ambulatory (52%), and 94% of these patients remained so. Paraparetic and paralyzed cases did not respond as well, with only 60% and 11%, respectively, being ambulatory after treatment. Median survival time was longer for those patients who remained ambulatory, for females, and for those individuals with favorable histologies such as myeloma and breast and prostate cancers. Again, the major conclusion drawn from this study is the importance of early diagnosis.

In a study at a cancer center, the outcome status of 166 patients with spinal cord compression was evaluated by looking at performance and neurological status.[32] More than 90% of the patients received radiation therapy; neurological status improved in 20% of patients, while performance status improved in only 16%. The majority of patients stayed the same, but 25% were worse after treatment. Radiation therapy, however, is quite effective in relieving pain. One large study found that pain was relieved in 85% of patients who received such treatment.[31]

Newer approaches to radiation therapy in the treatment of spinal cord compression include short-course radiotherapy, intensity-modulated radiotherapy, and stereotactic radiosurgery. Short-course radiotherapy includes one or two fractions of 800 cGy and has been found to be an effective treatment with tolerable side effects.[33] It is indicated for palliation and pain relief in those patients who have been paralyzed more than 24 hours and who have a very short life expectancy. Intensity-modulated radiotherapy and stereotactic radiosurgery are techniques that are geared toward treating the tumor while sparing surrounding healthy tissue.[34] Additional research is needed to fully evaluate these newer approaches and define their roles in the treatment of spinal cord compression.

Approximately 10% of individuals with spinal cord compression will experience a local recurrence, the majority within a couple of vertebrae of the initial site of cord compression.[21] Additional radiation may or may not be an option given the maximum amount the spinal cord can tolerate without injuring the healthy neural tissue. If excessive radiation is given, the cord may become damaged and result in further weakness, sensory changes, or autonomic dysfunction. The likelihood of radiation-induced myelopathy depends on the dose of radiation per fraction, total dose, size or volume of the field, and amount of time between courses of radiation.[30] If the maximum dose of radiation has been reached, then stereotactic radiosurgery or intensity-modulated radiotherapy may be indicated.

The side effects of radiation are minimal and relate to where on the spinal column the radiation is directed. Radiation is generally well tolerated, but patients with preexisting bone metastasis and less than optimal bone marrow function may incur further suppression of marrow function due to radiation effects. Skin reactions are usually very mild, and doses are delivered in such a fashion that surrounding tissue is minimally affected.

Surgical interventions

In the past, surgery was indicated only for those patients with neurological deficits that progressed during radiation or that presented acutely with rapid deterioration, with spinal instability, or with local recurrence after completion of radiation. The development of MRI, which provides detailed imaging of the tumor and neural structures, and new spine stabilization techniques have made surgery a more effective and earlier option. Historically, surgery involved a laminectomy and posterior approach because surgeons were unable to stabilize the spine, which would be required with an anterior approach. The laminectomy would partially resect the tumor and decompress the cord or nerve roots, but the outcome proved to be no more effective than radiation alone.[35] Most spinal cord metastases are located anteriorly, anterolaterally, or posterolaterally, and this surgical approach precludes complete resection.

A newer surgical approach, called circumferential decompression, completely resects the tumor, frees the thecal sac and nerve roots of malignant compression, and reconstructs the spine so that stability is achieved.[34] To accomplish this, surgery may include multiple approaches. Because the majority of tumors are anterior, an anterior approach is most often required. The diseased vertebral body is resected (corpectomy) and reconstructed with methylmethacrylate or other material, then the spine is further stabilized with either anterior or posterior devices that attach to healthy adjoining vertebral bodies. The spine can also be stabilized with bone grafting or fusion posteriorly. The anterior approach requires a thoracotomy for thoracic and some cervical vertebrae. For lumbar resection, a retroperitoneal approach is often used, whereas an anterolateral approach is required for most cervical lesions.[34,36]

The first study comparing circumferential surgery followed by radiation versus radiation alone was stopped prematurely because the results were so positive in the surgery arm.[37] Patients in the surgery arm were able to walk for a median of 126 days versus 35 days in the radiation arm. In addition, more than 50% of the nonambulatory patients in the surgical arm regained the ability to walk compared to 19% in the radiation arm. The surgical patients maintained continence and performance status significantly longer than the patients who received radiation. Pain was also significantly less in the surgery arm. While length of survival was not significant, quality of life was maximized. Surgery is usually followed by radiation therapy to achieve maximal results. Because radiation will interfere with bone grafting and wound healing, it must be timed appropriately and radiation should not be given before surgery if possible.[38]

Surgery, while it has many advantages, is not without risk. Surgical morbidity with resection and stabilization has been estimated to be as high as 48% and mortality to be about 6%.[33] Complications encountered postoperatively include wound dehiscence, infection, CSF leakage, progression of neurological deficits, instrumentation or stabilization failure, and hemorrhage.[32] Some tumors, such as sarcomas and renal and thyroid cancers, are particularly vascular and require preoperative embolization prior to surgery to reduce the risk of bleeding.[3,39]

Surgery must be carefully considered on a case-by-case basis, and the indications for this treatment approach are outlined in Table 39-2. Two important factors are the performance status of the individual prior to surgery and whether the benefit outweighs the risk. Surgery is indicated when tissue is needed for histologic diagnosis, especially if this is the only accessible area of disease. Extensive bone destruction, vertebral collapse, and spine instability (particularly when accompanied by intractable pain) may be best treated with a surgical approach. Paravertebral tumors, which are most common in lung cancer, are also best treated with a surgical approach. In addition, if the patient is currently receiving steroid and radiation therapy and experiences rapid neurological deterioration, surgery may be warranted but must be performed within 24 hours.[38] Paralysis beyond 24 hours eliminates surgery as an option. Surgery should also be considered in those cases of solitary recurrence in the spinal cord, given that intact surrounding vertebrae are required for the attachment of stabilization instruments. New techniques related to the attachment of these instruments, known as cages, are being investigated as part of surgery for patients with multilevel spinal metastases.[40] The desire to maintain and improve the quality of life for those patients with metastatic cancer initially motivated the use of this aggressive approach, which is now considered both effective and safe.

Table 39-2 Indications for Surgical Management of Spinal Cord Compression

- Spinal instability caused by pathological fracture
- Compression of the spinal cord by bone
- Histologic diagnosis required
- Radioresistant tumor
- Neurologic deterioration despite radiation
- Prior radiation to the site
- Intractable pain

Data from Fuller, Heiss, Oedfield[2]; Gerstzen, Welch[3]; Meyers.[5]

Chemotherapy

Chemotherapy may be a treatment option in extremely chemosensitive tumors such as Hodgkin's and non-Hodgkin's lymphoma, small cell lung cancer, neuroblastoma, and germ cell tumors.[2,12,41] It may also be used as an adjuvant therapy to surgery and radiation, but it has a limited role and usually is not the primary treatment in an acute situation. Hormone therapy is another option for those patients with prostate and breast cancer. Usually, these patients have had the disease a long time, and have been treated with hormone manipulation, and may be resistant. The hormone-sensitive cases may benefit from a trial in addition to standard therapy for spinal cord compression.

A new therapy that has emerged as a preventive measure for spinal cord compression is the administration of bisphosphonates. Bisphosphonates are bone resorption inhibitors that have been traditionally used to treat osteoporosis. They work by inhibiting osteoclast-mediated bone resorption, which slows bone remodeling and increases bone mineral density.[42] Recent research has shown that bisphosphonates delay the onset and reduce the frequency of skeletal-related episodes (SREs) such as pathologic fractures, bone pain, hypercalcemia, and spinal cord compression.[43,44] They also reduce the need for palliative radiotherapy and orthopedic surgery. When they were first introduced, these agents were used primarily with bone metastases from breast cancer and multiple myeloma. Their administration has since expanded to other cancers that have metastasized to bone, such as renal cell, prostate, and lung cancers. While bisphophonates have improved quality of life, prolonged survival has not been associated with their addition to supportive care.[45] Their efficacy is proven in patients with lytic bone metastasis and still being investigated in blastic metastases.[46]

Both pamidronate and, more recently, zoledronic acid have been used to treat bone metastases. They are associated with renal toxicity, which can be minimized by adhering to recommended dosing and infusion times.[47] If renal dysfunction does develop, bisphophonates should be held until renal function is restored. Hypocalcemia may develop as a result of the administration of bisphosphonates, so calcium supplements may be required. Mild side effects of bisphosphonates include arthralgias, myalgias, and fever lasting about 48 hours.[48]

Zoledronic acid has emerged as the bisphosphonate of choice because its administration time is significantly shorter than that of pamidronate, 15–30 minutes versus 2 hours.[42] Few long-term effects have emerged with pamidronate — specifically, ocular effects and mild anemia and thrombocytopenia.[45] Jaw necrosis leading to oral infections as well as tooth and bone loss have been observed in patients on long-term therapy with zoledronic acid.

Overall, bisphosphonates have had a profound impact on bone metastases and their effects on patients with cancer, but currently no evidence indicates that they reduce the incidence of spinal cord compression.[49]

Symptom Management

The nursing care of the individual experiencing spinal cord compression is primarily concerned with early detection and symptom management. Clinical problems evolve from the rapidity of onset, level and degree of compression, presenting symptoms, as well as type and response to treatment. Assessment is crucial throughout this emergency for evaluation of neurological status and preservation of maximal function. Assessment includes monitoring of sensory and motor function as well as of bowel and bladder function. Table 39-3 lists the problems most frequently associated with epidural spinal cord compression and management goals with interventions to help direct care.

Pain

Because more than 95% of patients with spinal cord compression have pain, knowledge of pain management is essential in caring for these individuals. Pain assessment is crucial to help identify intensity, location, factors that help or exacerbate pain, and other symptoms that accompany pain. Oncology nurses need extensive knowledge of the principles of analgesia, opioids, equianalgesia, cost analyses of various regimens, and nonpharmacological approaches. In addition, adjunct agents such as nonsteroidal anti-inflammatory drugs (NSAIDs), anticonvulsants, and antidepressants may be helpful in pain management.

An "analgesic ladder" approach has been developed by the Cancer Pain Relief and Palliative Care Program of the World Health Organization.[50] This approach helps clinicians select agents based on the patient's severity of pain and provides a standard for pain management. Many large institutions have "pain teams" that act as consultants for individuals with unusual or refractory pain and for whom standardized approaches, as outlined in the analgesic ladder, are ineffective.

NSAIDs are very useful in managing bone pain, but bleeding and renal problems may occur and individuals require close monitoring when these agents are used on a regular basis. Recently, anticonvulsants and antidepressants have emerged as useful agents to treat neuropathic pain that occurs when peripheral nerves or their roots are compressed or infiltrated.[46] This type of pain typically does not readily respond to opioids and requires adjunct agents for management. Epidural cord compression may also cause spastic reactions below the level of the compression and require the use of benzodiazepines. With affected patients, effective analgesia is established early and adjusted as steroids and radiation relieve pain. A variety of agents and types of administration are available to provide comfort.

Two new approaches to establish spine stabilization and pain relief in metastatic spinal disease are vertebroplasty and kyphoplasty. Both of these procedures have specific indications and contraindications, but offer an approach that may be adjunct to the tradition-

Table 39-3 Symptom Management

Problems	Patient Goals	Interventions
Pain due to irritation and compression of nerve roots and neural tissue and/or vertebral collapse as evidenced by localized or radicular pain	Maximum comfort as reported on a pain scale during rest and activity by appropriately using various types of analgesics and nonpharmacologic interventions	• Opioids — time release, immediate, transdermal release • Dexamethasone • NSAIDs • Anticonvulsants/antidepressants • Complementary medicine: capsicum cream, hydrotherapy, massage, accupressure • Vertebroplasty, kyphoplasty
Immobility due to compression of neural tissue, motor neurons as evidenced by proximal muscle weakness that progresses to motor loss	Maintain optimal level of mobility, range of motion, and strength through an activity and exercise program	• Referral to physical therapy • Obtain equipment and devices to preserve alignment, enhance mobility, and stabilize spine • Assist home care agency in organizing environment to be conducive to mobility
Risk of injury related to sensory loss, which includes paresthesia, loss of temperature, position and vibratory senses, and light touch	Safety will be preserved at all times	• Assess degree of sensory changes: touch, temperature, paresthesia • Assess environment for physical, thermal, chemical hazards and organize environment to minimize hazards • Assist patient with ADLs as indicated
Bladder dysfunction due to disruption of lower motor neurons (autonomic function) as evidenced by incontinence, frequency, and/or retention	Maintain adequate urinary elimination with early identification and treatment of urinary tract infections	• Fluid intake greater than 2 quarts/day • Adequate intake of juices to maintain acidity (e.g., cranberry) • Straight catheterization/indwelling catheter to maintain continence and empty bladder • Change indwelling catheter each week • Urinalysis/urine culture for pain, burning, foul-smelling/cloudy urine, fever, increased WBC count • Prompt treatment of urinary tract infection with antibiotic sensitive to the organism identified • Daily perineal hygiene
Bowel disturbances due to opioid use and disruption of lower motor neurons (autonomic function) as evidenced by constipation, incontinence, and/or difficulty expelling stool	Maintain adequate bowel elimination and prevent ileus from constipation	• Establish bowel regimen including stool softener (i.e., docusate sodium), intestinal lubricants, mineral oil, laxatives; senna products, magnesium-based products (i.e., milk of magnesia, magnesium citrate) • Dietary recommendations include fresh fruits, vegetables, high-fiber cereals • Adequate fluid intake greater than 2 quarts/day • Provide periodic perineal hygiene

Data from Wilkes.[16]

al treatment for spinal cord compression. Further research is needed to define their particular roles.

Vertebroplasty is a minimally invasive procedure performed under CT guidance or fluoroscopy in which a needle is inserted into the vertebral body and polymethylmethacrylate (PMMA) is injected. Once the vertebral body is strengthened and fortified, the patient experiences relief of pain and greater mobility. Theories as to how this procedure relieves pain include immobilization of microfractures, reduction of mechanical forces, destruction of nerve endings by PMMA, and a possible antitumor effect of PMMA. The complication rate for vertebroplasty is about 10%, and the major complications are related to trauma to surrounding vessels or organs and cement leakage.[51]

Kyphoplasty evolved from vertebroplasty and also uses PMMA to strengthen the vertebral body. This procedure, however, uses a balloon that is inserted into the vertebral body and slowly inflated to restore the height of that vertebral body. Once this is accomplished, PMMA is injected into the space created by the balloon using a cement filler. The advantage of this procedure is that it restores vertebral body height in addition to providing pain relief and stabilization.[52] Reversing kyphosis also prevents respiratory compromise, which can be imposed by the kyphotic shape of the chest.

Complementary medicine offers a unique approach to pain management through therapies that enhance well-being and control symptoms, such as yoga or traditional Chinese medicine. Warm baths and Jacuzzi as part of hydrotherapy promote muscle relaxation and overall relaxation. A professional massage can help relieve pain by working on specific muscle groups that are affected by the spinal cord compression. Capsicum cream contains a powerful pain-relieving chemical found in hot red peppers; it may help relieve the back pain associated with cord compression.

Mobility

Quality of life is deeply affected by changes in one's ability to ambulate and function independently. It is crucial, therefore, that the oncology nurse identify any motor or sensory changes early, before more profound loss is encountered. Preserving and maximizing function are a priority because many patients have rehabilitative potential after treatment is initiated.

If spine and vertebral instability is present at diagnosis, the patient should be fitted for a stabilization brace to provide support until surgery can be performed. This brace is worn whenever the patient is moved or gets out of bed and postoperatively until the stabilization materials or bone grafts heal and strengthen the structures surrounding the spine. If the patient undergoes a thoracotomy for anterior resection or a two-step procedure of anterior and posterior resection, postoperative care includes turning and positioning with special attention to preserving alignment and spine stabilization during recovery. Neurological assessment is critical in the postoperative phase as well as pain control, wound care, and preliminary rehabilitation.[53]

Physical therapy is essential for patients who experience any motor weakness. If recovery is realistic, therapy is directed toward regaining full mobility and strength. If there is permanent weakness or motor loss, the goals of therapy include maintaining existing function, strength, and range of motion. Assistive devices such as walkers, commodes, wheelchairs, and transfer boards may be required to maximize the patient's mobility. This equipment can be individualized to the patient's needs and physical environment.

Bowel and bladder dysfunction

Autonomic disturbances include bowel and bladder incontinence and retention. Weakness of sphincters can lead to incontinence, whereas paralysis of muscles associated with emptying the bladder and rectum can lead to retention and constipation. Establishment of daily elimination regimens will help manage any bowel and bladder dysfunctions.

If a patient is dexterous with a good prognosis, intermittent self-catheterization is the most effective method for urinary continence. It provides control and continence, offers ease of mobility without external devices, and reduces the incidence of urinary tract infections. Conversely, patients with advanced cancer would benefit from an indwelling urinary catheter.

Fluid intake, daily perineal hygiene, and catheter care with scheduled changes will reduce the incidence of urinary tract infections associated with indwelling catheters. Fluid intake should exceed 2 liters per day and contain liquids that maintain acidity (e.g., cranberry juice). Nurses must be vigilant about early diagnosis of urinary tract infections by watching for such symptoms as foul-smelling or cloudy urine, elevated white count on complete blood count (CBC), and fever. Treatment with a fluoroquinolone or sulfa-based antibiotic will usually cover most common organisms associated with urinary infections.

Bowel control can be established with the appropriate use of diet, stool softeners, lubricants, and laxatives. In addition to maintaining fluid intake, dietary adjustments to help reduce constipation and establish a regular pattern include increasing fiber consumption. For oncology patients, however, these goals are very difficult to accomplish due to anorexia and fatigue. A bowel regimen will reduce the incidence of constipation as well as establish continence. Stool seepage is less likely if the rectum is evacuated on a regular basis. If muscle tone and sphincter control are disrupted, medication can assist in developing regular bowel habits.

Many lubricants and laxatives are available. Compliance, degree of being palatable, ease of use, and individual preference are factors to consider when selecting laxatives and lubricants for each individual. The regimen usually consists of a stool softener and laxative. Lubricants (e.g., mineral oil) are essential if the patient has refractory constipation or impaction.

Laxatives are classified as saline, osmotic, or stimulant. Saline-type laxatives include magnesium citrate and magnesium hydroxide. The most common osmotic laxatives are lactulose and sorbitol. Senna products, bisacodyl (Dulcolax), and cascara are stimulant laxatives that are frequently prescribed.[54] A combination of these types of laxatives may be required to adequately establish regularity. Usually rectal suppositories and enemas are reserved for impaction and severe cases of constipation. In spinal cord compression, however, rectal suppositories may be needed to stimulate the intestinal nerve plexus so as to evacuate the rectum.[54]

Skin care

Skin care is essential during radiation therapy, particularly if the patient is receiving higher doses or treatment to a large port. The radiation oncology nurse should perform routine assessment so that skin problems are identified promptly. During radiation therapy, skin should not be washed with soap, and topical creams and oils should be avoided. Once radiation is completed, a water-soluble lotion such as Aquafor may be applied. Usual skin reactions are redness and mild discomfort similar to sunburn. While skin reactions from spine irradiation are rare, silver nitrate cream can be applied if an open area develops.

Conclusion

Spinal cord compression is one of the most common neurological emergencies facing the individual with cancer. Prompt recognition and treatment may preserve neurological function and prevent permanent deficits, such as paraplegia and bowel and bladder incontinence or retention. Magnetic resonance imaging has emerged as the safest and most clinically useful diagnostic tool in spinal cord compression. Although radiation therapy has been the primary treatment, new surgical techniques are emerging as feasible options to restore ambulation and relieve pain. Nurses play a pivotal role in identifying those patients at risk and early cases of spinal cord compression.

References

1. Quinn JA, DeAngelis LM: Neurologic emergencies in the cancer patient. *Semin Oncol* 27:311–321, 2000
2. Fuller BG, Heiss J, Oedfield EH: Spinal cord compression, in DeVita VT, Hellman S, Rosenberg SA (eds.): *Cancer Principles and Practice* (ed 6). Philadelphia, Lippincott-Raven, 2001, pp 2617–2633
3. Gerszten PC, Welch WC: Current surgical management of metastatic spinal disease. *Oncology* 14:1013–1024, 2000
4. Gilbert RW, Kim JH, Posner JB: Epidural spinal cord compression from metastatic tumor: diagnosis and treatment. *Ann Neurol* 3:40–51, 1978
5. Meyers JS: Oncologic complications, in Otto SE (ed.): *Oncology Nursing* (ed 4). St. Louis, Mosby, 2001, pp 513–581
6. Moore KL, Dalley AF: *Clinically Oriented Anatomy* (ed 4). Philadelphia, Lippincott, Williams and Wilkins, 1999
7. Henze R: Traumatic and vascular injuries of the central nervous system, in Bullock B, Henze R (eds.): *Focus on Pathophysiology*. Philadelphia, Lippincott, 2000, pp 938–978
8. Byrne TN, Waxman SG: Spinal cord compression: diagnosis and principles of treatment, in *Contemporary Neurology Series,* vol. 33. Philadelphia, F. A. Davis, 1990
9. Byrne TN: Spinal cord compression from epidural metastasis. *N Engl J Med* 325:614–619, 1992
10. Weinstein SM: Management of spinal cord and cauda equine compression, in Berger AM, Portnoy RK, Weissman DE (eds.): *Principles and Practice of Palliative Care and Supportive Oncology* (ed 2). Philadelphia, Lippincott, Williams and Wilkins, 2002, pp 532–543
11. Batson OV: The function of the vertebral veins and their role in the spread of metastasis. *Ann Surg* 112:138–149, 1940
12. Deangelis LM, Posner JB: Neurologic complications, in Holland JF, Frei E, Bast RC, et al (eds.): *Cancer Medicine* (ed 5). Baltimore, Williams and Wilkins, 2001, pp 2451–2467
13. Buckholtz, J: Metastatic epidural spinal cord compression. *Semin Oncol Nurs* 15:150–159, 1999
14. Perrin RG, Janjan NA, Langford LA: Spinal axis metastasis, in Levin V (ed.): *Cancer of the Nervous System.* London, Blackwell Science, 1997, pp 259–280
15. Helweg-Larsen S, Hansen SW, Sorenson PS: Second occurrence of symptomatic metastatic spinal cord compression and findings of multiple spinal epidural metastases. *Int J Radiat Oncol Biol Phys* 33:595–597, 1995
16. Wilkes GM: Neurological disturbances, in Yarbro CH, Frogge MH, Goodman M (eds.): *Cancer Symptom Management* (ed 2). Sudbury, MA, Jones and Bartlett, 1999, pp 344–381
17. Helweg-Larsen S, Sorenson PS, Kreiner S: Prognostic factors in metastatic spinal cord compression: a prospective study using multivariate analysis of variables influencing survival and gait function in 153 patients. *Int J Radiat Oncol Biol Phys* 46:1163–1169, 2000
18. Posner JB: *Neurologic Complications of Cancer.* Philadelphia, Davis, 1995
19. Hickey JV: *The Clinical Practice of Neurological and Neurosurgical Nursing* (ed 5). Philadelphia, Lippincott, Williams and Wilkins, 2003
20. Huff SJ: Neoplasms, spinal cord. *eMedicine Journal* 2, 2001. *www.emedicine.com/emerg/topic337.htm.* Accessed February 20, 2004
21. Schiff D: Spinal cord compression. *Neurol Clin* 21:67–86, 2003
22. Quint DJ: Indications for emergent MRI of the central nervous system. *JAMA* 283:853–860, 2000
23. Bilsky MH, Lis E, Raizer J, et al: The diagnosis and treatment of metastatic spinal tumor. *Oncologist* 4:459–464, 1999
24. Baba H, Uchida K, Sadato N, et al: Potential usefulness of ^{18}F-2–fluoro-deoxy-D-glucose positron emission tomography in cervical compressive myelopathy. *Spine* 24:1449–1457, 1999
25. Poggi M, Patronas N, Buttman A, et al: Intramedullary spinal cord metastasis from renal cell carcinoma: confirmation by positron emission tomography. *Clin Nucl Med (US)* 26:837–839, 2001
26. Byrne TN: Metastatic epidural spinal cord compression, in Black PH, Loeffler JS (eds.): *Cancer of the Nervous System.* London, Blackwell Scientific, 1997, pp 664–673
27. Sitton E: Central nervous system metastasis. *Semin Oncol Nurs* 14:210–218, 1998
28. Vecht CJ, Haaxma-Reiche H, van Putten W, et al: Initial bolus of conventional versus high dose dexamethasone in metastatic spinal cord compression. *Neurology* 39:1255–1257, 1989
29. Maranzano E, Latini P, Beneventi S, et al: Radiotherapy without steroids in selected metastatic spinal cord compression patients. A phase II trial. *Am J Clin Oncol* 19:179–183, 1996
30. Janjan NA, Delclos ME, Ballo MT, et al: Palliative care, in Cox JD, Ang KK (eds.): *Radiation Oncology* (ed 8). St. Louis, Mosby, 2003, pp 954–986
31. Maranzano E, Latini P: Effectiveness of radiation therapy without surgery in metastatic spinal cord compression: final results from a prospective trial. *Int J Radiat Oncol Biol Phys* 32:959–967, 1995
32. Cowap J, Hardy JR, A'Hearn R: Outcome of malignant spinal cord compression at a cancer center: implications for palliative care services. *J Pain Symptom Manage* 19:257–264, 2000
33. Maranzano E, Latini P, Perrucci E, et al: Short-course radiotherapy (8Gy × 2) in metastatic spinal cord compression: an effective and feasible treatment. *Int J Radiat Oncol Biol Phys* 38:1037–1044, 1997
34. Klimo P, Kestle JR, Schmidt MH: Treatment of metastatic spinal epidural disease: a review of the literature. *Neurosurg Focus* 15, 2003. *www.medscape.com/viewarticle/465359.* Accessed February 23, 2004
35. Young RF, Post EM, King GA: Treatment of spinal epidural metastases. Randomized prospective comparison of laminectomy and radiotherapy. *J Neurosurg* 53:741–748, 1980
36. Jacobs WB, Perrin RG: Evaluation and treatment of spinal metastases: an overview. *Neurosurg Focus* 11, 2001. *www.medscape.com/viewarticle/421516.* Accessed February 23, 2004
37. Patchell R, Tibbs PA, Regine WF, et al: A randomized trial of direct decompressive surgical resection in the treatment of spi-

nal cord compression caused by metastasis. *Proc Am Soc Clin Oncol* 22, 2003 (abstr)
38. Ghogawala Z, Mansfield FL, Borges LF: Spinal radiation before surgical decompression adversely affects outcomes of surgery for symptomatic metastatic spinal cord compression. *Spine* 26:818–824, 2001
39. Vrionis FD, Small J: Surgical management of metastatic spinal neoplasms. *Neurosurg Focus* 15, 2003. *www.medscape.com/viewarticle/465374*. Accessed March 1, 2004
40. Jang JS, Sang HL, Chang HR, et al: Polymethylmethacrylate-augmented screw fixation for stabilization in metastatic spinal tumors. *J Neurosurg (Spine 1)* 96:131–134, 2002
41. Daw HA, Markman M: Epidural spinal cord compression in cancer patients: diagnosis and management. *Clev Clin J Med* 67: 497–504, 2000
42. Viale PH, Yamamoto DS: Bisphosphonates: expanded roles in the treatment of patients with cancer. *Clin J Oncol Nurs* 7:393–401, 2003
43. Ali SM, Esteva FJ, Hortobagyi G, et al: Safety and efficacy of bisphosphonates beyond 24 months in cancer patients. *J Clin Oncol* 19:3434–3437, 2001
44. Van Poznak CH: The use of bisphosphonates in patients with breast cancer. *Cancer Control* 9:480–489, 2002
45. Hillner BE, Ingle JN, Berenson JR, et al: American Society of Clinical Oncology guideline on the role of bisphosphonates in breast cancer. *J Clin Oncol* 18:1378–1391, 2000
46. Lipton A, Zheng M, Seaman J: Zoledronic acid delays the onset of skeletal-related events and progression of skeletal disease in patients with advanced renal cell carcinoma. *Cancer* 98:962–969, 2003
47. Major P: The use of zoledronic acid, a novel, highly potent bisphosphonate, for the treatment of hypercalcemia of malignancy. *Oncologist* 7:481–491, 2002
48. Body JJ: Dosing regimens and main adverse events with bisphosphonates. *Semin Oncol* 28:49–53, 2001
49. Theriault RL, Lipton A, Hortobagyi GN, et al: Pamidronate reduces skeletal morbidity in women with advanced breast cancer and lytic bone lesions: a randomized, placebo-controlled trial. Protocol 18 Aredia Breast Cancer Study Group. *J Clin Oncol* 17:846–854, 1999
50. Ashby M, Jackson K: When the WHO ladder appears to be failing: approaches to refractory or unstable cancer pain, in Sykes N, Fallon MT, Patt RB (eds.): *Clinical Pain Management: Cancer Pain*. New York, Oxford University Press, 2003, pp 143–156
51. Pilitsis JG, Rengachary SS: The role of vertebroplasty in metastatic spinal disease. *Neurosurg Focus* 11, 2001. *www.medscape.com/viewarticle/421515*, accessed March 3, 2004
52. Linville DA: Vertebroplasty and kyphoplasty. *South Med J* 95:583–587, 2002
53. Wiggins GC, Mirza S, Bellabarba C, et al: Perioperative complications with costotransversectomy and anterior approaches to thoracic and thoracolumbar tumors. *Neurosurg Focus* 11, 2001. *www.medscape.com/veiw article/421505*. Accessed March 3, 2004
54. Curtiss CP: Constipation, in Yarbro CH, Frogge MH, Goodman M (eds.): *Cancer Symptom Management*. Sudbury, MA, Jones and Bartlett, 1999, pp 512–521

CHAPTER 40

Superior Vena Cava Syndrome

Susan Moore, RN, MSN, ANP, AOCN®

Scope of the Problem

Definitions

Obstruction of blood flow through the superior vena cava (SVC) can result in superior vena cava syndrome (SVCS). SVCS refers to the constellation of signs and symptoms indicative of venous congestion proximal to the occlusion. Increased venous pressures occur in the head, neck, upper extremities, and upper thorax and can result in restricted cardiac output. The most common cause of SVCS is compression of the upper central venous return by a malignant tumor in the mediastinum. Less common causes include thrombosis of the SVC, obstruction by a benign process, and direct tumor invasion of the SVC. Manifestations of compromise of the SVC generally develop gradually but may occur quickly. Unless there is respiratory distress or cerebral edema, SVCS is not considered an oncologic emergency. Prognosis is affected more by the underlying cause than by SVCS itself, which is rarely life-threatening.[1] Treatment decisions are determined by the underlying diagnosis.[2]

Incidence

A relatively uncommon condition, SVCS affects only 3%–4% of individuals with cancer.[3] However, 78%–95% of SVCS presents in individuals with cancer.[2,3] Any primary or metastatic tumor in the mediastinum can obstruct the SVC.

The incidence of SVCS not directly related to cancer appears to be increasing.[4–7] As many as 15%–22% of SVCS cases may be caused by nonmalignant conditions, including thrombus formation and compression. Thrombus formation related to vascular access devices, including hemodialysis catheters, central venous monitoring catheters, and cardiac pacemaker electrodes, accounts for 3%–5% of all SVCS cases. The SVC is easily compressed by benign tumor, mediastinal fibrosis, histoplasmosis, and thoracic aortic aneurysm.[8–10]

In the pediatric population, SVCS is a rare diagnosis, appearing at presentation in 12% of children with malignant mediastinal tumors. The most frequent malignancy causing SVCS in children is non-Hodgkin's lymphoma; other malignancies producing this syndrome in children include Hodgkin's disease and acute lymphoblastic leukemia.[11] Benign causes of pediatric SVCS are largely iatrogenic and include cardiac surgery and ventriculoatrial shunt for hydrocephalus. The most common nonmalignant cause is thrombosis from venous access catheterization.[12] In children, the trachea and right main stem bronchus are easily compressed and have small diameters. Respiratory symptoms such as cough, dyspnea, air hunger, and wheezing caused by tracheal compression often predominate in children.

Table 40-1 Cancer Etiology of SVCS

Type of Cancer	Percentage
Lung cancer	52–81
Lymphoma	2–21
Metastatic breast cancer	3–11

Etiology and Risk Factors

William Hunter first described SVCS in 1757. At that time, causes were generally reported as tuberculosis and syphilitic aortic aneurysms. Currently, malignant disease is the predominant etiology. Published series show that the types of cancer most commonly associated with SVCS are lung cancer (52%–81%), lymphoma involving the mediastinum (2%–21%), and metastatic breast cancer (3%–11%)[13] (see Table 40-1). Locally advanced bronchogenic carcinoma is the most common malignant etiology of SVCS. Thirty-eight percent of SVCS cases due to lung cancer is caused by small cell and 26% by squamous cell lung cancer. Ultimately, SVCS occurs in 3%–10% of all individuals with lung cancer. Individuals with cancer of the right lung are four times more likely to develop the syndrome than those with cancer of the left lung due to the location of the SVC nearer to the right lung.[5] This syndrome also occurs in 3%–8% of cases of lymphoma. High-grade lymphomas such as diffuse large cell and lymphoblastic lymphoma are more likely to cause SVCS than lower-grade lymphomas. SVCS is rarely caused by Hodgkin's lymphoma in spite of the high incidence of mediastinal involvement.[13]

Physiologic Alterations

Normal Anatomy and Physiology

The mediastinal space contains the SVC, aorta, pulmonary artery, sternum, vertebrae, trachea, right bronchus, and perihilar and paratracheal lymph nodes. The SVC is located in the right anterior superior mediastinum and begins at the junction of the right and left brachiocephalic veins (see Figure 40–1). The SVC extends to the right atrium, where it is anchored to the pericardial sac in a relatively fixed position. This thin-walled, large blood vessel (1.5–2.0 cm in diameter, 7–8 cm in length) carries venous blood from the head, neck, upper extremities, and upper thorax to the right

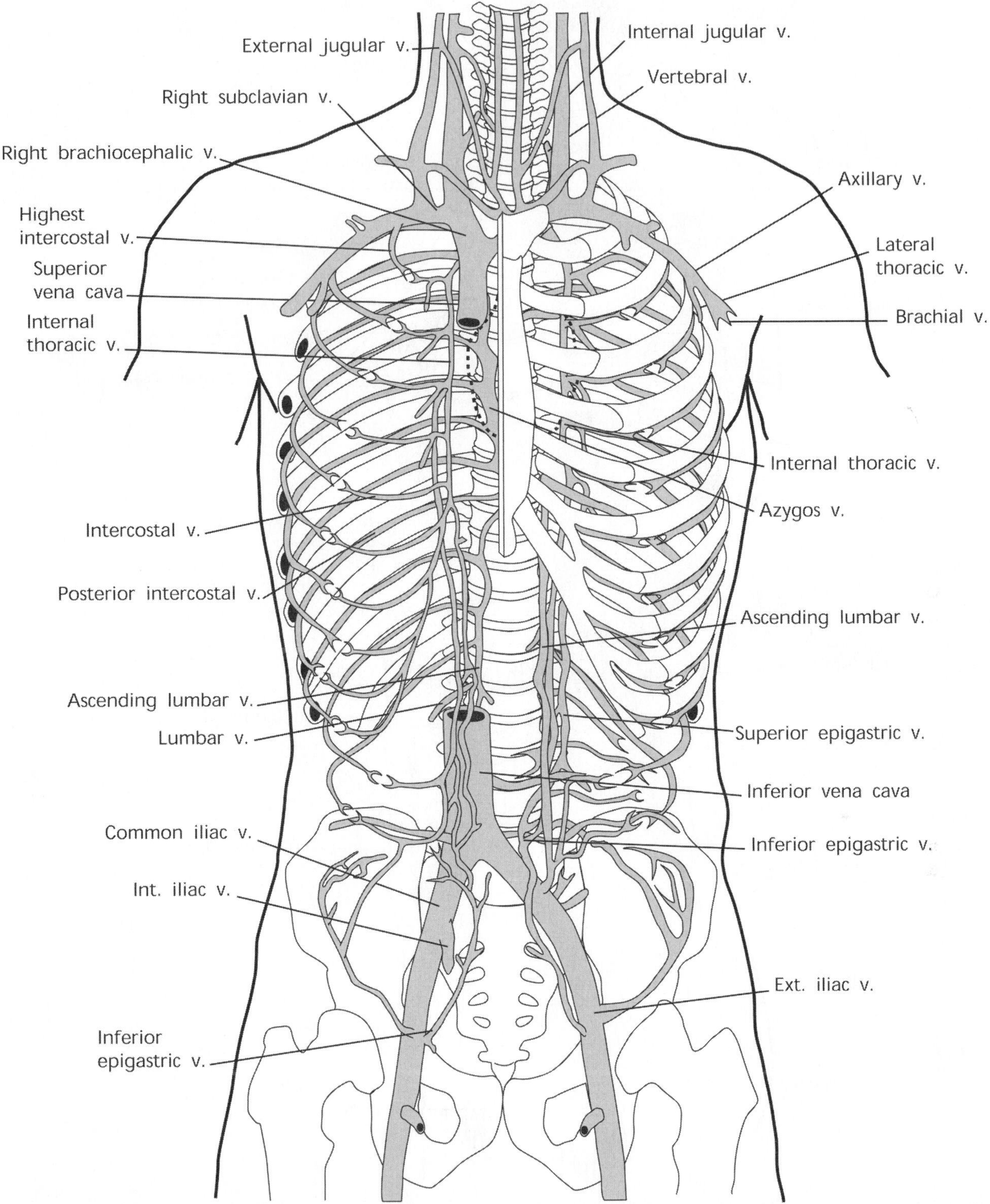

Figure 40–1 Anterior view of SVC and venous drainage.

atrium of the heart. Intravascular pressure in the SVC is low and may contribute to the formation of intraluminal thrombi. One major vein, the azygos vein, empties into the SVC at the level of the right main stem bronchus, carrying blood returned from the posterior torso (see Figure 40–2). Most structures in the mediastinum are relatively rigid except for the SVC, which can easily be compressed. Lymph nodes surround the SVC and can be a major factor in SVC obstruction when they are invaded by cancer (see Figure 40–3).

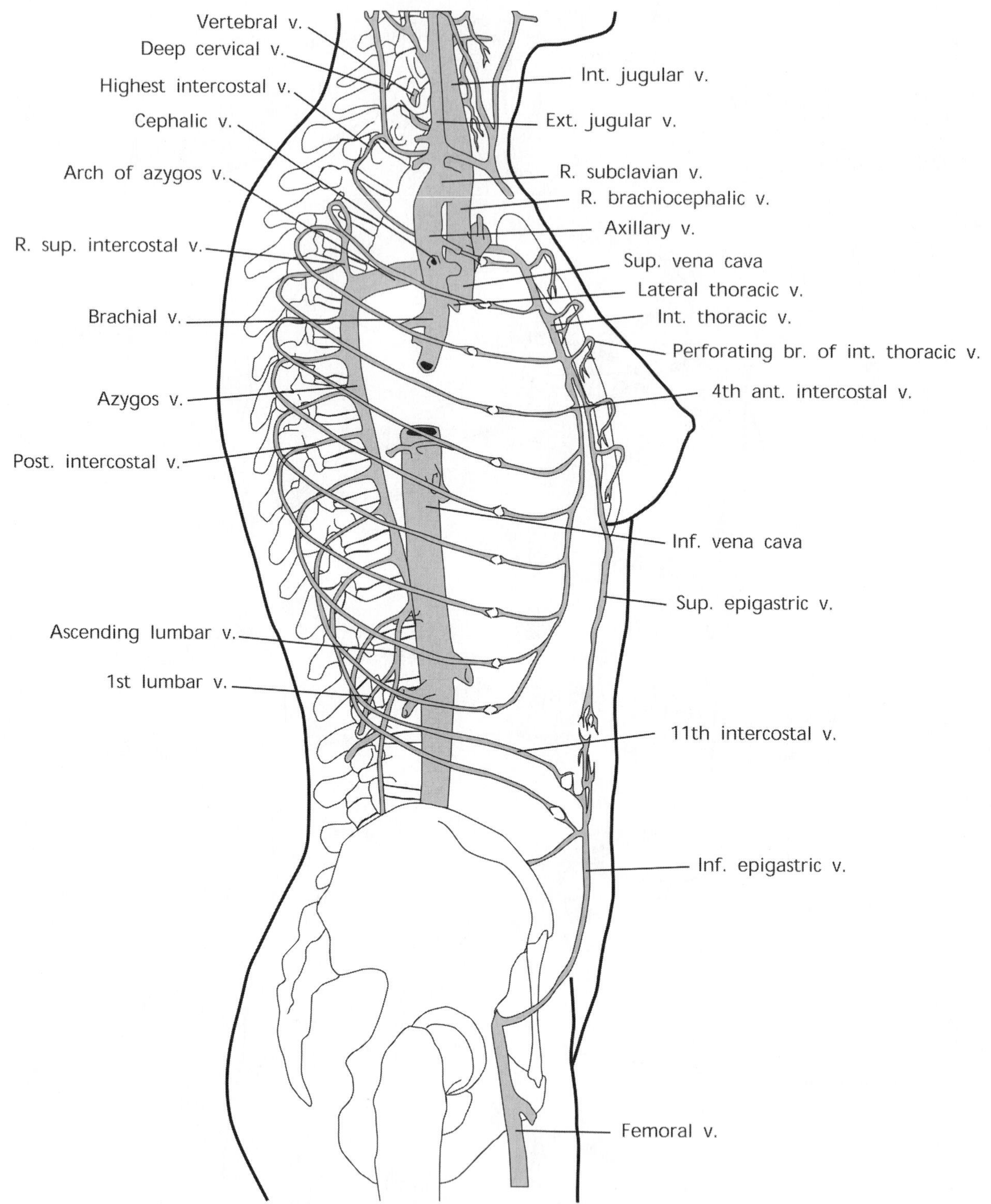

Figure 40–2 Lateral view of SVC and venous drainage.

Even moderate increase in lymph node size can produce SVC compromise.

Partial or complete occlusion of the SVC results in increased venous hypertension, leading to venous stasis and engorgement in the areas normally drained by the SVC. Blood from the upper body bypasses the SVC obstruction and is diverted into various collateral venous pathways in the area to return blood to the right atrium. The specific pathways develop in direct relation to the location and extent of obstruction of the SVC. Collateral circulation is generally associated with four interconnected venous pathways: (1) azygos

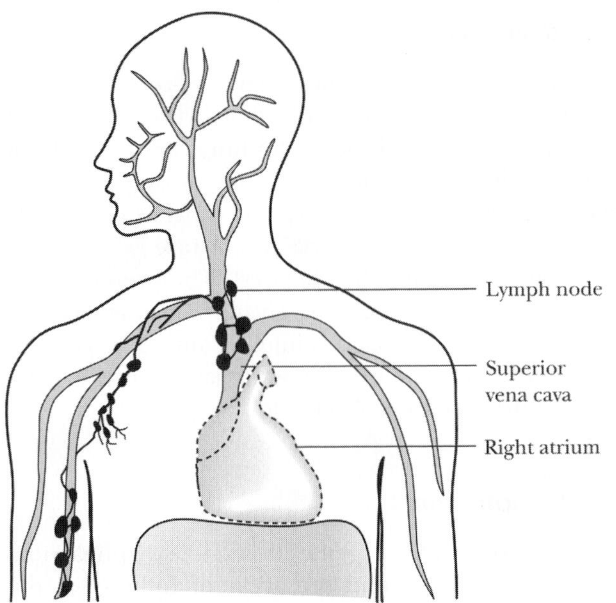

Figure 40–3 Lymph nodes near the SVC.

and hemiazygos; (2) internal mammary; (3) lateral thoracic and superficial thoracoabdominal; and (4) vertebral venous plexus.[13] The azygos pathway branches posteriorly from the SVC and is the most common venous collateral route. When the azygos vein is also obstructed as it enters the SVC, the other three routes develop to a higher degree. The azygos vein can also be compressed when lymph nodes are invaded by cancer.

Pathophysiology

Superior vena cava syndrome may be caused by external compression by primary or metastatic cancer, direct invasion by tumor, or thrombus formation within the vessel. Obstruction reduces venous blood return to the heart from the upper body, increases venous congestion, and decreases cardiac output. Venous hypertension may cause pleural or pericardial effusion and edema of the face, neck, upper thorax, and upper extremities. Tumor invasion or compression of other structures such as the esophagus, trachea, or pericardium interferes with the functioning of these organs.

Changes in blood composition, reduced blood flow, and damage to the vein wall contribute to intraluminal thrombus formation. Individuals with cancer often suffer from hypercoagulability states that can contribute to thrombus formation.[4,14] When a venous access device (VAD) is immobilized by an intraluminal thrombus, infusion of chemotherapeutic agents and other drugs may irritate the vessel wall. Indwelling central vascular catheters may cause mechanical slowing of blood flow and irritation and inflammation of the vessel wall, especially in the presence of infection. Mechanical trauma of the vein wall during central-line catheter placement can result in accumulated fibrin and aggregation of blood components, which in turn may cause the catheter to adhere to the vein wall and induce thrombus formation.[8,9,15,16]

Clinical Manifestations

Clinical manifestations of SVCS are related to the underlying disease process and SVC obstruction-related venous hypertension of the upper body, decreased cardiac output, and venous collateral circulation. The severity of SVCS depends on how quickly the obstruction occurs — rapid development may preclude the development of collateral circulation. Signs and symptoms are progressive if the underlying cause of the syndrome is not corrected. Initial signs and symptoms may be vague and barely noticeable, or they may develop rapidly. Early recognition and treatment of SVCS may prevent progression of life-threatening respiratory and cerebral complications.[4] In general, survival and symptom resolution depend on the ability to treat the underlying disease if SVCS is caused by malignancy or to reverse the obstructive process in nonmalignant SVCS. No explanation has been found for the fact that SVCS in small cell lung cancer is a positive prognostic indicator associated with higher 5-year survival rates than small cell lung cancer without SVCS.[5,17] Figure 40–4 describes an algorithm for evaluation and management of SVCS.

Assessment and Grading

A comprehensive history and physical examination are essential when assessing individuals at high risk for SVCS. High-risk individuals include those with lung cancer, mediastinal lymphoma, or long-term VAD placement. Subjective statements as to the severity and duration of symptoms should be obtained from the patient. Clinical manifestations are related to the extent and location of obstruction and the development of collateral circulation.[13] In many cases, signs and symptoms develop gradually and may be vague and difficult to attribute to a specific cause. Mild symptoms of head congestion, dyspnea, and facial or orbital edema may disappear after the individual has been upright for several hours. Gradual, slow progression of obstruction causes slow onset of symptoms due to the development of collateral circulation that compensates for the obstruction.[5] If the obstruction occurs too quickly for collateral circulation to develop, rapid presentation of

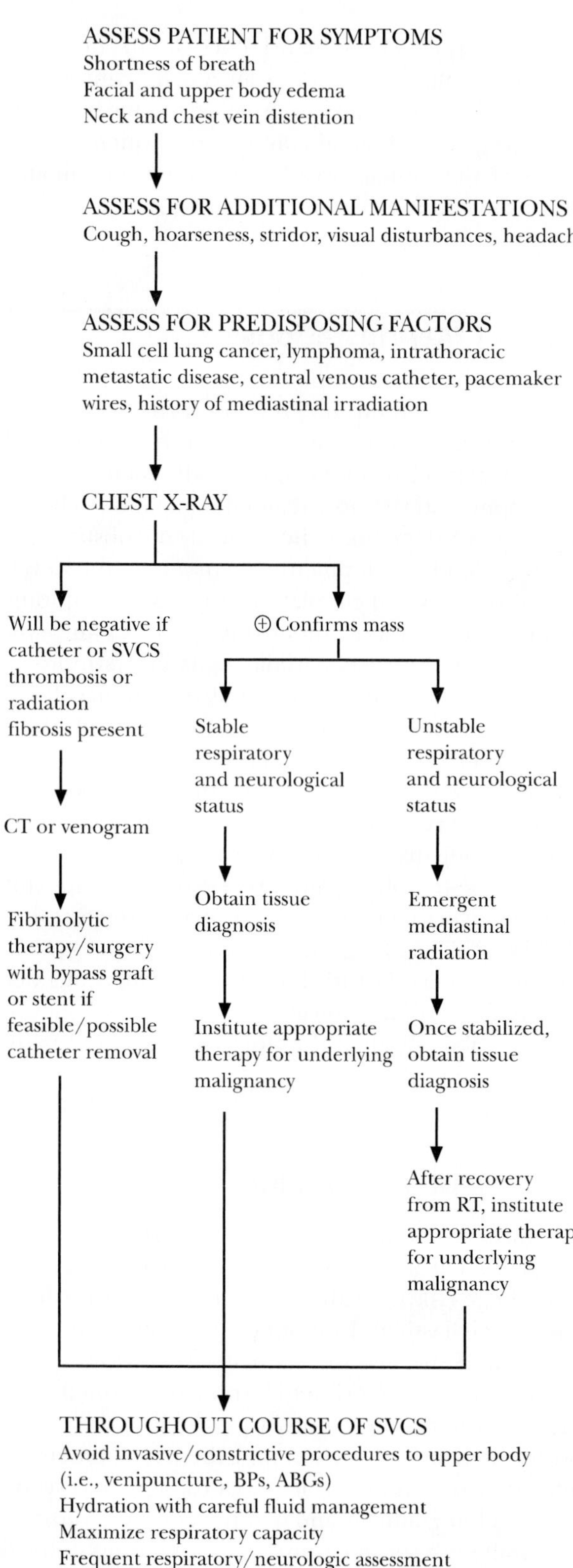

Figure 40–4 Evaluation and management of SVCS.

acute symptoms will result. Intravascular thrombosis may be associated with rapid onset of symptoms.[9]

Patient history

The primary etiology of malignancy-related SVCS is lung cancer; therefore individuals with a history of smoking or other risk factors for lung cancer may be at a relatively high risk for development of SVCS. Likewise, known metastatic or primary cancer in the mediastinum is a risk factor for SVCS. A rare risk factor is previous mediastinal irradiation.[18] The presence of a VAD should also be noted. Thrombosis may occur if the wall of the vena cava is injured during VAD insertion, and trauma to the vein wall may occur with infusion of drugs, especially chemotherapy.[8,9,19]

Physical exam

Symptoms of SVCS generally include dyspnea, nonproductive cough, and sensation of fullness of the face, neck, upper trunk, and extremities[14] (see Table 40-2). Bending over or lying flat may aggravate symptoms. Dyspnea is the most commonly encountered symptom of SVCS in individuals with lung cancer and lymphoma.[13] Classic clinical findings include neck vein distention, chest wall vein distention, edema of the face and upper extremities, and periorbital edema.[20] Dilated veins over the trunk and upper extremities may appear prominent and tortuous and are often palpable (see Figure 40–5). Physical assessment may also reveal facial flushing, cyanosis, and tachypnea. Infrequently, the individual may experience hoarseness, chest pain, dysphagia, dizziness, and hemoptysis. Signs that rarely occur are Horner's syndrome (unilateral ptosis, constricted pupil, and ipsilateral loss of sweating from pressure on the cervical sympathetic nerves) and a paralyzed vocal cord causing hoarseness or stridor (due to cervical sympathetic nerve compromise of recurrent laryngeal nerve entrapment or involvement by lymph nodes). Laryngeal edema may cause stridor, cyanosis, hoarseness, and use of accessory muscles for breathing.[4] Headache, visual disturbances, anxiety, irritability, lethargy, papilledema, confusion, and change in level of consciousness may indicate venous congestion severe enough to cause increased intracranial pressure. Cerebral or airway compromise negatively affects survival and is an indication for emergent treatment.[21,22]

Some patients found to have SVCS are diagnosed based on incidental findings during routine radiology examinations. For example, evidence of collateral circulation may be found on mammograms[23] or CT scans performed for cardiac screening. Visualization of compression of the SVC may occur during transesophageal echocardiography.[24] Masses may be incidental findings on routine chest x-ray (CXR).[25] Incidental findings of collateral circulation or mediastinal masses

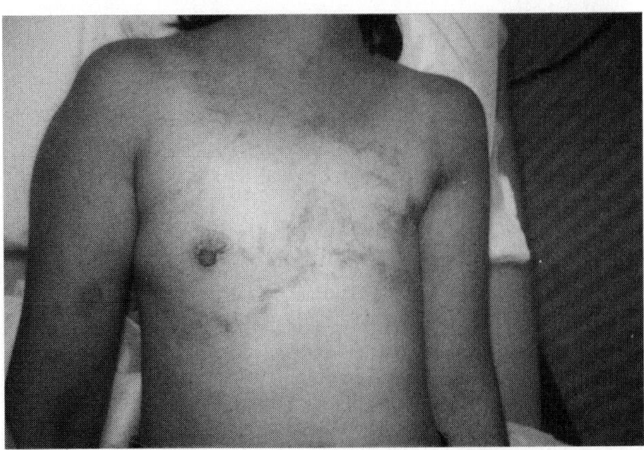

Figure 40–5 Clinical presentation of visible collateral circulation on chest wall. (Image courtesy of Rush University Medical Center, Division of Hematology and Oncology, Chicago, Illinois)

should be followed up with evaluation of the patient for the presence of SVCS and its underlying etiology.

Diagnostic studies

Because SVCS may be the presenting symptom of underlying pathology, determination of this syndrome's etiology is important prior to treatment.[13,22] In cases of suspected malignancy, accurate histologic diagnosis is necessary to plan appropriate anticancer treatment. Note that a significant number of cases are caused by nonmalignant etiologies. A CXR in an individual with SVCS will often indicate a mass, mediastinal widening, or pleural effusion.[25] If the etiology is an intravascular thrombus, the CXR will most likely be normal.

A spiral or helical computerized tomography (CT) scan provides detailed information related to mediastinal structures and the extent of disease involvement. Evaluation of critical structures such as the SVC, other vascular structures, lymph nodes, bronchi, and spinal cord provides information necessary for treatment planning. In particular, this type of imaging is useful in determining the location and extent of thrombi, vascular compression and invasion, and pathways of venous circulation including collaterals.[26] The presence of collateral vessels is a highly sensitive and specific CT sign of SVCS.[27] The CT is also used to localize a tumor for CT-guided biopsy and to determine radiation treatment fields.

Contrast venography can detect compromise in circulation and patterns of collateral development. It is especially useful when a surgical bypass procedure is considered. Similar information can be obtained from such studies as CT and magnetic resonance imaging (MRI); MRI as a noninvasive diagnostic tool to visualize vascular pathways as well as mediastinal structures is still being evaluated in clinical trials.

Table 40-2 Early and Late Signs and Symptoms of SVCS

Early	Late
Respiratory System	
• Vague breathing changes (e.g., heaviness; shortness of breath on exertion) • Dyspnea • Tachypnea (>30 per minute) • Orthopnea • Nonproductive cough • Hoarseness (secondary to paralysis of vocal cord) (laryngeal edema) • Fatigue	• Stridor • Respiratory distress • Facial flushing • Anxiety • Laryngeal changes (hoarseness, stridor due to edema or nerve compression)
Cardiovascular System	
• Neck vein distention • Blood pressure higher in upper than lower extremities • Facial swelling and conjunctival edema especially in the morning upon arising; may decrease as day progresses • Nasal stuffiness, epistaxis • Feeling of fullness in ears • Periobital edema • Redness and edema in conjunctiva • Fullness of face • Facial erythema • Swelling of neck, arms, and hands (tight collar, tight rings, tight watch) • Visible collateral veins on the chest and/or breast; veins tortuous, prominent, and dilated • Cyanosis of upper torso (due to venous stasis)	• Tachycardia • Decreased or absent peripheral pulses • Congestive heart failure • Chest pain (due to pleural effusion) • Decreased blood pressure • Cyanosis
Central Nervous System	
• Mild headache • Mood changes • Anxiety • Lethargy • Lightheadedness especially on exertion	• Severe headache • Irritability • Visual disturbances, blurred vision • Dizziness, syncope • Mental status changes: confusion, change in level of consciousness, stupor, coma • Seizures • Papilledema • Homer's syndrome (unilateral ptosis, unilateral constricted pupil, loss of sweating on same side forehead)
Gastrointestinal System	
• Nausea	• Dysphagia • Hemoptysis

If the underlying pathology remains indeterminate, the least invasive method to obtain a tissue diagnosis is used. Sputum cytology may identify underlying lung cancer. When pleural effusion is present, cytologic examination of pleural fluid obtained by thoracentesis will establish the diagnosis of cancer in approximately 70% of cases. Biopsy of a mass or palpable lymph node may be performed. Percutaneous transthoracic CT-guided fine-needle aspiration biopsy[28] and transbronchial needle aspiration[29] have emerged as safe and effective alternatives to mediastinoscopy or open thoracotomy. Bone marrow biopsy is indicated when bone marrow involvement is suspected, although it reveals only about 25% of cancers. Mediastinoscopy and thoracotomy are performed when other procedures have failed to yield a definitive diagnosis and lung cancer is suspected. Both risk disruption of chest wall collateral pathways. Invasive procedures have traditionally been avoided in patients with SVCS for fear of uncontrolled bleeding secondary to high venous pressures. Anecdotal and clinical reports of both standard and minimally invasive procedures report no increased risk of bleeding in patients with SVCS compared to those without the syndrome.[1]

Additional tests may include arterial blood gases, electrolytes, renal function tests, complete blood count, and coagulation studies. When prioritizing diagnostic procedures, those procedures that will help establish histologic diagnosis should be given priority over noncontributory procedures.[13]

Therapeutic Approaches and Nursing Care

Management

The treatment of SVCS takes into account the cause of the obstruction, severity of symptoms, prognosis, patient preferences, and goals of treatment (palliation or cure).[1] Historically SVCS was treated as a medical emergency with immediate mediastinal irradiation. Because SVCS is rarely a true oncologic emergency, current treatment supports histologic diagnosis prior to treatment. Administering radiation therapy before obtaining tissue for histologic diagnosis can interfere with subsequent diagnosis and treatment plan. Unless respiratory distress or cerebral edema is present, the treatment plan is determined after the diagnosis has been made. Nursing management includes measures to relieve symptoms of the SVCS and side effects of treatment (see Table 40-3).

Thrombolysis

A thrombus in the SVC presents the possibility of embolization or migration of the clot, possibly leading to pulmonary embolism. Cases of SVCS related to thrombosis in the presence of a central VAD catheter are treated with infusion of a thrombolytic agent followed by treatment with antithrombotic agents. Intravenous administration may be infused through the catheter or a peripheral venipuncture site.

Thrombolytic agents dissolve the thrombus by activating plasminogen to the active agent plasmin. Plasmin, in turn, degrades fibrin to soluble peptides. Thrombolytic agents currently approved for use in venous thromboembolism are streptokinase, urokinase, and recombinant tissue plasminogen activator (rt-PA). Use of thrombolytic therapy followed by heparin achieves more rapid resolution of thromboembolus compared with heparin alone.[30]

Thrombolytic agents are administered only intravenously. Extravasation into surrounding tissue can cause ecchymosis and/or inflammation. In case of extravasation, terminating the infusion and applying ice or cold packs is the appropriate intervention. The IV can be restarted at another site. Obviously, systemic administration will achieve thrombolysis throughout the vasculature, not just in the thrombus identified diagnostically. Tissue plasminogen activator appears somewhat more fibrin specific than streptokinase and urokinase; however, all three agents have the ability to lyse a fresh platelet–fibrin plug anywhere in the vasculature and cause bleeding at that site. Heparin should not be infused concurrently with streptokinase or urokinase. For rt-PA, concurrent use of heparin is optional.[30]

The use of rt-PA is associated with a decreased likelihood of hemorrhage, faster lysis of clot, and higher probability of success when administered more than 5 days after clot formation. Febrile reactions are more common with this agent, however, though they are generally managed effectively with acetaminophen. Serious adverse reactions to rt-PA have occurred, including anaphylaxis and angioedema; these events have been documented during the use of rt-PA in the management of acute thrombotic (ischemic) stroke and myocardial infarction.[31,32] Although allergic reactions to thrombolytics can occur, anaphylaxis is uncommon. Anaphylaxis and angioedema during rt-PA infusion is likely caused by activation of the complement and kinin cascades. Patients who are taking angiotensin-converting enzyme inhibitors (ACE-I) concurrently may be at increased risk of this complication based on recent case reports.[33] All patients receiving rt-PA should be closely monitored for signs of anaphylaxis or angioedema during and immediately after its administration.[33,34] Standard emergency treatment for

Table 40-3 SVCS Treatment Approaches: Management of Side Effects

Possible Side Effects of Treatment Approaches	Management of Side Effects
Thrombolytic and Anticoagulation Therapy • Hemorrhage related to anticoagulation or thrombolysis	• Bleeding precautions • Assess for bleeding (e.g., petechiae, bruising, epistaxis, gingival bleeding, hematuria, melena, mental status changes) • Monitor coagulation studies
Chemotherapy • Myelosuppression • Nausea • Vomiting • Stomatitis • Alopecia	• Myelosuppression: assess for infection and bleeding; minimize risk of infection; bleeding precautions • Nausea and vomiting: antiemetics; nonpharmacologic interventions; small, frequent meals; bland diet • Stomatitis: oral care; soft toothbrush; topical anesthetics; analgesics; avoid irritants; bland diet • Alopecia: assess perception of hair loss; provide resources for head coverings and support groups
Radiation Therapy • *Early*: esophagitis, cough, nausea, skin reaction, fatigue • *Late*: pneumonitis (depends on amount of lung treated), pulmonary fibrosis, esophageal sequelae (rare: stenosis, ulceration, fistula), cardiac changes (rare: pericardial effusion, constrictive pericarditis, cardiomyopathy), spinal cord myelopathy, brachial plexopathy	• Esophagitis: topical anesthetics such as viscous lidocaine; agents such as liquid antacids that coat mucosa; analgesics; avoid irritants; soft diet • Cough: antitussives possibly with codeine • Nausea: antiemetics; small, frequent meals; bland diet • Skin reactions: topical moisturizing creams; protect from irritants • Fatigue: balance rest/activity; prioritize and pace activities; plan rest PRN • Pneumonitis: bed rest; bronchodilators; corticosteroids
Stent Placement • Groin hematoma • Femoral-site deep-vein thrombosis • Access-site cellulitis • Pleuritic chest pain • Stent migration • Stent fracture • Shoulder pain • Occlusion • Pulmonary embolism • SVC perforation	• Catheter access site: assess for bleeding; infection; pain • Occlusion: assess for recurrent SVCS • Pulmonary embolism: assess breathing; assess pain • SVC perforation: assess for bleeding
Vein Graft Surgery • Infection • Postoperative complications	• Nursing care for postoperative thoracotomy

anaphylaxis should be administered if this reaction occurs; angioedema may be effectively treated with ranitidine, diphenhydramine, and epinephrine at the first signs of swelling of the tongue or throat.[33] Inspection of the tongue and oropharynx 30–45 minutes after the start of the rt-PA infusion should be performed to assess for signs of swelling. Case reports of angioedema associated with rt-PA note that the swelling is often unilateral early, progressing to involvement of the entire tongue and oropharynx.[33]

All individuals undergoing thrombolytic therapy should be monitored for signs of bleeding. Administrations of rt-PA for ischemic stroke is associated with increased risk of intracranial hemorrhage.[33,35] The concurrent use of aspirin or nonsteroidal anti-inflammatory drugs (NSAIDs) for febrile episodes is generally avoided during thrombolytic therapy due to alterations in platelet aggregation and the risk of gastrointestinal (GI) bleeding with NSAIDs. If aspirin or NSAIDs must be used, patients should be closely monitored for GI bleeding.

Anticoagulant therapy is required following thrombolytic therapy to prevent recurrence of the clot. Unfractionated heparin or low-molecular-weight heparin

(LMWH) should be continued for at least 5 days following thrombolytic therapy. Oral anticoagulants (warfarin) should be overlapped with heparin or LMWH for at least 4–5 days. For most patients, treatment with warfarin can be started together with heparin or LMWH. Heparin can be discontinued after the INR has been in a therapeutic range for two consecutive days. Therapeutic INR is generally considered to be between 2.0 and 3.0. An adjusted dose of subcutaneous heparin or LMWH would be the treatment of choice for pregnant women, patients with warfarin hypersensitivity, or those individuals for whom warfarin therapy monitoring is inadequate.[30]

Nursing care during thrombolytic or anticoagulation administration includes bleeding precautions. Assess for bleeding and monitor vital signs. Monitor for intracranial hemorrhage related to increased intracranial pressure secondary to venous hypertension. The effects of thrombolytic agents continue for several hours after infusion, so monitoring for bleeding must be continued after the therapy session ends. Coagulation studies during thrombolytic therapy are monitored with fibrinogen levels and partial thromboplastin times prior to thrombolytic therapy and every 6 hours during therapy. Coagulation studies during antithrombotic therapy include partial thromboplastin time (aPTT) during unfractionated heparin therapy and prothrombin time/International Normalized Ratio (PT/INR) during warfarin administration. LMWH therapy does not require coagulation monitoring.[30]

Treatment decisions include whether to save the catheter or remove it. The central line may be salvaged with successful thrombolysis. Removal of the catheter should be combined with anticoagulation to avoid embolization.[13] Thrombolytic agents are contraindicated in individuals with bleeding disorders, increased intracranial pressure, intracranial or intraspinal surgery, history of hemorrhagic stroke, and cerebral metastasis.

External compression or tumor invasion of the SVC may also cause intravascular thrombus formation. Because of ongoing venous stasis, anticoagulation with heparin or oral anticoagulants may be used to decrease the extent and prevent progression of thrombus formation.

Chemotherapy

When SVCS is caused by cancer, treatment generally involves multidrug chemotherapy and/or radiation therapy. Cancers that are chemotherapy- and radiation-sensitive often respond quickly to both methods of control. Other solid tumors may require a longer period of time to alleviate symptoms. If collateral circulation is sufficient to maintain homeostasis until treatment becomes effective, surgical intervention is not necessary. Venous hypertension, cerebral edema, or airway compromise may result if collateral circulation is insufficient. In these situations, surgical consultation should be requested both to relieve and to prevent progressive symptoms.

Multidrug chemotherapy is especially effective in the treatment of SVCS caused by small cell lung cancer and non-Hodgkin's lymphoma,[2,36] with relief of acute symptoms often occurring during the first week of treatment. Note that venous stasis may cause local drug concentration in the upper thorax if chemotherapy is infused through a peripheral line in the upper extremities or a VAD. A long-term venous access catheter or femoral vein catheter may be necessary to administer chemotherapy safely.

Several studies have demonstrated an advantage for combined chemotherapy and radiation therapy.[36] Neoadjuvant chemotherapy to decrease tumor volume may allow smaller subsequent radiation fields to be used. Combined chemotherapy and radiotherapy may be used to downstage malignant SVCS to resectable lesions in candidates with good functionality.[37] A combination of chemotherapy and radiation therapy is often used to treat non-Hodgkin's lymphoma. In individuals who have had previous mediastinal irradiation, chemotherapy is the treatment of choice. Current chemotherapy guidelines for small cell lung cancer (SCLC) include etoposide, cisplatin, carboplatin, ifosfamide, cyclophosphamide, doxorubicin, and vincristine. Several newer agents, including the taxanes and two topoisomerase I inhibitors, gemcitabine and vinorelbine, appear to have activity in SCLC.[36,38] Patients with advanced lung cancer should receive a two-drug regimen of chemotherapy.[36] Relief of SVCS in SCLC patients with either chemotherapy or radiation therapy alone is achieved in approximately 80% of cases.[14,39] Combined chemotherapy and radiotherapy achieves an SVCS response rate of approximately 90%.[39]

Nursing care of the individual receiving chemotherapy depends on the agents being administered. Combined chemotherapy and radiation therapy results in a higher incidence of esophagitis and neutropenia. Nursing management may be required for myelosuppression, nausea and vomiting, stomatitis, esophagitis, and alopecia. When deciding where chemotherapy will be administered, peripheral veins in the upper extremities should be avoided.[4] Venous stasis due to obstruction may result in local accumulation of the drug with poor absorption and irritation of the vessel wall. Because of the risk for extravasation and tissue damage, administering irritant or vesicant chemotherapy through lower-extremity peripheral veins is not recommended. Placement of a long-term

VAD into the inferior vena cava via the femoral vein may be necessary to administer chemotherapy safely.

Radiation therapy

Tumor histology, extent of tumor obstructing the SVC, any history of previous irradiation to the mediastinum or lungs, and performance status will determine the radiation dose prescribed. Radiation therapy for SVCS is often administered for 2–3 days as high-dose fractions of 4 Gy and subsequently as daily fractions of 1.8–2.0 Gy until the total prescribed dose is completed.[13] Higher initial daily doses are believed to result in more rapid decrease in symptoms than standard dose fractions.[40] Some investigators have found that symptom relief is not enhanced by the higher initial fractions and recommend standard fractionation throughout the treatment. Standard fractionation is generally 30–50 Gy administered over 2–5 weeks but may be as high as 60–70 Gy in 6–7 weeks. Lymphoma is more responsive to radiation and generally requires less therapy than other tumor types. Radiation fields for mediastinal treatment generally include mediastinal, hilar, and supraclavicular lymph nodes and any adjacent lung lesions. Most patients experience some symptom relief within a few days of starting radiotherapy,[5] with maximum relief occurring at 3 weeks.

Side effects of mediastinal radiation depend on the total dose, dose per fraction, volume of normal tissue included in the field, and whether chemotherapy is combined with radiation therapy. Side effects that occur during and for one month after radiation therapy are considered early side effects. Nursing management is often necessary for esophagitis, cough, nausea, skin reaction, and fatigue. Symptomatic treatment helps minimize these side effects. Late effects of radiation therapy to the mediastinum include pneumonitis, pulmonary fibrosis, esophageal ulceration or stenosis, cardiac changes, spinal cord myelopathy, and brachial plexopathy.

In SVCS caused by non-small cell lung cancer (NSCLC), radiation therapy is the treatment of choice, as NSCLC generally does not respond to chemotherapy. Although symptom relief is high, prognosis remains poor. Radiation therapy is also the treatment of choice in individuals without a histologic diagnosis in whom rapid deterioration in mental status due to increased intracranial pressure or severe upper airway compression occurs.

Stent placement

For many years, radiation therapy and chemotherapy were considered the standard treatments for SVCS. The intravascular placement of self-expanding stents to relieve SVC obstruction has increased in the past 10 years and has been shown to be at least equivalent to chemotherapy and radiation therapy, especially in tumors that are not particular chemotherapy- or radiotherapy-sensitive. Percutaneous stenting of the SVC is increasingly being used as a primary treatment modality.[3] Analysis of retrospective studies comparing stenting to radiation therapy and chemotherapy appears to indicate that stenting is the most effective and rapid treatment for the relief of symptoms. Because the numbers of patients participating in these studies are smaller than those receiving traditional therapies, and because the studies have not stratified patients by histologic type, generalization of their results is not possible; prospective randomized trials are needed to fully evaluate stenting as a therapeutic measure for SVCS.[39] Several nonrandomized studies have compared stent insertion to radiation therapy. Stent placement resulted in faster relief of symptoms and greater improvement in SVC obstruction, with many patients experiencing complete disappearance of symptoms within 24–72 hours.[41] Endovascular techniques may be used to revascularize the SVC after unsuccessful thrombolysis or in cases of tumor compression or invasion[42] but are increasingly being used as first-line therapy.[41]

The stent is generally placed by an interventional radiologist under local anesthesia. The most common approach in stenting for SVCS is through the basilic or subclavian veins. The common femoral vein could be used if needed. Subjective improvement in symptoms is reported in more than 90% of cases.[39,41] Resolution of peripheral edema generally occurs within 1–7 days. Low-pressure venous blood flow may contribute to thrombus formation in the stented area. Heparin is generally administered during the procedure and may be converted to oral warfarin therapy for 3–6 months after stent placement to prevent thrombus formation. Anticoagulant therapy after stent placement is controversial. When a thrombus is present, thrombolysis may be performed before stent placement. This procedure decreases the size of the thrombus and the amount of potential embolic material. Recurrent SVC obstruction often occurs, possibly due to malignant invasion through the stented area, compression by tumor, intimal thickening, or thrombus formation.[39,41,43] Stent placement is contraindicated in cases of tumor invasion of the vessel.

Nursing management after stent placement includes care for potential complications such as hematoma, infection, or deep-vein thrombosis (DVT). The nurse also evaluates the patient for pleuritic chest pain and shoulder pain and administers analgesics as needed. Pulmonary embolism (PE) is a life-threatening complication of DVT, occurring in 12% of patients. It presents as dyspnea, decrease in oxygen saturation, or chest pain. Bleeding can also occur due to vascular injury following stent placement; it most often presents as a localized hematoma, hypotension, or tachycardia. Other complications of stent placement include stent migration, fracture, and occlusion.

Surgical bypass

Intravascular stents have largely replaced surgical venous bypass to obtain rapid relief of SVCS caused by cancer.[14] Surgical bypass to relieve SVC obstruction utilizes a reconstructed saphenous vein graft that connects the brachiocephalic or left jugular vein with the right atrium, bypassing the obstructed SVC. This technique is rarely used in individuals in SVCS with a malignant etiology due to the expedient need to treat the underlying disease so as to prevent progression or recurrence of the obstruction. In benign etiologies, surgical bypass may be used if the individual is not a candidate for or has failed intravascular stenting. Bypass should be used when less invasive measures have failed or, in the case of an underlying malignancy, when other palliative efforts have failed to relieve acute symptoms.[13,44]

Nursing care

Oncology nurses play a major role in the management of patients experiencing SVCS. Assessment of cardiopulmonary, neurologic, and mental status can help prevent progressive symptoms. Taking adequate measures to maximize oxygenation and perfusion is of utmost importance. Elevating the head of the bed and encouraging patients to remain in a sitting position, as tolerated, will increase both patient comfort and oxygenation. Supplemental oxygen should be provided to dyspneic patients or those with decreased oxygen saturation. Comfort measures to relieve dyspnea and anxiety (see Table 40-4) will serve to reassure both patients and family members. In addition, minimizing activity level may reduce dyspnea. Baseline assessment includes vital signs, oxygen saturation by pulse oximeter, appearance, activity level, and mental status. Emergency action is required at the first signs of bronchial compression, laryngeal edema, or alterations in mental or neurologic status.

Individuals considered to be at high risk for SVCS should be monitored for early signs and symptoms of obstruction. In the individual diagnosed with lung cancer or mediastinal lymphoma, the nurse must remain alert for early signs and symptoms of SVCS. Often it is nurses caring for patients with VADs in ambulatory settings who note the early symptoms of SVCS; therefore, infusion center and clinic nurses should be mindful of the signs and symptoms of SVCS when tending to these patients.

Avoid peripheral upper extremity venipuncture and intravenous therapy. A femoral or central venous line with the tip past the obstruction may be necessary to administer drugs or chemotherapy.[4,5] Venous access of the involved extremity in the individual with SVCS should be avoided whenever possible. As an alternative, lower extremities can be used for venipuncture and blood pressure measurement.

Steroids are often used concomitantly with radiation therapy to relieve laryngeal and cerebral edema despite a lack of evidence to support their use. If steroids are to be used, high-dose therapy should be limited to a short period of time.[13,39] Diuretics and low-sodium diets are frequently prescribed, although their efficacy is not well documented. Efforts to reduce edema through diuretics and low salt intake must be done carefully to avoid an increased risk of thrombus formation with dehydration. Overhydration will exacerbate SVCS.[13]

The valsalva maneuver increases venous pressure and should be prevented by administration of medications such as stool softeners and cough suppressants when indicated. The sensations of breathlessness and head congestion may cause anxiety in the individual with SVCS. Providing a calm and restful environment, emotional support, and anxiolytics as necessary may help fearful individuals cope until symptoms begin to resolve with treatment. Remember that for some lung cancer patients, the appearance of SVCS heralds their lung cancer diagnosis; for these individuals and their families, coping with the symptoms of SVCS and a new diagnosis of lung cancer may prove overwhelming. Changes in physical appearance such as periorbital and facial edema will decrease with successful treatment.

Continuity of Care

Recovery from the symptoms of SVCS occurs rapidly when the underlying disease is controlled, although SVCS may recur when it is caused by an underlying malignancy. Follow-up for the diagnosis by the medical oncologist or oncology nurse practitioner should include surveillance of symptoms that suggest early signs of recurrence of SVCS. Prior to the patient's discharge from the hospital, the nurse provides self-care instructions to the individual and family and educates them about early signs of recurrence and symptoms to report to the oncologist. The individual recovering from SVCS should be made aware that the syndrome's recurrence may be related to progression of underlying disease. Individuals discharged on anticoagulant therapy must be educated on bleeding precautions, side effects of therapy, medication interactions, and any blood testing necessary to monitor therapy. Postra-

Table 40-4 Nursing Diagnoses for SVCS

Problem	Expected Outcomes	Nursing Interventions
Cardiac output, decreased, related to decreased venous return Tissue perfusion, ineffective, related to venous congestion and venous hypertension Breathing pattern, ineffective, related to airway compression by tumor Activity intolerance related to reduced cardiac output	Maintain adequate oxygenation Maintain airway Maintain optimal venous drainage Maintain adequate hydration Reduce edema Reduce fatigue	Assess respiratory system (cyanosis, hoarseness, stridor, dyspnea, tachypnea, cough, rales/rhonchi) Assess cardiac system (tachycardia, dysrhythmias, hypotension) Monitor blood pressure on lower extremity Administer oxygen Monitor oxygen saturation Administer corticosteroids for laryngeal edema Position upright Monitor for dysphagia Administer diuretics and fluids Monitor fluid balance Remove constrictive clothing and jewelry Avoid upper extremity venipuncture Avoid valsalva maneuver Avoid bending, stooping, lying flat, coughing Administer cough suppressants Administer analgesics
Injury, risk for, related to increased intracranial pressure Acute pain: headache related to increased intracranial pressure	Prevent neurologic complications Reduce discomfort	Assess central nervous system (altered mental status, lethargy, headache, vomiting, visual changes) Administer analgesics
Injury, risk for, related to thrombolytic and anticoagulant treatment	Prevent bleeding Reduce thrombus	Administer thrombolytics and anticoagulants Monitor coagulation studies Assess for bleeding Teach bleeding precautions
Anxiety related to respiratory distress	Relieve anxiety	Provide emotional support Assure relief of symptoms Maintain calm environment Teach relaxation techniques Administer anxiolytics or mild sedation
Fatigue related to disease process, treatment and reduced cardiac output	Minimize fatigue Perform activities of daily living	Teach energy conservation techniques Prioritize activities Assist with activities of daily living
Body image, disturbed, related to edema	Reduce edema Reassure that edema will resolve	Assure relief of symptoms with successful treatment
Knowledge deficit	Recognize early symptoms of SVCS	Educate individual and family to recognize signs and symptoms of recurrent SVCS Educate about treatment and side effects

Data from Carpenito-Moyet.[45]

diation therapy patients should be given information on management of localized symptoms such as esophagitis, skin changes, and fatigue.

Conclusion

Future trends in the diagnosis and treatment of SVCS will involve more sensitive radiologic modalities for diagnosis and refinement of endovascular techniques for stenting. Stents may be used as first-line therapy to provide almost immediate symptom relief, because stenting does not interfere with subsequent antitumor treatments. Conformational radiation therapy may allow targeted retreatment of the occluding mass in patients who have previously undergone radiation therapy. Prevention of SVCS will be significantly enhanced by new and more effective treatment of lung cancer and lymphoma, the malignancies most frequently associated with SVCS. Targeted therapies may be used concomitantly with cytotoxic therapy to reduce malignant thoracic masses. Individuals with long-term venous access devices may be treated prophylactically with low-dose rt-PA or other thrombolytic therapies in an effort to prevent SVCS. Investigational studies are currently under way to evaluate the safety and efficacy of this preventive approach.

Fortunately, SVCS is a relatively rare complication. Although it can develop rapidly and constitute a true oncologic emergency, more often it develops insidiously. Most often, SVCS is caused by an underlying malignancy; however, a significant number of cases result from nonmalignant causes. When the cause is unknown initially, every effort is made to establish the diagnosis prior to treatment, as appropriate treatment is based on the syndrome's etiology. Early detection and treatment of SVCS can prevent progression to severe complications.

References

1. Porte H, Metois D, Finzi L, et al: Superior vena cava syndrome of malignant origin. Which surgical procedure for which diagnosis? *Eur J Cardio-Thoracic Surg* 17:384–388, 2000
2. Markman M: Diagnosis and management of superior vena cava syndrome. *Cleveland Clin J Med* 66:59–61, 1999
3. Wudel LJ, Jr, Nesbitt JC: Superior vena cava syndrome. *Curr Treat Opt Oncol* 2:77–91, 2001
4. Flounders JA: Oncology emergency modules: superior vena cava syndrome. *Oncol Nurs Forum Online* 30:E84–E90, 2003
5. Haapoja IS, Blendowski C: Superior vena cava syndrome. *Semin Oncol Nurs* 15:183–189, 1999
6. Merrill P: Oncologic emergencies. *Lippincott's Prim Care Pract* 4:400–409, 2000
7. Nicolin G: Emergencies and their management. *Eur J Cancer* 38:1365–1377, discussion 1378–1369, 2002
8. Verso M, Agnelli G: Venous thromboembolism associated with long-term use of central venous catheters in cancer patients. *J Clin Oncol* 21:3665–3675, 2003
9. Morales M, Comas V, Trujillo M, et al: Treatment of catheter-induced thrombotic superior vena cava syndrome: a single institution's experience. *Support Care Cancer* 8:334–338, 2000
10. Stockton PA, Ledson MJ, Walshaw MJ: Persistent superior vena caval syndrome due to totally implantable venous access systems. *J Royal Soc Med* 94:584–585, 2001
11. Piastra M, Caresta E, Ruggiero A, et al: Management of critically ill children with mediastinal neoplasms: a 6–year survey from a single institution. *Med Pediat Oncol* 40:329–331, 2003
12. Journeycake J, Buchanan GR: Thrombotic complications of central venous catheters in children. *Curr Opin Hematol* 10:369–374, 2004
13. Yahalom J: Oncologic emergencies, in DeVita VT, Hellman S, Rosenberg SA (eds.): *Cancer: Principles and Practice of Oncology* (ed 6). Philadelphia, Lippincott, Williams and Wilkins, 2001, pp 2609–2616
14. Kvale PA, Simoff M, Prakash UB, et al: Palliative care. *Chest* 123:284S–311S, 2003
15. Aurora R, Milite F, Vander Els NJ: Respiratory emergencies. *Semin Oncol* 27:256–269, 2000
16. Morales M, Llanos M, Dorta J: Superior vena cava thrombosis secondary to Hickman catheter and complete resolution after fibrinolytic therapy. *Support Care Cancer* 5:67–69, 1997
17. Wurschmidt F, Bunemann H, Hellman HP: Small cell lung cancer with and without superior vena cava syndrome: a multivariate analysis of prognostic factors in 408 cases. *Int J Radiat Oncol Biol Phys* 33:77–82, 1995
18. Van Putten JW, Schlosser NJ, Vujaskovic Z, et al: Superior vena cava obstruction caused by radiation induced venous fibrosis. *Thorax* 55:245–246, 2000
19. Calderon MC, Lozano VM, Jaquez A, et al: Surgical repair of superior vena cava syndrome. *Ann Thoracic Surg* 71:1351–1353, 2001
20. Burgdorff T, Douwes KE, Bogenrieder T, et al: Superior vena cava syndrome: an important differential diagnosis in patients with facial edema. *Acta Dermato-Venereologica* 81:205–206, 2001
21. Brigden ML: Hematologic and oncologic emergencies. Doing the most good in the least time. *Postgrad Med* 109:143–146, 151–154, 157–158, 2001
22. Hemann R: Superior vena cava syndrome. *Clin Excel Nurse Pract* 5:85–87, 2001
23. Krishnan P, Uragoda L, Rao H, et al: Venous dilatation seen on routine mammography: a clue to superior vena cava obstruction. *Chest* 121:1361–1363, 2002
24. Behar DM, Reisner SA, Ben-Ami H: Superior vena cava syndrome diagnosed by transesophageal echocardiography. *Isr Med Assoc J* 3:457, 2001
25. Dhaliwal G, Schmidt KE, Gilden DJ, et al: True, true and related. *N Engl J Med* 350:60–65, 2004
26. Groves AM, Dixon AK: CT diagnosis of superior vena cava syndrome. *Br J Radiol* 75:645–647, 1993
27. Kim HJ, Kim HS, Chung SH: CT diagnosis of superior vena cava syndrome: importance of collateral vessels. *Am J Roentgenol* 161:539–542, 1993
28. Reyes CV, Thompson KS, Massarani-Wafai R, et al: Utilization of fine-needle aspiration cytology in the diagnosis of neoplastic superior vena caval syndrome. *Digest Cytopathol* 19:84–88, 1998
29. Selcuk ZT, Firat P: The diagnostic yield of transbronchial needle aspiration in superior vena cava syndrome. *Lung Cancer* 42:183–188, 2003
30. Hyers TM, Agnelli G, Hull RD, et al: Antithrombotic therapy for venous thromboembolic disease. *Chest* 119:176S–193S, 2001
31. Fayad PB, Albers GW, Frey JL, et al: Orolingual angioedema complicating rt-PA therapy for acute ischemic stroke. *Stroke* 30:242, 1999 (abstract)
32. Rudolf J, Grond M, Prince WS, et al: Evidence of anaphylaxy following alteplase infusion. *Stroke* 30:1142–1143, 1999
33. Hill MD, Barber PA, Takahashi J, et al: Anaphylactoid reactions and angioedema during alteplase treatment of acute ischemic stroke [see comment]. *CMAJ* 162:1281–1284, 2000
34. Chodirker WB: Reactions to alteplase in patients with acute thrombotic stroke [comment]. *CMAJ* 163:387–389, 2000
35. Parker C, Rode H: Alteplase (Activase; rt-PA) for acute ischemic stroke: special precautions for new indication. *CMAJ* 161:73–74, 1999
36. Spira A, Ettinger DS: Multidisciplinary management of lung cancer. *N Engl J Med* 350:379–392, 2004
37. Roberts JR, Bueno R, Sugarbaker DJ: Multimodality treatment of malignant superior vena caval syndrome. *Chest* 116:835–837, 1999
38. Network NCC. *Small Cell Lung Cancer. Practice Guidelines in Oncology.* Rockledge, PA, National Comprehensive Cancer Network, 2004
39. Rowell NP, Gleeson FV: Steroids, radiotherapy, chemotherapy and stents for superior vena caval obstruction in carcinoma of the bronchus: a systematic review. *Clin Oncol (Royal Coll Radiolog)* 14:338–351, 2002
40. Lonardi F, Gioga G, Agus G, et al: Double-flash, large-fraction radiation therapy as palliative treatment of malignant superior

vena cava syndrome in the elderly. *Support Care Cancer* 10:156–160, 2002

41. Lanciego C, Chacon JL, Julian A, et al: Stenting as first option for endovascular treatment of malignant superior vena cava syndrome. *Am J Roentgenol* 177:585–593, 2001
42. Sasano S, Onuki T, Mae M, et al: Wallstent endovascular prosthesis for the treatment of superior vena cava syndrome. *Japan Thoracic Cardiovasc Surg* 49:165–170, 2001
43. Miller JH, McBride K, Little F, et al: Malignant superior vena cava obstruction: stent placement via the subclavian route. *Cardiovasc Intervention Radiol* 23:155–158, 2000
44. Panneton JM, Andrews JC, Hofer JM: Superior vena cava syndrome: relief with a modified saphenojugular bypass graft. *J Vascular Surg* 34:360–363, 2001
45. Carpenito-Moyet LJ: *Handbook of Nursing Diagnosis.* Philadelphia, Lippincott, Williams and Wilkins, 2003

CHAPTER 41

Syndrome of Inappropriate Antidiuretic Hormone

AnnMarie K. McDonnell Keenan, RN/APN, MS, AOCN®

Scope of the Problem

Syndrome of inappropriate antidiuretic hormone (SIADH) is a paraneoplastic endocrine disorder most often associated with lung carcinomas. Typically, the disorder results from tumor secretion of an endocrine peptide (vasopressin) unrelated to tissue invasion or metastases. Besides ectopic vasopressin secretion by tumors, abnormal secretion of vasopressin is also related to intrathoracic infection, positive pressure ventilation, central nervous system disorders, acquired immunodeficiency syndrome (AIDS), and a variety of drugs. Although SIADH is frequently classified as an oncologic emergency, the majority of patients present with asymptomatic hyponatremia that is discovered upon routine chemistry evaluation, before or at the time of malignant diagnosis or during the course of treatment. Alternatively, some patients may develop chronic SIADH with exacerbations relating to the progression of the malignancy.

Definitions

Schwartz and colleagues originally described two patients with bronchogenic carcinoma who developed hyponatremia with elevated urine sodium levels, hypothesized to be due to inappropriate secretion of antidiuretic hormone (ADH).[1] Subsequent research suggested that tumor-derived ADH may cause SIADH.[2] SIADH is currently defined as the inappropriate production and secretion of ADH, also known as its biologically active form, arginine vasopressin (AVP), causing a syndrome of hyponatremia, urine osmolality disproportionately higher than plasma osmolality, and elevated urinary sodium concentrations.

Although ADH is the primary endocrine peptide involved in SIADH, the ectopic production of atrial natriuretic peptide (ANP) by cardiac atrial cells may independently cause SIADH.[3,4] In some patients, ectopic ADH and ANP secretion both contribute to the etiology of SIADH.

Incidence

SIADH is primarily associated with bronchogenic carcinoma, particularly small cell lung cancer (SCLC), which constitutes approximately 20% of all lung cancers. Nearly 10% of patients with SCLC will develop SIADH, with only a minority manifesting symptoms, ranging from anorexia, nausea, and weakness to life-threatening seizures and coma.[5,6,7] The presence of SIADH is unrelated to the stage and prognosis of disease.[8]

Etiology and Risk Factors

SIADH is caused by the ectopic production of vasopressin by malignant cells. While structurally identical to normal ADH, ectopic ADH is unregulated. In a series of 263 lung cancer patients, 21 of the 133 patients with SCLC were hyponatremic. Eleven of these patients had tumor cell lines assayed for the presence of ADH and ANP. Nine patients' tumors produced ANP, seven produced ADH, and five produced both ANP and ADH.[9] The more severe cases of hyponatremia are associated with ectopic ADH, rather than ANP, production.[10]

Apart from a paraneoplastic origin, SIADH is associated with pulmonary disease (pneumonia, tuberculosis, aspergillosis), central nervous system disorders (head trauma, acute psychosis, peripheral neuropathy), pain, stress, nausea, surgery, and pharmacologic agents, all of which may increase ADH secretion.[6,11–15] An increasing number of patients with AIDS have been reported to have hyponatremia, with SIADH as the underlying cause in up to 66% of these patients (see Table 41-1).[16]

Patients who are at risk for developing SIADH are primarily those with lung carcinomas, especially SCLC. Other patients at risk include those with head and neck carcinomas, particularly following neck dissection.[13] Gastrointestinal, gynecologic, prostatic, hematologic, and neurologic malignancies are also associated with SIADH; however, case reports include very few patients.[17–20] The patients at highest risk are those with tumors of squamous cell or neuroendocrine histology (see Table 41-2).

Physiologic Alterations

Normal Physiology and Scientific Principles

Understanding how the body maintains its fluid balance is necessary to comprehending the impact of ectopic ADH production. Constant regulation of body water within a very narrow range is achieved by the effect of ADH or AVP on the kidney. Arginine vasopressin is produced by the hypothalamus and stored in the posterior pituitary, where it is released in response to changes in plasma osmolality or volume. Normally, plasma osmolality is maintained within a narrow range of 286–294 mOsm/kg. Conditions such as dehydration, positive pressure breathing, and vasodilation result in an increase in plasma osmolality, which is detected by the osmoreceptors in the hypothalamus and the pressoreceptors in the left atrium and carotid sinus. These receptors stimulate the release of AVP,

Table 41-1 Nonparaneoplastic Causes of SIADH

Pulmonary
- Infection (tuberculosis, lung abscess, pneumonia, empyema)
- Chronic obstructive pulmonary disease

Central Nervous System
- Trauma (subdural hematoma, skull fracture, concussion, stroke, subarachnoid hemorrhage, cerebral vascular thrombosis)
- Intracranial space-occupying lesions (primary or metastatic tumors)
- Infection (encephalitis, meningitis)
- Guillain-Barré syndrome
- Vasculitis (lupus)
- Acute intermittent porphyria
- Pain and emotional stress
- Nausea

Drugs
- Chemotherapeutic agents (vincristine, vinblastine, vinorelbine, cyclophosphamide, ifosfamide, cisplatin, docetaxel)
- Narcotics (morphine, barbiturates)
- General anesthesia
- Nicotine
- Chlorpropamide (Diabinese)®
- Carbamazepine (Tegretol)®
- Tricyclic antidepressants
- Immunoglobulin therapy

Surgery
- Neck dissection
- Mitral stenosis correction

Other
- AIDS

Data from Arnold et al;[6] Turchin et al;[11] Flounders;[12] Zacay et al;[13] Langer-Nitsche et al;[14] Kao et al.[15]

Table 41-2 Malignancies Associated with SIADH

- Lung cancer
  - small cell
  - non-small cell
- Head and neck carcinoma
- Duodenal and pancreatic carcinoma
- Prostate carcinoma
- Lymphomas (Hodgkin's and non-Hodgkin's)
- Leukemias
- Gynecologic
  - Ovarian carcinoma
  - Cervical (small cell)
  - Ovarian teratoma (germ cell)
  - Papillary serous carcinoma peritoneum
- Neuroblastoma
- Thymoma

Data from Galesic et al;[17] Thompson, Adlam;[18] Bogdanos et al;[19] Robertson.[20]

which acts to conserve water and concentrate the urine by binding to the G-protein-coupled V_2 receptor on the surface of the principal cell of the renal collecting duct.[21] The resulting receptor-hormone complex activates adenylate cyclase and increases cyclic adenosine monophosphate (cAMP), causing activation of protein kinase A and subsequently the phosphorylation of aquaporin 2 (AQP2), a protein exclusively expressed in the collecting duct. Phosphorylation of AQP2 results in its transfer from the cytoplasm into the luminal (apical) membrane of the collecting duct cells. The insertion of AQP2 water channels leads to increased permeability to water. Other aquaporins, AQP3 and AQP4, located in the basolateral membranes of the collecting duct, facilitate water reabsorption. Water that enters the cell through AQP2 on the apical membrane leaves the cell through AQP3 and AQP4 on the basolateral membrane, with the overall results of water conservation and urine concentration.[22] Decreased circulating levels of ADH cause the water channels to be reinternalized back into the cytoplasm.

The presence of AVP increases the transfer of water from the collecting duct to the renal capillaries. At the same time, it increases the permeability of the collecting duct to urea and increases sodium absorption in the ascending limb of the loop of Henle. The resulting increase in plasma volume and normalization of plasma osmolality provides the feedback loop that inhibits AVP release. Cold temperatures, recumbency, and negative pressure breathing can also inhibit AVP release.

The release of AVP is also regulated by certain neurotransmitters and neuropeptides. Angiotensin II, histamine, and bradykinin all appear to stimulate the release of AVP. On the other hand, AVP release may be inhibited by the presence of dopamine, norepinephrine, and serotonin.[16]

Pathophysiology

The ability of neoplastic cells to synthesize, store, and release AVP results in excessive amounts of AVP, leading to a condition known as *water intoxication*. The presence of high levels of AVP causes water to be conserved in the kidney, with production of a concentrated urine (urine osmolality > 300 mmol/kg). The increase in free water in the extracellular fluid (ECF) leads to plasma hypo-osmolality and dilutional serum hyponatremia. Sodium continues to be excreted from the kidney in parallel to the sodium intake. Intracellular edema occurs as the plasma water follows an osmotic gradient, moving extracellular to intracellular.[23] Cerebral edema eventually occurs and leads to a disruption of neural function and death.

Clinical Manifestations

Water intoxication accounts for the symptomatology of SIADH. Since the excess water is distributed to the intracellular fluid compartment with only a slight expansion of intravascular volume, patients have normal extracellular volume and appear normovolemic with no edema. Moderate hyponatremia (serum sodium level of 115–120 mEq/L) may cause nausea, weakness, anorexia, fatigue, and muscle cramps. These vague, nonspecific complaints can easily be attributed to the primary malignancy or treatment regimens and are often not identified as early signs of hyponatremia. The symptoms that a patient exhibits depend upon the severity of the hyponatremia and the rate of development. Rapid-onset hyponatremia (48 hours or less) is associated with the most severe symptomatology.

As hyponatremia worsens, symptoms progress to include changes in mental status, such as confusion, lethargy, combativeness, or psychotic behavior. These signs and symptoms result from brain cell edema. Severe hyponatremia (100–110 mEq/L) is associated with generalized seizures, coma, and death.[7]

Assessment and Grading

Assessment of the patient with SIADH focuses on a skillful neurologic exam. Due to the nonspecificity and vagueness of the symptoms related to mild hyponatremia, SIADH may go undiagnosed until the hyponatremia becomes severe and cerebral edema produces neurologic changes. With regard to patients with SCLC, the presence of SIADH does not appear to negatively correlate with the stage of disease, response to chemotherapy, or survival.[6,8]

The diagnosis of SIADH is most frequently made concurrently with discovery of the malignancy. Ectopic SIADH is a diagnosis of exclusion. Other nonmalignant etiologies must be ruled out, such as infection, pneumothorax, or drug-related SIADH. The diagnosis of SIADH requires the presence of hyponatremia in addition to decreased plasma osmolality and inappropriately concentrated urine (see Table 41-3). Plasma osmolality must be less than 280 mOsm/kg, and concurrent urinalysis must show increased levels of sodium (> 20 mEq/L). Serum chemistries frequently show a low blood urea nitrogen (BUN), creatinine, albumin, and uric acid — a dilutional effect as a result of a modest increase in intravascular volume. Measurement of serum and urine AVP levels is possible by radioimmunoassay but is rarely done because these levels are an unreliable indicator of changes in secretion or plasma concentration of the hormone.[21]

Table 41-3 Criteria for the Diagnosis of SIADH

- Serum osmolality (< 275 mOsm/kg)
- Serum sodium (< 130 mEq/L)
- Urine osmolality (urine osmolality > serum osmolality)
- Urinary sodium (> 20 mEq/L)
- Euvolemia
- Decreased levels of blood urea nitrogen, uric acid, creatinine, and albumin
- Absence of edema
- Normal renal, adrenal, and thyroid function

Therapeutic Approaches and Nursing Care

The only potential cure for SIADH is successful treatment of the underlying malignancy. In the meantime, stabilization of the patient and correction of the hyponatremia is essential. The degree and rate of development of the hyponatremia, along with the presence or absence of symptoms, determine the treatment of SIADH. Fluid restriction to 800–1000 mL/day is the initial treatment of choice for mild hyponatremia (serum sodium between 125 and 134 mEq/L), and may be the only therapy necessary. Fluid restriction allows the plasma osmolality, and the sodium level, to gradually increase through eventual loss of free water.

Severe, symptomatic, acute hyponatremia (serum sodium concentration < 110–115 mEq/L) resulting from SIADH is an oncologic emergency requiring immediate attention. During the first few hours of correction, hypertonic (3%) saline given intravenously at a rate of 0.05 mL/kg/minute should increase the serum sodium by 2 mEq/L per hour.[20] Intravenous furosemide (1 mg/kg) is often used to expedite water loss. Such therapeutic endeavors are instituted only in carefully controlled situations, such as an intensive care setting. The patient must be monitored carefully and the serum sodium and electrolytes checked frequently, at least every 1–3 hours. Frequent neurologic assessments of the severely hyponatremic patient are essential. These assessments should include an evaluation of mental status and level of conciousness. Restriction of oral fluids should also be instituted. The patient's fluid balance is monitored, and the patient is weighed daily. The rate of total correction of the serum sodium should be no faster than 12 mEq/L during the first 24 hours.[7] Initial therapy is discontinued once the patient becomes mildly hyponatremic (serum sodium 125–130 mEq/L), in an effort to avoid neurologic complications. Correcting the serum sodium too rapidly may cause brain damage from brain cell dehydration. It can also lead to an irreversible neurodegenerative disorder known as *central pontine myelinolysis* (CPM),[24] which results from osmotic injury to

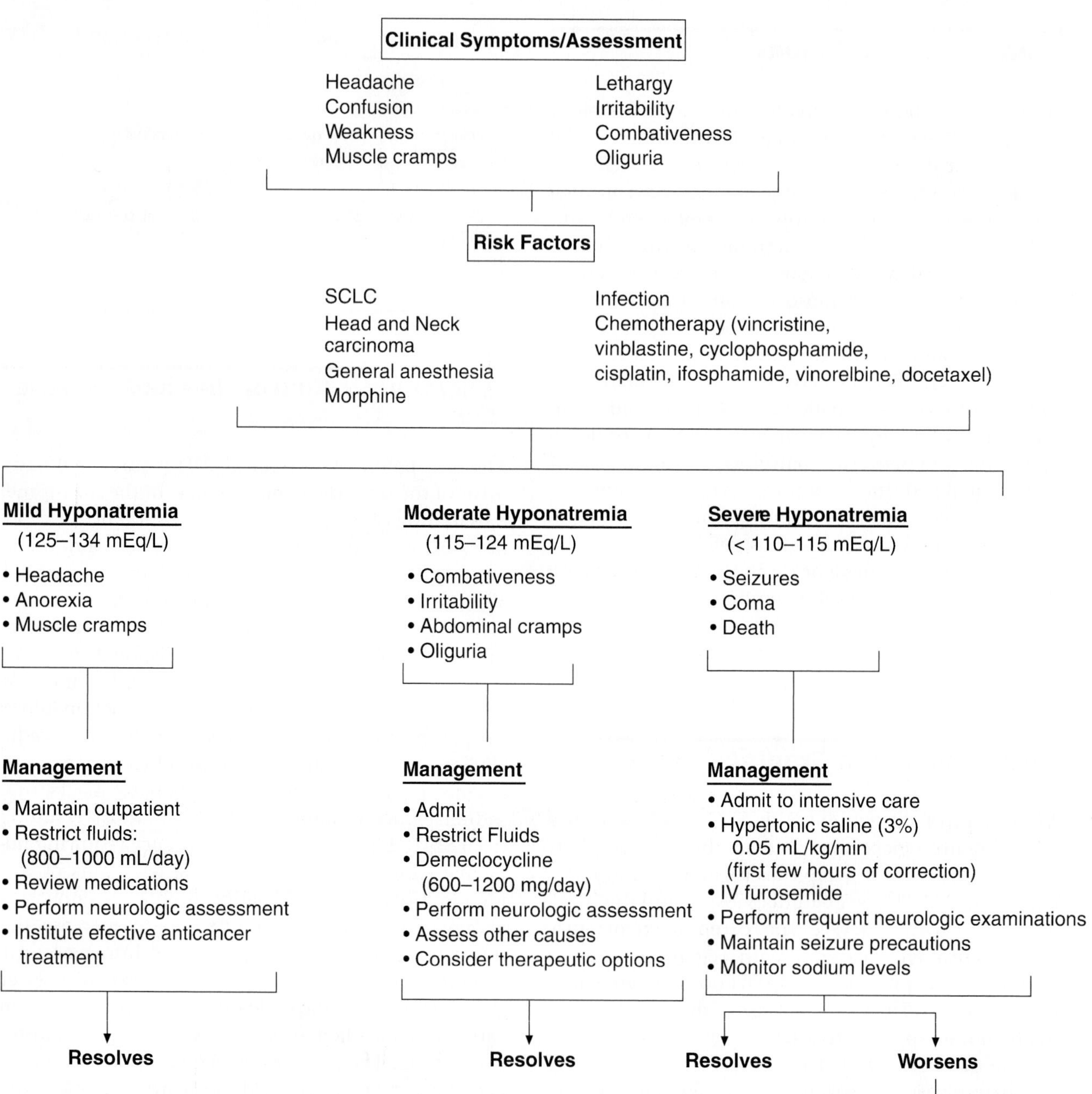

Figure 41-1 Phone triage for SIADH.

endothelial cells in the brain and a breakdown of the blood-brain barrier, primarily in the pons and thalamus. Severe edema develops, causing demyelination of white matter that can be seen on computerized tomography (CT) or magnetic resonance imaging (MRI). Symptoms of CPM range from dysphagia to quadraparesis.[25]

Chronic mild to moderate hyponatremia may be managed with oral medications. Demeclocycline (600–1200 mg daily) is an antibiotic that is most frequently used to treat chronic SIADH. It stimulates diuresis by inhibiting the effect of AVP on the renal tubule. Demeclocycline allows a normal daily intake of water and other fluids. Superinfections, azotemia, and hematologic changes may occur. Some patients develop diabetes insipidus. The patient's renal function should be monitored frequently while taking demeclocycline. Acute renal failure has occurred in patients with liver cirrhosis who were being treated for SIADH with demeclocycline. Other drugs occasionally used to treat SIADH include lithium carbonate, urea, and fludrocortisone.

Novel targeted approaches to treat SIADH involve the use of AVP, V2 receptor antagonists. Currently, nonpeptide AVP antagonists are being evaluated in phase 3 studies. These agents selectively and competitively inhibit the binding of AVP to V_2 receptors present predominantly in the collecting ducts, thus promoting free water excretion without inducing sodium loss. Advantages of nonpeptide antagonists include oral bioavailability, prolonged half-life, and minimal fluid restriction, hopefully resulting in a simpler and more effective therapy.[26]

Obtaining a complete patient history, conducting a careful nursing assessment, and reviewing serum chemistries assist with early diagnosis. Figure 41–1 describes clinical symptoms and phone triage for SIADH. Patients and their family members are instructed regarding the early symptoms of hyponatremia (nausea, weakness, muscle cramps, confusion, lethargy) and are encouraged to report these symptoms promptly. Communication between inpatient and outpatient nurses regarding the hospitalization course, current medications, and status at discharge is essential.

Conclusion

SIADH is a paraneoplastic endocrine syndrome primarily associated with SCLC that most frequently follows a chronic course but can present as an oncologic emergency. Nurses caring for oncology patients, especially those with small cell lung cancer, must have a high index of suspicion for the presence of SIADH. Early intervention can prevent serious complications resulting from hyponatremia.

References

1. Schwartz WB, Bennett W, Curelop S, et al: A syndrome of renal sodium loss and hyponatremia probably resulting from inappropriate secretion of antidiuretic hormone. *Am J Med* 23:529–542, 1957
2. Amatruda TT, Mulrow PJ, Gallagher JC, et al: Carcinoma of the lung with inappropriate antidiuresis. Demonstration of an antidiuretic-hormone-like activity in tumor extract. *N Engl J Med* 269:544–550, 1963
3. Shimizu K, Nakano S, Nakano Y, et al: Ectopic atrial natriuretic peptide production in small cell lung cancer with the syndrome of inappropriate antidiuretic hormone secretion. *Cancer* 68:2284–2288, 1991
4. Sorensen JB, Anderson MK, Hansen HH: Syndrome of inappropriate secretion of antidiuretic hormone (SIADH) in small-cell lung cancer. *J Intern Med* 238:97–110, 1995
5. Blumenschein GR: Chemotherapy in the treatment of extensive-stage small cell lung cancer, in Fossella FV, Komaki R, Putnam JB (eds.): *MD Anderson Cancer Series: Lung Cancer.* New York, Springer, 2003, pp 207–219
6. Arnold SM, Lowy AM, Patchell R, et al: Paraneoplastic syndromes, in DeVita VT, Hellman S, Rosenberg SA (eds.): *Cancer: Principles and Practice of Oncology* (ed 6). Philadelphia, Lippincott, Williams & Wilkins, 2001, pp 2511–2536
7. Gross P: Treatment of severe hyponatremia. *Kidney Int* 60:2417–2427, 2001
8. Vaporciyan AA, Kies M, Stevens C, et al: Cancer of the lung, in Kufe DW, Pollack RE, Weichselbaum RR, et al (eds.): *Cancer Medicine.* London, BC Decker Inc, 2003, pp 1385–1445
9. Gross AJ, Steinberg SM, Reilly JG, et al: Atrial natriuretic factor and arginine vasopressin production in tumor cell lines from patients with lung cancer and their relationship to serum sodium. *Cancer Res* 53:67–74, 1993
10. Marchioli CC, Graziano SL: Paraneoplastic syndromes associated with small cell lung cancer. *Chest Surg Clin North Am* 7:65–80, 1997
11. Turchin A, Seifter JL, Seely EW: Clinical problem solving: mind the gap. *N Engl J Med* 349:1465–1469, 2003
12. Flounders JA: Continuing education: oncology emergency modules: syndrome of inappropriate antidiuretic hormone. *Oncol Nurs Forum Online* 30, 2003 *http://ons.org/publications/journals/ONF/2003exclusives.shtml.* Accessed January 15, 2004
13. Zacay G, Bedrin L, Horowitz Z, et al: Syndrome of inappropriate antidiuretic hormone or arginine vasopressin secretion in patients following neck dissection. *Laryngoscope* 112:2020–2024, 2002
14. Langer-Nitsche C, Luck HJ, Heilmann M: Severe syndrome of inappropriate antidiuretic hormone secretion with docetaxel treatment in metastatic breast cancer (letter). *Acta Oncologica* 39:1001, 2000
15. Kao CD, Chen JT, Wu ZA, et al: SIADH and seizures associated with immunoglobulin therapy (letter). *Eur J Neurol* 10:748–749, 2003
16. Berl T, Verbalis J: Pathophysiology of water metabolism, in Brenner BM (ed.): *The Kidney* (ed 7). Philadelphia, Saunders, 2004, pp 865–919
17. Galesic K, Krizanac S, Vrkljan M, et al: Syndrome of inappropriate secretion of antidiuretic hormone due to malignant thymoma. *Nephron* 91: 752–754, 2002
18. Thompson M, Adlam DM: Syndrome of inappropriate antidiuretic hormone secretion associated with oral squamous carcinoma. *Br J Oral Maxillofac Surg* 40: 216–219, 2002
19. Bogdanos J, Karamanolakis D, Milathianakis C, et al: Syndrome of inappropriate antidiuretic hormone secretion in a patient with hormone refractory prostate cancer. *Anticancer Res* 23:1775–1756, 2003
20. Robertson GL: Neuroendocrinology: antidiuretic hormone, normal and disordered function. *Endocrinol Metab Clin North Am* 30:671–694, 2001
21. Robertson GL: Disorders of the neurohypophysis, in Braunwald E, Fauci AS, Kasper DL, et al (eds.): *Harrison's Principles of Internal Medicine* (ed 15). New York, McGraw Hill Professional, 2001, pp 2052–2060
22. Molina PE: The hypothalamus and posterior pituitary gland, in Molina PE (ed.): *Endocrine Physiology.* New York, Lange Medical Books/McGraw-Hill, 2004, pp 27–47
23. Hawthorne Maxson JL: Syndrome of inappropriate antidiuretic hormone secretion, in Chernecky C, Berger BJ (eds.): *Advanced and Critical Care Oncology Nursing: Managing Primary Complications.* Philadelphia, Saunders, 1998, pp 622–636
24. Gross P, Reimann D, Neidel J, et al: The treatment of severe hyponatremia. *Kidney Int* 53(suppl 64):S6–S11, 1998
25. Norenberg MD, Leslie KO, Robertson AS: Association between rise in serum sodium and central pontine myelinolysis. *Ann Neurol* 11:128–135, 1982
26. Verbalis JG: Receptor antagonists: vasopressin V_2 receptor antagonists. *J Mol Endocrinol* 29:1–9, 2002

CHAPTER 42

Tumor Lysis Syndrome

Jean Lydon, RN, MS, AOCN®

Scope of the Problem

Definition

Tumor lysis syndrome (TLS) is a metabolic complication of effective cancer therapy that occurs when large numbers of tumor cells are destroyed rapidly. Tumor cell destruction causes high levels of intracellular components — primarily potassium, phosphorus, and uric acid — to be released into the bloodstream. Metabolic abnormalities associated with TLS include hyperuricemia, hyperkalemia, hyperphosphatemia, and hypocalcemia. This syndrome can lead to life-threatening complications, including cardiac arrhythmias, renal failure, and acute respiratory distress syndrome. Although the most frequent cause of TLS is the administration of systemic chemotherapy, any form of cancer therapy that causes rapid cell lysis and necrosis of a tumor mass can induce this syndrome.

Incidence

The true incidence of TLS is not known. Since its first description in 1980 as a potential oncologic emergency,[1] several case reports and studies have been done to determine its incidence in children and adults. Two retrospective studies found that laboratory evidence of metabolic changes associated with TLS occurred frequently (42% [adults], 70% [children]), whereas life-threatening clinical TLS requiring specific additional interventions was infrequent (3% [children], 6% [adults]).[2,3]

TLS occurs more frequently in patients with aggressive hematologic malignancies, particularly acute leukemias and high-grade lymphomas, than in those with solid tumors. It is therefore not surprising that this syndrome occurs more frequently in the pediatric population. Hematologic malignancies commonly associated with TLS include Burkitt's lymphoma, acute lymphoblastic lymphoma (ALL), acute myeloid leukemia (AML), chronic lymphocytic leukemia (CLL), chronic myelogenous leukemia (CML), and non-Hodgkin's lymphoma (NHL). It has also been observed in patients with advanced myeloma, myelodysplastic syndrome (MDS), and refractory anemia.[4–6] A recent retrospective chart review of 755 cases of AML, ALL, and NHL patients revealed a 5% incidence of TLS despite preventive measures in many patients.[7] Although rare in patients with solid tumors, TLS has been reported in a variety of solid tumors, including breast cancer, testicular cancer, medulloblastoma, small cell and non-small cell lung cancer, Merkel cell carcinoma, hepatocellular carcinoma, melanoma, colorectal cancer, vulvar carcinoma, neuroblastoma, teratoma, and germ cell tumors.[4,8] In a review of the literature, a total of 45 cases of TLS were reported in solid tumors. Among these cases, 37 occurred in tumors sensitive to chemotherapy, whereas eight occurred in tumor types relatively insensitive to therapy.[8] Although it is thought that early recognition and prophylactic treatment have decreased the incidence and severity of TLS, particularly in high-risk patients, the incidence of TLS may increase as more sophisticated and targeted therapies are developed to manage previously untreatable diseases.[4,5]

Etiology and Risk Factors

Analysis of tumor, patient, and treatment characteristics can help identify those patients most likely to develop TLS (see Figure 42-1).[1,2,4,6,9–12] TLS can occur with any malignancy in which there is a large tumor burden, a high growth fraction, and/or effective therapy, usually chemotherapy. Additional risk factors for the development of TLS that are commonly seen in patients with large, bulky tumors include extensive lymph node involvement, enlarged spleen, multiple metastases, and elevated levels of lactic dehydrogenase (LDH), white blood cells (WBC), and uric acid.[1–4] Studies with ionizing radiation in both murine cell models and human malignancies utilizing flow cytometric techniques support the finding that TLS occurs more frequently in malignancies involving B cells and activated T cells.[9]

In addition to tumor-related factors, several patient-related factors increase the risk of TLS. Patients with pretreatment renal impairment as a result of dehydration, metabolic disturbances, or obstruction are at greater risk for TLS because they are less able to clear the products of cellular breakdown. Patients with preexisting metabolic disturbances are at increased risk for TLS. Significant hyperphosphatemia, hyperuricemia, and/or hyperkalemia may exist prior to initiating cytotoxic therapy. For example, the lymphoblasts of leukemia patients contain four times more phosphate than do normal mature lymphoblasts. Thus, the phosphate metabolism is increased in patients with high levels of lymphoblasts, causing significant hyperphosphatemia before initiating treatment. Serum uric acid and uric acid excretion can be affected by the degree of elevation in the WBC count; the degree of enlargement of the lymph nodes, spleen, and liver; dehydration; baseline renal insufficiency; acidic urine; and decreased urinary flow rate 24 hours prior to treatment.[8] In the patient with cancer, hyperkalemia may be present before initiating cytotoxic therapy, due to renal insufficiency, dehydration, adrenal insufficiency, acidosis, and/or medications.[4,5,10,11]

The primary treatment-related cause of TLS is chemotherapy. Specific chemotherapeutic agents more

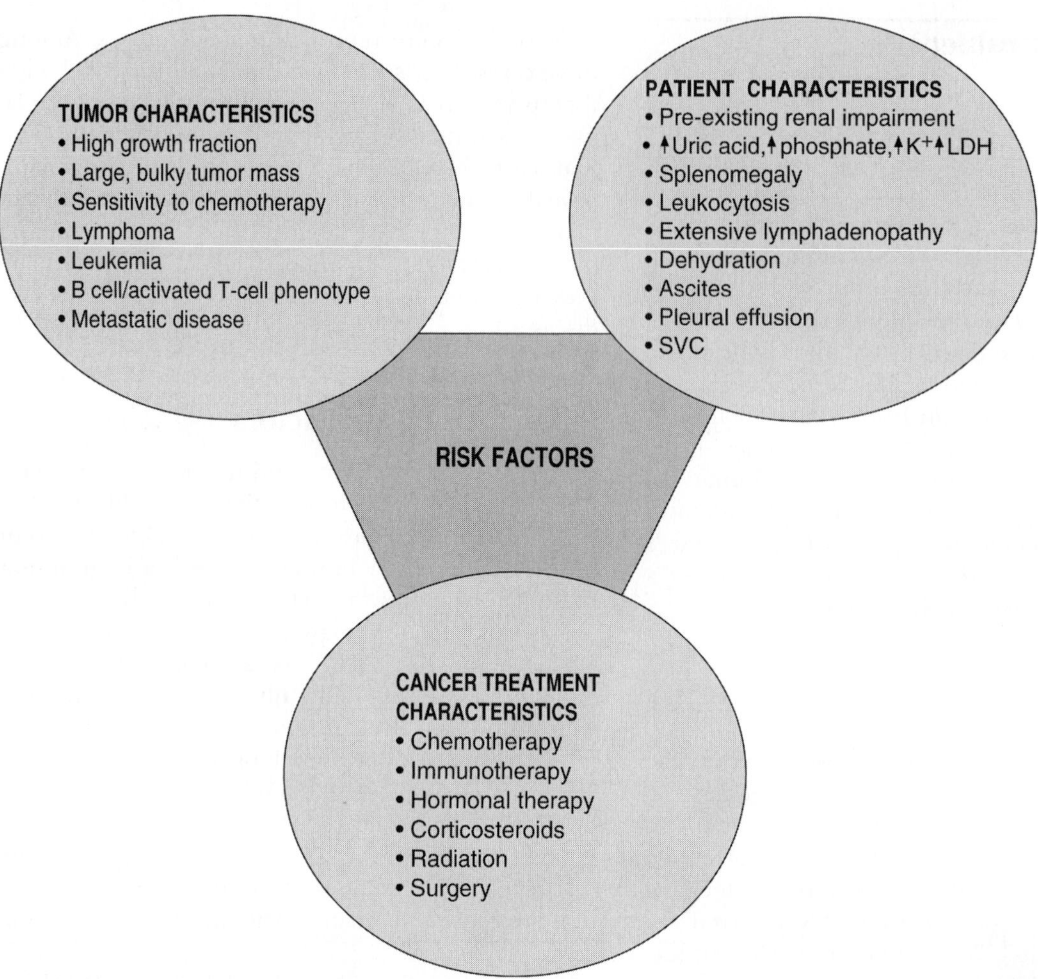

Figure 42-1 Risk factors for TLS.

commonly associated with TLS include cisplatin, etoposide, cytosine arabinoside, paclitaxel, fludarabine, intrathecal methotrexate, and hydroxyurea.[12–16] Immunotherapy such as interferons, interleukins, and tumor necrosis factor, as well as monoclonal antibodies including rituximab, gemtuzumab, alemtuzumab, and Gleevec have been associated with this syndrome. Additionally, radiation therapy, surgery, hormone therapy, particularly tamoxifen, and corticosteroids, either alone or in combination, have been shown to induce TLS.[4,17,18–21] Finally, acute spontaneous TLS unrelated to any form of treatment has been described in patients with leukemia and lymphoma and in one patient with inflammatory breast cancer.[21] The actual incidence of spontaneous TLS is difficult to ascertain. In one study of 16 patients with acute uric acid nephropathy, 4 developed this syndrome prior to treatment.[21] The important distinction between spontaneous TLS (STLS) and acute TLS (ATLS) is the lack of hyperphosphatemia in STLS. It is postulated that in STLS the tumor is able to reutilize the released phosphate to synthesize new tumor cells, whereas in ATLS cell destruction results in no new cancer cells that could potentially reutilize large amounts of phosphorus.[21,22] In summary, cytotoxic therapy in the patient with pretreatment hyperphosphatemia, hyperuricemia, and/or hyperkalemia increases the risk of TLS.[4,10,11]

Physiologic Alterations

The kidneys regulate fluid and electrolyte balance by filtering essential substances from the blood — selectively reabsorbing needed fluid and electrolytes and excreting those not needed into the urine. Normally, small and controlled amounts of potassium, phosphorus, and uric acid are present in the blood. In the intracellular fluid, potassium is the major cation and phosphorus is the major anion. When cells are destroyed, the DNA in the nucleus of the cell is released into the blood, and the purines are converted in the liver to uric acid. Uric acid production requires cell catabolism but relies on the kidney for excretion. At normal rates of production and excretion, excesses of potassium, phosphorus, and uric acid do not occur.[23] When massive amounts of cells are destroyed, however, these substances are released into the blood, causing abnormally high levels of these minerals. An inverse relationship exists between phosphorus and calcium whereby if one mineral increases, the other decreases in the same proportion. Thus, when tumor cells lyse, which results in the release of large amounts of phosphorus into the blood, there is a proportional decrease in serum calcium, resulting in hypocalcemia.

Patients with massive tumor burdens have rapidly dividing cells that may be more sensitive to chemotherapeutic agents that are cytotoxic to dividing cells. Effective cancer therapy—usually chemotherapy—can initiate TLS by causing the cell membrane to rupture, releasing the intracellular contents into the extracellular fluids and subsequently into the bloodstream. Tumor lysis syndrome usually occurs 6–72 hours following chemotherapy and lasts for 5–7 days. It is during this post-therapy time that increased tumor cytolysis occurs.[4,5,10] Pathophysiologically, these events can lead to acute renal failure and cardiac conduction abnormalities.

Acute renal failure secondary to TLS is primarily due to hyperuricemia and hyperphosphatemia. Uric acid nephropathy is a complication that can occur secondary to hyperuricemia whereby uric acid crystals form in the collective ducts of the kidneys and ureters. These crystallizations lead to obstructive uropathy, resulting in decreased glomerular filtration, increased hydrostatic pressure, obstructed urine flow, and eventually acute renal failure. Similarly, calcium phosphate salts secondary to hyperphosphatemia may precipitate in the renal tubules and cause renal failure. Although the kidneys normally can accommodate moderate elevations in uric acid and phosphorus by increasing excretion, continued tumor lysis overwhelms the body's homeostatic mechanisms, ultimately resulting in acute renal failure. Renal insufficiency in turn exacerbates the existing hyperkalemia and hypocalcemia.[4,5,10,23]

The cardiac conduction abnormalities related to TLS are due to hyperkalemia. Ninety-eight percent of the body's potassium (K+) is in the intracellular compartment. When cell lysis occurs, potassium is released from the intracellular compartment to the extracellular compartment and serum potassium levels increase. Hyperkalemia has a major depressant effect on cardiac function, resulting in bradycardia, heart block, and cardiac standstill. Electrocardiogram changes reveal widening of the QRS complex, tall T waves, and flat or absent P waves. At serum potassium concentrations of greater than 9 mEq K+, conduction is so delayed that the heart becomes flaccid and, if not recognized and treated immediately, cardiac arrest will result.[4,5,23]

Clinical Manifestations

The four major clinical manifestations of TLS are hyperuricemia, hyperkalemia, hyperphosphatemia, and hypocalcemia. These manifestations may occur individually, together, or in combination. The severity of these metabolic alterations is related to tumor burden and renal dysfunction, which determine the signs and symptoms observed in TLS.

The early manifestations of TLS include fatigue/lethargy, nausea, vomiting, anorexia, diarrhea, cloudiness of urine, flank pain, muscle weakness, and cramps. These initial symptoms can be vague, mild complaints easily attributed to a side effect of treatment. As the potassium level increases, elevations in blood pressure and heart rate may occur. A patient in the early phase of TLS may exhibit minimal renal symptoms. As the metabolic abnormalities increase, however, the patient will become more symptomatic and exhibit further TLS-related symptoms. Gastrointestinal symptoms will increase in severity, and the patient may experience severe abdominal cramping and pain. Neuromuscular symptoms will also increase from mild paresthesias and muscle irritability to tetany and convulsions. Specific electrocardiogram changes are evident in the early and late phases of TLS. Prolongation of the QT interval and ST segment, and lowering and inversion of the T wave are early electrocardiogram (ECG) changes associated with TLS. Late TLS-associated ECG changes include tall T waves, shortened QT interval, widened QRS, loss of P wave, and sine wave. Initially the patient may exhibit an increase in blood pressure and heart rate, but as these metabolic disturbances continue, a decrease in blood pressure and heart rate occurs. Persistent hypocalcemia and hyperkalemia result in neurologic changes, including memory loss, delirium, and hallucinations. Severe azotemia, which generally presents as increased serum urea and creatinine levels, and anuria due to progressive renal impairment are seen in the later phases of TLS. If TLS is unrecognized, untreated, or continues despite treatment, complete anuria, cardiac arrest, and death may occur. In summary, the physical consequences of TLS affect all body organs and frequently result in severe systemic effects. Figure 42-2 provides an overview of early and late signs and symptoms of TLS by body systems.[5,23,24]

Assessment and Grading

The diagnosis of TLS is based primarily on laboratory and clinical findings of four metabolic abnormalities: hyperuricemia, hyperkalemia, hyperphosphatemia, and hypocalcemia. An accurate assessment of the patient prior to initiating cytotoxic therapy is necessary to rule out pretreatment TLS and to establish baseline laboratory and clinical data. Initially, a complete history and physical is performed and risk factors for TLS are identified. In taking the patient's history, the healthcare provider will obtain information regarding weight, nutritional and hydration status, past and current medications, and history of chronic health problems or organ dysfunction. Assessment of risk factors is necessary for the prevention and management of TLS but can also assist the physician to determine the best setting for initiating cytotoxic therapy. Patients at high risk of developing TLS (e.g., those with high-grade lymphoma, acute leukemia, preexisting renal impairment, or elevated LDH pretreatment) may require hospitalization for their treatment, whereas those patients at low risk (e.g., those with solid tumor, low-grade lymphoma, adequate renal function, or normal pretreatment LDH) can be treated on an outpatient basis. Specific laboratory parameters evaluated prior to, during, and after treatment include serum potassium, phosphorus, calcium, uric acid, blood urea nitrogen (BUN), creatinine, LDH, complete blood count (CBC), platelet count, and urinary pH and sediment. Assessment of the physical signs and symptoms of TLS related to gastrointestinal, neuromuscular, neurologic, cardiovascular, and renal function is critical to TLS management (see Figure 42-2). Renal function is closely monitored by analyzing serum electrolytes, BUN, creatinine, and urinary pH and sediment every 4–6 hours, or more frequently if necessary. Cardiac function is evaluated by frequent vital signs, ECG, and, if necessary, a chest x-ray and multigated acquisition heart scan (MUGA) to assess for fluid overload and the heart's left ventricular ejection fraction (LVEF).

TLS has been broadly defined as the metabolic abnormalities that occur after rapid tumor cell destruction. However, a specific grading scale or guideline related to the degree or type of metabolic abnormality required to qualify for TLS is lacking. In the literature, two grading scales have been used to study patients with TLS. Razis and associates developed a grading scale for evaluating 41 patients with acute leukemia at high risk for TLS, which was divided into three grades (grades I, II, and III) based on the severity of metabolic parameters.[25] In Hande and Garrow's retrospective analysis of 102 patients receiving chemotherapy for intermediate to high-grade non-Hodgkin's lymphoma, TLS was divided into either "laboratory tumor lysis syndrome" (LTLS) or "clinical tumor lysis syndrome" (CTLS).[2] LTLS was defined as any two of the following metabolic changes occurring within four days of treatment: a 25% increase in serum phosphate, potassium, uric acid, or urea nitrogen concentrations or a 25% decline in the serum calcium concentration. CTLS was defined as LTLS plus one of the following: a serum potassium greater than 6 mEq/L, a creatinine level greater than 2.5 mg/dL, a calcium level less than 6 mg/dL, the development of a life-threatening arrhythmia, or sudden death.[2] Development of a standardized grading scale for TLS would increase our knowledge of the incidence, tumor types, risk factors, and morbidity and mortality rates associated with this syndrome. Furthermore, specific prevention and treatment programs based on the grade of TLS could be developed and evaluated.

Therapeutic Approaches and Nursing Care

The primary goal of TLS management is prevention. Recognition of patients at risk for this syndrome allows preventive measures to be instituted 24–48 hours prior to treatment, thereby decreasing the risk of severe electrolyte imbalances. Early identification of TLS requires frequent laboratory assessment of electrolytes and renal function, as well as careful assessment of the signs and symptoms associated with each metabolic abnormality. Laboratory evaluation of patients with TLS or at high risk of developing TLS requires monitoring of LDH, potassium, sodium, uric acid, BUN, creatinine, phosphorus, and calcium every 4 hours during the first 24 hours of treatment and every 6–8 hours thereafter.[4] Existing therapies and/or medications that could contribute to the electrolyte abnormalities associated with TLS should be minimized or eliminated. For example, ACE inhibitors, angiotensin II receptor blockers, heparin, and exogenous potassium sources such as oral supplements and dietary intake can contribute to hyperkalemia and therefore should be avoided where appropriate. While it is important to minimize or eliminate medications or conditions that could contribute to TLS, the implementation of prophylactic treatment regimens is crucial to preventing this syndrome.[26]

The established key elements of TLS prevention and intervention are (1) aggressive hydration and diuresis, (2) allopurinol, and (3) urinary alkalinization.[4,5,10,11,27] The recent development of a recombinant urate oxidase, rasburicase (Elitek), provides an alternative to the prevention and treatment of hyperuricemia. The rationale, use, and considerations for each of these element will be discussed in turn.

The most important mechanism for preventing uric acid nephropathy and acute renal failure is by aggressively hydrating a patient with at least 3 liters/

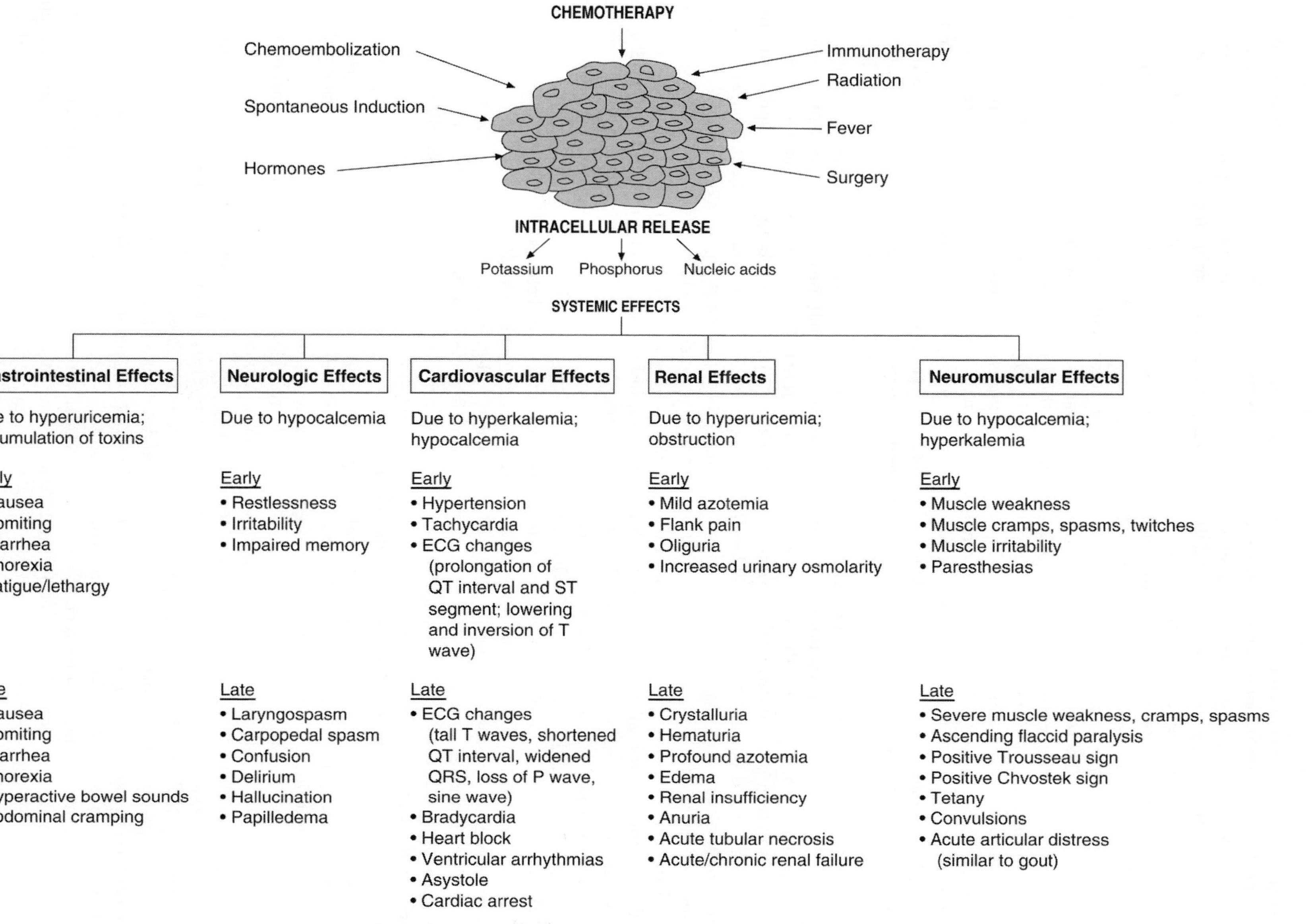

Figure 42-2 Systemic effects of TLS occurring early and late in the disease, and their treatment.

m^2/per day of a hypotonic or isotonic saline solution and ensuring an adequate urinary output of 100–125 mL/m^2/hour.[4,10] Expansion of plasma volume through aggressive hydration is an important intervention to induce diuresis, thereby decreasing renal insufficiency. Diuretics (loop or osmotic) are often used to maintain this urinary flow rate and to prevent renal tubular damage. The use of diuretics is particularly important for elderly patients and those at risk for fluid overload, such as patients with a large abdominal tumor or large mediastinal mass, or those with superior vena cava syndrome. These measures improve glomerular filtration; enhance excretion of potassium, phosphate, and uric acid; and inhibit calcium reabsorption. If necessary, dopamine at low doses (5μg/kg/min) can be given to further improve renal perfusion. It is important that aggressive hydration, with or without diuretics, begin 24–48 hours prior to treatment and continue for several days posttreatment.[4,10]

Allopurinol is the second key element of TLS prevention and intervention. Allopurinol inhibits the enzyme xanthine oxidase and prevents the formation of uric acid, which in turn prevents uric acid nephropathy. The standard oral dose of allopurinol is 300–600 mg per day for adults and 300 mg/m^2 per day in children, given for several days before, during, and after cytotoxic therapy.[1,4,10] An intravenous (IV) formulation of allopurinol is now available for patients who cannot take anything by mouth. The approved IV dose for adults is 200–400 mg/m^2/day and 200 mg/m^2/day for pediatric patients, with the maximum daily dose of 600 mg. IV allopurinol can be given as a single infusion or in equally divided doses administered at 6-, 8-, or 12-hour intervals. It is important to note that the efficacy, administration schedule, and adverse effects of IV allopurinol are similar to the oral formulation, with no superiority shown between the two routes.[11]

There are several limitations relative to the effectiveness of allopurinol in the prevention and treatment of hyperuricemia. First, it prevents the formation of new uric acid but does not affect the preexisting uric acid. Therefore, the reduction in urate levels occurs slowly, beginning 1–3 days after initiation and reaching maximum efficacy after 7–10 days. Second, it increases the level of xanthine, which can aggravate or induce obstructive nephropathy.[4,10,11,28] It may be necessary to reduce the dose of allopurinol based on creatinine clearance in patients with renal impairment. Although allopurinol is generally well tolerated, with skin rash being the most frequent side effect, 3% of patients will develop a hypersensitivity reaction, and some patients will develop a severe allergic reaction manifested as Stevens-Johnson syndrome. If allergic side effects occur, allopurinol should be discontinued immediately.[4] Finally, allopurinol can interfere with the metabolism of several drugs, including cyclophosphamide, 6 mercaptopruine, azathioprine, cyclosporin, chlorpropamide, dicumarol, and thiazide diuretics.[4] However, one advantage of allopurinol is its low cost as compared to the newer agent rasburicase.[7,28]

Rasburicase, a recombinant urate oxidase, converts uric acid into allantoin. Allantoin is 5–10 times more soluble than uric acid and is therefore rapidly excreted by the kidneys. The rationale for the development of rasburicase came from studies using nonrecombinant urate oxidase, initially conducted in France and Italy in the 1970s and 1980s, respectively, and later in the United States. The results of these studies demonstrated the effectiveness of urate oxidase in rapidly reducing urate levels and decreasing the need for dialysis during the early management of TLS. However, this form of urate oxidase was associated with a 5% rate of acute hypersensitivity reactions, including life-threatening anaphylaxis.[4,10] Thus, a recombinant form of urate oxidase was developed. Several studies have demonstrated that rasburicase can significantly decrease uric acid levels more rapidly and to a greater degree than allopurinol in both children and adults. In a randomized phase III trial of 52 children with leukemia and lymphoma at high risk of TLS, rasburicase decreased uric acid levels by 86% within 4 hours, as compared a to 12% reduction with allopurinol.[29] In general, rasburicase is well tolerated, with mild headache being the most commonly reported side effect. In summary, rasburicase provides an effective but costly alternative for the prevention and treatment of hyperuricemia (see Table 42-1).[4,7,10,11,29–32] However, at this time, there is insufficient clinical data to support replacing allopurinol with rasburicase as the standard of care in patients with TLS. The high cost alone may prohibit routine use of this agent. Additionally, there are many unanswered questions related to the use of rasburicase, including (1) identification of patients requiring rasburicase versus general supportive treatment with allopurinol, (2) duration of therapy, and (3) benefit/cost ratio.

The third key element of TLS prevention and intervention, alkalinization of the urine, is controversial. Urinary alkalinization increases the solubility of uric acid. However, alkalinization leads to precipitation of calcium and phosphate, which can increase the risk of renal failure and lead to calcium-phosphate deposits in other organs, such as the heart. Furthermore, alkalinization can cause hypocalcemia and increase the risk of xanthine nephropathy. Therefore, urinary alkalinization measures to prevent renal complications secondary to TLS must be individualized and used cautiously. Alkalinization of the urine can be achieved by adding 50–100 mEq of sodium bicarbonate to each

Table 42-1 Rasburicase

Indication	Prevention and management of hyperuricemia
Mechanism of action	Converts uric acid to allantoin in the final step of purine catabolism (allantoin is 5–10 times more soluble than uric acid[UA])
Type	Recombinant urate oxidase protein produced by a genetically modified *Saccharomyces corevisiae* strain, originally cloned from *Aspergillus flavus*
Dosage	• 0.20mg/kg/IV daily for 5–7 days for children and adults • Administration — dose in 50ml sterile normal saline and infused over 30 minutes (Note: In some studies, it was given every 12 hours for first 48–72 hours to keep UA down)
Adverse reactions	• Hypersensitivity reactions 5% • Fever 6.6% • Nausea 1.6% • Vomiting 1.3% • Rash 0.9% • Diarrhea 0.9% • Headache 0.9%
Interactions	None reported
Precautions	Contraindicated in patients with glucose-6-phosphate dehydrogenase (G6PD) deficiency (hydrogen peroxide is a byproduct of the transformation of uric acid into allantoin and can precipitate hemolytic anemia in patients with G6PD deficiency)
Advantages	• Rapid onset of action (can decrease UA within 2–4 hours of administration, thereby avoiding delays in chemotherapy administration) • High solubility of allantoin allows it to be easily excreted in urine • Lowers preexisting uric acid and prevents further accumulation of uric acid because it works at the end of the uric acid pathway • Does not have known drug–drug interactions, particularly with 6-mercaptopurine
Disadvantages	• Expensive (cost per 5-day therapy based on AWP: pediatric dose= $3,725–$5,587.50; adult dose= $11,175–$14,900 versus $12.00 for allopurinol 5-day treatment for adults or children) • No effect on other electrolyte or acid base disturbances associated with TLS
Nursing responsibilities	• Verify payment for drug with insurance company • Assess patients for history of anaphylactic reactions or severe allergic reactions (asthma, G6PF deficiency) — do not administer if patients have history of these • Have emergency drugs/equipment available (oxygen, diphenhydramine, steroids, epinephrine) • Weigh patient (may need to convert lbs to kgs (2.2 lb = 1 kg) • Verify correct dose calculation at 0.20 mg/kg • Administer rasburicase over 30 minutes • Closely monitor patient throughout administration, to include pulse, respiration, blood pressure, S/S of allergic/hypersensitivity reaction. Recommendation: Stay with patient for first 5 minutes of administration • Document treatment in medical record • Monitor and document side effects of treatment • Take special precautions when drawing blood to ensure accuracy of blood specimens. Precautions include: (1) obtain appropriate prechilled tube containing heparin, (2) after blood drawing, immediately put blood sample in EDTA tube on ice, (3) analyze specimen within 4 hours for uric acid evaluation

liter of intravenous (IV) hydration and/or administering acetazolamide, 250–500 mg IV daily.[4,10]

Early identification and correction of electrolyte imbalances is the key component of TLS prevention and management. Accurate phone triage is critical to the management of TLS on an outpatient basis (see Figure 42-3).[1–4,25] Prompt recognition and treatment of these metabolic abnormalities often reduces the need for hospitalization by preventing the development of clinical TLS. However, if TLS metabolic abnormalities and/or clinical symptoms persist for 48–72 hours despite aggressive preventive and treatment measures, hospitalization is necessary.

Laboratory values and the patient's clinical condition can change dramatically over a few hours, necessitating more intensive monitoring and treatment. The patient will be admitted to the intensive care unit if the laboratory and/or clinical signs and symptoms of TLS continue to worsen despite preventive and treatment measures, or if the patient develops renal, respiratory, or cardiac failure. These patients often require aggressive hemodynamic monitoring and mechanical ventilation. If the electrolyte abnormalities of TLS cannot be corrected or if renal failure worsens despite aggressive management, dialysis should be instituted. Dialysis has been particularly successful in treating obstructive

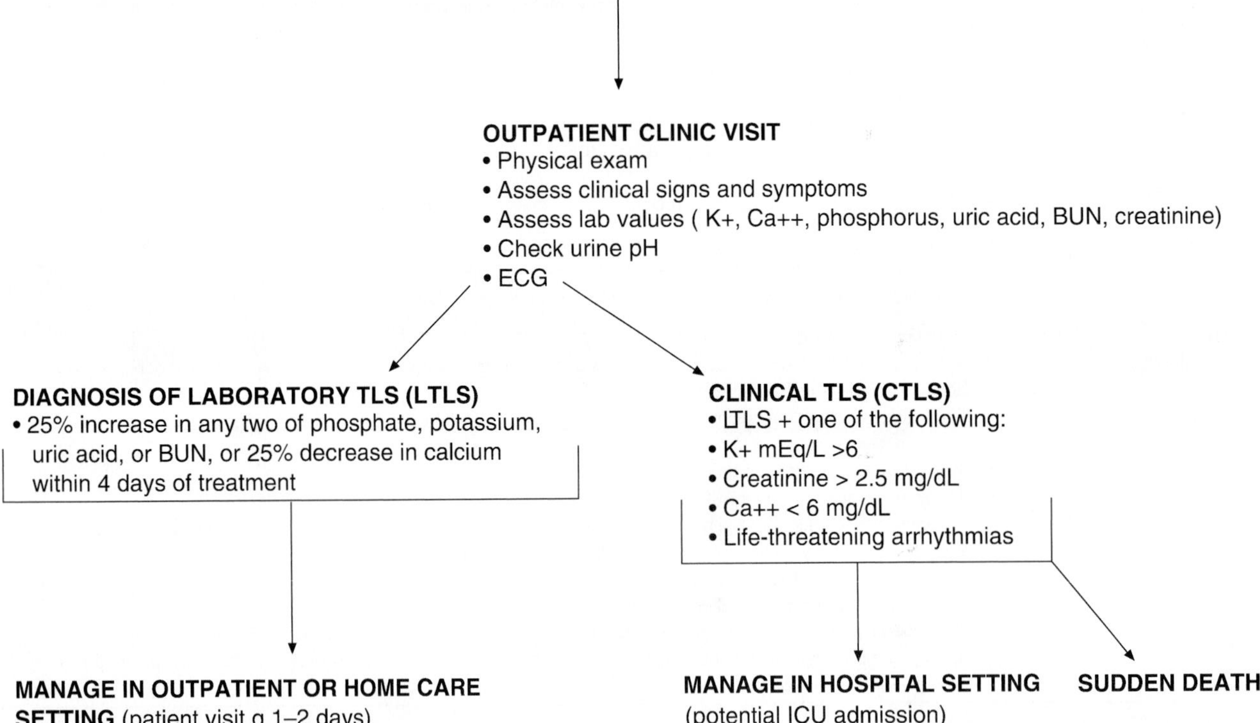

Figure 42-3 Phone triage assessment of TLS and patient disposition (S/S = signs and symptoms, ICU = intensive care unit)

nephropathy, acute renal failure, and accompanying metabolic abnormalities associated with TLS. Suggested criteria for dialysis therapy in TLS include patients who have the following serum blood levels: (1) potassium greater than 6 mEq/L, (2) phosphorus greater than 10 mg/dL, (3) uric acid greater than 10 mg/dL, or (4) creatinine greater than 10 mg/dL. Dialysis is also recommended for patients with fluid volume overload, renal insufficiency, or symptomatic hypocalcemia, and for those patients who do not respond to other corrective treatment measures. Hemodialysis, peritoneal dialysis (PD), and continuous hemofiltrations have been used in the treatment of both children and adults with TLS. Unfortunately, data comparing the various modalities are sparse. In general, hemodialysis is preferred because it can rapidly correct life-threatening electrolyte disturbances. Compared to hemodialysis, peritoneal dialysis is much less efficient in correcting metabolic abnormalities and can be technically difficult when hepatosplenomegaly or a large abdominal tumor is present. Continuous arteriovenous hemofiltration (CAVH) with a high dialysate flow rate and continuos venovenous hemofiltration (CVVH) have also been effectively used in TLS.[27–29,30,32] The duration of dialysis should be every 12 hours until renal function and metabolic abnormalities are corrected. Repeated dialysis procedure at 12- to 24-hour intervals may be necessary in patients with a large phosphate burden.[4,5] TLS resulting in renal failure and the requirement of dialysis has been reported to occur in 5%–25% of cases, depending on the histology of the hematologic malignancy and the degree of renal dysfunction at the time of diagnosis.[4] Studies with the nonrecombinant urate oxidase (Uricozyme), as well as the recombinant urate oxidase (rasburicase) have been shown to decrease the need for dialysis during the early phases of treatment. In comparing studies of pediatric patients with Stage IV NHL and ALL receiving chemotherapy, 2.6% of patients receiving either Uricozyme or rasburicase needed dialysis, as compared to 16% and 23% in the United Kingdom Children's Cancer Study Group and Pediatric Oncology Group protocol, respectively, using allopurinol.[33] In summary, the identification of, institution of prophylactic measures for, and early treatment of TLS prevent acute renal failure and the need for dialysis. Management and potential outcomes of TLS are presented in Figure 42-4.[1,2,4,5,10,11]

Currently, little information exists on the overall cost or medical resource utilization related to TLS. However, Farber reported the relatively low cost of preventive measures as compared to the cost of managing TLS. The high costs were associated with prolonged hospital stay, intensive care, and dialysis.[34] A retrospective chart review of 755 patients from different cities in Spain, the United Kingdom, Belgium, and the Netherlands revealed that the average cost of management in patients with TLS was approximately 11 times higher than the average cost of managing patients with hyperuricemia.[7] A recent Pan-European Multicenter economic evaluation of rasburicase concluded that the treatment of hyperuricemia/TLS with rasburicase is cost-saving in children and cost-effective in adults.[7] Further studies will need to be conducted to evaluate the cost-effectiveness between allopurinol and rasburicase whereby the cost of the drug is compared with the costs associated with hospital days, treatment in an intensive care unit, and dialysis.

Precise morbidity and mortality rates for patients who develop TLS are not known. Some authors report resolution of TLS with treatment, while others report death despite appropriate treatment. In the Hande and Garrow study of 102 patients with non-Hodgkin's lymphoma receiving chemotherapy, 42% of patients had LTLS and only 6% had CTLS. No deaths were reported in this study.[2] In 1192 patients with NHL or B-cell acute lymphoblastic leukemia treated in the therapeutic NHL-BFM trial between 1990 and 1997, mortality in patients with TLS was 14%. In the previously discussed retrospective chart review, 15 of 755 patients, or 1.9%, died from TLS-related complications.[7] A review of the literature of 45 patients with solid tumors who developed TLS found that 16 of the 45 patients, or one-third of the patients, died as a result of TLS due to either cardiac arrythmias or acute uremia. The authors concluded that the mortality rate among patients with TLS in solid tumors is higher than among those with hematologic malignancies, presumably due to the heightened awareness of this syndrome and the institution of prophylactic measures.[8] Further studies are needed to define morbidity and mortality associated with TLS. It seems likely, however, that the occurrence and resolution of TLS depend not only on specific risk factors but also on the early identification and initiation of preventive measures.

When caring for a patient at risk for TLS, a nurse's goal is prevention and minimization of the syndrome. Prevention of, early identification of, and intervention against TLS require a knowledge of risk factors, laboratory and clinical signs and symptoms of each metabolic abnormality, and treatment measures. Identification of patients who are at risk based on the type of malignancy, extent of disease, preexisting clinical condition, and baseline laboratory values can lead to a proactive management approach and implementation of preventive measures. Whether TLS is a potential problem for an individual or has already occurred, two major nursing responsibilities are education and assessment. Education of the patient and family regarding the risk factors, clinical manifestations, possible treatment measures, and when to seek medical help is key to preventing TLS. All patients at risk for TLS should receive both verbal and written information regarding the syndrome. Educating and encouraging patients and families to be involved in the prevention and treatment of TLS can increase the patient's sense of control, as well as highlight the importance of family involvement in caring for their loved one. The importance of educating patients and family members regarding the complications of cancer therapy has become increasingly clear, as the majority of cancer therapies are given on an outpatient basis and the complexity of cancer therapies has increased.

Another major responsibility of the nurse is the accurate and continual assessment of the patient before, during, and after cancer therapy. Baseline and ongoing assessment of laboratory parameters and clinical

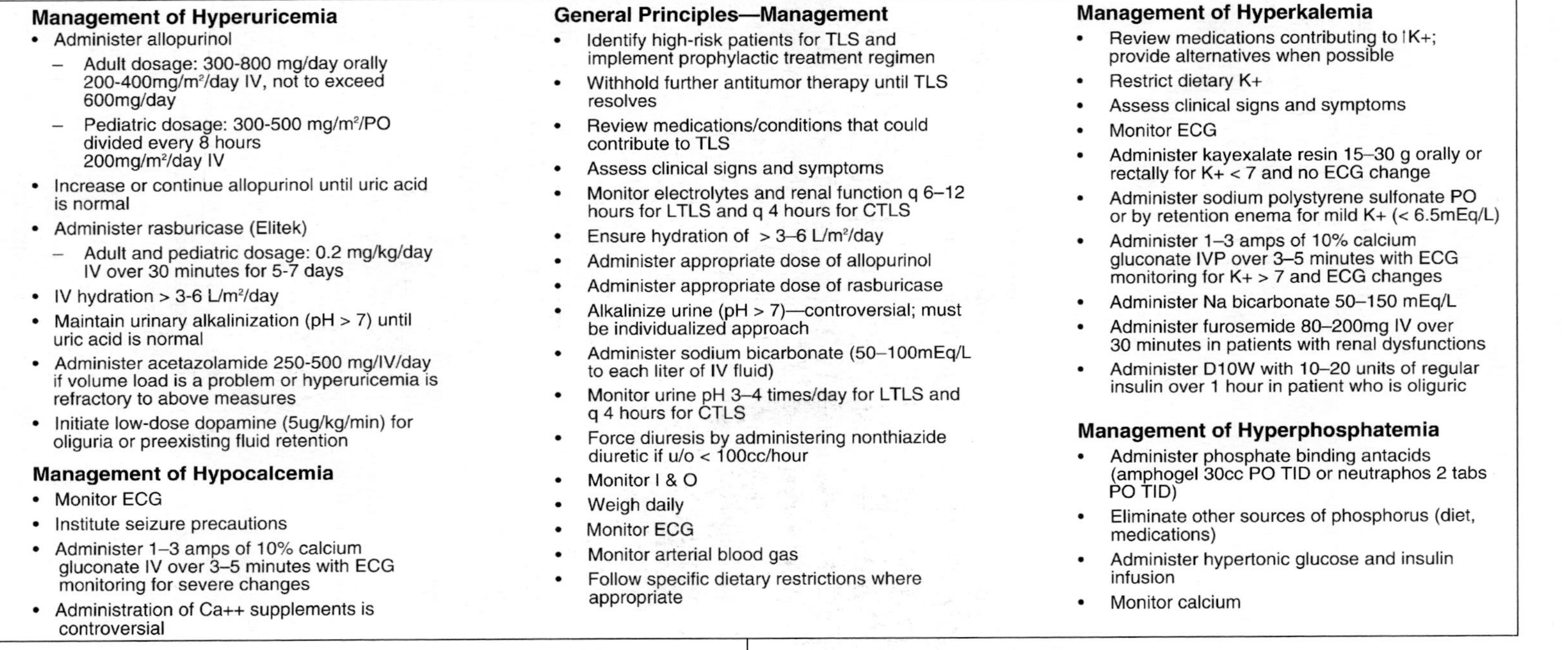

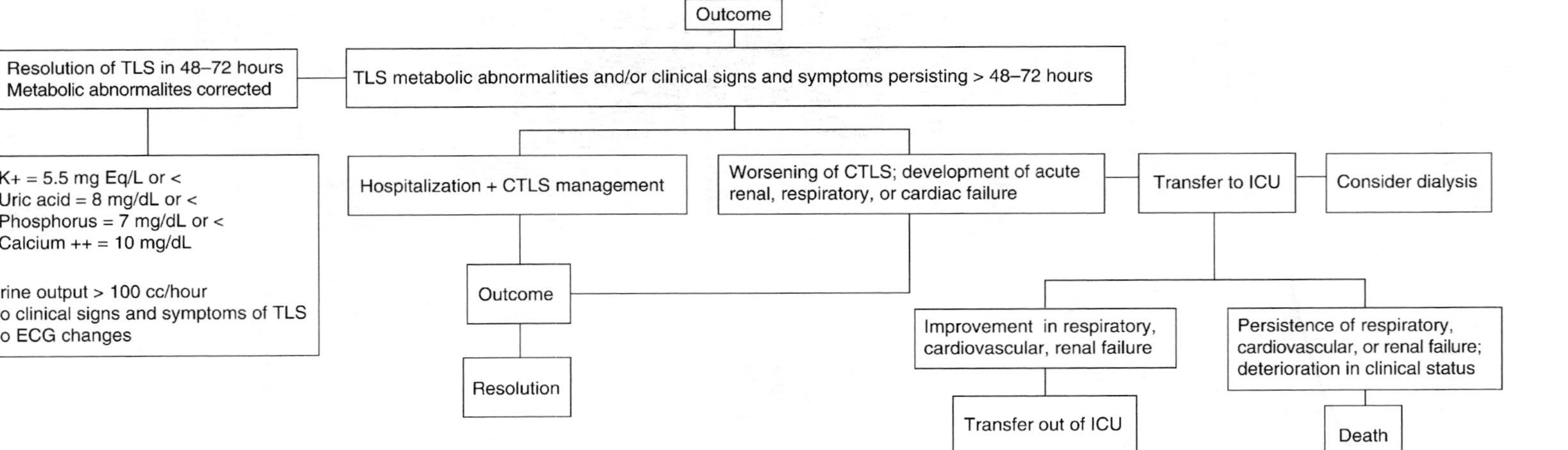

Figure 42-4 Principles of management of TLS.

manifestations will detect subtle changes, thereby preventing serious and life-threatening complications of TLS. A thorough physical assessment is conducted prior to, during, and after cancer therapy to determine the effect of the metabolic abnormalities on many organ systems. Certain diagnostic tests such as Chvostek's sign, Trousseau's sign, deep tendon reflexes, and ECG are useful in monitoring the clinical status of a patient with potential or actual TLS.

The medical management of TLS requires active participation of nurses in various healthcare settings. They are primarily responsible for the day-to-day management of the patient. Specific responsibilities include drawing of blood; administering of chemotherapy, hydration, electrolytes, diuretics, and blood products; and documenting of pertinent findings and interventions in the medical record. The development of new cancer therapies, prophylactic/therapeutic regimens for TLS, and alternative routes of administration for medications will significantly affect patient outcomes associated with TLS. Participation in research studies may lead to a better understanding of the incidence, prevention strategies, and management of this syndrome. Since patients with potential or actual TLS often traverse different healthcare settings in the treatment of their disease, the nurse serves as the liaison or coordinator to ensure continuity of care. Communication of all patient-related findings to physicians and other healthcare providers is necessary for prompt recognition and treatment of TLS. The importance of providing emotional support to the patient and family cannot be understated. It is often difficult for patients and families to understand how such a severe and life-threatening complication can occur when the treatment is working so well against the disease.

Conclusion

Although our knowledge of TLS risk factors, prevention measures, and management strategies has increased, the results of current studies indicate that despite available preventive measures, tumor lysis syndrome and its associated complications still occur. With advances in cancer therapy, particularly newer and more targeted therapies, the incidence of TLS may increase. The major clinical consequences, significant costs, and morbidity and mortality associated with TLS warrant the need for more effective preventive measures and treatment. Further study will be required to establish the role of rasburicase in the prevention and treatment of hyperuricemia caused by the treatment of malignancies. The oncology nurse plays a critical role in the prevention and management of TLS through assessments, careful monitoring, implementation of prophylactic treatment regimens, and collaboration with other members of the healthcare team. Oncology nurses' early recognition of TLS and prompt intervention may prevent this serious complication.

References

1. Cohen LF, Balow JE, Magrath IT, et al: Acute tumor lysis syndrome: a review of 37 patients with Burkitt's lymphoma. *Am J Med* 68:486–491, 1980
2. Hande KR, Garrow GC: Acute tumor lysis syndrome in patients with high-grade non-Hodgkin's lymphoma. *Am J Med* 94:133–139, 1993
3. Kedar A, Grow W, Neiberger RE: Clinical versus laboratory tumor lysis syndrome in children with acute leukemia. *Pediatr Hematol Oncol* 12:129–134, 1995
4. Navolanic PM, Pui C-H, Larson RA, et al: Elitek™-rasburicase: an effective means to prevent and treat hyperuricemia associated with tumor lysis syndrome: a meeting report, Dallas, Texas, January, 2002. *Leukemia* 17:499–514, 2003
5. Yarpuzlu AA: A review of clinical and laboratory findings and treatment of tumor lysis syndrome. *Clin Chim Acta* 333:13–18, 2003
6. Wössmann W, Schrappe M, Meyer U, et al: Incidence of tumor lysis syndrome in children with advanced stage Burkitt's lymphoma/leukemia before and after introduction of prophylactic use of urate oxidase. *Ann Hematol* 82:160–165, 2003
7. Annemans L, Moeremans K, Lamotte M, et al: Incidence, medical resource utilisation and costs of hyperuricemia and tumour lysis syndrome in patients with acute leukemia and non-Hodgkin's lymphoma in four European countries. *Leuk Lymphoma* 44:77–83, 2003
8. Baeksgaard L, Sorensen JB: Acute tumor lysis syndrome in solid tumors: a case report and review of the literature. *Cancer Chemother Pharmacol* 51:187–192, 2003
9. Fleming DR, Henslee-Downey PJ, Coffey CW: Radiation induced acute tumor lysis syndrome in the bone marrow transplantation. *Bone Marrow Transplant* 8:235–236, 1991
10. Ribeiro RC, Pui C-H: Recombinant urate oxidase for prevention of hyperuricemia and tumor lysis syndrome in lymphoid malignancies. *Clin Lymphoma* 3:225–232, 2003
11. Holdsworth MT, Nguyen P: Role of I.V. allopurinol and rasburicase in tumor lysis syndrome. *Am J Health Syst Pharm* 60:2213–2223, 2003
12. McCroskey RD, Mosher DF, Spencer CD, et al: Acute tumor lysis syndrome and treatment response, in patients treated for refractory chronic lymphocytic leukemia with short course, high dose cytosine arabinoside, cisplatinum and etoposide. *Cancer* 66:246–250, 1990
13. Hussain K, Mazza JJ, Clouse LH: Tumor lysis syndrome (TLS) following fludarabine therapy for chronic lymphocytic leukemia (CLL): case report and review of the literature. *Am J Hematol* 72:212–215, 2003
14. Seki JT, Al-Omar HM, Amato D, et al: Acute tumor lysis syndrome secondary to hydroxyurea in acute myeloid leukemia. *Ann Pharmacother* 37:675–677, 2003
15. Simmons ED, Somberg KA: Acute tumor lysis syndrome after intrathecal methotrexate administration. *Cancer* 65:2062–2065, 1991

16. Ustundag Y, Boyacioglu S, Haznedaroghi IC, et al: Acute tumor lysis syndrome associated with paclitaxel (letter). *Ann Pharmacother* 31:1548–1549, 1997
17. Dann EJ, Fineman R, Rowe JM: Tumor lysis syndrome after STI571 in Philadelphia chromosome-positive acute lymphoblastic leukemia. *J Clin Oncol* 20:354–355, 2002
18. Vora A, Bhutani M, Sharma A, et al: Severe tumor lysis syndrome during treatment with STI 571 in a patient with chronic myelogenous leukemia accelerated phase. *Ann Oncol* 13:1833–1834, 2002
19. Linck D, Basara N, Tran V, et al: Peracute onset of severe tumor lysis syndrome immediately after 4 GY fractionated TBI as part of reduced intensity preparative regimen in a patient with T-ALL with high tumor burden. *Bone Marrow Transplant* 31:935–937, 2003
20. Mourad YA, Taher A, Shamseddine A, et al: Acute tumor lysis syndrome in large B-cell non-Hodgkin's lymphoma induced by steroids and anti-CD 20. *Hematol J* 4:222–224, 2003
21. Yang SS, Chau T, Dai MS, Lin SH: Steroid-induced tumor lysis syndrome in a patient with preleukemia. *Clin Nephrol* 59:201–205, 2003
22. Vaisban E, Braester A, Mosenzon O, et al: Spontaneous tumor lysis syndrome in solid tumors: really a rare condition? *Am J Med Sci* 325:38–40, 2003
23. Hebert SC, Reilly RF, Kriz W: Structural-functional relationships in the kidney, in Schrier RW (ed.): *Diseases of the Kidney and Urinary Tract.* Philadelphia, Lippincott, Williams and Wilkins, 2001, pp 3–57
24. Weizstein GA: Tumor lysis syndrome: a treatment guide. *Oncology* 4:123–126, 2001
25. Razis E, Arlin ZA, Ahmed T, et al: Incidence and treatment of tumor lysis syndrome in patients with acute leukemia. *Acta Haematol* 91:171–174, 1994
26. Gobel BH: Management of tumor lysis syndrome: prevention and treatment. *Semin Oncol Nurs* 18 (suppl 3):12–16, 2002
27. Yim BT, Sims-McCallum RP, Chong PH: Rasburicase for the treatment and prevention of hyperuricemia. *Ann Pharmacother* 37:1047–1054, 2003
28. Cairo MS: Recombinant urate oxidase (rasburicase): a new targeted therapy for prophylaxis and treatment of patients with hematologic malignancies at risk of tumor lysis syndrome. *Clin Lymphoma* 3:233–234, 2003
29. Goldman SC, Holcenberg JS, Finklestein JZ, et al: A randomized comparison between rasburicase and allopurinol in children with lymphoma or leukemia at high risk for tumor lysis. *Blood* 97:2998–3003, 2001
30. Bosly A, Sonet A, Pinkerton CR, et al: Rasburicase (recombinant urate oxidase) for the management of hyperuricemia in patients with cancer: report of an internal compassionate use study. *Cancer* 98:1048–1054, 2003
31. Lee ACW, Li CH, So KT, et al: Treatment of impending tumor lysis with single-dose rasburicase. *Ann Pharmacother* 37:1614–1617, 2003
32. Goldman SC: Rasburicase: potential role in managing tumor lysis in patients with hematological malignancies. *Expert Rev Anticancer Ther* 3:429–433, 2003
33. Patte C, Sakiroglu C, Ansorborlo S, et al: Urate oxidase in the prevention and treatment of metabolic complications in patients with B-cell lymphoma and leukemia, treated in the Société Francaise d' Oncologie Pediatrique LMB89 protocol. *Ann Oncol* 13:789–795, 2002
34. Farber MS: Pharmacoeconomic considerations in the management of acute tumour lysis syndrome. *Semin Oncol* 28(suppl 5):19–22, 2001

PART VI

The Care of Individuals with Cancer

CHAPTER 43

AIDS-Related Malignancies

James C. Pace, DSN, RN, MDiv, ANP-CS
Laura E. Gallagher, MSN, RN, CNS

Introduction

An Overview of HIV Disease

The history of the acquired immunodeficiency syndrome (AIDS) pandemic in the United States began in 1981 when the first description of what would soon be referred to as AIDS appeared in the Centers for Disease Control's *Morbidity and Mortality Weekly Report* of June 5, 1981. This report described the occurrence of a rare type of pneumonia in five young men from Los Angeles. From that moment on, similar cases across the United States and Europe began to paint images of people who shared a clinical picture of severe immunosuppression. Over the next few years, the human immunodeficiency virus (HIV) was identified and named. Much has been learned since 1981.

HIV and AIDS are not synonymous terms. The term "AIDS" is used to indicate only the most severe clinical conditions and diseases observed in the continuum of HIV infection. The natural history of HIV infection spans a range of conditions, from an initial symptom-free period of ten years or more (with CD4+ T-cell counts greater than 500/mm^3) to clinically apparent disease states (CD4+ T-cell counts greater than 200/mm^3 and greater than 500/mm^3) with constitutional symptoms (including candidiasis [oral and/or genital], cervical dysplasia, herpes zoster, pelvic inflammatory disease, and peripheral neuropathy) to conditions characterized by severe immunodeficiency (CD4+ T-cell counts less than 200/mm^3), serious opportunistic infections, and malignancies.[1] Once advanced HIV disease occurs, with CD4+ T-cell counts less than 50/mm^3, death becomes likely within one year.[1] The last decade of the twentieth century led to many breakthroughs in the prevention, treatment, and understanding of HIV disease and AIDS; however, the discovery of a cure is hindered because HIV is able to change its genetic makeup rapidly, allowing for multiple mutations of the virus that are resistant to current treatment approaches.[1]

Malignancies and HIV Disease

Malignancies have long been associated with both congenital and acquired immunodeficiency disorders. For example, patients undergoing organ transplantation with subsequent receipt of immunosuppressive drugs developed Kaposi's sarcoma within two years of the time of transplant 400–500 times more frequently than expected.[2] Non-Hodgkin's lymphoma (NHL) occurs at an average of three years from time of transplant and is seen 25–50 times more frequently than expected, while anogenital cancers occur approximately eight years from transplantation, with a frequency of 100 times greater than expected.[2] In early 1981, AIDS was initially recognized from the outbreak of Kaposi's sarcoma along with another opportunistic infection, *Pneumocystis carinii* pneumonia (PCP), among young, previously healthy homosexual men.[3–5]

The model of transplant-related cancers is remarkably similar to the cancers that have been described in association with HIV: Kaposi's sarcoma became an AIDS-defining condition at the onset of the epidemic, while NHL and cervical cancer became AIDS-defining in 1985 and 1993, respectively.[2] The presence of an AIDS-defining condition indicates that the HIV infection has reached a level where it meets the Centers for Disease Control (CDC) criteria for AIDS. Additional malignancies associated with HIV/AIDS include anal cancer, Hodgkin's disease, seminoma, melanoma, oropharyngeal cancer, and multiple myeloma. As of December 2002, more than 886,975 cases of AIDS have been documented in the United States.[4] The most recent estimate of HIV prevalence since the beginning of this pandemic indicates that nearly one million people in North America are living with HIV.[6] Statistical models suggest that at least 40,000 persons in the United States are being infected each year, and roughly the same number die each year of HIV-related illness.[7] Because the number of persons infected each year has been roughly the same as the number who die each year, prevalence since 1992 has been stable. Recently, however, because of the use of highly active antiretroviral therapies (HAART), more persons with HIV are living longer, and the prevalence of AIDS increased from 1995 to 1996.[8] The implication is that this population is living longer in an advanced state of immunodeficiency that allows for the occurrence of some form of cancer. Of those persons now living with AIDS, it is postulated that approximately 40% will experience an AIDS-related malignancy. Ongoing research is required to determine if the incidence and variety of cancers will continue to increase as HIV-infected patients live longer due to effective treatment. To date, no cure or vaccine has been discovered for HIV infection, and predictions are that AIDS will continue long into the twenty-first century.

Kaposi's Sarcoma

In 1872 the Hungarian physician Moriz Kaposi first described the disease that would come to bear his name as "multiple idiopathic pigmented hemangiosarcoma."[9] He described the condition as localized, nodular, brown-red tumors that appeared first on the soles of the feet and then on the hands. He recognized the disease as rare, affecting men over age 40. He was aware of the multifocal nature of the disease, the occurrence of visceral involvement, and the vascular nature of the tumor (*classic* Kaposi's sarcoma).[9] In the 1950s and 1960s, *endemic* Kaposi's sarcoma (KS), a more aggressive form of the disease that occurred in younger individuals, was described in central Africa. During the 1970s, KS was reported among a new group of patients receiving immunosuppressive therapy for renal transplantation and other medical conditions.[10,11] Individuals infected with HIV, especially homosexual or bisexual men, are currently the group with the highest incidence of an aggressive form of KS known as *epidemic* or *AIDS-associated* KS.[5,12] Thus, variations in the pattern, clinical manifestation, and course of KS have contributed to the creation of four separate classifications: (1) classic or non-HIV related KS, usually in men of Mediterranean descent; (2) endemic KS, occurring in men, women, and children in certain areas of Africa; (3) KS associated with iatrogenic immunosuppression, sometimes referred to as *renal transplant* KS; and (4) epidemic or HIV-related KS, which occurs primarily in men who have sex with men (MSM).[13] The most notable characteristics that distinguish HIV-related KS from the other three classifications of KS are its fulminate, widely disseminated course and shorter survival.[13] Histopathologically, all four variations of KS are essentially the same.[13]

Epidemiology

Prior to the AIDS epidemic, KS was considered to be a rare disease with an annual incidence in the United States of 0.021–0.061 per 100,000 population.[14] Since the AIDS pandemic, more than 24,000 cases of AIDS-associated KS have been reported to the CDC. Throughout the course of HIV infection, KS has been reported in approximately 40% of homosexual/bisexual men, 11% of heterosexual men, and 2% of women who are infected.[15] The reasons for this predisposition in homosexual men is uncertain, although it has been historically postulated that there exists a sexually transmitted cofactor that might be spread via receptive anal sex. Consistent with this idea is that HIV-infected women who are diagnosed with KS are most likely to have acquired HIV by heterosexual contact with a bisexual male.[16] The incidence of AIDS-associated Kaposi's sarcoma has steadily decreased since the mid-1980s. To date, AIDS-associated KS is seen in approximately 14% of all cases of AIDS reported to the CDC.[17] This downward trend has been attributed to a number of explanations, several of which are widely disputed in current literature. Among the reasons given for the decreased incidence of KS are the decline in the use of unlabeled amyl nitrate, an inhalant recreational drug and possible mutagen,[18] and changes in sexual practices such as decreased anal lingus, anal intercourse, and anal fisting that may increase the chance for developing Kaposi's sarcoma.[19] Primarily, however, the decrease in KS is attributed to the use of HAART to decrease viral loads (HIV RNA quantification), to increase CD4+ T-cell counts, to offset future infections with opportunistic infections, and to improve the patient's prognosis in terms of life span.

While the incidence of KS as an AIDS-defining illness has declined in recent years, the disease is now more common in patients with more severe underlying immunosuppression and history of prior AIDS-defining illnesses.[20] Despite this fact, the median survival rate appears to have improved over time.[20]

Etiology and Related Pathophysiology

Several risk factors are implicated in the development of KS. First is the existence of underlying immunosuppression. It is interesting to note that among transplant recipients, once immunosuppressant therapy is discontinued, there is a resultant spontaneous regression of KS in approximately 20%–30% of cases.[2] There is also a relationship between *HLA-DQI* and the development of KS, as opposed to other AIDS-defining illnesses, and thus a genetic predisposition may exist.[21] A third factor may relate directly to the HIV virus. When the *tat* gene of HIV is inserted into the fertilized ova of inbred mice, skin tumors that closely resemble KS develop in approximately 15% of the male offspring. It is believed that the *tat* gene serves as the malignant event, transforming a normal mesenchymal cell, presumably of vascular endothelial origin, into the malignant phenotype. It is also believed that the tat protein functions as a growth factor for KS.[22]

KS-associated herpes virus (KSHV)/human herpes virus 8 (HHV-8)

Unique DNA sequences have been found in KS tissues that were absent in normal, uninvolved skin.[23] These DNA sequences were found to be similar to two known herpes viruses — the Epstein-Barr virus (EBV) and the herpes virus saimiri, which causes fulminate lymphoma in New World monkeys. This virus, dubbed KSHV (KS-associated herpes virus) and now termed HHV-8 (human herpes virus type 8), is present in almost all cases of KS, including classic Mediterranean KS, endemic KS from Africa, transplant-associated KS, and AIDS-associated KS.[24] HHV-8 has been found to have a very narrow spectrum of human illness, including KS and a newly described type of lymphoma known as body-cavity-based lymphoma.[25]

The Multicenter AIDS Cohort Study (MACS) provided further data indicating that HHV-8 may be etiologic in the pathogenesis of KS. MACS reported that in a study of 40 homosexual/bisexual men who developed KS, 80% were seropositive to HHV-8 prior to developing of KS. The median time between seroconversion to HHV-8 and the diagnosis of KS was 33 months, with a range of 6–75 months. These 40 men were matched to 40 control homosexual/bisexual men who eventually developed AIDS based on an illness other than KS. Only 18% of those in the control group were seropositive for HHV-8 prior to developing AIDS.[26] From this study, it can be deduced that HHV-8 is present in KS tissues from all forms of the disease and that infection by HHV-8 occurs prior to the development of KS. Studies are evaluating the role of therapy against HHV-8 and the prevention and treatment of KS. It is postulated that HHV-8 is present within prostatic tissues and secretions, and perhaps in sperm as well. The virus is also present in the nasal secretions and bronchoalveolar lavage fluids of patients who have pulmonary KS.

Growth factors and KS

HIV disease causes the infected mononuclear cell to synthesize a whole range of inflammatory cytokines and angiogenic factors, including interleukin 6 (IL-6), Oncostatin-M, tumor necrosing factor-alpha (TNFα), tumor growth factor-alpha (TGFα), and others.[27] These inflammatory cytokines actually function as growth factors for KS. The KS cell is also capable of synthesizing its own angiogenic and growth factors, including IL-6, vascular growth endothelial factor, basic fibroblast growth factor, transforming growth factor-beta, and others, which function in an autocrine fashion by up-regulating the growth of the cells from which they came. These angiogenic factors and cytokines constitute the climate in which the KS cells live and grow, which ensures the continued growth of surrounding vessels and KS cells. Based on these findings, new treatment protocols are aimed at down-regulating these cytokines in order to retard growth and development of disease.

Thus, the complete pathogenesis of KS involves the following steps:

- A genetic predisposition
- Relative immunodeficiency
- HHV-8 becoming activated, leading to a chain of events that causes the transformation of a normal vascular endothelial cell to a malignant phenotype
- In the HIV/AIDS environment, the associated inflammatory cytokines and angiogenic factors released from HIV-infected cells increase the growth of transformed KS cells, leading to eventual widespread clinical disease

Prevention, Screening, and Early Detection

A person with HIV should be continuously screened for the possibility of malignancies, via comprehensive histories and full-body assessments. As the patient's immune system becomes further compromised, the healthcare provider must be alert to any signs and symptoms of KS. Examination of the upper body (head, neck, and arms), the oral cavity, and the lower body (legs and feet) are the first steps in screening and detection. As of yet, there is no known way to prevent KS. Early detection, of course, leads to earlier treatment strategies and increased survival time. Since there is increasing evidence that KS is associated with an oncogenic virus that may be sexually transmitted, teaching safer sex strategies and related practices might contribute to decreased rates of transmission.

Clinical Manifestations

KS usually presents with the appearance of single or multiple pink, red, or violaceus macular papules or nodules that are nonblanching, painless, nonpruritic, and palpable.[28,29] In some persons, discrete patch-stage lesions appear and are often mistaken for bruises, purpura, or diffuse cutaneous hemorrhages.[13] These patches can form plaques that eventually coalesce and form nodular tumors. New, multifocal lesions can occur at any time, most frequently on the tip of the nose, eyelid, hard palate, posterior pharynx, glans penis, thigh, and sole of the foot (see Figure 43-1).[28,29] In rare circumstances, the skin over the tumor can break down, causing bleeding, necrosis, and pain. Lymphatic involvement at the site(s) can lead to lymphatic obstruction, resulting in lymphedema (severe in some circumstances) of the face, penis, scrotum, and lower extremities. These areas of edema are usually firm and nonpitting.[28]

Extracutaneous sites for AIDS associated KS involve the mucous membranes, gastrointestinal (GI) tract, lung, liver, spleen, adrenal gland, pancreas, and testis.[30] The most commonly affected extracutaneous site is the GI tract, although this site is often clinically unapparent. Pulmonary KS may be present, with related dyspnea, hemoptysis, or both, and may be difficult to distinguish clinically and radiologically from PCP.

Assessment

A complete history and physical examination of the patient includes past history of drug use; sexual practices; ethnic ancestry (paying close attention to those born in the Caribbean, Mexico, Central America, or Africa); and a close examination of the sclera, oral

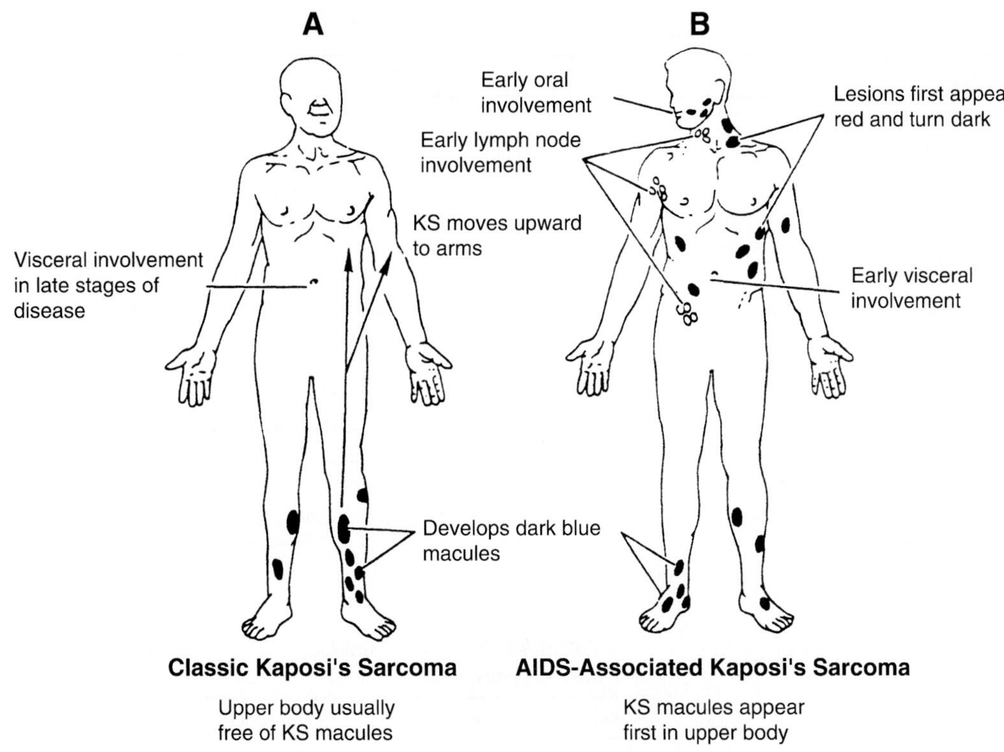

Figure 43-1 Classic and AIDS-associated Kaposi's sarcoma. **(A)** Patients with classic KS (non-AIDS-related) KS demonstrate violet to dark blue bruises, spots, or macules on their lower legs. Gradually, the lesions enlarge into tumors and begin to form ulcers. KS lesions may, with time, spread upward to the trunk and arms. The movement of KS appears to follow the veins and involves the lymph system. In the late stages of the disease, visceral organs may become involved. **(B)** For AIDS patients, initial lesions appear in greater numbers and are smaller than in classic KS. They first appear on the upper body (head and neck) and arms. The lesions first appear as pink or red oval bruises or macules that, with time, become dark blue and spread to the oral cavity and the lower body, legs, and feet. Visceral organs may be involved early on, and the disease is aggressive. However, death is usually caused by opportunistic infection. Reprinted with permission from Stine GJ: *AIDS Update 1998*. Englewood Cliffs, NJ, Prentice Hall, 1998, pp 127–158[29]

cavity (to include the hard palate, gum line, tongue, and tonsils), and skin (to include the soles of the feet, legs, abdomen, arms, palms of the hands, neck, and face). Suspicious lesions, after careful examination by experienced healthcare providers, are biopsied before a diagnosis of KS can be established. Suspected KS involvement of other organs will lead to such diagnostic procedures as bronchoscopy and endoscopy of the upper and lower GI tract.

Diagnosis

In terms of diagnosis, KS lesions are readily recognized by most clinicians. In 1987, the CDC revised the definition of AIDS to include the presumptive diagnosis of KS based on the characteristic gross appearance of any erythematous or violaceus plaquelike lesion on the skin or a mucous membrane.[31] However, the CDC urges clinicians to use caution with presumptive diagnoses and to make such decisions only when laboratory evidence supports the diagnosis of HIV infection. Definitive diagnosis is by punch biopsy of an accessible cutaneous lesion that can support a histiologic diagnosis. Such definitive diagnoses are usually required before treatment with chemotherapy or radiation.

Prognostic Factors for Survival and Staging System of AIDS-Related KS

Several factors are associated with a poorer prognosis in AIDS-related KS:

- CD4+ cell count < 200/mm^3
- History of AIDS prior to development of KS
- History of systemic "B" symptoms, such as fever, drenching night sweats, and/or weight loss[32]

The AIDS Clinical Trials Group (ACTG) has developed a staging system for AIDS-related KS known as TIS (see Table 43-1).[33] This acronym recognizes that factors related to the tumor (T), the immune system (I), and the presence of other associated illnesses (S) are all important in determining the stage and prognosis of the patient's KS. This staging system's validity

Table 43-1 Staging for AIDS-Related Kaposi's Sarcoma

	Good Risk	Poor Risk
Tumor (T)	Confined to skin and/or lymph nodes and/or minimal oral disease (confined to palate)	Tumor-associated edema or ulceration Extensive oral KS Gastrointestinal KS KS in visceral organs
Immune System (I)	CD4+ cells > 200/mm^3	CD4+ cells < 200/mm^3
Systemic Illness (S)	No history of opportunistic infection or thrush No systemic "B" symptoms* Karnofsky performance status > 70%	History of opportunistic infection or thrush Systemic "B" symptoms* Karnofsky performance status < 70% Other HIV-related illness

*Systemic "B" symptoms are unexplained fever, night sweats, > 10% involuntary weight loss, or diarrhea persisting for more than two weeks.

Reprinted with permission from Krown SE, Metroka C, Wernz JC, et al: Kaposi's sarcoma in AIDS: a proposal for a uniform evaluation, response, and staging criteria. *J Clin Oncol* 7:1201–1207, 1989.[33]

was confirmed in a study of 294 patients enrolled in eight ACTG-sponsored trials.[34]

Therapeutic Approaches for AIDS-Related KS

AIDS associated KS is a multicentric disease with wide dissemination at the outset despite the absence of visible lesions. The pace of the disease is variable — some patients progress extremely rapidly while others have disease states that remain quiet for years. Since there is no curative treatment at present, most clinicians find it reasonable to "watch and wait" in the initial phase of disease. The pace of the disease process is monitored and specific treatments are begun as necessary (see Table 43-2).[2]

Localized KS

Treatment for localized KS includes the use of cosmetics, surgical excision, cryotherapy, or laser therapy. In addition, local injections of vincristine (0.1 mg); vinblastine (0.1–0.2 mg) or interferon-α (1 million units) have all been used effectively in approximately 60%–90% of treated lesions.[2] Chemotherapeutic agents injected into the skin may be locally painful but are usually without systemic complications. Local radiotherapy has also been found useful. Local skin toxicities with "usual" doses of radiotherapy are common due to the extreme sensitivity of normal skin fibroblasts.[35] Lower-dose fractions of radiotherapy are often employed in AIDS-related KS with limited treatment periods. Following a week of rest, further radiation may be given if needed. In terms of edema and lymphedema, local radiation is helpful only with periorbital edema; it is less effective with lymphedema involving the upper or lower extremities.[2]

Table 43-2 Treatment Guidelines in AIDS-Related Kaposi's Sarcoma

Extent of Disease	Treatment
Few, small lesions	No treatment, "watch and wait"
Few lesions, cosmetically or psychologically unacceptable	Cosmetic makeup Surgical excision Local treatments: Local injections: IFN-α, vinblastine, vincristine, liquid nitrogen cryotherapy, argon laser therapy, hCG Experimental: β-hCG, topical 9 cis-retinoic acid
Extensive mucocutaneous KS +/– asymptomatic visceral disease	Radiation therapy IFN-α plus antiretrovirals
Limited lymphedema	Experimental protocol
Rapidly progressive mucocutaneous KS Symptomatic visceral disease Pulmonary KS Lymphedema	Systemic chemotherapy with single or multiple agents: ABV Doxil or DaunoXome Paclitaxel Experimental: 9 cis-retinoic acid; 9 AC topotecan; hCG

Data from Levine.[2]

Extensive disease

Biologic response modifiers. Local treatment is not effective with extensive disease. Among patients whose prognosis is poor, approximately 40% will respond to interferon-α; among those with good prognostic factors, 60% respond to interferon-α when combined with antiretroviral therapy.[36]

Antiretroviral drugs used in prescribed combinations have shown therapeutic results when combined with interferon-α at subcutaneous doses of 10 million units or less given each day.[36] Higher doses of interferon are required if not combined with antiretrovirals (up to 36 million units per day).[36] The higher the dosage of interferon, the greater the complaints of such side effects as fatigue, fever, and systemic symptoms. While interferon is effective, complete response is usually not achieved. Nevertheless, the use of such therapy is correlated with prolonged survival rates in those who do respond to such therapy.

Chemotherapy for AIDS-related KS

Since the use of chemotherapeutic drugs is associated in most cases with further immune compromise, the decision to treat KS with chemotherapy protocols requires thoughtful consideration. Indications for the use of chemotherapy include the following:

- Rapid progression of disease
- Presence of symptomatic visceral disease
- Presence of pulmonary KS
- Presence of significant lymphedema

Single agents such as vincristine, vinblastine, doxorubicin, bleomycin, and etoposide are usually quite effective.[37] ABV combination chemotherapy — doxorubicin 20 mg/m^2, bleomycin 10 mg/m^2, and vincristine 2 mg given intravenously (IV) every two weeks — was shown to be more effective than single-agent therapy, with response rates as high as 80%.[38] Recent trials with liposomes embedded with chemotherapeutic agents have demonstrated greater tumor penetration with decreased systemic toxicities. Liposomal anthracyclines have been compared with ABV therapy with similar or somewhat better results. Doxil (liposomal doxorubicin) every two weeks[39] and DaunoXome (liposomal daunomycin) every two weeks[40] have been associated with partial remission rates of 43% and 25%, respectively. The toxicities of these agents include neutropenia and a syndrome of back pain, chest tightness, and flushing. These symptoms usually occur during infusion of the drug and tend to resolve upon subsequent slowing of the infusion and end with the infusion's completion. In addition, the use of paclitaxel in patients with relapsed AIDS-related KS has been shown to be efficacious. Low doses of paclitaxel (100 mg/m^2) IV every two weeks were approved in 1997 for the treatment of relapsed KS and have demonstrated partial remissions with acceptable levels of toxicity (neutropenia and alopecia) in 57% of patients and complete remissions in 2% of patients studied.[41] In patients with advanced KS, paclitaxel in a regimen of 135 mg/m^2 IV every 3 weeks as a 3-hour infusion showed a response rate of 71% as reported by investigators at the National Cancer Institute, including all five patients in the study diagnosed with pulmonary KS.

Experimental therapies for AIDS-related KS

If HHV-8 is as instrumental in the pathogenesis of KS as is currently postulated, then agents that block HHV-8 will be an important potential treatment option. Several antiherpetic agents, including acyclovir, foscarnet, ganciclovir, and cidofovir, are being studied to evaluate their ability to prevent the development of KS.

Clinical trials are underway to determine whether IL-4 and cis-retinoic acid (to down-regulate IL-6), tecogalen, and fumagillan (to down-regulate the angiogenic factors necessary for KS growth) block angiogenic and/or growth factors that may be associated with AIDS-related KS. Initial trials have been promising. Gill and associates reported that the beta chain of human chorionic gonadotropin (hCG) is associated with the decreased growth of KS lines in vitro and complete remission in 83% of KS lesions after intralesional therapy. The mechanism of response appears to be apoptotic death.[42]

Nursing Care

Nursing care of the person with KS is first directed toward any potential knowledge deficit. The patient may not know what to look for or may believe simple nevi or bruises are indicative of KS long before the possibility of the actual occurrence of KS. For the patient who is diagnosed with KS, explaining treatment options and the availability of standard or investigational treatment and ensuring that the patient understands any and all drugs and modalities (including radiotherapy and the use of immunotherapy) that may be used is essential for the patient to feel informed and in control. All patients need counseling regarding safer sex techniques and how to avoid exposure to other infections. Teaching about the need for adequate rest, good nutrition, and stress reduction rounds out the educational/counseling needs of the patient. Answering the questions of family members and significant others helps establish a supportive "team" that is ready to rally around the patient whenever needed.

As KS progresses, the obstructive and compressive nature of the tumor dictates the range of nursing care measures needed. Small, frequent, high-protein and high-calorie meals may be necessary to maintain the patient's weight. Anorexia, diarrhea, and weight loss may necessitate various teaching strategies, dietary modifications and supplements, and nursing protocols for symptom management. Good oral hygiene and meticulous skin care of the mouth, lips, and gums are warranted. Soft toothbrushes and toothettes can spare the mucosa abrasion and further damage that may have been caused by the disease process itself or the effects of radiation. Frequent monitoring of the patient's intake and output, and the presence of nausea, vomiting, diarrhea, and anorexia will help to assess the patient's hydration and the potential need for intravenous fluid replacements. Continuous assessment of the patient's level of pain and the provision of comfort and pain relief measures is an essential aspect of care.

Cutaneous KS can lead to a breakdown of skin integrity if the lymphatic system is blocked due to tumor invasion. Such blockage can lead to chronic edema, ulceration, and constant weeping of the lesions themselves and the surrounding tissues. Nutritional irregularities, weight loss, and decreased mobility can lead to further tissue damage and breakdown. Meticulous skin inspection and care is essential. The skin must be kept clean and dry and free from possible contamination due to incontinence. The rectal area, the ankles, the elbows, and the heels of the feet should be continually assessed for their integrity and the potential for breakdown. Ointments, lamb's wool, and egg crate mattresses are all a part of the nurse's armamentarium in the quest to maintain skin integrity.

Pulmonary KS, which can cause severe respiratory compromise and resultant distress, is an indicator of an extremely poor prognosis. Assessing the patient's respiratory status includes evaluating chest sounds, presence of cough, respiratory rate and volume, and color of skin and nail beds, as well as assessing temperature and related vital signs. Oxygen and other ventilatory needs in home or hospital require education, planning, and assessment for the proper functioning, upkeep, and service of equipment.

Decreased mobility and functional status require the assessment of support systems and prevention of their "burnout" over time. Because of limitations in time, availability, and financial resources, persons with AIDS are often moved from caregiver to caregiver. When these supports can no longer provide the needed care and attention required by patients, they are often forced to return to the homes of their elderly parent(s) or other relatives for provision of care. This places multiple burdens on the caregivers over time, who may have various healthcare needs of their own. Securing help in the home, hospital, or long-term care facility may be necessary for those patients whose support systems are few or become incapacitated over time.

Above all else, the nurse must always be aware of how this diagnosis is affecting the patient's self-image. Body image disturbances are frequent when the lesions are visible on the face and extremities. Weight loss can give the appearance of being emaciated, wasted, or cachectic. Patients may experience a range of distressed reactions from others, including close friends and family, and may become extremely depressed and withdrawn. The nurse who fosters an atmosphere of acceptance combined with accurate and adequate information can promote the ventilation of feelings, fears, and frustrations.

All members of the interdisciplinary team should work to discover and plan for the patient's and family's full range of needs. Better healthcare outcomes in the long run are attained by making sure that the patient's legal needs are in order and by assessing the patient's and family's feelings regarding palliative and hospice care, including resuscitative measures, as early in the process as possible. Assessing the patient's spiritual/religious resources and potential areas of need ensures the incorporation of a holistic plan of nursing care.

Non-Hodgkin's (AIDS-Related) Lymphoma

Lymphoma is the second most common cancer in persons infected with HIV (following KS) and the seventh most common cause of death for people with AIDS. A lymphoma is a neoplastic disorder (cancer) of the lymphoid tissue. The two most common types of lymphoma are non-Hodgkin's lymphoma (NHL) and Hodgkin's disease. Burkitt's lymphoma is a rare variation of non-Hodgkin's lymphoma and is commonly reported in central Africa, where its distribution appears to be determined by climatic factors, suggesting an insect vector and an infectious agent. Aggressive B-cell lymphoma (a non-Hodgkin's lymphoma) occurs in about 1%–5% of HIV-infected people, and yet it makes up about 90%–95% of all lymphomas in people with HIV. The most common sites of non-Hodgkin's (AIDS-related) lymphoma are the brain, the heart, and the anorectal area. In this section, AIDS-related lymphoma is understood to refer to a non-Hodgkin's lymphoma when found in persons who are infected with HIV/AIDS.

As early as 1982, physicians in San Francisco, Los Angeles, and New York noted that their homosexual patients were at increased risk for non-Hodgkin's lymphoma. These same physicians also began to notice links between NHL and the immunodeficiency disease state that later became known as AIDS. In 1987, the CDC included systemic high-grade, B-cell NHL in

HIV-infected patients as a criterion for the diagnosis of AIDS.

Epidemiology

The incidence of NHL among persons with HIV/AIDS is much higher than in the general population. A study involving hemophiliacs found a 29-fold increase in the risk of NHL among hemophiliacs with AIDS, compared to hemophiliacs without HIV infection.[43] NHL is frequently the initial AIDS-defining diagnosis. In a series of studies of persons with AIDS, NHL was the initial AIDS-defining illness in 3.5% of the cases in Europe[43] and in 3.7% of persons with AIDS in studies conducted in the United States.[44,45] NHL may also develop after another initial AIDS-defining diagnosis such as recurrent pneumonia, wasting syndrome, esophageal candidiasis, or invasive cervical cancer. For example, one study reported that the rate of NHL among persons with AIDS was 2.4 per 100 patient-years.[45]

NHL occurs in all populations of persons with AIDS, regardless of the way HIV was contracted. Some studies have revealed that there is a slightly higher incidence of NHL among men who have sex with men compared with other HIV patient populations.[45–47] Pederson and colleagues, however, found a slightly higher incidence of NHL among those with a history of injecting drugs than among men who had sex with men.[44] It has also been postulated that white men and increasing age are associated with the risk of developing AIDS-related NHL.[43–47] Lymphoma appears to be a late manifestation of HIV infection and usually occurs after fairly prolonged immunosuppression. NHL is the cause of death in approximately 16%–20% of HIV-infected persons.[48]

Etiology and Related Pathophysiology

Lymphomas are cancers of the immune system and manifest in the growth of lymph tissue cells, with spread to other organs. Although AIDS-related NHL can originate as a malignancy of T cells, the vast majority begin as B-lymphocyte malignant neoplasms. Such neoplasms are heterogeneous, and their course can range from indolent to fulminant.[49] It is well known that HIV infection induces chronic B-cell stimulation, proliferation, and activation. HIV also indirectly causes B-cell stimulation in response to the inflammatory cytokines IL-6 and IL-10, which are released from HIV-infected mononuclear cells, resulting in further B-cell stimulation.[50,51] This B-cell stimulation/proliferation leads to the polyclonal hypergammaglobulinemia that is so common in HIV infection, as well as to the persistent generalized lymphadenopathy (PGL) that is also characteristic of HIV infection. In PGL, florid follicular (B-cell) hyperplasia is almost always seen. It has recently been demonstrated that the dendritic reticulum cells sequester HIV during the asymptomatic stages of infection and serve as sites from which uninfected CD4 cells, traveling through the node, are infected.[52]

It is also interesting to note that lymphocytes are the only cells that normally rearrange their DNA during the life span of an adult. Such DNA rearrangement allows the full range of antibody specificity that is required throughout the person's lifetime. In the milieu of chronic B-cell proliferation over a decade or more in the presence of HIV, it is not impossible to imagine genetic "errors" or "accidents" occurring over the course of normal DNA rearrangement. The translocation of even one piece of genetic information to a new site creates the distinct possibility of the activation or dysregulation of an oncogene or tumor suppressor gene. This event allows a particular clone of B lymphocytes a growth advantage; the resultant development of a monoclonal B-cell lymphoma, caused by an earlier reactive B-cell response, would be exhibited.[53]

The brain is one of the most common sites of involvement; cerebral lymphoma accounted for 43% of all AIDS-related lymphomas.[45] In over 80% of AIDS-related NHL cases, the tumor is extranodal, making lymph-node-based tumors uncommon. Such extranodal disease is common to the GI tract, liver, orbit, gallbladder, jaw, rectum, earlobe, popliteal fossa, heart, lung, skin, pancreas, subcutaneous and soft tissue, epidural spaces, appendix, gingiva, parotid gland, paranasal sinuses, and bone marrow.[54]

It is postulated that two herpes viruses, EBV and HHV-8, may play a role in the pathogenesis of AIDS-related NHL. In studies that examined pathologic tissue from patients with AIDS-related NHL, Morgello found EBV DNA in 50% of the cases;[55] Levine and colleagues found EBV DNA in 68% of AIDS-related NHL but in only 15% of non-HIV lymphomas.[54] In the case of HHV-8, one particular type of lymphoma seems to be more common — namely, body-cavity-based lymphoma (BCBL), which exhibits itself as lymphomatous effusions involving the pleura, pericardium, peritoneal cavity, and other sites without any evidence of solid tumor. In these cases, morphologic studies demonstrate a high proportion of BCBL cells containing HHV-8 DNA.[45,56–58] This disorder seems to be quite aggressive, with a median survival of only about 60 days.

Prevention, Screening, and Early Detection

No recommendations exist for primary prevention of NHL in HIV-infected persons. The key to improved outcome remains early detection. Educating persons infected with HIV to make them aware of the need to identify early neurologic changes or unexplained abdominal pain so that they can obtain imaging studies such as computerized tomography (CT) or magnetic resonance imaging (MRI) scans may allow them to detect the disease early in its course. Rapidly enlarging peripheral lymph nodes should be evaluated by tissue biopsy as soon as possible. Assessing fevers of unknown origin and frequently testing for any sudden elevation of the serum lactate dehydrogenase level are also ways to be cautiously suspicious for occult lymphoma.

Clinical Manifestations

Approximately 74% of persons with AIDS-related NHL present with nonspecific symptoms of weight loss, unexplained fever, and drenching night sweats.[54] It is also quite common to see elevations in the serum lactate dehydrogenase levels. Depending on where the tumor is located, associated signs and localized symptoms may also occur. NHL of the brain is associated with focal neurologic deficits such as hemiparesis, mental status changes, seizures, and headache.[45] GI tract lymphoma presents with abdominal pain, tenderness, weight loss, and GI bleeding.[59,60] Small bowel lymphoma may elicit the unusual manifestations of obstructive jaundice and small-bowel intussusception.[61,62]

Assessment

A patient with NHL will often present to the healthcare provider with complaints of fatigue, weight loss, fevers, and newly found swollen, often tender lymph nodes. On physical exam, the nurse may note the presence of enlarged cervical, axillary, and/or groin lymph nodes. Since such lymphadenopathy may already be present by virtue of the HIV infection, a careful history as to whether these areas have increased in size, number, and tenderness over time is important. The patient's current CD4+ T-cell count and viral load (and their current trends) can yield a measure of "risk" for lymphoma. The associated presence of fever or systemic complaints might suggest the possibility of lymphoma and may lead to biopsy and definitive diagnosis. Prior to the workup required for staging, a careful history is taken to ascertain the presence or absence of "B" symptoms (fever, sweats, and weight loss of more than 10% of body weight). The physical exam must carefully note the size of the liver and spleen as well as the presence of abdominal tenderness. Laboratory data include complete blood count (CBC), differential cell and platelet count, sedimentation rate, serum chemistries, and liver function tests in order to screen for such conditions as hypercalcemia, hyperphosphatemia, and hyperuricemia. A chest x-ray and CT scan of the chest, abdomen, and pelvis are indicated to assess the extranodal involvement that is characteristic of HIV-related NHL. The clinician may also order a bone marrow biopsy and lumbar puncture to assist with staging and the planning of therapy.

The prognosis for HIV-infected individuals with lymphoma is usually very poor. Lymphoma is a late-stage manifestation of HIV/AIDS, is usually accompanied by a low CD4+ T-cell count, and necessitates treatments (such as radiation and chemotherapy) that can themselves further weaken the immune system. Factors associated with decreased survival for persons with AIDS-related NHL include an elevated serum lactate dehydrogenase, stage III or IV disease, age over 35 years, poor performance status (Karnofsky scores less than 50%), a CD4+ T-cell count less than 100/mm^3, and a history of an AIDS-defining illness prior to the lymphoma.[63,64] The best prognosis is for the patient in whom the disease has not yet spread to the bone marrow and who has a CD4+ T-cell count over 200/mm^3, a Karnofsky score over 70%, and no prior opportunistic infections. Median survival for those with even the best prognosis is usually less than one year, compared with four months for those with a poor prognosis.[63,64]

Diagnosis

As was mentioned earlier, a definitive diagnosis is arrived at with the pathologic examination of biopsy specimens or resected tissue or the cytologic examination of tissue fluid. Once lymphoma is diagnosed, a thorough staging evaluation is performed. Staging is done based on evaluations of the following parameters: CT scan of chest, abdomen, and pelvis; gallium-67 scan; lumbar puncture; bone marrow aspirate and biopsy; and a culture to exclude other opportunistic infections in the presence of fever, night sweats, or weight loss. Such tests reveal the possibility for any of the following: lymphomatous masses, enlarged abdominal lymph nodes or extranodal masses, pleural effusions, lung nodules, axillary adenopathy, or interstitial lung disease.[65] Since many infections often present as "masses" or effusions, care must be taken to differentiate such infections from lymphoma. As was mentioned previously, methods of obtaining specimens for definitive diagnosis include surgical biopsy and needle aspiration of tissue fluid. In the case of cerebral lymphoma, stereotactic biopsies reveal the cause of masses to the brain in a high percentage of cases.[66] Patients with neurologic symptoms should be evaluated as soon as possible with either CT or MRI scans of the brain; lumbar punctures should also be performed if not contraindicated by such scanning. Because of the dangers posed by brain biopsies and the reluctance of many patients to undergo them, a two-week trial of empiric antitoxoplasmosis therapy is often attempted, and actual biopsy of the brain is reserved for those patients whose lesions do not exhibit a decrease in size with this therapy. Because toxoplasmosis is rare in those with negative toxoplasmosis serologies, brain biopsy should be performed in a timely fashion.[49] Several scanning devices have been developed in an effort to differentiate central nervous system (CNS) lymphoma from infection. Single positron emission computed tomography (SPECT) and positron emission tomography (PET) have shown a high degree of sensitivity and specificity for diagnosing cerebral malignant lesions in persons with AIDS.[67–71]

Therapeutic Approaches for Non-Hodgkin's Lymphoma

Treating AIDS-related lymphoma is difficult because of the underlying presence of immunosuppression, poor bone marrow reserve, and increased risk for opportunistic infections. In those patients who have CNS lymphoma, the treatment of choice is usually radiotherapy. Although the prognosis is generally poorer than for those patients with similar cancers who are not HIV positive, survival has improved significantly since the advent of HAART. Multimodal therapy involving chemotherapy and radiotherapy is an option in patients with primary CNS lymphoma.[45,72]

Systemic AIDS-related lymphoma is usually treated with chemotherapy, which in itself is problematic since it suppresses the immune system and may accelerate the course of HIV disease. Sparano and colleagues[73] found that patients with AIDS-related lymphoma who were treated with combination chemotherapy had a progressive decline in CD4 count, a twofold increase in the incidence of opportunistic infections, and short survival times. In response to these occurrences, Levine and colleagues[74] evaluated a low-dose chemotherapy regimen of methotrexate, bleomycin, doxorubicin, cyclophosphamide, vincristine, and dexamethosone (m-BACOD). The regimen was given over four months, as opposed to the standard ten-month schedule. This low-dose regimen, given with intrathecal cytosine arabinoside to prevent CNS relapse, resulted in a complete remission rate of 51%. Responders usually survived for a median of 18 months; the cause of death was usually an opportunistic infection.

In a 1995 study,[75] patients with AIDS-related lymphoma were stratified by prognostic category and then randomized to receive either low dose m-BACOD or a standard-dose m-BACOD regimen given with granulocyte-macrophage colony-stimulating factor (GM-CSF) support. The results of this study ($n = 198$) reveal that complete remission rates were similar in the groups—median time to recurrence was greater than 190 weeks for those patients receiving the low-dose therapy and 106 weeks for patients receiving standard-dose chemotherapy. Median survival was 35 weeks in the low-dose group and 31 weeks in the standard-dose group. Thus, low-dose chemotherapy regimens became the treatment of choice for the majority of patients with AIDS-related lymphoma.

In a recent study, Spina and colleagues[76] compared the clinical characteristics and outcomes of 100 patients with HIV-associated NHL treated with HAART with those of 82 HIV-negative patients with aggressive NHL. The three-year overall survival (OS) was 37% among patients with HIV-associated NHL and 74% among HIV-negative patients with NHL ($P < .0001$). However, because the response-adjusted OS was similar in the two groups, the achievement of complete remission should be the main goal in the treatment of patients with HIV-associated NHL.

The administration of colony-stimulating factors (CSFs) such as G-CSF and GM-CSF is effective in reducing associated bacterial and fungal infections.[77] It is currently believed that antiretroviral therapy may enhance the clinical response of the patient to chemotherapy and that their combined efforts may exhibit antineoplastic effects. Preliminary results of studies[52,73,78] comparing regimens of combination chemotherapy with combination chemotherapy combined with antiretroviral drugs indicate that the combination of chemotherapy and antiretrovirals is associated with an increase in mucositis, anemia, and neurotoxicities. Protease inhibitors such as indinavir and saquinavir may alter the metabolism of such chemotherapeutic drugs (such as the cyclophosphamide, doxorubicin, vincristine, prednisone regimen), leading to heretofore unexplained toxicities such as anemia and neurotoxicity.[52]

Treatment for Relapsed or Refractory Disease

Few options exist for those patients who fail initial therapy. A response rate of about 20% to 25% has been reported in patients with multiple relapses of AIDS-related lymphoma who were treated with mitoguazone.[52] Mitoguazone is not associated with bone marrow suppression and easily crosses the blood-brain barrier in levels that are potentially therapeutic; it is being studied as a first-line agent for those newly diagnosed with AIDS-related lymphoma. Other treatment modalities that have been used include (1) an infusional chemotherapy regimen of cyclophosphamide, doxorubicin, and etoposide,[79] (2) monoclonal antibodies conjugated to toxins such as B4-blocked ricin, (3) IL-2, and (4) protocols that seek to determine if certain latent EBV proteins can be modulated in an attempt to render the tumor immunogenic and susceptible to the normal mechanisms of immune surveillance.[52]

Nursing Care

AIDS-related lymphoma is treated with radiation therapy, chemotherapy, or both. Essential areas for nurses to cover in their discussions with patients are the nature of the illness, the management of side effects, how to avoid infections when neutropenic, how to care for the skin and mucous membranes, and the importance of adequate rest, nutrition, and sleep. In addition, some patients may be prone to tumor lysis syndrome if they are being treated for a bulky tumor. In the case of CNS lymphoma, the nurse must deal with safety issues related to the patient's potential for motor incoordination and cognitive deficits. As with KS, the patient's home environment must be assessed for the type and extent of support systems necessary for adequate and comprehensive care in the home setting. If these resources are not available or have been exhausted, transfer to a skilled nursing facility may be necessary. Providing emotional support to the patient and to the family and significant others is essential. Making decisions related to complex care management issues can oftentimes be challenging. The competence of the patient must be ascertained at each step of the treatment plan. Next of kin may step in and attempt to make decisions on the patient's behalf and may totally disregard those of the patient's long-term partner if there is not an authorized power of attorney in place. Such legal and ethical issues as "who is in charge" when the patient cannot make such decisions should be explored early in the palliative care trajectory, rather than waiting until it is too late.

If the mental deterioration is such that the patient becomes moribund or comatose, decisions related to placing the patient on life support (or the discontinuation of such therapy), starting intravenous or tube feedings, or the withdrawal of such support may surface. Once again, planning for the eventual likelihood of these circumstances with the patient and those close to the patient is best done early in the illness.

Cervical Cancer

Women represent the fastest-growing population group at risk for HIV/AIDS in the United States.[80] Consistent with this statistic is the fact that cervical cancer became an AIDS-defining condition in 1993.[45]

Epidemiology

The true incidence of invasive cervical cancer in women with AIDS is unknown. In 1993, 1.3% of women with AIDS reported to the CDC had an initial AIDS diagnosis of invasive cervical cancer. This rate is thought to capture only a small portion of those women who actually have invasive cervical cancer.[45]

Etiology and Related Pathophysiology

Cervical intraepithelial neoplasia (CIN), also known as *cervical dysplasia*, is characterized by precursor lesions. In an HIV-positive woman, the progression of CIN to invasive cancer is a slow process, often taking several years. On average, CIN occurs in women ages 45 to 50.[45] When CIN is detected by a Papanicolaou (Pap) smear in the early stages, treatment outcomes are favorable. However, in HIV-positive women, the occurrence of CIN has been noted to be more likely to progress rapidly, to be more advanced, to be more likely to occur between ages 16 and 48, to be less responsive to standard treatments, and to yield a poorer prognosis than in women not infected with HIV.[81]

The CDC reports multiple risk factors for the development of CIN and cervical cancer in HIV-infected women. These risk factors include:

- Early age at first intercourse
- Multiple sex partners
- Sex with men who have sex with multiple partners
- Dietary deficiencies
- Cigarette smoking
- Use of oral contraceptives
- Immunosuppression
- Low socioeconomic status
- Lack of access to healthcare
- History of sexually transmitted diseases, especially human papillomavirus (HPV)
- Exposure to diethylstilbestrol (DES) in utero[82–84]

According to Klevens and associates,[85] there appears to be a greater incidence of AIDS-defining cervical cancer in women who are black, live in the South, are injecting drug users, and have a higher mean CD4 cell count than in women with other AIDS-defining illnesses.

A strong correlation exists between HPV, HIV, and cervical dysplasia. There are multiple types of HPV, including HPV 6 and HPV 11, that are associated with either viral condyloma or mild dysplastic changes (CIN I) and rarely progress to frank neoplasia. However, certain other types of HPV — HPV 16, 18, 31, 33, and 35, among others — are often associated with the more advanced precursor lesions (CIN II and CIN III) and are found in most of the cases of invasive carcinoma. HPV types that are associated with high risk of cervical cancer produce viral proteins termed E6 or E7, which are crucial for malignant transformation. Studies have shown that HPV is detected in more than 95% of all cervical cancers.[45] As the CD4 cell count drops below 500/mm^3, there also appears to be an increase in oncogenic HPV types as well as greater severity and prevalence of cervical dysplasia.[45] It is believed that approximately 50% of HIV-infected women with CD4 cell counts less than 200/mm^3 are infected with HPV 18.[86] Furthermore, it is now known that the HIV *tat* gene activates HPV.[2]

Pathogenesis and Staging

The early stage of cervical disease involves the microinvasion of the lesion into the basement membrane of the cervix. This microinvasion involves small fingerlike processes that extend into the stroma and, if left undetected, produce measurable lesions that increase in size, developing and extending into the endometrium and adjacent areas.[83] Cervical cancer is staged according to the standards of the International Federation of Gynecology and Obstetrics. The staging sequences range from 0 to IV, depending on the extent of tissue or organ involvement (see Chapter 48). CIN and carcinoma of the cervix have been conceptualized as a continuum progressing from mild dysplasia (grade I) to moderate dysplasia (grade II) to severe dysplasia and carcinoma in situ (grade III). A complete assessment involves a gynecologic oncologist and a radiation oncologist to determine the best individualized treatment plan possible.

Clinical Manifestations

There are no symptoms in the early stages of CIN. In such cases, CIN is usually discovered on Pap smears. The most common symptom of cervical cancer is vaginal bleeding, usually postcoital. Also present may be metorrhagia and a malodorous, blood-tinged vaginal discharge. With disease progression, there may be abdominal, pelvic, back, or leg pain; anorexia; weight loss; anemia as a result of vaginal bleeding; and edema of the leg(s) caused by the obstruction of lymph nodes. In advanced disease, there may be hematuria or rectal bleeding due to possible involvement of the bowel, bladder, or both.[87]

Assessment

When taking the patient's history, the nurse should inquire about the occurrence and duration of the last normal menses. If the patient has a history of vaginal bleeding, she is asked how current bleeding deviates from the usual flow. A check to determine whether the woman is ovulating can be accomplished in part by asking about premenstrual symptoms, midcycle increase in mucus from the vagina, and biphasic temperatures. Questions related to abdominal pain, vaginal discharge, dysuria, birth control measures, sexual practices, use of oral contraceptives, recent trauma, potential family violence, past pregnancies, and past medical history, to include endocrine, hematologic, and gynecologic problems, are essential. For women born between 1940 and 1974, the nurse should ask whether the patient's mother took DES during pregnancy. During the physical exam, the nurse should attempt to discover whether blood loss (if present) is significant by obtaining orthostatic blood pressure and pulse readings. The skin should be inspected for bruising, petechia, or purpura. A pelvic and speculum exam are performed, checking for foreign bodies, infection, or organic pathology such as visible tumors. Diagnostic tests that may prove helpful include a urine or serum hCG, Pap smear with maturation index, saline vaginal wet prep, cervical culture for *Neisseria gonorrhoeae*, cervical culture for *Chlamydia trachomatis*, hemoglobin/hematocrit, and CBC.

Diagnosis

The Pap smear is the primary screening tool to ascertain the presence of abnormal cells, visible lesions, or both. Women with abnormal Pap smears are referred for a colposcopic examination and cervical biopsy to determine whether HPV and CIN are present.[83] In the case of the nonpregnant patient, an endocervical curettage is performed to obtain cervical cells. Conization is indicated if the lesion extends into the cervical canal and cannot be evaluated by colposcopy. Conization, or cone biopsy, is both a diagnostic and treatment method, as it establishes the severity of CIN and removes a cone-shaped wedge of abnormal tissue. If invasive cervical cancer is found, the patient is usually anesthetized and the disease is staged to determine the spread of disease beyond the cervix.[83]

At the present time, many researchers are questioning the value of routine Pap smear screening in the HIV-positive woman. It is a known fact that such Pap smears are associated with false-negative readings, while true CIN is confirmed by colposcopy and biopsy. Some investigators believe that all HIV-infected women should undergo baseline colposcopy with assessment of HPV status. Routine Pap screening would then be indicated for some patients, while others whose baseline evaluation revealed an abnormal lesion or the presence of certain types of HPV would need to undergo serial colposcopy. Further study is needed before standards of care related to the optimal method for CIN screening in HIV-infected women can be established.

Prevention and the HIV-Positive Patient

Cervical cancer is preventable given adequate screening and early treatment of cervical dysplasia, which can halt neoplastic progression. Current recommendations are that HIV-infected women have two Pap smears during the first year after diagnosis. Provided that both of these are negative, yearly Pap smears are then recommended. If a woman has a history of abnormal Pap smears before diagnosis with HIV, she should be referred for colposcopic examination with the appropriate treatment and follow-up.[87–89] There is some suspicion of an underdiagnosis of cervical cancer in women infected with HIV. Reasons for such underdiagnosis include fragmentation of care, limited access to such care (particularly in women of color), and the tendency to overlook gynecologic care and screening in the presence of more life-threatening care needs.[45,83,87] It goes without saying, therefore, that women diagnosed with CIN whose HIV status is unknown should be offered HIV counseling and testing.

Therapeutic Approaches for Cervical Cancer

Approximately 40% of HIV-infected women have abnormal Pap smears and/or colposcopic evidence of CIN (a precancerous lesion) when evaluated during routine gynecologic testing.[45] Low-grade CIN lesions (CIN I) are expected to regress spontaneously in seronegative women. High-grade CIN lesions — CIN II and III — eventually progress to invasive cervical cancer even in seronegative women. Well-established, definitive therapy for CIN II or III in such seronegative women includes the use of cryotherapy/cryosurgery, carbon dioxide (CO_2) laser therapy, cone biopsy or loop excision, and simple hysterectomy. Such therapies usually result in complete resolution of disease, with eventual relapse in only 10%–15% of patients treated. In HIV-infected women with CIN I or II, such definitive therapy is associated with relapse in approximately 50% of patients after only one to two years.[89,90] In the HIV-infected population, optimal therapy for invasive cervical cancer is not yet known. Treatment may include single or combination strategies that include surgery, radiation, or chemotherapy. Chemotherapy often has limited effectiveness because cervical cancer responds poorly to chemotherapy. However, response rates of up to 70% have been reported with treatment that includes cisplatin, methotrexate, bleomycin, and doxorubicin.[83]

In most circumstances, when compared to their seronegative counterparts, HIV-positive women with cervical cancer present with a higher grade of disease, a higher stage of disease, and early evidence of metastatic disease. In such cases, the relapse rate after definitive therapy is 100%, with a median survival of less than one year.[91] In view of such relapse rates, several studies are attempting to discover an agent that might prolong response. Such experimental approaches include the use of topical fluorouracil (5–FU) cream, oral difluoromethylornithine (DFMO), and HPV vaccines.[92] Also of note is the National Cancer Institute alert of February 22, 1999, urging physicians to begin treating metastatic cervical cancer with a combination of chemotherapy and radiation, which will significantly reduce the death rate by 30% to 50%. The implications of this government-sponsored recommendation for the HIV-positive patient with metastatic cervical cancer continues to await further study and guidelines.

Nursing Care

Women infected with HIV have specific gynecologic needs that must be met to be assured of quality and comprehensive care. Some healthcare protocols require Pap smears every six months, others every year. Routine pelvic exams, and explorations of the patient's sexual practices and habits acquaint the nurse with the specific and sometimes unique care needs of each patient. Continually assessing for such signs and symptoms as vaginal bleeding; dyspareunia; malodorous vaginal discharges; pelvic, back, or leg pain; and/or the presence of edema in the legs assures the patient that the nurse is not only interested in her full range of healthcare needs but is available to discuss potentially sensitive and embarrassing subjects and questions.

Treatment of CIN and cervical carcinoma requires the nurse to educate the patient about the range of treatment modalities, including the possible side effects of radiation therapy and chemotherapy. Counseling the patient as to when to avoid sex, how to participate safely in sexual activities before and after therapies, and potential decisions regarding pregnancy and childbirth foster an environment of trust, openness, and compassionate understanding.

Cervical cancer is considered to be a preventable cancer when adequate screening is provided and cervical dysplasia is treated. It is often the nurse who is at the forefront of making sure that all avenues are explored when it comes to comprehensive screening and detection and consistent healthcare over time.

Other Malignancies

In the past few years, several other cancers have been noted in persons with HIV. Lyter and colleagues[93,94] reported an increase in the incidence of anal cancer, Hodgkin's disease, seminoma, melanoma, oropharyngeal cancer, and multiple myeloma in HIV-infected homosexual/bisexual men, as compared to their HIV-seronegative counterparts. Anal intraepithelial neoplasia (AIN) among HIV-positive men has increased substantially now that persons with HIV and AIDS are living longer. Palefsky[95] studied 348 HIV-positive men and 260 HIV-negative men over a four-year period. The risk for high-grade AIN was 19% among HIV-negative men, 30% among HIV-positive men with a CD4 cell count greater than 500 mm^3, and 52% among those with a CD4 cell count less than 200 mm.[3,95] Routine screening for AIN by obtaining samples and smears through anoscopy should be considered in populations that are at risk.

Unlike non-Hodgkin's lymphoma, Hodgkin's disease (HD) is not an AIDS-defining illness. However, HD occurs with greater frequency among HIV-infected individuals, is significantly more aggressive, and has poorer therapeutic outcomes in the HIV-positive population. Frequent opportunistic infections and a depleted bone marrow reserve make it difficult to treat these individuals with chemotherapy regimens. Much like the treatment measures used in NHL, those used in HD have resulted in poor response rates and short survival times.

As persons with AIDS continue to live longer, it remains to be seen if the incidence and varieties of cancers they experience will continue to increase. It may be difficult to determine if there is a direct relationship between these cancers and the HIV infection itself. Nevertheless, monitoring the HIV-infected population for cancer is important. If a malignancy is encountered in a patient who may be at risk for HIV/AIDS, exploration into HIV testing may indeed be warranted, as an underlying immune deficiency will certainly influence future treatment plans.

The Double Trauma: AIDS *and* Malignancy

The stigma of AIDS involves a terrifying series of events and images: young people dying before their time; a link between sex and death; fear and homophobia; loss of insurance and career status; potential loss of disapproving family members and friends who find out that their child or loved one is a homosexual, bisexual, and/or drug user; discrimination and alienation/isolation; loss of self-control and functional status; loss of income; and a new-found dependency on drug-assistance programs and AIDS-related programs and charities. The social meaning of AIDS intimately touches our ideas and feelings about religion, sexuality, social responsibility, individual privacy, health, promiscuity, and the prospect of living a "normal" lifespan. AIDS is a disease marked by a slow, progressive, and permanent course characterized by ever-increasing occurrences of a wide range of infections, drug side effects, and eventual wasting, loss of independence, and death. This worst-case scenario of AIDS lurks in the deepest recesses of the patient's consciousness at all times. There is no cure on the horizon.

When the diagnosis of a malignancy is added to that of AIDS, the addition of yet another "terminal" illness only reinforces the sense of living under a death sentence for those who strive to maintain a positive attitude, take care of themselves, and strictly adhere to complex medication regimens. There is the potential fear of utter vulnerability — having no resistance and no reserves to combat new infections currently held at bay. Issues regarding the additional expenses related to cancer treatments and the medical and nursing care needed only compound already strained financial reserves and plans for recovery or stabilization. One grieves for another aspect of the self that has been rendered sick, and an even deeper sense of helplessness is experienced as another domain of the medical establishment (the realm of oncology and hematology) must now become a part of the patient's culture. If the malignancy involves visible lesions, the HIV-infected individual encounters further issues related to body image and physical attractiveness.

The nurse can make an enormous difference in the care of the patient with AIDS who is diagnosed with a malignancy. The nurse who is comfortable with his or her own sense of sexuality and who keeps an open mind and heart can offer humane care to a person in need of human comfort and support. During the worst and best of times, the nurse can provide much-needed encouragement and a sense of worth and value to a patient population in need of hope, dignity, courage, and a sense of control.

Conclusion

HIV causes severe cellular immunodeficiency, which renders the infected individual vulnerable to opportunistic infections and neoplasms. The three most common cancers associated with AIDS are Kaposi's sarcoma, AIDS-related lymphoma, and, in women, cervical cancer. The nursing care of patients with these malignancies is oriented toward screening and prevention, assessment, diagnosis, treatment, provision of emotional support, symptom management, discharge planning, home care, short-term hospital and outpatient care, sometimes skilled facility care, and, finally, terminal care and follow-up support to the family. The more compassionate, expert, and understanding the nursing care, the more humane and comfortable will be the healthcare experiences of the person with HIV/AIDS.

References

1. Flaskerud JH, Ungvarski PJ: Overview and update of HIV disease, in Ungvarski PJ, Flaskerud JH (eds.): *HIV/AIDS: A Guide to Primary Care Management* (ed 4). Philadelphia, Saunders, 1999, pp 1–25
2. Levine A: AIDS-related malignancies. *Clin Care Options HIV* 2(3):1–10, 1996
3. Safai B, Schwartz JJ: Kaposi's sarcoma and the acquired immunodeficiency syndrome, in Devita VT, Hellman S, Rosenberg SA (eds.): *AIDS: Etiology, Diagnosis, Treatment, and Prevention.* Philadelphia, Lippincott, 1997, pp 210–228
4. Centers for Disease Control and Prevention: Pneumocystis pneumonia — Los Angeles. *Morb Mortal Wkly Rep* 30:250, 1981
5. Centers for Disease Control and Prevention: Kaposi's sarcoma and Pneumocystis pneumonia among homosexual men — New York and California. *Morb Mortal Wkly Rep* 30:305, 1981
6. Centers for Disease Control and Prevention: *HIV/AIDS Surveillance Report.* Atlanta, CDC, October 27, 2003
7. Centers for Disease Control and Prevention: *HIV and AIDS Trends: The Changing Landscape of the Epidemic: A Closer Look.* Atlanta, GA, Centers for Disease Control and Prevention, 1997
8. Centers for Disease Control and Prevention: Update: trends in AIDS incidence — United States, 1996. *Morb Mortal Wkly Rep* 46:861–866, 1997
9. Braun M: Classics in oncology: idiopathic multiple pigmented sarcoma of the skin by Kaposi. *CA Cancer J Clin* 32:340–347, 1982
10. Myers BD, Kessler E, Levi J, et al: Kaposi's sarcoma in kidney transplant recipients. *Arch Int Med* 133:307–311, 1974
11. Gange RW, Wilson JE: Kaposi's sarcoma and immunosuppressive therapy: an appraisal. *Clin Exp Dermatol* 3:135–146, 1978
12. Haverkos HW, Curran JW: The current outbreak of Kaposi's sarcoma and opportunistic infections. *CA Cancer J Clin* 32:330–339, 1982
13. Friedman-Kien AE, Ostreicher R, Saltzman B: Clinical manifestations of classical, endemic, African, and epidemic AIDS-associated Kaposi's sarcoma, in Riedman-Kien AE (ed.): *Color Atlas of AIDS.* Philadelphia, Saunders, 1989, pp 11–48
14. Rothman S: Remarks on sex, age, and racial distribution of Kaposi's sarcoma and on possible pathogenetic factors. *Acta Unio Int Contra Cancrum* 18:326–329, 1962
15. Beral V, Peterman TA, Berkelman RL, et al: KS among persons with AIDS: a sexually transmitted infection? *Lancet* 335:123–128, 1990
16. Lassoued K, Caluvel JP, Fegueux S, et al: AIDS associated Kaposi's sarcoma in female patients. *AIDS* 5:877–880, 1991
17. Centers for Disease Control: *HIV/AIDS Surveillance Report.* Atlanta, CDC, January 1990
18. Haverkos HW, Pinsky PF, Dortman DP, et al: Disease manifestation among homosexuals with acquired immunodeficiency syndrome: a possible role of nitrites in Kaposi's sarcoma. *Sex Transm Dis* 12:203–208, 1985
19. Kaldor JM, Tiondall B, Williamson P, et al: Factors associated with Kaposi's sarcoma in a cohort of homosexual and bisexual men. *J Acquir Immune Defic Syndr* 6:1145–1149, 1993
20. Miles SA, Wang H, Elashoff R, et al: Improved survival for patients with AIDS related Kaposi's sarcoma. *J Clin Oncol* 12:1910–1916, 1994
21. Mann DL, Murray C, O'Donnell M, et al: HLA antigen frequencies in HIV-1 related Kaposi's sarcoma. *J Acquir Immune Defic Syndr* 3:51–55, 1990
22. Vogel J, Hinrichs SH, Reynolds RK, et al: The HIV *tat* gene induces dermal lesions resembling Kaposi's sarcoma in transgenic mice. *Nature* 335:606–611, 1988
23. Chang Y, Cesarman E, Pessin MS, et al: Identification of herpesvirus-like DNA sequences in Kaposi's sarcoma. *Science* 266:1865–1869, 1994
24. Moore PS, Chang Y: Detection of herpesvirus-like DNA sequences in Kaposi's sarcoma in patients with and those without HIV infection. *N Engl J Med* 332:1181–1185, 1995
25. Cesarman E, Chang Y, Moore PS, et al: Kaposi's sarcoma-associated herpesvirus-like DNA sequences in AIDS-related body-cavity-based lymphomas. *N Engl J Med* 332:1186–1191, 1995
26. Gao SJ, Kingsley L, Hoover DR, et al: Seroconversion to antibodies against Kaposi's sarcoma-associated herpesvirus-related latent nuclear antigens before the development of Kaposi's sarcoma. *N Engl J Med* 335:233–241, 1996
27. Ensoli B, Nakamura S, Salahuddin SZ, et al: AIDS-Kaposi's sarcoma derived cells express cytokines with autocrine and paracrine growth effects. *Science* 243:223–226, 1989
28. Kaplan LD: Malignancies associated with HIV disease: Kaposi's sarcoma, in Cohen PT, Sande MA, Volberding PA (eds.): *The AIDS Knowledge Base* (ed 3). Philadelphia, Lippincott, Williams and Wilkins, 1999, pp 803-805
29. Stine GJ. *AIDS Update 1998.* Englewood Cliffs, NJ, Prentice Hall, 1998, pp 127–158
30. Safai B, Dias BM: Kaposi's sarcoma and cloacogenic carcinoma associated with AIDS, in Broder S, Merigan TC, Bolognesi D (eds.): *Textbook of AIDS Medicine.* Baltimore, Williams and Wikins, 1994, pp 401–415
31. Centers for Disease Control: Revision of the CDC surveillance case definition for acquired immunodeficiency syndrome. *Morb Mortal Wkly Rep* 36(1S):3S–15S, 1987
32. Chachoua A, Krigel R, Lafleur F, et al: Prognostic factors and staging classification of patients with epidemic Kaposi's sarcoma. *J Clin Oncol* 7:774–780, 1989

33. Krown SE, Metroka C, Wernz JC, et al: Kaposi's sarcoma in AIDS: a proposal for a uniform evaluation, response, and staging criteria. *J Clin Oncol* 7:1201–1207, 1989
34. Krown SE, Testa MA, Huang J. AIDS-related Kaposi's sarcoma: prospective validation of the AIDS Clinical Trials Group Staging Classification. *J Clin Oncol* 75:3085–3092, 1997
35. Chak LY, Gill PS, Levine AM, et al: Radiation therapy for AIDS-related KS. *J Clin Oncol* 6:863–867, 1988
36. Mitsuyasu RT: Interferon alpha in the treatment of AIDS related KS. *Br J Haematol* 79:69–73, 1991
37. Lilenbaum RC, Ratner L: Systemic treatment of KS: current status and future directions. Editorial review. *AIDS* 8:141–151, 1994
38. Gill PS, Rarick MU, McCutchan JA, et al: A systemic treatment of AIDS-related KS: results of a randomized trial. *Am J Med* 90:427–433, 1991
39. Northfelt DWQ, Dezube B, Miller B, et al: Randomized comparative trial of doxil vs. Adriamycin, bleomycin, and vincristine (ABV) in the treatment of severe AIDS related KS. *Blood* 86:382a, 1995 (abstr)
40. Gill PS, Wernz J, Scadden DT, et al: A randomized trial of liposomal daunorubicin (Daunoxome) versus Adriamycin, bleomycin, and vincristine (ABV) in 232 patients with advanced AIDS related KS. *Proc Am Soc Clin Oncol* 14:291, 1995 (abstr)
41. Welles L, Saville W, Lietzau J, et al: Phase II trial with dose titration of paclitaxel for the therapy of human immunodeficiency virus-associated Kaposi's sarcoma. *J Clin Oncol* 16:1112–1121, 1998
42. Gill PS, Lunardi-Iskandar Y, Louis S, et al: The effect of preparation of human chorionic gonadotropin on AIDS-related KS. *N Engl J Med* 335:1261–1269, 1996
43. Ragni MV, Bele SH, Jaffee RA, et al: Acquired immunodeficiency syndrome-associated non-Hodgkin's lymphomas and other malignancies in patients with hemophilia. *Blood* 81:1889–1897, 1993
44. Pedersen C, Barton SE, Cjiesi A, et al: HIV related non-Hodgkin's lymphoma among European AIDS patients: AIDS in Europe Study Group. *Eur J Haematol* 55:245–250, 1995
45. Staats JA, Sheran M, Herr R: Adolescents and adults. Care management of AIDS-indicator diseases, in Ungvarski PJ, Flaskerud JH (eds.): *HIV/AIDS: A Guide to Primary Care Management* (ed 4). Philadelphia, Saunders, 1999, pp 194–254
46. Cote TR, Manns A, Hardy CR, et al: Epidemiology of brain lymphoma among people with or without acquired immunodeficiency syndrome: AIDS/Cancer Study Group. *J Natl Cancer Inst* 88:675–679, 1996
47. Serriano D, Salamina G, Franceschi S, et al: The epidemiology of AIDS-associated non-Hodgkin's lymphoma in the World Health Organization European Region. *Br J Cancer* 66:912–916, 1992
48. Peters BS, Beck EJ, Coleman DG, et al: Changing disease patterns in patients with AIDS in a referral centre in the United Kingdom: the changing face of AIDS. *Br Med J* 302:203–207, 1991
49. Kaplan LD, Northfelt DW: Malignancies associated with AIDS, in Sande MA, Volberding PA (eds.): *The Medical Management of AIDS* (ed 5). Philadelphia, Saunders, 1997, pp 413–439
50. Emile D, Coumbaras J, Raphael M, et al: Interleukin-6 production in high-grade B lymphomas: correlation with the presence of malignant immunoblasts in acquired immunodeficiency syndrome and in human immunodeficiency seronegative patients. *Blood* 80:498–504, 1992
51. Masood R, Zhang Y, Bond MW, et al: Interleukin 10 is an autocrine growth factor for AIDS related B cell lymphoma. *Blood* 85:3423–3430, 1995
52. Levine A: Oncologic disorders and cytokines. *Clin Care Options for HIV* 4(2):1–19, 1998.
53. Ballerini P, Gaidano G, Gon JZ, et al: Molecular pathogenesis of HIV associated lymphomas. *AIDS Res Hum Retroviruses* 8:731–735, 1992
54. Levine AM, Shibata D, Sullivan-Hurley J, et al: Epidemiological and biological study of acquired immunodeficiency syndrome-related lymphoma in the County of Los Angeles: preliminary results. *Cancer Res* 52(suppl 19):5482s–5484s, 1992
55. Morgello S: Epstein-Barr and human immunodeficiency viruses in acquired immunodeficiency syndrome-related primary central nervous system lymphoma. *Am J Pathol* 141:441–450, 1992
56. Carbone A, Gloghini A, Vaccher E, et al: Kaposi's sarcoma-associated herpesvirus DNA sequences in AIDS related and AIDS-unrelated lymphomatous effusions. *Br J Haematol* 94:533–543, 1996
57. Gessain A, Briere J, Angelin-Duclos C, et al: Human herpes virus 8 (Kaposi's sarcoma herpes virus) and malignant proliferations in France: a molecular study of 250 cases including two AIDS-associated body cavity lymphomas. *Leukemia* 11: 266–272, 1997
58. Nador RG, Cesarman E, Chadburn A, et al: Primary effusion lymphoma: a distinct clinicopathologic entity associated with the Kaposi's sarcoma-associated herpes virus. *Blood* 88: 645–656, 1996
59. Beck PL, Gill MJ, Sutherland LR: HIV-associated non Hodgkin's lymphoma of the gastrointestinal tract. *Am J Gastroenterol* 91:2377–2381, 1996
60. Cappell MS, Botros N: Predominantly gastrointestinal symptoms and signs in 11 consecutive AIDS patients with gastrointestinal lymphoma. *Am J Gastroenterol* 89:545–549, 1994
61. Danin JD, McCarty M, Coker R: Case report: lymphoma causing small bowel intussusception in a patient with the acquired immune deficiency syndrome. *Clin Radiol* 46:350–351, 1992
62. Schoeppner HL, Wong DK, Bresalier RS: Primary small bowel lymphoma manifested as obstructive jaundice in a patient with AIDS. *South Med J* 88:583–585, 1995
63. Levine AM, Seneviratne L, Espina BM, et al. Evolving characteristics of AIDS-related lymphoma. *Blood* 96:4084–4090, 2000
64. Matthews GV, Bower M, Mandelia S, et al: Changes in AIDS-related lymphoma since the introduction of highly active antiretroviral therapy. *Blood* 96:2730–2734, 2000
65. Sider L, Melany M: Thoracic AIDS-related lymphoma: CT appearance and CD4 counts. *AJR Am J Roentgenol* 160(suppl 4):97–102, 1993
66. Iacoangeli M, Roselli R, Antinor A, et al: Experience with brain biopsy in acquired immune deficiency syndrome-related focal lesions of the central nervous system. *Br J Surg* 81:1508–1510, 1994
67. Hoffman JM, Waskin A, Schifter T, et al: FDG-PET in differentiating lymphoma from nonmalignant central nervous system lesions in patients with AIDS. *J Nucl Med* 34:567–575, 1993
68. Lorberboym M, Estok L, Machac J, et al: Rapid differential diagnosis of cerebral toxoplasmosis and primary central nervous system lymphoma by thallium-201 SPECT. *J Nucl Med* 37:1150–1154, 1996
69. O'Malley JP, Ziessman HA, Kuman PN, et al: Diagnosis of intracranial lymphoma in patients with AIDS: value of 201Tl single-photon emission computed tomography. *AJR Am J Roentgenol* 163:417–421, 1994
70. Pierce MA, Johnson MD, Maciunas RJ, et al: Evaluating contrast-enhancing brain lesions in patients with AIDS by using positron emission tomography. *Ann Int Med* 123:594–598, 1995
71. Ling SM, Roach M, Larson DA, et al: Radiotherapy of primary central nervous system lymphoma in patients with and without

human immunodeficiency virus: ten years of treatment experience at the University of California San Francisco. *Cancer* 73:2570–2582, 1994

72. Forsyth PA, Yahoalom J, DeAngelis LM: Combined-modality therapy in the treatment of primary central nervous system lymphoma in AIDS. *Neurology* 44:1473–1479, 1994
73. Sparano JA, Wiernik PH, Hu S, et al: Pilot trial of infusional cyclophosphamide, doxorubicin, and etoposide plus didanosine and filgrastim in patients with non-Hodgkin's lymphoma. *J Clin Oncol* 14:3026–3035, 1996
74. Levine AM, Tulpule A, Expina B, et al: Low dose methotrexate, bleomycin, doxorubicin, cyclophosphamide, vincristine, and dexamethasone with zalcitabine in patients with acquired immunodeficiency syndrome related lymphoma: effect on human immunodeficiency virus and serum interleukin-6 levels over time. *Cancer* 78:517–526, 1996
75. Kaplan L, Staus D, Testa M, et al: Randomized trial of standard dose mBACOD with GM-CSF vs. reduced dose mBACOD for systemic HIV-related lymphoma. *Proc Am Soc Clin Oncol* 14:288, 1995 (abstr)
76. Spina M, Carbone A, Vaccher E, et al: Outcome in patients with non-Hodgkin's lymphoma and with or without human immunodeficiency virus infection. *Clin Infect Dis* 38:142–144, 2004
77. Newell M, Goldstein D, Milliken S, et al: Phase I/II trial of filgrastim (r-metHuG-CSF), CEOP chemotherapy and antiretroviral therapy in HIV-related non-Hodgkin's lymphoma. *Ann Oncol* 7:1029–1036, 1996
78. Levine AM, Tulpule A, Espina B, et al: Low dose m-BACOD with zalcitabine in patients with AIDS-related lymphoma: effect on HIV and serum interleukin-6 levels over time. *Cancer* 78:517–526, 1996
79. Sparano JA, Wiernik PH, Strack M, et al: Infusional cyclophosphamide, doxorubicin, and etoposide in HIV and HTLV-1 related non-Hodgkin's lymphoma: a highly active regimen. *Blood* 81:2810–2815, 1993
80. Centers for Disease Control: Characteristics of, and HIV infection among, women served by publicly funded HIV counseling and testing services: USA, 1989–1990. *Morb Mortal Wkly Rep* 40:195–203, 1991
81. Maimon M, Fruchter RG, Guy L, et al: Human immunodeficiency virus infections and invasive cervical carcinoma. *Cancer* 71:402–406, 1993
82. Centers for Disease Control: Risk for cervical disease in HIV infected women. *Morb Mortal Wkly Rep* 39:846–849, 1990
83. Peel KR: Premalignant and malignant disease of the cervix, in Whitefield CR (ed.): *Dewhurst's Textbook of Obstetrics and Gynecology for Postgraduates* (ed 6). London, Blackwell Scientific, 1999, pp 572-581
84. Richart RM, Wright TC: Controversies in the management of low-grade cervical intraepithelial neoplasia. *Cancer* 71(suppl 4):1413–1421, 1993
85. Klevens MR, Fleming PL, Mays MA, et al: Characteristics of women with AIDS and invasive cervical cancer. *Obstet Gynecol* 88:269–273, 1996
86. Vermund SH, Kelley KF, Kelin RS, et al: High risk of human papillomaviruses infection and cervical squamous intraepithelial lesions among women with symptomatic HIV infection. *Am J Obstetric Gynecol* 165:392–400, 1991
87. Hatch KD, Fu YS: Cervical and vaginal cancer, in Berek JS, Adashi EY, Hillard PA (eds.): *Novak's Gynecology* (ed 12). Baltimore, Williams and Wilkins, 1996, pp 1111–1122
88. Centers for Disease Control: USPHS/IDSA guidelines for the prevention of opportunistic infections in persons infected with human immunodeficiency virus. *Morb Mortal Wkly Rep* 46(RR-12):1–13, 1997
89. Denenberg R. Cervical cancer and women with HIV. *GMHC: Treatment Issues* 11(7/8):10–18, 1997
90. Maiman M, Fruchter RF, Serur E, et al: Recurrent cervical intraepithelial neoplasia in HIV seropositive women. *Obstet Gynecol* 82:170–174, 1993
91. Maiman M, Fruchter RG, Sedlis A, et al: Prevalence, risk factors, and accuracy of cytologic screening for cervical intraepithelial neoplasia in women with the human immunodeficiency virus. *Gynecol Oncol* 68:233–239, 1998
92. Levine A: Oncologic disorders and cytokines. *Clin Care Options for HIV* 4(2):1–19, 1998
93. Lyter DW, Bryant J, Thackeray R, et al: Incidence of human immunodeficiency virus related and nonrelated malignancies in a large cohort of homosexual men. *J Clin Oncol* 13: 2540–2546, 1995
94. Lyter DW, Kingsley LA, Rinaldo CR, et al: Malignancies in the Multicenter AIDS Cohort Study (MACS) 1984–1994. *Proc Am Soc Clin Oncol* 15:305, 1996 (abstr)
95. Palefsky JM. Anal human papillomavirus infection and anal cancer in HIV positive individuals: an emerging problem. *AIDS* 8:283–295, 1994

CHAPTER 44

Bone and Soft-Tissue Sarcomas

Jayne K. Sumner, RN, BA, PCRM

Introduction

Sarcomas of the bone and soft tissue are rare neoplasms. A practicing orthopedic surgeon may see fewer than one primary bone or soft-tissue sarcoma every three years.[1] These forms of cancer affect both genders and all age groups. The orthopedic oncologist, cytologist, vascular surgeon, plastic surgeon, thoracic surgeon, physical therapist, nurse, social worker, rehabilitation physician, and prosthetist are the essential team members who guide the patient and family through diagnosis and treatment. Advances in the understanding of the biology of sarcomas, new surgical techniques, and a multidisciplinary approach to treatment have improved the outcome for the sarcoma patient.

Epidemiology

Malignant bone and soft-tissue tumors that present as primary tumors are exceptionally small in number. The American Cancer Society, which keeps track of newly diagnosed cases and deaths by cancer type, estimated 2440 new cases of bone cancer in 2004, with a slightly higher proportion of males than females. The estimate for soft-tissue cancer was approximately 8680, again with a slightly higher proportion of males. The number of deaths was estimated to be 1300 from bone sarcomas and 3660 from soft-tissue sarcomas.[1]

Etiology

The cause of primary bone and soft-tissue tumors, for the most part, eludes the medical community, and as a result, prevention is problematic. Risk factors have been isolated in some instances. Patients with a diagnosis of Ollier's disease, a disease involving multiple enchondromas, may deteriorate to a low-grade chondrosarcoma. Neurofibromatosis patients have a low but very real risk of their tumor deteriorating into a neurofibrosarcoma. Finally, Paget's disease has been linked to osteosarcoma.

Environmental factors related to sarcomas, according to the American Cancer Society, include smoking, chemicals, infectious disease, and radiation. Factors such as tobacco use, physical inactivity, and a diet high in saturated fat and low in fiber have a greater influence on an individual's risk of cancer than low concentrations of pollutants in the air, food, or drinking water.[1] Smoking, diet, and inactivity are controllable variables. Exposure in the workplace to higher concentrations of certain chemicals, metals, and ionizing radiation provides a greater risk, which increases substantially with prolonged exposure, more intense exposure, and higher concentrations of pollutants. Examples of workplace carcinogens include radon and asbestos. Tobacco use greatly increases these risks.

Certain chemicals increase one's risk of cancer, including Agent Orange (a defoliant used in the Vietnam War), vinyl chloride gas, dioxin, and arsenic. Previous cancer treatment with high-dose radiation has been associated with the development of both bone and soft-tissue sarcomas. Alkylating agents used in chemotherapy have also been associated with the development of sarcomas.

Molecular genetics may provide clues to the underlying cause of sarcomas. Cancer as a whole is viewed as a sequence of genetic alterations that result in damage to growth regulation.[2] Tumor-suppressor genes lose their function and, with this loss, contribute to the development of a tumor. Tumor-suppressor genes often serve as cell-cycle regulators.[3] The tumor-suppressor gene *p53* and the retinoblastoma *Rb* gene are often mutated in osteosarcoma. The cell-cycle regulator *Rb* has the capability to induce programmed cell death, or apoptosis. It can trigger the repair of genetic damage or cause apoptosis in the cell if restoration is not feasible. A flaw in this gene or its protein could possibly lead to an explosion of DNA-damaged progeny.[3] The *p53* gene is thought to be the predominant gene that is altered in human cancers.[2] These genetic alterations are thought to be the origin of neoplasms.

Screening and Early Detection

Primary malignant bone and soft-tissue sarcomas are very rare, which contributes to the lack of routine screening to detect these conditions, as is done for prostate cancer or breast cancer. Patients with a family history of sarcomas should be vigilant in watching for presenting symptoms and should be certain that their routine physicals are comprehensive. Li-Fraumeni syndrome is a primarily inherited malady that is identified by the early development of tumors. This is an example of a familial cancer syndrome. The medical community does not advocate routine radiographs as a screening tool. The only exception to this principle would be a chest x-ray at the discretion of the physician during a comprehensive physical examination. Symptoms such as unexplained bone pain, especially at night, or a palpable mass should be investigated, even if there is no family history of cancer.

Pathophysiology

Primary bone and soft-tissue tumors originate from the mesoderm germ layer of the cell. These tumors are characterized by their ability to form certain types of cells. Osteosarcoma is characterized by the formation of bone or osteoid. Primary chondrosarcoma is characterized by the formation of cartilage by tumor cells. Marrow tumors or round-cell tumors are composed of densely packed small cells with rounded nuclei. Ewing's sarcoma falls into this category. Vascular tumors, such as angiosarcomas, are characterized by asymmetric vascular channel formations. These channels are lined with atypical epithelial cells and solid accumulations of poorly differentiated cells. The vascular formations can occur in any of the blood vessels of the bone. Collagen-producing tumor cells structure the osteogenic, chondrogenic, and fibrogenic tumors.

Bone and soft-tissue tumors can affect almost the entire skeleton and its adjacent soft-tissues. One diagnostic tool the physician utilizes is that certain tumors have a predilection for certain bones and locations. Soft-tissue tumors occur most often in the extremities. They are also found in the retroperitoneal area and the neck and head. Bone and soft-tissue sarcomas metastasize most commonly to the lungs. The lymphatic system, bone, soft tissues, and liver are other sites of metastatic disease. The theory regarding why this phenomenon occurs is that a microinvasion of cancer cells into the venous system takes place, and the cells then circulate to the lungs. The pulmonary metastases cannot be detected until the nodule reaches 3 mm.[3] Chest computed tomography is used to diagnose the presence of distant disease.

Clinical Manifestations

Bone and soft-tissue tumors can present as one or more of the following:

- A palpable mass, painful or not painful
- Pain that wakes the patient at night
- Change in function or ambulation

Assessment

Patient and Family History

Physical symptoms are often the defining motivation for a patient to seek the advice and expertise of a physician. These may include pain, a palpable mass, or change in function. Family history may also induce a patient to seek medical help. Pain evaluation is an important diagnostic tool in the diagnosis differential. Pain that alters in intensity, worsening at night or at rest, is often a signal of a malignant process. The initial symptom of Ewing's sarcoma is pain. The presenting pain symptom is often associated with minor trauma, with pain that has not improved over time; this is the motivation to seek medical help.[4] A change in function is often another symptom that motivates a patient to consult a physician. In the case of bone tumors, microfractures through the involved portion of the bone or the compression of juxtaposed neurovascular structures may be the cause of pain.[3] The clinical picture may also involve a palpable mass, which may be masked in an area such as the pelvis or groin area.

The most critical component of the differential diagnosis is the age of the patient, which is used in conjunction with the interpretation of the radiographic findings.[5] In the evaluation of a bone lesion in a patient, male or female, over the age of 40, metastatic disease is the likely diagnosis. Bone tumors tend to develop in a span of approximately two decades. Osteosarcoma usually develops between the ages of 10 and 30, while Ewing's sarcoma generally occurs between the ages of 5 and 15.

Some tumors affect one sex more commonly than the other. Osteosarcomas occur more frequently in males, with a ratio varying from 1.3 to 1 to 1.7 to 1. The exception is parosteal osteosarcoma, which has a female-to-male ratio of 2 to 1.[2]

Soft-tissue sarcomas often present as a painless mass that increases in size. As the mass increases in bulk, pain may appear as the tumor impinges on surrounding neurovascular structures. It is critical to evaluate the patient's account of when the mass was initially found and how rapidly it enlarged. A family history of cancer, the treatment, and outcome is of importance to the emerging clinical picture. Additional signs such as café-au-lait spots, hemangiomas, or asymmetrical edema can be beneficial in the diagnostic process. Prior orthopedic conditions (i.e., Paget's disease, neurofibromatosis, or Ollier's disease); exposure to known carcinogens; and other presenting systemic symptoms must be noted, along with fever or other areas of pain.

It is critical at this time to evaluate for problems, potential or immediate, with regard to social and financial support systems. If a patient receives a diagnosis of a sarcoma, it is crucial to know what support systems are available to the patient and family. The inability to pursue one's livelihood as well as leisure activities can be of great importance to a patient facing a life-threatening diagnosis. If a patient is the carrier of the primary medical insurance, the inability to work is

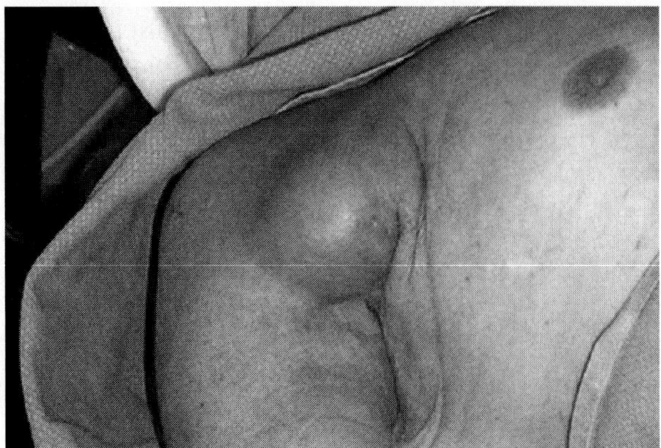

Figure 44-1 Leiomyosarcoma soft tissue mass with superficial veins.

very stressful. The continued dignity of a patient and family is an important facet in the patient's treatment and overall well-being. Educating the patient concerning the diagnosis is important; this education will need to be reinforced and expanded as the treatment evolves. It is crucial for a patient to receive accurate explanations from physicians and other involved healthcare professionals.

Physical Examination

The physical examination of the patient with an alleged bone or soft-tissue sarcoma entails observation and palpation of the affected region. These findings are often nonspecific but, when combined with radiographic findings, lead to a more complete diagnostic picture. If a mass is evident, there may be a locally elevated temperature and possibly a network of dilated superficial veins. (See Figure 44-1.) The mass may be firm and fixed. When a soft-tissue mass is evident, a physician should suspect the possibility of an aggressive bone lesion.[5] Physical inspection may also reveal café-au-lait spots or hemangiomas. The patient may report some form of neurologic deficit; this is probably a result of the tumor exerting pressure on surrounding nerves and vessels. Unilateral edema may result from a bone tumor's expansive spread to soft-tissue. The contralateral side is examined for symmetry with the affected side. Joint involvement may result in limited motion, which may lead to muscle atrophy. If one of the lower extremities is involved, the patient may favor the affected limb, which would result in an antalgic gait or limp. The physician should also assess for adenopathy or hepatomegaly. A soft-tissue mass would also be assessed for any appreciable bruit or thrill, which would indicate vascular involvement.

Diagnostic Studies

Laboratory tests are routinely ordered to form a complete diagnostic picture. These have been found to have limited value in the diagnosis and staging of both bone and soft-tissue sarcomas, however. A differential diagnosis must be formed using every feasible diagnostic tool. The erythrocyte sedimentation rate (ESR) is a somewhat vague value that is found to be elevated in the presence of bone infection. Marrow-cell tumors (Ewing's sarcoma, multiple myeloma, lymphoma of the bone, leukemia, and histiocytosis) often show a marked increase in the ESR value.[6] Patients who are diagnosed with Ewing's sarcoma or lymphoma and are found to have an elevated ESR generally have a poor prognosis. It must be noted that other conditions may also elevate this blood test, including infection, pregnancy, or recent surgery.[2]

An elevated alkaline phosphatase level is evident in approximately one half of osteosarcoma patients. In other primary malignant bone tumors, this level is smaller. The prognostic value of this test has been widely debated due to natural variations related to adolescent growth surges, the peak age for developing osteosarcoma. The possibility of Paget's disease and metastatic osteosarcoma must also be examined.

The remaining laboratory tests that may be ordered include complete blood count, metabolic count, and prothrombin time, if a biopsy is scheduled. Serum protein electrophoresis is ordered for the patients if the physician is concerned about a diagnosis of myeloma.

Radiographic correlation is a very important aspect of the diagnostic process. The multidisciplinary collaboration among the orthopedic oncology surgeon, radiologist, and pathologist provides the expertise needed for the proper diagnosis and treatment of both bone and soft-tissue sarcomas. A patient's medical history is used in conjunction with computed tomography (CT), magnetic resonance imaging (MRI), plain radiographs, bone scans, positron-emission tomography (PET), and ultrasound. These tests each have their value in the diagnosis of sarcomas.

Plain x-rays are valued as a cost-conscious procedure to obtain the total pathological features of a bone tumor. This assessment provides valuable information with respect to the intraosseous extent of a bone tumor, except when there is a rather vague zone of transition that makes the medullary extent of the tumor difficult to determine. If the zone of transition is narrow or well demarcated, the host bone responds by forming new bone in reaction to the lesion. In this instance, the lesion is most likely benign.[2] The vast majority of diagnoses are made with plain radiographs alone.

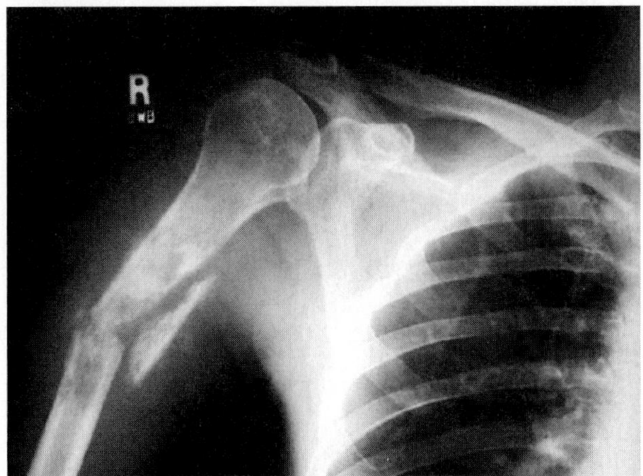

Figure 44-2 A destructive lesion is producing bone in the metaphysis of the humerus. There is a pathologic fracture at the tumor site.

Radiographs also produce evidence as to the distinction between ossification and calcification. The mineralization of matrix is ossification, which has a semblance of order. Calcification is viewed as chaotic mineralization; its appearance is compressed and random. Lesions with calcified areas usually indicate a cartilaginous process. Ossification in the substance of the lesion indicates bone formation by a tumor.[2] Cortical destruction or periosteal formation of new bone is considered a red flag for an aggressive tumor. (See Figure 44-2 and Figure 44-3.)

CT scans are invaluable in evaluating the intraosseous extent of primary bone tumors and the destruction of bone cortex by soft-tissue sarcomas. They show mineralization, subtle fractures, and calcification or ossification of bone far better than MRI scans do. CT scans provide cross-sectional images and greater contrast resolution to delineate bony details.[5] They also show heterogeneous fat density, which is invaluable in the diagnosis of soft-tissue tumors (i.e., liposarcoma) and are beneficial in discerning the dimensions and the approximation of juxtaposed anatomical structures (i.e., neurovascular). CT scans are used to diagnose metastatic disease to the lungs, pelvis, and abdomen.

MRI scans are far superior to CT scans in the diagnosis of soft-tissue tumors. They are excellent for demonstrating the relationship between a soft-tissue mass and the cortex of a bone. MRI offers a concise picture of cortical as well as medullary bone. It can also visualize soft-tissue involvement as well as tumor necrosis and its relationship to neurovascular structures. It is thought to be the optimal choice for staging pelvic tumors.[8] MRI imaging is invaluable in assessing the salvageability of a limb, including the neurovascular structures, intramedullary bone and soft tissue involvement as well as the corruption of an immediate joint.[8]

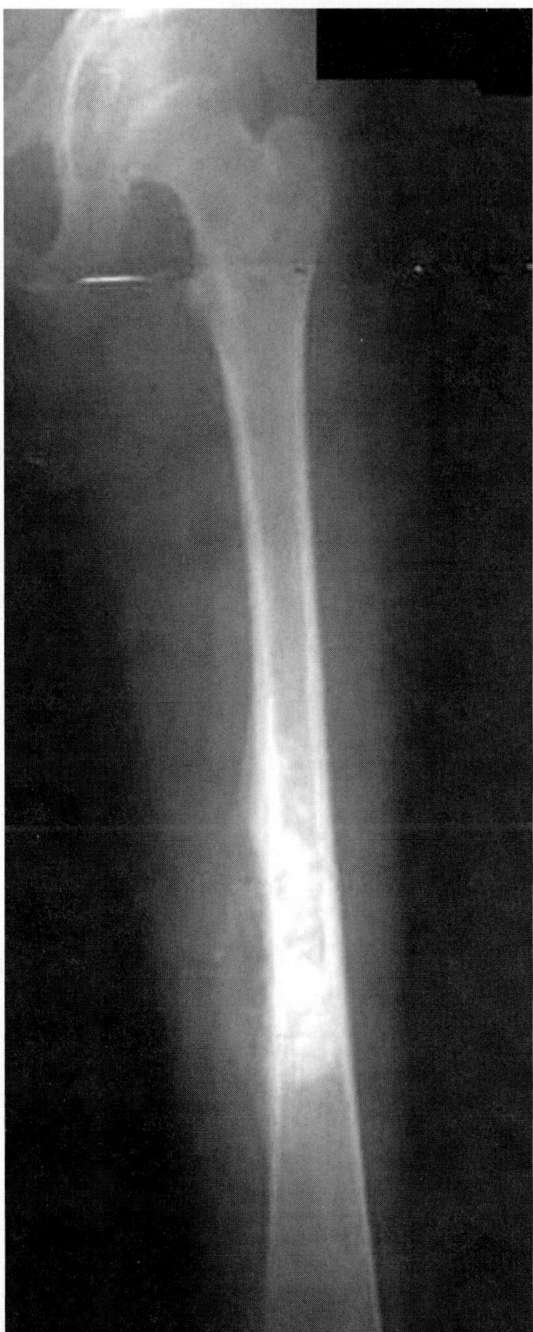

Figure 44-3 Midshaft femur osteosarcoma with cortical destruction.

MRI scans aid the physician in delineating the tumor and the affected areas, as well as bone marrow and cancellous bone.[9] This provides the orthopedic oncology surgeon with the blueprint needed for surgery, biopsy, and limb salvage, as well as amputation. This blueprint is critical to ensure that the entire tumor as well as any contaminated structures are identified. The axial views provide the optimal perspective.[3] The MRI is the best modality for observing the relationship

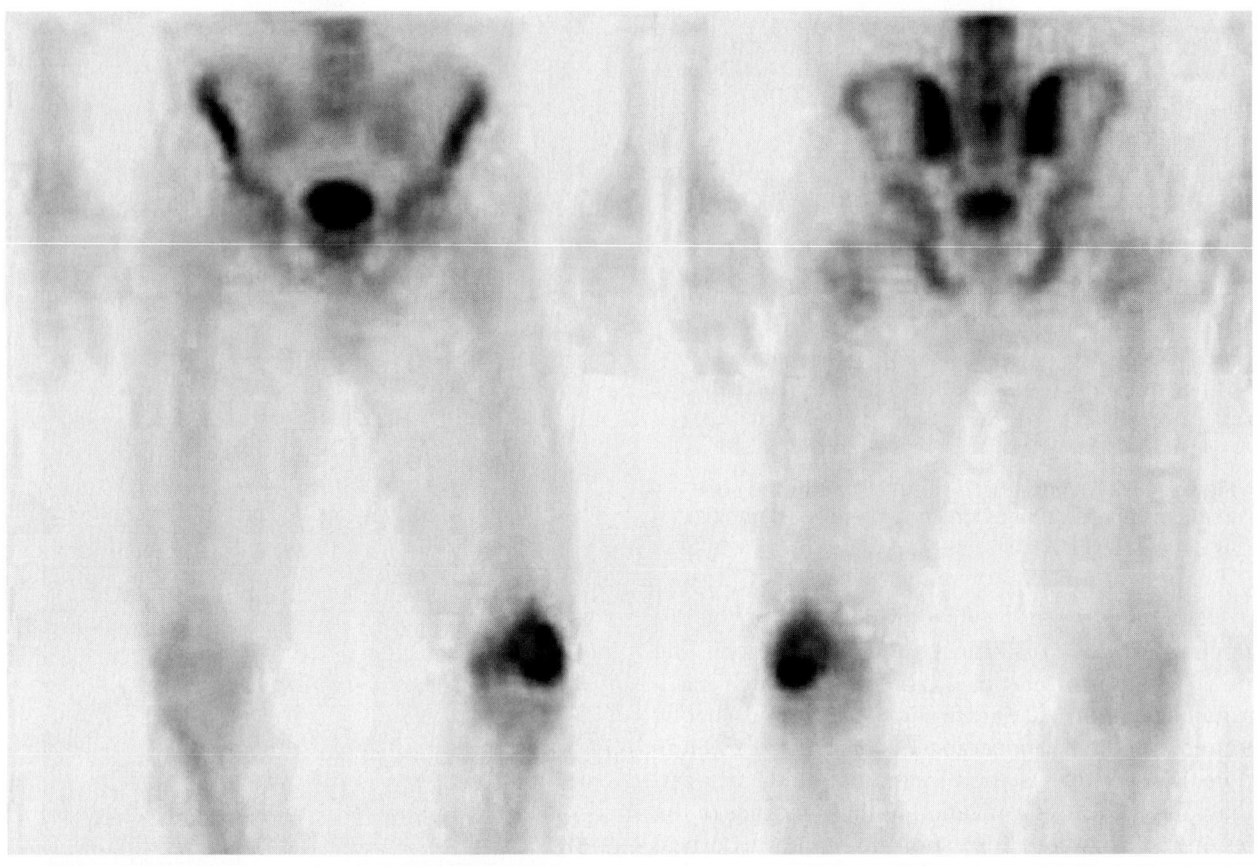

Figure 44-4 Bone scan of a distal femur osteosarcoma.

among the neurovascular structures, the intramedullary extent, and the tumor anatomy.

Bone scintigraphy or bone scans are a somewhat nonspecific exam that provide an excellent medium for evaluating and detecting bone metastasis. (See Figure 44-4.) Although bone scans are useful in accentuating abnormal bone, they do not differentiate between a benign and malignant process. They also will not provide the specifics of the dimension or extent of tumors.[10] Bone scans do not provide any conclusive diagnosis with regard to soft-tissue sarcomas. They will provide an indication of bone metastasis, which is prevalent with bone sarcomas.[10]

Positron-emission tomography (PET) is a new diagnostic tool that enables the physician to evaluate the metabolism and physiology of both normal and diseased tissues. The radiolabeled tracer most commonly used in PET imaging is F-18 fluorodeoxyglucose (FDG). This tracer has been shown to accumulate in certain cancer tissues. PET is still not accepted for differentiating between benign and malignant tissues.[11]

Fluoroscopy is another tool used to pinpoint bony lesions during a biopsy; this ensures a more accurate biopsy.

Utilization of all of the appropriate modalities available to the orthopedic oncologist ensures that the staging of the bone or soft-tissue tumor will be as accurate as possible. These tools are all employed to arrive at a differential diagnosis before a biopsy is performed.[10] Tumors that are large and deep are more likely to have a malignant diagnosis. It is critical that the biopsy be performed by a musculoskeletal oncologist; in the best scenario, the biopsy and ultimate surgery would be performed by the same surgeon.

The importance of performing a biopsy correctly cannot be stressed enough. A biopsy is performed open, with an incision, or closed, using a needles or a special biopsy instrument used for bone or soft tissue. A properly placed incision may prevent a postoperative hematoma or infection. This may mean the difference between salvaging the limb and amputation or the recurrence of the tumor.[8,10,12]

Biopsies can be performed in a variety of ways. Closed needle biopsies have approximately an 84% accuracy rate.[13] It is crucial to obtain diagnostic tissue — viable tumor cells, not necrotic tissue. Another mode of biopsy is the CT-guided core needle biopsy. This technique provides an excellent avenue for the diagnosis of bone and soft-tissue tumors. It allows for accurate penetration into the desired tissue, with the ability to avoid critical structures.[14]

If these biopsy types are nondiagnostic or inconclusive, an open biopsy, considered the gold standard, is then scheduled. The pathologist will take two types of sections during an open biopsy: frozen and permanent sections. Frozen sections are deemed preliminary; snap-freezing may alter the look of the cells under scrutiny. The final diagnosis is not rendered until the permanent section, which has been embedded in paraffin, has been evaluated. It should be noted that bone specimens take more time to diagnose, due to the need to decalcify the specimen and evaluate the tumor cells.

Prognostic Indicators

The prognosis for patients with a bone or soft-tissue sarcoma is determined by the size, location, histologic grade, and presence or absence of distant metastasis of the tumor. Large tumors that are deep, with distant metastasis, have a much poorer prognosis. Metastasis occurs in the lungs, in the lymph nodes, and in other bones.

Classification and Staging

A number of variables influence how a physician views a sarcoma. One variable is the grade of the tumor. This is a histologic calculation of a tumor and the tendency of the tumor to metastasize.[10] Enneking and colleagues provided a staging system that designates two grades: G1, which is low grade, and G2 which is high grade.[15] In this system, the high-grade sarcoma has a greater potential for metastasis than the lower grade. A second staging system, developed by the American Joint Committee on Cancer, designates four grades of sarcomas.[16] Well-differentiated sarcomas are graded as G1. Moderately well-differentiated sarcomas are designated as G2. Poorly differentiated sarcomas are designated as G3, and undifferentiated sarcomas as G4 (see Table 44-1). The main reasons for staging a tumor are to ascertain the patient's prognosis and to guide treatment.[17] The staging process begins at the time that a tumor is diagnosed as malignant. Restaging may take place if the sarcoma recurs or metastasis is discovered. The purpose of this restaging is to change the treatment if needed or to direct the patient to clinical trials.

Another important component in the diagnosis, classification, and staging of a sarcoma is the size of the mass.[18–21] A sarcoma that is larger than 5 cm is thought to have a poorer prognosis than one that is smaller.[22] Masses that grow quickly are more likely to be malignant than slower-growing tumors.[23,24] The location of the tumor, in conjunction with the size, is an important diagnostic tool. Tumors that are large have a greater risk for local recurrence and for distant metastasis.[2] Considerations for treatment are also influenced by these variables (see Table 44-2).

Table 44-1 Enneking System for the Staging of Soft-Tissue Sarcoma and Sarcoma of the Bone

Stage	Grade	Site	Metastases
IA	G1	T1	M0
IB	G1	T2	M0
IIA	G2	T1	M0
IIB	G2	T2	M0
IIIA	G1–G2	T1–T2	M1
IIIB	G1–G2	T1–T2	M1

The final and most significant component in the staging process is the presence or absence of metastases. A patient who presents with metastatic disease at the initial diagnosis has a poorer prognosis.[23]

Therapeutic Approaches and Nursing Care

The ultimate treatment goal for any patient with a primary bone or soft-tissue sarcoma is long-term survival. This would be accomplished by the complete eradication of the tumor to maintain optimal function and the best quality of life. This goal may or may not include amputation. Amputation may provide a more desirable level of function than a resection would. It should not be viewed as a failure in treatment, but as the best-informed choice for the patient's particular circumstance. Treatment strategies for patients with bone or soft-tissue sarcomas may include surgery, radiation therapy, chemotherapy, and a variety of supportive therapies. The medical regimen for sarcoma is a specialized program: each bone and soft-tissue sarcoma has an individualized protocol for treatment.

Surgery

Bone

The decision as to the type of surgery to perform is based on the anatomical site and on the specific neurovascular structures involved. The anatomical site is divided between intracompartmental and extracompartmental; these data are obtained from radiographic studies. The histopathological characteristics of the primary bone or soft-tissue sarcoma and its dimensions

Table 44-2 Anatomic Staging of Musculoskeletal Sarcomas

Rules for Classification

Clinical staging. Includes physical examination, clinical laboratory tests, and biopsy of the sarcoma for microscopic diagnosis and grading

Pathological staging. Consists of the removal of the primary tumor, nodes, or suspected metastases

Primary Tumors (T)				
TX	Primary tumor cannot be assessed			
T0	No evidence of primary tumor			
T1	Tumor 5 cm or less in greatest dimension			
T2	Tumor more than 5 cm in greatest dimension			
Regional Lymph Nodes (N)				
NX	Regional lymph nodes cannot be assessed			
N0	No regional lymph node metastasis			
N1	Regional lymph node metastasis			
Distant Metastasis (M)				
MX	Presence of distant metastasis cannot be assessed			
M0	No distant metastasis			
M1	Distant metastasis			
Tumor Grade (G)				
GX	Grade cannot be assessed			
G1	Well differentiated			
G2	Moderately well differentiated			
G3–4	Poorly differentiated, undifferentiated			
Stage Grouping				
Stage IA	G1	T1	N0	M0
Stage IB	G1	T2	N0	M0
Stage IIA	G2	T1	N0	M0
Stage IIB	G2	T2	N0	M0
Stage IIIA	G3–4	T1	N0	M0
Stage IIIB	G3–3	T2	N0	M0
Stage IVA	Any G	Any T	N1	M0
Stage IVB	Any G	Any T	Any N	M1

Data from Fleming et al.[16]

are also a primary concern. Critical data obtained from radiographic studies, lab studies, the history, and the physical examination of the patient are all incorporated to provide the best strategy for surgery.

Prior to the 1970s, amputation or disarticulation was the accepted treatment for primary bone tumors. These surgeries provided a very poor survival rate of 10% to 20%.[25,26] The treatment was aimed at completely eliminating the tumor, hence the acceptance of amputation or disarticulation. Tumors that, by virtue of their anatomical location, were not resectable were treated in a palliative manner. These locations included the pelvis, spine, and skull. Because such tumors were difficult to eradicate completely, they could recur or metastasize. The 1970s and 1980s brought chemotherapy, which provided an improved efficacy in the treatment of primary bone sarcomas. A combination of improved protocols and chemotherapeutic agents provided the surgeon with the option of limb preservation.[27]

When deciding whether to perform limb-sparing surgery, the surgical team must take certain considerations into account. The incidence of recurrence of the tumor should be no greater than it would be with amputation. Patient survival should be equal between both types of surgeries, and the initial surgery and any treatment of complications should in no way hinder the resumption of adjuvant chemotherapy. In addition, the function of the limb should be comparable to the function of the limb with an amputation. A patient may choose amputation over sparing the limb or vice versa depending on occupation, lifestyle, or self image.[28] It is important to maintain both a sensate and functional limb.[8] Contraindications exist that may preclude a limb salvage surgery, such as (1) a tumor that involves a neurovascular bundle that cannot be reconstructed; (2) surgical margins that do not include a cuff of normal tissue; (3) pathologic fractures with a hematoma; (4) limb length discrepancy of more than 8 cm, usually in children under the age of ten years; (5) severe infection within the area of surgery; (6) expansive implication of soft-tissue or muscle; (7) a biopsy that was performed in an inferior fashion or one with complications; and (8) a meager response to neoadjuvant chemotherapy.[26,29]

Radical resection with reconstruction

A radical resection with a reconstruction is a long process that will be unfamiliar to the patient and family. Therefore they must be provided a clear and concise picture of the surgery, postoperative management, and rehabilitation. Patients must be aware of the possibility of further surgeries for complications, including implant failure, infection, and the possible need for amputation. The postoperative course is directly related to the severity of the resection in terms of the amount of soft-tissue and bone involved. The management of physical therapy, mobility, the necessity for bracing equipment, and the progression of recovery depends on the individual surgery. Radical resections may involve the complete resection of major muscle groups, as well as reconstruction of a joint and soft tissue. Any limitation of motion, whether related to the surgery or to lack of resected tissue, must be dictated by the surgeon. Figure 44-5 demonstrates intraoperative placement of a megaprosthesis following resection of an osteosarcoma of the distal femur.

Radical reconstructive surgeries are lengthy procedures due to the extensive reconstruction of bone, connective tissue, and vascular structures. These complex procedures require an extensive perioperative period, which requires the patient to be under anesthesia for an extended period. Complications of these

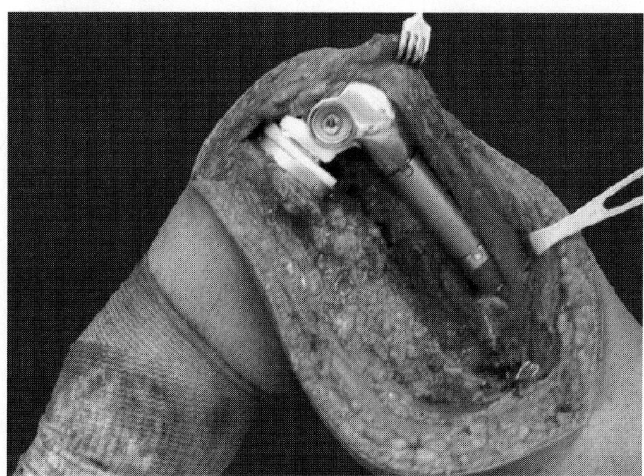

Figure 44-5 Megaprosthesis placement intraoperatively following the resection of osteosarcoma of the distal femur.

lengthy surgeries include pulmonary problems as well as possible venous stasis. Venous stasis may lead to deep vein thrombosis and pulmonary embolism. The physician may require the patient to wear sequential stockings and elastic antiembolic hose postoperatively. A low-molecular-weight heparin may also be initiated to prevent blood clots while the patient is hospitalized and warfarin for another six weeks after discharge. Pulmonary complications may involve atelectasis and related fevers, as well as pneumonia. These complications are often preventable if the healthcare team is vigilant in its baseline assessment and follow-up care. Pulmonary toilet must be stressed to the patient to facilitate the healing process. An ongoing assessment by the physician as well as the nurse and physical therapist is critical to evaluate the progress of motor function and any changes in sensation of the operative limb. The nature of the reconstruction may alter or damage the neurovascular structures, and it is imperative to observe the patient for any changes, positive or negative.

Lengthy surgeries may also result in extensive blood loss, which may lead to anemia. Patients with anemia will need blood transfusions postoperatively to normalize their hematocrit. It is critical that these patients have the stamina to participate in physical therapy and rehabilitation in a productive manner. Oncology patients, by nature of their illness, are unable to donate autologous blood. Patients may choose to have their family and friends donate blood or to utilize the hospital's blood bank program. Orthopedic oncology surgeries may require 2 to 6 units of blood, as well as fresh frozen plasma in some cases. Ferrous sulfate may be requested to help increase red blood cells. These patients may also have had neoadjuvant chemotherapy, which affects their healing and laboratory values. It is very important to observe for low hematocrit and infection, both of which are complications that may be evident after chemotherapy and extensive surgery. In addition, radical reconstructive surgeries may involve the resection of extensive amounts of bone and soft-tissue, which may leave large deficits in the operative field. Drainage tubes are placed during surgery to prevent seromas and hematomas, which may lead to complications such as infection. These tubes are left in place until the drainage is minimal. While these drainage tubes are intact, an antibiotic is administered to prevent infection complications.

Radical reconstructive surgeries may involve restrictions involving the position of the affected limb; these may include flexion, elevation of the limb, and precautions about extending the limb and using it to bear weight. These are all determined by the surgeon, with the goal of optimal function of the surgical limb. These precautions vary with the nature of the surgery and the extent of the resection. Pain management for the patient is handled by the pain service team, if available, and the orthopedic team. Surgical pain is managed by an epidural, patient-controlled analgesic pump, peripheral nerve sheath catheter, or a combination of these. As the pain decreases, the intravenous narcotics are withheld and oral narcotics are initiated. When the pain is under control with the oral medications, the intravenous medications, epidural, or nerve sheath catheter is discontinued. Patients are discharged to rehabilitation or to their homes with oral medications prescribed. Patients may also experience nerve pain, which is managed in a different manner than surgical pain. Gabepentin and amitriptyline are medications used to control nerve pain; this includes phantom pain in amputees.

An essential member of the multidisciplinary team is the plastic surgeon. The treatment of the patient may include chemotherapy and/or radiation therapy. These modalities may lead to the complication of insufficient soft-tissue coverage due to wound necrosis or the resection of radiated tissue. The tibia is a common location for lower-extremity sarcomas. This location has been particularly problematic due to poor soft-tissue coverage. Wound necrosis and infection can occur in the flaps used to close the surgical wound. This problem is exacerbated by irradiated skin, which is more fragile than healthy tissue. Plastic surgeons utilize local or free muscle flaps and split-thickness skin grafts to provide adequate soft-tissue coverage.

Surgical procedures are often performed in stages, with the soft-tissue coverage occurring two to three days after the initial surgery. A wound vacuum may be used to granulate the tissue before the grafts are secured. Figure 44-6A shows the shoulder at the time of excision; in 44-6B a skin graft is applied over the defect. Figure 44-6C shows the healing of the skin graft.

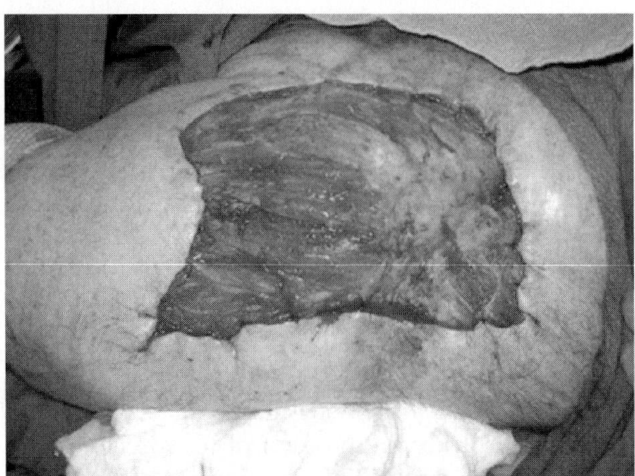

Figure 44-6A Shoulder with a soft-tissue mass excision.

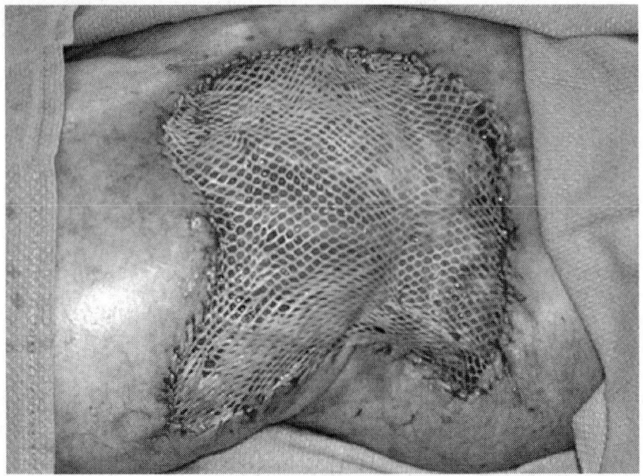

Figure 44-6B Skin graft covering the surgical defect after the excision.

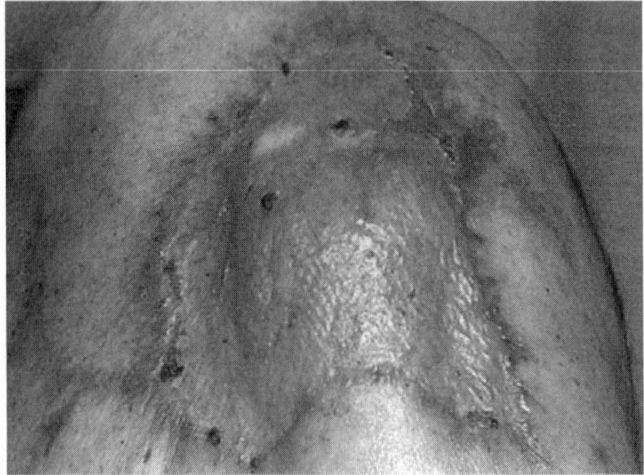

Figure 44-6C Skin graft healing.

Wound care is managed by the plastic surgeon. Complications may include wound necrosis, infection, seromas, and hematomas. Due to preoperative radiation therapy and neoadjuvant chemotherapy used in the treatment of sarcomas, wound infection is a prime concern of the surgeon. These therapies compromise the immunity of the patient, which may in turn lead to a wound infection. Metallic implants and allografts are used to replace the bone and joint that have been resected to remove the tumor. Deep infections following these surgeries may require the removal of the metallic hardware and possibly an amputation if the infection cannot be treated. If the infection can be identified and treated, antibiotic treatment is initiated. Intravenous antibiotic therapy usually is conducted for at least six weeks and as long as a year or more. Additional surgeries may include irrigation and debridement of the affected limb and may be performed in stages. It is critical that the patient be educated to watch for the signs and symptoms of infection and to report these immediately to the physician.

The primary goal of the orthopedic surgeon is to preserve life, and the next goal is to preserve the affected limb. Preoperative education concerning the functional independence of the patient is critical. Physical and occupational therapists, as well as prosthetists and orthotists, are instrumental in the rehabilitation of the surgical oncology patient. Social workers, psychologists, and possibly support groups can contribute to the patient's emotional growth and well-being. A patient's needs after surgery vary greatly with the type and extent of the surgical procedure. The patient may need braces and assistive walking devices, which may be permanent or temporary, and shoe lifts to compensate for discrepancies in limb length.

The reconstruction of a limb may involve an arthroplasty, which utilizes allografts and metal implants that replace the bone and the involved joint.[29] The allograft, which is procured from deceased donors, is selected by the surgeon according to the dimensions of the resected bone that it is to replace. The prosthesis is cemented, which permits a speedier rehabilitation and recovery. Complications include implant fracture and loosening, infection, and nonunion. This option does not permit the patient to engage in repetitive activities such as jogging, due to the artificial joint. Intercalary allograft reconstruction is another method that surgeons utilize. These allografts are secured with plates and screws, which ensure the stability of the reconstruction.

The third most utilized method of reconstruction is the arthrodesis or fusion. It provides a stable and durable joint, but one that is stiff. This surgical option is achieved with the use of an intercalary allograft, metallic implants, and possibly hardware to stabilize the joint. It is an excellent option for geriatric patients due to a lower expenditure of energy necessary for gait. Complications include nonunion and infection.

Nursing care for these surgeries, which can be varied, does have some standards of care. The assessment of neurovascular function in a reconstructed limb is of the utmost importance. Nerves may be sacrificed during the tumor resection. Patients must be aware of the possibility of insensate areas that may or may not be permanent. The patient may also experience referred pain or sensation related to transposed muscle in flaps. The viability of resected tissues must be constantly monitored to assess for wound necrosis and infection. Radical resections may make patients prone to hematomas and seromas, which could lead to infection. This infection could lead to further surgeries, including amputation. Another consideration with respect to surgical wound healing is the resumption of chemotherapy and radiation therapy. The surgeon has the final say as to when a wound is ready for radiation and chemotherapy. Follow-up appointments with the orthopedic oncology surgeon include possible serial plain x-rays to evaluate bone healing, wound evaluation and staple removal, and the progression of physical or occupational therapies.

Rotationplasty

Children present a challenging dilemma to the surgeon. Due to the fact that children are skeletally immature, surgery options for them are unique. One option is the Van Nes rotationplasty.[30] Rotationplasties in the lower extremities were first utilized in the treatment of infections and then with congenital deformities. The rotationplasty demands special planning and preparation by the entire surgical team. The first step is to fully educate the patient and family about all the options available to the patient; these include amputation or the use of an expandable prosthesis. One valuable mode of education is the use of videos to show other patients who have had the surgery and how they have adapted to everyday life. This is especially critical to young patients who still have the desire to have a more active lifestyle. The optimal educational tool is to have the patient personally meet other rotationplasty patients. This meeting allows a question-and-answer exchange that may help to put many concerns to rest. The patient is able to view firsthand how a prosthesis will fit and how well he or she will ambulate.

When the patient and family have made a firm decision to have the rotationplasty, the intensive planning begins. The surgical team must calculate the length of both lower limbs; this measurement is essential to ensure minimal length discrepancy. The child's age must be added to the equation; this varies with the amount of growth remaining. Another consideration by the surgeon is that the sciatic nerve must be salvageable. Vascular structures are preserved and coiled, but can be reconstructed if necessary. After a transtibial

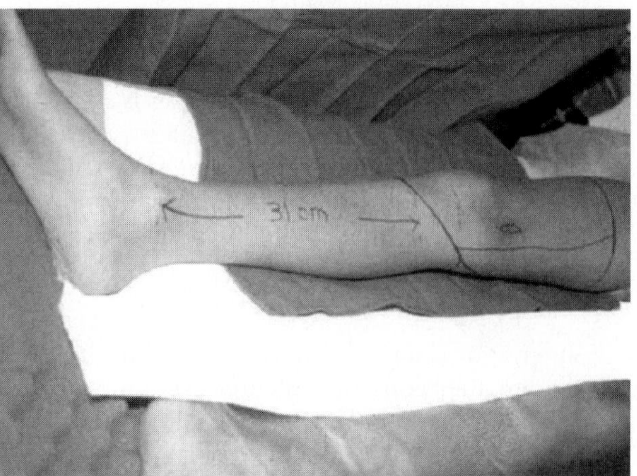

Figure 44-7 Incision planning for a rotationplasty.

and transfemoral incision is made, the soft-tissues are resected, maintaining the neurovascular bundle. Figure 44-7 shows the incision sites for a rotationplasty.

The malignant tumor in the distal femur and proximal tibia is removed by means of an osteotomy, and the tibia rotated 180 degrees. The calculations previously made by the surgeons become critical to ensure that the rotated ankle is at a similar level as the contralateral knee.[29] The rotated ankle now becomes the new knee joint, which in time will support a prosthesis. The osteotomy is secured with a compression plate and screws, aligning the distal femur to the proximal tibia.[2] Bone graft may also be used where the bones are aligned to aid the healing process. Postoperatively, the patient is placed in a spica cast to ensure stabilization of the mending bones. The healing of the bones is monitored with serial radiographs and takes about 12 weeks. After the surgeon is assured that the bone is sufficiently healed, a below-the-knee prosthesis is fitted and the long rehabilitation begins. Complications of this procedure include infection, nonunion, postoperative vascular occlusions, tibial to femur pseudarthrosis, and nerve palsies or osteopenia related to prolonged inability to bear weight on the leg.[31] Most patients have an excellent outcome with a very good level of function. In spite of the unusual appearance of the rotated limb, the patients are able to lead an active life. Extended follow-up studies show very good durability of the rotationplasty and good to excellent results after eight years.[30]

Expandable prosthesis

One challenge that the pediatric patient presents is that growth is still an ongoing process. To compensate for the length discrepancy between the operative and nonoperative limb, the expandable prosthesis was developed. One type of expandable prosthesis is the Lewis Expandable Adjustable Prosthesis (LEAP).[32]

The lengthening process is accomplished in steps; the average lengthening is 1.5 to 2 cm. The technology needed to perfect this type of prosthesis is still evolving. This surgery has many disadvantages, including the need for multiple surgeries, loosening or failure of the prosthesis, collapse of the prosthesis, nerve palsy, flexion contractures, and a lengthy rehabilitation.[2,26]

Allografts

Allograft or cadaver bone is harvested in the operating room after consent is secured from the donor's family, just as organ donation is obtained. Tissue banks, under the American Association of Tissue Banks, have aggressively pursued bone donations.[2] These allografts are procured in all sizes; skeletal reconstruction demands large as well as smaller allografts. Donors are carefully screened with a multitude of serologic tests that screen for most viral agents. This screening is done according to current blood bank parameters. The one additional test used to screen allografts is the polymerase chain reaction, which is used to detect the AIDS virus. This test is an added safety test that is not included in a routine antibody screen. Tissue banks irradiate the procured grafts with low-dose radiation, which decreases the bacteria of the grafts. Viruses are not eliminated by this process, but they are significantly reduced. HIV transmission is approximately the same in allografts as in blood: about one in every half-million units of blood.[2] Allografts are not tissue typed and have a very low rejection rate.

Allografts, by nature of the availability of various sizes, are very adaptable to the needs of the tumor surgeon. The surgeon must determine the strength and size needed for the bone replacement. Freeze-drying of the bone, as well as irradiation, affects the overall strength and torsion strength to some degree. The function of allografts is to heal the bone graft by the host bone to incorporate both bone elements into one union. The surgeon may use the allograft as an intercalary graft, which is secured between two sections of host bone by metallic screws and plates. These sections eventually heal to the allograft to form one contiguous bone. Studies involving the allograft replacement of long bones have met with encouraging results.[33–35]

Patients who have had a metallic implant as well as allograft surgery have similar restrictions. Weight-bearing restrictions are surgery specific, but the ability to bear weight is limited, and the surgery eliminates the possibility of high-impact exercise. During the healing period, the patient's mobility may be limited by a specialty brace or a cast. This healing process may take as long as a year. The complications of both procedures include infection, nonunion, and fracture at the site of the allograft. The reported incidence of infection is approximately 1 in 20 cases.[36–39] Oncology patients who must undergo chemotherapy may take longer to heal and have an increased risk of complications. Chemotherapy may lead to increases in infection and wound-healing problems, but the use of allografts is a promising alternative in tumor surgery.

Radical resection without reconstruction

Sarcomas in bones that are not essential for structure or stability are resected without the necessity of reconstruction. These bones include the clavicle, areas of the pelvis, and the fibula. The difference between this type of resection surgery and surgery with reconstruction is that nonreconstructive surgery lacks implants. The concern for infection is therefore less, as are other considerations related to implant surgery.

One difference between amputation and limb salvage is the difference in gait. Gait analysis is measured by the level of oxygen consumption during ambulation and the amount of muscle strength. Studies have shown that patients who have had limb salvage surgery involving the knee have a lower expenditure of energy than do patients with amputations.[40] Another consideration is the rate of complications in limb-sparing surgeries as opposed to amputation. One study found that complications occur in limb-sparing surgeries three to four times more often than in amputations.[41] Limb-sparing surgeries may eventually lead to amputation, if the complications are significant.

Amputation

Once a patient has been diagnosed and staged, the decision is made with the patient as to which type of surgical intervention should be performed. The decision to undergo an amputation is an extremely difficult one. The patient is faced with the prospect of possible death, disability, and body image disturbance, which is defined as a negative perception of oneself, making healthy function problematic.[39] The decision is irreversible and may affect the patient's ability to earn a living and to interact socially or to engage in recreational activities. Many patients may have problems with depression, anxiety, and low self-esteem. It is important to address these prospective problems before the day of surgery. Amputation must be viewed as an option and not as a failure; it is often the best choice when the involved limb would be flaccid or nonfunctioning if it was salvaged.[29]

When amputation is the surgical choice, the goal is to achieve wide margins in the surgical resection and to reconstruct the residual limb to provide optimal function. Amputation in a lower extremity is performed in one of five ways; transtibial amputation (below the knee amputation, or BKA), knee disarticulation, transfemoral amputation (above the knee amputation, or AKA), hemipelvectomy, and hip disarticulation. The bulk of amputations are of the AKA variety, due to the predilection of bone sarcomas for the distal femur.[29] Function is a prime concern in surgery, and the lower the amputation, the better the limb function; therefore, transtibial amputations have a better functional outcome than transfemoral amputations.[42–46]

Patients who must undergo a hemipelvectomy for tumors of the pelvis have special concerns regarding basic function, ambulation, and physical and emotional issues. Surgery varies from an internal hemipelvectomy, or partially resected pelvis, to a radical hemipelvectomy. These surgeries can produce a significant disability to the patient with regard to joint stability and compromised hip function. They present a special challenge to the prosthetist with regard to creating a prosthesis or a customized hip brace. Prosthetic devices have improved dramatically in both appearance and function. It is important that the patient meet with his or her prospective prosthetist before surgery. It is also beneficial for the patient to meet other patients with a similar amputation who have learned to cope with the challenges involved. Personal concerns regarding sexual adequacy and function must also be addressed. The age of the patient and the type of surgery will affect sexual function, as will nerve damage or resection. The alteration of the blood supply during surgery may also affect function, if only temporarily. Pregnancy and a vaginal delivery are possible after a hemipelvectomy, but the patient will not be able to use her prosthesis during pregnancy due to increased edema. Her gait and balance will also be altered due to her increasing girth. It is important that the patient discuss any concerns with regard to prospective pregnancies with her obstetrician.

A prosthesis can be a costly undertaking. Children constantly need their prostheses revamped due to growth. Many patients wish to return to the very active lifestyle that they enjoyed prior to their surgery. Patients must understand their limitations and use any adaptive devices that may make their lives as active as possible. Many amputees enjoy downhill skiing, cycling, basketball, soccer, and even karate with their prosthesis or a specialized recreational prosthesis. The range of recreational sporting activities enjoyed by amputees is growing. More than 20,000 amputees now participate in sporting activities, and more than 5000 participate in organized competition.[47] An amputation provides a special challenge to the elderly because of decreased strength and possible associated medical conditions. These patients may need to use adaptive devices, such as canes or walkers and even wheelchairs on a regular basis.

The social worker who is involved with the oncology group can provide the patient with answers regarding financial resources, rehabilitation programs, and support groups. Examples of these support groups include associations such as the American Cancer Society and the American Handicapped Association.

Rehabilitation is a crucial piece in the patient's recovery and return to a fulfilling and productive life. Physical and occupational therapy is a long process, requiring extensive physical energy, dedication, and a positive attitude. The patient must be certain to keep the avenues of communication open with all of the professionals involved in his or her care. Progress in rehabilitation depends on a prosthesis that is comfortable and on having enough physical reserves to participate in a demanding physical therapy program. A patient who has undergone chemotherapy or is still receiving therapy must relay any physical problems to his or her medical oncologist so that they can be addressed.

Phantom limb phenomenon. Patients who are scheduled for an amputation must be educated about phantom limb sensation and pain. This phenomenon is caused by the nerve pathway that has been transected during surgery. This transection results in the transmission of abnormal impulses. Patients may feel pain, burning, itching, cramping, and throbbing sensations in the limb that has been amputated. This is a strange and somewhat disconcerting experience that may occur approximately one to four weeks postoperatively. Phantom pain usually decreases substantially during the first year; however, some patients are troubled with it for years.[29] Any pain must be evaluated to differentiate between phantom pain and a possible neuroma, which is a possible complication of surgery. Phantom sensation can be exacerbated by stress, fatigue, and emotional stressors. It is managed in a variety of ways, including with a variety of medications. Gabapentin, which is an antiseizure medication, is prescribed postoperatively. Muscle relaxants and tranquilizers have also been used. Chronic pain specialists may be consulted to manage any ongoing problems. At times, simple measures such as the use of a stump shrinker, which exerts pressure; heat packs; or distraction measures may reduce or eliminate the problem. If the problem cannot be resolved, additional surgery may be warranted. The stump may need revision or possibly a higher-level amputation.

Amputation of the lower extremity. During the preoperative visit, the patient is told what to expect after surgery. Patients who are having a hemipelvectomy must have a bowel preparation to thoroughly clean the bowel to prevent contamination during surgery.

Patients will have a urethral catheter placed to measure urine output. Pain will be managed with an epidural, patient-controlled analgesic pump, peripheral nerve sheath catheter, or a combination of these methods. Compressive embolic devices, antiembolic stockings, and prophylactic anticoagulants are utilized postoperatively. Hospital beds should be equipped with a trapeze to aid the patient with mobility and strengthening in preparation for the use of crutches or a walker.

Prosthetic fitting may take place immediately postoperatively or may be delayed. The immediate postoperative fitting uses a fixed dressing and a cast. This type of prosthesis is utilized with younger, healthier patients, not the elderly or vascularly impaired patient. A pylon prosthesis is attached to the molded cast to provide stump shaping with appropriate compression.

If a delayed prosthesis is chosen as the better option, the patient will emerge from surgery with a compressive dressing and an Ace elastic wrap. The residual limb is kept wrapped and the patient is taught how to care for the limb until the postoperative edema has decreased. An early postsurgical fitting takes place three to six weeks after surgery, and the patient works with a physical therapist who will help with gait training. A permanent prosthesis is fitted approximately three months after surgery, if there are no postoperative complications. A prosthesis may need adjustment related to ongoing chemotherapy, which may affect the residual stump size; to weight gain or loss; or to other health-related problems.

Each type of prosthesis, immediate and delayed, has advantages and disadvantages. Postoperatively, the stump needs careful assessment related to neurovascular function and possible infection. It needs to be elevated to curtail edema and to encourage venous return. Care must be taken to prevent contractures of the hip. This is done by encouraging the patient to lie prone every six to eight hours and to sleep in this position. Physical therapy can encourage muscle tone, reduce edema, and strengthen the affected limb as well as the upper extremities for ambulation and can encourage range of motion of the hip and knee, if applicable.

Care of the amputated limb involves wrapping the stump with an Ace wrap or using an elastic stump shrinker to mold the stump and control edema. Physical therapists will work on the first day postoperatively to help the patient sit on the side of the bed and possibly stand with the aid of a walker or crutches and transfer to a chair. Patients who have had the more radical hemipelvectomy usually work with physical therapists on the third day after surgery, or earlier if the patient is progressing well. Hospital stays vary depending on the nature of the surgery, generally two days for BKA surgery, three days for AKA surgery, and five days for hip disarticulations and hemipelvectomy. These are estimates and are based on there being no postoperative complications.

Pelvic resections are divided into four different types. Type I includes the ilium, type II the acetabulum, type III the ischium, and type IV the sacrum. These types may be combined and in such cases are identified by both numbers. The resection of the pelvis is a challenge to the prosthetist due to the removal of the ischium, which is necessary for sitting balance. A patient who has undergone a hemipelvectomy must have a bucket prosthesis fashioned. This allows the patient to sit more comfortably without exerting undue pressure on the surgical region. Until the prosthesis is made, the surgical region is elevated with pillows or other nonirritating padding. Adults often do not use a prosthesis for ambulating but will wear one for cosmetic reasons. Children and more active younger adults are more likely to use a prosthesis. Care should be taken to encourage patients to take advantage of a prosthesis, if they are able to use one.[2]

The optimal progression of care after an amputation and hospital stay is for the patient to go to a rehabilitation hospital. The main focus of the rehabilitation stay is on mobility, to prevent complications that may develop with prolonged bed rest, such as deep vein thrombosis and muscle atrophy. Intensive education and training regarding gait, transfers, maneuvering stairs, muscle strengthening, and range of motion are all included in the postoperative period. Depending on the type of surgery, a patient may have special restrictions or a brace that requires special training for the activities of daily life. This training helps ensure that the patient adheres to all prescribed restrictions while taking care of daily activities. It also provides the opportunity to procure equipment that may be needed at home or at the patient's place of work. The return to work and to a more stable financial future provides a great incentive for the patient. This equipment may include environmental adaptive devices such as ramps, grab bars, elevated commode seats, and bathtub seats to ensure patient safety.[8]

Patients must also be taught to care for the stump. They must be taught to wash the stump with mild soap and water and to inspect the area for problems. Skin irritations, blisters, or abrasions could delay the wearing of the prosthesis. Patients need to avoid alcohol, which is drying, and skin creams or oil. Elastic wraps or stump socks should be fitted to ensure proper compression and should be changed daily. Patients need to be instructed in the importance of keeping edema at a minimum by wearing their prosthesis as soon as they rise in the morning. They will gradually increase their wearing time, which will also help keep edema at a minimum. During their hospital stay, patients should also be instructed in how to care for a prosthesis if it is an immediate rather than delayed one. Any malfunctions or discomfort in the prosthesis should be reported to the prosthetist, who should make any necessary adjustments. A patient's prosthesis is ordered via a prescription from the physician to the prosthetist. The prosthetist evaluates the patient physically and determines the patient's expectations regarding lifestyle needs. It is important to have a prosthetist who is certified by the American Board for Certification of Prosthetists to ensure optimal treatment. Prosthesis fitting is a dynamic endeavor that may need periodic adjustments. A lower-extremity prostheses has components that usually consist of a socket, knee joint, ankle joint, and various suspension systems. These suspension systems may involve a waistband and latex or suction sleeves that cover the stump sock. A wide variety of components provide the patient with many options. Gait is a very important element in the construction of the prosthesis. Mechanical or hydraulic knee joints control the elements of walking and ensure standing stability. A variety of prosthetic feet are available that aid in a smoother gait. The prosthesis is assembled and adjusted to fit the patient and to ensure as smooth a gait as possible. These various components may add additional weight, be costly, and increase maintenance problems. Careful thought must be given to the design and construction of the prosthesis. Variables include the patient's age, physical health, occupation, financial considerations, comfort, fit, alignment, appearance, and the user-friendliness of the prosthesis. This information is gathered by the healthcare professional, patient, and prosthetist.

Patients should be made aware of other outpatient programs that may prevent or improve some chronic problems, such as lymphedema and soft-tissue and joint contractures. Patients who are troubled with chronic pain should be evaluated and treated by pain management specialists. Other issues that may be addressed include scar massage, special exercises focusing on flexibility and endurance, and the protection and assessment of insensate skin. The final intervention may include counseling to cope with the patient's new lifestyle and necessary adaptations.

Rehabilitation is a long process, and it may take many months for the patient to complete physical therapy, prosthesis adjustment, and other medical treatments so that he or she can declare independence and satisfaction with his or her new body.

Amputation of the upper extremity. The patient who is about to undergo an upper-extremity amputation faces many of the same concerns as a lower-extremity amputee; however, the psychological impact of losing an arm is greater than that of losing part of a lower extremity. Preoperative and postoperative guidelines are similar, but the rehabilitation process presents some additional considerations. Lower-limb prostheses are far superior to those available for the upper-extremity amputee. Positive outcomes are directly influenced by the level of amputation necessary to resect the tumor with adequate margins. It is critical to retain adequate soft-tissue coverage and stump length. The primary concern is to eradicate the tumor and then to provide a stump that is sufficient in length to accommodate a prosthesis. A prosthesis with a longer stump has better function than one with a shorter stump.

Body-powered components use the mechanical transmission of muscular exertion (myoelectric transmission) that originates from another area of the body, not the amputation site. An active muscle provides a small amount of electrical potential, which acts as the source of control. This potential is electronically processed and is used to start the controller that sends power to the electric motor. This motor drives the prosthetic device. Electrodes on the surface of the body are used to pick up the electrical signal. These electrodes must be worn daily and for extended periods of time, meaning that the patient must be able to tolerate these electrodes without irritation. Testing is performed on the patient to evaluate the ability to produce and control myoelectric signals. Externally powered components use battery-powered electronic devices when the use of body power is not feasible or the power is insufficient. These units provide the best cosmetic appearance with less energy depletion, but they tend to be costly. Other problems pertain to electrical interference and involuntary muscle contractions (coughing, sneezing, or stretching) that interfere with function.

Although upper-extremity prostheses are improving with regard to function and appearance, lower-extremity prostheses are still superior. Function is often sacrificed for cosmesics, and vice versa. It is crucial that patients have all their questions answered and have the opportunity to see what options are available to them. Prosthetic rehabilitation is a long process, and it is important for the patient to understand what is involved. Questions are best addressed by a certified prosthetist, who can show the patient different options and explain their advantages and disadvantages.

Upper-extremity amputations are very similar to lower-extremity amputations with regard to postoperative care. The prosthesis can be applied directly after the amputation (immediate) or as a delayed procedure. Stump care is the same as in a lower-extremity amputation, including compression and a soft dressing with an elastic bandage. The postoperative hospital stay depends on any complications and the age and medical condition of the patient, but is usually one to two days. Home nursing may be needed for stump care, assessment, and occupational therapy for activities of daily living. The patient will also need vocational rehabilitation, which is usually a community resource, for possible employment changes or adjustments.

Soft-Tissue Surgery

Dramatic strides have been made in the treatment of soft-tissue sarcomas. Advances in imaging and meticulous biopsy techniques have improved the diagnostic process. MRIs are the preferred modality for imaging soft-tissue sarcomas. The treatments for soft-tissue sarcomas include adjuvant radiation therapy, surgery, brachytherapy, postoperative radiation, neoadjuvant chemotherapy, and adjuvant chemotherapy. These techniques are used in combination; not all treatments are necessarily effective with all soft-tissue sarcomas. As a rule, large, deep soft-tissue masses have a poorer prognosis.[17,22] This is due in part to the compromise of neurovascular structures and the ability of the mass to cause more harm with its increasing size.

The goal of the orthopedic surgeon is to resect the soft-tissue tumor with a clear margin of tissue and to save and protect the surrounding tissue from contamination. Function of the limb is protected, but not at the expense of the patient's survival. The resection of a large portion of a major muscle group is not uncommon to achieve tumor-free margins. Large tumors demand a sizable resection, which leaves a huge defect. The defect may need coverage by a plastic surgeon after the resection of the tumor. If the margins of the resection are suspect, brachytherapy may be used to eradicate the remaining tumor.

The biopsy is a crucial element in the diagnosis of a soft-tissue mass. A poorly placed biopsy, with inadequate hemostasis, will cause a larger excision and a more extensive defect. The diagnostic process is also crucial and, together with the biopsy, may mean the difference between a functioning limb and one that is suboptimal.

Metastatic Sarcoma

Metastatic disease is the spread or dissemination of cells from a primary tumor to local tissues through local blood vessels. The tumor cells are spread through the vascular and lymphatic systems. The cells then lodge in distant organs and bones, where they must establish a blood supply to survive. These cells must undergo numerous mutations to survive and then thrive.

Bone and soft-tissue sarcomas have a predilection for the pulmonary system as a site of metastasis. Seventy-five percent of the sarcoma patients who develop metastasis have pulmonary metastasis. This occurrence may be explained by the systemic venous circulation that carries the tumor cells.[2]

Pulmonary metastasis is managed by surgery or multiagent chemotherapy. Approximately 20% of patients who initially present with a high-grade bone or soft-tissue sarcoma have metastatic pulmonary disease. The prognosis for these patients is very poor if not treated. Untreated patients usually die within 18 months. Surgical management consists of a wedge resection or a video-assisted thoracic surgery (VATS). The cardiothoracic surgeon reviews the CT scan of the chest to determine whether surgery is a viable alternative and to decide which procedure is indicated. Another very critical factor is the control of the primary tumor. If the pulmonary surgery is to be effective, the primary tumor must be under control before the pulmonary nodules are resected. During surgery, the lungs are salvaged and the nodules resected. Patients who have pulmonary metastatic disease that has been successfully resected have a more promising survival rate at five years.[38]

Patients with bone and soft-tissue sarcomas have a CT scan at the initial staging and then every three months for the first two years. Musculoskeletal radiologists compared the scans to evaluate for metastatic disease and to follow the lesions that are less than 5 mm. These lesions are considered nonspecific until they are larger than 5 mm and deemed unresectable. Biopsies are performed only if these small lesions increase in size or multiply. Sarcomas that have a low potential for pulmonary metastasis are followed with plain chest x-rays instead of the more costly CT scan.

Radiotherapy

Radiation therapy is based on the premise that radiation will interfere with the tumor cells. The dosage of radiation must be sufficient to kill a significant number of cells and not permit the cells to repair. High doses can cause severe injury to normal, healthy tissue and are unlikely to produce tumor control. A balance must be sought to maintain healthy tissue and at the same time destroy malignant tissue. High-dose treatment has proved less effective than fractionated small-dose treatment. The notion of fractionation is based on the four Rs of radiobiology: repair, repopulation, redistribution, and reoxygenation (see Table 44-3).[48]

Table 44-3 Radiobiology Fractionation

Repair	Repopulation	Redistribution	Reoxygenation
Recovery of normal cells before the next dose; prevent the repair of malignant cells	Replacement of the killed cells by the surviving cells through growth and division; repopulation determines the radiosensitivity of some tissues	Radiation kill is more effective during certain phases of the cell cycle; redistribution is more effective on malignant cells than on normal cells	Well-oxygenated cells are more susceptible to radiation; hypoxic tumor cells can become reoxygenated between treatments

Treatment consists of an initial consultation, simulation, and the actual treatment.

Radiation therapy has its limits: malignant bone sarcomas are less responsive to it than are soft-tissue sarcomas. Radiation therapy is used in the palliative treatment of metastatic bone tumors. It is also used in conjunction with both surgery and chemotherapy. When used preoperatively, it is hoped that radiation will shrink the tumor bulk, preserve neurovascular structures, and provide adequate surgical margins. This may determine whether the mass is resectable. Radiation therapy performed preoperatively has the highest wound-healing complication rate, approximately 30%.[49] These complications are site dependent; areas may become burned and infected, and tissue can become fibrotic. Surgery should be scheduled three to four weeks after radiation treatment is completed. This permits the healing of soft-tissue before surgery yet does not allow time for tissue to become fibrotic, which would make resecting the vessels and nerves adjacent to the tumor more difficult.

Soft-tissue tumors are far more radiosensitive than bone tumors. Ewing's sarcoma is the exception; it is susceptible to radiation, and radiation is often utilized in pelvic tumors that are not resectable. Due to necrosis, these tumors form a covering or rind that aids the surgeon in the resection. Radiation of tumors is diagnosis specific, and the efficacy of treatment depends on this diagnosis. Brachytherapy permits the delivery of localized high-dose radiation while protecting adjacent structures. Surgeons use brachytherapy to ensure the radiation of margins and nearby structures. This method is used in previously radiated sites, with positive results.[50] The advantages of brachytherapy are that the overall treatment time is short, the radiation is restricted to the smallest and most efficacious area, and the treatment is made to the affected area when it remains well oxygenated.[49]

Teletherapy or external beam radiation therapy (EBRT) is the most commonly used type of radiation therapy. It is used for curative as well as palliative treatment. Positioning of the patient is crucial for effective treatment. The patient feels no heat, pain, tingling, or burning during treatment. Any discomfort felt by the patient is due mostly to the positioning. The radiation oncologist checks the periodic beam radiographs against the original simulation radiographs to ensure accuracy. Studies have shown that adjuvant brachytherapy gives acceptable morbidity as well as local control similar to that of external beam radiation.[51] Table 44-4 summarizes types of radiation therapy used in sarcomas.

Nursing care of the patient who is undergoing radiation therapy is dependent on the type of therapy. A patient who is receiving brachytherapy must be isolated in a specially constructed room, and both staff and visitors must observe radiation precautions. Education of the patient and family is an important aspect of treatment. It is important to maintain these precautions without making the patient feel isolated and alone. The side effects of radiation should be discussed with the patient before the start of therapy. Patients have varying degrees of side effects, especially skin reactions. These include itching, erythema, dryness, wet desquamation (similar to a second-degree burn), rash, loss of hair, radiation-induced necrosis, and general discomfort.[51,52] Post-therapy skin care must also be reviewed with the patient. The patient must protect his or her skin from sunlight; wear loose-fitting clothing; avoid alcohol, which is drying to the skin; use mild soap and water and a water-soluble moisturizer; and avoid cornstarch powder, which provides

Table 44-4 Types of Radiation Therapy Used in Sarcomas

Teletherapy/External Beam Radiation Therapy/EBRT	Brachytherapy/Internal Radiation
Beam of ionizing radiation from an external source Fixed source at a distance from the patient, with a designated target Palliative course is a lower dose and for a shorter period Curative treatment uses a maximum dose over a longer period 5- to 8-week treatment period	Source of radiation is on the body or placed at the time of surgery in the tumor bed Trocars are placed during surgery and radioactive wires inserted through the trocars after surgery Designated target for predetermined time period Wires are removed after surgery

Data from Alektiar et al.[51]

an excellent medium for fungus. The skin condition must be evaluated by the surgeon before the tumor can be resected. There is usually a three- to four- week hiatus between radiation therapy and surgery, which allows the skin to heal.

Chemotherapy

Responses rates in bone and soft-tissue sarcomas have shown marked improvement with the introduction of multiagent therapy instead of the use of a single agent. A careful balance between effectiveness and minimizing toxicity is the goal during treatment. Chemotherapy is administered intravenously; intraarterial dosing remains controversial. The duration of therapy ranges from 6 to 12 months, depending on the diagnosis and treatment plan. Protocols have been developed through careful monitoring of patients and their response to prescribed agents.

Neoadjuvant chemotherapy is given before surgery, with the desired effect of reducing tumor load and eliminating micrometastasis. If this goal is realized, limb salvage is more likely. After the prescribed cycles of neoadjuvant chemotherapy, new scans are taken to evaluate the effectiveness of the therapy. The definitive result of the chemotherapy cannot be evaluated until the tumor has been resected and the pathologist determines the extent of tumor kill.

Chemotherapy has proven effective in the treatment of osteosarcoma and Ewing's sarcoma, but not chondrosarcoma. The use of chemotherapy in soft-tissue sarcomas remains controversial, but it is sometimes done. The protocol used in soft-tissue sarcomas is known as MAID therapy. It consists of mesna (cystitis protectant), doxorubicin, ifosfamide, and dacarbazine. The Children's Oncology Group uses a multiagent chemotherapy, which is most frequently cisplatin, doxorubicin, high-dose methotrexate, and ifosfamide.[53]

The side effects of chemotherapy are far-reaching. Cells with a rapid turnover (skin, hair, mucous membranes, and hematopoietic stem cells) are affected. Skin reactions are usually temporary; erythema, pruritus, hyperpigmentation, photosensitivity, and dry desquamation are known side effects. Major side effects include immunosuppression (neutropenia), infection, thrombocytopenia, anemia, and renal and cardiac compromise. These conditions are all closely monitored, and doses may need to be adjusted. General physical well-being is also affected, with fatigue, constipation, and loss of appetite being reported.

Description of Selected Sarcomas

Osteosarcoma

Primary bone tumors are extremely rare. Osteosarcoma and Ewing's sarcoma are two of the most prevalent types that occur in the second decade of life.[3] Osteosarcoma has an annual incidence of 1000 new cases a year in the United States and 4.6 per million in Sweden (where records are better and more accurate). Ewing's sarcoma occurs at 0.8 per million.[54,55] A peak incidence occurs in the seventh decade, mostly associated with Paget's disease of the bone. The ratio of male to female incidence is approximately 3 to 2.

Presenting symptoms of osteosarcoma include pain related to strain and trauma, which is often what brings the patient to see the physician. Pain symptoms are evident at night in approximately 21% of the patients, and a palpable mass was found in about 39% of the patients in a study conducted in Sweden.[4] Patients with osteosarcoma who have a pathologic fracture at initial diagnosis have a decreased survival rate compared to patients without such a fracture.[56] Figure 44-8 depicts the destructive nature of osteosarcoma of the humerus.

The accepted definition of osteosarcoma is a malignant tumor originating from mesenchymal tissue that produces bone.[57] Osteosarcoma is a highly aggressive disease that rapidly metastasizes to distant sites. It is commonly found at the distal portion of long bones. In fact, the anatomic distribution of osteosarcoma has been reported in almost every skeletal bone. The preponderance, however is in the long tubular bones of the extremities, approximately 80% by report. Of these, 40% to 45% occur in the femur. The tibia is the second most affected site, with 15% to 20%. The humerus ranks third at approximately 10% to 15%.[2] This distribution shows a predominance of osteosarcomas in the metaphyseal portion of the long tubular bones.

Histologic patterns of osteosarcoma vary and are made up a variety of cells. Malignant cells produce osteoid and are mitotic. Some areas may exhibit tumor necrosis. Stroma in the background may exhibit a dominance of fibrous or chondroid tissue. Periosteal and parosteal osteosarcomas occur on the surface or juxtacortical surface of the bone. Parosteal lesions occur in the distal femoral metaphysis and appear on x-rays as radiodense lesions. These lesions have a predilection for females between 20 and 40 years of age.[3] These tumors are usually low grade and can be treated with surgery only and no chemotherapy. The long-term prognosis is very favorable, at 93%.[58] Periosteal osteosarcoma has been diagnosed as an intermediate-grade tumor with a preponderance for the diaphyseal portion of the tibia. The histiologic composition of the

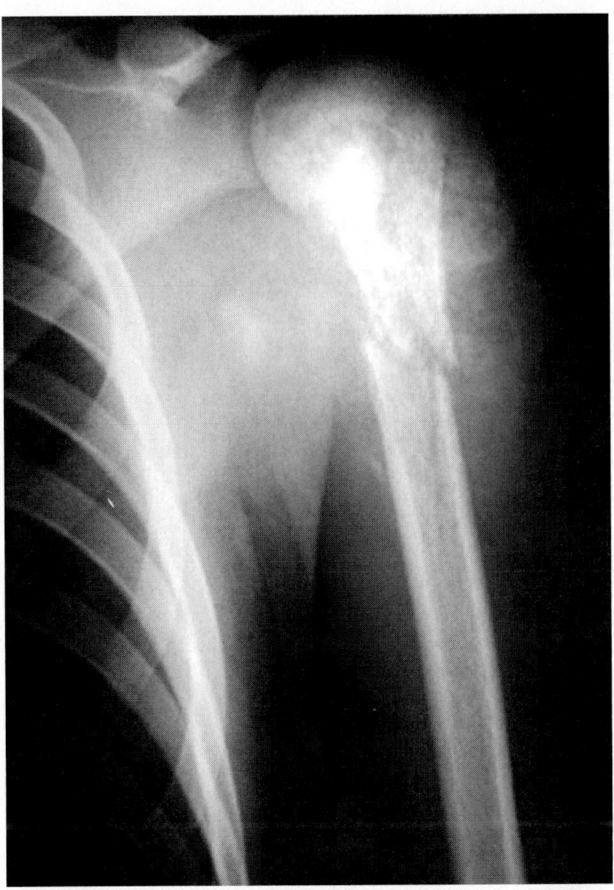

Figure 44-8 The destructive nature of osteosarcoma of the humerus is depicted on plain x-ray.

tumor is osteoid with a chondroid background.[3] Treatment usually consists of wide excision.[3]

Laboratory values have a very limited value in the diagnosis of osteosarcoma. Serum alkaline phosphatase, which measures osteoblastic activity, is elevated in some individuals with osteosarcoma. This level decreases postoperatively after the sarcoma resection. As a child matures and grows, these levels are normally elevated, so this laboratory value can be somewhat ambiguous. There does seem to be a correlation between patients who present with elevated serum alkaline phosphatase levels and a higher recurrence rate.[59]

Osteosarcoma metastasizes to the lungs more often than to any other site. Chest CT scans are therefore performed on a routine basis, usually every three months until five years after the initial diagnosis. The first two years are the critical period when lung metastatic disease usually occurs. Patients with osteosarcoma who have a pathologic fracture with their initial presentation or during chemotherapy have a decreased survival rate and an increased rate of local recurrence.[56] This factor must be evaluated with regard to limb salvage. Such factors as the patient's response to chemotherapy and whether the fracture has attained union are important in the patient's treatment plan.

Chemotherapy has proved an effective treatment, both preoperatively and postoperatively. After a preoperative chemotherapy regimen, surgery is performed and the tumor is evaluated for tumor kill, or tumor necrosis, which indicates the effectiveness of the chemotherapy. Tumor necrosis of 90% carries a better prognosis. The effectiveness of chemotherapy, the lack or presence of pulmonary metastasis, and the possibility of a pathological fracture are considerations for the surgeon when considering limb salvage versus amputation. Chemotherapy, if effective, can reduce the soft-tissue involvement of the tumor. It is also effective in destroying microscopic disease after the spread of tumor cells to the lungs. Chemotherapy may be important in treatment after lung resections for metastatic nodules.

The optimal treatment for osteosarcoma is preoperative or neoadjuvant chemotherapy, surgery, and then postoperative or adjuvant chemotherapy. Additional surgeries and alternative chemotherapy treatments are possible in the event of a recurrence. Radiation therapy is not a recognized treatment for osteosarcoma. It is only used in cases that present as inoperable. (See Table 44-5 for characteristics of common sarcomas.)

Chondrosarcoma

Chondrosarcoma is a malignant lesion composed of cartilage cells with a mesenchymal origin. This diagnosis is more prevalent in the middle decades of life. Histologically, the tumor appears very mitotic with plump nuclei and sheets of spindle cells that encompass lobules of chondroid.[60] It may arise from benign lesions that exist in the bones, from exostosis, and occasionally from an enchondroma. Tumors cells form cartilage cells that are of a higher cellularity and a greater pleomorphism than a benign chondroma. Nearly 75% of chondrosarcomas are primary lesions not associated with preexisting lesions, and 25% are secondary tumors, originating from benign preexisting cartilage lesions. Secondary tumors are related to diagnoses of Ollier's disease and Maffucci's syndrome, which are multiple enchondromatosis. An association exists between secondary tumors and multiple hereditary exostoses, Paget's disease, and fibrous dysplasia. Radiographically, the lesion is seen as a thick, irregular cartilage cap with an irregular pattern of mineralization. A cartilage cap thickness of more than 2 cm is considered a sign of malignancy in those patients with secondary exostoses.

Chondrosarcomas are also designated as central or peripheral. A central chondrosarcoma has its origin

Table 44-5 Characteristics of the Most Common Types of Sarcoma

	Osteosarcoma	Chondrosarcoma	Fibrosarcoma	Ewing's Sarcoma
Gender Predilection	Male 1.3 to 1 Female 1.7 to 1	Male 1.4 to 1	None	Male 1.3 to 1 Female 1.5 to 1
Symptoms	Pain, local soft-tissue edema (tumor extension through cortical bone destruction); soft-tissue masses may or may not be palpable (depending on location)	Pain, local tenderness, extraosseous soft-tissue mass, cortical destruction and calcification	Slow-growing, solitary mass, deep, ill-defined (3–8 cm)	Pain, edema, low-grade temperature, elevated ESR, anemia, elevated skin temperature, erythema; systemic symptoms mimic osteomyelitis (due to hemorrhage and tumor necrosis), venous dilation, palpable or tender mass
Location	Distal metaphyseal femur, bone surfaces, humerus, tibia	Pelvis, femur, hip girdle, shoulder girdle, ribs, sternum, craniofacial bones	Femur, tibia, humerus, radius, ulna, skull, facial bones, pelvic bones	Diaphyseal and metaphyseal long tubular bones, femur, tibia, fibula, pelvic girdle flat bones, ribs, scapula
Age	10 to 30 years	30 to 60 years	30 to 55 years	5 to 15 years
Radiographic Appearance	Soft tissue with mineral density, blastic on x-ray with bone destruction; skip lesions can occur in the same bone, matrix production, poor mineralization of bone lesion	Endosteal cortical erosion, thickening and expansion, soft tissue has popcorn-like calcifications	Radiolucent, permeative appearance on x-ray	Large soft-tissue mass, Codman's triangle (plain x-ray shows a trumpet-shaped area; elevated periosteum meets intact cortex at the apex; base of triangle is perpendicular to the shaft and mass is formed by tumor mass), motheaten appearance, little or no soft-tissue mineralization

within the medullary cavity of the bone. A peripheral chondrosarcoma originates on the outer surface of the bone cortex. The majority of primary chondrosarcomas, approximately 75%, are of the central variety. Secondary chondrosarcomas are classified mostly as peripheral tumors. Patients who present with a secondary chondrosarcoma have a significantly better survival rate than patients with a primary diagnosis.[60]

Chondrosarcoma occurs, in most cases, in the shoulder girdle, hip girdle, and trunk. The pelvis accounts for approximately 30%, of the reported cases, the femur about 20%, the shoulder girdle about 15%, and the ribs and sternum about 10%. The remaining cases are distributed among various bones.[2] The size of the tumor depends on the location; the pelvis has the largest tumors, which may grow for years before they are diagnosed. The grade is higher among the myxoid chondrosarcomas, dedifferentiated chondrosarcomas, and mesenchymal chondrosarcomas. There is a higher correlation between tumors with a higher grade and distant metastasis. In turn, distant metastasis increases the risk of death.

The treatment for chondrosarcoma is surgical resection, with the goal of adequate resection in conjunction with wide margins of normal tissue. Chemotherapy and radiation therapy used in the neoadjuvant or adjuvant mode have been shown to be ineffective.[61] These treatment modes are used only for patients with dedifferrentiated chondrosarcoma or mesenchymal chondrosarcoma, or in patients with a poor surgical outcome.

When a patient presents to the physician, it is usually with the complaint of pain, which may be intermittent and aching. Laboratory findings are usually normal, although occasionally the ESR may be elevated. All other lab values of serum and urine should present as normal. The physical examination may show subtle abnormalities, such as a mild antalgic gait and a possible decrease in the range of motion of adjacent joints. The affected extremity may also demonstrate mild atrophy.[62]

Primary central chondrosarcoma usually arises in the metaphysis, but it can also arise in the long bone diaphysis. Plain x-rays show bone destruction, with periosteal reaction and intralesional calcifications. Periosteal reaction is circumferential, and the cortex is thinned in an unequal fashion. CT scans are utilized to evaluate the intralesional calcifications. In a patient with a diagnosis of dedifferentiated chondrosarcoma, the aggressive nature of the disease is evident in the rapid rate of its growth and its destructive nature. An extraosseous portion of the tumor is often evident and can be detected by an MRI. MRIs are best for visualizing the intrameduallary portion of the tumor, which is evident on the T2-weighted image. It presents as a bright signal, which is the norm for cartilage.

Diagnosis can be established with a biopsy. When a definitive diagnosis is firmly established, surgery is the accepted form of treatment. Extremity chondrosarcomas that are central in nature are treated by wide resection and reconstruction if the cortex has not been breached. Limb salvage is a possibility if the neurovascular component is intact. Amputation is also an option if it would not be possible to reconstruct the extremity to provide a useful limb.

The five-year survival rate for pelvic chondrosarcoma has been shown to be approximately 65%, with a 54% survival at ten years. Chondrosarcoma of the entire skeleton is approximately 67%–79% at five years and 50%–66% at ten years.[60] Patients diagnosed with chondrosarcoma have a better prognosis than those with osteosarcoma.

Fibrosarcoma

Historically, fibrosarcoma has been one of the most common of the adult soft-tissue sarcomas. However, over the last 20 years, as diagnostic criteria have become more standardized, it has been replaced by malignant fibrous histiocytoma (MFH). The diagnosis of fibrosarcoma is now reserved for those tumors displaying the classic herringbone pattern of interlacing fascicles of spindle cells and not the whorled pattern of the more common MFH.

Ewing's Sarcoma

Ewing's sarcoma is the second most common primary malignant bone tumor in children. Approximately 10% of all primary bone tumors are the small, round-cell Ewing's sarcoma. Males under the age of 20 years account for a significant number of Ewing's sarcoma patients. This malignancy can occur in any bone, but the majority are in the lower extremities and the pelvic girdle.

Cytogenetic studies have made great strides in identifying an 11;22 translocation in 90% of the Ewing's sarcoma patients.[2,3] Patients present with pain, edema, or a palpable mass; a small number will also present with a fever, weight loss, or fatigue. Ewing's sarcoma is often mistaken for an infection; needle biopsy specimens will even have the appearance of pus. It is crucial to have a frozen section evaluated, as well as to test cultures for infection. Laboratory tests may show an elevated ESR or WBC. Specimens should be sent for cytogenetic and molecular studies to identify the t(11;22) translocation.

The radiographic appearance of Ewing's sarcoma demonstrates an extensive destructive bone lesion that includes the diaphyseal or metadiaphyseal section of the long tubular bone. An "onion skin" appearance on the periosteum is a common characteristic. There is often a soft-tissue component of varying size and extent. This component is best visualized with an MRI. Bone scans to evaluate the possibility of multiple sites, CT scans of the chest to evaluate for metastatic disease, and a bone marrow aspiration are all performed as part of the diagnostic process.

A microscopic examination of Ewing's sarcoma cells shows small, round cells that are uniform in appearance, with a sparse intercellular stroma. A chromatin pattern is also evident, but thin.

The treatment for Ewing's sarcoma includes chemotherapy, radiation, and possibly surgical resection, depending on the tumor location. The outcome of the operative treatment of Ewing's sarcoma that has not metastasized depends on the histologic response to preoperative chemotherapy and the size of the primary tumor. These outcomes should be used to identify patients who are at higher risk, so that they can look to a more aggressive approach or even clinical trials.[63] Neoadjuvant chemotherapy is used to address micrometastases in the lungs and bone and to shrink the tumor prior to surgery. Current studies in the administration of chemotherapeutic agents have focused on a more intensive therapy over a shorter period and on intensifying the alkylating agents (cyclophosphamide). The chemotherapeutic regimen includes vincristine, actinomycin D, cyclophosphamide, and doxorubicin. Ifosfamide and etoposide may also be added to increase the response rate to close to 50%.[64] The treatment course usually takes from six months to a year. Surgery and/or radiation are performed depending on the location of the tumor; pelvic tumors are often treated with chemotherapy and radiation only.

The 5% to 10% of patients who present with a pathologic fracture pose a unique dilemma: fracture hematoma. Fracture displacement may influence the possibility of limb-sparing surgery. Preoperative chemotherapy and the response of the tumor will be the determining factors in limb-sparing surgery for patients with pathologic fractures.

Ewing's sarcoma is extremely radiosensitive. Radiation therapy may be used in conjunction with chemotherapy as the only treatment. Doses of 45–60 Gy are used to shrink tumors. The higher doses may cause fibrosis of the soft-tissues and of the joints and may compromise pediatric growth plates. The combination of chemotherapy, radiation, and surgery with negative margins is the treatment used for cure. The patient who relapses is treated with an alkylating agent, ifosfamide, as a single-agent therapy. Currently, approximately 70% of Ewing's sarcoma patients are long-term survivors.[3]

Table 44-6 Bone Sarcoma Long-Term Follow-up

Initial staging	Physical exam	Plain x-ray	MRI and/or CT of affected area	Bone scan	CXR	Chest CT
2-year follow-up	Physical exam			Q 6 month		Q 3 month
2- to 5-year follow-up	Physical exam			Yearly	Q 3 months	Q 6 months alternate with CXR
5- to 10-year follow-up	Physical exam					Yearly

The treatment needed to provide a cure for Ewing's sarcoma involves a multidisciplinary approach; the orthopedic oncology surgeon, medical oncologist, and radiation oncologist are critical to the care of the patient (see Table 44-6).

Soft-Tissue Sarcomas

Classifications of soft-tissue sarcomas have been dramatically transformed in the last 30 years. These changes are due mainly to the use of the electron microscope, histologic analysis, and immunohistochemistry by the experienced pathologist.[40] The new classification system is based on the cell origin. The goal is to identify the patient population that may need more intensive therapy or less aggressive treatment. These finite classifications help to differentiate soft-tissue sarcomas with a low metastatic potential from those with a higher potential for metastasis.

One study looked at cases diagnosed between 1972 and 1994 and reviewed the pathology in accordance with the modern sarcoma classification system. The original recurrent diagnoses were malignant fibrous histiocytoma (MFH) at 26%, liposarcoma at 21%, fibrosarcoma at 11%, and leiomyosarcoma at 10%. The diagnoses using the new classification showed a dramatic swing in the proportions. Leiomyosarcomas increased to 20%, liposarcomas decreased to 17%, synovial sarcomas totaled 14%, and finally the sarcomas "not otherwise specified" (NOS) were at 11%. Of the original cases, 57% had a change in diagnosis. The diagnosis of fibrosarcoma decreased from 32 cases to 6, and the diagnosis of MFH was dramatically reduced from 72 cases to 2. The remaining cases included 22 that were renamed as myxofibrosarcomas, and another 20 (7%) were determined not to be sarcomas.[65] These changes were made due to advances in immunohistochemistry (IHC) in addition to the alterations in nonmenclature. The World Health Organization (WHO) published a classification of soft-tissue sarcomas in the fall of 2002.[66] This classification recognizes the inclusion of IHC in the diagnosis; in addition, molecular genetic results are often included.[65]

Patients with a soft-tissue mass present with a palpable mass but with little or no pain. Function of the affected area is usually not altered significantly. Benign soft-tissue masses outnumber sarcomas at a ratio of 100 to 1. One half of sarcomas are found in the extremities, with those in the lower extremities outnumbering those in the upper extremities. Soft-tissue sarcomas are also found in the retroperitoneum, head, and neck. Plain x-rays have little value in the diagnosis of soft-tissue sarcomas. Masses should be evaluated with a physical examination using percussion, which evaluates for a Tinel sign (a lesion that involves a nerve will cause a tingling sensation distally). Auscultation can assess for a bruit, which would indicate an aneurysm.[5] Ultrasound may be utilized to evaluate the depth and dimensions of the tumor and whether it is a solid mass or cystic. Bone scans are used to reveal bone metastasis. CT scans are used to provide the physician with information regarding the local extent of the tumor. They provide critical data with regard to adjacent anatomy, showing fat densities and cortical integrity of bone. MRIs are an excellent mode of imaging to demonstrate neurovascular involvement and the relationship to the tumor. They are capable of providing axial, sagittal, and coronal images, which produce different views of the tumor. The signals are weighted as T1 or T2, which also provide different data, aiding the physician in the diagnostic process.[5,17] MRI is the best imaging modality for the evaluation of soft-tissue masses.

The most critical portion of the diagnosis is the biopsy, which is performed after the scans are completed. A biopsy that is performed properly is paramount in the treatment of the patient. An improperly placed biopsy that is not a longitudinal incision will most certainly have an adverse affect on the patient. A biopsy that does not include meticulous hemostasis may contaminate the area and necessitate more-extensive surgery. An inferior biopsy may also make determining of the margins of the original mass very difficult. When the pathology is finalized, the treatment plan is implemented. It should be noted that in some cases a biopsy may need to be repeated if the specimen is insufficient or nondiagnostic.

Table 44-7 Soft-Tissue Sarcoma Long-Term Follow-Up

Initial Staging	Physical exam	Plain x-ray	MRI of affected area	Chest CT
2-year follow-up	Physical exam		MRI of affected area	Q3 month CT CAP
2- to 5-year follow-up	Physical exam		Yearly MRI of affected area	Q6 month CT CAP
5- to 10-year follow-up	Phyiscal exam			Yearly CT CAP

Patients with alveolar, rhabdomyosarcoma, synovial cell sarcoma, or epithelioid sarcoma should receive a CT of the chest, abdomen, and pelvis (CAP) during their initial staging, and those with upper-extremity involvement should receive a CT to include the axilla.

Soft-tissue tumors are divided into groups according to their histogenetic origins.[2] The most common types include leiomyosarcoma, liposarcoma, synovial sarcoma, rhabdomyosarcoma, and malignant fibrous histiocytoma. Fibrosarcoma was closed among the soft-tissue sarcomas until the reclassification changed many of the former diagnoses.

Leiomyosarcoma is a sarcoma that arises from smooth muscle fibers. It is usually seen in the viscera, but it is also seen in the extremities that arise from the walls of the major vessels. Liposarcoma arises from adipose tissue. The thigh is a common site; less common are the omentum, breast, and chest wall. Synovial sarcomas are histologically similar to normal or reactive synovium, but they do not arise from synovial tissue. Approximately 70% of synovial sarcomas occur in the lower extremities, 25% of patients present with upper-extremity masses, and the remaining 5% are located in the trunk.[2] Rhabdomyosarcoma, the most common childhood soft-tissue sarcoma, is often located in the head and neck (40%) and in the trunk and extremities (25%). The remaining tumors are found in the retroperitoneum and genitourinary tract. These tumors arise from striated muscle. Malignant fibrous histiocytoma arises from fibrous tissue. It is usually found in the lower extremities, often the thigh. These tumors are often large at diagnosis, from 5 cm to 30 cm.[2]

Treatment for soft-tissue sarcomas may include chemotherapy, radiation therapy, and surgical excision. The chemotherapy agents doxorubicin, cyclophosphamide, etoposide, and high-dose methotrexate are utilized in the treatment of soft-tissue sarcomas. Ifosfamide has also been used. Surgical resection includes the resection of the tumor, including any contaminated tissue and an uncontaminated margin. If the margins are smaller than 3 cm or are questionable, radiation is used to control the disease. The timetable for treatment depends on whether radiation is necessary. Radiation is given prior to surgery and the skin must then heal for three to four weeks before surgery can be performed. Wound complications are a significant concern when radiation is performed preoperatively. The rationale for preoperative radiation is to shrink the tumor and ensure a more definitive resection. If the surgical margins are not optimal, postoperative radiation may be ordered. Intraoperative radiation or brachytherapy may be ordered to ensure that the tumor bed and nearby neurovascular structures are disease free. This is especially effective for large, deep tumors. Metastasis in soft-tissue sarcomas has a hematogenous behavior. The primary site of metastasis is the lungs, with the liver and bone being only occasional sites. Lymph nodes are not common metastatic sites; the exception is in certain subtypes of synovial sarcomas, rhabdomyosarcomas, and epithelioid sarcoma. Lymph node involvement, larger masses, and deep or high-grade tumors have a poorer prognosis. Table 44-7 describes the recommended long-term follow-up following initial staging.

Metastatic Bone Tumors

Malignant tumors have the capability of spreading to distant sites and growing at those sites. It is difficult to determine the volume of cells that escape from the primary tumor in relation to the number that are able to thrive and form a clinical metastatic focus. The process of metastasis is accomplished in a progressive effect. First, the cells leave the primary tumor and invade adjacent normal tissue. The tumor cells then must invade a blood or lymphatic vessel and travel to a distant part of the vascular system. Therefore, the tumor cell must be capable of finding its way through the vessel wall and invading the nearby tissue. When the tumor cell reaches this tissue, it must establish its own blood supply and begin to divide. Metastases typically disseminate via a hematogenous route.

Patients with a history of cancer of the lung, breast, kidney, thyroid, or prostate commonly present with skeletal pain. The metastatic sites are the proximal long bones (femur and humerus), spine, pelvis, ribs, and skull. A patient who is over 40 years of age and who presents with skeletal pain and a prior history of cancer will have a bone scan to establish any other sites of disease. Pathologic fractures are a serious risk at any site of metastasis. Diagnosis is established with a biopsy and radiographic imaging. CT scans are valuable for evaluating cortical destruction. MRI scans are useful for evaluating compression fractures of the spine.

When the sites of metastasis are identified, the surgeon evaluates the risk of fracture. One treatment option includes the use of bisphosphonates, compounds that inhibit osteoclastic-mediated bone reabsorption.[67] Preventing this mechanism decreases the likelihood of pain and pathologic fractures.[68] Pamidronate is usually prescribed for breast cancer patients with bone metastasis. A new bisphosphonate, zoledronic acid or Zometa, is being prescribed for metastatic breast cancer, multiple myeloma, and renal cell carcinoma.[68] The new drugs have provided encouraging results for certain types of metastatic lesions.

External beam radiation therapy (EBRT) is a palliative treatment for pain in metastatic disease. It has been found to be more effective for patients with lung or breast cancer than those with renal cell carcinoma.[68] Newer technology in radiation oncology has provided the possibility of more-focused and directed doses, which allows a varying dose of fractionated treatments. This may allow the protection of the soft-tissues that surround the targeted lesion. The question then arises as to which lesions should be radiated and which need surgical intervention. CT scans are a useful tool for evaluating bone destruction.

Surgical intervention for bone metastasis is palliative. One advancement is in the use of radiofrequency ablation, which is especially effective in spine metastasis. This is an investigational therapy that is minimally invasive and that seems to have few adverse neurological effects at present.[68] Surgery would include curettage of the lesion, possible cementation (polymethylmethacrylate, or PMMA), and fixation of the lesion with nails, screws, and plates. Joint replacements are also performed for pain relief and to reestablish mobility. One concern of the surgical team is whether enough healthy bone exists to anchor the hardware. Intramedullary nails and rods are used in upper-extremity procedures. Proximal femurs and hip surgeries make use of long-stemmed prostheses.

Patients with renal cell metastasis and myeloma present a special concern with any surgical procedure. Metastasis from kidney cancer or myeloma is extremely vascular and must be embolized before surgery to prevent excessive blood loss. Pathologic fracture and biopsies at these sites are especially problematic due to the risk of hemorrhage.

The optimal outcome for the patient with metastatic disease is the reduction of pain and the stabilization of the affected areas. This may be accomplished with medications, radiation, surgery, or a combination of these modalities. Pain management may be an ongoing and evolving process for the patient and his or her healthcare team.

Symptom Management and Supportive Care

Pain

Bone sarcomas often cause pain, which often interferes with a patient's daily activities. Soft-tissue sarcomas may present with pain when the mass exerts pressure on surrounding tissue. Patients will start their pain management with over-the-counter medications such as ibuprofen, aspirin, or acetaminophen. The newer nonsteroidal anti-inflammatory medications may provide some pain relief for a period of time. Patients may later be obliged to seek stronger medications to control their pain. Physicians may prescribe mild opiates, such as codeine, for this purpose. As the patient's treatment progresses, stronger medications, including opiates, would be utilized. Multidisciplinary treatment may reduce pain; for example, radiation treatments may shrink tumors and, as a result, decrease pain. This also presents the challenge of which physician will handle the patient's pain management needs. As the patient pursues treatment, it is important to provide him or her with as much independence as possible. This may be accomplished with the use of mobility aids, such as a cane, walker, wheelchair, or motorized scooter, if applicable. The patient may need to see a social worker to assist with everyday responsibilities, such as transportation or child care.

Limitations of Mobility

The physician may instruct the patient not to place any weight on the affected limb to prevent further injury or pain. The patient may find it necessary to use crutches, a walker, or even a wheelchair for lower-extremity protection. An upper-extremity tumor may limit mobility and necessitate a sling or splint. Day-to-day activities may present a challenge for the patient during treatment. Impaired mobility, fatigue, and pain may also impede the patient's ability to continue a normal life. The patient may find it necessary to call upon friends and family to provide both emotional and physical support. Patients may benefit from assistive measures such as obtaining handicap parking permits, reducing work hours, and collecting disability insurance benefits.

Continuity of Care: Nursing Challenges

One of the greatest challenges facing both the patient and the orthopedic oncology team is the complex system of healthcare insurance. Health care is becoming more specialized, and patients with special needs will seek out those specialists. Many insurance companies penalize customers for seeking care that is out of their network. Oncology treatments are extremely costly and many are experimental, causing insurance companies to deny payment. Other logistical problems, such as allowing surgery at a tertiary facility but denying laboratory or radiographic studies at the same institution, cause needless delays in treatment. Problems may extend to rehabilitation care and home care after surgery, which may be denied by insurance companies. It is important to be certain that patients fully understand what benefits their insurance provides.

Hospital stays for complicated surgeries are becoming briefer. Insurance companies are encouraging shorter hospital stays, with possible skilled nursing or rehab stays afterward. Treatments such as radiation and some chemotherapy infusions are now performed on an outpatient basis. This provides the patient with the comfort of staying at home but presents the logistical problem of how to get to treatments once and sometimes twice a day. Continuity of care is crucial and must be stressed to the patient and family members; appointments must be kept to advance the progression of care in a positive direction.

Many insurance companies will provide home care for dressing changes, medication infusion, central venous line care, wound assessment, and physical and occupational therapy for a limited time. The ideal plan, according to the insurance companies, is to teach family members to assume these tasks after a short period of time. As was stated earlier, some insurance plans do not provide home care or any outpatient services. It is important that the healthcare team maintain an open line of communication with the patient to answer questions regarding pain, wound care, and any follow-up care that may be necessary.

Future Trends

Advances in the diagnosis and treatment of a very complex and often enigmatic disease have made great strides in the past few decades. The improvements in surgical techniques, neoadjuvant and adjuvant chemotherapy, and radiation therapy have contributed to a better prognosis for cancer patients. Impressive surgical advances such as limb salvage and the use of prosthetic implants have given patients the possibility of a fuller and longer life. Research in chemotherapy, advances in radiation therapy and new modalities from clinical trials provide additional hope in the treatment of sarcoma patients and in their long-term survival.

References

1. Jemal A, Tiwari RC, Murray T, et al: Cancer statistics 2004: estimated new cases and death by sex. *CA Cancer J Clin* 54: p 9, 2004
2. Simon MA, Springfield DS (eds.): *Surgery for Bone and Soft Tissue Tumors*. Philadelphia, Lippincott-Raven, 1998
3. Gibbs CP, Weber K, Scarborough MT: Malignant bone tumors. *AAOS Instr Course Lect* 51:413–428, 2002
4. Widhe B, Widhe T: Initial symptoms and clinical features in osterosarcoma and Ewing's sarcoma. *J Bone Joint Surg Am* 82:667–674, 2002
5. Simon MA, Finn HA: Diagnostic strategy for bone and soft tissue tumors. *AAOS Instr Course Lect* 43:527–536, 1994
6. Simon MA, Schaaf HW, Metz CE: Clinical utility of erythrocyte sedimentation rate in preoperative evaluation of solitary skeletal lesions. *J Orthop Res* 2:262–268, 1984
7. DeBeuckeleer LH, DeSchepper AM, Ramon F: Magnetic resonance imaging of pelvic bone tumors. *J Belge Radiol* 79:11–13, 1996
8. Yasko AW, Reece GP, Gillis TA, et al: Limb-salvage strategies to optimize quality of life: the M.D. Anderson Cancer Center experience. *CA Cancer J Clin* 47:226–238, 1997
9. Reiser M, Nagele M, Schuller H, et al: Malignant skin and soft-tissue tumors: diagnostic imaging. *Langenbecks Arch Chir Suppl II Verh Dtsch Ges Chir* xx:893–900, 1990, ISSN: 0173-0541
10. Peabody TD, Gibbs CP, Simon MA: Current concepts review: evaluation and staging of musculoskeletal neoplasms. *J Bone Joint Surg Am* 80:1204–1218, 1998
11. Aoki J, Endo K, Watanabe H, et al: FDG-PET for evaluating musculoskeletal tumors: a review. *J Orthop Sci* 8:1435–1441, 2003
12. Mankin HJ, Mankin CJ, Simon MA: The hazards of the biopsy, revisited. Members of the Musculoskeletal Tumor Society. *J Bone Joint Surg Am* 78:656–663, 1996
13. Springfield DS, Rosenberg A: Biopsy: complicated and risky. *J Bone Joint Surg Am* 78:639–643, 1996
14. Issakov J, Flusser G, Kollender Y, et al: Computed tomography-guided core needle biopsy for bone and soft-tissue tumors. *Isr Med Assoc J* 5:28–30, 2003
15. Enneking WF, Spanier SS, Goodman MA: A system for surgical staging of musculo-skeletal sarcoma. *Clin Orthop* 153:106–120, 1980
16. Fleming ID, Cooper JS, Henson DE, et al (eds.): *AJCC Cancer Staging Manual* (ed 5). Philadelphia, Lippincott-Raven, 1975, pp 149–156
17. Cheng EY, Thompson RC: New developments in the staging and imaging of soft-tissue sarcomas. *Inst Course Lect* 81:882–892, 1999
18. Collin C, Godbold J, Hajdu S, et al: Localized extremity soft-tissue sarcoma: an analysis of factors affecting survival. *J Clin Oncol* 5:601–612, 1987
19. Li XQ, Parkekh SG, Rosenberg AE, et al: Assessing prognosis for high-grade soft-tissue sarcomas: search for a marker. *Ann Surg Oncol* 3:550–557, 1996
20. Peabody TD, Monson D, Montag A, et al: A comparison of the prognoses for deep and subcutaneous sarcomas of the extremities. *J Bone Joint Surg Am* 76:1167–1173, 1994
21. Russell WO, Cohen J, Enzinger F, et al: A clinical and pathological staging system for soft-tissue sarcomas. *Cancer* 40:1562–1570, 1977
22. Rydholm A, Gutafson P: Should tumor depth be included in the prognostication of soft-tissue sarcoma? *BMC Cancer* 3:17, 2003
23. Raney RB Jr, Tefft M, Maurer HM, et al: Disease patterns and survival rate in children with metastatic soft-tissue sarcoma: a

report from the Intergroup Rhabdomyosarcoma Study (IRS)-1. *Cancer* 62:1257–1266, 1988
24. Gibbs CP, Peabody TD, Simon MA: Classification, clinical features, preoperative assessment and staging of soft-tissue tumors: mini-symposium: soft tissue tumors of the musculoskeletal system. *Current Orthopaedics* 11:75–82, 1997
25. Dahlin DC, Unni K: *Bone Tumors*. Springfield, IL, Charles Thomas, 1986
26. DiCaprio MR, Friedlander GE: Malignant bone tumors: limb sparing versus amputation. *J Am Acad Orthop Surg* 11:25–37, 2003
27. Eilber FR, Eckhardt J, Morton DL: Advances in the treatment of sarcomas of the extremity: current status of limb salvage. *Cancer 54* (11 suppl):2695–2701, 1984
28. Simon MA: Limb salvage for osteosarcoma in the 1980s. *Clin Orthop* 270:264–270, 1991
29. Nagarajan R, Neglia J, Clohisy DR, et al: Limb salvage and amputation in survivors of pediatric lower-extremity bone tumors: what are the long-term implications?: *J Clin Oncol* 20:4493–4501, 2002
30. Hanlon M, Krajbich JI: Rotationplasty in skeletally immature patients: long term follow-up results. *Clin Orthop* 358:75–82, 1999
31. Ozaki T, Nakatsuka Y, Kunisada T, et al: High complication rate of reconstruction using Ilizarov bone transport method in patients with bone sarcomas. *Arch Orthop Trauma Surg* 118:136–139, 1998
32. Kenan S, Bloom N, Lewis MM: Limb-sparing surgery in skeletally immature patients with osteosarcoma: the use of an expandable prosthesis. *Clin Orthop* 270:223–230, 1991
33. Wallace RD, Davoudi MM, Neel MD, et al: The role of a pediatric plastic surgeon in limb salvage surgery for osteosarcoma of the lower extremity: *J Craniofac Surg* 14:680–686, 2003
34. Weiner SD, Scarborough MT, Vander Griend RA: Resection arthrodesis of the knee with intercalary allograft. *J Bone Joint Surg* 78:185–192, 1996
35. Gebhardt M, Flugstad D, Springfield D, et al: The use of bone allografts for limb salvage in high-grade extremity osteosarcoma. *Clin Orthop* 270:181–196, 1991
36. Dion N, Sim FH: The use of allografts in orthopedic surgery, part I: the use of allografts in musculoskeletal oncology. *J Bone Joint Surg* 84:644–654, 2002
37. Tomford W, Thongphasuk J, Mankin H, et al: Frozen musculoskeletal allografts. *J Bone Joint Surg Am* 72A:1137–1150, 1990
38. Snyder C, Saltzman D, Ferrell K, et al: A new approach to the resection of pulmonary osteosarcoma metastases. *Clin Orthop* 270:247–253, 1991
39. Sparks SM, Taylor CM: *Nursing Diagnosis Reference Manual.* Springhouse, PA, Springhouse Corporation, 1991, pp 46–48
40. Gebhardt MC: What's new in musculoskeletal oncology. *J Bone Joint Surg Am* 84:694–701, 2002
41. Renard AJ, Veth RP, Schreuder HW, et al: Function and complications after ablative and limb-salvage therapy in lower extremity sarcoma of bone. *J Surg Oncol* 73:198–205, 2000
42. Thomas MD, Epps CH: Complications of amputation surgery, in Epps CH, Bowen JR (eds.): *Complications in Pediatric Orthopedic Surgery.* Philadelphia, Lippincott, 1995, pp 817–830
43. Persson B: Lower limb amputation, part 1: amputation methods — a 10-year literature review. *Prosthet Orthot Int* 25:7–13, 2001
44. Geertzen J, Martina J, Rietman H: Lower limb amputation, part 2: rehabilitation — a 10-year literature review. *Prosthet Orthot Int* 25:14–20, 2001
45. Leung E, Rush P, Devlin M: Predicting prosthetic rehabilitation outcome in lower limb amputee patients with the Functional Independence Measure. *Arch Phys Rehabil* 77:605–608, 1996
46. Treweek S, Condie M: Three measures of functional outcome for lower limb amputees: a retrospective review. *Prosthet Orthot Int* 22:178–185, 1998
47. Michael J, Gailey R, Bowker J: New developments in recreational prostheses and adaptive devices for the amputee. *Clin Orthop* 256:64–75, 1990.
48. American Cancer Society: *Cancer Manual* (ed 8). Boston, American Cancer Society, 1990, pp 85–98
49. Crownover RL, Marks KE: Adjuvant brachytherapy in the treatment of soft-tissue sarcomas. *Hematol Oncol Clin North Am* 13:595–607, 1999
50. Nori D, Shupak K, Shiu MH, et al: Role of brachytherapy in recurrent extremity sarcoma in patients treated with prior surgery and radiation. *Int J Radiat Oncol Biol Phys* 20:1229, 1991
51. Alektiar KM, Leung D, Zelefsky MJ, et al: Adjuvant brachytherapy for primary high-grade soft-tissue sarcoma of the extremity. *Ann Surg Oncol* 9:48–56, 2002
52. McGowan KL: Radiation therapy: saving your patient's skin. *RN* 52:24–27, 1989
53. Hawkins DS, Arndt CAS: Pattern of disease recurrence and prognostic factors with osteosarcoma treated with contemporary chemotherapy. *Cancer* 98:2447–2456, 2003
54. Larsson S-E, Lorentzon R: The incidence of malignant primary bone tumours in relation to age, sex and site: a study of osteogenic sarcoma, chondrosarcoma and Ewing's sarcoma diagnosed in Sweden from 1958 to 1968. *J Bone Joint Surg Br* 56:534–540, 1974
55. Vlasak R, Sim FH: Ewing's sarcoma. *Orthop Clin North Am* 27:575–581, 1996
56. Scully SP, Ghert MA, Zurakowski D, et al: Pathological fracture in osteosarcomas: prognostic importance and treatment implications. *J Bone Joint Surg Am* 84:49–57, 2002
57. Enneking WF: *Clinical Musculoskeletal Pathology.* Gainesville, FL, University Presses of Florida, 1990
58. Sheth DS, Yasko AW, Raymond AK, et al: Conventional and dedifferentiated parosteal osteosarcoma: diagnosis, treatment, and outcome. *Cancer* 78:2136–2145, 1996
59. Bacci G, Picci P, Ferrari S, et al: Prognostic significance of serum alkaline phosphatase measurements in patients with osteosarcoma treated with adjuvant or neoadjuvant chemotherapy. *Cancer* 71:1224–1230, 1993
60. Pring ME, Weber KL, Unni KK, et al: Chondrosarcoma of the pelvis. *J Bone Joint Surg Am* 83:1630–1642, 2001
61. Lee FY, Mankin HJ, Fondren G, et al: Chondrosarcoma of bone: an assessment of outcome. *J Bone Joint Surg* 81:326–338, 1999
62. Springfield DS, Gebhardt MC, McGuire MH: Chondrosarcoma: a review. *Instr Course Lect* 78:141–149, 1996
63. Wunder JS, Paulian G, Huvos AG, et al: The histological response to chemotherapy as a predictor of the oncological outcome of operative treatment of Ewing's sarcoma. *J Bone Joint Surg* 80:1020–1033, 1998
64. Wexler L, DeLaney T, Tsokos M: Ifosfamide and etoposide plus vincristine, doxorubicin and cyclophosphamide for newly diagnosed Ewing's sarcoma family of tumour. *Cancer* 78:901–911, 1996
65. Daugaard S: Current soft-tissue sarcoma classifications. *Eur J Cancer* 40:543–548, 2004
66. Fletcher CDM, Unni KK, Mertens F (eds.): *Pathology and Genetics of Tumours of Soft Tissue and Bone (World Health Organization Classification of Tumours).* Lyon, France, IARC Press, 2002
67. Green J: Bisphosphonates in cancer therapy. *Curr Opin Oncol* 14:609–615, 2002
68. Weber KL, Gebhardt MC: What's new in musculoskeletal oncology. *J Bone Joint Surg Am* 85:761–767, 2003

CHAPTER 45

Bladder and Renal Cancers

Laura S. Wood, RN, MSN, OCN®
Dorothy Calabrese, MSN, RN, CNP

Introduction

The two urinary tract cancers discussed in this chapter, bladder and renal cancer, account for approximately 9% of all cancers. Advances in detection and therapeutic management of bladder and kidney cancer are discussed here, providing the oncology nurse with a basis for the care and management of the person diagnosed with these cancers.

Bladder Cancer

Epidemiology

Bladder cancer is the second most common genitourinary cancer (following prostate cancer) in the United States, accounting for approximately 6% of all newly diagnosed cancers. Approximately 60,240 Americans will be diagnosed with bladder cancer in 2004 and an estimated 12,710 deaths from this cause will occur.[1] It is the fourth most common cancer and the ninth leading cause of cancer deaths in men. Less common in women, bladder cancer ranks tenth in incidence and is grouped in "all other sites" when death rates are calculated. Bladder cancer occurs 2.7 times more often in men than in women, it is more common in Caucasians than in blacks,[1] and the average age at diagnosis is 65 years.

Etiology

The neoplastic changes in the bladder lining, the urothelium, that occur in bladder cancer are a multistep phenomenon. Researchers believe that bladder tumors are the result of a combination of genetic events, including oncogene activation and antioncogene inactivation (an initiator induces an alteration in a single normal cell's DNA, allowing it to transform into a malignant cell; noncarcinogenic promoters bind to the cell-surface receptors, causing the transformed cells to proliferate).[1]

Cigarette smoking, which has been demonstrated to initiate and promote these events, is a risk factor that accounts for approximately 50% of bladder cancer among men and 31% among women. Risk of bladder cancer is associated with both lifetime consumption of cigarettes and duration of smoking.[2]

Occupational exposures to aniline dyes and aromatic amines, most commonly betanaphthylamine and benzidine, have also been identified as a risk factor for bladder cancer. For this reason, workers in the chemical, dye, rubber, petroleum, and printing industries have an increased risk for developing bladder cancer. The latency period between exposure and tumor development is often prolonged. Ingestion of other physical agents, such as coffee, alcohol, saccharine, and phenacetin, have also been proposed as risk factors, but studies have failed to confirm the association.[2]

Additional risk factors for bladder cancer include physical trauma of the urothelium due to infection, instrumentation, and calculi and the use of cyclosphosphamide, a chemotherapeutic agent.[2] A high incidence of squamous cell carcinoma of the bladder in many African countries, most notably Egypt, is linked to exposure to the parasite *Schistosoma haematobium,* which can be found in the water of these countries.

Pathophysiology

The urinary bladder is lined by a transitional epithelium called the *urothelium* that rests on a layer called the basement membrane (Table 45-1). Approximately 90% of bladder tumors diagnosed in people in North America arise in the epithelial layer and are called transitional cell carcinoma (TCC). The other 10% consist of squamous cell carcinoma and adenocarcinoma and originate below the basement membrane.

The growth rate of bladder tumors varies depending on histologic type, tumor grade, and depth of bladder wall invasion. Tumors have the potential to spread via the lymphatic system to the lymph nodes and the pelvis or hematogenously to the bones, liver, and lungs.[2]

Clinical Manifestations

Hematuria is the most common presenting symptom of bladder cancer, reported by 85%–90% of patients. The hematuria may be macroscopic or microscopic,

Table 45-1 Urinary Bladder Characteristics

- Hollow muscular organ that serves as a reservoir for urine
- Adult bladder has a normal capacity of 400–500 mL
- Lies behind the symphis pubis (pelvic organ)
- Layers (inner to outer): mucosa (lamina propria, epithelium), submucosa, muscle (deep longitudinal, middle circular, inner longitudinal), subserosa and perivesical fat

intermittent or continuous, and the degree of hematuria does not relate to the stage or extent of the disease. Additional symptoms that the patient may experience include dysuria, urinary frequency, and urgency. Symptoms of advanced disease can include flank, rectal, pelvic, or bone pain; bowel habit changes; decreased appetite or weight loss; lower extremity edema; and/or fever.

Assessment

Physical Examination and Diagnostic Studies

No early signs of bladder cancer are evident on physical examination, but an invasive mass in the trigonal area occasionally may be felt by rectal examination. Tests that may help to establish the presence of a bladder mass include urine cytology, excretory urogram, cystoscopy, ultrasound, computerized tomography (CT), and magnetic resonance imaging (MRI). Exfoliative urinary cytology is a relatively simple diagnostic tool that examines the cells shed by the urothelium; it is particularly useful in high-grade malignancies or carcinoma in situ, and may be used as a screening tool or to assess response to treatment. Bladder washings obtained through saline irrigation of the bladder produce even more reliable results.

Newer tests are being performed on voided urine specimens to validate their specificity and sensitivity for detected bladder cancer. These tests include the BTA test, the BTA stat test, the BTA TRAL assay, NMP22, Lewis, Xantigen, FDP, and BLCA-4. Currently, these tests are being utilized as a complement to traditional evaluation tools.[2]

An excretory urogram (IVP) is often done as part of an evaluation of hematuria to visualize the urinary tract and identify filling defects of the upper tract or bladder. This test will show the presence of hydronephrosis. In addition, CT scan and MRI are used to stage high-grade bladder tumors and assist in defining the extent of bladder wall invasion, extension beyond the bladder, lymph node involvement, or distant metastasis.

Cystoscopy and biopsy confirm the presence of a bladder tumor. The cystoscopy procedure directly visualizes the interior bladder and urethra. If a tumor is visualized, a biopsy is done to assess the depth of invasion into the bladder musculature. Multiple biopsies of the surrounding bladder wall, bladder neck, and trigone may be undertaken to diagnose carcinoma in situ or atypia. Bimanual palpation is performed under anesthesia when muscle invasion and/or extravesical extension is suspected.

Prognostic Indicators

Tumor grade and stage may not be reliable in predicting the course of many bladder tumors. Tumor markers may add information to help predict the response to treatment, recurrence, and progress of the bladder cancer. The identification of multiple markers may provide more accurate information regarding the multiple mechanisms that result in tumor recurrence or progression.

One such marker is the *p53* gene, a cell-cycle regulatory protein (tumor suppressor gene). Research demonstrates that the aberration of *p53* in bladder tumors may increase the rate of recurrence, but that adjuvant chemotherapy in these patients may increase survival.[2] Another marker is the blood group antigen. Angiogenesis, the growth of new blood vessels to feed the tumor, is necessary for tumor growth. Microvessel density, a useful prognostic indicator in bladder cancer, has been associated with lymph node metastases, disease progression, and overall survival in patients with invasive bladder cancer treated by radical cystectomy. The retinoblastoma (*Rb*) gene, a tumor suppressor gene, is expressed in TCC and may be associated with poorer prognosis and decreased overall survival.[2]

Classification and Staging

The classification and staging of bladder tumors provide information to estimate prognosis and to help in treatment decision making. Two staging systems are used for bladder cancer: the Jewett-Marshall system (modified in 1952 and based on the relationship of the depth of tumor penetration into the bladder wall to the incidence of lymph node or distant metastasis) and the TNM system developed by the American Joint Committee for Cancer Staging (AJCC) (Table 45-2). The TNM system provides a more accurate classification and definition of tumor types than does the Jewett-Marshall system. It also promotes collaboration in cancer research and facilitates comparison of data among national and international clinical investigators.[2] Either staging system gives a reasonable clinical estimate of a tumor's biological potential and need for treatment. Pathological staging following removal of the bladder and lymph nodes establishes an accurate staging of the cancer, however, understaging remains a problem.[2]

The grade or degree of cell differentiation of bladder tumors is an important factor that predicts the speed of recurrence, progression to invasion, and metastases. The grades for bladder cancer are referred to as grade I, II, III, or IV, with grade IV indicating poor differentiation.

Table 45-2 AJCC TMN Clinical Classification

T: Primary tumor
- TX: Primary tumor cannot be assessed
- TO: No evidence of primary tumor
- Ta: Noninvasive papillary carcinoma
- Tis: Carcinoma in situ
- T1: Tumor invades subepithelial connective tissue
- T2: Tumor invades muscle
- T2a: Tumor invades superficial muscle (inner half)
- T2b: Tumor invades deep muscle (outer half)
- T3: Tumor invades perivesical tissue
- T3a: Microscopically
- T3b: Macroscopically
- T4: Tumor invades any of the following: prostate, uterus, vagina, pelvic or abdominal wall
- T4b: Tumor invades prostate, uterus, or vagina
- T4b: Tumor invades pelvic or abdominal wall

N: Regional lymph nodes
- NX: Regional lymph nodes cannot be assessed
- NO: No regional lymph node metastasis
- N1: Metastasis in a single lymph node 2 cm or smaller (largest dimension)
- N2 Metastasis in a single lymph node 2 to 5 cm or multiple lymph nodes less than 5 cm in greatest dimension

M: Distant metastasis
- MX: Distant metastasis cannot be assessed
- MO: No distant metastasis
- M1: Distant metastasis

Therapeutic Approaches

Carcinoma in Situ

Carcinoma in situ (CIS) is a noninvasive lesion that has a high potential for invasion and recurrence. It appears as a flat, red, velvety lesion. It may present as diffuse or focal, symptomatic or asymptomatic, and it may or may not be associated with superficial papillary tumors. This type of bladder cancer requires aggressive follow-up after initial diagnosis and treatment to provide surveillance for tumor recurrence and invasive disease. Transurethral resection (TUR) and fulgeration are the most common and conservative forms of management of CIS. The TUR to obtain tissue for diagnosis is often sufficient to remove the tumor(s). Radical cystectomy is indicated for high-grade, poorly differentiated CIS.[3] Radiotherapy has not proven to be of benefit in the treatment of CIS.

Bacillus Calmette-Guérin (BCG) is a live, attenuated strain of *Mycobacterium bovis.* The first-line treatment for CIS, it has proven to be more effective in prevention of tumor recurrence and progression compared to the chemotherapeutic agents. This biological response modifier is believed to exert its antitumor effect by stimulating various immune responses in the host.[2] Although the frequency and dosage of BCG vary slightly from institution to institution, it is most commonly administered weekly for six treatments at a dosage of 120 mg per instillation. Maintenance treatments (given monthly or every three months) can be useful to increase disease-free survival.[2] Side effects of BCG treatments include dysuria, urinary frequency, and urgency. The patient may experience macroscopic or microscopic hematuria. Hemorrhagic cystitis is rare (affecting less than 2% of recipients).[2] Symptoms are treated with antibiotics and pyridium if appropriate.

Nurses play an important role in assessing the patient for side effects. Treatment may be withheld until any adverse effects have resolved. Care should be used in catheterizing the patient, as a traumatic catheterization may cause a systemic tuberculin (TB) infection. In addition, BCG sepsis may occur. Common symptoms of such sepsis include high fever, chills, confusion, hypotension, respiratory failure, and jaundice. Medications to treat TB (isoniazid, rifampin, and ethambutol) should be initiated promptly if BCG systemic infection is suspected.

Superficial, Low-Grade Tumors

More than 75% of people diagnosed with bladder cancer initially present with superficial tumors (stage T0, Tis, Ta, or Tb).[4] Superficial tumors of the bladder affect the innermost lining of the bladder (epithelium and lamina propria), and the majority of these cancers (approximately 80%) do not progress to muscle invasive disease. Treatment of these tumors usually comprises a TUR and fulgeration. In 40%–60% of cases, the tumor(s) recur, and intravesical chemotherapy is often given as adjuvant therapy to prevent the recurrence and to minimize the speed at which they recur.[4] Chemotherapeutic agents used to treat superficial, low-grade bladder tumors are either mitomycin C, thiotepa, or doxorubicin (Table 45-3).

Intravesical chemotherapy

Intravesical therapy with chemotherapeutic and immunotherapeutic agents has been shown to be effective in the treatment of superficial bladder cancer,

Table 45-3 Treatment for Superficial Bladder Cancer

- CIS: TUR followed by BCG
- Ta: TUR or TUR followed by intravesical therapy or immunotherapy
- T1: TUR followed by intravesical or immunotherapy therapy; with recurrence, more aggressive therapy

TUR = Transurethral resection.
BCG = Bacillus Calmette-Guérin.

Table 45-4 Information for Patients Undergoing BCG Treatment

- Do not drink liquids for 4 hours prior to your appointment.
- Empty your bladder prior to the treatment.
- The medication must stay in your bladder for 2 hours.
- Speak to your doctor if you cannot hold the medication for 2 hours; there are medications that may help.
- You should turn from side to side during the time the medication is in your bladder so that all the surfaces have contact with the medication.
- You should sit to urinate to get the medication out of your body (avoid splashing).
- Put 2 cups of chlorine bleach in the toilet following urination. Close the lid and wait 15 minutes before flushing.
- Clean your genital area and hands carefully with soap and water each time you void.
- Unless medically contraindicated, drink plenty of fluids to flush your system for at least 6 hours following your treatment.
- Talk to your doctor or the nurse about any concerns that you have during your treatment.

although no agent has demonstrated a clear advantage.[3] Treatment with BCG has delayed progression of disease, reduced recurrence, and prolonged survival. As a consequence, it is considered a successful adjuvant treatment of superficial bladder cancer. The typical regimen of BCG begins one to two weeks following the TUR or biopsy, and it is repeated weekly for 6 treatments. Approximately 6 weeks following completion of the BCG therapy, a cystoscopy is performed to evaluate the effectiveness of treatment. Additional treatments with BCG may be required. Most patients tolerate the BCG course reasonably well (Table 45-4).

Emerging data suggest that one perioperative dose of a chemotherapeutic agent given within 1–24 hours after the TUR may be of similar effectiveness to the 6-week course of BCG. Chemotherapeutic agents used include mitomycin, doxorubicin, and thiotepa. The use of maintenance (or extended) therapy with these drugs remains controversial.[5] Other agents less commonly used include epirubicin, epodyl, cisplatin, mitoxantrone, and pirarubicin.[6] Trials of interferon-alfa, bropirimine (an oral immunomodulator), and valrubicin (an anthracycline derivative), used alone or in combination with other chemotherapeutic agents, may be effective in high-risk patients or those who have failed to respond to the first-line therapy.[2]

Partial cystectomy

A partial cystectomy is recommended very selectively. It is appropriate for patients with a solitary infiltrating tumor along the posterior lateral wall or dome of the bladder; a diverticulum; diffuse unresectable tumors located away from the bladder neck or bladder base; or patients who have not responded to intravesical therapy. While this surgery is effective in many cases, local recurrence is common.

Invasive Tumors

Bladder cancer that invades the muscle wall of the bladder needs to be treated aggressively. In the United States, it is common to remove the bladder (radical cystectomy) and create a urinary diversion (continent or incontinent). Preservation of the bladder through the use of chemotherapy combined with radiation therapy is becoming an option for patients with muscle-invasive disease.

Radical cystectomy

Radical cystectomy with bilateral lymphadenectomy is the standard treatment for muscle-invasive bladder cancer. It is considered the most effective treatment for the local control of tumor recurrence, precise pathological staging, and optimal survival. In men, a radical cystoprostatectomy involves removing the bladder with perivesical fat, peritoneal attachments, prostate, prostatic urethra, and seminal vesicles. In women, a radical cystectomy (anterior exenteration) includes the removal of the bladder with perivesical fat, peritoneal attachments, proximal urethra, ovaries, fallopian tubes, uterus, cervix, anterior vaginal vault, and lymph nodes. In both men and women, the entire urethra is removed if evidence of disease is present.

Cystectomy with urinary diversion

Following the removal of the patient's bladder, a urinary diversion needs to be created to manage the urine. Diversions can be incontinent (ileal conduit) or continent (catheterizable or orthoptic).

Ileal conduit. Since the early 1950s, the Bricker ileoconduit has been the cornerstone treatment for diverting urine in the absence of the bladder. This procedure involves isolation of a section of the terminal ileum, the proximal end of this section is closed, and the distal end is brought out through an opening in the abdomen. The site should be selected and marked prior to surgery, taking into consideration the patient's body habitus.

The ileal segment is sutured to the skin, creating a stoma; the ureters are implanted into the ileal segment. Urine flows into the conduit, and peristalsis propels the urine out through the stoma. Ureteral stents or a red Robinson catheter (left in place for 5–7 days) are placed in the conduit to facilitate urinary drainage in the immediate postoperative period. Following this procedure, an external appliance is worn to collect urine.

Complications that may occur following the creation of an ileal conduit include a flushed or recessed stoma or placement of the stoma in skin creases or over bony prominences. The result may be difficulties in management of the stoma and leakage of urine. Late complications can include stomal stenosis, stone formation, and peristomal hernias. Chronic pyelonephritis and deterioration of kidney function may occur due to urinary reflux, ureter-ilial obstruction, or urinary infection.

Continent urinary diversions. In recent years, continent urinary diversions have become the procedure of choice for total cystectomy. Continent diversions were developed in an attempt to have a diversion that functions more like the original bladder. Ideally, the urinary diversion should be one of high volume and low pressure, and it should be able to store 300–400 mL of urine. Voiding should be under voluntary control and occur at intervals that approximate those of the original bladder. The upper urinary tract should be protected from urine reflux and obstruction. For many patients, a continent diversion provides both functional and psychological advantages over the ileal conduit procedure, because it approximates the original bladder.

Many parts of the bowel have been used to create a urinary diversion. Currently, the small intestine is utilized in many continent urinary diversions. The types of continent urinary diversions currently being constructed include diversions with a catheterized limb (Kock pouch, Indiana pouch, T-pouch) and the orthoptic neobladder (Studer pouch, Mainz pouch, Camey pouch). Differences between the reservoirs relate to the segment of intestine used to make the pouch, the antireflux mechanism, and the location of the urinary outlet (stoma or urethra).

Creation of a continent urinary reservoir is technically more complicated than construction of an ileal conduit. Patients remain hospitalized for 7–10 days and they must be taught management of the tubes and drains that will be in place for approximately three weeks following surgery. Because the segment of the intestine reconfigured for a bladder will continue to produce mucus, the patient is instructed to irrigate the tubes and catheter every four hours and as needed with 30–60 mL of normal saline. Prior to removal of the tubes, radiographic examination of the bladder is performed to determine the presence of extravasation. If the bladder is intact without extravasation, the patient's tubes are removed and he or she is taught to intubate the stoma or voiding techniques. Early postoperative complications may include any complication related to a major surgical procedure. Late complications may include metabolic disorders, stomal stenosis, pyelonephritis, and calculi.[5]

Radiation Therapy

External beam radiation therapy of approximately 60 Gy delivered in fractions to the pelvis in 5–8 weeks is an alternative to radical cystectomy in selected patients. Although this treatment remains controversial, studies have shown that radiation therapy for bladder cancer can be an option in certain cases. This treatment is generally well tolerated, although approximately 15% of patients will experience significant bowel, bladder, or rectal problems. Radiation therapy is generally offered to patients who are not candidates to have the bladder removed because local recurrence is common.[2] A combination of chemotherapy and radiation therapy may improve local recurrence rates.

Chemotherapy

The goals of chemotherapy for bladder cancer are to control the cancer, eradicate micrometastasis, downstage bladder tumors, and cure patients. Chemotherapy can be given neoadjuvantly followed by cystectomy or adjuvantly following radical cystectomy. A methotrexate, vinblastine, doxorubicin, and cisplatin (MVAC) regimen is often used for patients with metastatic bladder cancer, leading to a complete response in approximately 13%–35% of patients. The median survival is approximately one year, and the sustained survival rate is 20%–25%. Note that MVAC treatment is associated with substantial toxicity.[2]

Newer agents are demonstrating effectiveness in treating bladder cancer without the toxicity seen with MVAC. These agents include ifosfamide, gemcitabine, paclitaxel, and gallium nitrate. The advantages of using these drugs in combination include lower toxicity and improved tolerability.[2]

Nursing Care

Preoperative Nursing Care

Education and support before, during, and following surgery for bladder cancer is essential to help the patient and family deal with this potentially overwhelming experience. They are dealing with many unknowns, are anticipating a major surgical procedure that will have a significant impact on their future life, and may be struggling with the anticipation of an altered body image.

Some patients have anticipated the surgery for many years, as they have been undergoing cystoscopy procedures every 3 months with multiple intravesical regimens. Often they feel a sense of relief that they will no longer have to organize their life around the cystoscopy schedule. Yet as the surgery date approaches, the reality of the physical changes that will occur may become overwhelming. Other patients are confronted with the need to have their bladder removed following one episode of hematuria and its subsequent evaluation. Education and support are equally important for each group of patients.

The patient is often given a choice regarding the type of urinary diversion to be created. While a choice is viewed by healthcare professionals as a "positive" or "good" thing, it can cause much anxiety for the patient. Giving the patient and family written information to review in addition to the verbal explanation will be helpful as the patient tries to sort through the issues and come to a decision. This information should include material about the surgery and the urinary diversion's effects on future life. The patient may want to speak with another patient who has each type of diversion, gaining a better understanding of the procedure, recovery, and impact on quality of life.

In the period immediately before surgery, the patient will need to begin the physical preparation for surgery. While this preparation will vary according to physician preferences, it typically includes several steps. Approximately 2 days before surgery, the patient will begin a restricted diet (low-residue or full-liquid diet). The day prior to surgery, the diet is further restricted to clear liquids, and the patient will need to undergo a bowel preparation. That prep is usually a strong cathartic, but it may also include antibiotics.

During the preoperative period, the patient receives a lot of information, but stress may cause the patient or family to ask the same questions repeatedly. It is important to reinforce the information to help alleviate the stress. A description of the surgical procedure and a discussion of what will occur immediately prior to the surgery will help to familiarize the patient with the preoperative regimen. A description of the midline incision, as well as the tubes and drains that the patient can expect to have upon awakening in the recovery room, will help the patient know what to expect. An explanation of the postoperative care routines during hospitalization regarding pain management, activity (progressive ambulation), and diet progression will allow the patient to actively participate in his or her care. While the amount of information can seem to be overwhelming, a thorough education will help the patient to know what to expect and continued reinforcement during the hospitalization will let the patient judge how he or she is progressing.

General Postoperative Care

Postoperative care may vary slightly depending on the urinary diversion that is created. The general principles of caring for all patients undergoing cystectomy with urinary diversion are similar. These principles can be found in any medical-surgical text. They include pain management, respiratory toilet, fluid management, and prevention of postoperative complications. Issues specific to each of the patient populations will be addressed in the following sections.

Nursing Care of the Patient with an Ileal Conduit

An ileal conduit is an incontinent urinary diversion, one in which urine drains constantly into a pouch. The stoma is usually placed in the right abdomen in a position that is easily accessible for the patient but is not at the belt line or in abdominal creases. The stoma needs to be assessed frequently for viability (at least once per nursing shift) during the immediate postoperative period. Normal stoma color is a beefy, dark red. A stoma with a dusky appearance, ranging from purple to black, indicates circulatory impairment and should be reported immediately to the surgeon as reoperation to restore circulation may be indicated.

Stoma edema is normal in the immediate postoperative period due to surgical manipulation, but the edema should not interfere with the stoma function. In the immediate postoperative period, the stoma size is larger than it will ultimately be. This larger size is due to edema, and it will decrease as the edema subsides. The pouch size will need to be adjusted as this occurs, so as to prevent urinary leakage and/or peristomal skin irritation.

An enterostomal therapist (ET), a nurse with special education regarding stomas and wound and skin care, is a valuable resource to assist the patient and family in learning to manage the care of the ileal conduit. Some patients may become upset when they first view the stoma. It may be difficult for the patient to view this change to his or her body and body image. It is important to support and encourage the patient and family during this process. As the patient is physically and psychologically able, he or she should be encouraged to first observe the stoma care, and then begin to assist with the care. Ultimately, the goal is to have the patient assume care under supervision and then independently. Instructions should be given to the patient in writing to serve as a reference for the patient following hospital discharge. These instructions should include management of the peristomal skin, equipment being used, how and where to get supplies, and how to reach the resource person if questions or problems arise. The United Ostomy Association and the American Cancer Society are additional resources for the patient.

Follow-up Care for the Patient with an Ileal Conduit

Physician guidelines will direct the follow-up that the patient will need after the cystectomy and creation of the ileal conduit. Certain common items need to be assessed, including the kidney and its function. A basic metabolic panel (BMP) will assess the creatinine level, the indicator of how well the kidney is functioning. An excretory urogram (IVP) or renal ultrasound is done to evaluate for hydronephrosis. Untreated hydronephrosis can lead to kidney damage and decreased function. Other potential complications include ureteral stenosis, ureteral obstruction, and lithiasis. Regular evaluation and assessment can identify emerging problems, allowing for ready intervention to preserve kidney function.

There also needs to be a periodic evaluation of the stoma, the peristomal skin, and the stoma functioning. Potential problems may include a stoma that receeds (difficulty keeping an appliance intact without leakage), irritated or macerated peristomal skin (caused by an improperly fitting appliance), or encrustations around the stoma (due to alkaline urine). Stomal stenosis or narrowing interferes with urinary drainage and can lead to urinary stasis and/or infection. Education regarding potential problems is necessary so that appropriate interventions can be instituted to avoid long-term sequelae.

Nursing Care of the Patient with a Continent Urinary Diversion

Following surgery for a continent urinary diversion (catherizable stoma or orthoptic neobladder), the patient remains hospitalized for 7–10 days. In addition to routine postoperative care, the patient needs to learn to irrigate the tubes placed in the continent reservoir so as to facilitate drainage of urine and keep the reservoir empty. Irrigation is important because the bladder should not be overly distended until healing has occurred. The tubes that the patient has will vary according to physician preference, but may include stents, a suprapubic tube, as well as a catheter through the stoma (Indiana pouch) or a Foley catheter (orthoptic neobladder) (Table 45-5).

Table 45-5 Care of Tubes in the Immediate Postoperative Period for the Patient with a Continent Urinary Diversion

The purpose of the abdominal tube and Foley catheter (if present) is to keep the neobladder empty until it has healed following surgery.

- Inspect the skin and sutures around the abdominal tube daily.
- Wash the surrounding skin with mild soap and water, and dress with a gauze pad daily.
- Irrigate this tube with 30–60 mL normal saline every 3–4 hours. Irrigation may need to be repeated if the solution is not returning freely.
- It may be necessary to use gentle suction to remove the fluid, mucus plug, or blood clots.
- The tubes need to be irrigated at least once during the night.
- It is important to drink at least six 8-ounce glasses of fluids each day. Your tubes may have better drainage if at least half of your liquid intake is water.
- If you are unable to irrigate either of the tubes or if the fluid does not drain out, call your doctor's office.

Approximately 3 weeks after surgery, the patient shoud have an x-ray of the bladder to assess healing. If no extravasation of contrast occurs, the patient will proceed to learn how the new bladder will function.

For the patient with a catherizable stoma, he or she will be taught to intubate the reservoir with a 14 or 16 Fr. catheter. Once the patient is comfortable with this procedure, the tubes will be removed, and the patient will intubate the pouch according to a set schedule, increasing the time between intubations by an hour each week. The patient should not go longer than 5–6 hours between intubation procedures.

With an orthoptic neobladder, the patient is instructed on voiding technique. He or she is instructed to void by sitting on the commode, bearing down, and applying gentle pressure on the lower abdomen (Credé maneuver). The patient should begin a toileting regimen of voiding every two hours and increasing the time interval by 30–60 minutes per week (Table 45-6).

Following the removal of the tubes, patients with an orthoptic neobladder can expect to be incontinent for a period of time. Many products are available to help the patient manage the leakage until urinary control returns, including guards, undergarments, and briefs (diapers). Each person regains urinary control at a different rate. Control during the daytime usually returns first, and approximately 90% of patients eventually obtain complete urine control during the day. Complete night-time control returns in approximately 80% of patients, while the other 20% experience some amount of incontinence during the night.[7] Emptying the bladder at bedtime (either by voiding or by doing self-catheterization) or setting the alarm to awaken once during the night may help to alleviate the incontinence.

Table 45-6 Orthoptic Neobladder: Instructions After the Tubes Are Removed

- Urination is done slightly differently now. You should sit on the toilet, relax your pelvic muscles, and bear down using your abdominal muscles to empty your bladder. You may also use gentle pressure on your bladder with your hands to help empty the bladder. In time, this will become "second nature" to you.
- Follow this schedule for voiding:

  First week: Void every 2 hours during the day and every 3 hours at night.

  Second week: Void every 3 hours during the day and every 4 hours at night.

  Third week: Void every 4 hours during the day and every 4–5 hours at night.

  Fourth week and thereafter: Void every 4–5 hours during the day and every 4-6 hours at night
- It is important to drink 6–8 8-ounce glasses of fluids each day. Make it a habit to drink a glass of fluids with each meal and one glass of fluids between each meal every day for the rest of your life.
- You will leak urine when your Foley catheter is removed. Be patient with yourself. As your body heals, you will begin to regain urine control.
- You will always have mucus in your urine because your bladder is made from intestine. You will learn what is a normal amount of mucus for you.
- If something does not seem right to you, call your doctor's office.

The next follow-up appointment for the patient usually is in 4–5 weeks. At that time, the patient will have blood work to evaluate kidney function and an imaging study of the upper urinary tract to evaluate for hydronephrosis. Cancer follow-up evaluations with CT scans are per the physician's usual protocol.

Complications of continent urinary diversions can include metabolic and nutritional disorders (related to the part of the bowel that is used), pyelonephrits and renal deterioration (manifested by hydronephrosis or an increasing serum creatinine), and formation of renal or bladder calculi. The latter complication is related to persistent infection. Some patients may need suppressive antibiotics for the remainder of their lifetime.

Sexual functioning can be affected following removal of the bladder. Men may be impotent even if the procedure is a nerve-sparing one. Treatment options for these patients are the same as for men undergoing a radical prostatectomy. For women, the removal of the tubes and ovaries can lead to vaginal dryness, decreased libido, and discomfort with intercourse (because part of the vagina is removed). There can also be a psychological component to the changes in sexual functioning. A change in body image can affect the person's relationship with others.

Nurses working with these patients are in a unique position to help the patient, significant other, and family through major surgery and the changes that come along with the cystectomy and urinary diversion. By being open to the issues and concerns that patients voice, nurses can provide suggestions on how to deal with these issues and improve their quality of life.

Kidney Cancer

Epidemiology

Cancer of the kidney and renal pelvis are a heterogeneous group of diseases, accounting for less than 3% of the estimated new cancers and deaths in 2004.[1] Renal cancer incidence and death rates continue to rise steadily, with an estimated 35,710 new cases and 12,480 deaths in the United States in 2004, and a male-to-female ratio of 2:1.[1] Renal cancer is the third most common genitourinary malignancy. Its incidence rises steadily between the ages of 25 and 79, and reaches a peak between ages 40 and 70. The incidence of kidney cancer rose steadily between 1975 and 1995, increasing by 2.3% among Caucasian men, 3.9% among African American men, 3.1% among Caucasian women, and 4.3% among African American women.[8] Five-year relative survival rates have slowly improved to approximately 62% for patients with all stages of disease, 87% for patients with localized disease, and 9% for patients with stage IV disease.[1]

Renal malignancies include adenocarcinomas; transitional cell tumors of the renal pelvis, ureter, and urethra; and Wilms' tumor, which occurs in children. Differences between the types of renal cancers are related to molecular events leading to oncogenesis as well as the epithelial site targeted by these events, and reflect the disparate clinical course of renal cancer and its variable prognosis.[9] The highest incidences of this cancer are in North America and Scandinavia, with lower rates observed in Japan, China, and India. Improvements in diagnostic techniques, leading to earlier diagnosis and identification of smaller tumors, and advances in surgical techniques have produced modest increases in 5-year survival.

Etiology

Renal cell carcinoma arises from the proximal renal tubular epithelium. It occurs in sporadic, inherited, and noninherited forms, with 75%–80% of cases having a clear cell histology. Although many potential risk factors have been associated with renal cancer, strong associations have not been found, partly because renal cell carcinoma is a relatively rare disease and many associations fall short of statistical significance. Cigarette use, obesity, and hypertension or its medications have been associated with an increased risk of renal cancer. The combined effect of obesity and hypertension poses a greater risk for women compared to men. Several hereditary forms of renal cancer have been identified, including von Hippel-Lindau disease, tubular sclerosis, hereditary clear cell, hereditary papillary syndromes, and hereditary renal oncocytoma.[10] Associations have been made between sickle cell anemia and collecting duct carcinoma, and between end-stage renal disease and both clear cell and papillary type renal cancers. Genetic alterations associated with renal cancer have been studied with inconsistent results. Interpretation of the clinical value of some genetic alterations is challenging because of the difficulty in separating chromosomal changes of tumor initiation and proliferation compared to those occurring secondary to tumor growth.[11]

Von Hippel-Lindau (VHL) disease is a familial multiple-cancer syndrome in which the affected person has a predisposition to a variety of malignancies, including clear cell renal carcinoma, renal cysts, and other tumors. Clear cell renal carcinomas are characterized by abnormalities in chromosome 3, whereas VHL disease is not associated with papillary tumors. Individuals with VHL disease inherit a germ-line mutation that inactivates one of the VHL suppressor genes located on chromosome 3p25. Malignancies result when the remaining VHL allele is inactivated, and unregulated cell growth occurs.[12] Individuals present with multifocal or bilateral disease at an earlier age, often between 35 and 50 years, with a higher incidence being noted in males. The VHL mutations, which are seen in 60%–70% of clear cell renal carcinomas, result in aggressive biologic behavior and increased tumor vascularity.

Prevention, Screening, and Early Detection

Renal carcinoma is characterized by a lack of early-warning symptoms and variability of presenting symptoms that do not appear directly related to the kidney. This cancer is generally curable only when it is localized and amenable to surgical resection; approximately one-third of patients present with synchronous metastasis, and approximately 50% of patients surgically resected will develop metastatic disease. Von Hippel-Lindau disease is an autosomal dominant inherited disorder resulting in the potential to develop multiple types of cancer. Periodic clinical screening may benefit those who are clinically affected with VHL, individuals who carry the VHL gene mutation but do not have clinical manifestations, and family members who are at genetic risk for inheriting VHL.[13] Screening may also be beneficial in patients with end-stage renal disease, acquired renal cystic disease, hereditary papillary renal cancer, tuberous sclerosis, and autosomal dominant polycystic kidney disease.[14]

Table 45-7 Classification of Epithelial Tumors Arising in the Renal Parenchyma

Malignant tumors
Conventional (clear cell) RCC
Papillary RCC
Chromophobe RCC
Collecting duct carcinoma
"Bellini duct carcinoma"
Medullary carcinoma

Pathophysiology

The pathophysiology of renal cell carcinoma (RCC) represents the extreme heterogeneity of these tumors. The accumulation of germ-line or somatic mutations in critical gain-of-function or loss-of-function genes has been associated with the clonal evolution of most histologic phenotypes of renal cell carcinoma.[15] Because of the diversity in tumor types and the variability in the clinical progression of each type, a revised classification for renal neoplasms was developed in 1997 (Table 45-7).[16]

Most renal cell carcinomas are solid, with sinusoidal vessels that create a highly vascular tumor. Renal tumors are found most frequently in the superior pole, ranging from 3 to 15 cm in size, and averaging 7 cm. They may invade the renal capsule and perirenal fat, becoming large enough to fill the entire retroperitoneum.[17] Tumors have a tendency to invade the renal vein, appearing as a solid column of cells within the vessel, and can extend far along the inferior vena cava into the heart.[18–20] Advances in surgical techniques have made possible extensive surgical resection of both tumor and inferior vena caval thrombi.

Clear cell RCC accounts for 70% of renal cancers. It is sporadic, unilateral, and unifocal, and usually presents during the sixth or seventh decade of life.[21,22] The cytoplasms of these tumors consist of mixtures of cells with clear and granular cytoplasms, and occasionally a pure clear or granular carcinoma. Clear cell tumors have a delicate branching vasculature that can facilitate histologic diagnosis of metastatic lesions.[23] Papillary tumors account for 7%–14% of renal cancers and have a unique tumor pattern, in which cells aggregate in papillae supplied by a single fibrovascular stalk.[24] Chromophobe tumors account for 6%–11% of renal cancers and often arise from cells of the renal cortex. Chromophobe RCC may have an indolent course, although those cancers with a sarcomatoid component behave more aggressively.[22] Oncocytomas represent 7%–10% of renal neoplasms, occur in the seventh decade of life, are benign tumors, and are not graded. Collecting duct carcinoma (Bellini duct carcinoma) are rare tumors, accounting for 1% of renal neoplasms; they arise within the collecting ducts of the renal medulla and have an aggressive course.[16] Medullary renal carcinomas tend to affect young African Americans, originate in the renal medulla, may be associated with a sickle cell trait, and have an aggressive course.[19]

Grading of renal tumors is based on nuclear size, irregularity of the nuclear membrane (shape), and nucleolar prominence, which can be used to characterize the clinical behavior of tumors and serves as a prognostic factor.[20] Nuclear grade classifies cells from grades 1 to 4, with Fuhrman grade 4 tumors having a larger nucleus, a more irregular shape, and a more aggressive behavior, and being associated with a shorter survival.[21] Renal cancer metastasizes via the circulatory and lymphatic systems, involving the retroperitoneal lymph nodes, lungs, liver, bone, muscle, and brain. The most common sites of metastasis involve the lungs, pulmonary and retroperitoneal lymph nodes, liver, and bone. Paraneoplastic syndromes occur in renal cancer and may be the initial symptoms that lead to the diagnosis of renal cancer. These syndromes, which result from biologically active substances or hormones released by the malignant tumor, occur in 10%–14% of renal cancer patients (Table 45-8).

Table 45-8 Paraneoplastic Syndromes

Hypercalcemia
Erythrocytosis
Thrombocytosis
Anemia
Anorexia
Fever/night sweats
Hypertension
Cachexia
Polyneuromyopathy
Amyloidosis

Clinical Manifestations

Renal carcinoma is characterized by diverse symptoms, many of which may be unrelated to the kidney mass. The classic diagnostic triad of gross hematuria, costovertebral pain, and a flank mass is estimated to occur in only 10%–20% of patients. Additional presenting symptoms include weight loss, anorexia, or symptoms arising from metastatic sites and paraneoplastic syndromes. The lung is the most common site of metastatic disease in renal cancer (in approximately 50% of cases), while other sites of metastasis include the retroperitoneal lymph nodes, liver, bone, adrenal gland, and brain. Renal cancer metastasizes to other sites as well, including the pancreas, abdominal and pelvic muscles, diaphragm, and skin. Asymptomatic brain metastasis may be identified during diagnostic work-up or pretreatment staging studies, with symptomatic disease being diagnosed at any time during the disease. Lytic disease occurs in approximately 30% of patients, emphasizing the importance of early assessment and intervention to reduce the potential for significant functional impairment and morbidity.

Spontaneous regression of metastatic renal cell carcinoma occurs in a small percentage of patients, most often in those individuals with good-risk prognostic criteria and minimal disease, although the immunologic process occurring in such cases is unclear. Spontaneous regression occurs in 3%–5% of patients with metastatic disease following nephrectomy or during periods of observation.

Assessment

Diagnosis of renal cell carcinoma includes the exclusion of other malignant or nonmalignant processes, including benign inflammatory abscesses or pyelonephritis; hematomas within the structure of the kidney; various pseudotumors; and various cystic masses including benign cysts, polycystic kidney, cystic dysplastic kidney, and hydronephrosis. Incidental detection of renal tumors has resulted from increased use of imaging, including ultrasound, CT scan, and MRI for nonrenal symptoms.[22,23] A detailed review of symptoms, family history, and current physical exam will assist in determining appropriate radiology procedures to be completed. Intravenous urography is often the initial diagnostic procedure done to evaluate nonspecific symptoms including flank pain or hematuria; it assesses the urothelial tract.[23] Ultrasound is a noninvasive procedure that can differentiate between cystic and solid masses. Doppler ultrasound procedures can further evaluate the vascularity of a renal mass and assess the renal vein and inferior vena cava for the presence of tumor thrombus.[23] Computed tomography scans provide highly sensitive imaging, including scans obtained both before and after administration of intravenous contrast. Magnetic resonance imaging may be used in patients in whom intravenous ionic contrast is contraindicated due to allergy or impaired renal function. Demonstration of "enhancement" or increased density on CT scan or an increase in signal intensity on MRI after intravenous contrast is given is indicative of increased vascularity associated with a renal mass. Histologic confirmation of renal cell carcinoma can be obtained from ultrasound or CT-guided biopsy procedures. F-18 fluorodeoxyglucose positron emission tomography (FDG-PET) imaging provides information regarding the presence of metastatic lesions and may reduce the need for biopsy procedures.[24] Arteriography, venography, and three-phase renal helical CT scan provide information concerning the relationship of the tumor to the collecting system and adjacent normal parenchyma and the renal and tumor vascular supply; these data essential for preoperative planning and intraoperative management of renal lesions.[25] An inferior venacavogram can further delineate the presence and extent of tumor thrombus involvement of the vena cava. Three-phase renal helical scan provides data for three-dimensional volume rendering in a video format that enhances preoperative and intraoperative planning and management for nephron-sparing surgical procedures.[25]

The prognosis for individuals with renal cell carcinoma takes into account several variables, including grade, tumor histology, TNM staging, and various prognostic groupings. Important prognostic indicators include the TNM staging at diagnosis, tumor histology, tumor grade, and ECOG status.[21,26] Recent analysis has provided new information regarding prognostic indicators for previously untreated and previously treated patients with renal carcinoma. Several studies have identified various clinical features that can be used to predict survival for patients with advanced renal carcinoma (Table 45-9).[27–29] Five criteria (Karnofsky Performance Status (KPS), lactate dehydrogenase, hemoglobin, calcium, and nephrectomy status) were used to retrospectively analyze survival in 670 patients, demonstrating three-year survival rates of 31% for patients in the favorable-risk group (no risk factors), 7% for the intermediate-risk group (one to two risk factors), and 0% for the poor-risk group (three or more risk factors).[27] Analysis of another group of patients identified similar criteria, with the additional criteria related to the number of sites of metastatic disease (fewer than two sites or more than two sites).[28] The median overall survival in a group of 353 patients studied was 14.9 months, with a 32.2-month median survival for patients having a favorable risk (fewer than two risk factors), 17.6-month median survival for the intermediate-risk group (three to five risk factors), and 8.8-month median survival for the poor-risk group (more than five risk factors).[28] Further studies in untreated and treated patients with renal cancer will provide additional information relevant to determining appropriate therapeutic strategies and evaluation of outcomes for new anticancer agents.

Table 45-9 Prognostic Factors in Untreated, Advanced Renal Carcinoma

KPS < 80%
LDH > 1.5 × upper limit of normal
Hemoglobin < lower limit of normal
Corrected serum calcium > 10 mg/dL
Absence of prior nephrectomy
Metastasis-free interval
Number of sites of metastatic disease

Classification and Staging

Renal carcinoma has been previously classified according to the Robson classification system for RCC staging, but this system does not sufficiently differentiate stages that might have substantially different prognoses.[30] The fifth edition of the American Joint Committee on Cancer's TNM system altered staging criteria to mirror the improved results attained with the contemporary management of renal cancer.[31] The TNM staging system differentiates between tumor size, local invasion, vena caval involvement, regional lymph node status, and distant metastasis (Table 45-10).[32] The optimal breakpoint in tumor size for defining localized tumor stage remains controversial, as recent studies demonstrate prognostic differences between small tumors (3–4 cm) and larger tumors (4–7cm).[33,34]

Therapeutic Approaches

Surgery

Nephrectomy has long been the mainstay of treatment for renal carcinoma, but advances in surgical procedures have reduced the need for radical nephrectomy and potential surgical complications. Minimally invasive nephron-sparing surgery preserves functioning of renal parenchyma, with potentially comparable outcomes demonstrated when long-term data are analyzed.[35] Procedures include laparoscopic partial or radical nephrectomy (Figures 45-1 and 45-2), probe ablation (cryotherapy or radiofrequency ablation),

Table 45-10 TNM Staging of Renal Carcinoma

Primary Tumor (T)	
TX	Primary tumor cannot be assessed
T0	No evidence of primary tumor
T1	Tumor 7 cm or less in greatest dimension limited to the kidney
T2	Tumor more than 7 cm in greatest dimension limited to the kidney
T3	Tumor extends into major veins or invades the adrenal gland or perinephric tissues, but not beyond Gerota's fascia
T3a	Tumor invades the adrenal gland or perinephric tissues but not beyond Gerota's fascia
T3b	Tumor grossly extends into the renal vein(s) or vena cava below the diaphragm
T3c	Tumor grossly extends into the renal vein(s) or vena cava above the diaphragm
T4	Tumor invades beyond Gerota's fascia
Regional Lymph Nodes (N)*	
NX	Regional lymph nodes cannot be assessed
N0	No regional lymph node metastases
N1	Metastasis in a single regional lymph node
N2	Metastasis in more than one regional lymph node
Distant Metastasis (M)	
MX	Distant metastasis cannot be assessed
M0	No distant metastasis
M1	Distant metastasis

Stage Grouping			
Stage I	T1	N0	M0
Stage II	T2	N0	M0
Stage III	T1	N1	M0
	T2	N1	M0
	T3a	N0	M0
	T3a	N1	M0
	T3b	N0	M0
	T3b	N1	M0
	T3c	N0	M0
	T3c	N1	M0
Stage IV	T4	N0	M0
	T4	N1	M0
	Any T	N2	M0
	Any T	Any N	M1

* Laterality does not affect the N classification.

Date from American Joint Committee on Cancer, American Cancer Society, American College of Surgeons: Kidney cancer, in *AJCC Cancer Staging Handbook*. Philadelphia, Lippincott-Raven, 2002.[32]

and noninvasive ablation (high-intensity, focused ultrasound), all of which are associated with shorter hospital stays and fewer complications. Laproscopic partial nephrectomy procedures are evolving and demonstrate comparable surgical outcomes with minimally invasive techniques.[36,37] Laparoscopic renal cryoablation is appropriate for small (< 4 cm) exophytic lesions located away from the collecting system. Laparoscopic radical nephrectomy is appropriate for T_1–T_{3a} N_0M_0 lesions without perirenal, lymphatic, or vascular extension. Complications include hemorrhage, ureteral injury, urinary leakage, hematoma, hematuria, incisional hernia, and infection. Nursing care includes monitoring for signs and symptoms of postoperative complications, patient education regarding wound care, and preparation for discharge and home recovery.

Cytoreductive nephrectomy prior to or following immunotherapy can prolong survival and delay disease progression for many patients. Resection of metastatic disease following immunotherapy results in a significant disease-free period for patients who have a good performance status and minimal disease burden. Radiofrequency ablation of tumors is being investigated, but its role is yet to be determined.

Radiation

Radiation in renal cancer focuses on symptom management, with occasional use in the initial management of the disease. Intraoperative or postoperative radiotherapy should be considered only for cases in which there is a significant risk of local recurrence and should target the smallest possible volume. Palliative radiation for patients with lytic metastasis provides both pain relief and structural stabilization. It may be given following orthopedic surgery, including bone stabilization using rods or pins, and joint replacement for metastatic disease. Palliative radiation is used for pulmonary metastasis causing obstruction, which is often associated with cough and postobstructive pneumonia. Surgical intervention prior to radiation for spinal cord compression may improve functional outcome.

Complications of radiation therapy may include dermatological effects and gastrointestinal effects such as nausea, vomiting, diarrhea, or obstruction. Nursing care includes assessment and patient education regarding pain management, dermatological effects, and appropriate modifications in short-term and long-term mobility and activity, and management of gastrointestinal or urinary symptoms associated with treatment. Patients should be instructed to avoid the use of deodorant soaps and skin care products with fragrances, and be aware of specialized skin care products used during and following treatment. Small, frequent meals will maximize caloric intake, emphasizing the importance of adequate hydration to promote tissue hydration and to minimize dehydration, fatigue, nausea, and constipation.

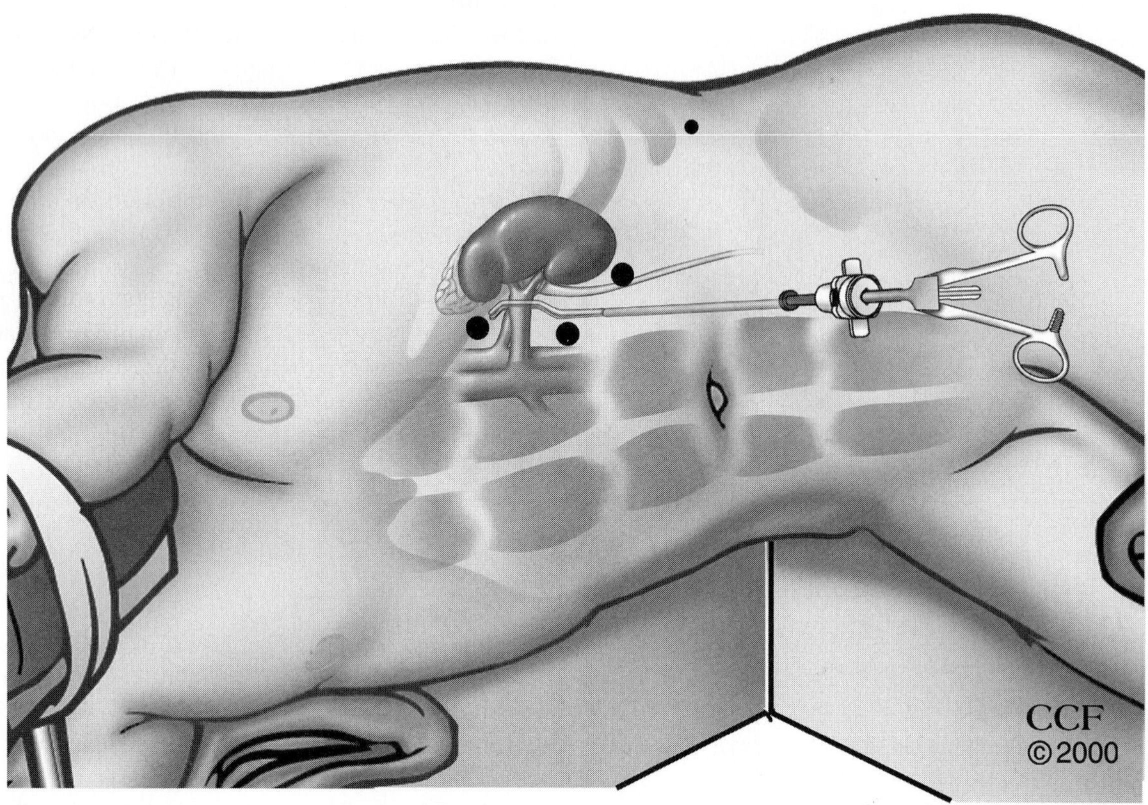

Figure 45-1 Transperitoneal technique for laparoscopic partial nephrectomy.

Chemotherapy

Renal cell carcinoma is generally chemoresistant. Agents including vinblastine, floxuridine, 5–fluorouracil, and gemcitabine have been investigated for its treatment and have demonstrated response rates of 5%–10%. Research continues to define the multidrug resistance observed in kidney cancer, the role of p glycoprotein and glutathione — S-transferase, and use of combination strategies.

Biotherapy

Cytokine therapy is the current ''standard'' systemic treatment for metastatic renal cancer. It stimulates various immune effector cells, including T cells and natural killer (NK) cells, to react to the tumor. Aldesleukin (interleukin-2) is the only FDA-approved therapy for metastatic renal cancer in the United States. High-dose intravenous interleukin-2 has demonstrated a 15% overall response rate; a 7% complete response rate, and an 8% partial response rate, both of which are durable; and a median survival of 16.3 months.[38] A three-arm study of high-dose IV, low-dose IV, and low-dose SC interleukin-2 found a higher response rate in the high-dose arm, but no difference in survival.[39] Nursing care focuses on effective management of toxicities, in the hospital or the outpatient setting. Side effects vary according to the dose, route of administration, and duration of therapy, but may include chills, fever, subcutaneous injection site reactions, fluid retention and capillary leak syndrome, and organ toxicities that are generally reversible. Clinical pathways have been established that provide detailed nursing assessments, interventions, and patient education strategies.[40] Interferon-α, -β, and -γ remain investigational therapies but provide additional options in clinical trials or for off-label use. The patient receiving high-dose interleukin-2 requires careful assessment and monitoring for cardiopulmonary toxicities including pulmonary edema, hypoxia, cardiac arrhythmia, and temporary renal impairment, which may require the use of vasopressor support. ''Constitutional symptoms,'' including chills, fever, myalgias, and arthralgias, are typically managed with the use of acetaminophen and anti-inflammatory agents. Nursing care

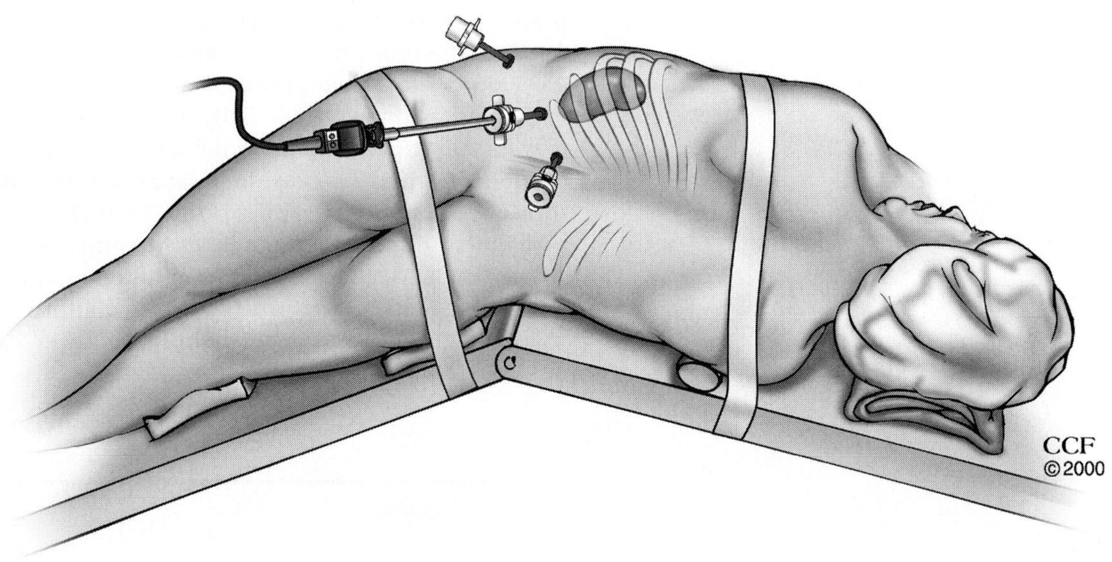

Figure 45-2 Retroperitoneal technique for laparoscopic partial or radical nephrectomy.

includes patient education for subcutaneous injection and management of side effects including chills, fever, fatigue, taste changes, and anorexia.

Nursing Care

Care of patients hospitalized for surgery, anticancer therapy, or symptom management includes patient and family education, support, and coordination of care. Discharge planning focuses on skin and wound care, maximization of nutritional intake, effective pain management, and follow-up care. Patient education should emphasize effective communication with healthcare providers so that early intervention can minimize the severity of side effects, enhance quality of life, and maximize therapeutic outcomes.

Symptom Management and Supportive Care

Comprehensive care of the patient with renal carcinoma results from detailed assessment of disease-related symptoms, prompt intervention, and ongoing evaluation of medical and nonmedical interventions. Patients may develop complex symptoms that often overlap with toxicities associated with treatment, and they often require a multidisciplinary approach for effective management (Table 45-11). Pain management includes the use of narcotic analgesic agents, radiation, surgery, and bisphosphonate therapy for bone metastasis to reduce the incidence of skeletal-related events. Early diagnosis and intervention will minimize the spinal cord compression associated with lytic vertebral involvement. Erythrocytosis is rare, and phlebotomy should be considered for a hematocrit greater than 55 g/dL. Management of complex disease-related gastrointestinal symptoms will allow patients to tolerate anticancer therapies that might otherwise result in dose modification or discontinuation in treatment. The management of brain metastasis is evolving, with advances in the use of steriotactic gamma knife radiosurgery and surgical interventions effectively managing brain metastasis, thereby delaying the need for and neurologic toxicities associated with whole-brain radiotherapy and providing for a shorter recovery

Table 45-11 Symptoms Associated with Renal Cancer

Pain
Tumor compression
Bone metastasis
Nerve root compression
Gastrointestinal
Nausea
Vomiting
Anorexia
Constipation
Diarrhea
Neurologic
Fatigue
Depression
Confusion due to brain metastasis
Impaired mobility due to bone metastasis or fracture
Hematological
Anemia
Erythrocytosis
Thrombocytosis

period. Whole-brain radiation is appropriate for patients who have disease progression following local intervention, have large tumors, or experience extensive metastasis.[41,42] Collaboration with palliative care specialists provides opportunities for coordination of multiple modalities so as to enhance therapeutic outcomes, ultimately improving quality of life.

Follow-up care for patients after nephrectomy includes surveillance reflecting the stage of disease at diagnosis. Patients with stage I disease should be monitored yearly with a physical exam and blood studies. Those with stage II disease should be monitored yearly with a physical exam, blood studies, chest x-ray, and CT scans every 2 years. Patients with stage III disease will typically be monitored every 6 months with blood studies, chest x-ray, and CT scans for several years, with the interval between procedures increasing after 2 years. Those with stage IV disease will be monitored every 2–3 months during treatment to assess the effectiveness and appropriateness of treatment.

Conclusion

Treatment options for renal carcinoma are expanding with additional studies involving adoptive immunotherapy, non-myeloablative allogeneic peripheral stem cell transplant, vaccine strategies, and novel targeted therapies. Translational research has led to identification of molecular processes and pathways leading to malignant cell proliferation. Renal carcinomas are highly vascular tumors, and targeting VEGF pathways with drugs such as bevacizumab, SU011248, or AG013736 as single agents or in combination may provide new directions in treatment strategies; these options are currently being investigated in clinical trials. Agents targeting raf and ras kinase pathways (BAY 43–9006), endothelial growth factor receptors (ABX-EGF) and pathways (OSI-779), and other pathways may further expand the potential therapeutic options. These strategies may provide an approach to reduce the development or delay the progression of metastatic disease. Continued efforts in the identification, development, and clinical application of tumor antigens and tumor markers will provide valuable information in the diagnosis and management of renal cell carcinoma.

References

1. Jamal A, Tiwari RC, Muuray T, et al: Cancer statistics 2004. *CA Cancer J Clin*, 54:2–29, 2004
2. Skinner DG: Management of invasive bladder cancer: a meticulous lymph node dissection can make a difference. *J Urol* 128:34–36, 1982
3. O'Donnell M: Intravesical therapy for superfical bladder cancer: a practical guide, in Kursh ED, Ulchaker JC (eds.): *Office Urology: The Clinician's Guide.* Totowa, NJ, Humana Press, 2001, pp 185–201
4. Droller MJ: Evaluation and management of low-grade, low-stage bladder cancer, in Kursh ED, Ulchaker JC (eds.): *Office Urology: The Clinician's Guide.* Totowa, NJ, Humana Press, 2001, pp 175–184
5. Carroll PR, Grossfeld GD, Barbour S: Urinary diversion and bladder substitution, in Tanagho EA, McAninch JW (eds.): *Smith's General Urology* (ed 16). New York, Lange Medical Books/McGraw-Hill, 2004, pp 400–415
6. Witjes JA, Debruyne FM: Intravesical chemotherapy, in Vogelzang NJ, et al (eds.): *Comprehensive Textbook of Genitourinary Oncology* (ed 2). Philadelphia, Lippincott, Williams and Wilkins, 2000, pp 394–408.
7. Montie JE, Marcovich R: Selecting and counseling patients for cystectomy or cystoprostatectomy, in Kursh ED, Ulchaker JC (eds.): *Office Urology: The Clinician's Guide.* Totowa, NJ, Humana Press, 2001, pp 203–212
8. Chow WH, Devesa SS, Warren JL, et al: The rising incidence of renal cell cancer in the United States. *JAMA* 281:1628–1631, 1999
9. Uzzo RG, Cairns P, Al-Saleem T, et al: The basic biology and immunobiology of renal cell carcinoma: considerations for the clinician. *Urol Clin North Am* 30:423–436, 2003
10. Enquist D, Zambrano N, Zbar B, et al: Molecular genetics of renal cell carcinoma, in Bukowski RM, Novick AC (eds.): *Renal Cell Carcinoma: Molecular Biology, Immunology, and Clinical Management.* Totowa, NJ, Humana Press, 2000, pp 79–92
11. Rini BI, Vogelzang NJ: Prognostic factors in renal carcinoma. *Semin Oncol* 27:213–220, 2000

12. Hwang JJ, Uchio EM, Linehan WM, et al: Hereditary kidney cancer. *Urol Clin North Am* 30:831–842, 2003
13. Middelton L, Lessick M: Inherited urologic malignant disorders: nursing implications. *Urol Nurs* 23:15–29, 2003
14. Cohn EB, Campbell SC: Screening for renal cell carcinoma, in Bukowski RM, Novick AC (eds.): *Renal Cell Carcinoma: Molecular Biology, Immunology, and Clinical Management.* Totowa, NJ, Humana Press, 2000, pp 93–110
15. Uzzo RG, Cairns P, Al-Saleem T, et al: The basic biology and immunobiology of renal cell carcinoma: considerations for the clinician. *Urol Clin North Am* 30:423–436, 2003
16. Reuter VE, Presti JC: Contemporary approach to classification of renal epithelial tumors. *Semin Oncol* 27:124–137, 2000
17. Levin HS, Myles JL: The pathology of renal neoplasms, in Bukowski RM, Novick AC (eds.): *Renal Cell Carcinoma: Molecular Biology, Immunology, and Clinical Management.* Totowa, NJ, Humana Press, 2000, pp 15–38
18. Weiss LM, Gelb AB, Medeiros LJ: Adult renal epithelial neoplasms. *Anatom Pathol* 103:624–635, 1995
19. Davis CJ, Mostofi FK, Sesterhenn IA: Renal medullary carcinoma. The seventh sickle cell nephropathy. *Am J Surg Pathol* 19:1–11, 1995
20. Pantuck AJ, Zisman A, Belldegrun A: Basic biology and clinical behavior of renal cell carcinoma, in Belldegrun A, Ritchie AWS, Figlin RA, et al (eds.): *Renal and Adrenal Tumors: Biology and Management.* New York, Oxford University Press, 2003, pp 81–89
21. Tsui K, Shvarts O, Smith RB, et al: Prognostic indicators for renal cell carcinoma: a multivariate analysis of 643 patients using the revised 1997 TNM staging criteria. *J Urol* 163:1090–1095, 2000
22. Israel GM, Bosniak MA: Renal imaging for diagnosis and staging of renal cell carcinoma. *Urol Clin North Am* 30:499–514, 2003
23. Hilton S: Imaging of renal cell carcinoma. *Semin Oncol* 27:150–159, 2003
24. Majhail NS, Urbain JL, Albani JM, et al: F-18 fluorodeoxyglucose positron emission tomography in the evaluation of distant metastases from renal cell carcinoma. *J Clin Oncol* 21:3995–4000, 2003
25. Derweesh IH, Herts B, Novick AC: Three-dimensional image reconstruction for preplanning of renal surgery. *Urol Clin North Am* 30:515–528, 2003
26. Russo P: Renal cell carcinoma: presentation, staging, and surgical treatment. *Semin Oncol* 27:160–176, 2000
27. Motzer RJ, Mazumdar M, Bacik J, et al: Survival and prognostic stratification of 670 patients with advanced renal cell carcinoma. *J Clin Oncol* 17:2530–2540, 1999
28. Abou-Jawde R, Mekhail T, Merhi GB, et al: Prognostic factors for survival in previously untreated metastatic renal cell cancer: a comprehensive evaluation and validation of established risk groups. *J Clin Oncol* 22:385, 2003 (abstr 1545)
29. Elson P: Prognostic factors in advance renal cell carcinoma, in Belldegrun A, Ritchie AWS, Figlin RA, et al (eds.): *Renal and Adrenal Tumors: Biology and Management.* New York, Oxford University Press, 2003, pp 186–194
30. Pantuck AG, Zisman A, Belldegrum AS: The changing natural history of renal cell carcinoma. *J Urol* 166:1611–1623, 2001
31. Leibovich BC, Pantuck AJ, Matthew HT, et al: Current staging of renal cell carcinoma. *Urol Clin North Am* 30:481–497, 2003
32. American Joint Committee on Cancer, American Cancer Society, American College of Surgeons: Kidney cancer, in *AJCC Cancer Staging Handbook.* Philadelphia, Lippincott-Raven, 2002
33. Hafez KS, Fergany AF, Novick AC: Nephron sparing surgery for localized renal cell carcinoma: impact of tumor size on patient survival, tumor recurrence and TNM staging. *J Urol* 162:1930–1933, 1999
34. Zisman A, Pantuck AH, Chao D, et al: Reevaluation of the 1997 TNM classification for renal cell carcinoma: T1 and T2 cutoff point at 4.5 rather than 7 cm better correlates with clinical outcome. *J Urol* 166:54–58, 2001
35. Gill IS: Minimally invasive nephron-sparing surgery. *Urol Clin North Am* 30:551–579, 2003
36. Gill IS, Desai MM, Kaouk JH, et al: Laparoscopic partial nephrectomy for renal tumor: duplicating open surgical techniques. *J Urol* 167:469–476, 2002
37. Gill IS, Matin SF, Desai MM, et al: Comparative analysis of laparoscopic versus open partial nephrectomy for renal tumors in 200 patients. *J Urol* 170:64–68, 2003
38. Fisher RI, Rosenberg SA, Sznol M, et al: High-dose aldesleukin in renal cell carcinoma: long-term survival update. *Cancer J* 3(suppl 1):S1–S4, 1997
39. Yang JC, Sherry RM, Steinberg SM, et al: Randomized study of high-dose and low-dose interleukin-2 in patients with metastatic renal cancer. *J Clin Oncol* 21:3127–3132, 2003
40. Mavroukakis SA, Muehlbauer PM, White RL, et al: Clinical pathways for managing patients receiving Interleukin 2. *Clin J Oncol Nurs* 5:207–217, 2001
41. Cannady SB, Cavanaugh KA, Lee SY, et al: Results of whole brain radiotherapy and recursive partitioning analysis in patients with brain metastases from renal cell carcinoma: a retrospective study. *Int J Radiat Oncol Biol Phys* 58:253–258, 2004
42. Sheehan JP, Sun MH, Kondziolka D, et al: Radiosurgery in patients with renal cell carcinoma metastasis to the brain: long-term outcomes and prognostic factors influencing survival and local tumor control. *J Neurosurg* 98:342–349, 2003

CHAPTER 46

Breast Cancer

Dianne D. Chapman, ND, RN, ANCP
Susan Moore, RN, MSN, CNP, AOCN®

Introduction

Breast cancer is the most common cancer in women, accounting for 32% of all cases of female cancers. It is the leading cause of death for women ages 20–59 and is second to lung cancer as the leading cause of cancer deaths in women.[1] The incidence of breast cancer increases with age, increases more slowly between the ages of 45 and 50,[2] then increases steadily with each year.[3] More than 70% of all breast cancer occurs in women who are 50 years of age or older. Screening methods, particularly mammography, have become more precise, permitting earlier diagnosis, which in part accounts for the dramatic increase in incidence in breast cancer between 1982 and 1987, and is likely responsible for the current slight decrease in mortality and incidence figures.[1,4]

Breast cancer incidence has increased among all races since 1980. It is highest among whites and African Americans, lower in American Indians, Alaska Natives, Asians and Pacific Islanders, and Hispanics. White women are increasingly being diagnosed with small (< 2cm) tumors that tend to be localized. The incidence rate for African American women stabilized during the 1990s, but a large proportion of these women will have larger tumors and more advanced disease at diagnosis. Similarly, women from other racial and ethnic groups are more likely to be diagnosed with more advanced disease.[4] More research in the area of chemoprevention, improved systemic therapies, and better access to preventive health care and early detection for the socioeconomically disadvantaged are needed to change the current mortality rates from this disease.[5,6]

The lifetime risk of breast cancer has increased from 5.5% (1 in every 18 women) to 13% (1 in every 8 women) in the past 40 years.[1,7] This increasing incidence affects predominantly women younger than 55 years of age and African American women younger than 45 years of age.[8] Possible reasons for this trend are that women are living longer into the cancer-prone years, statistical reporting is better, and better screening methods are available. In addition, changes in dietary and socioeconomic habits, and increasing exposure to carcinogens, may contribute to the higher incidence of breast cancer.[9,10]

While the incidence of breast cancer has increased over the past 30 years, the mortality rate has recently demonstrated a slight decrease (down 2.3% from 1990–2000),[1] reflecting better cure rates for earlier-staged lesions. This apparent progress may be related to a better understanding of the natural history of breast cancer as well as reflect the benefit of early detection methods. The disparity between survival rates for white women and African American women has increased in the last 20 years, however. In 2000, the death rate was 32% higher in African American women than in white women.[4] Several theories have been put forward to explain this survival disparity, ranging from diagnosis at a more advanced stage of disease to tumors with poor prognostic indicators due to biologic or hormonal differences.[8] It is imperative that nurses be acquainted with the various cultural and economic barriers that may keep women from utilizing screening tools and benefiting from community education programs.[11]

It is now widely accepted that breast cancer is not one disease but many diseases, differing in its histologic, biologic, and immunologic characteristics. It is considered systemic rather than localized disease, with the ability to exhibit early hematogenous spread prior to lymph node involvement. Phenotypic heterogeneity exists within individual breast neoplasms such that intrinsic and acquired drug resistance occurs, rendering unresponsive cell lines unopposed and capable of establishing metastatic sites. Whether the individual with breast cancer survives the disease is determined by numerous factors, but the outcome primarily depends on the intrinsic growth rate of the tumor, which varies dramatically; the age of the woman at diagnosis; and numerous biological parameters that ultimately define the natural history of the disease.

The interdisciplinary team utilizes a variety of clinical, histological, and pathological findings to define, as precisely as possible, the particular characteristics of a breast cancer that will determine the most appropriate treatment plan for a given patient. This approach integrates the physical examination with the histopathological characteristics of the tumor, and it incorporates the patient's personal bias based on her emotional needs and physical preferences. As a member of this team, the nurse must be aware of the factors affecting the selection of the treatment plan and appropriately educate the patient regarding the various treatment strategies in an effort to prevent and manage complications of the disease and its treatment.

Etiology

Experimental and clinical data indicate that the development of breast cancer is not a chance event. The genesis of breast cancer seems to be a multiphasic process involving many factors that are influential in the ongoing duel between tumor growth potential and host resistance. Attempts are being made to reveal the etiology of breast cancer through an intense study of its epidemiology. As populations are identified in whom the incidence of the disease is increased, a genetic, hormonal, or biochemical factor may be identified that is considered significant in etiology. Epidemiological features, when statistically correlated with incidence of disease, designate a particular factor as a "risk factor." Each risk factor merely serves as one piece of the puzzle, however, because so many different factors either increase or decrease a woman's risk of developing breast cancer. Table 46–1 groups current risk factors in terms of importance, according to our understanding of the etiology of breast cancer.

Table 46-1 Risk Factors for Breast Cancer

Primary	
Female	
Age > 50	
Country of origin	North America Northern Europe
Family history	Known *BRCA1*/*BRCA2* mutation Personal history of invasive breast cancer Two or more first-degree relatives with breast cancer Bilateral breast cancer or male breast cancer in relative
Ionizing radiation	Radiation to chest prior to age 30
Biopsy history	Atypical hyperplasia Carcinoma in situ (DCIS and LCIS)
Secondary	
Postmenopausal obesity	
Early menarche (<12 years) coupled with late menopause (> 55 years); onset of regular cycles within 1 year of menarche	
Nulliparity or first full-term pregnancy > 30 years of age	
Combined hormone replacement therapy	
Alcohol >2 drinks per day	
Other	
Estrogen replacement therapy	
Diet	

Hormonal Factors

The hormone environment has long been recognized as a major factor in the development of breast cancer. This relationship is well demonstrated in that gender is the most significant risk factor for the development of the disease. Women are 100 times more likely to develop breast cancer than men. Additionally, after a diagnosis of breast cancer has been made, the relationship of the tumor estrogen receptor with the response to hormonal manipulation strongly suggests a hormonal connection. Attempting to predict the effect of hormones on breast cancer, Cauley recently conducted a study that examined the serum concentrations of estradiol in women with breast cancer and a control group, and found that higher concentrations were associated with increased risk.[12] Early menarche (before age 12), nulliparity or parity after age 30, and late menopause (after age 55) are well-known events that are considered risk factors for development of breast cancer. All of these events are linked to the type and duration of exposure to endogenous hormones that may influence the development of breast cancer.

Pregnancy (full term) has been reported to exert a deterrent effect on the development of breast cancer. This relationship is generally thought to be based on the change in the hormonal milieu. The exact mechanism is unknown, but speculation includes the effects of the alteration of estrogens, especially estriol. A significant increase in estriol compared with estrone and estradiol occurs during pregnancy. Estriol is considered to have a protective effect against cancer genesis, whereas estrone and estradiol may act as initiators or promoters in breast tissue. Additionally, the protective effect related to an early first pregnancy may change the biological properties of the mammary cells, allowing the differentiated cells to spend more time on DNA repair, thereby reducing carcinogenesis.[13,14]

This preventive effect may be more pronounced with pregnancies at a young age (< 20 years) and is enhanced by subsequent pregnancies.[15] Additionally, the benefit conferred on these women continues to be a positive factor during the extent of their lifetime. Lactation and breast-feeding have historically been considered protective mechanisms against breast cancer development. Although the theory remains controversial and the benefit may be related to parity, several studies have found correlations between progressive risk reduction in premenopausal women and the number of breast-feeding years.[16–19]

A correlation between breast cancer and abortion, whether spontaneous or elective, has been suggested. Studies in the United States have compared the reproductive histories of women diagnosed with breast cancer and those of a matched control group and have either indicated a small overall increase in risk or negligible risk associated with abortion.[20–22] Conversely, a large Danish study (1.5 million women) used population registries to investigate this correlation and found no increased risk of breast cancer.[23] Because abortion is such a highly charged emotional issue, it is important for the nurse to properly assess reported modifiers of risk. All studies, especially those incorporating controversial issues, should meet the standards of validity and reliability.

The role that endogenous estrogens may play in the development of breast cancer suggests that exogenous therapy may be instrumental in the development of breast cancer. Exogenous hormones are given in various instances, but the primary reasons are pregnancy prevention in childbearing years and prophylaxis for osteoporosis and amelioration of hot flashes in menopausal women. While information on the use of hormone therapy is limited in its consistency, recent papers have addressed these correlations.

Oral contraceptives have been marketed since the 1960s. Although enough time has elapsed to study large numbers of women, the connection between oral contraceptives (OC) and breast cancer has resulted in inconsistent and controversial reports. Although studies investigating OC are often difficult to interpret, some basic risk information has been extrapolated. In general, nulliparous women who begin using contraceptives before age 18 and continue uninterrupted use for more than 8 years have a minimal increased risk of developing breast cancer. Current users have a slight increase in risk, which subsequently declines after stopping OC use, and returns to baseline after 10 years.[14] The literature also suggests that OC use during the middle reproductive years poses no additional risk. Another increase in risk has been associated with OC use during the perimenopausal years.[14] This risk may be due to the delay of menopause brought about by creating and maintaining a hormonal environment that mimics that of a menstruating woman.

While the question of risk in relation to hormone replacement therapy (HRT) has been difficult to ascertain, new evidence of risk associated with combined therapy has been documented. The Women's Health Initiative (WHI) is a large, ongoing, randomized study to investigate strategies to reduce heart disease, breast cancer, colorectal cancer, and fractures in postmenopausal women (161,809 women aged 50–79). The study is divided into several trials focusing on low-fat dietary patterns, calcium and vitamin D intake, and hormone use — two trials involving (1) either 0.625 mg estrogen plus 2.5 mg progestin or placebo (for women with a uterus) and (2) either estrogen alone or placebo (for women with a hysterectomy). The estrogen and progestin arm (16,608 women) was stopped after 5.2 years due to a small but statistical increased risk of breast cancer, coronary heart disease (CHD) events (fatal and nonfatal), stroke, and pulmonary embolism. Although there was a reduction in fractures and colorectal cancer and a smaller reduction in endometrial cancer, the results indicated that combined HRT is not a recommended intervention for primary prevention. Note that the increased risk in breast cancer applies only to current HRT users and those who stopped taking HRT less than 5 years earlier. The risk of breast cancer for women who stopped HRT use more than 5 years earlier is no different than that for women who never used HRT. Women seeking combined HRT for menopausal symptoms should be aware of their personal risk of CHD and breast cancer versus the potential benefits of risk reduction noted in the study.[24,25] The publicity surrounding this report on combined therapy motivated many women on HRT to consider discontinuing it. A study conducted by Ettinger and colleagues indicated that 50% of women who received WHI information through their health plan was likely to discontinue the therapy.[26] Additional information from the estrogen-only arm of the WHI trial was recently released. The estrogen-only trial was stopped in February 2004. A March 2004 release noted that the estrogen-only arm had been stopped due to the finding of an increased risk for stroke among participants as well as the failure to identify any cardioprotective properties.

The concern surrounding prescribing HRT for premenopausal breast cancer survivors remains a problematic issue for clinicians. The number of survivors has increased steadily and includes a growing population of women who are "forced" into menopause through chemotherapeutic agents. The premenopausal women who experience an acute, early menopause seem to report more severe symptoms than premenopausal women who experience gradual, natural hormonal decreases over time. Although a majority of these women will enjoy disease-free survival, their quality of life may be compromised by somatic complaints caused by the dramatic drop in estrogen levels (e.g., hot flashes, dyspareunia, labile mood swings) and physical manifestations (e.g., osteoporosis and possible heart disease). Observational studies have demonstrated that HRT may remedy or reduce osteoporosis, ischemic heart disease, vasomotor symptoms, and urogenital atrophy in these young women, but healthcare providers remain reluctant to prescribe it. Giving breast cancer survivors estrogen therapy is a controversial issue, as the current standard of practice generally precludes prescribing these hormonal agents and the WHI results will likely give added credence to existing practice. [27,28]

Several articles have addressed this problem in the past and the need for quantitative data to resolve it: Large, prospective, randomized studies are required to elucidate this complicated issue.[29] One study conducted by Vassilopoulou-Sellin and colleagues reported the results of a 5-year study of 299 women. The participants were randomized to either no treatment (n = 43) or conjugated estrogen replacement (n = 34) for a total of 77 patients. An additional group of 222 women who chose not to be randomized were observed; 22 of these women were already taking estrogen replacement therapy (ERT), giving a final participation of 56 women on ERT and 243 women not on ERT. Combined therapy with progesterone was not offered due to the possibility that progesterone may have an independent effect on recurrence or developing new breast cancers.[30,31] The preliminary and 5-year findings indicated no significant increase in the incidence of breast cancer for the ERT group. This study provided additional reinforcement and reassurance that ERT does not decrease disease-free survival.[32] Two other recent studies reported no increase in new or recurrent breast cancer for users of combined therapy or estrogen-only therapy.[29,33] Despite these favorable studies, the WHI findings may provide additional confirmation that the safety of using combined hormonal agents in breast cancer survivors has not been demonstrated and that use of these agents should be considered only when nonhormonal agents fail to remedy severe vasomotor symptoms. Practitioners counseling women who elect to take combined therapy must provide detailed information regarding the risks versus the potential benefits. In any event, the use of HRT should be limited to the lowest dose and shortest duration possible.[34]

Family History

Along with age and gender, family history of breast cancer is a contributing factor to the potential risk of developing the disease. Many people, including healthcare providers, estimate risk factors erroneously. This error is due to the wide range of risk associated with a family history of breast cancer dependent upon the age and known risk factors of the patient, the ages and number of first- and second-degree relatives with unilateral or bilateral breast cancer, and the presence of autosomal dominant gene mutations. Many studies have tried to extrapolate risk based on personal and family history.[35–37] The Gail model is an assessment tool that calculates the risk of invasive breast cancer within a specific time frame among white, African American, and Hispanic women. The risk factor data were initially extrapolated from the Breast Cancer Detection Demonstration project and modified for the National Surgical Breast and Bowel Program prevention trial (NSABP P-1). The Gail model is used as a screening tool but will not capture several elements of potential risk—namely, age of relatives' diagnosis, history of bilateral cancer, breast cancer in second-degree relatives, and history of ovarian cancer. The Claus model was developed to address some of these deficits.[37] Using data from the Cancer and Steroid Hormone Study, this model gives the age-specific risk for a woman with a family history of one or more relatives. BRCAPRO is a statistical model used to calculate the probability of a genetic mutation based on family history that includes second-degree relatives, bilateral breast cancer, and ovarian cancer.[35]

Most women (approximately 70%) who develop breast cancer have no known risk factors. Although 10%–20% of patients with either breast or ovarian cancer have a first- or second-degree relative with one of these cancers, hereditary breast cancer accounts for a very small proportion of the diagnosed cases (approximately 5%) and hereditary ovarian cancer is associated with approximately 10% of all cases.[38–40] The majority of breast cancers are considered to be sporadic, which is defined as no history of breast cancer through two generations. Familial breast cancer is described as a positive family history with one or more first- or second-degree relatives, which does not fit the hereditary risk definition. Hereditary or genetic breast cancer is defined as a positive family history, often with related cancers (e.g., ovarian), consistent with an autosomal dominant factor that includes onset at an early age (average 45), an excess of bilaterality, male breast cancer, and other multiple cancers.[40] Two autosomal dominant gene mutations have been isolated — one on chromosome 17q and another on chromosome 13q.[41,42] Research for new susceptibility genes continues, and the ultimate goal of gene mapping is to be able to identify a crucial gene, characterize it, and thereby gain an understanding of the molecular predisposition of breast cancer in families. The scientific advancements in molecular biology have begun to identify the interaction of genes and their mechanisms, distinguishing the cellular pathways that lead to malignancy and promote metastases. Application of these principles will revolutionize breast cancer therapy through the translation of bench research into clinical practice.

The genes responsible for inherited familial cancers are most often tumor suppressor genes that are actively involved in suppressing malignant growth during the cell cycle. The human genome consists of 23 pairs of chromosomes, 22 pairs of which are autosomes and 1 sex-linked pair. Mutation carriers are born with one normal functioning gene and one mutated gene, which may be from either the maternal or the paternal side. When the function of the normal gene is lost, the consequence is a loss of heterozygosity, causing abnormal proliferation and resulting in neoplastic and malignant cell growth.[43,44]

Epidemiologists and physician researchers began to look for patterns within families having an abnormal incidence of breast cancers among the members. Using linkage analysis, two breast/ovarian cancer susceptibilty gene mutations (*BRCA1* and *BRCA2*) have been mapped and cloned. The first mutation identified *BRCA1* (BReast CAncer 1), lies on the long arm of chromosome 17 (17q12–21); *BRCA2* is located on the long arm of chromosome 13 (13q12–13).[42,45]

Inheritance of the *BRCA1* and *BRCA2* susceptibility genes is often associated with a high penetrance (likelihood that the effect of the mutation will result in the disease) for families with multiple breast and ovarian cancers. These gene mutations follow an autosomal dominant pattern, meaning that the mutation can be passed from either parent to a child and that each child (male or female) has a 50% likelihood of inheritance. Given that the science of genetics is constantly evolving, risk estimates can vary depending on the locus of the mutation or ethnicity and should be interpreted with care. Women who have inherited a mutation on *BRCA1* or *BRCA2* may have up to an 85% risk of developing breast cancer by age 70. The risk for developing ovarian cancer varies from 26%–54% for *BRCA1* to approximately 27% for *BRCA2*.[46,47] Mutation carriers diagnosed with breast or ovarian cancer have additional risks of developing a second cancer (ovarian, contralateral breast, or primary breast cancer). They also have an increased risk for male breast cancer, prostate, pancreatic, and fallopian tube cancers.[48] The search continues for other genes that confer breast cancer susceptibility, but no probable candidate has been confirmed at this time.[49,50]

Some populations that have been isolated due to geographic, cultural, or religious considerations may exhibit a "founder effect" — that is, a deleterious mutation exists within one person and has been passed through the group and continues to be identified within the group. The Ashkenazi Jewish population exhibits this founder effect, which is estimated to affect 1 person in 40, a considerably higher rate than in the heterogenous groups, estimated to be 1 person in 300–500. Ashkenazi women with ovarian cancer have a 40%–50% likelihood of having a hereditary mutation.[51] Three mutations have been identified that are linked with Ashkenazi Jewish heredity, two on *BRCA1* and one on *BRCA2*. The risk of developing breast cancer for this group was initially estimated to be 56% by age 70, and the risk for ovarian cancer is estimated to be 16%.[52] These figures are considerably lower than those for more heterogenous populations. A recent report from King and colleagues examined 1008 index cases and reported that the lifetime risk for Ashkenazi women is 82% for breast cancer and 54% for ovarian cancer.[47] The disparities cannot be confirmed but may reflect data from the more general population of mutation carriers rather than the highly penetrant, linkage groups originally noted in the literature.

Although there does not appear to be any difference between the prognosis for sporadic and hereditary breast cancer, women with *BRCA*-linked ovarian cancer tend to survive longer.[43,53,54] Although the inherited gene mutation affects only a very small proportion of the breast cancer population (approximately 5%), the hope is that the information gleaned from this and other inherited genes will provide additional information with which to better understand the complex puzzle known as sporadic breast cancer, which affects approximately 95% of those diagnosed with breast cancer.

Current information indicates that *BRCA1* and *BRCA2* are responsible for most or all hereditary ovarian cancers, but not all hereditary breast cancers.[44] Other, presumably low-penetrance gene variants are thought to be responsible for moderate increases in breast cancer risk. Among these are mutations in *ATM* (ataxia telangiectasia mutated), *Chk2* (checkpoint kinase 2), *p53* (associated with Li-Fraumeni syndrome), and *PTEN* (associated with Cowden disease). *BRCA1* is phosphorylated by *ATM* and *Chk2* in response to DNA damage. All of these genes are components of the cell cycle repair pathway affecting *BRCA1* and *BRCA2*.[55–57]

For the woman who has breast cancer, there is a 0.7%–0.8% per year risk of developing a second primary breast cancer.[58] Variables that may alter the risk of developing a contralateral breast cancer include a personal early age of onset, having a first-degree relative with early-onset or bilateral disease, or a genetic mutation. Treatment with chemotherapy and/or hormones for breast cancer may reduce the development of a second breast cancer.

Diet

The wide range of variance in breast cancer rates worldwide and dramatic increases in migrant populations may reflect one or several factors that influence the risk of breast cancer. The risk of breast cancer is greatest in developed countries, especially those of North America and northern Europe. The risk is lowest in Asia and developing countries. Apart from a genetic influence, diet has been investigated as the most plausible variant, but direct correlations are yet to be proven through migration and international studies.

People emigrating from countries of low incidence to high incidence of breast cancer exhibit the higher rate of risk by the third generation. Some countries associated with low breast cancer risk are experiencing an increased incidence. Japan is known to have a low incidence of breast cancer, but the incidence of breast cancer has been rising there since the 1950s. The westernization of Japan has altered the Japanese culture, and increasing fat consumption has been implicated as a causal effect. Conversely, famine has been correlated with a decreased risk of breast cancer. Women who survived a famine in Norway had a 13% reduction in breast cancer risk, suggesting that decreases in dietary fat reduce breast cancer risk.[59]

While these data may suggest a correlation between breast cancer risk and dietary fat, the association may be in error because it is difficult to separate out a single aspect without considering other related factors. The westernized culture may provide accessibility to additional factors that were not previously present. Changes in exercise habits, alcohol and drug use, hormone therapy, and smoking may take place, which could confound the diet correlation. Additionally, the risk reduction in breast cancer in famine survivors may not be directly correlated with a lack of dietary fat intake without considering other factors, such as later onset of menarche and amenorrhea, which are associated with nutritional deprivation and may confound the breast cancer risk reduction.

The hypothesis that dietary fat influences breast cancer risk is based on the theory that fat acts as an indirect promoter of carcinogenesis through the action of hormonal pathways. Although the exact mechanism is unclear, estrogen may promote carcinogenesis by stimulating increased mitotic division resulting in cell proliferation. However, the hypothesis that diet acts as a causal factor in breast cancer has not been proven. Lee and Lin reviewed the literature of dietary studies between 1980 and 1990 and individual studies since 1990 and reported equivocal findings.[60] Dietary influences may be more pronounced at certain times in life, and it would be helpful to know when intervention would be most effective. Interest has been directed to the diet of children and adolescents, but relating diet to breast cancer that occurs decades later is a monumental task.[61,62] The identification of intermediate endpoints such as changes in serum markers may prove most helpful in determining the correlation of dietary fat with breast cancer.

The Women's Health Initiative, sponsored by the National Institutes of Health, may provide an answer to these dietary questions. This study is accruing data on approximately 100,000 women from a multitude of cultural and socioeconomic backgrounds. It is examining the effects of reducing dietary fat, adding calcium supplements, and hormone replacement to determine whether any intervention reduces the expected incidence of breast and colorectal cancer, osteoporosis, and heart disease. This will be accomplished through clinical trials, observational studies, and community educational programs.[62]

Obesity

Recent literature suggests that obesity is associated with an increased breast cancer risk for postmenopausal women and little or no increase in risk for premenopausal women.[63] The Nurses Health Study indicated that the risk is greatest for women who demonstrated a weight gain of 25 kg or more since age 18.[64,65] A possible explanation of the discrepancy between premenopausal and postmenopausal risk may be linked to hormonal influences. Obesity during childbearing years has been associated with a decrease in the level of progesterone, which reduces cell proliferation in the breast. Obese postmenopausal women have no ovarian function, are exposed to an extragonadal source of bioavailable estrogens stored in adipose tissue, and have higher rates of conversion of androstenedione to estrogen in adipose tissue and lower levels of sex hormone-binding globulin than do thinner women.[66] Additionally, the enzyme responsible for converting estrone to estradiol is present in adipose breast tissue, and the rate of conversion has been positively correlated to body weight.

Obesity is a modifiable risk factor. Nurses are instrumental in providing education, support, and encouragement to assist women with weight-reduction programs. Many versions of diet and exercise programs exist that can meet the particular needs of most women who are motivated to reduce their risk of breast cancer as well as improve cardiovascular status.

Alcohol

According to meta-analyses,[67,68] the literature favors a positive association between alcohol and breast cancer risk. The biological mechanisms of the association are not known. Whether the increased risk involves increased estrogen and androgen levels, decreased DNA repair, exposure to circulating cytotoxic by-products of alcohol, a possible alteration in the cell membrane permeability in breast tissue, or other mechanisms is yet to be determined.[69] The most compelling evidence suggests that the relationship between alcohol and breast cancer risk is greatest for women who consume more than two drinks per day and that this significant trend persists until age 50.[15,16,67,69] However, this connection is not strong enough at this point to conclude that a causality exists between the use of alcohol and breast cancer. Women who consume alcohol should be counseled regarding the potential cancer risks based on family history.

Radiation

The carcinogenic effects of both low- and high-dose ionizing radiation have been well documented. Survivors of atomic bombs exhibited an increase in breast as well as other cancers. A risk of breast cancer has been associated with radiation therapy for a broad spectrum of health problems, including chronic mastitis, tuberculosis, tinea capitis, thymus disorders, and adult and childhood cancers.[70] This risk increases with dosage, especially if a woman is exposed in the period of young adulthood. Mantle radiation for Hodgkin's disease (HD) is associated with an increased risk relative to age during treatment.

While those treated with radiation after age 30 carry a negligible risk, increases in risk have been reported for women who received radiation therapy before the age of 30 and additional risk is associated with therapy before the age of 15.[71] A recent study noted that the risk associated with mantle radiation can persist for 25 years after treatment.[70,72,73] A disturbing issue is that this long-term risk is not communicated to the patient. A recent study reported that 40% of women treated before the age of 30 did not perceive themselves to be at increased risk for breast cancer.[74] Survivors of HD should be made aware of their increased risk for developing breast cancer, and appropriate screening and prevention strategies should be discussed.

The concern about the effects of radiation has generated some apprehension regarding the potential harm of repeated mammograms and chest radiographs. A cumulative exposure greater than 100 cGy is associated with an increase in risk. The doses for these procedures are extremely small, and the potential benefit far outweighs the risk. A mammogram emits a dose of 0.2–0.4cGy per study, and a chest film generates approximately 0.002 cGy to each breast.[75,76] The radiation exposure from a mammogram is similar to the radiation exposure incurred from flying 400 miles in an airplane.

Aspirin

Preliminary evidence indicates that aspirin may reduce the risk of breast cancer in women prone to hormone-sensitive tumors. While the mechanism is unclear, laboratory studies suggest that aspirin may act by blocking an enzyme needed to produce estrogen, which can promote breast cancer in some women. In the study conducted by Terry and associates[77], women who took aspirin seven or more times a week had a 26% lower risk of developing breast cancer compared to women who did not take it.

Breast Biopsy

There is a presumed relationship between biopsy-proven benign breast change and breast cancer risk. The assessment of breast cancer risk varies according to histology. Nonproliferative lesions confer no increased risk and include simple cysts, apocrine change, and fibrosis.

Proliferative lesions indicate the presence of increased cell growth and are usually differentiated by the presence or absence of atypia. Cells without atypia are usually cytologically benign and vary in their size and shape. Usual hyperplasia, fibroadenoma, intraductal papilloma, and sclerosing adenosis are more common examples and are associated with an increase in risk of 1.5- to 2-fold.[78,79] A biopsy finding of atypical hyperplasia indicates that the cells no longer appear normal and are undergoing neoplastic change resembling the characteristics of carcinoma in situ. Atypical hyperplasia is associated with a 4- to 5-fold increase in risk.[69,79,80] Today both ductal and lobular atypical hyperplasia are being diagnosed more frequently, and they are often associated with mammographically detected microcalcifications. The risk statistics given here are not lifetime estimates, but apply to approximately 18 years after biopsy, which is the limit of most benign breast disease follow-up. A recent retrospective study by Page and Simpson indicated that invasive carcinoma is more likely to develop in the breast with atypical lobular hyperplasia, disputing the conventional thought that both breasts are at equal risk for invasive cancer.[78]

Carcinoma in Situ

Carcinoma in situ has been referred to as a "precancerous condition." This definition reflects the potential capabilities of the cells to be a predictor of later malignancy.[81] The nomenclature of "carcinoma in situ" refers to a localized process in which cells remain within the site of origin. In this condition, a malignant change has occurred without evidence of invasion in the basement membrane. A carcinoma in situ that remains in the breast is capable of transforming into an invasive cancer but does not necessarily do so.[82,83]

Ductal carcinoma in situ (DCIS) and lobular carcinoma in situ (LCIS) are characterized by an 8- to 10-fold increased risk of developing invasive cancer.[84,85] The incidence of DCIS lesions has increased in the past 25 years and currently accounts for 20% of all breast cancer diagnoses.[32] It can vary in mammographic, clinical, and histopathologic presentations.[83,86] While conservative treatment with local excision is an accepted treatment, simple mastectomy (breast tissue only — no removal of axillary nodes) may be the recommendation for multifocal disease.[87] There is controversy regarding whether a sentinel node biopsy should be done when the DCIS is high grade and/or large and extensive, as some papers have reported rates of positive sentinel nodes ranging from 6% to 12%.[88,89] Although DCIS is the most common form of noninvasive breast cancer in women, it occurs in approximately 5% of male breast cancer cases.

Lobular carcinoma in situ lesions are associated with increased risk within both breasts but this abnormality is not considered a *premalignant* condition.[90] This uncommon finding occurs predominately in premenopausal women, with an average age at diagnosis of 44–47 years.[91] LCIS is usually not detected by palpation or mammography, but rather is most often an incidental microscopic finding when breast tissue is removed for another reason. Current evidence suggests that LCIS functions as a marker of increased risk for developing an invasive ductal (more common) or lobular (less common) cancer.[92] Mastectomy for LCIS should be considered a prophylactic procedure rather than therapeutic.[84,93] Because many observations have concluded that most women with LCIS do not develop breast cancer, clinicians increasingly believe that LCIS may be treated with local excision and close follow-up that employs mammograms twice a year and clinical exam every three to four months. Improvements in mammography sensitivity have made this approach more feasible. Women who are unable or unwilling to comply with frequent monitoring may opt for a unilateral or bilateral mastectomy with or without reconstruction.

Patients are often confused about recommendations for a mastectomy for a noninvasive cancer. Nurses play a significant role in the management of these patients, educating them about the characteristics of their disease and reinforcing the rationale for the treatment options through discussion and printed information.

Prevention, Screening, and Early Detection

Assessment based on known risk factors can be used to determine the possibility of an individual developing breast cancer. The unknown etiology of breast cancer, coupled with conflicting data regarding the identification of risk factors as well as how these risk factors influence the genesis of breast cancer, makes preventive action difficult, however. As molecular studies move forward, there are clear indications that breast cancer has multiple causes, making it nearly impossible to predict with certainty who will develop the disease. As mentioned earlier in this chapter, some elements have been recognized to be primary risk factors in the development of breast cancer, whereas others may be secondary or possible risk factors. Even this information has limited utility, because 70% of women with breast cancer have no identifiable risk factors.

Research concerning prevention and early detection of breast cancer is critically important in the reduction of mortality from this disease. Current evidence indicates that the disease is often present in the breast six to eight years before it presents clinically or becomes evident through breast imaging. Of the nearly 216,000 women who will be diagnosed with breast cancer in 2004, only 50% will be diagnosed with stage I disease, and approximately 20% of all women with breast cancer will subsequently die of their disease.[1]

Ductal Lavage

The majority of breast cancers arise from ductal epithelial cells that have gone through progressive changes in morphology and molecular composition. In an attempt to provide accurate risk assessment, some centers have been evaluating ductal lavage as a predictor of risk.[94,95] Ductal lavage is a new method under investigation that samples the breast epithelium by collecting ductal cells without disrupting the breast parenchyma. Nipple aspiration is usually performed using a suction device to identify ducts that produce fluid; a microcatheter is inserted into the fluid-yielding duct and the duct is lavaged with normal saline. Cells are then analyzed for abnormal changes.[95]

While this method is safe and effective, it is fraught with potential problems. Limited information is available regarding the sensitivity of diagnosing atypia and malignancy as well as a treatment algorithm if malignant cells are found.[95,96] Ductal lavage may be useful for women who are deciding whether to employ a risk-reduction modality such as tamoxifen. Until more information is available regarding its optimal use, this procedure should be evaluated only in a clinical trial.[97]

Chemoprevention

Chemoprevention is the use of a chemical agent to prevent or alter the development of cancer. The development of a chemoprevention agent should be based on a disease model that identifies progressive development over several years and involves multiple factors that can be reversed. These interventions must be based on a biological rationale and have minimal toxic effects.

Chemoprevention for breast cancer has been utilized to alter the course of disease for those individuals with known risk factors. Several dietary micronutrients such as soy isoflavones have been promoted for their presumed protective capabilities, but data from randomized, prospective clinical trials are lacking and the true effect is still unknown.[98] Vitamin A and its retinoid derivatives offer some promise for chemoprevention by affecting the growth and differentiation of epithelial tissue. The evidence is stronger regarding the benefits of retinoid sources of vitamin A,[2] although studies have produced mixed results in breast cancer.[98] The antioxidant capabilities of vitamins A, E, and C in foods defend against free radicals and aid in stimulating the immune response. Their role in cancer prevention may be difficult to determine because it is impossible to attribute these qualities to specific micronutrients due to the multiple components of vegetables and fruits as well as varying preparation methods that may affect the bioavailability of micronutrients.[2,98]

The influence of hormones in breast cancer is uniformly recognized. Agents that mimic the effects of estrogen in selected tissues and act as estrogen antagonists in other tissues are referred to as *SERMs*—*s*elective *e*strogen *r*eceptor *m*odulators. Tamoxifen citrate, introduced in the 1970s, was the first SERM and is the most widely used drug for breast cancer in the United States. It was originally launched as a treatment for advanced breast cancer in postmenopausal women. Since then, tamoxifen has been found to be effective in the treatment of premenopausal women with advanced disease.[99–101] Tamoxifen has also been found to increase disease-free survival in node-negative, estrogen receptor (ER)–positive disease[102] as well as node-positive disease.[99,103] Women taking tamoxifen for primary breast cancer have experienced a reduction in the expected incidence of contralateral breast cancer. This finding strengthened the belief in tamoxifen's chemoprotective effect, and led to its use in a large U.S. prevention trial through the National Surgical Adjuvant Breast and Bowel Program (NSABP).

This breast cancer prevention study, NSABP P-1, also known as the Breast Cancer Prevention Trial (BCPT), was a randomized study using the standard daily dose of 20 mg of tamoxifen versus a placebo to determine whether breast cancer could be prevented in women with known high risk. The P-1 study was to have lasted for five years, but preliminary information indicated that the risk reduction was 49% for the tamoxifen group. This result was felt to be significant enough that the reports were published early to allow all high-risk women to have the opportunity to select this documented risk-reduction agent. The study did result in morbid events, which, though few, occurred more often in the tamoxifen group. Early-stage endometrial cancer was diagnosed twice as often in the tamoxifen group, and this group had an increased incidence of thromboembolic events, primarily deep-vein thrombosis (DVT). These events generally occurred in women over age 50.[104]

The P-1 study is being followed by NSABP P-2, a prevention trial examining the effects of breast cancer risk reduction and relative side effects using tamoxifen versus raloxifene; it has been dubbed the *STAR* (*s*tudy of *t*amoxifen *a*nd *r*aloxifene) trial. Eligibility for the STAR trial is essentially the same as for the P-1 trial, except that participants must be postmenopausal women. If women are currently taking HRT, they must stop for three months prior to enrollment. The goal is to enroll 22,000 women with no prior history of breast cancer. As with the P-1 trial, the participants will be expected to comply with the schedule for daily medication, clinical examinations, and mammography. The

STAR trial closed in 2004 and preliminary results should be available approximately 2006.

The *MORE* (*m*ultiple *o*utcomes of *r*aloxifene *e*valuation) trial examined the effects of raloxifene versus placebo on osteoporosis in 7705 postmenopausal women. Subjects were also followed for breast cancer incidence. The data showed a 76% reduction in relative risk for invasive breast cancer in the women who took raloxifene. Raloxifene has similar properties to tamoxifen's but does not appear to exert an estrogenic effect on the endometrium.[105]

Side effects are an important consideration when any drug is taken electively. The tamoxifen toxicities commonly reported are similar to menopausal symptoms: hot flashes, vaginal discharge, and irregular menses. Rare events include ocular changes, thromboembolic disease, and second primary cancers of the endometrium. The side effects of raloxifene are similar, without the expected increase in endometrial cancer.

Although tamoxifen is considered an antiestrogen and, therefore, an antagonist, it may also act as an agonist. As an antagonist, tamoxifen competes with estradiol for the receptor sites in the nucleus. This mechanism causes an estrogen blockade and impedes the growth of malignant cells. Although the drug's exact mechanism of action is unknown, several explanations have been postulated. Tamoxifen may alter the growth factors that regulate breast cell proliferation; bind to cytoplasmic antiestrogenic binding sites, thereby increasing intracellular drug levels; inhibit the amount of free estrogen available to the cell; stimulate natural killer cells; or affect the endocrine regulation of breast cancer cells.[104] This drug also exhibits agonist activity, which was recognized in the early trials. The agonist mechanism suggests beneficial action regarding osteoporosis and cardiovascular disease, both of which are significant factors of morbidity and mortality in postmenopausal women.[104]

The favorable outcomes of the P-1 and MORE trials will prompt the investigation of additional SERMs as more sources of tumor modulation are recognized. In the interim, tamoxifen continues to be used as the primary chemopreventive agent in clinical practice. Studies of the risks, benefits, and cost-effectiveness of tamoxifen have validated its use in the prevention of breast cancer for selected patients at high risk for such cancer and low risk for the most serious adverse events.[106–108]

Aromatase inhibitors (AIs) are also under study as chemopreventive agents in breast cancer. Rather than blocking estrogen from breast tissue, AIs prevent the action of the enzyme aromatase, which is needed by the body to convert two substrates, testosterone and androstenedione, to estradiol. Aromatase is present throughout the body. In premenopausal women, the highest levels of aromatase are found in ovarian tissue. In postmenopausal women, peripheral adipose tissue contains large amounts of aromatase.[109,110] Aromatase inhibitors have been used successfully in hormone-dependent metastatic breast cancer after the failure of first-line therapy such as tamoxifen. Trials to demonstrate the efficacy of AIs as chemopreventive agents in postmenopausal women with no history of breast are ongoing.

Biomarkers

Cancer is a heterogenous disease, and it has recently been hypothesized that all such diseases are the result of an evolving process of altered cells accumulating genetic mutations, either inherited or acquired. Identifying biomarkers that appear early in cell alterations theoretically would allow for repair of these alterations and prevention of disease. Endpoints may indicate later effects such as dysplasia. A more desirable endpoint would be earlier alterations such as cell proliferation. The ability of these mutated cells to express malignancy may develop from the genetic disposition of *SEBs* (*s*urrogate *e*ndpoint *b*iomarkers). An effective SEB should be a factor in the causal pathway of breast cancer. The identified SEB should be altered in the presence of a chemoprotective agent and should ultimately reduce the incidence of breast cancer. Some cellular changes that occur along histopathological pathway to malignancy have been identified as probable indicators of neoplasia. Certain proteins and genes are abnormally expressed or regulated in breast cancer. Changes in DNA, markers of cellular proliferation, and apoptosis (programmed cell death) are under consideration. Studies that do identify modulation of a known biomarker will enable the practitioner to shift the care paradigm by offering interventions directed at preventing the onset of breast cancer rather than hoping for early detection using standard methods of clinical and mammographic examinations.

Biomarkers may also assess the risk of disease development. In breast cancer, *BRCA1* and *BRCA2* serve as biomarkers for the risk of developing breast cancer. Biomarkers may predict the likelihood of response to a particular therapy, such as the evaluation of *HER2/NEU* status in regard to the administration of trastuzumab for patients whose tumors overexpress *HER2/NEU*.[111] Breast cancer may respond to biotherapeutics targeting the epidermal growth factor receptor (EGFR). Testing for overexpression of EGFR, especially in combination with *HER2/NEU* overexpression, may someday direct targeted therapy for certain women.

Table 46-2 Clinical Uses for Breast Cancer Biomarkers

Category of Biomarker	Example
Risk assessment	*BRCA1, BRCA2*
Prognostic, staging	Axillary lymph node status Tumor size
Predicting therapeutic response	ER/PR
Monitoring therapeutic response	CA125, CA15-3, CEA, CA27.29
Therapeutic target	*HER2/NEU*, EGFR

ER = estrogen receptor.
PR = progesterone receptor.
EGFR = epidermal growth factor receptor.

Still other biomarkers are generally referred to as tumor markers and may be used in some settings to monitor response to therapy. In breast cancer, common tumor markers are the surface proteins CA125, CA15.3, CA27.29, and carcinoembryonic antigen (CEA). While these tumor markers may increase and decrease during periods of disease exacerbation and remission, using tumor markers as the sole directive for modification or initiation of treatment is not generally recommended.[112–114] Table 46-2 lists the common biomarkers currently in use for breast cancer.

To date, the strongest predictive and prognostic factor in evaluating breast cancer has been the number of positive lymph nodes at diagnosis. Often, however, the clinical outcome is in conflict with the prognosis; that is, women with 10 or more positive lymph nodes may have an unexpectedly long survival, whereas women with node-negative disease may develop early distant metastases and succumb to the disease.[115] Many investigators are trying to find molecular markers in the form of gene expression signatures that may more accurately predict prognosis as well as response to therapy.[116]

Exercise

The role of exercise in the prevention of breast cancer has not been widely studied. The endorsement of exercise is usually presented in the context of reducing or counteracting known risk factors. Women who exercise tend to have less body fat, which influences their hormonal milieu. Strenuous exercising alters ovarian function, which may delay menarche or create irregular menses or an amenorrheic state. Exercising may reduce the risk of breast cancer for postmenopausal obese women by reducing the amount of free estrogen stored in body fat.

Early studies that looked at exercise as a protective agent have been generally inconclusive. This outcome may be related to the presence of confounding risk factors, inaccurate activity measures, or alteration of activity over time. Recently, a few studies have suggested that exercise confers a direct protective effect on the development of breast cancer. Bernstein and associates found that young women (menarche to early middle age) who vigorously exercised 3–8 hours or more per week, experienced a 58% reduction in risk.[117] Mittendorf and colleagues conducted a large case-controlled study, which showed a modest effect for young women who reported any strenuous activity and a 50% reduction for those who vigorously exercised daily.[118] A study by Rockhill and colleagues supported the protective effect of vigorous exercise (> 7 hours per week),[119] and a Canadian study determined that exercise conferred a risk reduction in postmenopausal women who exercised regularly.[120] While more studies are necessary, these similar findings support the hypothesis that physical activity may reduce the risk of breast cancer.

Prophylactic Mastectomy

A prophylactic mastectomy, the removal of the majority of breast tissue including the total breast, tail of Spence, and nipple–areola complex, may be warranted in certain high-risk women; however, controversy exists over how much risk is enough to justify performing this procedure. Women for whom a prophylactic mastectomy may be indicated have been identified as those with some or all of the following characteristics:[121,122]

1. A family history of documented hereditary breast cancer consistent with an autosomal dominant factor. Women who are presumed to be gene carriers may have a breast cancer risk ranging from 50% to 85% depending on their family history.
2. A personal risk of at least 50% for developing breast cancer.
3. A proven history of breast cancer in one breast and extreme nodularity or cystic changes in the opposite breast. The incidence of a second breast cancer in the opposite breast is estimated to be 15%–20%.
4. Chronic cystic mastitis or a diagnosis of atypical hyperplasia with repeated surgical biopsies.
5. An overwhelming fear of breast cancer such that the possibility of developing breast cancer interferes with daily life.

Because prophylactic mastectomies have been done for various reasons (not just for high risk), it is now possible to quantify the reduction in breast cancer risk. The most complete study to date investigated women who had bilateral prophylactic mastectomies performed at the Mayo Clinic. The women were evaluated according to a risk profile, and the results showed a 90% risk reduction for those who had a moderate or high risk for developing breast cancer. This is important information for women considering the surgery based on risk. Breast cancer has been known to occur in the chest wall or axillary region. It is therefore important for a woman to recognize that some risk of developing breast cancer exists after a prophylactic mastectomy, as breast cancer cells may extend to the clavicle, the latissimus, or the abdomen, and are not included in the mastectomy.[122] The risk reduction for *BRCA1* or *BRCA2* carriers appears to be equal or greater to these statistics.[123,124] It is well known that oophorectomy reduces the risk of developing ovarian cancer, but recent information indicates that oophorectomy also confers a 50% risk reduction for breast cancer for mutation carriers.[125,126] Women who have a mutation in *BRCA1* or *BRCA2* may opt for a prophylactic oophorectomy after completing childbearing either to increase the risk reduction for those not electing to have mastectomies or to gain optimal risk reduction in conjunction with bilateral mastectomy.[127]

The patient must be presented with a clear, in-depth evaluation of her current and potential risk, stressing that although she may have a dramatically increased risk of breast cancer, there is no guarantee that she will develop disease in her lifetime. It is important for women to take adequate time in weighing the risks versus benefits of these procedures. The complications of prophylactic mastectomies are similar to those for other mastectomies. However, if reconstruction is added to this procedure, capsular contracture is another possibility. Additionally, the woman should be evaluated by a gynecological oncologist if she is considering an oophorectomy.

Optimally, women at high risk for breast cancer should be followed by close surveillance utilizing mammogram and possibly MRI, along with frequent clinical examination, preferably through a comprehensive breast center. Provided such surveillance is feasible, this alternative is an important—even reassuring—alternative for the woman considering prophylactic mastectomy.

Multidisciplinary Breast Centers

The increasing public awareness of breast cancer treatment options and the recognized controversies in breast cancer detection and management, together with oncologists' and institutions' commitment to provide optimal care, have spearheaded the concept of the multidisciplinary breast center. The design of these centers represents a response to the reality that treatment of breast cancer has become a complicated process necessitating specialized, collaborative management that is often beyond the scope of an individual practitioner. The purpose and goals of a multidisciplinary breast center include, but are not limited to, the following:

1. To provide a comprehensive interdisciplinary evaluation and planning in the management of all aspects of breast disease
2. To provide prompt and timely evaluation and diagnosis of potential breast disease implementing current methodology and state-of-the-art diagnostic tools
3. To participate in and support national protocol studies that investigate new surgical and adjuvant treatment modalities as well as maintain a patient database for retrospective and prospective in-house studies
4. To provide risk assessment, genetic counseling referrals, and surveillance of women at high risk for breast cancer, thereby minimizing the anxiety associated with the knowledge that one has an increased risk for developing the disease as well as reducing the risk of patients being lost for follow-up
5. To provide educational materials and the opportunity to learn about early detection measures (e.g., breast self-examination) and the possibility of participating in breast cancer prevention studies as well as research studies aimed at early detection and management of malignant breast cancer
6. To provide educational opportunities for medical students, fellows, general practitioners, nurses, and others involved in the care of the woman with breast disease as well as a mechanism for peer review of the oncologist in practice
7. To provide highly specialized assessment and diagnostic procedures that enable prompt decision making in the evaluation of a breast mass, which may conceivably minimize unnecessary surgical biopsies
8. To provide the woman and family with the necessary information to allow her to make an informed decision regarding her choices for treatment in a prompt and timely manner
9. To offer educational programs to the community that include instruction in breast self-examination (BSE) and information on risk factors and the importance of utilizing the current methods available to promote early detection[128]

Ideally, the comprehensive breast center should have a full complement of disciplines available to provide an expert opinion regarding assessment of diagnostic and histopathological data; prognostic indicators; genetic assessment and evaluation; and surgical diagnostic and treatment options, including systemic chemotherapy/endocrine therapy, radiation treatment, and surgical reconstructive techniques, when warranted. A psycho-oncologist and social worker may provide counseling regarding body image issues, sexual concerns, and anticipated changes in lifestyle for those patients dealing with a potentially life-threatening disease.[129]

The oncology clinical nurse specialist is often viewed as the coordinator of the comprehensive breast center. It is imperative that this professional possess specialized knowledge in all aspects of breast cancer and its treatment as well as a compassionate, yet controlled approach to the evaluation of a suspected breast cancer. It is not uncommon for women to telephone the breast center, frantic with fear and apprehension, expressing a need to be seen as soon as possible. Regardless of the schedule, this is exactly what needs to occur if possible. Such understanding and prompt attention to the woman's needs and concerns will help to establish a trusting and caring relationship, which is vital considering the possible diagnostic outcome. This approach to patient management is critical to the success of a comprehensive breast center.

The nurse coordinator ensures that all materials (e.g., slides, x-rays) necessary for a comprehensive evaluation are present at the time of the consultation. The nurse informs the patient and family of the sequence of events once the appointment is established. This information includes which doctor(s) the patient will see and when, how materials will be reviewed, and how the patient plays a critical role in the decision-making process. Emphasis is placed on the fact that often more than one approach to management of the problem exists and that, once informed of her options, the patient is the ultimate decision maker. The nurse can be instrumental in ensuring that information is delivered in a manner that will enhance the patient's understanding and ability to make an informed decision.

In addition to facilitating the process of informed consent and decision making, the nurse is instrumental in providing BSE instruction to all patients. The nurse also will be called on to answer questions regarding diagnostic tests, therapy regimens, clinical trials, postoperative events, and potential complications of treatment. Ideally, this professional will be able to provide exercise instruction prior to surgery and evaluate understanding and potential for compliance during the period following hospitalization. Additionally, the nurse utilizes every opportunity to lecture to professionals and the public concerning breast cancer as a health issue and methods available for early detection. Finally, time should be set aside to accept or return phone calls concerning questions related to breast cancer risk and other pertinent issues.

The design of a comprehensive breast center should reflect the goals of providing a complete, efficient, yet personal evaluation of the patient. The exam rooms should be large enough to accommodate the patient, family or significant other, and team of physicians. The clinical area should have additional smaller consult rooms where the patient may be seen by individual consultants based on her particular concerns and needs.

A physician conference room should be available to provide an area for viewing films, pathology slides, and reports. Diagnostic tests and outpatient surgery suites positioned on site facilitate a quick and efficient diagnostic process.

These centers are successful because they meet a growing need for a multidisciplinary and comprehensive approach to the care of the woman with breast disease and because they are philosophically based on the premise that women are entitled to all the information available to make an informed decision regarding their choice of treatment.[130]

Genetic Counseling Programs

As science and biotechnology continue to identify chromosomal abnormalities that confer a high probability for developing breast cancer, the need to provide more comprehensive risk assessment for families as well as genetic counseling and testing will direct practitioners and the public to seek genetic counseling programs. The data emanating from the Human Genome Project may overwhelm and will definitely challenge a primary care physician in assessing and referring patients for genetic abnormalities. The primary physician will often be responsible for referring a patient for further evaluation and, therefore, must possess a basic working knowledge of the personal and familial histories that may suggest a genetic link. According to Stopfer,[131] genetic counseling should assist the patient and family in understanding the medical information pertinent to the disease(s), comprehending how heredity causes or predisposes one to disease and the personal risk of developing a condition, and creating a plan for follow-up that may include several treatment modalities.[132] Another important consideration is the psychological impact of genetic counseling and testing. A recent study addressed this issue and found no increase in psychological distress from such counseling.[133] Additionally, Braithwaite and colleagues reviewed controlled trials and prospective studies evaluating the psychological impact of genetic testing and reported no apparent adverse effect on cancer-specific worry or anxiety.[134]

Table 46-3 Cancer Risk Evaluation Program: Breast and Ovarian Screening Guidelines

LOW RISK ≤ 15% LIFETIME CUMULATIVE RISK	
Follow standard ACS recommendations	
Mammography	Baseline at age 35 Every other year age 40–50 Every year age 50 and on
Clinical breast exam	Every year
Breast self-examination	Every month
MODERATE RISK 15%–30% LIFETIME CUMULATIVE RISK	
Start following the standard ACS guidelines at any age when breast cancer risk is ≥ to the risk of an average 50-year-old woman (1 in 50 or 2%)	
HIGH RISK ≥ 30% LIFETIME CUMULATIVE RISK	
Mammography	Baseline at age 30 Next mammogram depending on informativeness
Clinical breast exam	Every 6 months
Breast self-examination	Every month

Table 46-4 Screening Guidelines for *BRCA1/BRCA2* Mutation Carriers

Type of Cancer	Screening Procedure	Starting Age	Frequency
Screening for Women with Mutations in *BRCA1* or *BRCA2*			
Breast	Mammograms Physician breast exam Breast self-exam Breast MRI	25 years 25 years 20 years 25 years	Every 12 months Every 6 months Once every month Every 12 months
Ovarian	CA125 blood test Ovarian ultrasound *(Note: these tests have never been proven to reduce the risk of dying from ovarian cancer.)*	25 years, until childbearing complete, then removal of ovaries (prophylactic oophorectomy)	Every 6–12 months
Colon	Colonoscopy	50 years	Every 3–5 years
Uterine/Cervical	Pelvic exam/Pap smear	18 years	Every 12 months
Screening for Men with Mutations in *BRCA1* or *BRCA2*			
Breast	Physician breast exam	50 years	Once every year
Prostate	Prostate exam and PSA blood test	45 years	Once every year
Colon	Colonscopy	50 years	Every 3–5 years

Reprinted with permission from: Cancer Risk Evaluation Program, University of Pennsylvania Cancer Center. These guidelines may change as new data become available, and must be individualized.

The creation and implementation of a breast cancer genetic counseling program must include the following elements: a database and an assessment model based on known and accepted risk factors; genetic counselors who carefully interview, screen, and educate patients and families; psychosocial support staff to address the emotional and physical consequences of the counseling and testing process; and clinicians, nurses, and researchers who share clinical responsibilities and actively participate in treatment protocols and prevention trials for breast cancer. Once risk has been established, the patient and family members should also receive specific recommendations tailored to the needs of the individual (see Tables 46-3 and 46-4).

Technological advances historically precede the ethical and moral issues that may arise from such data. Confidentiality, informed consent, potential discrimination, and insurance issues should be carefully addressed by the counseling program staff. The institution's risk management team may play an active or consultant role, providing advice and counsel for current problems and future dilemmas. The Ethical, Legal, and Social Implications branch of the Human Genome Project has a major role in addressing the basic rights of the individual seeking counseling, the role of the government, and moral and religious conflicts that will arise from such testing.

The American Society of Clinical Oncology (ASCO) issued a revised position paper regarding genetic testing for cancer susceptibility.[135] The ASCO paper recognizes that identifying those individuals with the highest risk will certainly increase early detection and may ultimately lead to the prevention of many cancers. However, ASCO also cites the importance of addressing the actual and potential risks of testing in a setting that offers extensive patient/family counseling and education. Additionally, ASCO endorses pre- and post-test counseling and testing within a research protocol format that includes a national registry, long-term outcomes, and psychological ramifications.

The Internet has become a valuable source of information for both professionals and patients. Patients may inquire about Web sites that provide basic genetic information, and care must be taken to review any site before making a recommendation. A new search engine designed to assist health professionals and the public with genetic information is *http://search.info.nih.gov/grow/*. Some other appropriate sites for patients and families are *www.cdc.gov/genomics/*, listing information about genetic testing and testing centers as well as links to similar sites; the National Center for Biotechnology Information, *www.ncbi.nlm.nih.gov*, which offers a primer about the biology of genetics and links to the Human Genome Project; and the National Human Genome Institute's Spanish-language talking glossary, *www.genome.gov/sglossary.cfm*. A peer-support hotline has been established at the University of Pennsylvania; it is staffed by volunteers located across the country who have undergone genetic testing and can be reached at 866-824-RISK (866-824-7475). Nurses may wish to access other sites of interest: *www.geneclinics.org* has a directory of genetic abnormalities and testing sites. The International Society of Nurses in Genetics (ISONG) site, *www.isong.com*, lists education, nursing, and genetics resources and standards of practice. Additional sites include *www.geneticnurse.org*; *www.nchpeg.org*, the web site of the National Coalition for Health Education in Genetics; and *www.geneticalliance.org*.

An oncology nurse who receives additional education in the field of genetics will provide a wealth of information for the patient and family. All individuals who seek genetic counseling for breast cancer may not necessarily be at high risk. It is important for the staff to educate the patient and family as well as the referring physician regarding family and personal history assessments.

Pathophysiology

Cellular Characteristics

The majority of primary breast cancers are adenocarcinomas located in the upper outer quadrant of the breast (Figure 46-1). The most common histologic types of breast tumors are summarized in Table 46-5.

Infiltrating ductal adenocarcinoma may take various histological forms: well differentiated and slow growing; poorly differentiated and infiltrating; or undifferentiated with many mitoses and highly malignant. Adenocarcinoma can occur at any age, but highly malignant varieties with rapidly dividing cells affect more women in their early fifties. The overall ten-year survival rate is 50%–60%.

Invasive lobular carcinoma occurs in the same age range as ductal carcinoma, accounts for 10%–15% of

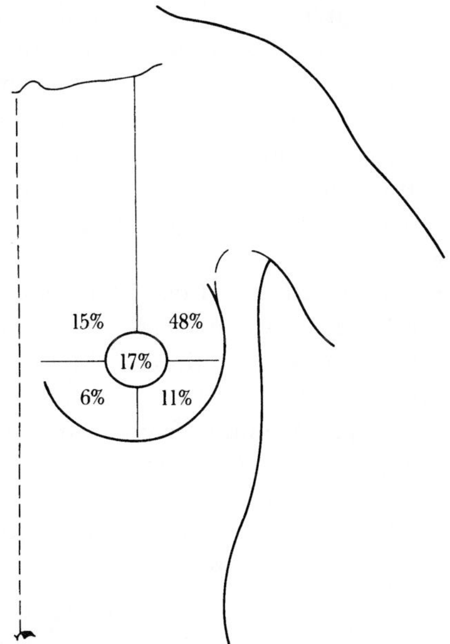

Figure 46-1 Incidence of breast cancer according to location.

Table 46-5 Histological Types of Invasive Breast Cancers

Histological Type	Percentage of Occurrence	Clinical Features	Metastatic Pattern	Prognosis
Infiltrating ductal carcinoma	70	Stony hardness to palpation Prominent lump Malignant cells have invaded through the walls of the duct May have a spiculated appearance on mammogram	Axillary lymph nodes (common) Bone Lung Liver Brain	Poor
Infiltrating lobular carcinoma	10–15	Diffuse, ill-defined thickness Multicentric Bilaterality (30%)	Axillary lymph nodes (common) Occult lymph node micrometastasis may occur	Poor
Tubular	2	May be quite large	Axillary lymph nodes (uncommon) Distant metastases uncommon	Favorable
Medullary	5–7	Well circumscribed Rapid growth rate Bilaterality	Approximately 40% of cases demonstrate lymph node involvement at diagnosis	Favorable
Mucinous (colloid)	3	Slow growing, bulky	Axillary lymph node involvement in less than one-third of cases at diagnosis	Favorable

Data from Schnitt, Guidi.[136]

all breast cancers, and is frequently bilateral. The prognosis is similar to ductal carcinoma.

Tubular carcinoma is fairly uncommon and represents a well-differentiated adenocarcinoma of the breast. These cancers typically occur in women age 55 and older. The presence of microcalcifications is characteristic and facilitates early mammographic discovery. Axillary metastasis is uncommon.

Medullary carcinomas account for 5%–7% of malignant breast tumors, occurring most commonly in women younger than age 50. These tumors may be quite large and circumscribed, and may be bilateral.

Mucinous or colloid carcinoma is uncommon, typically occurring in women aged 60–70. This tumor type is characterized by the presence of large pools of mucin interspersed with small islands of tumor cells. Metastasis to axillary lymph nodes occurs in about one-third of patients, and distant metastasis occurs late in the course of disease.

Inflammatory breast cancer occurs infrequently and accounts for less than 4% of breast cancers. This type of cancer often presents with skin edema, redness, warmth, and induration of the underlying tissue and may be mistaken for cellulitis. Even though it appears to be localized, it is associated with a poor prognosis.

Other malignant tumors of the breast include sarcomas, papillary carcinoma, apocrine, invasive cribiform, and Paget's disease.[136]

Patterns of Metastasis

Breast cancer is a heterogenous, highly variable disease. Even among women with the same histological type, clinical stage, and treatment, some will be cured while others develop metastatic disease within six months of therapy. The development of aberrant cell clones, with diverse growth rates and metastatic potential, may in part account for the differences seen in clinical behavior. While the process of metastasis is a complex and poorly understood phenomenon, a growing body of evidence suggests that angiogenesis (neovascularization) of the tumor plays an important role in the biological aggressiveness of breast cancer.[137–139]

Breast cancer metastasizes widely and to almost all organs of the body, but primarily to the bone, lungs, lymph nodes, liver, and brain. Patients with metastatic disease may present with symptoms specific to that organ. For instance, women with metastatic disease to bone often complain of bone pain. Those with liver metastases may report anorexia, weight loss, malaise, and occasionally right upper quadrant pain. Central nervous system (CNS) metastases may present with specific neurological symptoms such as headache that is more severe in the morning or is accompanied by nausea, or relate to specific neurological damage such as cranial nerve palsies (double vision), motor dysfunction, or spinal cord symptoms.

Clinical Manifestations

Diagnostic Studies

Routine mammography may reveal a large spectrum of breast pathology, ranging from equivocal benign conditions, to those that may mimic suspicious or ma-

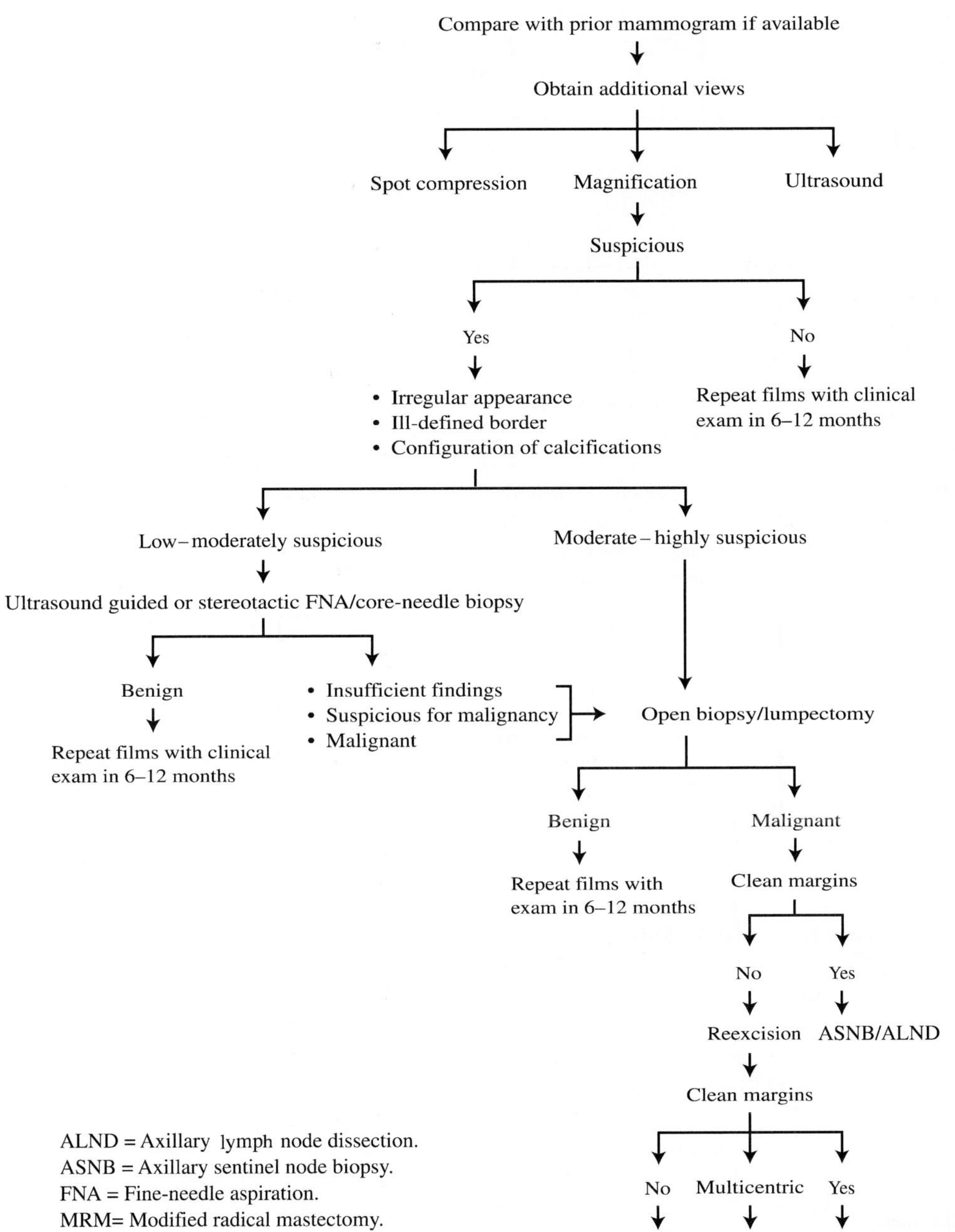

Figure 46-2 Evaluation of a nonpalpable mass found on mammogram.

lignant processes, to those that are considered malignant until proven otherwise. The appearance of these lesions is often a coincidental finding on a screening mammogram of an asymptomatic woman. However, if a palpable abnormality is present, additional diagnostic tools will be utilized to isolate the abnormality and provide more specific information for the clinician.

The diagnostic evaluation of breast lesions may be a simple one-step procedure or may progress to a multilevel process. Several noninvasive and minimally invasive diagnostic tools may aid the clinician in identifying lesions within the breast. The standard "triple test" approach to a reliable diagnosis of a breast abnormality calls for correlating the clinical, imaging, and cytologic findings, resulting in a sensitivity and specificity greater than 97% for diagnosing breast cancer. Of the three modalities, the two that combine to be most reliable are imaging and cytology.[140] A series of steps may be taken before determining which lesions actually need open (excisional) biopsy. Figures 46–2 and 46–3 describe the steps involved in the diagnostic evaluation of a nonpalpable and a palpable breast mass.

Clinical manifestations that are more suspicious of malignant disease include nipple retraction or elevation, which may be due to tumor fixation or infiltra-

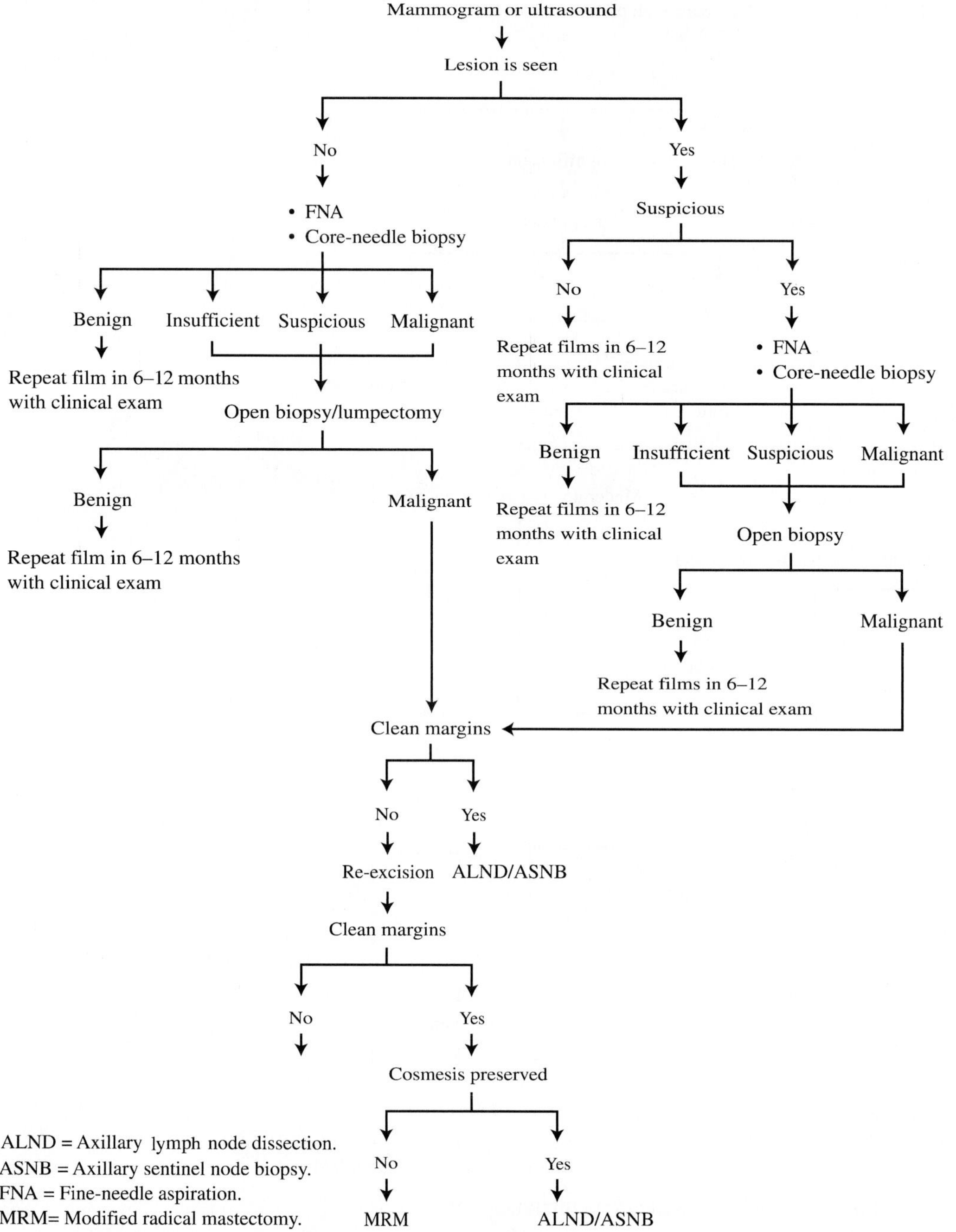

Figure 46-3 Evaluation of a palpable breast mass.

tion into the underlying tissues. Skin dimpling or retraction also may be present and is possibly due to invasion of the suspensory ligaments and fixation to the chest wall. Heat and erythema of the breast skin may be related to inflammation, but they are also signs of inflammatory breast carcinoma. Skin edema, or peau d'orange, the French term for "skin of the orange" (Figure 46-4), is characteristic of malignant disease. The edema is thought to be due to the invasion and obstruction of dermal lymphatics by tumor. Ulceration of the skin with secondary infection may be present. The presence of isolated skin nodules indicates invasion of blood vessels and lymphatics. It often results in implantation of tumor emboli in adjacent tissues and indicates that distant metastases are likely. Clinical presentation may also include, or be limited to, signs of local or distant metastatic disease.

Mammograms

Screening mammograms are used for routine breast surveillance for the asymptomatic patient. The

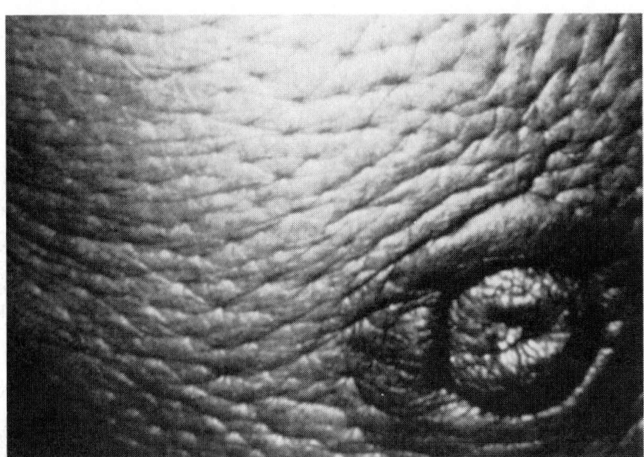

Figure 46-4 *Peau d'orange;* characteristic of lymphatic and dermal invasion by adenocarcinoma (inflammatory carcinoma).

consensus recommendation is that such mammography should begin at age 40[141–143] (Table 46-6). The goal of screening mammography is to detect a malignancy before it becomes clinically apparent. A woman who adheres to the screening mammography and clinical breast examination recommendation increases the likelihood that any cancer noted on mammogram will be an in situ carcinoma or early-stage invasive cancer with an excellent prognosis.

Clinical detection through the use of BSE generally occurs when a tumor is approximately the size of a walnut, which is by no means early in the biological history of the cancer. Therefore, mammography is an important consideration in the triad of early detection of breast cancer.

The routine screening mammogram provides a high-sensitivity study at the lowest possible cost. A highly sensitive study enables the radiologist to detect any discrete abnormality, thereby reducing the number of false-negative reports. Film-screen mammography allows for a high-quality image with a minimum of radiation.

A woman should consider the institution where the mammogram is performed. Since 1994, all facilities except Veterans Administration hospitals have been required to comply with standards regarding equipment, personnel, and record keeping, and must be certified by the FDA through an FDA-accredited body, such as the American College of Radiology. One can call 800-ACR-LINE or visit *www.acr.org* for current information on accredited hospital and clinics.

Screening mammography

The screening mammogram usually consists of four views, two per breast (Figures 46-5 and 46-6). A mediolateral oblique view and a craniocaudal view of each breast enable the technologist to image as much breast as possible (i.e., the axillary tail and pectoralis muscle).

A screening mammogram allows the radiologist to detect characteristic benign and malignant masses. Benign masses include cysts, fibroadenomas, and inframammary lymph nodes, all of which have defined borders. Malignant lesions may present as spiculated or ill-defined masses, architectural distortion, asymmetric densities, and microcalcifications (Figures 46-7 and 46-8). Additionally, subtle abnormalities may be noted by the radiologist that require further studies to determine whether pathology exists.[144]

Digital mammography records the radiographic image in a digital format that can be stored in a computer. This image can be displayed on a monitor or transferred on to film. The advantages of digital tech-

Table 46-6 American Cancer Society Guidelines for Early Breast Cancer Detection

Women at average risk	Begin mammography at 40 with a yearly clinical breast examination. Beginning at approximately age 20, women should be told about the benefits and limitations of breast self-examination (BSE). Prompt reporting of any new breast symptom to a healthcare professional should be emphasized. Women who choose to perform BSE should have the technique reviewed during a periodic health examination. It is acceptable for women to choose not to do BSE or to do BSE irregularly. Women should have an opportunity to become informed about the benefits, limitations, and potential harms associated with regular screening.
Older women	Screening considerations in older women should be individualized by considering the potential risks and benefits of mammography in the context of current health status and estimated life expectancy. As long as a woman is in reasonably good health and would be a candidate for treatment, she should continue to be screened with mammography.
Women at increased risk	Women at increased risk of breast cancer might benefit from additional screening strategies beyond those offered to women at average risk, such as earlier initiation of screening, shorter screening intervals, or the addition of screening modalities other than mammography and physical examination such as ultrasound or magnetic resonance imaging. However, the evidence currently available is insufficient to justify recommendations for any of these screening approaches.

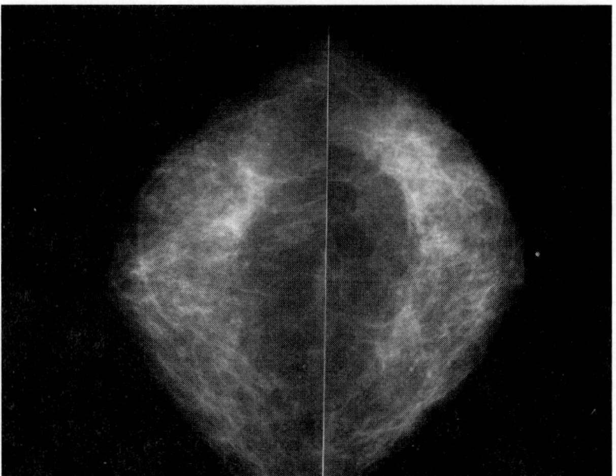

Figure 46-5 Screening mammography of an asymptomatic breast from above (craniocaudal view).

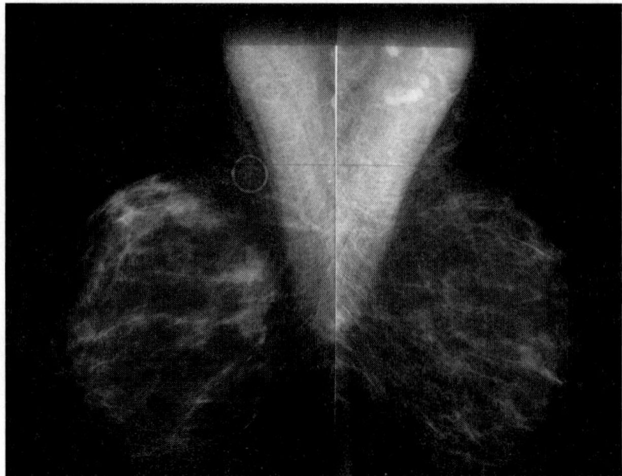

Figure 46-7 The mediolateral views show the appearance of an asymmetric density.

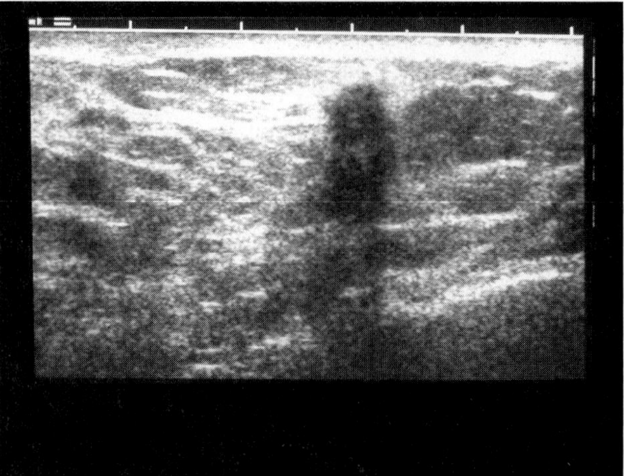

Figure 46-6 Screening mammography of an asymptomatic breast from the side (mediolateral view). Note the inclusion of the axilla and the pectoralis muscle, which ensures that the entire breast is imaged.

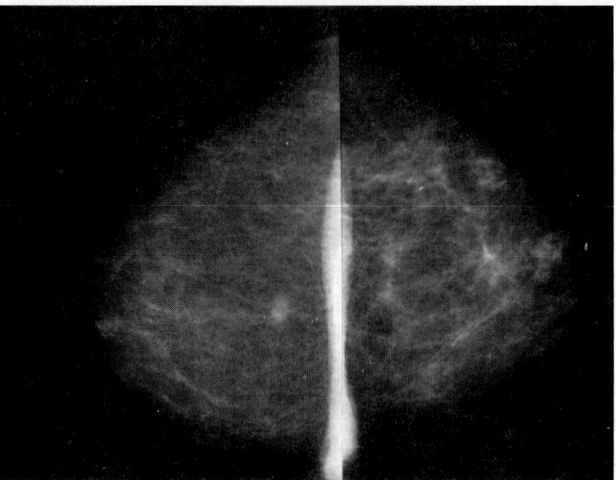

Figure 46-8 A craniocaudal view demonstrates the presence of spiculated nodules.

nology over screen-film mammography were listed by Adler and Wahl[145] and Schmidt and Nishikawa[146] in an early study:

1. Digital technology allows for more variations in exposure.
2. The radiologist's performance is increased by virtue of a second look.
3. Differences in tissue contrast are more easily seen.
4. Images can be transmitted and easily stored.

A more recent comparison of screen-film and digital mammography by Lewin and colleagues reported no statistical difference in detecting cancers, and there were fewer false-positive and true-positive examinations with digital imaging.[147] More studies must be conducted to determine whether digital mammography is superior to screen-film mammography. An answer may be forthcoming from the Digital Mammographic Imaging Screening Trial (DMIST), begun in 2001, which is comparing digital mammography with screen-film mammography. This National Cancer Institute (NCI)–sponsored study, with a proposed enrollment of 49,500 women, is being conducted by the American College of Radiology Imaging Network (ACRIN; *www.acrin.org*).

Computer-assisted detection (CAD) utilizes a software program to target potentially suspicious lesions for the radiologist to review and interpret. The computer identification involves an algorithm from a preset database generated from probability tables. Several recent reports have demonstrated improved detection using computer-aided detection systems,[148–150] but one large study noted no such improvement in detection, suggesting that more studies need to be conducted.[151] Several promising outcomes may result from this method of imaging. The specificity of the image is enhanced by real-time evaluation on a screen, allowing for manipulation of contrast that enhances detection and permits more rapid interventional procedures. The goal of CAD is to reduce the number of false-negative results and unnecessary biopsies. Mastering all of the technology available in breast imaging can pose a challenge to the general radiologist who is responsible for interpreting a variety of radiographic studies in his or her department. Given that specialist radiologists have higher cancer detection rates and lower recall rates, CAD may prove most useful for general radiologists.[144] Additionally, this real-time evaluation will enhance the use of mobile systems in remote areas. Expert consultation may be immediately accessed via satellite, while the unit is still on site.[152]

Nevertheless, digital imaging has some limitations and potential problems. Whole-breast images equal to the quality of film-screen mammography are only recently available for large-breasted women, and it is difficult to do an adequate comparison of previous film-screen studies with the digital images. The major limitation of digital mammography is that the luminance range and spatial resolution are less than those available with film-screen mammography. Cost is a another limiting factor for digital imaging and CAD. A basic digital mammographic unit is priced in the range of $500,000, much more than the standard film-screen unit price (approximately $90,000), and CAD devices are approximately $150,000. Additional expense will be incurred as accessory equipment is acquired to fully utilize the capabilities of digital imaging.

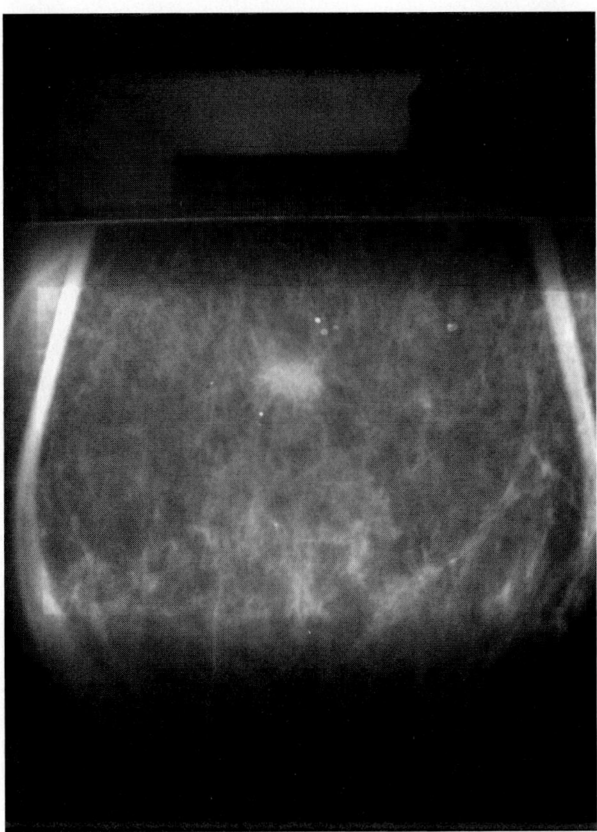

Figure 46-9 Magnification of the nodule provides a more accurate picture of the irregular border noted on screening mammogram. Note that the border is not clearly defined, but appears fuzzy or hazy, which is especially demonstrated on the left side. The irregular appearance and spiculations make this nodule suspicious for cancer.

Diagnostic mammography

A diagnostic mammogram is performed when the patient reports specific symptoms, suspicious clinical findings exist, or an abnormality has been found on a screening mammogram. A diagnostic film uses additional views of the affected breast as well as the possibility of localized compression and magnification views to increase the specificity when trying to identify the abnormality. The area in question is locally compressed and/or magnified, which enables the radiologist to comment more accurately on the lesion (Figure 46-9). The radiologist should be present during the diagnostic study. The ongoing evaluation of the additional films is crucial for rendering a diagnosis or recommending a plan of care.

Diagnostic mammography provides the radiologist with additional detail with which to render a more specific diagnosis, which may preclude the need for an open biopsy. However, if the diagnosis is nonspecific and the lesion has a low-suspicion threshold and is felt to be benign, the radiologist may recommend repeat films in six months to ensure that the area in question has not changed. This information must be discussed with the patient, as some people are uncomfortable waiting to be reexamined mammographically and may prefer to have the abnormality sampled or excised.

Sonogram

A sonogram or ultrasound has primarily been used as an adjunct to mammography to determine whether a lesion is solid or cystic.[153] In recent years, the use of ultrasound has been expanded to guide interventional procedures such as cyst aspiration, abscess drainage, FNA, core-needle biopsies, or presurgical localization; in the future, advances in high-resolution technology will continue to refine new methods of diagnosing breast abnormalities.[154]

Ultrasound is appropriate to investigate palpable lesions in young women whose breasts have dense fibroglandular tissue that may obscure a lesion in the breast or to evaluate suspected implant rupture. It is are also useful in pregnant women, who need to be spared radiation when an abscess or galactocele is sus-

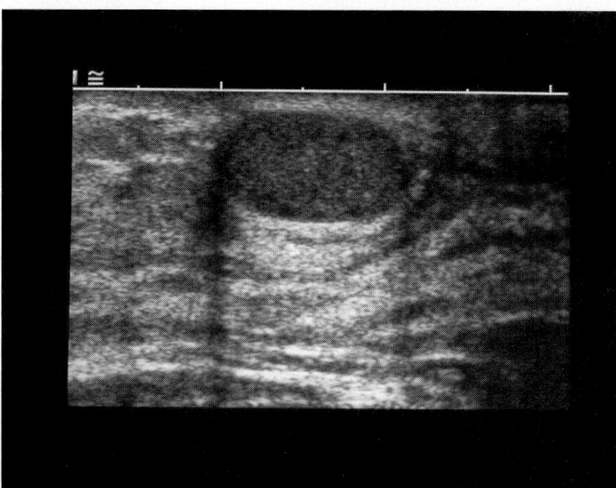

Figure 46-10 An ultrasound of a palpable mass reveals the characteristics of a fibroadenoma, which is a benign nodule.

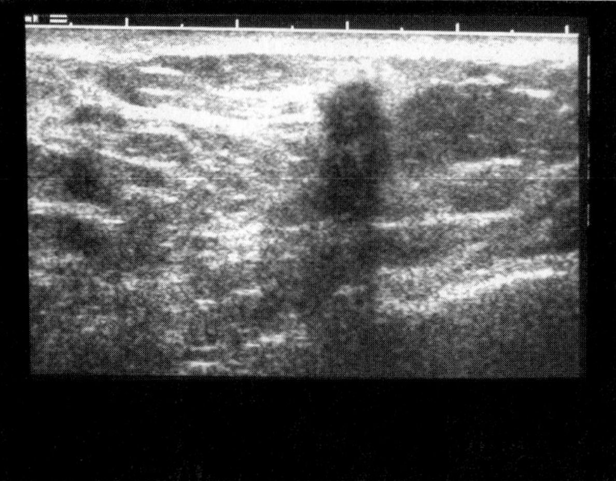

Figure 46-11 This ultrasound demonstrates two characteristics of a suspicious mass: (1) irregular shape and (2) ill-defined borders and spiculations.

pected, or in recently lactating women, whose breasts are extremely dense.

Sonogram is useful in determining whether a lesion is solid or cystic, and can assist in diagnosing breast cancer in certain instances. However, its sensitivity and specificity are not the same caliber as found in mammograms. Sonograms should generally not be used for screening purposes (Figures 46-10 and 46-11).

Magnetic resonance imaging

Magnetic resonance imaging (MRI; also known an magnetic resonance mammography [MRM]) of the breast is a relatively new procedure that may allow for earlier detection based on its ability to identify smaller lesions and provide finer detail. This technology has become a highly accurate, albeit costly, diagnostic tool, now that its specificity is enhanced by contrast infusion. It is not currently used for routine screening, however. MRI is superior to ultrasound in imaging the parenchyma, axilla, or chest wall and may aid in staging.[155] Potential advantages are that MRI emits no ionizing radiation, may improve diagnosis of benign and malignant lesions, and is not hampered by breast density, suggesting that it may be better suited for high-risk younger women.[155] Disadvantages include its high cost, unreliable identification of microcalcifications, and lack of standards for use in breast imaging. Additionally, some women may not be able to complete the study due to claustrophobia or indwelling metal devices.[154] Magnetic resonance imaging evaluates the rate at which the contrast initially enters the breast tissue and the intensity of enhancement. Malignant lesions tend to exhibit an increased enhancement within the first two minutes. Absence of uptake and areas of slow enhancement are considered negative findings.[156] In some cases, however, MRI findings may confound rather than clarify the issue. Areas of enhancement that are not classically benign may result in a biopsy or a repeat MRI in six months, adding to the financial and emotional burden of the patient. For these reasons, MRI may be best viewed as a complement to mammography and clinical exam to distinguish between a benign or malignant lesion in the high-risk population, with the goal of preventing benign biopsies and diagnosing cancer as early as possible. It may also be utilized to identify occult lesions, pinpoint recurrences, evaluate implant integrity, and biopsy suspicious areas not imaged on other studies.[155,157,158]

Positron emission tomography

Positron emission tomography (PET) employs metabolic activity to image the breast tissue. A glucose radiopharmaceutical, 2–deoxy-2–[18F]-fluoro-D-glucose (FDG), has been reported most useful as a metabolic tracer; it quantifies the overconsumption of glucose by a tumor cell and emits a metabolic ''hot spot.''[159,160]

PET may be superior to MRI in identifying viable tumor versus scar tissue, benign and malignant axillary nodes, and tumors that are 0.5–1.0 cm in size. It may also be utilized to locate primary, regional, and systemic metastases, and could eventually play a role in surgery and chemotherapy planning.[160] The major limitations of this technology are the high cost of the scanners and limited availability, as well as the short half-life of the radiopharmaceuticals. To date, PET has been approved for imaging of various cancers, including breast cancer, and its clinical applications continue to be evaluated in the research setting. PET will not be accepted as a routine screening tool until more definitive data become available.[160]

Scintimammography

Scintimammography uses a variety of radioisotopes to scan the axilla and supraclavicular area while imaging the breast,[161] but the most commonly used radiopharmaceutical tracer is technetium-99M sestamibi (MIBI). The tracer is injected intravenously and the rate of tissue absorption is then calculated, with higher rates being suspicious for malignancy. Scintimammography was introduced as a tool with superior specificity compared to mammography, with the suggestion that it would reduce the rate of benign biopsy. Liberman and colleagues reviewed 83 papers evaluating scintimammography and reported that the overall sensitivity and specificity was significantly higher than with mammography (> 85%), but the rate of detection of nonpalpable masses was significantly lower (67%) and the sensitivity for detecting cancers smaller than 1 cm was also poorer.[162] Scintimammography could eventually improve the accuracy of breast cancer diagnosis and decrease the number of unnecessary biopsies performed when used as an adjunct to mammography.

Fine-needle aspiration

Fine-needle aspiration (FNA) is employed to determine whether a palpable lesion is a cyst or a solid mass, and if solid, to determine whether it is benign or malignant. This technique may also be used to confirm a clinically apparent positive diagnosis. Newer immunochemical techniques allow the analysis of steroid receptors, ploidy, and proliferation index.[163] FNA is a simple office procedure that can be performed with or without local anesthesia using a small 21- or 23-gauge needle and 10 mL or larger syringe.[163,164]

If the lump in question is a cyst, it should disappear after the aspiration is completed. The decision to discard the cyst contents or to send them to cytopathology involves several factors: the clinical evaluation of the mass, the appearance of fluid (straw-colored, green, and cloudy are typical presentations), the number of previous aspirations, and the risk of breast cancer. Some practitioners routinely send any fluid aspirated from the breast for analysis, while others have a higher threshold for discarding the aspirates. Cysts may return in the same area or in other areas of the breast, and the patient may have repeated aspirations over time. If a previously aspirated cyst refills more than once in a short period of time (6–8 weeks), the decision to excise may be made, based on the patient's history of previous aspirations and personal risk of breast cancer. If a lump is solid, one can obtain a sample by making several passes into the lesion using the same entry point. This method will retrieve small cell samples from several sites within the lesion and reduce the chance of a false-negative result. Complications are rare, but hematoma, ecchymosis, and pneumothorax have occurred.

The usefulness of FNA cytology can vary, and the practitioner makes a decision about its value based on several factors: the quality of the sample; confidence in the skill of the cytopathologist; knowledge that the sample may not render a definitive diagnosis; and recognition that a malignant cytology cannot distinguish between in situ or invasive cancer.

Given that the major problem with FNA is false-negative results, it should be mentioned that a lesion that does not demonstrate a malignant histology may remain clinically suspicious to the physician. In such cases, a biopsy will often be recommended.

Core-needle biopsy

Core-needle biopsy is generally used for presumably solid, palpable masses that have some suspicion for cancer. Such biopsies are performed with a spring-action "gun," which automatically advances the needle to the lesion and obtains a specimen. The needle gauge is larger than in FNA, 14 or 16 gauge, thereby producing a small core of tissue. The gun may be used several times, so as to ensure an adequate sampling. Core-needle biopsy is felt to be superior to FNA for several reasons: The diagnosis is based on pathology interpretation, rather than cytopathology; a definitive diagnosis is usually rendered; and in situ carcinomas can be distinguished from invasive cancers, although some in situ cancers with microinvasion or small foci of invasion may be missed.[154]

Stereotactic needle-guided biopsy

The increasing acceptance of mammography as a diagnostic tool has fostered advances in minimally invasive biopsy techniques. The stereotactic needle-guided biopsy (SNB) is mainly used to target and identify mammographically detected nonpalpable lesions in the breast and is most often employed to identify the morphology of microcalcifications. It is appropriate for sampling most nonpalpable lesions, but is less suitable for very small lesions or areas of calcification, superficial lesions, those close to the chest wall, or those on the extreme medial or lateral area of the breast.[165] Patients who have cervical or shoulder pain may not be able to tolerate the positioning, and individuals who weigh 300 pounds or more are not eligible for SNB as the tables are not licensed to exceed this limit.[166]

While mammography offers the best detection of early breast cancer, mammography often cannot distinguish between benign and malignant tumors. Approximately 60%–80% of recommended biopsies are for benign abnormalities. The stereotactic biopsy permits diagnosis of benign disease without the trauma or

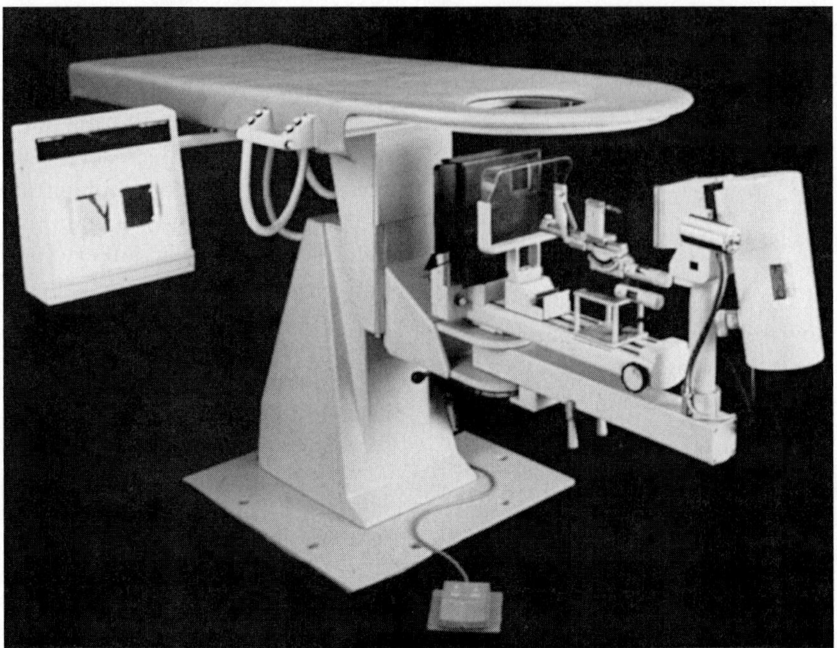

Figure 46-12 The stereotactic table allows for localization of the nonpalpable lesion between the Plexiglas plates below the opening from which the breast hangs down. Some machines allow for the procedure to be done in a sitting position, which is less favorable due to the possibility of syncope. (Photo courtesy of Fisher Imaging, Denver, CO.)

scarring of an open biopsy. This procedure has been improved over time and now yields sufficient tissue for diagnosis more than 97% of the time when performed by an experienced practitioner. It also results in a definite cost saving over excisional biopsy.[167] The basic principle of stereotactic biopsy is to immobilize the breast from fixed horizontal and vertical coordinates so as to calculate the exact position of the lesion within a three-dimensional field.[168]

The procedure takes place in a specially equipped operating room and generally takes about an hour. The most common position is prone, but some systems can accommodate an upright position. The room contains breast-imaging equipment and an examination table that has an opening at the front end through which the breast is suspended as the patient lies in a prone position. This positioning facilitates examining and targeting the precise area to be sampled. (See Figure 46-12.)

After proper placement is confirmed by stereoradiographs or digital mammograms, the breast is locally anesthetized and a small incision is made to penetrate the subcutaneous fibrous tissue. A needle (14–20 gauge) is placed in an automated needle biopsy gun that is mounted and stabilized. The gun emits a loud "pop," so it is helpful to fire the gun before placing the needle to reduce the risk of startling the patient. An alternative method is the vacuum-assisted biopsy technique that uses a larger-gauge needle (11–14 gauge).[166,169] The needle is inserted several times, which allows two or three core biopsy samples to be taken. Histology samples are then sent to the pathology department, and results are usually reported in one to two days. Cytology specimens may also be taken at this time.

Stereoradiographs are repeated to identify the exact area from which the samples are taken to ensure adequate sampling. If microcalcifications are the target, a specimen radiograph is used to confirm removal.[166]

After the procedure, pressure with or without an ice pack is applied for five minutes. The area is then cleaned and a sterile bandage is applied. The patient may shower the next day, but should avoid bathing for two days. The patient is also given instructions regarding notification of results.

Wire localization biopsy

The preparation for the wire-localized biopsy is somewhat similar to the stereotactic method. The difference lies in the goal of the procedure. The aim of this biopsy procedure is to radiographically assist the surgeon in locating the nonpalpable lesion for the purpose of excisional biopsy and to minimize the volume of tissue removed to avoid unnecessary deformity.[163] The character of the abnormality is identified after biopsy. (See Figure 46-13.)

The needle-localized biopsy targets the area via mammography, typically using a 90-degree view to determine the depth of the abnormality, possibly in conjunction with craniocaudal and mediolateral oblique

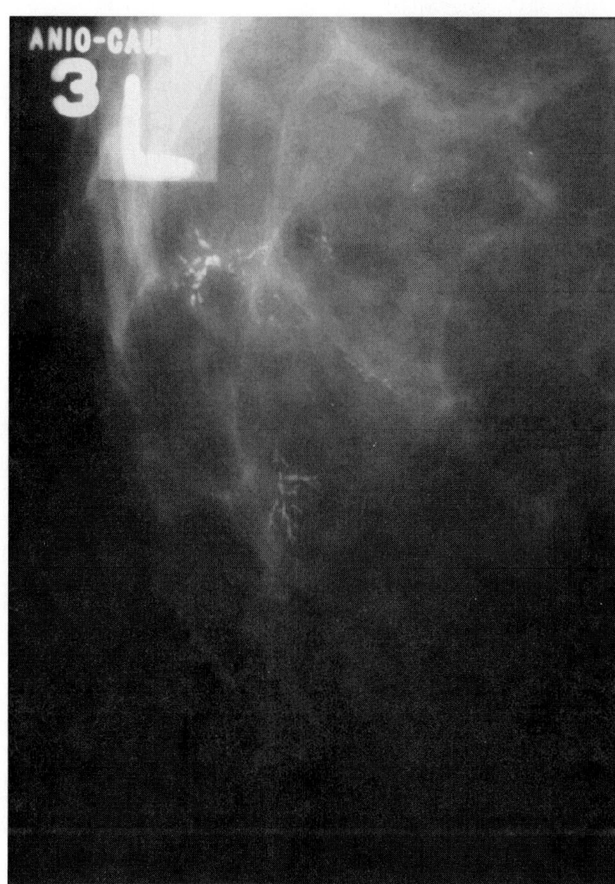

Figure 46-13 Magnification view of two areas of suspicious microcalcifications.

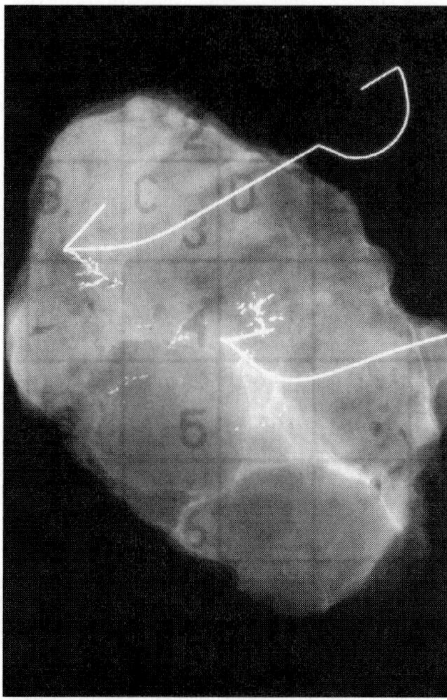

Figure 46-14 Specimen mammogram: Hook-wires were placed in each area of calcification. They were removed with good margins of surrounding tissue.

views. Once the area is anesthetized, a double-lumen needle is inserted into the area that has been calculated by the planes of the mammograms. Multiple lesions may be localized at one time using several wires. A set of repeat mammograms is then taken to ensure proper placement.

Once proper placement has been determined, the outer needle is removed, leaving a thin hook wire marking the area of concern (Figure 46-14). This wire is then taped to the skin of the breast to prevent dislodgement. The patient is sent to the operating room with the mammograms that note the area to be excised.[170] After the biopsy is complete, a specimen mammogram of the tissue is taken to ensure the abnormality has been removed.

Excisional biopsy/lumpectomy

The excisional biopsy is the most invasive diagnostic procedure. There are several reasons for recommending an excisional biopsy:

1. Sonogram findings show the lesion to be solid and indeterminate.
2. The cytology and/or histology results are insufficient.
3. The clinical or mammographic findings are suspicious.
4. The patient with a probable low-risk lesion requests a biopsy to allay her anxiety.

The objective of this biopsy is to remove the lump or area identified, along with a small amount of surrounding normal tissue. The potential for breast conservation should be considered during the planning for the biopsy. This is done by placing the incision above the lesion, using the most appropriate incision to follow the lines of tension, and avoiding tunneling. After the tumor is removed, the skin is closed without approximating breast tissue or fat. This method results in less deformity at the biopsy site. The excised tissue is identified and sent to the pathology lab for histopathological diagnosis.

An incisional biopsy that removes only part of the lesion is rarely performed. If the tumor is very large and a diagnosis and/or additional tumor markers are needed, core-needle biopsy is usually sufficient and an incisional biopsy is not necessary.

Prognostic Indicators

When breast cancer is diagnosed and found to be localized without evidence of metastatic spread, it is critical to identify patients who are at a substantial risk of recurrence, either locally or systemically. Identification of variables that are associated with disease recurrence may make it possible to design the most appropriate treatment for the individual based on the biological aggressiveness of the cancer. Most women with node-negative disease, representing approximately 60% of women diagnosed with breast cancer today, will be cured by surgery alone. Thirty percent of women will develop recurrent disease within ten years of their initial therapy. The identification of various prognostic indicators helps to define the natural history of breast cancer, establish prognosis with increasing accuracy, and, most important, identify those subsets of women who may be cured by local therapy alone versus those who would most benefit from adjuvant systemic therapies.[171]

Valuable parameters for determining the prognosis for patients with breast cancer include the status of the axillary lymph nodes, size of the tumor, invasive nature of the neoplasm, multicentricity, nuclear grade, hormone receptor levels, *HER2/NEU* oncogene, and histological type. Cell proliferative indices, DNA ploidy, and vascular endothelial growth factor (VEGF) protein — currently areas of investigation — are considered to be of high prognostic value in breast cancer, especially for women who have node-negative disease.[172] Age at diagnosis and menopausal status remain controversial prognostic indicators. It is generally recognized, however, that breast cancer patients younger than age 35 have a worse prognosis than older patients.[172]

Axillary lymph node status

The involvement of axillary nodes by tumor is a key feature in determining prognosis in breast cancer (Figure 46-15). Clinical assessment of the axillary nodes carries 30% false-positive and false-negative rates. Pathological staging of the lymph nodes is mandatory, including examination for microscopic metastases of the nodes.[173] Once involvement is determined, important issues are whether the metastases are microscopic or macroscopic, the number of nodes involved, the levels of involvement, and whether the lymph node capsule has been invaded. Extranodal extension is significant prognostically only when the metastases are confined to one to three nodes. Recovery of a small number of negative lymph nodes during a traditional axillary node dissection may understage disease and lead to an increased rate of regional relapse and poorer survival.[174]

Seventy percent of patients with negative nodes survive ten years. Prognosis worsens as the number of positive lymph nodes increases. Recurrence of disease is seen in approximately 75% of women with many positive nodes. Table 46-7 demonstrates the correlation between survival and number of involved nodes in a large population of women.[175] Metastases to the internal mammary nodes have the same significance as metastases to the axillary nodes. Internal mammary node metastasis occurs more readily in patients who have medial lesions. Although internal mammary nodes are not commonly sampled, they are invaded in 10% of patients when axillary nodes are negative. This phenomenon may help to explain the recurrence patterns in some axillary node–negative women.[176]

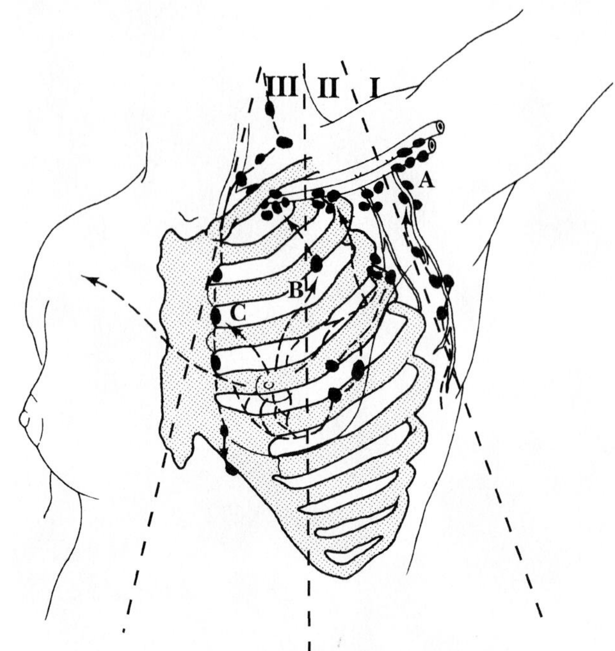

Figure 46-15 Lymphatics of the breast leading to **(A)** axillary nodes, which are distributed over a large area from the lateral aspects of the breast proper to the axillary vessels; **(B)** interpectoral chain leading to interpectoral node (circle detail) and to high nodes in the axilla; and **(C)** chain of the internal mammary leading frequently to nodes in second interspace and to supraclavicular and cervical nodes. The levels of lymph nodes (I, II, III) are defined by the pectoralis minor muscle.

Table 46-7 Recurrence Rates in 20,547 Women with Breast Cancer According to the Number of Histologically Involved Axillary Nodes

Number of Positive Nodes	Recurrence at 5 Years
0	25%
1–3	40%
4–6	49%
7–9	58%
10 +	78%

Data from Nemoto, Vana, Bedwani.[175]

Table 46-8 Five-Year Disease-Free Survival by Tumor Size for Node-Negative Patients

Tumor Size (cm)	Five-Year Disease-Free Survival (%)
1–2	79
2–3	77
3–4	72
4–5	74
5–6	72
> 6	57

Data from Clark.[172]

Tumor size

Women with node-negative breast cancer and tumors smaller than 1 cm in diameter have a relative overall five-year survival rate of nearly 99%. Patients with tumors measuring 1–3 cm have a relative five-year survival rate of approximately 91%, while those with tumors measuring more than 3 cm have a five-year survival rate of 85%.[176,177] Survival rates for patients with tumors larger than 3 cm is less than 50%.

Table 46-8 demonstrates a clear relationship between systemic risk of recurrence and tumor size in node-negative patients.[172] In addition, the presence of peritumoral vascular invasion is a marker of both local recurrence and future distant metastases. Consideration of other prognostic indicators is often necessary to determine the appropriate approach to systemic therapy.

Hormone receptor status

Normal breast epithelium contains hormone receptors and responds specifically to the stimulatory effects of estrogen and progesterone. A majority of breast cancers will retain estrogen receptors; for these tumors, estrogen will retain proliferative control over the malignant cells. The major benefit to knowing a woman's hormone receptor status concerns its value in predicting which patients will respond to hormone manipulation. Tumors that are more well differentiated or are of a lower grade tend to be positive for estrogen and progesterone receptors (ER and PR) and have a better than 75% response rate to endocrine therapy; in comparison, tumors that are positive only for ER have a response rate less than 35%. Tumors that lack receptor activity will not respond to hormonal therapy and tend to be of higher histologic grades. Postmenopausal women tend to be ER positive, while premenopausal women tend to be ER negative.

Cell proliferative indices and DNA ploidy

Research indicates that assessment of cell proliferative potential may have important prognostic significance, especially in node-negative breast cancer. Using flow cytometry, it is possible to measure the DNA content and proliferative activity (S-phase fraction) of a tumor. Patients whose tumors have an abnormal amount of DNA are aneuploid; those with normal DNA are diploid. A high S-phase fraction predicts a poorer outcome compared to a low S-phase calculation. Tumors that are ER negative tend to have a high S-phase fraction, reflecting a more aggressive metastatic potential.[172]

Histopathological considerations

The more well differentiated the tumor cells, the better the prognosis. Tumors are generally classified according to their histopathological grade, which takes into account the nuclear pattern and morphology and mitotic activity. Tumors that are well differentiated (grade I) have ductal/glandular features, uniform nuclear shape and staining characteristics, and low mitotic counts; such tumors are considered low grade. Tumors without these features and with markedly pleomorphic hyperchromic nuclei and abundant mitotic activity as evidenced by a high S-phase fraction are considered high-grade carcinomas. Such factors as nuclear size and shape, mitotic figures, and degree of tubule formation determine differentiation and likewise predict aggressiveness and metastatic potential of tumor cells. Approximately 10% of patients have low-grade tumors. Of these patients, more than 90% have ER-positive tumors; the majority have diploid DNA, low mitotic activity, and smaller tumors. Other important histopathologic considerations of tumor behavior are the amount of tumor necrosis, lymphatic/vascular invasion, and the extent of involvement of the surgical resection margin. Evidence of tumor involvement of either the microcapillary or lymphatic channels is considered nearly as predictive of recurrence as lymph node involvement.[172]

Molecular and biological factors

A variety of molecular markers have been studied in breast cancer to determine whether pretreatment clinical features and molecular markers can predict treatment response and survival in patients with primary breast cancer.[178]

Under normal circumstances, *p53* is a tumor suppressor gene that codes for a nuclear transcription factor that is involved with cell-cycle regulation and programmed cell death. The loss of functioning of this tumor suppressor gene may be associated with increased aggressive tumor behavior. Mutation of the *p53* gene appears to be an independent prognostic marker of early relapse and could be an important factor in identifying node-negative patients who have a poor prognosis and would therefore benefit from adjuvant systemic therapy.[179,180]

The *HER2/NEU* proto-oncogene encodes for a transmembrane protein that appears to be a receptor for a peptide growth factor. Amplification of this gene occurs in approximately 30% of women with breast cancer, resulting in overexpression of the gene product. It appears that overexpression of *HER2/NEU* is associated with worse disease-free and overall survival, especially for those patients with node-positive disease. Further, in women with metastatic breast cancer, high levels of *HER2/NEU* are correlated with poor response to endocrine therapy and favorable response to chemotherapy—especially cisplatin, doxorubicin and paclitaxel.[171,181] Current clinical research is focusing on gene expression profiling, which may someday enable clinicians to determine an individual patient's potential for relapse with reasonable certainty.[115,182–186]

Overexpression of VEGF is thought to be involved in tumorigenesis and metastasis in primary breast cancer. Increased expression of this growth factor is associated with decreased overall survival in women with node-negative breast cancer. The degree of intratumoral vascularization in primary breast cancer is a significant independent prognostic indicator that correlates with metastasis and shortened survival.[187] Primary tumors and metastases will not grow beyond 2 mm in diameter without an enhanced vascular supply. Chemical signals (cytokines) from tumor cells are thought to stimulate resting vascular endothelial cells to begin a rapid growth phase, thereby supporting the growth and spread of the tumor. VEGF is an angiogenic factor that stimulates proliferation of vascular endothelial cells. Tumor-induced neovascularization appears to be a critical step in the oncogenic and metastatic cascades and may have important implications for the evaluation and treatment of women with breast cancer, especially those with node-negative disease. Research in the development of monoclonal anti-VEGF antibody (rhuMAbVEGF) is an exciting development in breast cancer. Clinical trials are currently under way to test the safety and efficacy of rhuMAbVEGF in combination with chemotherapy.

Assessment

Classification and Staging

Once breast cancer has been diagnosed, a complete evaluation of the disease is initiated to establish the stage of disease and the most appropriate approach to treatment. Such planning and evaluation are optimally orchestrated through the auspices of a comprehensive breast center, where all disciplines consult with the patient and family concerning decisions about therapy.

In the initial evaluation, the diagnostic mammogram is utilized to look for evidence of tumor multicentricity or bilaterality. The history and physical exam; routine blood work including complete blood counts, liver function tests, and a complete metabolic profile; and a chest x-ray are completed prior to the initial planning session. A bone scan is generally considered part of the basic work-up if the tumor is larger than 1 cm or if the patient has an elevated alkaline phosphatase level. Bone films or a dedicated bone window computerized tomography (CT) scan are indicated if a suspicious area suggests tumor involvement. Likewise, a CT scan of the chest and liver would be indicated if the primary tumor were inflammatory in nature or larger in size, or if liver function tests or chest x-ray were abnormal.

Clinical staging is based on the characteristics of the primary tumor, the physical examination of the axillary nodes, and the presence or absence of distant metastases. As previously mentioned, the clinical evaluation is less accurate than pathological evaluation. Because of the prognostic significance of axillary node involvement, a pathological stage is necessary to determine stage of disease. The pathological staging recommended by the American Joint Committee on Cancer (AJCC)[188,189] is presented in Table 46-9.

The 2003 staging updates take into account the latest cancer research and changes in clinical practice. Recent changes consider micrometastatic axillary nodes and classification changes for the number of involved lymph nodes. Stage reclassification using the new AJCC staging system for breast cancer will result in significant changes in reported outcome by stage.[190] This system is somewhat complicated and can be simplified in terms of the most critical components—that is, whether nodes are involved and whether distant metastases are known to be present:

Stage I	Tumor 0–2 cm in size; negative lymph nodes and no evidence of metastasis
Stage II	Small tumor with positive lymph nodes or larger tumor with negative lymph nodes
Stage III	More advanced locoregional disease with suspected but undetectable distant metastases
Stage IV	Distant metastases are known to be present

Table 46-9 American Joint Committee on Cancer Staging for Breast Cancer Tumor–Node–Metastasis (TNM) Classifications

Primary Tumor (T)		Regional Lymph Nodes (N)	
T0	No tumor evident	N0	No regional lymph node metastasis
T1s	Carcinoma in situ	pN1	Metastasis to 1–3 axillary lymph nodes and/or internal mammary nodes identified by sentinel node biopsy
T1mic	Less than 1 mm in greatest dimension	pN2	Metastasis to 4–9 ipsilateral axillary lymph nodes or clinically apparent internal mammary nodes
T1a	1–5 mm	PN2	Metastases to 10 or more ipsilateral axillary nodes; clinically apparent internal mammary nodes and 1 or more axillary nodes; or ipsilateral supraclavicular lymph nodes
T1b	6–10 mm	NX	Regional lymph nodes cannot be assessed
T1c	11–20 mm		Node staging modified by presence of disease identified by immunohistochemistry or molecular studies: see *AJCC Staging Manual* for full details
T2	21–50 mm (2–5 cm)	**Distant Metastases**	
T3	Larger than 50 mm (> 5 cm)	M0	No distant metastases
T4	Tumor of any size with direct extension to chest wall or skin	M1	Distant metastases
T4a	Extension to chest wall	MX	Distant metastases cannot be assessed
T4b	Edema or ulceration of the skin of the breast or satellite skin nodules on the same breast		
T4c	Both T4a + T4b		
T4d	Inflammatory carcinoma		
TX	Primary tumor cannot be assessed		

Stage	TNM (Tumor–Nodes–Metastasis)	10-Year Overall Survival (%)
0	Tis N0 M0	95
I	T1 N0 M0	88
IIA	T0 N1 M0 T1 N1 M0 T2 N0 M0	62
IIB	T2 N1 M0 T3 N0 M0	62
IIIA	T0 N2 M0 T1 N2 M0 T2 N2 M0 T3 N1 M0 T3 N3 M0	29
IIIB	T4 N0 M0 T4 N1 M0 T4 N2 M0	29
IIIC	Any T N3 M0	29
IV	Any T, Any N, M1	7

Used with permission of the American Joint Committee on Cancer (AJCC), Chicago, Illinois. The original source for this material is *AJCC Cancer Staging Manual* (ed 6). New York, Springer-Verlag, *www.springer-ny.com, 2002.*[188]

Therapeutic Approaches and Nursing Care

Women today are discriminating health consumers who actively seek information regarding their treatment options. It is not uncommon for the nurse to be asked for advice about where a woman might go for a consultation concerning how a suspicious mass should be investigated. If one is available in the area, patients should be referred to a comprehensive breast center for an opinion. Women should not delay in seeking medical attention for evaluation of a palpable mass or abnormal mammographic finding. While a breast cancer diagnosis causes significant emotional, social, and economic/vocational upheaval, such distress eases over time as therapy is planned and carried out. Most women actively participate in the decision-making process and are able to clearly articulate their need for information throughout treatment planning and months of therapy. To be a supportive advocate for the woman and her family, the nurse must be knowledgeable concerning the options for therapy, the goals of therapy, the measures to minimize complications of treatment, and the various resources that may need to be mobilized throughout the treatment period and beyond.

For rehabilitation to be optimal, the nurse should pay careful attention to the woman's expressed need for information at each juncture of treatment. Seeking information is a valuable coping device and yet rarely useful unless the woman recognizes the need for it. The right amount of accurate information will help the woman formulate questions and will facilitate decision making, decrease anxiety, and enhance overall adjustment to the illness and treatment.

A woman's psychological and social adjustment to diagnosis and treatment will depend on her previous coping strategies and emotional stability. In addition, social support has consistently been found to influence a woman's adjustment through treatment.[191] The threat to emotional, social, sexual, and physical well-being is multifaceted, and the relative impact of these factors on adjustment varies from patient to patient and assumes varying degrees of importance at different stages of treatment.[192]

A strong source of social support will be extremely valuable throughout all phases of treatment. While the most important sources of social support are the woman's spouse, family, and friends, other sources of support may be needed to maintain a strong social network. The roles of the psycho-oncologist, the social worker, and various support groups are important resources in the care of these women and their families.

The patient's need for information will vary considerably throughout each phase of treatment. It is not uncommon for the treatment plan to include surgery, radiation, and chemotherapy. For many women, the time of active treatment lasts at least six months and most do not feel rehabilitated for up to a year following their diagnosis. If reconstruction is planned, this rehabilitation phase will be extended.

Surgery

Primary breast cancer

Local–regional disease. Intraductal carcinoma or DCIS generally presents as clustered microcalcifications on mammography and rarely carries a risk of axillary node involvement. Options for treatment include total mastectomy, wide excision followed by radiation, or wide excision alone. Because ductal carcinoma in situ frequently extends beyond the area of microcalcification, a wide excision should include tumor-free margins around the area.

While it is true that nearly 60% of women diagnosed with breast cancer today will have localized node-negative breast cancer and therefore be highly curable, many women with primary breast cancer, stages I–II, will have metastatic disease from which they will die, regardless of local or systemic treatment. Furthermore, numerous clinical trials have demonstrated that breast-conserving treatment, consisting of removal of the primary tumor by lumpectomy with radiation therapy, results in a survival rate that is comparable to that associated with more extensive local therapy, such as mastectomy or modified radical mastectomy.[82,193–195] Currently, more than one-third of women with breast cancer in the United States are managed by lumpectomy and radiation therapy. Breast-conserving surgery would not be appropriate for women with larger tumors, tumors involving the nipple–areola complex, or tumors with extensive intraductal disease appearing to be multicentric, or for women who are unable or unwilling to undergo adjuvant radiation therapy.

An extensive intraductal component is a predictor of recurrence and is generally considered a contraindication to conservative surgery. Selection of the most appropriate surgical procedure is critical to local control of the primary cancer so as to reduce the risk of local failure and systemic disease. The cosmetic result of breast-conserving surgery is generally considered to be acceptable, as body image is maintained. Scar tissue may form and cause some contracture over time, but most women find the cosmetic result acceptable, especially when wearing a bra. Complications following breast-conserving surgery include arm edema, seroma formation and wound infection, shoulder dysfunction, upper extremity weakness, fatigue, and limitations in mobility.

A modified radical mastectomy involves the removal of all breast tissue and the nipple–areola complex, plus level I and II axillary node dissection (see Figure 46-15). The pectoralis muscle is preserved. A horizontal incision is made because it is cosmetically more acceptable. Modified radical mastectomy is indicated for larger, multicentric disease or where cosmesis could not be achieved with conservative surgery. Modified radical mastectomy may also be employed as definitive treatment following local recurrence in patients who fail conservative surgery and radiation. In general, patients with noninvasive or locally invasive tumors have excellent prognoses following salvage mastectomy. However, patients with predominantly invasive recurrent tumors are at significant risk for further relapse.

Postoperative complications following mastectomy include wound infection, flap necrosis, and seroma formation. A transverse incision is associated with less skin flap necrosis. Seromas occur in approximately 10% of patients and generally resolve following aspiration. Antibiotics may be indicated. Nursing care of the postmastectomy patient centers on wound care, with special attention being paid to maintaining functioning wound drains. If drains become blocked, the wound is more likely to develop a seroma/hematoma, leading to infection and possibly flap necrosis. To maintain suction and an adherent flap, drains may be "milked" to remove small clots. Drains are usually removed within two to four days following surgery. Patients may be discharged with drains intact.

Postmastectomy exercises to maintain shoulder and arm mobility may begin as early as 24 hours after surgery. The woman is instructed to maintain the affected arm in the adducted position but to perform limited exercises involving the wrist and elbow. Flexing fingers and touching the hand to the shoulder are encouraged. Squeezing a ball is discouraged, as it increases blood flow and, if done too vigorously, leads to swelling in the early postoperative period (Tables 46-10 and 46-11).

Prior to discharge, the patient should have clear instructions regarding wound care and drain management. Initial care of the wound involves maintaining a clean incision with dressing changes daily if indicated. A return appointment is usually made to assess the wound and, if necessary, remove stitches. At that time, the patient should receive specific instructions regarding postmastectomy exercises. A mild analgesic may be indicated to promote arm mobility during exercises and to prevent shoulder dysfunction.

Complaints of a stiff shoulder are common and are due primarily to postoperative immobility. It is not uncommon for a tightness to develop under the axilla extending to the elbow. This cord-like substance is thought to comprise sclerosed lymphatics that gradually dissipate two to three months after surgery. Range of motion (ROM) exercises and massage therapy are beneficial. Care of the axilla involves avoiding the use of depilatory creams, strong deodorants, and shaving under the arm for approximately two weeks following surgery.

Instructions regarding breast self-exam and follow-up are usually given during the first outpatient visit after surgery. Introducing the patient to various prostheses and mastectomy bras can occur in the hospital, but women are generally more ready to receive this information once the surgery is behind them. Most are advised not to wear a prosthesis until the wound has healed completely (six to ten weeks). During this period, the woman may want to meet with a Reach to Recovery or Y-ME volunteer who will assist her in learning about resources in her area for purchasing a prosthesis. Many different kinds of prostheses exist: Some are foam filled, others are liquid silicone filled, or still others are the more permanent, self-adhering variety. It is important that the prosthesis fit properly and that the weight be similar to the remaining breast. Insurance pays for most prostheses provided a prescription or letter demonstrating medical necessity is submitted.

Table 46-10 Patient Information: Hand and Arm Precautions

Do not permit injections (chemotherapy), blood samples, or vaccinations to be done on your affected arm unless approved by your physician.
When trimming cuticles, take extra care not to tear hangnails. Professional manicures *are* recommended.
Wear heavy gloves when gardening and digging or handling thorny plants.
Always use a thimble when sewing to avoid pinpricks, and wear rubber gloves while washing dishes.
Protect your arm from burns, especially from small appliances such as irons or frying pans, and from the sun.
Be sure your hand and arm are well protected with an elbow-length mitt when reaching into a hot oven.
Always have blood pressure measurements taken on the opposite arm.
Avoid arm constriction from tight elastic, sleeves, or jewelry.
Do not carry a heavy purse or other objects — especially grocery bags or luggage — with your affected arm.
Avoid strenuous upper body aerobics unless arm is supported by a properly fitted antilymphedema compression sleeve. Lifting weights of any kind is not recommended.
Apply a good lanolin cream several times daily if your skin appears dry.
Treat cuts and scratches by washing the area well and applying an antiseptic. Contact your physician if signs of infection, redness, warmth, or swelling occur.

Table 46-11 Postmastectomy Exercises

When to Begin	Purpose	Exercises: Perform Exercises 5–10 Times Each, Three Times a Day
Postoperatively days 1–5	Prevent and/or reduce swelling	• Position arm against your side in a relaxed position. Elbow should be level with your heart, and the wrist just above the elbow when resting. • Rotate wrist in a circular fashion. • Touch fingers to shoulder and extend arm fully.
After drains are removed	Promote muscle movement without stretching	• While standing, brace yourself with your other arm and bend over slightly, allowing your affected arm to hang freely. Swing the arm in small circles and gradually increase in size. Make 10 circles — rest — repeat in the opposite direction. • Swing arm forward and back as far as you can without pulling on the incision. • While standing, bend over slightly and swing arms across the chest in each direction. • While sitting in a chair, rest both arms at your side. Shrug both shoulders, then relax. • While sitting or standing, pull shoulders back, bring the shoulder blades together.
After sutures are removed	Stretch and regain full range of motion; to gain mobility of your shoulder, you must move it in *all* directions, several times a day	• While lying in bed with arm extended, raise arm over your head and extend backward. • While lying in bed, grasp a cane or short pole with both hands across your lap. Extend arms straight up and over your head and return. • Repeat, rotating the cane clockwise and then counterclockwise while over your head. • While standing, extend arm straight over your head and down. • Extend your elbow out from your side at a 90° angle — hold it for 10 seconds — relax. • Extend your arm straight out from your side even with your shoulder — extend arm straight up toward the ceiling. • Stand at arm's length facing a wall. Extend arms so your fingertips touch the wall. Creep fingers up the side of the wall, stepping forward as necessary. Repeat the procedure going down the wall — keep arms extended. • Stand sideways to the wall. Extend arm out so fingers touch the wall. Creep up the wall a little more each day. • Use hand and arm normally (see Table 46-10).
After 6 weeks	Strengthen arm and shoulder and regain total use of arm and shoulder	• Begin water aerobics. • Begin overall fitness program. • Begin aerobics, Jazzercise, or other resistive exercises. • Avoid using weights as these may increase arm edema and subsequent swelling.

The woman alone or together with her husband, partner, or significant other should have the opportunity to discuss any physical or emotional concerns regarding sexual relations. Evidence is mounting to support the contention that, while the diagnosis of breast cancer and the loss of a breast are certainly emotionally distressing for all concerned, they do not result in an increased prevalence of psychiatric disorders or sexual dysfunction.[192] The woman's overall psychological health, relationship satisfaction, and prior sexual relations are far stronger predictors of sexual health than the extent of breast surgery. Younger women may experience more episodes of depression, anger, resentment, sexual problems, and fears of recurrence compared to older women.

Axillary and sentinel lymph node dissection. Axillary lymph node dissection (ALND) is not a therapeutic procedure, as the overall survival, disease-free survival, and rate of distant metastasis are the same for those patients who have axillary dissection as for those who do not.[92,196,197] The principal reason to perform this procedure is to help determine prognosis and risk for recurrence, and to decide whether adjuvant chemotherapy — specifically, a doxorubicin-containing regimen — is indicated. Because lymph node dissection is responsible for significant morbidity associated with breast surgery, there is increasing interest in finding alternative methods to obtain prognostic information. Lymphatic mapping and sentinel node biopsy are two of the most promising techniques.

The first node in the lymphatic basin that receives primary lymphatic flow is the sentinel lymph node. The histological characteristic of the sentinel lymph node is thought to predict the histological characteristics of the remaining lymph nodes in the axilla. Sentinel lymph node mapping involves the injection of a radioactive substance or blue dye into the area around the tumor, which later drains into the ipsilateral axilla. The axilla is explored through a small incision, and the lymph node that takes up the blue dye or technetium-labeled sulfur colloid — that is, the sentinel node — is excised. If the sentinel node is positive for tumor, then the patient undergoes an axillary dissection, but only if doing so will contribute to decisions regarding therapy. If the sentinel node is negative, the remaining axilla is negative 92%–95% of the time.[198] Many women — but especially those with small primary tumors and clinically negative axillary lymph nodes — could potentially be spared an axillary dissection if the sentinel node is found to be negative. Axillary node dissection would then be reserved for women for whom more information is required to determine the need for chemotherapy and for those with larger primary tumors.

Axillary lymph node dissection is not without complications. Despite its advantages, ALND is often associated with pain, numbness, swelling, weakness and stiffness, lymphedema, and a decreased quality of life. An option for women with newly diagnosed breast cancer is sentinel lymph node biopsy (SLNB). Several clinical trials designed to assess the safety and predictive value of this procedure have found that SLNB performed by a surgeon with sufficient experience is as accurate as a full axillary dissection if the nodes are found to be negative. Current practice suggests that a full axillary dissection be performed if the sentinel node is malignant but is not required if the sentinel node is negative. Debate continues over whether micrometastases in the sentinel node dictate a full axillary dissection. Results of ongoing trials and increasing experience with SLNB may eventually make SLNB the standard for assessing the axilla, so that women can potentially be spared unnecessary axillary dissection and avoid the risk of lymphedema, without sacrificing disease-free and overall survival.[197–199]

Radiation Therapy

The role of radiation in the treatment of localized breast cancer has evolved over the years to the point where such therapy is now considered standard treatment. In fact, with an equivalent survival rate and preservation of the breast, conservative surgery plus radiation is considered preferable to mastectomy for the majority of women. The major criteria for selecting patients for breast-conserving surgery and radiation therapy (RT) are (1) the size of the tumor and the feasibility of resecting the primary tumor without causing major cosmetic deformity, and (2) the likelihood of tumor recurrence in the breast. Local failure following breast-conserving surgery and radiation occurs in 13% of patients at ten years.[92] Every effort should be made to decrease the local failure rate, mainly by obtaining clear surgical margins and possibly by adding chemotherapy and antiestrogen therapy.

When radiation and chemotherapy are given following breast-conserving surgery, patients experience higher survival rates overall. For women who are at high risk for local or regional recurrence (patients with large tumors, patients with tumors that invade the skin of the breast or the chest wall, or those with many positive axillary nodes), radiation and chemotherapy are indicated postmastectomy. In patients whose tumors overexpress the *HER2/NEU* proto-oncogene and are eligible for Herceptin therapy, Herceptin therapy may be given weekly during the radiation course to enhance the radiation effect.

The role of RT postmastectomy is less well established owing to the risks associated with radiation to the chest wall, particularly when it is given for left-sided breast cancer. There appears to be a higher risk for fatal myocardial infarction 10–15 years later in left-sided cases compared with adjuvant radiation for right-sided cases,[200] although a retrospective study by Vallis and colleagues found no evidence of excess morbidity and mortality from coronary artery disease among women treated with RT to the left breast at 10.2 years of follow-up.[201] Postmastectomy radiotherapy is routinely considered for premenopausal patients with involved axillary nodes, particularly those with four or more involved nodes and/or tumors larger than 5 cm. The value of specific nodal irradiation in patients who undergo adequate axillary dissection is much less clear, especially considering the potential for long-term complications of lymphedema.

Radiation generally begins within three to four weeks following chemotherapy if a doxorubicin or taxane regimen is used. If CMF or methotrexate, 5-FU, and leucovorin are used, radiation usually begins following day 8 of cycle 3. Radiation doses to the breast are delivered using supervoltage equipment and tangential fields to minimize lung and heart exposure. The whole-breast dose ranges from 45 to 50 Gy delivered over five to six weeks. Whether a boost is given depends on the type of local excision and risk for local recurrence. The morbidity associated with a boost of moderate size and dose delivered either by electron beam or interstitial implantation is small.[202] The cosmetic result following partial mastectomy and radiation therapy is generally considered to be good.

Women undergoing external beam therapy commonly experience fatigue and some nausea, but primarily skin changes and arm and breast swelling. Immediate side effects of external beam RT may include transient breast edema, erythema, and dry or wet desquamation. Later effects include telangiectasia, which is seen less often, and arm edema, which usually results from radiating the axilla for multiple positive nodes. Breast edema is unique to patients undergoing breast-conserving surgery and radiation and usually appears during or within the first six months after treatment. It is more common in women who have had an axillary dissection where more than 11 nodes are removed and in those patients receiving adjuvant chemotherapy. Skin reactions occur in all patients and generally present as itching, dryness, scaling, redness, and tenderness. The breast may feel sore and warm to touch. Patients are instructed not to use soap to wash the area and to pat it dry. Dry desquamation can progress to a moist desquamation with infection.

Arm edema occurs more commonly in patients who have axillary dissection followed by RT to the axilla. Symptomatic pneumonitis characterized by a dry cough and low-grade fever is infrequent, but can appear within two to three months of therapy and is more common in women receiving methotrexate and 5-FU concurrently with RT. Brachial plexopathy manifesting as paresthesias, with or without arm and hand weakness, may be transient or permanent, but is an infrequent complication. Rib fractures and cardiac complications are also rare and relate to dose and whether concurrent chemotherapy is given.

An alternative to external beam therapy for early-stage breast cancer is high dose rate (HDR) brachytherapy. It can be delivered in two ways: through the intraoperative placement of a balloon catheter in the lumpectomy site, or via rod placement in the lumpectomy site after completion of adjuvant chemotherapy, if chemotherapy was given. In both regimens, fractionated therapy is given twice daily for five days, after which the rods or balloon catheter is removed.[203,204] The patient undergoing brachytherapy may find it more convenient to stay in the hospital for the duration of treatment, or she may travel from home twice daily for treatment. The radioactive material is removed after each fraction and reinserted for the next fraction. Early single-institution trials have found that HDR partial-breast irradiation has similar outcomes to standard whole-breast external beam therapy.[205,206] If HDR brachytherapy is to follow adjuvant chemotherapy containing an anthracycline, the start of the brachytherapy should be delayed for approximately six weeks to avoid radiation recall in the irradiated skin.

Table 46-12 Histologic Subtypes of Male Breast Cancer

Type	Incidence (%)
Infiltrating ductal carcinoma	> 80%
Papillary carcinoma	5%
Lobular carcinoma	1%
Inflammatory carcinoma	1%
Paget's disease	1%
Medullary, tubular, mucinous	< 1%

Data from Giordano, Buzdar, Hortobagyi.[208]

Breast Cancer in Special Populations

Males

An estimated 1300 new cases of breast cancer were diagnosed in men in 2003 and 400 men were expected to die of their disease.[1] Male breast cancer accounts for less than 1% of all breast cancer cases and 0.2% of all malignancies in men.[207] The anatomical structures of the male breast are the same as those of the female breast. It is the hormonal stimulation present in the female breast but absent in the male that accounts for the developmental and physiological differences between the male and female breast. This lack of hormonal stimulation also may explain the comparatively low incidence of male breast cancer. Nevertheless, the disease is similar in both sexes in terms of epidemiology, natural history, and response to therapy.

The strongest risk factor for male breast cancer is Klinefelter's syndrome, in which the male has inherited an additional X chromosome (47, XXY karyotype). Gynecomastia, atrophic testis, high levels of gonadotropins, and low testosterone levels are characteristic of Klinefelter's syndrome. The risk of breast cancer in males with Klinefelter's syndrome is as much as 50 times that of males in the general population.[208]

Other risk factors include chronic liver disorders, administration of exogenous estrogen to treat prostate cancer[209] or to maintain female characteristics in transsexuals; obesity; *BRCA2* mutations; and a family history of breast cancer in female relatives.[207,210]

Breast cancer occurs most frequently in men after age 60, with the peak incidence noted between 60 and 69 years. The majority of male breast cancers (81%) are known to be ER positive; however, receptor positivity does not increase with advancing age as it does in women.[208] Male breast cancer typically arises from ductal elements and presents as infiltrating ductal carcinoma (Table 46-12). Analysis of tumor cells for overexpression of *HER2/NEU* by FISH suggests that breast cancer in males has a very low rate (< 1%) of protein overexpression.[211] The remaining prognostic factors are the same as in female breast cancer.

A moderately tender, centrally located subareolar mass is usually the first symptom that brings the man to seek medical attention. Pectoral fixation, involvement of skin, nipple changes, and discharge are commonly present, often because of delay in seeking medical attention. These factors may account for the increased frequency with which advanced disease and early invasion of local and regional lymphatics are diagnosed in men. Ulceration may occur early in the course of the disease and carries a relatively poor prognosis. Because of its relatively central location, male breast cancer can be expected to metastasize to the internal mammary nodes. The lungs and bony skeleton are the most common metastatic sites.

Because of the low incidence of male breast cancer and relatively small number of male patients, it is difficult to conduct controlled clinical trials to aid in establishing appropriate therapy. Giordano and colleagues conducted a population-based sample of 2524 men with breast cancer in an attempt to characterize the disease.[212] Men were found to be significantly older at diagnosis, more likely to present with later-stage disease, more likely to have larger tumors, and more likely to have nodal involvement, ductal histology, and estrogen receptor–positive tumors than women.[212]

The treatment of male breast cancer is based on the treatment of female breast cancer. The modified radical mastectomy has been the mainstay of therapy. Because male breast cancer is often diagnosed at a later stage, the skin and underlying fascia are frequently involved. Skin grafting may be required to adequately close the surgical wound. Adjuvant radiotherapy, hormonal manipulation using SERMs or AIs, and chemotherapy are also part of the approach to treatment.[207,213,214]

Orchiectomy appears to remove the source of estrogen and androgen in recurrent male breast cancer and can result in a prompt remission. With recurrent disease, further hormonal manipulation using tamoxifen, anastrazole, and progestin may be helpful. Anastrazole, tamoxifen, and other forms of hormone manipulation are relatively ineffective without orchiectomy. However, goserelin acetate effectively reduces testosterone to castration levels and may be an important alternative for men who refuse orchiectomy.

Young Women

Breast cancer is a rare occurrence in young women. The incidence of breast cancer in 20- to 24-year-olds is 1.4 per 100,000 women; the incidence increases to 8.1 per 100,000 for women 25–29 years of age and 24.8 per 100,000 for women 30–34 years of age.[215] When breast cancer occurs in young women, it is generally more aggressive biologically and has an unfavorable prognosis compared with older, postmenopausal patients. Tumors in young women tend to present with a higher grade, higher proliferative fraction, and more vascularization than in older women.[216] Younger women are more likely to present with more advanced disease at diagnosis, and the risk of death from breast cancer is highest among the youngest and oldest cohorts as compared with women of intermediate age.[99]

Adjuvant chemotherapy is a nearly universal recommendation for younger women diagnosed with invasive breast cancer. The role of ovarian suppression in the management of localized breast cancer in premenopausal women has been a controversial issue for some time. In premenopausal women, evidence appears to support a dual mechanism of action of chemotherapy, involving both direct cytotoxicity and ovarian suppression resulting from chemotherapy-induced ovarian failure. Tamoxifen plus ovarian function suppression may be sufficient in node-negative women, but few prospective clinical trials have been completed to address this issue. Early studies of ovarian suppression indicate that it is a viable treatment alternative for premenopausal women with ER-positive breast cancer.[217]

Questions of timing of surgery with respect to the menstrual cycle, appropriate use of endocrine therapy in premenopausal women, ovarian function suppression, and duration and intensity of chemotherapy remain to be answered. The majority of clinical trials upon which treatment decisions are based report data for women age 40 and older. There is a need for clinical investigations of the younger population given that chemotherapy is invariably recommended for these high-risk patients.[218]

In addition to issues related to the poor prognosis and appropriate medical management of young breast cancer patients, issues of early menopause, sexual functioning, childbearing, and dealing with the young family require support from the physician, nurse, and psychosocial staff. The possibility of pregnancy after treatment for breast cancer remains controversial. Most studies have utilized case-control designs and have shown that pregnancy following breast cancer is not detrimental to survival and, in fact, often linked to an improvement in survival.[219] Some sources recommend waiting until two years postsurgery before attempting conception, but this recommendation is based on limited data from a small and selectively obtained group of patients. Based on available data gleaned largely from retrospective case-control studies, no definitive recommendations can be made with regard to local recurrence, risk of distant metastasis, or survival.

Cancer is generally viewed to be a disease of aging, and the diagnosis of breast cancer in a very young woman can be devastating to the woman, her partner, and her family. Many breast cancer support groups, such as Y-ME and Gilda's Club, now include groups specifically geared toward young breast cancer survivors.

Elders

Cancer is largely a disease of aging; that is, the incidence and mortality rates of breast cancer increase with age. The size of the geriatric population is increasing annually. Barring any unforeseen breakthrough in cancer prevention, the number of breast cancer cases will increase exponentially as well. More than 50% of breast cancer cases occur in women older than age 65.[1]

A common question raised during the physical assessment of the healthy older woman is how long to continue annual mammographic screening for breast cancer. Breast cancer is a leading cause of cancer death in women older than 65 years of age. Unfortunately, mammographic screening is underutilized in elderly women in the United States, with only one-third of women in the 65–69 age group undergoing routine screening mammography.[220] Life expectancy in the United States is approximately 83 years for women; therefore, a 65-year-old woman can expect to live another 18 years. Women who are otherwise healthy and would choose to treat breast cancer if it were found should continue mammographic screening and annual breast exams until their situation changes.[221,222] Women whose life expectancy due to co-morbid conditions or advancing age is less than 5 years would probably not realize a survival benefit from early diagnosis of breast cancer and therefore should stop screening.[221]

Caring for the elder with breast cancer poses a challenge. Postmenopausal women are generally diagnosed with stage I or II, hormone receptor–positive, infiltrating ductal carcinoma. Breast cancer in the older woman is associated with a more favorable tumor biology, and survival rates for older women are similar to survival rates for the general population.[223] Small tumor size and negative nodes mean that treatment can be effectively confined to endocrine therapy — that is, a SERM or AI, both of which are generally well tolerated by elders.[224] Treatment issues arise when the prognosis is poor and recurrence seems likely due to a large tumor or positive axillary nodes or when the tumor is hormone receptor negative or positive for *HER2/NEU*. Recent studies indicate the use of an AI may be more effective than tamoxifen in women who overexpress *HER2/NEU*.[225] When chemotherapy is indicated, an accurate assessment of the older patient's co-morbidities, tumor biology, functional status, and support systems is necessary. It is difficult to determine optimal treatment regimens for older patients as few clinical trials in the past have included a sizable number of older subjects.

Chronic co-morbidities increase with aging, and breast cancer patients are no less likely than the general population to have one or more co-morbid conditions. Evaluating the status of the co-morbid conditions, the effect of chemotherapy, and the availability of supportive care is necessary before making treatment decisions.[226] Chemotherapy doses may require modification for the appearance of side effects; the side effects may be more or less pronounced in elders or may be masked by symptoms from preexisting conditions. Most chemotherapy dosage adjustments relate only to decreases in creatinine clearance; renal function should be monitored in all older patients receiving chemotherapy.[226] Table 46-13 lists issues to be considered when contemplating chemotherapy in elders.

Many older patients lack sufficient social support systems, and providing the necessary support may become a trying issue for the nurse and family alike. Family caregivers usually play an essential role in caring for patients with cancer. Lack of financial support and physical access to treatment facilities may represent barriers for many older women. Referral to a community-based senior center or psychologist may provide support not otherwise available for the family in an effort to offset the negative aspects of caregiving.[227] Many older women are overwhelmed by the prospect of several surgical procedures to obtain a full diagnosis, chemotherapy, radiation therapy, and continuing follow-up care. These women may benefit from the presence of a nurse case manager to assist in directing and obtaining care.[228]

When preparing to care for an older woman with suspected or confirmed breast cancer, several concepts should guide clinical decision making and choice of treatment: (1) average life expectancy of the patient; (2) co-morbidities and their impact on diagnostic and therapeutic options as well as life expectancy; and (3) the trade-off between potential treatment benefits and risks, taking into account survival as well as quality of life.[222] Older women who are contemplating treatment should be encouraged to enter clinical trials and should be active participants in the decision-making process.

African American Women

For many years, the disparities in cancer incidence and survival between African Americans and whites

Table 46-13 Chemotherapy Considerations in Older Breast Cancer Patients

Agent or Regimen	Side Effects of Concern	Considerations	Co-morbid Condition Alert
Anthracyclines	Cardiotoxicity	Obtain MUGA prior to treatment	Congestive heart failure
		Avoid use with history of cardiac disease	Coronary artery disease History myocardial infarction
	Nausea/vomiting	Fluid loss/dehydration	
	Myelosuppression	Consider use of growth factor support	
Cyclophosphamide	Nephrotoxicity	Monitor urinary function	Renal insufficiency
	Nausea/vomiting	Fluid loss/dehydration	
Taxanes	Peripheral neuropathy	Monitor motor/sensory function	Diabetes mellitus
	Peripheral edema	Monitor fluid retention (docetaxel)	Congestive heart failure
	Hand–foot syndrome	Monitor skin changes (docetaxel)	Psoriasis; eczema
Vinorelbine	Constipation	Prophylactic bowel regimen	
Capecitabine	Hand–foot syndrome	Monitor skin changes	Psoriasis; eczema
	Nausea/diarrhea	Fluid loss/dehydration	

MUGA = multiple gated acquisition.

have been the subject of study and controversy. African American women are more likely to die of breast cancer, even though they are less likely to get this disease.[4] Whether African American women have biologically more aggressive breast cancer than white women and whether race acts as a significant independent prognostic factor for survival have not been determined by any large-scale clinical trial. A meta-analysis of articles reporting on overall survival for black and white patients treated similarly for cancer reported only modest cancer-specific survival differences, highlighting the need for further research into differences in treatment, presentation stage, and mortality from other diseases.[229]

Some researchers believe that biology may be responsible for the higher mortality rates among African American breast cancer patients. One-third of African American women with breast cancer are diagnosed premenopausally (before age 50) compared to 23% of white women. Estrogen receptor–negative breast cancer is also more common among African American women (40%) compared to white women (23%).[230] These two factors, however, are linked for all women: Premenopausal women of all races tend to have hormone receptor–negative breast cancers.

Continuing genomic research seeking a biologic variable that may account for these survival differences recently identified a gene, *BP1*, that may be responsible for the differing survival outcomes between African American and white women treated for breast cancer. The expression of *BP1* in tissue was closely correlated with both ER-negative tumors and race: 89% of tumors from African American women were *BP1* positive, whereas only 57% of tumors from white women expressed *BP1*. *BP1* could provide a useful target for therapy or early diagnosis, if activation of *BP1* proves to be an early event in carcinogenesis.[231]

Other researchers support the theory that socioeconomic status (SES) replaces race as a predictor of poorer outcome after women are diagnosed with breast cancer.[232] This factor has been correlated with increased risk of disease and poorer health outcomes. Poorer populations have higher incidence and mortality from all kinds of disease, but especially a number of cancers. African American women with breast cancer have disproportionately more high-grade disease at diagnosis as compared with white women. Comparisons between these groups that account for SES find little difference in outcome. It is conceivable, however, that genetic causes of certain cancers may be more prevalent in populations whose members originate from certain geographic areas, such as Africa,[233] but it is most likely that any genetic causes are due to a combination of genes, not just one. The issue of population genetics may assume increasing importance in this post-genomic age as we gain the ability to investigate the origin of certain diseases in depth. Population genetics deals with certain diseases that are more prevalent in certain ethnic populations, such as sickle cell anemia among people of African descent and Tay-Sachs disease among Ashkenazi Jews.

Whatever the cause, nurses need to be aware that survival of breast cancer is less likely for African American women than for white women. African American women generally present with later-stage disease. The incidence of small tumors and localized disease is consistently higher in white women; the incidence of tumors larger than 5 cm and distant-stage disease is higher among African American women.[4] Higher relative survival rates and greater improvement in survival over time are observed in white women than in African American women.[215,234]

Access to adequate, high-quality mammographic screening and clinical breast examination remains the goal for early detection of breast cancer in all women, but especially so for African American women, who are currently diagnosed with larger tumors and at later stages of the disease. Although federally funded programs for mammographic screening have been available for many years, adequate funding to treat women diagnosed through these screening programs had been lacking. Passage of the Breast and Cervical Cancer Prevention Act of 2000 provides medical assistance through federally funded, state-run Medicaid programs to eligible women who were screened through the Centers for Disease Control and Prevention's National Breast and Cervical Cancer Early Detection Program.[235] African American women who are diagnosed with breast cancer should be evaluated for participation in clinical trials that may provide access to state-of-the-art cancer care that might otherwise be unavailable to them.

Breast Reconstruction

Modern breast reconstruction began in the 1960s with the advent of silicone implants. Prior to that time, surgery was regarded as a primary curative modality with the emotional and psychological effects being virtually ignored or regarded as the "price a woman must pay." Consequently, many women experienced feelings of loss, depression, and alterations in body image. These responses may be lessened now that breast reconstruction has come to be regarded as a viable and acceptable component in the treatment of breast cancer. In the past two decades, improved procedure techniques, advances in autologous tissue reconstruction, and the manufacture of implants have enabled many women to retain their self-confidence and body image, thereby enhancing their quality of life. Before plastic surgery became an acceptable procedure for the treatment of breast cancer, many women found the external prostheses cumbersome and consequently felt it necessary to alter their activities and/or selection of clothing due to fear of displacement or discomfort of the prosthesis.

Despite the recent findings equating the two surgical procedures (mastectomy versus lumpectomy plus radiation) in terms of survival, many women either choose or are advised to have a mastectomy. This decision may be based on a variety of circumstances, including histological findings, emotional or body image issues, financial considerations, or accessibility of medical resources.

A woman who presents with diffuse microcalcifications or multicentric disease throughout the breast is not considered a suitable candidate for breast preservation. Some patients are troubled by the fact that, although the cancer appears to have been removed, an occult lesion may remain; consequently, they will choose to remove the breast. Additionally, cosmesis may be compromised because too great a proportion of breast tissue needs to be removed to ensure clear margins. Patients who are responsible for a substantial portion of their medical bills may forego the cost of radiation treatments and choose mastectomy. Other women find that suitable medical facilities for radiation treatments may require extensive travel time or are geographically unavailable. Cost may also determine the type of reconstruction a woman chooses, if a portion is not covered by insurance. Spear and colleagues reviewed costs and reported that the average total cost for implant reconstruction was $15,497 versus $19,607 for transverse rectus abdominus muscle (TRAM) reconstruction.[236]

Implants are considered to be safe and effective treatment despite recent media comments to the contrary.[237] Citing the potential harmful effects of silicone implants revealed in an ongoing investigation, the FDA imposed a moratorium on the use of silicone implants for augmentation and issued guidelines to limit the use of silicone implants for reconstruction.

To qualify for placement of silicone implants, certain criteria must be met. The surgeon must inform the patient of the possible side effects as well as document that the patient has an "urgent need" as previously defined by the FDA. Additionally, the patient must be enrolled in a registry to aid in the long-term tracking of these patients.

Initially, the criteria were very stringent, but the revised guidelines issued in August 1992 expanded the eligibility regulations and have not been amended. The patient must be 18 years of age or older. Women who have experienced cancer, other disease, or trauma may have immediate or delayed reconstruction. Implants may be placed in any woman who currently has silicone implants and needs replacement or revision for medical or health reasons resulting from augmentation or mastectomy surgery. Women with congenital defects or severe asymmetry are considered candidates for silicone implants. Additionally, women who require augmentation of the unaffected breast for any of the preceding reasons may have an implanted silicone prosthesis. Additional information on current guidelines issued by the FDA is available from the American Society for Aesthetic and Plastic Surgery or the American Society of Plastic and Reconstructive Surgeons at 888-475-2784 (*www.plasticsurgery.org*).

The patient exclusion criteria include pregnancy or lactation, tissue abnormalities, and increased risk due to other treatment or psychological issues. Women who demonstrate active infection, lupus, scleroderma, or uncontrolled diabetes are not candidates for the procedure. Patients who are experiencing radiation damage, who have problems with vascularization, or who have inadequate tissue available are considered to be ineligible.[238–241] The surgeon may declare any patient unsuitable who possesses any other physical or psychological condition that will compromise compliance and/or success of the surgical procedure. Because of the adverse publicity about silicone gel implants, many women and physicians today choose saline-filled implants, which reduces the risk of silicone contamination if rupture should occur. These implants, however, do not have the same suppleness and natural feel of silicone gel implants.

Although implants are considered a viable and acceptable choice, other avenues continue to be explored for breast reconstruction. Autologous transplants have provided a suitable alternative to the inert prosthesis in certain circumstances. These procedures include lattissimus dorsi flap, deep inferior epigastric perforator (DIEP) flap, TRAM flap, and the less frequently used gluteal tissue flap. The TRAM and latissimus dorsi flaps are most commonly used, and most of these autologous surgeries may be performed as a tissue transfer or free flap.[242–247]

The silicone implant was introduced in the 1960s, and the basic design remains relatively unchanged today, although the use of silicone implants has been dramatically reduced from 95% of breast implants at its peak to 10% today. The saline tissue expander was introduced in the 1980s as an alternative to silicone. It is used as a temporary device or may function as a more permanent implant to remain in place until the woman decides on a permanent saline implant or more is known regarding the potential risk of the silicone implants. Virtually every patient who chooses a mastectomy is a candidate for some form of expander/implant reconstruction. Although most women are reconstructed using the two-step method (placement of an expander for inflation, followed by its replacement with a permanent implant), some are able to have the permanent implant placed immediately (one-step method) if they are very small breasted and adequate skin is available for an acceptable breast mound.

The timing of the consultation is very important because of the myriad of considerations to be addressed prior to surgery. In the past, the rule of thumb was to delay reconstruction, sometimes waiting months to years. Currently, surgeons who recognize that the psychological trauma associated with the loss of a breast may be lessened by more timely reconstruction will, after careful assessment, offer the patient immediate reconstruction. Immediate reconstruction is often preferred to reduce the potential morbidity of the process, as it allows the woman to avoid an additional bout of general anesthesia. However, the woman's general health or treatment plan may dictate that a delay in reconstruction be considered.

The ideal candidate is one who has early-stage disease. However, the absolute limiting factor for this surgery is the presence of any medical conditions that may compromise the patient's safety during or after surgery. Patients who have undergone prior abdominal surgery may not be eligible for abdominal flap surgery. Morbidly obese women will be discouraged from abdominal flap surgery, as larger flaps have a greater tendency to develop fat necrosis.[248,249] Heavy smokers may be advised to quit smoking for at least three to four weeks prior to surgery to ensure an adequate blood supply.[240] The surgeon will also attempt to identify those patients who may be subject to additional problems such as hypotension or hypoxia, which may compromise circulation and influence the success of the surgical procedure.[240,249] Patients who present with extensive local or metastatic disease may need further evaluation regarding chemotherapy or radiation therapy, which may necessitate a minor or significant delay in reconstruction due to immunosuppression or skin changes.

During the initial consultation, the surgeon evaluates and addresses the patient's and family's expectations of surgery. This may be done through the use of before and after pictures as well as the surgeon's frank explanation of the expected outcome. A patient with realistic expectations is well informed and more likely to accept the expected imperfections when these aspects are known prior to surgery. The goals of reconstructive surgery are to achieve "acceptable" symmetry and softness, correct any deformity caused by prior treatment, and construct an adequate nipple–areola complex. Some women are apprehensive about the thought of mastectomy because they have never seen a reconstructed breast, and may envision a poor cosmetic outcome. A helpful visual tool to assuage their initial anxiety before the visit to the plastic surgeon is the *Show Me* book, published by the Breast Cancer Support Group from Penn State at the Geisinger Health System Women's Center, Hershey, Pennsylvania (717-531-5867). The book collects photos of survivors who have had mastectomies with and without reconstruction and lumpectomies, and can be ordered for $25.

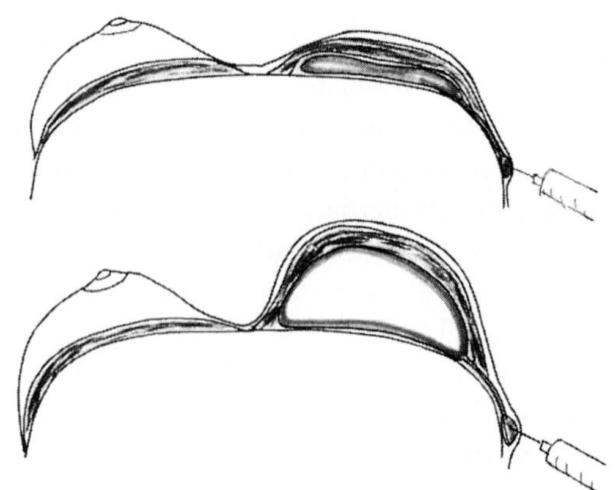

Figure 46-16 The horizontal view illustrates the overexpansion that is needed to allow for a more natural suppleness when the permanent prosthesis is implanted. (Courtesy of Dr. Craig Bradley, MD, Senior Attending, Plastic and Reconstructive Surgery, Rush University Medical Center, Chicago.)

Saline Tissue Expanders

Saline expanders are used when an inadequate supply of skin is available at the mastectomy site or when a large and/or ptotic breast is required. Tissue expansion is the most frequently used reconstructive procedure. The expander is placed behind the chest wall muscles using the lines of the mastectomy incision. Mastectomy plus reconstruction surgery will last 3–4 hours and require a hospital stay of 1–2 days.

The expanders have a filling port that is located either remotely or on the anterior of the implant. After allowing sufficient time for wound healing, a series of injections is performed as an office procedure. The saline expanders, which are partially filled at the time of insertion, usually require 60–200 mL injections on a weekly or biweekly basis. The expansion continues until the device is overinflated by approximately 50%, usually in 6–8 weeks,[250] but may take longer for those patients who are unable to tolerate standard expansion. The overfilled expander is left in place for several months to allow for accommodation of the stretched tissue. This overfilling helps to promote a more natural, supple contour of the reconstructed breast (Figure 46-16). The expander is then removed and a permanent prosthesis of equal or lesser fluid volume is placed.

Migration of the implant upward is a concern postoperatively. This possibility is minimized by proper placement of the dressing under the axillae, which exerts a downward pressure on the implant.[238] Although contracture helps provide shape to the breast, excessive contracture will distort the appearance and may hinder or prevent further expansion. Deflation can occur spontaneously or as a result of needle puncture. Expanders with remote ports are less likely to be accidentally deflated.

Permanent Saline Prostheses

Class-action litigation and the influence of wary consumers have led to the widespread preference for saline implants over those containing silicone, although studies have failed to directly correlate collagen disease with silicone implants. Although saline expanders have no silicone in the pocket, the outer casing contains silicone. When Hoshaw and colleagues conducted a meta-analysis of human and animal studies, they concluded that breast implants constructed of whole or part silicone posed no additional risk for breast cancer.[251] The surgery for the permanent saline prosthesis is usually done in stages: The expander is placed during the mastectomy, the permanent implant is placed after desired expansion has been attained, the nipple–areola complex is constructed during another procedure, and some additional surgery may be needed subsequently to attain the desired cosmetic result.

Exchanging the expander for the permanent prosthesis is an outpatient procedure. Just prior to surgery, the patient stands before a mirror as saline is removed to match the opposite breast. In the operating room, the surgeon incises along the mastectomy scar, and opens the wound with cautery to expose the expander. Cautery is used to protect the wall of the expander. The expander is removed and the volume of saline is measured to determine the size required for the permanent implant. The permanent implant is placed behind the muscle in the pocket created by the expander. Placing the implant beneath the chest wall muscles helps counteract the expected firmness due to capsular contraction and supports the implant.[250]

Complications that may arise include progressive contracture, hematoma, infection, and flap necrosis. Contracture is an expected sequela of implants and is the result of scar tissue enveloping the prosthesis. However, some patients will experience increasing contracture that alters and deforms the breast. New implants are being designed in an attempt to reduce the incidence of contracture, which has decreased from a peak of 35%–55% to 2%–11% today. Approximately 5% of implants need to be removed due to severe contracture.[239] Hematoma occurs infrequently and is most often surgically drained. Infections happen rarely and are most often successfully treated with antibiotics or removal of the implant in extreme cases. Flap necrosis can be serious and, if extensive, may necessitate the removal of the prosthesis. Usually, the necrosis involves a small amount of tissue that is excised.[238,239]

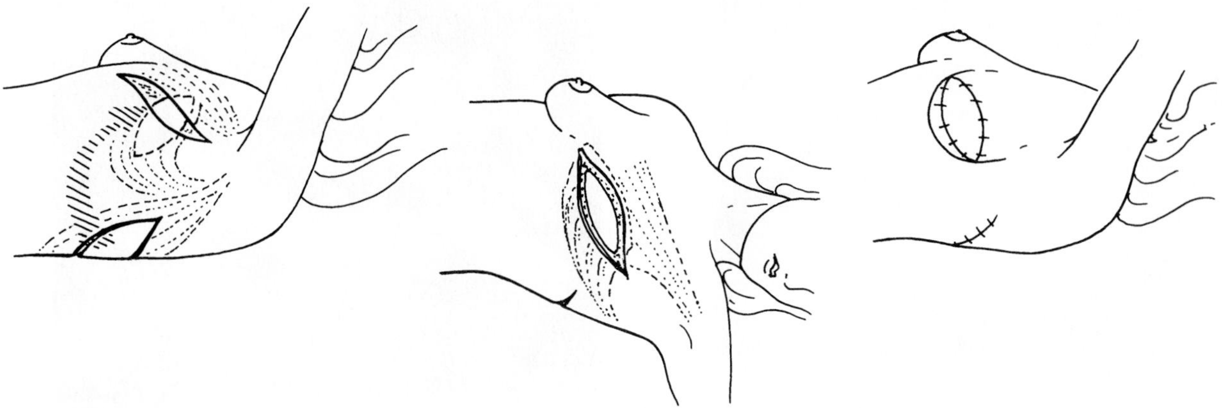

Figure 46-17 A diagram of the lastissimus dorsi procedure. (Courtesy of Dr. Craig Bradley, MD, Senior Attending, Plastic and Reconstructive Surgery, Rush University Medical Center, Chicago.)

Latissimus Dorsi Flap

The latissimus dorsi is a large, fan-shaped muscle that is considered an expendable unit because alternative muscle groups are able to adduct the humerus and posteriorly rotate the shoulder. Upper extremity weakness may result from this procedure, however — a consideration for athletic women and those who have jobs that require upper body strength.[245] The latissimus dorsi flap is used when inadequate skin is available at the mastectomy site or if additional tissue is needed to fill the supraclavicular hollow and create an anterior axillary fold following a radical mastectomy (Figure 46-17). In this procedure, an ellipse of skin along with the latissimus dorsi muscle is rotated onto the mastectomy site. The viability of the tissue is maintained through the thoracodorsal vessels. The latissimus dorsi flap may also include a prosthesis for symmetrical cosmesis.

Flap necrosis is rare due to the abundant vascularization of the area. The donor defect is often unnoticeable because the scar is located beneath the bra line.[245] This surgery takes three to four hours, approximately double the time needed for an implant procedure.

TRAM Flap

The transverse rectus abdominus muscle (TRAM) flap, commonly referred to as the "tummy tuck," is considered the gold standard for breast reconstruction due to the usual excellent cosmetic outcome. This surgical procedure and recovery from it are protracted and often difficult, however. The surgery may require transfusions, and the recovery time is often 6–8 weeks. During this procedure, a low transverse ellipse incision is made and abdominal muscle and fat are tunneled under the abdominal skin to the mastectomy site. Segments of artery, vein, fat, skin, and muscle are then molded by the surgeon to create a breast mound that is attached to the chest wall. Tissue viability and perfusion are retained by the abdominal rectus muscle (Figures 46-18, 46-19, and 46-20).[245]

Potential complications include hernia at the donor site, which can be remedied by the placement of synthetic mesh, and flap necrosis, which may be largely avoided by careful selection of surgery candidates. Extremely thin women, morbidly obese patients (> 20% overweight), those with circulatory problems, those with diabetes mellitus, those with prior history of liposuction or abdominal surgery, heavy smokers, and those older than age 65 generally are not considered eligible for this procedure.[240,245,248,249,252]

DIEP Flap

The deep inferior epigastric perforator (DIEP) flap is a new procedure that employs the same technique as the TRAM, but spares the muscle and is said to improve the strength and contour of the abdominal wall, resulting in improved patient satisfaction.[253,254] Results in reducing complications such as muscle weakness and hernia are encouraging, although the rate of fat necrosis complication is slightly increased with DIEP, possibly as a result of altered perfusion.[243,254] One limiting factor appears to be related to the volume of tissue. According to Nahabedian and colleagues, patients requiring more than 1000 cm^3 are better served with a TRAM flap, and careful patient selection predicts the best outcome.[248] The contraindications for this procedure are similar to those for the TRAM flap.

Free Flap

The free flap represents the newest technique in reconstructive surgery. This procedure entails removing a portion of skin and fat from the lower abdomen that may also include a portion of muscle, and grafting it to

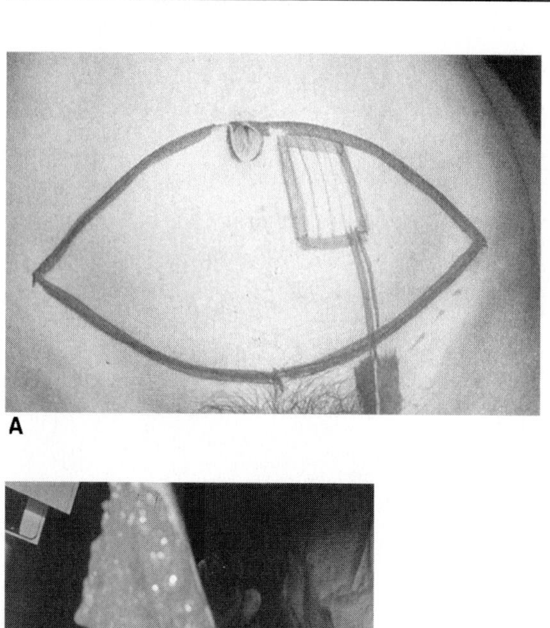
A

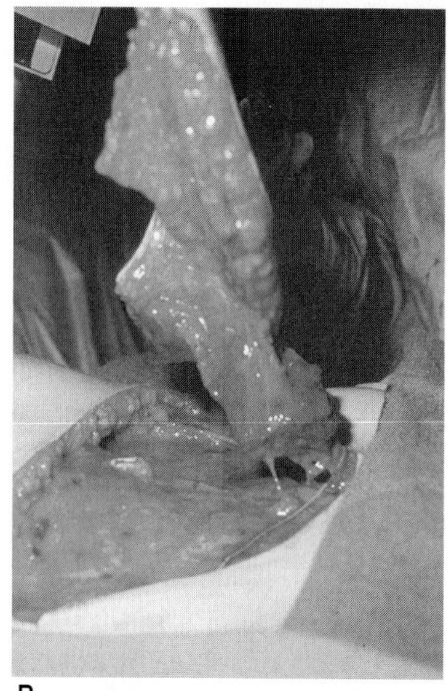
B

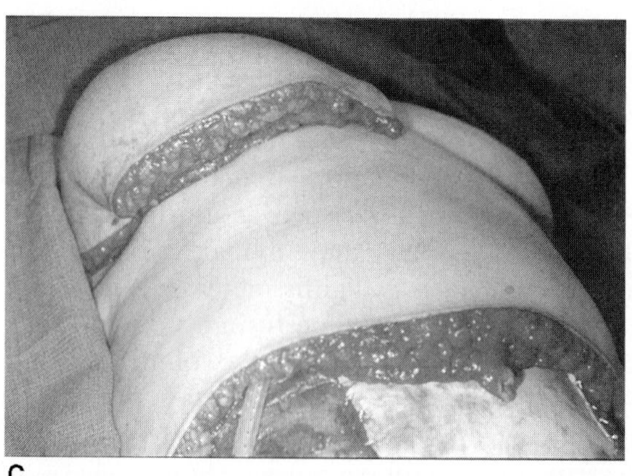
C

Figure 46-18 Three pictures illustrate (**A**) mapping the amount of tissue to be taken, (**B**) lifting the flap from the abdomen, and (**C**) the new mound prior to closing the incisions. Note that the abdomen needs placement of a reinforcement material (white area) to prevent hernia or other complications. (Courtesy of Dr. Craig Bradley.)

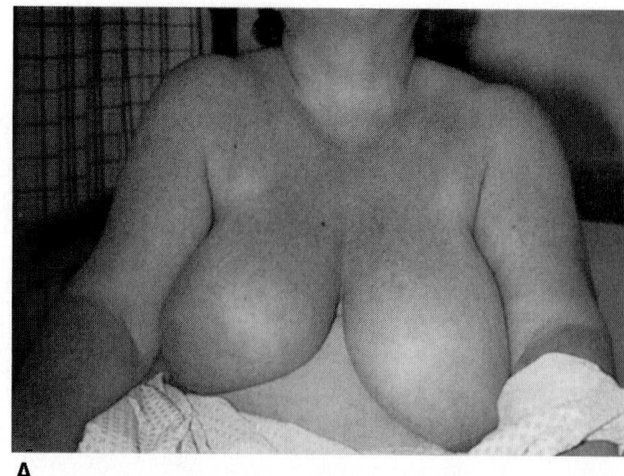
A

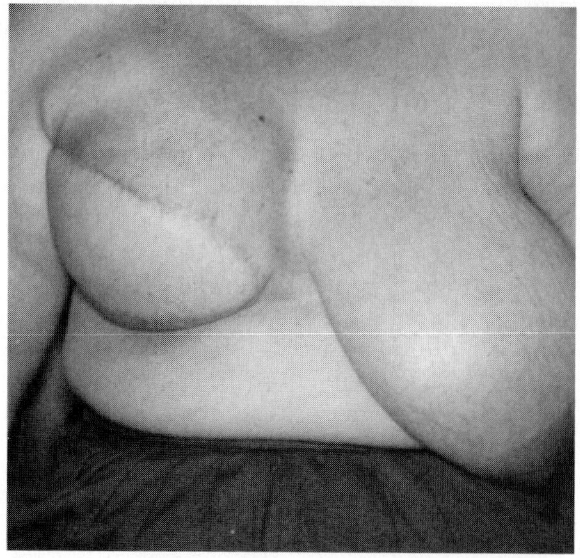
B

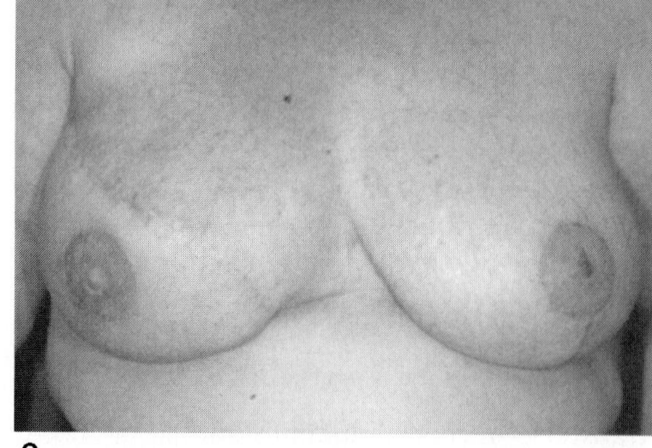
C

Figure 46-19 Three pictures illustrate a large woman (**A**) before the procedure, (**B**) after the mastectomy and latissimus dorsi flap, and (**C**) after mastopexy was performed to reduce the size of the other breast. Note the appearance of the tattooed nipple, which closely resembles the reduced breast. (Courtesy of Dr. Craig Bradley, MD, Senior Attending, Plastic and Reconstructive Surgery, Rush University Medical Center, Chicago.)

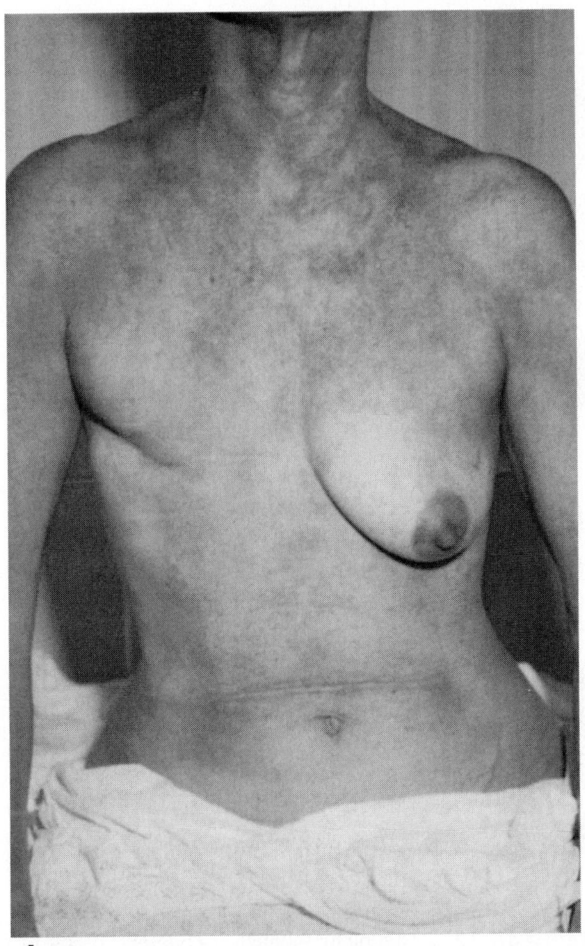

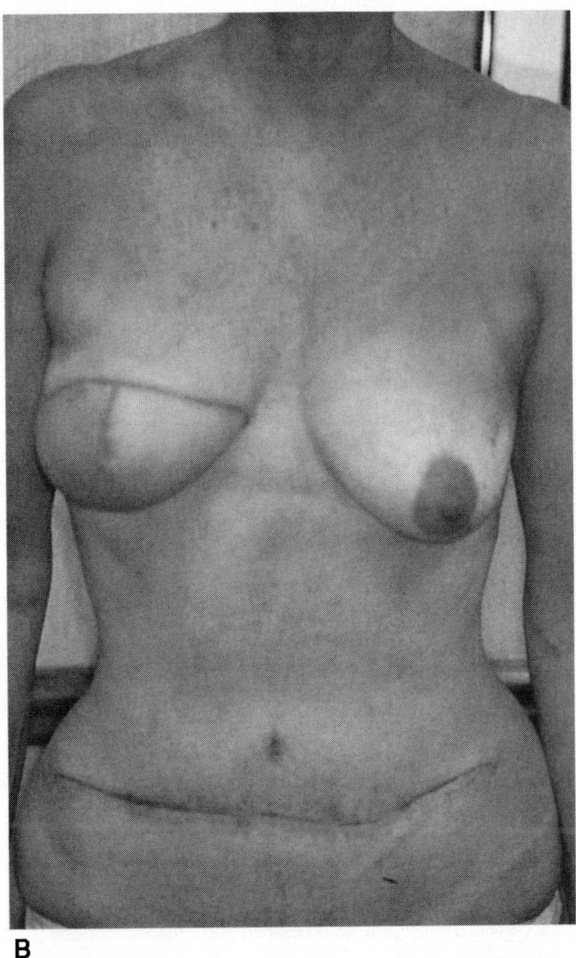

A B

Figure 46-20 First picture shows a patient **(A)** after mastectomy and before the TRAM flap. The second and third pictures show the **(B)** anterior and **(C)** continued on next page: lateral view of the same patient shortly after the procedure. The scars will fade with time. (Courtesy of Dr. Craig Bradley, MD, Senior Attending, Plastic and Reconstructive Surgery, Rush University Medical Center, Chicago.)

the mastectomy site with microvascular anastomoses. A complicated procedure, it demands microsurgical technique from two teams of surgeons — one to remove the flap and one to prepare the recipient vessels. The free flap has been reported to reduce complications, require shorter hospitalizations, and enhance the cosmetic outcome over pedicled tissue.[245]

The success of this operation depends on the reliability of the anastomoses of the vessels to ensure adequate nourishment of the tissues. The main complication is failure to maintain sufficient perfusion in the postoperative period. Tissue death will ensue within six hours if flow is interrupted and cannot be sustained.[245] Nursing assessment is crucial during the immediate postoperative period. The donor site is examined for petechiae, loss of color, and mottling — all signs of poor venous return or arterial insufficiency that will necessitate a return to the operating room. The flow within the flap is monitored hourly by Doppler flow and clinical appearance for the first 24 hours, and then every 2–4 hours according to hospital policy. Another potential complication is thrombosis, the risk of which is decreased by administering heparin.[245] Patients are usually discharged within 4–5 days after being given detailed instructions for wound care and flap assessment.

Nipple–Areolar Construction

Construction of the nipple–areola complex is the final phase of the breast reconstruction process. The symmetry and cosmetic result of the breast mound should be satisfactory before this procedure is performed. The nipple should closely match the opposite side in size and pigment.

Tissue may be taken from the opposite breast if an adequate supply is available or if mastopexy has been performed. Previously, the nipple was often "banked" to the patient's thigh or groin to be used later. This

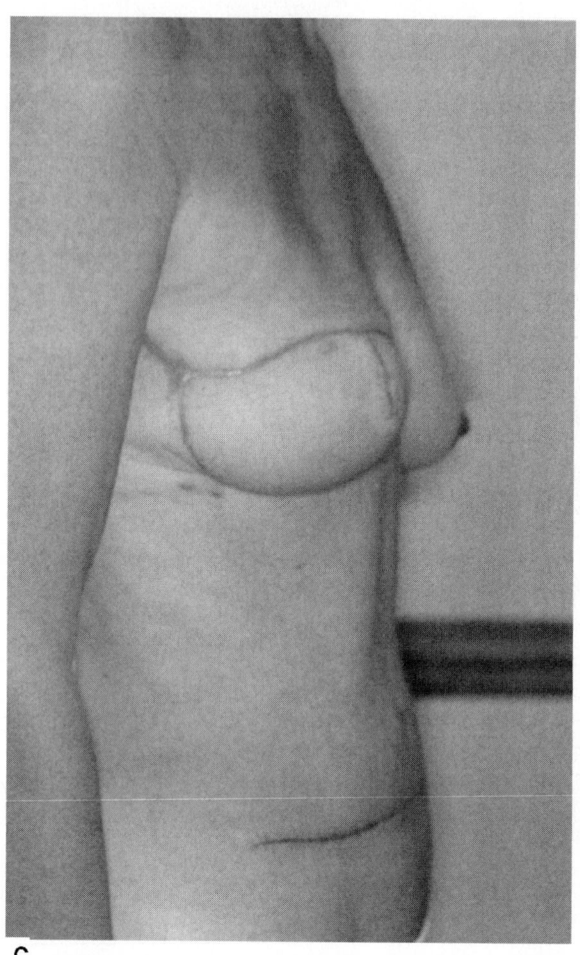

C

Figure 46-20 (Continued)

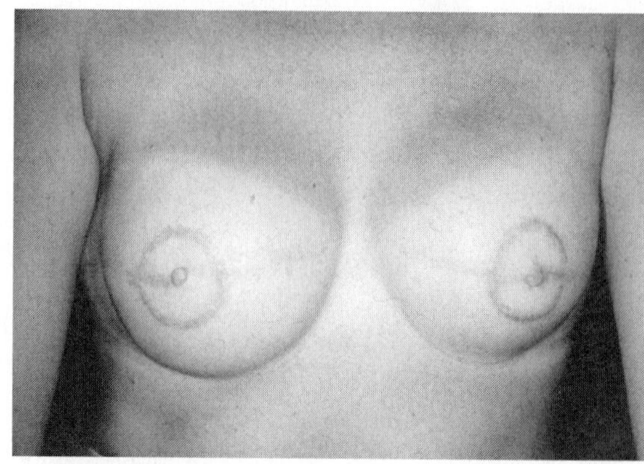

A

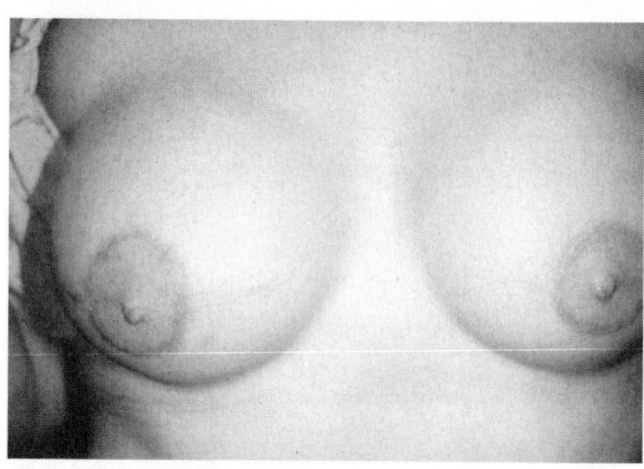

B

Figure 46-22 Two pictures illustrate bilateral nipple reconstruction **(A)** shortly after tattooing and **(B)** a few months later.

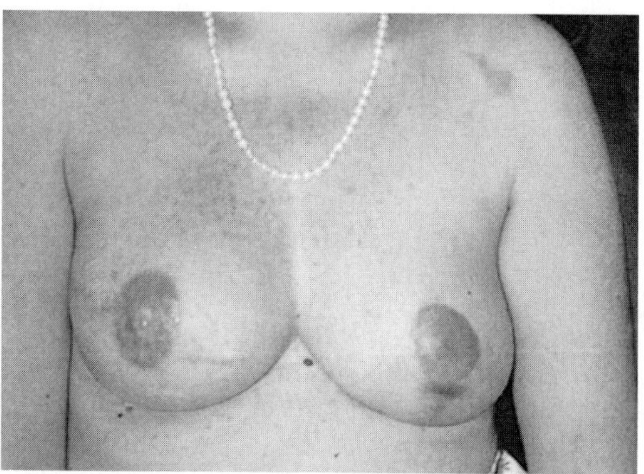

Figure 46-21 Right breast reconstruction following a modified radical mastectomy. Unilateral nipple tattoo on the right is compared to the patient's own unaffected nipple on the left following mastopexy. (Courtesy of Dr. Craig Bradley, MD, Senior Attending, Plastic and Reconstructive Surgery, Rush University Medical Center, Chicago.)

method has fallen out of favor due to the risk of introducing potentially malignant tissue to the disease-free breast.

Tattooing is the primary method for creating the darker pigment of the areola. Another option is a skin graft from the inner thigh. However, grafts are uncomfortable and can fade, requiring tattooing, so most women prefer to forgo this surgery and have the area tattooed.[255] (See Figures 46-21 and 46-22.)

Maintaining projection is a challenge that has been met by construction of pedicle flaps. These techniques fold the skin to achieve a slightly protuberant nipple. The most popular methods are the skate flap and the c-v flap technique, in which the skin is raised and folded to achieve a natural nipple profile.[256] A study conducted by Jabor and colleagues noted increased patient satisfaction with the keyhole flap, in which the superior portion of the keyhole is left as pedicle for flap perfusion.[255]

Complications are rare with nipple–areolar reconstruction, but may include failure to maintain suitable projection of the nipple, graft failure, and fading of the pigmented areas.

Table 46-14 Systemic Adjuvant Therapy: Node-Negative Breast Cancer

	Number of Patients	Reduction in Recurrence (%)	Mortality (%)
Tamoxifen	12,900	26	17
Chemotherapy	2700	26	18

Data from Carlson, Edge, Theriault, et al.[257]

Systemic Adjuvant Therapy

Local–Regional Breast Cancer

Much of the research in breast cancer has concentrated on finding optimal regimens of systemic therapy that can potentially destroy circulating tumor cells. The need for such research is paramount, given that nearly 90% of women newly diagnosed with breast cancer are potentially curable. Of that group, nearly 60% will have node-negative disease. The results of prospective clinical trials suggest that the rate of disease recurrence in patients with node-negative breast cancer can be reduced 20%–50% by administration of adjuvant therapy. This led to the conclusion at the NIH Consensus Development Conference on Early Stage Breast Cancer that, although the majority of patients with node-negative breast cancer are cured by breast-conserving treatment or total mastectomy and axillary node dissection, the rate of local and distant relapse following local therapy for node-negative breast cancer is decreased both by combination cytotoxic chemotherapy and by tamoxifen.[257] (See Table 46-14.)

Adjuvant therapy

The benefits of adjuvant treatment of primary breast cancer can be estimated from the meta-analyses reported by the Early Breast Cancer Trialists' Collaborative Group, updated in 1998.[258] This large statistical analysis demonstrated that optimal use of adjuvant therapy can significantly improve long-term survival in women with stage I and II breast cancer and has the potential to save more lives from this disease than any other malignancy. In women younger than age 50, adjuvant chemotherapy alone reduces the annual odds of recurrence by 35% and the annual odds of death by 27%. Adjuvant chemotherapy is less effective in postmenopausal women older than age 50. Treatment for this group reduces the annual odds of recurrence by 20% and the annual odds of death by 11%.[258]

For patients with tumors smaller than 1 cm in diameter and negative nodes, the chance of recurrence is less than 10% at ten years if no chemotherapy is given. It may be reasonable not to offer these patients systemic adjuvant therapy. In certain subsets of women with node-negative breast cancer, however, the incidence of metastatic disease approaches 50%.[259] Combination chemotherapy can effectively reduce the annual odds of recurrence by at least 30% in this population but to achieve this rate, 70% of patients will receive therapy unnecessarily because they would have been cured by surgery alone. Recent trials in the field of genomics conducted with NSABP have led to approval of a DNA microarray (OncotypeDX Breast Cancer Assay, Genomic Health Inc., Redwood City, California) that uses a scoring system to assign a numeric risk to individual women based on the particular genetic profile of their breast cancer. Use of this test along with assessment of existing risk factors for recurrence may allow oncologists to prospectively determine who needs chemotherapy and who does not.[260]

Although prognostic indicators such as ploidy, proliferative indices, and tumor grade may help to determine a woman's risk of recurrence, no one parameter is completely predictive of recurrence. Most clinicians agree that many women with node-negative breast cancer should receive adjuvant chemotherapy, especially those with larger tumors. Women with the lowest risk of recurrence are those with tumors smaller than 1 cm, a low-grade malignancy, positive estrogen/progesterone receptors, negative *HER2/NEU* status, and a low proliferative rate. In contrast, those with tumors larger than 2 cm, a high-grade malignancy, negative estrogen/progesterone receptors, positive *HER2/NEU* status, and a high rate of proliferation are at highest risk for tumor recurrence.

For women with local–regional breast cancer, a number of regimens are known to be effective. One regimen involves methotrexate followed in 1 hour by 5-FU (M-F). Oral leucovorin calcium (L) is begun 24 hours after the methotrexate. When this regimen was compared to standard cyclophosphamide, methotrexate, and 5-FU (CMF) therapy, it was found that both regimens offer at least a 30% risk reduction for recurrence. The M-F + L regimen appears to be less toxic in terms of myelosuppression and hair loss and does not have the leukemogenic potential of an alkylating agent–containing regimen. In premenopausal women, M-F + L does not affect gonadal function.

Adjuvant tamoxifen significantly reduces the risks of recurrence and death from breast cancer in women in all age groups. Tamoxifen is a viable choice in women who present with advanced tumors when chemotherapy is contraindicated. (See Figure 46-23.) The benefit is greatest when tamoxifen is administered for five years and when it is given to women with estrogen receptor–positive tumors. Tamoxifen has been shown to significantly reduce the incidence of contralateral breast cancer in women whose primary breast cancer was hormone receptor positive. Aromatase inhibitors (AIs) can be used for postmenopausal women for

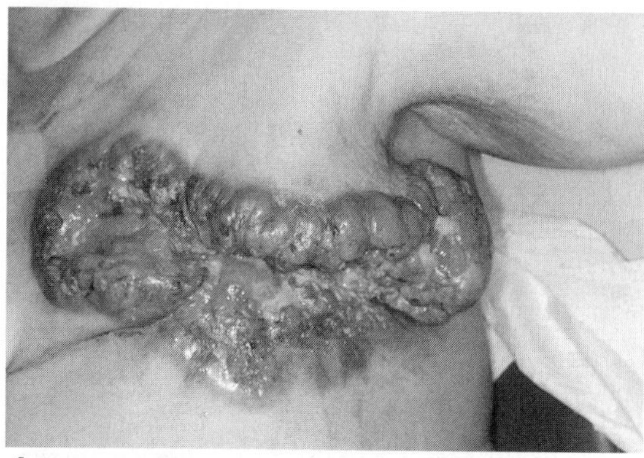

A

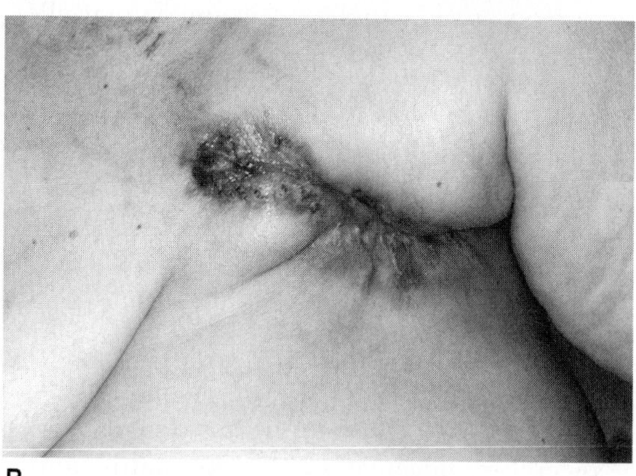

B

Figure 46-23 Two pictures depict (**A**) a patient with a long-neglected breast cancer who was placed on tamoxifen 20 mg/qd and (**B**) the improvement after six months of therapy.

whom tamoxifen is contraindicated due to history of thromboembolic disorders or gynecologic cancer. A large, randomized clinical trial investigating the use of anastrozole or tamoxifen alone or in combination in the adjuvant setting—*a*nastrazole, *t*amoxifen *a*lone or in *c*ombination (ATAC)—showed anastrozole to be an effective and well-tolerated endocrine option in early breast cancer.[261] AIs may also be used as extended adjuvant therapy following five years of tamoxifen therapy.

Women with tumors involving the lymph nodes are recognized as having a greater risk of distant recurrence and death. Adjuvant chemotherapy, especially for premenopausal women age 50 and younger, is widely accepted. One approach to node-positive breast cancer is CMF for 6 months. The combination of doxorubicin and cyclophosphamide (AC) every 3 weeks for 4 cycles is another approach. In clinical trials, patients receiving 4 cycles of AC did as well as those who received CMF for 6 months. While patients receiving AC experienced more immediate and profound hair loss, they suffered less nausea over time, visited health professionals one-third as often, and completed their therapy in less time compared to those patients receiving CMF. Another option as adjuvant therapy for the woman with node-positive breast cancer is the combination of cyclophosphamide orally for 14 days, plus epirubicin and 5-FU (CEF) on days 1 and 8 every 28 days, for 6 cycles.

For women with localized disease that also carries with it less favorable prognostic indicators, the addition of 4 cycles of paclitaxel to 4 cycles of AC may improve both disease-free survival and overall survival rates, although early clinical trial results report marginal increases in disease-free survival to date.[262,263] In women whose tumors overexpress the *HER2/NEU* proto-oncogene, the addition of weekly trastuzumab during the duration of the paclitaxel therapy is thought to increase the sensitivity and efficacy of the paclitaxel, due to the synergism between the two agents. Clinical trials continue to evaluate the safety and efficacy of trastuzumab in adjuvant treatment.[181]

Locally Advanced Breast Cancer

Efforts to improve outcome in patients with more-advanced stage, node-positive cancer have focused on the development and application of new drugs, many utilizing targeted molecular therapeutics, in combination with systemic therapy. Dose-dense regimens in which treatment with myelosuppressive agents is given every two weeks, rather than every three weeks, may effectively increase intracellular drug concentration. With the addition of colony-stimulating factors, it may be possible to ameliorate the dose-limiting toxicity of myelosuppression in the dose-dense regimens, possibly preventing the need for dose reductions or treatment delays. Giving optimal doses at regular, frequent intervals is an important strategy in preventing resistance and ultimate recurrence of disease. An intergroup clinical trial that evaluated dose-dense versus standard AC followed by paclitaxel showed that, after a median follow-up of 36 months, there was a 26% relative risk reduction in the odds of recurrence. Four-year disease-free survival was 82% for the dose-dense treatment versus 75% for the standard, every-three-week regimen. Dose-dense treatment was associated with a 31% proportional reduction in mortality.[264,265]

The goal of treating patients with operable breast cancer using neoadjuvant (i.e., preoperative) chemotherapy is twofold: The early treatment of micrometastases is hoped to improve survival and to achieve reduction of disease stage, thereby allowing breast conservation in patients who would otherwise be treated with mastectomy. In terms of survival, there is no apparent advantage to preoperative chemotherapy as compared with postoperative chemotherapy.[266]

Locally advanced breast cancer is associated with a high risk of developing distant metastases. The larger the size of the primary tumor and the greater the number of histologically positive lymph nodes, the greater the risk of metastasis and death. Clinical characteristics of locally advanced disease include large (> 5 cm) or unresectable primary tumors, fixed axillary nodes, and the classic inflammatory carcinoma. While distant metastases are presumed to be present, they are not clinically apparent at staging.

If the tumor is fixed to the chest wall, inflammatory carcinoma is present, significant ulceration exists, or the axillary nodes are fixed to one another or other structures, the situation is generally considered to be inoperable due to the almost certain risk of recurrence. The presence of positive supraclavicular lymph nodes is considered locally advanced breast cancer.[188]

The prognosis of patients with locally advanced disease is rarely improved by local therapy alone. While many physicians approach these patients with a purely palliative intent, the role of systemic therapy in their care is becoming more widely accepted. Results are superior when chemotherapy and radiation are included in the treatment plan.[267] The use of neoadjuvant chemotherapy has resulted in significant tumor regression in 60%–90% of women.[268] The advantage of this approach includes in vivo assessment of response. Significant tumor shrinkage may permit resection in previously unresectable disease, allowing for less extensive surgical procedures. In addition, primary chemotherapy provides immediate treatment to presumed metastasis that would otherwise be delayed by local therapy. It also avoids the postsurgery growth spurt of metastatic disease observed in the laboratory. Combined modality therapy employing chemotherapy, surgery, and radiation may result in complete disappearance of disease in many patients, including those with inflammatory cancer.[266,269]

High-dose chemotherapy (HDC) with peripheral blood stem cell autologous bone marrow transplant and hematopoietic growth factor support has been viewed as an option for treatment of women with high-risk advanced or metastatic disease. The relative efficacy of HDC remains a source of controversy due partly to discredited South African studies and partly to issues of patient selection. Short-term follow-up of the evaluable studies shows modest progression-free survival but no difference in overall survival.[270–272] Several more years of maturation of the existing studies and continued enrollment into ongoing trials are needed to determine outcomes. Rodenhuis conducted a multicenter trial of 540 women with at least ten involved ipsilateral axillary lymph nodes randomized to conventional adjuvant chemotherapy either with or without HDC and autologous stem cell transplantation, and found no significant differences in disease-free survival, overall survival, or time to recurrence between the two groups.[273] Until definitive results are available, HDC followed by transplantation should be undertaken only in the context of a randomized clinical trial.

Metastatic Breast Cancer

Despite improved screening techniques and increased awareness of breast cancer as a major health threat, approximately 10% of women diagnosed with breast cancer have metastatic disease at clinical presentation. Approximately 30% of women diagnosed with early-stage, node-negative disease and roughly 60% with node-positive disease will relapse despite adjuvant therapy. The majority of patients who relapse (80%) do so within two years of the diagnosis. Excessive physical examination and testing (x-ray, CT, MRI) to identify disease recurrences and metastases in an effort to institute aggressive treatment have not altered the clinical course of women with metastatic breast cancer.[114,274,275]

Most recurrences or metastases are diagnosed on the basis of symptoms and physical findings. Often a biopsy of a local recurrence will turn out to be cancer and the metastatic work-up ensues. Instead of an obvious physical finding, a patient may complain of loss of appetite and a slightly swollen abdomen, which on CT scan reveals liver metastasis. An assessment of the extent of disease is carried out, first to document the recurrence of disease and second to determine the most appropriate therapeutic approach. Typically, a chest x-ray, bone scan, CT scan of the chest and liver, and serum chemistries are done at the time of known or suspected recurrence to identify any abnormalities and the need for further investigation of extent of disease. Tumor markers may be done as a baseline, as they may parallel the clinical course. If the tumor has not been tested for overexpression of the *HER2/NEU* proto-oncogene, the biopsy or archival tumor specimen is sent to pathology so that analysis of *HER2/NEU* gene amplification and expression can be carried out. Only women whose tumors are *HER2/NEU* positive would be candidates for trastuzumab therapy.[111]

The median survival time for stage IV disease is two to three years; however, reports of five-year survival range from 12% to 35% and ten-year survival from 5% to 22%.[234] The goal of treatment is to control symptoms and provide the best quality of life possible given the fact that metastatic breast cancer is currently not curable.

Routes of Metastasis

Breast cancer most commonly metastasizes to bone (more than 50% of patients), specifically, the spine, ribs, and proximal long bones. Affected patients may complain of localized, deep-seated, unrelenting pain. Pathological fracture of the proximal femur may occur spontaneously despite efforts to protect the weakened bone. Likewise, persistent back pain may herald a compression fracture and possible neurological impairment. Hypercalcemia may reflect bone resorption due to tumor growth and resultant osteoclastic stimulation. Bone marrow metastasis occurs frequently in patients with extensive multifocal bone disease, generally presenting as either pancytopenia or nocturnal pain. Pancytopenia in patients with a history of breast cancer should be evaluated by bone marrow aspiration and biopsy to rule out bone marrow infiltration by breast cancer cells, myelodysplastic disease, or acute leukemia.

Loss of appetite and abnormal liver function tests are early symptoms of liver involvement. Late symptoms include pain, abdominal distention, nausea, emesis, periodic fever, jaundice, and generalized weakness. Pulmonary involvement may begin as a subtle, nonproductive cough or shortness of breath. Lymphangitic pulmonary spread is an ominous sign of rapidly progressive disease. Pleural effusions can progress slowly over time but may respond temporarily to drainage and sclerosing. Renal involvement generally presents as oliguria or uremia in a woman with deteriorating mental status. Brain metastasis usually occurs in the supratentorial region, in multiple sites, or as carcinomatous meningitis presenting as cranial nerve palsies, altered mentation, seizures, or focal paresis.

Local cancer that has spread to the chest wall usually presents as a painless subcutaneous nodule along the mastectomy scar and adjacent chest wall areas. These lesions may respond well to local therapy, but distant disease is presumed to be present.[276] If the disease recurs locally after breast-conserving surgery plus radiation, mastectomy may be indicated, provided that the cancer is present just in the breast tissue and not in the skin. Evidence of disease in a supraclavicular node or recurrence in the scar or chest wall after mastectomy generally indicates metastatic spread beyond the breast, warranting systemic therapy.

The management of patients with metastatic breast cancer is aimed at judicious use of local and systemic measures that control and/or palliate symptoms and improve quality of life. The initial choice of therapy is generally the one that is the least toxic and carries with it the highest response rate. (See Figure 46-24.) The basic strategy seeks to achieve optimal control of the disease and temporize it for as long as possible. Local and systemic therapies are added periodically as needed until they have outworn their usefulness. For many women, especially those with hormone receptor–positive disease, this can mean many years with better quality of life. Clinical trials of investigational agents should be considered for women with progressive metastatic breast cancer.

It may be difficult for a woman with metastatic disease to understand why her oncologist is not recommending more aggressive treatment. The idea that a new or different treatment is introduced only with evidence of disease or troublesome symptoms causes some women to ask why the treatment was not given to prevent the problem before it occurred. The answer is based on the desire not to make the woman more ill than her disease is making her and the knowledge that these therapies, including chemotherapy, have only a small effect on the median survival of women with metastatic disease. The goal is to get the maximum benefit from each therapy without compromising quality of life unless temporarily and absolutely necessary.

Chemotherapy

Women who have had a disease-free interval of less than two years, have hormone receptor–negative disease, are refractory to hormone therapy, or have aggressive disease in the liver or pulmonary system are candidates for chemotherapy. Response rates for first-line therapy vary from 30% to 70% and can last for 9–12 months. The rate of complete response (percentage of individuals in whom all evidence of disease disappears) consistently has been only 10%–20% of cases.[277–280]

Currently, cyclophosphamide–methotrexate–5-FU, cyclophosphamide–epirubicin–5-FU, cyclophosphamide–doxorubicin–5-FU, and taxane-containing regimens are among the more commonly used treatment approaches. Doxorubicin-containing regimens have shown a 10%–20% better response rate, but currently offer no significant survival advantage over combinations not containing doxorubicin. For women who are elderly and prefer a regimen that does not cause hair loss or significant nausea or vomiting, methotrexate–5-FU plus leucovorin is available. All women who overexpress the *HER2/NEU* oncogene should be given trastuzumab at the time of recurrence, either as a single agent or in combination with a cytotoxic chemotherapy. Capecitabine, a fluoropyrimidine prodrug of 5–fluorouracil, offers a 20% response rate and is preferred because it is taken orally.[281,282] For women who experience disease recurrence following therapy that included an anthracycline or a taxane, vinorelbine, gemcitabine, and liposomal-encapsulated doxorubicin are second- and third-line choices with minimal toxicity.[278,279]

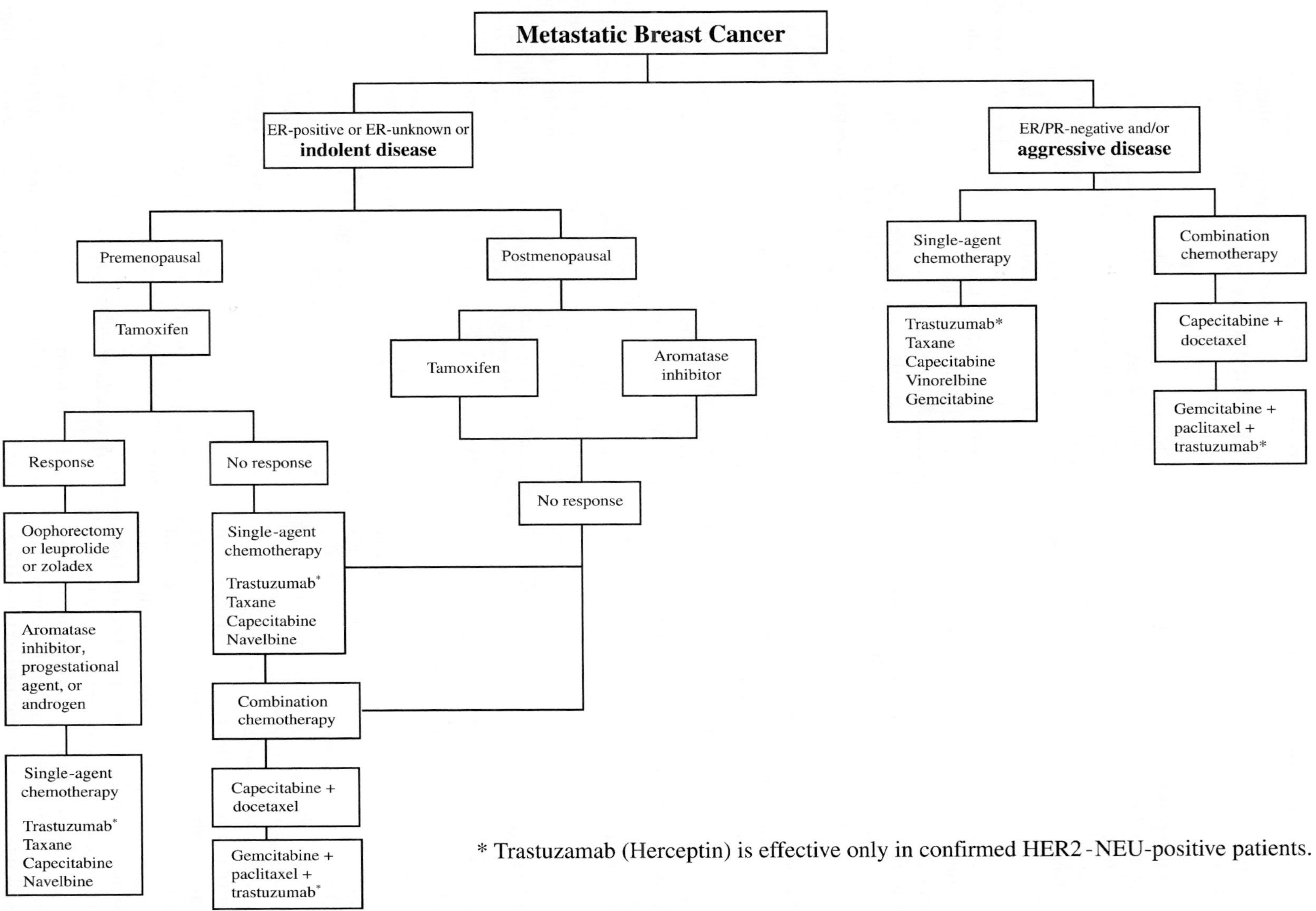

Figure 46-24 Metastatic breast cancer: systemic approaches to management.

Women with metastases to bone only should be placed on a bisphosphonate to slow disease progression, decrease the rate of bone loss, and protect against pathologic fracture. Women with bone metastases who are hormone receptor–positive should also receive appropriate endocrine therapy. The bisphosphonate therapy should continue for life, regardless of progression or change in other therapies.

The response of women to cytotoxic agents is not significantly related to the predominant site of disease. Women with visceral metastases as well as those with bony involvement will respond. Although radiological evidence of bone healing may take as long as six months to appear, subjective improvement occurs within a shorter time. For women who have lytic bony disease, zoledronic acid given as an infusion over 15–30 minutes once a month has proved useful to promote bone healing; prevent new disease in bone; and decrease the fracture rate, the need for palliative radiation, and the use of narcotic analgesics in patients with metastatic disease in bone.[283] Pamidronate, an alternative to zoledronic acid, is given as an infusion over two hours once a month. Renal function should be monitored monthly for patients receiving zoledronic acid or pamidronate, as renal insufficiency has been known to occur in patients receiving long-term intravenous bisphosphonate therapy.[284–286]

Endocrine Therapy

Antiestrogen therapy

Women who have ER-positive breast cancer demonstrate a consistently superior survival after recurrence compared to women who have ER-negative disease. It is generally accepted that the greater the ER content, the greater the response rate. Similarly, the presence of both the ER and the progesterone receptor (PR) on the tumor confers a higher response rate than the presence of only the ER.

The choice of hormonal therapy is based on several factors. When possible, tissue from the recurrent tumor should be tested for hormone receptors. Loss of the ER at relapse is a highly significant predictor of poor response to second-line endocrine therapy. Hormone receptor expression is a better predictor for second-line response to AIs than is prior tamoxifen response.[287] For the patient who has not experienced prior hormonal manipulation, the use of tamoxifen, selective estrogen receptor modulator (SERM), currently represents the standard of care, although recent clinical trials have demonstrated superior efficacy for aromatase inhibitors (AIs) and strong evidence exists to choose an AI over tamoxifen in the first-line metastatic setting.[288] Approximately 40%–50% of patients who relapse after an initial response to tamoxifen therapy respond to second-line endocrine therapy.[289]

The SERM drugs bind the ER and modulate the functions mediated by this receptor system. Tamoxifen is a nonsteroidal antiestrogen that binds competitively to the ER present in tumor cells. By blocking the binding of estrogen, it blocks cell cycle transit in the G_1 phase and inhibits tumor growth. Raloxifene is similar to tamoxifen in its antibreast cancer activity as well as in its pro-estrogenic effects on bone and serum lipids. One difference may be its neutral effects on the uterus; in contrast, tamoxifen is well established as a uterotrophic agent that increases the risk of uterine cancer. Although raloxifene is active as an antiosteoporosis agent, little is known about its cardioprotective effects. At this time, raloxifene is not approved for use in treatment of metastatic breast cancer. A new antiestrogen, fulvestrant, degrades and down-regulates the ER but does not bind to DNA; as a result, it has no estrogenic activity. Side effects are minimal. Fulvestrant is indicated when disease has progressed despite tamoxifen therapy.[290]

Undesirable consequences of the estrogen-like effects of SERMs include stimulation of the endometrium. Although tamoxifen may promote endometrial cancer due to its estrogen agonist effects, the benefits of preventing disease recurrence or progression usually outweigh the risk of developing endometrial cancer. The risk of endometrial cancer is greater in postmenopausal women than in those still experiencing regular menses.[259,291–293] Approximately 15% of women on tamoxifen reported severe hot flashes, compared with 3% of a group that received placebo. Vaginal discharge and irregular menses are also associated with tamoxifen therapy. Ocular toxicity (retinopathy or keratophy) has been reported in women taking conventional doses of tamoxifen, but in general ocular toxicity is not a clinically significant danger of tamoxifen therapy.[294] After tamoxifen withdrawal, ocular abnormalities are usually found to be reversible. Currently, the recommendation is to continue treatment unless visual symptoms are present. Patients might benefit from routine eye examination, especially those with preexisting ophthalmologic conditions.[294–296]

Aromatase inhibitors

The conversion of adrenal androgens to estrogens occurs primarily in adipose, muscle, ovarian, brain, and liver tissue, and is the primary source of estrogen in postmenopausal estrogen-dependent breast cancer. Aromatase inhibitors reversibly bind to the aromatase enzyme that is responsible for the conversion of androstenedione to estrone. Randomized clinical trails have established the role of third-generation AIs (letrozole, anastrozole, and exemestane) as standard treatment for patients with hormone-sensitive metastatic breast cancer who have experienced disease progression despite antiestrogen therapy.[287]

Aromatase inhibitors prevent the peripheral aromatization of other steroids to estrogen, primarily in body fat. The aromatase enzyme acts at the last step in the estrogen-synthesis pathway, catalyzing the conversion of androgens to estrogens. Nonsteroidal AIs, such as letrozole and anastrozole, work by reversible inhibition of aromatase and subsequent reduction of estrogen synthesis.[287] Exemestane, a steroidal aromatase inactivator, is indicated for the treatment of advanced breast cancer in women who have recurrent disease following tamoxifen therapy. This agent is of particular interest because it irreversibly binds to and inactivates aromatase.

The side effects most commonly reported with AIs include bone loss and hot flashes. Bone loss appears to increase during the first two years of therapy, with declining loss thereafter. In a phase III study of letrozole versus megestrol acetate by Buzdar and colleagues, hair thinning, headache, nausea, and diarrhea were reported more frequently in the letrozole arm.[297]

Androgens

Androgens are most effective in women who are five or more years postmenopause. The overall response rate to these agents is 20%. Androgens block pituitary gonadotropin secretion, thereby opposing endogenous estrogens. This type of therapy may be added to oophorectomy in women younger than age 35, but response rates are low. In postmenopausal women, androgens are indicated for the treatment of soft tissue or bone metastases and may result in "tumor flare" with initiation of treatment. Danazol is a synthetic steroid and is more commonly used because it has fewer virilizing effects (hirsutism, hair loss, acne, deepening of the voice, and increased libido) compared to testosterone or fluoxymesterone (Halotestin). Generally, because of their toxicity profile, androgens are reserved for use after most other forms of hormonal manipulation are exhausted.[298]

Progestins

Although the precise mechanism of action of progestins is unclear, they appear to inhibit the stimulator effect of estradiol on tumor growth. Megestrol acetate is a progestational agent with a response rate of 12%–16% and a median duration of up to 18 months as second-line therapy.[287,297] The standard dose of this progestin is 160 mg per day. Dyspnea, hypertension, sweating, vaginal hemorrhage, and weight gain are all observed more commonly in megestrol acetate-treated patients compared with those receiving AIs.[287,297] This

Table 46-15 Hormonal Agents for Breast Cancer

Agent	Category
Tamoxifen	SERMs
Estradiol	Estrogen
DES	Estrogen
Progestins	Megestrol acetate Medroxyprogesterone acetate
Fulvestrant	ER down-regulator
Anastrozole (nonsteroidal)	Aromatase inhibitors
Letrozole (nonsteroidal)	
Exemestane (steroidal)	
Goserelin	LHRH analogs
Fluoxymesterone	Androgens

drug is generally well tolerated and is typically prescribed only after the patient has failed on tamoxifen. Its mechanism of action is thought to include interference in binding of estrogen to the estrogen receptor as well as interference with the aromatization of androgens to estrogens. Megestrol acetate effectively decreases levels of follicle-stimulating hormone (FSH) and luteinizing hormone (LH) as well as estradiol.

Antiprogestins, including RU486 (mifepristone), are investigational agents. Mifepristone blocks progesterone receptors and may also regulate expression of VEGF mRNA.[299] This drug is generally well tolerated. Its common side effects include mild nausea, hot flashes, and dizziness. Studies of mifepristone in breast cancer are hindered by the societal implications of this drug's use as an abortifacient. The most important side effect is weight gain, which occurs in as many as 50% of patients. This weight gain is related primarily to increased food intake and increases with higher doses. Other side effects include vaginal bleeding, hypercalcemia, tumor flare, and thrombophlebitis.[300] Table 46-15 summarizes the hormonal agents currently employed for treatment of breast cancer.

Symptom Management and Supportive Care

Women with breast cancer often experience menopausal symptoms as a consequence of chemotherapy, following hormone therapy, or as a function of aging. Permanent ovarian failure occurs in 63%–85% of women treated with CMF and 50% or more of women treated with anthracycline-containing regimens.[301] Women older than age 40 develop ovarian failure after a shorter duration of chemotherapy; the risk of ovarian failure is increased for any woman older than age 35 who undergoes chemotherapy. For most, menses cease during therapy or become erratic over two to three years, and amenorrhea occurs. Levels of follicle-stimulating hormone (FSH) increase gradually and remain elevated for two to five years; FSH levels greater than 30 ng/L are usually considered diagnostic for ovarian failure.

Premenopausal women who receive chemotherapy should be clearly informed of their risk for temporary or permanent ovarian failure. Women with ovarian failure generally experience less subjective desire and arousability, vaginal dryness, vulvar/vaginal soreness, a burning pain, and light spotting after intercourse. They should be encouraged to use a water-soluble lubricant during vaginal intercourse to minimize discomfort. Localized estradiol therapy in the form of a vaginal tablet or estradiol-impregnated silastic ring can safely be used to lessen the effects of vaginal atrophy in breast cancer survivors, as it delivers the hormone to the vaginal tissues only and is not absorbed systemically.[302]

Other menopausal symptoms that commonly occur in women receiving chemotherapy or hormonal therapy include hot flashes, night sweats, and irregular menses. Hot flashes and profuse perspiration may be most troublesome at night and may interfere with sleep. Some women may benefit from lowering the thermostat in the home, especially where they sleep. Avoiding highly seasoned foods, caffeine, and alcohol may minimize the frequency of hot flashes. Dressing in loose-fitting cotton clothing and in layers, so that a sweater or jacket can be removed during a hot flash, is advised.

Some selective serotonin reuptake inhibitor (SSRI) antidepressants have been effective in reducing the number and severity of hot flashes in some women. The effective dose of venlafaxine for hot flash relief is considered to be 75 mg daily.[303] Primary side effects of SSRIs include decreased appetite, nausea, and dry mouth. Fluoxetine was evaluated in a double-blind, randomized, crossover trial as treatment for hot flashes in women with a history of breast cancer. A dose of 20 mg per day was well tolerated and showed modest improvement in hot flashes.[303] Bellergal-S, a long-acting combination of belladonna, ergotamine, and phenobarbital used for seizure control, may be effective especially when used at bedtime in women who experience hot flashes or sweats at night. Clonidine, an α-adrenergic agonist primarily used as an antihypertensive, may be effective for hot flashes in the transdermal or oral form. Somnolence and dizziness upon beginning therapy are the most frequently reported side effects at this dose, but they generally disappear as the body becomes accustomed to the medication.[304]

Gabapentin, a gamma-aminobutyric acid (GABA) analog that is indicated for treatment of epilepsy, neuropathic pain, restless leg syndrome, migraine prophylaxis, and other neurologic disorders, has been studied for management of hot flashes as well. A randomized, double-blind, placebo-controlled trial was conducted in 59 postmenopausal women with seven or more hot flashes per day examining the effects of gabapentin on hot flash frequency after 12 weeks of treatment. Gabapentin 900 mg per day was associated with a 45% reduction in hot flash frequency and a 54% reduction in hot flash composite score (frequency and severity combined into one score) from baseline, compared with 29% ($P = .02$) and 31% ($P = .01$) reductions, respectively, for placebo.[305] A dose of 900 mg per day reduced hot flashes and was found to be well tolerated. The primary side effects reported were mild dizziness and drowsiness.[306]

Debate continues on the use of herbal products containing soy, black cohosh, other herbal products, or vitamin E to relieve hot flashes. Randomized clinical trials have not supported the efficacy of these nonpharmacologic approaches to menopausal symptom management. The placebo effect is often in the range of 26%–30% and, therefore, may make interpretation of any clinical findings related to alternative therapies difficult to interpret.[304,307]

Recent findings from the Women's Health Initiative linking an increase in the incidence of breast cancer to prolonged use (> 5 years) of certain hormone replacement therapy (HRT) regimens strongly suggests that HRT may not be a safe option for breast cancer survivors.[24,34] Studies of women who have used HRT long term — specifically in excess of 10 years — or who have used combination HRT show an increased risk of developing breast cancer.[308–310] A review of the literature by Colditz concludes that a causal relationship exists between HRT use and breast cancer in postmenopausal women, especially among women who use HRT over the long term.[311]

Awareness of the underlying physiology of menopause, the patient's perceptions, and response to symptoms are important considerations for the nurse to adequately manage the symptoms of menopause. Research indicates that breast cancer survivors generally exhibit levels of physical, emotional, and social well-being that are similar to age-matched healthy women and are superior to those seen for patients with other chronic diseases. Likewise, there appears to be little disturbance in sexual functioning for most women who are in a partnered relationship.

Weight gain is a troublesome side effect of therapy. Menopausal status, nodal status, and adjuvant treatment appear to be significant predictors of weight gain. Furthermore, women who receive cyclophosphamide orally with methotrexate and 5-FU have been found to gain more weight than women who receive adjuvant doxorubicin and cyclophosphamide. Women commonly relate their weight gain following breast cancer to their tamoxifen treatment, but research indicates that the moderate weight gain observed in this patient population is comparable to that found in the general aging disease-free population and may not be related to the tamoxifen. Significant correlations do exist between weight gain and subjective feelings of unhappiness, worry, and increased distress regarding appearance when these women are compared to women who lost or maintained their weight. Factors contributing to weight gain include prednisone, oral cyclophosphamide, taste changes, increased appetite, depression, mild nausea that is relieved by eating, and psychological distress.[312] Kumar and colleagues suggest that cytotoxic agents may influence thyroid function in breast cancer patients.[313] Evidence of weight gain, especially when accompanied by fatigue, should prompt a thyroid-stimulating hormone (TSH) test to assess thyroid function. Women should receive nutritional counseling regarding the avoidance of weight gain at the outset of therapy.

Fatigue is a common subjective complaint associated with adjuvant therapy, and symptoms such as total body tiredness, forgetfulness, and wanting to rest increase over time throughout therapy. Women should be encouraged to interject rest periods into their normal schedule and, if possible, to begin a regular exercise program such as walking or water aerobics.

Nausea and vomiting with chemotherapy are predictable effects based on the type of chemotherapy or hormone therapy treatment. Patients on methotrexate and 5-FU experience less nausea and vomiting than women receiving CMF. Oral cyclophosphamide is associated with more prolonged nausea compared to intravenous cyclophosphamide. Women on higher doses of doxorubicin and cyclophosphamide experience intense nausea and vomiting for 48–72 hours following therapy if appropriate antiemetics are not employed.

Most women will not experience nausea and vomiting on the first day of their therapy, especially when given a 5-HT_3 serotonin antagonist plus 20 mg of dexamethasone as a single dose. However, the nausea and vomiting are worse on the second and third days post-treatment. Therefore, patients need a clear plan for managing these unpleasant symptoms for at least 72 hours post-treatment. Use of oral 5-HT_3 serotonin antagonists, such as prochlorperazine and lorazepam, for three days following therapy, are effective in minimizing these symptoms. A new class of antiemetics, substance P/neurokinin 1 (NK1) receptor antagonists (aprepitant), has recently been approved for treatment of chemotherapy-induced, delayed nausea and vomiting. Aprepitant is given orally one hour before chemotherapy and daily for the next two days following chemotherapy. Palonosetron, a long-acting second-generation 5-HT_3 receptor antagonist, is given intravenously 30 minutes prior to moderately or highly emetic chemotherapy regimens. It has a higher binding affinity for the 5-HT_3 receptor and a longer half-life than other available 5-HT_3 antagonists. Phase III trials have found a greater efficacy for palonosetron versus ondansetron in preventing both acute and delayed (through 120 hours post-treatment) chemotherapy-induced nausea and vomiting.[314]

Certain regimens used primarily in adjuvant treatment, such as doxorubicin and cyclophosphamide (AC), will cause many women to experience total alopecia within two to three weeks of beginning therapy. This side effect is highly distressing and contributes greatly to feelings of loss and body image changes. Women need to be aware of when and how hair loss will occur and have a management plan. Some women prefer shaving their heads or cutting the hair very short to minimize the constant and annoying shedding of their hair. The American Cancer Society's "Look Good, Feel Better" program is an excellent support and resource for women experiencing not just hair loss but body image changes in general.

Women on methotrexate–5-FU therapy do not lose significant amounts of hair and rarely require a wig. Those receiving CMF experience gradual thinning over the six to eight months of therapy and may require a wig only toward the end of treatment. Hair begins to grow back within a month of ending therapy at a rate of about ¼ inch per month. Women, especially younger ones, often are able to go without a wig or head covering within four months of therapy.

Chronic Lymphedema

Lymphedema is the accumulation of a protein-rich lymph fluid resulting in an increased interstitial colloid oncotic pressure that attracts water molecules, creating a chronic build-up of fluid in the extremity. The increase in size of the arm contributes to pain, immobility, cellulitis, and even lymphosarcoma. Lymph is an excellent culture medium, and infections such as cellulitis can flourish in it. Prevention of lymphedema is of primary concern because any fluid accumulation that goes unchecked merely leads to further edema. The longer the edema persists, the more difficult it is to manage. Once lymphedema is established it can be managed, but it cannot be entirely reversed.

The overall incidence of lymphedema in breast cancer is 15%–20%. The extent of the surgery including axillary dissection is a primary factor in the occurrence of lymphedema. Lymphedema occurs in as many as 22% of women following radical mastectomy and 10% of women who have modified radical mastectomy. Breast-conserving surgery such as partial mastectomy or lumpectomy results in lymphedema in 5%–8% of cases.[315] Because of research concerning the role of adjuvant chemotherapy in early-stage breast cancer, some would argue that an axillary lymph node dissection (ALND) should be performed only when the primary tumor is larger than 5 mm. Others contend that there is no survival benefit associated with ALND and women with larger tumors should be spared any potentially damaging effects of ALND because adjuvant chemotherapy will be given regardless of whether the women has positive nodes.

Axillary lymph node dissection, which is associated with pain, numbness, swelling, and weakness/stiffness of the ipsilateral arm or shoulder, is a diagnostic and staging procedure, not a therapeutic procedure. As newer, more advanced sampling procedures such as sentinel lymph node biopsy (SLNB) prove to be diagnostic as well as provide for accurate staging with minimal morbidity compared to ALND, then these procedures should be preferred relative to ALND. SLNB contributes less to physical morbidity because it involves less nerve damage and a smaller surface area of tissue damage. Lymphedema leads to physical impairment and diminished quality of life. Pain in the affected arm has at least a moderate impact on the daily life functioning of many breast cancer patients.[315]

Younger women tend to report more intense pain than older women. Women with a greater extent of axillary dissection — that is, more than 13 nodes removed — report more pain than women who have fewer nodes removed. Overall, researchers have found that women who undergo ALND for breast cancer experience enduring surgery-related symptoms, the most predominant of which is numbness. Obviously, more invasive surgery to the axilla causes greater damage to surrounding tissue and nerves, including the intercostobrachial nerve, so more pain and numbness would be anticipated. Surgeons should be encouraged to preserve the intercostobrachial nerve whenever possible.

Lymphedema can develop weeks, months, or years after axillary dissection. Lymph node dissection, radiation therapy, infection and delayed wound healing, obesity, and age all are considered risk factors for this condition. Lymphedema is most common in women who have undergone axillary dissection followed by radiation in excess of 46 Gy. The most common causes of late or chronic edema are infection and tumor recurrence, or tumor enlargement in the axilla.[316]

Prevention includes avoidance of medical procedures such as blood draws, IVs, injections, and blood pressure measurements on the affected arm. The patient should avoid heavy lifting and vigorous, repetitive movements of the arm against resistance. Anything that increases blood flow to the affected arm contributes to the incidence and degree of lymphedema. Heat, strenuous exercise, or lifting objects weighing more than 10 pounds may contribute to lymphedema. Women who have undergone an axillary dissection are instructed not to lift weights, for instance, because that repetitive strenuous motion increases blood flow and can contribute to edema. Note, however, that a pilot study of the effect of exercise on arm lymphedema reported no change in women who exercised their arms after axillary node dissection.[317] Carrying a suitcase or grocery bags should be avoided because the dependent arm has increased blood flow and muscle strain that ordinarily would promote lymph drainage, but does not because of the dependent nature of the arm as it carries the heavy object. Heavy handbags with shoulder straps should not be carried on the affected arm. Tight jewelry impedes venous blood flow and contributes to swelling. The patient should be instructed to avoid cuts, bruises, sunburns, sports injuries, insect bites, and pet scratches or bites. An electric razor should be used to shave under the arm, especially given that this area is usually numb. The woman should be instructed to keep the wrist higher than the elbow and the elbow higher than or even with the heart whenever possible. A compression sleeve with 20–30 mm Hg of pressure may be recommended for the arm. It is important that the patient or significant other inspect the arm and hand daily for warmth, redness, swelling, or pain. Any rashes, blistering, or redness of the arm or increased temperature, pain, or discomfort should be reported immediately to the medical care team.

The most effective treatment for lymphedema is complex decongestive physiotherapy (CDP), which combines manual lymph drainage, compression bandaging, and exercise. The first step is manual lymph drainage. This procedure stimulates the healthy lymphatics and increases lymph transport of the involved extremity. The arm is then wrapped with compression bandages to decrease resorption of fluid back into the extremity. The wrapping is most snug distally to promote a graded fluid drainage. Initially the arm is wrapped 24 hours a day until the appropriate size is reached; at that point, it is wrapped only at night.[315] The exercise component of CDP involves strengthening exercises and aerobic exercises with the compression bandaging in place. Strengthening exercises create a muscle-pumping action that increases lymph flow. Aerobic activity elevates the heart rate and respiratory rate, further stimulating the lymph transport.[317] Women with breast cancer should consume a well-balanced, low-sodium, high-fiber diet. Patients are also encouraged to achieve or maintain ideal body weight.

The edematous arm is cosmetically unattractive and can be functionally useless if lymphedema is severe. The arm can place a tremendous strain on the neck and shoulder muscles, which can result in pain. The woman may have difficulty adjusting her wardrobe to provide for the increasing size of her arm. Furthermore, the edematous arm can rarely be concealed adequately and can renew feelings of disfigurement and depression associated with the mastectomy that the woman may have resolved before the lymphedema occurred. When function of the arm is affected, the woman may not be able to work or perform activities of daily living. Efforts should be made to discuss the goals and rationale of management with the woman, thereby enlisting her cooperation and participation in the planned treatment regimen. Maximal effectiveness may be realized by referring the woman with lymphedema to a lymphedema specialist who can design a program to minimize fluid accumulation early, at the first sign of fluid accumulation. To find the nearest lymphedema center, contact the National Lymphedema Network at *www.lymphnet.org* or contact physical rehabilitation or comprehensive breast centers in your area for names of certified lymphedema specialists.

Continuity of Care

Support Systems

Women with breast cancer may find a need for a variety of support systems as they maneuver through the different phases of their diagnosis, treatment, and survival. Initially, the prediagnosis worry is often shared with friends and family, who then continue to provide ongoing support. A multitude of patients find support through their faith and the people with whom they worship. Many people have found comfort, validation, and information by joining a support group. Support groups are recognized as valuable sources of hope, encouragement, and education for the individual with breast cancer as well as other chronic diseases.[191]

Although the prognosis for breast cancer is constantly improving, the psychological impact of the disease may result in feelings of anxiety, depression, insomnia, and fear of recurrence and death and may directly affect the patient's ability to function. Seeking out and participating in a support group often helps to reduce and alleviate some of these feelings of loss of control and vulnerability.

Most cancer support groups rely on mutual aid or interdependence to attain a common goal, and individual participation is usually grounded in the needs of the individual and the goals that she hopes to accomplish. Many successful groups, such as Y-ME and Gilda's Club, use the common bond shared by their members to provide a forum where common needs such as assistance, personal insights, support, and belonging can be addressed. Break-out groups stress needs and goals that are more specific to the concerns of their particular members (e.g., type of surgery or current disease status). These smaller groups may deal with concerns of the spouse or partner, be conducted in languages other than English, or address concerns of women at varying stages of breast cancer by stratifying groups accordingly: Women who have been treated with mastectomy have concerns and questions that differ from those of women who have had breast preservation; women with metastatic disease have needs and issues beyond those of women who are disease-free.

Other recent advances in information and support include telephone support lines and online Web pages, which allow women who are isolated by geographic or physical constraints to communicate with others even on an international basis.[318] Valuable information is provided by a wide spectrum of healthcare workers as well as patients and families, whose sharing of stories and experiences can create a helpful and inspiring chronicle. Internet message boards may also serve a useful purpose by allowing patients to exchange information on a more personal basis.[319] Patients who utilize online web pages should be reminded that not all information posted on the Internet is medically valid. They should be encouraged to ask questions of the nurse or physician instead of making decisions based solely on Internet information.

Nursing Challenges

Possibly the greatest challenge in the care of the patient with breast cancer is to recognize appropriate patient goals throughout the continuum of the disease as the individual woman experiences it. When the woman is first diagnosed with breast cancer, her initial fear of the disease may be eased with the task of formulating a plan of care by consulting with a team of experts including a surgeon, plastic surgeon, medical oncologist, radiation oncologist, and clinical nurse specialist. When managed through the auspices of a comprehensive breast center, she and her family may come to value the combined efforts of the team assembled to help manage her disease. With a thorough explanation of the disease and treatment plan, she may choose to proceed or to seek other opinions before making her decision. The task of seeking other opinions for treatment is worthwhile because it allows the individual to learn more about her disease and to feel confident in her decision once she has had time to evaluate all treatment options. Of course, this time may also be particularly stressful because of the number of treatment options from which she is expected to choose. The nurse can be particularly helpful in clarifying the differences among the various approaches to management, explaining why such differences exist, and giving the woman and her family the opportunity to explore all options including appropriate research studies. Throughout this endeavor, the nurse concentrates on helping the woman find information and make contact with individuals who will help her make her own decision regarding treatment.

Once the plan of care is decided, the nurse formulates rehabilitation goals that are accomplished by further education regarding what the woman can expect and by teaching her self-care measures. Initially these goals will include postoperative care of the wound and appropriate exercises to regain optimal function of the arm and shoulder. Such instructions are written with personalized directions regarding how to perform the exercises and minimize pain through adequate use of analgesics. Some women will benefit from the assistance of a physical therapist trained specifically in the rehabilitation of the woman who has had a mastectomy. Women need frequent follow-up in the postoperative period to be certain that they are progressing to the best of their abilities.

In the initial six weeks following mastectomy, the patient will be instructed not to wear a prosthesis. Instead, she usually wears a soft cotton form in her bra that will not irritate the incision. During this time she can be fitted for a prosthesis and explore the type she prefers. Because women need referrals to stores that specialize in these garments and breast forms, nurses must keep up-to-date records on such specialty stores because surgeons rarely address this issue with their patients. The American Cancer Society's "Look Good, Feel Better" program is especially helpful to these women to help them look and feel their best. The Y-ME organization is another invaluable resource for women experiencing breast cancer and looking for advice concerning prostheses.

When chemotherapy is incorporated into the treatment plan, the nurse will instruct the patient and family regarding the side effects of chemotherapy and management strategies. Depending on the plan, this instruction can include prevention and management of nausea and vomiting, ways to minimize fatigue, management of hair loss, oral hygiene, and prevention of infection. Eventually other problems may arise, including difficulty in sleeping, complaints of fatigue and lack of energy, and menopausal symptoms.

The primary goal for the woman with localized breast cancer is to finish therapy and resume her life goals and activities she enjoyed prior to her illness. For most women this process takes about a year, at which time the individual is likely to feel more energetic and experience fewer sleepless nights. Often her hair has grown back and she feels more like herself. She may begin to inquire about breast reconstruction if she has not already done so. Most women should realize that reconstruction is major surgery and will again require an extended time period for recovery. It is often associated with a six-month period of fatigue and complaints of exhaustion. This is normal, however, and should not in any way discourage a woman from having the reconstructive procedures done.

While most women fear recurrence of their disease, seeing the medical oncologist, surgeon, or oncology nurse practitioner every three months for the first year, every six months for two years, and then yearly after that usually is frequent enough to be reassuring. Some patients may prefer to be seen more frequently.

If the cancer does recur, it is devastating. The disappointment and fears are often more intense than with the initial diagnosis. The patient feels betrayed by her own body. Most breast cancer patients work very hard to achieve wellness and to comply with all of their doctors' and nurses' recommendations. When the disease comes back, the woman feels she has little control and begins initially to lose hope in her ability to once again be courageous. At this time many will need the counsel of a psycho-oncologist trained specifically in the care of the cancer patient. The recurrence is just as devastating to the family as it is to the woman, and family members may also need to talk about their fears as therapy is once again discussed.

Goals for the person with recurring cancer center on helping her and her family understand the treatment goals and recognize how the treatment is helping. Remaining hopeful and supportive throughout, with emphasis on the success of therapy and numerous options available, is reassuring. Few women will need home care at this time because most recurrences are not debilitating unless the individual is elderly and the disease recurs in the brain or liver. When the cancer begins to affect a woman's ability to perform activities of daily living, the idea for home care should be brought up to determine the woman's options for insurance coverage. The family needs to be encouraged to identify their needs and decide whether they need assistance in her care on a daily basis or two or three times per week. Establishing a relationship with a nursing service that also has a hospice component is worthwhile because it ensures a smooth transition when hospice is deemed appropriate. Hospice should be introduced as an option for care once treatment is felt to be strictly palliative and the woman is thought to have less than six months to live.

Bereavement counseling is a component of hospice care and usually continues for at least a year. The nurse also can play a pivotal role in helping the family through the grieving process, thereby providing the patient and family with continuity of care from diagnosis through end of life.

Future Trends

The future of cancer care lies in the prevention of disease. Breast cancer is not one disease but rather an amalgam of many heterogenous manifestations of disease. If scientists are unable to identify the cause of breast cancer, it will be impossible to isolate suitable targets for preventing the initial steps that cause a normal cell to avoid immune surveillance and apoptosis and become malignant. One of the most exciting areas of current research is the search for a molecular signature that is unique to each breast cancer. The Human Genome Project has revealed detailed information about the human gene structure. From this information, new molecular analysis techniques have been developed. DNA microarrays allow simultaneous analysis of tens of thousands of genes in a single experiment, permitting identification of single genes as prognostic indicators or therapeutic targets. Once it has been established that these molecular targets are valid therapeutic targets, the same information may be used to screen women deemed at high risk for development of breast cancer. Identification of a target gene may open the door to drugs that will disable the gene and serve as true chemoprevention.

Prognosis based on molecular signature appears, in early studies, to be a more accurate predictor of prognosis than the standard parameters of lymph node status and tumor size. The molecular signature does appear to be associated with patient age, tumor histologic grade, and estrogen receptor status.[185] Van de Vijver and colleagues.[115] studied 295 subjects with both lymph node–positive and –negative breast cancer and found that expression levels of the 70 predictor genes identified subjects as having good or poor prognosis. Interestingly, nodal status was found to be equally distributed between the two groups. In this study the probability of remaining free of distant metastases at ten years was 85.2% in the good-prognosis group and 50.6% in the poor-prognosis group. Prognosis profiles were also predictive of overall survival. Ten-year survival in the good-prognosis group was 94.5%; overall survival was 54.6% in the poor-prognosis group. This study also revealed that the development of lymph node metastases and distant metastases were independent properties of the tumor. Other investigators have found microarrays to be predictive of recurrence in node-negative women, a group that has generally been considered to be at low risk of recurrence,[260] as well as in women with ten or more positive lymph nodes, a group that is viewed as being at high risk of recurrence.[320]

Monoclonal antibodies are rapidly becoming the treatment of choice for women with metastatic breast cancer and are currently under investigation as treatment in the adjuvant setting. Trastuzumab is an example of a monoclonal antibody targeted therapy; antiangiogenesis monoclonal antibodies are also being investigated for their use in metastatic breast cancer. As microarrays become part of the diagnostic work-up for breast cancer patients, researchers will strive to find treatments targeting the variety of genes that appear to play a part in breast cancer. As a result of their work, new and effective monoclonal antibodies may someday replace the systemic chemotherapeutic agents currently in use. It is not unreasonable to anticipate monoclonal antibody treatments custom-designed for each newly diagnosed breast cancer patient based on the molecular profile of the individual's particular tumor. This approach is currently under investigation in a new type of laboratory in which cell engineering is a key component of the work.

Progress in the treatment of breast cancer has dramatically improved survival rates, but until breast cancer is eradicated, more advanced surgical techniques, diagnostic tools, and evaluation strategies will be proposed. Imaging technologies that will predict even earlier detection of breast cancer, allow image-guided ablation of malignant tumors, provide presurgical evaluation of regional or distant disease, and assess response to therapy are currently being investigated.

Women with dense breasts pose a challenge for mammographers. Breast density is noted predominantly in younger women, but breast density may persist into old age in some women. Higher density has the potential to obscure potential pathologic areas and is a source of anxiety for many women. Although MRI is a better imaging modality, it is very costly compared to mammography and insurers are unlikely to reimburse for MRI as a screening tool. A small study, conducted by Jong and colleagues, used IV contrast material with digital mammography to enhance the detection of breast lesions. The technique was limited in that only the craniocaudal view could be used, but initial findings were promising. The report indicated the morphology correlated with the pathology, suggesting that this imaging tool may prove useful for diagnosing women with dense breasts.[321]

Building on the fact that breast conservation and mastectomy provide equal survival rates, researchers are investigating less invasive local therapy. There has been recent interest in using high-intensity focused ultrasound (HIFU), interstitial laser photocoagulation (ILP), and radiofrequency ablation (RFA) to treat breast cancer through nonsurgical methods. A study by Gianfelice and others evaluated MRI-guided ultrasound ablation of breast cancers.[322] Women who had a single focus of breast cancer (< 3.5 cm in diameter), which had been identified and diagnosed using standard imaging and percutaneous core biopsy, were treated with HIFU beams directed by a specialized transducer. The ablation was accomplished through absorbed energy, which raises the temperature in the tissue and creates protein denaturation and tissue necrosis. Each patient also had a surgical excision of the area after ablation to evaluate the efficacy of the ablation. The percentage of variability in identifying the tumor ranged from 46% to 95%, indicating that the total targeted area needed to be increased for better margin assessment. The authors suggest that this noninvasive procedure is well tolerated and has potential as a future breast cancer treatment.[322]

Interstitial laser photocoagulation delivers laser light energy directly into the tumor via optical fibers inserted into the tumor, causing cell death through hyperthermia. Dowlatshahi and colleagues published a work in progress describing stereotactic-guided laser ablation on 36 women with tumors ranging in size from 0.5 mm to 2.00 cm. All patients underwent wire-localized biopsy, and those with invasive cancer had an axillary sampling after the laser procedure. The results indicated that 66% of the patients had complete necrosis of their tumors with negative margins and 33% had residual tumors. The authors postulate that ILP may be appropriate for in situ and well-defined lesions.[323]

Radiofrequency ablation uses an electrode to delineate the ablation field. It causes cell death by thermal destruction, resulting in coagulation necrosis.[100] Several small studies have addressed the feasibility of using this therapy for small breast tumors with promising results, and the M. D. Anderson Cancer Center is conducting a study to evaluate the efficacy of RFA and determine whether its survival and recurrence rates are equal or better than those for breast conservation surgery.[90] A preliminary report of this study reinforced the feasibility of RFA for small (< 2 cm) breast tumors.[324]

Patients with locally advanced breast cancer often select neoadjuvant chemotherapy to reduce the size of the tumor and allow for a better surgical outcome. Evaluating the response to treatment has been limited to imaging studies assessing for reduction in tumor bulk. Looking for additional methods to determine tumor characteristics and response to therapy, Mankoff and colleagues evaluated the blood flow of tumors in women with locally advanced breast cancer before and during treatment, comparing (Tc-99m)-sestamibi uptake with (0-15)-water PET serial imaging.[325] The change in MIBI correlated with blood flow uptake and washout: Faster uptake and faster washout were associated with higher blood flow. Based on these preliminary findings, the authors created a model of the MIBI kinetics of breast tumors to be used to further assess tumor characteristics.[325]

The Human Genome Project has made a significant contribution to the body of scientific knowledge, but much remains to be done. Despite the many advances in understanding the molecular basis of oncologic diseases, considerable gaps exist in our knowledge of pathogenesis, affecting the development of effective prevention and treatment strategies. The idea that gene therapy would follow the identification of disease-linked mutations has not yet come to fruition.[326] There is a growing realization that cancer heterogeneity is more the result of complex biologic interactions and factors than an alteration of a single genetic marker.

While research will continue to provide data on the genetic links to disease processes, proteomics offers the potential of altering disease by effecting change in one or more proteins. Proteins are constantly changing, fluctuating with the sleep/wake cycle, health/illness continuum, and satiety/hunger and are responsible for the structure and function of organs and tissue. Although serum contains a vast repository of information that indicates the current physiological state of the body, current serum markers cannot detect preclinical or early-stage disease. Scientists have begun examining proteins by using two methods: detection proteomics and functional proteomics. Detection proteomics compares protein expression in diseased cells and normal cells, while functional proteomics evaluates the role of the protein in the cell and interventions to alter the protein function.

One promising area of proteomics research relates to ovarian cancer, which is often diagnosed at an advanced stage due to a lack of specific diagnostic symptoms. Improving survival for ovarian cancer will require a better method of detecting early-stage disease. Petricoin and colleagues have developed and are investigating "serum-based proteomic pattern diagnostics." The proteins were identified by artificial intelligence (AI)–based systems that used genetic algorithms to find 5–20 proteins that are expressed differently in healthy and diseased women. The AI tool constantly adapts to new information, and consequently multiple pattern combinations may be generated. The sensitivity and specificity were both 95% in the initial pilot study, which sought to evaluate the tool's predictive ability in diagnosing recurrent ovarian cancer (50 women with ovarian cancer and a control group of 66 healthy women). This research will continue through the NCI-sponsored Gynecological Oncology Group study, which will enroll women at high risk for developing ovarian cancer based on personal history of breast cancer, family history of breast or ovarian cancer, or being a *BRCA1* or *BRCA2* mutation carrier. The study will evaluate serum CA-125 and protein profiling, determining if one is superior over the other, as well as diagnostic tools and histopathologic tissue assays. The hope is that proteomics will be more specific and predictive than genetic testing and will cost significantly less.

The diagnosis and treatment of breast cancer is no longer based on a traditional hierarchical model, but has become a complex plan designed by the multidisciplinary team. The continuing influx of innovative diagnostic tools and therapies will continue to challenge the knowledge base of all healthcare providers. It is imperative that nurses belong to professional organizations and participate in continuing education courses addressing novel therapies and techniques. Understanding the basic scientific principles of these new tools and therapies will enable nurses to remain integral members of the team that actively participates in the education, treatment, and support of the patient and family.

References

1. Jemal A, Tiwari RC, Murray T, et al: Cancer statistics, 2004. *CA Cancer J Clin* 54:8–29, 2004
2. Willett WC, Rockhill B, Hankinson SE, et al: Epidemiology and nongenetic causes of breast cancer, in Harris JR, Lippman ME, Morrow M, et al (eds.): *Diseases of the Breast* (ed 2). Philadelphia, Lippincott, Williams and Wilkins, 2000, pp 175–220
3. La Vecchia C, Brinton LA, McTiernan A: Cancer risk in menopausal women. *Best Pract Res* 16:293–307, 2002
4. Ghafoor A, Jemal A, Cokkinides V, et al: Cancer statistics for African Americans. *CA Cancer J Clin* 52:326–341, 2002
5. Ghafoor A, Jemal A, Ward E, et al: Trends in breast cancer by race and ethnicity. *CA Cancer J Clin* 53:342–355, 2003
6. Ward E, Jemal A, Cokkinides V, et al: Cancer disparities by race/ethnicity and socioeconomic status. *CA Cancer J Clin* 54:78–93, 2004
7. Shimkin MB: Cancer of the breast. *JAMA* 183:358–361, 1963
8. Swanson GM, Haslam SZ, Azzouz F: Breast cancer among young African-American women. *Cancer* 97:273–279, 2003
9. Baquet CR, Commiskey P: Socioeconomic factors and breast carcinoma in multicultural women. *Cancer* 88:1256–1264, 2000
10. Jatoi I, Becher H, Leake CR: Widening disparity in survival between white and African-American patients with breast carcinoma treated in the U.S. Department of Defense healthcare system. *Cancer* 98:894–899, 2003
11. Guidry JJ, Matthews-Juarez P, Copeland VA: Barriers to breast cancer control for African-American women: the interdependence of culture and psychosocial issues. *Cancer* 97:318–323, 2003
12. Cauley JA, Lucas FI, Kuller LH et al: Elevated serum estradiol and testosterone levels are associated with a high risk for breast cancer. *Ann Intern Med* 130:270–277, 1999
13. Sharpe CR: A developmental hypothesis to explain the multicentricity of breast cancer. *C MAJ* 159:55–59, 1998
14. Vogel V: Epidemiology of breast cancer, in Bland KI, Copeland EM 3rd (eds.): *The Breast: Comprehensive Management of Benign and Malignant Disorders*. St. Louis, Saunders, 2004, pp 341–354
15. Wrensch M, Chew T, Farren G, et al: Risk factors for breast cancer in a population with high incidence rates. *Breast Cancer Res* 5:R88–R102, 2003
16. Newcomb PA, Storer BE, Longnecker MP, et al: Lactation and a reduced risk of premenopausal breast cancer. *N Engl J Med* 330:81–87, 1994
17. Yang C, Weiss N, Band P, et al: History of lactation and breast cancer risk. *Am J Epidemiol* 138:1050–1056, 1993
18. Yoo K, Tajima K, Kuroishi T, et al: Independent protective effect of lactation against breast cancer: a case-control study in Japan. *Am J Epidemiol* 135:726–733, 1992
19. Beral V, Collaborative Group on Hormonal Factors in Breast Cancer: Breast cancer and breastfeeding: collaborative reanalysis of individual data from 47 epidemiological studies in 30 countries, including 50302 women with breast cancer and 96973 women without the disease. *Lancet* 360:187–195, 2002
20. Mahue-Giangreco M, Ursin G, Sullivan-Halley J, et al: Induced abortion, miscarriage, and breast cancer risk of young women. *Cancer Epidemiol, Biomarkers Prevent* 12:209–214, 2003
21. Newcomb PA, Mandelson MT: A record-based evaluation of induced abortion and breast cancer risk (United States). *Cancer Causes Control* 11:777–781, 2000
22. Lazovich D, Thompson JA, Mink PJ, et al: Induced abortion and breast cancer risk. *Epidemiology* 11:76–80, 2000
23. Melbye M, Wohlfahrt J, Olsen JH, et al: Induced abortion and the risk of breast cancer. *N Engl J Med* 336:81–85, 1997
24. Writing group for the Women's Health Iniative Randomized Controlled Trial: Risks and benefits of estrogen plus progestin in healthy postmenopausal women: principal results from the Women's Health Initiative randomized controlled trial. *JAMA* 288:321–333, 2002
25. Kim C, Kwok YS: Decision analysis of hormone replacement therapy after the Women's Health Initiative. *Am J Obstet Gynecol* 189:1228–1233, 2003
26. Ettinger B, Grady D, Tosteson AN, et al: Effect of the Women's Health Initiative on women's decisions to discontinue postmenopausal hormone therapy. *Obstet Gynecol* 102:1225–1232, 2003
27. Cyr MG, Moulton AW: Menopausal hormone therapy: benefits, risks, and alternatives, in Bland KI, Copeland EM 3rd (eds.): *The Breast: Comprehensive Management of Benign and Malignant Disorders*. St. Louis, Saunders, 2004, pp 1533–1544
28. Col NF, Hirota LK, Orr RK, et al: Hormone replacement therapy after breast cancer: a systematic review and quantitative assessment of risk. *J Clin Oncol* 19:2357–2363, 2001
29. DiSaia PJ, Brewster WR, Ziogas A, et al: Breast cancer survival and hormone replacement therapy: a cohort analysis. *Am J Clin Oncol* 23:541–545, 2000
30. Vassilopoulou-Sellin R, Theriault R, Klein MJ: Estrogen replacement therapy in women with prior diagnosis and treatment for breast cancer. *Gynecol Oncol* 65:89–93, 1997
31. Vassilopoulou-Sellin R, Cohen DS, Hortobagyi GN, et al: Estrogen replacement therapy for menopausal women with a history of breast carcinoma: results of a 5-year, prospective study. *Cancer* 95:1817–1826, 2002
32. Vassilopoulou-Sellin R, Asmar L, Hortobagyi GN, et al: Estrogen replacement therapy after localized breast cancer: clinical outcome of 319 women followed prospectively. *J Clin Oncol* 17:1482–1487, 1999
33. O'Meara ES, Rossing MA, Daling JR, et al: Hormone replacement therapy after a diagnosis of breast cancer in relation to recurrence and mortality [see comment]. *J Natl Cancer Inst* 93:754–762, 2001

34. Chlebowski RT, Hendrix SL, Langer RD, et al: Influence of estrogen plus progestin on breast cancer and mammography in healthy postmenopausal women: the Women's Health Initiative randomized trial. *JAMA* 289:3243–3253, 2003
35. Berry D, Parmigiani G, Sanchez J, et al: Probability of carrying a mutation of breast–ovarian cancer gene BRCA1 based on family history. *J Natl Cancer Inst* 89:227–238, 1997
36. Gail M, Brinton L, Byar D, et al: Projecting individualized probabilities of developing breast cancer for white females who are being examined annually. *J Natl Cancer Inst* 81:1879–1886, 1989
37. Claus EB, Risch N, Thompson WD: Autosomal dominant inheritance of early-onset breast cancer: implications for risk prediction. *Cancer* 73:643–651, 1994
38. Wooster R, Weber BL: Breast and ovarian cancer. *N Engl J Med* 348:2339–2347, 2003
39. Shattuck-Eidens D, Oliphant A, McClure M, et al: BRCA1 sequence analysis in women at high risk for susceptibility mutations. Risk factor analysis and implications for genetic testing [see comment]. *JAMA* 278:1242–1250, 1997
40. DeMichele A, Weber B: Inherited genetic factors, in Harris JR, Lippman ME, Morrow M, et al (eds.): *Diseases of the Breast* (ed 2). Philadelphia, Lippincott, Williams and Wilkins 2000, pp 221–236
41. Wooster R, Bignell G, Lancaster J, et al: Identification of the breast cancer susceptibility gene BRCA2 [see comment] [erratum appears in Nature 379:749, 1996]. *Nature* 378:789–792, 1995
42. Miki Y, Swensen J, Shattuck-Eidens D, et al: A strong candidate for the breast and ovarian cancer susceptibility gene BRCA1. *Science* 266:66–71, 1994
43. Boyd J, Sonoda Y, Fedreici MG, et al: Clinicopathologic features of BRCA-linked and sporadic ovarian cancer. *JAMA* 283:2260–2265, 2000
44. Rahman N, Stratton MR: The genetics of breast cancer susceptibility. *Ann Rev Genet* 32:95–121, 1998
45. Collins N, McManus R, Wooster R, et al: Consistent loss of the wild type allele in breast cancers from a family linked to the BRCA2 gene on chromosome 13q12–13. *Oncogene* 10:1673–1675, 1995
46. Ford D, Easton DF, Stratton M, et al: Genetic heterogeneity and penetrance analysis of the BRCA1 and BRCA2 genes in breast cancer families. The Breast Cancer Linkage Consortium. *Am J Hum Genet* 62:676–689, 1998
47. King MC, Marks JH, Mandell JB, et al: Breast and ovarian cancer risks due to inherited mutations in BRCA1 and BRCA2 [see comment]. *Science* 302:643–646, 2003
48. Breast Cancer Linkage Consortium T: Cancer risks in BRCA2 mutation carriers. *J Natl Cancer Inst* 91:1310–1316, 1999
49. Gayther SA, Russell P, Harrington P, et al: The contribution of germline BRCA1 and BRCA2 mutations to familial ovarian cancer: no evidence for other ovarian cancer-susceptibility genes. *Am J Hum Genet* 65:1021–1029, 1999
50. Thompson D, Szabo CI, Mangion J, et al: Evaluation of linkage of breast cancer to the putative BRCA3 locus on chromosome 13q21 in 128 multiple case families from the Breast Cancer Linkage Consortium. *Proc Natl Acad Sci USA* 99:827–831, 2002
51. Lynch HT, Snyder CL, Lynch JF, et al: Hereditary breast–ovarian cancer at the bedside: the role of the medical oncologist. *J Clin Oncol* 21:740–753, 2003
52. Struewing JP, Hartge P, Wacholder S, et al: The risk of cancer associated with specific mutations of BRCA1 and BRCA2 among Ashkenazi Jews [see comment]. *N Engl J Med* 336:1401–1408, 1997
53. Verhoog LC, Brekelmans CTM, Seynaeve C, et al: Survival and tumour characteristics of breast-cancer patients with germline mutations of BRCA1. *Lancet* 351:316–321, 1998
54. Verhoog LC, Brekelmans CTM, Seynaeve C, et al: Survival in hereditary breast cancer associated with germline mutations of BRCA2. *J Clin Oncol* 17:3396–3402, 1999
55. Marsh D, Dahia P, Caron S, et al: Germline PTEN mutations in Cowden syndrome-like families. *J Med Genet* 35:881–885, 1998
56. Varley J, Haber D: Familial breast cancer and the Hchk2 1100delc mutation: assessing cancer risk. *Breast Cancer Res* 5:123–125, 2003
57. Chenevix-Trench G, Spurdle AB, Gatei M, et al: Dominant negative ATM mutations in breast cancer families. *J Natl Cancer Inst* 94:205–215, 2002
58. Samant RS, Olivotto IA, Jackson JS, et al: Diagnosis of metachronous contralateral breast cancer. *Breast J* 7:405–410, 2001
59. Tretli S, Gaard M: Lifestyle changes during adolescence and risk of breast cancer: an ecologic study of the effect of World War II in Norway. *Cancer Causes Control* 41:507–512, 1996
60. Lee MM, Lin SS: Dietary fat and breast cancer. *Ann Rev Nutrition* 20:221–248, 2000
61. Frazier AL, Ryan CT, Rockett H, et al: Adolescent diet and risk of breast cancer. *Breast Cancer Res* 5:R59–R64, 2003
62. Willett WC: Diet and breast cancer. *J Intern Med* 249:395–411, 2001
63. van den Brandt PA, Spiegelman D, Yaun SS, et al: Pooled analysis of prospective cohort studies on height, weight, and breast cancer risk. *Am J Epidemiol* 152:514–527, 2000
64. Trentham-Dietz A, Newcomb PA, Egan KM, et al: Weight change and risk of postmenopausal breast cancer (United States). *Cancer Causes Control* 11:533–542, 2000
65. Huang Z, Hankinson SE, Colditz GA, et al: Dual effects of weight and weight gain on breast cancer risk. *JAMA* 278:1407–1411, 1997
66. Deslypere JP: Obesity and cancer. *Metabolism* 44:24–27, 1995
67. Smith-Warner SA, Spiegelman D, Yaun S-S, et al: Alcohol and breast cancer in women: a pooled analysis of cohort studies. *JAMA* 279:535–540, 1998
68. Singletary KW, Gapstur SM: Alcohol and breast cancer: review of epidemiologic and experimental evidence and potential mechanisms. *JAMA* 286:2143–2151, 2001
69. Singletary ES: Rating the risk fators for breast cancer. *Ann Surg* 237:474–482, 2003
70. John EM, Kelsey J: Radiation and other environmental exposures and breast cancer. *Epidemiol Rev* 15:157–162, 1993
71. Wahner-Roedler DL, Nelson DF, Croghan IT, et al: Risk of breast cancer and breast cancer characteristics in women treated with supradiaphragmatic radiation for Hodgkin's lymphoma: Mayo Clinic experience. *Mayo Clin Proc* 78:708–715, 2003
72. Travis LB, Hill DA, Dores GM, et al: Breast cancer following radiotherapy and chemotherapy among young women with Hodgkin's disease. *JAMA* 290:465–475, 2003
73. Travis LB, Curtis R, Boice JD, Jr: Late effects of treatment for Hodgkin's disease. *N Engl J Med* 95:971–980, 2003
74. Diller L, Nancarrow CM, Shaffer K, et al: Breast cancer screening in women previously treated for Hodgkin's disease: a prospective cohort study. *J Clin Oncol* 20:2085–2091, 2002
75. Osuch JR: Breast health and disease over a lifetime. *Clin Obstet Gynecol* 45:1140–1161, 2002
76. Kruger RL, Schueler BA: A survey of clinical factors and patient dose in mammography. *Med Phys* 28:1449–1454, 2001
77. Terry MB, Gammon MD, Zhang FF, et al: Association of frequency and duration of aspirin use and hormone receptor status with breast cancer risk. *JAMA* 291:2433–2440, 2004
78. Page D, Simpson JF: Benign, high-risk, and premalignant lesions of the breast, in Bland KI, Copeland EM 3rd (eds.): *The Breast: Comprehensive Management of Benign and Malignant Disorders.* St. Louis, Saunders, 2004, pp 175–198

79. Schnitt SJ: Benign breast disease and breast cancer risk: morphology and beyond. *Am J Surg Pathol* 27:836–841, 2003
80. Morrow M, Schnitt SJ: Lobular carcinoma in situ, in Harris JR, Lippman ME, Morrow M, et al (eds.): *Diseases of the Breast* (ed 2). Philadelphia, Lippincott, Williams and Wilkins, 2000, pp 377–381
81. Simpson JF, Page DL: Pathology of preinvasive and excellent-prognosis breast cancer. *Curr Opin Oncol* 11:442–446, 2001
82. Kricker A, Armstrong B: Surgery and outcomes of ductal carcinoma in situ of the breast: a population-based study in Australia. *Eur J Cancer* 40:2396–2402, 2004
83. Adamovich TL, Simmons RM: Ductal carcinoma in situ with microinvasion. *Am J Surg* 186:112–116, 2003
84. Lakhani SR: In-situ lobular neoplasia: time for an awakening. *Lancet* 361:96, 2003
85. Page DL, Simpson JF: Pathology of preinvasive and excellent-prognosis breast cancer. *Curr Opin Oncol* 12:526–531, 2000
86. Silverstein MJ: Current controversies in ductal carcinoma in situ of the breast: summary from the Lynn Sage Breast Cancer Symposium. *J Am Coll Surg.* 108:115–118, 2003
87. Kotwall C, Brinker C, Covington D, et al: Local and national trends over a decade in the surgical treatment of ductal carcinoma in situ. *Am J Surg* 186:723–728, discussion 728–729, 2003
88. Klauber-DeMore N, Tan LK, Liberman L, et al: Sentinel lymph node biopsy: is it indicated in patients with high-risk ductal carcinoma-in-situ and ductal carcinoma-in-situ with microinvasion? *Ann Surg Oncol* 7:636–642, 2000
89. Pendas S, Dauway E, Giuliano R, et al: Sentinel node biopsy in ductal carcinoma in situ patients. *Ann Surg Oncol* 7:15–20, 2000
90. Singletary ES: Radiofrequency ablation of breast cancer. *Am Surgeon* 69:37–40, 2003
91. Camus MG, Joshi MG, Mackarem G, et al: Ductal carcinoma in situ of the male breast. *Cancer* 74:1289–1293, 1994
92. Morrow M, Harris JR: Local management of invasive breast cancer, in Harris JR, Lippman ME, Morrow M, et al (eds.): *Diseases of the Breast* (ed 2). Philadelphia, Lippincott, Williams and Wilkins, 2000, pp 515–560
93. Fisher ER, Land SR, Fisher B, et al: Pathologic findings from the National Surgical Adjuvant Breast and Bowel Project: twelve-year observations concerning lobular carcinoma in situ. *Cancer* 100:238–251, 2004
94. Morrow M, Gradishar W: Breast cancer. *BMJ* 324:410–414, 2002
95. Morrow M, Vogel V, Ljung B-M, et al: Evaluation and management of the woman with an abnormal ductal lavage. *J Am Coll Surg* 194:648–656, 2002
96. Brogi E, Robson M, Panageas KS, et al: Ductal lavage in patients undergoing mastectomy for mammary carcinoma: a correlative study. *Cancer* 98:2170–2176, 2003
97. Lynch HT, Marcus JN, Lynch JF, et al: Breast cancer genetics, in Bland KI, Copeland EM 3rd (eds.): *The Breast: Comprehensive Managemant of Benign and Malignant Disorders.* St. Louis, Saunders, 2004, pp 375–411
98. Fairfield KM, Fletcher RH: Vitamins for chronic disease prevention in adults. *JAMA* 287:3116–3126, 2002
99. Hortobagyi GN: Progress in systemic chemotherapy of primary breast cancer: An overview. *J Natl Cancer Inst Monogr* 30:72–79, 2001
100. Miyoshi Y, Taguchi T, Tamaki Y, et al: Current status of endocrine therapy for breast cancer. *Breast Cancer* 10:105–111, 2003
101. Cummings FJ: Evolving uses of hormonal agents for breast cancer therapy. *Clin Ther* (suppl) 24:C3–C25, 2002
102. Anonymous: Tamoxifen for early breast cancer: an overview of the randomised trials. Early Breast Cancer Trialists' Collaborative Group. *Lancet* 351:1451–1467, 1998
103. Gradishar WJ, Jordan VC: The evolving role of endocrine therapy for the treatment and prevention of breast cancer. *Cancer Chemother Biol Response Modif* 20:227–238, 2002
104. Fisher B, Costantino JP, Wickerham DL, et al: Tamoxifen for prevention of breast cancer: report of the National Surgical Adjuvant Breast and Bowel Project P-1 study. *J Natl Cancer Inst* 90:1371–1388, 1998
105. Cummings SR, Eckert S, Krueger KA, et al: The effect of raloxifene on risk of breast cancer in postmenopausal women: results from the more randomized trial. Multiple outcomes of raloxifene evaluation. *JAMA* 281:2189–2197, 1999
106. Kinsinger LS, Harris R, Woolf SH, et al: Chemoprevention of breast cancer: a summary of the evidence for the U.S. Preventive Services Task Force. *Ann Intern Med* 137:59–69, 2002
107. Vogel VG: Breast cancer prevention: a review of current evidence [comment]. *CA Cancer J Clin* 50:156–170, 2000
108. Hershman D, Sundararajan V, Jacobson JS, et al: Outcomes of tamoxifen chemoprevention for breast cancer in very high-risk women: a cost-effectiveness analysis. *J Clin Oncol* 20:9–16, 2002
109. Santen RJ, Yue W, Naftolin F, et al: The potential of aromatase inhibitors in breast cancer prevention. *Endocrine-Related Cancer* 6:235–243, 1999
110. Smith IE, Dowsett M: Aromatase inhibitors in breast cancer. *N Engl J Med* 348:2431–2442, 2003
111. Yamauchi H, Stearns V, Hayes DF: When is a tumor marker ready for prime time? A case study of c-erb-2 as a predictive factor in breast cancer. *J Clin Oncol* 19:2334–2356, 2001
112. American Society of Clinical Oncology Expert Panel: Clinical practice guidelines for the use of tumor markers in breast and colorectal cancer: report of the American Society of Clinical Oncology expert panel. *J Clin Oncol* 14:2843–2877, 1996
113. American Society of Clinical Oncology Expert Panel: 1997 update of recommendations for the use of tumor markers in breast and colorectal cancer. *J Clin Oncol* 16:793–795, 1998
114. Bast RC Jr, Ravdin P, Hayes DF, et al: 2000 update of recommendations for the use of tumor markers in breast and colorectal cancer: clinical practice guidelines of the American Society of Clinical Oncology. *J Clin Oncol* 19:1865–1878, 2001
115. van de Vijver MJ, He YD, van't Veer LJ, et al: A gene-expression signature as a predictor of survival in breast cancer. *N Engl J Med* 347:1999–2009, 2002
116. Ahr A, Karn T, Solbach C, et al: Identification of high risk breast-cancer patients by gene expression profiling. *Lancet* 359:131–132, 2002
117. Bernstein L, Henderson BE, Hanisch R, et al: Physical exercise and reduced risk of breast cancer in young women. *J Natl Cancer Inst* 86:1403–1408, 1994
118. Mittendorf R, Longnecker MP, Newcomb PA, et al: Strenuous physical activity in young adulthood and risk of breast cancer (United States). *Cancer Causes Control* 6:347–353, 1995
119. Rockhill B, Willett WC, Hunter DJ, et al: A prospective study of recreational physical activity and breast cancer risk. *Arch Intern Med* 159:2290–2296, 1999
120. Friedenreich CM, Bryant HE, Courneya KS: Case-control study of lifetime physical activity and breast cancer risk. *Am J Epidemiol* 154:336–347, 2001
121. Bilimoria MM, Murrow M: The woman at increased risk for breast cancer: evaluation and management strategies. *CA Cancer J Clin* 45:263–278, 1995
122. Bland KI, Chang HR, Chandler GS, et al: Modified radical and total (simple) mastectomy, in Bland KI, Copeland EM 3rd (eds): *The Breast: Comprehensive Managemant of Benign and Malignant Disorders.* St. Louis, Saunders, 2004, pp 865–884
123. Hartmann LC, Sellers TA, Schaid DJ, et al: Efficacy of bilateral prophylactic mastectomy in BRCA1 and BRCA2 gene mutation carriers [see comment]. *J Natl Cancer Inst* 93:1633–1637, 2001

124. Rebbeck TR, Friebel T, Lynch HT, et al: Bilateral prophylactic mastectomy reduces breast cancer risk in BRCA1 and BRCA2 mutation carriers: the Prose Study Group. *J Clin Oncol* 22:1055–1062, 2004
125. Kauff ND, Satagopan JM, Robson ME, et al: Risk-reducing salpingo-oophorectomy in women with a BRCA1 or BRCA2 mutation. *N Engl J Med* 346:1609–1615, 2002
126. Rebbeck TR, Lynch HT, Neuhausen SL, et al: Prophylactic oophorectomy in carriers of BRCA1 or BRCA2 mutations. *N Engl J Med* 346:1616–1622, 2002
127. Haber D: Prophylactic oophorectomy to reduce the risk of ovarian and breast cancer in carriers of BRCA mutations. *N Engl J Med* 346:1660–1662, 2002
128. Link JS: History and overview of comprehensive interdisciplinary breast centers. *Surg Oncol Clin North Am* 9:147–157, 2000
129. Rabinowitz B: Psychologic issues, practitioners' interventions, and the relationship of both to an interdisciplinary breast center team. *Surg Oncol Clin North Am* 9:347–365, 2000
130. Kolb GR: Disease management is the future: breast cancer is the model. *Surg Clin North Amer* 9:217–232, 2000
131. Stopfer JE: Genetic counseling and clinical cancer genetics services. *Semin Surg Oncol* 18:347–357, 2000
132. Croyle RT, Lerman C: Risk communication in genetic testing for cancer susceptibility. *J Natl Cancer Inst Monogr* 30:59–66, 1999
133. Schwrtz MD, Peshkin BN, Hughes C, et al: Impact of BRCA1/BRCA2 mutation testing on psychological distress in a clinic-based sample. *J Clin Oncol* 20:514–520, 2002
134. Braithwaite D, Emery J, Walter F, et al: Psychological impact of genetic counseling for familial cancer: a systematic review and meta-analysis. *J Natl Cancer Inst* 96:122–133, 2004
135. Anonymous: American Society of Clinical Oncology policy statement update: Genetic testing for cancer susceptibility. *J Clin Oncol* 21:2397–2406, 2003
136. Schnitt SJ, Guidi AJ: Pathology of invasive breast cancer, in Harris JR, Lippman ME, Morrow M, et al (eds.): *Diseases of the Breast.* (ed 2). Philadelphia, Lippincott, Williams and Wilkins, 2000, pp 425–470
137. Folkman J: Angiogenesis in breast cancer, in Bland KI, Copeland EM (eds.): *The Breast.* Philadelphia, W. B. Saunders, 1998, p 586
138. Fox SB, Harris AL: Angiogenesis as a diagnostic and therapeutic target, in Harris JR, Lippman ME, Morrow M, et al (eds.): *Diseases of the Breast* (ed 2). Philadelphia, Lippincott, Williams and Wilkins, 2000, pp 799–809
139. Elkin M, Orgel A, Kleinman HK: An angiogenic switch in breast cancer involves estrogen and soluble vascular endothelial growth factor receptor 1. *J Natl Cancer Inst* 96:875–878, 2004
140. Anonymous: The uniform approach to breast fine-needle aspiration biopsy. NIH consensus development conference [see comment]. *Am J Surg* 174:371–385, 1997
141. Smith RE: A review of selective estrogen receptor modulators and National Surgical Adjuvant Breast and Bowel Project clinical trials. *Semin Oncol* 30:4–13, 2003
142. Anonymous: Screening for breast cancer: Recommendations and rationale. U.S. Preventative Services Task Force. *Arch Intern Med* 137:344–346, 2002
143. Smith RA, Saslow D, Andrews Sawyer K, et al: American Cancer Society guidelines for breast cancer screening: update 2003. *CA Cancer J Clin* 53:141–169, 2003
144. Sickels EA, Wolverton DE, Dee KE: Performance parameters for screening and diagnostic mammography: specialist and general radiologists. *Radiology* 224:861–869, 2002
145. Adler DD, Wahl RL: New methods for imaging the breast: techniques, findings, and potential. *AJR Am J Roentgenol* 164:19–30, 1995
146. Schmidt RA, Nishikawa RM: Clinical use of digital mammography: the present and the prospects. *J Digital Imag* 8:74–79, 1995
147. Lewin JM, Hendrick RE, D'Orsi CJ, et al: Comparison of full-field digital mammography with screen-film mammography for cancer detection: results of 4,945 paired examinations. *Radiology* 218:873–880, 2001
148. Zheng B, Ganott MA, Britton CA, et al: Soft-copy mammographic readings with different computer-assisted detection cuing environments: preliminary findings. *Radiology* 221:633–640, 2001
149. Brem RF, Baum J, Lechner M, et al: Improvement in sensitivity of screening mammography with computer-aided detection: a multiinstitutional trial. *AJR Am J Roentgenol* 181:687–693, 2003
150. Taylor GA, Champness J, Reddy M, et al: Reproducibility of prompts in computer-aided detection of breast cancer. *Clin Radiol* 58:733–738, 2003
151. Gur D, Sumkin JH, Rockett H, et al: Changes in breast cancer detection and mammography recall rates after the introduction of a computer-aided detection system. *J Natl Cancer Inst* 96:185–190, 2004
152. Newman L: Developing technologies for early detection of breast cancer: a public workshop summary, in Institute of Medicine (ed.): *Early Detection of Breast Cancer.* Washington, DC, National Academy Press, 2000, pp 1–24
153. Flobbe K, Bosch AM, Kessels AG, et al: The additional diagnostic value of ultrasonography in the diagnosis of breast cancer. *Arch Intern Med* 163:1194–1199, 2003
154. Bassett LW, Shiroishi M: Breast imaging, in Bland KI, Copeland EM 3rd (eds.): *The Breast: Comprehensive Management of Benign and Malignant Disorders.* St. Louis, Saunders, 2004, pp 611–665
155. Warner E, Plewes DB, Shumak RS, et al: Comparison of breast magnetic resonance imaging, mammography, and ultrasound for surveillance of women at high risk for hereditary breast cancer [see comment]. *J Clin Oncol* 19:3524–3531, 2001
156. Teifke A, Lehr HA, Vomweg TW, et al: Outcome analysis and rational management of enhancing lesions incidentally detected on contrast-enhanced MRI of the breast. *AJR Am J Roentgenol* 181:655–662, 2003
157. Inoue M, Sano T, Watai R, et al: Dynamic multidetector CT of breast tumors: diagnostic features and comparison with conventional techniques. *AJR Am J Roentgenol* 181:679–686, 2003
158. Lehman CD, Eby PR, Chen X, et al: MR imaging-guided breast biopsy using a coaxial technique with a 14-gauge stainless steel core biopsy needle and a titanium sheath. *Am J Radiol* 181:183–185, 2002
159. Lobrano MB, Singha P: Positron emission tomography in oncology. *Clin J Oncol Nurs* 7:379–385, 2003
160. Haberkorn U: [The role of diagnostic PET in treatment planning before tumor surgery]. *Chirurg* 72:1010–1019, 2001
161. Chen J, Wu H, Zhou J, et al: Using TC-99m MIBI scintimammography to differentiate nodular lesions in breast and detect axillary lymph node metastases from breast cancer. *Chinese Med J* 116:620–624, 2003
162. Liberman M, Sampalis F, Mulder DS, et al: Breast cancer diagnosis by scintimammography: a meta-analysis and review of the literature. *Breast Cancer Res Treat* 80:115–126, 2003
163. Sakorafas GH: Breast cancer surgery — historical evolution, current status and future perspectives. *Acta Oncol* 40:5–18, 2001
164. Daltrey IR, Lewis CE, McKee GT, et al: The effect of needle gauge and local anaesthetic on the diagnostic accuracy of breast fine-needle aspiration cytology. *Eur J Surg Oncol* 25:30–33, 1999
165. King TA, Fuhrman GM: Image-guided breast biopsy. *Semin Surg Oncol* 20:197–204, 2001

166. Robinson DS, Sundaram M: Stereotactic imaging and breast biopsy, in Bland KI, Copeland EM 3rd (eds.): *The Breast: Comprehensive Managemant of Benign and Malignant Disorders.* St. Louis, Saunders, 2004, pp 685–697
167. Bold RJ: Surgical management of breast cancer: today and tomorrow. *Cancer Biother Radiopharm* 17:1–9, 2002
168. Liberman L: Percutaneous image-guided core breast biopsy. *Radiol Clin North Am* 40:483–500, vi, 2002
169. Hoorntje LE, Peeters PH, Mali WP, et al: Vacuum-assisted breast biopsy: a critical review. *Eur J Cancer* 39:1676–1683, 2003
170. Chung K, Velanovich V: Patient-perceived cosmesis after biopsy: comparison of stereotactic incisional, excisional, and wire-localized biopsy testniques. *Surgery* 131:497–501, 2002
171. Clark GM: Interpreting and integrating risk factors for patients with primary breast cancer. *J Natl Cancer Inst Monogr* 30:17–21, 2001
172. Clark GM: Prognostic and predictive factors, in Harris JR, Lippman ME, Morrow M, et al (eds.): *Diseases of the Breast* (ed 2). Philadelphia, Lippincott, Williams and Wilkins, 2000, pp 489–514
173. Baker M, Gillanders WE, Mikhitarian K, et al: The molecular detection of micrometastatic breast cancer. *Am J Surg* 186:351–358, 2003
174. Weir L, Speers C, D'yachkova Y, et al: Diagnostic significance of the number of axillary lymph nodes removed in patients with node-negative breast cancer. *J Clin Oncol* 20:1793–1799, 2002
175. Nemoto T, Vana J, Bedwani RN: Management and survival of female breast cancer: results of a national survey by the American College of Surgeons. *Cancer* 45:2917–2924, 1980
176. Hellman S, Harris JR: Natural history of breast cancer, in Harris JR, Lippman ME, Morrow M, et al (eds.): *Diseases of the Breast* (ed 2). Philadelphia, Lippincott, Williams and Wilkins, 2000, pp 407–423
177. Carter C, Allen C, Henson D: Relation of tumor size, lymph node status and survival in 24,740 breast cancer cases. *Cancer* 63:181–186, 1989
178. Chang J, Powles TJ, Allred DC, et al: Biologic markers as predictors of clinical outcome from systemic therapy for primary operable breast cancer. *J Clin Oncol* 17:3058–3063, 1999
179. Jerry DJ, Minter LM, Becker KA, et al: Hormonal control of p53 and chemoprevention. *Breast Cancer Res* 4:91–94, 2002
180. Marchetti P, Cannita K, Ricevuto E, et al: Prognostic value of p53 molecular status in high-risk primary breast cancer. *Ann Oncol* 14:704–708, 2003
181. Tan-Chiu E, Piccart M: Moving forward: Herceptin in the adjuvant setting. *Oncology* 63:57–63, 2002
182. van 't Veer LJ, Dai H, van de Vijver MJ, et al: Gene expression profiling predicts clinical outcome of breast cancer. *Nature* 415:530–536, 2002
183. West M, Blanchette C, Dressman H, et al: Predicting the clinical status of human breast cancer by using gene expression profiles. *Proc Acad Sci USA* 98:11462–11467, 2001
184. Colpaert C, Vermeulen P, Jeuris W, et al: Early distant relapse in "node-negative" breast cancer patients is not predicted by occult axillary lymph node metastases, but by the features of the primary tumour. *J Pathol* 193:442–449, 2001
185. Kallioniemi A: Molecular signatures of breast cancer — predicting the future [comment]. *N Engl J Med* 347:2067–2068, 2002
186. Stephenson J: Study indicates utility for new breast cancer prognostic marker. *JAMA* 285:3077–3078, 2001
187. Cobleigh MA, Langmuir VK, Sledge GW, et al: A phase I/II dose-escalation trial of bevacizumab in previously treated metastatic breast cancer. *Semin Oncol* 30:117–124, 2003
188. AJC: Breast, in Greene FL, Page DL, Fleming ID, et al (eds.): *AJCC Cancer Staging Handbook.* (ed 6). Philadelphia, Lippincott, Raven, 2002, pp 255–282
189. Singletary SE, Allred C, Ashley P, et al: Revision of the American Joint Committee on Cancer staging system for breast cancer. *J Clin Oncol* 20:3628–3636, 2002
190. Woodward WA, Strom EA, Tucker SL, et al: Changes in the 2003 American Joint Commission on Cancer staging for breast cancer dramatically affect stage-specific survival. *J Clin Oncol* 21:3244–3248, 2003
191. Sammarco A: Psychosocial stages and quality of life of women with breast cancer. *Cancer Nurs* 24:272–277, 2001
192. Rowland JH, Massie MJ: Psychosocial issues and interventions, in Harris JR, Lippman ME, Morrow M, et al (eds.): *Diseases of the Breast* (ed 2). Philadelphia, Lippincott, Williams and Wilkins, 2000, pp 1009–1031
193. Fisher B, Anderson S, Bryant J, et al: Twenty-year follow-up of a randomized trial comparing total mastectomy, lumpectomy, and lumpectomy plus irradiation for the treatment of invasive breast cancer. *N Engl J Med* 347:1233–1241, 2002
194. Poggi MM, Danforth DN, Sciuto LC, et al: Eighteen-year results in the treatment of early breast carcinoma with mastectomy versus breast conservation therapy. *Cancer* 98:697–702, 2003
195. Veronesi U, Cascinelli N, Mariani L, et al: Twenty-year follow-up of a randomized study comparing breast-conserving surgery with radical mastectomy for early breast cancer. *N Engl J Med* 347:1227–1232, 2002
196. Veronesi U, Paganelli G, Viale G, et al: A randomized comparison of sentinel-node biopsy with routine axillary dissection in breast cancer. *N Engl J Med* 349:546–553, 2003
197. Guenther JM, Hansen NM, DiFronzo LA, et al: Axillary dissection is not required for all patients with breast cancer and positive sentinel nodes. *Arch Surg* 138:52–56, 2003
198. Bonnema J, van de Velde CJH: Sentinel lymph node biopsy in breast cancer. *Ann Oncol* 13:1531–1537, 2002
199. Weaver DL: Sentinel lymph nodes and breast carcinoma: which micrometastases are clinically significant? *Am J Surg Pathol* 27:842–845, 2003
200. Paszat LF, Mackillop WJ, Groome PA, et al: Mortality from myocardial infarction after adjuvant radiotherapy for breast cancer in the surveillance, epidemiology, and end-results cancer registries. *J Clin Oncol* 16:2625–2631, 1998
201. Vallis KA, Pintilie M, Chong N, et al: Assessment of coronary heart disease morbidity and mortality after radiation therapy for early breast cancer. *J Clin Oncol* 20:1036–1042, 2002
202. Bartelink H, Horiot JC, Poortmans P: Recurrence rates after treatment of breast cancer with standard radiotherapy with or without additional radiation. *N Engl J Med* 345:1378–1387, 2001
203. Hevezi JM: Emergeing technology in cancer treatment: radiotherapy modalities. *Oncology* 17:1445–1456, 2003
204. Truong MT, Hirsch AE, Formenti SC: Novel approaches to postoperative radiation therapy as part of breast-conserving therapy for early-stage breast cancer. *Clin Breast Cancer* 4:253–263, 2003
205. Kuske RRJ: Breast brachytherapy. *Hematol Oncol Clin North Am* 13:543–558, 1999
206. Gordils-Perez J, Rawlins-Duell R, Kelvin JF: Advances in radiation treatment of patients with breast cancer. *Clin J Oncol Nurs* 7:629–636, 2003
207. Buzdar AU: Breast cancer in men. *Oncology* 17:1361–1364, 2003
208. Giordano SH, Buzdar AU, Hortobagyi GN: Breast cancer in men. *Ann Intern Med* 137:678–687, 2002
209. Thellenberg C, Malmer B, Tavelin B, et al: Second primary cancers in men with prostate cancer: an increased risk of male breast cancer. *J Urol* 169:1345–1348, 2003

210. English JC 3rd, Middleton C, Patterson JW, et al: Cancer of the male breast. *Int J Dermatol* 39:881–886, 2000
211. Bloom K, Reddy V, Green L, et al: Male breast carcinomas do not show amplification of the *HER-2/neu* gene. *Breast Cancer Res Treat* 64:127, 2000
212. Giordano SH, Cohen DS, Buzdar AU, et al: Breast carcinoma in men: a population-based study. *Cancer* 101:51–57, 2004
213. Giordano SH, Valero V, Buzdar AU, et al: Efficacy of anastrozole in male breast cancer. *Am J Clin Oncol* 25:235–237, 2002
214. Peate I: Caring for men with breast cancer: causes, symptoms and treatment. *Br J Nurs* 10:975–981, 2001
215. Institute NC. Surveillance, epidemiology, and end results (SEER) program CD ROM (1973–1997). Bethesda, MD, National Cancer Institute, DCCPS, 2000
216. Mintzer D, Glassburn J, Mason B, et al: Breast cancer in the very young patient: A multidisciplinary case presentation. *Oncologist* 7:547–554, 2002
217. IBCSG: Adjuvant chemotherapy followed by goserelin versus either modality alone for premenopausal lymph node-negative breast cancer: a randomized trial. *J Natl Cancer Inst* 95:1833–1845, 2003
218. Goldhirsch A, Gelber RD, Yothers G, et al: Adjuvant therapy for very young women with breast cancer: need for tailored treatments. *J Natl Cancer Inst Monogr* 30:44–51, 2001
219. Upponi SS, Ahmad F, Whitaker IS, et al: Pregnancy after breast cancer. *Eur J Cancer* 39:736–741, 2003
220. Field LR, Wilson TE, Strawderman M, et al: Mammographic screening in women more than 64 years old: a comparison of 1- and 2-year intervals. *Am J Radiol* 170:961–965, 1998
221. Kimmick GG, Balducci L: Breast cancer and aging. Clinical interactions. *Hematol Oncol Clin North Am* 14:213–234, 2000
222. Holmes CE, Muss HB: Diagnosis and treatment of breast cancer in the elderly. *CA Cancer J Clin* 53:227–244, 2003
223. Diab SG, Elledge RM, Clark GM: Tumor characteristics and clinical outcome of elderly women with breast cancer. *J Natl Cancer Inst* 92:550–556, 2000
224. Muss HB: Factors used to select adjuvant therapy of breast cancer in the United States: an overview of age, race, and socioeconomic status. *J Natl Cancer Inst Monogr* 30:52–55, 2001
225. Ellis MJ, Coop A, Singh B, et al: Letrozole is more effective neoadjuvant endocrine therapy than tamoxifen for ErbB-1–and/or ErbB-2–positive, estrogen–receptor positive primary breast cancer: evidence from a phase III randomized trial. *J Clin Oncol* 19:3808–3816, 2001
226. Aapro MS: Progress in the treatment of breast cancer in the elderly. *Ann Oncol* 13:207–210, 2002
227. Haley WE: Family caregivers of elderly patients with cancer: understanding and minimizing the burden of care. *J Support Oncol* 1:25–29, 2003
228. Goodwin JS, Satish S, Anderson ET, et al: Effect of nurse case management on the treatment of older women with breast cancer. *J Am Geriatr Soc* 51:1252–1259, 2003
229. Bach PB, Schrag D, Brawley OW, et al: Survival of blacks and whites after a cancer diagnosis. *JAMA* 287:2106–2113, 2002
230. Joslyn SA, West MM: Racial differences in breast carcinoma survival. *Cancer* 88:114–123, 2000
231. Fu SW, Schwartz A, Stevenson J, et al: Correlation of expression of BP1, a homeobox gene, with estrogen receptor status in breast cancer. *Breast Cancer Res* 5:R82–R87, 2003
232. Cross CK, Harris J, Recht A: Race, socioeconomic status, and breast carcinoma in the U.S. *Cancer* 95:1988–1999, 2002
233. Brawley OW: Some perspective on black–white cancer statistics. *CA Cancer J Clin* 52:322–325, 2002
234. Ries LA, Eisner MP, Kosary CL, et al: *SEER Cancer Statistics Review, 1975–2000.* Bethesda, MD, National Cancer Institute, 2003
235. Cancer Prevention and Control: *Guidance and Summary of Actions on the Breast and Cervical Cancer Prevention and Treatment Act of 2000.* Atlanta, GA, CDC, 2003
236. Spear SL, Mardini S, Ganz J: Resource cost comparison of implant-based breast reconstruction versus TRAM-flap reconstruction. *Plast Reconstruct Surg* 112:101–105, 2003
237. Brinton L, Lubin J, Burich MC, et al: Breast cancer following augmentation mammoplasty. *Cancer Causes Control* 11:819–827, 2000
238. McCraw JB, Papp C, Cramer A, et al: Breast reconstruction following mastectomy, in Bland KI, Copeland EM 3rd (eds.): *The Breast: Comprehensive Managemant of Benign and Malignant Disorders.* St. Louis, Saunders, 2004, pp 901–940
239. Fine NA, Mustoe TA, Fenner G: Breast reconstruction, in Harris JR, Lippman ME, Morrow M, et al (eds.): *Diseases of the Breast* (ed 2). Philadelphia, Lippincott, Williams and Wilkins, 2000, pp 561–575
240. Chang DW, Reece GP, Wang B, et al: Effect of smoking on complications in patients undergoing free TRAM flap breast reconstruction. *Plast Reconstruct Surg* 105:2374–2380, 2000
241. Kronowitz SJ, Robb GL, Youssef A, et al: Optimizing autologous breast cancer reconstruction in thin patients. *PlasT Reconstruct Surg* 12:1768–1778, 2003
242. Apffelstaedt J: Indications and complications of latissimus dorsi myocutaneous flaps in oncologic breast surgery. *World J Surg* 26:1088–1093, 2002
243. Blondeel PN, Arnstein M, Verstraete K, et al: Venous congestion and blood flow in free transverse rectus abdominis myocutaneous and deep inferior epigastric perforator flaps. *Plast Reconstruct Surg* 106:1295–1299, 2000
244. Garcia-Tutor E, Murillo J: The ideal patient for the first breast reconstruction using a DIEP flap. *Plast Reconstruct Surg* 111:947–948, 2003
245. Sandau KE: Free TRAM flap breast reconstruction. *Am J Nurs* 102:36–43, quiz 44, 2002
246. Gurunluoglu R, Spanio S, Rainer C, et al: Skin expansion before breast reconstruction with the superior gluteal artery flap. *Ann Plast Surg* 50:475–479, 2003
247. Kaplan JL, Allen RJ, Guerra A, et al: Anterolateral thigh flap for breast reconstruction. *J Reconstruct Microsurg* 19:63–68, 2003
248. Nahabedian MY, Momen B, Galdino G, et al: Breast reconstruction with the free TRAM or DIEP flap: patient selection, choice of flap, and outcome. *Plast Reconstruct Surg* 110:466–475, discussion 476–467, 2002
249. Chang DW, Wang B, Robb GL, et al: Effect of obesity on flap and donor-site complications in free transverse rectus abdominis myocutaneous flap breast reconstruction. *Plast Reconstruct Surg* 105:1640–1648, 2000
250. Noone RB: Adjustable implant reconstruction, in Spear SL (ed.): *Surgery of the Breast: Principles and Art.* Philadelphia, Lippincott-Raven, 1998, pp 357–374
251. Hoshaw S, Klein P, Clark B, et al: Breast implants and cancer: causation, delayed detection, and survival. *Plast Reconstruct Surg* 107:1393–1408, 2001
252. Nahabedian MY, Dooley W, Singh N, et al: Contour abnormalities of the abdomen after breast reconstruction with abdominal flaps: the role of muscle preservation. *Plast Reconstruct Surg* 109:91–101, 2002
253. Nahabedian MY, Momen B, Galdino G, et al: Breast reconstruction with the free TRAM or DIEP flap: patient selection, choice of flap, and outcome [see comment]. *Plast Reconstruct Surg* 110:466–475, discussion 476–467, 2002
254. Kroll SS: Fat necrosis in free transverse rectus abdominis myocutaneous and deep inferior epigastric perforator flaps [see comment]. *Plast Reconstruct Surg* 106:576–583, 2000

255. Jabor MA, Shayani P, Collins DR Jr, et al: Nipple–areola reconstruction: satisfaction and clinical determinants. *Plast Reconstruct Surg* 110:457–463, discussion 464–455, 2002
256. Losken A, Mackay GJ, Bostwick JI: Nipple reconstruction using the c-v flap technique: a long term evaluation. *Plast Reconstruct Surg* 108:361–369, 2001
257. Carlson RW, Edge SB, Theriault RL, et al: NCCN: breast cancer. *Cancer Control* 8:54–61, 2001
258. Group EBCTC: Polychemotherapy for early breast cancer: an overview of the randomized trials. *Lancet* 352:930–942, 1998
259. Fisher B, Jeong JH, Dignam J, et al: Findings from recent National Surgical Adjuvant Breast and Bowel Project adjuvant studies in stage I breast cancer. *J Natl Cancer Inst Monogr* 30:62–66, 2001
260. Paik S, Shak S, Kim C, et al: *Multi-gene RT-PCR Assay for Predicting Recurrence in Node Negative Breast Cancer Patients — NSABP studies B-20 and B-14.* San Antonio Breast Cancer Symposium, San Antonio TX, 2003 (abstr 16)
261. Buzdar AU: Role of anastrozole in adjuvant therapy for postmenopausal patients. *Semin Oncol* 30:21–29, 2003
262. Goble S, Bear HD: Emerging role of taxanes in adjuvant and neoadjuvant therapy for breast cancer: the potential and the questions. *Surg Clin North Am* 83:943–971, 2003
263. Henderson IC, Berry DA, Demetri GD, et al: Improved outcomes from adding sequential paclitaxel but not from escalating doxorubicin dose in an adjuvant chemotherapy regimen for patients with node-positive primary breast cancer. *J Clin Oncol* 21:976–983, 2003
264. Citron ML, Berry DA, Cirrincione C, et al: Randomized trial of dose-dense versus conventionally scheduled and sequential versus concurrent combination chemotherapy as postoperative adjuvant treatment of node-positive primary breast cancer: First report of Intergroup Trial C9741/Cancer and Leukemia Group B trial 9741. *J Clin Oncol* 21:1431–1439, 2003
265. Hudis C: Dose-dense chemotherapy for breast cancer: the story so far. *Br J Cancer* 82:1897–1899, 2000
266. Buchholz TA, Hunt KK, Whitman GJ, et al: Neoadjuvant chemotherapy for breast carcinoma: multidisciplinary considerations of benefits and risks. *Cancer* 98:1150–1160, 2003
267. Baum M: The changing face of breast cancer — past, present and future perspectives. *Breast Cancer Res Treat* 75:S1–S5; discussion S33–S35, 2002
268. Ikeda T, Jinno H, Matsu A, et al: The role of neoadjuvant chemotherapy for breast cancer treatment. *Breast Cancer* 9:8–14, 2002
269. Recht A, Edge SB: Evidence-based indications for postmastectomy irradiation. *Surg Clin North Am* 83:995–1013, 2003
270. Dicato M: High-dose chemotherapy in breast cancer: where are we now? *Semin Oncol* 29:16–20, 2002
271. Antman K: Randomized trials of high-dose chemotherapy in breast cancer: fraud, the press and the data (or lessons learned in medical policy governing clinical research). *Trans Am Clin Climatol Assoc* 113:56–66, discussion 66–57, 2002
272. Nieto Y: The verdict is not in yet. Analysis of the randomized trials of high-dose chemotherapy for breast cancer. *Haematologica* 88:201–211, 2003
273. Rodenhuis S: High-dose chemotherapy in breast cancer — interpretation of the randomized trials. *Anti-Cancer Drugs* 12:85–88, 2001
274. Loprinzi CL, Hayes D, Smith T: Doc, shouldn't we be getting some tests? *J Clin Oncol* 18:2345–2348, 2000
275. Hayes DF: Evaluation of patients after primary therapy, in Harris JR, Lippman ME, Morrow M et al (eds.): *Diseases of the Breast* (ed 2). Philadelphia, Lippincott, Williams and Wilkins, 2000 pp 709-730
276. Moore S: Cutaneous metastatic breast cancer. *Clin J Oncol Nurs* 6:255–260, 2002
277. Danova M, Porta C, Ferrari S, et al: Strategies of medical treatment for metastatic breast cancer. *Int J Oncol* 19:733–739, 2001
278. Ellis MJ, Hayes DF, Lippman ME: Treatment of metastatic breast cancer, in Harris JR, Lippman ME, Morrow M, et al (eds.): *Diseases of the Breast* (ed 2). Philadelphia, Lippincott, Williams and Wilkins, 2000, pp 749–797
279. Nabholtz JM, Reese DM, Lindsay MA, et al: Combination chemotherapy for metastatic breast cancer. *Exp Rev Anticancer Therap* 2:169–180, 2002
280. Perez EA: Update on metastatic breast cancer. *Curr Oncol Rep* 1:11–15, 1999
281. O'Shaughnessy J: Clinical experience of capecitabine in metastatic breast cancer. *Eur J Cancer* 38:10–14, 2002
282. Gerbrecht BM: Current Canadian experience with capecitabine: partnering with patients to optimize therapy. *Cancer Nurs* 26:161–167, 2003
283. Rosen LS, Gordon DH, Dugan WJ, et al: Zoledronic acid is superior to pamidronate for the treatment of bone metastases in breast carcinoma patients with at least one osteolytic lesion. *Cancer* 100:36–43, 2003
284. Rosen LS, Gordon D, Tchekmedyian S, et al: Zoledronic acid versus placebo in the treatment of skeletal metastases in patients with lung cancer and other solid tumors: A phase III, double-blind, randomized trial — the Zoledronic Acid Lung Cancer and Other Solid Tumors Study Group. *J Clin Oncol* 21:3150–3157, 2003
285. Ali SM, Esteva FJ, Hortobagyi G, et al: Safety and efficacy of bisphosphonates beyond 24 months in cancer patients. *J Clin Oncol* 19:3434–3437, 2001
286. Hillner BE, Ingle JN, Chlebowski RT, et al: American Society of Clinical Oncology 2003 update on the role of bisphosphonates and bone health issues in women with breast cancer. *J Clin Oncol* 21:4042–4057, 2003
287. Rose C: A comparison of the efficacy of aromatase inhibitors in second-line treatment of metastatic breast cancer. *Am J Clin Oncol* 26:S9–S16, 2003
288. Ingle JN: Sequencing of hormonal therapy in breast cancer. *Breast J* 8:332–337, 2002
289. Johnston SR, Smith IE, Dowsett M: Place of aromatase inhibitors in the endocrine therapy of breast cancer, in Miller WR, Santen RJ (eds.): *Aromatase Inhibition and Breast Cancer.* New York, Marcel Dekker, 2001, pp 29–49
290. Jones SE: Fulvestrant: an estrogen receptor antagonist that downregulates the estrogen receptor. *Semin Oncol* 30:14–20, 2003
291. Gail MH: The estimation and use of absolute risk for weighing the risks and benefits of selective estrogen receptor modulators for preventing breast cancer. *Ann NY Acad Sci* 949:286–291, 2001
292. Osborne CK, Zhao H, Fuqua SA: Selective estrogen receptor modulators: structure, function, and clinical use. *J Clin Oncol* 18:3172–3186, 2000
293. Roe EB, Chiu KM, Arnaud CD: Selective estrogen receptor modulators and postmenopausal health. *Adv Intern Med* 45:259–278, 2000
294. Sadowski B, Kriegbaum C, Apfelstedt-Sylla E: Tamoxifen side effects, age-related macular degeneration (AMD) or cancer associated retinopathy (CAR)? *Eur J Ophthalmol* 11:309–312, 2001
295. Noureddin BN, Seoud M, Bashshur Z, et al: Ocular toxicity in low-dose tamoxifen: a prospective study. *Eye* 13:729–733, 1999
296. Alwitry A, Gardner I: Tamoxifen maculopathy. *Arch Ophthalmol* 120:1402, 2002
297. Buzdar A, Douma J, Davidson N, et al: Phase III, multicenter, double-blind, randomized study of letrozole, an aromatase in-

hibitor, for advanced breast cancer versus megestrol acetate. *J Clin Oncol* 19:3357–3366, 2001

298. Kimmick GG, Muss HB: Endocrine therapy in metastatic breast cancer. *Cancer Treat Res* 94:231–254, 1998
299. Hyder SM, Murthy L, Stancel GM: Progestin regulation of vascular endothelial growth factor in human breast cancer cells. *Cancer Res* 58:392–395, 1998
300. Lanari C, Molinolo AA: Progesterone receptors — animal models and cell signalling in breast cancer. Diverse activation pathways for the progesterone receptor: possible implications for breast biology and cancer. *Breast Cancer Res* 4:240–243, 2002
301. Lower EE, Blau R, Gazder P, et al: The risk of premature menopause induced by chemotherapy for early breast cancer. *J Women Health Gender-Based Med* 8:949–954, 1999
302. Rioux JE, Devlin C, Gelfand MM, et al: 17beta-estradiol vaginal tablet versus conjugated equine estrogen vaginal cream to relieve menopausal atrophic vaginitis. *Menopause* 7:156–161, 2000
303. Loprinzi CL, Sloan JA, Perez EA, et al: Phase III evaluation of fluoxetine for treatment of hot flashes. *J Clin Oncol* 20:1578–1583, 2002
304. Moore S: Menopausal symptoms, in Yarbro CH, Frogge MH, Goodman M (eds.): *Cancer Symptom Management* (ed 3). Sudbury, MA, Jones and Bartlett, 2003, pp 571–575
305. Guttuso T Jr, Kurlan R, McDermott MP, et al: Gabapentin's effects on hot flashes in postmenopausal women: a randomized controlled trial. *Obstet Gynecol* 101:337–345, 2003
306. Guttuso TJ Jr: Gabapentin's effects on hot flashes and hypothermia. *Neurology* 54:2161–2163, 2000
307. Graf MC, Geller PA: Treating hot flashes in breast cancer survivors: a review of alternative treatments to hormone replacement therapy. *Clin J Oncol Nurs* 7:637–640, 2003
308. Schairer C, Lubin J, Triosi R: Menopausal estrogen and estrogen-progestin replacement therapy and breast cancer risk. *JAMA* 283:485–491, 2000
309. Snyder G, Sielsch E, Reville B: The controversy of hormone-replacement therapy in breast cancer survivors. *Oncol Nurs Forum* 25:699–706, 1998
310. Chen WT, Colditz GA, Rosner B, et al: Use of postmenopausal hormones, alcohol, and risk for invasive breast cancer. *Ann Intern Med* 137:798–804, 2002
311. Colditz GA: Hormones and breast cancer: evidence and implications for consideration of risks and benefits of hormone replacement therapy. *J Women Health* 8:347–357, 1999
312. Demark-Wahnefried W, Peterson BL, Winer EP, et al: Changes in weight, body composition, and factors influencing energy balance among premenopausal breast cancer patients receiving adjuvant chemotherapy [comment]. *J Clin Oncol* 19:2381–2389, 2001
313. Kumar N, Allen KA, Riccardi D, et al: Fatigue, weight gain, letharge and amenorrhea in breast cancer patients on chemotherapy: Is subclinical hypothyroidism the culprit? *Breast Cancer Res Treat* 83:149–159, 2004
314. Gralla R, Lichinitser M, Van der Vegt S, et al: Palonosetron improves prevention of chemotherapy-induced nausea and vomiting following moderately emetogenic chemotherapy: results of a double-blind randomized phase III trial comparing single doses of palonosetron with ondansetron. *Ann Oncol* 14:1570–1577, 2003
315. Petrek JA, Pressman PI, Smith RA: Lymphedema: current issues in research and management. *CA Cancer J Clin* 50:292–307, 2000
316. Erickson VS, Pearson ML, Ganz PA, et al: Arm edema in breast cancer patients. *J Natl Cancer Inst* 93:96–111, 2001
317. McKenzie DC, Kalda AL: Effect of upper extremity exercise on secondary lymphedema in breast cancer patients: a pilot study. *J Clin Oncol* 21:463–466, 2003
318. Gustafson DH, Hawkins R, Pingree S, et al: Effect of computer support on younger women with breast cancer. *J Gen Intern Med* 16:435–445, 2001
319. Schultz PN, Stava C, Beck ML, et al: Internet message board use by patients with cancer and their families. *Clin J Oncol Nurs* 7:663–667, 2003
320. Cobleigh MA, Bitterman P, Baker J, et al: *Tumor Gene Expression Predicts Distant Disease-Free Survival (DDFS) in Breast Cancer Patients with 10 or More Positive Nodes: High Throughput RT-PCR Assay of Paraffin-Embedded Tumor Tissues.* ASCO Annual Meeting 2003. Chicago, IL, ASCO, 2003, p 850
321. Jong RA, Yaffe MJ, Skarpathiotakis M, et al: Contrast-enhanced digital mammography: initial clinical experience. *Radiology* 228:842–850, 2003
322. Gianfelice D, Khiat A, Amara M, et al: MR imaging-guided focused US ablation of breast cancer: histopathologic assessment of effectiveness — initial experience. *Radiology* 227:849–855, 2003
323. Dowlatshahi K, Fan M, Gould V, et al: Stereotactically guided laser therapy of occult breast timors. *Arch Surg* 135:1345–1352, 2000
324. Fornage BD, Sneige N, Ross MI, et al: Small (2-cm) breast cancer treated with US-guided radiofrequency ablation: feasibility study. *Radiology* 231:215–224, 2004
325. Mankoff DA, Dunnwald LK, Gralow JR, et al: [Tc-99m]-sestamibi uptake and washout in locally advanced breast cancer are correlated with tumor blood flow. *Nucl Med Biol* 29:719–727, 2002
326. Winslow RL, Boguski MS: Genome informatics: current status and future prospects. *Circulation Res* 92:953–961, 2003
327. Petricoin EF, Zoon KC, Kohn EC, et al: Clinical proteomics: translating benchside promise into bedside reality. *Nat Rev Drug Discov* 1(9):683–695, 2002

CHAPTER 47

Central Nervous System Cancers

Karen Belford, RN, MS, AOCN®

Introduction

Cancer of the central nervous system (CNS) includes primary and metastatic tumors of the brain and spinal cord. CNS cancers are not uncommon and are associated with significant morbidity and mortality. Whether benign or malignant, primary or secondary, CNS tumors can drastically affect an individual's life and impede the ability to function. Knowledge of the various tumor types and their differences, associated neuroanatomy and neurophysiology, and the many issues related to treatment is essential to provide accurate assessment, ongoing intervention, and supportive management for these individuals.

Brain Tumors

Epidemiology

Primary CNS cancers represent approximately 2% of all reported malignancies. Approximately 39,550 new cases of primary benign and malignant brain tumors were diagnosed in the United States in 2002.[1] An estimated 18,400 new cases of malignant primary brain tumors were expected to be diagnosed in 2004.[2] However, any intracranial tumor, regardless of its histological behavior, can potentially invade and displace critical areas of the brain, causing devastating effects. The incidence is slightly higher in men than in women with the exception of meningiomas, which occur more often in women. Brain cancer is the second most common cancer diagnosed in children, second only to leukemia.

Malignant CNS tumors are responsible for approximately 2.5% of all cancer-related deaths. An estimated 12,690 deaths in 2004 were attributable to primary brain tumors.[3] The majority of these deaths result from malignant gliomas. Brain tumors are found in persons of all ages. In men and women younger than age 20, brain and other nervous system tumors are the leading cause of cancer mortality and in men ages 20–39, they are the second.[2] Most intracranial tumors, however, occur in individuals older than age 45.[4] The median age at diagnosis is 57 years.[1] Over the past three decades, the incidence of primary brain tumors appears to have increased in the elderly.[5] The increasing incidence of brain tumors with age could result from the length of exposure required for cells to become malignant or from the aging immune system's decreasing ability to protect against disease. It also may be attributed to environmental carcinogens found in industrialized nations, improved diagnostic capabilities, better access to specialized care, changing attitudes toward the care of the elderly, medical support programs,[6] and the increasing size of the elderly population.[7] The increased incidence is truly established only for primary central nervous system lymphoma (PCNSL).

Historically, it has been difficult to estimate the true epidemiology of CNS tumors. Fifteen cell types can potentially give rise to CNS tumors,[4] and many of these tumors consist of more than one cell type. In addition, not all cancer registries report nonmalignant histologies such as meningioma. The overall number of CNS tumors in the United States may be substantially underestimated.[8] The most common primary brain tumor is the malignant glioma, accounting for more than half of all primary CNS cancers. The most prevalent CNS malignancy is the metastatic brain tumor, which is increasing in frequency and occurs ten times more often than primary brain tumors. Brain metastasis is the most common neurological complication of systemic cancer.

Etiology

Genetic Factors

Specific causes and risk factors for the majority of CNS tumors have not been identified. Fewer than 5% of CNS tumors are associated with specific genetic disorders. Individuals with specific autosomal dominant disorders (i.e., neurofibromatosis, tuberous sclerosis, Li-Fraumeni syndrome, Turcot syndrome, and von

Hippel-Lindau disease) have a higher incidence of brain tumors than the general population.

Neurofibromatosis type 1 (NF-1), also called von Recklinghausen's disease, occurs in 1 out of 3000 individuals.[9] The most common brain tumors associated with NF-1 are optic nerve gliomas, astrocytomas, ependymomas, meningiomas, and neurofibromas.[10,11] Neurofibromatosis type 2 (NF-2) occurs less frequently and is characterized by an increased incidence of schwannomas, meningiomas, ependymomas, and astrocytomas.[10,12] Tuberous sclerosis, or Bourneville disease, has a reported incidence ranging from 1 in 10,000 to 1 in 50,000. Approximately one-half of individuals with this disorder develop subependymal giant cell astrocytomas.[13] The Li-Fraumeni syndrome has been studied in more than 100 families and is associated with an increased incidence of many different types of cancer, including astrocytomas and primitive neuroectodermal tumors (PNETs).[12] Gliomas, medulloblastomas, and pituitary adenomas have been observed in individuals with Turcot syndrome, a syndrome of CNS tumors in individuals with adenomatous polyposis coli (APC). Approximately 5% of families with APC have this syndrome.[9] Finally, those with von Hippel-Lindau disease are at risk for developing cerebellar hemangioblastomas.[14]

As with other cancers, CNS tumor pathogenesis is a multistep process in which tumor suppressor gene inactivation and oncogene activation and overexpression play a part, along with alterations in cell cycle progression, abnormalities in signal transduction pathways, glial cell invasion, and angiogenesis.[12] Genetic changes during the pathogenesis of CNS tumors can occur either at the chromosomal level or at the gene expression level. These changes can result from the loss of a major portion of a chromosome or from mutations within a single gene.[15] Growth factors also appear to be involved in the pathogenesis of CNS cancers. Mutation of growth factors or their receptors may result in tumor cell proliferation and transformation. These include epidermal growth factor receptor (EGFR), platelet-derived growth factor receptor (PDGFR), vascular endothelial growth factor (VEGF), and fibroblast growth factor receptor (FGFR). However, the genetic alterations are not present in all tumors of a particular histological type. For example, mutations of the *p53* tumor suppressor gene that are present in a majority of glioblastoma multiforme (GBM) cases are not present in all glioblastomas.[16] This indicates that tumors that are histologically identical under the microscope may have significantly different genetic origins. Also, these tumors are extremely heterogeneous. Each tumor cell may not have the same identified genetic change. For example, EGFR overexpression is found in 40% of GBM,[17] but it is not present in all glioblastoma tumor cells.[16]

Radiation

Ionizing radiation and immunosuppression are the only two definitive risk factors related to the development of CNS cancers. Scalp irradiation, once used for the treatment of tinea capitus, has led to an increase in meningiomas,[18] gliomas, and nerve sheath tumors.[19] Brain irradiation, used in the treatment of pituitary tumors,[20,21] head and neck cancers, and leukemia, has led to an increase in gliomas, meningiomas, and sarcomas.[22]

Immunosuppression and Viral Factors

Viruses have been directly implicated in the development of CNS tumors in animals. Acquired immunosuppression, such as results from human immunodeficiency virus (HIV) infection and the use of immunosuppressive agents after organ transplant, has led to an increased incidence of PCNSL.[23,24] Tumor cells from individuals with acquired immune deficiency syndrome (AIDS)–related PCNSL usually contain the Epstein-Barr virus (EBV).

Chemical and Environmental Factors

Although many chemicals are carcinogenic in animals and produce brain tumors, the possible association of chemical exposure and brain tumors has not truly been established. Some studies suggest a relationship between brain tumors and such industries as synthetic rubber, petrochemical, aeronautics, drug manufacturing, nuclear energy, and those associated with precision metal work. Substances that have been investigated include polyvinyl chloride, pesticides, herbicides, fertilizers, organic solvents, phenols, formalin, polycyclic aromatic hydrocarbons, hair dyes, and N-nitroso compounds.

Electromagnetic Fields

Concern has existed over the possible association between extremely low-frequency electromagnetic fields (ELF-EMFs) and the development of brain tumors, particularly exposure from cellular telephones. Exposure to ELF-EMFs is almost universal today in industrialized nations. In addition to cellular telephones, other sources of ELF-EMF include residential heating, electrical appliances, hand-held radios, electric power lines, transformers, and computer terminals. Some

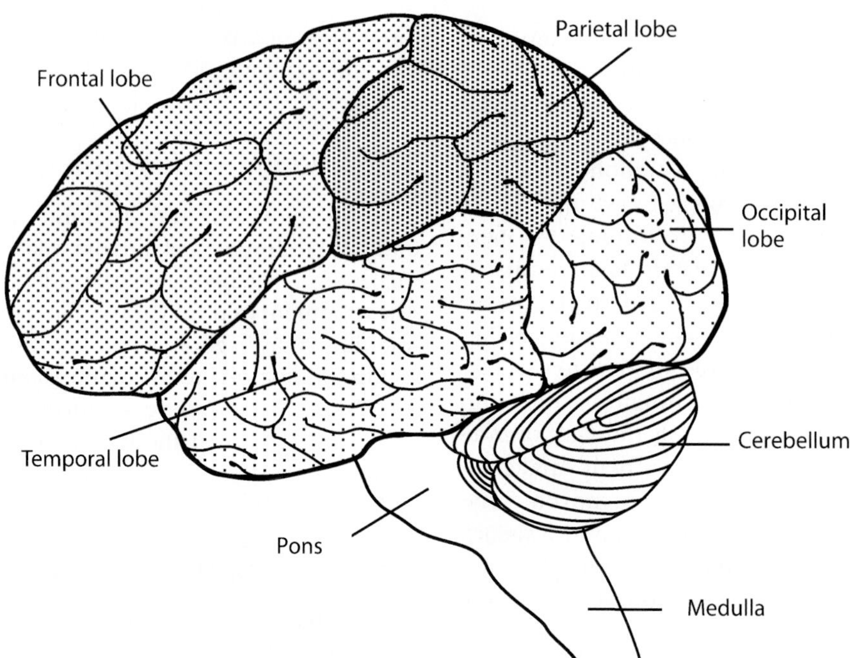

Figure 47-1 Lobes of the cerebral hemispheres.

studies have reported a higher than expected incidence of brain tumors, particularly gliomas,[25] among electricians, electronics and communications workers,[26,27] railway workers, and welders.[28] At this point, most of the now extensive research fails to support ELF-EMF as a risk factor for brain tumors.[29-33]

Pathophysiology

Anatomy and Physiology

The nervous system contains two types of cells: neurons and glial cells. The neurons are the basic anatomical and functional unit of the nervous system. The glial cells provide structural support, nourishment, and protection for the neurons. Approximately 40% of the brain and spinal cord is composed of glial cells. In the CNS, glial cells are subdivided into four main types: astrocytes, oligodendrocytes, ependymal cells, and microglia. In the peripheral nervous system (PNS), Schwann cells form myelin sheaths.[34] Unlike neurons, glial cells in the adult nervous system retain their capacity to divide. They can undergo anaplasia and are the major source of primary tumors of the CNS. The specific tumor type is derived from the glial cell of origin. For example, astrocytomas arise from astrocytes, and ependymomas arise from ependymal cells.

The brain is divided into three main areas: the cerebrum, the brain stem, and the cerebellum. The cerebrum contains the two cerebral hemispheres and the diencephalon. The cerebral hemispheres are connected by a large area of white matter, the corpus callosum, which allows each portion of one hemisphere to connect with the corresponding portion of the other hemisphere. It essentially allows communication between the two hemispheres.[35] Each cerebral hemisphere is divided into four lobes: frontal, parietal, temporal, and occipital (Figure 47-1). The diencephalon is composed of the thalamus, hypothalamus, and basal ganglia. The pituitary gland is connected to the hypothalamus. The brain stem is made up of the midbrain, pons, and medulla. The cerebellum has two hemispheres and is connected to the brain stem by the cerebellar peduncles. The functions of these areas are listed in Table 47-1.[36,37]

Cranial nerves. The 12 pairs of cranial nerves (CNs) are part of the PNS. They have fiber pathways entering and exiting the brain. Cranial nerves I and II are located in the cerebral hemispheres, cranial nerves III and IV in the midbrain, cranial nerves V–VIII in the pons, and cranial nerves IX–XII in the medulla (Figure 47-2). They are responsible for motor and sensory function of the head and neck; their functions are listed in Table 47-2. Symptoms of cranial nerve dysfunction (cranial nerve palsy) can provide valuable information for localizing an intracranial tumor.

Meninges. The meninges are the membranes covering the brain and spinal cord. The cranial meninges are shown in Figure 47-3. There are three layers of meninges: the dura mater, arachnoid, and pia mater.

Table 47-1 Clinical Manifestations of Intracranial Tumors

Location	Function	Abnormality
Frontal lobes	Intellect Personality Judgment Abstract thinking Mood and affect Long-term memory Voluntary motor activity (contralateral) Secondary urinary control Language expression (dominant side)	Intellectual deterioration Personality changes Impaired judgment Emotional lability, flat affect Memory loss Muscle weakness or paralysis Babinski sign Increased deep-tendon reflexes Incontinence Expressive aphasia (Broca's aphasia) Seizures
Parietal lobes	Sensory integration (contralateral) Sensory interpretation (contralateral) Ability to carry out and understand special constructs	Decrease or loss of sensation (pain, temperature, pinprick, light touch, proprioception, vibration, two-point discrimination, stereognosis, graphesthesia) Inability to write, calculate Construction apraxia Seizures
Temporal lobes	Hearing Short-term memory Language comprehension (dominant side) Interpretation of memory Emotion	Hearing changes, hallucinations Memory loss Receptive aphasia (Wernicke's aphasia) Intellectual impairment Emotional lability Seizures
Occipital lobes	Vision Visual interpretation	Visual field defects (contralateral homonymous hemianopsia), blindness Hallucinations Inability to identify objects or symbols or meaning of written words Seizures
Thalamus	Sensory relay station Conscious awareness of pain Sleep–wake cycle Focusing of attention Emotion	Sensory abnormality Neuropathic pain Inattentiveness Emotional lability Hydrocephalus, increased ICP
Hypothalamus	Coordination of autonomic nervous system function Temperature regulation Regulation of water metabolism Regulation of hormone secretions Regulation of appetite Control of thirst center Regulation of part of sleep–wake cycle Mediation of affective and sexual behavior	Abnormalities in sweating, vasodilation, hypotonia, pulse Hypothermia or hyperthermia Abnormalities in absorption of free water Endocrine dysfunction Increase or decrease appetite Increase or decrease thirst Flat affect Emotional lability
Basal ganglia	Fine motor control	Weakness or paralysis Intention tremors, Parkinsonism
Brain stem Midbrain Pons Medulla	Point of origin for cranial nerves III through XII Vital reflex centers Maintenance of consciousness	Cranial nerve dysfunction Abnormalities of reflex activities (heart rate, respirations, blood pressure, coughing, sneezing, swallowing, vomiting) Change in level of consciousness
Cerebellum	Coordination Fine motor control Balance (ipsilateral)	Ataxia, dysarthria Action tremor, nystagmus, Loss of balance, wide-based gait Hydrocephalus

The outermost layer, the dura mater, lines the interior of the skull. The outer layer of the dura is the periosteum of the cranial bone.[34] There is a potential space between the dura and the skull called the *epidural space.* The inner dural layer extends throughout the skull and folds in on itself to create anatomical compartments. The falx cerebri, the tentorium cerebelli, and the falx cerebelli are three such dural folds. The falx

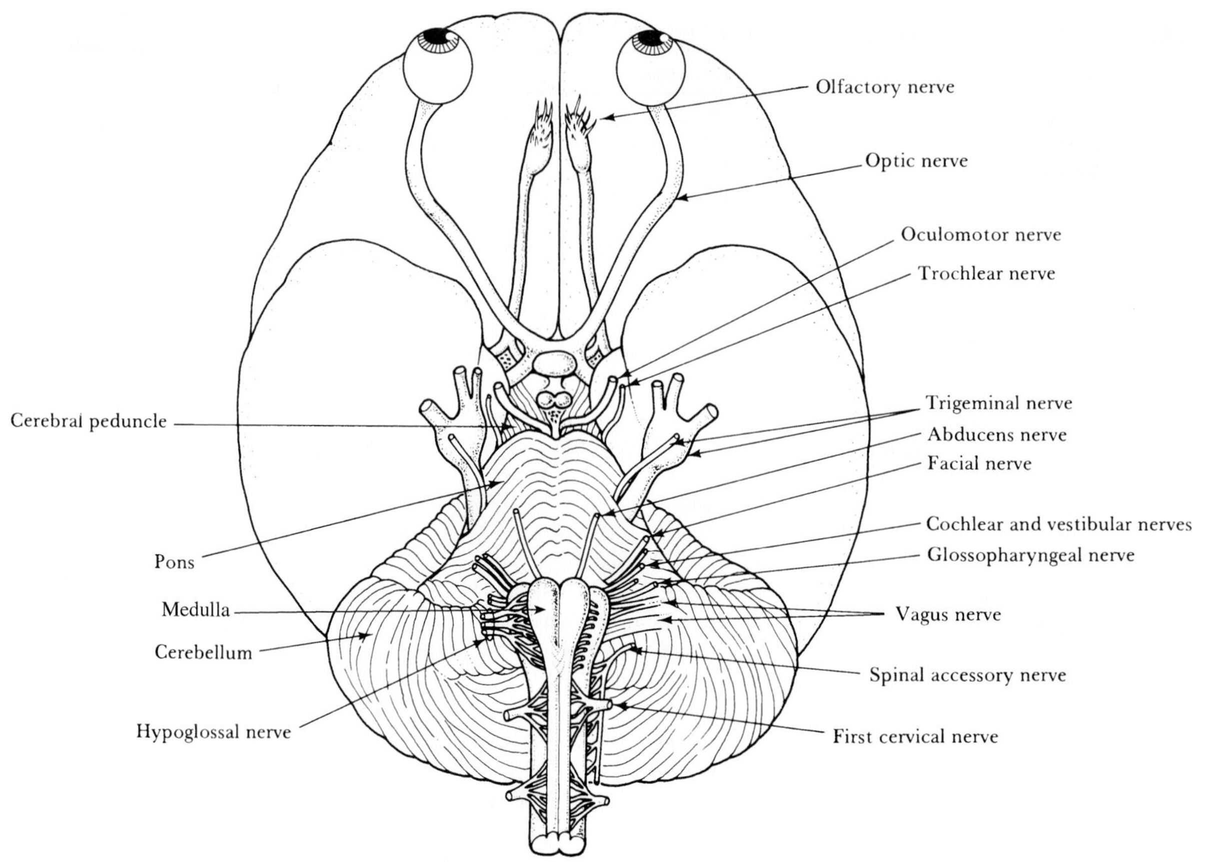

Figure 47-2 Cranial nerves from the base of the brain.

cerebri descends vertically between the two cerebral hemispheres to partially separate the two hemispheres. The tentorium cerebelli divides the skull into the supratentorial space and the infratentorial space. Structures and tumors that lie above the tentorium (cerebral hemispheres, diencephalon, and basal ganglia) are located in the supratentorial compartment; those lying below the tentorium (cerebellum and brain stem) are in the infratentorial compartment, also known as the posterior fossa. An opening in the tentorium—the tentorial notch—allows the brain stem, blood vessels, and nerves to pass through the tentorium. A third fold of dura, the falx cerebelli, separates the two lobes of the cerebellum.

The middle meningeal layer, the arachnoid, is a thin, delicate, transparent membrane that loosely surrounds the brain. There is a potential space between the dura and the arachnoid—the subdural space—which is a common site of hematomas. The pia mater is the innermost meningeal layer. The meshlike, vascular membrane adheres directly to the surface of the brain, dipping down between the convolutions of the brain surface. The pia mater and the arachnoid together are referred to as the *leptomeninges*. The space between the arachnoid and the pia mater, the subarachnoid space, is where cerebrospinal fluid (CSF) circulates.

Ventricular system. The ventricular system consists of a series of interconnected chambers and pathways responsible for the production and circulation of CSF around the brain and spinal cord[38] (Figure 47-4). The majority of CSF is formed in the choroid plexuses. Approximately 20–25 mL of CSF is produced hourly, and the volume of CSF found in the ventricular system at any one time is 125–150 mL. In addition, CSF may be aspirated in expanded areas of the subarachnoid space called *cisterns*. The major cisterns are the cisterna magna, located between the medulla and the cerebellar region, and the lumbar cistern, between vertebrae L-2 and S-2.[34]

Cerebrovascular circulation. The cerebral arterial circulation is the body's most complex vascular network. The brain receives approximately 20% of the body's resting cardiac output. This large amount of blood flow reflects the brain's tremendous metabolic requirements, particularly for oxygen and glucose.[38] An adequate cerebral blood flow (CBF) is necessary to deliver oxygen, glucose, and other nutrients to the brain, and to remove carbon dioxide and other

Table 47-2 Examination of Cranial Nerves

Cranial Nerve	Major Function	Method of Testing	Desired Response
I. Olfactory	Smell	Inhalation of commonly recognized aromatic substance such as cloves; avoid use of ammonia or alcohol as these stimulate the trigeminal nerve and evoke a pain response	Correct identification of the substance with each nostril
II. Optic	Vision	Direct ophthalmoscopy; use finger movement and eye charts to test visual acuity and fields	Note the appearance of the optic disc, vessels, and retina; correct eye movement and chart identification with each eye separately
III. Oculomotor	Movement of eyes in four of the six cardinal directions of gaze (inward, upward, downward, and outward); pupillary constriction and accommodation; elevation of upper eyelid	Individual follows the examiner's finger with the eyes while not moving head to test eye movement; check pupil response to light; observe for ptosis of the eyelid	Movement of eyes should be equal in the cardinal directions of gaze; pupils react equally and briskly to light; consensual response and accommodation to light is present; eyes are symmetrical at rest and move conjugately
IV. Trochlear	Movements of eyes (downward and inward)	Individual follows the examiner's finger with the eyes to test eye movement	Movement of eyes should be equal
V. Trigeminal	Muscles of mastication and eardrum tension; general sensations from anterior half of head including face, nose, mouth	Individual clamps the jaw, opens the mouth against resistance and masticates to check motor division of the nerve; touch both sides of the person's face, checking for pain, touch, and temperature response; gently touch the person's cornea with a cotton wisp to check the corneal reflex	Jaw movement is strong and symmetrical; correct identification of sensations; rapid blinking
VI. Abducens	Lateral movement of eyes	Individual follows the examiner's finger to test eye movement (oculomotor, trochlear, and abducens are tested together)	Movement of eyes should be equal
VII. Facial	Muscles of facial expression and tension on ear bones; lacrimination and salivation; taste to anterior two-thirds of tongue	Observe for facial symmetry and the individual's ability to contract muscles to check motor division; individual tastes sweet, sour, salty, and acidic flavor	Individual smiles, frowns, wrinkles nose and brow, closes eyes tightly with symmetry; correct identification of tastes
VIII. Acoustic (cochlear and vestibular)	Hearing; balance and equilibrium	Test hearing ability with the use of whispered voice and tuning fork at various distances from the ear to check the cochlear nerve; check the vestibular nerve by having the individual stand on one foot with eyes closed	Recognition of sound; maintenance of balance
IX. Glossopharyngeal	Gag and swallowing, salivation, taste to posterior third of tongue	Have individual say "ah"; check the gag reflex by touching the pharynx with a tongue depressor; have individual taste different flavors	Soft palate and uvula elevate in the midline; gag response is present; correct identification of tastes
X. Vagus	Gag and swallowing, laryngeal control, parasympathetic to thoracic and abdominal viscera	Check the individual's swallowing ability; ask individual to cough and speak; glossopharygeal and vagus nerves are examined together because of overlapping innervation of the pharynx	No dysphagia present; speak without hoarseness or weakness
XI. Spinal accessory	Movement of head and shoulders	Ask the individual to elevate the shoulders, turn the head, and resist the examiner's attempts to pull the chin back to midline; check the symmetry of the trapezius and sternocleidomastoid muscles	Equal bilateral strength; atrophy may indicate nerve dysfunction
XII. Hypoglossal	Movement of tongue	Ask the individual to protrude the tongue and move from side to side and up and down	Absence of deviations, atrophy, or tremors

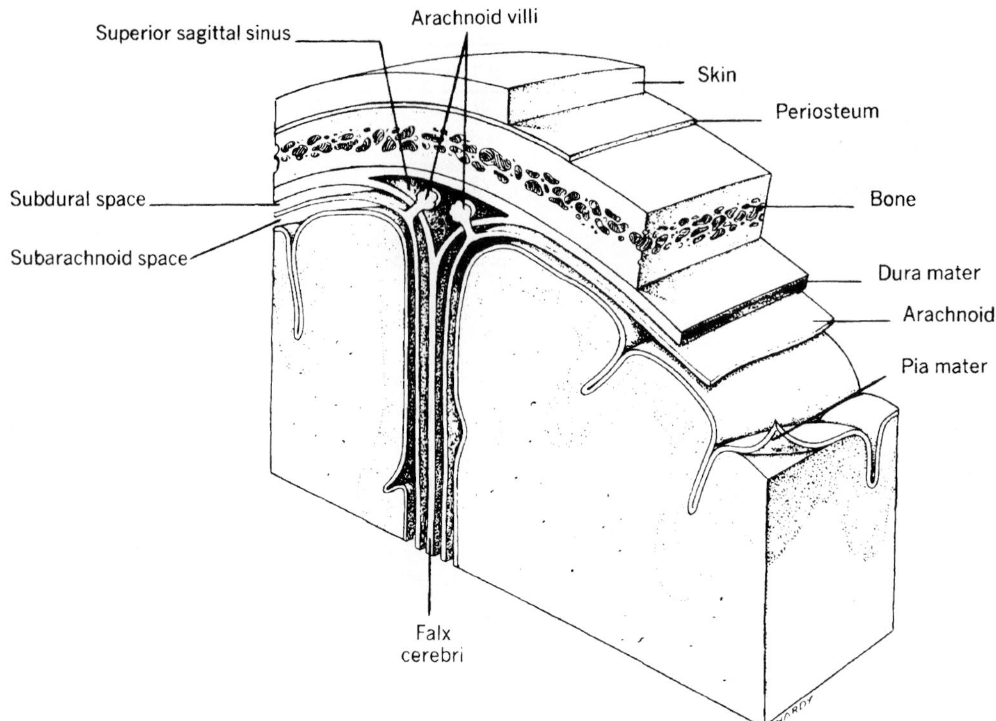

Figure 47-3 The cranial meninges. (Reprinted with permission from Hickey JV: Overview of neuroanatomy and neurophysiology, in Hickey JV (ed.): *The Clinical Practice of Neurological and Neurosurgical Nursing* (ed 4). Philadelphia, Lippincott, 1997, pp 35–79. Originally published in Chaffee EE, Lytle IM: *Basic Physiology and Anatomy.* Philadelphia, Lippincott, 1980[34]).

metabolic products from the brain. The CBF must remain relatively constant because the CNS has little ability to store oxygen and glucose in its tissue. Even brief circulation failure may result in temporary or permanent loss of neurological function.

Arterial blood flow to the anterior brain is supplied by the two internal carotid arteries and to the posterior brain by the two vertebral arteries. The cerebral venous circulation consists of veins located on the surface of the brain and vascular channels or sinuses located between the two dural layers. The superior sagital sinus is one of the dural venous sinuses and is a major site of CSF reabsorption. The cerebral veins drain into the cerebral sinuses, empty into the jugular veins, and return blood to the heart. Obstruction of venous outflow can result in increased intracranial pressure (ICP).

Physiology of Intracranial Pressure

Intracranial pressure is exerted within the skull and meninges by brain tissue, CSF, and cerebral blood volume (CBV). The skull and meninges form a rigid compartment holding these three major components: brain tissue (representing 80% of the total volume), CSF (constituting 10%), and the blood volume (accounting for the remaining 10%). According to the Monro-Kellie hypothesis, the rigid vault formed by the skull and meninges is filled to capacity with essentially noncompressible contents, which remain relatively constant, and therefore is unyielding to any increases in volume. If any one component increases in volume, a concomitant decrease in the volume of one or both of the remaining components must occur to maintain normal ICP. If the reciprocal compensation does not occur, ICP rises. The normal ICP is 0–15 mm Hg (80–180 cm H_2O).

The mechanism by which this secondary decrease in volume occurs is called *compensation.* Brain tumors increase the brain mass, and the often-accompanying edema can further increase the volume. To maintain a normal ICP, the compensatory mechanisms reduce the amount of CSF, blood volume, or both. The volume of CSF is decreased by displacing CSF from the cranial subarachnoid space to the spinal subarachnoid space, and by increasing the amount of CSF absorbed into the venous circulation by the arachnoid villi. When ICP is elevated for prolonged periods, the choroid plexuses can decrease the amount of CSF they produce. The CBV decreases by shunting the venous blood away from the affected area into the venous sinuses. These compensatory mechanisms are finite, however, and eventually become exhausted. Once all the compensatory mechanisms are depleted, relatively

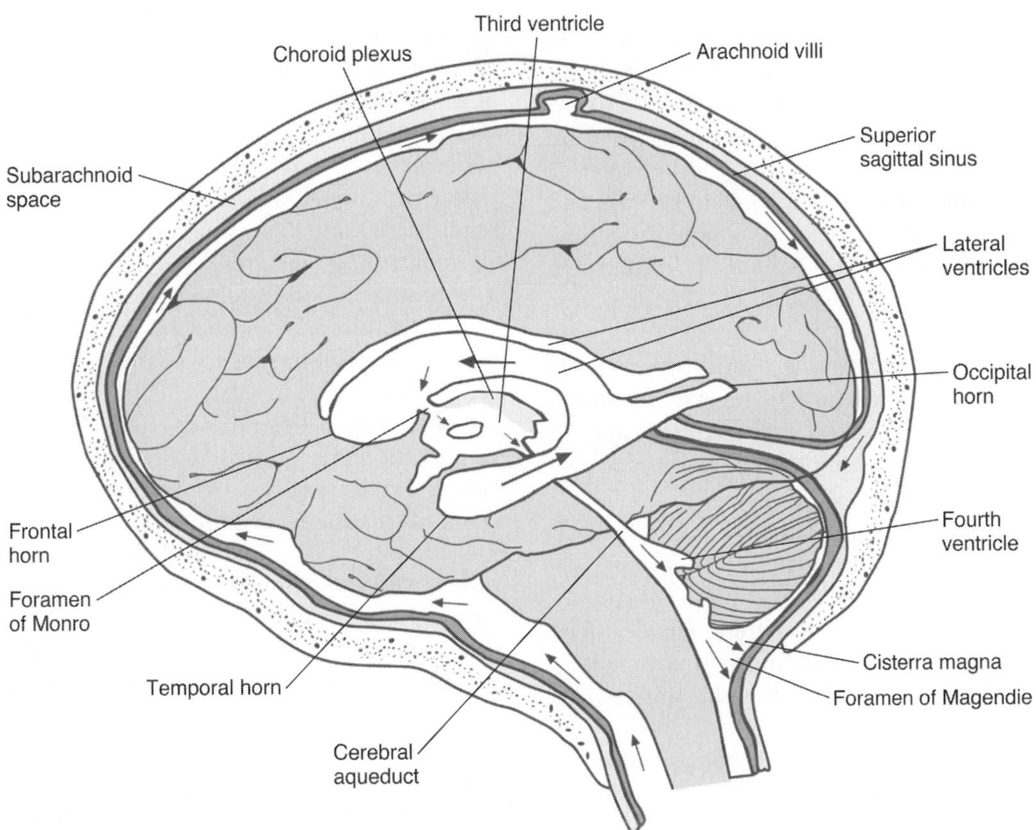

Figure 47-4 Circulation of cerebrospinal fluid.

small increases in volume result in large increases in ICP.

Small volume increments can be compensated for far more readily than large volume increments. Increases in volume made over long periods can be accommodated more easily than a comparable quantity introduced within a much shorter interval. An individual with an acute subdural hematoma, for example, will develop signs and symptoms of increased ICP much more rapidly than a person with a large, slow-growing, low-grade brain tumor.

Another important concept relating to ICP is autoregulation, which provides a constant CBF despite fluctuations in systemic arterial pressure (SAP) by adjusting the diameter of blood vessels. However, when the SAP falls below 60 mm Hg or above 160 mm Hg, or when ICP is sustained above 30 mm Hg, the autoregulatory mechanisms fail and the CBF becomes passively dependent on changes in SAP.[39,40]

The autoregulatory mechanism also responds to certain metabolic factors. The cerebral blood vessels vasodilate in response to increased $PaCO_2$ and decreased pH, leading to an increased CBF and CBV. Decreased $PaCO_2$ and increased pH lead to constriction of cerebral blood vessels, resulting in decreased CBF and CBV. The cerebral blood vessels are less sensitive to changes in the PaO_2. Vasodilation leading to increased CBF and CBV generally does not occur until the PaO_2 falls to the hypoxic range.

Another consideration relating to ICP is the cerebral venous system. The cerebral veins do not have valves as do other venous vessels in the body. Any condition that obstructs or compromises the venous outflow may also increase CBV because more blood is backed up in the intracranial cavity.[39] Activities such as coughing, sneezing, or performing the valsalva maneuver increase intrathoracic and intraabdominal pressures that increase ICP by decreasing cerebral venous outflow via the jugular veins.[40] Rotation and extreme flexion or extension of the neck may also obstruct venous outflow and arterial inflow. Positive end-expiratory pressure (PEEP) treatments, hip flexion, and lying on the abdomen also increase thoracic and abdominal cavity pressures.[37] Elevating the head of the bed facilitates venous drainage.

Gliomas

Gliomas are the most common primary brain tumor in adults. They include the astrocytomas, oligodendrogliomas, ependymomas, and mixed gliomas.

Astrocytomas. The majority of gliomas are astrocytomas, accounting for approximately 60% of all primary brain tumors. These tumors are graded to describe their degree of malignancy. Grade is based on the tumor's microscopic appearance and indicates its similarity to normal cells, its tendency to spread, and its growth rate. A four-grade system describes these tumors as grades I through IV: pilocytic astrocytoma (grade I), low-grade astrocytoma (grade II), anaplastic astrocytoma (grade III), and glioblastoma multiforme (grade IV). In this system, grade I tumors tend to be benign and grade IV tumors are the most malignant. A three-grade system is also used, dividing this group of tumors into astrocytoma, anaplastic astrocytoma, and glioblastoma multiforme (GBM).

Increasing grades of malignancy within the astrocytoma group are often associated with increasing patient age. Approximately 75% of pilocytic astrocytomas occur in individuals younger than age 20.[16] The mean age at diagnosis of a low-grade astrocytoma is 34 years, an anaplastic astrocytoma 40 years, and a GBM 53 years.[41,42] Low-grade astrocytomas rarely occur in those older than 50, whereas glioblastomas can occur in younger individuals and children. There is a slightly higher incidence of astrocytomas in males than in females.

Pilocytic astrocytomas represent 5% of the gliomas. Although typically pediatric tumors, 25% occur in individuals older than 18 years.[43] These tumors are usually found in the cerebellum, optic tracts, and diencephalon, but can occur in the cerebral hemispheres and brain stem.[44] On imaging, they are well circumscribed, and often cystic, are enhanced with contrast, and usually lack the surrounding edema commonly seen in higher-grade tumors.[16,42] Malignant transformation rarely occurs. Whenever possible, surgical resection is the preferred treatment, leading to cure or long-term survival in most cases. Overall 15-year survival is 80%.[45] For individuals with completely resected tumors in the cerebellum, survival is 95%.[43]

Low-grade astrocytomas generally arise in the cerebral hemispheres. The lobar distribution of these tumors is similar to the amount of white matter present in each lobe, with the highest frequency occurring in the frontal lobes. Low-grade astrocytomas show an increased cellularity and have mild nuclear pleomorphism compared with normal brain tissue. Other features of anaplasia, such as mitotic activity, vascular proliferative changes, and necrosis, are absent. Some astrocytomas may be cystic, and microcalcifications can be present. They are diffusely infiltrative tumors, although their invasion is largely limited to white matter. These tumors account for approximately 10% of the gliomas.[15]

Controversy exists with regard to the optimal management of low-grade astrocytomas.[46-48] Because much of the available retrospective literature suggests a survival benefit with aggressive surgical resection,[47] the general recommendation is to have as complete an excision of tumor as possible without compromising function.[48] Some low-grade astrocytomas present with well-controlled seizures and are relatively small, asymptomatic, and indolent lesions. Many individuals with these tumors can be safely observed and closely monitored without surgery or other treatment. Intervention would be indicated if the tumor progressed, the radiographic appearance changed (such as the development of new contrast enhancement), or the individual developed new or uncontrolled symptoms.[49] Delayed treatment postpones the risks of surgery and the side effects of radiation therapy (RT). Most individuals with low-grade astrocytomas are prescribed RT, although the timing of treatment is still debated.[47,50] A prospective randomized study evaluating the prognostic effect of RT in low-grade gliomas showed an improved progression-free survival for patients who received early postoperative RT compared to those who received RT at tumor recurrence.[51] However, overall survival was similar for both groups. Radiation treatment options include RT immediately after surgery, for only incompletely resected tumors, and at the time of tumor recurrence or progression. Currently, there is no established role for chemotherapy in the standard treatment of these tumors.

Low-grade astrocytomas are rarely cured because they cannot be completely excised. In addition, a large percentage of these tumors undergo malignant transformation to a higher tumor grade over time. Some individuals with low-grade astrocytomas may survive for many years, whereas others experience a malignant course with short survival time. No specific therapy has been identified that can reliably prevent malignant transformation of a low-grade astrocytoma.[50] The median survival for individuals with low-grade astrocytoma is 5–8 years with 15%–20% surviving for 10 years.[16]

Anaplastic astrocytoma and GBM are usually grouped together under the classification of malignant glioma or high-grade glioma. Also included in this group are tumors referred to as gliomatosis cerebri which diffusely infiltrate all or much of the brain without necessarily forming a mass lesion. Malignant gliomas account for approximately half of all primary brain tumors. Anaplastic astrocytomas represent 10%–30% of gliomas, whereas GBM is the most common adult primary brain tumor and accounts for more than 50% of all gliomas. The histological features of anaplastic astrocytoma are similar to those of low-grade astrocytoma but are more abundant and exaggerated. Cellularity is increased, as are nuclear and cellular pleomorphism. Mitotic activity and proliferative vascular changes are found within the tumor. Necrosis is not present. Glioblastoma multiforme has these characteristics plus necrosis, which distinguishes it from anaplastic astrocytoma. These tumors infiltrate the brain extensively but rarely spread to distant locations. Individuals with anaplastic astrocytoma have a better prognosis than those with glioblastoma. With conventional therapy, median survival for anaplastic astrocytoma is approximately 3 years, with 10%–15% of individuals surviving 5 years. Median survival for GBM is 12 months, with 15%–20% surviving 2 years.[16] Conventional treatment for these high-grade gliomas includes surgery, RT, and chemotherapy.

Oligodendrogliomas. Reports suggest that the incidence of oligodendrogliomas has been largely underestimated[16,47,52–54] and that they may represent as many as 25%–33% of all gliomas. Oligodendrogliomas arise from oligodendrocyte cells, which are responsible for the development and maintenance of the myelin sheath. Many of these tumors contain oligodendrocytes, astrocytes, and ependymal cells and are referred to as *mixed gliomas.* Oligodendrogliomas frequently arise in young individuals, with a peak incidence occurring at age 30.[16]

These tumors are usually located in the frontal or temporal lobes of the cerebral hemispheres. Many oligodendrogliomas have calcifications within the tumor and adjacent brain tissue and have a cystic component.[4] The classification of oligodendrogliomas distinguishes between two grades. Low-grade tumors are well differentiated and have cells that appear to be only slightly abnormal. They tend to be slow growing and are often present for many years before diagnosis. Anaplastic oligodendrogliomas have highly abnormal-looking cells and usually grow more quickly. Anaplastic features include high cellularity, nuclear pleomorphism, frequent mitosis, areas of necrosis, and proliferation of blood vessels.[48] The majority of oligodendrogliomas are low grade at diagnosis.

Clinically, these tumors present in the same fashion as other similarly located tumors. However, two features separate the oligodendrogliomas: the antecedent (prodromal) history, averaging 7–8 years, tends to be longer, and seizures are more common, occurring in 70%–90% of patients by the time of diagnosis.[4,55] The standard treatment for oligodendrogliomas has been surgery, when a good neurological outcome is possible, and RT. Postoperative RT may be held off for completely resected tumors.[48] Anaplastic oligodendrogliomas have been found to be chemosensitive tumors. Dramatic and prolonged responses to chemotherapy have been seen in tumors whose genetic analysis has shown a loss of heterozygosity on the long arm of chromosome 19 and the short arm of chromosome 1.[56–58] Treatment may eventually be tailored according to the genetic profile, as anaplastic oligodendrogliomas appear to not be a homogeneous group to tumors.[42] The PCV (procarbazine, lomustine [CCNU], and vincristine) regimen has produced the longest and most reliable response to date[54,55,59] and has become standard therapy for these tumors, although responses have also been seen with carmustine (BCNU). The PCV regimen as neoadjuvant therapy has been reported to have a good response and is currently being evaluated in randomized trials in combination with RT. Responses to PCV have also been reported in low-grade oligodendrogliomas.[56,60,61] Median survival is approximately 15 years for low-grade oligodendrogliomas and 4 years for anaplastic oligodendrogliomas.[57,58]

Ependymomas. Ependymomas represent approximately 9% of gliomas.[62] They occur in all age groups but are most often seen in young adults and children. Ependymomas arise from the ependymal cells, which form the lining of the ventricles and the central canal of the spinal cord.

Most intracranial ependymomas are infratentorial and arise from the fourth ventricle. Supratentorial tumors develop from the ependymal lining of the third and lateral ventricles or may be located deep in the cerebral hemispheres without visible connection to the ventricles. Ependymomas may be differentiated and low grade or anaplastic and high grade. The characteristic histological pattern of low grade ependymomas consists of epithelial-like arrangements of cells around an irregular open space or a radiating, tapering process of tumor cells surrounding a blood vessel.[62] In addition to the typical pattern of low-grade tumors, anaplastic ependymomas also have cellular pleomorphism, necrosis, mitoses, and multinucleation.[63] The majority of these tumors are low grade.

Infratentorial and high-grade tumors are more likely to spread through the CSF pathways. Signs and symptoms vary depending on the location of the tumor. Ependymomas are often associated with obstructive hydrocephalus, and a ventriculoperitoneal (VP) shunt may be required to relieve the increased ICP.

Standard treatment of ependymomas is surgery and then RT. Maximal surgical resection should be performed when possible because outcome is closely associated with extent of surgical resection. Individuals with totally resected tumors have the best prognosis.[48] Tumor location often makes complete resection impossible, especially when structures at the floor of the fourth ventricle are involved.[16] Unless evidence of disseminated disease is present, ependymomas are treated with local radiation because the majority of tumors recur at the primary site. Craniospinal radiation is reserved for those individuals with either radiographic or pathologic evidence of craniospinal seeding. Chemotherapy does not appear to be very effective against ependymomas,[43] so it is used primarily for recurrent tumors. Individuals with infratentorial tumors have higher survival rates than those with supratentorial tumors.[64] Low-grade ependymomas are associated with higher survival rates than anaplastic ependymomas.[65] Overall five- and ten-year survival rates are approximately 80% and 50%, respectively.[16]

Meningiomas

Meningiomas, the most common benign brain tumor, account for 20% of all adult intracranial tumors. They arise from the meninges and are often located near major venous sinuses, large cerebral blood vessels, and the skull base.[66,67] They may occur as single or multiple lesions. Meningiomas occur twice as often in women as in men and tend to occur in those aged 50–80 years. The incidence of meningiomas is higher in women with breast cancer.[68]

Most meningiomas are differentiated with low proliferative capacity, limited invasiveness, and well-defined borders. The traditional classification divides meningiomas into various subtypes, but this distinction has little prognostic significance with the exception of the malignant meningioma, which contains abundant mitoses, nuclear pleomorphism, necrosis, high nuclear-to-cytoplasmic ratio, loss of normal architecture, and invasion of surrounding brain tissue.[69] Malignant meningiomas account for less than 10% of all meningiomas, occur more often in men, are frequently multifocal, cause systemic metastases, and generally have a high recurrence rate.[70,71]

Meningiomas produce symptoms by compression of surrounding brain tissue rather than by infiltration as the gliomas do. The precise clinical features vary depending on the exact location of the tumor.

The primary treatment modality for meningiomas is surgery, with the extent of surgical resection being the primary factor that influences the recurrence rate. Factors that may prevent complete resection include tumor location, size, consistency, vascular and cranial nerve involvement, and, in the case of recurrence, prior surgery, radiotherapy, or both. Improved neurosurgical techniques allow many previously unresectable meningiomas to be surgically excised today. Preoperative embolization can decrease the size and vascularity of the tumor, making the surgical procedure easier and safer. The risk of recurrence for completely resected benign meningiomas is small, and postoperative radiation is usually not recommended. Recurrence rates for completely resected meningiomas are approximately 3% at 5 years and 20% at 20 years.[43] Radiation is indicated for individuals with inoperable, partially resected, and recurrent meningiomas. Postoperative radiation prolongs the interval to recurrence, prevents tumor regrowth, and improves the survival of some individuals with incompletely resected tumors.[4] Those with malignant meningiomas should receive adjuvant radiation regardless of the extent of resection.[72–74] Although chemotherapy and hormonal therapies have played only a limited and investigational role in the management of meningiomas,[75] there have been some responses to alfa-interferon[76] and hydroxyurea.[77] Other systemic treatment options under investigation include angiogenesis inhibition, meningioma cell growth inhibition, blockage of growth factor effects, inhibition of intracellular secondary pathways, and gene therapy.[78]

Vestibular Schwannomas (Acoustic Neuromas)

Vestibular schwannomas, traditionally called *acoustic neuromas*, are benign tumors arising from the Schwann cells at the vestibular portion of the eighth cranial nerve (vestibulocochlear or acoustic nerve). They account for approximately 8% of all intracranial tumors, occur twice as often in woman, and are found in individuals aged 30–60. With these very slow-growing tumors, symptoms are related to compression and stretching of cranial nerves, causing interference with their function.[79] As the tumor expands from its origin on the vestibular nerve, it extends into the area between the cerebellum, pons, and medulla known as the *cerebellopontine angle*. The cochlear, trigeminal, and facial nerves are compressed. As the tumor continues to grow, it ultimately compresses the cerebellar peduncles, cerebellum, brain stem, and cranial nerves IX, X, and XI (glossopharyngeal, vagus, and spinal accessory nerves).[70] The most common presenting symptom is a unilateral sensorineural hearing loss. Other initial symptoms are tinnitus, vertigo, and disequilibrium. Late clinical features are facial palsy, facial numbness, headache, ataxia, diplopia, dysphagia, and hydrocephalus.[69,70]

Diagnostic tests include audiometry and brain stem auditory evoked potentials followed by magnetic resonance imaging (MRI) with gadolinium. Surgery and radiosurgery are the primary treatment modalities for most individuals with vestibular schwannomas. The goal of surgery is to completely remove the tumor while preserving facial nerve function and hearing. Factors that predict the success of postoperative hearing preservation are preoperative hearing level and tumor size.[80] Because most of these tumors lie around the vestibular portion of the eighth cranial nerve, the nerve may be severed during surgery in an effort to remove the entire tumor;[81] vertigo occurs as a result. For those tumors not completely resected or in individuals who do not undergo surgery, radiosurgery may be used.

Primary Central Nervous System Lymphomas

PCNSL is an aggressive non-Hodgkin's lymphoma that arises within and is confined to the CNS.[82] Until recently, PCNSL had been a rare tumor, accounting for 2% of all intracranial cancers.[83,84] A recent analysis from the Central Brain Tumor Registry reveals that it now represents 6%–7% of all intracranial tumors.[1] Its incidence is increasing in both immunocompetent and immunosuppressed individuals. The number of cases of PCNSL in otherwise healthy individuals has increased sevenfold in recent years.[85] This increase cannot be attributed solely to new and improved diagnostic techniques, the adoption of a uniform classification system, or a similar rise in the number of systemic lymphomas diagnosed.[83,86,87] PCNSL is often associated with acquired or congenital immunosuppression. The highest incidence occurs in patients with AIDS, in whom PCNSL develops in as many as 6% of cases.[82,88] This number may actually be higher, because approximately 40% of AIDS-related PCNSLs are diagnosed only at autopsy.[89–91] PCNSL is the second most common brain lesion and the fourth most common cause of death in AIDS patients.[84] Other populations at risk include organ transplant recipients, individuals with collagen vascular diseases, those with congenital immunodeficiencies, and patients with a previous history of cancer.[92,93]

PCNSL is almost always disseminated within the CNS. The sites involved may include the brain, leptomeninges, eyes, and (rarely) the spinal cord. Ninety-five percent of patients diagnosed with PCNSL have a brain lesion, and 50% of these lesions are multifocal. The lesions are often periventricular and involve the leptomeninges. As a result, seeding within the CSF often occurs. Positive cytology is found in approximately 30% of patients at diagnosis[48], and an additional one-third have a suspicious cytology.[94] The eyes are a direct extension of the nervous system and are involved in as many as 20% of patients at diagnosis. PCNSL may develop in the eye only. Eventually 60%–80% of these patients will go on to develop PCNSL in the brain.[94–96]

These lymphomas are primarily of B-cell origin and are of the intermediate- to high-grade type. PCNSL is a stage I_E lymphoma; that is, it is confined to a single extranodal site. Affected patients show no evidence of a systemic lymphoma. Epstein-Barr virus has been found in pathology specimens of AIDS patients with PCNSL, but it is not yet known what role this pathogen plays in the development of PCNSL.

Most PCNSLs involve the frontal lobes. Diagnostic work-up includes MRI, CSF analysis, ophthalmologic exam, and a work-up to rule out systemic lymphoma. In immunocompetent individuals, PCNSL has a typical appearance on MRI that can help distinguish it from other processes. The lesions are usually multifocal, are uniformly enhanced with contrast, and are located near the ventricles, basal ganglia, and corpus callosum. If a diagnosis is made from positive CSF cytology or a positive biopsy of the vitreous of the eye, a brain biopsy is unnecessary.

PCNSL does not respond well to the standard chemotherapy regimens used in systemic lymphoma.[97] High-dose methotrexate is the single most effective agent against PCNSL and is currently the standard treatment.[48] The most successful regimen to date in immunocompetent individuals has included methotrexate (high-dose and intra-Ommaya), vincristine, and procarbazine followed by focal RT and high-dose cytarabine, for which median survival was reported to be 60 months.[98] Other treatments include a variety of high-dose methotrexate-based regimens, blood–brain barrier (BBB) disruption with mannitol followed by intraarterial and systemic chemotherapy without RT,[99] and the combination of PCV chemotherapy,[100] yielding a mean survival of approximately 3.5 years. High-dose chemotherapy with stem cell rescue has been tried in relapsed patients and produced some responses but a high rate of complications.[101] The combination of cranial RT with chemotherapy, particularly methotrexate, carries an increased risk of delayed neurological toxicity, especially in older individuals. In a follow-up report of individuals treated with intra-Ommaya and high-dose methotrexate, cranial irradiation, and high-dose cytarabine, nearly 80% of one-year survivors older than age 60 developed progressive leukoencephalopathy.[102] It is therefore recommended to avoid the addition of RT to methotrexate in patients older than 60 years, if possible.[48]

Brain Metastases

Brain metastases occur in 20%–40% of individuals with cancer.[48] The incidence of brain metastases is increasing as patients are living longer, better control of systemic cancer becomes possible, and the incidence of cancers that commonly metastasize to the brain (e.g., lung and breast) continues to rise. Other factors contributing to this phenomenon are advances in neuroimaging, use of routine staging tests that assess the CNS, and perhaps the sanctuary effect provided by the

BBB, which may isolate the nervous system tissue from the antitumor effects of systemic chemotherapy.[103]

Brain metastases occur at three sites: the brain parenchyma itself, the skull and dura, and the leptomeninges. Parenchymal brain metastases are found most frequently and occur ten times more often than primary brain tumors.[48] Approximately 170,000 new cases will be diagnosed annually.[104] The majority of brain metastases are a result of hematogenous spread from the primary tumor. Although most cancers can metastasize to the brain, melanoma and cancers of the lung, breast, kidney, colon, and thyroid have a particular propensity to do so.[105] The lung is the most common site of origin. If the primary tumor is not pulmonary, it may have metastasized to the lungs before reaching the brain. In addition, the majority of metastatic brain tumors of unknown primary cancer are of the lung. From the lungs, cancer cells may enter the pulmonary veins and reach the left atrium and ventricle. Tumor cells transported in this manner are widely dispersed and are ultimately deposited in the arterial circulation, where the tumor cells can readily travel to the brain. Breast and lung cancers are prevalent in the population, whereas melanoma accounts for only 1% of all cancers diagnosed. Nevertheless, melanoma has the highest propensity of all systemic cancers to metastasize to the brain. Almost 40% of patients with melanoma develop brain metastases,[106,107] making it — despite the rarity of melanoma as a primary tumor — the third most frequent cause of brain metastases.

When neurological symptoms of brain metastases develop, the individual often has widespread systemic disease. Brain metastases are characterized by severe peritumoral edema, which contributes to the neurological symptoms. The presenting signs and symptoms of metastatic brain disease are dependent upon the lesion's location in the brain and can be identical to those of other space-occupying lesions.

The majority of metastatic brain lesions occur in the cerebral hemispheres (80%), with 15% being found in the cerebellum and 5% in the brain stem.[48] Between 50% and 70% of individuals with brain metastases have multiple lesions.[48,107] Multiple metastatic lesions are often found in melanoma and lung cancer, whereas single lesions tend to occur in colon, breast, and renal cell cancers.[107,108] With early diagnosis and management, brain metastases may respond to therapy. Most individuals benefit from palliative treatment, and an increasing number of patients experience a prolonged remission. Neurological function may be preserved and quality of life maintained. Thus, systemic cancer, rather than neurological disease, usually limits life expectancy.[103,109]

Treatment of brain metastases depends on the number and location of the lesions, the particular type of primary tumor, and the extent of systemic disease present. For many years, whole-brain RT (WBRT) had been the standard treatment for both single and multiple brain metastases. Two randomized prospective studies compared surgery plus WBRT with WBRT alone in patients with single metastases.[110,111] Those patients who underwent surgery plus WBRT lived longer, maintained a higher performance status and improved quality of life for a longer period of time, and had fewer recurrences compared to those receiving WBRT alone. Surgery is now considered the first therapeutic option for single brain metastases when feasible.[105,106] Postoperative RT is often recommended. Patients with multiple (2–4) lesions may also be considered for surgery. Bindel and colleagues compared a group of individuals who had multiple lesions resected to a group who had some lesions left unresected.[112] Survival in patients who had all metastases resected was longer than in the group who had lesions left unresected. Surgery should be considered if one lesion is causing a life-threatening herniation, hemorrhage, or hydrocephalus. Unfortunately, nearly 50% of patients are not candidates for surgery because of the inaccessibility of the tumor(s), extensive systemic disease, or other factors.[48] These individuals are generally treated with radiosurgery or WBRT. Retrospective comparisons suggest that survival is comparable for individuals treated with radiosurgery and those who receive the combination of surgery and WBRT,[104,113,114] although no prospective randomized trials have examined the two on a head-to-head basis. Some physicians advocate radiosurgery instead of surgery. Although multiple metastases have been treated effectively with radiosurgery,[115] this option is contraindicated for large tumors. At times, radiosurgery may be used as a planned boost therapy after WBRT or may be used to treat recurrences or new metastases after prior WBRT. For individuals whose extent of systemic or intracranial cancer makes them poor candidates for either surgery or radiosurgery, WBRT may be indicated as a palliative measure.[104]

Chemotherapy is rarely used as primary therapy for brain metastases.[48] Many tumors that metastasize to the brain, such as non-small cell lung cancer, melanoma, and unknown primary cancer, are often resistant to chemotherapy.[48,105] Adjuvant chemotherapy may be considered for individuals with more chemosensitive tumors (e.g., germ cell, breast, and small cell lung cancers). Chemotherapy has been combined with WBRT in an attempt to improve the outcome compared with either modality alone. Survival was longer in patients with brain metastases from small cell lung cancer treated with teniposide and WBRT compared to WBRT alone,[116] and in patients treated with temozolomide and WBRT compared to temozolomide alone.[117]

Chemotherapy may also be useful in the setting of recurrent brain metastases.[118]

Tumors that metastasize to bone—particularly metastatic tumors of the breast, prostate, and lung+1—may infiltrate the skull or dura by direct extension and compress the venous sinuses or underlying brain tissue. Treatment may consist of RT, surgical resection, or both.

Leptomeningeal metastasis, once thought to be a rare complication of cancer, is increasing in frequency. Also known as meningeal carcinomatosis, it entails a diffuse or multifocal seeding of cancer cells throughout the meninges and CSF. The seeding pattern of growth covers the surface of the brain and spinal cord. Leptomeningeal metastasis is usually an indication of progressive systemic cancer.

Although the exact incidence of leptomeningeal metastasis is difficult to determine, studies have found an overall incidence as high as 8%.[107] While any systemic cancer can seed the meninges, the cancers most commonly leading to meningeal carcinomatosis are leukemia, lymphoma, melanoma, and breast, lung, and gastrointestinal (GI) cancers. The incidence of meningeal involvement from leukemia has decreased, while the incidence of leptomeningeal metastasis from breast and lung cancer is increasing. Diagnosis is established by close examination of the CSF and MRI of the brain and spinal cord. Repeated lumbar punctures (LPs) are often required to identify malignant cells in the CSF. Treatment includes radiation to symptomatic areas only, because radiation to the entire neuroaxis leads to bone marrow depression. This RT is followed by chemotherapy administered directly into the CSF. Chemotherapy can be injected directly into the lateral ventricle of the brain by using an Ommaya reservoir, thereby ensuring optimal consistent CSF levels. Common chemotherapeutic agents include methotrexate, cytarabine, and thiotepa. Reports of median survival range from 7 to 24 weeks.[107]

Pattern of Spread

The pattern of spread noted with brain tumors differs from that found with other cancers. While brain tumors may spread to other parts of the CNS, metastases outside the brain and spinal cord are rare. Metastases outside the CNS may occur when tumor cells are transferred to the scalp, cerebral blood vessels, or dural sinus during an operative procedure. Once they invade the cerebral blood vessels, tumor cells enter the circulation. The CNS does not contain lymphatic vessels,[107,119] but once the tumor cells have traveled outside the CNS, they can spread by way of the lymphatic system.[120] The spread of glial tumor cells through ventriculopleural and VP shunts has also been reported.

Brain tumors grow by expansion, infiltration, or both. Although gliomas invade locally, cells can sometimes be found at intracranial sites distant from the main tumor, making many of these lesions seem multifocal. Brain tumors may seed the CSF and spread through the subarachnoid space. Seeding occurs along the surface of the brain and spinal cord, and "drop metastases" can occur. Some tumors, including PCNSLs, ependymomas, and medulloblastomas, seed the CSF more often than others.

Most metastatic brain tumors develop from hematogenous spread of tumor cells, usually through the arterial circulation. In some cases, tumor cells may reach the brain by way of Batson's plexus, which is a valveless system of veins that runs the length of the vertebral column from the pelvic veins to the large venous sinuses of the skull.[37]

Clinical Manifestations

The clinical manifestations of a brain tumor can vary tremendously from one individual to another and among different types of tumors. The particular signs and symptoms with which an individual presents depend on the location, size, type, method of expansion, and rate of tumor growth. The clinical manifestations can be divided into three major categories: generalized effects of increased ICP, focal effects, and effects caused by displacement of brain structures. Often a combination of these effects produces signs and symptoms simultaneously.

Generalized Effects of Increased Intracranial Pressure

Brain tumors increase ICP by their size, cerebral edema, or obstruction of CSF pathways. The presence of increased ICP and the speed at which it develops can vary. In some locations of the brain, a very small tumor can lead to marked elevations of ICP. In other areas of the brain, by contrast, large, extensive tumors may not initially cause ICP to rise. A rapidly developing tumor with extensive edema will raise ICP sooner than a slower-growing lesion with little edema.

Signs and symptoms result from the effects of increasing pressure on nerve cells, blood vessels, and the dura. Sustained increases in ICP ultimately cause nerve cell damage and cell death. An expanding tumor (or other space-occupying lesion) can create a vicious cycle of intracranial hypertension (Figure 47-5). After the brain's normal compensatory mechanisms have been exhausted, the increased ICP results in a decreased CBF. A reduction in the brain's blood

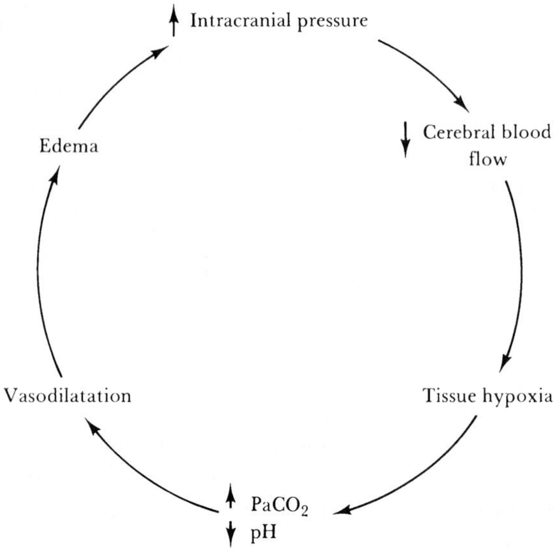

Figure 47-5 Cycle of intracranial hypertension.

supply leads to tissue hypoxia because the brain does not receive sufficient oxygen. The diminished blood supply also interferes with the removal of CO_2 and lactic acid. These metabolic by-products act as potent vasodilators. Vasodilation of the cerebral blood vessels leads to further edema. As a result, the total volume within the cranium increases, ICP rises further, and the cycle repeats itself.[37]

The signs and symptoms of increased ICP include change in the level of consciousness or cognition, headache, motor and sensory deficits, pupillary changes and papilledema, vomiting, and changes in vital signs.

Level of consciousness can be an extremely sensitive index of neurological status[35] and ranges from alert and oriented, restless, confused, unable to follow simple commands, lethargic, to comatose. An individual may have short-term memory loss, impaired judgment, difficulty concentrating, or be forgetful. He or she may be drowsy or exhibit personality changes or diminished cognitive ability. Sleeping more is the most commonly reported early sign of the tumor. Many of the initial changes have a gradual onset and can be so subtle that they are evident only to the family or a skilled observer.[37] Families report that the individual just isn't himself or herself.

Headache is a common presenting symptom. The location and characteristics of the headache must be evaluated to distinguish them from other common types of headache. The headache is usually bilateral in the frontal, temporal, or retroorbital areas. Typically, the pain occurs in the early morning, subsides after arising, and recurs the following morning. The pain can be described as dull, sharp, or throbbing. Some individuals complain of an uncomfortable feeling in the head rather than a headache. Bending over, coughing, or performing a valsalva maneuver often aggravates or initiates the pain. The headaches gradually increase in frequency, duration, and severity until, in the later stages, they are almost constant.

Motor signs of increased ICP may include hemiparesis or hemiplegia on the contralateral (opposite) side of the tumor, diminished reflexes, or development of pathological reflexes. Decorticate and decerebrate posturing can occur in the late stages of increased ICP when the diencephalon and brain stem become compressed. Decorticate posturing is an abnormal flexion of the arms with extension of the legs. Decerebrate posturing is an abnormal extension of the arms and legs. Sensory symptoms consist of impaired sensation, inability to interpret sensory information, or both.

Papilledema is considered a cardinal sign of increased ICP, but it may be a late finding. The edema of the optic disk results from compression around the optic nerve impeding the outflow of venous blood. A trained individual using an ophthalmoscope should assess for the presence of papilledema. Other visual signs and symptoms can occur including blurry vision, visual field deficits, and changes in pupillary size and reaction to light.

Vomiting as a sign of increased ICP occurs more commonly in children and in those with infratentorial tumors.[4] It may be preceded by nausea, or it may be sudden, unexpected, and projectile. Vomiting is not related to eating. Increased pressure on the medulla is believed to precipitate this symptom.[37]

Changes in vital signs occur late in the course of increased ICP. They result from increased pressure on the medulla. Systolic blood pressure (SBP) rises and diastolic blood pressure (DBP) drops, widening the pulse pressure. Bradycardia and an abnormal respiratory pattern (usually slowed and irregular respirations) develop. This combination of hypertension, bradycardia, and abnormal respirations, referred to as *Cushing's triad,* is a very late sign of increased ICP. By the time Cushing's triad is identified, the patient is usually already comatose.

Focal Effects

Intracranial tumors may also cause localized or focal signs and symptoms of neurological dysfunction. Specific anatomical areas in the CNS have unique functions, and the neurological deficits produced are directly related to the area involved. Performing a careful neurological examination and possessing knowledge of neuroanatomy and neurophysiology help in identifying the location of a lesion based on the neurological findings (see Table 47-1).

Tumors of the frontal lobe can lead to inability to concentrate, inattentiveness, difficulty with abstraction, impaired memory, personality changes, quiet flat affect, inappropriate behavior, lack of social control, indifference, emotional lability, and loss of initiative. To complicate the situation, the individual may be unaware that his or her behavior has changed or is inappropriate.[121] Tumors in the posterior portion of the frontal lobe can result in hemiparesis or hemiplegia on the contralateral side of the tumor. Deep-tendon reflexes increase on the paretic side, and a positive Babinski sign is present. Broca's area is located in the frontal lobe. Damage to this area in the dominant hemisphere results in the inability to express oneself in words even though the individual may comprehend speech and language. Broca's aphasia has been referred to as *expressive aphasia* and can be extremely frustrating for individuals.

Most people have one cerebral hemisphere that is more developed or dominant than the other with respect to language. In right-handed and most left-handed individuals, the dominant hemisphere is the left. This is important to distinguish because the left side of the brain controls language. The right hemisphere is the nonverbal or perceptual hemisphere, which processes temporospatial information.

Parietal lobe tumors affect sensory and perceptual functions more than motor function, although mild hemiparesis is sometimes seen with these tumors.[4] Common symptoms include impaired sensation, paresthesias, loss of two-point discrimination, inability to recognize an object by feeling its size and shape (astereognosis), inability to locate or recognize parts of the body (autotopagnosia), loss of awareness or denial of a motor or sensory defect in the affected body part (anosognosia), inability to write (agraphia) or to calculate numbers (acalculia), and inability to execute learned movements in the absence of weakness or paralysis (apraxia).

Tumors of the temporal lobe can cause impairment of recent memory, aggressive behavior, and psychomotor seizures. Involvement of the dominant side can lead to an inability to recall names (dysnomia), impaired perception of verbal commands, and Wernicke's or receptive aphasia. In this type of aphasia, the patient speaks easily, appears to be making an effort to communicate, and is easily engaged in conversation. However, little meaning is conveyed. The individual does not understand what is being said. He or she may speak in phrases or complete sentences, but the listener is usually unable to make sense of the content. *Receptive aphasia* can make patient teaching extremely difficult. The meeting point of the temporal, occipital, and parietal lobes is called the *interpretive area.* Cognitive function will be significantly altered by damage to this area in the dominant hemisphere.[121]

Occipital lobe tumors produce visual symptoms, including homonymous hemianopsia (visual loss in half of each visual field on the contralateral side of the lesion) and visual hallucinations. Tumors located in this area can also interfere with the ability to interpret what is seen. Tumors located in or near the thalamus can lead to hydrocephalus, sensory disturbances, paresthesias, neuropathic pain, emotional lability, and sleep pattern disturbances. Hypothalamic tumors lead to endocrine dysfunction. These tumors can also affect water metabolism, appetite, sexual behavior, and regulation of body temperature, the sleep-wake cycle, and the autonomic nervous system.

Brain stem tumors can produce dire consequences, because the centers that control respiration and heart rate are located here. The points of origin of cranial nerves III through XII are also located here, and dysfunction is common. Multiple nerve fiber tracts in the brain stem allow transmission of nerve impulses between the cerebral hemispheres and the spinal cord.

Tumors located in the cerebellum have a classic presentation. Individuals may have a wide-based ataxic gait, a dysarthric speech pattern, and nystagmus. They may exhibit clumsiness, balance difficulty, or tremors. Symptoms of increased ICP are often present.

Seizures — another common clinical manifestation in both primary and metastatic brain tumors — are seen primarily with supratentorial tumors. They may occur in 70%–90% of individuals with low-grade astrocytomas and oligodendrogliomas, 50% of individuals with melanoma, and 20%–30% of individuals with other tumor types. Seizures may be the initial presenting symptom in a number of patients, sometimes occurring months to years before the clinical diagnosis is made. Focal or partial seizures involve a particular area of the brain, whereas generalized seizures involve both cerebral hemispheres. Focal seizures can aid in localizing the tumor, depending on the pattern of seizure activity.

Displacement of Brain Structures

Pressure is normally distributed equally between the supratentorial and infratentorial compartments. A growing tumor mass and the associated edema cause pressure to increase within the compartment. Once the brain's compensatory mechanisms are exhausted, the increased pressure can cause the brain tissue in the high-pressure compartment to protrude into the lower-pressure compartment. This process, called *herniation,* is a life-threatening neurological emergency.[37]

The shifting brain tissue compresses other neural tissue and structures, further increases the edema, causes ischemia from damage to blood vessels, and can obstruct CSF pathways, leading to hydrocephalus. These compressive, ischemic, vascular, and obstructive changes all add to and aggravate the original problem of increased ICP.

Abnormal clinical signs usually follow an orderly progression. Careful neurological assessment in patients at risk for herniation may facilitate early identification of this potentially life-threatening complication. However, herniation can occur with little warning. A sudden change in the ICP or contents (as in an acute hemorrhage or the performance of an LP) will rapidly lead to brain stem compression.

There are two major classifications of herniation: supratentorial and infratentorial. Supratentorial tumors can lead to cingulate, uncal, or central transtentorial herniation. Herniation of the cingulate gyrus under the falx cerebri compresses the contralateral frontal lobe and the anterior cerebral arteries. Such herniation can cause bilateral frontal lobe ischemia, urinary incontinence, leg weakness, and mental status changes. The diencephalon is shifted to the contralateral side, compresses itself and the third ventricle, and leads to diminished consciousness.[107]

Uncal herniation, usually occurring with expanding temporal lobe tumors, forces the temporal lobe (the uncus) into the tentorial notch. The midbrain is compressed laterally. The third cranial nerve, the posterior cerebral artery, and the diencephalon are compressed. Compression of the third cranial nerve, the oculomotor nerve, initially causes the ipsilateral pupil to sluggishly react to light. With further compression, the pupil dilates and becomes unreactive. With midbrain compression, the motor pathways of the cerebral peduncle produce a contralateral hemiparesis. A positive Babinski sign may be seen with the hemiparesis. The enlarging mass also shifts the diencephalon, leading to a progressive loss of consciousness beginning with drowsiness and proceeding to stupor and finally to coma.[107] Compression of the posterior cerebral artery can cause ischemia or infarction of the ipsilateral occipital lobe. Later findings in uncal herniation include decorticate followed by decerebrate posturing, and impaired oculocephalic and oculovestibular reflexes. Oculocephalic reflexes are tested by holding the patient's eyelids open and briskly rotating the head from side to side or by briskly flexing and extending the neck (doll's eyes phenomenon). Oculovestibular reflexes are tested by injecting ice water into the external ear canal. In the comatose patient, testing these reflexes assesses for the presence of brain stem function.

Central or transtentorial herniation results from the downward displacement of the cerebral hemispheres and basal ganglia onto the diencephalon and midbrain, which are then forced through the tentorial notch. Initially, there will be a change in the level of consciousness or behavior. The person becomes drowsy, inattentive, or agitated. Pupil size is reduced. There may be deep sighing or yawning with respirations.[35] As the tumor continues to displace tissue downward, the individual becomes stuporous and eventually comatose. Pupils become nonreactive, eye movements disconjugate, and, as the brain stem becomes compressed, decorticate posturing deteriorates to decerebrate in response to noxious stimuli. Oculocephalic and oculovestibular reflexes may be absent.

Both central and uncal herniations cause changes in the respiratory pattern. Irregular depth and rhythm often are more significant than changes in respiratory rate alone. Initially, respirations may be irregular with occasional pauses, sighs, or gasps. Later respiratory pattern changes include Cheyne-Stokes breathing, sustained hyperventilation, ataxic breathing, apnea, and finally respiratory arrest.[37] The classic vital sign changes of Cushing's triad are seen during the terminal phase of herniation.

Infratentorial herniation results from tumors of the posterior fossa, leading to displacement of the cerebellum either upward through the opening in the tentorium cerebelli or downward through the foramen magnum. In upward transtentorial herniation, the cerebellum compresses the midbrain. Obstruction and blockage of CSF pathways may occur. The individual may lose consciousness immediately. This event may be accompanied by hyperventilation; pinpoint, fixed, and unequal pupils; upward-gaze paralysis; vomiting; and decerebration.[35]

Downward cerebellar tonsillar herniation is more common and results in the downward protrusion of the cerebellar tonsils through the foramen magnum. The lower brain stem is compressed; when the compression is acute, it can cause sudden loss of consciousness followed by respiratory arrest. This may be precipitated by events causing a sudden rise in ICP such as sneezing, coughing, or performing a valsalva maneuver. The outflow of CSF from the fourth ventricle becomes blocked, leading to obstructive hydrocephalus. Other signs include lower cranial nerve dysfunction, suboccipital headache, vomiting, and neck pain. Altered consciousness with resulting coma may be an early sign. Later signs of medullary compression include abnormal respiratory patterns, fluctuating blood pressure and heart rate, and cardiac dysrhythmias. In both types of infratentorial herniation, respiratory arrest, cardiac arrest, or both will occur if the condition goes untreated. Figure 47-6 illustrates the herniation syndromes.

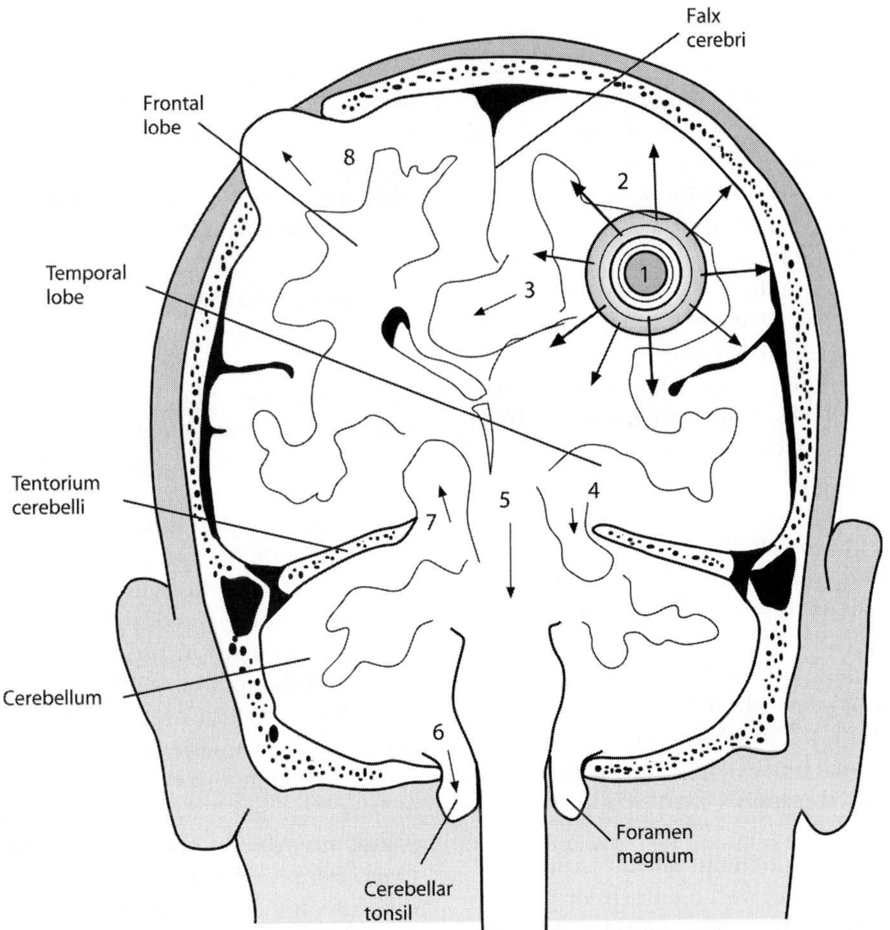

Figure 47-6 Herniation syndromes. (1) Tumor. (2) Edema. (3) Cingulate herniation. (4) Uncal herniation. (5) Central transtentorial herniation. (6) Downward cerebellar tonsillar herniation. (7) Upward herniation of the cerebellum. (8) Herniation through a cranial defect.

Assessment

Assessment of the individual with a known or suspected brain tumor begins by obtaining the individual's medical history. The description and duration of symptoms, when they occur, the presence of exacerbating or relieving factors, and the order of their appearance are assessed. This assessment is followed by a complete neurological examination. An initial neurological assessment is essential because it provides a baseline knowledge of the individual's neurological function. Future assessments will be evaluated in comparison with the initial examination, allowing the detection of any changes or abnormalities.

The neurological exam begins with an assessment of the patient's level of consciousness and mental status. In most instances the first, earliest, and most sensitive indicator of dysfunction will be a change in the level of consciousness. The individual whose level of consciousness is impaired must be sufficiently stimulated to be able to appropriately describe the degree of alteration. Levels of alteration ranging from full consciousness to deep coma may occur. Common descriptions include alert and oriented, confused, lethargic, stuporous, obtunded, semicomatose, and comatose. Many institutions have included components of the Glasgow Coma Scale, a tool that assesses neurological function in comatose patients, as part of their neurological assessment form.

Conversing with and observing the individual evaluates mental status and cognitive ability. One should note the person's behavior, appearance, mood, and affect. Observation of actions, posture, facial expressions, and responses to the conversation and environment provide information regarding general cerebral function. Orientation, general knowledge, recent and remote memory, attention span, immediate recall, abstract reasoning, and judgment are also part of the assessment of cognitive function. Language is evaluated for content, flow of speech, speech patterns, and comprehension. The presence of aphasia (the inability to understand or express one's own language), agnosia (the inability to recognize common objects through the senses of sight, touch, and sound), and apraxia (the inability to perform a skilled motor act in the absence of weakness or paralysis) is noted. Mental status changes often go unnoticed by patients. For this reason, family members, significant others, or work colleagues may initially identify a problem. They can often provide valuable information regarding the onset and progression of symptoms.

Motor and sensory functions are also evaluated. A motor exam assesses whether the individual moves normally or abnormally, what the level of response is, and how strong both the upper and lower extremities are against gravity and resistance. This exam also tests gait, posture, and reflexes. Sensation is assessed by introducing various stimuli to different parts of the body with the eyes closed. Light touch, pain, temperature, and position sense are evaluated bilaterally.

Assessment of cerebellar function focuses on the ability to coordinate movement and to maintain normal muscle tone and equilibrium. The person is asked to perform the finger-to-finger, finger-to-nose, hand patting, Romberg, and tandem walking tests.

Testing of cranial nerve function can be the most intimidating portion of the neurological assessment. The 12 pairs of cranial nerves, their function, method of testing, and desired response are listed in Table 47-2.

The performance of the initial assessment is equally important for the person with recurrent or progressive disease. Changes in the neurological assessment, the development of new symptoms, or both can indicate increased ICP, recurrent disease, or side effects of treatment. Any change in symptom characteristics should be identified, along with possible exacerbating or relieving factors. Seizures are another area that warrants investigation. The nurse determines whether the individual has experienced seizures, what the frequency and pattern of occurrence are, and whether the person experiences an aura before the seizure.

Diagnostic Studies

Developments in neuroimaging have dramatically improved the ability to diagnose, localize, and treat individuals with brain tumors. Computerized tomography (CT) and MRI are the standard imaging techniques. Positron emission tomography (PET) and single-photon emission computed tomography (SPECT) are being used to distinguish tumor from radiation necrosis and to increase the understanding of the metabolism of malignant tumors.[122]

Computerized tomography. CT scan allows differentiation between bone, brain tissue, and CSF.[35,123] It is highly sensitive to blood within the brain and is the technique of choice for evaluating the presence of acute hemorrhage. A CT scan can be used to evaluate skull metastases and other bony pathology,[124] because bony structures are extremely well visualized on CT. This type of study can be performed more rapidly than MRI, an important consideration in emergency situations or when sedation may be contraindicated.[37,125]

Magnetic resonance imaging. MRI is the more definitive and preferred imaging study for the individual with a brain tumor. It provides much better resolution than a CT scan and more clearly differentiates between solid tumor, edema, and fluid collection. MRI provides superior definition of the borders of a brain tumor, and the extent of the tumor and its invasiveness can be better demonstrated by MRI.[125] The use of paramagnetic agents such as gadolinium-DTPA allows for contrast scanning with minimal risk of allergic complications or renal toxicity,[12] results in remarkable improvement in the image resolution, and illustrates BBB breakdown.[123,126]

MRI also demonstrates an increased sensitivity for small (< 1 cm) lesions[37] and can detect CT-occult tumors.[103] Such a study may show multiple metastatic lesions that the CT demonstrated as a single one. MRI is also superior to CT scan in imaging the posterior fossa, because bone artifact is not present in MRI. Likewise, it can more readily identify leptomeningeal metastases.

Positron emission tomography. PET is a functional imaging technique that may also be used in individuals with brain tumors, specifically malignant gliomas. This technique provides dynamic information on CBF and metabolism rather than the precise anatomical localization seen in MRI. PET combines the properties of nuclear scanning with physical characteristics of positron-emitting isotopes of naturally occurring atoms.[37,124] Radioactive isotopes produced in a cyclotron are incorporated into a chosen brain metabolite and injected intravenously. These isotopes disintegrate and form a positively charged electron (a positron). The positron travels until it comes together with an electron; the pair are then converted to a pair of photons traveling in opposite directions. A ring of collimators surrounding the individual's head records these events, computers calculate measurements, and a reconstruction algorithm produces an axial view of brain uptake. Also, by monitoring the arterial concentration of radioactivity via an arterial line, the absolute metabolic rate of areas in the brain can be calculated.[124]

Most PET studies have used ^{18}F-fluorodeoxyglucose (FDG), a fluorinated glucose analog, to measure glucose metabolism, which is increased in tumor cells.[122,127] The amount of FDG uptake correlates with the degree of malignancy— that is, low-grade gliomas tend to have lower uptake (hypometabolic) and malignant gliomas have higher uptake (hypermetabolic). In addition to determining tumor grade, this technique has become the standard imaging modality to distinguish between tumor recurrence and radiation necrosis. PET scans are useful in guiding stereotactic needle biopsies and, in the future, may provide a more relevant measure of early treatment response.[128]

Single-emission photon computed tomography. SPECT, another functional imaging technique, is used to differentiate high-grade from low-grade tumors and malignant from nonmalignant brain lesions.[128] This technique involves the IV administration of isotopes taken up by the brain and tumor cells. These isotopes emit photons, which are then detected by a rotating gamma camera. Regions of intense thallium uptake usually represent active solid tumor recurrence, whereas low thallium uptake generally indicates the presence of radiation necrosis. This technique has also been shown to be effective in distinguishing the presence of infiltrating tumor from solid tumor[124] and in differentiating between tumor and infection in HIV-positive individuals.[43]

Functional magnetic resonance imaging. Specific areas of brain function can be identified using functional MRI (fMRI). This type of study identifies focal changes in cerebral blood flow in response to repetition of specific tasks so as to accurately localize specific areas of the brain in relation to the tumor. The changes result in an increased signal intensity on MRI.[129] This technique is helpful for presurgical planning to enable maximal tumor resection while avoiding areas of critical neurological function such as language, motor, and sensory areas.

Angiography. Cerebral angiography may be used to confirm that the lesion in question is a vascular malformation or an aneurysm rather than a neoplasm. In other situations (e.g., with large meningiomas), angiography may be useful before surgery to determine the blood supply so that it can be embolized during the angiography procedure, obliterated during the surgical procedure, or both.[4] Cerebral angiography involves percutaneous puncture of the femoral artery with injection of radiopaque medium to visualize the cerebral vasculature. Magnetic resonance angiography (MRA) has largely replaced invasive intraarterial angiography.

Lumbar puncture. CSF is often examined for malignant cells in individuals with tumors such as medulloblastomas, ependymomas, and PCNSLs, all of which have the propensity to seed the subarachnoid space and spread throughout the CSF pathways. Such studies are also evaluated in individuals with known or suspected leptomeningeal metastases. An LP should be performed after neuroimaging studies such as MRI and CT scan, especially in an individual with a suspected tumor, because of the risk of herniation.[130]

Prognostic Indicators

The prognosis for an individual with a brain tumor varies considerably depending on the specific type and location of the tumor. Generally, the prognosis for an intracranial malignant glioma, the most common adult primary brain tumor, is dismal. However, several important prognostic factors have been identified that may affect the eventual outcome. Young age, lower histological grade, and high performance status are favorable prognostic indicators for astrocytomas.[131] In adults, younger patients do better and live longer than older patients even when adjusted for the other prognostic factors. Age appears to be a more important prognostic indicator than even histology.[132] The more aggressive tumors, or those with a higher histological grade, have a poorer prognosis. For example, individuals with anaplastic astrocytoma have a significantly better prognosis than those with GBM. The prognosis of individuals with high-grade gliomas, as with most of the CNS tumors, decreases as their functional status decreases. Those who have severe neurological deficits or are debilitated generally do not tolerate treatment as well as those with a higher performance status. They are also more susceptible to complications.

The extent of surgical resection may be another important prognostic factor. Most of the retrospective studies have demonstrated a delay in tumor recurrence and an increased survival for those individuals undergoing a complete surgical resection compared with those having a partial resection or biopsy alone.[131,133] Although this may not be universally accepted, the recent trend in the literature has been to support the strategy of removing as much tumor as possible in both malignant gliomas[134] and low-grade gliomas.[135] The extent of tumor resection is also an important prognostic indicator for other types of tumors. For example, completely excised meningiomas and acoustic neuromas have lower recurrence rates.

Approximately 2% of patients with glioblastoma have been reported to survive at least five years.[136–138] In these patients, long-term survival was associated with young age, good preoperative and postoperative KPS, extensive tumor resection, multimodality therapy, and a prolonged relapse-free period. Currently, no clinical or pathological characteristics identify GBM patients destined for long-term survival;[137] however, the importance of patient age suggests that the biological features of GBM, such as a specific set of genetic abnormalities, could be the main determinant of survival.[138]

Brain metastases are generally associated with a poor prognosis. However, more favorable outcomes are associated with a high KPS, absent or controlled primary tumor, age younger than 60, metastatic spread limited to the brain, and a single surgically accessible lesion.[130,139]

Classification and Staging

CNS neoplasms represent a diverse heterogeneous group of primary and metastatic tumors of the brain and spinal cord. The classification of CNS tumors is based on the premise that each type of tumor results from the abnormal growth of a specific cell type. The consistent naming and grouping of similar tumor types are extremely important when gathering information and statistics on the incidence, etiology, effectiveness of treatment, and prognosis of CNS tumors.

The most critical feature in the classification of CNS tumors is histopathology.[140] The World Health Organization (WHO) first characterizes a CNS tumor histologically by its cell of origin and then designates a grade based on its similarity to normal cells. Grading assesses the degree of malignancy or aggressiveness of the tumor cells by comparing the cellular anaplasia, differentiation, and mitotic activity with those of the cells' normal counterparts.[141,142] Tumor classification has clinical implications, dictates the choice of therapy, and predicts prognosis.

Therapeutic Approaches and Nursing Care

Conventional treatment of the high-grade gliomas is usually a combination of surgery, RT, and chemotherapy. Low-grade gliomas and most benign tumors are generally treated with surgery and, in some cases, RT. The therapy for recurrent tumors is based on the types of therapy that the individual has already received.

Surgery

Surgery remains the initial treatment for the majority of individuals with brain tumors. Recent technical advances in neuroanesthesia, neuroimaging, and instrumentation have made the surgical treatment of brain tumors safer and more effective. The goal of surgery is often multipurpose: to establish a diagnosis by providing tissue for histological examination; to provide relief of symptoms by quickly reducing the tumor bulk; and to alleviate ICP and the mass effect caused by compression or infiltration of brain tissue. As a result of the decreased mass effect, patients may tolerate RT better and experience fewer side effects[143] because room now exists for the edema that may develop with RT and tumor recurrence.[144] Decreasing the tumor burden may also increase the effectiveness of adjuvant therapies by decreasing the number of tumor cells that must be treated, altering cell kinetics, removing radioresistant hypoxic cells, and removing areas of the tumor inaccessible to chemotherapy.[145] Because low-grade tumors often evolve into higher-grade tumors, reducing the tumor bulk decreases the number of tumor cells remaining that may be at risk for malignant transformation.[143]

When evaluating an individual for surgery, many factors must be considered: size and location of the tumor, relationship of the tumor to functional brain regions, presence of widespread or multiple sites of disease, and the individual's age and neurological status. For example, a tumor with well-defined margins or one that is encapsulated in the nondominant hemisphere lends itself to an extensive resection. A rapidly growing infiltrative tumor that extends across the midline and is located in a deep vital structure or within the motor or sensory cortex may not be completely excised. In such a case, a biopsy or partial resection may be a safer option than a radical procedure. PCNSL, a tumor often widely disseminated throughout the CNS, is not usually surgically resected. This tumor is often best managed by biopsy only, followed by adjuvant therapy. Careful preoperative planning is the most important factor in minimizing neurological complications.[146]

Biopsy. The goal of biopsy is to provide the neuropathologist with a representative sampling of the lesion with which to establish a histological diagnosis. Stereotactic biopsy is the most precise means of obtaining a tissue sample and is the most widely used method today. Stereotaxis precisely locates areas in the brain using three-dimensional coordinates without direct visual access. Using a stereotactic frame (Figure 47-7),[147] the patient's head is secured to the head ring, with four percutaneous skull pins to provide rigid skull fixation. A localizing cage composed of vertical and diagonal graphite rods is secured in the head ring, and a CT or MRI is performed. The lesion is referenced to the nine *x*- and *y*-coordinates of the localizing cage, and these points are transformed to create a three-dimensional space. The localizing cage is removed, and in the operating room a sterile arc

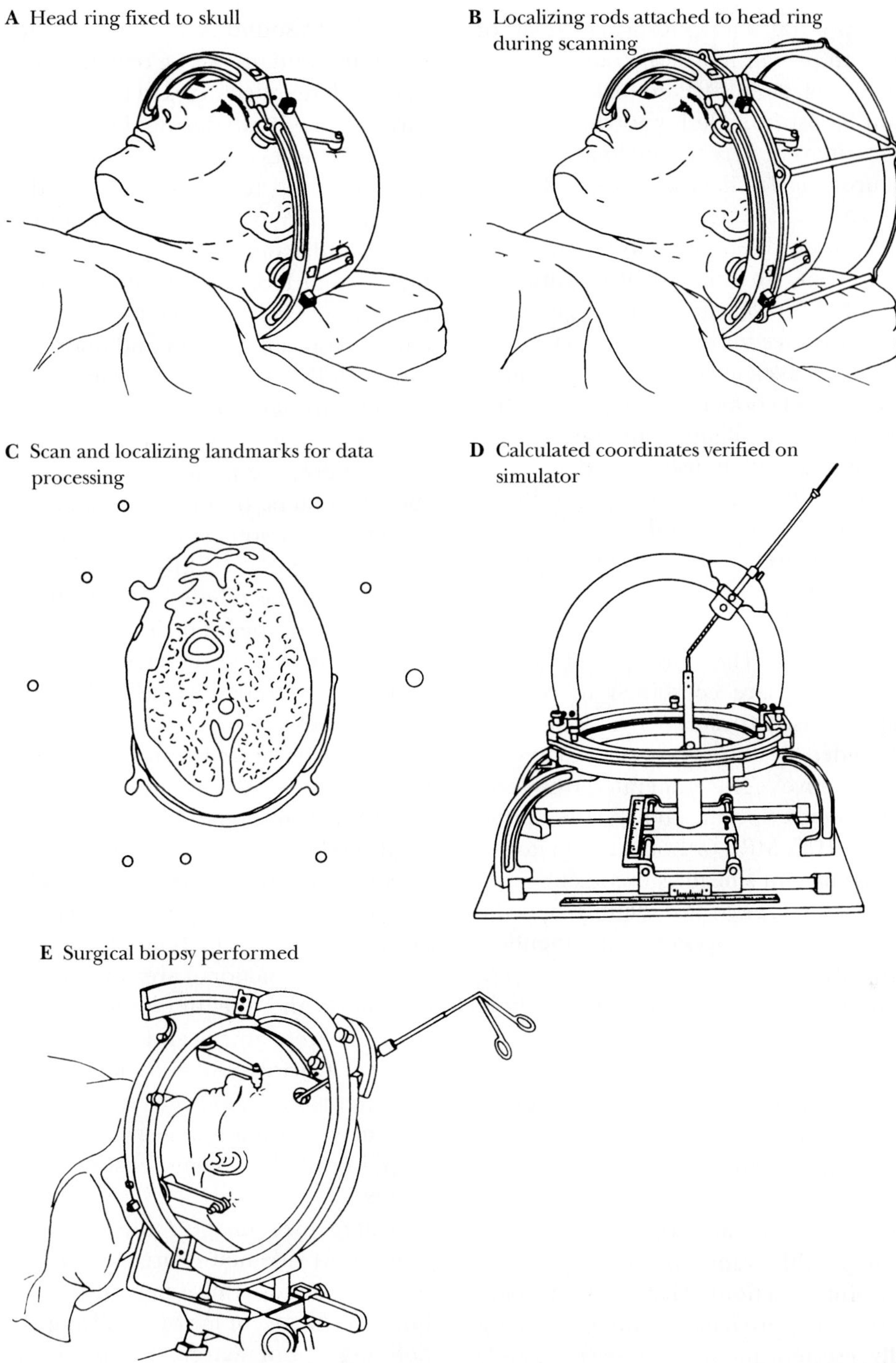

Figure 47-7 Stereotaxic surgery. Diagrams show the sequence of steps using the BRW stereotaxic guidance system. **(A)** The head ring is fixed to the skull. **(B)** The localizing rod system is attached to the head ring for scanning. **(C)** A sample localizing scan from which *x-y* coordinates of nine localizing rod and intracranial target images are determined for computation by the calculator. **(D)** Computed arc settings are verified for correct trajectory and depth to target on the simulator. **(E)** Arc guidance system is attached to the head ring, and intracranial procedure is performed. (Reprinted with permission from Heilbrun MP, Roberts TS, Apuzzo MLJ, et al: Preliminary experience with Brown-Roberts-Wells (BWR) computerized tomography stereotaxic guidance system. *J Neurosurg* 59:217-222, 1983.[147])

guidance system is fixed to the head ring. The center of the arc depicts the target lesion, which can be approached from any angle or point on the arc quadrant. The biopsy probe or needle is accurately directed to within 1–2 mm of the target.[126,134] In this way, the needle or probe can be guided to the target along the safest pathway (i.e., one that avoids major vascular and functional structures).[144]

Stereotactic biopsy has a diagnostic accuracy of greater than 95%, an overall morbidity rate of 3.2%, and a mortality rate of 0.6%.[148] Potential complications after a brain biopsy include hemorrhage at the biopsy site, exacerbation of cerebral edema, development of a new neurological deficit, seizures, and infection.

Because they report discomfort with the head frame during placement, patients usually require premedication. In adults, stereotactic biopsy is generally performed under local anesthesia. This approach may decrease complications associated with general anesthesia but requires patient cooperation to perform the procedure. The need for patient cooperation with these systems discourages their use in pediatric patients and patients with dementia,[149] who typically require general anesthesia. Associated mortality and morbidity may be decreased with stereotactic procedures and hospital stays may be shorter.

Stereotactic resection. The concepts of stereotaxis and radical surgery are combined to remove tumors in computer-assisted stereotactic resection. The surgeon is guided by three-dimensional reconstructions of the operative region generated from preoperative imaging studies. Specific coordinates on the preoperative images (CT, MRI, or both) are matched to landmarks on the patient's head (stereotactic registration), allowing the surgeon to identify specific points on the image as corresponding to identical points in the operative field.[105] Stereotactic craniotomies may be useful for small deep tumors or multiple brain metastases.

Craniotomy. The goal of brain tumor surgery is to remove the tumor completely while preserving neurological function.[150] Surgical cure is often not possible, however, as in the case of most gliomas. Recent advances in neurosurgical and monitoring techniques allow most individuals with brain tumors today to safely undergo successful resections. Many tumors traditionally considered unapproachable are now being biopsied, partially resected, and sometimes completely removed with success. The advances that make these successes possible include intraoperative monitoring; interactive, image-guided, frameless stereotactic systems; and intraoperative MRI. Major neurological morbidity has been reduced to 8.5% and mortality to 1.7% for patients undergoing craniotomy for tumor removal.[143]

Intraoperative monitoring includes intraoperative ultrasound (IOUS) and brain mapping techniques. With IOUS, the surgeon receives immediate feedback during the craniotomy and views images that assist in the maximal resection of the tumor. A major advantage of ultrasound is its ability to portray an image of the tumor and operating field in real time, allowing visual tracking of changes in the tumor and shifts in the surrounding brain during the operation. Preoperative imaging studies are unable to precisely define the margins of a solid tumor, the surrounding areas of infiltrating tumor cells and peritumoral edema, and the normal adjacent brain.[145] IOUS helps to define the tumor's borders by delineating both the tumor and its transition toward normal tissue and by differentiating edema from solid tumor and normal brain.[145,151] In addition, IOUS is useful in planning the route or approach through normal tissue to reach the tumor.

Brain mapping is useful in surgery in the dominant hemisphere, the motor and sensory regions, and the speech centers. Brain mapping techniques use either direct stimulation of the cerebral cortex or sensory evoked potentials (SEPs). In direct cortical stimulation, the dura is opened and electrodes are placed on the surface of the brain. The patient is then awakened and, by stimulating the electrodes and having the patient perform repetitive tasks, the motor cortex can be located. Broca's area is located by detecting a speech arrest during stimulation of the cortex while asking the patient to count forward and backward or to identify pictures of familiar objects. Wernicke's area is localized by stimulation of the cortex while asking the patient to complete simple phrases by naming a missing word or to repeat phrases. Successful localization is associated with an inability to complete these tasks.[146] Once these functional areas are located, the resection continues and the tumor is removed, keeping the mapped areas intact and reducing the neurological deficits. During SEP monitoring, sensory structures are stimulated and the electrical responses of the areas are analyzed on a monitor.[152] This technique permits mapping of the somatosensory, auditory, and visual cortex.

Interactive, image-guided, frameless stereotactic systems provide neurosurgeons with precise preoperative and intraoperative patient information. They can improve the accuracy of localizing lesions and aid in defining tumor margins. This allows the surgeon to perform a safe, more effective, and less invasive tumor excision. Before surgery, the patient undergoes a CT or MRI and markers or fiducials, which will be visible on the images, are applied to the patient's head. Some systems do not require markers to be placed but instead use previously referenced surface points on the patient's head. A computer transforms the data into a three-dimensional image for use in the operating room. Before the surgery, the surgeon can plan each step of the procedure and the ideal access to the tumor via the three-dimensional image on the computer screen. The tumor and its surroundings can be viewed from different angles and in relation to landmark structures. Once in the operating room, the patient's fiducials or coordinates are integrated to the image. A pointing device, such as the viewing wand, is used to quickly communicate surgical locations to the computer system.[149] Some systems use a mechanically linked arm; others communicate through sonic, optical, or magnetic digitizers.[153] At any time during the surgery, the surgeon can place the probe on a structure and, by viewing the screen, determine its location in relation to surrounding structures within 1–2 mm.[145] The main limitation of such a system is its reliance on preoperative images. During the surgery, anatomical changes occur. These changes may be related to CSF, edema, or the resection itself. Their occurrence can make the data derived from preoperative images somewhat outdated. Only intraoperative imaging can provide the updated information required to maintain accurate navigation during surgery.[150]

Intraoperative imaging was developed to overcome the limitations of using navigation systems that are based on preoperative images and to provide updated images during the actual procedure. With updated intraoperative images, the course of the surgery may be affected. For example, unrecognized tumor that otherwise would have been seen only on a postoperative MRI done outside the operating room can be removed, allowing for a more complete tumor resection. Unnecessary further dissection may be avoided, thereby decreasing the risk of neurological injury.[150] In addition, once the procedure is complete, a final image may be obtained to evaluate for a hematoma or other complication. Intraoperative MRI (iMRI) designs range from dedicated units requiring the construction of a special operating room,[154] to MRI suites that can be transformed into sterile surgical areas,[155] to iMRI devices designed specifically to work in neurosurgical operating rooms.[156,157]

Surgery also provides access for other adjuvant therapies. A stereotactic surgical procedure may be used to place radioactive sources within the tumor. Chemotherapy wafers may be implanted surgically within a tumor cavity and then slowly and continuously release chemotherapy directly into the brain. Ommaya reservoirs may be placed to deliver chemotherapy directly into the CSF.

Nursing care. Nursing interventions for patients undergoing neurosurgical procedures begin preoperatively in the outpatient setting. A baseline neurological examination is essential. Preoperative teaching consists of education in the planned surgical procedure, postoperative routines, measures to prevent complications, and medications that will be administered. Patients must be instructed to refrain from taking aspirin, aspirin-containing products, and nonsteroidal anti-inflammatory drugs (NSAIDs) preoperatively. Postoperative recovery practices vary among institutions. Neurological assessment is conducted on an ongoing basis to identify any variations that may signify potential complications. If no complications occur, patients undergoing craniotomy are usually hospitalized for 3–5 days, while those having a stereotactic biopsy require a 24- to 48-hour hospital stay. Some patients will initially be cared for in a postoperative step-down or an intensive care unit. Others will not require intensive monitoring beyond the postanesthesia care unit.

Postoperatively, patients may have new or worsened neurological deficits. Neurological deficit occurs in approximately 10% of patients.[158] The plan of care must be individualized, reflecting the specific deficits encountered. Safety measures assume the utmost importance for all personnel involved in the patient's care. Family members may not truly understand the severity of the potential risks related to deficits such as impaired judgment, memory loss, weakness or paralysis, and visual field disturbances, and will require frequent reinforcement.

Postoperative complications. Complications after neurosurgery may include intracranial bleeding, cerebral edema, further neurological impairment, electrolyte imbalance, infection, seizures, venous thromboembolism, and hydrocephalus. Hemorrhage at the operative site can occur within hours after surgery. Bleeding may also occur from traction on the bridging veins between the brain and the dura, leading to a subdural hematoma.[37] Additional areas where bleeding may occur are the epidural space, the subarachnoid space, or within the ventricles. Patients usually present with a new or worsening of a preoperative neurological deficit or seizures and often require surgery to evacuate the hematoma.

Postoperative cerebral edema is especially severe when residual tumor is present, but it occurs even after complete tumor removal. This complication results from the surgical manipulation of the surrounding brain tissue, changes in regional blood flow, or brain injury caused by excessive retraction.[145] The amount of edema varies in each individual but generally reaches its maximum peak at 48–72 hours postoperatively. Cerebral edema is treated with corticosteroids, usually dexamethasone; careful fluid management; and osmotherapy when necessary. Other techniques for controlling ICP include hyperventilation, CSF drainage, and the use of anesthetic agents. Activities that can exacerbate ICP should be avoided. The head of the bed is generally elevated 30°.

Electrolyte imbalance — namely, hyponatremia — can occur and may be treated with fluid restriction.

Some patients require fluid restriction, although most are kept euvolemic. Hyponatremia can decrease the seizure threshold, exacerbate cerebral edema, and increase neurological deficits. Infection is often prevented by the prophylactic use of antibiotics for 24–48 hours postoperatively.

Seizures are managed with prophylactic anticonvulsants and maintenance of therapeutic serum levels. Controversy persists concerning the use of prophylactic anticonvulsants in individuals who have not previously had a seizure.[16] Phenytoin (dilantin) is the most commonly used agent. A CT scan is indicated after a postoperative seizure to rule out hematoma, increased cerebral edema, or pneumocephalus.

Venous thromboembolism is a particular concern in neurosurgery patients because of the length of surgery, immobility of some postoperative patients, hemiparesis, and tumor-related hypercoagulable states.[145] Early ambulation is encouraged whenever possible. The risk of venous thromboembolism is reduced by the use of pneumatic compression devices and prophylactic anticoagulation. This complication may occur early or late in the postoperative period.

Postoperative hydrocephalus may be caused by tumor, periventricular swelling, or intraventricular blood. When severe, it is usually treated with ventriculostomy or VP shunting.

Radiation Therapy

Radiation therapy plays a central role in the treatment of adult brain tumors.[159] Early randomized studies by the Brain Tumor Cooperative Group (BTCG) firmly established the role of postoperative RT in patients with malignant gliomas. Individuals who received postoperative RT had a significantly prolonged survival compared with those who received only postoperative supportive care.[160] These studies were so convincing that subsequent clinical trials evaluating adjuvant therapy for malignant brain tumors have included RT in all treatment arms.[161] Likewise, RT plays an important role in the treatment of patients with low-grade gliomas; inoperable, partially resected, or recurrent benign brain tumors; and metastatic brain tumors.

Conventional radiotherapy. Radiotherapy for malignant gliomas historically was delivered to the whole brain. Neuroimaging studies have shown that the majority of tumors recur within 1–2 cm of their original location. In addition, many individuals who survive for extended periods after WBRT develop significant treatment-related morbidity. Therefore, partial brain irradiation or local-field radiotherapy (LFRT) is now accepted as the standard treatment approach.[162,163] With this approach, radiation is delivered to the tumor and a 3-cm margin of tissue surrounding the perimeter[159,162,164] in divided doses (fractions), generally once daily over 5–6 weeks, to deliver 60 Gy to the involved field.[48] WBRT is usually reserved for multifocal disease.

Attempts to improve responses to conventional RT while preserving normal tissue have included further manipulation of the dose and schedule of RT by hyperfractionation and accelerated treatment schedules and the use of radiosensitizers. However, these attempts have not improved the outcome and in some cases have led to increased toxicity.

Other primary brain tumors may be treated with RT. In benign brain tumors such as meningiomas and pituitary adenomas that cannot be completely excised or that recur despite aggressive resection, RT is an important adjuvant therapy. Completely resected tumors have a low risk of recurrence, and postoperative RT is not generally recommended. In contrast, the risk of recurrence in partially resected tumors is much higher, and studies have suggested that postoperative RT may delay recurrence, prevent tumor regrowth in some patients and provide a cure, and improve survival. A dose of 54 Gy is recommended for benign tumors. Individuals with malignant meningiomas generally receive postoperative RT, regardless of the extent of resection, and the dose is increased to 60 Gy.[4]

Radiation therapy is administered to most individuals with low-grade gliomas, although no consensus exists regarding its appropriate timing.[47,48,50] The rationale for immediate postoperative RT is based on the poor long-term survival in these individuals, the likelihood that low-grade tumors will be transformed into high-grade tumors, and the decreased morbidity of modern RT.[165,166] Other researchers have reported no increase in survival in individuals who received postoperative RT.[167,168] Those in favor of observation alone base their opinion on the lack of proven benefit, the potential long-term effects of RT in these patients,[134] and the fact that some low-grade gliomas are remarkably indolent.[50] Immediate postoperative RT to prevent neurological deterioration may be appropriate for patients with poor prognostic factors (older age, bulky residual disease, astrocytoma pathology versus oligodendroglioma). Delayed RT to avoid or postpone the possibility of the neurotoxic effects of RT may be appropriate for patients with favorable prognostic factors (younger age, complete resection, oligodendroglioma pathology).[48,50] The standard radiation dose for these tumors is generally 54 Gy.[48]

Three-dimensional conformal radiation therapy. In most centers, the RT plan for primary brain tumor patients uses three-dimensional treatment planning (3D-CRT). This method of high-precision RT utilizes MRI, CT information, or both, plus powerful computer technology, to plan and deliver external beam radiation treatments that shape the prescription dose distribution to conform to the anatomical boundaries of the tumor in its entire three-dimensional configuration while minimizing the dose to the surrounding tissue.[162] It requires reproducible and precise head immobilization.[169] Comparative two-dimensional and three-dimensional treatment planning studies in brain tumor patients have demonstrated a 30% reduction in the amount of normal brain irradiated when the 3D-CRT method is used.[162,170] In addition, 3D-CRT may allow higher than traditional doses to be safely administered to selected individuals.[16]

Intensity-modulated RT (IMRT) is an advanced form of 3D-CRT that offers an additional refinement of the dose configuration. Dose distributions in this method exquisitely conform to the shape of the target volume and sculpt around adjacent critical structures.[16]

Stereotactic radiosurgery. Stereotactic radiosurgery (SRS) uses an imaging-compatible stereotactic device to precisely localize an intracranial target and provides a high radiation dose in a single session without delivering significant radiation to the surrounding normal brain tissue.[162] This technique is performed using a modified linear accelerator or gamma knife unit. A noninvasive, single-day procedure, SRS is usually performed in an outpatient setting. It was initially used for small arteriovenous malformations (AVMs), benign brain tumors, and brain metastases. Malignant tumors were not considered appropriate for SRS because of their invasiveness and large size. However, the use of SRS in the treatment of primary and recurrent malignant brain tumors has increased. Shrieve and associates reported on a group of individuals with recurrent GBM treated with SRS.[164] The median survival was 10.2 months, with a 19% two-year survival. In another study, 69 newly diagnosed individuals with GBM received SRS as a boost following surgery and external beam RT. Median survival was 19.7 months, and two- and three-year survival rates were 31% and 20%, respectively.[159,171] Unfortunately, the majority of individuals with malignant gliomas are not eligible for this type of therapy because of the size or shape of their tumors. Tumors larger than 4 cm cannot be treated with SRS, for example. Patients with previously irradiated small lesions have been safely treated with SRS.[162,172]

Stereotactic radiotherapy. Stereotactic radiotherapy uses the planning technology and precision of SRS but delivers the treatment using standard fractionation doses, combining the focal advantages of SRS with the radiobiological advantage of fractionation.[16] SRS hardware, software, and head frames can be relocalized daily in a nontraumatic and reproducible fashion.[162] Standard fractionation avoids the toxicities associated with large single doses, and tumors located near critical structures may be more successfully treated with the precision of the stereotactic technique. This approach is being used for some benign tumors and gliomas.

Interstitial brachytherapy. Brachytherapy involves the temporary high-activity or permanent low-activity implantation of radioactive sources directly into the brain tumor. Catheters are placed into the tumor using stereotactic surgical techniques, and the radiation seeds or pellets are then inserted in the catheters. The implants are removed either after a few days or several months, or are left in permanently, depending on the source used. Iodine-125 (^{125}I) and iridium-192 (^{192}I) are the most commonly used sources for both temporary and permanent implants. The area of tumor receives the highest dose but the surrounding normal brain tissue is spared because there is a rapid fall-off in dose as the distance from the radiation source increases.[159]

Only about 30% of individuals with malignant gliomas are eligible for brachytherapy. Individuals with tumors that are large or multifocal, that cross the midline, that are inaccessible or located in functionally vital areas, or whose performance status is low are not candidates for this form of therapy. The initial studies using brachytherapy demonstrated an increased survival in individuals with recurrent GBM. These results led to trials with ^{125}I implants as a component of primary therapy along with conventional external beam RT.[173,174] A significant finding was the increased two-year survival — as high as 39%. Although the outcomes for brachytherapy and SRS are similar in terms of survival, SRS offers several advantages. It is a noninvasive, single-day treatment usually scheduled on an outpatient basis, allowing a prolonged hospitalization with the risk of hemorrhage and infection to be avoided. Therefore, SRS has become the preferred focal therapy for recurrent GBM except in cases of large or irregularly shaped tumors. For large tumors that cannot be treated with SRS, brachytherapy can be used.

Permanent sources may be implanted at the time of initial surgery. Advantages of this approach are that the tumor burden can be decreased at the same time, irradiation to high doses occurs over a long period of time, and the rate of subsequent radiation necrosis may be lower.[173,175]

Alternative methods of local radiation administration under investigation involve the placement of radioactive colloid or radiolabeled antibody into a cystic tumor cavity[43] and administration of an aqueous iodinated radiation source by way of a balloon catheter system into a tumor cavity.[176] Such therapy is designed to deliver intracavitary brachytherapy to the resection margins.

Brain metastases. Radiation is standard treatment for metastatic brain tumors. As many as 50% of individuals with metastatic brain tumors will not be surgical candidates. These individuals and those with multiple metastases typically undergo RT. Patients who undergo surgery generally receive postoperative WBRT. Two randomized studies reported a prolonged survival in which patients who received postoperative WBRT maintained a higher performance status and had fewer intracranial recurrences.[110,111] Traditionally WBRT has been preferred over partial-field RT because multiple metastases may be present even if some are too small to be detected on imaging studies. Typical radiation treatment schedules for metastatic brain tumors consist of a total dose of 30 Gy delivered over 10 fractions.[48] Lower daily fractions and a more protracted course may be indicated in individuals with a better prognosis.[107] As with primary tumors, response rates vary with the histological characteristics of the primary tumor. For example, metastases from breast and small cell lung cancers respond better to RT than do metastases from melanoma, renal, or colon cancers.[37,107]

Many metastatic brain lesions are now being treated with SRS. Unlike with surgery, few lesions are inaccessible to SRS because of their location in the brain. Because metastatic tumors are generally small in size and tend not to invade adjacent brain tissue, the individual with brain metastases is an ideal candidate for radiosurgery.[177] Uncontrolled primary disease, uncontrolled or progressing nonbrain metastases, tumors larger than 4 cm, tumors associated with significant mass effect and neurological symptoms, and, in some cases, low KPS scores are considered contraindications to SRS.[177] Median survival for patients with brain metastases treated with SRS has generally been reported at 7–10 months,[177] although Young and colleagues found more than 30% of patients surviving beyond one year and 15%–20% beyond two years.[178] SRS may be used alone, may be used with WBRT, or may be used to treat recurrent or new metastases after prior WBRT[48] or SRS.[172] Multiple lesions may be treated as long as they are small. The disadvantages of radiosurgery relate to its high cost, increased risk of radiation necrosis, and failure to control micrometastases elsewhere in the brain.[178,179]

Side effects. Side effects of RT can be classified as acute, subacute, or delayed. Acute reactions occur during the course of treatment and are temporary. They are manifested as signs of increased ICP or worsening of neurological deficits. These effects result from an increase in cerebral edema; the administration of corticosteroids usually decreases or alleviates symptoms. Steroids are generally administered during the course of therapy to prevent this problem. Other acute adverse effects include nausea, vomiting, anorexia, fatigue, alopecia, and skin irritation. Alopecia lasting several months occurs after 54 Gy; it is often permanent after 60 Gy.[169] Acute reactions have been reported to occur in one-third of patients undergoing stereotactic radiosurgery and include headaches, nausea, vomiting, dizziness and vertigo (more commonly with acoustic neuromas), worsening neurological deficit, and seizures.[180]

Subacute reactions generally develop 1–3 months after completion of therapy. These, too, are of a temporary nature. Symptoms include anorexia, sleepiness, lethargy, and an increase in neurological deficits. These effects are thought to result from the temporary disruption of myelin formation, which helps speed the relay of nerve signals. It takes approximately 6 weeks for myelin to be fully repaired.

Delayed effects of RT usually occur 6–24 months after completion of treatment. These effects are irreversible and often progressive. They result from direct injury to brain tissue and blood vessels. Leukoencephalopathy — that is, degeneration of the white matter — occurs at the tumor site and surrounding irradiated brain. The risk of developing leukoencephalopathy increases with a higher total dose, higher dose per fraction, and concomitant use of neurotoxic chemotherapeutic agents, particularly methotrexate. The clinical manifestations range from mild cognitive neurological impairment to dementia to death. The onset and progression can be quite variable. Radiation necrosis occurs more commonly after brachytherapy and radiosurgery but can occur after conventional RT as well. Individuals at increased risk for long-term radiation effects include children younger than age 2 and adults older than 60. Long-term effects can be initially managed to some degree with corticosteroids and surgery to remove necrotic tissue. Other long-term effects include loss of vision, development of secondary malignancies, and endocrine disturbances. The major complication of both brachytherapy and radiosurgery is the development of symptomatic radiation necrosis requiring prolonged administration of steroids and reoperation. The rate of reoperation is 30%–40%, usually within six months.

Nursing care. Nursing management of the individual receiving RT includes neurological assessment and evaluation of side effects, and patient and family education regarding treatment schedules, routines, possible side effects, and management of these effects. Additional interventions focus on the specific irradiation method used. The most common method, conventional external beam, is usually administered on an outpatient basis. Assistance may be necessary for transportation arrangements. Most patients will be on steroids to reduce the cerebral edema that occurs during brain irradiation. Education is necessary regarding these agents' many adverse effects. Brain irradiation causes the skin to become dry and peel, and moist desquamation may occur, most often behind the ears.[181] Individuals should be instructed on appropriate skin care and creams, and they must avoid sun exposure. Extreme fatigue occurs during and after treatment, and patients require support and encouragement to manage this distressing symptom.

Chemotherapy

Although it does not produce a cure, chemotherapy plays an important adjuvant role in the treatment of adult primary brain tumors. The most widely studied group of tumors has been the malignant glioma because it is the most common adult primary brain tumor and accounts for the majority of deaths in individuals with brain tumors. Many studies have evaluated a variety of single chemotherapeutic agents and multiple-drug regimens. BCNU; the combination of procarbazine, procarbazine, and vincristine (PCV); and the most recently approved agent, temozolomide,[43] remain the most commonly used agents for both newly diagnosed and recurrent malignant gliomas.[182]

Of the malignant gliomas, GBM responds the least well to chemotherapy, anaplastic astrocytoma responds somewhat better, and oligodendrogliomas may be the most chemosensitive.[183] Unfortunately, no one prognostic factor or clinical feature reliably predicts which individuals will benefit most from adjuvant chemotherapy. In a meta-analysis by Fine and associates,[161] 16 randomized clinical trials were evaluated to determine whether adjuvant chemotherapy did, indeed, improve survival in individuals with malignant gliomas. The authors found a statistically significant but still modest survival advantage for those who received adjuvant chemotherapy.

The delivery of adequate concentrations of intravenous chemotherapy to tumors within the CNS is limited by the presence of the BBB. The BBB is made of a continuous lining of endothelial cells that are connected by tight junctions.[37] Large, water-soluble, charged particles and compounds bound to plasma proteins are unable to penetrate the BBB. This vascular barrier normally protects the brain by limiting the entry of potentially toxic substances into brain tissue. Unfortunately, it also prevents the majority of chemotherapeutic agents from entering brain tissue.

Although the BBB can be a potential obstacle to the delivery of chemotherapy, the most malignant brain tumors are often associated with marked BBB disruption. Water-soluble contrast agents administered with CT or MRI are able to cross the normally impermeable BBB and enter the brain in the region of the tumor. The surrounding normal brain, however, continues to exclude the contrast material because its BBB remains intact. Thus, the enhancing masses seen on CT and MRI represent regions of tumor with a substantially disrupted BBB. Malignant cells, however, often infiltrate adjacent tissue and spread to distant sites. Contrast enhancement usually does not occur in the surrounding normal brain that typically contains micrometastatic disease.[184] The BBB is, therefore, at least partially intact in many brain tumors, particularly in the periphery of the tumor and around infiltrating tumor cells.

After years of study and many trials, no other chemotherapeutic agent or combination of agents has been shown to be more effective than BCNU for those with GBM. In some studies, the combination of PCV has been found to be more effective than BCNU for those with anaplastic astrocytoma. Levin and colleagues demonstrated an increased median survival of 151 weeks in individuals with anaplastic astrocytoma treated with PCV as opposed to 82 weeks for those who received BCNU.[55] Subsequent analyses, however, suggest that there is little difference between PCV and BCNU.[185] The nitrosoureas (BCNU and CCNU) cause delayed and cumulative myelosuppression, pulmonary fibrosis, nausea, vomiting and, during administration of BCNU, facial flushing and pain and burning along the IV site. Side effects of procarbazine include rash, myelosuppression, encephalopathy, peripheral neuropathy, hepatotoxicity, and hypertensive crisis with consumption of foods containing tyramine. Side effects of vincristine include peripheral neuropathies, constipation, myelosuppression, alopecia, nausea, and vomiting.

Temozolomide is the most recently approved agent for malignant gliomas—specifically, recurrent anaplastic astrocytoma. It appears to be active in approximately 20% of patients with malignant glioma.[16] This drug has produced responses in individuals with recurrent anaplastic astrocytoma and anaplastic oligoastrocytoma[186] and in individuals with recurrent GBM.[187] An oral alkylating agent, temozolomide has mild toxicities including nausea, vomiting, and noncumulative myelosuppression, making this agent an attractive alternative for glioma treatment. Other agents that have shown some activity against gliomas include thiotepa, cisplatin, carboplatin, etoposide, cyclophosphamide, paclitaxel, and tamoxifen.

Anaplastic oligodendrogliomas have been found to be chemosensitive tumors. The PCV combination has been the most widely studied regimen for these tumors, and positive results have been obtained in both newly diagnosed and recurrent tumors. This regimen is now standard therapy.[188] Mixed gliomas[189,190] and nonanaplastic oligodendrogliomas[191] also appear to respond to these agents. Abrey and colleagues reported that intensive PCV chemotherapy followed by high-dose thiotepa and autologous stem cell transplantation resulted in prolonged tumor control in some patients, and median survival has not yet been reached at almost 5 years.[61] Durable responses to chemotherapy are associated with loss of heterozygosity of the long arm of chromosome 19 and short arm of chromosome 1.[55–58] This raises the possibility that molecular analysis of tumor tissue will guide treatment decisions and identify a subgroup of patients who are more likely to benefit from intensive chemotherapy.[61] Other agents to which these tumors seem to respond include BCNU, diaziquone (AZQ), and melphalan.[192]

Unfortunately, the addition of adjuvant chemotherapy has not dramatically improved the survival of individuals with malignant brain tumors, particularly those with GBM. New approaches have been explored in an attempt to increase the efficacy of the currently available chemotherapeutic agents. These options include IV continuous-infusion chemotherapy, intrathecal or intraventricular chemotherapy, intraarterial chemotherapy, high-dose chemotherapy with autologous bone marrow or stem cell rescue, and interstitial chemotherapy. Such strategies can selectively deliver higher concentrations of chemotherapy to the tumors.

Continuous infusion. As mentioned previously, water-soluble contrast agents used to image tumors on CT or MRI scan are able to pass through the disrupted BBB near the area of tumor, producing contrast enhancement at the outer ring of the tumor. The inner portion of the tumor is not initially enhanced. Bolus infusions of water-soluble agents with short plasma half-lives might treat the contrast-enhancing tumor ring but may never reach therapeutic concentrations within the center of the tumor. The observation that contrast enhancement, after hours of sustained blood levels, can reach the center of the tumor suggests that continuous infusions of water-soluble chemotherapeutic agents might result in a more uniform drug distribution within brain tumors.[184] In one study, combination of BCNU and cisplatin (a lipid- and water-soluble agent) continuously administered over three days demonstrated an objective response greater than 60%, with some complete radiographic responses.

Intrathecal/intraventricular. The instillation of chemotherapy directly into the CSF is an important method of administering chemotherapy for individuals with leptomeningeal metastases, leukemic or lymphomatous meningitis, PCNSL, and primary CNS tumors such as medulloblastomas where the subarachnoid space is involved. An LP for intrathecal chemotherapy administration has been performed safely in selected individuals. Nevertheless, chemotherapy instilled directly into the ventricular CSF by way of an Ommaya reservoir has been found to produce better drug distribution throughout the CSF and more consistent drug levels. As a consequence, the Ommaya reservoir is the preferred method of delivering chemotherapy into the CSF. It allows for greater ease of administration and less discomfort for the patient. Complications occurring with the use of this device may include infection, catheter blockage, catheter leakage, and, after the administration of chemotherapy, chemical meningitis. Chemotherapeutic agents administered via this method include methotrexate, cytarabine, and thiotepa.

Intraarterial. Intraarterial chemotherapy involves the catheterization of the carotid or vertebral arteries, which provide the arterial supply to brain tumors for the administration of chemotherapeutic agents. Agents that have been evaluated using this approach include BCNU, cisplatin, carboplatin, CCNU, and methotrexate. Intraarterial delivery can increase the amount of chemotherapy delivered to the tumor by as much as ten times[193] while decreasing systemic toxicity. This method of drug delivery still has significant toxicities, however.

Blood–brain barrier disruption. Another approach to intraarterial chemotherapy is to transiently disrupt the BBB with an osmotic agent such as mannitol just before the administration of intraarterial chemotherapy. Hypertonic mannitol stimulates a loss of fluid from the capillary endothelial cells, causing the endothelial cells to shrink and the tight junctions to break, thereby resulting in osmotic shrinkage.[194] Large molecular-sized materials or water-soluble agents may then diffuse through the opened junctions into the surrounding brain. Gumerlock and associates treated GBM patients with IV cyclophosphamide followed by intraarterial mannitol, methotrexate, and oral procarbazine and described a 22-month median survival rate.[194] Unfortunately, BBB disruption can be associated with significant toxicity. Worsening neurological deficits occurred in as many as 56% of patients and seizures in 44% of patients. One reason for this toxicity is that mannitol enhances the permeability of normal capillaries, which significantly increases the vulnerability of the normal brain tissue to the toxic effects of chemotherapy.

Autologous transplantation. High-dose chemotherapy followed by autologous stem cell rescue has been evaluated in individuals with malignant gliomas. Most of the studies have used BCNU alone or in combination with other agents, including thiotepa and etoposide, as the preparative regimen. Although some long-term survivors were noted, median survival for newly diagnosed patients undergoing this procedure was 12–17 months. This approach was also associated with significant morbidity.

Interstitial. Interstitial chemotherapy—the use of biodegradable polymers impregnated with chemotherapeutic agents—is a promising approach in chemotherapy delivery for brain tumors. These polymers are placed intraoperatively in the walls of the tumor cavity after resection and continuously release high local concentrations of chemotherapeutic agents. Chemotherapy delivered directly to the tumor bypasses the variably disrupted BBB, results in high local drug concentrations, and minimizes systemic toxicity. Implantation of BCNU wafers was found to prolong median survival in patients with recurrent high-grade gliomas.[195–198] This new route of administration may facilitate the use of new and established chemotherapeutic agents that previously could not be efficiently, safely, or effectively delivered to the brain.

To date, progress in the development of new chemotherapeutic agents for malignant brain tumors has been slow. Neoadjuvant chemotherapy is being increasingly used to evaluate new agents.[199] This approach permits the precise evaluation of tumor response while avoiding the confounding effects of RT.

Nursing care. Nursing management of the individual receiving chemotherapy depends on the method of chemotherapy administration and the specific agents used. It includes assessment and evaluation of side effects; patient and family education regarding treatment schedules, routines, and possible side effects; and interventions to enhance tolerance and maintain functional ability.

Biotherapy

To date, biotherapy has had little success in the treatment of malignant brain tumors. Methods investigated include the use of cytokines (interferons, interleukins, and tumor necrosis factor), adoptive immunotherapy with lymphokine-activated killer (LAK) cells and interleukin-2 (IL-2), and monoclonal antibodies. Research continues as improved methods of administration are developed and new agents are identified. Eventually, these agents may be used in combination with other treatment modalities. Additional areas of investigation that appear promising include gene therapy, antiangiogenesis, inhibition of signal transduction, growth factor inhibitors, and molecular genetics.

Gene therapy. Most gene therapy studies have focused on the insertion of the herpes simplex thymidine kinase gene into tumor cells. The tumor cell becomes genetically like the herpes virus, divides, and produces more such cells. The patient is then treated with an antiviral drug (ganciclovir), and the tumor cells are killed. Brain tumors appear to be a good choice for gene therapy because they are relatively localized, they rarely metastasize outside the CNS, and well-established methods of drug delivery directly into the tumor (stereotactic injection, Ommaya reservoir, and intraarterial injection) already exist.

Another application for gene therapy would be to try to normalize the mutated genes in tumor cells. Therapeutic studies using the wild-type *p53* gene, which should cause tumor cells that lack the gene to stop reproducing, are currently in progress.[16] The tumor suppressor gene, when carried to the tumor by a virus, can restore normal function to existing but altered tumor suppressor genes or replace missing genes.[200]

Antiangiogenesis. Angiogenesis is the growth of new blood vessels. Tumor growth is dependent on the development of a new vascular supply, and endothelial proliferation is a characteristic feature of astrocytomas. The inhibition of tumor-associated new-vessel growth (antiangiogenesis) could retard tumor growth and become a potentially useful treatment modality. Antiangiogenic agents in clinical trials include thalidomide and PTK787.

Signal transduction inhibition. Inhibition of signal transduction is another area of research. The inhibition of protein kinase C (PKC) is one such strategy. Malignant gliomas express very high PKC activity as compared to nonmalignant glial cells.[170] Tamoxifen inhibits PKC activity and growth in some malignant glioma cell lines,[201] suggesting that high-dose tamoxifen may have a role in the adjuvant therapy of individuals with malignant gliomas.[202]

Growth factor inhibition. Inhibitors of growth factors involved in tumorigenesis are being investigated. Most brain tumors are dependent on growth factors such as epidermal growth factor (EGF), platelet-derived growth factor (PDGF), and vascular endothelial growth factor (VEGF) for both angiogenesis and tumor growth. A number of agents that inhibit growth factors are currently undergoing clinical trials, including Gleevec (PDGF receptor tyrosine kinase inhibitor), Iressa (EGF receptor tyrosine kinase inhibitor), and Tarceva (erlotinib EGF receptor tyrosine kinase inhibitor).[203]

Molecular genetics. Current research is focused on identifying the molecular and genetic alterations associated with the development and progression of gliomas. Gliomas may soon be classified according to their intrinsic molecular alterations, and treatments will likely be tailored to target the genetic alterations that generated the tumors.[204]

Spinal Cord Tumors

Epidemiology

Primary spinal cord tumors occur less frequently than primary brain tumors, accounting for only 15% of all primary CNS tumors. Approximately 2700 of these tumors are diagnosed each year. They occur most often in individuals aged 20–60. With the exception of meningiomas, which occur more often in women, spinal cord tumors are found with equal frequency in men and women. Metastatic tumors are much more common than primary spinal cord tumors, reportedly afflicting 5%–10% of individuals with systemic cancer.

Etiology

The etiology of the majority of primary spinal cord tumors is unknown. Individuals with NF-1 may develop neurofibromas and astrocytomas of the spinal cord[205] Spinal nerve root tumors (schwannomas) and ependymomas may be present in patients with NF-2, and individuals with von Hippel-Lindau disease are at risk for developing spinal hemangioblastomas.[205,206]

Pathophysiology

Anatomy and Physiology

The spine is a flexible column formed by a series of vertebrae, each stacked one upon another to support the head and trunk. The vertebral column shown in Figure 47-8 consists of 33 vertebrae: 7 cervical, 12 thoracic, 5 lumbar, 5 sacral, and 4 coccygeal. The five sacral vertebrae fuse to form the sacrum, and the four coccygeal vertebrae fuse to form the coccyx.

The spinal cord, housed within the vertebral column, is an elongated mass of nerve tissue less than 1 inch in diameter and approximately 17–18 inches in length. It arises from the medulla oblongata, beginning at the top of the first cervical vertebra, and extends down to the lower border of the first lumbar vertebra, where it ends in a tapered, conelike structure called the *conus medullaris.* The spinal cord is about 10 inches shorter than the vertebral column, and the lower segments of the spinal cord, therefore, are not aligned opposite corresponding vertebrae. Thus, the lumbar and sacral spinal nerves have very long roots. These roots descend in a bundle from the conus, and because of its resemblance to the tail of a horse, this formation is called the *cauda equina.*[207]

There are 31 pairs of spinal nerves exiting from the spinal cord through the intervertebral foramina: 8 cervical, 12 thoracic, 5 lumbar, 5 sacral, and 1 coccygeal. The intervertebral foramina are narrow, and the nerves may easily be compressed at this site by a protruding disk or arthritic spurring.[38] Each spinal nerve has a dorsal root by which afferent (sensory) impulses enter the cord and a ventral root by which efferent (motor) impulses leave the spinal cord. The dorsal roots convey sensory input from skin segments that represent specific areas of the body known as *dermatomes.*[208] Interruption of one sensory nerve root may result in paresthesias or pain in that dermatomal area. The ventral roots convey motor impulses from the spinal cord to the body, innervating specific areas of muscle groups called *myotomes* (Table 47-3).

The cranial meninges are contiguous within the spinal canal to support and protect the spinal cord. The spinal dura is a continuation of the inner layer of the cerebral dura. The outer dural layer ends at the foramen magnum, being replaced by the periosteal lining of the vertebral canal. The spinal dura encloses the spinal nerves and terminates at the level of the sacrum. The arachnoid layer of the spinal meninges is a continuation of the cerebral arachnoid. The pia mater in the spinal cord is thicker, firmer, and less vascular than that of the brain.[34] The spinal meninges are illustrated in Figure 47-9.

A cross section of the spinal cord shows that it is arranged as a butterfly-shaped area of gray matter sur-

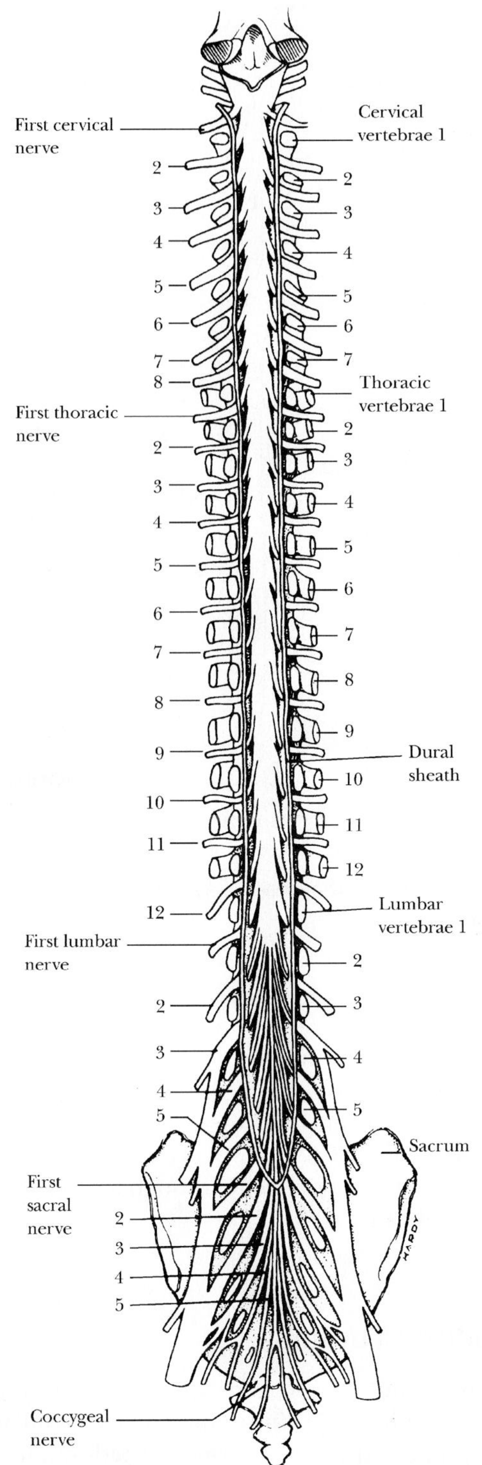

Figure 47-8 The spinal cord lying within the vertebral column. Spinal nerves are numbered on the left side, and the vertebrae are numbered on the right side. (Reprinted with permission from Hickey JV: Overview of neuroanatomy and neurophysiology, in Hickey JV (ed.): *The Clinical Practice of Neurological and Neurosurgical Nursing* (ed 4). Philadelphia, Lippincott, 1997, pp 35–79. Originally published in Chaffee EE, Lytle IM: *Basic Physiology and Anatomy*. Philadelphia, Lippincott, 1980[34]).

Table 47-3 Motor Nerve Roots (Myotomes) and Areas They Innervate

Spinal Cord Segment	Muscle Action
C-1 to C-4	Flexion, lateral flexion, extension, and rotation of neck
C-3 to C-5	Diaphragm (inspiration); elevation of upper thorax and scapula
C-5 to C-6	Shoulder movement; flexion of elbow
C-5 to C-7	Forward thrust of shoulder
C-5 to C-8	Adduction of arm from front to back
C-6 to C-8	Extension of forearm and wrist
C-6 to T-1	Thumb and index finger (C-6), middle finger (C-7), ring finger (C-8), and pinky finger (T-1)
C-7 to T-1	Flexion of wrist
T-1 to T-12	Control of thoracic, abdominal, and back muscles
L-1 to L-3	Flexion of hip
L-2 to L-4	Extension of leg; adduction of thigh
L-4 to S-2	Flexion, abduction, and rotation of thigh; flexion of lower leg; extension, flexing, and spreading of toes
L-4 to L-5	Dorsal flexion of foot
L-5 to S-2	Plantar flexion of foot
S-2 to S-4	Perineum and sphincters

rounded by white matter. The gray matter consists of cell bodies, axon, and dendrites. The white matter consists of longitudinally running fiber tracts. The white matter in each half of the cord is divided into columns. These columns are further divided into tracts, which are the sensory and motor pathways of the spinal cord. Impulses are conducted up the spinal cord via ascending tracts (sensory) to the brain, and the descending tracts conduct impulses from the brain down to the spinal cord (motor). The specific motor and sensory symptoms seen in spinal cord tumors depend on the tumor's involvement of these specific tracts.

Extradural Tumors

Spinal cord tumors are also classified by their cell of origin and anatomical location. The major anatomical consideration of spinal cord tumors relates to the tumor's location in relation to the spinal dura mater (Figure 47-10). Extradural tumors lie outside the dura. Most of these tumors are caused by metastatic cancer to the vertebral column, a common site of bone metastasis. Metastases can occur in multiple contiguous vertebrae and in multiple sites of the vertebral column. Metastatic spinal cord tumors most often originate from cancers of the breast, lung, prostate, and

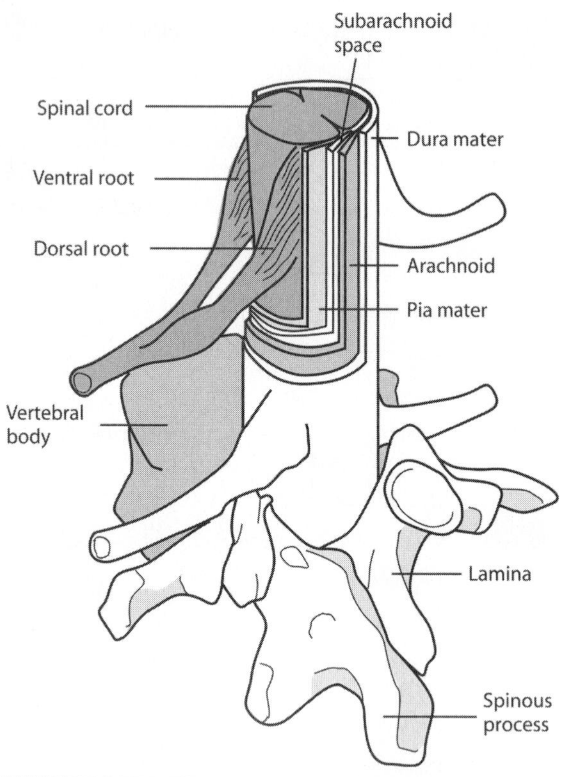

Figure 47-9 Spinal meninges.

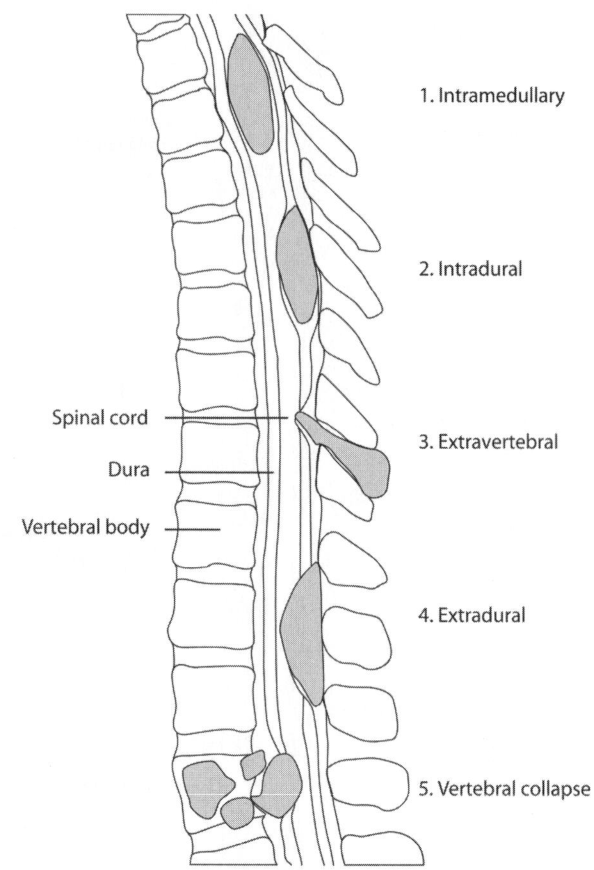

Figure 47-10 Anatomical location of spinal cord tumors.

kidney and from multiple myeloma. Less common are cancers of the GI tract, thyroid, and melanoma. The neurological symptoms seen with extradural tumors result from compression rather than invasion of the spinal cord. The spinal cord is usually compressed anteriorly, which leads to edema and ischemia of the spinal cord and mechanically distorts and damages the nervous tissue. Spinal cord compression (SCC) occurs either by direct extension of the tumor into the epidural space, by vertebral collapse and displacement of bone into the epidural space, or by direct extension through the intervertebral foramina. The thoracic spine is the most frequent location of epidural SCC, followed by the lumbosacral and cervical spine. Lung and breast cancer most often cause thoracic compression, whereas prostate, renal, and GI tumors are more likely to affect the lower thoracic or lumbosacral vertebrae.

Lymphomas may be a cause of SCC because they can extend directly through the intervertebral foramina. Other tumors such as sarcoma and chordoma may arise as primary extradural tumors. The chordoma is a slow-growing but highly invasive tumor. It often occurs in the sacrum but can also be found in the cervical spine and intracranially at the base of the skull. This tumor erodes bone and soft tissue extensively; even though it is histologically benign, it is difficult to remove in its entirety.[209]

Epidural SCC is a relatively common neurological complication of cancer and is considered an oncological emergency. The incidence of SCC may actually be increasing because patients are living longer and the incidence of cancers that commonly spread to bone is rising. Epidural SCC usually occurs late during the course of metastatic cancer, although it can also be the first sign of cancer.[107]

Intradural Tumors

Intradural tumors arise from the nerve roots or coverings of the spinal cord (intradural, extramedullary) or develop in the spinal cord itself (intradural, intramedullary). Intradural, extramedullary tumors account for almost 90% of primary spinal cord tumors. Schwannomas are the most common extramedullary tumor and often are located in the lumbar spine on one of the many nerve roots of the cauda equina.[210] Meningiomas are the second most frequently occurring extramedullary tumor. They commonly arise in the thoracic spine. Both spinal schwannomas and meningiomas can often be completely removed by surgery, and recurrence is rare with complete resection.

Sarcomas can also arise as extramedullary tumors. Other less common intradural extramedullary tumors are vascular tumors, chordomas, and epidermoids.[4]

Intradural, intramedullary tumors arise from the same cell as their intracranial counterparts; however, the grade of malignancy is often lower, making the majority of primary spinal cord tumors benign. The majority of intramedullary tumors are ependymomas (60%),[211] followed by astrocytomas (30%).[212] Less common histologies include hemangioblastomas and various hemangiomas, oligodendrogliomas, gangliogliomas, and medulloblastomas.[4] Most ependymomas are located in the lumbosacral area. Spinal cord ependymomas located in the cauda equina can often be removed without functional sacrifice.[64] Treatment usually includes maximal surgical resection and RT. Ependymomas that involve the CSF are treated with craniospinal RT. Chemotherapy is usually reserved for recurrent tumors.[211] Astrocytomas are more commonly located in the cervical and thoracic spinal cord.[213] As treatment for them, surgical resection is often attempted followed by RT. As many as 20% of spinal cord astrocytomas are malignant; such high-grade tumors are generally treated only with RT. Hemangioblastomas are vascular tumors evenly distributed throughout the spinal cord except for those associated with von Hippel-Lindau syndrome, in which they are predominantly located in the cervical cord.[210]

Spinal cord tumors are also anatomically described based on their location in relation to the vertebral column. Approximately 50% of spinal tumors are located in the thoracic spine, 30% are located in the lumbosacral region, and 20% involve the cervical spine. Knowledge of the specific level of involvement is helpful in understanding the signs and symptoms in relation to the specific dermatomes and myotomes involved.

Pattern of Spread

The most common mechanism of spread for extradural spinal metastases is thought to involve hematogenous arterial spread. A second mechanism is direct invasion through the intervertebral foramina by a paravertebral mass. Another possible mechanism of metastatic epidural spinal cord metastases is retrograde venous spread from the primary site by way of Batson's plexus.[214]

Intradural, intramedullary metastases may occur through CSF pathways. Ependymomas can involve the CSF. A higher incidence of distant spread has been reported in high-grade spinal astrocytomas. This increased propensity for dissemination of malignant spinal cord astrocytomas compared to intracranial astrocytomas is thought to result from the close proximity of tumor cells to the subarachnoid space and CSF pathways.[215] In contrast, primary spinal cord tumors rarely metastasize outside the CNS.

Clinical Manifestations

The clinical manifestations associated with spinal cord tumors result from compression and, much less frequently, invasion of the spinal cord. Extramedullary tumors affect the cord by compression, causing traction on or irritation of the spinal nerve roots, displacement of the spinal cord itself, interference with the spinal blood supply, or obstruction of CSF circulation. Intramedullary tumors invade and destroy the spinal cord itself. When spinal cord compression occurs, the normal physiology involved in providing an adequate blood supply, maintaining stable cellular membranes, and facilitating afferent and efferent impulses for specific sensory, motor, and reflex functions of the spinal cord and related spinal nerves is altered.[216] Edema results, causing additional deficits.

The clinical manifestations seen with spinal cord tumors depend on the tumor's rate of growth and the level of the spinal cord affected. Symptom duration prior to diagnosis is often in the range of 3–4 years.[217] A slow-growing, benign tumor better allows the cord to accommodate the mass. Tumors can compress the cord into a thin, ribbonlike structure without causing significant neurological deficits. By contrast, the spinal cord cannot accommodate a sudden mass or rapidly growing lesion such as a hematoma or a malignant tumor. It has little ability to compensate for such lesions, which increase pressure and create extensive edema causing sudden neurological dysfunction. The signs and symptoms of spinal cord tumors include pain, motor weakness, sensory impairment, and autonomic dysfunction involving bowel and bladder function.

Pain is the most common presenting symptom of a spinal cord tumor. In epidural metastases, back or neck pain may be present for weeks or months, and intradural tumors can cause pain for years before the correct diagnosis is established. Often the pain is initially dismissed as arthritis, back strain, or disc disease, and until other more obvious neurological manifestations appear, the diagnosis of a spinal cord tumor is usually not considered. Back or neck pain in cancer patients, especially those with tumor types that commonly metastasize to bone, should be evaluated for spinal metastases.

The pain may be localized or radicular. Localized pain and tenderness are common over the involved area, particularly with epidural metastases. Radicular pain may be described as bandlike and follows the distribution of the spinal nerve roots (dermatomes). The pain can vary from mild to severe and from dull to sharp or burning, and almost always becomes more severe with time. Pain may be worse at night; a recumbent position often aggravates it. Pain that is aggravated by movement and relieved with immobility may indicate spinal instability. Activities that produce a valsalva maneuver, such as sneezing, coughing, and straining, increase the spinal pressure and cause intensification of pain.

Weakness is the most readily identified objective finding and may follow the appearance of sensory symptoms. The level of impairment determines the muscle groups involved (myotomes). The weakness is often associated with hyperreflexia, spasticity, and a positive Babinski sign. It will eventually progress to complete paraplegia unless treatment is initiated. Specific motor symptoms will vary depending on where the tumor is located on a cross section of the spinal cord. A lateral tumor will affect voluntary movement in the arms and legs, muscle tone, coordination, and posture. Tumors in the anterior cord will affect voluntary movement of the trunk muscles, equilibrium, and posture.

Specific sensory deficits will depend on where the tumor is located on a cross section of the spinal cord. A lateral tumor will affect pain and temperature, causing symptoms of coldness, numbness, and tingling. Awareness of vibration and proprioception of body parts are affected if the posterior aspect is involved. Touch and pressure on the opposite side of the body will be affected if the tumor is anterior. Compression affects function below the lesion; therefore, it is important to determine the highest functional level. A sensory assessment begins at the toes and moves upward to determine the level at which function remains, which is generally the level of the tumor. However, there may be a discrepancy between the level of remaining function and apparent tumor location. The lesion may be one or two vertebrae above the level of compression. A narrow band of hyperesthesia directly above often accompanies the tumor level.[216]

The effects may be symmetrical and bilateral, asymmetrical, and even unilateral. A combination of sensory and motor deficits may also be seen. A loss of touch, vibration, position sense, and motor ability on the same side as the lesion with contralateral loss of pain and temperature is called the Brown-Séquard syndrome. This syndrome occurs in approximately 20% of patients with spinal cord tumors.[4]

Later symptoms may involve bowel dysfunction, bladder dysfunction, or both, and include constipation, fecal incontinence, urgency, difficulty in initiating urination, urinary retention, and urinary incontinence. These symptoms may be present earlier with an intramedullary tumor.

Assessment

Assessment of the individual with a known or suspected spinal cord tumor begins by obtaining a history. The description and duration of symptoms, the presence of exacerbating or relieving factors, and the order of their appearance must be established. A neurological examination, especially of motor and sensory function, gait, and reflexes, is performed. In addition, the possible presence of bowel or bladder dysfunction must be established, and a pain assessment is performed. This initial assessment provides a baseline from which all future assessments will be compared. This neurological assessment should attempt to determine where the tumor is likely to be located (cervical, thoracic, or lumbar).

Diagnostic Studies

The diagnostic procedure of choice for the evaluation of both intramedullary and extramedullary spinal cord tumors is MRI. It provides superb anatomical detail of the spinal cord, is noninvasive, and carries fewer risks than myelography. Use of contrast is standard when evaluating spinal cord tumors, as the majority of intramedullary tumors demonstrate enhancement despite the histologic grade.[213] MRI is also helpful for planning radiation therapy and surgery.

For imaging spinal cord tumors, MRI has largely replaced CT myelography. In CT myelography, contrast medium is injected into the subarachnoid space, usually by means of a lumbar puncture, and CT images of the spinal cord and vertebral column are taken to determine whether a partial or a complete obstruction is present. When the level of a complete block identified by lumbar myelography is uncertain, a cisternal myelogram should be performed to determine the extent of the lesion or to identify multiple levels of involvement. CT myelography may be useful where the complete extent of a block is unable to be determined by MRI or the individual has stabilization hardware already in the spine, which may interfere with obtaining a good MRI image, or if MRI is contraindicated. This procedure also allows for examination of the CSF.

After a CT myelogram has been performed, the individual must be assessed for any neurological changes and positioned appropriately (usually supine, with the head of the bed elevated at a prescribed level). Possible complications include allergic reaction to the contrast agent, meningeal irritation, headache, nausea, vomiting, infection, and seizure.

Spine x-rays may be performed in individuals suspected of epidural metastases. It is estimated, however, that 30%–50% of the vertebral body must be destroyed before changes are seen on a plain radiograph.[107]

Bone scans are sensitive in identifying vertebral disease, but they are not always specific and may identify pathology other than cancer.

Prognostic Indicators

The majority of extradural spinal tumors result from metastatic disease, which generally carries a poorer prognosis because of the more advanced stage of disease. Many patients with metastases survive less than a year, and death is often a result of the widespread systemic cancer rather than the epidural tumor. However, patients with limited systemic disease and radiosensitive tumors may survive for longer periods.

Rapid onset and quick progression are worse prognostic factors for recovery. Tumors causing neurological dysfunction that develop over hours to days carry a worse prognosis than those that evolve more slowly. When SCC develops rapidly, neurological recovery is less likely after treatment. The outcome of SCC relates to the individual's neurological status at the time of treatment. The severity of weakness is the most significant prognostic factor for neurological recovery. Eighty percent of those patients who are ambulatory at the time of diagnosis remain so after treatment. As the neurological dysfunction increases, the likelihood of recovery diminishes. Only 30%–45% of patients who are initially paraparetic and nonambulatory become ambulatory, and those who are paraplegic at diagnosis are likely to remain so, with only 5% regaining the ability to walk.[214]

Favorable prognostic factors for intradural tumors include extent of surgical resection, histological grade, performance status, age, and, as in extradural tumors, slow onset of neurological dysfunction. Schwannomas, meningiomas, and ependymomas have a low recurrence rate if completely resected. The same cannot be said for astrocytomas, where the available literature has failed to demonstrate a significant correlation between prognosis and degree of surgical resection.[218,219] A patient's preoperative level of neurological function is the strongest prognostic indicator of postoperative functional outcome.

Classification and Staging

Spinal tumors are classified by their cell of origin and their anatomical location. The types of spinal cord tumors are similar to those tumors found in the brain. Histologically, however, they tend to be less malignant. The major anatomical consideration with spinal cord tumors relates to the tumor's location in relation to the spinal dura mater.

Therapeutic Approaches and Nursing Care

Surgery

In the treatment of spinal cord tumors, the goals of surgery include provision of a diagnosis and partial or complete removal of the tumor. For most intradural, extramedullary tumors, surgery is the primary treatment. Schwannomas and meningiomas can often be completely resected with modern microsurgical techniques and neurosurgical instruments. As in brain tumor surgery, intraoperative monitoring assists the surgeon in maximizing the resection while protecting the spinal cord. In most cases, these tumors can be removed through a posterior (laminectomy) approach. The risk of recurrence is estimated at 10% for complete resections, while recurrence rates increase to 20% for incompletely resected tumors.[218] When possible, recurrences are generally treated with repeat surgical resection.

Surgery is the initial treatment for intramedullary tumors (ependymomas and astrocytomas) with the exception of the malignant astrocytomas. The determining factor in the successful surgical treatment of these tumors is the degree of tumor infiltration of the surrounding spinal cord. As with intracranial glial tumors, indistinct tumor margins and microscopic infiltration can prevent complete tumor removal. Attempts at complete removal often risk loss of neurological function. Astrocytomas are less clearly demarcated from the surrounding spinal cord tissue than ependymomas.[210] Some astrocytomas are treated with biopsy only, followed by RT. For well-delineated astrocytomas, surgical removal can provide long-term tumor control, and sometimes, cure. Ependymomas of the spinal cord have a longer natural history than astrocytomas. Recurrence of ependymomas may be delayed up to 12 years, whereas astrocytomas that recur generally do so within 3 years.[220,221]

For extradural tumors, surgery is generally indicated only in cases where the cause of SCC is unknown, there is spinal instability or bone collapse into the spinal canal, a recurrence cannot be retreated with additional RT, the tumor is known to be radioresistant, or the individual is rapidly deteriorating neurologically, perhaps during the course of RT. Two surgical procedures often performed in this setting are posterior decompressive laminectomy and anterior vertebral body resection.

A laminectomy generally only decompresses the spinal cord. The surgeon may be unable to remove the bulk of the tumor with this approach because the tumor is usually located anterior to the spinal cord. If the tumor has invaded posterior to the epidural space, a modified approach can sometimes allow considerable tumor removal. In a vertebral body resection, most or the entire tumor can be removed, and the resected vertebra is replaced with either bone or a synthetic substance such as methylmethacrylate. The spinal column is often further stabilized anteriorly, for example, with Steinmann pins or plates screwed into intact bone, or posteriorly with instruments such as Harrington rods or hooks.[107] Stabilization procedures require intact bone above and below the site of compression to accept, support, and maintain the fixation devices.[218] Patients with spinal instability typically must remain in bed until they can undergo a stabilization procedure or be fitted for a brace.

Complications related to surgical intervention include the standard surgical risks as well as the development of neurological deficits, CSF leak, and wound dehiscence. The individual with significant or long-standing preoperative neurological deficits is likely to show no improvement or even progression after surgery. The most significant complication requiring treatment is a new neurological deficit in which the neurological function often may not return. The onset of a new deficit is typically related to vascular insult of or manipulation of the spinal cord during surgery.[220] A CSF leak may develop because the dura is not completely sealed or a tear was not repaired. Such a leak is usually treated with lumbar drainage for several days. If the leakage continues, surgery may be required to repair it.

Radiation Therapy

Radiation therapy is generally not recommended for completely resected intradural (intramedullary and extramedullary) spinal cord tumors. Both intramedullary and extramedullary tumors may be treated with RT if incompletely resected or on recurrence if repeat surgical resection is not feasible. Doses of 50–55 Gy are generally used.[4] Ependymomas are radiosensitive tumors. In patients with ependymomas who received adjuvant RT, five- and ten-year survival rates are 60%–100% and 68%–95%, respectively.[221,222] The five- and ten-year survival rates for low-grade astrocytomas who received RT are 60%–90% and 40%–90% respectively.[220] For individuals with high-grade astrocytomas, RT is the only therapy available; even with RT, the prognosis is poor. Survival in such cases is 6–8 months.[220]

RT and steroids are the most widely used therapies for extradural tumors. The usual dose of radiation administered is 30 Gy in 300-cGy fractions.[107] Often, higher doses are administered for the initial treatments, especially if evidence of neurological dysfunction is present.

Spinal RT does not cause acute clinical symptoms. The major complication of spinal cord radiation — radiation myelopathy — results from demyelination and white matter necrosis or intramedullary microvascular injury. Radiation myelopathy may present as a subacute or more severe delayed reaction. A transient subacute myelopathy is clinically manifested by momentary electrical shock-like paresthesias or numbness radiating from the neck down to the extremities, and it is precipitated by flexing the neck (Lhermitte's sign). This syndrome develops after an average of 3–4 months following treatment and resolves within 3–6 months without the need for intervention.[4]

The more severe delayed radiation myelopathy generally occurs 12–28 months following RT, but can take up to 4 years to appear. The clinical manifestations are irreversible; they begin with weakness and can progress to a complete functional loss from the level of the radiation portal down. It is estimated that for doses in the range of 57–61 Gy with conventionally fractionated RT, the incidence of myelopathy is 5%.[221] Risk factors for myelopathy include both the total dose and the dose per fraction.

Chemotherapy

Chemotherapy does not play a large role in the treatment of spinal cord tumors. It may be considered for metastatic extradural tumors in individuals with chemosensitive tumors. Although there have been no trials of chemotherapy for primary spinal cord tumors, drugs active against intracranial gliomas might potentially be effective against these same histologies in the spinal cord. Anecdotal evidence indicates that patients have been treated with nitrosourea-based regimens.[4]

Symptom Management and Supportive Care

Individuals with CNS tumors frequently suffer from disabling symptoms that dramatically affect their ability to function. Many of these symptoms are directly related to the tumor, but other symptoms are only indirectly related to the cancer — for example, side effects of medications used for symptom relief, such as corticosteroids and anticonvulsants, and the psychological symptoms resulting from the devastating effects of the nervous system tumor itself (e.g., aphasia, paralysis, incontinence, cognitive dysfunction).[222] The care of these patients continues to shift to the home and community, regardless of prognosis. Supportive nursing measures assume importance in all areas of patient care.[37] Table 47-4 describes common nursing diagnoses, suggests causes of the problems, and offers some of the associated nursing interventions for the care of these individuals.

Cerebral edema is often managed with corticosteroids such as dexamethasone. Dramatic improvements in neurological function are often seen along with reduction in ICP within hours to days following the initiation of steroids, particularly in those individuals with tumors producing substantial edema.[223] In situations where ICP is acutely elevated, steroids alone are insufficient and osmotic diuretics, also referred to as *hyperosmolar agents*, are required. The high concentration of the drug causes water to be drawn from the normal tissue. Diuresis occurs within one to three hours and lasts up to approximately eight hours. An indwelling urinary catheter, strict recording of intake and output, and monitoring of electrolytes are necessary. Other methods to help control increased ICP include fluid restriction, hyperventilation, sedation, and temperature control. Valsalva maneuvers, isometric muscle contractions, coughing, sneezing, straining, and the use of positive-end expiratory pressure (PEEP) should be avoided, as they can further aggravate increased ICP. A decrease in venous outflow will increase the total blood volume within the intracranial space, leading to elevated ICP. Head and neck positions that impair venous outflow include jugular compression, head rotation, neck flexion, and neck extension. The head of the bed should be elevated to promote venous drainage. Lying prone and flexing the hips should be avoided because these positions increase intraabdominal and intrathoracic pressures, also leading to elevations in ICP. When turning or positioning in bed, the head and neck should be maintained in a neutral position. Alert individuals should be instructed not to turn themselves. Many patients unintentionally perform a valsalva maneuver or grab the side rails tightly (isometric muscle contraction) when turning.[37]

Unfortunately, many nursing interventions, although necessary, can aggravate the already increased ICP. Although many of these activities cannot be avoided, they can be better spaced over time. It is a common practice to group these activities together. For example, when a patient is bathed, he or she is turned several times, receives range-of-motion exercises and pulmonary toileting, and is repositioned. The patient is probably suctioned, is medicated, and may have a dressing or two changed before the nurse leaves the room to attend to other patients or responsibilities. While this practice is often considered necessary to manage the nurse's time and remain efficient and organized, it is not always in the best interest of the patient with increased ICP. Spacing out these activities and care can decrease sustained elevations of increased ICP.

Blocked CSF pathways may lead to hydrocephalus. In such cases, a VP shunt or temporary ventriculostomy may be required. A ventriculostomy is indicated when the etiology of the hydrocephalus is believed to be of a temporary nature. Patients with a ventriculostomy require correct head positioning in relation to the level of the drainage system. The drainage system drip chamber level is ordered by the physician and is usually positioned level with the external auditory meatus. The level is changed based on the patient's clinical condition and the amount of CSF drainage. The procedure of leveling the drip chamber at, above, or below the external auditory meatus minimizes the risk of both excessive CSF drainage leading to collapse of the ventricles and insufficient CSF drainage leading to hydrocephalus. The level of the drip chamber is continuously monitored, the amount and consistency of CSF are assessed hourly, and the patient is evaluated for any neurological changes and signs of infection.

Individuals with spinal cord tumors also receive steroids, especially when SCC has developed. Once the condition is determined or even clinically suspected, steroids are initiated immediately. Steroids decrease the edema of the spinal cord and rapidly relieve back pain in many patients. For patients without neurological symptoms except for pain, low doses of steroids can be administered — usually 4 mg given four times daily. For patients with severe pain or with neurological symptoms, high doses are given, usually 100 mg as an IV bolus followed by 24 mg every six hours for several days.[107] The dose is tapered as the patient is treated with other modalities.

More than 95% of individuals with SCC report having pain. While the administration of steroids provides pain relief for many individuals, others require additional analgesics. Effective analgesia needs to be established early on and dosages adjusted as the steroids and treatment further reduce the pain.

Neurological symptoms of SCC other than pain usually evolve quickly. If prompt treatment is not initiated, weakness leading to paralysis will occur. If diagnosis and treatment are delayed until the patient becomes paraplegic, functional recovery is rare. However, patients who are ambulatory at the onset of treatment will most likely retain that ability. Individuals are taught to report signs and symptoms so as to ensure prompt treatment. The goal of treatment is to preserve and maintain existing neurological function. Patient assessment is therefore crucial throughout this period to evaluate neurological status. Changes in the neurological exam or the development of new deficits must be followed up immediately.

Glucocorticoid hormones are the most widely used drugs in neurooncology.[214] Unfortunately, they have many unwanted side effects. Some of the common side

Table 47-4 Nursing Management of an Individual with a CNS Tumor

Nursing Diagnosis	Possible Cause	Nursing Interventions
Altered cerebral tissue perfusion	Tumor size Cerebral edema Obstruction of CSF pathways Decreased cranial venous outflow Increased intraabdominal and intrathoracic pressure Increased systemic arterial blood pressure	Neurological assessment Corticosteroid administration ICP monitoring Avoid cumulative activities Ventriculostomy Elevate head of bed Avoid head rotation, neck flexion, and extension Avoid hip flexion and prone position Avoid valsalva maneuvers, isometric muscle contractions, coughing, emotional arousal
High risk for seizures	Disturbance of intracranial contents Electrolyte abnormality	Prophylactic anticonvulsants Institute seizure precautions Maintain safe environment Be aware of concurrent medications that interfere with anticonvulsant action, absorption, or both Correct electrolyte abnormalities
Impaired cognition Memory Judgment Thought processes	Frontal tumor Cerebral edema Hydrocephalus Radiation therapy Medication effects	Maintain safe environment Reorient individual Utilize calendars, clocks, labels, photographs, etc., as visual cues or reminders Maintain as close to normal function as possible Encourage use of remaining functional ability Encourage social activities Instruct family members Provide written instructions
Impaired physical mobility Hemiparesis Hemiplegia Paraparesis Paraplegia Ataxic gait Level of consciousness	Frontal tumor Parietal tumor Spinal tumor Spinal RT Steroids	Maintain maximal activity level Provide assistance as necessary for ambulation, transfer, ADLs Encourage proper footwear (nonskid soles that enclose the foot) Maintain safe environment Keep needed objects close at hand Physical and occupational therapy Range-of-motion exercises Teach proper use of assistive devices (brace, cane, walker) Institute measures to prevent complications such as DVT, pressure ulcer, foot drop, pneumonia Develop specific interventions to compensate for deficits Instruct patient and family in safety measures and above techniques When preparing for discharge, obtain necessary equipment for home (wheelchair, bed, commode, walker, guardrail for bathroom, stool for shower) Assess home for physical setup and safety (stairs, rugs)
Alteration in sensory/perceptual ability	Occipital tumor Parietal tumor Frontal tumor Spinal cord tumor Peripheral neuropathy	Monitor sensory function Identify highest level of intact sensory function Instruct patient and family on methods of compensation (checking position of involved areas visually, turning head completely to scan area) Occupational therapy for assistive devices Instruct patient and family in safety measures, proper clothing, and footwear
Knowledge deficit Disease Treatment Medications Discharge	New diagnosis Anxiety	Provide education to patient and family appropriately Encourage questions Clarify misconceptions Refer to resources as needed Provide written materials and written instructions
Alteration in comfort Headache Back pain	Intracranial tumor Increased ICP Spinal cord compression Steroid withdrawal	Assess for verbal and nonverbal indicators of pain Have patient rate pain using 0–10 scale, if possible Administer analgesics, steroids, or other non-narcotic agents and evaluate effectiveness Encourage relaxation techniques or meditation Encourage diversional activities
High risk for impaired skin integrity	Immobility Sensory changes Poor nutrition	Assess skin condition frequently Position changes Frequent, thorough skin care Use of pressure-relieving devices Maximize nutrition Instruct patient and family on measures to prevent skin breakdown (proper positioning techniques, lotion, massage, bathing, nutritious snacks, and meals)

(continued)

Table 47-4 Nursing Management of an Individual with a CNS Tumor (continued)

Nursing Diagnosis	Possible Cause	Nursing Interventions
Alteration in urinary elimination Retention	Immobility Spinal cord tumor	Monitor intake and output Assist into effective position to void Assess for bladder distention Encourage increased fluids Intermittent catheterization If necessary, instruct patient or family member in catheterization technique
Incontinence	Overflow due to retention Frontal tumor Spinal cord tumor Diminished LOC	Assess for urinary retention Skin care Attempt toileting schedule Bladder training
Alteration in bowel elimination Constipation	Decreased mobility Spinal cord tumor Narcotics Steroids Inadequate diet	Assess bowel sounds and normal pattern of elimination Institute bowel regimen Encourage increased fluids and foods high in fiber Allow sufficient time and privacy Assist to proper position
Anxiety Individual Family	New diagnosis Treatment protocols Functional loss Anticipatory grieving Poor prognosis	Assess for verbal and nonverbal signs of anxiety Allow individual, family, or both, to verbalize feelings and source of anxiety Provide emotional support Keep individual and family updated on treatment plans, condition, etc. Refer to appropriate resources as necessary
Other possible nursing diagnoses Self-care deficit High risk for falls Alteration in nutrition Ineffective individual coping Ineffective family coping Alteration in comfort: nausea and vomiting Alteration in oral mucosa Fatigue Altered protective mechanisms: myelosuppression Anticipatory grieving		

effects, while distressing to the individual, are considered mild: insomnia, fatigue, increased appetite, hiccups, blurry vision, behavioral changes, acne, edema, abdominal bloating, and the characteristic moon face. Other effects can be more serious: GI bleeding, bowel perforation, hyperglycemia, hallucinations, psychosis, myopathy manifested by proximal leg weakness, osteoporosis, and acute adrenal insufficiency resulting from steroid withdrawal. Immunosuppression caused by prolonged steroid administration can lead to opportunistic infections, particularly *Pneumocystis carinii* pneumonia (PCP). For this reason, many individuals on prolonged steroid therapy also receive PCP prophylaxis with either trimethoprim and sulfamethoxazole (Bactrim) or pentamadine. PCP prophylaxis generally continues for one month after the steroids have been discontinued.

Ongoing assessment is necessary because neuro-oncology patients often receive steroids for prolonged and repeated periods of time. Patients and families need to be educated regarding the medications, including the side effects to observe for and interventions to take, indications to call their physician, and the absolute necessity of taking the prescribed dose. Sudden withdrawal of steroids can lead to adrenal insufficiency. Symptoms of this condition include fatigue, muscular weakness, joint pain, fever, anorexia, nausea, and orthostatic hypotension.[37] Steroid dosages are tapered slowly to prevent these symptoms of withdrawal. Patients should be given written instructions about the schedule of the steroid taper and should be monitored for increased neurological symptoms as the dose is decreased. Some individuals may become steroid-dependent and do not tolerate even a slow taper. It is also important to be familiar with the drug interactions of steroids and other medications that the individual may be taking. Drugs such as dilantin, phenobarbital, and perhaps carbamazepine (Tegretol) increase the metabolic clearance of steroids and may decrease their therapeutic effect.

Anticonvulsants commonly used to prevent seizures in individuals with primary and metastatic brain tumors include dilantin, phenobarbital, Tegretol, and valproate (Depakene). All of these agents cause drowsiness and cognitive dysfunction. Worsening neurological symptoms occur at toxic therapeutic levels and can add to existing neurological dysfunction. Patients receiving these agents should have their blood levels assessed periodically for therapeutic range. Seizures may be controlled at levels below the therapeutic range; conversely, seizures may occur despite therapeutic levels. Also, some individuals may not exhibit signs of toxicity at high therapeutic levels. Individuals should be encouraged to obtain and wear a medic alert bracelet.

Many individuals with CNS cancers experience anxiety and depression. The psychological impact of the diagnosis, with its relatively poor prognosis, can be devastating. While considered natural responses to the illness with its disabling neurological deficits, anxiety and depression are sometimes overlooked. Antidepressants and antianxiolytics may help improve the psychological symptoms. Counseling can be of benefit to both the individual and his or her family who are grieving the loss of the "person they once knew." The debilitating effects of CNS cancers are not limited to obvious neurological deficits; perhaps more devastating are the effects on the "persona." The personality of the individual is often permanently changed due to the disease, treatment, or both.

Continuity of Care: Nursing Challenges

Discharge planning for the individual with a CNS tumor should begin on the day of hospital admission and evolve during the hospitalization. An accurate assessment of neurological deficits and functional limitations is made. A family member or caregiver should be involved in discharge teaching, as brain tumors frequently cause cognitive disabilities. Anxiety alone may impair an individual's ability to retain new information. The patient and family may be faced with many new issues in the home care setting, and they should be assisted in setting realistic goals. For example, the paraplegic patient will not be able to walk up stairs. Rehabilitation potential is always viewed with realistic hope and optimism. A modified program of home physical therapy is often available for those with CNS cancers even though they may be considered to have a shortened survival. Some individuals may benefit from speech therapy as well. Rehabilitation is especially important for the individuals with low-grade primary CNS tumors because many of them have extended periods of time between recurrences. Vocational rehabilitation may be necessary.

The home should be assessed for its physical setup and safety. Maintaining a safe environment must be constantly reinforced. Continuous supervision may become necessary to prevent harm. Stairs, rugs, and the shower are often a potential source of injury for individuals with CNS cancers. Obstacles should be cleared from common pathways to avoid falls. The individual may need to remain on the ground floor, making room changes necessary. Reality-orientation devices (clocks, calendars, written instructions, photographs) need to be readily visible. Daily roles and routines may need to be altered to accommodate the individual who now has neurological deficits. A thorough assessment of healthcare benefits, family, community, and agency support is essential.

Once the individual with a CNS tumor is discharged, coordination of care assumes an even greater role. Just as the primary nurse in the inpatient setting coordinated the patient's care among the many disciplines involved, the nurse in the outpatient setting must do the same. Follow-up appointments, diagnostic tests, travel arrangements, treatment schedules, special instructions, side effects of medications and treatments, home care issues, insurance company issues, and communication between the various disciplines involved are some of the many issues that the outpatient nurse manages daily. It is important that the patient and family know the person who is familiar with the patient history and disease management. This familiarity provides a sense of continuity and can often allay anxiety. Many of these individuals develop progressive disease, and as their neurological deficits increase, they will require additional support. Many may travel a great distance for their cancer therapy. These individuals then must have a local physician who can provide emergency care and manage the day-to-day issues and problems that arise. For example, many individuals on steroids develop diabetes and require frequent insulin dosage adjustments as the steroids are tapered.

Many persons with CNS tumors will rapidly deteriorate as their disease advances. As a consequence, their neurological function, physical status, and support systems will need to be reevaluated frequently. Adjustments in the plan of care may be necessary. The coping mechanisms of caregivers should be evaluated as they deal with the patient's increasing disability as the disease progresses. There may be issues related to young children at home, employment, and finances. New goals and plans should be formulated. Family members may need to take on added responsibilities such as physical care of the individual and medication administration. Additional resources may need to be accessed, such as other family members, friends, community agencies, local community programs, and support groups. Given that life expectancy at home may not be of long duration, hospice care is an appropriate resource for families struggling with both physical and emotional concerns.

Conclusion

Malignancies of the CNS present tremendous challenges for individuals, families, and caregivers. Because the clinical manifestations, course of treatment, and complications vary with the type and site of tumors, individuals with CNS cancers require highly individualized plans of care. Supportive care takes on a role of utmost importance and encompasses the entire course of illness from diagnosis through the terminal phase of disease. Even with advances in overall therapeutic modalities, successful treatment of CNS cancers remains elusive.[199] Outcomes can range from cure to permanent disability to life prolonged by a few days, weeks, or months. The ongoing physical and emotional support necessary for both the individual and the family create a challenging role for oncology nurses. The neurological symptoms and complications produced by CNS cancers are, unfortunately, profoundly disabling and severely affect quality of life. Assisting the individual to manage problems of daily living, maintain normal function to the best of his or her ability, and attain quality of life are nurses' ultimate goals.

References

1. Central Brain Tumor Registry of the United States Statistical Report: *Statistical Report: Primary Brain Tumors in the United States 1995–1999.* Chicago, Central Brain Tumor Registry of the United States, 2003
2. Jemal A, Tiwari RC, Murray T, et al: Cancer statistics, 2004. *CA Cancer J Clin* 54:8–29, 2004
3. American Cancer Society: *Cancer Facts and Figures 2004.* Atlanta, American Cancer Society, 2004
4. Levin VA, Leibel SA, Gutin PH: Neoplasms of the central nervous system, in Devita VT Jr, Hellman S, Rosenberg SA (eds.) *Cancer: Principles and Practice of Oncology* (ed 6). Philadelphia, Lippincott, Williams and Wilkins, 2001, pp 2100–2160
5. Legler JM, Ries LAG, Smith MA, et al: Brain and other central nervous system cancers: recent trends in incidence and mortality. *J Natl Cancer Inst* 91:1382–1390, 1999
6. Modan B, Wagener DK, Feldman JJ, et al: Increased mortality from brain tumors: a combined outcome of diagnostic technology and change of attitude toward the elderly. *Am J Epidemiol* 135:1349–1357, 1992
7. Riggs JE: Rising primary malignant brain tumor mortality in the elderly. *Arch Neurol* 52:571–575, 1995
8. Gurney JG, Kadan-Lottick N: Brain and other central nervous system tumors: rates, trends, and epidemiology. *Curr Opin Oncol* 13:160–166, 2001
9. Watkins D, Rouleau GA: Genetics, prognosis and therapy of central nervous system tumors. *Cancer Detect Prev* 18:139–144, 1994
10. Bondy M, Wiencke J, Wrensch M, et al: Genetics of brain tumors: a review. *J Neurooncol* 18:69–81, 1994
11. Bohnen NI, Radhakrishnan K, O'Neill BP, et al: Descriptive and analytic epidemiology of brain tumors, in Black PM, Loeffler JS (eds.): *Cancer of the Nervous System.* Cambridge, Blackwell Science, 1997, pp 3–24
12. Prados MD, Berger MS, Wilson CB: Primary central nervous system tumors: advances in knowledge and treatment. *CA Cancer J Clin* 48:331–360, 1998
13. National Brain Tumor Foundation (NBTF): *Brain Tumors: A Guide.* Oakland, National Brain Tumor Foundation, 1994
14. Martz CH: von Hippel-Lindau disease: a genetically transmitted multisystem neoplastic disorder. *Semin Oncol Nurs* 8:281–287, 1992
15. Sehgal A: Molecular changes during the genesis of human gliomas. *Semin Surg Oncol* 14:3–12, 1998
16. DeAngelis LM, Gutin PH, Leibel SA, Posner JB (eds.): *Intracranial Tumors Diagnosis and Treatment.* London, Martin Dunitz, 2002
17. Prados MD, Levin V: Biology and treatment of malignant glioma. *Semin Oncol* 27:1–10, 2000
18. Sadetzki S, Modan B, Chetrit A, et al: An iatrogenic epidemic of benign meningioma. *Am J Epidemiol* 151:266–272, 2000
19. Ron E, Modan B, Boice JD, et al: Tumors of the brain and nervous system after radiotherapy in childhood. *N Engl J Med* 319:1033–1039, 1988
20. Tsang RW, Laperriere NJ, Simpson WJ, et al: Glioma arising after radiation therapy for pituitary adenoma. *Cancer* 72:2227–2233, 1993
21. Alexander MJ, DeSalles AA, Tomiyasu U: Multiple radiation-induced intracranial lesions after treatment for pituitary adenoma. *J Neurosurg* 88:111–115, 1998
22. Walter AW, Hancock ML, Pui CH, et al: Secondary brain tumors in children treated for acute lymphoblastic leukemia at St. Jude Children's Research Hospital. *J Clin Oncol* 16:3761–3767, 1998
23. Schiff D, Suman VJ, Yang P, et al: Risk factors for primary central nervous system lymphoma. *Cancer* 82:975–982, 1998
24. Schabel M: Epidemiology of primary CNS lymphoma. *J Neurooncol* 43:199–201, 1999
25. Heath CW: Electromagnetic field exposure and cancer: a review of epidemiologic evidence. *CA Cancer J Clin* 46:29–44, 1996
26. Berleur MP, Cordier S: The role of chemical, physical, or viral exposures and health factors in neurocarcinogenesis: implications for epidemiologic studies of brain tumors. *Cancer Causes Control* 6:240–256, 1995
27. Sahl JD, Kelsh MA, Greenland S: Cohort and nested case-control studies of hematopoietic cancers and brain cancers among electric utility workers. *Epidemiology* 4:104–114, 1993
28. Floderus B, Persson T, Stenkind C, et al: Occupational exposure to electromagnetic fields in relation to leukemia and brain tumors: a case-control study in Sweden. *Cancer Causes Control* 4:465–476, 1993
29. Wrensch M, Yost M, Miike R, et al: Adult glioma in relation to residential power frequency electromagnetic field exposures in the San Francisco Bay area. *Epidemiology* 10:523–527, 1999
30. Gurney JG, van Wijngaarden E: Extremely low frequency electromagnetic fields (EMF) and brain cancer in adults and children: review and comments. *Neuro-oncology* 1:1–9,1999

31. Portier CJ, Wolfe MS (eds.): *Assessment of Health Effects from Exposure to Power-Line Frequency Electric and Magnetic Fields: NIEHS Working Group Report.* NIH Publication No. 98-3981. Research Triangle Park, NC, National Institute of Environmental Health Sciences, 1998
32. Muscat JE, Malkin MG, Thompson S, et al: Handheld cellular telephone use and risk of brain cancer. *JAMA* 284:3001–3007, 2000
33. Inskip PD, Tarone RE, Hatch EE, et al: Cellular telephone use and brain tumors. *N Engl J Med* 344:79–86, 2001
34. Hickey JV: Overview of neuroanatomy and neurophysiology, in Hickey JV (ed.): *The Clinical Practice of Neurological and Neurosurgical Nursing* (ed 4). Philadelphia, Lippincott, 1997, pp 35–79
35. Leahy NM: *Quick Reference to Neurological Critical Care Nursing.* Rockville, MD, Aspen, 1990
36. Chaffee EE, Lytle IM: *Basic Physiology and Anatomy.* Philadelphia, Lippincott, 1980
37. Wegmann JA: Central nervous system cancers, in Groenwald SL, Frogge MH, Goodman M, Yarbro CH (eds.): *Cancer Nursing: Principles and Practice* (ed 3). Sudbury, MA, Jones and Bartlett, 1993, pp 959–983
38. Marshall SB, Marshall LF, Vos HR, et al: *Neuroscience Critical Care.* Philadelphia, Saunders, 1990
39. Hickey JV: Intracranial pressure theory and management of increased intracranial pressure, in Hickey JV (ed.): *The Clinical Practice of Neurological and Neurosurgical Nursing* (ed 4). Philadelphia, Lippincott, 1997, pp 295–328
40. Andrus C: Intracranial pressure: dynamics and nursing management. *J Neurosci Nurs* 23:85–92, 1991
41. Shafqat S, Hedley-Whyte TE, Henson JW: Age-dependent rate of anaplastic transformation in low-grade astrocytoma. *Neurology* 52:867–869, 1999
42. Behin A, Hoang-Xuan K, Carpentier AF, et al: Primary brain tumors in adults. *Lancet* 361:323–331, 2003
43. Abrey LE, Mason WP (eds.): *Brain Tumors: Fast Facts Indispensable Guides to Clinical Practice.* Oxford, Health Press, 2003
44. Bampoe J, Bernstein A: The role of surgery in low-grade gliomas. *J Neurooncol* 42:259–269, 1999
45. Shaw EG, Scheithauer BW, O'Fallon JR: Supratentorial gliomas: a comparative study by grade and histologic type. *J Neurooncol* 31:273–278, 1997
46. Lote K, Egeland T, Hager B, et al: Survival, prognostic factors, and therapeutic efficacy in low-grade glioma: a retrospective study in 379 patients. *J Clin Oncol* 15:3129–3140, 1997
47. Keles GE, Lamborn KR, Berger MS: Low-grade hemispheric gliomas in adults: a critical review of extent of resection as a factor influencing outcome. *J Neurosurg* 95:735–745, 2001
48. National Comprehensive Cancer Network: *NCCN Practice Guidelines Central Nervous System Cancers.* Jenkintown, PA, National Comprehensive Cancer Network, 2003
49. Macdonald DR: Low-grade gliomas, mixed gliomas, and oligodendrogliomas. *Semin Oncol* 21:236–248, 1994
50. Leighton C, Fisher B, Bauman G, et al: Supratentorial low-grade glioma in adults: an analysis of prognostic factors and timing of radiation. *J Clin Oncol* 4:1294–1301, 1997
51. Karim ABMF, Afra D, Cornu P, et al; Randomized trial on the efficacy of radiotherapy for cerebral low-grade glioma in the adult: European Organization for Research and Treatment of Cancer Study 22845 with the Medical Research Council Study BR04: an interim analysis. *Int J Radiat Oncol Biol Phys* 52:316–324, 2002
52. Daumas-Duport C, Varlet P, Tucker ML, et al: Oligodendrogliomas. Part 1: patterns of growth, histological diagnosis, clinical and imaging correlations: a study of 153 cases. *J Neurooncol* 34:37–59, 1997
53. Coons SW, Johnson PC, Scheithauer BW, et al: Improving diagnostic accuracy and interobserver concordance in the classification and grading of primary gliomas. *Cancer* 79:1381–1393, 1997
54. Fortin D, Cairncross GJ, Hammond RR: Oligodendroglioma: an appraisal of recent data pertaining to diagnosis and treatment. *Neurosurgery* 45:1279–1291, 1999
55. Levin VA, Silver P, Hannigan J, et al: Superiority of post-radiotherapy adjuvant chemotherapy with CCNU, procarbazine, and vincristine (PCV) over BCNU for anaplastic gliomas: NCOG 6G61 final report. *Int J Radiat Oncol Biol Phys* 18:321–324, 1990
56. Cairncross JG, Ueki K, Zlatescu MC, et al: Specific genetic predictors of chemotherapeutic response and survival in patients with anaplastic oligodendroglioma. *J Natl Cancer Inst* 90:1473–1479, 1998
57. Bigner SH, Rasheed K, Wiltshire RN, et al: Morphologic and molecular genetic aspects of oligodendroglial neoplasms. *Neuro-oncology* 1:52–60, 1999
58. Ino Y, Betensky RA, Zlatescu MC, et al: Molecular subtypes of anaplastic oligodendroglioma: implications for patient management at diagnosis. *Clin Cancer Res* 7:839–845, 2001
59. Macdonald DR: New therapies of primary CNS lymphomas and oligodendrogliomas. *J Neurooncol* 24:97–101, 1995
60. Buckner JC, Gesme D, O'Fallon JR, et al: Phase II trial of procarbazine, lomustine, and vincristine as initial therapy for patients with low-grade oligodendroglioma or oligoastrocytoma: efficacy and associations with chromosomal abnormalities. *J Clin Oncol* 21:251–255, 2003
61. Abrey LA, Childs BH, Paleologos N, et al: High-dose chemotherapy with stem cell rescue as initial therapy for anaplastic oligodendroglioma. *J Neurooncol* 65:127–134, 2003
62. Schiff D, Wen PY: Uncommon brain tumors, in Wen PY, Black PM (eds.): *Neurologic Clinics: Brain Tumors in Adults.* Philadelphia, Saunders, 1995, pp 953–974
63. Cohen ME, Duffer PK: Ependymomas, in Cohen ME, Duffer PK (eds.): *Brain Tumors in Children* (ed 2). New York, Raven, 1994, pp 219–239
64. McLaughlin MP, Marcus RB, Buatti JM, et al: Ependymomas: results, prognostic factors and treatment recommendations. *Int J Radiat Oncol Biol Phys* 40:845–850, 1998
65. Guyotat J, Signorelli F, Desme S, et al: Intracranial ependymomas in adult patients: analysis of prognostic factors. *J Neurooncol* 60:255–268, 2002
66. DeMonte F: Current management of meningiomas. *Oncology* 9:83–96, 1995
67. Schrell UMH, Fahlbusch R, Adams EF: Meningiomas and neurofibromatosis for the oncologist. *Curr Opin Oncol* 6:247–253, 1994
68. Markopoulos C, Sampalalis F, Givalos N, et al: Association of breast cancer with meningioma. *Eur J Surg Oncol* 24:332–334, 1998
69. Black PM: Brain tumors. *N Engl J Med* 324:1555–1564, 1991
70. Black PM: Benign brain tumors, in Wen PY, Black PM (eds.): *Neurologic Clinics: Brain Tumors in Adults.* Philadelphia, Saunders, 1995, pp 927–954
71. Younis GA, Sawaya R, DeMonte F, et al: Aggressive meningeal tumors: review of a series. *J Neurosurg* 82:17–27, 1995
72. Wilson CB: Meningiomas: genetics, malignancy, and the role of radiation in induction and treatment. *J Neurosurg* 81:666–674, 1994
73. Dziuk TW, Woo S, Butler EB, et al: Malignant meningioma: an indication for initial aggressive surgery and adjuvant radiotherapy. *J Neurooncol* 37:177–188, 1998

74. Hug EB, DeVries A, Thornton AF, et al: Management of atypical and malignant meningiomas: role of high-dose, 3D-conformal radiation therapy. *J Neurooncol* 48:151–160, 2000
75. Kondziolka D, Levy EI, Niranjan A, et al: Long-term outcomes after meningioma radiosurgery: physician and patient perspectives. *J Neurosurg* 91:44–50, 1999
76. Kaba SE, DeMonte F, Bruner JM, et al: The treatment of recurrent unresectable and malignant meningiomas with interferon alpha-2B. *Neurosurgery* 40:271–275, 1997
77. Mason WP, Gentili F, Macdonald DR, et al: Stabilization of disease progression by hydroxyurea in patients with recurrent or unresectable meningioma. *J Neurosurg* 97:341–346, 2002
78. Ragel B, Jensen RL: New approaches for the treatment of refractory meningiomas. *Cancer Control* 10:148–158, 2003
79. Campbell C: Acoustic neuroma: nursing implications related to surgical management. *J Neurosci Nurs* 23:50–60, 1991
80. Koos WT, Day JD, Matula C, et al: Neurotopographic considerations in the microsurgical treatment of small acoustic neurinomas. *J Neurosurg* 88:506–512, 1998
81. Young JS: Acoustic neuroma: postoperative vertigo and the mechanisms of compensation. *J Neurosci Nurs* 24:194–198, 1992
82. DeAngelis LM: Primary central nervous system lymphoma. *Recent Results Cancer Res* 135:155–169, 1994
83. Eby NL, Grufferman S, Flannelly CM, et al: Increasing incidence of primary brain lymphoma in the US. *Cancer* 62:2461–2465, 1988
84. O'Neill BP, Illig JJ: Primary central nervous system lymphoma. *Mayo Clin Proc* 64:1005–1020, 1989
85. Cote TR, Manns A, Hardy CR, et al: Epidemiology of brain lymphoma among people with or without acquired immunodeficiency syndrome. *J Natl Cancer Inst* 88:675–679, 1996
86. Selch MT, Shimizu KT, DeSalles AF, et al: Primary central nervous system lymphoma. *Am J Clin Oncol* 17:286–293, 1994
87. Olson JE, Janney CA, Rao RD, et al: The continuing increase in the incidence of primary central nervous system non-Hodgkin's lymphoma. *Cancer* 95:1504–1510, 2002
88. Rosenblum ML, Levy RM, Bredesen DE, et al: Primary central nervous system lymphoma in patients with AIDS. *Ann Neurol* 23:513–516, 1988
89. Forsyth PA, Yahalom J, DeAngelis LM: Combined-modality therapy in the treatment of primary central nervous system lymphoma in AIDS. *Neurology* 44:1473–1479, 1994
90. Loureiro C, Gill PS, Meyer PR, et al: Autopsy findings in AIDS-related lymphoma. *Cancer* 62:735–739, 1988
91. Cornford ME, Holden JK, Boyd MC, et al: Neuropathology of the acquired immune deficiency syndrome (AIDS): report of 39 autopsies from Vancouver, British Columbia. *Can J Neurol Sci* 19:442–452, 1992
92. DeAngelis LM: Primary central nervous system lymphoma. *J Neurol Neurosurg Psychiatry* 66:699–701, 1999
93. Buggage RR, Chan CC, Nussenblatt RB: Ocular manifestations of central nervous system lymphoma. *Curr Opin Oncol* 13:137–142, 2001
94. DeAngelis LM: Current management of primary central nervous system lymphoma. *Oncology* 9:63–71, 1995
95. Peterson K, Gordon KB, Heinemann MH, et al: The clinical spectrum of ocular lymphoma. *Cancer* 72:83–89, 1993
96. Akpek EK, Ahmed I, Hochberg FH, et al: Intraocular-central nervous system lymphoma: clinical features, diagnosis, outcomes. *Ophthalmology* 106:1805–1810, 1999
97. Cheng AL, Yeh KH, Uen WC, et al: Systemic chemotherapy alone for patients with non-acquired immunodeficiency syndrome–related central nervous system lymphoma. *Cancer* 82:1946–1951, 1998
98. Abrey LA, Yahalom J, DeAngelis LM: Treatment for primary CNS lymphoma: the next step. *J Clin Oncol* 18:3144–3150, 2000
99. Dahlborg SA, Braziel R, Crossen JR, et al: Non-AIDS primary CNS lymphoma: first example of a durable response in a primary brain tumor using enhanced chemotherapy delivery without cognitive loss and without radiotherapy. *Cancer J Sci Am* 2:166–174, 1996
100. Chamberlain MC, Levin VA: Primary central nervous system lymphoma: a role for adjuvant chemotherapy. *J Neurooncol* 14:271–275, 1992
101. Soussain C, Suzan F, Hoang-Xuan K, et al: Results of intensive chemotherapy followed by hematopoietic stem-cell rescue in 22 patients with refractory or recurrent primary CNS lymphoma or intraocular lymphoma. *J Clin Oncol* 19:742–749, 2001
102. Abrey LE, DeAngelis LM, Yahalom J: Long-term survival in primary CNS lymphoma. *J Clin Oncol* 16:859–863, 1998
103. O'Neill BP, Buckner JC, Coffey RJ, et al: Brain metastatic lesions. *Mayo Clin Proc* 69:1062–1068, 1994
104. Young RF: Radiosurgery for the treatment of brain metastases. *Semin Surg Oncol* 14:70–78, 1998
105. Lang FF, Sawaya R: Surgical treatment of metastatic brain tumors. *Semin Surg Oncol* 14:53–63, 1998
106. DeAngelis LM: Management of brain metastases. *Cancer Invest* 12:156–165, 1994
107. Posner JB: *Neurologic Complications of Cancer.* Philadelphia, Davis, 1995
108. Sitton E: Central nervous system metastases. *Semin Oncol Nurs* 14:210–219, 1998
109. Posner JB: Surgery for metastases to the brain. *N Engl J Med* 322:544–545, 1990
110. Patchell RA, Tibbs PA, Walsh JW, et al: A randomized trial of surgery in the treatment of single metastases to the brain. *N Engl J Med* 322:544–545, 1990
111. Vecht CJ, Haaxma-Reiche H, Noordijk EM, et al: Treatment of single brain metastasis: radiotherapy alone or combined with neurosurgery? *Ann Neurol* 33:583–590, 1993
112. Bindel RK, Sawaya R, Leavens ME, et al: Surgical treatment of multiple brain metastases. *J Neurosurg* 79:210–216, 1993
113. Oben A, Moriarty TM, Loeffler JS: Radiosurgery for metastases. *J Neurooncol* 27:279–285, 1996
114. Muacevic A, Kreth FW, Horstmann GA, et al: Surgery and radiotherapy compared with gamma knife radiosurgery in the treatment of solitary cerebral metastases of small diameter. *J Neurosurg* 91:35–43, 1999
115. Hilliard VH, Shih LL, Chin S, et al: Safety of multiple stereotactic radiosurgery treatments for multiple brain lesions. *J Neurooncol* 63:271–278, 2003
116. Postmus PE, Haaxma-Reiche H, Smit EF, et al: Treatment of brain metastases of small-cell lung cancer: comparing teniposide and teniposide with whole-brain radiotherapy — a phase III study of the European Organization for the Research and Treatment of Cancer Lung Cancer Cooperative Group. *J Clin Oncol* 18:3400–3408, 2000
117. Antonadou D, Paraskevaidis G, Sarris N, et al: Phase II randomized trial of temozolomide and concurrent radiotherapy in patients with brain metastases. *J Clin Oncol* 20:3644–3650, 2002
118. Abrey LE, Olson JD, Raizer JJ, et al: A phase II trial of temozolomide for patients with recurrent or progressive brain metastases. *J Neurooncol* 53:259–265, 2001
119. Freilich RJ, DeAngelis LM: Primary central nervous system cancer, in Wen PY, Black PM (eds.): *Neurologic Clinics: Brain Tumors in Adults.* Philadelphia, Saunders, 1995, pp 901–914
120. Willis D: Intracranial astrocytoma: pathology, diagnosis and clinical presentation. *J Neurosci Nurs* 23:7–14, 1991
121. Schnell S, DeLeon MEM: Anatomy of the central nervous system. *Semin Oncol Nurs* 14:2–7, 1998
122. Byrne TN: Imaging of gliomas. *Semin Oncol* 21:162–171, 1994

123. Hickey JV: Diagnostic procedures and laboratory tests for neuroscience patients, in Hickey JV (ed.): *The Clinical Practice of Neurological and Neurosurgical Nursing* (ed 4). Philadelphia, Lippincott, 1997, pp 81–101
124. Schwartz RB: Neuroradiology of brain tumors, in Wen PY, Black PM (eds.): *Neurologic Clinics: Brain Tumors in Adults.* Philadelphia, Saunders, 1995, pp 723–756
125. Jaeckle KA: Neuroimaging for central nervous system tumors. *Semin Oncol* 18:150–157, 1991
126. Arbour RA: Stereotactic localization and resection of intracranial tumors. *J Neurosci Nurs* 25:14–21, 1993
127. Wen PY, Alexander E III, Black PM, et al: Long term results of stereotactic brachytherapy used in the initial treatment of patients with glioblastomas. *Cancer* 73:3029–3036, 1994
128. Hoffman JM: New advances in brain tumor imaging. *Curr Opin Oncol* 13:148–153, 2001
129. Forster BB, Mackay AL, Whittall KP, et al: Functional magnetic imaging: the basics of blood-oxygen-level dependent (BOLD) imaging. *Can Assoc Radiol* 49:329–339, 1998
130. Van den Bent MJ: The role of chemotherapy in brain metastases. *Eur J Cancer* 39:2114–2120, 2003
131. Laws ER, Parney IF, Huang W, et al: Survival following surgery and prognostic factors for recently diagnosed malignant glioma: data from the Glioma Outcomes Project. *J Neurosurg* 99:467–473, 2003
132. Wen PY, Fine HA, Black PM, et al: High-grade astrocytomas, in Wen PY, Black PM (eds.): *Neurologic Clinics: Brain Tumors in Adults.* Philadelphia, Saunders, 1995, pp 875–900
133. Hess KR: Extent of resection as a prognostic variable in the treatment of gliomas. *J Neurooncol* 42:227–231, 1999
134. Berger MS: Malignant astrocytomas: surgical aspects. *Semin Oncol* 21:172–185, 1994
135. Berger MS, Rostomily RC: Low grade gliomas: functional mapping resection strategies, extent of resection, and outcome. *J Neurooncol* 34:85–101, 1997
136. Chandler KL, Prados MD, Malec M, et al: Long-term survival in patients with glioblastoma multiforme. *Neurosurgery* 32:716–720, 1993
137. Morita M, Rosenblum MK, Bilsky MH, et al: Long-term survivors of glioblastoma multiforme: clinical and molecular characteristics. *J Neurooncol* 27:259–266, 1996
138. Salvati M, Cervoni L, Artico M, et al: Long-term survival in patients with supratentorial glioblastoma. *J Neurooncol* 36:61–64, 1998
139. Chidel MA, Suh JH, Reddy CA, et al: Application of recursive partitioning analysis and evaluation of the use of whole brain radiation among patients treated with stereotactic radiosurgery for newly diagnosed brain metastases. *Int J Radiat Oncol Biol Phys* 47:993–999, 2000
140. American Joint Committee on Cancer: *AJCC Cancer Staging Manuel* (ed 5). Philadelphia, Lippincott-Raven, 1997
141. O'Mary SS: Diagnostic evaluation, classification, and staging, in Groenwald SL, Frogge MH, Goodman M, Yarbro CH (eds.): *Cancer Nursing: Principles and Practice* (ed 4). Sudbury, MA, Jones and Bartlett, 1997, pp 175–199
142. Kleihues P, Cavanee WK: *World Health Organization Classification of Tumours: Tumours of the Nervous System — Pathology and Genetics.* Lyon, France, IRAC Press, 2000
143. Hentschel SJ, Sawaya R: Optimizing outcomes with maximal surgical resection of malignant gliomas. *Cancer Control* 10:109–114, 2003
144. Harbaugh KS, Black PM: Strategies in the surgical management of malignant gliomas. *Semin Surg Oncol* 14:26–33, 1998
145. Sawaya R, Rambo WM, Hammond MA, et al: Advances in surgery for brain tumors, in Wen PY, Black PM (eds.): *Neurologic Clinics: Brain Tumors in Adults.* Philadelphia, Saunders, 1995, pp 757–771
146. Vives KP, Piepmeier J: Complications and expected outcome of glioma surgery. *J Neurooncol* 42:289–302, 1999
147. Heilbrun MP, Roberts TS, Apuzzo MLJ, et al: Preliminary experience with Brown-Roberts-Wells (BRW) computerized tomography stereotaxic guidance system. *J Neurosurg* 59:217–222, 1983
148. Krieger MD, Chandrasoma PT, Zee CS, et al: Role of stereotactic biopsy in the diagnosis and management of brain tumors. *Semin Surg Oncol* 14:13–25, 1998
149. League D: Interactive, image-guided, stereotactic neurosurgery systems. *AORN J* 61:360–370, 1995
150. Schulder M, Carmel PW: Intraoperative magnetic resonance imaging: impact on brain tumor surgery. *Cancer Control* 10:115–124, 2003
151. Gooding GA, Edwards MS, Rabskin AE, et al: Intraoperative real-time ultrasound in the localization of intracranial neoplasms. *Radiology* 146:459–461, 1983
152. Bohan EM: Neurosurgical management of patients with central nervous system malignancies. *Semin Oncol Nurs* 14:8–17, 1998
153. Chen TC, Apuzzo MLJ: Principles of stereotactic neurosurgery, in Black PM, Loeffler JS (eds.): *Cancer of the Nervous System.* Boston, Blackwell Science, 1997, pp 156–177
154. Black P, Moriarty T, Alexander E III, et al: Development and implementation of intraoperative magnetic resonance imaging and its neurosurgical applications. *Neurosurgery* 41:831–845, 1997
155. Hall W, Liu H, Martin AJ, et al: Safety, efficacy, and functionality of high-field strength interventional magnetic resonance imaging for neurosurgery. *Neurosurgery* 46:632–642, 2000
156. Sutherland GR, Kaibara T, Louw D, et al: A mobile high-field magnetic resonance system for neurosurgery. *J Neurosurg* 91:804–813, 1999
157. Hadani M, Spiegelman R, Feldman Z, et al: Novel, compact, intraoperative magnetic resonance imaging–guided system for conventional neurosurgical operating rooms. *Neurosurgery* 48:799–809, 2001
158. Rambo WM, Sawaya RE: Neurosurgical treatment of brain tumors. *Cancer Bull* 45:320–325, 1993
159. Shrieve DC, Loeffler JS: Advances in radiation therapy for brain tumors, in Wen PY, Black PM (eds.): *Neurologic Clinics: Brain Tumors in Adults.* Philadelphia, Saunders, 1995, pp 773–793
160. Walker MD, Alexander E, Hunt WE, et al: Evaluation of BCNU and/or radiotherapy in the treatment of anaplastic gliomas. *J Neurosurg* 49:333–343, 1978
161. Fine HA, Dear KB, Loeffler JS, et al: Meta-analysis of radiation therapy with and without adjuvant chemotherapy for malignant gliomas in adults. *Cancer* 71:2585–2597, 1993
162. Leibel SA, Scott CB, Loeffler JS: Contemporary approaches to the treatment of malignant gliomas with radiation therapy. *Semin Oncol* 21:198–219, 1994
163. Vick NA, Paleologos NA: External beam radiotherapy: hard facts and painful realities. *J Neurooncol* 24:93–95, 1995
164. Shrieve DC, Alexander E III, Wen PY, et al: Comparison of stereotactic radiosurgery and brachytherapy in the treatment of recurrent glioblastoma multiforme. *Neurosurgery* 36:275–284, 1995
165. Shaw EG, Scheithauer BW, O'Fallon JR: Management of supratentorial low-grade gliomas. *Oncology* 7:97–111, 1993
166. Shaw EG: Low grade gliomas — to treat or not to treat? The radiation oncologist's perspective. *Arch Neurol* 47:1138–1139, 1990

167. Recht LD, Lew R, Smith TW: Suspected low-grade glioma: is deferring treatment safe? *Ann Neurol* 31:431–436, 1992
168. Philippon JH, Clemenceau SH, Fauchon FH, et al: Supratentorial low-grade astrocytomas in adults. *Neurosurgery* 32:554–559, 1993
169. Larson DA, Wara WW: Radiotherapy of primary malignant brain tumors. *Semin Surg Oncol* 14:34–42, 1998
170. Thorton AF, Hegarty TJ, Ten Haken RK, et al: Three-dimensional treatment planning of astrocytomas, a dosimetric study of cerebral irradiation. *Int J Radiat Oncol Biol Phys* 20:1309–1315, 1991
171. Addesa AE, Shrieve DC, Alexander A III, et al: Stereotactic radiosurgery as primary adjuvant treatment for glioblastoma: the JCRT update. *Proc Am Soc Clin Oncol* 14:144, 1995 (abstract 274A)
172. Bhatnagar A, Heron DE, Kondziolka D, et al: Analysis of repeat stereotactic radiosurgery for progressive primary and metastatic CNS tumors. *Int J Radiat Oncol Biol Phys* 53:527–532, 2002
173. McDermott MW, Sneed PK, Gutin PH: Interstitial brachytherapy for malignant brain tumors. *Semin Surg Oncol* 14:79–87, 1998
174. Gutin PH, Prados MD, Phillips TL, et al: External irradiation followed by an interstitial high activity iodine-125 implant "boost" in the initial treatment of malignant gliomas: NCOG study 6G-82-2. *Int J Radiat Oncol Biol Phys* 21:601–606, 1991
175. Halligan JB, Stelzer KJ, Rostomily RC, et al: Operation and permanent low-activity ^{125}I brachytherapy for recurrent high-grade astrocytomas. *Int J Radiat Oncol Biol Phys* 35:541–547, 1996
176. Tatter SB, Shaw EG, Rosenblum ML, et al: An inflatable balloon catheter and liquid ^{125}I radiation source (Gliasite Radiation Therapy System) for treatment of recurrent malignant glioma: multicenter safety and feasibility trial. *J Neurosurg* 99:297–303, 2003
177. Vermeulen SS: Whole brain radiotherapy in the treatment of metastatic brain tumors. *Semin Surg Oncol* 14:64–69, 1998
178. Young RF, Jacques DB, Duma C, et al: Gamma knife radiosurgery for treatment of multiple brain metastases: a comparison of patients with single versus multiple lesions. *Radiosurgery* 1:92–101, 1995
179. Sneed PK, Lamborn KR, Forstner JM, et al: Radiosurgery for brain metastases: is whole brain radiotherapy necessary? *Int J Radiat Oncol Biol Phys* 43:549–558, 1999
180. Werner-Wasik M, Rudoler S, Preston PE, et al: Immediate side effects of stereotactic radiotherapy and radiosurgery. *Int J Radiat Oncol Biol Phys* 43:299–304, 1999
181. Strohl RA: Radiation therapy in tumors of the central nervous system. *Semin Oncol Nurs* 14:26–33, 1998
182. Prados MD, Russo C: Chemotherapy of brain tumors. *Semin Surg Oncol* 14:88–95, 1998
183. Shapiro WR, Shapiro JR: Biology and treatment of malignant glioma. *Oncology* 12:233–246, 1998
184. Lesser GJ, Grossman SA: The chemotherapy of high-grade astrocytomas. *Semin Oncol* 21:220–235, 1994
185. Prados MD, Scott C, Curran WJ Jr, et al: Procarbazine, lomustine, and vincristine (PCV) chemotherapy for anaplastic astrocytoma: a retrospective review of radiation therapy oncology group protocols comparing survival with carmustine or PCV adjuvant chemotherapy. *J Clin Oncol* 17:3389–3395, 1999
186. Yung WKA, Prados MD, Yaya-Tur R, et al: Multicenter phase II trial of temozolomide in patients with anaplastic astrocytoma or anaplastic oligoastrocytoma at first relapse. *J Clin Oncol* 17:2762–2771, 1999
187. Yung WKA, Albright RE, Olson J, et al: A phase II study of temozolomide vs procarbazine in patients with glioblastoma multiforme at first relapse. *Brit J Can* 83:588–593, 2000
188. Conrad CA, Milosavljevic VP, Yung WK: Advances in chemotherapy for brain tumors, in Wen PY, Black PM (eds.): *Neurologic Clinics: Brain Tumors in Adults.* Philadelphia, Saunders, 1995, pp 795–812
189. Glass J, Hochberg FH, Gruber ML, et al: The treatment of oligodendrogliomas and mixed oligodendrogliomas-astrocytomas with PCV chemotherapy. *J Neurosurg* 76:741–745, 1992
190. Kyritsis AP, Yung WKA, Bruner J, et al: The treatment of anaplastic oligodendrogliomas and mixed gliomas. *Neurosurgery* 32:365–371, 1993
191. Mason WP, DeAngelis LM: Procarbazine, CCNU, vincristine (PCV) chemotherapy (CT) for benign oligodendroglioma. *Neurology* 44:A262–A263, 1994
192. Peterson K, Cairncross JG: Oligodendroglioma. *Cancer Invest* 14:243–251, 1996
193. Armstrong TS, Gilbert MR: Chemotherapy of astrocytomas: an overview. *Semin Oncol Nurs* 14:18–25, 1998
194. Gumerlock MK, Belshe BD, Madsen R, et al: Osmotic blood–brain barrier disruption and chemotherapy in the treatment of high grade malignant glioma: patient series and literature review. *J Neurooncol* 12:33–46, 1992
195. Olivi A, Brem H: Interstitial chemotherapy with sustained release polymer systems for the treatment of malignant gliomas. *Recent Results Cancer Res* 135:149–154, 1994
196. Brem H, Piantadosi S, Burger PC, et al: Intraoperative controlled delivery of chemotherapy by biodegradable polymers: safety and effectiveness for recurrent gliomas evaluated by a prospective multi-institutional placebo-controlled clinical trial. *Lancet* 345:1008–1012, 1995
197. Westphal M, Hilt DC, Bortey E, et al: A phase III trial of local chemotherapy with biodegradable carmustine (BCNU) wafers (Gliadel wafers) in patients with primary malignant glioma. *Neuro-oncology* 5:79–88, 2003
198. Giese A, Kucinski T, Knopp U, et al: Pattern of recurrence following local chemotherapy with biodegradable carmustine (BCNU) implants in patients with glioblastoma. *J Neurooncol* 66:351–360, 2004
199. Gruber ML, Glass J, Choudhri H, et al: Carboplatin chemotherapy before irradiation in newly diagnosed glioblastoma multiforme. *Am J Clin Oncol* 21:338–340, 1998
200. American Brain Tumor Association (ABTA): *A Primer of Brain Tumors.* Des Plaines, IL, ABTA, 1998
201. Couldwell WT, Hinton DR, Surnock AA, et al: Treatment of recurrent malignant gliomas with chronic oral high-dose tamoxifen. *Clin Cancer Res* 2:619–622, 1996
202. Mastronardi L, Puzzilli F, Couldwell WT, et al: Tamoxifen and carboplatin combinational treatment of high-grade gliomas. *J Neurooncol* 38:59–68, 1998
203. Tremont-Lukats IW, Gilbert MR: Advances in molecular therapies in patients with brain tumors. *Cancer Control* 10:125–137, 2003
204. Kitange GJ, Templeton KL, Jenkins RB: Recent advances in the molecular genetics of primary gliomas. *Curr Opin Oncol* 15:197–203, 2003
205. Parsa AT, Fiore AJ, McCormick PC, et al: Genetic basis of intramedullary spinal cord tumors and therapeutic implications. *J Neurooncol* 47:239–251, 2000
206. Thomas LT, Waxweiler JR: Brain tumors and occupational risk factors: a review. *Scand J Work Environ Health* 12:1–15, 1986
207. Gilman S, Newman SW: *Manter and Gatz's Essentials of Clinical Neuroanatomy and Neurophysiology* (ed 8). Philadelphia, Davis, 1992
208. Barr ML, Kiernan JA: *The Human Nervous System* (ed 5). Philadelphia, Lippincott, 1988
209. Kornblith PJ, Walker MD, Cassady JR: *Neurologic Oncology.* Philadelphia, Lippincott, 1987
210. Maher de Leon ME, Schnell S, Rozental JM: Tumors of the spine and spinal cord. *Semin Oncol Nurs* 14:43–52, 1998

211. Schild SE, Nisi K, Scheithauer BW, et al: The results of radiotherapy for ependymomas: the Mayo Clinic experience. *Int J Radiat Oncol Biol Phys* 42:953–958, 1998
212. Houten JK, Cooper PR: Spinal cord astrocytomas: presentation, management and outcome. *J Neurooncol* 47:219–224, 2000
213. Lowe GM: Magnetic resonance imaging of intramedullary spinal cord tumors. *J Neurooncol* 47:195–210, 2000
214. Grant R, Papadoppoulos SM, Sandler HM, et al: Metastatic epidural spinal cord compression: current concepts and treatment. *J Neurooncol* 19:79–92, 1994
215. Cohen AP, Wisoff JH, Allen JC, et al: Malignant astrocytomas of the spinal cord. *J Neurosurg* 70:50–54, 1989
216. Hickey JV, Armstrong TS: Spinal cord tumors, in Hickey JV (ed.): *The Clinical Practice of Neurological and Neurosurgical Nursing* (ed 4). Philadelphia, Lippincott, 1997, pp 527–539
217. Schwartz TH, McCormick PC: Intramedullary ependymomas: clinical presentation, surgical treatment strategies and prognosis. *J Neurooncol* 47:211–218, 2000
218. Abernathey CD: Spinal intradural extramedullary tumors, in Rengachary SS, Wilkins RH (eds.): *Principles of Neurosurgery*. London, Wolfe, 1994, pp 38-1–38-8
219. Minehan KJ, Shaw EG, Scheithauer BW, et al: Spinal cord astrocytoma: pathological and treatment considerations. *J Neurosurg* 83:590–595, 1995
220. Linstadt DE, Wara WM, Leibel SA, et al: Postoperative radiotherapy of primary spinal cord tumors. *Int J Radiat Oncol Biol Phys* 16:1397–1403, 1989
221. Waldron JN, Laperriere NJ, Jaakkimainen L, et al: Spinal cord ependymomas: a retrospective analysis of 59 cases. *Int J Radiat Oncol Biol Phys* 27:223–229, 1993
222. Whitaker SJ, Bessell EM, Ashley SE, et al: Postoperative radiotherapy in the management of spinal cord ependymoma. *J Neurosurg* 74:720–728, 1991
223. Schultheiss TE: Spinal cord radiation "tolerance": doctrine versus data. *Int J Radiat Oncol Biol Phys* 19:219–221, 1990
224. Posner JB: Supportive care of the neuro-oncology patient, in Hildebrand J (ed.): *Management in Neuro-Oncology*. Berlin, Springer-Verlag, 1992, pp 89–99
225. Byrne TN, Cascino TL, Posner JB: Brain metastasis from melanoma. *J Neurooncol* 1:313–317, 1983

CHAPTER 48

Cervical Cancer

Susan Vogt Temple, RN, MSN, AOCN®

Introduction

Cervical cancer is a sexually transmitted disease. Persistent infection with oncogenic human papillomavirus (HPV), most frequently contracted through vaginal intercourse, is necessary for the development of cervical cancer and high-grade precursor lesions. Virtually all cases of invasive squamous cell cervical cancer harbor HPV DNA integrated into the host genome. Fortunately, most women have transient HPV infections and clear the virus to undetectable or negligible levels. In the United States, the majority of cervical lesions are diagnosed in the preinvasive stages of intraepithelial neoplasia, when the disease is curable. Like many other cancers, cervical cancer can be cured when it is diagnosed in early stages. However, in developing nations and among older women, ethnic minorities, and the medically underserved in the United States, cervical cancer screening is unavailable or inaccessible.[1]

Epidemiology

Cervical cancer remains a significant source of morbidity and mortality for women worldwide, with more than 466,000 women being diagnosed with invasive disease. Approximately 200,000 deaths are attributed to progressive disease and concomitant complications yearly. Globally, cervical cancer ranks as the second most common cancer in women and is one of the leading causes of cancer-related deaths for women in developing nations. The highest incidence of invasive cervical cancer is reported in southern and eastern Africa, Central America, and southern Asia. A disproportionate share (more than 80%) of cervical cancer deaths occur in those nations that lack the necessary resources and infrastructure for ongoing screening, surveillance, and treatment of preinvasive and invasive lesions.[1–3]

According to the American Cancer Society, more than 10,500 new cases of invasive cervical cancer will have been diagnosed in the United States in 2004, and approximately 3900 women will die of the disease. Deaths from invasive cervical cancer decreased by 74% between 1955 and 1992, and they continue to decline by about 2% per year.[3] This dramatic decline can be attributed, in part, to increased utilization of the Pap test, which can identify premalignant changes in cervical cytology.[3–6] Cervical cancer rarely affects women younger than age 25.[3,7] Indeed, half of all women diagnosed with cervical cancer are between the ages of 35 and 55.[3,6] Nevertheless, invasive cervical cancer remains a significant health problem in women who are less likely to undergo regular screening and are at increased risk for cervical cancer, including women age 65 and older, minority populations, and those who are medically underserved.[3–5,7–9]

Although the incidence of invasive cervical cancer has decreased dramatically, the incidence of noninvasive disease or carcinoma in situ (CIS) in the United States has climbed since 1945; this type of cancer is currently about four times more common than invasive disease. The increased incidence is due, in part, to early detection of preinvasive disease through screening and surveillance. Women with premalignant/CIS lesions are usually 10–15 years younger, on average, than women with invasive cervical cancer. This prolonged natural history, representing progression from preinvasive disease or intraepithelial carcinoma to clinically invasive disease, can allow for effective screening and early intervention.[7,10–12]

Etiology

Epidemiologic studies have produced substantial evidence indicating that *persistent infection with oncogenic human papillomaviruses (HPV)* is the most significant risk factor for the development of preinvasive or invasive cervical cancer.[10–16] Human papillomavirus is the most prevalent sexually transmitted disease; more than 100 distinct types of HPV have been identified and more than 30 types of HPVs can be sexually transmitted.[17–20] Low-risk forms of HPV are implicated in the etiology of genital warts (condyloma) and rarely lead to carcinogenesis, whereas oncogenic HPVs are referred to as "high-risk" viruses.[17,19–22]

Sexually transmitted high-risk HPVs induce cellular hyperproliferation and are integrated into the host genome in carcinomas. High viral load appears to increase the risk of developing high-grade disease and, ultimately, progression to invasive cancer. In HPV infections, the E2 protein binds to numerous sites in the nucleus, blocks gene transcription, and probably regulates cell growth indirectly through down-regulation of the E6 and E7 oncogenes. The E6 and E7 viral oncoproteins from oncogenic types of HPV inactivate the cell-cycle regulators *p53* and retinoblastoma, providing the initiating event in abnormal cellular proliferation and carcinogenesis.[13,20–25] High-risk HPVs include types 16, 18, 31, 33, 35, 39, 45, 51, 52, 56, 58, 59, 68, and 82. Types 26, 66, and 73 may be carcinogenic.[20,22] In particular, HPV 16, 18, 31, 33, and 51 have been recovered from more than 95% of all invasive cervical neoplasms.[20,22] One 1999 study estimated that 99% of cervical cancers worldwide contain HPV DNA.[12] Based on available data, the World Health Organization's International Agency for Research on Cancer has classified HPV 16 and 18 as carcinogenic in humans.[20,22] HPV 18 is associated with 15%–50% of invasive

Table 48-1 Risk Factors for Oncogenic HPV Exposure, Cervical Cancer Precursors, and Cervical Cancer

Infection with oncogenic forms of HPV
Cigarette smoking
Large number of sexual partners
Immunosuppression
Unavailability/lack of screening
Ethnic minority
Older age
Long-term oral contraceptive use
History of sexually transmitted diseases
Early age at first coitus
Partner sexual behaviors/number of sexual encounters
Partner whose partner/first wife was diagnosed with cervical cancer
DES exposure in utero
Diet low in folate, carotene, and vitamin C
Multiparity

cervical cancer lesions and is the most common papillomavirus found in women with adenocarcinoma of the cervix. HPV 16 is more commonly associated with squamous cell carcinomas.[7,23]

All sexually active women are at risk for HPV infection.[16,26,27] The list of risk factors for cervical cancer includes behaviors that increase the potential for exposure to oncogenic HPV (Table 48-1) as well as demographic and gynecologic factors. An estimated 20 million people in the United States are infected with HPV, yet few of the women who have been exposed actually develop invasive cervical cancer.[28,29] Human papillomavirus infection is suppressed or cleared in the majority of cases; only a minority of women exposed to high-risk forms of HPV develop a latent or persistent infection.[17–20,22,24,25]

Data indicate that oncogenic HPV infection by itself is a necessary but insufficient factor for the development of cervical neoplasia.[11–14] Other host and environmental cofactors have yet to be fully elucidated. Cofactors that may play a role in carcinogenesis include immunosuppression (HIV/AIDS and transplant-related immunosuppresion);[19,30,31] age; smoking/exposure to tobacco products;[32–35] deficiencies in vitamin C, carotenoids, possibly vitamin E, and folate;[36,37] and the presence of other sexually transmitted diseases. Cigarette smoking and tobacco use have been identified as cofactors for squamous cell cervical cancer development, as nicotine and the tobacco-specific carcinogen cotinine have been isolated from the cervical mucus and genital tracts of both women who use tobacco products and women who are passively exposed to cigarette smoke.[32–35]

Squamous cervical carcinoma is rare in women who are nulliparous as well as in those who are lifetime celibates or in lifetime monogamous relationships. Females exposed to diethylstilbestrol (DES) in utero have a higher incidence of clear-cell adenocarcinoma of the cervix and vagina.[7]

Since 1993, cervical cancer has been designated as AIDS-defining illnesses by the Centers for Disease Control and Prevention, and cervical intraeptithelial neoplasia (CIN) has been designated as an HIV-related condition. Women with human immunodeficiency virus (HIV) infection are at higher risk for developing high-grade squamous intraepithelial lesions (HSIL) of the cervix; the increased risk may be due to an inability to effectively clear the virus. In HIV-infected females, cervical cancer may manifest itself in unusual ways, be more aggressive, and run a more fulminant course.[30,37]

Prevention, Screening, and Early Detection

Prevention of cervical cancer centers on modifying sexual behavior, thereby limiting a woman's exposure to oncogenic HPV. Risk-reducing behaviors include limiting the number of lifetime sexual partners, maintenance of a lifetime monogamous relationship by both sexual partners, limiting sexual activity in the teenage years, use of barrier contraceptives to reduce exposure to other sexually transmitted diseases, and an increased understanding and practice of safe sexual behavior. Additionally, screening (Pap test) at appropriate intervals and prompt treatment of cervical cancer precursors are integral to prevention and early detection. Women should also be encouraged to stop smoking and to avoid tobacco use.[1,2,38,39]

The Pap test is an effective, relatively accurate, and economical screening technique to detect cervical neoplasia. In the traditional Pap test, an Ayres spatula and cytobrush are used to collect squamous and endocervical cells. The collection/sample is then smeared on a glass slide, with the spatula used first, followed by the endocervical brush; the slide is then sprayed with a fixative. Accuracy of the Pap smear results depends on the sampling method, staining, and microscopic examination.[40–45] In 1999, the Agency for Health Care Policy and Research reported the results of a meta-analysis of 84 robust studies, which found that conventional Pap smears have a specificity of 98% and a sensitivity of 51%.[41]

Recently, liquid-based cytology has been introduced as an option for cervical cytology screening. This technique was developed to respond to five major limitations of conventional Pap tests: failure to capture the complete specimen; inadequate fixation/drying artifact; presence of elements that obscure evaluation; random distribution of abnormal cells; and technical variance in smear quality. When using liquid-based cytology, the cellular collection is not smeared on a slide but rather is transferred to a vial containing a liquid medium. Cells are separated from mucus and blood and placed in a single layer, which is then reviewed. Liquid-based cytology is more expensive than standard Pap tests but offers the advantages of greater accuracy and possibility of reflex HPV testing. The increased accuracy of the test results may reduce the need for repeat Pap tests and colposcopic evaluation. Additionally, liquid-based cellular collections allow for HPV typing; differentiating between the known oncogenic HPV subtypes and other low-risk viral types enables practitioners to plan interventions specific to high-risk and low-risk HPV subtypes.[46–48]

Automated interpreters can be useful in the detection of cervical abnormalities and can lower false-negative rates. High-resolution video scanners are able to distinguish between normal and abnormal cytologic specimens and can decrease mistakes due to human error.[7,49]

The National Cancer Institute, the Society of Gynecologic Oncologists, and the Society of Gynecologic Nurse Oncologists support recently revised guidelines on screening for cervical cancer and precursor lesions. The American Cancer Society released its revised guidelines in November 2002;[50] the United States Preventive Services Task Force published its recommendations in January 2003.[51] Summary points include:

- All women who are or have been sexually active should begin having Pap tests three years following initiation of vaginal intercourse but no later than at 21 years old.
- Screening should be done every year with the conventional Pap test or every two years when using the newer liquid-based Pap test.
- Beginning at age 30, women who have had three or more consecutive normal Pap tests in a row may be screened every two to three years with the conventional Pap test or liquid-based Pap test.
- Women with specific risk factors (e.g., immunosuppression, exposure to DES in utero) may need to be screened more frequently.
- Women 70 years of age or older who have had three or more normal Pap tests in a row and no abnormal Pap tests in the last 10 years may opt to stop cervical cancer screening. Women with a history of cervical cancer, DES exposure in utero, HIV infection, or immunosuppression should continue to be screened.
- Women who have had a total hysterectomy (including removal of the cervix) may choose to stop cervical cancer screening unless the surgery was done for cervical cancer or precursor lesions. Women who have a cervix should screen according to the preceding guidelines.

Preinvasive Disease

Squamous Intraepithelial Lesions

The cervix—the lower part of the uterus—extends from the isthmus into the vagina and is divided into two major parts: the endocervix and the exocervix. The endocervix is contiguous to the exocervix, which includes the external os and extends to the vaginal fornix. Squamous epithelial cells line the outside surface of the cervix and the vagina, while columnar epithelial cells line the rest of the cervix and the uterus. The *squamocolumnar junction* (often identified as the transformation zone) refers to the area where the columnar epithelium of the endocervix joins the squamous epithelium of the exocervix at the os (Figure 48–1). Cancer of the cervix is a culmination of a progressive disease that begins as a neoplastic alteration of the squamocolumnar junction. Over time, these abnormal cells can progress to involve the full thickness of the epithelium and invade the stromal tissue of the cervix.

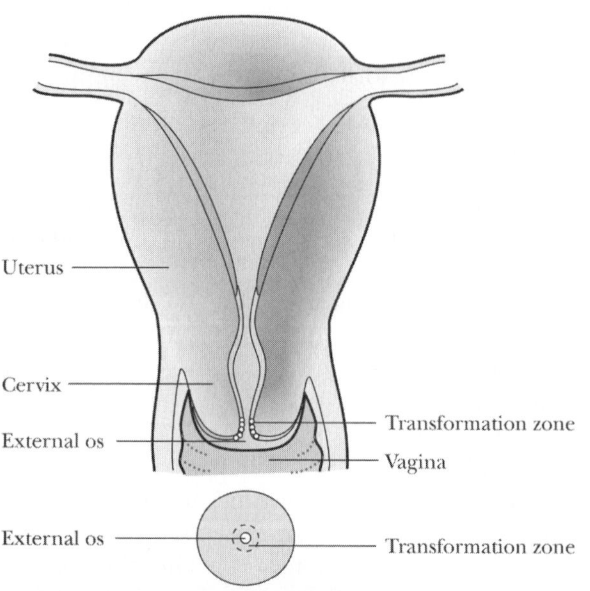

Figure 48-1 Cervical transformation zone.

The initial preinvasive or premalignant changes are called *cervical intraepithelial neoplasia* (CIN).[7,49]

Assessment

Despite the presence of CIN, no gross lesions or abnormality may be observed during the visual inspection of the cervix. Visual inspections are limited because only a portion of the cervix is visible for assessment.

The Pap smear is an effective, accurate, and economical screening and assessment tool. There have been many refinements made in this technology, but debates continue about the best approach, handling, and interpretation of Pap smears.

The terminology used to describe cervical cytology has changed since the original Papanicolaou numeric system was introduced. Originally, Pap smear findings were divided into five classes (I to V) that described atypical changes in cervical cells. In 1988, a workshop sponsored by the National Cancer Institute (NCI) was held in Bethesda, Maryland, to address problems inherent in the Papanicolaou system. The goal was to review existing terminology and to make recommendations for a more effective method of reporting. The outcome of this conference was the Bethesda system (TBS).[2,38,39,49,52,53]

The Bethesda system, proposed in 1988, updated in 1991, and revised in 2001, describes the type and adequacy of the specimen submitted, indicates the testing performed, and gives an interpretation of the results.[39,52–54] Under the 2001 Bethesda guidelines, the Pap test can be "negative for intraepithelial lesion" or it can evidence "epithelial cell abnormalities." Epithelial cell abnormalities are divided into squamous cell or glandular cell abnormalities. Squamous cell abnormalities include *atypical squamous cells of undetermined significance* (ASC-US), *atypical squamous cells—cannot exclude high-grade squamous intraepithelial abnormality* (ASC-H), *low-grade squamous intraepithelial lesion* (LSIL), *high-grade squamous intraepithelial lesion* (HSIL), and *squamous cell carcinoma.* Glandular cell abnormalities include *atypical glandular cells* (AGC), with qualifying statements being added to indicate the cellular origin of the atypical cells (endometrial, glandular, or endocervical). Atypical glandular cells detected on cervical Pap tests may indicate significant cervical or endometrial pathology, and additional testing is required in certain situations.[39,52–54]

When the Pap test report shows ASC-H or SIL, or if the patient is considered to be at high risk for cervical cancer, referral for colposcopic examination with endocervical assessment, biopsy, and/or treatment is indicated. Colposcopy is performed on an outpatient basis, using a stereoscopic, binocular microscope that illuminates and magnifies the view of the cervix. During this procedure, the cervix is swabbed with an acetic acid solution that accentuates the abnormalities and differentiates between normal or metaplastic areas. The epithelium of the cervix is visualized and the abnormal areas biopsied.[7,39,49,52,54]

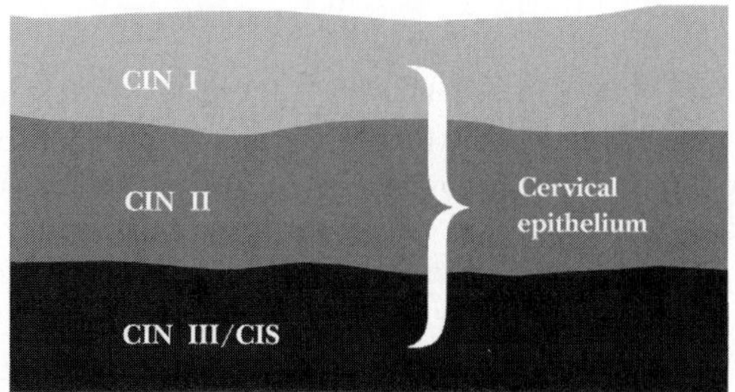

Figure 48-2 Atypical changes in the cervical epithelium.

While Pap test results describe cytologic findings, histopathologic findings are described using the term cervical intraepithelial neoplasia. The term "intraepithelial neoplasia" or "dysplasia," is used to describe premalignant changes in epithelial tissue. Controversy exists regarding the commonly held belief that the CIN classification demonstrates progression of the disease process rather than delineating distinctly different abnormalities. CIN is divided into three categories: CIN I, CIN II, and CIN III. LSIL includes CIN 1 and condyloma; HSIL, as defined by the Bethesda system, includes the categories of CIN 2 (moderate dysplasia) and CIN 3 (severe dysplasia or carcinoma in situ). CIN I describes dysplasia or atypical changes in the cervical epithelium involving less than one-third of the thickness of the epithelium. CIN II describes dysplastic changes involving as much as two-thirds of the thickness. CIN III, also known as severe dysplasia or carcinoma in situ, involves two-thirds to full thickness involvement of the epithelium with no areas of stromal invasion or metastases (Figure 48–2). Once the disease progresses beyond the basement membrane and invades the cervical stroma, it is considered invasive.[7,39,49,52,54]

Therapeutic Approaches and Nursing Care

Each type of SIL lesion can regress, persist, or become invasive. High-grade SIL (CIN III) is more likely to progress than the milder forms, which may regress spontaneously to normal. The rate of progression from LSIL to HSIL is less than 20%. Unlike LSIL, however, HSIL (CIN 2 and 3) has a greater potential to progress to invasive cervical cancer if left untreated. Because there is no way to predict which lesions will become invasive and which will not, patients with low-grade lesions are followed and high-grade lesions are treated when they are discovered.[7,28,29,49,52,54–57]

It is critical that the extent of the lesion be determined as accurately as possible before treatment begins. The Pap test, colposcopy, and colposcopically directed biopsies may determine the extent and severity of the cervical lesion, differentiating between SIL, carcinoma in situ, and invasive carcinoma of the cervix. Treatment for SIL includes a diagnostic excisional procedure such as a direct cervical biopsy, cryotherapy, laser surgery, electrosurgery, cone biopsy, or hysterectomy. The selection of therapy is based on the extent of the disease, patient compliance with follow-up, the patient's wishes to preserve ovarian and reproductive function, and the physician's recommendation. In general, complications of excisional therapies are related to the amount of endocervix that is removed.[7,38,39,49,52,54,57]

Cryotherapy has been used for more than 50 years and is an effective option for the treatment of CIN in selected patients. This technique uses liquid nitrogen to induce freezing of cervical tissue. A portable probe is placed on the lesion; the probe is then activated to initiate freezing, which in turn leads to tissue necrosis. Cryotherapy is a cost-effective and relatively painless treatment with low morbidity that can be performed on an outpatient basis. Patients most often complain of a watery discharge for two to four weeks after treatment. Reepithelialization is complete within three months of therapy. Serious complications secondary to cryotherapy are rare.[7,38,39,52,54,57]

Laser technology can also be used to eradicate SIL. The laser is mounted on the colposcope, and the beam is directed under colposcopic control. The advantage of using a laser is that significantly less disease-free tissue is removed with the entire lesion. Patients may experience a little more discomfort than with cryosurgery, but there is usually less vaginal discharge, and complete healing occurs in about two weeks. A primary disadvantage of laser treatment is that it may cause thermal damage to the tissue specimen, making it difficult for the pathologist to rule out invasive cancer.[7,38,39,49,52,54,57,58]

The most widespread excisional technique used in the treatment of SIL is the loop electrosurgical excision procedure (LEEP), or loop diathermy excision. LEEP uses a thin wire loop and a low level of electricity to excise affected cervical tissue with minimal ablation. Because very thin wires are used, greater control can be exercised over the amount of tissue removed; additionally, the excised tissue contains minimal thermal artifact that might hinder the histopathologic evaluation. The patient can expect a heavy, brown, and sometimes malodorous discharge for two to three weeks following the LEEP. Patients should avoid heavy lifting or strenuous activity for several weeks after the procedure and should not insert anything into the vagina for four weeks. Complications of loop excision therapy occur in 1%–2% of patients and include infection and heavy bleeding. Later complications may include delayed bleeding and cervical stenosis. In selected patients, use of LEEP may allow for diagnosis and treatment of SIL during one outpatient visit. The "see and treat" office visit avoids the usual two sessions (diagnosis at initial visit and biopsy during the second) and is particularly advantageous in situations where patient follow-up is episodic or inconsistent.[7,38,39,49,52,54,57,59–61]

Cold knife conization involves removal of a cone-shaped piece of tissue from the exocervix and endocervix. Performed under general anesthesia on an outpatient basis, conization can be used in four situations:

1. For diagnosis, if no lesion of the cervix is noted and an endocervical tumor is suspected
2. To determine the extent of the lesion if microinvasion is diagnosed on biopsy or if the entire lesion cannot be seen with the colposcope
3. If there are discrepancies between the cytologic report (Pap test) and the histologic appearance of the lesions on biopsy
4. When the patient cannot be relied upon for long-term follow-up

Major immediate complications of conization may include hemorrhage, uterine perforation, and complications of anesthesia. Delayed complications may include bleeding, cervical stenosis, infertility, cervical incompetence, and increased chances of preterm (low-birth-weight) delivery.[7,38,39,57,54,61,62]

Total vaginal hysterectomy (TVH) may be employed for treatment of individuals with HSIL (CIN III). This option is appropriate for individuals with HSIL who have completed childbearing. These individuals must be followed as closely for recurrence as those patients who are treated with more conservative measures.[7,38,39,57,61,62]

The primary nursing responsibilities for women with SIL relate to education. This educational process includes defining the disease, explaining the treatment, teaching the importance of close follow-up, and modifying high-risk behaviors.[38,39,54,57]

If the biopsy indicates the presence of SIL, the woman may erroneously think that she has invasive cancer. She may also blame herself, her past sexual behavior, and her sexual partners for exposure to oncogenic HPV and subsequent development of SIL. The nurse must assure the patient that she does not have cancer and that SIL is an easily treated premalignant condition. In women treated for SIL, self-esteem may drop and anxiety may increase during the initial and postsurgical visits. In addition, women may fear losing fertility and sexual function. The nurse should help the woman understand the type of treatment recommended, explain the nature and purpose of treatment, and describe the side effects of the therapy.[38,39,54,57]

Following treatment, the nurse instructs the woman on how to care for herself at home. Douching, tampons, and sexual intercourse are prohibited for at least two to four weeks, depending on the treatment. A return visit must be scheduled for two to four weeks, then every three months for a year, and every six months thereafter. The importance of this follow-up must be stressed, because there is a possibility of treatment failure or recurrence of the SIL. Minimal bleeding and vaginal discharge may be present for a week or longer after biopsy, cryosurgery, LEEP, or laser and for several weeks following conization.[38,39,54,57]

Information concerning sexual functioning and fertility should be discussed with women undergoing treatment for SIL, although electrocautery, cryosurgery, laser therapy, and conization rarely cause physiologic sexual dysfunction. Most women report no change in libido, orgasm, coital frequency, or overall satisfaction with their sex life. Fertility is usually maintained, but difficulty with conception may occur. Nurses should take time to educate women about reducing risk factors (e.g., HIV, multiple sexual partners) and preventive measures (e.g., smoking reduction, minimizing the number of sexual partners, and barrier protection) related to preinvasive disease. Table 48-2 summarizes issues specifically related to nursing management of patients with preinvasive disease.[38,39,54,57]

Although mortality rates for cervical cancer have decreased over the past 40 years, the rates among ethnic minorities, poor women, and elderly women of all races are higher due to decreased utilization of screening methods in these populations. Access to cervical cancer screening for African Americans, Hispanics, older women, and those who are economically disadvantaged should be a priority for healthcare professionals. Barriers that discourage women from taking advantage of cervical screening include embarrassment, discomfort, financial burden, fatalism, lack of access, lack of transportation, population mobility, opposition by partners, lack of education, lack of health insurance, and age.[5–9,38,39,63–70] Researchers have employed some creative approaches to increase cervical cancer screening and follow-up for underserved groups, including a screening program in a public hospital emergency room, Pap smear screening offered in an inpatient setting, the use of lay educators, the use of nurse practitioners for cervical screening in medically underserved areas, culturally based educational programs, and interventions based on socioeconomic status.[5–9,38,39,63–70]

Invasive Disease

Pathophysiology

Cellular Characteristics

Invasive cervical cancer types are divided into three major categories: squamous carcinoma, adenocarcinoma, and other types. Histologically, 80%–90% of cervical tumors are squamous cell carcinomas; 10%–20% are adenocarcinomas. A very small number of epithelial cervical cancers include adenosquamous and glassy cell carcinomas, and neuroendocrine variants including carcinoid, large cell neuroendocrine, and small cell cancers of the cervix. Squamous carcinomas originate in the squamocolumnar junction and are often associated with carcinoma in situ, microinvasive disease, and invasive carcinoma. They are assigned one of four grades: well differentiated (G1), moderately differentiated (G2), poorly differentiated (G3), or undifferentiated (G4).[6,62,71–73]

Adenocarcinomas generally occur in younger women and carry a greater risk because the tumor arises within the endocervical mucus-producing gland cells. The tumor can become quite bulky before it becomes clinically evident. The bulkiness makes the tumor harder to treat, so this type of cancer has a high rate of local recurrence. Adenocarcinomas appear to be increasing in prevalence and are more difficult to detect than squamous carcinomas. There is no consistent definition of this histological type, no uniform reporting method, and no clear-cut histological pattern for correlation of cytological features.[6,62,74] Oral contraceptives may be associated with higher rates of adenocarcinoma in younger women, especially if oral contraceptives are used during adolescence when the cervix has not fully matured.[7,62]

Primary sarcomas and lymphomas of the cervix have been described in the literature. The incidence of primary or secondary sarcomas and lymphomas is very rare.[7,62]

Progression of Disease

Initially, the invasive malignant process breaks through the basement membrane to invade the

Table 48-2 Treatment Modalities and Nursing Management of the Woman with Cervical Preinvasive or Invasive Disease

Treatment Modalities	Nursing Management
Local therapies (e.g., laser cryosurgery, electrocautery) for preinvasive (SIL, CIN) disease	Explain the disease. Assure patient that SIL (CIN) is not cancer.
	Explain treatment and possible complications of treatment.
	Discuss possibility of treatment failure.
	Instruct in self-care after treatment (no douching, tampons, sexual intercourse for 2–4 weeks).
	Stress importance of follow-up care (next appointment, call physician if fever, bleeding develops).
	Assess concerns related to sexual function (changes in libido, orgasm, coital frequency, fertility).
	Assess for anxiety, depression, changes in body, self-image.
	Assess for psychological issues associated with sexually transmitted disease (guilt, blame, mistrust).
Surgery	Instruct patient preoperatively in use of incentive spirometer, importance of turning, coughing, deep breathing, abdominal splinting, early ambulation, and use of antiemboletic stockings. Have patient do return demonstration as indicated.
	Review bowel preparation procedure.
	Review need for IV, urinary catheter, colostomy, ileal conduit as indicated.
	Begin ostomy teaching preoperatively as indicated.
	Stress availability of pain medication.
	Review use of patient-controlled analgesia as indicated.
	Explore nonpharmacologic pain relief measures with patient.
	Provide postoperative wound care.
	Encourage patient to participate in wound care as indicated.
	Assess concerns related to sexual function (changes in libido, orgasm, coital frequency, fertility).
	Assess cultural beliefs as they relate to treatment (blood transfusions, avoidance of drugs, dietary restrictions).
	Assess spiritual needs/concerns.
	Assess vital signs, body systems, lab values postoperatively.
	Assess for deep-vein thrombosis.
	Assess nutritional status, lymphedema, skin integrity hazards of immobility, alteration in sleep/rest patterns.
	Assess psychosocial functioning.
Radiotherapy	Review treatment procedure (e.g., external beam, intracavitary).
	Review side effects of therapy (e.g., to skin, effect on blood values, vaginal stenosis as indicated).
	Explain mobility restrictions with intracavity, interstitial radiotherapy as indicated.
	Assess for deep-vein thrombosis.
	Encourage diversional activities to relieve boredom.
	Emphasize availability of pain relief measures.
	Explore nonpharmacologic pain relief measures with patient.
	Assess concerns related to sexual function (changes in libido, orgasm, coital frequency, fertility).
	Assess cultural beliefs as they relate to treatment (blood transfusions, avoidance of drugs, dietary restrictions).
	Assess spiritual needs/concerns.
Chemotherapy	Explain treatment (rationale for chemotherapy, name of chemotherapy agents, nadir, method of administration, side effects).
	Assess psychological status of patient.
	Assess for anxiety, depression, changes in body, self-image.
	Assess effects of treatment on quality of life.
	Assess concerns related to sexual function.
	Assess cultural beliefs as they relate to treatment (blood transfusions, avoidance of drugs, dietary restrictions).
	Assess spiritual needs/concerns.
Clinical trials	Review information related to clinical trials if indicated.

cervical stroma. The lesion may infiltrate the endocervix, be exophytic and extend into the exocervix, or be visible as a superficial ulceration. The lesion may then spread in any direction by direct extension. For example, it may begin on the endocervix and spread through cervix, into the parametrial tissue, and through the vesicovaginal and rectovaginal septae into the bladder and rectum. The upper vagina and corpus of the uterus may also become involved.[7,62,75]

Involvement of the lymph nodes in the spread of cervical cancer is fairly predictable and includes paracervical and parametrial lymphatics. Obturator, hypogatric, and other external iliac nodes may be involved; the tumor may also metastasize to the common iliac or paraaortic lymph nodes. Parametrial lymph node metastasis occurs and may be correlated with involvement of iliac lymph nodes.[7,62]

Hematogenous spread through the venous plexus and the paracervical veins occurs less frequently than lymphatic spread but is relatively common in the more advanced stages of disease. The most common sites of distant metastasis are the mediastinal and supraclavicular nodes, lungs, liver, and bone.[7,62]

Clinical Manifestations

Cervical cancer is usually asymptomatic in its preinvasive and early stages, although women may notice a watery or muccoid vaginal discharge. In the majority of cases, the disease is discovered by Pap test during routine examination. Later symptoms that often prompt the woman to seek medical attention in cervical cancer include postcoital bleeding, intermenstrual bleeding, or heavy menstrual flow. If this bleeding is chronic, the woman may complain of symptoms related to anemia. A common complaint in advanced cervical malignancy is that of a foul-smelling, serosanguineous, or yellowish vaginal discharge.[7,62,75]

Other late symptoms, which are indicative of advanced disease, include pain in the pelvis, hypogastrium, lumbosacral or gluteal area, flank, or leg. This pain occurs secondary to involvement of the pelvic wall, ureters, lymph nodes, or sciatic nerve roots. Urinary and rectal symptoms may indicate invasion of these structures by tumor. End-stage disease may be characterized by edema of the lower extremities due to lymphatic and venous obstruction. Massive vaginal hemorrhage and development of renal failure may result from local invasion of blood vessels and bilateral ureteral obstruction by tumor.[7,62,75]

Assessment

Physical Examination

The most frequent physical finding for invasive cervical cancer is a lesion on the cervix. Suspicious lesions should be biopsied to an adequate depth to confirm the diagnosis of invasive carcinoma. Lesions that extend into the exocervix are termed exophytic; lesions may also be ulcerative or plaque-like. Cervical cancer is staged clinically by bimanual pelvic and recto-vaginal examination, with careful attention being paid to the size of the lesion and free space between the tumor and the pelvic sidewall. The tumor may extend into the adjacent vaginal fornices or to the paracervical and parametrial tissues; if untreated, it may invade the bladder, rectum, or both.[7,62,75]

Surgical staging to ascertain pelvic and paraaortic lymph nodes status prior to treatment has been evaluated in several clinical trials. Although surgical findings do not change the clinical stage, information obtained via surgery may influence therapeutic interventions.[7,62,75]

Diagnostic Studies

Diagnostic testing may include chest and skeletal radiographs, intravenous pyelogram, barium enema, complete blood count (CBC), and blood chemistries. If liver enzyme levels are elevated, a liver scan [or computerized tomography (CT) scan] is indicated. Ureteral obstruction has been found in 30% of patients with stage III disease and as many as 50% of women with stage IV disease; these patients will present with hydronephrosis on the affected side and may have concomitant elevations in BUN and creatinine levels. Cystoscopy and rectosigmoidoscopy are indicated in patients with advanced-stage disease.[7,62,75]

Additional studies that are helpful in defining the extent of disease but that do not alter clinical staging include CT and magnetic resonance imaging (MRI). Computerized axial tomograms may be used to determine the extent of pelvic disease, to define radiotherapy portals, and to evaluate lymph node status. However, CT and MRI are not effective in detecting small metastases. The main use of CT is to help identify enlarged lymph nodes in the pelvis and paraaortic areas. MRI offers no advantage over CT in evaluating lymph node metastasis or assessing the parametrium. Researchers have found, however, that MRI provides improved evaluation of tumor size, stromal invasion, and extent of disease as compared to CT. Both CT and MRI are generally able to evaluate lymph node metastasis (86% each). Although MRI has been used to assess the response of cervical cancer to neoadjuvant chemotherapy, it is not as precise as surgical staging. Verification of tumor volume (the most important prognostic factor for survival of the patient with cervical cancer) by MRI may help the physician to determine the best treatment modality. Positron emission tomography (PET) may be able to detect disease not seen on CT or MRI. In addition, PET, if used in conjunction with CT and MRI, may be better able to determine the extent of local disease and nodal involvement.[7,62,75]

A supraclavicular node biopsy is performed if one of these nodes is palpable or if paraaortic nodes are positive. The left node is most often positive—it is where the thoracic duct enters into the subclavian vein. Positive supraclavicular nodes are often associated with a positive aortic node. In such cases, a blind scalene node biopsy is recommended. If this biopsy is positive, systemic therapy is necessary. Following a thorough evaluation, the clinical stage is determined.[7,62,75]

Prognostic Indicators

Factors that influence prognosis include stage, tumor volume, tumor histology and grade, lymph node and endometrial involvement, and presence of lymphovascular space invasion in the pathologic specimen.[7,62,73,75–77] Coexpression of epidermal growth factor receptors and cyclooxygenase-2 portends a poorer prognosis in patients with stage IIB disease. Performance status and patient age are also significant in more advanced stages.[78] Both squamous cell antigens and tumor markers have been evaluated for their clinical significance; however, application of the information gleaned from these data has been limited to clinical studies. These measures are not readily available for screening or for ongoing clinical evaluation.[75]

Classification and Staging

Cervical cancer is staged clinically, with confirmation being obtained from bimanual pelvic and recto-vaginal examinations completed with the patient under anesthesia. This approach allows for more accurate staging, including visualization of the upper vagina and palpation of parametrial and lateral side wall tissues. Evaluation under anesthesia usually occurs at the same time as the planned surgical intervention or when radiation implants are inserted.[62,75,79–82] The clinical stage is not changed if disease recurs.

The most commonly used staging system used today is the International Federation of Gynecology and Obstetrics (FIGO) system (Table 48-3). This system was most recently revised in 1995. The American Joint Committee on Cancer staging system may also be used; both staging systems are applicable to all histologic types. The identifier microinvasion, however, is used only with squamous cell carcinoma.[62,75,79–81]

Disease that is confined to the cervix is defined as stage I. Stratification into particular substages is based on depth and breadth of invasion. Stage IA lesions are considered microinvasive, and risk of lymph node metastases and recurrent disease is low. Stage II disease includes lesions in which the tumor has extended beyond the cervix but has not extended to the pelvic wall. The tumor has extended to the pelvic wall in stage III disease. Tumors that involve the lower one-third of the vagina and all cases with hydronephrosis or nonfunctioning kidney are considered to be stage III (unless they are due to other co-morbid conditions). Spread to adjacent organs or a distant site is included in stage IV.[62,75,79–81]

Therapeutic Approaches and Nursing Care

Once invasive cervical cancer is diagnosed and the clinical stage is established, treatment is based on the woman's age, general medical condition including comorbidities, extent of the cancer, and the presence of any complicating abnormalities. Either surgery or radiation therapy can be used with equal efficacy for patients with early-stage disease.[6,62,75] With either radiation therapy or surgery, the five-year survival rate for early-stage cervical cancer is 85%.[7,62] In the past 20 years, outcomes for locally advanced disease have improved with radiation therapy. This trend reflects more adequate placement of intracavitary brachytherapy, higher paracentral doses, and reduction of overall treatment time. Radiation therapy can be used for all individuals, whereas surgery is indicated only for women who are considered good surgical candidates. In general, patients with more advanced disease (stages IIb to IV) are treated with radiation therapy.[7,62,83–85]

Several randomized trials have shown a survival advantage for cisplatin-based chemotherapy given concurrently with radiation therapy.[83–91] The positive trials vary in terms of disease stage, radiation dose, and schedule of chemotherapy/radiation therapy, yet all demonstrate a significant benefit of concurrent therapy. The risk of death from cervical cancer is reduced by 30%–50%, suggesting that cisplatin-based chemotherapy should be given to women who require radiation therapy for the treatment of cervical cancer.[83–91]

Table 48-3 Clinical Staging for Carcinoma of the Cervix

Stage		Description
0		Carcinoma in situ, intraepithelial carcinoma.
I		The carcinoma is strictly confined to the cervix.
	IA	Invasive cancer identified only microscopically. All gross lesions even with superficial invasion are stage IB cancers. Invasion is limited to measured stromal invasion with maximum depth of 5 mm and no wider than 7 mm.
	IA1	Measured invasion of stroma no greater than 3 mm in depth and no wider than 7 mm.
	IA2	Measured invasion of stroma greater than 3 mm and no greater than 5 mm in depth, and no wider than 7 mm.
	IB	Clinical lesions confined to the cervix or preclinical lesions greater than stage IA.
	IB1	Clinical lesions no greater than 4 cm in size.
	IB2	Clinical lesions greater than 4 cm in size.
II		The carcinoma extends beyond the cervix but has not extended to the pelvic wall. The carcinoma involves the vagina but not as far as the lower third.
	IIA	No obvious parametrial involvement.
	IIB	Obvious parametrial involvement.
III		The carcinoma has extended to the pelvic wall. On rectal examination, there is no cancer-fee space between the tumor and the pelvic wall.
		The tumor involves the lower third of the vagina. All cases with hydronephrosis or nonfunctioning kidney are included unless they are known to be due to other causes.
	IIIA	No extension to the pelvic wall.
	IIIB	Extension to the pelvic wall and/or hydronephrosis of nonfunctioning kidney.
IV		The carcinoma has extended beyond the true pelvis or has clinically involved the mucosa of the bladder or rectum. A bullous edema as such does not permit a case to be allotted to state IV.
	IVA	Spread of the growth to adjacent organs.
	IVB	Spead to distant organs.

Data from FIGO, International Federation of Gynecology and Obstetrics, 2000.

Stage IA

Stage IA disease (microinvasive carcinoma) has been subdivided into two stages, IA1 and IA2. Stage IA1 (≤3 mm depth of invasion, horizontal dimension < 7 mm, no lymphatic or vascular space involvement) should be treated by total abdominal hysterectomy (TAH) or total vaginal hysterectomy (TVH) if the patient is healthy and does not desire further childbearing. Conization can be done for those women who are poor surgical risks or who wish to preserve fertility, as long as the biopsy margins are free of disease and the patient is followed closely. Intracavitary radiation may also be utilized to treat cervical cancer in this stage.[7,62,75,77,92]

Stage IA2 disease is treated by TAH or TVH if invasion is less than 3 mm and there is no lymphovascular involvement. If the invasion is greater than 3 mm or lymphovascular invasion has occurred, the disease is managed the same way as stage IB disease. Five-year survival in patients with properly staged IA cervical cancer is close to 100%. Conservative measures are recommended to treat stage IA1 cervical cancer, whereas more aggressive measures (radical or modified radical hysterectomy with pelvic lymph node dissection) are indicated for stage IA2 because of the higher risk of lymphovascular involvement.[7,62,75]

Stages IB and IIA

In 1995, FIGO subdivided stage IB into stage IB1 (lesions ≤ 4 cm in size) and stage IB2 (lesions > 4 cm in size). The choice of therapy for patients with stage IB and IIA disease remains controversial, and the choice of surgery or radiation depends on the gynecologist and radiation oncologist involved as well as on the woman's condition and the characteristics of the lesion.[7,62]

Stage IB and IIA disease can be treated with radical abdominal hysterectomy and pelvic lymphadenectomy or with definitive radiation, which may include external beam and/or intracavitary insertions. Cure rates for stage IB disease using radiation or surgery are in the range of 80%–90%.[7,62,93,94]

Some gynecologic oncologists prefer surgery to radiotherapy because ovarian function may be preserved with the former approach. Radical hysterectomy involves removal of the uterus, upper third of the vagina, entire uterosacral and uterovesical ligaments, all of the parametria, and pelvic node lymphadenectomy. It is a complex procedure because the organs removed are proximal to many vital body structures—the bladder, ureters, rectum, and great vessels of the pelvis. The major complications of radical hysterectomy include ureteral fistulas, bladder dysfunction, pulmonary embolus, lymphocysts, pelvic infection, bowel obstruction, rectovaginal fistulas, and hemorrhage. The vagina usually remains more pliable after surgery than with radiation, the overall treatment time is shorter, and long-term radiation complications to pelvic tissue can be avoided. Postoperative bladder dysfunction is manifested by the loss of the sense to void and inability to empty the bladder. A suprapubic catheter is placed intraoperatively, and the patient is taught bladder training prior to discharge. Alternatively, the patient may be taught intermittent self-catheterization. Postoperatively, potential complications include bleeding, infection, pneumonia, pulmonary embolus, myocardial infarction, and deep-vein thrombosis. Patients should be ambulatory on the first postoperative day.

The upper portion of the vagina is removed in a radical hysterectomy; the vagina may be shorter but remains distensible. Psychosexual sequelae following radical hysterectomy include sexual dysfunction and infertility.[7,62,75]

Some patients who desire a fertility-sparing procedure may be candidates for radical vaginal or abdominal trachelectomy. This procedure is a conservative, yet radical approach in which the corpus uteri is left intact and fertility potential may be maintained. The cervix, parametrium, and vaginal cuff are excised; lymphadenectomy is accomplished laproscopically.[95,96]

Radiation therapy has the advantages of avoiding major intraoperative and postoperative complications and allowing the patient to receive the therapy as an outpatient. Acute and chronic complications following radiation therapy include diarrhea, abdominal cramping, desquamation of the skin, anemia, sexual dysfunction and infertility, fistulas, bowel obstructions, and vaginal stenosis. Patients should be instructed to engage in vaginal intercourse or use a vaginal dilator three times a week in an effort to delimit vaginal stenosis[6,75,76]

Patients with bulky disease (barrel-shaped cervix) have a higher incidence of central recurrence, pelvic and paraaortic lymph node metastases, and distant dissemination. An increased dose of radiation to the central pelvis followed six weeks later by radical hysterectomy, or both, have been advocated in patients with bulky disease. Radical surgery followed by radiation therapy remains controversial because the patient faces the prospect of complications associated with each treatment modality and the potential for concomitant toxicity from combination therapy.[7,62,75]

Stages IIB, III, and IVA

Women with stage IIB, III, or IV cervical cancer are usually treated with high doses of external pelvic radiation followed by brachytherapy. The initial dose of external radiation may help reduce tumor load and facilitate placement of vaginal applicators to enhance the effects of brachytherapy. Treatment is usually completed in approximately eight weeks. The five-year survival rate of patients with stage IIB cancer is 60%–79%, while those with stage III disease have a five-year survival rate of 25%–50%, and those with stage IVA disease have a five-year survival rate of 18%–34%. The advantages of radiation over surgery for advanced disease are that radiation can be given on an outpatient basis, it avoids surgery, and it is suitable for women who are poor surgical candidates.[7,62,75]

Morbidity resulting from properly administered radiotherapy in cervical cancer is usually manageable. Adverse reactions have been reported when poor technique is used, but these reactions occur infrequently in properly treated women. The higher the dose of radiation, the higher the rate of complications. Some morbidity attributed to radiation is secondary to uncontrolled tumor growth or the compounded effects of multiple therapies and is not a direct result of the radiation therapy. Major complication rates range from 3% to 5% for stage I and IIA disease and from 10% to 15% for stage IIB and III disease.[7,62,75]

The major complications related to radiotherapy include vaginal stenosis, fistula formation, sigmoid perforation or stricture, uterine perforation, rectal ulcer or proctitis, intestinal obstruction, fistulas, ureteral stricture, severe cystitis, pelvic hemorrhage, and pelvic abscess. Other problems related to radiation therapy include nausea, vomiting, diarrhea, and, rarely, radiation myelitis.[7,62,75]

Sexual dysfunction secondary to vaginal atrophy, stenosis, and lack of lubrication is a known effect of the radiation therapy. Radiation causes thinning of the vaginal epithelium, and the vagina may become shortened, less flexible, and partially obliterated. Vaginal intercourse may cause dyspareunia and bleeding. Women who are not sexually active experience a higher incidence of atrophy and stenosis than do sexually active women. The use of vaginal dilators and water-soluble lubricants can minimize the effects of radiation. Patients should be instructed to engage in vaginal intercourse and/or use a vaginal dilator three times a week in an effort to delimit vaginal stenosis.[7,62,75]

Surgical staging of advanced disease before initiating treatment is advocated in an attempt to gain a more precise evaluation of the extent of the disease. Arguments in favor of pretreatment laparotomy are that (1) the extent of the disease can be ascertained, (2) patients who have disease not curable by radiation may be offered palliative therapy, and (3) those patients most likely to benefit from extended-field radiation are identified. Arguments against pretreatment laparotomy are that (1) surgical staging can cause morbidity and mortality, (2) many patients with paraaortic nodal metastases also have systemic disease not detected by surgery, (3) there is only minimal improvement in net survival, and (4) surviving patients have high morbidity. Currently, surgeons choose to use alternative extraperitoneal staging methods to determine the extent of disease. One approach involves making a small incision near the umbilicus and outside the proposed radiation field. This strategy allows sampling of the aortic and/or common iliac nodes, collection of peritoneal fluids for cytology, and palpation of pelvic structures.[7,62,75,97]

Recurrent or Persistent Disease

Approximately 35% of women with invasive cervical cancer will have recurrent or persistent disease. Therefore, thorough, regular follow-ups after treatment are mandatory. Recurrent cervical cancer is difficult to diagnose. Clinical and cytological evaluation of an irradiated cervix is problematic because the cells and configuration of the cervix are distorted from the radiation. Therefore, histological confirmation of recurrence is essential.[7,62,75]

Almost 80% of recurrences become manifest within two years after therapy. The signs and symptoms may be subtle and varied, including unintentional weight loss; unilateral leg edema; pain in the buttock, pelvis, or thigh; serosanguinous vaginal discharge; ureteral obstruction; supraclavicular lymph node enlargement (usually of the left side); cough; hemoptysis; and chest pain. The triad of sciatic pain, hydronephrosis, and leg edema is particularly ominous. Evaluation following histologic confirmation generally includes a chest x-ray, intravenous pyelogram (IVP), CBC, and blood chemistries. A CT scan, lymphangiography, or fluoroscopically directed needle biopsies to evaluate the status of the regional lymph nodes, liver, and kidneys may be performed. These procedures have replaced more elaborate operative procedures to provide histological confirmation of recurrence, which may save the woman from unnecessary surgery. In general, the prognosis for women who have central recurrence of disease is better than for those who experience recurrence in the pelvic wall.[7,62,75]

Following surgery or radiotherapy as primary treatment for patients with cervical cancer, approximately half of all recurrences are local (cervix, uterus, vagina, parametrium, and regional lymph nodes). The remaining cases involve distant metastases to the lung, liver, bone, mediastinal, or supraclavicular lymph nodes.[7,62,75]

The prognosis for patients with persistent or recurrent carcinoma of the cervix is dismal. One-year survival rates are 10%–15%. Survival averages six to ten months once recurrent cervical cancer is diagnosed. The aim of treatment in recurrent disease is palliation because control or cure is rare.[7,62,75]

Surgery. Pelvic exenteration entails en bloc removal of the pelvic organs and is limited to those patients with a central recurrence of their disease. A total pelvic exenteration includes a radical hysterectomy, pelvic lymph node dissection, and removal of the bladder and rectosigmoid colon. The surgical procedure is aborted if the patient is found to have recurrent disease outside the pelvis, positive lymph nodes, or disease fixed to the pelvic side wall. Occasionally, a posterior exenteration (which preserves the bladder) or anterior exenteration (which preserves the rectum) can be performed. The number of total pelvic exenterations has decreased dramatically in the past 20 years, and today this procedure is performed only in a selected group of patients. It is important to ensure that patients will be psychologically able to adjust to the changes in body function and body image. Unfortunately, inoperable disease is found about 60% of the time in candidates for pelvic exenteration.[7,62,75,98]

Extensive preoperative evaluation must be done to ensure that no disease exists outside the pelvis and that renal function is adequate. Studies usually performed include chest x-ray, IVP, blood chemistries, creatinine clearance, CT scan, bone scan, and liver–spleen scan. Some clinicians also order lymphangiography as well as an abdominal CT scan to evaluate the regional lymph nodes. If lymphadenopathy is present, a needle aspiration of the nodes may be done. If the aspirate is positive for malignancy, the woman may be spared an unnecessary laparotomy. A blind scalene node biopsy may be recommended to complete the evaluation. Preoperative evaluation of nutritional status is also important in this population. As many as 60% of cancer patients may exhibit laboratory or clinical evidence of malnutrition.[7,62,75,98]

At laparotomy, the entire abdomen and pelvis are explored in search of metastases. A selective paraaortic lymphadenectomy, bilateral pelvic lymphadenectomy, and biopsies of the pelvic side walls are done and sent for frozen section. If any of these samples test positive, or if the patient has positive intraoperative washings for disease, the exenteration is abandoned as the disease is considered incurable.[7,62,75,98]

The use of the end-to-end anastomotic (EEA) stapling device has resulted in patients' not requiring a permanent colostomy after pelvic exenteration; the creation of a continent conduit may be a surgical alternative to a more traditional urinary diversion. The EEA reduces the risk of anastomotic leaks, fistula formation, and late strictures, and it decreases operative time. Permanent colostomy can also be avoided by using a segment of sigmoid colon as a rectal substitute.[7,62,75,98]

Immediate postoperative problems include pulmonary embolism, pulmonary edema, cerebrovascular accident, hemorrhage, myocardial infarction, sepsis, and small bowel obstruction. Long-term problems include fistula formation, urinary obstruction, infection, and sepsis. The use of pelvic exenteration has been limited to a very narrowly defined group of candidates, because reports indicate a five-year survival rate of 23%–50% and an operative mortality rate of approximately 9.8%. Women younger than age 35 have a better prognosis as compared to those older than age 35. Psychosexual and social rehabilitation of surviving patients is a major challenge. Vaginal reconstruction at the time of exenteration and psychological support in the postoperative period can help patients adjust. Survival statistics are worse for women who have recurrent disease greater than 3 mm, bladder involvement, positive pelvic lymph nodes, and recurrence less than a year after previous treatment.[7,62,75,98]

Radiation therapy. In previously irradiated individuals, metastatic disease outside the initial radiation field may be treated cautiously with radiation to provide local control and relieve symptoms. In selected cases, radiation within previously treated areas may be used. For women treated initially with surgery, full-dose radiotherapy using a combination of external and intracavitary implants may afford excellent palliation or even cure.[7,62,75,97]

Chemotherapy. In general, surgery or radiation will not be curative for most women who have recurrent cervical cancer. Previous radiation therapy to the pelvis alters the vascular supply, which limits potential drug delivery to tumor sites located in previously irradiated fields. Additionally, therapeutic doses of radiation therapy to the pelvis will compromise bone marrow reserve, and poor renal function secondary to previous radiation or surgery and ureteral obstruction from tumor or scarring may necessitate or delimit chemotherapeutic options.[6,75,76]

Response rates for patients with recurrent cervical cancer treated with single-agent and investigational chemotherapy range from 0% to 48%, with most studies reporting a response rate less than 20%. In general, there is no long-term benefit from chemotherapy, as responses last less than nine months with variable lengths of survival. Response rates are higher in patients who have received no prior radiation therapy or chemotherapy.[7,62,75]

Activity has been documented for a number of single agents, including cisplatin, ifosfamide, paclitaxel, vinorelbine, topotecan, and irinotecan.[99–110] Other agents with demonstrated activity include cyclophosphamide, chlorambucil, melphalan, doxorubicin, carboplatin, 5-fluorouracil, methotrexate, vincristine, vindesine, and hexamethylmelamine.[7,62] Recently, gemcitabine has exhibited antitumor activity against cervical cancer in phase II clinical trials.[111] Topotecan has also shown efficacy against cervical cancer in phase II trials.[107] Of the single agents, cisplatin remains the drug with the greatest antineoplastic activity, although carboplatin may be used as first-line treatment as well. Even so, objective response rates with cisplatin only range between 17% and 30% and the drug does not provide any increase in survival time for patients.[7,62,75]

Combination chemotherapy regimens have been reported to have marginal success.[108,112,113] Recently, the results of a study using combination chemotherapy with cisplatin and topotecan was presented at the 2004 Society of Gynecologic Oncologists meeting. The researchers concluded that the combination of cisplatin and topotecan improves survival compared with cisplatin alone. This is the first chemotherapy combination to demonstrate an improvement in survival over single-agent cisplatin.[114]

Complications of chemotherapy may manifest themselves in any organ system and depend on the agent, dose, and route utilized. In addition, chemotherapy may adversely affect psychological, emotional, and psychosocial aspects of the cancer patient's life. Side effects associated with cisplatin include nausea and vomiting, renal dysfunction, peripheral neuropathy, anemia, neutropenia, hypomagnesemia, and ototoxicity.[7,62,75]

Symptom Management and Supportive Care

Symptoms seen in patients with progressive cervical cancer include the development of ureteral obstruction, pain, cachexia, bleeding and anemia, and lymphedema. Patients with recurrent cervical cancer to the lung may complain of hemoptysis, cough, shortness of breath, and chest pain. Patients may have bony or brain metastases with the expected symptomatology associated with these lesions. Urinary diversion may be considered and is palliative in those patients with ureteral obstruction; embolization or additional radiation may be used for vaginal bleeding or hemorrhage. Spot radiation may be an option for metastatic lesions or areas of pain.[7,62,75]

Patients who are cured are seen every three months for the first two to three years with gradual lengthening of post-therapy evaluations. Those individuals receiving definitive radiation therapy should be instructed to engage in vaginal intercourse or use a vaginal dilator at least three times a week. Significant vaginal stenosis precludes optimal post-therapy follow-up and evaluation.[7,62,75]

Conclusion

The burden of cervical cancer incidence, morbidity, and mortality is felt primarily in developing nations. Cancer prevention efforts worldwide have focused on screening women using the Pap smear/test and treating precursor lesions prior to the development of a malignancy. Unfortunately, developing nations often do not have the necessary infrastructure to provide access to screening, educational programs to create awareness, or availability to provide Pap smear screening services and follow-up. Currently, screening efforts in areas with limited resources continue to focus on intermittent visual inspections of the cervix. The cervix is swabbed with an acetic acid solution which highlights differences in cell structure. Healthcare practitioners then visually inspect for evidence of cervical lesions. Clinical trials using magnification with visual inspections may be useful in identifying moderate to severe cervical lesions.[1,49]

Cervical cancer is preventable, as the vast majority of cases are caused, in part, by persistent infection with oncogenic human papillomaviruses. Primary prevention efforts have focused on the development of HPV vaccines to prophylax/prevent oncogenic HPV infection. Studies on HPV prophylaxis and prevention have been conducted and are currently under way in both the United States and developing nations.[115–119]

Cervical cancer accounts for significant morbidity and mortality worldwide. Of the gynecologic malignancies, only cervical cancer has an effective screening method for early detection. The potential for cure is enhanced when the disease is diagnosed in early stages. Treatment modalities for women with invasive disease can be very aggressive and may result in a variety of illness-related demands on the woman and her family. Additionally, when recurrences appear, expectations for cure may be unrealistic and effective palliation remains to be discovered. Risk factors in the development of preinvasive and invasive disease are well known, but it may take many years for invasive disease to develop. Additional research should target the goal of improving the percentage of women who receive regular screening in an effort to diagnose the disease in its earliest stages.

References

1. Department of Reproductive Health and Research, World Health Organization: *Outlook: Preventing Cervical Cancer in Low Resource Settings* 18:1–8, 2000
2. *Worldwide Cervical Cancer Issues. http://nccc-online.org/worldcancer.htm* Accessed March 15, 2004
3. American Cancer Society: *2004 Facts and Figures. www.cancer.org/statistics/selectcancers.htm/#cervix.* Accessed March 15, 2004
4. Cramer DW: The role of cervical cytology in the declining morbidity and mortality of cervical cancer. *Cancer* 34:2018–2027, 1974
5. Symonds RP: Screening for cervical cancer: different problems in the developing and developed world. *Eur J Cancer Care* 6:275–279, 1997
6. Brooks SE: Cervical screening and the older woman. *Cancer Pract* 4:125–129, 1996
7. DiSaia PJ, Creasman WT: *Clinical Gynecologic Oncology* (ed 6). St. Louis, Mosby, 2002
8. Borrayo EA, Thomas JJ, Lawsin C: Cervical cancer screening among Latinas: the importance of referral and participation in parallel cancer screening behaviors. *Women Health* 39:13–29, 2004
9. Reynolds D: Cervical cancer in Hispanic/Latino women. *Clin J Oncol Nurs* 8:146–150, 2004
10. Bosch FX, Manos MM, Munoz N, et al: Prevalence of human papillomavirus in cervical cancer: A worldwide perspective. International Biological Study on Cervical Cancer (IBSCC) study group. *J Natl Cancer Inst* 87:796–802, 1995
11. Schiffman MH, Brinton L: The epidemiology of cervical carcinogenesis. *Cancer* 76:1888–1901, 1995
12. Wallboomers JM, Jacobs MV, Manos MM, et al: Human papillomavirus is a necessary cause of invasive cervical cancer worldwide. *J Pathol* 189:12–19, 1999
13. Isom HC, Wigdahl B, Howett MK. Molecular pathology of human oncogenic viruses, in Sirica AE (ed.): *Cellular and Molecular Pathogenesis.* Philadelphia, Lippincott-Raven, 1996, pp 341–347
14. National Institute of Health: *Consensus Statement on Cervical Cancer.* National Institute of Health, Bethesda, MD, April 1–3, 1996
15. Schoell WM, Janicek MF, Mirhashem R: Epidemiology and biology of cervical cancer. *Semin Surg Oncol* 16:203–211, 1999
16. Wolf JK, Franco EL, Arbeit JM, et al: Innovations in understanding the biology of cervical cancer. *Cancer* 98:2064–2069, 2003
17. Ho GY, Bierman R, Beardsley L, et al: Natural history of cervicovaginal papillomavirus infection in young women. *N Engl J Med* 338:423–428, 1998
18. Evander M, Edlund K, Gustafsson A, et al: Human papillomavirus infection is transient in young women: a population based cohort study. *J Infect Dis* 171:1026–1030, 1995
19. Viscidi R: Epidemiology of genital tract human papillomavirus infections, in Apgar B, Brotzman G, Spitzer M (eds.): *Colposcopy: Principles and Practice.* Philadelphia, W.B. Saunders, 2002, pp 1–2

20. Schlossser BJ, Howett MK: Human papillomaviruses: molecular aspects of the viral life cycle and pathogenesis, in Apgar B, Brotzman G, Spitzer M (eds.): *Colposcopy: Principles and Practice.* Philadelphia, W.B. Saunders, 2002, pp 23–39
21. Lorincz AT, Reid R, Jenson AB, et al: Human papillomavirus infection of the cervix: relative risk associations of 15 common anogenital types. *Obstet Gynecol* 79:328–337, 1992
22. Munoz N, Bosch FX, de Sanjose S, et al: Epidemiologic classification of human papillomavirus types associated with cervical cancer. *N Engl J Med* 348:518–527, 2003
23. Burk RD, Terai M, Gravitt PE, et al: Distribution of human papillomavirus types 16 and 18 variants in squamous cell carcinomas and adenocarcinomas of the cervix. *Cancer Res* 63:7215–7220, 2003
24. Turek LP, Smith EM: The genetic program of genital human papillomavirus in infection and cancer. *Obstet Gynecol Clin North Am* 23:735–758, 1996
25. Franco EL, Villa LL, Sobrinho JP, et al: Epidemiology of acquisition and clearance of cervical human papillomavirus infection in women from a high risk area for cervical cancer. *J Infect Dis* 180:1415–1423, 1999
26. Bosch FX, Castellsague X, Munoz N, et al: Male sexual behavior and human papillomavirus DNA: key risk factors for cervical cancer in Spain. *J Natl Cancer Inst* 88:1060–1067, 1996
27. Burk RD, Ho GY, Beardsley L, et al: Sexual behavior and partner characteristics are the predominant risk factors for genital human papillomavirus infection in young women. *J Infect Dis* 174:679–689, 1996
28. Ostor AG: Natural history of cervical intraepithelial neoplasia: a critical review. *Int J Gynecol Pathol* 12:186–192, 1993
29. Melnikow J, Nuovo J, Willan AR, et al: Natural history of cervical squamous intraepithelial lesions: a metaanalysis. *Obstet Gynecol* 92:727–735, 1998
30. Maiman M, Fruchter RG, Guy L, et al: Human immunodeficiency virus infection and invasive cervical carcinoma. *Cancer* 71:402–406, 1993
31. Maiman M, Fruchter RG, Clark M, et al: Cervical cancer as an AIDS-defining illness. *Obstet Gynecol* 89:76–80, 1997
32. Prokopczyk B, Cox JE, Hoffmann D, et al: Identification of tobacco-specific carcinogen in the cervical mucus of smokers and nonsmokers. *J Natl Cancer Inst* 89:868–873, 1997
33. Castellsague X, Munoz N: Cofactors in human papillomavirus carcinogenesis — role of parity, oral contraceptives, and tobacco smoking. *J Natl Cancer Inst Monogr* 31:20–28, 2003
34. Harris TG, Kulasingam SL, Kiviat NB, et al: Cigarette smoking, oncogenic human papillomavirus, Ki-67 antigen, and cervical intraepithelial neoplasia. *Am J Epidemiol* 159:834–842, 2004
35. Plummer M, Herrero R, Franceschi S, et al: Smoking and cervical cancer: pooled analysis of the IARC multi-centric case-control study. *Cancer Causes Control* 14:805–814, 2003
36. Sedjo RL, Roe DJ, Abrahamsen M, et al: Vitamin A, carotenoids, and risk of persistent oncogenic human papillomavirus infection. *Cancer Epidemiol Biomarkers Prev* 11:876–884, 2002
37. Centers for Disease Control: 1993 revised classification system for HIV infection and expanded surveillance case definition for AIDS among adolescents and adults. *MMWR* 41:1–17, 1993
38. Spinelli A: Preinvasive diseases of the cervix, vulva, and vagina, in Moore-Higgs G, Almadrones LA, Colvin-Hoff B, et al (eds.): *Women and Cancer: A Gynecologic Oncology Nursing Perspective.* Boston, Jones and Bartlett, 2000, pp 50–81
39. Spinelli A: Preinvasive diseases of the cervix, vulva, and vagina. *Semin Oncol Nurs* 18:184–192, 2002
40. Soost HJ, Lange HJ, Lehamcher W, et al: The validation of cervical cytology. Sensitivity, specificity, and predictive values. *Acta Cytol* 35:8–14, 1991
41. Agency for Healthcare Policy and Research: *Evidence Report/Technology Assessment, Number 5. Evaluation of Cervical Cytology.* Bethesda, MD, AHCPR Publication No. 99–E010, 1999
42. DeMay RM: Common problems in Papanicolaou smear interpretation. *Arch Pathol Lab Med* 121:229–238, 1997
43. Cox JT: Advances in cervical cancer screening: Pap testing. *Contemp Obstet Gynecol* 46(suppl):3–18, 2001
44. Bernstein SJ, Sanchez-Ramos L, Ndubisi B: Liquid-based cervical cytologic smear and conventional Papanicolaou smears: a metaanalysis of prospective studies comparing cytologic diagnosis and sample adequacy. *Am J Obstet Gynecol* 185:308–317, 2001
45. Sptizer M, Johnson C: Terminology in cervical cytology: B. conventional cytology, in Apgar B, Brotzman G, Spitzer M (eds.): *Colposcopy: Principles and Practice.* Philadelphia, W.B. Saunders, 2002, pp 52–56
46. Bur M, Knowles K, Pekow P, et al: Comparison of ThinPrep preparations with conventional cervicovaginal smears. Practical considerations. *Acta Cytol* 39:631–642, 1995
47. Ferenczy A, Robitaille J, Franco E, et al: Conventional cervical cytologic smears vs ThinPrep smears. A paired comparison study on cervical cytology. *Acta Cytol* 40:1136–1142, 1996
48. Sptizer M, Johnson C: Terminology in cervical cytology: C. liquid-based thin-layer cytology, in Apgar B, Brotzman G, Spitzer M (eds.): *Colposcopy: Principles and Practice.* Philadelphia, W.B. Saunders, 2002, pp 56–68
49. Wright, T Jr: Pathogenesis and diagnosis of preinvasive lesions of the lower genital tract, in Hoskins WJ, Perez CA, Young RC (eds.): *Principles and Practice of Gynecologic Oncology* (ed 3). Philadelphia, Lippincott, Williams and Wilkins, 2000, pp 735–774
50. Saslovar D, Runowicz CD, Solomon D, et al: American Cancer Society guideline for the early detection of cervical neoplasia and cancer. *CA Cancer J Clin* 52:342, 2002
51. United States Preventive Services Task Force: Recommendations and Rationale: Screening for Cervical Cancer. *www.preventive services.ahrq.gov.* Accessed March 27, 2004
52. Wright TC Jr, Cox JT, Massad LS, et al: 2001 consensus guidelines for the management of women with cervical cytological abnormalities. *JAMA* 287:2120–2129, 2002
53. Sptizer M, Johnson C: Terminology in cervical cytology: A. the Bethesda system, in Apgar B, Brotzman G, Spitzer M (eds.): *Colposcopy: Principles and Practice.* Philadelphia, W.B. Saunders, 2002, pp 41–52
54. Apgar B, Brotzman G: High grade squamous intraepithelial lesion, in Apgar B, Brotzman G, Spitzer M (eds.): *Colposcopy: Principles and Practice.* Philadelphia, W.B. Saunders, 2002, pp 249–263
55. Schlecht NF, Platt RW, Duarte-Franco E, et al: Human papillomavirus infection and time to progression and regression of cervical intraepithelial neoplasia. *J Natl Cancer Inst* 95:1336–1343, 2003
56. The Atypical Squamous Cells of Undetermined Significance/Low-Grade Squamous Intraepithelial Lesions Triage Study (ALTS) Group. Human papillomavirus testing for triage of women with cytologic evidence of low-grade squamous epithelial lesions: baseline data from a randomized trial. *J Natl Cancer Inst* 92:397–402, 2000
57. Cox JT: Management of precursor lesions of cervical carcinoma: history, host defense, and a survey of modalities. *Obstet Gynecol Clin North Am* 29:751–785, 2002
58. Tsukamoto N: Treatment of cervical intraepithelial neoplasia with the carbon dioxide laser. *Gynecol Oncol* 21:331–336, 1985
59. Wright TC Jr, Gagnon S, Richart RM, et al: Treatment of cervical intraepithelial neoplasia using the loop electrosurgical excision procedure. *Obstet Gynecol* 79:173–178, 1992

60. Naumann RW, Bell MC, Alvarez RD, et al: LLETZ is an acceptable alternative to diagnostic cold-knife conization. *Gynecol Oncol* 55:224–228, 1994
61. Bloss JD: The use of electrosurgical techniques in the management of premalignant diseases of the vulva, vagina, and cervix: an excisional rather than ablative approach. *Am J Obstet Gynecol* 169:1081–1085, 1993
62. Stehman FB, Perez CA, Kurman RJ, et al: Uterine cervix, in Hoskins WJ, Perez CA, Young RC (eds.): *Principles and Practice of Gynecologic Oncology* (ed 3). Philadelphia, Lippincott, Williams and Wilkins, 2000, pp 841–918
63. Centers for Disease Control and Prevention: The National Breast and Cervical Cancer Early Detection Program: About the Program. *www.cdc.gov/cancer/NBCCEDP/about.htm.* Accessed February 1, 2004
64. Lovejoy NC: Multinational approaches to cervical cancer screening: a review. *Cancer Nurs* 19:126–134, 1996
65. Peragallo NP, Alba ML, Tow C: Cervical cancer screening practices among Latino women in Chicago. *Public Health Nurs* 14:251–255, 1977
66. Dignan M, Sharp P, Blinson K, et al: Development of a cervical cancer education program for Native American women in North Carolina. *J Cancer Educ* 9:235–242, 1994
67. Harmon MP, Castro FG, Coe K: Acculturation and cervical cancer: knowledge, beliefs, and behaviors of Hispanic women. *Women Health* 24:37–57, 1996
68. Jennings KM: Getting a Pap smear: focus group responses of African American and Latina women. *Oncol Nurs Forum* 24:827– 835, 1997
69. Jubelireer SJ, Blanton MF, Blanton PD: Assessment of knowledge, attitudes, and behaviors relative to cervical cancer and the Pap smear among adolescent girls in West Virginia. *J Cancer Educ* 11:230–237, 1996
70. Carpenter V, Colwell B: Cancer knowledge, self-efficacy, and cancer screening behaviors among Mexican-American women. *J Cancer Educ* 10:217–222, 1995
71. Gersell DJ, Mazoujian G, Mutch D, Rudloff MA: Small-cell undifferentiated carcinoma of the cervix: a clinicopathologic, ultrastructural, and immunocytochemical study of 15 cases. *Am J Surg Pathol* 12:684–698, 1988.
72. Stoler MH, Mills SE, Gersell DJ, et al: Small-cell neuroendocrine carcinoma of the cervix. A human papillomavirus type 18-associated cancer. *Am J Surg Path* 15:28–32, 1991
73. Bethwaite P, Yeong ML, Holloway L, et al: The prognosis of adenosquamous carcinomas of the uterine cervix. *Br J Obstet Gynaecol* 99:745–750, 1992
74. Widrich T, Kennedy AW, Myers TM, et al: Adenocarcinoma in situ of the uterine cervix: management and outcome. *Gynecol Oncol* 61:304–308, 1996
75. Fischer M: Cancer of the cervix. *Semin Oncol Nurs* 18:193–199, 2002
76. Stanley MA: Prognostic factors and new therapeutic approaches to cervical cancer. *Virus Res* 89:241–248, 2002
77. Creasman WT, Zaino RJ, Major FJ, et al: Early invasive carcinoma of the cervix (3 to 5 mm invasion): risk factors and prognosis. A Gynecology Oncology Group study. *Am J Obstet Gynecol* 178:62–65, 1998
78. Kim GE, Kim YB, Cho NH, et al: Synchronous coexpression of epidermal growth factor receptor and cyclooxygenase-2 in carcinomas of the uterine cervix: a potential predictor of poor survival. *Clin Cancer Res* 10:1366–1374, 2004
79. Shepherd JH: Cervical and vulva cancer: changes in FIGO definitions of staging. *Br J Obstet Gynaecol* 103:405, 1996
80. Creasman WT: New gynecologic cancer staging. *Gynecol Oncol* 58:157, 1995
81. Cervix uteri, in Greene FL, Page DL, Fleming ID, et al (eds.): *American Joint Committee on Cancer: AJCC Cancer Staging Manual* (ed. 6). New York: Springer, 2000, p 260
82. Hoffman MS, Cardosi RJ, Roberts WS, et al: Accuracy of pelvic examination in the assessment of patients with operable cervical cancer. *Am J Obstet Gynecol* 190:986–993, 2004
83. Thomas GM: Improved treatment for cervical cancer — concurrent chemotherapy and radiotherapy. *N Engl J Med* 340:1198, 1999
84. Thomas GM: Concurrent chemotherapy and radiation for locally advanced cervical cancer: the new standard of care. *Semin Radiat Oncol* 10:44–50, 2000
85. Rose PG, Bundy BN: Chemoradiation for locally advanced cervical cancer: does it help? *J Clin Oncol* 20: 891, 2002
86. Pearcey R, Brundage M, Drouin P, et al: Phase III trial comparing radical radiotherapy with and without cisplatin chemotherapy in patients with advanced squamous cell carcinoma of the cervix. *J Clin Oncol* 20:966–972, 2002
87. Whitney CS, Sause W, Bundy BN, et al: Randomized comparison of fluoruracil plus cisplatin versus hydroxyurea as an adjunct to radiation therapy in stage IIB — IVA carcinoma of the cervix with negative para-aortic lymph nodes: a Gynecology Oncology Group and Southwest Oncology Group study. *J Clin Oncol* 17:1339–1348, 1999
88. Morris M, Eifel PJ, Lu J, et al: Pelvic radiation with concurrent chemotherapy compared with pelvic and para-aortic radiation for high-risk cervical cancer. *N Engl J Med* 340:1137–1143, 1999
89. Rose PG, Bundy BN, Watkins EB, et al: Concurrent cisplatin-based radiotherapy and chemotherapy for locally advanced cervical cancer. *N Engl J Med* 340:1144–1153, 1999
90. Keys HM, Bundy BN, Stehman FB, et al: Cisplatin, radiation, and adjuvant hysterectomy compared with radiation and adjuvant hysterectomy for bulky stage I cervical carcinoma. *N Engl J Med* 340:1154–1161, 1999
91. Peters WA 3rd, Liu PY, Barrett RJ 2nd, et al: Concurrent chemotherapy and pelvic radiation therapy compared with pelvic radiation therapy alone as adjuvant therapy after radical surgery in high-risk, early stage cancer of the cervix. *J Clin Oncol* 18:1606-1613, 2000
92. Grigsby PW, Perez CA: Radiotherapy alone for medically inoperable carcinoma of the cervix: stage IA and carcinoma in situ. *Int J Radiat Oncol Biol Phys* 21:375–378, 1991
93. Delgado G, Bundy BN, Zaino R, et al: Prospective surgical-pathological study of disease-free interval in patients with stage IB squamous cell carcinoma of the cervix: a Gynecology Oncology Group study. *Gynecol Oncol* 38:352–357, 1990
94. Zaino R, Ward S, Delgado G, et al: Histopathologic predictors of behavior of surgically treated stage IB squamous cell carcinoma of the cervix. A Gynecology Oncology Group study. *Cancer* 69:1750–1758, 1992
95. Schlaerth JB, Spirtos N, Schlaerth AC: Radical trachelectomy and pelvic lymphadenectomy with uterine preservation in the treatment of cervical cancer. *Am J Obstet Gynecol* 188:29–34, 2003
96. Koiopoulos G, Sotiriadis A, Kyrgiou M, et al: Conservative surgical methods for FIGO stage IA2 squamous cervical carcinoma and their role in preserving women's fertility. *Gynecol Oncol* 93:469–473, 2003
97. Fine BA, Hempling RE, Piver MS, et al: Severe radiation morbidity in carcinoma of the cervix: impact of pretherapy surgical staging and previous surgery. *Int J Radiat Oncol Biol Phys* 31:717–723, 1995
98. Ruth-Sahd LA, Zulkosky KD: Cervical cancer: caring for patients undergoing total pelvic exenteration. *Crit Care Nurs* 19:46–57, 1999

99. Alberts DS, Kronmal R, Baker LH, et al: Phase II randomized trial of cisplatin chemotherapy regimens in the treatment of recurrent or metastatic squamous cell cancer of the cervix: a Southwest Oncology Group Study. *J Clin Oncol* 5:1791–1795, 1987
100. Thigpen JT, Blessing JA, DiSaia PJ, et al: A randomized comparison of a rapid versus prolonged (24 hr) infusion of cisplatin in therapy of squamous cell carcinoma of the uterine cervix: a Gynecologic Oncology Group study. *Gynecol Oncol* 32:198–202, 1989
101. Coleman RE, Harper PG, Gallagher C, et al: A phase II study of ifosfamide in advanced and relapsed carcinoma of the cervix. *Cancer Chemother Pharmacol* 18:280–283, 1986
102. Kudelka AP, Winn R, Edwards CL, et al: An update of a phase II study of paclitaxel in advanced or recurrent squamous cell cancer of the cervix. *Anticancer Drugs* 8:657–661, 1997
103. Thigpen JT, Vance RB, Khansur T: The platinum compounds and paclitaxel in the management of of carcinomas of the endometrium and uterine cervix. *Semin Oncol* 22(suppl 12):67–75, 1995
104. McGuire WP, Blessing JA, Moore D, et al: Paclitaxel has moderate activity in squamous cervix cancer. A Gynecologic Oncology Group study. *J Clin Oncol* 14:792–795, 1996
105. Morris M, Brader K, Levenback C, et al: Phase II study of vinorelbine in advanced and recurrent squamous cell carcinoma of the cervix.*J Clin Oncol* 16:1094–1098, 1998
106. Lacava JA, Leone BA, Machiavelli M, et al: Vinorelbine as neoadjuvant chemotherapy in advanced cervical carcinoma. *J Clin Oncol* 15:604–609, 1997
107. Coleman RL, Miller DS: Topotecan in the treatment of gynecologic cancer. *Semin Oncol* 24(suppl):S20–S55, 1977
108. Buxton EJ, Meanwell CA, Hilton C, et al: Combination bleomycin, ifosfamide, and cisplatin chemotherapy in cervical cancer. *J Natl Cancer Inst* 81:359–361, 1989
109. Verschraegen CF, Levy T, Kudelka AP, et al: Phase II study of irinotecan in prior chemotherapy-treated squamous cell carcinoma of the cervix. *J Clin Oncol* 15:625–631, 1997
110. Look KY, Blessing JA, Levenback CA, et al: A phase II trial of CPT-11 in recurrent squamous cell carcinoma of the cervix: a Gynecologic Oncology Group study. *Gynecol Oncol* 70:334–338, 1998
111. Carmichael J: The role of gemcitabine in the treatment of other tumors. *Br J Cancer* 78:21–25, 1998
112. Rose PG, Blessing JA, Gershenson DM, et al: Paclitaxel and cisplatin as first-line therapy in recurrent or advanced squamous cell carcinoma of the cervix: a Gynecologic Oncology Group study. *J Clin Oncol* 17:2676–2680, 1999
113. Burnett AR, Roman LD, Garcia AA, et al: A phase II study of gemcitabine and cisplatin in patients with advanced, persistent, or recurrent squamous cell carcinoma of the cervix. *Gynecol Oncol* 76:63–66, 2000
114. Long HJ, Bundy BY, Grendys EC, et al: Randomized Phase III trial of cisplatin (P) vs. Cisplatin plus topotecan (CT) vs MVAC in stage IVB recurrent or persistent carcinoma of the uterine cervix. A Gynecologic Oncology Group study. The Annual Meeting on Women's Cancer. Abst #9, pp 80, 2004.
115. Chu NR: Therapeutic vaccination for the treatment of mucosotropic human papillomavirus-associated disease. *Exp Opin Biol Ther* 3:477–486, 2003
116. Koutsky LA, Ault KA, Wheeler CM, et al: A controlled trial of human papillomavirus type 16 vaccine. *N Engl J Med* 347:1645–1651, 2002
117. National Cancer Institute: Future directions in epidemiologic and preventive research on human papillomavirus and cancer. *J Natl Cancer Inst Monogr*, 31, 2003
118. Mandic A, Vujkov T: Human papillomavirus vaccine as a new way of preventing cervical cancer: a dream or the future? *Ann Oncol* 15:197–200, 2004
119. Goldie SJ, Kohli M, Grima D, et al: Projected clinical benefits and cost-effectiveness of a human papillomavirus 16/18 vaccine. *J Natl Cancer Inst* 96:604–615, 2004

CHAPTER 49

Colon, Rectal, and Anal Cancers

Gail Wilkes, MS, RNC, ANP, AOCN®

Colon Cancer

Introduction

Colon and rectal cancers are combined in the term "colorectal cancer," and most available statistics on these cancers are also combined. Colorectal cancer is the second leading cause of death from cancer in men and women combined, and the third leading cause of cancer and third leading cause of death if women and men are considered separately, following lung and breast cancer in women and lung and prostate cancer in men. In 2004, the American Cancer Society (ACS) estimated that 106,370 people developed colon cancer (50,400 men and 55,970 women), and 40,570 developed rectal cancer (23,220 men and 17,350 women). ACS expected 56,730 people to die of colon and rectal cancers in 2004: 28,320 men and 28,410 women.[1] Clearly, colon and rectal cancers combined are a major public health problem. In terms of incidence, colon cancer is 2.5 times more common than rectal cancer, and anal cancers account for fewer than 4% of all lower gastrointestinal (GI) cancers.[2]

Despite the fact that colon and rectal cancers share a similar cellular path of carcinogenesis, they are two separate diseases. In this chapter, they will be discussed together and differences pointed out in their epidemiology, as many of the studies and statistics discuss both cancers concurrently. The chapter will then discuss them separately in terms of treatment. Anal cancer is histologically different and is discussed in a separate subsection.

Colon cancer is a *preventable and curable disease,* which is known to be inflenced by genetic as well as environmental factors such as micronutrients, exercise, and obesity. Strong evidence of these relationships is emerging, and counseling about exercise and elimination of obesity is included in prevention regimens. For both colon and rectal cancers, 90% of disease occurs in individuals who are age 50 and older. Many reasons explain the high incidence and mortality figures, ranging from cultural aversions to discussion of bowel function, primary care providers' lack of compliance with standard recommended screening, and lack of access to standard care among socioeconomically disadvantaged populations. Screening and early detection activities are critical for all individuals aged 50 years or older, and for younger individuals who are at risk for the development of colon cancer. As the twenty-first century unfolds, it will bring a better genetic understanding of cancer with the deciphering of the human genome. It is therefore imperative that we understand the changes that occur in the malignant transformation in colon and rectal cancers.

Colon cancer is the most extensively studied of the GI malignancies, particularly in terms of its genetic, molecular, biological, environmental, and dietary aspects. Because this cancer may be silent until it reaches an advanced stage, screening and early detection have become the primary methods for reducing morbidity and mortality. Advances in endoscopy, specialty radiology, and surgical resection for primary as well as metastatic disease, together with improvements in chemotherapy and radiation therapy over the last decade, have helped to diminish the mortality and morbidity of colon cancer. Nurses, physicians in primary care, and members of the healthcare team can help increase awareness that screening is available and that prevention methods are effective and valuable. More than 30,000 lives could be saved each year if the general public, primary care physicians, and managed care companies were more aware of and promoted methods of early detection and treatment.[3] State-of-the-art treatment and care can be provided by healthcare professionals as genetic mapping, clinical trials, advancements in the management of side effects, and alternative methods of treatment and support are developed.

Epidemiology and Etiology

Approximately 6% of the U.S. population will at some point develop colorectal cancer.[1] Colon and rectal cancers combined are one of the leading causes of cancer-related deaths in the Western world. They account for approximately two-thirds of all cancers arising in the GI tract. Their peak incidence occurs in the sixth and seventh decades of life. Approximately 7% of colorectal cancer occurs in persons younger than age 40.[4] More women than men develop colon cancer, but more men than women develop rectal cancer.[5] Adenocarcinomas of the colon can be hereditary or sporadic. Inherited colon cancers account for about 6% of colon cancers, either familial adenomatous polyposis (FAP) or hereditary nonpolyposis colorectal cancer (HNPCC). Of the sporadic colon cancers, 25% arise in individuals at risk for developing colon cancer due to a personal or family history of colon cancer: having had colon cancer or adenomatous polyps, or having a first-degree relative who had colon cancer or adenomatous polyps before the age of 60.

Colon cancer develops as the result of an accumulation of genetic mutations. For example, initially an epithelial cell of the colon acquires the characteristics of an adenoma that eventually acquires the characteristics of invasive cancer. With or without familial risk, colon cancers seem to develop from a similar set of genes and a similar progression of accumulated mutations.[6] The most commonly mutated genes in colon cancer are the adenomatous polyposis coli genes, the *K-ras* oncogene, the *p53* tumor suppressor gene, the deleted-in-colon-cancer gene, and the DNA mismatched pair genes. Other molecular characteristics that are associated with an aggressive phenotype are mutation in p27, a cyclin-dependent kinase inhibitor that helps balance active cell division with no cell division based on the body's needs, especially in stage II colon cancer and in cancers that lack this protein (turned off and not expressed); epidermal growth factor receptor (EGFR) overexpression, which inhibits apoptosis (programmed cell death) and leads to the formation of new blood vessels (angiogenesis) and metastatic spread; and DNA aneuploidy (an incorrect number of chromosomes), which is associated with recurrence of colon cancer and poor outcomes. Hereditary nonpolyposis colorectal cancer arises from mutations in one of the four genes that participate in mismatch repair, or the repair of defective DNA strands. When mismatch repair does not function, mutations occur in one or more of the genes that are important to the control of cell growth, and the mutations are perpetuated in subsequent generations of colon mucosal epithelial cells.[6] The mutated genes in cancer syndromes have been identified, and genetic testing is available for patients and their first-degree relatives.

Some 95% or more of colon cancers develop outside of the previously described syndromes and are referred to as *sporadic* or *common* cancers. About 10% of adults in Western countries have a first-degree relative who is affected by colon cancer. These persons have a twofold to threefold increased risk of acquiring the disease. Having multiple relatives with colon cancer or relatives with a diagnosis at a younger age further increases the risk.[7] Colon cancers are generally known to evolve through a multistep process involving a benign adenomatous polyp that eventually becomes cancerous. This entire process can take approximately 10 years. Early colon and rectal carcinomas confined to the mucosa or submucosa usually produce a polypoid mass. Cancers smaller than 1.5 cm have a noticeable absence of lymph node metastasis.[4] There is generally no risk of invasive malignancy in polyps smaller than 5 mm. There is a 1% risk in polyps 5–19 mm, a 10% risk in polyps 1–2 mm, and a 30%–50% risk in polyps larger than 2 mm.[4]

Incidence and mortality rates among racial and ethnic groups differ, perhaps as the result of differences in socioeconomic status, especially in terms of access to standard health care and as the role of micronutrients becomes clearer — purchasing fresh fruits and vegetables and eating a healthy diet are costly.[8] Among African Americans, the incidence of colon cancer has increased by 30% since 1973 and is now higher than in Caucasians.[2] In ACS statistics for the period 1996–2000, the incidence rate (per 100,000) among African American males was 72.4 compared to 64.1 in white males and 56.2 for African American females versus 46.2 for white females.[1] Death rates (per 100,000) are also higher: 28.5 for African Americans versus 20.7 for Caucasians. The incidence and death rates of colon and rectal cancers for the same period among Asians/Pacific Islanders, American Indians/Alaskan Natives, and Hispanics/Latinos (although not mutually exclusive from all others such as Caucasian) are lower than those among whites.

The higher incidence and mortality rates in African Americans are believed to be due to reduced access to regular screening such that patients present with more advanced disease and, in some cases, due to poorer access to timely, high-quality treatments.[1] For example, ACS statistics show that 38% of white patients present with localized colon and rectal cancers, while only 34% of African Americans do; 19% of whites present with distant disease compared to 24% of African Americans. The question of whether colon and rectal cancers have a more aggressive biology has been raised, but a study by McCollum and colleagues showed that with equal staging (high-risk stage II and stage III colon cancer) and similar access to healthcare resources and treatment with adjuvant chemotherapy, Caucasians and African Americans with colon cancer have similar five-year survival and overall survival rates.[9] In addition, health beliefs of inner-city patients pose challenges: many black Americans use emergency rooms for evaluation of health problems, rather than prevention; fatalism with the belief that cancer means death, together with an aversion to discussion of any aspects of bowel elimination; and inability to buy healthy foods so that canned foods and high-fat foods form much of the diet, resulting in obesity.

The incidence of colorectal cancer decreased from 1985 to 1995, a trend believed to be related to improved public education and professional awareness and accountability.[10] Increased screening and polyp removal translated to a 7% decrease in incidence and a 21% decrease in mortality during this period.[11] ACS statistics reveal that mortality rates decreased by 1.9% per year for men and 1.5% per year for women between 1990 and 1994.[8] However, the incidence of colon and rectal cancers stabilized in the mid-1990s and remains unchanged since then. With the aging of the "baby boomers," it is expected that by 2050, the number of individuals with all cancers will double.[12]

About 70% of individuals who have colon and rectal cancers present with apparently localized disease; the remaining 30% have advanced disease at diagnosis.[2] Twenty-five percent of the latter patients have distant metastatic disease and 5% have locally advanced disease. Metastasis to adjacent organs or lymph nodes reduces the survival rate to approximately 67%.[2] If the cancer has spread to distant sites, survival becomes much less likely.[2] The Digestive Health Initiative, a national study published in 1997, estimated the five-year survival rate from colorectal cancer to be 52%–55%.[3] In 1999, the five-year survival rate for colorectal cancer increased to greater than 90% when it is diagnosed in the early localized stage, and to greater than 60% after spread to adjacent organs or nodes.[2] Although colon and rectal cancers are preventable and curable cancers, progress in treatment has enabled slightly more than half of patients in the United States to achieve five-year disease-free status in 2004.

One-fourth of combined colon and rectal cancers are found in the rectum; the remainder are located in the colon.[4] Surveillance, Epidemiology, and End Results (SEER) studies reveal that the incidence of right-sided (proximal) colon tumors is increasing slowly. The incidence of right-sided (proximal) colon cancer was 54.7% in 1993 compared to 50.9% in 1988.[13] In African Americans, the incidence of right-sided adenomas approaches 65%.[14] While right-sided cancers appear to be increasing in young African Americans, it is hypothesized that this trend may reflect an increase in type II diabetes incidence related to obesity.[15] According to this hypothesis, insulin-like growth factor may play a role in the development of proximal, right-sided colon cancer.[16,17]

The incidence of colon and rectal cancers is high in industrialized regions like North America, northwestern Europe, and Australia. Incidence is low in less developed regions such as Asia, Africa, and South America. Residents of high-risk countries typically consume diets that are high in total fat, animal fat, and protein, and that are relatively low in fruits, vegetables, and fiber. Individuals moving from a low-risk country to a high-risk one assume the higher risk of their new country. In addition to diet, many lifestyle habits are related to a higher risk of colorectal cancer.[8]

The incidence of colon cancer increases with age —not surprising given that the colonic mucosal epithelium is continually exposed to all the things an individual eats over the lifetime. Factors that have been identified as contributing to the development of colon cancers include fecal carcinogens, bile acids, lifestyle, diet, alcohol intake, inflammatory bowel conditions, radiation exposure, cholecystectomy, and family and genetic factors.[18] Most important are age, obesity, familial/genetic factors, and diet (micronutrient deficiency, and factors that slow bowel transit time).

Familial/genetic and lifestyle factors

Lieberman and colleagues studied 3121 asymptomatic patients aged 50–75 years from 13 Veterans Affairs medical centers over the period 1994–1997, all of whom had an adenoma greater than 10 mm in diameter, villous adenoma, an adenoma with high-grade dysplasia, or invasive cancer.[19] They found positive associations for history of a first-degree relative with colorectal cancer, current smoking, and current moderate or heavy alcohol use. Inverse or protective associations were found for cereal fiber intake (more than 4.2 g per day), vitamin D intake (greater than 645 IU per day), and daily use of nonsteroidal anti-inflammatory drugs (NSAIDS). The authors reported that slight or marginal factors were physical activity, daily multivitamin use, intake of calcium, and consumption of fat derived from red meat. No association was found with body mass index (BMI) or prior cholecystectomy. For patients for whom hyperplastic polyps were the only finding at colonoscopy, risk was similar to that of patients with no polyps, except that current or past smoking increased the risk for hyperplastic polyps.

A decrease in physical activity or sedentary lifestyle leads to a decrease in intestinal tract transit time and allows potential carcinogens to have longer contact with gut mucosa. A number of studies have shown that vigorous exercise is associated with a decreased risk of colon cancer.[20,21] There is a noted association between obesity, or increased caloric intake in excess of energy expenditure, and an increased risk for colon cancer.[2]

Diets high in fat increase the production and change the composition of bile salts. These altered bile salts are converted into potential carcinogens by intestinal flora. While the exact mechanism by which bile salts act as a promoter for colon and rectal cancers is unknown, researchers suggest that the process is mediated by diacylglycerol.[22] Phospholipids are converted to diacylglycerol by intestinal bacteria. Diacylglycerol then enters the epithelial cells of the colon and activates protein kinase C, which plays a role in cell growth and tumor promotion. Of interest, the inflammatory response is regulated by eicosanoids, which are derived from the omega-6 fatty acid arachidonic acid.

Through a complex relationship, cyclooxygenase (COX) exerts an inflammatory effect. Colorectal cancers often express COX-2, and this expression correlates with tumor angiogenesis, more invasive tumor phenotype, resistance to apoptosis, and systemic immunosuppression.[23] Cyclooxygenase-2 inhibitors can reduce the growth of colorectal polyps. For this reason, the drug celecoxib is indicated for the prevention of FAP in high-risk individuals. COX-2 inhibitors are also being studied for their anticancer effect.[24]

Studies have produced conflicting results regarding the role of dietary fiber in reducing risk. The protective mechanism of dietary fiber is exerted in a number of ways. For example, it increases fecal bulk, which changes the bacterial composition of the feces and accelerates the transit time in the intestinal tract.

Heavy alcohol consumption has been considered a factor in the development of colon and rectal cancers.[25,26] Alcohol is thought to stimulate gastrointestinal cell proliferation and promote carcinogenesis secondary to an excess of unabsorbed carcinogens such as the nitrosamines found in beer and whiskey.[27] However, the body's demand for folate increases with alcohol consumption, and low folate levels may actually confer the risk.[28] Uterosigmoidostomy is performed for a number of malignant conditions. Reports in the literature show a 5%–10% increase in incidence of colon carcinoma occurring 15 years after the initial surgery.[29] In these cases, the most common site of the colon cancer is distal to the surgical site where there has been chronic exposure of the intestinal mucosa to both urine and feces. Persons with a history of colorectal carcinoma are also at increased risk of developing a second primary colon cancer. Women with a history of endometrial, ovarian, or breast cancer have an increased chance of developing colorectal cancer.[2] Patients who have undergone a cholecystectomy have also been noted to have a higher incidence of colon cancers, but studies conflict as to the exact level of risk.[2]

Studies show that the only definite risk factor is obesity (BMI > 27 increases the relative risk to 1.5, whereas BMI < 21 carries a risk of 1.0). Alcohol (drinking more than one drink per day versus none) probably increases the relative risk to 1.4, eating red meat (consumption by the top 25% compared to the lower 25%) probably increases the relative risk to 1.5, smoking (25 or more cigarettes per day compared to none) possibly increases the risk to 1.5, and high vegetable consumption (five or more servings per day) possibly reduces the risk to 0.7.[30]

Inflammatory bowel disease (IBD) increases the risk of colon cancer.[31] In general, cancer that develops in individuals with IBD begins with dysplasic changes in the intestinal mucosa and occurs at site of active disease. The relative risk of colon cancer increases with the duration of IBD. Of note, risk of colon cancer is increased in patients who have sites of IBD in the small bowel.

Over the last two decades, mortality rates for colorectal cancer in many developed countries have declined in women but not in men. A possible explanation for the decrease in women is the use of oral contraceptives and hormone replacement therapy. A 20%–40% risk reduction is reported among users of hormone replacement therapy. The apparent protection is related to estrogen, and tended to be stronger among recent users.[32]

Other risk factors for colorectal cancer can be broadly classified as environmental and genetic. Environmental factors include occupational exposure to asbestos, acrylonitrile, ethyl acrylate, synthetic fibers, halogens, printing materials, and fuel oils. Genetic risk factors are related to inherited germ-line mutations (FAP or HNPCC), or inherited risk conferred by a first-degree relative having colon cancer.

Several genetic polyposis syndromes are associated with a high risk of colon and rectal cancers. Familial adenomatous polyposis coli is an inherited autosomal dominant trait that results in the development of polyps throughout the colon and rectum. This process generally starts in late adolescence. Persons with this syndrome have a 100% risk of developing colorectal cancer.[18] Hereditary nonpolyposis colorectal cancer is an inherited autosomal dominant condition characterized by the occurrence of colorectal cancer at an average age of 45 years.[33] Affected persons have one or few adenomatous polyps, but no polyposis.

Hereditary nonpolyposis colon cancer occurs as type A (Lynch type I) or type B (Lynch type II). Type A is familial, site-specific, nonpolyposis colon cancer. Type B is also nonpolyposis colon cancer but is found in association with other forms of cancer such as breast, endometrial, gastric, and ovarian cancer. Once an individual at risk for HNPCC develops cancer, a subtotal colectomy should be performed. Prophylactic hysterectomy and/or bilateral salpingoophorectomy should be considered for women with HNPCC who are diagnosed with cancer or who are genetic carriers.

A variant of FAP consists of multiple, flat adenomas that have an increased risk of becoming cancerous.[34,35] Other genetic premalignant polyposis syndromes associated with a high risk of colorectal cancer include hamartomatous polyposis syndromes [Peutz-Jeghers, juvenile polyposis, Cowden's disease (multiple hamartoma syndrome), and neurofibromatosis] and types of adenomatous polyposis (Gardener's syndrome and Turcot's syndrome).[2]

Inherited risk conferred by a first-degree family member with colorectal cancer has been established. Fuchs and colleagues[36] reported results of a prospective study of 32,085 men and 87,031 women, and determined risk for individuals who had a family history of first-degree relatives with colon or rectal cancer. Compared to a relative risk of 1.0 for an individual without a first-degree relative who had colon or rectal cancer, the relative risk for an individual who had an affected first-degree relative was 1.72 (95% confidence interval, 1.34–2.19); if an individual had two or more first-degree relatives with colon or rectal cancers, the relative risk was 2.75 (95% confidence interval, 1.34–5.63); and if the individual was younger than age 45 and had one or more affected first-degree relatives, the relative risk was 5.37 (95% confidence interval, 1.98–14.6). Risk decreased with increasing age ($p < 0.001$).

Studies on primary prevention are summarized in Table 49-1. There is still controversy about which factors directly or indirectly cause colon cancer. At this time, it is known that the following factors definitely increase risk and play a role in the development of colon cancer: familial/genetic factors, obesity, inflammatory bowel disease (IBD), and micronutrient deficiency.

Prevention, Screening, and Early Detection

While family history or history of colon adenomas or colon cancer cannot be changed, much can be done to reduce an individual's risk. Two types of prevention are recognized for colorectal cancer: primary and secondary. Work is currently being done to gather more evidence in support of many of the primary prevention strategies. *Primary prevention* involves minimizing external risk factors such as obesity, exercise,[37] and fat intake, and increasing elements that will decrease the likelihood of polyp formation and transformation, such as inclusion of fruits and vegetables, other high-fiber foods, and certain micronutrients in the diet, increasing physical activity, and use of COX-2 inhibitors. Table 49-1 describes the numerous studies, their findings, and references for further reading.[38–73] It is estimated that as many as 80% of colon cancers can be prevented by dietary change. *Secondary prevention*, or the identification and modification of risk factors following the development of a colonic polyp, involves surgical removal of suspicious adenomatous or malignant polyps to prevent the development of colon cancer.

Table 49-1 Primary Prevention Strategies

Prevention Strategy	Study, Findings, or Article	Reference
Dietary fiber	Prospective study of 88,757 women age 34–59 years without a history of cancer or colon cancer risk factors, who were followed for 16 years. No association was found between the intake of dietary fiber and development of adenoma or risk of colon or rectal cancer.	Fuchs et al.[38]
High-fiber cereal	No effect on the recurrence of colorectal adenomas.	Alberts et al.[39]
Low-fat, high-fiber diet	No effect on the recurrence of colorectal adenomas.	Schatzkin et al.[40]
Cereal fiber supplementation	No protective effect against the development of recurrent colon or rectal adenomas, regardless of intake of fruit, vegetables, or grains, including wheat bran fiber.	Jacobs et al.[41]
Diet high in vegetables, fruits, grains	Increased risk in men for the development of colorectal adenoma from a diet high in saturated fat and low in fiber. Diet of chicken and fish instead of red meat, and increased intake of vegetables, fruits, and grains are protective against colorectal cancer in men.	Giovonnucci et al.[42]
Cereal fiber, vitamin D, daily use of NSAIDs	Inverse or protective association for cereal fiber intake (> 4.2 g/day), vitamin D intake greater than 645 IU/day, and daily use of NSAIDs.	Lieberman et al.[19]
Dietary fiber	Randomized study of 33,971 subjects [Prostate, Lung, Colorectal and Ovarian (PLCO) Cancer Screening Trial]: high intake of dietary fiber was associated with a lower risk of colon and rectal adenomas. Individuals ingesting the highest amounts of fiber had a 27% lower risk of distal colonic adenoma as compared to the lowest quintile, with fiber from grains, cereals, and fruits conferring the most protection. No reduction in risk for rectal adenomas.	Peters et al.[43]
Dietary fiber	Large (519,978 subjects) prospective study of the association between dietary fiber intake and the incidence of colorectal cancer [European Prospective Investigation into Cancer and Nutrition (EPIC)]. Highest-intake group (mean fiber intake 35 g/day) had a 27% lower incidence of adenoma ($p = 0.002$) after an average follow-up of 4.5 years. Dietary fiber intake was inversely proportional to incidence of colon cancer, and the protective effect was greatest for left-sided colon cancer and least for rectal cancer.	Bingham et al.[44]
Fruit and vegetables	Inverse relationship between the amount of fruit and vegetables consumed and the risk of colorectal cancer.	Terry et al.[45]
Red meat	Diets high in animal fats and red meat were associated with an increased risk of colonic adenomas and colon cancer in women and men, respectively.	Willett et al.[46]; Giovannucci et al.[42]
Red meat	Meta-analysis of articles published during 1973–1999 showed that high intake of red meat, and especially processed meat, was associated with a moderate but significant increase in colorectal cancer risk. Total meat intake was not significantly associated with colorectal cancer risk.	Norat et al.[47]
Red meat	Cohort studies of vegetarians in developed countries do not show low death rates from colon and rectal cancers, so meat is probably not the key factor leading to high rates of colon and rectal cancers in developed countries.	Key et al.[48]
Meat	No evidence that mutagenic heterocyclic amines and polycyclic aromatic hydrocarbons produced when meat is cooked at high temperatures, or nitrites and related compounds in smoked and processed meats, play a significant role in the development or progression of colon and rectal cancers.	Key et al.[48]

(continued)

Table 49-1 Primary Prevention Strategies (continued)

Prevention Strategy	Study, Findings, or Article	Reference
Micronutrients	Nurses' Health Study data from 88,756 women showed that women who had taken multivitamins containing folic acid for at least 15 years had a significant reduction in the risk of developing colon cancer but not of developing rectal cancer.	Giovannucci et al.[49]
Folate	Folic acid or folate intake was found to be inversely proportional to colorectal cancer risk in women participating in the Canadian National Breast Screening Study (N = 56,837), with a 40% risk reduction in the women with the highest folate intake compared to women with the lowest. The risk reduction was not statistically significant.	Terry et al.[45]
Folate	Significant risk reduction using a case-control study when subjects with the highest folate intake were compared to those with the lowest intake.	LaVecchia, et al.[50]
Folate	Nurses with and without a family history of colon cancer in first degree relatives. Women without a positive family history for colon cancer who took > 400 mcg/day of folate had a relative risk of 0.81, compared to 0.48 in those with a positive family history. The authors hypothesized that those with a family history of colon cancer may be vulnerable to folate deficiencies.	Fuchs et al.[51]
Folate	Hypothesize that folate deficiency may lead to DNA hypomethylation, which may then lead to the activation of proto-oncogenes and trigger carcinogenesis.	Duthie[52]; Pufulete et al.[53]
Folate, aspirin	Aspirin/Folate Polyp Prevention Study in progress.	Baron et al.[54]
Folate	Low folate levels increase the risk of malignancy by reducing DNA methylation and cause uracil to be substituted for thymine in DNA synthesis.	Chen et al.[55]
Folate	DNA in adenomas was hypomethylated compared to controls who did not have adenomas, and patients with colorectal cancer had a significantly lower folate status than controls. Patients who had a high folate status, as determined by dietary intake, plasma, and erythrocyte folate concentrations, had a significantly reduced risk of developing colon cancer.	Pufulete et al.[53]
Folate	Decreased dietary folate intake leads to decreased methionine pools, which directly provide methyl groups for DNA methylation.	Wu et al.[56]
Folate	Hypothesize role of folate: Folate lies at the intersection of metabolic pathways involved in DNA methylation and biosynthesis. Methyl groups are needed for normal cellular metabolism. If there are insufficient methyl groups available for dietary intake, new methyl groups are synthesized using one carbon group donated by folate. If there is insufficient folate, methylation does not occur or occurs slowly. Methylation refers to the process by which methyl groups are added to certain nucleotides in the DNA helix. The areas of DNA that are methylated are difficult to transcribe, and thus are not expressed. Low levels of folate in the body may cause malignant transformation by altering the normal DNA-methylation process (where genes that are not needed are not expressed), altering the steady-state level of DNA precursors. This results in aberrant DNA synthesis and repair, and causes changes in chromosome and chromatin in the genome.	Lamprecht and Lipkin.[57]

(continued)

Table 49-1 Primary Prevention Strategies (continued)

Prevention Strategy	Study, Findings, or Article	Reference
Calcium and vitamin D	Hypothesize extracellular calcium exerts anticancer effects by activating calcium-sensing receptors, resulting in increased levels of intracellular calcium. Vitamin D, when binding to a nuclear receptor, influences gene expression, either up-regulating (turning on) or down-regulating (turning off) specific gene expression. Vitamin D also participates in cross-talk with growth factors/cytokines, inhibiting activation of the cell cycle (cell division), and stimulating apoptosis (programmed cell death when the cell's DNA has mutations that cannot be repaired).	Lamprecht and Lipkin[57]
Calcium	Nurses' Health Study and Health Professionals' Follow-up Study. Higher calcium intake was associated with a significantly lower risk of cancer in the distal colon, but not in the proximal colon.	Wu et al.[56]
Calcium	In a prospective study, 930 patients with a history of colorectal adenomas were randomly assigned to receive either 3 g of calcium carbonate daily or placebo. The group receiving the calcium carbonate had a significantly reduced number of adenomas compared to the placebo group (p = 0.03) at 1 and 4 years.	Baron et al.[58]
Ursodeoxycholic acid	In a small group of patients with ulcerative colitis and primary sclerosing cholangitis, risk of developing colonic dysplasia or colon cancer was significantly reduced in the group receiving ursodeoxycholic acid.[59] A secondary bile acid, deoxycholic acid is absorbed in the colon; it has been found to be significantly elevated in men with adenomas of the colon, and is associated with rates of colonic mucosal cell proliferation.[22] Thus, treatment with the synthetic bile acid urosdeoxycholic acid results in reduced levels of deoxycholic acid and, it is hoped, will reduce the incidence of adenomas. This is now being studied in individuals at risk for developing sporadic adenomas.[60]	Pardi et al.[59]; Brentnall[60]
Exercise	Harvard University alumni studied. Those who were highly active (energy expenditure of 25,000 kilocalories per week) had 50% the risk of developing colon cancer than those who were not physically active (< 1000 kilocalories per week).	Lee et al.[61]
Exercise	Nurses' Health Study data. Vigorous exercise reduced the risk for developing colon adenoma and cancer in both men and women. Women in the highest energy expenditure quintile had 57% of the risk of developing large adenoma of sedentary women.	Giovannucci et al.[62,63]
Exercise	Lack of lifetime vigorous leisure-time physical activity was associated with increased risk for the development of colon cancer (63% for men and 59% for women).	Slattery[64]
Exercise	Strongest protection is conferred by high levels of physical activity maintained over a long period of time.	Hardman et al.[65]
Exercise	Review of the literature showing a relationship between exercise and reduced risk of colon cancer: 50% reduction in incidence of colon cancer in individuals with the highest level of activity, which persisted when controlled for diet and other factors that might reduce or increase risk for colon cancer.	Colditz et al.[20]
Aspirin and NSAIDs	Reduces incidence of premalignant adenomas and colon cancer.	Kune et al.[66]; Muscat et al.[67]

(continued)

Table 49-1 Primary Prevention Strategies (continued)

Prevention Strategy	Study, Findings, or Article	Reference
Aspirin and NSAIDs	Protective effect due to inhibition of COX-2. COX-2 regulates prostaglandins, which are known to regulate intestinal epithelial cell growth and proliferation. COX-2 can be induced by cytokines, growth factors, and tumor promoters. It regulates the synthesis of prostaglandin E^2, which has been associated with tumorigenesis. It is believed that COX-2 is involved in converting carcinogen precursors to carcinogens and thus is a key player in tumorigenesis. COX-2 inhibits apoptosis and induces angiogenesis. It is involved early in the formation of adenomas, and is overexpressed in colonic adenomas and adenocarcinomas. Aspirin and NSAIDs exert their anti-inflammatory effect by inhibiting COX-1 and COX-2 enzymes; selective COX-2 inhibitors inhibit only COX-2. Arachnoidonic acid is critical in apoptosis, and aspirin and NSAIDs inhibit the metabolism of arachnoidonic acid so it accumulates and stimulates apoptosis.	Dixon,[68]; Courtney et al.[69]; Prescott and Fitzpatrick[70]; Cao et al.[71]
Selective COX-2 inhibitors	Reduction in the mean number of polyps by 28% in patients with familial adenomatous polyposis.	Gwyn and Sinicrope[72]
Aspirin 325 mg qd	Prospective study of 635 patients with a history of colon cancer who were randomized into groups taking aspirin 325 mg daily or placebo. The aspirin group had significantly fewer adenomas than did the placebo group, and a longer time to adenoma detection as compared to the placebo group	Sandler et al.[73]
Aspirin 81 mg versus 325 mg daily	Placebo-controlled trial of 1121 patients with a history of adenoma, who were randomized into one of three groups: aspirin 81 mg daily, aspirin 325 mg daily, or placebo. Only the group receiving aspirin 81 mg daily had a significantly reduced risk of developing adenomas, compared to the placebo group. While 7 patients in the aspirin group had a stroke, this number was not statistically significant. Some have questioned the cost–risk benefit in patients who have had either colon cancer or adenomas, as these patients will have close endoscopic follow-up with early identification and removal of adenomas.	Baron et al.[54]

Primary Prevention

The data shown in Table 49-1 continue to underscore the importance of diet. Ingested foods that undergo digestion continually bathe the colonic mucosa. The only definite modifiable risk factor for colon cancer is obesity, where a BMI greater than 27 is associated with a relative risk of 1.5 times the risk of a normal individual (1.0), defined as an individual with a BMI less than 21.[30] Weight reduction is important to achieve and maintain normal body weight. It is hypothesized that obesity and lack of exercise together may be responsible for altering the metabolism of insulin and insulin-like growth factors. Insulin regulates energy metabolism and anabolic signals related to hyperinsulinemia can promote tumorigenesis (stimulating cell proliferation and inhibiting apoptosis).[37] Dietary fiber has long been touted as a way to protect the colonic and rectal carcinogens through increasing the transit rate of fecal material containing carcinogens. General daily dietary recommendations for fiber intake are 20–30 g per day or more, especially wheat bran,[1] and eating at least five fruits and vegetables each day. Exercise appears to be an important preventive factor, and many studies have consistently shown a decreased risk for development of adenoma in individuals who exercised vigorously as measured in energy expenditure, after controlling for other factors such as diet and body mass index (BMI). Today, the most important primary prevention strategies are weight reduction to appropriate weight for height; regular exercise; eating five or more fruits and vegetables per day; including micronutrients such as folate, calcium, and vitamin D in the diet; and taking a baby aspirin or NSAIDs daily if at risk and appropriate.

Secondary Prevention and Screening

It is well known that certain polyps are precursors to colon and rectal cancers. Secondary prevention involves removing premalignant polyps, thereby preventing the evolution of colon cancer in most cases. Polyps commonly form in the colon and rectum as an individual ages, with risk increasing beyond 50 years of age. Screening goals are to identify polyps before they become malignant. Often polyps bleed as they enlarge, and bleeding can be identified by use of the fecal occult blood test (FOBT). It is estimated that deaths from colon and rectal cancer could be reduced by 50% or more if Americans age 50–80 years followed the current screening guidelines.[74] Based on reports by the Congressional Office of Technology Assessment and the National Cancer Institute, the cost per year of lives saved by colon and rectal cancer screening renders the mass screening cost-effective and could save as many as 30,000 lives per year.[3]

ACS recommends the following screening for individuals age 50 and older: FOBT annually, and sigmoidoscopy every 5 years or colonoscopy every 10 years or double-contrast barium enema every 5 years.[75] While controversy remains regarding the equivalence of double-contrast barium enema plus flexible sigmoidoscopy or colonoscopy, it is quite clear that if an individual has any increased risk in the development of colon cancer, then a colonoscopy should be performed (see Table 49-2). In addition, if there is any suggestion the tumor may be on the right (proximal) side, or if distal adenomas are found at sigmoidoscopy, a colonoscopy must be performed.

Persons with an inherited risk for colorectal cancer, such as family history of FAP, should begin screening by colonoscopy between the ages of 10 and 12, at puberty (see Table 49-2). Individuals with one or more first-degree relatives who developed colon cancer before the age of 55 should have an annual fecal occult blood test and a colonoscopy or double-contrast barium enema every 5 years starting 10 years before the age of onset in the relative. Persons with lower levels of risk (one relative with colorectal cancer diagnosed at an age more than 60 years) should have standard screening with FOBT and flexible sigmoidoscopy performed starting at age 50. The Society of Gastroenterology Nurses and Associates supports routine screening using flexible sigmoidoscopy performed by trained nurses as a way to increase access to screening.[76]

The FOBT and periodic flexible sigmoidoscopy are two easy methods of screening. Most studies, including randomized trials, show that periodic FOBT reduces the risk of death from colon and rectal cancer by 15%–33%.[77–80] Mandel and colleagues[77] studied the effect of FOBT screening on the incidence of colorectal cancer. They found that (1) the number of positive FOBT slides was associated with a positive predictive value for both colorectal cancer and adenomatous polyps at least 1 cm in diameter, and (2) use of either annual or biennial FOBT significantly reduced the incidence of colorectal cancer. In screening general populations, it is estimated that 1%–16% of patients have positive FOBT, depending on age, whether the sample is rehydrated, and the purpose of the test. Following colonic evaluation, the rate of finding colon or rectal cancer is only 2%–17%, and the rate of finding early colon or rectal cancer is 2%–14%.[81] However, once a positive FOBT is found, there must be adequate evaluation of the colon and follow-up.

Digital rectal examinations are simple but can detect abnormalities only up to 7 cm from the anal verge. Thus they are not useful for colon cancer screening. FOBT should not be obtained via a digital rectal exam.

Sigmoidoscopy using a flexible, fiber-optic sigmoidoscope is easy to perform, requires no sedation, and detects as many as 65% of colorectal tumors within 60 cm from the anal verge.[82] If adenomas are found in the distal colon, then colonoscopy is usually performed to examine the proximal colon. Advanced proximal lesions are more likely if the individual is older than age 65, and if villous or tubulovillous distal adenomas were found, or there is a family history of colon or rectal cancer or multiple distal polyps.[83] If adenomas can be found and removed early, colon cancer can be prevented. A number of noncontrolled studies have suggested that sigmoidoscopy can reduce mortality from colon cancer. In two case-controlled trials, one showed a decreased incidence of fatal colon and rectal cancers in the groups screened compared to those not screened.[84,85] Schoen and colleagues[86] reported on data from the Prostate, Lung, Colorectal and Ovarian (PLCO) Cancer Screening trial showing that a repeat sigmoidoscopy 3 years following a negative sigmoidoscopy found a polyp or lesion in the rectum or distal sigmoid in 13.9% of patients (1292 out of 9317 subjects). Most of the polyps were benign, but 2.3% of subjects (214 out of 9317) had nonadvanced adenomas, and 0.8% (78 out of 9317) had advanced adenoma or cancer. Of patients with advanced adenoma or malignancy, 80% had a thorough examination 3 years earlier. The PLCO is a large, randomized, prospective study that will continue to accrue patients through 2015.

According to Gatto and colleagues[87] there is a risk of perforation during sigmoidoscopy (incidence = 0.88/1000 procedures), especially in elderly patients with two or more co-morbidities. The risk is less than that of colonoscopy, although the risk of perforation with colonoscopy is decreasing.

Most sigmoidoscopies are performed by physicians, but evidence indicates that nurse endoscopists are equally able to do effective examinations. Maule[88]

Table 49-2 American Cancer Society Guidelines for Screening and Surveillance for Early Detection of Colorectal Polyps and Cancer

Risk Category*	Recommendation†	Age to Begin	Interval
AVERAGE RISK			
All people 50 years or older who are not in the categories below	One of the following: FOBT plus flexible sigmoidoscopy‡ or TCE¶	Age 50	FOBT every year and flexible sigmoidoscopy every 5 y Colonoscopy every 10 y or DCBE every 5–10 y
MODERATE RISK			
People with single, small (< 1 cm) adenomatous polyps	Colonoscopy	At time of initial polyp diagnosis	TCE within 3 y after initial polyp removal; if normal, as per average-risk recommendations (above)
People with large (≥ 1 cm) or multiple adenomatous polyps of any size	Colonoscopy	At time of initial polyp diagnosis	TCE within 3 y after initial polyp removal; if normal, TCE every 5 y
Personal history of curative-intent resection of colorectal cancer	TCE§	Within 1 y after resection	If normal, TCE in 3 y; if still normal, TCE every 5 y
Colorectal cancer or adenomatous polyps in first-degree relative younger than 60 y or in two or more first-degree relatives of any age	TCE	Age 40 or 10 y before the youngest case in the family, whichever is earlier	Every 5 y
Colorectal cancer in other relatives (not included above)	As per average risk recommendations (above); may consider beginning screening before age 50		
HIGH RISK			
Family history of familial adenomatous polyposis	Early surveillance with endoscopy, counseling to consider genetic testing, and referral to a specialty center	Puberty	If genetic test positive or polyposis confirmed, consider colectomy; otherwise, endoscopy every 1–2 y
Family history of hereditary nonpolyposis colon cancer	Colonoscopy and counseling to consider genetic testing	Age 21	If genetic test positive or if patient has not had genetic testing, colonoscopy every 2 y until age 40, then every year
Inflammatory bowel disease	Colonoscopies with biopsies for dysplasia	8 y after the start of pancolitis; 12–15 y after the start of left-sided colitis	Every 1–2 y

*Approximately 70%–80% of cases are from average-risk individuals, 15%–20% are from moderate-risk individuals, and 5%–10% are from high-risk individuals.

†Digital rectal examination should be done at the time of each sigmoidoscopy, colonoscopy, or DCBE.

‡Annual FOBT has been shown to reduce mortality from colorectal cancer, so it is preferable to no screening. However, the ACS recommends that annual FOBT be accompanied by flexible sigmoidoscopy to further reduce the risk of colorectal cancer mortality.

§This assumes that a perioperative TCE was done.

¶TCE includes either colonoscopy or DCBE. The choice of procedure should depend on the medical status of the patient and the relative quality of the medical examinations available in a specific community. Flexible sigmoidoscopy should be performed in those instances in which the rectosigmoid colon is not well visualized by DCBE. DCBE would be performed when the entire colon has not been adequately evaluated by colonoscopy.

DCBE = double-contrast barium enema; FOBT = fecal occult blood testing; TCE = total colon examination; y = years.

Reprinted with permission from Byers I, Levin B, Rothenberger D, et al: ACS guidelines for screening and surveillance for early detection of colorectal polyps and cancer. *CA Cancer J Clin* 47:154–160, 1997.[75]

described a comparative study of nurse performance of sigmoidoscopy compared to physicians: Nurses performed 1881 independent exams compared to 730 by physicians. The mean depth of insertion of the sigmoidoscope was significantly greater by physicians (48 cm versus 46 cm in men, and 41 cm versus 38 cm in women). There was no significant difference in the number of adenomas or cancer found, or in the complications (none) between nurses and physicians. There was however, a highly significant difference between the number of patients who returned for follow-up sigmoidoscopy: More patients examined by nurses returned as compared to those examined by physicians ($p = 0.001$).

Combining FOBT and flexible sigmoidoscopy should increase early detection of advanced adenomas or early-stage cancers, but two studies showed no significant difference between both modalities compared to sigmoidoscopy (or colonoscopy as a surrogate) alone.[89,90] Winawer and colleagues[91] compared colonoscopy and double-contrast barium enema for surveillance after polypectomy as part of the National Polyp Study Work Group, and found that colonoscopy was a more effective method of surveillance than double-contrast barium enema. Colonoscopy is a more sensitive tool for detecting tumors throughout the entire colon. Biopsy specimens can be obtained and polyps removed during the actual procedure. The accuracy of the colonoscopy examination depends on the ability of the endoscopist to reach the cecum and to negotiate blind corners and mucosal folds. To achieve a satisfactory examination, patient teaching for preparation and support during the procedure itself are crucial.

Lieberman and colleagues[92] studied 3121 veterans and found that patients with distal polyps were also more likely to have proximal polyps. However, Imperiale and colleagues[93] showed that all patients with proximal neoplastic lesions do not have distal polyps; hence, if colonoscopy was reserved only for high-risk patients or those with distal polyps, then 46% or more of patients with proximal lesions will be missed. The authors developed an index to assess risk for advanced proximal colon cancer to try to tailor endoscopic screening, so that patients could be triaged after sigmoidoscopy.[94] Risk for advanced proximal colon cancer was defined as adenoma 1 cm or larger or with villous histology, severe dysplasia, or malignancy. The authors tested the index on 1031 subjects and found 0.4% to be at risk. The index identified 92% of the subjects who actually had advanced proximal colon cancers. The authors suggest further validation of this index, and offer that its adoption could reduce the need for colonoscopy in low-risk individuals by 40%. Incidence of perforation after colonoscopy in one study was 1.9 per 1000 procedures, with the risk increasing as the age of the patient increased and with two or more co-morbidities.[87] The authors concluded that the risk of perforation from colonoscopy is double that of sigmoidoscopy, but the difference between the two modalities is decreasing.

Virtual colonoscopy or colonography. Recently, much attention has been focused on virtual colonoscopy or colonography as a means to examine the colon. Virtual colonoscopy uses computer-generated images from abdominal computed tomography (CT) or magnetic resonance imaging (MRI) to simulate colonoscopic examination. At this time, this procedure has not been perfected to a point where it can replace conventional colonoscopy. The procedure is as uncomfortable for the patient as is colonoscopy. In addition, it is unclear whether virtual colonoscopy provides the same accuracy in identifying polyps, especially if they are smaller than 1 cm, or if it can provide the same reliability when used for follow-up of lesions as does conventional colonoscopy. Finally, because the procedure is visual only, as many as 30% of patients will eventually require colonoscopy for polypectomy.

A number of important studies have examined this technology. Yee and colleagues[95] evaluated 300 patients and found a sensitivity of 90% for lesions measuring greater than 10 mm, and 80% for lesions 5.0–9.0 mm. In this study, there were false-positive findings for lesions smaller than 10 mm. Miao and colleagues[96] found lower sensitivity values in their study of 201 patients with symptoms suggestive of colon cancer or surveillance for a resected prior colon cancer—namely, sensitivity of 73% and specificity of 94% for identification of colon cancer lesions or polyps 10.0 mm or larger. Mascari and colleagues[97] compared thin-section, multidetector CT colonography with conventional colonoscopy to detect colon/rectal polyps and cancer in average-risk, asymptomatic subjects. The authors found 98 polyps in 39 patients; only 21 (21.4%) were detected by CT colonography. They found a sensitivity of 11.5% for polyps 1–5 mm, 52.9% for polyps 6–9 mm, and 100% for polyps that were 10 mm or larger. The CT colonography image was interpreted fairly quickly (mean time = 9 minutes). Thus, it appears that CT colonography is sensitive and specific in detecting polyps 10 mm or larger, but these measures decrease as the size of the polyp decreases. Unfortunately, virtual colonoscopy does not permit excision of polyps once found; patients still need to have a conventional colonoscopy for polypectomy. Perhaps virtual colonoscopy will be used for patients at low risk and in mass screenings, and colonoscopies will be reserved for individuals who are at high risk or who, either on blood test or DNA stool analysis, show mutations in colonic mucosa. However, additional studies must be done to validate the effectiveness and role for virtual colonoscopy.

Other screening technologies. Laboratory tests for gene mutations are now available, thus making it possible to screen individuals at increased risk for developing colorectal cancer as a result of inherited mutations. Genetic analysis of populations at risk could result in more specific measures to reduce risk and earlier identification of the colorectal malignancy. Unfortunately, persons at high risk who should be genetically tested are potentially more likely to lose their insurance coverage. The role of the nurse and/or the genetic counselor in this situation is to provide the necessary information needed for the patient to be

Table 49-3 Colorectal Cancer Screening of Adults Aged 50 and Older by Age, 1992–1997

	FOBT	FOBT	FOBT	Sigmoidoscopy or Colonoscopy	Sigmoidoscopy or Colonoscopy	Sigmoidoscopy or Colonoscopy
	Total	Male	Female	Total	Male	Female
50–59 yr	15.6%	13.4%	17.6%	26.2%	28.8%	23.8%
60–69 yr	23.3%	21.4%	24.8%	37.2%	41.9%	33.4%
70–79 yr	26.0%	25.1%	26.6%	40.9%	45.7%	37.5%
80–84 yr	24.0%	22.8%	24.7%	39.1%	48.7%	34.5%
85+ yr	17.3%	16%	17.9%	30.6%	33.9%	29.2%

FOBT = Fecal occult blood test.
Data from *Behavioral Risk Factor Surveillance System (BRFSS) Summary*, National Center for Disease Pevention and Health Promotion, Centers for Disease Control and Prevention, 2000.[101]

able to make an informed decision. Many patients pay out of pocket for genetic testing to avoid insurance cancellation or loss of employment. Genetic testing and clinical screening usually should not be undertaken until 10–12 years of age.[3]

New ways to identify asymptomatic patients at risk are emerging, and clinical testing of these technologies is ongoing. The Colorectal Alert test uses metabolic abnormalities in mucosal cellular sugars to identify early colon and rectal cancers when they are easily curable. For mass screenings, colonoscopy, although the most effective option, is too expensive when only a small subset of patients will develop the disease. The colorectal alert test provides an inexpensive tool to screen large numbers of asymptomatic individuals and identify those few who require colonoscopy. In clinical studies of 1787 subjects, the test identified 54% of early-stage colon and rectal cancers and 49% of all cancers, and patients with a positive Colorectal Alert test had a 3.5 times greater likelihood of having cancer than those who tested negative.[98]

Theoretically, by analyzing colonic mucosal cells sloughed into the feces during normal cellular wear and tear, mutational changes in the DNA of the colonic cells could identify those patients at risk for advanced adenomatous polyps or malignancy. Dong and colleagues[99] demonstrated that three genetic markers were able to detect the majority of colorectal cancers when analyzed in stool DNA. Traverso and colleagues[100] studied the feasibility of detecting the first mutation in the series, that of the adenomatous polyposis coli (APC) gene, in fecal DNA using the new method. The APC gene is a tumor suppressor gene that, when mutated, begins to lose control over cell division, allowing uncontrolled cell division to occur. The authors found APC mutations in 26 of the 46 patients with colon or rectal cancer (57%) and in none of the control subjects. They concluded that the APC gene mutation could be detected in fecal DNA from patients with early colorectal tumors. A benefit of this test is that it could identify individuals for whom colonoscopy should be used, in addition to those known to be at high risk. This type of a test—if future tests establish its reliability, sensitivity, and specificity—would permit early identification of patients at risk based on DNA mutations and consequent development of adenomas or early cancers, would not require dietary preparation (unlike stool guaiac testing), and would be painless for the patient.

Despite the ability to identify premalignant polyps and early colon cancer lesions and to remove them, fewer than 40% of colon cancers are identified when they are localized and easily curable. Unfortunately, as shown in Tables 49-3, 49-4, and 49-5, few Americans aged 50 years and older received adequate screening in 1992–1997. Patients presenting with advanced disease have lower rates of survival. When queried about the lack of screening for individuals age 50 and older, the following reasons were cited:[101]

- Lack of discussion between the physician and the patient about colorectal cancer screening
- Patient's lack of knowledge about the importance of colorectal cancer screening
- Limitations in health insurance coverage for screening tests

Table 49-4 Stage of Colorectal Cancer at Diagnosis, 1992–1997

	White	African American	All Races
Localized	37%	33%	37%
Regional	38%	36%	38%
Distant	20%	24%	20%
Unstaged	6%	7%	6%

Data from American Cancer Society: *Cancer Facts and Figures — 2002*. Atlanta, American Cancer Society, 2002.[11]

Table 49-5 Relative Five-Year Survival Rates for Colorectal Cancer in the United States, 1992–1997

	White	African American	All Races
Localized	90.6%	82.7%	89.7%
Regional	65.3%	56.2%	64.4%
Distant	8.5%	7.1%	8.3%
Unstaged	35.5%	33.6%	34.9%
All stages	62%	51.5%	61.1%

Data from American Cancer Society: *Cancer Facts and Figures — 2002.* Atlanta, American Cancer Society, 2002.[11]

Data from the Centers for Disease Control and Prevention (CDC) have shown that low utilization of screening correlates to low income levels, limited or absent health insurance coverage, and fewer years of education.[102] In addition, some authors believe that in clinical practice, providers may not complete the work-up for occult bleeding, including colonoscopy or flex sigmoidoscopy with barium enema.[103]

Early Detection Efforts

Symptoms are usually absent in colon and rectal cancer and appear only when large polyps or lesions bleed or cause cramping, abdominal pain, and obstructive symptoms. It is imperative that colon cancer be detected early, so that the lesion can be removed before invasion and metastases. As expected, early detection of colon and rectal cancer improves survival. Table 49-4 shows the stage at which individuals with colon and rectal cancers were diagnosed in the United States during 1992–1997. Only 37% of patients were diagnosed with early-stage disease. Also, it appears that more African Americans were diagnosed with later-stage disease as compared to white Americans.[101]

Table 49-5 shows how inadequate screening and later stage at diagnosis translate into low five-year survival rates for Americans. Five-year survival for all stages is about 60%. At least 90% of people diagnosed with colon cancer could be cured of their disease if currently available screening, prevention, and early detection techniques were used routinely.[101]

Pathophysiology

Cellular Characteristics

In colorectal cancers, a series of mutations occurs in the epithelial cells of the colonic and rectal mucosa. Carcinogens that stimulate these changes include fecal mutagens, meat intake, bile acids, altered vitamin and mineral intake, and fecal pH.[18] These mutations affect the genes of *somatic* cells of the body (but not the reproductive cells), and involve both proto-oncogenes (genes that encourage the cell to go through active division) and suppressor genes (genes that discourage the cell from going into active division, thereby balancing cell division so that cell birth equals cell death). In some individuals, the mutations occur in the *germ-line* (reproductive) proto-oncogenes and some germ-line tumor suppressor genes, which affect all cells that arise from the reproductive cells. This genetic predisposition accounts for only 7%–8% of patients with colon or rectal cancer. Familial colorectal cancer is the only cancer where the sequential mutations leading to malignant transformation are known (see Figure 49-1).[104]

Kinzler and Vogelstein[104] were able to trace the genetic mutations from the time that the initial mutation occurred in the colonic mucosa, to the formation of an adenoma on the mucosal surface, and continuing to an adenocarcinoma during the period of 10–20 years it took for an invasive adenocarcinoma to develop. The intestinal mucosal epithelial cells are constantly bathed by carcinogens, such as fecal mutagens, meat breakdown products, bile acids, altered vitamin

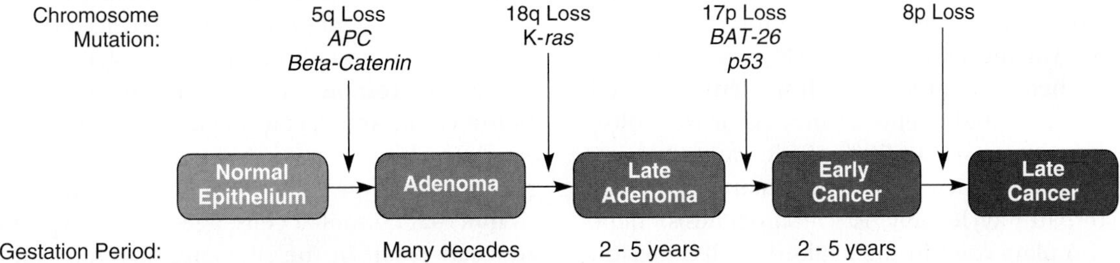

Figure 49-1 Genetic sequence of mutations in malignant transformation of familial colorectal cancer (HNPCC). The initial mutation occurs in the colonic mucosal epithelial cells in gene 5, called the adenomatous polyposis coli (APC), with loss of expression leading to the formation of an adenoma, which then, with additional mutations, leads to malignant transformation. The mutation of *p53* leads to invasive characteristics and metastases. (Reprinted with permission from Kinzler K, Vogelstein B: Lessons from hereditary colorectal cancer. *Cell* 87:159–170, 1996.[104])

and mineral intake, and fecal pH.[18] These cause mutations, but normally the body cells are able to repair themselves using functional DNA repair genes. At some point, a mutation occurs in the APC gene, a tumor suppressor gene. When the mutation in the APC gene is not corrected, the mutation is carried through the cell division cycle, and the DNA mutation passes into each of the two daughter cells. This mutation results in the loss of a portion of the APC gene (5q21, long arm of chromosome 5). Loss of a portion of a chromosome is called loss of heterozygosity (LOH). This initial genetic mutation occurs in somatic cells in 80% of the sporadic cancers, and is the inherited (germ-line) mutation in individuals with FAP HNPCC. There are two alleles for this gene. When both are mutated, the gene is inactivated. This removes the tumor suppressor function, so that no force opposes the continual cell division. In addition, the APC gene makes a protein that regulates cell–cell adhesion, cell migration, and possibly apoptosis. Genetic analysis shows that both APC alleles are inactivated in most colon and rectal adenomas, and in all colon and rectal adenocarcinomas.

Another gene that is mutated and often associated with the mutation in the APC gene is beta-catenin, which keeps cells attached to the cytoskeleton. Both mutations in the APC and beta-catenin genes activate the same signaling pathway. In a Japanese study of patients with HNPCC, tumors had either the APC gene or the beta-catenin gene mutated in 65% of tumors.[105] The mutation occurs on the short arm of chromosome 3 (3p21), which is an area often mutated in many cancers. The mutation removes the regulation of the cell adhering to the cytoskeleton, so cells can, over time, grow away from the cytoskeleton and move away, which normally cause them to die (automatically go into programmed cell death, or apoptosis). In malignant cells, this phenomenon allows the cell to become invasive and metastasize. In addition, there appear to be two general morphologically distinct types of colon and rectal cancers, both of which involve the APC mutation: *polypoid,* involving *K-ras* (proto-oncogene) mutations, and *ulcerative,* where beta-catenin plays a much larger role. Chaing and colleagues[106] found that expression of beta-catenin in the cell nucleus occurred in 26.9% of polypoid adenocarcinomas of the colon and rectum, compared to 72% of ulcerative lesions. Today we have a much better understanding of the molecular pathway leading to carcinogenesis: Beta-catenin also plays roles in the cadherin cell adhesion complex and in the essential signaling pathway.[107]

After the mutations in the APC and beta-catenin genes, with continued exposure to carcinogens, an early adenomatous polyp forms. The next mutation involves the loss of 18q (portion of long arm of chromosome 18) and later mutation of the proto-oncogene *K-ras,* forming an oncogene. The *K-ras* oncogene is found in many solid tumors, when it is turned on, the adenoma continues to grow because the mucosal cells tell themselves to keep dividing. The next gene that becomes mutated is a tumor suppressor gene, the deleted-in-colon-cancer (DCC) gene. As there is no opposition to the activated oncogene, cell division continues and results in a late adenoma. The tumor suppressor gene, *p53,* "the brakes of the cell cycle," is then mutated. This mutation removes the final opposing force to uncontrolled cell division, and moves the late adenoma into malignant transformation. An adenocarcinoma is born.

This information has helped to divide colon tumors into two general classes: those with chromosomal instability (CIN) and those with microsatellite instability (MSI). Eighty-five percent of sporadic colon cancers are CIN, and 15% are MSI. Characteristics of CIN include nonrandom chromosome losses (long or short arms of chromosomes 5q, 12p, 18q, 17p in APC, beta-catenin, *K-ras,* and DCC genes). MSI characteristics are related to defects in mismatched repair (MMR) genes; are common in HNPCC; have an increased mutation rate in APC, beta-catenin, and *K-ras* genes due to defects in MMR genes so the cell cannot correct the DNA mistakes; and produce replication errors in transforming growth factor-beta (TGF-β) and BAT-26 gene loci.

Interestingly, patients with MSI tumors have an increased response to chemotherapy. MSI often involves *MLH1* (one of the DNA mismatch repair genes that, when mutated, prevents certain types of DNA repair). In HNPCC, *MLH1* is an inherited mutation; in the sporadic cancers, it is brought about by epigenetic (involving a mutation or change in the chromatin structure in the gene) silencing by *hypermethylation* of the promoter region. Both avenues result in the same MSI phenotype.[108] DNA methylation is a normal process that allows the cell to shut off or silence gene expression, so that the gene no longer is transcribed to make a specific protein that the body no longer needs. For example, during embryogenesis, the embryo cells must differentiate into specific body tissues; once the fetus is formed, the responsible genes are silenced or shut off. As the colon and rectal mucosa ages, methylation of the DNA slowly occurs. Although a small amount of gene methylation is found in normally aging colorectal mucosal epithelial cells, age-related hypermethylation may result in the silencing of tumor suppressor genes, leading to malignant transformation.[109] It is believed that abnormal DNA methylation occurs early in the formation of an adenoma, especially villous adenomas. Unfortunately, DNA methylation by itself in colon and rectal cancers is associated with a worse outcome as compared to methylated tumors showing MSI characteristics.[110]

Inherited colon cancer

Familial adenomatous polyposis. FAP involves a mutation in the APC tumor suppressor gene. Normally, this gene brings about death of the colonic cells once their usefulness is finished. It also helps to keep the protein beta-catenin in check. If the beta-catenin protein is allowed to accumulate in the cell, it stimulates genes that turn on cell division. The *APC* gene is an autosomal dominant gene — that is, this gene on one of the nonsex chromosomes is always expressed or turned on, even if only one copy of the gene or allele is present. The mutation renders the gene inactive. When a person with this mutation has children, the chance of passing the gene to offspring is 50% for each pregnancy. Every cell in the affected person's colonic and rectal mucosa has one normal copy of the gene and one mutated copy of the gene that was inherited (it is a germ-line mutation). A second mutation in the normal allele will inactivate the tumor suppressor function, leading to development of an adenomatous polyp. The more frequently the cells divide, the more likely another mutation will occur, thereby initiating the process of malignant transformation depicted in Figure 49-1. The mutation of the *APC* gene is *highly penetrant:* If a person inherits the gene, the likelihood of developing colon or rectal cancer over the individual's lifetime is 100%. FAP affects about 1 in 8000 individuals, with polyps usually beginning at age 16, with malignant transformation usually occurring between the ages of 30 and 40 years. FAP represents 0.5% of all colon and rectal cancers. The affected individual develops hundreds to thousands of polyps in the colon and rectum. Thus, screening begins at puberty and genetic counseling is important to prevent or detect at an early stage any malignant transformation so that curative resection can occur. Prophylactic total colectomy may be offered, or celecoxib may be indicated for the prevention of polyp formation in individuals with FAP. When celecoxib 400 mg po bid was used to prevent polyps, it was found to reduce the polyp burden (sum of polyp diameters) by 30.7% in subjects with FAP ($p = 0.001$).[24]

Hereditary nonpolyposis colorectal cancer. This hereditary condition is also known as Lynch I syndrome. In contrast to patients with FAP, individuals with HNPCC do not present with multiple polyps. These genetic mutations are also autosomal dominant, but the penetrance is incomplete, so only 80% of individuals with the genetic mutations develop the colon or rectal cancer. HNPCC affects about 1 in 1000 individuals, and 1 in 100 individuals with colon or rectal cancer. This disease accounts for about 7% of all colorectal cancers.[111]

Table 49-6 Revised Bethesda Criteria for Hereditary Nonpolyposis Colorectal Cancer Diagnosis (Only one criteria needs to be met)

- Diagnosed with CRC before the age of 50 years old.
- Synchronous or metachronous colorectal or other HNPCC-related tumors, including stomach, bladder, ureter, renal pelvis, biliary tract, brain (glioblastoma), sebaceous gland adenomas, keratoacanthomas, and carcinoma of the small bowel, regardless of age.
- CRC with high MSI morphology that was diagnosed before the age of 60 years.
- CRC with one or more first-degree relatives with CRC or other HNPCC-related tumors. One of the cancers must have been diagnosed before the age of 50 years, including adenoma, which must have been diagnosed before the age of 40 years.
- CRC with two or more relatives with CRC or other HNPCC-related tumors, regardless of age.

CRC = Colorectal cancer.
HNPCC = Hereditary nonpolyposis colorectal cancer.
MSI = Microsatellite instability.
Data from Umar, Risinger, Hawk, Barrett.[112]

The germ-line genetic mutations (passed on in the reproductive cells of the parent), appear in one of the five DNA mismatch repair genes (proofreading molecules on DNA — *MSH2, MLH1, PMS1, PMS2,* and *MSH6*).[112] The mismatch repair genes ensure that the cell's genes are identical to the parent cells' genes (genomic fidelity). The mismatch repair genes repair base–base mismatches, insertion–deletion loops, and mistakes that occur during DNA replication and recombination, as well as activation of cell-cycle checkpoint function and induction of apoptosis if the DNA mutation cannot be repaired.[113] These cancers tend to be MSI and occur in the right, proximal colon. Originally, the Amsterdam criteria defined the syndrome: At least three family members must have had colorectal cancer, the history must involve at least two generations, and one individual must have been diagnosed before the age of 50 years old. These criteria were replaced in 1997 by the Bethesda criteria. As more became known about the genetic changes, this standard was revised again.[112] The current standard for diagnosis is known as the revised Bethesda criteria (see Table 49-6). There appear to be some racial and ethnic variations in HNPCC, and other countries such as Japan and China have slightly different criteria. In the United States, Lynch and colleagues[111] suggest that when an individual undergoes genetic testing for HNPCC, the primary DNA sequence of the *MSH2* gene should be tested first; if it is positive for a mutation, then the rest of the genes should be tested as the individual most likely has HNPCC.

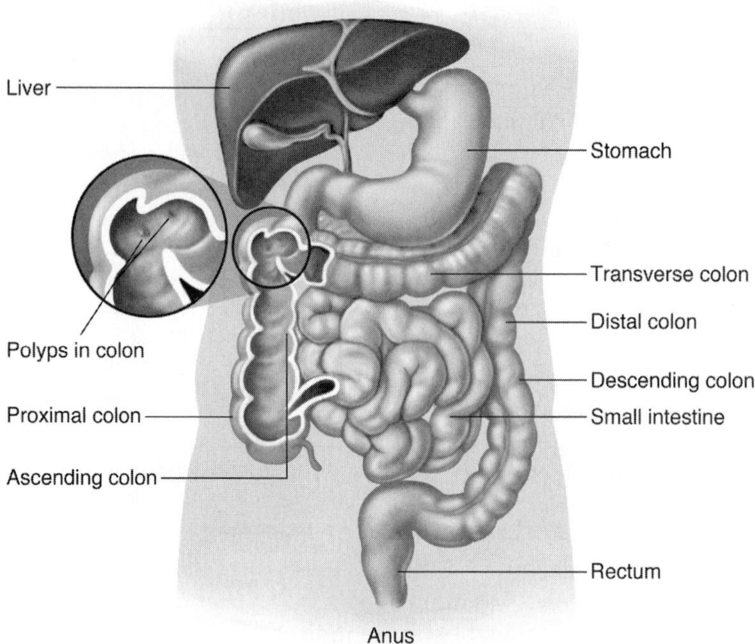

Figure 49-2 Anatomy of the colon.

Lynch II syndrome refers to the development of extracolonic cancers such as ovarian, endometrial, breast, and biliary cancers. A woman with HNPCC has a 60% lifetime risk of developing endometrial cancer.

Progression of Disease and Patterns of Spread

The colon is made up of four layers: the mucosa, the submucosa, the muscularis, and the serosa. The mucosa and submucosa are divided by the muscularis. Reproduction of cells in the colon takes place in the crypts of Lieberkuhn, which are located in the mucosal layer. As new cells are produced, old cells mature, migrate out of the crypt, and are shed. Damage to the crypts will affect reproducing cells and cause the crypts to become prone to errors and to the formation of early adenomas.[114]

The large intestine consists of the cecum, ascending colon, transverse colon, descending colon, sigmoid colon, and rectum, as shown in Figure 49-2. The ascending colon and descending colon are considered extraperitoneal organs because they lie in the anterior pararenal space and are covered by a single layer of the posterior peritoneum. The transverse and sigmoid colon are suspended in the peritoneal cavity by the mesocolon that is formed by two layers of peritoneal linings. The ceum is attached to the ileocolic mesentery in the right iliac fossa. The arterial supply to the cecum, ascending colon, and transverse colon derives from the superior mesenteric artery. The blood supply to the sigmoid colon and descending colon comes from the inferior mesenteric artery. The superior mesenteric vein drains the cecum, ascending colon, and transverse colon. The artery and vein supplying and draining each segment of the colon accompany each other in the mesocolon. The venous system of the colon drains into the portal circulation.

Nodal spread from each segment of the colon follows the blood vessels in the mesocolon.[115] Invasion of the venous system yields a poor prognosis. Once tumor cells invade the vascular system, widespread dissemination of the disease follows; it is not amenable to surgical resection, and chemotherapy and radiation therapy have only limited effects. Local invasion into the neighboring structures is more common in the cecum and rectosigmoid areas. The liver is the most frequent site of metastatic involvement. Solitary pulmonary metastasis is rare. Other areas of metastasis include the brain (cerebellum), bones, kidneys, and adrenals.[114] By the time of diagnosis, approximately 25% of colon cancers will have extended through the bowel wall.[2] Implantation of tumor cells at other sites can occur as a result of surgical manipulation of the tumor, intraluminal spread, or shedding of tumor cells into the peritoneum. Intraperitoneal seeding and carcinomatosis may occur even without lymphatic or visceral spread.

Histology

The most common histological type of colon cancer is adenocarcinoma. The degree of differentiation of the tumor is based on the appearance of well-formed glands, and poorly differentiated tumors do not show well-defined glandular structures.[116] Most adenocarcinomas are moderately well differentiated. If cells are poorly differentiated or high grade, the cancer is more aggressive and often associated with lymphatic or vascular invasion. Many tumors produce mucin, which either stays inside the cells or is secreted. Secreted mucin helps the cells move away into neighboring cells. If more than 50% of the tumor mass is made up of extracellular mucin, it is called a mucinous carcinoma. These are found principally in the sigmoid (descending) colon and rectum, account for 11%–17% of colon and rectal cancers, and often are diagnosed at a more advanced stage of disease.[116] If mucin stays inside the cell in more than 50% of the tumor mass, it is called a signet ring carcinoma. These cancers are rare, accounting for 1%–2% of colon and rectal cancers, but are very aggressive. In one study, more than 93% of patients with signet ring carcinoma presented with stage III or IV disease at diagnosis, and 64% of patients had peritoneal spread.[117] Some distal colon cancers may include areas of squamous cells, so the cancers are called adenosquamous carcinomas.[118] Rarely, there may be small areas of neuroendocrine cells, especially in poorly differentiated tumors. When these are present in larger amounts in non-gland-forming tumors, they are called small cell carcinomas and have a poor prognosis.[116] Lastly, medullary carcinoma is a type of non-gland-forming colon cancer that is characterized by tumor-infiltrating lymphocytes, microsatellite instability, and HNPCC.[116]

Other tumors may involve the colon rarely, such as Kaposi's sarcoma, primary non-Hodgkin's lymphoma (cecum, right colon, or rectum), and carcinoid (cecum or rectum). Sometimes the primary tumor is unclear. Adenocarcinomas of colorectal origin are almost always cytokeratin 20 positive and cytokeratin 7 negative by immunohistochemistry.[119] While molecular diagnosis is still being clinically explored, eventually microarray gene profiling may permit rapid diagnosis and treatment planning.

Previously the most common sites of colon cancers were the sigmoid and descending colon, but the proximal colon is now the site of highest incidence at 54.7%.[13] Evidence indicates that sporadic left colon tumors differ genetically from right-sided or proximal tumors. Olesen and colleagues[120] found 44 different abnormal gene expressions between right- and left-sided colon cancer lesions when genes were analyzed using microarray technology. These differences in gene expression were not based on microsatellite instability. The researchers also found both right- and left-sided cancers share 30 genes that are not present in normal colonic mucosa, which can be used as tumor markers. Therefore, in developing molecular-targeted therapy against colon cancer using gene expression as a guide, separate strategies will be needed for targeting right-versus left-sided colon adenocarcinomas.

Adenocarcinomas of the colon and rectum develop initially in the mucosa. The tumor then locally invades into the lumen of the bowel wall. When it has traversed the muscularis mucosa and infiltrated the serosa, it is termed *invasive.* Further infiltration by way of the lymph and vascular system occurs next, and direct extension may occur into the peritoneal surfaces as well.

Depending on their location in the bowel, colon lesions may exhibit different characteristics. Tumors in the ascending (proximal or right-sided) colon present as cauliflower-like fungating masses that progress to become ulcerative and necrotic. They are usually well differentiated and have a better prognosis. Tumors in the descending and sigmoid colon present as ulcerative tumors that tend to infiltrate the bowel wall and have a poorer prognosis than those in the ascending colon, especially those at or below the peritoneal reflection (rectosigmoid). Distal colon tumors commonly are annular or lesions that encircle the bowel, called "apple-core" or "napkin ring" lesions. Rectosigmoid tumors present as villous, frond-like lesions.

In the United States, an individual's risk of developing colon cancer increases with age, with most cases (90%) being diagnosed in individuals older than 50 years of age.[101] At age 60, about 50% of individuals will have at least one polyp. Initially, polyps form when the intestinal glandular epithelium undergoes mutation. Most polyps are adenomatous polyps or adenomas. In fact, about 75% of all polyps are adenomas. Other types of polyps are always benign: hyperplastic, inflammatory, and hamartomatous polyps. Adenomatous polyps or adenomas have the ability to become malignant. Two factors influence the likelihood that an adenoma will become malignant: histology and size. Histologically, adenomas can be tubular (shaped like a tube), villous (tiny projections), or tubulo-villous (tubes and fingerlike projections) adenomas. Most adenomas are tubular polyps, which represent 70% of adenomas. Villous adenomas confer the highest risk, and tubular adenomas have the lowest risk of transformation. As the polyp becomes larger, the risk of malignant transformation increases. When a polyp reaches 2 cm or larger, the risk of malignant transformation is 20%. This relationship between size and malignancy underscores the importance or removing polyps when they are small. It mirrors the molecular change occurring as the polyp undergoes another mutation and becomes dysplastic, characterized by abnormal differentiation; in so doing, it moves one step closer to malignant transformation. As shown in Figure 49-1, the time from polyp formation to malignant transformation can be as long as 10 years. At age 50, the incidence of adenomas is 25%; by age 70, the risk increases to 50%.[121] Further, inflammatory conditions near the polyp increase the risk of malignant transformation. Ulcerative colitis (UC) increases the risk of colorectal cancer by 20 times, related to the chronic cycles of mucosal injury, with subsequent regrowth resulting in dysplasia.[122]

Polyps are either pedunculated (stalk-like) or sessile (flat). Sessile polyps are closer to the bowel wall, so as they enlarge, they can more easily invade the bowel mucosa as compared to pedunculated polyps. They are also more difficult to remove. Sometimes they are flat, plaque-like polyps that are difficult to visualize except on colonoscopy, as they may lie slightly below the surface of the bowel mucosa. Figure 49-3 shows a pedunculated polyp.

Polyps are removed at colonoscopy, with the site marked. Superficial adenomatous polyps with malignant transformation are simply removed with close follow-up. If they have deep invasion into the stalk, are high grade [poorly differentiated (grade 3) or undifferentiated (grade 4)], or show lymphatic invasion, or if the surgical margins show residual tumor, then a colectomy with en bloc removal of the regional lymph nodes is performed.[123]

If the polyp is a villous adenoma or villoglandular adenoma with cancer, during colonoscopy the polyp is removed and the site marked. An in situ malignancy

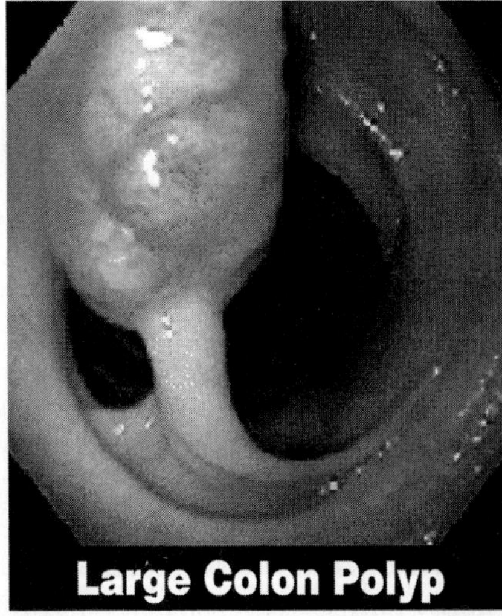

Figure 49-3 Pedunculated polyp. (Image courtesy of Dr. Robert Fusco. http://www.gihealth.com. Reprinted with permission.)

Table 49-7 Clinical Manifestations of Colon Cancer

- Progressive fatigue
- Black tarry stools with or without mucus or bright red blood in the stool
- A feeling of incomplete stooling
- Change in bowel habits, such as constipation, diarrhea, or one alternating with the other
- Change in size of the size or shape of the stool, such as pencil or ribbon-like
- Cramping, pain, or discomfort in the stomach or abdomen
- Abdominal distention or bloating
- Jaundice

with negative margins is removed, and the patient closely followed. If the tumor specimen is fragmented, is high grade, or has penetrated to the submucosa or deeper, or if the margins are involved with tumor, then a colectomy with en bloc removal of the regional lymph nodes is performed.[123]

An adenomatus polyp smaller than 1 cm can transform into an invasive cancer over a ten-year period.[1,4] Patients with a history of colorectal cancer are at increased risk of developing a second primary colon cancer or other malignancy, especially at the site where an anastomotic connection was made by the previous surgery. Patients with UC are also at increased risk of developing colorectal cancer, depending on the extent of colitis, the development of mucosal dysplasia, and the duration of symptoms. Colorectal cancer risk is also higher than normal in patients with Crohn's disease, an inflammatory disease usually involving all layers of the intestinal mucosa. Although the risk is less, persons with Crohn's disease can develop adenocarcinoma at a younger age.

Clinical Manifestations

General signs and symptoms of colon cancer are listed in Table 49-7. Clinical manifestations of tumors in the colon vary depending on location.

Tumors in the *cecum and ascending or right colon* occur in 54% of patients, and may be large and bulky if not detected early. As ingested food that has been digested moves down the gastrointestinal tract, liquid or semi-liquid material enters the ascending colon. Thus, there is no change in bowel habits as a presenting sign. However, there can be intermittent or chronic bleeding, which, over time, leads to iron-deficiency anemia. Symptoms generally include those of anemia (fatigue, weakness, shortness of breath, and exercise intolerance), melena, anorexia, and vague, dull pain or aching. Signs include a palpable mass in the right lower quadrant on physical exam and weight loss. There is an increasing incidence of proximal or right-sided colon cancers, especially in the cecum.

The *transverse colon* is the site of water absorption, where the fecal material begins to become formed and firm. About 10% of colon cancers appear here. Signs and symptoms of a malignant lesion in the transverse colon include a change in bowel habits, gas, abdominal cramping, partial or complete obstruction, possible perforation of the bowel, and blood in the stool. Signs and symptoms of anemia may also occur.

About 36% of colon cancers are found in the *descending and sigmoid colon*. Here, a lesion may partially occlude the lumen, causing a change in bowel habits as well as a change in caliber of the stool, so the stool may be pencil-like or ribbon-like and narrow. Partial obstruction of the bowel lumen can cause constipation alternating with diarrhea, abdominal pain, cramps, flatulence, bright red blood on stooling, a feeling of incomplete stooling, and obstructive symptoms such as nausea and vomiting; melena may occur, as may bowel perforation. In 3%–5% of patients, synchronous lesions will appear in two different places in the colon, and the clinical manifestions will reflect the locations of both tumors.

Early in the course of malignancy, the individual may be asymptomatic. Early signs and symptoms may include vague abdominal pain, flatulence, and minor changes in bowel movements with or without (rectal) bleeding. This is in contrast to signs and symptoms of late cancer, which include severe pain, anorexia and weight loss, sacral or sciatic pain, jaundice, pruritus, ascites, hepatomegaly, and renal impairment.[2,124] Carcinoma of the colon or rectum during pregnancy is rare, but has been noted. Early diagnosis is difficult because symptoms can be related to pregnancy.[125]

Assessment

Patient and Family History

Assessment includes a thorough history, focusing on the symptoms bringing the patient in for an evaluation, as well as a full review of systems and family history, and physical exam. Specifically, the history should include a symptom analysis focusing on presenting signs and symptoms: recent weight loss or gain; changes in appetite; changes in the size, shape, caliber, or color of stools; difficulty passing stool; nausea and/or vomiting; blood in the stools; abdominal pain; bloating; fatigue; palpitations; skin color changes; and unusual itching. Social history should include lifestyle factors such as smoking and alcohol intake, occupational history, diet, exposure to chemicals or radiation, and prior medical and surgical procedures. Medical history should include history of inflammatory bowel disease such as ulcerative colitis or Crohn's disease, adenoma or cancer in the colon, any other malignancy such as those associated with HNPCC (colon or rectum, uterus, ovary, ureter, bladder), and hemorrhoids. The family history should be as complete as possible, including first-degree relatives for two generation and the age at onset of cancer in each family member who has had colon or rectal cancer. The review of systems will elicit symptoms or changes in function outside the gastrointestinal system and help to give a full picture of the extent of disease. For example, the neurological exam would identify changes in mobility, balance, and cognition, suggesting brain metastases.

Physical Examination

Sweed and Meropol[126] note key features of the physical examination: abdomen, breasts, rectum, and lymph nodes to identify any abnormalities that reflect the status of primary or metastatic colon cancer. Initially, general features are assessed, such as temperature and vital signs, weight for size, and functional and mental ability, as well as overall nutritional status of facial muscles (wasting of the temporal or masseter muscles), which may signify advanced disease.

Auscultation of the abdomen reveals bowel status: high-pitched bowel sounds reflect hypermotility and possible partial bowel obstruction, while faint-pitched or absent bowel sounds suggest complete bowel obstruction. Observe the abdomen for distention and any abnormalities. A Sister Mary Joseph nodule at the umbilicus suggests metastatic disease (Figure 49-4).

Palpation is useful in identifying masses, especially of right-sided or proximal lesions; areas of tenderness; ascites; and rebound tenderness that may signal bowel perforation. Bowel perforation may be acute or chronic. Acute perforation is accompanied by pain, fever, and a palpable mass, and the differential diagnosis will include appendicitis or diverticulitis depending on the patient's history. In chronic perforation, acute signs are absent and fistulae may form, with resulting signs and symptoms. If a sigmoid cancer develops a fistula into the bladder, the patient will develop symptoms of chronic urinary tract infection and hematuria. Percussing and palpating the right upper quadrant will give information about possible liver metastases, the most common metastatic site of colon cancer. Approximately 10%–15% of patients will have liver metastases at presentation. To augument assessment of liver metastases, assess the eye sclera for icterus, which preceeds jaundice related to biliary obstruction.

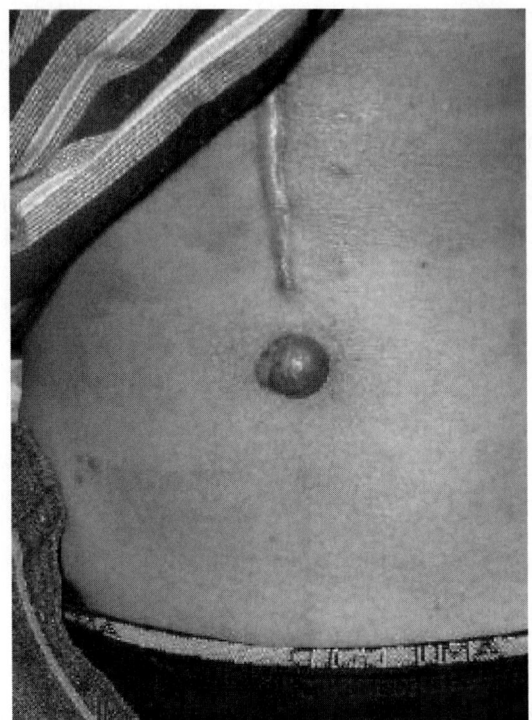

Figure 49-4 Sister Mary Joseph nodule. This firm, red, nontender nodule at the umbilicus was named after Sister Mary Joseph, Head Nurse for Dr. William Mayo, who first associated the nodule with advanced malignant disease. The nodule is the result of metastases from the falciform ligament, most commonly from adenocarcinomas of the ovary, stomach, colon, and pancreas. (Reprinted with permission. Courtesy of *http://www.surgical-tutor.org.*)

Systematically assess the lymph nodes. If a female patient has pelvic pain, a pelvic exam should be done to identify metastases to the ovary or cul-de-sac. The neurologic exam gives information about possible brain metastases or metastases to the spinal cord with spinal cord compression. Rarely, patients may present with paraneoplastic symptoms, such as superficial or deep-vein thrombosis related to hypercoagulability. Patients with advanced disease are most likely to have a history of right upper quadrant pain, abdominal distention, early satiety, and, on exam, supraclavicular or umbilical/periumbilical nodules. The physical exam elucidates and confirms suspicions aroused in the detailed review of systems.

Diagnostic Studies

Initial tests attempt to determine whether colon cancer is the most likely of the differential diagnoses. A definitive biopsy confirms the diagnosis, often done via colonoscopy. Complete blood count, electrolytes, renal and liver function studies, and coagulation assays are done. A baseline carcinoembryonic antigen (CEA) level is drawn once a diagnosis of colon cancer is made. Computerized tomography (CT) scans of the chest, abdomen, and pelvis are performed to evaluate metastases in the lungs, liver, and extracolonic tissue. A chest x-ray may be done instead of CT for patients undergoing colon resection.[127] Magnetic resonance imaging (MRI) is used to further explore questionable areas found on CT or to evaluate recurrence. Positron emission tomography (PET) scans provide whole-body evaluation and highlight active tumors within the body. Malignant tumors have an increased rate of glycolysis, shown by an increased uptake of a glucose analog tracer, which is then trapped in the tumor cells. PET scan is not the standard diagnostic test at this time for initial diagnosis and staging, but is commonly performed for determination of resectable metastases in the liver and lung.[127] A bone scan should be done to identify bony metastases, as their presence will affect the treatment plan. If the patient is young and has a profile suggestive of FAP or HNPCC, genetic testing should be offered. If positive, then genetic counseling should be offered to siblings and children.

Spiral CT scans allow identification of all layers of the tumor's circumference and assist in the prognosis, surgical management, and adjuvant therapy.[128] Virtual colonoscopy is a new technology that permits a noninvasive evaluation through use of spiral CT volume imaging with virtual-reality computer technology. It is not as sensitive as colonoscopy, however, and if polyps or lesions are found, a colonoscopy still must be performed for biopsy or removal. Potential limitations of colonography include the possibility of a false-positive diagnosis secondary to residual stool,[128] and the fact that the patient requires the same bowel clean-out as with regular colonoscopy. CT portography enables clinicians to detect small focal hepatic metastases 1–2 cm in diameter that cannot be appreciated on a conventional CT scan with contrast. It works on the principle that hepatic metastases derive their blood supply from the hepatic artery whereas normal hepatocytes are supplied predominantly by the portal circulation.[129] During CT portography, contrast medium is infused through an angiography catheter introduced into the superior mesenteric or splenic artery. Seconds after injection of the contrast, dynamic-sequence CT scanning of the liver begins. As the dye passes into the portal vein, the normal hepatic parenchyma infused by the portal blood circulation is enhanced with contrast; the hepatic metastases, which receive no blood via the portal route, are visualized as dark spots that indicate solid lesions.[130]

In addition to the previously mentioned diagnostic tests, patients with recurrent or metastatic disease may have other tests to evaluate the extent of disease. Immunoscintigraphy has been shown to exhibit a high positivity rate in cases of local recurrence and can detect metastases simultaneously at multiple sites. Two types of immunoscintigraphy are available: satumomab pendetide and the CEA scan. The former is used to determine the extent of extrahepatic malignant disease and to detect pelvic tumors as well as extrahepatic abdominal metastasis. In patients with occult cancer, combining the CEA scan with conventional imaging techniques significantly increases diagnostic accuracy.[2] MRI may also be done for patients who are unable to tolerate the CT scan or who are allergic to the contrast material. Fine-needle aspiration, with or without other diagnostic tests, is generally indicated to confirm the recurrence of disease.

Prognostic Indicators

Stage of disease at presentation is the most important prognostic factor in colon cancer. Patients who are symptomatic at diagnosis have a worse prognosis.[131] The prognosis is dependent on depth of invasion or penetration through the wall of the colon, involvement of local and regional lymph nodes, and presence of disease in distant sites. Another factor that affects prognosis is whether the lesion causes obstruction or perforation in patients with stage II and III colon cancers. Many years ago, the National Surgical Adjuvant Breast and Bowel Project (NSABP) showed that disease-free survival was negatively associated with obstruction and bowel perforation in Duke's B2 and C, or stage II and III, colon cancer.[132] Rectal bleeding had a positive impact on survival. Location of tumor — either right, left, or rectosigmoid — did not correlate with survival or disease-free survival. This study was replicated by Steinberg and colleagues[133] as part of the Gastrointestinal Tumor Study Group, with similar findings. Other, more recent studies have found a difference in survival related to right or left colon cancer location. Halvorsen and Johannesen[134] found that for each stage of disease, those patients with lesions located at or below the peritoneal reflection (rectosigmoid and rectum) had a shorter survival compared to patients with a more proximal lesion. Another prognostic factors is pretreatment level of CEA, where a high CEA level confers a poor prognosis.[135]

Following the development of microarray technology and further elucidation of the sequence of genetic mutations in colon cancer, many molecular markers have been identified as prognostic indicators. Microsatellite instability (MSI) is associated with improved survival, as well as the presence of tumor-infiltrating lymphocytes.[136] It means there are a high number of mistakes in DNA replication and instability of 30 or more microsatellite loci that result in expansion or contraction of short, repeated DNA sequences caused by insertion or deletion of repeated units.[116] Even though tumors with MSI are often poorly differentiated, patients are more likely to respond to chemotherapy and have longer survival.

Loss of heterozygosity (LOH) confers a poor prognosis. It refers to the loss of an allele or copy of chromosome 18q, which, when lost, is involved in tumorigenesis. The DDC gene is located on this arm of this chromosome. When this tumor suppressor gene is mutated, it takes the brakes off uncontrolled cell division. In one study, patients with stage II colon cancer who had LOH 18q had the same risk as patients with stage III disease.[137]

Other interesting factors that have not been adequately studied to date include DNA content (aneuploidy or abnormal DNA content in cells is associated with a poor prognosis); molecular markers such as LOH in tumor suppressor genes; the oncogenes *K-ras, c-myc; bcl-2,* and *BAX*; DNA synthesis–related genes; growth factors and growth factor receptor genes; cell-cycle regulator genes *p27* and *p21*; and angiogenesis-related genes for vascular endothelial growth factor (VEGF), among others.[116]

As mentioned earlier, although racial differences in overall survival are reported in ACS statistics, there has been equivalent survival after adjuvant therapy when patients were compared stage for stage. Thus it appears that other factors, such as co-morbid conditions, need to be explored.[138]

Classification and Staging

The prognosis for persons with colon cancer is directly related to the stage of the disease at the time of diagnosis. Stage is determined by the depth of penetration (invasion) of the tumor into and through the intestinal wall, the number of regional lymph nodes involved, and the presence or absence of distant metastases.

There are three staging systems available, but most clinicians use the American Joint Committee on Cancer (AJCC) staging system. Colon cancer stage is determined by the T (tumor depth of invasion), N (lymph node involvement), and M (metastastic spread to distant organs) system (Table 49-8).[139] Lymph nodes are extensive over the large bowel and are the first barrier that malignant cells traverse after leaving the colon. The more lymph nodes removed at colon cancer surgery, the more accurate the nodal staging, and the more appropriate the treatment plan. The portal venous system brings embolized colon malignant cells to the liver, and cells can be disseminated by tumors that penetrate through the full thickness of the bowel

Table 49-8 TNM Staging of Colon Cancer, and Comparison to Duke's and Astler-Coller Staging Groups

Stage	T	N	M	Duke's	Modified Astler-Coller
0	Tis	N0	M0	—	—
I	T1	N0	M0	A	A
	T2	N0	M0	A	B1
IIA	T3	N0	M0	B	B2
IIB	T4	N0	M0	B	B3
IIIA	T1–T2	N1	M0	C	C1
IIIB	T3–T4	N1	M0	C	C2/C3
IIIC	Any T	N2	M0	C	C1/C2/C3
IV	Any T	Any N	M1	—	D

T0: No evidence of primary tumor
Tis: Carcinoma in situ: intraepithelial or invasion of lamina propria
T1: Tumor invades submucosa
T2: Tumor invades muscularis propria
T3: Tumor invades through the muscularis propria into the subserosa, or into nonperitonealized pericolic or perirectal tissues; V and L substaging are used to identify the presence or absence of vascular or lymphatic invasion
T4: Tumor directly invades other organs or structures, and/or perforates visceral peritoneum; V and L substaging are used to identify presence or absence of vascular or lymphatic invasion
N1: Metastases in 1–3 regional lymph nodes
N2: Metastases in 4 or more regional lymph nodes
M1: Distant metastases
Histologic Grade
G1: Well differentiated
G2: Moderately differentiated
G3: Poorly differentiated
G4: Undifferentiated

Data from Greene FL, Page DS, Fleming ID, et al, American Joint Committee on Cancer: *AJCC Cancer Staging Manual*, (ed 6). New York, Springer-Verlag, 2002.[139]

wall and onto the periotoneal surface. The recognition of this phenomenon has led to improved staging classification of T3 and T4 tumors (stage II) as well as subdivisions in stage III, as there are significant differences in survival based on the stratification: The five-year survival rate for stage IIIA is 59.8%, IIIB is 42%, and IIIC is 27.3%.[139]

The sixth edition of the *AJCC Cancer Staging Manual* contains a number of additions:[139]

1. Smooth metastatic nodules in the pericolic fat are considered lymph node metatastases (N).
2. Irregularly shaped metastatic nodules in the peritumoral fat are considered vascular invasion.
3. Stage II is subdivided into IIA (T3 lesions) and IIB (T4 lesions).
4. Stage III is subdivided into IIIA (T1–2, N1, M0), IIIB (T3–4, N1, M0), and IIIC (any T, N2, M0).
5. The surgeon should mark the specimen where the tumor penetration is the deepest so the radial margin can be evaluated, and also should indicate whether the tumor was completely resected with negative margins (R0), incompletely resected with microscopic margins (R1), or incompletely resected with gross residual tumor (R2).

Following surgical resection of colorectal tumors, pathologic stage is the single most important prognostic factor. The prognosis for stage I and II disease is more favorable, whereas stage III and IV disease have a poorer prognosis. In the TNM classification, each of the three subsets of tumor, nodal, and metastatic categories does not make any assumptions about the status in another part of the system. Two areas in staging are of particular concern: (1) lymph node sampling to determine accurate staging must be adequate, and (2) T4 tumors (stage IIB) have biologic characteristics that allow them to invade through the bowel wall and into contiguous tissues.

In past practice, the number of lymph nodes sampled during standard colectomy for colon cancer varied, with the average being 8 lymph nodes. Esser and colleagues[140] estimated that to correctly classify lymph node status with 95% confidence, the surgeon needed to sample 20 lymph nodes for T1 lesions, 17 nodes for T2 lesions, and 15 nodes for T3 lesions. They found that patients with stage I disease who had fewer than

10 lymph nodes sampled had shorter survival than patients who had 10 or more lymph nodes evaluated ($p < 0.01$). Thus, a number of patients have been incorrectly staged because insufficient lymph nodes were sampled, and the patient's stage was therefore underestimated. Le Voyer and colleagues[141] performed a secondary analysis and found that survival decreased with increasing numbers of lymph nodes involved with tumor, and survival increased as more lymph nodes were analyzed. Other studies have shown that often patients with stage II colon cancer are understaged, with too few lymph nodes being removed at the time of definitive surgery. Swanson and colleagues[142] found that patients with T3 lesions (penetration through the bowel wall but not invading lymph nodes or contiguous organs) who had only 1–2 lymph nodes removed and examined had a 64% five-year survival rate, as compared to an 86% survival rate if more than 25 lymph nodes were examined. The stratification distinctions that influenced five-year survival are 1–7, 8–12, and 13 or more nodes. Thus, the current standard is that a minimum of 13 lymph nodes should be examined to identify a T3 colon cancer lesion as node negative.

Lennon and colleagues[143] studied patients with stage II disease after excluding those with perforation or tumor involving adjacent organs at the time of surgery. They found that the peritoneal space contained tumor cells in 13.6% of patients and that these patients had high rates of lymphovascular invasion and neural invasion (69% and 44%, respectively). Of this group of patients, 60% died of recurrent disease within three years of initial surgery. The AJCC's Prognostic Factors Group has recommended that T4 lesions be subgrouped into T4a (tumor invading adjacent structures or organs) and T4b (tumor involves the visceral peritoneum).[144] It is well recognized that patients with stage II colon cancer who have obstruction, perforation, or ulceration have a poorer prognosis than patients without these complications. For this reason, patients, with obstruction, perforation, or ulceration are encouraged to consider adjuvant chemotherapy or entry into a clinical trial.

Therapeutic Approaches and Nursing Care

Surgery

The National Comprehensive Cancer Network (NCCN) has developed practice guidelines for the management of advanced adenomas and colon cancer.[127] Surgery is the primary treatment for colon cancer. The goal of surgery is to eliminate disease in the colon, nodal basins, and contiguous organs. The tumor location, blood supply, and lymph node pattern in the involved region will define the extent of surgical resection.

The procedure of choice for resectable colon cancer is a colectomy with en bloc removal of regional lymph nodes.[127] Laparoscopic colectomy has been studied, and in Europe, a small study showed a survival advantage.[127,145] At this time, laparoscopic colectomy is not recommended since studies to date have shown increased cost and similar recovery time, but outcome data are still maturing.[127] The various surgical options as well as their indications and major morbidities are briefly discussed below and illustrated in Figure 49-5.

Right hemicolectomy involves removal of the distal 5–8 cm of the ileum, right ascending colon, hepatic flexure, and transverse colon proximal to the middle colic artery. This procedure is indicated for cecal, ascending colon, and hepatic flexure lesions. Major morbidities include ureteral injury, duodenal injury, and bile acid deficiency. Bile acid deficiency is rarely seen and only with extensive resection of the terminal ileum.

Right radical hemicolectomy involves the removal of the transverse colon (including resection of the middle colic artery at its origin) in addition to structures removed in the right hemicolectomy. Indications for this procedure are lesions of the hepatic flexure or transverse colon. In addition to the complications associated with right hemicolectomy, morbidities include anastomotic dehiscence and diarrhea.

Transverse colectomy is the segmental resection of the transverse colon. This procedure is indicated for mid-transverse colon lesions. The major morbidity is anastomotic dehiscence. This procedure is rarely performed because of the difficulty of achieving a tension-free anastomosis with adequate blood supply, as the marginal artery of Drummond is sacrificed. Surgeons prefer to perform an extended right radical hemicolectomy with an ileosigmoid anastomosis.

Left hemicolectomy includes the removal of the transverse colon distal to the right branch of the middle colic artery and the descending colon up to, but not including, the rectum, plus division and ligation of the inferior mesenteric artery (IMA). Indications for this procedure are left colon lesions. Anastomotic dehiscence is the major morbidity.

Low anterior resection involves the removal of the descending colon distal to the splenic flexure, sigmoid colon, upper two-thirds of the rectum, and ligation of IMA and inferior mesenteric vein either at the origin or just distal to the origin of the left colic artery. This procedure is indicated for lesions of the sigmoid colon and proximal rectum. Morbidities include anastomotic dehiscence and bowel ischemia secondary to inadequate flow through the marginal artery of Drummond.

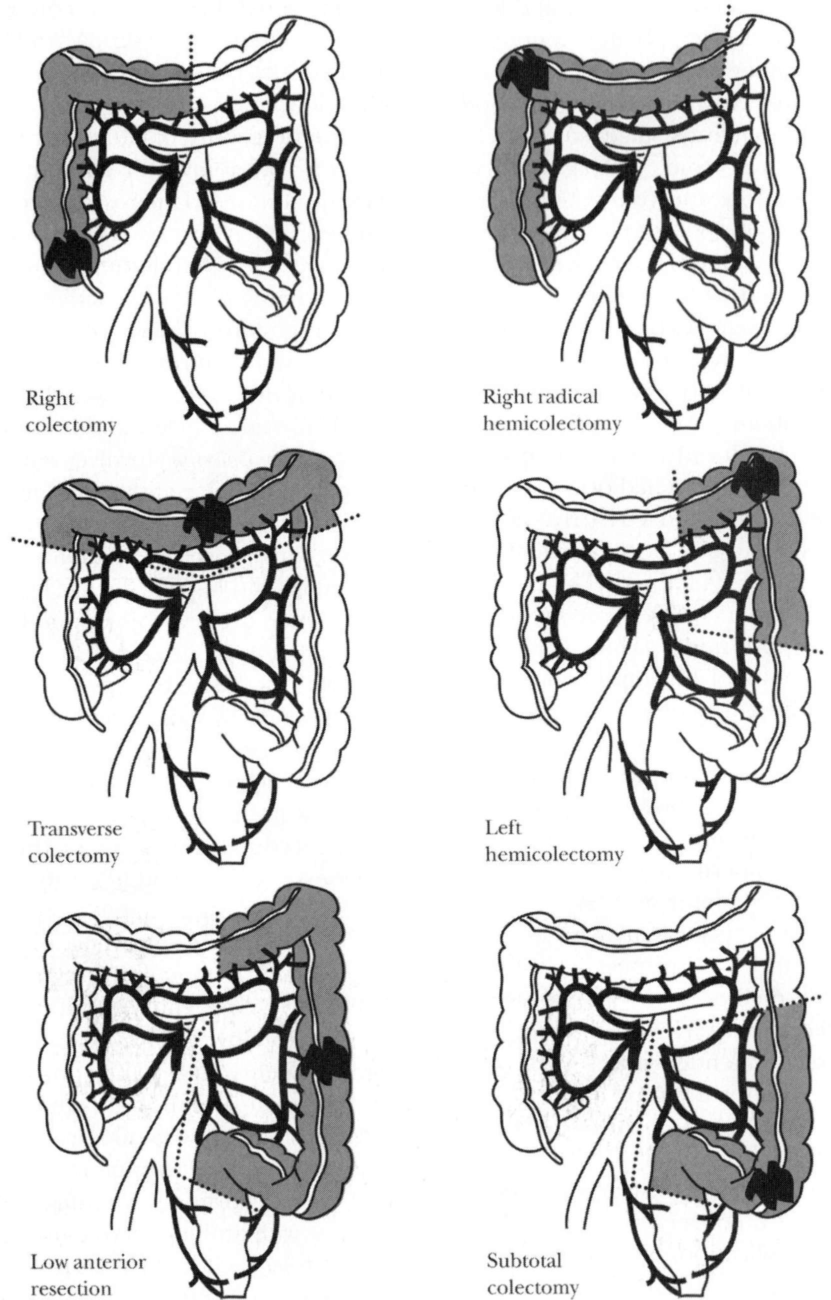

Figure 49-5 The procedure selected relates to the location and extent of the tumor.

Subtotal colectomy is the removal of the right, transverse, descending, and sigmoid colon with ileorectal anastomosis. This procedure is indicated for multiple synchronous colon tumors and distal transverse colon lesions particularly in a patient with a clotted IMA. Morbidities include diarrhea, perineal excoriation, and anastomotic dehiscence.[146]

The role of sentinel lymph node (SLN) mapping and biopsy in staging remains under investigation. Sentinel lymph node mapping follows the template established for melanoma and breast cancer. Sentinel lymph nodes that are the first lymph nodes to be reached by malignant cells are identified by dye or labeling, and then biopsied to see if they contain tumor. If tumor is found, then it is likely more lymph nodes are involved. If the biopsy is negative, then it is likely that none of the remaining lymph nodes are involved. Dye is injected around the tumor, and the sentinel lymph nodes are identified by their uptake of the dye. Esser and colleagues reported on their use of SLN mapping and found at least one sentinel lymph node in 58% of patients, sensitivity of 67%, specificity and positive predictive values of 100%, and a negative predictive value of 94% in those patients in whom a sentinel lymph node was found.[140] Saha and colleagues[147] described their multi-institutional study of 203 patients and found that SLN mapping (1–4 lymph nodes) was 98% successful. In this study, 14% of patients had micrometastases and were upstaged from stage I/II to stage III. Skipped metastases were found in 0.03% of patients. The authors concluded that SLN was simple and cost-effective.

SLN mapping has brought benefits of improving the accuracy of lymph node evaluation in lymph node–negative patients, as approximately one-third of patients with lymph node–negative cancer develop recurrent disease. Bilchik and colleagues[148] studied lymphatic mapping followed by focused analysis of sentinel nodes using molecular profiling. They found that 8 of 31 patients with lymph node–negative disease had micrometastases using molecular profiling, and were upstaged to stage III. This change in stage has important implications, as these patients would otherwise not have received adjuvant chemotherapy.

Feig and colleagues[149] at M. D. Anderson Cancer Center cautioned surgeons about the value of SLN mapping in colon and rectal cancer. They reported that they were successful in finding sentinel lymph nodes in 98% of patients. They found a false-negative rate of 38%, however, and recommended large prospective studies to evaluate the accuracy and potential of SLN mapping in colon cancer.

Liver metastases

An estimated 20% of patients will present with liver metastases, another 20%–30% will develop liver metastases as a site of recurrence following primary treatment, and as many as 70% of patients who are not cured will ultimately develop liver metastases. For some patients, however, resection of isolated metastases can result in cure. The usual criteria for resection of liver metastases are surgically accessible lesion(s), small (1–2 cm in diameter), three or fewer lesions, and no other distant disease.[150] Fong and colleagues found that seven factors were significant and independent predictors of poor long-term outcome: positive surgical margins, extrahepatic disease, node-positive primary tumor, disease-free interval from primary tumor to metastases less than 12 months, more than one hepatic tumor, largest hepatic tumor more than 5 cm, and CEA level greater than 200 ng/mL.[151] The authors recommended that if a patient has two or fewer of the factors, there is a favorable outcome; however, if the patient has three or more factors, the individual should consider experimental adjuvant trials following resection. Of patients who undergo hepatic resection, 25%–40% are alive at five years.[151]

The NCCN recommends adjuvant chemotherapy following potentially curable hepatic resection.[127] The liver and any liver metastatic lesions receive their blood supply from the hepatic artery; hepatic artery infusional (HAI) chemotherapy via an implanted infusion pump has offered promise for many years.[152] Kemeny and colleagues[153] compared hepatic artery floxuridine plus systemic 5-fluorouracil (5-FU) chemotherapy with systemic 5-FU chemotherapy alone in patients who had undergone hepatic resection. They found improved two-year disease-free and overall survival for 86% of patients in the combination arm compared to 72% in the 5-FU monotherapy arm ($p = 0.03$). No difference in median survival was observed. A meta-analysis conducted by the Meta-Analysis Group in Cancer demonstrated that floxuridine HAI has a significantly increased response rate compared to systemic therapy, but there is significant improvement in survival.[154] Kemeny and colleagues[155] presented Cancer and Leukemia Group B (CALGB) data showing superior response (48% versus 25%, $p = 0.009$) and survival (22.7 months versus 19.8 months, $p = 0.027$) of patients with liver-only metastases from colon and rectal cancer receiving HAI fluoxouridine, leucovorin, and dexamethasone as compared to patients receiving 5-FU and leucovorin (5-day Mayo regimen). Median time to progression was not significantly different. Quality of life as measured by physical functioning was similar at 9 months, but poorer at 12 months in the group receiving systemic chemotherapy. Of interest, the patients who did best had lower gene expression of thymidylate synthase and p21 (cyclin-dependent kinase inhibitor). Finally, in the cost-benefit analysis, the lifetime cost for HAI was $157,800 compared to $97,600 for systemic therapy; some of the greater cost for HAI was related to longer survival.

Radiofrequency ablation is an option for patients who are not eligible for resection of liver metastases. It uses ultrasound guidance to deliver high temperatures to the hepatic tumor and provides long-term control for some patients. Another treatment technique is chemo-embolization, in which drug is directly injected into the tumor, and then the vessel is embolized to keep the drug in that specific location. Cryotherapy is also used to freeze the hepatic lesions, thereby killing the tumor cells. Both radiofrequency and cryotherapy ablation techniques are being studied with combination intrahepatic artery and systemic chemotherapy. These techniques are not options in patients with widespread liver metastases or other systemic disease.

Peritoneal metastases

Peritoneal carcinomatosis may occur in patients with colon cancer. Studies have defined the lymphatic and portal dissemination of malignant cells, where the cells may or may not successfully become implanted and begin to divide and establish a blood supply of their own as a metastatic site (metastatic inefficiency).[156,157] In contrast, colon cancer cells that are disseminated into the peritoneum metastasize efficiently and are able to implant successfully. Unfortunately, positive peritoneal washings in such cases confer a uniformly dismal prognosis. Malignant cells reach the peritoneum through invasion through the bowel wall (T3 and T4 lesions) as well as a possible iatrogenic introduction via surgery itself. If tumor contaminates the surgical site, the healing process, including angiogenesis, enhances tumor growth and metastatic efficiency.[157] The recommended treatment options are limited colon resection for nonobstructing abdominal/peritoneal metastases, or for impending obstruction, limited resection, diverting colostomy, or bypass of the impending obstruction followed by salvage chemotherapy are treatment options.[127]

In an effort to minimize the growth of metastatic cells in the peritoneum, new combination techniques using peritonectomy plus intraperitoneal chemotherapy are being studied. All visible tumor is removed at surgery, and heated intraoperative intraperitoneal chemotherapy is used to kill the remaining tumor cells. The heated intraperitoneal chemotherapy may be repeated if well tolerated during the first five postoperative days.[157] Chemotherapy drugs used are fluorouracil, mitomycin C, doxorubicin, cisplain, paclitaxel, gemcitabine, and oxaliplatin.

Pulmonary metastases

While endobronchial metastases are rare, colorectal carcinoma is one of the most common primary tumors with pulmonary metastases.[158] Colorectal tumors that metastasize to the lungs may present as solitary masses or multiple nodules. Individuals who experience pulmonary metastases from a colorectal primary tumor may present with symptoms of dyspnea, but it has been estimated that 85% of such patients are asymptomatic for pulmonary problems.[158] Most colorectal metastases to the lungs are detected by routine chest x-ray. More definitive evaluation can be accomplished by a CT scan of the chest, which further defines the number and location of the lesions.

Pulmonary resection of the metastatic area provides the best long-term survival. Pulmonary wedge resection is undertaken if the lesion is isolated. Individuals with four or fewer metastatic pulmonary lesions have a better prognosis than individuals with four or more lesions.[159] Individuals with metastatic lung involvement from colon cancer have been found to have a 31% five-year survival rate after surgical resection of the metastatic lesion.[160]

Table 49-9 Potential Complications of Colorectal Surgery

Complication	Signs and Symptoms
Anastomotic leak	Abdominal pain, post-operative fever, ileus, elevated white count
Intra-abdominal abcess	Persistent, recurring post-operative fever; elevated white count
Bowel obstruction	Abdominal distention and pain, constipation, nausea/vomiting, high pitched (partial) to absent (complete) bowel sounds
Alterations in bowel elimination pattern	Irregular bowel elimination, constipation; diarrhea, fecal incontinence (uncommon); temporary or permanent stoma
Alteration in urinary elimination	Urgency; bladder dysfunction, with injury to bladder or ureters, urine can leak through incision; oliguria
Sexual dysfunction	Impotence, difficulty with ejaculation; short-or long-term problems depend upon nerve preservation
Stoma dysfunction	Skin breakdown, stomal prolapse, hernia, infection of peristomal skin, bleeding

Complications of colorectal surgery

Some of the options for colon and rectal surgery are listed in Table 49-9. The primary surgical procedure may produce both anatomical and functional alterations. If the patient requires a diverting colostomy, he or she will require preoperative teaching and a visit by the Certified Wound, Ostomy, Continence Nurse (CWOCN; also known as an enterostomal therapist or ET nurse), as well as postoperative teaching and follow-up. Emotional as well as physical self-care strategies will need to be supported so the patient will be able to function as independently as possible.

Radiation Therapy

Radiation poses significant toxicity potential to the cells of the gut due to the rapid turnover of mucosal cells. However, in some studies postoperative radiation combined with chemotherapy improves survival in patients with bulky, locally advanced disease (T4, N0, M0; T4, N1–2, M0; or T3, N0, M0 disease with perforation, close indeterminate resection margins, or positive resection margins).[161,162] Radiation provides local and regional control, while systemic chemotherapy theoretically attacks metastatic cells that have embolized. Rarely, whole-abdomen radiation is used for patients at risk for abdominal recurrence.[163] Potential side effects of radiation for locoregional control include enteritis, diarrhea (small bowel), nausea and vomiting (stomach, liver), and flank pain (kidneys).[164]

As another option, a clinical trial or observation could be selected as a treatment choice.[127]

Concurrent chemotherapy, usually continuous infusion, during radiation increases the cells' sensitivity to radiation damage, called radiosensitization. 5-fluorouracil is most commonly used.[164–166] The dose-limiting toxicities of continuous 5-FU infusion are mucositis and diarrhea. Palmar-plantar erythrodysesthesia (hand–foot syndrome) has also been noted with protracted infusions of 5-FU.[2] In a study of patients with locally advanced colon cancer, Schild and colleagues[165] found that patients with locally advanced colon cancer had improved local control after external beam radiation and 5-FU chemotherapy. For patients with residual disease at resection, intraoperative electron radiotherapy improved local control and survival.

Chemotherapy

Chemotherapy plays a significant role in the management of colon cancer. While patients with stage I disease are considered cured with surgery alone, one-third of patients with stage II disease will have recurrence following surgery. For this reason, patients with stage II disease with obstruction, perforation, or residual disease are offered adjuvant chemotherapy or entry into a clinical trial. Survival in patients with stage III disease (lymph node involvement) is significantly improved with adjuvant chemotherapy.

For years, the standard adjuvant therapy for stage III colon cancer was 5-FU plus levamisole. In 1988, studies that added leucovorin to 5-FU demonstrated stabilization of the 5-FU–thymidylate–synthase complex, thereby increasing the period of tumor inhibition. While overall survival was not increased with leucovorin and 5-FU therapy, the response rate was increased significantly. Studies comparing dual therapy with 5-FU and levamisole to the combination of 5-FU and leucovorin, demonstrated that 12 months of adjuvant therapy offered no significant improvement over 6 months of such therapy. The MOSAIC study demonstrated the superiority of 5-FU, leucovorin, and oxaliplatin (FOLFOX) compared to 5-FU and leucovorin, the prior standard. The current standard adjuvant therapy is FOLFOX as it demonstrated a superior relapse-free survival at 3 years.[167]

For patients with stage II colon cancer, the answers are not as clear. The five-year survival rate without chemotherapy for stage II colon cancer is 75%–80%. In the future, molecular profiling may determine that subset of patients who will benefit from adjuvant chemotherapy. Table 49-10 describes adjuvant therapy and treatment options for advanced colon and rectal cancers.[168–184]

Within the last decade, significant advances in the management of advanced colon cancer have occurred related to chemotherapy. As is well known, the most effective chemotherapeutic agents in the management of colon cancer are 5-FU and its modulator, leucovorin. Together, they result in a response rate of 20%–25%, with an overall median survival of 11–12 months.[167] In Europe, the de Gramont regimen demonstrated an increased response, but equivalent overall survival with significantly reduced toxicity using infusional 5-FU with bolus leucovorin (LV).[174] Irinotecan (Camptosar) was available as a second-line treatment option in 1996, and then received FDA approval in 2000 as a first-line therapy in combination with bolus or infusional 5-FU/LV (when given as bolus, it is known as IFL, when given with infusional 5-FU, it is known as the Douillard regimen or FOLFIRI). The doses are listed in Table 49-10. Phase III studies demonstrated a favorable effect on survival, quality of life, and amelioration of disease-related symptoms compared to best supportive care. However, the dose of irinotecan often needs to be reduced to prevent severe toxicities, such as fatal diarrhea and sepsis.[182,185]

The cornerstone for future combination studies uses the de Gramont infusional regimen plus either oxaliplatin or irnotecan. The combination of oxaliplatin, 5-FU (continuous infusion), and leucovorin known as FOLFOX 4 was found to be superior to 5-FU and LV, so both IFL and FOLFOX 4 are FDA approved as first-line treatment for advanced colon and rectal cancers. The acronym FOLFOX is derived from FOLinic acid (leucovorin), F (fluorouracil or 5-FU), and OX (oxaliplatin). FOLFOX 4 was shown to increase overall response rate to 45% compared to IFL (31%), and overall survival to 19.5 months compared to IFL (15.0 months).[186] In addition, capecitabine was shown to be equivalent in terms of overall survival to 5-FU and LV, so the drug is FDA approved for this first-line indication as well, when fluoropyrimidines alone are preferred. FOLFOX has a number of iterations, such as FOLFOX 6 and 7. These iterations combine the two 22-hour 5-FU infusions into a single 46-hour infusion, which minimizes patient clinic visits.

Bevacuzimab, a monoclonal antibody against VEGF, prevents the mobilization of endothelial cells and their migration to form new blood vessels for the developing malignancy. Solid tumors cannot grow beyond about 2 mm, the size of a pencil point, without forming new blood vessels to provide nourishment and the removal of waste products. The addition of bevacuzimab to IFL increased the objective response rate in newly diagnosed patients with metastatic colon cancer to 45% (compared to 35% with IFL) and median survival of 20.3 months (compared to 15.6 with IFL).[187] Bevacuzimab (Avastin) is the first antiangiogeneis

Table 49-10 Chemotherapeutic Regimens for Adjuvant Therapy and Treatment of Advanced Colon and Rectal Cancers

Regimen Name	Regimen Dosages	Reference
Adjuvant Therapy		
5-FU/LV Mayo	5-FU 425 mg/m^2 IV days 1–5, LV 20 mg/m^2 IV days 1–5 prior to 5-FU; repeat every 4–5 weeks × 6 cycles	O'Connell MJ, Mailliard JA, Kahn MJ, et al: Controlled clinical trial of fluorouracil and low-dose leucovorin given for 6 months as postoperative adjuvant therapy for colon cancer. *J Clin Oncol* 81:213–215, 1997[168]
Roswell Park (high dose)	5-FU 500 mg/m^2 IV q week × 6 administered midway through LV; LV 500 mg/m^2 IV q week × 6 over 2 hours; repeat week cycle q 8 weeks × 4 cycles	Wolmark N, Rockette H, Fischer B, et al: The benefit of leucovorin-modulated fluorouracil as postoperative adjuvant therapy for primary colon cancer: results from National Surgical Adjuvant Breast and Bowel Project Protocol C-03. *J Clin Oncol* II: 1879–1887, 1993[169]
5-FU/ LV (low dose)	5-FU 500 mg IV q week × 6 weeks; LV 20 mg/m^2 IV q week × 6 weeks given before 5-FU; repeat cycle q 8 weeks × 4–6 cycles	Benson AB, Choti MA, Cohen AM, et al: NCCN practice guidelines for colorectal cancer. *Oncology* 14:203–212, 2000[170]
FOLFOX 4	**Day 1**: oxaliplatin 85 mg/m^2 day IV over 2 hours, through 1 of 2 Y arms, simultaneously with leucovorin 200 mg/m^2 IV over 2 hours of second arm, followed by D5W flush, then 5-FU 400 mg/m^2 IVP, then 600 mg/m^2 infusion over 22 hours **Day 2**: leucovorin 200 mg/m^2 IV over 2 hours, 5-FU 400 mg/m^2 IVP, then 600 mg/m^2 infusion over 22 hours. Cycle repeated q 2 weeks	de Gramont A, Boni C, Navarro C, et al: Oxaliplatin/5-FU/LV in adjuvant colon cancer: results of the international randomized mosaic trial. *Proc Am Soc Clin Oncol* 22:253, 2003 (abstr 1015)[171]
Capecitabine	1250 mg po bid × 14 day, q 21 days, × 6 months	Cassidy J, Scheithauer J, McKendrick H, et al: Capecitabine (X) vs bolus 5-FU/leucovorin (LV) as adjuvant therapy for colon cancer (the X-ACT study): efficacy results of a phase III trial. *J Clin Oncol* 14S(suppl):3509, 2004[172]
Metastatic Treatment		
Capecitabine	1250 mg/m^2 po bid days 1–14 q 21 days (usual dose is 1000 mg/m^2 po bid days 1–14)	Hoff P, Ansari R, Batist G, et al: Comparison of oral capecitabine versus intravenous fluorouracil plus leucovorin as first-line treatment in 605 patients with metastatic colorectal cancer: results of a randomized phase III study. *J Clin Oncol* 19:2282–2292, 2001[173]
De Gramont	**Day 1**: leucovorin 200 mg/m^2 IV over 2 hours, 5-FU 400 mg/m^2 IVP, then 5-FU 600 mg/m^2 IV infusion over 22 hours **Day 2**: 200 mg/m^2 IV over 2 hours, 5-FU 400 mg/m^2 IVP, then 5-FU 600 mg IV infusion over 22 hours Cycle repeated every 2 weeks	de Gramont A, Bassett JF, Milan C, et al: Randomized trial comparing monthly low-dose leucovorin and fluorouracil bolus with bimonthly high-dose leucovorin and fluorouracil bolus plus continuous infusion for advanced colorectal cancer: a French intergroup study. *J Clin Oncol* 15:808–815, 1997[174]
Douillard	**Day 1:** Irinotecan 180 mg/m^2 IV over 90 min, at same time as leucovorin 200 mg IV over 2 hours, followed by 5-FU 400 mg/m^2 IVP, then 5-FU 600 mg/m^2 IV infusion over 22 hours **Day 2:** leucovorin 200 mg/m^2 IV over 2 hours, 5-FU 400 mg/m^2 IVP, then 5-FU 600 mg IV infusion over 22 hours Cycle repeated every 2 weeks	Douillard JY, Cunningham D, Roth AD, et al: Irinotecan combined with fluorouracil compared with fluorouracil alone as first-line treatment for metastatic colorectal cancer: a multicentre randomized trial. *Lancet* 355:1041–1047, 2000[175]
Floxuridine (hepatic artery infusion, HAI)	Floxuridine (FUDR) 0.3 mg/kg/day plus dexamethasone 20 mg, plus heparin 50,000 units as HAI on days 1–14, repeat cycle every 14 days	Kemeny N, Conti JA, Cohen A, et al: Phase II study of hepatic arterial floxuridine, leucovorin, and dexamethasone for unresectable liver metastatses from colorectal carcinoma. *J Clin Oncol* 12:2288–2295, 1994[176]
FOLFOX 4	**Day 1**: oxaliplatin 85 mg/m^2 day IV over 2 hours, through 1 of 2 Y arms, simultaneously with leucovorin 200 mg/m^2 IV over 2 hours of second arm, followed by D5W flush, then 5-FU 400 mg/m^2 IVP, then 600 mg/m^2 infusion over 22 hours **Day 2**: leucovorin 200 mg/m^2 IV over 2 hours, 5-FU 400 mg/m^2 IVP, then 600 mg/^{2} infusion over 22 hours Cycle repeated q 2 weeks	de Gramont A, Figer A, Seymour M, et al: Leucovorin and fluorouracil with and without oxaliplatin as first-line treatment in advanced colorectal cancer. *J Clin Oncol* 18:2938–2947, 2000[177]

(continued)

Table 49-10 Chemotherapeutic Regimens for Adjuvant and Treatment of Advanced Colon and Rectal Cancers (continued)

Regimen Name	Regimen Dosages	Reference
FOLFOX 6	Oxaliplatin 100 mg/m² IV over 2 hours through 1 arm of Y-set, leucovorin 400 mg/m² IV over 2 hours through second arm of Y-set, flush with D5W, 5-FU 400 mg/m² IVB, then 5-FU 2.4-3.0 g/m² IV over 46 hours, cycle repeated q 2 weeks	Tournigand C, Louvet C, Quinaux E, et al: FOLFIRI followed by FOLFOX versus FOLFOX followed by FOLFIRI in metastatic colorectal cancer (MCRC): final results of a phase III study. *Proc Am Soc Clin Oncol* 20:124a, 2001 (abstr 494)[178]
FOLFOX 7	Oxaliplatin 130 mg/m² IV over 2 hours through 1 arm of Y-set, leucovorin 400 mg IV through second arm of Y-set over 2 hours, flush with D5W, 5-FU 2.4 g/m² IV over 46 hours, repeat cycle q 2 weeks	Andre T, Figer A, Cervanteo G, et al: FOLFOX7 compared to FOLFOX4. Preliminary results of the randomized optimox study. *Proc Am Soc Clin Oncol* 22:254, 2003 (abstr 1016)[179]
FOLFIRI	Irinotecan 180 mg/m² IV over 90 min, at same time as leucovorin 200 mg IV over 2 hours, followed by 5-FU 400 mg/m² IVP, then 5-FU 2.4–3.0 g/m² IV infusion over 46 hours, repeat cycle q 2 weeks	Andre T, Louvet C, Maindrault-Goebeal F, et al: CPT-11 (irinotecan) addition to bimonthly, high-dose leucovorin and bolus and continuous-infusion 5-fluorouracil (FOLFIRI) for pretreated metastatic colorectal cancer GERCOR. *Eur J Cancer* 35:1343–1347, 1999[180]
FUFOX	Weekly oxaliplatin 50 mg/m² IV over 2 hours, leucovorin 500 mg/m² IV over 2 hours, then 5-FU 2000 mg/m² as 24-hour continuous infusion, repeated d1, 8, 15, 22, q 5 weeks	Grothey A, Deschler B, Kroening H, et al: Phase III study of bolus 5-fluorouracil (5-FU)/ folinic acid (FA) (Mayo) vs weekly high-dose 24h 5-FU infusion/ FA + oxaliplatin (OXA) (FUFOX) in advanced colorectal cancer (ACRC). *Proc Am Soc Clin Oncol* 21:254, 2002 (abstr 512)[181]
IFL	Irinotecan 125 mg/m² IV over 90 min, IV bolus 5-FU 500 mg/m², LV 20 mg/m² q week × 4 every 6 weeks	Saltz LB, Cox JV, Blanke C, et al: Irinotecan plus fluorouracil and leucovorin for metatatic colorectal cancer. *N Engl J Med* 343:905–914, 2000[182]
IROX	Oxaliplatin 85 mg/m² IV day 1, irinotecan 200 mg/m² repeated q 3 weeks	Wasserman E, Sutherland N, Critkovic E, et al: Irinotecan plus oxaliplatin: a promising combination for advanced colorectal cancer. *Clin Colorectal Cancer* 1:149–153, 2001[183]
XELOX	**Day 1:** oxaliplatin 130 mg/m² as 2-hour infusion **Days 1–14:** capecitabine 1000 mg/m² po bid × 14 days, repeated q 3 weeks	Tabernero J, Butts CA, Cassidy J, et al: Capecitabine and oxaliplatin in combination (Xelox) as first-line therapy for patients with metastatic colorectal cancer (MCRC): results of an international muticenter phase II trial. *Proc Am Soc Clin Oncol* 21:133a, 2002 (abstr 531)[184]

agent approved by the FDA. It is indicated for first-line treatment of advanced colon and rectal cancers in combination with a 5-FU–based regimen. Bevacuzimab is currently being studied in other combinations, such as with FOLFOX 4.

Colon and rectal cancers overexpress the epidermal growth factor receptor (EGFR), prompting cells to continually divide, become invasive, block apoptosis (programmed cell death), and make new blood vessels. Cetuximab, a monoclonal antibody directed against EGFR, when given in combination with irinotecan resulted in an improved response in previously treated, refractory patients with advanced colon and rectal cancers. Patients must test positive to EGFR to respond to the drug. The overall response rate in the cetuximab-treated arm of one study was 22.9% compared to 10.8% in the irinotecan monotherapy arm, and overall survival was 8.6 months compared to 6.9 months in the single-agent irinotecan arm.[188] Cetuximab is being studied in combination with FOLFOX 4 and FOLFOX 6.

Exciting advances have occurred in the adjuvant setting as well. Two national studies explored combinations of irinotecan or oxaliplatin with 5-FU/LV, and the results of the NSABP C-07 (5-FU/LV versus FLOX in patients with stage II and III disease) and the CALGBC89803 (5-FU/LV versus IFL in stage III) are anxiously awaited. In Europe, de Gramont and colleagues completed the MOSAIC study, a multinational study of 2246 patients with stage II and III resected colon cancer, and presented three-year follow-up data: Disease-free survival was significantly better for FOLFOX 4 (77.8%) versus 5-FU/LV (72.9%), $p < 0.01$, and FOLFOX 4 reduced risk of recurrence by 23%.[167] Overall survival data are still maturing, but FOLFOX 4 has become the standard of care for adjuvant chemotherapy. The X-ACT trial, a multi-institutional, randomized, controlled trial of 1987 patients, compared capecitabine (a 5-FU prodrug) with 5-FU/LV in the adjuvant setting. This phase III trial showed equivalence of the comparators in achieving disease-free survival.[172] In addition, national clinical trials groups are exploring the use of bevacuzimab as an adjuvant treatment for colon cancer. For example, NSABP C-08 is comparing FOLFOX 6 +/– bevacuzimab.

Side effects from chemotherapy can be severe. The nurse's role is critical in safely administering the drug(s), but, even more importantly, nurses must provide education about potential side effects, self-assessment, and self-care measures to minimize toxicity and maximize quality of life, as most side effects occur once the patient has returned home. The oncology nurse uses the Oncology Nursing Society (ONS) standards to ensure that the patient's physical, psychosocial, and educational needs are being addressed. Educating patients about adverse treatment effects helps them to manage symptoms and helps alleviate the serious or life-threatening treatment complications. Irinotecan combinations are perhaps the most challenging. During one clinical trial, the arm containing irinotecan was stopped pending further investigation. Although it was found that the mortality rate was not significantly higher, clinicians were reminded that patients receiving IFL require close monitoring for febrile neutropenia and the late onset of diarrhea.[189] Diarrhea can be severe, and a suggested approach to its management is a 4 mg loading dose of loperamide at the first sign of diarrhea, then 2 mg doses every 2 hours until diarrhea abates, for at least 12 hours. The major toxicities of each drug are shown in Table 49-11. The dose-limiting toxicities for irinotecan are diarrhea and neutropenia; for oxaliplatin, persistent neurotoxicity; for bevacuzimab, hemorrhage and hypertension; and for cetuximab, severe acne-like rash and diarrhea. Potential side effects from the combination of 5-FU and leucovorin include nausea, vomiting, diarrhea, mucositis, fever, leukopenia, thrombocytopenia, and hypotension. Oncology nurses play a critical role in assessing and managing patients who are receiving chemotherapy, as well as teaching them self-care measures.

Table 49-11 Toxicities of Major Agents Used in the Treatment of Colon and Rectal Cancers

Drug	Major toxicities
5-FU/LV	Bone marrow suppression, nadir days 10–14; mucositis, diarrhea, dry skin and photosensitivity, nausea, blepharitis (tear duct stenosis), hand–foot syndrome (palmar-plantar erythrodysesthesia), rare cerebellar toxicity and angina
Irinotecan	Diarrhea (acute and late), bone marrow suppression especially febrile neutropenia, mucositis, mild alopecia, asthenia, fever, vascular syndrome
Oxaliplatin	Rare hypersensitivity reactions; acute and chronic/persistent neuropathy, mild bone marrow suppression, nausea and vomiting, diarrhea
Bevacuzimab	Uncommon: hemorrhage, gastrointestinal perforation, delayed wound healing (delay until ≥ 21 days from or before surgery) More common: asthenia, pain, abdominal pain, headache, hypertension, diarrhea, nausea, vomiting, anorexia, stomatitis, constipation, upper respiratory infection, epistaxis, dyspnea, exfoliative dermatitis, proteinuria
Cetuximab	Rare: severe infusion reaction and pulmonary toxicity More common: acne-like rash, diarrhea, pain, fever, nausea, vomiting, anorexia, constipation, headache

Molecular Targeted Therapy

Two major molecular targeted therapies have been approved for use in advanced colon and rectal cancers: bevacuzimab and cetuximab, both monoclonal antibodies. Bevacuzimab, which targets the VEGF receptor, has shown efficacy in combination with irinotecan, 5-FU, and leucovorin (IFL) in extending survival in patients with advanced colon and rectal cancers. The drug has recently been granted FDA approval for administration in combination with a 5-FU–based regimen. In addition to levamisole, alpha- and gamma-interferon have shown activity in colon cancer cell lines but have not resulted in improved clinical outcomes. A large study is investigating the murine monoclonal antibody 17-1A (edrecolomab), which is marketed in Europe as Panorex.[190]

Significant advances have been made in the management of colon cancer. The current treatment options are summarized in Table 49-12.

Symptom Management and Supportive Care

Many patients have uncomplicated, curative surgery for colon cancer. For others, their course may be complicated by several expected and unexpected developments. Symptoms produced by disease and progression can affect quality of life, self-care and symptom management needs, and educational needs for self-care. Bowel obstruction and fistula formation require supportive care and symptom management, as does palliative care for patients with progressive disease.

Bowel Obstruction

Bowel obstruction is a common complication in patients with abdominal or pelvic cancers, such as those arising in the colon, ovary, and stomach. Although bowel obstruction may develop at any time, it is more common and may evolve more rapidly in patients with

Table 49-12 Management of Colon Cancer

Pathology and Extent of Disease	Surgical Management	Follow-up and Adjuvant Therapy
Polyps		
Pedunculated polyp with invasive cancer: • Adenoma with deep invasion into stalk • Adenoma with margins that cannot be assessed, high-grade lesion (3–4), vascular or lymphatic invasion, positive margins	Colectomy with excision of regional lymph nodes (en bloc)	Superficial, completely removed polyps: no further surgery Follow-up depends on pathological stage
Sessile adenomatous polyp, villous adenoma, or villoglandular adenoma with invasive cancer with high risk for recurrence: • Fragmented specimen, tissue margins that cannot be assessed, or adverse pathology) • ≥ T1 or positive margins	Colectomy with excision of regional lymph nodes (en bloc)	Single specimen, Tis, with negative margins, completely removed: no further surgery Follow-up depends upon pathological stage
Colon Cancer		
Nonobstructing lesion	Colectomy with excision of regional lymph nodes (en bloc)	Adjuvant chemotherapy based on stage: Stage I: none Stage IIA (T3): clinical trial or observation, or 5-FU/LV, FOLFOX, capcitabine if high risk for recurrence (high grade, LVI, vascular invasion, bowel obstruction) Stage IIB (T4) or T3 with high risk of recurrence (positive margins, perforation): 5-FU/LV with or without XRT, FOLFOX or capecitabine chemotherapy; clinical trial, or observation Stage III: FOLFOX, 5-FU/LV, or capecitabine; consider addition of XRT for T4 lesion if high risk
Resectable, obstructing lesion (unprepped)	Colectomy with excision of regional lymph nodes (en bloc) if possible; otherwise resection with diversion or stent	
Unresectable lesion	Palliative resection, diversion or stent	Salvage chemotherapy: First line: FOLFOX, FOLFIRI, bevacizumab + 5-FU–based regimen *if patient can tolerate aggressive therapy*; if not, capecitabine, 5-FU/LV, or 5-FU CI Second line: FOLFOX or FOLFIRI (depending on first line chemotherapy), irinotecan +/– cetuximab
Metastatic Disease		
Liver metastases		
• Isolated, resectable	Resection of primary lesion, excision of regional lymph nodes (en bloc), with liver resection or later, staged liver resection; neoadjuvant chemotherapy as needed to make resection possible with FOLFOX or FOLFIRI	6 months of adjuvant chemotherapy using 5-FU/LV (bolus or CI), capecitabine, FOLFOX, FOLFIRI, hepatic artery infusion +/– 5-FU/LV (bolus or CI), or FU CI, or observation
• Unresectable	Palliative colectomy if at high risk for obstruction	Salvage chemotherapy: First line: FOLFOX, FOLFIRI, bevacizumab + 5-FU–based regimen *if patient can tolerate aggressive therapy*; if not, capecitabine, 5-FU/LV, or 5-FU CI Second line: FOLFOX or FOLFIRI (depending on first line chemotherapy), irinotecan +/– cetuximab
Lung metastases		
• 1–3 nodules, resectable	Resection of primary tumor with excision of regional lymph nodes (en bloc), then resection of pulmonary lesions	6 months of adjuvant chemotherapy using 5-FU/LV (bolus or CI), capecitabine, FOLFOX, FOLFIRI, hepatic artery infusion +/– 5-FU/LV (bolus or CI), or FU CI or observation
• Multiple nodules, unresectable	Palliative resection of primary tumor is an option	Salvage chemotherapy: First line: FOLFOX, FOLFIRI, bevacizumab + 5-FU–based regimen *if patient can tolerate aggressive therapy*; if not, capecitabine, 5-FU/LV, or 5-FU CI Second line: FOLFOX or FOLFIRI (depending upon first line chemotherapy), irinotecan +/– cetuximab.

(continued)

Table 49-12 Management of Colon Cancer (continued)

Pathology and Extent of Disease	Surgical Management	Follow-up and Adjuvant Therapy
Abdominal/peritoneal metastases	Option of limited resection of primary tumor, diverting colostomy or bypass if impending obstruction	Salvage chemotherapy: First line: FOLFOX, FOLFIRI, bevacizumab + 5-FU-based regimen *if patient can tolerate aggressive therapy*; if not, capecitabine, 5-FU/LV, or 5-FU CI Second line: FOLFOX or FOLFIRI (depending upon first line chemotherapy), irinotecan +/– cetuximab.
Local recurrence		
• Resectable	PET scan shows no further metastatic disease so resection	Adjuvant therapy for 6 months if not already received
• Unresectable or multiple lesions	Treatment plan based on performance status	Salvage chemotherapy or best supportive care based on performance status

5-FU = 5-fluorouracil; LV = leucovorin; XRT = radiation therapy; H+P = history and physical exam; CI = continuous infusion; LVI = lymphatic invasion
Data from National Comprehensive Cancer Network[127]; Meyers[128]; Change[129]; Brandt et al.[130]; Kemeny, Huang, et al.[153]; Kemeny, Niedzwiecki, et al.[155]; McCormick, Martini[158]; Avis[159]; Willett et al.[162]; Minsky[164]; Meta-analysis Group in Cancer[167]; deGramont[171,174,177]; Cassidy, et al.[172]; Andre et al.[179]; Goldberg et al.[186]; Hurwitz, et al.[187]; Cunningham, et al.[188]; Peters, Haller[190]; Greene.[209]

advanced disease. If the patient presents with an obstructing lesion, and the bowel cannot be adequately prepped for resection, a flexible stent may be placed temporarily, or it may be placed for palliation.[191,192]

Bowel obstruction secondary to advanced colon or rectal carcinoma may be extrinsic or intrinsic. Extrinsic compression of the bowel may occur as a result of abdominal carcinomatosis or tumor studding along the bowel wall. Intrinsic compression of the bowel can result from growth and progression of the tumor within the lumen of the bowel itself. Signs and symptoms of bowel obstruction include nausea and vomiting, abdominal pain, progressive constipation, and the absence of bowel sounds over the affected area. Initially, there is sporadic vomiting, but it increases progressively until its prevalence is in the range of 68%–100% of the time.[193] Vomiting can remain intermittent or become continuous. It develops early and in large amounts with obstruction of the gastric outlet or small intestine, but develops later in large bowel obstruction.[58] Biliary vomiting is almost odorless and indicates an obstruction in the upper part of the abdomen. The presence of foul-smelling, fecaloid vomiting can be the first sign of an ileal or colonic obstruction.

Diagnosis of a bowel obstruction is made via radiologic assessment. An abdominal x-ray is taken in a supine or standing position to document dilated loops of bowel, air–fluid interfaces, or both. An x-ray following the ingestion of contrast dye can distinguish obstruction from metastases, radiation injury, or adhesions. A more definitive examination can be done with colosigmoidoscopy.[194]

The usual treatment for symptom control is nasogastric suction and administration of parenteral fluids. This inpatient treatment decompresses the stomach and/or intestine and corrects fluid and electrolyte imbalances before surgery or while the decision for surgery is being made. To prevent the tube from becoming occluded, periodic flushing or replacement is needed.

If the obstruction continues for more than a few days, a gastrostomy tube is a much more acceptable and well-tolerated route for decompression than nasogastric intubation.[195] Intermittent venting of the gastrostomy tube allows the patient to continue oral intake and maintain an active lifestyle without the inconvenience of a nasogastric tube. The two options currently available are surgically placed gastrostomy and percutaneous endoscopic gastrostomy (PEG). A gastrostomy tube placed at the time of surgical exploration is the traditional method of long-term gastric decompression. It should be done whenever the surgeon's intraoperative impression is that complete bowel obstruction is imminent or may be prolonged or imminent. PEG entails the insertion of a tube into the stomach through the abdominal wall under fluoroscopic or endoscopic guidance. It can be performed safely as a venting procedure for patients with advanced cancer who are suffering from nausea and vomiting due to bowel obstruction.

Colicky pain occurs in 72%–76% of patients, and continuous abdominal pain is present in more than 90% of cancer patients with bowel obstruction.[195] Pain may be due to abdominal distention, tumor mass, or hepatomegaly, as well as the obstruction itself.

Initially described 14 years ago, the pharmacological management of bowel obstruction due to advanced cancer focuses on the treatment of nausea, vomiting, pain, and other symptoms without the use of nasogastric tube or intravenous hydration. Palliative care units worldwide now use this approach. Somatostatin or octreotide can be used to minimize intestinal secretions.

Antiemetic and pain regimens are well established.[195] The average survival of patients who have inoperable bowel obstruction and are treated with drugs ranges from 2 to 50 days.[196]

Fistula

Solid tumors may extend into the bowel from adjacent organs or may spread from the bowel to create fistulous openings to the skin, the vagina, or other organs. Fistulas also may occur as a result of anastomotic breakdown following a surgical procedure on the bowel or as a complication of radiation therapy.

Initial interventions for the patient with a fistula involving the intestinal tract include fluid and electrolyte stabilization and control of infection.[197] Specific fluid and electrolyte needs depend on the type and volume of fistula output; for example, small bowel fistulas usually produce high volumes of effluent containing significant amounts of sodium, potassium, and bicarbonate.[197] The patient with high-output fistula (more than 500 mL in 24 hours) requires close monitoring of fluid–electrolyte balance, with replacement titrated in response to the type and volume of output and laboratory indices. Initial management also involves careful evaluation for any intraabdominal infectious process. Abscesses are drained via open surgical exploration and irrigation or via percutaneous catheter placement.[197]

Fistula closure is typically achieved either through medical management promoting spontaneous closure or through surgical resection or bypass of the fistulous tract. Usually, conservative medical management is tried first, assuming no intraabdominal infection is present and the distal bowel is patent. This conservative medical approach is based on studies indicating that in the absence of distal obstruction about 50% of fistulas will close spontaneously within four to six weeks and on the fact that surgical closure is frequently ineffective until the underlying factors contributing to fistula development have been corrected.[197] The two major principles on which conservative management is based are (1) provision of nutritional support and (2) bowel rest for the involved segment of the intestine. The goal is to ensure the adequate intake and absorption of calories and protein to support the healing process while minimizing the volume of drainage through the segment of bowel containing the fistula.

Recently, a number of studies have demonstrated a significant reduction in fistula output and in the time required for spontaneous fistula closure with the administration of somatostatin or its analog, octreotide acetate. Somatostatin is a naturally occurring intestinal hormone that reduces the volume of intestinal secretions.[198]

A major component of effective fistula management is the containment of the effluent and odor and the protection of the surrounding skin, as these aspects of care have a profound impact on the patient's quality of life. Many products and techniques are now available for achieving and maintaining these goals.

Progressive Disease

Symptoms of progressive disease relate to the areas of metastases. The most common metastatic sites in colon cancer are the lymph nodes, liver, and lungs, with metastases to the brain and bone occurring less commonly. The patient with colon cancer metastatic to the liver is likely to receive or has received chemotherapy for advanced disease, such as combination therapy with irinotecan, 5-fluorouracil, and leucovorin or FOLFOX 4. The liver is a large organ and can accommodate many metastatic tumors before the patient experiences signs and symptoms of an obstructed liver. Ultimately, however, the malignant clones develop resistance and the disease progresses. As the liver becomes replaced with tumor, liver function tests start to become abnormal. Often patients develop nausea, anorexia, cachexia, and ascites as the serum albumin falls, decreasing the colloidal osmotic pressure in the blood vessels. Fluid shifts into the third space, with pedal edema that becomes pitting, and which may progress up the calf and thigh. Dyspnea on exertion occurs as the peritoneal fluid pushes up the diaphragm, shrinking the area of lung expansion. Nurses work with the patient and family to minimize, manage, or prevent complications.

In terms of nausea, the nurse discusses antiemetics with the physician and teaches the patient and family how to administer them. The challenging anorexia–cachexia syndrome often requires the assistance of the dietitian, but focuses on helping the patient eat small, frequent feedings of foods and fluids that are pleasing and calorie dense, because the stomach fills quickly. Loss of appetite can be distressing to patients. Despite the fact that this loss does not affect survival, it may affect quality of life. As a consequence, appetite stimulants may be prescribed, such as megestrol acetate. It is important to avoid using total parenteral nutrition for the patient with progressive disease unless there is a chance of reversing the disease with aggressive therapy.

Dyspnea can be distressing, so the nurse focuses on teaching the patient positioning to help the diaphragm descend and increase space for lung expansion, such as using 2–3 pillows, a high Fowler's position, or a cardiac recliner. Although the administration of salt-poor albumin should theoretically reverse the colloidal osmotic pressure in the blood vessels, or paracentesis should reduce ascites, unfortunately the fluid often quickly reaccumulates following salt-poor albumin or paracentesis, so these measures are not the standard of care. A trial of diuretic therapy may be effective in reducing painful peripheral edema, together with elevation of the lower extremities. Nurses teach self-administration of diuretics, evaluate responses, and teach other self-care activities to prevent skin breakdown.

Patients may have visceral pain, requiring opioid analgesics. The nurse works closely with both the patient and family to achieve established pain–comfort goals, with care to prevent constipation or other opioid-induced complications. Nursing care and teaching focus on helping the patient ''live with cancer.'' As the disease advances, talking with the patient, about advanced directives can be challenging, but rewarding as the patient makes important decisions, such as making a will while still feeling well enough. Many patients wish to die at home surrounded by their family, so involving the hospice team can be critical to ensure that symptoms are managed, and that the patient maintains the highest quality of life until death. The nurse is a catalyst, stimulating the healthcare team to continue to strive for management and control of symptoms, and an advocate, ensuring that, given the particular set of circumstances, the highest quality of life for each patient is achieved. For information on palliative care measures, see symptom-specific chapters Chapters 71 and 72.

Long-Term Monitoring and Follow-up

In today's healthcare environment, the delivery of care takes place in an accelerated fashion. The time span between presentation, physiological work-up, diagnosis, acute intervention, and follow-up treatment can be compressed into a month. Often a multitude of healthcare professionals are involved in the individual's care, which makes communication and coordination of the treatment plan paramount. It has been estimated that 62% of whites and 53% of blacks diagnosed with colon cancer will attain the five-year survival rate.[1] Continuity of care during the disease trajectory is critical to assure regular follow-up and intervention as needed.

The average length of stay for someone who has undergone a surgical resection secondary to colorectal carcinoma is less than five days. At the time of admission, the appropriate referrals need to be made. Should the individual have a colostomy, the CWOCN nurse needs to be involved. A registered dietitian lends support for caloric calculations, hyperalimentation guidelines, and dietary specifics. Social service may be needed as dictated by the individual's home and support situation. Home care is also a consideration to meet specific healthcare needs once the individual is discharged.

At discharge, the individual needs to be clear about when to call the physician for problems such as fever, chills, shortness of breath, or hemoptysis. Should any change occur with the incision, such as erythema, drainage, or wound separation, the surgeon also needs to be notified. Information about discharge medications and resuming previous medications must be reviewed and clarified. Optimally, the name and telephone number of the same healthcare professional should be given to the individual and family as a contact for questions or difficulties that may arise before the return appointment to the surgeon.

Upon the patient's return for the postoperative check, an overall physical assessment takes place and the final pathology is shared with the individual and family if the tissue diagnosis was not available at the time of discharge. The general plan for follow-up treatment can be discussed as well. While additional adjunctive therapy may not begin for another few weeks, the appropriate referrals to the radiation oncologist or medical oncologist need to be made in a timely fashion.

Post-treatment surveillance is important and a schema is shown in Table 49-13. Some controversy exists regarding the exact sequence and measures, however, and outcome studies are being conducted. Coordination of all these services and the provision for continuity of care is imperative. For the individual confronted with a diagnosis of cancer, recovery from surgery, and treatment follow-up, the nurse can provide invaluable assistance in organizing, scheduling, interpreting, and managing the treatment plan.

If the disease is advanced, palliation of symptoms is part of the spectrum of care. The individual and family should be educated regarding the gradual progression of the disease, what to expect from a physiological standpoint, and options available for the treatment of these symptoms. The individual and family can be offered the services and support of hospice. Discussion about advanced directives should occur in a supportive environment. Options for interventions need to be explored so that an informed decision can be made. Most symptoms can be handled within the comfort of the individual's home if so desired. Should a hospital admission become necessary, however, decisions regarding life-support measures need to be explored with the individual and family prior to the hospitalization.

Table 49-13 Post-treatment Surveillance for Colon Cancer

Curative resection, and NED	H+P q 3 months × 2 years, then q 6 months for the next 5 years. Colonoscopy within 1 year of resection or 3–6 months postoperatively; repeat annually if malignant polyp(s) found; otherwise repeat colonoscopy at least every 3 years.
≥ T2 or greater lesions	CEA blood test baseline then q 3 months × 2 years, then q 6 months for the next 2–5 years if curative. Aggressive surgery for detected recurrence is feasible. Colonoscopy within 1 year of resection or 3–6 months postoperatively; repeat q year if neoplastic polyps found; otherwise at least every 3 years.
Increasing CEA level after resection	Colonoscopy; CT (chest, abdominal, pelvic), H+P. If scans WNL despite increasing CEA, repeat scans every 3 months if symptoms occur. PET scan may be helpful in identifying isolated metastases, and should be done to establish whether recurrence is resectable.

CEA = carcinoembryonic antigen; NED = no evidence of disease, H+P = history and physical exam; WNL = within normal limits.
Data from *NCCN Practice Guidelines in Oncology: Colon Cancer v.2.2004*,[127]; Meyers[128]; Chang.[129]

Conclusion

The last decade has seen an awakening realization of the importance of prevention and early detection of colon cancer. However, much work remains to be done to ensure that basic screening tests are offered and made accessible to Americans, especially those age 50 years or older. A number of diagnostic tests, such as DNA stool testing, are under study and offer promise for more precise screening. Although public education efforts in primary prevention have increased, obesity—a known risk factor for colon cancer—remains an enormous problem in the United States. Great strides have been made in the management of advanced colon cancer, especially in terms of chemotherapy, and similar advances need to be made in adjuvant therapy so that patients with colon cancer can, indeed, be cured. Colon cancer should be a preventable and curable cancer.

Rectal Cancer

Introduction

In 2004, the ACS estimated that 40,570 people would develop rectal cancer (23,220 men and 17,350 women).[1] The ACS estimated that 56,730 people would die from colon and rectal cancers in 2004: 28,320 men and 28,410 women. Similar to colon cancer, rectal polyps can be found early and removed so that rectal cancer in most cases can be prevented, or detected early so it can be cured through regular, routine screening. For both colon and rectal cancers, 90% of disease occurs in individuals who are age 50 or older.

Epidemiology and Etiology

Rectal cancer is seen more frequently in men than in women.[2] The mortality from rectal cancer has decreased during the last 30 years.[199] Risk factors for rectal cancer that are shared with colon cancer are age (risk increases with age more than 50 years old), genetic history of FAP, family history (first-degree relative with adenomas or invasive rectal carcinoma), and history of ulcerative colitis.

Prevention, Screening, and Early Detection

Peters and colleagues[43] studied 33,971 subjects in the randomized Prostate, Lung, Colorectal and Ovarian (PLCO) cancer screening trial, and found that a high intake of dietary fiber was associated with a lower risk of colon but not rectal adenomas. Individuals ingesting the highest amounts of fiber had a 27% lower risk of distal colonic adenoma as compared to the lowest quintile, with fiber from grains, cereals, and fruits conferring the most protection. The researchers did not find a reduction in risk for rectal adenoma.[43] Giovannucci and colleagues[49] reviewed the Nurses' Health Study data from 88,756 women, and found that women who had taken multivitamins containing folic acid for at least 15 years had a significant reduction in the risk of developing colon cancer but not the risk of developing rectal cancer.[49] Exercise does not appear to reduce the risk of rectal cancer.[61]

Digital rectal examination allows exploration of the rectum as far as 7 cm from the anal verge. Herrinton and colleagues[200] used a case-controlled study to show that routine digital rectal exam did not significantly reduce mortality from rectal cancer.[200] Thus, patients age 50 or older should be screened using the same standard as those with colon cancer, shown in Table 49-2.

Bleeding from the anus is often an early sign of rectal cancer, and leads to prompt intervention and likelihood of cure. This underscores the need for colon and rectal cancer screening as part of the annual physical exam in all individuals age 50 or older, and starting at age 40 for individuals at risk as discussed previously.

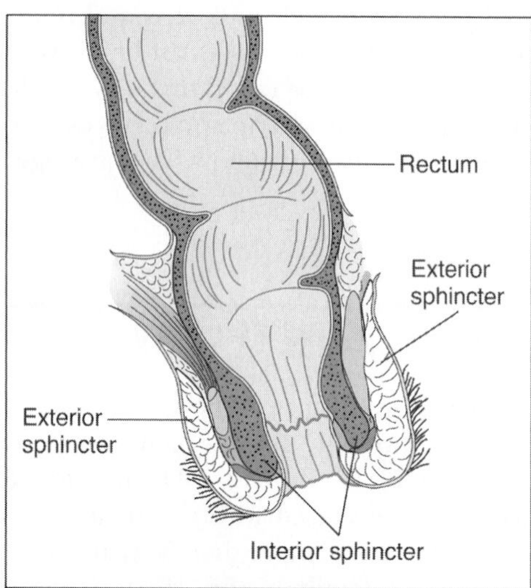

Figure 49-6 Anatomy of the rectum.

Later symptoms occur when large polyps or lesions bleed or cause tenesmus or incomplete evacuation of stool, cramping, abdominal pain, and obstructive symptoms. These cases have a lower chance of cure.

Pathophysiology

The rectum is divided into three sections:

- Lower rectum, 3–6 cm from the anal verge; extraperitoneal
- Midrectum, 6–10 cm from anal verge; extraperitoneal
- Upper rectum, 10–15 cm above the anal verge but with the upper limit of the rectum approximately 12 cm from the anal verge; surrounded by peritoneum on its anterior and lateral surfaces

The rectum temporarily stores fecal waste from which water, electrolytes, and nutrients have been removed as it travels down the intestines. When stimulated, it propels the waste into the anus for evacuation. The rectal mucosa secretes mucus that helps move the waste to the anus. The rectum, together with the muscles in the pelvic floor, help maintain continence. As the rectum fills with fecal waste, sensory nerves stimulate conscious or unconscious tightening of the external anal sphincter until it is appropriate to evacuate the stool, when the sphincter is relaxed. See Figure 49-6.

Skibber and colleagues[18] help explain the lymphatic and nervous innervation of the rectum. The rectum has a number of lymphatic channels, and most of the lymphatic drainage follows the hemorrhoidal artery toward the mesenteric artery, as does the drainage from the perirectal lymph nodes that lie mid-rectum and above. The lower perirectal lymph nodes drain laterally, and the hypogastric and iliac lymph node drainage is carried along the aorta. The autonomic nervous system innervates most of the pelvic organs and is important to sexual and bladder function. The sympathetic nerves form the hypogastric plexus; the nerve trunks lie under the pelvic peritoneum, lateral to the mesorectum (the fold of mesentery or peritoneum that is attached to the rectum). These nerve fibers lie close to the arteries supplying the pelvic organs. Parasympathetic fibers leave the 2–4 sacral nerve roots to innervate the pelvic viscera, and join the sympathetic fibers at the pelvic plexus. It is critical that the autonomic nerves be preserved during resection of the mesorectum so as to preserve sexual and bladder function.[201]

The location of a rectal tumor is identified by the distance from the lower edge of the tumor to the anal verge, dentate line, or anorectal ring. Progress in surgical technique has led to the selection of patients for whom sphincter-sparing resection of the rectum is a viable option. This choice is discussed in greater detail in the ''Therapeutic Approaches and Nursing Care'' section.

Cellular Characteristics

Rectal and colon cancers appear to share the same mutational sequence, which results first in adenomatous polyp formation, then malignant transformation. Most cancers of the rectum are adenocarcinomas, or carcinomas arising in glandular cells in the mucosa. Adenocarcinomas can be either mucinous (colloid) or signet ring types. Other histologic types are scirrhous, neuroendocrine (which confers a poorer prognosis than pure adenocarcinoma), and carcinoid tumors. Squamous cell carcinomas and adenosquamous and undifferentiated carcinomas have been found in the rectum as well.[2] Rarely, carcinoid tumors may arise in the rectum, often appearing as submucosal nodules, and may be indolent; in contrast, colonic carcinoid tumors are aggressive and metastasize.[202] Uncommonly, small cell histologies have been described in the rectum, in some cases associated with ulcerative colitis.[203]

Adenocarcinomas of the rectum develop initially in the mucosa, then locally invade into the lumen of the bowel wall. When the tumor has traversed the muscularis mucosa and infiltrated the submucosa, it is termed *invasive*. Further infiltration by way of the lymph and vascular systems occurs next, and direct extension may occur onto the peritoneal surfaces as well. If the tumor secretes large amounts of mucin so that more than 50% of the tumor mass is made up of extracellular mucin, it is called a mucinous carcinoma.

Progression of Disease and Patterns of Spread

The large intestine consists of the cecum, ascending colon, transverse colon, descending colon, sigmoid colon, and rectum. The rectum is surrounded by extraperitoneal perirectal fat in the pelvis. The blood supply to the sigmoid colon, descending colon, and upper rectum comes from the inferior mesenteric artery. The lower rectum is supplied by the internal iliac arteries. The rectum is drained by two routes: the superior hemorrhoidal veins, which empty into the portal venous system, and the middle and inferior hemorrhoidal veins, which empty into the inferior vena cava.[18]

By the time of their diagnosis, rectal cancers will have penetrated through the wall in 50%–77% of patients and will have metastasized to lymph nodes in 50%–60% of cases.[2] Implantation of tumor cells at other sites can occur as a result of surgical manipulation of the tumor, intraluminal spread, or shedding of tumor cells into the peritoneum. Intraperitoneal seeding and carcinomatosis may occur even without lymphatic or visceral spread. The most common sites of distant metastases for rectal cancer are the liver and lung. Solitary pulmonary metastasis is rare, but may occur with distal rectal cancers.[2] Other areas of metastasis include the brain (cerebellum), bones, kidneys, and adrenals.[116]

The most common sites of rectal cancer recurrence are (1) anterior local recurrence—anastomotic site, prostate and seminal vesicles in men, and vagina, uterus, or bladder in women; and (2) posterior local recurrence—sacrum, pyriformis muscle, sciatic nerve, and pelvic sidewalls.[18]

Clinical Manifestations

Signs and symptoms of rectal cancer relate to the location of the tumor near the end of the descending (sigmoid) colon in the rectum. As discussed earlier, most rectal cancers begin as polyps that grow slowly, then undergo malignant transformation with successive mutations. As the malignancy increases in size, signs and symptoms reflect the degree of obstruction in the rectum, such as changes in bowel elimination patterns. In contrast to right-sided colon cancers, which may cause anemia, left-sided colon cancers and rectal cancers have a higher incidence of bright red bleeding.[18] Early signs are bleeding from the anus and painful defecation. Other symptoms include a change in bowel habits such as new onset of constipation or diarrhea, or constipation with diarrhea where diarrhea occurs due to the partial obstruction created by the tumor; changes in the caliber of stool; increased pain on defecation; and a feeling of incomplete stooling or fullness after defecation.

Late signs of rectal cancer are tenesmus, or urgent feeling of having to defecate, but inability to empty the rectum because of circumferential growth and transmural penetration by the rectal tumor;[18] abdominal pain; jaundice; malaise; pelvic pain; anorexia; weight loss; pruritus; ascites; and hepatomegaly. In cases where bleeding from the rectum has continued for a long period of time, signs and symptoms of anemia (fatigue, shortness of breath) can occur. If the tumor locally invades neighboring organs, such as the prostate, bladder, or high sacral nerve roots, the patient will have dysuria, hematuria, or other urinary symptoms. If the tumor locally invades posteriorly, the patient will complain of buttock or perineal pain.[18]

Very late signs are urinary signs related to local invasion of neighboring organs such as the prostate or bladder, and destruction of sacral nerve roots causing sacral or sciatic pain, and buttock or perineal pain.[18]

The sensation of a mass in the rectum is often mistakenly attributed to hemorrhoids or anal fissures and may require a rectal examination and biopsy for accurate diagnosis. A proctosigmoidoscopy will provide an adequate examination to secure biopsy and provide a baseline for surgical assessment. Instructing the patient, assisting with the examination, and providing support and privacy for the patient during the procedure are crucial to a successful examination.

Assessment

Patient and Family History

The history should include patient and family history, with attention being paid to a personal history of FAP or HNPCC; rectal or colon adenomas; rectal, colon, uterine, ovarian, bladder, or other cancers; and a history of inflammatory bowel diseases. Family history of adenomas or rectal, colon, or other cancers, and their age at onset, should be elucidated. Social history of smoking or alcohol consumption should be queried. In addition, a systems review should be done, with a careful exploration of bowel habits, changes, rectal sensation of fullness or incomplete stooling, bleeding, and hemorrhoids.

Physical Examination

Key features of the physical examination are assessment of the abdomen, breasts, rectum, and lymph nodes to identify any abnormalities that reflect the status of primary or metastatic rectal cancer.[126] Initially, general features are assessed, such as weight for size, functional and mental ability, and nutritional status, with a focus on wasting of the temporal or masseter wasting. If the rectal cancer invades the bladder or develops a fistula into the bladder, the patient will develop symptoms of chronic urinary tract infection and hematuria. Percussing and palpating the right upper quadrant will give information about possible liver metastases, the most common metastatic site of rectal cancer. To augment assessment of liver metastases, assess the eye sclera for icterus, which preceeds jaundice related to biliary obstruction. A digital rectal exam should be performed to locate masses and identify tenderness. In men, it should include a prostate exam. In women, a bimanual vaginal exam should be performed.

Diagnostic Studies

Diagnostic studies include a biopsy of the suspicious lesion with pathological analysis of invasion of the muscularis mucosa, a chest x-ray, abdominal and pelvic CT, serum CEA level,[199] and endorectal ultrasound or MRI, which provides information about depth of invasion and lymph node status.[204] These studies provide adequate information to identify clinical stage and treatment of choice. Endoscopic ultrasound (EUS) clarifies surgical options and contributes to choosing a sphincter-saving procedure. EUS is superior to CT scan in evaluating the depth of wall invasion and the involvement of adjacent soft tissues, but it may not be sensitive enough to detect microinvasion of the submucosa. This imaging modality has up to 95% accuracy in identifying the correct stage, and 74% accuracy in identifying perirectal lymph node involvement.[205] When MRI is used in preoperative staging, it can detect pelvic sidewall and ascral involvement, so it complements the information gained from EUS.[126]

MRI is also useful in diagnosing advanced disease and can detect recurrent rectal cancer or tumors too small to be evaluated on CT scan. MRI may also be done for patients who are unable to tolerate the CT scanner or who are allergic to the contrast material. Fine-needle aspiration, with or without the above diagnostic tests, is generally indicated to confirm the recurrence of disease.

Prognostic Indicators

In rectal cancer, as in colon cancer, staging of the tumor is based on depth of invasion rather than size of the tumor as with other solid tumors such as breast cancer, because depth of tumor penetration has been shown to independently influence survival.[206] The most important predictors of long-term survival of patients with rectal cancer are pathologic stage at diagnosis, presence of distant metastases, extent of local tumor, number of positive lymph nodes, and residual disease after definitive therapy.[207] As the molecular basis of carcinogenesis has become better understood, other biologic, genetic, molecular, and tissue factors have been identified, in addition to TNM staging, that influence survival for the patient with rectal cancer. Seven prognostic indicators are supported by multiple, statistically robust clinical trials:[207]

1. Local extent of tumor defined as *depth of tumor penetration*
2. Serosal involvement by tumor
3. Regional lymph node involvement
4. Nodal micrometastases, where lymph nodes that contain a tumor measuring 3 mm or larger in diameter are considered positive, while those containing tumor measuring 0.2 mm or smaller or identified by nonhistologic means such as polymerase chain reaction or immunostaining are considered micrometastases
5. Lymphatic or vascular invasion (LVI), which predicts local or regional recurrence regardless of tumor status
6. Residual tumor following definitive therapy
7. Elevated preoperative serum level of CEA $\geq$ 5.0 ng/mL, which predicts reduced survival

Classification and Staging

TNM staging is the most widely accepted form of staging for rectal cancer, yet some clinicians may use Duke's stage (see Table 49-14). The most important predictor of survival is stage at presentation. Five-year survival rates by stage are as follows: stage I, 79%; stage II, 52%; stage III, 37%; and stage IV, 4%. Each stage has a lower five-year survival rate than the comparable stage of colon cancer.[208] Stage III rectal cancer patients are now stratified into three subsets, each with a different prognosis.[209] Stage IIIA patients with T1–2, N1 lesions have a five-year survival rate of 39% when treated with surgery alone, compared to 55.1% (relative survival, 67.2%) when surgery is followed by adjuvant chemotherapy and radiation therapy. Stage IIIB patients with T3–4, N1 lesions have a five-year survival rate of 21.7% when treated with surgery alone, com-

Table 49-14 Staging for Rectal Cancer

Stage	Tumor	Nodal Status	Metastases	Duke's Stage
0	Tis (in situ intraepithelial or invades lamina propria)	N0 (no metastasis in the lymph nodes)	M0 (no distant metastasis)	—
I	T1 (invades submucosa)	N0	M0	A
	T2 (invades muscularis propria)	N0	M0	A
IIA	T3 (through muscularis propria into subserosa or into nonperitonealized pericolic or perirectal tissue)	N0	M0	B
IIB	T4 (directly invades other organs or structures, and/or perforates visceral peritoneum)	N0	M0	B
IIIA	T1–T2	N1 (metastasis to 1–3 regional lymph nodes)	M0	C
IIIB	T3–T4	N1	M0	C
IIIC	Any T	N2 (metastasis to 4 or more regional lymph nodes)	M0	C
IV	Any T	Any N	M1 (distant metastasis)	D

Data from Greene FL, Page DS, Fleming ID, et al, American Joint Committee on Cancer: *AJCC Cancer Staging Manual*, (ed 6). New York, Springer-Verlag, 2002.[139]

pared to 40.9% with surgery plus adjuvant therapy. Stage IIIC patients have any T, N2 disease and a 12.2% five-year survival rate, which increases to 28.9% when treated with surgery combined with chemotherapy and radiation. Staging is done preoperatively as clinical staging (''c'' prefix) and postoperatively by the pathologist (indicated with a ''p'' prefix). If neoadjuvant therapy is given, such as preoperative chemotherapy, a ''y'' prefix is used, and an ''r'' prefix signifies cancers that have recurred.[199]

Therapeutic Approaches and Nursing Care

Table 49-15 details strategies developed by leading experts for the management of rectal cancer. The approaches have become widely adopted as the standard of care.

Surgery

The successful management of rectal cancer has five goals: cure, local control, restoration of intestinal continuity, preservation of anorectal sphincter function, and preservation of the patient's sexual and urinary function. Because of the anatomical constraints of the bony pelvis, it may be difficult in some cases to achieve adequate sphincter, sexual, and urinary function without compromising cure and local control.[210]

Local control is an extremely important aspect of treatment. As many as 25% of the patients who die of rectal cancer will have local recurrence only; another 50% will have local recurrence in addition to distant disease. For patients with local recurrence after initial treatment for rectal cancer, additional surgery rarely has advantages. Many of these patients with advanced disease experience significant problems with bone and nerve pain, hemorrhage, pelvic sepsis, and bowel and urinary obstruction.

The surgical procedure employed for rectal cancer depends on the stage and depth of tumor invasion of the mucosa. Total mesorectal excision is the standard, in which the tumor, blood vessels, and lymphatics are removed to decrease the risk of locoregional recurrence, since lymphatic spread from rectal cancers occurs upward, lateral, and distal. Criteria for a local, transanal excision are that the tumor is less than 30% of the bowel circumference, smaller than 3 cm in size, resectable with clear margins (T1 lesion), mobile, within 8 cm of the anal verge, without LVI (lymphatic or vascular invasion); well to moderately well differentiated; and grade 1–2.[199] A low anterior resection (LAR) or coloanal anastomosis (CAA) is appropriate for uncomplicated lesions in the mid and upper rectum.[18] Either procedure will preserve the sympathetic and parasympathetic nerves as long as there is adequate blood supply, sphincter muscle function, and no tension at the anastamosis.[211]

If the sphincter muscles are involved or the tumor extends to within 2 cm of the dentate line, abdominoperineal resection (APR) with sacrifice of the sphincter is necessary. This radical surgical approach involves transabdominal resection of the rectum and mesorectum from the level of the inferior mesenteric vessels to the levator muscles, in combination with transperineal excision of the anus and distal rectum.[146] APR is

Table 49-15 Management of Rectal Cancer

Stage of Disease	Primary Treatment	Adjuvant Treatment
T1–2, N0		
• T1–2, N0, M0	Abdominoperineal resection, low anterior resection, or coloanal anastomosis (total mesorectal excision)	Observe
• pT3, N0, M0 or T1–3, N1–2	Abdominoperineal resection, low anterior resection, or coloanal anastomosis (total mesorectal excision)	5-FU +/– LV, then CI 5-FU/XRT or capecitabine/XRT, then 5-FU +/– LV
• T1, NX, negative margins after primary treatment	Transanal excision (if tumor < 30% of bowel circumference, < 3 cm in size, clear margins, mobile, within 8 cm of anal verge, no LVI, well- to moderately well differentiated, grade 1–2.	Observe
• T1–2, NX, positive margins, LVI, grade 3–4 after primary treatment	Transanal excision (if tumor < 30% of bowel circumference, < 3 cm in size, clear margins, mobile, within 8 cm of anal verge)	Abdominoperineal resection, low anterior resection, or coloanal anastomosis (total mesorectal excision)
• T2, NX, margins clear	Transanal excision (if tumor < 30% of bowel circumference, < 3 cm in size, clear margins, mobile, within 8 cm of anal verge, no LVI, well- to moderately well differentiated, grade 1–2)	Abdominoperineal resection, low anterior resection, or coloanal anastomosis (total mesorectal excision) or 5-FU/XRT
T3, N0 or T any, N1–2	Preoperative 5-FU/XRTfor lymph node–positive patients, or capecitabine/XRT; then abdominoperineal resection, low anterior resection, or coloanal anastomosis (total mesorectal excision.	5-FU +/– LV or FOLFOX
	Abdominoperineal resection, low anterior resection, or coloanal anastomosis using mesorectal excision alone	pT1–2, N0, M0: observe pT3, N0, M0 or pT1–3, N1-2: 5-FU +/– LV or FOLFOX; then CI 5-FU/XRT or capecitabine/XRT, then 5-FU +/– LV or FOLFOX
T4	CI IV 5-FU/XRT or capecitabine/XRT, followed by resection if possible	5-FU +/– LV
T any, N any, M1 resectable	CI IV 5-FU/XRT followed by resection of tumor and metastasic lesion(s), or	5-FU +/– LV or FOLFOX or FOLFIRI
	FOLFOX or FOLFIRI for 2–3 months, followed by resection of tumor and metastatic lesions, or	Optional 5-FU/pelvic XRT
	Resection of tumor and metastatic lesion(s)	T1–2, N0, M1: 5-FU +/– LV or FOLFOX or FOLFIRI for 4–6 months
		T3–4, any N, or any T, N1–2: 5-FU +/– LV or FOLFOX, then CI 5-FU/XRT or capecitabine/XRT, then 5-FU +/– LV
T any, N any, M1 unresectable	Options include resection of tumor, diverting colostomy, stenting, laser photocoagulation, 5-FU/XRT, single-modality chemotherapy	Chemotherapy regimens: First line: FOLFOX, FOLFIRI, bevacizumab + 5-FU–based regimen *if patient can tolerate aggressive therapy*; if not, capecitabine, 5-FU/LV, or 5-FU CI Second line: FOLFOX or FOLFIRI (depending on first-line chemotherapy), irinotecan +/– cetuximab

Data from de Gramont et al[171,174,177]; Goldberg et al[186]; Hurwitz et al[187]; Cunningham et al,[188]; Peters et al, [190]; *NCCN Practice Guidelines in Oncology: Rectal Cancer*, v. 3.2004[199]; Tominaga et al, [206]; Jessup et al[208]; Greene et al[209]; Minsky, [210]; Kodner et al.[211]

NX = nodal status unknown; LVI = lymphovascular invasion; XRT = radiation therapy; pTNM = pathological TNM staging; 5-FU = 5-fluorouracil; LV = leucovorin; XRT = radiation therapy; CI = continuous infusion currently indicated for tumors of the distal third of the rectum within 3 cm of the anal verge, tumors involving the anal–sphincter musculature, tumors of the recto-vaginal septum, patients with poor continence preoperatively, and patients with diarrheal disorders.[146]

In recent years, the use of adjuvant therapy, the introduction of circular stapling devices, and the demonstrated adequacy of 2 cm distal margins have allowed safe use of sphincter-preserving surgery for resection of midrectal and some distal rectal cancers.[146] In low anterior resection, as described earlier, the dissection and anastomosis are performed below the peritoneal reflection.

A coloanal anastomosis preserves the sphincter mechanism in patients with low-lying rectal tumors whose negative distal margin of resection is up to, but does not include, the anal–sphincter musculature. The operative dissection is similar to that of LAR and APR, with transection of the distal margin at the level of the levator ani muscles within the abdomen. Through a perineal approach, the remaining anal mucosa is stripped and an anastomosis is made between the colon and the anus to restore intestinal continuity.[146] Some surgeons will hand suture the anastomosis at this level rather than using a stapling device. To provide adequate bowel length and a tension-free anastomosis, the splenic flexure of the colon is completely mobilized. The vascular supply of the left colon is then based on the middle colic artery. The surgeon will perform a protective diverting ileostomy in all patients who have coloanal anastomosis. Contraindications for an LAR or coloanal anastomosis include tumors involving the anal–sphincter musculature, tumors involving the rectovaginal septum, patients with poor continence preoperatively, patients with diarrhea disorders, and unfavorable anatomical constraints (e.g., obesity, narrow pelvis).

The success and options presented to patients for surgical management of rectal cancers depend on the skill of the surgeon. Meyerhardt and colleagues[212] studied the impact of hospital procedure volume on surgical operation and long-term outcomes in high-risk (stage II and III), curatively resected patients with rectal cancer. They found a significant difference in the rates of APR as a function of hospital procedure volume: a 46% rate in low-volume hospitals compared to a 31.8% rate in high-volume hospitals.

Radiation Therapy

Combined modality therapy with chemotherapy and radiation therapy has a significant role in the management of patients with rectal cancer (below the peritoneal reflection). Randomized clinical trials have shown that adjuvant chemotherapy combined with radiation therapy improves survival for patients with stage II and III rectal cancer.[213] In clinical practice, there is considerable variation in physicians offering this option to their patients with rectal cancer, based on age, race, marital status, hospital volume, and individual hospital.[213] Three-dimensional, conformal radiation treatment planning is used in many centers for more precise targeting of radiation, because it yields an improved ability to plan and localize the target and normal tissues of treatment volume as compared to traditional radiation therapy. In one study, however, it provided only a marginal benefit in sparing normal tissues.[18]

When considering preoperative radiation, it is important to note that tumor cells are often well oxygenated because the blood supply to the tumor has not been surgically manipulated. Well-oxygenated cells are believed to have increased radiosensitivity; as a consequence, tumor cell killing by radiotherapy may be increased.[214] Despite these radiobiologic advantages, preoperative radiation has not affected overall rates of survival, distant recurrence, or cure rates.[210] However, locoregional tumor control rates have improved with preoperative radiation. Randomized studies have shown a significant decrease in local recurrence rates when preoperative doses of radiotherapy were higher than 34.5 Gy.[210] Additionally, one study reported a 91% sphincter preservation rate for patients with T3 and T4 lesions treated with 45 Gy of preoperative radiotherapy.[215] Local control and overall survival have reached acceptable levels with this approach, and 10% of patients in this series achieved a complete pathological response.[214]

Radiotherapy is most commonly used following surgical resection. The advantages of pursuing postoperative radiotherapy are that (1) adequate pathology data are available to evaluate the extent of disease, (2) patients who will not benefit from therapy are not treated, and (3) surgical treatment is not delayed. Despite the multiple research approaches, the rates of survival, local pelvic control, and extrapelvic recurrence have not been improved consistently with postoperative radiation of 45–50 Gy.[214,215] In a large cohort study comparing preoperative to postoperative radiotherapy, a significant decrease in local recurrence was found in the group that received preoperative therapy compared to the postoperative therapy group.[216]

Intraoperative radiation therapy (IORT) and stereotactic radiation therapy are innovative approaches to the treatment of colorectal cancer. IORT provides high-dose radiation therapy during an operative procedure directly to a localized area, such as an inoperable colorectal tumor, locally recurrent colorectal cancer, and residual disease after resection. High-energy radiation can be delivered while significantly reducing radiation exposure to adjacent tissues. To provide IORT, the facility must have a designated operating room or radiation suite, radiation equipment that is able to deliver electron or orthovoltage beams, computer planning equipment, and extensive coordination by the multidisciplinary healthcare team.

Patient selection for IORT is usually based on the following criteria:

1. Surgery alone will not achieve local control.
2. An external beam radiation therapy (EBRT) dose of 60–70 Gy or greater is needed for a curative attempt.
3. IORT will be performed at the same time as a planned operative procedure.
4. The IORT plus EBRT technique would theoretically result in a more suitable therapeutic ratio between cure and complications.
5. There is no evidence of distant metastases or peritoneal seeding.[217]

IORT requires extensive preoperative planning and intraoperative collaboration between the radiation oncologist and the surgeon. The procedure starts with the surgical exposure of the tumor. IORT may be delivered prior to excision of the tumor or after the mass is removed. Specialized electron cones are placed within the surgical cavity where a 15–20 Gy dose of radiation will be delivered. Potential complications and nursing implications are reviewed in a later section of this chapter.

Stereotactic radiation (SRT) is a precise method for the delivery of focused radiation beams for small, well-defined lesions. It enables the radiation oncologist to treat a limited area within an organ and minimizes or prevents the radiation dose being delivered to adjacent normal tissue. There are three primary treatment delivery methods for SRT: (1) gamma knife: cobalt-60 gamma radiation; (2) linear accelerator: high-energy photon; and (3) heavy charged particle beams (e.g., proton, helium, neon).[218]

For rectal tumors, the rate of locoregional recurrence has been reduced by the use of radiation therapy. Preoperative radiation therapy has demonstrated a reduction in local tumor recurrence, but has not affected overall survival for patients with stage II or III rectal cancers. A combination of 5-FU–based chemotherapy and radiation given postoperatively is the most effective adjuvant therapy for patients with stage II or III rectal cancer. Radiation doses of 45–55 Gy are recommended in combination with 5-FU–based chemotherapy. Preoperative chemoradiation may be more effective than postoperative adjuvant treatment, especially in patients with T3 or T4 lesions. Such treatment may improve resectability and produce fewer complications compared to the postoperative treatment.[2] IORT can be used to treat advanced, recurrent, or inoperable rectal cancer. Unresectable rectal tumors may be treated with palliative radiation.

Injury to the bowel may occur as a result of radiation therapy. Some side effects of radiation may require surgical intervention, but most such effects subside when radiation therapy is stopped. Chronic radiation enteritis can lead to bowel mucosal thinning and inflammation, eventually resulting in ulceration.

Radiation therapy is used as palliation for advanced rectal cancer symptoms. The pain from the local recurrence of rectal cancer is very difficult to control. Advanced rectal cancer is treated with 5-FU combinations, either by bolus injection or by continuous infusion, in combination with oxaliplatin or irinotecan as shown in Table 49-10. The dose-limiting toxicities of continuous 5-FU infusion are mucositis and diarrhea. Palmar-plantar erythrodysesthesia (hand–foot syndrome) has also been noted with protracted infusions of 5-FU.[185] The dose-limiting toxicity of oxaliplatin is chronic, persistent sensory neuropathy, while the comparable toxicities of irinotecan are diarrhea and neutropenia.

Chemotherapy

Adjuvant chemotherapy is recommended for patients with tumors having positive circumferential or radial margins (CRM). For rectal cancers without a peritonealized surface, the external surface is considered a CRM.[207] It is positive when the distance from the tumor to this margin surface is less than 1 mm. Because of the bony pelvis limitation, surgeons may find it difficult to achieve wide resection margins. A positive margin is one of the most important predictive factors for both local and distant recurrence. In addition, patients with stage II and III rectal cancers are at high risk of recurrence. Thus, aggressive adjuvant chemotherapy combined with radiotherapy is used to reduce local recurrence and increase overall survival. For patients with metastatic rectal cancer, the NCCN guidelines suggest that single, isolated metastases may be resected together with the primary rectal lesion, followed by adjuvant chemotherapy and radiotherapy to the pelvis. For patients with unresectable metastases, FOLFOX 4 is one of several treatment options that is effective as palliative therapy.

Molecular Targeted Therapy

See the discussion for colon cancer on bevacuzimab and cetuximab, both of which are indicated in combination with chemotherapy for the treatment of advanced rectal cancer.

Symptom Management and Supportive Care

Patients who have an APR will have a permanent sigmoid or descending colostomy; those who undergo a LAR or CAA, may have a temporary ileostomy. All of these patients will benefit from consultation with a CWOCN (i.e., ET nurse) from the first visit when they are told the diagnosis through the preoperative and postoperative phases. Nursing management focuses on early recognition of potential problems.

Postoperative care is focused on facilitating an uncomplicated recovery with healing of the operative site and recovery of baseline function and patterns. If the patient has a stoma, another goal is to empower the individual to effectively care for it. Nurses play a critical role in providing patient education, emotional support, and coordination of care across care boundaries.

Perineal Wound Healing

The perineal wound or incisional site may be closed immediately following the removal of the rectum, anus, muscle, and fatty tissue, or it may be left open to heal by secondary intention. Primary closure of the perineal wound site at the time of surgery is the preferred technique, because it is more comfortable for the patient and requires much less care. Closed suction drains are inserted at the time of surgery and exit either through the incisional area or through a separate stab wound in the buttocks. The drains are removed on the third or fifth postoperative day. Primary closure is contraindicated when fecal spillage occurs, the bowel is perforated, an infected hematoma is present, or there is perineal disease such as abscess or fistula.

Perineal wound healing by secondary intention prolongs the healing process, which may take as long as four months. The wound requires packing and meticulous care to promote granulation and to avoid infection or sepsis. Irrigations and sitz baths facilitate wound healing. The drainage and healing process must be carefully monitored by the nurses, and any untoward signs and symptoms of infection must be reported to the primary surgeon. Nursing care can range from complex dressing changes to washing the area with soap and water, monitoring intake and output, and checking for patency of drainage tubes.

Stoma and Colostomy Management

Careful selection of the stoma site by the CWOCN and surgeon is an important step toward ensuring the patient's quality of life after surgery. By assessing the patient's abdomen in lying, sitting, and standing positions, the healthcare provider can ensure that the selected stoma site is within the rectus muscle and is in an area that can physically support ostomy equipment. It is important that the patient is able to visualize the proposed stoma site so that self-care will be easier.[219] Scars, folds, bony prominences, belt and waistlines, and the umbilicus need to be avoided to ensure proper fit of the ostomy equipment. The anatomical location of the stoma influences the abdominal quadrant placement as well as the surgical technique employed.

The stoma must be evaluated for viability, condition, size, and shape, and it must be determined whether all sutures are holding the everted stoma onto the abdomen. A red, shiny, moist, budded, or flush stoma with all sutures and peristomal skin intact is the desired outcome. Deviations from this finding should be reported to the surgeon, as they may indicate early problems and require immediate surgical intervention.[219]

Psychological support of the patient begins preoperatively with an explanation of the surgery to be performed and introduction to the pouching system and equipment. After surgery, support shifts to coping and adaptation, particularly when the patient first looks at his or her stoma, which can be very upsetting. The initial size of the stoma will depend on the portion of the bowel segment involved and any bowel obstruction that existed prior to surgery. The initial bowel edema gradually subsides following surgery, and the actual stoma size is established in six to eight weeks.[219] This is an important variable to remember when preparing the pouch opening to ensure proper sizing.

Initially the patient will have serosanguineous fluid in the pouch. The time at which the stoma begins to function depends on the preoperative cleansing and prior obstruction. If this was an emergent surgery or poor cleansing was performed, stool will be present almost immediately. Once peristalsis returns and flatus is passed, food is introduced. Stool will soon be expelled from the stoma. Usually, the more proximal a stoma is in the bowel, the sooner it functions and the more liquid the stool content.

The key principles in stoma management include the containment of the effluent and odor and the protection of the peristomal skin. The degree of skin protection required is dictated by the characteristics of the effluent. Effluent that is proteolytic, highly acidic, or highly alkaline (ileostomy, cecostomy, ascending colostomy) requires meticulous protection of peristomal skin. Nonenzymatic effluent with a pH that is essentially neutral primarily requires protection against pooling of drainage that can macerate the skin (descending/sigmoid colostomies).

Equipment costs vary but are reimbursable to some degree by Medicare and most private insurers. Certain agencies help with the costs for those individuals who have particular needs; however, these groups differ across the country. A CWOCN is usually aware of various groups that provide assistance in a specific region. Patient teaching proceeds in a stepwise fashion from the simple to the complex. Asking the patient what he or she wants to learn first may relieve some of the patient's anxiety. With a family member or significant other present to serve as a backup caregiver when the patient is at home, the teaching usually proceeds from removing or applying the pouch closure clamp, to looking at and cleansing the stoma, to applying and emptying the pouch. The goal is for the patient to independently manage the pouch changing and stoma care prior to discharge.

The shorter length of stay in hospitals has made it difficult to include colostomy irrigation teaching prior to discharge. Individuals usually learn to perform colostomy irrigation and thus regulate evacuation from their clinic or home health nurse.[219]

Case managers coordinating the discharge plan for the patient should be encouraged to recommend home health agencies with CWOCN consultants to ensure continuity of care and management of any peristomal complications. Many hospital-based CWOCN consultants will also see outpatients for postdischarge care and instruction. Individualized patient education materials, mail-order catalogs and a list of the supplies, names of community vendors, and support groups at the United Ostomy Association or the American Cancer Society are available to facilitate patients' self-care.

Sexual Dysfunction

Early-stage rectal cancer treated with resection of the rectal lesion may interfere with an individual's potential for orgasm, although erectile dysfunction is less common. In contrast, patients who undergo more extensive surgery have a far higher incidence of sexual dysfunction, especially males. A study of 60 men who were sexually active prior to pretreatment and who received either high anterior resection, low anterior resection, or abdominoperineal resection demonstrated that patients in the APR arm had the highest percentage of sexual problems. Sixty-five percent became sexually inactive, 50% were unable to ejaculate, and 45% reported erectile dysfunction.[220]

Patients with ostomies can become concerned with their body image as they worry about stoma appearance, stool collecting in the pouch, pouch leakage, sounds, and odors. These can all cause the person to feel unattractive and to have a diminished libido. Fear of rejection by one's significant other can cause stress in the relationship and have a negative impact on the patient's self-concept. Support for the patient and significant other includes the following:[221]

1. *Depression or anxiety.* Antidepressants may be useful but some drugs can interfere with erectile function; prescribing physicians should consult with a pharmacist.
2. *Fatigue.* Napping prior to sexual activity as well as avoiding heavy meals and alcohol can be helpful. Trying different positions during sexual activity that require minimal effort, such as the side-lying position, may be helpful.
3. *Pain.* Timing of medication is important to provide pain control without drowsiness. Relaxation techniques, warm baths or soaks, and massage may decrease pain and can be an opportunity for sexual foreplay when done as a couple.
4. *Nausea.* Meditating prior to sexual activity is often suggested. A light meal or crackers prior to activity may also be helpful. Usual accoutrements of sexual activity, such as perfumes, colognes, and scented candles, may have to be avoided if smells cause nausea.
5. *Odors.* Elimination ostomies should be emptied prior to sexual activity. Deodorizers or odor eliminators are available if odors are a concern. Pouch covers are also available to shield the pouch contents.

Ureteral Obstruction

With advanced rectal cancer, bilateral ureteral obstruction can occur as a result of direct tumor compression of the ureters. Individuals with ureteral obstruction present with oliguria and elevated serum creatinine. A cystoscopy and bilateral retrograde pyelogram are the most reliable diagnostic tools for determining ureteral obstruction. These exams also determine whether the obstruction is intrinsic to the ureter or extrinsic, as would be seen with an advancing colorectal lesion.

Treatment of ureteral obstruction may be accomplished at the time of the retrograde pyelogram. Urinary stents can be inserted into the ureters to establish patency and prevent further compression by the tumor. Stents can circumvent the need for a surgical procedure. If the ureteral stents become occluded, they can be usually changed via cystoscopy. In some situations, however, urinary stents cannot be utilized because of ureteral strictures or inability to visualize the ureters. In such cases, percutaneous nephrostomy tubes can be used to treat the obstruction. Nephrostomy tubes placed directly into the kidney via a percutaneous approach allow adequate urinary drainage from the renal pelvis.

Liver Metastases

Similar to the symptoms experienced by a patient with advanced colon cancer, a patient with rectal cancer metastatic to the liver may develop nausea, vomiting, anorexia, referred pain in the shoulder, abdominal pain, ascites with increasing shortness of breath, dyspnea on exertion, pruritus, cachexia, peripheral edema, and fatigue. Patients with rectal cancer may experience symptoms of intermittent obstruction, as well as pain and dysfunction depending on the organs involved by local invasion. Nursing care is directed toward support and symptom management to help the patient maximize the quality of life for the time remaining. Community resources such as hospice should be consulted early in the period of advanced disease so that relationships can be established, and a symptom management plan can be instituted when needed.

Follow-up

Approximately 60% of whites and 52% of blacks diagnosed with rectal cancer will be alive at the five-year mark.[76] Because the course of treatment and follow-up for rectal carcinoma including follow-up can span many years, there must be provision for continuity of care.

The NCCN identifies recommended follow-up based on stage of disease and treatment.[199] Patients should have a history and physical every 3 months for 2 years, then every 6 months for a total of 5 years. CEA measurements should generally be repeated every 3 months for 2 years; for patients with T2 or greater lesions, they should be repeated every 6 months for 2–5 years. Colonoscopy should be performed in 1 year following treatment, then repeated in 1 year if abnormal or at least every 2–3 years if negative for polyps. If the patient did not have a preoperative colonoscopy due to obstruction, then it should be performed 3–6 months after initial treatment.

Conclusion

Screening and early detection strategies must be perfected so that patients will be diagnosed earlier, especially in minority communities. Adenomatous polyps can be removed to prevent rectal cancer. If a tumor is not prevented, it can be cured when diagnosed early and removed by endoscopy. In addition, fecal DNA testing offers more efficient screening. In terms of treatment, prospective clinical trials of pathologic predictors such as molecular flaws and genetic mutations will produce mature data in the next few years, which will help stratify patients requiring aggressive adjuvant therapy. Continued improvements in combination chemotherapy, radiation therapy, and molecular targeted therapy will offer improved control in both the adjuvant and the metastatic settings.

Anal Cancer

Introduction

Anal canal cancer is an uncommon yet curable cancer. Several subcategories of disease with different risks and etiologies exist. In HIV-positive men and women who have receptive anal intercourse, cancer results from sexually transmitted human paillomavirus (HPV) infection. The incidence of this disease increased markedly in the 1980s in relation to HIV infection, and it appears to be increasing with the prolongation of longevity in HIV-positive men who have sex with men. Diamond and colleagues[222] found that since the arrival of highly active antiretroviral therapy (HAART), HIV-infected men who had sex with men had an increasing annual incidence from 1996 (when HAART was introduced) to 2000. In non-HIV-positive populations, the etiology of anal cancer is less clear. Effective combination chemotherapy and radiation treatment results in an 80% five-year survival rate for most patients, with sphincter preservation.[223] For patients with recurrence or progression, APR may result in cure.

Epidemiology and Etiology

Anal cancer represents less than 4% of all gastrointestinal cancers, but, as noted earlier, its incidence is increasing. ACS estimated that 4010 people would develop anal cancer in 2004, resulting in 580 deaths: 1890 men (210 deaths) and 2120 women (370 deaths).[1] More women (17%) are expected to die of anal cancer than men (11%)[1]. In a study of patients who were diagnosed during the period 1988–1993, more women than men were diagnosed, most patients were white, most patients had squamous cell histology (75%–80%), and 75% had stage II or II tumors.[223] About 80% of anal cancers are diagnosed in patients age 60 or older, but in patients younger than age 35, men are more frequently affected than women.[224] Anal cancer in HIV-infected men and women appears to be related to the sexual transmission of HPV-16 by receptive anal intercourse, resulting in the initial mutational event. The incidence of anal cancer among single men is said to be six times higher than that among married men.[2] A history of genital warts (condylomata) is also associated with anal cancer, again suggesting that HPV may be a causative factor. Pfister and Fuchs[225] showed that HPV-16 infection is associated with high-grade anal intraepithelial neoplasia (AIN) and risk of anal cancer, but many patients with HPV-16–positive cytologies do not develop anogenic cancer.[223] Other sexually transmitted diseases besides genital warts have been linked to increased risk for anal cancer. Daling and colleagues[226] showed an association between seropositivity for herpes simplex type I and *Chlamydia trachomatis* infections in women, and gonorrhea in men. Anal fissures and fistulae have been studied, but greater risk may exist only in the first year following their development. In one study, smoking was seen as a risk factor independent of sexual behavior.[227]

Immunosuppression, either induced by radiation therapy or by pharmacologic means such as that for to prevent transplant rejection, increases one's risk for the development of anal cancer.[228] Patients who have undergone renal transplant have 100-fold higher risk. Patients with HIV infection have a 15–30 times higher risk, with risk increasing as CD4 levels fall below 200/μL.[223] Another study showed that homosexual men who were HIV positive had a 13.9 relative risk, which jumped to 84.1 when the infection evolved into AIDS.[223] Thus the two main risk factors that have been highly correlated with the development of anal cancer are HPV infection (especially HPV-16) and immunosuppression.[223]

Prevention, Screening, and Early Detection

Prevention strategies are based on known etiology. Because the risk for anal cancer appears to be related to receptive anal intercourse in many patients, especially HIV-infected patients, protective sexual practices and screening should be encouraged. In one study involving female subjects, Friis and colleagues[229] found that (1) women with more than 10 lifetime sexual partners had a five times greater risk for anal cancer compared to women with one lifetime partner; (2) women who had more than four partners before the age of 20 had a three times higher risk than women who had not had intercourse before age 20; and (3) women with anal warts had a tenfold increased risk, while women with a prior history of sexually transmitted diseases or cervical neoplasia also had increased risk. As has been the practice for more than two decades, all individuals who are sexually active should be encouraged to use condoms during sexual activity. Indeed, for those who engage in receptive anal intercourse, condoms are critical. This information should be provided to all sexually active individuals, as some may be engaging in anal intercourse and not be HIV infected.

For those individuals at risk (i.e., those with immunosuppression and the possibility of HPV-16 infection), screening for anal cancer should begin early. The standard for screening is an anal Pap smear followed by high-resolution anoscopy. The value of screening for AIN in homosexual and bisexual HIV-infected individuals has been shown to be cost-effective and results in improved survival.[230,231] In Canada, the risk for developing anal cancer in HIV-positive men is 163-fold compared to non-HIV infected men. Salit and colleagues[232] reported preliminary data for their anal cancer screening program in HIV-positive men. Seventy-five of a total of 680 HIV-positive men were screened using anal Pap smears, HPV detection, and high-resolution anoscopy. High-risk oncogenic HPV was found in 80% of patients; Pap smears were abnormal in 70% of the patients, with high-grade changes (high-grade squamous intraepithelial lesions, HSIL) in 17% and low-grade changes (low-grade squamous intraepithelial lesions, LSIL) in 38%; anal biopsies were abnormal in 56% of the patients, with a distribution of 25% LSIL, 28% HSIL, and 1% anal cancer. As shown in this emerging study, anoscopists and pathologists must agree on the diagnostic criteria when analyzing anoscopic digital images, histopathology, and cytopathology. In addition, large, prospective studies remain to be done.[233] Often symptoms of anal cancer, such as bleeding, pain, and a sensation of fullness, are attributed to hemorrhoids or anal fissure, with resulting delay in evaluation and diagnosis.

Pathophysiology

The anus is the terminal 4–6 cm of the gastrointestinal tract, and the anal canal connects the rectum to the perianal skin (see Figure 49-6). It is lined by an epithelial mucous membrane that covers the internal sphincter[227] and is responsible for maintaining continence. The anal canal is that region extending from the anal verge to the rectal mucosa. Another way of describing this area is as the area between the anal verge and the anorectal ring. The anorectal ring is easily palpable and corresponds to the junction of a portion of the levator muscle with the external anal sphincter. The dentate line is located at the transition zone, where the columnar epithelium of the proximal canal meets the stratified squamous epithelium of the lower canal. The anal glands empty here.[223] Squamous cell tumors may develop in the anal canal or the anal margin. Cloacogenic carcinomas develop above the dentate line. Adnocarcinomas arise from the glands located at the dentate line. Anal margin tumors may consist of squamous cell, basal cell, Bowen or Paget's disease, verrucous carcinoma, or Kaposi's sarcoma. Melanomas tend to develop below the dentate line.[223]

The arteries supplying the distal rectum and anal canal are the superior, middle, and inferior hemorrhoidal arteries; venous drainage parallels the arteries. Sympathetic nerves innervate the internal rectal sphincter muscles, while parasympathetic fibers in sacrum sense distention of the rectum and anus. Lymphatic vessels drain the anal canal via the inguinal, pelvic visceral, and hypogastric nodes, which are interconnected, and ultimately empty into the para-aortic nodes.[223]

Cellular Characteristics

Most anal cancers are squamous cell (epidermoid) carcinomas. Less common cell types are cloacogenic, basaloid, transitional, and mucoepidermoid carcinomas.[2] Tumors in the anal canal are keratinized squamous cell carcinomas, whereas those arising in the transitional zone or above are nonkeratinizing transitional cell or cloacogenic carcinomas.[234] Unusual tumors arising in the anal canal include small cell carcinomas, melanomas, and adenocarcinomas. Small cell carcinomas of the anal canal are aggressive and signal early distant metastases; adenocarcinomas carry a poor prognosis and should be managed aggressively with multimodality treatment.[223]

Non-oncogenic human papillomavirus types 6 and 11 are implicated in the formation of genital warts, in contrast to the oncogenic HPV-16, which is associated with both cervical and anal cancers. HPV-16 is responsible for about 50% of cervical cancers, and with HPV-18, -31, and -45 in another 20% of cervical cancers.[235] The malignant transformation may be related to the two viral proteins E7 and E6 which bind to the tumor suppressor gene products *Rb* and *p53* in the anal epithelial mucosal cells. The proteins E7 and E6 help the virus divide and infect the epithelial cell DNA. Likewise, *Rb* and *p53* protect against uncontrolled cell growth and the inclusion of mutated DNA into the cell's DNA. Once the viral genetic material is incorporated into the anal mucosal cells' DNA, cell division results in E6 and E7 proteins being transcribed, causing the cell to move from premalignant to malignant. HPV genetic material is commonly found in the DNA of anal cancer cells.[236] HIV apparently enhances the malignant transformation, a result that is believed to be due to the HIV tat protein, which helps to produce more E6 and E7.[237]

The first changes seen clinically are similar to those found in HPV-induced cervical cancer. HPV first causes dysplasia in the epithelial mucosal cells: low-grade squamous intraepithelial lesions are called LSIL while high-grade lesions are called HSIL (which includes moderate and severe dysplasia, as well as carcinoma in situ). HIV infection, history of receptive anal intercourse, and lower CD4 levels are associated with HSIL. Analogous to the location of cervical dysplastic changes, dysplasia occurs in the transition zone, where the columnar epithelial cells (tall, narrow cells) in the upper part of the anal canal meet the squamous (flat) cells of the lower part of the anal canal, and where the columnar cells are continually changed into squamous cells. There is hyperplasia, angiogenesis, and loss of apoptosis (programmed cell death).[238] As in cervical cancer, the Pap smear in the anal canal is performed here at the transition zone.

The risk for developing anal cancer in HIV-positive men doubles from 15 to 30 times as the CD4 levels falls, and is increased if the patient is also infected with other oncogenic strains of HPV. It is unknown how rapidly the progression from HSIL occurs, if it occurs at all. Nevertheless, it appears that for HIV-infected patients, as their survival increases thanks to HAART, patients with unknown HSIL will progress to invasive squamous cell cancer.[239] Use of the Pap test in screening may identify dysplastic changes in the anal epithelial cells.

Progression of Disease

The distribution of anal and perianal cancers can be predicted based on the anatomy because the tumor usually spreads by direct extension, through the lymphatic system, and via the bloodstream. Proximal tumors may spread upward for 5–6 cm before ulcerating into the rectum. Tumors extending locally rarely invade the bladder, sacrum, prostate, or vagina. While tumors in the anal margin are unlikely to metastasize, those in the anal canal may. Tumors developing on or above the dentate line tend to metastasize by the venous route into the portal system, with the ensuing development of liver, lung, or bone metastases in a small number of patients. Lymph node metastases are more common, with inguinal lymph node involvement in 15%–63% of patients.[223] Lymphatic drainage for anal cancer above the dentate line goes into the perirectal and paravertebral nodes similar to rectal adenocarcinoma, while tumors below this line drain into the inguinal and femoral lymph nodes.[220] Proximal lesions above the dentate line are more likely to involve the mesenteric nodes than distal lesions.

Clinical Manifestations

Many of the signs and symptoms of anal cancer are attributed to benign conditions such as hemorrhoids, even by primary care physicians. Common signs and symptoms are change in bowel elimination patterns, bleeding, anal discharge, anal mass, tenesmus, tenderness on palpation, pain on defecation, pruritus, and rarely inguinal lymph node swelling.

Assessment

Patient and Family History

A systematic history is taken, beginning with patient factors including present and past medical history, social history including sexual practices, history of sexually transmitted diseases (STDs), benign anal diseases such as fissure, and perineal condylomata. A complete symptom analysis should be performed of the presenting symptoms, asking about anal pruritus, bleeding, tenesmus, changes in bowel habits, anal discharge, and pain. In women, signs and symptoms should be elicited that would suggest tumor infiltration of the vagina. A detailed review of systems should follow.

Physical Examination

Physical examination includes a full examination, including digital rectal exam palpating for any lesions. An intraluminal mass should be described in terms of location, size, extent, and relationship to dentate line (Minsky). Most tumors are hard, indurated, and, as they enlarge, become fixed. Palpation for lymph nodes should be performed, especially the inguinal area. If lymph nodes are enlarged, a biopsy or fine-needle aspiration should be done.[234] In women, a vaginal exam should be done to rule out tumor infiltration.

Diagnostic Studies

The NCCN recommends that anoscopy as well as pelvic CT scan or MRI be performed as part of the workup for evaluation of anal canal cancers.[234] Pelvic CT or MRI may help determine whether pelvic or inguinal lymph nodes are involved with tumor. Transrectal ultrasound may prove helpful in defining depth of invasion and involvement of adjacent organs.[223] For more advanced lesions, an abdominal CT should also be performed to evaluate for liver metatastases and a chest x-ray should be obtained.[223] Anal lesions often appear flat or slightly raised with indurated borders and should be biopsied.[223] HIV testing should be performed, and, if positive, CD4 should be assessed.[234]

Prognostic Indicators

The most important prognostic factors in anal canal cancer are the size of the primary tumor and the extent of lymph node involvement.[2] If the tumor is 2 cm or smaller, the patient has a 80% likelihood of cure; by comparison, a patient with a tumor larger than 5 cm has a 50% chance of cure. However, if metastasis is present, then these factors no longer are important. Patients with T3 and T4 tumors (larger than 5 cm) have a 50% likelihood of recurrence even after combined modality therapy.[223] Anal margin cancers behave much like skin cancers and rarely metastasize.

Classification and Staging

Most anal cancers are squamous cell cancers and are treated with combined modality therapy, which is reflected in the staging. Table 49-16 depicts the AJCC staging for anal canal cancers.

Therapeutic Approaches and Nursing Care

The most common approaches to the management of anal cancer are reviewed in Table 49-17.[240–242] Early, in situ lesions may be curable by surgery alone, but most require multimodality therapy. Patients with stage IIIB anal canal cancer having positive inguinal nodes have a poor prognosis, although some may be cured. Available clinical trials should be discussed with these patients.

Surgery

Surgical resection alone is indicated only for small, in situ lesions that do not involve the anal sphincter, when it is expected that adequate surgical margins can be obtained. Unfortunately, most anal canal cancers are not detected at this early stage.[243] In the past, APR for anal canal tumors was considered the treatment of choice for stage I and II lesions, and resulted in a five-year survival rate of approximately 70%; today, survival is at least as likely using lower-dose radiation and chemotherapy with sphincter preservation.[244] Surgical resection is also indicated for the treatment of residual or recurrent anal canal cancer following nonsurgical

Table 49-16 Staging of Anal Canal Cancer

Stage	Tumor	Nodal Status	Metastases
0	Tis (carcinoma in situ)	N0 (no metastasis in the lymph nodes)	M0 (no distant metastasis)
I	T1 (tumor ≤ 2 cm in greatest dimension)	N0	M0
II	T2 (tumor > 2cm and < 5 cm in greatest dimension)	N0	M0
	T3 (tumor > 5 cm in greatest dimension)	N0	M0
IIIA	T1	N1 (metastasis in perirectal lymph nodes)	M0
	T2	N1 (metastasis in perirectal lymph nodes)	M0
	T3	N1 (metastasis in perirectal lymph nodes)	
	T4 (tumor of any size invades adjacent organ(s), such as vagina, urethra, or (bladder)	N0	M0
IIIB	T4	N1 (metastasis in perirectal lymph nodes)	M0
	Any T	N2 (metastasis in unilateral internal iliac and/or inguinal lymph nodes)	M0
	Any T	N3 (metastasis in perirectal and inguinal lymph nodes and/or bilateral internal iliac and/or inguinal lymph nodes)	M0
IV	Any T	Any N	M1

Data from Greene FL, Page DS, Fleming ID, et al, American Joint Committee on Cancer: *AJCC Cancer Staging Manual*, (ed 6). New York, Springer-Verlag, 2002.[139]

primary therapy.[234] Palliative surgery may be indicated for stage IV anal canal cancer.

In the care of HIV-infected patients with HSIL, Chang and colleagues[244] reported their prospective study of surgical treatment (excision and cautery) using high-resolution anoscopy. The procedure was effective in eliminating HSIL in HIV-negative patients, but the HIV-positive group showed a high degree of HSIL persistence and recurrence.

Radiation Therapy

Chemoradiation is the preferred treatment for anal cancers. Approximately 80%–90% of patients will achieve a complete response with combination therapy.[224] Stage I, II, and III anal canal cancers are treated with mitomycin/5-FU infusional therapy plus external beam radiotherapy as definitive therapy. A major clinical trial involving the Eastern Cooperative Oncology Group (ECOG) and the Radiation Therapy Oncology Group (RTOG) demonstrated that the addition of chemotherapy to radiation alone increased the disease-free survival rate from 51% to 73% (p = 0.0003) and resulted in a lower colostomy rate (9% compared to 22%, p = 0.002).[241] Five-year survival rates exceeding 70% have been noted.[2] Selected patients with small residual disease may be treated with a radiation boost plus chemotherapy or interstitial iridium-192, to achieve a complete response.[245] Palliative radiotherapy may be indicated alone, or in combination with chemotherapy, for treatment of stage IV anal canal cancer.

Chemotherapy

Flam and colleagues[241] demonstrated the efficacy of mitomycin together with 5-FU continuous infusion for anal canal cancer, in combination with external beam radiotherapy. However, mitomycin C has potentially severe side effects. Its principal toxicities are delayed myelosuppression with cumulative neutropenia and thrombocytopenia, nausea and vomiting, anorexia and fatigue, mucositis. The drug can also cause hemolytic–uremic syndrome that may be fatal, and interstitial pneumonitis. Hung and colleagues demonstrated in a phase II study that cisplatin in combination with 5-FU produced equivalent results with less toxicity.[242] Chemotherapy regimens are described in Table 49-18.

Molecular Targeted Therapy

Biotherapeutic approaches have not been used in the treatment of anal canal cancer. In one study by Sobhani and colleagues,[248] the authors found that HPV infection increased the number of dendritic cells in the anal mucosa in HIV-negative patients with anal condylomata. HIV-infected patients have significantly fewer dendritic cells, which may contribute to the development of invasive anal canal cancer. Dendritic cells are

Table 49-17 Management of Anal Canal Cancer

Stage	Primary Treatment	Comments
Tis	Local excision	Re-excision If inadequate margins or local XRT +/– 5-FU based chemotherapy
T1, N0	Mitomycin/5-FU plus XRT	PE including DRE at 8-12 weeks post-therapy; biospy if suspicious lesion or signs/symptoms of progressive disease -If recurrence, APR, +/– preceeded by 5-FU/cisplatin chemotherapy
T2-4, N0 or N+	Mitomycin/5-FU plus XRT (45-59 Gy)	PE including DRE at 8-12 weeks post-therapy; biospy if suspicious lesion or signs/symptoms of progressive disease -If recurrence, APR, +/– preceeded by 5-FU/cisplatin chemotherapy; if LN+ on groin dissection, XRT if not previously given -If distant metastasis, platinum-containing chemotherapy regimen

Data from: Allal et al[240]; Ellenhorn et al[224]; Flam et al[241]; Hung et al[242]; Minsky et al[223]; *NCCN Practice Guidelines in Oncology: Anal Canal Cancer*,[234]; Ryan DP et al[227]

NX = nodal status unknown; PE = physical exam; DRE = digital rectal exam; APR +c abdominoperineal resection; LVI = lymphovascular invasion; XRT = radiation therapy; pTNM = pathological TNM staging; 5-FU = 5-fluorouracil; LV = leucovorin; CI = continuous infusion

special, powerful immune cells that are antigen-presenting cells, responsible for activing T lymphocytes. Dendritic cell vaccines are being studied in melanoma and renal cell cancer and have a promising future in the treatment of cancers with identifiable, specific antigens. Unfortunately, there are no known specific antigens on anal cancer cells.

As molecular profiling is applied to anal canal cancer, the specific mutations and intracellular flaws may become the focus of molecularly targeted therapy. These efforts include determining overexpression of epidermal growth factor.

Symptom Management and Supportive Care

Nurses play a very important role in the care of patients at risk for anal canal cancer. HIV-infected individuals, as well as other individuals who practice anal receptive intercourse, are at higher risk for this cancer. Nurses help teach patients and their partners about risk, protective precautions, and screening methods. Once HSIL is diagnosed, the patient requires definitive treatment and close follow-up.

Once a patient has developed anal canal cancer, symptoms relate to bowel elimination. The nurse provides support and teaching prior to definitive treatment. Ideally, symptoms will resolve with aggressive combined chemotherapy and radiotherapy. For those patients with residual or recurrent disease, APR is the treatment of choice and may cure some patients.

Symptoms of progressive disease relate to metastases in the liver, lung, and bone. Symptom management and care of patients with liver metastases from anal cancer is the same as that for colon cancer with liver metastases. Lung metastases result in dyspnea, cough, and shortness of breath. The nurse works with the patient and family to help reduce anxiety, improve pulmonary status, and maximize coping. The nurse collaborates with the physician on self-care measures, the prescription of antianxiety agents such as lorazepam, and agents that may reduce the effort of breathing. Safety and comfort are the goals in caring for the patient with bony metatastases. The nurse assesses risk for injury through falls, monitors the effectiveness of current analgesics, and collaborates with the physician regarding the prescription of analgesics for bony pain, agents that may reduce the incidence of skeletal events, and stabilization of any unstable bony fractures in weight-bearing areas.

Long-Term Monitoring and Follow-up

For many patients, anal canal cancer is a curable cancer. Unfortunately, some patients — especially those with large, bulky tumors — may develop local recurrence, which can be effectively treated by resection and salvage therapy. Following definitive therapy, anal cancer will continue to regress for as long as 3 months or more.[224] A biopsy should be done of the tumor site at least 3 months following completion of combined treatment, and repeated until either a complete response or a need for residual therapy is determined. Recurrence usually occurs within the first 3 years.[223] According to NCCN guidelines, follow-up and long-term monitoring should included examinations every 3 months for 2 years, with a digital rectal exam, anoscopy, and inguinal node palpation.[234] If post-defini-

Table 49-18 Chemotherapy Regimens Used in the Treatment of Anal Canal Cancer

Therapy		Reference
Wayne State 5-FU/Mitomycin/Radiation		
5-Fluorouracil	1,000 mg/m²/day IV CI days 1–4, 29–32	Nigro ND, Seydel HG, Considine B, et al: Combined preoperative radiation and chemotherapy for squamous cell carcinoma of the anal canal. *Cancer* 51:1826–1829, 1983[246]
Mitomycin C	15 mg/m² IV day 1	
Radiation therapy	200 cGy/day on days 1–5, 8–12, and 5–19 Total Dose 3000 cGy	
EORTC 5-FU/Mitomycin/Radiation		
5-Fluorouracil	750/m²/day IV CI days 1–5, 29–33	Bartelink H, Roelofsen F, Eschwege F, et al: Concomitant radiotherapy and chemotherapy is superior to radiotherapy alone in the treatment of locally advanced anal cancer: results of a phase III randomized trial of the European Organization for Research and Gastrointestinal Cooperative Groups. *J Clin Oncol* 15:2040–2049, 1997[247]
Mitomycin C	15 mg/m² IV day 1	
Radiation therapy	180 cGy/day over 5 weeks Total dose 4500 cGy	
Chemotherapy Given Concurrently with Radiation Therapy		
If PR or CR,		
Radiation boost	1500–2000 cGy	
M. D. Anderson 5-FU/Cisplatin/Radiation		
5-Fluorouracil	250/m²/day IV CI days 1–5, each week of radiation	Hung A, Crane C, Delclos M, et al: Cisplatin-based combined modality therapy for anal carcinoma: a wider therapeutic index. *Cancer* 97:1195–1202, 2003[242]
Cisplatin	4 mg/m²/day IV CI days 1–5 each week of radiation	
Radiation Therapy	180 cGy/day over 6 weeks+ Total dose 5500 cGy	
Chemotherapy given concurrently with radiation therapy.		
Metastatic/Salvage 5-FU and Cisplatin		
5-Fluorouracil	1000 mg/m²/day IV CI days 1–5, repeat every 21–28 days	Flam M, John M, Pajak TF, et al: Role of mitomycin in combination with fluorouracil and radiotherapy, and of salvage chemoradiation in the definitive nonsurgical treatment of epidermoid carcinoma of the anal canal: results of a phase III randomized intergroup study. *J Clin Oncol* 14:2527–2539, 1996[241]
Cisplatin	100 mg/m² IV on day 2	

IV = intravenous; CI = continuous infusion; 1cGy = 1/100 Gy, the international system unit of absorbed dose of radiation; 1 Gy = 100 rad.

tive treatment biopsy shows persistent disease, or if the patient recurs, APR is effective in providing long-term control and survival in 40%–50% of patients.[240]

Conclusion

Clinical trials are exploring advances in screening and early detection in HIV-infected patients and immunologically suppressed patient populations. Given that the majority of anal canal cancers are virally induced, vaccines could prevent malignant transformation. Vaccines for cervical cancer have been developed, and similar work in anal cancer could provide protection for individuals who are unable or unwilling to change their high-risk behaviors. Research into the molecular flaws leading to malignant transformation is needed to help new therapies target anal canal malignancy and to improve treatment of large, bulky tumors. Improved chemotherapy regimens with greater efficacy for achieving a complete response for T4 and lymph node–positive patients are needed as well.[223] Finally, more than one-third of patients who present with large anal canal lesions have been told by their providers that the bleeding or sensation of a fullness was related to benign anal problems, so education of primary care providers is needed to improve the early detection of anal malignancies.

Over the past 30 years, there has been a downward trend in the incidence, morbidity, and mortality associated with colon and rectal cancers. Current screening mechanisms, diagnostic techniques, surgical interventions, and adjuvant therapy regimens have enabled individuals diagnosed with such malignancies to experience improved long-term survival and enhanced quality of life. However, despite the fact that colon and rectal cancers are preventable in most situations through removal of polyps, and otherwise highly curable if found early, colon and rectal cancers combined remain the third leading cause of incidence and mortality from cancer. Anal cancer, although uncommon, has shown an increase in incidence which appears to correlate with HPV infection and high-risk sexual behaviors. Although highly curable when found early, many patients delay seeking a diagnosis due to assumptions that symptoms relate to benign anal conditions such as hemorrhoids.

Factors that contribute to the pathogenesis of colon and rectal cancers are multifactorial. Age, genetics, diet, alcohol use, environment, inflammatory bowel conditions, prior radiation therapy, and surgery are all risk factors for colorectal cancer. The genetic mutational sequence for colon and rectal cancers is providing direction in the development of novel screening and early detection strategies.

Surgery continues to be the mainstay of therapy for adenocarcinoma of the colon and rectum. To accurately stage these malignancies, sufficient numbers of lymph nodes must be sampled, so that appropriate adjuvant therapy can be delivered. Chemotherapy, radiation therapy, and molecularly targeted therapy are utilized preoperatively, intraoperatively, postoperatively, and in patients with advanced disease to achieve better long-term survival. In instances when APR is indicated for optimal treatment, nurses contribute much to the patient preparation, supportive management, and prevention of complications for patients who require an ostomy.

Today's healthcare environment continues to change rapidly; more is accomplished on an outpatient basis and hospital lengths of stay continue to dwindle. A multitude of specialized nurses and physicians will care for the individual with colon, rectal, or anal carcinoma. The coordination and quality of care delivered is paramount as we move toward earlier diagnosis and better long-term survival for this disease.

References

1. American Cancer Society: *Cancer Facts and Figures — 2004.* Atlanta, American Cancer Society, 2004
2. Ellerhorn JDI, Cullinane CA, Coia LR, et al: Colorectal and anal cancers, in Pazdur R, Coia LR, Hoskins WJ, et al (eds.): *Cancer Management: A Multidisciplinary Approach* (ed 7). San Francisco, Oncology Publishing Group, 2003, pp 323–353
3. Bond J, Levin B: *Prevention and Early Detection of Colorectal Cancer: A Clinical Update of the Digestive Health Initiative.* Washington, DC, Colorectal Cancer Education Company, American Digestive Health Foundation, 1997
4. Kelvin F: Diagnosis of colorectal cancer by conventional radiology, in Myers M (ed.): *Neopla of the Digestive Tract: Imaging, Staging, and Management.* Philadelphia, Lippincott-Raven, 1998, pp 219–235
5. Jemal A, Tiwari RC, Murray T, et al: Cancer statistics, 2004. *CA Cancer J Clin* 54:8–29, 2004
6. Burt R: Update on genetic advances in colorectal cancer. *Pract Gastroenterol* 21:9–15, 1997
7. Burt R, Peterson G: Familial colorectal cancer: diagnosis and management, in Young G, Rozen P, Lein B (eds.): *Prevention and Early Detection of Colorectal Cancer.* Philadelphia, Saunders, 1998, pp 171–192
8. Landis SH, Murray T, Bolden S, et al: Cancer statistics in 1998. *CA Cancer J Clin* 48:6–30, 1998
9. McCollum AD, Catalano PJ, Haller DG, et al: Outcomes and toxicities in African-American and Caucasian patients in a randomized adjuvant chemotherapy trial for colon cancer. *J Natl Cancer Inst* 94:1160–1167, 2002
10. Ries LA, Eisner MP, Kosary CL, et al: *SEER Cancer Statistics Review 1973–1998.* Bethesda, MD, National Cancer Institute, 2001, pp 1–5
11. American Cancer Society: *Cancer Facts and Figures, 2002.* Atlanta, GA, American Cancer Society, 2002
12. Edwards BK, Howe HL, Ries LA, et al: Annual report to the nation on the status of cancer, 1973–1999, featuring implications of age and aging on U.S. cancer burden. *Cancer* 94:2766–2792, 2002
13. Jessup JM, McGinnis LS, Steele GD, et al: The national cancer data base: report on colon cancer. *Cancer* 78:918–926, 1996
14. Rex DK, Khan AM, Shah P, et al: Screening colonoscopy in asymptomatic average-risk African Americans. *Gastrointest Endosc* 51:524–527, 2000
15. Cheng X, Chen V, Steele B, et al: Subsite-specific incidence rate and stage of disease in colorectal cancer by race, gender, and age group in the United States, 1992–1997. *Cancer* 92:2547–2554, 2001
16. Nishi T, Kono S, Abe H, et al: Glucose intolerance, plasma insulin levels, and colon adenomas in Japanese men. *Jpn J Cancer Res* 92:836–840, 2001
17. Nakagawa H, Chadwick R, Peltomaki P, et al: Loss of imprinting of the insulin-like growth factor II gene occurs by biallelic methylation in a core region of H19-associated CTCF-binding sites in colorectal cancer. *Proc Natl Acad Sci USA* 98:591–596, 2001
18. Skibber JM, Minsky BD, Hoff PM: Cancer of the colon, in DeVita VT, Hellman S, Rosenberg SA (eds.): *Cancer: Principles and Practice of Oncology* (ed 6). Philadelphia, Lippincott, Williams and Wilkins, 2001, pp 1216–1319
19. Lieberman DA, Prindiville S, Weiss DG, et al: Risk factors for advanced neoplasia and hyperlastic polyps in asymptomatic individuals. *JAMA* 290:2959–2967, 2003
20. Colditz GA, Cannuscio CC, Frazier AL: Physical activity and reduced risk of colon cancer: implications for prevention. *Cancer Causes Control* 8:649–667, 1997
21. Giovannucci E, Ascherio A, Rimm EB, et al: Physical activity, obesity and risk for colon cancer and adenoma in men. *Ann Intern Med* 122:327–334, 1995
22. Ochsenkuhn T, Bayerdorffer E, Meining A, et al: Colonic mucosal proliferation is related to serum deoxycholic acid levels. *Cancer* 85:1664–1669, 1999
23. Blanke CD, Benson AB, Dragovich T, et al: A phase II trial of celecoxib (CX), irinotecan (I), 5-fluorouracil (5FU), and leucovorin (LCV) in patients with unresectable or metastatic colorectal cancer (CRC). *Proc Am Soc Clin Oncol* 38:2002, (abstr 505)
24. Steinbach G, Lynch PM, Phillips RK, et al: The effect of celecoxib, a cyclo-oxygenase inhibitor, in familial adenomatous polyposis. *N Engl J Med* 342:1946–1952, 2000
25. Kune GA, Vitetta L: Alcohol consumption and the etiology of colorectal cancer: a review of the scientific evidence from 1957 to 1991. *Nutr Cancer* 18:97–111, 1992
26. Newcomb PA, Storer BE, Marcus PM: Cancer of the large bowel in women in relation to alcohol consumption — a case control study in Wisconsin. *Cancer Causes Control* 4:405–411, 1993
27. Meyer F, White E: Alcohol and nutrients in relation to colon cancer in middle-aged adults. *Am J Epidemol* 138:225–236, 1993
28. Baron JA, Sandler RSH, Mandel JS, et al: Folate intake, alcohol consumption, cigarette smoking and risk of colorectal cancer. *J Natl Cancer Inst* 90:57–62, 1998

29. Mayer RJ: Tumors of the large and small intestine, in Isselbacher K, Braunwald E, Wilson J, et al: *Harrison's Principles of Internal Medicine* (ed 13). New York, McGraw-Hill, 1994, pp 1424–1429
30. Colditz, GA, Atwood KA, Emmons K, et al, for the Risk Index Working Group, Harvard Center for Cancer Prevention: Harvard report on cancer prevention volume 4: Harvard Cancer Risk Index. *Cancer Causes Control* 11:477–488, 2000
31. Itzkowitz S: Colon carcinogenesis in inflammatory bowel disease: applying molecular genetics to clinical practice. *J Clin Gastroenterol* 36(suppl):S70–S74, S94–S96, 2003
32. Franceschi S, LaVecchia C: Colorectal cancer and hormone replacement therapy: an unexpected finding. *Eur J Cancer Prev* 7:427–438, 1998
33. Lynch H, Smyrk T, Watson P, et al: Genetics, natural history, tumor spectrum, and pathology of hereditary nonpolyposis colorectal cancer: an updated review. *Gastroenterology* 104:1535–1549, 1993
34. Lynch H, Smryk T, McGinn T, et al: Attenuated familial adenomatous polyposis (AFAP): a phenotypically and genotypically distinctive variant of FAP. *Cancer* 76:2427–2433, 1995
35. Stollman N, Raskin J: Diverticular disease of the colon. *Lancet* 363:631–639, 2004
36. Fuchs CS, Giovannucci EL, Colditz GA, et al: A prospective study of family history and the risk of colorectal cancer. *N Engl J Med* 331:1669–1674, 1994
37. Kaaks R, Lukanova A: Energy balance and cancer: the role of insulin and insulin-like growth factor. *Proc Nutr Soc* 60:91–98, 2001
38. Fuchs CS, Giavannucci EL, Colditz GA, et al: Dietary fiber and decreased risk of colorectal cancer and adenoma in women. *N Engl J Med* 340:169–176, 1999
39. Alberts DS, Martinez ME, Roe DJ, et al: Lack of effect of a high-fiber cereal supplement on the recurrence of colorectal adenomas, Phoenix Colon Cancer Prevention Physician's Network. *N Engl J Med* 342:1156–1162, 2000
40. Schatzkin A, Lanza E, Corle D, et al: Lack of effect of a low-fat, high-fiber diet on the recurrence of colorectal adenomas. Polyp Prevention Trial Study Group. *N Engl J Med* 342: 1149–1159, 2000
41. Jacobs ET, Guiliano AR, Roe DJ, et al: Intake of supplemental and total fiber and risk of colorectal adenoma recurrence in the wheat bran fiber trial. *Cancer Epidemiol Biomark Prev* 11:906–914, erratum 11:1699, 2002
42. Giavonnucci E, Stampfer MJ, Colditz GA, et al: Relationship of diet to risk of colorectal adenoma in men. *J Natl Cancer Inst* 84:91–98, 1992
43. Peters U, Sinha R, Chatterjee N, et al: Dietary fibre and colorectal adenoma in a colorectal cancer early detection programme. *Lancet* 361:1491–1495, 2003
44. Bingham SA, Day NE, Luben R, et al: Dietary fibre in food and protection against colorectal cancer in the European Prospective Investigation into Cancer and Nutrition (EPIC): an observational study. *Lancet* 361:1496–1501, erratum 362:1000, 2003
45. Terry P, Giovannucci E, Michels KB, et al: Fruit, vegetables, dietary fiber, and risk of colorectal cancer. *J Natl Cancer Inst* 93:525–533, 2001
46. Willett WC, Stampfer MJ, Colditz GA, et al: Relation of meat, fat, and fiber intake to the risk of colon cancer in a prospective study among women. *N Engl J Med* 323:1664–1672, 1990
47. Norat T, Lukanova A, Ferrari P, et al: Meat consumption and colorectal cancer risk: dose-response meta-analysis of epidemiological studies. *Int J Cancer* 98:241–256, 2002
48. Key TJ, Allen NE, Spencer EA, et al: The effect of diet on risk of cancer. *Lancet* 360:861–868, 2002
49. Giovannucci E, Stampfer MJ, Colditz GA, et al: Multivitamin use, folate, and colon cancer in women in the Nurses' Health Study. *Ann Intern Med* 129:517–524, 1998
50. LaVecchia C, Negri E, Pelucchi C, et al: Dietary folate and colorectal cancer. *Int J Cancer* 102:545–547, 2002
51. Fuchs CS, Willett WC, Colditz GA, et al: The influence of folate and multivitamin use on the familial risk of colon cancer in women. *Cancer Epidemiol Biomarkers Prev* 11:227–234, 2002
52. Duthie SJ: Folic acid deficiency and cancer: mechanisms of DNA instability. *Br Med Bull* 55:578–592, 1999
53. Pufulete M, Alghnaniem R, Leather AJ, et al: Folate status, genomic DNA hypomethylation, and risk of colorectal adenoma and cancer: a case control study. *Gastroenterology* 124: 1240–1248, 2003
54. Baron JA, Cole BF, Sandler RS, et al: A randomized trial of aspirin to prevent colorectal adenomas. *N Engl J Med* 348:891–899, 2003
55. Chen J, Giovannucci EL, Hunter DJ: MTHFR polymorphism, methyl-replete diets and the risk of colorectal carcinoma and adenoma among US men and women: an example of gene–environment interactions in colorectal cancer tumorigenesis. *J Nutr* 129(suppl): 560S–564S, 1999
56. Wu K, Willett WC, Fuchs CS, et al: Calcium intake and risk of colon cancer in women and men. *J Natl Cancer Inst* 94:437–446, 2002
57. Lamprecht SA, Lipkin M: Chemoprevention of colon cancer by calcium, vitamin D and folate: molecular mechanisms. *Nat Rev Cancer* 3:601–614, 2004
58. Baron JA, Beach M, Mandel JS, et al: Calcium supplements for the prevention of colorectal adenomas: Calcium Polyp Prevention Study Group. *N Engl J Med* 340:101–107, 1999
59. Pardi DS, Loftus EV Jr, Kremers WK, et al: Ursodeoxycholic acid as a chemopreventive agent in patients with ulcerative colitis and primary sclerosing cholangitis. *Gastroenterology* 124:889–893, 2003
60. Brentnall TA: Ursodiol: good drug makes good. *Gastroenterology* 124:1139–1140, 2003
61. Lee IM, Paffenbarger RS Jr, Hsieh C: Physical activity and the risk of developing colorectal cancer among college alumni. *J Natl Cancer Inst* 83:1324–1329, 1991
62. Giovannucci E, Ascherio A, Rimm EB, et al: Physical activity, obesity, and risk for colon cancer and adenoma in men. *Ann Intern Med* 122:227–263, 1995
63. Giovannucci E, Colditz GA, Stampfer MJ, et al: Physical activity, obesity and risk of colorectal adenoma in women (United States). *Cancer Causes Control* 7:253–263, 1996
64. Slattery ML, Potter J, Caan B, et al: Energy balance and colon cancer beyond physical activity. *Cancer Res* 57:75–80, 1997
65. Hardman AE: Physical activity and cancer risk. *Proc Nutr Soc* 60:107–113, 2001
66. Kune G, Kune S, Watson L: Colorectal cancer risk, chronic illness, operations, and medications: case control results for the Melbourne colorectal cancer study. *Cancer Res* 48:4399–4404, 1988
67. Muscat JE, Stellman SD, Wynder EL: Nonsteroidal anti-inflammatory drugs and colorectal cancer. *Cancer* 74:1847–1854, 1994
68. Dixon DA: Regulation of COX-2 expression in human cancer. *Prog Exper Tumor Res* 37:70–89, 2003
69. Courtney EDJ, Melville DM, Leicester RJ: Chemoprevention of colorectal cancer. *Aliment Pharmacol Ther* 19:1–24, 2004
70. Prescott SM, Fitzpatrick FA: Cyclooxygenase-2 and carcinogenesis. *Biochem Biophys Acta* 1470:69–78, 2000
71. Cao Y, Pearman AT, Zimmerman GA, et al: Intracellular unesterified arachidonic acid signals apoptosis. *Proc Natl Acad Sci* 97:280–285, 2000
72. Gwyn K, Sinicrope FA: Chemoprevention of colorectal cancer. *Am J Gastroenterol* 97:13–21, 2002

73. Sandler RS, Halabi S, Baron JA, et al: A randomized trial of aspirin to prevent colorectal adenomas in patients with previous colorectal cancer. *N Engl J Med* 348:883–890, 2003
74. Levin B: Colorectal cancer screening: sifting through the evidence. *J Natl Cancer Inst* 91:389–394, 1999
75. Byers I, Levin B, Rothenberger D, et al: American Cancer Society guidelines for screening and surveillance for early detection of colorectal polyps and cancer. *CA Cancer J Clin* 47:154–160, 1997
76. American Gastroenterological Association: *Colorectal Cancer Screening: Clinical Guidelines and Rationale — Executive Summary.* Philadelphia, Saunders, 1997
77. Mandel JS, Church TR, Bond JH, et al: The effect of fecal occult-blood screening on the incidence of colorectal cancer. *N Engl J Med* 343:1603–1607, 2000
78. Mandel JS, Bond JH, Church TR, et al: Reducing mortality from colorectal cancer by screening for fecal occult blood. Minnesota Cancer Control Study. *N Engl J Med* 328:1365–1371, 1993
79. Lang CA, Ransohoff DF: Fecal occult blood screening for colorectal cancer. Is mortality reduced by chance selection for screening colonoscopy? *JAMA* 271:1011–1013, 1994
80. Ederer F, Church TR, Mandel JS: Fecal occult blood screening Minnesota study: role of chance detection of lesions. *J Natl Cancer Inst* 89:1423–1428, 1997
81. Ransohoff DR, Lang CA: Screening for colorectal cancer with the fecal occult blood test: a background paper. American College of Physicians. *Ann Intern Med* 126:811–812, 1997
82. Fath RB, Winawer SJ: Endoscopic screening by flexible fiberoptic sigmoidoscopy. *Front Gastrointest Res* 10:102–111, 1986
83. National Cancer Institute: Colorectal cancer. *www.cancer.gov/cancerinfo/pdq/screening/colorectal/healthprofessional/#Reference3.20.* Accessed March 13, 2004
84. Newcomb PA, Norfleet RG, Storer BE, et al: Screening sigmoidoscopy and colorectal cancer mortality. *J Natl Cancer Inst* 84:1572–1575, 1992
85. Slattery ML, Edwards SL, Ma KN, et al: Colon cancer screening, lifestyle, and risk of colon cancer. *Cancer Causes Control* 11:555–563, 2000
86. Schoen RE, Pinsky PF, Weissfeld JL, et al: Results of repeat sigmoidoscopy 3 years after a negative examination. *JAMA* 290:41–50, 2003
87. Gatto NM, Frucht H, Sundararajan V, et al: Risk of perforation after colonoscopy and sigmoidoscopy: a population-based study. *J Natl Cancer Inst* 95:230–236, 2003
88. Maule WF: Screening for colorectal cancer by nurse endoscopists. *N Engl J Med* 330:183–187, 1994
89. Lieberman DA, Weiss DG: Veterans Affairs Cooperative Study Group 380: One time screening for colorectal cancer with combined fecal occult-blood testing and examination of the distal colon. *N Engl J Med* 345:550–560, 2001
90. Gondal G, Grotmol T, Hofstad B, et al: The Norwegian Colorectal Cancer Prevention (NORCAPP) screening study: baseline findings and implementations for clinical work-up in age groups 50–64 years. *Scand J Gastroenterol* 38:635–644, 2003
91. Winawer SJ, Stewart ET, Zauber AG, et al: A comparison of colonoscopy and double-contrast barium enema for surveillance after polypectomy. National Polyp Study Work Group. *N Engl J Med* 342:1766–1772, 2000
92. Lieberman DA, Weiss DG, Bond JH, et al: Use of colonoscopy to screen asymptomatic adults for colorectal cancer. Veterans Affairs Cooperative Study Group 380. *N Engl J Med* 343:162–168, 2000
93. Imperiale TF, Wagner DR, Lin CY, et al: Risk of advanced proximal neoplasms in asymptomatic adults according to the distal colorectal findings. *N Engl J Med* 343:169–174, 2000
94. Imperiale TF, Wagner DR, Lin CY, et al: Using risk for advanced proximal colonic neoplasia to tailor endoscopic screening for colorectal cancer. *Ann Intern Med* 139:959–965, 2003
95. Yee J, Akerkar GA, Hung RK, et al: Colorectal neoplasia: performance characteristics of CT colonography for detection in 300 patients. *Radiology* 219:685–692, 2001
96. Miao YM, Amin Z, Healy J, et al: A prospective single centre study comparing computed tomography pneumocolon against colonoscopy in the detection of colorectal neoplasms. *Gut* 47:832–837, 2000
97. Mascari M, Bini EJ, Jacobs SL: Colorectal polyps and cancers in asymptomatic average-risk patients: evaluation with CT colonography. *Radiology* 230:629–636, 2004
98. Evelegh MJ: A novel method for the quantification of the galactose oxidase — Schiff's reaction and its use in cancer detection. *J Clin Ligand Assay* 25:91–94, 2002
99. Dong SM, Traverso G, Johnson C, et al: Detecting colorectal cancer in stool with the use of multiple genetic targets. *J Natl Cancer Inst* 93:858–865, 2001
100. Traverso G, Shuber A, Levin B, et al: Detection of APC mutations in fecal DNA from patients with colorectal tumors. *N Engl J Med* 346:311–320, 2002
101. Behavioral Risk Factor Surveillance System (BRFSS) Summary, National Center for Disease Prevention and Health Promotion, Centers for Disease Control and Prevention, 2000
102. Centers for Disease Control and Prevention Trends in screening for colorectal cancer: United States 1997 and 1999. *MMWR* 50:162–166, 2001
103. Baig NA, Weinberg DS, Myers R, et al: Inadequate follow-up of positive fecal occult blood test results: survey of physician-reported reasons. *Gastroenterology* 120:A-66, 2001 (abstr 350)
104. Kinzler K, Vogelstein B: Lessons from hereditary colorectal cancer. *Cell* 87:159–170, 1996
105. Miyaki M, Iijima T, Kimura J, et al: Frequent mutations of beta-catenin and APC genes in primary colorectal tumors from patients with hereditary nonpolyposis colorectal cancer. *Cancer Res* 59:4506–4509, 1999
106. Chiang JM, Chou YH, Chen TC, et al: Nuclear beta-catenin expression is closely related to ulcerative growth of colorectal carcinoma. *Br J Cancer* 86:1124–1129, 2002
107. Aberle H, Bauer A, Stappert J et al: Beta-catenin is a target for the ubiquitin–proteasome pathway *EMBO J* 16:3793–3804, 1997
108. Klein G: Cancer, apoptosis, and non-immune surveillance. *Cell Death Differ* 11:13–17, 2004
109. Toyota M, Issa JP: CpG island methylator phenotypes in aging and cancer. *Semin Cancer Biol* 9:349–357, 1999
110. Ward RL, Cheong K, Ku SL, et al: Adverse prognostic effect of methylation in colorectal cancer is reversed in microsatellite instability. *J Clin Oncol* 21:3729–3736, 2003
111. Lynch HT, Coronel SM, Okimoto R, et al: A founder mutation of the *MSH2* gene and hereditary nonpolyposis colorectal cancer in the United States. *JAMA* 291:718–724, 2004
112. Umar A, Risinger JI, Hawk ET, et al: Testing guidelines for hereditary non-polyposis colorectal cancer. *Nat Rev Cancer* 4:153–158, 2004
113. Cortellino S, Turner D, Masciullo V, et al : The base excision repair enzyme MED1 mediates DNA damage response to antitumor drugs and is associated with mismatch repair system integrity. *Proc Natl Acad Sci* 100:15071–15076, 2003
114. Savoca P, Wong W: Anal carcinoma: anatomy, staging, and prognostic variables, in Cohen A, Winawer S (eds.): *Cancer of the Colon, Rectum, and Anus.* New York, McGraw-Hill, 1995, pp 1013–1020
115. Chuselp C: Pathways of nodal metastasis from cancer of the colon, in Meyers MA (ed.): *Neoplasms of the Digestive Tract: Imag-*

ing, Staging, and Management. Philadelphia, Lippincott-Raven, 1998, pp 257–267

116. Compton CC, Fielding LP, Burgart LJ: Prognostic factors in colorectal cancer. College of American Pathologists consensus statement. *Arch Pathol Lab Med* 124:979–994, 1999
117. Psathakis D, Schiedeck TH, Krug F, et al: Ordinary colorectal adenocarcinoma vs. primary colorectal signet-ring cell carcinoma: study matched for age, gender, grade and stage. *Dis Colon Rectum* 42:1618–1625, 1999
118. Frizelle FA, Hobday KS, Batts KP, et al: Adenosquamous and squamous carcinoma of the colon and upper rectum: a clinical and histopathologic study. *Dis Colon Rectum* 44:341–346, 2001
119. Chu P, Wu E, Weiss LM: Cytokeratin 7 and cytokeratin 20 expression in epithelial neoplasms: a survey of 435 cases. *Mod Pathol* 13:962–972, 2000
120. Olesen SH, Frederiksen CM, Sorensen FB, et al: Differential gene expression in right and left sided colon cancers identified by microarray analysis. *Am Assoc Cancer Res,* 94th annual meeting, July 11–14, 2003, Washington, DC, (abstr R1481)
121. Winawer SJ, Fletcher RH, Miller L, et al: Colorectal cancer screening: clinical guidelines and rationale. *Gastroenterology* 112:594–602, erratum 112:1060, 1997
122. Lewis JD, Deren JJ, Lichtenstein GR: Cancer risk in patients with inflammatory bowel disease. *Gastroenterol Clin North Am* 28:459–464, 1999
123. National Comprehensive Cancer Network: *Practice Guidelines in Oncology: Colorectal Screening,* v.1.2003. Jenkintown, National Comprehensive Cancer Network, 2003
124. Strohl R: Nursing care of the client with cancer of the gastrointestinal tract, in Itano J, Taoka K (eds.): *Core Curriculum for Oncology Nursing* (ed 3). Philadelphia, Saunders, 1998, pp 470–483
125. Colecchia G, Nardi M: Colorectal cancer in pregnancy. *Giornal Chirurgia* 20:159–161, 1999
126. Sweed MR, Meropol NJ: Assessment, diagnosis and staging, in Berg DT: *Contemporary Issues in Colorectal Cancer.* Sudbury, MA, Jones and Bartlett, 2001, pp 65–79
127. National Comprehensive Cancer Network: *Practice Guidelines in Oncology: Colon Cancer,* v.2.2004. Jenkintown, National Comprehensive Cancer Network, 2004
128. Meyers MA: Overview, colorectal carcinoma: imaging, staging, and management, in Meyers MA (ed.): *Neoplasms of the Digestive Tract: Imaging, Staging, and Management.* Philadelphia, Lippincott-Raven, 1998, pp 203–217
129. Chang AE: Colorectal cancer, in Greenfield LJ, Mulholland MW, Oldham KT, et al (eds.): *Surgery: Scientific Principles and Practice.* Philadelphia, Lippincott-Raven, 1997, pp 1139–1146
130. Brandt B, DeAntonio P, Dezort M, et al: Hepatic cryosurgery for metastatic colorectal carcinoma. *Oncol Nurs Forum* 23:29–37, 1996
131. Polissar L, Sim D, Francis A: Survival of colorectal cancer patients in relation to duration of symptoms and other prognostic factors. *Dis Colon Rectum* 24:364–369, 1981
132. Wolmark N, Wieand HS, Rockette HE, Fisher B: The prognostic significance of tumor location and bowel obstruction in Dukes B and C colorectal cancer. Findings from the NSABP clinical trials. *Ann Surg* 198:743–748, 1983
133. Steinberg SM, Barkin JS, Kaplan RS, et al: Prognostic indicators of colon tumors. The Gastrointestinal Tumor Study Group experience. *Cancer* 57:1866–1870, 1986
134. Halvorsen TB, Johannesen E: DNA ploidy, tumor site, and prognosis in colorectal cancer. *Scand J Gastroenterol* 25:141–146, 1990
135. Filella X, Molina R, Grau JJ, et al: Prognostic value of CA 19.9 levels in colorectal cancer. *Ann Surg* 216:55–59, 1992
136. Gryfe R, Kim H, Hsieh ET, et al: Tumor microsatellite instability and clinical outcome in young patients with colorectal cancer. *N Engl J Med* 342:69–77, 2000
137. Jen J, Kim H, Piantadosi S: Allelic loss of chromosome 18q and prognosis in colorectal cancer. *N Engl J Med* 331:213–221, 1994
138. Dignam JJ, Colangelo L, Tian W, et al: Outcomes among African-Americans and Caucasians in colon cancer adjuvant therapy trials: findings from the National Surgical Adjuvant Breast and Bowel Project. *J Natl Cancer Inst* 91:1933–1940, 1999
139. Greene FL, Page DS, Fleming ID, et al, American Joint Committee on Cancer: *AJCC Cancer Staging Manual* (ed. 6). New York, Springer-Verlag, 2002
140. Esser S, Reilly WT, Riley LB, et al: The role of sentinel lymph node mapping in staging of colon and rectal cancer. *Dis Colon Rectum* 44:850–854, 2001
141. Le Voyer TE, Sigurdson ER, Hanlon AL, et al: Colon cancer survival is associated with increasing number of lymph nodes analyzed: a secondary survey of intergroup trial INT-0089. *J Clin Oncol* 21:2912–2919, 2003
142. Swanson RS, Compton CC, Stewart AK, et al: The prognosis of T3N0 colon cancer is dependent on the number of lymph nodes examined. *Ann Surg Oncol* 10:65–71, 2003
143. Lennon AM, Mulcahy HE, Hyland JMP: Peritoneal involvement in stage II colon cancer. *Am J Clin Pathol* 119:108–113, 2003
144. Compton C, Fenoglio-Preiser CM, Pettigrew N, et al: American Joint Committee on Cancer Prognostic Factors Consensus Conference: Colorectal Working Group. *Cancer* 88:1739–1757, 2000
145. Lacy AM, Garcia-Valdecasa JC, Delgado S, et al: Laparoscopy assisted colectomy versus open colectomy for treatment of non-metastatic colon cancer: a randomized trial. *Lancet* 359:2224–2229, 2002
146. Hurd T, Gutman H: Cancer of the colon, rectum and anus, in Berger DH, Feig BW, Fuhrman GM (eds.): *The M. D. Anderson Surgical Oncology Handbook.* Boston, Little, Brown, 1995, pp 160–177
147. Saha S, Bilchik A, Wiese D, et al: Ultrastaging of colorectal cancer by sentinel lymph node mapping technique — a multicenter trial. *Ann Surg Oncol* 8(suppl):94S-98S, 2001
148. Bilchik AJ, Nora DT, Saha S, et al: The use of molecular profiling of early colorectal cancer to predict micrometastases. *Arch Surg* 137:1377–1383, 2002
149. Feig BW, Curley S, Lucci A, et al: A caution regarding lymphatic mapping in patients with colon cancer. *Am J Surg* 182:707–712, 2001
150. Fong Y, Cohen AM, Fortner JG, et al: Liver resection for colorectal metastases. *J Clin Oncol* 15:938–946, 1997
151. Fong Y, Fortner J, Sun RL, et al: Clinical score for predicting recurrence after hepatic resection for metastatic colorectal cancer: analysis of 1001 consecutive cases. *Ann Surg* 230:309–318; discussion 318–321, 1999
152. Mulay M: Treatment decision making, in Berg DT (ed.): *Contemporary Issues in Colorectal Cancer: A Nursing Perspective.* Sudbury, MA, Jones and Bartlett, 2001, pp 81–104
153. Kemeny N, Huang Y, Cohen AM, et al: Hepatic arterial infusion of chemotherapy after resection of hepatic metastases from colorectal cancer. *N Engl J Med* 341:2039–2048, 1999
154. Meta-Analysis Group in Cancer: Reappraisal of hepatic arterial infusion in the treatment of nonresectable liver metastases from colorectal cancer. *J Natl Cancer Inst* 88:252–258, 1996
155. Kemeny NE, Niedzwiecki D, Hollis DR, et al: Hepatic arterial infusion (HAI) versus systemic therapy for hepatic metastases from colorectal cancer: a CALGB randomized trial of efficacy, quality of life (QOL), cost effectiveness, and molecular markers. *Proc Am Soc Clin Oncol* 22:2003 (abstr 1010)

156. Weiss L: Metastatic inefficiency: causes and consequences *Cancer Metastasis Rev* 3:1–24, 1986
157. Sugarbaker PH: Managing the peritoneal surface component of gastrointestinal cancer. Part I. Patterns of dissemination and treatment options. *Oncology* 18:51–59, 2004
158. McCormick PM, Martini N: A current view of surgical management of pulmonary metastases, in Economou SG, Witt TR, Deziel DJ, et al (eds.): *Adjuncts to Cancer Surgery*. Philadelphia, Lea and Febiger, 1991, pp 246–251
159. Avis F: Surgical treatment of isolated metastases to the liver, lungs, brain, in Wittes RE (ed.): *Manual of Oncologic Therapeutics*. Philadelphia, Lippincott, 1991, pp 308–309
160. Mountain CF, McMurtrey MJ, Hermes KF: Surgery for pulmonary metastases: a 20 year experience. *Ann Thorac Surg* 38:323–330, 1984
161. Willett CG, Fung CY, Kaufman DS, et al: Postoperative radiation therapy for high-risk colon cancer. *J Clin Oncol* 11:1112–1117, 1993
162. Willett CG, Goldberg S, Shellito PC, et al: Does postoperative irradiation play a role in the adjuvant therapy of stage T4 colon cancer? *Cancer J Sci Am* 5: 242–247, 1999
163. Gosselin TK: Radiation therapy, in Berg DT (ed.): *Contemporary Issues in Colorectal Cancer*. Sudbury, MA, Jones and Bartlett, 2001, pp 135–157
164. Minsky B: Colon cancer, in Leibel SA, Phillips TL (eds.): *Textbook of Radiation Oncology*, (ed 3). Philadelphia, W. B. Saunders, 1998, pp 686–702
165. Schild SE, Gunderson LL, Haddock MG, et al: The treatment of locally advanced colon cancer. *Int J Radiat Oncol Biol Phys* 37:51–58, 1997.
166. Martenson J, Willett C, Sargent D, et al: A phase III study of adjuvant radiation therapy (RT), 5-fluorouracil (5-FU), and levamisole (LEV) vs 5-FU and LEV in selected patients with resected high risk colon cancer: initial results of Int 0130. *Proc Am Soc Clin Oncol* 18:A-904, 1999 (abstr 235a)
167. Meta-analysis Group in Cancer: Efficacy of intravenous continuous infusion of fluorouracil compared with bolus administration in advanced colorectal cancer. *J Clin Oncol* 16:301–308, 1998
168. O'Connell MJ, Mailliard JA, Kahn MJ, et al: Controlled clinical trial of fluorouracil and low-dose leucovorin given for 6 months as postoperative adjuvant therapy for colon cancer. *J Clin Oncol* 81:213–215, 1997
169. Wolmark N, Rockette H, Fisher B, et al: The benefit of leucovorin-modulated fluorouracil as postoperative adjuvant therapy for primary colon cancer: results from National Surgical Adjuvant Breast and Bowel Project Protocol C-03. *J Clin Oncol* 11:1879–1887, 1993
170. Benson AB, Choti MA, Cohen AM, et al: NCCN practice guidelines for colorectal cancer. *Oncology* 14:203–212, 2000
171. de Gramont A, Boni C, Navarro C, et al: Oxaliplatin/5-FU/LV in adjuvant colon cancer: results of the international randomized mosaic trial. *Proc Am Soc Clin Oncol* 22:253, 2003 (abstr 1015)
172. Cassidy J, Scheithauer J, McKendrick H, et al: Capecitabine (X) vs. bolus 5-FU/leucovorin (LV) as adjuvant therapy for colon cancer (the X-ACT study): efficacy results of a phase III trial. *J Clin Oncol* 22:3509, 2004
173. Hoff PM, Ansari R, Batist G, et al: Comparison of oral capecitabine versus intravenous fluorouracil plus leucovorin as first-line treatment in 605 patients with metastatic colorectal cancer: results of a randomized phase III study. *J Clin Oncol* 19:2282–2292, 2001
174. de Gramont A, Bossett JF, Milan C, et al: Randomized trial comparing monthly low-dose leucovorin and fluorouracil bolus with bimonthly high-dose leucovorin and fluorouracil bolus plus continuous infusion for advanced colorectal cancer: a French intergroup study. *J Clin Oncol* 15:808–815, 1997
175. Douillard JY, Cunningham D, Roth AD, et al: Irinotecan combined with fluorouracil compared with fluorouracil alone as first-line treatment for metastatic colorectal cancer: a multicentre randomized trial. *Lancet* 355:1041–1047, 2000
176. Kemeny N, Conti JA, Cohen A, et al: Phase II study of hepatic arterial floxuridine, leucovorin, and dexamtheasone for unresectable liver metastases from colorectal carcinoma. *J Clin Oncol* 12:2288–2295, 1994
177. de Gramont A, Figer A, Seymour M, et al: Leucovorin and fluorouracil with and without oxaliplatin as first-line treatment in advanced colorectal cancer. *J Clin Oncol* 18:2938–2947, 2000
178. Tournigand C, Louvet C, Quinaux E, et al: FOLFIRI followed by FOLFOX versus FOLFOX followed by FOLFIRI in metastatic colorectal cancer (MCRC): final results of a phase II study. *Proc Am Soc Clin Oncol* 20:124a, 2001 (abstr 494)
179. Andre T, Figer A, Cervanteo G, et al: FOLFOX7 compared to FOLFOX4. Preliminary results of the randomized optimox study. *Proc Am Soc Clin Oncol* 22:254, 2003 (abstr 1016)
180. Andre T, Louvet C, Maindrault-Goebel F, et al: CPT-11 (irinotecan) addition to bimonthly, high-dose leucovorin and bolus and continuous-infusion 5-fluorouracil (FOLFIRI) for pretreated metastatic colorectal cancer GERCOR. *Eur J Cancer* 35:1343–1347, 1999
181. Grothey A, Deschler B, Kroening H, et al: Phase III study of bolus 5-fluorouracil (5-FU)/folinic acid (FA) (Mayo) vs weekly high-dose 24h 5-FU infusion/FA + oxaliplatin (OXA) (FUFOX) in advanced colorectal cancer (ACRC). *Proc Am Soc Clin Oncol* 21:254, 2002 (abstr 512)
182. Saltz LB, Cox JV, Blanke C, et al: Irinotecan plus fluorouracil and leucovorin for metastatic colorectal cancer. *N Engl J Med* 343: 905–914, 2000
183. Wasserman E, Sutherland N, Critkovic E, et al: Irinotecan plus oxaliplatin: a promising combination for advanced colorectal cancer. *Clin Colorectal Cancer* 1:149–153, 2001
184. Tabernero J, Butts CA, Cassidy J, et al: Capecitabine and oxaliplatin in combination (Xelox) as first-line therapy for patients with metastatic colorectal cancer (MCRC): results of an international multicenter phase II trial. *Proc Am Soc Clin Oncol* 21:133a, 2002 (abstr 531)
185. Sargent DJ, Niedzwiecki D, O'Connell MJ, et al: Recommendation for caution with irinotecan, fluorouracil and leucovorin for colorectal cancer. *N Engl J Med* 345:144–146, 2001
186. Goldberg RM, Sargent DJ, Morton RF, et al: A randomized controlled trial of fluorouracil plus leucovorin, irinotecan, and oxaliplatin combinations in patients with previously untreated metastatic colorectal cancer. *J Clin Oncol* 22:23–30, 2004
187. Hurwitz H, Fehrenbacher L, Cartwright T, et al: Bevacizumab (a monoclonal antibody to vascular endothelial growth factor) prolongs survival in first-line colorectal cancer (CRC): results of a phase III trial of benacizumab in combination with bolus IFL (irinotecan, 5-fluorouracil, leucovorin) as first-line therapy in subjects with metastic CRC. *Pro Am Soc Clin Oncol* 22:2003 (abstr 3646)
188. Cunningham D, Humblet Y, Siena S, et al: Cetuximab (C225) alone or in combination with irinotecan (CPT-11) in patients with epidermal growth factor receptor (EGFR)–positive, irinotecan refractory metastatic colorectal cancer (MCRC). *Proc Am Soc Clin Oncol* 22:252, 2003 (abstr 1012)
189. Rothenberg ML, Meropol NJ, Poplin EA, et al: Mortality associated with irinotecan plus bolus fluorouracil/leucovorin: summary findings of an independent panel. *J Clin Oncol* 19:3801–3807, 2001
190. Peters M, Haller D: Therapy for early-stage colorectal cancer. *Oncology* 13:307–315, 1999

191. Vrazas JI, Ferris S, Bau S, Faragher I: Stenting for obstructing colorectal malignancy: an interim or definitive procedure. *ANZ J Surg* 72:392–394, 2002
192. Gregorio MA, Mainar A, Teiero E, et al: Acute colorectal obstruction: stent placement for palliative treatment: results of a multicenter study. *Radiology* 209:117–120, 1998
193. Baines M: The pathophysiology and management of malignant intestinal obstruction, in Doyle D, Hanks GWC, MacDonald N (eds.): *Oxford Textbook of Palliative Medicine* (ed 2). Oxford, UK, Oxford University Press, 1998, pp 526–534
194. Markowitz SK: Radiologic diagnosis: colon, in Welch JP (ed.): *Bowel Obstruction.* Philadelphia, Saunders, 1990, pp 108–118
195. Ripamonti C: Management of bowel obstruction in advanced cancer patients. *J Pain Symptom Manage* 9:193–200, 1994
196. Ventafridda V, Ripamonti C, Caraceni A, et al: The management of inoperable gastrointestinal obstruction in terminal cancer patients. *Tumori* 76:389–393, 1990
197. Kimbrough T: Intraabdominal abscesses and fistulas, in Yamada T (ed.): *Textbook of Gastroenterology.* Philadelphia, Lippincott, 1995, pp 2289–2298
198. Berry SM, Fischer JE: Classification and pathophysiology of enterocutaneous fistulas. *Surg Clin North Am* 76:1009–1017, 1996
199. National Comprehensive Cancer Network: *Practice Guidelines in Oncology: Rectal Cancer,* v.1.2004. Jenkintown, National Comprehensive Cancer Network, 2004
200. Herrinton LJ, Selby JV, Friedman GD, et al: Case-control study of digital-rectal screening in relation to mortality from cancer of the rectum *Am J Epidemiol* 142:961–964, 1995
201. Havenga K, Enker WE, McDermott K, et al: Male and female sexual and urinary function after total mesorectal excision with autonomic nerve preservation for carcinoma of the rectum. *Am Coll Surg* 182:495–502, 1996
202. Ono A, Fujii T, Saito Y, et al: Endoscopic submucosal resection of rectal carcinoid tumors with a ligation device. *Gastrointest Endoscopy* 57:583–587, 2003
203. Yaziji H, Broghamer WJ: Primary small cell undifferentiated carcinoma of the rectum associated with ulcerative colitis. *Southern Med J* 89:177–186, 1996
204. Bartram C, Brown G: Endorectal ultrasound and magnetic resonance imaging in rectal cancer staging. *Gastroenterol Clin North Am* 31:827–839, 2002
205. Snady H, Merrick MA: Improving the treatment of colorectal cancer: the role of EUS. *Cancer Invest* 16:572–581, 1998
206. Tominaga T, Sakabe T, Koyama Y, et al: Prognostic factors for patients with colon or rectal carcinoma treated with resection only: five year follow-up report. *Cancer* 78:403–407, 1996
207. Compton CC: Colorectal carcinoma: diagnostic, prognostic and molecular features. *Mod Pathol* 16:376–388, 2003
208. Jessup JM, Stewart AK, Menck HR: The National Cancer Data Base report on patterns of care for adenocarcinoma of the rectum, 1985–1995. *Cancer* 83:2408–2418, 1998
209. Greene FL, Stewart AK, Norton HJ: A new TNM staging strategy for node-positive (stage III) rectal cancer. An analysis of 5,988 patients. *Proc Am Soc Clin Oncol* 22:251, 2003 (abstr 1007)
210. Minsky BD: Sphincter preservation in rectal cancer. Preoperative radiation therapy followed by low anterior resection with coloanal anastomosis. *Semin Rad Oncol* 8:30–35, 1998
211. Kodner IJ, Fry RD, Fleshman JW, et al (eds.): *Principles of Surgery* (ed 7). New York, McGraw-Hill, 1999
212. Meyerhardt JA, Tepper JE, Niedzwiecki D, et al: Impact of hospital procedure volume on surgical operation and long-term outcomes in high-risk curatively resected rectal cancer: findings from the Intergroup 0114 study. *J Clin Oncol* 22:166–174, 2003
213. Ayanian JZ, Zaslavsky AM, Fuchs CS, et al: Use of adjuvant chemotherapy and radiation therapy for colorectal cancer in a population-based cohort. *J Clin Oncol* 21:1293–1300, 2003
214. Perez CA, Brady LW, Roti JL: Overview, in Perez CA, Brady LW (eds.): *Principles and Practice of Radiation Oncology* (ed 3). Philadelphia, Lippincott-Raven, 1998, pp 1–78
215. Marks G, Mohiuddunm M, Masoni L: The reality of radical sphincter preservation surgery for cancer of the distal 3 cm of rectum following high-dose radiation. *Int J Radiat Oncol Biol Phys* 27:779–783, 1993
216. Mohiuddin M, Marks G: Long-term results of "selective sandwich" adjunctive radiotherapy for cancer of the rectum. *Am J Clin Oncol* 17:264–268, 1994
217. Grunderson LL, Willett CG, Harrison LB, et al: Intraoperative irradiation: current and future status. *Semin Oncol* 24:715–731, 1997
218. Iwamoto RJ: Emerging strategies in radiation therapy for colorectal cancer: intraoperative radiation therapy and sterotactic radiation therapy, in *Colorectal Cancer: Balancing Therapeutic Interventions and Quality of Life Symposium.* Philadelphia, Meniscus Educational Institute, 1998, pp 14–23
219. Turnbull GW, Erin-Toth P: Ostomy care: foundation for teaching and practice. *Ostomy/Wound Management* 1A(suppl): 235–305, 1999
220. Koukouras D, Spiliotis J, Scopa C, et al: Radical consequences in the sexuality of male patients operated for colorectal carcinoma. *Eur J Surg Oncol* 17:285–288, 1991
221. Ellis C, Saddler DAH: Colorectal cancer, in Yarbro CH, Frogge MH, Goodman M, Groenwald SL (eds.): *Cancer Nursing Principles and Practice* (ed 5). Sudbury, MA, Jones and Bartlett, 2000, pp 1117–1137
222. Diamond C, Taylor TH, Anton-Culver H: Dramatic increase in anal cancer diagnoses in the era of highly active antiretroviral therapy. *Conference on Retroviruses and Opportunistic Infections.* San Francisco, CA, February 2–11, 2004 (*www.retroconference.org/2004/cd/PDFs/778.pdf.* Accessed March 24, 2004)
223. Minsky BD, Hoffman JP, Kensen DP: Cancer in the anal region, in DeVita VT, Hellman S, Rosenberg SA (eds.): *Cancer: Principles and Practice of Oncology* (ed 6). Philadelphia, Lippincott, Williams and Wilkins, 2001, pp 1319–1342
224. Ellenhorn JD, Cullinane CA, Coia LR, et al: Colorectal and anal cancers, in Pazdur R, Hoskins WJ, Coia LR, et al (eds.): *Cancer Management: A Multidisciplinary Approach,* (ed 6). Philadelphia, Oncology Group, 2003, pp 323–353
225. Pfister H, Fuchs PG: Relation of papillomavirses to anogenital cancer. *Dermatol Clin* 9:267–270, 1991
226. Daling JR, Weiss NS, Hislop TG: Sexual practices, sexual transmitted diseases, and the incidence of anal cancer. *N Engl J Med* 317:973–979, 1987
227. Ryan DP, Compton CC, Mayer RJ: Carcinoma of the anal canal. *N Engl J Med* 342:792–800, 2000
228. Penn I: Cancer of the anogenital region in renal transplant recipients. *Cancer* 58:611–616, 1986
229. Friis S, Kjaer SK, Frisch M, et al: Cervical intraepithelial neoplasia, anogenital cancer, and other cancer types in women after hospitalization for condyloma acuminata. *J Infect Dis* 175:743–748, 1997
230. Goldie SJ, Kuntz KM, Weinstein MC, et al: The clinical effectiveness and cost-effectiveness of screening for anal intraepithelial lesions in homosexual and bisexual HIV-positive men. *JAMA* 281:1822–1826, 1999
231. Goldie SJ, Kuntz KM, Weinstein MC, et al: The cost-effectiveness of screening for anal squamous intraepithelial lesions in HIV-negative homosexual and bisexual men. *Am J Med* 108:634–641, 2000
232. Salit IE, Tinmouth J, Lytwyn A, et al: Screening for anal cancer. *Community Alliance for Health Research,* Canadian Institutes of Health Research, Ottawa, Ontario, 2004 (abstr 158)
233. Klencke BJ, Palefsky JM: Anal cancer: an HIV associated cancer. *Hematol Oncol Clin North Am:* 17:859–872, 2003

234. National Comprehensive Cancer Network: *Practice Guidelines in Oncology: Anal Canal Cancer,* v.1.2004. Jenkintown, National Comprehensive Cancer Network, 2004
235. Palefsky JM, Holly EA, Hogeboom CJ, et al: Virologic, immunologic and clinical parameters in the incidence and progression of anal squamous intraepithelial lesions in HIV-positive and HIV-negative homosexual men. *J Acquir Immune Defic Syndr Hum Retrovirol* 17:314–319, 1998
236. Haga T, Kim SH, Jensen R, et al: Detection of genetic changes in anal intraepitnelial neoplasia (AIN) of human immunodeficiency virus (HIV)-positive and HIV-negative men. *J AIDS* 26:256–262, 2001
237. Vernon SD, Hart CE, Reeves WC, et al: The HIV-1 tat protein enhances E-2 dependent human papillomavirus 16 transcription. *Virus Res* 27:133–135, 1993
238. Little VR, Leavenworth JD, Darragh TM, et al: Angiogenesis, proliferation and apoptosis in anal high grade squamous intraepithelial lesions (HSIL). *Dis Colon Rectum* 43:346–352, 2000
239. Palefsky JM, Holly EA, Ralston ML, et al: High incidence of anal high-grade squamous intraepithelial lesions among HIV-positive and HIV-negative homosexual and bisexual men. *AIDS* 12:495–503, 1998
240. Allal AS, Laurencet FM, Reymond MA, et al: Effectiveness of surgical salvage therapy for patients with locally uncontrolled anal carcinoma after sphincter-conserving treatment. *Cancer* 86:405–409, 1999
241. Flam M, John M, Pajak TF, et al: Role of mitomycin in combination with fluorouracil and radiotherapy, and of salvage chemoradiation in the definitive nonsurgical treatment of epidermoid carcinoma of the anal canal: results of a phase III randomized intergroup study. *J Clin Oncol* 14:2527–2539, 1996
242. Hung A, Crane C, Delclos M, et al: Cisplatin-based combination modality therapy for anal carcinoma: a wider therapeutic index. *Cancer* 97:1195–1202, 2003
243. Fuchshuber PR, Rodriguez-Bigas M, Weber T, et al: Anal canal and perianal epidermoid cancers. *J Am Coll Surg* 185:494–505, 1997
244. Chang GJ, Berry JM, Jay N, et al: Surgical treatment of high-grade anal squamous intraepithelial lesions: a prospective study. *Dis Colon Rectum* 45:453–458, 2002
245. Flam M, Sandhu AP, Symonds RP, et al: Interstitial iridium-192 implantation combined with external radiotherapy in anal cancer: ten years experience. *Int J Radiat Oncol Biol Phys* 40:575–581, 1998
246. Nigro ND, Seydel HG, Considine B, et al: Combined preoperative radiation and chemotherapy for squamous cell carcinoma of the anal canal. *Cancer* 51:1826–1829, 1983
247. Bartelink H, Roelofsen F, Eschwege F, et al: Concomitant radiotherapy and chemotherapy is superior to radiotherapy alone in the treatment of locally advanced anal cancer: results of a phase III randomized trial of the European Organization for Research and Gastrointestinal Cooperative Groups. *J Clin Oncol* 15:2040–2049, 1997
248. Sobhani I, Walker F, Aparicio T, et al: Effect of anal epidermoid cancer-related viruses on the dendritic (Langerhans') cells of the human anal mucosa. *Clin Cancer Res* 8:2862–2869, 2002

CHAPTER 50

Endocrine Malignancies

Michelle Goodman, RN, MS
Rita Wickham, PhD, RN, AOCN®

Introduction

In 2004, approximately 25,520 new cases of endocrine cancers were diagnosed in the United States and 2440 individuals died of their disease, accounting for less than 0.21% of all cancer deaths.[1] More than 90% of endocrine cancers occur in the thyroid gland. The extreme discrepancy between the incidence of endocrine cancers and the small percentage of deaths exemplifies the indolent nature of thyroid cancer and the long-term survival associated with this malignancy.

Endocrine malignancies arise from endocrine glands that elaborate and secrete hormones (chemical signals) into the bloodstream and exert their effects at distant sites. The classic endocrine glands of interest for this chapter include the pituitary, the thyroid, the parathyroids, and the adrenal glands. This chapter focuses on malignancies arising in these tissues, as well as multiple endocrine neoplasia (MEN) syndromes.

Thyroid Tumors

The thyroid is a small organ that lies below the cricoid cartilage at the base of the neck and around either side of the trachea. The functional units of the thyroid are follicles, composed of epithelial cells interspersed with parafollicular cells (also known as *C cells*). Groups of follicles are bound tightly together to form lobules. The follicular cells produce the thyroid hormones thyroxine (T_4) and triiodothyronine (T_3), and the C cells produce calcitonin. The thyroid synthesizes its hormones, all of which hold large amounts of iodine, in response to thyroid-stimulating hormone (TSH) released by the anterior pituitary gland.[2]

Virtually all body cells and tissues require thyroid hormones for optimal functioning. For example, thyroid hormone is required for the production of growth hormone (GH), and acts as a growth factor to promote bone formation and skeletal maturation. Thyroid hormones also play a critical role in the maturation of the central nervous system (CNS) in infants and modulate the actions of the autonomic nervous system throughout life.[3] Furthermore, they play roles in oxidative metabolism, help maintain a steady body temperature by heat production or conservation, and positively affect carbohydrate and lipid metabolism, as well as the synthesis and degradation of body proteins.

Epidemiology

The incidence of thyroid cancer has been increasing over the last decade.[4] These malignancies usually occur between the ages of 25 and 65, but are most common in persons older than age 45 and in women, who in a Japanese study were three times as likely as men to develop a thyroid tumor.[5] In contrast, the radiation-induced tumors that occurred in children exposed in the Chernobyl nuclear plant disaster affected males and females equally.[6] Differentiated thyroid cancers account for more than 90% of all thyroid tumors.

The overall survival and outcome in patients with differentiated thyroid cancer are excellent. The long-term survival rates in low-, intermediate-, and high-risk groups are approximately 99%, 87%, and 57%, respectively.[7] Patients in the high-risk group would include those individuals who have differentiated thyroid tumors larger than 4 cm with extrathyroidal extension and who are older than age 45. Age is an important determinant of prognosis. Patients younger than 45 years of age do remarkably well compared with those older than 45 years. This is the only cancer in which age is included in the staging system by the American Joint Committee on Cancer (AJCC) and the Union Internationale Contre le Cancer (UICC). (See Table 50-1.) Also, no thyroid cancer of stage III or IV occurs in patients younger than 45 years of age, because younger patients — even with distant metastasis — do extremely well. Likewise, the presence of nodal metastasis has no bearing on prognosis.[8]

Table 50-1 AJCC TNM Staging for Thyroid Carcinomas

PRIMARY TUMOR (T)	
All categories may be subdivided: (a) solitary; (b) multifocal tumor (the largest determines classification)	
TX	Primary tumor cannot be assessed
T0	No evidence of primary tumor
T1	Tumor 1 cm or less in greatest dimension limited to the thyroid
T2	Tumor more than 1 cm but not more than 4 cm limited to the thyroid
T3	Tumor more than 4 cm in greatest dimension limited to the thyroid
T4	Tumor of any size extending beyond the thyroid capsule
REGIONAL LYMPH NODES (N)	
Regional nodes are cervical and upper mediastinal lymph nodes	
NX	Regional lymph nodes cannot be assessed
N0	No regional lymph node metastasis
N1	Regional lymph node metastasis
N1a	Metastasis in ipsilateral cervical lymph node(s)
N1b	Metastasis in bilateral, midline, or contralateral cervical or mediastinal lymph nodes
DISTANT METASTASIS (M)	
MX	Presence of distant metastasis cannot be assessed
M0	No distant metastasis
M1	Distant metastasis

STAGING GROUPING

Papillary or Follicular

	Under 45 Years	45 Years and Over
Stage I	Any T, Any N, M0	T1, N0, M0
Stage II	Any T, Any N, M1	T2, N0, M0
		T3, N0, M0
Stage III		T4, N0, M0
Stage IV		Any T, Any N, M1

	Medullary	Undifferentiated
Stage I	T1, N0, M0	All cases are classified as Stage IV
Stage II	T2, N0, M0	**Stage IV** Any T, Any N, Any M
	T3, N0, M0	
	T4, N0, M0	
Stage III	Any T, N1, M0	
Stage IV	Any T, Any N, M1	

Based on data from American Joint Committee on Cancer Staging.

Etiology

Ionizing radiation to the head and neck is the only clearly identified etiologic agent for papillary thyroid cancer.[2,9] Other risk factors include benign thyroid disease and consumption of a diet deficient in iodine.[10] Both the age at radiation exposure and the dose of radiation appear to be important factors in determining the latency period prior to the detection of thyroid cancer. The carcinogenic risk of radiation is dose-dependent: Minimal risk exists with exposure to very small doses (6.5–80 cGy), and risk increases linearly to a dose of 2000 cGy. At doses greater than 2000 cGy, the risk for thyroid cancer falls off as the thyroid cells die and the gland becomes sterile.[9] The carcinogenic effect of radiation has been demonstrated in adults who were treated as children with radiation for benign head and neck conditions such as enlarged thymus glands, tonsillitis, adenoid hypertrophy, pharyngitis, or acne.[2,11] Risk is inversely related to age; hence infants and young children are more susceptible to the carcinogenic effects of radiation to the neck region than are older children.

The carcinogenic effects of radiation may persist for as long as four decades after exposure, and are also more pronounced in persons who received therapeutic or accidental radiation to the thyroid as younger children.[10,11] For instance, children who receive total body irradiation in preparation for allogeneic bone marrow transplant are at increased risk for developing papillary thyroid malignancy, and they require regular follow-up for thyroid tumors. Likewise, the incidence of thyroid cancer has increased dramatically in children exposed to high levels of radioactive fallout from the Chernobyl nuclear plant disaster.[12] The thyroid glands of very young children (< 5 years) may be more sensitive to the carcinogenic effects of radiation than those of older children (> 5 years) and adults. In evaluating outcomes of the Chernobyl nuclear accident, the average latency period was 8 years before the development of benign tumors and 7.2 years before the development of malignant thyroid tumors. The latency period prior to the detection of papillary carcinomas was only 6.3 years.

The commonly held theory that papillary thyroid cancers and follicular carcinomas arise from follicular adenomas has recently been disputed. In their evaluation of the relationship between latency period and radiation-induced thyroid neoplasia, Kikuchi and colleagues surmise the following:[12]

1. Adenomas and carcinomas probably develop independently and not sequentially.
2. Multiple mutations probably occur simultaneously and not sequentially.

Thus, the idea that a malignant thyroid tumor occurs as a progression from a benign nodule is probably invalid.

Pathophysiology

At least 94% of thyroid carcinomas are differentiated carcinomas that derive from the follicular epithelial cells and are either papillary thyroid carcinomas or follicular thyroid carcinomas. Another 5% involve medullary thyroid carcinoma, a neuroendocrine tumor, and the remaining 1% are anaplastic thyroid carcinomas arising from differentiated papillary or follicular tumors. Prognosis and therapy decisions are mainly related to the patient's age, size of tumor, presence of extrathyroidal tumor extension, and characterization of the tumor as well, intermediate, or poorly differentiated.[4]

Papillary and Follicular Tumors

Papillary carcinomas include tumors consisting only of papillary cells and those consisting of mixed papillary and follicular cells, which behave similarly. In regions of iodine insufficiency, follicular thyroid carcinoma is more common than papillary thyroid carcinoma. Differentiated carcinoma can be inherited as a component of familial adenomatous polyposis, Gardner's syndrome, and Cowden's disease.[10] Familial nonmedullary carcinoma has been reported in 5% of all patients with papillary thyroid carcinoma, and it might herald a more aggressive disease course. Potential loci of susceptibility have been identified on chromosomes 1q21, 2q21, and 19p13.2.[13]

Papillary tumors usually are multifocal and infiltrate local tissues, and 40% of patients have regional lymph node metastases at time of diagnosis. Vascular invasion and metastasis to distant site, such as bone and lung, are more common in papillary tumors than in follicular tumors. Women are three times more likely than men to develop papillary carcinomas. Although papillary carcinomas are typically well differentiated, are usually indolent, and have a good prognosis, males and older patients more often have aggressive tumors. Histological subtypes that might signal poor prognosis include tall cell and columnar cell variants of papillary type carcinoma; Hurthle cell cancer, which often occurs in older patients who may retain the ability to synthesize thyroid hormones and thus present with hyperthyroidism; and poorly differentiated variants of the follicular type.[14] Patients may survive for decades even when they have metastatic disease.

Follicular thyroid cancer, which accounts for approximately 20% of all cases, is more aggressive than papillary cancer. Age, tumor size, and blood vessel invasion are significant prognostic indicators. Follicular cancer is most often diagnosed in persons in their fifties, but individuals younger than age 40 have the best prognosis. Indicators of poor prognosis include large tumor size (> 6 cm) and blood vessel invasion.

Medullary Tumors

Medullary thyroid carcinoma (MTC) occurs in equal numbers of men and women older than age 50. This type of cancer derives from the neuroendocrine C cells of the thyroid. The majority of cases of MTC are sporadic, while the remainder occur because of an inherited gene mutation that increases susceptibility for multiple endocrine neoplasia (MEN).[15] Many patients have tumor spread to their cervical lymph nodes at time of diagnosis. Regional lymph node spread is an ominous prognostic sign; the ten-year survival rate is only 42% in patients with involved lymph nodes but is 90% in patients with negative regional lymph nodes. For patients who have known family members with inherited medullary thyroid carcinoma, prospective family screening to identify gene carriers is recommended in view of the 90%–95% penetrance of the disease. Patients with multiple endocrine neoplasia type 2B are more likely than those with either type 2A or familial medullary thyroid carcinoma to have locally aggressive disease.[16] MTC tumors metastasize via the blood stream and lymphatics to lung, liver, and bone.

Anaplastic Tumors

Anaplastic thyroid carcinoma occurs in women slightly more often than in men and rarely occurs in persons younger than 50 years of age. The most serious complication of well-differentiated thyroid carcinoma is anaplastic transformation. Approximately half of all patients with anaplastic cancer have previous or coexistent differentiated thyroid carcinoma with some evidence of dedifferentiation, often associated with loss of the p53 tumor suppressor protein.[17,18] Patients typically present with a rapidly growing, firm or hard, ill-defined neck mass accompanied by dysphagia, and dysphonia caused by invasion or extension into neck structures. Completely resectable tumors have the best prognosis. Unfortunately, complete resection is not the usual case, and most patients live for only 4–12 months following diagnosis. Patients often present with metastatic disease to the lungs, pleura, bone, and brain. Radiation therapy and chemotherapy do not significantly alter survival rates.

Clinical Manifestations

Thyroid malignancies often do not cause symptoms until the disease is advanced. The patient may seek medical attention when the individual or someone else notices that the person's neck looks larger, or because a neck mass becomes painful and is noticeably enlarging. Symptoms or signs that are highly suspicious of cancer include rapid tumor growth, a very firm nodule, fixation to adjacent structures, vocal cord paralysis, and enlarged regional lymph nodes. A manifestation unique to medullary thyroid tumors is the ability of the tumor to oversecrete measurable quantities of calcitonin, along with other hormonally active peptides such as adrenocorticotropic hormone, which leads to unexplained diarrhea, symptoms of Cushing's syndrome, or facial flushing in approximately 20%–30% of patients.

Assessment

Diagnostic procedures for thyroid malignancies include history and physical examination, laboratory tests, and imaging procedures followed by biopsy to confirm the diagnosis. The history may provide clues to the diagnosis, especially information about radiation exposure to the neck in early childhood. A thorough family history is important, especially if familial MTC or MEN2 is suspected.

At presentation, young patients with thyroid masses most often have painless anterior cervical adenopathy, whereas older individuals usually have regional lymph node metastasis or, rarely, distant metastasis. An asymptomatic thyroid nodule is commonly found by patients themselves or by an examiner during routine physical examination. Gentle palpation of the normal neck reveals thyroid lobes that are small, smooth, and free of nodules, and a thyroid that freely rises with swallowing. Any deviations from normal require further investigation. It is not uncommon for patients with papillary thyroid cancer to have involvement of cervical lymph nodes at the time of diagnosis, whereas lymph node metastasis in follicular thyroid cancers is much less common. Hurthle cell neoplasms are similar to follicular thyroid cancers in terms of survival and natural history, but tend to spread to the cervical lymph nodes more frequently.

Thyroid function tests may not be included as part of the work-up for thyroid cancer because most patients are euthyroid and cancer of the thyroid does not alter the thyroid's functional capacity. One exception is elevated serum calcitonin levels, which are strongly suggestive of medullary hyperplasia or MTC. Medullary tumor cells continue to secrete calcitonin, which may serve as a useful tumor marker to monitor the effectiveness of treatment and disease recurrence.[19] Postoperative calcitonin levels are correlated with survival, and normalization is associated with long-term, complication-free survival. Patients whose calcitonin does not normalize typically survive for less than five years and often have extensive metastases.[19] A patient with a suspicious thyroid nodule may receive a trial of TSH-suppressive drugs. These agents may cause benign nodules to shrink but will have no effect on malignant nodules. The drugs, however, have adverse effects and suppression of growth does not guarantee that the nodule is benign.

Current research is focusing on identifying biochemical markers or gene mutations that might aid in the work-up of thyroid tumors. For instance, *p53* status and germ-line point mutations in RET exon 8 in familial medullary thyroid cancer may someday assist clinicians in determining the diagnosis and extent of disease.[20,21] Although ultrasonography or radionuclide scanning alone cannot distinguish benign and malignant nodules, these or other imaging procedures—such as computerized tomography (CT), magnetic resonance imaging (MRI), and positron emission tomography (PET)—may provide useful diagnostic information regarding primary or metastatic disease. Ultrasonography, which can distinguish between cystic, solid, and mixed lesions, is safe for children and pregnant women because it does not use ionizing radiation. Radionuclide scans following injection of radioiodine (usually ^{123}I) or technetium (^{99m}Tc) are used to visualize the thyroid. A suspicious nodule can trap and incorporate iodine, while ^{99m}Tc can only demonstrate a nodule's ability to trap iodine. However, ^{99m}Tc may be more sensitive than ^{131}I in identifying metastatic lesions. Radionuclide scans usually show that malignant lesions are hypofunctioning or cold, but this finding is nonspecific and nondiagnostic. Conversely, ultrasound has been shown to have an increased sensitivity compared with thyroid scintigraphy, is of relatively low cost, and is easily accessible.[22] In the presence of poorly defined margins and a thick halo with evidence of fine internal calcifications on ultrasound, a malignant thyroid nodule would be highly suspected.

Biopsy and histopathologic examination of tumor tissue are ultimately necessary, and fine-needle aspiration (FNA) and biopsy is the procedure of choice to confirm thyroid malignancy. When done by an experienced and proficient surgeon, FNA biopsy is highly sensitive and accurately diagnoses thyroid malignancy 95% of the time. Under these circumstances, the false-negative rate is only 5%–10%. FNA helps eliminate unnecessary surgery for benign lesions and allows appropriate treatment to be selected when a malignant tumor is found. If the FNA is negative, it may be repeated with ultrasound guidance to confirm that the lesion is, indeed, benign.[22] Other advantages of FNA are that it is relatively inexpensive, can be performed in the outpatient setting, causes minimal complications, and allows sufficient tissue to be obtained for DNA analysis, which may provide further information about the malignant potential of the tumor. Of interest is the fact that the FNA biopsy is of limited value in determining the malignant potential of follicular neoplasms. A suspected follicular lesion is nearly always classified as indeterminate via this technique, requiring definitive surgical resection to establish the diagnosis. Only by identifying capsular or vascular invasion may follicular cancer be diagnosed, because cells from follicular adenomas and follicular carcinomas appear identical pathologically.[2]

Classification and Staging

Histological diagnosis and age are the two most important determinants of prognosis. As noted earlier, these factors are incorporated into the American Joint Committee on Cancer (AJCC) staging system for thyroid cancer (Table 50-1). Prognosis is most favorable for patients younger than age 40 whose tumors have not invaded local structures or blood vessels.

Therapeutic Approaches and Nursing Care

Surgery

Treatment decisions regarding thyroid tumors are controversial, and they are complicated by the fact that most tumors are indolent. Because of this protracted clinical course, some clinicians do not recommend treatment until the patient becomes symptomatic.[10] Surgery is the agreed-upon treatment of choice for thyroid tumors, but no consensus exists regarding the extent of surgical resection for well-differentiated tumors. Studies comparing total, subtotal, and partial thyroidectomy have found that subtotal resection of tumors less than 1 cm in patients younger than age 45 results in similar recurrence and survival rates as more extensive surgery.[2,23] The risk of surgical complications is lower with lobectomy, but the risk for recurrence is 5%–10% higher than with total resection of the thyroid. When cure is possible, more aggressive surgery (near-total thyroidectomy, tumor resection, and neck dissection) has been advocated for medullary and anaplastic tumors.[24] Table 50-2 summarizes the recommended therapeutic approaches in the management of thyroid tumors.

Overall considerations in the management of thyroid cancer indicate that 80% of patients will do well with lobectomy alone, 15% will require a total thyroidectomy (based on the extent of the disease and the need for radioactive iodine or external radiation therapy), and 5% will die regardless of the extent of thyroidectomy or adjuvant treatment. The latter individuals are usually elderly with locally aggressive poorly differentiated thyroid cancer.[25]

Postoperative complications of thyroidectomy include recurrent laryngeal nerve paralysis, vocal cord paralysis with subsequent respiratory embarrassment, thyroid storm, hemorrhage, and hypothyroidism.[26] Thyroid storm, or thyrotoxic crisis, is an acute episode of thyroid overactivity that is characterized by high fever, tachycardia, delirium, dehydration, and extreme excitability. Patients may experience temporary postoperative hoarseness, which is related to

Table 50-2 Recommended Treatment Approaches for Thyroid Tumors

Tumor Type	Recommended Surgery	Comments	Postoperative
Papillary and follicular		Choice of surgery is based on age and size of nodule	Exogenous thyroid hormone (thyroxine) therapy is administered to suppress TSH
Stage I	Lobectomy	Lower incidence of complications Abnormal lymph nodes are biopsied and selectively resected 5%–10% local recurrence	Papillary: ^{131}I may decrease recurrence Follicular: Remaining disease may compromise effectiveness of ^{131}I ablative therapy
Stage II	Total thyroidectomy	Higher incidence of hypoparathyroidism Facilitates follow-up thyroid scanning	
Stage III	Total thyroidectomy or lobectomy	High incidence of local recurrence in patients with extrathyroidal extension	Local radiation therapy may be used to control symptoms
Stage IV	Total thyroidectomy and removal of lymph nodes/extrathyroid disease		Patients are monitored for metastasis to lung and bone Treatment for metastases: ^{131}I, external beam radiation therapy, TSH suppression
Medullary	Total thyroidectomy with modified neck dissection if extrathyroidal disease present, unless patient has distant metastasis	Surgery is curative when disease is confined to the thyroid	Chemotherapy leads to occasional responses in metastatic disease
Anaplastic	Total thyroidectomy to reduce mass-induced symptoms and facilitate the radioactive iodine ablation	Tracheostomy is often necessary	Radiation therapy may be used for patients whose tumors are not surgically resectable or who cannot undergo surgery Chemotherapy may induce partial responses in some patients

intubation and local swelling. Permanent hoarseness is rare but more serious, and is caused by damage to the laryngeal nerve during surgery that leads to vocal cord paralysis. Hemorrhage is another possible postoperative complication, so the nurse monitors for local hematoma (which may compromise the patient's airway) as well as for output from drains and symptoms of impending shock. With the adoption of minimally invasive surgical techniques utilizing endoscopic technology, the surgical complications following throidectomy should become less problematic.[27]

Postoperative nursing management also requires keen assessment for the signs and symptoms of tetany, for hypocalcemia, and for other complications (Table 50-3). Calcium levels are monitored daily, because 1% of patients undergoing near-total thyroidectomies and as many as 6%–8% of those undergoing total thyroidectomies will experience temporary or permanent hypoparathyroidism. Hypothyroidism results in hypocalcemia, so patients must take exogenous thyroid hormone to prevent the clinical effects of hypothyroidism.[28]

Radiation Therapy

Radioiodine therapy is used to treat some cases of papillary and follicular tumors but not medullary or anaplastic tumors, which do not concentrate and retain iodine. Four to six weeks after surgery, oral ^{131}I is administered to ablate any remaining functioning thyroid tissue as well as residual local and metastatic tumor. A whole-body scan is performed two to three months after treatment to determine whether any tumor and functioning thyroid tissue remain, it is repeated at four- to six-month intervals as necessary.[9] If any tumor remains, ^{131}I therapy is repeated until the whole-body scan is negative.

Side effects of ^{131}I include nausea and vomiting, fatigue, headache, bone marrow suppression, salivary gland inflammation, and infrequently leukemia and radiation-induced pulmonary fibrosis. Nursing care focuses on minimizing the patient's sense of isolation and providing radiation safety for staff and visitors. Patient and family education is extremely important to clarify misconceptions regarding ^{131}I treatment (Figure 50-1).

External beam radiation occasionally results in local control of anaplastic tumors that do not take up ^{131}I, but tumors are usually radioresistant. Because most patients with these tumors die from local progression with airway or esophageal obstruction, treatment with radiation results in increased morbidity and is reserved for palliation of painful bone metastases.

Chemotherapy

Clinical trials with chemotherapeutic drugs have produced only rare and limited positive responses in thyroid cancer.[29–31] There are very few reports of chemotherapy for refractory, metastatic, and anaplastic thyroid cancers, and the results of those that exist are generally discouraging. Doxorubicin, epirubicin, and

Table 50-3 Care Plan for Patient Undergoing Thyroid Surgery

Problem/Diagnosis	Nursing Observations/Actions	Comments
Potential for ineffective airway clearance related to: • Hematoma • Vocal cord paralysis	Assess respiratory status every hour for 12 hours, then every 4 hours for 48 hours Assess vital signs every 4 hours for 48 hours Observe for: • Hoarseness • Inability to speak • Retraction of neck muscles • Crowing respirations • Dyspnea • Cyanosis • Hematoma formation Keep head of bed elevated to < 45 degrees at all times Maintain neck support by placing hand behind neck with elbows raised when moving or sitting Turn, cough, and deep breathe every 2 hours	Notify MD immediately for: • Signs and symptoms of vocal cord paralysis • Respiratory distress • Patient reports of neck tightness, fullness, or pressure (indicates possible internal bleeding)
Potential for decreased serum calcium level related to impaired parathyroid function, secondary to removal or reimplantation	Observe for signs and symptoms of tetany every 4 hours for 7 days Monitor daily serum calcium Administer calcium gluconate, as ordered Teach patient to avoid foods that suppress calcium absorption (e.g., spinach, Swiss cheese, beets, bran, and whole-grain cereals)	Symptoms of hypocalcemia: • Numbness, tingling, cramps in extremities or around mouth • Stiffness, twitching, or spasms in hands or feet • Positive Chvostek sign • Positive Trousseau sign
Potential for thyrotoxic crisis (thyroid storm) related to partial thyroidectomy	Observe patient for signs and symptoms of thyroid storm every 4 hours In case of thyroid storm administer: • Prescribed IV fluid, vitamins, and glucocorticoids • Prescribed antithyroid medication (propylthiouracil) • Prescribed iodine medication Employ measures to reduce body temperature, such as cooling blanket, tepid sponge bath	Manifestations of thyroid storm: • Sudden increase in temperature • Extreme restlessness or irritability • Delirium • Tachycardia • Widening pulse pressure followed by hypotension • Nausea and vomiting, diarrhea, and warm, flushed skin Notify MD immediately if temperature rises to > 99°F orally or 100°F rectally (may be first sign of thyroid storm)

carboplatin have shown the greatest activity against thyroid malignancies. Response rates vary, ranging from 14% to 31% for anaplastic tumors and well-differentiated medullary tumors, respectively. Chemotherapy for thyroid carcinoma is commonly performed under TSH suppression, aimed to block proliferation of thyroid cells. This approach contradicts the idea that cell-cycle–specific agents are most effective on tumors with a high growth fraction. The use of TSH-suppressive therapy could potentially counteract the efficacy of chemotherapeutic drugs and narrow their therapeutic index.[32]

Parathyroid Tumors

The parathyroid glands are located on the posterior thyroid, and lie at the surface or are embedded in the thyroid. Most people have four glands, but the normal range is two to eight. Chief cells are the major functional cells of the parathyroid glands and produce parathyroid hormone (PTH), which is critical to maintain normal serum calcium balance. PTH is secreted to increase calcium resorption from bone when serum calcium is low; when the serum calcium level is high, it is not secreted.[33]

What is ^{131}I?
^{131}I is radioactive iodine that goes to the thyroid gland and thyroid cancer cells. It is toxic to these cells, and the aim of treatment is to kill cancer cells. It will also kill normal thyroid cells.

Where will I go to get the ^{131}I treatment?
You will have to go to the hospital to get this treatment. While in the hospital, you will wear only hospital gowns, robe, and slippers. Do not bring things from home.

How will I take the ^{131}I?
You will be given a special container of ^{131}I, and you will drink it through a straw.

Will I be able to have visitors while I am in the hospital?
You may have adult visitors while you are in the hospital, but because you will be radioactive there are some rules:

1. No pregnant women can visit.
2. Visitors will only be able to stay for 30 minutes or less for the first 48 hours.

Will I have any side effects from the ^{131}I?
Possible side effects may include nausea and vomiting, tiredness, headache, a sore mouth, and a lowered white blood count after you get the treatment. Your nurse will give you medicine for the nausea or the headache if you have them, and your doctor may want you to get a blood test after you go home. You may also have a metallic taste in your mouth for several days after taking ^{131}I.

Will I still be radioactive when I go home?
Yes, you will be radioactive for a few days. For three days after you go home, you should:

1. Sleep alone.
2. Not hold children close.

How can I help my body get rid of the ^{131}I?
You need to drink as much fluid as you can (at least 2 quarts) for several days after getting the ^{131}I. This can include water, juices, sodas, and so forth. The ^{131}I will pass out of your body in your urine, so when you go to the bathroom you should:

1. Sit on the toilet to urinate so urine does not splash anywhere.
2. Flush the toilet three times after you pass urine.

How will my doctor know if the thyroid cancer is gone?
Your doctor will schedule you for a body scan in about three to six months. If the scan shows that there aren't any more thyroid cancer cells, you will not need any more ^{131}I. If there are any thyroid cancer cells that show up on the scan, you will get another ^{131}I treatment.

If you have any other questions, please write them down so you remember to ask your doctor or your nurse.

Figure 50-1 Teaching sheet for the patient receiving ^{131}I treatment.

Epidemiology

The majority of parathyroid tumors are benign. Parathyroid carcinoma is an uncommon cause of PTH-dependent hypercalcemia and accounts for less than 0.1%–5% of primary hyperparathyroidism.[33] Tumors occur with equal frequency in males and females, who are usually diagnosed in their forties and fifties. Parathyroid tumors most commonly occur in individuals who have familial MEN1, and less frequently in those with MEN2A.[34]

Etiology

No definitive risk factors have been identified for the development of parathyroid carcinoma. For instance, only rare individuals diagnosed with parathyroid adenoma or carcinoma have received radiation to or near the neck area. Parathyroid carcinoma has been associated with chronic renal failure and dialysis. One suggestion proposes a relationship between parathyroid carcinoma and chronic hypocalcemia caused by renal insufficiency, hypovitaminosis D, malabsorption of calcium in the gut, or PTH resistance.[11]

Pathophysiology

It is often difficult to establish that a tumor is benign or malignant, or even that hyperplasia is present, because all such cells appear histopathologically similar. However, adenomas usually involve only one parathyroid gland and are surrounded by a rim of normal parathyroid tissue. Hyperplasia occurs in multiple glands, while carcinomas may have more mitoses and may be surrounded by a thick and irregular capsule.[35] Ultimately, local infiltration, invasion into blood vessels, and metastases characterize malignant tumors. When discovered, carcinomas may be hard, lobulated, and larger than benign tumors, and they will eventually invade adjacent structures. The clinical features of parathyroid carcinoma primarily reflect the effects of excessive secretion of PTH by the functioning tumor leading to hyperparathyroid bone disease, and nephrolithiasis or nephrocalcinosis due to renal involvement.[33]

Carcinomas tend to be indolent, so tumors may be discovered late. The recurrence of hypercalcemia or elevated serum PTH after surgery signals that a tumor, which may have been diagnosed as benign, is malignant. When parathyroid carcinoma is diagnosed, 20% of patients have cervical lymph node metastases and 16% have distant metastases—most commonly to the lungs, bone, or liver.

Clinical Manifestations

Symptoms of hypercalcemic effects on the kidney, bone, and other organs and sometimes a palpable neck mass (30%–75% of patients), hoarseness, or recurrent laryngeal nerve palsy in a patient with primary hyperparathyroidism who has not had previous neck surgery are very suggestive of parathyroid cancer. Typically, a patient's serum calcium exceeds 14 mg/dL (3.5 mmol/L). Prolonged hypercalcemia may lead to rheumatologic symptoms, renal calculi, and calcification of the cornea and other soft tissues. Recurrent severe pancreatitis, peptic ulcer disease, and anemia occur with greater frequency in patients with malignant disease than in those with benign primary hyperparathyroidism.

Assessment

The pathognomic signs and symptoms essentially confirm the diagnosis of parathyroid tumor. The patient may initially notice nonspecific symptoms such as fatigue, irritability, and difficulty concentrating. In some cases, these progress to symptoms of worsening hypercalcemia, which is characterized by nausea, anorexia, weight loss, and dehydration.

When unexplained hypercalcemia is discovered, a search for parathyroid carcinoma begins with an immunoassay for immunoassayable parathyroid hormone (iPTH). In the case of parathyroid tumor, levels are usually markedly increased. The majority of patients do not have a palpable mass, so visualization procedures (ultrasonography, nuclear scan, CT, and MRI) are used to localize and evaluate tumor masses after surgery.[36] For instance, a 99m-technetium sestamibi (MIBI) radionuclide scan can aid in determining whether disease is confined to one or more glands, which may direct the extent of surgery.[37] Radiographs or bone scans are useful to confirm bone metastases, but the lung is the most frequent site of distant disease.[34]

Research continues in an effort to find more effective measures to confirm that a parathyroid tumor is malignant. For example, one study found that the expression of *p27* is greatly reduced in carcinomas as compared to hyperplasia and benign adenomas.[35] It is likely that *p27* is a tumor suppressor gene, which codes for a cyclin-dependent kinase that regulates the progression of a cell from G_1 to the S phase of cell division. Assaying for reduced levels might, therefore, be useful in diagnosis.

Therapeutic Approaches and Nursing Care

Surgery

Surgery is the recommended treatment for parathyroid tumors. In general, performance of the appropriate surgical procedure during the initial operation is critical and is one of the most important prognostic factors. Most patients who have recurrences after initial surgery will ultimately die of cancer-related causes, usually the metabolic complications of hypercalcemia.[38] Radiotherapy and chemotherapy are ineffective to treat primary and metastatic disease.

The primary tumor is resected en bloc with the ipsilateral thyroid lobe and isthmus. The surgeon must be careful to avoid rupture of the parathyroid capsule, which may result in local seeding of tumor. Surgery for localized parathyroid adenomas and carcinomas may include unilateral neck dissection if local structures are involved.[39] Extensive surgery may be necessary to remove all tumor from the trachea, involved central lymph nodes, and any contiguous tissues to which the tumor adheres. If the recurrent laryngeal nerve is involved, it must also be resected. Parathyroid tumors are usually indolent, and patients typically benefit from further resection of metastatic disease, such as lung metastases. Recurrent disease is rarely curable.

In some situations where multiglandular disease is not suspected, localizing the tumor using sestamibi scanning may be possible. Sestamibi scanning offers both high sensitivity and high specificity; therefore, minimally invasive radioguided parathyroidectomy may be performed with a shorter operative time, low morbidity, and decreased duration of hospital stay.[37,40]

The focus of postoperative nursing care is to monitor calcium levels, prevent hemorrhage, and teach the patient and family self-care management (see Table 50-3). As calcium and phosphorus are deposited into the skeleton, symptomatic hypocalcemia (''hungry bone'' syndrome) occurs and provides evidence of successful tumor removal. The patient will require supplemental intravenous calcium and calcitrol until the remaining parathyroid glands recover. Serum calcium and PTH levels are monitored every three months for elevation, which signifies recurrent local or metastatic disease. Hemorrhage is another potential and serious complication, particularly for patients undergoing parathyroid reexploration surgery.

Chemotherapy

Parathyroid malignancy is so rare that there are no reported chemotherapy studies, but a few case reports document limited success and remissions of metastatic disease. Combination regimens—including 5-FU, cyclophosphamide, and methotrexate, doxorubicin, cyclophosphamide, and paclitaxel—have been used. Overall, however, chemotherapy has been judged ineffective for treatment of parathyroid carcinomas.

Palliative Care

Control of hypercalcemia in patients with parathyroid tumors is often difficult because it is caused by tumor recurrence. When surgery is not feasible, recurrent hypercalcemia is treated with the same drugs used to treat other instances of hypercalcemia. Calcitonin, bisphosphonates, or other antiresorptive therapies may be partially effective for a limited time, but calcium levels may remain persistently elevated despite attempts to inhibit the effects of tumor PTH. Chronic, uncontrolled hypercalcemia, which leads to uncontrollable nausea, vomiting, and dehydration, remains the cause of death for most patients with parathyroid tumors.

Pituitary Tumors

Pituitary tumors are the most commonly encountered intracerebral lesion.[41] The majority of pituitary tumors express and secrete pituitary hormones producing a variety of endocrinological syndromes, including hyperprolactinemia, Cushing's syndrome due to adrenocorticotrophin excess, acromegaly due to growth hormone hypersecretion, and other less common disorders. While isolation of a single, causatory factor in sporadic pituitary tumorigenesis is difficult, mutations of the tyrosine kinase receptor, RET, have been recently implicated in the pathogenesis of a subset of pituitary tumors.[42] As more is learned concerning the targets of these markers, the closer researchers will come to prediction of tumor behavior and potential therapeutic interventions.

The pituitary is a 1 cm organ that lies at the base of the brain in the sella turcica, a bony cavity in sphenoid bone. It consists of the anterior pituitary and the posterior pituitary, which are anatomically and physiologically distinct. The anterior pituitary cells are hormone-secreting or nonsecreting cells. Secreting cells differ in that each synthesizes a different hormone that controls the physiologic function of the thyroid, adrenal glands, gonads, or mammary glands. Secreting cells give rise to pituitary tumors. The anterior pituitary also controls growth by secreting trophic hormones, including thyroid-stimulating hormone (TSH), adrenocorticotropin, prolactin, and growth hormone (GH). TSH controls the rate of thyroxine secretion by the thyroid, adrenocorticotropin controls some adrenocortical hormones, prolactin promotes breast tissue development and milk production, and GH promotes growth and affects multiple metabolic processes. Secretion of trophic hormones is regulated by negative feedback loops that are influenced by the target organs and by the CNS, particularly the hypothalamus, which is connected to and communicates with the pituitary by means of the pituitary stalk. The hypothalamus plays a critical role in pituitary function by secreting releasing and inhibitory hormones that are carried through the hypothalamic-hypophysial portal vessels directly to the pituitary. Nonsecreting cells synthesize cytokines, which may play roles in regulating hypothalamo-pituitary-adrenal axis functions.[43]

Epidemiology

Approximately 10% of brain tumors are pituitary tumors.[44] These tumors usually remain small and hormonally silent, and as many as 11% of individuals are discovered to have evidence of a pituitary carcinoma at autopsy or upon CT or MRI scans done for other reasons.[45] Female-to-male incidence varies by tumor type. Women are four times more likely than men to develop a prolactinoma, and are at three times greater risk of developing Cushing's disease. In contrast, acromegaly occurs at an equal rate in women and men. Although 70% of pituitary adenomas occur in persons aged 30–50, these tumors can also develop in children and teenagers.

Etiology

The pathogenesis of pituitary tumors is unknown. Studies have shown that most pituitary tumors are monoclonal in origin; that is, they arise from repeated division of a single mutated cell, which probably occurs because of some key somatic mutation. A pituitary tumor–transforming gene (*PTTG*) has recently been cloned and is thought to play a role in tumorigenesis and progression.[46] *PTTG* is expressed in some nonfunctioning and functioning pituitary tumors, but not in normal pituitary tissues. As a consequence, it may be a useful marker for pituitary tumor aggressiveness. Many genetic mutations in tumor suppressor genes and oncogenes have been identified in pituitary tumors, which further demonstrates that pituitary tumorigenesis is a multistep process. These alterations accumulate, causing tumors to become increasingly aggressive over time. For example, mutations in the *p53* gene are found only in invasive pituitary adenomas and carcinomas.[47] It is important to recognize that currently there are no accepted genetic markers for predicting biological behavior in pituitary gland tumors.[43]

Pathophysiology

Both benign and malignant pituitary tumors express altered gene products for neurotransmitters and hypothalamic hormones that cause physiological effects. Carcinomas may invade the subarachnoid space and metastasize to the brain and spinal cord through lymphatic or vascular channels, and to the liver and bone through the cervical lymphatics.

Clinical Manifestations

In most cases, the signs and symptoms of pituitary adenomas result from secretion or depression of particular hormones, and from mass effects in rarer instances. A variety of tumors can arise, so a corresponding number of syndromes may occur. These relate to the hypersecretion of prolactin, growth hormone, adrenocorticotropic hormone (ACTH), or less commonly, other hormones. Because prolactinomas arise most frequently, oligomenorrhea, or amenorrhea, and galactorrhea are the most frequent hormone effects documented. The most frequent symptoms of mass effects include headaches in 40%–60% of patients and visual changes (e.g., blurred vision, loss of peripheral vision or changes in particular visual fields, double vision, changes in visual acuity) in 60% of affected individuals.

Hormone Effects

Prolactinomas. Prolactinomas constitute 40% of all pituitary tumors.[48] Women are more likely to have small tumors (microadenomas), which cause galactorrhea, menstrual irregularities including amenorrhea, oligomenorrhea, or infertility, and in some instances osteoporosis. Men are more likely to have large tumors (macroadenomas), and high prolactin levels produced by these tumors may cause men to have decreased libido or impotence, and in some cases galactorrhea.[49] Women tend to notice their symptoms and seek medical attention earlier than men, who may attribute their symptoms to advancing age.

Growth hormone–secreting tumors. Almost all cases of GH-secreting tumors arise in the pituitary. These tumors induce acromegaly in adults and gigantism in prepubescent children. They progress slowly, with the average time from onset of symptoms to diagnosis being 6.5 years and perhaps as long as 10 years.[50,51] Early symptoms are nonspecific and include fatigue or lethargy, paresthesia, and headache. As tumors grow, the excessive GH levels lead to enlargement of bone, organs, and soft tissues. The result is arthropathies and neuropathies (from soft tissue swelling) that interfere with normal activities, and the characteristic disfigurement of the face. Other signs and symptoms include weight gain, excessive perspiration, insulin resistance, and decreased glucose tolerance leading to diabetes.[52] Cardiovascular and cerebrovascular disease, hypertension, respiratory and metabolic dysfunction, and GI malignancy may shorten life expectancy and increase mortality by twofold to threefold compared with two to three times higher than in age-matched individuals.[53] Death often results from cardiac complications, cerebrovascular accidents, or infection.

Cushing's syndrome. Sustained hypersecretion of ACTH by a pituitary adenoma is the major cause of Cushing's syndrome, resulting in 70%–80% of all cases.[54] The most frequent manifestations of Cushing's syndrome include the characteristic moon face, experienced by more than 90% of affected individuals; 80%–90% have truncal obesity, hypertension, impaired glucose tolerance, and hypogonadism (menstrual irregularities, loss of libido).[55] Other common symptoms in severe Cushing's syndrome include congestive heart failure (CHF), purple striae, muscular weakness, pedal edema, skeletal pain, and psychological changes. In addition, women may develop hirsutism. Less common symptoms are easy bruising, infection, poor wound healing, osteoporosis and fractures, polyuria, polydipsia, and renal calculi.

The onset of the symptoms of Cushing's syndrome is often subtle, so there is usually a long period between symptom onset and diagnosis. Patients are frequently treated for individual symptoms such as obesity, menstrual irregularities, or depression before the pattern of symptoms is noted. Cushing's syndrome is a severe disease, even if it is caused by a benign adenoma. As many as 50% of patients will die within five years from cardiovascular disease, infection, or suicide secondary to severe depression if treatment is not instituted.

Assessment

Confirmation of a pituitary tumor includes a history and physical examination, endocrinology testing, radiologic findings, and histopathologic examination. Because most pituitary tumors progress slowly, the history focuses on identifying subtle changes that have occurred over a long period. The medication history is also important because many drugs, including dopamine antagonist antiemetics, tricyclic antidepressants, opioids, and antihypertensives, as well as physical conditions (e.g., chronic renal failure, cirrhosis, hypothyroidism, exercise), can elevate serum prolactin, albeit to a lesser degree than elevations induced by tumors. Physical examination includes testing of peripheral visual fields and cranial nerve function.

Diagnostic procedures for all patients with suspected pituitary tumor focus on tests for the most frequently encountered tumors, but may also include evaluation of gonadal, thyroid, and adrenal functioning. Thus prolactinomas are assessed at baseline and after therapy by measurement of serum prolactin levels.[53] In women, gonadal function evaluation includes luteinizing hormone, follicle-stimulating hormone, and plasma estradiol; in men, plasma testosterone is assessed. When indicated, thyroid function tests, including T_3, T_4, and TSH, are checked, and adrenal functioning is evaluated by sampling basal plasma or urinary steroids. More specific tests for stimulation and suppression of pituitary hormones are done in some cases to detect tumors and to evaluate response to therapy (Table 50-4).[56–58]

Radiologic tests may confirm abnormalities in and around the pituitary. Plain radiographs of the head can show only gross enlargement of the sella turcica. MRI and CT may more clearly demonstrate in three dimensions the tumor size and extension both preoperatively and after surgery. Some tumors, such as those that cause Cushing's disease, may be so small as to elude detection. PET may also be useful to evaluate pituitary tumors.

Classification and Staging

Pituitary adenomas are classified by the hormone secreted, secretory ability, size, and invasiveness. Most tumors are functioning, meaning that they secrete a given hormone and cause the corresponding clinical syndrome. Other tumors do not secrete an excessive amount of hormone, or they secrete biologically inactive molecules or hormone precursors, and are thus considered to be nonfunctioning. Prolactinomas are most common and account for 60% of all functioning tumors, GH-secreting tumors (acromegaly) occur in 20% of cases, and ACTH-secreting tumors (Cushing's disease) are found in 10% of patients.

Microadenomas are tumors that are smaller than 10 mm in diameter, while macroadenomas are larger than 10 mm. Signs and symptoms often predict tumor size. For example, women of childbearing age are more likely to report symptoms of a prolactinoma, whereas men may attribute decreased libido to normal aging. Thus women are more likely to have a microadenoma, while macroadenomas are diagnosed more often in men. ACTH-secreting tumors tend to be diagnosed while they are microadenomas, whereas 70% of GH-secreting tumors are macroadenomas. Tumors are also characterized as intrasellar and extrasellar, depending on their ability to expand outside the sella turcica, and as noninvasive or invasive, depending on whether they can infiltrate into the dural and osseous walls.[59]

Therapeutic Approaches and Nursing Care

The goals of medical management are to normalize pituitary secretion, alleviate signs and symptoms of hormone hypersecretion, reduce tumor size so as to relieve compression on vital structures, preserve or restore residual anterior pituitary function, and prevent tumor recurrence. The primary treatment approach depends on the tumor type, and may include surgery, radiation therapy, and drug therapy either alone or in combination with other measures. Treatment decisions are based on the immediacy of need to relieve mass effect or endocrinologic abnormalities, the likelihood of long-term control from a particular therapy, and the adverse effects associated with each therapy. If the tumor is small and not producing excess hormone, the physician may choose to monitor the patient with MRI or CT scans at yearly intervals.[60]

Surgery

Surgery is the treatment of choice for almost all tumors. An exception is prolactinomas, which are usually managed with medications. However, surgical resection is used if the patient is resistant to dopamine antagonists, has an invasive macroadenoma, or is experiencing compromised vision. A potential benefit of surgery for patients with prolactinomas is that their serum prolactin levels will normalize and their symptoms will be alleviated without lifelong medication. The primary purposes of surgery are to resect or debulk large tumors that are compressing vital structures about the sella (optic chiasm or cranial nerves) and to confirm the histologic diagnosis.[43,49,60] In other instances, surgery is performed to evacuate a cyst about the tumor, to decompress a hemorrhagic tumor, or to reduce obstructive hydrocephalus.

The surgical approach used most often is the transsphenoidal procedure, because it allows the tumor to be removed and pituitary function to be preserved. The neurosurgeon makes an incision behind the upper lip, displaces the maxillary sinus and nasal septum, opens the sella, and microsurgically resects the tumor (Figure 50-2).[60] The surgeon then packs the sella with adipose tissue harvested from the abdomen

Table 50-4 Laboratory Tests for Pituitary Tumors

Diagnostic Test/Tumor	Normal Values	Test Procedure	Comments
Glucose tolerance test/ GH-secreting (acromegaly)	• Growth hormone = 2–6 ng/mL (in morning after 8 hr of sleep) • GH suppressed to < 2 ng/m after glucose tolerance test	• Fasting test (do in morning) • Administer 75–100 g of oral glucose (lemon juice may increase palatability) • Blood samples collected 1, 2, and 3 hr later	• In normal individuals GH causes increased blood glucose, which increases resistance to insulin; hypoglycemia leads to GH release and hyperglycemia to GH suppression • Acromegaly: GH not suppressed to < 0.5 μg within 20–120 min • 60% of acromegalics have a paradoxical increase of GH
Urinary excretion of GH/GH-secreting (acromegaly)		• 24-hour urine collection • Store collection bottle in refrigerator to decrease bacterial growth	• Increased in some patients with acromegaly
Plasma insulin-like growth factor I (ILGF-I/ Somatomedin C)/GH-secreting (acromegaly)	• Normal values vary in males and females; children, adolescents, and adults	• Blood sample	• Normal values Males: preadolescent, 60.8–724 ng/mL; adolescent, 112.5–450 ng/mL; adult, 141.8–389.3 ng/mL Females: preadolescent, 65.5–841 ng/mL; adolescent, 83.3–378.5 ng/mL; adult, 54.0–328.5 ng/mL
Dexamethasone suppression test/ACTH-secreting (Cushing's syndrome)	• Serum cortisol suppressed to < 5 μ/dL • Fasting, 8 A.M.–noon, 5–25 μ/dL	• Administer 1 mg po dexamethasone at 11 P.M. • Draw plasma cortisol at 9 A.M. the following morning	• In normal individuals increased corticosteroid suppresses ACTH release and subsequently cortisol production • To confirm results, test may be repeated for 3 days while administering larger doses of dexamethasone • Sensitive test, but not specific for tumors only
Urinary free cortisol/ ACTH-secreting tumor	• 20–70 μ/24 hr • 25–95 ng/mg of creatinine	• Give dexamethasone 0.5 mg q 6 hr for 2 days • Then collect 24-hour urine sample (refrigerate)	• More specific than dexamethasone suppression test • Single best screening test for ACTH-secreting tumor • Spironolactone and quinacrine may affect accuracy
Plasma prolactin/ prolactinoma	• Women (nonlactating): 0.48–0.9 IU/L or 0–15 ng/mL • Values increase during pregnancy • Values increase during lactation • Men: 0–15 ng/mL		• Values < 1 U/L are rarely clinically significant • Values < 2.5 U/L usually indicate nonfunctioning tumor • Values > 6 U/L usually indicate a macroprolactinoma • Tests repeated because of normal variations in serum prolactin levels

Data from Molitch[56]; Samuels[57]; Corbett.[58]

or other body site, muscle, and fibrin glue to decrease the risk of CSF leak. The septum and maxillary sinus are then reapproximated and the nares packed. An advantage of transsphenoidal surgery over the transcranial route is that the procedure is usually well tolerated by elderly patients and those individuals with cardiac or pulmonary disease or diabetes. In addition, body image is preserved because there is no visible scar; risks for infection and bleeding are lower; and the surgery is shorter and less traumatic, so patients are mobilized and discharged from the hospital earlier.

Radiation Therapy

External beam radiation is used for patients who refuse or who cannot tolerate surgery, for tumor recurrence, in some cases of subtotal resection, or as part of the treatment plan with surgery. Radiation plus surgery may increase rates of long-term control of pituitary adenomas.[61] Stereotactic radiosurgery by gamma knife is an attractive therapeutic option after failure of microsurgical removal in patients with pituitary adenomas. In these tumors or remnants of them,

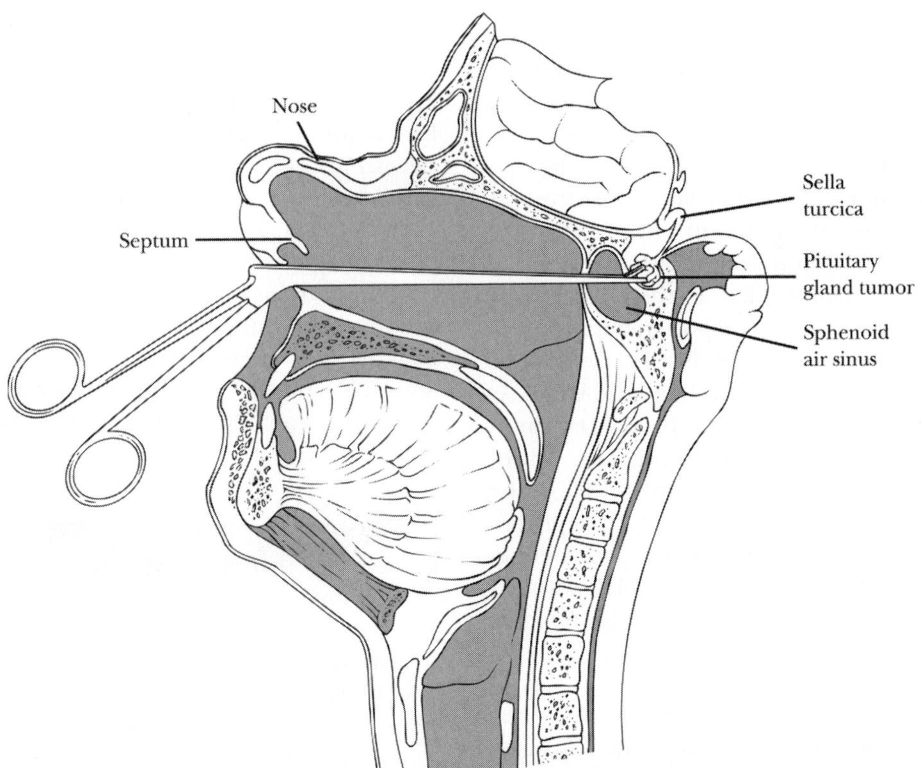

Figure 50-2 Transsphenoidal surgical resection of a pituitary tumor. The upper lip is retracted and an incision is made in the gingival mucosa. After displacing the septal cartilage, the surgeon removes the anterior wall of the sphenoid sinus and the floor of the sella turcica. The pituitary tumor is removed using the microsurgery technique in an attempt to preserve normal pituitary structure and function.

this approach aims to obtain the arrest of cell proliferation and hormone hypersecretion using a single, precise, high dose of ionizing radiation, thereby sparing surrounding structures.[51] In most instances, standard radiation therapy is used and treatment fields are calculated so as to treat the tumor and minimize scatter to adjacent structures. Potential disadvantages of radiation therapy are that a therapeutic effect is achieved too slowly in tumors that secrete excessive hormone, hypopituitarism or injury to the optic nerves/chiasm may occur, and in rare instances there is radiation-induced secondary CNS malignancy. Patients may complain of nausea and headache following the procedure. Although visual deterioration might seem to be a risk for people undergoing this procedure, its incidence is low.

Drug Therapy

Antineoplastic chemotherapy is not used for pituitary tumors. Other drugs are indicated as first-line therapy for microadenomas or macroadenomas before surgery or radiation in some instances, and post-therapy in others. Dopamine agonists and octreotide are used to treat hormone oversecretion.[50] Bromocriptine, a long-acting dopamine agonist, is universally considered to be the primary therapy for prolactinomas. Sixty to seventy percent of treated patients experience decreased tumor size, normalization of serum prolactin level, and improved vision.[53] Dopamine agonists bind to D_2 dopamine receptors in the anterior pituitary, inhibit the synthesis and secretion of prolactin, and inhibit the proliferation of lactotroph cells in the pituitary. Women who have small prolactinomas may be treated only with estrogen or oral contraceptives to restore ovulation and menses. Estrogen is less expensive and prevents bone loss, unlike bromocriptine.

Octreotide is an effective agent to reduce GH secretion in patients with acromegaly. Octreotide, octreotide LAR, and lanreotide may be administered before surgery to reduce tumor size and increase resectability, and to strengthen diminished cardiac functioning.[62–64] Either dopamine agonists or octreotide may be helpful for gonadotropin-secreting pituitary tumors.

Nursing Care

Nursing care for patients with pituitary tumors begins during diagnosis and is an active part of surgical treatment and post-hospitalization follow-up. Patient teaching is particularly important during all phases. For example, during the diagnostic phase, the nurse explains the purposes of tests and how they are done, and provides written teaching materials to patients and families. Patients are cared for in a neurosurgical or surgical intensive care unit immediately after surgery. Nurses monitor them for postoperative complications, which are usually transient but may be long lasting. The most common complication is surgical trauma–related transient swelling of the pituitary and pressure on the pituitary stalk or posterior pituitary.[65] It causes temporary diabetes insipidus (DI), with resultant excretion of large volumes of dilute urine and sodium retention. Manifestations of DI include urinary output greater than 200 mL per hour for at least three hours, a decreased urine specific gravity (< 1.005), and increased serum sodium (> 145 mEq/L). If DI occurs, fluid losses are replaced, on a milliliter per milliliter basis each hour, until DI improves. Mild DI is usually managed with isotonic intravenous fluids. Vasopressin is administered in more severe cases, with the usual dose being 5 units given subcutaneously every four to six hours until urine volume becomes normal. If the patient develops *hyponatremia*, fluids are restricted until DI resolves, usually within ten days. Desmopressin (DDAVP), 0.1-mL intranasal, is administered once or twice a week in patients in whom DI persists.

Another major complication of transsphenoidal surgery is CSF fistula and leak, which can lead to meningitis or tension pneumocephalus. The nurse monitors the patient for signs and symptoms of meningitis, and checks the patient's mustache-type dressing for glucose in any drainage, which indicates CSF fluid. CSF leak presents as persistent postnasal drip, so affected patients may notice a salty taste in their mouth, may swallow frequently, and may notice increased drainage when they bend over. If CSF leak is confirmed, elevating the head of the bed and maintaining bed rest to decrease pressure are indicated.

Other major complications include prolonged epistaxis; vascular injury to the carotid artery; damage to cranial nerves III, IV, V, and VI; optic nerve or optic chiasm damage; anterior pituitary insufficiency; and death. Damage to cranial nerves, optic nerves, or the optic chiasm may lead to complete or partial visual loss or visual field defects. In addition, sinusitis can occur from the intranasal trauma or if the nasal packing is left in too long. To avoid this problem, the nasal packing is removed within 24–48 hours unless the patient has epistaxis. Other nursing assessments include neurologic checks and visual field and acuity checks (e.g., blurred or double vision).

Patients who undergo transsphenoidal surgery may be discharged from the hospital in as few as three or four days and require clear, written discharge instructions regarding signs and symptoms of infection, medications to be taken, and diet and activity restrictions. They are instructed to notify the surgeon for any fever greater than 101°F, any symptoms of meningitis (e.g., headache, stiff neck), persistent clear nasal drainage, persistent headache, visual changes, and excessive thirst.[66] The nurse also reinforces the importance of physician follow-up after the postsurgical period. Patients must be carefully monitored at regular intervals because complications of therapy — especially hypopituitarism and tumor recurrence — can occur as late as 30 years after treatment. In addition, surgery and radiation therapy may result in moderate to severe memory loss that can affect patients' daily lives.[66]

Adrenal Tumors

The adrenal glands lie atop each kidney and comprise a cortex and a medulla, which are both critical to homeostasis. The adrenal cortex constitutes approximately 90% of the adrenal gland, and it synthesizes several corticosteroids essential to life in response to signals from the pituitary gland or other systems. The most important are the glucocorticoid cortisol (hydrocortisone) and the mineralocorticoid aldosterone, as well as small amounts of androgens (including testosterone) and estradiol. Corticosteroids play critical roles in many body processes, such as glucose, protein, and lipid metabolism, as well as in wound healing, myocardial contractility, and arteriolar tone. In addition, they oppose the inflammatory response by reducing the formation of inflammatory mediators (e.g., prostaglandins, leukotrienes, histamine); cause an overall general immunosuppression — specifically, inhibiting interleukins-1 and -2 (IL-1 and IL-2); and may inhibit the synthesis of antibodies and B lymphocytes. Mineralocorticoids are critical to maintaining normal serum sodium balance and, to a lesser degree, potassium balance. Although the primary stimulus for the synthesis of aldosterone is fluid loss, the pituitary plays a small role as well. Aldosterone induces the kidney to secrete renin and continue production of angiotensin. Adrenal cortical hormones are released slowly, but their actions are long-lived.

The adrenal medulla is actually part of the sympathetic nervous system (SNS), which is responsible for the "fight or flight" reaction. The functional cells of the medulla are chromaffin cells, which are modified postganglionic neurons. Chromaffin cells synthesize catecholamines — mainly epinephrine and norepinephrine — that have positive and inhibitory effects on almost all body tissues.[67] The medulla acts rapidly, secreting catecholamines within seconds of encountering a stressful event (internal or external). When the stressor is abolished, the catecholamine effects disappear rapidly, as catecholamines return to sympathetic nerve endings via a reuptake mechanism. The medulla and the cortex thus act in concert, with medullary hormones rapidly responding to changes in the environment and the cortical hormones amplifying and sustaining the stress response.

Several types of adrenocortical tumors arise from the cortex, and pheochromocytomas arise from the medulla. Most of these tumors are benign, but both adenomas and carcinomas can alter quality of life and may be life-threatening. Because they occur in essentially different organs, adrenocortical tumors and pheochromocytomas will be discussed separately.

Adrenocortical Tumors

Epidemiology

Adrenocortical carcinomas are extremely rare. The estimated risk of tumor development is approximately 0.6–2.0 new cases per 1 million population, and only 0.05%–0.2% of all malignant tumors in adults and less than 0.5% in children occur in the adrenal cortex.[68–70] Adrenocortical tumors have a bimodal peak occurrence, arising most frequently in children younger than age 5 and in adults in their forties and fifties. Females of all ages are more likely than males to develop adrenal tumors; children and women most often have hypersecreting tumors, whereas men more often have nonfunctioning tumors.[68,70] Incidence of adrenocortical tumors is typically sporadic, but some people have an increased risk of developing tumors because of inherited mutations in predisposition genes for Li-Fraumini syndrome, Wiedemann-Beckwith syndrome, Carney complex, or MEN1.[68,71]

Etiology

There are no known risk factors for adrenocortical tumors. Pathogenesis is a multistep process and is probably related to some chronic stimulation of the adrenal cortex by pituitary hormones that initiates a random mutation in a single cell. It is not clear whether benign tumors progress to malignant ones or if each type of tumor arises independently. It has been confirmed that the DNA of adrenocortical carcinomas becomes increasingly less stable as tumors become larger.[72] Genetic analysis of tumors confirm loss of heterozygosity (LOH) or allelic imbalance (AI) related to losses or gains of genetic material in multiple protooncogenes and tumor suppressor genes, most commonly 11q, 18p, 2q, 11p, and 4p. One mutation, LOH in 2p16, is encountered frequently in carcinomas but never found in adenomas, which indicates that this region is probably critical in malignant progression. Other genes that are highly expressed in carcinomas but rarely found in adenomas are the multidrug resistance gene (*MDR-1*) and overexpression of an insulin-like growth factor.[73,74] Similarly, mutations of the *p53* tumor suppressor gene have been documented in adults and children with adrenal cortical carcinomas.[71]

Pathophysiology

Adrenocortical tumors may be functional or nonfunctional — that is, hormone secreting or nonsecreting. Functional tumors are further characterized in terms of the hormones they produce in excess. Thirty to fifty percent of adrenocortical carcinomas hypersecrete cortisol to cause Cushing's syndrome; 20%–30% secrete estradiol or testosterone to cause feminizing or masculinizing effects, respectively; and rare tumors secrete aldosterone to cause Conn's syndrome.[68] Nonfunctional incidentalomas do not produce adrenocortical hormones and are usually serendipitously discovered on radiologic scans done for unrelated reasons or at autopsy. It is often difficult to histopathologically differentiate adrenocortical adenomas and carcinomas. Tumors do not synthesize hormones as efficiently as normal adrenal glands, and tend to become large by the time they cause symptoms and are detected. If on initial imaging characteristics suggestive of malignancy — such as intratumor necrosis, irregular margins, and local metastasis — are present, then a malignant cancer should be suspected. Generally, adrenal tumors with malignant potential grow faster than those with a benign phenotype. However, it should be noted that even adrenal tumors smaller than 2 cm at detection might already be metastatic.[71,75] As many as one-third of all patients may have thrombus extension of tumor into the vena cava that may lead to ascites, nephrotic syndrome, hepatomegaly, or acute tricuspid valve failure, or that may be asymptomatic. Tumor thrombi are friable and gelatinous, and can result in massive hemorrhage, intravascular collapse, and death if preoperative planning does not take place.[76]

Clinical Manifestations

The signs and symptoms of adrenal cortical tumors vary depending on the hormone or hormones secreted, as do symptoms from local mass effects. Among patients who have adrenocortical carcinomas, 50%–80% have an endocrine syndrome when they present (usually Cushing's syndrome) and 30%–40% have metastases.[68,77]

Benign or malignant adrenal cortical tumors are the cause of 20%–25% of all cases of Cushing's syndrome and result in symptoms in multiple body systems (similarly to pituitary tumors). Patients with aldosterone-hypersecreting tumors (Conn's syndrome) have hypertension, hypokalemia (serum potassium usually less than 3.5 mEq/L), hypernatremia, and suppressed renin activity. Hypokalemia may cause the most serious effects, such as cardiac arrhythmias, abnormal changes on electrocardiogram (ECG), digitalis toxicity, weakness, polydipsia, and visual disturbances.

Women are likely to have virilizing tumors and experience symptoms reflecting hypersecretion of androgen. Progressive hirsutism (increased hair on the face, trunk, and limbs) is the most frequent symptom. Acne, clitoral hypertrophy, menstrual abnormalities, deepening of the voice, frontal baldness, and increased libido may also occur. Tumors that hypersecrete estradiol are the rarest adrenal tumors and generally occur in young to middle-aged men, who experience diminished libido, testicular atrophy, and gynecomastia. Sex hormone–secreting tumors in children are manifested by pseudosexual precocious puberty in boys and virilization in girls, with the development of pubic hair, tall stature, accelerated growth and bone maturation, and clitoral or penile enlargement.[70] The most common symptoms experienced by patients whose tumors do not hypersecrete hormones are fever, weight loss, symptoms related to the abdominal mass (pain or discomfort, abdominal fullness), and rarely symptoms from distant metastases.[77]

Assessment

Diagnosis of adrenocortical tumors is often protracted and delayed because symptoms are typically nonspecific and slowly progressive. In addition, these tumors are exceedingly rare and thus are not likely to be high on an initial list of differential diagnoses. Diagnosis is confirmed by correlating physical findings with laboratory values and localization procedures. Laboratory tests focus on abnormally high adrenal cortical hormones in the blood and high amounts of their metabolites in the urine. Even patients without symptoms of hormone overproduction should be evaluated by biochemical evaluation for hormone-functioning tumors, because of the importance of early diagnosis of adrenocortical carcinoma. Urinary excretion tests are frequently done because hormone metabolites are excreted in the urine, and these noninvasive tests are highly sensitive. Because no test is 100% sensitive or specific, two or more tests may be done to confirm the diagnosis (Table 50-5).[58,71,78,79]

Localization or imaging procedures to examine the adrenal cortex may include CT or MRI.[68] CT scans are useful to visualize adipose tissue surrounding the adrenal glands; to define the size of large, unilateral, irregular masses; and to identify the homogeneity, calcification, areas of necrosis, and local invasion of masses. MRI, in contrast, can confirm whether a tumor is invading into blood vessels (inferior vena cava, adrenal and renal veins) and can differentiate whether an adrenal mass is a primary adenoma or carcinoma, or a pheocromocytoma.

Classification and Staging

It is often difficult to determine whether an adrenocortical tumor is benign or malignant at initial diagnosis. If the patient does not have regional spread or distant metastases — to lung, liver, or peritoneum, and (rarely) brain or lung — no single finding confirms a diagnosis. While small tumors are more likely to be benign and large masses (greater than 100 g) are more likely to be malignant, considerable overlap occurs, so size alone is not a reliable indicator of pathology. Several histologic features are characteristic of carcinomas: a high mitotic rate (which correlates with poor prognosis), atypical mitoses, aneuploidy, high nuclear grade, hyperchromatic nuclei, low proportion of clear cells, grossly lobulated tumor, areas of necrosis, calcifications, capsular or vascular invasion, and steroid production.[68,71] Immunohistochemistry tests, such as MiB-1 activity and *p53* expression, may aid in diagnosis. The MiB-1 antibody reacts with an antigen expressed only in proliferating cells (not in G_0). In one study, the majority (66%) of primary adrenocortical carcinomas were positive for *p53*, whereas all adenomas were negative for *p53*.

Adrenocortical tumors are staged using the TNM system. Stage I tumors (< 5 cm) and stage II tumors (> 5 cm) are considered localized. Advanced disease includes stage III (positive regional lymph nodes) and stage IV (metastases present). The overall prognosis for individuals with adrenocortical carcinomas is poor: Median survival is 4–30 months, and fewer than 25% of patients survive for five years.[80] Of patients who have advanced disease at time of diagnosis, fewer than 50% survive for one year, and fewer than 10% are alive at ten years.[81]

Table 50-5 Laboratory Values of Adrenal Tumors

Tumor/Syndrome	Test	Implications/Comments
Cushing's disease	• Dexamethasone suppression test (see Table 50-4)	• Tumor-induced cortisol or metabolites will not be suppressed by feedback mechanisms • Plasma cortisol will be elevated the morning after administration
	• 24-hour urine for free cortisol	• Will be elevated to > 80–100 μg
	• 2-day, high-dose dexamethasone suppression test	• Metabolites of adrenocortical steroids, 17 ketosteroids, are not suppressed; normal values vary with gender and age
	• Plasma ACTH immunoassay	• Suppressed to less than normal because of negative feedback loop (increased adrenal cortisol leads to decreased ACTH release by pituitary); normal: 6–76 ng/mL
Virilizing	Basal serum testosterone	• Elevated; nonsuppressible with dexamethasone administration (usually suppresses adrenocortical hormone production); normal: women, 20–90 ng/dL, men, 250–1000 ng/dL
Conn's syndrome (aldosterone-secreting)	• Plasma aldosterone	• Elevated with tumor or hyperplasia, which increase production; normal: 7 A.M. supine < 16 ng/mL, 9 A.M. upright 4–316 ng/mL
	• Urinary aldosterone	• Elevated > 20 μg in 24 hr
	• Plasma renin activity	• Suppressed because increased plasma aldosterone has not been induced by low extracellular fluid volume-induction of renin/angiotensin system; normal: supine, 0.5–1.6 ng/mL; upright, 1.9–3.6 ng/mL
Pheochromocytoma	• Plasma catecholamines (dopamine, epinephrine, norepinephrine)	• Elevated by tumor production • Antihypertensives and antidepressants may invalidate test; confirm drug history
	• 24-hour urine for metanephrines or for normetanephrines	• Metabolites of catecholamines, elevated to 1.5 to 2 times greater than normal; normal: 0.0–0.9 μ/24 hr • Elevated to 1.5–2 times greater than normal • HCl is added to urine specimen bottle to maintain pH ≤ 3 • BP, height, and weight are recorded on laboratory requisition • Patient must be instructed to collect entire 24-hour collection, or results may be false-negative

Data from Corbett[58]; Koch, Pacak, Chrousos[71]; Hes, Hoppener, Lips[78]; Sawka, Jaeschke, Singh, et al.[79]

Therapeutic Approaches and Nursing Care

Surgery

Surgery offers the only chance for cure of malignant adrenal tumors, so resection of local (and sometimes metastatic) disease is recommended whenever possible. Excisions of hormone-secreting tumors, hormone-nonsecreting masses larger than 5 cm, and ''suspicious'' masses smaller than 5 cm are recommended, because surgery may increase the chance of cure or prolong survival for patients with localized disease. En bloc resection offers the best chance of cure. Large tumors and those suspected or confirmed to be malignant are resected during laparotomy, whereas adenomas smaller than 6 cm may be resected via laparoscopic adrenalectomy.[82] Even with surgery, almost 80% of patients develop recurrent regional disease or distant metastases.[77] Virtually all patients with stage III disease develop recurrent disease and metastases within five years of surgical resection.[68]

Chemotherapy

Chemotherapy is given in some instances for cortical tumors. Mitotane controls hormone hypersecretion in 75% of treated patients and is the usual first-line agent given after resection of stage III and IV carcinomas.[77] This drug may act by reversing the multidrug resistance mediated by *MDR-1*.[74] Phase II and other clinical trials have demonstrated that response rates to mitotane are approximately 35%, but responses are rarely prolonged or complete, and survival does not increase.

Mitotane often causes significant and unacceptable dose-related side effects. Approximately 50% of patients experience neurologic effects including weakness, somnolence, confusion, lethargy, and headache. In addition, most patients experience GI symptoms, which can include anorexia, nausea and vomiting, and diarrhea. Uncommon reactions include skin rash and toxic retinopathy with papilledema. Side effects are greatest when a dose of 6–10 mg/day is administered; smaller doses (1.5–3 mg/day) that have been used as adjuvant therapy after surgery are well tolerated and may decrease the risk for recurrence. Fewer patients experience prolonged bleeding times, ataxia or dysarthria, or depression progressing to suicidal ideation.[80]

Antineoplastic therapy is indicated for patients whose tumors progress during mitotane therapy. There are few prospective trials or anecdotal reports of either chemotherapy alone or of chemotherapy plus mitotane. Cisplatin is the most widely tested antineoplastic agent and, when given as single-agent therapy, leads to response rates of about 30%. Cisplatin plus etoposide, with or without mitotane, is considered "standard" chemotherapy but does not generally result in greater response rates than cisplatin or mitotane alone (e.g., 33% versus 30%), and median survival is less than 12 months.[81]

Symptom Management and Supportive Care

Because of delays in diagnosis, many patients with adrenal tumors have progressive disease that does not respond to treatment. Palliative treatment for these individuals includes medications to reduce symptoms produced by hormone excess. Thus patients who have Cushing's syndrome may be treated with drugs that block steroid synthesis (aminoglutethimide, metyrapone, ketoconazole) or block steroid actions in target organs (mefipristone), which may control symptoms but not tumor growth. Patients experiencing Conn's syndrome may be treated with spironolactone, a potassium-sparing diuretic, which is administered to correct tumor-induced hypokalemia.

Pheochromocytoma

Epidemiology

Pheochromocytomas arise from chromaffin cells (pheochromocytes). Although 85%–95% of such tumors arise in the adrenal medulla, they may also arise from the abdominal aortic paraganglia (and rarely within the thorax or urinary bladder) and hence be termed *paragangliomas.* Both benign and malignant tumors synthesize, store, and release catecholamines, which are not regulated by the nervous system.[83] The unregulated release of massive amounts of catecholamines during stressful periods often causes life-threatening crises that may lead to death from myocardial infarction, cardiac arrhythmia or arrest, or shock. While most patients are symptomatic, some individuals have pheochromocytomas that are discovered incidentally.[84]

Pheochromocytomas are rare tumors. The estimated incidence is less than five cases per 1 million population, and pheochromocytomas constitute only 0.3%–0.95% of all neuroendocrine tumors and affect less than 1% of all hypertensive patients.[85,86] Approximately 90% of affected adults have a benign pheochromocytoma, but individuals younger than age 50 and children are at greater risk to have malignant tumors.[86] Males and females are at equal risk to develop a sporadic pheochromocytoma, most frequently in their thirties to fifties, and affected children frequently have a familial risk.

Etiology

Almost nothing is known about the etiology of pheocromocytomas, though hyperplasia precedes tumor development. Approximately 90% of tumors occur sporadically, and the remainder occur as part of MEN2A, MEN2B, or another neuroectodermal syndrome. It has also been demonstrated that in comparison to normal adrenal tissue, tumor tissue has increased expression of three genes for catecholamine-synthesizing enzymes, whereas one gene is expressed at a decreased level.[78]

Pathophysiology

Diagnosis of a benign or a malignant tumor depends on the absence or presence of metastases. Microscopic features have little predictive value for the biologic nature of the tumor, and both benign and malignant tumors may have aneuploid DNA, cellular hyperchromatism, and bizarre mitotic figures, as well as capsular and vascular invasion.[87] Although malignant tumors have been noted to be larger in some instances, such differences have not been quantified and cannot be used to determine malignant status. Both benign and malignant pheocromocytomas hypersecrete the catecholamines norepinephrine and, less often, epinephrine. Altered gene expression may explain why the predominant catecholamines in tumor (90% norepinephrine) and normal tissues (90% epinephrine) are reversed.[83,88]

A problem in determining pathologic status is that after an initial diagnosis of benign or malignant tumor, a pheochromocytoma may recur in the tumor bed, in regional lymph nodes, or as distant metastases as long as 10–15 years later.[86,87] Malignant tumors can metastasize to lymph nodes, bone, lung, liver, brain, and omentum.

Clinical Manifestations

Intermittent catecholamine release usually causes the typical manifestations of pheochromocytoma, and tumors that produce large amounts of epinephrine cause many symptoms in all organ systems. Hypertension (diastolic blood pressure greater than 110–120 mm Hg), whether persistent or paroxysmal (intermittent), is considered the cardinal symptom and is experienced by 82% of patients. Other frequently reported symptoms include sudden throbbing or pounding headache (58%), palpitations (48%), profuse and generalized perspiration (37%), and shortness of breath (28%). Some patients also experience, anxiety, nausea and vomiting, pallor, and chest or abdominal pain.

Symptoms usually occur during life-threatening crises, when excessive catecholamines are being released into the bloodstream, and are spontaneously triggered by changes in position, increased abdominal pressure, exercise, passing urine or stool, intercourse, pain, pressure on or palpation of the abdomen, trauma, labor, anesthesia, surgery, or chemotherapy. In addition, anticholinergic drugs may cause perilous tachycardias, and other drugs such as dopamine antagonists (metoclopramide and phenothiazines), tricyclic antidepressants, and naloxone may precipitate extreme hypertension. The most severe complication is pheochromocytoma crisis. It may lead to encephalopathy that can progress to coma, shock, and multiple organ system failure including renal and hepatic failure, disseminated intravascular clotting (DIC), seizures, and possibly death. Crisis episodes vary: They may last from a few minutes to an hour, and they may occur daily or sporadically.[89] Afterward, the patient may have tremor and feel short of breath, weak, or exhausted.

Assessment

The diagnosis of pheochromocytoma is often delayed because hypertension is much more likely to be caused by other factors. Diagnosis is confirmed by correlating physical findings with laboratory values and localization procedures. Some clinicians advocate taking at least two 24-hour urine collections for total and fractionated catecholamines, metanephrines, and vanillylmandelic acid (VMA), and plasma epinephrine and norepinephrine. However, urinary excretion tests for the catecholamine metabolite metanephrine, which is a direct tumor marker and indirect marker of catecholamine release, is most sensitive to detect pheochromocytomas (see Table 50-5). Test accuracy may be affected by the procedure for collecting the sample and the analysis technique. That is, if the collection period is less than or greater than 24 hours, the test result may be falsely negative or falsely positive, respectively. High-performance liquid chromatography and indexing urinary metanephrine levels by urinary creatinine levels increase test sensitivity and eliminate false-positive results related to consumption of food or drugs. In addition, urinary catecholamine evaluation may be inaccurate in patients who have advanced renal insufficiency.[89] Measurement of the serum catecholamines is not as useful because catecholamines have a short half-life and may not be present in measurable quantities if a sample is obtained when the patient is not hypertensive. Patients are followed after surgery with regularly scheduled measurements of plasma catecholamines and blood pressure checks for the duration of their lives.

Localization studies before surgery are imperative to prepare the patient for surgery and to minimize the risk for cardiovascular morbidity during surgery. Ultrasound, CT, MRI, and iodine^{131}–meta-iodobenzylguanidine (MIBG) scans are all useful to localize pheochromocytomas, but there is no universal agreement regarding which should be included and in what order procedures should occur. Ultrasonography can detect about 90% of tumors and is widely available and inexpensive; a CT scan is highly sensitive and can more precisely image and localize tumors; and MRI can delineate tissue characteristics and extent of tumor localization. MIBG injection is followed by a nuclear scan and is advantageous to determine the functional characteristics of a tumor and locate occult secondary or metastatic sites.

Classification and Staging

As mentioned earlier, most pheochromocytomas are benign in adults, and the presence of metastases is the only reliable indicator of malignancy. Patients with benign or malignant tumors may succumb from complications related to excessive catecholamine effects on normal systems, such as cardiovascular disease, hypertension, cerebral vascular accident, renal disease, or diabetes mellitus.

Therapeutic Approaches and Nursing Care

Surgery

The treatment of choice for pheochromocytoma is surgery, which may cure resectable disease, and is indicated to resect or debulk recurrent disease and metastases.[85] Surgery or other invasive procedures can precipitate severe and uncontrolled hypertension, however, so treatment to induce alpha-adrenergic blockade is commonly started at least one to two weeks before surgery or chemotherapy in an attempt to control arterial hypertension and decrease the risk of crisis during surgery and of postoperative hypotension. Phenoxybenzamine or another selective postsynaptic alpha-1-adrenergic receptor antagonist (e.g., prazosin, terazosin) is administered. Calcium-channel blockers also prevent paroxysmal hypertension, do not cause overshoot or orthostatic hypotension, and may prevent cardiovascular complications.[90] If the patient has persistent tachycardia (pulse greater than 140 per minute), extrasystoles, or a history of arrhythmias, then propranolol, atenolol, or metoprolol may be added only after the alpha blockade is complete to induce beta-adrenergic blockade (e.g., control tachycardia).

Preoperative nursing care focuses on ensuring adequate hydration, monitoring blood pressure, and patient teaching.[88] The patient's weight is checked daily; he or she is prescribed a liberal-salt diet and may be given 1–2 L of IV fluids each day. In addition to concerns about hypertension, the nurse must be aware that the patient may experience postural hypotension. Patient teaching includes avoidance of straining and rapid changes in position, and medication may be given to decrease stress.

Cardiovascular and hemodynamic status are monitored continuously during surgery, and hypertension and arrhythmias are treated promptly. During surgery, IV nitroprusside, nitroglycerin, and pentalomine are administered to control hypertension, and esmolol, a short-acting beta blocker, may be used to control tachyarrhythmias. Immediate postoperative concerns include monitoring vital signs, hemodynamic status, fluid and electrolyte status, and urinary output. The nurse also monitors for other postoperative complications such as bleeding and infection, which are rare, and pain. Patients may be hypotensive and receive IV fluid replacement for a few days after surgery, and they may experience hypoglycemia. Blood pressure is usually normal by the time the patient is discharged from the hospital, but may remain elevated for four to eight weeks. A 24-hour urine collection for catecholamines is done about two weeks after surgery to monitor for residual disease (local or metastatic) and is checked annually for at least five years.[88]

Radiation Therapy

The indication for radiation therapy is to palliate metastatic disease.[89] Total doses of 3000–5000 cGy may reverse neurologic deficit from CNS metastases and provide symptomatic relief from metastases to lymph nodes or bone. In addition, some patients may experience long-term control of disease with radiation therapy.[91]

Chemotherapy

Chemotherapy is generally considered to be ineffective for pheochromocytomas, but it has been suggested that patients may respond to drugs that have been found to be effective for other neuroendocrine neoplasms. The reason for this recommendation is that few reports of chemotherapy for this tumor are found in the literature, perhaps because of the rarity of malignant pheochromocytomas.

Chemotherapy is a stressor and may precipitate severe hypertension as well as possible headache, vomiting, or chest pain within a few hours after administration. For example, hypertension was documented in two patients after treatment with cyclophosphamide, vincristine, and dacarbazine.[92] A possible explanation is that chemotherapy induces tumor lysis and rapid release of tumor-stored catecholamines into the circulation. Patients therefore require adequate blood pressure control before chemotherapy starts, and their hemodynamic status must be closely and continuously monitored, particularly during the first cycle of therapy. Nifedipine 10-mg tablets are administered sublingually or orally to abort hypertensive crisis on a temporary basis.

Symptom Management and Supportive Care

Some patients who have unresectable metastatic disease will experience recurrent hypertension, which is usually managed with phenoxybenzamine, propranolol, or labetolol.[88] Phenoxybenzamine, an irreversible, long-acting, alpha-adrenergic antagonist, has adverse effects including postural hypotension, tachycardia, miosis, nasal congestion, inhibited ejaculation, diarrhea, and fatigue. Administration of this agent starts at a low dose, which is gradually increased. Other patients may receive metyrosine, which prevents the conversion of catecholamine precursors to catecholamines. A benefit of metyrosine is that it allows the use

Table 50-6 Multiple Endocrine Neoplasia Syndromes

Syndrome	Major Organ Tumors	Presenting Symptoms/Comments
MEN1	Parathyroid (hyperplasia), 80%–100% Pancreas (insulinoma), 40%–85% Duodenum (gastrinoma, VIPoma), 25% Pituitary (prolactinoma, growth hormone–secreting adenoma), 30%–65% Neuroendocrine (carcinoids), other sites, 5%–9%	• Presenting symptoms depend on organs involved and whether tumor secretes hormone. May include: Hypercalcemia, urolithiasis Hypoglycemia Peptic ulcer, diarrhea Galactorrhea, acromegaly • Other, less common tumors: thymus, stomach, carcinoid, lipoma, spinal cord ependymoma • Prediagnostic manifestations: 50% of patients have cutaneous manifestations, including angiofibromas, café-au-lait spots, pipomas, confetti-like hypopigmented macules, multiple gingival papules
MEN2		
MEN2A	Thyroid (medullary thyroid carcinoma), 70% Adrenal medulla (pheochromocytoma), > 50% Parathyroid (adenoma), 15%–30%	• Presenting symptoms depend on organs involved and whether tumor secretes hormone. May include: Diarrhea Hypertension, palpitations Hypercalcemia, urolithiasis
MEN2B	Thyroid (medullary thyroid carcinoma), 100% Adrenal medulla (pheochromocytoma)	• Onset of MTC is 10 years earlier than MEN2A, most aggressive • Developmental abnormalities accompany syndrome: typical facies, marfanoid appearance, oral mucosa, conjunctiva, intestinal mucosa • Ganglioneuromas may cause difficult swallowing, vomiting, constipation, diarrhea • Parathyroid adenomas are noted to be rare to absent • Hypercalcemia, urolithiasis
Familial MTC	Thyroid (medullary thyroid carcinoma) 100%	• More benign than MEN2A or MEN2B, good prognosis

Data from Yip, Gilbert, Shapiro, et al.[93]; Komminoth, Heitz, Kloppel[94]; Marx[95]; Gibril, Schumann, Pace, et al[96]; Hermans, Lips, Bravenboer.[97]

of lower doses of alpha-adrenergic blockers, which minimizes the potential side effects of those agents.

Multiple Endocrine Neoplasia

Individuals affected with a multiple endocrine neoplasia (MEN) syndrome develop two or more characteristic benign or malignant endocrine tumors simultaneously or sequentially over their lifetimes (Table 50-6).[93–97] To date, two broadly defined syndromes, MEN1 and MEN2, have been identified. Sporadic MEN syndromes are rarely diagnosed, and are almost always caused by an inherited gene mutation. MEN tumors produce the same symptoms as sporadic tumors but share the cardinal features of all hereditary cancers: early age of onset of hyperplasia, benign or malignant neoplasia, multiple primary tumors that occur in particular combinations, portending physical signs in some individuals, distinctive pathologic features, more severe disease and poorer prognosis than sporadic tumors, and a Mendelian pattern of tumor transmission.[98]

Patients with familial MEN1 or MEN2 develop tumors because of an inherited, autosomal dominant mutated gene that codes for a particular tumor suppressor or proto-oncogene. This gene, which is present in the germ line of one parent, is passed on to affected offspring and is thus found in all of those individuals' cells. These persons are predisposed to earlier and more frequent (but less than 100%) tumor development because these mutations have a high degree of expressivity but a variable rate of penetrance. For instance, an estimated 35% of the children who have the *MEN2* gene will develop clinically significant disease.[96] Point mutations, which result in the substitution of a single nucleotide (codon) for another, cause missense mutations that change a single amino acid, thereby leading to activation and gain of function of a proto-oncogene or loss of function of a suppressor gene. A second mutation in the normal allele inherited from the unaffected parent occurs some time after birth and is necessary for tumor transformation. Mutations of several other genes that code for suppressor genes, oncogenes, and growth factors are undoubtedly involved in progression to malignancy.

Multiple Endocrine Neoplasia 1

The estimated incidence of MEN1 varies from 1:10,000 to 1:100,000.[99] The most frequently encountered endocrine manifestations of MEN1 are diffuse or nodular parathyroid hyperplasia, anterior pituitary adenomas (most often prolactin or GH-secreting tumors), and enteropancreatic neuroendocrine tumors.[94,95] It is not possible to predict how these conditions will present, but patients may have one, two, or all three tumors. Parathyroid neoplasms are diagnosed in 80%–100% of all patients at a mean age of 19, whereas 30%–65% of patients develop a single, pituitary adenoma that is usually clinically insignificant. These tumors, often diagnosed in patients in their forties, may or may not secrete hormones, and they are frequently discovered only at autopsy.[100] Sixty-six percent of patients develop numerous microadenomas throughout the pancreas, and 30%–75% of these patients are symptomatic secondary to tumor secretion of one of the pancreatic peptides. Gastrin is the most frequently secreted peptide and causes hypersecretion of gastric acid (Zollinger-Ellison syndrome). Fewer patients also develop carcinoids or neuroendocrine lung tumors, and other nonendocrine tumors (e.g., duodenum, stomach, thymus, adrenal hyperplasia, lipomas, spinal cord ependymomas).

Manifestations of MEN1 vary depending on which organs are involved and whether tumors secrete hormones. Approximately 50% of affected individuals die at a younger age (mean 51 years) than non-MEN1-affected family members, and prognosis is affected by which sites are involved with tumor. For example, thymic tumors are aggressive, while pancreatic and duodenal tumors are usually low grade.[94] The majority of patients with MEN1 who are not diagnosed early die from GI bleeding or metastatic pancreatic cancer in their sixties.

Etiology

Linkage analysis located the gene for MEN1 on the long arm of chromosome 11, and it has now been confirmed to lie at 11q13. This gene, which was designated *Mu* among the original candidate genes, has been cloned and codes for a protein that is called *menin*.[101] The function of the *MEN1* gene is not known, and at least 12 mutations (including frameshift, nonsense, inframe deletions, and missense) have been identified. The genotype/phenotype implications of mutations in this large gene are not clear, and the implications for clinical management have not yet been defined. Tumors occur because of a second mutation in the normal allele that results in the loss of that allele (loss of heterozygosity), suggesting that *MEN1* is a tumor suppressor gene. Inactivation of both alleles may not be sufficient to induce tumors, and other genes are likely to be involved.[95]

Multiple Endocrine Neoplasia 2

The estimated incidence of MEN2 is 1:500,000.[99] Individuals with MEN2 develop hyperplasia or tumors of the thyroid, parathyroid, and adrenal glands. Among the subcategories of MEN2, MEN2A is most common and accounts for more than 90% of cases, whereas MEN2B accounts for about 5% of cases. Some individuals develop only familial medullary thyroid cancer (FMTC).

MEN2A

The hallmark tumor of MEN2A is hyperplasia of thyroid C cells that progresses to MTC. The *RET* gene is not completely penetrant; 70% of carriers develop tumors by age 70, and more than 95% of patients develop only MTC. Long-term prognosis depends on the success of treatment for MTC. More than 50% of patients with MEN2A develop pheochromocytomas, most of which are benign and cause symptoms by overproducing hormones.[95] Hypertension is the most frequently encountered symptom, as with sporadic pheochromocytoma, and is a major cause of death. Fifty to eighty percent of patients present with bilateral disease, and another 10% require adrenalectomy of the remaining gland within five years.[78] Parathyroid adenomas develop in 15%–30% of persons with MEN2A, albeit much later than in individuals with MEN1. These tumors are not usually significant and patients appear physically normal.

MEN2B

The onset of MEN2B, which is more aggressive than MEN2A and FMTC, occurs approximately ten years earlier than the onset of MEN2A. Virtually all patients with MEN2B develop MTC, and the average age of death is 21 in untreated patients.[93] Affected individuals may be identified by their typical physical appearance, including marfanoid appearance (85%), facial features, and proximal muscle wasting. Patients often have musculoskeletal abnormalities including pes cavus, or an abnormally high arch of the foot (persons who have Marfan syndrome have pes planus, or flat feet), kyphosis, scoliosis, lordosis, and increased joint looseness.[102] Characteristic facial features include enlarged, blubbery lips from mucosal neuromas that are located throughout the entire GI tract, from anterior and dorsal tongue to colon. Neuromas can occur on other mucosal surfaces, such as the eyelids, which makes the patient look wide-eyed. In addition, the eyebrows are large, and an elongated face and prominent jaw are common. Puberty is delayed in patients with MEN2B, and their reproductive rates are low secondary to mortality, impotence, and infertility. These findings support the idea that new mutations are common in MEN2B, and as many as 50% of cases of MEN2B arise from new mutations.

Etiology

RET, a proto-oncogene located on the long arm of chromosome 10 (10q11.2), has been confirmed to be responsible for MEN2 and FMTC.[93] This proto-oncogene is expressed during fetal development of neural crest structures as well as postnatally in neural crest–derived tissues including parathyroid glands, thyroid C cells, adrenal medulla, enteric ganglia, and the urogenital system. *RET* is a dominant transforming gene for cancer/neoplasia, and a mutation in it results in a permanently activated mutant receptor that responds to its intrinsic tyrosine kinase enzyme activity.[103] Mutation of a single codon is sufficient to cause neoplastic transformation and gain of function. More than 92% of patients in MEN2 families have mutations in *RET.* Eight mutations account for all cases. For instance, 85% of all cases of MEN2A are associated with a mutation at codon 634 (TGC to CGC, which changes cysteine to arginine), which is strongly associated with the development of pheochromocytoma and hyperparathyroidism. In addition, a point mutation at codon 919 (ATG to ACG, which results in the substitution of threonine for methionine) is implicated in more than 95% of all cases of MEN2B.[104]

Assessment and Screening

Baseline and ongoing screening for affected individuals in families known to express MEN-related genes is the major focus of management. Current recommendations for MEN1 and MEN2 vary because of the differences in availability of genetic screening and therapy options. Annual screening may include serum tests for laboratory evidence of hypersecreting tumors, but negative tests do not guarantee that a person does not have the syndrome. Because tumors may arise at any age, a negative test merely indicates that the individual does not yet have detectable disease.

MEN1 is most commonly diagnosed when patients are in their forties, but can be identified when patients are in their teens or twenties by periodic evaluations of serum hormones secreted by constituent tumors (calcium, parathyroid hormone, fasting gastrin, insulin, glucose, prolactin, and GH). It is recommended that annual biochemical testing begin between ages 8 and 15. If a patient does not convert to positive by age 30, the risk of being a gene carrier decreases to 10%, but testing continues because the maximal age for conversion is not known.[95] In addition, patients may be clinically monitored for premonitory cutaneous manifestations of MEN1, such as multiple facial angiofibromas, collagenomas, café-au-lait macules, lipomas, and multiple gingival papules, which may aid in presymptomatic diagnosis. Clinical genetic testing is not standard for several reasons: *Mu* is a large gene and identified mutations are spread across it; new mutations are being discovered; and no testing "shortcuts" (e.g., protein truncation assay) are available because of the nature of gene mutations. In addition, MEN1 is a rare tumor, so there is limited demand for a genetic test, and confirmation would not lead to major therapeutic interventions.

Genetic testing for *RET* mutations in family members with a known risk for MEN2A and MEN2B is the diagnostic method of choice. DNA testing is simple and routine because of the small number of *RET* mutations and the high likelihood that one of these mutations will be detected in more than 90% of cases.[104] Confirmation of genetic status eliminates the need for screening in noncarriers and identifies patients who should have an early thyroidectomy without waiting for abnormal biochemical tests. Advantages of genetic tests over previously used pentagastrin provocation are that the test is practical (it requires just one blood sample), has no side effects, and is cost-effective because repeated, expensive biochemical testing for all potential tumors is necessary only in carriers. Furthermore, patients who require early surgery are identified when cure is most likely. DNA analysis of *RET* gene for mutations is highly reliable, having no false-positive or false-negative results.[93] Persons in whom the mutation exists will require annual screening, as outlined earlier, starting in early childhood. Annual screening for MEN2A/FMTC gene mutation carriers—which includes plasma calcitonin after IV pentagastrin or calcium stimulation, blood pressure, urinary or plasma catecholamines, serum calcium, and perhaps imaging of the adrenal glands—is recommended to start by age 4–5 and continue to age 20. The recommended screening for older patients is controversial, and some clinicians opt to screen them at wider intervals until age 35.

Provocative tests for calcitonin involve the injection of pentagastrin or calcium and the measurement of serum calcitonin at three points: at baseline, two to three minutes post-injection, and five to ten minutes post-injection. Reproducible serum calcium elevations above a normal range indicate the need to proceed to total thyroidectomy, and patients whose calcitonin levels are borderline are retested within three to six months. Calcitonin provocation tests are problematic in that both false-negative results, which erroneously lull the patient into a sense of security, and false-positive results, which may result in an unnecessary total thyroidectomy, can occur.

Therapeutic Approaches and Nursing Care

A multidisciplinary team — physicians, nurses, a genetic counselor, and a psychologist — that is knowledgeable and experienced in inherited cancer syndromes is required to care for patients with MEN syndromes.[99] Oncology nurses should be skilled in gathering a family history that includes the history of cancer at other sites and in constructing a pedigree.[98] These data are useful in medical interpretation of risk and identification of the need for further diagnostic testing. In addition, knowledgeable nurses can play a key role in patient and family teaching, counseling, and support before and following genetic testing. Some of the issues surrounding genetic risk testing that the nurse should consider include family members' emotional responses and concerns, and potential areas of dissatisfaction, such as a lack of knowledge on the part of healthcare providers, who therefore cannot provide accurate information about genetic testing, support, and genetic counseling.[105] Waiting for the results of a genetic test is difficult, and finding out what the results are — whether normal or carrier — causes shock and anxiety that may decrease over time.

Treatment of constituent tumors may vary with MEN syndromes as opposed to sporadic tumors. For instance, one major difference in the treatment of parathyroid hyperplasia or tumors is that most individuals with MEN1 have tumor in all four glands, whereas those with sporadic tumors do not. Thus, the surgical exploration is always bilateral and includes extensive exploration of the tissues surrounding the thyroid so that all of the parathyroid tissue is located. Three and one-half parathyroid glands are removed, and the remaining half gland is autotransplanted to an accessible site (e.g., a neck muscle or the forearm) to maintain calcium homeostasis. Tissue in these sites is easier to monitor and is important because even when the small amount of parathyroid appears normal, patients are most likely to experience remission and not cure. That is, hyperplasia and hyperparathyroidism recur in 67% of patients within eight years after surgery.[106] Thus, periodic screening of serum calcium will always be required in these patients.

MEN2-affected individuals undergo prophylactic thyroidectomy, usually no later than age 4–5, especially MEN2A patients who have a mutation at codon 634 and MEN2B patients, whose disease is highly aggressive and often metastasizes by age 6–10.[102] Patients whose adrenal glands or thyroid are resected will require lifelong hormone replacement.

Conclusion

Several rare endocrine tumors occur. While most often they are benign, both benign and malignant tumors may cause significant morbidity, shorten life expectancy, and negatively affect quality of life. As with other malignancies, early detection of small tumors that are surgically resectable affords the best prognosis. The relative rarity of these tumors has hampered our ability to test the effectiveness of chemotherapy in most instances. Many endocrine tumors are detected late in their course and cause the affected person's death because of mass effects or because of physiologic effects induced by hypersecretion of an endocrine hormone. Nursing care for patients with endocrine tumors requires knowledge of the hormones secreted, and of their effects on body systems, and, in cases of inherited genes that increase tumor risk, knowledge of etiology. The focus of care is often on symptom assessment and management.

References

1. Jemal A, Tiwari RC, Murray T, et al: Cancer statistics, 2004. *CA Cancer J Clin* 54:9, 2004
2. Fraker DL, Skarulis M, Livolsi V: Thyroid tumors, in DeVita VT, Hellman S, Rosenberg SA (eds.): *Cancer Principles and Practice of Oncology* (ed 6). Philadelphia, Lippincott, Williams and Wilkins, 2001, pp 1740–1762
3. Goodman HM: Thyroid gland, in: *Base Medical Endocrinology* (ed 3). New York, Raven Press, 2003, pp 77–109
4. Sywak M, Pasieka JL, Ogilvie T: A review of thyroid cancer with intermediate differentiation. *J Surg Oncol* 86:44–54, 2004
5. Mizukami Y, Noguchi M, Michigishi T, et al: Papillary thyroid carcinoma in Kanazawa, Japan: prognostic significance of histological subtypes. *Histopathology* 20:243–250, 1992
6. Nikiforov Y, Gnepp DR: Pediatric thyroid cancer after the Chernobyl disaster. Pathomorphologic study of 84 cases (1991–1992) from the Republic of Belarus. *Cancer* 74:748–766, 1994
7. Shaha AR: Implications of prognostic factors and risk groups in the management of differentiated thyroid cancer. *Laryngoscope* 114:393–402, 2004
8. Shaha AR: Controversies in the management of thyroid nodule. *Laryngoscope.* 110(Pt 1):183–193, 2000

9. Grigsby PW: Thyroid, in Perez CA, Brady LW, Halperin EC, et al (eds.): *Principles and Practice of Radiation Oncology* (ed 4). Philadelphia, Lippincott-Raven, 2004, pp 1179–1200
10. Sherman SI: Thyroid carcinoma. *Lancet* 361:1–26, 2003
11. Stratakis CA, Chrousos GP: Endocrine tumors, in Pizzo PA, Poplack DG (eds.): *Principles and Practice of Pediatric Oncology* (ed 4). Philadelphia, Lippincott-Raven, 2002, pp 1115–1148
12. Kikuchi S, Perrier ND, Ituarte P, et al: Latency period of thyroid neoplasia after radiation exposure. *Ann Surg* 239:536–543, 2004
13. McKay JD, Lesueur F, Jonard L, et al: Localization of a susceptibility gene for familial nonmedullary thyroid carcinoma to chromosome 2q21. *Am J Hum Genet* 69:440–446, 2001
14. Burman KD, Ringel MD, Wartofsky L: Unusual types of thyroid neoplasms. *Endocrinol Metab Clin North Am* 25:49–68, 1996
15. Brandi ML, Gagel RF, Angeli A, et al: Guidelines for diagnosis and therapy of MEN type 1 and type 2. *J Clin Endocrinol Metabol* 86:5658–5671, 2001
16. Hyer SL, Vini L, A'Hern R, et al: Medullary thyroid cancer: multivariate analysis of prognostic factors influencing survival. *Eur J Surg Oncol* 26:686–690, 2000
17. Machens A, Niccoli-Sire P, Hoegel J, et al: Early malignant progression of hereditary medullary thyroid cancer. *N Engl J Med* 346:1517–1525, 2003
18. McIver B, Hay ID, Giuffrida DG, et al: Anaplastic thyroid carcinoma: a 50 year experience at a single institution. *Surgery* 130:1028–1034, 2001
19. Hanna FWF, Cunningham RT, Ardill JES, et al: Prognostic factors in medullary carcinoma of the thyroid. *Endocrine Related Cancer* 5:49–53, 1998
20. Da Silva AMA, Rui MBM, Magnus RD, et al: A novel germ-line point mutation in RET exon 8 in a large kindred with familial medullary thyroid carcinoma. *J Clin Endocrinol Metabol* 88:5438–5443, 2003
21. Hunt JL, Tometsko M, LiVolsi VA, et al: Molecular evidence of anaplastic transformation in coexisting well-differentated and anaplastic carcinomas of the thyroid. *Am J Surg Pathol* 27:1559–1564, 2003
22. Staren ED: Thyroid and parathyroid ultrasonography, in Gagner M, Inabnet WB (eds.): *Minimally Invasive Endocrine Surgery*. Lippincott, Williams and Wilkins, 2002, pp 21–29
23. Song JI, Myers EN: Throidectomy, in Pellitteri PK, McCaffery TV (eds.): *Endocrine Surgery of the Head and Neck*. Australia, Thomson Delmar Learning, 2003, pp 103–111
24. Shah MD, Hall FT, Eske SJ, et al: Clinical course of thyroid carcinoma after neck dissection. *Laryngoscope* 113:2102–2107, 2003
25. Shaha AR: Risk and prognostic factors in thyroid cancer, in Pellitteri PK, McCaffery TV (eds.): *Endocrine Surgery of the Head and Neck*. Australia, Thomson Delmar Learning, 2003, pp 131–139
26. Kloos RT, Mazzaferri EL: Thyroid cancer, in Molitch ME (ed.): *Challenging Cases in Endocrinology*. Totowa, NJ, Humana Press, 2002, pp 81–118
27. Inabnet WB, Gagner M: Endoscopic thyroidectomy: supraclavicular approach, in Gagner M, Inabnet WB (eds.): *Minimally Invasive Endocrine Surgery*. Philadelphia, Lippincott, Williams and Wilkins, 2002, pp 45–54
28. Barengolts EI, Kukreja SC: Hypoparathyroidism and hypocalcemia, in Molitch ME (ed.): *Challenging cases in endocrinology*. Totowa, NJ, Humana Press, 2002, pp 201–215
29. Hanna MM, McGrath PC, Sloan DA, Kenady DE: Advances in the pathogenesis and treatment of thyroid cancer. *Curr Opin Oncol* 11:42–47, 1999
30. Haigh PI: Anaplastic thyroid carcinoma. *Curr Treat Oncol* 1:353–357, 2000
31. Haigh PI, Ituarte PH, Wu HS, et al: Completely resected anaplastic thyroid carcinoma combined with adjuvant chemotherapy and irradiation is associated with prolonged survival. *Cancer* 91:2335–2342, 2001
32. Ferruccio S, Botticі V, Elisei R, et al: Cytotoxic effects of carboplatinum and epirubicin in the setting of an elevated serum thyrotropin for advanced poorly differentiated thyroid cancer. *J Clin Endocrin Metabol* 87:4160–4165, 2002
33. Shane E: Parathyroid carcinoma. *J Clin Endocrin Metabol* 86:485–493, 2001
34. Grau AM, Evans DB, Hoff AO, et al: Carcinoma of the parathyroid glands, in Pellitteri PD, McCaffery TV (eds.): *Endocrine Surgery of the Head and Neck*. Australia, Thomson Delmar Learning, 2003, pp 429–440
35. Erickson LA, Jin L, Wollan P, et al: Parathyroid hyperplasia, adenomas, and carcinomas; differential expression of p27 protein. *Am J Surg Pathol* 23:288–295, 1999
36. Sloan DA, Scheartz RW, C,Grath PC, et al: Diagnosis and management of thyroid and parathyroid hyperplasia and neoplasia. *Curr Opin Oncol* 7:47–55, 1995
37. Goldstein RE, Billheimer D, Martin WH, et al: Sestamibi scanning and minimally invasive radioguided parathyroidectomy without intraoperative parathyroid hormone measurement. *Ann of Surg* 237:722–731, 2002
38. Obara T, Okamoto T, Kanbe M, et al: Functioning parathyroid carcinoma: clinicaopathologic features and rational treatment. *Semin Surg Oncol* 13:134–141, 1997
39. Kebebew E, Cumhur A, Duh QY, et al: Localization and reoperation results for persistent and recurrent parathyroid carcinoma. *Arch of Surg* 136:878–885, 2001
40. Sidiropoulos N, Vento J, Malchoff C, et al: Radioguided tumorectomy in the management of parathyroid adenomas. *Arch Surg* 138:716–720, 2003
41. McCabe CF, Heaney AP: Pituitary tumor transforming gene in endocrine cancer. *Clin Endocrinol* 58:673–682, 2003
42. Japon MA, Urbano AG, Saez C, et al: Glial-derived neurotropic factor and RET gene expression in normal human anterior pituitary cell types and in pituitary tumors. *J Clin Endocrin Metabol* 87:1879–1884, 2002
43. Ironside JW: Pituitary gland pathology. *J Clin Pathol* 56:561–568, 2003
44. Barker FG, Klibanski A, Swearingen B: Transsphenoidal surgery for pituitary tumors in the United States, 1996–2000: mortality, morbidity, and the effects of hospital and surgeon volume. *J Clin Endocrin Metabol* 88:4709–4719, 2003
45. Nieuwenhuijzen D: Structure and function of the hypothalamus and pituitary, in Grossman A (ed.): *Clinical Endocrinology* (ed 2). Boston, Blackwell Science, 1998, pp 83–89
46. Ezzat S: Editorial: pituitary tumor pathogenesis — the hunt for novel candidate genes continues. *J Clin Endocrin Metabol* 88:5116–5118, 2003
47. Thapar K, Scheitauer BW, Kovacs K, et al: p53 expression in pituitary adenomas and carcinomas: correlations with invasiveness and tumor growth fractions. *Neurosurgery* 38:765–771, 1996
48. Schlechte JA: Prolactinoma. *N Engl J Med* 349:2035–2041, 2003
49. Shimon I, Melmed S: Management of pituitary tumors. *Ann Intern Med* 129:472–483, 1998
50. Ben-Shlomo A, Melmed S: The role of pharmacotherapy in perioperative management of patients with acromegaly. *J Clin Endocrin Metabol* 88:963–968, 2003
51. Attanashio R, Epaminonda P, Motti E, et al: Gamma-knife radiosurgery in acromegaly: a 4 year follow-up study. *J Clin Endocrin Metabol* 88:3105–3112, 2003
52. Lamberts SWJ: Acromegaly, in Grossman A (ed.): *Clinical Endocrinology* (ed 2). Boston, Blackwell Science, 1998, pp 170–183

53. Shimon I, Melmed S: Management of pituitary tumors. *Ann Intern Med* 129:472–483, 1998
54. Molitch ME: Clinical manifestations of acromegaly. *Endocrinol Metab Clin North Am* 21:597–614, 1992
55. Von Werder K, Muller OA: Cushing's syndrome, in Grossmann A (ed.): *Clinical Endocrinology* (ed 2). Boston, Blackwell Science, 1998, pp 415–431
56. Molitch ME: Hypothalamic and pituitary tumors: general principles, in Grossman A (ed.): *Clinical Endocrinology* (ed 2). Boston, Blackwell Science, 1998, pp 129–137
57. Samuels MH: Cushing's syndrome, in McDermott MT (ed.): *Endocrinology Secrets*. Philadelphia, Hanley and Belfus, 1995, pp 102–105
58. Corbett JV: *Laboratory Tests and Diagnostic Procedures with Nursing Diagnoses*. Stamford, CT, Appleton and Lange, 1996
59. Melmed S: Mechanisms for pituitary tumorigenesis: the plastic pituitary. *J Clin Invest* 112:1603–1618, 2003
60. Ciric I, Rosenblatt Sami, Zhao JC: Transsphenoidal microsurgery. *Neurosurgery* 51:161–169, 2002
61. Cornett MS, Paris KJ, Spanos WJ, et al: Radiation therapy for pituitary adenomas: a retrospective study of the University of Louisville experience. *Am J Clin Oncol* 19:292–295, 1996
62. Colao A, Cuocolo A, Marzullo P, et al: Effects of 1 year treatment with octreotide on cardiac performance in patients with acromegaly. *J Clin Endocrinol Metabol* 84:17–23, 1999
63. Colao A, Marzullo P, Ferone D, et al: Cardiovascular effects of depot long-acting somatostatin analog sandostatin LAR in acromegaly. *J Clin Endocrinol Metabol* 85:3132–3140, 2000
64. Hradec J, Kral J, Janota T, et al: Regression of acromegalic left ventricular hypertrophy after lanreotide (a slow release somatostatin analog). *Am J Cardiol* 83:1506–1509, 1999
65. Ciric I, Ragin A, Baumgartner C, et al: Complications of transsphenoidal surgery: results of a national survey, review of the literature, and personal experience. *Neurosurgery* 40:225–237, 1997
66. Guinan EM, Lowy C, Stanhope N, et al: Cognitive effects of pituitary tumors and their treatments: two case studies and an investigation of 90 patients. *J Neurol Neurosurg Psychiatry* 65:870–876, 1998
67. Vinson GP, Whitehouse BJ, Hinson JP: The adrenal cortex, in Grossman A (ed.): *Clinical Endocrinology* (ed 2). Boston, Blackwell Science, 1998, pp 395–414
68. Latronico AC, Chrousos GP: Extensive personal experience; adrenocortical tumors. *J Clin Encocrinol Metabol* 82:1317–1324, 1997
69. Vargas MP, Vargas HI, Kleiner DE, et al: Adrenocortical neoplasms: role of prognostic markers MIB-1, P53, and RB. *Am J Surg Pathol* 21:556–562, 1997
70. Wolthers OD, Cameron FJ, Scheimbeg I, et al: Androgen secreting adrenocortical tumors. *Arch Dis Child* 80:46–50, 1999
71. Koch CA, Pacak K, Chrousos GP: The molecular pathogenesis of hereditary and sporadic adrenocortical and adrenomedullary tumors. *J Clin Endocrinol Metabol* 87:5367–5384, 2002
72. Kjellman M, Roshani L, The BT, et al: Genotyping of adrenocortical tumors: very frequent deletions of the MEN1 locus in 11Q13 and of a 1-centimorgan region in 2p16. *J Clin Endocrinol Metabol* 84:730–735, 1999
73. Gicquel C, Bertagna X, Schneid H, et al: Rearrangements at the 11p15 locus and over expression of insulin-like growth factor-11 gene in sporadic adrenocortical tumors. *J Clin Endocrinol Metabol* 78:1444–1453, 1994
74. Berruti A, Terzolo M, Pia A, et al: Mitotane associated with etoposide, doxorubicin, and cisplatin in the treatment of advanced adrenocortical carcinoma. *Cancer* 83:2194–2200, 1998
75. Barnett CC Jr, Varma DG, El-Naggar AK, et al: Limitations of size as a criterion in the evaluation of adrenal tumors. *Surgery* 128:973–982, 2000
76. Figueroa AJ, Stein JP, Lieskowvky G, et al: Adrenal cortical carcinoma associated with venous tumor thrombus extension. *Br J Urol* 80:397–400, 1997
77. Gicquel C, Baudin E, Lebouc Y, et al: Adrenocortical carcinoma. *Ann Oncol* 8:423–427, 1997
78. Hes FJ, Hoppener JWM, Lips CJM: Pheochromocytoma in von Hippel-Lindau disease. *J Clin Endocrinol Metabol* 88:969–974, 2003
79. Sawka AM, Jaeschke R, Singh RJ, et al: A comparison of biochemical tests for pheochromocytoma: measurement of fractionated plasma metanephrines compared with the combination of 24-hour urinary metanephrines and catecholamines. *J Clin Endocrinol Metabol* 2:53–558, 2003
80. Haake HR, Hermans J, Van De Veld CJH, et al: Optimal treatment of adrenocortical carcinoma with mitotane: results in a consecutive series of 96 patients. *Br J Cancer* 69:947–951, 1994
81. Bonacci R, Gigliotti A, Baudin E, et al: Cytotoxic therapy with etoposide and cisplatin in advanced adrenocortical carcinoma. *Br J Cancer* 78:546–549, 1998
82. Ushiyama T, Suzuki K, Kageyama S, et al: A case of Cushing's syndrome due to adrenocortical carcinoma with recurrence 19 months after laparoscopic adrenalectomy. *J Urol* 157:2239, 1997
83. Isobe K, Nakai T, Ykimasa N, et al: Expression of mRNA coding for four catecholamine-synthesizing enzymes in human adrenal pheochromocytomas. *Eur J Endocrinol* 138:383–387, 1998
84. Eisenhofer G, Goldstein DS, Walther MM, et al: Biochemical diagnosis of pheochromocytoma: how to distinguish true from false postitive test results. *J Clin Endocrinol Metabol* 88:2656–2666, 2003
85. Sandur S, Das Gupta A, Shapiro JL, et al: Thoracic involvement with pheochromocytoma: a review. *Chest* 115:511–521, 1999
86. Vassilopoulou-Sellin R: Clinical outcome of 50 patients with malignant abdominal paragangliomas and malignant pheochromocytomas. *Endocrine Related Cancer* 5:59–68, 1998
87. Goldstein RE, O'Neill JA, Holcomb GW, et al: Clinical experience over 48 years with pheochromocytoma. *Ann Surg* 53(suppl 64): S2–S5, 1998
88. Gavaghan M: Surgical treatment of pheochromocytomas. *AORN* 65:1041–1071, 1997
89. Young WF: Pheochromocytoma: issues in diagnosis and treatment. *Compr Ther* 23:319–326, 1997
90. Ulchaker JC, Goldfarb DA, Bravo EI, et al: Successful outcomes in pheochromocytoma surgery in the modern era. *J Urol* 161:764–767, 1999
91. Yu L, Fleckman AM, Chadha M, et al: Radiation therapy of metastatic pheochromocytoma: case report and review of the literature. *Am J Clin Oncol* 19:389–393, 1996
92. Wu L-T, Dicpinigaitis P, Bruckner H, et al: Hypertensive crisis induced by treatment of malignant pheochromocytoma with combination of cyclophosphamide, vincristine, and dacarbazine. *Med Pediatr Oncol* 22:389–393, 1996
93. Yip L, Gilbert JC, Shapiro SE, et al: Multiple endocrine neoplasia type 2: evaluation of the genotype–phenotype relationship. *Arch Surg* 138:409–416, 2003
94. Komminoth P, Heitz PU, Kloppel G: Pathology of MEN-1: morphology, clinicopathologic correlations and tumor development. *J Intern Med* 243:455–464, 1998
95. Marx SJ: Multiple endocrine neoplasia type 1, in Vogelstein B, Kinzler KW (eds.): *The Genetic Basis of Human Cancer*. New York, McGraw-Hill, 1998, pp 489–506
96. Gibril F, Schumann M, Pace A, et al: Multiple endocrine neoplasia type 1 and Zollinger-Ellison syndrome: a prospective

study of 107 cases and comparison with 1009 cases from the literature. *Medicine* 83:43–83, 2004
97. Hermans MMH, Lips CJM, Bravenboer B: Growth hormone overproduction in a patient with multiple endocrine neoplasia type 1. *J Intern Med* 248:525–530, 2000
98. Anderson RJ, Lynch HT: Familial neuroendocrine tumors as a model for hereditary cancer. *Curr Opin Oncol* 9:45–54, 1997
99. de la Chapelle A, Eng C: Molecular genetic diagnosis for hereditary cancer, in Perry MC (ed.): *American Society of Clinical Oncology. 1999 Educational Book.* Alexandria, VA, American Society of Clinical Oncology, 1999, pp 445–453
100. Marx S, Spiegel AM, Skarulis MC, et al: Multiple endocrine neoplasia type 1: clinical and genetic topics. *Ann Intern Med* 129: 484–494, 1998
101. Chandrasekharappa SC, Guru SC, Manickam P, et al: Positional cloning of the gene for multiple endocrine neoplasia-type 1. *Science* 276:404–407, 1997
102. Takami H: RET proto-oncogene mutation analysis for multiple endocrine neoplasia, type 2. *Arch Surg* 133:679, 1998
103. Falchetti A, Brandi ML: Genetic testing for multiple endocrine neoplasias. *Endocrine Related Cancer* 5:37–44, 1998
104. Eng C, Clayton D, Schuffenecker I, et al: The relationship between specific RET proto-oncogene mutations and disease phenotype in multiple endocrine neoplasia type 2: International RET Mutation Consortium analysis. *JAMA,* 276:1575–1579, 1996
105. Grosfeld FJM, Lips CJM, Beemer FA: Psychosocial consequences of DNA analysis for MEN type 2. *Oncology* 10:141–146, 1996
106. Burgess JR, Reuben D, Parameswaran V, et al: The outcome of subtotal parathyroidectomy for the treatment of hyperparathyroidism in multiple endocrine neoplasia type 1. *Arch Surg* 133:126–129, 1998

CHAPTER 51

Endometrial Cancer

Lois Almadrones, RN, MS, CFNP, MPA

Introduction

Endometrial cancer is the fourth leading cause of cancer in women and the predominant cancer of the female genital tract (see Table 51-1).[1] It may be most curable when diagnosed early. Endometrial carcinomas make up 97% of all cancers of the corpus uteri and are the subject of this chapter. The remaining 3% are uterine sarcomas.[2]

Epidemiology

In 2004, an estimated 40,320 new cases of endometrial cancer were diagnosed in the United States, while it is estimated that only 7,090 women died of the disease.[1] Incidence and mortality rates have been relatively stable over the last 25 years. During that span, approximately 21 new cases of endometrial cancer were diagnosed per 100,000 women each year, with approximately 3.3 deaths per 100,000 white women and 6 deaths per 100,000 black women.[3] Endometrial cancer is also among the five most frequent cancers in women of all races and ethnicities (except in Korean, Vietnamese, and Alaskan native women).[4]

The racial disparity with regard to incidence and mortality rates—white women are twice as likely to have the disease although black women are twice as likely to die from it—has been of great concern and the focus of several epidemiologic studies. Black women are diagnosed at a more advanced stage, have more aggressive histologic types, and have more comorbid illnesses than white women.[1,5] Even after controlling for clinicopathologic and socioeconomic factors, black women are still associated with a significantly worse outcome.[6]

The low overall mortality rate reflects the fact that most women are diagnosed with localized disease (74% of white women and 53% of black women).[3,4,7] Relative five-year survival rates for endometrial cancer, regardless of race, are 82% for all stages, 96% for localized disease, 65% for regional disease, and 26% for distant disease at the time of diagnosis.[3]

Table 51-1 Leading Sites of Cancer in U.S. Women in 2004

Site	Incidence
Breast	215,990
Lung and bronchus	80,660
Colon and rectum	73,320
Endometrium	40,320
Ovary	25,580

Data from Jemal et al.[1]

Table 51-2 Risk Factors for Endometrial Cancer

Characteristic	Increased Risk
Obesity	
> 30 lb	3 ×
> 50 lb	10 ×
Nulliparity	2 ×
Late menopause	2.4 ×
"Bloody" menopause	4 ×
Diabetes mellitus	2.8 ×
Hypertension	1.5 ×
Unopposed estrogen	9.5 ×
Complex atypical hyperplasia	29 ×

Reprinted with permission from Barakat RR, Grigsby PW, Sabbatini P, et al: Corpus: epithelial tumors, in Hoskins WJ, Perez CA, Young RC (eds.): *Principles and Practice of Gynecologic Oncology* (ed 3). Philadelphia, Lippincott, Williams and Wilkins, 2000, p 920.

Endometrial cancer is primarily a disease of postmenopausal women. The median age at diagnosis is 61 years. Approximately 5% of women will be diagnosed with the disease before the age of 40, and 20%–25% will be premenopausal when diagnosed.[7,8]

Etiology

Multiple risk factors have been associated with the development of endometrial cancer (see Table 51-2).[9] These include obesity (being more than 30 pounds overweight or more than 50 pounds overweight increases one's risk by three- and tenfold, respectively), nulliparity, late menopause (after age 52), ''bloody'' menopause, anovulation, irregular menses, diabetes mellitus, hypertension, unopposed estrogen (no opposing progesterone), tamoxifen use, complex atypical hyperplasia, and family history of endometrial, colorectal, breast, or ovarian cancer. There are two hypotheses for the development of endometrial cancer.[9,10] The more common type of endometrial cancer, grade 1 or 2 adenocarcinoma, is thought to be related to unopposed estrogen exposure, either endogenous or exogenous. These high estrogenic states are found in women who are obese, who are nulliparous, or who experience early menarche, late menopause, chronic anovulation, endometrial hyperplasia, diabetes, or hypertension. The second type of endometrial cancer includes more undifferentiated cell types (serous, clear cell, adenocarcinoma with squamous differentiation [formerly adenosquamous], and grade 3 cancers). The risk factors related to these more aggressive endometrial cancers with poorer prognoses are less well defined.[9,10]

Obesity, defined as a body mass index (BMI) — the ratio of measured weight (in kg) divided by measured height (in m^2) — of 30 or greater, has increased to epidemic proportions in the United States, with the prevalence of age-adjusted obesity increasing from 22.9% in 1988–1994 to 30.5% in 1999–2000 among U.S. adults.[11–13] Obesity at the time of diagnosis (but not at younger ages) has been associated with risk for endometrial cancer.[14] A prospective study in Sweden found that the relative risk (RR) for endometrial cancer in obese women versus the general population was 2.9, consistent with the literature in the United States (which finds an RR ranging from 2 to 4).[15] An obese, nulliparous woman who experiences menopause after age 59 appears to have a fivefold increased risk of developing endometrial cancer.[7,8] Additionally, Feldman and associates found that nulliparous, diabetic women over the age of 70 who present with abnormal vaginal bleeding have an 87% risk of developing endometrial cancer or hyperplasia, while women who present with abnormal bleeding and have none of the other factors have only a 3% risk.[16] Diabetes and hypertension are no longer considered independent risk factors but may be present as cofactors related to endocrine imbalances. Similarly, these factors tend to be more prevalent in older, obese women.[7,17]

Excessive endogenous estrogen metabolism or production or inadequate progesterone levels have also been implicated in the development of endometrial cancer. Several hormonal aberrations can be linked to obesity. Increased body size plays a role in androgen conversion to estrogen.[2,18] As was mentioned previously, women who are more than 50 pounds overweight have a tenfold increased risk of developing endometrial cancer.[2] Additionally, women with an upper-body-fat pattern have a 5.8-fold increase in risk over women who are not obese or who have a lower-body-fat pattern.[19] Fat cells are an excellent storage depot for estrogen, and the chronic slow release of estrogen from these cells may account for the increased risk. In obese, postmenopausal women, secretion of serum sex-hormone-binding globulin (SHBG) is depressed, leaving higher concentrations of free estradiol in the blood. Obese women tend to have endocrine malfunctions, such as inadequate progesterone levels that cause anovulatory cycles with irregular menses. Chronic anovulation, such as in polycystic ovarian disease, results in the failure of progesterone to oppose chronic estrogen effects on the endometrium. Another source of endogenous estrogen can be feminizing ovarian tumors (e.g., granulosa cell tumors).[2]

The use of unopposed estrogen therapy has been linked to an increased incidence of endometrial cancer since the mid 1970s.[20,21] This problem can be virtually eliminated by cycling or combining estrogen and progesterone. Progesterone should be administered a minimum of 12 days per month.[8,22] Results of the Women's Health Initiative (WHI) study reported that women who took 0.625 mg of conjugated equine estrogen and 2.5 mg of medroxyprogesterone acetate daily were not more likely to develop endometrial cancer than placebo group patients who did not take hormones (hazard ratio [HR] 0.81). However, there was an increased risk of ovarian cancer (HR 1.58), and more endometrial biopsies to assess vaginal bleeding were required in the estrogen with progesterone group. Therefore, the authors suggest caution in the use of continuous combined hormones.[23]

Tamoxifen, which acts as an antiestrogen on breast tissue, has a weak estrogenic effect on endometrial tissue and has been associated with thickening of the endometrium and changes from polyps to hyperplasia and cancer.[24–27] As early as 1989, Fornander and colleagues reported a 6.4-fold increase in women with breast cancer receiving tamoxifen 40 mg daily versus the placebo group.[25] Data from the National Surgical Adjuvant Breast and Bowel Project (NSABP) in breast cancer prevention demonstrated a 2.53% increase in risk for endometrial cancer in women taking tamoxifen (95% confidence interval = 1.35–4.97). The greatest risk was in women over the age of 50. All endometrial cancers among the study group were diagnosed as stage I.[28]

Either exogenous or endogenous estrogen may lead to endometrial hyperplasia. While adenomatous hyperplasia is considered a risk factor for endometrial cancer, it is unclear whether it is a precursor, unless atypia accompanies the hyperplasia.[16]

A genetic link also exists for a predisposition to develop endometrial cancer. Lynch II or HNPCC (hereditary nonpolyposis colorectal cancer) syndrome is associated with a lifetime risk of 40% to 60% for the development of endometrial cancer.[29,30] A woman should be referred to genetic counseling if she has three family members who have had an HNPCC-associated cancer — one being a first-degree relative and one of the other two having been diagnosed before the age of 50 — in at least two successive generations.[10] Overall, a family history of endometrial cancer is present in about 5% of all cases and a family history of colorectal cancer in about 2%.[2,22,31]

Prevention, Screening, and Early Detection

Two factors appear to have a protective effect against the development of endometrial cancer — oral contraceptives and cigarette smoking. Use of oral contraceptives, which since the 1970s have consisted mostly of progesterone, decreases a woman's risk of developing endometrial cancer for at least 12 months; this protection seems to persist for up to 15 years in nulliparous women. Similarly, smoking has been correlated with a reduction in risk, especially in women over the age of 50. The biologic mechanism underlying the association between smoking and prevention of endometrial cancer remains unclear, but it is thought to be the antiestrogenic effect of cigarette smoking on circulating estrogen concentrations, a reduction of body weight, and an earlier age of menopause among cigarette smokers. However, the risks of developing lung cancer and other health problems well outweigh any protection gained against endometrial cancer.[8,32]

A review of the evidence-based policy recommendations on cancer screening and prevention in both Canada and the United States found the following recommendations for preventing endometrial cancer: using progesterones to prevent cancer associated with estrogenreplacement; using combination oral contraceptives; avoiding tamoxifen; controlling obesity, diabetes, and hypertension; avoiding a high-fat diet; and increasing breast feeding and physical activity.[33]

Endometrial atypical hyperplasia has a risk of progression to carcinoma of approximately 25%, and the standard treatment recommendation is hysterectomy. Although the incidence of endometrial cancer is 3% to 5% in women under 40 years of age, fertility preservation may be desired in the younger patient population.[7,34] Recent studies indicate that women with either atypical hyperplasia or well-differentiated adenocarcinoma confined to the endometrium may be offered the option of progesterone therapy with successful regression of their hyperplasia or early endometrial cancers in up to 75% of cases, with subsequent pregnancies reported.[35,36] Women who are compliant with treatment and careful monitoring, including repeat endometrial biopsies, to evaluate response may benefit from this option.[9]

Unfortunately, there is no sensitive and specific screening test for endometrial cancer. The Papanicolaou (Pap) smear will only occasionally detect an endometrial cancer. Although endometrial biopsy is 90% effective in detecting a cancer and can be accomplished in the outpatient setting, the procedure is not without morbidity and cost and is not recommended at this time as a screen for the general population. The American Cancer Society currently recommends that women with an average or increased risk should be informed about the risks and symptoms of endometrial cancer at the onset of menopause and should be strongly encouraged to report any unexpected vaginal bleeding or spotting to their physicians. Women with a genetic risk for endometrial cancer should have annual screenings beginning at age 35, although this recommendation is based on expert opinion without definitive scientific evidence.[37] Special screenings of asymptomatic women on tamoxifen with either periodic endometrial biopsies or pelvic ultrasounds have shown no proven benefit.[38–40] Annual gynecologic examinations are recommended for these women, as well as for the population at large.[7,28] Other screening techniques, such as transvaginal ultrasonography, endometrial biopsy, and the monitoring of serum melatonin levels, have been investigated but are not currently recommended as appropriate for screening in asymptomatic women.[2,22,41]

Pathophysiology

Cellular Characteristics

The uterine corpus is a muscular, hollow, pear-shaped organ with an endometrial lining composed of ciliated epithelial cells. Throughout the epithelium are small, tubular glands that extend to the myometrium, or muscle wall of the corpus. Endometrial cancer develops in the tubular glands of the epithelial layer. Tumors that arise in the lower uterine segment involve the cervix sooner and have a higher incidence of pelvic and paraaortic lymph node involvement than do tumors that arise higher in the fundus or other locations in the uterus. Similarly, tumors that have deep myometrial invasion tend to be more aggressive and have a poorer survival rate.[8,9]

Endometrial hyperplasia, primarily the atypical type, is a premalignant cytologic change that can progress to malignancy. However, simple or complex hyperplasia without atypia rarely progresses to cancer.[34,42]

The majority of endometrial cancers are adenocarcinomas. Three types of adenocarcinomas account for more than 80% of histologic patterns — pure endometrioid adenocarcinoma, adenocarcinoma with a squamous metaplasia (formerly adenoacanthoma), and adenocarcinoma with squamous differentiation (formerly adenosquamous). The less frequent patterns include clear cell (mesonephroid) carcinomas, undifferentiated carcinomas, and papillary serous carcinomas. The clear cell and serous patterns are more aggressive than the other carcinomas.[8,9]

Progression of Disease and Patterns of Spread

Multiple factors affect the natural history and prognosis of endometrial cancer (see Table 51-3). These include histologic type and differentiation (grade), stage of disease, myometrial invasion, peritoneal cytol-

Table 51-3 Prognostic Indicators for Endometrial Cancer

Indicator	Good Prognosis	Poor Prognosis
Stage of disease	I	II, III, IV
Histology	Adenocarcinomas: nonserous, non–clear cell	Serous or clear cell
Tumor differentiation	Grade I	Grades 2, 3
Myometrial invasion	Superficial or none	Deep (> 50%)
Nodal metastasis	None	Present
Peritoneal cytology	Negative	Positive

ogy, isthmus-cervix extension, pelvic and aortic lymph node metastasis, intraperitoneal spread, and adnexal metastasis.[8,9,43,44]

Endometrial cancer usually starts in the fundus and can spread to involve the entire endometrium. Through direct extension and infiltration, the cancer spreads to the myometrium, endocervix, cervix, fallopian tubes, and ovaries. Adnexal spread is infrequent but is found during surgery in approximately 6% of women with clinical stage I and occult stage II disease. Recurrence appears in 38% of women with adnexal spread compared to 11% in women without such involvement.[8,44]

Metastatic spread is usually to the pelvic and paraaortic lymph nodes and has been positively correlated with tumor differentiation, stage of disease, and amount of myometrial invasion. Pelvic and paraaortic lymph node metastases can be present even in women with stage I disease (see Figure 51-1),[45] among which approximately 10% will have positive pelvic nodes, and stage II disease, among which 36% will have positive nodes.[8] Less common sites of metastases include the vagina, peritoneal cavity, omentum, and inguinal lymph nodes. Hematogenous spread often involves the lung, liver, bone, and brain. The size of the uterus, measured by uterine sound, has been used as an indicator of survival. However, because large uterine size can be secondary to concomitant disease, such as fibroids, uterine size is no longer included in the staging and prognosis of endometrial cancer.[8,9,44]

Histologic differentiation is one of the most sensitive indicators of metastases and prognosis. The less differentiated the tumor, the poorer the prognosis. Grade 1 tumors are highly differentiated, grade 2 tumors are moderately differentiated, and grade 3 tumors are mostly solid or undifferentiated carcinomas.[9,46] Overall five-year survival rates are 96% for patients with grade I tumors, 79% for those with grade II tumors, and 70% for those with grade III tumors.[7–9]

The degree of myometrial invasion, another prognostic indicator, is generally classified as none (localized to the endometrium), superficial (invasion that is less than 50%), or deep (greater than 50%).[7–9] The greater the invasion, the poorer the prognosis. Additionally, the less differentiated the tumor, the greater the chance of myometrial invasion. Thus, the grade of the tumor is combined with the degree of myometrial invasion to estimate survival.

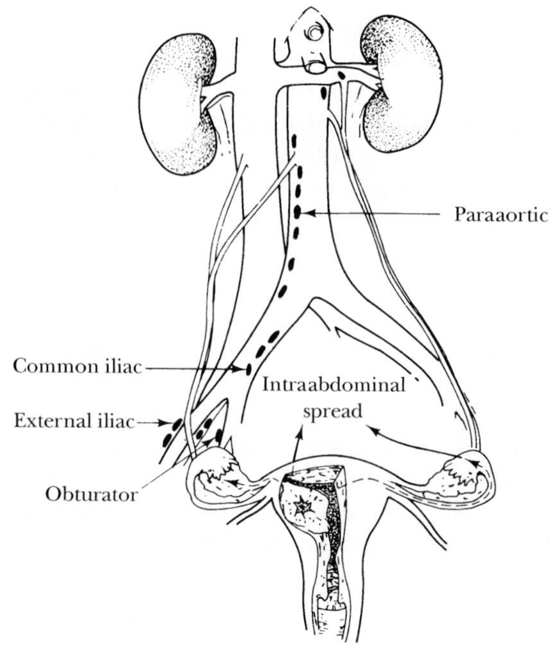

Figure 51-1 Spread pattern of endometrial cancer, with particular emphasis on potential lymph node spread. Pelvic and paraaortic nodes are at risk, even in stage I disease. (Reprinted with permission from DiSaia PJ, Creasman WT: *Clinical Gynecologic Oncology*. St Louis, Mosby, 1993.[45])

During surgery, in addition to biopsies or resection, samples of peritoneal fluid or washings of the peritoneal cavity are obtained for staging purposes, but the significance of positive results on prognosis is unclear. Women with positive peritoneal washings associated with extrauterine disease usually have a more aggressive disease and a worse prognosis. [9,47]

Endometrial cancer tends to recur within the first three years following surgery. It can recur locally in the pelvis, regionally in the abdomen, or at distant sites outside the abdominal–peritoneal cavity. Patients whose tumors have good prognostic indicators rarely have distant metastases, while women with poorer prognoses more frequently have distant metastases.[9,42]

Clinical Manifestations

Abnormal vaginal bleeding, an early symptom associated with endometrial cancer, usually prompts women to seek medical attention. Postmenopausal bleeding should always be evaluated, even though only 20% of women with this symptom will have cancer. Any serosanguinous vaginal discharge or new heavy bleeding should also be evaluated. Premenopausal onset of irregular or heavy menstrual flow may be significant, especially if the patient is infertile with anovulatory cycles. Other less frequent symptoms include pyometria and hematometria, particularly in older women, and lumbosacral, hypogastric, and pelvic pain in women with more advanced disease.[9,10,46]

Assessment

Patient and Family History

In women suspected of having endometrial cancer, a thorough history is taken. First, an in-depth description of the presenting symptom, such as postmenopausal bleeding, is obtained, including onset of symptoms, duration, amount, intensity, color, consistency, and cramping. Other pertinent history information involves risk factors, such as reproductive history, estrogen use, weight change, tamoxifen use, and dietary habits. History questions should be focused on determining the extent of disease through a review of systems to identify symptoms, such as abdominal pain, change in bowel or bladder function, and weight loss. Family and personal history of cancer, particularly breast, ovarian, endometrial, and colorectal cancer, should also be obtained.[42]

Physical Examination

Physical examination includes nodal surveillance (particularly supraclavicular and inguinal lymph nodes), lungs, abdomen for evidence of disease and organomegaly, and a complete pelvic examination (external genitalia, vagina, cervix, uterine size, adnexa, and rectovaginal bimanual examination) to evaluate the parametria and rectovaginal area.[42]

Diagnostic Studies

A Pap smear will only occasionally detect an endometrial cancer. A more reliable diagnostic technique is endometrial biopsy, which allows histologic rather than cytologic examination. Endometrial biopsy, endocervical curettage, or Pap smears done in the outpatient setting have shown a 99% rate of detection of cancer in postmenopausal women. If the endometrial biopsy is negative and symptoms persist, a fractional dilatation and curettage (D & C) should be performed to obtain a differential diagnosis.[10,48]

Other diagnostic tests include transvaginal ultrasound, chest x-ray, stool guaiac, complete blood count (CBC), and blood chemistry profiles, including liver function studies. Cystoscopy, barium enema, and proctoscopy are performed if bladder or rectal involvement is suspected. Though not routinely recommended, other studies that may be used to evaluate the status of pelvic, abdominal, and nodal disease include hysterography, hysteroscopy, lymphangiography, magnetic resonance imaging (MRI), and computerized axial tomogram scan.[2] A CA-125 level may be drawn and, if elevated, may indicate the presence of advanced or metastatic disease.[49] Although an MRI cannot distinguish benign from malignant neoplasms, it is effective in detecting the degree of myometrial invasion.[50,51] An MRI that shows no myometrial invasion may be of value in the decision to recommend progesterone therapy for women with early-stage endometrial cancer or atypical endometrial hyperplasia who desire to preserve fertility.

Prognostic Indicators

Prognostic indicators in endometrial cancer are obtained through surgical staging and pathologic information. Good prognostic indicators include having risk factors that relate to endogenous or exogenous estrogen levels, such as obesity, estrogen use without progesterone, nulliparity, and late menopause; estrogen-related risk factors; histologic grade 1 or 2; superficial myometrial invasion; no nodal metastasis; and stage I disease. In contrast, a poor prognosis involves histologic grade 3, deep myometrial invasion, nodal metastasis, high stage, and aggressive histologic behavior (usually clear cell or papillary serous).[2,9]

Classification and Staging

Endometrial cancer is staged surgically (see Table 51-4),[52] if medical conditions and intraabdominal disease permit the woman to be a candidate for surgery. Staging helps to define primary tumor size, location, and the extent of spread beyond the uterus.[52] Approximately 73% of tumors are diagnosed in stage I, 12% in stage II, 12% in stage III, and 3% in stage IV.[9]

The standard surgical staging and treatment of endometrial cancer includes bimanual examination under anesthesia, laparotomy through an adequate abdominal incision (usually vertical), exploration of the peritoneal cavity, peritoneal cytology, biopsies of suspicious areas, selective pelvic and paraaortic

Table 51-4 Staging for Carcinoma of the Corpus Uteri

FIGO Stages			TNM Category
		Primary tumor cannot be assessed	TX
		No evidence of primary tumor	T0
0		Carcinoma in situ (preinvasive carcinoma)	Tis
I		Tumor confined to corpus uteri	T1
	IA	Tumor limited to endometrium	T1a
	IB	Tumor invades up to less than half of myometrium	T1b
	IC	Tumor invades more than half of myometrium	T1c
II		Tumor invades cervix but does not extend beyond uterus	T2
	IIA	Endocervical glandular involvement only	T2a
	IIB	Cervical stromal invasion	T2b
III		Local and/or regional spread as specified in IIIA, B, C	T3 and/or N1
	IIIA	Tumor involves serosa and/or adnexa (direct extension or metastasis) and/or cancer cells in ascites or peritoneal washings	T3a
	IIIB	Vaginal involvement (direct extension or metastasis)	T3b
	IIIC	Metastasis to pelvic and/or paraaortic lymph nodes	N1
IVA		Tumor invades bladder mucosa and/or bowel mucosa*	T4
IVB		Distant metastasis (excluding metastasis to vagina, pelvic serosa, or adnexa, including metastasis to intra-abdominal lymph nodes other than paraaortic and/or inguinal nodes)	M1

*Note: The presence of bullous edema is not sufficient evidence to classify a tumor as T4.
Data from *FIGO News*.[52]

lymphadenectomy, total abdominal hysterectomy (TAH), bilateral salpingo-oophorectomy (BSO), and possible omentectomy and resection of tumor implants.[8,10,52] The best-trained physician to treat any gynecologic cancer is a gynecologic oncologist. The Society of Gynecologic Oncologists recommends referral of women with known or suspected endometrial cancer to a gynecologic oncologist for surgery and subsequent surveillance.[53]

Therapeutic Approaches and Nursing Care

Early-Stage Disease

The goals of treatment in stage I and II disease are for cure and long-term survival; thus, nursing care must focus on managing the side effects of treatment and promoting health maintenance behaviors.

Surgery

Treatment of endometrial cancer includes surgical staging, TAH, BSO, selective pelvic and paraaortic lymphadenectomy, omentectomy, and peritoneal washings. Surgical staging is initially done on all women who are surgical candidates so that adjuvant radiation, if needed, can be tailored to the individual's extent of disease. Many women with early-stage disease will not need additional therapy beyond the initial surgery, thus avoiding the time, effort, and morbidity associated with adjuvant radiation therapy. Also, the pathologist is better able to evaluate untreated tissue for the histologic indicators of prognosis (histologic type, grade, and myometrial invasion).

An alternative method for surgical staging of endometrial cancer that has gained popularity is minimally invasive surgery (see Figure 51-2).[54] Childers and associates first reported successful laparoscopically assisted vaginal hysterectomies (LAVHs) in women with early-stage endometrial cancer.[55] Laparoscopy is associated with few complications, shorter hospital stays and recovery time, cosmetically better outcomes, and lower overall hospital charges. Women also report a higher level of satisfaction with laparoscopy compared to women treated with laparotomy.[56,57] Barakat and associates reported that the median number of lymph nodes sampled during surgery increased with laparoscopy, which led to fewer women requiring whole abdominal radiation postoperatively. This change in the treatment paradigm also seems to decrease morbidity and overall cost.[58] LAVH must be done by a physician who is well trained in this technique, including laparoscopic lymph node dissections. One con-

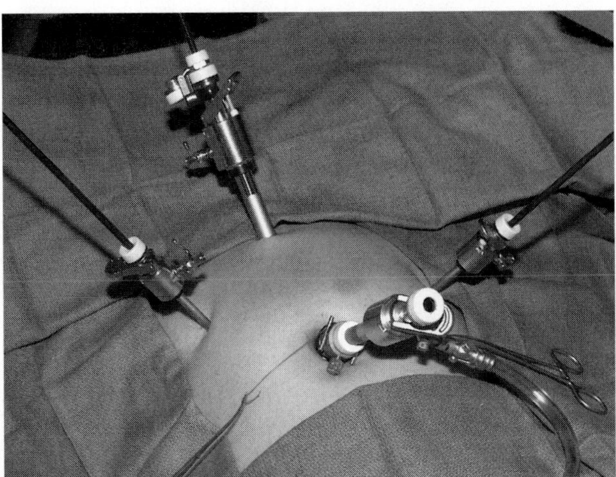

Figure 51-2 Minimally invasive surgical staging procedure using reusable or disposable trocars. (Courtesy of Levine DA, Barakat RR, Hoskins WJ [© 2003 Memorial Sloan-Kettering Cancer Center]: *Atlas of Procedures in Gynecologic Oncology*. London, Martin Dunitz, 2003.)

traindication for laparoscopic surgery may be the obese patient, with a BMI greater than 28—a relative weight greater than 120% of the desirable weight.[59] The Gynecologic Oncology Group (GOG) is currently conducting a randomized trial comparing LAVH to the standard laparotomy to determine equivalency in cancer outcomes and quality of life.

Prior to undergoing surgery for endometrial cancer, women must be thoroughly informed about surgical procedures, recovery, and self-care issues. (see Table 51-5). Postoperative care includes fluid and electrolyte monitoring, progressive ambulation, and cardiopulmonary monitoring and intervention. Since many of these women may be overweight and over the age of 60, they may have concurrent medical problems, such as hypertension, diabetes, or renal compromise, that will require careful assessment and monitoring. Due to shortened hospital stays, discharge planning must begin early, even in the preoperative period. Assessment includes identifying the need for home care, ongoing monitoring, and follow-up care. Because hysterectomy is still associated with a loss of femininity and sexuality, psychosocial support is an important part of follow-up care. Sexual alterations may be particularly important when the woman is still of childbearing age and premenopausal, since the surgery itself will render her sterile and place her abruptly into menopause. Mobilization of support resources, such as family, friends, social workers, spiritual counselors, and home care nurses, may assist the woman in coping with these changes. Some of the most common postoperative complications that the nurse should anticipate and assess include wound infection, deep venous thrombosis, pulmonary atelectasis and pneumonia, and bleeding.

Radiation

The need for adjuvant radiation therapy for endometrial cancer is determined by stage and pathologic risk factors (see Tables 51-2 and 51-4).[9] Women with Stage IA, grade 1 or 2 disease and no myometrial invasion are considered at low risk for recurrence and require no further treatment.[60] The vagina is the most common site of local recurrence; therefore, adjuvant intravaginal brachytherapy may be recommended for women with intermediate risk—less than 50% myometrial invasion. Intravaginal brachytherapy is administered in the outpatient setting in three divided fractions delivered every two weeks. Morbidity is minimal and consists of mild gastrointestinal and urinary symptoms and vaginal dryness.[61,62] The role of external pelvic radiation added to intravaginal brachytherapy remains controversial in women with adequate surgical staging and no extrauterine disease because it adds to morbidity and cost. It has also been demonstrated that women can be treated at the time of recurrence with no negative effect on overall survival.[10,62,63]

Indications for pelvic external-beam radiation therapy (which allows treatment of all pelvic tissue, including nodes and lymphatics) usually include disease localized to the pelvis, a high-grade tumor, and greater than 50% myometrial invasion. Women with stage IC or IIA disease are recommended to receive whole pelvis radiation; stage IIB treatment adds intravaginal or intracavitary radiation to the regimen; stage III therapy includes whole pelvis, paraaortic (if positive), and possibly whole abdominal radiation; and stage IV treatment may include pelvic and abdominal radiation as well as chemotherapy.[2,8,10,22,42,43,64] Finally, in women who are poor surgical candidates, radiation is a justifiable option with good overall five-year survival.[65]

Before receiving radiation therapy women should be educated about the treatment plan, side effects, monitoring, and self-care issues. During therapy, the patient is monitored closely for side effects of the treatment so that timely intervention can occur. These side effects of pelvic and abdominal radiation will be directly related to the organs or systems included in the radiation port. Potential side effects include nausea, diarrhea, urinary urgency or burning, myelosuppression, and skin changes, such as erythema, dryness, itching, burning, and desquamation. Vaginal atrophy and stenosis resulting from radiation therapy can lead to sexual dysfunction. The use of moisturizers will help minimize dryness. If the woman is sexually active, water-based lubricants can be used liberally during intercourse. If the woman is not sexually active, the use of vaginal dilators with lubricants may help prevent va-

Table 51-5 Information Needs Related to Endometrial Cancer

Topic	Information
Health maintenance issues that affect risk	
Estrogen replacement therapy (ERT)	Indications: Vaginal atrophy with infection or sexual dysfunction Loss of pelvic support with incontinence Perimenopausal emotional lability Early surgical or radiation castration Vasomotor instability Estrogen cycled with progesterone Annual pelvic exam Annual mammogram Seek medical attention if any abnormal vaginal bleeding occurs, including postmenopausal bleeding (PMB)
Breast self-examination (BSE)	Importance of BSE in conjunction with ERT Determine schedule to aid in compliance Technique for performing BSE and demonstration of skill
Diet and weight control	Low-fat, calcium-rich diet, calcium supplements, diphosphonate therapy for osteopenia Maintain weight within normal range Large amounts of caffeine and fiber may decrease calcium absorption Weight-bearing exercises to decrease bone loss (e.g., walking)
Abnormal vaginal bleeding	Seek medical attention for new onset of abnormal bleeding, including intramenstrual and PMB PMB and abnormal bleeding in the infertile patient with anovulatory cycles must be evaluated, even though only 20% of PMB is associated with malignancy Evaluation of abnormal bleeding includes pelvic exam and endometrial biopsy
Therapeutic interventions	
Surgery	Types of surgery planned, what will be removed, change in anatomy and function anticipated Clarify, reinforce informed consent Role in postoperative care to facilitate recovery, e.g., progressive ambulation, respiratory care Discharge planning related to self-care issues, need for assistance, and appointment for postoperative follow-up
Radiation	Type of therapy planned Associated morbidity, e.g., GI, GU Appointments for follow-up
Hormonal	Schedule for medications Expected side effects
Chemotherapy	Types of drugs and regimen planned Side effects and toxicities of drugs Inpatient versus outpatient versus home chemotherapy Duration of therapy Need for venous access device Regular appointments to monitor response
Psychosexual concerns	
Role functioning	Dispel myths related to perceived loss of femininity due to removal of uterus, tubes, and ovaries, e.g., weight gain, loss of sexual interest/enjoyment, aging, mental deterioration Help redefine self in terms other than reproduction
Sexual functioning	Review anatomy, physiology, and sexual functioning preoperatively Complete sexual assessment Alteration in sexual response secondary to hysterectomy: Cervix contributes to but is not essential for orgasm Uterus elevates during excitement phase and contracts rhythmically during orgasm Alteration in sexual functioning secondary to radiation: Vaginal dryness and stenosis may result in patient who is not sexually active, unless vaginal dilators and lubricants are employed Use of water-soluble lubricants during intercourse, such as Astroglide® or nonhormonal moisturizers used three times a week, such as Replens® Use of low-dose estrogen vaginal pellets (Vagifom®) or ring device (Estring®) that release minimal systemic estrogen Nonhormonal therapy for menopausal symptoms: Low-dose antidepressants — vasomotor instability Layered cotton, light wool clothing Paced respirations/relaxation techniques Cool environment Avoid hot baths, hot tubs, hot food before bedtime Regular exercise

ginal stenosis.[66,67] For specific radiation therapy issues and nursing care, see Chapters 13 and 14.

Advanced or Recurrent Disease

Treatment goals for stage III or IV or for recurrent disease include controlling the disease and associated symptoms. Long-term survival is rare unless the disease is confined to the vagina. Palliation and supportive care are important nursing management goals in order to maximize the patient's quality of life.

Surgery and radiation

Endometrial cancer is difficult to treat if it has metastasized or recurred. Women with isolated vaginal recurrences can be treated successfully with radiation therapy, with a salvage rate of 40%.[68] However, women with recurrences outside the upper vagina (pelvis or distant) require multimodal therapy, and the five-year progression-free survival is only approximately 20%.[10] Radical surgery with pelvic exenteration has been attempted in women with central pelvic recurrences after radiation, but morbidity is high and overall long-term survival is only 20% to 45%.[68,69] A newer approach to central recurrence is the combination of exenteration (total, anterior, or posterior) with intraoperative radiation therapy delivered directly to the site with the highest risk of local failure. Although morbidity is high with this combined therapy, local control and salvage are possible in patients who would otherwise be offered only palliative treatment.[70] Palliative radiation can be used to control heavy vaginal bleeding in patients with advanced, incurable disease.

Hormonal therapy

The most commonly used systemic therapy for recurrent endometrial cancer has been synthetic progestational agents. A GOG study reported a response rate of 25% with low-dose medroxyprogesterone acetate. Responses were higher in women with histologically well-differentiated and progesterone-receptor-positive tumors.[71] Receptor status can also predict which tumors will respond to progesterones. Positive progesterone receptor status correlates with a better response to progesterone therapy regardless of the grade of the tumor. If both receptors are positive, a 77% response rate is associated with progesterone therapy, compared with only a 9% response rate if both receptors are negative.[2]

Single-agent tamoxifen has also been studied; the overall response is only 10%, but when combined with megestrol acetate responses increased to 27%.[72,73] Oral preparations of megestrol acetate or intramuscular medroxyprogesterone acetate are effective agents against endometrial cancer and are continued until the disease progresses. At that time, chemotherapy is considered.

Patient education, close assessment, and monitoring for side effects of the progestational agents are important components of care. The side effects include fluid retention, phlebitis, and thrombosis. Feelings of well-being, as well as weight gain, while taking progesterones are also possible. Side effects are usually minimal, unless high doses are employed.[46]

Chemotherapy

Cytotoxic agents have a limited role in the treatment of advanced-stage endometrial cancer after women have failed to respond to hormonal therapy. Only a few agents have demonstrated activity equal to or greater than progesterone therapy. Drugs that have shown activity in women who have not had prior chemotherapy include doxorubicin (37% response rate), cisplatin (up to 46%), ifosphamide (24.3%), and paclitaxel (35%).[74,75]

Combination chemotherapy using doxorubicin and cisplatin has become the standard of care following the results of a randomized trial that showed improved response rates for the combination compared to doxorubicin alone.[76] Another GOG study incorporating the standard plus paclitaxel showed a better response rate (57%) but only a small improvement in overall survival.[77] Studies of other combinations with additional drugs, such as vinblastine and methotrexate, have shown little additional improvement in response rates, with increased side effects.[78,79]

Initially, the woman will need intensive education regarding the chemotherapy regimen, schedule, and side effects of the drugs. Once treatment has been started, ongoing assessment and monitoring for side effects will permit early recognition of problems and prompt intervention. Continuous psychosocial support is needed to assist the woman and her family in coping with the side effects of treatment, such as nausea, vomiting, hair loss, myelosuppression, and peripheral neuropathy. For specific issues and side effects of chemotherapy, refer to Chapters 15, 16, and 17.

Symptom Management and Supportive Care

The woman with early-stage endometrial cancer can expect long-term, disease-free survival. Since the majority of women with endometrial cancer fall into this favorable category, health maintenance will be a major focus of their ongoing care. It is important to note that this population of women will live their remaining lives without the potential health benefits of endogenous estrogen because of surgical hormonal ablation, and they may experience uncomfortable menopausal symptoms.

Estrogen replacement therapy (ERT) without progesterone is often discussed as an important factor for quality of life and relief of menopausal symptoms, but the issue is controversial, especially after the results of the WHI showed no added cardiac benefit and an increase in both breast and ovarian cancers in women who took hormones.[23] A randomized study was done by the GOG to evaluate the effect of ERT on recurrence-free survival and overall survival in women with Stage I or II endometrial cancer. Unfortunately, the study was closed early due to decreased enrollment after publication of the WHI. Although the number of participants in the study before it closed reached only 1240 of the proposed 2107 patients needed for statistical validity, reported results at a median follow-up of 30.8 months suggested that ERT in Stage I/II endometrial cancer patients did not increase either recurrence of their endometrial cancer or new malignancy.[80]

Even without the current data from the GOG, in 1993 the American College of Obstetricians and Gynecologists (ACOG) issued a statement that estrogen therapy may be used in women with endometrial cancer, using the same criteria as are used with the general population, but that special consideration should be given to the individual prognostic indicators and the risks that the woman is willing to accept.[81] Currently, ACOG has not issued any specific recommendations for women with endometrial cancer treated with TAH/BSO requiring only estrogen therapy. As for short-term use of estrogen/progesterone therapy for the relief of menopausal symptoms, "ACOG continues to recommend that this be a personal, individualized decision made after consultations between a woman and her physician and taking into account a woman's individual benefits and risks from such use."[82]

Additionally, as younger women develop endometrial cancer, conservative fertility-sparing therapy for early-stage, low-grade disease has demonstrated efficacy, but long-term outcomes are still unknown. Another major area for assessment and intervention is knowledge related to health-maintenance behaviors, therapeutic interventions, and psychosocial concerns.

For those women who present with advanced-stage disease or who have a recurrence, the challenges of care will vary according to the location and extent of disease. Women with local, pelvic recurrence will have symptoms related to the structures that are involved, such as hematuria (if the bladder is involved), fecal incontinence (if a rectovaginal fistula is present), or pain (if nerves are involved). Regional recurrence in the abdominal cavity can include ascites, a change in bowel habits due to compression or involvement of the bowel, or right upper quadrant pain from liver involvement. Finally, distant recurrence can involve respiratory compromise with lung metastases/effusions or central nervous system morbidity with brain metastases. The type of therapy used will depend on the specific recurrence. Although surgery or radiation may be used in selected situations, such as when removing an isolated mass or treating an area that did not previously receive any radiation, chemotherapy is usually offered. Researchers are just beginning to explore the use of selective estrogen receptor modulators and other novel endocrine therapies in endometrial cancer.

Important considerations include the side effects of therapy and how to manage them; self-care issues, such as care of a venous access device, nutritional intake, and pain control; and community resources for assistance, including home care resources, support groups, and counseling. Quality of life is also an important issue to discuss with the woman and her family, particularly focusing on physical changes and functional status, psychosocial concerns (such as changes in roles within the family), economic concerns, and spiritual and religious concerns. When the goal of treatment is supportive care, hospice care and bereavement counseling are the focus.

For the vast majority of women with endometrial cancer, the major nursing challenges relate to compliance and regular follow-up. Since most patients will be cured with their primary surgery, regular follow-up will be the focus of their care. Follow-up usually involves regular pelvic examinations, at least quarterly in the initial years after diagnosis. Other tests and scans are performed as clinically indicated. Education about the importance of follow-up, as well as of a healthy lifestyle, must be stressed. A healthy lifestyle includes weight reduction, if appropriate, a diet low in fat, regular exercise, and regular screening for other cancers, including mammography, Pap smears, and colonoscopy.

For women who have advanced disease, mobilization of resources will be important in order to maximize care and quality of life. Coordination of care or case management is important to ensure that all physical and psychosocial needs are being addressed, either at the time of discharge from the hospital or when care requirements change. Local ambulatory and home care resources, including nursing, social work, support groups, and spiritual counseling, can help the woman remain at home during ongoing care for advanced-stage disease, whether the goal is cure, palliation, or comfort measures.

Although the majority of women are diagnosed with early-stage endometrial cancer, women still die from recurrent or advanced-stage disease. Ongoing efforts strive to define appropriate screening techniques, adjuvant therapy, and new cytotoxic agents and regimens to improve survival. Comprehensive, holistic nursing management will assist the woman and her family to achieve optimal health and quality of life.

Future Trends

One of the biggest challenges faced by healthcare providers is educating women about the correlation between obesity and endometrial cancer. Obesity is a growing epidemic, especially in the United States, and can be prevented with a healthy diet and exercise. Nurses can have a significant role in educating and empowering women about the benefits of good nutritional habits, which may help to prevent many medical conditions, including endometrial cancer.

Economics and reimbursement issues continue to influence the delivery of health care. Laparoscopic surgery reduces the length of hospital stays; therefore, the results of the GOG randomized trial of laparoscopy versus standard laparotomy for the initial treatment of early-stage endometrial cancer are eagerly awaited. If laparoscopy is shown to be equivalent to laparotomy in clinical outcomes and improves a woman's quality of life, it may become a new standard surgical approach for this disease.

The role of genetics in endometrial cancer will continue to be explored and may lead to the discovery of a gene linked to endometrial cancer. A gene would identify women at higher risk for this form of cancer, which may lead to early intervention.

References

1. Jemal A, Tiwari R, Murray T, et al: Cancer statistics, 2004. *CA Cancer J Clin* 54:8–29, 2004
2. Rose P: Endometrial carcinoma. *N Engl J Med* 335:640–649, 1996
3. Ries LAG, Eisner MP, Kosary CL, et al (eds.): SEER Cancer Statistics Review, 1975–2000. *http://seer.cancer.gov/csr/1975–2000.* Accessed October 28, 2004
4. Parker SL, Davis JK, Wingo PA, et al: Cancer statistics by race and ethnicity. *CA Cancer J Clin* 48:31–48, 1998
5. Hill HA, Coates RJ, Austin H, et al: Racial differences in tumor grade among women with endometrial cancer. *Gynecol Oncol* 56:154–163, 1995
6. Connell PP, Rotmensch, J, Waggoner SE, et al: Race and clinical outcome in endometrial cancer. *Obstet Gynecol* 94:713–720, 1999
7. Creasman WT: Endometrial cancer: incidence, prognostic factors, diagnosis, and treatment. *Semin Oncol* 24(suppl 1):140–150, 1997
8. DiSaia PJ, Creasman WT: *Clinical Gynecologic Oncology* (ed 6). St. Louis, Mosby, 2002
9. Barakat R, Grigsby PW, Sabbatini P, et al: Corpus: epithelial tumors, in Hoskins WJ, Perez CA, Young RC (eds.): *Cancer Principles and Practice of Gynecologic Oncology* (ed 3). Philadelphia, Lippincott, Williams, and Wilkins, 2000, pp 919–959
10. Sonoda Y: Optimal therapy and management of endometrial cancer. *Expert Rev Anticancer Ther* 3:37–47, 2003
11. Mokdad AH, Bowman, BA Ford ES, et al: The continuing epidemics of obesity and diabetes in the United States. *JAMA* 286:1195–1200, 2001
12. Flegal KM, Carroll MD, Ogden CL, et al: Prevalence and trends in obesity among US adults 1999–2000. *JAMA* 288:1723–1727, 2002
13. Polednak AP: Trends in incidence rates for obesity-associated cancers in the US. *Cancer Detect Prevent* 27:415–421, 2003
14. Persson I, Adami HO: Endometrial cancer, in Adami HO, Hunter D, Trichopulos D (eds.): *Textbook of Cancer Epidemiology.* New York, Oxford University Press, 2002, pp 359–377
15. Wolk A, Gridley G, Svensson M, et al: A prospective study of obesity and cancer risk in Sweden. *Cancer Causes Contr* 12:13–21, 2001
16. Feldman S, Cook EF, Harlow BL, et al: Predicting endometrial cancer among older women who present with abnormal vaginal bleeding. *Gynecol Oncol* 56:376–381, 1995
17. Shoff SM, Newcomb PA: Diabetes, body size, and risk of endometrial cancer. *Am J Epidemiol* 148:234–240, 1998
18. Goodman MT, Hankin JH, Wilkens LR, et al: Diet, body size, physical activity, and the risk of endometrial cancer. *Cancer Res* 57:5077–5085, 1997
19. Elliott EA, Matonoski GM, Rosenshein NB, et al: Body fat patterning in women with endometrial cancer. *Gynecol Oncol* 39:253–258, 1990
20. Persson I, Adami HO, Bergkvist L, et al: Risk of endometrial cancer after treatment with oestrogens alone or in conjunction with progestogens: results of a prospective study. *Br Med J* 298:147–151, 1989
21. Antunes CMF, Stolley PD, Rosenshein MB, et al: Endometrial cancer and estrogen use. *N Engl J Med* 300:9, 1979
22. Yamada SD, McGonigle KF: Cancer of the endometrium and corpus uteri. *Curr Opin Obstet Gynecol* 10:57–60, 1998
23. Anderson GL, Judd HL, Kaunitz AM, et al: Effects of estrogen plus progesterone on gynecologic cancers and associated diagnostic procedures: the Women's Health Initiative randomized trial. *JAMA* 13:1739–1748, 2003
24. Fisher B, Costantino JP, Redmond CK, et al: Endometrial cancer in tamoxifen-treated breast cancer patients: findings from the National Surgical Adjuvant Breast and Bowel Project (NSABP) B-14. *J Natl Cancer Inst* 86:527–537, 1994
25. Fornander T, Rutquist LE, Cedarmark B, et al: Adjuvant tamoxifen in early breast cancer: occurrence of new primary cancers. *Lancet* 1:117–129, 1989
26. Barakat RR, Wong G, Curtin JP, et al: Tamoxifen use in breast cancer patients who subsequently develop corpus cancer is not associated with a higher incidence of adverse histologic features. *Gynecol Oncol* 55:164–168, 1994
27. Cuzick J, Powles T, Veronesi U, et al: Overview of the main outcomes in breast cancer prevention trials. *Lancet* 361:296–300, 2003
28. Fisher B, Costantino JP, Wickerham DL, et al: Tamoxifen for prevention of breast cancer: report of the National Surgical Adjuvant Breast and Bowel Project P-1 study. *J Natl Cancer Inst* 90:1371–1388, 1998

29. Aarnio M, Sankila R, Pakkala E, et al: Cancer risk in mutation carriers of DNA mismatch-repair genes. *Int J Cancer* 81:214–218, 1999
30. Dunlop MG, Farrington SM, Carothers AD, et al: Cancer risk associated with germline DNA mismatch repair gene mutations. *Hum Mol Genet* 6:105–110, 1997
31. Zawacki KL, Phillips M: Cancer genetics and women's health. *J Obstet Gynecol Neonatal Nurs* 31:208–216, 2002
32. Terry PD, Rohan TE, Franceschi S, et al: Cigarette smoking and the risk of endometrial cancer. *Lancet* 3:470–480, 2002
33. Franco EL, Duarte-Franco,E, Rohan TE: Evidence-based policy recommendations on cancer prevention and screening. *Cancer Detect Prevent* 26:350–361, 2002
34. Kurman RJ, Kaminski PE, Norris HJ: The behavior of endometrial hyperplasia: a long term study of untreated hyperplasia in 170 patients. *Cancer* 56:403–412, 1985
35. Randall TC, Kurman RJ: Progesterone treatment of atypical hyperplasia and well-differentiated carcinoma of the endometrium in women under age 40. *Obstet Gynecol* 90:434–440, 1997
36. Kaku T, Yoshikawa H, Tsuda H, et al: Conservative therapy for adenocarcinoma and atypical endometrial hyperplasia of the endometrium in young women: central pathologic review and treatment outcome. *Cancer Letters* 167:39–48, 2001
37. Smith RA, von Eschenbach AC, Wender R, et al: American Cancer Society guidelines for the early detection of cancer: update of early detection guidelines for prostate, colorectal, and endometrial cancers. *CA Cancer J Clin* 51:38–53, 2001
38. Barakat RR, Gilewski A, Almadrones LA, et al: Effect of adjuvant taomoxifen on the endometrium in women with breast cancer: a prospective study using office endometrial biopsy. *J Clin Oncol* 18:3459–3463, 2000
39. Burgmann S, Goodman A: Surveillance for endometrial cancer in women receiving tamoxifen. *Ann Int Med* 131:137–135, 1999
40. Gerber B, Krause A, Muller H, et al: Effects of adjuvant tamoxifen on the endometium in postmenopausal women with breast cancer: a prospective long-term study using transvaginal ultrasound. *J Clin Oncol* 18:3464–3470, 2000
41. Grin W, Grunberger W: A significant correlation between melatonindeficiency and endometrial cancer. *Gynecol Obstet Invest* 45:62–65, 1998
42. Greven KM, Corn BW: Endometrial cancer. *Curr Probl Cancer* 21:72–127, 1997
43. Hacker NF: Uterine cancer, in Berek JS, Hacker NF (eds.): *Practical Gynecologic Oncology* (ed 3). Philadelphia, Lippincott, Williams, and Wilkins, 2000, pp 407–455
44. Creasman WT, Morrow CP, Bundy BN, et al: Surgical pathologic spread patterns of endometrial cancer: a Gynecologic Oncology Group study. *Cancer* 60:2035–2041, 1987
45. DiSaia PJ, Creasman WT: *Clinical Gynecologic Oncology*. St. Louis, Mosby, 1993
46. Burke TW, Eifel PJ, Muggia FM: Cancers of the uterine body, in DeVita VT Jr, Hellman S, Rosenberg SA (eds.): *Cancer: Principles and Practice of Oncology* (ed 6). Philadelphia, Lippincott, Williams, and Wilkins, 2001, pp 1573–1594
47. Hirai Y, Takeshima N, et al: Malignant potential of positive peritoneal cytology in endometrial cancer. *Obstet Gynecol* 97:725–728, 2001
48. Dijkhuizen FP, Mol BW, Brolmann HA, et al: The accuracy of endometrial sampling in the diagnosis of patients with endometrial carcinoma and hyperplasia: a meta-analysis. *Cancer* 89:1765–1772, 2000
49. Sood AK, Buller RE, Burger RA, et al: Value of preoperative CA 125 level in the management of uterine cancer and prediction of clinical outcome. *Obstet Gynecol* 90:441–447, 1997
50. Atsukawa H, Saski H, Tada S: A multivariate analysis of assessment of myometrial invasion of endometrial carcinoma by magnetic resonance imaging. *Gynecol Oncol* 54:298–306, 1994
51. Barakat RR, Hricak H: What do we expect from imaging? *Radiol Clin North Am* 40:521–526, 2002
52. FIGO, International Federation of Gynecology and Obstetrics: Corpus cancer staging: FIGO news. *Int J Gynecol Obstet* 70:207–312, 2000
53. Society of Gynecologic Oncologists: Referral guidelines in gynecologic oncology. *Gynecol Oncol* 78:S1–13, 2000
54. Sonoda Y: Laparoscopic staging procedures, in Levine DA, Barakat RR, Hoskins WJ (eds.): *Atlas of Procedures in Gynecologic Oncology*. London, Martin Dunitz, 2003, p 105
55. Childers JM, Brzechffa PR, Hatch KD, et al: Laparoscopically assisted surgical staging of endometrial cancer. *Gynecol Oncol* 51:33–38, 1993
56. Gemignani ML, Curtin JP, Zelmanovich J, et al: Laparoscopic-assisted vaginal hysterectomy for endometrial cancer: clinical outcomes and hospital charges. *Gynecol Oncol* 73:5–11, 1999
57. Spiritos NM, Schlaerth JB, Gross GM, et al: Cost and quality-of-life analyses of surgery for early endometrial cancer: laparotomy versus laparoscopy. *Am J Obstet Gynecol* 174:1795–1799, 1996
58. Barakat RR, Lev G, Hummer A, et al: Ten-year experience in the management of 1032 women with uterine cancer: a change in treatment paradigm. Society of Gynecologic Oncologists Annual Meeting on Women's Cancer; February 7–11, 2004, San Diego, CA. (Abstr 432)
59. Eltabbakh GH, Sahmonki MI, Moody JM, et al: Hysterectomy for obese women with endometrial cancer: laparoscopy or laparotomy? *Gynecol Oncol* 78:329–335, 2000
60. Straughn JM, Huh WK, Kelly FJ, et al: Conservative management of Stage I endometrial carcinoma after surgical staging. *Gynecol Oncol* 84:194–200, 2002
61. Chadha MP, Nanavati PJ, Liu P, et al: Patterns of failure in endometrial carcinoma Stage IB, grade 3 and IC patients treated with postoperative vaginal vault brachytherapy. *Gynecol Oncol* 75:103–107, 1999
62. Sabbatini P, Alektiar KM, Barakat RR: Endometrial cancer, in Barakat R, Bevers MN, Gershenson DM, et al (eds.): *Handbook of Gynecologic Oncology*. London, Martin Dunitz, 2000, pp 265–278
63. Creutzberg CL, van Putten WL, Koper PC, et al: Surgery and postoperative radiotherapy versus surgery alone for patients with Stage I endometrial carcinoma: multicenter randomized trial. PORTEC Study Group. Post Operative Radiation Therapy in Endometrial Carcinoma. *Lancet* 355:1405–1411, 2000
64. Small W, Mahadevan A, Roland P, et al: Whole abdominal radiation in endometrial carcinoma: an analysis of toxicity, patterns of recurrence and survival. *Cancer J* 6:394–400, 2000
65. Kupelian PA, Eifel PJ, Tornos C, et al: Treatment of endometrial carcinoma with radiation therapy alone. *Int J Radiat Oncol Biol Phys* 27:817–824, 1993
66. Denton AS, Maher EJ: Interventions for the physical aspects of sexual dysfunction in women following pelvic radiotherapy. *Cochrane Database Systematic Rev* 3:3, 2003
67. Wilmoth MC, Spinelli A: Sexual implications of gynecologic cancer treatments. *JOGNN — Obst, Gyn and Neonat Nurs* 29:413–421, 2000
68. Morris M, Alvarez RD, Kinney WK, et al: Treatment for recurrent adenocarcinoma of the endometrium with pelvic exenteration. *Gynecol Oncol* 60:288–291, 1996
69. Barakat RR, Goldman NA, Patel DA, et al: Pelvic exenteration for recurrent endometrial cancer. *Gynecol Oncol* 75:99–102, 1999

70. Gemignani ML, Alektiar KM, Leitao M, et al: Radical surgical resection and high-dose intraoperative radiation therapy in patients with recurrent gynecologic cancers. *Int J Rad Oncol Biol Phys* 3:687–694, 2001
71. Thigpen JT, Brady MF, Alvarez RD, et al: Oral medroxyprogesterone acetate in the treatment of advanced or recurrent endometrial carcinoma: a dose-response study by the Gynecologic Oncology Group. *J Clin Oncol* 17:1736–1744, 1999
72. Thigpen T, Brady MF, Homesley HD, et al: Tamoxifen in the treatment of advanced or recurrent endometrial carcinoma: a Gynecologic Oncology Group study. *J Clin Oncol* 19:364–367, 2001
73. Fiorica J, Brunetto V, Hanjani P, et al: A phase II study (GOG 153) of recurrent and advanced endometrial carcinoma treated with alternating courses of megestrol acetate and tamoxifen citrate. *Proc Am Soc Clin Oncol* 19:379, 2000 (abstr)
74. Ball HG, Blessing JA, Lentz SS, et al: A phase II trial of taxol in advanced or recurrent adenocarcinoma of the endometrium: a Gynecologic Oncology Group study. *Gynecol Oncol* 62:278–281, 1996
75. Sutton GP, Blessing JA, DeMars LR, et al: A phase II Gynecologic Oncology Group trial of ifosphamide and mesna in advanced or recurrent adenocarcinoma of the endometrium. *Gynecol Oncol* 63:25–27, 1996
76. Thigpen JT, Blessing J, Homesley H, et al: Phase III trial of doxorubicin +/− cisplatin in advanced or recurrent endometrial carcinoma: a Gynecologic Oncology Group (GOG) study. *Proc Am Soc Clin Oncol* 12:261, 1993 (abstr)
77. Fleming GF, Brunetto VL, Mundt AJ, et al: Randomized trial of doxorubicin plus cisplatin versus doxorubicin plus cisplatin plus paclitaxel in patients with advanced or recurrent endometrial carcinoma: a Gynecologic Oncology Group study. *Proc Am Soc Clin Onc* 807, 2002 (abstr)
78. Long HJ, Langdon RM Jr, Cha SS, et al: Phase II trial of methotrexate, vinblastine, doxorubicin, and cisplatin in advanced/recurrent endometrial carcinoma. *Gynecol Oncol* 58:240–243, 1995
79. Burke TW, Gershenson DM, Morris M: Postoperative adjuvant cisplatin, doxorubicin, cyclophosphamide (PAC) chemotherapy in women with high risk endometrial carcinoma. *Gynecol Oncol* 55:47–50, 1994
80. Barakat RR, Bundy BN, Spiritos NM, et al: A prospective randomized double-blind trial of estrogen replacement therapy versus placebo in women with Stage I or II endometrial cancer: a Gynecologic Oncology Group (GOG) study. Society of Gynecologic Oncologists Annual Meeting on Women's Cancer, February 7–11, 2004; San Diego, CA (abstr 439)
81. American College of Obstetricians and Gynecologists: *Estrogen Replacement Therapy and Endometrial Cancer*. Washington, DC, ACOG Committee Opinion No. 126. 1993
82. American College of Obstetricians and Gynecologists: Statement on the estrogen plus progestin trial of the Women's Health Initiative by the American College of Obstetricians and Gynecologists (July 9, 2002). *www.acog.org/fromhome/publications/press_releases/nr07–09–02.cfm*. Accessed February 25, 2004.

CHAPTER 52

Esophageal Cancer

Nancy D. Tsottles, RN, BSN
Anita M. Reedy, RN, MSN, OCN®

Introduction

The esophagus is a tube that extends from the pharynx at the area of the cervical spine and ends at the junction connecting it to the stomach. It lies posterior to the trachea and is divided into the cervical (proximal) esophagus and the thoracic (mid and distal) esophagus (see Figure 52-1).[1] Its function is to facilitate the swallowing process by peristaltic movements so that food and liquid can pass from the mouth to the stomach. The esophagus is made up of four layers; from innermost to outermost, they are the (1) mucosal, (2) submucosal, (3) muscularis propria, and (4) adventitia layers. The mucosal layer is convoluted, is lined with epithelial tissue, and secretes mucus and other substances to keep the surface moist and flexible, features necessary for swallowing. Beneath the epithelium are the lamina propria, where the exocrine glands are located, and the muscularis mucosae, which is a thin layer of muscular tissue. Between the mucosa and submucosa are located major blood and lymphatic vessels. The submucosa, the second layer, consists of the submucus nerve plexus, an area rich in nerve fibers. The third layer, the muscularis propria, consists of both circular and longitudinal muscles as well as nerve tissue. The adventitia is the fourth and outer layer. There is no serosal layer in the esophagus.

Because of its location and function, the esophagus is subject to both internal and external factors that may affect its health. For example, the type and temperature of foods consumed, overflow of substances inhaled into the trachea, and acid refluxed from the stomach are all factors that are potentially harmful and damaging to the cells of the esophagus. One of the possible adverse outcomes of this cellular damage is the development of cancer of the esophagus.

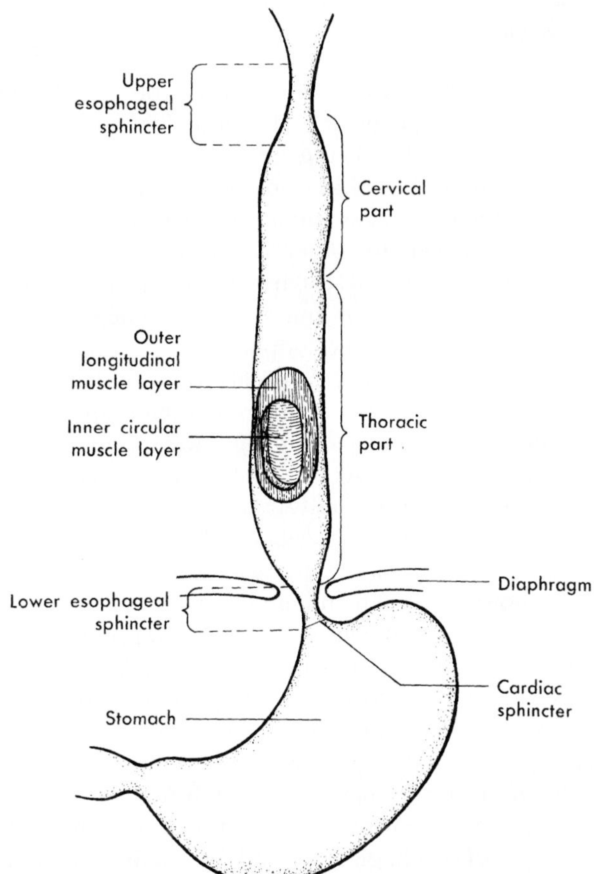

Figure 52-1 Normal anatomy of the esophagus with cutaway to show muscle layer.

Epidemiology

In the United States, an estimated 14,250 new cases of esophageal cancer were expected in 2004.[2] This accounts for approximately 1.5% of all cancers diagnosed in the United States.[3,4] Almost the same number of deaths occur from this cancer each year (13,300) as the number of new cases diagnosed.[2] Esophageal cancer is ranked as the ninth most common malignancy[4] and the sixth leading cause of death from cancer worldwide.[5] In the United States, the incidence of esophageal cancer is higher in the eastern part of the country and in major urban centers.[6,7] Cancer of the esophagus is more prevalent in men than in women and occurs more frequently in those over age 50. There are two major histologic types of esophageal cancer: squamous cell carcinoma (SCC) and adenocarcinoma (AC). SCCs are most often found in the proximal and midesophagus, whereas ACs are most often found in the distal esophagus and esophagogastric junction. SCC is more prevalent among Asians and blacks, while AC is more prevalent among whites.[6,7,8] SCC is the leading type of esophageal cancer in such countries as Japan, China, and Iran. In Western countries like the United States, the incidence of AC has increased by 350% between 1976 and 1994.[9] Thus adenocarcinoma of the esophagus is one of the most rapidly increasing types of cancer today. Currently, about 50% of new cases are AC.[10] The reason for this increase is not clear. It may be linked to the increasing prevalence of obesity and gastroesophageal reflux disease (GERD), and the decreasing prevalence of *Helicobacter pylori* infection in the population.[9,11,12] Obesity is felt to increase intraabdominal pressure and GERD[5] and may be associated with a fourfold increase in risk of AC.[9] *Helicobacter pylori* infection may provide protection against the development of AC,[5] as it can lead to the development of chronic atrophic gastritis and reduction of gastric acidity.[9] In the United States, the decrease in SCC of the esophagus may be linked to the decline in smoking, especially among men.[9]

Etiology

The cause of esophageal cancer is not completely known but is probably multifactorial. The major risk factors associated with the development of SCC are cigarette smoking and alcohol consumption. Caustic injury to the esophagus and a prior diagnosis of head and neck cancer are other risk factors.[5] The most noted risk factor for AC is Barrett's esophagus,[3] which is a condition caused by injury from chronic reflux of gastric contents into the esophagus, resulting in the squamous epithelium in the distal esophagus being replaced by columnar epithelium. Heitmiller and Sharma[13] noted that Barrett's esophagus was found in 64% of the patients with resected AC. Other risk factors for AC may be smoking, obesity, and poor nutritional intake of substances such as vitamin A, vitamin C, magnesium, selenium, and zinc.[14] Hiatal hernia has also been shown to be an independent risk factor and, when found in combination with reflux symptoms, can lead to an eightfold increase in risk of AC.[15] Medications such as beta-blockers, aminophyllines, and anticholinergic agents that may decrease lower esophageal sphincter (LES) pressure, possibly increasing reflux, have also been associated with AC.[5,16]

Dietary links may play a role in the development of both types of esophageal cancer. Diets low in fruits and vegetables[6] and foods high in nitrosamine concentrations such as pickled and fermented foods may increase the risk. An increased risk has also been associated with diets high in vitamin B_{12}, animal protein, total fat, saturated fat, and cholesterol.[9] In contrast, diets high in vitamins C, B_6, and E, folate, beta carotene, and fiber are associated with a reduced risk.[9]

Another possible risk factor for developing esophageal cancer is viral infection. Human papilloma virus was found in up to 70% of patients with SCC of the esophagus.[17] These viruses can disable tumor-suppressor genes such as the *p53* gene located on chromosome 17p13, which may lead to the overgrowth of tumor cells.[3] There may, in fact, be genetic components that contribute to the development of esophageal cancer. Both tumor-suppressor genes such as *p53* and *APC* and proto-oncogenes including *EGFR* and *ERB-2* may be involved. The *p53* gene mutations are frequently found in high-grade dysplasia and adenocarcinoma[18] and may play a role in the tumor's resistance to chemotherapy.[19]

Prevention, Screening, and Early Detection

Flexible upper endoscopy is the most reliable screening tool for detecting esophageal cancers, since it allows direct visualization of the esophagus and gastroesophageal junction.[20] However, this procedure is generally done under conscious IV sedation, and it is not practical to use to screen large populations. Recently, transnasal endoscopy has been introduced and may be more useful for population screening in the future. This method does not require sedation, can be done in an office, requires less time, and is reportedly equally tolerable and effective for patients.[20]

There are no current recommendations in the United States for screening and early detection programs for esophageal cancer. The relatively small number of patients diagnosed with esophageal cancer each year may make developing and using a mass-screening program impractical. Screening programs used in clinical practice usually concentrate on high-risk candidates with tobacco and alcohol use, poor dietary habits, and history of GERD. Individuals should be educated about the role of tobacco, alcohol, and diet in the potential development of esophageal cancer.

The presence of risk factors such as long-standing, frequent symptoms of gastroesophageal reflux; obesity; and male gender may identify individuals who should undergo screening for Barrett's esophagus. Unfortunately, screening does not reduce the rate of progression of Barrett's esophagus to AC,[20] nor does it decrease cancer mortality.[21]

Once cellular changes associated with Barrett's esophagus are detected, it is recommended that regular endoscopic surveillance be conducted. Studies suggest that individuals with Barrett's esophagus who have regular endoscopic surveillance may present with smaller, lower-grade tumors at an earlier stage than individuals who do not receive surveillance and who usually present with tumor-related symptoms of more advanced disease, such as dysphagia and weight loss.[20,21] Therefore, for those with Barrett's esophagus that eventually develops into esophageal cancer, the five-year survival rate is close to 60% if they had ongoing surveillance for Barrett's esophagus, versus 20% or less for individuals without previously documented Barrett's esophagus.[20,22]

A person who reports frequent, chronic gastric reflux symptoms should be evaluated for the presence of Barrett's esophagus and should be medically managed with antireflux therapy. Even though antireflux medications are highly effective in controlling the symptoms of GERD, they are not proven to reduce the risk of AC.[23]

Prevention of esophageal cancer must focus on reducing the risk factors associated with developing the disease. The risk of SCC may be reduced by eliminating smoking, limiting alcohol intake, and increasing intake of fruits and vegetables.[5,24] The risk of AC may be reduced by eliminating smoking, reducing obesity, increasing intake of fruits and vegetables, and reducing GERD.[24] Nurses can play a key role in educating patients and the public regarding ways to reduce risk factors.

Pathophysiology

Cellular Characteristics

The esophagus is lined in a continuous manner with squamous epithelium until the gastroesophageal junction, where it is lined with columnar tissue. Although a range of cellular differentiation is found in esophageal tumors, SCCs are generally better differentiated at diagnosis than ACs.[25] SCCs are most frequently found in the proximal esophagus or midesophagus. Cellular atypia usually precedes the development of SCC and is found more often in smokers than nonsmokers.[5] SCCs of the esophagus can be classified as polypoid, ulcerative, or infiltrative.[26] Tumor growth in the esophagus that is infiltrative in nature thickens the wall and leads to luminal narrowing. Frequently, the tumor is a polypoid mass that projects into the lumen of the esophagus. If not detected and removed, the tumor will grow until the esophagus is completely obstructed. Tumors that are ulcerative in nature are elevated with irregular, nodular edges. These ulcerative tumors expand into the submucosa and can be elevated to the point of obstruction. Some of these tumors will remain localized, while others will extend throughout large areas of the esophagus.

ACs frequently arise from the columnar epithelium of the distal esophagus. The cellular changes in the columnar epithelium are most often attributed to Barrett's esophagus, discussed in detail later in this chapter.

Progression of Disease

Because the esophagus does not have a serosal outer layer, it is easy for tumors to spread into adjacent tissues early in the disease. Frequently, the disease has spread to adjacent tissue and/or regional lymph nodes before it is detected. More than 50% of patients have either metastatic disease or unresectable tumors at the time of diagnosis.[5] Tumors of the cervical esophagus can involve the left main stem bronchus, thoracic duct, aortic arch, or pleura. Tumors of the more distal areas of the esophagus can penetrate into the pericardium, pleura, descending aorta, and diaphragm. Invasion into these adjacent structures can make the tumor unresectable. The presence of a rich lymphatic system makes it easy for the tumor to metastasize to distant sites, and such tumors are incurable.

Patterns of Spread

The area surrounding the esophagus is rich in lymph nodes and vessels. These lymph nodes begin at the cervical esophagus and include the scalene, internal jugular, upper cervical, periesophageal, supraclavicular, and cervical nodes. Biopsy-proven, positive nodes in these areas are considered to be localized disease for cervical esophageal tumors but are considered distant disease for more distal tumors of the esophagus.

More distally located nodes surrounding the esophagus include the tracheobronchial, superior mediastinal, peritracheal, carinal, hilar, periesophageal, perigastric, pericardial, and mediastinal nodes. Positive nodes in these areas are considered localized disease for tumors of the thoracic esophagus but distant disease for tumors of the proximal esophagus.

The most distal nodes are the celiac axis nodes. When the celiac axis nodes are positive, it is considered localized disease for tumors of the distal and esophagogastric junction but distant disease for tumors of the proximal esophagus and midesophagus.

Common distant metastatic sites beyond the esophageal area are the liver, lungs, pleura, and kidneys.[7] Other metastatic sites include bone, adrenal, peritoneum, and brain.[7,26,27] Following treatment for esophageal cancer, SCC tends to recur locally, whereas AC tends to recur in abdominal nodes and distant organ sites.[27]

Clinical Manifestations

Weight loss and dysphagia are the most common presenting symptoms of esophageal cancer.[7,10] The dysphagia is gradually progressive and may be described as foods "sticking" or getting caught, throat fullness, chest discomfort, or a feeling of obstruction.[7] Loss of appetite, malaise, and painful swallowing may also be present. An individual may be unable to swallow or clear salivary secretions if the esophagus is obstructed. There may also be pain if a bone metastasis is present, or the person may have elevated liver enzymes if a liver metastasis is present.

Assessment

It is important to accurately determine the extent of the disease and the overall health status of the individual in order to provide the proper therapy. The first step in this assessment process is an extensive history and physical examination. Diagnostic studies and prognostic indicators all contribute to a comprehensive assessment for esophageal cancer. A multidisciplinary assessment by an experienced team is beneficial, since the management and treatment of esophageal cancer requires the involvement of many disciplines. Evaluation by medical oncology, radiation oncology, thoracic surgery, endoscopy, nutrition, nursing, and social work may all be a part of the assessment process.[27]

History

The history should include information on any tobacco and alcohol use; diet; weight loss and over what period of time this loss has occurred; presence of dysphagia; pain, especially with swallowing; heartburn; or gastric reflux, as well as the presence of co-morbid conditions such as heart disease, pulmonary disease, and diabetes. Any family history of cancer is also obtained. Performance status is a reliable indicator of general condition. For example, is the person able to carry on the usual activities of daily living, or is he or she staying in bed the majority of the day? Performance status usually correlates with the length of time the individual has experienced dysphagia, weight loss, and other symptoms. It is also important to determine what medications the individual is taking. Since alternative therapies are becoming more common, the use of any natural remedies to treat the disease or control symptoms should be included in the general history.

Physical Examination

Physical examination alone may not be particularly helpful in detecting esophageal cancer. However, the overall assessment of the person's condition is useful to determine the ability to tolerate treatment. A thin, emaciated appearance could indicate more advanced disease. Weight loss in excess of 10% of body mass is indicative of a poor prognosis.[5] Other foci of the physical examination might include assessment for the presence of lymph nodes in the cervical and supraclavicular areas, focal tenderness, abdominal masses, or an enlarged or nodular liver.

Diagnostic Studies

Endoscopy with biopsy is the only definitive method for diagnosing the presence of esophageal cancer. Histologic examination of biopsied tissue will also determine cellular differentiation. Cancer cells are classified as well differentiated, moderately differentiated, poorly differentiated, or undifferentiated. Most esophageal cancers are determined to be of the moderately differentiated grade.

Several tests and procedures are utilized to determine the extent or stage of the disease. The endoscopic ultrasound (EUS) and computerized tomography (CT) are used to identify tumor location, size, depth of invasion, and lymph node metastasis.[27] EUS is superior to CT in staging local lymph node involvement and for staging the depth of invasion into the esophagus (T staging).[28] EUS can also be used to determine response to neoadjuvant therapy. In a study by Chak and colleagues, EUS was the only predictor of prognosis in patients with AC.[29] The location of the tumor at the time of endoscopy is noted by measuring the distance in centimeters from the front teeth (or incisors) to the tumor. The cervical esophagus is approximately 18 cm from the upper incisor teeth; the midthoracic esophagus extends approximately 24–32 cm from the upper incisor teeth; the distal thoracic esophagus and esophagogastric junction extend to approximately 40 cm from the incisors.

CT scans are useful for detecting regional lymph node involvement as well as distant metastatic disease.[30] They are effective in detecting metastasis to the liver and adrenals and are also used to plan for radiation therapy and to monitor tumor response to treatment.[31] Areas of the chest, abdomen, and pelvis need to be radiographically examined for thorough assessment.

Positron emission tomography (PET) is a newer technology that uses the uptake of a radiolabeled glucose analogue by tumors to detect the presence and extent of disease. Unlike CT scans, which have a structural-based technology, PET has a metabolism-based technology. Previously used in the assessment of lung cancer, PET has been shown in research trials to be more accurate than CT in detecting metastatic disease.[32,33] One study conducted by Flamen and colleagues found the PET scan to have superior accuracy over CT or EUS in diagnosing Stage IV disease.[28] Therefore, PET scans are also useful in the preoperative staging process to determine resectability.

Another method for determining the presence or absence of metastatic disease is the exploratory laparoscopy. Through small abdominal incisions, the area is visually explored for the presence of nodes or tissue that appear suspicious. If something suspicious is observed, a biopsy is taken so a definitive diagnosis can be made. Intraperitoneal metastases and/or small liver metastases that may not have previously been identified by imaging studies may be detected during laparoscopy.

When the tumor involves the upper two thirds of the esophagus, bronchoscopy should be performed to rule out invasion into the trachea or formation of a tracheoesophageal fistula.[10] These findings may preclude the patient from having esophageal surgery.

Thorough staging involves the combination of all these diagnostic procedures to ensure the most accurate staging of the disease. This extensive assessment is extremely important in order to determine the best treatment approach.

Prognostic Indicators

The prognosis for patients with esophageal cancer is poor. This is partly due to the absence of a serosal layer in the esophagus that makes it easier for a tumor to extend beyond the esophageal wall. Also, the rich lymphatic system in the esophageal area lends itself to early metastasis of the disease. Another factor contributing to the poor prognosis is the difficulty in eradicating the tumor at the primary site with surgery or radiation.[30]

Prognostic factors include stage, performance status, sex, age, anatomic location of the tumor, degree of weight loss, depth of tumor invasion, and involvement of lymph nodes.[6] Two key prognostic indicators for esophageal cancer are the depth of tumor invasion into or through the esophageal wall (T3 or T4) and the presence or absence of abdominal metastasis (M1).[34] Patients with T3N0 (stage IIA) disease have a 30%–40% five-year survival rate post-surgical resection.[5,7] The five-year survival rate drops to less than 20% for T3N1 (stage III) disease.[5,7] The median survival is less than one year for patients with metastatic disease treated with chemotherapy.[5]

Classification and Staging

Staging for esophageal cancer involves both clinical and pathologic staging of the disease. Clinical staging, conducted prior to treatment, involves disease that can be examined objectively. Included are history, physical examination, biopsy of the tumor, laboratory results, endoscopic examination, and radiologic imaging.[34]

Pathologic staging is based on surgical exploration, such as exploratory laparoscopy, and the examination of the surgically resected tissue and associated lymph nodes. Involvement of adjacent structures and detection of any distant metastatic sites must be documented in order to treat the disease appropriately.

Classification (Table 52-1) is based on the TNM system and includes the depth of invasion of the primary tumor, invasion into surrounding tissue, nodal involvement, and the presence or absence of metastasis.[34] *T* indicates the presence and depth of invasion of the primary tumor, *N* indicates the presence of positive lymph nodes, and *M* indicates the presence of metastatic disease. The majority of people with esophageal cancer present with disease classified as either T3N1 (invasion of the adventitia and spread to regional nodes) or T4 (penetration into adjacent structures).[35]

Table 52-1 AJCC TNM Staging for Esophageal Cancer

Primary Tumor (T)

TX	Primary tumor cannot be assessed
T0	No evidence of primary tumor
Tis	Carcinoma *in situ*
T1	Tumor invades lamina propria or submucosa
T2	Tumor invades muscularis propria
T3	Tumor invades adventitia
T4	Tumor invades adjacent structures

Regional Lymph Nodes (N)

NX	Regional lymph nodes cannot be assessed
N0	No regional lymph node metastasis
N1	Regional lymph node metastasis

Distant Metastasis (M)

MX	Distant metastasis cannot be assessed
M0	No distant metastasis
M1	Distant metastasis

Tumors of the lower thoracic esophagus

M1a	Metastasis in celiac lymph nodes
M1b	Other distant metastasis

Tumors of the midthoracic esophagus

M1a	Not applicable
M1b	nonregional lymph nodes and/or other distant metastasis

Tumors of the upper thoracic esophagus

M1a	Metastasis in cervical nodes
M1b	Other distant metastastis

STAGE GROUPING

Stage 0	Tis	N0	M0
Stage I	T1	N0	M0
Stage IIA	T2	N0	M0
	T3	N0	M0
Stage IIB	T1	N1	M0
	T2	N1	M0
Stage III	T3	N1	M0
	T4	Any N	M0
Stage IV	Any T	Any N	M1
Stage IVA	Any T	Any N	M1a
Stage IVB	Any T	Any N	M1b

Therapeutic Approaches and Nursing Care

Treatment for esophageal cancer is varied and depends on the stage of the disease and upon the general health status of the patient. For instance, tumor invasion into the aorta or tracheobronchial tree or T4 classification makes the tumor unresectable.[31] The presence of metastatic disease eliminates surgery (except for palliation) as an option. Presence of co-morbid conditions may also preclude certain treatments. It is therefore important to have thorough staging and evaluation of the individual's condition, and to make sure that he or she understands the risks and benefits of the various therapies before proceeding.

Nursing care for an individual with esophageal cancer is complex and sometimes difficult. Aggressive measures for symptom control and support of the patient and family throughout treatment need to be coordinated and implemented. Because treatment may cross many settings—inpatient, outpatient, home care, and hospice—and requires the use of many resources, coordination is a critical component of care. The number and severity of side effects of treatment and the nursing care to manage these side effects depends on the extent of disease and the treatment given.

Barrett's Esophagus

Barrett's esophagus is a premalignant condition resulting from GERD that may be exacerbated by obesity or hiatal hernia.[27] Barrett's esophagus develops in 5%–20% of patients with chronic GERD.[22] Symptoms associated with GERD can include heartburn, regurgitation, chest pain, hoarseness, sore throat, and asthma/cough.[36] An endoscopy with esophageal biopsy is needed to diagnose Barrett's esophagus.[21] Normal squamous lining is pale and glossy in appearance, whereas the characteristic lining of Barrett's esophagus is dull and reddish in color.[21] If the area of abnormal columnar epithelium is less than 3 cm, it is characterized as short-segment Barrett's esophagus, and if the area is 3 cm or larger, it is characterized as long-segment Barrett's esophagus.[21,22] Varying degrees of cellular dysplasia are associated with Barrett's esophagus, and thus varying approaches are taken to its treatment. Barrett's esophagus with low-grade dysplasia may be treated with intensive medical antireflux therapy for 8–12 weeks and repeated endoscopic examination. If the condition persists, intensive antireflux therapy is continued with periodic surveillance; if the condition improves with therapy, periodic surveillance is still conducted.[3]

The duration of the surveillance interval remains controversial due to the lack of data from randomized trials. Gopal and colleagues report patient age and the segment length of involved Barrett's esophagus as risk factors for the development of dysplasia.[22] The authors note an increase in the risk of dysplasia by 3.3% per year in persons over 40 years of age and a 14% increase in risk per 1 cm increase in the segment length of involved Barrett's esophagus.[22] The American College of Gastroenterology recommends that patients with Barrett's esophagus have regular surveillance endoscopy with biopsies to detect dysplasia every three years for patients who have had two consecutive endoscopies without evidence of dysplasia.[21] For patients found to have low-grade dysplasia, annual endoscopy is recommended.[21] Patients with high-grade dysplasia should have repeat endoscopy with multiple biopsies to rule out invasive cancer. If the high-grade dysplasia is focal or limited, the condition should be monitored at three-month intervals with endoscopic surveillance.[21] For patients with multifocal high-grade dysplasia, surgical resection may be considered.[21] It is estimated that patients with Barrett's esophagus have an annual cancer incidence ranging from 0.1 to 0.5%.[22]

The treatment for Barrett's esophagus with high-grade dysplasia is more controversial and involves three options: esophagectomy, endoscopic ablative therapy, or intensive surveillance.[21,23] An important rationale supporting surgical resection is the prevalence of AC in as many as 30% of specimens surgically removed from people with high-grade dysplasia.[19,37] Esophagectomy is the only treatment that can definitively prevent the progression from dysplasia to cancer.[21,23] Several nonsurgical treatment options have been developed for patients who are not surgical candidates. Endoscopic mucosal resection can be used to treat superficial cancers found by endoscopy.[20] Endoscopic laser therapy in combination with a proton pump inhibitor is another nonsurgical option for patients with high-grade dysplasia or early AC.[20] Proton pump inhibitors such as omeprazole, lansoprazole, rabeprazole, pantoprazole, and esomeprazole are potent acid-suppressive drugs.[36] In some patients with Barrett's esophagus, the combination of administering a proton pump inhibitor and endoscopic ablation may result in the abnormal mucosa returning to normal squamous mucosa.[5] However, no study has shown that ablative therapy decreases the long-term risk for developing cancer in the presence of Barrett's esophagus.[21]

Photodynamic therapy has also been studied for the treatment of Barrett's esophagus, but it is not a commonly accepted approach to treatment at this time[38] and is best used in the setting of an approved research protocol.[21] Another option is a more conservative treatment similar to that for lower grades of dysplasia as described earlier, with intense surveillance at three-month intervals. However, limited data exist on the safety and efficacy of this approach.[23] Invasive carcinoma may develop within three years in up to 50% of patients with untreated high-grade dysplasia.[5]

Nursing care for people with Barrett's esophagus is focused on education about the disease process and the risk of the disease progressing to AC. The person must understand the importance of scheduled follow-up evaluations and appropriate treatment with antireflux medications such as histamine-2 receptor antagonists and proton pump inhibitors. For many individuals, reflux symptoms may have been present for lengths of time varying from months to years prior to the diagnosis of Barrett's esophagus or esophageal cancer. Reflux symptoms may also recur following esophagectomy surgery. In addition to using medications, patients need to be taught lifestyle modifications to assist in controlling reflux symptoms. They need to be aware of foods that may increase reflux, such as coffee, alcohol, chocolate, fat, onions, citrus, and tomato products, and should limit their intake of these foods.[21,36] Avoiding meals for three hours prior to bedtime, elevating the head of the bed, and sleeping on the left side can improve clearance of esophageal acid and reduce nighttime exposure.[36] Loose-fitting clothing should be worn, since tight clothing may increase intragastric pressure.[36] Obesity should be avoided, as it has been shown to correlate with reflux and decreased LES pressures.[36] Smoking should also be avoided, as it has been documented to increase esophageal acid exposure.[36] The care of the individual with a surgically resected esophagus is discussed in the following section.

Local and Locoregional Esophageal Cancer

Surgery alone

Surgical resection of the esophagus is the primary treatment for local and locoregional cancer for people with resectable disease whose co-morbid conditions do not prohibit surgical treatment. This has been the standard treatment, particularly in settings where clinical trials are not available. Several different resection approaches have been developed. The approach selected depends on the location of the tumor and the preference and expertise of the surgical team. The different approaches are radical en bloc esophagectomy, left thoracoabdominal approach, combined abdominal and right thoracotomy approach (Ivor-Lewis), and transhiatal approach.[4,6,10]

The radical esophagectomy involves complete resection of the esophagus 10 cm above and below the tumor, with resection of adjacent structures including arterial and venous supplies of the tumor as well as selected tissues. This radical procedure is associated with a high mortality rate. The combined abdominal and right thoracotomy is used for cancers of the upper esophagus and midesophagus because it allows better visualization of the involved area. The left thoracoabdominal and transhiatal approaches are typically used for cancers of the distal esophagus and gastroesophageal junction or for resection of Barrett's esophagus. The thoracoabdominal approach involves making an incision across the left abdomen and thorax and then resecting the distal esophagus and the proximal stomach. The remaining stomach is prepared as a conduit and attached to the esophageal stump with an intrathoracic or cervical anastomosis.[4]

The transhiatal esophagectomy (Figure 52-2) has become more extensively used in recent years. Upper-midline abdominal and cervical incisions are made.[39] The intrathoracic esophagus is removed, the stomach is repositioned in the posterior mediastinum where the esophagus was located, and the gastric fundus is anastomosed to the cervical esophagus above the level of the clavicles. The advantages of this approach include the ability to avoid a thoracotomy, with its attendant complications, such as pain leading to ineffective breathing and atelectasis. Since the anastomosis site is in the neck as opposed to the chest, there is also a decreased risk of delayed detection should leakage at the anastomosis site occur. One disadvantage of transhiatal esophagectomy is the limited surgical view or exposure of the site, which makes it more difficult to mobilize the midesophagus and could increase the risk of bleeding. Nodal resection is completed at the time of surgery, depending on the location of the tumor.[40]

Complications of surgery include esophageal leak at the anastomosis site, cardiac and pulmonary complications, and wound infection.[8] People who have undergone esophagectomy have an altered gastric passageway that changes the way they swallow and digest. A patient can experience gastric stasis, steatorrhea, diarrhea, early satiety, and regurgitation following esophagectomy.[41] Initially, people are fed by tube or vein following esophagectomy. After performing a swallowing test to determine whether there is leakage, the individual is advanced from a liquid to a soft diet to a regular diet as tolerated. Because the stomach is small as a result of the partial gastrectomy, the person must eat frequent small meals. This is quite often a struggle for people, and they commonly lose weight after surgery until they are able to take in enough calories to maintain nutritional requirements. It is usually a trial-and-error process for the person to find the foods that can be eaten and tolerated best. Eventually the individual is able to eat in a more normal way and maintain or even regain some weight. However, stenosis caused by scar tissue can occur at the surgical site, which may require mechanical dilatation at intervals following surgery. This stenosis and dilatation process can be very frustrating for the person who expected to be free of

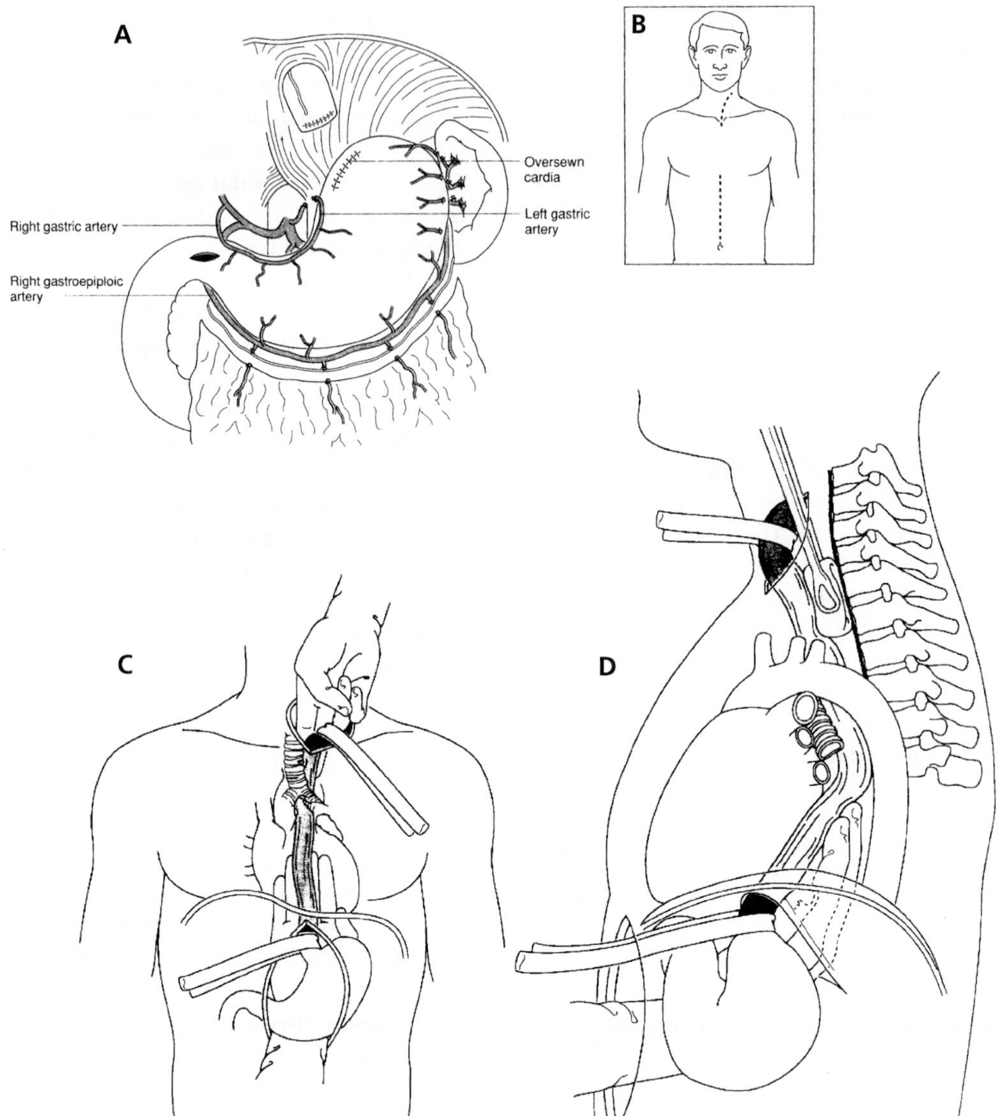

Figure 52-2 **(A)** Standard mobilization of the stomach for esophageal replacement either in the posterior mediastinal or substernal position. The left gastric artery and left gastroepiploic vessels have been divided. The mobilized stomach is based on the remaining right gastric and right gastroepiploic arteries that are preserved. A pyloromyotomy and generous Kocher maneuver are performed. **(B)** Left cervical incision and upper midline abdominal incision used for transhiatal esophagectomy and esophageal replacement with stomach in the posterior mediastinum. **(C)** Transhiatal mobilization of the thoracic esophagus from the posterior mediastinum using blunt dissection and traction on rubber drains placed around the esophagogastric junction and the cervical esophagus. The volar aspects of the fingers are kept against the esophagus to reduce the risk of injury to adjacent structures. **(D)** Lateral view showing transhiatal mobilization of the esophagus away from the prevertebral fascia using a half sponge on a stick inserted through the cervical incision and advanced until it makes contact with the hand inserted from below through the diaphragmatic hiatus. Arterial pressure is monitored as the heart is displaced forward by the hand in the posterior mediastinum. (Reprinted with permission from Orringer MB: Tumors, injuries, and miscellaneous conditions of the esophagus, in Greenfield LJ, Mulholland M, Oldham KT, et al (eds.): *Surgery: Scientific Principles and Practice* (ed 2). Philadelphia, Lippincott-Raven, 1997, pp 694–735.[39])

swallowing problems once recovered from surgery. Additionally, patients may fear that difficulty in swallowing is indicative of a recurrence of cancer.

Initially there are drainage tubes at the incision site. The tubes are usually discontinued three to four days postsurgery.[42] The wound is then left open to air to heal. The patient also has a nasogastric tube in place until oral intake is initiated. He or she may also have a jejunostomy feeding tube in place until adequate nutrition can be taken orally. The inpatient hospital stay following esophagectomy is generally 7 to 14 days.[7]

Nursing care involves educating the person about what to expect following surgery. Expectations play a major role in how the patient and family view postsurgical status and progress. Aggressively evaluating weight and fluid balance postsurgery is important, since these elements are being maintained via a feeding tube or intravenous route. Cardiac assessment is important following the surgical procedure, since atrial fibrillation due to irritation of the vagus nerve during surgery may occur early in the postoperative period. It may be necessary to administer medications to control this dysrhythmia. Pulmonary assessment is also important to detect postsurgical fluid overload and the development of pneumonia. Once the patient is extubated, usually 24 hours postsurgery, aggressive pulmonary management is needed.[42] Frequent turning, coughing, and deep breathing as well as spirometry are employed. After discharge from intensive care, physical therapy is initiated to gradually increase mobility. Pulmonary complications are less likely with the transhiatal esophageal approach, since a thoracotomy is not performed. Drainage tubes need to be maintained for patency and the drainage assessed for signs of bleeding, infection, or anastomotic leak. Surgical wounds need to be monitored for signs and symptoms of infection. Once oral intake is initiated, assessment of the ability to swallow is important, since the person may need encouragement to try different positions and approaches to swallowing. Initiating a nutritional consult to further educate the individual regarding dietary needs and possible supplements is helpful. The individual needs assurance that there will be gradual improvement in his or her ability to tolerate varied and larger quantities of food.

The patient may experience the dumping syndrome following surgery, which results from the unusually rapid passage of food from the mouth to the intestine due to removal of the esophagus. This syndrome improves with dietary correction, including the amount eaten and the frequency of meals. Dietary supplements such as Ensure® that were helpful prior to surgery often exacerbate the dumping syndrome postsurgery. Antidiarrheal drugs may also be useful. Other symptoms include fatigue and tension.[43] People should be encouraged to keep their follow-up appointments and to call the surgeon if there are problems after discharge.

Unfortunately, the prognosis following the surgical treatment approach alone is poor. Most people die of distant metastasis within two years. Following surgical resection, the five-year survival is reported to be anywhere from 10%–25%.[24,44,45] Other approaches need to be explored to improve survival.

Combined therapy

Since the late 1970s, clinical trials have been conducted to evaluate the use of multimodal or combined therapy in the treatment of esophageal cancer.[35,45] Strategies that have evolved to increase the survival rate in this population include combined chemotherapy and radiation alone without surgery, neoadjuvant chemotherapy given prior to surgery, and neoadjuvant chemotherapy and radiation therapy given concurrently prior to surgery.

Combined chemoradiation (without surgery). Combined chemoradiation (without surgery) for the treatment of esophageal cancer has been shown to be more effective than radiation alone. The Intergroup (RTOG 85-01) study reported by Herskovic and colleagues proved that radiation alone was not curative and established chemoradiotherapy as a curative option.[27,46,47] Patients were randomized to receive either radiation alone (64 Gy at 2 Gy/d) or four cycles of fluorouracil (5-FU) 1000 mg/m^2/day for four days and cisplatin 75 mg/m^2 on day 1 given in weeks 1, 5, 8, and 11 with radiation (50 Gy at 2 Gy/d).[45–47] Five-year survival was 0% in the patients receiving radiation alone and 27% in those receiving combined modality therapy.[27,45–47] Long-term survival has been reported in approximately 25% of patients treated with combined chemoradiation utilizing cisplatin- and fluorouracil-based regimens.[5] This is comparable to the survival rate with surgery alone.[5] Combined chemoradiation alone can be utilized for patients who have localized, potentially curable disease and either decline surgery or have comorbid conditions that make them nonsurgical candidates. Chemoradiotherapy is also the preferred treatment for cancers located in the cervical esophagus,[4,27] thereby avoiding an extensive surgical procedure.

Neoadjuvant therapy prior to surgery. Neoadjuvant therapy is used to debulk or downstage the tumor, thus facilitating surgical resection. This approach provides local and systemic therapy. Accurate staging prior to treatment is used to identify areas of locoregional disease so the radiation port can be adjusted accordingly. The most active agents for treating esophageal cancer are cisplatin, fluorouracil (5-FU), vindesine, mitomycin, and paclitaxel. The most active single agent is cisplatin.[30,35] Vinblastine and methotrexate have also been used. Agents such as docetaxel, irinotecan, oxaliplatin, and gemcitabine have been incorporated into clinical trials for the treatment of esophageal cancer. These agents not only provide systemic treatment but also act as sensitizing agents for radiotherapy. Cisplatin and 5-FU, as combined therapy, have been shown to double or triple radiosensitivity.[44] Trials using various cisplatin-based chemotherapy regimens without radiation prior to surgery in comparison to surgery alone showed that approximately 50% of tumors responded to chemotherapy; however, pathologic complete remissions were rare.[45] No survival advantage was demonstrated by administering chemotherapy prior to surgery.[35,45]

The use of both chemotherapy and radiation as neoadjuvant therapy prior to surgery may offer the most promising approach to treatment, since the radiation allows for direct treatment of both the primary site and surrounding nodes along with the systemic treatment provided by chemotherapy. However, randomized trials comparing preoperative chemoradiotherapy to surgery alone have produced conflicting results regarding survival benefit.[5,27] The studies are difficult to compare due to differences in study design, chemotherapy and radiation sequencing, chemotherapy dosing, types and schedules, and radiation and surgical outcomes.[27] Therefore, despite widespread use of preoperative chemoradiotherapy, this approach cannot yet be considered the standard of care and is best used in the setting of a clinical trial.[27]

In clinical trials at Johns Hopkins, it was found that patients who had undergone combined chemoradiation and had no residual tumor (a pathologic complete response) at surgical resection had the best prognosis.[42,48] Two sequential protocols utilizing cisplatin, protracted infusion 5-FU, and 44 Gy radiotherapy followed by transhiatal esophagectomy resulted in a pathologic complete response rate of 33%.[48] The five-year survival rate was 67% for patients with a pathologic complete response and 27% for the remainder of the patients.[48] Other experts also report a survival benefit for patients achieving a pathologic complete response following neoadjuvant therapy.[27,49,50] The pathologic complete response rate is approximately 25% for patients treated with standard cisplatin/5-FU-based preoperative chemoradiotherapy regimens.[27,45]

Various doses and schedules have been used to deliver cisplatin and 5-FU concomitantly with radiation to patients with esophageal cancer. Some typical protocols follow. Cisplatin and 5-FU has been given for 15 days with 5-FU given over 16 hours on days 1–5 and cisplatin infused over 8 hours on day 7. This chemotherapy treatment was repeated in week 6 of the cycle. Radiotherapy was begun on the first day of the first course of therapy and given on days 1–5, 8–12, and 15–19, for a total of 15 days. The radiation dose was 40 cGy per day using a three-field technique (anterio-posterior, right-posterior, and left-posterior oblique fields).[25] Another regimen for delivering 5-FU and cisplatin has been to give cisplatin 100 mg/m^2 on days 1 and 21 and 5-FU 600 mg/m^2 by continuous infusion on days 2–5 and days 22–25. With this regimen, a total radiation dose of 2000 cGy in 10–200 cGy fractions was given on days 8–19, followed by surgery.[40] Another treatment regimen used to administer cisplatin, 5-FU, and radiation is 5-FU 1000 mg/m^2/day as a continuous infusion over 96 hours on days 1–4 and days 29–32 of irradiation. Cisplatin 100 mg/m^2 was administered on day 1 of irradiation only. Radiation was delivered in 25 (5 days per week) fractions over a 33-day period for a total dose of 45 Gy (39.6 Gy was given anteroposteriorly and 5.4 Gy through opposed lateral fields). One of the most effective treatment regimens is cisplatin 100 mg/m^2 given on day 1 and infusional 5-FU 1000 mg/m^2/day for four or five days at three-week intervals.[35] Protracted infusion of low dose 5-FU given with cisplatin enhances the radiosensitizing effect because of the continual presence of the drug with each fraction of radiation given. Neoadjuvant 5-FU 225–300 mg/m^2/day given as a continuous infusion for 30 days along with cisplatin 20–26 mg/m^2 on days 1–5 and 26–30 given concomitantly with a total of 44 Gy of radiotherapy are treatment approaches that have been researched in clinical trials at Johns Hopkins.[40,48] A clinical trial at the University of Michigan Medical Center reported by Urba and colleagues utilized cisplatin 20 mg/m^2/day on days 1–5 and 17–21, protracted infusion 5-FU 300 mg/m^2/day on days 1–21, and vinblastine 1 mg/m^2/day on days 1–4 and 17–20.[51] Radiotherapy was given twice daily, 5 days per week, over 21 days for a total dose of 45 Gy.[51]

At the time of this writing, the Eastern Cooperative Oncology Group (ECOG) is enrolling patients with operable adenocarcinoma of the esophagus or gastroesophageal junction in a randomized study of radiotherapy with pre- and post-operative cisplatin plus paclitaxel versus cisplatin plus irinotecan. These regimens may eliminate some of the gastrointestinal (GI) toxicities found with concurrent use of 5-FU and radiation therapy, while maintaining efficacy.[52]

Although the combined approach may result in a better tumor response and longer survival, it also has more associated toxicities, and thus more complex nursing care is required. There are the postesophagectomy complications discussed earlier, plus the toxicities associated with chemotherapy and radiation administered prior to surgery. One of the more serious complications of chemotherapy includes myelosuppression, resulting in decreased levels of white blood cells (WBCs), red blood cells (RBCs), and platelets. Routine monitoring of blood counts needs to be done so that the specific type of deficiency can be treated appropriately. Individuals may need transfusions of RBCs and platelets during the course of treatment. Colony-stimulating factors, such as erythropoietin to stimulate RBC growth and filgrastim to stimulate WBC growth, can also be used in some clinical situations. The American Society of Clinical Oncology (ASCO) has developed clinical practice guidelines to follow when using hematopoietic colony-stimulating factors.[53] Sufficient iron stores must be available for stimulation of RBCs to be effective. Growth-stimulating factors are given on varying schedules from daily to every other week, depending on the medication being used. They are usually given by subcutaneous injection, either during a clinic visit or at home by the patient or a family member who has been trained to do so. The patient may need to be started on prophylactic antibiotics should neutropenia develop (usually when the absolute neutrophil count [ANC] drops to less than 1000/mm^3). The patient will also need to monitor his or her temperature and should be advised to call if a fever of 100.5°F (38.3°C) or greater develops. Combining the use of growth factors and prophylactic antibiotics may enable the patient who has previously experienced a neutropenic fever to tolerate chemotherapy treatments at higher and more effective doses. Growth-stimulating factors are expensive, and the patient's insurance benefits and financial status need to be take into consideration before initiating treatments with these medications.

GI complications are another serious and common side effect of chemotherapy and radiation therapy. Prior to any treatment, people with esophageal cancer typically experience dysphagia and weight loss. In order to provide adequate nutritional support through treatment, it is often necessary to place a gastrostomy or jejunostomy feeding tube for aggressive supplementation. A nutritional consult will be needed once the tube is placed and the person educated as to the amount and type of feeding to be used. Caloric requirements are increased during treatment, and often a daily intake of 2000 calories or more is necessary to maintain weight.[42] Home nursing visits may need to be initiated once the tube is placed to educate the individual and family regarding the care of the tube as well as how to deliver the feedings. Chemotherapy, particularly cisplatin-based regimens, can cause nausea, vomiting, diarrhea, constipation, taste changes, mucositis, and loss of appetite. All of these side effects make it difficult to manage a patient's nutritional and fluid status. Antiemetics are utilized to prevent and control nausea and vomiting. The use of the 5HT3 blockers such as granisetron, dolasetron, and ondansetron have been particularly helpful for patients receiving highly emetogenic chemotherapies such as cisplatin. These antiemetics should be administered around the clock for 24 to 72 hours following administration of chemotherapy.[54] Combining a steroid, such as dexamethasone, with a 5HT3 blocker provides a synergistic effect and improves efficacy.[54] Other antiemetics, such as prochlorperazine, promethazine, metoclopramide, and lorazepam, can be used on an as-needed basis. Diarrhea and constipation are managed with medications and by adjusting activity level and fluid intake, particularly if the patient is nutritionally supported with tube feedings. Diarrhea associated with irinotecan can be severe but is usually controlled with aggressive use of loperamide.

Quite often, foods served at room temperature are better tolerated than heated foods and have fewer odors that people undergoing chemotherapy may find intolerable. Adding spices such as cinnamon or ginger may help improve the taste of foods. Tobacco and alcohol use should be avoided, since they further irritate the GI lining.

Radiation side effects can include esophagitis, stenosis, and fistula formation that further contributes to difficulty swallowing, pain, and increased risk of aspiration.[55] Analgesics, which are usually required at some point in treatment, are more easily given transdermally or through a feeding tube, since the patient may have difficulty swallowing. Transdermal and sustained-release analgesics provide continuous blood levels of analgesia and improved pain control. Patients and their families must be educated about the use and side effects of analgesic medications and how to apply the transdermal medications or give medications through the feeding tube. People are sometimes concerned about taking narcotics and need to be supported and educated about their proper use and effectiveness.

Fatigue is present in nearly 100% of people with esophageal cancer who are receiving chemoradiation. It is often distressing to patients and their families because they may perceive that fatigue is an indicator of their disease status and because fatigue interferes with the routines of daily life. This type of treatment-induced fatigue may not be relieved by rest, and people need to learn new ways to manage it. Exercise has been shown to be effective in decreasing fatigue in people with breast cancer.[56] It is important to maintain a balance between activity and rest. For example, daily walks and afternoon naps help establish a routine that can be managed by most people staying at home. Daily fatigue diaries can help identify times during the day when the person is most fatigued so that the day's activities can be adjusted accordingly. Priorities may need to be set and limits established, since patients often do not feel up to their pretreatment activity level.

Anxiety, fear, worry, and depression are understandable and expected reactions to the diagnosis and treatment of esophageal cancer. Patients and their families may need counseling to help them cope with the challenges of therapy and outcomes of the disease. A social work or psychologic consult may be necessary. Financial burdens brought on by the cost of treatment or the inability to work may be a major source of stress. A social work consult may be helpful in assisting the individual and family to apply for disability benefits or other areas of financial assistance. Patients may find it beneficial to utilize self-care approaches such as massage therapy or other relaxation techniques to manage anxiety and stress. Patients and their families may also benefit from talking to others who have successfully undergone similar treatments for esophageal cancer.

Other side effects of chemotherapy include cardiac toxicity manifested by irregular cardiac rhythms, particularly with the taxanes. Hepatic toxicity is evidenced by an increase in liver enzyme levels. Pulmonary toxicity is particularly associated with mitomycin. Nephrotoxicity and ototoxicity can occur with cisplatin. Peripheral neuropathy is a side effect associated with cisplatin and the taxanes that is manifested by numbness and tingling of the fingers and toes. 5-FU can produce "hand/foot" syndrome, which is a redness and peeling of the skin that will resolve over time. The use of lotions and protection from the elements are usually adequate treatments. Alopecia, rashes, and dry skin are other common side effects associated with chemotherapy. While not a serious side effect, alopecia can be very difficult for people because of the visible change in appearance that results. Wigs, hats, or turbans may be used depending on cost and personal preference. Patients should be educated regarding which side effects to expect with their particular chemotherapy regimen and how to assess themselves for early signs of complications throughout treatment. Cardiac and pulmonary assessments need to be made during clinic visits and hospitalizations. If severe enough, side effects may limit the scope of the treatment plan.

Educating the individual and family about the disease process and side effects of treatments can involve verbal instruction, written information, and audiovisual material to help the patient and family assimilate the information. Frequent review of the educational information is necessary, since high stress levels may make it difficult for the patient and family to remember much of the information initially provided. Often, talking to someone else who has had the disease and experienced similar treatments may be helpful. Support groups where people can talk about their experiences and share with others can also be helpful. Many patients find using the Internet helpful when looking for information. The National Cancer Institute (NCI) sites *www.nci.nih.gov* and *cancertrials.nci.nih.gov* contain information about the NCI and its programs and information on clinical trials. Other Web sites patients and families may find useful are: *cancernet.nci.nih.gov*, *rex.nci.nih.gov*, and *chid.nih.gov/ncichid/*, to name a few.

Follow-up for patients who have undergone treatment for locoregional disease includes a complete history and physical examination, with labs and radiological evaluations as clinically indicated, every three to four months for one year, then every 6 months for two years, and yearly thereafter.[4]

Nonresectable or Metastatic Disease

Tumors may be considered to be nonresectable for various reasons. Patients may have co-morbid conditions that preclude surgical resection. The location of the tumor may be such that resection is not feasible. This is often the case with tumors located in the proximal cervical esophagus, as they require an extensive surgical procedure, which may include a total laryngectomy. Nonresectable tumors are often treated with radiation alone or with radiation combined with chemotherapy. This combination has been shown to be more effective than radiation alone.[30] It is the treatment of choice in people with localized disease that is considered nonresectable either because of comorbid conditions or the location of the tumor.

The presence of metastatic disease eliminates the option of surgery except as a palliative procedure. Treatment approaches utilized in patients with metastatic disease are palliative in intent. The type of treatment given depends on the type and location of the tumor, the overall condition of the person, accessibility, cost, and the individual's and physician's preference.[55] In the setting of metastatic disease, radiation may be used to relieve dysphagia or to relieve symptoms associated with conditions such as lytic bone lesions and brain metastases. Chemotherapy is utilized to decrease the size of the tumor in order to provide symptom relief. Although SCC and AC are both responsive to chemotherapy, the duration of response is usually short, lasting only a few months.[5] Tumor shrinkage may occur in 35%–55% of patients with metastatic disease.[5] Combinations of usually two chemotherapy drugs that may include cisplatin, 5-FU, a taxane (docetaxel or paclitaxel), or irinotecan are used.[5] Capecitabine may also be used as a single agent for patients with a reduced performance status or an inability to tolerate combination chemotherapy.[27] The use of capecitabine combined with agents such as docetaxel, cisplatin, or oxaliplatin is also being studied. Clinical trials are ongoing to evaluate these and other drug combination regimens.

Brachytherapy, alone or in combination with external beam radiation, is one treatment option for patients with nonresectable tumors or metastatic disease. Brachytherapy has been shown to improve dysphagia due to obstruction by the tumor. An advantage of brachytherapy is the ability to directly treat the nonresectable tumor while limiting exposure to surrounding tissue. Side effects of brachytherapy to the esophagus include ulceration, stricture, and fistula formation. Endoscopic esophageal dilatation with surgical instruments can also help alleviate dysphagia but must be repeated frequently or performed in conjunction with other treatments such as radiation. Serious side effects include bleeding and perforation and occur in about 0.5% of all esophageal dilation procedures.[21] It is also possible to place an esophageal stent during an endoscopic procedure that can be performed during an outpatient visit or overnight stay and usually provides relief longer than dilatation. Raltz and Kozarek conducted a study using metallic expandable stents and found that 77% of patients experienced symptom relief after stent placement.[57] Stent placement is associated with less risk of perforation and bleeding than dilatation. Other complications can occur, however, including tumor overgrowth of the stent and migration or erosion of the stent.[57] A barium swallow may be performed after stent placement to assess for perforation.

Laser therapy is another treatment option for people with tumors in locations amenable to laser therapy and for those who have a completely obstructed esophagus. The complication rate of the laser procedure is low, with perforation and bleeding being the most common complications. Photodynamic therapy (PDT) is a more recent treatment option and can be used to treat total or partial obstructed esophageal lesions. A chemical sensitizer is given intravenously and is selectively taken up by the tumor. Via endoscopy, the chemical sensitizer is activated in the presence of molecular oxygen by a laser light source using a specific wavelength that damages the tumor. The PDT process can be repeated as often as needed to open the obstructed esophagus. Complications of PDT include fistula and stricture formation and photosensitivity that can last four to six weeks and may be mild to severe in nature. Patients need to be taught that sunscreen is ineffective and that it is important to wear full body cover when outdoors during daylight hours.[58] Body cover needs to include the use of a ski mask, gloves, long-sleeved shirts, long pants, and sunglasses. Sunglasses may be needed at night because bright lights, such as car headlights, may cause ocular pain. When possible, fluorescent lights should be used when indoors. Patients may also experience chest pain as a result of tissue damage and will need this pain managed. One patient satisfaction study reported that odynophagia and dysphagia were the patients' most significant reported problems following PDT.[59] This may result in a decrease in nutritional and fluid status, which will need to be managed. For most patients with obstruction due to an unresectable tumor, the use of PDT and placement of a self-expanding stent provides the most effective palliation.[4] Sclerotherapy can also be used to treat total or partial obstructing tumors. Sclerotherapy is less expensive to use and has a relatively low complication rate.

Nursing care of the patient with advanced disease involves the management of physiologic side effects of treatment as well as the psychosocial issues that are most often present. The patient and family must make difficult decisions about whether to undergo a particular treatment, when to stop treatment, financial matters associated with treatment, and how they wish the dying process to occur. Support through social work consult, open discussions with individuals and families, and referral to hospice care are all appropriate approaches that depend on personal preference, cultural differences, and social supports. Pain control and nutritional support are ongoing care needs.

Symptom Management and Supportive Care

Dysphagia and weight loss are the most common clinical symptoms associated with esophageal cancer.[7,10] Therefore, nutritional needs are often the most pressing initial problems to address. Assessment of swallowing capabilities of the individual and nutritional consults should be made. Patients who are able to swallow soft and liquid foods may be able to supplement their diet with high-calorie liquids such as Ensure®, Ensure Plus®, or Scandi Shakes®. If the patient is unable to swallow adequately and maintain nutritional requirements, feeding tubes can be placed and the individual started on tube feedings as a means of achieving complete nutrition. Nutrition can also be provided by parenteral infusions if alternative strategies fail. The patient may also be dehydrated, so fluid requirements must be taken into account.

Patients who have problems with nutritional intake and are fed through tubes often have other GI complications such as diarrhea or constipation. Often the type and amount of enteral solution and fluids will need to be adjusted. Patients may need to take medications to control diarrhea or constipation. Those persons with jejunostomy tubes may experience the dumping syndrome, and the types, amounts, and frequency of feedings may need to be adjusted. Patients will need to be followed closely for weight changes and dehydration until tube feedings are adequately adjusted.

Individuals who have tumors that occlude the esophagus are not able to adequately clear their secretions. Consequently, they expectorate frequently. This is often frustrating and embarrassing for them. They may also be fearful of choking on the secretions, especially at night while sleeping. It may be helpful for the person to sleep with the head of the bed elevated so the risk of aspiration is decreased. Individuals with obstructing esophageal tumors need to have palliative treatment such as stent placement or dilatation as soon as possible to open up the area so secretions can be cleared adequately.

Tumors that are extensive can erode into surrounding tissue and vasculature, causing hemorrhage. Emergency surgery may be required. Esophagothoracic fistulas may form, especially after radiation to the site of the primary tumor. Esophageal tumors can also invade surrounding organs or structures such as the lung and mediastinum, causing pain and respiratory complications.

Distant metastatic disease can result in impairment of organ function such as hepatic failure. Elevated liver enzymes can lead to impaired mental function. The person with advanced esophageal cancer may also experience pain associated with bone metastasis. Supportive care includes home nursing, pain and nutritional management, respite care for the family, and hospice care.

Complications of esophageal cancer as well as of the treatments delivered are multifaceted, and the nursing care required to manage them is complex. Thorough physical and psychosocial assessments must be made in order to develop a plan of care optimal for the patient and family. Symptom management is necessary in order to help the individual tolerate treatment. Coordination of various resources to provide care across the continuum and at the various stages of the disease is essential in addressing the needs of this population. Educating and supporting the individual and family so they can make informed decisions about treatments and life issues helps them to maintain some measure of control at one of the most difficult times in their lives.

Conclusion

While the incidence of esophageal cancer is relatively low, it is one of the more rapidly increasing types of cancer today. The prognosis for esophageal cancer is generally poor; however, if the disease is diagnosed early there are options for treatment that may increase the likelihood for survival. While management of Barrett's esophagus is controversial, there is reason to consider prophylactic surgery for people with high-grade dysplasia in order to prevent the development of AC. For people with locoregional disease, a combined approach using neoadjuvant chemoradiation followed by esophagectomy continues to be controversial and has not yet been proven to be more effective than the standard of care, which is surgery.[27] For people with unresectable disease, various options are available, but the combination of radiation and chemotherapy seems to be superior. The person with metastatic disease also has several options for treatment and palliation, depending on such factors as complications the person is experiencing, performance status, and personal preferences.

Prevention and early detection of esophageal cancer may be key factors in reducing the incidence and mortality of this devastating disease. Public education regarding known risk factors and efforts to reduce these factors may affect the increasing incidence. Improved screening for persons at risk for developing cancer and standardized surveillance programs for persons with Barrett's esophagus may lead to earlier diagnosis of the disease and improved survival. New chemotherapeutic agents including antiangiogenic agents, gene therapy, vaccines, and antireceptor agents may lead to future advances in treatment and thereby affect survival.[4] Incorporating targeted therapies with chemotherapy regimens, particularly those that target epidermal growth factor receptors or cyclooxygenase-2 inhibitors warrant further study.[5] Identifying and using biological markers to predict response to therapy may allow for adjusting therapies to the individual patient's tumor in the future.[50] It is clear that much progress is needed to improve patient survival for this often lethal disease.

References

1. Given BA, Simmons SJ: *Gastroenterology in Clinical Nursing.* St Louis, Mosby, 1979, p 942
2. Jemal A, Tiwari R, Murray T, et al: Cancer statistics, 2004. *CA Cancer J Clin* 54:8–29, 2004
3. Spechler SJ: Barrett's esophagus and adenocarcinoma of the esophagogastric junction: epidemiology, surveillance, and management. *Proc Am Soci Clin Oncol* 7:11-17, 1997 (abstr)
4. National Comprehensive Cancer Network: Esophageal cancer. *Clinical practice guidelines in oncology* version 1, 2003. *www.nccn.org.* Accessed December 12, 2003
5. Enzinger PC, Mayer RJ: Esophageal cancer. *N Engl J Med* 349:2241–2252, 2003
6. Coia LR, Sauter ER: Esophageal cancer. *Curr Probl Cancer* 18:189–247, 1994
7. Brooks-Brunn JA: Esophageal cancer: an overview. *Medsurg Nurs* 9:248–254, 2000
8. Blot WJ: Esophageal cancer trends and risk factors. *Semin Oncol* 21:104–109, 1994
9. Mayne ST, Navarro SA: Diet, obesity and reflux in the etiology of adenocarcinomas of the esophagus and gastric cardia in humans. *J Nutr* 132(11 suppl):3467–3470, 2002
10. McCarthy N, Grem J: Esophageal cancer, in Abraham J, Allegra C (eds.): *Bethesda Handbook of Clinical Oncology.* Philadelphia, Lippincott, Williams, and Wilkins, 2001, pp 59–69
11. Holtmann G: Reflux disease: the disorder of the third millennium. *Eur J Gastroenterol Hepatol* 1(13 suppl):S5–11, 2001 (abstr)

12. Brown LM, Devesa SS: Epidemiologic trends in esophageal and gastric cancer in the United States. *Surg Oncol Clin North Am* 11:235–256, 2002 (abstr)
13. Heitmiller RF, Sharma RR: Comparison of prevalence and resection rates in patients with esophageal squamous cell carcinoma and adenocarcinoma. *J Thorac Cardiovasc Surg* 12:130–136, 1996
14. Brown LM, Swanson CA, Gridley G, et al: Adenocarcinoma of the esophagus: role of obesity and diet. *J Natl Cancer Inst* 87:104–109, 1995
15. Wu AH, Tseng CC, Bernstein L: Hiatal hernia, reflux symptoms, body size, and risk of esophageal and gastric adenocarcinoma. *Cancer* 98:940–948, 2003 (abstr)
16. Corley DA, Buffler PA: Oesophageal and gastric cardia adenocarcinomas: analysis of regional variation using the Cancer Incidence in Five Continents database. *Int J Epidemiol* 30:1415–1425, 2001
17. Suzuk L, Noffsinger AE, Hui YZ, et al: Detection of human papilloma virus in esophageal squamous cell carcinoma. *Cancer* 78:704–710, 1996
18. Moskaluk CA, Heitmiller R, Zahurak M, et al: *p53* and *p21* (WAF1/CIP1/SDI1) gene products in Barrett esophagus and adenocarcinoma of the esophagus and esophagogastric junction. *Hum Pathol* 27:1211–1220, 1996
19. Nabeya Y, Loganzo F, Maslak P, et al: The mutational status of p53 protein in gastric and esophageal adenocarcinoma cell lines predicts sensitivity to chemotherapeutic agents. *Int J Cancer* 64:37–46, 1995
20. Gerson LB, Triadafilopoulos G: Screening for esophageal adenocarcinoma: an evidence-based approach. *Am J Med* 113:499–505, 2002
21. Spechler SJ: Clinical manifestations and esophageal complications of GERD. *Am J Med Sci* 326:279–284, 2003
22. Gopal DV, Lieberman DA, Margaret N, et al: Risk factors for dysplasia in patients with Barrett's esophagus (BE): results from a multicenter consortium. *Dig Dis Sci* 48:1537–1541, 2003
23. Spechler SJ: Barrett's esophagus. *N Engl J Med* 346:836–842, 2002
24. Engel LS, Chow WH, et al: Population attributable risks of esophageal and gastric cancers. *J Natl Cancer Inst* 95:1404–1413, 2003
25. Walsh TN, Noonan N, Hollywood D, et al: A comparison of multimodal therapy and surgery for esophageal adenocarcinoma. *N Engl J Med* 335:462–467, 1996
26. Livinstone EM, Skinner DB: Tumors of the esophagus, in Berk JE (ed.): *Gastroenterology*. Philadelphia, Saunders, 1985, pp 818–840
27. Gibson MK, Forastiere AA: Cancer of the esophagus, in Bayless T (ed.): *Advanced Therapy of Gastroenterology and Liver Disease*. Toronto, BC Decker, 2004, pp 5–68
28. Flamen P, Lerut A, Van Cutsem E, et al: Utility of positron emission tomography for the staging of patients with potentially operable esophageal carcinoma. *J Clin Oncol* 18:3202–3210, 2000
29. Chak A, Canto MI, Cooper GS, et al: Endosonographic assessment of multimodality therapy predicts survival of esophageal carcinoma patients. *Cancer* 88:1788–1795, 2000 (abstr)
30. Kelsen DP, Ilson DH: Chemotherapy and combined modality therapy for esophageal cancer (review). *Chest* 107(suppl 6):224–232, 1995
31. Saunders HS, Wolfman NT, Ott DJ: Esophageal cancer. Radiologic staging: review. *Radiol Clin North Am* 35:281–294, 1997
32. Luketich JD, Schauer PR, Meltzer CC, et al: Role of positron emission tomography in staging esophageal cancer. *Ann Thorac Surg* 64:765–769, 1997
33. Block MI, Patterson GA, Sundaresan RS, et al: Improvement in staging of esophageal cancer with the addition of positron emission tomography. *Ann Thorac Surg* 64:770–777, 1997
34. Greene FL, Page DL, Fleming ID, et al: *AJCC Cancer Staging Handbook* (ed 6). New York, Springer-Verlag, 2002, pp 101–109
35. Forastiere AA, Heitmiller RF, Kleinberg L: Multimodality therapy for esophageal cancer. *Chest* 112(suppl 4):195–200, 1997
36. Tutuian R, Castell DO: Management of gastroesophageal reflux disease. *Am J Med Sci* 326:309–318, 2003
37. Heitmiller RF, Redmond M, Hamilton SR: Barrett's esophagus with high-grade dysplasia: an indication for prophylactic esophagectomy. *Ann Surg* 224:66–71, 1996
38. Overholt BF, Panjehpour M: Photodynamic therapy in Barrett's esophagus: reduction of specialized mucosa, ablation of dysplasia, and treatment of superficial esophageal cancer. *Semin Surg Oncol* 11:372–376, 1995
39. Orringer MB: Tumors, injuries, and miscellaneous conditions of the esophagus, in Greenfield LJ, Mulholland M, Oldham KT, et al (eds.): *Surgery: Scientific Principles and Practice* (ed 2). Philadelphia, Lippincott-Raven, 1997, pp 694–735
40. Flood WA, Forastiere AA: Esophageal cancer. *Curr Opin Oncol* 7:381–386, 1995
41. Sigley T: Nutritional problems, in Ziegfeld CR, Lubejko BG, Shelton BK (eds.): *Oncology Fact Finder: Manual of Cancer Nursing*. Philadelphia, Lippincott-Raven, 1998, pp 349–368
42. Quinn KL, Reedy AM: Esophageal cancer: therapeutic approaches and nursing care. *Semin Oncol Nurs* 15:17–25, 1999
43. Brooks JA, Kesler KA, Johnson CS, et al: Prospective analysis of quality of life after surgical resection for esophageal cancer: preliminary results. *J Surg Oncol* 81:185–194, 2002
44. Girvin GW, Matsumoto GH, Bates DM, et al: Treating esophageal cancer with a combination of chemotherapy, radiation, and excision. *Am J Surg* 5:557–559, 1995
45. Schrump D, Altorki N, Forastiere A, et al: Cancer of the esophagus, in DeVita VT Jr, Hellman S, Rosenberg SA (eds.): *Cancer Principles and Practice of Oncology*. Philadelphia, Lippincott, Williams, and Wilkins, 2001, pp 1051–1091
46. Herskovic A, Martz K, Al-Sarraf M, et al: Combined chemotherapy and radiotherapy compared with radiotherapy alone in patients with cancer of the esophagus. *N Engl J Med* 326:1593–1598, 1992
47. Cooper JS, Guo MD, Herskovic A, et al: Chemoradiotherapy of locally advanced esophageal cancer: long-term follow-up of a prospective randomized trial (RTOG 85–01). Radiation Therapy Oncology Group. *JAMA* 281:1623–1627, 1999
48. Kleinberg L, Knisely J, Heitmiller R, et al: Mature survival results with preoperative cisplatin, protracted infusion 5–fluorouracil, and 44–Gy radiotherapy for esophageal cancer. *Int J Radiat Oncol Biol Phys* 56:328–334, 2003
49. Swanson SJ, Batirel HF, Bueno R, et al: Transthoracic esophagectomy with radical mediastinal and abdominal lymph node dissection and cervical esophagogastrostomy for esophageal carcinoma. *Ann Thorac Surg* 72:1918–1924, 2001 (abstr)
50. Refaely Y, Krasna MJ: Multimodality therapy for esophageal cancer. *Surg Clin North Am* 82:729–746, 2002 (abstr)
51. Urba SG, Orringer MB, Turrisi A, et al: Randomized trial of preoperative chemoradiation versus surgery alone in patients with locoregional esophageal carcinoma. *J Clin Oncol* 19:305–313, 2001
52. Carlson R: Less toxicity in new regimens for esophageal cancer. *Oncol Times* 7:7, 2004
53. Ozer H, Armitage JO, Bennett CL, et al: 2000 update of recommendations for the use of hematopoietic colony-stimulating factors: evidence-based, clinical practice guidelines. *J Clin Oncol* 18:3558–3585, 2000

54. Violette KM: Nausea and vomiting, in Shelton BK, Ziegfeld CR, Olsen MM (eds.): *The Sidney Kimmel Comprehensive Cancer Center at Johns Hopkins Manual of Cancer Nursing*. Philadelphia, Lippincott, Williams, and Wilkins, 2004, pp 393–406
55. Reed CE: Comparison of different treatments for unresectable esophageal cancer (review). *World J Surg* 19:828–835, 1995
56. Mock V, Dow KH, Meares CJ, et al: Effects of exercise on fatigue, physical functioning, and emotional distress during radiation therapy for breast cancer. *Oncol Nurs Forum* 24:991–1000, 1997
57. Raltz SL, Kozarek RA: Do age, gender, or tumor location affect outcomes when using metallic stents in the palliative treatment of esophageal carcinoma? *Gastroenterol Nurs* 22:249–253, 1999
58. Durkin S: Photodynamic therapy: a cancer treatment for the 21st century. *Gastroenterol Nurs* 22:115–120, 1999
59. Hemminger LL, Wolfsen HC: Photodynamic therapy for Barrett's esophagus and high grade dysplasia: results of a patient satisfaction survey. *Gastroenterol Nurs* 25:139–141, 2002

CHAPTER 53

Gallbladder and Bile Duct Cancer

JoAnn Coleman, RN, MS, ACNP, AOCN®

Gallbladder Cancer

Introduction

The two most common malignancies of the biliary tree are adenocarcinoma of the gallbladder and of the bile duct (cholangiocarcinoma). Although there is some overlap in the diagnosis and treatment of these two cancers, they are distinct enough to require separate discussions. Carcinoma of the gallbladder, which we consider first, is a rare form of cancer and as such has a distinct etiology, pathophysiology, clinical presentation, and treatment. In most patients, the disease is not suspected clinically and is found at an advanced stage, often during surgery for cholelithiasis.

Table 53-1 Risk Factors for Gallbladder Cancer

Risk Factors
Gallstones (single gallstone usually larger than 3 cm)
Choledochal cyst
Anomalous pancreatobiliary duct junction
Carcinogens
Rubber plant workers
Azotoluene
Nitrosamines
Obesity
Estrogens
Typhoid carriers
Porcelain gallbladder (calcification of the gallbladder wall)
Gallbladder polyps

Epidemiology

Although gallbladder cancer is a rare form of cancer, it is the most common malignancy of the biliary tract and the sixth most common cancer of the gastrointestinal (GI) tract.[1] Approximately 6000 cases are diagnosed in the United States each year. The incidence of gallbladder cancer in the United States is 2.5 per 100,000 residents.[2] Wide variations in incidence exist throughout the world and in different regions of the United States. In the United States, the incidence is highest in the Southwest, where the occurrence is most common among Native Americans and Hispanic Americans.[3] Other countries with high rates of gallbladder cancer include Israel, Mexico, Bolivia, Chile, and northern Japan. In contrast, gallbladder cancer rates are low in India, Nigeria, and Singapore.[4]

Women develop gallbladder cancer *three* times more often than men, which is similar to the incidence of gallstones.[3,5] Studies have also shown that female sex, age, postmenopausal status, and cigarette smoking are risk factors. Gallbladder cancer is rare in individuals under age 50, with most cases occurring among those in their late sixties and early seventies.[6]

Etiology

Several factors are associated with an increased risk for gallbladder cancer (see Table 53-1). Gallstones are the most common etiologic factor, probably due to their high prevalence in the general population. More than 90% of individuals with gallbladder cancer have coexistent chronic cholecystitis (inflamed gallbladder) and cholelithiasis (gallstones). Gallbladder cancer is more likely to occur in individuals with a single large gallstone than in those with multiple smaller stones. It is presumed that the large gallstones have been present for a long period of time, causing chronic irritation of the gallbladder wall and thus predisposing it to the development of carcinoma.[7]

Individuals with a choledochal cyst may develop carcinoma throughout the biliary tree, but most tumors arise in the gallbladder. The chance of developing an associated gallbladder or bile duct cancer increases with age.[8] Recent studies have suggested that an anomalous pancreatobiliary duct junction (APBDJ) is associated with an increased incidence of gallbladder cancer in individuals with a choledochal cyst.[6,8] This common channel abnormality between the common bile duct and pancreatic duct allows reflux of pancreatic juice into the biliary tree. The question still remains whether it is the regurgitation of pancreatic juice or the relationship of the abnormal junction to bile stasis and the subsequent retention of carcinogens within the biliary tree that causes gallbladder cancer.[9,10]

Various chemical carcinogens have been suspected to cause biliary cancers because excretion via the bile is a common way of clearing toxic metabolites. Exposure to chemicals used in the rubber, automobile, wood finishing, and metal fabricating industries has been associated with an increased risk of gallbladder carcinoma.[11,12] Further, animal studies have suggested that azotoluene and nitrosamines can cause gallbladder cancer, and an association between gallbladder cancer and obesity and estrogens has been suggested in epidemiological studies.[13]

Typhoid carriers have an increased risk of gallbladder and bile duct cancer. The higher incidence of gallbladder cancer in chronic typhoid carriers is also thought to result from chronic irritation.[14] Calcification of the gallbladder wall, the so-called porcelain gallbladder, is associated with sustained chronic cholecystitis and gallbladder cancer.[15] Gallbladder polyps are also a risk factor for cancer. Polyps larger than

1 cm are most likely to become malignant and are an indication for cholecystectomy.[16]

Prevention, Screening, and Early Detection

At present there is no effective screening method for gallbladder cancer, as it is a rare tumor that is often confused with other biliary cancers. The presenting symptoms of gallbladder cancer usually occur with advanced disease, making early detection almost impossible. Effective ways to eliminate the formation of gallstones in the general population, and especially in high-risk individuals, would be beneficial for many reasons, one of which is decreased gallbladder cancer. Consideration may be given to more aggressive screening of high-risk individuals and early resection of the gallbladder with any findings suggestive of gallbladder cancer.[17] Heightened awareness of the incidence of gallbladder cancer through education of high-risk individuals may lead to routine surveillance and early detection. Wide geographical, ethnic, and cultural variations exist in the incidence of gallbladder cancer, which suggests that there are major genetic and environmental influences on the development of the disease, including diet and lifestyle. Identifying and eliminating these factors could lead to prevention and control of gallbladder cancer.

Carcinoembryonic antigen (CEA), alpha-fetoprotein (AFP), and carbohydrate antigen 19-9 (CA 19-9) are serum markers that may raise suspicion of malignancy associated with gallbladder carcinoma, but more recent studies have shown no diagnostic or prognostic significance for this cancer.[18] Novel tumor markers are being investigated to determine whether they are expressed in gallbladder and biliary cancers. The existence of such markers would be useful in developing diagnostic tests and treatment paradigms for these tumors.[19]

Pathophysiology

Cellular characteristics

The vast majority of gallbladder cancers are adenocarcinomas, which occur in 85% of patients, followed in frequency by papillary carcinoma and mucinous adenocarcinoma. Cancers of the gallbladder can be one of several histologic types, including papillary, nodular, tubular, and combinations. Histologic grades of gallbladder carcinoma include well differentiated, moderately differentiated, poorly differentiated, and undifferentiated.[4]

Progression of disease

Since most individuals with cancer of the gallbladder present with disease at an advanced stage, it is difficult to know the exact progression of the disease. Gallbladder cancer is a locally invasive tumor that can extend directly into the gallbladder bed of the liver, extrahepatic bile ducts, duodenum or transverse colon, portal vein, hepatic artery, or pancreas. A tumor may originate anywhere in the gallbladder, with the most common site being the fundus, although the site of origin may be difficult to determine because most gallbladder cancers have grown beyond the limits of resectability before they are discovered.[20]

The patterns of spread predictably follow lymphatic and venous drainage of the gallbladder and peritoneal "drop" metastases. Venous drainage of the gallbladder is directly into the adjacent liver, and the most common pattern of spread of gallbladder cancer is through direct extension into the liver. The lymphatic drainage of the gallbladder is to the cystic duct lymph nodes and periportal lymph nodes, and then to the celiac and superior mesenteric lymph nodes. These tumors can spread into and around the cystic duct and can extend into the common bile duct, causing biliary obstruction (Figure 53-1). Thus, jaundice may be the first clinical manifestation of a problem. Diffuse peritoneal seeding and distant metastasis are less common and occur late in the course of the disease.[21]

Clinical Manifestations

In its early stages, carcinoma of the gallbladder is usually asymptomatic. This fact contributes to the low curability rate of gallbladder carcinoma, since the lack of symptoms precludes the early diagnosis of the disease.

When signs and symptoms of gallbladder cancer manifest, they usually resemble those of benign gallbladder disease. Common symptoms are pain in the right upper abdominal quadrant, nausea, vomiting, an intolerance of fatty food, chills, and fever. A change in the pattern of pain and advanced age should raise the index of suspicion.[22] Individuals with gallbladder cancer commonly have advanced disease and present with nonspecific signs of malaise, anorexia, weight loss, abdominal distention, jaundice, and pruritus. Most individuals have multiple symptoms. Almost half of individuals with gallbladder cancer will present with jaundice in addition to the clinical symptoms suggestive of biliary tract disease. This usually denotes advanced disease. Tumor invasion of the cystic duct can cause cystic duct obstruction, resulting in the development of acute cholecystitis. In advanced stages of the disease, individuals may present with a palpable mass in the right upper quadrant resulting from obstruction and

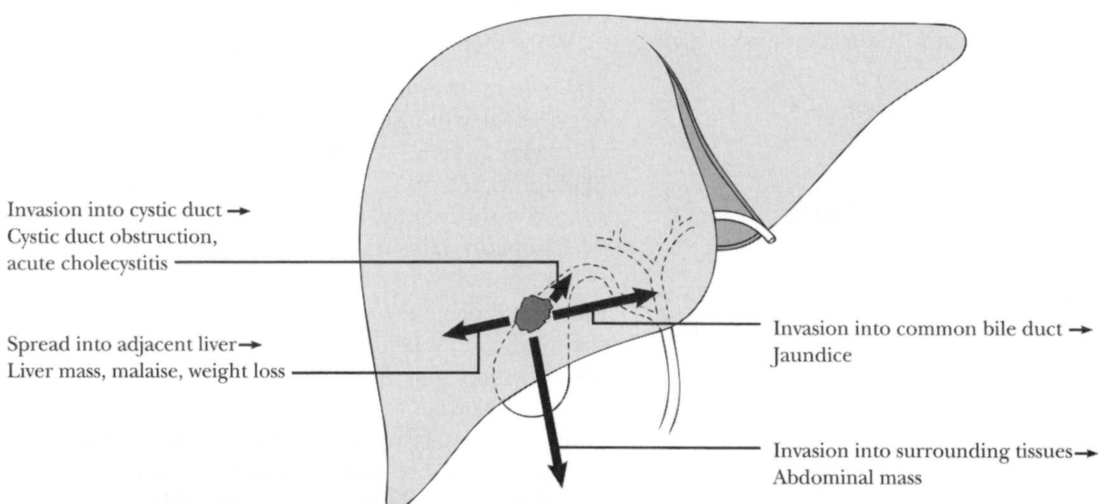

Figure 53-1 Tumor spread and presenting signs in gallbladder cancer. Gallbladder cancer commonly spreads by direct extension into surrounding tissues. This tumor extension results in the clinical presentations of jaundice, acute cholecystitis, abdominal mass, and weight loss. (Adapted with permission from Norwold DL, Dawes LG: Biliary neoplasms, in Greenfield LJ, et al (eds.): *Surgery: Scientific Principles and Practice* (ed 2). Philadelphia, Lippincott-Raven, 1997, pp 1056-1067.[21])

distention of the gallbladder. Hepatomegaly, jaundice, cachexia, fever, and ascites may also be present as evidence of progressive disease and liver failure. Definitive diagnosis often is made at the time of surgery for jaundice or acute cholecystitis.[21]

Assessment

Patient and family history

The individual may have had no previous symptoms or may have vague, chronic complaints of right upper quadrant pain. A change in the character of the symptoms may prompt the person to seek medical attention. Any individual who is at high risk for gallbladder cancer or who has a family history of the disease should receive a thorough evaluation.

Physical examination

Jaundice with pruritus may be evident in individuals with an obstructing gallbladder cancer. In advanced carcinoma of the gallbladder, an individual with severe weight loss may have a visibly palpable gallbladder when supine.

Diagnostic studies

With the exception of jaundice, no specific laboratory abnormalities may be seen. Some individuals present with acute cholecystitis manifested by fever and leukocytosis on complete blood count (CBC). Other laboratory findings may include anemia, elevated sedimentation rate, and reduced serum albumin. In more advanced cases, elevated transaminase and coagulation abnormalities may reflect liver failure.

Radiographic imaging is used to determine the extent of liver invasion, invasion of adjacent organs, vascular involvement, extent of biliary involvement, presence of nodal metastases, and presence of peritoneal metastases. The finding of a nonuniform mass replacing all or part of the gallbladder is most suspicious for a gallbladder cancer.

Ultrasonography (US), computerized tomography (CT) scan, magnetic resonance imaging (MRI), cholangiography, and angiography may all be helpful in evaluating individuals with suspected gallbladder cancer. US is used to identify a thickened gallbladder wall or a mass protruding into the gallbladder, either filling or replacing the gallbladder. It also may show tumor invasion of the liver or porta hepatis and may visualize adjacent adenopathy. A dilated biliary tree and hepatic metastasis may also be evaluated by ultrasound.[23] A CT scan can demonstrate a gallbladder cancer as an intraluminal mass, a mass replacing the gallbladder, or a mass extending from the gallbladder. CT scans also allow accurate assessment of the spread of the disease. Direct invasion of the liver or porta hepatis, involvement of adjacent lymph nodes, liver metastases, and invasion of adjacent structures can also be evaluated by CT.[24]

New magnetic resonance cholangiography and vascular enhancement techniques make it possible to visualize biliary obstruction, encasement of the portal vein, and hepatic involvement.[25] Cholangiography can be useful for diagnosing gallbladder cancer in an individual with jaundice. Percutaneous transhepatic cholangiography (PTC) or endoscopic retrograde cholangiopancreatography (ERCP) may both be beneficial. The typical finding with either study is a long stricture of the common hepatic duct.[26] Direct cholangiography may allow brush sampling or biopsy of the areas of tumor invasion for cytologic diagnosis but also carries the risk of introducing bacteria into an obstructed biliary tree, which may cause infection and sepsis. Angiography may be used to determine resectability through assessment of vascular encasement if the individual has had previous surgery in the area or if a CT scan and/or MRI fail to provide an adequate vascular image. However, new spiral CT scan and MRI techniques, including MR cholangiopancreatography and MR angiography, have replaced invasive procedures for staging gallbladder cancer by defining the presence of tumor in the gallbladder, the extent of biliary involvement, and encasement of the portal vein or hepatic artery.[27]

If radiologic studies suggest that the gallbladder cancer may be resectable or if palliative surgery is considered, tissue diagnosis is not required before surgery. However, if resection is deemed not possible due to extensive liver invasion, liver or peritoneal metastases, or encasement of the main portal vein, a biopsy of the tumor is necessary to help establish a diagnosis and confirm the stage of tumor. A percutaneous fine needle biopsy with US or CT scan guidance can assist in establishing the diagnosis.[28] The advent of endoscopic ultrasound (EUS) has become another means of obtaining tissue diagnosis.[29] Brushings of obstructed bile ducts or bile cytology via PTC or ERCP have a low yield of samples for diagnosis.[28] Laparoscopy may also be used to obtain a biopsy of the liver, peritoneum, or tissue around the gallbladder.[30]

Prognostic indicators

The histologic grade of gallbladder cancer has significant prognostic implications. The presence or absence of metaplasia is an important prognostic factor. Individuals with metaplasia, which is more common in women, have a better prognosis.[31] Poorly differentiated infiltrating tumors have a strong association with gallstones, lymph node metastases, and direct extension into the liver. Papillary cell tumors are less likely to invade the liver directly and have a lower incidence of lymph node metastasis. They are also less likely to have associated gallstones. Nodular forms of tumor are more likely to infiltrate early, to invade the liver, and to have lymph node metastases along with a higher incidence of gallstones. Tubular tumors are in the midrange with respect to their aggressive metastatic behavior.[4]

The degree of invasion by the tumor is predictive of survival. Tumors with the best prognosis are those found incidentally at the time of cholecystectomy for symptomatic gallstone disease.[32] This serendipitous finding emphasizes the importance of surgically opening the gallbladder at the time of cholecystectomy so that any suspicious lesion can be examined immediately. Unfortunately, carcinoma is an incidental finding in approximately 1%–3% of all patients undergoing routine cholecystectomy for cholelithiasis and in 8%–10% of specimens from patients over age 70.[4]

The majority of individuals with gallbladder cancer have advanced-stage tumors at the time of diagnosis. Fewer than 15% of all individuals with gallbladder cancer are alive after five years. Individuals with unresectable stage III tumors have a median survival of six months. The median survival for an individual with stage IV gallbladder cancer with liver or peritoneal metastases at the time of presentation is only one to three months.[3]

Classification and Staging

The American Joint Committee for Cancer Staging (AJCC) has established the TNM classification presented in Table 53-2.[33] Alternative classification schemes are currently used in Europe and Japan. Histologic grading on the basis of differentiation and the degree of invasion of the tumor are both important factors in staging gallbladder cancer and determining survival. Almost all known survivors of gallbladder cancer have had well-differentiated tumors. The higher the histologic grade, the greater the association with advanced stage and rapid disease progression. No ideal staging system exists that adequately correlates all aspects of gross and histologic pathology of cancer of the gallbladder.

Therapeutic Approaches and Nursing Care

The individual and the stage of the tumor must be considered when deciding on the appropriate treatment for gallbladder cancer. An individual's general medical condition is more important than his or her chronological age. When surgery is contemplated, several factors must be considered. Special attention must be given to any liver problems, as cirrhosis and portal hypertension will increase surgical risk. Obstructive jaundice may alter organ and immune function and should be treated preoperatively if liver resection is being considered. Altered renal function, poor nutritional status, and sepsis are other parameters that increase the risk for a poor surgical outcome in individuals who are jaundiced.[7] The majority of patients undergoing treatment for gallbladder cancer are in

Table 53-2 AJCC TMN Staging for Gallbladder Cancer

Primary Tumor (T)

TX Primary tumor cannot be assessed

T0 No evidence of primary tumor

Tis Carcinoma in situ

T1 Tumor invades lamina propria or muscle layer

T1a Tumor invades lamina propria

T1b Tumor invades muscle layer

T2 Tumor invades perimuscular connective tissue; no extension beyond serosa or into liver

T3 Tumor perforates the serosa (visceral peritoneum) and/or directly invades the liver and/or one other adjacent organ or structure, such as stomach, duodenum, colon, or pancreas, omentum or extrahepatic bile ducts

T4 Tumor invades main portal vein or hepatic artery or invades multiple extrahepatic organs or structures

Regional Lymph Nodes (N)

NX Regional lymph nodes cannot be assessed

N0 No regional lymph node metastasis

N1 Regional lymph node metastasis

Distant Metastasis (M)

MX Distant metastasis cannot be assessed

M0 No distant metastasis

M2 Distant metastasis

Stage Grouping

Stage 0	Tis	N0	M0
Stage IA	T1	N0	M0
Stage IB	T2	N0	M0
Stage IIA	T3	N0	M0
Stage IIB	T1	N1	M0
	T2	N1	M0
	T3	N1	M0
Stage III	T4	Any N	M0
Stage IV	Any T	Any N	M1

Data from Greene FL, Page DL, Fleming ID, et al: *AJOC Cancer Staging Manual* (ed 6). New York, Springer-Verlag, 2002, pp 139–144.[33]

their seventh decade of life and may be at increased risk for major surgery as a consequence of concomitant medical problems.

Local invasion of the liver is a common finding that can sometimes be managed with a wedge resection of the liver. More extensive liver involvement may require a larger liver resection. Extension of the tumor into the colon may require a colon resection. Progression of tumor into the duodenum or pancreatic head can be resected with a pancreaticoduodenectomy. Multiple metastases in both lobes of the liver or peritoneum or distant metastases are considered contraindications to resection of the primary gallbladder tumor.

Surgery

Although fewer than 25% of cancers of the gallbladder are resectable, the most effective treatment for this form of cancer is resection of the primary tumor and areas where it has locally invaded. With improving safety of liver resections and biliary reconstructions, major resections are being performed and have shown a curative potential even for advanced disease.[34]

Cholecystectomy is the primary treatment for Stage I gallbladder carcinoma. Many gallbladder cancers are found incidentally at the time of elective cholecystectomy. Reexploration to perform an extended resection may then be recommended within a few weeks of the original cholecystectomy.[34,35]

The treatment approach also depends on the depth of invasion of the gallbladder wall. If the tumor is limited to the mucosa, a simple cholecystectomy is sufficient therapy and has a very good prognosis. If the tumor penetrates the serosa, however, a simple cholecystectomy is not adequate. The position of the tumor within the gallbladder wall may also dictate further therapy. If the tumor is next to the liver bed, with minimal invasion, the recurrence rate may be high. Likewise, if the tumor is superficial and away from the liver, cholecystectomy may be an adequate operation.[34,35]

Laparoscopic removal of known gallbladder cancer is not recommended. Tumor implantation at the port sites has been found when gallbladder cancer was removed laparoscopically. Laparoscopic manipulation of the tumor could also lead to tumor dissemination in the abdomen.[36]

When the cancer involves deeper layers of the gallbladder wall, the prognosis is grim. A radical or extended cholecystectomy has been recommended in the hopes of improving survival. The extended procedure consists of a cholecystectomy with a wide resection of the liver around the gallbladder bed and a major lymph node dissection[37] (Figure 53-2). If the tumor is near the cystic duct or if the bile duct is involved with the tumor, a bile duct resection may be performed at the time of the extended cholecystectomy. Studies have shown a five-year survival of 70%–85% with this extended cholecystectomy approach. Even when the serosa is involved, extended cholecystectomy provides a better survival advantage over simple cholecystectomy. This extensive resection should be considered the therapy of choice for preoperatively recognized and potentially resectable gallbladder cancer.[38,39] More extensive resections that include both the liver and the

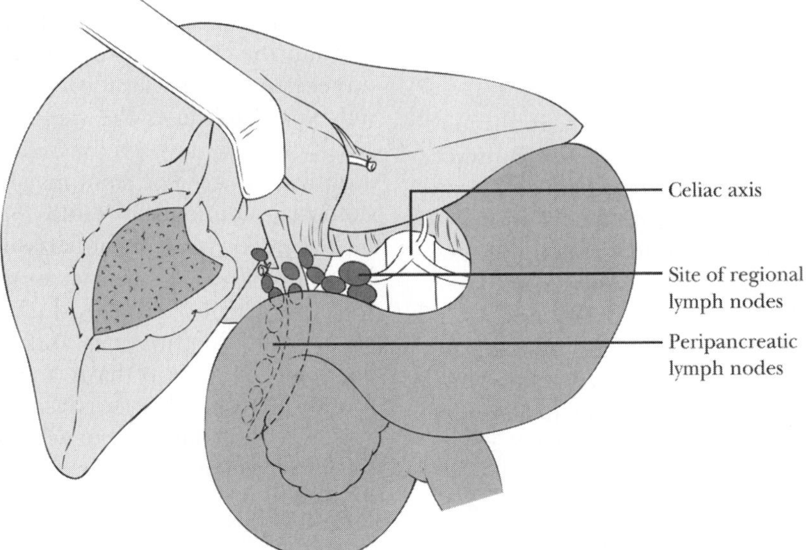

Figure 53-2 Treatment for invasive gallbladder cancer is cholecystectomy and a wedge resection of the liver along with a regional lymphadenectomy. The wedge resection of the liver is illustrated along with the lymph node regions that drain the gallbladder and that should be removed during the operation for gallbladder cancer. (Adapted with permission from Norwold DL, Dawes LG: Biliary neoplasms, in Greenfield LJ, et al (eds.): *Surgery: Scientific Principles and Practice* (ed 2). Philadelphia, Lippincott-Raven, 1997, pp 1056-1067.[21])

duodenum or pancreas have been advocated by some researchers, but considerable morbidity and mortality occurs with these radical operations.[40,41]

Survival after surgical resection depends on tumor stage and the operation performed. For stage I tumors, the five-year survival after routine cholecystectomy is greater than 85%. For stage II, III, and IV tumors, five-year survival is approximately 25%, 10%, and 2%, respectively. Individuals with stage II tumors treated with an extended cholecystectomy may be expected to have a five-year survival of better than 65%.[42] The best survival for individuals with advanced tumors has been attained in Japan with more radical surgery, including removal of adjacent liver, lymph nodes, and/or involved adjacent viscera.[43] Results from major hepatobiliary centers in the United States are revealing improved survival with reoperation after an incidental finding of gallbladder cancer during cholecystectomy and radial resection in patients with advanced disease.[38]

Postoperative care. Routine postoperative care is necessary for an individual having a simple cholecystectomy. The surgery may be done on an outpatient basis or with a hospitalization of only a few days. For an extensive surgery involving the removal of any part of the liver or surrounding tissues, more intensive monitoring and assessment are needed. The nursing care for these individuals is the same as for anyone having a major liver resection. The main concerns in the care of an individual following hepatic surgery are control of hemorrhage, replacement of blood loss, prevention of infection and pneumonia, and appropriate supportive care. Postoperative complications include hemorrhage, biliary fistula, infection, transient metabolic consequences, subphrenic abscess, pneumonia, atelectasis, portal hypertension, and clotting defects. Careful attention to any wound, tubes, and drains, along with critical analyses of the appearance of drainage, is also vital. Knowledge of the potential complications, expected reactions, and anticipatory nursing care will aid greatly in the postoperative period.

Adjuvant treatment modalities are limited. It can be disconcerting to the individual to learn that there is little treatment to offer with any proven benefit for advanced cancer of the gallbladder. The nurse should review and explain postoperative treatment. Listening and supporting patients during their perioperative care helps them and their families during a stressful time. Whereas hospitalization is often minimal after surgery, patients are faced not only with attempting to recover from a physical insult but also with the psychological impact of a cancer with a grim prognosis.

Palliative therapy

Most therapies for gallbladder cancer are palliative. Palliative management for gallbladder cancer is directed at the relief of jaundice, treatment of sepsis, and palliation of pain. The majority of gallbladder tumors are unable to be resected with negative margins. If a tissue diagnosis can be obtained through percutaneous liver biopsy or by laparoscopy, nonoperative palliation should be considered.

Nonoperative management. Many individuals with gallbladder cancer will have obstructive jaundice, which can be relieved and managed with an endoscopic biliary stent or percutaneous transhepatic biliary stent.[44] If metastatic disease is found, the jaundice may be relieved with a percutaneous transhepatic biliary stent, which may be left in place or changed to an internal stent. Patients with a percutaneous transhepatic biliary stent may develop acute cholecystitis, which subsequently may require percutaneous drainage of the gallbladder and intravenous antibiotics.[45] Recurrent jaundice and cholangitis are problems that may recur during the course of the disease due to tumor obstruction of the biliary tree or biliary stent. However, when a patient has a biliary stent placed that resolves jaundice and pruritus, an improvement in appetite, nausea, and quality of life also occur.[46]

Unfortunately, individuals who require nonoperative palliation usually do not survive more than three months. Pain should be treated aggressively to improve the individual's quality of life. Opiates are given as indicated. Radiation therapy may help to reduce the pain. Percutaneous celiac nerve block may also be helpful for this purpose.

Operative palliation. Surgery may be performed to obtain a tissue diagnosis, remove the gallbladder to prevent acute cholecystitis, relieve or prevent pain, and treat or prevent gastric outlet obstruction. A gastrojejunostomy bypass may be performed to relieve or prevent gastric outlet obstruction.

For a tumor that is locally unresectable without extension to adjacent organs (duodenum or pancreas), a Roux-en-Y choledochojejunostomy (anastomosis of a loop of jejunum to the common bile duct proximal to the obstruction) may be performed. At the time of exploration, the tumor margins should be marked with radiopaque clips if external beam radiotherapy is being considered. Nursing care is the same as for any abdominal surgery.

The addition of an internal-external percutaneous transhepatic biliary stent depends on the extent of the disease and the choice of the physician in treating jaundice. The individual and the family will need to be taught how to care for and flush the stent, as it may be left in place for the rest of the person's life. The stent is usually flushed twice a day with sterile normal saline solution. Daily cleansing of the stent site is required. A patient may require right and left biliary stents to drain both lobes of the liver if the tumor is obstructing the bifurcation of the biliary tree into the liver. Signs and symptoms of complications related to the stent must be reviewed to enable the individual and family to notify the clinician promptly to avoid problems and unnecessary hospitalization. The use of an internal self-expandable metallic stent to palliate obstructive jaundice is now favored for individuals with only a few months to live.[47] The stent may be placed by an interventional radiologist or endoscopist.

The majority of individuals with gallbladder cancer have advanced-stage tumors at the time of diagnosis. Fewer than 15% of all individuals with gallbladder cancer are alive after five years. Individuals with unresectable stage III tumors have a median survival of six months. The median survival for an individual with stage IV gallbladder cancer with liver or peritoneal metastases at the time of presentation is only one to three months.[3]

Radiation therapy

Radiation therapy has been used to treat individuals with resected gallbladder cancer as well as those with unresectable tumors. There has been no proven, survival advantage with external beam radiation, alone or after surgery. In unresectable cancer, external beam radiation has been used to help relieve pain or to relieve biliary obstruction. Intraoperative radiation has also been used, but the advantage of this technique combined with resection and/or external beam radiotherapy has not been proven, and further trials regarding this modality are necessary.[48] Likewise, the role of radiation sensitizers, such as fluorouracil (5-FU), and the addition of leucovorin to intraoperative or external beam radiation therapy has yet to be conclusively studied in individuals with gallbladder cancer.[49] Overall, the data in support of using radiotherapy are meager but hopeful.[50] The curative potential of an operation may be enhanced by postoperative radiotherapy. Palliation, including relief from obstruction, may be achieved for a period in patients with advanced disease.[51]

Chemotherapy

Chemotherapy agents for the treatment of gallbladder cancer have been limited due to poor tumor response. Mitomycin C and 5-FU have been most commonly used. Gemcitabine has shown promise for treatment of advanced gallbladder carcinoma, but its effectiveness must be assessed in clinical trials.[32] In individuals suspected of having microscopic disease after resection, chemotherapy may be considered as adjuvant therapy, but its effectiveness has been difficult to document. Intraarterial and intraperitoneal delivery of chemotherapeutic agents has been tried, with varying results. Chemotherapy combined with radiation therapy has not been effective in the treatment of gallbladder cancer.[52]

The rarity of gallbladder cancer limits the ability to perform prospective, randomized studies of therapy, as the majority of cases present at an advanced stage. Since there is no standard therapy for advanced gallbladder cancer, individuals should be offered the opportunity to participate in controlled clinical trials.

Symptom Management and Supportive Care

Individuals with advanced cancer of the gallbladder usually have disease involving the liver and biliary tree. Obstructive jaundice, liver abscess, and liver failure are potential complications. The patient and his or her family must be taught how to manage any drain or percutaneous transhepatic biliary stent. Teaching them the signs and symptoms of potential problems resulting from the tumor or any tubes and drains may allow for earlier intervention and less need for hospitalization. Persistent pain, fever, chills, and recurrent jaundice may be symptoms of a liver abscess caused by obstructed bile ducts, or of a malfunctioning endoscopic or percutaneous biliary stent.

With progressive liver failure, ascites and increased abdominal girth may cause pain, discomfort, and dyspnea. Supportive measures include aggressive pain management and proper body positioning. Ascites can be controlled by fluid and sodium restriction along with diuretic therapy. A peritoneal tap may be necessary to relieve abdominal distention and provide comfort and easier breathing. Intraabdominal spread of tumor can cause pain and palpable or visible tumor.

Nutritional intake is poor in the individual with gallbladder cancer and jaundice. Elevated bilirubin levels cause changes in taste, leading to a decrease in appetite and weight loss. Cold foods may be better tolerated. Food prepared with spices that enhance taste can be tried. Plastic silverware can be used if the individual complains of a metallic taste in the mouth. Small, frequent snacks and a change in the environment may be helpful. Nausea, vomiting, and anorexia can also hinder nutrition. Antiemetics prior to eating may assist in controlling nausea and vomiting. Megestrol acetate and cannabinoids may help to manage anorexia.

Liver failure usually develops as the disease progresses and follows a progression of lethargy and weakness to encephalopathy and hepatic coma. Renal failure is also common at this time. The nurse can assist the family by explaining what to expect as the symptoms develop. Individual and family support is the major goal of nursing care.

Most individuals with gallbladder cancer present with advanced disease and rapid decline. Palliative care should be initiated early with transition to hospice care. Communication from the inpatient or outpatient nurse to home care, palliative care, and hospice nurses can be invaluable in providing quality care to an individual with a rapidly changing condition. Attention to individual and family needs is made easier when the nurses who know the most about the individual share information. The burden to the family and their experience with cancer can be greatly eased by anticipatory management and supportive care.

Future Trends

Advances in the understanding of the genetics of gallbladder cancer may help in diagnosing this form of cancer, screening patients at risk, and developing new therapies. The use of noninvasive radiographic imaging will continue to enhance the diagnosis of carcinoma of the gallbladder. Surgical innovations for gallbladder cancer will continue to be a challenge for the surgeon and nurses caring for these patients. Multi-institutional clinical trials are needed before routine use of any neoadjuvant or adjuvant chemotherapy and/or radiation therapy for gallbladder cancer can be recommended.

Bile Duct Cancer

Introduction

Adenocarcinoma of the bile duct is also referred to as *cholangiocarcinoma.* It is a rare malignancy that can occur anywhere in the biliary tree. The spectrum of cholangiocarcinoma is best classified into three anatomic groups: (1) perihilar, (2) distal, and (3) intrahepatic. Perihilar lesions are the most common, accounting for approximately 70% of these tumors. Distal tumors are the second most common, and intrahepatic cholangiocarcinomas occur least frequently (Figure 53-3).[53] Cholangiocarcinoma occurs with conditions in which bile is stagnant, infected, or both, and with the formation of bile duct stones. A diagnosis of cholangiocarcinoma should be considered in every case of obstructive jaundice. Diagnosis and management of cholangiocarcinoma are often challenging and complex. Ideally, diagnosis of an early cholangiocarcinoma may reveal a small, localized tumor that may be amenable to an aggressive multidisciplinary approach.

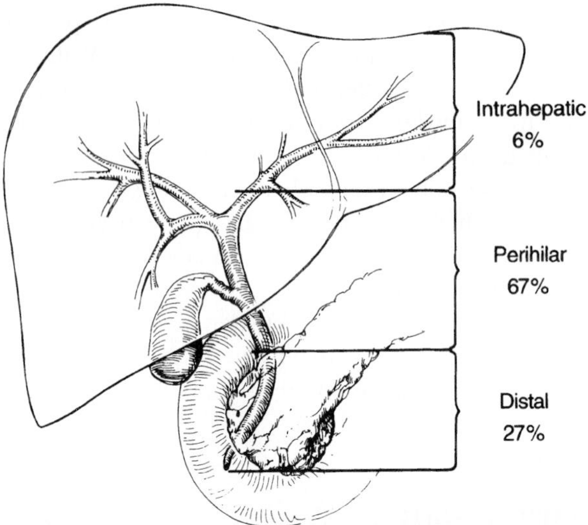

Figure 53-3 Distribution of 294 cholangiocarcinomas into intrahepatic, perihilar, and distal subgroups. (Used with permission from Nakeeb A, Pitt HA, Sohn TA, et al: Cholangiocarcinomas: a spectrum of intraphepatic, perihilar, and distal tumors. *Annals of Surgery* 224:463-475, 1996.[53])

Table 53-3 Risk Factors for Bile Duct Cancer

High Risk	Possible Increased Risk
Cystic dilation of bile duct Choledochal cyst Caroli's disease	Asbestos Dioxin (Agent Orange)
Clonorchis	Isoniazid
Hepatolithiasis	Methyldopa
Sclerosing cholangitis	Nitrosamines
Thorium dioxide (Thorotrast)	Opisthorchiasis
Ulcerative colitis	Oral contraceptives
	Polychlorinated biphenyls

Epidemiology

Approximately 19,000 new cases of liver and intrahepatic bile duct cancer are diagnosed annually in the United States.[2] Intrahepatic cholangiocarcinoma is much less common than liver cancer and also occurs less frequently than extrahepatic cholangiocarcinoma. Surveillance, Epidemiology, and End Results (SEER) data report the total number of cancers of the extrahepatic bile duct to have been approximately 4000 in 1995.[3] The U.S. incidence approaches 1 per 100,000 people each year, with a higher incidence in specific groups at high risk for the disease.[54] The incidence of cholangiocarcinoma increases with age, with the mean age at presentation being over 65 years. These tumors occur with similar frequency in men and women.[55]

Increased frequency of cancers of the biliary tract have been reported in Southeast Asia, Japan, Eastern Europe, Central and South America, and among American Indians and Hispanic Americans.[56,57]

Etiology

Several risk factors have been linked to cholangiocarcinoma (Table 53-3). Factors common to a number of these etiological parameters include biliary stasis and infection with and without intrahepatic or common bile duct stones. Only a small proportion of individuals with cholangiocarcinoma typically have these risk factors.

Strong associations have been seen in individuals with cystic dilatation of the bile duct, including both choledochal cyst disease and Caroli's disease. Individuals with cholangiocarcinoma associated with choledochal cysts are usually diagnosed in the fourth decade of life.[58] The origin of choledochal cysts and subsequent formation of cholangiocarcinoma has been explained by an anomalous pancreatic biliary duct junction (APBDJ) where there is a high entry of the pancreatic duct into the extrahepatic biliary tree. This finding suggests that reflux of pancreatic exocrine secretions into the bile duct may lead to malignant transformation of the biliary epithelium. Other factors that may lead to malignant transformation in choledochal cysts include bile stasis within the cyst, stone formation, chronic inflammation, and bacterial infection.[59] These same factors may play a role in the high incidence of cholangiocarcinoma in individuals with congenital dilatation of the intrahepatic bile ducts (Caroli's disease).[60]

In East Asia, a clear association has been recognized between cholangiocarcinoma and infection with the liver fluke *Clonorchis sinensis.* This infection results from consuming infected raw fish. The parasite usually occupies the intrahepatic bile ducts, obstructing the flow of bile. Another liver fluke, *Opisthorchis viverrini,* is endemic to Thailand and is also associated with cholangiocarcinoma.[61] The combination of liver fluke infestation and a diet high in nitrosamines may explain the high incidence of cholangiocarcinoma in this region.[62] It has been suggested that the presence of *Opisthorchis viverrini* may induce DNA damage and mutation in the intrahepatic biliary epithelium.[63]

The cause-and-effect relationship between cholelithiasis and cholangiocarcinoma has not been established. Yet a recent study showed that the risk of biliary tract cancer among women was significantly associated with a history of cholelithiasis and postmenopausal status.[64,65]

Individuals with hepatolithiasis, which is commonly found in Southeast Asia, have a 5%–10% risk of developing cholangiocarcinoma during their lifetime. Bile stasis, infected bile, and cystic dilatation of the intrahepatic biliary tree may all be risk factors for the development of bile duct cancer.[66]

Individuals with sclerosing cholangitis are also at increased risk for developing cholangiocarcinoma. Primary sclerosing cholangitis is an idiopathic disease characterized by multiple intrahepatic and extrahepatic inflammatory bile duct strictures that cannot be attributed to specific causes.[67] Cholangiocarcinoma that develops in individuals with sclerosing cholangitis is often manifested by rapid clinical deterioration and progressive jaundice.[68] The majority of individuals with sclerosing cholangitis have coexisting ulcerative colitis. The prevalence of cholangiocarcinoma in individuals with ulcerative colitis is significantly greater than the risk for the general population.[4] Ulcerative colitis is often quiescent in individuals who develop sclerosing cholangitis and can go unrecognized. The colitis precedes the cholangiocarcinoma by an average of five years. Individuals with sclerosing cholangitis or ulcerative colitis who develop bile duct cancer are usually in their fifth decade, approximately 20 years younger than individuals without these risk factors.[69]

The radiocontrast agent thorium dioxide (Thorotrast) has also been shown to cause hepatic and bile duct malignancies. Thorotrast was used as a contrast agent for radiography from the late 1920s until the 1940s. It emits energy as alpha particles and, when injected intravenously, is retained in the reticuloendothelial system for life. Cholangiocarcinomas have been diagnosed in individuals an average of 35 years after exposure.[70] A number of chemicals and several other drugs have been associated with cholangiocarcinoma, including asbestos, dioxin (Agent Orange), isoniazid, methyldopa, oral contraceptives, and polychlorinated biphenyls. Dietary nitrosamines, which are present in cured meats, have also been suspected.[4] A clustering of persons with cholangiocarcinoma has been reported in certain geographical areas of the United States, underscoring the importance of environmental factors in the pathogenesis of cholangiocarcinoma.[71,72]

Prevention, Screening, and Early Detection

At present there is no effective screening for cancer of the biliary tree. Studies are needed to develop a serum or a bile marker for early detection of cholangiocarcinoma in high-risk individuals with hepatolithiasis, choledochal cysts, sclerosing cholangitis, or ulcerative colitis. Further genetic, dietary, occupational, and environmental analysis of clusters of people with cholangiocarcinoma may provide additional clues to the pathogenesis of these rare tumors.

The role of prevention is important, as there is limited benefit from surgery in these patients, and other therapies are even less effective. Early detection with timely resection is necessary to improve the survival rate of persons with biliary carcinoma. Screening and removal of stone-containing gallbladders may gain acceptance with the advent of innovative surgical techniques.

Pathophysiology

Cellular characteristics

Cholangiocarcinomas arise from the epithelium of the intrahepatic and extrahepatic bile ducts. They appear as firm, gray-white tumors. Central necrosis may be observed. The majority of bile duct cancers are adenocarcinomas, with papillary adenocarcinoma and mucinous and mucin-producing adenocarcinomas the next largest groups. Extrahepatic bile duct papillary adenocarcinomas have the best prognosis, while mucinous adenocarcinomas have the poorest outcome.[73]

The tumors range from well-differentiated to poorly differentiated varieties that exhibit glandular or acinar structures. Mucin is almost always found within the cytoplasm of the cells. Cells tend to be cuboidal or low columnar and resemble biliary epithelium, though bile production is not usually seen.[4]

Other histologic types of bile duct cancers include squamous, mucoepidermoid, leiomyosarcoma, rhabdomyosarcoma, cystadenocarcinoma, carcinoid, and granular cell carcinoma.[4] The pathologic determination of malignancy may be difficult, especially if there is cholangitis, hepatolithiasis, biliary obstruction, and stents. The pathologic diagnosis is supported by any additional finding of (1) a positive reaction to carcinoembryonic antigen (CEA), (2) nuclear size variation, (3) distended intracytoplasmic lumina, or (4) neural invasion. Most cholangiocarcinomas will stain positively for CEA as well as for the carbohydrate antigens CA 50 and CA 19-9.[74]

Progression of disease

Cholangiocarcinoma originating within the hepatic parenchyma is usually a solitary and large mass. Tumor invasion of the large portal or hepatic veins may occur. Intrahepatic tumors tend to present as solitary masses. Perihilar cholangiocarcinoma may present as an infiltrative mass that extends from the hilum into the parenchyma of the liver as a sclerotic mass that encircles a large bile duct, or as a polypoid tumor that invades the lumen of a large bile duct. Distal bile duct cancers tend to infiltrate locally.[69]

In both the gallbladder and extrahepatic bile ducts, areas of dysplasia and carcinoma in situ may be found adjacent to invasive carcinoma, suggesting such a sequence in the development of these tumors.[69]

Extrahepatic metastases occur more frequently through the lymphatic system than through the hematogenous route. Peripancreatic and hilar lymph nodes are involved in approximately half of the cases. Metastases to the liver or peritoneal cavity are common in cholangiocarcinoma. Perineural and periductal spaces and portal tracts tend to be invaded by tumor. Lung, bone, and other sites are much less likely to be involved. When the tumor causes chronic biliary obstruction, the liver may develop secondary biliary cirrhosis.[4]

Clinical Manifestations

The majority (more than 90%) of individuals with cholangiocarcinoma present with jaundice. Pruritus, mild abdominal pain, fatigue, anorexia, and weight loss occur less frequently. Cholangitis is rarely a presenting symptom but commonly occurs following endoscopic or percutaneous biliary tract manipulation. Except for jaundice and multiple excoriations of the skin from pruritis, the physical examination is usually normal. A mass may be palpable or the liver may be enlarged with intrahepatic biliary tumors. A person with perihilar cholangiocarcinoma typically presents with mild upper abdominal pain and unilobular hepatic enlargement, as the tumor may be obstructing the intrahepatic biliary tree in either the right or left lobe of the liver.[4]

An individual who presents with upper abdominal symptoms or abnormal hepatic function without jaundice will require diagnostic studies to assist in the early diagnosis of possible bile duct carcinoma. Bile duct carcinoma without jaundice can be regarded as being in a relatively early stage and is likely to have a more favorable outcome than most bile duct carcinomas with jaundice.[75]

Assessment

Patient and family history

The individual diagnosed with cholangiocarcinoma may have had subtle weight loss, malaise, indigestion, and vague abdominal pain; or there may have been no previous symptoms. Pruritus along with the appearance of tea-colored urine and clay-colored (acholic) stools may be noticed before jaundice is evident.

Cholangiocarcinoma is difficult to diagnose in the presence of primary sclerosing cholangitis. Rapid elevation of bilirubin associated with weight loss and abdominal discomfort in an otherwise stable person with primary sclerosing cholangitis should alert the clinician to the possibility of cholangiocarcinoma.[76,77] Individuals should be questioned regarding any conditions that predispose them to cholangiocarcinoma.

Physical examination

Apart from jaundice, the physical examination is usually normal in individuals with perihilar tumors. A mass may be palpable or the liver may be enlarged with an intrahepatic bile duct tumor. In an individual with a distal bile duct tumor, a distended, nontender gallbladder may be palpable.

Diagnostic studies

Laboratory data. Laboratory evaluation reveals elevation of total serum bilirubin (greater than 10 mg/dL) in most individuals with cholangiocarcinoma at the time of presentation. Marked elevations of alkaline phosphatase and gamma-glutamyl transferase levels reflect bile duct epithelial cell injury. Markers of hepatocyte injury such as alanine amino transferase and aspartate amino transferase may be only slightly elevated. Individuals with chronic biliary obstruction may have laboratory evidence of depressed hepatocyte function, such as low albumin or prolonged prothrombin time.[4]

Serum tumor markers such as CEA and AFP are usually normal. Serum CA 19-9 and CA 50 may be elevated in individuals with cholangiocarcinoma, and they may be useful in screening those individuals at high risk of developing cholangiocarcinoma. The use of serum and bile tumor markers has been shown to improve the early detection of cholangiocarcinoma in persons with primary sclerosing cholangitis.[76,78–79] Other serum tumor markers are being investigated. High levels of interleukin 6 (IL-6) have been found in individuals with cholangiocarcinoma and correlate with tumor burden. In association with other tumor markers such as AFP, CEA, and CA 19-9, IL-6 may be useful in distinguishing among hepatic neoplasms.[80] Currently, no accurate serum or bile screening test for bile duct cancer exists.

Radiologic evaluation. The goal of radiologic evaluation for individuals with cholangiocarcinoma is delineation of the extent of the tumor, including involvement of the bile ducts, liver, portal vessels, and distant metastases. An ordered sequence of studies will achieve this goal. Cholangiocarcinoma is suspected on the basis of an abnormal US or CT scan. An intrahepatic tumor is visualized as a liver mass, with or without peripherally dilated bile ducts. A perihilar cholangiocarcinoma produces a picture of dilated intrahepatic bile ducts, a normal or collapsed gallbladder, and a normal pancreas. A distal cholangiocarcinoma causes dilation of intrahepatic and extrahepatic bile ducts as well as of the gallbladder, with or without a mass in the head of the pancreas.

US and CT scans have comparable accuracy in depicting the level of biliary obstruction.[81,82] CT is more useful than US for determining resectability because of its greater sensitivity in depicting the actual tumor mass, vascular invasion, spread to adjacent organs, and distant metastases.[83] However, a primary tumor mass often does not visualize on a standard CT scan or US. The newer helical 3-dimensional CT techniques and even MRI are better at detecting the parenchymal extent of the tumor. Magnetic resonance cholangiopancretography is a noninvasive method for detecting the existence and extent of a bile duct tumor, and MR angiography is effective in assessing vascular invasion by a tumor.[84–86]

In some institutions, after documentation of bile duct dilation, biliary anatomy may be better defined cholangiographically through either the percutaneous transhepatic or endoscopic retrograde route. The proximal extent of the tumor is the most important feature in determining resectability. In tumors of the perihilar region/hepatic hilum, percutaneous transhepatic cholangiography is favored because it best defines the proximal (uppermost) extent of tumor involvement. This approach also allows the preoperative placement of percutaneous transhepatic biliary stents to drain the obstructed biliary tree for partial or complete relief of jaundice. For neoplasms involving the proximal common hepatic duct or the bifurcation of the bile duct, both the left and right hepatic ducts may be intubated with transhepatic biliary stents to drain both lobes of the liver.[87,88] A noninvasive approach is now favored in the diagnosis of bile duct cancer, as it prevents biliary instrumentation and infection associated with preoperative morbidity.

For tumors of the distal common bile duct, the use of ERCP may allow visualization of both the proximal and distal extent of the tumor within the extrahepatic biliary tree. Decompression of the obstructed biliary tree can be performed by the placement of a biliary endoprosthesis.[89]

Biopsy/cytology. Percutaneous needle aspiration biopsy, brush or scrape biopsy, or cytologic examination of bile may determine a tissue diagnosis.[90] The use of needle biopsy to establish a diagnosis may be required only when the tumor is deemed unresectable. In this setting, punch biopsies from the lumen of the bile duct before placement of transhepatic biliary stents may yield the best diagnostic information.[4] These techniques are not performed in persons with presumed bile duct cancer to confirm diagnosis, as those individuals will ultimately be explored for resection or palliation.[53]

Classification and Staging

In the United States, cholangiocarcinoma is staged by the TMN classification developed by the AJCC (Table 53-4).[91] In this system, stage I tumors are confined to the bile duct mucosa or muscular layer, whereas stage II tumors invade periductal tissues. Stage III tumors have spread to regional lymph nodes and stage IV tumors either invade adjacent structures or have distant metastases. In Europe, the International Union Against Cancer classifies cholangiocarcinomas in a similar fashion. In Japan, a more complex system devised by the Japanese Cancer Society takes into account invasion of specific adjacent organs or blood vessels.

A combination of CT scan, MR imaging, and endoscopy *may be* used to stage cholangiocarcinoma. CT scan findings of bilobar peripheral hepatic metastases or extrahepatic disease preclude curative resection. Atrophy of the lobe containing the tumor with hypertrophy of the other lobe is also a sign that resection may not be possible. Cholangiography findings of extensive bilobar intrahepatic duct involvement are another indicator of unresectability. Radiographic evidence of encasement or occlusion of the common hepatic artery or main portal vein by tumor is also indicative of unresectability.[92]

As imaging technology improves, more patients with unresectable disease will be identified avoiding the need for laparotomy. The importance of staging laparoscopy in abdominal malignancies has been increasingly recognized.

Therapeutic Approaches and Nursing Care

Surgery

Surgical resection is the most effective therapy for cancer of the bile duct. It is the appropriate option for prolonged survival and potential cure. Diagnostic imaging may not provide enough accuracy for a definitive decision regarding resectability. Obtaining a histologically proven diagnosis of malignancy may not be possible. Specialized hepatobiliary surgeons should be consulted in most cases.[93] Laparoscopy is becoming a major tool for better predicting the resectability of hepatobiliary malignancies. A staging laparoscopy may

Table 53-4 AJCC TNM Staging for Extrahepatic Bile Duct Tumors

Primary Tumor (T)

TX Primary tumor cannot be assessed

T0 No evidence of primary tumor

Tis Carcinoma in situ

T1 Tumor confined to the bile duct histologically

T2 Tumor invades beyond the wall of the bile duct

T3 Tumor invades the liver, gallbladder, pancreas, and/or unilateral branches of the portal vein (right or left) or hepatic artery (right or left)

T4 Tumor invades any of the following: main portal vein or its branches bilaterally, common hepatic artery, or other adjacent structures, such as colon, stomach, duodenum, or abdominal wall

Regional Lymph Nodes (N)

NX Regional lymph nodes cannot be assessed

N0 No regional lymph nodes metastasis

N1 Regional lymph node metastasis

Distant Metastasis (M)

MX Distant metastasis cannot be assessed

M0 No distant metastasis

M1 Distant metastasis

Stage Grouping

Stage 0	Tis	N0	M0
Stage IA	T1	N0	M0
Stage IB	T2	N0	M0
Stage IIA	T3	N0	M0
Stage IIB	T1	N1	M0
	T2	N1	M0
	T3	N1	M0
Stage III	T4	Any N	M0
Stage IV	Any T	Any N	M1

correctly identify unresectable disease and prevent unnecessary laparotomy.[94]

The type of surgical resection performed depends on the anatomic location of the tumor. A pancreaticoduodenectomy, or Whipple procedure, is usually the surgical operation for a distal bile duct carcinoma (see Chapter 61). The median survival rate has been reported to be 22 months. Intrahepatic cholangiocarcinoma is managed optimally with hepatic resection (see Chapter 56).[95] The prognosis for resectable intrahepatic cholangiocarcinoma is more favorable than that for perihilar cholangiocarcinoma, with a median survival rate of 9–30 months.[96] Incidental bile duct carcinomas may be found at the time of liver transplantation performed for primary sclerosing cholangitis.[97]

Percutaneous transhepatic biliary stents may be inserted preoperatively in individuals undergoing surgical exploration for perihilar cholangiocarcinoma. The stents assist in the technical aspects of hilar dissection by allowing palpation of the catheter within the biliary tree to identify and dissect the hepatic duct bifurcation at the time of exploration. The stents also aid in the reconstruction of the biliary tract during the removal of the tumor and facilitate the placement of larger, softer silastic transhepatic biliary stents at the time of surgery.[98] Perihilar bile duct carcinomas may be removed with a hilar resection at the hepatic duct bifurcation combined with a hepaticojejunostomy (biliary enteric anastomosis).[72]

Perihilar cholangiocarcinoma may extend along either the right or left hepatic duct into the hepatic parenchyma. A hepatic lobectomy may be considered in addition to the hilar resection.[99] The role of total hepatectomy and liver transplantation in treating intrahepatic cholangiocarcinoma has been disappointing as a result of early and widespread recurrence and the critical shortage of available organs for transplant.[100] However, there is a select group of patients with early-stage tumors that may potentially benefit from liver transplantation. Combination neoadjuvant chemotherapy and radiation may further improve results after liver transplantation.[101]

Factors shown to be predictors of survival in patients with resection for bile duct carcinomas include negative margin status, preoperative albumin level, postoperative sepsis, serum bilirubin concentration, preoperative jaundice, and tumor grade. Nutritional status and underlying sepsis may also play an important role in the eventual outcome.[102,103]

The care of the patient after surgery for bile duct cancer is the same as for any major abdominal procedure. Expert nursing care is essential in managing stents and potential complications. Patients and their families are helped throughout the perioperative period by education and support provided by the nurse.

Palliative therapy

Although much progress has been made in the diagnosis and management of perihilar cholangiocarcinoma, complete surgical resection is usually impossible because of local tumor invasion. Most patients can be managed only by palliative drainage.

Palliative therapy in patients with cholangiocarcinoma can include both nonoperative and operative procedures. Patients who need nonoperative palliation may have biliary decompression performed using stents placed by either the percutaneous or endoscopic route.[104] Most patients with unresectable perihilar

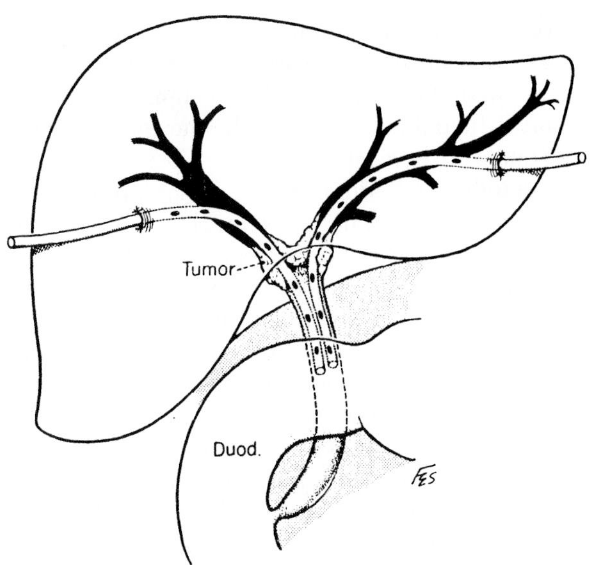

Figure 53-4 Transhepatic stents are placed in both the right and left hepatic ductal system for palliation of an obstructing proximal tumor. The internal ends of the tubes are left in the distal common bile duct. (Used with permission from Rossi RL, Gordon M, Braasch JW: Intubation techniques in biliary tract surgery. *Surgical Clinics of North America* 60:297-312, 1980.)

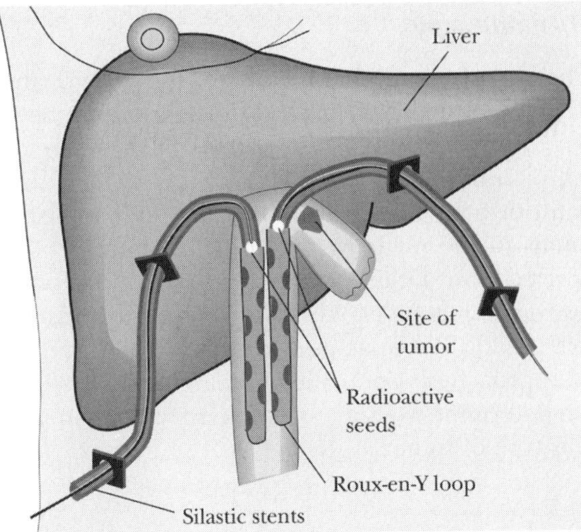

Figure 53-5 Transhepatic silastic stents can be used as conduits for delivering radioactive ^{192}Ir seeds to the site of tumor.[105]

tumors are not candidates for endoscopic biliary stents. The placement of percutaneous transhepatic biliary stents and subsequent placement of self-expandable metallic stents is the palliative procedure of choice for these patients. Percutaneous transhepatic biliary stents are left in place and may be exchanged for larger-diameter, softer silastic transhepatic stents by interventional radiology (Figure 53-4).[105] Transhepatic biliary stents may also be placed to facilitate the delivery of high doses of local radiation (brachytherapy). Radioactive seeds on long guidewires are placed directly adjacent to the site of the tumor through the transhepatic stent (Figure 53-5).[98]

A patient who is found at laparotomy to have a widespread intraperitoneal tumor will have his or her gallbladder removed to prevent the subsequent development of acute cholecystitis, which may result from the preoperative placement of percutaneous transhepatic biliary stents causing obstruction of the cystic duct.[46]

A patient with a locally advanced unresectable perihilar tumor may have a Roux-en-Y choledochojejunostomy with intraoperative placement of larger silastic transhepatic stents. A segment III bypass to the left intrahepatic ducts may be performed for biliary decompression.[106] For distal bile duct tumors, a double bowel bypass, choledochojejunostomy, and gastrojejunostomy are usually the procedures of choice (see Chapter 61).

Newer therapies such as photodynamic therapy, transarterial embolization, and intraluminal brachytherapy have also been employed in the treatment of patients with unresectable perihilar bile duct cancer.[107,108] Preoperative portal vein embolization has been used to provide safer liver surgery and to make these difficult perihilar tumors more resectable.[109]

Chemotherapy or radiation or both have offered generally poor results as palliative therapy for unresectable bile duct carcinoma. Patients may elect to participate in novel therapies and embark on an unknown journey. Educating and supporting the patient and the family throughout the diagnosis, treatment, and disease trajectory is the hallmark of nursing care.

Radiation therapy

Experience with adjuvant and multimodal treatment in randomized prospective trials is limited. Reports in the literature discuss combining external and internal brachytherapy via iridium wires, and intraoperative radiotherapy with systemic chemotherapy.[110] Radiotherapy combined with chemotherapy may be used for those patients with positive resection margins and unresectable tumors to relieve pain and contribute to biliary decompression.[111] Neoadjuvant radiation and chemoradiation have also been investigated. The small number of patients in these studies makes it difficult to draw any conclusions.[112–114]

Retrospective studies suggest that patients who receive external beam radiation therapy combined with self-expanding metallic stents have improved survival and stent patency compared with those receiving stenting alone.[115]

Chemotherapy

The use of chemotherapy alone, using 5-FU and multiple other chemotherapeutic drugs, has not been shown to improve survival in patients with either resected or unresected bile duct carcinoma. 5-FU and cisplatin or 5-FU and gemcitabine may be promising regimens in the palliative treatment of unresectable bile duct cancer. Other drugs — including hormones, antiestrogens, cholecystokinin, somatostatin, and antibiotics used as cytotoxic agents — have been tried as novel approaches.[4] Controlled human trials are necessary to determine whether any of these have an impact on this type of tumor.

Symptom Management and Supportive Care

The symptom management of individuals with advanced bile duct cancer parallels that of individuals with gallbladder cancer. Palliation of obstructive jaundice by endoscopic or percutaneous stents may be a primary objective. Internal metallic, expandable stents placed in the biliary ducts to maintain lumen patency may be the optimal intervention for patients with only a couple of months to live. Liver abscess due to obstruction of the biliary ducts, as well as liver failure are potential complications. The symptoms of persistent pain, fever, chills, and recurrent jaundice may indicate a liver abscess, which can be treated by percutaneous drainage and antibiotics. Malfunctioning endoscopic or percutaneous biliary stents can also present as fever, chills, and recurrent jaundice. Internal, metallic expandable stents may become occluded with debris or tumor. A percutaneous transhepatic biliary stent may need to be placed to relieve the obstruction from a metallic stent.

Erosion of tumor into a major blood vessel, such as the portal vein or hepatic artery, is another potential problem that can cause a massive bleed and death. Support for the family is important, as the individual may unexpectedly meet a rapid demise. The nurse can assist the patient and family by explaining what to expect as symptoms develop.

Maintenance of nutrition is a challenge, as individuals with obstructive jaundice have major interference of their taste buds and decreased appetite due to lack of bile in the GI system. Different food preparations or appetite stimulants can be tried to help bolster an individual's intake.

Individuals who succumb to progressive liver failure usually lapse into hepatic coma. Progressive liver failure must be recognized and supportive nursing care rendered. The major goals of nursing care in individuals with carcinoma of the biliary tree are recognition of overt as well as subtle symptoms and their impact as the disease progresses. Comfort measures are paramount in these patients. Family support is also important to help them cope with the inevitable loss of a loved one.

Most individuals with bile duct cancer present at an advanced stage and rapidly decline. For those individuals who have surgical intervention, and whose length of survival may be extended, the outcome of the disease is the same. The nurse must be aware of how the individual and the family are coping. Not only the physical status of the patient but also the psychosocial welfare must be considered. Whatever treatment modality the patient embarks upon, there is always a reason to provide hope and encouragement. When the patient truly declines and enters the terminal stage of the disease, palliative care with emphasis on quality of life becomes paramount.

Future Trends

Therapy for cholangiocarcinoma is limited. Surgery remains the principal treatment modality and the only potential for cure. Laparoscopy is an increasingly important modality in determining the resectability of these tumors. The role of chemotherapy and radiation remains controversial, as there are no data supporting a survival advantage for patients. As most patients present with advanced disease, relief of biliary obstruction via biliary stents, with or without photodynamic therapy, constitute the only palliative options. The continued investigation into newer agents and novel therapies may hold promise in the treatment of these difficult malignancies. Any further advances in the therapy of cholangiocarcinoma will most likely be based on a molecular understanding of the disease.

Conclusion

Significant advances in the pathogenesis, diagnosis, and treatment of malignancies of the biliary tract have been made in recent years. Most patients with carcinoma of the gallbladder and bile duct, however, continue to have a poor prognosis. Identification of the gene responsible for biliary anomalies and the development of serum or bile tumor markers may make early detection and prevention of these cancers possible for persons at risk. Dietary, occupational, environmental, and further genetic analysis of clusters of patients may provide more clues to the pathogenesis of these rare tumors.

Advances in technology will allow less-invasive imaging diagnostic studies. Quality of life and length of survival will continue to be assessed in both palliated and aggressively surgically resected patients. New chemotherapeutic agents and novel therapies need to be tested. Advances in our understanding of the genetics of the disease will help in diagnosing bile duct cancer, as well as in screening patients at risk and developing new therapies. Safer surgeries and more effective adjuvant therapy are needed to improve the outlook for future patients with malignancies of the gallbladder and biliary tract. Further innovations will require multidisciplinary collaboration to treat these patients based on the foundation of nursing care.

References

1. Jemal A, Tiwari RC, Murray T, et al: Cancer statistics, 2004. *CA Cancer J Clin* 54:8–29, 2004
2. American Cancer Society: *Cancer Facts and Figures, 2004*. Atlanta, American Cancer Society, 2004
3. Carriaga MT, Henson DE: Liver, gallbladder, extrahepatic bile ducts, and pancreas. *Cancer* 75:171–190, 1995
4. Levin B: Gallbladder carcinoma. *Ann Oncol* 10 (suppl 4):129–130, 1999
5. Donohue JH, Stewart AK, Menck HR: The National Cancer Data Base report on carcinoma of the gallbladder, 1989–1995. *Cancer* 83:2618–2628, 1998
6. Khan ZR, Neugut AI, Chabot JA: Risk factors for biliary tract cancers. *Am J Gastroenterol* 94:149–152, 1999
7. Pitt HA, Dooley WC, Yeo CJ, et al: Malignancies of the biliary tree. *Curr Probl Surg* 32:11–36, 1995
8. Bismuth H, Krissat J: Choledochal cystic malignancies. *Ann Oncol* 10(suppl4):94–98, 1999
9. Yoshida T, Shibata K, Matsumoto T, et al: Carcinoma of the gallbladder associated with anomalous junction of the pancreaticobiliary duct in adults. *J Am Coll Surg* 189: 557–562, 1999
10. Matsumoto T, Fujii H, Itakura J, et al: Recent advances in pancreaticobiliary maljunction. *J Hepatobiliary Pancreat Surg* 9:45–54, 2002
11. Bond GG, McLaren EA, Sabel FL, et al: Liver and biliary tract cancer among chemical workers. *Am J Ind Med* 18:19–24, 1990
12. Mancuso TF, Brennan MJ: Epidemiological consideration of cancer of the gallbladder, bile ducts and salivary glands in the rubber industry. *J Occup Med* 12:333–341, 1970
13. Strom BL, Soloway MD, Rios-Dalenz JL, et al: Risk factors for gallbladder cancer: an international collaborative case-control study. *Cancer* 76:1747–1756, 1995
14. Nath G, Singh H, Shukla VK: Chronic typhoid carriage and carcinoma of the gallbladder. *Eur J Cancer Prev* 6:557–559, 1997
15. Stephen AE, Berger DL: Carcinoma in the porcelain gallbladder: a relationship revisited. *Surgery* 129:699–703, 2001.
16. Myers RP, Shaffer EA, Beck PL: Gallbladder polyps: epidemiology, natural history and management. *Can J Gastroenterol* 16:187–194, 2002
17. Misra S, Chaturvedi A, Misra NC, et al: Carcinoma of the gallbladder. *Lancet Oncol* 4:167–175, 2003
18. Vij U, Baskaran V: Value of serum CEA and AFP in the diagnosis and prognosis of carcinoma gallbladder. *Trop Gastroenterol* 22:227–229, 2001
19. Swierczynski SL, Maitra A, Abraham SC, et al: Analysis of novel tumor markers in pancreatic and biliary carcinomas using tissue microarrays. *Hum Pathol* 35:357–366, 2004
20. Levy AD, Murakata LA, Rohrmann CA: Gallbladder carcinoma: radiologic-pathologic correlation. *Radiographics* 21:295–314, 2001
21. Norwold DL, Dawes LG: Biliary neoplasms, in Greenfield LJ, Mulholland M, Oldham KT, et al (eds.): *Surgery: Scientific Principles and Practice* (ed 2). Philadelphia, Lippincott-Raven, 1997, pp 1056–1067
22. Liu KJ, Richter HM, Cho MJ, et al: Carcinoma involving the gallbladder in elderly patients presenting with acute cholecystitis. *Surgery* 122:748–754, 1997
23. Bach AM, Loring LA, Hann LE, et al: Gallbladder cancer: can ultrasonography evaluate extent of disease? *J Ultrasound Med* 17:303–309, 1998
24. Levy AD, Murakata LA, Rohrman CA: Gallbladder carcinoma: radiologic-pathologic correlation. *Radiographics* 21:295–314, 2001
25. Tseng JH, Wan YL, Hung CF, et al: Diagnosis and staging of gallbladder carcinoma: evaluation with dynamic MR imaging. *Clin Imaging* 26:177–182, 2002
26. Curley SA: Biliary tract cancer. *Cancer Treat Res* 90:273–307, 1997
27. Kim JH, Kim TK, Eun HW, et al: Preoperative evaluation of gallbladder carcinoma: efficacy of combined use of MR imaging, MR cholangiography, and contrast-enhanced dual-phase three-dimensional MR angiography. *J Magn Reson Imaging* 16:676–684, 2002
28. Shukla VK, Pandey M, Kumar M, et al: Ultrasound-guided fine needle aspiration cytology of malignant gallbladder masses. *Acta Cytol* 41:1654–1658, 1997
29. Jacobson BC, Pitman MB, Brigge WR: EUS-guided FNA for the diagnosis of gallbladder masses. *Gastrointest Endosc* 57:251–254, 2003
30. Corvera CU, Weber SM, Jarnagin WR: Role of laparoscopy in the evaluation of biliary tract cancer. *Surg Oncol Clin North Am* 11:877–891, 2002.
31. Yamamoto M, Nakajo S, Tahara E: Carcinoma of the gallbladder: the correlation between histogenesis and prognosis. *Virchows Arch A Pathol Anat Histopathol* 414:83–90, 1989
32. Misra S, Chaturvedi A, Misra NC, et al: Carcinoma of the gallbladder. *Lancet Oncol* 4:167–176, 2003
33. Greene FL, Page DL, Fleming ID, et al: *AJCC Cancer Staging Manual* (ed 6). New York, Springer Verlag, 2002, pp 139–144
34. Shoup M, Fong Y: Surgical indications and extent of resection in gallbladder cancer. *Surg Oncol Clin North Am* 11:985–994, 2002
35. Dawes LG: Gallbladder cancer. *Cancer Treat Res* 109:145–155, 2001
36. Lundberg O, Kristoffersson A: Port site metastases from gallbladder cancer after laparoscopic cholecystectomy: results of a Swedish survey and review of published reports. *Eur J Surg* 165:215–222, 1999
37. Shirai Y, Ohtani T, Tsukuda K, et al: Radical surgery is justified for locally advanced gallbladder carcinoma if complete resection is feasible. *Am J Gastroenterol* 92: 181–182, 1997
38. Fong Y, Malhotra S: Gallbladder cancer: recent advances and current guidelines for surgical therapy. *Adv Surg* 35:1–20, 2001
39. Tsukada K, Hatakeyama K, Kurosaki I, et al: Outcome of radical surgery for carcinoma of the gallbladder according to the TNM stage. *Surgery* 120:816–821, 1996
40. Shirai Y, Ohtani T, Tsukada K, et al: Combined pancreaticoduodenectomy and hepatectomy for patients with locally advanced gallbladder carcinoma: long term results. *Cancer* 80:1904–1909, 1997
41. Doty JR, Cameron JL, Yeo CJ, et al: Cholecystectomy, liver resection, and pylorus-preserving pancreaticoduodenectomy for

gallbladder cancer: report of five cases. *J Gastrointest Surg* 6:776–780, 2002

42. Pradeep R, Kaushik SP, Sikora SS, et al: Predictors of survival in patients with carcinoma of the gallbladder. *Cancer* 76:1145–1149, 1995
43. Nimura Y: Extended surgery in bilio-pancreatic cancer: the Japanese experience. *Semin Oncol* 29 6 (Suppl 20):17–22, 2002
44. Feng GH, Cai Y, Jia Z, et al: Interventional therapy of malignant obstructive jaundice. *Hepatobiliary Pancreat Dis Int* 2:300–302, 2003
45. Lillemoe KD, Pitt HA, Kaufman HS, et al: Acute cholecystitis occurring as a complication of percutaneous transhepatic drainage. *Surg Gynecol Obstet* 168:348–352, 1989
46. Luman W, Cull A, Palmer KR: Quality of life in patients stented for malignant biliary obstructions. *Eur J Gastroenterol Hepatol* 9:481–484, 1997
47. Lee BH, Choe DH, Lee JH, et al: Metallic stents in malignant biliary obstruction: prospective long-term clinical results. *AJR Am J Roentgenol* 168:741–745, 1997
48. Lindell G, Holmin T, Ewers SB, et al: Extended operation with or without intraoperative (IORT) and external (EBRT) radiotherapy for gallbladder carcinoma. *Hepatogastroenterology* 50:310–314, 2003
49. Kresl JJ, Schild SE, Henning GT, et al: Adjuvant external beam radiation therapy with concurrent chemotherapy in the management of gallbladder carcinoma. *Int J Radiat Oncol Biol Phys* 52:167–175, 2002
50. Houry S, Barrier A, Huguier M: Irradiation therapy for gallbladder carcinoma: recent advances. *J Hepatobiliary Pancreat Surg* 8:518–524, 2001
51. Macdonald OK, Crane CH: Palliative and postoperative radiotherapy in biliary tract cancer. *Surg Oncol Clin North Am* 11:941–954, 2002
52. Yee K, Sheppard BC, Domreis J, et al: Cancers of the gallbladder and biliary ducts. *Oncology (Huntingt)* 16:939–946, 2002
53. Nakeeb A, Pitt HA, Sohn TA, et al. Cholangiocarcinomas: a spectrum of intraphepatic, perihilar, and distal tumors. *Ann Surg* 224:463–475, 1996
54. Yeo CJ: Bile duct cancer, in Cameron JL (ed.): *Current Surgical Therapy* (ed 5). St. Louis, Mosby-Year Book, 1995, pp 380–386
55. Shaib Y, El-Serag HB: The epidemiology of cholangiocarcinoma. *Semin Liver Dis* 24:115–125, 2004.
56. Hsing AW, Gao YT, Devesa SS, et al: Rising incidence of biliary tract cancers in Shanghai, China. *Int J Cancer* 75:368–370, 1998
57. Fraumeni JF, Devesa SS, McLaughlin JK, et al: Biliary tract cancer, in Schottenfeld D, Fraumeni JD (eds.): *Cancer Epidemiology and Prevention.* New York, Oxford University Press, 1996, pp 683–691
58. Lipsett PA, Pitt HA, Colombani PM, et al: Choledochal cyst disease. A changing pattern of presentation. *Ann Surg* 220:644–652, 1994
59. Benjamin IS: Biliary cystic disease: the risk of cancer. *J Hepatobiliary Pancreat Surg* 10:335–339, 2003
60. Dagli U, Atalay F, Sasmaz N, et al: Caroli's disease: 1977–1995 experiences. *Eur J Gastroenterol Hepatol* 10:109–112, 1998
61. Watanapa P: Cholangiocarcinoma in patients with opisthorchiasis. *Br J Surg* 83:1062–1064, 1996
62. Watanapa P, Watanapa WB: Liver fluke-associated cholangiocarcinoma. *Br J Surg* 89:962–970, 2002
63. Shirai T, Pairojkul C, Ogawa K, et al: Histomorphological characteristics of cholangiocellular carcinomas in northeast Thailand, where a region infection with the liver fluke, *Opisthorchis viverrini,* is endemic. *Acta Pathol Jpn* 42:734–739, 1992
64. Okuda K, Nakanuma Y, Miyazaki M: Cholangiocarcinoma: recent progress, part 1: epidemiology and etiology. *J Gastroenterol Hepatol* 17:1049–1055, 2002
65. Khan ZR, Neugut AI, Ahsan H, et al: Risk factors for biliary tract cancers. *Am J Gastroenterol* 94:149–152, 1999
66. Su CH, Shyr YM, Lui WY, et al: Hepatolithiasis associated with cholangiocarcinoma. *Br J Surg* 84:969–973, 1997
67. Thuluvath PJ, Rai R, Venbrux AC, et al: Cholangiocarcinoma: a review. *Gastroenterologist* 5:306–315, 1997
68. Stiehl A: Primary sclerosing cholangitis: neoplastic potential in bile ducts and the pancreas? *J Hepatol* 36:433–435, 2002
69. Molmenti EP, Marsh JW, Dvorchik I, et al: Hepatobiliary malignancies: primary hepatic malignant neoplasms. *Surg Clin North Am* 79:43–57, 1999
70. Lipshutz GS, Brennan TV, Warren RS: Thorotrast-induced liver neoplasia: a collective review. *J Am Coll Surg* 195:713–718, 2002
71. Gores GJ: Cholangiocarcinoma: current concepts and insights. *Hepatology* 37:961–969, 2003
72. Ahrendt SA, Nakeeb A, Pitt HA: Cholangiocarcinoma. *Clin Liver Dis* 5:191–218, 2001
73. Lim JH: Cholangiocarcinoma: morphologic classification according to growth pattern and imaging findings. *AJR Am J Roentgenol* 181:819–827, 2003
74. Yoon JH, Gores GJ: Diagnosis, staging, and treatment of cholangiocarcinoma. *Curr Treat Options Gastroenterol* 6:105–112, 2003
75. Sugiyama M, Atomi Y, Kuroda A, et al: Bile duct carcinoma without jaundice: clues to early diagnosis. *Hepatogastroenterology* 44:1477–1483, 1997
76. Hultcrantz R, Olsson R, Danielsson A, et al: A 3-year prospective study on serum tumor markers used for detecting cholangiocarcinoma in patients with primary sclerosing cholangitis. *J Hepatol* 30:669–673, 1999
77. Boberg KM, Schrumpf E: Diagnosis and treatment of cholangiocarcinoma. *Curr Gastroenterol Rep* 6:52–59, 2004
78. Ramage JK, Donaghy A, Farrant JM, et al: Serum tumor markers for the diagnosis of cholangiocarcinoma in primary sclerosing cholangitis. *Gastroenterology* 108:865–869, 1995
79. Nakeeb A, Lipsett PA, Lillemoe KD, et al: Biliary carcinoembryonic antigen levels are a marker for cholangiocarcinoma. *Am J Surg* 171:147–153, 1996
80. Goydos JS, Brumfield AM, Frezza E, et al: Marked elevation of serum interleukin-6 in patients with cholangiocarcinoma: validation of utility as a clinical marker. *Ann Surg* 227:398–404, 1998
81. Yarmenitis SD: Ultrasound of the gallbladder and the biliary tree. *Eur Radiol* 12:270–282, 2002
82. Gandolfi L, Torresan F, Solmi L, et al: The role of ultrasound in biliary and pancreatic diseases. *Eur J Ultrasound* 16:141–159, 2003
83. Mortele KJ, Ji H, Ros PR: CT and magnetic resonace imaging in pancreatic and biliary tract malignancies. *Gastrointest Endosc* 56 (suppl):S206–S212, 2002.
84. Worawattanakul S, Semelka RC, Noone TC: Cholangiocarcinoma: spectrum of appearances on MR images using current techniques. *Magn Reson Imaging* 16:993–1003, 1998
85. Yeh TS, Jan YY, Tseng JH, et al: Malignant perihilar biliary obstruction: magnetic resonance cholangiopancreatographic findings. *Am J Gastroenterol* 95:432–440, 2000
86. Kim JH, Kim MJ, Chung JJ: Differential diagnosis of periampullary carcinomas at MR imaging. *Radiographics* 22:1335–1352, 2002
87. Morgan RA, Adam AN: Malignant biliary disease: percutaneous interventions. *Tech Vasc Interv Radiol* 4:147–152, 2001
88. Hatzidakis A, Adam A: The interventional radiological management of cholangiocarcinoma. *Clin Radiol* 58:91–96, 2003

89. Baron TH, Mallery JS, Hirota WK, et al: The role of endoscopy in the evaluation and treatment of patients with pancreaticobiliary malignancy. *Gastrointest Endosc* 58:643–649, 2003
90. Mansfield JC, Griffin SM, Wadehra V, et al: A prospective evaluation of cytology from biliary strictures. *Gut* 40:671–677, 1997
91. Szklaruk J, Tamm E, Charnsangavej C: Preoperative imaging of biliary tract cancers. *Surg Oncol Clin North Am* 11:865–876, 2002
92. Greene FL, Page DL, Fleming ID, et al: *AJCC Cancer Staging Manual* (ed 6). New York, Springer Verlag, 2002, pg 145–150
93. Pichlmayr R, Weimann A, Klempnauer J, et al: Surgical treatment in proximal bile duct cancer: a single-center experience. *Ann Surg* 224:628–638, 1996
94. Corvera CU, Weber SM, Jarnagin WR: Role of laparoscopy in the evaluation of biliary tract cancer. *Surg Oncol Clin North Am* 11:877–891, 2002
95. Martin R, Jarnagin W: Intrahepatic cholangiocarcinoma: current management. *Minerva Chir* 58:469–478, 2003
96. Gores GJ: Cholangiocarcinoma: current concepts and insights. *Hepatology* 37:961–969, 2003
97. Goss JA, Shackleton CR, Farmer DG, et al: Orthotopic liver transplantation for primary sclerosing cholangitis: a 12-year single center experience. *Ann Surg* 225:472–481, 1997
98. Ahrendt SA, Cameron JL, Pitt HA: Current management of patients with perihilar cholangiocarcinoma. *Adv Surg* 30:427–452, 1996
99. Sarmiento JM, Nagorney DM: Hepatic resection in the treatment of perihilar cholangiocarcinoma. *Surg Oncol Clin North Am* 11:893–908, 2002
100. Jeyarajah DR, Klintmalm GB: Is liver transplantation indicated for cholangiocarcinoma? *J Hepatobiliary Pancreat Surg* 5:48–51, 1998
101. Pascher A, Jonas S, Neuhaus P: Intrahepatic cholangiocarcinoma: indication for transplantation. *J Hepatobiliary Pancreat Surg* 10:282–287, 2003
102. Pitt HA, Nakeeb A, Abrams RA, et al: Perihilar cholangiocarcinoma. Postoperative radiotherapy does not improve survival. *Ann Surg* 221:788–798, 1995
103. Washburn WK, Lewis WD, Jenkins RL: Aggressive surgical resection for cholangiocarcinoma. *Arch Surg* 130:270–276, 1995
104. Madoff DC, Wallace MJ: Palliative treatment of unresectable bile duct cancer: which stent? which approach? *Surg Oncol Clin North Am* 11:923–939, 2002
105. Rossi RL, Gordon M, Braasch JW: Intubation techniques in biliary tract surgery. *Surg Clin North Am* 60:297–312, 1980.
106. Jarnagin WR, Burke E, Powers C, et al: Intrahepatic biliary enteric bypass provides effective palliation in selected patients with malignant obstruction at the hepatic duct confluence. *Am J Surg* 175:453–460, 1998
107. Berr F, Wiedmann M, Tannapfrel A, et al: Photodynamic therapy for advanced bile duct cancer: evidence for improved palliation and extended survival. *Hepatology* 31:291–298, 2000
108. Vogl TJ, Balzer JO, Dette K, et al: Initially unresectable hilar cholangiocarcinoma: hepatic regeneration after transarterial embolization. *Radiology* 208:217–222, 1998
109. Shimamura T, Nakajima Y, Une Y, et al: Efficacy and safety of preoperative percutaneous transhepatic portal embolization with absolute ethanol: a clinical study. *Surgery* 121:135–141, 1997
110. Foo ML, Gunderson LL, Bender CE, et al: External radiation therapy and transcatheter iridium in the treatment of extrahepatic bile duct carcinoma. *Int J Radiat Oncol Biol Phys* 39:929–935, 1997
111. Erickson BA, Nag S: Biliary tree malignancies. *J Surg Oncol* 67:203–210, 1998
112. Lee CK, Barrios BR, Bjarnason H: Biliary tree malignancies: the University of Minnesota experience. *J Surg Oncol* 65:298–305, 1997
113. McMasters KM, Tuttle TM, Leach SD, et al: Neoadjuvant chemoradiation for extrahepatic cholangiocarcinoma. *Am J Surg* 174:605–608, 1997
114. Hishinuma S, Ogata Y, Matsui J, et al: Preoperative radiotherapy for cancer of the extrahepatic bile duct. *Am J Clin Oncol* 21:203–208, 1998
115. Yoon JH, Gores GJ: Diagnosis, staging, and treatment of cholangiocarcinoma. *Curr Treat Options Gastroenterol* 6:105–112, 2003

CHAPTER 54

Head and Neck Malignancies

Ellen Carr, RN, MSN, AOCN®

Introduction

For many years, the standard treatment for head and neck cancers has consisted of surgery and radiation. In the past 20 years, chemotherapy regimens have improved and have been a welcome addition to the list of available combined modality treatments.

This chapter provides an overview of head and neck cancers — their etiology, treatment, and rehabilitation issues.

Epidemiology

In 2004, more than 55,000 Americans developed cancer of the head and neck, and nearly 13,000 died from their disease.[1] Most of these tumors were preventable. The majority of head and neck tumors occur in the oral cavity (48%), larynx (25%), and oropharynx (10%).[2]

Tobacco is the most preventable cause of these deaths. In the United States, as many as 200,000 people die each year from smoking-related illnesses.[1] The rate at which new cases of head and neck cancer are diagnosed has increased in recent years. Although the rate of smoking has declined, some former smokers have switched to smokeless or spit tobacco, assuming it is a safe alternative. Because of this trend, incidence rates have not dramatically declined.[1]

Oral cancer is a serious public health problem, with more than 200,000 new cases reported annually worldwide, two-thirds of which occur in developing countries.[3] According to the American Cancer Society (ACS), oral cancer accounts for 3% of all cancers in the United States. In 2004, the incidence rate was 28,260 with 7930 deaths.[4] The death rate has declined since the 1970s, with the largest decline occurring in the 1990s.

New cases of oral cancer are twice as common in men as in women. In men, 3% of all cancer cases are oral cancers. Men older than 40 years are at the highest risk. According to the American Dental Association, oral cancer is the sixth leading site of cancer globally. More than 90% of those diagnosed with oral cancer use tobacco.[5] African Americans are more likely than whites to be diagnosed with oral cancer. Moreover, those with oral cancer have a 10%–15% rate of developing additional primary cancers in the head or neck area, especially in the esophagus.[6] Malignant lymphomas of the oral region accounted for 3.5% of all oral malignancies.[7]

In 2003, for patients with oral cavity or pharyngeal malignancies, the one-year survival in the United States was 84%. The five-year survival rate for this group of patients was 57% and the ten-year survival rate was 45%.[4] The five-year survival rate was 82.1% for tumors that were localized at the time of diagnosis. For tumors spreading regionally, the five year survival rate was 47.9% and 26.1% for distant tumors. The overall five-year survival rate for oral and pharyngeal malignancies is 57.2%.[4]

Nasopharyngeal cancer accounts for about 0.25% of all cancers and approximately 2% of all head and neck cancers. At diagnosis, patients are generally 30–50 years old. This type of cancer is most common in Asia and North Africa. In southern China, it represents 18% of all cancers.[8] In Southeast Asia, 273

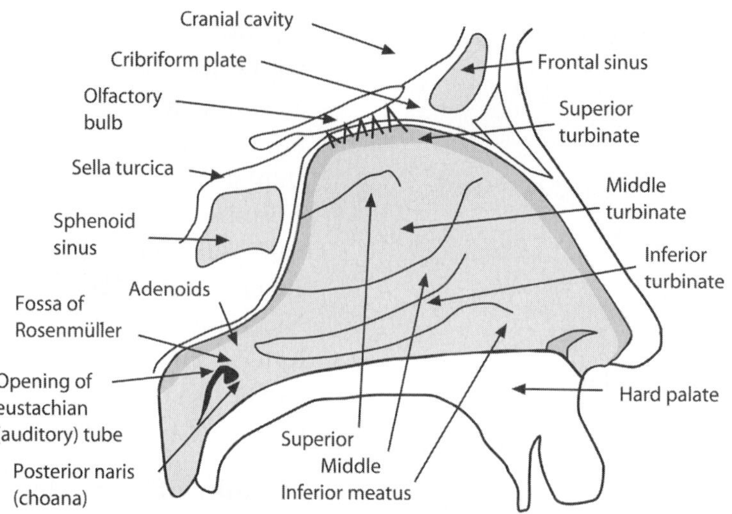

Figure 54-1 Structures of the nose and nasopharynx.

of every 100,000 individuals are diagnosed with nasopharyngeal cancer; in the United States, 1 in 100,000 persons is diagnosed with nasopharyngeal cancer.[9]

Cancer of the hypopharynx is uncommon. Approximately 2500 new cases are diagnosed in the United States each year, with peak incidence occurring in those 60 years or older. More men than women are diagnosed with hypopharyngeal cancer. In the United States, 65%–85% of hypopharyngeal cancers involve the pyriform sinuses.[10] Overall mortality is 32%. Only 1% of those individuals diagnosed with nasopharyngeal cancer are nonsmokers. Patients present with regional metastasis 25% of the time and with distant metastasis 10% of the time.[11]

Malignant salivary gland tumors represent less than 0.5% of all malignancies, making up 3%–5% of all head and neck cancers. They mostly occur in people aged 50–60.[12]

For neck cancers of unknown primary, the primary tumor eventually will be detected in approximately 40% of patients. Approximately 80% of cancers initially designated as cancer of unknown primary of the head and neck are eventually found to be from the base of the tongue or tonsillar fossa. The five-year survival rate for tumors of the neck with unknown primary is approximately 50%.[13]

Anatomy

Nasal Fossa and Paranasal Sinuses

The nasal cavity (Figure 54-1) is supported by the hard palate and soft palate (floor), divided by the septum, and topped by the ethmoid bone, which separates the superior aspect of the nasal fossa from the cranial cavity. Three curving, scroll-like bones form the lateral walls of the nasal cavity. These bones are the superior turbinate, middle turbinate, and inferior turbinate. Each of these bones has a tiny meatus (opening) for drainage to specific sinus regions. The masolacrimal duct drains into the inferior meatus. The middle turbinate meatus drains the maxillary, anterior ethmoid, and frontal sinuses (Figure 54–2). The superior turbinate drains the posterior ethmoid and sphenoid sinuses. The four paired, paranasal sinuses are the maxillary, ethmoid, frontal, and sphenoid sinuses. Each pair of sinuses is named according to the skull bone housing it. The majority of sinus malignancies occur in the maxillary sinuses.

Skull Base

The skull base is divided into three regions—anterior, middle, and posterior. The anterior region includes the ethmoid sinuses, frontal sinuses, and superior hemispheres of the orbits. The middle region includes the greater and lesser wings of the sphenoid bone, infratemporal bone, infratemporal fossa, optic apex, and optic chiasm. The posterior skull base region contains the clivis, posterior fossa, jugular foramen, and interior auditory canal. Tumors can originate intracranially and extend into head and neck sites. Malignancies also can spread from the nasal fossa, paranasal sinuses, nasopharynx, or infratemporal fossa.

Nasopharynx

The nasopharynx is bordered anteriorly by the posterior naris/choana and posteriorly by the adenoids, body of the sphenoid, and basilar process of the occipital

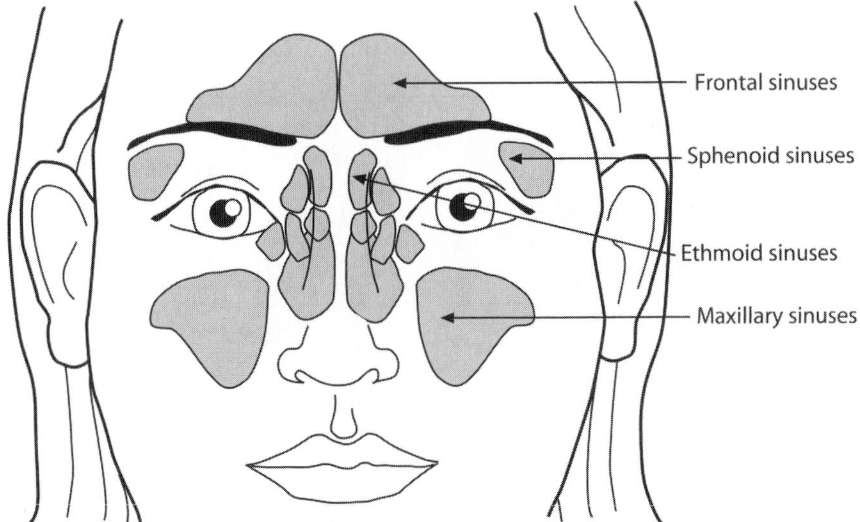

Figure 54-2 The paranasal sinuses.

bones (Figure 54-1). Interiorly, the nasal passage merges with the oropharynx at the level of the soft palate. The eustachian tube orifice is just anterior to the fossa of Rosenmüller, which is also called the pharyngeal recess. The majority of nasopharyngeal malignancies occur in the fossa of Rosenmüller. Anterior to the fossa of Rosenmüller are the adenoids (pharyngeal tonsils).

Lymphatic drainage is abundant, with spread going to ipsilateral and contralateral retropharyngeal nodes. Regional spread usually occurs early as nasopharyngeal cancer progresses. Due to the abundant capillary lymphatic system, spread initially involves the cervical triangle, upper/middle/lower jugular chains, or supraclavicular nodes. The common carotid provides the blood supply.

Oral Cavity

The boundaries of the oral cavity are the upper and lower alveolar processes. The oral cavity extends from the anterior vermilion border of the lips superiorly to the posterior border of the hard palate and superior maxillary bone. Inferiorly, the oral cavity extends to the circumvallate papillae of the base of the tongue (BOT) and the floor of mouth (FOM) muscle. Lateral boundaries are the palatine arches or cheeks and include the muscle of the cheek. The oral cavity includes the lips, tongue, salivary glands, FOM, mesopharynx, and hypopharynx. The most commonly encountered tumors involve the lips, tongue, and FOM (Figure 54-3). Of the head and neck cancers, oral cancers are the least likely to spread to the cervical lymph nodes.

Oropharynx

The oropharyngeal region borders the facial arch, which includes the inferior surface of the soft palate, the uvula, and the anterior border of the tonsillar pillar as well as the lingual tonsils, also called the pharyngeal tonsils; posterior one-third of the tongue; and the adjacent pharyngeal wall (Figure 54-4). All structures of the oropharynx contribute to aerodigestion, including mastication, deglutition, phonation, and respiration. Malignancies of the oropharynx are infrequent and difficult to diagnose because they tend to be hidden. Carcinoma of the tonsil (tonsillar fossa or pillars) is the most common oropharyngeal malignancy. These tumors usually begin in the tonsil, soft palate, or tonsil-like tissue of the tongue base.

Salivary Gland

The three paired salivary glands are the submandibulars, sublinguals (submentals), and parotids (Figure 54-5). The parotids are in the preauricular areas, the sublinguals are within the FOM, and the submandibulars are deep and inferior to the mandible.

Major salivary glands include the parotid, submandibular, and sublingual. Minor salivary glands include the oral mucosa, palate, uvula, FOM, posterior tongue, retromolar and pretonsillar areas, pharynx, larynx, and paranasal sinuses.

The most common type of salivary tumor is mucoepidermoid cancer, representing 10% of all salivary gland tumors. Malignancy of the salivary gland is estimated to account for 35% of cases, with the most frequent location in the parotid gland. The palate is the most common site of minor salivary gland tumors

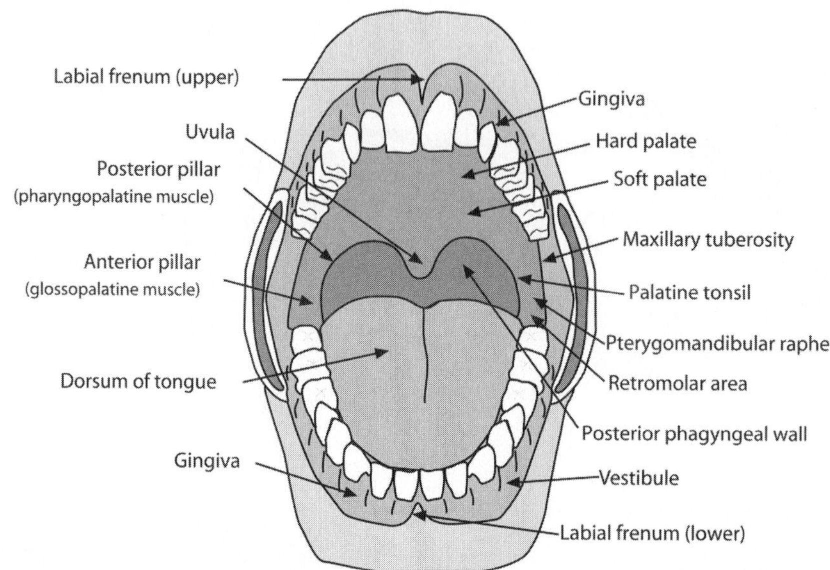

Figure 54-3 The oral cavity.

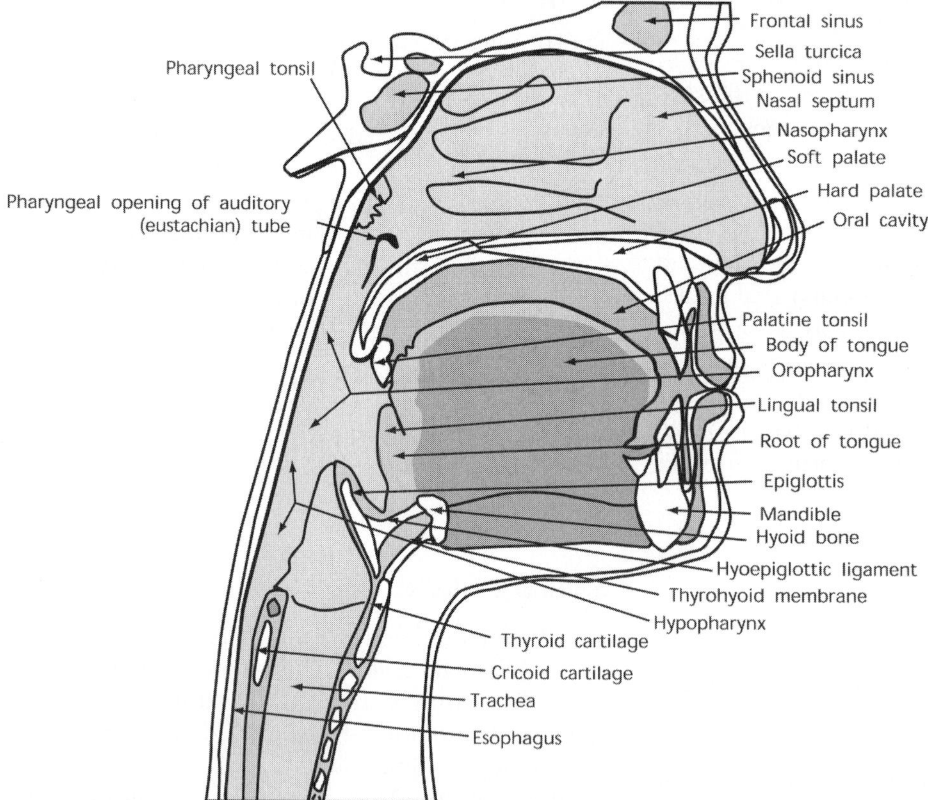

Figure 54-4 Structures of the oropharynx, hypopharynx, trachea, and larynx.

(70%–80% of all salivary gland tumors start in the parotid gland).[12]

Larynx

The larynx lies between the epiglottis, cricoid cartilage, and carotid arteries. It is located posterior to the thyroid gland (Figure 54-6). Its three regions are the supraglottic, the glottis, and the subglottis. The supraglottic region is inferior to the posterior one-third of the tongue, and includes the epiglottis, aryepiglottic folds, arytenoid cartilages, and false vocal cords (FVC). The glottis includes the true vocal cords (TVC), rima glottis, and glottic slit, which separates the TVC. The

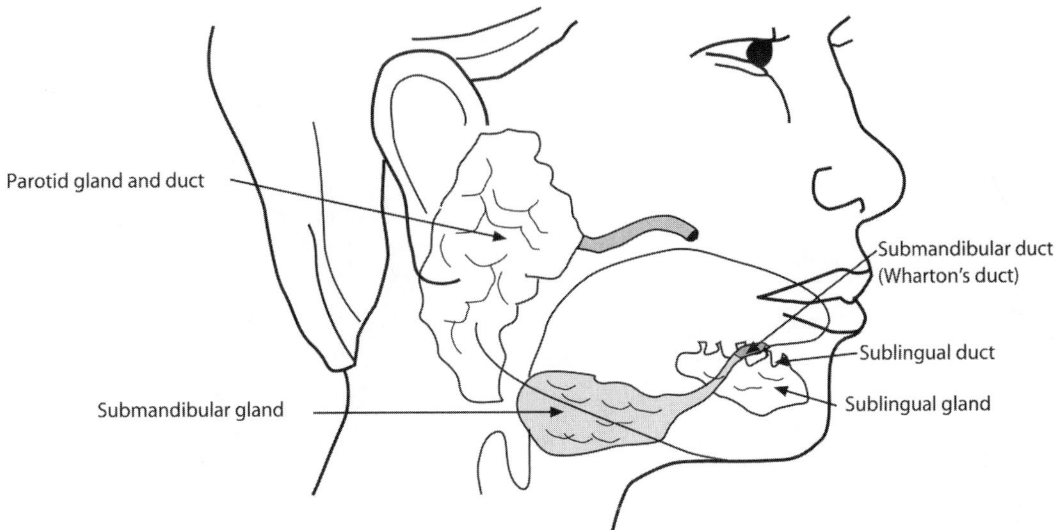

Figure 54-5 Major salivary glands and ducts.

subglottis extends 1 cm below the TVC to the cricoid cartilage or first tracheal ring. Recurrent and superior laryngeal nerves innervate the area; they are branches of the vagus nerve (CN X). Glottic carcinoma is the most common laryngeal malignancy. The subglottic site is the least common location for cancer.

Hypopharynx and Neck

The hypopharynx (Figure 54-4), also called the laryngopharynx, connects the oropharynx from the hyoid bone to the esophageal introitus. The lower end is at the level of the sixth cervical vertebra. The hypopharynx is divided into three regions: (1) the paired pyriform sinuses, (2) the posterior pharyngeal walls, and (3) the postcricoid area (lower pharyngeal wall). The majority of hypopharyngeal lesions start in one of the pyriform sinuses. Once cancer cells have penetrated the mucosa of the pharynx, they can easily spread regionally. The neck nodes (Figure 54-7) provide avenues for lymphatic drainage from the base of skull to the clavicle. The level of lymph node involvement is indicative of the location of the primary tumor.

Etiology and Risk Factors

Tobacco abuse has been implicated as a risk factor for all head and neck tumor sites. Cigarettes, pipes, cigars, smokeless tobacco, and habitual use of marijuana are all considered to be physical carcinogens. Tobacco use increases the risk of developing head and neck cancer 25-fold.[2]

Every type of tobacco has been connected to dysplastic injuries and carcinogenic changes in all head and neck primary malignancy sites. Upper hypopharyngeal cancer is associated with heavy drinking and smoking.[10] In adults who neither smoke nor drink, cancer of the mouth and throat are nearly nonexistent.[1] Risk increases with the amount smoked per day.[5]

The strongest link between alcohol and cancer is evident with cancers of the oral cavity, esophagus, larynx, pharynx, and liver.[14] Excessive alcohol intake increases the risk of developing oral or pharyngeal cancer nine-fold.[2] The risk is associated with more alcohol consumed — two drinks per day for men and one drink per day for women — and increases when the number of drinks per day rises. The carcinogenic effect of alcohol is thought to make cells vulnerable to other carcinogens (especially tobacco related) or to increase certain hormone levels associated with cancer growth.[14]

Carcinoma of the Nasal Cavity and Paranasal Sinuses

Exposure to tobacco, alcohol, chemicals (such as nickel), and chemical inhalants (such as those found in furniture making, shoe leather working, and textile work) have been associated with increased incidence of cancers of the nasal cavity and paranasal sinuses. In addition, chronic sinusitis has been linked with carcinoma of the maxillary sinus.

Carcinoma of the Nasopharynx

Nasopharyngeal carcinoma risk factors — unlike risk factors for other head and neck cancers — are not primarily linked to tobacco and alcohol. They include (1) infection by the Epstein-Barr virus (EBV), which is

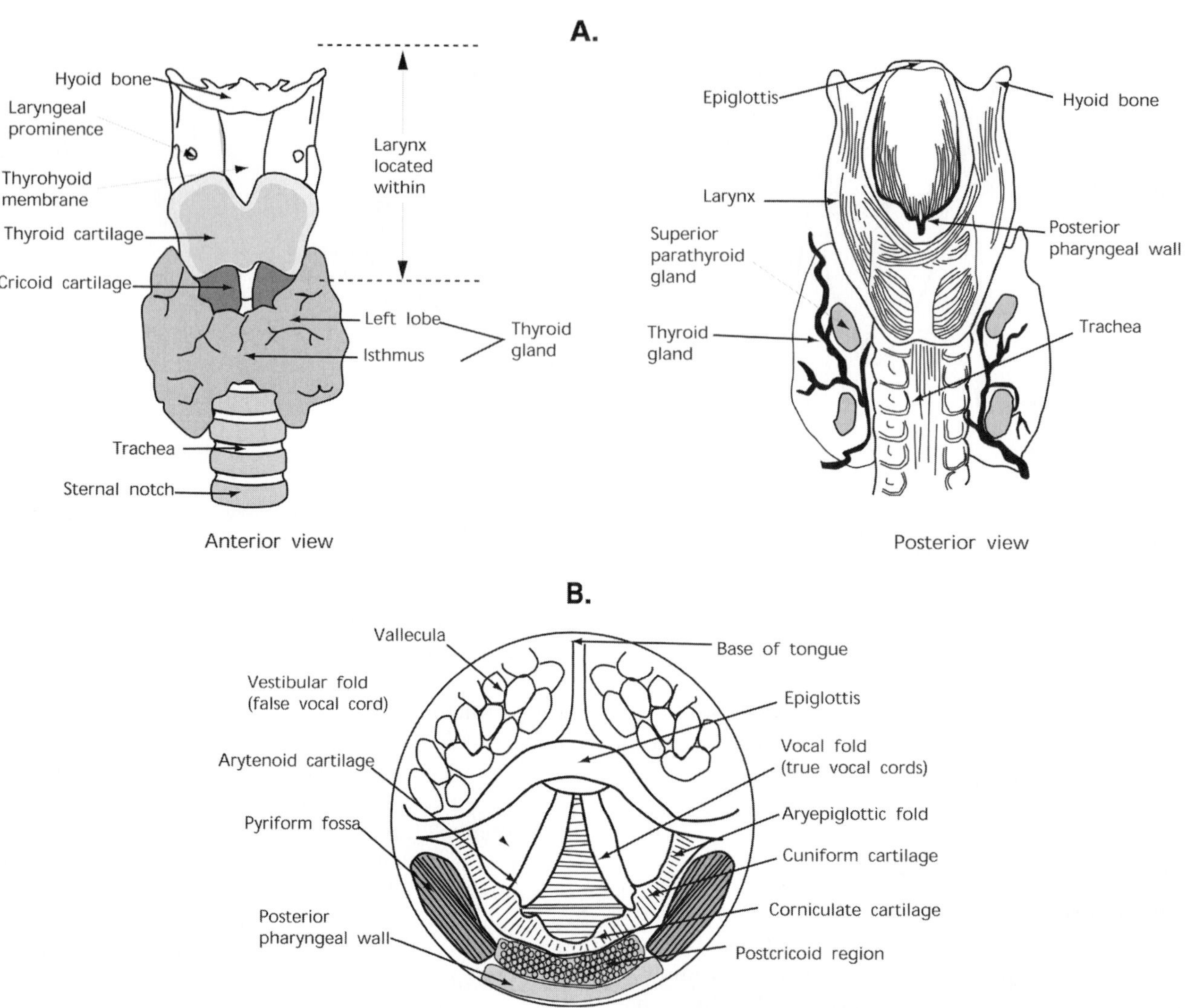

Figure 54-6 **(A)** Larynx, trachea, thyroid, and parathyroid glands (anterior and posterior). **(B)** Vocal cords and cartilages of the larynx and epiglottis (mirror view).

applicable for all ethnic cultures; (2) routine inhalation of the nitrosamines in salt-cured, steamy foods such as meats, fish, eggs, and leafy vegetables, especially for Chinese and other Asian cultural groups; and (3) inhalation of toxic chemicals, such as those encountered in woodworking.[15]

Carcinoma of the Major or Minor Salivary Glands

The etiology of most salivary gland tumors is not clearly known, although there are some associations with environmental factors—rubber products manufacturing, asbestos mining, plumbing, some types of woodworking and ionizing radiation.[12] Many types of salivary gland carcinomas and mixed tumors are found in salivary glands: mucoepidermoid, adenoic cystic, adenocarcinomas, malignant mixed. Also, lymphomas of major salivary glands can occur; they are usually non-Hodgkin's lymphomas.[12]

Carcinoma of the Oral Cavity

Tobacco use is responsible for 90% of oral cancers in men and 60% of cases in women.[5] The risk of oral cancer decreases by as much as 50% within 3–5 years after a person stops smoking. It returns to a normal level within 10 years of stopping smoking. Heavy cigar smoking is particularly closely associated with oral cancer.[5]

The synergistic effects of tobacco use and alcohol consumption increase the risk for developing oral cancer, compared to exposure to either risk factor alone.[5] Alcohol users are six times more likely to develop oral cancer than nonusers.[14] The risk of developing cancer

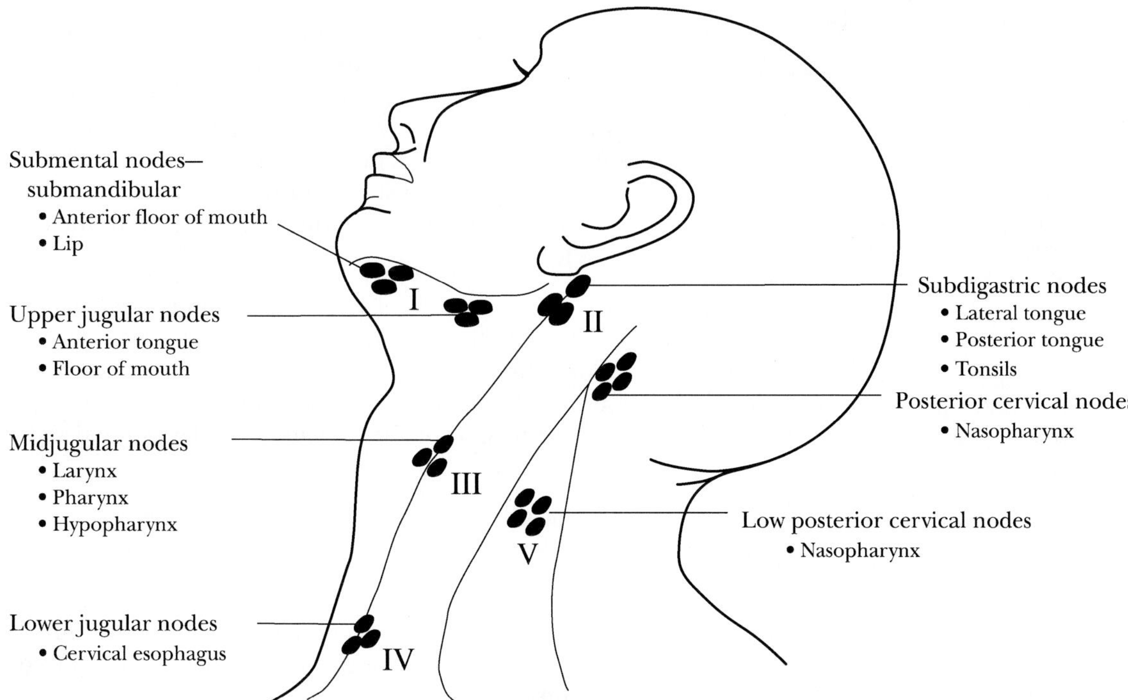

Figure 54-7 Lymphadenopathy of the head and neck area provides important clues to the location of the primary site.

with tobacco use increases when the person drinks and continues to smoke or chew tobacco.[16]

Approximately 75%–80% of patients with oral cancer drink alcohol frequently, and 90% of patients with oral cancer use tobacco.[17] The risk of developing such cancer increases with combined tobacco and alcohol use with oral leukoplakia. Ethanol is oxidized to acetaldehyde and then to acetate by alcohol dehydrogenase (ADH) and aldehyde dehydrogenase (ALDH), both of which have genetic polymorphisms. A review of case-control studies of the effects of *ALDH2, ADH2,* and *ADH3* genotypes shows associations with the risk for head and neck cancer in moderate-to-heavy-drinking Japanese individuals.[18]

For oropharyngeal cancer, an often-quoted study showed that the high alcohol content in mouthwash was associated with a 40%–60% increase in the incidence of oral cancer.[16] A study published in 2003 looked at the risk of developing oropharyngeal cancer because of the use of alcohol-containing mouthwash. It concluded that previous studies suggesting such an association were incorrect and that use of a mouthwash containing alcohol does not increase one's risk of developing oropharyngeal cancer.[19]

For oral cancer, additional risk factors include poor oral hygiene, mechanical irritation, and Plummer-Vinson syndrome. Oral cancer has also been linked to human papillomavirus (HPV), and precancerous oral lesions, called leukoplakia. The body of knowledge about etiological factors is growing, especially relating to genetics. Studies have shown that oral cancer tumors have missing chromosome arms — specifically, 3, 17, and 19. Future treatments will likely focus on the genetic basis for these tumors, expanding our knowledge of gene suppressor proteins.[20]

Carcinoma of the Lip

Prolonged exposure to sunlight is linked with cancer of the lip and is an established major cause of skin cancer.[1] (See Chapter 63.) Squamous cell carcinoma (SCC) and basal cell carcinoma are the major nonmelanomatous skin cancers of the head and neck area. Lip malignancies occur most frequently on the lower lip. The carcinogenic effect on the skin is compounded if the individual is fair-skinned.

Carcinoma of the Larynx

The majority of individuals who develop laryngeal cancer have a long history of habitual tobacco use and alcohol abuse. Other etiologic factors may include constant irritation of the vocal cords due to chronic laryngitis or an overprojection of the voice, sometimes called voice abuse.

Table 54-1 Symptoms of Head and Neck Malignancies

Tumor Site	Symptoms
Oral cavity (including lip, floor of mouth, tongue, hard palate	Nonhealing white, red, or white/red patch on gums, tongue, tonsil, or lining of the mouth; pain; loosening teeth, ill-fitting dentures; gingival swelling; hyperplasia; dysplasia; difficulty chewing or moving the tongue; sore throat (feels that something is caught)
Nose and parnasal sinuses	Unilateral obstruction of naris; nonhealing ulcer; intermittent epistaxis
Nasopharynx	Nasal obstruction; pain; may present without mucosal changes; painless, enlarged lymph node(s) in neck; recurrent otitis media
Oropharynx (base of tongue, tonsil, soft palate)	Asymmetry; dull ache; pain; dysphagia; superficial diffuse erythroplakia; refered otalgia; trismus; muffled voice; neck mass
Trachea	Not a primary tumor site (distant spread from larynx, lung, or esophagus)
Larynx, hypopharynx	Voice changes (early stage when lesion is on vocal cord); leukoplakia or erythroplakia; stridor or dyspnea; skip lesions
Supraglottic	Dysphagia; sore throat; aspiration; referred ear pain; tickling sensation in throat; change in vocal quality; hoarseness; enlarged neck nodes
Glottic	In addition, stridor with large tumors
Subglottic	In addition, hemopstysis
Salivary gland	Unilateral symptoms; impaired jaw mobility; neurological changes (numb lower lip); face numbness or persistent facial pain; painless gland swelling

Carcinoma of the Hypopharynx

Plummer-Vinson syndrome, a type of chronic iron-deficiency anemia, is a risk factor for tongue and postcricoid tumors in nonsmoking, premenopausal women. With this condition, before malignant changes occur, a thin web grows that coats the mucosal to submucosal esophagus. The patient experiences dysphagia related to the degeneration of esophageal muscle. Another metabolic deficiency — malabsorption of vitamin B_{12} — is also a risk factor. Hypopharyngeal tumors are a risk factor for the occurrence of other primary tumors.

Clinical Manifestations

Cancer of the head and neck is curable if caught early. Many of these malignancies are associated with early symptoms, which have been present for a while before the patient presents for evaluation (Table 54-1). Unfortunately, the majority of head and neck cancers are diagnosed at more advanced stages.[1]

The symptoms of the various head and neck cancers correspond to changes in function caused by tissue injury to the specific anatomical site. Common symptoms for all sites include weight loss and a persistent unilateral lump or mass. A neck mass is highly suspicious of regional spread of the carcinoma.

Other general symptoms of tumor growth include the following:

- *Expectorating blood.* This symptom is often caused by something other than cancer. However, tumors in the nose, mouth, throat, or lungs can cause bleeding. Individuals who have blood in their saliva or phlegm for more than a few days should see a physician.[1]
- *Swallowing problems.* Cancer of the throat or esophagus may make swallowing solid foods difficult.
- *Persistent earache.* Constant pain in or around the ear when swallowing can be a sign of infection or tumor growth in the throat.
- *A lump in the neck.* When the lump lasts more than two weeks, the person should be seen by a physician as soon as possible. Not all lumps are cancer, but a lump in the neck can be the first sign of cancer of the mouth, throat, larynx, or thyroid gland, or of certain lymphomas or leukemias. Most masses are painless and enlarged on physical exam.

Skull Base Malignancies

Epidermoid, mucoepidermoid, and adenoid cystic adenocarcinoma skull base tumors are rare. Presenting symptoms include otalgia, facial pain, epistaxis, headaches, changes in vision or hearing, and recurrent sinus infections. Abnormalities commonly correlate with cranial nerve (CN) involvement.

Nasal Cavity, Paranasal Sinuses, and Nasopharyngeal Malignancies

In the United States, nasal cavity SCC occurs rarely, and the majority of nasal tumors are of a low grade at diagnosis. The most common paranasal sinus malignancies involve the maxillary sinus. Symptoms of a malignancy of the nasal cavity or paranasal sinus may include nasal obstruction, epistaxis, localized pain, facial swelling, trismus, loosened teeth, localized mass, and facial nerve (CN VII) dysfunction. Malignant changes of the nasopharynx may present with symptoms similar to those noted with cancer of the nasal cavity, such as epistaxis, nasal obstruction, and impaired CN VII function. Additional signs are enlarged but pain-free

Table 54-2 Examination Techniques by Cranial Nerve Distribution

Region	Evaluates	Assessment
Head	CN V–Trigeminal	
	Sensory: maxillary sinus, teeth	Place hands on temporal muscles and then masseter muscles to palpate muscle contractions for symmetry
	Motor: chewing action	
	CN VII–Facial	
	Motor: assess symmetry	Ask patient to lift both eyebrows, tightly close eyes, make exaggerated frown and then wide smile, puff cheeks
	Sensory: taste	Taste test
Auditory	CN VIII–Acoustic	
	Sensory: hearing	Refer to audiologist to evaluate unilateral changes in hearing
	CN IX–Glossopharyngeal	
	Sensory: middle ear	
Nose and paranasal sinuses	CN I–Olfactory	
	Sensory: smell	Test smell with scratch card if possible, alcohol swab may be used
	Nasal structure	Inspect with headlight and nasal speculum
	Frontal sinuses	Palpate sinuses bilaterally for lumps, tenderness; transilluminate sinuses
	Maxillary sinuses	
	Ethmoid sinuses	
Mouth and pharynx	Parotid	Palpate for unilateral mass
	Mucosa	Inspect oral cavity for leukoplakia, erythroplakia, ulcer, mass
	CN IX–Glossopharyngeal	Test on both sides of back of tongue with tongue blade for gag reflex
	CN X–Vagus	Watch for rise of uvula/soft palate when patient says "ah"
	Mucosal changes	
Hypopharynx and larynx	CNX-Vagus	Apply local anesthetic spray to oropharynx, ask to breathe through mouth, stick out tongue, and repeat vowels "a" and "e" while examining, using laryngeal mirror and headlight or fiber-optic equipment
Neck		Palpate for masses, tenderness or pain, swelling along the cervical lymph node chains
	CNXI-Accessory	Gently hold neck and have patient turn head from side to side against resistance Direct patient to shrug shoulders against resistance

lymph nodes of the neck, tinnitus, recurrent otitis media, headache, and other symptoms associated with cranial nerve compression. (See Table 54-2.) Sinus cancers are associated with a poor prognosis due to early perineural and skull base invasion.

Oral Cavity and Oropharynx Malignancies

Structures of the oral cavity that may be affected by malignant changes include the lip, upper and lower buccal mucoses, upper and lower alveolar ridges, retromolartrigone, hard palate, anterior two-thirds of the tongue, and floor of the mouth.

Abnormalities of any of these structures may include a nonhealing ulcer versus a painless, firm mass, and they may involve either leukoplakia or erythroplakia. The individual's first symptom may be that dentures no longer fit comfortably. Malignancies of the oropharynx are difficult to diagnose, as the same symptoms can readily be ascribed to nonmalignant conditions. Generalized symptoms may include mild but persistent dull ache and sore throat, referred otalgia, dysphagia with ongoing weight loss, and worsening airway obstruction.

Most cancers of the mouth or tongue cause a sore or swelling that does not go away. These sores and swellings may be painless unless they become infected. Bleeding may occur, but often not until late in the disease. If an ulcer or swelling is accompanied by lumps in the neck it is considered a particularly ominous sign.

Laryngeal Malignancies

Most cancers of the larynx cause some change in voice. Any hoarseness or other voice change lasting more than two weeks is significant.

Symptoms of laryngeal carcinomas are associated with the region of the larynx where the tumor originated. The larynx is divided into three areas: supraglottic, glottic, and subglottic. Early on, presenting symptoms can be masked due to the persistent irritation that the person has experienced over many years of habitual tobacco use or occupational exposure to irritants such as petroleum products or wood dust. The presence of a neck mass indicates regional lymph node spread. Presenting symptoms will be determined by the anatomical structures involved.

Hypopharyngeal Malignancies

Because of the anatomical location of the hypopharynx, tumors in this area are often detected late, after they have invaded muscle and adjacent structures. As with laryngeal carcinomas, early symptoms are often masked by years of chronic irritation from tobacco and alcohol use. Pyriform sinus lesions may present with otalgia, which is usually described as dull ear pain. Voice changes and dysphagia tend to occur late, when advanced disease is present. Posterior pharyngeal wall lesions may present as a sore throat or with a feeling of mucous retention after swallowing.

Pathophysiology

Cellular Characteristics

More than 90% of head and neck tumors are SCC in origin. These tumors arise from the epilethium. Those that do not originate in squamous cells arise in white blood cells (lymphoma) or glandular cells (adenocarcinoma).[21,22]

An invasive carcinoma will be either well differentiated, moderately well differentiated, poorly differentiated, or undifferentiated. Other categories used include infiltrative (originating within the epithelium), exophytic (originating on the surface of the epithelium), and verrucous (wart-like) carcinomas. Microscopic variants of SCCs are further classified as keratinizing (well-differentiated and moderately well-differentiated changes) or nonkeratinizing (anaplastic). Nonkeratinizing cells include the less common lymphoepithelioma, transitional cell, and spindle cell SCCs of the head and neck.

Adenocarcinomas of the major and minor salivary glands include poorly differentiated, high- or low-grade mucoepidermoid, adenoid cystic, acenic cell, and malignant mixed adenocarcinomas (which include more than one of the adenocarcinoma tumor types). Thyroid cancer, a head and neck malignancy, is discussed with endocrine conditions (see Chapter 50).

For oral cancers, no statistically significant correlation exists between the degree of differentiation and the biologic behavior of the cancer. However, vascular invasion is a negative prognostic factor.[20]

When the carcinoma is noninvasive, it is called "carcinoma in situ." In oral cancer, "leukoplakia" is a clinically descriptive term indicating a white patch that does not rub off. The significance of leukoplakia is based on its histology. Leukoplakia can range from hyperkeratosis to early invasive carcinoma, or it may merely represent a fungal infection, lichen planus, or other benign oral disease.[20]

Progression of Disease

Head and neck tumors tend to recur locally. The basement membrane, which underlies the squamous epithelium, provides an important natural barrier to local tumor cell invasion. However, primary head and neck lesions are locally invasive because specific neoplastic receptors can advance tumor growth into the basement membrane.

In establishing a treatment plan, the intensity of therapy takes into account several prognostic factors. Among these prognostic parameters are the T (tumor), N (node), and M (metastatic) stage, the presence of extranodal growth (extracapsular spread); tumor volume; lymph node burden; extent of tumor necrosis; and histologic grading.

The incidence of spread to regional lymph nodes at diagnosis is high. Based on the tumor's location, there may be either early or late spread to one or more of the adjacent superficial or deep cervical lymph node chains (Figure 54-7). Lymph node involvement is predictable and based on the anatomical location of the tumor. When there is involvement of distant lymph nodes, such as mediastinal nodes, the cancer is considered metastatic.

Lymph node metastasis is an important factor in head and neck cancer prognosis. Lymph node involvement indicates stage III or IV disease.[21] The most common area of lymph node spread is bilaterally along the internal jugular vein underneath the sternocleidomastoid muscle, especially along the angle of the jaw. The risk of distant metastasis is increased if the tumor has spread to the neck lymph nodes and multiple lymph nodes are involved. Lymph node involvment in the lower neck is more ominous than involvement of lymph nodes in the upper neck. As a general rule, as tumor cells proceed from the lips posterior to the hypopharynx, prognosis worsens. Tumor thickness correlates with lymph node spread as well as poor survival rates. Patients with head and neck cancers have an increased chance of developing a second primary tumor in the upper aerodigestive tract.[20]

In oral cancers, a positive margin or tumor depth greater than 5 mm increases the risk of local recurrence in oral/lip cancer. No statistically significant correlation between the degree of differentiation of the cell and the spread of the tumor has been found.[20,23]

For salivary tumors, tumor size appears to be more important than histologic grade in terms of prognosis. Approximately 80% of metastasis to the major salivary glands originates from other primary head and neck tumors, especially those of squamous cell origin and melanoma. The remainder of metastases to the salivary glands come from the lung, kidney, and breast. The parotid gland is the site of 80%–90% of metastases.[12]

The prognosis for small laryngeal cancers that have not spread to lymph nodes is good. Cure rates range from 75%–90%, depending on tumor size, site, and degree of infiltration. In laryngeal cancer, 25%–50% patients present with involved lymph nodes.[24] Locally advanced lesions are difficult to treat and distant metastasis is common, even if primary laryngeal cancer is controlled. For laryngeal cancer, the most adverse prognostic factor is higher T and N stage. Other prognostic factors include sex, age, performance status, and pathology. Laryngeal cancer patients are at highest risk of recurrence after treatment in their first 2–3 years after diagnosis. Recurrences after 5 years are rare. If cancer is found in and around the larynx 5 years after treatment, it is generally considered a new primary.[24]

For patients with hypopharyngeal tumors, 50% present with cervical lymph node involvement and one-fourth have a second primary tumor. Hypopharyngeal tumors tend to spread within the mucosa, beneath intact epithelium, and can skip metastasis, resurfacing at various remote locations. When diagnosed, these tumors are at an advanced stage.[25] The most important features determining prognosis are the size and extent of local spread of the primary carcinoma and the extent of involvement of regional lymph nodes. These tumors have a relatively high incidence of delayed regional spread (two or more years after completing primary therapy) and distant metastasis.[26–28]

Nasopharyngeal cancer prognosis is associated with the size of the tumor, T stage, and neck node involvement. Other factors include the patient's age, diminished immune function at diagnosis, and incomplete excision of the initial tumor.[15]

Tumors of the paranasal sinuses present at advanced stages and cure rates are poor (<50%).[26] Most tumors spread directly into vital areas of the skull or rapidly recur as local disease, especially in the first two years after treatment; therefore, lifetime follow-up is necessary.

Assessment

Once a clinical evaluation is suspicious for a malignancy, further diagnostic testing follows. For many head and neck evaluations, more sophisticated scoping is possible with a flexible fiber-optic nasopharyngoscope, which is an office-based examination. This examination allows the physician to see the patient's nasal cavity, nasopharynx, oropharynx, and larynx. Before the exam, the patient's nasal area is sprayed with a topical anesthetic. The patient remains able to respond to verbal requests during the exam, such as making the sound "a" or "e" to see movement of the vocal cords. After being scoped, the patient is advised to avoid eating or drinking for 30 minutes until the gag reflex returns.

To stage the tumor, tissue is biopsied (incisional, excisional, needle biopsy) to establish a histopathic diagnosis. Pathologic review of biopsied tissue is the only way to establish a definitive diagnosis.[21] Some biopsies can be performed in the clinic office with the biopsy area anesthetized with an oral spray. A fine-needle aspiration (FNA) can be attempted in the clinic in an effort to evaluate a gland or neck mass.

If the suspected tumor in the oral cavity or pharynx cannot be viewed easily with the fiber-optic nasopharyngoscope, then the physician will view the area with a esophagoscope. The patient is under general anesthesia during the procedure. A direct laryngoscopy (DL) is also called a *panendoscopy*. During the procedure, the surgeon will take excisional samples for a biopsy, then send them to the pathology laboratory for histological evaluation.

Radiological studies are crucial in the evaluation of tumor size, invasion, and lymph node spread so that the best treatment option can be determined.[29] Computed tomography (CT) and magnetic resonance imaging (MRI) are often complementary to determine the extent of disease. Both MRI and CT view the oral cavity and the parotids equally well.[30,31]

Magnetic Resonance Imaging

The MRI technique is superior to CT for showing the depth of primary tumor invasion in soft tissues and fatty areas. It shows malignant changes from inflammation and better illuminates metastasis to the lymph nodes.[6,30] MRI is the preferred diagnostic film for tumors of the paratoid, parpharyngeal, retropharyngeal, and prevertebral spaces, as it can show greater contrast resolution.[30–33] It also provides better soft tissue contrast in images of the tongue, oropharynx, and tonsil.[32]

For most head and neck tumors, MRI is more capable than CT for identifying mature scarring, bony involvement, tumor recurrence, and postradiation complications.[30] For nasopharyngeal cancer, CT is widely used because it offers greater availability, is less expensive, and is less time-consuming. However, MRI is becoming the preferred imaging modality. In some nasopharyngeal cancer cases, MRI cannot reliably demonstrate mucosal recurrence or differentiate tumor recurrence from postradiation tissue changes.[33]

Newer MRI techniques include dynamic contrast-enhanced MRI for evaluating soft tissue masses and cervical lymph nodes. Ultra-small superparamagnetic iron oxide contrast agents are used in this application. Additionally, functional techniques — such as in vivo and in vitro MRI spectroscopy of head and neck cancer — are under development. Another technique focuses on mapping of the lymph nodes and the apparent diffusion coefficient mapping of parotid glands. These techniques can help to differentiate nonmalignant tissue from malignant tumors and lymph nodes and can aid in differentiating residual malignancies from postradiation changes.[34]

Further technical development of MRI is necessary to improve the accuracy of lymph node metastases in patients with clinically negative (N0) nodes. Development of new tissue-specific MRI contrast agents and functional imaging studies to address the biologic activity of lymph nodes are essential to bring about future improvements in imaging.[35]

Computed Tomography

For malignancies of the pharynx (nasopharynx, oropharynx, and hypopharynx) as well as the sinuses, computerized tomography (CT) is superior to x-rays in distinguishing inflammation from tumor. It also can show cartilage invasion, bony destruction or erosion, and the extent of disease for most of the head and neck malignancies.[30] CT may be more reliable and accurate than MRI in revealing metastatic invasion.[32] In the oral cavity, CT accuracy in showing tumor and its changes ranges from 81%–94%. Lymph node infiltration can be represented 15%–20% of the time with negative images.[29]

Positron Emission Tomography

Positron emission tomography, or a PET scan, is a diagnostic examination that shows physiologic images of the entire body based on the detection of biochemical changes. The value of a PET scan is enhanced when it is part of a larger diagnostic work-up with CT or MRI.

A PET scan is indicated in head and neck cancer patients (1) to guide biopsy or local resection at the initial stage of an unknown primary; (2) to prevent unnecessary further treatment in high-risk patients; (3) to monitor tumor response before full-dose irradiation; (4) to detect residual, recurrent, or secondary neoplasms after definitive radiotherapy; (5) in patients with no known nodal disease, to evaluate the necessity of neck treatment; and (6) in cases when laryngeal cancer recurrence is suspected with no objective findings, to determine if a biopsy is warranted.[36,37]

PET scans can better show lymphadenopathy. When used with CT images, the PET scan can help to determine the origin of disease locally, which is especially important in the case of an unknown primary. Reports estimate that PET scans were able to establish the location of the primary cancer 25% of time.[32]

In a study of 26 patients with histologically confirmed stage III–IV squamous cell carcinoma of the head and neck (SCCHN), patients underwent PET scan before and approximately 6 weeks after the end of combined radiation and chemotherapy. The PET findings were confirmed by histologic analysis and a 6-month clinical follow-up. For detection of locoregional residual cancer and distant metastases or secondary tumors, the PET findings had a sensitivity of 90.9% and a specificity of 93.3%.[38]

In another study involving 97 patients with oral SCC, the overall sensitivity of a PET scan did not exceed 90%, and its specificity varied from 67% for local disease recurrence/second primaries to 99% for lymph node metastasis. The researchers concluded that PET scans are highly valuable for diagnosing oral SCC recurrence in a postoperative setting.[39]

For T1 to T2 laryngeal tumors, videostroboscopy is used for early detection. Videolaryngoscopy permits assessment of larger lesions. If the individual has a hypopharyngeal or pyriform sinus malignancy, a barium sulfate cinefluoroscopy or upper GI is ordered to assess tracheo-esophageal function and to detect a second primary tumor.

Angiography is another radiological test that can define collateralization, especially when the tumor is adjacent to or invading the carotid artery. Following the angiogram, the patient will undergo frequent neurological checks. When resection of the carotid artery is anticipated, cerebral contralateral blood flow is evaluated using a balloon test occlusion (BTO) with single-photon emission computerized tomography (SPECT) scans.

Advances in head and neck cancer imaging include use of thallium-201 chloride (Tl-201) scintigraphy and gallium-67 citrate (Ga-67) scintigraphy to differentiate between malignant tumors and benign tumors.[40,41] High-resolution sonography and color (power) Doppler sonography can be used as the first-line modality for evaluating cervical soft tissue masses and when performing sentinel node radiolocalization to solid tumors of the head and neck.[41–44]

Classification and Staging

Staging of head and neck cancers is key to treatment decisions, providing a baseline for the evaluation of treatment outcomes and prognosis.

The American Joint Committee on Cancer (AJCC) has established a staging criteria for lip and oral, nasal cavity and paranasal, nasopharynx, major salivary, hypopharynx, and laryngeal cancers.[45] Table 54-3 provides the criteria for lip and oral cancers.[46]

The latest revision of the AJCC staging criteria (2002) takes into account detailed local anatomical features, recognizing that the degree of locoregional tumor involvement of these structures may be as important as distant metastasis. The latest revision includes criteria of more advanced cases (T4 categories and stage IV disease), which better clarify the goal of cure or palliation.[47]

Therapeutic Approaches and Nursing Care

Surgery

Surgery alone for early-stage disease is the standard of care in most patients with squamous cell carcinoma of the head and neck (SCCHN). For stage I and stage II disease, when no cervical nodes are involved, surgical resection can remove the tumor with clear margins. (*Note:* Radiation therapy alone is another treatment option for certain stage I and II malignancies and is also a standard of care for early disease.) Negative margins predict high probability of tumor control at stage I or II.

With stage III and IV malignancies, the tumor is surgically removed. Then adjuvant treatment is given —chemotherapy and/or radiation treatment. Most

Table 54-3 Lip and Oral Cavity Staging

TNM Definitions

Primary tumor (T)

TX:	Primary tumor cannot be assessed
T0:	No evidence of primary tumor
Tis:	Carcinoma in situ
T1:	Tumor 2 cm or less in greatest dimension
T2:	Tumor more than 2 cm but not more than 4 cm in greatest dimension
T3:	Tumor more than 4 cm in greatest dimension
T4:	(lip) Tumor invades through cortical bone, inferior alveolar nerve, floor of mouth, or skin of face (i.e., chin or nose)
T4a:	(oral cavity) Tumor invades adjacent structures (e.g., through cortical bone, into deep [extrinsic] muscle of tongue [genioglossus, hyoglossus, palatoglossus, and styloglossus], maxillary sinus, skin of face)
T4b:	Tumor invades masticator space, pterygoid plates, or skull base and/or encases internal carotid artery (*Note:* Superficial erosion alone of bone/tooth socket by gingival primary is not sufficient to classify a tumor as T4.)

Regional lymph nodes (N)

NX:	Regional lymph nodes cannot be assessed
N0:	No regional lymph node metastasis
N1:	Metastasis in a single ipsilateral lymph node, 3 cm or less in greatest dimension
N2:	Metastasis in a single ipsilateral lymph node, more than 3 cm but not more than 6 cm in greatest dimension; or in multiple ipsilateral lymph nodes, none more than 6 cm in greatest dimension; or in bilateral or contralateral lymph nodes, none more than 6 cm in greatest dimension
N2a:	Metastasis in a single ipsilateral lymph node more than 3 cm but not more than 6 cm in dimension
N2b:	Metastasis in multiple ipsilateral lymph nodes, none more than 6 cm in greatest dimension
N2c:	Metastasis in bilateral or contralateral lymph nodes, none more than 6 cm in greatest dimension
N3:	Metastasis in a lymph node more than 6 cm in greatest dimension

In clinical evaluation, the actual size of the nodal mass should be measured and allowance should be made for intervening soft tissues. Most masses larger than 3 cm in diameter are not single nodes but are confluent nodes or tumors in soft tissues of the neck. There are 3 stages of clinically positive nodes: N1, N2, and N3. The use of subgroups a, b, and c is not required but recommended. Midline nodes are considered homolateral nodes.

Distant metastasis (M)

MX:	Distant metastasis cannot be assessed
M0:	No distant metastasis
M1:	Distant metastasis

AJCC Stage Groupings

Stage 0	Tis, N0, M0
Stage I	T1, N0, M0
Stage II	T2, N0, M0
Stage III	T3, N0, M0
	T1, N1, M0
	T2, N1, M0
	T3, N1, M0
Stage IVA	T4a, N0, M0
	T4a, N1, M0
	T1, N2, M0
	T2, N2, M0
	T3, N2, M0
	T4a, N2, M0
Stage IVB	Any T, N3, M0
	T4b, any N, M0
Stage IVC	Any T, any N, M1

Data from American Joint Committee on Cancer: *AJCC Cancer Staging Manual* (ed 6). New York, Springer, 2002.[46]

surgeries are performed before radiation and chemotherapy are begun. Surgery after radiation therapy has been shown to benefit selected patients with regional advanced disease.[48] When straightforward surgical excisions and resections are not adequate because of cervical lymph node involvement, the surgeon can perform a radical neck dissection (RND) or a modified neck dissection (MND).[49]

Elective neck dissections (unilateral or bilateral, radical or selective, as appropriate) are performed when occult nodal metastases is suspected even if patient has a relatively small T1 or T2 tumor. Dissections are part of treatment plans because imaging has proven to be unreliable in identifying patients with occult cervical metastasis. The false-negative rate in imaging is too high, with unacceptably low sensitivity.

Surgery of the neck

Preoperatively, teaching should review tasks and capabilities that eventually will become the responsibility of the patient: short-term and long-term airway management, nutritional support, wound care, pain management, and communication. Depending on the procedure, some patients will undergo placement of both a temporary tracheostomy tube and a temporary gastric tube.

After surgery, attentive tracheostomy suctioning and care will help promote tissue oxygenation as well as improve pulmonary functioning. With a total laryngectomy plus neck dissection, there are increased risks for postoperative complications such as fistula formation, carotid rupture, wound infection, and pharyngeal stenosis. These risks are especially of concern when the tumor is recurrent and the individual has received prior radiation treatments to the tumor site. The healing of a fistula to the laryngeal region requires meticulous management of fistula drainage, with scheduled irrigations and packing of the wound.

Salivary drainage from a fistula, when there is insufficient tissue coverage of the carotid, can result in the most dreaded critical complication — carotid artery rupture. If the patient is at risk for this condition, "carotid artery blowout precautions" are in order. For carotid blowout, supplies kept at the bedside include gloves, a cuffed tracheostomy tube of the correct size, sterile saline, and towels for padding.

Should a carotid rupture occur, the nurse, following standard precautions, assists the medical team in securing the airway with the inflation of the cuffed tracheostomy tube, engaging the suction, and applying pressure to the site (using saline-soaked gauze for intraoral bleeding and padding to the neck for an external rupture). Later laryngeal complications, which can require surgical repair, include tracheostomal stenosis and hypopharyngeal stricture.

Paranasal surgery

One month postresection, the patient may be taught to use a 50% solution of 3% hydrogen peroxide and water to loosen crusting. A sponge-tipped applicator is used to gently scrub the skin graft, followed by rinsing of the oral cavity with a salt-and-soda solution. These patients are at risk for infection, due to the decreased blood supply with postoperative tissue contraction. The irrigation solution should be changed daily and the equipment is regularly cleaned with soap and water.

If the sinus tumor has invaded the patient's orbit, a radical maxillectomy with orbital exteneration will need to be performed. Following this procedure, the oral cavity is checked for displacement of packing, which is replaced if necessary.

The head of the patient's bed should remain elevated to promote nasal drainage, minimize edema, and improve nasal breathing. The patient will need time to accommodate proprioceptively to the loss of vision in one eye and is at increased risk for falls during the postoperative phase.

Prior to discharge, the patient must be taught oral irrigation and hygiene skills and instructed in care of the prosthetic device.

Salivary gland surgery

When facial nerve injury has occurred because of surgery, the cornea needs protection from eye abrasions. Eye drops and ophthalmic ointments are used to provide moisture to the cornea. If facial numbness occurs, the skin is protected from sun, wind, and cold damage.

Postoperative care: care of flaps and grafts

Skin grafts and flaps allow blood flow to and from the affected area, allowing nutritional support, oxygenation, thermoregulation, and transport of metabolic waste. To ensure proper healing, the donor and recipient sites are frequently assessed and the conditions documented.

Full-thickness (FTSG) and split-thickness skin grafts (STSG) are secured by suturing the graft into the recipient defect. Full-thickness grafts are usually harvested from areas of the body which have natural creases, such as the preauricular, supraclavicular, or lower lateral regions of the neck. STSGs may also be taken from the lateral thigh.

When the recipient site is the floor of mouth, the area is bolstered in the operating room with gauze saturated with bismuth tribromophenate (XeroForm). This bolus packing is not disturbed until it is removed in approximately five days. Regular oral care cannot begin until the bolus dressing is removed. While the dressing remains in place, the patient's oral cavity is assessed frequently for drainage, odor, and infection. Once the dressing is removed, the patient receives instruction on oral hygiene.

In the operating room, donor sites for skin grafts are often covered with a transparent adhesive film product that is occlusive to liquids and bacteria. The film product provides a moist environment that promotes healing (and limits scarring), allowing for observation and assessment. The transparent dressing conforms to the patient's wound and may stay in place, undisturbed, for as long as seven days. Once the dressing is ready to be removed, it causes less discomfort to the patient.

If the surgeon uses a dry dressing, generally it is padded with a circular gauze dressing and stays in place for several days after surgery. Sterile technique is used when changing the dressing. If it becomes dry and adheres to the wound, saline-soaked gauze is applied to the area for several minutes to release it. Gentle manipulation is used when removing the dressing to prevent damage to viable tissue and bleeding which delays healing.

The patient is more likely to complain of pain at the donor site than at the recipient defect. Analgesics are administered every three to four hours. Friction of any sort on the donor graft can increase the individual's discomfort during the early postresection days. With flaps, it is important to avoid placing pressure on the flap from tracheostomy ties or dressings so that they do not restrict blood flow and promote venous congestion in the flap.

If ischemia of the graft occurs, there may be decreased perfusion pressure and lowered platelet activation following thrombus development at the level of the anastomoses. If lymphatic drainage is obstructed, then interstitial pressure may increase, causing edema.

When myocutaneous flaps are used, the surgeon provides instruction about how to maintain proper positioning to prevent tension or entanglement of the pedicle of the graft. The incision sites are to be kept clean, typically by using a 50% hydrogen peroxide and 50% normal saline solution, three or four times per day. Fibrin build-up on the suture line interferes with granulation and provides an avenue for infection.

Surgical restoration: reconstruction

Microvascular free tissue transfer (reconstruction flaps) has gained worldwide acceptance as a means to reconstruct post-oncologic surgical defects in the head and neck region.[50–52]

With a wide resection, reconstruction involves pedicle flaps and grafts to close defects.[53,54] Recent advances in reconstructive surgical techniques include neovascularization, microvascular soft tissue transfer, and delivery of sufficient blood flow through the flap or graft. Full-thickness skin grafts (epidermis and dermis) may cover large defects. Such grafts to cover facial defects (nasal tip, eyelid, or auricle) are harvested from preauricular or postauricular areas.

STSGs are nearly transparent, with a thickness between 0.006 and 0.02 inch. The lateral thigh is a common site for the STSG harvest. This type of graft has limited use in facial reconstruction, because the thin graft can shrink or shift as it contracts and wrinkles following radiation therapy.[55] Complications after graft surgery are associated with the type of graft, with revascularized flaps showing some diminished rate of complications. Functional outcomes after reconstruction flap surgery have been promising.[55–57]

Radiation Therapy

Early-stage cancer of the head and neck can be treated with radiation or surgery. Radiation has been used successfully alone for early-stage tumors (T1, T2) and for cases when resection is not advisable (i.e., neck dissection is not feasible based on the extent of the tumor, the patient's general medical condition, or an anticipated unacceptable deficit).[23]

For locally advanced tumors (T3, T4) and for patients at high risk of local recurrence, radiation therapy follows surgery in the combined treatment of choice. High-risk cases include T4 tumors, close or positive margins, perineural/perilymphatic/vascular invasion of the same tumor, positive multiple nodes, and extracapsular invasion. Studies have established a dose of up to 60 Gy (200 cGy/day) in 5–6 weeks as standard adjuvant treatment for locally advanced cancers of the mouth and throat. Relapse rates are 11% with negative margins, and 26% with positive margins.[58]

After surgery, if the residual tumor burden is minimal, then postoperative radiation is effective. If the risk of relapse is high without postoperative irradiation (i.e., the margin of resection is unsatisfactory, extracapular extension is present, or the morbidity of irradiation is low), salvage treatment is possible.

Advancements in surgery have made it possible to resect cancers that had previously been regarded as incurable. Similarly, new developments in radiation oncology have improved the outlook for patients with locally advanced or recurrent head and neck cancers. Among these advancements are refinements in altered fractionation, three-dimensional conformal radiotherapy, intensity-modulated radiotherapy, stereotactic radiosurgery and fractionated stereotactic radiotherapy, neutron-beam radiotherapy, charged-particle radiotherapy, and intraoperative radiotherapy. These developments have allowed radiation oncologists to escalate the dose of radiation delivered to tumors while minimizing the dose delivered to surrounding normal tissue.[59]

Adjuvant treatment strategies

Postoperative radiation therapy reduces the risk of local–regional failure and probably improves survival. Patients who are at high risk for recurrence after surgery may benefit from more aggressive dose-fractionation schedules that may include altered fractionation to decrease the overall time from surgery to the completion of radiation thearpy. Adjuvant chemotherapy also appears to improve the probability of cure in high-risk patients.[23,48]

In an effort to increase the effectiveness of radiation therapy while at the same time minimizing toxicity, different schedules of radiation therapy have been tested. For example the randomized controlled trial of CHART (continuous hyperfractionated accelerated radiotherapy) was compared to conventional scheduled radiotherapy in 918 patients. Mucositis in the CHART cohort was found to start and peak earlier but also ended earlier than in those patients who received conventional therapy. For a given dose and overall treatment time, highly significant increases in incidence and severity of both mucositis and erythema were seen with increasing field size.[60] These data prove that altered fractionation increases acute side effects.[61]

Despite the use of conformal techniques, the prognosis of patients who have recurrent or new primary head and neck cancer and who receive re-irradiation is poor, and complications are not infrequent. Nevertheless, some clinicians argue that a subset of patients is salvageable, and high-dose re-irradiation may be appropriate in selected patients.[61,62]

Brachytherapy and interstitial implantation

Interstitial and endocavitary brachytherapy are well-accepted modes of radiotherapy that are commonly used in recurrent head and neck cancer. Successful brachytherapy treatment of head and neck tumors uses low dose rate brachytherapy.[63]

Brachytherapy for head and neck tumors places radioactive material in close proximity to or directly into the tumor on a temporary basis. The treatment is generally well tolerated. A commonly used radioisotope for this treatment is cesium-137, which is used for both intercavitary and interstitial implants. Other radioisotopes used for head and neck tumors include iridium-192 and gold-198. The determination of a specific radionuclide for brachytherapy is based on its half-life. For example, the half-life of cesium-137 is 30 years, while iridium-192 has a half-life of 74 days.

Implants are most often placed in the operating room, under general anesthesia. When surgery is not an option, brachytherapy may be combined with external beam therapy to boost the total dose of radiation to the tumor.

Primary tumor sites that are more often treated with implants are the tongue, lip, floor of mouth, skin, nasal vestibule, and buccal mucosa. Implants are generally uncomfortable. BOT lesions, for example, may be treated with needles placed into the dorsum and through the tongue to the BOT region. Pain must be managed and nutritional status monitored. Oral intake may be too uncomfortable for the patient. Also, brachytherapy may adversely affect the individual's ability to speak and enunciate.

Only limited experiences exist with high dose rate brachytherapy (HDRBT) in patients with head and neck cancers. One report suggests that HDRBT with ^{192}Ir, is an effective treatment modality in locoregional recurrent head and neck cancer. In cases of persistent or residual tumor after primary radiochemotherapy, a local boost with brachytherapy can improve the patient's chance for cure.[63]

Another study reported that radioactive iodine-125 sources can boost treatment to the region of primary tumor after resection and external beam irradiation.[64,65]

Intensity-modulated-radiation-treatment (IMRT)

Locoregional recurrence remains a major obstacle to achieving cure of locally advanced head and neck cancers despite maximal resection and postoperative external beam radiation therapy. Locoregional failure occurs in 30%–40% of high-risk resected head and neck cancer patients after standard postoperative external radiation.[66]

One strategy suggested to improve radiation delivery is intensity-modulated radiation treatment (IMRT).[67–69] The definitive benefit of IMRT is not yet established, because a sufficient body of prospective trial data has not yet been accumulated. However, the expectations for this modality are high. IMRT is the next evolutionary step for three-dimensional conformal radiotherapy (3–DCRT). IMRT plans are generated with computer-optimized nonuniform radiation beam focused on a narrowly defined target or field. The technique better regulates and controls the dosage given by fractionation so that higher doses are possible without more intense side effects. The tumor receives higher doses; lower doses go to areas of subclinical disease.[67]

Intraoperative radiation therapy (IORT)

Another approach to increase the effectiveness of radiotherapy is intraoperative radiation therapy (IORT). High-dose rate IORT delivers a single, large dose of radiation (17.5 Gy) at the time of surgery when the tumor bed is exposed.[69] Trials of this modality have focused on recurrent disease. Some researchers have also added external beam radiation therapy after high-dose IORT.[70]

In addition to aggressively treating the tumor bed during surgery, high-dose IORT has the potential to allow reduction of subsequent doses of external beam radiation therapy, shortening overall treatment time and to provide a means for dose escalation. Planning is key in the successful delivery of high-dose IORT. Special attention is needed to properly treat lymph nodes and subclinical disease fields adjoining the gross tumor bed.[71]

Chemotherapy

When organ preservation is the goal, induction chemotherapy followed by radiation therapy may be indicated for locally advanced tumors (larynx and hypopharynx). This form of chemoradiation has smiliar rates of overall survival when compared to surgery plus induction chemotherapy followed by radiation therapy. Even so, local failure can occur, so options for salvage surgery need to be preserved.[23] A typical induction regimen is cisplatin 100 mg/m^2 IV on day 1 with 5-FU, 1000 mg/m^2 per day as continuous infusion for 5 consecutive days, repeating every 3 weeks.

Chemotherapy as single therapy for advanced, distant head and neck cancer has demonstrated limited effectiveness. In patients with metastatic or recurrent disease who are given the standard induction regimen (cisplatin and 5-FU), the five-year survival rate is approximately 30%. Alternative protocols have combined paclitaxel with carboplatin as treatment for recurrent or metastatic SCCHN. Tumor response, time to progression, and survival advantages were modest at best, with significant toxicities being noted.[28]

Other combination therapy trials currently use cisplatin or methotrexate plus fluorouracil (5-FU). These protocols generally include a total of three or four chemotherapy drugs.

Adjuvant chemotherapy is being evaluated in clinical trials, but is not considered a standard treatment strategy. So far, patients who are at low risk of disease recurrence (i.e., negative resection margins, one or no positive nodes, no extracapsular spread of the tumor), have not been shown to benefit from adjuvant chemotherapy.[23]

Chemoradiation: the RADPLAT protocol

Based on clinical studies reported in the 1990s, protocols that combine simultaneous chemotherapy and radiation therapy have been shown to be effective in advanced head and neck cancers. These studies showed a significant improvement in response rates, especially when cisplatin-based chemotherapy regimens were used. However, the disease-free survival benefit of these regimens has produced mixed results.[72]

A protocol was developed in the late 1990s to provide more durable survival rates while preserving organ function. The novel protocol—called RADPLAT—involved weekly administration of high dose cisplatin directly to the tumor site (150 mg/m^2) with simultaneous intravenous thiosulfate (9 g/m^2). Radiation therapy was also given during the treatment period.[72]

Patients receiving treatment under the RADPLAT protocol had better survival rates with organ preservation. A study published in 2000 reported on 213 patients with stage III/IV head and neck cancer who were treated in conformance with the RADPLAT protocol. In the study, 80% of the patients had a complete response in the primary site of tumor and 62% had a complete response in the regional site. Coupled with neck dissection, 98% of the patients showed no regional disease. The recurrence rate was 26%, and the five-year survival rates were calculated at 38.8% overall and 53.6% cancer related.[73]

Additional studies using the cisplatin-intraarterial protocol with radiation therapy reported a complete or partial response rate of 91% with durable disease-free survival rates for both previously untreated and recurring treated patients.[74] Although providing excellent treatment of locoregional disease, RADPLAT has shown to have limited effectiveness for patients with subclinical metastases or micrometastases at distant sites.[73]

Since the initial promising reports of RADPLAT as a concurrent chemoradiation, clinicians have developed variations of salvage protocols for local and regionally advanced SCCHN. Because the intraarterial scheduling of RADPLAT has proved to be operationally difficult, chemoradiation schedules—with chemotherapy delivery through regular intravenous and oral routes—are more prevalent. These strategies have resulted in high response rates, significant complete response rates, and improved survival. In addition to cisplatin, chemotherapy agents given with radiation therapy include docetaxel, 5-FU, Tegafur, carboplatin, bleomycin, paclitaxel, and hydroxyurea).[75–81] The total radiation dose to the primary tumour site and neck lymph nodes is 63–74 Gy, given in fractionated daily doses.[77,80] Protocols have included induction chemotherapy of carboplatin and paxlitaxel followed by weekly chemotherapy and high-dose radiation courses to increase response rates, decrease distant failure, and increase survival rates.[80,81]

Variations of the chemoradiation schedule have included 3-week multiple fractionated daily doses of radiation therapy rather than daily doses, which lasted 7 weeks. The condensed radiation schedule allowed for a higher daily dose of cisplatin, with acute and late toxicities being similar in both schedules and equal, if not better, response rates being observed. In a study of 86 patients with recurrent SCCHN who were treated with radiation with concurrent hydroxyurea and 5-FU, results showed a moderate mean increase and one-year survival advantage compared with systemic chemotherapy.[82]

No matter what the combination protocol, significant toxicities have been reported, especially mucositis and moist desquamation of the skin. In an attempt to minimize toxicity, chemotherapy and radiation have been given on an alternating basis.[83–85] Nevertheless, to achieve optimal therapy strategies, further trials need to address the choice of drugs, their schedule, and the radiation dose and schedule coupled with surgery.[83–90] For an updated list of NIH sponsored clinical trials, the reader is referred to the NIH: Clinical trials Website.

Other protocol variations have been tried. For example, the neo-RADPLAT protocol consisted of four weekly intraarterial infusions of cisplatin (150 mg/m^2) and intravenous infusions of sodium thiosulfate (9 g/m^2), and concurrent radiation therapy (2 daily doses of 50 Gy) followed by tumor resection at 8 weeks.[85] Published results from this protocol for patients with oral cancer showed that 80% had a complete response to chemoradiation in the primary site and 79% had a complete response in the neck. The five-year estimates for overall survival, disease-specific survival, and locoregional control were 54%, 64%, and 74%, respectively.[85]

Treatment Strategies for Specific Head and Neck Cancers

Nasal fossa and paranasal sinuses

Small tumors can be treated by either surgery or radiation therapy. Surgery and postoperative radiation therapy may result in improved local control and survival with no evidence of disease recurrence, but complications are more severe when compared with radiation therapy alone.[91] Elective neck irradiation has been seen as unnecessary for patients with early-stage disease.

Tumor spread commonly occurs along the lateral walls of the nasal cavity. Local spread is to the maxillary sinus or nasopharynx and may be present upon initial diagnosis. Concomitant or sequential multimodal treatment can provide improved local and regional control.

For maxillary sinus lesions, when the tumor is confined to the sinus, a maxillectomy will usually be performed. Prior to surgery, a consultation with the maxillofacial prosthodontist will be scheduled. The prosthodontist will make impressions of the hard and soft palates and then create an obturator that will be used to fill the surgical defect. Following resection of the cancer, a skin graft may be required to cover the surgical defect. The graft also counters contraction of the tissue, which is a normal part of the healing process. The obturator will be wired into place in the operating room following resection, after the defect is packed with petroleum-based gauze or nonadhering intermediate reline resin.

The ability to speak and to complete the oral phases of swallowing are restored for the patient with placement of the obturator, so there may be no need for a nasogastric tube postoperatively. After about five days, the surgeon removes the obturator and gauze and examines the surgical site. A removable obturator is designed by the prosthodontist. The patient is taught how to remove, clean, and replace the obturator. It can take as many as six months of revisions before the fit of the obturator is satisfactory, depending on the size of the defect and the healing necessary following chemotherapy and radiation. The patient is taught to remove the obturator after every meal and at bedtime. The patient then irrigates the cavity with a solution of normal saline and baking soda, which cleanses the area without causing irritation.

Skull base

Large lesions are treated with a combination of surgery and chemotherapy, while small tumors can be treated with radiation therapy alone. Surgery can involve the head and neck surgeon, neurosurgeon, microvascular surgeon, and plastic surgeon. For patients with stage III or IV tumors, chemotherapy is combined with radiation therapy.

In addition to the risk of standard complications following surgery (aspiration pneumonia, pulmonary edema, congestive heart failure, myocardial infarction, and sepsis), postsurgical complications may include cerebral spinal fluid (CSF) leak, increased intracranial pressure (cerebral edema), artery thrombosis, seizure, and stroke.

Close monitoring of intracranial pressure (ICP) assists in detecting subtle changes requiring immediate interventions to correct bleeding or promote adequate ventilation. Headache is an early sign of increasing ICP. Fluid balance can be erratic. Wide fluctuations in blood pressure can occur postoperatively as a result of vasoconstriction and insufficient cerebral perfusion.

As the patient recovers from treatment, he or she may need rehabilitation for impaired vision and for defects in swallowing, hearing, mobility, and balance.

Nasopharynx

Treatment of small nasopharyngeal cancers with radiation is the treatment of choice and yields 80%–90% survival rates.[15] Surgery is generally not recommended due to the difficulty in accessing this location.

Intracavitary brachytherapy has been effective in salvaging early-stage locally persistent or first-recurrence nasopharyngeal carcinoma.[92]

Patients with positive lymph nodes, cranial nerve involvement, and bone destruction have more advanced disease and are generally resistant to multimodality treatment.[15] Most recurrences occur in the first five years post-treatment. Studies have looked at the benefits of multisegmental IMRT with or without chemotherapy for treating nasopharyngeal patients. A recent study of 83 patients showed that there was high locoregional control for nasopharyngeal carcinoma with multisegmental IMRT. However, distant metastases proved to have a negative impact on survival.[93]

For nasopharyngeal radiation treatment, both sides of the patient's neck are usually treated, even when there is no current evidence of lymph node spread. This is because the risk is high for undetectable neck disease. The delivery of radiation therapy to this site is complex, with critical attention being paid to protect the spinal cord from injury.

Serous otitis media, with obstruction of the eustachian tube, is associated with treatment of nasopharyngeal malignancies. Prior to any radiation treatment, in anticipation of serous drainage during treatment, the surgeon may perform a myringotomy with ventilation tube insertion.

For locoregional control of advanced disease (T3, T4), chemotherapy is given in conjunction with radiation therapy. One effective regimen combines epirubicin, cisplatin, and infusional fluorouracil (5-FU) chemotherapy followed by radiation with concurrent cisplatin.[94]

Oral cavity

Early-stage cancers (stages I and II) of the lip and oral cavity are highly curable by surgery or by radiation therapy. For early-stage oral cancer, external beam radiation therapy and brachytherapy have been used successfully. The presence of a positive margin or a tumor depth greater than 5 mm significantly increases the risk of local recurrence and suggests the need for combined modality treatment.

With oral cavity tumors, depending on the clinical stage, a continuous or discontinuous ipsilateral neck dissection is performed to prevent regional spread, followed by adjuvant radiation therapy. Chemoradiation protocols are used for patients with advanced, recurrent, and metastatic head and neck cancer,[19] although evidence is limited regarding their survival benefit.[95]

Salvage surgery after treatment with radiation or chemotherapy has been shown to have limited survival benefit except when recurrent locoregional tumors were initially staged at stage I or II.[96] Early reports indicate that IMRT may benefit these patients by allowing the option of reradiating fields when locoregional relapses occur while reducing the toxicities associated with standard radiation treatment.[97]

Oropharynx

Stage I and II tumors of the oropharynx are managed similarly to early-stage oral cavity malignancies.

Early carcinoma of the tonsil can effectively be treated using single modality therapy. Local regional control and survival are similar following surgery or radiotherapy. Radiation therapy is used for recurrent disease. Advanced disease warrants multimodality therapy.[98]

Base of the tongue (BOT) cancers can be treated with surgery and postoperative radiation. These strategies offer patients a high probability of locoregional control, survival, and good quality of life.[99]

A surgical resection of the BOT carcinoma is the most difficult site of the oropharynx to manage postoperatively. Therefore, primary high-dose irradiation, often with brachytherapy, is added. A higher level of tumor control may be achieved with a local surgical resection plus a neck dissection.

For advanced (T4) BOT tumors, treatment is usually a total laryngectomy in conjunction with total resection of the tongue base. A laryngectomy is necessary when the adjacent preepiglottic space, which is separated by only a thin membrane from the tongue base, has tumor invasion.

A total laryngectomy removes the entire tumor. With the recent advances in combination therapy, however, tumor control may be accomplished without the need for a laryngectomy. This organ-sparing treatment involves a hyperfractionated (twice daily) schedule of radiation therapy and may include brachytherapy as part of the treatment plan.

Adjuvant chemotherapy can maintain local tumor control.[90,100] Results from selected studies regarding the benefit of concomitant chemotherapy with radiation therapy appear promising.[101,102] For advanced oropharyngeal tumors, concomitant chemotherapy with radiation therapy has been shown to be more effective than radiation therapy alone in terms of disease-free survival. Nevertheless, overall survival has not been shown to improve.[103]

Salivary gland

For patients with parotid tumors, the standard treatment is a superficial parotidectomy with facial nerve dissection. This procedure may be both diagnostic (with the biopsy confirming the histology) and therapeutic (removal of the tumor).

Distant metastasis is the most common cause of treatment failure. Total parotidectomy with neck dissection and adjunctive radiation therapy remains the preferred treatment for local and regional control of disease.[104]

Radiation may be a treatment option for inoperable locoregional disease. Surgery, radiation, and repeat radiation are treatment options for local relapse, whereas radical neck dissection is indicated for regional relapses. Metastastic disease may be either treated with radiotherapy or palliative chemotherapy, depending on the site of metastasis.[105]

Glottis and larynx

Unlike supraglottic tumors, glottic carcinomas initially remain localized. Lymphatic supply is limited in this region, resulting in a lower percentage of early spread to the cervical neck nodes. Glottic tumors are also more likely to be detected early, because the individual promptly develops symptoms of hoarseness.

In situ tumors can be treated with laser vaporization, microexcision, or radiation therapy.[106] The advantage of laser excision and irradiation to the glottis over surgical treatment is the retention of a near-normal voice. With microexcision surgery, the voice changes the least.

Patient's with T2 glottic carcinomas with fixed, immobile vocal cords may be treated with irradiation alone or by a vertical hemilaryngectomy. For the vertical hemilaryngectomy, the surgeon removes a part or all of the true vocal cord and false vocal cord, as well as the associated half of the thyroid cartilage. If the vocal cord is fixed and evidence of tumor extension or invasion is found, generally a total laryngectomy will be necessary.

In advanced cases of glottic carcinomas, patients with T3 or T4 tumors are treated with either a total laryngectomy plus neck dissection and adjuvant radiation therapy or radiation therapy followed by surgical salvage as necessary for persistent disease.[107]

For early-stage laryngeal cancer, both surgery and radiotherapy are effective treatment modalities, offering a high rate of local control.[108,109] Radiation therapy as a choice for treatment is based on the locoregional extent of the malignancy, efforts to maintain the patient's functioning vocal cords, and expected disease-free and survival outcomes of disease.[105,108] Factors in the multivariate analysis that contributed to the choice of treatment included the independent prognostic factors of gender, region of origin, T stage, nodal involvement, differentiation, and hemoglobin.

The mainstay treatment for advanced-stage laryngeal cancer is conservation laryngeal surgery.[111] Efforts to improve the treatment and prognosis of advanced-stage laryngeal cancer have focused on combination chemotherapy and radiation regimens.[109] A multivariate analysis of prognostic factors in 1252 patients with laryngeal SCC treated with primary radical radiotherapy was reviewed. The study revealed that 10% of patients had positive neck nodes. Most of the patients (48%) had stage I disease; 24% had stage II disease; 18% had stage III disease, and 10% had stage IV disease. Of these patients, 60% were controlled by primary treatment and 40% had residual tumor or recurrent disease. The larynx was preserved in 62% of patients. The five-year actuarial values for disease-specific and overall survival were 78% and 60%, respectively.[110]

Future Management Strategies

Developments in the prevention or treatment of head and neck cancers focus on better understanding of the molecular and genetic bases of the diseases as well as novel treatment approaches. As our understanding of the inherited genetic factors for head and neck cancers grows, agents can be targeted those who show genetic susceptibility. Emerging data (both phenotypic and genotypic) point to differences in DNA repair ability, carcinogen metabolism, and cell-cycle control as the systems that are important to the risk of tobacco-induced malignancies.[112]

Epidermal growth factor receptor (EGFR) has been shown to be a transmembrane glycoprotein that is highly expressed in SCCHN. Agents in development block the effects of growth factors, which are proteins that promote cell growth, thereby triggering cancer cell growth. These agents are directly injected into the cancer cell or blood vessel.[17] Increased expression of EGFR is associated with enhanced tumor invasiveness, resistance to chemotherapy, and a lower patient survival rate.[113] Therapies that incorporate two categories of treatment using EGFR inhibitors — monoclonal antibodies and tyrosine kinase inhibitors — may potentiate chemotherapy and radiation therapy.[114]

Among those agents in trials is the anti-EGFR monoclonal antibody IMC-C225, which competitively binds to the extracellular receptor site and prevents binding by the natural EGFR ligands EGF and transforming growth factor-alpha. Phase I studies of IMC-C225 combined with chemotherapy or radiation showed promising response rates in patients with recurrent or refractory SCCHN. This monoclonal antibody's clinical efficacy appears to involve multiple mechanisms, including inhibition of cell-cycle progression, induction of apoptosis, inhibition of angiogenesis, inhibition of metastasis, and enhancement of the response to chemotherapy and radiation therapy. Phase II and III trials of IMC-C225, are ongoing.[113]

The human papillomavirus (HPV) has been a focus of study since it was found to be associated with SCCHN. Vaccines are in development that seek to stimulate HPV-specific immune responses. Two HPV oncogenic proteins, E6 and E7, have been targeted in experimental vaccine systems.[115]

Alteration of the *p53* tumor suppressor gene has been shown to be associated with a high risk of developing SCCHN. Thus *p53* appears to play an important role in the pathogenesis and progression of head and neck cancers. Further understanding of the role of *p53* gene mutations might clarify the diagnosis, prognosis, and treatment of high-risk patients.[116] For example, local recurrence is the most common cause of mortality after SCCHN surgery; *p53* gene mutations have been observed in tissue adjacent to the tumor, and constitute a good prognostic marker of tumor recurrence. Resected tumors with negative margins have been shown to have residual tumor cells with persistent *p53* mutations at the margins. This finding suggests that patients with submicroscopic marginal involvement may have a worse prognosis than patients with negative margins.[116,117]

Using *p53* as a foundation, clinicians may eventually be able to determine the most appropriate therapeutic strategy, especially for chemotherapy and radiation, in the individual patients.[118,119] A 2002 meta-analysis, which included studies of patients with head and neck cancer, looked at immunohistochemically detected *p53* mutations in epithelial tumors. The analysis reported that *p53* overexpression had a nearly significant negative effect on outcome of treatment with cytotoxic drugs and radiation.[119]

Given that the mutation of *p53* is one of the most frequent genetic changes found in human cancer, gene therapy that capitalizes on the effects of *p53* has been targeted in treatments that seek to use radiotherapy and thermotherapy to treat head and neck cancers.[120–122]

For oral cancers, photodynamic therapy has been shown to be clinically useful, with improvements in photosensitizers and technology being anticipated.[123]

Symptom Management and Supportive Care

Rehabilitation is key to a patient's recovery and continued stability after head and neck cancer treatment. Rehabilitation programs and services involve a team of multidisciplinary professionals, who can help a patient learn and adapt to his or her new lifestyle after surgery.[124] The rehabilitation period begins before treatment, and continues throughout the therapeutic period until complete recovery is achieved.

Before therapy begins, the patient needs to establish ways to communicate that will sustain him or her after treatment. Simple means to continue communication include pads of paper and pens or pencils, a computer or other electronic device, an erasable whiteboard, or a picture book, that shows commonly used phrases or items.

Swallowing

Preservation and/or restoration of swallowing is a primary rehabilitation goal after most head and neck surgeries.[125] A speech pathologist in partnership with a radiologist helps evaluate and treat patients who have diminished or no swallowing function (dysphagia) due to their disease or treatment.[126]

It is not uncommon that swallowing function for patients following radiation treatment for nasopharyngeal cancer continues to deteriorate over time, even many years after radiation therapy has ended.[127] Poorer outcomes of voice and swallowing function may also be observed for patients with the glottic and supraglottic cancer.[126]

Before a patient takes food or fluid orally, swallowing function is evaluated and rehabilitation efforts are put in place. For example, a patient who has had a tongue resection will need to learn how to use the remainder of the tongue to propel a bolus of food back to and through the anterior faucial arches for the first phase of swallowing. The swallow trigger is affected when the cranial nerves have been impaired or damaged by disease or treatment. Cranial nerves that can be affected are the trigeminal (V), facial (VII), glossopharyngeal (IX), vagus (X), spinal accessory (XI), or hypoglossal (XII) nerves (Table 54-2).

To assess an individual's degree of dysphagia it is important to determine the presence or absence of aspiration, any voice impairment, ease of movement of the larynx, any evidence of gurgling with respiration, and the degree of fatigue. Further assessment by video-fluoroscopy or modified barium swallow shows how liquid or food travels. Evaluation includes the presence or absence of aspiration, the amount of pharyngeal residue post-swallow, and the amount of time it takes to complete all three phases of swallowing.

Swallow Therapy

The action of swallowing requires mobility of pharyngeal structures, which allow liquid or food boluses to move through the patient's oral cavity, fauces, pharynx, and esophagus, and into the stomach. For example, a supraglottic laryngectomy affects the pharyngeal phase of swallowing, decreasing protection of the glottis. Until swallowing techniques are learned, the patient is at risk of aspiration. When structures in the oral cavity and oropharynx undergo extensive resections (requiring flap reconstruction), swallowing phases change, creating difficulties such as drooling of saliva, decreased mastication, aspiration, and pooling of food and fluids. In addition, radiation therapy to this area causes xerostomia, with loss of lubrication of the food bolus and taste changes.

The speech therapist works with patients in anticipation of the first oral intake, Normally, aspiration is prevented during the pharyngeal phase of swallowing by spontaneous, sequential actions: (1) the epiglottis closes to protect the laryngeal inlet; (2) the true vocal cords come together; (3) the larynx rises and moves forward; (4) the cricopharyngeus opens in response to the laryngeal pull; and (5) the bolus travels above the larynx to the open cricopharyngeus and on to the esophagus.

Supraglottic swallowing is a technique that protects the airway from aspiration. It includes the following steps:

1. Prepare the bolus of food in the oral preparatory phase.
2. Before initiating the swallow, hold one's breath to close the vocal cords.
3. Swallow while still holding one's breath.
4. Cough while exhaling after the swallow to expectorate remaining food or fluids on top of vocal cords, thereby preventing aspiration.

Additional compensatory strategies that the speech pathologist may recommend include postural changes that facilitate passage of food into the oral cavity and pharynx (head elevated); changes in food consistency (i.e., thin versus thick fluids, semisolid versus pureed foods—Jello, applesauce, or mashed potatoes); indirect swallowing therapy—jaw and tongue range of motion exercises; and adduction of tongue exercises; to improve laryngeal closure.

Table 54-4 Dysphagia in Head and Neck Cancer Patients: Exercises and Compensatory Swallow Techniques

Problem	Technique
Oral Preparatory Phase Problems	
Decreased lip closure	Labial strength/ROM
Decreased mandibular ROM	ROM exercises
Decreased tongue ROM	ROM exercises/head tilt Palatal augmentation prosthesis Effortful swallow Reduce each bolus volume Head back position
Pharyngeal Phase Problems	Alternate liquids/solids Limit diet to liquids/pureed foods Multiple swallows per bolus Turn head toward affected side Tilt head toward stronger side
Laryngeal Protection Problems	Mendelsohn maneuver Supraglottic swallow Chin tuck maneuver Laryngeal adduction exercises

ROM = range of motion.

Data from Stephen Goldman, M.A.C.C., Speech Pathology Associates, 2004.

Table 54-4 provides an example of a plan of care for dysphagia, which a speech therapist might follow during the patient's rehabilitation.

Speech

Rehabilitation efforts that concentrate on improving or restoring the patient's ability to speak are key to a patient's continued progress in recovery and beyond. Research indicates that the communication needs, communication methods, and perception of voice quality among patients with head and neck cancer are often ignored by professionals during the in-hospital period.[128] Moreover, a study of patients with nonlaryngeal head and neck cancer reported significant objective and subjective changes in vocal function (articulation and phonation) long after their radiation treatments ended.[129]

To offset the limitations affecting communication ability post-treatment, standards for rehabilitation of individuals who use laryngeal speech have been created.[130,131] These standards include support and plans of care that prescribe speech therapy. As part of these care plans, speech pathologists recommend exercises to increase strength, range of motion, coordination, and accuracy of tongue movement. In addition, these plans support the use of oral prostheses to compensate for tissue loss and allow for greater contact of the tongue with the palate, thereby creating more intelligible speech.

In esophageal speech, air that is swallowed becomes trapped in the esophagus, then is released. This technique allows air to vibrate against the walls of the esophagus. The puff of air is like a burp. It vibrates the walls of the throat, making sound for the new voice. The tongue, lips, and teeth form words as the sound passes through the mouth. This type of speech sounds low pitched and gruff, but it usually more closely resembles a natural voice than speech made by a mechanical larynx.[131,132]

A tracheoesophageal prosthesis or puncture (TEP) uses an opening created by the surgeon, called a tracheoesophageal fistula. A small plastic or silicone valve fits into this opening. The valve keeps food out of the trachea. After a TEP, patients can cover their stoma with a finger and force air into the esophagus through the valve. The air produces sound by making the walls of the throat vibrate. Sound is formed by air from the lungs, creating a better quality of esophageal speech.[131–133]

Mechanical speech using a hand-held, battery-operated electrolarynx or pneumatic larynx transmits the vibration of sound when the patient holds the device to his or her neck or near the mouth. A pneumatic larynx is held over the stoma and uses air from the lungs instead of batteries to make it vibrate.

Young patients may have the worst result, and vocal dysfunction may increase with time.[134] Voice function decline is well documented after radiation therapy. Nevertheless, because voice function has been shown to decline with age, the additional impact of postradiation therapy changes can be equal to dystonia that comes with age.[135]

Mucositis

Oral mucositis remains the most common complication among patients with head and neck cancer.[136,137] Radiation and/or chemotherapy (e.g., methotrexate and 5-FU) can destroy the rapidly regenerating epithelial cells on the mucous membrane. With this damage comes oral mucositis, an inflammation that is both progressive and painful.[137]

Tissues that are at risk of mucositis include the buccal mucosa, soft palate, tonsillar pillars, lateral tongue, pharyngeal walls, and larynx. Mucositis can appear as early as the first week of radiation treatment, and its severity can increase over time.[138] Clinical reports indicate that mucositis can be more severe with altered fractionation of radiation therapy.[139] This trend may be associated with late effects of radiotherapy, characterized by a decreased number of blood vessels and by significantly different expression patterns of the adhesion and of integrins and macrophage subpopulations.[139]

Patients report that pain is the worst part of their treatment experience and that the mucositis accompanying a sore throat is more than just a sore mouth.[140] Mucositis affects the patient's ability to eat and enjoy a full quality of life. When eating is difficult (no taste, dry mouth), patients report that their quality of life is significantly compromised. They need additional emotional and psychosocial support because the sequelae from mucositis may extend beyond physical or pharmaceutical treatment of the mucositis.[140]

Table 54-5 describes a scoring system that takes into account mucositis as well as xerostomia.

Oral Care

Oral care is key to management of mucositis. Therapies have been designed to interfere with the causative factors of mucositis, thereby protecting normal mucosa either through direct radioprotection or by manipulation of growth factors and cytokines that are involved in mucosal repopulation. Other therapies have tried to counter inflammation or infection.[141] Weak evidence suggests that local antibiotics have a clinically significant ability to prevent acute radiotherapy side effects. There is insufficient evidence that radioprotective agents offer clinically significant protection of parotid glands.[142]

Patients are cautioned to use only the recommended mouth rinses and to avoid using solutions containing alcohol. Individuals also should be taught to avoid spicy and acid-containing fruits, vegetables, and juices (e.g., oranges, grapefruits, lemons, and tomatoes). Both hot and cold foods can induce pain. Systemic analgesics such as hydrocodone or acetaminophen alone or with codeine may be necessary on an around-the-clock schedule or as needed.

Although a number of strategies and products are being investigated for oral care of patients with head and neck cancer, none are clearly superior to traditional regimens.[139] Most treatment protocols to prevent mucositis are based on clinical experience, but alternatives based on fundamental basic and clinical research are becoming more widely available.[143]

The results of studies that have evaluated prophylactic and ongoing treatment for oral mucositis are summarized in Table 54-6. Agents that have shown positive benefits include benzydamine oral rinse[144] and fluconazole for candida mucositis, allopurinal, and vitamin E.[145] In the *Cochrane Review*of interventions for treating oral mucositis, several agents — benzydamine HCl, tetracholorodecaoxide, chlorhexidine, and "magic" (lidocaine solution, diphenhydramine

Table 54-5 RTOG Scoring for Skin, Mucosal, and Tongue Reactions

	1	2	3	4
Acute skin reaction	Follicular, faint or dull erythema, epilation, dry desquamation, decreased sweating	Tender or bright erythema, patchy moist desquamation, moderate edema	Confluence, moist desquamation other than skin folds, pitting edema	Ulceration, hemorrhage, or necrosis
Acute mucous membrane reaction	Inflammation, may experience mild pain not requiring analgesic	Patchy mucositis that may produce an inflammatory serosanguineous discharge, may experience moderate pain requiring analgesics	Confluent fibrinous mucositis, may include severe pain requiring narcotic	Ulceration, hemorrhage, or necrosis
Acute salivary gland reaction	Mild mouth dryness, slightly thickened saliva may have slightly altered taste such as metallic taste, these changes not reflected in baseline feeding behavior, such as increased liquid with meals	Moderate mouth dryness, thick sticky saliva, markedly altered taste	Complete mouth dryness, markedly altered taste or absence of taste	Acute salivary gland necrosis
Acute pharynx reaction	Mild dysphagia or odynophagia, may require topical anesthetic or non-narcotic analgesics, may require soft diet	Moderate dysphagia or odynophagia, may require narcotic analgesics, may require soft or liquid diet	Severe dysphagia or odynophagia with dehydration or weight loss (>15% from pretreatment baseline) requiring NG feeding tube, IV fluids, or hyperalimentation	Complete obstruction, ulceration, perforation, fistula
Actue larynx reaction	Mild or intermittent hoarseness, cough not requiring antitussive, erythema of mucosa	Persistent hoarseness but able to vocalize, referred ear pain, sore throat, patchy fibrinous exudate or mild arytenoids, edema not requiring narcotic, cough requiring antitussive	Whispered speech, throat pain or referred ear pain requiring narcotic, confluent fibrinous exudate, marked arytenoids edema	Marked dyspnea, stridor or hemoptysis with tracheostomy or intubation necessary
Acute tongue reaction	Mild erythema, may have slightly altered taste not affecting nutritional intake	Tender, bright erythema, coated, loss of papillae with shiny appearance, markedly altered taste, moderate pain requiring analgesia	Blistered, cracked appearance, markedly altered taste or absence of taste, severe pain requiring narcotic	Ulceration, hemorrhage, or necrosis

Data from Radiation Therapy Oncology Group, 1995.

hydrochloride, and aluminum hydroxide suspension) —were not found to be effective.[146]

The most effective way to treat radiation-induced mucositis in patients with head and neck cancer remains frequent oral rinsing with a bland mouthwash, such as saline or a sodium bicarbonate rinse, to reduce the amount of oral microbial flora. Dental care, consistent oral assessments, and the initiation of a standardized oral hygiene protocol before cancer treatment begins are the most effective approaches for oral mucositis.[136,146]

Patients benefit most when they cleanse the oral cavity every three to four hours during the day and at night if possible. Cleansing the oral cavity with a soft bristle brush, using toothpaste with baking soda or saline/soda rinses, and flossing regularly are important components of oral care.[136,137,146,147] Despite such rigorous oral hygiene, white or yellow patches may appear as a result of epithelial tissue destruction. A sore throat or mouth closely follows, and by the fourth to fifth week of treatment, the discomfort has been building and the tissue is vividly erythemic.

After treatment ends, late complications are common, especially in elderly patients. Repeat irradiation may induce serious complications (additional mucositis, xerostomia, malnutrition, pain) because of overdosage to previously irradiated areas. There are reports of severe late complications developing 3–10 months after re-irradiation.[148]

Pain can be managed topically by a pharmaceutical mixture of anesthetic and anti-inflammatory medications along with an antacid, which provides a coating action to promote its adherence to tissues. Patients are taught to swish this mixture for two to three minutes, then expectorate or swallow (if allowed) four times a day (e.g., after meals and at bedtime). Coating agents

Table 54-6 Treatment for Oral Mucositis

Category	Agent	Efficacy	Comments
Saliva stimulant	Pilocarpine	Mixed results, may be more efficacious for nonradiation-induced xerostomia	Can take up to 12 weeks for effect in radiotherapy patients; can cause sweating, headache, urinary frequency
	Artificial saliva (mucin or carboxymethylcellulose based)	Short duration	Mucin (porcine derivative) unsuitable for Muslims, religious Jews, other groups
	Vitamin C	Limited data, subjective findings demonstrate superiority over artificial saliva only	Local irritation, demineralization of teeth make it unsuitable for long-term use in dentate patients
	Citric acid	Limited data demonstrating efficacy in non-RT-related xerostomia only	May cause burning sensation, demineralization of teeth
Oral rinse, antimicrobial	Chlorhexidine	Overall no significant change in severity or suppression	Reports of rinse-induced discomfort, taste alteration, teeth staining
Oral rinse, antiseptic	Hydrogen peroxide	Mixed results in clinical trials	Long-term use discouraged; breaks down granulation tissue, disrupts flora
	Providone-iodine	Data indicate possible advantage over hydrogen peroxide in terms of severity and duration	Should be diluted; full-strength formulation damages new granulated tissue
	0.9% saline solution	No formal evaluation available	Relatively innocuous, economical
	Sodium bicarbonate	No formal evaluation available	Creates alkaline environment that promotes bacterial microflora; unpleasant taste; NCI recommended
	0.9% saline/sodium bicarbonate	No formal evaluation available	NCI recommended

(continued)

may also be topically applied in the event of breakthrough discomfort.

Because mucositis represents the dose-limiting acute toxicity and xerostomia ranks as the most common long-term quality of life complaint, a reduction of the External Beam Radiation Therapy (EBRT) dose may provide an important benefit in reducing toxicity, especially when combined with the radioprotectant amifostine. Amifostine as a treatment for mucositis is currently a component of a clinical trial that combines High dose radiation–intraoperative radiation treatment (HDR-IORT) with a reduced dose of postoperative EBRT to improve locoregional control and quality of life outcomes in patients with advanced-stage, resected head and neck cancer.[149]

Xerostomia

Radiation injury can cause permanent, noncorrectable xerostomia or the lack of saliva. Because radiation treatment can damage the salivary glands, the patient's production of saliva may decrease by as much as 50% during the first one to two weeks of treatment. As treatment progresses, the saliva becomes thick, tenacious, ropey, or even nonexistent. Without saliva, the patient experiences burning sensations or ulcerations, difficulty swallowing, and oral friction that is associated with tongue adherence to the palate or buccal mucosa. Various studies have reported that xerostomia is one of the major patient-reported distresses from therapy.[150,151]

Xerostomia is commonly measured and graded using objective measures of major salivary gland output and observer-rated toxicity grading.[152] Additional elements of grading have better defined functional deficits.

Although artificial saliva products are available, the soothing effect is costly and only temporary. Xerostomia may be equally relieved with frequent small sips of water. Patients are advised to carry a water bottle with them. Hard candies and sugarless gum are other ways to moisten the oral mucosa. It is usually recommended

Table 54-6 Treatment for Oral Mucositis[136–156] (Continued)

Category	Agent	Efficacy	Comments
Coating agent, mucosal protectant	Sucralfate suspension	Most data demonstrate no statistically significant difference in severity, pain intensity scores, and other subjective symptoms (taste alterations, dry mouth)	May offer little or no benefit compared to oral hygiene, symptomatic treatment
	Hydroxypropyl cellulose film	Initial studies are mostly open label; some products provide relief for at least 3 hours	Further study needed
	Kaolin pectate	Limited data, usually mixed in "cocktail"	NCI recommended
	Aluminum hydroxide	Limited data, usually mixed in "cocktail"	Coating may interfere with oral assessment
Mucosal protectant cytokine-like agent	Granulocyte-macrophage colony-stimulating factor	Some data indicate reduction in severity, pain;	May prove especially beneficial for chemotherapy or radiotherapy patients; with use, patients discontinue due to intolerable side effects: local skin reactions, fever, bone pain, nausea when administered subcutaneously
	Granulocyte colony-stimulating factor	Limited data, some indication of significant reductions in bone marrow transplant patients; occurrences less in radiotherapy patients when used as prophylactic	Further study needed
Anti-inflammatory, immunity promotion	Immunoglobulin	Limited data, may lessen severity in patients receiving radiation and chemotherapy	Further study needed
Topical anesthetic	Viscous lidocaine	Limited data, may provide significant relief of limited duration	Further study needed
	Benzocaine sprays/gels; Dyclonine rinse; Diphenhydramine solution	See viscous lidocaine	See viscous lidocaine

that dentures not be worn. The use of either tobacco or alcohol further dries and irritates the mucosa.

Sodium bicarbonate toothpaste and swabs will help to thin the saliva and can partially correct the acidic effect of xerostomia. Zinc sulfate may play a role in the perception of taste by the patient who receives radiation.

The combination of partial salivary gland sparing and radiation protectors/stimulants may provide additive or synergistic gains in reducing the severity of xerostomia.[152,153] To increase secretions from the remaining portions of the salivary gland, a few medications may help. Pilocarpine may be prescribed either upon beginning or following radiation therapy.[154] To offset the diaphoresis as a side effect of pilocarpine, patients are encouraged to increase fluid intake.

Along with pilocarpine, antholetrithione promotes saliva secretion. The radioprotectant amifostine, shown to be effective in reducing mucositis and dysphagia following radiation therapy,[155] has also been shown to reduce acute and chronic xerostomia, especially when the radiation field is limited.[156]

Loss of Taste

Diminished saliva flow results in changes to taste and smell, especially when taste or olfactory cells are in the radiation field. Taste changes are typically first reported by the second week of radiation treatment and become most pronounced two months after treatment begins. The alterations to the taste of salty and bitter foods are the most pronounced changes, while the taste of sweets is the least affected.[157]

Dental Prophylactic Care

A dental evaluation should precede radiation therapy, with extractions as necessary. A preradiation oral examination and treatment[158] will identify existing oral disease, the potential risk of oral disease, remove infectious dental/oral areas, and establish an adequate standard of ongoing oral hygiene and care.[159] Among the effects of radiation therapy are reduced vascularity and oxygen tension of the oral hard and soft tissues and salivary gland dysfunction. These changes increase the risk of dental decay and oral infections and may lead to reduced healing capacity following oral surgery procedures. An additional severe complication of radiation therapy is osteoradionecrosis of the jaw bone.[160] To improve mastication, speech, and saliva control for patients with osteoradionecrosis, the patient can benefit from acrylic/rubber prosthetics.[161] Patients are commonly instructed on appropriate oral hygiene and the use of fluoride trays.

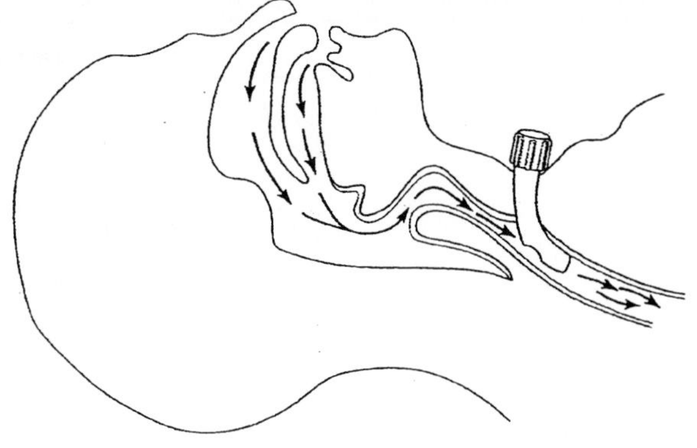

Figure 54-8 Airway using a fenestrated trache tube. (Data from Nelcor Puritan Bennett, 2004.)

Trismus

Patient treatment involving the oral cavity (e.g., surgery or grafts) can affect muscles for mastication and the posterior mandible. When the oral cavity opening is tightly restricted, the condition called trismus results. With trismus, the patient is at risk of developing fibrosis of oral cavity muscles. With time, exercises can stretch the interarch of the oral cavity. An example of such an exercise is increasing the number of stacked tongue blades to stretch the opening. This exercise should be done three or four times a day.

Pain Management

Pain is a significant problem for patients with head and neck cancer during treatment as their tumors grow.[162] Pain can occur because of surgery. For example, severed superficial nerves may cause numbness in the initial postoperative period. Subsequent edema may cause feelings of pressure. When the jugular vein has been ligated or occluded, the increase in spinal fluid pressure may cause the patient to experience throbbing, pounding, and pressure sensations in the head.

Pain from mucositis and skin erythema, as well as toxicities from radiation and chemotherapy treatment, can build as treatment courses progress. In a study of patients with nasopharyngeal cancer, the pain from radiation treatment was often severe and undertreated, affecting swallowing and talking more than sleeping or other general activities.[163] In a similiar study of individuals who had pain post-treatment, 31% of the patients had pain at diagnosis. Later, 74% reported some degree of pain at 6–12 months following treatment.[162] A significant number of patients rejected regular pharmacological management and employed a variety of other pain-relieving methods. The authors concluded that this patient population has a unique pain experience and attitudes toward pain management.

Tracheostomy Care

When the airway is compromised by tumor or postoperative edema, the surgeon will perform a tracheostomy. The procedure is needed if an airway obstruction is anticipated or to manage an existing, compromised pulmonary function. The tracheostomy may be temporary or permanent.

As a form of treatment, the surgeon may perform a total laryngectomy (TL). A TL results in a complete separation of the pharynx from the trachea. It removes the cricoid and thyroid cartilage, both arytenoids, both true vocal cords, both false vocal cords, the epiglottis, the preepiglottic and paraglottic spaces, and the hyoid bone.

Care for laryngeal cancer patients includes ongoing attention to tracheostomy care and suctioning. Individuals with a total laryngectomy will require only a temporary laryngectomy tube, which is short and wide in comparison to the conventional tracheostomy tube. The laryngectomy tube helps to shape the stoma. Table 54-7 lists ways to troubleshoot problems that may arise for individuals with a tracheostomy tube.

Individuals with altered airways have lost their ability to moisten, warm, or filter the air they breathe. This results in thick, tenacious, dry tracheal secretions

Table 54-7 Tracheostomy Tubes: Solving Problems

Symptom	What May Have Happened	What to Do
Excessive air leak through nose and mouth	Insufficient air in cuff (cuffed tubes only)	Deflate and reinflate the cuff with the proper amount of air
	Leak in cuff, inflation line, pilot balloon, or luer valve (cuffed tubes only)	Replace the tube
	Tube too small for trachea	Call doctor
	Uncuffed versus cuffed tube	Call doctor
	Fenestrated inner cannula is in tube (see Figure 54-8)	Remove and replace with nonfenestrated inner cannula
Tube comes out of neck opening	Excessive pull or weight at the connector	Readjust tubing to reduce pulling
	Trache tube ties are too loose or are tied incorrectly	Retie and secure
Difficulty when removing inner cannula for fenestrated tube	Tracheal lining may be pushing through the fenestration	Call doctor
	Trache tube alignment has changed	Call doctor
Tube or part of tube breaks or does not work	Excessive use or wear on the tube	Replace tube
	Trach tube was cleaned using wrong cleaning agents	Replace tube; use recommended cleaning agents
	Excessive pulling or weight on connector	Readjust tubing to reduce pulling
	Trache tube ties are too loose or are tied incorrectly	Retie and secure
Unable or difficult to pass suction catheter through trache tube	Mucous plug	Remove inner cannula and clean it if reusable; replace it if disposable
	Catheter is too large for tube size	Replace with correct size
	Tube is not properly positioned in the trachea	Reposition the tube
	Fenestrated inner cannula is in the tube	Replace with a nonfenestrated inner cannula

that are a challenge to clear by coughing. If they cannot be cleared, the secretions may create mucous plugs that obstruct the tracheostomy tube and can block breathing.

To avoid developing these plugs, supplemental humidity is necessary. In the hospital, warm, humidified oxygen should be administered via tracheostomy collar when the patient is at rest. At home, a large (ten-gallon) humidifier in the living area and a small bedside humidifier in the sleeping room are useful to provide needed humidity. Patients can apply moistened gauze pads at the trache site and foam or crocheted stoma covers to collect the moisture of exhaled air and optimize humidity. Also, they can instill up to 5 mL of normal saline or spray four to five puffs of normal saline into the stoma using a nasal atomizer.

Nutritional Management

Nutritional support provides the calories for healing after surgical resection and during intensive radiation or chemotherapy treatments. Before their diagnosis, many patients with head and neck cancer already have nutritional deficits. When the malignant process starts or treatment begins, cancer-related weight loss is common because diseases of the head and neck cause impairments in mastication and/or deglution.[164] Patients can become malnourished after surgery or during treatment, increasing their risk of complications — specifically, infection and delayed wound healing.[165] Loss of appetite and weight contribute to weakness and lethargy and predict a poor prognosis for cancer patients.[143,166] In addition, patients with these malignancies may be severely malnourished because of years of tobacco or substance abuse, which can contribute to liver disease.

With cancer-related weight loss, caregivers can be realistic in setting eating goals and, when appropriate, provide pharmacologic interventions with progestational agents or corticosteroids — both of which are aimed at managing anorexia. Other pharmacologic interventions include thalidomide (Thalomid), adenosine triphosphate, and nonsteriodal anti-inflammatory drugs. These interventions promise to replenish lean tissue but require further investigation before they can be recommended as standard clinical practice.[166]

Enteral Therapy

If the upper GI tract is compromised or fully obstructed because of disease or treatment, the patient's ability to swallow is impaired. In such cases, enteral feedings may be necessary through a nasogastric feeding tube (NG tube) or a gastrostomy tube (G-tube), which is placed by a surgeon. Another option is the percutaneous puncture (PEG tube), a gastrostomy tube with a small diameter, which is placed by an interventional radiologist. Before it is used, its placement is checked by x-ray.

Tube feeding can start when the patient has bowel sounds. For either the NG tube or the G-tube, the patient assumes a sitting position or elevates the head of the bed. Generally feedings start at the slow rate of 25–30 mL/hour, increasing to 25 additional mL/hour per day to meet volume and calorie goals.

Tube feedings can occur via gravity or pump (bolus every 4–6 hours or continuous flow). Changes to the nutritionals used or the feeding schedule may be necessary if side effects develop, such as diarrhea. Diarrhea can be caused by certain antibiotics and medications containing sorbital.

Psychosocial Support

Head and neck malignancies can be devastating. Some of the key senses — including sight, taste, smell, hearing, and sense of touch — may be permanently impaired.

Survivors of head and neck cancer face many challenges that jeopardize their psyche. Researchers reports that these patients deal with a long list of issues, which may be categorized as treatment side effects, self-image disturbance, depression, and pain.[167] The rate of depression appears to remain higher with postlaryngectomy patients compared to the general population.[168] Also, these patients may possess risk factors for depression even before treatment begins.[168] Laryngectomy patients have been reported to be at increased risk of psychosocial stressors, depression, and suicide.[169] These patients also report problems with trismus, xerostomia, speech and swallowing disorders, fatigue, and self-image. Supporting these patients by recognizing and addressing their challenges has been shown to help with coping and improved patient-perceived quality of life.[170] When the social, emotional, and physical ways a person relates to others are changed by a deformity, the individual may feel isolated or rejected. It is clear that the need is great to support patients' coping strategies and to help them maintain their involvement in important relationships, activities, and interests.[169]

Table 54-8 Selected Web-Based Sources of Information and Support for Patients with Head and Neck Cancer

Source	Website
Support for People with Oral and Head and Neck Cancer	*www.spohnc.org*
Let's Face It USA	*www.faceit.org*
National Cancer Institute	*www.nci.nih.org*
International Association of Laryngectomees	*www.larynxlink.com*
Head and Neck Cancer Community	*www.headandneckcancer.org*

During the first weeks of treatment, the person is coping with self-image changes. Furthermore, while dealing with fatigue, the individual must learn complex self-care rituals such as dressing changes, tracheostomy care, and suctioning, as well as enteral feeding techniques. Conscientious assessment of coping, social situations, risk factors, systematic rehabilitation efforts, ongoing counseling, and support may improve outcomes for patients.[169]

Signs of effective coping immediately after surgery include the patient's attention to self-care and resocialization.[169] Appropriate interventions to help patients and their families will support their skill building, set boundary limits, help them focus on dealing with current problems, and support their coping mechanisms. A 2001 study prospectively documented anxiety in surgical patients with head and neck cancer. The findings suggest that at a specific point in time (postoperative day 5), self-care precedes a reduction in anxiety, and that this negative relationship increases over time.[171]

To boost psychosocial support, a visit by a recovered patient with a similar diagnosis may be requested from the Lost Chord Club, American Cancer Society, or another community support group. Such a visit may be well received about seven days after surgery. Contact with Internet support groups may also benefit the patient (Table 54-8). Nevertheless, it is important to provide continued clinical support and follow-up to augment Internet resources and connections.[169]

Quality-of-Life Issues

As treatments for head and neck cancer have improved, preserving organ function and extending disease-free periods, researchers have focused on the patient's quality of life. In addition to the psychological challenges of treatment and survivorship, frequently cited problems that patients must address following treatment include pain, xerostomia, speech and swallowing disorders, trismus, fatigue, weakness, and weight loss.[137]

Increased symptoms, observed over the six months after therapy, are associated with decreased quality of life.[172] Although quality of life is multifactorial and subjective, studies show that some improvement may be achieved when healthcare professionals recognize and address symptom and coping problems during the course of treatment.[170] Quality of life can also be improved when social and family well-being are addressed.[149]

Studies indicate that pain and the functional impairment of chewing and swallowing are the most important parameters before treatment. Immediately after surgical treatment, other variables that are fundamental to quality of life are speech intelligibility and mobility disorders in the head, neck, and shoulder regions.[173,174] Yet studies indicate that no amount of preoperative counseling prepares patients and families for the aftermath of laryngectomy surgery. One study reported that the period for the highest level of stress within families is 6 months after surgery, plateaus by 12 months, and reaches a level of stabilized and improved quality of life measured at 2 years after treatment.[168]

In a study of post-treatment oropharyngeal patients, when physical, role, emotional, cognitive, and social functioning can be addressed and problem-solved, quality of life is rated as generally good.[175] Yet head and neck cancer involves very distinct sites, which researchers caution must be taken into account when assessing quality of life. Morton and Izzard found that organ-preservation techniques do not necessarily lead to better quality of life outcomes, especially in laryngeal cancer.[176] Moreover, not much is known about the co-morbidity of continued alcohol abuse and tobacco use after surgery in laryngectomy patients.[169]

Healthcare providers commonly perceive disfigurement, alternation in function (loss of voice), and disease control as the most relevant issues in the postoperative period. Patients and families give high ratings to management of physical symptoms, social reintegration, participation in enjoyed activities, vocation issues, and communications impairment. Patients may be able to meet rehabiltation goals (talk and eat) but cannot cope with day-to-day living (relationships with family, spouse, finances, work, sexual interest and performance).[173]

Continuity of Care

Care of the patient with head and neck cancer is challenging for more reasons than just clinical issues. Barriers to providing the care, which requires many disciplines and resources, reside in a healthcare system that is already taxed by many demands. Patients expect optimal care even when insurance coverage is limited. With many patients being underinsured or lacking any insurance, the challenges become even greater.[177]

Many components in the patient's delivery of care are affected by dwindling healthcare resources. Surgical procedures now performed in same-day units limit the opportunity for presurgical and postprocedure teaching. Chemotherapy and radiation treatments are usually outpatient procedures. Even if the patient requires a hospital admission, the stay is usually short. Therefore, the opportunity to provide adequate teaching and support is limited. Due to the risk factors that are associated with these patients, their compliance with ongoing and after-care may be shaky.[178] These patients tend to be less health conscious and to have less social support than most other groups of cancer patients.

Integrating the rehabilitation team in after-care is another challenge. Among the multidisciplinary team members who come together for a patient with head and neck cancer are the oncologist, head and neck surgeon, dentist, nurse, dietician, physical therapist, social worker, and, in some instances, plastic surgeon, prosthodontist, and psychologist. Their services need coordination for these patients — specifically, in managing follow-up appointments, supplies and equipment, therapy sessions, dental care, symptom management, and psychosocial support.

References

1. American Academy of Otolaryngolog — Head and Neck Surgery: *Head and Neck Cancer. www.entnet.org/healthinfo/tobacco/cancer.cfm*(accessed March 20, 2004)
2. Haggood AS: Head and neck cancers, in Otto S (ed.): *Oncology Nursing* (ed 4). St. Louis, Mosby, 2001, pp 285–325
3. Walker DM, Boey G, McDonald LA: The pathology of oral cancer. *Pathology* 35:376–383, 2003
4. American Cancer Society: *Cancer Facts and Figures 2004.* Atlanta, American Cancer Society, 2004
5. National Cancer Institute: Oral Cancer (PDQ): Prevention, February 20, 2004. *www.nci.nih.gov/templates/doc_pdq.aspx?cdrid=62837.* Accessed March 15, 2004
6. National Cancer Institute: Oropharyngeal Cancer (PDQ): Treatment *www.nci.nih.gov/cancerinfo/pdq/treatment/oropharyngeal/healthprofessional.* Accessed March 15, 2004
7. Epstein JB, Epstein JD, Gorsky M: Characteristics of oral and paraoral malignant lymphoma: a population-based review of 361 cases. *Oral Surg Oral Med Oral Pathol Oral Radiol Endodont* 92:519–525, 2001

8. American Cancer Society: Detailed Guide: Nasopharyngeal CA: What Are the Key Stats about Nasopharyngeal Cancer? *www.cancer.org/docroot/CRI/content/CRI_2_4_1X_What_is_naso pharyngeal_cancer_17.asp?sitearea=CRI.* Atlanta, ACS, Accessed March 20, 2004
9. Ondrey FG, Wright SK: Neoplasms of the nasopharynx, in Snow JB (ed.): *Manual of Ororhinolaryngology Head and Neck Surgery.* Ontario, BC Decker, 2003, pp 484–495
10. National Cancer Institute: Hypopharyngeal Cancer (PDQ): Treatment, *www.nci.nih.gov/cancerinfo/pdq/treatment/hypopharyngeal/healthprofessional.* Accessed March 15, 2004
11. Weisman R, Moe K, Orloff L: Neoplasms of the larynx and laryngopharynx, in Snow JB (ed.): *Manual of Ororhinolaryngology Head and Neck Surgery.* Ontario, BC Decker, 2003, pp 470–483
12. National Cancer Institute: Salivary Gland Cancer (PDQ): Treatment *www.nci.nih.gov/cancerinfo/pdq/treatment/salivarygland/healthprofessional.* Accessed March 15, 2004
13. Mendenhall WM, Mancuso AA, Amdur RJ, et al: Squamous cell carcinoma metastatic to the neck from an unknown head and neck primary site. *Am J Otolaryngol* 22:261–267, 2001
14. American Cancer Society: *Alcohol and Cancer.* Atlanta, ACS, 2002
15. National Cancer Institute: Nasopharyngeal Cancer (PDQ): Treatment *www.nci.nih.gov/cancerinfo/pdq/treatment/nasopharyngeal/healthprofessional.* Accessed March 15, 2004
16. National Cancer Institute: Lip and Oral Cancer (PDQ): Treatment *www.nci.nih.gov/cancerinfo/pdq/treatment/lip-and-oral-cavity/healthprofessional.* Accessed March 15, 2004
17. American Cancer Society: *Oral Cancer.* Atlanta, ACS, 2002
18. Yokoyama A, Omori T: Genetic polymorphisms of alcohol and aldehyde dehydrogenases and risk for esophageal and head and neck cancers. *Jpn J Clin Oncol* 33:111–21, 2003
19. Cole P, Rodu B, Mathison A: Alcohol-containing mouthwash and oropharyngeal cancer: a review of the epidemiology. *J Am Dent Assoc* 134:1079–1087, 2003
20. Silverman S: *Oral Cancer: American Cancer Society, Atlas of Clinical Oncology.* Ontario, BC Decker, 2002
21. Koch W: Do I have a tumor of the oropharynx? Website of the American Head and Neck Society, *www.headandneckcancer.org/patienteducation/docs/oropharynx.php.* Accessed March 20, 2004
22. Fang B, Forastiere A: Head and neck cancer, in Abraham J, Allegra C (eds.): *Bethesda Handbook of Clinical Oncology,* New York, Lippincott, Williams and Wilkins, 2001, pp 3–28
23. Sheahan P, O'Keane C, Sheahan JN et al: Predictors of survival in early oral cancer. *Otolaryngol Head Neck Surg* 129:571–576, 2003
24. National Cancer Institute: Laryngeal Cancer (PDQ): Treatment *www.nci.nih.gov/cancerinfo/pdq/treatment/laryngeal/healthprofessional.* Accessed March 15, 2004
25. Helliwell TR: ACP best practice no 169. Evidence based pathology: squamous carcinoma of the hypopharynx. *J Clin Pathol* 56:81–85, 2003
26. National Cancer Institute: Paranasal Sinus and Nasal Cavity Cancer (PDQ): Treatment. *http://cancer.gov/cancerinfo/pdq/treatment/paranasalsinus/healthprofessional.* Accessed March 15, 2004
27. Monnerat C, Faivre S, Temam S, et al: End points for new agents in induction chemotherapy for locally advanced head and neck cancers. *Ann Oncol* 13:995–1006, 2002
28. Clark JI, Hofmeister C, Choudhury A, et al: Phase II evaluation of paclitaxel in combination with carboplatin in advanced head and neck carcinoma. *Cancer* 92:2334–2340, 2001
29. Hurt C, Yousem DM, Beauchamp N: Imaging neoplasms of the central nervous system, head and neck, in Holland JF, Frei E, et al (eds.): *Cancer Medicine* (ed 6, vol. 1) Hamilton, Ontario, BC Decker, 2003, pp 509–517
30. Loevner LA, Sonners AI: Imaging of neoplasms of the paranasal sinuses. *Magn Reson Imaging Clin North Am* 10:467–493, 2002
31. Chong VF, Khoo JB, Fan YF: Imaging of the nasopharynx and skull base. *Magn Reson Imaging Clin North Am* 10:547–571, 2002
32. Weber AL, Romo L, Hashmi S: Malignant tumors of the oral cavity and oropharynx: clinical, pathologic, and radiologic evaluation. *Neuroimaging Clin North Am* 13:443–447, 2003
33. Ng SY, Songra A, Ali N, et al: Ultrasound features of osteosarcoma of the mandible — a first report. *Oral Surg Oral Med Oral Pathol Oral Radiol Endodont* 92:582–586, 2001
34. Shah GV, Fischbein NJ, Patel R, et al: Newer MR imaging techniques for head and neck. *Magn Reson Imaging Clin North Am* 11:449–469, 2003
35. Ishikawa M, Anzai Y: MR imaging of lymph nodes in the head and neck. *Magn Reson Imaging Clin North Am* 10:527–542, 2002
36. Sheikholeslam-zadeh R, Choufani G, Goldman S, et al: Unknown primary detected by FDG-PET. A review of the present indications of FDG-PET in head and neck cancers. *Acta Otorhinolaryngol Belg* 56:77–82, 2002
37. Perez CA, Bradley J, Chao CK, et al: Functional imaging in treatment planning in radiation therapy: a review. *Rays* 27:157–173, 2002
38. Goerres GW, Schmid DT, Bandhauer F, et al: Positron emission tomography in the early follow-up of advanced head and neck cancer. *Arch Otolaryngol Head Neck Surg* 130:105–109; discussion 120–121, 2004
39. Kunkel M, Forster GJ, Reichert TE, et al: Detection of recurrent oral squamous cell carcinoma by [18F]-2-fluorodeoxyglucose — positron emission tomography: implications for prognosis and patient management. *Cancer* 98:2257–2265, 2003
40. Sato T, Indo H, Kawabata Y, et al: Dynamic scintigraphy with thallium-201 chloride (TI-201) for the diagnosis of tumors of the head and neck *Oral Surg Oral Med Oral Pathol Oral Radiol Endodont.* 92:228–235, 2001
41. Ahuja A, Ying M: Sonography of neck lymph nodes. Part II: abnormal lymph nodes. *Clin Radiol* 58:359–366, 2003
42. Gritzmann N, Hollerweger A, Macheiner P, et al: Sonography of soft tissue masses of the neck. *J Clin Ultrasound* 30:356–373, 2002
43. Alex JC: The application of sentinel node radiolocalization to solid tumors of the head and neck: a 10-year experience. *Laryngoscope* 114:2–19, 2004
44. von Buchwald C, Bilde A, Shoaib T, et al: Sentinel node biopsy: the technique and the feasibility in head and neck cancer. *ORL J Otorhinolaryngol Relat Spec* 64:268–274, 2002
45. American Joint Committee on Cancer: *AJCC Cancer Staging Manual* (ed 6). New York, Springer, 2002
46. Lip and oral cavity, in American Joint Committee on Cancer: *AJCC Cancer Staging Manual* (ed 6). New York, Springer, 2002, pp 23–32
47. O'Sullivan B, Shah J: New TNM staging criteria for head and neck tumors. *Semin Surg Oncol* 21:30–42, 2003
48. Mendenhall W, Amdur R, Hinerman R, et al: Postoperative radiation therapy for squamous cell carcinoma of the head and neck. *Am J Otolaryngol* 24:41–50, 2003
49. Samant S, Robbins KT, Kumar P, et al: Bone or cartilage invasion by advanced head and neck cancer: intra-arterial supradose cisplatin chemotherapy and concomitant radiotherapy for organ preservation. *Arch Otolaryngol Head Neck Surg* 127:1451–1456, 2001
50. Makitie AA, Beasley NJ, Neligan PC, et al: Head and neck reconstruction with anterolateral thigh flap. *Otolaryngol Head Neck Surg* 129:547–555, 2003
51. Nakatsuka T, Harii K, Asato H, et al: Analytic review of 2372 free flap transfers for head and neck reconstruction following cancer resection. *Reconstr Microsurg* 19:363–368, 2003

52. Rosenthal EL, Dixon SF: Free flap complications: when is enough, enough? *Curr Opin Otolaryngol Head Neck Surg* 11:236–239, 2003
53. Couch ME: Laryngopharyngectomy with reconstruction. *Otolaryngol Clin North Am* 35:1097–1114, 2002
54. Sabri A: Oropharyngeal reconstruction: current state of the art. *Curr Opin Otolaryngol Head Neck Surg* 11:251–254, 2003
55. Chepeha DB, Annich G, Pynnonen MA, et al: Pectoralis major myocutaneous flap vs revascularized free tissue transfer: complications, gastrostomy tube dependence and hospitalization *Arch Otolaryngol Head Neck Surg* 130:181–186, 2004
56. Hudgins PA: Flap reconstruction in the head and neck: expected appearance, complications, and recurrent disease. *Eur J Radiol* 44:130–138, 2002
57. Butler CE, Lewin JS: Reconstruction of large composite oromandibulomaxillary defects with free vertical rectus abdominis myocutaneous flaps. *Plast Reconstr Surg* 113:499–507, 2004
58. Laramore GE, Scott CB, Al-Sarraf M, et al: Adjuvant chemotherapy for respectable squamous cell carcinomas of the head and neck. Report on Intergroup Study 0034. *Int J Radiat Oncol Biol Phys* 23:705–713, 1992
59. Chou RH, Wilder RB, Wong MS, et al: Recent advances in radiotherapy for head and neck cancers. *Ear Nose Throat J* 80:704–707, 711–714, 716, 2001.
60. Bentzen SM, Saunders MI, Dische S, Bond SJ: Radiotherapy-related early morbidity in head and neck cancer: quantitative clinical radiobiology as deduced from the CHART trial. *Radiother Oncol* 60:123–135, 2001
61. Zackrisson B, Mercke C, Strander H, et al: A systematic overview of radiation therapy effects in head and neck cancer. *Acta Oncol* 42:443–461, 2003
62. Ng SH, Liu HM, Ko SF, et al: Posttreatment imaging of the nasopharynx. *Eur J Radiol* 44:82–95, 2002
63. Glatzel M, Buntzel J, Schroder D, et al: High-dose-rate brachytherapy in the treatment of recurrent and residual head and neck cancer. *Laryngoscope* 112(pt 1):1366–1371, 2002
64. Nag S, Cano ER, Demanes DJ, et al: American Brachytherapy Society. The American Brachytherapy Society recommendations for high-dose-rate brachytherapy for head-and-neck carcinoma. *Int J Radiat Oncol Biol Phys* 50:1190–1198, 2001
65. Beitler JJ, Smith RV, Silver CE, et al: Close or positive margins after surgical resection for the head and neck cancer patient. The addition of brachytherapy improves local control. *Int J Radiat Oncol Biol Phys* 40:313–317, 1998
66. Hu K, Ship JA, Harrison LB: Rationale for integrating high-dose rate intraoperative radiation (HDR-IORT) and postoperative external beam radiation with subcutaneous amifostine for the management of stage III/IV head and neck cancer. *Semin Oncol* 30(suppl 18):40–48, 2003
67. Penagaricano JA, Papanikolaou N: Intensity-modulated radiotherapy for carcinoma of the head and neck. *Curr Oncol Rep* 5:131–139, 2003
68. Chao KS, Ozyigit G, Thorsdad WL: Toxicity profile of intensity-modulated radiation therapy for head and neck carcinoma and potential role of amifostine. *Semin Oncol* 30(suppl 18):101–108, 2003
69. Ng SH, Liu HM, Ko SF, et al: Posttreatment imaging of the nasopharynx. *Eur J Radiol* 44:82–95, 2002
70. Huang D, Xia P, Akazawa P, et al: Comparison of treatment plans using intensity-modulated radiotherapy and three-dimensional conformal radiotherapy for paranasal sinus carcinoma. *Int J Radiat Oncol Biol Phys* 56:158–168, 2003
71. Eisbruch A, Foote RL, O'Sullivan B, et al: Intensity-modulated radiation therapy for head and neck cancer: emphasis on the selection and delineation of the targets. *Semin Radiat Oncol* 12:238–249, 2002
72. Argiris A: Update on chemoradiotherapy for head and neck cancer. *Curr Opin Oncol* 14:323–329, 2002
73. Doweck I, Robbins K, Viera F: Analysis of risk factors predictive of distant failure after targeted chemoradiation for advanced head and neck cancer. *Arch Otolaryngol Head Neck Surg* 127:1315–1318, 2001
74. Wilson WR, Siegel RS, Harisiadis LA, et al: High-dose intra-arterial cisplatin therapy followed by radiation therapy for advanced squamous cell carcinoma of the head and neck. *Arch Otolaryngol Head Neck Surg* 127:809–812, 2001
75. Katori H, Tsukuda M, Mochimatu I, et al: Phase I trial of concurrent chemoradiotherapy with docetaxel, cisplatin and 5–fluorouracil (TPF) in patients with locally advanced squamous cell carcinoma of the head and neck (SCCHN). *Br J Cancer* 90:348–352, 2004
76. Nabell L, Spencer S: Docetaxel with concurrent radiotherapy in head and neck cancer. *Semin Oncol* 30(suppl 18):89–93, 2003
77. Nagy B, Molnar J, Rovo L, et al: Effective chemoradiotherapy without additive toxicity in locoregionally advanced head and neck cancer. *Anticancer Res* 23:4329–4332, 2003
78. Tishler RB, Norris CM Jr, Colevas AD, et al: A Phase I/II trial of concurrent docetaxel and radiation after induction chemotherapy in patients with poor prognosis squamous cell carcinoma of the head and neck. *Cancer* 95:1472–1481, 2002
79. Suntharalingam M, Haas ML, Van Echo DA, et al: Predictors of response and survival after concurrent chemotherapy and radiation for locally advanced squamous cell carcinomas of the head and neck. *Cancer* 91:548–554, 2001
80. Vokes EE, Stenson K, Rosen FR, et al: Weekly carboplatin and paclitaxel followed by concomitant paclitaxel, fluorouracil, and hydroxyurea chemoradiotherapy: curative and organ-preserving therapy for advanced head and neck cancer. *J Clin Oncol* 12:320–326, 2003
81. Hainsworth JD, Meluch AA, McClurkan S, et al: Induction paclitaxel, carboplatin and infusional 5-FU followed by concurrent radiation therapy and weekly paclitaxel/carboplatin in the treatment of locally advanced head and neck cancer: a phase II trial of the Minnie Pearl Cancer Research Network. *Cancer J* 8:311–321, 2002
82. Spencer S, Wheeler R, Peters G, et al: Phase 1 trial of combined chemotherapy and reirradiation for recurrent unresectable head and neck cancer. *Head Neck* 25:118–122, 2003
83. Datta NR, Nagar YS, Singh S, et al: Loco-regional failures in head and neck cancer: can they be effectively salvaged by non-surgical therapeutic modalities? *Int J Clin Oncol* 8:31–39, 2003
84. Gemmete JJ: Complications associated with selective high-dose intraarterial cisplatin and concomitant radiation therapy for advanced head and neck cancer. *J Vasc Interv Radiol* 14:743–748, 2003
85. Robbins KT, Samant S, Vieira F, et al: Presurgical cytoreduction of oral cancer using intra-arterial cisplatin and limited concomitant radiation therapy (Neo-RADPLAT). *Arch Otolaryngol Head Neck Surg* 130:28–32, 2004
86. Haddad R, Tishler RB, Norris CM, et al: Docetaxel, cisplatin, 5-fluorouracil (TPF)–based induction chemotherapy for head and neck cancer and the case for sequential, combined-modality treatment. *Oncologist* 8:35–44, 2003
87. Harari PM, Mehta MP, Ritter MA: Clinical promise tempered by reality in the delivery of combined chemoradiation for common solid tumors. *Semin Radiat Oncol* 13:3–12, 2003
88. Kies MS, Haraf DJ, Rosen F, et al: Concomitant infusional paclitaxel and fluorouracil, oral hydroxyurea, and hyperfractionated radiation for locally advanced squamous head and neck cancer. *J Clin Oncol* 19:1961–1969, 2001

89. Sunwoo JB, Herscher LL, Kroog GS, et al: Concurrent paclitaxel and radiation in the treatment of locally advanced head and neck cancer *J Clin Oncol* 19:800–811, 2001
90. Adelstein DJ: Oropharyngeal cancer: the role of chemotherapy. *Curr Treat Options Oncol* 4:3–13, 2003
91. Katz TS, Mendenhall WM, Morris CG, et al: Malignant tumors of the nasal cavity and paranasal sinuses. *Head Neck* 24:821–829, 2002
92. Law SC, Lam WK, Ng MF, et al: Reirradiation of nasopharyngeal carcinoma with intracavitary mold brachytherapy: an effective means of local salvage. *Int J Radiat Oncol Biol Phys* 54:1095–1113, 2002
93. Liu MT, Hsieh CY, Chang TH, et al: Prognostic factors affecting the outcome of nasopharyngeal carcinoma. *Jpn J Clin Oncol* 33:501–508, 2003
94. Rischin D, Corry J, Smith J, et al: Excellent disease control and survival in patients with advanced nasopharyngeal cancer treated with chemoradiation. *J Clin Oncol* 20:1845–1852, 2002
95. Day TA, Davis BK, Gillespie MB, et al: Oral cancer treatment. *Curr Treat Options Oncol* 4:27–41, 2003
96. Wong LY, Wei WI, Lam LK, et al: Salvage of recurrent head and neck squamous cell carcinoma after primary curative surgery. *Head Neck* 25:953–959, 2003
97. Claus F, Duthoy W, Boterberg T, et al: Intensity modulated radiation therapy for oropharyngeal and oral cavity tumors: clinical use and experience. *Oral Oncol* 38:597–604, 2002
98. Genden EM, Ferlito A, Scully C, et al: Current management of tonsillar cancer. *Oral Oncol* 39:337–342, 2003
99. Harrison LB, Ferlito A, Shaha AR, et al: Current philosophy on the management of cancer of the base of the tongue. *Oral Oncol* 39:101–105, 2003
100. Kovacs AF, Ghahremani MT, Stefenelli U, et al: Postoperative chemotherapy with cisplatin and 5-fluorouracil in cancer of the oral cavity and the oropharynx — long term results. *J Chemother* 15:495–502, 2003
101. Denis F, Garaud P, Bardet E: Final results of the 94–01 French Head and Neck Oncology and Radiotherapy Group randomized trial comparing radiotherapy alone with concomitant radiochemotherapy in advanced-stage oropharynx carcinoma. *J Clin Oncol* 22:69–76, 2004
102. LoTempio MM, Wang MB, Sadeghi A: Treatment of advanced oropharyngeal cancers with chemotherapy and radiation. *Ear Nose Throat J* 82:367–370, 2003
103. Olmi P, Crispino S, Fallai C, et al: Locoregionally advanced carcinoma of the oropharynx: conventional radiotherapy vs. accelerated hyperfractionated radiotherapy vs. concomitant radiotherapy and chemotherapy — a multicenter randomized trial. *Int J Radiat Oncol Biol Phys* 55:78–92, 2003
104. Hosal AS, Fan C, Barnes L, et al: Salivary duct carcinoma. *Otolaryngol Head Neck Surg* 129:720–725, 2003
105. Licitra L, Bernier J, Grandi C, et al: Cancer of the larynx. *Crit Rev Oncol Hematol* 47:65–80, 2003
106. Flint PW: Minimally invasive techniques for management of early glottic cancer. *Otolaryngol Clin North Am* 35:vi–vii, 1055–1066, 2002
107. Bhalavat RL, Fakih AR, Mistry RC, et al: Radical radiation vs surgery plus post-operative radiation in advanced (resectable) supraglottic larynx and pyriform sinus cancers: a prospective randomized study. *Eur J Surg Oncol* 29:750–756, 2003
108. Hinerman RW, Mendenhall WM, Amdur RJ, et al: Early laryngeal cancer. *Curr Treat Options Oncol* 3:3–9, 2002
109. Lefebvre JL, Lartigau E: Preservation of form and function during management of cancer of the larynx and hypopharynx. *World J Surg* 27:811–816, 2003
110. Johansen LV, Grau C, Overgaard J: Laryngeal carcinoma — multivariate analysis of prognostic factors in 1252 consecutive patients treated with primary radiotherapy. *Acta Oncol* 42:771–778, 2003
111. Strome SE, Weinman EC: Advanced larynx cancer. *Curr Treat Options Oncol* 3:11–20, 2003
112. Sturgis EM, Wei Q: Genetic susceptibility — molecular epidemiology of head and neck cancer. *Curr Opin Oncol* 14:310–311, 2002
113. Herbst RS, Hong WK: IMC-C225, an anti-epidermal growth factor receptor monoclonal antibody for treatment of head and neck cancer. *Semin Oncol* 29(suppl 14):18–30, 2002
114. Tortochaux J, Aunoble B, Rolhion C, et al: [Targeting of epidermal growth factor receptor and applications in ORL cancer]. *Bull Cancer* 90:S220–S227, 2003
115. Devaraj K, Gillison ML, Wu TC: Development of HPV vaccines for HPV-associated head and neck squamous cell carcinoma. *Crit Rev Oral Biol Med* 14:345–362, 2003
116. Lopez-Martinez M, Anzola M, Cuevas N, et al: Clinical applications of the diagnosis of *p53* alterations in squamous cell carcinoma of the head and neck. *Med Oral* 7:108–120, 2002
117. Thames HD, Petersen C, Petersen S, et al: Immunohistochemically detected *p53* mutations in epithelial tumors and results of treatment with chemotherapy and radiotherapy. A treatment-specific overview of the clinical data. *Strahlenther Onkol* 178:411–421, 2002
118. Shinagawa Y, Kawamata H, Omotehara F, et al: Evaluation of the chemosensitivity of head and neck cancer cells based on the diverse function of mutated-p53. *Int J Oncol* 22:383–389, 2003
119. Vokes EE, Stenson K, Rosen FR, et al: Weekly carboplatin and paclitaxel followed by concomitant paclitaxel, fluorouracil, and hydroxyurea chemoradiotherapy: curative and organ-preserving therapy for advanced head and neck cancer. *J Clin Oncol* 21:320–326, 2003
120. Higuchi Y, Asaumi J, Murakami J, et al: Effects of *p53* gene therapy in radiotherapy or thermotherapy of human head and neck squamous cell carcinoma cell lines. *Oncol Rep* 10:671–677, 2003
121. Xi S, Grandis JR: Gene therapy for the treatment of oral squamous cell carcinoma. *J Dent Res* 82:11–16, 2003
122. Levitan DA, Nanda R, Rowley JD: Recurring chromosome rearrangements in human cancer, in Holland JF, Frei E, et al (eds.): *Cancer Medicine* (ed 6. vol. 1.) Hamilton, ON, BC Decker, 2003, pp 107–136
123. Date M, Sakata I, Fukuchi K, et al: Photodynamic therapy for human oral squamous cell carcinoma and xenografts using a new photosensitizer, PAD-S31. *Lasers Surg Med* 33:57–63, 2003
124. Papadas T, Charokopos N, Karamouzis MV, et al: Rehabilitation after laryngectomy: a practical approach and guidelines for patients. *J Cancer Educ* 17:37–39, 2002
125. Samlan RA, Webster KT: Swallowing and speech therapy after definitive treatment for laryngeal cancer. *Otolaryngol Clin North Am* 35:1115–1133, 2002
126. Jepsen MC, Gurushanthaiah D, Roy N, et al: Voice, speech, and swallowing outcomes in laser-treated laryngeal cancer. *Laryngoscope* 113:923–928, 2003
127. Chang YC, Chen SY, Lui LT, et al: Dysphagia in patients with nasopharyngeal cancer after radiation therapy: a videofluoroscopic swallowing study. *Dysphagia* 18:135–143, 2003
128. Happ MB, Roesch T, Kagan SH: Communication needs, methods, and perceived voice quality head and neck surgery: a literature review. *Cancer Nurs* 26:346–354, 2003
129. Perry AR, Shaw MA, Cotton S: An evaluation of functional outcomes (speech, swallowing) in patients attending speech pathology after head and neck cancer treatments: results and analysis at 12 months post intervention. *J Laryngol Otol* 117:368–381, 2003

130. Eadie TL: The ICF: a proposed framework for comprehensive rehabilitation of individuals who use alaryngeal speech. *Am J Speech Lang Pathol* 12:189–197, 2003
131. National Cancer Institute: What You Need to Know About Cancer of the Larynx. NIH Publication No. 02–1568, May 5, 2003. *www.nci.nih.gov/cancerinfo/wyntk/larynx*
132. Eksteen EC, Rieger J, Nesbit M, et al: Comparison of voice characteristics following three different methods of treatment for laryngeal cancer. *J Otolaryngology* 32:250–253, 2003
133. Koch WM: Total laryngectomy with tracheoesophageal conduit. *Otolaryngol Clin North Am* 35:1081–1096, 2002
134. Fung K, Yoo J, Leeper HA, et al: Effects of head and neck radiation therapy on vocal function. *J Otolaryngol* 30:133–139, 2001
135. Behrman A, Abramson AL, Myssiorek D: A comparison of radiation-induced and presbylaryngeal dysphonia. *Otolaryngol Head Neck Surg* 125:193–200, 2001
136. Shih A, Miaskowski C, Dodd MJ, et al: A research review of the current treatments for radiation-induced oral mucositis in patients with head and neck cancer. *Oncol Nurs Forum* 29:1063–1080, 2002
137. Rose-Ped AL, Bellm L, Epstein J, et al: Complications of radiation therapy for head and neck cancers. *Cancer Nurs* 6:461–467, 2002
138. Ohrn KE, Wahlin YB, Sjoden PO: Oral status during radiotherapy and chemotherapy: a descriptive study of patient experiences and the occurrence of oral complications. *Support Care Cancer* 9:247–257, 2001
139. Borbasi S, Cameron K, Questead B, et al: More than a sore mouth: patients' experience of oral mucositis. *Oncol Nurs Forum* 7:1051–1057, 2002
140. Prott FJ, Handschel J, Micke O, et al: Long-term alterations of oral mucosa in radiotherapy patients. *Int J Radiat Oncol Biol Phys* 54:203–210, 2002
141. Garden AS: Mucositis: current management and investigations. *Semin Radiat Oncol* 13:267–273, 2003
142. Zackrisson B, Mercke C, Strander H, et al: A systematic overview of radiation therapy effects in head and neck cancer. *Acta Oncol* 42:443–461, 2003
143. Vissink A, Burlage FR, Spijkervet FK, et al: Prevention and treatment of the consequences of head and neck radiotherapy. *Crit Rev Oral Biol Med* 14:213–225, 2003
144. Epstein JB, Silverman S Jr, Paggiarino DA, et al: Benzydamine HCl for prophylaxis of radiation-induced oral mucositis: results from a multicenter, randomized, double-blind, placebo-controlled clinical trial. *Cancer* 92:875–885, 2001
145. Koc M, Aktas E: Prophylactic treatment of mycotic mucositis in radiotherapy of patients with head and neck cancers. *Jpn J Clin Oncol* 33:57–60, 2003
146. Worthington HV, Clarkson JE, Eden OB: Interventions for treating oral mucositis for patients with cancer receiving treatment (Cochrane Review), in: *The Cochrane Library*. Issue 1. Chichester, UK, John Wiley and Sons, 2004
147. Dodd MJ, Miaskowski C, Greenspan D, et al: Radiation-induced mucositis: a randomized clinical trial of micronized sucralfate versus salt and soda mouthwashes. *Cancer Invest* 21:21–33, 2003
148. Ohizumi Y, Tamai Y, Imamiya S, Akiba T: Complications following re-irradiation for head and neck cancer. *Am J Otolaryngol* 23:215–221, 2002
149. Yu CL, Fielding R, Chan CL: The mediating role of optimism on post-radiation quality of life in nasopharyngeal carcinoma. *Qual Life Res* 12:41–51, 2003
150. Seikaly H: Xerostomia prevention after head and neck cancer treatment. *Arch Otolaryngol Head Neck Surg* 129:250–251, 2003
151. Nguyen NP, Sallah S, Karlsson U: Combined chemotherapy and radiation therapy for head and neck malignancies: quality of life issues. *Cancer* 94:1131–1141, 2002
152. Eisbruch A, Rhodus N, Rosenthal D, et al: How should we measure and report radiotherapy-induced xerostomia? *Semin Radiat Oncol* 13:226–234, 2003
153. Vissink A, Burlage FR, Spijkervet FK, et al: Prevention and treatment of the consequences of head and neck radiotherapy. *Crit Rev Oral Biol Med* 14:213–225, 2003
154. Haddad P, Karimi M: A randomized, double-blind, placebo-controlled trial of concomitant pilocarpine with head and neck irradiation for prevention of radiation-induced xerostomia. *Radiother Oncol* 64:29–32, 2002
155. Antonadou D, Pepelassi M, Synodinou M, et al: Prophylactic use of amifostine to prevent radiochemotherapy-induced mucositis and xerostomia in head-and-neck cancer. *Int J Radiat Oncol Biol Phys* 52:739–747, 2002
156. Gosselin TK, Mautner B: Amifostine as a radioprotectant. *Clin J Oncol Nurs* 6:175–176, 180, 2002
157. Maes A, Huygh I, Weltens C, et al: De Gustibus: time scale of loss and recovery of tastes caused by radiotherapy. *Radiother Oncol* 63:195–201, 2002
158. Hancock PJ, Epstein JB, Sadler GR: Oral and dental management related to radiation therapy for head and neck cancer. *J Can Dent Assoc* 69:585–590, 2003
159. Schiodt M, Hermund NU: Management of oral disease prior to radiation therapy. *Support Care Cancer* 1:40–43, 2002
160. Kanatas AN, Rogers SN, Martin MV: A practical guide for patients undergoing exodontia following radiotherapy to the oral cavity. *Dent Update* 29:498–503, 2002
161. Sykes LM: An interim extraoral prosthesis used for the rehabilitation of a patient treated for oseoradionecrosis of the mandible: a clinical report. *J Prosthetic Dentist* 86:130–134, 2001
162. Whale Z, Lyne PA, Papanikolaou P: Pain experience following radical treatment for head and neck cancer. *Eur J Oncol Nurs* 5:112–120, 2001
163. Huang HY, Wilkie DJ, Chapman CR, et al: Pain trajectory of Taiwanese with nasopharyngeal carcinoma over the course of radiation therapy. *J Pain Symptom Manage* 25:247–255, 2003
164. Dawson ER, Morley SE, Robertson AG, et al: Increasing dietary supervision can reduce weight loss in oral cancer patients. *Nutrition Cancer* 41:70–74, 2001
165. Porock D, Nikoletti S, Cameron F: The relationship between factors that impair wound healing and the severity of acute radiation skin and mucosal toxicities in head and neck cancer. *Cancer Nurs* 27:71–78, 2004
166. Jatoi A, Loprinzi CL: Current management of cancer-associated anorexia and weight loss. *Oncology* 15:497–502, 508–510, 2001
167. Fritz DJ: Life experiences of head and neck cancer survivors: a pilot study. *ORL Head Neck Nurs* 19:9–13, 2001
168. de Leeuw J, de Graeff A, Ros W, et al: Prediction of depression 6 months to 3 years after treatment of head and neck cancer. *Head Neck* 23:892–898, 2001
169. Cady J: Laryngectomy: beyond loss of voice — caring for the patient as a whole. *Clin J Oncol Nurs* 6:347–351, 2002
170. Talmi YP: Quality of life issues in cancer of the oral cavity. *J Laryngol Otol* 116:785–790, 2002
171. Dropkin MJ: Anxiety, coping strategies and coping behaviors in patients undergoing head and neck cancer surgery. *Cancer Nurs* 24:143–148, 2001
172. Sweed MR, Schiech L, Barsevick A: Quality of life after esophagectomy for cancer. *Oncol Nurs Forum* 29:1127–1131, 2002
173. Gellrich NC, Schimming R, Schramm A, et al: Pain, function, and psychologic outcome before, during, and after intraoral tumor resection. *J Oral Maxillofac Surg* 60:772–777, 2002

174. Laverick S, Lowe D, Brown JS, et al: The impact of neck dissection on health-related quality of life. *Arch Otolaryngol Head Neck Surg* 130:149–154, 2004
175. Tschudi D, Stoeckli S, Schmid S: Quality of life after different treatment modalities for carcinoma of the oropharynx. *Laryngoscope* 113:1949–1954, 2003
176. Morton RP, Izzard ME: Quality-of-life outcomes in head and neck cancer patients. *World J Surg* 27:884–889, 2003
177. Mignogna MD, Fedele S, Lo Russo L, et al: Costs and effectiveness in the care of patients with oral and pharyngeal cancer: analysis of a paradox *Eur J Cancer Prev* 11:205–208, 2002
178. Specht L: Oral complications in the head and neck radiation patient. Introduction and scope of the problem. *Support Care Cancer* 10:36–39, 2002

CHAPTER 55

Leukemia

Debra Wujcik, RN, MSN, AOCN®

Introduction

Leukemia is the name given to a group of hematologic malignancies affecting the bone marrow and lymph tissue. First described by the German pathologist Virchow in 1847 as simply "white blood," the term *leukemia* now includes abnormalities of proliferation and maturation in lymphocyte and myeloid (nonlymphocyte) cell lines. The acute leukemias are marked by an abnormal proliferation of immature blood cells with a short natural history (one to five months), while the chronic leukemias have an excessive accumulation of more mature-appearing but still ineffective cells and a slower, progressive course (two to five years). The excessive proliferation of the leukemia cells results in an overcrowding of the bone marrow, causing a decreased production and function of normal hemopoietic cells.

In the last decade, much has been learned about the biology of leukemia through cytogenetic and molecular analysis. This has led to an era of risk-adapted therapy where the identification of specific genetic abnormalities determines the aggressiveness of treatment and the expected prognosis.[1,2]

Epidemiology

Leukemia represents 2% of the cancer incidence in the United States, with an estimated 33,440 new cases and 23,300 deaths in 2004.[3] More than one-half of the cases are acute; the remaining cases are chronic. The most common types of leukemia in adults are acute myelogenous leukemia (AML) and chronic lymphocytic leukemia (CLL). The incidence of leukemia rose steeply in the years between 1900 and the 1940s. Since then, the incidence of AML has continued to increase steadily, both in the United States and developing countries, suggesting the influence of occupational and environmental exposure.[4]

Etiology

The cause of leukemia is not known. The etiologic factors most commonly considered are genetic predisposition, radiation, chemicals, drugs, and viruses.

Genetic Factors

The relationship of genetic factors to the incidence of leukemia has been suggested in certain high-risk families and specific hereditary syndromes. There is some evidence of familial clustering, with a fourfold to sevenfold increased risk being noted in individuals with a family member diagnosed with leukemia.[5] Additionally, 10%–20% of monozygous twins of individuals with leukemia develop the disease.[5,6]

Certain genetic disorders are associated with increased incidence of leukemia. Children with Down's syndrome (trisomy 21) have an 18-fold to 20-fold increased incidence of acute leukemia.[6,7] Other disorders with chromosomal abnormalities or fragilities also associated with acute leukemia are Bloom's syndrome, Fanconi's anemia, Klinefelter's syndrome, and Ellis-Van Creveld syndrome.[4]

Acquired clonal chromosomal abnormalities are found in 55%–78% of adult patients with acute leukemia and in 90% of patients with secondary leukemias.[2] Evidence suggests that some individuals who appear to have normal cytogenetics (karyotyping) actually have submicroscopic aberrations of genetic material that can be detected only by molecular genetic techniques such as Southern Blot analysis. The cytogenetic and molecular analysis of leukemia gene abnormalities will be discussed in detail later in this chapter.

Radiation

Populations exposed to ionizing radiation have an increased incidence of leukemia, especially AML. Japanese survivors of the atomic bomb experienced a 20-fold increased incidence of AML and chronic myelogenous leukemia (CML). There appeared to be a direct relationship between increased incidence and distance from the center of the explosion. The peak incidence was at five to seven years following exposure, and increased risks continued for 20 years.[5,8] In addition, early radiologists exposed to excessive irradiation experienced a higher incidence of leukemia.[9] Also, patients treated for benign disorders such as ankylosing spondylitis, menorrhagia, and other gynecologic disorders have increased risk of AML.[5] Radiation remains the most conclusively identified leukemogenic factor in humans.

Chemicals

Chronic exposure to certain chemicals has been associated with an increased incidence of pancytopenia and subsequent AML. Benzene, an aromatic hydrocarbon, is produced by natural processes and by industry (unleaded gasoline, rubber cement, cleaning solvents).[7,10] It was first implicated in the development of acute leukemia in Turkish cobblers in the early 1900s. Since then, other populations have been identified as being at risk, including workers with explosives, distillers, dye users, painters, and shoemakers.

Drugs

Drugs that have demonstrated a relationship to the etiology of acute leukemia include certain alkylating agents, the antibiotic chloramphenicol, and phenylbutazone.[11,12] AML is the most frequently reported second cancer following aggressive chemotherapy and is associated with treatment for Hodgkin's disease, multiple myeloma, ovarian cancer, non-Hodgkin's lymphoma, and breast cancer. The epipodophyllotoxin etoposide and topoisomerase II inhibitors have also been implicated as being leukemogenic.[7]

Secondary leukemias induced by alkylators are characterized by chromosome translocations such as t(9;22) or t(4;11), while leukemias arising after epipodophyllotoxin therapy are identified with 11q abnormalities. Therapy-related leukemia now represents 20%–25% of all cases of AML patients, and overall median survival is four to eight months.[13] The time of greatest risk appears to be the first ten years after treatment.

Viruses

The role of viruses in the etiology of human leukemia remains unclear. Adult T-cell leukemia in Japan and the Caribbean is associated with the human T-cell leukemia virus (HTLV-I). There is evidence for a role of HTLV-I in the etiology of adult T-cell leukemia in the United States.[5,14]

Table 55-1 Manifestations of Leukemia

Etiology	Manifestation
Granulocytopenia	Fever Abdominal pain Respiratory infection Perirectal abscess Adenopathy Mucositis
Thrombocytopenia	Purpura, petechiae, ecchymoses Bleeding gums Epistaxis Retinal hemorrhage Intracranial bleeding
Anemia	Fatigue or malaise Pallor Dyspnea
Leukemia infiltrates	Pain or swelling in bones and joints Hepatomegaly Splenomegaly

Pathophysiology

In the normal bone marrow, efficient regulatory mechanisms ensure that cell proliferation and maturation are adequate for the needs of the individual. In leukemia, control is missing or abnormal. The results are (1) arrest of the cell in an early phase of its maturation process, causing the accumulation of immature cells; (2) an abnormal proliferation of these immature cells; and (3) crowding of other marrow elements, resulting in inhibited growth and function of these elements and eventual replacement of the marrow by leukemic cells.

Clinical Manifestations

Manifestations of leukemia are related to three factors: (1) excessive proliferation of immature leukocytes within blood-forming organs such as the bone marrow, spleen, and lymph nodes, resulting in destruction of tissue; (2) infiltration of proliferating leukocytes into various organs of the body; and (3) decrease in the number of normal leukocytes, erythrocytes, and thrombocytes as a result of crowding of the bone marrow by proliferating leukemic cells. Table 55-1 summarizes possible leukemic manifestations, although these vary considerably with each type of leukemia.[15] The presenting manifestations, complications, course of disease, and treatment for each major type are discussed separately (Table 55-2).

Table 55-2 Comparative Features of the Leukemias at Presentation

Description	Median Age	Initial Remission Rate	Median Survival with Treatment	Splenomegaly	Infection	Adenopathy	Hemoglobin	White Blood Cell Count	Platelets
Acute myelogenous leukemia	50–60	60%–70%	10–15 mo	No	Yes	No	Low	Variable	Low
Acute lymphoblastic leukemia	4	Adult 65%–85%; children 90%	Adult 2 yr; children 5 yr	Yes	Yes	Yes	Low	Variable	Low
Chronic myelogenous leukemia	49	90%	3 yr	Yes	No	No	Low	100,000–300,000/mm^3 granulocytes	Normal or low
Chronic lymphocytic leukemia	60	90%	4–6 yr	Yes	Yes	Yes	Low	20,000/mm^3 lymphocytes	Low

Assessment of Acute Leukemia

Factors that influence the symptoms and physical findings are (1) the type of leukemic cell, (2) the degree of leukemic cell burden (early-stage or advanced disease), (3) the involvement of organs or systems outside of the bone marrow or peripheral circulation, and (4) the depression of normal marrow elements by the leukemic process. Because the presenting symptoms of AML and ALL are similar, the assessment parameters of acute leukemia are discussed first. The classification and treatment of AML and ALL are discussed individually. The chronic leukemias, CML and CLL, are then discussed separately.

Patient History

Acute leukemia presents with a large and rapidly growing population of leukemic cells. Usually, signs and symptoms have been present for less than three months, and perhaps for only a few days. Although the diagnosis cannot be made from the patient's history alone, many of the findings are typical and essential in guiding the diagnostic work-up.

The most common complaints of the patient are nonspecific — for example, fatigue, malaise, weight loss, and fever. The presenting symptoms are the manifestations of the effects of leukemic cells on the normal marrow elements. Infections are recurrent in commonly affected sites such as the skin, gingiva, perianal tissue, lung, and urinary tract. The patient may complain of sore throat and describe fever with or without signs of localized infection. Unexplained bleeding may occur with nosebleeds, gingival bleeding, mid-cycle menstrual flow, or heavy bleeding with menses. Symptoms of progressive anemia include fatigue, palpitations, shortness of breath, and anorexia. Pain may arise from several sources — bones such as the sternum, enlarged lymph nodes, and hepatosplenomegaly.

Neurological complaints are frequent and may signal either leukemia infiltration (especially in ALL) or intracerebral hemorrhage. These include a history of headache, vomiting, visual disturbances, or seizures.

Review of the individual's past medical history may be noncontributory. However, it is of etiologic importance to note a history of recurrent infections or bleeding tendencies as well as the type and time of any drug exposure to try to document the approximate onset of leukemia. Similarly, occupational (especially chemical and radiation) exposure and family history of genetic abnormalities or cancer will contribute to the total epidemiologic picture.

An essential part of the initial history that serves as a baseline for understanding the individual and planning for his or her care is the psychosocial profile. Questions that elicit details concerning past and present coping strategies with illness or other crises should be asked. Determination of significant others can be made by asking such questions as "Who can you talk to most easily about your illness?" Finally, the nurse must ascertain how the patient and family perceive the illness and what their previous experience with hospitalization has been.

Physical Examination

The physical findings of acute leukemia usually relate directly to the effects of pancytopenia. Vital signs may demonstrate fever, tachycardia, and tachypnea. The skin and mucous membranes generally appear pale, with readily apparent ecchymoses or petechiae. Generalized or localized adenopathy may be present due to leukemic infiltration or infection.

A comprehensive physical examination validates findings elicited in the complete history and review of

Table 55-3 Chromosomal and Molecular Abnormalities in Acute Myelogenous Leukemia

Abnormality	Karyotype	FAB	Molecular Change	Complete Response Rate
Transcription	t(6;11)(q27;q23)	M4, M5	AF6(6q27)	Low
	t(8;21)(q22;q22)	M2	ET0(8q22)	High
	t(10;11)(p12;p23)	M4, M5	AF10(p12)	Low
	t(11;17)(q23;q21)	M5	ALL 1(11q23)	Low
	t(11;19)(q23;p13)	M4, M5	ELL(19p13.1)	Low
	t(15;17)(q22;q11)	M3	PML-RARα	High
	t(16;16)(p13;q22)	M4Eo	MYHI 1(16p13)	High
	t(3;3)(q23;q26)	M1, M2, M4, M6	Gene activation	Low
	t(9;11)(p22;q23)	M5a	AF9(9p22)	Low
Inversion	inv(16)(p13;q22)	M4Eo	MYHI 1 (16p13)	High
	inv(3)(q21;q26)	M0, M1, M4, M5, M6, M7	Gene activation	Low
Loss or deletion	5			Low
	7			High
	del(16)(q22)	M4Eo		

symptoms. Ophthalmoscopic examination may reveal retinal capillary hemorrhage or papilledema due to leukostatic or thrombocytopenic-induced bleeding and/or increased intracranial pressure. An oral infection with *Candida albicans* may be present. Examination of the lungs and heart may reveal the effects of anemia (cardiac murmurs) or infection (abnormal lung sounds). Abdominal palpation may demonstrate hepatosplenomegaly or enlarged kidneys due to leukemic infiltration, especially in children with ALL. Perirectal tissue may be tender and swollen and the only evidence of an abscess or a fistula. Finally, gentle palpation of bones and joints may reveal swelling and elicit pain.

Diagnostic Studies

Laboratory and radiographic studies are essential for proper diagnosis. It is important to distinguish between AML and ALL, because the treatment and prognosis for these conditions differ markedly. An ongoing explanation to the patient and family of the plan and purpose of the exhaustive diagnostic work-up will facilitate cooperation, decrease anxiety, and create an atmosphere of confidence and trust.

The diagnosis is suggested by the peripheral smear but requires a full examination of the bone marrow. The white blood cell count may be low, normal, or high, and 90% of patients have blast cells present in the peripheral blood. Neutropenia (absolute granulocyte count less than 1000 cells/mm^3) is frequent, and thrombocytopenia is present in 40% of patients. Blood chemistry studies may reveal hyperuricemia and increased lactic dehydrogenase as well as altered serum and urine muramidase (greatly increased with monocyte and myelomonocytic leukemia, but normal to low in lymphoblastic leukemia). If acute promyelocytic leukemia (M^3) is suspected, laboratory evaluation should include plasma fibrinogen, fibrin split products, and prothrombin time.

Bone marrow contents are usually hypercellular, with 60%–90% blasts in the differential blood count. Auer rods are diagnostic of AML, as are special stains (Sudan black and peroxidase).

Improved techniques of cytogenetics (chromosome analysis) can provide information confirming the diagnosis and specific classification of the leukemia. More than two-thirds of patients with de novo acute leukemia exhibit nonrandom chromosome abnormalities.[16] These abnormalities in the leukemic cells serve as tumor markers that disappear during remission and reappear with recurrence of the leukemia.[17,18]

Cytogenetic analysis is performed at the time of diagnosis and is rapidly becoming the standard for establishing diagnosis and prognosis in acute leukemia.[19] These chromosome abnormalities are described as translocations, inversions, or loss or gain in chromosome number. Specific aberrations are related to a favorable or unfavorable outcome[16–19] (Tables 55-3 and 55-4). The results of chromosome analysis are usually available within four weeks. As the patient is also recovering from induction therapy at this time, the information is useful in planning further treatment.

Structural chromosomal abnormalities produce protein products of genes that are inappropriately activated or altered. Gene activation occurs when the transcription regulatory elements of one gene become juxtaposed (placed side by side) with another gene. Under the control of the new promoter/enhancer re-

Table 55-4 Chromosomal and Molecular Abnormalities in Acute Lymphocytic Leukemia

Abnormality	Karyotype	FAB	Molecular Change	Complete Response Rate
B-lineage translocations	t(8;14)(q24;Q32)	L 3	IGH, cMYC	Moderate
	t(1;19)(q23;p13)	L 1	EZA, PBX1	Low
	t(17;19)(q22;p13)	L 1	EZA, PBX1	Low
	t(9;22)(q34;q11)	L 1	cABL, BCR	High
	t(4;11)(q21;q23)	L 1	MLL, AF4	High
T-lineage translocations	t(8;14)(q24;q11)	L 3		Low

gion, the expression pattern is disrupted, leading to leukemogenesis.[16,18] Gene fusion occurs when segments from two genes become fused to create a new structure. Most chromosomal aberrations result in gene fusions. Genetic alterations in AML give rise to fusion genes. The majority of genetic alterations seen in ALL result in transfer of regulatory elements from one gene to another, causing dysregulated expression from an otherwise normal gene. Further information is provided by differentiating primary alterations (one karyotype abnormality) from secondary alterations (extra alterations thought to be later genetic events). Secondary alterations may be present at diagnosis or appear at the time of relapse.[16]

Additional information is obtained from immunologic studies. More that 100 antigen groups known as *clusters of differentiation (CDs)* reside on the surface of hematopoietic cells.[7] Monoclonal antibodies reactive to immature cells can identify the predominant cell type and stage of arrested development in the leukemic cell line. The use of surface marker antigens in patients with ALL has revealed the presence of markers for both lymphoid and myeloid cells.[20] Mixed lymphoid and myeloid surface markers are found in 21% of patients with de novo ALL.[21] These hybrid leukemias may be biphenotypic, in which one cell line expresses characteristics of two lineages, or bilineal, in which two distinct populations may express either myeloid or lymphoid characteristics separately.[7] In general, patients with mixed lineage leukemia have a poor response to treatment and should be considered candidates for other investigational therapies.

Classification

Leukemias are classified as either chronic or acute and as either myeloid or lymphoid. In chronic leukemia, the predominant cell is mature appearing but does not function normally. The disease has a gradual onset, prolonged clinical course, and a relatively longer survival time. The predominant cell in acute leukemia is undifferentiated or immature, usually a "blast" cell. The abrupt onset and rapid disease progression result in a short survival time. However, as progress is made in the treatment of children with acute lymphocytic leukemia and longer survival occurs, it may no longer be appropriate to describe acute leukemia as having a short survival.

Figure 55-1 presents the major classification of leukemia according to the type of cell that predominates and the location of arrested cellular maturation. All cell lines arise from the same totipotent stem cell. From this cell, which has the potential to differentiate into a variety of cells, the myeloid and lymphocyte series are derived. The myeloid stem cell is pluripotent and gives rise to erythrocyte, thrombocyte, granulocyte, and monocyte progenitors, or committed cells. These immature forms eventually mature into fully functional red blood cells, platelets, and white blood cells. The lymphoid stem cell matures in the thymus to form T-cell progenitors, or in the bone marrow to form B-cell progenitors.

The type of leukemia is named according to the point at which cell maturation is arrested. Although the terms *lymphocytic* and *myelogenous* (nonlymphocytic) leukemia are most commonly used, further specification within each class (e.g., *promyelocytic, myelocytic*) describes the exact point at which arrest of maturation seems to occur.

In 1976, the French-American-British (FAB) Cooperative Group developed criteria for the classification of the acute leukemias[22] (Table 55-5). The goal was to provide a systematic, objective system that would be feasible for use in most hematologic laboratories. The system, based on morphology and number of cells, was later revised and updated and is still used today to distinguish lymphoid and myeloid lineages and to assign initial treatment.[23–25] The additional information obtained through cytogenetics, identification of surface markers, and histochemical staining provides important therapeutic and prognostic information.

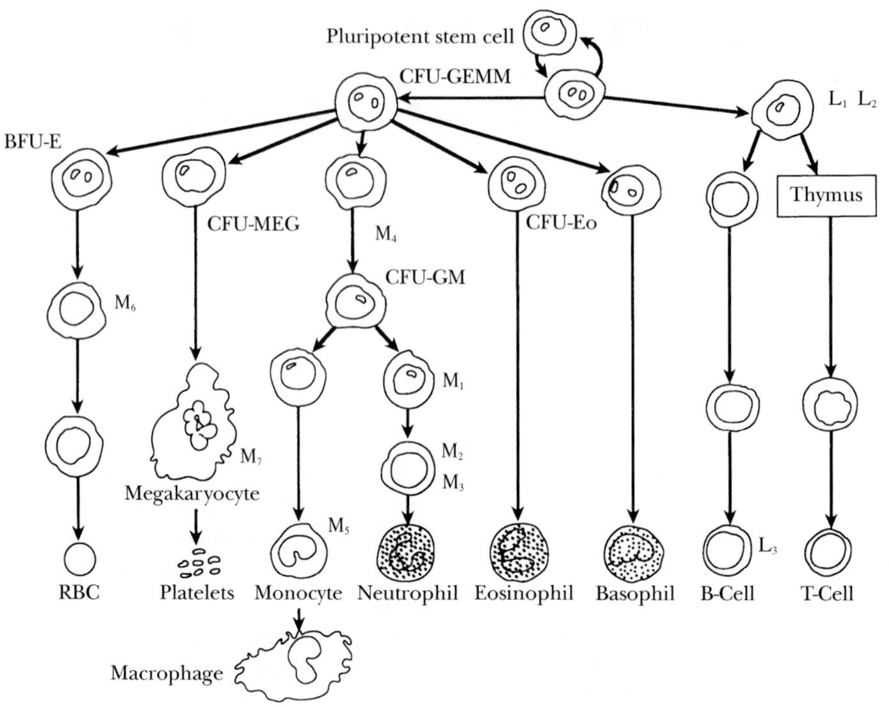

Figure 55-1 Hematopoietic cascade with FAB classifications of acute nonlymphocytic leukemia and acute lymphocytic leukemia at proposed levels of arrested cell maturation. BFU = burst-forming unit; CFU = colony-forming unit; GM = granulocyte, macrophage; GEMM = granulocyte, erythrocyte, macrophage, megakaryocyte; Epo = erythropoietin; MEG = megakaryocyte; Eo = eosinophil; E = erythrocyte; M_1 = undifferentiated myelocytic; M_2 = myelocytic; M_3 = promyelocytic; M_4 = myelomonocytic; M_5 = monocytic; M_6 = erythroleukemia; M_7 = megakaryocytic; L_1 = childhood; L_2 = adult; L_3 = Burkitt's type.

Table 55-5 French-American-British (FAB) Classification of Acute Leukemia

Myeloid		Lymphocytic
M0	Minimally differentiated	
M1	Undifferentiated myelocytic	L1, childhood (Pre B- and T-cell)
M2	Myelocytic	
M3	Promyelocytic	L2, adult (Pre B- and T-cell)
M4	Myelomonocytic	L3, Burkitt's type (B-cell)
M5	Monocytic	
M6	Erythroleukemia	
M7	Megakaryocytic	

Data from Bennett, Catovsky, Daniel, et al.[22]

Acute Myelogenous Leukemia

Classification

Acute myelogenous leukemia (AML), also referred to as acute nonlymphocytic leukemia (ANLL), is a disease of the pluripotent myeloid stem cell. The malignant clone arises in the myeloid, monocyte, erythroid, or megakaryocyte lines. The exact event that triggers the malignant transformation is not known.

The leukemic cells have more abundant cytoplasm, and granulation in the cytoplasm is usually but not always present. Auer rods, which are abnormal lysosomal granules, are present and pathognomonic for AML. Multiple nucleoli are present and tend to vary in size.

As previously stated, the type of leukemia is named for the predominant cell. The most common myeloid leukemia is acute myelocytic leukemia (M_1). Acute promyelocytic leukemia (APL; M_3) is associated with an increased risk of disseminated intravascular coagulation. This is due to the release of procoagulants from granules within the leukemic promyelocyte, especially during remission induction therapy.[15] Patients with acute monocytic (M_5) or myelomonocytic (M_4) leukemia often exhibit extramedullary leukemic infiltration with gingival hypertrophy, cutaneous leukemia, and liver, spleen, and lymph enlargement.[5]

Erythroleukemia (M_6), which was first described by DiGugliolmo, has both chronic and acute forms.[4] As the erythroleukemia progresses, the morphologic picture resembles that of myelocytic or myelomonocytic leukemia. Megakaryocytic leukemia (M_7) is quite rare and less responsive to chemotherapy.[1] By the time an individual is diagnosed with AML, the bone marrow and peripheral blood may contain as many as 10^{12} leukemic cells.[26] Their accumulation within the bone marrow space results in inhibition and crowding out of normal marrow stem cells and infiltration of other organs by myeloblasts. Anemia, thrombocytopenia, and neutropenia result. If the disease is left untreated, death occurs within a few months due to infection or uncontrolled bleeding.

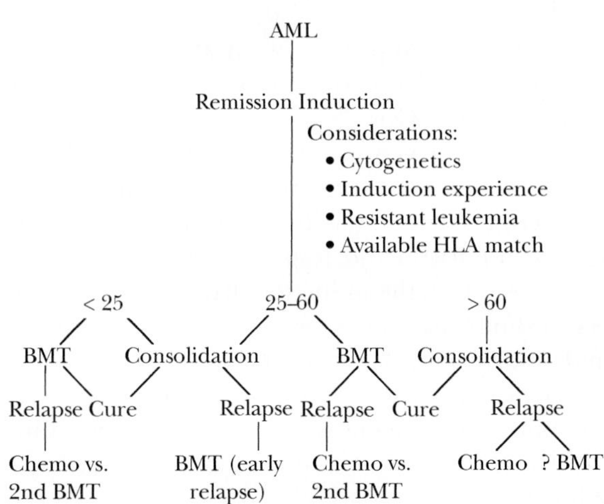

Figure 55-2 Treatment considerations and options for patients with acute myelogenous leukemia.

Therapeutic Approaches

The goal of antileukemic treatment for AML is the eradication of the leukemic stem cells. Complete remission is defined as the restoration of normal peripheral counts and less than 5% blasts in the bone marrow.[20] Treatment regimens capable of inducing a complete remission comprise several drugs, each of which is known to be effective against leukemic myeloblasts. The course of therapy is divided into two stages: (1) induction, and (2) postremission therapy.

Induction Therapy

The goal of induction therapy is to cause severe bone marrow hypoplasia. At diagnosis, the leukemic cells are proliferating more slowly than the normal myeloid precursors. As a consequence, the myeloid stem cells repopulate the depleted marrow faster than leukemic cells. The cornerstone of remission induction is the cell cycle–specific antimetabolite cytosine arabinoside plus an anthracycline (daunorubicin, doxorubicin, mitoxantrone, amsacrine, or idarubicin).[27–29] It is theorized that a drug that is not cycle specific will act synergistically when given sequentially with a cell cycle–specific drug, causing proliferating cells to enter the cell cycle concurrently. Cytosine arabinoside is administered continuously for seven days, and the anthracycline is given for three days. The continuous infusion of cytosine arabinoside ensures that slowly cycling leukemia cells are adequately exposed to the drug during the synthesis phase of the cell cycle. This protocol is called *7 + 3*, but variations include five- or ten-day infusions of cytosine arabinoside. Bishop[28] summarized the results of eight clinical studies, reporting a complete response rate of 64%, with the best results in the protocols with seven days of cytosine arabinoside. Idarubicin is the most common anthracycline used.[7,30]

The effectiveness of the chemotherapy is assessed at one week after the completion of therapy with a bone marrow biopsy and aspiration on the fourteenth day. If residual leukemia is present, a second course is begun. Bone marrow recovery usually takes 14–21 days after the end of the chemotherapy, with median time to complete recovery being 28–32 days. Complete response rates are now observed in 65%–80% of patients. Unfortunately, despite improving remission rates, only 20% of patients remain in complete remission. Relapse occurs in the remaining cases within one to two years.[30–32] Thus, postremission therapy is essential.

Postremission Therapy

By the addition of postremission therapy, the median duration of remission can be increased from 4–8 months to 10–60 months, and disease-free survival (DFS) of four years from 30% to 40%.[33] Leukemia cells have certain biologic properties that allow them to be distinguished from normal cells. Certain chromosomal aberrations are detected by polymerase chain reaction (PCR) or by fluorescence in situ hybridization (FISH). RNA transcript errors are detected by reverse transcription PCR (RT-PCR). Patterns of antigen coexpression are detected by flow cytometry.[34] All of these technologies are used to detect minimal residual disease (MRD).

Postremission therapies include consolidation, intensification, maintenance, and allogeneic or autologous bone marrow transplant.[30] None has emerged as the clear-cut, optimal therapy (Figure 55-2).

Consolidation therapy consists of one or two courses of very high doses of the same drugs used for induction. Up to 30 times induction doses of cytosine arabinoside are used to consolidate the remission. Although the patient is in a healthier state for this part of the treatment, the toxicities are substantial, with extended myelosuppression, cerebellar dysfunction, dermatitis, hepatic dysfunction, and conjunctivitis. The longest remissions appear to occur after two or more courses of consolidation therapy, with a median remission of one to two years.[30]

Intensification may be initiated immediately following remission induction (early intensification) or several months later (late intensification). Different drugs are used with the hope that they will not be cross-resistant with the induction drugs. Mitoxantrone is less cardiotoxic and has less extramedullary toxicity than daunorubicin. With a steep dose-response curve, mitoxantrone is good for dose intensification.[35] Another combination being used for postinduction therapy is ICE (idarubicin, cytosine arabinoside, and etoposide).[35]

Maintenance therapy entails treatment with lower doses of the same or other drugs given monthly for a prolonged period of time. Maintenance therapy is not currently recommended in the treatment of AML.[30]

Patients who relapse after induction and postinduction chemotherapy have a 30%–60% likelihood of achieving a second remission.[32] Leukemic cells acquire increasing resistance to chemotherapy. The cellular kinetics change due to an increased growth fraction and shortened generation time, resulting in a decreased doubling time.[20] As a result, the second and subsequent remissions are influenced by prior treatment, length of remission, and the initial response to therapy. Patients who relapse quickly or who have resistant leukemia should be considered for clinical trials or bone marrow transplant (BMT).

The role of BMT in the treatment of AML has been studied for more than 20 years.[36] The first issue is the availability of an HLA-matched donor. In the general population, a potential donor exists in less than 40% of cases. Other options may include a matched unrelated donor BMT obtained through the National Marrow Donor Program. Increased risks of graft-versus-host disease (GVHD) and lack of engraftment from these histocompatible but unrelated cells occur, however. A purged autologous BMT may be performed in a young patient with no HLA match. In patients younger than age 30, BMT may offer a higher cure rate than standard treatment. In patients in the fourth decade of life, the results of chemotherapy versus BMT vary. Transplant centers usually do not admit patients older than age 60. Non-myeloblative transplants, also known as mini-transplants, are currently used in patients with poor performance status or older age.[37]

Because allogeneic BMT carries the risk of GVHD, interstitial pneumonia, and infection with cytomegalovirus, the decision to undertake BMT is not easy.[38] The question of the optimal timing for transplant remains unanswered. Patients who relapse after allogeneic BMT can be treated with a second BMT or an infusion of donor buffy coat to stimulate the graft-versus-leukemia effect. (See Chapter 21 for an in-depth discussion of bone marrow transplantation.)

Another consideration in the treatment of AML is the significance of prognostic indicators, which may be useful in determining the best course of therapy. For example, patients with unfavorable factors such as older age or multiple chromosomal abnormalities may be treated with high-dose or investigational drugs. Patients who had a poor response to initial therapy and other medical problems are unlikely to benefit from reinduction therapy. These individuals may benefit from a less aggressive approach, with transfusion support and oral hydroxyurea to control the white blood cell (WBC) count. In younger patients with unfavorable morphologic subtypes, BMT may be preferred to consolidation therapy.

APL is biologically distinct from other subtypes of AML. All-*trans* retinoic acid (RA), a derivative of vitamin A, is now used to induce remissions through differentiation.[39,40] The break point for the chromosome region abnormality characteristic in APL, t(15;17)(q22;q12), is clustered near the location of the retinoic acid receptor–alpha. The administration of RA seems to induce terminal differentiation and subsequent death of the previously arrested leukemic cells. Recently, RA was approved for remission induction in patients with APL who are refractory to chemotherapy or who have relapsed after prior chemotherapy. Once remission is obtained, treatment switches to chemotherapy because patients quickly develop resistance to RA.[15] Patients who are unable to tolerate conventional chemotherapy (older individuals or those with concomitant illness) may also benefit from RA therapy. The most commonly used dosage is 45 mg/m^2/day, administered orally in two evenly divided doses, for remission induction. Approximately half of all patients experience the complications of disseminated intravascular coagulopathy, but few hemorrhagic deaths occur. Common side effects include headache, dry skin, xerostomia, cheilitis (cracking at the corners of the lips), and bone pain.

Approximately 25%–30% of patients will relapse after RA and anthracycline-based chemotherapy.[40] Arsenic trioxide (Trisonex, Cell Therapeutics Inc., Seattle, Washington) was approved for induction of remission and consolidation in patients who are refractory to or who have relapsed after RA and anthracycline chemotherapy and whose APL is characterized by the presence of the t(15;17) translocation or PML-RARα gene expression. The dose for induction is 0.15 mg/kg/day IV over 1–2 hours until the bone marrow is cleared of leukemia cells or for a maximum of 60 days. Consolidation therapy is 0.15 mg/kg/day IV for 25 doses or a maximum of 5 weeks. Adverse events associated with arsenic trioxide include APL differentiation syndrome and EKG abnormalities, including prolongation of QT interval and complete atrioventricular block. The symptoms of APL differentiation syndrome are fever, dyspnea, weight gain, pulmonary infiltrates, pleural or pericardial effusion, and leukocytosis; steroids are the recommended treatment.[41]

FLT3 is a transmembrane tyrosine kinase growth factor receptor that is selectively expressed on the hematopoietic cells of 80% of AML patients.[42,43] In normal cells, FLT3 mediates stem cell proliferation and differentiation. Activation of the FLT3 receptor in AML precursor cells appears to stimulate proliferation and inhibit apoptosis. In 30% of patients an FLT3 mutation results in auto-activation of the receptor in the absence of ligand. This, in turn, leads to independent activation of all growth mediated by the Ras and STAT5 signaling pathways. An FLT3 mutation is present in as many as 36% of older AML patients and indicates a poor outcome. Several FLT3 inhibitors are currently under investigation. CEP-701, MLN 518, and PKC 412 are all oral agents and are well tolerated.

Treatment of AML in older adults is challenging but essential: 60%–70% of adult AML occurs in patients older than 60 years.[44] Co-morbidities limit treatment tolerance, and increased age suggests a more aggressive tumor biology and greater incidence of unfavorable karyotypes. Gemtuzumab ozogamicin, (Mylotarg, Wyeth-Ayerst Laboratories, Philadelphia, Pennsylvania) was approved in May 2000 for the treatment of adults with AML who are more than 60 years old. Side effects include infusion-related reactions, infection, tumor lysis syndrome, myelosuppression, venoocclusive disease, pulmonary events (dyspnea, hypoxia, or infiltrates), and liver and renal impairment.[45,46]

Acute Lymphocytic Leukemia

Acute lymphocytic leukemia (ALL) is a malignant disease of the lymphoid progenitors. The abnormal clone originates in the marrow, thymus, and lymph nodes, but the exact etiologic event is unknown. The leukemic lymphoblast is nongranular, with little cytoplasm. The round nucleus resembles a normal lymphoblast. Although the defect does not involve the myeloid cell lines, the secondary effect of the high leukemic cell burden on the bone marrow interferes with normal hematopoietic activity.

Classification

The FAB classification for ALL is based on several cell properties: size ratio of nucleus to cytoplasm; number, size, and shape of nucleoli; and amount and basophilia of the cytoplasm[22,25] (see Table 55-5). In childhood ALL, 85% of cases demonstrate L_1 morphology, whereas the majority of adults with ALL have L_2 morphology. Patients with L_3 ALL, which resembles Burkitt's lymphoma, are rare.

Lymphoblasts have a propensity for organ infiltration and may remain sequestered in sanctuary sites even after remission has been achieved. Leukemic cells infiltrate into the central nervous system (CNS) early in the disease.[47] Because the drugs used for treatment penetrate poorly into the cerebrospinal fluid, the leukemic cells remain sheltered from the cytotoxic effects of the drugs. Over time, the leukemic cells proliferate and cause relapse. Cells can also be harbored in the testes. In addition, 80% of patients have lymphadenopathy and/or splenomegaly at the time of diagnosis due to the infiltration of these organs by leukemic cells.[26]

The prognosis for long-term survival is more favorable for individuals with ALL than with AML because drugs are available that are uniquely effective against lymphocytes — for example, prednisone. CNS prophylaxis is used in ALL and has proven successful.

As with AML, long-term survival and cure for individuals with ALL is possible only if a complete remission is achieved. This is documented by a bone marrow aspirate containing less than 5% lymphoblasts and the disappearance of all peripheral manifestations of the disease.

Therapeutic Approaches

In contrast to AML, current chemotherapeutic regimens proven effective against ALL contain drugs that are selectively toxic to lymphoblasts and relatively sparing of normal hematopoietic stem cells. Therefore, the patient experiences hypoplasia that is less severe and of shorter duration with greater leukemic cell kill. In addition, relapses may be more effectively treated because the marrow is better able to recover.

The goals of therapy for ALL are to eradicate all leukemic cells from the marrow and lymph tissue and to eliminate any residual foci of disease within the CNS. Treatment is divided into three stages: (1) induction, (2) CNS prophylaxis, and (3) postremission therapy (Figure 55-3).

Induction Therapy

Although current therapy for ALL induces complete remission in 65%–85% of adults, only 20%–30% are cured of the disease.[48,49] Induction regimens usually comprise five drugs, including vincristine, prednisone,

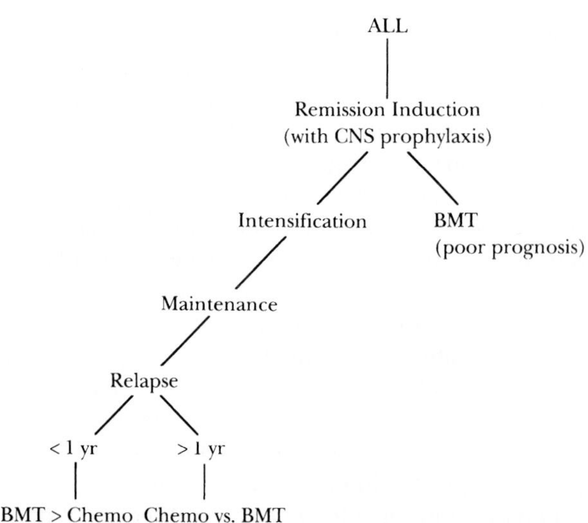

Figure 55-3 Treatment considerations and options for patients with acute lymphocytic leukemia.

an anthracycline, cyclophosphamide, and/or asparaginase.[50] Some 35%–40% of patients achieve long-term, disease-free survival.[49] Therapy usually begins in the hospital, but hypoplasia is shorter than with AML treatment. Once remission is documented, the therapy is completed on an outpatient basis.

CNS Prophylaxis

Meningeal leukemia is present at diagnosis in 5%–10% of patients and is known to occur in as many as 35% of patients with ALL in the absence of CNS prophylaxis.[26,47] By comparison, the incidence is less than 5% in patients with AML. Leukemic lymphoblasts enter the leptomeninges either by direct extension from the blood of the meningeal vessels or by seeding from thrombocytopenic bleeding. The cells extend deeply into the cerebral sulci and nerve sheaths, causing a mechanical obstruction of the cerebral spinal fluid (CSF). If left unchecked, hydrocephaly and death occur. Signs and symptoms of CNS leukemia include headache, blurred vision, nausea/vomiting, and cranial nerve palsies.[47]

CNS prophylaxis should start within a few weeks of the initiation of therapy. Previously, treatment included intracranial radiation and intrathecal methotrexate. Due to the high morbidity associated with this combination, current protocols recommend only intrathecal methotrexate.[47,51]

Postremission Therapy

As in AML, even after complete remission, patients with ALL harbor remaining leukemic cells. Relapse occurs in two to three months if there is no continuing therapy. Prolonged chemotherapy may lead to a 40% overall cure rate, but the type and duration are not completely defined.[26,47] Currently, many patients receive some type of intensification with high-dose chemotherapy or the use of multiple new drugs.[49] Methotrexate and 6-mercaptopurine may be added to the drugs used during induction. Maintenance therapy often continues for two to three years.

The outlook for patients in whom relapse occurs during therapy is quite poor, and younger patients with an HLA-matched donor should be immediately referred for BMT.[35] If relapse occurs after the completion of therapy, treatment is continued with high-dose methotrexate, tenoposide, and cytarabine, or high-dose cytosine arabinoside with an anthracycline or amsacrine. Second remission can be achieved in as many as 72% of cases.[49]

Chromosomal aberrations (summarized in Table 55-4) are also important in planning treatment for ALL.[20,52] Because patients treated with allogeneic BMT show a trend toward longer survival if the transplant is performed during the first remission, it is important to identify patients with an unfavorable prognosis in the early stages of disease.

Myelodysplastic Syndromes

Myelodysplastic syndromes (MDS) are a group of hematologic disorders with an increased risk of transformation to AML. They are characterized by a change in the quantity and quality of bone marrow products. Hematologic disorders that preceded acute leukemia were first reported in the late 1940s and referred to as *preleukemia anemia*.[53] Other terms used are *preleukemia, hematopoietic dysplasia, refractory anemia with excessive myeloblasts, subacute myeloid leukemia, oligoblastic leukemia,* and *dysmyelopoietic syndromes*.[54]

Currently, MDS are divided into five subtypes according to the FAB group classification: refractory anemia (RA); refractory anemia with ringed sideroblasts (RARS); refractory anemia with excessive blasts (RAEB); refractory anemia with excessive blasts in transformation (RAEB-t); and chronic myelomonocytic leukemia (CMML).[55] The FAB classification has limited usefulness, however, because it does not include such variables as the wide range of marrow blast cells within certain subgroups, marrow cytogenetics, and the degree of morbidity-associated cytopenias. The World Health Organization has proposed a new classification system that recognizes multilineage dysphasia and adds a new subgroup, 5q- syndrome. It remains to be seen how this new system will be incorporated into clinical practice.[56] Table 55-6 lists each type, along with diagnostic criteria, risk of evolution into acute leukemia, and average survival time.[54,55]

Table 55-6 Classification of Myelodysplastic Syndrome with Percentage of Blast Cells, Leukemia Risk, and Average Survival

Category	BLASTS (%) Blood	Bone Marrow	Risk of Evolution to Acute Leukemia (%)	Survival (months)
RA	< 1	< 5	0–25	18–71
RARS	< 1	< 5	8	14–76 +
RAEB	< 5	≥ 5	20–44	7–16
RAEB-t	> 5	20–30	27–60	2.5–20
CMML	< 5	1–20	14	9–60
	> 10^9 monocytes			

RA = refractory anemia; RARS = refractory anemia with ringed sideroblasts; RAEB = refractory anemia excess blasts; RAEB-t = refractory anemia with excess blasts in transformation; CMML = chronic myelomonocytic leukemia.

Data from Kouides and Bennett[54]; Bennett, Catovsky, Daniel, et al.[55]

An International Prognostic Scoring System (IPSS) for MDS has been developed that categorizes risk as low, intermediate-1, intermediate-2, or high[57,58] (Table 55-7). Therapeutic decision making is guided by the patient's IPSS risk category, age, and performance status.

MDS are believed to occur as the result of altered stem cells. The cause of this alteration is unknown. Chromosome abnormalities are present at the level of the stem cell in 50% of patients with primary MDS and 75% of patients with therapy-related MDS. None is exclusively associated with MDS but commonly encountered abnormalities involve chromosomes 5, 7, 8, 11, 12, and 20[54,55,57] (Table 55-8).

Approximately 30% of patients diagnosed with AML initially present with preleukemic syndrome.[7] MDS may be considered to be different stages of the same disease. Even if the evolution to acute leukemia never occurs, life-threatening anemia, thrombocytopenia, and/or neutropenia invariably occur. The defect is usually noted in the erythrocyte line first, then in the granulocytes and megakaryocytes.

As with other hematologic disorders, chromosomal aberrations are proving to be significant. Chromosome region 12–13 contains myeloid leukemia factor-2 gene (*MLF2*), which has the same structure as myeloid leukemia factor-1 gene (*MLF1*) on region 3q25.1. *MFL1* is associated with several subtypes of AML and MDS.[58] Another variable in MDS is the inability to repair DNA damage. The p53 protein is expressed by a tumor suppressor gene with a central link between DNA damage events, control of the cell cycle, and net cellular metabolism. When stimulated by certain types of DNA damage, it triggers pathways that culminate in apoptosis. Loss of p53 function may determine the net drug resistance of a malignant cell population. This loss is associated with secondary MDS more frequently than with de novo MDS.[55] Several agents are being studied for their ability to overcome drug resistance by blocking P-glycoprotein activity. These include verapamil, quinine, cyclosporine, and its nonimmunosuppressive analog PSC 833. The mutation and abnormal expression of *ras* oncogenes are also detected in 10%–15% of MDS and are common in patients undergoing transformation to leukemia.[58]

The observation of increased programmed cell death (apoptosis) in the presence of rapid hyperproliferation of marrow cells has caused a major advance in understanding the pathogenesis of MDS.[59,60] Increased apoptosis may be related to apoptosis-related gene products such as *MYC,* which enhances apoptosis, and *BCL-2,* which diminishes apoptosis. Other cy-

Table 55-7 International Prognostic Scoring System for Myelodysplastic Syndromes

Score	Subgroup	Median Survival (Years)	Bone Marrow Blasts (%)	Karyotype	Cytopenias
0	Low	5.7	< 5	Good	0–1
0.5–1.0	Intermediate-1	3.5	5–10	Intermediate	2–3
1.5–2.0	Intermediate-2	1.2	11–30	Poor	
≥ 2.5	High	0.4	> 30		

Karyotype: Good = normal, -Y, del(5q), del(20q); intermediate = other abnormalities; poor = complex (> 3 abnormalities) or chromosome 7 abnormalities; cytopenias = anemia, thrombocytopenia, and/or neutropenia.

Table 55-8 Chromosomal Abnormalities in Myelodyspastic Syndromes

Abnormality	Description	Comment
Loss or deletions		
Monosomy 7	Loss of one of two chromosomes 7	Target for environmental or occupational toxins; DNA-damaging agents associated with de novo AML
del 5q	Loss of small arm of chromosome 5	Associated with elderly women with macrocytic anemia; relatively benign
del 11q	Loss of small arm of chromosome 11	Associated with ringed anemia MDS
del 20q	Loss of small arm of chromosome 20	Associated with ringed anemia MDS
Chromosomal gain		
Trisomy 8	Gain of one extra chromosome 8	Poor prognosis and short survival
Rearrangements		
3q	inv(3)(q21;q26) t(3;5)(q26;q34) t(3;3)(q21;q26)	40% therapy related; poor response to chemotherapy and poor survival
12p	t(5;12)(q33;p12)	Associated with topisomerase II activators; 50% RAEB, 50% RAEB-t, 10% CMML

tokines that may be involved are TNF alpha, transforming growth factor beta, and interleukin 1-beta converting enzyme. This finding explains the opposing clinical findings of most MDS patients — marrow hypercellularity and peripheral blood pancytopenia.[61] Researchers are looking for new ways to interfere with this pathway.

Eighty to ninety percent of patients diagnosed with MDS are older than age 50. The incidence is slightly higher in males than in females.[56] A bone marrow biopsy and aspirate usually reveal dyshematopoiesis in all cell lineages. Ringed sideroblasts, abnormal nuclear shapes, cytoplasmic abnormalities, and maturation defects of red blood cells (RBCs) indicate dyserythropoiesis. Evidence of dysmegakaryocytopoiesis includes atypical shapes; multiple, small nuclei; and increased or decreased numbers of platelets. Dysgranulocytopoiesis is seen with hypogranular cells, nuclear abnormalities, and maturation defects of granulocytes. A hypocellular bone marrow with one or more of these lineage defects prompts a diagnosis of MDS.

About half of patients with MDS develop AML. Historically, patients with MDS have not responded as well to antileukemic therapy as did those individuals with de novo AML. However, a subset of patients with MDS (RAEB and RAEB-t) do respond to AML-type chemotherapy.[62] Survival for MDS ranges from several months to years, with median survival of 28 months. Poor prognostic indicators include excessive blast cells in the bone marrow, small clusters of immature myeloid precursors, pancytopenia, and complex chromosomal abnormalities.[57,58] Death usually occurs within two years from complications related to bone marrow depression or transformation to acute leukemia.

Treatment for MDS is as aggressive as the course of the disease.[63] Serial bone marrow and peripheral blood examinations allow the physician to monitor the pace of the disease's progression. Treatment for high-risk or intermediate-2 patients includes bone marrow ablation, suppression, or differentiation. Ablation of the abnormal clone of cells is accomplished with BMT, which is curative if the marrow comes from an HLA-matched donor and the patient is younger than age 55. Success with BMT is limited by the morbidity and mortality of the procedure. High-dose chemotherapy for ablation can induce remission in 40%–60% of patients, but it is of short duration.[59]

Agents administered to stimulate differentiation of cells so that they can mature and die include retinoic acids, vitamin D_3, and interferon-alfa. A newly developed retinoid, CD437, inhibits AML cell growth independent of retinoic acid receptor–based pathways and activates multiple pathways that may reverse the premature apoptosis problem.[64]

Options for the low-risk or intermediate-1 group focus on the cytopenia. Supportive therapy includes replacement of RBCs if the hematocrit is less than 28%–30% or platelets if the level is less than 50,000/mm^3. Antibiotics are used to treat infection and hematopoietic growth factors are given to avoid recurrent infections.

Chronic Myelogenous Leukemia

Chronic myelogenous leukemia (CML), also called *chronic granulocytic leukemia*, is a disorder of the myeloid stem cells characterized by marked splenomegaly and an increased production of granulocytes, especially neutrophils.[65] Approximately 90% of patients with CML have a diagnostic marker, the Philadelphia chromosome (Ph^1). The G group chromosome, number 22, is missing a portion of the long arm (q), which has been translocated to the long arm of chromosome 9.

The significance of the marker[3] is that a proto-oncogene is activated. When the proto-oncogene *ABL* is translocated from chromosome 9 to 22, a new oncogene, *BCR-ABL*, is formed. This gene produces a protein that is associated with triggering growth factor receptors.[66] It is speculated that this gene may induce uncontrolled growth of leukemic cells. Patients with Ph1-negative CML have been found to have activation of this same gene even though no visible chromosome change is present.[67] In addition, as long as the marker is present, the patient is not cured of the disease.

There is no known specific cause for CML except exposure to ionizing radiation.[66] Its peak incidence occurs in the third and fourth decades of life, and both sexes are affected equally.

The natural course of CML is divided into chronic and terminal phases. The initial chronic phase is characterized by excessive proliferation and accumulation of mature granulocytes and precursors. There is an absence of lymphadenopathy, but 90% of patients have palpable splenomegaly. Within 30–40 months, the disorder evolves into a terminal phase consisting of accelerated and blastic phases. The accelerated phase includes progressive leukocytosis with increasing myeloid precursors (including blasts), increasing basophils, splenomegaly, weight loss, and weakness. There is increasing resistance to therapy, and serial cytogenetic studies indicate progressive chromosomal abnormalities.[65]

The blastic phase resembles AML, with 30%–40% of the bone marrow cells being blasts or promyelocytes. A crisis occurs as blast cell counts rise rapidly, often exceeding 100,000/mm^3. Leukostatic lesions caused by the high cell count result in occlusion in the microvasculature of the CNS or lungs. The majority of patients have myeloblastic transformation, but some have lymphoblastic transformation, evidenced by the presence of TdT or cALLa. Median survival after the onset of the terminal phase is three months.[68]

Assessment

In as many as 20% of affected individuals, CML is diagnosed in the absence of any symptomatology.[65] Most patients, however, present with a history that reflects the gradual accumulation of a WBC mass that is 10–150 times the normal level.

Patient History

The initial symptoms or illness typically are related to massive splenomegaly due to infiltration of the spleen by leukemic cells. Left upper quadrant pain, early satiety, and vague abdominal fullness may be the presenting complaints. Leukemic infiltration of joints may also cause bone and joint pain. A history of malaise, fatigue, weight loss, and fever caused by a gradually worsening hypercatabolic state may precede more acute symptoms of anemia.[66]

To a lesser extent than with acute leukemia, epidemiologic clues may be provided by a complete past medical and family history, such as a history of exposure to ionizing radiation or a positive family history for leukemia.

Physical Examination

The vast majority of people with CML are diagnosed during the chronic phase of their disease. The anemic individual appears pale, and examination of the eyes, ears, nose, and throat may reveal leukemic infiltration. Splenomegaly and hepatomegaly are common.

The physical examination of the patient in blast crisis is similar to that of the patient with acute leukemia. In blast crisis, blastic transformation of the leukemic granulocytes has replaced the bone marrow, causing an acute illness with pancytopenia, infection, and hypercatabolism. Rapid diagnosis and treatment to reduce the number of proliferating blasts are essential.

Diagnostic Studies

A complete blood count in the chronic phase reveals anemia and severe leukocytosis (WBC > 100,000/mm^3). The differential count of the leukocytes demonstrates WBCs in every stage of maturation, with a predominance of more mature cells. The presence of functional but leukemic granulocytes in affected individuals accounts for the low incidence of infection during the chronic phase. There is usually moderate anemia and thrombocytosis. The anemia is normocytic and normochromic with a median hemoglobin of 9–10 g/dL.[65]

Other laboratory studies reveal high serum B_{12} levels and a low leukocyte alkaline phosphatase level (LAP).[65] Both may return to normal with successful therapy. Bone marrow biopsy demonstrates hyperplasia, with a myeloid-to-erythroid ratio of 15:1 and normal to increased megakaryocytes (platelet precursors). If the abnormal Ph^1 chromosome is found in the granulocytic, erythrocytic, and megakaryocytic series of the marrow, the diagnosis of CML is confirmed.[17]

Another tool that has become useful in confirming the diagnosis of CML is polymerase chain reaction (PCR) probes, which are used to separate RNA from viable cells for analysis.[17] This process of reverse transcriptase PCR (RT-PCR) is used to detect the fusion genes that result from chromosome translocations. In the case of patients with CML, RT-PCR detects the

BCR-ABL fusion gene. In some cases, the PCR data may show the presence of the *BCR-ABL* fusion gene after successful response was indicated by the Ph chromosome negativity. Hypermetaphase fluorescent in situ hybridization (FISH) is a newer technique thought to be more sensitive in detecting the Ph chromosome.[69]

Therapeutic Approaches

The only chance for cure of CML is with ablation of the Ph[1] chromosome and absence of the *BCR-ABL* fusion gene. Currently, this occurs after high-dose therapy followed by allogeneic BMT. In most cases, CML is a chronic disease and usually is suppressed by chemotherapy with hydroxyurea or busulfan. Late in the disease or at blastic crisis, investigational drugs are used. Interferon is approved for treatment of patients with chronic-phase CML.[70]

Chronic Phase

The standard therapy during the chronic phase of CML has been single-agent oral chemotherapy with hydroxyurea or busulfan. Although both of these drugs decrease the leukemic cell mass and improve the quality of life, the progression to a terminal, refractory stage is not altered.

Interferon-alfa (IFN) is approved for previously untreated or pretreated patients with chronic-phase, Ph-positive CML. The dose is 9 million international units (MIU) daily, administered subcutaneously or intramuscularly.[70] Patients who achieve a hematologic response (defined as a normalization of blood counts) and a cytogenetic response (absence of the *ABL-BCR* gene) continue with treatment until disease progression. Those who achieve only hematologic response continue therapy for as long as two years to maximize the possibility of achieving a cytogenetic response.

Side effects associated with IFN therapy in this population are similar to others previously reported. The most common are flu-like symptoms such as fever, chill, malaise, fatigue, headache, and myalgias.[71] Lowered blood counts occur with neutropenia (22%), thrombocytopenia (27%), and anemia (15%) that quickly reverses when therapy is withheld.

The new standard of care for chronic CML is imatinib mesylate.[72] This agent inhibits the *BCR-ABL* tyrosine kinase, interfering with the signaling pathway that leads to proliferation of malignant cells.[73] Imatinib mesylate was approved in 2001 for treatment of chronic, acute, and blastic-phase CML after IFN-α therapy failure and for treatment of newly diagnosed Ph-positive CML in 2003.[74] Phase I and II trial results were superior to those found in previous trials with IFN-α and hydroxyurea even in accelerated and blast phases of CML.[73,75,76] Efficacy was documented in three international open-label, one-arm studies in patients who had failed IFN-α therapy.

The common adverse events encountered with imatinib mesylate are nausea (55%–68%), vomiting (28%–54%), edema (52%–68%), and muscle cramps (25%–46%). Patients are monitored for pleural effusions, ascites, pulmonary edema, and rapid weight gain. Managing edema includes interruption of therapy and diuretics. Gastrointestinal irritation associated with ingesting the medication can be decreased by taking it with food and three full glasses of water.[46] If the patient has difficulty swallowing, the capsules can be opened and their contents mixed with mineral water or apple juice. Drug interactions may occur due to imatinib mesylate metabolism through the CYP3A4 pathway. The dose is 400 mg/day for chronic-phase CML and 600 mg/day for accelerated- or blastic-phase CML. The dose can be increased to a maximum of 400 mg BID.

Terminal Phase

CML is a chronic neoplasm with a 100% incidence of blastic transformation.[65] Serial cytogenetic analyses can reveal signs of blastic transformation three to four months before clinical signs become evident. Bone marrow aspirations are required, however, which are costly and uncomfortable for the patient. The current trend is to treat the accelerated phase by continuing chronic-phase therapy until evidence of the blastic phase appears. Because the transformation from a benign to a malignant condition appears to be random in length, it is difficult to predict survival, although average life expectancy is less than one year.

Blast crisis after imatinib mesylate therapy requires intensive chemotherapy, similar to that used in the treatment of AML. If the transformation is myeloblastic, therapy includes cytosine arabinoside, an anthracycline, and thioguanine. If lymphoblastic transformation has occurred, vincristine and prednisone are added. Patients who develop lymphoblastic transformation are more responsive to treatment and tend to live longer.[65]

Although BMT remains the only chance for cure, only 25% of patients with CML have an HLA-matched, related donor.[77] The best results have been obtained in patients receiving allogeneic BMT during the chronic phase, with 55%–70% being disease free at three to five years. Transplants from unrelated, matched donor transplants and autologous transplants are being evaluated as other options.[78–80]

Table 55-9 Three Systems for the Classification of Chronic Lymphocytic Leukemia

Rai	Binet	IWCLL*	Prognosis
0	A	A(0), A(I), A(II)	Good: > 10 yr
I	B	B(I), B(II)	Intermediate: < 7 yr
II	C	C(III), C(IV)	Poor: < 2 yr
III			
IV			

* International Workshop on Chronic Lymphocytic Leukemia.
Data from Cheson.[82]

The addition of imatinib mesylate to the armamentarium has greatly changed the treatment of CML patients. It is not clear, however, how long the drug remains effective in keeping the disease arrested and at what point BMT is to be considered.

Chronic Lymphocytic Leukemia

A progressive accumulation of morphologically normal but functionally inert lymphocytes is found in chronic lymphocytic leukemia (CLL). As the disease progresses, the abnormal lymphocytes accumulate in the bone marrow, spleen, liver, and lymph nodes. The median age at diagnosis is 70 years; the majority of cases occur in males.[65]

The pathologic cells are usually small lymphocytes with markers of B lymphocytes and surface IgM or IgD. The malignant cells express a characteristic phenotype with antigens such as CD5, CD19, CD20, and CD23.[81] Approximately one-half of individuals with CLL experience frequent viral and fungal infections due to hypogammaglobulinemia. For more than 95% of patients, the diagnosis is an incidental finding during routine examination. Anemia, lymphadenopathy, or infection may be present. Coomb's positive autoimmune hemolytic anemia occurs in 25% of patients.[26]

The clinical course is variable, and, as with other hematologic malignancies, many attempts have been made to correlate a staging system with prognosis.[65] The two most commonly used systems are Rai and Binet. The Rai staging system, which is accepted in the United States, has five levels based on the extent of tissue involvement and compromise of bone marrow function. The Binet system distinguishes among three groups — A to C — on the basis of worsening prognosis; it is used in Europe. The International Workshop on CLL (IWCLL) attempt to combine the two systems has not gained wide acceptance (Table 55-9). In general, treatment is withheld until the patient shows evidence of hemolytic anemia, cytopenia, disfiguring or painful lymphadenopathy, symptomatic organomegaly, or marked systemic symptoms.

Assessment

One-fourth of individuals with CLL are diagnosed during a routine physical examination. Clues that alert the clinician early on, however, may be provided by a complete health history.

Patient History

Early CLL may be asymptomatic. However, because CLL is a disease of immunoglobulin-secreting cells, a history of recurrent infections, especially of the skin and respiratory tract, may be elicited. The onset, location, duration, and response to treatment for infection should be documented.

Progressive infiltration and accumulation in nodal structures and the bone marrow gradually produce the symptoms that are typical of more advanced disease. Vague complaints of malaise, anorexia, and fatigue are common, as is noticeable and bothersome lymphadenopathy. Splenomegaly may cause early satiety and abdominal discomfort. The past medical history should focus on the documentation of any underlying autoimmune or immune-deficiency diseases, bleeding tendencies, and infectious episodes.

Physical Examination

The individual with early CLL appears well. Splenomegaly may be the only clinical finding. In advanced disease, there may be evidence of infection, fever, and rashes. Lymphadenopathy occurs in 60% of patients, especially in the cervical, axillary, inguinal, and femoral nodes. The nodes are described as mobile, discrete, and nontender.[65]

Diagnostic Studies

Peripheral blood examination reveals lymphocytosis with normal or immature lymphocytes. The lymphocyte count is greater than 20,000/mm^3 in early disease and may exceed 100,000/mm^3 in advanced disease.[81] Protein electrophoresis documents the hypogammaglobulinemia that occurs in approximately 50% of patients. Bone marrow aspirate reflects the lymphocytosis seen peripherally, with varying degrees of infiltration. The severity of infiltration depends on the severity of the disease. Although early CLL causes patchy or focal infiltrates of the mature-appearing lymphocytes, progressive disease leads to a "packed marrow" with few normal hematopoietic cells.

As in the other hematologic disorders, cytogenetic analysis is important for making the diagnosis and determining prognosis. Chromosomal abnormalities are present in 50% of patients with CLL. Early-stage disease is indicated by 20% abnormalities, while 70% abnormalities are present in later disease.[82,83]

Therapeutic Approaches

A consensus group sponsored by the National Cancer Institute has published guidelines for diagnosis and treatment of CLL.[83] In general, treatment consists only of observation until the patient becomes symptomatic with cytopenias or organomegaly.[82,84] The rate of progressive lymphocytosis directs the frequency of observation and start of therapy. The lymphocyte doubling time (LDT) is important to assess. For patients with a LDT of less than 12 months, the median survival is 12 months.[81]

Chlorambucil and cyclophosphamide are two alkylating agents used to treat CLL; they provide a response rate of 60%, with complete remission in 10%–20% of patients.[82,85] Corticosteroids are used to control leukocytosis and immune-mediated cytopenias. When the patient no longer responds to steroid therapy, splenectomy may provide relief of symptoms. Radiation therapy may be used to treat lymphadenopathy or painful splenomegaly.

For untreated patients with advanced disease (stage III or IV) and either anemia or thrombocytopenia, treatment with fludarabine is recommended.[86,87] Fludarabine, which produces an 80% response rate, is the newest agent approved for use in B-cell CLL. It is given as a daily 30-minute infusion for five days and is generally well tolerated.[82] For patients refractory to fludarabine alone, cyclophosphamide is added.[84]

Alemtuzumab (Campath, Berlex Laboratories, Wayne, New Jersey) is the first monoclonal antibody (MoAb) approved for B cell CLL.[88,89] This recombinant MoAb is directed against CD52 surface antigens expressed on the surface of normal and malignant B and T lymphocytes, natural killer cells, and monocytes. Alemtuzumab has produced a 33% response rate in patients who were refractory to fludarabine. The starting dose is 3 mg in a two-hour daily infusion. The dose is increased to 10 mg three times per week for 12 weeks. As with other MoAbs, more than 80% of patients develop fever and rigors. Premedication with diphenhydramine and acetaminophen decreases infusion reactions. Side effects of alemtuzumab include profound bone marrow depression, including lymphopenia. As a consequence, patients have an increased risk of developing serious bacterial, fungal, viral, and protozoan infections.[46]

Rituximab (Rituxan, IDEC Pharmaceuticals, San Diego, California) is used alone and in combination with fludarabine or cyclophosphamide for CLL. This MoAb is directed at CD20 receptors and is given intravenously 1–3 times per week. Although there are also risks of infusion reactions with this agent, the bone marrow depression is much less than with alemtuzumab.[46]

Hairy Cell Leukemia

Etiology

An unusual variant of the chronic leukemias is hairy cell leukemia (HCL), so named for the prominent cytoplasmic projections on circulating mononuclear cells. HCL is also called *leukemic reticuloendotheliosis.* Clinically, HCL may be difficult to distinguish from CLL or malignant lymphoma. No genes have been found to be directly related to HCL. The distinguishing characteristics are massive splenomegaly and little or no adenopathy. The characteristic hairy cells stain positively for tartrate-resistant acid phosphatase.[26] Two-thirds of individuals with HCL have pancytopenia, with symptomatic anemia, bleeding, and infection.

Therapeutic Approaches

The goal of therapy in HCL has progressed from palliation to cure, thanks to the use of nucleoside analogs and interferon. Historically, patients without cytopenias required no immediate treatment. Because infection is the primary cause of death, however, patients with HCL are monitored closely. Splenectomy has been the treatment of choice for patients with marked pancytopenia, recurrent infections, massive splenomegaly, or rapid disease progression; it may allow prolonged survival of up to 15 years. However, complete remissions have been obtained in HCL with 2′-deoxycoformycin and 2-chlorodeoxyadenosine.[89–91] Normalization of peripheral blood counts occurs with absence of hairy cells in the bone marrow, and long-term results are positive. Recombinant interferon-alfa is considered the treatment of choice for those in whom the disease progresses.[86] Administered daily by intramuscular or subcutaneous injection, interferon-alfa decreases the need for transfusions, reduces the risk of infection, and improves overall quality of life.

White blood cells fight infection	Red blood cells carry oxygen	Platelets control bleeding
If bone marrow is not producing enough cells:		
1. may develop infection	1. anemia	1. may have nosebleeds
2. may develop sore mouth	2. feel out of breath	2. gums may bleed
	3. feel weak or tired	3. may notice bruises
		4. blood in urine or stool
Treatment:		
1. prevent infection	1. transfusions	1. prevent bleeding
		2. transfusions
Report to doctor or nurse:		
1. fever over 100°F	1. feeling out of breath	1. nosebleed that will not stop
2. excess cough and sputum production	2. increasing weakness	2. blood in stool
3. burning with urination		3. cloudy urine

Figure 55-4 Patient teaching sheet for blood cell function.

Supportive Care

The increase in the length and quality of survival experienced by most individuals with leukemia is due not only to advances in antileukemic therapy but also to improved blood product and antimicrobial support and specialized nursing care. The complex means of providing effective supportive care include medical management to maintain physiologic homeostasis as well as an interdisciplinary approach to the healthcare plan.

Effective nursing participation in the supportive care of any patient with leukemia depends on an understanding of the staging and natural history of each type of leukemia. From this base of knowledge, the nurse contributes to the care of the patient with leukemia in the areas of education, physical care, symptom management, and psychosocial adaptation.

Education

Providing information related to the disease process and treatment is clearly a standard in oncology nursing.[92] The nurse caring for the patient with AML has a unique opportunity to provide information to the patient and family because the patient is usually hospitalized throughout the course of therapy. The teaching plan for all patients includes pertinent information about the diagnosis, strategies for self-care in the prevention and treatment of side effects both in the hospital setting and at home, and methods to facilitate coping and adaptation to the illness.

For all patients with leukemia, it is helpful to include the basic physiology of the bone marrow in the teaching plan. A hematologic malignancy is not as easy to understand as the concept of a solid tumor. Describing the bone marrow as the center of the bone where all blood products are made is a simple start. Further explanation includes the type, function, and abnormalities of the blood cells (Figure 55-4). From this base, individualized instruction related to the specific leukemia is given. Educational materials can be obtained from the Leukemia Society, American Cancer Society, and the National Cancer Institute.

Physical Care

The physical care needs of patients with leukemia require nurses who are skilled in physical assessment. Patients with AML receive intensive therapy aimed at producing bone marrow aplasia for several weeks. Those with ALL have defective lymphocytes that lead to altered immunocompetence. The drugs received are cytotoxic. The hypogammaglobulinemia associated with CLL increases the patient's susceptibility to viral and fungal infections. In any type of leukemia the incidence of infection is high, but the usual signs and symptoms of infection may be diminished or absent. Therefore, the nurse must regularly conduct a thorough physical examination to detect any evidence of infection. Subtle changes in vital signs and mentation may indicate early sepsis. Oozing of blood from gums and intravenous sites may be the first sign of disseminated intravascular coagulation. Cerebellar toxicity related to chemotherapy may be manifested as slightly altered responses in the neurological examination. Each of these situations may be life-threatening, and the astute skills of the experienced nurse may be the crucial factor in initiating appropriate treatment.

In addition to having good assessment skills, the nurse caring for the patient with acute leukemia must be experienced in the use of right atrial catheters (RACs) and vascular access devices (VADs).[93,94] Patients undergoing aggressive induction therapy in the hospital often have a double- or triple-lumen RAC placed prior to the start of therapy. This catheter is used for blood sampling as well as for the infusion of fluids, chemotherapy, antibiotics, total parenteral nutrition, and blood products.[94,95] Patients who require ongoing treatment but less frequent blood sampling and no simultaneous infusion of multiple fluids may have a VAD placed subcutaneously.[96] The advantages, disadvantages, and nursing procedures associated with RACs and VADs are beyond the scope of this chapter. However, given that most patients with acute leukemia have one of these devices, it is important for the nurse to become familiar with them.

Symptom Management

Certain side effects associated with antileukemic therapy and disease-related complications can best be ameliorated if they are detected early and treated promptly. Knowing which side effects are expected and when they may occur allows the nurse to focus care appropriately.

Bone marrow depression

The desired effect of cytotoxic therapy is bone marrow hypoplasia. The duration of pancytopenia is variable, depending on the type of therapy and the person's ability to recover. However, individuals with acute leukemia in the induction phase or individuals with CML in blast crisis may remain severely hypoplastic for months.

Neutropenia. It takes nine to ten days for immature cells formed in the bone marrow to become mature granulocytes. Because granulocytes circulate for only six to ten hours, any interruption in their production quickly places the patient at risk for developing an infection. Infection is the major complication for leukemia patients, with mortality as high as 20%–30%.[97,98] Neutropenia is commonly defined as an absolute neutrophil count less than 1000/mm^3. Because the neutrophils are responsible for phagocytosis, neutropenia eliminates one of the body's first lines of defense against infection. The patient with leukemia is particularly at risk due to a rapid drop in WBCs with the initiation of therapy, a continuing decrease until the nadir (lowest point) is reached, and a prolonged time for recovery.[99]

Approximately 60% of neutropenic individuals develop infection. One-third have documented bacteremia, another third have documented infection without bacteremia, and the rest have apparent infection with no microbiologically documented pathogen. The most frequent cause of bacteremia is coagulase-negative staphylococci and *viridans* streptococci.[97] The risk of infection increases as the neutrophil count decreases, with 100% incidence of infection if the neutrophil count remains less than 100/mm^3 for three weeks. Other factors that add to the risk of infection are corticosteroids, hospital environment, antibiotic usage leading to increased colonization, and mucosal alteration.[97]

Adrenal corticosteroids are frequently used as part of the chemotherapeutic regimen or as supportive therapy. Steroids cause lysis of lymphocytes, suppression of antibody production, protein malnutrition, and suppression of inflammatory responses. As a result, the use of corticosteroids predisposes the patient to infection.

Most infections are caused by organisms that are endogenous to the host or present in the environment.[99] The most common sites of infection are the alimentary tract (pharynx, esophagus, anorectum), sinuses, lungs, and skin.[100,101] The alimentary mucosa is directly damaged by chemotherapy, and neutropenia subsequently allows colonization with yeasts and/or gram-negative bacilli. Perianal infection occurs in 25% of patients with AML. The only signs may be induration, erythema, and pain on defecation. Pneumonia can be caused by gram-negative organisms such as *Pseudomonas aeruginosa, Klebsiella pneumonia,* or *Escherichia coli.* The most common gram-positive organism causing infection is *Staphylococcus epidermidis.*[100,101]

More serious infections associated with prolonged neutropenia are fungal infections such as *Candida tropicalis, Aspergillus* spp., *Fusarium* spp., and *Trichosporon* spp. or protozoa such as *Pneumocystis carinii.*[102] When these infections occur during severe aplasia and immune depression, recovery of the blood counts offers the best hope for survival.

Empiric antibiotic therapy is used to treat high-risk (neutropenic and febrile) patients until an infecting organism is identified. Early empiric antibiotic therapy includes drugs to cover both gram-negative and gram-positive organisms. The usual combinations include an aminoglycoside plus an extended-spectrum cephalosporin or a broad-spectrum antipseudomonal penicillin.[103,104]

Amphotericin B is used to treat life-threatening fungal infections in myelosuppressed, immunosuppressed individuals. It is indicated if fever continues for five to seven days after the start of antibiotic therapy, if there is no identified source of infection, and if continued neutropenia is expected.[105] Common side effects of this toxic therapy include fever, chills, rigors, nephrotoxicity, headache, anorexia, vomiting, and anemia. Because anaphylaxis is a risk, a test dose of 1 mg is administered over 30 minutes. If the patient does not experience cardiopulmonary or mental changes, the starting dose is given. Fever is not a contraindication when the patient has recurrent fevers prior to the therapy. The dose is escalated daily until the desired dose is reached, and therapy continues for weeks to months, depending on the organism being treated and the patient's response.

Symptom management includes the following interventions to prevent or treat fever, chills, or rigors: premedication with corticosteroids, acetaminophen, or diphenhydramine, and adding 10–15 mg hydrocortisone sodium succinate to the infusion. Intravenous meperidine 25–50 mg is given at the onset of chills or as a premedication. Increasing the room temperature, adding extra covers, using relaxation and hypnosis, and isometric leg and arm movements are other suggested comfort measures.[99] Potential nephrotoxicity due to a decreased glomerular filtration rate requires close monitoring of blood urea nitrogen, creatinine, sodium, and magnesium as well as evaluation of fluid balance.[106] Peripheral phlebitis can be avoided by adding heparin to the solution. The anemia associated with amphotericin B is reversible and problematic only in that it compounds the existing myelosuppression.

New lipid formulations of amphotericin B are available. Liposomal amphotericin B is less nephrotoxic and has fewer infusion-related side effects. Due to their higher cost, the liposomal amphotericins are generally used only when the patient has renal insufficiency or cannot tolerate of infusion-related toxicities.[107]

Because the neutropenic patient does not produce an adequate inflammatory response to infection, the usual signs and symptoms are absent.[99] Fever is usually the first sign of infection that prompts closer inspection of high-risk areas (perirectal area, oral mucosa, IV sites). Patients are often unable to produce sputum; thus, the early indications of pneumonia are shortness of breath or cough. Vital signs are assessed every four hours. At the onset of fever more than 100°F in the neutropenic patient, blood, urine, and sputum cultures are obtained and empiric antibiotic therapy is initiated. The importance of prompt reporting of fever and initiation of therapy cannot be overemphasized, as delay of only a few hours can allow the patient to go into septic shock.

Prevention of infection focuses on restoring host defenses, decreasing invasive procedures, and decreasing colonization of organisms. Treatment and remission induction will restore normal defenses against infection. Decreasing invasive procedures includes avoiding the use of Foley catheters. If catheterization is necessary, the smallest lumen possible should be used, and the catheter should be anchored. Other helpful measures include meticulous care of IV or RAC exit sites and aseptic technique for any invasive procedures.

To decrease the number of gram-negative organisms encountered by the patient, uncooked fruits and vegetables are avoided, especially salads. *P. aeruginosa* can be decreased by removing aerators from faucets, using ice machines in which the ice falls directly into the cup, and frequently changing stagnant water sources such as oxygen humidifiers. Proper handwashing techniques by everyone who comes in contact with the patient can eliminate the main source of gram-positive organisms. Fungi that are found in food or the air can also be decreased by cooking foods and eliminating live plants or flowers from the patient's room. A private room is necessary, and visitors are restricted. All of these measures are to be practiced by the healthcare team and taught to the patient and family. Further information is provided in Chapter 28. In certain circumstances such as BMT, total reverse isolation may be used. The patient is kept in a sterile laminar air-flow room. Nonabsorbable antibiotics are used to sterilize the alimentary canal. Normal skin flora are decreased by frequent cleansing with hexachlorophene or an iodine-base soap.

Granulocyte transfusions may be indicated for patients with profound neutropenia and documented infections not responding to antibiotics.[108,109] However, the hazards of this therapy (increased alloimmunization and refractoriness to platelet transfusions) and its high cost make it a controversial choice.

Hematapoietic growth factors (HGFs) have been used in the treatment of patients with leukemia as part of supportive care and for priming effects.[110,111] Both granulocyte colony-stimulating factor (G-CSF) and granulocyte-macrophage colony-stimulating factor (GM-CSF) have been administered to patients after completion of standard induction therapy to shorten the period of neutropenia. Because myeloid leukemia cells have receptors for CSFs and have demonstrated increased growth in response to CSFs in vitro, supportive use of HGFs are recommended for high-risk patients only, such as those older than age 60. There is concern about administering myeloid CSFs to patients with AML.

Erythrocytopenia. Individuals undergoing intensive chemotherapy develop a tolerance for chronic, low-grade anemia. However, in severe cases of hypoplasia, sudden blood loss due to bleeding, or symptomatic anemia, support with transfusions of RBCs is provided. Premedication with acetaminophen and diphenhydramine can decrease the febrile response to antibodies to WBCs that occurs after multiple transfusions. Leukocyte-poor RBCs may be used to decrease the antibody production against antigens on the leukocytes.[112,113]

Thrombocytopenia. Thrombocytopenia is an abnormal decrease in the number of circulating platelets. The potential for bleeding occurs when levels are less than 50,000 platelets/mm^3, and spontaneous bleeding occurs at levels of less than 20,000 platelets/mm^3.[112] The first evidence of bleeding may be petechiae or ecchymoses on the skin of dependent limbs or on mucous membranes or oozing from gums, nose, or IV site.

Random donor platelets are given to keep the platelet count above 20,000/mm^3. Once antibodies to the platelets develop, refractoriness to random-donor platelets occurs. When blood counts one hour post-transfusion reveal poor increments, the patient may require HLA-matched, single-donor platelets.[112] Because chills and fever can destroy circulating platelets, the patient is premedicated with acetaminophen and diphenhydramine. Additional measures used to prevent bleeding include maintaining skin integrity, preventing trauma, and avoiding medications that have the potential to induce or prolong bleeding. Stool softeners will prevent the Valsalva maneuver and rectal tears. Further detail is given in Chapter 29.

Complications

Certain complications of the specific leukemic process or therapy may be singled out as untoward but not unexpected side effects. Knowledge of these occurrences assists the nurse in anticipating problems in high-risk individuals. These complications include leukostasis, disseminated intravascular coagulation, retinoic acid–APL (RA-APL) syndrome, oral complications, and cerebellar toxicity.

Leukostasis. Individuals with extremely high numbers of circulating blasts are at risk of developing leukostatic-induced hemorrhage. This problem occurs most often in patients with ALL. Leukostasis arises when leukemic blasts accumulate and invade vessel walls, causing rupture and bleeding. Because of the extensive capillary network and the limited vasculature space of the brain, intracerebral hemorrhage is the most common and most lethal manifestation of this complication. Therefore, early detection of patients at risk (WBC > 50,000 cells/mm^3) and immediate efforts to reduce the number of circulating cells are imperative. Treatment consists of high doses of cytotoxic drugs to reduce the burden of circulating cells. Leukapheresis and cranial irradiation may be used to provide immediate treatment.[47]

Disseminated intravascular coagulation. Disseminated intravascular coagulation (DIC) is most frequently associated with acute promyelocytic leukemia, although it may occur with any acute leukemia.[15,41] During induction therapy, excessive release of procoagulants from granules within the leukemic promyelocyte occurs. (See Chapter 37 for a discussion of the pathophysiology of DIC.)

Correction of the coagulopathy in DIC depends on the successful treatment of the leukemia. Therapy usually includes heparin and replacement of plasma factors and platelets. Nursing care focuses on the prevention of injury, administration of prescribed therapy, and monitoring of the appropriate laboratory results.[112]

Retinoic acid–APL syndrome. Another toxicity associated with treatment of APL is RA-APL syndrome. This syndrome appears clinically similar to the capillary leak syndrome associated with interleukin-2 therapy and is characterized by fever, respiratory distress, pulmonary infiltrates on chest x-ray, and weight gain. Its incidence is 40% among patients with APL, and its etiology is unknown. Early identification and treatment with high-dose intravenous steroids has decreased the mortality associated with this syndrome.[46] Nursing care focuses on early detection of fluid retention (with measurement of weight, abdominal girth, orthostatic blood pressure, and intake and output), fever (vital signs), and pulmonary distress.[46]

Oral complications. Oral complications of leukemia may result from either the disease or the therapy. Gingival hypertrophy due to massive infiltration by leukemic cells is associated with acute myelomonocytic and monocytic leukemia.[7] The gingiva may be swollen, necrotic, and/or superinfected. The most effective treatment is therapy for the leukemia. Stomatitis due to the direct toxicity of chemotherapeutic agents such as the anthracyclines or methotrexate, combined with prolonged neutropenia and antibiotic therapy, renders the patient at high risk for oral infection.

Oral care consists of regular cleansing with a solution of one quart of water with one teaspoon each of salt and sodium bicarbonate or 1.5% hydrogen peroxide, treatment of infection with nystatin mouth rinses, and appropriate analgesia as needed.[114]

Cerebellar toxicity. Cerebellar toxicity is a CNS toxicity associated with the administration of high-dose cytosine arabinoside (HDCA).[115] Conventional dosages are 100–200 mg/m^2, whereas HDCA consists of doses greater than 3 g/m^2. The incidence of neurotoxicity is 11%–28% at dosages of 3 g/m^2 and as high as 67% in dosages up to 4.5 g/m^2. This toxicity is also age-related, with an increased risk in patients older than age 50. The syndrome may begin with signs of ataxia and nystagmus, then progress to dysarthria (difficulty in articulating words) and adiadochokinesis (inability to perform rapid alternating movements). This toxicity may be irreversible if not detected early. Therefore, it is essential that prior to each dose of HDCA the nurse completes a full neurological assessment. Any changes are reported and the dosage is held until the physician evaluates the patient.

Psychosocial Support

Individuals and their significant others are at risk for ineffective coping both during the diagnostic work-up for malignancy and during subsequent treatments.[116] A primary objective of supportive care must be to facilitate the most effective coping mechanisms for the individual and family as well as to enable the patient to live as full and normal a life as possible. Several factors should be taken into consideration as the nurse coordinates the care plan for psychological and physical rehabilitation.

The age of the individual at the time of diagnosis may vary from infancy to old age. Issues may range from concern about fertility or the risk of a second malignancy in the young adult to fear of job stigma in the middle-aged individual. The elderly patient may be dealing with increasing physical decline in addition to the debilitating effects of cancer. Assessment of the individual's needs and degree of stress will facilitate the planning of suitable interventions.[117]

The stage and "curability" of the disease must also be considered. It is imperative that the nurse understand the implications of the planned therapy and assist the patient in making appropriate decisions. For example, a young mother undergoing intensive chemotherapy for AML may need to make arrangements for child care and housekeeping for six to eight weeks. A patient undergoing BMT may need to discuss with his or her employer the need to take extended sick leave. The emotional ups and downs related to multiple remission inductions and relapses are exhausting to the patient and family. As survival with leukemia increases, patients must deal with many issues such as fear of relapse, return to an independent state, and an uncertain future.[118] Ongoing support from the healthcare team is essential to overcome these fears. Education and reassurance by consistent nursing staff can help the individual regain a sense of control and hopefulness.

Conclusion

The care of the individual with a diagnosis of leukemia requires a multidisciplinary approach that considers many factors. Currently, classification, stage of disease, and age are the best predictors of response. As more becomes known about the molecular biology of leukemia and its genetic markers, the treatment plan will be customized for each patient. Targeted therapies will be added earlier in the treatment continuum as additional risk factors are identified.

The role of the nurse in providing direct care for patients with leukemia includes education, physical care, symptom management, and psychosocial support. Care in the future will require increased knowledge of the diagnostic tests and treatments so as to appropriately educate and support patients and their families. Nurses must continue to participate in research trials of new antileukemic therapies and to develop nursing care strategies needed for symptom management and emotional support.

References

1. Miller K, Daoust P: Clinical manifestations of acute myeloid leukemia, in Hoffman R, Benz E, Shattil S, et al (eds.): *Hematology Basic Principles and Practice.* Philadelphia, Churchill Livingstone, 2000, pp 999–1024
2. Mrozek K, Heinomen K, Bloodfield CD: Prognostic value of cytogenetic findings in adults with acute myeloid leukemia. *Int J Hematol* 72:261–271, 2000
3. Jemal A, Riwari RC, Murray T, et al: Cancer statistics, 2004. *CA Cancer J Clin* 54:8–29, 2004

4. Hutton JJ: The leukemias and polycythemia, in Stein JH (ed.): *Internal Medicine* (ed 5). St. Louis, Mosby, 1998, pp 682–691
5. Stone R, Mayer R: Acute myeloid leukemia in adults, in Abeloff M, Armitage J, Lichter A, et al (eds.): *Clinical Oncology*. New York, Churchill Livingstone, 2000, pp 2490–2510
6. Sandler DP: Epidemiology of acute leukemia in children and adults. *Semin Oncol* 24:3–16, 1997
7. Stock W, Thirman M: Pathobiology of acute myeloid leukemia, in Hoffman R, Benz E, Shattil S, et al (eds.): *Hematology Basic Principles and Practice*. Philadelphia, Churchill Livingstone, 2000, pp 979–999
8. Preston DI, Kusumi S, Tomonaga M, et al: Cancer incidence in atomic bomb survivors: part III. Leukemia, lymphoma, and multiple myeloma, 1950–1987. *Radiat Res* 137 (suppl): S68–S97, 1994
9. Matanowski GM, Seltser R, Sartwell PE: The current mortality rates of radiologists and other physician specialists: specific causes of death. *Am J Epidemiol* 101:199–210, 1975
10. Paustenbach DJ, Bass RD, Price P: Benzene toxicity and risk assessment, 1972–1992: implications for future regulation. *Environ Health Perspect* 101 (suppl 6):177–200, 1993
11. Dougan L, Woodleff AJ: Acute leukemia associated with phenylbutazone treatment. *Med J Aust* 1:217–219, 1965
12. Brauer MJ, Dameshek W: Hypoplastic anemia and myeloblastic leukemia following chloramphenicol therapy. *N Engl J Med* 277:1003–1005, 1967
13. Karp JE, Smith ME: The molecular pathogenesis of treatment induced (secondary) leukemias: foundations for treatment and prevention. *Semin Oncol* 24:103–113, 1997
14. Farias de Carvalho SM, Pombo de Oliveira MS, Thuler LC, et al: HTLV-I and HTLV-II infections in hematologic disorder patients, cancer patients and healthy patients from Rio de Janeiro, Brazil. *J Acquir Immune Defic Syndr Hum Retrovirol* 15:238–242, 1997
15. Fenaux P, Chomienne C, Degos L: Acute promyelocytic leukemia: biology and treatment. *Semin Oncol* 24:92–102, 1997
16. Caligiuri MA, Strout MP, Gilliland DG: Molecular biology of acute myeloid leukemia. *Semin Oncol* 24:32–44, 1997
17. Rowley JD: Cytogenetic analysis in leukemia and lymphoma: an introduction. *Semin Hematol* 37:315–319, 2000.
18. Stolzfus PK, Rust, D, Ried T: Molecular cytogenetics and gene analysis: implications for oncology nurses. *Clin J Oncol Nurs* 5:201–206, 2001
19. Bloomfield CD, Caligiuri MA: Molecular biology of leukemias, in DeVita VT, Hellman S, Rosenberg SA (eds.): *Cancer: Principles and Practices of Oncology*. Philadelphia, Lippincott, Williams and Wilkins, 2001, pp 2389–2404.
20. Ferrando AA, Look AT: Clinical implications of recurring chromosomal and associated molecular abnormalities in acute lymphoblastic leukemia. *Semin Hematol* 37:381–395, 2000
21. Matutes E, Morilla R, Farahat N, et al: Definition of acute biphenotypic leukemia. *Haematologia* 82:64–66, 1997
22. Bennett JM, Catovsky D, Daniel MT, et al: Proposals for the classification of the acute leukemias. *Br J Haemat* 33:451–458, 1976
23. Bennett JM, Catovsky D, Daniel MT, et al: Criteria for the diagnosis of acute leukemia of megakaryocyte lineage (M7). *Ann Intern Med* 103:460–462, 1985
24. Bennett JM, Catovsky D, Daniel MT, et al: Proposed revised criteria for the classification of acute myeloid leukemia. *Ann Intern Med* 103:626–629, 1985
25. Catovsky D, Matukis E, Buccheri V, et al: A classification of acute leukemia for the 1990s. *Ann Hematol* 62:16–21, 1991
26. Champlin R, Golde DW: The leukemias, in Braunwald E, Isselbacher KJ, Petersdorf RG, et al (eds.): *Harrison's Principles of Internal Medicine* (ed 14). New York, McGraw-Hill, 1998, pp 1541–1550
27. Lowenberg G, Downing JR, Burnett A: Acute myeloid leukemia. *N Engl J Med* 341:1051–1062, 1999
28. Bishop JF: The treatment of adult acute myeloid leukemia. *Semin Oncol* 24:57–69, 1997
29. Ravandi F, Kantarjian H, Giles F, et al: New agents in acute myeloid leukemia and other myeloid disorders. *Cancer* 100:441–454, 2004
30. Leopold LH, Willemze R: The treatment of acute myeloid leukemia in first relapse: a comprehensive review of the literature. *Leuk Lymphoma* 43:1715–1727, 2002
31. Schiller G, Gajewski J, Territo M, et al: Long-term outcome of high dose cytarabine based consolidation therapy for adults with acute myelogenous leukemia. *Blood* 80:2977–2982, 1992
32. Baer MR: Assessment of minimal residual disease in patients with acute leukemia. *Curr Opin Oncol* 10:17–22, 1998
33. Estey E, Thall P, Giles F, et al: Gemtuzumab ozogamicin with or without interleukin 11 in patients 65 years or older with untreated acute myeloid leukemia and high risk myelodysplastic syndrome: comparison with idarubicin plus continuous infusion high-dose cytosine arabinoside. *Blood* 99:43–49, 2002
34. Zittoun RA, Mandelli F, Willemze R, et al: Autologous or allogeneic bone marrow transplantation compared with intensive chemotherapy in acute myelogenous leukemia. *N Engl J Med* 332:217–223, 1995
35. Tabbara IA, Zimmerman K, Morgan C, et al: Allogeneic hematopoietic stem cell transplantation: complications and results. *Arch Intern Med* 162:1558–1566, 2002
36. Devine H, DeMeyer E: Hematopoietic cell transplantation in the treatment of leukemia. *Semin Oncol Nurs* 19:118–132, 2003
37. Degos L, Dombret H, Chomienne C, et al: All-*trans* retinoic acid as a differentiating agent in the treatment of acute promyelocytic leukemia. *Blood* 85:2643–2653, 1995
38. Dombret H, Fenaux P, Soignet S, et al: Established practice in the treatment of patients with acute promyelocytic leukemia and the introduction of arsenic trioxide as a novel therapy. *Semin Hematol* 39:8–13, 2002
39. Roche Laboratories: Vesanoid (tretinoin) capsules (package insert). Nutley, NJ, 2000
40. Davison K, Mann K, Miller W: Aresenic trioxide: mechanism of action. *Semin Hematol* 39 (suppl 1):3–7, 2002
41. Liu P, Han ZC: Treatment of acute promyelocytic leukemia and other hematologic malignancies with arsenic trioxide: review of clinical and basic studies. *Int J Hematol* 78:32–39, 2003
42. Kottaridis PD, Gale RE, Linch DC: Prognostic implications of the presence of FLT3 mutations in patients with acute myeloid leukemia. *Leuk Lymphoma* 44:905–913, 2003
43. Levis M, Small D: FLT3: it does matter in leukemia. *Leukemia* 17:1738–1752, 2003
44. Lowenberg B: Managing therapy in older patients with AML. *Semin Hematol* 38 (suppl 6):10–16, 2001
45. Berger MS, Leopold LH, Dowell JA, et al: Licensure of gemtuzumab ozogamicin for the treatment of selected patients 60 years of age or older with acute myeloid leukemia in first relapse. *Invest New Drugs* 20:395–406 2002.
46. Stull DM: Targeted therapies for the treatment of leukemia. *Semin Oncol Nurs* 19:90–99, 2003
47. Stock W, Byrd J, Frankel S, et al: Adult acute lymphoblastic leukemia, in Abeloff M, Armitage J, Lichter A, Niederhuber J (eds.): *Clinical Oncology*. New York, Churchill Livingstone, 2000, pp 2451–2489
48. Linker C, Damon L, Ries C, et al: Intensified and shortened cyclical chemotherapy for adult acute lymphoblastic leukemia. *J Clin Oncol* 20:2462–2471, 2002

49. Hoelzer D, Gokbuget N, Ottmann O, et al: Acute lymphoblastic leukemia. *Hematology (Am Soc Hematol Educ Program)* 2002:162–192, 2002
50. Federl S, Jeha S, Kantarjian HM: The biology and therapy of adult acute lymphoblastic leukemia. *Cancer* 98:1337–1354, 2003
51. Cortes J: Central nervous system involvement in adult acute lymphocytic leukemia. *Hematol Oncol Clin North Am* 15:145–161, 2001
52. Thomas X, Le QH: Prognostic factors in adult acute lymphoblastic leukemia. *Hematology* 8:233–242, 2003
53. Hamilton-Paterson JL: Preleukemia anemia. *Acta Haematology* 2:309–316, 1949
54. Kouides PA, Bennett JM: Morphology and classifcation of myelodysplastic syndromes. *Hematol Oncol Clin North Am* 6:485–499, 1992
55. Bennett JM, Catovsky D, Daniel MT, et al: The French-American-British (FAB) Cooperative Group: proposals for the classification of the myelodysplastic syndromes. *Br J Haematol* 51:189–199, 1982
56. Komrokji R, Bennett JM: The myelodysplastic syndromes: classification and prognosis. *Curr Hematol Rep* 2:179–185, 2003
57. Sanz G, Sanz M, Greenberg P: Prognostic factors and scoring systems in myelodysplastic syndromes: recent advances in myelodysplastic syndromes. *Haematologica* 83:358–376, 1998
58. Karp J: Molecular pathogenesis and targets for therapy in myelodysplastic syndromes (MDS) and MDS-related leukemias. *Curr Opin Oncol* 10:3–9, 1998
59. Erba HP: Recent progress in the treatment of meylodysplastic syndrome in adult patients. *Curr Opin Oncol* 15:1–9, 2003
60. Magill MK, Macfarlane E, McMullin MF: Intramedullary apoptosis may simply be a correlate of ineffective hematopoiesis. *Br J Haematol* 97 (suppl 1):17–23, 1997
61. Koides PA, Bennett JM: Understanding the myelodysplastic syndromes. *Oncologist* 2:389–401, 1997
62. Steensma DP, Tefferi A: The myelodysplastic syndrome(s): a perspective and review highlighting current controversies. *Leuk Res* 27:95–120, 2003
63. National Cancer Center Network: NCCN practice guidelines for the myelodysplastic syndromes. *Oncology* 12:53–80, 1998
64. Hsu CA, Rishi AK, Su-Li X, et al: Retinoid induced apoptosis in leukemic cells through a retinoic acid nuclear receptor–independent pathway. *Blood* 89:4470–4479, 1997
65. Miller KB, Grodman HM: Leukemia, in Lenhard RE, Osteen RT, Gansler T (eds.): *Clinical Oncology*. Atlanta, American Cancer Society, 2001, pp 527–551
66. Sawyers CL: Chronic myeloid leukemia. *N Engl J Med* 340:1330–1340, 1999
67. Deininger MWN, Goldman JM, Melo JV: The molecular biology of chronic myeloid leukemia. *Blood* 96:3343–3356, 2000
68. Shet AJ, Jahagirdar BN, Verfaillie CM: Chronic myelogenous leukemia: mechanisms underlying disease progression. *Leukemia* 16:1402–1411, 2002
69. Wujcik D: Molecular biology of leukemia. *Semin Oncol Nurs* 19:83–89, 2000
70. Kantarjian HM, Giles FJ, O'Brien SM, et al: Clinical course and therapy of chronic myelogenous leukemia with interferon-alpha and chemotherapy. *Hematol Oncol Clin North Am* 12:31–80, 1998
71. Rieger PT: Interferon-alpha: a clinical update. *Cancer Pract* 3:356–365, 1996
72. Faderl S, Kantarjian HM, Talpaz M, et al: New treatment approaches for chronic myeloid leukemia. *Semin Oncol* 27:578–586, 2000
73. Savage DG, Antman KH: Imatinib meslylate: a new oral targeted therapy. *N Engl J Med* 346:645–652, 2002
74. O'Brien SG, Guilhot F, Larson RA, et al: Imatinib compared with interferon and low-dose cytarabine for newly diagnosed chronic-phase chronic myeloid leukemia. *N Engl J Med* 348:994–1004, 2003
75. Druker BJ, Talpaz M, Resta DJ, et al: Efficacy and safety of a specific inhibitor of BCR-ABL tyrosine kinase in chronic myeloid leukemia. *N Engl J Med* 344:1031–1037, 2001
76. Kantarjian MD, Sawyers CL, Hochhaus A, et al: Hematologic and cytogenetic responses to imatinib mesylate in chronic myelogenous leukemia. *N Engl J Med* 356:645–652, 2002
77. Pasweg JR, Rowlings PA, Horowitz MM: Related donor bone marrow transplantation for chronic myelogenous leukemia. *Hematol Oncol Clin North Am* 12:81–92, 1998
78. McGlave P: Unrelated donor transplant therapy for chronic myelogenous leukemia. *Hematol Oncol Clin North Am* 12:93–106, 1998
79. Bhatia R, Forman J: Autologous transplantation for the treatment of chronic myelogenous leukemia. *Hematol Oncol Clin North Am* 12:151–172, 1998
80. Kantarjian HM, Giles FJ, O'Brien S, et al: Therapeutic choices in younger patients with chronic myeloid leukemia. *Cancer* 89: 1647–1658, 2000
81. Zwiebel JA, Cheson BD: Chronic lymphocytic leukemias: staging and prognostic factors. *Semin Oncol* 25:42–59, 1998
82. Cheson BD: Therapy for previous untreated chronic lymphocytic leukemia: a reevaluation. *Semin Hematol* 35:14–21, 1998
83. Dohner H, Stilgenbauer S, Benner A, et al: Genomic aberrations and survival in chronic lymphocytic leukemia. *N Engl J Med* 343:1902–1916, 2000
84. Chronic Lymphocytic Leukemia Trialists' Collaborative Group: Chemotherapeutic options in chronic lymphocytic leukemia: a meta-analysis of the randomized trials. *J Natl Cancer Inst* 91:861–868, 1999
85. Keating MJ: Chronic lymphocytic leukemia in the next decade: where do we go from here? *Semin Hematol* 35:27–33, 1998
86. Byrd JC, Rai KR, Sausville EA, et al: Old and new therapies in chronic lymphocytic leukemia: now is the time for reassessment of therapeutic goals. *Semin Oncol* 25:65–74, 1998
87. Rai KR, Peterson BL, Appelbaum FR, et al: Fludarabine compared with chlorambucil as primary therapy for chronic lymphocytic leukemia. *N Engl J Med* 343:1799–1801, 2000
88. Lynn A, Williams ML, Sickler J, et al: Treatment of chronic lymphocytic leukemia with alemtuzumab: a review for nurses. *Oncol Nurs Forum* 30:689–694, 2003.
89. Cheson BD, Sorenson JM, Vena DA, et al: Treatment of hairy cell leukemia with 2-chlorodeoxyadenosine via the Group C protocol mechanism of the National Cancer Institute: a report of 979 patients. *J Clin Oncol* 16:3007–3015, 1998
90. Casselith PA, Cheuvart B, Spiers AS, et al: Randomized comparison of pentostatin versus interferon alpha-2a in previously untreated patients with hairy cell leukemia: an intergroup study. *J Clin Oncol* 13:974–982, 1995
91. Goodman GR, Beutler E, Saven R: Cladaribine in the treatment of hairy-cell leukaemia. *Best Pract Res Clin Haematol* 16:101–116, 2003.
92. Somerville ET: Knowledge deficit related to chemotherapy, in McNally JC, Stair JC, Somerville ET (eds.): *Guidelines for Cancer Nursing Practice*. Philadelphia, Saunders, 1985, pp 57–61
93. Intravenous Nurses Society: The Registered Nurse' role in vascular access device selection. *J Intravenous Nurs* 20:71–72, 1997
94. Voit M: Intravenous access: related problems in oncology. *Int J Antimicrob Agents* 16:165–168, 2000
95. Douard MC, Arlet G, Loguet P, et al: Diagnosis of venous access port–related infections. *Infect Dis* 29:1197–1202, 1999

96. Moran AB, Camp-Sorrell D: Maintenance of venous access devices in patients with neutropenia. *Clin J Oncol Nurs* 6:126–130, 2002
97. Segal BH, Walsh TJ, Holland SM: Infections in the cancer patient, in DeVita VT, Hellman S, Rosenberg SA (eds.): *Cancer: Principles and Practice of Oncology* (ed 6). Philadelphia, Lippincott, Williams and Wilkins, 2001, pp 2815–2868
98. Pizzo PA: Fever in immunocompromised patients. *N Engl J Med* 341:893–900, 1999
99. Wujcik D: Infection, in Yarbro CH, Frogge MH, Goodman M (eds.): *Cancer Symptom Management* (ed 3). Sudbury, MA, Jones and Bartlett, 2004, pp 252–275
100. Zinner SH: New pathogens in neutropenic patients with cancer: an update for the new millennium. *Int J Antimicrob Agents* 16:97–101, 2000
101. Zinner SH: Changing epidemiology of infections in patients with neutropenia and cancer: emphasis on gram-positive and resistant bacteria. *Clin Infect Dis* 29:490–494, 1999
102. Faveri AD: Management of fungal infections in neutropenic patients: more doubts than certainties. *Int J Antimicrob Agents* 16:135–137, 2000
103. Cruciani M: Antibacterial prophylaxis. *Int J Antimicrob Agents* 16:123–125, 2000
104. Klatersky J: Empirical treatment of sepsis in neturopenic patients. *Int J Antimicrob Agents* 16:131–133, 2000
105. Donnelly JP: Febrile neutropenia: antifungal prophylaxis. *Int J Antimicrob Agents* 16:127–130, 2000
106. Mayer J, Doubek M, Varlick J: Must we really fear toxicity of conventional amphotericin B in oncological patients? *Support Care Cancer* 7:51–55, 1999
107. DePauw BE: New antifungal agents and preparations. *Int J Antimicrob Agents* 16:147–150, 2000
108. Hubel K, Dale DC, Conrad W: Granulocyte transfusion therapy: update on potential clinical applications. *Curr Opin Hematol* 8: 161–164, 2001
109. Dale DC, Liles WC, Price TH: Return of granulocyte transfusions. *Curr Opin Pediatr* 12:18–22, 2000
110. Buchner T, Wolfgang H, Wormann B, et al: Hematopoietic growth factors in acute myeloid leukemia: supportive and priming effects. *Semin Oncol* 24:124–131, 1997
111. American Society of Clinical Oncology: 2000 update of recommendations for the use of hematopoietic colony-stimulating factors: evidenced based clinical practice. *J Clin Oncol* 18:3358–3585, 2000
112. Friend PH, Pruett J: Bleeding and thrombotic complications, in Yarbro CH, Frogge MH, Goodman M (eds.): *Cancer Symptom Management* (ed 3). Sudbury, MA, Jones and Bartlett, 2004, pp 233–251
113. Gordon MS: Managing anemia in the cancer patient: old problems, future solutions. *Oncologist* 7:331–341, 2002
114. Beck SL: Mucositis, in Yarbro CH, Frogge MH, Goodman M (eds.): *Cancer Symptom Management* (ed 3). Sudbury, MA, Jones and Bartlett, 2004, pp 276–292
115. Wilkes GM: Cerebellar syndromes, in Yarbro CH, Frogge MH, Goodman M (eds.): *Cancer Symptom Management* (ed 3). Sudbury, MA, Jones and Bartlett, 2004, pp 389–398
116. Doublisky J: Ineffective individual coping, in McNally JC, Stair JC, Somerville ET (eds.): *Guidelines for Cancer Nursing Practice.* Philadelphia, Saunders, 1985, pp 66–72
117. Barsevick AM, Much JM: Depression, in Yarbro CH, Frogge MH, Goodman M (eds.): *Cancer Symptom Management* (ed 3). Sudbury, MA, Jones and Bartlett, 2004, pp 668–692
118. Shannon-Dorcy K, Wolfe V: Decision making in the diagnosis and treatment of leukemia. *Semin Oncol Nurs* 19:142–149, 2003

CHAPTER 56

Liver Cancer: Primary and Metastatic Disease

Nina N. Grenon, MS, APRN, BC, CCRN, AOCN®

Introduction

Primary and secondary cancers of the liver constitute a significant challenge to the multidisciplinary oncology team. Worldwide, hepatocellular carcinoma (HCC) is among the most frequent causes of death from malignancy. The liver is the second most commonly involved organ by metastatic disease.

HCC is the most common cell type among primary malignancies of the liver and accounts for as many as half a million deaths annually worldwide.[1] In some parts of the world, HCC is the most common malignancy and the most common cause of death from cancer. Although HCC is less common in most of the developed Western world, over the past three decades its incidence has increased by about 80% in the United States and Western Europe.[2] This increase has been attributed to the high prevalence of chronic infection with hepatitis C virus (HCV) within these populations. Patients usually present with advanced disease, so treatment options are limited, prognosis is poor, and survival is relatively short. Because of the availability of new forms of therapies for early-stage HCC, a growing emphasis is being placed on recognition of risk factors, screening programs, and early diagnosis. Additionally, efforts are being made to prevent HCC by using antivirals to treat chronic viral hepatitis.

In the United States, a focal liver lesion is more likely to represent a metastatic deposit than a primary malignancy. The liver may be the site of metastasis from virtually any primary cancer. Common primary sources of metastases to the liver are cancers of the eye, colon, stomach, pancreas, breast, and lung. Colorectal carcinoma (CRC) is the single most common primary malignancy that results in hepatic metastasis. If liver metastases are found early in the course of colon cancer, surgical resection for metastases is more common than for primary liver cancer.

Epidemiology

Hepatocellular Carcinoma

HCC is the most common cell type among primary malignant tumors of the liver, ranking fifth in incidence among all malignancies in the world. Approximately 90% of all cases of primary liver cancer are HCC.[1] In the United States, an estimated 18,920 new cases of liver and intrahepatic bile duct cancer occurred in 2004, with an annual mortality of 14,270 cases, which reflects the rapid course and grave prognosis of the disease.[3]

The incidence of HCC varies considerably in different parts of the world.[4–6] High-incidence regions (more than 15 cases per 100,000 population per year) include sub-Saharan Africa, the People's Republic of China, and Taiwan. In these areas, causative factors associated with HCC are chronic hepatitis B virus (HBV) infection acquired predominately through perinatal infection and a high incidence of HBV carriers who acquired the virus early in life. North and South America, Europe, Australia, and parts of the Middle East are low-incidence areas, with fewer than 3 cases reported per 100,000 population per year. In the United States, the incidence of HCC has increased over the past two decades, probably due to the existence of a large pool of people with a history of chronic HCV. Intermediate-incidence areas (more than 5 cases per 100,000 of the population per year) include several countries in eastern and southern Europe, Thailand, Indonesia, Jamaica, Haiti, New Zealand (Maoris), and Alaska (Eskimos).[1] The extreme differences in distribution of HCC are probably due to regional variations in exposure to HBV, HCV, and environmental pathogens.

Males are two to three times more likely to develop HCC than females. The differences in sex distribution may reflect variations in chronic hepatitis carriers, exposure to environmental toxins, and the trophic effects of androgens.[7,8] Rates of HCC incidence also increase with age. Although cases can be identified in childhood, this disease typically begins to occur in substantial numbers by the third and fourth decades of life.[9] The majority of HCC cases occur in people with chronic liver disease or cirrhosis. In countries with the highest rate of occurrence, HCC tends to affect people at an earlier age, almost invariably due to HBV infection, such as occurs in China and southern Africa.[9]

Liver Metastases

The true incidence of liver metastases is unknown because most data are from autopsy series that reflect the end-stage disease. Depending on the site of the primary tumor, 30%–70% of patients who die of cancer have liver metastasis.[10]

Gastrointestinal malignancies are prone to spread to the liver, facilitated by the portal venous system. Metastases to the liver from primary colorectal cancer are common, with 15% of patients presenting with synchronous metastasis at the time of diagnosis and an additional 60% of patients developing metastasis later in the course of their disease.[11,12] Other tumors metastasize to the liver less often, including breast cancer (4%), lung cancer (15%), and melanoma (25%).[12]

Etiology

Hepatocellular Carcinoma

Unlike most cancers, a number of causative factors for the development of HCC have been identified. Common risk factors include chronic viral hepatitis and underlying liver disease in the form of cirrhosis. Some environmental and chemical toxins, hormones, alcohol and smoking, and a number of hereditary disorders may also play a role in the development of HCC. Nevertheless, HCC can occur in individuals without any known risk factors.[9,12,13]

HBV was the first virus identified as causing tumors in humans, and it is currently believed to be — along with tobacco — the most important carcinogen to which humans are exposed. Worldwide, HBV is the most frequent underlying cause of HCC. A strong positive correlation exists between HCC incidence rates and the prevalence of hepatitis B surface antigen (HBsAg) in the population, especially in regions where the incidence of HCC is very high.[1] In areas of endemic HBV infection such as Southeast Asia and sub-Saharan Africa, 10%–20% of the population is seropositive for HBsAg with a lifetime risk of developing HCC as high as 80%.[14,15] The majority of HBV infections are acquired in the neonatal period and early childhood and then become chronic; the lifetime relative risk of developing HCC is 70%–90%.[1] As many as 45% of HBV-infected individuals will die from the tumor, from the infection, or from both. Because of neonatal exposure to HBV, the age of onset of HCC in these countries is younger than that found in Europe and North America.[15,16]

HBV infection in Europe and North America is more commonly the result of sexual or parenteral exposure, occurring later in life than in endemic areas. As a result, HCC in Europe and North America is typically diagnosed after the fourth decade of life. The risk of HCC climbs after several decades of exposure to HBV, typically after cirrhosis has developed.[16]

Hepatitis C virus (HCV) is the leading cause of HCC in the United States, Europe, and Japan. The annual risk of developing HCC increases as the duration of cirrhosis due to HCV increases. The development of HCC in HCV-infected persons has also been linked to several risk factors, such as age greater than 60 years, histologic grade of HCC, injury to the liver paranchyma from cirrhosis, viral load, severity of transaminase elevation, and failure to respond to interferon treatment. Among HCV-infected individuals, a history of alcohol abuse and HBV infection increase the risk of HCC by twofold. Concomittant infection with both HBV and HCV is associated with a 3–5 times greater risk of developing HCC than infection with either virus alone.[16,17]

The mechanism by which chronic viral hepatitis causes HCC is not known. HBV has a DNA genome that can become incorporated within the genomes of infected cells. These integration events may lead to the development of cancer.[18] In contrast, HCV has an RNA genome that does not become integrated with host chromosomes. It is believed that HCV infection leads to HCC through the chronic inflammation and regeneration that are commonly encountered with cirrhosis.[9]

In some parts of the world, high levels of dietary aflatoxin intake have been associated with HCC. Aflatoxin is a mycotoxin produced by molds (*Asperigillus flavus* and *Asperigillus paraseticus*) that contaminate stored foodstuffs such as corn, soybeans, and peanuts.[19,20] Mutations of the *p53* tumor suppressor gene have been identified in patients with HCC who have been chronically exposed to aflatoxin.[5,21] The blue-green algal toxin *Microcycstin*, which commonly contaminates ponds in rural China, is thought to be a strong promoter of HCC.[22] In this geographic area, there is a higher mortality rate from HCC among people who drink pond ditch water compared to those who drink well water (100 deaths versus fewer than 20 deaths per 100,000 population per year).[23]

Chemical carcinogens linked to primary liver cancer include nitrites, hydrocarbons, solvents, organochlorine pesticides, primary metals, and polychlorinated biphenals.[22] Ethanol is the chemical most closely linked to the development of HCC. Both alcohol abuse and the subsequent development of hepatic cirrhosis are predisposing factors for HCC. Alcohol can also act as a synergistic carcinogen with other agents such as HBV, HCV, hepatotoxins, and tobacco.[24]

It has been suggested that androgenic steroids (in men) and estrogenic steroids (in women) may increase the risk of HCC. A statistically significant link exists between the prolonged use of oral contraceptive steroids and the development of HCC in patients without cirrhosis who are serology negative for HBV and HCV.[25,26]

In addition, some rare hereditary disorders are associated with an increased risk of developing HCC. Hemochromatosis and alpha-1-antitrypsin deficiency usually cause cirrhosis and are believed to be major contributors to the neoplastic transformation into HCC. Likewise, Wilson's disease, primary biliary cirrhosis, type 1 glycogen storage disease, and porphyria are all thought to increase the risk of HCC.[27,28]

A minor risk factor for the development of HCC is membranous obstruction of the inferior vena cava, thought to be either a congenital abnormality or the result of vena cava thrombosis. HCC develops in 46% of South African blacks and 36% of Japanese with this abnormality.[29]

Recently, diabetes mellitus (DM) and obesity have been suggested to be risk factors for HCC. DM has been associated with nonalcoholic fatty liver disease (NAFLD), including the most severe form, nonalcoholic steatohepatitis (NASH).[30] NASH is a chronic necroinflammatory condition that can lead to liver fibrosis, cirrhosis, and subsequently HCC.[31] Whether the development of HCC is related to obesity and diabetes or to underlying NAFLD-related changes is not clear.[32] In a series of patients who underwent surgical resection for cryptogenic liver disease–related HCC, the study revealed that these patients frequently exhibited the same risk factors as those for NAFLD. These results support the contention that NAFLD is also a significant risk for HCC.[33]

Liver Metastases

The liver has a rich blood supply from both the hepatic artery and the portal circulation. As a consequence, metastases can reach the liver from any organ. The direct passage of blood from the gastrointestinal tract to the portal circulation explains the high rate of liver metastases. Differences are seen in the natural history of the liver metastases from gastrointestinal tumors. Liver metastases found in patients with gastric or pancreatic cancer usually indicate widespread metastatic disease. In contrast, a significant number of patients with colorectal cancer may have isolated liver metastases.

Prevention, Screening, and Early Detection

Primary prevention aims at reduction of the risk of developing a disease by implementing strategies such as lifestyle modifications, chemoprevention, and vaccination. In the case of HCC, primary prevention of the infection seeks to prevent viral hepatitis and control disease in those already infected with HBV and HCV. In Taiwan, a vaccination program for HBV was established in the mid-1980s; after ten years, the percentage of HBsAg-positive children declined from 10% to less than 2%. The incidence of HCC among children between the ages of 6 to 9 was reduced by 80%.[34] Vaccination for HBV will most likely reduce the risk of HCC in the next decade.[14] In the United States, the current recommendation is that all newborns be vaccinated against HBV. In contrast, no vaccine for HCV is available, and it may be some time before any such vaccine is developed. However, vigorous screening of blood used for transfusions has greatly reduced the incidence of HCV infection.

In those individuals who are already infected with HBV and HCV, prevention of HCC has focused on using chemoprevention to treating the viral infection. Interferon has been the primary means of chemoprevention. Several reports have demonstrated the ability of interferon-alpha to lower the incidence of HCC.[35] However, these reports have primarily relied on retrospective nonrandomized data, so their results should be interpreted with caution. Recent reports of large, prospective, randomized trials using the combination of interferon and ribavirin in patients with HCV infection show that this regimen can slow the progression of fibrosis, decrease viral load, and lessen histologic and biological markers of inflammation. The impact on the reduction of cirrhosis and HCC remains to be determined. Of interest, these reports indicate that people who do not respond to interferon are at a higher risk for developing HCC.[36,37]

Currently, COX-2 inhibitors are used as chemoprevention agents in patients with documented cirrhosis from viral hepatitis, alcohol abuse, hemachromatosis, or other causes. Cirrhosis represents a premalignant state for HCC, and increased COX-2 expression is noted in both cirrhosis and dysplasias. It is also believed that angiogenesis inhibitors may represent a potential novel strategy to prevent HCC, and COX-2 inhibitors are known to have some antiangiogenic effects. Clinical trials are currently attempting to determine the actual role of COX-2 in human hepatocarcinogenesis and to identify whether COX-2 inhibitors may have a potential role in the primary or secondary prevention of HCC.[38]

Strategies for prevention of HCC in nonviral cirrhosis include decreasing iron overload in patients with hemochromatosis by the regular use of phlebotomy, and decreasing hepatotoxin exposure to agents such as alcohol and aflatoxins.[14]

Regular screening of patients at risk for developing HCC remains controversial; data demonstrating a survival advantage are inconsistent.[39,40] Nevertheless, HCC may be diagnosed at an earlier stage in patients who undergo screening at regular intervals. When the disease is caught early, liver transplantation and resection, which offers the best chance for a cure, are more likely to be treatment options.[41,42] Recommendations from two consensus conferences are that healthy HBsAg carriers older than age 35 or with a family history of HCC should be screened once a year using alpha-fetoprotein (AFP) analysis. Patients with cirrhosis from any cause should be screened with AFP and ultrasound every six months.[43,44] Patients with chronic hepatitis C do not warrant screening unless they have cirrhosis, as HCC is rare in the early stages of chronic HCV infection.

Pathophysiology

Cellular Characteristics

Primary liver cancers are commonly adenocarcinomas that arise from epithelial cells.[45] Among the cell types that are sources of HCC are hepatocytes, which account for the majority of primary liver cancers. The remainder are cholangiocarcinomas, which arise from the bile duct epithelium. In rare cases, there is a mixed type pattern that is usually poorly differentiated. Fewer than 3% of primary liver cancers arise from mesenchymal cells; these malignancies include sarcomas, angiosarcomas, epithelioid tumors, and hemangioendotheliomas.[46]

Fibrolamellar carcinoma is a variant of HCC that generally occurs in young persons in Western countries and presents in the absence of cirrhosis. The tumor is well demarcated and often encapsulated. Also, the AFP level is not usually elevated and is associated with prolonged survival when compared to the typical HCC. This tendency most likely reflects the fact that the tumor is well demarcated and that a wider range of treatment options are available in the absence of cirrhosis.[47]

The gross appearance of HCC can be characterized as a single mass, multiple nodules, or diffuse liver involvement, referred to as *massive, nodular*, and *diffuse* forms, respectively. The carcinomas may range from well-differentiated lesions to highly anaplastic undifferentiated lesions. In well- and moderately well-differentiated tumors, hepatocystic cells assume a trabecular (the most common histologic variant), acinar, or pseudoglandular pattern (often characterized by bile-filled strictures).[48,49] It is important to determine the differential diagnosis for well-differentiated HCC, which includes liver cell adenomas and dyplastic nodules.[49] In poorly differentiated tumors, cells take on a pleomorphic appearance characterized by numerous anaplastic, giant cells as well as small, completely undifferentiated cells, and sometimes can resemble a spindle cell sarcoma.[48]

Well- and moderately well-differentiated HCC can be easily diagnosed, while poorly differentiated tumors may need to be distinguished from primary HCC or metastatic disease to the liver from another primary site. Liver cancer can be distinguished from other metastatic tumors by examining the production of bile and the presence of albumin mRNA. Staining studies for the expression of AFP, biliary glycoprotein-1, and CD10 may also help identify HCC. In 67% of HCCs, the immunostain is positive for AFP.[49]

Progression of Disease

The natural course of primary liver cancer can be progressive with enlargement of the primary mass until it encroaches on hepatic function or metastasizes. Hematogenic tumor spread most commonly occurs to the lungs, followed by the adrenal glands, bones, gastrointestinal tract, gallbladder, and pancreas. Lymphatic metastases can be found in approximately 25% of patients with HCC and usually occur in hilum or paripancreatic nodes. More distant lymph nodes, such as perigastric and periaortic nodes, can be involved with advanced disease in distant lymph nodes.[49,50–52]

Death from HCC usually occurs less than 12 months after the diagnosis due to cachexia, gastrointestinal or esophageal varices bleeding, liver failure with hepatic coma, or rarely fatal hemorrhage from tumor rupture.[6]

Clinical Manifestations

Most patients with liver cancer will be asymptomatic. The most common symptom of HCC is abdominal pain in the right upper quadrant. It is most often felt in the right hypochondrium and epigastrium and sometimes in the back and lower abdomen. The pain is described as a constant dull ache, which may become severe in the advanced stages of the disease. It rarely radiates through the back or refers to the right shoulder. The pain may cause the patient to become aware of an upper abdominal mass.[52] The patient may present with increased abdominal girth from ascites, which may be the source of pain, though it is a different pain than that generated by the liver tumors. Weight loss, anorexia, and early satiety often indicate advanced lesions.[53] Fever may be present with infection; it may be accompanied by leucocytosis, which may be misleading by suggesting that the patient has an infection. Pyrexia is thought to be the result of pyrogens released into the bloodstream from the malignant necrotic liver cells. Typically, the fever is intermittent and self-limited.[52]

Obstructive jaundice can be caused by compression of the major intrahepatic ducts from the primary tumor, by obstruction of the common bile duct from nodal metastasis in the porta hepatis, by direct invasion of the biliary tree, or rarely as the result of hemobilia.[52] Diarrhea can occur and may be severe and intractable, leading to electrolyte and fluid imbalance. Diarrhea may result from the HCC tumor behaving as a carcinoid tumor (see the discussion of paraneoplastic syndromes). Other gastrointestinal symptoms include nausea, vomiting, indigestion, and constipation. Gastrointestinal bleeding may occur in the later stages of the disease or in patients with known cirrhosis. It is most likely due to portal hypertension causing gastroesophageal varices, and is frequently a terminal event.[52]

Pain can result from bone metastases localized to the vertebrae, sacrum, ribs, femur, or skull. Dyspnea may be related to pleural effusion, a markedly elevated hemidiaphragm, or extensive lung metastasis.

Occasionally, patients with HCC may develop paraneoplastic syndromes. Hypoglycemia can occur in advanced HCC as a result of the tumor's high metabolic need. Although typically the hypoglycemia is mild, in some instances the decrease in serum glucose can be severe, resulting in lethargy and confusion. In a small percentage of patients, hypoglycemia can occur early in the disease when the tumor secretes insulin-like growth factor, which acts as an insulin agonist and causes severe symptomatic hypoglycemia.[52,54,55]

Erythrocytosis in HCC is thought to be due to secretion of erythropoietin by the tumor. Raised serum erythropoietin levels may be found in as many as 23% of patients with HCC, elevations in packed cell volume and hemoglobin concentration are uncommon, and the majority of the patients are anemic.[56]

Hypercalcemia can occur as a result of osteolytic metastases, which are uncommon in HCC. Most often, hypercalcemia is due to secretion of parathyroid hormone–related protein.[52,57] The patient with hypercalcemia may be severely symptomatic and require urgent treatment.

Watery diarrhea is significantly more common in patients with cirrhotic HCC. The diarrhea may be severe and intractable. Although the mechanism involved is not well understood, the diarrhea may be caused by the expression of peptides that cause increased intestinal secretions.[58]

Metastatic disease in the liver usually remains asymptomatic. Many patients with liver metastasis from colorectal cancer are diagnosed through routine surveillance laboratory tests, such as elevated CEA or serum alkaline phosphatase. Early symptoms of liver metastases may include fatigue and abdominal pain. If the metastases involve extensive liver tissue, the patient may present with the same symptoms as for primary HCC.

Assessment

Patient and Family History

To assess for primary liver cancer or metastases, the history should identify any potential risk factors, such as HBV or HCV infection, cirrhosis, or exposure to toxins. The history should also identify possible risk factors for the development of cancer that could prompt metastasis to the liver, such as a history of any genetic syndrome that might increase an individual's risk for the development of primary liver cancer, colorectal cancer, or breast cancer. Other disease states should also be considered — for example, a history of inflammatory bowel disease and the subsequent risk of developing colorectal cancer. Most important, investigating a family history of cancer and recognizing the development of various carcinomas within each generation will provide information regarding a possible genetic mutation. This information may prompt genetic counseling that can recommend screening the individual who is deemed to be at risk of developing other cancers.

Physical Examination

The most frequent finding on physical examination in patients with HCC is an enlarged liver. One or both lobes may be enlarged, and the surface may be nodular. The liver may be hard or just firm. Focal or generalized tenderness may be present on palpation. Often an elevated right hemidiaphragm may be found on the exam due to the enlarged liver. A bruit caused by compression of the aorta over the liver may be occasionally heard.[52,59,60] Ascites is present in more than 50% of patients with HCC and indicates decompensated cirrhosis.[52,53] Splenomegaly is another common finding as a result of chronic portal hypertension from cirrhosis. Often the enlarged spleen is difficult to feel due to tense ascites and an enlarged left lobe of the liver.[52,53] Muscle wasting becomes evident as the disease runs its course and may be evident at presentation with large, rapidly growing tumors. Slight to moderate jaundice may be observed at initial diagnosis. A sudden onset of acute abdominal pain, accompanied by hypovolemic shock, abdominal distention, absent bowel sounds, and diffuse abdominal tenderness, can result from tumor rupture. This is a rare and usually catastrophic event. The rupture is typically confirmed by radiological exam, which reveals a liver mass and free intraperitoneal blood.[52,61]

Patients with liver metastases will present with a different physical exam from the preceding profile. The liver may be extensively replaced by disease in the advanced state. Although any of the above findings may be present on exam, the most commonly encountered are liver enlargement, ascites, jaundice, and muscle wasting.

Diagnostic Studies

Laboratory studies

In the early stages of liver cancer, laboratory data such as liver function tests may be normal. After a significant volume of the liver parenchyma is involved by tumor, abnormalities in liver function tests (LFTs) may be seen. In the setting of cirrhosis, elevated bilirubin and lowered albumin levels are indicative of a poor survival. Serum gamma-glutamyl transferase (GGT) is elevated in most cases of HCC, and alkaline phosphatase can be slightly elevated in metastatic disease. Laboratory evaluation should include hepatitis B and C virus titers and serology alpha-fetoprotein (AFP).

The serum AFP measurement is helpful in the diagnosis and management of HCC. The AFP level is elevated to greater than 20 ng/mL in more than 70% of patients with HCC. Elevation to 500–1000 ng/mL can be seen in patients with viral hepatitis who do not have HCC.[62,63] In patients with known chronic hepatitis, persistently elevated AFP values indicate a higher risk of developing HCC.[63] Note that AFP does not correlate to tumor size or growth rate. The lack of specificity limits the use of the AFP value except in those patients in whom the level is elevated to greater than 400 ng/mL. However, AFP is useful in monitoring response to treatment and detecting recurrence after treatment of HCC, if it was elevated before treatment.[62]

Carcinoembryonic antigen (CEA) is widely used in the detection of colorectal cancer recurrences. Mildly elevated levels of CEA can be detected among smokers and in many benign conditions including peptic ulcer disease, pancreatitis, and prostatitis. Additionally, CEA levels can be elevated in a number of malignancies, including colon, breast, pancreas, liver, and gastric cancer. Due to its lack of specificity, CEA cannot be used as a diagnostic or screening test. Nevertheless, CEA levels are monitored after resection of a primary colorectal cancer or resection of liver metastases. A rise in CEA usually predicts recurrence 6–8 months before the patient is symptomatic or findings of disease recurrence appear on radiologic tests.[64]

One large study revealed that measurement of CEA level appeared to be more sensitive for hepatic metastases and less sensitive for focal or peritoneal disease. Overall, 75%–90% of patients with hepatic colorectal metastases have elevated CEA levels.[64]

Imaging studies

Imaging studies play a key role in the diagnosis of lesions in the liver and can differentiate between a primary liver cancer and metastatic disease to the liver. The imaging tests most commonly used to diagnose HCC are ultrasound (US), computed tomography (CT), magnetic resonance imaging (MRI), and in some rare instances angiography, CT hepatic arteriography, and arterial portography. In metastatic liver disease, CT scans of the abdomen and liver, MRI of the liver, and positron emission tomography (PET) scans can be useful. Additionally, CT scan of the chest is routinely performed with staging to detect pulmonary metastasis.

The HCC lesions detected by *ultrasound* have different echogenecity from the surrounding liver tissue. Small HCC tumors are typically hypoechoic but may be hyperechoic as the lesions enlarge and can be difficult to distinguish from normal surrounding tissue.[62,65] Visualization of lesions under the right hemidiaphragm, with overlying gas, or in obese patients can be difficult. Although US cannot distinguish HCC from other solid tumors in the liver, it can be used as a screening tool for HCC. An added benefit of US is its use in the assessment of the patency of the hepatic blood supply and the presence of vascular invasion by the tumor in the portal vein. It can also be used intraoperatively to detect small tumor nodules during hepatic resection. The diagnosis of HCC may be improved with the use of new contrast agents.[66] However, CT and MRI have largely replaced US in the diagnosis of HCC.

Computed tomography is often performed to evaluate an abnormality of the liver that was detected on US. It can also be used as a primary screening modality for HCC in patients with cirrhosis. Developments in helical CT imaging include spiral scanners that allow rapid imaging of the liver after infusion of intravenous contrast agents, and the adaptation of scanning protocols that delineate the vascularity of the tumors. HCC derives its blood supply primarily from the hepatic artery; the remainder of the liver receives its blood supply from both the arterial and portal veins. On CT exam, liver carcinomas appear enhanced early during the infusion of dye in the arterial phase (the first 20–40 seconds), allowing for detection of hypervascular HCC as small as 3 mm.[62,67] The liver parenchyma is enhanced during the portal venous phase (50–90 seconds after the infusing contrast). The term *triphasic CT scan* is used to describe the process of enhancement before contrast, during the arterial phase, and the portal venous phase.[62] Tumors that isoattenuate on both arterial- and portal-phase imaging can be missed, but may be detected in delayed-phase imaging.[67] The sensitivity of helical CT for detecting HCC has been reported to be as high as 90%.[67] Metastases from colorectal cancer are typically hypovascular and are best identified as nonenhancing lesions on portal-phase imaging.[68] Lipiodol is a contrast agent that can increase sensitivity, but it must be given by intrarterial injection.[69]

Magnetic resonance imaging is another imaging modality that can distinguish HCC from normal liver tissue.[53,65] Although MRI has a similar sensitivity for the diagnosis of HCC as helical CT, it has a better sensitivity and specificity as compared to CT and US in patients with cirrhotic livers.[70] MRI is also superior in distinguishing benign vascular lesions such as hemangioma and focal fatty changes within the liver. Likewise, MRI is the preferred imaging test in patients with renal insufficiency or in those patients with an allergy to contrast media agents.

To improve the detection and characterization of HCC, angiography can be combined with CT and MRI in a technique known as *CT hepatic arteriography and arterial portography*.[71,72] Immediately prior to MRI or CT, contrast dye is injected intraarterially in the superior mesenteric, hepatic, or splenic artery; images are then obtained during the arterial and portal venous phases. This technique can detect HCC smaller than 1 cm in diameter.[73] Hepatic arteriography delineates the hepatic arterial anatomy and has been used for preoperative evaluation of HCC, chemoembolization, or infusion of antineaoplastic drugs directly into the hepatic artery.[53] This diagnostic technique is not commonly used in the United States. The benefit of CT hepatic arteriography and arterial portography as compared to MRI is unclear due to the former's invasiveness without added benefit of accuracy.[73]

Positron emission tomography is the latest advance in imaging techniques. PET evaluates cell metabolism using a glucose analog, F-flurodeoxyglucose (FDG). Tumors typically have higher rates of glucose uptake and metabolism than surrounding tissues. When FDG is given to the patient, the increased uptake of the glucose analog by the tumor can be detected by the PET scanner.[74] This imaging modality can be used to detect recurrent or metastatic disease, and it can be an accurate imaging technique for differentiating hepatic metastasis, although it may not detect lesions smaller than 1 cm.

Future imaging modalities for HCC include a technetium–99m (^{99m}Tc) — labeled anti-alpha-fetoprotein (AFP) Fab imaging kit.[75] *Gallium scanning* was a common imaging technique for the diagnosis of HCC prior to the advent of CT and MRI. It can still play a role in patients where a diagnosis remains unclear after other noninvasive testing and where more aggressive diagnostics may be inappropriate.[76]

Liver biopsy

Tissue examination is usually recommended and commonly performed in patients with focal liver lesions in whom the diagnosis is uncertain. The routine use of needle biopsy in HCC in controversial, especially in patients with HCC who are candidates for resection and transplantation, because the risks of biopsy include bleeding and spreading of tumor cells along the needle track. Some reports suggest local spread of HCC can occur in as many as 1% of patients after a needle biopsy.[62,77,78] A biopsy may not be needed if the diagnosis is obvious, such as in the case of a large mass found in the liver associated with elevated serum AFP.

Several methods are available for biopsy procedures. Fine-needle aspiration (FNA) biopsy can be performed under US or CT radiological guidance.[79] Directed core biopsy is more useful than FNA, because more tissue can be obtained.[79] If the tumor is massive or spread extensively throughout the liver, a blind biopsy is performed by palpating the mass. Open surgical biopsy procedure is usually indicated if the tumor cannot be radiologically located with precision.[62]

Table 56-1 Child-Pugh Classification of Severity of Liver Disease

Parameter	Points Assigned		
	1	2	3
Ascites	Absent	Slight	Moderate
Bilirubin (mg/dL)	< 2	2–3	> 3
Albumin (g/dL)	> 3.5	2.8–3.5	< 2.8
Prothrombin time			
Seconds over control	1–3	4–6	> 6
INR	< 1.7	1.8–2.3	> 2.3
Encephalopathy	None	Grade 1–2	Grade 3–4

Grade A, 5-6 points; Grade B, 7-9 points; Grade C, 10-15 points.
Data from Child, Turcotte.[82]

Classification and Staging

Staging is essential for the management of HCC. The purpose of staging is to group patients based on the characteristics of their disease to determine the most appropriate treatment.[80] The prognosis for HCC, unlike for other cancers, depends on both the functional state of the liver and the extent of tumor growth.[62,81] The functional status of the liver in a patient with cirrhosis is usually assessed by the Child-Pugh classification (Table 56-1).[82]

The two most popular HCC staging systems are the Okuda system and the tumor-node-metastasis (TNM) classification of the International Union Against Cancer. The Okuda staging system takes into account the extent of the tumor; the patient is evaluated on the four criteria of ascites, serum albumin, serum bilirubin, and tumor size, then staged as I, II, or III (Table 56-2).[83] Survival with no therapy for patients with stages I, II, and III disease are 8.3, 2.0, and 0.7 months, respectively.[83] The TNM staging system classifies

Table 56-2 Okuda Staging System for HCC

Criterion	Positive	Negative
Tumor size	> 50%	< 50%
Ascites	Clinically detectable	Clinically undetectable
Serum albumin	< 3 g/dL	> 3 g/dL
Serum bilirubin	> 3 mg/dL	< 3 mg/dL
Stage		
I	No positive	
II	One or two positives	
III	Three or four positives	

Data from Okuda, Ohtuki, Obata, et al.[83]

patients from stages I through IV based solely on tumor size and number, lobar involvement, and nodal and distant metastasis (Table 56-3).[84] The TNM staging system is based primarily on imaging studies. It is generally felt that this approach leads to the risk of understaging of patients, especially preoperatively.[80]

More recently, the Cancer of the Liver Italian Program (CLIP) group proposed a new prognostic score that includes the Child-Pugh score, tumor morphology and extension, presence of portal vein thrombosis, and AFP level (Table 56-4).[85] Prospective validations of the CLIP score include more accurate prognostic information and better survival prediction than found with the Okuda system.[86,87]

Therapeutic Approaches and Nursing Care

Hepatocellular Carcinoma

A number of therapeutic interventions are available for the treatment of primary liver cancer with the goal of either cure or palliation (Table 56-5).[88] Of the treatment options available, surgical resection with partial hepatectomy and/or liver transplantation offers the only potential for a cure. Patients with unresectable HCC have a number of palliative treatment modalities available, including regional therapy, ablative/cytoreductive therapy, external beam radiation, and systemic chemotherapy. All treatment options may affect normal liver paranchyma and, ultimately, liver function. Supportive care includes pain management, nutritional support, control of nausea and vomiting, management of ascites, minimizing discomfort of jaundice, management of encephalopathy, and attempts to minimize psychosocial distress and disturbances in body image.

Once a diagnosis of HCC is established through a combination of history, physical assessment, imaging, studies, and laboratory tests, a decision is made whether to biopsy. Once the disease is appropriately staged, treatment options will be based on the extent of liver involvement, size of the tumor, portal vein involvement, performance status, co-morbid conditions, and

Table 56-3 TNM for HCC: Stage Grouping

Stage I	T1	N0	M0
Stage II	T2	N0	M0
Stage IIIA	T3	N0	M0
Stage IIIB	T4	N0	M0
Stage IIIC	Any T	N1	M0
Stage IV	Any T	Any N	M2

Data from Greene, Page, Fleming, et al.[84]

Table 56-4 CLIP Score: Cancer of the Liver Italian Program

Variable	Score
Child-Pugh Stage	
A	0
B	1
C	2
Tumor Morphology	
Uninodular and extension < 50%	0
Multinodular and extension < 50%	1
Massive or extension > 50%	2
Alpha-fetoprotein (AFP)	
< 400 ng/mL	0
> 400 ng/mL	1
Portal Vein Thrombosis	
No	0
Yes	1

Data from Cancer of the Liver Italian Program (CLIP) Investigators.[85]

Table 56-5 Treatment Modalities for HCC

Potentially Curative Treatments
- Hepatic resection
- Liver transplantation

Palliative Treatments
- Chemoembolization
- Hepatic artery infusion
- Percutaneous interstitial ablation
  - Percutaneous ethanol injection
  - Radiofrequency ablation
  - Microwave coagulation therapy
- Cryosurgery
- Radiation therapy
  - External beam radiation
  - Internal radiation
- Systemic chemotherapy
- Hormonal therapy
- Immunotherapy
- Gene therapy

Data from Bruix.[88]

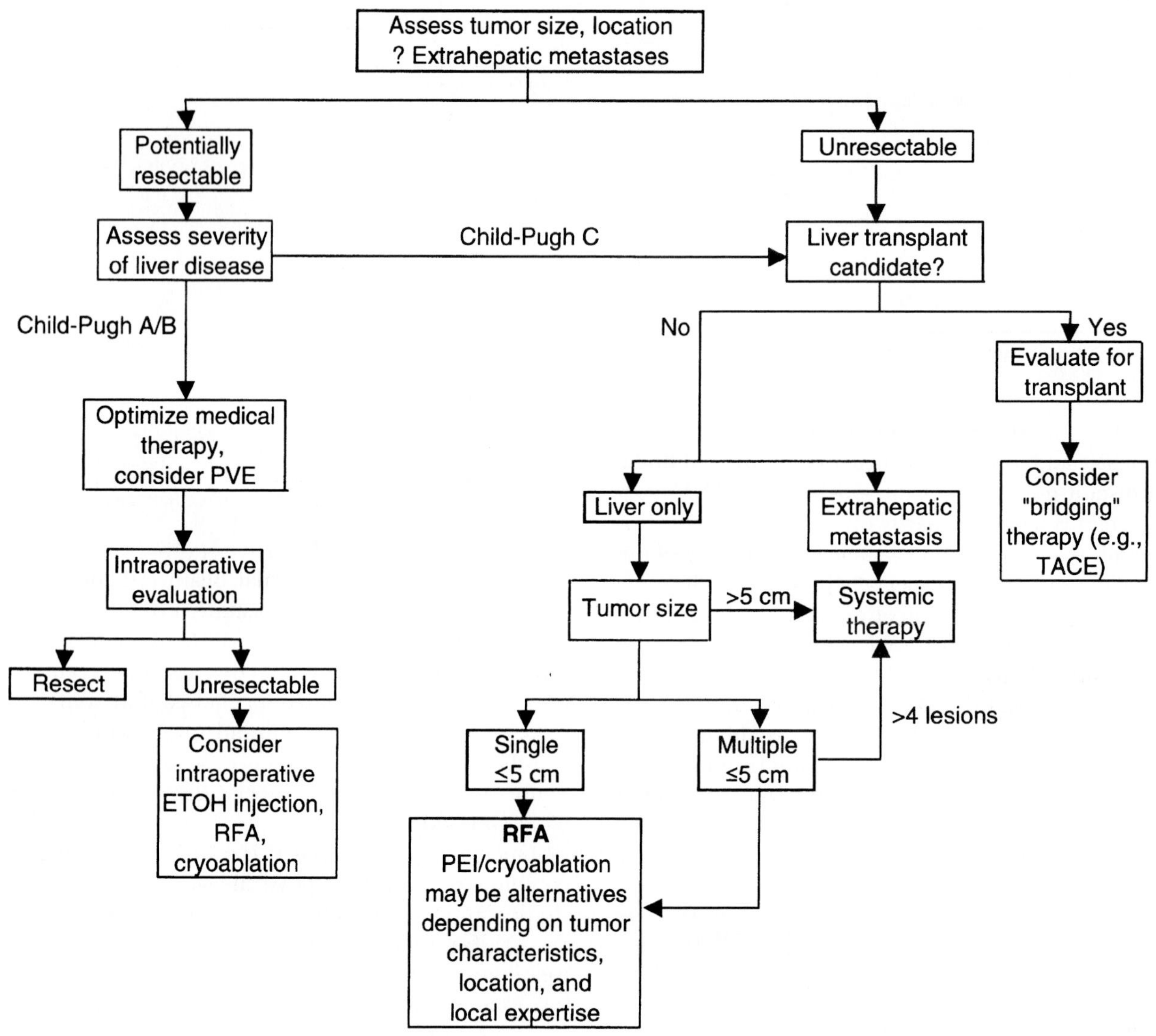

Figure 56-1 Treatment algorithm for hepatocellular carcinoma.

patient preference. Figure 56-1 provides a treatment algorithm for HCC.[89]

Partial hepatectomy

Partial hepatectomy offers the best option for cure in patients with HCC. The ideal candidate for resection will have disease confined to the liver, with a solitary lesion usually smaller than 5 cm, and no nodal metastasis. Radiological evidence should confirm the lack of hepatic vascular involvement, and the patient should have normal LFTs and no ascites, portal hypertension, or coagulopathies.[90–92] Surgical resection is attempted in patients with Child-Pugh stage A, TNM stages I and II, and Okuda stage 1 lesions.[93] Unfortunately, most patients do not fall into this category. In geographic areas with a high incidence of HCC, only 10%–15% of patients are potentially curable; in low-incidence areas, 15%–30% of patients may be suitable candidates for resection.[94–97] Resection is associated with a five-year survival rate of 30%. In patients with no cirrhosis, the mortality rate associated with surgical liver resection is less than 5%.[98]

Intraoperative staging via laparoscopy and intraoperative ultrasound (IOUS) can improve the selection of patients who can be potentially cured by resection. IOUS can accurately determine the size of the primary tumor and identify portal and hepatic vein involvement. Additionally, IOUS can be used to identify major intrahepatic vascular structures and can guide segmental and anatomical resection.[99]

For patients with cirrhosis, liver resection is associated with a number of additional risks, leading to increased morbidity and mortality in this population. Typically, patients with cirrhosis have rigid liver parenchyma with varices, making it difficult to resect during surgery. Many of these patients also have thrombocytopenia and coagulation abnormalities that place them at even greater risk for hemorrhage. Postoperative complications may include liver failure due to the liver not being able to regenerate, and exaggeration of portal hypertension leading to ascites and variceal bleeding.

The type and extent of resection undertaken depend on tumor location. The type of incision used to perform liver resection is usually subcostal; with this approach, the incision can be extended farther if the tumor is bulky or invades the diaphragm. Resections will be as extensive as needed to eradicate the tumor. Resections can be classified as either minor or major. Major resections include hepatic lobectomy or extended hepatic lobectomy, also referred to as trisegmentectomy. Minor resection includes nonanatomical wedge resection or anatomical resection of a specific segment. An example of a more difficult resection would involve removing a lesion located within the posterior segment of the right lobe, which is complicated by the location of the hepatic veins.

Liver transplantation

In patients with localized HCC and no distant metastasis, liver transplation (LT) can offer the best chance for long-term survival, as it can eradicate the cancer as well as the underlying disease (cirrhosis). Over the past decade, reports have shown that survival in carefully selected patients with HCC who undergo LT is the same as survival for those patients who undergo LT for nonmalignant causes.[100–102] The criteria used to identify a suitable candidate include size of a single tumor — smaller than 5 cm or smaller than 3 cm if there are one to three tumors; the number of tumor nodules — less than three; the absence of vascular invasion; and a well-differentiated histology. These criteria are merely guidelines; they are not mandatory. An overall five-year survival rate of 70% has been reported.[100]

Studies using intravenous doxurubicin both before and after transplantation are ongoing.[103] Additional studies are evaluating pretransplant chemoembolization.[104–106] As yet, these strategies remain to be proven in terms of their ability to affect overall survival. Another factor complicating LT for patients with HCC is the waiting period for an available donor. Patients who are candidates for LT should be entered in clinical trials that offer adjuvant therapy such as chemoembolization pending transplant. When possible, the application of adult living donors for LT in HCC may offer an opportunity for earlier transplantation, which decreases the chance that the disease will progress.

Liver Metastases

Initial resection. Resection of liver metastases from stomach or pancreatic cancer is not an option due to the aggressive biologic nature of these two cancers. Occasionally, solitary lesions from breast cancer metastases can be resected with good results. However, resection of liver metastases is done only when strong evidence indicates that the liver is the only site of metastasis. Generally, such resection is not advisable because breast cancer is usually a systemic disease. The role of hepatic resection in metastatic neuroendocrine cancers is not known due to the rarity of these tumors. Resection of hepatic metastases is most often appropriate in CRC. The liver can often be the only site of metastases in patients with CRC. Results from autopsy studies have shown that in patients who died from CRC, as many as 38% had metastases limited to only the liver.[10] Based on this data, if liver metastases in patients with CRC are found early, surgical resection can offer effective therapy for a significant number of patients.[10] Over the past three decades, perioperative mortality rates in experienced centers have been reported to range between 4% and 6%. Five-year survival rates have been reported to range between 25% and 38%.[107]

Guidelines for resection of liver metastases include the following: there should be no distant metastases or extrahepatic intraabdominal metastases; if the periportal lymph nodes have metastatic disease present, the resection is typically aborted. The extent of the resection can range from a small nodule to a trisegmentectomy, where as much as 75% of the liver is removed. If a patient has cirrhosis, extensive resection is typically not performed because it is not possible to predict which patients can survive with 75% of the liver removed. Patients with poor performance status are typically not good candidates for liver resection. Age alone is not a contraindication for a patient's eligibility for liver resection.[11]

Resectable synchronous liver lesions can be found at the time of the resection of the primary colorectal tumor. Typically, the liver lesions are biopsied at the time of the colorectal resection with a plan to resect the metastases at a later date. Intraoperative ultrasonography is utilized to confirm resectability.

Repeat surgical resection. Among the patients who have undergone primary liver resection for metastatic CRC, 50%–60% will have recurrence within the liver.[108] Repeat hepatectomy to remove the recurrence is possible because the liver regenerates almost to the original mass within four to six weeks.[109,110] Repeat resection within the liver is technically more difficult due to adhesions and the adherence of the surface of the previous resection to neighboring organs. Regeneration of the liver also changes the shape of the organ and vascular structures, creating a more difficult resection. In some cases, there may be a greater risk of bleeding.[111] Perioperative mortality is similar to that for initial hepatic resections, although the morbidity rates are higher. The Repeat Hepatic Metastases Registry noted 20% higher postoperative morbidity with repeat resection compared to the first resection.[112] Nonetheless, repeat resection for liver metastases should be considered a treatment option if the disease is resectable.

Postoperative Care

Following major hepatic resection, the patient typically requires close monitoring in an intensive care setting for a period of 24 hours to manage intravascular volume and perfusion changes. Fluid restriction and/or transfusion may be necessary.

Individuals with cirrhosis are at increased risk for complications during the postoperative period compared to the noncirrhotic individual. Knowledge of the potential complications, signs of impending problems, and aggressive treatment are vital in caring for a patient postoperatively.

Monitoring liver function tests (LFT), phosphate, and glucose frequently is important until a downward trend in transaminase levels is noted. Hypophosphatemia is commonly seen postoperatively, and replacement of phosphate may be necessary. The levels seen in liver function tests rise immediately postoperatively but will usually return to normal within seven to ten days postoperatively. The degree of elevation depends on the extent of liver resected and intraoperative ischemic time. If LFT results are extraordinarily high in the early postoperative period, they may indicate an injury to vascular inflow or outflow in the retained liver segment. In this case, a Doppler ultrasound of the liver should be performed to rule out portal vein thrombosis. In addition, it is important to monitor an individual's glucose level, as it may also be indicative of hepatic failure. Decreased albumin levels are also noted following liver resection, related to protein loss in the abdomen. No benefit from administration of albumin has been noted.[113] The patient's diet is slowly advanced with resolution of a postoperative ileus. Drainage tubes, if placed, are discontinued when the biliary output tapers off and no bile leak is evident.

If the patient develops ascites, it may interfere with nutritional intake and ventilation. Therefore, it is important to restrict sodium intake to 1000–1500 mg per day and fluid intake to 1500 mL per day. Addition of a loop diuretic and spironolactone will likely decrease the patient's weight by 0.5–1.0 kg. With this particular intervention, the patient's potassium, BUN, and creatinine should be monitored closely, with potassium being replaced as necessary.

Following hepatic resection, potential complications include hemorrhage, biliary leak or biloma, subphrenic abscess, infection, pneumonia, pleural effusion, transient metabolic consequences, portal hypertension, clotting defects, and hepatic failure. See Table 56-6.

Table 56-6 Postoperative Complications Following Liver Resection

Liver-Related Complications
Hemorrhage
Bile fistula
Biloma
Subphrenic abscess
Ascites
Liver failure
Portal hypertension
Coagulopathy
Infections
Wound
Urinary tract
Pneumonia

Hemorrhage. The liver is a vascular organ and with hepatic resection, a raw surface area of the liver could produce bleeding in the first 24 hours postoperatively. Bleeding may be indicated by hypotension, tachycardia, and increasing abdominal girth. A decrease in hematocrit and hemoglobin will be evident. Intraabdominal hemorrhage will require immediate exploratory laparotomy to repair the bleeding area. Nursing observations and assessment should include frequent monitoring of vital signs and central venous pressure; assessing skin for adequate perfusion; measuring abdominal girth; assessing for bleeding from the incision site; assessing urine and stool; and serial monitoring of hemoglobin and hematocrit. In addition, cirrhotic individuals are at increased risk for bleeding complications and should be evaluated for overt and subclinical signs of bleeding disorders.

Biliary leak or biloma. Wound drains — typically Jackson-Pratt drains — are placed to prevent bile accumulation. A subhepatic drain is placed and a small amount of bile may be noted from necrosis on the edge of the liver. When no drains are present or when the bile leak does not resolve following drain placements, a collection of bile, called biloma, may develop. Fever, pain, and a distended abdomen may also indicate a biliary leak or biloma. The drain remains until a leak is no longer noted. If the leak persists, the patient may require further percutaneous drainage.

Subphrenic abscess. Perihepatic infection or necrosis of the remaining liver may precipitate a subphrenic abscess. Warning signs include sharp, piercing right upper quadrant pain and low-grade fever. Auscultation of the base of the lungs may detect fluid and possible abscess. Given the short length of the typical hospital stay, patients will be at home and need to notify the physician of these symptoms as they appear later in the postoperative course.

Infection. Individuals with cirrhosis are at increased risk for infection following hepatic resection as a result of decreased protein stores. The mortality rate associated with infection is high.[114] Continued assessment of vital signs, wound healing, and drain patency is crucial. Aggressive intervention is required early.

Pleural effusion and pneumonia. Pleural effusion is common following liver resection, most often after right hepatectomy. In most cases, patients are asymptomatic and should not be treated for the effusion. Aggressive pulmonary toilet with incentive spirometry and deep breathing can prevent pneumonia. Individuals are often reluctant to perform respiratory exercises due to the pain experienced with a subcostal incision, so they need encouragement. In addition, frequent ambulation and administration of analgesics prior to conducting respiratory exercises are important nursing measures.

Transient metabolic consequences. A transient elevation in liver function tests occurs postoperatively. Concern arises when a persistent upward trend is noted in the bilirubin and liver function tests. If accompanied by jaundice and signs of hepatic failure, mechanical obstruction and portal vein thrombosis must be ruled out.

Portal hypertension. Portal hypertension results from the surgical rerouting of the portal venous flow through a small remnant of liver. This leads to sequestration of blood in the splanchic circulation. Fortunately, the liver has a great potential for increasing blood flow if it has adequate time to compensate. Central venous pressure monitoring is a reliable indicator of blood volume. Bleeding from a puncture site, wound, or cavity requires immediate attention.

Clotting defects. A slight rise in the prothrombin time may be noted postoperatively. Severe coagulopathies may develop and need to be treated with fresh frozen plasma. The nurse can detect complications from deficiencies in clotting mechanisms by observing puncture sites for bleeding, monitoring abdominal girth, and testing urine and stool for blood.

Hepatic failure. Hepatic failure following hepatic resection can occur as a result of portal vein thrombosis or insufficient hepatic parenchyma. Insufficient parenchyma is more frequently the cause of hepatic failure in a cirrhotic individual. A continued rise in bilirubin and liver function tests will occur if hepatic failure is developing. In addition, the patient may display mental confusion with an increase in serum ammonia levels. Other systems — for example, renal, neurologic, and cardiac systems — may be also compromised. Frequent monitoring of mental status, vital signs, and laboratory studies are important nursing measures.

Post-Transplantation Care

Postoperative care following transplantation is similar initially to care following hepatic resection. However, the most important aspect of postoperative care in LT is the administration of immunosuppressive therapy to prevent organ rejection. Ongoing support to patients is critical because they are overwhelmed with the number of medications that must be taken on a daily basis. Studies of post-transplant improvement in emotional well-being have found that male spouses demonstrate more family cohesion with less conflict, whereas female spouses experience a higher level of stress. At one year, patients' and families' overall quality of life is generally improved.[115]

Palliative Treatments

Regional therapy

Hepatic artery infusion (HAI) for hepatocellular cancer. HAI is a treatment modality used for unresectable HCC confined only to the liver. The hepatic artery is the main supply of blood flow to the liver.[93] Chemotherapy with effective first-pass hepatic extraction can be delivered selectively to the tumor via the hepatic artery. Thus, HAI can, in theory, result in a higher concentration of drug to the tumor tissue with fewer systemic side effects.[116] Complications of HAI may include impaired liver function, biliary sclerosis, liver abscess, and dislodgment of the infusion catheter tip. An implantable pump is placed surgically for continuous delivery of the drugs. Chemotherapy agents used for HAI include 5-fluorouracil (5-FU) and floxuridine (FUDR), 5-FU/cisplatin, FUDR/mitomycin, doxorubicin, and FUDR/leucovorin/doxorubicin/platinol (FLAP).[93] Tumor response rates in various studies have been reported to be 40%, with a modest survival advantage of a few months.[116]

However, the studies on HAI for the most part have been small and patients selected for the studies have had less advanced liver disease, good performance status, and the ability to withstand abdominal surgery for pump placement. Potential selection bias needs to be taken into account when interpreting the results of improved survival.[88]

In summary, HAI therapy does not seem to offer a greater survival advantage than systemic therapy. Additionally, the risks associated with performing a major surgical procedure for pump placement need to be taken into account. HAI therapy is not to be considered standard therapy for unresectable HCC confined to the liver, but it may be considered in a clinical trial setting.

HAI for liver metastasis. Regional chemotherapy via HAI is a treatment option that is used mostly for unresectable hepatic metastases from colorectal cancer. The principle utilized in the delivery of HAI chemotherapy is that normal hepatic parenchyma derives the majority of its blood supply from the portal system, whereas metastatic lesions in the liver derive most of their afferent blood supply from the hepatic artery.[116,117] Therefore, high doses of chemotherapeutic agents are delivered directly into the hepatic artery, increasing the concentration of drug to which the tumor is exposed, while limiting both normal liver and systemic exposure and toxicity. The systemic toxicities are limited because the chemotherapeutic agents delivered have short half-lives and are extracted by the liver on the first pass. Most commonly, floxuridine is used for HAI, because of the high percentage of first-bypass extraction.

Regional chemotherapy delivers drugs via the hepatic artery with an implantable pump. Preoperative angiography with selective injection of the celiac and superior mesenteric arteries should be performed to assure proper placement of the catheter. The standard anatomy is classified as the common hepatic artery arising from the celiac artery.[118]

The patient then undergoes exploratory laparotomy via right subcostal incision and exploration of the abdomen to rule out extrahepatic metastases. An implantable pump is placed in a subcutaneous pocket in the lower abdominal wall, and the catheter is attached to a subcutaneously implanted port. Fluroscein injection is performed intraoperatively with an ultraviolet lamp to determine adequate perfusion of both lobes of the liver. Cholecystectomy is routinely performed at the time of pump implant, to prevent potential complications related to chemotherapy. Postoperatively, a nuclear scan is used to assess the perfusion of the liver. Bilobular flow must be documented and extrahepatic perfusion ruled out.

Surgical expertise is a key factor to the implantation of hepatic arterial pumps, especially when variant anatomy of the liver is present. An inadequate surgical technique can result in both gastroduodenal ulceration and inadequate liver perfusion.[119,120] In addition, medical oncologists must be familiar with the management of HAI chemotherapy in terms of determining the need for decreased dosage versus discontinuation of therapy, because HAI treatment may trigger the beginning of sclerosing cholangitis. Medical management includes close follow-up of biweekly laboratory tests, and close attention to rising liver function tests, especially bilirubin and alkaline phosphatase. CEA levels are also measured monthly. Fluoropyrimidines — for example, 5-FU and FUDR — are utilized to treat hepatic metastases. Regional chemotherapy can be delivered every two weeks or weekly on a protracted basis. Therefore, the tumor cells are exposed to the drug throughout the vulnerable phase of their mitotic cycle.[121]

Regional chemotherapy can produce a variety of side effects related to the toxicity of the specific drug. In the early development of hepatic intraarterial infusion of FUDR, a high incidence (10%–56%) of gastroduodenal ulceration occurred.[122–124] With increased expertise in surgical technique, this complication has been seen less frequently.

Other complications from HAI chemotherapy can include partial or complete thrombosis of the hepatic artery, occlusion or displacement of the catheter, hemorrhage, infection of the device or catheter, and acalculous cholecystitis.[125]

Another complication of regional chemotherapy with the delivery of FUDR is "chemical hepatitis," which is demonstrated by a rise in the levels of liver enzymes and bilirubin.[122] Bilirubinemia and strictures of the bile duct may indicate biliary sclerosis.[126] To distinguish this condition from biliary obstruction as a result of nodal metastases in the porta hepatitis or stricturing of the bile ducts, a cholangiography should be conducted.

To detect sclerosing cholangitis early, it is important to frequently monitor serum bilirubin. A slight elevation of serum bilirubin should prompt temporary discontinuation of FUDR treatment. Also, dexamethasone has been given through the hepatic artery to normalize alkaline phosphotase and persistent bilirubin elevation in those patients undergoing hepatic arterial chemotherapy. Patients with extensive liver involvement may experience diarrhea due to impaired fluoropyrimidine hepatic metabolism.[127] Overall, complications of HAI therapy can vary and chemotherapy may need to be discontinued.[128]

Hepatectomy rarely can be performed following intraarterial chemotherapy unless the tumor volume has been reduced enough to render it surgically resectable.[129] It may be difficult to quantify the size and number of lesions due to the steatosis (fatty degeneration) that can result from intraarterial therapy. It may also be more difficult to determine whether enough functional hepatic parenchyma remains to prevent postoperative hepatic failure. Technically, it is more difficult to perform hepatectomy because the hepatic artery has been ligated and multiple collateral vessels may have developed.[130] Emerging data from randomized trials suggest a potential benefit of combined regional and systemic chemotherapy following liver resection due to metastatic colorectal cancer.[131]

The use of HAI therapy plus systemic chemotherapy after a hepatic resection has been found to decrease the rate of hepatic recurrence. In addition, it improves two-year survival rates when compared to systemic chemotherapy alone.[132]

Embolization/chemoembolization. Chemoembolizaton is a local regional treatment option involving drugs or devices to restrict blood flow to certain areas of the liver. The majority of tumors receive blood flow from the hepatic artery, and normal hepatic parenchyma receives its blood supply from the portal vein.[133] Studies have shown that chemotherapy given during surgery achieves a ten times higher intratumoral concentration when it is given through the artery rather than through the portal vein.[134] As a consequence, arterially directed embolization can make the tumor ischemic while uninvolved liver is spared. Chemoembolization is best for treating hypervascular tumors (e.g., HCC and neuroendocrine liver metastases). CRC lesions are hypovascular and limit the ability to deliver adequate chemotherapy and embolic agents. Patient selection criteria required for possible chemoembolization include adequate hematologic and renal function, well-preserved hepatic function, and portal vein patency. On a case-by-case basis, patients with focal tumors with partial portal vein occlusion may still be feasible candidates for chemoembolization.[135,136]

Prior to the chemoembolization procedure, tissue diagnosis should be obtained in addition to CT or MRI to exclude extrahepatic disease. Laboratory studies include complete blood count, liver function tests, tumor markers, partial thromboplastin, and prothrombin time. Patient education should focus on side effects related to the postembolization syndrome.

The chemoembolization procedure is performed in the angiography suite with the patient under conscious sedation. A catheter is inserted in the common femoral artery; alternatively, the brachial artery may be used. A diagnostic mesenteric and hepatic arteriography is performed to determine arterial blood supply to the liver and mesentery and to confirm patency of the portal vein. A catheter is then introduced into the right or left hepatic artery depending on which lobe contains the tumor.[137] A coil is introduced into the gastroduodenal artery to protect the stomach and duodenum from potential reflux of the embolic agent.

With the catheter in the appropriate vessel supplying the tumor, the chemotherapy mixture is then injected. Some centers use a single agent, such as doxorubicin, while others add different drugs such as cisplatin, mitomycin, or 5-FU. Lipiodol (ethiodized oil), a cottonseed oil–based contrast agent, is frequently added to form a chemoemulsion, which suspends droplets of chemotherapy in an oil matrix. When embolic emulsions are added, this agent increases the response rate. Embolization creates an impedance to arterial blood flow and increases the exposure of chemotherapy to the metastatic lesions.

A gelatin sponge, mixed with the chemotherapy, is inserted to block hepatic artery flow that induces ischemic necrosis of bulky tumors. The sponge also retains ethiodized oil for a period of time and maintains a high concentration of chemotherapeutic agents. The drug concentration delivered to the tumor is 10–25 times higher than that achieved by systemic infusion.[138] Various centers administer antibiotics before and after the procedure to decrease the risk of infection and abscess formation.[139]

The patient is typically admitted following the chemoembolization procedure, for a period of 24–48 hours. Side effects from the treatment are common but self-limited. Most patients will experience post-embolization syndrome, characterized by fever, dull right upper quadrant pain, nausea, and vomiting due to transient liver capsule stretching. The symptoms are treated with antipyretics and hydrocortisone, which achieve good control in most cases.[116] Transient elevation in liver function tests is common in patients treated with chemoembolization. Rarely, patients may develop bacteremia, pneumonia, ascites, renal dysfunction, pleural effusions, or encephalopathy.[140] More serious but rare complications include liver failure, cerebral hemorrhage, liver abscess, tumor lysis syndrome, gallbladder ischemia, pancreatitis, and gastric and duodenal ulcers.[140]

For an individual with cirrhosis, a rising bilirubin level is a warning sign of potential irreversible liver necrosis. To reduce significant hepatic toxicity, chemoembolization is typically restricted to one lobe or major branch of the hepatic artery. The patient is then brought back in four weeks, once toxicities and laboratory values return to normal, to complete the procedure in the opposite lobe. Retreatment of new lesions is possible if the patient continues to meet eligibility criteria.[141]

A recent study showed that chemoembolization with gelfoam and doxorubicin improved survival in selected patients with unresectable HCC. The study was eventually stopped because of continued observations of improved survival with this intervention.[142] The benefits in survival in this study can be attributed to the strict inclusion criteria, which excluded those patients who had factors associated with treatment intolerance, such as diffuse tumor, renal failure, and poor performance status related to the tumor-associated symptoms.[143] The strict patient selection for this study precludes generalization of its results but highlights the need for selective recruitment to obtain a survival advantage.[142,144]

Ablative/cytoreductive therapy

Percutaneous ethanol injection. Percutaneous ethanol injection (PEI) is an appropriate treatment modality for patients with HCC who have solitary tumors smaller than 2 cm in diameter and who do not have the hepatic reserve to withstand a surgical resection. Because local recurrences are common, PEI is generally not recommended for patients with tumors larger than 5 cm.[145] PEI may also be performed for patients who are transplantation candidates and may be on a long waiting list, as a means of controlling disease while awaiting a transplant.

Injection of 95% ethanol into a tumor induces tumor necrosis and shrinkage. The mechanism of action is cytoplasmic dehydration with subsequent intracellular coagulation, leading to necrosis. Ethanol also affects endothelial cells, causing platelet aggregation, thrombosis, vascular occlusion, and fibrosis — all of which can decrease the blood supply to the tumor.[146]

PEI may be performed as an outpatient procedure for smaller lesions, with multiple separate injections of 1–8 mL ethanol being administered twice weekly, for a total of 4–12 sessions.[147,148] The survival rates for patients with Child-Pugh A cirrhosis (no ascites or encephalopathy, well-preserved liver function) and tumors smaller than 5 cm at one, three, and five years have been reported to be 98%, 79%, and 47%, respectively.[147,148] Poorer results have been reported in less stringently selected patients.[146–150]

In general, PEI is well tolerated. Common side effects include localized pain due to tumor necrosis and peritoneal irritation due to ethanol leakage. Rare complications occurring in less than 5% of patients may include intraperitoneal hemorrhage, hepatic insufficiency, bile duct or biliary fistula, hepatic infarction, hypotension, and renal failure.[151]

Cryoablation. Cryoablation is an ablative therapy for patients with unresectable HCC who have multifocal lesions, typically fewer than five total lesions, with each being smaller than 5 cm in diameter. The cryoablation technique involves inserting a cryoprobe, driven by circulating liquid nitrogen to achieve subzero temperature to less than −35°C; it leads to the death of both tumor and normal cells, either immediately or during the subsequent thawing period. Using multiple freeze–thaw cycles increases the percentage of tumor cells killed.[152] To achieve adequate margins, ultrasound guidance is used to direct the site of the freezing procedure. Cryoablation has not been compared prospectively to hepatic resection in noncirrhotic patients. In patients with HCC, survival rates have been reported to approach 20%.[153]

Postoperatively, patients are monitored in the intensive care unit with frequent serial laboratory evaluation, including complete blood count, coagulation profile, electrolytes, BUN, serum creatinine, and myoglobin. Alkaline hydration is administrated until the urine is free of myoglobin.[154–156] Complications arise frequently with cryoablation. They may include cracking of the ice ball, liver surface fracture,[154–156] hypothermia and associated coagulopathy, cardiac arrhythmia, consumptive coagulopathy,[157] thrombocytopenia,[156] biliary fistula,[158] bleeding,[155,158,159] electrolyte disturbance,[153,154] iatrogenic probe injury, cryogenic shock,[154,156] abscess, pleural effusion,[158] myoglobinuria,[155,156,158] and acute renal failure.[159] Due to the relatively high rate of complications associated with cryoablation, radiofrequency ablation is currently favored over cryoablation, as the former treatment is associated with lower rates of both recurrences and complications.

Radiofrequency ablation. Radiofrequency ablation (RFA) is another type of ablative modality used in treating patients with HCC (Figure 56-2), liver metastases from CRC, and neuroendocrine tumors. RFA is typically used in those patients who do not meet the criteria for surgical resection, but who are candidates for liver-directed procedures based on the absence of extrahepatic disease. The RFA technique uses high-

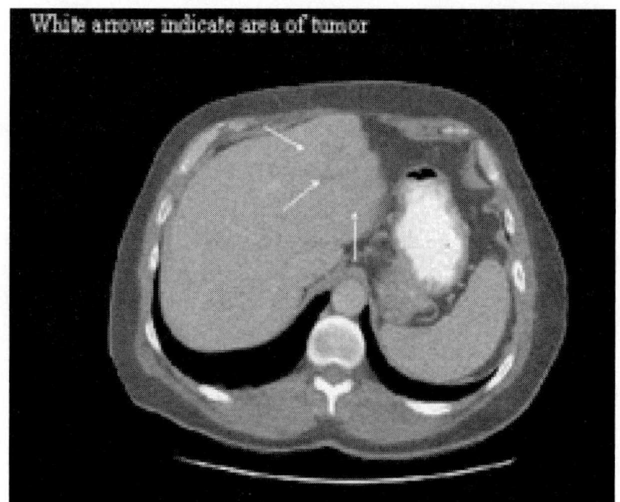

Figure 56-2 HCC of right medial lobe. CT scan pre-radiofrequency ablation. (Photo courtesy of the Massachusetts General Hospital Department of Interventional Radiology.)

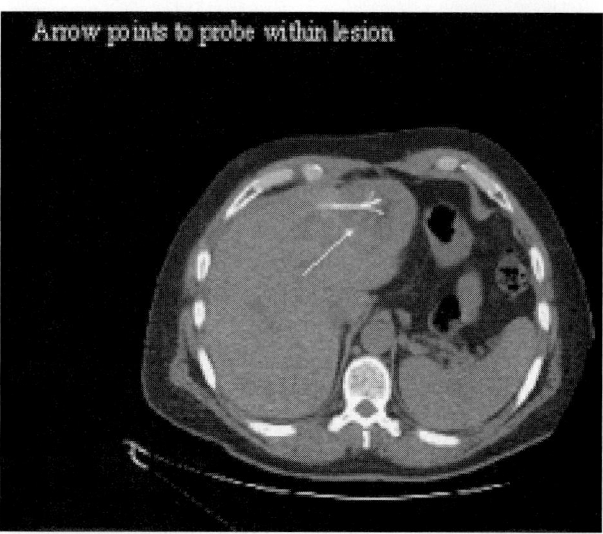

Figure 56-3 RFA probe within the lesion. (Photo courtesy of the Massachusetts General Hospital Department of Interventional Radiology.)

energy heat greater than 60°F to produce cell destruction and tissue necrosis.[160,161] The RFA procedure may be done percutanously under US or CT guidance, laparoscopically, or as an open laparotomy procedure. US is used to guide placement of a needle electrode, which is then advanced into the area of the tumor to be treated. The needle electrode is attached to a radiofrequency generator, and the treatment is delivered (Figure 56-3). To obtain a tumor-free margin, the thermal electrode is used to produce a thermal lesion encompassing the entire treated area, including not only the tumor but also nondiseased liver tissue of 1 cm around the tumor.[162] The patient is monitored with CT to determine whether additional therapy is necessary (Figure 56-4).

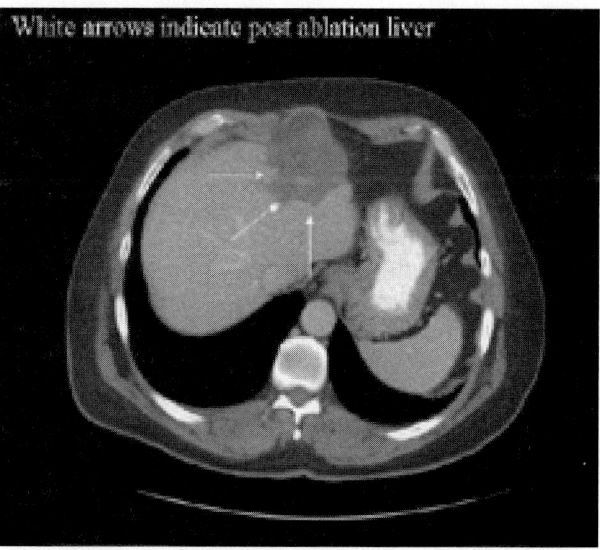

Figure 56-4 Post-RFA of HCC lesion CT scan. The goal of treatment with RFA is complete destruction of the tumor and a surrounding margin of hepatic parenchyma. Post-ablation CT scan (four weeks) shows lesions larger than original tumor. (Photo courtesy of the Massachusetts General Hospital Department of Interventional Radiology.)

Radiation Therapy

External beam radiotherapy has limited use in the treatment of HCC because normal liver tissue has low tolerance for radiation. A dosage of greater than 50 Gy has been recommend to kill HCC cells, but this dosage will provoke radiation-induced hepatitis and liver failure.[163] Survival following radiation therapy is short, with most patients dying within six months.[164] Conventional radiotherapy in the range of 30–35 Gy can be used in patients who require palliation of painful liver lesions.

Larger doses of radiation can be delivered via linear accelerator and proton beam therapy because of the better targeting of the radiation to the tumor. Large doses of radiation are directed at the tumor lesion via three-dimensional radiation ports. A 50% reduction in tumor size has been reported with minimal side effects and good quality of life.[163] Radiotherapy can be used safely in patients with Child-Pugh A cirrhosis and tumors smaller than 8 cm or in patients with Child-Pugh B and tumors smaller than 5 cm. This approach, however, does not work with micrometastatic or multifocal disease.[93]

Intraarterially administered yttrium-90 glass microspheres have also been used in HCC.[164,165] Clinical trials of this procedure in the United States are ongoing. Like many other treatment options, radiation therapy has yet to be defined in regard to unresectable HCC. It can be an option in patients with localized disease who have failed other local therapies, have no extrahepatic disease, and have limited tumor burden and good liver function.

Systemic Chemotherapy

Chemotherapy may be the only potential treatment option for patients with advanced HCC, because the majority of these patients are not candidates for curative resection. To date, many chemotherapy agents have been studied to treat advanced HCC without much success, because several limitations exist in treating the disease. For example, HCC is known to be a chemotherapy-refractory tumor. This tendency could be due to its high rate of expression of drug-resistant genes, and the heterogenous nature of the tumor.[146,166–168] Additionally, patients with advanced HCC who have significant liver dysfunction cannot tolerate systemic chemotherapy.[153] In one study, no objective responses were found in patients with poor performance status, ascites, portal vein thrombus, or serum bilirubin greater than 2 mg/dL.[169]

Single- and combination-agent chemotherapies have been studied. Doxorubicin is usually given as a single agent. A number of small studies have reported partial response rates of less than 20%.[170–172] One small trial suggested a survival benefit compared to best supportive care (median survival of 10.6 months versus 7.5 months).[173,174]

Another agent with a low toxicity profile and broad antitumor activity is 5-FU. Despite the fact that 5-FU is extensively metabolized by the liver, adequate doses can be administered in the setting of liver dysfunction. When it is given as a single agent, response rates are low. When it is given in combination with leucovorin, response rates can be as high as 28%.[173]

Oral agents such as capecitabine[175] or the angiogenic agent thalidomide[176] have been associated with minor objective tumor activity and, in some patients, with stablization of disease growth. A complete response on radiologic examination has been observed in one patient with HCC after receiving capecitabine.[175]

Combination chemotherapy agents have been studied in patients with advanced HCC. These studies have not shown a survival benefit. Of the combination regimens, cisplatin-based regimens have produced higher objective response rates as compared to non-cisplatin-based regimens. Cisplatin-containing regimens include a combination of cisplatin and epirubicin; cisplatin and infusional 5-FU; sequential low-dose infusional cisplatin plus infusional 5-FU; and gemcitabine and cisplatin. Median survival in all studies of these agents was 4.4–11 months.[177–183]

Interferon-alfa (IFN-α) has been studied as a single agent with three times weekly subcutaneous injections achieving a response rate of 31% and improved median survival benefit when compared to the best-supportive-care group. Tolerability was good, with fatigue being cited as the major toxicity.[184]

Combination regimens with interferon-alfa (IFN-α), such as IFN-α and 5-FU or IFN-α and cisplatin, when compared to best supportive care, have better one-year survival rates.[185] Additionally, the regimen toxicity profile is acceptable. The combination regimen of cisplatin, IFN-α, doxorubicin, and infusional 5-FU (PIAF) resulted in response rates of approximately 26%, with some patients achieving complete response.[186] However, this regimen is associated with significant toxicity. It may be an appropriate choice in young patients with adequate liver function.[186]

Gene Therapy

Gene therapy represents an exciting and promising approach for the treatment of HCC, although currently it is largely confined to the preclinical and experimental settings. Gene therapy can produce a biologic effect by the transfer of foreign genes into the target cells using viral or nonviral vectors.[187] Gene therapies that have been studied for the treatment of HCC include gene replacement therapy with *p53,* a tumor suppressor gene; antisense therapy against the *K-ras* oncogene; drug sensitization with a suicide-gene encoding a foreign enzyme that transforms a nontoxic prodrug into a toxic compound in transfected cells; and genetic immunotherapy that seeks to stimulate a more effective response against tumor antigens. Technical problems need to be overcome prior to successful clinical application of gene therapy, including better gene delivery, improved tumor specificity, more stable transgene expressions, and larger therapeutic windows.[188]

Symptom Management and Supportive Care

At diagnosis, the clinical course of primary liver cancer and metastatic liver cancer may vary widely. However, as the disease in the liver and the metastatic process progress, their clinical courses will be very similar. Palliative approaches for treating patients with advanced or metastatic liver cancer may rely on systemic chemotherapy, regional therapy, or radiation therapy. Patients may initially present with advanced disease and impaired liver function that is not possible to treat. Regardless of the stage of the disease, comfort measures and management of distressing symptoms should be provided.

Pain can be a common symptom of advanced disease. The etiology of pain in this patient population may include pain caused by abdominal fullness, stretching of the liver capsule, ascites, or intraabdominal disease metastasis. The three-step analgesic ladder developed by the World Health Organization should guide pain management therapy.[189] Initially, pain may be controlled with anti-inflammatory drugs and acetaminophen. Due to their gastrointestinal, hepatotoxic, and hematological side effects, these drugs often have limited long-term use. Transdermal and long-acting oral opioids are used along with short-acting narcotics for breakthrough pain. A bowel regimen should be instituted to avoid or treat constipation. If pain cannot be adequately controlled, external beam radiation with or without chemotherapy may be used to palliate the pain of advanced liver cancer.

As the liver fails and secretes less bile, bilirubin will accumulate in the blood. Clinically jaundice becomes apparent when bilirubin levels exceed 3mg/dL. Hemolysis of red blood cells may add to the jaundice. Pruritus can become distressing to the patient. Management of pruritus may include avoiding hot baths and hot drinks that can cause blood vessel dilation; applying local ice pack to areas of most severe itching; taking starch or oatmeal baths; and applying moisturizing agents with topical lotions containing menthol, camphor, phenol, zinc oxide, calamine, doxepin, and/or corticosteroids. Systemic oral antihistamines may be effective when given in high doses at bedtime. Cholestyramine may be used to remove bile acids if the patient is able to tolerate oral intake.

With advanced disease, ascites can cause pain and dyspnea. Paracenteses can lead to loss of albumin, volume depletion, hypotension, and the risk of peritonitis. Low doses of morphine may help with the dyspnea, and pain management intervention as discussed previously should be instituted. Diuretics, such as furosemide and spironolactone, can be used as needed. Last, peritoneovenous catheter or shunts are sometimes used for palliation of ascites depending on the patient's goals.

Nausea, vomiting, and early satiety may be present and should be treated with antiemetics such as prochloperazine and haloperidal. Allowing the patient to self-regulate oral intake and consume small frequent meals may help.

Psychological distress should be assessed. If present, clinical depression should be treated. There is no particular class of antidepressants that is especially advantageous for this patient population. Selective serotonin reuptake inhibitors (SSRIs) may be a good choice because they have fewer side effects and the potential to improve energy levels. The use of psychostimulants may also be indicated to improve mood, increase appetite, and counter the sedation of opioid treatments. Counseling and a support group for patients and caretakers may be benefit these individuals as well.

Generalized debilitation, fatigue, weight loss, and cachexia will be present in advanced disease. Supportive nutritional management initially may include caloric supplementation and oral hydration. Enteral or parental nutrition is usually not preferred in most cases of the anorexia/cachexia syndrome in patients with advanced cancer because it does not yield any prolonged benefit.[190] Appetite stimulants such as megesterol acetate at doses of 200–800 mg/day and corticosteroids can be used to treat anorexia.[191,192] Another class of drugs that may be used alone or in conjunction with other agents to stimulate appetite are the cannabinoids. Dronabinol has been proven to improve chemotherapy-induced nausea and vomiting in 65% of cancer patients.[192] It also improves appetite in HIV-associated cachexia. Fatigue is a persistent symptom with many causes including the disease itself, side effects of treatment, and depression. Fatigue may be reduced by aggressively treating contributing factors such as depression, anxiety, and uncontrolled pain. Anemia may be a contributing factor to fatigue anywhere along the disease trajectory. Once diagnosed, it should be treated with blood transfusion. If appropriate, recombinant human erythropoietin can also be used to promote adequate hemoglobin levels.

Clinical indicators of end-stage liver failure include hepatic encephalopathy, hepatorenal syndrome, recurrent variceal bleeding, ascites, and coagulopathies refractory to indicated therapies. Hepatic encephalopathy is considered an early stage of hepatic coma. Due to the inability of the liver to perform detoxifying functions, ammonia and other toxic substances to the brain will be present in the circulation.

Clinical features of hepatic encephalopathy include drowsiness, confusion, irritability, and characteristic flapping tremors (asterixis). Treatment may include diazepam and haloperidal for agitation and hallucinations. Ammonia levels can be decreased by administering lactulose 30 mL every 8 hours, titrated to produce 2–3 stools daily. Likewise, neomycin 1 g daily can be used to decrease ammonia levels.

Anticipatory management of rapidly developing symptoms of the patient and family support are major goals in advanced and end-stage disease. Psychosocial, spiritual, and symptom management are all equally paramount concerns. The person dying from liver failure, whatever its cause, is dying from multisystem failure. For some patients, death may be precipitated by an acute event such as gastrointestinal bleeding, respiratory failure, hypovolemic shock, sepsis, or pneumonia. For others, death may occur quietly, with the patient lapsing into a coma.

Conclusion

Oncology nurses caring for patients with primary liver cancer and metastatic liver disease face a tremendous challenge. Treatment options in patients with HCC are generally limited due to the presence of underlying severe liver disease, advanced tumor stage, and restricted options for transplantation. In the future, improved screening tools and treatment for HCC, as well as the discovery of new treatments such as gene therapy, hold promise for improving survival of patients with HCC. Continued refinements in the surgical management of patients with CRC liver metastasis and regional therapies such as HAI infusion pump and RFA will contribute to improved survival rates.

Preventive strategies will most likely make the greatest impact. As in the case of hepatitis B, vaccination of children in Taiwan resulted in a decline in HCC incidence. Additionally, using antiviral therapy in patients with HBV and HCV infection should contribute to the prevention of HCC. Further primary prevention aimed at public health measures to reduce food contamination with aflatoxins and to eliminate excessive alcohol use should also reduce the incidence of liver disease, cirrhosis, and hence HCC.

Oncology nurses can play a key role within the multidisciplinary team caring for patients with HCC and liver metastases. Providing education to patients about disease prevention, screening options for early disease, and treatment options can empower patients and their families in making decisions regarding their treatment and care. Additionally, oncology nurses play a key role in providing expert care in the area of symptom assessment and management of pain, nutrition, functional status, and spiritual well-being. In the future, nursing research related to the care of patients with HCC and liver metastases and focused on quality of life, symptom experience from the disease, and treatment can contribute to improving patient outcomes and quality of care.

References

1. El-Serag HB: Hepatocellular carcinoma: an epidemiologic view. *J Clin Gastroenterol* 35:S72–S78, 2002
2. El-Serag HB, Mason AC: Rising incidence of hepatocellular carcinoma in the United States. *N Engl J Med* 340:745–750, 1999
3. Jemal A, Tiwari RC, Murray T, et al: Cancer statistics, 2004. *CA Cancer J Clin* 54:8–29, 2004
4. Parkin DM, Pisani P, Ferlay J: Estimates of worldwide incidence of 25 major cancers in 1985. *Int J Cancer* 80:827–841, 1999
5. Bosch FX, Ribes J, Borras J: Epidemiology of primary liver cancer. *Semin Liver Dis* 19:271–285, 1999
6. Parkin DM, Muir CS, Whelan SL, et al (eds.): *Cancer Incidence in Five Continents, vol 6.* Lyon, France: International Agency for Research on Cancer, 1997
7. Kew MC: Epidemiology of hepatocellular carcinoma. *Toxicology* 181–182:35–38, 2002
8. Bosch FX: Global epidemiology of hepatocellular carcinoma, in Okuda K, Tabor E (eds.): *Liver Cancer.* New York, Churchill Livingstone, 1997, pp 13–28
9. DiBisceglie AM: Epidemiology and clinical presentation of hepatocelluar carcinoma. *J Vascul Intervention Radiol* 13:S169–S171, 2002
10. Gilbert HA, Hakagn AR: Metastases: incidence, detection. An evaluation without histologic confirmation, in Weiss L (ed.): *Fundamental Aspects of Metastasis.* Amsderdam, North-Holland Publishing, 1976, pp 385–405
11. Kelvin JF, Scagliola J: Metastases involving the gastrointestinal system. *Semin Oncol Nurs* 14:187–198, 1998
12. Kemeny NE, Kemeny M, Lawrence TS: Liver metastases, in Abeloff MD, Armitage JO, Lichter AS, et al (eds.): *Clinical Oncology* (ed 2). Philadelphia, Harcourt Brace, 2000, pp 886–921
13. Kew M: Hepatocellular cancer: epidemiology and risk factors, in Kelsen DP, Daly JM, Kern SE, et al (eds.): *Gastrointestinal Oncology, Principles and Practice.* Philadelphia, Lippincott, Williams and Wilkins, 2002, pp 529–538
14. Bralet MP, Regimbeau JM, Pineau P, et al: Hepatocellular carcinoma occurring in nonfibrotic liver: epidemiologic and histopathologic analysis of 80 French cases. *Hepatology* 32:200–204, 2000
15. Beasley RP, Hwang L-Y: Epidemiology of hepatocellular carcinoma, in Vyas GN, Dienstag JL, Hoofnagle JH (eds.): *Viral Hepatitis and Liver Disease.* Orlando, FL, Grune and Stratton, 1984, pp 209–244
16. International Agency for Research on Cancer: Hepatitis virus. *IARC Monographs on the Evaluation of Carcinogenic Risks,* 159:66–97, 1994
17. Nissen NN, Martin P: Hepatocellular carcinoma, the high-risk patient. *J Clin Gastroenterol* 13(suppl 2):79–85, 2002
18. Monto A, Wright TL: The epidemiology and prevention of hepatocelllullar carcinoma. *Semin Oncol* 28:441–449, 2001
19. Chen CJ, Wang LY, Lu SN, et al: Elevated aflatoxin exposure and increased risk of hepatocellular carcinoma. *Hepatology* 24:38–42, 1996
20. Wang JS, Huang T, Su J: Hepatocellular carcinoma and aflatoxin exposure in Zhuqing village, Fusui county, People's Republic of China. *Cancer Epidemiol Biomarker Prevent* 10:143–146, 2001
21. Szymanska K, Hainaut P: TP53 and mutations in human cancer. *Acta Biochimica Polonica* 50:231–238, 2003
22. Ueno Y, Nagata S, Tsutsumi T, et al: Detection of microcystins, a blue-green algal hepatotoxin, in drinking water sampled in Haimen and Fusui, endemic areas of primary liver cancer in China, by highly sensitive immunoassay. *Carcinogenesis* 17:1317–1321, 1996
23. Tabor E, DiBisceglie AM: Hepatocellular carcinoma. *Clin Liver Dis* 3:327–348, 1999
24. Donato F, Tagger A, Gelatti U, et al: Alcohol and hepatocellular carcinoma: the effect of lifetime intake and hepatitis virus

infections in men and women. *Am J Epidemiol* 155:323–331, 2002

25. Collaborative MILTS Project Team: Oral contraceptives and liver cancer. Results of a Multicentre International Liver Tumor Study (MILTS). *Contraception* 56:275–284, 1997
26. Granata OM, Carruba G, Montalato G: Altered androgen metabolism eventually leads hepatocellular carcinoma to an impaired hormone responsiveness. *Mol Cell Endocrinol* 193:51–58, 2002
27. Niederau C, Fischer R, Sonnenberg A, et al: Survival and causes of death in cirrhotic and non-cirrhotic patients with primary hemochromatosis. *N Engl J Med* 313:1256–1262, 1985
28. Mandioshona E, MacPhail AP, Gordeuk VK, et al: Dietary iron overload as a risk factor for hepatocellular carcinoma in black Africans. *Hepatology* 27:1563–1567, 1998
29. Simson IM: Membranous obstruction of the inferior vena cava and hepatocellular carcinoma in South Africa. *Gastroenterology* 82:171–178, 1998
30. Regimbeau JM, Colombat M, Mognol P, et al: Obesity and diabetes as a risk factor for hepatocellular carcinoma. *Liver Transpl* 10(suppl 2):S69–S73, 2004
31. El-serag HB, Tran T, Everhart JE: Diabetes increases the risk of chronic liver disease and hepatocellular carcinoma. *Gastroenterology* 126:460–468, 2004
32. Yang S, Lin HZ, Hwang H, et al: Hepatic hyperplasia in noncirrhotic fatty livers: obesity steatosis, a premalignant condition? *Cancer Res* 61:5016–5023, 2001
33. Poonawala A, Nair S, Thuluvath P: Prevalance of obesity and diabetes in patients with cryptogenic cirhhosis: a case control study? *Hepatology* 32:689–692, 2000
34. Huang K, Lin S: Nationwide vaccination: a success story in Taiwan. *Vaccine* 1:S35–S38, 2000
35. Effect of interferon-alpha on progression of cirrhosis to hepatocellular carcinoma: a retrospective cohort study. International Interferon-alpha Hepatocellular Carcinoma Study Group. *Lancet* 352:1230, 1998
36. Tanaka H, Tsukuma H, Kasahara A, et al: Effect of interferon therapy on the incidence of hepatocellular carcinoma and mortality of patients with chronic hepatitis C: a retrospective cohort study of 738 patients. *Int J Cancer* 87:741–749, 2000
37. Hayashi K, Kumada T, Nakano S, et al: Incidence of hepatocellular carcinoma in chronic hepatitis C after interferon therapy. *Hepatogastroenterology* 49:508–512, 2002
38. Koga H: Hepatocellular carcinoma: is there a potential for chemoprevention using cylooxygenase-2 inhibitors? *Cancer* 98: 661–667, 2003
39. Collier J, Sherman M: Screening for hepatocellular carcinoma. *Hepatology* 27:273, 1998
40. Larcos G, Sorokopud H, Berry G, et al: Sonographic screening for hepatocellular carcinoma in patients with chronic hepatitis or cirrhosis: an evaluation. *AJR Am J Roentgenol* 171:433–435, 1998
41. Okuda K: Hepatocellular carcinoma. *J Hepatol* 32(suppl 1):225-237, 2000
42. Schafer DF, Sorrell MF: Hepatocellular carcinoma. *Lancet* 353:1253-1257, 1999
43. Nguyen MH, Keeffe EB: Screening for hepatocellular carcinoma. *J Clin Gastroenterol* 35(suppl 2):S86–S91, 2002
44. Colombo M: Early diagnosis of hepatocellular carcinoma in Italy. A summary of a Consensus Development Conference held in Milan, 16 November 1990, by the Italian Association for the Study of the Liver (AISF). *J Hepatol* 14:401, 1992
45. Bisgard HC, Thorgeirsson SS: Hepatic regeneration: the role of regeneration in pathogenesis of chronic liver disease. *Clin Lab Med* 16:325–329, 1996
46. Yuman F, Kemeny N, Lawrence TS, et al: Cancer of the liver and biliary tree, in DeVita VT, Hellman S, Rosenberg SA (eds.): *Cancer: Principles and Practice of Oncology* (ed 6). Philadelphia, Lippincott, Williams and Wilkins, 2001, pp 1162–1177
47. Rolfes DB: Fibrolamellar carcinoma of the liver, in Okuda K, Shak KG (eds.): *Neoplasms of the Liver.* Tokyo, Springer-Verlag, 1987, p 137
48. Nakanuma Y: Pathology of hepatocellular cancer, in Rustgi AK (ed.): *Gastrointestinal Cancers.* New York, Saunders, 2003, pp 593–604
49. Crawford JM: The liver and the biliary tract, in Cotran RS, Kumar V, Collins T (eds.): *Robbins Pathologic Basis of Disease* (ed 6). Philadelphia, W.B. Saunders, 1999, pp 845–901
50. Katyal S, Oliver JH, Peterson MS, et al: Extrahepatic metastases of hepatocellular carcinoma. *Radiology* 216:698–703, 2000
51. Okazaki N, Yoshino M, Yoshida T, et al: Bone metastases in hepatocellular carcinoma. *Cancer* 56:1991–1994, 1985
52. Kew MC: Clinical aspects of hepatocellular cancer, in Rustgi AK (ed.): *Gastrointestinal Cancers.* New York, Saunders, 2003, pp 564–574
53. Kew MC: Hepatocellular cancer a century of progress. *Clin Liver Dis* 4:257–259, 2000
54. Eastman RC, Carson RE, Orloff DG, et al: Glucose utilization in a patient with hepatoma and hypoglycemia. Assessment by a positron emission tomography. *J Clin Invest* 89:1958–1963, 1992
55. Tietge UJ, Schofl C, Ocran KW, et al: Hepatoma with severe non-islet tumor hypoglycemia. *Am J Gastroenterol* 93:997–1000, 1998
56. Kew MC, Fisher JW: Serum erythropoietin concentration in patients with hepatocellular carcinoma. *Cancer* 58:2486–2488, 1986
57. Yen TC, Hwang SJ, Wang CC, et al: Hypercalcemia and parathyroid hormone-related protein in hepatocellular carcinoma. *Liver* 13:311–315, 1993
58. Bruix J, Castells, Calvet X, et al: Diarrhea as a presenting symptom of hepatocellular carcinoma. *Dig Dis Sci* 35:681–685, 1990
59. Watkins KT, Curley SA: Liver and bile ducts, in Abeloff MD, Armitage JO, Lichter SA, et al (eds.): *Clinical Oncology* (ed 2). New York, Churchill Livingstone, 2000, pp 1681–1748
60. Gonzalez KB, Woodall M: Hepatocellular carcinoma: surgical treatment options. *Nurs Clin North Am* 36:593–603, 2001
61. Yeh CN, Lee WC, Jeng LB: Spontaneous tumour rupture and prognosis in patients with hepatocellular carcinoma. *Br J Surg* 89:1125–1129, 2002
62. Befeler AS, Di Disceglie AM: Hepatocellular carcinoma: diagnosis and treatment. *Gastroenterology* 122:1609–1619, 2002
63. Chen DS, Sung JL, Lai MY, et al: Serum alpha-fetoprotein in the early stage of hepatocellular carcinoma. *Gastroenterology* 86:1404–1409. 1984
64. Moertel CG, Fleming TR, Macdoald JS, et al: An evaluation of the carcinoembryonic antigen (CEA) test for monitoring patients with resected colon cancer. *JAMA* 270:943–947, 1993
65. Ishiguchi T, Shimamoto K, Fukatsu H, et al: Radiologic diagnosis of hepatocellular carcinoma. *Semin Surg Oncol* 12:164–169, 1996
66. Whittingham TA: New and future developments in ultrasonic imaging. *Br J Radiol* 70:S119–S132, 1997
67 Lim JH, Choi D, Kim SH, et al: Detection of hepatocellular carcinoma: value of adding delayed phase imaging to dual-phase helical CT. *AJR Am J Roentgenol* 179:67–73, 2002
68. Miller FH, Butler RS, Hoff FL, et al: Using triphasic helical CT to detect focal hepatic lesions in patients with neoplasms. *AJR Am J Roentgenol* 171:643–649, 1998
69. Veltri A, Robba T, Anselmetti GC, et al: Computerized tomography with lipiodol in hepatocarcinoma. Assessment of its diag-

nostic accuracy with anatomo-pathological control. *Radiol Med* 96:81–86, 1998

70. Libbrecht L, Bielen D, Verslype C, et al: Focal lesions in cirrhotic explant livers: pathologic evaluation and accuracy of pretransplantation imaging examinations. *Liver Transpl* 8:749–761, 2002
71. Heiken JP, Weyman PJ, Lee JK, et al: Detection of focal hepatic masses: prospective evaluation with CT, delayed CT, CT during arterial portography, and MR imaging. *Radiology* 171:47–51, 1989
72. Yu AS, Kim KW, Lee JT, et al: MR imaging during arterial portography for assessment of hepatocellular carcinoma: comparison with CT during arterial portography. *AJR Am J Roentgenol* 170:1501–1506, 1998
73. Choi D, Kim S, Lim J, et al: Preoperative detection of hepatocellular carcinoma: ferumoxides-enhanced MR imaging versus combined helical CT during arterial portography and CT hepatic arteriography. *AJR Am J Roentgenol* 176:475–482, 2001
74. Wudel LJ, Delbeke D, Morris R, et al: The role of [18F] fluorodeoxyglucose positron emission tomoraphy imaging in the evaluation of hepatocellular carcinoma. *Am Sur* 69:117–124, 2003
75. Dresel S, Kirsch CM, Tatsch K, et al: Detection of hepatocellular carcinoma with a new alpha-fetoprotein antibody imaging kit. *J Clin Oncol* 15:2683–2690, 1997
76. Serafini AN, Jeffers LJ, Reddy KR, et al: Early recognition of recurrent hepatocellular carcinoma utilizing gallium-67 citrate scintigraphy. *J Nucl Med* 29:712–716, 1998
77. John TG, Garden OJ: Needle track seeding of primary and secondary liver carcinoma after percutaneous liver biopsy. *HPB Surgery* 6:199–203, 1993
78. Durand F, Regimbeau JM, Belghiti J, et al: Assessment of the benefits and risks of percutaneous biopsy before surgical resection of hepatocellular carcinoma. *J Hepatol* 35:254–258, 2001
79. Kuo FY, Chen WJ, Lu SN, et al: Fine needle aspiration cytodiagnosis of liver tumors. *Acta Cytol* 48:142–148, 2004
80. Nguyen MH, Keeffe EB: Treatment of hepatocellular cancer, in Rustgi AK (ed.): *Gastrointestinal Cancers*. New York, Saunders, 2003, pp 605–622
81. Yu AS, Keeffe EB: Management of hepatocellular carcinoma. *Rev Gastroenterol Disord* 3:8–24, 2003
82. Child CG III, Turcotte JG: Surgery in portal hypertension, in Child CG III (ed.): *The Liver and Portal Hypertension*. Philadelphia, W.B. Saunders, 1964, p 50
83. Okuda K, Ohtuki T, Obata H, et al: Natural history of hepatocellular carcinoma and prognosis in relation to treatment: study of 850 patients. *Cancer* 56:918-928, 1985
84. Greene FL, Page DL, Fleming ID, et al (eds.): *AJCC (American Joint Committee on Cancer) Cancer Staging Manual* (ed 6). New York, Springer-Verlag, 2002, p 148
85. Cancer of the Liver Italian Program (CLIP) Investigators: A new prognostic system for hepatocellular carcinoma: a retrospective study of 435 patients. *Hepatology* 28:751, 1998
86. Levy I, Sherman M: The Liver Cancer Study Group of the University of Toronto. Staging of hepatocellular carcinoma: assessment of the CLIP, Okuda, and Child-Pugh staging systems in a cohort of 257 patients in Toronto. *Gut* 50:881–885, 2002
87. Farinati F, Rinaldi M, Gianni S, et al: How should patients with hepatocellular cancer be staged? Validation of a new prognostic system. *Cancer* 89:2266–2273, 2000
88. Bruix J: Treatment of hepatocellular carcinoma. *Hepatology* 25:259, 1997
89. Curley SA, Barnett CC, Abdalla EK: Treatment algorithm for hepatocellullar carcinoma. *www.uptodate.com* (accessed December 18, 2003)
90. Bruix J, Castells A, Bosch L, et al: Surgical resection of hepatocellular carcinoma in cirrhotic patients: prognostic value of preoperative portal pressure. *Gastroenterology* 111:1018–1022, 1996
91. Aguayo A, Patt YZ: Liver cancer. *Clin Liver Dis* 5:479–507, 2001
92. Tung-Ping PR, Fan ST, Wong J: Risk factors, prevention, and management of postoperative recurrence after resection of hepatocellular carcinoma. *Ann Surg* 232:10–24, 2000
93. Poon RT, Fan ST: Hepatectomy for hepatocellullar carcinoma: patient selection and postoperative outcome. *Liver Transpl* 10(suppl 1):S39–S45, 2004
94. Nagorney DM, vanHeerden JA, Ilstrup DM, et al: Primary hepatic malignancy: surgical management and determinants of survival. *Surgery* 106:740–748, 1989
95. Kaibori M, Matsui Y, Kitade H, et al: Hepatic resection for hepatocellular carcinoma in severely cirrhotic livers. *Hepatogastroenterology* 50:491–496, 2003
96. Llovert JM, Bruix J, Gores GJ: Surgical resection versus transplantation for early hepatocellullar carcinoma: clues for the best strategy. *Hepatology* 31:1019–1021, 2000
97. Yoo HY, Patt CH, Geshwind JF, et al: The outcome of liver transplantation in patients with hepatocellular carcinoma in the United States between 1988 and 2001: 5-year survival has improved significantly with time. *J Clin Oncol* 21:4329–4335, 2003
98. Little SA, Fong Y: Hepatocellular carcinoma: current surgical management. *Semin Oncol* 28:474–486, 2001
99. Lo CM, Lai EC, Liu CL, et al: Laparoscopy and laparoscopic ultrasonography avoid exploratory laparotomy in patients with hepatocellular carcinoma. *Ann Surg* 227:527–532, 1998
100. Figueras J, Jaurrieta E, Vallas C, et al: Survival after liver transplantation in cirrhotic patients with and without hepatocellular carcinoma: a comparative study. *Hepatology* 25:1485–1489, 1997
101. Mazzaferro V, Regalia E, Doci R, et al: Liver transplantation for the treatment of small hepatocellular carcinomas in patients with cirrhosis. *N Engl J Med* 334:693–699, 1996
102. Yao FY, Ferrell L, Bass NM, et al: Liver transplantation for hepatocellular carcinoma: expansion of the tumor size does not adversely impact survival. *Hepatology* 33:1394–1403, 2001
103. Schwartz JD, Schwartz M, Mandeli J, et al: Neoadjuvant and adjuvant therapy for resectable carcinoma: review of randomized clinical trials. *Lancet Oncol* 3:593–603, *2002*
104. Venhook AP, Ferrell LD, Roberts, JP, et al: Liver transplantation for hepatocellular carcinoma: results of preoperative chemoembolization. *Liver Transpl Surg* 1:242–248, 1995
105. Majno PE, Adam R, Bismuth H, et al: Influence of preoperative transarterial lipiodol chemoembolization on resection and transplantation for hepatocellular carcinoma in patients with cirrhosis. *Ann Surg* 226:688-701, 1997
106. Harnois DM, Steers J, Andrews JC, et al: Preoperative hepatic artery chemoembolization followed by orthotopic liver transplantation for hepatocellular carcinoma. *Liver Transpl Surg* 5:192–199, 1999
107. Fong Y, Cohen AM, Fortner JG, et al: Liver resection for colorectal metastases. *J Clin Oncol* 15:938–946, 1997
108. Bismuth H, Adam R, Navarro F, et al: Re-resection for colorectal metastases. *Surg Oncol Clin North Am* 5:353–363, 1996
109. Kin T, Nakajima Y, Kanehiro H, et al: Repeat hepatectomy for recurrent colorectal metastases. *World J Surg* 24:620–621, 1998
110. Fong Y, Blumgart LH, Cohen A: Repeat hepatic resections for metastatic colorectal cancer. *Ann Surg* 220:657–662, 1994
111. Chu QD, Vezeridis MP, Avaradopoulos KA, et al: Repeat resection for recurrent colorectal cancer. *World J Surg* 21:292–296, 1996

112. Adam R, Bismuth H, Castaing D, et al: Repeat hepatectomy for colorectal liver metastases. *Ann Surg* 225:51–62, 1997
113. Degremont AC, Ismail M, Arthaud M, et al: Mechanisms of postoperative prolonged plasma volume expansion with low molecular weight hydroxethy (HES 200/0.62, 6%). *Intensive Care Med* 21:577–583, 1995
114. Vauthey JN, Klimstra D, Franceschi D, et al: Factors affecting long-term outcome after hepatic resection for hepatocellular carcinoma. *Am J Surg* 169:28–34, 1995
115. Tarter RE: Quality of life following liver transplantation. *Hepatogastroenterology* 45:1398–1403, 1998
116. Colleoni M, Audisio RA, De Braud F, et al: Practical considerations in the treatment of hepatocellular carcinoma. *Drugs* 55:367, 1998
117. Watkins E, Khazei AM, Nahra KS: Surgical basis for arterial infusion chemotherapy of disseminated carcinoma of the liver. *Surg Gynecol Obstet* 130:581–605, 1970
118. Lin G, Lunderquist A, Hagerstrand I, et al: Postmortem examination of the blood supply and vascular pattern of small liver metastases in man. *Surgery* 96:517–526, 1984
119. Campbell KA, Burns RC, Sitzmann JV, et al: Regional chemotherapy devices: effect of experience and anatomy on complications. *J Clin Oncol* 11:822–826, 1993
120. Daly J, Kemeny N, Sigurdson E, et al: Regional infusion of colorectal hepatic metastases: a randomized trial comparing the hepatic artery versus the portal vein. *Arch Surg* 122:1273–1277, 1987
121. Mavlight GM, Patt YZ, Haynie TP, et al: Differential tumor progression in patients with bilobar hepatic metastases and dual arterial supply: evidence supporting the advantage of intra-arterial over intravenous route of drug delivery. *Sel Cancer Ther* 5:37–45, 1989
122. Hohn DC, Stagg RJ, Price DC, et al: Avoidance of gastroduodenal toxicity in patients receiving hepatic arterial 5-fluoro-2′-deoxyuridine. *J Clin Oncol* 3:1257–1260, 1985
123. Ensminger WD: Intrahepatic arterial infusion of chemotherapy: pharmacologic principles. *Semin Oncol* 29:119–125, 2002
124. Kemeny N, Daly J, Oderman P, et al: Hepatic artery pump infusion: toxicity and results in patients with metastatic colorectal carcinoma. *J Clin Oncol* 2:595–600, 1984
125. Lorenz M, Müller HH: Randomized, multicenter trial of fluorouracil plus leucovorin administered either via hepatic arterial or intravenous infusion versus fluorodeoxyuridine administered via hepatic arterial infusion in patients with nonresectable liver metastases from colorectal carcinoma. *J Clin Oncol* 18:243–254, 2000
126. Kemeny MM, Goldberg DA, Browning S, et al: Experience with continuous regional chemotherapy and hepatic resection as treatment of hepatic metastases. *Cancer* 55:1265–1270, 1985
127. Kemeny MM, Hogan JM, Goldberg DA, et al: Continuous hepatic artery infusion with an implantable pump: problems with hepatic artery anomalies. *Surgery* 99:501–504, 1986
128. Kemeny MM, Baltifora H, Douglas W, et al: Sclerosing cholangitis after continuous hepatic artery infusion of FUDR. *Ann Surg* 202:176–181, 1985
129. Kemeny N, Seiter K, Conti JA, et al: Hepatic arterial floxuridine and leucovorin for unresectable liver metastases from colorectal carcinoma. *Cancer* 73:1132–1142, 1994
130. Elias D, Lasser P, Rougier P, et al: Frequency, technical aspects, results and indications of major hepatectomy after prolonged intra-arterial hepatic chemotherapy for initially unresectable tumors. *J Am Coll Surg* 180:213–219, 1995
131. Cohen AD, Kemeny NE: An update on hepatic arterial infusion chemotherapy for colorectal cancer. *Oncologist* 8:553–566, 2003
132. Kemeny N, Huang Y, Cohen A: Hepatic arterial infusion of chemotherapy after resection of hepatic metastases from colorectal cancer. *N Engl J Med* 341:2039–2048, 1999
133. Yamaguchi A, Taniguchi H, Kunishima S, et al: Correlation between angiographically assessed vascularity and blood flow in hepatic metastases in patients with colorectal cancer. *Cancer* 89:1236–1244, 2000
134. Shankar A, Loizidou M, Taylor I: The vascularity of colorectal liver metastases. *Eur J Surg Oncol* 22:389–396, 1996
135. Perry LJ, Stuart KE: Hepatic chemoembolization, in Saini S, Gazelle GS, Mueller PR (eds.): *Hepatobiliary and Pancreatic Radiology*. New York, Thieme, 1998, pp 448–469
136. Stuart K: Chemoembolization in the management of liver tumors. *Oncologist* 8:425–437, 2003
137. Venook AP, Stagg RJ, Lewis JL, et al: Chemoembolization for hepatocellular carcinoma. *J Clin Oncol* 8:1108-1114, 1990
138. Konno T: Targeting cancer chemotherapeutic agents by use of lipiodol contrast medium. *Cancer* 66:1897–1903, 1990
139. Castells A, Ayusu C, Bru C, et al: Transarterial embolization for hepatocellular carcinoma: antibiotic prophylaxis and clinical meaning of postembolization fever. *J Hepatol* 22:410–415, 1995
140. Venhook AP: Treatment of hepatocellular carcinoma: too many options? *J Clin Oncol* 12:1323–1334, 1994
141. Ernst O, Sergent G, Mizrahi D, et al: Treatment of hepatocellular carcinoma by transcatheter arterial chemoembolization: comparison of planned periodic chemoembolization and chemoembolization based on tumor response. *Am J Roentgenol* 172:59–64, 1999
142. Llovet JM, Real MI, Montana X, et al: Arterial embolisation or chemoembolisation versus symptomatic treatment in patients with unresectable hepatocellular carcinoma: a randomised controlled trial. *Lancet* 359:1734–1739, 2002
143. Vetter D, Wenger JJ, Bergier JM, et al: Transcatheter oil chemoembolization in management of advanced hepatocellular carcinoma in cirrhosis: results of a Western comparative study in 60 patients. *Hepatology* 13:427–433, 1990
144. Llovet JM, Bustanmante J, Castells A, et al: Natural history of untreated hepatocellular carcinoma: rationale for the design and evaluation of therapeutic trials. *Hepatology* 29:62–67, 1999
145. Livraghi T, Benedini V, Lazzaroni S: Long term results of single session percutaneous ethanol injection in patients with large hepatocellular carcinoma. *Cancer* 83:48–57, 1998
146. Livraghi T, Giorgio A, Marin G, et al: Hepatocellular carcinoma and cirrhosis in 746 patients: long-term results of percutaneous ethanol injection. *Radiology* 197:101–108, 1995
147. Livraghi T, Bolondi L, Lazzaroni S, et al: Percutaneous ethanol injection in the treatment of hepatocellular carcinoma in cirrhosis. A study of 207 patients. *Cancer* 69:925–929, 1992
148. Livarghi T, Bolondi L, Buscarini L, et al: No treatment, resection, and ethanol injection in hepatocellular carcinoma: a retrospective analysis of survival in 391 patients with cirrhosis. Italian Cooperative HCC Study Group. *J Hepatol* 22:522–526, 1995
149. Hasegawa S, Yamaski N, Hiwaki T, et al: Factors that predict intrahepatic recurrence of hepatocellular carcinoma in 81 patients initially treated by percutaneous ethanol injection. *Cancer* 86:1682–1690, 1999
150. Khan KN, Yatsuhashi H, Yamasaki K, et al: Prospective analysis of risk factors for early intrahepatic recurrence of hepatocellular carcinoma following ethanol injection. *J Hepatol* 32:269–278, 2000
151. Kurokohchi K, Masaki T, Miyauchi, et al: Percutaneous ethanol and lipiodol injection therapy for hepatocellullar carcinoma. *Int J Oncol* 24:381–387, 2004
152. Ravikumar TS, Steele GD: Hepatic cryosurgery. *Surg Clin North Am* 69:433–440, 1989

153. Zhou XD, Tang ZY, Yu YQ, et al: Clinical evaluation of cryosurgery in the treatment of primary liver cancer. Report of 60 cases. *Cancer* 61:1889-1892, 1988
154. Onik GM, Atkinson D, Zemel R, et al: Cryosurgery of liver cancer. *Semin Surg Oncol* 9:309–317, 1993
155. Onik G, Rubinsky B, Zemel R, et al: Ultrasound-guided hepatic cryosurgery in the treatment of metastatic colon carcinoma. *Cancer* 67:901–907, 1991
156. McKinnon JG, Temple WJ, Wiseman DA, et al: Cryosurgery for malignant tumours of the liver. *Can J Surg* 39:401–406, 1996
157. Morris DL, Ross WB: Australian experience of cryoablation of liver tumors: metastases. *Surg Oncol Clin North Am* 5:391–397, 1996
158. Weaver ML, Atkinson D, Zemel R: Hepatic cryosurgery in treating colorectal metastases. *Cancer* 76:210–214, 1995
159. Ross WB, Horton M, Bertolino P, et al: Cryotherapy of liver tumours — a practical guide. *HPB Surg* 8:167–173, 1995
160. Barnett CC, Curley SA: Ablative techniques for hepatocellular carcinoma. *Semin Oncol* 28:487–496, 2001
161. McGahan JP, Dodd GD III: Radiofrequency ablation of the liver. *AJR Am J Roentgenol* 176:3–16, 2001
162. Curley SA: Radiofrequency ablation of malignant liver tumors. *Oncologist* 6:14–23, 2001
163. Aguayo A, Patt YZ: Nonsurgical treatment of hepatocellular carcinoma. *Semin Oncol* 28:503–513, 2001
164. Ho S, Lau JW, Leung TW: Intrahepatic (90)Y-microspheres for hepatocellular carcinoma. *J Nucl Med* 42:1587–1589, 2001
165. Lau W, Ho S, Leung T, et al: What determines survival duration in hepatocellular carcinoma treated with intraarterial yttrium-90 microspheres. *Hepatogastroenterology* 48:338–340, 2001
166. Soini Y, Virkajarvi N, Raunio H, et al: Expression of P-glycoprotein in hepatocellular carcinoma: a potential marker of prognosis. *J Clin Pathol* 49:470–473, 1996
167. Huang CC, Wu MC, Xu GW, et al: Overexpression of the NDR1 gene and P-glycoprotein in human hepatocellular carcinoma. *J Natl Cancer Inst* 84:262, 1992
168. Caruso ML, Valentini AM: Overexpression of p53 in a large series of patients with hepatocellular carcinoma: a clinicopathological correlation. *Anticancer Res* 19:3853–3856, 1999
169. Nagahama H, Okada S, Okusaka T, et al: Predictive factors for tumor response to systemic chemotherapy in patients with hepatocellular carcinoma. *Jpn J Clin Oncol* 27:321–324, 1997
170. Plweny CL, Toya T, Katongole-Mbidde E, et al: Treatment of hepatocellular carcinoma with adriamycin. Preliminary communication. *Cancer* 36:1250–1257, 1975
171. Chelbowski RT, Brzechwa-Adjukiewicz A, Cowden A, et al: Doxorubicin (75 mg/m^2) for hepatocellullar carcinoma: clinical and pharmacokinetic results. *Cancer Treat Rep* 68:487–491, 1984
172. Ihde DC, Kane RC, Cohen MH, et al: Adriamycin therapy in American patients with hepatocellular carcinoma. *Cancer Treat Rep* 61:1385-1387, 1977
173. Nerenstone SR, Ihde DC, Friedman MA: Clinical trials in primary hepatocellular carcinoma: current status and future directions. *Cancer Treat Rev* 15:1-31, 1988
174. Lai CL, WU PC, Chan GC, et al: Doxorubicin versus no antitumor therapy in inoperable hepatocellular carcinoma. A prospective randomized trial. *Cancer* 62:479–483, 1988
175. Lozano RD, Patt YZ, Hassan MM, et al: Oral capecitabine for the treatment of hepatobiliary cancers. *Proc Am Soc Clin Oncol* 19:264a, 2000 (abstr)
176. Patt YZ, Hassan MM, Lozano RD, et al: Phase II trial of thalidomide for treatment of non-resectable hepatocellular carcinoma. *Proc Am Soc Clin Oncol* 19:266a, 2000 (abstr)
177. Porta C, Moroni M, Nastasi G, et al: 5-Fluorouracil and d,1-leucovorin calcium are active to treat unresectable hepatocellular carcinoma patients: preliminary results of a phase II study. *Oncology* 52:487–491, 1995
178. Yang TS, Wang CH, Hsieh RK, et al: Gemcitabine and doxorubicin for the treatment of patients with advanced hepatocellular carcinoma: a phase I–II trial. *Ann Oncol* 13:1771–1778, 2002
179. Okada S, Okusaka T, Ueno H, et al: Phase II trial of cisplatin, mitoxantrone, and continuous infusion 5-fluorouracil (5-FU) (FMP therapy) for hepatocellular carcinoma (HCC). *Proc Am Soc Clin Oncol* 18:248a, 1999 (abstr)
180. Ellis PA, Norman A, Hill A, et al: Epirubicin, cisplatin and infusional 5-fluorouracil (5-FU) (ECF) in hepatobiliary tumors. *Eur J Cancer* 31A:1594–1598, 1995
181. Rai K, Tsuji A, Morita S, et al: Continuous infusion of 5-FU and low-dose consecutive CDDP therapy in advanced hepatocellular carcinoma: a phase II study. *Proc Am Soc Clin Oncol* 21:164a, 2002 (abstr)
182. Yang TS, Chang WC, Lin YC, et al: A phase II study of gemcitabine and cisplatin for patients with advanced hepatocellular carcinoma. *Proc Am Soc Clin Oncol* 22:336a, 2002 (abstract)
183. Boucher E, Corbinais S, Brissot P, et al: Treatment of hepatocellular carcinoma (HCC) with systemic chemotherapy combining epirubicin, cisplatinum and infusional 5-fluorouracil (ECF regimen). *Cancer Chemother Pharmacol* 50:305–308, 2002
184. Llovet JM, Sala M, Castellas L, et al: Randomized controlled trial of interferon treatment for advanced hepatocellular carcinoma. *Hepatology* 31:54–58, 2000
185. Chung YH, Song IH, Song BC, et al: Combined chemotherapy consisting of intraarterial cisplatin infusion and systemic interferon-alpha for hepatocellular carcinoma patients with major portal vein thrombosis or distant metastasis. *Cancer* 88:1986–1991, 2000
186. Leung TW, Tang AM, Zee B, et al: Factors predicting response and survival in 149 patients with unresectable hepatocellular carcinoma treated by combination cisplatin, interferon-alpha, doxorubicin and 5-fluorouracil chemotherapy. *Cancer* 94:421–427, 2002
187. Qian C, Drozdzik M, Caselmann WH, et al: The potential of gene therapy in the treatment of hepatocellular carcinoma — review. *J Hepatol* 32:344–351, 2000
188. Sangiro B, Qian C, Schmitz V, et al: Gene therapy of hepatocellular carcinoma and gastrointestinal tumors. *Ann NY Acad Sci* 963:6–12, 2002
189. Levy M: Pharmacology treatment of cancer pain. *N Engl J Med* 335:1124–1132, 1996
190. Loprinzi C: Anorexia and cachexia, in Loprinzi C (ed.): *Cancer Management: A Multidisciplinary Approach* (ed 6). Melville, NY, Publishers Research and Representation, 2002, pp 831–834
191. Inui A: Cancer anorexia–cachexia syndrome: current issues in research and management. *CA Cancer J Clin* 52:72–91, 2002
192. Gagnon B, Breura E: A review of the drug treatment associated with cancer. *Drugs* 55:675–688, 1998

CHAPTER 57

Lung Cancer

Carol S. Knop, RN, AOCN®

Introduction

Lung cancer remains the leading cause of cancer-related death in both men and women. It is one of the few diseases in which a carcinogen has been directly linked to the development of cancer. Smoking avoidance could nearly completely eliminate this disease. Tobacco prevention education needs to begin as early as the elementary school years. Recent advances in technology have allowed earlier diagnosis of lung cancer, but its effect on overall survival is yet to be determined. Advances in surgery, radiation therapy, and chemotherapy have provided better response rates but not significantly affected overall survival.

Molecular targets on lung cancer cells are rapidly being discovered, and promising new targeted therapy agents are in various stages of development and testing for both treatment and chemoprevention of lung cancer. It is the molecular biology of this deadly disease that will ultimately lead to the discovery of therapy that will affect both response and survival.

Epidemiology

Lung cancer was a rare disease until about 1930, when a sharp rise in incidence in men occurred, making lung cancer the leading cause of cancer death among men by the mid-twentieth century. In women, a corresponding rise in lung cancer rates has occurred from the 1960s to the present.[1] The increase in incidence followed the introduction of manufactured cigarettes with addictive properties in the beginning of the twentieth century.[1] In 2004, an estimated 173,770 new cases of lung cancer were expected to be diagnosed: 93,110 men and 80,660 women, accounting for 13% of all cancer diagnoses.[2] Lung cancer is the second most commonly occurring cancer in both men and women.[3] More than 50% of all new lung cancer cases will involve ex-smokers.[4] Lung cancer rates have been declining in men since 1984, but are still increasing in women, albeit at a slower rate of increase than in recent years.[2,3] The frequency in African American males is about 50% higher than that in white males in the United States.[1] Peak incidence for both males and females is in the age range of 60–79, when the disease affects 1 in 17 males and 1 in 25 females.[3] Over time, increased incidence rates have reflected increased smoking rates, with a lag time of less than 2 years and up to 20 years between smoking incidence and development of cancer.[1]

Lung cancer remains the leading cause of cancer death in both men and women in the United States and worldwide. It surpassed breast cancer as the leading cause of cancer death in women in 1987.[3] In 2004, an estimated 160,440 lung cancer deaths were expected to account for 28% of all cancer deaths: 91,930 men and 68,510 women.[2] Death rates have declined by 1.8% per year in men since 1991, but death rates in both white and African American females have continued to increase, albeit at a slower rate since the early 1990s.[3] A recent study investigated death rates among people aged 30–39 and found a decrease over two time intervals (1990–1994 and 1995–1999) in states that have put tobacco control measures in place.[5] Table 57-1 shows the dismal five-year survival rates by gender and stage of disease at presentation; these rates have not shown any substantial change in the last 30 years.[6]

Table 57-1 Five-year Relative Survival Rates by Stage of Disease from SEER Program Data, 1990–1999

	Male	Female
All stages	13%	17%
Stage I	53%	60%
Stage II	31%	33%
Stage III	9%	10%
Stage IV	2%	2%
Unknown stage	13%	19%

Data from Gloeckler, Reichman, Lewis, et al.[7]

Etiology

Tobacco

An estimated 46.2 million adults in the United States were current smokers in 2001, or 22.8% of the population. By gender, 25.2% of men and 20.7% of women were smokers. Among high school students in the same year, 22% smoked a whole cigarette before the age of 13 and 64% had tried cigarette smoking. Among middle school students, 8% had smoked a whole cigarette by the age of 11, with 36% having tried cigarette smoking. In total, 15% of middle schoolers reported using some form of tobacco, including cigarettes, cigars, smokeless tobacco, tobacco in pipes, bidis, or kreteks.[3] Peak prevalence for smoking occurred in 1955 at 55% for men and in 1966 at 35% for women.[8]

The association of smoking with the development of lung cancer is one of the strongest and most thoroughly documented causal relationships in biomedical research.[1] In a study of 70 nations, tobacco use was ranked as the fourth most *preventable* health risk, behind malnutrition, unsafe sex, and high blood pressure;[9] it is now the leading cause of preventable disease and death in women.[10] Some 85%–90% of all lung cancers can be linked directly to tobacco exposure.[6] Smokers have a 20-fold increased risk of developing lung cancer than never-smokers.[1] The risk for the development of lung cancer increases with younger age at initiation of smoking, greater number of years of smoking, and greater number of cigarettes smoked per day. Age at initiation and number of years of smoking are more important risk factors than the number of cigarettes smoked per day.[4] Other factors contributing to a higher risk include use of nonfiltered cigarettes and deep inhalation.[1] Women smoking the same amount as men have a two times higher risk of developing lung cancer.[10] Smokers who choose products advertised as having lower tar and nicotine levels tend to smoke more cigarettes and inhale more deeply, thereby negating any beneficial features of these products.[1] Smokers who do not inhale more deeply or who smoke an increased number of low tar or low nicotine cigarettes experience a lung cancer mortality that is approximately 80% the mortality rate for those who do inhale deeply and increase the number of cigarettes smoked.[1] Since 1993, cigar smoking has increased in popularity, especially among young adult men. Along with this increased popularity has come a relative risk of dying from lung cancer of 5.1 compared to never-smokers.[11]

The scientific basis for the relationship between smoking and lung cancer is still being elucidated. Approximately 3500 different chemical substances contain at least 20 proven pulmonary carcinogens. These include three major groups of chemical compounds: polycyclic aromatic hydrocarbons [e.g., benzo (a)pyrene], aromatic amines, and N-nitrosamines [e.g., 4-(methylnitrosamino)-1- (3-pyridyl)-1-butanone (NNK)].[6] Tar is the condensable residue of cigarette smoke; this complex mixture includes many chemicals that are initiators and/or promoters in the development of lung cancer. Therefore, tobacco is a complete carcinogen.[1]

West and colleagues[12] showed activation of serine/threonine kinase Akt (protein kinase B) by two components of cigarette smoke: nicotine and the tobacco-specific carcinogen 4-(methylnitrosamino)-1-(3-pyridyl)-1-butanone (NNK). Akt controls cellular processes such as glucose metabolism, cell-cycle progression, and apoptosis; it is found within the airway epithelial cells as well as in lung tumors of smokers. Activation of Akt by nicotine or NNK contributes to tumorigenesis by inhibiting apoptosis in normal airway epithelial cells and by decreasing contact inhibition, dependence on exogenous growth factors, and adherence to the extracellular matrix.[12] Nicotine can also stimulate endothelial cell growth and angiogenesis.[13] In addition, etoposide-induced apoptosis is decreased by 61% in the presence of nicotine in vitro.[12] The tumor suppressor gene *p53* has been implicated in the development of lung cancer as well. It normally functions to provide cell-cycle control, DNA synthesis and repair, cell differentiation, gene transcription, and apoptosis. Carcinogens in tobacco smoke are associated with mutations in the *p53* gene. Tumors in women exhibit more tobacco-related mutations than those in men.[14]

Cannabis

No strong epidemiologic or research evidence indicates that cannabis smoking causes lung cancer. Nevertheless, strong qualitative similarities exist between the carcinogens found in cannabis and those found in tobacco smoke. Cannabis contains cannabinoids instead of tobacco, but otherwise proffers many of the same carcinogens and mutagens as tobacco. Histopathologic examination of bronchial mucosa in cannabis smokers demonstrates changes typically seen preceding carcinoma development in tobacco smokers. Case-controlled studies would now be very timely, as the cannabis users of the "baby boomer" generation are now approaching their sixties, the peak age for the diagnosis of lung cancer.[15]

Environmental Tobacco Smoke

Environmental tobacco smoke (ETS) is a complex mixture of smoke that was classified as a known human (class A) carcinogen in 1992 by the U.S. Environmental Protection Agency (EPA).[1] Exposure to ETS accounts for approximately 3000 deaths annually in the United States.[1,16] In one recent study, 82% of never-smokers who presented with lung cancer had exposure to ETS. In addition, never-smokers had a higher exposure than smokers to ETS in childhood.[16] In another study, urinary metabolites of NNK were measured in nonsmoking women who were married to smoking men. These levels were found to be statistically significantly higher in exposed women than in nonexposed women.[17]

Radon

Radon was classified as a human carcinogen by the EPA, World Health Organization (WHO), and U.S. Department of Health and Human Services in 2000.[18] This colorless, odorless, radioactive gas is produced as a result of uranium and radium decay. Exposure to radon can occur in homes where there is minimal indoor air turnover and ventilation. Radon enters the home through the lower levels of the dwelling via cracks in the foundation; sump pits; gaps in suspended floors, around service pipes, and inside walls; and crawl spaces.[18] It is also an occupational hazard for individuals who work in underground mines.[19] When radon progeny become attached to airborne particles and are inhaled, the alpha particles they emit lodge in the bronchioles, where they continually emit ionizing radiation to the surrounding epithelial tissue, thereby increasing the risk for lung cancer.[18,19] Tobacco and radon act synergistically in the development of lung cancer.[20] Data from the National Research Council's report on the Sixth Committee on Biological Effects of Ionizing Radiation in 1998 suggested that indoor radon exposure is the second leading cause of lung cancer (after cigarette smoking), accounting for 10% of cases and 3000–32,000 deaths per year in the United States.[1,18] Radon detection and mitigation strategies are modes of primary prevention that nurses can easily initiate in the community.[18]

Asbestos

Epidemiologic evidence of asbestos's role as a carcinogen dates back to the 1950s, before regulations to limit asbestos dust in factories were implemented. Reports of an association between asbestos and lung cancer date back to the 1800s. Asbestos itself may be the carcinogen or it may cause cancer through an indirect mechanism of chronic inflammation. Asbestos and cigarette smoking act synergistically in the development of lung cancer, potentially by enhancing the retention of the asbestos fibers within the airways.[1] Asbestos is most closely associated with the development of pulmonary mesothelioma.

Occupational Agents

Occupational exposures to carcinogens account for 9%–15% of lung cancer cases.[1] Occupations with a known risk of lung cancer include uranium mining (source of radon) and quarrying; chemical exposures and chemical processes; asbestos production (insulators, textile, cement products); refineries, foundations, and activities that entail handling metals [chromium, nickel, copper (arsenic), and cadmium]; construction; painting [*bis*(chlormethyl)ether, BCME]; shipbuilding and motor vehicle manufacturing; wood-related activities; rubber industry; ceramic and brick industry; and exposure to diesel exhaust (taxi and bus drivers). The risk for the development of lung cancer sharply increases when exposure in these occupations is combined with smoking.[6,20]

Indoor Pollution

Indoor air pollution includes tobacco smoke, building materials, radon, household products, and combustion from heating and cooking. In developed countries, radon and ETS are of the greatest concern; in developing countries, the use of unprocessed solid fuels, especially coal, for cooking and space heating are of higher concern.[1]

Genetic Susceptibility

Because only 15% of heavy smokers develop lung cancer, genetic polymorphisms that cause carcinogens to accumulate to a greater or lesser degree in any individual are highly suspect in contributing to the development of lung cancer.[6] The genes most associated with lung cancer are *CYP1A1, CYP2D6,* and *GSTM1.* Family history of lung cancer has also been associated with an increased risk. The risk of developing this disease is higher in people younger than age 59 with a history of lung cancer among their first-degree blood relatives. First-degree blood relatives of any cancer sufferer have a 2.4-fold increased risk of developing lung cancer. Lung cancer is also more common in those families with a history of breast or ovarian cancer.[6]

Dietary Factors

Retinoid (β-carotene) and vitamin E (α-tocopherol) supplementation were associated with an increased risk for the development of lung cancer in heavy smokers in three chemoprevention trials that were completed between 1994 and 1996: the α-Tocopherol β-Carotene Cancer Prevention Study (ATBC), the Carotene and Retinal Efficacy Trial (CARET), and the Physicians' Health Study.[1,4] The overall conclusion from these and other studies was that heavy smokers should eat a balanced diet rich in fruits and vegetables while avoiding high-dose beta-carotene supplementation.[21]

Other Risk Factors

Alkylating agents and radiation therapy for Hodgkin's disease lead to a higher risk of lung cancer in a dose-dependent fashion: the higher the dose of either therapy, the higher the risk of lung cancer. In studies of this relationship, tobacco use increased risk by 20 times; risks from treatment were multiplied by smoking.[22] Preexisting pulmonary disease such as tuberculosis (TB), chronic obstructive pulmonary disease (COPD; 8.8% of patients with COPD develop lung cancer within 10 years), and silicosis increases the risk of lung cancer.[6] Patients with COPD have inflamed lung mucosa, and the most important cause of this inflammation is cigarette smoking. NNK, a tobacco-specific carcinogen, is a beta-adrenergic receptor agonist that releases arachidonate, up-regulates COX-2 expression, and stimulates proliferation in lung adenocarcinoma cell lines in vitro. Nicotine induces angiogenesis and reduces cell-mediated immune responses, which could facilitate the survival and proliferation of mutated cells transformed by carcinogens such as NNK. Nicotine also may induce COX-2 expression.[23]

Prevention

Smoking Prevention and Cessation

The benefits of smoking cessation were outlined in 1990 by the U.S. Surgeon General: People who quit smoking live longer than those who continue to smoke, and smokers who quit before age 50 cut their risk of dying in the next 15 years in half compared to those who continue to smoke.[3] With smoking cessation, the risk of lung cancer decreases over time. The amount of time it takes to reach the risk of a never-smoker depends on the number of years of smoking cessation as well as the number of cigarettes smoked per day. The more cigarettes smoked per day, the longer it takes to reach a level of risk close to that of a never-smoker. Ex-smokers never reach the same low level of risk as a nonsmoker.[1,8] At each encounter with a healthcare provider, all smokers should be encouraged to quit smoking.[24] Guidelines are available for healthcare providers through the U.S. Department of Health and Human Services and can be ordered on the Agency for Healthcare Research and Quality National Guideline Clearinghouse Web site, *www.guidelines.gov.* Strategies available to assist with cessation include nicotine replacement therapies, drug therapy such as bupropion (see Table 57-2), and psychosocial therapies that include social support in a group setting.[8,25–28] A combination of strategies with the inclusion of psychosocial support has proven to be the most successful approach.

Efforts at tobacco control should have stemmed from the 1998 Master Settlement Agreement with the tobacco industry. This agreement prohibited tobacco advertising aimed at youth younger than age 18 and provided $28.35 per capita to the average state.[29,30] In reality, the average state dedicated only $3.49 per capita toward tobacco control programs, and in the year after the settlement, the tobacco industry spent $8.24 billion on marketing, a 24% increase in marketing expenditures compared to pre-settlement levels and the highest spending ever reported.[30,31]

An example of a successful state initiative is California's Tobacco Control Program, which was established in 1989. Successes to date include a decrease in adult smoking prevalence from 11% lower than the rest of the nation in 1988 to 20% lower in 1996; a decrease in per capita cigarette consumption by more than 50%; a higher rate of decline in California's lung cancer incidence than for the rest of the nation; and significant declines in youth smoking rates. The strategy to "denormalize" tobacco was implemented by countering pro-tobacco influences, reducing exposure to ETS, reducing access to tobacco products, and promoting cessation through a toll-free quit-line number.[32]

Table 57-2 Pharmacologic Smoking Cessation Interventions

Pharmacologic Intervention	Estimated OR (95% CI)	Estimated Abstinence Rate (95% CI)	Dose	Duration	Adverse Effects/Contraindications
Bupropion	2.1 (1.5–3.0)	30.5 (23.2–37.8) Placebo = 17.3	150 mg every morning for 3 d. then 150 mg bid (begin treatment 1–2 weeks pre-quit)	7–12 weeks, maintenance up to 6 months	Insomnia, dry mouth. Caution: history of seizures, eating disorders
Nicotine gum	1.5 (1.3–1.8)	23.7 (20.6–26.7) Placebo = 17.1	1–24 cigarettes/d: 2 mg gum (up to 24 pieces); > 25 cigarettes/d: 4 mg gum (up to 24 pieces)	Up to 12 weeks	Mouth soreness, dyspepsia
Nicotine inhaler	2.5 (1.7–3.6)	22.8 (16.4–29.2) Placebo = 10.5	6–16 cartridges/d	Up to 6 months	Local irritation of mouth and throat
Nicotine nasal spray	2.7 (1.8–4.1)	30.5 (21.8–39.2) Placebo = 13.9	8–40 doses/d	3–6 months	Nasal irritation
Nicotine patch	1.9 (1.7–2.2)	17.7 (16.0–19.5) Placebo = 10.0	1–25 cigarettes/d 21 mg/24 h 14 mg/24 h 7 mg/24 h > 25 cigarettes/d can start with 21–42 mg/24 h	 4 weeks 2 weeks 2 weeks	Local skin irritation, insomnia
Clonidine	2.1 (1.4–3.2)	25.6 (17.7–33.6) Placebo = 13.9	0.15–0.75 mg/d	3–10 weeks	Dry mouth dizziness, sedation. Caution: Rebound hypertension
Nortriptyline	3.2 (1.8–5.7)	30.1 (18.1–1.6) Placebo = 11.7	75–100 mg/d	12 weeks	Sedation, dry mouth. Caution: Risk of arrhythmias

OR, odds ratio; CI, confidence internal; bid, twice daily.
Data from Ahuja, Weibel, Leone.[8]

The American Society of Clinical Oncology published an updated policy statement on tobacco control in July 2003. Its recommendations to reduce tobacco use are:

- Restrict access by children and teenagers
- Increase tobacco excise taxes
- Allocate state tobacco settlement funds for tobacco prevention and cessation
- Restrict advertising and promotion
- Require disclosure of ingredients
- Enhance public education
- Create more effective tobacco cessation services
- Target use of noncigarette tobacco products
- Eliminate public exposure to secondhand smoke
- Assist tobacco farmers through government aid for loss of income related to tobacco
- Enhance research efforts
- Enhance global tobacco control
- Take responsibility as healthcare professionals[33]

All oncology practitioners are charged with contributing to this effort, with the goal of ultimately eliminating 90% of lung cancer cases in men and 79% of lung cancer cases in women.[8]

Chemoprevention

Primary chemoprevention

Chemoprevention is defined as the use of natural or chemically synthesized compounds to prevent, inhibit, or reverse the process of carcinogenesis.[4] The principles of chemoprevention in lung cancer are built on two concepts: field cancerization, characterized by diffuse injury of the epithelial surface from

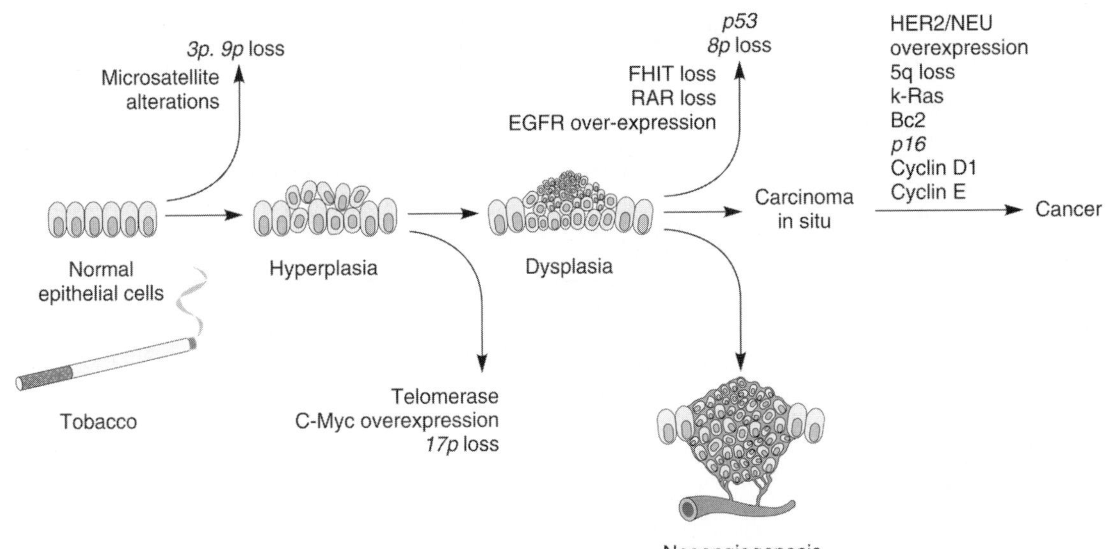

Figure 57-1 The multistep carcinogenesis model for development of lung cancer. (Reprinted from Soria, Kim, Fayette, et al.[35])

long-term carcinogenic exposure, and multistep carcinogenesis.[4] Primary chemoprevention is prevention in healthy high-risk smokers. Phase III trials with retinoids and α-tocopherol (vitamin E) have demonstrated negative results, as mentioned previously. However, high blood levels of vitamin E in younger men with fewer years of smoking were associated with a lower lung cancer incidence. This finding suggests that if high serum levels of α-tocopherol are present during the early stages of carcinogenesis, the development of lung cancer may be inhibited.[4]

The New York University Women's Health Study analyzed data in a case-control study of lung cancer nested within the larger study. The researchers looked at the risk of lung cancer in women who regularly take aspirin. The results suggested that women who use aspirin three or more times weekly have a decreased risk of developing lung cancer, with an adjusted odds ratio of 0.66, and an even lower risk of developing non-small cell lung cancer, with an adjusted odds ratio of 0.39.[34] Currently, studies are investigating the ability of nonsteroidal anti-inflammatory drugs (NSAIDs), such as celecoxib, to prevent the development of lung cancer in high-risk smokers. The rationale: increased amounts of COX-2 have been found in both premalignant and malignant tumors of the lung; genetic and pharmacologic studies have shown a mechanistic link between COX-2 and the development of cancer; NNK and possibly nicotine up-regulate COX-2 expression and stimulate proliferation in lung adenocarcinoma cell lines; and COX-2 appears to inhibit apoptosis and enhance angiogenesis.[4,23]

Secondary chemoprevention

Secondary chemoprevention aims to prevent the development of cancer in people with precancerous lesions. As noted earlier, the carcinogenesis of lung cancer is a multistep process through which a series of molecular changes accumulate and progress to preinvasive and invasive disease. It has been suggested that 10–20 or more genetic events must take place for lung cancer to develop (Figures 57–1 and 57–2).[35]

Along the carcinogenic pathway, there are multiple targets for inhibiting this progression. Four Phase IIb trials have evaluated the ability of α-tocopherol, β-carotene, retinol, retinyl palmitate, or isotretinoin to reverse changes in smokers with metaplasia or sputum atypia. Only smoking cessation was correlated with a significant reduction in metaplasia and cell proliferation; isotretinoin plus smoking cessation further reduced metaplasia.[4] In a randomized phase IIb study, 112 current or former smokers with bronchial dysplasia were randomized to receive 25 mg of anethole dithiolethione (ADT), an organosulfur compound found in many vegetables, or placebo for 3 months. Although no response difference was observed between the two groups, the progression rate in the ADT group was significantly lower than that in the placebo group. This suggests that ADT may be a potentially effective chemopreventive agent in smokers.[4,35]

Loss of expression of the retinoic acid receptor beta (RAR-β) in the bronchial epithelium is considered a biomarker of preneoplasia. Retinoids can restore expression of this receptor. A study was done to evaluate whether either of two retinoid-based regi-

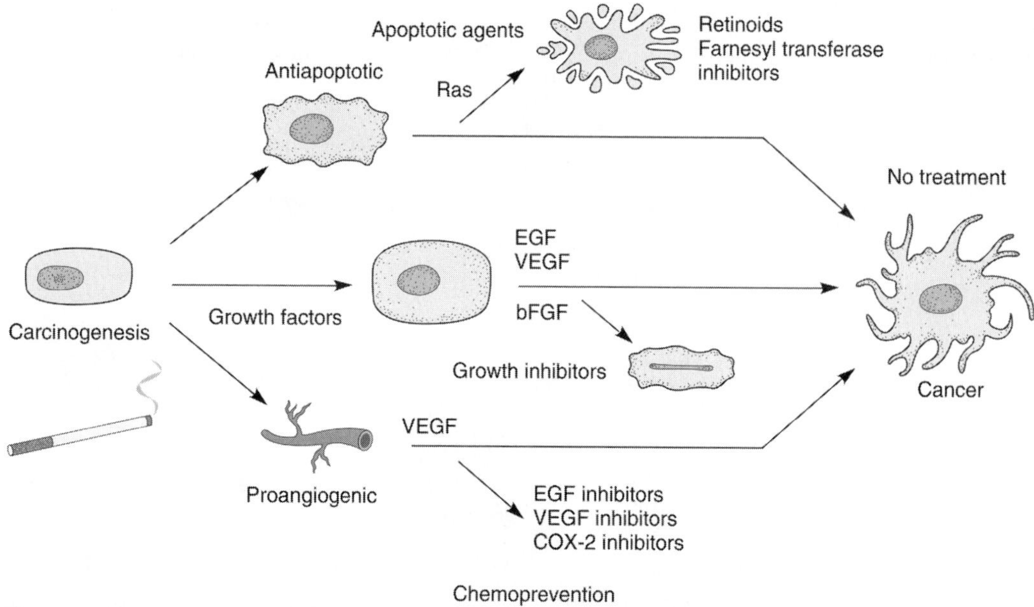

Figure 57-2 Detouring carcinogenesis. (Reprinted from Soria, Kim, Fayette, et al.[35])

mens, 9-*cis*-retinoic acid (RA) or 13-*cis*-RA plus α-tocopherol could reverse RAR-β expression loss in former smokers after 3 months of treatment. The group who received 9-*cis*-RA experienced restoration of RAR-β expression and reduction of metaplasia, implying that this compound might have chemopreventive effects.[36] Trials targeting intermediate biological markers aimed at reversing damage are the current focus of research in secondary chemoprevention of lung cancer.[4,35]

Tertiary chemoprevention

Tertiary chemoprevention targets individuals who have previously had lung cancer with the goal of preventing recurrence or the development of a second primary tumor. Because of the multistep nature of carcinogenesis and the field cancerization concept, patients who have been successfully treated for lung cancer are at risk for developing second primary tumors at the rate of 2%–4% per year.[35] A large phase III study of 1166 patients with pathologic stage I non-small cell lung cancer that randomized patients to receive isotretinoin (13-*cis*-RA) or placebo for 3 years found no significant differences between the two arms related to overall rates of second primary tumors, recurrences, or mortality. Secondary multivariate and subset analyses revealed that isotretinoin was harmful in current smokers and beneficial in never-smokers.[37]

New classes of chemopreventive agents are on the horizon. These therapies take advantage of the unfolding molecular biology of lung cancer and use the identified targeted pathways to inhibit the development of lung cancer. Table 57-3 lists oncogenes and tumor suppressor genes implicated in the development of lung cancer as well as substances that may potentially be candidates for chemoprevention. The erbB family of receptors is important in the proliferation of epithelial cancers.[4,38] Preneoplastic bronchial lesions have demonstrated expression of epidermal growth factor receptor (EGFR), thus making that receptor a target for an EGFR inhibitor in both the chemoprevention and the treatment arenas. NNK also increases EGFR expression.[39] A clinical trial investigating the use of gefitinib (Iressa) in the adjuvant setting to prevent the development of second primary tumors and recurrence for early-stage lung cancer is under way.[40] New data suggest that a combination strategy of EGFR inhibition and RAR modulation might potentially be more successful as a cancer prevention strategy.[41] A dual inhibitor that takes advantage of the heterodimerization of the erbB receptors is in development. These oral agents are both convenient and well tolerated.[4] Currently, an intergroup clinical trial (ECOG-E5597) is evaluating the effectiveness of selenium in preventing second primary lung tumors. Selenium has been shown to have anticarcinogenic properties and to play a role in cellular defense against oxidative stress.[4]

Screening and Early Detection

Although lung cancer is the second most common type of cancer and the leading cause of cancer death in both men and women, currently there are no stan-

Table 57-3 Genes Implicated in the Development of Lung Cancer

	Oncogenes	Tumor Suppressor Genes	Potential Chemopreventive Agents
Non-small cell lung cancer	*ras*	*p53*	EGFR inhibitors
	c-myc	*RB*	COX-2 inhibitors
	EGFR	*p16*	Lipooxygenase inhibitors
	her2/neu	*9p*	Prostacyclin analogs
	Cyclins D1, E, B1	*8p*	Farnesyltransferase inhibitors
	raf	*3p*	*ras* inhibitors
	bcl1, bcl2	FHIT	Retinoids
	igf1	*p21*	Angiogenesis inhibitors
	Telomerase	*RASSF1*	Cell-cycle inhibitors
	c-met		Proteasome inhibitors
	pten		mTOR inhibitors
Small cell lung cancer	*c-myc*	*p53*	Protein kinase C inhibitors
	raf	*RB*	Demethylation agents
	myb	*p16*	DFMO combination
	EGFR	*9p*	Budenoside
	Telomerase	*8p*	
		3p	
		PTEN	
		RASSF1	

Data from Winterhalder, Hirsch, Kotantoulas, et al[4]; Soria, Kim, Fayette, et al[35]; Wistuba, Gazdar, Minna.[42]

dard screening guidelines for it. This lack of guidelines is due largely to earlier trials that failed to show survival advantages for screening using chest x-ray and/or sputum cytology. In the future, technological, pathological, and molecular biologic advances will almost certainly be instrumental in developing successful screening and early detection guidelines.

Sputum Cytology

Examination of sputum has been documented as far back as the 1930s. Papanicolaou applied his famed pelvic Pap test to diagnose lung cancer, and this application was later perfected by Saccomanno.[43] Sputum cytology has not become the standard for screening for lung cancer because of negative trials performed in the 1970s, which had unmistakable flaws in their research designs. Petty, a known advocate for screening sputum cytology examination for patients at high risk for the development of lung cancer, defines these patients as heavy smokers with spirometric evidence of air flow obstruction, personal or strong family history of lung cancer, or an occupational exposure risk such as asbestos.[43] Sputum is collected spontaneously or induced and then placed in Saccomanno's fixative. A specimen is considered representative if alveolar macrophages or bronchial epithelial cells are present, as their existence indicates that the cells come from deep within the lung. The chance of detecting abnormal cells increases for large, centrally located, squamous cell carcinomas and with an increased number of collected specimens.[44]

The rationale for the use of this tool relates directly to the multistep process involved in the carcinogenesis of lung cancer. At any step prior to the development of carcinoma in situ or invasive carcinoma, sputum cytology may be able to diagnose preinvasive changes. It is more sensitive in detecting squamous cell carcinomas, which tend to originate centrally in the bronchial tree, as opposed to adenocarcinomas, which typically originate in the periphery.[45] Early genetic and epigenetic analysis (related to loss of heterozygosity in the bronchial epithelium of smokers), detection of methylation of genes, nuclear image analysis, and the development of molecular markers (microsatellite alterations of DNA or promoter hypermethylation of tumor suppressor genes), and a search for autologous antibodies that recognize human lung cancer antigens all show potential in improving and refining diagnosis beyond the currently available techniques.[46] Once these techniques have been adequately tested, detection of lung cancer will improve.[44,47]

Chest X-ray

Chest x-ray is a primitive screening modality, usually detecting lung cancer at later, incurable stages.[48] Screening trials between 1960 and 1980 with or without sputum cytology included a trial in London, the Mayo Lung Project, the Czech Study on Lung Cancer, the Johns Hopkins Lung Project, and the Memorial Sloan-Kettering Lung Cancer Screening Program. None of these trials demonstrated a survival difference or mortality reduction, although updated reanalysis of the Mayo Lung Project has shown superior survival in the screened population.[49,50]

In modern trials, chest computed tomography (CT) is showing superiority over chest x-ray in the early detection of lung cancer. Chest x-ray continues to be used for surveillance and screening even without good evidence, because it is inexpensive, it is easy, and it exposes an individual to a low dose of radiation.

Low-Dose Spiral Chest CT

Spiral (or helical) high-resolution computed tomography (HRCT) was introduced in the early 1990s. These CT scanners can noninvasively obtain images of the chest in 5–10 seconds with only one breath-hold, which promotes patient comfort.[51] Studies from Japan and the United States have demonstrated a greater detection of lung nodules larger than 5 mm with spiral CT than with chest x-ray but have failed to show improvement in survival.[51–53] The Anti-Cancer Lung Association (ALCA) in Japan published the results of the first trial using low-dose CT (LDCT) screening. Out of 9993 CT scans on 1669 individuals, 22 of 24 peripheral cancers detected were stage IA. In the United States, the Early Lung Cancer Action Project (ELCAP) screened 1000 moderate- to high-risk patients, finding 27 cancers out of 233 CT-detected nodules; 85% were stage I.[49]

A limitation of LDCT is its inability to image clearly the tissues of the mediastinum, where lymph node disease may be detected.[54] If a nodule is demonstrated in the lung parenchyma, a complete clinical work-up would need to include a CT with contrast to adequately image the mediastinum, which increases radiation exposure and cost. Another limitation is inherent in the population screened. In these high-risk individuals, who include current and past smokers older than age 50, CT has a strong chance of detecting small nodules created by past infection or trauma. The challenge is to sort out which nodules require tissue evaluation and which should be reimaged and at what interval.[48] Morbidity and mortality are associated with the invasive work-up of these nodules.

In addition to nodular densities, HRCT detects infiltrative changes referred to as ground-glass opacities (ggo), which are now recognized as noninvasive precursor lesions for bronchioloalveolar carcinoma (BAC).[55] Recent clinical trial evidence has established that the ggo lesions of BAC are reversible with Iressa. This represents the first example of actual modulation of a preinvasive carcinogenesis paradigm (decreasing BAC) using a site-directed therapy (EGFR inhibition) resulting in a spatially defined change on a radiology-driven exam (HRCT).[56–58] Chemoprevention trials are currently testing this paradigm of combining RAR and EGFR modulation as a chemoprevention strategy.[41]

LDCT has been prematurely popularized because of the ready availability of the technology, the lower radiation dose delivered, the superiority of images over chest x-ray, and the promising results of phase II trials. The lack of randomized phase III clinical trials has prevented a firm recommendation for its routine use as a screening tool from organizations such as the American Society of Clinical Oncologists, the American Cancer Society, the Society of Thoracic Radiology, and the American College of Chest Physicians. They do, however, recommend enrollment of high-risk individuals in phase III trials. Randomized phase III trials are under way in Europe as well as the United States. The National Cancer Institute (NCI) Lung Screening Study successfully enrolled 3000 people into a pilot study, randomizing participants to undergo either chest x-ray or LDCT. The purpose of this study was to determine whether people would be willing to be randomized with the availability of LDCT to the community at large. On the heels of the success of this pilot program, the NCI has begun accrual into a large study, which will randomize 50,000 individuals with a smoking history to undergo annual LDCT or chest x-ray. Completion of this study is expected in 2009.[59]

Bronchoscopy and Fluorescence Bronchoscopy

Bronchoscopy is the most commonly used diagnostic tool for obtaining a tissue diagnosis of cancer, but it has limitations in detecting premalignant lesions.[60] Premalignant lesions rarely show visual changes that would be detected on bronchoscopy. Light-induced fluorescence endoscopy (LIFE) takes advantage of the difference in the ability of normal tissues and abnormal tissues to fluoresce when exposed to blue light. Invasive and preinvasive lesions such as dysplasia and carcinoma in situ exhibit slightly weaker red and much weaker green fluorescence than normal tissues.[61] Studies comparing white-light bronchoscopy (WLB) to LIFE bronchoscopy report that LIFE has a higher diagnostic sensitivity in the detection of premalignant and early malignant lesions but a lower specificity.[60] Overall, LIFE is able to detect twice as many lesions that represent moderate to severe dysplasia and carcinoma in situ as compared to WLB.[61]

With the LIFE bronchoscope, a new morphological entity has been recognized. Angiogenic squamous dysplasia (ASD) may be an important biomarker and target for antiangiogenic chemoprevention.[60] This technology continues to evolve.

Pathophysiology

Cellular Characteristics

Lung cancer is classified into two major categories: non-small cell lung cancer (NSCLC) and small cell lung cancer (SCLC). NSCLC is further classified into adenocarcinoma, squamous cell carcinoma, and large cell carcinoma. In planning treatment for lung cancer, it is important to identify the cell type.

Non-small cell lung cancer

Adenocarcinoma arises from alveolar surface epithelium or bronchial mucosal glands, forms glands, and produces mucin.[62] It is currently the most commonly occurring NSCLC, representing 40% of primary tumors, and is the subtype most commonly found in nonsmokers and women.[62,63] Adenocarcinoma is subdivided into six categories: acinar, papillary, bronchioloalveolar (BAC), solid adenocarcinoma with mucin formation, mixed, and variants. Variants include mucinous, signet ring, and clear cell.[64,65] BAC is a distinctive subtype that spreads along alveolar septae but does not invade lung parenchyma.[63] Areas of BAC are often found within areas of other invasive disease. BAC is currently a topic undergoing further definition through basic research due to an observed response to Iressa.[56–58] Estrogen receptors are present on some adenocarcinomas. In this setting, it is important to distinguish a primary lung cancer from a metastatic breast cancer so as to provide the most effective treatment approach.[66] Tumors of the adenocarcinoma subtype are often located in the periphery of the lung parenchyma and therefore present with fewer symptoms. Adenocarcinomas progress more slowly than squamous cell carcinomas but tend to invade lymphatic and blood vessels earlier. This invasion accounts for a higher rate of distant metastasis and a poorer survival rate.[62] Gene expression profiles are beginning to define different prognostic factors based on different gene and enzyme profiles.[67]

Squamous cell carcinoma, once the predominant type of NSCLC, now represents 30%–35% of cases. One theory is that filtered cigarettes cause smokers to inhale more deeply, thereby exposing the deeper, more peripheral airways to the carcinogens.[62] Squamous cell carcinomas arise in the more centrally located areas of the lungs. They progress from noninvasive metaplasia and dysplasia to carcinoma in situ. Once a carcinoma in situ penetrates the basement membrane, involving the lamina propria, it becomes invasive and has the ability to metastasize.[62] Squamous cell carcinoma is the most amenable to early detection through cytologic examination of sputum and bronchial brushes and washes because of its central location.[63] Histologic features key to the diagnosis include keratin formation, keratin pearl formation, and intercellular bridges.[62] Because of the central airway involvement of this type of cancer, symptoms of cough or hemoptysis or obstructive symptoms often cause patients to seek medical attention. Necrosis and cavitation occur in approximately 10% of squamous cell tumors.[62] These tumors tend to be more slow growing, with progression from in situ to the invasive stage occurring in 3–4 years.[62]

Large cell carcinoma represents approximately 15% of all lung cancers. This undifferentiated tumor displays no evidence of squamous or glandular maturation. The diagnosis is made by exclusion. Its incidence has decreased in recent years because better histopathologic techniques are now able to distinguish those adenocarcinomas and squamous cell carcinomas that were previously defined as large cell undifferentiated tumors.[62,63] Large cell tumors are usually found in the periphery of the lung, invading into airways. The cells more frequently contain neuroendocrine features, which are associated with a poorer prognosis.[62] Giant cell carcinoma is a subtype that also tends to have a poorer prognosis.[62]

Small cell lung cancer

Approximately 98% of SCLC is associated with cigarette smoking.[68] This disease's incidence has declined from a peak at 20%–25% of all lung cancers to as low a share as 13.8% in 1998, presumably because of downward trends in cigarette smoking 20 years ago.[68,69] SCLC is an aggressive cancer that usually arises from the large central airways and frequently metastasizes early.[62] Survival in patients with extensive disease is strictly related to performance status and can be as short as only 5 weeks without treatment. Mixed NSCLC/SCLC carries the same prognosis as SCLC.[69]

SCLC probably arises from Kulchitsky cells, neuroendocrine cells that secrete peptide hormones.[62] The pathologic criteria for the diagnosis of SCLC include the following characteristics: small size; scant cytoplasm; finely granular nuclear chromatin; absent or faint nucleoli; high mitotic rate (which accounts for its high rates of response to chemotherapy); and frequent necrosis.[70] Crush artifact is a frequent finding because the cells are fragile.[62]

Progression of Disease

Lung cancers spread within the lung to areas such as the pleura and lymph nodes; by lymphatic invasion, which then leads to metastasis via the lymph channels; and via hematogenous routes, which lead to distant metastases. In NSCLC, spread by direct extension (squamous cell) or lymphatic invasion (adenocarcinoma) may cause occlusion of the airway and compression of pulmonary structures, such as major blood vessels, nerves, and alveolar structures. Extension to the pleurae, chest wall, and diaphragm also occurs. The lung possesses a rich network of lymph nodes and vessels that facilitate spread to local (intrapulmonary and hilar), regional (hilar and mediastinal), and distant (supraclavicular) nodal sites. Common sites of metastatic disease in NSCLC include the brain, bone, adrenal gland, contralateral lung, liver, pericardium, and kidney. At the time of presentation, SCLC is much more likely to have undergone hematogenous spread to distant sites including the bone, liver, adrenal gland, CNS, lymph nodes, pleura, and subcutaneous tissue.[71]

Phenotypes of metastatic disease on the molecular level include matrix metalloproteinases (MMP), enzymes produced by lung cancer cells. Cells use these enzymes to destroy the basement membrane of surrounding tissues to allow for invasion into that adjacent tissue. Matrix metalloproteinase inhibitors (MMPIs) may affect or decrease the invasive properties and are currently under investigation.[38] Lung cancers are also associated with increased expression of vascular endothelial growth factor (VEGF) and increased angiogenesis. Antiangiogenesis agents are under investigation as potential therapies as well.[38]

Clinical Manifestations

Clinical features of lung cancer can be classified into four groups of symptoms and signs related to the primary tumor; intrathoracic, extrapulmonary extension of the primary tumor; extrathoracic metastases; and indirect attributes.[72]

Signs and Symptoms Related to the Primary Tumor

Cough is the most common presenting symptom, occurring in 8%–75% of patients on diagnosis. It occurs most frequently in the setting of centrally occurring tumors. The mechanism of the cough may result from an irritative effect of the tumor, poor drainage due to an obstructive tumor, secondary infection, or pleural or pericardial effusion.[72,73]

Hemoptysis occurs in 6%–35% of patients at diagnosis.[73] The amount of blood found ranges from blood-streaked sputum to frank blood clots. This symptom is also most commonly associated with centrally located tumors in the following decreasing frequency: SCLC, squamous cell, adenocarcinoma.[72] The mechanism of bleeding is related to ulceration of the tumor into bronchial mucosa or, rarely, direct invasion of a blood vessel.

Dyspnea is reported as a presenting symptom in 3%–60% of patients.[73] It results from hypoxemia related to airway obstruction, atelectasis, post-obstructive pneumonitis, or lymphatic carcinomatosis (often related to BAC). It can also result from a pleural or pericardial effusion.[72] Patients with phrenic nerve paralysis can complain of breathlessness. Evidence of this problem can be seen on a chest x-ray as the presence of a raised hemidiaphragm.[73]

Signs and Symptoms Related to Intrathoracic Extrapulmonary Spread

Chest pain or discomfort can result from direct spread of the primary tumor to the pleural surface or from direct invasion into the mediastinum or bony structures surrounding the pleural space. Approximately 50% of patients present with chest pain or discomfort.[73] Pain is usually dull, persistent, poorly localized, and unrelated to coughing or breathing. Retrosternal pain may be present with hilar and mediastinal node involvement. Pain in the shoulder or arm may be due to brachial plexus infiltration from a superior sulcus (Pancoast) tumor. Brachial plexus involvement may also result in weakness, atrophy, or paresthesia in the upper extremity.[72] Pleuritic chest pain often disappears with the development of a pleural effusion and is related to neoplastic pleural invasion.[73]

Pleural effusions, especially unilateral, are suspicious for malignancy. Exudative or bloody effusions are usually due to extension of a peripheral tumor or metastases to the pleura.

Superior vena cava syndrome (SVCS) is a presenting sign in 0%–4% of patients, but lung cancer accounts for 46%–75% of all cases of SVCS[73] and this sign most frequently occurs in patients with SCLC.[74] The superior vena cava is vulnerable to compression from tumor because of low intraluminal pressures and thin vessel walls. Its location also renders it vulnerable to enlarged mediastinal lymph nodes, right-sided tumors, and superior sulcus tumors.[74] Presenting symptoms result from interrupted blood flow through this vessel and include edema of the face, neck, upper torso, and breasts; headache; dizziness; drowsiness; visual distortion; conjunctival edema and erythema; and dilation of collateral veins on the upper torso, shoulders, and arms.[72,73] See Chapter 40 for complete information on this syndrome.

Lymphadenopathy in the hilar and mediastinal lymph nodes usually represents the initial spread of lung cancer.[72] Palpable lymph nodes in the axilla, supraclavicular, and scalene regions can be biopsied percutaneously to obtain a relatively noninvasive diagnosis in the clinic or physician's office.[72] This step is critical because a positive test result implies stage IV unresectable disease.

A presenting symptom in only 2.2% of patients, *dysphagia* occurs because of compression of the esophagus by tumor in the posterior mediastinal compartment and generally represents unresectable disease.[72]

Pericardial effusion/tamponade may be evidenced by a new-onset arrhythmia or EKG abnormality.[75] Symptoms include palpitations, dyspnea, cough, light-headedness, chest pain, and diaphoresis.[72] Physical exam may reveal jugular venous distention, diminished heart sounds, a pericardial rub, or knock on auscultation.[72] See Chapter 36 for a complete discussion of this oncologic emergency.

Symptoms Related to Extrathoracic Spread

Central nervous system symptoms include seizures, headache, hemiplegia, personality changes, cerebellar disturbances, or difficulty speaking. The symptom displayed relates to the area of the brain affected, with the exception of seizure, which is a more global symptom.[72] Lung cancer is responsible for 70% of brain metastases, which are present in 10% of patients on presentation.[73]

Bone pain represents bone metastases until proven otherwise in a patient with lung cancer, especially squamous cell. Approximately 25% of patients present with bone pain.[73] Spinal cord compression is an oncologic emergency that can result from bone metastases to the vertebral bodies that impinge on the spinal cord.[76] Lung cancer is the most common cause of spinal cord compression, with the thoracic spine most often being affected.[72] Localized back pain is the most common symptom progressing to neurologic changes, which may include findings two vertebra below the site of compression — namely, loss of sensation to pinprick or temperature, followed by motor changes and loss of deep-tendon reflexes. Without immediate intervention, spinal cord compression can result in permanent loss of nerve function. It is best diagnosed with MRI; treatment includes corticosteroids, radiation, chemotherapy, and, in rare cases, surgery.[72]

Weakness and weight loss are often the result of hepatic involvement or the disease itself.

Paraneoplastic Syndromes: Signs and Symptoms Indirectly Related to Tumor

Paraneoplastic syndromes are not directly related to the physical effects of the primary or metastatic tumors. In some cases, the mechanism is well understood; more often, it is not. A paraneoplastic syndrome may be the presenting symptom of disease. Indeed, in some cases a malignancy is never found. Most such syndromes resolve with treatment of the underlying disease, but some are indicative of a poor prognosis. Table 57-4[77–80] lists the common paraneoplastic syndromes present in lung cancer along with their associated symptoms. See Chapter 33 for a more detailed discussion of these syndromes.

Assessment

History

A health history may provide important clues for making a diagnosis of lung cancer. It can also contribute to the body of knowledge when included in formalized databases. Some institutions have developed lung cancer databases so that demographic, risk factor, health history, and symptom information are available when performing other research activities. Coupled with this effort are tumor banks where tissue is stored and can later be used to correlate patient and tissue characteristics with treatment and survival outcomes via molecular studies. Tissue is obtained at the time of surgery and placed in freezer banks, where it is saved until there are an adequate number of tissue specimens on which to perform molecular studies.

A family history includes information about cancer (specifically lung cancer) as well as smoking history in family members. The patient history includes all body systems. Specific to this patient population are important questions about tobacco, which includes cigarettes, cigars, pipes, smokeless tobacco, and recreational drugs such as marijuana, age at initiation, average number of cigarettes per day, number of years smoked, and number of years since quitting. In addition, information is solicited about exposure to ETS (how many years), radon, and occupational exposures. Specifics related to a history of underlying respiratory illness are ascertained: bronchitis, COPD, emphysema, asthma, pneumonia, TB, frequent respiratory infections. Specific respiratory symptom issues to be explored include questions about the frequency, duration, and severity of symptoms such as cough, sputum expectoration (and its characteristics), hemoptysis, dyspnea, wheezing, and chest pain or discomfort. Constitutional and general symptoms include pain, fatigue, weight loss, and appetite changes as well as neurological changes including gait disturbances, memory changes, dizziness, headache, vision changes,

Table 57-4 Paraneoplastic Syndromes Associated with Lung Cancer

Syndrome	Type of Lung Cancer	Signs/Symptoms
		Skeletal
Clubbing	NSCLC, SCLC	• Sponginess of soft tissue at base of nail • Pericuticle skin smooth, flushed, glossy • Palpable fingernail at proximal edge • Shape of fingernail altered: "parrot's beak," watch glass," "drumstick"
Hypertrophic osteoarthropathy	NSCLC, SCLC	• Achiness/stiffness relieved by elevation • Periosteal new-bone formation • Symmetric arthritic changes in joints and periarticular tissues • Thickening of soft tissues in face or distal one-third of arms and legs • Neurovascular changes: chronic erythema, paresthesia, increased sweating
		Systemic/Constitutional
Anorexia, cachexia, weight loss (Poor prognosis)	NSCLC, SCLC	• Disappearance of subcutaneous fat • Loss of skin turgor
Fatigue	NSCLC, SCLC	
		Neuromuscular Syndromes: Central Nervous System Syndromes
Subacute cortical cerebellar degeneration	SCLC, adenocarcinoma	• Bilateral and symmetrical neurologic findings • Difficulty walking • Incoordination of arms, legs • Dysarthria • Nystagmus • Noncerebellar deficits: sensorineural hearing loss, peripheral neuropathy, dementia
Visual paraneoplastic syndromes	SCLC	• Rapidly progressive binocular vision loss • Photosensitivity • Ring-scotomatous visual field loss • Attenuated retinal arteriole caliber
		Neuromuscular Syndromes: Peripheral Nervous System Syndromes
Eaton-Lambert syndrome	SCLC, adenocarcinoma, undifferentiated	• Fatigue and weakness disproportionate to physical findings • Proximal extremity weakness, legs > arms • Decreased to absent deep-tendon reflexes • Increasing muscle strength with repeated muscle movement
Sensory neuropathy/encephalomyelitis	SCLC	Rapidly progressive • Pain • Paresthesia • Loss of sensation to temperature, vibration, pressure • Hypotension • Impotence • Constipation Presence of Anti-Hu antibody

(continued)

seizures, and changes in sensation. All other systems are evaluated for significant past medical or surgical history. An assessment of the patient's level of emotional disturbance related to the diagnosis of lung cancer is made, with emotional support being provided to the patient and family and referral to psychology or social services being offered as needed. During the history interview, opportunities abound for providing smoking cessation information and counseling, radon detection and mitigation strategies, and other health education information.[81]

Physical Exam

The physical exam focuses on the respiratory system, lymph system, abdomen, and other areas where specific symptoms were identified in the history. The thorax is observed for obvious signs of abnormality: abnormal retraction of the intercostal spaces, impaired respiratory movement of one or both lungs, or deformities or asymmetry such as a tracheal shift. Palpation focuses on locating areas of tenderness, testing chest expansion, and feeling for tactile fremitus (which is decreased in COPD, pleural effusion, or infiltrating

Table 57-4 Paraneoplastic Syndromes Associated with Lung Cancer (continued)

Syndrome	Type of Lung Cancer	Signs/Symptoms
		Endocrine Syndromes
Hypercalcemia (Poor prognosis)	Squamous cell	• High serum calcium levels • Weakness • Lethargy • Nausea and vomiting • Constipation • Abdominal pain • Renal insufficiency at levels > 13mg/dL
Syndrome of inappropriate ADH (Poor prognosis)	SCLC	• Elevated arginine vasopressin (AVP, antidiuretic hormone) • Slow onset: anorexia, nausea, vomiting • Acute onset: cerebral edema, irritability, confusion, lethargy, seizures • Decreased serum osmolality • Urine osmolality increased
Cushing's syndrome (Poor prognosis)	SCLC	• Elevated cortisol levels • Hyperglycemia • Hypokalemia • Metabolic acidosis
		Cutaneous Syndromes
Dermatomyositis–polymyositis	NSCLC, SCLC	• Women > men • Pain/weakness in proximal muscles of extremities • Dysphagia • Skin rash: heliotrope-colored erythema about the face, neck, arms, and hands • Telangiectasia surrounding eyes or fingernails • Elevated serum creatine kinase, LDH, SGOT
Acanthosis nigrans	NSCLC, SCLC	• Velvety hyperpigmentation in neck, groin, flexor surfaces
Sign of Leser-Trelat	Squamous, adenocarcinoma	• Sudden appearance of seborrheic keratosis on shoulder or trunk

Data from Feinstein, Stover[72]; Beckles, Spiro, Colice, et al[73]; Mazzone, Arroliga[77]; Douglas, Ellershaw[78]; Flounders[79]; Langfeldt, Cooley.[80]

tumor). Decreased unilateral chest expansion can be related to pleural effusion, lobar pneumonia, and unilateral bronchial obstruction. Percussion can reveal abnormalities such as pleural effusion (flatness), lobar pneumonia (dullness), chronic bronchitis (resonance), emphysema or pneumothorax (hyperresonance), or a large pneumothorax (tympany). Auscultation may reveal adventitious sounds such as crackles (pneumonia, fibrosis, CHF, bronchitis), wheezes from narrowed airways (asthma, COPD, bronchitis), and rhonchi (secretions).

The remainder of the physical exam focuses on evaluating for distant disease. The lymph nodes are palpated in the axillary, supraclavicular, scalene, submandibular, and cervical regions as well as the groin. The abdomen is palpated for abnormal enlargement of the liver or spleen. Any areas of pain noted in the history are examined, and a brief neurologic exam is performed evaluating for areas of changed strength and sensation. Gentle percussion of the spine may reveal focal areas of abnormalities suggestive of metastatic disease. The skin and joints are inspected for evidence of paraneoplastic disorders.[81]

Preoperative Evaluation

If a patient is being considered for surgery, additional testing is completed to determine perioperative risk and long-term risks of pulmonary disability.[82] A thorough cardiopulmonary evaluation should include pulmonary function tests measuring the forced expiratory volume (FEV_1) and diffusion capacity (DLCO), which measures carbon monoxide and is a reflection of gas exchange. If the FEV_1 is greater than 80% of the predicted normal value or greater than 2 L, the patient is a suitable candidate for pneumonectomy. If the FEV_1 is greater than 1.5 L, a lobectomy would most likely be tolerated. A DLCO of less than 40% is indicative of an increased risk for perioperative complications and mortality.

The extent of cardiac evaluation depends on the individual's risk factors.[82] Elderly patients require multidisciplinary evaluation for surgery. Cardiac and pulmonary function needs to be carefully evaluated. Functional status, co-morbid conditions, nutritional status, cognitive status, psychological state, and social support as well as a thorough prescription and over-the-counter medication review are essential in identifying suitable elderly surgical candidates.[83] Elderly patients should not be denied surgery based on age alone, as surgery has been found to be both feasible and effective in the appropriate elderly candidate.[83]

Diagnostic Studies

Diagnostic studies for lung cancer in any given individual patient are planned to obtain the most information using the least invasive tests. They can range from a simple tissue diagnosis using a fine-needle aspiration (FNA) obtained in the physician's office to multiple noninvasive imaging studies to a surgical procedure. During the diagnostic studies, staging and classification of the patient is completed. Staging determines treatment and is indicative of prognosis.

Imaging studies

Chest x-ray is the oldest imaging modality for the radiographic diagnosis of lung cancer. Many lung nodules are initially recognized incidentally when a chest x-ray is done in a preoperative evaluation. These studies are useful in detecting pneumonia, in evaluating resolution after treatment, and in evaluating congestive heart failure (CHF), pulmonary edema, and pleural effusions.[84] The limitation of the chest x-ray in the diagnosis of lung cancer is that it provides a two-dimensional picture of a three-dimensional person. This characteristic makes anatomical structures difficult to delineate, and structures such as ribs, the heart, hilar structures, and the aortic arch often hide small abnormalities, such as lung tumors.[84] The chest x-ray is also not a useful tool in evaluating the mediastinum for tumor invasion or lymph node involvement or for detecting invasion of the chest wall or diaphragm.[85,86]

Computed axial tomography (CAT or CT) is now the standard radiographic examination for staging lung cancer.[86] Introduced in the 1970s, it has made many developmental advances since then. This technology immediately led to improvements in staging and analysis of survival curves.[87] CT of the chest allows visualization of structures behind the heart as well as those anterior and posterior to the hilar region.[84] It has a much higher sensitivity than chest x-ray for the detection of small pulmonary nodules (> 5 mm in size) as well as accompanying infiltrative changes such as ground-glass opacities.[88,89] CT provides gross information regarding mediastinal lymph node involvement and serves as a good guide to determine the optimal approach to biopsy the nodes (mediastinoscopy, mediastinotomy, or transbronchial or percutaneous biopsy) but is limited because it reveals anatomy and size only. For example, it cannot distinguish between malignant and inflammatory lymph nodes.[86,90] On pathologic examination, lymph nodes that appeared normal in size on CT can be shown to harbor microscopic disease and nodes that were enlarged can prove pathologically benign. The addition of intravenous contrast enhances the visualization of mediastinal lymph nodes, especially right paratracheal and aortopulmonary (AP) window nodes and hilar lymph nodes. With spiral CT imaging at 5-mm and 7-mm intervals, contrast may not be routinely required for visualizing the mediastinal lymph nodes.[86]

CT imaging of the chest usually includes the upper abdomen, which images the liver and adrenal glands. The American Society of Clinical Oncology (ASCO) 2003 guidelines for the diagnostic staging of locoregional disease recommends a chest x-ray and a CT with intravenous contrast, which is to include the liver and adrenal glands.[91] A normal CT of the adrenal glands does not necessarily rule out metastatic disease, but an abnormal scan can lead to more definitive studies.[92] Metastatic disease to the liver is identifiable within the full chest CT, with better definition in the setting of a scan using IV contrast.[92] Although CT of the brain with intravenous contrast is very accurate in the detection of metastatic disease, it has been superceded by magnetic resonance imaging (MRI), which is more sensitive for the detection of CNS metastases.[92]

Magnetic resonance imaging is useful in detecting pericardial involvement,[90] evaluating superior sulcus tumors for invasion into the brachial plexus in the chest,[85] evaluating vertebral invasion in the spinal cord, defining adrenal masses that remain indeterminate on CT, differentiating benign from malignant tumors in the liver, and identifying brain metastases. It is superior to all other imaging modalities for the diagnosis of CNS lesions, including parenchymal and menningeal carcinomatosis.[92]

Bone scintigraphy (bone scan) is more sensitive than plain x-rays or CT for the detection of bone metastases. A study of potentially operable NSCLC cases demonstrated positive bone metastases in only 3.4% of patients. In another study, 94% of the patients with a true-positive scan were symptomatic.[92] Because false-positive results are common due to focal areas of increased uptake in degenerative disease, a plain film may be recommended to evaluate an abnormality on a bone scan in an effort to exclude traumatic or degenerative lesions. Bone scans have 50% sensitivity and 92% specificity.[92]

Positron emission tomography (PET) uses the radionuclide F-18 Fluorodeoxyglucose (FDG) as a radiotracer. Areas of high FDG intake are indicative of tumor growth — malignant tumors use glucose at a higher rate than healthy tissues.[93] Because PET is a metabolic examination, correlation with the CT to elucidate anatomical detail is essential. Used in the lung cancer diagnostic and staging period, whole-body PET has been shown to change the initial management plan in 41% of cases.[92] Management was changed either because lesions that had gone undetected with standard imaging were revealed or because lesions that had looked suspicious on standard imaging proved negative on PET. The ability of PET to improve the preoperative staging of NSCLC patients is critical in distinguishing stage IIIA from stage IV disease, as it represents the difference between resectable and unresectable disease.

An area of ongoing controversy is the use of PET in staging the mediastinum. In a meta-analysis of 19 studies and 1111 patients, PET demonstrated both higher sensitivity and specificity than CT. Because of the imperfect nature of these diagnostic tests, both ASCO and the American College of Chest Physicians recommend obtaining a tissue biopsy from image-positive mediastinal lymph nodes.[85,86,91] PET is more accurate than conventional imaging (MRI, CT, bone scan) for metastases at all sites except the brain. The sensitivity of PET for the brain is only 60%, largely because of the high background uptake of glucose in the normal brain.[94] PET is an effective tool to further characterize adrenal lesions found on CT. Sensitivity for the detection of metastatic disease has been reported to be as high as 100%.[92] Data on liver imaging are still being gathered but suggest that PET is more specific than conventional imaging.[92] PET is far superior to bone scan, demonstrating 92% sensitivity and 99% specificity.[94] The current recommendation from ASCO is for PET to be performed on anyone who is potentially a surgical candidate and shows no evidence of metastatic disease on the CT scan of the chest.[91]

Many patients present with solitary pulmonary nodules (SPNs) that are difficult to define on CT alone, especially given the increased use of the LDCT as a screening tool. PET has been found to be highly accurate in evaluating these SPNs, with the added benefit that a full staging work-up may be performed at the time of the PET scan if the nodule is malignant.[95,96] PET is also gaining favor as a modality for staging and planning for radical radiotherapy, assessing response to radical radiotherapy or chemoradiotherapy, and assessing response to neoadjuvant therapy prior to surgery.[95] Current limitations of this imaging modality include access, cost, and inconvenience (the scan takes 4 hours to perform). False-positive results can occur if the patient has inflammation, rheumatoid arthritis, infection, pneumonia, abscess, histoplasmosis, aspergillosis, blastomycosis, active TB, granulomas, tumor necrosis, radiation pneumonitis, airway inflammation associated with asthma, hyperplasia, sarcoid, or anthracotic lymph nodes. False-negative results can occur with hyperglycemia (because hyperglycemia interferes with uptake, it is a contraindication to PET), microscopic tumor deposits, and biologically indolent neoplasms such as BAC.[86,90,92] Future directions with this modality include development of radioisotopes that will decrease scan time and the use of CT/PET fusion scans, which will combine anatomy and function into one scan.[95]

Diagnostic tissue sampling

Tissue sampling is used to define the type of lung cancer a patient has, aid in the diagnosis of metastatic disease, and identify radiographically abnormal mediastinal lymph nodes as malignant or benign. The results obtained from such tests will determine the initial treatment plan for any given patient. Tissue sampling is done in the least invasive way possible to obtain the most information.

Tissue sampling of the primary tumor. The level of invasiveness required to obtain tissue from the primary tumor depends on its size and location. As noted previously, bronchoscopy is one of the procedures most commonly used to obtain tissue. Tissue biopsies, brushings, and washings can be diagnostic in lesions located above the segmental bronchus.[97] Bronchial biopsies, brushings, and washings have a much lower sensitivity in the case of peripheral tumors.[97] In the presence of abnormal CT or PET findings, a negative bronchoscopy should not be considered definitive and further attempts to confirm tissue identification should be made.[98] Bronchoscopy is well tolerated and performed on an outpatient basis with sedation.

Transthoracic needle aspiration (TTNA) gains sensitivity with CT guidance and increasing tumor size (> 2 cm). A nonspecific result requires further tissue evaluation.[98] This procedure is associated with minimal complications, which may include pneumothorax and bleeding. The TTNA can be performed in the interventional radiology suite or in the operating room, and the patient is usually sent home after the procedure.

A definitive thoracoscopy or thoracotomy may be the first procedure performed to obtain tissue in a patient who has a small inaccessible tumor or a solitary pulmonary nodule that is suspicious for malignancy on CT or PET scan in the absence of evidence for metastatic disease.[98]

Sputum cytology, the least invasive method of obtaining cells, is most useful in diagnosing centrally located lesions in patients who present with hemoptysis. Unfortunately, most institutions do not have an established program for sputum collection and processing.[98]

With all of the previously described modalities, a positive pathologic or cytologic diagnosis of a non-small cell type of lung cancer is reliable. Because of the fragility of SCLC cells in cytology specimens, a diagnosis of SCLC must be correlated with the clinical and radiographic findings.[98]

Tissue sampling of the mediastinum. The evaluation of mediastinal lymph node involvement in NSCLC is the most important aspect of staging related to treatment planning and prognosis. The most important distinction is between stage IIIA and IIIB disease: the former may be operable; the latter is not.[99] As discussed previously, the noninvasive methods of evaluating the mediastinum for malignant lymph nodes have improved but still fail to provide a definitive tissue diagnosis.[99] The ASCO guideline recommends biopsy for any lymph nodes larger than 1 cm on CT.[91] Factors to consider in deciding to perform more invasive testing include the patient's co-morbid conditions, the degree of suspicion for metastatic disease, and the results' effect on the treatment plan.[99]

Endobronchial ultrasound (EUS) is a newer technique used in the evaluation of the mediastinum. It is widely used for staging and sampling gastrointestinal (GI) tumors and can be safely performed on an outpatient basis with the use of sedation.[100] The procedure itself involves the insertion of an endoscope with an attached real-time ultrasound probe into the GI tract and performance of an ultrasound examination of the liver, adrenal glands, and structures of the mediastinum. Fine-needle aspirates of abnormal lymph nodes in the aortopulmonary (AP) window (level 5), subcarinal region (level 7), and inferior mediastinum can be obtained through the endoscope (see Figure 57-3).[101] A major advantage of this procedure is that it can image lesions as small as 3 mm and can sample lesions as small as 5 mm. A major limitation is the inability to assess nodes in the anterior mediastinum.[102] These nodes can be sampled bronchoscopically with a transbronchial-needle aspiration (TBNA).

Cervical mediastinoscopy and anterior mediastinotomy (Chamberlain procedure) remain the gold standards for pathologic staging of mediastinal lymph nodes; they offer the highest negative predictive value as compared to EUS/FNA.[99,103] Cervical mediastinoscopy involves an incision above the suprasternal notch, insertion of a mediastinoscope along the trachea, and biopsy of accessible lymph nodes: the left and right high and low paratracheal nodes (levels 2R, 2L, 4R, and 4L), pretracheal nodes (1 and 3), and anterior subcarinal nodes (7). Nodes that cannot be assessed include the posterior subcarinal (7), inferior mediastinal (8 and 9), and AP window (5 and 6). (See Figure 57-3.) Left upper lobe tumors tend to favor the AP window nodes as metastatic sites, and these nodes can be sampled through the anterior mediastinotomy approach. This approach involves an incision in the second or third intercostal space just to the left of the sternum.[103] These procedures are performed in the operating room under general anesthesia: The cervical mediastinoscopy is done on an outpatient basis, whereas the anterior mediastinotomy usually requires overnight observation.[103] The complication rate is about 1.7% in the experienced thoracic surgeon's hands; potential complications include pneumothorax, left recurrent laryngeal nerve injury, bleeding, and infection.[90]

Tissue sampling of metastatic disease. According to the ASCO 2003 guideline, suspected metastatic disease in the adrenal glands or liver should be confirmed by biopsy in patients who would otherwise be considered operative candidates.[91] These tissue specimens are obtained in the least invasive manner possible. Generally, a percutaneous procedure is performed on an outpatient basis with local anesthesia and under some type of radiographic guidance: CT, fluoroscopy, or ultrasound. In some cases, a palpable lymph node can be accessed with FNA to provide the necessary pathologic information.

Prognostic Indicators

Overall lung cancer has a poor prognosis, with only 10%–15% of patients surviving five years.[104] Non-small cell lung cancer and small cell lung cancer behave differently and thus have different prognostic variables, although tumor stage is the most important prognostic factor identified for both types of lung cancer.[104]

Non-small cell lung cancer

Squamous cell carcinoma has the best prognosis stage for stage followed by adenocarcinoma. The prognosis for adenocarcinoma is dependent on the particular subgroup involved, with resected early stage nodular bronchioloalveolar carcinomas having the best five-year survival rate of 75%–100%. The prognosis for large cell carcinoma is generally poor, as the disease often demonstrates characteristics similar to SCLC.[104]

Between 1990 and 2000, 169 prognostic indicators for NSCLC were identified in more than 887 articles.[105] The large number of prognostic indicators identified speaks to the heterogeneity of lung cancers. Several subgroups have been identified based on stage of disease. For resected stage I disease, important indicators of poorer survival include tumor extension and volume, multiple and/or macroscopic N1 lymph node involvement,[106,107] microscopic involvement of mar-

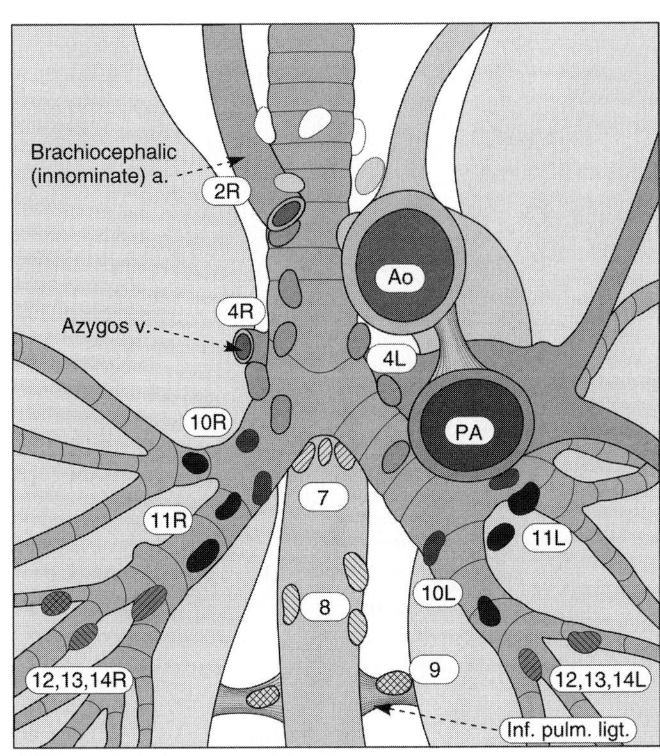

Figure 57-3 Regional lymph node stations for lung cancer staging. (Reprinted from Mountain, Dresler.[101])

gins with tumor,[105] extensive tumor necrosis,[108] EGFR overexpression,[109] COX-2 overexpression,[110] LDH level, bone marrow metastases, poor performance status, weight loss, and clinical symptoms.[107] In relation to histopathology, grade of tumor differentiation does not seem to play a role in prognosis and remains a controversial factor. Lymphatic and vascular invasion as well as the presence of mucin and a high mitotic index are all indicative of a poorer prognosis.[107] An example of a molecular marker that shows promise in

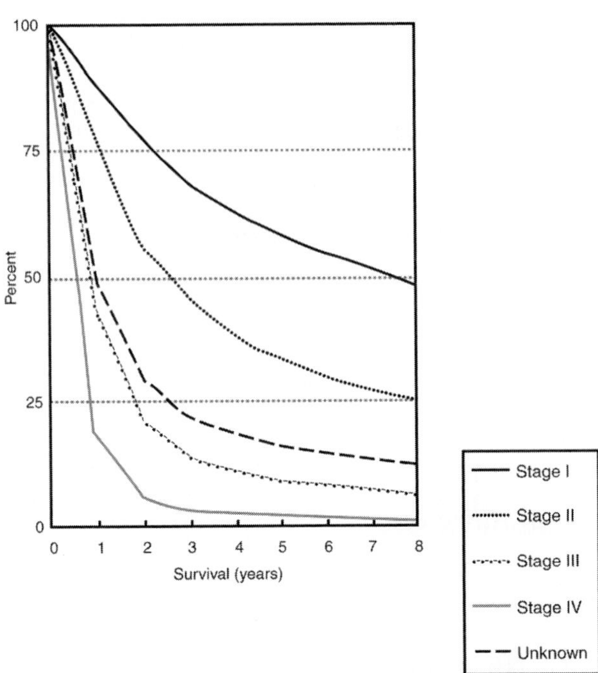

Figure 57-4 Survival curves by stage of disease. (Reprinted from Beadsmoore, Screaton.[104])

predicting disease recurrence and decreased survival is *CYP1A1* status. This gene is responsible for the metabolic activation of benzopyrene, a chemical found in cigarette smoke. High susceptibility to smoking-related lung cancer has been found in the presence of a polymorphism of the *CYP1A1* gene.[105] Patients with resectable tumors who are not candidates for resection have a poorer prognosis if they have symptoms, a poor performance status, a low hemoglobin level, and a higher stage of disease.[105] Recently, correlations of survival by stage with tissue molecular markers have been reported but require clinical trial verification.[111,112]

Advanced disease is subdivided into locally advanced disease and advanced disease, reflecting the difference in prognosis. The most predictive indicators of survival in these patients are extent of disease, weight loss, and performance status. Patients with locally advanced disease who are symptomatic, have experienced weight loss, and have a poor performance status fall under the same prognostic umbrella as those with advanced disease.[105] Favorable prognostic indicators in patients with advanced disease are female gender, good performance status, and age younger than 70.[105] Patients with single sites of metastatic disease have a better prognosis than those with multiple sites of disease.[107] Molecular markers that have significance in terms of prognosis in this group are more difficult to define because of the paucity of tissue available for study. Markers that have been implicated but remain under investigation include markers of angiogenesis, *p21*, cytokeratin 19, argyrophilic nucleolar organizing region, *p185*, *ki67*, VEGF, and *p53*.[105] In locally advanced disease, two subgroups experience a better prognosis. First, patients with a good performance status, no weight loss, and no systemic symptoms have a better prognosis with a combination of chemotherapy and radiation therapy than with radiation therapy alone.[105] Second, poor prognostic indicators in T3N0M0 tumors, otherwise known as superior sulcus or Pancoast tumors, include nerve and vertebral body involvement.[105]

Small cell lung cancer

Stage of disease is also an important prognostic indicator for SCLC. Small cell lung cancer is classified as limited stage (confined to one hemithorax) or extensive (disease beyond the hemithorax). Because SCLC is a rapidly growing tumor, 75% of affected patients are diagnosed with extensive-stage disease and have a poorer outcome. Pleural effusion, performance status, gender, elevated LDH or alkaline phosphatase, low sodium, and potentially paraneoplastic syndromes are all poor prognostic indicators.[113] The number and location of metastatic sites contribute to prognosis. The brain as the only metastatic site has the same prognosis as limited disease, whereas liver and bone marrow metastases have a poorer prognosis.[104]

Classification and Staging

Non-Small Cell Lung Cancer

The treatment of NSCLC depends on the stage of disease at presentation. The staging system applied to NSCLC is the T (tumor), N (lymph node), and M (metastasis) system applied to many solid tumors. Table 57-5 details this system. The stage groupings are displayed in Table 57-6.[114,115]

The TNM staging system accounts for anatomical stage only. Clinical staging has improved with the use of functional imaging (i.e., PET); further improvements are expected with the use of combination CT-PET. In the future, biological aspects of this heterogenous group of tumors will be incorporated with staging to determine the optimal treatment for any individual patient.

Small Cell Lung Cancer

SCLC is classified according to the Veterans Administration Lung Study Group (VALG) definitions. Limited-stage disease is confined to one hemithorax with or without contralateral mediastinal or supraclavicular lymph node involvement. This is roughly defined as

Table 57-5 AJCC TNM Definitions for Lung Cancers

Primary Tumor (T)	
TX	Primary tumor cannot be assessed, or tumor proven by the presence of malignant cells in sputum or bronchial washings but not visualized by imaging or bronchoscopy
T0	No evidence of primary tumor
Tis	Carcinoma in situ
T1	Tumor 3 cm or less in greatest dimension, surrounded by lung or visceral pleura, without bronchoscopic evidence of invasion more proximal than the lobar bronchus (The uncommon superficial tumor of any size with its invasive component limited to the bronchial wall, which may extend to the main bronchus, is also classified as T1)
T2	Tumor with any of the following features of size or extent: • More than 3 cm in greatest dimension • Involves main bronchus, 2 cm or more distal to the carina • Invades visceral pleura • Associated with atelectasis or obstructive pneumonia that extends to the hilar region but does not involve the entire lung
T3	Tumor of any size that directly invades any of the following: chest wall (including superior sulcus tumors), diaphragm, mediastinal pleura, parietal pericardium; or tumor in the main bronchus less than 2 cm distal to the carina; or associated atelectasis or obstructive pneumonitis of the entire lung
T4	Tumor of any size that invades any of the following: mediastinum, heart, great vessels, trachea, esophagus, vertebral body, carina; or separate tumor nodules in the same lobe; or tumor with malignant plural effusion (Most pleural effusions associated with lung cancer are due to tumor. However, in a few patients multiple cytopathologic examinations of pleural fluid are negative for tumor. In these cases, fluid is nonbloody and is not an exudate. Such patients may be further evaluated by video-thoracoscopy and direct pleural biopsies. When these elements and clinical judgment dictate that the effusion is not related to the tumor, the effusion should be excluded as a staging element and the patient should be staged T1, T2, or T3.)
Regional Lymph Nodes(N)	
NX	Regional lymph nodes cannot be assessed
N0	No regional lymph node metastasis
N1	Metastasis to ipsilateral peribronchial (levels 14, 13, 12, 11) and/or ipsilateral hilar lymph nodes (level 10), and intrapulmonary nodes including involvement by direct extension of the primary tumor
N2	Metastasis to ipsilateral mediastinal (levels 9, 8, 6, 5, 4, 3, 2, 1) and/or subcarinal (level 7) lymph nodes
N3	Metastasis to contralateral mediastinal, contralateral hilar, ipsilateral or contralateral scalene, or supraclavicular lymph nodes
Distant Metastasis (M)	
MX	Distant metastasis cannot be assessed
M0	No distant metastasis
M1	Distant metastasis present [(includes separate tumor nodule(s) in a different lobe (ipsilateral or contralateral)]

disease within a tolerable radiation therapy port. Extensive disease is everything outside of this tolerable radiation port.[104,115] Institutions are beginning to apply the TNM system to SCLC.

Therapeutic Approaches

Treatment of lung cancer is determined by stage (see Table 57-7). Surgery, photodynamic therapy, and radiation therapy are local therapies; chemotherapy and targeted therapy are systemic treatment modalities. In addition, combinations of local and systemic therapies are often used. Because of the mutimodality approach to the treatment of lung cancer, multidisciplinary programs provide an efficient method through which care is planned and delivered.

Multidisciplinary Thoracic Oncology Programs

People with lung cancer require complex care, often receiving mutimodality therapy from multiple specialists. Unique to the lung cancer population are tobacco-related issues such as cardiovascular and pulmonary diseases. To receive coordinated care and minimize duplication of services, it is recommended that institutions develop some form of multidisciplinary program to care for patients with lung cancer, although no studies prove the benefits of such a program.[116] This program can include a multidisciplinary clinic, a virtual network, and minimally should include a weekly conference. Such a conference allows the specialists involved to prospectively discuss patients' initial treatment plans, design of adjuvant treatment, second-line therapy, and palliative care. To accomplish this goal, the following medical specialists must be involved: pulmonologist, thoracic surgeon, medical oncologist, radiation oncologist, radiologist, pathologist,

Table 57-6 Stage Grouping for Lung Cancer

Stage Group	TNM			One-I Year Survival (%)	Five-Year Survival (%)
Local					
Occult carcinoma	TX	N0	M0		
Stage 0	Tis	N0	M0		
Stage IA	T1	N0	M0	94	67
Stage IB	T2	N0	M0	87	57
Stage IIA	T1	N1	M0	89	55
Locally Advanced					
Stage IIB	T2	N1	M0	73	39
	T3	N0	M0		
Stage IIIA	T1	N2	M0	64	23
	T2	N2	M0		
	T3	N1	M0		
	T3	N2	M0		
Stage IIIB	Any T	N3	M0	32	3
Advanced					
Stage IIIB	T4	Any N	M0	37	7
Stage IV	Any T	Any N	M1	20	1

Data from American Joint Committee on Cancer[114]; Wood.[115]

and primary care physician. To provide consistency in care, NCCN or ASCO guidelines can be incorporated into the patient care decision-making process. Clear and consistent written communication is essential in this mode. Components that should be included in this communication include the stage of disease, treatments and their efficacy, results of follow-up studies, changes in the treatment, and the patient's tolerance of the plan. Additional healthcare providers who are involved in both the conference and a multidisciplinary clinic include social work, psychology, psychiatry, pastoral care, and dietary support.

Nursing support is essential to this model. The role of the Clinical Nurse Specialist (CNS) is to coordinate and triage patients to the appropriate specialists for the initial consultation in a manner that allows patients to enter the treatment arena in a timely and efficient manner. Although no studies suggest that delay in treatment by a matter of weeks leads to a poor outcome,[116] studies do indicate that patients with lung cancer present with the highest amount of psychological distress as compared to patients with other malignancies.[117] It behooves the healthcare team to initiate a plan of treatment quickly to manage psychological stress. The patient with stage I or II disease is sent directly to the thoracic surgeon if the patient is a surgical candidate. All specialists who will be involved in the individual's care initially see the patient with stage IIIA disease who is to receive neoadjuvant therapy. The patient with unresectable stage IIIB or IV disease is sent directly to the medical oncologist.[116] The CNS provides support and a point of contact for the patient and family throughout the care trajectory. Other nursing involvement includes the oncology nurse practitioner, clinical trials nurse, and clinic or primary nurse.[117]

Surgery

Surgery represents the best hope of cure for the patient with NSCLC and is the recommended treatment for stage I and II disease. It is also an option after neoadjuvant chemotherapy and radiation therapy in stage IIIA disease and for the patient with a stage IIIB Pancoast tumor. In stage IIIB and IV disease, its use is limited to palliation in the least invasive manner possible. Surgery is rarely a consideration for SCLC.

Non-small cell lung cancer

The goal of surgery for NSCLC is cure and long-term survival, so patient selection is critical. Surgery is the treatment of choice for suitable candidates who have clinical stage I and II lung cancer. The type of procedure depends on the tumor location, the patient's co-morbidities, and the effect of the procedure on long-term pulmonary function. A lobectomy is ideal for a tumor confined to a single lobe. It involves removal of the lobe as well as the lymph nodes draining that lobe. Studies are under way to determine whether mediastinal lymph node dissection or systematic sampling of mediastinal lymph nodes provides the optimal benefit.[118] Studies are also ongoing to determine the feasibility of identifying a sentinel lymph node intraoperatively and its usefulness in determining the extent of lymph node dissection that will be necessary for a resection to be considered complete.[118,119] Pneumonectomy is utilized for central tumors involving the main stem bronchus or invading the pulmonary artery. A sleeve segmentectomy is an alternative to pneumonectomy in some tumor types.[120] Less extensive resections include wedge resection and segmentectomy. These procedures are performed on patients who have inadequate pulmonary function and elderly patients with prohibitive co-morbidities; they carry a higher likelihood of local recurrence.[120]

The choice of incision is based on tumor location, size, and patient co-morbidities. Video-assisted thoracic surgery (VATS) is best utilized for limited resection but is under investigation for lobectomy.[121] It is a very attractive option for elderly patients, as it seems to be associated with less postoperative morbidity.[122] The ax-

Table 57-7 Treatment of Lung Cancer by Stage and Histology of Disease

Stage	Treatment Modalities*
Non-small Cell Lung Cancer	
IA	Surgery Chemotherapy Radiation therapy if not a surgical candidate
IB, IIA, IIB	Surgery Adjuvant chemotherapy +/- radiation therapy
IIIA resectable	Neoadjuvant chemotherapy followed by surgery or Surgery alone Adjuvant radiation therapy +/- Chemotherapy
IIIA unresectable, IIIB due to involvement of contralateral or supraclavicular lymph nodes	Concurrent chemoradiotherapy or Chemotherapy followed by radiation therapy
IIIB with pleural effusion, IV	Chemotherapy Surgical resection of solitary brain metastasis + surgical resection of primary T1 tumor
Small Cell Lung Cancer	
Limited stage	Chemotherapy + concurrent radiation therapy
Extensive stage	Chemotherapy

* Treatment modalities are listed in the order they should be given.

Data from Wood.[115]

illary thoracotomy is the incision most often utilized, and the posterolateral thoracotomy is necessary when better exposure and visualization is required. No difference in quality of life was found between patients who had VATS and those who had a thoracotomy.[123]

Small cell lung cancer

Surgery plays a very limited and still controversial role in the treatment of SCLC. Potential roles for surgery in this usually systemic disease include resection of small peripheral tumors diagnosed as small cell by needle aspiration; treatment of tumors that responded poorly to chemotherapy and are suspected to be of a mixed type (i.e., small cell plus non-small cell disease) in potentially resectable patients; and adjuvant to chemotherapy and radiation.[124] Patients with SCLC who are under consideration for resection need to undergo a thorough preoperative evaluation to include mediastinoscopy as well as a complete metastatic work-up, even in small, clinically stage I tumors. Clinical trials evaluating the role of surgery in SCLC have yielded conflicting results. The only prospective randomized trials evaluating the role of surgery failed to show a benefit, whereas retrospective analyses and prospective nonrandomized trials showed longer disease-free survival and higher rates of long-term survival than did chemoradiotherapy alone.[124] Elderly patients with SCLC may be considered for surgery just as their younger counterparts, with special consideration being paid to cardiac and pulmonary function as well as performance status and co-morbidities.[122,125]

Complications and nursing management

Pulmonary. Pulmonary morbidities are the most common complication after thoracic surgery for lung cancer. A 2.7 times higher incidence of major pulmonary morbidity [i.e., pneumonia and adult respiratory distress syndrome (ARDS)], has been noted in patients who were still smokers within one month of pneumonectomy. Risk of death is also significantly higher in this group compared to never-smokers and smokers who quit more than four weeks before surgery.[126] Another study investigated pulmonary morbidities in patients who underwent resections ranging from limited wedge resections to pneumonectomy. The results revealed higher morbidity and mortality for smokers and showed that patients who quit smoking more than 10 weeks before surgery had the same incidence of morbidity and mortality as people who had never smoked.[127] Therefore, the necessity to implement smoking cessation strategies prior to scheduling a thoracic resection is critical.

The benefits of smoking cessation include prompt reductions in carboxyhemoglobin nicotine blood levels and improvement of mucociliary function.[127] During the first few weeks after smoking cessation, mucus production increases in tandem with improvement in the protective mechanisms of the ciliary system throughout the respiratory tract. This increased mucus production can lead to pulmonary complications when the patient has quit smoking fewer than four weeks before surgery.

Other risk factors for pulmonary complications include advanced age, obesity, type of resection, type of anesthesia, and history of pulmonary or cardiac disease. Nursing care related to the prevention of pulmonary complications includes good pain management, early and frequent ambulation, the use of incentive spirometry followed by coughing, and referral to respiratory therapy for nebulizer treatments and chest physiotherapy.

Cardiac. Atrial arrhythmias are common in the patient who has undergone a lung resection because of irritation to the vagus nerve. Stroke is a complication of atrial fibrillation. Patients are monitored closely during the postoperative period, and beta blockers are initiated if atrial fibrillation persists. Patients who have had a myocardial infarction (MI) within three months of resection are at risk of another MI, and the mortality from this complication increases with increasing age. Patients older than 70 have a higher incidence of heart failure in the postoperative period.[128]

Pain. Pain is an inevitable phenomenon following thoracic surgery. The nursing goal for pain management is to provide pain relief that allows the patient to actively participate in pulmonary exercises. Epidural analgesia is commonly utilized for thoracic surgery. It produces a neuroaxial sensory block of the trunk while sparing motor function. This allows the patient to participate in pulmonary hygiene activities and early ambulation with minimal discomfort, as does patient-controlled analgesia (PCA).[129] PCA is applied via both the intravenous and the epidural routes. Analgesics commonly employed include opioids and nonsteroidal anti-inflammatory drugs. Acute pain generally is at a level that does not require pain medication approximately 4–6 weeks after surgery, but chronic post-thoracotomy pain may last for months to years.

Radiation Therapy

The goal for radiation therapy (RT) in lung cancer is to prevent local recurrence of disease by eliminating small deposits of tumor cells near the primary site and to provide palliation of symptoms from both local and metastatic disease. A limiting factor in RT has been the inability to precisely target tumor tissue and to avoid undesirable side effects such as radiation pneumonitis and esophagitis. The advent of new technology in the delivery of radiation, such as three-dimensional conformal RT (3D-CRT) allows for the use of increasing doses while decreasing toxicity to surrounding normal tissue and minimizing the risk of underdosing or missing portions of tumor. Intensity-modulated RT (IMRT) allows for even more precise planning and the ability to safely escalate doses of radiation.[130]

Methods to minimize "tumor motion" are under investigation. The goal is to decrease radiation damage to nearby structures and to target the tumor more specifically. One such method coordinates delivery of the radiation to a specified phase in the patient's breathing cycle by gating the linear accelerator while the patient breathes normally.[130] A second approach employs active breathing control (ABC), which is controlled either by the patient or by an occlusion valve.

Biologic imaging with the use of PET augments CT imaging in planning the target volume. This approach better defines the tumor volume that needs to be treated and optimizes the dose delivered to the tumor while preventing the overdose of surrounding tissues. Stereotactic radiosurgery is frequently used for metastatic brain lesions and is currently under investigation for use extracranially.[130]

Non-small cell lung cancer

In NSCLC, RT can be utilized with a curative or palliative intent. In resected stage I disease, RT does not play a role in adjuvant treatment. A meta-analysis published in 1998 suggested that adjuvant RT could be detrimental; however, this trial was completed prior to the development and widespread use of more refined RT delivery techniques.[115] Patients not considered resectable, even though the tumor is, based on co-morbidities or patient refusal, should receive RT. In such cases, the survival rates with RT are lower than those obtained with surgical resection.[83] Similar overall and recurrence-free survival rates as well as equal tolerance of therapy was noted in patients more than 70 years old and those younger than 70.[83]

Implantation of iodine-125 brachytherapy seeds has been done investigationally in patients who had limited resection due to co-morbidities. This approach resulted in a decrease in local recurrence. Further studies need to be performed to determine whether survival will be positively affected.[131]

The recommendation for patients found to have N2 disease at resection and/or positive surgical margins is that they receive adjuvant RT. This recommendation is based on a study that showed a decrease in local recurrence but no improvement in overall survival in this group of patients.[115] Studies investigating neoadjuvant RT with chemotherapy have shown a survival advantage.

In stage IIIB and IV disease, RT is utilized for symptom palliation. The aim of treatment at this point is controlling symptoms and optimizing quality of life.[132]

Elderly patients may be eligible to receive the same therapy as younger patients but are frequently not evaluated with that intent. ASCO guidelines recommend definitive thoracic RT for those patients with performance status of 0, 1, or possibly 2; adequate pulmonary function; and disease confined to the thorax. Patients with pleural effusions and/or distant metastases should not be considered for definitive RT. The recommended dose is 60Gy in 1.8–2.0 Gy fractions.[91]

Three randomized trials and five nonrandomized trials have shown that prophylactic cranial irradiation (PCI) in NSCLC decreases or delays the incidence of CNS failure. The Radiation Therapy Oncology Group (RTOG) has an ongoing trial randomizing patients who have completed definitive therapy for locally advanced NSCLC and show no evidence of progressive disease or distant metastases to PCI or observation. The purpose of the study is to prove that PCI improves survival by safely preventing the development of CNS metastases.[133]

Other strategies under investigation to enhance the effects of radiation include use of COX-2 inhibitors,[134] epidermal growth factor inhibitors, and antiangiogenesis agents as radiation sensitizers.[135]

Small cell lung cancer

Combined chemotherapy and RT administered concurrently within a six-week period offer the best hope for long-term survival in patients with limited-stage SCLC. This strategy decreases the probability of metastatic events, resistance to chemotherapy and RT, and repopulation of tumor cells.[136] PCI at a total dose of 25–36 Gy given in 2–3 Gy daily fractions has proven to provide a survival benefit in both limited- and extensive-stage disease for patients who have attained a complete remission in the chest with chemotherapy and/or RT.[137] In patients with extensive-stage disease, RT is reserved for palliative efforts.

Complications and nursing management

Complications of thoracic RT include fatigue, radiation pneumonitis, and esophagitis, which increases with concurrent chemotherapy.[132] Esophagitis is managed symptomatically with systemic and local pain medications as required, as well as with antibiotics and antivirals.

Nutritional status must be maintained and can be the most challenging issue. Weight must be monitored and the patient coached on maximizing protein and caloric intake. Nutritionists should become involved early in the treatment phase, if not before the initiation of treatment, to assist in strategies to minimize weight loss. Elderly patients who lose weight during therapy have poorer outcomes.

Radiation pneumonitis is an inflammation of the lungs. Radiation causes alveolitis from injury to the endothelial and epithelial cells. Alveolitis results in an accumulation of inflammatory and immune cells in the alveolar spaces.[138] Pneumonitis can occur two weeks to six months after RT, with its severity depending on the dose and volume of lung radiated as well as the concurrent use of chemotherapy. Patients present with vague symptoms including dyspnea, chest pain, exertional shortness of breath, cough, wheezing, and fatigue. Steroids are the mainstay of treatment.[138]

Studies investigating neurocognitive deficits after PCI have failed to show a relationship. In patients who received concurrent chemotherapy and PCI, neurocognitive changes were present.[137]

Other Local Therapies

Photodynamic therapy (PDT) and neodymium: yttrium-aluminum-garnet laser (Nd-YAG) are local therapies for the treatment of early-stage lung cancer as well as palliation of obstructive symptoms from endobronchial tumors. Either of these therapies can be incorporated into the multimodality management of lung cancer.

PDT utilizes a photosensitizing agent, porfimer sodium (Photofrin), and laser application via bronchoscopy to destroy tumor through a photochemical reaction. Bronchoscopy is then used to remove tissue debris. Although PDT has been mainly used for NSCLC, a few studies have documented its success with SCLC as well.[139] The success rate in relieving obstructive symptoms has been reported to be as high as 70%.[139] Common events after the procedure include dyspnea and cough with expectoration of necrotic debris. Adverse events that can occur with the PDT procedure include hemorrhage, scarring, fibrosis, and airway perforation.[140] The patient must receive thorough instructions on staying out of direct sunlight to

Table 57-8 Chemotherapeutic Agents Used in Lung Cancer

Platinum Agents
Cisplatin
Carboplatin
Nonplatinum Agents
Etoposide
Topotecan
Irinotecan
Gemcitabine
Paclitaxel
Docetaxel
Vinorelbine
Vincristine
Doxorubicin
Cyclophosphamide
Ifosfamide

avoid severe sunburn related to the photosensitizing agent.[141]

Nd:YAG laser therapy produces direct thermal ablation of tissue and is used to coagulate or vaporize tumors. Procedural complications include hypoxia, hemorrhage, cardiac arrhythmia, myocardial infarction, and cardiac arrest. Both PDT and the laser therapy have similar efficacy.[142]

Chemotherapy

Several chemotherapy agents have been studied in the treatment of lung cancer (Table 57-8). Studies involving patients with all stages of disease have investigated single and combination chemotherapy regimens, as well as chemotherapy in conjunction with radiation therapy or surgery. Current trials are also incorporating targeted therapy with chemotherapy.

Elderly patients have generally been underrepresented in clinical trials. In the trials where elderly patients were included, however, age was not a prognostic indicator.[143] Special considerations for the elderly include performance status, presence of co-morbidities, renal function, cardiac function, and psychosocial issues such as living situation and support system. These patients may be more susceptible to the myelosuppressive effects of chemotherapy because of a more rapid depletion of pluripotent hematopoietic cells in response to stress.[143] Overall, stage for stage, good performance status elderly patients should receive the same consideration for chemotherapy as their younger counterparts.[143]

Non-small cell lung cancer

Cisplatin-based adjuvant chemotherapy for resected stage I, II, and III NSCLC was shown to yield a survival improvement of 4.1% over no adjuvant therapy in a trial that enrolled 1867 patients from 148 participating centers in 33 countries.[144] This survival benefit is consistent with that found with adjuvant therapy for other cancers, such as breast, colon, ovarian, and bladder cancers.[145,146] Investigators at each site were allowed to choose which agent to combine with cisplatin; the agents used were vindesine, vinblastine, vinorelbine, and etoposide. Additionally, radiation therapy was added at the discretion of the investigator. Grade 4 toxic effects occurred in 22.6% of patients and included neutropenia, thrombocytopenia, and vomiting.[144] Previous trials investigating adjuvant therapy in this population had failed to demonstrate any survival advantage. The results of this trial have the potential to change standard therapy for resected patients from observation to adjuvant therapy.[145,146]

Neoadjuvant chemotherapy followed by surgery is given with curative intent, as is chemoradiotherapy without surgery for stage IIIA disease. The rationale for neoadjuvant therapy is that it provides early treatment of systemic disease and can promote shrinkage of the primary tumor, leading to a more complete surgical resection.[115] Trials investigating platinum-based chemotherapy followed by surgery with or without RT show conflicting results. Three randomized trials demonstrated a survival benefit, whereas a larger trial failed to show a significant survival benefit but did have lower risk of distant recurrence in the chemotherapy group, indicating that microscopic metastases may have been eradicated by chemotherapy.[115,146] The most aggressive approach is chemoradiotherapy followed by surgery. Three large, prospective, cooperative group trials successfully demonstrated the ability to safely perform lobectomy or pneumonectomy after neoadjuvant chemoradiotherapy, although the RT dose in these trials was limited to 45 Gy.[115,146,147] Three separate trials have utilized higher doses of RT, with two of them experiencing a higher rate of mortality after pneumonectomy (42% and 33%).

The Bimodality Lung Oncology Team (BLOT) completed a phase II trial investigating the use of neoadjuvant chemotherapy (carboplatin and paclitaxel) followed by surgery and adjuvant chemotherapy in stage I and II disease. Although only half of the patients were able to complete the prescribed dose of chemotherapy after surgery, an overall survival rate of 85% was achieved at one year and 56% at two years.[148] A second trial using gemcitabine and cisplatin obtained similar results.[149] Ongoing randomized phase III trials are attempting to confirm the utility of this approach in patients with early-stage disease. Another important question addressed in these trials is which chemotherapy agents to use. Combinations of carboplatin/paclitaxel, gemcitabine/cisplatin, and gemcitabine/carboplatin have all been studied and are well tolerated. A study comparing cisplatin/paclitaxel and carboplatin/paclitaxel has shown a slight but significant survival advantage for cisplatin,[150] as did a study comparing cisplatin/docetaxel and carboplatin/docetaxel.[151] Studies comparing cisplatin/gemcitabine with carboplatin/gemcitabine are ongoing.

Chemotherapy is the mainstay of treatment for unresectable stage III and IV NSCLC. Because advanced disease is rarely curable, the goal of treatment is prolonged survival and enhanced quality of life. The ASCO 2003 guidelines recommend 2–4 cycles of platinum-based chemotherapy with RT for performance status 0, 1, and possibly 2 patients with unresectable stage III disease. The treatment should start soon after the diagnosis is made.[91]

In stage IV disease, treatment with chemotherapy has been proven superior to best supportive care with an increased survival of 2–4 months and a 1-year survival benefit in 10%–20% of patients.[115] These benefits, however, are restricted to patients with good performance status (i.e., 0, 1, or possibly 2). Single-agent cisplatin was the treatment of choice until the 1990s, when several new agents were introduced. A study published in 2000 was the first to report better response rates with paclitaxel/cisplatin versus the older standard of etoposide/cisplatin.[152] The ASCO guidelines for unresectable NSCLC now recommend a two-drug combination that may or may not include a platinum agent.[91] A 2002 report of four different two-drug combinations (cisplatin/paclitaxel, cisplatin/gemcitabine, cisplatin/docetaxel, carboplatin/paclitaxel) failed to show that any one combination was superior to another with regard to survival and adverse events, and all of the regimens resulted in response rates that were better than historical controls.[153] The 2003 ASCO guidelines recommend a duration of first-line therapy of no more than four cycles in those patients who are not responding and no more than six cycles in responders.[91] Studies have shown nothing more than increased toxicity for three versus six cycles.[151]

The ASCO guidelines recommend docetaxel as second-line therapy for patients with advanced NSCLC.[91] Several randomized studies suggest that docetaxel may provide a survival benefit in the second-line setting when compared with best supportive care and other agents.[154,155] Agents such as vinorelbine and gemcitabine are also reasonable second-line options.

Patients who have a single site of metastasis with a solitary lesion should be considered for resection of the tumor. Resection of solitary brain metastasis followed by whole-brain RT can yield a 10%–20% five-year survival rate.[115]

Small cell lung cancer

Because of its growth kinetics, SCLC is initially sensitive to therapy, with response rates as high as 70%–80% and complete response rates as high as 50% in patients with limited-stage disease who receive combination therapy.[156] The rate of relapse is high as demonstrated in five-year survival rates of 15%–25% for treated limited-stage SCLC and less than 5% for treated extensive-stage disease.[115]

When a patient has an undiagnosed lung cancer, is taken to surgery for resection, and the pathology comes back as SCLC, the recommendation is to provide adjuvant platinum-based therapy with RT if mediastinal nodes contained microscopic disease. If the SCLC is diagnosed with a biopsy, surgery is not recommended and the patient is treated with chemotherapy with or without RT.[115] Limited-stage SCLC is initially treated with an induction therapy consisting of cisplatin or carboplatin plus etoposide for 4–6 cycles with concurrent RT.[156] Combination therapy is superior to single-agent therapy, nonplatinum regimens are inferior to platinum-based regimens, and carboplatin and cisplatin are equally effective in treating SCLC.[115,157] Concurrent therapy is superior to sequential chemotherapy followed by RT.[115] A survival advantage has been proven for a regimen alternating carboplatin/etoposide with cyclophosphamide/doxorubicin/vincristine.[156] Attempts to prolong the progression-free interval may focus on maintenance therapy, dose intensity, dose density, and autologous bone marrow transplantation. All of these approaches have increased toxicity without improving survival.[156,157]

The goals of therapy when the patient relapses are palliation and prolonged quality survival.[158] Considerations for choosing second-line therapy include survival advantages; palliation (symptom control versus toxicities); quality of life (improved quality of life versus toxicities and inconvenience of therapy); and patient selection based on performance status (greater than or less than 2), co-morbidities (renal, hepatic, cardiac, pulmonary), progression-free interval (less than 3 months or greater than 3–6 months), and age (greater or less than 65 years). Topotecan is an agent that has been well characterized for use as second-line therapy alone and in combination therapy. It provides a good response rate of 33% for those patients who responded to first-line therapy and an overall response rate of 21% as well as symptom palliation with a noncumulative manageable toxicity profile.[158] Docetaxel provides an overall response rate of 25%; irinotecan demonstrates an overall response rate of 33%.[156] Gemcitabine, paclitaxel, and combination cyclophosphamide, doxorubicin, and vincristine have also demonstrated response rates in the relapsed setting ranging from 12% to 28%.[158]

Performance status is the most important prognostic indicator for patients who present with extensive-stage SCLC. Therapy is designed based on this variable, and many of the same combination regimens that are employed in limited-stage disease are also used in patients with a good performance status and extensive-stage disease. Carboplatin/etoposide is the standard for patients with a good performance status. A recent Japanese study investigating cisplatin/irinotecan demonstrated improved two-year survival and less hematologic toxicity but increased diarrhea. This study is currently being replicated in cooperative groups in the United States.[115] Other newer agents studied as first-line therapy for extensive-stage SCLC include gemcitabine (27% overall response rate) and vinorelbine (16% overall response rate). Ifosfamide has also demonstrated a 48% overall response rate.[156]

Considerations for elderly patients with either limited- or extensive-stage disease revolve around performance status and co-morbidities. Patients with a performance status of 2 or greater will receive palliative therapy, while those with performance status of 0, 1, or possibly 2 can receive the same therapy as their younger counterparts. Elderly patients treated with combination chemotherapy and RT have demonstrated equal response rates but an increased treatment-related mortality in the first six months after therapy.[83] It is especially important to base carboplatin dosing on renal function in this group of patients, as renal function normally declines in the elderly.[83]

Complications and nursing management

Patients with lung cancer who receive chemotherapy experience the common side effects from chemotherapy. Due to underlying tobacco-related pulmonary and cardiovascular disease, side effects of fatigue, loss of appetite, weight loss, and anemia may be more severe, be less tolerable, and ultimately lead patients to refuse treatment. Issues of dyspnea and hypoxia contribute to the severity of side effects experienced. This group of patients may realize more benefit from administration of erythropoietic agents early in the treatment course. Nursing management includes the usual strategies to mange side effects, additional coaching to encourage the patient to continue therapy if the intent is cure, and emotional support if therapy is no longer providing palliation.

Biologic Therapy

The use of targeted biologic therapy in lung cancer is adding an exciting dimension to the treatment of a dismal disease. Targeted therapy differs from chemotherapy in a number of ways. First, it employs tumor-selective killing, whereas chemotherapy nonselectively kills proliferating cells. Second, toxicities are lower than with conventional chemotherapy. Third, it is dosed at biologically active levels rather than at the maximum tolerated dose. Fourth, there is not only a tumor response and survival benefit such as occur with chemotherapy, but also novel clinical benefits.[159] Nursing's role in targeted therapy is to educate patients about these novel agents, to monitor for adverse events, and to ensure enrollment in clinical trials.

Non-small cell lung cancer

The epidermal growth factor receptor (EGFR) HER-1 (erbB-1) is expressed in 40%–80% of NSCLC cases. Selective EGFR tyrosine kinase inhibitors (EGFR TKI) inhibit signal transduction pathways that are implicated in proliferation and survival of cancer cells.[160]

ZD1839 (gefitinib, Iressa), an orally administered small-molecule tyrosine kinase inhibitor, received approval from the FDA in May 2003 as monotherapy for patients with locally advanced or metastatic NSCLC after failure of both platinum-based and docetaxel chemotherapies[161] and has been integrated into the ASCO guidelines for unresectable NSCLC for use within this indication.[91] The IDEAL 1 and IDEAL 2 (IDEAL = Iressa Dose Evaluation in Advanced Lung Cancer) studies, which led to this approval, showed not only survival and response benefits but also clinical benefits in which symptoms improved. Partial tumor responses (PR) were shown in 14% of patients receiving the subsequently approved dose of 250 mg/day and were more frequent in females and nonsmokers. The median duration of response was 7 months. The drug was well tolerated; side effects included grade 1 or 2 rash, acne, and diarrhea.[162] The clinical benefit was measured using the FACT-L (Functional Assessment of Cancer Therapy—Lung), which is a validated, sensitive, and reliable patient questionnaire evaluating quality of life. Symptoms measured include shortness of breath, weight loss, cognitive function, cough, appetite, and chest tightness. Symptoms as well as quality of life showed improvement in both trials.[163] Trials investigating gefitinib with either gemcitabine/cisplatin (INTACT 1; INTACT = Iressa NSCLC Trial Assessing Combination Treatment) or carboplatin/paclitaxel (INTACT 2) failed to show additional benefit with regard to response rate, time to progression, or survival over chemotherapy alone.[164,165]

A second EGFR TKI is still in clinical trials. Single-agent OSI-774 (erlotinib, Tarceva) has also shown activity in NSCLC in phase II trials and is currently being tested in phase II and III trials.[166] The use of Iressa in the treatment of BAC as a precursor to invasive NSCLC has been reported and is now being assessed in ongoing chemoprevention trials.[56–58] IMC-C225 (erbitux, Cetuximab), a monoclonal antibody against EGFR, is currently in phase II clinical trials.[160]

Several other targets are under investigation in the treatment of NSCLC. Farnesyl transferase inhibitors (FTIs) inhibit a critical enzymatic step in the expression of mutated *ras* genes. SCH66336 (Sarasar), BMS-214662, and R115777 (Zarnestra) are all in varying stages of development in phase I to phase III trials.[167]

The enzyme COX-2 is seen at increased levels in NSCLC. COX-2 inhibitors are currently under investigation in both treatment and preventive trials.

Vascular endothelial growth factor receptor (VEGFR) is under investigation as a target for both monoclonal antibodies and VEGFR inhibitors. RhuMAb-VEGF (bevacizumab, Avastin) is a human monoclonal antibody targeted against VEGF that has been tested in combination with chemotherapy in a phase II trial involving patients with stage IIIB or IV NSCLC. The addition of the monoclonal antibody increased response rates by 10% and prolonged time to tumor progression by three months. Four of six patients who developed severe hemoptysis died. The risk factors specific to these fatalities were a squamous histology and the use of the monoclonal antibody. Further studies with this agent are restricted to those patients who have a nonsquamous histology.[160] Drugs that block endothelial cell signaling via VEGF and its receptor (ZD6474, SU6668, SU5416, CP547,632, and ZD4190) are currently in phase I clinical trials.[168]

Trials of drugs targeting the different steps of angiogenesis, including drugs that inhibit matrix breakdown, the matrix metalloproteinases (marimistat, prinomastat, BMS275291, BAY12–9566, and neovastat), have all yielded negative results to date.[168] Bortezomib (Velcade) is a proteasome inhibitor that targets many pathways relevant to tumor progression and therapy resistance; in lung cancer, it can directly modulate expression of cyclins D, E, A (oncogenic); *p27*^{Kip1} (tumor suppressor); *p53* (tumor suppressor, therapy resistance); NFκB *bcl-2* (cell survival, therapy resistance); and *Bax* (promotes apoptosis).[169] It is currently in phase I and II trials in NSCLC and has a biologic rationale for its testing in SCLC due to the high *bcl-2* expression in this disease.[169] Cancer vaccine strategies currently being studied include GM-CSF gene-modified cancer cells, liposomal MUC1 peptide, anti-idiotype antibody targeting GD3, Mage-3 peptide, and mutant *p53* pulsed dendritic cells. Gene therapy has focused on intratumoral *p53* gene replacement therapy in locoregional NSCLC.[170]

Small cell lung cancer

Although the biologic targets are as numerous in SCLC as they are in NSCLC, far fewer targeted therapy trials have been undertaken for the former disease. Trials investigating MMPIs and interferons have failed to demonstrate any benefit. A vaccine trial called SILVA (Survival in an International Phase III Prospective Randomized Limited Disease Small Cell Lung Cancer Vaccination Study with Adjuvant BEC2 and BCG) is randomizing patients with limited-stage SCLC who have completed induction therapy to receive BEC2 vaccine or not. The vaccine group in a previous pilot study showed improved survival compared to historical controls. Planned trials in SCLC include trials targeting c-kit imatinib (Gleevec), VEGF, VEGFR, EGFR (Iressa), *bcl-2,* proteasome bortezomib (Velcade), and mTOR.[171]

Symptom Management and Supportive Care

Pain, fatigue, and dyspnea in advanced lung cancer all influence a patient's ability to perform daily activities. Dyspnea and fatigue have been noted to interfere with at least one daily activity in more than half of patients; pain interferes in about 40% of affected individuals. Dyspnea and fatigue interfere with physical activities such as walking and work, while pain interferes with almost all activities. Even symptoms rated 1–3 on a 10-point scale were severe enough to interfere with at least one activity.[172] At least 32 documented symptoms have been reported by lung cancer patients.[173] Symptom management is clearly a priority throughout the lung cancer experience. The discussion here focuses on pain, dyspnea, and cough.

Pain

The reported prevalence of pain in lung cancer ranges from 28% to 51%.[173] Because the majority of patients present with advanced disease, lung cancer has become known as a disease for which palliative treatment of symptoms is common. Pain in this population can be caused by the cancer or may be related to treatment; it is compounded by other factors such as dyspnea, fatigue, psychological distress, and insomnia. The most common sites of pain are the chest and back, especially the lumbar area, but multiple unrelated sites of pain are common. Approximately 60% of patients experience nociceptive pain, and 30% experience visceral or neuropathic pain. Patients older than ages 70–80 are significantly less likely to report pain symptoms than those younger than age 40.[174] Recommended treatment of pain in lung cancer patients follows the guidelines developed by the Agency for Healthcare Research and Quality.[175] Treatment of side effects of pharmacologic treatment is essential to optimize the benefits of analgesic therapy. These side effects include constipation, nausea, and sedation.

Lytic bone metastases are a common source of pain in the patient with lung cancer. The prognosis for patients with bone metastases is approximately 6 months of survival.[176] The primary treatment goal is to palliate pain and prevent complications such as pathologic fractures. Treatments available for bone metastases that are both palliative and antineoplastic include RT, chemotherapy, and bisphosphonates. Surgery may be employed to stabilize a fracture or vulnerable and painful site of bone metastases. Sites that require surgery for prevention of pathologic fractures include the femur, tibia, hip, vertebrae, and humerus.[175] Serious consideration of risk versus benefit as well as expected prognosis must be undertaken before a surgical procedure is performed. Surgery is not recommended in those patients whose prognosis is less than four weeks or who have a poor performance status.[175] In patients with SCLC, response to chemotherapy may be fairly rapid but RT is generally the therapy of choice, with some level of pain relief achieved in as many as 90% of patients.[175] The addition of the bisphosponate pamidronate to RT has recently demonstrated an improved response rate over chemotherapy plus pamidronate, or RT or pamidronate alone.[175]

Spinal cord compression is another cause of pain related to lung cancer. A patient presenting with back pain is considered to have a spinal cord compression until proven otherwise. Prompt diagnosis and treatment are essential to prevent permanent neurologic deficits. Immediate use of steroids with RT is recommended in symptomatic patients, whereas RT alone may be employed for asymptomatic patients. Surgery is required for spinal instability, bony compression, or paraplegia at the time of presentation.[175]

Dyspnea

Dyspnea has been described as a pain equivalent in that it is a subjective, complex, sensory, and affective experience resulting from the interaction of factors that influence that experience.[177] Approximately 65% of patients with lung cancer experience dyspnea at some point during their illness.[175] Causes of dyspnea in this population include direct tumor involvement of the lung parenchyma or airways, indirect complications such as pleural effusion and pneumonia, complications of chemotherapy or RT such as pneumonitis, co-morbid conditions such as COPD and heart failure, and respiratory complications that are more common to this population, such as pulmonary embolism.[175] Factors that contribute to the sensation of dyspnea include anxiety, fear of impending death, and pain.

Treatment of dyspnea utilizes both pharmacologic and nonpharmacologic therapies. Therapies are selected based on the suspected underlying mechanism of dyspnea. Opioids, bronchodilators, steroids, and benzodiazepines have all been used to treat dyspnea. Supplemental oxygen may be helpful even if the patient is not hypoxic. In patients with normal oxygen saturations, it may produce a placebo effect and air may be equally helpful. Use of this measure remains an area of controversy.[175,177] Nonpharmacologic therapies include positioning and posture, breathing control, pursed-lip breathing, moving fresh air across the face, activity pacing, relaxation techniques, and psychosocial support.[175,177] Complementary techniques that have demonstrated usefulness include acupuncture, acupressure, and progressive muscle relaxation.[177]

The major indication to treat a pleural effusion is to relieve dyspnea. If thoracentesis for either diagnostic or therapeutic purposes provides relief, definitive strategies to resolve the effusion may be considered. These include repeated thoracenteses as needed in patients with a poor performance status, chest tube or thoracoscopic pleuredesis, or placement of an indwelling pleural catheter that is managed by the patient on an outpatient basis.[175,178]

Cough

A new cough or a change in a chronic cough is often the presenting and most distressing symptom in patients with lung cancer. Among the initial symptoms, cough is present in more than 65% of patients, with more than 25% of patients experiencing a productive cough. Hemoptysis is the presenting symptom in 7%–10% of patients. Approximately 20% of all patients will develop hemoptysis, and 3% will have fatal massive hemoptysis.

Therapies aimed at relieving cough are symptomatic. Nonopioid cough suppressants will work in a small percentage of patients. Opioids, however, are the best cough suppressants. Bronchodilators are helpful in the presence of bronchospasm and underlying pulmonary disease such as COPD. Steroids may prove beneficial if the cough is related to inflammatory causes such as radiation pneumonitis. If cough is due to an obstructing tumor, palliation may be accomplished via bronchoscopic interventions such as Nd-YAG laser therapy, PDT, cryotherapy, or placement of stents. Interventions for hemoptysis initially consist of airway management, followed by bronchoscopic or surgical interventions to stop the bleeding.[175]

Surveillance and Long-Term Follow-up

Recurrence after a curative lung cancer resection can be locoregional, distant, or both. In the five years after a resection, 20%–30% of patients with stage I disease, 50% with stage II disease, and 70%–80% with stage III disease will experience a recurrence. In total, 50% and 90% of cases will have recurrence within the first two and five years, respectively.[179] Once recurrence is diagnosed, survival rates at two years are 37% for stage I disease, 20% for stage II disease, and 14% for stage III disease. *Local recurrence* is defined as new evidence of disease in the same hemithorax as the primary tumor; *regional recurrence* occurs in the lymph system draining the mediastinum and neck; *distant disease* is metastatic outside the previously defined parameters, most commonly in the brain, bone, liver, and adrenal glands. Approximately 60% of recurrences fall into the "distant disease" category, where hope for cure is dismal.[179] The purpose of surveillance is to detect recurrence at a stage where cure or control will be possible.[91]

The 2003 guidelines ASCO for follow-up of NSCLC patients treated with curative intent recommend a history and physical every 3 months during the first 2 years, every 6 months through year 5, and annually thereafter. In asymptomatic patients, there is no clear role for routine diagnostic studies but an annual chest x-ray may be reasonable. The routine use of annual low-dose chest CT needs further investigation to determine its usefulness and cost-effectiveness in surveillance. Other studies are performed as warranted by abnormal results on history or physical.[180] Similar guidelines have been developed by the National Comprehensive Cancer Network (NCCN), Association of Community Cancer Centers (ACCC), and American College of Radiology (ACR).[181] The NCCN and ACCC make the following recommendations for SCLC patients treated with curative intent: history, physical, and chest x-ray with or without CBC and blood chemistry every 2–3 months for the first 2 years, every 6 months for 3–5 years, and annually thereafter; ASCO recommends chest x-ray annually throughout the surveillance period.[181]

For patients with advanced disease, the 2003 ASCO guidelines recommend a history and physical every 3 months for 2 years, and every 6 months through year 5, and annually thereafter. Other diagnostic studies are performed as warranted by abnormalities found on exam.[91]

Patients, families, and often physicians typically feel more secure performing many diagnostic studies despite the lack of evidence supporting this practice. Investigation into current practice indicates that many more tests are performed at more frequent intervals than the guidelines suggest.[180] Patients require emotional support with each surveillance visit and follow-up test due to the anxiety related to the high risk of recurrence and its implications. It is important to educate patients about the evidence-based guidelines in a manner that does not drain hope from their lives.

Conclusion

Future directions in the prevention, diagnosis, and treatment of lung cancer include smoking prevention strategies; primary, secondary, and tertiary chemoprevention; early detection with LDCT; more accurate staging with CT-PET; and targeted therapy individualized to a patient's tumor phenotype. Exciting research is under way to better define tumor characteristics and viable targets for therapy. Hope exists for better therapy responses and improved survival. Nevertheless, the best treatment remains prevention.

References

1. Alberg AJ , Samet, JM: Epidemiology of lung cancer. *Chest* 123:21S-49S, 2003
2. Jemal A, Tiwari RC, Murray T, et al: Cancer statistics 2004. *CA Cancer J Clin* 54:8–29, 2004
3. American Cancer Society: *Cancer Facts and Figures — 2004*. Atlanta, American Cancer Society, 2004
4. Winterhalder RC, Hirsch FR, Kotantoulas GK, et al: Chemoprevention of lung cancer — from biology to clinical reality. *Ann Oncol* 15:185–196, 2004
5. Jemal A, Cokkinides VE, Shafey O, et al: Lung cancer trends in young adults: an early indicator of progress in tobacco control (United States). *Cancer Causes Control* 14:579–585, 2003
6. Ruano-Ravina A, Figueiras A, Barros-Dios JM: Lung cancer and related risk factors: an update of the literature. *Public Health* 117:149–156, 2003
7. Gloeckler LA, Reichman ME, Lewis DR, et al: Cancer survival and incidence from the Surveillance, Epidemiology, and End Results (SEER) program. *Oncologist* 8:541–552, 2003
8. Ahuja R, Weibel SB, Leone FT: Lung cancer: the oncologist's role in smoking cessation. *Semin Oncol* 30:94–103, 2003
9. Twombly R: Tobacco use a leading global cancer risk, report says. *J Natl Cancer Inst* 95:11–12, 2003
10. Siegfried JM: Women and lung cancer: does oestrogen play a role? *Lancet Oncol* 2:506–513, 2001
11. Shapiro JA, Jacobs EJ, Thun MJ: Cigar smoking in men and risk of death from tobacco-related cancers. *J Natl Cancer Inst* 92:333–337, 2000
12. West KA, Brognard J, Clarl AS, et al: Rapid Akt activation by nicotine and a tobacco carcinogen modulates the phenotype of normal human airway epithelial cells. *J Clin Invest* 111:81–90, 2003
13. Heeschen C, Jang JJ, Weis M, et al: Nicotine stimulates angiogenesis and promotes tumor growth and atherosclerosis. *Nat Med* 7:833–839, 2001

14. Toyooka S, Toshihide T, Gazdar, AF: The P53 gene, tobacco exposure, and lung cancer. *Hum Mutat* 21:229–239, 2003
15. Hall W, MacPhee D: Cannabis use and cancer. *Addiction* 97:243–247, 2002
16. de Andrade M, Ebbert JO, Wampfler JA, et al: Environmental tobacco smoke exposure in women with lung cancer. *Lung Cancer* 43:127–134, 2004
17. Anderson KE, Carmella SG, Ye M, et al: Metabolites of a tobacco-specific lung carcinogen in nonsmoking women exposed to environmental tobacco smoke. *J Natl Cancer Inst* 93:378–381, 2001
18. Duckworth LT, Frank-Stromberg M, Oleckno WA, et al: Relationship of perception of radon as a health risk and willingness to engage in radon testing and mitigation. *Oncol Nurs Forum* 29:1099–1107, 2002
19. Frumkin H, Samet JM: Radon. *CA Cancer J Clin* 51:337–344, 2001
20. Bach PB, Ginsberg RJ: Epidemiology of lung cancer, in Ginsberg RJ (ed.): *American Cancer Society Atlas of Clinical Oncology: Lung Cancer.* Hamilton, ON, BC Decker, 2002, pp 1–10
21. Epstein KR: The role of carotenoids on the risk of lung cancer. *Semin Oncol* 30:86–93, 2003
22. Travis LB, Gospodarowicz M, Curtis RE, et al: Lung cancer following chemotherapy and radiotherapy for Hodgkin's disease. *J Natl Cancer Inst* 94:182–192, 2002
23. Richardson CM, Sharma RA, Cox G, et al: Epidermal growth factor receptors and cyclooxygenase-2 in the pathogenesis of non-small cell lung cancer: potential targets for chemoprevention and systemic therapy. *Lung Cancer* 39:1–13, 2003
24. Fiore MC, Bailey WC, Cohen SJ, et al: *Treating Tobacco Use and Dependence. Quick Reference Guide for Clinicians.* Rockville, MD, U.S. Department of Health and Human Services, Public Health Service, October 2000
25. Hughes JR: New treatments for smoking cessation. *CA Cancer J Clin* 50:143–151, 2000
26. Cox LS, Patten CA, Ebbert JO, et al: Tobacco use outcomes among patients with lung cancer treated for nicotine dependence. *J Clin Oncol* 20:3461–3469, 2002
27. Carter CL, Key J, Marsh L, et al: Contemporary perspectives in tobacco cessation: what oncologists need to know. *Oncologist* 6:496–505, 2001
28. Brandon TH: Behavioral tobacco cessation treatments: yesterday's news or tomorrow's headlines? *J Clin Oncol* 19:64s–68s, 2001
29. King C, Siegel M: The master settlement agreement with the tobacco industry and cigarette advertising in magazines. *N Engl J Med* 345:504–511, 2001
30. Gross CP, Soffer B, Bach PB, et al: State expenditures for tobacco-control programs and the tobacco settlement. *N Engl J Med* 347:1080–1086, 2002
31. Schultz J: Tobacco programs wither as states divert settlement revenue. *J Natl Cancer Inst* 94:1598–1599, 2002
32. Bal DG, Lloyd JC, Roeseler A et al: California as a model. *J Clin Oncol* 19:69s–73s, 2001
33. American Society of Clinical Oncology Policy Statement Update: Tobacco control-reducing cancer incidence and saving lives. *J Clin Oncol* 21:2777–2786, 2003
34. Akhmedkhanov A, Toniolo P, Zeleniuch-Jacquotte A, et al: Aspirin and lung cancer in women. *Br J Cancer* 87:49–53, 2002
35. Soria JC, Kim ES, Fayette J, et al: Chemoprevention of lung cancer. *Lancet Oncol* 4:659–669, 2003
36. Kurie JM, Lotan R, Lee JJ, et al: Treatment of former smokers with 9–*cis*-retinoic acid reverses loss of retinoic acid receptor-β expression in the bronchial epithelium: results from a randomized placebo-controlled trial. *J Natl Cancer Inst* 95:206–214, 2003
37. Lippman SM, Lee JJ, Karp DD, et al: Randomized phase III intergroup trial of isotretinoin to prevent second primary tumors in stage I non-small cell lung cancer. *J Natl Cancer Inst* 93:605–618, 2001
38. Aberle MF, McLeskey SW: Biology of lung cancer with implications for new therapies. *Oncol Nurs Forum* 30:273–280, 2003
39. Dragnev KH, Stover D, Dmitrvsky E: Lung cancer prevention: the guidelines. *Chest* 123:60s–71s, 2003
40. Schiller JH: New directions for ZD1839 in the treatment of solid tumors. *Semin Oncol* 30(suppl 1):49–55, 2003
41. Averbuch SD: Lung cancer prevention: retinoids and the epidermal growth factor receptor — a phoenix rising? *Clin Cancer Res* 8:1–3, 2002
42. Wistuba II, Gazdar AF, Minna JD: Molecular genetics of small cell lung carcinoma. *Semin Oncol* 28(suppl 2):3–13, 2001
43. Petty TL: Sputum cytology for the detection of early lung cancer. *Curr Opin Pulm Med* 9:309–312, 2003
44. Thunnissen FBJM: Sputum examination for early detection of lung cancer. *J Clin Pathol* 56:805–810, 2003
45. Bach PB, Kelley MJ, Tate RC, et al: Screening for lung cancer: a review of the current literature. *Chest* 123:72s–82s, 2003
46. Jett JR: Screening for lung cancer: no longer a taboo subject. *J Clin Oncol* 20:1959–1961, 2002
47. Chen Y, Okunieff P, Ahrendt SA: Translational research in lung cancer. *Semin Surg Oncol* 21:205–219, 2003
48. Mulshine JL: Screening for lung cancer: in pursuit of pre-metastatic disease. *Nat Rev Cancer* 3:65–73, 2003
49. Wilkinson NW, Loewen GM, Klippenstein DL, et al: The evolution of lung cancer screening. *J Surg Oncol* 84:234–238, 2003
50. Strauss GM: The Mayo Lung Cohort: a regression analysis focusing on lung cancer incidence and mortality. *J Clin Oncol* 20:1973–1983, 2002
51. Giarelli E: To screen or not to screen: using spiral computerized tomography in the early detection of lung cancer. *Clin J Oncol Nurs* 6:223–224, 2002
52. Henschke CI, Naidich DP, Yankelevitz DF, et al: Early Lung Cancer Action Project: initial findings on repeat screening. *Cancer* 92:153–159, 2001
53. Henschke CI, Yankelevitz DF: Early Lung Cancer Action Project: annual CT screening for lung cancer. *Lung Cancer Princip Pract Update* 2:1–6, 2002
54. Prasad SR, Wittram C, Shepard JA, et al: Standard-dose and 50%-reduced-dose chest CT: comparing the effect on image quality. *AJR Am J Roentgenol* 179:461–465, 2002
55. Gaeta M, Blandino A, Pergolizzi S, et al: Patterns of recurrence of bronchioloalveolar cell carcinoma after surgical resection: a radiological, histological, and immunohistochemical study. *Lung Cancer* 42:319–326, 2003
56. Franklin WA, Gumerlock PH, Crowley J, et al: EGFR, HER-2 and ERB-B pathway activation in bronchioloalveolar carcinoma (BAC): analysis of SWOG 9417 and lung SPORE tissue samples. *Proc Am Soc Clin Oncol* 22:260, 2003 (abstr)
57. Miller VA, Patel J, Shah N, et al: The epidermal growth factor receptor tyrosine kinase inhibitor erlotinib (OSI-774) shows promising activity in patients with bronchioloalveolar cell carcinoma (BAC): preliminary results in a phase II trial. *Proc Am Soc Clin Oncol* 22:619, 2003 (abstr)
58. Onn A, Correa AM, Gilcrease M, et al: Synchronous overexpression of epidermal growth factor receptor and HER-2 *neu* protein is a predictor of poor outcome in patients with stage I non small cell lung cancer. *Clin Cancer Res* 10:136–143, 2004
59. Bach PB, Niewoehner DE, Black WC: Screening for lung cancer: the guidelines. *Chest* 123:83s–88s, 2003
60. Hirsch FR, Franklin WA, Gazdar AF, et al: Early detection of lung cancer: clinical perspectives of recent advances in biology and radiology. *Clin Cancer Res* 7:5–22, 2001

61. Banerjee AK, Rabbitts PH, George J: Lung cancer 3: fluorescence bronchoscopy: clinical dilemmas and research opportunities. *Thorax* 58:266–271, 2003
62. Ross J: Biology of lung cancer, in Haas M (ed.): *Contemporary Issues in Lung Cancer: A Nursing Perspective.* Sudbury, MA, Jones and Bartlett, 2003, pp 11–23
63. Zakowski MF: Pathology, in Ginsberg R (ed.): *American Cancer Society Atlas of Clinical Oncology: Lung Cancer.* Hamilton, ON, BC Decker, 2002, pp 23–42
64. Bambilla E, Travis WD, Colby TV, et al: The new World Health Organization classification of lung tumours. *Eur Respirat J* 18:1059–1068, 2001
65. Franklin WA: Diagnosis of lung cancer: pathology of invasive and preinvasive neoplasia. *Chest* 117:80s–89s, 2000
66. Dabbs DJ, Landreneau RJ, Liu Y, et al: Detection of estrogen receptor by immunohistochemistry in pulmonary adenocarcinoma. *Ann Thorac Surg* 73:403–406, 2002
67. Bunn PA: Molecular biology and early diagnosis in lung cancer. *Lung Cancer* 38:S5–S8, 2002
68. Krug LM: Small cell lung cancer, in Ginsberg R (ed.): *American Cancer Society Atlas of Clinical Oncology: Lung Cancer.* Hamilton, ON, BC Decker, 2002, pp 153–163
69. Spira A, Ettinger DS: Extensive stage small cell lung cancer. *Semin Surg Oncol* 21:164–175, 2003
70. Zakowski MF: Pathology of small cell carcinoma of the lung. *Semin Oncol* 30:3–8, 2003
71. Ingle R: Lung cancers, in Yarbro CH, Frogge MH, Goodman M, Groenwald SL, (eds.): *Cancer Nursing: Principles and Practice* (ed 5). Sudbury, MA, Jones and Bartlett, 2000, pp 1298–1328
72. Feinstein MB, Stover D: Clinical features of lung cancer, in Ginsberg R (ed.): *American Cancer Society Atlas of Clinical Oncology: Lung Cancer.* Hamilton, ON, BC Decker, 2002, pp 43–55
73. Beckles MA, Spiro SG, Colice GL, et al: Initial evaluation of the patient with lung cancer: symptoms, signs, laboratory tests, and paraneoplastic syndromes. *Chest* 123:97s–104s, 2003
74. Flounders JA: Superior vena cava syndrome. *Oncol Nurs Forum* 30:E84–E90, 2003
75. Flounders JA: Cardiovascular emergencies: pericardial effusion and cardiac tamponade. *Oncol Nurs Forum* 30:E48–E55, 2003
76. Flounders JA: Oncol emergency modules: spinal cord compression. *Oncol Nurs Forum* 30:E17–E23, 2003
77. Mazzone PJ, Arroliga AC: Endocrine paraneoplastic syndromes in lung cancer. *Curr Opin Pulm Med* 9:313–320, 2003
78. Douglas CA, Ellershaw J: Anti-Hu antibodies may indicate a positive response to chemotherapy in paraneoplastic syndrome secondary to small cell lung cancer. *Palliat Med* 17:638–639, 2003
79. Flounders JA: Syndrome of inappropriate antidiuretic hormone. *Oncol Nurs Forum* 30:E63–E70, 2003
80. Langfeldt LA, Cooley ME: Syndrome of inappropriate antidiuretic hormone secretion in malignancy: review and implications for nursing management. *Clin J Oncol Nurs* 7:425–430, 2003
81. Bickley LS, Szilagyi PG: *Bates' Guide to Physical Examination and History Taking* (ed 8). Philadelphia, Lippincott, Williams and Wilkins, 2003
82. Beckles MA, Spiro SG, Colice GL, et al: The physiologic evaluation of patients with lung cancer being considered for resectional surgery. *Chest* 123:105S–114S, 2003
83. Hurria A, Kris MG: Management of lung cancer in older adults. *CA Cancer J Clin* 53:325–341, 2003
84. Akhurst T, Heelan R: Imaging work-up of lung cancer: utility and comparison of computed tomography and FDG positron emission tomography, in Ginsberg R (ed.): *American Cancer Society Atlas of Clinical Oncology: Lung Cancer.* Hamilton, ON, BC Decker, 2002, pp 71–93
85. Silvestri GA, Tanoue LT, Margolis ML, et al: The noninvasive staging of non-small cell lung cancer: the guidelines. *Chest* 123:147s–156s, 2003
86. MacDonald SLS, Hansell DM: Staging of non-small cell lung cancer: imaging of intrathoracic disease. *Eur J Radiol* 45:18–30, 2003
87. Feinstein AR, Sosin DM, Wells CK: The Will Rogers Phenomenon. Stage migration and new diagnostic techniques as a source of misleading statistics for survival in cancer. *N Engl J Medicine* 312:1604–1608, 1985
88. Diederich S, Wormanns D, Heindel W: Lung cancer screening with low dose CT. *Eur J Radiol* 45:2–7, 2003
89. Gaeta M, Caruso R, Barone M, et al: Ground glass attenuation in nodular bronchioloalveolar carcinoma: CT patterns and prognostic value. *J Comput Assist Tomogr* 22:215–219, 1998
90. LeBlanc JK, Espada R, Ergun G: Non-small cell lung cancer staging techniques and endoscopic ultrasound: tissue is still the issue. *Chest* 123:1718–1725, 2003
91. Pfister DG, Johnson DH, Azzoli CG, et al: American Society of Clinical Oncology treatment of unresectable non-small cell lung cancer guideline: update 2003. *J Clin Oncol* 22:1–24, 2004
92. Pope RJE, Hansell DM: Extra-thoracic staging of lung cancer. *Eur J Radiol* 45:31–38, 2003
93. Lobrano MB, Singha P: Positron emission tomography in oncology. *Clin J Oncol Nurs* 7:379–385, 2003
94. Marom EM, McAdams HP, Erasmus JJ, et al: Staging non-small cell lung cancer with whole body PET. *Radiology* 212:803–809, 1999
95. MacManus MP, Hicks RJ: PET scanning in lung cancer: current status and future directions. *Semin Surg Oncol* 21:149–155, 2003
96. Gould MK, Maclean CC, Kuschner WG, et al: Accuracy of positron emission tomography for diagnosis of pulmonary nodules and mass lesions: a meta-analysis. *JAMA* 285:914–924, 2001
97. Schreiber G, McCrory DC: Performance characteristics of different modalities for diagnosis of suspected lung cancer: summary of published evidence. *Chest* 123:115s–128s, 2003
98. Rivera MP, Detterbeck F, Mehta AC: Diagnosis of lung cancer. *Chest* 123:129s–136S, 2003
99. Toloza EM, Harpole L, Detterbeck F, et al: Invasive staging of non-small cell lung cancer: a review of the current evidence. *Chest* 123:157S–166S, 2003
100. Wallace MB, Fritscher-Ravens A, Savides TJ: Endoscopic ultrasound for the staging of non-small cell lung cancer. *Endoscopy* 32:606–610, 2003
101. Mountain CF, Dresler CM: Regional lymph node classification for lung cancer staging. *Chest* 111:1718–1723, 1997
102. Fritscher-Ravens A: Endoscopic ultrasound evaluation in the diagnosis and staging of lung cancer. *Lung Cancer* 41:259–267, 2003
103. Detterbeck FC, DeCamp MM, Kohman LJ, et al: Invasive staging: the guidelines. *Chest* 123:167S–175S, 2003
104. Beadsmoore CJ, Screaton NJ: Classification, staging, and prognosis of lung cancer. *Eur J Radiol* 45:8–17, 2003
105. Brundage MD, Davies D, Mackillop WJ: Prognostic factors in non-small cell lung cancer: a decade of progress. *Chest* 122:1037–1057, 2002
106. Osaki T, Nagashima A, Yoshimatsu T, et al: Survival and characteristics of lymph node involvement in patients with N1 non-small cell lung cancer. *Lung Cancer* 43:151–157, 2004
107. Danesi R, DeBraud F, Fogli S, et al: Pharmacogenetics of anticancer drug sensitivity in non-small cell lung cancer. *Pharmacol Rev* 55:57–103, 2003
108. Swinson DEB, Jones JL, Richardson D, et al: Tumour necrosis is an independent prognostic marker in non-small cell lung

cancer: correlation with biological variables. *Lung Cancer* 37:235–240, 2002
109. Meert AP, Martin B, Paesmans M, et al: The role of HER-2/neu expression on the survival of patients with lung cancer: a systematic review of the literature. *Br J Cancer* 89:959–965, 2003
110. Castelao JE, Bart RD, DiPerna CA, et al: Lung cancer and cyclooxygenase-2. *Ann Thorac Surg* 76:1327–1335, 2003
111. Brabender J, Danenberg KD, Metzger R, et al: Epidermal growth factor receptor and HER-2 neu mRNA expression in non-small cell lung cancer is correlated with survival. *Clin Cancer Res* 7:1850–1855, 2001
112. Piyathilake CJ, Frost AR, Manne U, et al: Differential expression of growth factors in squamous cell carcinoma and precancerous lesions of the lung. *Clin Cancer Res* 8:734–744, 2002
113. Komaki R: Combined treatment for limited small cell lung cancer. *Semin Oncol* 30(suppl 9):56–70, 2003
114. American Joint Committee on Cancer: *AJCC Cancer Staging Manual* (ed 6). New York, Springer, 2002
115. Wood AJJ: Multidisciplinary management of lung cancer. *N Engl J Med* 350:379–392, 2004
116. Alberts WM, Bepler G, Hazelton T, et al: Practice organization. *Chest* 123:332S–337S, 2003
117. Davies MJ: Multidisciplinary clinic approach to lung cancer, in Haas M (ed.): *Contemporary Issues in Lung Cancer: A Nursing Perspective.* Sudbury, MA, Jones and Bartlett, 2003, pp 93–107
118. Haigentz M, Keller SM: Concepts in the intraoperative staging of lymph nodes in non-small cell lung cancer and the role of mediastinal lymph node dissection. *Lung Cancer Princip Pract Updates* 2:1–12, 2002
119. Liptay MJ, Grondin SC, Fry WA, et al: Intraoperative sentinel lymph node mapping in non-small cell lung cancer improves detection of micrometastases. *J Clin Oncol* 20:1984–1988, 2002
120. Thomas CR, Williams TE, Cobos E, et al: Lung cancer, in Lenhard RE, Osteen RT, Gansler (eds): *Clinical Oncology.* Atlanta, American Cancer Society, 2001, p 269–295
121. Lin J, Iannettoni MD: The role of thoracoscopy in the management of lung cancer. *Surg Oncol* 12:195–200, 2003
122. Jaklitsch MT, Mery CM, Audisio RA: The use of surgery to treat lung cancer in elderly patients. *Lancet Oncol* 4:463–471, 2003
123. Li WWL, Lee TW, Lam SSY, et al: Quality of life following lung cancer resection: video-assisted thoracic surgery versus thoracotomy. *Chest* 122:584–589, 2002
124. Szczesny TJ, Szczesna A, Shepherd FA, et al: Surgical treatment of small cell lung cancer. *Semin Oncol* 30:47–56, 2003
125. Weinmann M, Branislav B, Bamberg M, et al: Treatment of lung cancer in elderly part II: small cell lung cancer. *Lung Cancer* 40:1–16, 2003
126. Vaporciyan AA, Merriman KW, Ece F, et al: Incidence of major pulmonary morbidity after pneumonectomy: association with timing of smoking cessation. *Ann Thorac Surg* 73:420–426, 2002
127. Nakagawa M, Tanaka H, Tsukuma H, et al: Relationship between the duration of the preoperative smoke-free period and the incidence of postoperative pulmonary complications after pulmonary surgery. *Chest* 120:705–710, 2001
128. Quinn KL: Managing patients through thoracic surgery, in Haas M (ed.): *Contemporary Issues in Lung Cancer: A Nursing Perspective.* Sudbury, MA, Jones and Bartlett, 2003, pp. 33–48
129. Bush NJ, Griffin-Sobel JP: Acute postoperative pain management and malfunctioning epidural catheter. *Oncol Nurs Forum* 30:217–218, 2003
130. Rosenzweig KE, Amols H, Ling CC: New radiotherapy technologies. *Semin Surg Oncol* 21:190–195, 2003
131. Lee W, Daly BDT, DiPetrillo TA, et al: Limited resection for non-small cell lung cancer: observed local control with implantation of I-125 brachytherapy seeds. *Ann Thorac Surg* 75:237–243, 2003
132. Toy E, Macbeth F, Coles B, et al: Palliative thoracic radiotherapy for non-small cell lung cancer: a systematic review. *Am J Clin Oncol* 26:112–120, 2003
133. Gore EM: Prophylactic cranial irradiation for patients with locally advanced non-small-cell lung cancer. *Oncology* 17: 775–779, 2003
134. Saha D, Pyo Hongryull, Choy H: COX-2 inhibitor as a radiation enhancer: new strategies for the treatment of lung cancer. *Am J Clin Oncol* 26(suppl 2):S70–S74, 2003
135. Herbst RS, O'Reilly MS: The rationale and potential of combining novel biologic therapies with radiotherapy: focus on non-small cell lung cancer. *Semin Oncol* 30:113–123, 2003
136. Erridge SC, Murray N: Thoracic radiotherapy for limited-stage small cell lung cancer: issues of timing, volumes, dose, and fractionation. *Semin Oncol* 30:26–37, 2003
137. Yang GY, Matthews RH: Prophylactic cranial irradiation in small cell lung cancer. *Oncologist* 5:293–298, 2000
138. McManamen L: Interstitial densities following radiotherapy. *Clin J Oncol Nurs* 7:209–211, 2003
139. Moghissi K, Dixon K: Is bronchoscopic photodynamic therapy a therapeutic option in lung cancer? *Eur Respirat J* 22:535–541, 2003
140. Inzeo D, Haughney A: Laser therapy in the management of lung cancer. *Clin J Oncol Nurs* 8:94–95, 2004
141. Bruce S: Photodynamic therapy: another option in cancer treatment. *Clin J Oncol Nurs* 5:95–99, 2001
142. Ost D: Photodynamic therapy in lung cancer. *Oncology* 14:379–391, 2000
143. Hinton S, Sandler A: Lung cancer in the elderly: current and future therapeutic options. *Drugs Aging* 19:365–375, 2002
144. International Adjuvant Lung Cancer Trial Collaborative Group: Cisplatin-based adjuvant chemotherapy in patients with completely resected non-small-cell lung cancer. *N Engl J Med* 350:351–360, 2004
145. Blum RH: Adjuvant chemotherapy for lung cancer — a new standard of care. *N Engl J Med* 350:404–405, 2004
146. Edelman MJ: Neoadjuvant chemotherapy and chemoradiotherapy for non-small cell lung cancer: current status and future prospects. *Exp Opin Pharmacother* 4:843–852, 2003
147. Rusch VW, Giroux DJ, Kraut MJ, et al: Induction chemoradiation and surgical resection for non-small cell lung carcinomas of the superior sulcus: initial results of Southwest Oncology Group Trial 9416 (intergroup trial 0160). *J Thorac Cardiovasc Surg* 121:472–483, 2001
148. Pisters KNW, Ginsberg RJ, Giroux DJ, et al: Induction chemotherapy before surgery for early stage lung cancer: a novel approach. *J Thorac Cardiovasc Surg* 119:429–439, 2000
149. Van Zandwijk N, Smith EF, Kramer GW, et al: Gemcitabine and cisplatin as induction regimen for patients with biopsy proven stage IIIA N2 non-small-cell lung cancer: a phase II study of the European Organization for Research and Treatment of Cancer Lung Cancer Cooperative Group (EORTC 08955). *J Clin Oncol* 18:2658–2664, 2000
150. Rosell R, Gatzmeir U, Betticher DC, et al: Phase III randomized trial comparing paclitaxel/carboplatin with paclitaxel/cisplatin in patients with advanced non-small cell lung cancer: a cooperative multinational trial. *Ann Oncol* 13:1539–1549, 2002
151. Rodriguez J, Pawell J, Pluzanska A, et al: A multicenter randomized phase III study of docetaxel + cisplatin and docetaxel + carboplatin versus vinorelbine + cisplatin in chemotherapy naïve patients with advanced and metastatic non-small cell lung cancer. *Proc Am Soc Clin Oncol* 20:314a, 2001 (abstr 1252)
152. Bonomi P, Kim K, Fairclough D, et al: Comparison of survival and quality of life in advanced non-small-cell lung cancer patients treated with two dose levels of paclitaxel combined with

cisplatin versus etoposide with cisplatin: results of an Eastern Cooperative Oncology Group trial. *J Clin Oncol* 18:623–631, 2000

153. Schiller JH, Harrington D, Belani CP, et al: Comparison of four chemotherapy regimens for advanced non-small-cell lung cancer. *N Engl J Med* 346:92–98, 2002
154. Shepherd FA, Dancey J, Ramlau R, et al: Prospective randomized trial of docetaxel versus best supportive care in patients with non-small cell lung cancer previously treated with platinum-based chemotherapy. *J Clin Oncol* 18:2095–2103, 2000
155. Fosella FV, DeVore R, Kerr RN, et al: Randomized phase III trial of docetaxel versus vinorelbine or ifosfamide in patients with advanced non-small-cell lung cancer previously treated with platinum containing chemotherapy regimens. *J Clin Oncol* 18:2354–2362, 2000
156. Sandler AB: Chemotherapy for small cell lung cancer. *Semin Oncol* 30:9–25, 2003
157. Traynor AM, Schiller JH: First-line therapy in the treatment of advanced lung cancer. *Lung Cancer Princip Pract Update* 3:1–16, 2003
158. Eckardt JR: Second-line treatment of small-cell lung cancer. *Oncology* 17:181–188, 191, 2003
159. Rowinsky EK: The pursuit of optimal outcomes in cancer therapy in a new age of rationally designed target-based anticancer agents. *Drugs* 60(suppl 1):1–14, 2000
160. Kim ES: Targeted therapies in non-small cell lung cancer. *Lung Cancer Princip Pract Update* 3:1–19, 2003
161. Cohen MH, Williams GA, Sridhara R, et al: FDA drug approval summary: gefitinib (ZD1839) (Iressa) tablets. *Oncologist* 8:303–306, 2003
162. Herbst RS, Kies MS: ZD1839 (Iressa) in non-small cell lung cancer. *Oncologist* 7(suppl 4):9–15, 2002
163. Cella D: Impact of ZD1839 on non-small cell lung cancer-related symptoms as measured by the functional assessment of cancer therapy-lung scale. *Semin Oncol* 30(suppl 1):39–48, 2003
164. Giaccone G, Herbst RS, Manegold C, et al: Gefitinib in combination with gemcitabine and cisplatin in advanced non-small-cell lung cancer: a phase III trial — INTACT 1. *J Clin Oncol* 22:777–784, 2004
165. Herbst RS, Giaccone G, Schiller JH, et al: Gefitinib in combination with paclitaxel and carboplatin in advanced non-small-cell lung cancer: a phase III trial — INTACT 2. *J Clin Oncol* 22:785–794, 2004
166. Bonomi P: Erlotinib: a new therapeutic approach for non-small cell lung cancer. *Exp Opin Investig Drugs* 12:1395–1401, 2003
167. Adjei AA: An overview of farnesyltransferase inhibitors and their role in lung cancer therapy. *Lung Cancer* 41:S55–S62, 2003
168. Shepherd FA, Sridhar SS: Angiogenesis inhibitors under study for the treatment of lung cancer. *Lung Cancer* 41:S63–S72, 2003
169. Mack PC, Davies AM, Lara PN, et al: Integration of the proteasome inhibitor Ps-341 (Velcade) into the therapeutic approach to lung cancer. *Lung Cancer* 41:S89–S96, 2003
170. Hege KM, Carbone DP: Lung cancer vaccines and gene therapy. *Lung Cancer* 41:S103–S113, 2003
171. Bunn PA, Shepherd FA, Sandler A, et al: Ongoing and future trials of biologic therapies in lung cancer. *Lung Cancer* 41:S175–S186, 2003
172. Tanaka K, Akechi T, Okuyama T, et al: Impact of dyspnea, pain, and fatigue on daily life activities in ambulatory patients with advanced lung cancer. *J Pain Sympt Manage* 23:417–423, 2002
173. Gift AG, Jablonski A, Stommel, et al: Symptom clusters in elderly patients with lung cancer. *Oncol Nurs Forum* 31:203–212, 2004
174. Potter J, Higginson IJ: pain experienced by lung cancer patients: a review of prevalence, causes and pathophysiology. *Lung Cancer* 43:247–257, 2004
175. Kvale PA, Simoff M, Prakash UBS: Palliative care. *Chest* 123:284S–311S, 2003
176. Viale PH, Yamamoto DS: Bisphosphonates: expanded roles in the treatment of patients with cancer. *Clin J Oncol Nurs* 7:393–401, 2003
177. Wickham R: Dyspnea: recognizing and managing an invisible problem. *Oncol Nurs Forum* 29:925–933, 2002
178. Brubacher S, Gobel BH: Use of the Pleurx pleural catheter for the management of malignant pleural effusions. *Clin J Oncol Nurs* 7:35–38, 2003
179. Downey RJ: Follow-up after lung cancer resection, in Ginsberg RJ (ed.): *American Cancer Society Atlas of Clinical Oncology: Lung Cancer.* Hamilton, ON, BC Decker, 2002, pp 121–129
180. Smith TJ: Evidence-based follow-up of lung cancer patients. *Semin Oncol* 30:361–368, 2003
181. Colice GL, Rubins J, Unger M: Follow-up and surveillance of the lung cancer patient following curative-intent therapy. *Chest* 123:272S–283S, 2003

CHAPTER 58

Lymphomas

Sharon D. Manson, RN, MS, ACNP
Carlene Porter, RN, MSN, ACNP

Introduction

Hodgkin's lymphoma (HL) and non-Hodgkin's lymphoma (NHL) constitute a diverse group of cancers of the immune system. Arising from a single malignant lymphoid clone, the lymphoma may be B cell, T cell, or NK cell in origin. It is thought that lymphomagenesis results from a genetic change or series of changes that allows the cell to evade programmed cell death (apoptosis) or to grow uncontrollably. The subtype of lymphoma and its degree of aggressiveness depend on the precise genetic changes and the stage of lymphocyte maturation at which these changes occurred. During the disease course, a lymphoma can acquire additional abnormalities that may change its aggressiveness and prognosis.

The National Cancer Institute (NCI) predicted that there would be 62,250 new cases of lymphoma in the United States in 2004, with 20,730 deaths being attributed to this disease.[1] NHL was expected to account for 54,370 of the cases, while the much rarer HL was predicted to account for 7880 cases.[1] In the United States, the incidence of lymphoma increases with age and tends to show a male predominance. Since the 1970s, the incidence of NHL has almost doubled.[2] According to the NCI's Surveillance, Epidemiology, and End Result (SEER) program, the following subgroups have experienced a steady increase in NHL: young whites (age 15–24 years), older blacks (age ≥ 55 years), and females (age 25–54 years). Suspected reasons for these increases include a compromised immune system [e.g., from human immunodeficiency virus (HIV), infection, and the use of immunosuppressive drugs], environmental carcinogens, other infectious agents, and genetic predisposition. Unfortunately, the majority of people who will be diagnosed with lymphoma have no known risk factors.

Lymphoid Tissues and the Immune System

The immune system is a highly integrated, complex mechanism that has evolved to help the body protect itself against invading microbes such as viruses, bacteria, fungi, and parasites. Another important function of the immune system is to differentiate "self-antigens" from "nonself" or foreign antigens and to orchestrate specific and nonspecific measures to destroy the foreign antigens. The main organs of the immune system are scattered throughout the body and are referred to as the lymphatics or lymphoid tissues. Malignant lymphomas arise from these tissues.

The lymphoid tissues can be divided into primary and secondary lymphoid organs (see Figure 58-1). The primary organs are represented by the bone marrow, where the lymphocytes originate, and the thymus, where T lymphocytes mature. The thymus is a large organ located in the mediastinum that grows rapidly in the first two years of life, grows more slowly through puberty, and then slowly involutes. Adipose and connective tissue replace thymic tissue, and the thymus shrinks in size. Once the maturation of T lymphocytes is complete, the lymphocytes migrate to the secondary lymphoid tissues through the circulation. B lymphocytes derive their name from the bone marrow and T lymphocytes from the thymus.

The lymph nodes, spleen, and mucosa-associated lymphoid tissues (MALTs) form the secondary lymphatics. The MALTs are clumps of lymphocytes that protect the respiratory and gastrointestinal epithelium. These tissues include the tonsils, adenoids, appendix, and Peyer's patches, which are found in the small intestine. Those tissues associated with the gut have been named gut-associated lymphoid tissues (GALTs); and those associated with the bronchial tree are called

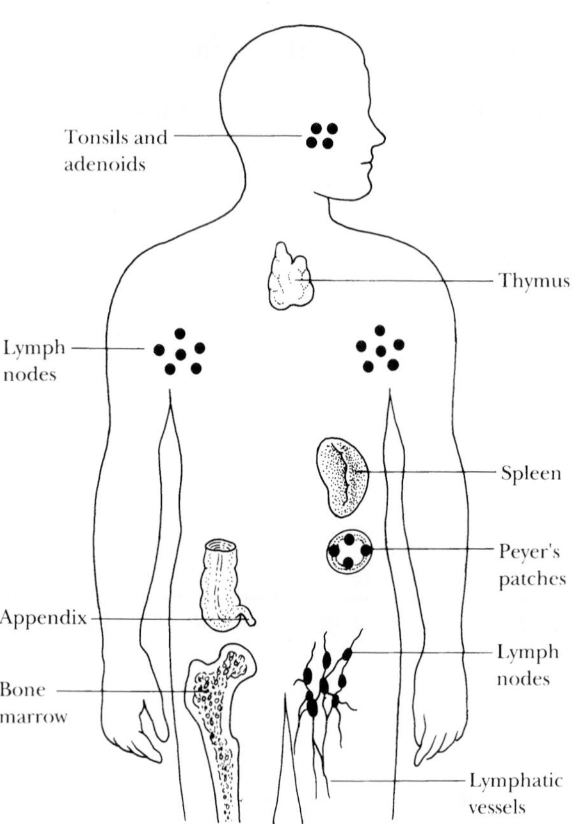

Figure 58-1 Organs of the immune system. (Illustrated by J. Thommen.)

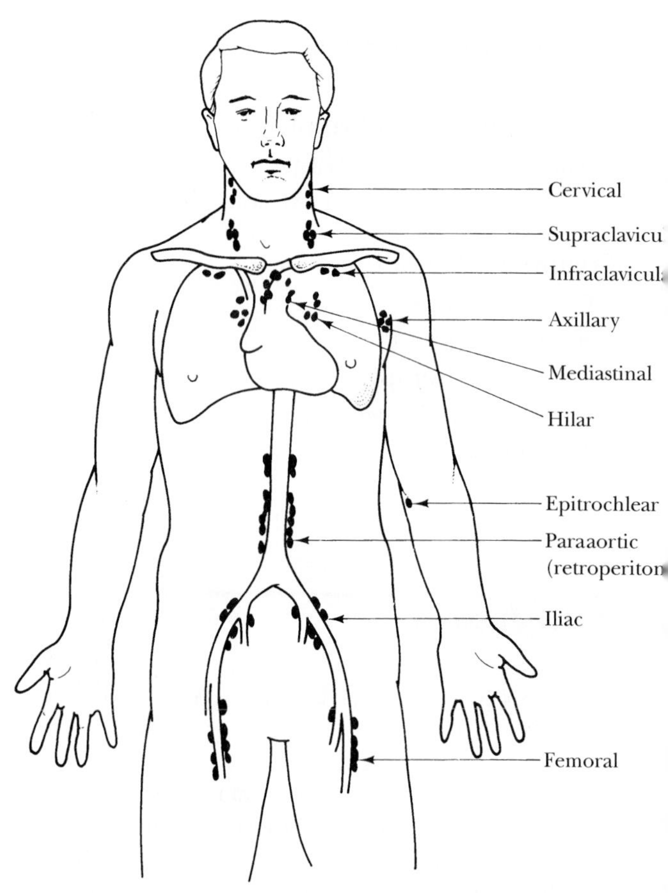

Figure 58-2 Major lymph node groups.

bronchial-associated lymphoid tissues (BALTs). Singular lymph nodules are found in and below the mucosa of the respiratory tract, the gastrointestinal tract, the urinary tract, and the vagina.[3] The blood and the lymphatic vessels that transport lymphocytes can also be considered part of this system.

Extracellular fluid, known as lymph, is drained via the afferent lymphatics to the lymph nodes. This fluid also carries antigens from sites of infection to the lymph nodes. Lymph nodes are encapsulated, highly organized structures that facilitate lymphocyte maturation and differentiation. They are found scattered throughout the body in the neck, axilla, chest, abdomen, and groin (Figure 58-2). The lymph node has an outer cortex and an inner medulla. The cortex contains follicles comprising largely B lymphocytes and a small number of T cells that facilitate B-cell differentiation. Some follicles contain germinal centers and are called secondary follicles. Deeper paracortical areas selectively concentrate T lymphocytes and dendritic cells. The medulla contains strands of T and B lymphocytes, macrophages, and antibody-secreting plasma cells. The architecture of the lymph node can be seen in Figure 58-3.

Lymph leaves the lymph node through the efferent lymphatics in the medulla and is transported to the thoracic duct. This duct returns the lymph to the circulatory system through the left subclavian vein. The organization of the spleen is similar to that of a lymph node; however, antigens enter the spleen through the blood, not the lymph.

Lymphomas are preeminently a malignancy of the lymphocytes, and the process by which a lymphoid neoplasm is generated may be envisioned as a series of cellular changes in which a normal lymphoid cell (or cell clone) becomes refractory to the regulation of its differentiation and proliferation. The unregulated growth is due to genetic mutations, chromosomal translocations, deletions, and insertions of foreign genes into the cell. Translocations occur when genetic material from one chromosome becomes rearranged with another chromosome, altering the expression of adjacent genes. This alters the expression and function of the genes, disrupting control of cell growth. Genes that result in the development of cancer when their expression and function are altered are called oncogenes. Deletions result in a loss of genetic material in a particular gene, whereas insertions result in the addition of other genetic material into a particular chromosome. These alterations may also result in deficiencies of cell growth and function. Follicular

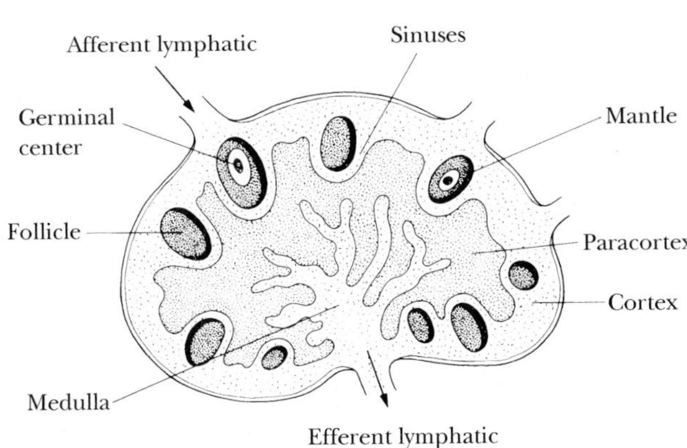

B-CELL LYMPHOMAS
Follicle
- Nodular lymphoma
- Large cell lymphoma
- Burkitt's lymphoma

Germinal Center/Mantle Zone
- Lymphocytic lymphoma
- Mantle zone lymphoma (intermediate differentiation)

Medulla
- Chronic lymphocytic leukemia
- Well-differentiated lymphocytic lymphoma
- Waldenström's macroglobulinemia

T-CELL LYMPHOMAS
Paracortex
- Peripheral T-cell lymphoma
- Mycosis fungoides
- Sézary syndrome
- Acute lymphoblastic leukemia
- T-cell lymphoblastic lymphoma

Miscellaneous Malignancies
Sinus Region
- Malignant histiocytosis
- Kt-1 large cell lymphoma

Figure 58-3 Sites of lymphocyte transformation in the lymph node. (Illustrated by J. Thommen.)

lymphomas are believed to be tumors of germinal center B cells in which the cells fail to undergo programmed death (apoptosis) because they have a chromosome translocation. Translocations, deletions, and insertions may be identified microscopically when dividing cells (metaphases) are analyzed.

Once transformed, the new clone of malignant cells follows the behavior pattern of the stage at which lymphocyte alteration took place. For example, if the function of the maturing lymphocyte is secretion of an antibody protein, the tumor cells will continue to secrete the antibody, albeit in abnormal quantities. The neoplasms' tendency to mimic the normal cells' differentiation serves as the basis for their classification.

The association of certain malignancies with congenital or acquired immunodeficiency states and the bimodal distribution of cancer in the very young and the very old suggest that an immature or debilitated immune system predisposes an individual to developing neoplasia.[4] Malignant lymphomas are strongly linked with congenital immunodeficiency disorders such as Wiskott-Aldrich syndrome, Klinefelter syndrome, and ataxia telangiectasia and in acquired diseases such as HIV infection. Patients who have had prior organ or stem cell transplantation are at higher risk for the development of lymphomas. The etiology of these post-transplant lymphoproliferative disorders is thought to be multifactorial, including immunosuppression (often drug induced) and the presence of Epstein-Barr virus (EBV). Epstein-Barr and other viruses have been implicated in the etiology of lymphoma. Likewise, some bacteria or the immunologic response to the antigens found on the bacteria may contribute to the formation of malignant cells. This relationship has been best identified with the *Helicobacter pylori* bacteria. The chronic inflammatory process activated by many autoimmune diseases (e.g., rheumatoid arthritis, systemic lupus erythematosus, and Sjogren syndrome) and the immunosuppressive treatment of these disorders may predispose these individuals to lymphoma.

Lymphocytes, like other blood cell types, originate in the bone marrow from the pluripotent stem cells. Pluripotent stem cells have the ability to self-replicate and differentiate into myeloid stem cells or lymphoid stem cells. Immature lymphocyte precursors arise from the commitment of the lymphoid stem cells. Subsequent maturation of these primitive cells leads to the development of mature T lymphocytes and B lymphocytes, as illustrated in Figure 58-4.

Lymphocytes are responsible for cellular and humoral immunity—both important immunologic defenses. An early step in the differentiation of the maturing lymphocyte occurs when the cell is programmed either by the bone marrow (bursa equivalent) or the thymus to become a B lymphocyte or T lymphocyte. Plasma cells develop from B lymphocytes and produce circulating antibodies against foreign antigens upon exposure. These B lymphocytes serve as the basis of humoral immunity. Memory cells are also produced to establish long-lasting immunity. Cellular immunity consists of circulating T lymphocytes that

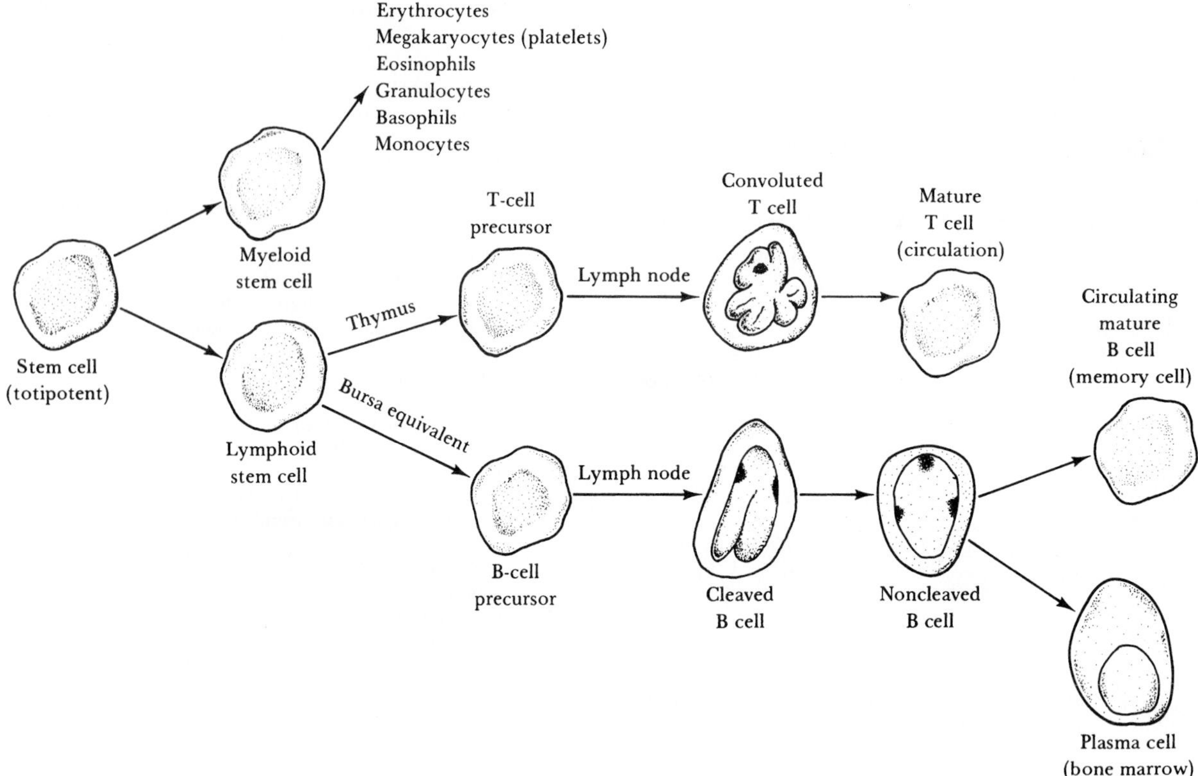

Figure 58-4 Maturation sequence of the lymphocyte. (Illustrated by J. Thommen.)

have developed specificity against foreign antigens. T lymphocytes, when stimulated, will clone into subsets of cells that include cytotoxic, suppressor, helper, and memory T cells. These subsets work together to kill identified targets and to regulate the immune process. Although the humoral and cellular arms of the immune system are distinct entities, they have a high degree of interaction and together protect the host against foreign proteins.

Approximately 90% of lymphomas worldwide have a B-cell origin, and most patients initially present with disease involving the lymph nodes or bone marrow and, to a lesser degree, the liver and spleen.[5] Extranodal disease — either extension from a node or an isolated site — can be observed either at the time of diagnosis or during the course of the disease. If the extranodal involvement occurs as the only site of the lymphoma, it is called primary extranodal lymphoma. This condition can include tissues such as the central nervous system (CNS), eye, paranasal sinuses, skin, lung, pericardium, gastrointestinal tract, testicle, spleen, bone, bone marrow, genitourinary tract, and, rarely, the heart, salivary glands, adrenals, and thyroid.

Lymphomas with a T-cell origin are less frequently observed but often present with more aggressive features. They are known to be among the most aggressive of all hematological neoplasms, although variability is seen. T-cell lymphomas are often grouped with neoplasms that arise from natural killer (NK) cells. Mature T-lymphocyte malignancies arise from post-thymic T cells. Because NK cells are closely related and share many properties, the two types of cancers are often considered together.

Diagnosis

The diagnosis of Hodgkin's or non-Hodgkin's lymphoma is made based on biopsy and histopathology of the tumor. The clinical presentation and subsequent assessment of the patient are often quite similar between these two malignancies and lead to a staging work-up. In this section, the diagnostic evaluation will be discussed in general terms. Each pathological subtype of lymphoma may have unique characteristics, which will be noted in the discussion of that specific disease entity.

Clinical Manifestations

Lymphadenopathy is the most common presentation in patients with lymphoma. It may be unilateral or bilateral. Characteristic nodes are nontender, firm, and rubbery. Some patients with HL report pain at involved lymph node sites with alcohol consumption.

The size of the lymph node varies, as does the growth pattern. Patients may report a slow, insidious growth of the node or even a waxing and waning pattern. Patients with a more aggressive lymphoma may report rapid growth of the mass and spread to contiguous or noncontiguous nodes. Lymph nodes of the same region may coalesce, forming a fixed mass. In such a case, individual nodes may be impossible to distinguish and measure.

Hodgkin's lymphoma presents most commonly in the cervical and supraclavicular area, with involvement of axillary and inguinal nodes being reported in less than 10% of the patients. Mediastinal lymphadenopathy may be noted on routine chest x-ray, or complaints of cough and dyspnea may have led to a chest radiograph being performed.

Patients with NHL are more likely to present with extranodal disease. Approximately 25%–50% of NHL cases show evidence of extranodal disease and may present with signs and symptoms related to its presence.

The liver or spleen may be involved in both HL and NHL. Related symptoms include pain, abdominal complaints, anorexia, early satiety, and even signs of bowel obstruction.

Lymphoma can occasionally infiltrate the skin. These lesions appear as red or purplish nodules, primarily in the head and neck region. Lytic bone lesions may be seen in the femurs, pelvis, vertebrae, ribs, and skull. Affected patients frequently complain of bone pain, which leads to the diagnosis of lymphoma. These lesions must be differentiated from bone metastasis, from solid tumors, or the lytic lesions observed in multiple myeloma. On rare occasions, lymphomas may present as oncologic emergencies such as cardiac tamponade, superior vena cava syndrome, spinal cord compression, increased intracranial pressure, or sepsis. These presentations are often due to the growth of aggressive lymphomas resulting in obstruction of lymphatic or circulatory vessels. Solitary brain lymphomas are being reported with increasing frequency and are associated with AIDS or iatrogenic immunosuppression. These mass lesions may result in headaches, seizures, and changes in mental status. Another common central nervous system manifestation is leptomeningeal spread, which results in cranial nerve palsies, meningeal irritation, and increased intracranial pressure. Replacement of the bone marrow by lymphoma can lead to a deficiency of the normal white blood cells, red blood cells, and platelets, resulting in a picture similar to that seen with leukemia.

It is important to determine whether the patient has experienced night sweats, fever, or nonintentional weight loss resulting in a loss of more than 10% of body weight within six months of presentation. The presence of these "B" symptoms (two of the three symptoms noted here) has an unfavorable prognostic significance. Patients with NHL are more likely than patients with HL to present with "B" symptoms, but these events have less prognostic significance in NHL. Other characteristic symptoms of lymphoma include generalized pruritus and fatigue, but the significance of these symptoms is unclear. Pruritis is found in as many as 30% of patients with HL prior to diagnosis.[6] Occasionally, patients with HL may complain of cyclical fevers, called Pel Ebstein fevers.

Biopsy

Few areas of pathology have evoked as much controversy and confusion as the classification of lymphoma. Nevertheless, following history and physical examination, pathological diagnosis is required. A biopsy of the involved tissue is done to formulate the diagnosis of lymphoma. In most situations, morphology (the way the cell looks) and immunophenotyping (the markers identified on the tumor) done via flow cytometry are sufficient for diagnosis of the subtype of lymphoma. In addition, immunoglobulin and T-cell receptor gene rearrangements are often performed on the involved tissues.

Other studies include polymerase chain reaction (PCR) for *BCL-1* and *BCL-2*, immunohistochemistry studies, and cytogetics. Cytogenetic studies assess for translocations, insertions, and deletions, which may be reflective of a particular subclassification of lymphoma or may have prognostic significance. Florescent in situ hybridization (FISH) is a method of analyzing large numbers of cells to assess for a particular genetic abnormality. This test may be employed if a specific type of lymphoma is suspected and can aid in diagnosis or monitoring for disease status following treatment. All available data are utilized to define the disease, predict response, and refine treatment plans.

Staging

Accurate staging is critical in the management of patients with lymphoma. It directs the intensity of treatment and allows for less toxic therapy to be administered when minimal disease is present, decreasing the risk of secondary malignancies and improving quality of life.[7] Clinical, pathological, and radiographic data are utilized to determine the stage of disease. Staging laporatomy, considered controversial for years, is rarely indicated today. On rare occasions, surgery may be required to relieve an obstruction or to obtain pathological diagnosis.

Table 58-1 Cotswold Modification of Ann Arbor Staging System

Stage	Criteria
I	Involvement of a single lymph node region
	or
I_E	Involvement of a single extranodal organ or site
II	Involvement of two or more lymph node regions on the same side of the diaphragm
	or
II_E	Involvement of a contiguous extranodal organ or site
III	Involvement of lymph node regions on both sides of the diaphragm
	or
III_S	Involvement on both sides of diaphragm including the spleen
	or
III_E	Involvement on both sides of the diaphragm with a contiguous extranodal organ or site
	or
III_{ES}	Involvement on both sides of the diaphragm including the spleen and a contiguous extranodal organ or site
IV	Multiple or disseminated sites of disease; may involve multiple extranodal organs or sites with or without lymphatic involvement

All cases should be subclassified with either "A" to indicate the absence of B symptoms or "B" to indicate the presence of B symptoms.

Clinical staging (CS) is determined by history, physical examination, biopsy, and laboratory and radiographic tests. Pathological staging (PS) is determined by biopsy of strategic sites and histopathological information.

The Ann Arbor staging classification system was created for the staging of HL.[8] Although it is not optimal for the staging of NHL, it has been viewed for years as the gold standard. The Ann Arbor staging system identifies four specific stages based on the number and location of lymph node regions or extranodal tissues determined to be involved. A modification of the Ann Arbor staging system was made to include the identification of those individuals with extranodal or splenic involvement. Known as the Cotswold modification of the Ann Arbor system, it is outlined in Table 58-1.[9] The absence of "B" symptoms is denoted with an "A" after the appropriate stage; the presence of "B" symptoms is indicated with a "B".

Laboratory Tests

Laboratory studies performed as initial staging include blood chemistries and a complete blood count. Elevations of the hepatic transaminase levels (AST and ALT) and, more specifically, an alkaline phosphatase level greater than twice the normal limit suggest liver involvement.[10] Fractionation of alkaline phosphatase may be useful in identifying the source of disease (i.e., liver versus bone). Unfortunately, these laboratory findings are nonspecific and may be elevated without radiographic evidence of disease. Bone marrow involvement may result in a deficiency of the normal mature cells produced in the marrow, leading to anemia and thrombocytopenia. Leukocytosis is often noted at presentation or at other points of disease activity. Lymphopenia is found in 50% of individuals diagnosed with HL and is a poor prognostic factor. Eosinophilia may also be seen. The erythrocyte sedimentation rate (ESR) is characteristically elevated in HL and may be used as a crude marker for disease activity. This test has been employed more commonly in Europe than in the United States.[10] The *BCL-2* (B-cell lymphoma) gene, present in some lymphomas, corresponds to a poor response to chemotherapy and reduced survival. The tumor or the blood can be analyzed for the presence of this gene.

Due to patchy infiltration of lymphoma, bilateral bone marrow aspirate and biopsies are performed to assess for evidence of disease. Flow cytometry and cytogenetic studies are often done on the bone marrow specimens to further characterize the tumor.

Radiographic Tests

Computerized tomography (CT) scans of the chest, abdomen, and pelvis are completed at diagnosis to delineate sites of disease that may not be clinically evident. A CT scan or magnetic resonance imaging (MRI) of the brain may be performed as well as a lumbar puncture with analysis of the CNS, if symptoms dictate it. Gallium scans have historically been performed as part of staging of lymphomas. If the tumor is positive for gallium, this scan will detect areas of disease and may be used in follow-up to determine response.

Positron emission tomography (PET) scan is a novel imaging technique that uses a radiolabeled glucose analog. The glycolytic activity is greater in tissues with metabolic activity. A higher uptake is observed in malignant tissues and, to a lesser degree, in areas of inflammation. PET scans appear to detect more disease sites above and below the diaphragm than gallium scans and have better sensitivity in detecting disease in the spleen. They may identify lymphomatous organ involvement that would otherwise not be documented by CT or MRI.[11,12] The reliability of PET scans in detecting malignant disease is greater than 90% in classical Hodgkin's disease, diffuse B-cell lymphoma, follicular lymphoma, and mantle cell lymphoma. They are less reliable (50%–90% positive) in marginal zone or mucosa-associated lymphoma tissue (MALT) lymphoma and small lymphocytic lymphoma.[12] Some lymphomas may have poor sensitivity to PET scanning. In one study, only 40% of cases with peripheral T-cell lymphomas were detected by PET scanning and bone marrow disease correlated poorly when compared to bone marrow biopsies in all subtypes.[13] PET scans, like gallium scans, cannot quantify the dimensions of the tumor and may be used only as an adjunct to CT scanning. The cost and the limited number of PET scanning units may impact the use of this technology.

International Prognostic Index

Sixteen institutions and cooperative groups in the United States, Canada, and Europe participated in a project to develop a model for prognostic factors for patients with aggressive NHL.[14] Patients with aggressive NHL, who were treated with similar regimens between 1982 and 1987, were evaluated for clinical and laboratory features that were predictive for overall survival and relapse-free survival. This analysis resulted in the development of an International Prognostic Index (IPI) based on age, stage of disease, serum LDH, performance status, and number of extranodal disease sites. Four risk groups were identified, with 5-year survival rates of 73%, 51%, 43%, and 26%, respectively.[14] While the IPI was originally developed for NHL patients with aggressive tumors, it has since been analyzed with various types of lymphoma.[15] The model has been successful in identifying patients with high- and low-risk follicular lymphoma, and other indolent, low-grade disease.[16–18] A working group in the Netherlands validated the IPI in low-, intermediate-, and high-grade lymphoma.[19] Table 58-2 details the IPI scoring.

Table 58-2 International Prognostic Index

Clinical Feature	Points
Age	
Age ≤ 60 years	0
Age > 60 years	1
Performance Status	
ECOG 0–1	0
ECOG 2–4	1
Ann Arbor Stage	
I to II	0
III to IV	1
Extranodal Involvement	
< 2 sites	0
≥ 2 sites	1
Serum LDH	
LDH normal	0
LDH elevated	1

To obtain IPI, add points from each category.

Low risk = 0–1
Low-intermediate risk = 2
High-intermediate risk = 3
High risk = 4–5

Hodgkin's Disease

Historical Perspective

In 1832, Thomas Hodgkin, an English physician, described clinical data and postmortem findings of seven patients with a relentlessly progressive, ultimately fatal, tumorous enlargement of the lymph nodes, liver, and spleen.[20] His recognition that these pathological changes represented a primary proliferation inherent in the nodal tissues themselves rather than a reactive, inflammatory process was extremely important and insightful. Prior to that time, lymphomas often were mistaken for a common infectious disease, tuberculosis of the lymph nodes.

More than three decades after Hodgkin's paper was presented, Samuel Wilks rediscovered the original manuscript. After further clinical clarification and elaboration, he attached the eponym *Hodgkin's disease* to the phenomenon in 1865.[21] A review of the original tissues nearly 100 years later demonstrated that Hodgkin's cases actually represented examples of what we now call Hodgkin's disease (HD) as well as non-Hodgkin's lymphoma. All lymphomas were called HD until around the turn of the century, when the giant, multinucleated cells in the nodal material of HD patients were characterized by Reed[22] and Sternberg,[23] and their names have been associated with the pathognomonic cell of HL ever since. Subsequently, those lymphomas demonstrating the Reed-Sternberg cell were classified as HL and those in which the cell was absent were called lymphosarcoma or reticulum cell sarcoma and later NHL. Although the precise nature and origin of the Reed-Sternberg cell remain uncertain, it is believed that this cell is B cell in origin and useful in predicting prognosis. Lymphocytic malignancies that are similar in pathological appearance behave differently depending on the presence or absence of this cell.

Today, diagnosis of HD requires two components. First, the presence of Reed-Sternberg cells must be documented. Second, the diagnostic cells must be identified within an appropriate cellular background that is composed of a polymorphous mixture of apparently normal inflammatory cells in various proportions.

Epidemiology

Hodgkin's disease accounts for less than 1% of all new cancers in the Unites States and approximately 15% of all lymphomas. Approximately 7880 new cases of Hodgkin's disease were expected to be diagnosed in 2004. The number of new cases of Hodgkin's lymphoma has declined since the late 1980s at the rate of 0.9% per year.[24] Although a relatively uncommon disease, it has been one of the most widely studied over the years and is considered one of the most curable, with a five-year survival of 84%. There is a slightly higher incidence in males than in females over all age spans (3:2 ratio), but 85% of childhood HL is observed in males.[24]

In Western countries, Hodgkin's lymphoma has a bimodal age distribution. The rates rise through early life, peak in the third decade, and decline through age 45, at which time the incidence again increases. Geographic patterns have been identified in the three major age groups: childhood, young adult, and older adults. In childhood, mixed cellular Hodgkin's lymphoma is seen commonly in less developed countries. More favorable subtypes are seen in developed countries in young adulthood. Several studies have supported the increased risk of Hodgkin's disease in young adults with high socioeconomic status.[25–27] High intelligence, higher education, small family size, early birth order, and single-family dwellings have all been identified as factors associated with higher risk.[28,29] There is a clear association between infectious exposure with Epstein-Barr virus and HL, with a threefold increased risk in patients with a history of mononucleosis. This linkage exemplifies the association between socioeconomic and environmental factors in the risk of developing Hodgkin's lymphoma.

Etiology

Many reports have suggested an infectious etiology of HL. "B" symptoms such as fever and chills, as well as leukocytosis and pathological changes similar to a granulomatous process, support this theory. Clusters of reported cases have even led to the question of infectious transmission. Significant controversy remains regarding this hypothesis, and many believe that statistical analyses show that these cases likely occurred by chance.[28] Nevertheless, it is has clearly been documented that a prior history of mononucleosis with serologically confirmed Epstein-Barr virus (EBV) results in a threefold increased risk of Hodgkin's lymphoma in young adults. In developing countries, exposure to EBV occurs in early childhood. In several studies, 85%–100% of pediatric patients diagnosed with HL had associated EBV exposure. One study reported that HIV-infected individuals who developed HL had a high frequency of EBV with the Reed-Sternberg cells.[30]

Evidence supports a genetic basis for increased susceptibility to Hodgkin's lymphoma. It has been difficult to distinguish genetic influences from environmental factors in these situations, however, and both may contribute to the increased risk of developing lymphoma. There is a sevenfold increased risk for the development of HL in siblings of patients with known disease, with a higher incidence in same-sex siblings.[31]

Cytogenetic clonal abnormalities have been demonstrated in more than half of cases of HL studied.[32–34] The most common breakpoints reported are similar to those found in NHL, which supports a lymphoid origin for HL. The various cytogenetic abnormalities identified suggest that genetic instability is a significant component of the etiology of HL.

Histological Classification and Patient Presentation

Two distinct disease entities make up Hodgkin's disease: classical Hodgkin's lymphoma and nodular lymphocyte-predominant Hodgkin's lymphoma. These two lymphomas share the feature that only a minority of the involved tissues contain the Hodgkin and Reed-Sternberg cells, while the majority of the cells appear to be inflammatory and accessory cells. A distinction has been made between these two because the epidemiology, clinical manifestations, natural history, immunophenotyping, genetics, and association with EBV differ for each entity.

In 1966, Lukes and Butler established a histologic classification system for Hodgkin's lymphoma, which appeared to correlate well with the known clinical characteristics of the disease. This system was later simplified into the Rye classification and has been widely used.[35] The World Health Organization (WHO) classification mimics the Rye classification with the exception of the establishment of the nodular lymphocyte-predominant Hodgkin's lymphoma category. The classical Hodgkin's lymphomas represent the same four subclassifications noted in the Rye system: nodular sclerosis, mixed cellularity, lymphocyte rich, and lymphocyte depleted. Many differences in their clinical features and characteristics distinguish these subtypes, but all four variants share the same immunophenotyping.

Nodular Lymphocyte-Predominant Hodgkin's Lymphoma

Nodular lymphocyte-predominant Hodgkin's lymphoma (NLPHL) accounts for only about 5% of all cases of HL. It affects predominantly males, and the most common age at diagnosis ranges from 30 to 50 years.[36] Most patients present with localized disease involving the cervical, axillary, or inguinal nodes. Only 5%–20% of patients present with advanced disease. This subtype of HL, if diagnosed at an early stage (I or II), is very responsive to therapy and rarely proves fatal. However, advanced-stage disease has an unfavorable prognosis.

A small percentage of these patients will have transformation to large B-cell NHL. Morphologically, this monoclonal B-cell neoplasm has a nodular or nodular and diffuse distribution of lymphocytic and/or histiocytic Reed-Sternberg cell variants called L & H cells. Due to the appearance of these large cells, which have folded or multilobulated nuclei, they have also been called "popcorn" cells.[36] The cells phenotypically are positive for CD20, CD79a, BCL-6, and CD45 in nearly all cases.[37–39]

Classical Hodgkin's Lymphoma

The four histological types of classical HL account of 95% of all cases of HL.[40] The cervical lymph nodes are involved in 75% of cases; approximately 60% of cases involve mediastinal nodes. Involvement of axillary and paraaortic nodes is less common. The spleen is involved in about 20% of patients and the bone marrow in only 5%. Approximately half of the patients present with localized disease (stage I or II) and half with advanced disease (III or IV). B symptoms are reported to be present in approximately 40% of patients.

Nodular sclerosis HL is the most common subtype of HL, accounting for approximately 70% of all cases. The median age at presentation is 28 years, and this disease is unique in that it has no male or female predominance.[40] Mediastinal involvement is very common (approximately 80% of cases), and bulky disease is noted in half of the cases. Bulky mediastinal adenopathy is an adverse risk factor. The spleen is involved in about 10% of cases and the bone marrow in 3% of cases.[41,42] The majority of patients present with stage II disease, and B symptoms are noted in 40% of cases.[43,44] A nodular growth pattern consistent with classical HL is observed morphologically. Collagen bands surround at least one nodule, resulting in fibrosis and thickening of the lymph node capsule. The presence of the lucunar cell, a variant of the Hodgkin Reed-Sternberg cells, is observed, giving this tumor a unique appearance morphologically.[40] The prognosis for patients with nodular sclerosing HL is better than that for patients with mixed-cellularity or lymphocyte-depleted subtypes.

Mixed cellularity HL represents 20%–25% of classical HL. It is observed more commonly in patients with HIV infection and in developing countries. The median age at presentation is 37 years, and males account for 70% of the cases.[40] Mixed cellularity HL presents more commonly as advanced-stage disease, and B symptoms are common. Mediastinal lymph node involvement is uncommon, but the spleen and the bone marrow are involved in approximately 30% and 10% of cases, respectively.[40] Morphologically, the lymph node structure is obliterated. There is no thickening of the lymph node capsule, as is observed in nodular sclerosing HL. Typical Hodgkin Reed-Sternberg cells are found. The background cells are a mixture of cell types including eosinophils, neutrophils, histiocytes, and plasma cells — hence the name mixed cellularity HL. The prognosis with mixed cellularity HL has historically been slightly worse than that with nodular sclerosis HL and better than that with lymphocyte-depleted HL. New treatment regimens, however, have minimized the differences in prognosis.

Lymphocyte-rich classical HL accounts for approximately 5% of all cases of HL. As with mixed cellularity HL, males account for 70% of the cases, but the median age at diagnosis for this variant is the highest of all subtypes of HL.[40] Most patients present with peripheral lymphadenopathy resulting in stage I or II disease. Mediastinal adenopathy and bulky disease are uncommon.[45] The morphology of the lymph node can appear as a nodular pattern or (uncommonly) a diffuse one.[46,47] Scattered Hodgkin Reed-Sternberg cells are present and small lymphocytes are abundant. Eosinophils and neutrophils are either absent or in small number. Lymphocyte-rich classical HL is often difficult to distinguish morphologically from NLPHL, and immunophenotyping is critical to demonstrate the classical Hodgkin Reed-Sternberg cells.[47] Prognosis is slightly better than that for other subtypes of classical HL and similar to that for NLPHL. Relapse is less common than in NLPHL; if relapse occurs, however, prognosis is less favorable.[45,47]

Lymphocyte-depleted HL is the rarest of all subtypes of HL, accounting for less than 5% of all cases.[40] The median age at diagnosis is similar to that of most other forms of HL (37 years), with 75% of cases being found in males.[48] Like mixed cellularity HL, this subtype is more common in individuals with HIV and in developing countries.[49] Peripheral lymphadenopathy is rarely seen. Disease is often found in the abdominal organs, retroperitoneal lymph nodes, and bone marrow. Diagnosis is usually made while the disease is in a more advanced stage with B symptoms present.[50] Morphologically, the appearance of lymphocyte-depleted HL is quite variable, but there is generally a predominance of Hodgkin Reed-Sternberg cells and a paucity of lymphocytes in the background cells. Prognosis is now thought to be similar to that for other subtypes of HL, although patients with HIV often experience a more aggressive course.[48]

Treatment Modalities

HL has one of the highest cure rates found among adult cancers, but only if appropriate and full-dose therapy is given on schedule. It is reported that more than 80% of patients can be cured with first-line therapy.[51] Treatment of this disease entails a balance between sufficient therapy to cure the disease but no more than is required to prevent unnecessary long-term consequences. This balance continues to inspire debate in the literature today. It is important to understand the history of HL treatment, as some survivors have undergone various treatments that are no longer considered standard therapy today. It is imperative to monitor these individuals for long-term side effects particular to their HL treatment.

HL must be staged carefully to determine appropriate therapy. In the past, a staging laparotomy and splenectomy were performed to definitively identify those patients with limited versus advanced disease. Curative radiation therapy was originally used as treatment. After World War II, a plethora of chemotherapy drugs became available and many were studied as single agents in HL. Eventually combinations of chemotherapy evolved and the MOPP regimen was developed. Originally used as salvage therapy, it was later employed as first-line therapy. This combination therapy produced a 54% disease-free survival rate at 20 years and demonstrated effective long-term management of HL with systemic treatment.[52]

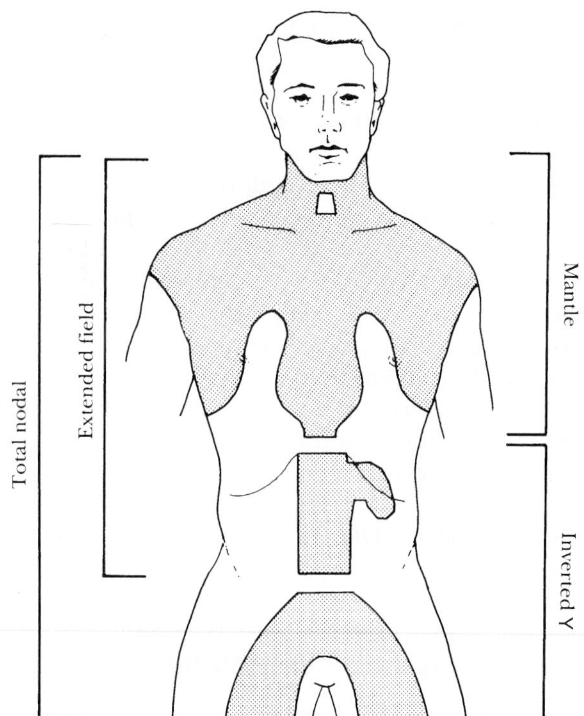

Figure 58-5 Standard radiation fields for Hodgkin's disease. Mantle – from mandible to diaphragm. Lungs, heart, spinal cord, and humeral heads are shielded. Inverted Y – from diaphragm to ischial tuberosities, including the spleen if not removed; spinal cord, kidneys, bladder, rectum, and gonads are shielded. Extended field – involves mantle zone and uppermost inverted Y zone; does not include the pelvic, inguinal, or femoral nodes. Total nodal – mantle zone and completed inverted Y zone.

Radiation Therapy

Prior to the 1960s, radiation therapy was the initial, and sometimes only, treatment for HL. When it was discovered that HL spread via contiguous lymph node chains, radiation for early-stage disease often was given as extended field. This included one lymph node group beyond those that were positive. The three classic areas of radiation fields were the mantle, paraaortic, and pelvic regions. (See Figure 58-5.) The mantle field consisted of the cervical, supraclavicular, infraclavicular, axillary, mediastinal, and hilar lymph node groupings. The paraaortic field included the spleen, if present. The pelvic field included the pelvic, inguinal, and femoral nodes. Subtotal lymphoid radiation encompassed all of the fields, while the extended field included the mantle and paraaortic regions. Finally, the inverted Y field consisted of the paraaortic region in addition to the pelvic area. Many vital organs fall within these fields, and blocks needed to be devised to provide protection. Therapy typically consisted of 3500–4400 cGy given to affected areas, with 3000–3500 cGy going to uninvolved areas.

Advances in radiotherapy have helped make these treatments less toxic, but this approach is still associated with significant long-term side effects. Currently, the extent and dose of radiation depend on the stage of disease as well as the residual tumor, if any, that remains after combination chemotherapy. Positron emission tomography results are now being taken into consideration in the determination of radiation therapy.

Chemotherapy

With the advent of effective combination chemotherapy, staging laparotomies with splenectomies have fallen by the wayside based on the presumption that chemotherapy will clear any occult disease. Early-stage HL is typically treated with four (sometimes fewer) cycles of combination chemotherapy followed by involved-field radiation. More advanced disease is often treated with six to eight cycles of combination chemotherapy. Radiation may or may not be given to sites of bulky disease. A recent study from Europe investigated the use of randomized involved-field radiation for advanced disease. The researchers concluded that involved-field radiation did not improve outcomes in patients who were in complete remission (CR) after combination therapy, but it was useful for those who were in partial remission (PR).[53] Typically, patients are restaged after three to four cycles of chemotherapy to gauge their response and to finalize the treatment plan.

Prior to 1960, chemotherapy agents were used only for palliative purposes. In 1964, MOPP combination chemotherapy was investigated and became the first treatment that cured patients with advanced disease.[54] Several years later, Italian researchers developed the ABVD protocol. It was first considered to be a non-cross-resistant treatment for MOPP failures, but later proved to be superior in efficacy with less long-term toxicity than MOPP.[55] Table 58-3 describes the chemotherapy regimens used to treat HL. MOPP has fallen out of favor as standard treatment for HL due to the increased risk of secondary malignancies associated with it. A recent randomized, multicenter trial compared a MOPP/ABV hybrid to ABVD, reporting results after five years.[56] The two regimens appear to be equally effective, but the MOPP/ABV therapy is associated with increased pulmonary and hematologic toxicity as well as an increased incidence of secondary leukemia.

Other combination therapies currently used include the 12-week Stanford V treatment as well as the European BEACOPP and escalated BEACOPP. As mentioned earlier, ongoing debate in the literature focuses on the balance between cure and toxicity. The German Hodgkin's Lymphoma Study Group recommends that patients with advanced, high-risk disease receive aggressive treatment upfront, rather than multiple chemotherapy regimens, including stem cell transplant, at time of relapse.[51] These researchers report that standard BEACOPP is equivalent to COPP/ABVD, but produces higher toxicities. Escalated BEACOPP, by comparison, appears to be more effective than either therapy.[57] Currently, an international trial is comparing six to eight cycles of ABVD to four cycles of escalated BEACOPP plus four cycles of standard BEACOPP in patients with advanced disease. Radiation will be given to those patients who achieve a PR after chemotherapy.

Table 58-3 Combination Chemotherapy Regimens Used to Treat Hodgkin's Lymphoma

MOPP

Mechlorethamine 6 mg/m^2 IV days 1 and 8
Vincristine (**O**ncovin) 1.4 mg/m^2 IV on days 1 and 8—not to exceed 2.5 mg/dose
Procarbazine 100 mg/m^2 PO days 1 through 14
Prednisone 40 mg/m^2 PO days 1 through 14 (cycles 1 through 4 only)
Cycle repeated every 28 days

ABVD

Doxorubicin (**A**driamycin) 25 mg/m^2 IV days 1 and 15
Bleomycin 10 units/m^2 IV days 1 and 15 (on cycle 1, 1 mg of the dose is administered as a test dose)
Vinblastine 6 mg/m^2 IV days 1 and 14
Dacarbazine 375 mg/m^2 IV days 1 and 15
Cycle repeated every 28 days

MOPP/ABV

Mechlorethamine 6 mg/m^2 IV day 1
Vincristine (**O**ncovin) 1.4 mg/m^2 IV on day 1—not to exceed 2.5 mg/dose
Procarbazine 100 mg/m^2 PO days 1 through 7
Prednisone 40 mg/m^2 PO days 1 through 14
Doxorubicin (**A**driamycin) 25 mg/m^2 IV day 8
Bleomycin 10 units/m^2 IV day 8 (on cycle 1, 1 mg of the dose is administered as a test dose)
Cycle repeated every 28 days

Stanford V

Vinblastine 6 mg/m^2 IV weeks 1, 3, 5, 7, 9, and 11
Doxorubicin (Adriamycin) 25 mg/m^2 IV weeks 1, 3, 5, 7, 9, and 11
Vincristine (Oncovin) 1.4 mg/m^2 IV (not to exceed 2 mg/dose) weeks 2, 4, 6, 8, 10, and 12
Bleomycin 10 units/m^2 IV (on cycle 1, 1 mg of the dose is administered as a test dose) weeks 2, 4, 6, 8, 10, and 12
Mechlorethamine 6 mg/m^2 IV weeks 1, 5, and 9
Etoposide 60 mg/m^2 IV daily × 2 on weeks 3, 7, and 11
Prednisone 40 mg/m^2 PO every other day on weeks 1 through 10 with tapering on weeks 11 and 12
All therapy is over in 12 weeks; no "cycles"

BEACOPP

Bleomycin 10 mg/m^2 IV day 8
Etoposide 100 mg/m^2 IV days 1 through 3
Doxorubicin (**A**driamycin) 25 mg/m^2 IV day 1
Cyclophosphamide 650 mg/m^2 IV day 1
Vincristine (**O**ncovin) 1.4 mg/m^2 IV day 8 (maximum dose 2 mg)
Procarbazine 100 mg/m^2 PO days 1 though 7
Prednisone 40 mg/m^2 PO days 1 through 13
Cycles repeated every 21 days

Increased BEACOPP

Bleomycin 10 mg/m^2 IV day 8
Etoposide 200 mg/m^2 IV days 1 through 3
Doxorubicin (**A**driamycin) 35 mg/m^2 IV day 1
Cyclophosphamide 1250 mg/m^2 IV day 1
Vincristine (**O**ncovin) 1.4 mg/m^2 IV day 8 (maximum dose 2 mg)
Procarbazine 100 mg/m^2 PO days 1 though 7
Prednisone 40 mg/m^2 PO days 1 through 13 with cytokine support
Cycles repeated every 21 days

Stem Cell Transplant

Stem cell transplant remains a potentially curative option for relapsed HL with chemotherapy-sensitive disease. Over the last 20 years, it has been established as the most effective treatment for patients not cured by initial multidrug regimens. Candidates for stem cell transplant include patients who progress through initial treatment, those who respond to treatment but fail to achieve a complete response, and those who relapse post-treatment. Despite the availability of high-dose therapy, prognosis remains poor for these patients, with an overall survival rate of 34% and a disease-free survival rate of 29% at ten years.[58] Two subsets of patients with a better prognosis have been identified: those who have relapsed at original lymph node sites that were not irradiated and those whose relapse occurred more than one year after completion of initial therapy. Patients receiving allogeneic (rather than autologous) transplants are more likely to remain relapse free after transplant, but the increased morbidity and mortality of allogeneic transplants may offset the benefits achieved by donation from an autologous marrow source. Negative prognostic factors for disease progression after stem cell transplantation include chemotherapy resistance prior to transplant, advanced-stage disease, and greater number of chemotherapeutic regimens prior to transplant.

Future Directions

Many clinical trials are looking for a nontoxic agent or regimen that is effective. As the biology of HL becomes better understood, it is hoped that new therapies will emerge. Targeted immunotherapy, an important adjuvant to treatment of NHL, is now being investigated in the management of HL. Preliminary data suggest that rituximab (anti-CD20 therapy) may have efficacy in some patients, with response rates for it exceeding 50%.[59]

Important questions still need to be answered. How little therapy can be used and still cure low-risk, early-stage disease? How much should we treat high-risk, advanced disease? What is the role of radiation therapy at all stages of disease? It is recommended that patients be offered enrollment in clinical trials to help answer these questions. Close follow-up for efficacy, acute toxicity, and long-term complications is necessary to discern the best options over the long term.

Prognosis

Hodgkin's disease has historically been one of the most "curable" cancers. Patients with early-stage disease (stage I and II) have a ten-year survival rate exceeding 80%.[28] Negative prognostic factors were determined by an international consortium.[60] Seven factors associated with poor prognosis were identified: stage IV disease; male sex; age greater than or equal to 45 years; hemoglobin < 10.5 g/dL; white blood cell count greater than or equal to 15,000/μl; lymphocyte count < 800/μl or < 6%, and albumin < 4 g/dL. Eighty-four percent of patients with no factors were estimated to be free of disease at five years. The rates declined steadily, however, with patients with five to seven factors having an estimated progression-free survival rate of 42%.[60]

Non-Hodgkin's Lymphoma

Historical Perspective

Non-Hodgkin's lymphoma (NHL) encompasses a diverse group of neoplasms of the immune system involving B or T lymphocytes. Although these malignancies share many characteristics, they also reflect the diversity of their normal counterpart cells and exhibit a wide range of immunological and biological characteristics. No precise, universally accepted definition of NHL exists. Although many disease entities meet the criteria that have been proposed, others lurk in a nebulous area between benign lymphoproliferation and true malignancy. Furthermore, the classification of lymphoma has long been a controversial issue and continues to undergo change.

In the past, pathologists used a variety of terms (e.g., giant follicle lymphoma, lymphosarcoma, and reticulum cell sarcoma) to categorize these tumors, and "pseudoleukemia" became a catchall term for describing a host of conditions that exhibited lymphadenopathy and splenomegaly. Technological refinements have enabled pathologists and clinicians to classify NHL according to a number of individual determinants, including cytoarchitecture (follicular versus diffuse), cell size (small or large), nuclear characteristics (cleaved or noncleaved, convoluted or cerebriform), immunological ontogeny (T-cell or B-cell lymphocytes), and maturity of the cell (precursor or mature). Today, the identity of the lymphoma is also determined with the aid of cytogenetic and immunological markers.

Epidemiology

An estimated 54,370 new cases of NHL were expected to be diagnosed in 2004, accounting for approximately 87% of all lymphomas.[24] The incidence of lymphoma climbed rapidly in the 1970s and 1980s, nearly doubling the number of new cases identified. Better detection and diagnosis accounted for some of this increase. The climbing incidence of AIDS and AIDS-related NHL, as well as the expanding use of immunosuppressive treatments, accounted for a substantial portion of these cases. In the 1990s, the incidence rates stabilized, a trend that has been attributed to the decline in AIDS-related NHL. An estimated 19,410 deaths were expected to occur in 2004 due to NHL. The prognosis for NHL is highly variable, but the overall five-year survival rate is approximately 56%.[24]

The incidence of NHL increases with age, and is slightly higher in males than in females. A male younger than age 40 has a 1 in 739 chance of developing NHL, whereas a male aged 60–79 has a 1 in 79 chance. The incidence also increases with age in females: 1 in 1258 chance prior to age 40, and 1 in 102 chance for ages 60–79.[24] The reduction in immune function during the aging process may explain the increasing rate of NHL. This theory is supported by other patients who are known to be at increased risk for the development of NHL — patients post-transplant who receive immunosuppressive therapy and those with HIV infection.

Etiology

An increased incidence of lymphoma has been reported in individuals with exposure to toxins, such as chemists, farmers, and those working with rubber production, asbestos, and arsenic.[61-68] Japanese survivors of the atomic bomb and patients receiving ionizing radiation for congenital disorders and HD also face increased neoplastic potential.[69,70] Other investigators report minimal or no risk associated with ionizing radiation and the risk of lymphoma.[71] Controversy has existed since 1975 over the risk associated with hair dyes. While many studies do not substantiate greater risk associated with the use of hair dyes, either personally or occupationally, a subset of individuals who use permanent dyes, dark in color, for prolonged periods (> 20 years) may have an increased risk of lymphoma.[72]

Chromosomal abnormalities are common in NHL. Investigators have identified cytogenetic abnormalities in more than 90% of cases.[73,74] The impact of chromosomal translocations may be significant. For example, the translocation t(14:18)(q32;q21), which is commonly found in follicular lymphoma, results in overexpression of *BCL-2*. The accumulation of BCL-2 protein results in inhibition of apoptosis (programmed cell death).[75–78] These alterations in the expression of genes affect normal cell function and regulation and are implicated in the process of malignant transformation.

Infectious agents have been implicated in the etiology of NHL as well as HL. The clearest evidence for this role is seen in the etiology of adult T-cell leukemia/lymphoma which arises in patients infected with human T-cell leukemia/lymphoma virus 1 (HTLV-1). Yet, not all individuals who are exposed and infected with HTLV-1 develop lymphoma. There appear to be host factors, potentially genetic, that result in the transformation of normal lymphocytes to lymphoma. The greatest incidence of adult T-cell leukemia/lymphoma is found in an island of Japan. Ten to fifteen percent of the population of this island is found to have antibody (signifying prior exposure) to HTLV-1. Other endemic areas include the Caribbean and southeastern United States.

The Epstein-Barr virus (EBV) has also been implicated in the development of NHL, especially Burkitt's lymphoma. Burkitt's lymphoma has been endemic in some communities in Africa and New Guinea; EBV is present in more than 95% of these cases. Malaria is thought to play a role in the stimulation of lymphocytes that then undergo transformation; this disease is commonly seen in endemic areas of Burkitt's lymphoma. Of note, EBV is present in only 20% of nonendemic cases of Burkitt's lymphoma.[79,80]

There is clear evidence that *H. pylori*, a gram-negative bacillus that induces gastric ulceration, can result in MALT lymphoma of the stomach. In its early stages, it may be cured by eradication of the bacteria with antibiotics.[81] It has also resulted in the development of large cell lymphomas in the gastric region, either de novo or due to transformation from a MALT lymphoma.[82–84]

Immunosuppression has also been identified as a significant risk factor for the development of NHL. Clear evidence exists that individuals with primary (genetic) immunodeficiency states have a greater incidence of lymphoma. It has been estimated that 25% of these individuals will develop cancer during their lifetime, with more than 50% of those cases resulting in NHL.[85] Secondary exposure, generally associated with immunosuppressive therapy in the setting of organ transplantation, also is linked to a substantially greater risk for the development of NHL. Although etiology is not entirely clear, it has been proposed that the immunosuppression and the chronic antigenic stimulation by the graft result in the lymphoma.[86] Likewise, individuals with autoimmune disorders have been linked to a higher risk of developing NHL. Patients with rheumatoid arthritis have a two to three times higher risk. When treated with immunosuppressive therapy, the risk increases by tenfold.[87]

Histological Classification Systems

Rappaport Classification

No malignancy has undergone more changes in terms of its classification system than NHL. The first widely accepted classification was proposed by Rappaport and associates in 1956.[88] This system distinguished lymphomas on the basis of the pattern and growth within the lymph node (nodular or diffuse) and the degree of cytological differentiation of the predominant malignant cells. Tumors composed of cells similar in size and morphology to normal lymphocytes were denoted as "well differentiated," while those composed of irregularly shaped lymphocytes were referred to as "poorly differentiated." If the tumor cells were two to three times larger than small lymphocytes and had abundant cytoplasm, they were called histiocytes because of their resemblance to macrophages. Undifferentiated lymphomas were composed of intermediate-sized cells that failed to demonstrate evidence of either lymphoid or histiocytic origin. Mixed lymphomas were tumors formed by poorly differentiated lymphocytes and histiocytes.

International Working Formula

A study funded by the National Cancer Institute developed what was hoped to be the international standard for classifying lymphomas. The International Working Formula (IWF) was proposed in 1982, and was built upon the foundation of the Rappaport classification. The term "histiocytic" was replaced by "large cell" and the histiocytic group was divided into large cell and immunoblastic large cell categories. This division created a split, with large cell disease falling into the intermediate grade and immunoblastic disease becoming the high grade.[89] At that time, six different classifications systems were in use, making it impossible to analyze and compare results of clinical investigations using different systems. The IWF proposed three major NHL categories: low-, intermediate-, and high-grade lymphomas. These categories were based on both clinical (response to treatment) and pathological findings. Letter designations from A to J were assigned, corresponding roughly to aggressiveness of the disease and decreasing survival rates.

As a group, low-grade lymphomas have a long natural history, with an average survival of seven to ten years. These diseases, however, show a relatively poor response to treatment, with few complete remissions, and are considered incurable. Low-grade lymphoma commonly affects the elderly. Patients tend to present with stage III or IV disease, and the bone marrow is often involved. During progression of the disease, the low-grade lymphoma will often become transformed into an intermediate- or high-grade lymphoma. At this time, the lymphoma becomes more aggressive and requires more intensive therapy.

Intermediate-grade lymphomas include B-cell neoplasms that present largely in adults, most often with nodal presentation. These subtypes frequently involve extranodal progression to the gastrointestinal tract, skin, and bone. These lymphomas are responsive to chemotherapy and curative therapy is possible. Although they demonstrate an intermediate aggressiveness, if left untreated they are often rapidly fatal.

High-grade lymphomas are highly aggressive and are B cell or T cell in origin. These malignancies exhibit rapid tumor growth and a high mitotic index. They may present in children or adults. Some subsets of high-grade lymphomas share many characteristics with acute leukemia. Affected patients require rapid diagnosis and treatment. If left untreated, high-grade lymphomas will frequently develop large lymph nodes, creating compression and obstruction of other organs and oncologic emergencies. Despite the aggressive nature of these diseases, they are sensitive to treatment and cure is possible.

REAL Classification

The International Lymphoma Study Group met in 1994 and proposed the Revised European–American Classification of Lymphoid Neoplasms (REAL) system.[90] This classification system was constructed by integrating all known information about the tumor to define the lymphoma: morphology, immunophenotyping, genetics, etiology, epidemiology, and clinical features.[89,91] It relies on recognition of the cell of origin (T cell or B cell) and the stage of differentiation (precursor versus peripheral). The REAL system acknowledges that a distinct lymphoma subtype may vary in histological grade and clinical aggressiveness. The follicle center (follicular) lymphomas exemplify this point. Three grades of this disease entity have been identified: I (predominantly small cleaved), II (mixed small cleaved and large cell), and III (predominantly large cell).

The JWF, Rappaport, and REAL classification systems are compared in Table 58-4.

WHO Classification

The World Health Organization (WHO) classification of hematopoietic and lymphatic tumors is the result of several years of discussions and consensus meetings, which began in 1995 and involved more than 50 hematopathologists from around the world. The classifica-

Table 58-4 Non-Hodgkin's Lymphoma Nomenclature: Comparative Classifications

Working Formulation	Rappaport System	Real Classification*
	Low-Grade	
A Small lymphocytic	Diffuse, well-differentiated lymphocytic	Chronic lymphocytic leukemia
B Follicular, small cleaved	Nodular, poorly differentiated lymphocytic	MALT† follicle center cell, follicular grade I
C Follicular, mixed small cleaved, and large cell	Nodular, mixed lymphocytic and histiocytic	Follicle center cell, follicular grade II
	Intermediate-Grade	
D Follicular, large cell	Nodular histiocytic	Follicle center cell, follicular grade III
E Diffuse, small cleaved	Diffuse, poorly differentiated lymphocytic	Mantle cell‡
F Diffuse, mixed small and large	Diffuse, mixed lymphocytic and histiocytic	Follicle center cell, diffuse small cell Large B cell rich in T cells
G Diffuse, large cell	Diffuse histiocytic	Diffuse large B cell
	High-Grade	
H Immunoblastic, large cell	Diffuse histiocytic	Diffuse large B cell
I Lymphoblastic	Lymphoblastic	Precursor B lymphocytic
J Small, noncleaved Burkitt's	Undifferentiated, Burkitt's and non-Burkitt's	Burkitt's high-grade B cell, Burkitt's-like

*The REAL classification separated B-cell and T-cell lymphomas. Most of the T-cell lymphomas are not shown here except for chronic lymphocytic leukemia.

†MALT tumors are extranodal indolent and usually follicular, but some were previously classified in groups A, B, C, E, and rarely F.

‡Mantle cell tumors are defined by *BCL-1* overexpression and sometimes have a morphology similar to groups AB and F.

tion of NHL is just one group of disease entities addressed. The WHO classification system is built upon the principles of the REAL classification system. As in the REAL system, the lymphoma is defined by its morphology, immunophenotype, genetic, and clinical features. The lineage of the cell and the cell of origin are important features. The cell of origin in many lymphoid neoplasms is determined at the stage of differentiation of the malignant cells seen in the tissues, not based on the cell in which the initial transforming event occurred. Two categories of NHL are recognized: B-cell neoplasms and T- and NK-cell neoplasms. Lymphoid leukemias, both chronic and acute, as well as multiple myeloma and related disorders, are now categorized within the classification of NHL, as they are of T- or B-cell lineage, but discussion of these diseases will be minimal here as they are discussed in other chapters of this book. Characteristics and management of the more common subtypes of NHL as classified by the WHO system will be discussed, followed by a review of treatment modalities. Table 58-5 outlines the WHO classification for NHL.[92]

Characteristics and Management of B-Cell NHL

Small Lymphocytic Lymphoma/Chronic Lymphocytic Leukemia

Small lymphocytic lymphoma (SLL)/chronic lymphocytic leukemia (CLL) is a neoplasm of small, round B cells found in the peripheral blood, bone marrow, and lymph nodes. By definition, CLL entails bone marrow and peripheral blood involvement and a lymphocyte count greater than 10×10^9/L.[93] SLL can be diagnosed without CLL if the morphology of the cells meets the criteria, but the blood and bone marrow are not involved. Historically, a monoclonal lymphocytosis of greater than 5×10^9/L was required for the diagnosis of CLL, and this parameter continues to be used as a criterion by many clinicians. The proportion of prolymphocytes is usually small, less than 2%. Increasing proportions are associated with a more aggressive form of the disease. The pattern of malignant cells seen in the bone marrow may be described as nodular, interstitial, diffuse, or a combination of these. The nodular and interstitial patterns are usually associated with early disease. Advanced disease is associated with the interstitial pattern. It is estimated that 61%–90% of patients with SLL present with stage IV disease, and

Table 58-5 WHO Classification of NHL

Precursor B-Cell and T-Cell Neoplasms
Precursor B-lymphoblastic leukemia/lymphoblastic lymphoma (precursor B-cell acute lymphoblastic leukemia)
Precursor T-lymphoblastic leukemia/lymphoblastic lymphoma (precursor T-cell acute lymphoblastic leukemia)

Mature B-Cell Neoplasms
Chronic lymphocytic leukemia/small lymphocytic lymphoma
B-cell prolymphocytic leukemia
Lymphoplasmacytic lymphoma
Splenic marginal zone lymphoma
Hairy cell leukemia
Plasma cell myeloma
Monoclonal gammopathy of undetermined significance (MGUS)
Solitary plasmacytoma of bone
Extraosseous plasmacytoma
Primary ameloidosis
Heavy-chain diseases
Extranodal marginal zone B-cell lymphoma of mucosa-associated lymphoid tissue (MALT lymphoma)
Nodal marginal-zone B-cell lymphoma
Follicular lymphoma
Mantle cell lymphoma
Diffuse large B-cell lymphoma
Mediastinal (thymic) large B-cell lymphoma
Intravascular large B-cell lymphoma
Primary effusion lymphoma
Burkitt's lymphoma/leukemia

B-cell Proliferations of Uncertain Malignant Potential
Lymphatoid granulomatosis
Post-transplant lymphoproliferative disorder, polymorphic

Mature T-Cell and NK Cell Neoplasms
Leukemic/disseminated
T-cell prolymphocytic leukemia
T-cell large granular lymphocytic leukemia
Aggressive NK cell leukemia
Adult T-cell leukemia/lymphoma

Cutaneous
Mycosis fungoides
Sezary syndrome
Primary cutaneous anaplastic large cell lymphoma
Lymphomatoid papulosis*

Other extanodal
Extranodal NK/T-cell lymphoma, nasal type
Enteropathy-type T-cell lymphoma
Hepatosplenic T-cell lymphoma
Subcutaneous panniculitis-like T-cell lymphoma

Nodal
Angioimmunoblastic T-cell lymphoma
Peripheral T-cell lymphoma, unspecified
Anaplastic large cell lymphoma

Neoplasm of uncertain lineage and stage of differentiation
Blastic NK lymphoma

* Not clinically considered a neoplastic disorder.

69%–82% of these patients have bone marrow involvement at diagnosis.[94–96]

Immunoglobulin gene rearrangements of both heavy- and light-chain variable regions are noted in SLL/CLL in 50% of patients. Approximately 80% of patients have abnormal karyotypes as determined by FISH analysis.[97] Deletion of 13q14 and trisomy 12 are the cytogenetic abnormalities most commonly noted. Those with deletion 13q14 more frequently have mutated variable genes, and those with trisomy 12 have predominantly unmutated genes. Malignant cells express IgM or IgM and IgD, CD5, CD23, and CD43. CD20 and CD22 also express weak activity. CD5 and CD23 markers are positive in SLL/CLL and negative in other B-cell leukemias with the exception of mantle cell lymphoma, which expresses CD5.

SLL/CLL accounts for 6.7% of cases of NHL.[98] The majority of patients are more than 50 years old, with a median age of 65 years. There is a male-to-female predominance of approximately 2:1. Many patients with CLL are asymptomatic at diagnosis and a lymphocytosis is found on a routine complete blood count (CBC). Because the SLL subtype does not have a significant lymphocytosis, diffuse lymphadenopathy or lymph node masses' effects on normal organ function often lead to diagnosis. The spleen and liver are often enlarged, and extranodal disease is not uncommon. Patients may complain of fatigue. Autoimmune disorders are often observed, with the most common being autoimmune hemolytic anemia and idiopathic thrombocytopenia. Hypogammaglobulinemia is identified in 75% of patients at some point during their disease, contributing to an increased risk of infection.

Treatment is often deferred in early-stage SLL/CLL unless there is an indication to treat. The following criteria have been identified as indications to treat: (1) patient eligibility for a clinical trial, (2) presence of autoimmune cytopenias, (3) recurrent infections, (4) significant symptomatology, (5) cytopenias, (6) massive bulky disease at presentation, (7) steady progression over at least 6 months, (8) lymphocyte number doubling in less than 12 months, and (9) patient preference.[99]

Single-agent therapy with a purine analog or alkylating agent may be administered or combination therapy may be initiated. It is recommended that anthracycline use be avoided in combination regimens. Fludarabine has been associated with higher response rates and longer progression-free survival than anthracycline-containing regimens.[100] It has not, however, been shown to improve survival. Current acceptable combinations include CVP (cyclophosphamide, vincristine, prednisone) and CF (cyclophosphamide, fludarabine). Rituximab is often added to combination therapy. If the disease continues to progress, treatment options include purine analog for fludarabine-sensitive or -naïve patients or alkylator-based therapy for fludarabine-resistant disease. Rituximab or alemtuzumab may also be used as second-line therapy. Alemtuzumab has been approved for use in fludarabine-refractory patients and is being investigated earlier in the disease course.

Locoregional radiotherapy may be utilized for adenopathy that may be localized and producing significant symptomatology. Although stem cell transplantation remains controversial, it may be utilized as treatment at this time. Small numbers of patients appear in long-term follow-up to be cured of their disease following stem cell transplantation.

Detection of minimal residual disease (MRD) following treatment is of growing interest in this disorder. Flow cytometry has been utilized to detect cells that coexpress CD5 and CD19. Polymerase chain reaction (PCR) for the identification of immunoglobulin heavy gene rearrangement appears to be a sensitive test for identifying MRD. In one study, patients without evidence of MRD who demonstrated a complete response following therapy with alemtuzumab had a longer time to treatment failure than those who were MRD positive.[101]

The clinical course for SLL/CLL is indolent (slow growing), but the disease is not considered curable. The five year survival rate for SLL in one study was 51%, with a disease-free survival rate of 25%.[98] The Rai and Binet staging systems are the best predictors of survival.[102] Abnormalities of 13q14 are associated with prolonged survival. Negative prognostic indicators include a rapid doubling time, increased proportion of prolymphocytes, trisomy 12, nonmutated variable gene rearrangements, and expression of CD38. Transformation to a high-grade lymphoma is seen in as many as 15% of these individuals, and is known as Richter's syndrome.[103] Although diffuse large B cells are most commonly associated with this disorder, patients treated with purine analogs may develop a lymphoma resembling HL.

Follicular Lymphoma

Follicular lymphoma (FL) is a neoplasm of follicle-center (germinal-center) B cells. The neoplastic follicles are poorly defined due to the closely packed lymphocytes. The pattern is reported as follicular if more than 75% of cells are follicular, follicular and diffuse if 25%–75% are follicular and minimally follicular if less than 25% are follicular. Two types of cells are normally found in the follicle centers — centrocytes (small, cleaved follicle-center cells) and centroblasts (large, noncleaved follicle-center cells) — but centrocytes typically dominate. One of three possible grades is assigned based on the number of centroblasts counted. Grade 1 has 0–5 centroblasts per high-power field (predominantly small cell), grade 2 has 6–15 centroblasts (mixed small and large cell), and grade 3 has more than 15 centroblasts (large cell). Grade 3 has also been subdivided into grade 3a, in which centrocytes are present, and grade 3b, in which solid sheets of centroblasts are observed.[104] Grades 1 and 2 tend to be indolent in nature, consistent with low-grade NHL; grade 3 is more aggressive, with a natural history similar to diffuse large cell NHL.

Follicular lymphoma accounts for approximately 35% of all cases of NHL in adults in the United States. It is less common elsewhere in the world, representing about 22% of NHL worldwide. This disease is the most frequent subtype of "low-grade" lymphoma observed. Follicular lymphoma is seen predominantly in adults and is characterized by a male-to-female ratio of 1:1.7 and a median age at diagnosis of 59 years. Patients often present with widespread disease. Approximately two-thirds of cases involve stage III or IV lymphoma at diagnosis.[98] Diffuse adenopathy may be present, but patients are frequently asymptomatic.

The BCL-2 protein is commonly expressed in FL. Lai and associates report that the incidence of BCL-2 expression ranges from 100% in grade 1 FL to 75% in grade 3 FL.[105] Because most low-grade lymphomas express BCL-2, it is not a useful tool for differentiating FL from other lymphoma subtypes but it can help differentiate neoplastic lymph nodes from reactive nodes. BCL-6 abnormalities can also be observed. The malignant cells also are $CD10^{+/-}$, $CD23^{+/-}$, Sig^{+}, $CD5^{-}$, and $CD43^{-}$. B-cell–associated antigens are expressed, including CD19, CD20, CD22, and CD79a. Cytogenetic abnormalities are almost universally found in FL. The most common abnormality, t(14;18)(q32;q21), is associated with the rearrangement of the *BCL-2* gene. This genetic abnormality does not appear to either positively or negatively impact prognosis.

Treatment of FL depends on the stage and grade of disease. Grade 1 and 2 disease are more indolent, with a median survival of 7–10 years, which has been relatively unchanged over the last 20 years despite increasing treatment options.[106] Observation — the "watch and wait" approach — is a valid option. Patients may receive local radiotherapy. Stage III or IV disease or stage II with bulky abdominal disease may be treated if indicated. The National Comprehensive Cancer Network recommends treatment if the patient has significant symptomatology, end-organ function is threatened, cytopenias are present due to the lymphoma, bulky disease is present, there has been steady progressive disease over the last six months, or the patient prefers it.[99] Due to the inability to cure this disease, participation in clinical trials is strongly advised.

Initial therapies may include single-agent or combination therapy with or without rituximab. Patients with FL appear to be highly responsive to rituximab when it is combined with chemotherapy. Autologous or allogeneic stem cell transplants may be considered. Grade 3 disease and histological transformation to diffuse large B-cell lymphomas are treated more aggressively with anthracycline-based chemotherapy with or without radiotherapy. The use of anthracyclines has resulted in improved survival.[104,107] If a complete or partial response is obtained, stem cell transplantation, participation in a clinical trial, or observation may be considered.

Radioimmunotherapy is an option if the patient shows no response or progressive disease. Two radioimmunoconjugates, ^{90}Y-ibritumomab tiuxetan (Zevalin) and ^{131}I-tositumomab (Bexxar), are approved in the United States for the treatment of relapsed, refractory follicular NHL, with or without transformation.

Grade I and II FL, while indolent in nature, are generally not curable. Grade III disease is more aggressive, but its curative potential is similar to that for diffuse large cell NHL. Transformed disease is also aggressive and associated with rapid decline. Approximately 60% of patients treated with various chemotherapeutic regimens demonstrated complete remission in analysis of multiple trials sponsored by the Southwestern Oncology Group (SWOG). Historically, responses have been observed with follicular lymphomas but relapses are frequent. While this malignancy is sensitive, multiple relapses are common, with response time decreasing as the number of therapies increases.[108]

It has been reported that clinical factors identified in the International Prognostic Index are as important as the grade in predicting outcome in follicular lymphoma.[14,98] In 1999, an international cooperative group developed the Follicular Lymphoma International Prognostic Index, commonly known by the acronym FLIPI. Adverse prognostic factors included in FLIPI are Ann Arbor stage III/IV disease, greater than or equal to five nodal sites involved, serum LDH greater than normal, age greater than or equal to 60 years, and hemoglobin < 12 g/dL. The good-risk group (36% of patients) had zero to one negative prognostic factor; the intermediate-risk group (37% of patients) had two negative factors; and the poor-risk group (27% of patients) had three or more factors. The 10-year overall survival rates reported were 70.7%, 50.9%, and 35.5%, respectively.[109]

MALT Lymphoma

MALT lymphoma, also known as maltoma, is an extranodal lymphoma of the mucosa-associated lymphoid tissues. Morphologically, the cells appear as heterogeneous, small B cells of various cell types. They include centrocyte-like cells known as marginal zone cells. The infiltrate of malignant cells is observed in the marginal zone of reactive B-cell follicles extending into the interfollicular region.

Eight percent of B-cell non-Hodgkin's lymphomas and 50% of primary gastric lymphomas are classified as MALT lymphoma.[98,110,111] It is primarily a disease of adults, with a median age at diagnosis of 61. The male-to-female ratio is 1:1.2. A higher incidence of gastric MALT lymphoma has been reported in northeast Italy.[110] Chronic inflammatory states, frequently involving autoimmune disorders, often precede the development of MALT lymphoma. In addition, *H. pylori* infection has been strongly implicated in the development of gastric maltomas. Wotherspoon and associates reported that *H. pylori* was found in more than 90% of gastric maltomas.[112] Others have reported a lower incidence. In any event, the rate of detection of *H. pylori* diminishes as the lymphoma evolves; indeed, there is an inability to detect the bacteria even when the patient is seropositive.

The gastrointestinal system is the most common site of disease, accounting for 50% of all MALT lymphomas. Of those cases, the stomach is involved in 85%.[110] When the intestine or colon is involved, patients typically are found to have a special subtype of MALT lymphoma known as immunoproliferative small intestine disease (IPSID), previously known as α-chain disease. IPSID is more commonly found in the Middle East and the Cape region of South Africa. Other less common sites of disease, in descending order of frequency, include the lung, head and neck, ocular adnexae, skin, thyroid, and breast.[113]

Patients frequently present with stage I or II disease. Overall, only 20% of patients have disease involving the bone marrow, but the incidence varies with the primary site of involvement. Gastric cases have a low frequency of marrow involvement, while cases of ocular adnexal and pulmonary origin have a higher incidence.[114,115] Multiple extranodal or nodal sites are uncommon, occurring in less than 10% of patients.[113] Even when multiple extranodal sites exist, they may not reflect the existence of disseminated disease and poorer prognosis, making the staging systems less useful in this lymphoma.

Malignant cells typically express IgM, although IgA or IgG may be observed. Light-chain restriction is noted in MALT lymphomas, which is significant because it differentiates benign lymphoid infiltrations. Typical cells are $CD10^-$, $CD5^-$, $CD20^+$, $CD23^-$, $CD79a^+$, and $CD43^{+/-}$ (weak). Cycin D1 is negative and *BCL-2* follicles are negative.[116] Immunoglobulin heavy- and light-chain rearrangement occurs. Two cytogenetic abnormalities are commonly observed in this subtype: Trisomy 3 is found in 60% of cases and t(11:18) (q21;q21) is seen in 25%–50% of cases. A t(11;18) alteration is a predictor for lack of disease response to antibiotic therapy.[117]

Patients with stage I E gastric MALT lymphoma may receive currently accepted antibiotic therapy for *H. pylori* as sole treatment for their disease if they lack the previously noted translocation and test positive for *H. pylori*. If they are *H. pylori* negative or have stage II disease, antibiotic therapy may still be considered or radiotherapy may be added to the treatment plan. Advanced-stage disease may involve chemotherapy, such as alkylating agents or anthracyline-containing regimens, with or without regional radiotherapy. Failure to eradicate the *H. pylori* infection occurs in approximately 10% of cases, so that an alternative antibiotic regimen is required.[118]

Serial endoscopies are recommended to follow the disease. Regression of the lymphoma may require several months, and chemotherapy is usually required only to treat recurrent or persistent disease. Regimens utilized to treat follicular lymphoma are often considered appropriate therapy for maltomas.[99] Surgical resection of gastric MALT lymphoma is reserved for life-threatening disease. Early-stage nongastric MALT lymphomas are generally treated with surgical resection and local radiotherapy. Advanced-stage disease is treated similarly to follicular lymphoma. The presence of diffuse large cell lymphoma, either primary gastric or coexistent with a MALT lymphoma, requires more aggressive management.

MALT lymphomas are indolent and do not disseminate rapidly. Extranodal recurrences are more often observed. Prognosis does not seem to be affected by the existence of multiple extranodal sites or even bone marrow involvement.[115] This disease is sensitive to antibiotic therapy, and successful eradication of the *H. pylori* infection frequently leads to regression of the lymphoma. MALT lymphomas have demonstrated sensitivity to radiotherapy often resulting in prolonged complete responses. Transformation to diffuse large B-cell lymphomas may occur, resulting in a need for more aggressive treatment.

Mantle Cell Lymphoma

Mantle cell lymphoma (MCL) is a relatively uncommon B-cell neoplasm consisting of small to medium-sized cells that resemble cleaved follicular-center cells or centrocytes. A monoclonal lymphoid proliferation destroys the architecture of the lymph node. A nodular, diffuse, or mantle zone growth pattern is observed. It is uncommon for a true follicular growth pattern to be seen. Blastoid and other variants have been identified.

Mantle cell lymphomas have strong surface IgM. The typical immunophenotyping is $CD20^+$, $CD5^+$, $CD3^-$, $CD10^-$, $CD23^-$ (or weakly positive), $CD43^+$, and *BCL-6* negative. $CD5^-$ cases do exist. These lymphomas tend to demonstrate a more indolent nature. All mantle cell lymphomas are *BCL-2* positive, and the vast majority express cyclin D1.[119–121]

Conventional cytogenetics demonstrate the t(11:14) (q13;q32) mutation between the immunoglobulin heavy-chain gene on chromosome 14 and the *BCL-1* gene on chromosome 11 in 70%–75% of cases of MCL.[122,123] However, this translocation is virtually universal if FISH testing is performed to identify it.[124] Many other cytogenetic abnormalities have been reported in low frequencies. Some have been associated with variants of MCL, whereas others are associated with SLL/CLL.[125]

Mantle cell lymphoma accounts for only 3%–10% of all cases of NHL. The median age of individuals at diagnosis is 60 years, and the disease shows a male-to-female predominance of 2:1. Although lymph nodes are most commonly involved, the spleen, liver, and bone marrow also have a high frequency of involvement. Hepatomegaly and splenomegaly are common findings on physical examination. Abnormalities of the peripheral blood, which may include a marked lymphocytosis, are seen in approximately 20% of patients. The most common extranodal sites reported include the gastrointestinal tract (about 30% of patients) and the Waldeyer's ring found in the tonsils. Multiple lymphomatous polyposis, a disorder involving multiple lymphomatous lesions of the GI tract, is usually a form of MCL.[126,127] Unfortunately, patients tend to present with advanced-stage disease.

Many treatments for MCL have been tried, albeit with limited success. Clinical trials are therefore highly encouraged. Treatment with chemotherapeutic combinations such as CHOP is often undertaken if the patient does not participate in a clinical trial. Rituximab is frequently added to the chemotherapy regimen, as MCL is a CD20+ lymphoma.

The disease course for mantle cell lymphoma is aggressive and cure is rare. Median survival is 3–5 years. Adverse prognostic indicators include a high mitotic rate, blastoid variant, peripheral blood involvement, and trisomy 12.[128]

Diffuse Large B-Cell Lymphoma

Diffuse large B-cell lymphoma (DLBCL), the most common type of NHL, encompasses a diffuse group of large, neoplastic B lymphocytes with large nuclei. The predominant cell is either a large noncleaved cell or an immunoblast, or a mixture of both types of cells.[129] Destruction of the normal architecture of the involved lymph node occurs in a diffuse pattern. Multiple variants of DLBCL with different cytological features exist, but there is poor reproducibility among pathologists. No definitive immunophenotypic or genetic markers are available by which to distinguish the variants. Morphologic variants include centroblastic, immunoblastic, T-cell/histiocytic-rich, and anaplastic subtypes. DLBCL can occur de novo or it can represent transformation from a more indolent lymphoma. Lymphoma subtypes known to cause this transformation include SLL/CLL, follicular lymphoma, marginal-zone B-cell lymphoma, and nodular lymphocyte-predominant Hodgkin's lymphoma.

Diffuse large B-cell lymphomas frequently express pan-B-cell markers such as CD19, CD20, CD22, and CD79a, but they may not express all markers. Surface or cytoplasmic immunoglobulin can be observed in one-half to two-thirds of these malignancies, with IgM being the most frequently seen, and IgG and IgA encountered in decreasing incidence. DLBCL is typically $CD45^-$ and $CD3^-$; CD5, CD30, and CD10 may be expressed. Cyclin D1 is negative; it is a biomarker that distinguishes this subtype from blastoid variants of mantle cell lymphoma. CD5 and CD10 markers are typically not observed. The CD5 marker may be noted in de novo DLBCL but is not observed in transformed SLL/CLL.[130] Translocation of the *BCL-2* gene resulting in the t(14;18) mutation commonly observed in follicular lymphoma is noted in 20%–30% of DLBCL, and there is a high frequency of *BCL-6* positivity.[131,132] Heavy- and light-chain, immunoglobulin gene rearrangements as well as multiple cytogenetic abnormalities are commonly observed.

Thirty to forty percent of NHL cases involve DLBCL in Western countries, and an even greater percentage of cases in developing countries represent DLBCL. These lymphomas may be noted in a wide range of individuals, including children, but the median age at diagnosis is 64 years. It has a slightly higher incidence in males. The incidence of DLBCL has been increasing over the last few decades.[133] Immunodeficiency is a risk factor for this lymphoma, and in this setting may be associated with EBV infection.

Diffuse large B-cell lymphoma presents either as primary lymph node disease or at extranodal sites. Forty to fifty percent of patients have extranodal involvement at presentation, with 15%–20% of patients having the gastrointestinal tract involved and another 15%–20% having bone marrow involvement.[129,134] The disease often grows rapidly and is symptomatic. Many patients present with disseminated, advanced-stage disease. Disease may involve any organ. Without biopsy, the diagnosis of lymphoma may be missed. Lymphomas often have a much more favorable prognosis than the primary malignancy of the involved organ. Diffuse large cell lymphoma of the brain as the primary site of disease is being diagnosed with increased frequency.[134] Mediastinal (thymic) large B-cell lymphoma is a subtype of DLBL that arises in the mediastinum. Affected patients generally present with localized disease and symptoms related to large mediastinal masses. These masses may impede on the superior vena cava, resulting in obstruction. Patients are typically young adult females.

Treatment of DLBCL usually involves a multidrug, anthracycline-based chemotherapy regimen, such as CHOP, which is administered for 4–8 cycles, depending on the stage and IPI. The number of cycles may be decreased and locoregional radiotherapy administered to sites of involvement in earlier-stage disease. Rituximab has activity against this disease and is frequently added to the chemotherapy regimen, especially in patients older than age 60. Significant research is now seeking to determine the best method of incorporating rituximab into the treatment plan. Radioimmunotherapy has been investigated in patients with transformed DLBCL (as well as relapsed or refractory low-grade FL). It has been suggested that ^{90}Y-ibritumomab tiuxetan (Zevalin) is more effective when given earlier in the course of this disease. Because hematologic toxicity is the most significant toxicity, this treatment is recommended only when the patient has adequate bone marrow reserves and less than 25% of the marrow is involved with lymphoma.[135] Peripheral blood stem cell transplantation has been used for patients who have failed to obtain a complete response or have relapsed.

Diffuse large B-cell lymphoma is aggressive but curable with appropriate multidrug chemotherapy. The IPI is strongly predictive of outcome in this disease.[114] Disease-free survival rates are approximately 60% for patients with an IPI of 0/1, 35% for those with an IPI of 2/3, and 20% for those with an IPI of 4/5.[136] *BCL-2* overexpression has been associated with a higher incidence of relapse.[137,138] Conversely, the *BCL-6* translocation has been associated with a better prognosis.

Burkitt's Lymphoma

Burkitt's lymphoma (BL) is the most aggressive lymphoma, involving 100% of the cells in cell cycle at any time.[139] The malignancy is composed of monomorphic medium B-cells and divides rapidly. Three variants of Burkitt's lymphoma exist: endemic, sporadic, and immunodeficiency associated. Each of the variants demonstrates a different morphology and clinical history. Burkitt's lymphoma may also present as leukemia.

Endemic Burkitt's lymphoma is found in Africa and Papua, New Guinea. It is the most common malignancy in childhood there, occurring in a male-to-female ratio of 2:1 and with a peak age incidence of 4–7 years.[140,141] There appears to be a possible link between the climatic factors that are associated with malaria in the endemic regions. In addition, EBV is found in nearly all patients with endemic BL.[142,143] Multiple bacterial, viral, and parasitic infections (especially malaria) result in polyclonal B-cell activation and proliferation. The EBV-infected B cells are noted to have defective T-cell regulation, which supports the development of lymphoma.[143]

Sporadic Burkitt's lymphoma may be found throughout the world, affecting mainly children and young adults It is rare in adults. Thus it accounts for only 1%–2% of all lymphomas but is responsible for 30%–50% of childhood lymphomas.[144] This variant also has a higher incidence in males than in females (2–3:1 ratio), and the average age of adults at diagnosis is 30 years. There is an association with EBV infection, but it is observed in only 15%–20% of patients with BL in Europe and North America. Low socioeconomic status and early EBV infection are associated with increased risk of EBV-positive Burkitt's lymphoma. Fifty to seventy percent of patients with these risk factors are EBV positive.[145]

Both the endemic and the sporadic forms of BL occur in immunocompetent hosts. Tumor growth is not related to malfunction of the individual's immunity. Rather, the BL cell is thought to escape immune rejection because cell factors resemble resting B cells. In contrast, immunodeficiency-associated Burkitt's lymphoma is primarily seen in patients with HIV infection, but may be observed in other immunodeficiency states. It may be the initial AIDS-defining illness.[146] EBV is reported in 25%–40% of immunodeficiency-associated Burkitt's lymphoma.[146,147]

Burkitt's lymphoma commonly presents at extranodal sites. Patients with all three variants are at risk for CNS disease.[148] In endemic disease, the jaw, orbit, or other facial bones are involved approximately 50% of the time. Other potentially affected sites include the small intestine, omentum, ovaries, kidneys, and breast. Most patients with sporadic Burkitt's lymphoma present with abdominal masses. The ileo-cecal region is the most common site of involvement. Retroperitoneal masses may compress the spinal cord, resulting in sensory and motor loss. The ovaries, kidneys, and breasts may also be involved. Breast involvement is usually bilateral and is associated with the onset of puberty, pregnancy, or lactation. Lymph node involvement may occur but is more common in adults than children. A leukemic phase of this lymphoma may be observed, especially in patients with bulky disease. Rarely, patients present with bone marrow infiltration without other sites of disease. In such cases, the cells observed in the bone marrow resemble Burkitt cells. If more than 5% but less than 25% of the cells in the bone marrow are involved, the patient is classified as having stage IV Burkitt's lymphoma. If the bone marrow has more than 25% infiltration, the condition may be classified as acute lymphocytic leukemia (ALL), L3, or Burkitt's leukemia. Both nodal disease and marrow involvement are more common in immunodeficiency-associated Burkitt's lymphoma.

The morphology of classical Burkitt's lymphoma is observed in endemic BL and most sporadic cases of BL, especially in children. The cells are medium in size and diffusely infiltrate the tissue. These cells have multiple mitotic figures suggestive of a high proliferative rate. Two variants may be observed: the BL variant with plasmacytoid differentiation and the atypical Burkitt/Burkitt-like variant. The BL variant with plasmacytoid differentiation lacks the monotonous morphology of the classical BL cells and most commonly arises in immunodeficiency states.[149] The atypical Burkitt/Burrkitt-like variant is composed of cells similar to Burkitt cells except for their greater variety of nuclear size and shape. Diagnosis is dependent on a growth fraction of nearly 100% and evidence or strong suggestion of *MYC* translocation.[150] Some individuals with BL or Burkitt-like lymphoma demonstrate a strong granulomatous reaction. It has been postulated that it may represent an immune response to the disease and is associated with an excellent prognosis.[151]

B-cell associated antigens are expressed on BL cells (CD19, CD20, CD22) as well as CD10, CD77, and *BCL-6.* The cells are negative for CD5, CD23, TdT, and *BCL-2.* Blasts of BL presenting with a leukemic phase are consistent with a mature B cell, unlike precursor B-ALL. They are CD34 negative and usually TdT negative. CD45 is brightly expressed. Clonal rearrangements of the immunoglobulin heavy- and light-chain genes are seen. All cases have a *MYC* translocation [t(8;14)] or, less commonly, t(2;8) or t(8;22). The *MYC* translocation plays a significant role in the pathology of this disease, increasing the rate of cell cycling, activating genes involved in apoptosis, and enhancing the lymphogenicity.[152,153] The *MYC* translocation is present in all BL variants, regardless of EBV status.

Patients typically present with rapidly growing, bulky disease. Elevated serum uric acid and LDH levels are commonly found due to the rapid cell turnover. Patients are at risk for tumor lysis syndrome during institution of therapy and require close monitoring. Burkitt's lymphoma has a unique staging system developed by Murphy and associates and modified by Magrath.[154,155] See Table 58–6.

Table 58-6 Staging System for Burkitt's Lymphoma

Stage	Definition
I	A single nodal or extranodal mass with the exclusion of the mediastinum or abdomen.
II	A single extranodal tumor with regional lymph node involvement. Two or more nodal areas on the same side of the diaphragm. Two extranodal tumors with or without regional node involvement on the same side of the diaphragm. Primary gastrointestinal tract tumor, with or without involvement of the mesenteric nodes only.
II R	Completely resected abdominal disease.
III	Two single extranodal tumors on opposite sides of the diaphragm. Two or more nodal areas above and below the diaphragm. All mediastinal, pleural, or thymic tumors (primary intrathoracic tumors). All paraspinal or epidural tumors, regardless of other sites. All extensive primary intraabdominal disease.
IIIA	Localized but nonresectable abdominal tumors.
IIIB	Widespread multiorgan abdominal disease.
IV	Any of the above with initial CNS and/or bone marrow involvement < 25%.

Both endemic and sporadic BL are extremely aggressive but curable. Endemic BL is very sensitive to multidrug regimens. Treatment should be initiated as soon as possible because of the rapid doubling time of the tumor. Intensive regimens result in cure in as many as 90% of patients with early-stage disease and 60%–80% of patients with advanced disease.[139,144,155] Children have a more favorable prognosis than adults. Negative prognostic indicators include stage IV disease (CNS or bone marrow involvement), unresected tumor larger than 10 cm, and an elevated serum LDH level. Relapse, if it occurs, is likely to take place within the first year of diagnosis. Relapse-free survival for two years is considered a cure.[154] Burkitt's leukemia is treated with very intensive regimens but for short durations. Regimens must include intensive alkylating agents with an anthracyline and high-dose methotrexate. Traditional CHOP therapy, often prescribed for other lymphomas, is not adequate therapy for BL. Treatment is also considerably different than that for other subtypes of acute lymphocytic leukemia; as a consequence, accurate diagnosis is essential. Intrathecal therapy is recommended for all patients, possibly with the exception of those with stage I disease. Methotrexate and cytarabine are often administered intrathecally, sometimes including systemic high- or moderate-dose methotrexate.

The use of radiotherapy to prevent CNS involvement is controversial in this disease. No clear evidence proves that it benefits patients without known disease involving the CNS. Clearly, there is an increased risk of neurotoxicity associated with the addition of cranial irradiation. Even without radiotherapy, intrathecal chemotherapy in addition to systemic high-dose cytarabine and methotrexate may increase neurotoxicity. With appropriate treatment, 80%–90% of patients with BL survive.[139,156, 157]

AIDS-Related Lymphoma

The high frequency of AIDS-related NHL was first recognized in 1985. It is the second most common malignancy in patients with AIDS. Primary lymphoma of the brain, in patients younger than age 60, was included as an AIDS-defining diagnosis in 1982; three years later, systemic large cell lymphoma in an HIV-positive patient was added as a criterion for diagnosis of AIDS. Several types of HIV-associated lymphomas exist. The most common include Burkitt's lymphoma (50% of such cases); diffuse large B-cell lymphoma, which often involves the CNS (25%); primary effusion lymphoma (< 5%); and plasmablastic lymphoma of the oral cavity. Burkitt's lymphoma often develops in patients who are less immunosuppressed and earlier in their HIV disease course, whereas DLBCL tends to develop in patients with longstanding AIDS. There is also up to an eight-fold increased incidence of Hodgkin's lymphoma in patients with HIV.[158] Lymphoma is now believed to be the first AIDS-defining illness in approximately 3%–5% of patients.

The National Cancer Institute followed a group of patients with AIDS or symptomatic HIV infection beginning in 1985. In the study, 116 patients were started on treatment for HIV and followed through 1991. Nineteen percent of the patients developed NHL after three years, with an incidence rate of 5.6% per patient-year compared to 0.015% in the general population. The risk increased with time.[159] HIV does not seem to cause NHL, but rather the immune compromise due to HIV infection appears to be a significant risk factor for this lymphoma's development.

The role of EBV in the development of these high-grade, aggressive lymphomas remains controversial. Levine and colleagues reported that 68% of HIV-positive lymphoma patients had the EBV genome present, compared with 15% of HIV-negative patients.[160] Nearly all patients with primary CNS lymphoma and primary effusion lymphoma and 30%–70% of Burkitt's lymphoma have experienced EBV infections.

Most of these malignancies are monoclonal B-cell neoplasms. Immunophenotyping is consistent with the histological subtype of lymphoma that develops. Immunoglobulin gene rearrangements are commonly observed, while the minority of T-cell cases have clonal rearrangement of the T-cell receptor genes. Numerous genetic abnormalities involving the *MYC* and *BCL-6* oncogenes as well as tumor suppressor genes are recognized in HIV-related lymphomas. Abnormalities of the *MYC* gene are observed in HIV-related BL, similar to other cases of BL. Similarly, rearrangements of *BCL-6* are observed in DLBCL, while mutations of the non-coding region of the *BCL-6* can be detected in both DLBCL and BL. They represent the most common genetic alteration seen in HIV-related lymphoma.[160] Fifteen percent of cases demonstrate mutation of the *Ras* family proto-oncogenes. These mutations are unique to HIV-related lymphomas and are not normally found in lymphomas developing in immunocompetent hosts.[161] Tumor suppressor gene mutations and deletions are observed in 50%–60% of BL cases and 40% of DLBCL cases, leading to inactivation of this gene.[162]

Patients with HIV-associated lymphomas generally present with advanced-stage and bulky disease. B symptoms are observed in 80% of individuals and often lead to diagnosis. These early symptoms may prompt a work-up for opportunistic infection. HIV-related lymphomas commonly present in extranodal sites such as the CNS (30%) gastrointestinal tract (25%), bone marrow (20%–30%), and liver (9%–26%).[163–166] Unusual sites of disease, such as the oral cavity, jaw, and body cavities, may be involved as well. These tumors often meet the criteria of plasmablastic lymphomas of the oral cavity. As localized tumors, they grow rapidly and have a high mitotic index. The myocardium, testes, rectum, anus, gallbladder fossa, skeletal muscle, skin, soft tissue, ear lobes, adrenals, and other organs have been reported as sites of involvement. Only one-third of patients have lymph node disease at presentation. The serum LDH is elevated. Primary effusion lymphoma typically presents as either a pleural or peritoneal effusion. It can present as a solid tumor mass, most commonly involving the gastrointestinal tract or soft tissue.[167]

A dilemma exists over treatment of AIDS-related lymphoma. Aggressive chemotherapy regimens are typically utilized to treat the high-grade disease that is manifested as Burkitt's lymphoma. Due to the immunosuppression caused by the underlying HIV infection, patients often develop significant toxicity and a high incidence of opportunistic infections. This outcome has led to the administration of reduced-dose chemotherapy in patients with low CD4 counts. Patients with minimal risk factors can usually tolerate full-dose chemotherapy. Less aggressive treatment regimens, such as CHOP, with or without rituximab, may be used to treat DLBCL. Treatment is comparable to that given to patients without HIV infection. Prophylaxis of the CNS must be strongly considered for this population, however. Complete remission can be achieved in approximately 50%–60% of patients, many of them durable. Although CNS lymphoma has been treated with radiotherapy or high-dose methotrexate, survival in affected patients is poor.

Long-term survival can be achieved in approximately one-third of patients with HIV-related lymphomas with good prognostic indicators. Overall, the complete remission rate is about 50%, but the two-year survival is better in patients with BL than in those with DLBCL.[168] Although primary effusion lymphoma responds poorly to treatment and has a poor prognosis, the worst prognosis is associated with primary CNS lymphoma. The level of immunosuppression is a significant indicator of prognosis and correlates well with the IPI.[168] Negative independent prognostic indicators include age greater than 35 years, intravenous drug use, advanced-stage disease (III or IV), and CD4 counts less than $100 \times 10^6/L$. A multivariate analysis of prognostic factors was performed in 60 patients with newly diagnosed AIDS lymphoma. Four factors were associated with shorter survival: the diagnosis of AIDS made prior to the diagnosis of lymphoma, a low CD4 count, Karnofsky performance status less than 70%, and stage IV disease (with bone marrow involvement).[169] Primary CNS lymphoma may respond to radiotherapy, improving the patient's quality of life, but survival is in the range of 2–3 months.

Lymphoblastic Lymphoma: Precursor B- or T-Cell Lymphoblastic Leukemia/ Lymphoma

Sternberg first recognized lymphoblastic lymphoma (LL) in 1905, when a case of lymphoma of the mediastinum evolved into acute leukemia. At that time, this disease entity was known as Sternberg sarcoma. Lymphoblastic lymphoma — now classified by the World Health Organization as precursor B- or T-cell lymphoblastic leukemia/lymphoma — has had significant advances in therapy. In particular, recognition of low- and high-risk groups, as determined by cytogenetics and immunophenotyping, has permitted more specified therapeutic regimens.

The distinction between the terms "lymphoblastic leukemia" and "lymphoblastic lymphoma" is a blurry one. If the disease process presents with a mass lesion (nodal or extranodal) with minimal or no evidence of bone marrow and blood involvement, the term "lymphoma" is generally used. The cell of origin, either a precursor B lymphoblast or T lymphoblast, will further classify the disease. Precursor B-cell lymphoma accounts for approximately 10%–20% of lymphoblastic lymphoma, while precursor T-cell lymphoma represents 80%–90% of cases. Lymphoblastic lymphoma is rare in adults, accounting for only 4% of all cases of

NHL, but represents one-third to one-half of all cases of pediatric lymphoma.[170–172]

Precursor T-lymphoblastic lymphoma (T-LBL) is composed of small to medium-sized blasts. Morphologically, the cells look similar to those found in precursor B-lymphoblastic lymphoma (B-LBL). They diffusely infiltrate the lymph node and invade capsular and pericapsular tissues. Azurophilic granules may be observed in about 10% of B-LBL cases. Mitotic figures are generally more numerous in T-LBL. Immunophenotyping is required to distinguish these diseases. The lymphoblasts in T-LBL are positive for Tdt and for CD7, CD5, CD2, and CD3. The presence of CD3 is considered specific to the T-cell lineage. Other markers may be variably expressed, including CD1a, CD4, and CD8. Findings are negative for CD10.

Abnormal cytogenetic findings have been reported in 94% of lymphoblastic lymphomas. The abnormalities are similar to those found in T-cell acute lymphocytic leukemia (T-ALL) and support the belief that these diseases are different manifestations of the same disorder.[173] Certain translocations [such as t(9;17)], however, have been identified only in patients with T-LBL. At this time, the cytogenetic changes in T-LBL do not have any significant prognostic relevance. Burkitt's lymphoma must be ruled out, particularly in children presenting with lymphoblastic lymphoma. In adults, the blastoid variant of mantle cell lymphoma is included in the differential diagnosis. Evidence of Tdt rapidly distinguishes these other types of lymphoma.

The lymphoblasts in B-LBL are positive for Tdt and are almost always positive for CD10 (CALLA), CD19, and CD24. A cytogenetic abnormality, t(4;11) (q21;q23), may be seen. These mutations often account for those cases that do not express CD10 and CD24. Cytogenetic abnormalities in B-cell acute lymphoblastic leukemia/lymphoma are classified into multiple groups. These groups have significant prognostic significance and influence treatment planning, especially in the pediatric populations. Groups with a good prognosis include individuals with hyperdiploidy between chromosomes 59 and 65 and t(12;21) (p12;q22). Abnormalites including del(6q), del(9p), del(12p), hyperploidy < 51, near triloidy, and near tetraploidy denote an intermediate risk. Groups with a poor prognosis include those that have t(9;22) (Philadelphia chromosome), t(4;11), t(1;19), and hypoploidy. T-LBL is frequently found in adolescent males.

T-ALL is frequently characterized by its presentation of a rapid-growing mass in the mediastinum (50% of cases), with associated pleural effusions. Other sites of involvement include peripheral lymph nodes, skin, liver, spleen, Waldeyer's ring, central nervous system, and gonads.[174]

Historically, lymphoblastic lymphoma was associated with a poor prognosis. Today, thanks to more aggressive treatment regimens stratified by prognostic features and the availability of CNS prophylaxis, it is considered one of the most curable lymphomas. Intensive induction and consolidation regimens are used, similar or identical to leukemia regimens. Treatment regimens typically include higher doses of cyclophosphamide and anthracyline, standard-dose vincristine and asparaginase, and intrathecal chemotherapy.[100] Adults with advanced age, high serum LDH levels, bone marrow involvement, and CNS involvement have a poorer prognosis.

B-LBL is most commonly found in pediatric and young adult patients. Seventy-five percent of cases involve individuals who are younger than 18 years of age.[175] While most patients with B-cell leukemia/lymphoma present with leukemia, a small number (approximately 10%) present without significant marrow involvement. The most frequent sites of involvement in this subtype are the skin (may manifest as multiple nodules), bone, soft tissue, and lymph nodes.[176] Mediastinal masses in B-LBL are rare, in contrast to T-LBL. Treatment is similar to that identified for T-LBL. There is a high remission rate in patients with B-LBL, and a high cure rate in disease that remains limited to lymph nodes. Negative prognostic indicators include a high white blood cell count, symptomatic CNS disease, and unfavorable cytogenetic abnormalities.

Post-Transplant Lymphoproliferative Disorder

Post-transplant lymphoproliferative disorder (PTLD) is a lymphoma or lymphoid proliferation that develops due to immunosuppression in a recipient of a solid organ or peripheral blood (or bone marrow) stem cell transplant. These lymphomas have a high association with EBV infection (80% positive) and typically develop sooner after transplant than they do in EBV-negative cases.[177,178] The majority of PTLD cases that occur more than 5 years after transplant are EBV negative. Although PTLDs resulting in B-cell lymphomas are far more common, T-cell lymphomas represent approximately 12%–14% of the lymphomas.

Post-transplant lymphoproliferative disease comprises a spectrum of disorders that range from early lesions with reactive plasmacytic hyperplasia or infectious mononucleosis-like disease to monomorphic B- or T-cell neoplasms or Hodgkin's lymphoma. Table 58-7 outlines the categories of PTLD. The early lesions seen in PTLD are characterized by a diffuse proliferation of plasma cells and immunoblasts that do not

Table 58-7 Categories of Post-Transplant Lymphoproliferative Disease

1. Early lesions
   - Reactive plasmacytic hyperplasia
   - Infectious mononucleosis-like
2. Polymorphic PTLD
3. Monomorphic PTLD
   - B-cell neoplasms
     - Diffuse large B-cell lymphoma
     - Burkitt's/Burkitt-like lymphoma
     - Plasma cell myeloma
     - Plasmacytoma-like lesion
   - T-cell neoplasms
     - Peripheral T-cell lymphoma
     - Other
4. Hodgkin's lymphoma and Hodgkin's-like lymphoma

completely destroy the architecture of the affected lymph node or tissue. These lesions tend to occur in children and young adults and are often EBV negative. They may regress spontaneously with withdrawal or reduction of the immunosuppression or they may progress to monomorphic or polymorphic PTLD.

Polymorphic PTLD consists of destructive lesions affecting immunoblasts, plasma cells, and lymphoid cells. Unlike the early lesions, these lesions may efface the architecture of the lymph nodes or form destructive extranodal tumors. They are considered polymorphic because they demonstrate the full maturation of B cells. As with the early lesions, withdrawal or reduction of immunosuppressive agents is the treatment of choice, but it may lead to regression of the PTLD or progression to lymphoma. Monomorphic PTLDs have sufficient changes to diagnose lymphoma and express either B- or T-cell antigens. Although the majority of B-cell PTLDs are diffuse large B-cell lymphomas, Burkitt's lymphoma may be diagnosed in a minority of cases. Plasma cell myeloma is uncommon, but is important in that it appears to be unresponsive to withdrawal of immunosuppression.[179,180]

Plasmacytoma-like PTLD is also rare and its clinical behavior is not well studied. The extramedullary plasmacytomas occur in the gastrointestinal tract, lymph nodes, or other extranodal sites. Monomorphic T-cell lymphomas account for 12%–14% of PTLD. A broad spectrum of T-cell neoplasms are reported. The development of T-cell PTLD is generally longer than that for the B-cell PTLDs. Response to withdrawal or reduction of immunosuppression is less likely. Some reports have cited cases involving both Hodgkin's lymphoma and Hodgkin's-like lymphoma. Classical HL has been reported after allogeneic stem cell transplants with a threefold increase over its expected frequency.[181]

The genetic features of PTLDs vary depending on the category of lesion found. The monomorphic B-PTLDs consistently demonstrate clonal immunoglobulin gene rearrangement, typically containing EBV genomes. Conversely, the monomorphic T-PTLDs demonstrate clonal T-receptor gene rearrangements, and only 25% have EBV genomes.

Fewer than 2% of organ transplant recipients develop PTLD, but the risk of lymphoma depends on the type of organ transplanted and the immunosuppressive regimen used to prevent rejection. The highest risk is associated with transplantation of heart and lung or liver and bowel. Five percent of these patients develop PTLD. Those with a liver or heart allograft have an intermediate risk (1%–2%). Renal allografts have the lowest risk (< 1%).

Allogeneic stem cell transplant recipients have a low overall risk of developing PTLD (< 1%), but risk factors have been identified that may substantially increase the incidence in this group. In one study, more than 18,000 patients who underwent allogeneic bone marrow transplant at 235 centers throughout the world were followed for development of PTLD. The disease ultimately developed in 78 recipients. Eighty-two percent of these cases arose within one year of transplant, the other 18% occurred between 1 and 8.6 years post-transplant. The peak incidence of PTLD development was during the third month post-transplant. Eighty-six percent of patients who had a confirmed PTLD died during the survey period; rapid disease progression was noted in this group. Nine patients with early PTLD are alive with a range of follow-up of 3–131 months (median = 88 months).[182] Identified risk factors for early-onset PTLD (< 1 year) included receipt of HLA-mismatched, unrelated, or T-cell–depleted marrow; use of antithymocyte globulin; or use of anti-CD3 monoclonal antibody. As many as 20% of the patients with three or four of these risk factors developed a PTLD. A weaker association was noted with grade II–IV graft-versus-host disease (GVHD). The significance of these risk factors diminished after one year, and only extensive chronic GVHD was identified as a strong risk factor.

Clinical manifestations of PTLD vary depending on the immunosuppressive agent administered. Patients receiving azothioprine-based therapy tend to present with extranodal disease, whereas those receiving cyclosporine- or tacrolimus-based regimens present with lymph node and gastrointestinal tract involvement. The time to diagnosis post-transplant also correlates to the immunosuppressant used, the type of allograft, and EBV status. The mean interval to the development of PTLD post-transplant is 48 months when azathioprine is used and 15 months with cyclosporine therapy.[183] The majority of PTLDs develop within 5 months of stem cell transplant and new cases of the disease are relatively uncommon among survivors more than 1 year after transplant.[182] The median interval for the development of EBV-positive PTLD is 10 months, compared to 4–5 years for EBV-negative cases.[178,184]

Treatment of many PTLDs is often directed at reduction of immunosuppressant. This feat must be accomplished without rejection of the transplanted organ and control of GVHD in stem cell transplant recipients. It is often successful in early lesions and in children. Cases that fail to respond to withdrawal of immunosuppression require chemotherapy. The mortality among solid-organ transplant recipients who develop PTLD is approximately 60%, and among stem cell transplant recipients is 80%. The use of rituximab is being investigated in these transplant patients. Curtis and colleagues have reported that careful monitoring for EBV reactivation following bone marrow transplantation may provide warning of early PTLD development.[182]

Characteristics and Management of T-Cell NHL

Cutaneous T-Cell Lymphoma

Cutaneous T-cell lymphomas (CTLs) encompass a group of lymphomas of T-cell origin that involve primarily the skin and affect other sites secondarily. The subtypes of lymphoma that make up this group include mycosis fungoides (MF), Sezary syndrome (SZ), primary cutaneous anaplastic large cell lymphoma, and lymphomatoid papulosis. Lymphomatoid papulosis is not clinically considered a neoplastic disease.

Mycosis fungoides is a mature T-cell lymphoma. It has no relationship to a fungal etiology but received its name because of the mushroom-like appearance of the malignant lesions.[185] Infiltration of the epidermis and dermis with small to medium-sized T cells results in the characteristic cutaneous patches/plaques. Mycosis fungoides is the most common of the CTLs, but is still a rare disease, accounting for 0.5%–3% of all cases of NHL. It is primarily a disease of the elderly (median age at diagnosis is 55–60) and strikes males twice as often as females.[186] Mycosis fungoides is a slow-growing disease. Although the etiology of this cutaneous lymphoma is unknown, some reports have implicated recreational or occupational exposure to some chemicals as an origin. These reports have been refuted by two studies, one based on the Surveillance, Epidemiology, and End Results (SEER) program.[187,188] Whittemore and colleagues hypothesize that chronic antigeneic stimulation from contact allergens may be an initiating factor in the development of mycosis fungoides.[188]

Patients may report a history of scaly skin lesions for years prior to diagnosis. The skin may be the only

Table 58-8 Clinical Staging System for Mycosis Fungoides

Stage	Description
Stage I	Disease confined to the skin
Ia	Limited plaques/patches
Ib	Disseminated plaques/patches
Ic	Skin tumors
Stage II	Lymph nodes enlarged, but histologically uninvolved
Stage III	Lymph node involved documented histologically
Stage IV	Visceral dissemination

site of involvement for many years, with lesions initially seen on the trunk. The palms and soles may be either heavily involved or spared. These plaques usually become more generalized and eventually progress to tumor formation. At later stages, extracutaneous dissemination may occur involving the lymph nodes, liver, spleen, lungs, and blood. This spread is seen most frequently in patients who have developed cutaneous tumors (30%), compared to only 8% of those with limited plaques.[189] Involvement of bone marrow is rare. A simple clinical staging system has been developed for MF and is important in determining prognosis; Table 58-8 outlines this staging system.[190]

Lymph nodes are categorized when they become enlarged. Category I represents no involvement by MF; category II reflects early involvement; and category III entails massive involvement by MF. Clonal T cells are present occasionally in category I lesions, and in most category II and III lesions. These clonal cells may be associated with a unfavorable outcome. Immunophenotyping is usually $CD2^+$, $CD3^+$, $CD5^+$, $CD4^+$, and $CD8^-$.[190] No specific cytogenetic abnormality is associated with MF, but numerous, complex karyotypes are present in advanced disease. One or more subunits of the interlukin-2 (IL-2) receptor are often expressed in CTL; existing in three affinities: low, intermediate, or high.

Treatment depends on the stage of disease. Phototherapy, topical chemotherapy, radiotherapy, and occasionally systemic therapy are all used in the treatment of MF. Topical corticosteroids may be sufficient to relieve symptoms of early disease. This therapy does not provide long-term control, however, nor does it affect survival.

Phototherapy is performed by providing the patient with an oral photosensitizing drug, followed by ultraviolet light exposure (PUVA). Until the lesions clear, patients require treatment two to three times per week. Approximately 50% of patients will see the disease clear with phototherapy. The combination of PUVA with interferon has resulted in a complete response in as many as 80% of patients.[191] If clearance is achieved, a maintenance program is continued, with variable frequencies of treatment. Erythema and blistering are common acute side effects of PUVA. Cataract development and secondary skin malignancies are long-term concerns.

Topical chemotherapy is an effective, but less intrusive therapy on the patient's lifestyle. Topical nitrogen mustard is the most common agent administered. There is no absorption of the drug, which limits the toxicity and the follow-up needed. The drug is generally mixed in a water or ointment base and applied daily until the lesions clear. The concentration of the nitrogen mustard may be altered depending on the response of the lesions and the patient's tolerance. Self-administration may be impossible depending on the location of the lesions. The average time to clearance is approximately 6 months, and maintenance therapy is used for another 6 months.[185] A cutaneous hypersensitivity reaction develops in approximately 30% of patients receiving the aqueous solution and 5% receiving the ointment.[192] Desensitization has proved successful in overcoming this problem. Complete responses range from 32% to 61%, depending on the initial extent of skin involvement.[192] Only 10%–15% of patients maintain a long-term complete response after discontinuation of the topical nitrogen mustard. Topical BCNU has also been utilized for this disease. Although the response rate is similar to that with nitrogen mustard, BCNU is systemically absorbed. Its toxicity is also greater and hematologic monitoring is required.

Mycosis fungoides is very sensitive to radiotherapy, and ionizing irradiation is a most effective single-agent treatment for it. A complete response is generally obtained with doses greater than 20 Gy, but higher doses are often necessary to ensure long-term control. Electron therapy is more effective than photon therapy. Acute complications include erythema, desquamation, and temporary loss of hair and nails. For 6–12 months, patients experience an inability to sweat. Similar to other treatments for MF, an increased risk of secondary skin malignancies exists. Complete response rates have been reported to be as high as 98% in patients with limited plaques and approximately 35% in patients with generalized erythroderma or skin tumors. However, only about half of these complete responders demonstrated long-term responses.[185]

Systemic chemotherapy has limited value in the treatment of MF. Although multiple agents have been utilized, complete responses have been documented in only about 25% of cases with limited durations. Only 10%-20% of patients with MF require systemic treatment. Denileukin diftitox (Ontak) is a new antineoplastic agent, produced by genetically fusing protein from the diphtheria toxin to the interleukin-2 receptor. This biotherapeutic agent targets cells with IL-2 receptors. Nearly 60% of patients with CTLs have IL-2 receptors, and Ontak has demonstrated activity in this population of patients. Ontak is indicated for the treatment of persistent or recurrent CTL whose malignant cells express the CD25 subunit of the IL-2 receptor.[193] Acute hypersensitivity reactions have been reported in 69% of patients during or within the 24 hours of the Ontak infusion. These reactions were frequently associated with the first dose of a treatment cycle. Twenty-seven percent of the patients in clinical trials developed vascular leak syndrome manifested by hypotension, edema, and hypoalbuminemia.[193] Because patients with CTL are at risk for infection and Ontak affects normal lymphocytes, patients must be monitored closely for this complication.

Prognosis depends on the extent of the MF. Limited disease generally has an excellent prognosis, and survival is not affected by the disease. Prognosis is poor in advanced stages of MF, however. Negative prognostic features include age more than 60 years, skin tumors, extracutaneous dissemination, and elevated LDH. Transformation to a large T-cell lymphoma may be seen as a terminal event. Ulcerated tumors may develop a supra-infection. Sepsis is the leading cause of death in mycosis fungoides.

Sezary syndrome is often considered a variant of MF, but the clinical behavior is much more aggressive. This mature CTL is characterized by erythroderma, lymphadenopathy, and malignant T lymphocytes in the blood. These cells have the same morphology, immunophenotyping and cytogenetic characteristics as the cells that infiltrate the epidermis.[194] Despite the presence of neoplastic cells in the blood, the bone marrow is rarely involved. In advanced stages of disease, the visceral organs may be involved. Intense pruritis, cold intolerance, and skin pain are common complaints and can be very debilitating.

Sezary syndrome is an extremely rare disease and is found only in adults. There is a question of association of this disease with HTLV-1 infection. Morphologically, the cutaneous infiltrates are similar to those seen in MF. However, the density of dermal involvement and the extent of epidermal involvement may be significantly less, making diagnosis difficult. Topical use of corticosteroids may diminish the changes in the epidermis, further complicating diagnosis. The presence of neoplastic cells in the blood is the hallmark sign of SZ. The size of these cells may be small, large, or a combination of the two. Small cells are called Lutzner cells, while large cells are known as classical Sezary cells.[190] The immunophenotype of the malignant cells is typically $CD3^+$, $CD4^+$, $CD5^+$, and $CD7^-$, and $CD8^-$. T-cell receptor gene rearrangement is found.[191]

Sezary syndrome is an aggressive disease. Treatment requires a systemic approach due to its disseminated nature. Chemotherapy may clear systemic disease or may prove useful in relief of symptoms. Alternative approaches, such as PUVA or topical nitrogen mustard, may be utilized, with or following systemic therapy. As in MF, Ontak is indicated for refractory or relapsed SZ that expresses the CD25 component of the IL-2 receptor.[193] Temezolomide is a new oral alkylating agent that is in clinical trials for the treatment of relapsed SZ or MF. Transformation to large T-cell lymphoma may be seen as a terminal event. Five-year survival rates are reported to be between 10% and 20%.[186,190]

Primary cutaneous CD30-positive T-cell lymphoproliferative disorder [anaplastic large cell lymphoma (ALCL)] is a CTL that consists of anaplastic large T-lymphoid cells, most of which are CD30+.[190] This subtype of lymphoma must be distinguished from systemic anaplastic large cell lymphoma with skin involvement. It is found primarily in adults, and shows an increased incidence in males relative to females.

At diagnosis, nearly all patients have only skin involvement. Presentation commonly occurs with a solitary or localized skin lesion. Such lesions appear as a tumor, a nodule, or, uncommonly, a papule.[190] In approximately 20% of cases, multiple lesions or a lesion with satellites of tumor in surrounding tissues (multicentric) can be found. Dissemination to regional lymph nodes may occur, but involvement of other organs is rare.[194]

Morphologically, the features are similar to those of systemic anaplastic large cell lymphoma. Giant cells and Reed-Sternberg-like cells are often numerous. The infiltrates are diffuse and may involve all layers of the dermis as well as the subcutaneous tissue. Cells usually express CD4 in addition to the T-cell antigens. More than 75% of the cells are CD30+.[194] T-cell rearrangement is recognized in the majority of cases.

Partial or complete regression of the lesions of ALCL may occur, even without intervention. However, relapse is common. Dissemination, primarily to regional lymph nodes, occurs in approximately 10% of cases. It is seen more frequently in patients who present with multicentric disease. Treatment of limited disease is usually restricted to radiotherapy or surgical excision. Multidrug chemotherapeutic regimens are withheld unless evidence of overt extracutaneous involvement is found. Cutaneous anaplastic large cell lymphoma is considered indolent but incurable. The five-year survival rate is approximately 90%.[195] Spontaneous regression of the disease has been identified as a positive prognostic factor, whereas extracutaneous disease is associated with a poorer outcome.

Lymphomatoid papulosis is a generally benign disorder characterized by the spontaneous appearance and regression of papules and/or nodules infiltrated with atypical T lymphocytes. This disorder is limited to the skin. Dissemination of the disease can occasionally occur, resulting in progression to lymphoma in 10%–20% of patients.[190,195] Various lymphoma subtypes have been reported following lymphomatoid papulosis, including MF, cutaneous anaplastic large cell lymphoma, and Hodgkin's lymphoma.

Anaplastic Large Cell Lymphoma

Anaplastic large cell lymphoma is a T-cell lymphoma accounting for 2%–3% of adult and 10%–30% of childhood lymphomas.[196] It is characterized by large, lymphoid cells with abundant cytoplasm. These cells express CD30, also known as Ki-1 antigen. Most ALCLs express cytotoxic granule-associated proteins and are positive for anaplastic large cell lymphoma kinase (ALK) protein. It is important to distinguish this subtype of NHL from cutaneous anaplastic large cell lymphoma and from other NHL subtypes with anaplastic features.

Anaplastic large cell lymphoma is most commonly seen in younger patients, often younger than age 30. There is a male predominance to its incidence, especially during the second and third decades of life, for which the male-to-female ratio is reported to be 6.5:1.0. Patients who present with ALK-negative ALCL are often older, and this form of the disease demonstrates an almost even distribution between males and females.[196]

Fifty to seventy percent of patients present with stage III to IV disease, and most report B symptoms. High fevers are common. Serum LDH is elevated in approximately 50% of cases.[134] Peripheral and/or abdominal lymph nodes often present with extranodal disease and bone marrow involvement. The skin (21%), bone (17%), soft tissue (17%), lung (11%), and liver (8%) are the most common extranodal sites of involvement.[197] The bone marrow is found to be involved in almost one-third of cases when special stains are utilized to detect CD30 and ALK.[198] Bone marrow disease, however, is difficult to detect with morphological examination only due to the small number of scattered neoplastic cells.

Morphologically, considerable variability exists among cases of ALCL. However, all cases contain some cells with characteristic horse-shoe or kidney-shaped nuclei; these cells are found in all variants of ALCL.[199] The cells are often large, with a greater cytoplasm than is observed in most lymphomas. When the architecture of the involved lymph node is only partially destroyed, the neoplastic cells grow within the sinus, resembling a metastatic tumor.

Several variants of ALCL have been identified, including a lymphohistiocytic variant found in 10% of cases and a small cell variant found in 5%–10% of cases. The lymphohistiocytic variant occurs when malignant cells are found with a large number of histiocytes. The numerous histiocytes often mask the neoplastic cells, making morphologic diagnosis difficult. Special stains and testing to identify CD30, ALK, and/or cytotoxic granule-associated proteins are important aids in diagnosing this variant of ALCL. The small cell variant features a predominant population of small to medium-sized neoplastic cells. Hallmark cells can always be found, and are often seen in highest concentration around blood vessels.[199] When diagnosis is made without the use of specialized testing, this variant may be confused with peripheral T-cell lymphoma.

The large neoplastic cells are most strongly positive for CD30. Smaller cells may be negative or weakly positive. ALK is expressed in 60%–85% of cases. ALK staining is extremely specific for ALCL. Other than ALCL, only rare cases of diffuse large B-cell lymphoma express ALK. Clonal T-cell receptor rearrangement is seen in approximately 90% of ALCL cases. The ALK expression is due to genetic abnormalities of the *ALK* locus on chromosome 2. The most frequent and characteristic abnormality is a translocation between the *ALK* gene on chromosome 2 and the nucleophosmin gene on chromosome 5.[200] Translocations between the *ALK* gene on chromosome 2 and other genes on chromosomes 1, 2, 3, and 17 may also be seen.

Aggressive treatment regimens, such as those used to treat patients with diffuse large B-cell lymphoma, are appropriate for treatment of ALCL. The most important prognostic factor is ALK positivity, which is associated with a favorable outcome. The various genetic translocations seem to lack prognostic significance. The five-year survival rate is close to 80% in ALK-positive cases compared to 40% in ALK-negative cases.[195]

Peripheral T-Cell Lymphoma, Unspecified

Unspecified peripheral T-cell lymphomas (PTLs) encompass a group of heterogeneous, unspecified, mature T-cell neoplasms, which lack the distinct characteristics for a specific diagnosis. The neoplastic cells are typically a combination of small and large atypical lymphocytes. While some features of this group may lead the pathologist toward diagnosis of other specific T-cell subtypes, clear evidence of diagnosis is lacking and there is poor inter-observer and intra-observer reproducibility.[201] Anaplastic large cell lymphoma, MF, SZ and other subtypes of NHL are identified as specific types of PTL.[202] T-cell antigens are generally observed on immunophenotyping. Most nodal disease is $CD4^+$ and $CD8^-$. Most large cell variants express CD30. While anaplastic large cell lymphomas express cytotoxic granule-associated proteins, the unspecified PTLs rarely do so. Frequent cytogenetic abnormalities have been noted, but no consistent karyotypes have been associated with this group of malignancies.

Unspecified peripheral T-cell lymphomas are common, representing 7%–10% of all cases of NHL in the United States. They are typically found in adults with a median age near 60, and patients frequently present with systemic disease.[203] Most patients present with generalized lymphadenopathy. Involvement of the bone marrow, liver, spleen, and extranodal tissues—especially the skin—is common. Leukemic presentation may be seen with malignant cells in the peripheral blood. B symptoms are usually present.[202,204] Other common manifestations include eosinophilia and pruritus. The disease is aggressive and relapses are common. Treatment is similar to that of diffuse large B-cell lymphoma. With adequate treatment, this disease may be curable in some patients.

In an analysis of 92 cases of peripheral T-cell lymphoma by Arrowsmith and colleagues, 28 patients (30%) had what the WHO classifies as an unspecified peripheral T-cell lymphoma.[203] The median age of this group was 57.5 years and the male-to-female ratio was 3:1. Two-thirds of the patients presented with advanced (stage III/IV) disease, and 70% had either a low-intermediate or high-intermediate IPI. Twenty-three of the 28 patients received combination chemotherapy, with 74% achieving a complete remission. However, at 5 years, the estimated progression-free survival was only 17%, with an estimated survival of 42%. It was suggested that many of these cases acted similarly to a low-grade lymphoma.[203] Another analysis by Lopez-Guillermo and colleagues of 95 cases of unspecified PTL yielded a complete remission rate of 45% after treatment with an adriamycin-containing regimen. Median survival was 20 months.[204] Others have reported 5-year failure-free survival rates of 20%–30%. Only stage and IPI have demonstrated significant prognostic value with PTLs.[204]

Treatment Modalities

The treatment of NHL usually requires a multimodal approach to effect optimal treatment. This approach is determined by several key factors: histology of the tumor, stage of the disease, and the physiologic condition of the patient. These, in turn, help predict the curability of the tumor and guide treatment decisions. The WHO classification system encompasses a wide variety of lymphomas: Some are very indolent and may not need treatment for several years, while more aggressive disease may require immediate attention.

Unlike HL, NHL is often widely disseminated at diagnosis. Treatment to cure NHL is often multimodal and can be quite toxic. The armamentarium of the hematologist has never been greater. New chemotherapeutic drugs and combinations are being developed, radiation therapy is becoming more precise, monoclonal antibodies are increasing therapy responses, transplant technology is becoming less toxic, and many new approaches are in clinical study.

Chemotherapy

Depending on the curative intent, chemotherapy for NHL may consist of single-agent therapy or multidrug regimens. With indolent NHL, there exist a wide range of treatment options, from watchful waiting to chemotherapy. Depending on the disease and patient characteristics, single-agent oral therapy or treatment with a purine analog may be offered. Patients may undergo combination chemotherapy with or without a stem cell transplant, or they may be enrolled in a clinical trial utilizing a novel agent.

In the more aggressive lymphomas, mutidrug regimens are the standard of care. Several common regimens are listed in Table 58-9. It must be stressed that variations of the same combination of chemotherapy agents may be in use at individual institutions or cooperative groups. A randomized study conducted by the Southwestern Oncology Group (SWOG) and the Eastern Cooperative Oncology Group (ECOG) compared standard CHOP therapy to third-generation combination therapies such as Pro-MACE-CytaBOM in aggressive NHL. With a six-year follow-up, they concluded that there were no differences in response or survival rates, but that toxicity and cost were much higher with the newer therapies.[205]

Chemotherapy is myelotoxic. Many growth factors are used in conjunction with chemotherapy in an attempt to decrease transfusion requirements and to avoid delays in administration. One must be vigilant to observe side effects. Given that patients are now living longer, latent effects of chemotherapy, such as myelodysplastic syndrome (MDS), are becoming evident. Alkylating agents have been particularly implicated in the higher incidence of MDS, and treatment-related MDS is almost universally fatal.

If NLH returns or proves resistant to the above regimens, cure may still be attained in some subtypes through the use of stem cell transplantation. The source of the stem cells may be the patient (autologous) or another individual (allogeneic). If no family match is available, stem cell donor registries may be used to find an appropriate donor. Stem cell transplant works best in patients who have low amounts of chemotherapy-responsive disease. Salvage regimens are used to attempt to achieve this state prior to transplant or to decrease disease in patients who are resistant or refractory to initial therapy (See Table 58-10).

Two large, randomized studies have attempted to guide decision making about who should be offered a stem cell transplant. One trial examined autologous transplant in chemosensitive patients with relapsed aggressive NHL.[206] The five-year survival rate was 46% in the transplant group versus 12% in the chemotherapy group ($p = 0.001$). It is uncertain whether high-risk patients should be offered stem cell transplant as part of their initial treatment or only if they relapse. A large, cooperative group study is currently looking at this issue.

The second trial is the CUP trial from Europe, which randomized patients with follicular lymphoma who responded with three cycles of chemotherapy to either autologous stem cell transplant or more chemotherapy.[207] The transplant arm was further subdivided into purged and unpurged marrow. The researchers concluded that stem cell transplant significantly improved both progression-free survival and overall survival. They did not see a benefit in purging but, due to technical issues related to purging, could not generalize their data. Gribbin and colleagues, however, reported less relapse if the stem cell product was free of tumor.[208]

Radiation Therapy

Unlike HL, NHL typically does not spread via contiguous lymph nodes. Radiation therapy is frequently combined with chemotherapy and is targeted to areas of bulky disease, but not to entire zones of lymph nodes as it is in HL. Rarely, for stage I indolent NHL, radiation may be used alone in a curative attempt. Symptomatic lymphadenopathy can be treated with palliative doses of radiation for incurable disease.

Targeted Therapy

In 1997, rituximab became the first monoclonal antibody approved for cancer treatment. The mechanism for manufacturing monoclonal antibodies, which was devised in 1975 by Kohler and Milstein, involved making a hybridoma by fusing murine antibody-producing lymphocytes with a myeloma cell line. This technique allowed large-scale production of specific monoclonal antibodies.[209] Monoclonal antibodies can be naked or conjugated with radioisotopes or toxins. With naked monoclonal antibodies, the anticancer effect is thought to be induced by antibody-dependent cellular cytoxicity, complement-dependent cytotoxicity, and direct apoptosis. The attached radioisotope or toxin in

Table 58-9 Selected Combination Chemotherapy Regimens for NHL

Regimen	Dose and Route	Day	Frequency
CHOP			21 days
Cyclophosphamide	750 mg/m^2 IV	1	
Doxorubicin (Adriamycin)	50 mg/m^2 IV	1	
Vincristine (Oncovin)	1.4 mg/m^2 IV (max 2 mg)	1	
Prednisone	100 mg PO	1–5	
CNOP			21 days
Cyclophosphamide	750 mg/m^2 IV	1	
Mitoxantrone (Novantrone)	10 mg/m^2 IV	1	
Vincristine (Oncovin)	1.4 mg/m^2 IV (max 2 mg)	1	
Prednisone	100 mg PO	1–5	
CVP			21 days
Cyclophosphamide	400–600 mg/m^2 IV	1	
Vincristine (Oncovin)	1.4 mg./m^2 IV (max 2 mg)	1	
Prednisone	100 mg PO	1–5	
CVP 2			21 days
Cyclophosphamide	400 mg/m^2 PO	1–5	
Vincristine (Oncovin)	1.4 mg./m^2 IV (max 2 mg)	1	
Prednisone	100 mg PO	1–5	
COPP			28 days
Cyclophosphamide	400–650 mg/m^2 IV	1 and 8	
Vincristine (Oncovin)	1.4 mg./m^2 IV (max 2 mg)	1 and 8	
Procarbazine	100 mg/m^2 PO	1–14	
Prednisone	100 mg PO	1–14	
FN +/– D			28 days
Fludarabine	25 mg/m^2 IV	1–3	
Mitoxantrone (Novantrone)	10 mg/m^2 IV	1	
Dexamethasone	20 mg IV/PO	1–5	
FC			28 days
Fludarabine	25 mg/m^2 IV	1–3	
Cyclophosphamide	250 mg/m^2 IV	1–3	
Hyper-CVAD (alternating cycles up to total of 8)			When counts recover
Odd cycles (1, 3 ,5, 7)			
Cyclophosphamide	300 mg/m^2 IV q 12h	1–3	
Mesna	600 mg/m^2 IV over 24h	1–3	
Vincristine	2 mg IV	4 and 11	
Doxorubicin (Adriamycin)	50 mg/m^2 IV	4	
Dexamethasone	40 mg PO/IV	1–4 and 11–14	
Even cycles (2, 4, 6, 8)			
Methotrexate	1 g/m^2 IV over 24h	1	
Leucovorin	50 mg IV then 15 mg IV q 6h	1 (12h after methotrexate) until MTX level < 0.05 × 10^{-6} M	
Cytarabine (ARA-C)	3 g/m^2 IV q 12h × 4 doses	2 and 3	
Intrathecal therapy given with Hyper-CVAD			
Methotrexate	12 mg	Day 2 every cycle	
ProMACE/CytaBOM			21 days
Cyclophosphamide	650 mg/m^2 IV	1	
Doxorubicin (Adriamycin)	25 mg/m^2 IV	1	
Etoposide	120 mg/m^2 IV	1	
Cytarabine (ARA-C)	300 mg/m^2 IV	8	
Bleomycin	5 units/m^2 IV	8	
Vincristine (Oncovin)	1.4 mg/m^2 IV	8	
Methotrexate	120 mg/m^2 IV	8	
Leucovorin	25 mg/m^2 PO q 6h × 4 doses)	9	
Prednisone	60 mg/m^2 PO	1–14	

(continued)

Table 58-9 Selected Combination Chemotherapy Regimens for NHL (continued)

Regimen	Dose and Route	Day	Frequency
MACOP-B			One 12 week cycle
Methotrexate	400 mg/m² IV	8, 36, 64	One 12-week cycle
Leucovorin	15 mg/m² PO q 6h × 6 doses	9, 37, 65	
Doxorubicin (Adriamycin)	50 mg/m² IV	1, 15, 29, 43, 57, 71	
Vincristine (Oncovin)	1.4 mg/m² IV	8, 22, 36, 50, 64, 78	
Bleomycin	10 mg/m² IV	22, 50, 78	
Prednisone	75 mg/m² PO	1-84 (tapered days 70-84)	
COMLA			91 days
Cyclophosphamide	1500 mg/m² IV	1	
Vincristine (Oncovin)	1.4 mg/m² IV	8, 22, 36, 50, 64, 78	
Methotrexate	120 mg/m² IV	22, 29, 36, 43, 50, 57, 64, 71	
Leucovorin	25 mg/m² PO × 4	24h after each methotrexate	
Cytarabine (ARA-C)	300 mg/m² IV	Same days as methotrexate	

Many regimens are slightly different according to institution or country.
Vincristine (Oncovin) is sometimes capped at a 2 mg total dose.
Rituximab is often added

Table 58-10 Selected Salvage Chemotherapy Regimens for Lymphomas

Regimen	Dose and Route	Day	Frequency
ESHAP			21–28 days
Etoposide	40–60 mg/m² IV	1–4	
Methylprednisolone	500 mg IV	1–4	
Cytarabine (ARA-C)	2 g/m² IV	5	
Cisplatin	25 mg/m² IV over 24	1–4	
DHAP			21–28 days
Dexamethasone	40 mg PO/IV	1–4	
Cisplatin	100 mg/m² IV over 24h	1	
Cytarabine (ARA-C)	2 g/m² IV q 12h × 2	2	
ICE			21–28 days
Ifosfamide	1g/m2 IV	1–3	
Etoposide (VP16)	150 mg/m² IV q 12h (4 total)	1 and 2	
Carboplatin	200 mg/m² IV	1 and 2	
Mesna	333 mg/m² IV	30 min before and 4 and 8 h after every ifosfamide dose	

Rituximab is often added to these regimens.

conjugated monoclonal antibodies delivers extra killing ability. Although the monoclonal antibody was first developed in mice, there are now versions that are chimeric (60% human, 40% murine) and humanized (95% human). Infusional toxicity and the duration of time the drug remains in the bloodstream depend on the subtype of monoclonal antibody. Typically, the more humanized the antibody, the lower the frequency of side effects and the longer it remains in circulation.[210]

Rituximab may be used alone or in conjunction with chemotherapy in the treatment of B-cell lymphomas. The standard dose is 375 mg/m² weekly for four weeks. Premedication with acetaminophen and diphenhydramine is standard, and there should be easy access to emergency drugs and equipment. Reactions to rituximab are typically infusional in nature and may involve chills, dyspnea, myalgias, or hives. These side effects are more common during the first infusion. If a reaction occurs, the drug is stopped and medication is given. Once the symptoms resolve, rituximab is restarted at a lower rate. Caution must be exercised in patients with high amounts of circulating lymphocytes such as those with CLL. They are at risk for life-threatening infusional reactions from cytokine release and tumor lysis.[211]

When early phase I/II studies examined the pharmacokinetics of rituximab, they found that circulating B cells were promptly cleared and the effects lasted three to six months. In some patients, rituximab was still measurable in the blood several months after therapy completion.[212] The phase II pivotal trial used rituximab to treat relapsed, indolent disease. It reported an overall response rate of 48%, but found that the response was delayed and occurred at a median of 50 days. Time to progression was 13 months. Patients with CLL or chemotherapy-resistant disease did not respond as well as chemosensitive patients.[213] Retreatment is possible in responding patients and can lead to a 40% response.[214]

Rituximab is also used in conjugation with chemotherapy. Coiffier and the GELA group in France explored the use of rituximab combined with CHOP chemotherapy in the treatment of diffuse large cell NHL in patients 60–80 years old. They found a significant difference in CR and improved event-free survival and overall survival rates at two years.[215] These results have tended to be generalized to all patients with this type of NHL, and the combination is now a popular first-line therapy. Many questions remain to be answered, however, and investigators are currently exploring the optimal dose and scheduling of rituximab, the day on which combination chemotherapy should be given, the role of maintenance rituximab, the usefulness of extended treatment, ways to combine rituximab with other monoclonal antibodies and substances, and factors influencing rituximab sensitivity or resistance.

Aletuzumab (Campath-1H) is a humanized monoclonal antibody that targets the CD52 antigen; it was approved by the FDA in 2001. CD52 is found on the surface of most normal and malignant T and B cells, as well as on NK cells, macrophages, monocytes, and male reproductive system cells. Aletuzumab has been used in the treatment of autoimmune disorders, solid-organ transplants, graft-versus-host disease, and both T- and B-cell malignancies.[216] It has been used most often in the treatment of CLL. The pivotal trial in fludarabine-resistant patients with CLL showed a 33% response rate, with a time to progression of more than 9 months.[217] This drug appears to have more of an effect in the blood, bone marrow, and spleen compared with lymph nodes.[218]

Aletuzumab is typically given three times per week for a total of 12 weeks using an escalating dose. Infusional reactions are common, and pretreatment with acetaminophen and diphenhydramine is necessary. The drug may be given as a subcutaneous injection with less toxicity.[219] Because of its effect on many cells in the immune system, prolonged immunosuppression can occur that may last as long as 18 months and lead to opportunistic infections such as *Pneumocystis carinii*. Prophylaxis with trimethoprim/sulfamethoxole and an antiviral agent is indicated.[220]

Radioimmunotherapy

Although naked monoclonal antibodies have added much to the treatment of NHL, all patients do not respond to them. Linking a radioactive molecule to a monoclonal antibody provides a number of advantages, as lymphoma cells are very radiosensitive, and cell kill would not have to depend on the presence of an intact immune system. Many different combinations of radionucleotides and monoclonal antibodies are being tested in a variety of cancerous and noncancerous diseases. Two radioconjugates currently on the market used for NHL, Iodine 131 tositumomab (Bexxar) and Ibritumomab tiuxetan (Zevalin), are both attached to a CD20 monoclonal antibody. These beta-particle emitters lead to fatal DNA damage in both the cells they target via the CD20 antigen and cells in close proximity to them (the bystander effect).[221] Bexxar also emits gamma particles that can be used to determine dose.

Bexxar and Zevalin share many similarities, and both require a dedicated team to safely administer them. Physicians and nurses along with nuclear medicine, radiation pharmacy, and radiation safety personnel are all needed. A cold antibody is first administered to deplete B cells in the peripheral blood; it has been shown to improve the distribution of the radioimmunotherapy at the target sites. Depending on the drug, dosing is based on weight (Zevalin) or on gamma elimination of a test dose (Bexxar). Because it is important to clear the radiation from the body in a timely manner, the monoclonal antibody of both drugs is murine in derivation. Human antimouse antibodies (HAMA) and human antichimeric antibodies (HACA) may be tested. Patients with high titers of these antibodies tend to respond poorly and can experience severe infusion reactions.[222]

Other safety issues important in patient selection are ensuring low tumor burden in the marrow and adequate marrow function. Patients who receive these drugs are at high risk for prolonged cytopenias and marrow dysfunction following treatment. Surrogate markers for marrow dysfunction are prior myeloablative therapy, external beam radiation to greater than 25% of the marrow, failed stem cell harvest, platelets $< 100{,}000/mm^3$, absolute neutrophil count $< 1500/mm^3$, and a hypocellular marrow (< 15%). The marrow should be 25% or less involved with disease.[223] Depending on the drug, radiation safety precautions must occur for patients after therapy. For both drugs, body secretions are contaminated with radiation for about one week after dosing. Body fluids must be cleaned promptly, and condoms should be worn during this time. Because Bexxar is also a gamma emitter with a longer path length of radiation, patients must remain in semi-isolation for about one week. They need to avoid prolonged contact with others and avoid young children and pregnant women. In the United States, radiation safety is regulated by both the state and federal governments. The Nuclear Regulatory Commission publishes regulations and guidelines that must be followed.

Because of the radiation, these drugs are myelotoxic. Peripheral blood count nadirs are more delayed and prolonged than with conventional chemotherapy. With Bexxar therapy in low-grade or transformed NHL, nadirs occur between 4 and 6 weeks and generally begin to recover by weeks 8 to 9. The incidence of grade III/IV hematologic toxicity is 30%–40%.[223]

Both Bexxar and Zevalin have produced remissions in 60%–80% of patients with indolent NHL and relapsed/refractory disease. The results are even better in treatment-naïve patients, with 97% RR and 63% CR.[210] Many remissions are durable, and patients who relapse after Bexxar can still have a 56% response with repeat dosing.[223] Investigations are currently looking at the precise role of immunotherapy in the treatment of NHL as well as examining the long-term side effects of these compounds.

New Therapies

With today's standard therapies, 50% or fewer patients with advanced diffuse large cell lymphoma are cured; rarely are those with low-grade NHL or CLL cured.[224] To compound the problem, many patients with NHL are older, have co-morbidities, and/or have decreased marrow reserves from the myelotoxicity of prior regimens. Clearly, new agents are needed. As we learn more about the biology and cellular activities of lymphoma cells, novel ways to fight the disease may become apparent. A chromosomal abnormality or an adverse marker for a lymphoma might be turned into an area for investigation. The therapies described next are in clinical trials either alone or in combination with approved treatments in an attempt to increase response and eventually cure rates.

New monoclonal antibodies: epratuzumab (anti-CD22) and galiximab (anti-CD80). CD20 is a well-known B-cell antigen targeted by the monoclonal antibody rituximab, but there are concerns that resistance to it may develop. As a consequence, other targets on B cells are under investigation for monoclonal antibody development. CD22 is an attractive target expressed in 60%–80% of B-cell lymphomas. This transmembrane protein, unlike rituximab, is internalized when it binds to antibody. It appears to be involved with numerous B-cell operations, including homing, intracellular adhesion, and receptor signaling thresholds.[225] Several human studies are looking at epratuzumab's use in naked form as well as conjugated with radiation molecules. Responses were seen in relapsed/refractory follicular and diffuse large cell lymphoma with the naked antibody. Toxicities were mild and no dose-limiting toxicities were observed.[225] Studies are also looking at epratuzumab's use in combination with rituximab as well as chemotherapy. Because the CD22 molecule internalizes, this monoclonal antibody is being investigated as a potential combination therapy with an immunotoxin.

CD80 is another target under investigation. It is found on the surfaces of activated B cells and other antigen-presenting cells.[226] Unlike in normal B cells, CD80 is highly expressed on malignant B cells and is thought to lead to deregulated growth. The monoclonal antibody galiximab, which targets CD80, has been given as a continuous intravenous infusion over seven days either alone or in combination with R-CHOP. Reported side effects include fatigue, cough/dyspnea, nausea, and rash.[226]

Vaccine therapy: tumor-specific idiotype vaccines. On the surface of each B lymphocyte is a unique immunoglobulin molecule that is produced by shuffling of gene segments during the lymphocyte's development. B-cell lymphomas frequently express this unique molecule on all cells in the malignancy. Thus the individual with a B-cell lymphoma has an idiotype unique to his or her tumor cells—and a potential target for vaccine therapy. Upon vaccination, the immune system can prime T cells to reject the tumor. Anti-idiotype vaccines can be made via hybridoma technology or via dendritic cells. Trials of such vaccines are currently under way in human patients. Upon diagnosis, a piece of tumor is sent to the laboratory for idiotype amplification and vaccine manufacture. The patient is then given therapy to achieve a minimal residual disease state. The vaccine is attached to KLH (keyhole limpet hemocyanin) and given to the patient on a set schedule, typically in conjunction with an adjuvant such as GMCSF that is used to prime the immune system. Some patients develop induration at the injection site. In one trial, several responders with follicular lymphoma are 12 years from diagnosis with no evidence of disease.[227] Current trials are emphasizing ways to augment the patient's immune response and strategies to make vaccine technology available to more people.

Antisense oligonucleotides: olimersen sodium (Genesense). Programmed cell death (apoptosis) is regulated by a balance of pro- and anti-apoptotic proteins within the cell. One event that occurs when a cell receives a death signal is the release of cytochrome c from mitochondria, which activates enzymes called capsases. These enzymes cause cell destruction and degradation. BCL-2 is an anti-apoptotic protein that resides in the mitochondrial membrane and blocks the release of cytochrome c. It was first reported at the t(14;18) breakpoint in follicular NHL, and is often overexpressed in other NHL and cancers. BCL-2 is an adverse predictor of response to antineoplastic therapies. Olimersen sodium (Genesense) is a drug that has been devised to block the messenger RNA that encodes for BCL-2. This, in turn, allows the cell to respond appropriately to apoptotic signals, leading to cell death. Genesense is given as a continuous infusion and is currently in clinical trials both alone and in combination for many different cancers. Common side effects seen in phase I/II studies include low-grade fever, fatigue, and a transient decrease in platelets.[228]

Gallium nitrate. Gallium nitrate was first discovered in 1875. More than 30 years ago, it was noticed that, when this compound was injected into patients with NHL, it concentrated preferentially in tumor involved areas. This discovery led to its use in the familiar gallium scan to detect active lymphoma.[229] Gallium nitrate was investigated by the NCI as one of the Group III "near metals" with potential anticancer activity,[230] and is currently used as an antihypercalcemic agent because it promotes bone resorption.[231] The precise mechanism of action of gallium nitrate as an antitumor drug is not fully clear. Gallium binds to transferrin, an iron transport protein, and is taken up in the cell, where it leads to cellular iron deprivation. It ultimately inhibits ribonucleotide reductase—a step needed in DNA synthesis leading to growth arrest and possibly apoptosis. It is known that lymphomas with higher concentrations of transferrin receptors are more aggressive.[232]

Gallium nitrate is currently being evaluated in clinical trials both as a single agent and in combination with other therapies. Because of its unique mechanism of action, it has shown promise in refractory disease. It is given as a continuous, seven-day intravenous infusion by a portable infusion pump. Common side effects include hypocalcemia, hypophosphatemia, hypomagnesemia, and anemia. Rarer reactions include conjunctivitis, renal insufficiency, and skin rash. Optic neuritis, paresthesias, and thrombocytopenia have been noted in very rare patients.[233] An ophthalmology exam is indicated prior to initiating therapy, and patients are encouraged to maintain adequate oral hydration to decrease the risk of nephrotoxicity. Patients require monitoring of their CBC and electrolytes.

Proteosome inhibition: bortezomib (Velcade). The ubiquitin–proteosome pathway regulates the breakdown of many intracellular proteins involved with cell homeostasis, proliferation, and apoptosis in both normal and cancerous cells. This pathway is responsible for the control of key cell-cycle regulatory activities such as the p53 protein, NF-κB system, and BCL-2.[234] Malignant cells are thought to be more sensitive to disruption of this pathway than are normal cells. Bortezomib (Velcade) inhibits this pathway. Now on the market for the treatment of multiple myeloma, it is under investigation in NHL both as a single agent and in combination therapy. Bortezomib is typically given in 21-day cycles, with twice-weekly infusions administered on days 1, 4, 8, and 11. Its toxicities include fatigue, malaise, nausea, diarrhea, thrombocytopenia, and anemia. In a phase II trial in relapsed/refractory lymphoma, it produced a 53% response rate.[235]

Fusion toxins: denileukin diftitox (Ontak). Fusion toxins combine, via recombinant DNA technology, a toxin with a delivery system to a specific target. Denileukin diftitox (Ontak) is a fusion protein that combines a diphtheria toxin with an IL-2 sequence. It thereby targets the diphtheria toxin to IL-2 receptor–bearing cells, which include activated T cells, B cells, and macrophages. Ontak is currently FDA approved for use in CD25-positive cutaneous T-cell lymphoma, but also shows promise in B-cell NHL. Phase I/II clinical trials have demonstrated responses in diffuse large cell and follicular NHL, with the median time to response being two months. Its use has been associated with acute infusional toxicities such as fever, rash, and hypotension as well as low-grade vascular leak syndrome.[236] Phase II trials of this drug are in progress.

Acute Complications of Therapy

The individual therapies or combined modalities used in the treatment of HL and NHL will invariably result in acute and chronic side effects. The precise complications of therapy depend on the subtype of lymphoma, tumor burden, treatment, and patient variances. The medical team must be prepared to assess and manage these toxicities in a timely manner. Preparation and education of the patient and family are critical to effective treatment.

Radiotherapy may cause local or systemic toxicities depending on the site or sites being irradiated. Mantle radiation is often associated with loss of taste, dry mouth, dysphagia, erythema of the skin, and a characteristic loss of hair at the nape of the neck. Due to the decrease in saliva production, individuals who undergo such treatment are at increased risk for dental caries. Instructions regarding oral care should be provided. Acute radiation pneumonitis may be clinically observed 3–4 months following mantle radiotherapy.[237] Inverted Y-port irradiation usually results in anorexia, nausea, vomiting, diarrhea, and malaise. Bone marrow depression may occur and must be monitored by frequent complete blood counts. Localized radiotherapy to a specific lymph node or extranodal mass is often delivered at higher doses. As a consequence, local skin reactions may become a significant problem. In addition, toxicity to underlying or nearby organs may be more pronounced — for example, radiation of the cervical lymph node chain may result in more severe mucositis and dysphagia.

Total nodal irradiation may result in the previously mentioned side effects. Suppression of bone marrow function may be pronounced. The use of total-body irradiation is limited to myeloablative therapy followed by stem cell transplantation. The gastrointestinal tract and bone marrow are exquisitely sensitive to radiotherapy, and most acute side effects are related to toxicity of these organs. Stomatitis, esophagitis, gastritis, parotitis, nausea, vomiting, and diarrhea may be observed. The profound suppression of the bone marrow, resulting in aplasia, is a desired effect in this treatment.

Acute toxicities of chemotherapeutic agents vary widely, depending on the agent or combination of agents given and the dosage administered. The most common acute side effects occur due to damage of the gastrointestinal tract, hair, skin, bladder, kidneys, peripheral nervous system, and bone marrow. Emphasis on prevention and/or control of nausea and vomiting has been the focus of the healthcare team over the years, particularly in the management of Hodgkin's lymphoma. MOPP therapy, for example, was associated with severe nausea and vomiting, resulting in quality of life issues and poor compliance with completion of therapy. Given that Hodgkin's lymphoma has historically been considered one the most curable malignancies, early discontinuation of therapy had a life-threatening impact.

The use of vinca alkaloids in the treatment of lymphoma has resulted in many patients experiencing some degree of peripheral neuropathy. Preexisting hypertension and diabetes mellitus have been identified as risk factors for the development of peripheral neuropathy during treatment.[238] Acute myocardial injury may occur, and congestive heart failure may be observed as an acute or a chronic toxicity. Congestive heart failure may be precipitated by the use of aggressive hydration, corticosteroids, and anthracyline therapy. An analysis by Sonnen and colleagues found that congestive heart failure was observed only in patients with prior heart disease.[238]

The inclusion of prednisone as part of the chemotherapy regimen (such as in CHOP) or the administration of dexamethasone as part of the antiemetic regimen may result in hyperglycemia. Corticosteroid-induced hyperglycemia does not respond well to oral antihyperglycemic agents but rather usually requires management with insulin. Patients who receive these agents — and particularly those with a history of glucose intolerance — must be monitored closely for hyperglycemia.[238]

Psychological stress is common in patients with lymphomas, sometimes resulting in anxiety or a depressive disorder. This development affects quality of life and may jeopardize therapy completion. Ongoing nursing support, close monitoring for signs of psychological decompensation, and early intervention are critical to the overall care of the patient.

Immunotherapy including monoclonal antibodies and radioimmunotherapy are frequently associated with infusion-related toxicities. Fever, chills, hypotension, dyspnea, hypoxia, and signs of hypersensitivity reactions are common side effects. The initial doses of agents such as rituximab, anti-CD52 monoclonal antibody (Campath), and Ontak are associated with the greatest risk of reaction. The frequency of reactions to rituximab has been associated with the white blood cell count, number of CD20$^+$ cells in the blood, and intensity of CD20 staining. Premedication with diphenydramine and acetaminophen is standard with many of these agents, and close monitoring during the infusion is mandatory. Agents such as anti-CD52 monoclonal antibody therapy (Campath-1H) suppress both humoral and cellular immunity, and opportunistic infections are well documented with their use.[239]

Oncologic emergencies such as superior vena cava syndrome, tumor lysis syndrome, and sepsis may be observed in patients with lymphoma. These may occur independent of therapy or as a toxicity related in part to therapy.

Obstruction of the superior vena cava may result from the presence of a mass on the right side of the superior mediastinum, which serves to compress this large blood vessel. Obstruction of blood return to the heart produces a characteristic syndrome of edema in the upper half of the body that is associated with prominent collateral circulation. Lymphoma is second only to lung cancer as the leading malignancy contributing to superior vena cava obstruction. This oncologic emergency necessitates prompt therapy aimed at eliminating the obstruction. External beam radiation therapy has been the traditional approach to rapidly restore normal flow, especially when the signs and symptoms are rapidly progressive.

Prophylaxis for hyperuricemia is provided in many patients with lymphoma, especially those with elevated serum uric acid levels prior to initiation of therapy, those with intermediate- or high-grade lymphomas, and those with significant tumor burden. Adult patients with normal renal function may be prescribed 300 mg of allopurinol daily. It is important to stress the need for maintaining adequate hydration to all patients before starting therapy. Control of nausea and vomiting is necessary for patients who receive outpatient chemotherapy and will self-hydrate orally. Patients should be instructed to contact their healthcare team if hydration is jeopardized. Inadequate hydration will result in uric acid crystal deposition in the kidneys with subsequent renal dysfunction. The risk for tumor lysis syndrome is greatest after initiation of therapy in patients with high-grade lymphomas, such as those with acute lymphoblastic lymphoma and Burkitt's lymphoma, and those with large tumor burdens. Tumors that are extremely sensitive to treatment will result in a rapid breakdown of cells. The intracellular contents are then released in the bloodstream, increasing the potential for electrolyte abnormalities and renal insufficiency or failure. Measures commonly employed to prevent tumor lysis syndrome include hydration, alkalinization of the urine, and administration of allopurinol. Despite these measures, approximately 20% of patients at high risk for tumor lysis syndrome will require dialysis, delaying chemotherapy. Recombinant urate oxidase (Resburicase), an intravenous agent, has demonstrated superior efficacy in prevention of hyperuricemia, tumor lysis syndrome, and renal failure.[240]

Bone marrow depression, resulting in neutropenia and an increased subsequent risk of infection, is a well-recognized toxicity of aggressive combination chemotherapy. Neutropenia is the dose-limiting toxicity of many regimens that are used to treat patients with HL and NHL. Age, poor performance status, and increased intensity of chemotherapy doses are the major risk factors for neutropenia.[241] Because NHL is commonly found in elderly individuals (more than 60% of patients are older than age 60), the incidence of this complication is substantial. Colony-stimulating factors, when administered prior to the onset of chemotherapy-induced neutropenia, are effective in reducing the incidence and severity of neutropenia and related complications.[242] Debate persists over the administration of colony-stimulating factors, however. The most widely accepted approach is to administer these costly agents on subsequent cycles if the patient experiences neutropenia and/or infection during a course of therapy. Others suggest that administration of these agents, without first waiting for an infectious event to occur, can help prevent neutropenia and facilitate the delivery of antineoplastic agents on the proposed schedule.[241]

Bacterial infections are most frequently encountered following chemotherapy for HL and NHL. Opportunistic infections from organisms such as *Pneumocystis carinii* (protozoan), *Aspergillus* or *Candida* species (fungal), and cytomegalovirus (CMV) and herpes (viral) may be seen in individuals treated with dose-intensive therapy. Therapies that lead to prolonged neutropenia, that suppress cellular and humoral immunity, and that incorporate corticosteroids in the regimen result in the highest incidence of bacterial and opportunistic infections. Anemia and thrombocytopenia may also be observed either secondary to the lymphoma or secondary to therapy. Epoietin alfa (Procrit) or darbopoieitin (Aranesp) are indicated for patients with anemia related to chemotherapy. Subcutaneous administration of these agents may negate or minimize the need for red blood cell transfusions, decrease fatigue, and improve quality of life.

Chronic Complications of Therapy

Survivors of Hodgkin's lymphoma and childhood leukemias have provided substantial information regarding the long-term complications of their therapies. However, therapies continue to change, and the unknowns about treatments may outweigh the knowns. The advancements in the treatment of all lymphomas now means that many patients face a future in which long-term survival is a reasonable expectation.

It is important to emphasize that no organ system is exempt from potential long-term toxicity. Nevertheless, much of the emphasis has been on the incidence of cardiovascular effects, reproduction impact, and the development of secondary malignancies.

Fatigue

Fatigue is a common complaint in the normal population and is multifactorial in nature. It may be a presenting manifestation of cancer or it may reflect advanced disease. In addition, treatment may produce or worsen symptoms of fatigue. While fatigue is accepted as an acute toxicity of therapy, long-term fatigue is more disturbing to the patient. An analysis of 116 survivors of Hodgkin's disease reported that pulmonary dysfunction — most commonly manifested by impairment of gas transfer — was highly associated with chronic fatigue.[243]

Pulmonary Dysfunction

Radiation fibrosis may follow mantle field acute radiation pneumonitis, stabilizing 9–12 months following completion of treatment. Patients often present with dyspnea and exercise intolerance. Most chemotherapeutic agents do not cause long-term damage to the lungs. The exception is bleomycin, which may cause pulmonary damage in as many as 40% of patients or enhance radiation-induced toxicity.[244]

Thyroid Dysfunction

Thyroid dysfunction is a relatively common finding in the general population, with 2% of all people having diagnosed hypothyroidism. The true incidence is likely much higher, as the condition often goes unrecognized. Subsets of patients treated for lymphoma are at greater risk for hypothyroidism. More than 50% of long-term survivors of HL who received mantle field radiation therapy eventually develop thyroid dysfunction and require synthetic supplementation.[245] Iodine-131 tositumobab (Bexxar) therapy may result in hypothyroidism due to a high level of radiation-absorbed dose. Patients must receive thyroid-blocking agents prior to its administration and should be evaluated clinically and through laboratory assessment on an annual basis.

Cardiovascular Toxicity

Pericarditis, a form of accelerated coronary artery disease that may lead to myocardial infarction, and valvular dysfunction are major complications following radiation therapy for HL,[245,246] and for NHL if the heart is within the radiation field. Exposure to even a low dose of radiation may increase atherosclerotic changes 20–30 years later.[247] The incidence of coronary artery disease has been estimated to be 4%–11% following radiation therapy for HL. The relative risk of fatal cardiovascular events after mediastinal irradiation for HL ranges between 2.2 and 7.2.[248] Ultimately, 76% of patients who receive mediastinal radiotherapy develop pericardial toxicity.[249] A retrospective review of patients who underwent mediastinal irradiation and required valve replacement concluded that radiation injury was the major factor responsible for the development of mitral valve disease and was a contributing factor in aortic valve disease.[249] Chemotherapy regimens that include anthracyclines also result in an increased risk for cardiac damage. Anthracylcine-related cardiotoxicity is dose related and cumulative. The risk of cardiotoxicity, secondary to doxorubicin therapy, substantially increases when the cumulative dose exceeds 550 mg/m^2. Six to ten percent of adults who received a total doxorubicin dose of 550 mg/m^2 reported signs of symptomatic congestive heart failure. Synergistic toxic effects on the myocardium have been reported in patients receiving radiation and doxorubicin.[247]

Reproductive Changes

Reproductive changes will vary significantly with the therapy and the intensity of the treatment used. During radiotherapy, men will experience transient aspermia, but recovery of spermatogenesis has been documented when careful testicular shielding is employed. Reproductive concerns have largely focused on HL because this disease strikes a younger group of patients, but patients treated for NHL with alkylating agents may also be at risk for sterility. Premature menopause may occur following treatment for HL or more aggressive NHL treatment. The use of MOPP therapy for HL frequently results in sterilization for both males and females. Approximately 75% of women became amenorrheic, and more than 50% require hormone replacement therapy following MOPP therapy.[250] The rate of premature menopause during therapy is significant, with women older than age 25 likely to have cessation of menses.[251] More than 80% of men develop azospermia and testicular atrophy with elevated serum follicle-stimulating hormone.[252] Total-body irradiation, which is used as a conditioning regimen for stem cell transplantation, may result in sterility in both males and females. Sperm banking should be considered, if time permits, prior to therapy that is known or suspected to diminish spermatogenesis. Reproductive counseling and procreative alternatives are essential components of nursing care to consider for this patient population. Reports of successful pregnancies following egg donation are reported.[253]

Secondary Myelodysplasia and Malignancies

Myelodysplastic syndrome (MDS) is a group of disorders characterized by abnormal cell morphology in the bone marrow and a deficiency of normal blood cells in the peripheral blood. Although not a cancer, MDS may progress to acute myeloid leukemia. Exposure to alkylating agents and possibly radiotherapy, as well as other toxins, are risk factors for the development of MDS and AML. Dose intensity and advanced age are associated with a higher frequency of AML following treatment for lymphoma. The risk of MDS and AML is increased following therapy for HL and NHL, especially when bone marrow/stem cell transplantation has been performed. The development of secondary AML occurs within 10 years of treatment for HL. Myelodysplasia may precede the development of leukemia, and is often characterized by unexplained anemia or thrombocytopenia. Cytogenetic findings often demonstrate abnormalities of chromosomes 5 and 7 in treatment-related secondary MDS and AML. The standard treatment for AML is recommended; however, prognosis is poor. At the Mayo Clinic, 64 patients with HL and 166 patients with NHL who underwent autologous (self-donor) stem cell transplantation were followed for evidence of MDS or AML. Of the 230 consecutive patients followed, 10 developed MDS or AML (incidence of 4.3%) at a median time of 40 months following transplant and 75 months from original lymphoma diagnosis. None of these patients survived.[254]

Following radiotherapy for HL, carcinomas, sarcomas, and NHL have also been observed. An increased incidence of breast cancer is seen approximately 15 years after treatment. Girls younger than age 15 years who receive mantle field irradiation have more than a 100-fold increased risk for the development of breast cancer; those 15–25 years old have a 20-fold increased risk; those 25–29 years old have a sevenfold increased risk; and those older than age 30 have no increased risk.[255] Patients receiving more than 9 Gy of radiotherapy for HL have a statistically increased incidence of lung cancer. Patients who smoked more than 10 pack-years after the diagnosis of HL was established have a sixfold increased risk of lung cancer compared to those who had less than a 1-pack-year history.[256] These data support the need for education of patients and close follow-up following therapy.

Conclusion

The diagnosis, classification, and treatment of Hodgkin's lymphoma and non-Hodgkin's lymphoma have undergone significant changes over the last five years. The identification of immunologic or cytogenetic markers is extremely important to the continued expansion of treatment options. Many treatment options now exist for the patient with lymphoma. Because it is one of the most curable malignancies, the acute and chronic toxicities of these treatments are important factors in decision making. Ideally, the use of targeted therapy will result in improved survival and decreased long-term toxicity.

References

1. Jemal A, Tiwari R, Murray T, et al: Cancer statistics, 2004. *CA Cancer J Clin* 54:8–29, 2004
2. American Cancer Society: *Cancer Facts and Figures 2003*. Atlanta, American Cancer Society, 2003, pp 14-15
3. Kipps TJ: The lymphoid tissues, in Beutler E, Lichtman MA, Coller BS, et al (eds.): *Williams Hematology* (ed 6). New York, McGraw-Hill, 2001, pp 59–66
4. Appelbaum JW: The role of the immune system in the pathogenesis of cancer. *Semin Oncol Nurs* 8:51–62, 1992
5. Harris NL: Mature B-cell neoplasms: introduction, in Jaffe ES, Harris NL, Stein H, et al (eds.): *Pathology and Genetics of Tumours of Haematopoietic and Lymphoid Tissues*. Lyon, ARC Press, 2001, pp 121–126
6. Moses, S: Pruritis. *Am Fam Physician* 68:1135–1142, 1145–1146, 2003
7. Ng AK, Bernardo MV, Weller E, et al: Decision analysis on alternative treatment strategies for favorable-prognosis, early stage Hodgkin's disease (comments). *J Clin Oncol* 17:3577–3585, 1999
8. Carbone P, Kaplan H, Musshoff K: Report of the committee on the Hodgkin's disease staging. *Cancer Res* 31:1860–1861, 1971
9. Lister TA, Crowther D, Sutcliffe SB, et al: Report of a committee convened to discuss the evaluation and staging of patients with Hodgkin's disease: Cotswolds meeting. *J Clin Oncol* 7:1630–1636, 1989
10. Rosenberg SA, Cannellos GP: Hodgkin's disease, in Cannellos GP, Lister TA, Sklar JL (eds.): *The Lymphomas*. Philadelphia, W.B. Saunders, 1998, pp 305–331
11. Golder W: Positive emission tomography and lymphoma therapy. *Oncologie* 24:496–498, 2001
12. Friedberg JW, Chengazi V: PET scans in the staging of lymphoma: current status. *Oncologist* 8:438–447, 2003
13. Elmstrom R, Guan L, Baker G, et al: Utility of FDG-PET scanning in lymphoma by WHO classification. *Blood* 101:3875–3876, 2003
14. Anonymous: A predictive model for aggressive non-Hodgkins' lymphoma. The International Non-Hodgkin's Lymphoma Prognostic Factors Project. *N Engl J Med* 329:987–994, 1993
15. Ship MA: Prognostic factors in aggressive non-Hodgkin's lymphoma: who has "high-risk" disease? *Blood* 83:1165–1173, 1994
16. Coiffier B, Bastion Y, Berger F, et al: Prognostic factors in follicular lymphomas. *Semin Oncol* 20(suppl 5):89–95, 1993
17. Lopez-Guillermo A, Montserrat E, Rozman C: The International Prognostic Index (IPI) for large-cell lymphomas is also useful when applied to patients with low-grade lymphoma. Lugano, Switzerland, Fifth International Conference on Malignant Lymphoma: 59, 1993
18. Bastion I, Coiffier B: Is the International Prognostic Index for aggressive lymphoma patients useful for follicular lymphoma patients? *J Clin Oncol* 12:1340–1342, 1994
19. Hermans J, Krol ADG, van Groningen PhM, et al: International Prognostic Index for aggressive non-Hodgkin's lymphoma is valid for all malignancy grades. *Blood* 86:1460–1463, 1995
20. Hodgkin T: On some morbid appearances of the absorbent glands and spleen. *Med Chir Tran* 17:69–114, 1832
21. Wilks S: Cases of enlargement of the lymphatic glands and spleen, or Hodgkin's disease. *Guy's Hosp Rep* 11:56–67, 1865
22. Reed DM: On the pathological changes in Hodgkin's disease, with especial reference to tuberculosis. *Johns Hopkins Rep* 10:133–196, 1902
23. Sternberg C: Uber eine eigenartige unter dem Bilde der Pseukoleukamie verlaufende: tuberculose des lymphatischen apparates. *Z Heilkd* 19:21–90, 1898
24. American Cancer Society: Cancer Facts and Figures. *www.cancer.org*: 1–56. Accessed March 4, 2004
25. MacMahon B: Epidemiology of Hodgkin's disease. *Cancer Res* 26:1189–1201, 1966

26. Abramson JH, Pridan H, Sacks MI, et al: A case-controlled study of Hodgkin's disease in Israel. *J Natl Cancer Inst* 61:307–314, 1978
27. Gutensohn N, Cole P: Childhood social environment and Hodgkin's disease. *N Engl J Med* 304:135–140, 1981
28. Horning S: Hodgkin lymphoma, in Beutler E, Coller BS, Lichtman MA, et al (eds.): *Williams Hematology* (ed 6). New York, McGraw-Hill, 2001, pp 1215–1235
29. Paffenbarger R Jr, Wing AL, Hyde RT: Characteristics in youth indicative of adult onset Hodgkin's disease. *J Natl Cancer Inst* 58:1489–1491, 1977
30. Herndier BG, Sanchez HC, Chang KL, et al: High prevalence of Epstein-Barr virus in the Reed-Sternberg cells of HIV-associated Hodgkin's disease. *Am J Pathol* 142:1073–1079, 1993
31. Grufferman S, Cole P, Smith PG, Lukes RJ: Hodgkin's disease in siblings. *N Engl J Med* 296:248–250, 1977
32. Cabanillas F, Pathak S, Trjillo J, et al: Cytogenetic features of Hodgkin's disease suggest possible origin from a lymphocyte. *Blood* 71:1615–1617, 1988
33. Schouten HC, Sanger WG, Duggan M, et al: Chromosomal abnormalities in Hodgkin's disease. *Blood* 73:2149–2154, 1989
34. Tilly H, Bastard C, Delastre T, et al: Cytogenetic studies in untreated Hodgkin's disease. *Blood* 77:1298–1304, 1991
35. Craver LF, Hall TC, Rappaport H, et al: Report of the nomenclature committee. *Cancer Res* 26:1311, 1966
36. Stein H, Delsol G, Pileri S, et al: Nodular lymphocyte predominant Hodgkin lymphoma, in Jaffe ES, Harris NL, Stein H, et al (eds.): *World Health Organization Classification of Tumors, Pathology and Genetics of Tumours of Haematopoietic and Lymphoid Tissue.* Lyon, ARC Press, 2001, pp 240–243
37. Coles FB, Cartun RW, Pastuszak WT: Hodgkin's disease, lymphocyte-predominant type: immunoreativity with B-cell antibodies. *Mod Pathol* 1:274–278, 1988
38. Pinkus GS, Said JW: Hodgkin's disease, lymphocyte predominance type, nodular — a distinct entity? Unique staining profile for L & H variants of Reed-Sternberg cells defined by monoclonal antibodies to leukocyte common antigen, granulocyte-specific antigen, and B-cell-specific antigen. *Am J Pathol* 118:1–6, 1985
39. Poppema S: The diversity of the immunohistological staining pattern of Sternberg-Reed cells. *J Histochem Cytochem* 28:788–791, 1980
40. Stein H, Delsol G, Pileri S, et al: Nodular lymphocyte predominant Hodgkin lymphoma, in Jaffe ES, Harris NL, Stein H, et al (eds.): *World Health Organization Classification of Tumors, Pathology and Genetics of Tumours of Haematopoietic and Lymphoid Tissue.* Lyon, ARC Press, 2001, pp 244–253
41. Diehl V, Franklin J, Sextro M, Mauch P: Clinical presentation and treatment of lymphocyte predominance Hodgkin's disease, in Mauch P, Armitage JO, Diehl V (eds.): *Hodgkin's Disease.* Philadelphia, Lippincott, Williams and Wilkins, 1999, pp 563–582
42. Colby TV, Hoppe RT, Warnke RA: Hodgkin's disease: a clinicopathologic study of 659 cases. *Cancer* 49:1848–1858, 1982
43. Von Spronsen DJ, Vrints LW, Hofstra G, et al: Disappearance of prognostic significance of histopathological grading of nodular sclerosing Hodgkin's disease for unselected patients. *Br J Haematol* 96:322–327, 1997
44. MacLennan KA, Bennett MH, Vaughan HB, et al: Diagnosis and grading of nodular sclerosing Hodgkin's disease: a study of 2190 patients. *Int Rev Exp Pathol* 33:27–51, 1992
45. Diehl V, Sextro M, Franklin J, et al: Clinical presentation, course, and prognostic factors in lymphocyte-predominant Hodgkin's disease and lymphocyte-rich classical Hodgkin's disease: report from the European Task Force on Lymphoma Project on Lymphocyte-Predominant Hodgkin's Disease. *J Clin Oncol* 17:776–783, 1999
46. Ashton-Key M, Diss TC, Pan L, et al: Follicular Hodgkin's disease. *Am J Surg Pathol* 19:1294–1299, 1995
47. Anagnostopoulos I, Hansmann ML, Franssila K, et al: European Task Force on Lymphoma Project on Lymphocyte Predominance Hodgkin Disease: histologic and immunohistologic analysis of submitted cases reveals 2 types of Hodgkin disease with a nodular growth pattern and abundant lymphocytes. *Blood* 96:1889–1899, 2000
48. Kant JA, Hubbard SM, Longo DL et al: The pathologic and clinical heterogeneity of lymphocyte-depleted Hodgkin's disease. *J Clin Oncol* 4:284–294, 1986
49. Tirelli U, Errante D, Dolcetti R, et al: Hodgkin's disease and human immunodeficiency virus infection: clinicopathologic and virologic features of 114 patients from the Italian Cooperative Group on AIDS and Tumors. *J Clin Oncol* 13:1758–1767, 1995
50. Neiman RS, Rosen PJ, Lukes RJ: Lymphocyte-depletion Hodgkin's disease. A clinicopathological entity. *N Engl J Med* 288:751–755, 1973
51. Josting A, Wiedenmann S, Franklin J, et al: Secondary myeloid leukemia and myelodysplastic syndromes in patients treated for Hodgkin's disease: a report from the German Hodgkin's Lymphoma Study Group. *J Clin Oncol* 21:3440–3446, 2003
52. Longo DL, Young RC, Wesley M, et al: Twenty years of MOPP therapy for Hodgkin's disease. *J Clin Oncol* 4:1295–1306, 1986
53. Aleman BMP, Raemaekers JM, Trelli U, et al: Involved field radiotherapy for advanced Hodgkin's lymphoma. *N Engl J Med* 348:2396–2406, 2003
54. DeVita VT, Serpick AA, Carbone PP: Combination chemotherapy in the treatment of advanced Hodgkin's disease. *Ann Intern Med* 73:881–895, 1970
55. Bonadonna G, Zucali R, Monfardini S, et al: Combination chemotherapy of Hodgkin's disease with adriamycin, bleomycin, vinblastine, and imidazole carboxamide versus MOPP. *Cancer* 36:252–259, 1975
56. Duggan DB: Randomized comparison of ABVD and MOPP/ABV hybrid for the treatment of advanced Hodgkin's disease: report of an intergroup trial. *J Clin Oncol* 21:607–614, 2003
57. Diehl V, Franklin J, Pfreundschuh M, et al: Standard and increased dose BEACOPP chemotherapy compared with COPP-ABVD for advanced Hodgkin's disease. *N Engl J Med* 348:2386–2395, 2003
58. Popat U, Hosing C, Saliba RM, et al: Prognostic factors for disease progression after high-dose chemotherapy and autologous hematopoietic stem cell transplantation for recurrent or refractory Hodgkin's lymphoma. *Bone Marrow Transplant* 33:1015–1023, 2004
59. Lucas JB, Hoppe RT, Horwitz SM, et al: Rituximab is active in lymphocyte predominance Hodgkin's disease. *Blood* 96:831a, 2000
60. Hasenclever D, Diehl V: A prognostic score for advanced Hodgkin's disease. International Prognostic Factors Project on Advanced Hodgkin's Disease. *N Engl J Med* 339:1506–1514, 1998
61. Olin GR: The hazards of chemical laboratory environment: a study of the mortality in two cohorts of Swedish chemists. *Am Ind Hyg Assoc J* 39:557–562, 1978
62. Wong O: An industrywide mortality study of chemical workers occupationally exposed to benzene: II. Dose response analyses. *Br J Indust Med* 44:382–395, 1987
63. Pearce NE, Sheppard RA, Smith AH, et al: Non-Hodgkin's lymphoma and farming: an expanded case-control study. *Int J Cancer* 39:155–161, 1987

64. Morrison HI, Wilkins K, Semenel WR, et al: Herbicides and cancer. *J Natl Cancer Inst* 84:1866–1874, 1992
65. Li FP, Fraumeni JR, Mantel N, et al: Cancer mortality among chemists. *J Natl Cancer Inst* 43:1159–1164, 1969
66. Cantor KP: Farming and mortality from non-Hodgkin's lymphoma: a case-control study. *Int J Cancer* 29:239–247, 1982
67. Axelson O, Dahlgren E, Jansson CD, et al: Arsenic exposure and mortality: a case-referent study from a Swedish copper smelter. *Br J Ind Med* 35:8–15, 1978
68. Ross R, Dworsky R, Nichols P, et al: Asbestos exposure and lymphomas of the gastrointestinal tract and oral cavity. *Lancet* 2:1118–1120, 1982
69. Urba WJ, Longo DL: Lymphocytic lymphomas: epidemiology, etiology, pathology, and staging, in Moosa AR, Schimpff SC, Robson MC (eds.): *Comprehensive Textbook of Oncology, vol. 2* (ed 2). Baltimore, Williams and Wilkins, 1991, pp 1268–1276
70. Beebe GW, Kato H, Land C: Studies of the mortality of A-bomb survivors. Mortality and radiation dose. 1950–1974. *Radiat Res* 75:138–201, 1978
71. Boice JJ: Radiation and non-Hodgkin's lymphoma. *Cancer Res* 52:5489S–5491S, 1992
72. Thun MJ, Altekruse SF, Namboodiri MM, et al: Hair dye use and the risk of fatal cancers in U.S. women. *J Natl Cancer Inst* 86:210–215, 1994
73. Yunis JJ, Oken MM, Kaplan ME, et al: Distinctive chromosomal abnormalities in histologic subtypes of non-Hodgkin's lymphoma. *N Engl J Med* 307:1231–1236, 1982
74. Yunis JJ, Oken MM, Theologides A, et al: Recurrent chromosomal defects are found in most patients with non-Hodgkin's lymphoma. *Cancer Genet Cytogenet* 13:17–28, 1984
75. Ngan BY, Chen-Levy Z, Weiss LM, et al: Expression in non-Hodgkin's lymphoma of the bcl-2 protein associated with the t(14;18) chromosomal translocation. *N Engl J Med* 318:1638–1644, 1988
76. Korsmeyer SJ: Bcl-2 initiates a new category of oncogenes: regulators of cell death. *Blood* 80:879–886, 1992
77. Hockenbery D, Zutter M, Hickey W, et al: Bcl-2 protein is topographically restricted in tissues characterized by apoptotic cell death. *Proc Natl Acad Sci USA* 88:6961–6965, 1991
78. McDonnell T, Deanne N, Platt F, et al: BCL-2 immunoglobulin transgenic mice demonstrate extended B-cell survival and follicular proliferation. *Cell* 57:79–88, 1989
79. Grogan TM, Lippman SM, Spier CM, et al: Independent prognostic significance of a nuclear proliferation antigen in diffuse large cell lymphomas as determined by the monoclonal antibody Ki-67. *Blood* 71:1157–1160, 1988
80. Levine EG, Arthur DC, Frizzera G, et al: Cytogenetic abnormalities predict clinical outcome in non-Hodgkin's lymphoma. *Ann Inten Med* 108:14–20, 1988
81. Doll DC: Introduction: extranodal lymphomas. *Semin Oncol* 26:249–250, 1999
82. Isaacson PG, Spencer J: Gastric lymphoma and *Helicobacter pylori. Important Adv Oncol* 111–121, 1996
83. Nakamura S, Yao T, Aoyagi K, et al: *Helicobacter pylori* and primary gastric lymphoma: a histopathologic and immunohistochemical analysis of 237 patients. *Cancer* 79:3–11, 1997
84. Savio A, Franzin G, Wotherspoon AC, et al: Diagnosis and posttreatment follow-up of *Helicobacter pylori*-positive gastric lymphoma of mucosa associated lymphoid tissue: Histology, polymerase chain reaction, or both? *Blood* 87:1255–1260, 1996
85. Filipovich AH, Mathur A, Kamat D, et al: Primary immunodeficiencies: genetic risk factors for lymphoma. *Cancer Res* 52:5465s–5467s, 1992
86. Gridley G, Klippel JH, Hoover RN, et al: Incidence of cancer among men with Felty syndrome. *Ann Intern Med* 120:35–39, 1994
87. Kinlen L: Immunosuppressive therapy and acquired immunological disorders. *Cancer Res* 52:5474s–5476s, 1992
88. Rappaport H, Winter WJ, Hick EB: Follicular lymphoma: a reevaluation of its position in the scheme of malignant lymphomas, based on a survey of 253 cases. *Cancer* 9:792–821, 1956
89. Jaffe ES: Histopathology of the non-Hodgkin's lymphomas and Hodgkin's disease, in Canellos GP, Lister TA, Sklar JL (eds.): *The Lymphomas.* Philadelphia, W.B. Saunders, 1998, pp 77–106
90. Pileri SA, Leoncini L, Falini B: Revised European-American Lymphoma Classification. *Curr Opin Oncol* 7:401–407, 1995
91. Harris NL, Jaffe ES, Kiebold J, et al: Lymphoma classification — from controversy to consensus: the REAL and WHO classification of lymphoid neoplasms. *Ann Oncol* 11:s3–s10, 2000
92. Jaffe ES, Harris NL, Stein H, Vardiman JW (eds.): *World Health Organization Classification of Tumours. Pathology and Genetics. Tumours of Haematopoietic and Lymphoid Tissues.* Lyon, ARC Press, 2001
93. Muller-Hermelink HK, Catovsky D, Monserrat E, et al: Chronic lymphocytic leukaemia/small lymphocytic lymphoma, in Jaffe ES, Harris NL, Stein H, et al (eds.): *World Health Organization Classification of Tumours. Pathology and Genetics. Tumours of Haematopoietic and Lymphoid Tissues.* Lyon, ARC Press, 2001, pp 127–130
94. Ben-Ezra J, Burke JS, Swartz WG, et al: Small lymphocytic lymphoma: a clinicopathologic anlysis of 268 cases. *Blood* 73:579–587, 1986
95. Icli F, Ezdinli EZ, Costello W, et al: Diffuse well-differentiated lymphocytic lymphoma (DLWD): response and survival. *Cancer* 42:1936–1942, 1978
96. Morrison WH, Hoppe RT, Weiss LM, et al: Small lymphocytic lymphoma. *J Clin Oncol* 7:598–606, 1989
97. Dohner H, Stilgenbauer S, Dohner K, et al: Chromosome aberrations in B-cell chronic lymphocytic leukemia: reassessment based on molecular cytogenetic analysis. *J Mol Med* 77:266–281, 1997
98. Anonymous: A clinical evaluation of the International Lymphoma Study Group classification of non-Hodgkin's lymphoma. The Non-Hodgkin's Lymphoma Classification. *Blood* 89:3909–3918, 1997
99. National Comprehensive Care Network: *NCCN Clinical Practice Guidelines in Oncology. Non-Hodgkin's Lymphoma.* Jenkintown, PA Version 1, 2003
100. Leporrier M, Chevret S, Cozin B, et al: Randomized comparison of fludarabine, CAP, and CHOP in 938 previously untreated stage B and C chronic lymphocytic leukemia patients. *Blood* 98:2319–2325, 2001
101. Moreton P, Kennedy DB, Rawstron AC, et al: Achieving a MRD negative response after alemtuzumab for CLL is the best predictor for prolonged survival. *Blood* 102:2003 (abstr 5290)
102. Rai KR, Sawitsky A, Cronkite EP, et al: Clinical staging of chronic lymphocytic leukemia. *Blood* 46:219–234, 1975
103. Long JC, Aisenberg AC: Richter's syndrome: a terminal complication of chronic lymphocytic leukemia with distinct clinicopathologic features. *Am J Clin Pathol* 63:786–795, 1975
104. Nathwani BN, Harris NL, Weisenburger D, et al: Follicular lymphoma, in Jaffe ES, Harris NL, Stein H, et al (eds.): *World Health Organization Classification of Tumours. Pathology and Genetics. Tumours of Haematopoietic and Lymphoid Tissues.* Lyon, ARC Press, 2001, pp 162–167
105. Lai R, Arber DA, Chang KL, et al: Frequency of bcl-2 expression in non-Hodgkin's lymphoma: a study of 778 cases with comparison of marginal zone lymphoma and monocytoid B-cell hyperplasia. *Mod Pathol* 11:864–869, 1988
106. Fisher RI: Overview of non-Hodgkin's lymphoma: biology, staging, and treatment. *Semin Oncol* 30(suppl 4):3–9, 2003

107. Weisenburger DD, Anderson J, Armitage J, et al: Grading of follicular lymphoma: diagnostic accuracy reproducibility, and clinical relevance. *Mod Pathol* 11:142a, 1998
108. Gallagher CJ, Gregory WM, Jones AE, et al: Follicular lymphoma: prognostic factors for response and survival. *J Clin Oncol* 4:1470–1480, 1986
109. Solal-Celigny P: Follicular Lymphoma International Prognostic Project (FLIPP). *Ann Oncol* 13(suppl 2):18, 2002 (abstr 054)
110. Radaszkiewicz T, Dragosics B, Bauer P: Gastrointestinal malignant lymphomas of the mucosa-associated lymphoid tissues: factors relevant to prognosis. *Gastroenterology* 102:1628–1638, 1992
111. Doglioni C, Wotherspoon AC, Moschini A, et al: High incidence of primary gastric lymphoma in northeastern Italy. *Lancet* 339:834–835, 1992
112. Wotherspoon AC, Ortiz-Hidaglgo C, Falzon MR, et al: *Helicobacter pylori*-associated gastritis and primary B-cell gastric lymphoma. *Lancet* 338:1175–1176, 1991
113. Thieblemont C, Bastion Y, Berger F, et al: Mucosa-associated lymphoid tissue gastrointestinal and nongastrointestinal lymphoma behavior: analysis of 108 patients. *J Clin Oncol* 15:1624–1630, 1997
114. Armitage, JO, Weisenburger DD: New approach to classifying non-Hodgkin's lymphomas: clinical features of the major histologic subtypes. Non-Hodgkin's Classification Project. *J Clin Oncol* 16:2780–2795, 1998
115. Thieblemont C, Berger F, Dumontet C, et al: Mucosa-associated lymphoid tissue lymphoma is a disseminated disease in one third of 158 patients analyzed. *Blood* 95:802–806, 2000
116. Isaacson PG, Muller-Hermelink HK, Piris MA, et al: Extranodal marginal zone B-cell lymphoma of mucosa-associated lymphoid tissue (MALT lymphomas), in Jaffe ES, Harris NL, Stein H, et al (eds.): *World Health Organization Classification of Tumours. Pathology and Genetics. Tumours of Haematopoietic and Lymphoid Tissues.* Lyon, ARC Press, 2001, pp 157–160
117. Liu H, Ruskon-Formestraux A, Lavergne-Slove A, et al: Resistance of t(11:18) positive gastric-mucosa–associated lymphoid tissue lymphoma to *Helicobacter pylori* eradication therapy. *Lancet* 357:39–40, 2001
118. Foon KA, Fisher RI: Lymphomas, in Beutler E, Coller BS, Lichtman MA, et al (eds.): *Williams Hematology* (ed 6). New York, McGraw Hill, 2001, pp 1237–1261
119. Yang WI, Zukerberg LR, Motokura T, et al: Cyclin D1 (Bcl-1, PRAD1) protein expression in low-grade B-cell lymphomas and reactive hyperplasia. *Am J Pathol* 145:86–96, 1994
120. Zukerberg LR, Yang WI, Arnold A, et al: Cyclin D1 expression in non-Hodgkin's lymphomas. Detection by immunohistochemistry. *Am J Clin Pathol* 103:756–760, 1995
121. De Boer CJ, Schurring E, Dreef E, et al: Cyclin D1 protein analysis in diagnosis of mantle cell lymphoma. *Blood* 86:2715–2723, 1995
122. Vandenberge E, Wolf-Peeters C, van Den OJ, et al: Translocation (11;14): a cytogenetic anomaly associated with B-cell lymphomas of non-follicle centre cell lineage. *J Pathol* 163:13–18, 1991
123. William ME, Swerdlow SH, Rosenberg CL, Arnold A: Chromosome 11 translocation breakpoints at the PRAD1/cyclin D1 gene locus in centrocytic lymphoma. *Leukemia* 7:241–245, 1993
124. Vaandrager JW, Schuuring E, Zwikstra E, et al: Direct visualization of dispersed 11q13 chromosomal translocations in mantle cell lymphoma by multicolor DNA fiber fluorescence in situ hybridization. *Blood* 88:1177–1182, 1996
125. Caligaris-Cappio F: B-chronic lymphocytic leukemia: a malignancy of anti-self B cells. *Blood* 87:2615–2620, 1996
126. Kumar S, Krenacs L, Otsuki T, et al: Bcl-1 rearrangement and cyclin D1 protein expression in multiple lymphomatous polyposis. *Am J Clin Pathol* 105:737–743, 1998
127. Obriain DS, Kennedy MJ, Daly PA, et al: Multiple lymphomatous polyposis of the gastrointestinal tract. A clinicopathologically distinctive form of non-Hodgkin's lymphoma of B-cell centrocytic type. *Am J Surg Pathol* 13:691–699, 1989
128. Swerdlow SH, Berger F, Isaacson PI, et al: Mantle cell lymphoma in Jaffe, ES, Harris NL, Stein H, et al (eds.): *World Health Organization Classification of Tumours. Pathology and Genetics. Tumours of Haematopoietic and Lymphoid Tissues.* Lyon, ARC Press, 2001, pp 168–170
129. Harris NL, Jaffe ES, Stein H, et al: A revised European–American classification of lymphoid neoplasms: a proposal from the International Lymphoma Study Group. *Blood* 84:1361–1392, 1994
130. Matolcsy A, Chadburn A, Knowles DM, et al: De novo CD5-positive and Richter's syndrome–associated diffuse large B cell lymphomas are genotypically distinct. *Am J Pathol* 147:207–216, 1995
131. Weiss LM, Warnke RA, Sklar J, et al: Clonal T-cell populations in lymphomatoid origin for a clinically benign disease. *N Engl J Med* 315:475–479, 1986
132. Lipford E, Wright JJ, Urba W, et al: Refinement of lymphoma cytogenetics by the chromosome 18q21 major breakpoint region. *Blood* 70:1816–1823, 1987
133. Gatter KC, Warnke, RA: Diffuse large B-cell lymphoma, in Jaffe ES, Harris NL, Stein H, et al (eds.): *World Health Organization Classification of Tumours. Pathology and Genetics. Tumours of Haematopoietic and Lymphoid Tissues.* Lyon, ARC Press, 2001, pp 171–174
134. Armitage JO, Longo DL: Malignancies of lymphoid cells, in Braunwald E, Fauci SA, Kasper DL, et al (eds.): *Harrison's Principles of Internal Medicine* (ed 15). New York, Mc-Graw Hill, 2001, pp 715–726
135. Gregory SA: Selecting patients for treatment with 90Y ibritumomab tiuxetan (Zevalin) [Review]. *Semin Oncol* 30(suppl 17):17–22, 2003
136. Shipp MA, Harrington DP, Anderson JR, et al: A predictive model for aggressive NHL: the International Non-Hodgkin's Lymphoma Prognostic Factors Project. *N Engl J Med* 329:987–994, 1993
137. Hermine O, Haioun C, Lepage E, et al: Prognostic significance of bcl-2 protein expression in aggressive non-Hodgkin's lymphoma. Groupe d'Etude des Lymphomes de l'Adulte (GELA). *Blood* 87:265–272, 1996
138. Hill ME, MacLennan KA, Cunningham DC, et al: Prognostic significance of BCL-2 expression and bcl-2 major breakpoint region rearrangement in diffuse large cell non-Hodgkin's lymphoma: a British National Lymphoma Investigation Study. *Blood* 88:1046–1051, 1996
139. Soussain C, Patte C, Ostronoff M, et al: Small noncleaved cell lymphoma and leukemia in adults. A retrospective study of 65 adults treated with the LMB pediatric protocols. *Blood* 85:664–674, 1995
140. Wright DH: Burkitt's lymphoma: a review of the pathology, immunology and possible aetiological factors, in Sommers SC: *Pathology Annual.* New York, Appleton-Century-Crofts, 1971, pp 337–363
141. Klein G: Epstein-Barr virus (EBV) strategy in normal and neoplastic B cells [minireview]. *Cell* 77:791–793,1994
142. Magrath K: The pathogenesis of Burkitt's lymphoma. *Adv Cancer Res*, 55:133–270, 1990
143. Facer CA, Playfair JH: Malaria, Epstein-Barr virus, and the genesis of lymphomas. *Adv Cancer Res* 53:33–72, 1989

144. Divine M, Casassus P, Koscielny S, et al: Small non-cleaved cell lymphoma. A prospective multi-center study of 51 adults patients treated with the LMB pediatric protocol. *Blood* 10(suppl 1):523a, 1999
145. Cavdar AO, Gozdasoglu S, Yavuz G, et al: Burkitt's lymphoma between African and American types in Turkish children. Clinical, viral (EBV), and molecular studies. *Med Pediatr Oncol* 21:36–42, 1993
146. Raphael M, Gentihomme O, Tulliez M: Histopathologic features of high-grade non-Hodgkin's lymphomas in acquired immunodeficiency syndrome. The French Study Group of Pathology for Human Immunodeficiency Virus-Associated Tumors. *Arch Pathol Lab Med* 115:15–20, 1991
147. Hamilton-Dutroit SJ, Raphael M, Audouin J: In situ demonstration of Epstein-Barr virus small RNAs (EBER 1) in acquired immunodeficiency syndrome–related lymphomas: correlation with tumor morphology and primary site. *Blood* 82:619–624, 1993
148. Ziegler JL, Bluming AZ, Morrow RH, et al: Central nervous system involvement in Burkitt's lymphoma. *Blood* 36:718–728, 1970
149. Hui PK, Feller AC, Lennert K: High-grade non-Hodgkin's lymphoma of B-cell type. I. Histopathology. *Histopathology* 12:127–143, 1988
150. Spina D, Leoncini L, Megha T, et al: Cellular kinetic and phenotypic heterogeneity in and among Burkitt's and Burkitt-like lymphomas. *J Pathol* 182:145–150, 1997
151. Hollingsworth HC, Longo DL, Jaffe ES: Small noncleaved cells with florid epithelioid granulomatous response: a clinicopathologic study of seven patients. *Am J Surg Pathol* 17:51–59, 1993
152. Gaidano G, Ballerini P, Gong JZ, et al: p53 mutations in human lymphoid malignancies: association with Burkitt lymphoma and chronic lymphocytic leukemia. *Proc Natl Acad Sci USA* 88:5413–5417, 1991
153. Yano T, Sander CA, Clark HM, et al: Clustered mutations in the second exon of the MYC gene in sporadic Burkitt's lymphoma. *Oncogene* 8:2741–2748, 1993
154. Murphy SB, Hustu HO: A randomized trial of combined modality therapy of childhood non-Hodgkin's lymphoma. *Cancer* 45:630–637, 1980
155. Magrath IT, Janus C, Edwards BK, et al: An effective therapy for both undifferentiated (including Burkitt's) lymphomas and lymphoblastic lymphomas in children and young adults. *Blood* 63:1102–1111, 1984
156. Weitzman S, Greenberg ML, Thorner P: Treatment of non-Hodgkin's lmphoma in childhood, in Wiernik PH, Canellos GP, Kyle RA, et al (eds.): *Neoplastic Disease of Blood* (ed 2). New York, Churchill Livingstone, 1991, pp 753–768
157. Magrath IT: Burkitt's lymphoma. The small noncleaved cell lymphomas, in Canellos GP, Lister TA, Sklar JL (eds.): *The Lymphomas.* Philadelphia, W.B. Saunders, 1998, pp 423–437
158. Goedert JJ: The epidemiology of acquired immunodeficiency syndrome malignancies. *Semin Oncol* 27:390–401, 2000
159. Pluda JM, Venzon DJ, Tosato G, et al: Parameters affecting the development of non-Hodgkin's lymphoma in patients with severe human deficiency virus infection receiving antiretroviral therapy. *J Clin Oncol* 11:1099–1107, 1993
160. Levine AM, Shibata D, Sullivan HJ, et al: Epidemiological and biological study of acquired immunodeficiency syndrome–related lymphoma in the County of Los Angeles: preliminary results. *Cancer Res* 52:5482s–5484s, 1992
161. Ballerini P, Gaidano G, Gong JZ, et al: Multiple genetic lesions in acquired immunodeficiency syndrome–related non-Hodgkin's lymphoma. *Blood* 81:166–176, 1993
162. Martin A, Flaman JM, Frebourg T, et al: Functional analysis of the p53 protein in AIDS-related non-Hodgkin's lymphomas and polymorphic lymphoproliferations. *Br J Haematol* 101:311–317, 1998
163. Levine AM, Gill PS, Meyer PR, et al: Retrovirus and malignant lymphoma in homosexual men. *JAMA* 254:1921–1925, 1985
164. Knowles DM, Chamulak GA, Subar M, et al: Lymphoid neoplasia associated with the acquired immunodeficiency syndrome (AIDS): the New York University experience. *Ann Intern Med* 108:744–753, 1988
165. Lowenthal DA, Straus DJ, Campbell SW, et al: AIDS-related lymphoid neoplasia: the Memorial Hospital experience. *Cancer* 61:2325–2337, 1988
166. Kaplan LD, Abrams DI, Feigal E, et al: AIDS-associated non-Hodgkin's lymphomas in San Francisco. *JAMA* 261:719–724, 1989
167. Bekkenk MW, Geelen FA, Voorst Vader PC, et al: Primary and secondary cutaneous $CD30^+$ lymphoproliferative disorders: a report from the Dutch Cutaneous Lymphoma Group on the long-term follow-up data of 210 patients and guidelines for diagnosis and treatment. *Blood* 95:3653–3661, 2000
168. Gisselbrecht C, Spina M, Gabarre J, et al: Dose adjusted treatment in human immuno-deficiency virus related lymphoma. *Blood* 94(suppl 1):599a, 1999
169. Levine AM, Sullivan-Halley J, Pike MC, et al: HIV-related lymphoma: prognostic factors predictive of survival. *Cancer* 68:2466–2472, 1992
170. Rosenberg SA: The Non-Hodgkin's Lymphoma Pathologic Classification project: the National Cancer Institute–sponsored study of classifications of non-Hodgkin's lymphomas. *Cancer* 49:2112, 1982
171. Simon R, Durrleman S, Hoppe RN, et al: The Non-Hodgkin's Lymphoma Classification project: long-term follow-up of 1153 patients with non-Hodgkin's lymphoma. *Ann Intern Med* 109:939–945, 1988
172. Murphy SB: Classification, staging and end results of treatment of childhood non-Hodgkin's lymphomas: dissimilarities from lymphomas in adults. *Semin Oncol* 7:332–339, 1980
173. Carroll AJ, Crist WM, Link MP, et al: The t(1;14)(p34;q11) is nonrandom and restrict to T-cell acute lymphoblastic leukemia: a Pediatric Oncology Group study. *Blood* 76:1220–1224, 1990
174. Brunning RD, Borowitz M, Matutes E, et al: Precursor T lymphoblastic leukaemia/lymphoblastic lymphoma (precursor T-cell acute lymphoblastic leukaemia), in Jaffe ES, Harris NL, Stein H, et al (eds.): *World Health Organization Classification of Tumours. Pathology and Genetics. Tumours of Haematopoietic and Lymphoid Tissues.* Lyon, ARC Press, 2001, pp 115–117
175. Brunning RD, Borowitz M, Matutes E, et al: Precursor B lymphoblastic leukaemia/lymphoblastic lymphoma (precursor B-cell acute lymphoblastic leukaemia), in Jaffe ES, Harris NL, Stein H, et al (eds.): *World Health Organization Classification of Tumours. Pathology and Genetics. Tumours of Haematopoietic and Lymphoid Tissues.* Lyon, ARC Press, 2001, pp 111–114
176. Lin P, Jones D, Dorfman DM, Medeiros LJ: Precursor B-cell lymphoblastic lymphoma: a predominantly extranodal tumor with low propensity for leukemic involvement. *Am J Surg Pathol* 24:1480–1490, 2000
177. Ferry JA, Jacobson JO, Conti D, et al: Lymphoproliferative disorders and hematologic malignancies following organ transplantation. *Mod Pathol* 2:583–592, 1989
178. Nelson BP, Nalesnik MA, Bahler DW, et al: Epstein-Barr virus–negative post-transplant lymphoproliferative disorders: a distinct entity? *Am J Surg Pathol* 24:375–385, 2000
179. Knowles DM, Cesarman E, Chadburn A, et al: Correlative morphologic and molecular genetic analysis demonstrates three

distinct categories of posttransplantation lymphoproliferative disorders. *Blood* 85:552–565, 1995

180. Chucrallah AE, Crow MK, Rice LE, et al: Multiple myeloma after cardiac transplantation: an unusual form of posttransplant lymphoproliferative disorder. *Hum Pathol* 25:541–545, 1994
181. Rowlings PA, Curtis RE, Passweg JR, et al: Increased incidence of Hodgkin's disease after allogeneic bone marrow transplantation. *J Clin Oncol* 17:3122–3127, 1999
182. Curtis RE, Travis LB, Rowlings PA, et al: Risk of lymphoproliferative disorders after bone marrow transplantation: a multi-institutional study. *Blood* 94:2208–2216, 1999
183. Penn I: The changing pattern of post transplant malignancies. *Transplant Proc* 23:1101–1103, 1991
184. Leblond V, Davi F, Dorent R, et al: Post transplant lymphoproliferative disorders not associated with Epstein-Barr virus: a distinct entity? *J Clin Oncol* 16:2052–2059, 1998
185. Hoppe RT: Mycosis fungoides and other cutaneous lymphomas, in Canellos GP, Lister TA, Sklar JL (eds.): *The Lymphomas.* Philadelphia, W.B. Saunders, 1998, pp 495–506
186. Kim YH, Hoppe RT: Mycosis fungoides and the Sezary syndrome. *Semin Oncol* 26:276–289, 1999
187. Weinstock MA, Horm JW: Mycosis fungoides in the United States: increasing incidence and descriptive epidemiology. *JAMA* 260:42–46, 1988
188. Whittemore AS, Holly EA, Lee IM, et al: Mycosis fungoides in relation to environmental exposures and immune response: a case control study. *J Natl Cancer Inst* 81:1560–1567, 1989
189. van Doorn R, Van Haselen CW, Voorst Vader PC, et al: Myclosis fungoides: disease evolution and prognosis of 309 Dutch patients. *Arch Dermatol* 136:504–510, 2000
190. Willemze R, Kerl H, Sterry W, et al: EORTC classification for primary cutaneous lymphomas: a proposal from the Cutaneous Lymphoma Study Group of the European Organization for Research and Treatment of Cancer. *Blood* 90:354–371, 1997
191. Querfeld C, Guitart J, Kuzel TM, et al: Primary cutaneous lymphomas: a review with current treatment options. *Blood Rev* 17:131–142, 2003
192. Hoppe RT, Abel EA, Deneau DG, et al: Mycosis fungoides: management with topical nitrogen mustard. *J Clin Oncol* 5:1796–1803, 1987
193. Ligand Pharmaceuticals Incorporated: Ontak package insert. 2003
194. Weiss LM, Wood GS, Hu E, et al: Detection of clonal T-cell receptor gene rearrangements in the peripheral blood of patients with mycosis fungoides and dermatopathic lymphadenopathy. *N Engl J Med* 313:539–544, 1985
195. Bekkenk MW, Geelen FA, Voorst Vader PC, et al: Primary and secondary cutaneous CD30+ lymphoproliferative disorders: a report from the Dutch Cutaneous Lymphoma Group on the long-term follow-up data of 219 patients and guidelines for diagnosis and treatment. *Blood* 95:3653–3661, 2000
196. Delsol G, Ralfkiaer E, Stein H, et al: Anaplastic large cell lymphoma, in Jaffe ES, Harris NL, Stein H, et al (eds.): *World Health Organization Classification of Tumours. Pathology and Genetics. Tumours of Haematopoietic and Lymphoid Tissues.* Lyon, ARC Press, 2001, pp 230–235
197. Brugieres L, Deley MC, Pacquement H, et al: CD30+ anaplastic large-cell lymphoma in children: analyses of 82 patients enrolled in two consecutive studies of the French Society of Pediatric Oncology. *Blood* 92:3591–3598, 1998
198. Fraga M, Brousset P, Schlaifer D, et al: Bone marrow involvement in anaplastic large cell lymphoma. Immunohistochemical detection of minimal disease and its prognostic significance. *Am J Clin Pathol* 103:82–89, 1995
199. Benharroch D, Meguerian-Bedoyan Z, Lamant L, et al: ALK-positive lymphoma: a single disease with a broad spectrum of morphology. *Blood* 91:2076–2084, 1998
200. Wellman A, Otsuki T, Vogelbruch M, et al: Analysis of the t(2;5)(p23;q35) by RT-PCR in CD 30-positive anaplastic large cell lymphomas, in other non-Hodgkin's lymphomas of T-cell phenotype and in Hodgkin's disease. *Blood* 86:2321–2328, 1995
201. Hastrup N, Hamilton-Dutoit S, Ralfkiaer E, et al: Peripheral T-cell lymphomas: an evaluation of reproducibility of the updated Kiel classification. *Histopath* 18:99–105, 1991
202. Lee HF, Im FG, Goo FM, et al: Peripheral T-cell lymphoma: spectrum of imaging findings with clinical and pathologic features. *Radiogr* 23:7–26, 2003
203. Arrowsmith ER, Macon WR, Kinney MC, et al: Peripheral T-cell lymphomas: clinical features and prognostic factors of 92 cases defined by the Revised European American Lymphoma Classification. *Leuk Lymph* 44:241–249, 2003
204. Lopez-Guillermo A, Cid J, Salar A, et al: Peripheral T-cell lymphomas: initial features, natural history, and prognostic factors in a series of 174 patients diagnosed according to the R.E.A.L. Classification. *Ann Oncol* 9:849–855, 1998
205. Fisher RI, Gaynor ER, Dahlberg S, et al. Comparison of standard regimen CHOP with three intensive chemotherapy regimens for advanced non-Hodgkin's lymphoma. *N Engl J Med* 328:1002–1006, 1993
206. Philip T, Guglielmi C, Hagenbeek A, et al: Autologous bone marrow transplantation as compared to salvage chemotherapy in relapses of chemotherapy-sensitive non-Hodgkin's lymphoma. *N Engl J Med* 333:1540–1545, 1995
207. Schouten HC, Qian W, Kvaloy S, et al: High dose therapy improves progression-free survival and survival in relapsed follicular non-Hodgkin's lymphoma: results from the randomized European CUP trial. *J Clin Oncol* 21:3918–3927 2003
208. Gribbin JG, Freedman AS, Neuberg D, et al: Immunologic purging of marrow assessed by PCR before autologous bone marrow transplantation for B-cell lymphoma. *N Engl J Med* 325:1525–1533, 1991
209. Forero A, LoBulio AF: History of antibody therapy for non-Hodgkin's lymphoma. *Semin Oncol* 30(suppl 17):1–5, 2003
210. Press OS: Radioimmunotherapy for non-Hodgkin's lymphomas: a historical perspective. *Semin Oncol* 30(suppl 4):10–21, 2003
211. Byrd JC, Waselenko JK, Maneatis TJ, et al: Rituximab therapy in hematologic malignancy patients with circulating blood tumor cells: association with increased infusion-related side-effects and rapid tumor clearance. *J Clin Oncol.*17:791–795, 1999
212. Maloney DG, Liles TM, Czerwinski DK, et al: Phase I clinical trial using escalating single-dose infusion of chimeric anti-CD20 monoclonal antibody (IDEC-C2B8) in patients with recurrent B-cell lymphoma. *Blood* 84:2457–2466, 1994
213. McLaughlin P, Grillo-Lopez AJ, Link BK, et al: Rituximab chimeric anti-CD20 monoclonal antibody therapy for relapsed indolent lymphoma: half of patients respond to a four-dose treatment regimen. *J Clin Oncol* 16:2825–2833, 1998
214. Davis TA, Grillo-Lopez AJ, White CA, et al: Rituximab anti-CD20 monoclonal antibody therapy in non-Hodgkin's lymphoma: safety and efficacy of re-treatment. *J Clin Oncol* 18:3135–3143, 2000
215. Coiffier B, LePage E, Briere J, et al: CHOP chemotherapy plus rituximab compared with CHOP alone in elderly patients with diffuse large-B-cell lymphoma. *N Engl J Med* 346:235–242, 2002
216. Leonard JP, Coleman M, Matthews JC, et al: Phase I/II trial of abratuzumab (humanized anti CD22 antibody) in non-Hodgkin's lymphoma. *Blood* 358a(suppl 1), 2002 (abstract 1388)

217. Keating MJ, Byrd J, Rai K, et al: Multicenter study of CAMPATH-1H in patients with chronic lymphocytic leukemia (B-CLL) refractory to fludarabine. *Blood* 94:705a, 1999
218. Khorana A, Bunn P, McLaughlin P, et al: A phase II multicenter study of CAMPATH-1H antibody in previously treated patients with non-bulky non-Hodgkin's lymphoma. *Leuk Lymph* 41:77–87, 2001
219. Osterborg A, Vassas AS, Anagnostopoulos A, et al: Humanized CD52 monoclonal antibody Campath-1H as first line treatment in chronic lymphocytic leukemia. *Br J Haematol* 93:151–153, 1996
220. Kennedy B, Rawstron A, Richards S, et al: CAMPATH-1H in CLL: immune reconstitution and viral infections during and after therapy. *Blood* 96:164a, 2000
221. Vose JM, Chiu BC, Cheson BD, et al: Update of epidemiology and therapeutics for non-Hodgkin's lymphoma. *Hematology (Am Soc Hematol Educ Prog)* 241–262, 2002
222. Witzig TE. Efficacy and safety of 90Y ibratumomab tiuxetan (Zevalin) radioimmunotherapy for non-Hodgkin's lymphoma. *Semin Oncol* 30(suppl 17):11–16, 2003
223. Kaminski MS, Gregory SA, Fehrenbacher L, et al: Acute and delayed hematologic toxicities associated with Bexxar therapy are modest: overall experience in patients with low-grade or transformed low-grade non-Hodgkin's lymphoma (NHL). *Blood* 98:339a, 2001
224. National Comprehensive Cancer Network (NCCN): *Non-Hodgkin's Lymphoma. Practice Guidelines in Oncology*. Rockledge, PA, NCCN, V1, 2002. *www.nccn.org*
225. Siegal AB, Goldenberg DM, Cesano A, et al: CD22-directed monoclonal antibody therapy for lymphoma. *Semin Oncol* 30:457–464, 2003
226. Leonard JP, Coleman M, Vose J, et al: Phase II study of oblimersen sodium (G3139) alone and with R-CHOP in mantle cell lymphoma. *Pro Am Soc Clin Oncol* 22:566, 2003 (abstr 2276)
227. Liang L, Sha WC: The right place at the right time: novel B7 family members regulate effector T cell responses. *Curr Opin Immunol* 14:384–390, 2002
228. Rai KR, O'Brien S, Cunnignham C, et al: Genasense (BCL2 Antisense) monotherapy in patients with relapsed or refractory CLL: phase 1 and 2 results. *Blood* 100:384a, 2002
229. Rehm PK: Gallium-67 scintigraphy in the management of Hodgkin's disease and non-Hodgkin's lymphoma. *Cancer Biother Radiopharm* 14:251–262, 1999
230. Hart MM, Adamson RH: Antitumor activity and toxicity of salts of inorganic Group IIIa metals: aluminum, gallium, indium, and thallium. *Proc Natl Acad Sci USA* 68:1623–1626, 1971
231. Leyland-Jones B: Treatment of cancer-related hypercalcemia: the role of gallium nitrate. *Semin Oncol* 30(suppl 5):13–19, 2003
232. Habeshaw JA, Lister TA, Stansfield AG: Correlation of transferrin receptor expression with histological class and outcome in non-Hodgkin lymphoma. *Lancet* 1:498–501, 1983
233. Straus DJ: Gallium nitrate in the treatment of lymphoma. *Semin Oncol* 30(suppl 5):1–4, 2003
234. Wang CY, Mayo MW, Korneluk RG, et al: NF-κB antiapoptosis: induction of TRAF1 and TRAF2 and c-IAP1 and cIAP2 to suppress capsase-8 activation. *Science* 281:1680–1683, 1998
235. O'Connor OA, Wright L, Moskwitz C, et al: Promising activity of the proteosome inhibitor bortezomib (Velcade) in the treatment of indolent non-Hodgkin's lymphoma and mantle cell lymphoma. *Blood* 102, 2003 (abstr 2346)
236. LeMaistre CF, Saleh MN, Kuzel TM, et al: Phase I trial of a ligand fusion protein (DAB389-IL2) in lymphomas expressing the receptor for interleukin-2. *Blood* 91:399–405, 1998
237. Knobel H, Loge JH, Lund MB, et al: Late medical complications and fatigue in Hodgkin's disease survivors. *J Clin Oncol* 19:3226–2322, 2001
238. Sonnen R, Schmidt W-P, Kuse R, Schmitz N: Treatment results of aggressive B non-Hodgkin's lymphoma in advanced age considering comorbidity. *Br J Haematol* 119:634–639, 2002
239. Pangalis GA, Dimopoulou MN, Angelopoulou MK, et al: Campath-1H (anti-CD52) monoclonal antibody therapy in lymphoproliferative disorders. *Med Oncol* 18:99–107, 2001
240. Wossmann W, Schrappe M, Meyer U, et al: Incidence of tumor lysis syndrome in children with advanced stage Burkitt's lymphoma/leukemia before and after introduction of prophylactic use of urate oxidase. *Ann Hematol* 82:160–165, 2003
241. Zelenetz AD: Risk models for chemotherapy-induced neutropenia in non-Hodgkin's lymphoma. *Oncology* 17(suppl 11):21–26, 2003
242. Dale D: Current management of chemotherapy-induced neutropenia; the role of colony-stimulating factors. *Semin Oncol* 30(suppl 13):3–9, 2003
243. Knobel H, Loge JH, Lund MB, et al: Late medical complications and fatigue in Hodgkin's disease survivors. *J Clin Oncol* 19:3226–3233, 2001
244. Peerboom PF, Hassink EAM, Melkert R, et al: Thyroid function 10–18 years after mantle field irradiation for Hodgkin's disease. *Eur J Cancer* 28A:1716–1718, 1992
245. Cosset JM, Henry-Amar M, Pellae-Cosset B, et al: Pericarditis and myocardial infarctions after Hodgkin's disease therapy at the Institute of Gustave-Roussy. *Int J Radiat Oncol Biol Phys* 21:447–449, 1992
246. Hancock SL, Tucker MA, Hoppe RT: Factors affecting late mortality from heart disease after treatment of Hodgkin's disease. *JAMA* 270:1949–1955, 1993
247. Basavaraju SR, Easterly CE: Pathophysiological effects of radiation on atherosclerosis development and progression, and the incidence of cardiovascular complications. *Am Assoc Phys Med* 29:2391–2403, 2002
248. Adams MJ, Hardenbergh PH, Constine LS, Lipshultz SE: Radiation-associated cardiovascular disease. *Crit Rev Oncol-Hematol* 45:55–75, 2003
249. Handa N, McGregor CGA, Danielson TA, et al: Coronary artery bypass grafting in patients with previous mediastinal radiation therapy. *J Thorac Cardovasc Surg* 117:1136–1143, 1999
250. Clark ST, Radford JA, Crowther D, et al: Gonadal function following chemotherapy for Hodgkin's disease: a comparative study of of MVPP and a seven-drug hybrid regimen. *J Clin Oncol* 13:134–139, 1995
251. Andrieu JM, Ochoa-Molina ME: Menstrual cycle, pregnancies and offspring before and after MOPP therapy for Hodgkin's disease. *Cancer* 52:435–438, 1983
252. Yarbro CH, Perry MC: The effect of cancer therapy on gonadal function. *Semin Oncol Nurs* 1:3–8, 1985
253. Anselmo AP, Cavalieri E, Aragona C, et al: Successful pregnancies following an egg donation program in women with previously treated Hodgkin's disease. *Haematology* 86:624–628, 2001
254. Howe R, Micaleff INM, Inwards DJ, et al: Secondary myelodysplastic syndrome and acute myelogenous leukemia are significant complications following autologous stem cell transplantation for lymphoma. *Bone Marrow Transplant* 32:317–324, 2003
255. Hancock SL, Tucker MA, Hoppe RT: Breast cancer after treatment. *J Natl Cancer Inst* 85:25–31, 1993
256. Kaldor JM, Day NE, Bell J, et al: Lung cancer following Hodgkin's disease: a case control study. *Int J Cancer* 52:677–681, 1992

CHAPTER 59

Multiple Myeloma

Joseph D. Tariman, RN, APN, MN, APRN-BC, OCN®

Introduction

Multiple myeloma (MM) is a B-cell malignancy of the plasma cells. One of its hallmarks is the presence of a serum or urine monoclonal immunoglobulin, commonly known as M-protein or paraprotein. MM cells are usually responsive to radiotherapy and chemotherapy, but relapse is inevitable. The need for novel therapeutic agents that can prolong and improve overall survival has remained high.[1]

Major advances have been seen in approaches to management of patients with MM in the last five years. The refinement in the delivery of high-dose chemotherapy with growth factor support with or without stem cell transplantation, the use of bisphosphonates, and the discovery of a novel proteasome inhibitor, bortezomib (Velcade, Millennium Pharmaceutical, Inc., Cambridge, Massachusetts), are among the most encouraging areas of progress. The role of angiogenesis in MM continues to evolve with promising results of thalidomide (Thalomid, Celgene Corporation, Warren, New Jersey) in newly diagnosed multiple myeloma. Revimid (Celgene Corporation, Warren, New Jersey), a thalidomide analog and an immunomodulatory derivative (IMiD), is now entering phase III clinical trials after showing promising antitumor activity against MM in an earlier clinical trial.[2] New developments in imaging, immunology, cytogenetics, transplantation, molecular biology, and gene microarray expression profiling have also contributed to a significant understanding of MM and eventually will lead to better disease management.[3,4] A stepwise approach in targeting not only the MM cells but also their microenvironment, using novel biologically based therapeutic agents alone or in combination with conventional chemotherapy, has shown that drug resistance can be overcome and better survival can be achieved.[5,6]

Epidemiology

In the general population, MM accounts for 1% of all malignancies and approximately 10% of all hematologic malignancies. Within the United States, it represents approximately 14% of all hematologic malignancies and is the second most common of all hematologic malignancies, after non-Hodgkin's lymphoma.[7] The incidence of MM is approximately 15,270 new cases each year, including 8090 male and 7180 female cases. An estimated 11,070 deaths occur annually due to the disease — 5430 males and 5640 females.[7] A male predominance in incidence is noted, with a male-to-female ratio of 3:2, although black females have a higher incidence than white males in the United States. Approximately 40,000 people have a diagnosis of multiple myeloma at any one time.[8] The reported increase in incidence during the past several decades in the United States is probably due to increased availability and use of medical facilities for the elderly and improved diagnostic techniques, rather than a true increase in incidence.[9,10]

Age and race are among the demographic factors that have been shown to have a consistent relationship with MM. Persons affected by MM are often elderly, with a median age at diagnosis of 66 years. Thirty-eight percent of patients are 70 years or older, and 2% are younger than 40 years.[9] The disease affects African Americans twice as much as Caucasian Americans. MM is one of the leading causes of cancer death among African Americans. The black–white differential in incidence has been found to be substantially related to socioeconomic status.[11] Worldwide, incidence of MM is relatively low among Asian and Hispanic populations.

The median duration of survival is approximately 33 months, and no improvement in overall survival was realized from 1985 to 1998.[9] Approximately 25% of patients survive five years or longer, but fewer than 8% live more than ten years.[12] Racial differences continue to be noted in the five-year relative survival rate for myeloma. For all Caucasian Americans diagnosed during the years 1974–1976 and 1992–1999, there was a statistically significant increase in the relative five-year survival rate (24%–31%, $p < 0.05$). Although a slight improvement was found in the relative five-year survival rate (28%–33%) for African Americans diagnosed with multiple myeloma during this same period, it did not reach statistical significance.[7]

Etiology

The cause of MM is unknown. Although several epidemiological studies have been conducted, no single cause is directly associated with the pathogenesis of MM. In 1997, human herpes virus 8 (HHV-8), also called Kaposi's sarcoma–associated human virus (KSHV), was reported to be present in dendritic cells of patients with MM,[13] but its role in the pathogenesis of MM remains controversial. No case-control and cohort studies have supported a consistent relationship of this virus in the majority of patients with MM. Further epidemiological studies, serologic data, and polymerase chain reaction (PCR) assays did not implicate KSHV in the pathogenesis of MM.[14]

There are a few reports of a possible link between human immunodeficiency virus (HIV) and MM.[15–17] Also, patients with acquired immune deficiency syndrome (AIDS) have a higher risk of developing MM compared with the normal population.[17] Conversely, little evidence suggests that chronic antigenic stimulation (i.e., exposure to viruses) plays a role in myeloma pathogenesis.[18] Despite extensive epidemiological studies, the etiology of MM remains unclear.[19]

Risk Factors

The most recognized and most common risk factor for the development of MM is the presence of a monoclonal gammopathy of undetermined significance (MGUS). It is a common precursor to MM. Patients with MGUS have an MM incidence rate of roughly 1.5%.[20] As with MM, the etiology of MGUS just remains unknown.

Several risk factors have been identified in association with MM. One is high doses of ionizing radiation.[19] Other risk factors include occupational exposures such as agricultural exposure, which includes fuels and pesticides;[21] diesel exhaust;[22] metal working;[23,24] working in the paint industry;[25] and employment in the leather[26] and textile industries.[27]

Employment in the petroleum industry does not increase an individual's risk of developing MM, but one recent study utilizing geographic information system analysis determined that there is a slight increase in risk among people who reside near a large chemical waste dump.[28] No association has been found between a history of asbestos exposure and MM[22,29] except in one report.[30] Diagnostic x-rays have a negligible impact, if any, on one's risk of developing MM.[31] Benzene exposure is also not a likely risk factor for developing MM.[32] The risk of having familial MM is relatively small, although an increased incidence of MM in certain families has been reported.[33,34]

In studies, some of the risk factors mentioned previously lacked the criteria of strength of association, consistency of association, and exposure–risk relationship. It is fair to say that in the vast majority of patients, no obvious explanation for the occurrence of the disease is available at this time.[19]

Prevention, Screening, and Early Detection

In the absence of known causative agents, identified tumor markers, or definitive diagnostic tests, the ability to apply prevention and early detection strategies to MM remains elusive. MM should be suspected when a patient presents with bone pain in which lytic lesions are discovered on radiographic films. An increase in serum total protein or presence of M protein in the serum or urine, new-onset renal failure without an obvious cause, or hypercalcemia strongly suggests the diagnosis of MM, and a comprehensive diagnostic workup must be performed.[35]

Pathophysiology

New insights into the pathophysiology of multiple myeloma have been reported. Recent findings support the hypothesis that MM pathogenesis involves genetic and molecular defects in the early development of malignant plasma cells.[36–38] The nonrandom, recurrent nature of chromosomal abnormalities in myeloma suggests that they play a role in disease pathogenesis. One study reported that translocation of immunoglobulin heavy-chain (IgH) locus (14q32) and deletion of chromosome 13 were found in 75% and 45% of patients with plasma cell disorders, respectively, and were not randomly distributed but rather interconnected.[39] In contrast to certain hematologic malignancies such as chronic myelogenous leukemia, no single genetic anomaly has been implicated in the pathogenesis of MM.

The initial transformation is thought to occur in a postgerminal center (earliest stage of cell) B-lineage cell, carrying a somatically hypermutated IgH gene.[37] This plasmablastic (stem cell of plasma cell) cell colonizes the bone marrow, propagates clonally (originating from one cell) and then differentiates into a slowly proliferating myeloma cell population, all under the influence of specific cell adhesion molecules such as intracellular adhesion and vascular adhesion molecules and cytokines such as IL-6.[40] Cytogenetic analysis of myeloma cells frequently demonstrates multiple mutations and chromosomal aberrations. The most common cytogenetic abnormality found in MM involves the dysregulation of proto-oncogenes by rearrangement with the IgH locus of the plasma cell, commonly called translocation of IgH locus,[39,41] which could be among the earliest genetic events.[37] Translocation of IgH locus and deletion of chromosome 13 can be determined by using the fluorescent in situ hybridization (FISH) technique during bone marrow biopsy. Researchers also found that there is high correlation between deletion of chromosome 13 in these patients and their immunological status and clinical presentation, which may also be useful in prognostication.

Aberrant expression of antiapoptotic oncogenes such as *bcl-2*, *bcl-x₁*, and fibroblast growth factor receptor 3 (FGFR-3) has been identified in MM as well. Researchers believe that plasma cells are likely to require a mitogenic signal (a signal inducing the nucleus of the cell to divide, resulting into two nuclei) to promote malignancy. A study demonstrated that disease progression in patients with MM is associated with a concurrent alteration in the expression of both oncogenes and tumor suppressor genes, supporting the existence of a genetic abnormality in MM.[42] A recent study showed that deletion of the *TP53* gene predicted resistance to chemotherapy, highlighting its importance in the MM disease process.[43] There is high interest in studying the molecular and cytogenetic alterations in MM, but the precise causes of these abnormalities remain largely unknown.[44]

A good understanding of the nature of plasma cells, the immunoglobulins secreted by plasma cells, features of the malignant clone, and changes induced by the bone marrow microenvironment could lead to better understanding of the pathophysiology of MM. Plasma cell development originates in the bone marrow, then progresses through a number of sequential stages defined primarily by the status of the immunoglobulin rearrangements.[45] Most circulating B lymphocytes are naïve cells that have not been exposed to an activating antigen. Their life span is about one week in the absence of antigenic activation. Plasma cells are derived from B lymphocytes that have been activated by antigenic stimuli.[46] Because a plasma cell is derived from the B lymphocyte, it has been thought to be the identifiable malignant cell in MM; MM is therefore considered a B-cell malignancy of the plasma cell.[47]

Immunoglobulins or antibodies constitute the humoral immune response to a foreign antigen. They are secretory products of plasma cells, and each immunoglobulin molecule has two heavy and two light chains.[48] The five types of heavy chains are denoted by the Greek letters μ, δ, γ, α, and ϵ. The type of heavy chain present determines the class of the immunoglobulin: IgM, IgD, IgG, IgA, or IgE, respectively. The two types of light chains are denoted by the Greek letters κ (kappa) and λ (lambda). Each heavy-chain immunoglobulin molecule has either a κ or a λ subtype of light chain in association with one of the types of heavy chain (i.e., IgG kappa or IgG lambda).

Because MM is a neoplastic clonal process, the malignant cells and the secreted immunoglobulins are either κ- or λ-restricted. Because only two types of immunoglobulin expression are possible, this restriction readily enables determination of clonality. To determine clonality, one may perform immunohistochemistry staining of the plasma cell population during bone marrow biopsy. Most patients have more than 10% plasma cells in the bone marrow, with an average of 30%–40%,[46] and most of these cells are present in sheets or aggregates. It is important to note how much of the plasma cell population has either kappa or lambda restriction during immunohistochemistry staining to distinguish normal (polyclonal) from abnormal (monoclonal) plasma cells. Monoclonal plasma cells can express only either kappa or lambda restriction in immunohistochemistry studies.

The monoclonal proliferation of plasma cells produces a homogeneous immunoglobulin fraction detectable in the serum and/or urine, called myeloma protein or M-spike. Bone destruction due to the production of osteoclastic factors by the malignant plasma cells is the most characteristic feature of the disease, and bone pain is the predominant presenting symptom.[49] Although most patients have serum proteins with or without associated urinary proteins, 20% of affected individuals have only urinary proteins (Bence-Jones or light-chain proteins). Even though an excessive amount of immunoglobulin is being produced, these immunoglobulins are unable to effectively produce the antibodies required for maintaining humoral immunity, thereby placing patients with MM at higher risk for infections. Immunofixation (the most sensitive test for M protein) of the serum and urine shows M-protein in 97% of patients diagnosed with myeloma and only 3% are nonsecretory (no detectable M-protein).[9,50] Individuals who present with bone pain, numerous lytic lesions in their skeletal survey, hypercalcemia and low blood counts with no detectable M-protein either in blood or urine most likely have a nonsecretory type of MM (monoclonal plasma cells are not producing the homogenous immunoglobulin).

Role of Cytokines

Cytokines are believed to play a major role in the pathogenesis and pathophysiologic changes of myeloma cells. Cytokines are extracellular signaling molecules that activate a cascade of intracellular pathways and that regulate growth and differentiation of cells. These growth factors bind to specific cell-surface receptors, thereby establishing communication between malignant precursors and their environment.[51]

Plasma cell proliferation in MM is influenced by cytokines and certain biologic variables. Plasma cells produce interleukin-6 (IL-6), a major proliferative cytokine for malignant plasma cells,[51] as well as vascular endothelial growth factor (VEGF), one of the most important cytokines for angiogenesis.[46] In addition, myeloma cells express interleukin-1β and tumor necrosis factor alpha (TNF-α), which are potent osteoclast-activating factors (OAF). Notably, IL-6 does not induce proliferation of normal B lymphocytes or normal plasma cells, but rather has a significant proliferative and antiapoptotic effect on myeloma cells that confers resistance to conventional chemotherapy.[52] Although controversy surrounds the exact source of IL-6 in myeloma, some evidence suggests both autocrine (stimulates the myeloma cells itself for production of growth factor) and paracrine (stimulates other cells that are closest to the myeloma cells) production. IL-6 mediation of paracrine myeloma cell growth is supported by observations that bone marrow stromal cells (BMSC) are the major source of IL-6 in myeloma.[51] Studies have also found that freshly isolated myeloma cells cultured without exogenous IL-6 rapidly stop proliferating[53] and that adhesion of myeloma cells to BMSC up-regulates IL-6 secretion by BMSC.[54]

VEGF is also expressed by plasma cells and is a potent angiogenic cytokine.[55] Studies have shown that bone marrow angiogenesis is increased in MM and has prognostic value. Normal plasma cells do not produce IL-1β, whereas plasma cells from almost all MM patients produce it.[46] This aberrant production of IL-1β can induce the expression of genes for IL-6, colony-stimulating factors,[46] and various adhesion molecules, as well as mediate IL-6 production by bone marrow stromal cells.[56] IL-1β has potent OAF activity, and it may be the predominant factor responsible for the development of osteolytic lesions in myeloma.[51]

Several cytokines are implicated in the development of bone disease (lytic lesions) in patients with MM. Besides IL-6 and other members of the gp130 cytokine family, osteoclast-stimulating factors (OSF) or bone-resorbing activity has been detected in the supernatants of both myeloma cell lines and fresh patient cells; macrophage inflammatory protein 1-alpha (MIP-1α) has also been found to induce osteoclast formation.[51,57]

Granulocyte-macrophage colony-stimulating factor (GM-CSF), IL-3, stem cell factor (SCF), TNF-α, hepatocyte growth factor (HGF), insulin-like growth factors 1 and 2 (IGF-1 and -2),[58–60] and VEGF are all potential myeloma growth factors. All have been shown to stimulate growth or specific intracellular signaling events of myeloma cells or cell lines in vitro.[61,62]

Interferon-alpha (IFN-α) is another cytokine that has been used in patients with myeloma because of its antiproliferative action but clinical data have shown variable responses to it. This variation may be due to the dual role played by IFN-α in cytokine growth inhibition as well as proliferation. A study involving cell-cycle regulatory genes revealed that differential induction of cyclin D2 and $p19^{INK4D}$ may be one of the key mechanisms underlying these variable responses.[63]

IL-10 is also a growth factor for myeloma cells, increasing the proliferation of malignant plasma cells.[64] This interleukin increases the responsiveness of some myeloma cells to IL-11 (one of the cytokines responsible for the development of bone lesions in myeloma patients) by up-regulating the expression of IL-11 receptors.[65]

Recent advances in our understanding of the complex cytokine interactions between tumor cells and their microenvironment have already resulted in the development of novel therapeutic agents. Further research leading to a better understanding of the roles played by cytokines in the pathogenesis of MM may soon open up even more therapeutic targets, adding more potent and selective treatments in the armamentarium against MM (Table 59-1).[51]

Table 59-1 Cytokines under Investigation in the Pathogenesis of Multiple Myeloma

Interleukin-1β (IL-1β)	Insulin-like growth factor-1 and -2 (IGF-1 and -2)
Interleukin-3 (IL-3)	Vascular endothelial growth factor (VEGF)
Interleukin-6 (IL-6)	Osteoclast-stimulating factor (OSF)
Viral IL-6	Hepatocyte growth factor (HGF)
Interleukin-10 (IL-10)	Leukemia inhibitory factor (LIF)
Interleukin-11 (IL-11)	Granulocyte-macrophage colony-stimulating factor (GM-CSF)
Alfa-interferon	Granulocyte colony-stimulating factor (G-CSF)
Oncostatin M (OSM)	Tumor necrosis factor (TNF)
	Tumor growth factor-β (TGF-β)

Clinical Manifestations

Bone pain, particularly in the back and chest, is present at diagnosis in more than two-thirds of patients with myeloma and is the most predominant presenting symptom.[35] Other symptoms at presentation may include anemia, uremia, recurrent infection, and, less commonly, hypercalcemia, hyperviscosity, polyneuropathy, and spinal cord compression.[49] In most patients presenting with symptomatic disease, the classic triad of MM consists of multiple lytic bone lesions, high serum M protein, and extensive bone marrow plasmacytosis (> 30%) is present.

Some individuals with MM may have a long prodromal, indolent or asymptomatic period (Durie-Salmon stage 1 or smoldering myeloma). These patients do not need primary treatment because they can do well for many months to years before the disease progresses. Patients should be initially observed; if their disease progresses to stage II or higher, then they should be treated according to the guidelines for advanced MM.[50] Disease progression is defined as a sustained 25% or greater increase in serum or urine M-protein or development of new sites of lytic disease or hypercalcemia.[50,66]

Skeletal Involvement

Destructive, painful osteolytic lesions are one of the major clinical manifestations of myeloma.[49] In fact, patients who respond to chemotherapy may still have progression of skeletal disease, and recalcification of osteolytic lesions is slow and rare.[67] This bone destruction could lead to pathologic fractures, spinal cord compression, hypercalcemia, bone pain, and loss of height (if the vertebral spine is affected).[68] These complications are major causes of morbidity and mortality in patients with multiple myeloma. The osteolytic lesions in MM are due to rapid bone turnover, wherein increased osteoclastic bone resorption is not accompanied by a comparable increase in bone formation. A recent report has found an association between the myeloma cell production of DKK1, an inhibitor of osteoblast differentiation, and the presence of lytic bone lesions in patients with multiple myeloma.[69]

Conventional radiography (metastatic skeletal survey) reveals osteolytic lesions, osteopenia, or fractures in 80% of patients with MM at diagnosis.[35] Comparative studies have repeatedly shown that conventional radiographic surveys can detect more lytic lesions than bone scanning.[70] Bone scan is usually negative in MM. For this reason, radiographic studies continue to be used almost universally in the initial evaluation and widely in the follow-up of patients with myeloma. Subsequent follow-up skeletal surveys during and after treatment help determine worsening of myeloma status based on the occurrence of new lytic lesions and/or increases in their size. One disadvantage of this simple test is its lack of sensitivity, particularly in determining response to treatment.[71]

In cases of unequivocal response to treatment, magnetic resonance imaging (MRI) can supplement conventional radiographs. It offers clinicians an additional tool not only for determining response to treatment but also for assessing the extent of the disease and detecting disease progression in patients with no measurable M-protein.[71,72] Likewise, MRI is useful in patients with suspected cord compression and solitary plasmacytoma of the spine,[50] and in patients with MM who have bone pain but no abnormalities found on the radiographs.[35]

Infection

Infection plays an important role in the morbidity and mortality associated with MM.[73] Fever caused by viral and bacterial infections is the presenting symptom in about 10% of patients with MM. The incidence of infection in patients with MM is 15 times higher than in normal individuals,[49] and approximately 70% of patients will die from infection.[73] The predominant pathogens isolated from patients with MM are bacterial in nature, which reflects the defect in humoral immunity seen in myeloma. This defect is demonstrated in the reduction of polyclonal immunoglobulin (the immunoglobulins produced by myeloma cells are monoclonal and defective) synthesis and a failure to make antibody responses post immunization.[73]

Streptococcus pneumoniae and *Haemophilus influenzae* are the most frequently isolated bacteria during the early course of the disease, and the respiratory and urinary tracts are common sites of infection. Other infections occurring later during the course of the disease may involve gram-negative organisms and *Staphylococcus aureus.* This biphasic pattern of bacterial infections in patients with MM is related to the stage of the disease,[74] treatment modalities such as high-dose therapy and transplantation leading to neutropenia, high-dose corticosteroids, and the use of central venous catheters.[49]

Systemic, fungal, protozoal, and mycobacterial infections are uncommon in patients with MM. The only viral infection that has been consistently reported in patients with myeloma is herpes zoster.[73] Prophylactic use of antiviral agents is recommended particularly in post-transplant patients or other severely immunocompromised patients.

Impairment of T-cell function is commonly seen in MM, although it is clinically not as important as the B-cell deficiency.[49] The intensive corticosteroid therapy found in regimens such as vincristine, doxorubicin, dexamethasone (VAD) or high-dose pulsed dexamethasone suppresses T-cell function markedly, and there are incidental reports of *Pneumocystis carinii* infections.[73] Prophylactic use of antibiotic agents such as the trimethoprim/sulfamethoxazole combination may prove highly useful in preventing these opportunistic infections.[49]

Bone Marrow Involvement

Approximately two-thirds of patients with MM have anemia at presentation.[9] It is usually normocytic, normochromic, and clinically manifested by fatigue and weakness. This problem is typically associated with depressed erythropoietin levels due to an inadequate erythropoietin response to anemia. Other contributing factors to the development of anemia include impaired availability of storage iron and overproduction of cytokines such as IL-1, IL-6, and TNF-α that can inhibit erythropoiesis. Determining the level of endogenous erythropoietin may help to select patients who may benefit from treatment with recombinant erythropoietin.[10] A recent study reported that anemia in patients with multiple myeloma is related to a pathogenetic mechanism whereby malignant plasma cells express very high levels of apoptogenic receptors, which triggers apoptosis of immature erythroblasts. This persistent erythroblast cytotoxicity within the bone marrow leads to progressive destruction of the erythroid matrix.[75]

As myeloma cells infiltrate the bone marrow or if the patient is treated with systemic chemotherapy, both qualitative and quantitative defects in neutrophil and platelet function can occur. Impaired serum opsonic activity (release of a substance that renders microbes more vulnerable to being engulfed by phagocytes) in the neutrophils of patients with MM can result in a quantitative defect in the function of circulating neutrophils. Decreased platelets can be attributed to M-protein's effect on clotting factors or to nonspecific coating of platelets with immunoglobulins resulting in platelet dysfunction and bleeding. Leukopenia usually occurs in very advanced disease or after chemotherapy.[76]

Renal Insufficiency

Multiple myeloma is frequently associated with renal dysfunction. In addition, it has been shown that the presence of renal failure indicates a higher tumor burden and consequently more aggressive disease.[77] Patients who are diagnosed with renal insufficiency should be treated aggressively because reversal of renal insufficiency results in survival outcomes similar to those for patients who have normal renal function at diagnosis. The reported incidence of renal disease at presentation or during the course of MM ranges from 20% to 60%. Most renal disease is found in patients who produce excess light chains and IgD myeloma. These groups include patients with cast nephropathy, renal tubular dysfunction (acquired Fanconi syndrome), amyloidosis, and light-chain deposition disease. A spectrum of renal syndromes, including proteinuria, progressive renal failure, acute renal failure (ARF), and various acid–base and electrolyte disorders, may be seen in patients with multiple myeloma.[78]

Cast nephropathy or myeloma kidney is the most common histological diagnosis found in refractile tubular casts surrounded by multinucleated giant cells located in the distal and collecting tubules.[79] These large, dense, tubular casts could lead to the formation of precipitates in the tubules that might obstruct or rupture the tubular epithelium. Tubulointerstitial damage may appear as flattened tubular cells, varying degrees of degeneration with necrosis, and denudation of the tubular basement membrane, leading to tubuloepithelial cell atrophy and interstitial fibrosis.[78]

Light-chain deposition disease (LCDD) occurs in 5%–10% of patients with myeloma. It is characterized by the deposition of light chains in the kidney and other vital organs (liver, heart, peripheral nerves).[78] The primary renal presentation involves elevated serum creatinine and nephrotic range proteinuria in 25% of the cases. Symptomatic management of these patients with correction of volume depletion and hypercalcemia, plus chemotherapy for control of the underlying malignancy, may improve renal function in as many as 50% of cases.[78] LCDD in the proximal tubules of the kidney can cause tubular dysfunction with an acquired Fanconi syndrome. Fanconi syndrome is a generalized disorder of proximal tubular transport dysfunction, leading to urinary excretion of amino acids, glucose, bicarbonate, uric acid, phosphate, potassium, and low-molecular-weight proteins.[80] The presence of hypophosphatemia, hypokalemia, hypouricemia, and a normal anion gap metabolic acidosis point to the possibility of Fanconi syndrome. Glycosuria in a patient with normal serum glucose may be also seen. LCDD has a poor prognosis. Apart from age, prognostic factors that have been identified include degree of renal insufficiency at presentation affecting the renal prognosis, underlying hematologic disorder, and extrarenal LC deposition affecting the patient prognosis. Dialysis is worth performing in uremic LCDD patients.[81]

Primary (AL) amyloidosis can occur in as many as 10% of patients with myeloma. It results from tissue infiltration with immunoglobulin light chains. In contrast, secondary amyloidosis (AA protein) is commonly associated with chronic infectious, inflammatory, immune, genetic, and neoplastic disorders. AL amyloidosis is most commonly associated with IgD myeloma and light-chain disease.[82] Patients with AL amyloidosis present with renal impairment and proteinuria often in the nephrotic range (> 3.5 g/24 hr). Renal insufficiency was observed in approximately 50% of patients, while proteinuria was seen in 90% of cases at diagnosis of myeloma with coexisting amyloidosis.[78] Coexisting amyloidosis in patients with MM is a strong adverse prognostic factor, and treatment-related mortality with autologous stem cell transplant (ASCT) remains high.[83]

ARF is a common feature of MM, and as many as half of patients with MM have potentially reversible and quick identifiable factors.[78] Dehydration, hypercalcemia, and infection are the most important precipitating factors, and are found in 50%–95% of patients with myeloma-associated renal failure.[49] Dehydration leads to decreased renal perfusion, resulting in prerenal azotemia. In addition, enhanced reabsorption of fluids in response to fluid depletion results in an increased concentration of paraproteins in the distal tubules, promoting aggregation and cast formation. Hypercalcemia, by contrast, can cause dehydration due to osmotic diuresis induced by the high serum calcium level, hypercalcemia-induced emesis, and nephrogenic diabetes insipidus.[78] Hypercalcemia can also cause a decrease in the glomerular filtration rate (GFR) secondary to renal vasoconstriction and alteration in the glomerular permeability coefficient. Lastly, hypercalcemia may increase the toxicity of light chains by increasing the aggregability of Bence-Jones protein (BJP) and Tamm-Horsfall protein (THP).[78] BJPs are immunoglobulin light chains synthesized by plasma cells independently of heavy chains that combine in the endoplasmic reticulum to form immunoglobulin molecules. When excess light chains are synthesized, they escape into circulation and appear in the urine as light-chain proteins or BJPs.[84] BJPs and THPs are components of casts in patients with cast nephropathy secondary to myeloma.[78] Infections such as bacteremia without hemodynamic compromise or full-blown sepsis can decrease renal perfusion, resulting in acute tubular necrosis (ATN).

Other reversible factors producing ARF include nephrotoxic antibiotics like aminoglycosides and amphotericin B, acyclovir, nonsteroidal anti-inflammatory drugs (NSAIDs), radiographic contrast, hyperuricemia, and tumor lysis syndrome. Aminoglycosides and amphotericin B can cause ATN, while acyclovir can cause acute interstitial nephritis, acute tubular necrosis, and obstruction secondary to tubular deposition of crystals.[78] NSAIDs block the production of vasodilatory prostaglandins, cause a reduction in renal blood flow and GFR, and can lead to ARF. Several reports cite the risk of ARF due to NSAIDs intake in patients with MM, and the use of these drugs should be avoided in such individuals.[85,86] The contrast agents with high protein binding commonly used in the 1950s and 1960s were predisposed to precipitate and obstruct tubular fluid flow, leading to increased incidence of contrast-induced ARF.[78] Consequently, the use of contrast agents that could potentially damage the kidney should be minimized. Hyperuricemia results from rapid cell turnover, especially after chemotherapy, or tumor lysis syndrome after combination chemotherapy or high-dose chemotherapy (HDC) with hematopoietic stem cell transplantation (HSCT). Aggressive hydration, alkalinization of urine, and allopurinol are helpful in addressing this condition. Hemodialysis may be considered in patients with severe hyperuricemia who become oliguric.[78]

Careful evaluation for potentially reversible factors in patients with MM who present with or develop renal insufficiency is critical. Treatment should be directed toward preventing or correcting the factor that contributed to the renal insufficiency and reducing the concentration and/or risk for precipitation of light-chain proteins in the renal tubules.

In the past, patients with MM who developed renal insufficiency were considered to have a worse prognosis. Today, due to advances in intensive supportive therapy, overall survival is not dramatically changed by the presence of renal failure but rather is determined by the response of the underlying disease to chemotherapy regardless of kidney function.[78]

Metabolic Syndromes

Hypercalcemia may be observed in 20%–30% of patients with MM, but a high proportion of patients with hypercalcemia may be totally asymptomatic.[49] The severity of signs and symptoms will vary depending on the degree of hypercalcemia. Typical symptoms include polydipsia (increased thirst), nausea, constipation, irritability, confusion, and precoma. As described earlier, hypercalcemia can precipitate renal insufficiency through multiple mechanisms and must be reversed quickly to prevent serious permanent kidney damage.

Hyperuricemia is frequently found in patients with MM and is related to a combination of factors, including high tumor cell turnover, tumor cell kill, and impairment of renal function.[87] Symptomatic hyperuricemia (gout) is rare, but prophylaxis is indicated, because a raised serum uric acid may contribute to renal impairment.[49] Usually, the really symptomatic patient is dehydrated and has a severely impaired renal function. Uric acid–induced nephropathy is caused by the precipitation and crystallization of uric acid in the distal tubules, where the urine pH is low and the concentration of uric acid is high. Aggressive hydration, alkalinization of urine, allopurinol, and hemodialysis may be instituted as indicated.

Other uncommon metabolic disturbances associated with MM that have been reported include hyperviscosity and hyperammonaemia. The latter is manifested as central nervous system symptoms such as somnolence and precoma. Hyperviscosity syndrome is rare, occurring in 2%–6% of patients with MM. It can occur in individuals with IgM myeloma (< 0.01% of all MM cases), and occasionally in those with IgA and IgG MM. This syndrome is caused by a high concentration of macroglobulins (e.g., IgA and IgM immunoglobulins) that increase serum viscosity and result in vascular sludging. Symptoms usually appear when the relative serum or plasma viscosity exceeds 5 (normal range, 1.4–1.8 cp).[88] The most common sign of hyperviscosity is hemorrhagic diathesis resulting in gingival and mucosal bleeding, ecchymosis, and epistaxis.[49] Ophthalmic changes, such as visual disturbances, diplopia, and retinal abnormalities, are also common. Neurologic signs include headache, dizziness, vertigo, drowsiness, coma, and seizures. Vascular sludging may also occur in the kidney, further compromising renal perfusion and increasing the risk of renal insufficiency. Other symptoms related to hyperviscosity may include malaise and cardiac insufficiency. Plasmapheresis is an effective—albeit temporary—measure for patients in whom rapid reduction in the concentration of circulating macroglobulins is deemed essential, such as those with acute renal failure.[88] Effective tumor kill is necessary to eventually decrease the circulating macroglobulins produced by plasma cells, thereby decreasing serum viscosity.[78]

Neurologic Involvement

The most well-known and dramatic presenting symptom of MM is the sudden onset of paraplegia due to spinal cord compression.[89] Signs of spinal cord compression on examination were found in 12% of newly diagnosed patients with myeloma. Other studies reported incidence of presentation with neurologic symptoms at a lower rate, less than 5%.[49] Other neurologic complications include cauda equina syndrome, radicular pain, peripheral neuropathy, and cranial nerve palsies usually due to local encroachment by tumor cells near the exit foraminae of the skull floor. A careful neurologic history and examination are done at presentation and during follow-up so that early signs of cord compression will be recognized and adequately treated.

Peripheral neuropathy associated with MM is a well-known entity. It is rare, with an incidence rate of less than 5% in patients with overt MM.[90] In most patients with MM, it is a late complication. The axonal, mixed sensorimotor symptoms are usually symmetrical, distal, mild, and progressive. Peripheral neuropathy may or may not be associated with amyloid deposits in the nerves.[49] Its exact mechanism is unknown, but it may be related to paraprotein, weight loss, or other metabolic or toxic factors associated with the malignancy.[90] In some cases, hyperviscosity syndrome has been identified as a causative factor; other studies have shown that neuropathy could be related to an autoimmune mechanism, with the IgM monoclonal antibody being directed at peripheral nerve antigens. There is no known effective treatment for peripheral neuropathy associated with MM. In particular, removing the paraprotein by plasmapheresis has no consistent effect on the neuropathy.[91]

Neuropathic symptoms developing during therapy may result from administration of drugs such as vincristine, cisplatin, thalidomide, and bortezomib.[92–94] Neuropathy arising from treatment is considered chemotherapy-induced peripheral neuropathy (CIPN). Pharmacologic agents (e.g., mild analgesics, opioids, tricyclic antidepressants, and anticonvulsants) and nonpharmacologic agents (e.g., capsaicin cream, exercise, relaxation techniques, transcutaneous electronic nerve stimulation, and occupational therapy) may be helpful in alleviating chemo-induced peripheral neuropathy.[92]

Assessment

Patient and family history are obtained during the initial visit. Clinicians should look for any history of MGUS, as it is a well-known predisposing factor for MM. It is also important to obtain a work history, because certain occupational exposures predispose individuals to developing MM. Family history should be assessed for any occurrence of MM among the patient's relatives.

The most common physical finding related to MM is pallor. The liver and spleen are palpable in a minority of patients. Extramedullary (nonbony) plasmacytomas are rare but may be found late in the disease course. They appear as large, purplish, subcutaneous masses.[35] Mental status changes such as disorientation, decreased level of consciousness, or coma can be related to hypercalcemia, hyperviscosity syndrome, or renal insufficiency.[49] Limitations in range of motion, inability to bear weight, loss of height, or abnormal curvature of the spine may be seen on initial presentation or later in the disease course and could be related to bone disease associated with MM. Routine chemistry laboratory values may be significant for elevations in blood urea nitrogen (BUN), creatinine, uric acid, and calcium. Serum and urine protein electrophoresis (SPEP) may reveal monoclonal spikes. Immunofixation, which is more sensitive than electrophoresis, can confirm specific, small residual monoclonal protein; this technology is particularly helpful in identifying the presence of abnormal immunoglobulin in the hyposecretory type of myeloma.[76]

True nonsecretors (no detectable M-protein) are often misdiagnosed or undiagnosed because of the absence of monoclonal protein. In some cases, severe complications from myeloma, such as pathologic fracture, may have already occurred before the patient with nonsecretory myeloma is diagnosed. It is also important that a 24-urine specimen for urine protein electrophoresis and urine immunofixation be checked during the initial work-up to assess for urine M-spike and to identify the specific monoclonal light chain, respectively. Twenty percent of myeloma cases have urinary light-chain proteins only (kappa- or lambda-type multiple myeloma), which may not be detectable by serum protein electrophoresis.[9]

The National Comprehensive Cancer Network (NCCN) recommends specific laboratory tests as part

Table 59-2 Diagnostic Work-up for Multiple Myeloma

Tests	Purpose
Bone marrow aspirate/biopsy	Check percentage of plasma cells
Serum protein electrophoresis (SPEP)	Check for the presence of serum M-protein
Quantitative immunoglobulins	Identify specific elevated immunoglobulin level
Serum immunofixation electrophoresis (SIFE)	Identify specific monoclonal immunoglobulin
Serum chemistry	Check for evidence of hypercalcemia, renal dysfunction
Complete blood count	Check for evidence of anemia, thrombocytopenia
24 hour urine for urine protein electrophoresis (UPEP)	Check for urine M-protein (Bence-Jones protein)
Urine immunofixation electrophoresis (UIFE)	Identify specific monoclonal light-chain (κ or λ) immunoglobulin
Skeletal survey	Check for osteolytic lesions
Plasma cell labeling index	Check for proliferative rate of plasma cells, prognostication purpose
Beta-2 microglobulin	Prognosis
Magnetic resonance imaging	Check for occult osteolytic lesions, spinal cord compression

of a multiple myeloma diagnostic work-up (Table 59-2).[50] Some tests may be needed in most patients, including plasma cell labeling index (PCLI), popularized by the Mayo Clinic, to identify the fraction of the myeloma cell that is proliferating; C-reactive protein, a surrogate marker for IL-6; lactic dehydrogenase (LDH), which can serve as a measure of tumor burden in lymphoma-like or plasmablastic myeloma; cytogenetic tests, to detect chromosomal abnormalities—particularly deletions—which may suggest a worse prognosis; and bone marrow flow cytometry, used to quantify the number of phenotypically abnormal plasma cells and help confirm the diagnosis. Additional tests under some circumstances include MRI for suspected spinal cord compression or solitary plasmacytoma of the bone; computerized tomography (CT) scan for evaluation of extradural extraosseous plasmacytomas; serum viscosity if hyperviscosity is suspected; tissue biopsy through fine-needle aspiration to confirm the presence of plasmacytomas; evaluation of the erythropoietin level or hemoglobin to help determine the necessity of erythropoietin therapy; and bone marrow immunohistochemistry to confirm the clonality of the plasma cells.

Table 59-3 Negative Prognostic Factors in Multiple Myeloma

Older age
High labeling index
High lactic dehydrogenase (LDH)
High beta-2 microglobulin
High C-reactive protein (CRP)
Chromosomal aberration
Abnormal cytogenetics
Poor immune status
Poor performance status
Refractory to induction chemotherapy
Plasmacytosis (> 50%) in the bone marrow
High level (> 20%) of circulating plasma cells (plasma cell leukemia)

Prognostic Factors

A number of negative prognostic factors (Table 59-3)[95] have been identified in the literature in patients who have been treated with conventional chemotherapy, defined as treatment that has been validated and routinely offered outside clinical trial. As these prognostic factors were identified during conventional therapy, the roles of prognostic factors need to be reassessed in the context of high-dose therapy[95] and new targeted therapies.

The poor prognostic factors identified in MM include poor performance status, older age, high tumor burden, poor immune status, high β_2M levels, elevated LDH, plasmacytosis (> 50%) in the bone marrow,[96] high level of circulating plasma cell,[97] plasmablastic morphology of tumor cells, high PCLI,[9] or high proliferative activity (S-phase plasma cells > 3%).[95,98]

Other poor prognostic factors include abnormal cytogenetics,[38,99] chromosomal aberrations (deletion of chromosome 13),[100] molecular abnormality such as presence of a *p53* deletion,[101] C-reactive protein (CRP) level greater than 6 mg/L, low albumin (< 3 g/dL) combined with high β_2M (> 6 mg/L),[102] and high soluble IL-6 receptor (sIL-6R > 185 mg/L).[95]

Several attempts have been made to combine prognostic factors with disease staging. Some authors have introduced new staging systems. Three prognostic factors are commonly used: β_2M and albumin, β_2M and CRP, and β_2M and PCLI. To date, none of these factors has superseded the "old and simple" parameters of tumor burden and clinical and laboratory findings associated with multiple myeloma such as the Durie-Salmon staging system.[49]

One reason for studying prognostic factors is to identify high-risk groups so that the patient treatment can be adapted to the expected outcome. Among the prognostic factors identified, the initial β_2M level appears to be more accurate, as its prognostic value has been shown in a number of clinical trials with conventional chemotherapy and confirmed in studies on autologous transplantation. Cytogenetics may emerge as an important prognostic factor for the future. Likewise, the combination of β_2M and cytogenetics might help to define therapeutic strategies. Patients with low β_2M and without unfavorable cytogenetics could benefit from intensive strategies with autologous transplantation, while new approaches are needed for patients with high β_2M and/or unfavorable cytogenetics.[5]

Diagnostic Criteria

Several diagnostic systems are used to diagnose and classify patients with plasma cell dyscrasias, including the Durie-Salmon, Kyle and Greipp, and British Columbia Cancer Agency (BCCA) systems.[49] The BCCA criteria were thought by most clinicians to be the easiest to use since they require just one of the following for diagnosis: presence of a paraprotein in serum or urine, lytic bone lesions, or bone marrow plasma cell infiltrate in excess of 10% of the cells present.[49] The Durie and Salmon diagnostic criteria are widely used in the United States because a number of parameters included in other diagnostic systems have not yet been validated by large multicenter trials and are not easily accessible in the majority of hematology-oncology clinics.[95]

The diagnosis of MM can be confirmed utilizing the Durie and Salmon diagnostic criteria, which are divided into two categories: "major" and "minor." In most cases, one major criterion plus one minor criterion are sufficient to diagnose myeloma (Table 59-4). In patients who satisfy the diagnostic criteria for MM, the Durie-Salmon clinical staging system is commonly applied to determine the stage of disease based on the presence or absence of bone lesions, anemia, hypercalcemia, and paraproteinemia levels.

Table 59-4 Diagnostic Criteria: Durie and Salmon

Myeloma

Major Criteria	Minor Criteria
1. Plasmacytoma on tissue biopsy	a. Bone marrow plasmacytosis with 10%–30% plasma cells
2. Bone marrow plasmacytosis with 30% plasma cells	b. Monoclonal globulin spike present, but lower levels than defined in the major criteria
3. Monoclonal globulin spike (M-protein) on SPEP: IgG > 3.5 g/dL, IgA > 2.0 g/dL, light-chain excretion on UPEP ≥ 1 g/24 hr in the absence of amyloidosis	c. Lytic bone lesions d. Normal IgM > 50 mg/dL, IgA > 100 mg/dL, or IgG > 600 mg/dL

The diagnosis of myeloma requires a minimum of one major criterion and one minor criterion (although 1 + a is not sufficient) or three minor criteria that must include a + b

Indolent Myeloma

Criteria for myeloma with the following limitations:

a. Absent or only limited bone lesions (≤ 3 lytic lesions), no compression fractures

b. Stable paraprotein levels: IgG level < 700 mg/dL, IgA < 500 mg/dL

c. No symptoms or associated disease features: Karnofsky performance status > 70%, hemoglobin > 10 g/dL, normal serum calcium, normal serum creatinine, no infections

d. Plasma cell labeling index ≤ 0.5%

Data from Lokhorst H: Clinical features and diagnostic criteria, in Mehta J, Singhal S (eds): Myeloma. London, Martin Dunitz, 2002, p. 155. Reprinted with permission.[49]

Classification and Staging

The Durie-Salmon clinical staging system for MM has been the most widely used system in the United States. This simple and reproducible system is based on easily accessible data. However, its usefulness in MM prognostication has been demonstrated only in the context of conventional chemotherapy, and has not been confirmed in the context of autologous transplantation.[95] This staging system incorporates both the Durie-Salmon system proposed in 1975 and the labeling index proposed by Durie and associates in the 1980s (see Table 59-5).[103,104] It integrates both clinical and laboratory findings associated with MM.

In 1980, Durie and associates identified a process to quantitate the total-body myeloma cell mass.[104] This number is calculated by dividing the total-body M-component synthetic rate per myeloma cell. In examining a large series of individuals with MM, the authors identified three stages of the disease. Stage I disease, or low cell mass, consists of less than 0.6×10^{12} cells/m^2. Stage II disease, or intermediate cell mass, reflects more than $0.6–1.2 \times 10^{12}$ cells/m^2. Stage III disease, or high cell mass, consists of more than 1.2×10^{12} cells/m^2.

Further staging is done based on renal status at the time of diagnosis. Group A includes individuals with a normal renal function (creatinine level less than 2.0 mg/dL), and group B includes individuals with evi-

Table 59-5 Myeloma Staging System

Criteria	Estimated Myeloma Mass (Cells × $10^{12}/m^2$)
Stage I	
All of the following:	
Hemoglobin value > 10 g/dL	
Normal serum calcium	
Normal bone structure	< 0.6 (low burden)
Low M-protein production:	
IgG value < 5.0 g/dL	
IgA value < 3.0 g/dl	
Urine kappa or lambda < 4.0 g/24/hours	
Stage II	
Overall data fit in neither stage I nor stage III	0.6–0.12 (intermediate burden)
Stage III	
One or more of the following:	
Hemoglobin value < 8.5 g/dL	
Serum calcium value > 12.0 mg/dL	
More than 3 lytic bone lesions	
High M-protein production	>1.2 (high burden)
IgG value > 7.0 g/dL	
IgA value > 5.0 g/dL	
Urine kappa or lambda > 12.0 g/24/hours	
Subclassification	
A = creatinine value < 2.0 mg/dL	
B = creatinine value ≥ 2.0 mg/dL	

IgA, = immunoglobulin A; IgG = immunoglobulin G.

Source: Reprinted with permission from Durie BG, Salmon SE: A clinical staging system for multiple myeloma: correlation of measured myeloma cell mass with presenting clinical features, response to treatment and survival. *Cancer* 36: p 855, 1975[103]

dence of renal dysfunction (creatinine level greater than 2.0 mg/dL).

Other attempts have been made to simplify the staging system for MM. The simple staging system developed by Southwest Oncology Group (SWOG) is based on two common measures with prognostic significance in multiple myeloma: serum β_2M and serum albumin. The proponents of the SWOG staging system believe that this scheme could provide an alternative to Durie-Salmon staging for patients with previously untreated MM based on easily obtained laboratory measures.[105] More studies in another population of patients with MM are needed to confirm these data and might eventually increase acceptance of this new staging system among clinicians.

Table 59-6 Conventional Chemotherapy Commonly Used in Multiple Myeloma

Primary Therapy
Melphalan/prednisone (MP)
Vincristine/BCNU/melphalan/cyclophosphamide/prednisone (VBMCP)
Vincristine/carmustine/doxorubicin/prednisone (VBAP)
Vincristine/doxorubicin/dexamethasone (VAD)
High-dose pulsed dexamethasone (D)
Vincristine/melphalan/cyclophosphamide/prednisone (VMCP)/VBAP alternating therapy
Doxorubicin/carmustine/cyclophosphamide/melphalan (ABCM)
Relapsed/Refractory Multiple Myeloma
Repeat primary conventional therapy (if relapse at > 6 months)
Cyclophosphamide-VAD (hyper-VAD)
Etoposide/dexamethasone/cytarabine/cisplatin (EDAP)
High-dose cyclophosphamide
Thalidomide (Thal)
Thalidomide/dexamethasone (Thal/Dex)
Cyclophosphamide/dexamethasone/etoposide/cisplatin (CDEP)
Dexamethasone/thalidomide/cisplatin/doxorubicin/cyclophosphamide/etoposide (DT-PACE)
Maintenance Therapy
Steroids
Interferon

Therapeutic Approaches and Nursing Care

Primary Conventional Treatment (Patients without Transplant Options)

Conventional chemotherapy is defined by the NCCN guidelines as therapy where the safety and efficacy have been validated and, as a result, the therapy is routinely offered outside the context of a clinical trial. It is classified into three categories: primary, salvage and maintenance. Primary conventional therapies utilized in MM are outlined in Table 59-6.[50]

Not all patients who fulfill the minimal criteria for diagnosis of MM should be treated.[35] Individuals with indolent, asymptomatic, smoldering multiple myeloma should be observed initially for months and may do well without treatment over many years.[50] No evidence indicates that early treatment of patients with asymptomatic MM offers an overall survival advantage.[50] A recent review of randomized controlled trials with a parallel design that compared early versus deferred treatment of patients with early-stage MM based on the Durie-Salmon staging system concluded that early treatment of early-stage MM inhibits disease progression and may reduce vertebral compression, but no significant effects on response rates or overall survival were seen.[106]

When disease progression is evident, as demonstrated by a sustained 25% or greater increase in M-protein in serum or urine or by development of new sites of lytic disease or hypercalcemia, treatment should be started immediately.[50] Exposure to myelotoxic agents (alkylating agents—that is, mustards such as melphalan and cyclophosphamide, and nitrosureas, such as carmustine or lomustine) and pelvic irradiation should be limited to avoid compromising the stem cell reserve prior to stem cell harvest in patients who may be candidates for transplant.[50,107] Systemic therapy is the preferred initial approach to symptomatic MM. The use of radiation therapy in this disease should be limited to discrete lesions because it does not benefit the patient with systemic disease and could further deplete the bone marrow reserve.

If the individual is 70 years of age or younger, the clinician should discuss the possibility of autologous stem cell transplantation.[35] Ideally, the hematopoietic stem cells should be collected before the patient is exposed to alkylating agents. High-dose chemotherapy (HDC) followed by autologous stem cell transplant (ASCT) has been recommended by the NCCN myeloma panel as a primary treatment in patients with symptomatic MM, with the consensus being based on high-level evidence.[50]

In patients with symptomatic MM who are older than 70 years of age or in younger patients in whom transplant is not feasible, intermittent systemic oral melphalan and prednisone (MP) combination therapy has been the first-line choice for the last three decades.[35,108,109] Numerous regimens have been tested in an attempt to improve mean survival from the time of diagnosis, but none has proved superior to systemic oral MP.[110] After three decades of anticipated benefits of combination chemotherapy, not a single combination regimen appears to be better than MP.[107] In 1998, the Myeloma Trialists' Collaborative Group conducted an overview of MM clinical trials, which included data on 6623 patients entered in 27 trials worldwide. The group declared MP and combination therapy to be of comparable effectiveness, although the response to combination therapy may occur more rapidly.[111] This group's findings supported an earlier meta-analysis of 18 clinical trials, which suggested that there was no survival difference between the two approaches, either overall or within any patient subgroup.[107,112]

Melphalan and prednisone

Prior to the advent of high-dose chemotherapy with or without stem cell rescue, the MP oral regimen was the most frequent treatment for newly diagnosed MM.[113] Its response rate ranges from 50% to 60%, and the mean survival rate with this regimen is 24–36 months.[114] The survival rates at 5 and 10 years are 25% and 8%, respectively.[12] Standard MP chemotherapy consists of melphalan 8 mg/day for 7 days and prednisone 20 mg three times daily for the same 7 days every 6 weeks.[35] It can also be given as melphalan 8 mg/m^2 daily for 4 consecutive days and prednisone 60 mg/m^2 daily by mouth, also for 4 consecutive days.

Oral melphalan must be taken on an empty stomach at least 2 hours before meals or 3 hours after eating, because food reduces its absorption by at least 50%;[115] in contrast, prednisone needs to be taken with meals. Patients may take an H_2 histamine receptor antagonist to prevent the gastric distress associated with steroids. White blood cells and platelets are checked every 3 weeks after beginning each cycle of therapy. The dosage of melphalan must be adjusted until modest midcycle cytopenia occurs.[35] If the serum creatinine level is more than 2 mg/dL, the dose of melphalan should be reduced by 25% to prevent severe myelosupression. If cytopenias do not occur, the dose of melphalan should be increased in a stepwise escalation by 2–3 mg/m^2.[35,107]

Unless the disease progresses rapidly, at least three courses of MP should be given before therapy is discontinued because delayed responses are common. An objective response may not be seen for 6–12 months or even longer in some patients. If the pain is alleviated and no evidence of progressive disease is present (no increase in serum or urine M-protein, no new bone lesions, no hypercalcemia), the regimen should be continued.

The relative importance of the two active agents in the MP regimen has been debated because of conflicting results when using either the MP combination or intermittent melphalan alone. Analysis has clearly shown the usefulness of steroids by correlating survival with prednisone dose intensity and not with the total melphalan dose.[116] In general, corticosteroids as part of primary treatment of MM demonstrate high activity in plasma cells, with concomitant sparing of normal hematopoietic elements. Corticosteroids may increase the speed of response without added myelosuppression while improving the well-being of patients.[107] Older individuals who are at risk for infectious or gastrointestinal complications must be monitored closely.

Vincristine, doxorubicin, and dexamethasone (VAD) therapy

Infusional VAD came into use in the early 1980s, when it was developed at the M. D. Anderson Cancer Center in Houston, Texas. The reported response rate in chemotherapy-naïve patients with MM is approximately 60%–80% with a 10%–15% complete remission (CR) response rate.[117,118] When VAD was compared with standard alkalyting agent–based therapies, researchers found no obvious survival benefit in the VAD arm.[119] Clinically, the VAD regimen may be preferable for patients in whom rapid tumor control is desired, such as those with hypercalcemia, renal failure, or widespread painful bone lesions. It is especially indicated in patients with plasma cell leukemia (myeloma associated with > 20% circulating plasma cells), because standard alkylating agents are ineffective in such cases.[120] VAD is also useful in patients with renal failure because none of its components are excreted through the renal system and dose adjustments are not necessary. No more than three courses of VAD are usually needed to confirm partial response (50% reduction of M-protein) or resistance to this regimen.[118] Monitoring the total dose of doxorubicin and treating patients to a maximum tolerated dose of 450 mg/m^2 are typical.

The major drawbacks of this regimen are the side effects associated with high-dose steroids, particularly among elderly patients, who may have more steroid-related toxicity,[121] and the need for central intravenous access. The use of pegylated liposomal doxorubicin (nonvesicant) avoids the inherent risks (extravasation of a vesicant) that result from the use of central venous catheters, and the treatment regimen appears to be effective and well tolerated as first-line treatment.[122] Monitoring for signs and symptoms of steroid toxicity (e.g., severe dyspepsia, fluid and sodium retention, corticosteroid myopathy, acute pancreatitis, insulin-dependent hyperglycemia, and steroid psychosis) is important. Patient and family education will include signs and symptoms of steroid-induced gastritis; if these persist or worsen (including nausea and vomiting with or without hematemesis), the clinician is usually contacted to prevent serious complications such as gastric ulceration and bleeding.

Elderly patients require close monitoring, particularly those with concurrent diseases such as congestive heart failure, because steroid-associated sodium and water retention can exacerbate symptoms.[121] Monitoring the patient for weight gain and peripheral edema on a daily basis will help in detecting pulmonary rales and compromise. Instructing the patient to report to the clinician any weight gain greater than 5 pounds in one day is also important. Individuals with preexisting diabetes require close monitoring for signs and symptoms of steroid-induced hyperglycemia. Teaching patients how to monitor blood sugar and when to report side effects to the clinician are important aspects of treatment. Home care visits by a registered nurse may be initiated to monitor blood pressure, blood sugar level, and other steroid-related side effects, as clinically indicated. Dose reductions or change of treatment regimen may be required in patients who develop steroid-related psychosis, when side effects become more pronounced, and when the risks outweigh the benefits of treatment.

VAD produces much less myelosupression than do other alkylating agent combinations, and it may be conveniently used in cases presenting with neutropenia or thrombocytopenia secondary to bone marrow infiltration.[107] In some patients, prolonged thrombocytopenia and granulocytopenia may be observed and require a reduction in the dose of doxorubicin. If the doxorubicin cannot be administered due to prolonged bone marrow suppression, the entire cycle may be delayed for one week and therapy resumed once the platelet count exceeds 50,000/mm^3 and the absolute neutrophil count (ANC) exceeds 750/mm^3. Hepatic toxicity characterized by a bilirubin level greater than 2.0 mg/dL requires reduction or discontinuation of both doxorubicin and vincristine, depending on the severity. If the bilirubin level is greater than 5.0 mg/dL, both doxorubicin and vincristine should be discontinued.

High-dose pulsed dexamethasone

High-dose pulsed dexamethasone (D) is another primary treatment regimen in patients with MM, offering response and survival rates that are similar to those achieved with other standard regimens, such as VAD.[123] Dexamethasone alone could be an alternative regimen for VAD, and it provides the convenience of oral administration. It is usually dosed at 40 mg on days 1–4, 9–12, and 17–20 with a one-week break (28-day cycle) or two-week break (35-day cycle). Because dexamethasone is not associated with myelosuppression, this agent is indicated when radiotherapy is needed for the treatment of painful bone lesions, and it may be the primary treatment of choice in the occasional patient who presents with pancytopenia.[107] Prophylactic antacids or proton pump inhibitors and anti-infectives are usually given to prevent the side effects common with steroids.

Interferon plus conventional chemotherapy

Interferon was introduced into the treatment of patients with MM more than two decades ago,[124] but its role is still not clearly defined. It has been added to standard chemotherapy in previously untreated patients with myeloma because it has antitumor activity and because it may have a different mechanism of action from conventional chemotherapeutic regimens.[125] The specific mechanisms of action employed by interferons (alpha, beta, and gamma) have not been clearly elucidated, but they may have direct antitumor effects through induction of apoptosis and indirect effects mediated through the host, inhibition of angiogenesis, or immunomodulation.[126] A recent meta-analysis of trials of interferon therapy in patients with MM revealed a 6% higher response rate and a six-month prolongation of the recurrence-free interval for the IFN-α–containing induction regimens.[127] This report lacked compelling data to support the addition of IFN-α to standard alkylating agent regimens, however, the minor benefits, if any, should be weighed against possible bone marrow or systemic toxicities and the cost.[107]

The toxicities associated with IFN-α require thorough assessment and consistent interventions to manage side effects. They may include flu-like syndrome, anorexia, progressive fatigue, depression, hepatotoxicity, thrombocytopenia, granulocytopenia, neurological, and renal/metabolic toxicity.[126] A patient on IFN-α needs close monitoring by the clinician for evidence of interferon toxicity so that appropriate dose reduction can be initiated in a timely manner. The dose reduction schedule and plan to discontinue IFN-α depend on the patient's response to the severity of the toxicity. Nurses play a key role in assessing and grading treatment-related toxicities and in assisting patients and their families in managing side effects.

Many attempts have been made to define the role of interferons in the treatment of MM so that they may be utilized to maximum effect. Controversy continues regarding the in vitro studies showing that, under various conditions, IFN-α can either stimulate or inhibit the growth and proliferation of myeloma cells. Overall, the interferons' use appears beneficial, and IFN-α currently plays a role as part of standard myeloma treatment, mostly as maintenance therapy and not with standard alkylating agent regimens.[126] Additional studies involving large patient numbers will clarify the areas where interferons can have maximum impact on survival.

Primary Treatment (Patients with Transplant as an Option)

Autologous stem cell transplantation

The efficacy of high-dose chemotherapy (HDC) and autologous stem cell transplant (ASCT) is well established in MM and both are considered effective first-line treatments for patients with MM.[128] HDC has been used for more than 10 years for the treatment of MM, either alone or with ASCT. HDC with ASCT treatment has improved remission rates, event-free survival, and overall survival in patients with MM compared to conventional chemotherapy.[129] This procedure is suitable for patients younger than 70 years without significant co-morbid conditions and for selected older patients. Alkylating agents such as regimens containing melphalan should not be administered to newly diagnosed patients with MM to avoid damage to stem cells. Patients who have received standard treatment for less than one year and/or a total melphalan dose of less than 200 mg/m^2 retain a good chance of mobilizing sufficient numbers of stem cells to provide for ASCT.[128]

Early ASCT appears to be the approach of choice rather than late autotransplantation.[128] A large French study reported that although overall survival was not influenced by the time of ASCT, the early-transplant group had superior event-free survival.[130]

Induction. The nonmyelotoxic VAD therapy is the preferred induction regimen because a rapid response is desirable and it causes less damage to bone marrow progenitor cells. Vincristine, doxorubicin, melphalan, and prednisone (VAMP) or VAMP plus weekly cyclophosphamide (C-VAMP)[131] may be an alternative that provides an enhanced response without affecting cumulative toxicity or compromising subsequent stem cell collection. A vincristine, melphalan, cyclophosphamide, and prednisone (VMCP)/vincristine, carmustine, doxorubicin, and prednisone (VBAP) with IFN-α regimen has also been utilized as induction therapy to produce remission prior to stem cell collection and transplantation (Table 59-7).[132] Dexamethasone, thalidomide, cisplatin, doxorubicin, cyclophosphamide, and etoposide (DT-PACE) may be also utilized as an induction therapy before ASCT, especially in patients with high-risk characteristics such as those with high LDH or chromosome 13 abnormality, and in those patients who are refractory to standard therapy.[133]

Recently, a thalidomide and dexamethasone combination has been considered a possible alternative to infusional VAD as induction therapy in autotransplantation. One study reported promising results using thalidomide and dexamethasone as induction therapy in transplant-candidate patients who were newly diagnosed with MM.[134] A lower incidence of major complications and an absence of stem cell collection problems among this group of patients were also reported. A similar study reported thalidomide and dexamethasone to be a possible alternative induction regimen.[135] Both of these studies demonstrated that the use of thalidomide in combination with dexamethasone in

Table 59-7 Treatment Schema of European Bone Marrow Transplant Trial in Multiple Myeloma

Conventional treatment: VMCP/BVAP*		
VMCP		
	Vincristine	1 mg IV; day 1
	Melphalan	5 mg/m² PO; days 1–4
	Cyclophosphamide	110 mg/m² PO; days 1–4
	Prednisone	60 mg/m² PO; days 1–4
VBAP		
	Vincristine	1 mg IV; day 1
	Carmustine	30 mg/m² IV; day 1
	Doxorubicin	30 mg/m² IV; day 1
	Prednisone	60 mg/m² PO; days 1–4
Recombinant alfa-interferon (3 million units/m² SQ 3 times/week from cycle 9 until relapse)		
High-Dose treatment (as above)		
Autologous bone marrow was collected after cycle 4 (200 million nucleated cells/kg body weight).		
All patients received 4–6 cycles VMCP/VBAP; if their WHO (World Health Organization) performance status was < 3 and a transplant facility was available, the individual was transplanted.		
Preparative regimen:	Melphalan 140 mg/m² Total-body irradiation (8 Gy in 4 fractions over 4 days with no lung shields)	
Unpurged autologous bone marrow was readministered.		
Alfa-interferon was administered from cycle 9 until relapse; after bone marrow transplantation hematologic recovery occurred (granulocyte count > 1500/mm³; platelet count > 75,000/mm³).		

* Alternating cycles (every 3 weeks for 12 months; total 18 cycles).

Data from Attal, Harousseau, Stoppa, et al.[132]

newly diagnosed patients with symptomatic myeloma can induce a high frequency of response, rapid onset of remission, low incidence of serious irreversible toxicities, and no substantial effect on stem cell collection. An earlier study on the use of thalidomide plus dexamethasone with doxorubicin in patients with untreated, symptomatic myeloma reported similar findings.[136] Thromboembolic events were reported but patients receiving therapeutic doses of warfarin or low-molecular-weight heparin did not experience thrombotic episodes.[135]

Collection of peripheral blood stem cells. In general, collection and cryopreservation of blood stem cells should be initiated as soon as the best possible response is confirmed (reduction of M-protein from baseline).[107] The use of another chemotherapeutic agent prior to stem cell collection and cryopreservation is a common practice (chemomobilization) to further reduce tumor burden. Use of growth factor alone (i.e., granulocyte colony-stimulating factor [G-CSF] or granulocyte-macrophage colony-stimulating factor [GM-CSF]) without chemotherapy prior to stem collection to mobilize stem cells (G-mobilization) may be used in a selected group of patients. Older age adversely affects CD34+ cell yield even with limited premobilization therapy, indicating that early collection is especially important in elderly patients.[137] Sequential administration of VAD followed by high-dose cyclophosphamide and consolidated by the combination of etoposide, dexamethasone, cytarabine, and cisplatin (EDAP) has improved the CR rate and allowed for the collection of an adequate number of stem cells to support two autologous transplants.[138] Other chemomobilization regimens include high-dose cyclophosphamide and cyclophosphamidel/dexamethasone/etoposide/cisplatin (CDEP).

Purging (removal of lingering malignant plasma cells) with monoclonal antibodies or 4-hydroperoxycyclophosphamide (4-HC) and positive selection of CD34+ progenitor cells (myeloma cells do not express the CD34 antigen) has been performed to obtain tumor-free stem cells and improve the response rate and overall survival. A long-term follow-up of a randomized study[139] showed no survival benefit from CD34+ selection. Thus the benefits of purging and positive selection of stem cells remain questionable.[128]

Conditioning regimen. High-dose melphalan appears to be the most active conditioning regimen and is considered the standard method for ablating the bone marrow of patients with multiple myeloma. Other combination regimens containing busulfan or etoposide proved to be complex and showed no obvious additional benefit.[128] High-dose melphalan at 200 mg/m² given in one dose or at 100 mg/m² on two consecutive days followed by reinfusion of stem cells 24 hours after the completion of melphalan administration is commonly utilized in clinical practice.

The reinfusion of stem cells 24 hours after high-dose melphalan administration is safe based on pharmacokinetic studies suggesting that the terminal half-life of melphalan ranges from 50 to 170 minutes.[128] The dose of melphalan is sometimes reduced depending on the age of the patient (i.e., age > 70 years) and presence of co-morbid conditions. A reduced dose of melphalan at 140 mg/m² is commonplace in the elderly patient population to avoid high mortality.[140]

In the past, age older than 65 years and co-morbid conditions such as renal compromise were considered negative factors in the selection of transplant candidates. Recently, studies have shown that neither of these factors is an important adverse parameter affecting the outcome following high-dose therapy and autologous transplantation.[141–145] These reports have led to an increase in the number of older patients who are deemed eligible for ASCT for the treatment of MM.[107]

A number of studies have shown that the attainment of a complete response is an independent favorable prognostic factor for overall survival and event-free survival after HDC.[128] Several other variables have been found to be predictive of prognosis in patients undergoing high-dose therapy. These include high tumor burden (based on M-protein and plasma cells in the marrow), chromosomal aberrations, abnormal karyotype (cytogenetic abnormality), high β_2M at the time of initial presentation, and duration of standard therapy prior to high-dose therapy.[128] Gender is the only patient factor that has prognostic significance; age was found to be a nonsignificant factor, except in patients with renal failure.[144] Response to previous therapy was once thought to be a poor prognostic factor[128] but recent reports have contradicted this conclusion, so patients who showed a lack of response to induction therapy should not be disqualified from undergoing ASCT.[146]

Long-term sequelae. Patients with MM who underwent ASCT may develop secondary acute myeloid leukemia (AML) or myelodysplastic syndrome (MDS).[128,147,148] One study reported that these complications were seen exclusively in patients treated with conventional-dose alkylating agent chemotherapy.[147] The actuarial five-year probabilities of developing cytogenetic MDS and combined cytogenetic MDS-MM are 5% and 10%, respectively. It is also possible that this high rate of myelodysplastic changes results from undergoing two ASCTs in comparison with a single transplant.[128] Another study reported that prolonged duration of pretransplant chemotherapy was the most important risk factor for the development of MDS, followed by older age and a low number of infused CD34$^+$ cells.[149] Reported risks for treatment-related malignancies range between 1.3-fold and 20-fold higher in patients with MM in comparison to the general public. Clearly, monitoring patients with multiple myeloma for evidence of acute leukemia and treatment-related MDS is crucial. As patients with MM continue to undergo intensive regimens requiring transplant support, clinicians will need to incorporate attention to the risk for the development of AML and MDS into the informed consent process, the ongoing management, and the long-term follow-up of these patients.

In the controversial field of myeloma disease management, HDC with autologous stem cell transplant seems to be an approach with tangible benefits such as longer overall survival.

Maintenance Therapy

The role of maintenance therapy in patients with MM remains controversial. It is usually initiated following induction remission therapy (conventional chemotherapy)[150] or 8–12 weeks after HDC with ASCT.[151]

Interferon

The role of IFN-α as maintenance therapy in patients with MM has been well studied.[126] Unfortunately, IFN-α treatment trials in MM have yielded discordant results regarding response rate, maintenance duration, and survival times. Despite the fact that these studies have shown conflicting results, most investigators suggested that the role of IFN-α in the management of patients with MM is mainly as maintenance therapy to prolong the plateau phase of remission.[126]

Steroids

Steroids play a significant role as single agents or in combination with chemotherapy as induction remission treatment for myeloma. Studying their role as maintenance therapy, therefore, has merit. The use of alternate-day prednisone 50 mg as an effective maintenance treatment for patients with MM who achieve a response to induction chemotherapy has been reported.[150]

Conventional and Novel Therapies for Relapsed and Refractory Myeloma

At least one-third of patients with MM fail to respond to induction chemotherapy and those who initially achieve remission even with high-dose chemotherapy may eventually relapse and require additional treatment.[152] Patients with MM treated with HDC and hematopoietic stem cell transplantation are considered to have disease progression when the serum or urine paraprotein has increased by 25%.[153] Patients with relapsed myeloma are usually divided into two groups: drug-resistant and relapsing. The drug-resistant group has the poorest overall prognosis, and only a few respond to alternative treatments.[154] For simplicity, refractory myeloma indicates disease unresponsive to the most recent therapy administered. Patients with refractory multiple myeloma are usually encouraged to participate in clinical trials.

For treatment of patients with relapsed MM, therapeutic agents typically include the same drugs used in initial induction therapy. The appropriate therapy for a given situation depends on the nature of the disease, age, organ function, prior treatment, availability of stem cell donors, and access to novel agents. Broadly, these options include bortezomib, thalidomide and

Table 59-8 Potential Effects of Bortezomib in Cancer

Induce cancer cell apoptosis
Limit tumor survival, growth, spread, and angiogenesis
Affect cellular signals involved in resistance to standard chemotherapies
Affect ability of myeloma cells to interact with bone marrow microenvironment

thalidomide-based therapies, high-dose dexamethasone, high-dose chemotherapy with ASCT, allogeneic hematopoietic stem cell transplantation, combination chemotherapy such as etoposide-based regimens, and novel/investigational agents.[155]

Approximately 40% of patients with resistant and relapsing MM may achieve second remission with glucocorticoids[154] and 40%–50% of patients with relapsing MM respond to VAD.[156] Second-line combination chemotherapy regimens (primarily including alkylating agents) may help a small percentage of patients: 8% of resistant patients, 22% of refractory patients, and a slightly higher percentage of patients receiving doxorubicin-based regimens may respond, but the duration of second response may be less than one year.[154]

Bortezomib

Bortezomib, formerly known as PS-341, is a novel, first-in-class agent that inhibits the 26S proteasome (simply called "the proteasome").[157] The mechanism of action of this proteasome inhibitor in MM has been described, and its potential effects in myeloma and other types of cancer are outlined in Table 59-8.[158] In clinical trials, patients with relapsed and refractory MM treated with bortezomib showed an overall response rate of 59%.[159] The median duration of response was 14 months and median overall survival was 17 months.[160]

Patients on bortezomib therapy should be closely monitored for any adverse effects. Failure to assess for them and lack of appropriate early interventions may jeopardize the patient's health. Peripheral neuropathy needs close monitoring, and appropriate dose reduction based on patient's degree of neuropathy is recommended. Monitoring of complete blood counts before each dose and weekly chemistries are done to check for any electrolyte imbalance and creatinine abnormality.[94] Transfusion support and use of growth factors may be clinically indicated. Grade 4 hematologic toxicities will require dose reduction, and the dose is usually withheld until it returns to the grade 2 level (based on National Cancer Institute toxicity criteria) with or without transfusion and/or use of growth factors. Antidiarrheals and antiemetics may be used as clinically indicated. Oncology nurses play a vital role in the assessment and monitoring of these adverse effects and in initiating immediate interventions before serious health problems or irreversible damage occur.[161]

Multiple options are available in the management of relapsed and refractory MM, but no randomized, controlled trial data are available to guide clinicians regarding what approach to take first. A systematic review of randomized studies in MM concluded that the overall quality of the body of evidence for myeloma management was poor and has ample room for improvement.[129] These findings support the recommendation that the best management of any cancer patient occurs in clinical trials and patient participation should therefore be encouraged.[50]

Radiation Therapy

Radiation therapy (RT) has long been recognized as an important therapeutic option to palliate symptoms associated with MM. Approximately 70% of patients will eventually benefit from this therapy.[154] MM is considered a disseminated disease with evidence of distant organ involvement at the time of diagnosis requiring systemic combination chemotherapy, rather than focal treatment such as radiation. In rare instances (fewer than 5% of cases), the disease may be localized and present as a solitary plasmacytoma of bone or SPB (approximately 70% of cases) or extramedullary plasmacytoma or EMP (approximately 30% of cases). On biopsy, the individual's bony lesion will show evidence of plasma cells. Bone marrow aspiration and biopsy, peripheral counts including blood counts, and serum chemistry will be unremarkable and show no evidence of other organ involvement. The diagnosis of osseous plasmacytoma, defined as a plasmacytoma emanating from bone without other evidence of disease, requires a thorough evaluation to rule out the presence of systemic disease, because many patients presumed to have solitary plasmacytomas are eventually found to have occult disease.[162] MRI of the spine may be very useful in these conditions.[50]

Radiation therapy of a solitary plasmacytoma in doses of 40 Gy or more demonstrates local control rates of 88%–100% in osseous sites and 80%–100% in soft tissue sites.[162] These data support the contention that MM is an extremely radiosensitive malignancy. The NCCN recommends delivering doses of 45 Gy or more to involved field in both osseous and tissue plasmacytomas. For soft tissue plasmacytoma, surgery may be required plus CT or MRI every 6 months for two cycles, then as clinically indicated. Follow-up and surveillance in osseous plasmacytoma includes quantitative immunoglobulin tests plus quantification of M-protein after RT, complete blood counts, differential assessment, platelets, bone survey annually or for symptoms, bone marrow biopsy as clinically indicated, and M-protein measurement every 3–6 months as clinically indicated.[50]

The outcome following RT for a solitary plasmacytoma of the bone or an extramedullary plasmacytoma should be discussed thoroughly with the patient and family. Nearly all patients presenting with SPB will progress to myeloma, with a median myeloma-free interval of approximately 10 years with adequate local therapy. Because true solitary plasmacytoma is a rare event,[162] it is important that patients understand the need for continued follow-up and surveillance. SPB has higher risk of conversion of 54% at 10 years after adequate treatment, compared with a conversion rate of 11% for patients with EMP.[163] Moreover, patients presenting with SPB have a poorer prognosis following progression to myeloma than do patients with EMP. The disappearance of M-protein following RT of SPB has been found to be a significant prognostic indicator.[164]

In MM, just as in solitary plasmacytoma, RT is a very effective palliative modality for symptomatic osseous or extramedullary manifestations. Palliative RT for MM must be individualized. The palliative regimen of 30 Gy given in 10 fractions, which is commonly used to treat metastatic lesions, may not be appropriate for all patients. Lower doses of 10–20 Gy will produce palliation in the majority of patients, while allowing for retreatment in those few in whom it is required. Higher total doses may be recommended in two situations: neurologic compromise from tumor impingement on the spinal cord or cranial nerve and involvement of weight-bearing bones with impending pathologic fracture. In these cases, it is recommended that higher doses of 30–40 Gy be given in standard fractionation (usually 2 Gy per fraction) to obtain the best probability of durable reversal of symptoms in the former case and tumor eradication and bone healing in the latter.[162]

Hemibody irradiation

Hemibody irradiation has been used in patients with advanced or refractory MM because of the disseminated nature and radiosensitivity of myeloma.[165] In this technique, a single dose of radiation (500–800 cGy) is administered to a large body area at one time. This approach allows the potential treatment of both halves of the body sequentially using doses that are higher than could be delivered with total-body irradiation. It can provide pain relief in 24–48 hours, and this time frame is taken into consideration by clinicians when ordering and administering narcotic analgesics to manage pain. Treatment fields include the upper hemibody field — head to the fourth lumbar vertebrae; the midbody field — the abdomen and pelvis from the top of the diaphragm to the obturator foramina; and the lower hemibody — the torso below the iliac crest and extending to the ankles. Complications may be significant particularly in patients receiving upper-half-body irradiation and may include pnuemonitis, infection or sepsis, pancytopenia, bleeding, and treatment-related death.[165] Patient education is very important regarding the potential side effects depending on the field of treatment. Proper coordination and administration of premedications such as corticosteroids, antiemetics, and narcotic analgesics is important to maintain the patient's comfort and facilitate compliance with the plan of treatment.

Bisphosphonates

Bisphosphonates are potent inhibitors of osteoclast-mediated bone resorption and accumulate in the mineralized bone matrix, making it more resistant to dissolution by osteoclasts. Moreover, bisphosphonates directly inhibit the osteolytic activity of osteoclasts and reduce their survival. They have been shown to provide supportive benefits to multiple myeloma patients with lytic bone disease.[166]

Pamidronate, a second-generation amino-bisphosphonate, has been evaluated in a randomized, double-blind trial focusing on advanced MM.[167] Bone pain and analgesic requirements were significantly reduced in the pamidronate group. The total number of skeletal events and episodes of hypercalcemia was reduced by half. Pamidronate is currently used at a dose of 90 mg once a month in a 2-hour intravenous infusion indefinitely; long-term use with this agent has been shown to be safe and efficient.[168] In comparison with ibandronate, pamidronate was found to be superior in reducing osteoclast activity, bone resorption, IL-6, and possibly tumor burden in MM.[169]

A more potent third-generation bisphosphonate, zoledronic acid (Zometa, Novartis Pharmaceutical Corporation, East Hanover, New Jersey), has proven superior to pamidronate in the treatment of hypercalcemia and skeletal metastasis.[170] Also, preclinical studies have demonstrated that this agent has a direct antitumor activity in myeloma cells.[171] Zoledronic acid is currently used at a dose of 4 mg once a month in a 15- to 30-minute intravenous infusion, indefinitely. Although concerns over the nephrotoxicity of zoledronic acid have arisen,[166] one study reported that in patients with mildly to moderately reduced renal function, dosage adjustment of zoledronic acid is likely not necessary.[172] Both zoledronic acid and pamidronate can reduce the risk of vertebral, wrist, and hip fractures by 30%–50%.[173] Zoledronic acid is contraindicated in patients who have renal impairment and patients who are experiencing fluid and electrolyte imbalance.

As with pamidronate, its prolonged use seems to be well tolerated and safe.[168,174]

Common side effects from IV bisphosphonates include bone pain, nausea, fatigue, fever, vomiting, diarrhea, and myalgia.[174] Supportive care measures include assessing for dehydration, measurement of electrolyte level, and administration of antiemetics, antipyretics, antidiarrheals, and analgesics as clinically indicated.[175] Chemistry results are usually reviewed before intravenous bisphosphonate administration, and serum creatinine is monitored on a regular basis. An increase in creatinine of 0.5 mg/dL in patients with normal baseline and of 1.0 mg/dL in patients with abnormal baseline creatinine would require the dose to be held until the creatinine returns to within 10% of the baseline value. Patients who are receiving any bisphosphonate therapy for malignant bone disease are instructed to take daily calcium (500 mg) and vitamin D (400 IU) supplements.[175]

The American Society of Clinical Oncology (ASCO) has published clinical practice guidelines for the use of bisphosphonates in the prevention and treatment of lytic bone disease in patients with MM. The committee has recommended intravenous pamidronate or zoledronic acid only for the prevention of skeletal events. The superiority of one agent relative to the other cannot be definitively established. As a consequence, the choice between pamidronate and zoledronic acid will depend on balancing the higher cost of zoledronic acid, with its shorter, more convenient infusion time (15 minutes), against the lower cost of pamidronate, with its longer infusion time (2 hours).[166]

Investigational Novel Therapeutic Agents

Thalidomide

Thalidomide reentered the oncology clinical setting in 1998. Since then, it has demonstrated significant activity against relapsed and refractory MM.[176] Several studies confirmed the finding that thalidomide has antitumor properties against relapsed and refractory multiple MM, with response rates averaging 30%–35% (minimal response of less than 50% reduction of M-protein was not included).[177–179] The median duration of response is approximately 8–9 months. Individual responses were maintained from as little as 2 months to more than 30 months.[180]

The exact mechanism of the antineoplastic action of thalidomide is unclear. Researchers believe that angiogenesis inhibition, immunomodulation, and cytokine modulation, individually or in combination, likely underlie the drug's antitumor activity.[176,181–184] The mechanisms of action of thalidomide are outlined in Table 59-9.[185]

Table 59-9 Mechanisms of Action of Thalidomide

Inhibition of angiogenesis
Inhibition of TNF-α
Inhibition of cyclooxygenase-2 (COX-2)
Down-regulation of IL-6
Inhibition of TNF-α–induced interleukin-8 (IL-8)
Increased IL-10
Enhancement of Interleukins (IL-4, IL-5, and IL-12)
Stimulatory effect on T-cell activity

The most common reported side effects of thalidomide are constipation, somnolence, and fatigue. Fairly common to least common side effects include peripheral neuropathy, skin rash, and deep-vein thrombosis.[93] In addition, thalidomide is highly teratogenic. Clinicians and patients must strictly adhere to the STEPS (System for Thalidomide Education and Prescribing Safety) program.[186] Therapeutic anticoagulation may be also essential during thalidomide therapy in newly diagnosed patients[134,135] and when the drug is combined with cytotoxic chemotherapy such as doxorubicin, CDEP, and DT-PACE given that deep-vein thrombosis incidence was reported to be higher.[187]

The optimal dose and duration of treatment with thalidomide for patients with relapsed or refractory MM remain unresolved. Various titrations and dosing have been employed. One study reported that the best-tolerated dose of thalidomide is 400 mg/day in patients with relapsed or refractory MM.[188] Furthermore, a reasonable approach for use of thalidomide in MM is to initiate therapy at 50–100 mg nightly and escalate the dose every two weeks in 50–100 mg increments as tolerated; efforts should be made to titrate the dose up to 600 mg/day for patients with poor prognostic features.[188,189]

Several trials are currently under way to determine the clinical benefit of thalidomide in newly diagnosed patients with MM. The optimal dose of thalidomide in relapsed and refractory myeloma still needs to be defined, and its role in the post-transplant setting as consolidation therapy or maintenance therapy merits further investigation. Therapeutic use of thalidomide in a well-designed study will further clarify its effect on long-term toxicity, best timing of therapy, event-free remission, and overall survival in patients with MM.

Arsenic trioxide

Research into the mechanism by which arsenic targets malignant cell types led to the discovery that arse-

Table 59-10 Nursing Care of the Patient with Multiple Myeloma

System	Signs and Symptoms	Patient Education
Neuromuscular	Pain (acute/chronic) Hypercalcemia Hyperviscosity syndrome Spinal cord compression Pathological fracture Depression	Pain control measures Signs and symptoms of hypercalcemia Prevention of pathological fractures Immediate reporting of signs and symptoms of cord compression Cognitive strategies Counseling
Immunosuppression	Anemia Neutropenia Thrombocytopenia	Exercise Energy conservation activities Prevention of infection Avoiding contact with individuals with known infection Prevention of bleeding Self-administration of prescribed hematopoietic growth factors
Respiratory	Pneumonia	Prevention of pooling of pulmonary secretions Increase gas exchange Use of incentive spirometer Strict adherence to antibiotic treatment
Gastrointestinal	Constipation	Preventive measures Change in fluid and dietary intake Exercise
Genitourinary	Renal insufficiency	Increase fluid intake Avoidance of nephrotoxic drugs Recognition of signs of urinary tract infection

nic affects a myriad of pathways that contribute to the cellular transformation process.[190] This greater understanding of the mechanisms by which arsenic affects cellular pathways and arsenic trioxide's efficacy in treating acute promyelocytic leukemia (APL) provided a rationale for investigating the compound's use in treating other hematologic malignancies, such as MM.[191] The achievement of clinical responses marked by molecular conversion of the malignant phenotype and remissions in patients who had failed to respond to multiple courses of conventional chemotherapy provided the impetus to explore its use in multiple myeloma.[192] Several clinical trials are now investigating arsenic trioxide alone or in combination with other agents.[93]

The adverse effects associated with arsenic trioxide administration in patients with MM during clinical trials were usually manageable and well tolerated by patients. In cases involving APL, careful monitoring of the patient's complete blood counts two times per week and chemistries including potassium and magnesium levels at least once per week are essential throughout the therapy period. These tests are needed to assess for severe myelosupression and electrolyte imbalances during treatment. Patients should also have a weekly electrocardiogram and be monitored for possible prolongation of the QTC interval and atrioventricular block.

Symptom Management and Nursing Care

During the course of their disease, patients with MM experience a number of complications that occur secondary to the widespread immunologic, hematologic, and hormonal/cytokine abnormalities seen in this disorder. These problems include infections, hypercalcemia, anemia, pain, and fractures. Nursing interventions are directed toward addressing these clinical issues, which in some cases, could be fatal. Rice and Sheridan have identified some aspects of care for the patient with MM that may have a significant impact on the medically underserved and underrepresented minority—namely, pain, polypharmacy, renal insufficiency, transfusion dependency, and HDC with ASCT. These authors have suggested specific nursing actions and collaboration with other disciplines to address these clinical issues.[193] In planning the nursing care, the entire treatment team must be knowledgeable about the patient's prognosis. It is also critical to include the patient and family when discussing therapeutic goals and treatment options. Goals may include intensive treatment, preventing or delaying life-threatening complications, prolonging disease-free survival, palliation, or end-of-life care. Regardless of the goal, a symptom management approach to nursing care with a review of systems is useful in organizing assessment and interventions (Table 59-10).[194]

Neuromuscular Symptoms

Bone pain is one the most common symptoms of MM and is caused mainly by bone lesions. Other causes of pain in patients with MM include nerve or root compression, post-herpetic neuralgia and unrelated causes.[195] The degree of pain may vary from moderate to severe in intensity. The pain can be acute, characterized by a specific trauma and lasting less than six months in duration, or chronic, having no specific obvious initiation point and occurring over a protracted period. Optimal pain control is essential in maintaining satisfactory quality of life. One study found that pain and mood disturbance were significant predictors of quality of life in patients with MM.[196]

Oncology nurses play a significant role in facilitating an ongoing, adequate pain assessment and effective management. Specific nursing interventions for pain include assessment and documentation of the individual's severity of pain (0–10 scale), proper positioning of affected limbs, use of supports and braces (cervical collar, back brace, sling) to prevent additional stress on bones, and consultation with physical or occupational therapists. Effective pain control is possible in patients with multiple myeloma utilizing the WHO pain treatment ladder, a three-step treatment plan that has been widely used for the treatment of tumor pain.[197] The use of a clinical algorithm may also assist the nurse in identifying bone metastases and managing clinical sequelae, such as pain.[198] Pain management should incorporate nonpharmacological therapies such as aromatherapy, massage, heat, cold, relaxation, and immobilization as necessary.[199]

Mental status changes can be an initial sign of hypercalcemia, hyperviscosity syndrome, or drug toxicity. Any change in mental status requires careful assessment to determine its etiologic factors so that appropriate treatment can be promptly initiated. When hypercalcemia occurs, adequate intravenous hydration (3–6 L daily) is started immediately. Patients who are at risk of developing hypercalcemic crisis may require calcitonin for rapid reduction of calcium levels. The use of saline replenishment and bisphosphonates such as pamidronate or zoledronic acid has become the standard of treatment for hypercalcemia.[200,201] Corticosteroids, which are part of most chemotherapy regimens for the treatment of myeloma, inhibit bone resorption to some degree: they also exert an inhibitory effect on intestinal calcium absorption. They are often used as part of the combination therapy of hypercalcemia.[195] Plasmapheresis is indicated for hyperviscosity syndrome.[202] Effective tumor kill is necessary to correct both hypercalcemia and hyperviscosity. The nursing plan should include prevention of injury and maintenance of patient safety.

Psychosocial Issues

Depression, anxiety, and insomnia are but a few of the psychological responses that patients may exhibit in response to their disease and treatment.[203] Listening, cognitive restructuring, assisting with problem solving, giving information in small amounts, and expressing care and concern are among the strategies that oncology nurses can employ to assist patients in the adaptation to their cancer diagnosis. It is reasonable to experience and show genuine sadness about a patient's situation. Mood disturbances are more severe in patients with MM than in other cancers and objectively affect their quality of life.[196] Because MM is an incurable disease with a median survival of 3–5 years, it places a significant psychological burden on patients, especially the elderly. Oncology nurses play a vital role in ensuring that patients receive the optimal psychological support necessary to promote their well-being and overall quality of life. Information about support groups and multiple myeloma organizations is beneficial when patients and families desire it (Table 59-11). These organizations provide individual and group support, as well as written materials describing the disease and its treatment. Many of these organizations can be accessed via the Internet.

Protective Mechanisms

Infection, particularly of bacterial origin, is the leading cause of death in patients with multiple myeloma. Their susceptibility to infection stems mainly from granulocytopenia and deficiencies in humoral and/or cellular immunity. Guidelines for the care of neutropenic patients are principally aimed at the early recognition and prevention of infection. Prophylactic use of antibiotics during the first two months of induction chemotherapy was found to decrease the frequency and severity of bacterial infections significantly in a randomized clinical trial.[204] Routine use of hematopoietic colony-stimulating factors as an adjunct therapy for the treatment of uncomplicated fever and neutropenia is not generally recommended because it has little impact on disease-free and overall survival.[205] However, clinicians may use poor performance status and advanced form of cancer as risk factors when assessing patients prior to ordering hematopoietic growth factors for primary prophylaxis of febrile neutropenia after myelosupressive therapy.[205]

Blood product support will consist mainly of packed red blood cells and platelet transfusions. The clinical use of hematopoietic growth factors in the prevention of febrile neutropenia after myelosuppressive therapy, in the treatment of anemia in cancer patients receiving chemotherapy, in patients undergoing pe-

Table 59-11 Patient Education Support Services

Counseling and Support	Patient Resources
Bone Marrow Transplant Family Support Network P.O. Box 845 Avon, CT 06001 800-826-9376	American Cancer Society (ACS) 1599 Clifton Road, NE Atlanta, GA 30329-4251 404-329-7623 (patient services) 800-ACS-2345 *www.cancer.org*
Cancer Care, Inc. 275 Seventh Avenue New York, NY 10001 212-712-8354 *www.cancercare.org*	International Myeloma Foundation (IMF) 2129 Stanley Hills Drive Los Angeles, CA 90046 800-452-CURE *www.myeloma.org*
National Coalition for Cancer Survivorship (NCCS) 1010 Wayne Avenue, Suite 505 Silver Spring, MD 20910 301-650-8868	Leukemia Society of America (LSA) 600 Third Avenue New York, NY 10016 212-573-8484 800-955-4LSA *www.leukemia.org*
	Multiple Myeloma Research Foundation (MMRF) 3 Forest Street New Canaan, CT 06840 203-972-1250 *www.multiplemyeloma.org*

ripheral blood progenitor cell (PBPC) collection, and in patients receiving bone marrow or stem cell transplant, is now well established as supportive therapy in managing individuals with MM.[205–209]

The supportive care of cancer patients with anemia, thrombocytopenia, and neutropenia is well documented in the nursing literature. Guidelines for the care of patients with anemia, infection, and bleeding are provided in this book in Chapters 23, 28, and 29, respectively.

Respiratory Symptoms

The respiratory system is the most frequent site of infection in patients with MM. As a result, nursing care is directed toward teaching patients and their families about ways to decrease pooling of pulmonary secretions and increase gas exchange (e.g., coughing and deep breathing exercises, use of incentive spirometers, avoiding contact with individuals who show signs and symptoms of upper respiratory tract infection). Patient and family instructions — for example, immediate notification of the healthcare team when the patient develops fever, cough, sore throat, and sputum production — are important. Vaccination with live organisms is contraindicated in patients with MM due to their defective humoral immunity and exposure to others who may have received live organism vaccines should be avoided (i.e., children immunized with oral polio and measles/mumps/rubella vaccines).[210] All patients with MM, and in particular those older than age 65, should be immunized with a single dose of the 23-valent pneumococcal vaccine.[211]

Gastrointestinal Symptoms

Constipation is a problem experienced by many patients with MM, especially the elderly. It usually results from decreased activity or lack of exercise due to bone pain/pathologic fractures, dehydration, opioids analgesic use, spinal cord compression, or use of vinca alkaloids. Although not a life-threatening problem, constipation can influence nutritional intake, comfort, and quality of life.[212] Nursing management includes assessment of past and present bowel habits, increasing dietary fiber, adequate hydration, use of a stool softener, judicious use of mild laxatives, encouraging the patient to increase his or her physical activity, facilitating home-based exercise therapy,[213] and patient and family education.

Genitourinary Symptoms

Renal insufficiency can be exacerbated as a result of the primary disease, fluid and electrolyte abnormalities (hyperuricemia, hypercalcemia), dehydration, or infection that could lead to renal failure. The NSAIDs frequently employed in the treatment of bone pain have been associated with the development of acute renal failure in patients with multiple myeloma.[214,215] Amphotericin B and acyclovir can also be nephrotoxic and should be used cautiously or avoided in patients with MM unless no other alternatives are available.[214,216,217] When acute renal failure occurs, nursing care is directed toward reversing renal insufficiency. Prevention and immediate intervention in case of known reversible causes such infection, dehydration, hypercalcemia, hyperuricemia, and use of nephrotoxic drugs should be one of the goals of care. Patients require close monitoring for early signs and symptoms of urinary tract infection (e.g., fever, dysuria, frequency, urgency). Patient and family education directed toward recognition of these signs and symptoms is important, and prompt reporting of such events to the healthcare team is crucial.

Conclusion

New treatments have recently been developed that target the MM cell, the MM cell–host interaction, and the bone marrow microenvironment to overcome drug resistance and have shown clinical activity in patients with multiple myeloma. These include trisenox oxide and immunomodulatory drugs (IMiDs), such as Revimid (CC5013), Actimid (CC-4047), and ENMD 099. Better understanding of the biology of myeloma cells and the bone marrow microenvironment has led to the development of these novel agents. Numerous clinical trials are under way to identify their exact roles in the management of patients with MM.

Two sequential autologous transplants (tandem transplantation) have been used in an attempt to improve response rates and survival in patients with MM. Insufficient evidence exists to support this practice, as the only study showing a benefit from two transplants over one transplant was handicapped by the use of a conditioning regimen known to be associated with inferior outcomes. Tandem ASCT is recommended to those patients who have responded to the first ASCT but are not in CR or near-CR.[218] For those patients with high-risk features defined by chromosomal abnormalities (usually involving chromosomes 11 and 13) and high β_2M levels, novel therapies should be offered as an option during induction therapy.

Despite its curative potential, allogeneic transplantation had been used sparingly in MM until recently because of poor results.[219] The factors responsible for the poor outcomes are related to the underlying disease, the patient's condition, and the treatment regimen, including supportive therapy: advanced Durie-Salmon stage, extensive prior therapy, high β_2M, high LDH, long diagnosis–transplant interval, low albumin, prior autograft, refractory disease, and renal dysfunction. It is also believed that poor patient selection (e.g., including patients with poor performance status and terminal disease) has contributed to the poor results.[219] The role of nonmyeloablative transplantation is currently being investigated in MM management because of its lower mortality rate and possible therapeutic benefit.

Several other biologically based therapeutic agents are currently under preclinical and clinical investigation for MM. These include NF-κB inhibitor (PS-1145), 2-methoxyestradiol (2ME2), tyrosine kinase inhibitor (PTK787), histone deacetylase inhibitor (NVP-LAQ824), farnesyl transferase inhibitor (R115777), and osteoprotegerin (OPG).[220–229]

The last decade has witnessed dramatic improvements in the overall response rates for patients with MM. Therapeutic options have increased, patient outcomes have improved, and further insight has been gained into the biology and genetics of MM.[5] ASCT using high-dose melphalan as a conditioning regimen is now considered standard therapy for myeloma, at least for younger patients.[5,132,230] Evidenced-based guidelines that address the initial work-up, ongoing surveillance, and supportive care of patients with MM have been established by NCCN and could guide clinical practice, clinical trials, and areas for future nursing research.[50]

We are also witnessing increasing utilization of new technologies and biologically based novel therapeutics.[220] The use of tumor- and host-directed nongenocidal therapies (i.e., glucocorticoids, bisphosphonates, anti-IL-6, proteasome inhibitors, immunomodulatory agents) may be important adjuncts in effecting a traditional cure or a return to a chronic benign state akin to MGUS or smoldering myeloma.[5] The role of immunotherapy in MM remains under investigation, and it is hoped that future strategies will further improve overall survival of patients with MM.[231,232] Systematic application of cytogenetics and molecular genetics, especially gene expression profiling, may soon aid in a molecular classification of MM.[4,233,234]

The nursing care of patients with MM and their families offers the nurse an opportunity to interact with patients who are experiencing both acute and chronic sequelae of the disease. Nursing care can have a direct effect by ensuring early recognition of complications and management of treatment-related toxicity. Patient and family education regarding the disease, conventional and novel treatment, and early recognition of signs and symptoms of complications can contribute to an overall improvement in quality of life. Nurses play important roles not only as direct caregivers, but also as patient advocates and educators. It is imperative that they keep abreast of the recent changes and advances related to multiple myeloma. Promising areas for nursing research include clinical demonstration projects that produce evidence that specific nursing interventions enhance patients' quality of life and event-free and overall survival.[235]

References

1. Tariman JD: Understanding novel therapeutic agents for multiple myeloma. *Clin J Oncol Nurs* 7:521–528, 2003
2. Richardson P, Jagannath S, Schlossman RL, et al: A multi-center, randomized, phase II study to evaluate the efficacy and safety of two CDC-5013 dose regimens when used alone or in combination with dexamethasone for the treatment of relapsed or refractory multiple myeloma. *Blood* 100:104a, 2002 (abstr)
3. Anderson KC, Shaughnessy JDJ, Barlogie B, et al: Multiple myeloma. *Hematology* (Am Soc Hematol Educ Prog) 1:214–240, 2002
4. Claudio JO, Masih-Khan E, Stewart AK: Insights from the gene expression profiling of multiple myeloma. *Curr Hematol Report* 3:67–73, 2004
5. Barlogie B, Shaughnessy J, Tricot G, et al: Treatment of multiple myeloma. *Blood* 103:20–32, 2004
6. Anderson KC: Moving disease biology from lab to the clinic. *Cancer* 97(suppl 3):796–801, 2003
7. Jemal A, Tiwari RC, Murray T, et al: Cancer statistics, 2004. *CA Cancer J Clin* 54:8–29, 2004
8. Sjak-Shie NN, Vescio RA, Berenson JR: Recent advances in multiple myeloma. *Cur Opin Hematol* 7:241–246, 2000
9. Kyle RA, Gertz MA, Witzig TE, et al: Review of 1027 patients with newly diagnosed multiple myeloma. *Mayo Clin Proc* 78:21–33, 2003
10. Anderson KC: Multiple myeloma: How far have we come? *Mayo Clinic Proc* 78:15–17, 2003
11. Baris D, Brown LM, Silverman DT, et al: Socioeconomic status and multiple myeloma among US blacks and whites. *Am J Public Health* 90:1277–1281, 2000
12. Munshi N, Desikan K, Barlogie B: Clinical experience with thalidomide in multiple myeloma: phase II trials in refractory disease and ongoing studies. *Semin Hematol* 37(suppl 3):15–21, 2000
13. Rettig MB, Ma HJ, Vescio RA, et al: Kaposi's sarcoma–associated herpes virus infection of bone marrow dendritic cells from multiple myeloma patients. *Science* 276:1851–1854, 1997
14. Tarte K, Klein B: The role of viruses in the pathogenesis of plasma cell disorders, in Mehta J, Singhal S (eds.): *Myeloma.* London, Martin-Dunitz, 2002, pp 39–51
15. Yee TT, Murphy K, Johnson M, et al: Multiple myeloma and human immunodeficiency virus-1 (HIV-1) infection. *Am J Hematol* 66:123–125, 2001
16. Pantanowitz L, Dezube BJ: Editorial comment: multiple myeloma and HIV infection — causal or casual coincidence? [comment]. *AIDS Reader* 13:386–387, 2003
17. Grulich AE, Li Y, McDonald A, et al: Rates of non-AIDS-defining cancers in people with HIV infection before and after AIDS diagnosis. *AIDS* 16:1155–1161, 2002
18. Morgan GJ, Davies FE, Linet M: Myeloma aetiology and epidemiology. *Biomed Pharmacother* 56:223–234, 2002
19. Joshua DE, Gibson J: Epidemiology of plasma cell disorders, in Mehta J, Singhal S (eds.): *Myeloma.* London, Martin Dunitz, 2002, pp 139–150
20. Kyle RA, Therneau TM, Rajkumar SV, et al: A long-term study of prognosis in monoclonal gammopathy of undetermined significance. *N Engl J Med* 346:564–569, 2002
21. Lee WJ, Hoppin JA, Blair A, et al: Cancer incidence among pesticide applicators exposed to alachlor in the Agricultural Health Study. *Am J Epidemiol* 159:373–380, 2004
22. Lee WJ, Baris D, Jarvholm B, et al: Multiple myeloma and diesel and other occupational exposures in Swedish construction workers. *Int J Cancer* 107:134–138, 2003
23. Fritschi L, Siemiatycki J: Lymphoma, myeloma and occupation: results of a case-control study. *Int J Cancer* 67:498–503, 1996
24. Costantini AS, Miligi L, Kriebel D, et al: A multicenter case-control study in Italy on hematolymphopoietic neoplasms and occupation. *Epidemiology* 12:78–87, 2001
25. Lundberg I, Milatou-Smith R: Mortality and cancer incidence among Swedish paint industry workers with long-term exposure to organic solvents. *Scand J Work Environ Health* 24:270–275, 1998
26. Mikoczy Z, Schutz A, Hagmar L: Cancer incidence and mortality among Swedish leather tanners. *Occup Environ Med* 51:530–535, 1994
27. Miligi L, Seniori Costantini A, Crosignani P, et al: Occupational, environmental, and life-style factors associated with the risk of hematolymphopoietic malignancies in women. *Am J Ind Med* 36:60–69, 1999
28. Speer SA, Semenza JC, Kurosaki T, et al: Risk factors for acute myeloid leukemia and multiple myeloma: a combination of GIS and case-control studies. *J Environ Health* 64:9–16, 2002
29. Satin KP, Bailey WJ, Newton KL, et al: Updated epidemiological study of workers at two California petroleum refineries, 1950–95. *Occup Environ Med* 59:248–256, 2002
30. Raffn E, Lynge E, Juel K, et al: Incidence of cancer and mortality among employees in the asbestos cement industry in Denmark. *Br J Industrial Med* 46:90–96, 1989
31. Hatcher JL, Baris D, Olshan AF, et al: Diagnostic radiation and the risk of multiple myeloma (United States). *Cancer Causes Control* 12:755–761, 2001
32. Sonoda T, Nagata Y, Mori M, et al: Meta-analysis of multiple myeloma and benzene exposure. *J Epidemiol* 11:249–254, 2001
33. Hemminki K, Li X, Czene K: Familial risk of cancer: data for clinical counseling and cancer genetics. *Int J Cancer* 108:109–114, 2004
34. Lynch HT, Sanger WG, Pirruccello S, et al: Familial multiple myeloma: a family study and review of the literature.[see comment]. *J Natl Cancer Inst* 93:1479–1483, 2001
35. Kyle RA: Diagnosis and treatment of multiple myeloma in the elderly. *Clin Geriat* 10:47–56, 2002
36. Saez B, Martin-Subero JI, Guillen-Grima F, et al: Chromosomal abnormalities clustering in multiple myeloma reveals cytogenetic subgroups with nonrandom acquisition of chromosomal changes. *Leukemia* 18:654–657, 2004
37. Seidl S, Kaufman H, Drach J: New insights into the pathophysiology of multiple myeloma. *Lancet Oncol* 4:557–564, 2003
38. Debes-Marun CS, Dewald GW, Bryant S, et al: Chromosome abnormalities clustering and its implications for pathogenesis and prognosis in myeloma. *Leukemia* 17:427–436, 2003
39. Avet-Loiseau H, Facon T, Grosbois J, et al: Oncogenesis of multiple myeloma: 14q32 and 13q chromosomal abnormalities are not randomly distributed, but correlate with natural history, immunological features, and clinical presentation. *Blood* 99:2185–2191, 2003

40. Kastrinakis NG, Gorgoulis VG, Foukas PG, et al: Molecular aspects of multiple myeloma. *Ann Oncol* 11:1217–1228, 2000
41. Avet-Loiseau H, Li JY, Facon T, et al: High incidence of translocations t(11;14)(q13;q32) and t(4;14)(p16;q32) in patients with plasma cell malignancies. *Cancer Res* 58:5640–5645, 1998
42. Pope B, Brown R, Luo XF, et al: Disease progression in patients with multiple myeloma is associated with a concurrent alteration in the expression of both oncogenes and tumor suppressor genes and can be monitored by the onco-protein phenotype. *Leuk Lymphoma* 25:545–554, 1997
43. Elnenaei MO, Gruszka-Westwood AM, A'Hernt R, et al: Gene abnormalities in multiple myeloma: the relevance of TP53, MDM2, and CDKN2A. *Haematologica* 88:529–537, 2003
44. Elnenaei MO, Hamoudi RA, Swansbury J, et al: Delineation of the minimal region of loss at 13q14 in multiple myeloma. *Genes Chromosomes Cancer* 36:99–106, 2003
45. Rudin CM, Thompson CB: B-cell development and maturation. *Semin Oncol* 25:435–446, 1998
46. Rajkumar SV, Greipp PR: Plasma cells and immunoglobulins, in Mehta J, Singhal S (eds.): *Myeloma*. London, Martin Dunitz, 2002, pp 3–23
47. Varterasian ML: Biologic and clinical advances in multiple myeloma. *Oncology* 9:417–424, 1995
48. Kyle RA, Lust JA: Immunoglobulins and laboratory recognition of monoclonal proteins, in Kyle RA (ed.): *Neoplastic Diseases of the Blood*. New York, Churchill Livingstone, 1996, pp 453–475
49. Lokhorst H: Clinical features and diagnostic criteria, in Mehta J, Singhal S (eds.): *Myeloma*. London, Martin Dunitz, 2002, pp 151–168
50. National Comprehensive Cancer Network (NCCN): NCCN 2003 multiple myeloma clinical practice guidelines in oncology, in: *The Complete Library of NCCN Clinical Practice Guidelines in Oncology* [CD-ROM]. Rockledge, PA, NCCN, 2004
51. Raje N, Anderson KC: Cytokine abnormalities in plasma cell disorders, in Mehta J, Singhal S (eds.): *Myeloma*. London, Martin Dunitz, 2002, pp 54–64
52. Hideshima T, Nakamura N, Chauhan D, et al: Biologic sequelae of interleukin-6 induced P13–K/Akt signaling in multiple myeloma. *Oncogene* 20:5991–6000, 2001
53. Zhang XG, Klein B, Bataille R: Interleukin 6 is a potent myeloma cell growth factor in patients with aggressive multiple myeloma. *Blood* 74:11–13, 1989
54. Chauhan D, Uchiyama H, Akbarali Y, et al: Multiple myeloma cell adhesion-induced interleukin-6 expression in bone marrow stromal cells involves activation of NF-κB. *Blood* 87:1104–1112, 1996
55. Dankbar B, Padro T, Mesters RM, et al: VEGF is expressed by myeloma cells and stimulates IL-6 secretion by microvascular endothelial and marrow stromal cells. *Blood* 92(suppl 1):681a, 1998
56. Lauta VM: A review of the cytokine network in multiple myeloma: diagnostic, prognostic, and therapeutic implications. *Cancer* 97:2440–2452, 2003
57. Abe M, Hiura K, Wilde J, et al: Role for macrophage inflammatory protein (MIP)-1alpha and MIP-1beta in the development of osteolytic lesions in multiple myeloma. *Blood* 100:2195–2202, 2002
58. Tai YT, Podar K, Catley L, et al: Insulin-like growth factor-1 induces adhesion and migration in human multiple myeloma cells via activation of beta1–integrin and phosphatidylinositol 3′-kinase/AKT signaling. *Cancer Res* 63:5850–5858, 2003
59. Mitsiades CS, Mitsiades N, Poulaki V, et al: Activation of NF-kappaB and upregulation of intracellular anti-apoptotic proteins via the IGF-1/Akt signaling in human multiple myeloma cells: therapeutic implications. *Oncogene* 21:5673–5683, 2002
60. Qiang Y-W, Yao L, Tosato G, et al: Insulin-like growth factor I induces migration and invasion of human multiple myeloma cells. *Blood* 103:301–308, 2004
61. Hideshima T, Chauhan D, Schlossman R, et al: The role of tumor necrosis factor alpha in the pathophysiology of human multiple myeloma: therapeutic applications. *Oncogene* 20:4519–4527, 2001
62. Podar K, Tai YT, Davies FE, et al: Vascular endothelial growth factor triggers signaling cascades mediating multiple myeloma cell growth and migration. *Blood* 98:428–435, 2001
63. Arora T, Jelinek DF: Differential myeloma cell responsiveness to interferon-alpha correlates with differential induction of p19INK4D and cyclin D2 expression. *J Biol Chem* 273:11799–11805, 1998
64. Klein B, Tarte K, Jourdan M, et al: Survival and proliferation factors of normal and malignant plasma cells. *Int J Hematol* 78:106–113, 2003
65. Otsuki T, Yata K, Sakaguchi H, et al: IL-10 in myeloma cells. *Leuk Lymphoma* 43:969–974, 2002
66. Blade J: Criteria for disease progression. *Br J Haematol* 102:1115–1123, 1998
67. Berenson JR: Bone disease in myeloma, in Mehta J, Singhal S (eds.): *Myeloma*. London, Martin Dunitz, 2002, pp 97–117
68. Berenson JR: Advances in the biology and treatment of myeloma bone disease. *Semin Oncol* 29(suppl 6):11–16, 2002
69. Tian E, Zhan F, Walker R, et al: The role of the Wnt-signaling antagonist DKK1 in the development of osteolytic lesions in multiple myeloma. *N Engl J Med* 349:2483–2494, 2003
70. Woolfenden JM, Pitt MJ, Durie BGM, et al: Comparison of bone scintigraphy and radiography in multiple myeloma. *Radiology* 134:723–728, 1980
71. Angtuaco EJ, Moulopoulos A, Hronas T, et al: Imaging studies, in Mehta J, Singhal S (eds.): *Myeloma*. London, Martin Dunitz, 2002, pp 297–309
72. Tariman JD: Clinical applications of magnetic resonance imaging (MRI) in patients with multiple myeloma. *Clin J Oncol Nurs* 8:317-318, 2004
73. Kelleher P, Chapel H: Infections: principles of prevention and therapy, in Mehta J, Singhal S (eds.): *Myeloma*. London, Martin Dunitz, 2002, pp 223–239
74. Savage DG, Lindenbaum J, Garrett TJ: Biphasic pattern of bacterial infection in multiple myeloma. *Ann Intern Med* 96:47–50, 1982
75. Silvestris F, Tucci M, Quatraro C, et al: Recent advances in understanding the pathogenesis of anemia in multiple myeloma. *Int J Hematol* 78:121–125, 2003
76. San Miguel JF, Almeida J, Orfao A: Laboratory investigations, in Mehta J, Singhal S (eds.): *Myeloma*. London, Martin Dunitz, 2002, pp 243–268
77. Pandit SR, Vesole DH: Management of renal dysfunction in multiple myeloma. *Curr Treat Options Oncol* 4:239–246, 2003
78. Shaver-Lewis MJ, Shah SV: The kidney in plasma cell disorders, in Mehta J, Singhal S (eds.): *Myeloma*. London, Martin Dunitz, 2002, pp 203–221
79. Chim CS, Li FK, Chan KW: Cast nephropathy in multiple myeloma. *Haematologica* 89:EIM08, 2004
80. Messiaen T, Deret S, Mougenot B, et al: Adult Fanconi syndrome secondary to light chain gammopathy. Clinicopathologic heterogeneity and unusual features in 11 patients. *Medicine (Baltimore)* 79:135–154, 2000
81. Pozzi C, D'Amico M, Fogazzi GB, et al: Light chain deposition disease with renal involvement: clinical characteristics and prognostic factors. *Am J Kidney Dis* 42:1154–1163, 2003
82. Sinclair D: IgD myeloma: clinical, biological and laboratory features. *Clin Lab* 48:617–622, 2002

83. Mollee PN, Wechalekar AD, Pereira DL, et al: Autologous stem cell transplantation in primary systemic amyloidosis: the impact of selection criteria on outcome. *Bone Marrow Transpl* 33:271–277, 2004
84. Baumal R, Scharff MD: Synthesis, assembly and secretion of mouse immunoglobulin. *Transplant Rev* 14:163–183, 1973
85. Guo X, Nzerue C: How to prevent, recognize, and treat drug-induced nephrotoxicity. *Cleve Clin J Med* 69:289–290, 293–294, 296–297, 2002
86. Perazella MA: Drug-induced renal failure: update on new medications and unique mechanisms of nephrotoxicity. *Am J Med Sci* 325:349–362, 2003
87. Fuente N, Mane JM, Barcelo R, et al: Tumor lysis syndrome in a multiple myeloma treated with thalidomide. *Ann Oncol* 15:537, 2004
88. Mehta J, Singhal S: Hyperviscosity syndrome in plasma cell dyscrasias. *Semin Thromb Hemost* 29:467–471, 2003
89. Yeshurun M, Laporte JP, Lesage S, et al: Spinal cord compression of dual etiology, multiple myeloma and spinal tuberculosis. *Leuk Lymphoma* 43:427–428, 2002
90. Gorson KC, Ropper AH: Neuropathy in plasma cell disorders, in Mehta J, Singhal S (eds.): *Myeloma*. London, Martin Dunitz, 2002, pp 185–201
91. Kelly JJJ, Kyle RA, Miles JM, et al: The spectrum of peripheral neuropathy in myeloma. *Neurology* 31:24–31, 1981
92. Marrs J, Newton S: Updating your peripheral neuropathy "know-how." *Clin J Oncol Nurs* 7:299–303, 2003
93. Tariman JD: Thalidomide: current therapeutic uses and management of its toxicities. *Clin J Oncol Nurs* 7:143–147, 2003
94. Tariman JD, Lemoine C: Bortezomib. *Clin J Oncol Nurs* 7:687–689, 2003
95. Harousseau JL, Moreau P: Prognostic factors in myeloma, in Mehta J, Singhal S (eds.): *Myeloma*. London, Martin Dunitz, 2002, pp 169–183
96. Blade J, Rozman C, Cervantes F, et al: A new prognostic system for multiple myeloma based on easily available parameters. *Br J Haematol* 72:507–511, 1989
97. Witzig TE, Gertz MA, Lust JA, et al: Peripheral blood monoclonal plasma cells as a predictor of survival of patients with multiple myeloma. *Blood* 88:1780–1787, 1996
98. San Miguel JF, Garcia-Sanz R, Gonzalez M, et al: A new staging system for multiple myeloma based on the number of S-phase plasma cells. *Blood* 85:448–455, 1995
99. Lai JL, Zandecki M, Mary JY, et al: Improved cytogenetics in multiple myeloma: a study of 151 patients including 117 patients at diagnosis. *Blood* 85:2490–2497, 1995
100. Perez-Simon JA, Garcia-Sanz R, Tabernero MD, et al: Prognostic value of numerical chromosome observation in multiple myeloma: a FISH analysis of 15 different chromosomes. *Blood* 91:3366–3371, 1998
101. Drach J, Ackerman J, Fritz E, et al: Presence of a p53 gene deletion in patients with multiple myeloma predicts for short survival after conventional-dose chemotherapy. *Blood* 92:802–809, 1998
102. Bataille R, Durie BG, Grenier J, et al: Prognostic factors and staging in multiple myeloma: a reappraisal. *J Clin Oncol* 4:80–87, 1986
103. Durie BG, Salmon SE: A clinical staging system for multiple myeloma: correlation of measured myeloma cell mass with presenting clinical features, response to treatment and survival. *Cancer* 36:842–854, 1975
104. Durie BG, Salmon SE, Moon TE: Pretreatment tumor mass cell kinetics and prognosis in multiple myeloma. *Blood* 55:364–372, 1980
105. Jacobson JL, Hussein MA, Barlogie B, et al: Southwest Oncology Group. A new staging system for multiple myeloma patients based on the Southwest Oncology Group (SWOG) experience. *Br J Haematol* 122:441–450, 2003
106. He Y, Wheatley K, Clark O, et al: Early versus deferred treatment for early stage multiple myeloma. *Cochrane Database Syst Rev* 1:CD004023, 2003
107. Zomas A, Dimopoulos MA: Conventional treatment of myeloma, in Mehta J, Singhal S (eds.): *Myeloma*. London, Martin Dunitz, 2002, pp 313–326
108. Anderson KC, Hamblin TJ, Traynor A: Management of multiple myeloma today. *Semin Hematol* 36:3–8, 1999
109. Rajkumar SV, Gertz MA, Kyle RA, et al: Current therapy for multiple myeloma. *Mayo Clin Proc* 77:813–822, 2002
110. Hjorth M, Holmberg E, Rodjer S, et al: Survival in conventionally treated younger (<60 years) multiple myeloma patients: no improvement during two decades. Nordic Myeloma Study Group (NMSG). *Eur J Haematol* 62:271–277, 1999
111. Myeloma Trialists' Collaborative Group: Combination chemotherapy versus melphalan plus prednisone as treatment for multiple myeloma: an overview of 6633 patients from 27 randomized trials. *J Clin Oncol* 16:3832–3842, 1998
112. Gregory WM, Richards MA, Malas JS: Combination chemotherapy versus melphalan and prednisone in the treatment of multiple myeloma: an overview of published trials. *J Clin Oncol* 10:334–342, 1992
113. Sonneveld P, Segeren CM: Changing concepts in multiple myeloma: from conventional to high-dose treatment. *Euro J Cancer* 39:9–18, 2003
114. Bataille R, Harousseau JL: Multiple myeloma. *N Engl J Med* 336:1657–1664, 1997
115. Albert DS, Chang SY, Chen HS, et al: Oral melphalan kinetics. *Clin Pharmacol Ther* 26:737–745, 1979
116. Palmer M, Belch A, Hanson J, et al: Dose intensity analysis of melphalan and prednisone in multiple myeloma. *J Natl Cancer Inst* 80:414–418, 1988
117. Samson D, Gaminara E, Newland A, et al: Infusion of vincristine and doxorubicin with oral dexamethasone as first-line therapy for multiple myeloma. *Lancet* 2:882–885, 1989
118. Alexanian R, Barlogie B, Tucker S: VAD-based regimens as primary treatment for multiple myeloma. *Am J Hematol* 33:86–89, 1990
119. Monconduit M, Menard JF, Michaux JL, et al: VAD or VMBCP in severe multiple myeloma: The Groupe d'Etudes et de Recherche sur le Myelome (GERM). *Br J Haematol* 80:199–204, 1992
120. Dimopoulos MA, Palumbo A, Delasalle KB, et al: Primary plasma cell leukemia. *Br J Haematol* 88:754–759, 1994
121. Gautier M, Cohen MJ: Multiple myeloma in the elderly. *J Am Geriatr Soc* 42:653–664, 1994
122. Hussein M: Pegylated liposomal doxorubicin, vincristine, and reduced-dose dexamethasone as first-line therapy for multiple myeloma. *Clin Lymphoma* 4 (Suppl 1):S18–S22, 2003
123. Alexanian R, Dimopoulos MA, Delasalle K, et al: Primary dexamethasone treatment of multiple myeloma. *Blood* 80:887–890, 1992
124. Mellstedt H, Aahre A, Bjorkholm M, et al: Interferon therapy in myelomatosis. *Lancet* 2:697, 1979
125. Quesada JR, Alexanian R, Hawkins M, et al: Treatment of multiple myeloma with recombinant alpha-interferon. *Blood* 67:275–278, 1986
126. Sirohi B, Treleaven J, Powles R: Role of interferon, in Mehta J, Singhal S (eds.): *Myeloma*. London, Martin Dunitz, 2002, pp 383–396
127. Wheatley K: A meta-analysis of trials of interferon as therapy for myeloma. Abstract book of the VIIth International Multiple Myeloma Workshop 973, 1999

128. Singhal S: High-dose therapy and autologous transplantation, in Mehta J, Singhal S (eds.): *Myeloma*. London, Martin Dunitz, 2002, pp 327–347
129. Kumar A, Loughran T, Alsina M, et al: Management of multiple myeloma: a systematic review and critical appraisal of published studies. *Lancet Oncol* 4:293–304, 2003
130. Fermand JP, Ravaud P, Chevret S, et al: High-dose therapy and autologous peripheral blood stem cell transplantation in multiple myeloma: upfront or rescue treatment? Results of a multicenter sequential randomized clinical trial. *Blood* 92:3131–3136, 1998
131. Raje N, Powles R, Kulkarni S, et al: A comparison of vincristine and doxorubicin infusional chemotherapy with methylprednisolone (VAMP) with the addition of weekly cyclophosphamide (C-VAMP) as induction treatment followed by autografting in previously untreated myeloma. *Br J Haematol* 97:153–160, 1997
132. Attal M, Harousseau JL, Stoppa AM, et al: A prospective randomized trial of autologous bone marrow transplantation and chemotherapy in multiple myeloma. Intergroupe Francais du Myelome. *N Engl J Med* 335:91–97, 1996
133. Lee CK, Barlogie B, Munshi N, et al: DTPACE: an effective, novel combination chemotherapy with thalidomide for previously treated patients with myeloma. *J Clin Oncol* 21:2732–2739, 2003
134. Rajkumar SV, Hayman S, Gertz MA, et al: Combination therapy with thalidomide plus dexamethasone for newly diagnosed myeloma. *J Clin Oncol* 20:4319–4323, 2002
135. Weber D, Rankin K, Gavino M, et al: Thalidomide alone or with dexamethasone for previously untreated multiple myeloma. *J Clin Oncol* 21:16–19, 2003
136. Osman K, Frank R, von Hassel M, et al: Thalidomide, Adriamycin, and dexamethasone as initial therapy in patients with multiple myeloma [abstract #P227]. VIIIth International Myeloma Workshop, Banff, Canada, 2001
137. Morris CL, Siegel E, Barlogie B, et al: Mobilization of CD34+ cells in elderly (>/= 70 years) with multiple myeloma: influence of age, prior therapy, platelet count and mobilization regimen. *B J Haematol* 120:413–423, 2003
138. Barlogie B, Jagannath S, Vesole D, et al: Superiority of tandem transplantation over standard therapy for previously untreated multiple myeloma. *Blood* 89:789–793, 1997
139. Vescio R, Schiller G, Stewart AK, et al: Multicenter phase III trial to evaluate CD34(+) selected versus unselected autologous peripheral blood progenitor cell transplantation in multiple myeloma. *Blood* 93:1858–1868, 1999
140. Badros A, Barlogie B, Siegel E, et al: Autologous stem cell transplantation in elderly multiple myeloma patients over the age of 70 years. *Br J Haematol* 114:600–607, 2001
141. Siegel DS, Desikan KR, Mehta J, et al: Age is not a prognostic variable with autotransplants in multiple myeloma. *Blood* 93:51–54, 1999
142. Terpos E, Apperley JF, Samson D, et al: Autologous stem cell transplantation in multiple myeloma: improved survival in nonsecretory multiple myeloma but lack of influence of age, status at transplant, previous treatment and conditioning regimen. A single center experience in 127 patients. *Bone Marrow Transplant* 31:163–170, 2003
143. Magagnoli M, Castagna L, Balzarotti M, et al: Feasibility and toxicity of high-dose therapy (HDT) supported by peripheral blood stem cells in elderly patients with multiple myeloma and non-Hodgkin's lymphoma: survey from a single institution. *Am J Hematol* 73:267–272, 2003
144. Badros A, Barlogie B, Siegel E, et al: Results of autologous stem cell transplant in multiple myeloma patients with renal failure. *B J Haematol* 114:822–829, 2001
145. Sirohi B, Powles R, Mehta J, et al: The implication of compromised renal function at presentation in myeloma: similar outcome in patients who receive high-dose therapy: a single-center study of 251 previously untreated patients. *Med Oncol* 18:39–50, 2001
146. Singhal S, Powles R, Sirohi B, et al: Response to induction chemotherapy is not essential to obtain survival benefit from high-dose melphalan and autotransplantation in myeloma. *Bone Marrow Transplant* 30:673–679, 2002
147. Govindarajan R, Jagannath S, Flick JT, et al: Preceding standard therapy is the likely cause of MDS after autotransplant for multiple myeloma. *B J Haematol* 95:349–353, 1996
148. Saso R, Kulkarni S, Powles R, et al: Secondary MDS/AML in patients treated for myeloma. *Blood* 92(suppl 1):455a, 1998
149. Drach J, Ayers D, Govindarajan R, et al: MDS-associated cytogenetic abnormalities (CGA) in both hematopoietic and neoplastic cells after autotransplants (AT) in 868 patients with multiple myeloma (MM). *Blood* 92(suppl 1):97a, 1998
150. Berenson JR, Crowley JJ, Grogan TM, et al: Maintenance therapy with alternate-day prednisone improves survival in multiple myeloma patients. *Blood* 99:163–168, 2002
151. Santos ES, Goodman M, Byrnes JJ, et al: Thalidomide effects in the post-transplantation setting in patients with multiple myeloma. *Hematology* 9:35–39, 2004
152. Kyle RA: Multiple myeloma, macroglobulinemia, and the monoclonal gammopathies. *Cur Pract Med* 2:1131–1137, 1999
153. Samson D: Criteria for evaluating disease response and progression in patients with multiple myeloma treated by high-dose therapy and hematopoietic stem cell transplantation. *Br J Haematol* 102:1115–1123, 1998
154. Munshi NC, Tricot G, Barlogie B: Plasma cell neoplasms, in DeVita VT, Hellman S, Rosenberg SA (eds.): *Principles and Practice of Oncology* (ed 6). Philadelphia, Lippincott-Raven, 2001, pp 2465–2493
155. Singhal S, Mehta J: Treatment of relapsed and refractory multiple myeloma. *Curr Treat Opts Oncol* 4:229–237, 2003
156. Zaidi AA, Vesole DH: Multiple myeloma: an old disease with new hope for the future. *CA Cancer J Clin* 51:273–285, 2001
157. Adams J: The proteasome: structure, function, and role in the cell. *Cancer Treat Rev* 29(suppl 1):3–9, 2003
158. Adams J: Potential for proteasome inhibition in the treatment of cancer. *Drug Discovery Today* 8:307–315, 2003
159. Richardson P, Barlogie B, Berenson J, et al: A phase 2 study of the proteasome inhibitor bortezomib in relapsed, refractory myeloma. *N Engl J Med* 348:2609–2617, 2003
160. Millennium Pharmaceuticals Inc. Bortezomib (Velcade) for injection. Data on file. Cambridge, MA, Millennium Pharmaceuticals, Inc., 2003.
161. Colson K, Doss DS, Swift R, et al: Bortezomib, a newly approved proteasome inhibitor for the treatment of multiple myeloma: nursing implications. *Clin J Oncol Nurs* 8:473–480, 2004.
162. Shrieve DC: The role of radiotherapy, in Mehta J, Singhal S (eds.): *Myeloma*. London, Martin Dunitz, 2002, pp 367–381
163. Bolek TW, Marcus RB, Mendenhall NP: Solitary plasmacytoma of bone and soft tissue. *Int J Radiat Oncol Biol Phys* 36:329–333, 1996
164. Liebross RH, Ha CS, Cox JD, et al: Solitary plasmacytoma: outcome and prognostic factors following radiotherapy. *Int J Radiat Oncol Biol Phys* 41:1063–1067, 1998
165. Singer CR, Tobias JS, Giles F, et al: Hemibody irradiation. An effective second-line therapy in drug-resistance multiple myeloma. *Cancer* 63:2446–2451, 1989
166. Berenson JR, Hillner BE, Kyle RA, et al: American Society of Clinical Oncology clinical practice guidelines: the role of bisphosphonates in multiple myeloma. *J Clin Oncol* 20:3719–3736, 2002

167. Berenson JR, Lichtenstein A, Porter L, et al: Efficacy of pamidronate in reducing skeletal events in patients with advanced multiple myeloma. *N Engl J Med* 334:488–493, 1996
168. Ali SM, Esteva FJ, Hortobagyi G, et al: Safety and efficacy of bisphosphonates beyond 24 months in cancer patients. *J Clin Oncol* 19:3434–3437, 2001
169. Terpos E, Viniou N, de la Fuente J, et al: Pamidronate is superior to ibandronate in decreasing bone resorption, interleukin-6 and beta 2–microglobulin in multiple myeloma. *Eur J Haematol* 70:34–42, 2003
170. Major P, Lortholary A, Hon J, et al: Zoledronic acid is superior to pamidronate in the treatment of hypercalcemia of malignancy: a pooled analysis of two randomized, controlled clinical trials. *J Clin Oncol* 19:558–567, 2001
171. Derenne S, Amiot M, Barille S, et al: Zolendronate is a potential inhibitor of myeloma cell growth and secretion of IL-6 and MMP-1 by the tumoral environment. *J Bone Mineral Res* 14:2048–2056, 1999
172. Skerjanec A, Berenson J, Hsu C, et al: The pharmacokinetics and pharmacodynamics of zoledronic acid in cancer patients with varying degrees of renal function. *J Clin Pharmacol* 43:154–162, 2003
173. Body JJ: Zoledronic acid: an advance in tumour bone disease therapy and a new hope for osteoporosis. *Exp Opin Pharmacother* 4:567–580, 2003
174. Rosen LS, Gordon D, Kaminsky M, et al J: Long-term efficacy and safety of zoledronic acid compared with pamidronate disodium in the treatment of skeletal complications in patients with advanced multiple myeloma or breast carcinoma: a randomized, double blind, multicenter, comparative trial. *Cancer* 98:1735–1744, 2003
175. Maxwell C, Swift R, Goode M, et al: Advances in supportive care of patients with cancer and bone metastasis: nursing implications of zoledronic acid. *Clin J Oncol Nurs* 7:403–408, 2003
176. Singhal S, Mehta J, Desikan R, et al: Antitumor activity of thalidomide in refractory multiple myeloma. *N Engl J Med* 341:1565–1571, 1999
177. Yakoub-Agha I, Attal M, Dumontet C, et al: Thalidomide in patients with advanced multiple myeloma: a study of 83 patients — report of the Intergroupe Francophone du Myelome (IFM). *Hematology J* 3:185–192, 2002
178. Kyle RA, Rajkumar SV: Therapeutic application of thalidomide in multiple myeloma. *Semin Oncol* 28:583–587, 2001
179. Barlogie B, Tricot G, Anaissie E: Thalidomide in the management of multiple myeloma. *Semin Oncol* 28:577–582, 2001
180. Durie B, Stepan D: Low dose thalidomide alone and in combination: long term follow-up. *Blood* 98:163a, 2001 (abstract 688)
181. Haslett PA, Corral LG, Albert M, et al: Thalidomide costimulates primary human T lymphocytes, preferentially inducing proliferation, cytokine production, and cytotoxic responses in the CD8+ subset. *J Exp Med* 187:1885–1892, 1998
182. McHugh SM, Rifkin IR, Deighton J, et al: The immunosupressive drug thalidomide induces T helper cell type 2 (Th2) and concomitantly inhibits Th 1 cytokine production in mitogen-and antigen-stimulated human peripheral blood mononuclear cell cultures. *Clin Experiment Immunol* 99:160–167, 1995
183. Moreira AL, Friedlander DR, Shif B, et al: Thalidomide and a thalidomide analogue inhibit endothelial cell proliferation in vitro. *J Neurooncol* 43:109–114, 1999
184. Rowland TL, McHugh SM, Deighton J, et al: Differential effect of thalidomide and dexamethasone on the transcription factor NF-kappa B. *Int Immunopharmacol* 1:49–61, 2001
185. Singhal S, Mehta J: Thalidomide in cancer. *Biomed Pharmacother* 56:4–12, 2002
186. Zeldis JB, Williams BA, Thomas SD, et al: S.T.E.P.S.: a comprehensive program for controlling and monitoring access to thalidomide. *Clin Ther* 21:319–330, 1999
187. Zangari M, Barlogie B, Thertulien R, et al: Thalidomide and deep vein thrombosis in multiple myeloma: risk factors and effect on survival. *Clin Lymphoma* 4:32–35, 2003
188. Thompson JL, Hansen LA: Thalidomide dosing in patients with relapsed or refractory multiple myeloma. *Ann Pharmacother* 37:571–576, 2003
189. Barlogie B, Desikan K, Eddlemon P, et al: Extended survival in advanced and refractory multiple myeloma after single-agent thalidomide: identification of prognostic factors in a phase 2 study of 169 patients. *Blood* 98:492–494, 2001
190. Novick SC, Warrell RP: Arsenicals in hematologic cancers. *Semin Oncol* 27:495–501, 2000
191. Soignet SL, Maslak P, Wang ZG, et al: Complete remission after treatment of acute promyelocytic leukemia with arsenic trioxide. *N Engl J Med* 339:1341–1348, 1998
192. Anderson KC, Boise LH, Louie R, et al: Arsenic trioxide in multiple myeloma: Rationale and future directions. *Cancer J* 8:12–25, 2002
193. Rice D, Sheridan CA: Nursing care of patients with multiple myeloma: A paradigm for the needs of special population. *Clin J Oncol Nurs* 5:89–93, 2001
194. McDaniel RW, Rhodes VA: Symptom experience. *Semin Oncol Nurs* 11:232–234, 1995
195. Ludwig H, Fritz E: Supportive therapy, in Mehta J, Singhal S (eds.): *Myeloma.* London, Martin Dunitz, 2002, pp 397–412
196. Poulos AR, Gertz MA, Pankratz VS, et al: Pain, mood disturbance, and quality of life in patients with multiple myeloma. *Oncol Nurs Forum* 28:1163–1172, 2001
197. World Health Organization: *Cancer Pain Relief and Palliative Care: Report of a WHO Expert Panel.* WHO Technical Report 804. Geneva, WHO, 1990
198. Struthers C, Mayer D, Fisher G: Nursing management of the patient with bone metastasis. *Semin Oncol Nurs* 14:199–209, 1998
199. Fellowes D, Barnes K, Wilkinson S: Aromatherapy and massage for symptom relief in patients with cancer. *Cochrane Database Syst Rev* CD002287, 2004
200. Body JJ: Dosing regimens and main adverse events of bisphosphonates. *Semin Oncol* 28(suppl 11):49–53, 2001
201. Major PP, Coleman RE: Zoledronic acid in the treatment of hypercalcemia of malignancy: Results of the International Clinical Development Program. *Semin Oncol* 28(suppl 3):17–24, 2001
202. Lawrence J: Critical care issues in the patient with hematologic malignancy. *Semin Oncol Nurs* 10:198–207, 1994
203. Redeker NS, Lev EL, Ruggiero J: Insomnia, fatigue, anxiety, depression, and quality of life of cancer patients undergoing chemotherapy. *Sch Inq Nurs Pract* 14:275–290, discussion 291–298, 2000
204. Oken MM, Pomeroy C, Weisdorf DJ, et al: Prophylactic antibiotics for the prevention of early infection in multiple myeloma. *Am J Med* 100:624–628, 1996
205. Ozer H, Armitage JO, Bennett CL, et al: ASCO 2000 update of recommendations for the use of hematopoietic colony-stimulating factors: evidence-based, clinical practice guidelines. *J Clin Oncol* 18:3558–3585, 2000
206. Rizzo JD, Lichtin AE, Woolf SH, et al: Use of epoetin in patients with cancer: Evidence-based clinical practice guidelines of the American Society of Clinical Oncology and the American Society of Hematology. *J Clin Oncol* 20:4083–4107, 2002
207. Desikan KR, Barlogie B, Jagannath S, et al: Comparable engraftment kinetics following peripheral blood stem cell infusion mobilized with granulocyte colony stimulating factor with

or without cyclophosphamide in multiple myeloma. *J Clin Oncol* 16:1547–1553, 1998

208. Alegre A, Diaz-Mediavilla J, San Miguel J, et al: Autologous peripheral blood stem cell transplantation for multiple myeloma: a report of 259 cases from the Spanish Registry. Spanish Registry for Transplant in MM (Grupo Espanol de Trasplante Hematopoyetico-GETH) and PETHEMA. *Bone Marrow Transplant* 21:133–140, 1998
209. Weaver CH, Zhen B, Schwartzberg LS, et al: Phase I–II evaluation of rapid sequence tandem high-dose melphalan with peripheral blood stem cell support in patients with multiple myeloma. *Bone Marrow Transplant* 22:245–251, 1998
210. Wong DL: Health promotion of the infant and family, in Wilson D (ed.): *Nursing Care of Infants and Children.* St. Louis, Mosby, 1995, pp 514–573
211. MMWR: Prevention of pneumococcal disease: recommendations of the Advisory Committee on Immunization Practices (ACIP). MMWR 46:1–24, 1997
212. Lynch MP: *Oncology Nursing Essentials.* New York, Professional Publishing Group, 2002, pp 112
213. Coleman EA, Coon S, Hall-Barrow J, et al: Feasibility of exercise during treatment for multiple myeloma. *Cancer Nurs* 26:419–419, 2003
214. Hoitsma AJ, Wetzels JF, Koene RA: Drug-induced nephrotoxicity. Aetiology, clinical features and management. *Drug Safety* 6:131–147, 1991
215. Shpilberg O, Douer D, Ehrenfeld M, et al: Naproxen associated fatal acute renal failure in multiple myeloma. *Nephron* 55:448–449, 1990
216. Rashed A, Azadeh B, Abu Romeh SH: Acyclovir-induced acute tubulo-interstitial nephritis. *Nephron* 56:436–438, 1990
217. Becker BN, Fall P, Hall C, et al: Rapidly progressive acute renal failure due to acyclovir: case report and review of the literature. *Am J Kidney Dis* 22:611–615, 1993
218. Attal M, Harousseau JL, Facon T, et al: Single versus double autologous stem-cell transplantation for multiple myeloma. *N Engl J Med* 349:2495–2502, 2003
219. Mehta J: Allogeneic hematopoietic stem cell transplantation in myeloma, in Mehta J, Singhal S (eds.): *Myeloma.* London, Martin Dunitz, 2002, pp 349–365
220. Anderson KC: Novel therapies for multiple myeloma. *Br J Haematol* 120:10–17, 2003
221. Mooberry SL: New insights into 2–methoxyestradiol, a promising antiangiogenic and antitumor agent. *Curr Opin Oncol* 15:425–430, 2003
222. Chauhan D, Catley L, Hideshima T, et al: 2–Methoxyestradiol overcomes drug resistance in multiple myeloma cells. *Blood* 100:2187–2194, 2002
223. Lin B, Podar K, Gupta D, et al: The vascular endothelial growth factor receptor tyrosine kinase inhibitor PTK787/ZK222584 inhibits growth and migration of multiple myeloma cells in the bone marrow microenvironment. *Cancer Res* 62:5019–5026, 2002
224. Catley L, Weisberg E, Tai YT, et al: NVP-LAQ824 is a potent novel histone deacetylase inhibitor with significant activity against multiple myeloma. *Blood* 102:2615–2622, 2003
225. Santucci R, Mackley PA, Sebti S, et al: Farnesyl transferase inhibitors and their role in the treatment of multiple myeloma. *Cancer Control* 10:384–387, 2003
226. Ochiai N, Uchida R, Fuchida S, et al: Effect of farnesyl transferase inhibitor R115777 on the growth of fresh and cloned myeloma cells in vitro. *Blood* 102:3349–3353, 2003
227. Alsina M, Fonseca R, Wilson EF, et al: The farnesyl transferase inhibitor Zanestra is well tolerated, induces stabilization of disease and inhibits farnesylation and oncogenic/tumor survival pathways in patients with advanced multiple myeloma. *Blood Online* DOI 10. 1182/Blood-2003-08–2764, 2004
228. Mitsiades CS, Mitsiades NS, McMullan CJ, et al: Transcriptional signature of histone deacetylase inhibition in multiple myeloma: biological and clinical applications. *Proc Natl Acad Sci USA* 101:540–545, 2004
229. Vanderkerken K, De Leenheer E, Shipman C, et al: Recombinant osteoprotegerin decreases tumor burden and increases survival in murine model of multiple myeloma. *Cancer Res* 63:287–289, 2003
230. Attal M, Harousseau JL, Facon T, et al: Double autologous transplantation improves survival of multiple myeloma patients: final analysis of a prospective randomized study of the Intergroupe Francophone du Myelome (IFM 94). *Blood* 100:5a, 2002 (abstr 7)
231. Yi Q: Immunotherapy in multiple myeloma: current strategies and future prospects. *Expert Rev Vaccines* 2:391–398, 2003
232. Gallucci BB, McCarthy D: The immune system, in Reiger PT (ed.): *Biotherapy: A Comprehensive Overview.* Sudbury, MA, Jones and Bartlett, 1995, pp 15–42
233. Zhan F, Hardin J, Kordsmeier B, et al: Global gene expression profiling multiple myeloma, monoclonal gammopathy of undetermined significance, and normal bone marrow plasma cells. *Blood* 99:1745–1757, 2002
234. Bumm K, Zheng M, Bailey C, et al: CGO: utilizing and integrating gene expression microarray data in clinical research and data management. *Bioinformatics* 18:327–338, 2002
235. Skeel RT: Measurement of outcomes in supportive oncology, in Weissman DE (ed.): *Principles and Practices of Supportive Oncology.* Philadelphia, Lippincott-Raven, 1998, pp 875–888

CHAPTER 60

Ovarian Cancer

Virginia R. Martin, MSN, RN, AOCN®

Introduction

Remarkable progress has been made in the understanding and management of ovarian cancer. It is now known that there is a genetic basis for hereditary ovarian cancer and screening efforts can target those at high risk; the roles of cytoreductive surgery and accurate staging of the disease are now well defined; and effective adjuvant chemotherapy treatment is available for advanced disease. Yet considerable work remains before the origin and biology of the disease are completely elucidated and, more important, before specific and sensitive tests to detect the disease in its early curable stages can be developed. For years ovarian cancer has been characterized as a "silent killer." Patients with ovarian cancer have recently found a powerful voice through coalition and advocacy groups, which speak out for research funding and other issues. For example, the Ovarian Cancer Coalition accurately describes the early stages of ovarian cancer by its motto: "It whispers . . . so listen." The advocacy conference held in 1998 by the Ovarian Cancer National Alliance titled its program "SILENT NO MORE." Both groups are working diligently to change both public and professional views about the disease.

The ovaries are located in the pelvis lateral to the uterus, and slightly posterior and caudal to the fallopian tubes (Figure 60-1).[1] Due to endocrine stimulation, the ovaries change size, shape, position, and histology during the monthly menstrual cycle and during their lifetime.[1]

Epidemiology

Ovarian cancer is the most lethal of the gynecologic cancers. Its incidence is about one-half that of endometrial cancer; however, its mortality rate in the Western world exceeds that of cervical and endometrial cancers combined. In 2004, 25,580 new cases were predicted in the United States and 16,090 deaths.[2] This disease accounts for only 4% of all cancer cases in women but, more notably, is the fourth leading cause of cancer death in women. Over a lifetime, 1 in every 55 women will develop ovarian cancer. The lifetime risk of this disease in the general population is 1.8%; unfortunately, three-fourths of those individuals will have advanced disease at diagnosis.[3] Ovarian cancer occurs primarily in women ages 40–70. The mean age of occurrence is 61, but the mean age of diagnosis for women with a family history is 54.[4] The incidence rate increases sharply in women as they age until the eighth decade of life, when incidence plateaus (see Figure 60-2).

Table 60-1 Risk Factors and Preventive Factors in Ovarian Cancer

Risk Factors	Preventive Factors
Nulliparity	Parity
Use of infertility drugs	Lactation
Pelvic inflammatory disease	Oral contraceptives
Low serum gonadotropin	Tubal ligation
Use of talc	Oophorectomy
Family history of breast or ovarian cancer	
Living in industrialized Western countries	
Being of Jewish descent	

Ovarian cancer has a wide variation in international incidence rates, with the highest rates found in North America, Scandinavia, and Israel. The lowest incidence is in Japan and in developing countries. Caucasians develop ovarian cancer almost 1.5 times more frequently than African-Americans.[5] There has been little change in the incidence of ovarian cancer in the United States over the past 20 years.

Etiology

Hormonal, environmental, and genetic factors all play roles in the development of ovarian cancer. The major risk and preventive factors for ovarian cancer are summarized in Table 60-1. The factors that attract the most attention are those that related to hormonal and reproductive issues.

Reproductive and Hormonal

The monthly ovulatory cycle in women and its effects on the ovarian epithelium are the focus of the hormonal etiology. Two long-standing hypotheses have been put forth: the incessant ovulation theory and the gonadotropin theory.

The incessant ovulation hypothesis postulates that the uninterrupted cell division and regeneration of the ovarian epithelium provides an opportunity for mutation and malignant transformation without pregnancy-induced rest periods, which contributes to neoplasia of the ovary.[6] Some laboratory experiments have supported this theory by showing that higher ovulatory activity is associated with more inclusion cysts and other changes in the surface of the ovary.[7] Recent studies of the ovaries of women with significant family

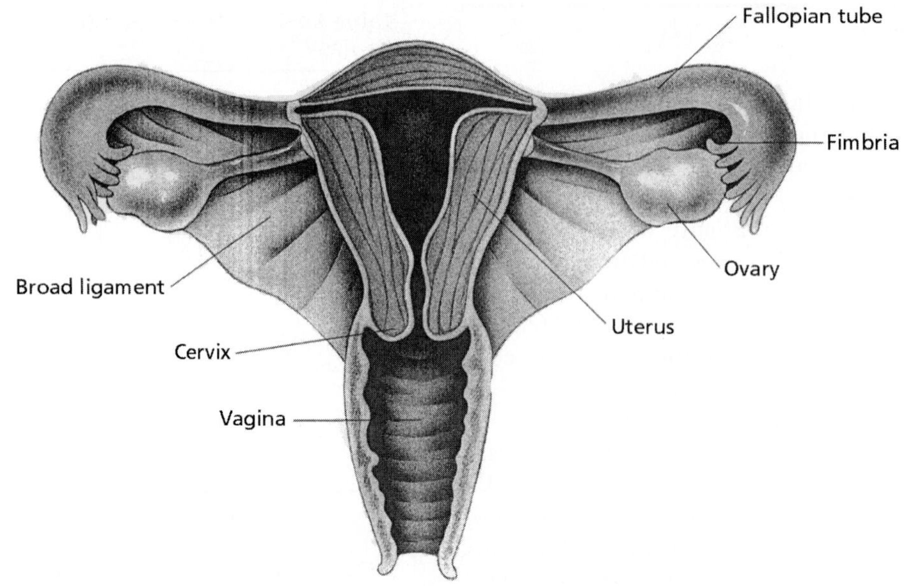

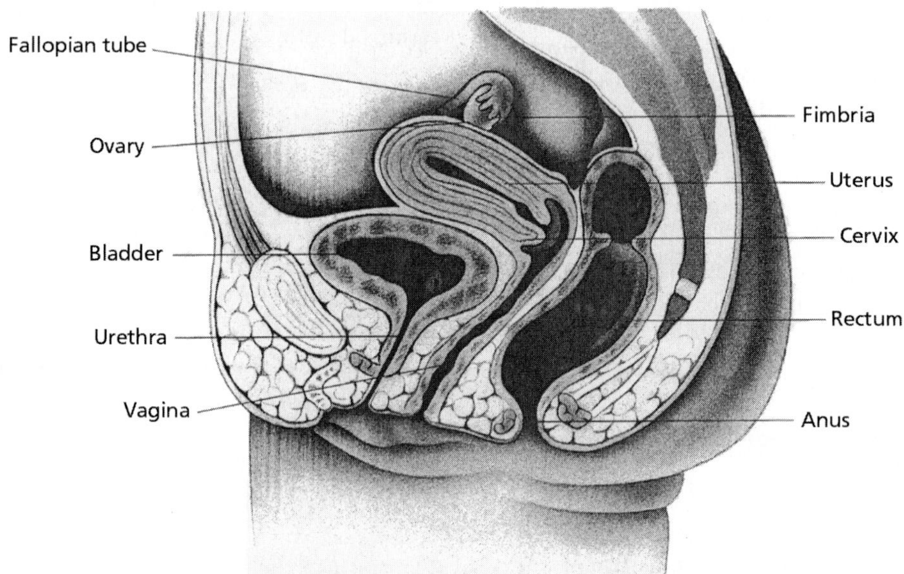

Figure 60-1 Female reproductive system. The ovaries are located deep in the pelvis, which makes it difficult to detect ovarian cancer at an early stage. (Reprinted with permission from Erikson JH, Frazier SR: Epithelial cancers of the ovary and fallopian tube, in Moore GJ (ed): *Women and Cancer: A Gynecologic Oncology Nursing Perspective.* Sudbury, MA., Jones and Bartlett, 1997.[1])

histories have reported more changes in the surface epithelium compared to control ovaries.[8]

The gonadotropin theory postulates that the ovarian epithelium repeatedly invaginates throughout life to form clefts and inclusion cysts within the ovary. It suggests that, under excessive gonadotropin stimulation of the ovarian stroma and resulting stimulation by estrogen or estrogen precursors, the epithelium may undergo proliferation and malignant transformation.[9]

Several newer theories are being investigated regarding the etiology of ovarian cancer. Risch theorizes that androgens and progestins play a role in ovarian cancer etiology.[10] Ness and Cottreau suggest that inflammation may have a role in disease development.[11] Inflammation may help explain the increased risk associated with environmental factors and may increase the cancer risk by causing mutations in epithelial cells. Cramer and colleagues hypothesize that oral contraceptives may reduce stromal hyperactivity.[12] Although no single unifying hypothesis exists, these new directions will shape the future of ovarian cancer investigation.

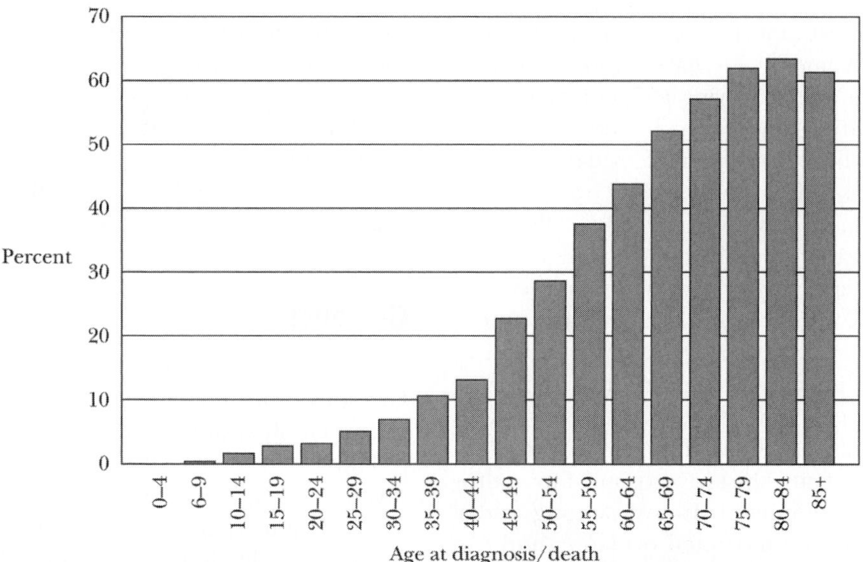

Figure 60-2 Incidence and mortality rates per 100,000 population by age for ovarian cancer in the United States. Median age of occurrence is 55 years. (Data from SEER Cancer Statistics Review, 1993–1996. Surveillance, Epidemiology, and End Results Program. National Cancer Institute, Bethesda, MD, Section XX.)

Parity, infertility, and lactation

Pregnancy has been associated with a protective effect in ovarian cancer risk. Women who are multiparas have a 10%–30% reduction in ovarian cancer compared to nulliparas.[13] A large prospective study showed a 45% decrease in ovarian cancer risk in parous women, as well as a 16% decrease in risk with each subsequent birth.[14] Most studies have concluded there is no significant effect from age at menarche, age at first birth, or age at menopause with regard to risk of ovarian cancer.[15] Infertility may be associated with risk, as childless women who have been pregnant have the same risk as nulliparas.[16] An increased risk is noted among women who have used fertility drugs because ovulation stimulation has probably been used as part of the treatment. Drugs such as clomiphene increase the risk of ovarian cancer twofold to threefold when used more than 12 cycles.[17] Evidence also suggests that pelvic inflammatory disease, which may result in infertility, may stimulate proliferation of the surface epithelium of the ovary and increase the risk for those women.[13] Lactation is known to suppress ovulation in some women, and pregnancy with lactation appears protective. Whittemore reported that the risk of ovarian cancer decreased 1% for each month of lactation, with the most significant protective effect occurring in the first six months after delivery.[16]

Exogenous hormones

Combined oral contraceptives decrease a woman's risk of ovarian cancer by 30%–60% depending on the duration of use.[13] In a meta-analysis report, five years of contraceptive use by nulliparous women reduced their risk to that of parous women and ten years of oral contraceptive use in women with a positive family history reduced their risk to a level below that of women with a negative family history.[18] A meta-analysis of 20 studies found that any use of oral contraceptives was associated with a relative risk of 0.64 compared to women who had never used them.[19] Narod and colleagues studied the use of oral contraceptives in *BRCA1* and *BRCA2* gene carriers and found that women who took oral contraceptives for six or more years had a 60% risk reduction.[20] Conversely, another study of Jewish women in Israel who were *BRCA1* and *BRCA2* gene carriers did not show any risk reduction with the use of oral contraceptives.[21] It is theorized that the progestin in the oral contraceptives induces damaged ovarian cells to die before they turn malignant.[22] Some studies have shown a modest increase in risk of ovarian cancer or ovarian cancer mortality with postmenopausal estrogen use, whereas other studies have not.[23–25]

Endogenous hormones

Women with low serum gonadotropin levels (follicle-stimulating hormone (FSH) and luteinizing hormone (LH)) are at an increased risk of ovarian cancer, as are women with high androstenedione and dehydroepiandrosterone (DHEA) levels.[26] Furthermore, women with a history of polycystic ovary syndrome and elevated androstenedione levels may be at increased risk of developing ovarian cancer.[27] Women with endometriosis experience a variety of hormone and immunologic abnormalities and are thus at increased risk, as are women with more total ovulatory cycles in their lifetime.[28] Women who have more ovulatory cycles are at higher risk for having *p53*-positive tumors if they develop ovarian cancer, which lends support to the theory that a higher number of ovulatory cycles may lead to increased DNA damage.[29]

A tubal ligation or hysterectomy physically interrupts the utero-ovarian circulation, thereby decreasing the risk of ovarian cancer.[30] It appears that because the route from the vagina to the ovaries is disrupted, exposure to exogenous toxins is likely to be diminished. The role of hormones in the etiology of ovarian cancer likely reflects a composite of factors. For example, among younger women with fewer menstrual cycles, aside from a family history, exposure to androgens may be the dominant factor; among older women, continuous uninterrupted ovulation and the greater number of menstrual cycles may be the most critical factor.[13]

Environmental

Industrialized countries, with the exception of Japan, have a higher incidence of ovarian cancer, which suggests the as-yet-unproven conclusion that environmental factors are somehow related to the etiology of ovarian cancer. Multiple dietary influences have been studied, however, and the results are not clear. Galactose metabolism has been proposed as a risk factor for ovarian cancer based on data showing that galactose is toxic to oocytes. Galactosemic women have premature menopause and increased gonadotropin levels. One study[31] has supported this theory; others have not.[32,33] Although consumption of a diet rich in vegetables and fruits may have a protective effect, the relationship between diet and risk of ovarian cancer is not yet settled.

Increased activity and vigorous physical exercise may increase the number of anovulatory cycles, which may provide a protective effect against ovarian cancer. However, in direct contrast to this finding, women reporting regular leisure physical activity have a 1.5-fold greater risk, and women who exercise vigorously (more than four times per week) have been found to have a 2.5-fold greater risk of developing ovarian cancer.[34] Daly and Obrams theorize that the rigorous activity has a negative effect on circulating estrogen feedback and produces increased serum gonadotropins.[13]

Cosmetic talc use in dusting the perineum, in feminine hygiene sprays, or on sanitary napkins, condoms, or diaphragms has also been suggested as a possible risk. Studies have reported a significant risk of ovarian cancer with the use of talc.[35–37] In another study, however, a significant association between the use of talcum powder and the risk of developing ovarian cancer was not demonstrated even with prolonged exposure.[38] In the Nurses Health Study, no association was found between using talc and ovarian cancer incidence.[39]

More research in the area of exercise, diet, and other potential environmental factors related to ovarian cancer is needed before final conclusions can be drawn.

Genetics

Of all the factors associated with increased risk of ovarian cancer, nothing alters the magnitude of risk more than a family history of ovarian cancer.[13] The number of family members with ovarian cancer defines the individual's degree of risk. If one family member has ovarian cancer, there is a twofold to threefold increased risk, leading to a lifetime risk of 4%–5%.[40] If two or more family members have the disease, the lifetime risk increases to 7%.[40] Family history and hereditary ovarian cancer are two separate risk categories. Familial risk does not approach the significant elevation of risk that occurs with hereditary ovarian cancer syndromes, where lifetime risk ranges from 16% to 60% for *BRCA1* and *BRCA2* mutation carriers.[7]

Three syndromes of genetic predisposition for ovarian cancer exist: (1) hereditary breast–ovarian cancer (HBOC), (2) site-specific ovarian cancer, and (3) hereditary nonpolyposis colorectal cancer (HNPCC). The Breast Cancer Linkage Consortium has defined hereditary breast–ovarian cancer as including at least three cases of early-onset (before age 60) breast cancer or ovarian cancer, and each family has to have at least one case of ovarian cancer.[4] Site-specific ovarian cancer syndrome may be a subset of the breast–ovarian cancer syndrome. It is distinguished from the latter by appearing in families with three or more cases of ovarian cancer occurring at any age and no cases of breast cancer diagnosed at an age younger than 50 years.[4] Breast–ovarian cancer is the more common syndrome.

The HBOC cancer trait is dominantly inherited. A link has been identified between a locus on chromosome 17q and breast cancer.[41] This same locus on chromosome 17q is responsible for HBOC syndrome.[42] The gene is known as *BRCA1*.[43] *BRCA1* is a tumor suppressor gene whose normal function is to inhibit the development of cancer. Mutations in this gene destroy its protective function and increase the chance of developing breast or ovarian cancer. A second breast cancer susceptibility locus on the long arm of chromosome 13q is the *BRCA2* gene.[44,45] *BRCA2* is associated with ovarian cancer, breast cancer, prostate cancer, head and neck cancer, malignant melanoma, and pancreatic cancer. Mutations in *BRCA1* and *BRCA2* are present in 50% of ovarian cancer patients with at least one first-degree relative having the disease and in 70% of patients with two or more affected relatives.[46] Additionally, women of Ashkenazi Jewish descent have *BRCA1* and *BRCA2* mutations that are carried by 1 in 40 women, as compared to by 1 carrier in 280 women in the general population.[47,48] Serous adenocarcinomas are part of the phenotype of *BRCA* germ-line mutation ovarian malignancies; mucinous and borderline tumors are not.[46]

In HNPCC or the family cancer syndrome known as Lynch II, DNA mismatch repair genes appear to be the underlying risk factor for developing cancer and have been identified: *hMSH2, hMLH1, hPMS2, hMSH3,* and *hMSH6.*[49] Ovarian cancer occurs in 5%–10% of HNPCC patients with a germ-line mutation.[50]

Prevention, Screening, and Early Detection

The ovaries are located anatomically deep in the pelvis (see Figure 60-1), which is one reason why it is difficult to detect ovarian cancer at an early stage. An ovarian tumor can grow undiscovered until it becomes large and is detected on pelvic exam. Along with the pelvic exam, serum tumor markers and ultrasonography may be useful for screening in certain circumstances. Overall, however, these tests fail to detect ovarian cancer at an earlier, more curable stage. Neither ultasound nor the CA-125 tumor marker has been shown to reduce morbidity or mortality of the disease, and neither is specific or sensitive enough to be recommended for general population screening.[51] Two ongoing trials, one in the United States and one in the United Kingdom, are assessing the effectiveness of screening techniques for ovarian cancer.[52]

Pelvic Examination

An annual physical exam, including a pelvic examination with bimanual rectovaginal exam, is part of routine health care for women. The palpation of the ovaries during this exam is not established as a useful screening procedure for ovarian cancer. Pap smear should be performed during the exam, although this test does not provide valuable screening information in this disease. The size of the ovaries in premenopausal women can change. Palpation of a pelvic mass on pelvic exam is abnormal in postmenopausal women and is an indication for a diagnostic ultrasound.

Table 60-2 Conditions Associated with an Increased CA-125 Level

Ovarian cancer
Endometriosis
Fibroids
Hemorrhagic ovarian cysts
Menstruation
Pelvic inflammatory disease (acute)
Pregnancy (first trimester)
Acute pancreatitis
Colitis
Chronic active hepatitis
Cirrhosis
Diverticulitis
Pericarditis
Renal disease (serum creatinine > 2.0)
Polyarteritis nodosa
Sjogren syndrome
Systemic lupus erythematosus
Other malignancies: bladder, breast, endometrium, lung, liver, non-Hodgkin's lymphoma, pancreas

Used with permission from Rosenthal A, Jacobs I: Ovarian cancer screening. *Semin Oncol* 25:315–323, 1998.[61]

CA-125

CA-125 is a tumor antigen that is commonly elevated in ovarian cancer. Eighty percent or more of women with epithelial ovarian cancers have been found to have serum CA-125 titers greater than 35 U/mL, whereas just 1% of healthy women have serum CA-125 titers at this level.[53] However, population screening studies found that only 50% of primary ovarian carcinomas confined to the ovary (stage I) are associated with elevated CA-125 levels.[54-56] Serum CA-125 determinations, while encouraging, are not sufficiently sensitive or specific enough to recommend them as a single test for population screening, particularly for premenopausal women.[54-59] Therefore, CA-125 is not helpful in the screening of the general population, although 75%–90% of women diagnosed with ovarian cancer will have an elevated CA-125 level.[53,60] An elevated CA-125 level in asymptomatic women may indicate the presence of cancer; if the CA-125 level is normal in women with an ovarian mass, however, it does not rule out ovarian cancer. This level can be elevated in multiple benign or other malignant diseases (Table 60-2).[61]

The rate of change of the CA-125 level over time appears to be a more specific screening method. A large prospective study in postmenopausal women with two or more longitudinal measurements of the CA-125 level found an improvement in sensitivity for the detection of ovarian cancer.[62] This finding led to the development of the Risk of Ovarian Cancer Algorithm (ROCA). It is currently being studied in a multicenter trial where high-risk women have the blood test performed every three months.[51,52]

If the CA-125 level is elevated prior to diagnosis, it is an important indicator of early treatment failure during front-line therapy. Further, this biomarker is of proven value in confirmation of disease relapse, and its measurement during treatment can serve as a tool to evaluate response to therapy.[63,64]

Ultrasonography

Although transabdominal ultrasound provides information on the characteristics of an ovarian mass and the presence or absence of ascites, it does not provide a definitive diagnosis. Ultrasound is unable to differentiate between a benign, functional, or malignant mass.

The transabdominal method has been replaced by the transvaginal method, which allows a closer evaluation of the ovaries via a probe placed in the vagina. Transvaginal ultrasound (TVS) permits superior visualization with shorter examination times, more comfort, and greater patient acceptance. Although color Doppler imaging is sometimes used with ultrasound to measure the blood flow patterns in ovarian vessels, the early enthusiasm for the addition of color Doppler imaging has not been supported.[65] A large study of TVS screening of 14,469 asymptomatic women is ongoing. A recent update reported that 180 patients with persistent abnormal ultrasound results had undergone surgery and 17 ovarian cancers had been detected.[66] The sensitivity and specificity of TVS were reported to be 81% and 98.9%, respectively.[66]

Routine screening with pelvic examination, CA-125, and ultrasound is not recommended for the general population. However, intensive screening using a combination of the methods available should be used for women with familial or hereditary risk factors. Pedigree analysis, linkage studies, and/or DNA testing are done to determine genetic risk.[50] The process of determining genetic risk begins with information about the availability of DNA testing. Genetic counseling is mandatory prior to DNA testing and at the time of disclosure of the findings. It is the clinician's role to provide detailed information regarding the inheritance and natural history of ovarian cancer as well as advantages and limitations of genetic testing, surveillance, and management strategies.

If a patient does not have an increased genetic risk based on the DNA testing, then she should return to the general population screening recommendations. For those women with a defined risk profile, one of the following is recommended: increased surveillance, surgical prophylaxsis, pharmacologic interventions (chemoprevention), or lifestyle changes. Screening and surveillance with baseline and interval multiple serum tumor markers and pelvic TVS are recommended for women at high risk. The National Comprehensive Cancer Network (NCCN) has published screening guidelines with criteria for identifying women with HBOC. The screening measures include an annual pelvic exam and TVS, plus a CA-125 level on an annual or semi-annual basis starting at age 25–35. Prophylactic oophorectomy should be considered on a case-by-case basis.[52] The International Collaborative Group on HNPCC have published the following guidelines for screening: (1) colonoscopy starting at age 20-25, repeat every two years to age 35, then annually; (2) annual endometrial curretage beginning at age 30; and (3) ovarian cancer screening with TVS, Doppler color blood flow, and serum CA-125 annually after the age of 30.[50]

Women should be counseled to eat a balanced diet, restrict fat and carbohydrate intake, and maintain a reasonable weight. High-risk women may also elect to take medicine to suppress ovulation or consider prophylactic oophorectomy at the completion of childbearing. Evidence from prospective and retrospective studies of women with *BRCA1* and *BRCA2* mutations demonstrated a reduction in subsequent ovarian and breast cancers in women who had prophylactic oophorectomy compared to those under surveillance alone.[67,68] In spite of prophylactic oophorectomy, the risk for a primary peritoneal carcinomatosis remains 2%–5%.[69–71]

A newer trend in screening seeks to identify novel molecular markers, including genomic and proteomic markers or panels of markers used in combination with ultrasound to improve the predictive value of screening. Proteomics is the study of proteins inside cells. A recent study using surface-enhanced laser desorption and ionization time-of-flight mass spectroscopy to discover a proteomic pattern in samples of blood with women with ovarian cancer and without the disease reported 100% sensitivity and 95% specificity.[72] In total, 18 of 18 stage I cancers and 63 of 66 healthy controls were accurately identified.[72] Until testing is both 100% specific and sensitive, it is not considered ready for the general population.

Video laparoscopy is an excellent method to examine the undersurfaces of the diaphragm, the peritoneum, serosal surfaces, and the pelvic contents. Members of families that have autosomal dominant hereditary cancer syndrome are encouraged to participate in studies to detect early precancerous and cancerous changes in their ovaries through programs that test and evaluate the screening methods now available.[46]

In the past, it was recommended that women in families vulnerable to HBOC and HNPCC syndrome take combined estrogen–progestin oral contraceptives before plans for conception and between pregnancies.[49] Oral contraceptives have since been linked to an increased risk for breast cancer among younger women, so it is no longer recommended for the HBOC syndrome families. Oral contraceptives are recommended for HNPCC families not genetically at risk for breast cancer.[49] Other agents in chemoprevention pilot studies include retinoids, progestational agents, and COX-2 inhibitors.

Women with hereditary ovarian cancer are usually diagnosed at an earlier age (early forties and younger) than women with sporadic ovarian cancer. The mean age for developing ovarian cancer in HBOC families is 51 years, compared to 43 years for HNPCC syndrome.[50] The youngest age observed was 26 years for HBOC, and 24 years for HNPCC syndrome.[50] For these reasons, genetic counseling of high-risk females should begin in their teenage years.

At present, the recommendations for the general population state that any woman older than age 18 should see a physician yearly for a thorough physical examination that should include a bimanual rectovaginal examination. With the tests currently available, routine screening for ovarian cancer is not recommended.[40] Asymptomatic women may consider discussing with their practitioner the use of oral contraceptives and tubal ligation for increased protection. Although a very personal decision, another method of risk reduction is parity.

Pathophysiology

Biology

The molecular events that underlie ovarian cancer development remain to be discovered. Although the exact mechanism of transformation is not clear, ovarian cancer appears to arise from a multistep process that entails the accumulation of mutations in multiple combinations of genes.[73] The normal ovarian epithelial cell has mechanisms that control its growth and differentiation. Cancer development involves alterations in many specific genes, including proto-oncogenes, tumor suppressor genes, and DNA repair genes. Ovarian cancer has demonstrated defects in genes such as *AKT, EGFR, ERBB2, RAS, PIK3CA, MYC, DOC-2/BAB2,* y-synuclein (*SNCG*), and *TP53*.[7,74] Penetration of the tumor cells through the basement membrane is a prerequisite for metastatic disease. The combination of genetic changes that determine the malignant phenotype, with its ability to invade and metastasize, accounts for the lethality of the disease.

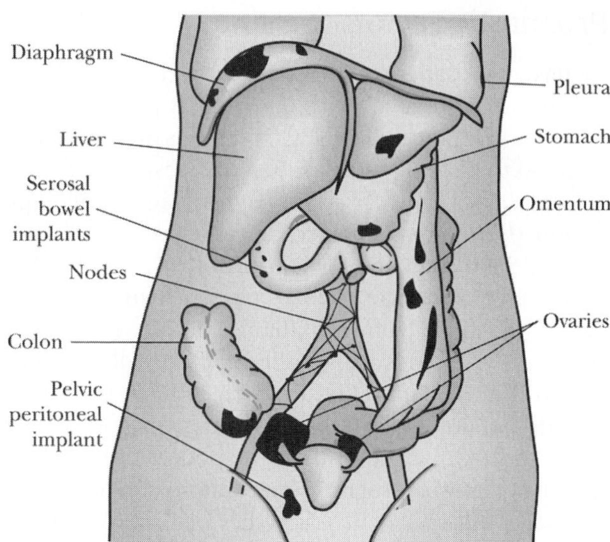

Figure 60-3 Typical sites of metastases. (Adapted with permission from DiSaia PJ: Diagnosis and management of ovarian cancer. *Hosp Pract* 22:235-250, 1987.)[75]

The most common type of ovarian cancer is the epithelial type, which accounts for 90% of the disease. Germ cell or sex-cord stromal cell tumors constitute the majority of nonepithelial tumors. Ovarian tumors range from benign, to tumors of low malignant potential, to invasive cancer. Epithelial cancer is further classified according to its behavior — either as borderline or invasive — and the cell type. Serous or mucinous types are the most common classifications of epithelial tumors. The epithelial type originates from the cells on the surface of the germinal epithelium or the mesothelium of the ovary. The remaining tumors arise from the germ or stromal cells. Germ cells are precursors of the ova; the most common type of malignancy is dysgerminoma. Sex-cord stromal cells secrete hormones and connect the different components of the ovary together; the most common tumor is the granulosa cell tumor.

Metastasis in epithelial ovarian cancer can often occur by direct extension. The malignancy penetrates the capsule of the ovary and invades the structures next to it. It can also spread by lymphatic dissemination, most frequently the pelvic or aortic lymph nodes. Rarely it spreads by blood-borne metastases. The continuous circulation of the peritoneal fluid in the peritoneal cavity facilitates the widespread dissemination of the malignant cells. This process may be referred to as *peritoneal seeding*. Disease spreads to the liver, diaphragm, bladder, or intestines by this route (Figure 60-3).[75]

Prognostic Factors

In terms of patient characteristics, age and performance status correlate with outcome. A patient with a good performance status (ECOG 0–2) is more likely to respond to treatment and experience less toxicity and a better outcome.[76–78] The Gynecology Oncology Group (GOG) has reported age as a prognostic variable in 2000 patients participating in six trials.[79] Patients older than age 69 had a poorer survival compared to those younger than age 50. Histologic subtypes and grades are significant, clear cell, and mucinous. Poorly differentiated tumors have the worst prognosis. The volume of disease after surgery is also significant: The more disease, the poorer the prognosis. The standard prognostic indicators are subjective and far from sufficient to predict prognosis. Abnormalities of oncogenes, such as *p53, MYC, RAS, ERB-2,* and tumor suppressor genes, have been reported to have prognostic importance; likewise, the expression of certain growth factors may be associated with poor prognosis.[80] The prognostic significance of *p53* mutations and overexpression was examined in 125 patients and *p53* alterations were found to be common. A mutation in *p53* was associated with a short-term survival benefit.[80,81] Other prognostic factors under investigation include DNA ploidy, proliferation activity (S-phase fraction), tumor markers, flow cytometry, and factors regulating transformation and growth. It is still too early to completely understand the significance of these findings related to the development of ovarian cancer or the progression of the disease and to apply the findings to clinical practice.

Clinical Manifestations

Ovarian cancer occurs most frequently in women older than age 50. Most patients with the disease are 50–59 years old, and approximately 70% of patients present with advanced stage III or IV disease. The initial signs and symptoms are often dismissed or ignored. Abdominal bloating or discomfort is the most common sign and symptom, followed by vaginal bleeding, gastrointestinal symptoms, or urinary tract symptoms. A study of 50 patients with ovarian cancer reported the following symptoms among more than one-half of the participants: fatigue, abdominal swelling, indigestion, lower abdominal pressure or heaviness, abdominal pain, back pain, early satiety, and constipation.[82] (See Table 60-3). A survey of 1725 women with ovarian cancer confirmed that the majority of women are symptomatic and frequently have delays in diagnosis.[83] Only 5% of women surveyed reported no symptoms before their diagnosis of ovarian cancer.[83] The duration of symptoms was reported as 2 months or less by 30%, 3–6 months for 35%, 7–12 months by 20%, and longer than 12 months by 15% of women.[83]

In Gilda Radner's book, *It's Always Something*, she described the frustrations she encountered in getting to the diagnosis of ovarian cancer.[84] The popularity of this book has helped other women become aware of the importance of recognizing their symptoms early and insisting that medical professionals interpret these symptoms appropriately. Another woman with ovarian cancer has developed and published a business card with the symptoms listed and would like it to be made available in physicians' offices to increase awareness of the disease (Figure 60-4).[85]

Table 60-3 Common Signs and Symptoms of Ovarian Cancer

Early Signs	Late Signs
Lower abdominal pressure: discomfort or pain	Ascites
	Pleural effusion
Abdominal distention	Anorexia
Change in bowel or bladder habits	Nausea or vomiting
	Abdominal, pelvic, ovarian, omental mass
Early satiety	
Indigestion, dyspepsia	
Back pain	

Ovarian Cancer Risk Factors

Risk Factors	Facts
• Genetic predisposition • Personal or family history of breast, ovarian or colon cancers • Increasing age • Undesired infertility	• All women are at risk • Symptoms do exist and can be extremely vague, yet increase over time • Early detection increases survival rate of early stage disease • A Pap Smear DOES NOT detect ovarian cancer

National Ovarian Cancer Coalition
www.ovarian.org • 1-888-OVARIAN

Potential Ovarian Symptoms

- Pelvic or abdominal pain or discomfort
- Vague, but persistent gastrointestinal upsets such as gas, nausea, and indigestion
- Frequency and/or urgency of urination in absence of an infection
- Unexplained weight gain or weight loss
- Pelvic and/or abdominal swelling, bloating and/or feeling of fullness
- Ongoing unusual fatigue
- Unexplained changes in bowel habits

Figure 60-4 Ovarian cancer risk factors and symptoms. (Source: National Ovarian Cancer Coalition)[85]

Assessment

During a physical assessment, the most important finding is the presence of an ovarian mass. A mass is considered suspicious if it is immobile and painless, if it is irregular, if there is bilateral ovarian involvement, or if any other mass is found on exam.[1] In premenopausal women, enlarged ovaries are common due to functioning ovarian cysts or benign ovarian cysts. It is common practice for the physician to observe an ovarian mass through several menstrual cycles because it may typically regress in one to three cycles. If the mass measures 8 cm or less on exam, observation is indicated. If the mass is greater than 10 cm or enlarges beyond 5 cm while under observation, further evaluation is indicated.[1] A physician may also prescribe oral contraceptives for these patients, expecting the mass to disappear. Masses that persist need investigation, including a CA-125 and a transvaginal ultrasound. Ultrasound should reveal if the mass has irregular borders, presence of solid components with papillary projections, or bilateral involvement or multiple dense irregular septae. If any of these characteristics are present, a malignancy is suspected.[1]

After these studies document an abnormality, a computerized tomography (CT) scan of the abdomen and pelvis with oral and intravenous contrast is ordered to assess the entire area. Particular attention is paid to the lymph nodes in the retroperitoneal and paraaortic areas. A barium enema or colonoscopy may be ordered if cancer is present or suspected or if the patient has symptoms. A chest x-ray, mammogram, and a baseline CA-125 complete the metastatic work-up prior to surgery. The patient should be referred to a gynecologic oncologist. Research has demonstrated that patients experience increased disease-free and overall survival when a gynecologic oncologist is part of the management team.[86–88]

Classification and Staging

The more than 30 types of ovarian cancer are classified by their cells of origin. The World Health Organization (WHO) and the International Federation of Gynecology and Obstetrics (FIGO) histologic classification is presented in Table 60-4.[89] This classification system reflects the cell type, the location of the tumor, and the degree of malignancy.

Ovarian cancer is a surgically staged disease and the FIGO staging system is used universally (Table 60-5).[90] FIGO stage is the most important prognostic variable—hence the need for rigorous surgical staging. Table 60-6[91] outlines survival based on FIGO stage.[92] The volume of residual tumor after surgery is another

Table 60-4 World Health Organization Classification of Malignant Ovarian Tumors

Common Epithelial Tumors
Malignant Serous Tumors
Adenocarcinoma, papillary, papillary cystadenocarcinoma
Surface papillary carcinoma
Malignant adenofibroma, cystadenofibroma
Malignant Mucinous Tumors
Adenocarcinoma, cystadenocarcinoma
Malignant adenofibroma, cystadenofibroma
Malignant Endometrioid Tumors
Carcinoma
Adenocarcinoma
Adenoacanthoma
Malignant adenofibroma, cystadenofibroma
Endometrioid stromal sarcomas
Mesodermal (müllerian) mixed tumors; homologous and heterologous
Clear cell (mesonephroid) tumors, malignant carcinoma and adenocarcinoma
Brenner tumors, malignant
Mixed epithelial tumors, malignant
Undifferentiated carcinoma
Unclassified
Sex-Cord Stromal Tumors
Granulosa–Stromal Cell Tumors
Granulosa cell tumor
Tumors in the thecoma-fibroma group
Fibroma
Unclassified
Androblastomas: Sertoli-Leydig Cell Tumors
Well differentiated
Tubular androblastoma, Sertoli cell tumor (tubular adenoma of Pick)
Tubular androblastoma with lipid storage, Sertoli cell tumor with lipid storage (folliculoma lipidique of Lecene)
Sertoli-Leydig tumor, hilus cell tumor of intermediate differentiation
Poorly differentiated (sarcomatoid) with heterologous elements
Gynandroblastoma
Unclassified
Lipid (Lipoid) Cell Tumors
Germ Cell Tumors
Dysgerminoma
Endodermal sinus tumor
Embryonal carcinoma
Polyembryoma
Choriocarcinoma
Teratomas
Immature
Mature dermoid cyst with malignant transformation
Monodermal and highly specialized
Struma ovarii
Carcinoid
Struma ovarii and carcinoid
Others
Mixed forms
Gonadoblastoma
Pure
Mixed with dysgerminoma or other form of germ cell tumor

Table 60-5 Staging for Ovarian Cancer: International Federation of Obstetrics and Gynecology.

Stage	Description
Stage I	Growth limited to the ovaries
Stage IA	Growth limited to one ovary, no ascites; no tumor on the external surface, capsule intact
Stage IB	Growth limited to both ovaries, no ascites; no tumor on the external surface, capsules intact
Stage IC*	Tumor stage IA or IB but with tumor on the surface of one or both ovaries, with capsule ruptured, with ascites present containing malignant cells, or with postitive peritoneal washings
Stage II	Growth involving one or both ovaries with pelvic extension
Stage IIA	Extension or metastases to the uterus or tubes
Stage IIB	Growth involving one or both ovaries with pelvic extension
Stage IIC*	Tumor either stage IIA or IIB with tumor on the surface of one or both ovaries, with capsules ruptured, with ascites present containing malignant cells, or with positive peritoneal washings
Stage III	Tumor involving one or both ovaries with peritoneal implants outside the pelvis or positive retroperitoneal or inguinal nodes; superficial liver metastases equal stage III; tumor limited to the true pelvis but with histologically verified malignant extension to small bowel or omentum
Stage IIIA	Tumor grossly limited to the true pelvis with negative nodes but with histologically confirmed microscopic seeding of abdominal peritoneal surfaces
Stage IIIB	Tumor of one or both ovaries with histologically confirmed implants of abdominal peritoneal surfaces, none exceeding 2 cm diameter; nodes negative
Stage IIIC	Abdominal implants greater than 2 cm in diameter, or positive retroperitoneal or inguinal nodes
Stage IV	Growth involving one or both ovaries with distant metastases; if pleural effusion is present, there must be positive cytologic test results to allot a case to stage IV; parenchymal lower metastases equals

* To evaluate the impact on prognosis of the different criteria for allotting cases to stage IC or IIC, it would be of value to know whether rupture of the capsule was spontaneous or caused by the surgeon, and what the source of malignant cells detected was — peritoneal washings or ascites.

very important prognostic variable, with an inverse relationship existing between the size of residual tumor and patient outcome.[92] Griffths and colleagues defined optimally debulked primary cytoreductive surgery as leaving no tumor larger than 1.5 cm.[93] An even better outcome has been demonstrated by several studies for patients with tumors less than 0.5 cm left behind.[94,95] The Gynecologic Oncology Group (GOG) defines optimally debulked disease as no tumor larger than 1 cm left behind.

Although histologic subtype is important to determine, only clear cell and mucinous types of tumors are of independent prognostic significance. Grade is more important prognostically than histologic subtype, although there is no universally accepted grading system. Well-differentiated tumors are grade I, moderately differentiated tumors are grade II, and poorly differentiated tumors are grade III. As the tumor grade increases, the survival rate decreases within each cell type. Grade is especially important in determining treatment. For example, grade I and II tumors need no further therapy.[96] Numerous studies have shown a high degree of intraobserver and interobserver variability associated with grading. Pathologists are interested in developing a more quantitative and reproducible grading system, such as molecular markers or DNA cytometry.[97]

A newer grading system that is reproducible, simple, and useful for all histologic subtypes and clinical stages of ovarian cancer has been developed.[98] With the new system, tumors are graded on architectural patterns, nuclear pleomorphism, and mitotic activity. The tumor grades correlate with survival in early and advanced disease for all histologic cell types except clear cell.[98] Staging, however, is commonly documented using the FIGO staging system that was revised in 1987 (see Table 60-5).[90] Surgical staging during cytoreductive surgery provides the basis of treatment decisions for ovarian cancer.

Therapeutic Approaches and Nursing Care

Surgery

Surgery is the mainstay of treatment in ovarian cancer. The aim of surgery is to provide a definitive diagnosis, determine the exact stage, and remove as much tumor as possible so as to improve survival and relieve symptoms. The National Institutes of Health (NIH) consensus conference concluded that aggressive efforts at maximal cytoreduction are important because minimal residual tumor is associated with improved survival.[40] The surgical procedures used include total abdominal hysterectomy, bilateral salpingoophorecto-

Table 60-6 Five-Year Survival of Ovarian Cancer Patients

Stage	Five-Year Survival (%)
I	85
II	60
III	30
IV	18

Data from Partridge, Phillips, Menck.[91]

my, peritoneal cytology, omentectomy, scraping of the undersurface of the right diaphragm, multiple peritoneal biopsies, pelvic and paraaortic lymph node sampling, and multiple random biopsies. A vertical midline incision from the symphysis pubis to above the umbilicus is essential. The goal is to leave no tumor greater than 1 cm (i.e., optimally debulked disease).

A gynecologic surgical oncologist is specially trained to perform ovarian cancer surgery. Gynecologic oncologists are concerned about adequate surgical staging in ovarian cancer. In a study of 785 women diagnosed with stage I or II ovarian cancer, only 10% of the women received optimal debulking surgery according to the NIH treatment guidelines.[99,100] The study revealed that women older than age 65 typically received incomplete surgical staging compared with those younger than 65.[100] When performed by those optimally trained to provide complete surgical cytroreduction, surgery is associated with a significant increase in survival.[101]

The gynecologic surgeon should discuss with the patient and family the goals of surgery, potential outcomes, and complications. Surgery is the initial approach to treatment in stages I–III of ovarian cancer. Surgical debulking is more controversial in stage IV disease. In a study by Curtin and associates, optimal debulking resulted in a 40-month median survival in stage IV patients versus an 18-month median survival in those suboptimally debulked.[102] There is an apparent survival benefit for women with stage IV disease who are aggressively debulked. This approach is supported by the NIH consensus conclusions, which stress the importance of aggressive surgical debulking.[40]

Surgery has a role at other times in the ovarian disease process. Procedures can include secondary cytoreductive surgery, second-look surgery, laparoscopic surgery, and palliative surgery. The timing of cytoreductive surgery remains an area of controversy and research. If the initial surgery was not successful, additional cytroreductive surgery may prove beneficial. Clinical trials are currently evaluating this approach.

Secondary cytoreductive surgery used at time of relapse is an approach whose value is unknown at this time. Second-look surgery, or exploratory surgery at the end of primary treatment, remains controversial. It is not appropriate for stage I and II disease but remains an option for stage III and IV disease. The patient with stage III or IV disease who had cytoreductive surgery followed by standard chemotherapy and is in a complete remission with a normal CA-125 and a negative CT scan is a potential candidate for second-look surgery. The goal would be to explore the entire abdomen and pelvis and do a series of biopsies to provide the most accurate assessment of the response to induction chemotherapy. Unfortunately, a negative second-look surgery does not mean the patient is cured. In fact, negative second-look surgery may be followed by relapse in as many as 50% of patients.[103] Additionally, if a patient is found to have disease at second-look surgery, the treatment available at this time is not effective in obtaining a cure.[103,104] No prospective randomized trials have confirmed any benefit from second-look surgery, and it is not routinely recommended outside of a clinical trial.

Laparoscopic surgery is not standard practice but is an acceptable alternative in a research setting.[99] Controversy exists because this type of surgery may facilitate rupture of the ovarian mass and studies have documented the adverse effects of rupture in patients with early-stage ovarian cancer.[105,106] Neoadjuvant chemotherapy treatment prior to surgery continues to be investigated, especially in stage IV disease. The goal of neoadjuvant therapy is to shrink the tumor so that debulking surgery will be more effective.

In recurrent disease, surgery has a role in promoting the patient's comfort. Patients who develop a recurrence following a long disease-free interval may benefit from a secondary debulking. Surgery is often effective in the palliative setting — for example, when a bowel obstruction occurs from peritoneal carcinomatosis. Surgery is an important treatment component in improving a patient's quality of life and providing relief of adverse symptoms in the palliative setting.

Treatment of Epithelial Ovarian Cancer

Early-stage disease

Once surgery has been performed, patients with early-stage (I and II) disease are further classified into the low-risk (favorable) category or the high-risk (unfavorable) category based on grade, cytology, presence or absence of ascites, differentiation of the tumor, rupture of the capsule, or growth outside the ovaries (Table 60-7).[107] Early-stage, low-risk (IA, IB, well or moderately well differentiated) patients require no further treatment after a comprehensive staging surgery.[96,108,109] Their five-year survival rate is greater than 90%.[96]

The recurrence rate for high-risk patients is 30%–40%. Vergote and colleagues reported on an analysis of 1000 high-risk patients with early-stage disease and established that the four most important risk factors for this group were degree of differentiation, FIGO stage (IA or IB), rupture of the capsule, and age.[110]

The perspective on treatment for the high-risk group began to evolve with a GOG trial of 81 patients randomized to melphalan versus observation that resulted in five-year survival rates of 91% and 98%,

Table 60-7 Classification of Risk of Early-Stage Ovarian Cancer

Favorable or Low Risk	Unfavorable or High Risk
Stage IA or IB disease with well- or moderately well-differentiated tumor	Stage IA or IB with poorly differentiated tumor All stage II
No ascites	Ascites
No tumor on external surface of the ovary	Tumor on external surface of ovary
Negative peritoneal cytology	Positive peritoneal cytology
Growth confined to ovaries	Growth outside the ovaries Ruptured capsule

Adapted with permission from Ozols RF, Rubin SC, Thomas G, et al: Epithelial ovarian cancer, in Hoskins WJ, Perez CA, Young RC (eds): *Principles and Practices of Gynecologic Oncology* (ed 2). Philadelphia, Lippincott-Raven, 1997, pp 919–986.

respectively, and defined the good-prognosis patients who required no further therapy.[95] High-risk (IC, high-grade IA2 or IB2, II), early-stage disease has a 25%–40% recurrence rate, and the role of immediate treatment and the type of therapy remains controversial. Those in the high-risk group have a 30%–40% risk of relapse and a 25%–30% chance of dying within the first five years after surgery.[111] When a high-risk group was treated with therapy in a trial randomizing them to either melphalan or p32, an intraperitoneal (IP) radioisotope, the result was an equivalent five-year survival rate of 80% in both arms.[96] Melphalan's risk of a second malignancy and severe myelosuppression eliminated this drug from further trials and p32 was the preferred treatment. The high-risk patients were then randomized in the next set of trials to intraperitoneal p32 versus cisplatin and cyclophosphamide (CP). Because p32 was difficult to administer and bowel complications occurred, the standard treatment became a platinum-based regimen for the high-risk group. The ten-year incidence of recurrence was 35% for the patients receiving p32 and 28% for the patients receiving CP.[112] Patients had a lower cumulative recurrence rate with CP, but no significant difference in survival was found. The authors concluded that platinum-based therapy was the preferred adjuvant treatment.[112]

Cisplatin and CP were replaced with carboplatin and paclitaxel after the results of the GOG-111 trial. A recently completed GOG trial is looking at whether three cycles versus six cycles of this regimen is significant. For now, it is too early to interpret data. European investigators explored a strategy of delaying treatment for high-risk individuals until recurrence. The results reported a 7% improvement in five-year survival for patients treated with immediate chemotherapy compared with patients who were treated when the disease recurred.[113] The current GOG trial is studying three cycles of carboplatin and paclitaxel, at standard doses, followed by observation, versus 24 weekly injections of paclitaxel at 40 mg/m^2. In conclusion, the treatment of the high-risk group of early-stage disease patients remains under investigation but currently includes combination chemotherapy consisting of a platinum-based regimen.

Advanced disease

Advanced-stage disease is routinely managed with a combination of surgery and postoperative chemotherapy. Complete cytoreductive surgery is feasible about 50% of the time and maximizes survival in patients with advanced ovarian cancer. Survival appears to be directly affected by the initial cytoreductive surgery in advanced disease.[93] Numerous studies have demonstrated a clear clinical benefit for patients in the optimal category having a higher complete response rate, prolonged progression-free survival, and improved median survival.[99] Therefore, the goal of cytoreductive surgery in this stage is to minimize the residual tumor to less than 1 cm in maximum diameter.

Chemotherapy — especially with anthracyclines, platinum-based compounds, and taxanes — is critically important in ovarian cancer treatment.[114-117] Five meta-analyses incorporating data from 45 randomized trials, including 10,000 patients, helped clarify the role of platinum-based chemotherapy in this indication. Immediate platinum-based therapy was better than nonplatinum-based therapy, platinum in combination was better than the single agent when used at the same doses, and there was no difference between carboplatin and cisplatin either as single agents or when substituted for one another in combination regimens.[118] Substitution of carboplatin, a less toxic analog, for cisplatin has been compared in multiple combination regimen clinical trials.[119-121] Results obtained by the Southwest Oncology Group (SWOG) and the National Cancer Institute of Canada showed no survival differences.[119,120] However, a European trial found a higher complete remission rate in the cisplatin arm.[121]

Anthracyclines were included in the early combination regimens in this disease. Controversy still exists as to whether the inclusion of anthracyclines is superior to non-anthracycline-containing regimens. Two meta-analyses in the 1990s focused on including doxorubicin in chemotherapy. One showed the three-drug regimen consisting of cyclophosphamide, doxorubicin, and cisplatin was superior to the two-drug regimen consisting of cyclophosphamide and cisplatin. There was a 7% improvement in both two- and five-year survival rates.[122] Two meta-analyses did demonstrate a modest survival benefit in the doxorubicin arms of the trials.[123,124] The early 1990s saw the development of a new class of drugs, the taxanes. The first drug from this group to be used in clinical trials, paclitaxel, was very active in women with advanced recurrent ovarian cancer.[125] Due to the drug's activity in recurrent disease, it was quickly included in clinical trials as initial therapy to be compared to the standard combination at that time, cisplatin and cyclophosphamide.

Several pivotal clinical trials occurred in the mid-1990s. First, in the GOG-111 trial, standard cyclophosphamide and cisplatin combination therapy was compared to paclitaxel and cisplatin. All patients participating in this clinical trial had suboptimal surgical debulking or stage IV disease. In the paclitaxel arm, there was improvement in response rate of 73% versus 60% for the standard therapy.[126] The paclitaxel-containing regimen led to a 4-month improvement in progression-free survival and a 14-month improvement in median survival.[126] A large clinical trial that confirmed these findings was titled "OV-10," and involved the Ovarian Group from Canada and Europe. Of the 600 patients enrolled in this trial, 35% had low-volume disease at entry or were optimally debulked. The treatment arms consisted of cyclophosphamide and cisplatin versus paclitaxel and cisplatin; paclitaxel was given at 175 mg/m^2 over three hours, a change from the GOG-111 protocol. Similar to the GOG-111 results, the response rate was significantly improved in the paclitaxel arm, 59% versus 45% for the cyclophosphamide arm, and the complete clinical response rates were 41% and 27%, respectively.[127] Longer progression-free survival (15.5 months versus 11.5 months) and longer overall survival (35.6 months versus 25.8 months) were found in the paclitaxel arm, but there was a large crossover rate from the cyclophosphamide arm to the paclitaxel arm at the first detection of progressive disease.[127] In both studies, the cisplatin and paclitaxel regimen proved superior; similar results were also achieved with 24-hour versus 3-hour paclitaxel. There was, however, significant neurotoxicity noted in the 3-hour paclitaxel regimen, with 18% grade III toxicity.

The GOG trial compared the cisplatin/paclitaxel combination with paclitaxel alone and cisplatin alone. Although no significant difference in median overall survival was noted between the three arms, cisplatin alone or in combination yielded superior response rates and progression-free survival.[128] The second and third International Collaborative Ovarian Neoplasm group studies (ICON-2, ICON-3) have provided further insight. ICON-2 compared carboplatin to cyclophosphamide, doxorubicin, and cisplatin (CAP) and found no difference in survival between the two groups.[129] The CAP arm was more toxic. ICON-3 compared carboplatin versus carboplatin and paclitaxel versus carboplatin plus paclitaxel with CAP. A total of 2074 patients were enrolled. The follow-up at 51 months did not show any difference in overall survival between the three arms of the trial.[130] Some of the challenges in interpreting this study are that it recruited a wide range of patient types (stages I–IV), 46% of patients had tumor bulk greater than 2 cm, 30% had absent or microscopic disease, and 55% had poorly differentiated disease.[131] In all of these studies, some patients did cross over and receive a taxane. As these data mature, they may offer an opportunity for review and refinement of current treatment guidelines.

Today the standard for ovarian cancer treatment with chemotherapy is a platinum compound and paclitaxel for first-line treatment. Clinical guidelines have been published to support the use of this regimen.[132] Three trials have now been completed using carboplatin/paclitaxel compared to cisplatin/paclitaxel.[133–135] The GOG-158 trial studied debulked stage III patients and compared cisplatin and pacliltaxel (R1) versus carboplatin and paclitaxel (R2). Patients were randomized to second-look surgery or no second-look surgery at the time of enrollment. The results showed no difference in median overall survival (48.8 months for R1 versus 56.7 months for R2) and no difference in progression-free survival or overall survival in the second-look surgery patients versus the no second-look surgery patients.[136] The researchers concluded that carboplatin/paclitaxel is not less effective than cisplatin/paclitaxel, carboplatin/paclitaxel is less toxic and easier to administer, and second-look surgery does not influence recurrence-free survival.[135] Two more studies confirmed this result by comparing carboplatin plus paclitaxel versus cisplatin plus paclitaxel and found no difference in progression-free survival or overall survival between the treatment arms.[133,134] The conclusion drawn from these studies is that the carboplatin/paclitaxel combination is the preferred regimen because it is equally effective, less toxic, and easy to administer in the outpatient setting.

Docetaxel has been studied as a single-agent therapy, in combination with the platinum drugs, and as front-line therapy in ovarian cancer; it demonstrated activity in all settings.[137–139] Docetaxel also has activity in paclitaxel-resistant ovarian cancer. A recent trial compared docetaxel/carboplatin with paclitaxel/carboplatin and found no significant difference between the regimens in terms of response or median progression-free survival.[139] The toxicity profiles are different, however: Docetaxel/carboplatin produces more mylosuppression, whereas paclitaxel/carboplatin is associated with more peripheral neuropathy. All of these studies have supported the use of docetaxel as an alternative to paclitaxel in front-line therapy.

The definition of the most effective carboplatin dose (AUC 7.5 or lower), the optimal number of platinum-based cycles of therapy, and the value of

Arm I	
Carboplatin AUC 6 (d1)	× 8 cycles
Paclitaxel 175 mg/m^2 (d1)	
Arm II	
Carboplatin AUC 5 (d1)	× 8 cycles
Paclitaxel 175 mg/m^2 (d1)	
Gemcitabine 800 mg/m^2 (d1, 8)	
Arm III	
Carboplatin AUC 5 (d1)	× 8 cycles
Paclitaxel 175 mg/m^2 (d1)	
Doxil 30 mg/m^2 (d1 every other cycle)	
Arm IV	
Carboplatin AUC (d3)	× 4 cycles
Topotecan 1.25 mg/m^2 (d1–3)	
Arm V	
Carboplatin AUC 6 (d8)	× 4 cycles
Gemcitabine 1 g/m^2 (d1, 8)	
Arms IV and V are followed with:	
Carboplatin AUC 6 (d1)	× 4 cycles
Paclitaxel 175 mg/m^2 (d1)	

Figure 60-5 Treatment schema for GOG-0182/ICON-5.

combined versus sequential therapy with taxanes are all questions that remain unanswered. The current phase III GOG intergroup trial includes four experimental arms to evaluate the addition of three new drugs (topotecan, gemictabine, and PEG-liposomal doxorubicin) using two different strategies for drug administration (sequential doublets and triplet combinations). The treatment schema for this current trial is depicted in Figure 60-5.

Paclitaxel administration poses several nursing challenges, the most significant of which is hypersensitivity reactions. Prevention of the hypersensitivity reaction involves a premedication regimen, including dexamethasone, given orally the evening before and morning of treatment or intravenously immediately before treatment. Most patients who have hypersensitivity reactions experience itching, shortness of breath, a tightness in the chest, and perhaps back pain. In such cases, the infusion is stopped immediately and routine anaphylactic measures are employed. The infusion may be restarted at half the rate. Olson and associates found that in the case of paclitaxel hypersensitivity, rapid retreatment was safe and cost-effective.[140] Platinum hypersensitivity reactions are also seen with ovarian cancer treatment. Hypersensitivity arises most frequently with subsequent treatment for recurrent disease and after primary therapy with platinum agents. One author describes skin testing for carboplatin hypersensitivity and concludes that a negative skin test seems to reasonably predict the absence of a hypersensitivity, whereas the effectiveness of a positive test result remains uncertain.[141]

To summarize, the majority of women with clinically curable ovarian cancer will receive primary debulking surgery and combination chemotherapy. The overall ten-year survival rate for ovarian cancer is approximately 20%; therefore, continued efforts must be directed at improving the results obtained with primary therapy.[142] The phase III clinical trial now under way may help define a new standard regimen for ovarian cancer if the progression-free interval and overall survival found in it are improved.

Maintenance therapy

Once a patient has completed primary therapy and achieves a complete remission, there is controversy regarding the role of maintenance therapy. Between 50% and 75% of patients with advanced disease who achieve a clinical complete remission following primary therapy will ultimately relapse.[143] Maintenance or consolidation therapy is commonly used to decrease the relapse rate and increase survival. Such therapy in women who achieve a clinical complete response has been studied using high-dose therapy with stem cell transplant, intraperitoneal therapy, administration of the radioactive isotope of phosphorous (^{32}P), hormone therapy, whole-abdominal radiotherapy, or prolonged administration of single-agent chemotherapy. Interest in maintenance therapy has intensified due to the results of a recent study evaluating 12 monthly cycles of single-agent paclitaxel compared to 3 monthly cycles following primary therapy; the former regimen provided improved progression-free survival (28 months versus 21 months).[144] No overall difference in survival was reported and the trial was stopped early. Controversy surrounds the issue of maintenance therapy, as its additional toxicity cannot be underestimated and no true clinical benefit has been established. Ideally, future studies will include research on quality of life, symptom control, and survival factors.

Intraperitoneal therapy

Intraperitoneal (IP) therapy can provide a large pharmacologic advantage — that is, the high ratio of the peak peritoneal drug levels compared to plasma levels. The drugs administered via the IP route will also enter the systemic circulation and achieve a 50%–75% uptake of IV administration exposure via the lymphatic channels or by passive diffusion. Because ovarian cancer is predominantly confined to the abdomen, there has been a great deal of interest in pursuing the IP method of drug administration. IP therapy has been investigated as consolidation therapy after a negative second-look laparotomy, as second-line treatment for resistant disease, and as first-line therapy in ovarian cancer. Numerous phase I and II trials over the last four decades have studied single agents including methotrexate, fluorouracil doxorubicin, carboplatin, cisplatin, and paclitaxel.

Cisplatin is the drug most frequently used in IP therapy in ovarian cancer. A GOG/SWOG trial enrolled optimal stage III patients with no tumor larger than 2 cm. These patients received IP or IV cisplatin (100 mg/m^2) and IV cyclophosphamide (600 mg/m^2).[145] More than 600 women participated, and the complete response rate for IP therapy was 47% compared to an IV rate of 36%; overall median survival was 49 months versus 41 months, respectively. A subsequent GOG trial randomized patients to six months of IV cisplatin (75 mg/m^2) and paclitaxel 135 mg/m^2 over 24 hours versus two doses of carboplatin (AUC = 9) followed by six cycles of IP cisplatin (100 mg/m^2) and IV paclitaxel 135 mg/m^2 over 24 hours.[146] There were statistically significant differences in progression-free survival (28 months versus 22 months) and overall survival (63 versus 52 months).[146] A third randomized trial examined first-line therapy of IV paclitaxel (135 mg/m^2 for 24 hours day 1) plus IP cisplatin (100 mg/m^2 day 2) and IP paclitaxel (60 mg/m^2 day 8) versus the control arm of cisplatin (75 mg/m^2) plus paclitaxel (135 mg/m^2 for 24 hours) every 21 days. A progression-free survival improvement was noted in the preliminary results reported.[147]

Another area of interest is the use of IP therapy as a consolidation treatment. Barakat and associates completed a phase II trial of IP cisplatin and etoposide as consolidation therapy in advanced disease.[148] At 36-month follow-up, 39% of patients who had consolidation therapy with three courses experienced recurrence compared to 54% of those in the observation arm.[148] Recently, records were reviewed for 433 patients who received IP therapy between 1984 and 1998 for consolidation or recurrent or persistent disease treatment. The authors concluded that prolonged survival was observed in selected patients receiving IP-based platinum therapy, and a relationship between size of disease at the initiation of IP therapy was demonstrated.[149] Toxicity profiles for IP therapy continue to be significant. Additionally, the use of cisplatin, by either the IV or the IP route, has been supplanted by the drug carboplatin, which has an equal effect but much less toxicity. Carboplatin has been studied using an IP delivery route, and data suggest that the uptake of this drug using the IP route may be less than that of cisplatin.[150]

In conclusion, IP therapy has shown an ability to improve progression-free or overall survival in multiple clinical trials. The therapy also produces significant toxicity. More clinical trials are needed to explore the use of IP therapy in front-line management of ovarian cancer.

Radiotherapy

Early trials suggested that control of pelvic disease was superior with radiotherapy. When this treatment was compared to chemotherapy, the survival rates were similar but the complication rates were higher in patients who had whole-abdominal radiation (WAR) therapy. Clinical trials have demonstrated that abdominopelvic or WAR radiotherapy is superior to limited pelvic radiotherapy. WAR is a toxic treatment because the entire abdomen is included in the radiation field; however, current techniques and new fractionation schedules appear to reduce toxicity.[151] It appears that WAR therapy has no role in curative management of the patient with optimally debulked, early-stage, low-risk ovarian cancer. Possible roles for radiotherapy include following chemotherapy for early-stage, high-risk patients as part of consolidation therapy; for advanced-disease patients with minimal or no residual disease; in the salvage setting with minimal residual disease; and in palliative therapy.[152]

Patients with platinum-resistant tumors were studied to determine the palliative benefit of radiation therapy. When 47 patients received palliative therapy, 39% obtained relief of their symptoms for longer than 12 months, and 30% obtained relief of their symptoms for 6–12 months. The authors concluded that radiation could provide effective and durable palliation of symptoms in patients with platinum-refractory ovarian cancer.[153]

Drug resistance

Drug resistance in ovarian cancer is a major problem. Fifty to seventy-five percent of patients with ovarian cancer achieve a complete response but then go on to relapse and develop resistance to further chemotherapy. About 20% of patients are intrinsically resistant to chemotherapy. Understanding the molecular basis for multidrug resistance (MDR) is important for the design of new treatment strategies.[154-156] Some of the identified mechanisms of MDR resistance include host factors (altered pharmacokinetics), host-tumor factors, cellular factors, DNA repair, tolerance to DNA repair, and altered cellular targets.[154] Decreased drug accumulation, metabolic drug inactivation, and repair or tolerance to drug-induced cellular injury contribute to resistance at the cellular level.[154] Resistance is a multifactorial problem in this disease, especially as it relates to alkylating agents and platinum compounds.[143]

Ovarian cancer drug resistance has been associated with decreased susceptibility to apoptosis. A recent study has identified the *BCl-xl* gene involved in ovarian cancer, which may be responsible for the resistance to chemotherapy-induced apoptosis.[157] Gene therapy, both related to tumor biology and overcoming drug resistance, represents a promising new strategy for improving survival in this disease. Progress has been made in MDR, from in vitro studies to the thorough study of cell lines from relapsed patients; an understanding of why ovarian cancer cells become resistant to treatment is emerging.[153]

Disease recurrence

An elevated level of the tumor marker CA-125 is predictive of a recurrence of ovarian cancer. The median time for CA-125 to become elevated is two to four months prior to obvious symptoms or definitive clinical disease progression. Thus, a rising CA-125 level has clouded the definition of time of recurrence because the patient often does not have clinically detectable disease. No evidence indicates that immediate chemotherapy is beneficial in recurrence. Patients follow this tumor marker closely, however, and they usually want treatment as soon as it is elevated. A rising CA-125 level is definitely associated with increased stress in patients. An alternative approach may be to use tamoxifen, a nontoxic but active drug, until clinical evidence of disease recurrence emerges.[132,158,159] Many clinicians feel that there is no reason to start chemotherapy in a patient with a serologic marker of recurrence as long as the patient is asymptomatic, has a normal pelvic exam, and is without evidence of definitive disease recurrence.

Patients with documented recurrent disease frequently respond to salvage therapy; however, the duration of response is brief. Roland and colleagues found that the tumor response to initial paclitaxel/platinum therapy was predictive of tumor response to second-line treatment.[152] The current salvage therapy appeared to have little benefit for resistant tumors and produced a 24% increase of significant complications. Most clinicians feel that patients must be classified into one of three categories prior to salvage therapy: (1) drug sensitive — time to recurrence is longer than six months; (2) drug resistant — time to recurrence is less than six months; or (3) drug refractory — no response to initial therapy. (See Table 60-8.) In treatment of recurrence, the drug-sensitive patients have a high response rate to drugs used in the initial regimen; the longer the treatment-free interval, the higher the chance of response when recurrence is treated.[160] Rechallenging patients with their original primary treatment does not appear to be any better than using new agents.

Recurrent disease treatment might start with single-agent paclitaxel or single-agent carboplatin. Some evidence suggests that combination therapy in the platinum-sensitive group is superior to single-agent therapy.[161,162] Two trials tested this theory, and both demonstrated a more favorable response rate with the combined therapy that included paclitaxel. These investigators concluded that the regimen containing both a taxane and a platinum agent may be superior to platinum alone. Other results point to the lack of survival benefit and the increased toxicity as evidence that single-agent therapy is superior.[163–165]

Table 60-8 Category of Response and Time to Recurrence for Ovarian Cancer

Category of Response	Time to Recurrence
Drug sensitive	> 6 months
Drug resistant	< 6 months
Drug refractory	No response to therapy

In conclusion, combination chemotherapy in drug-sensitive patients produces higher response rates but no evidence that long-term survival or quality of life is improved.[161] The drug-sensitive patient will probably show a higher response rate to new drugs as well. Drug-resistant patients are usually treated with new agents. Patients whose disease progresses while on treatment, called the *drug-refractory group*, should be offered investigational therapy. All patients should be considered candidates for clinical trials.

With disease recurrence, the challenge is that while second-line treatment is beneficial, it cannot produce a cure. Several chemotherapy agents demonstrate cytotoxic activity in patients with recurrent disease, but the response is not durable. The likelihood of benefit must be weighed against the toxicity of the treatment. The patients most likely to benefit from second-line treatment include those with small-volume disease, good performance status, a long treatment-free interval, serous histology, and a small number of sites of disease. Numerous chemotherapy agents may be utilized when the disease recurs. See Table 60-9.[160] Some critical parameters when choosing a treatment for recurrent disease include prior response, toxicity of prior treatment, quality of life, toxicity profile, age, co-morbid illness, extent of disease, cost, and patient preference. The standard approach is to treat the patient for two to three cycles and then reevaluate the patient to determine whether there has been a clinical benefit before continuing. If no response occurs, an alternative regimen is selected. Palliative support is used through to the end stages of the disease.

Molecular-targeted therapies are currently being investigated and appear to represent the future direction of therapy in ovarian cancer. The most studied

Table 60-9 Chemotherapy Agents Utilized in the Treatment of Recurrent Ovarian Cancer

Altretamine
Carboplatin or cisplatin
Docetaxel
Epirubicin
Etoposide
Gemcitabine
Ifosfamide
Liposomal doxorubicin
Paclitaxel
Tamoxifen
Topotecan
Vinorelbine

target for therapy is epidermal growth factor receptor (EGFR), which is expressed in 30%–70% of epithelial ovarian cancers.[7] Receptor function can be inhibited by blocking the binding of ligand to the receptor by a monoclonal antibody (cetuximab, ABX-EGF) or by inhibition of the enzyme activity of the receptor tyrosinase kinase with small molecules (gefitinib or erlotinib).[7] These drugs have been evaluated in clinical trials in patients with ovarian cancer and have produced responses; they are now being studied in combination with chemotherapy.[166,167]

Vascular endothelial growth factor (VEGF) plays a key role in ascites formation in ovarian cancer. Research conducted with an antibody against VEGF in preclinical murine models bearing human ovarian carcinoma xenografts prevented and even reversed ascites formation, but did not correlate with tumor response.[168]

Replacing defective genes that cause the malignant behavior of cancer cells represents another interesting approach in research.[7] One targeted gene is mutated *TP53,* which is detected in more than half of ovarian cancer cases. In one clinical trial, women with previously untreated disease were randomized to receive either standard treatment or the same therapy with IP administration of adenovirus carrying wild-type p53.[169] This study was closed after the first interim analysis when it failed to yield any signs of efficacy. These new forms of therapy remain in the early stages of research. Clearly, the presence of a target on a tumor by itself may not be sufficient for drugs to have activity. There may be a subset of patients in whom the target has a critical biological role in the growth of the cancer, and this group is most likely to benefit from targeted therapy. New tools that will allow highly specific tumor profiling such as genomic microarray and proteomic analysis will help facilitate the selection of those patients who are most likely to benefit from these techniques.[170] Overall, preclinical studies have demonstrated that molecular-targeted therapies have a synergistic effect with chemotherapy and are likely to have the greatest benefit in patients with small-volume disease.[171]

Primary Treatment of Other Ovarian Tumors

Ovarian germ cell tumors

Ovarian germ cell tumors are uncommon and occur in women in their teens and twenties.[172] The critical distinction to make during diagnosis is between dysgerminoma tumors and nondysgerminoma tumors (all others). Dysgerminoma is analogous to seminoma and is a radiosensitive tumor; it may be associated with pregnancy. The signs and symptoms of germ cell tumors include abdominal pain and a palpable pelvic or abdominal mass. Some 10% of patients present with acute abdominal pain usually caused by rupture, hemorrhage, or torsion of the ovarian mass.[172] Abdominal distention, fever, and vaginal bleeding are less common signs and symptoms. An abnormal HCG or alphafetoprotein level, or both, may be found, and the level of the marker CA-125 may be elevated. The staging system used for germ cell tumors is identical to that employed for epithelial ovarian cancer.

Initial treatment is surgery for both definitive diagnosis and treatment. A vertical midline incision is made, and the type of surgical procedure depends on the findings when the abdomen is explored. All attempts will be made to save the uterus and the other ovary if one goal is to preserve childbearing. At a minimum, it is important to remove the tumor and inspect the entire peritoneal cavity. Any suspicious lesions should be biopsied. If metastatic disease is present, cytoreductive principles apply as in epithelial ovarian cancer.

Treatment after surgery for nondysgerminoma includes three cycles of bleomycin, etoposide, and platinum (BEP) chemotherapy. Dysgerminoma patients will have the same chemotherapy but only if their disease stage is greater than IA. Stage IA patients are followed with observation only. Most cases of dysgerminoma are curable and have a good prognosis.

Sex-cord stromal tumors

Sex-cord stromal tumors arise from the sex cords or ovarian stroma and constitute 5%–8% of ovarian malignancies. These tumors consist of granulosa and theca cells as well as Sertoli and Leydig cells; the most common type is granulosa cell. Granulosa-theca cell tumors are low grade and secrete estrogen or testosterone. Women with sex-cord stromal tumors are typically younger than age 40. The symptoms include irregular periods in premenopausal women and vaginal bleeding in postmenopausal women. Sertoli-Leydig tumors are low-grade malignancies that occur usually in the third or fourth decade of life. These tumors present with signs of virilization due to androgen production.

The staging process for sex-cord stromal tumors is the same as for epithelial tumors, a surgical staging process. If the disease is diagnosed early, treatment consists of surgery alone. The surgical procedure depends on the extent of the tumor, the age of the patient, and whether the desire for fertility preservation is important. If chemotherapy is indicated, it is usually a combination such as BEP or cisplatin, bleomycin, and vinblastine. A GOG trial with these drugs showed a 37% response rate.[173] Prognosis is good, with a five-year disease-free rate of 85%–90%.[53] The majority of these tumors are diagnosed early, but advanced and recurrent disease may be found and granulosa cell tumors can recur 5–30 years after diagnosis.[174]

Ovarian cancer of low malignant potential

Epithelial tumors account for 90% of all ovarian cancers. Of the epithelial tumors, 10%–15% will have low malignant potential (LMP) or be borderline tumors or atypical proliferating epithelial tumors. Borderline or LMP designation means that although the cells of the tumor appear malignant, the cells have not invaded the underlying tissue. These tumors tend to occur in younger patients, in earlier stages, and have an excellent overall survival rate of 80%–90%.[175,176] These are intermediate tumors, between cystadenomas and frankly invasive disease. Lu and colleagues found that bilateral and advanced borderline tumors were multifocal in origin, whereas epithelial ovarian cancer is unifocal.[177] In 1971, FIGO called this group *low malignant potential*; in 1973, WHO labeled it *borderline tumors*.[178,179]

The surgical procedure and staging for LMP ovarian cancer are similar to those for epithelial ovarian cancer. Overall, the most important characteristic to note is that these tumors are not invasive. Surgery alone cures the majority, and adjuvant therapy is not indicated.

Extraovarian peritoneal carcinoma

Primary peritoneal carcinomas are characterized by their diffuse involvement of the peritoneal surfaces with a neoplasm appearing identical to papillary serous carcinoma but without a primary ovarian tumor. This disease can occur in women with intact ovaries or after an oophorectomy. The tumors are frequently advanced at presentation. Surgical cytoreductive surgery is less successful due to the diffuseness of the metastasis. The tumors are sensitive to platinum-based therapy after surgery.

Table 60-10 Common Problems Following Laparotomy for Tumor Debulking

Bleeding/hemorrhage
Thromboembolic event
Infection/sepsis
Fluid and electrolyte imbalance
Atelectasis/pneumonia
Bowel dysfunction
Bladder dysfunction

Reprinted with permission from Eriksson JH, Frazier SR: Epithelial cancers of the ovary and fallopian tube, in Moore GJ (ed.): *Women and Cancer: A Gynecologic Oncology Nursing Perspective.*Sudbury, MA, Jones and Bartlett, 1997, pp 205–256.[1]

Symptom Management and Supportive Care

Nursing care and support of patients with ovarian cancer occurs in three major phases: (1) during surgical therapy, (2) during chemotherapy, and (3) during advanced disease. The nurse plays critical roles in delivery and management of care, in patient education, as an advocate for the patient, and for emotional support.

In the first phase of care, nursing care focuses on the patient's preparation for surgery, the acute postoperative period and prevention of postsurgical complications, and the psychosocial support for a cancer diagnosis. Initially, the nurse will explain the plan with the patient and emphasize the prevention of possible postoperative complications (Table 60-10). Preadmission testing is done, and the patient is given a bowel prep to cleanse the bowel entirely prior to surgery. The family must be educated about the operative procedure itself and the length of time it takes. Nursing clinical pathways, a step-by-step outline of the components of care, can be developed to ensure that all aspects of care are considered.[180] These tools help increase the nurse's efficiency and decrease costs by providing specific outcomes to follow. The diagnosis and surgical intervention phase usually covers five to seven days in the hospital and a short recuperative break before the next phase of treatment, chemotherapy. However, many clinicians administer the first course of treatment during the postoperative period.

The second phase of nursing care targets the chemotherapy treatment plan. The nursing care focus is mainly one of education and information regarding the treatment regimen, and support and assessment for potential problems from chemotherapy toxicities. The specifics of nursing care in this phase depend on the treatment administered to the patient. The current standard for chemotherapy involves a taxane and a platinum compound. Possible side effects include alopecia, an allergic reaction, myelosuppression, nausea, vomiting, arthralgias, and myalgias. If a woman receives information about side effects of treatment and ways to manage them, she is more likely to successfully reduce her physical and emotional distress from treatment effects.[181] Nurses provide vital links to patients by performing telephone triage roles in the ambulatory or office setting for questions, problems, or support during this phase of care.

Unfortunately, the majority of patients with advanced ovarian cancer will have a recurrence of their disease. Nurses are critical caregivers during this final phase of care. Ovarian cancer, which is usually spread throughout the abdomen, can cause dysfunction in many different organ systems. Women often present with a multitude of gastrointestinal complaints at diagnosis, and these symptoms may continue or reoccur during treatment or recurrence. Metastases can appear in any organ and site; the most frequently occurring metastatic sites include the intestines, liver, diaphragm, or lungs. The major problems that nurses confront in caring for women with advanced recurrent disease include ascites, intestinal obstruction, malnutrition, lymphedema, and pleural effusion. Each of these potential problems is discussed here along with relevant nursing management strategies.

Ascites

One-third of women with ovarian cancer will present with ascites at diagnosis; two-thirds will have ascites present at their death. The parietal peritoneum lines the abdominopelvic wall, the diaphragm, and the visceral peritoneum that covers the abdominal organs and encloses the peritoneal cavity. Peritoneal fluid is normally present in a small volume to constantly lubricate the cavity and prevent abdominal organs from adhering to abdominal walls; 80% of this fluid is drained by the lymphatic system.[182,183] Ascites occurs when the fluid produced is greater than the amount of fluid cleared, usually caused by tumor obstructing the diaphragmatic or abdominal lymphatic channels or the tumor itself producing excessive fluid.[183,184] A fluid increase of greater than 500 mL produces symptoms that include weight gain, abdominal bloating, feeling full after small meals, indigestion, peripheral edema, altered bowel habits, inability to bend or sit upright, and lack of appetite. Early symptoms of ascites may progress if no intervention is instituted to eliminate its source. Profound ascites will have a devastating effect on the individual's ability to function. Gastrointestinal function, nutrition, ambulation, breathing, sleeping, and psychosocial sequelae are all affected by this condition. Nursing assessment could reveal any or all of the following physical findings: shiny or tense abdominal skin, everted umbilicus, diminished bowel sounds, dullness over flank area, or midabdomen tympany.[185,186] The presence of ascites in the abdomen may create a compression phenomenon that could contribute to bowel obstruction.

A diagnosis of ascites is confirmed with an abdominal flat plate x-ray or abdominal ultrasound. Paracentesis is used most often to remove the fluid without altering the hemodynamic equilibrium of the peritoneum. Blood chemistries should be drawn—specifically, serum protein, potassium, and sodium—and the ascitic fluid may be sent for gross inspection, cytology, cell count, chemistries, and microbiology. Paracentesis is a temporary measure. Unless the underlying reason for fluid accumulation is addressed, the ascitic fluid will recur.

Other approaches for fluid removal include intraperitoneal infusion therapy or peritoneovenous shunting, which is used less frequently. Intracavitary or intraperitoneal infusion therapy involves direct instillation of a drug into the abdominal cavity through a temporary or implanted catheter. The Pleurx catheter was used in one small study to improve patient comfort.[187] Radioactive colloids, chemotherapy, or biologic response modifiers can be administered through the intraperitoneal route. Once a catheter is placed, it offers a means of draining the fluid. A Tenckhoff catheter or an abdominal port is commonly utilized.

Peritoneovenous shunting entails placement of a continuous shunt that rechannels ascites fluid from the peritoneal cavity to the superior vena cava and eventually into the venous circulation. The shunt consists of a length of tubing, one end of which is placed in the peritoneal cavity; the other is tunneled subcutaneously and inserted into the superior vena cava.[186] The fluid flows upward into the superior vena cava via a one-way valve that opens with each inhalation as the intraperitoneal pressure increases and the intrathoracic pressure decreases.[183,188] Shunt malfunctions such as kinking or occlusion, pulmonary edema from rapid intravascular infusion of large quantities of fluid, disseminated intravascular coagulation, infection, and pulmonary embolus are all potential complications of this procedure. Shunting is reserved for untreatable disease and is appropriate if the time to reaccumulation of ascites is less than one month. It is usually reserved for those patients with a reasonable life expectancy where symptom relief is anticipated.[189] Mild diuretics are often prescribed but are usually not effective in diminishing ascites fluid.

Nursing care includes educating the patient to notify the physician or nurse when fluid starts to reaccumulate by measuring weight daily or abdominal girth daily or weekly. A bowel regimen may be needed to relieve constipation. Nursing care is aimed at relieving symptoms associated with ascites and minimizing further accumulation of the fluid. Instruct the patient to alternate activity with rest periods in an effort to conserve energy. Encourage the patient to lay on her left side with her feet elevated to alleviate pressure on the internal organs, improve vascular return from the lower extremities, facilitate lymphatic flow, and improve diuresis. Ascites can make it physically uncomfortable to eat, so consuming small frequent snacks or meals is suggested. An adequate protein intake and calories are needed to help increase low serum albumin levels. Families should offer calorie-rich beverages and encourage adequate fluids, especially after the paracentesis procedure, to restore fluid and electrolyte balance. Fluid restrictions may be imposed in some circumstances to minimize ascites reaccumulation. Ascites affects self-esteem, body image, and the ability to function. Assisting patients to take an active part in the management of ascites will lessen anxiety and help restore control.

Table 60-11 Signs and Symptoms of Intestinal Obstruction

Location	Signs and Symptoms
Small intestine	Colicky pain Vomiting Severe dehydration Minimal or absent distention
Lower small intestine	Less acute presentation Moderate vomiting Dehydration Some distention Lack of feces or flatus Severe electrolyte imbalances
Large intestine	Insidious Pronounced distention Lack of feces or flatus Overflow diarrhea Vomiting

Data from Martin.[185]

Intestinal Obstruction

The incidence of bowel obstruction is reported between 5.5% and 42% of patients with ovarian cancer.[190] With more advanced-stage disease, there is a higher probability of obstruction. Tumor or adhesions may cause extrinsic compression of the bowel. Obstruction can involve either the small or large intestine, can be acute or chronic, and can be partial or complete. Signs and symptoms depend on the location of the obstruction and are summarized in Table 60-11.[185]

When obstruction occurs, the bowel responds by increasing the force of peristalsis and attempting to move the bowel contents beyond the obstruction, so the first sounds are hyperactive bowel sounds.[191] After time the bowel tires and the peristalsis process slows. Hypoactive bowel sounds are then present.[191] A bowel obstruction with ovarian cancer most frequently tends to be an insidious process that progresses over weeks to months. An acute presentation of obstruction, such as perforation, is a rare complication. Accumulation of fluid in the bowel near the obstruction, increased gas from swallowed air, and overgrowth of bowel flora can all contribute to the compression problem.[188]

The most common presenting symptom is colicky abdominal pain. Abdominal distention usually occurs once the obstruction is established. Stools gradually become more infrequent and vomiting can occur with small bowel obstruction. If intestinal strangulation with ischemia is found, fever, rebound tenderness, and leukocytosis may be present.[188] A diagnosis is made based on presenting signs, physical findings, and a flat and upright x-ray film of the abdomen. The film will reveal dilated loops of bowel, increased gas and fluid accumulation, and multiple air–fluid levels.[188,191] Further testing might include a barium swallow with small bowel follow-through or a barium enema, an endoscopy, or a CT scan. A thorough assessment of the patient by the nurse includes evaluation for pain or abdominal tenderness, fever, distention, nausea, vomiting and quality of emesis, bowel pattern, history, bowel sounds, peritoneal signs, and fluid status.[188,190]

Medical treatment consists of relieving the distention, correcting the fluid imbalances, and removing the source of obstruction. Initial treatment may involve decompression of the bowel with a nasogastric tube or long intestinal tube or venting gastrostomy tube or simple bowel rest for 24–48 hours without oral intake. A retrospective chart review of 24 patients' records was done to examine the effectiveness of managing a bowel obstruction with a percutaneous endoscopic gastrostomy (PEG) tube. Seventy-five percent of the patients did not have nausea or vomiting at discharge, 92% resumed a clear liquid diet, 83% were discharged from the acute care setting, and 70% did not require readmission.[192] The PEG tube intervention effectively palliated the obstruction in these patients with advanced ovarian cancer. Intravenous fluids are administered simultaneously, if needed. Analgesics, antiemetics, anticholinergics, antihistamines, and somatostatin analogs are prescribed to manage pain, nausea, and vomiting, and to reduce gastrointestinal secretions. If no significant improvement occurs, surgery is considered. Intestinal stenting using colonic stents may provide a nonsurgical alternative for relief of the obstruction.

Decisions about surgery for advanced cancer are always difficult. Quality of life considerations and potential complications after surgery are significant factors that must be weighed against possible gains, because as many as one-third of patients with a bowel obstruction will develop another bowel obstruction from their advanced disease.[193] On the other side, the mortality rate from an ischemic bowel is 30% and patients who develop perforation, peritonitis, or bowel strangulation will likely require emergency surgery.[194] As part of an assessment for surgery, certain prognostic factors should be considered: the patient's age, tumor burden, nutritional status, and ability to tolerate additional chemotherapy after surgery to prevent further recurrence.[1] Surgery may involve lysis of the adhesions or a bypass procedure with a proximal diverting colostomy or ileostomy if the obstruction is in the colon. The goals of surgical intervention are to alleviate the obstruction, remove ischemic and necrotic tissue, prevent gangrene, and prevent sepsis.

Long-term medical management for patients who are not surgical candidates is achieved with placement of a gastrostomy tube. A gastrostomy tube is comfortable and patients can maintain adequate hydration by consuming small, low-residue fluid meals. Additionally, total parental nutrition may be initiated for temporary or permanent nutritional supplement. In advanced ovarian cancer, conservative management of a bowel obstruction through restricted oral intake is indicated and can be achieved while the patient is at home. Patients are instructed to begin taking small amounts of clear liquids after several hours of bowel rest and slowly advance their diet as tolerated. A low-fiber diet may be indicated because of profound narrowing of the small or large intestine.

Malnutrition

Anorexia and cachexia both lead to malnutrition.[195,196] The anorexia–cachexia syndrome can be caused by a bowel obstruction or dysfunction; excessive protein or fluid loss from the bowel; gastrointestinal symptoms such as nausea, vomiting, diarrhea, or early satiety; complications of chemotherapy; or psychologic factors.[1] Appetite and the ability to eat are closely linked to a patient's quality of life.[197] It is important to understand that the meaning of being able to eat is more significant than the nutritional or biological loss of food.[198] Unfortunately, the anorexia–cachexia symptom progresses as the ovarian cancer progresses.

Weight loss in cancer patients can influence both response to therapy and duration of survival.[197] In an Eastern Cooperative Oncology Group (ECOG) analysis of 3047 cancer patients on nine treatment protocols, median survival was significantly shorter for patients with weight loss compared with patients with no weight loss.[199] Patients should be evaluated first for reversible causes of decreased appetite, such as xerostomia and depression. Symptoms contributing to weight loss can include nausea, vomiting, diarrhea, fatigue, dyspnea, pain, and taste changes.[200]

Anorexia–cachexia syndrome is a major concern for nurses because its impact on patients is tremendous, coupled with disease and treatment side effects, physical weakness, fatigue, altered physical appearance, and loss of control over everyday life. The greater the degree of weight loss and malnutrition, the greater the degree of functional deficit and the higher the risk of complications.[201] Additionally, anorexia is most distressing to patients and their family members because those who have prepared the food may feel that they—not the food—are being rejected; as a consequence, tremendous struggles can develop over eating.[189]

An assessment of anorexia–cachexia involves subjective and objective measures including a food diary, daily weight measurements, tools to assess nutritional status and appetite, and blood tests. Severe weight loss is defined as an involuntary loss of more than 10% of usual body weight in six months or a 5% loss of usual body weight in one month; it is associated with poorer outcomes.[202,203] Early intervention is essential. The oral route of intervention is preferred because it is known that significant atrophy of intestinal villi occurs within days of decreased enteral stimulation.[194] Provide information on maintaining a well-balanced, high-calorie diet, enlist the help of a dietitian, and use nutritional supplements. Instruction includes tips on enhancing the flavor of foods, attention to the likes and dislikes of the patient, and avoiding foods with disturbing odors or tastes. Management of symptoms interfering with appetite may also be necessary.

Pharmacologic intervention for anorexia–cachexia include corticosteroids, appetite stimulants, metoclopramide, or cannabinoids. Corticosteroids may produce short-term improvements in appetite but are associated with adverse effects. Megestrol acetate demonstrated a dose-related benefit on appetite, caloric intake, body weight gain, and sensation of well-being with an optimal dose of 800 mg/day orally.[204–206]

A study of megesterol acetate versus dronabinol versus combination therapy found 75%, 49%, and 66% appetite increases, respectively.[207] Megesterol alone was the superior approach and had an improvement on the patients' quality of life.[207] Newer agents being studied include drugs to increase muscle mass, omega-3 fatty acids, growth hormones, and anticytokine therapies.[208] Nurses should assess food intake every 4 weeks and allow 8–12 weeks for weight gain. Successful intervention for anorexia–cachexia must focus on both the physiologic and psychologic factors influencing the development of the problem.

If adequate calories cannot be consumed by mouth, then nutritional support via the enteral route may be necessary. Enteral tube placement, such as a PEG tube (percutaneous endoscopically placed gastrostomy or jejunostomy tube), is an option. Total parental nutrition (TPN) should be reserved for those patients who are undergoing aggressive surgery, chemotherapy, or radiotherapy with severe gastrointestinal toxicity, or severely malnourished patients who are receiving active therapy. The difficult decision to initiate TPN must be made with the consensus of the entire medical team regarding its ethical appropriateness for a given patient.

Lymphedema

In ovarian cancer, lymphedema usually arises secondary to an obstruction or blockage of the lymph system caused by tumor or trauma to the lymphatic channels.[209] The dominant site for lymphedema in ovarian cancer is in the lower extremities because of blockage of the pelvic or inguinal lymph nodes. In the early stages of obstruction, compensatory mechanisms such as collateral lymphatic flow are activated, but often they prove insufficient and excessive accumulation of a protein-rich fluid in the tissue spaces ensues. Patients experience discomfort or pain, a fullness or heaviness of the extremity, numbness, weakness, and limited mobility. Clothing becomes increasingly tight and ambulation more difficult. Assessment is usually by patient self-report and measurement of the swollen limb. The current methods for assessing the extent of the lymphedema in the extremity are water displacement, circumferential measurements, calculation of the volume using the formula for a truncated cone, biometric impedance analysis, and comparative circumferential measurements.[210] CT scan or magnetic resonance imaging (MRI) can confirm a diagnosis of lymphedema and provide measures to characterize the degree of involvement: mild (stage I), moderate (stage II), or severe (stage III).[211] Management of lymphedema is related to the primary treatment of the cancer. With systemic chemotherapy, the lymph node involvement will shrink and the fluid will subsequently drain.

The stages of lymphedema, a description of the swollen limb's appearance and physical findings, and treatment are found in Table 60-12. Complex decongestive physiotherapy is a five-part regimen critical to successful management of lymphedema. It consists of skin care, manual lymphatic drainage (MLD), bandaging the affected limbs, exercises, and wearing a compression garment.[212] The mainstay of symptomatic lymphedema treatment is MLD performed by a physical therapist trained in lymphedema management. MLD entails light stimulation of the dermal lymphatomes and the lymphatic vessels; it is not to be confused with deep massage, which concentrates on the muscles.[211,213] By stimulating the lymphatic vessels, a therapist is able to redirect the protein-rich fluid around the affected area and increase the reabsorption of lymphatic fluid. Compression therapy is applied at the end of the one-hour session, wrapping the extremity with a low-pressure stretch bandage while carefully distributing pressure in a distal-to-proximal direction.[213] Patients are also instructed to perform exercises to increase flexion of the muscle, which creates resistance against the bandage to stimulate additional lymphatic flow. Patients are treated daily for four to five weeks during the initial phase. Maintenance therapy frequency is determined by the patient's response and the therapist's judgment. Compression garments should be worn continuously between treatments. Meticulous instructions regarding skin care are a component of the therapy plan, because skin of the edematous limb is at risk for breakdown and infection. If MLD no longer helps, gradient pressure pneumatic pumps may be prescribed. The pumps require a two-hour daily commitment and should be provided by a company that requires therapists and home counseling in conjunction with the treatment.

Limitations of mobility are difficult for patients to deal with because many people try to maintain their normal activities despite progressive disease. Diuretics are of limited benefit in the treatment of edema due to advanced disease. The nurse needs to engage women in protecting their legs from infection or trauma, provide nursing care that includes educating women about the early signs and symptoms of lymphedema, and provde information on how to access specialists early so that effective management can be initiated.[214] Lower limb lymphedema has an impact on appearance, mobility, finances, and self-image in many women.[214]

Table 60-12 Management of Lymphedema

Stages of Lymphedema	Findings	Treatment
Stage I (reversible)	Skin smooth, textured	Elevate extremity
	Pitting edema	Compression garment
	2–3 cm difference between limb circumference	Massage
	Limb feels heavy, throbbing	Physical therapy
Stage II (chronic, does not reverse spontaneously)	Limb is swollen	Same as stage I; if ineffective begin complex decongestive physiotherapy
	Edema, NOT pitting	
	Skin stretched, shiny	
	Tissue soft	
	3–5 cm difference in limb circumference	
Stage III (severe)	Extreme increase in swelling until the limb is column shaped, NOT pitting	Aggressive treatment
	Hand or foot massively swollen	May use gradient
	Skin dark or purple colored	Pneumatic pressure
	Skin stretched, tissue firm	Pump therapy
	Rough textured	Pain management
	Lymph leaks directly through the skin	
	> 5 cm difference in limb circumference	

Data from Martin.[185]

Pleural Effusion

Pleural effusions are an accumulation of fluid in excess of the normal 25 mL of fluid within the intrapleural space.[215] Approximately 25%–30% of patients with metastatic ovarian cancer develop pleural effusions.[1,216] They develop when the flow of pleural fluid from the parietal pleura to the visceral pleura is interrupted by tumor. The effusion may be exudate or transudate in nature. Two major pathophysiologic processes are associated with exudative effusion: an inflammatory process and neoplastic disease. Dyspnea caused by the accumulating effusion is the most commonly reported symptom.[215,217,218] Sharp pleuritic chest pain, if present, may or may not be accompanied by a pleural rub.[215,217] Other symptoms associated with a pleural effusion include fever (if inflammatory), dry irritating cough, and hypoxia.[215] Effusions are diagnosed by a posterior, anterior, and lateral chest x-ray. On physical exam, findings include decreased breath sounds and dullness to percussion, most often in the lung base.

Once the diagnosis of pleural effusion is made, a thoracentesis may be required to remove the excess fluid if it is causing significant impairment. An ultrasound is often used to locate the fluid for removal during a thoracentesis. The patient must be prepared for the procedure and its possible complications, which include pain, infection, pneumothorax, and pulmonary edema. The nurse must observe for any pain or discomfort, increased respiratory rate or dyspnea, increased pulse rate, vertigo, or uncontrollable cough during the procedure.[1] The fluid is removed and sent for diagnostic studies. A chest x-ray is performed after the procedure to rule out a pneumothorax. The fluid will usually rapidly reaccumulate in four to five days, unless the underlying cause of the problem, the ovarian cancer, is effectively treated with systemic chemotherapy.

The Pleurx pleural catheter is a new treatment option that allows patients to be treated on an outpatient basis for weeks or months.[219] The catheter is a 66-cm, 15.5-French, flexible silicone catheter that is surgically inserted into the pleural space and held in place by a polyester cuff. It remains in place and the family members are taught how to drain it on an intermittent basis.

Insertion of a chest tube or thoracostomy and the addition of a sclerosing agent or pleurodesis may also be performed if pleural fluid reaccumulates. The sclerosing procedure requires hospitalization; the chest tube is inserted at the bedside and the tube is connected to suction for several days. As the drainage diminishes, the pleural space is obliterated using a sclerosing agent to prevent the fluid reaccumulation. In women whose effusion cannot be adequately drained or in whom the lung does not reexpand, but who have a reasonable life expectancy, open pleurodesis or a pleuroperitoneal shunt may be considered.[188]

The severe dyspnea caused by a pleural effusion can be controlled in sedentary patients who have advanced disease with oxygen and/or opioids.[188] Opioids decrease the intensity of dyspnea and the sense of respiratory effort.[220] Morphine, hydromorphone, and fentanyl are all used and can be given via any route. The use of nebulized opiods can assist with dyspnea. By providing information concerning palliative measures to manage this distressing side effect, the nurse can help lessen anxiety, because pleural effusion is an undeniable indicator of disease progression. Relaxation exercises are helpful in decreasing anxiety and may include guided imagery, progressive relaxation with controlled breathing, listening to relaxing music, mild massage, and range-of-motion exercises.[221] Exercises to help with breathlessness include sitting upright and leaning forward, leaning over a table, or resting elbows on knees to promote lung expansion and help the patient breathe easier.[221] Patients must modify their activities of daily living and plan frequent rest periods for increased support.

Stress and Support

The impact of ovarian cancer on quality of life has been examined in a few studies.[222–226] High rates of anxiety and depression have been noted during chemotherapy treatment and high distress levels continue for one-third of long-term survivors.[222,223,227] Guidozzi found significant psychological distress in patients that impaired physical function.[227] For these distressed women, relief came from psychological counseling and support and improvement in their physical symptoms. Women who experienced pain and fatigue lost the ability to enjoy life, engage in normal relationship activities, and maintain employment status.[228] Increased family stress arose from anxiety about the diagnosis and treatment, sexual changes, and fears about prognosis.[223,225] Women reported problems with pain, appetite, fatigue, and finances that had a significant impact on their quality of life, and these symptoms worsened as the disease progressed.[222,226]

Positive changes have also been reported about the way some women's have changed after the diagnosis.[223] A new appreciation of life and adoption of a "live for the moment" philosophy have been reported.[223]

One qualitative study describing the concerns of women with ovarian cancer found increased distress because of the compressed time frame in which to confront life-threatening issues.[229] The group expressed overwhelming feelings of helplessness and uncertainty while facing mortality and redefining goals and expectations. Another study examined 21,806 letters, cards, and e-mails reflecting correspondence between ovarian cancer survivors and the editor of an ovarian cancer newsletter between 1994 and 2000. These authors identified major themes during all phases of the disease trajectory. Unique psychological factors found included: The women experienced profound isolation living with ovarian cancer; they contended with anxiety resulting from the genetic association of the disease and fear for their daughters more often than fear for themselves; and the stress of living with periods of recurrence created considerable stress and uncertainty.[230] The investigators hope to use the coping strategies identified in this study to build interventions that healthcare providers can use to assist women with ovarian cancer.[230]

Because ovarian cancer is a disease that commonly recurs, research looking at the time period after primary therapy and during disease recurrence has added to the knowledge base of the disease. The continual monitoring of the CA-125 level serves as a constant reminder of the potential for recurrence. Hamilton noted that women identified their CA-125 levels as evidence of disease status and that their emotions were governed by the value of the marker.[231]

In another study, 263 women returned surveys eliciting important issues associated with ovarian cancer. The respondents included 93 women who had experienced recurrent disease and 170 who had not. A greater proportion of the women with recurrent disease reported bowel problems, fear of dying, pain, problems getting around, and feelings of self-blame.[232] Overall, women with recurrent disease reported experiencing more problems since diagnosis than those without recurrent disease.[232] A particular concern raised in this study was that a significant proportion of women felt they had not received adequate help for the problems they experienced. Two specific areas of inadequate assistance were difficulties with bowels and sexual function.[232] These women perceived nurses as being helpful to them, thereby creating opportunities for nurses to provide more support.

In a more recent study, 18 women with ovarian cancer were interviewed and identified the following major challenges: living with uncertainty, lack of control, fear of the unknown, the stigma of cancer, and facing death.[233] These authors outline the implications of their findings for nursing practice: family-centered care to help deal with the adjustments in roles and relationships; a sensitivity to financial issues; the ability to express fears and anxieties about death; and assistance in planning for the future.[233] As these women faced recurrent disease, four primary themes surfaced: waiting for recurrence, facing the diagnosis of recurrence, managing treatment-related concerns, and attempting to regain control.[228] More important, these women described changed communication with their healthcare providers when recurrent disease was found. They felt increased hopelessness as a result of their perception that the provider was not listening to their symptoms and had no treatment options to present.[228] The message these patients received was that symptom management rather than prolongation of life had become the goal, and this caused them distress.

Finally, studying women without active disease has yielded additional information. In one study, 200 women who had ovarian cancer, were without evidence of active disease, and were not on treatment for at least two years were surveyed. Most respondents reported good physical, psychological, social, and spiritual health. However, the cancer experience did have a detrimental effect (57% reported) on the women's sex lives.[234] Nurses therefore have an opportunity to educate these women about their sexual health.

Patient support groups offer another way to provide emotional support to ovarian cancer patients. In a support group for patients with ovarian cancer, over a two-year period 30 women discussed two consistent themes: "fate versus freedom" (the struggle to face the real possibility of dying versus the freedom to enjoy life) and "despair versus hope" (the struggle to give in to loss, pain, and dejection versus maintaining optimism).[235] Struggling with these existential issues stood out as the most important therapeutic factor in this support group.

Information gained from surveys and interviews of patients with ovarian cancer, provides nurses with valuable insight into the experience of living with this disease. Nurses can help patients understand the information and meaning of monitoring for disease recurrence and provide more sensitive communication about their treatment options. They play key roles in helping women with ovarian cancer by providing both physical and emotional care during the disease trajectory and improving quality of life.

Patient Resources

Following the path established by the successful breast cancer and AIDS advocacy groups, ovarian cancer now has a public voice. The Ovarian Cancer National Alliance (OCNA), formed in 1997, is an organization with a mission of uniting organizations and individuals in the fight to overcome ovarian cancer. The National Ovarian Cancer Coalition (NOCC) was founded by a group of ovarian cancer survivors in April 1995. It now has more than 2000 members and 23 state chapters. The mission of NOCC is to raise awareness about ovarian cancer and to promote education about the disease. The alliance and coalition succeeded in having September 1998 designated as the first National Ovarian Cancer Awareness Month. President Clinton designated September 13–19, 1998, as the first Ovarian Cancer Awareness Week. OCNA held the initial national advocacy conference on ovarian cancer called "Silent No More" in September 1998, with other founding partner and member organizations.

In 1994, the NCI held the first consensus development conference devoted to screening, prevention, diagnosis, and treatment of ovarian cancer. Funding increased steadily for women's health from 1987 to 1996.[236] Today, ovarian cancer research and education initiatives seem to be close to getting an appropriate share of NCI monies budgeted for women's health. Bills remain before Congress asking for $90 million dollars for ovarian cancer research, and one Special Program of Research Excellence (SPORE) grant application has been approved.[236]

The Web sites *www.ovarian.org* and *www.ovariancancer.org* offer a multitude of information and include a chat forum and an "Ask the Experts" page. Other general information resources include the American Cancer Society, National Cancer Institute Cancer Information Service; Society of Gynecologic Oncologists; Gilda Radner Familial Ovarian Cancer Registry; and Gynecologic Cancer Foundation Information Hotline. Resources focusing on support include CancerCare; National Coalition for Cancer Survivorship; Gilda's Club; SHARE; and the Wellness Community. Addresses, phone numbers, and Internet addresses are provided in Table 60-13.

A new diagnosis of an unfamiliar disease prompted one woman to launch her own network of support. She was desperate to talk with another woman like herself, specifically a survivor, which led to the birth of a newsletter titled *Conversations*, for women fighting ovarian cancer.[237] *Conversations* started with a circulation of ten, but has grown considerably over the last ten years. Unfortunately, the editor lost her battle with ovarian cancer in 2003, but her family has continued to produce the newsletter for other women with ovarian cancer. The newsletter is filled with tips for dealing with treatment side effects and the latest clinical trials available for patients seeking treatments. The address for subscribing to this newsletter is P.O. Box 7948, Amarillo, Texas, 79114-7948.

Continuity of Care

Because no effective screening methods for ovarian cancer exist, this disease is often discovered in its late stages. Continuity of care during the long and chronic course of treating ovarian cancer is an area warranting concentration by the nurse. The trajectory of primary treatment and then management of the complications

Table 60-13 Resources for Ovarian Cancer Information

National Ovarian Cancer Coalition (NOCC) 500 N. E. Spanish River Boulevard, Suite 14 Boca Raton, Florida 33431 888-OVARIAN *www.ovarian.org*
National Ovarian Cancer Alliance 910 17th Street N. W. Suite 413 Washington, DC 20006 202-331-1332 *www.ovariancancer.org*
Women's Cancer Network c/o Gynecologic Cancer Foundation 401 N. Michigan Avenue Chicago, IL 60611 312-644-6610 *www.wcn.org*
CancerCare, Inc. 275 Seventh Avenue New York, NY 10001 800-813-HOPE *www.cancercare.org*
Gilda Radner Ovarian Cancer Familial Registry Roswell Park Cancer Institute Elm and Carlton Streets Buffalo, NY 14263 800-OVARIAN *www.ovariancancer.com*
Conversations! The Newsletter for Those Fighting Ovarian Cancer P.O. Box 7948 Amarillo, Texas 79114-7948 806-355-2565 *www.ovarian-news.com*
Marsha Rivkin Ovarian Cancer Research Center 1221 Madison St. Seattle, Washington 98104 206-215-6200 *www.marsharivkin.org*
National Ovarian Cancer Association 27 Park Rd. Toronto, Canada 877-413-7970 *www.ovariancanada.org*
Ovarian Cancer Research Fund, Inc. One Pennsylvania Plaza, Suite 1610 New York, NY 10119 800-873-9569 *www.ocrf.org*
SHARE: Self-help for Women with Breast or Ovarian Cancer 1501 Broadway, Ste 1720 New York, NY 10036 212-719-1204 *www.sharecancersupport.org*

in advanced disease are often centered in the outpatient or home setting. The acute phase of care in an inpatient setting usually occurs during the early phase of the disease treatment or briefly during a crisis of treatment or advanced disease. Nurses are in the key position to educate patients on the prevention and control of the side effects from treatment or disease progression so that their quality of life can be maintained. The plan for continuity of care must include seamless access to necessary care as needs arise, and information must flow between caregivers irrespective of their practice settings.

Ambulatory and office nurses are critical links to support and guide ovarian cancer patients. For example, the patient typically uses self-care measures to monitor the reaccumulation of ascites fluid and the nurse is informed when weight gain or discomfort reaches an unacceptable level. The nurse consults with the physician and a plan is developed to relieve the existing problem. In other instances, surgical intervention for a partial intestinal obstruction may not be possible in an advanced disease case. It is then the nurse who helps the patient and family cope with the problem until the end of life.

Addressing emotional needs is as important a component of nursing care as managing symptoms. Helping the patient and family cope with the end of life is central to the role and skills of the oncology nurse. Dealing with anxiety and depression and preventing feelings of abandonment or despair are a few of the psychosocial needs of both the patient and family during the final stages of the disease. Involvement of the hospice team when appropriate will add support at a critical phase of need for the patient and family. At each phase and step along the trajectory of ovarian cancer care, collaboration between healthcare team members, the patient, and the family is critical.

Future Trends

The five-year survival rate for ovarian cancer has improved from 37% in the 1970s to 53% in 1998. Ovarian cancer is now considered a chronic disease.[238] Much still remains to be discovered regarding its development, although it is believed to be a multistep process that involves alterations in several genes.[239] Two gene mutations have been identified in hereditary forms of the disease but how their discovery fits together with nonhereditary ovarian cancer is not yet known.[239] Several identified factors may increase an individual's risk, and attention has turned to identifying molecular markers (genomic and proteomic) to improve the predictive value of screening.[239] Future directions for treatment of ovarian cancer include research aimed at screening and prevention, finding a molecular basis for ovarian cancer, identifying high-risk individuals, and targeted therapy with molecular profiling. Chemotherapy will continue to have a major role in the treatment of ovarian cancer in the future, with clinical trials helping to establish the regimen of choice. Subsequent trials will combine chemotherapy with molecular-targeted biologic agents as initial treatment for ovarian cancer patients. New targeted therapy in ovarian cancer appears particularly promising. The current treatment regimens induce a state where minimal disease is present. In this situation the newer therapies may be at their most effective, and they may ultimately be continued as maintenance therapy to prevent or delay recurrences.[239] Drug resistance mechanisms and pharmacologic techniques to reverse the resistance are also major areas of clinical research.

Nursing research has made gains in increasing our knowledge base about living with ovarian cancer and some of the most important challenges faced by patients. Ovarian cancer is particularly difficult due to its advanced stage at diagnosis, the repetitive cycles of aggressive treatment with little respite, and the dismal survival statistics that serve as a constant reminder of the disease's seriousness to patients. Patients need to be assessed more thoroughly and given more information throughout the treatment trajectory. Support group referrals may be particularly helpful.[240] Nurses are key in improving awareness of the disease so that education is available and no delay in diagnosis occurs. The chronic nature of ovarian cancer challenges providers to balance quality of life issues with treatment toxicities.[240] The healthcare team will continue to be challenged to keep pace as new treatments for ovarian cancer enter the clinical arena and new patient care strategies unfold. The nurse on the healthcare team has the opportunity to make an invaluable contribution.

References

1. Eriksson JH, Frazier SR: Epithelial cancers of the ovary and fallopian tube, in Moore GJ (ed.): *Women and Cancer: A Gynecologic Oncology Nursing Perspective.* Sudbury, MA, Jones and Bartlett, 1997, pp 205–256
2. Jemal A, Tiwari RC, Murray T, et al: Cancer statistics 2004. *CA Cancer J Clin* 54:8–29, 2004
3. Surveillance, Epidemiology, and End Results Program: *SEER Cancer Statistics Review, 1975–2001.* National Cancer Institute, Bethesda, MD, 2004
4. Piver MS: Hereditary ovarian cancer. *Gynecol Oncol* 85:9–17, 2002
5. Whittemore AS, Harris R, Intyre J: Characteristics relating to ovarian cancer risk: collaborative analysis of 12 US case-control studies. IV. The pathogenesis of epithelial ovarian cancer. Collaborative Ovarian Cancer Group. *Am J Epidemiol* 136:1184–1203 1992.
6. Fathalla MF: Incessant ovulation — a factor in ovarian neoplasia? *Lancet* 2:163, 1971
7. Ozols RF, Bookman MA, Connolly DC, et al: Focus on epithelial ovarian cancer. *Cancer Cell* 5:19–24, 2004
8. Schlosshauer PW, Coeh CJ, Penault-Liorca F, et al: Prophylactic oophorectomy: a morphologic and immunohistochemical study. *Cancer* 98:2599–2606, 2003
9. Cramer DW, Welch WR: Determinants in ovarian cancer risk. II. Inferences regarding pathogenesis. *J Natl Cancer Inst* 49:717–721, 1983
10. Risch HA: Hormonal etiology of epithelial ovarian cancer, with a hypothesis concerning the role of androgens and progesterone. *J Natl Cancer Inst* 90:1774–1786, 1998
11. Ness RB, Cottreau C: Possible role of ovarian epithelial inflammation in ovarian cancer. *J Natl Cancer Inst* 91:1459–1467, 1999
12. Cramer DW, Barbieri RL, Faer AR, et al: Determinants of early follicular phase gonadotropin and estradiol concentrations in women of late reproductive age. *Hum Reprod* 17:221–227, 2002
13. Daly M, Obrams GI: Epidemiology and risk assessment for ovarian cancer. *Semin Oncol* 25:255–264, 1998
14. Hankinson SE, Colditz GA, Hunter DJ, et al: A prospective study of reproductive factors and risk of epithelial ovarian cancer. *Cancer* 76:284–290, 1995
15. Adami HO, Hsieh CC, Lambe M, et al: Parity, age at first childbirth, and risk of ovarian cancer. *Lancet* 344:1250–1254, 1994
16. Whittemore AS: Characteristics relating to ovarian cancer risk: implications for prevention and detection. *Gynecol Oncol* 55:515–519, 1994
17. Rossing MA, Daling JR, Weiss NS, et al: Ovarian tumors in a cohort of infertile women. *N Engl J Med* 52:161–183, 1994
18. Gross TP, Schlesselman JJ: The estimated effect of oral contraceptive use on the cumulative risk of epithelial ovarian cancer. *Obstet Gynecol* 83:419–424, 1994
19. Hankinson SE, Colditz GA, Hunter DJ, et al: A quantitative assessment of oral contraceptive use and risk of ovarian cancer. *Obstet Gynecol* 80:708–714, 1992
20. Narod SA, Risch P, Moslehi R, et al: Oral contraceptives and the risk of hereditary ovarian cancer. *N Engl J Med* 339:424–428, 1998
21. Modan B, Hartge P, Hirsh-Yechezel G, et al: Parity, oral contraceptives, and the risk of ovarian cancer among carriers and noncarriers of a BRCA1 and BRCA 2 mutation. *N Engl J Med* 334:235–240, 2001
22. Research Reports: Progestin may prevent ovarian cancers by triggering death of damaged ovarian cells. *Oncology* 12:1666–1667, 1998
23. Anderson GL, Judd HL, Kaunitz AM, et al: Effects of estrogen plus progestin on gynecologic cancers and associated diagnostic procedures: the Women's Health Initiative randomized trial. *JAMA* 290:1739–1748, 2003
24. Coughlin SS, Giustozzi A, Smith SJ, et al: A meta-analysis of estrogen replacement therapy and risk of epithelial ovarian cancer. *J Clin Epidemiol* 53:367–375, 2000
25. Sit AS, Modugno F, Weissfeld JL, et al: Hormone replacement therapy formulations and risk of epithelial ovarian carcinoma. *Gynecol Oncol* 86:118–123, 2002
26. Helzlsouer KJ, Alberg AJ, Gordon GB, et al: Serum gonadotropin and steroid hormones and the development of ovarian cancer. *JAMA* 274:1926–1930, 1995
27. Schildkraut J, Schwingl PJ, Bastos E, et al: Epithelial ovarian cancer risk among women with polycystic ovarian syndrome. *Obstet Gynecol* 88:554–559, 1996

28. Brinton LA, Gridley G, Persson I, et al: Cancer risk after a hospital discharge of endometriosis. *Am J Obstet Gynecol* 176:572–579, 1997
29. Schildkraut JM, Bastos E, Berchuck A: Relationship between lifetime ovulatory cycles and overexpression of mutant p53 in epithelial ovarian cancer. *J Natl Cancer Inst* 89:932–938, 1997
30. Hankinson SE, Hunter DJ, Colditz GA, et al: Tubal ligation, hysterectomy, and risk of ovarian cancer: a prospective study. *JAMA* 270:2813–2818, 1993
31. Cramer DW, Muto MG, Reichardt JK, et al: Characteristics of women with a family history of ovarian cancer. I. Galactose consumption and metabolism. *Cancer* 74:1309–1317, 1994
32. Risch HA, Jain M, Marrett LD, et al: Dietary lactose intake, lactose intolerance, and the risk of ovarian cancer in southern Ontario (Canada). *Cancer Causes Control* 5:540–548, 1994
33. Herrinton LJ, Weiss NS, Beresford SA, et al: Lactose and galactose intake and metabolism in relation to the risk of epithelial ovarian cancer. *Am J Epidemiol* 141:407–416, 1995
34. Mink PJ, Folsom AR, Sellers TA, et al: Physical activity, waist-to-hip ratio, and other risk factors for ovarian cancer: a follow-up study of older women. *Epidemiology* 7:38–45, 1996
35. Harlow BL, Cramer D, Bell DA, et al: Perineal exposure to talc and ovarian cancer risk. *Obstet Gynecol* 80:19–26, 1992
36. Cramer D, Welch WR, Scully RE, et al: Ovarian cancer and talc — a case control study. *Cancer* 50:372–376, 1982
37. Wong C, Hempling RE, Piver MS, et al: Perineal talc exposure and subsequent epithelial ovarian cancer: a case control study. *Obstet Gynecol* 93:372–376, 1999
38. Cramer DW, Liberman RF, Titus-Ernstoff L, et al: Genital talc exposure and risk of ovarian cancer. *Int J Cancer* 81:351–356, 1999
39. Gertig DM, Hunter DJ, Cramer DW, et al: Prospective study of talc use and ovarian cancer. *J Natl Cancer Inst* 92:249–252, 2000
40. National Institutes of Health Consensus Development Conference Statement: Ovarian cancer: screening, treatment, and follow-up. April 5–7, 1994. *Gynecol Oncol* 55:S4–S14, 1994
41. Hall JM, Lee MK, Neuman B, et al: Linkage of early-onset breast cancer to chromosome 17q21. *Science* 250:1684–1689, 1991
42. Narod SA, Feunteun J, Lynch HT, et al: Familial breast–ovarian cancer locus on chromosome 17q12–q23. *Lancet* 388:82–83, 1991
43. Miki Y, Swensen J, Shattuck-Eidens D, et al: A strong candidate for the breast and ovarian cancer susceptibility gene BRCA1. *Science* 266:66–71, 1994
44. Wooster R, Neuhausen SL, Mangion J, et al: Localization of a breast cancer susceptibility gene, BRCA2, to chromosome 13q12–13. *Science* 265:1088–2090, 1994
45. Wooster R, Bignell G, Lancaster J, et al: Identification of the breast cancer susceptibility gene BRCA2. *Nature* 378:789–792, 1995
46. Reedy M, Gallion H, Fowler JM, et al: Contribution of BRCA 1 and BRCA 2 to familial ovarian cancer: a Gynecologic Oncology Group study. *Gynecol Oncol* 85:255–259, 2002
47. Struewing JP, Abeliovich D, Peretz T, et al: The carrier frequency of the BRCA1 185delAG mutations is approximately 1 percent in Ashkenazi Jewish individuals. *Nat Genet* 11:198–200,1995
48. Abeliovich D, Kaduri L, Lerer I, et al: The founder mutations in 185delAG and 5382insC in BRCA1 and 617delIT in BRCA2 appear in 60% of ovarian cancer and 30% of early-onset breast cancer patients among Ashkenazi women. *Am J Hum Genet* 60:505–514, 1997
49. Lynch HT, Casey MJ, Shaw TG, et al: Hereditary factors in gynecologic cancer. *Oncologist* 3:319–338, 1998
50. Lynch HT, Casey MJ, Lynch J, et al: Genetics and ovarian carcinoma. *Semin Oncol* 25:265–280, 1998
51. Modugno F, Ovarian Cancer and High-Risk Women Symposium presenters: Ovarian cancer and high-risk women — implications for prevention, screening, and early detection. *Gynecol Oncol* 91:15–31, 2003
52. Cherry C, Vacchiano SA: Ovarian cancer screening and prevention. *Semin Oncol Nursing* 18:167–173, 2002
53. Bast R, Klug T, St John E, et al: A radioimmunoassay using a monoclonal antibody to monitor the course of epithelial ovarian cancer. *N Engl J Med* 309:883–887, 1993
54. Bast RC, Xu FJ, Yu YH, et al: CA 125: the past and the future. *Int J Biol Markers* 13:179–187, 1998
55. Jacobs I: Combinations of markers in screening for ovarian cancer. *Int J Gynecol Obstet* 46:83–86, 1994
56. Woolas RP, Xu FJ, Jacobs IJ, et al: Evaluation of multiple serum markers in patients with stage I ovarian cancer. *J Natl Cancer Inst* 85:1748–1751, 1993
57. Berek JS, Bast RC Jr: Ovarian cancer screening: the use of serial complementary tumor markers to improve sensitivity and specificity for early detection. *Cancer* 76:2092–2096, 1995
58. Cane P, Azen C, Lopez E, et al: Tumor marker trends in asymptomatic women at risk for ovarian cancer: relevance for ovarian cancer screening. *Gynecol Oncol* 57:240–245, 1995
59. Skates SJ, Xu FJ, Yu YH, et al: Toward an optimal algorithm for ovarian cancer screening with longitudinal tumor markers. *Cancer* 76:2004–2010, 1995
60. Nagele F, Petru E, Medl M, et al: Preoperative CA 125; an independent prognostic factor in patients with stage I epithelial ovarian cancer. *Obstet Gynecol* 86:259–264, 1995
61. Rosenthal A, Jacobs I: Ovarian cancer screening. *Semin Oncol* 25:315–323, 1998
62. Skates SJ, Menon U, MacDonald N, et al: Calculation of the risk of ovarian cancer from serial CA-125 values for preclinical detection in postmenopausal women. *J Clin Oncol* 21:206–210, 2003
63. Van Der Burg MEL, Lammes FB, Van Putten WLJ, et al: Ovarian cancer: the prognostic value of the serum half life of CA 125 during induction chemotherapy. *Gynecol Oncol* 30:307–312, 1988
64. Rustin GJS, Nelstrop AE, McClean P, et al: Defining response of ovarian carcinoma to initial chemotherapy according to serum CA 125. *J Clin Oncol* 14:1545–1551, 1996
65. Shy K, Dubinsky T: Is color Doppler ultrasound useful in diagnosing ovarian cancer? *Clin Obstet Gynecol* 42:902–915, 1999
66. van Nagell JR, DePriest PD, Reedy MB, et al: The efficacy of transvaginal ultrasonographic screening in asymptomatic women at risk for ovarian cancer. *Gynecol Oncol* 77:350–356, 2000
67. Kauff ND, Satagopan JM, Robson ME, et al: Risk-reducing salpingo-oophorectomy in women with a BRCA1 or BRCA2 mutation. *N Engl J Med* 346:1609–1615, 2002
68. Rebbeck TR, Lynch HT, Neuhausen SL, et al: Prophylactic oophorectomy in carriers of BRCA1 or BRCA2 mutations. *N Engl J Med* 346:1616–1622, 2002
69. Tobacman JK, Greene MH, Tucker MA, et al: Intra-abdominal carcinomatosis after prophylactic oophorectomy in ovarian cancer–prone families. *Lancet* 2:795–797, 1982
70. Piver MS, Jishi MF, Tsukada Y, et al: Primary peritoneal carcinoma after prophylactic oophorectomy in women with a family history of ovarian cancer: a report of the Gilda Radner Familial Ovarian Cancer Registry. *Cancer* 71:2751–2755, 1993
71. Struewing JP, Watson P, Easton DF, et al: Prophylactic oophorectomy in inherited breast/ovarian cancer families. *J Natl Cancer Inst Monogr* 17:33–35, 1995

72. Petricoin EF, Ardekani AM, Hitt BA, et al: Use of proteomic patterns in serum to identify ovarian cancer. *Lancet* 359:572–577, 2002
73. Bast RC Jr, Boyer CM, Jacobs I: Cell growth regulation in epithelial ovarian cancer. *Cancer* 71:1597–1601, 1993
74. Prowse A, Frolov A, Godwin AK: The genetics of ovarian cancer, in Ozols RF (ed.): *American Cancer Society Atlas of Clinical Oncology*, Hamilton, Ontario: BC Decker, 2003 pp 49–82
75. DiSaia PJ: Diagnosis and management of ovarian cancer. *Hosp Pract* 22:235–250, 1987
76. Omura GA, Brady MF, Homesley HD, et al: Long term follow up and prognostic factor analysis in advanced ovarian carcinoma: the Gynaecological Oncology Group experience. *J Clin Oncol* 9:1138–1150, 1991
77. van Houwelingen JC, ten Bokkel Huinink W, van der Burg ATM, et al: Predictability of the survival of patients with ovarian cancer. *J Clin Oncol* 7:769–773, 1989
78. Voest EE, van Houwelingen JC, Nejit JP: A meta-analysis of prognostic factors in advanced ovarian cancer with median survival and overall survival measured with the log (relative risk) as main objectives. *Eur J Cancer Clin Oncol* 28A:1328–1330, 1989
79. Thigpen T, Brady MF, Omura GA, et al: Age as a prognostic factor in ovarian carcinoma: the Gynaecological Oncology Group experience. *Cancer* 71:(suppl)606–614, 1993
80. Havrilesky L, Darcy KM, Hamdan H, et al: Prognostic significance of p53 mutation and p53 overexpression in advanced epithelial ovarian cancer: a Gynecologic Oncology Group study. *J Clin Oncol* 21:3814–3825, 2003
81. van der Zee AGT, Hollema H, Suurmeijer AJH, et al: Value of p-glycoprotein, glutathione s-transferase pi, c-erbB-2, and p53 as prognostic factors in ovarian carcinomas. *J Clin Oncol* 13:70–78, 1995
82. Igoe BA: Symptoms attributed to ovarian cancer by women with the disease. *Nurse Pract* 22:122–144, 1997
83. Goff B, Mandel L, Muntz HG, et al: Ovarian cancer diagnosis. *Cancer* 89:2068–2075, 2000
84. Radner G: *It's Always Something.* New York, Avon Books, 1989
85. National Ovarian Cancer Coalition: 500 NE Spanish River Blvd, Suite 14, Boca Raton FL
86. Mayer AR, Chambers SK, Graves E, et al: Ovarian cancer staging: does it require a gynecologic oncologist? *Gynecol Oncol* 47:223–227, 1992
87. Nguyen HN, Averette HE, Hoskins W, et al: National survey of ovarian carcinoma. Part V. The impact of physicians' specialty on patients' survival. *Cancer* 72:3663–3670, 1993
88. Eisenkop SM, Spirtos NM, Montag TW, et al: The impact of subspecialty training on the management of advanced ovarian cancer. *Gynecol Oncol* 47:203–209, 1992
89. Scully RE: Tumors of the ovary and maldeveloped gonads, in Rosai J, Sobun LH (eds.): *Atlas of Tumor Pathology.* Washington, DC, Armed Forces Institute, 1998, pp 340-358.
90. International Federation of Gynecology and Obstetrics: Changes in definition of clinical staging for carcinoma of the cervix and ovary. *Am J Obstet Gynecol* 156:263–264, 1987
91. Partridge EE, Phillips JL, Menck HR: The National Cancer Database report on ovarian cancer treatment in the United States hospitals. *Cancer* 78:2239–2246, 1996
92. Friedlander ML: Prognostic factors in ovarian cancer. *Semin Oncol* 25:305–314, 1998
93. Griffths CT, Park LM, Fuller AF: Role of cytoreductive surgery in the management of advanced ovarian cancer. *Cancer Treat Rep* 63:235–240, 1979
94. Hogberg T, Carstensen J, Simonsen E: Treatment results and prognostic factors in a population-based study of epithelial ovarian cancer. *Gynecol Oncol* 48:38–49, 1993
95. Eisenkop S, Nalick R, Teng N: Peritoneal implant excision or ablation during cytoreductive surgery. The impact on survival. *Gynecol Oncol* 45:97, 1993 (abstr)
96. Young RC, Walton L, Ellenberg SS, et al: Adjuvant therapy in stage I and II epithelial ovarian cancer. Results of two prospective randomized trials. *N Engl J Med* 322:1021–1027, 1990
97. Bertelson K, Holund B, Anderson E: Reproducibility and prognostic value of histologic type and grade in early epithelial ovarian cancer. *Int J Gynecol Cancer* 3:72–79, 1993
98. Shimizu Y, Kamai S, Amada S, et al: Toward the development of a universal grading system for ovarian epithelial carcinoma. *Cancer* 82:893–901, 1998
99. Boente MP, Chi DS, Hoskins WJ: The role of surgery in the management of ovarian cancer: primary and interval cytoreductive surgery. *Semin Oncol* 25:326–334, 1998
100. Munoz KA, Harlan CC, Trimble EL: Patterns of care for women with ovarian cancer in the United States. *J Clin Oncol* 15:3408–3415, 1997
101. Mutch DG: Surgical management of ovarian cancer. *Semin Oncol* 29(suppl 1):3–8, 2002
102. Curtin JP, Malik R, Venkatraman ES, et al: Stage IV ovarian cancer: impact of surgical debulking. *Gynecol Oncol* 18:161-163, 1997
103. Rubin SC, Hoskins WJ, Hakes TB, et al: Recurrence after negative second look laparotomy for ovarian cancer: analysis of risk factors. *Am J Obstet Gynecol* 159:1094–1098, 1988
104. Nicoletto MO, Tumolo S, Talamini R, et al: Surgical second look in ovarian cancer: a randomized study in patients with laparoscopic complete remission — a Northeastern Oncology Cooperative Group — Ovarian Cancer Cooperative Group Study. *J Clin Oncol* 15:994–997, 1997
105. Webb MJ, Decker DG, Mussey E, et al: Factors influencing the survival in stage I ovarian cancer. *Am J Obstet Gynecol* 116:222–228, 1973
106. Purola E, Nieminim U: Does rupture of cystic cancer during operation influence the prognosis? *Ann Chir Gynaecol* 57:615–617, 1968
107. Ozols RF, Rubin SC, Thomas G, et al: Epithelial ovarian cancer, in Hoskins WJ, Perez CA, Young RC (eds.): *Principles and Practices of Gynecologic Oncology* (ed 2). Philadelphia, Lippincott-Raven, 1997, pp 919–986
108. Schwartz PE: Surgical management of ovarian cancer. *Arch Surg* 116:99–106, 1981
109. Young RC, Decker DG, Wharton JT, et al: Staging laparotomy in early ovarian cancer. *JAMA* 250:3072–3076, 1983
110. Vergote I, DeBrabanter J, Fyles A, et al: Prognostic importance of degree of differentiation and cyst rupture in stage I invasive epithelial ovarian carcinoma. *Lancet* 357:176–182, 2001
111. Young RC, Pecorelli S: Management of early ovarian cancer. *Semin Oncol* 25:335–339, 1998
112. Young RC, Brady MF, Nieberg RK, et al: Adjuvant treatment for early ovarian cancer: a randomized phase III trial of intraperitoneal 32P or intravenous cyclophosphamide and cisplatin — a Gynecologic Oncology Group study. *J Clin Oncol* 21:4350–4355, 2003
113. Trimbos JB, Parmar M, Vergote I, et al: International collaborative ovarian neoplasm trial 1 and adjuvant chemotherapy in ovarian neoplasm trial: two parallel randomized phase III trials of adjuvant chemotherapy in patients with early-stage ovarian carcinoma. *J Natl Cancer Inst* 95:105–112, 2003
114. Young R, Chabner B, Hubbard S, et al: Advanced ovarian adenocarcinoma: a prospective clinical trial of melphalan (L-PAM) versus combination chemotherapy. *N Engl J Med* 299:1261–1266, 1978

115. Omura G, Blessing JA, Ehrlich CE, et al: A randomized trial of cyclophosphamide and doxorubicin, with or without cisplatin, in advanced ovarian carcinoma. *Cancer* 56:1725-1730, 1987
116. Decker DG, Fleming TR, Malkasian GD, et al: Cyclophosphamide plus *cis*-platinum in combination: treatment program for stage II or IV ovarian carcinoma. *Obstet Gynecol* 60:481–487, 1982
117. Neijt JP, ten Bokkel Huinink WW, van der Burg ME, et al: Randomized trial comparing combination chemotherapy regimens CHAP-5 versus CP in advanced ovarian carcinoma. *J Clin Oncol* 5:1157–1168, 1987
118. Stewart LA, for the Advanced Ovarian Cancer Trials Group (AOCTG): Chemotherapy in advanced ovarian cancer: an overview of randomized clinical trials. *BMJ* 303:884–893, 1991
119. Alberts DS, Green S, Hannigan EV, et al: Improved therapeutic index of carboplatin plus cyclophosphamide versus cisplatin plus cyclophosphamide: final report by the Southwest Oncology Group of a phase III randomized trial in stages III and IV ovarian cancer. *J Clin Oncol* 10:706–717, 1992
120. Swenerton K, Jeffrey J, Sturat G, et al: Cisplatin–cyclophosphamide versus carboplatin–cyclophosphamide in advanced ovarian cancer: a randomized phase III study of the National Cancer Institute of Canada Clinical Trials Group. *J Clin Oncol* 10:718–726, 1992
121. ten Bokkel Huinink WW, van der Burg MEL, van Oosterom AT, et al: Carboplatin in combination therapy for ovarian cancer. *Cancer Treat Rev* 15:9–15, 1988
122. The Ovarian Cancer Meta-Analysis Project: Cyclophosphamide plus cisplatin versus cisplatin plus cyclophosphamide, doxorubicin, and cisplatin chemotherapy of ovarian carcinoma. *J Clin Oncol* 9:1668–1674, 1991
123. West RJ, Zweig SF: Meta-analysis of chemotherapy regimens for ovarian carcinoma: a reassessment of cisplatin, cyclophosphamide and doxorubicin versus cisplatin and cyclophosphamide. *Eur J Gynaecol Oncol* 18:343–348, 1997
124. Fanning J, Bennett TZ, Hilgers RD: Meta-analysis of cisplatin, doxorubicin, and cyclophosphamide chemotherapy of ovarian carcinoma. *Obstet Gynecol* 80:954–960, 1993
125. Trimble EL, Adams JD, Vena D, et al: Paclitaxel for platinum-refractory ovarian cancer: results from the first 1,000 patients registered to National Cancer Institute Treatment Referral Center 9103. *J Clin Oncol* 11:2405–2410, 1993
126. McGuire WP, Hoskins WJ, Brady MR, et al: Cyclophosphamide and cisplatin compared with paclitaxel and cisplatin in patients with stage III and IV ovarian cancer. *N Engl J Med* 334:1–6, 1996
127. Piccart Mj, Bertelsen K, James K, et al: Randomized intergroup trial of cisplatin–paclitaxel vs cisplatin–cyclophosphamide in women with advanced epithelial ovarian cancer: three year results. *J Natl Cancer Inst* 92:699–708, 2000.
128. Muggia FM, Braly PS, Brady MF, et al: Phase III randomized study of cisplatin vs paclitaxel vs cisplatin and paclitaxel in patients with suboptimal stage III or IV ovarian cancer: a Gynecologic Oncology Group study. *J Clin Oncol* 18:106–115, 2000
129. ICON (International Collaborative Ovarian Neoplasm Group): ICON 2: randomized trial of single agent carboplatin against three-drug combination of CAP (cyclophosphamide, doxorubicin, and cisplatin) in women with ovarian cancer. *Lancet* 352:1571–1576, 1998
130. ICON (International Collaborative Ovarian Neoplasm Group): Paclitaxel plus carboplatin versus standard chemotherapy with either single-agent carboplatin or cyclophosphamide, doxorubicin, and cisplatin in women with ovarian cancer. The ICON 3 randomized trial. *Lancet* 360:505–515, 2002
131. McGuire WP, Markman M: Primary ovarian cancer chemotherapy: current standards of care. *Br J Cancer* 89(suppl 3):S3–S8, 2003
132. Ozols RF: Ovarian cancer practice guidelines. *Oncology* 11:95–105, 1997
133. Neijt JP, Engelholm SA, Tuxen MK, et al: Exploratory phase III study of paclitaxel and cisplatin versus paclitaxel and carboplatin in advanced ovarian cancer. *J Clin Oncol* 18:3084–3092, 2000
134. duBois A, Luck HJ, Meier W, et al: Cisplatin/paclitaxel vs carboplatin/paclitaxel in ovarian cancer. An update of an Arbeitsgemeinschaft Gynakologie (AGO) Study Group trial. *Proc Am Soc Clin Oncol* 18:A1374, 1999 (abstr)
135. Ozols RF, Bundy BN, Greer BE, et al: Phase III trial of carboplatin and paclitaxel compared with cisplatin and paclitaxel in patients with optimally resected stage III ovarian cancer: a Gynecology Oncology Group study. *J Clin Oncol* 21:3194–3200, 2003
136. Bookman MA, Greer BE, Ozols RF: Optimal therapy of advanced ovarian cancer: carboplatin and paclitaxel vs cisplatin and paclitaxel (GOG 158) and an update on GOG0 182-ICON5. *Int J Gynecol Cancer* 13:735–740, 2003
137. Rose PG: Chemotherapy for newly diagnosed and relapsed advanced ovarian cancer. *Semin Oncol Nurs* 19(suppl 2):25–35, 2003
138. Vasey P, for Scottish Gynaecological Cancer Trials Group: Preliminary results of the SCOTROC trial: a phase III comparison of paclitaxel–carboplatin (PC) and docetaxel–carboplatin (DC) as first-line chemotherapy for stage Ic–IV epithelial ovarian cancer (EOC). *Proc Am Soc Clin Oncol* 20:202a, 2001 (abstr 804)
139. Vasey PA, for Scottish Gynaecological Cancer Trials Group: Survival and long-term toxicity results of the SCOTROC study: docetaxel–carboplatin (DC) vs paclitaxel–carboplatin (PC) in epithelial ovarian cancer (EOC). *Proc Am Soc Clin Oncol* 21:202a, 2002 (abstr 804)
140. Olson JK, Sood AK, Sorosky JI, et al: Taxol hypersensitivity: rapid retreatment is safe and cost effective. *Gynecol Oncol* 68:25–28, 1998
141. Markman M: Hypersensitivity reactions to carboplatin. *Gynecol Oncol* 84:353–354, 2002
142. Thigpen JT, Vance RB, Khansu T: Second line chemotherapy for recurrent carcinoma of the ovary. *Cancer* 71:1559–1564, 1993
143. Ozols RF, Schwartz PE, Eifel PJ: Ovarian cancer, fallopian tube carcinoma, and peritoneal carcinoma, in DeVita VT, Hellman S, Rosenberg SA (eds.): *Cancer Principles and Practice of Oncology* (ed 5). Philadelphia, Lippincott-Raven, 1997, pp 1502–1539
144. Markman M: Role of intraperitoneal chemotherapy in the front-line setting. *J Clin Oncol* 21:134s–148s, 2003
145. Alberts DS, Liu PY, Hannigan EV, et al: Intraperitoneal cisplatin plus intravenous cyclophosphamide versus intravenous cisplatin plus intravenous cyclophosphamide for stage III ovarian cancer. *N Engl J Med* 335:1950–1955, 1996
146. Markman M, Bundy BN, Alberts DS, et al: Phase III trial of standard-dose intravenous cisplatin plus paclitaxel versus moderately high-dose carboplatin followed by intravenous paclitaxel and intraperitoneal cisplatin in small-volume stage III ovarian carcinoma: an intergroup study of the Gynecologic Oncology Group, Southwestern Oncology Group, and Eastern Cooperative Oncology Group. *J Clin Oncol* 19:1001–1007, 2001
147. Alberts DS, Markman M, Armstrong D, et al: Intraperitoneal therapy for stage III ovarian cancer: a therapy whose time has come! *J Clin Oncol* 20:3944-3946, 2002
148. Barakat R, Almadrones L, Venkatraman E, et al: A phase II trial of intraperitoneal cisplatin and etoposide as consolidation therapy in patients with stage II–IV epithelial ovarian cancer following negative surgical assessment. *Gynecol Oncol* 64:294, 1997

149. Barakat RR, Sabbatini P, Bhaskaran D, et al: Intraperitoneal chemotherapy for ovarian carcinoma: results of long-term follow-up. *J Clin Oncol* 20:694–698, 2002
150. Markman M: Intraperitoneal antineoplastic drug delivery: rationale and results. *Lancet Oncol* 4:277–283, 2003
151. Lanciano R, Reddy S, Corn B, et al: Update on the role of radiotherapy in ovarian cancer. *Semin Oncol* 25:361–371, 1998
152. Roland PY, Barnes MN, Niwas S, et al: Response to salvage treatment in recurrent ovarian cancer treated initially with paclitaxel and platinum based combination regimens. *Gynecol Oncol* 68:178–182, 1998
153. Gilblum D, Mychalczak B, Almadrones L: Palliative benefit of external-beam radiation in the management of platinum refractory epithelial ovarian cancer. *Gynecol Oncol* 69:36–41, 1998
154. Auersperg N, Edelson MI, Mok SC, et al: The biology of ovarian cancer. *Semin Oncol* 25:281–304, 1998
155. Ozols RF: Treatment of recurrent ovarian cancer: increasing options — "recurrent" results. *J Clin Oncol* 15:2177–2180, 1997
156. Lehnert M: Clinical multidrug resistance in cancer: a multifactorial problem. *Eur J Cancer* 32A:927–944, 1996
157. Liu JR, Fletcher B, Page C, et al: BCl-xl is expressed in ovarian carcinoma and modulates chemotherapy induced apoptosis. *Gynecol Oncol* 70:398–403, 1998
158. Markman M, Iseminger K, Hatch KD, et al: Tamoxifen in platinum-refractory ovarian cancer. A Gynecologic Oncology Group ancillary report. *Gynecol Oncol* 62:4–6, 1996
159. van der Velden J, Gitsch G, Wain GV, et al: Tamoxifen in patients with advanced epithelial ovarian cancer. *Int J Gynecol Cancer* 5:301–305, 1995
160. Markham M: Second-line chemotherapy of epithelial ovarian cancer. Expert Rev. *Anticancer Ther* 3:31-36, 2003
161. Rose PG, Fusco N, Fluellen L, Rodriguez M: Second-line therapy with paclitaxel and carboplatin for recurrent disease following first-line therapy with paclitaxel and platinum in ovarian or peritoneal carcinoma. *J Clin Oncol* 16:1494–1497 1998
162. Gronlund B, Hogdall C, Hansen HH, et al: Results of reinduction therapy with paclitaxel and carboplatin in recurrent epithelial ovarian cancer. *Gynecol Oncol* 83:128–134, 2000
163. Kurtz JE, Deplanque G, Duclos B, et al: Paclitaxel–anthracycline combination chemotherapy in relapsing advanced ovarian cancer after platinum-based chemotherapy: a pilot study. *Gynecol Oncol* 70:414–417, 1998
164. Bolis G, Scarfone G, Giardina G, et al: Carboplatin alone vs carboplatin plus epidoxorubicin as second-line therapy for cisplatin or carboplatin-sensitive ovarian cancer. *Gynecol Oncol* 81:3–9, 2001
165. Cantu MG, Buda A, Parma G, et al: Randomized controlled trial of single-agent paclitaxel versus cyclophosphamide, doxorubicin, and cisplatin in patients with recurrent ovarian cancer who responded to first-line platinum-based regimens. *J Clin Oncol* 20:1232–1237, 2002
166. Finkler N, Gordon A, Crozier M, et al: Phase 2 evaluation of OSI-774, a potent oral antagonist of the EGFR-TK in patients with advanced ovarian carcinoma. *Proc Am Soc Clin Oncol* 20:208a, 2001 (abstr)
167. Schilder RJ, Kohn E, Sill MW, et al: Phase II trial of gefitinib in patients with recurrent ovarian or pirmary peritoneal cancer: Gynecology Oncology Group 170C. *Proc Am Soc Clin Oncol* 22:451, 2003 (abstr)
168. Hu L, Hofmann J, Zaloudak C, et al: Vascular endothelial growth factor immunoneutralization plus paclitaxel markedly reduces tumor burden and ascites in athymic mouse model of ovarian cancer. *Am J Pathol* 161:1917–1924, 2002
169. Zeimet AG, Marth C: Why did p53 gene therapy fail in ovarian cancer? *Lancet Oncol* 4:415–422, 2003
170. Sawiris GP, Sherman-Baust CA, Becker KG, et al: Development of a highly specialized cDNA array for the study and diagnosis of epithelial ovarian cancer. *Cancer Res* 62:2923–2928, 2002
171. Ozols RF: Update on the management of ovarian cancer. *Cancer* 8:S22–S30, 2002
172. Williams SD: Ovarian germ cell tumors: an update. *Semin Oncol* 25:407–413, 1998
173. Homesley HD, Bundy BN, Hurteau JA, et al: Bleomycin, etoposide, and cisplatin combination therapy of ovarian granulose cell tumors and other stromal malignancies: a Gynecologic Oncology Group study. *Gynecol Oncol* 72:131–137, 1999
174 Door A: Less common gynecologic malignancies. *Semin Oncol Nurs* 18:207–222, 2002
175. Aure JC, Hoeg K, Kolstad P: Clinical and histologic studies of ovarian carcinoma. Long term follow up of 990 cases. *Obstet Gynecol* 37:1–9, 1971
176. Trimble CL, Trimble EL: Management of epithelial ovarian tumors of low malignant potential. *Gynecol Oncol* 55:552–561, 1994
177. Lu KH, Bell DA, Welch WR, et al: Evidence for multifocal origin of unilateral and advanced human serous borderline ovarian tumors. *Cancer Res* 58:2328–2330, 1998
178. Ingelman-Sandberg A: Classification and staging of malignant tumours of the female pelvis. *Acta Obstet Gynecol Scand* 50:1–7, 1971
179. Serov SF, Scully RE, Solun LH: Histologic typing of ovarian tumours, in *International Histologic Classification of Tumours no. 9.* Geneva, World Health Organization, 1973
180. Tucci RA, Bartels KL: Ovarian cancer surgery: a clinical pathway. *Clin J Oncol Nurs* 2:65–66, 1998
181. Ferrell BR, Dow KH, Leigh S, et al: Quality of life in long-term cancer survivors. *Oncol Nurs Forum* 22:915–922, 1995
182. Walczak JR, Heckman CS: Ascites, in Yarbro CH, Frogge MH, Goodman M (eds.): *Cancer Symptom Management* (ed 2). Sudbury, MA, Jones and Bartlett, 1999, pp 405–415
183. Collins CA: Ascites. *Clin J Oncol Nurs* 5:43–45, 2001
184. Puls LE, Duniho T, Hunter JE, et al: The prognostic implication of ascites in advanced-stage ovarian cancer. *Gynecol Oncol* 61:109–112, 1996
185. Martin VR: *Managing Symptoms Associated with Ovarian Cancer, Negotiating Optimal Ovarian Cancer Care: A Clinician's Guide* (Monograph). Bala Cynwyd, PA, Meniscus Educational Institute, 1999, pp 18–26
186. Kraemer K, Lynch MP: Ascites, in Preston FA, Cunningham RS (eds.): *Clinical Guidelines for Symptom Management in Oncology.* New York, Clinical Insights Press, 1998, pp 115–119
187. Iyengar TD, Herzog TJ: Management of symptomatic ascites in recurrent ovarian cancer patients using an intra-abdominal semi-permanent catheter. *Am J Hosp Palliat Care* 19:7–8, 2002
188. Kelvin JF, Scagliola J: Metastases involving the gastrointestinal system. *Semin Oncol Nurs* 14:187–198, 1999
189. Abrahm JL: Promoting symptom control in palliative care. *Semin Oncol Nurs* 14:95–109, 1998
190. Murphy-Ende K: Bowel obstruction. *Clin J Oncol Nurs* 4:291–293, 2000
191. Waldman AR: Bowel obstruction. *Clin J Oncol Nurs* 5:281–286, 2001
192. Jolicoeur L, Faught W: Managing bowel obstruction in ovarian cancer using a percutaneous endoscopic gastrostomy (PEG) tube. *Can Oncol Nurs J* 13:212–219, 2003
193. Chang AE, August DA: Acute abdomen, bowel obstruction, and fistula, in Abeloff MD, Armitage JO, Lichter AS, et al (eds.): *Clinical Oncology.* New York, Churchill Livingstone, 1995, pp 583–597

194. Summers RW, Lu CC: Approach to the patient with ileus and obstruction, in Yamada T (ed.): *Textbook of Gastroenterology* (ed 2). Philadelphia, Lippincott, 1995, pp 796–812
195. Rust DM: Anorexia and cachexia, in Yasko JM (ed.): *Management of Symptoms Associated with Chemotherapy.* Bala Cynwyd, PA, Meniscus Health Care Communications, 1998, pp 35–54
196. Grant MM, Rivera LM: Anorexia, cachexia, and dysphagia: the symptom experience. *Semin Oncol Nurs* 11:266–271, 1995
197. Cunningham R, Bell R: Nutrition in cancer: an overview. *Semin Oncol Nurs* 16:9098, 2000
198. Gwilliam B, Bailey C: The nature of terminal malignant bowel obstruction and its impact on patients with advanced cancer. *Int J Palliat Nurs* 7:474–481, 2001
199. Dewys WD, Begg C, Lavin PT, et al: Prognostic effect of weight loss prior to chemotherapy in cancer patients. *Am J Med* 69:491–497, 1980
200. Grant M, Kravits K: Symptoms and their impact on nutrition. *Semin Oncol Nurs* 16:113–121, 2000
201. Levy MH, Rosen SM, Ottery FD, et al: Supportive care in oncology. *Curr Probl Cancer* 16:335–385, 1992
202. American Society for Parental and Enteral Nutrition: Standards for nutrition support: hospitalized patients. *Nutr Clin Pract* 10:208–219, 1995
203. Ottery FD: Supportive nutrition to prevent cachexia and support quality of life. *Semin Oncol* 22(suppl 3):98–111, 1995
204. Loprinzi CL, Schaid DJ, Dose AM, et al: Body-composition changes in patients who gain weight while receiving megesterol acetate. *J Clin Oncol* 11:152–154, 1993
205. Oster MH, Enders SR, Samuels SJ, et al: Megesterol acetate in patients with AIDS and cachexia. *Ann Intern Med* 121:400–408, 1994
206. Loprinzi CL, Michalak JC, Schaid DJ: Phase three evaluation of four doses of megesterol acetate as therapy for patients with cancer anorexia and/or cachexia. *J Clin Oncol* 11:762–767, 1993
207. Jatoi A, Windschitl HE, Loprinzi CL, et al: Dronabinol versus megesterol acetate versus combination therapy for cancer-associated anorexia: a North Central Cancer Treatment Group study. *J Clin Oncol* 20:567–573, 2002
208. Bloch A: Nutrition support in cancer. *Semin Oncol Nurs* 16:122–127, 2000
209. Joyce M, Cunningham RS: Metastases that interfere with circulation. *Semin Oncol Nurs* 14:230–239, 1998
210. Brown J: A clinically useful method for evaluating lymphedema. *Clin J Oncol Nurs* 8:35–38, 2004
211. Ascherl P: Lymphedema. *Soc Gynecol Oncol Nurs J* 8:9–11, 1998
212. Kalinowski BH: Lymphedema, in Yarbro CH, Frogge MH, Goodman M (eds.): *Cancer Symptom Management* (ed 2). Sudbury, MA, Jones and Bartlett, 1999, pp 457–486
213. Cutter K, Atkins B: Freedom from lymphedema. *Soc Gynecol Oncol Nurs J* 6:11–13, 1996
214. Ryan M, Stainton MC, Jaconelli C, et al: The experience of lower limb lymphedema for women after treatment for gynecologic cancer. *Oncol Nurs Forum* 30:417–423, 2003
215. Shuey KM: Heart, lung, and endocrine complications of solid tumors. *Semin Oncol* 10:177–188, 1994
216. Rubin SC, Sutton GP: *Ovarian Cancer.* New York, McGraw-Hill, 1993, pp 361–373
217. McCoy AM, Mierzewski A: Acute oncologic disorders, in Kinney MR, Packa DR, Dunbar SB (eds.): *AACN's Clinical Reference for Critical Care Nursing* (ed 3). St. Louis, Mosby, 1993, pp 1077–1097
218. Harwood KV: Dyspnea, in Yarbro CH, Frogge MH, Goodman M (eds.): *Cancer Symptom Management* (ed 2). Sudbury, MA, Jones and Bartlett, 1999, pp 45–57
219. Brobacher S, Gobel BH: Use of the Pleurx pleural catheter for the management of malignant pleural effusions. *Clin J Oncol Nurs* 7:35–38, 2003
220. Wickham R: Dyspnea: recognizing and managing an invisible problem. *Oncol Nurs Forum* 29:925–933, 2002
221. Smith EL: Pulmonary metastasis. *Semin Oncol Nurs* 14:178–186, 1998
222. Kornblith AB, Thaler HT, Wong G, et al: Quality of life of women with ovarian cancer. *Gynecol Oncol* 59:231–242, 1995
223. Ersek M, Ferrell BR, Dow KH, et al: Quality of life in women with ovarian cancer. *West J Nurs Res* 19:334–350, 1997
224. Montazeri A, McEwen J, Gillis CR: Quality of life in patients with ovarian cancer: current state of research. *Support Care Cancer* 4:169–179, 1996
225. Jenkins B: Patients' reports of sexual changes after treatment for gynecological cancer. *Oncol Nurs Forum* 15:231–242, 1998
226. Lakusta CM, Atkinson MJ, Robinson JW, et al: Quality of life in ovarian cancer patients receiving chemotherapy. *Gynecol Oncol* 81:490–495, 2001
227. Guidozzi F: Living with ovarian cancer. *Gynecol Oncol* 50:202–207, 1993
228. Howell D, Fitch MI, Deane KA: Impact of ovarian cancer perceived by women. *Cancer Nursing* 26:1–9, 2003
229. Powell L, Midler A, Steiner A: Concerns of women with ovarian cancer: a qualitative investigation. *Quality of Life — A Nursing Challenge* 6:92–101, 1998
230. Ferrell B, Smith SL, Cullinane CA, et al: Psychological well being and quality of life in ovarian cancer survivors. *Cancer* 98:1061–1071, 2003
231. Hamilton AB: Psychological aspects of ovarian cancer. *Cancer Invest* 17:335–341, 1999
232. Fitch MI, Gray RE, Franssen E: Women's perspective regarding the impact of ovarian cancer. *Cancer Nurs* 23:359–366, 2000
233. Howell D, Fitch MI, Deane KA: Women's experience with recurrent ovarian cancer. *Cancer Nurs* 26:10–17, 2003
234. Stewart DE, Wong F, Duff S, et al: "What doesn't kill you makes you stronger": an ovarian cancer survivor survey. *Gynecol Oncol* 83:537–541, 2001
235. Sivesind D, Baile WF: An ovarian cancer support group. *Cancer Pract* 5:247–251, 1997
236. Burnett CB: Ovarian cancer: advocacy, quality of life, and politics. *Quality of Life — A Nursing Challenge* 4:73–77, 1996
237. Melancon C: From victim to victor: a personal perspective of ovarian cancer. *Quality of Life — A Nursing Challenge* 4:78–81, 1996
238. Jemal A, Murray T, Samuels A, et al: Cancer statistics 2003. *CA Cancer J Clin* 53:5–26 2003
239. Ozols RF: Future directions in the treatment of ovarian cancer. *Semin Oncol* 29(suppl 1):32–42, 2002
240. Martin VR: Ovarian cancer. *Semin Oncol Nurs* 18:174–183, 2002

CHAPTER 61

Pancreatic Cancer

JoAnn Coleman, RN, MS, ACNP, AOCN®

Introduction

Pancreatic cancer accounts for 2% of new cancer cases each year in the United States as well as worldwide.[1] The current estimate of 30,000 new cases of pancreatic cancer each year has stabilized since the end of the twentieth century. Approximately the same number of deaths from pancreatic cancer occur annually in the United States.[1,2] The disease has a poor prognosis and is considered by many to be one of the deadliest malignancies. Fewer than 20% of affected individuals survive one year after diagnosis, and the overall five-year survival rate is only 4%.[1] The majority of pancreatic cancers are metastatic at the time of diagnosis. Surgical resection offers the best possibility for cure, with the five-year survival rate approaching 40% when it is performed at specialized major medical institutions.[3,4]

Pancreatic cancer is one of the most difficult tumors to detect or diagnose because of the anatomical location of the pancreas. It is also difficult to treat due to the biologic nature of the tumor. Its onset is insidious, with signs and symptoms that occur late, are vague and misleading, and mimic other diseases. The individual with pancreatic cancer typically will ignore the initial signs and symptoms or rely on self-treatment for months until jaundice or other prominent and intolerable signs appear.

Recent advances in basic science and improved technology have provided a better understanding of the pathogenesis and clinical management of cancer of the pancreas.[5] It is hoped that a growing understanding of the biology and molecular genetics and the influence of growth factors on the progression of pancreatic cancer will provide opportunities for advances in prevention, earlier tumor detection, and more effective and novel therapies.

Epidemiology

The demographics of pancreatic cancer have been widely investigated (Table 61-1). Age is the strongest risk factor for pancreatic cancer, with the peak incidence occurring between the ages 60 and 80.[6] Pancreatic carcinoma incidence is slightly higher in men than in women.[1] The incidence rate is 30%–40% higher in African American men. Persons of Ashkenazi Jewish heritage have a higher risk of pancreatic cancer related to germ-line mutations.[3] Geography has been considered a possible risk factor. The incidence rates of pancreatic cancer are highest in Western and industrialized countries, and lowest in underdeveloped nations. Studies have been inconclusive regarding the risk of pancreatic cancer and socioeconomic status and migrant status.[6]

Table 61-1 Risk Factors for Pancreatic Cancer

Demographic Factors	Advancing age Black race Male gender Jewish religion Geography
Environmental Factors	Tobacco Radiation
Dietary Factors	Carbohydrate Cholesterol Meat Salt Dehydrated food Fried food Refined sugar Soybeans Nitrosamines
Occupational Factors	Chemists Coal gas workers Metal industries Aluminum milling Leather tanning Textile industry Building trades Transportation Butchers Flour industry Ethylene chlorhydrin Halogenated hydrocarbons Chlorinated water DDT
Host Factors	Diabetes Chronic pancreatitis Genetic syndromes

Etiology

Numerous environmental factors may be associated with increased risk of pancreatic cancer, including personal cigarette smoking, environmental tobacco smoke (tobacco smoke exposure), and chemical exposures. It has been estimated that tobacco smoking contributes to the development of 20%–30% of pancreatic cancers.[3,7] The strongest associations with cigarette smoking and pancreatic cancer were found when the pack-years smoked occurred within the previous 15 years. Environmental tobacco smoke contains the same toxins, irritants, and carcinogens as cigarettes and is known to cause cancer in humans. At this time, the exact contribution of environmental tobacco smoke to the development of pancreatic cancer has not been characterized, but it is thought to have a definite association, especially in persons with a lower education level.[8] Exposure to radiation has also been investigated as a risk for pancreatic carcinogenesis. Persons irradiated in infancy for skin hemangioma have been reported to have an increased risk of pancreatic cancer.[9]

Many epidemiological studies have examined the role of diet and pancreatic cancer, but the relationship remains unclear.[6,10] A number of studies have reported an association between pancreatic cancer and increasing ingestion of carbohydrate, cholesterol, meat, salt, dehydrated food, fried food, refined sugar, soybeans, and nitrosamines. The studies do not support an association with pancreatic cancer and excess intake of dietary fat or beta-carotene.[10] A decreased risk or perhaps a protective effect has been reported for fiber, vitamin C, fruits, vegetables, preservative-free foods, raw foods, and the use of pressure cooking and microwave cooking.[6]

Obesity as a risk factor for pancreatic cancer suggests that energy balance may play an important role in pancreatic carcinogenesis.[11] High body mass index, increased weight, and a low level of physical activity all increase the risk of pancreatic cancer.[12]

Numerous studies have examined certain occupational exposures. Cancer of the pancreas has been reported to occur among chemists and coal gas workers and among individuals working in metal industries, aluminum milling, and the leather tanning industry. There have been reports of increased risk associated with exposure to welding materials, paint thinners, refuse and detergents, and floor cleaning agents as well as petroleum products. Butchers, transportation workers, and workers in flour mills where pesticides were used more frequently than in other segments of the industry are occupations considered to be a possible risk. Workers exposed to DDT during the manufacturing process were at risk. Those workers exposed during production of ethylene chlorhydrin, halogenated hydrocarbons, and consumption of chlorinated water have also been implicated between exposure and disease.[6,13]

A meta-analysis of the relationship between diabetes and the development of pancreatic cancer confirmed that the relative risk in persons who have had diabetes for five years is double the risk of persons without diabetes. Diabetes may be an early symptom of pancreatic cancer as the tumor itself can destroy pancreatic parenchyma, causing pancreatitis and diabetes.[14]

Peptic ulcer surgery and cholecystectomy have also been linked to pancreatic cancer. The initial symptoms of pancreatic cancer can mimic biliary tract disease, which in turn may lead to cholecystectomy and subsequent discovery of pancreatic cancer.

Genetics

With advances in the understanding of human genetics, it is now known that cancer of the pancreas is a disease of acquired and inherited mutations in cancer-causing genes. The development of cancer of the pancreas has been associated with the activation of the oncogene, *K-ras*, the inactivation of multiple tumor suppressor genes, and DNA mismatch repair.[15] Specifically, the *p16* tumor suppressor gene is inactivated in approximately 95% of pancreatic cancers.[16] The second most important tumor suppressor gene is *p53*, which is inactivated in 50%–70% of pancreatic cancers.[17] The *DPC4* (deleted in pancreatic cancer on locus 4) gene is specific for pancreatic cancer and is inactivated in approximately 50% of pancreatic cancers.[18] The *BRCA2* gene is inactivated in only 7% of pancreatic cancers, but is noteworthy because the mutations in *BRCA2* associated with pancreatic cancer are inherited mutations.[19]

K-ras is the most frequently activated oncogene in pancreatic cancer. More than 90% of pancreatic cancers harbor activating mutations in *K-ras*, and most of these mutations affect codon 12 of the gene. The localization of these mutations to a single codon makes them relatively easy to detect.[20]

The DNA mismatch repair genes are the last group of cancer-causing genes that have been found to play a role in the development of pancreatic cancer. When these DNA repair genes do not function appropriately, errors in DNA replication are not repaired. Approximately 4% of pancreatic cancers have been found to contain genetic alterations in DNA mismatch repair genes. This subgroup of cancers may arise through a pathway separate from that of the usual ductal carcinomas and therefore may have a more favorable prognosis.[21]

Cancer of the pancreas has been shown to cluster within families. Two broad groups of familial aggregation of pancreatic cancer exist: those associated with known syndromes and those without such an association.[22] Six genetic syndromes are associated with an increased risk of developing pancreatic cancer. These syndromes account for less than 10% of the familial aggregation of pancreatic cancer. (See Table 61-2.)

Table 61-2 Genetic Syndromes Predisposing an Individual to Pancreatic Cancer

Hereditary pancreatitis
Hereditary nonpolyposis colorectal cancer (HNPCC)
Familial breast cancer (linked to *BRCA2* tumor suppressor gene)
Familial atypical multiple mole melanoma syndrome (FAMMM)
Ataxia–telangiectasia syndrome
Peutz-Jeghers syndrome

Hereditary pancreatitis is a rare disease characterized by recurrent episodes of severe epigastric pain and hyperamylasemia, with an onset usually before age

10. Individuals affected with this disease are at increased risk for the development of pancreatic pseudocysts, pancreatic exocrine insufficiency, chronic pancreatitis, diabetes mellitus, and a 50-fold increased risk of pancreatic cancer.[22,23]

Hereditary nonpolyposis colorectal cancer (HNPCC) can predispose some families to the development of pancreatic cancer, but the contribution of this syndrome to the number of individuals with pancreatic cancer appears to be small.[24] Familial breast cancer with germ-line mutations in the *BRCA2* gene are the most common mutations in persons with hereditary pancreatic cancer.[25] *BRCA2* has been found to be associated not only with an increased risk of breast cancer but also cancer of the ovary, prostate, colon, and pancreas.[19,26]

Familial atypical multiple mole melanoma syndrome (FAMMM) is characterized by multiple nevi, atypical nevi, and multiple melanomas. The gene responsible for the FAMMM syndrome is the *p16* tumor suppressor gene.[27,28]

The ataxia–telangiectasia syndrome is associated with disabling cerebellar ataxia, oculocutaneous telangiectasia, and humoral and cellular immune deficiencies. The *ATM* gene is responsible for this syndrome, and individuals who carry this genetic mutation are also at increased risk of leukemia, lymphoma, and cancer of the breast, ovary, biliary tract, stomach, and pancreas.[15]

Peutz-Jeghers syndrome is characterized by hamartomatous polyps of the gastrointestinal tract and by melanin deposits on the lips and around and inside the mouth. Affected individuals are at an increased risk of developing multiple cancers and have a 100-fold greater incidence of pancreatic cancer than expected.[29] The gene responsible for this syndrome has been found on a region of chromosone 19p.[30]

Studies of families without a genetic syndrome in which an aggregation of pancreatic carcinoma exists help researchers understand the genetic alterations associated with the development of cancer of the pancreas. A recent analysis of familial pancreatic tumor data looked at similarities and differences between familial and sporadic cases. There was no difference in the age at which pancreatic cancer was diagnosed between the two groups of cases, with both groups having a mean age at diagnosis of 65 years.[15]

Growth Factors

Various growth factors and their receptors are important in the regulation of pancreatic cancer cell growth. Overexpression of specific growth factors and their receptors may contribute to the biologic aggressiveness of pancreatic cancer.[31]

The epidermal growth factor receptor (EGFR) binds a family of peptides that includes epidermal growth factor (EGF), transforming growth factor alpha (TGF-α), heparin-binding EGF-like growth factor, amphiregulin, betacellulin, and epiregulin. These growth factors may all contribute to pancreatic cell growth. Overexpression of EGFR has been linked to enhanced metastatic potential and increased tumor invasiveness.[31]

The transforming growth factor beta (TGF-β) polypeptide family has been implicated in the development of pancreatic cancer. Overexpression of TGF-β enhances tumor development by promoting tumor angiogenesis, altering the extracellular array/matrix, and enhancing adhesiveness that facilitates tumor metastasis.[31] Overexpression of TGF-β has been associated with a shorter postoperative survival or worse prognosis in individuals with pancreatic adenocarcinoma.[32]

The fibroblast growth factor (FGF) family consists of many polypeptide growth factors that have an affinity for heparin, which results in changes in cell differentiation and tissue repair.[33] A current hypothesis suggests that FGFs enhance pancreatic cell growth and may contribute to abnormal epithelial–mesenchymal interactions inside the growing tumor.[34]

The insulin-like growth factor I (IGF-I) is also overexpressed in pancreatic cancer cells and enhances the growth of those cells.[35]

Other analyses that illuminate genetic alterations in pancreatic cancer–causing genes are karyotyping, comparative genomic hybridization (CGH), and allelotyping. Karyotyping can help to identify specific chromosomes lost or gained in pancreatic cancer. Comparative genomic hybridization has been used to screen for gains or losses of chromosomal material within the tumor DNA. Allelotyping has allowed for improved precision in identifying genetic material. Examination of pancreatic adenocarcinomas has revealed high frequencies of losses at specific chromosome arms.[36]

Prevention, Screening, and Early Detection

Prevention of pancreatic cancer will require definitive identification of factors demonstrated to cause or place individuals at a high risk of developing this disease. Then reduction or elimination of these risk factors may prevent cancer of the pancreas. It is an insidious disease with little known about the best treatment, much less the cause.

The general hypothesis currently being tested is that adenocarcinoma of the pancreas represents a

Table 61-3 Pathology of Exocrine Pancreatic Cancer

Solid tumors
Ductal adenocarcinoma
Adenosquamous carcinoma
Acinar cell carcinoma
Giant cell carcinoma
Cystic tumors
Serous cystic neoplasms
Mucinous cystic neoplasms
Intraductal papillary mucinous neoplasms (IPMN)
Solid and cystic papillary neoplasms (Hamoudi tumor)

multi-step disease involving progressive, acquired genetic rearrangements in cancer-causing genes. These mutations are detectable in stool, duodenal fluid, pancreatic juice samples, bile, and blood, and they may become an accurate screening marker for pancreatic cancer to easily detect persons at risk.[36] An ideal approach would be the use of an imaging test along with molecular markers of neoplastic disease to diagnose a benign, dysplastic precancerous lesion or an early, localized cancer.[3]

Pathophysiology

Pancreatic cancer is most commonly an adenocarcinoma that originates from the cells lining the pancreatic duct. Tumors of the pancreas develop in both the endocrine and the exocrine parenchyma (see Table 61-3). Approximately 90% of tumors arise from the exocrine pancreas, which contains two major types of epithelium: acinar and ductal. The acinar cells of the pancreas produce digestive enzymes, whereas the cells lining the pancreatic duct are responsible for the secretion of fluid and electrolytes and the conveyance of pancreatic juice to the duodenum.

Cellular Characteristics

Adenocarcinomas of the pancreas usually are whitish-yellow, hard, nodular, poorly defined, firm masses surrounded by dense reactive fibrous tissue that often obstruct and dilate the distal common bile duct and pancreatic ducts. Tumors may vary from well differentiated to undifferentiated, and exhibit variable gland formation, irregular cell size, and variable nuclear changes. Because of the tumor's infiltrative nature, visualizing the complete extent of the disease is difficult. Many ductal adenocarcinomas of the pancreas infiltrate into vascular spaces, lymphatic spaces, and perineural spaces, which can be appreciated only on microscopic examination.

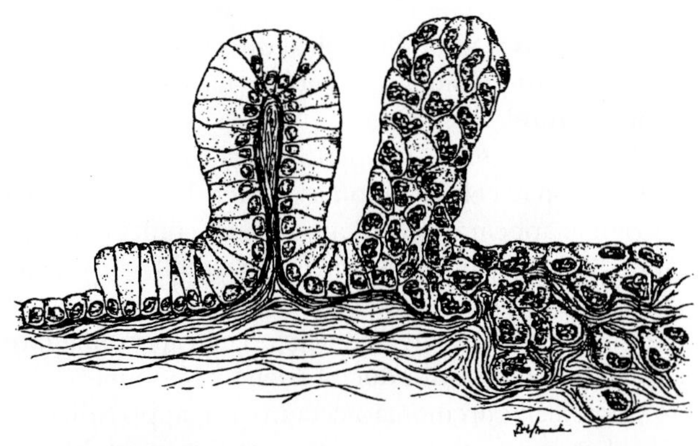

Figure 61-1 Progression from normal duct epithelium (left) to low-grade pancreatic intraepithelial neoplasia (PanIN) to high-grade PanIN to infiltrating cancer (right). (Used with permission from Wilentz RE, Hruban RH: Pathology of cancer of the pancreas. *Surg Oncol Clin North Am* 7:47, 1998.[38])

Precursors to Ductal Adenocarcinoma

Lesions in the small pancreatic ducts frequently are first found on histologic examination in resected pancreatic specimens. These lesions are now referred to as PanINs. Precursor lesions may progress from flat duct lesions (PanIN-1A), to papillary duct lesions without atypia (PanIN-1B), to papillary duct lesions with atypia (PanIN-2), and finally to carcinoma in situ of the pancreas (PanIN-3).[37] (See Figure 61-1.)[38] The lesions occur equally in both men and women in their sixties to seventies and can be found anywhere throughout the pancreas.[3]

Mucinous cystic neoplasms (MCNs) can be precursors of infiltrating ductal adenocarcimonas of the pancreas. These tumors differ from PanINs in that they are grossly visible and do not involve the ducts of the pancreas. It is important to differentiate MCNs from ductal adenocarcinomas, as MCNs have a better prognosis.[39] These neoplasms are found mostly in women in their forties to fifties and can be located in the body or tail of the pancreas.[3]

Intraductal papillary mucinous neoplasms (IPMNs) are grossly visible tumors that grow in the large ducts of the pancreas and have varying degrees of atypia.[40] They occur with approximately equal frequency in both sexes in their sixties to seventies; they are found mostly in the head of the pancreas but can infiltrate throughout the entire pancreas.[3] Patients with IPMNs usually have favorable outcomes after resection, but metastases can occur.[41]

Adenosquamous carcinoma of the pancreas is a rare variant of ductal adenocarcinoma that shows both glandular (adeno) and squamous differentiation. This variation is more common in individuals who have received previous chemotherapy or radiation therapy. The biologic behavior of adenosquamous carcinoma is the same as that of the typical ductal adenocarcinomas. Adenosquamous carcinoma has an especially poor prognosis.[38]

A small percentage of pancreatic cancers are classified as acinar cell carcinomas, which have a distinct histologic appearance and an unusual clinical presentation. Most individuals with acinar cell carcinoma have biliary or gastrointestinal obstruction because of the tumor. Individuals with acinar cell carcinoma fare better than those with ductal adenocarcinoma.[42]

Giant cell carcinoma accounts for approximately 5% of primary nonendocrine pancreatic malignancies. Giant cell carcinomas arise with equal frequency in the head, body, and tail regions of the pancreas. These pancreatic carcinomas are associated with a poorer prognosis than ductal adenocarcinomas.[38]

Cystic neoplasms of the pancreas, arising from the exocrine pancreas, are classified as either benign serous cystadenomas, potentially malignant mucinous cystadenomas, or malignant cystadenocarcinomas. Most serous cystic neoplasms are benign, and the prognosis for individuals with resected mucinous cystadenomas is excellent.[38]

Solid and cystic papillary neoplasms of the pancreas, also called *Hamoudi tumors,* occur primarily in women in their third and fourth decades of life. These tumors have solid, cystic, and papillary components when viewed microscopically. Most individuals are cured after surgical resection.[43] Pancreaticoblastoma is a neoplasm that occurs primarily in children younger than 15 years of age. The survival rate for patients with resected pancreaticoblastomas is relatively good.[44]

The most common tumor sites that may metastasize to the pancreas are breast, lung, colorectal, melanoma, and renal cell carcinoma. Systemic neoplasms such as leukemia and lymphoma can involve the pancreas. The pancreas may be the presenting site for these cancers. Most pancreatic lymphomas are non-Hodgkin's lymphomas.[36] Pancreatic lymphomas are rare, but early recognition is important because of their dramatic response to chemotherapy.[45]

Endocrine or islet cell tumors constitute the remainder of pancreatic malignant tumors. These uncommon tumors account for approximately 5% of all pancreatic neoplasms. Many islet cell tumors secrete excessive hormones, resulting in significant clinical manifestations. Nonfunctional islet cell tumors do not produce obvious clinical manifestations and are usually detected because of their space-occupying characteristics or as an incidental finding.[46]

Islet cell tumors arise from the endocrine parenchyma. They usually occur as small, well-circumscribed, reddish-orange tissue that rarely extends beyond the pancreas. On microscopy, islet cell tumors are well vascularized and encapsulated, usually compressing adjacent parenchyma. Fibrosis and calcification may be seen. Malignant islet cell tumors are difficult to distinguish because they closely resemble normal islet cells and retain secretory or synthetic functions. The presence of metastases is the most reliable criterion for establishing malignancy.[47] Chapter 50 presents a more detailed discussion of endocrine tumors.

Progression of Disease

Tumors of the head of the pancreas are those arising to the right of the left border of the superior mesentric vein. The uncinate process is part of the head of the pancreas. Tumors of the body of the pancreas are those arising between the left border of the superior mesenteric vein and the left border of the aorta. Tumors of the tail of the pancreas are those arising between the left border of the aorta and the hilum of the spleen.

Pancreatic cancer arises in the head, neck, or uncinate process of the pancreas in 60%–70% of cases. About 15% of tumors develop in the body and tail of the gland, and the remaining 20% diffusely involve the entire gland.[36]

Tumors in the head of the gland are often detected at a small size (2–3 cm). The bile duct is invaded early in the course of the disease, causing obstruction of the distal common bile duct. This obstruction accounts for easily recognized symptoms, such as jaundice, which enable detection of smaller tumors. Extension beyond the pancreas is the rule rather than the exception. Ductal adenocarcinomas usually infiltrate into vascular, perineural, and lymphatic spaces. These tumors tend to invade local structures, such as the duodenum and retroperitoneum, either directly or along the course of autonomic nerves of the celiac plexus. Some degree of perineural invasion is present in 90% of cases. The portal or superior vein may also be invaded. Venous invasion or encasement by tumor growth may result in obstruction, thrombosis, ascites, and portal hypertension. Vascular encasement and neural infiltration can contribute to severe back pain. Involvement of the mesenteric vessels may preclude resection of these tumors.[36]

In the body and tail of the pancreas, tumors often reach sizes larger than 5 cm before they produce symptoms. Tumors of the body and tail of the pancreas can invade the splenic vein, resulting in thrombosis and gastric varices.[3]

At the time of detection, the tumor may be fixed to tissues behind the pancreas or to the vertebral column. The tumor may directly invade surrounding organs, such as kidney, spleen, or diaphragm. Invasion of the celiac nerve plexus may account for unrelenting pain. Other sites of local invasion, which tends to occur later, include the superior mesenteric and splenic arteries, transverse colon, stomach, kidneys, and left adrenal gland.[3] Obstruction of the portal vein and tributaries can lead to portal hypertension and esophageal varices.

Characteristically, tumors of the pancreas grow slowly, with late signs and symptoms of pathology. At the time of diagnosis, 90% of cases have perineural invasion, 70%–80% have lymphatic spread, 50% have venous involvement, and 20%–25% have duodenal invasion. The liver, peritoneum, and regional lymph nodes are the most commonly involved structures.[48] Supraclavicular nodes (Virchow nodes) may be involved more frequently with carcinoma of the body and tail of the pancreas. Metastatic deposits reach the liver through the portal bloodstream or lymphatics. Peritoneal seeding by metastatic deposits also occurs.[3] The frequency of lymph node metastasis correlates with the size of the primary tumor.[49]

Table 61-4 Clinical Manifestations of Cancer of the Pancreas

Location of Tumor	Stage	Clinical Manifestation
Head	Early	Weight loss Jaundice Pain Anorexia Diarrhea Weakness Indigestion Depression
Body	Late	Palpable mass Severe pain Early satiety Indigestion Vomiting Weight loss
Tail	Late	Severe pain Indigestion Anorexia Weight loss GI bleeding Splenomegaly

Clinical Manifestations

The early signs and symptoms of pancreatic cancer are vague, nonspecific, and gradual, which often contributes to a delay in diagnosis by both the individual and the physician. Specific symptoms usually develop late and only after invasion or obstruction of a nearby structure. Careful assessment and extensive inquiry into the character, onset, duration, and modulators of presenting signs and symptoms is important. Manifestations of disease differ according to the location of the tumor (see Table 61-4). A clinical suspicion of pancreatic cancer must be high to identify the presence of a tumor. Individuals who have resectable pancreatic cancer tend to present with few symptoms.

Weight loss and clinical wasting are classic symptoms of cancer of the pancreas, particularly when the tumor is located in the head of the gland. Initially, the weight loss may not cause concern and may be attributed to gastric maladies. As the cancer advances, significant weight loss is common and often accelerated by pain, anorexia, flatulence, nausea, and vomiting. Duodenal obstruction, with nausea and vomiting, is a late manifestation of pancreatic cancer. Tumor involvement of the pancreas prevents secretions of the digestive pancreatic enzymes and may diminish insulin production. Malabsorption can lead to diarrhea, constipation, steatorrhea, and muscle weakness.[3] New-onset diabetes may be the first clinical feature in 10%–20% of individuals.[50] The onset of glucose intolerance in an elderly person with vague gastrointestinal symptoms should alert the clinician to the possibility of pancreatic cancer. Metabolic disturbances such as hyperglycemia, glycosuria, and hypoalbuminemia may occur.

A combination of factors probably causes the weight loss associated with pancreatic cancer. An increase in resting energy expenditure, a decrease in consumption of calories, and fat malabsorption exist in individuals with this disease.[51]

Pain is often vague and nonspecific. A dull, intermittent, diffuse, upper abdominal or back discomfort is initially experienced by most individuals. The discomfort may be attributed to other causes such as indigestion or gaseous distention. The discomfort or pain may become more distinctive. It may progress to continuous midepigastric pain and frequently radiates to the back or right upper quadrant of the abdomen, often becoming most pronounced during the evening or night. It may be colicky, dull, or vague. The intensity of the pain is affected by activity, eating, and posture. The pain is often ameliorated when the individual sits or leans forward, called *proning*, or lies in the fetal position on their right side with both knees drawn up to the chest.[52] The pain can be caused by invasion of the tumor into the splanchnic plexus and retroperitoneum, as well as by obstruction of the pancreatic duct.

Pain is a more prevalent symptom in individuals who have tumors in the body and tail of the pancreas. These tumors are larger at presentation and are located in the retroperitoneum, which contributes to nerve involvement, resulting in pain. Although intractable pain is associated with pancreatic cancer, seldom is it

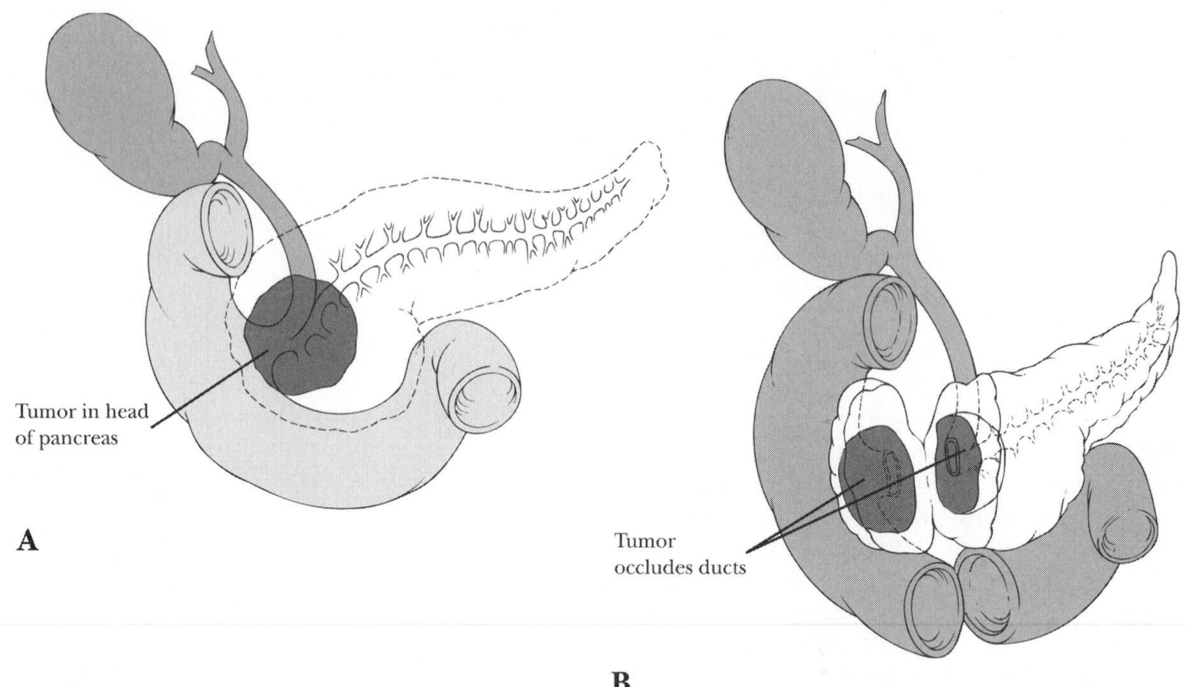

Figure 61-2 Pancreatic cancers originate in the duct and when they are located in the head of the pancreas **(A)** they will occlude the distal common bile duct **(B)**. Note the proximity of the pancreatic duct and common bile duct, explaining the characteristic cutoff on cholangiography at the "knee" of the distal bile duct. (Used with permission from Bastidas VA, Neiderhuber JE: Pancreas, in Abeloff MD, Armitage JD, Lichter AS, Neiderhuber JE (eds.): *Clinical Oncology*. New York, Churchill Livingstone, 1995, pp 1373–1403.[54])

an early manifestation. Recent studies suggest that fewer than one-third of individuals with cancer of the pancreas report moderate to severe pain. Severe pain usually indicates invasion of splanchnic nerves and is suggestive of advanced disease.[53]

Acute pancreatitis may be the presenting sign of a pancreatic neoplasm. It is caused by the partial obstruction of the pancreatic duct. Consideration must be given to the diagnosis of a pancreatic tumor in patients who are initially seen with pancreatitis, especially when there is no obvious cause for acute pancreatitis, such as gallstones or alcohol abuse.[36]

Head of Pancreas

When carcinoma involves the head of the pancreas, the signs and symptoms often appear earlier than with a tumor in the body or tail of the pancreas (Figure 61-2).[54] A classic triad of symptoms is seen in individuals with cancer of the head of the pancreas: jaundice, pain, and weight loss.

Jaundice, caused by obstruction of the distal common bile duct as it passes through the head of the pancreas, is the presenting symptom in most cases of cancer of the head of the pancreas. Regardless of whether jaundice is the initial symptom or follows the onset of pain, it is the symptom that invariably causes individuals to seek medical attention. Jaundice accompanied by abdominal pain is far more common than painless jaundice.[55] Obstructive jaundice leads to severe pruritus; dark, tea-colored urine; and clay-colored (acholic) stools. Jaundice does not necessarily indicate extensive disease and unresectability.

Other symptoms are less common and nonspecific. They include weakness, food intolerance, and anorexia. Two unusual symptoms are depression and superficial thrombophlebitis. Depression and anxiety may be part of the initial presentation of pancreatic cancer, independent of pain and other somatic symptoms. These symptoms predate the diagnosis of a pancreatic tumor in approximately 50% of individuals. A triad of depression, anxiety, and feelings of impending doom has been described.[56] The increased incidence of depression is significantly higher than that seen in individuals with other intraabdominal malignancies.[57] The triad of depression, anxiety, and feelings of doom may indicate the presence of neuroendocrine agents in pancreatic cancer that circulate and target the central nervous system. Thromboembolism (Trousseau syndrome) occurs in fewer than 5% of individuals with pancreatic cancer.[58]

Body of Pancreas

Tumors in the body of the pancreas produce signs and symptoms late in the disease process, making early detection virtually impossible. By the time it is brought to the attention of a clinician, the tumor may be large enough to palpate. Severe epigastric pain usually is the predominant symptom. The individual may experience intense epigastric pain three to four hours after a meal, caused by the space-occupying tumor displacing the stomach or by encroachment at the ligament of Treitz. The pain often is excruciating and accompanied by vomiting. Relief is brought about by sitting up, leaning forward (proning), or lying on the right side with both knees drawn up to the chest (fetal position). These episodes of pain are short in duration and are most severe at night.[53] Cancer located in the body and tail of the pancreas produce more pain and weight loss than lesions in the head of the pancreas.[36] There is no jaundice with tumors of the body and tail of the pancreas. An enlarged spleen may be found on palpation, caused by tumor pressing on the splenic vein and resulting in splenic vein thrombosis and splenomegaly.

Tail of Pancreas

Cancer in the tail of the pancreas has the most silent and insidious progression of disease. Individuals with such a carcinoma may complain of left upper quadrant abdominal pain, generalized weakness, vague indigestion, anorexia, and unexplained weight loss. Metastatic disease is usually present when cancer in the tail of the pancreas is diagnosed. Upper gastrointestinal bleeding, splenomegaly, and signs of portal hypertension and ascites may result from thrombosis of the portal system or extensive liver damage.

In advanced carcinoma of the pancreas, hepatomegaly and a palpable gallbladder (Courvoisier sign) may also be found. There may be evidence of cachexia, muscle wasting, and a nodular texture of the liver consistent with metastatic disease. Other physical findings that serve as markers in disseminated tumor include left supraclavicular adenopathy (Virchow node), periumbilical lymphadenopathy (Sister Mary Joseph nodes), and drop metastases in the pelvis encircling the perirectal region (Blumer shelf).[36]

Assessment

Patient and Family History

Careful attention to an individual's presenting symptoms and risk factors as well as a heightened awareness of the possibility of pancreatic cancer by the clinician are important. Eliciting a family history of pancreatic cancer or related genetic syndromes could help to detect genetic abnormalities, perhaps aid in surveillance, and provide better prophylactic treatments for family members at risk in the future.

Physical Examination

Physical examination of the pancreas is virtually impossible because it is an inaccessible organ, lying behind the stomach and in front of the vertebral column. It has been called the *hermit organ* because of its hidden location in the abdomen. Few signs are evident on presentation except in those individuals presenting with obstructive jaundice. A palpable liver is the most common finding on physical exam in 30%–50% of individuals. A hard, well-defined mass that is palpable in the left upper quadrant of the abdomen is found in individuals presenting with lesions in the body and tail of the pancreas but is uncommon in lesions in the head of the pancreas. Any finding of lymphadenopathy on physical examination may warrant a lymph node biopsy.

Diagnostic Studies

A number of diagnostic studies are available to assist in the identification of pancreatic cancer, to accurately define the extent of disease, to direct appropriate therapy, and to avoid unnecessary interventions in a cost-efficient fashion (Table 61-5). If definitive diagnosis cannot be made with these studies, diagnostic laparoscopy may be necessary, with exploratory laparotomy being performed as a last resort.

As the knowledge base of the molecular genetic abnormalities in pancreatic cancer accumulates, the importance of specific oncogenes, tumor suppressor genes, and genome maintenance genes will be elucidated and may play a role in the staging of the disease.

Diagnostic procedures

Ultrasonography (US) of the abdomen can be used as an initial diagnostic test when pancreatic cancer is suspected, especially for lesions in the head of the pancreas. It is a marginal study for visualization of the body, tail, and uncinate process of the pancreas. US can detect intrahepatic and extrahepatic bile duct obstruction, a pancreatic mass, liver metastases larger than 1 cm in diameter, and ascites. It is not sensitive in defining local nodal spread or involvement of the major blood vessels in the area.[59] This imaging modality has largely been replaced by computerized tomography (CT).

Table 61-5 Techniques for Assessment of Cancer of the Pancreas

Imaging	Laboratory	Tumor Markers	Surgery
Ultrasound	Total bilirubin	CA 19-9	Laparoscopy
Computerized tomography	Alkaline phosphatase	CA 494	Percutaneous fine-needle aspiration biopsy
Magnetic resonance imaging	Gamma glutamyl transpeptidase	CA 50	
Cholangiography Endoscopic Percutaneous	Alanine aminotransferase (ALT)	DU-PAN-2	
	Aspartate aminotransferase (AST)	CA 125	
Angiography	Hemoglobin	CA 72-4	
Endoscopic ultrasound	Hematocrit	Span-1	
Positive emission tomography	Albumin		
Magnetic resonance cholangiopancreatography	Total protein		
	PT, aPTT		
	Glucose		

A high-quality spiral or helical multidetector CT with three-dimensional reconstruction using thin-cut examination is the noninvasive diagnostic and staging procedure of choice for the jaundiced individual with a suspected pancreatic malignancy, especially in older individuals. Multidetector CT incorporates dual-phase imaging in both the arterial and venous phases of enhancement.[60] CT is superior in defining the level of obstruction. It can also demonstrate the presence of a pancreatic mass and enlarged lymph nodes adjacent to the pancreas, as well as detect liver metastases, local vascular invasion, or thrombosis. Likewise, CT is more accurate in the diagnosis of unresectability. CT findings that indicate the tumor is unlikely to be resected for cure include liver metastases, ascites, vascular invasion, and tumor spread to adjacent retroperitoneal structures.

Pancreatic cancer usually appears as a hypoechoic mass that differs in consistency from the normal surrounding tissue. The use of intravenous iodine contrast enhances the imaging of the pancreas and liver. Both venous- and arterial-phase imaging is necessary for the most complete evaluation of the pancreas and its adjacent structures. Improved CT imaging has diminished the role of visceral angiography and endoscopic retrograde cholangiopancreatography (ERCP) in the diagnosis and staging of cancers of the pancreas.

Recent advances in magnetic resonance imaging (MRI), including high-resolution imaging and magnetic resonance cholangiopancreatography (MRCP), have led to an improved quality of MRI for diagnosing and staging pancreatic cancer. CT is usually more cost-effective and less time-consuming.[61] MRI may be used if CT is inconclusive. It may also be used if the patient has a contraindication to CT, such as an allergy to iodine contrast. Positron emission tomography (PET) is a newer technique that may provide additional imaging of the pancreas. Major indications for MRI and PET include the detection of small neoplasms, characterization of metastatic disease, and particularly differentiation between pancreatic carcinoma and chronic pancreatitis.[62] Because of their limited availability and higher cost, MRI and PET continue to play complementary roles to CT in the evaluation of pancreatic malignancies.[63,64]

Cholangiography is indicated in the evaluation of the jaundiced individual to define the site of biliary obstruction, by either the endoscopic or the percutaneous approach. Using ERCP, both biliary and pancreatic ductal systems can be visualized. In addition to delineating the site of obstruction, biopsy specimens for cytologic analysis can be obtained. A diagnostic ERCP may be important if the differential diagnosis includes chronic pancreatitis and clinical deterioration. In most cases of pancreatic carcinoma, the pancreatic ductal system will be obstructed with the finding of a long, irregular stricture in an otherwise normal pancreatic duct—a finding not usually seen in pancreatitis. ERCP may be most useful to evaluate the nonjaundiced individual with vague gastrointestinal symptoms in whom an early nonobstructing cancer is suspected or in the person with obstructive jaundice presumed to have pancreatic cancer but in whom no mass is evident on CT.[55,65]

The percutaneous transhepatic cholangiographic (PTC) approach to the biliary tree is technically easier if a dilated biliary tree is present. It is most helpful in defining the proximal biliary system in cases of bile duct cancer (cholangiocarcinoma). PTC with percutaneous transhepatic biliary drainage (PTBD) is usually reserved for those individuals who fail endoscopic biliary drainage or when there is a delay in definitive treatment.

Preoperative angiography is performed selectively to determine vascular invasion and to delineate the important vascular anomalies that might alter the operative approach. The study may also be done when the CT scan suggests vascular abnormalities or in persons who have undergone previous operative palliation or chemoradiation. Assessment of the vascular anatomy may be difficult because of previous operation or radiation-induced scar formation.[36] Modern CT and MRI, including magnetic resonance angiography (MRA), have replaced angiography in the staging of pancreatic tumors.[61]

Endoscopic ultrasonography (EUS) is useful in staging pancreatic tumors because it can establish the size of the tumor, its extension into adjacent structures, local and regional nodal involvement, and any vascular involvement such as the celiac axis, superior mesenteric artery, and mesenteric venous structures. It is most useful in the detection of small pancreatic lesions, smaller than 3 cm, which are not visualized on CT or ERCP. EUS has also been found to be superior to both dynamic, nonspiral CT and MRI for staging pancreatic tumors. This technique is useful in the assessment of the pancreas in the case of failed ERCP, or in the evaluation of ductal structures seen at ERCP with a brush cytology sample that tests negative for malignancy. The development of EUS-guided fine-needle aspiration is a safe and effective approach for confirming the diagnosis of a pancreatic malignancy.[66]

Laparoscopy and direct visualization are best used for staging cancer of the pancreas. Laparoscopic examination allows direct visualization of intraabdominal contents and can identify hepatic and peritoneal metastases not visualized by other modalities. Biopsy of metastatic peritoneal or omental lesions or liver implants can be performed at the same time. Enlarged lymph nodes can also be sampled with needle biopsy. Laparoscopic ultrasound has also been used for the detection of metastases not seen on the surface of the liver, vascular invasion, or deep lymph node involvement. This minimally invasive procedure can help prevent an unnecessary laparotomy for diagnosis and staging of pancreatic cancer, particularly in individuals with advanced disease and limited survival prospects. Laparoscopy can be performed as an outpatient procedure, or it may be done as an initial procedure at the time of proposed resection to evaluate for resectability.[67] Peritoneal washings at the time of laparoscopy have detected micrometastases in individuals who had no other evidence of metastatic spread. This finding predicted advanced disease in which the individual would not benefit from aggressive surgical therapy.[68]

Percutaneous fine-needle aspiration biopsy (FNAB) of pancreatic tumors is useful in selected individuals, especially when guided by CT or US. This technique is safe and reliable, but it is not indicated in individuals who are candidates for resection or surgical palliation. FNAB may not be useful in potentially resectable tumors because a negative result cannot exclude malignancy, and it is the smaller and more curable tumors that are most likely to be missed by the needle.[3] Some reports have noted neoplastic cells seeding along the tract of the needle, raising concerns regarding tumor dissemination within the abdominal cavity.[69] The pancreas is a vascular organ with a rich lymphatic network. Unnecessary manipulation can disseminate a cancer that already has a high propensity for local invasion and vascular permeation.[55] FNAB is primarily used in individuals with unresectable cancer based on preoperative staging in whom nonoperative palliation is appropriate. The results of the biopsy may then help to direct palliative chemoradiation therapy. This technique is also useful in individuals with cancer in the head of the pancreas who are not surgical candidates and for whom neoadjuvant protocols are being considered. FNAB may be most useful in individuals whose clinical presentation and imaging studies do not suggest pancreatic adenocarcinoma. Uncommon pancreatic malignancies may be treated differently after diagnosis by FNAB, such as pancreatic lymphoma, which is best managed with chemotherapy, and pancreatic islet cell carcinoma may need further testing and consideration for aggressive surgery for tumor debulking.[70]

Laboratory tests

Routine laboratory tests are generally within the normal range in the setting of pancreatic cancer, except for those individuals presenting with obstructive jaundice. Increased serum total bilirubin, alkaline phosphatase, gamma glutamyl transpeptidase, and often elevated levels of hepatic aminotransaminases are found. Normochromic anemia and hypoalbuminemia may reflect chronic neoplastic disease and its nutritional sequelae. When liver function test abnormalities occur in individuals with cancer of the body and tail of the pancreas, it indicates metastatic disease with liver involvement. Coagulation parameters should be checked in persons with deep jaundice because prolonged absence of bile from the gastrointestinal tract leads to malabsorption of fat-soluble vitamins and decreased production of vitamin K–dependent clotting factors.[36]

New-onset diabetes mellitus may be found in an individual with elevated glucose levels, which may or may not be controlled with oral hyperglycemic agents. A pancreatic problem should be investigated in an individual with previously controlled diabetes who exhibits any unexplained changes in glucose control.

Table 61-6 AJCC TNM Staging for Exocrine Pancreas Cancer

Primary Tumor (T)

TX	Primary tumor cannot be assessed
T0	No evidence of primary tumor
Tis	Carcinoma in situ
T1	Tumor limited to pancreas and 2 cm or less in greatest dimension
T2	Tumor limited to pancreas and more than 2 cm in greatest dimension
T3	Tumor extends beyond pancreas but does not involve celiac axis or superior mesentery artery
T4	Tumor invades the celiac or the superior mesentery artery (unresectable primary tumor)

Regional Lymph Nodes (N)

NX	Regional lymph nodes cannot be assessed
N0	No regional lymph node metastasis
N1	Regional lymph node metastasis

Distant Metastasis (M)

MX	Distant metastasis cannot be assessed
M0	No distant metastasis
M1	Distant metastasis

Stage Grouping

Stage 0	Tis	N0	M0
Stage IA	T1	N0	M0
Stage IB	T2	N0	M0
Stage IIA	T3	N0	M0
Stage IIB	T1–T3	N1	M0
Stage III	T4	Any N	M0
Stage IV	Any T	Any N	M1

Tumor markers

No serum tumor marker is sufficiently sensitive or specific to be considered cost-effective and 100% reliable for screening of pancreatic cancer. Instead, a wide variety of serum tumor markers have been proposed for use in the diagnosis and follow-up of pancreatic carcinoma. The carbohydrate antigen 19-9 (CA 19-9) is tumor associated, not tumor specific, and has been a useful tool in the diagnosis and management of individuals with pancreatic cancer. Several factors can influence interpretation of CA 19-9: reference value, positive Lewis blood phenotype, jaundice, and prior use of interferon.[71] There is a lack of consensus concerning a useful reference value for the diagnosis of carcinoma of the pancreas. A reference value of CA 19-9 greater than 90 U/mL reaches an accuracy of 85% for diagnosis; the accuracy improves to 95% with a level greater than 200 U/mL.[72] CA 19-9 is not produced by individuals who lack the Lewis antigen (5%–10% of the Western population). Jaundice in an individual can cause a false increase in serum levels of CA 19-9. In addition, interferon significantly elevates CA 19-9 levels.[73]

CA 19-9 has not proved useful as a screening test, as levels are normal in early-stage, potentially curable tumors. Use of CA 19-9 measurements combined with either US, CT, or ERCP improves diagnostic accuracy. Elevated levels may help differentiate benign diseases from pancreatic cancer. After resection of pancreatic cancer, CA 19-9 levels fall. The antigen may then prove useful for prognosis and follow-up surveillance for tumor recurrence. A high preoperative CA 19-9 level usually indicates a large pancreatic neoplasm and greater probability of unresectability.[36] This biomarker is used to monitor response to treatment, as increasing levels of CA 19-9 reflect progression of disease. Stable or declining levels of CA 19-9 are associated with a stable tumor burden and an improved prognosis.[74]

Several other tumor markers have been evaluated, either alone or in combination, as ways to screen for pancreatic cancer but thus far have not proved as reliable as CA 19-9 in the disease's diagnosis and monitoring. The use of molecular genetic markers as a mechanism for screening for genetic abnormalities in individuals with pancreatic cancer continues to evolve.

Classification and Staging

The goal when staging cancer of the pancreas is to select the optimal treatment for each individual with minimal risks in a cost-effective manner. The aim is to determine whether the individual has potentially resectable disease, locally advanced disease, or metastatic disease, because therapeutic options and ultimate prognosis differ in each case. The definition of "resectability" can vary and reflects both the expertise and philosophy of the individual surgeon and institution.[75]

The staging of pancreatic carcinoma is based on the tumor-node-metastasis (TNM) system. Four stages have been described for use in the diagnosis of exocrine cancer of the pancreas by the American Joint Committee on Cancer (AJCC; see Table 61-6).[76] These parameters represent the most important factors influencing resectability and prognosis of exocrine tumors of the pancreas.

Therapeutic Approaches and Nursing Care

Every individual diagnosed with cancer of the pancreas should be carefully evaluated prior to initiation of any therapy. An individual must also be adequately prepared physiologically and psychologically before undergoing any therapy. Historically, the poor prognosis of individuals with pancreatic cancer has caused many clinicians to have a dismal outlook and thus be reluctant to treat the disease aggressively. However, recent reports on surgical outcomes are encouraging,[77,78] and the overall perspective on the disease appears to be changing.

Surgery, radiotherapy, and chemotherapy are the principal treatment modalities used for pancreatic cancer. Surgical resection remains the best therapeutic option, even though few individuals are cured. Most surgical procedures are palliative as nonresectable pancreatic cancer predominates. Only about 10% of malignancies of the head of the pancreas are resectable and potentially curable at surgery.[36] The three-year and five-year survival rates after resection of the head of the pancreas are only 35% and 21%, respectively.[79] The resection and survival rates for tumors in the body and tail of the pancreas are much lower.

Available therapeutic interventions include surgery, usually in combination with radiation therapy, and chemotherapy with single agents or a combination of agents for either cure or palliation. Various regimens of chemotherapeutic agents alone or combinations of agents with or without radiation therapy are also used for nonoperative cancer of the pancreas. Experimental vaccines and drugs that target the genes involved with pancreatic cancer are being investigated and may soon be a routine part of multimodal therapies.[80] Palliation for longer periods is usually achieved with combined modalities.

Once a diagnosis has been made, the extent of the tumor involvement established, and complete assessment of the individual's physical status made, a treatment plan will be presented to the individual. If surgery is an option, the patient's physical ability to undergo general anesthesia and a major abdominal operation must be considered; advanced age is not necessarily a negative factor.[81] Nutritional status, hematologic status, liver function, concomitant disease, and skill of the principal clinicians all contribute to the choice of therapy.

Prior to surgery, a biliary stent to alleviate jaundice may be placed through the obstructing lesion by either the endoscopic or the percutaneous approach. Current studies suggest that the use of routine preoperative biliary stenting leads to an increase in postoperative surgical complications.[82,83] In selected individuals with severe malnutrition, sepsis, and/or correctable medical conditions, or in whom there is a time delay before surgery, preoperative biliary drainage may be useful. Theoretically, the internal drainage of biliary secretions may provide an immunological advantage, leading to decreased perioperative complications of sepsis. An endoscopic stent or a percutaneously placed biliary stent can be used in the operative management of individuals with pancreatic cancer either for resection or for palliation. An ERCP with stent placement is performed under conscious sedation, and the person can be discharged the same day. Antibiotics are usually administered intravenously as prophylaxis against cholangitis due to manipulation within the biliary tract. The benefit of an internal stent for drainage is that there is no external tube to manage. The individual needs to be taught the signs and symptoms of possible complications of the stent, such as recurrent jaundice and cholangitis (shaking chills and fever). Any manifestation of these signs or symptoms needs to be reported to the health care provider immediately, as the individual may be prone to bacteremia and sepsis.

The individual having a PTC with placement of a PTBD stent needs to be taught about the procedure as well as the care and management of the external biliary stent. This interventional radiological procedure is performed under conscious sedation. An internal–external stent is placed. Prophylactic antibiotics are given to prevent biliary sepsis. Individuals are usually monitored for 24 hours to assess patency of the stent and to ensure bile drainage. Initially, the biliary stent is attached to a bile bag, for external drainage, to allow the obstructed biliary tree to decompress. The bile bag is then removed, and the biliary stent is capped off with a one-way valve to allow internal drainage and the free flow of bile into the bowel.

Care of a percutaneously placed biliary stent to maintain a properly functioning tube is an important aspect of patient teaching. Signs and symptoms of any complications — such as fever, chills, recurrent jaundice, bleeding at the exit site or through the biliary stent, dislodgment of the catheter from its original site, or inability to flush the stent — must be reported immediately to the health care provider to prevent problems. Teaching protocols are important for consistent and correct information. Written instructions given to the individual as a handout or a video to take home may be helpful.[82,83]

Cure is the objective if the tumor is small, localized, and not fixed to other structures, and if there is no evidence of regional or distant metastases. Complete resection of the tumor will be performed and supplemented with adjuvant therapy.

Control or palliation is the goal of therapy if the tumor is unresectable or has metastasized to regional or distant nodes or to other organs. Unfortunately, approximately 90% of all cases of pancreatic carcinoma are diagnosed as unresectable. In a significant number of individuals, operative palliation for obstructive jaundice or gastric outlet obstruction may be indicated for optimal long-term management. Other treatments aimed at relieving devastating symptoms may include radiotherapy, chemotherapy, percutaneous pain block, percutaneous or endoscopic biliary decompression to relieve obstruction and pressure, and gastric decompression for gastric outlet obstruction. Nutritional supplementation to achieve adequate total protein levels helps to decrease surgical risk, puts the individual in a better metabolic state for having any treatment modality, and increases the patient's overall well-being.

It is important to understand the individual's goal and plan for therapy, method of family coping, and pattern of communication. When all members of the health care team, along with the patient, agree upon a course of treatment, communication is enhanced and issues or problems can be identified and addressed. Illness has a special meaning to each person. Living with cancer of the pancreas and dealing with the knowledge that the disease has a poor prognosis, regardless of what treatment is undertaken, can create many unforeseen problems. Comprehensive education about diagnostics and modes of therapy, along with physical and emotional support to the patient with a new diagnosis of pancreatic carcinoma, is the hallmark of nursing care.

Surgery

Surgical resection of pancreatic cancer remains the best therapeutic option and the only opportunity for cure. Most surgical procedures for this disease are palliative. Only about 10%–20% of carcinomas of the head of the pancreas are resectable and potentially curable at surgery. The survival rate for individuals with tumors in the body and tail is much lower. There is limited prospective research evaluating surgical procedures for cancer of the pancreas.

Recent reports from institutions with large series of patients have reported increasing survival periods following resection and operative mortality rates that have decreased to less than 5%.[4,78,84–86] Decreased complications are attributed to refinements in surgical technique, anesthesia, critical care, and preoperative and postoperative care. Other reasons for the improvements in surgical outcome include the operations being performed by surgeons who are experienced in the surgical management of pancreatic carcinoma, concentration of patients in centers of excellence, and improved methods to diagnose and treat complications.[87] Most surgical results report collective overall outcomes; however, individuals with small (less than 2 cm) tumors have five-year survival rates of 30%, and survival rates increase for those with no residual disease or without lymphatic involvement.[85] The crux of the problem is late detection of pancreatic tumors. Until advances in early detection and diagnosis are made, curative surgery will be limited to very few candidates and palliative measures will continue as the mainstay of therapy.

When cure is the objective, the surgical approach most frequently used for neoplasms of the head of the pancreas is a pancreaticoduodenectomy (Whipple procedure). Total pancreatectomy may be performed for tumor involving the entire gland, tumor that extends across the neck and body of the gland, or when the pancreatic remnant is too soft and friable to allow a safe pancreatic–enteric anastomosis. An extended or radical pancreaticoduodenectomy has also been performed as an alternative or modification of the original regional pancreatectomy. Regional pancreatectomy has been found to have higher morbidity and mortality rates, with no improvement in survival over the standard pancreaticoduodenectomy.[88] Controversy exists regarding the advantages, disadvantages, and long-term results of each operation.[89] (See Table 61-7.)[5] To determine the best operation for resectable pancreatic cancer, data from prospective randomized studies comparing standard versus radical pancreaticoduodenectomy in individuals are being evaluated.

Despite sophisticated preoperative staging methods, many individuals with adenocarcinoma of the head of the pancreas that preoperatively appears to be resectable are ultimately found to have metastatic or locally invasive disease. During surgical exploration, it is possible to encounter local spread of tumor into adjacent major vascular structures (portal vein, superior mesenteric vein, superior mesenteric artery, or abdominal aorta). The tumor can encase and grow into these vessels, precluding surgical resection. The tumor may also have metastasized to the liver or peritoneal surfaces. If unresectable or metastatic disease is discovered, surgical palliation can be used to treat or prevent the major symptoms of obstructive jaundice, duodenal obstruction, and pain.

Pancreaticoduodenectomy (Whipple procedure). The Whipple procedure is the most commonly performed operation for carcinoma of the head of the pancreas (Figure 61-3A).[90] The classic Whipple procedure includes resection of the distal stomach, gallbladder, distal common bile duct, head of the pancreas,

Table 61-7 Comparison of Types of Pancreatic Resections for Malignancy

	Indications	Tissues Removed	Potential Advantages	Potential Disadvantages
Classic pancreaticoduodenectomy (Whipple)	Periampullary or localized carcinoma of head, neck, or uncinate process of pancreas	Head, neck, and uncinate process Duodenum Gastric antrum and pylorus Common bile duct Gallbladder Lymph nodes in pancreaticoduodenal groove	Pancreatic remnant may prevent diabetes and malabsorption Better cancer operation compared with pylorus preservation	Partial pancreatic resection may leave residual tumor in body or tail of gland Issue of multicentricity Dumping syndrome secondary to loss of pylorus Nutritional problems Leak at pancreatic anastomosis
Pylorus-preserving pancreaticoduodenectomy (Whipple)	Periampullary or localized carcinoma of head, neck, or uncinate process of pancreas	Head, neck, and uncinate process Duodenum (except most proximal portion) Common bile duct Gallbladder Lymph nodes in pancreaticoduodenal groove	Pancreatic remnant may prevent diabetes and malabsorption Normal gastric reservoir Less disruption of digestion compared with classic Whipple Reduced marginal ulceration at duodenojejunostomy	Partial pancreatic resection may leave residual tumor in body or tall of gland Leak at pancreatic anastomosis Delayed gastric emptying
Extended or radical pancreaticoduodenectomy	Periampullary or localized carcinoma of head, neck, or uncinate process of pancreas	Head, neck, and uncinate process Duodenum Gastric antrum and pylorus Common bile duct Gallbladder Extensive lymph node and retroperitoneal tissue dissection Vascular resection may be included	Extensive regional nodal dissection Pancreatic remnant may prevent diabetes and malabsorption Better cancer operation?	Partial pancreatic resection may leave residual tumor in body or tail of gland Leak at pancreatic anastomosis Dumping syndrome secondary to loss of pylorus Nutritional problems Chylous leak Longer operation with potential for increased blood loss and complications
Total pancreaticoduodenectomy (may be classic or pylorus-preserving)	Diffuse carcinoma of entire gland or a multicentric tumor	Entire pancreas Duodenum Gastric antrum and pylorus Common bile duct Gallbladder Spleen Peripancreatic nodes Lymph nodes in pancreaticoduodenal groove	Excision of entire pancreas may remove multifocal tumor More complete peripancreatic nodal dissection No pancreatic enteric anastomosis	Insulin-dependent diabetes and complete exocrine absence Need for insulin and enzyme replacement Postsplenectomy state
Distal pancreatectomy	Carcinoma localized to body or tail of gland	Distal pancreas Spleen Peripancreatic lymph nodes	Pancreatic remnant may prevent diabetes and malabsorption No pancreatic or billiary enteric anastomosis	Limited resection may leave residual tumor Postsplenectomy state

Source: Reprinted with permission from Sauter PK, Coleman J: Pancreatic cancer: a continuum of care. *Semin Oncol Nurs* 15:36–47, 1999.[5]

and duodenum. Gastrointestinal continuity is restored by anastomosing the common bile duct and the remaining pancreas to the jejunum proximal to the gastrojejunostomy. Some surgeons anastomose the remaining pancreas to the back of the stomach because they believe it is safer and decreases the potential for pancreatic fistula formation.[91] The gastrojejunostomy is performed to allow alkaline bile and pancreatic

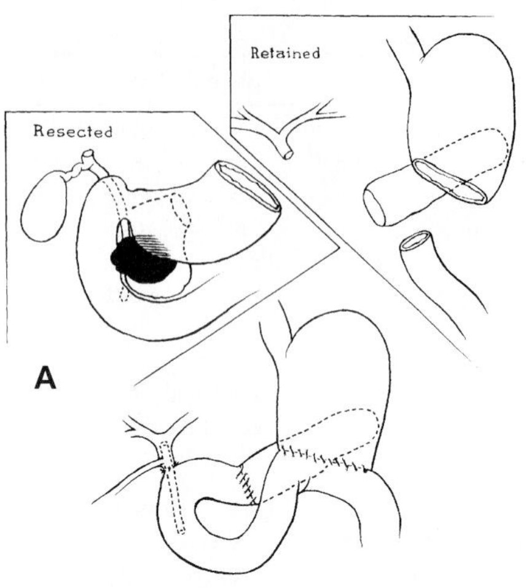

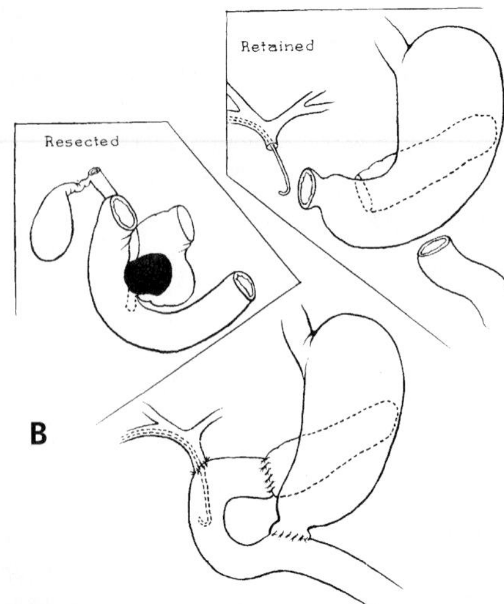

Figure 61-3 Classic pancreaticoduodenectomy (**A**) and pylorus-preserving pancreaticoduodenectomy (**B**), showing the resected specimens, the structures retained, and one method of reconstruction by way of pancreaticojejunostomy. (Used with permission from Yeo CJ, Cameron JL: The pancreas, in Hardy JD (ed.): *Hardy's Textbook of Surgery* (ed 2). Philadelphia, PA Lippincott-Raven, 1988, pp 695-725.[90])

juices to enter the jejunum before acidic gastric secretions.[92] This step decreases the potential for ulceration at the gastrojejunostomy. The distal gastrojejunostomy also reduces reflux of intestinal contents into the bile duct and pancreas. The risk of ulceration has been greatly reduced by the use of postoperative prophylactic acid antisecretory agents such as H_2-receptor antagonists and proton pump inhibitors.

A modification of the original or classic Whipple procedure, called a *pylorus-preserving pancreaticoduodenectomy*, is preferred by some surgeons (Figure 61-3B).[90] This procedure preserves the entire stomach, including the pylorus, and a small cuff of proximal duodenum. It has the advantage of maintaining a normal gastric reservoir and environment, thereby avoiding potential nutritional problems associated with the classic Whipple procedure such as weight loss, dumping syndrome, diarrhea, and anastomotic ulcer at the gastrojejunostomy site. This procedure requires less time and is technically easier to perform.[93] Delayed gastric emptying that may occur following this operation generally resolves over time with conservative treatment (gastric decompression, parenteral or enteral nutrition, and prokinetic agents). Erythromycin, a motilin agonist, also has been prescribed to improve gastric emptying after surgery.[94] Concern has arisen that the pylorus-preserving pancreaticoduodenectomy may not be an adequate cancer operation because of the limited surgical margins and inadequate removal of lymph nodes in the area draining the cancer, which may compromise cure. Studies have shown that pylorus preservation appears to be associated with no consistent adverse sequelae, and it has equivalent survival and quality of life as compared to classic pancreaticoduodenectomy.[84,86,95,96]

Table 61-8 Complications After Pancreaticoduodenectomy

Pancreatic fistula
Delayed gastric emptying
Wound infection
Intraabdominal abscess
Hemorrhage
Diabetes
Pancreatic exocrine insufficiency

Pancreatic fistula and delayed gastric emptying are the most common serious complications after a pancreaticoduodenectomy. The pancreas, attached to the jejunum, is technically the most difficult of the anastomoses. If it does not heal properly, a pancreatic fistula may develop. Although fistulae and leaks were previously associated with significant mortality because pancreatic juices eroded into major blood vessels, the incidence and severity of pancreatic anastomotic leaks appear to have decreased with improved surgical technique, intravenous nutritional support, modern antibiotics, and appropriate wound drainage systems.[81,96] The use of the somatostatin analog octreotide, which decreases pancreatic secretions, may also prove useful in the management of postoperative pancreatic fistulae. Intraabdominal infection, gastrointestinal bleeding, wound infection, diabetes, and pancreatic exocrine insufficiency occur less frequently.[93,97,98] (See Table 61-8.)

It is important for the nurse to know exactly what surgical procedure was performed so as to know what to assess from various drains and tubes placed at the time of surgery. Bile duct-to-jejunum anastomosis may be stented with a preoperatively placed percutaneous transhepatic biliary stent to ensure decompression of the jejunum and to allow the free flow of bile. This stent also provides direct access into the biliary tree postoperatively to assess for an anastomotic leak, obstruction, or stricture. Likewise, wound drains may be placed adjacent to the pancreatic and biliary anastomoses to enable rapid assessment of bile or pancreatic juice leakage or bleeding. The use of various feeding tubes placed at the time of surgery depends on the preference of the surgeon.

Nutritional assessment is important to establish that the person has adequate protein and calories for wound healing. Most individuals will receive postoperative adjuvant therapy; therefore, good nutritional status along with physical and psychological readiness are essential. Immediate postoperative pain management can be successfully provided by intravenous or epidural patient-controlled analgesia (PCA).

Extended (radical) pancreaticoduodenectomy. This operation consists of a pancreaticoduodenectomy or sometimes a total pancreatectomy, along with an extensive retroperitoneal lymph node and soft tissue resection. Resection of the superior mesenteric vein, portal vein, or superior mesenteric artery may also be performed. The extended pancreaticoduodenectomy has been advocated by some Japanese and European researchers because lymph node involvement is an important prognostic factor in individuals with carcinoma of the head of the pancreas. No published prospective randomized studies demonstrate a consistent survival advantage for individuals undergoing extended pancreaticoduodenectomy.[36]

Total pancreatectomy. A total pancreatectomy entails an en bloc resection of the distal stomach, duodenum, gallbladder, and distal common bile duct, along with the entire pancreas, spleen, and a wide margin of peripancreatic tissue including lymph nodes. It eliminates the problem of residual tumor at the margins of the pancreas, tumor spillage when the pancreas is divided, and pancreatic fistula. This operation has shown no reduction in mortality or morbidity nor evidence of any increase in survival when it is performed routinely.[3] Individuals who have a total pancreatectomy develop pancreatic endocrine and exocrine insufficiency and become brittle diabetics with glucose levels that may be difficult to control. Pancreatic enzyme supplementation is necessary for a lifetime. This operation is usually reserved for selected cases, particularly when there is evidence of tumor throughout the entire pancreas or when the pancreas is considered to be unsafe for anastomosis. Reasons for an unsafe anastomosis are that the pancreas is too soft and friable, or acute edematous pancreatitis develops during surgery after manipulation of the gland.[3,88]

Distal pancreatectomy. In rare cases, tumors of the body and tail of the pancreas are detected early enough to be considered curable. A distal pancreatectomy with a splenectomy is performed in these patients. The prognosis is poor, with few patients surviving for more than two years. Lesions of the body and tail rarely cause gastrointestinal obstructive symptoms and as a result are not recognized until the tumor has become unresectable.[99] Most individuals with adenocarcinomas of the body or tail of the pancreas are unresectable and survive for only a short period. The only change in the management of these individuals has been a diminished need for exploratory laparotomy to establish tissue diagnosis. The use of laparoscopy and FNAB to determine metastatic or unresectable disease spares these individuals an unnecessary laparotomy.[3]

Palliative procedures. Only about 10% of individuals with pancreatic cancer are resectable for cure at the time of presentation. Therefore, palliation of symptoms to maximize quality of life is the primary goal for most patients who are not curable.[99] These individuals present challenging management problems because optimal palliation of symptoms is difficult. Obstructive jaundice, duodenal obstruction, and pain are the symptoms most frequently requiring aggressive intervention using operative and nonoperative techniques.[3] Management can be tailored to the individual's clinical presentation, prognosis, and overall medical condition.[99] A choice must be made between operative and nonoperative palliation. Operative palliation is used for those patients who are deemed appropriate surgical candidates, have a good performance status, and are expected to survive for longer than six months. Individuals in poor health or those not expected to live for a prolonged time should be considered for nonoperative palliation.[3]

Conventional surgical palliation for an individual with a tumor in the head of the pancreas is done to relieve obstructive jaundice, avoid or treat duodenal obstruction, relieve tumor-associated pain, and improve quality of life. Operative procedures designed for palliation include biliary-enteric drainage, gastrojejunostomy, and chemical splanchnicectomy. Individuals with body and tail lesions of the pancreas are less likely to have jaundice or duodenal obstruction, and pain is the major symptom.

Obstructive jaundice is the most common presenting symptom in the majority of cancers of the head of the pancreas. If left untreated, it results in progressive liver dysfunction, culminating in liver failure and early death. In addition, the pruritus associated with obstructive jaundice can be unbearable and is seldom responsive to medications. The jaundiced individual usually experiences anorexia, nausea, and progressive malnutrition.[36] Relief of jaundice can provide improvement in an individual's overall well-being.

The surgical options for palliation of obstructive jaundice include an internal biliary bypass by means of a choledochojejunostomy (common bile duct to jejunum) or a cholecystojejunostomy (gallbladder to jejunum). Bypass of the obstructed biliary tree to the jejunum is preferred and is necessary if the gallbladder is surgically absent.

Minimally invasive surgery is now being used for palliation of biliary and duodenal obstruction with laparoscopic cholecystojejunostomy and gastrojejunostomy.[100] The preliminary results have shown technical success, low morbidity, and satisfactory outcomes. Palliative pancreaticoduodenectomy may also offer some advantages to those individuals with seemingly unresectable disease. This major operation would be performed on selected patients considered to have low perioperative morbidity and mortality.[101]

Nonoperative palliation of obstructed jaundice by either percutaneous or endoscopic drainage methods is also effective. Placement of a stent through the area of biliary obstruction facilitates the free flow of bile. Compared with operative decompression, a biliary stent reduces the length of initial hospitalization, is associated with lower complication rates and lower procedure-related mortality, and is significantly less expensive.[36]

Endoscopically placed biliary stents offer an advantage over the percutaneous technique, with fewer procedure-related complications and better patient acceptance. The major complication is stent occlusion associated with recurrent jaundice and sepsis. This problem can require stent replacement every three to four months or sooner. Prolonged stent patency is now being achieved with the use of large-diameter, expandable metallic stents. These stents appear to remain patent for a time that closely approximates the length of survival of the individual.[102] Endoscopic stents are also preferred for individuals with ascites to prevent the external leakage of ascites and avoid being a portal for infection.

Percutaneous biliary drainage is indicated when endoscopic biliary drainage is unsuccessful and with recurrent jaundice following surgical bypass.[103] An internal–external drainage stent is placed by an interventional radiologist. The biliary stent requires daily maintenance by the individual or caregiver—in particular, daily stent flushing and dressing of the stent entry site. The presence of the external stent serves as a constant reminder to the patient of the disease. Bile leakage around the stent, skin irritation, stent dislodgment, and stent occlusion may occur. In individuals with ascites, leakage of ascitic fluid around the stent almost always occurs and is difficult to control. Because all stents placed within the biliary tree eventually will occlude, percutaneous biliary stents are exchanged approximately every three months to prevent development of stent obstruction, recurrent jaundice, or cholangitis. This exchange can be easily performed as an outpatient procedure. Complications related to percutaneous biliary drainage include transient bacteremia or sepsis, hemobilia, and bile peritonitis.

Duodenal obstruction occurs in a significant number of individuals when unresectable disease progresses. Obstruction from cancer in the head of the pancreas typically occurs at the duodenal C loop, causing nausea and vomiting. A large tumor in the body or tail of the pancreas will usually obstruct the junction of the duodenum and jejunum at the ligament of Treitz.[104] A retrocolic gastrojejunostomy can be performed to treat or prevent gastric outlet obstruction. The procedure, when implemented as a prophylactic measure and combined with a biliary bypass, has been shown to be of value as the individual's morbidity or mortality is not increased when gastrojejunostomy is performed as either a therapeutic or a prophylactic measure.[105] If the patient is not a surgical candidate because of recurrent tumor or is in the terminal stage of disease, duodenal obstruction can be alleviated by placement of a percutaneous endoscopic gastrostomy (PEG) decompression tube. This tube is not used for feeding, but it is effective in relieving gastric distention and may improve the comfort of the individual in the terminal stages of the disease.

Endoscopically placed metallic stents within the native duodenum at the site of tumor infiltration or at the site of an obstructed gastrojejunostomy have provided an alternative nonoperative option for individuals with malignant duodenal obstruction. This novel approach continues to be assessed as an appropriate palliative management device to allow the patient to resume enteral nutrition until death.[106]

Pain is the most significant symptom for individuals with pancreatic cancer. For many patients, pain is poorly managed and remains so until death. The severity and persistence of pain correlate with the stage of the disease. For most individuals with pancreatic cancer who are not surgical candidates, the appropriate use of oral agents can successfully manage pain.[107] Chemical splanchnicectomy (alcohol nerve block) is an alternative therapy available to those patients who

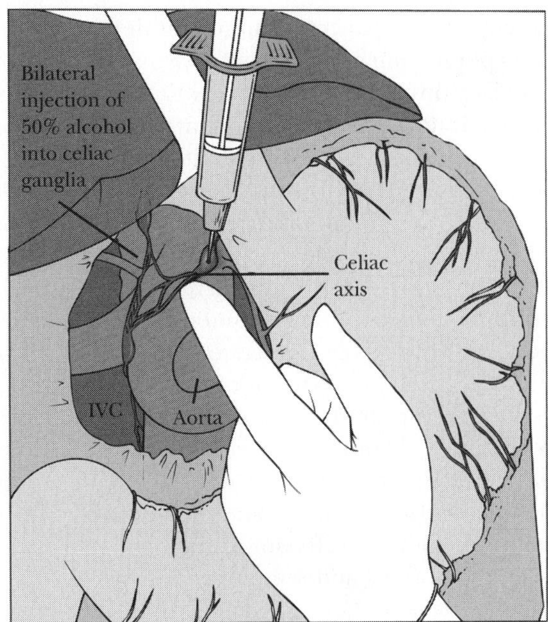

Figure 61-4 Chemical splanchnicectomy was performed using a syringe and a 20- or 22-gauge spinal needle. Solution (20 mL) was injected on each side of the aorta at the level of the celiac axis. (Used with permission from Lillemoe KD, Cameron JL, Kaufman HS, et al: Chemical splanchnicectomy in patients with unresectable pancreatic cancer: a prospective randomized trial. *Ann Surg* 217:447–457, 1993.[108])

do not benefit from oral analgesia or who cannot tolerate oral intake due to gastric outlet obstruction. It is performed using a spinal needle to inject alcohol on each side of the aorta at the level of the celiac axis (Figure 61-4).[108] Percutaneous celiac nerve block, with either fluoroscopic or CT guidance, can be performed to reduce pain and to decrease the need for oral narcotics. Nerve blocks can be done as an outpatient procedure or at the time of surgery for those individuals undergoing a palliative operation. Percutaneous nerve blocks can be repeated in individuals with previous blocks that have subsequently worn off. Orthostatic hypotension is the most common complication after the block. Intraoperative injection of alcohol into the celiac nerves has been shown to both relieve pain and prevent the development of pain. Improvement in pain control is associated with prolonged survival and enhanced quality of life.[108,109]

Another modality used for control of pain due to unresectable pancreatic cancer is external beam radiation therapy.[36] Finally, transthoracic splanchnicectomy and endoscopic chemical splanchnicectomy with the aid of US guidance have been performed to relieve pain due to unresectable pancreatic cancer in selected individuals.[109]

Postoperative care

Postoperative medical and nursing management of individuals who undergo pancreatic resection is critical for reducing surgical morbidity and mortality. Careful assessment, anticipatory management, and complete patient and family teaching will greatly enhance recovery and rehabilitation.[109,110] Hemorrhage, hypovolemia, and hypotension pose the greatest threats in the immediate postoperative period.

Following a pancreatic resection, individuals may be admitted to an intensive care unit, where hemodynamic monitoring is performed. Stabilizing and maintaining fluid requirements are essential. Careful attention is given to signs of bleeding, security and patency of wound drains, and pain management. Pain management can be achieved with opiates delivered by intravenous or epidural patient-controlled analgesia (PCA). Following endotracheal extubation, aggressive pulmonary toilet is needed to reduce the risk of respiratory problems. Ideally, patients should be out of bed and sitting in a chair within a few hours following extubation.

Hemorrhage in the early postoperative period can be life-threatening. This complication can occur from failure of surgical hemostasis, from leakage at the anastomosis, or from generalized coagulopathy. Abdominal distention, shock, hematemesis, bloody drainage from gastrointestinal decompression tubes, wound drains, or bloody stool warrant immediate attention. Successful management requires correction of the coagulation abnormalities and prompt reoperation if a surgical cause is suspected.

Hypovolemia can develop from fluids lost during extensive surgery, through decompression tubes and wound drains, or from the shift of fluid from the vascular space to the interstitial space (third spacing). Low levels of circulating plasma proteins secondary to malnutrition and hypoalbuminemia usually account for the third spacing syndrome. The first phase of fluid compartment shifting begins immediately after surgery and can last 48–72 hours. Signs of fluid shift are as follows:

- Decreased blood pressure
- Increased pulse rate
- Low central venous pressure
- Decreased urine output
- Increased specific gravity
- Low levels of serum albumin
- Hemoconcentration

When the plasma protein is replaced and levels return to normal, fluid reabsorption follows. Urine output will dramatically increase and will greatly exceed intake. The individual is closely monitored for signs of circulatory overload. The reabsorption phase will reach equilibrium within 24–48 hours.

Hypotension is a potential postoperative complication that is believed to result from severance of the sympathetic nerve fibers of the mesenteric complex. Vital signs and urine output should be monitored frequently to detect alterations. Vasopressor drugs and liberal intravenous fluids may be administered.

Pulmonary complications following surgery usually result from immobility and inadequate lung expansion secondary to pain and splinting. In addition, those individuals who are malnourished and protein deficient are susceptible to pneumonia. The importance of vigorous pulmonary hygiene and early ambulation cannot be overemphasized. Parenteral nutrition may also be needed to correct nutritional deficiencies.

Careful attention is given to wound drains for any sudden change in amount, color, or consistency of drainage. Abdominal wound drains are observed for evidence of bile or clear pancreatic juice that would suggest anastomotic leakage. Pancreatic juice that changes color to milky or brown with a foul odor suggests a pancreatic fistula. The somatostatin analog octreotide may be given to reduce pancreatic secretion and thereby allow the pancreatic anastomosis to heal.[97,98]

Prolonged ileus and delayed gastric emptying are other potential complications. These problems can generally be resolved by taking a conservative approach with nasogastric suction, maintenance of parenteral or enteral nutrition, and use of prokinetic agents, such as metoclopramide, or a motilin agonist, such as erythromycin.[94] The surgical incision must be examined routinely for any signs of infection, as this complication can be synergistic with a pancreatic fistula or delayed gastric emptying.[97]

Following resection of the pancreas, exocrine and endocrine functions will be temporarily or permanently altered, depending on the amount of viable pancreatic tissue remaining. In the immediate postoperative period, laboratory tests are useful for monitoring protein, fat, and glucose levels. Prior to discharge, the patient and family must become familiar with and be able to recognize the signs and symptoms of exocrine and endocrine abnormalities such as hyperglycemia, hypoglycemia, steatorrhea, stupor, and lethargy, especially in those patients who have undergone a total pancreatectomy.

Endocrine function, the secretion of insulin, and the production of glucagon may be altered after a pancreatic resection. Usually, a nondiabetic individual will not develop diabetes after a pancreaticoduodenectomy (occurring in less than 10% of cases).[111] Individuals who have a total pancreatectomy will develop significant hyperglycemia and are usually managed in the immediate postoperative period with an insulin drip infusion. Endocrinology consultants should be contacted soon after surgery to assist with glucose management and insulin adjustment, particularly when the patient is taking oral foods and fluids. Serum glucose levels are monitored at least every six hours, and a sliding-scale insulin dose is administered as needed if the individual can take nothing by mouth. These patients generally require only moderate amounts of insulin and are not prone to ketoacidosis. However, they are particularly brittle and readily develop life-threatening hypoglycemia. Maintaining tight glucose control is now advocated for postoperative and lifelong management. Discharge teaching and home therapy programs — including self-administration of insulin, knowledge of signs and symptoms of hyper- or hypoglycemia, diabetic diet, meticulous hygiene, and the importance of routine follow-up with an endocrinologist or a medical physician for diabetes management — are the same as for individuals with diabetes. Inability to control glucose levels may indicate recurrence of disease.

Alteration of exocrine function by removal of pancreatic tissue can result in a malabsorption syndrome characterized by an inability to use ingested forms of fat and protein. The caloric requirements of the individual following surgery exceed 3000 calories per day; therefore, adequate nutritional intake is essential to recovery. Oral ingestion of food is the best means of maintaining essential nutrients, but ileus or delayed gastric emptying may prohibit this mode. Parenteral or enteral alimentation may be necessary to replace calories lost as a result of the surgically induced malabsorption of fats and proteins until the individual can be advanced to an oral diet. Pancreatic enzymes are replaced with oral enzyme supplements, which contain lipase, amylase, and trypsin. The most frequently used forms are pancreatin and pancrelipase. Pancreatin and pancrelipase supplements are made from extracts of porcine or bovine pancreas enriched with bile salts and plant and fungal enzymes. The usual therapeutic dose is two to four tablets with each meal and one to two tablets with a fatty snack. The enzymes are taken with or during the meal.[112] It may require several adjustments before the most appropriate dosage for each person is determined, because eating patterns and individual responses vary.[113]

When the patient is able to tolerate food, several small feedings consisting of foods that are low in fat and high in carbohydrates and protein are tolerated better than large meals. Restrictions include overindulgence (which places a great demand on the pancreas), caffeine, and alcohol. It is advantageous for the clinical dietitian to consult with the patient to select the most agreeable diet plan based on individual needs and lifestyle. The patient and family should be instructed on how to monitor the individual's tolerance to the diet and pancreatic enzyme replacement therapy. Stool should be examined daily for the characteristic signs of steatorrhea: frothy, floating, foul-smelling stool with greasy, fat particles floating in the water, crampy abdominal pain, or bloating. If these characteristics are observed, they should be reported to the healthcare provider for dietary and/or pancreatic enzyme dosage adjustment.[112] The individual should be informed that steatorrhea will decrease but may not be eliminated.

Chemotherapy

Because most individuals present with unresectable cancer of the pancreas and are already in a debilitated state, benefit from antineoplastic therapy is unlikely. Individuals with pancreatic cancer exhibit precarious physiologic conditions, which makes it difficult to differentiate the side effects of therapy from the natural progression of the disease. Response to therapy is also difficult to evaluate.

Although the only curative therapy for pancreatic cancer is surgical resection, most studies document high rates of both local recurrence and distant metastases.[114] The benefit of using adjuvant combined chemotherapy and radiation therapy after surgical resection for pancreatic cancer was demonstrated by the Gastrointestinal Tumor Study Group (GITSG).[115] Radiation therapy is directed at the region from which the tumor was resected or where the greatest tumor burden lies; chemotherapy addresses the smaller or microscopic residual tumor. With the recent surge in interest in treatments for cancer of the pancreas, the role of multimodality therapy for patients with potentially resectable pancreatic cancer continues to evolve. Many different combinations of chemotherapeutic agents and radiation therapy are being investigated. Adjuvant therapy is now recommended for all individuals after resection for pancreatic cancer.

Neoadjuvant therapy. Trials exploring neoadjuvant chemoradiation were prompted by the observation of a prolonged recovery in some patients after pancreaticoduodenectomy, leading to a delay or cancellation of adjuvant therapy. This approach has both advantages and disadvantages. However, there are no objective data from a randomized trial demonstrating superior survival results.[116]

Treatment for locally advanced pancreatic cancer. Locally advanced pancreatic cancer is defined as arterial involvement or superior mesenteric artery or superior mesenteric–portal vein confluence occlusion. These patients are deemed unresectable due to invasion of the portal or mesenteric vessels even in the absence of metastatic disease. Studies have examined patients with locally unresectable pancreatic cancer who received neoadjuvant chemoradiation followed by surgery but suggest that it is unlikely to convert a locally, advanced, unresectable pancreatic cancer to a resectable one.[117] Intraoperative electron beam radiation (IOERT) has been used in an attempt to enhance local–regional control achieved by conventional external beam radiation and chemotherapy. No significant improvement in long-term survival was found using IOERT.[118]

Treatment of metastatic and recurrent disease. Minimal success has been achieved in identifying effective chemotherapy for metastatic pancreatic cancer. The median survival for patients with metastatic disease remains less than nine months. Chemotherapy with 5-fluorouracil (5-FU) remains the most widely used regimen in pancreatic cancer.[119]

Recently, gemcitabine has been studied in patients with locally advanced and metastatic pancreatic cancer.[120] Gemcitabine is a cytotoxic agent that was developed specifically for patients with advanced-stage disease. Clinical benefit response was the objective of treatment with this new drug rather than measuring tumor shrinkage. Clinical benefit response is a novel approach to assess the clinical effectiveness of gemcitabine based on marked improvement in pain control, analgesic consumption, and performance status. Prolonged survival was a secondary benefit. Gemcitabine is usually well tolerated, with a relatively mild toxicity profile. Studies have shown that gemcitabine confers a modest survival advantage as compared to treatment with 5-FU.[121] The results of these trials helped gemcitabine to become accepted as first-line therapy for patients with advanced or metastatic pancreatic carcinoma in the United States.

Both gemcitabine and 5-FU are now standard therapy as single agents for the treatment of metastatic and recurrent disease. More recent studies have incorporated gemcitabine into combined modality therapy. Other combination partners with gemcitabine under investigation include the antimetabolite 5-FU, the topoisomerase-I inhibitor irinotecan, the taxane docetaxel, the platinum agent oxaliplatin, the multitargeted antifolate pemetrexed, the farnesyl transferase inhibitor R-115777, the anti-*HER2/NEU* antibody trastuzumab, and the epidermal growth factor inhibitor cetuximab. Combined modality approaches with gemcitabine and radiation are also under investigation.[122]

Small-molecule therapy. Matrix metalloproteinases (MMPs) are a family of enzymes capable of degrading the components of the extracellular matrix. A high concentration of MMP enzymes has been detected in tumors, and the enzymes are considered to be important in invasion, angiogenesis, and metastasis. Matrix metalloproteinase inhibitors (MMPIs) bind to and inactivate MMPs. Marimastat, the first of the new class of MMPIs, is an oral agent that has been investigated in patients with advanced pancreatic cancer. Initial results did not establish marimastat as a treatment option for patients with unresectable disease when the drug was compared to gemcitabine.[123] Important conclusions of the study suggested that marimastat should be further investigated in patients with nonoperable, nonmetastatic pancreatic cancer.[124]

Pancreatic cancer arises from cells exhibiting a complex, multiple genetic aberrant state; in addition, selective genes are known to be involved in some sporadic and heritable tumors.[125] Potential therapeutic targets are the oncogene and tumor suppression gene pathways involved in the neoplastic transformation of the pancreas. The *K-ras* oncogene is one of the mutated genes most frequently found in pancreatic cancer, which makes it an attractive target. Targeting *ras* by using farnesyl-transferase inhibitors is one strategy being explored.[126] Tumor suppressor genes being investigated include *p53, p16, DPC4,* and *BRCA2*; DNA mismatch repair genes (*MLH1* and *MSH2*) and mitochondrial DNA mutations are also under study.[117]

A large number of growth factors and their receptors are overexpressed in pancreatic cancer, including epidermal growth factor (EGF) and fibroblast growth factor (FGF) and their receptors (EGFRs and FGFRs) and ligands. Inhibitors of these new targeted compounds are being studied, including members of the erbB family, HER1 (or EGFR) and HER2.[117]

Inhibitors of angiogenesis, also called antiangiogenetic agents, are another group of compounds offering promise in cancer research. These drugs block angiogenesis, the development of new blood cells. Solid tumors cannot grow beyond the size of a pinhead (1–2 mm^3) without causing the formation of new blood vessels to supply the nutritional needs of the tumor. Blocking the development of new blood vessels ensures that oxygen and nutrients are not supplied to the tumor, thereby preventing the continued growth and spread of the tumor. Vascular endothelial growth factor (VEGF) is up-regulated in pancreatic cancer;[127] TPN-470, derived from the fungus *Aspergillus,* has been found to have antiangiogenic properties;[128] and angiostatin, a peptide fragment of plasminogen, and endostatin, a fragment from collagenase,[129] are novel agents being studied for their effect on pancreatic carcinoma.

New therapeutic approaches for systemic disease. Treatment strategies have been developed in an attempt to modulate or interrupt growth factors and signal transduction pathway. Perilly alcohol is a nontoxic, naturally occurring substance that may enhance tumor apoptosis by increasing the ability of tumor cells to activate and respond to transforming growth factor beta.[130]

Immunotherapy

Immunotherapy of pancreatic cancer is an exciting therapeutic approach that focuses on activating the patient's immune system in an attempt to eradicate malignancy. Novel treatment strategies that capitalize on gene transfer technology have become possible through recent developments in molecular biology. Modern gene therapeutics, incorporating the use of recombinant DNA technology and more efficient gene delivery systems, have led to the development of new anticancer protocols.

Immunotherapeutic strategies that use recombinant DNA technology constitute the largest group of anticancer gene therapies. Immunotherapy has the potential to provide an alternative systemic treatment for adenocarcinoma of the pancreas. Having such an option is an important consideration in the treatment of pancreatic cancer as most individuals with pancreatic cancer present with locally unresectable or metastatic disease. Even for those individuals who have surgery that removes all evidence of gross disease, most will die of locally recurrent or metastatic disease within five years, and almost all eventually die as a direct result of their disease. Any effective treatment regimen against pancreatic cancer must address both its aggressive local growth and its propensity to metastasize.[131]

Immunotherapy has an advantage over chemotherapy and radiation because it can act specifically against the tumor without causing normal tissue damage. Vaccines are a form of immunotherapy. Pancreatic cancer vaccines have been developed using the whole tumor cell as the antigen source because it is not known which proteins expressed by pancreatic cancers are recognized by the immune system. Research is currently studying the genetic modification of pancreatic tumor cells to better present their tumor antigens to the immune system, which it is hoped will result in potent activation of a systemic antitumor immune response. In addition, tumor-associated antigens mixed with defined adjuvant therapy administered systemically are being developed that will result in new and more potent vaccines. Antigen-based vaccines may eliminate the need for the genetic manipulation of tumor cells.[75]

A phase I trial of an allogenic GM-CSF–secreting tumor vaccine for pancreatic cancer was assessed in patients with stage 1, 2, or 3 carcinoma of the pancreas. The vaccine was found to be safe and lacked treatment-related toxicity; it produced improvements in systemic antitumor immunity as measured by increased post-vaccination delayed-type hypersensitivity responses against autologous tumors.[132]

The effects of gene therapy and vaccine strategies on survival in individuals with pancreatic cancer are currently unknown. Immunotherapy has the potential to provide a mechanism of antitumor activity that may be integrated with surgery, chemotherapy, and radiation therapy.

Radiation Therapy

Radiation therapy has been used for both palliation and curative therapy of pancreatic cancer. Directed radiation to the pancreas is difficult because of the limited radiation tolerance of adjacent organs in the upper abdomen, including the kidney, liver, stomach, small bowel, and spinal cord. The technique typically used to treat pancreatic cancer is external beam radiotherapy. Newer techniques, such as conformal radiation and intensity-modulated radiation therapy, have the advantage of being able to precisely localize the radiation dose to the target volume while reducing the dose to critical structures.[133] More specialized methods of radiotherapy have been employed as well, such as intraoperative radiotherapy and brachytherapy, but no benefit over external beam irradiation has been found.[118,134]

The use of radiation-sensitizing agents is now being studied. Preliminary data demonstrate that gemcitabine may be a potent radiation sensitizer of human pancreatic cancer cells. It appears that DNA synthesis is prolonged in tumor cells as compared with normal tissues when gemcitabine is combined with irradiation.[135] For those individuals with unresectable pancreatic cancer, radiation therapy may palliate symptoms of local disease, especially pain.[136] Other radiosensitizing chemotherapy agents being investigated include capecitabine, which is more convenient than infusional 5-FU; cyclooxygenase-2 (COX-2) inhibitors, as there is a high degree of overexpression of COX-2 in pancreatic cancer; paclitaxel; and cisplatin.[137,138]

Newer combinations and techniques of administering radiation therapy and chemotherapy may provide better local control and survival for patients with resectable and locally unresectable disease. The development of more promising neoadjuvant and adjuvant therapies, such as combining chemoradiation with immunotherapy, may further enhance survival of individuals with pancreatic cancer.

Symptom Management and Nursing Care

The individual who has undergone surgery for pancreatic cancer usually dies of locally recurrent disease and/or metastatic disease. The most common harbingers of imminent death are recurrence of pain, jaundice from obstruction or intrahepatic metastases, and development of ascites. These symptoms require symptomatic or palliative treatment. Likewise, the individual who is diagnosed with advanced cancer of the pancreas, either locally or due to metastases, may present with the following:

- Pain
- Obstructive jaundice, which can lead to intrahepatic abscess
- Infection
- Ascites
- Liver failure
- Hemorrhage
- Malnutrition from bowel obstruction
- Anorexia
- Early satiety
- Cachexia
- Nausea and vomiting
- Change in bowel habits (constipation or diarrhea)
- Dyspnea

The goal of palliative therapy is to reduce the debilitating symptoms of the disease and to improve the quality of remaining life. This is best accomplished by treating the individual with respect to his or her wishes and not just treating the tumor.[139]

Relief of pain is a primary objective, particularly in advanced disease. The pain syndrome associated with cancer of the pancreas is usually related to the anatomical location of the tumor in the organ and subsequent impingement on other structures: tissues, blood vessels, bile or pancreatic ducts, or body organs. The complex nerve fibers and ganglions that affect the pancreas and related organs and structures contribute to the pain associated with pancreatic cancer.[140] Pain associated with tumors in the head of the pancreas may be due to pancreatitis. Tumors located in the body and tail of the pancreas often present later, are larger, and tend to cause pain by invading the stomach, retroperitoneum, and nerves.

The nature of pain will evolve and change throughout the progression of the disease. Treatment approaches must address the current, specific complaints of pain using all available modalities. Eliminating the source of the pain is the first objective, as in bile duct decompression or relief of duodenal obstruction. The most effective approach to pain therapy in individuals with advanced disease is to prevent the pain from peaking by routinely administering the selected relief measures. Oral, parenteral, or transdermal opiates, sedatives, nerve blocks, relaxation therapy, and proper positioning may provide pain relief. The administration of continuous subcutaneous opiate infusions by means of a PCA pump has the advantage of delivering analgesics to individuals with impaired gastrointestinal function and for whom oral analgesics are not appropriate. The pump can also provide optimal analgesia in those patients who develop a bowel obstruction and are not able to take food or liquids by mouth. Radiotherapy in combination with chemotherapy has also been used to reduce pain. Concomitant use of analgesics, celiac nerve blocks, and radiotherapy should be considered as palliative treatments. An aggressive pain treatment plan should be devised and started immediately. The goal of pain management should be to permit an acceptable level of functioning and to allow the individual to die as free of pain as possible.[141] Continuous pain assessment facilitated by good communication and trust between the individual and the clinician is necessary for effective pain management.

Nutritional status affects an individual's quality of life in regard to self-image, ability to perform activities of daily living, and overall life satisfaction. An individual's ability to socialize and interact with friends and family is affected by his or her ability or desire to eat. Malnutrition, cachexia, muscle weakness, and fatigue all contribute to depression, causing a cycle of difficulties.[142] Reduced activity and bedrest lead to constipation and more muscle wasting.[143,144]

Nutritional support may pose a difficult problem as a result of the obstructive nature of advanced pancreatic cancer. Supportive nutritional efforts for individuals undergoing active treatment can decrease complications, shorten hospital stays, reduce costs, and improve patients' sense of well-being. Oral feedings should be maintained as long as the individual can meet caloric requirements. Frequent, small feedings and supplemental mixtures may be tolerated better than larger meals. Adminstering antiemetics prior to eating may assist in controlling nausea and vomiting. Metoclopramide, megestrol acetate, and cannabinoids are some of the pharmacologic agents used to manage anorexia by stimulating the appetite.[145,146] Many individuals with pancreatic cancer complain of sensory changes that interfere with food intake. The sense of smell may be profoundly affected. Sensitivity to food odors as well as aversions to perfumes and soaps can also occur. Serving food cold instead of hot may be helpful in decreasing the aroma. Cooking odors can be minimized by using covered pots, boiling bags, or a kitchen fan. Taste changes are common, particularly complaints that food has a metallic taste. The use of plastic eating utensils and nonmetal cooking containers can help alleviate this problem. The use of parenteral nutrition in end-stage disease is controversial due to the high cost, high risk of complications, and lack of proven benefit.[145,146]

If the patient is diagnosed with a bowel obstruction, the cause must be elicited. Bowel obstruction can derive from a mechanical or a functional problem. Immediate management consists of nasogastric suction for control of nausea and large-volume emesis along with hydration by intravenous fluids. Bowel obstruction caused by tumor may necessitate the placement of a gastric tube — either surgically or endoscopically — for decompression. Removal of a nasogastric tube and allowing small amounts of liquids by mouth are the most humane course after a gastrostomy tube has been placed. Metallic expandable stents are under investigation as a palliative measure to maintain duodenal opening and allow unobstructed flow through this part of the small bowel. Somatostatin has also been used in treating individuals with bowel obstruction, as it reduces intestinal secretions and the dose can be titrated to control the volume of secretions. Prokinetic agents should not be used in patients with known bowel obstruction.

Opiate-induced bowel obstruction must also be considered. This complication can be avoided by the aggressive use of laxatives and an established bowel regimen along with appropriate education of the individual and family for symptoms suggestive of bowel obstruction: pain, nausea, vomiting, abdominal distention, and change in bowel elimination.

The cause of constipation can usually be delineated by a careful bowel history and abdominal examination. Prevention of opioid-induced constipation can best be accomplished by the use of an established bowel program.[147] Diarrhea is associated with tumors in the head of the pancreas; its management depends on identifying the cause. Malabsorption may result from steatorrhea and pancreatic exocrine insufficiency. Lactose intolerance may also be seen. Treatment consists of a diet high in protein and carbohydrate and replacement of pancreatic enzymes.

Individuals with cancer of the pancreas frequently have liver involvement, resulting in abdominal distention from malignant ascites. The treatment is difficult, but symptom control can be accomplished with the careful use of diuretics. Spironolactone and furosemide can reduce ascites, improve the person's comfort, and decrease the need for paracentesis.[139] Dyspnea may result not directly from the tumor itself but rather from disease complications, as seen in an individual with ascites and a diminished lung capacity. Patients with dyspnea from pancreatic cancer will have a shortened survival.

Jaundice due to bile duct obstruction or liver damage is a debilitating symptom that occurs in the majority of individuals with pancreatic cancer. It causes severe pruritus and dry skin. The individual should be instructed to use soap sparingly, preferably using mild soaps and oil-based lotions, calamine lotion, or cocoa butter, or to bathe in sodium bicarbonate to relieve pruritus.

Palliation of obstructive jaundice can be provided with endoscopic or percutaneous procedures. Insertion of internal biliary stents by endoscopy can relieve jaundice and its concomitant symptoms. Percutaneously placed internal–external biliary stents also can provide relief of jaundice. The stent and insertion site must receive daily care and stent flushing. Unrelieved biliary obstruction can cause recurrent infection in the biliary tree as well as lead to liver abscess that can cause pain and sepsis. Liver abscesses are treated by percutaneous insertion of a drain and intravenous antibiotics.

Jaundice that is not relieved by biliary decompression is usually a sign of liver failure. Liver failure results in progressive weakness, lethargy, encephalopathy, and eventual coma with imminent death of the individual. Renal failure usually occurs as the liver fails (hepatorenal failure). Patients are more prone to coagulation problems and bleeding as the liver continues to fail. Hemorrhage may also occur from metastatic tumor eroding into blood vessels in the liver or local tumor eroding into nearby vessels. Affected individuals die of massive internal hemorrhage.

Almost 90% of individuals with pancreatic cancer die within a year of their diagnosis. The course of the disease can be rapid. Patients should be assured that many treatments can be used aggressively to maintain their comfort and independence for as long as possible. They should be encouraged to inform their healthcare providers of any discomfort or medical or psychological problems they are experiencing. Timely referral to a palliative care service and hospice can have significant beneficial impact on the total care of the patient and on the home-based caregiver.[148]

Whatever the course of treatment chosen by the individual, both physiological and psychological preparation are necessary. By discerning patterns of family support, coping, and communication, the nurse can adopt a teaching style that suits the individual. Listening is vital to good communication, so as to understand and be sensitive to the patient's needs. Education by the nurse can increase compliance as well as prepare the individual and family for side effects of both the disease and its treatment. The nurse is the constant figure of hope, understanding, and support through all of the diagnostic tests, from the time the patient is told of the diagnosis of cancer of the pancreas, continuing through whatever treatment modalities are performed as the disease progresses, assisting with symptom management, and helping the individual and his or her family in the terminal stages of the disease.

The individual with terminal pancreatic cancer can be cared for at home by family or a caregiver with hospice support. The hospice nurse assists the patient and the caregiver in the terminal stages of the disease by educating them about what to expect and helping to manage symptoms. Individuals in the terminal stage of pancreatic cancer may not wish to eat, may become extremely cachectic, and may have decreased or no urine output as hepatorenal failure ensues. Helping the family—and especially the caregiver—to deal with the eventuality of the disease is a primary nursing concern.

Future Trends

Molecular genetics will play an increasingly important role in targeted therapy for pancreatic carcinoma. Knowledge of genetic alterations in individual tumors may allow selection of optimal therapeutic strategies for individual patients. Molecular detection of oncogene and tumor suppressor gene mutations may find application in the form of screening tests for pancreatic adenocarcinoma, at least in high-risk populations. Immunotherapy represents an exciting therapeutic approach that opens new perspectives in the treatment of pancreatic cancer.

Advances in prevention and screening for pancreatic cancer lie on the horizon. Innovations continue to emerge in diagnostic studies as well as in surgery, chemotherapy, and radiation therapy. Combined modalities will continue to be employed as treatment for pancreatic cancer. Collaboration and communiation among all healthcare providers, including oncology nurses, will ensure optimal care for patients with pancreatic carcinoma.

Much research is now being done on all aspects of pancreatic cancer. Discoveries in the field of molecular genetics hold promise for earlier detection. The ability to predict tumor biology and subsequently customize the treatment of patients with pancreatic cancer brings hope for improved survival. New vaccines aimed at activating an individual's immune system to fight his or her cancer are currently being developed and tested.

Superior outcomes have been reported for high-volume centers incorporating a multidisciplinary approach to treatment. Adjuvant chemotherapy and radiation therapy should be considered in patients with successfully resected pancreatic cancer. Combined modality treatment with chemotherapy and radiation should be considered for locally advanced, unresectable tumors.

Many advances have been made in the management of pancreatic cancer in the past several decades. Emerging techniques in the fields of surgery, radiation therapy, chemotherapy, and immunotherapy offer hope for greater locoregional control, improved survival, and enhanced quality of life for these patients. All patients with pancreatic cancer should be encouraged to enter clinical trials of new therapies.

References

1. Jemal A, Tiwari RC, Murray T, et al: Cancer statistics, 2004. *CA Cancer J Clin* 54:8–29, 2004
2. American Cancer Society: Cancer Facts and Figures — 2004. Altanta, American Cancer Society, 2004
3. Yeo TP, Hruban RH, Leach SD, et al: Pancreatic cancer. *Curr Probl Cancer* 26:176–275, 2002
4. Sohn TA, Yeo CJ, Cameron JL, et al: Resected adenocarcinomas of the pancreas — 616 patients: results, outcomes, prognostic indicators. *J Gastrointest Surg* 4:567–579, 2000
5. Sauter PK, Coleman J: Pancreatic cancer: a continuum of care. *Semin Oncol Nurs* 15:36–47, 1999
6. Gold EB, Goldin SB: Epidemiology of and risk factors for pancreatic cancer. *Surg Oncol Clin North Am* 7:67–91, 1998
7. Lowenfels AB, Maisonneuve P: Environmental factors and risk of pancreatic cancer. *Pancreatology* 3:1–8, 2003
8. Stamatakis K, Brownson R, Luke D: Risk factors for exposure to environmental tobacco smoke among ethnically diverse women in the United States. *J Women's Health Gender Based Med* 11:45–51, 2002
9. Lundell M, Holm LE: Risk of solid tumors after irradiation in infancy. *Acta Oncol* 34:727–734, 1995
10. Howe GR, Burch JD: Nutrition and pancreatic cancer. *Cancer Causes Control* 7:69–82, 1996
11. Silverman DT, Swanson CA, Gridley G, et al: Dietary and nutritional factors and pancreatic cancer: a case-control study based on direct interviews. *J Natl Cancer Inst* 90:1710–1719, 1998
12. Michaud DS, Giocannucci E, Willett WC, et al: Physical activity, obesity, height, and the risk of pancreatic cancer. *JAMA* 286:921–929, 2001
13. Ojajarvi J, Partanen T, Ahlbom A, et al: Occupational exposures and pancreatic cancer: a meta-analysis. *Occup Environ Med* 57:316–324, 2000
14. Everhart J, Wright D: Diabetes mellitus as a risk factor for pancreatic cancer: a meta-analysis. *JAMA* 273:1605–1609, 1995
15. Hruban RH, Petersen GM, Ha PK, et al: Genetics of pancreatic cancer. From genes to families. *Surg Oncol Clin North Am* 7:1–23, 1998
16. Schutte M, Hruban RH, Geradis J, et al: Abrogation of the Rb/p16 tumor-suppressive pathway in virtually all pancreatic carcinomas. *Cancer Res* 57:3126–3130, 1997
17. Rozenblum E, Schutte M, Goggins M, et al: Tumor-suppressive pathways in pancreatic cancinoma. *Cancer Res* 57:1731–1734, 1997
18. Hahn SA, Schutte M, Hogue ATMS, et al: *DPC4*, a candidate tumor suppressor gene at human chromosone 18q211. *Science* 271:350–353, 1996
19. Goggins M, Schutte M, Lu J, et al: Germline BRCA2 gene mutations in patients with apparent sporadic pancreatic carcinomas. *Cancer Res* 56:5360–5364, 1996
20. Wilentz RE, Chung CH, Sturm PDJ, et al: K-*ras* mutations in the duodenal fluid of patients with pancreatic carcinoma. *Cancer* 82:96–103, 1998
21. Goggins M, Offerhaus GJ, Hilgers W, et al: Pancreatic adenocarcinomas with DNA replication error (RER+) are associated with wild-type K-ras and characteristic histopathology. Poor differentiation, a syncytial growth pattern, and pushing borders suggest RER+. *Am J Pathol* 152:1501–1507, 1998
22. Whitcomb DC, Gorry MC, Preston RA, et al: Hereditary pancreatitis is caused by a mutation in the cationic trypsinogen gene. *Nat Genet* 14:141–145, 1996
23. Lowenfels AB, Maisonneuve EP, Dimagno YE, et al: International Hereditary Pancreatitis Study Group: hereditary pancreatitis and the risk of pancreatic cancer. *J Natl Cancer Inst* 89:442–446, 1997
24. Kinzler KW, Vogelstein B: Lessons from hereditary colorectal cancer. *Cell* 87:159–170, 1996
25. Breast Cancer Linkage Consortium: Cancer risks in BRCA2 mutation carriers. *J Natl Cancer Inst* 91:1310–1316, 1999
26. Phelan CM, Lancaster JM, Tonin P, et al: Mutation analysis of the BRCA2 gene in 49 site-specific cancer families. *Nat Genet* 13:120–122, 1996
27. Borg A, Sandberg T, Nilsson K, et al: High frequency of multiple melanomas and breast and pancreas carcinomas in CDKN2A mutation-positive melanoma families. *J Natl Cancer Inst* 92:1260–1266, 2000
28. Lynch HT, Brand RE, Hogg D, et al: Phenotypic variation in eight extended CDKN2A germline mutation familial atypical multiple mole melanoma–pancreatic carcinoma–prone families: the familial atypical mole melanoma–pancreatic carcinoma syndrome. *Cancer* 94:84–96, 2002
29. Giardiello FM, Welsh SB, Hamilton SR, et al: Increased risk of cancer in Peutz-Jeghers syndrome. *N Engl J Med* 316:1511–1514, 1987
30. Hemminki A, Tomlinson I, Markie D, et al: Localization of a susceptibility locus for Peutz-Jeghers syndrome to 19p using comparative genomic hybridization and targeted linkage analysis. *Nat Genet* 15:87–90, 1997
31. Kroc M: Role of growth factors in pancreatic cancer. *Surg Oncol Clin North Am* 7:25–41, 1998
32. Friess H, Yamanaka Y, Buchler M, et al: Enhanced expression of transforming growth factor beta isoforms in human pancreatic cancer correlates with decreased survival. *Gastroenterology* 105:1846–1856, 1993
33. Mason IJ: The ins and outs of fibroblast growth factors. *Cell* 78:547–552, 1994
34. Leung HY, Gullick WJ, Lemoine NR: Expression and functional activity of fibroblast growth factors and their receptors in human pancreatic cancer. *Int J Cancer* 59:667–675, 1994
35. Bergmann U, Funatomi H, Yokoyama M, et al: Insulin-like growth factor I overexpression in human pancreatic cancer: ev-

idence for autocrine and paracrine roles. *Cancer Res* 55:2007–2011, 1995
36. Yeo CJ, Cameron JL: Pancreatic cancer. *Curr Prob Surg* 36:57–152, 1999
37. Hruban RH, Adsay NV, Albores-Saavedra J, et al: Pancreatic intraepithelial neoplasia (PanIN): a new nomenclature and classification system for pancreatic duct lesions. *Am J Surg Pathol* 25:579–586, 2001.
38. Wilentz RE, Hruban RH: Pathology of cancer of the pancreas. *Surg Oncol Clin N Am* 7:43–65, 1998
39. Wilentz RE, Albores-Saavedra J, Zahurak M, et al: Pathologic examination accurately predicts prognosis in mucinous cystic neoplasms of the pancreas. *Am J Surg Path* 23:1320–1327, 1999
40. Z'graggen K, Rivera JA, Compton CC, et al: Prevalence of activating K-ras mutations in the evolutionary stages of neoplasia in intraductal papillary mucinous tumors of the pancreas. *Ann Surg* 22:491–500, 1997
41. Sohn TA, Yeo CJ, Cameron JL, et al: Intraductal papillary mucinous neoplasms of the pancreas: an increasingly recognized clinicopathologic entity. *Ann Surg* 234:313–322, 2001
42. Chiou YY, Chiang JH, Hwang JI, et al: Acinar cell carcinoma of the pancreas: clinical and computed tomography manifestations. *J Comput Assist Tomogr* 28:180–186, 2004
43. Abraham SC, Klimstra DS, Wilentz RE, et al: Solid-pseudopapillary tumors of the pancreas are geneticaly distinct from pancreatic ductal adenocarcinomas and almost always harbor mutations in the beta-catenin gene. *Am J Pathol* 160:1361–1369, 2002
44. Kataria R, Bhatnagar V, Agarwala S, et al: Clinical course and management of pancreaticoblastoma in children. *Trop Gastroenterol* 19:67–69, 1998
45. Boni L, Benevento A, Dionigi G, et al: Primary pancreatic lymphoma. *Surg Endosc* 16:1107–1108, 2002
46. Chun J, Doherty GM: Pancreatic endocrine tumors. *Curr Opin Oncol* 13:52–56, 2001
47. Somogyi L, Mishra G: Diagnosis and staging of islet cell tumors of the pancreas. *Curr Gastroenterol Rep* 2:159–164, 2000
48. Vogel I, Kalthoff H, Henne-Bruns D, et al: Detection and prognostic impact of disseminated tumor cells in pancreatic carcinoma. *Pancreatology* 2:79–88, 2002
49. Lillemoe KD: Current management of pancreatic carcinoma. *Ann Surg* 221:133–148, 1995
50. Rosa JA, Van Linda BM, Abourizk NN: New onset diabetes mellitus as a harbinger of pancreatic carcinoma. A case report and literature review. *J Clin Gastroenterol* 11:211–215, 1989
51. Barber MD: Cancer cachexia and its treatment with fish-oil–enriched nutritional supplementation. *Nutrition* 17:751–755, 2001
52. Ventafridda GV, Caraceni AT, Sbanotto Am, et al: Pain treatment in cancer of the pancreas. *Eur J Surg Oncol* 16:1–6, 1990
53. Hudis C, Kelsen D, Niedzwieck D, et al: Pain is not prominent in most patients with early pancreatic cancer. *Proc Am Soc Clin Oncol* 10:326, 1991 (abstr)
54. Bastidas VA, Neiderhuber JE: Pancreas, in Abeloff MD, Armitage JD, Lichter AS, et al (eds.): *Clinical Oncology*. New York, Churchill Livingstone, 1995, pp 1373–1403
55. Moossa AR, Gamagami PA: Diagnosis and staging of pancreatic neoplasms. *Surg Clin North Am* 75:871– 890, 1995
56. Green AI, Austin CP: Psychopathology of pancreatic cancer. A psychobiologic probe. *Psychosomatics* 34:208–221, 1993
57. Fras I, Litin EM, Pearson JS: Comparison of psychiatric symptoms of carcinoma of the pancreas with those in some other intra-abdominal neoplasms. *Am J Psychiatry* 123:1553–1562, 1967
58. Lin JT: Thromboembolic events in the cancer patient. *J Womens Health* (Larchmt) 12:541–551, 2003
59. Brand RE, Matamoros A: Imaging techniques in the evaluation of adenocarcinoma of the pancreas. *Dig Dis* 16:242–252, 1998
60. Horton KM: Multidetector CT and three-dimensional imaging of the pancreas. State of the art. *J Gastrointest Surg* 6:126–128, 2002
61. Bluemke DA, Fishman EK: CT and MR evaluation of pancreatic cancer. *Surg Oncol Clin N Am* 7:103–124, 1998
62. Reinhold C: Magnetic resonance imaging of the pancreas in 2001. *J Gastrointest Surg* 6:133–135, 2002
63. Mortele KJ, Ji H, Ros P: CT and magnetic imaging in pancreatic and biliary tract malignancies. *Gastrointest Endosc* 56:S206–S212, 2002
64. Alazraki N: Imaging of pancreatic cancer using fluorine-18 fluorodeoxyglucose positron emission tomography. *J Gastrointest Surg* 6:136–138, 2002
65. Hawes RH: Diagnostic and therapeutic uses of ERCP in pancreatic and biliary tract malignancies. *Gastrointest Endosc* 56:S201–S205, 2002
66. Wiersema MJ: Endoscopic ultrasonography. *J Gastrointest Surg* 6:129–132, 2002
67. Conlon KC, Minnard EA: The value of laparoscopic staging in upper gastrointestinal malignancy. *Oncologist* 2:10–17, 1997
68. Fernandez-del Castillo C, Warshaw AL: Laparoscopic staging and peritoneal cytology. *Surg Oncol Clin North Am* 7:135–142, 1998
69. Rashleigh-Belcher HJ, Russell RC, Lees WR: Cutaneous seeding of pancreatic carcinoma by fine-needle aspiration biopsy. *Br J Radiol* 59:182–183,1986
70. Centeno BA: Fine needle aspiration biopsy of the pancreas. *Clin Lab Med* 18:401–427, 1998
71. Ritts RE, Pitt HA: CA 19–9 in pancreatic cancer. *Surg Oncol Clin North Am* 7:93–101, 1998
72. Forsmark CE, Lambiase L, Vogel SB: Diagnosis of pancreatic cancer and prediction of unresectability using tumor-associated antigen CA 19–9. *Pancreas* 9:731–734, 1994
73. Fabris C, Basso D, Piccoli A, et al: Role of local and systemic factors in increasing serum glycoprotein markers of pancreatic cancer. *J Med* 22:145–146, 1991
74. Abrams RA, Grochow LB, Chakravarthy A, et al: Intensified adjuvant therapy for pancreatic and periampullary adenocarcinoma: survival results and observations regarding patterns of failure, radiotherapy dose and CA 19-9 levels. *Int J Radiat Oncol Biol Phys* 44:1039–1046, 1999
75. Yeo CJ: Pancreatic cancer: 1998 update. *J Coll Surg* 187:429–442, 1998
76. Greene FL, Page DL, Fleming ID, et al: *AJCC Cancer Staging Manual* (ed 6). New York, Springer, 2002, pp 157–164
77. Yeo CJ, Cameron JL, Sohn A, et al: Six hundred fifty consecutive pancreaticoduodenectomies in the 1990's: pathology, complications, and outcomes. *Ann Surg* 226:248–260, 1997
78. Yeo CJ, Sohn TA, Cameron JL, et al: Periampullary adenocarcinoma: analysis of 5-year survivors. *Ann Surg* 227:821–831, 1998
79. Yeo CJ, Cameron JL, Lillemoe KD, et al: Pancreaticoduodenectomy for cancer of the head of the pancreas: 201 patients. *Ann Surg* 221:721–733, 1995
80. Jaffee EM, Schutte M, Gossett J, et al: Development and characterization of cytokine-secreting pancreatic adenocarcinoma vaccine from primary tumors for use in clinical trials. *Cancer J Sci Am* 4:194–203, 1998
81. Sohn TA, Yeo CJ, Cameron JL, et al: Should pancreaticoduodenectomy be performed in octogenarians? *J Gastrointest Surg* 2:207–216, 1998
82. Heslin MJ, Brooks AD, Hochwald SN, et al: A preoperative biliary stent is associated with increased complications after pancreaticoduodenectomy. *Arch Surg* 133:149–154, 1998

83. Povoski SP, Karpeh MS, Conlon KC, et al: Preoperative biliary drainage: impact on intraoperative bile cultures and infectious morbidity and mortality after pancreaticoduodenectomy. *J Gastrointest Surg* 3:496–505, 1999
84. Yeo CJ, Cameron JL, Sohn TA, et al: Pancreaticoduodenectomy with or without extended retroperitoneal lymphadenectomy for periampullary ademocarcinoma: comparison of morbidity and mortality and short-term outcome. *Ann Surg* 229:613–624, 1999
85. Cohen SJ, Pinover WH, Watson JC, et al: Pancreatic cancer. *Curr Treat Options Oncol* 1:375–386, 2000
86. Yeo CJ, Cameron JL, Lillemoe KD, et al: Pancreaticoduodenectomy with or without distal gastrectomy and extended retroperitoneal lymphadenectomy for periampullary adenocarcinoma, part 2: randomized controlled trial evaluating survival, morbidity and mortality. *Ann Surg* 236:355–378, 2002
87. Sosa JA, Bowman HM, Gordon TA, et al: Importance of hospital volume in the overall management of pancreatic cancer. *Ann Surg* 228:424–438, 1998
88. Yeo CJ, Cameron JL: Alternative techniques for performing the Whipple operation. *Adv Surg* 30:293–310, 1996
89. Yeo CJ, Cameron JL: Pancreatic cancer: current controversies, in Schein M, Wise L (eds.): *Clinical Controversies in Surgery*. Basel, Karger Landes, 1998, pp 70–77
90. Yeo CJ, Cameron JL: The pancreas, in Hardy VD (ed.): *Hardy's Textbook of Surgery* (ed 2). Philadelphia, Lippincott-Raven, 1988, pp 695–725
91. Pikarsky AJ, Muggia-Sullam M, Eid A, et al: Pancreaticogastrostomy after pancreaticoduodenectomy: a retrospective study of 28 patients. *Arch Surg* 132:296–299, 1997
92. Yamamoto J, Shimamura Y, Nakahara H, et al: Simple technique for pancreaticogastrostomy and the histological findings of pancreaticogastric anastomosis. *Arch Surg* 132:785–788, 1997
93. Yeo CJ: Pylorus-preserving pancreaticoduodenectomy. *Surg Oncol Clin North Am* 7:143–156, 1998
94. Yeo CJ, Barry MK, Sauter PK, et al: Erythromycin accelerates gastric emptying after pancreaticoduodenectomy. A prospective, randomized, placebo-controlled trial. *Ann Surg* 218:229–238, 1998
95. Nyugen TC, Sohn TA, Cameron JL, et al: Standard versus radical pancreaticoduodenectomy for periampullary adenocarcinoma: a prospective, randomized trial evaluating quality of life in pancreaticoduodenectomy survivors. *J Gastrointest Surg* 7:1–11, 2003
96. Yeo CJ: The Whipple operation: is a radical resection of benefit? *Adv Surg* 37:1–25, 2003
97. Yeo CJ: Management of complications following pancreaticoduodenectomy. *Surg Clin North Am* 75:913–924, 1995
98. Halloran CM, Ghaneh P, Bosommet L, et al: Complications of pancreatic cancer resection. *Dig Surg* 19:138–146, 2002
99. Sohn TA, Lillemoe KD: Surgical palliation of pancreatic cancer. *Adv Surg* 34:249–271, 2000
100. Burdiles R, Rossi RL: Laparoscopy in pancreatic and hepatobiliary cancer. *Surg Oncol Clin N Am* 10:531–555, 2001
101. Lillemoe KD, Cameron JL, Yeo C, et al: Pancreaticoduodenectomy. Does it have a role in the palliation of pancreatic cancer? *Ann Surg* 223:718–728, 1996
102. Baron TH, Mallery JS, Hirota WK, et al: The role of endoscopy in the evaluation and treatment of patients with pancreaticobiliary malignancy. *Gastrointest Endosc* 58:643–649, 2003
103. Arguedas MR, Heudebert GH, Stinnett AA, et al: Biliary stents in malignant obstructive jaundice due to pancreatic carcinoma: a cost-effective analysis. *Am J Gastroenterol* 97:898–904, 2002
104. Sohn TA, Lillemoe KD, Cameron JL, et al: Surgical palliation of unresectable periampullary adenocarcinoma in the 1990s. *J Am Coll Surg* 188:658–669, 1999
105. Lillemoe KD, Cameron JL, Hardacre JM, et al: Is prophylactic gastrojejunostomy indicated for unresectable periampullary cancer? A prospective randomized trial. *Ann Surg* 230:322–330, 1999
106. Das A, Sivak MV: Endoscopic palliation for inoperable pancreatic cancer. *Cancer Control* 7:452–457, 2000
107. Levy MH: Pharmacologic treatment of cancer pain. *N Engl J Med* 335:1124–1132, 1996
108. Lillemoe KD, Cameron JL, Kaufman HS, et al: Chemical splanchnicectomy in patients with unresectable pancreatic cancer. A prospective randomized trial. *Ann Surg* 217:447–457, 1993
109. Lillemoe KD: Palliative therapy for pancreatic cancer. *Surg Oncol Clin N Am* 7: 199–216, 1998
110. Coleman J: Supportive management of the patient with pancreatic cancer: role of the oncology nurse. *Oncology* 10(suppl):23–24, 1996
111. Doty JE, Fink AS, Meyer JH: Alterations in digestive function caused by pancreatic disease. *Surg Clin North Am* 69:447–465, 1989
112. Ottery F: Supportive nutritional management of the patient with pancreatic cancer. *Oncology* 10(suppl):26–32, 1996
113. Held-Warmkessel J, Volpe H, Waldman AR: Treatment for pancreatic cancer. *Clin J Oncol Nurs* 2:127–134, 1998
114. Evans DB, Abbruzzese JL, Willett CG: Cancer of the pancreas, in DeVita VT Jr, Hellman S, Rosenberg SA (eds.): *Cancer: Principles and Practice of Oncology* (ed 6). Philadelphia, Lippincott, Williams and Wilkins 2001, pp 1126–1161
115. Gastrointestinal Tumor Study Group: Further evidence of effective adjuvant combined radiation and chemotherapy following curative resection of pancreatic cancer. *Cancer* 59: 2006–2010, 1987
116. Spritz FR, Abbruzzese JL, Lee JE: Preoperative and postoperative chemoradiation strategies in patients treated with pancreaticoduodenectomy for adenocarcinoma of the pancreas. *J Clin Oncol* 15:928–937, 1997
117. Akerele CE, Rybalova I, Kaufman HL, et al: Current approaches to novel therapeutics in pancreatic cancer. *Invest N Drugs* 21:113–129, 2003
118. Crane CH, Beddar AS, Evans DB: The role of intraoperative radiotherapy in pancreatic cancer. *Surg Oncol Clin North Am* 12:965–977, 2003
119. Glimelius B, Hoffman K, Sjoden PO, et al: Chemotherapy improves survival and quality of life in advanced pancreatic and biliary cancer. *Ann Oncol* 7:593–600, 1996
120. Casper ES, Green MR, Kelsen DP, et al: Phase II trial of gemcitabine (2,2′-difluorodeoxycytidine) in patients with adenocarcinoma of the pancreas. *Invest N Drugs* 12:29–34, 1994
121. Burris HA, Moore MJ, Andersen J, et al: Improvements in survival and clinical benefit with gemcitabine as first-line therapy for patients with advanced pancreas cancer: a randomized trial. *J Clin Oncol* 15:2403–2413, 1997
122. Haller DG: Future directions in the treatment of pancreatic cancer. *Semin Oncol* 29:31–39, 2002
123. Bramhall SR, Rosemurgy A, Brown PD, et al: Marimastat as first-line therapy for patients with unresectable pancreatic cancer: a randomized trial. *J Clin Oncol* 19:3447–3455, 2001
124. Hess KR, Abbruzzese JL: Matrix metalloproteinase inhibition of pancreatic cancer: matching mechanism of action to clinical trial design. *J Clin Oncol* 19:3445–3446, 2001
125. Mangray S, King TCL: Molecular pathobiology of pancreatic adenocarcinoma. *Front Biosci* 3:D1148–D1160, 1998
126. Adjei A: Blocking oncogenic Ras signaling for cancer therapy. *J Natl Cancer Inst* 93:1062–1074, 2001

127. Jayson GC, Mulatero C, Ranson M, et al: Anti-VEGF antibody HuMV833: an EORTC biological treatment development group phase 1 toxicity, pharmacokinetic and pharmacodynamic study. *Proc Am Soc Clin Oncol* 20:4a, 2001 (abstract 14)
128. Kudelka AP, Verschraegen CF, Edwards CL, et al: A phase 1 study of TNP-470 administered to patients with advanced squamous cell cancer of the cervix. *Clin Cancer Res* 3:1501–1505, 1997
129. Wolff RA: Novel therapies for pancreatic cancer. *Cancer J* 7:3349–3358, 2001
130. Ariazi EA, Satomi Y, Ellis MJ, et al: Activation of the transforming growth factor beta signaling pathway and induction of cytostasis and apoptosis in mammary carcinomas treated with anticancer agent perillyl alcohol. *Cancer Res* 59:1917–1928, 1999
131. Clary BM, Lyerly HK: Gene therapy and pancreatic cancer. *Surg Oncol Clin North Am* 7:217–237, 1998
132. Jaffee EM, Hruban RH, Biedrzycki B, et al: Novel allogeneic granulocyte-macrophage colony-stimulating factor–secreting tumor vaccine for pancreatic cancer: a phase I trial of safety and immune activation. *J Clin Oncol* 19:145–156, 2001
133. Pennerthy DR, Rich TA, Adams RB: Postoperative adjuvant therapy for pancreatic cancer. *Semin Oncol* 21:256–260, 2003
134. Abrams RA: Adjuvant therapy for pancreatic adenocarcinoma. *J Gastrointest Surg* 5:6–7, 2001
135. Li D, Xie K, Abbruzzese JL: Pancreatic cancer. *Lancet* 363:1049–1057, 2004
136. Dobelbower RR, Battle JA: Radiotherapy, in Howard JM, Idezuki Y, Ihse I, Prinz RA (eds.): *Surgical Diseases of the Pancreas* (ed 3). Baltimore, Williams and Wilkins, 1998, pp 587–595
137. Rich TA, Shepard R: COX-2 inhibitors as radiation sensitizers for upper GI tract cancers: esophagus, stomach, and pancreas. *Am J Clin Oncol* 26:S110–S113, 2003
138. Tsai JY, Iannitti DA, Safran H: Combined modality therapy for pancreatic cancer. *Semin Oncol* 30(suppl 9):71–79, 2003
139. Walsh D: Palliative management of the patient with advanced pancreatic cancer. *Oncology* 10:40–44, 1996
140. Alter CL: Palliative and supportive care of patients with pancreatic cancer. *Semin Oncol* 23:229–240, 1996
141. Moynihan TJ: Use of opioids in the treatment of severe pain in terminally ill patients — dying should not be painful. *Mayo Clin Proc* 78:1397–1401, 2003
142. Padilla GV: Psychological aspects of nutrition and cancer. *Surg Clin North Am* 66:1121–1135, 1986
143. Palesty JA, Dudrick SJ: What we have learned about cachexia in gastrointestinal cancer. *Dig Dis* 21:198–213, 2003
144. Tisdale MJ: Loss of skeletal muscle in cancer: biochemical mechanisms. *Front Biosci* 6:D164–D174, 2001
145. Watanabe S, Bruera E: Anorexia and cachexia, asthenia and lethargy. *Hematol Oncol Clin North Am* 10:189–206, 1996
146. Albrecht JT, Canada TW: Cachexia and anorexia in malignancy. *Hematol Oncol Clin North Am* 10:791–800, 1996
147. McNicol E, Horowicz-Mehler N, Fisk RA, et al: management of opioid side effects in cancer-related and chronic noncancer pain: a systematic review. *J Pain* 4:231–256, 2003
148. Ellison NM, Chevlen E, Still CD, et al: Supportive care for patients with pancreatic adenocarcinoma: symptom control and nutrition. *Hematol Oncol Clin North Am* 16:105–121, 2002

CHAPTER 62

Prostate Cancer

Jeanne Held-Warmkessel, RN, MSN, AOCN®, APRN, BC

Epidemiology

Each year, thousands of men are diagnosed with prostate cancer. Prostate cancer is the most commonly diagnosed solid tumor in U.S. males and the second-leading cause of cancer-related deaths. In 2004, an estimated 230,110 new cases of prostate cancer were predicted along with 29,900 deaths from the disease.[1] The incidence of prostate cancer increased rapidly in the years between 1976 and 1993,[2] declined between 1993 and 1995, and has been increasing slowly since 1995 although the death rate has declined.[3,4] Prostate-specific antigen (PSA) screening was largely responsible for the initial increase in the number of newly diagnosed patients. With the new availability of PSA testing in 1986, large numbers of men were diagnosed. As time passed, the pool of potential patients dwindled and fewer men were potentially diagnosable; as a consequence, the incidence of disease fell.[5,6] Prior to 1990, the death rate from prostate cancer was on the rise.[7] The death rate from prostate cancer fell from 26.5 to 17.3 deaths per 100,000 men in the years 1990–1995.[8] Possible causes underlying this trend include screening over the prior 20 years, improved documentation of cause of death, changes in treatment modalities, and diagnosis of disease at an earlier, more treatable stage.[7] The current increased incidence may be related to the increasing age and size of the population and ongoing screening efforts.

Black males have the highest incidence of prostate cancer, with a mortality rate twice that for white males. Among black Africans living in Africa, there is wide variability in the incidence of prostate cancer.[2] Racial and ethnic groups living in the United States with a lower prostate cancer incidence include men of Korean descent, for whom prostate cancer ranked as the fifth most common cause of cancer. Japanese men who emigrate to the United States have a similar incidence of prostate cancer as compared to white men living in the United States, even though Japanese men living in Japan have the world's lowest incidence of prostate cancer.[2,9,10]

Prostate cancer is a major health problem throughout the world. Countries with incidence rates higher than that found in the United States include Trinidad, Tobago, and Sweden. Countries with rates lower than that of the United States (in addition to Japan) include China and the Russian Federation.[11] The risk of prostate cancer continues to rise throughout the world even in countries characterized by a relatively low risk of prostate cancer.[12]

Etiology

The cause of prostate cancer is unknown. Risk factors have been identified and relate primarily to lifestyle, age, and heredity.

Lifestyle factors include nutrition and exposure to carcinogens. Fat consumption appears to be related to the risk of the development of prostate cancer[13] or the diagnosis of cancer at an advanced stage.[14] Diets higher in animal fat may alter the hormonal environment and predispose a man to an increased cancer risk.[15] Beef and butter are high in α-linolenic acid, and increased consumption of this essential fatty acid may increase the risk of prostate cancer.[16] Reducing one's consumption of animal fats and increasing one's consumption of fiber may reduce the risk of prostate cancer.[17] Obesity may contribute to the higher incidence of prostate cancer among black men.[18]

Soy products contain elevated levels of phytoestrogens that have been hypothesized to play a role in the reduced prostate cancer rates in Asia but the data supporting this concept are limited.[19,20] Tomatoes and tomato products may reduce the risk of prostate cancer,[21] as may consumption of beans, lentils, and peas.[22] More research is needed on the relationship between these foods and prostate cancer carcinogenesis.

The relationship between vitamins and risk of prostate cancer is being investigated in preclinical and clinical trials. Vitamin E is an antioxidant, proapoptotic, antiproliferative agent being studied in combination with selenium for the prevention of prostate cancer.[23] Selenium is a trace element found in plants and the animals that eat the plants grown in soil containing selenium.[24] Prostate antioxidant enzymes contain selenium, which suggests that this element may play a role in disease prevention. Vitamin D is metabolized by the body to the active form of the vitamin called calcitriol,[25] which inhibits cancer cell growth and induces apoptosis.[26] Weekly high-dose calcitriol is being studied in combination with chemotherapy for the treatment of metastastic prostate cancer with promising results.[27] Beta-carotene (a vitamin A precursor) and retinol (vitamin A) may play roles in prostate cancer as well. More study of them is needed, as a recent study failed to demonstrate an association between carotenoid serum levels and prostate cancer.[28] Vitamin A is an essential fat-soluble vitamin that promotes normal cellular growth.

Exposure to carcinogens such as chlorinated pesticides and methyl bromide, smoking, and heavy alcohol abuse may play a role in prostate cancer development.[15,29] Further research is needed into the roles that diet, animal fat, fiber, vitamins, and trace elements play in prostate carcinogenesis.

The use of bilateral vasectomy for birth control was studied extensively during the early 1990s and was initially thought to increase the risk of prostate cancer. However, this hypothesis has now been disproven and vasectomy is not considered a risk factor for prostate cancer development.[30] Sexual activity has been studied as a possible etiologic factor, along with infection with gonorrhea and having multiple female sexual partners.[31]

Prostate cancer is predominantly a disease of the older male. Before age 50, clinically evident prostate cancer is rare. The incidence after age 50 increases on a yearly basis to reach approximately 1000 cases per 100,000 males age 65–69.[32] By age 80–84, the incidence per 100,000 males is greater than 3000. Prostate cancer in younger men often behaves in a more aggressive manner.

Hereditary prostate cancer is characterized by an early onset of disease and the presence of an autosomal dominant pattern of inheritance; it accounts for approximately 8%–9% of prostate cancer diagnoses by age 85 but 43% of cases diagnosed in men younger than age 55.[33–35] A meta-analysis performed on 33 epidemiologic studies of family members of patients with prostate cancer revealed that the risk of cancer for a particular individual may be greater if the family member with cancer is a first-degree relative (brother affected implies greater risk than father affected).[36] The risk may be greatest if both first-degree and second-degree relatives (grandfather, uncle) had prostate cancer.[37] Also, family history is a greater risk factor for patients younger than age 55 than it is for older patients (70–85 years)[38] and for black and white men than for Asian American men.[39]

Black males have the highest incidence of prostate cancer in the world,[40] averaging more than a 50% higher incidence and poorer survival rates than whites.[41] Multiple factors may cause this higher incidence, including higher prevalence of high-grade prostatic intraepithelial neoplasia (PIN), a possible cancer precursor, and the reluctance of black males to participate in screening programs.[42,43] Generally poor attitudes held about the system of health care by black males represent an additional barrier to health care. Black males have more advanced tumors at the time of diagnosis, and their tumors may follow a more aggressive course.[44,45] It was thought that when patients have equal access to the same healthcare system, the survival rates for both groups would be similar.[45] However, in a study of health maintenance organization patients, black men had poorer survival because they experienced more aggressive disease.[46] More recent Surveillance, Epidemiology and End Results (SEER) program data found that PSA testing has altered the incidence, survival, and mortality rates of prostate cancer, such that the rates are now similar for white and black males.[47]

Testosterone levels are regulated by the hypothalamus and the anterior pituitary gland. The hormones from these glands cause the testicles to produce testosterone. The enzyme 5-alpha-reductase in the prostate converts testosterone into dihydrotestosterone (DHT), which has a potent direct effect on prostate development.[39] Research into the influence of hormones on prostate cancer development has been inconclusive.[48] Men without androgens do not develop prostate cancer.[2] A study of four different ethnic groups revealed that in all groups, older men have lower testosterone levels than younger men but the DHT:testosterone ratio was different among ethnic groups.[49] The ratios were highest in blacks and next highest in white men. These ratios are comparable to the incidence of disease in these groups and may be related to 5-alpha-reductase activity and the differences in enzyme activities among racial groups.[49] Testosterone levels were higher in black men but the results were not statistically significant.[49] Additional research on circulating testosterone levels did not support the finding that high levels of testosterone promoted cancer growth.[48]

Multiple genetic changes may play a role in the development of prostate cancer, the development of PIN, the incidence of localized disease, and a tumor's metastatic potential. The change from androgen dependence to androgen independence is associated with additional genetic alterations. Changes occur in oncogene expression, deletion of chromosome arms, suppression of apoptosis activation of oncogenes, and inactivation of tumor suppressor genes.[50] Variants of the human *SRD5A2* gene are found in high-risk black males.[51] This gene is responsible for 5-alpha-reductase activity, and its alteration may help explain the higher incidence of prostate cancer in this group. The prostate cancer susceptibility loci [hereditary prostate cancer 1 (*HPC1*)] is found on chromosome 1q.[52] Patients with this mutation may experience a prostate cancer diagnosis at an earlier age.[53] Other chromosome abnormalities have been discovered, including changes in the X chromosome and on chromosomes 8, 17, and 20.[54,55] It is thought that multiple genetic changes are needed for the development of prostate cancer, similar to the situation in other solid tumors; at least nine changes have been found in the *HPC1* gene.[50,56]

Prevention, Screening, and Early Detection

As the etiology of prostate cancer is unknown, specific recommendations regarding prevention of the disease cannot be made. Rather, based on the known risk factors, several suggestions can be put forth. Consuming a low-fat, high-fiber diet may reduce the risk of developing prostate cancer. Maintaining normal weight for height would also seem reasonable. Obtaining vitamins and trace minerals from vegetable sources and avoiding known carcinogens such as cigarette smoke may also reduce one's risk of prostate cancer. Participating in screening would be another important intervention.

The Prostate Cancer Prevention Trial (PCPT) opened to enrollment in 1993 and closed in 1996 after 18,882 men without prostate cancer were randomized. The men received either placebo or 5 mg finasteride daily for seven years. Finasteride is a 5-alpha-reductase inhibitor that interferes with the formation of dihydrotestosterone.[57] Each year, the participants underwent digital rectal exam (DRE) and analysis of PSA using a cutoff of 3 ng/mL as the maximum level. Seven years later, at the end of the drug intervention, the men had prostate biopsies performed if their PSA level was greater than 4.0 ng/mL or if an abnormality was found on DRE.[57] In the final analysis, there were 4368 men in the finasteride group and 4692 men in the placebo group. Of these men, 803 (18.4%) in the finasteride group and 1147 (24.4%) men in the placebo group developed prostate cancer.[58] Men in the finasteride group with prostate cancer were more likely to have high Gleason scores (7–10) than the men in the placebo group with prostate cancer (37% versus 22.2%). Side effects observed more commonly in the finasteride group included reduced libido, erectile dysfunction, reduced volume of ejaculate, and gynecomastia. The placebo group experienced more symptoms related to an enlarged prostate such as urgency, frequency, retention, and urinary tract infections. Finasteride is the first agent that has demonstrated the ability to reduce the risk of prostate cancer development, although multiple questions remain regarding its use.[57]

Vitamin E and selenium are also being investigated in a prostate cancer prevention trial.[58] This study aims to recruit 32,400 men without prostate cancer to be randomized to one of four arms, three of which include placebo. After a PSA test and DRE are completed, patients will receive placebo, selenium plus placebo, vitamin E plus placebo, or vitamin E plus selenium. The doses of agents are 200 μg of 1-selenomethionine, 400 mg of racemic α-tocopheros, and an optional vitamin pill that does not include either ingredient. Final study results will not be available for ten years. Many other agents are also under investigation for the chemoprevention of prostate cancer.

Screening for prostate cancer involves the use of DRE, PSA level, and, if appropriate, evaluation of the gland using transrectal ultrasound (TRUS). DRE involves palpation of the prostate gland. The posterior and lateral glandular tissue is evaluated by the examiner's finger.[59] DRE is the most commonly performed screening exam for prostate diseases[60] and assists in evaluating for lesions, texture, and symmetry of the gland. Limitations of DRE include its failure to locate tumors in the anterior and midline of the prostate, where approximately 40% of cancers may be found.[61,62] DRE is recommended as part of an annual physical exam for men beginning at age 50 who are expected to live ten years or more.[63]

Men considered to be at high risk for prostate cancer are those who have relatives diagnosed with prostate cancer before age 65. Those with higher risk factors, such as black men, should begin screening at a younger age (45), and those with the highest risk factors (more than one first-degree relative with prostate cancer) should begin at age 40. Ongoing follow-up after the first screening is dependent of the PSA result. It is also important that the man being screened is educated as to the risks versus the benefits of screening.[63]

PSA is a serine protease, a member of the kallikrein family that is found in prostate luminal epithelial cells.[64] The protein occurs in higher concentrations within the prostate gland than in the blood. A barrier of three tissue layers separates the blood and the PSA found in prostate ducts.[65] Anything that destroys this natural tissue barrier allows PSA to enter the bloodstream, where it can be collected and evaluated in a laboratory. Procedures that can falsely elevate PSA levels, such as biopsy, urethral instrumentation, catheterization, and possibly rectal examination, should be avoided prior to obtaining PSA blood specimens.[66]

The androgen receptor controls PSA production.[67] The normal reference range for PSA is 0–4 ng/mL.[5] Serial PSA levels provide more valuable information than a single reading. Relying on a single value of PSA greater than 4 ng/mL for performing biopsies on men of all ages will miss a number of clinically significant prostate cancers,[67] because not all men with prostate cancer secrete enough PSA to raise the level. The human prostate gland continues to grow in the adult male after the completion of puberty. As the prostate increases in size, the PSA level also increases. For this reason, benign prostatic hyperplasia (BPH) tissue can be expected to produce a higher serum concentration of PSA both in the absence and presence of prostate cancer. Also, conditions other than prostate cancer can give rise to elevated PSA levels. Men with prostate cancer have been found to have higher PSA levels even when variables such as tumor volume, stage, age, and tumor grade are controlled.[68]

To identify race-related and age-related PSA values, 3475 men (1802 white, 1673 black) were randomly selected from a pool of 14,826 military men to form a study group. The goal was to identify the PSA ranges in

Table 62-1 Summary of Recommendations Regarding Prostate Cancer Screening

Test	Frequency	Beginning at Age	How Test Is Performed
Digital rectal exam	Annual	50*	The examiner's gloved and lubricated finger is inserted into the rectum while the patient bends over the examining table
Prostate exam	Annual	50*	

*High-risk patients may begin screening at an earlier age. Age 45 for men with a first-degree relative diagnosed age < 65 or of African ancestory. Age 40 for men with more than one first-degree relative diagnosed age < 65.

Normal Results		Significance
DRE PE	No palpable abnormality prostate gland symmetry, texture, and no masses felt	Able to detect abnormal gland symmetry and texture and abnormal lesions in posterior and lateral areas of gland

Age	PSA Range — Whites [PSA Results (normal 0–4.0 ng/mL)]	PSA Range — Blacks
40–49	0–2.5 ng/mL	0–2.0 ng/mL
50–59	0–3.5 ng/mL	0–4.0 ng/mL
60–69	0–3.5 ng/mL	0–4.5 ng/mL
70–79	0–3.5 ng/mL	0–5.5 ng/mL

Results are age and race related. All abnormal results require additional diagnostic studies.
Data from Smith, Cokkinides, Eyre[63]; Morgan, Jacobsen, McCarthy, et al.[69]

white and black men. As a result of their study, the authors recommended a new range for PSA values based on patient age and race.[69] The new ranges will improve the usefulness of PSA in identifying important cancers in younger and older patients in both races (see Table 62-1).

Of course, PSA tests are not foolproof. Approximately 25% of cancers do not secrete PSA, and an elevated PSA level does not guarantee that a man has cancer. Additional diagnostic tests using PSA have been developed to more clearly identify men with prostate cancer and avoid unnecessary biopsies in those who do not have cancer.

Cancerous prostate cells and normal prostate cells produce the same amount of PSA. Total PSA includes free PSA and conjugated (unbound) PSA. Conjugated PSA is bound to alpha$_1$-antichymotrypsin, and this level is higher in patients with prostate cancer. Free PSA has been evaluated for its ability to enhance differentiation of benign and malignant disease. Free PSA levels are lower in patients with prostate cancer than in patients without prostate cancer.[70] Studies have determined that free PSA is useful in reducing the number of biopsies in men with PSA ranges of 4–10 ng/mL.[70] For cancer detection, the amount of free PSA as a percentage of total PSA should be 25% when the total PSA ranges between 4 and 10 ng/mL and DRE evaluation indicates benign disease.[71] The use of free PSA may also be helpful when evaluating men with PSA values of 2.6–4.0 ng/mL and a benign prostate exam.[72] Free PSA can be used with individual patients to help determine the need for biopsy or follow-up biopsy.[70] Patients with more than 25% free PSA are more likely to have benign disease, whereas those with 25% or less free PSA need to undergo biopsy to assess for cancer.

PSA density (PSAD) describes the ratio of serum PSA to prostate volume as determined by TRUS.[70] A PSAD level exceeding 0.15 ng/mL is indicative of prostate cancer (sensitivity of 72%, specificity of 95%).[70] PSA velocity describes how much PSA values increase over time. An increase of 0.75–0.80 ng/mL per year is significant in men with a PSA value of less than 10 ng/mL[70] and may be useful in identifying cancers. Specimens should be obtained over a two-year period to detect a trend in PSA changes.[73,74] As noted earlier, finasteride (a 5-alpha-reductase inhibitor used to treat BPH) reduces PSA levels by 50%. Thus a PSA level of 2 ng/mL should be used when screening for prostate cancer in men who are taking finasteride.[75]

A subject of recent debate is the issue of whether the threshold for PSA values should be lowered to increase the specificity and sensitivity of PSA testing. In one clinical trial focusing on PSA testing, a large number of prostate cancers were missed in men both older and younger than 60.[76] Even though PSA has been available as a diagnostic test for more than 15 years, its use is still being studied extensively in clinical trials.

TRUS is used to follow up abnormal DRE or elevated PSA levels. The test can evaluate prostate volume and identify suspicious areas of 5 mm or larger for biopsy.[77] Its role in screening programs is not yet defined.[78] In this imaging study, an ultrasound probe is inserted into the rectum and can reveal hypoechoic areas and other abnormalities in the prostate. Needle biopsies of suspicious areas are then obtained under ultrasonic guidance. Three additional directed biopsies from each lobe of the prostate are routinely obtained.

No area of cancer research continues to be as hotly debated as the issue of whether mass public screenings to detect prostate cancer are justified. The number of important cancers diagnosed at an early stage by PSA screening has certainly increased.[79] Finnish researchers reported on the 8975 men in their arm of the European Randomized Study of Screening for Prostate Cancer. Using a prospective randomized clinical trial format, 5975 men served as controls and 3707 men were asked to participate in the study of which 75% (2781) agreed. The men were screened using PSA testing. If the PSA level was 4 μg/L or higher, they were referred to a urologist, if the PSA level was 3–4 μg/L, they were offered DRE. Additional screening included TRUS and biopsy. Biopsy was repeated every three months if the initial work-up for cancer was negative. There were 56 cancers (2%) in the PSA-screened group and 21 cancers (0.32%) in the control group. The tumors identified in the PSA-screened group were more aggressive than those in the control group.[79]

In another study of PSA screening, a prospective randomized trial of 46,193 men was conducted in Canada. Men assigned to the screening arm underwent PSA testing (0–3 ng/mL was defined as normal) and DRE on the first evaluation. If either test was abnormal, TRUS was performed. On follow-up, TRUS was completed if the PSA level exceeded 3 ng/mL or had increased by 10% from the last visit. In the unscreened arm of 38,056 men, there were 137 prostate cancer–related deaths; 5 prostate cancer–related deaths occurred in the screening arm of 8137 men. This was a statistically significant difference and represented a 69% reduction in the rate of death due to prostate cancer.[80]

Additional clinical trials are needed to validate the benefits of screening. Several large-scale randomized studies are currently under way in both the United States and Europe, but it will be many years until their results are known.[81] Until then, the American Cancer Society (ACS) guidelines should be utilized. Black males, because of their higher risk of prostate cancer, should be encouraged by nurses to participate in annual prostate cancer screening provided by their family physicians. Men who have first-degree relatives with prostate cancer should also be educated regarding the need to participate in earlier screening.

The cost of screening to both the individual and society cannot be ignored. From a financial perspective, do the dollars spent on screening prolong life or prevent unnecessary deaths? Currently no research trials can answer the question of whether prostate cancer screening is cost-effective.[81] Screening identifies not only clinically important cancers that require treatment but also clinically insignificant prostate cancers that may not shorten survival or threaten the patient's life. The individual needs to understand that treatment may not influence survival and may cause important side effects including impotence and incontinence.

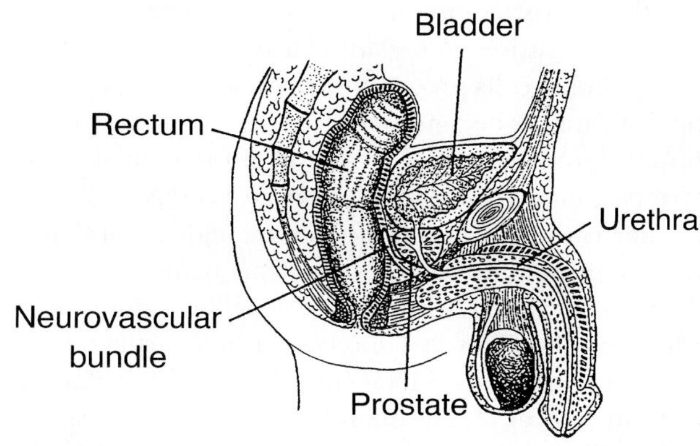

Figure 62-1 Prostate anatomy.

Pathophysiology

The prostate gland, which is approximately the size of an inverted, triangularly shaped walnut, sits beneath the bladder and anterior to the rectum. The section of the urethra that passes through the prostate is known as the *prostatic urethra.* Draining into the prostatic urethra are the prostatic ducts. Prostatic fluid drains into the prostatic ducts from the glandular elements of the prostate. This fluid aids in the fertilization process (Figure 62–1).

The prostate gland is composed of three major sections: the central zone, the peripheral zone, and the transitional zone. The larger peripheral zone that surrounds the central zone is the most common site for cancer.[81]

The prostate is well vascularized. Its major blood supply originates from the inferior vesical artery.[81] Venous drainage occurs through the inferior hypogastric venous system and the presacral prevertebral venous plexus; lymphatic drainage occurs via the external and internal iliac groups and obturator lymph nodes. These nodes and lymphatics then drain into the common iliac and preaortic lymph nodes.

Cellular Characteristics

The vast majority (95%) of prostate cancers are adenocarcinomas. Of the 5% of prostate cancers that are not adenocarcinomas, greater than 90% are transitional cell carcinomas. Rarely, squamous cell carcinoma—

the third most common type—may occur. All prostate cancers arise from glandular epithelial cells.[82]

Epithelial cells proceed through a variety of stages on their way to becoming malignant. As already mentioned, premalignant changes in prostate tissue are termed *prostatic intraepithelial neoplasia (PIN)*.[82] PIN is further categorized as low grade or high grade[82] and may be present for ten or more years before cancer is diagnosed.[83] Currently, it is not possible to determine whether PIN will evolve into cancer in a particular patient, but high-grade PIN is considered a risk factor for prostate cancer and as many as 94% of autopsy specimens will have both prostate cancer and PIN.[84] High-grade PIN should be further evaluated for the presence of invasive cancer; on rebiopsy, the incidence of prostate cancer increases over time.[82]

Prostate tissue specimens are subjected to a type of pathologic scoring based on cellular architecture known as the *Gleason score*. The majority of the tumor is occupied by cells with one type of histologic feature that is given a number (grade) of 1 to 5 based on the severity of the cellular changes. The lower numbers are assigned to cellular patterns that are similar to prostatic tissue (well differentiated). The higher numbers designate cellular patterns with more bizarre architectural features that look less like normal prostatic tissue (poorly differentiated).[85] This primary number is added to a secondary number, which reflects the second most common type of cellular structure using the same grading format. The sum of the two numbers gives the total Gleason score. Not all studies utilize the summed format. Tumors graded 1–3 are considered well differentiated, whereas those graded 4 or 5 are considered poorly differentiated carcinomas. When the entire prostate gland is available for pathologic review, the volume of tissue and the Gleason grade may be able to predict the presence of extracapsular spread and lymph node metastases.[85] When the Gleason grade is 4–5 (poorly differentiated), the risk of nodal metastases increases when the volume of cancer exceeds 3.2 cm^3.[86] The risk of nodal metastases is less than 1% when the cancer volume is less than 3.2 cm^3. Nodal metastases are correlated with Gleason grade, PSA, and clinical stage.[87]

Prostate cancers can also be divided into those that are clinically important (significant) and those that are clinically unimportant.[88] Clinically important cancers include features such as large tumor volume; Gleason grade 3–5 (moderate to poor differentiation); an invasive, proliferative pattern of growth, elevated PSA level; and origination in the peripheral zone. These cancers threaten the patient's life because they progress to fatal metastatic cancers. Cancers that do not threaten the patient's life are termed *indolent* and considered clinically unimportant. These indolent cancers, which constitute the vast majority of prostate cancers, are small with a Gleason grade of 1–2 (well differentiated), are noninvasive in their pattern of growth, do not elevate the PSA level, originate in the transitional zone, and tend to fail to progress into invasive metastatic cancers.[88] Patients with low Gleason score tumors require follow-up on a regular basis to monitor the status of the tumor, monitor for any progression of the disease, and determine whether therapy should be initiated.

Progression of Disease

Prostate cancer is generally characterized by a slow pattern of growth. The tumor grows locally along tissue planes such as the prostatic capsule and may penetrate through junctional areas of the capsule that include the bladder neck, ejaculatory ducts, and prostatourethral area.[77] Cancers of the prostate apex and base are more likely to have spread beyond the capsule due to inherent structural weaknesses in these areas.[77] Perineural invasion may accompany capsular invasion.[77] Surrounding structures such as the bladder may be involved with tumor growth. When lymphatic metastases occur, they may involve the obturator, presacral, presciatic, internal, and external iliac nodes.[77] After lymph node metastases, the next most commonly involved metastatic site is bone, especially the lumbar spine, pelvis, femur, and skull. The cancer cells spread to these distant sites via the bloodstream after gaining access to the Batson plexus of presacral veins.[74] Other distant sites of metastasis include the lungs, bladder, and liver.

Clinical Manifestations

Prostate cancer is usually asymptomatic in its early stages. As the disease progresses, patients may present with urinary tract obstructive symptoms similar to BPH, such as frequency, incomplete bladder emptying, hesitancy, nocturia, and urgency especially if the tumor lies in the central zone or near the urethra.[89] The closer the proximity of the tumor to the urethra, the more likely it is to produce symptoms of bladder outlet obstruction. Symptoms may be abrupt in their onset but otherwise are similar to those seen with BPH. Other symptoms may include a change in erectile capability.

Advanced prostate cancer may be evidenced by the appearance of ureteral obstruction caused by ureterovesical junction compression by tumor or nodal metastases.[89] Hydronephrosis can then ensue, threatening the function of the associated kidney. Back pain may reveal the presence of vertebral body metastases with the potential for spinal cord compression.[77] In addition, local pain may occur due to the presence of the cancer in the prostate gland and invasion into surrounding structures, as well as referred pain to the legs and abdomen. Bone pain can be problematic and is related to the presence of additional skeletal metastases. The hip, legs, neck, shoulders, and ribs are the next most common areas to be affected.[90] Additional symptoms related to advanced prostate cancer growth include weight loss, rectal obstruction from local growth, coagulation deficits related to the release of procoagulant into the bloodstream from the prostate cancer cells, hypercalcemia, leg edema from nodal metastases, and pancytopenia from marrow metastases.[89] In the past, patients often presented to the physician with symptoms of advanced disease, including back and hip pain or inability to void. It is now uncommon for patients to present with these symptoms of advanced disease without a prior diagnosis of prostate cancer.

Table 62-2 Questions Useful in Assessing Urinary Symptoms Associated with Prostate Cancer and Other Urologic Disorders

Symptom	Assessment
Dysuria	Does the patient have difficulty initiating urination? If so, how often?
	Does the patient have difficulty maintaining or ending the urine stream?
	Does the patient need to apply pressure to the bladder to initiate urination?
	Does dribbling occur at the end of urination?
	Is there pain on urination? If so, how does the pain feel? Does it persist or is it intermittent?
	Are there bladder spasms?
Frequency	How often does the patient need to urinate?
	What is the volume of each voiding?
	Does the patient void and then need to void again a few minutes later?
	Is there a reduction in the urine volume produced?
Nocturia	How many times does the patient get out of bed each night to urinate?
	Is there incontinence at night?
Hematuria	Is there blood in the urine? Clots?
	What is the color of the urine?
Other	Does the urine have an odor?
	Is particulate matter present in the urine?
	When did the patient void most recently?
	Can the patient feel his bladder through the abdominal wall?
	Is there flank pain?
	How many urinary tract infections has the patient had in the last 12 months?
	Has there been a change in the strength of penile erections?

Data from Degler[91]; McAninch[92]; Bates.[93]

Assessment

Patient and Family History

Nursing assessment of patients at risk for or with a diagnosis of prostate cancer should begin by questioning the patient about past medical problems or prior diagnoses of prostate disorders. The presence of a prostate cancer diagnosis in first- and second-degree relatives should be ascertained, and exposure to potential prostate carcinogens or risk factors needs to be determined.

The nurse should evaluate the patient's voiding pattern and ask if the patient has problems with dysuria, frequency, nocturia, hematuria, and other signs of bladder outlet obstruction (Table 62-2).

Physical Exam

The patient is examined for evidence of local and distant metastases. Early prostate cancer does not usually produce symptoms. The pelvic and suprapubic areas should be percussed and palpated for bladder distention. A postvoid residual measurement may be ordered by the physician or nurse practitioner to evaluate the volume of residual urine in the bladder. Inguinal nodes are assessed, and the patient is queried regarding bone pain, specifically back pain. If back pain is present, the patient is questioned about signs of spinal cord compression, such as numbness, tingling, and other indications of sensory loss, motor weakness, or bowel or bladder incontinence.[94] Other potential areas of pain include the rectum and local pelvic area. The patient is asked for information about any pain medications he has been using, their effectiveness, and side effects. The patient's legs should be examined for edema and its severity and for indications of deep-vein thromboses, such as unilateral leg edema, pain, local heat, and redness. The skin should be checked for petechiae and ecchymoses. The patient is weighed and asked how much weight he has lost since the illness began.

Diagnostic Studies

Once a presumptive diagnosis of prostate cancer is made, the patient will have a PSA level drawn and a DRE performed if these tests have not previously been ordered. As PSA levels often reflect the amount of the patient's disease,[95,96] samples may be drawn before and after therapeutic interventions and then periodically to monitor the status of the cancer. Additional blood tests include serum chemistries, including calcium, liver function tests, blood urea nitrogen (BUN), creatinine, and complete blood count (CBC). A urine analysis is performed and a chest x-ray is completed. Magnetic resonance imaging (MRI) scans of the abdomen and pelvis may be done to evaluate local and nodal metastasis and to determine the proper treatment for the patient. A bone scan is frequently performed to evaluate bone pain and may be carried out as part of the staging workup. Bone scans are usually negative in patients with a PSA level of less than 20 ng/mL.[90] TRUS is used to assist in evaluating the extent of localized prostate cancer[97] and in guiding prostate biopsies. In patients who are being considered for curative surgery and who have a Gleason score greater than 7 ng/mL, a laparoscopic pelvic lymph node dissection may be performed to evaluate the presence of nodal metastasis. One study examined 1091 men who had a radical retropubic prostatectomy performed, 695 of whom had a bilateral pelvic lymph node dissection. A PSA level of 15 ng/mL or higher, or a Gleason grade of 4–5 on four or more of the biopsy specimens, or a Gleason grade of 4–5 as the predominant architecture on the pathology specimen predicted lymph node metastasis.[98]

Prognostic Indicators

PSA levels may reflect the extent of disease and the amount of cancer found in the prostate gland.[95,96] They increase in a logarithmic fashion with the patient's stage of disease.[92] PSA levels are used to assess the effectiveness of treatment and to monitor the patient for disease recurrence. Unfortunately, not all prostate cancers produce PSA, so other diagnostic studies — such as MRI, computerized tomography (CT) scan, or ProstaScint scan — may be needed to monitor disease status. Baseline blood levels are obtained before and after treatment and usually are monitored every 3 months after treatment for one year and then every 6–12 months. Levels greater than 80 ng/mL reflect a large disease burden and, often, metastatic cancer.

After undergoing primary therapy for any stage of prostate cancer, an increasing PSA level reflects disease activity.[99] After undergoing curative resection for prostate gland–confined cancer, PSA levels should be undetectable.[99]

When external beam radiation therapy is used to treat prostate cancer, PSA levels should be normal 3–18 months after completion of therapy. Failure of PSA to normalize often reflects persistent disease.[96] For all of these reasons, PSA is a highly useful tool for the monitoring of disease response to therapy and monitoring the patient for cancer relapse.

Classification and Staging

Two commonly used staging systems for prostate cancer are the American Urologic Association (AUA) system,[90] which was originally developed by Whitmore and then updated by Jewett, and the tumor-node-metastasis (TNM) system (Table 62-3) developed by the American Joint Committee on Cancer (AJCC). Table 62-4 presents a comparison of these two staging systems.

Small cancers found on transurethral resection of the prostate for BPH are often asymptomatic and are staged as A. When the cancer involves less than one lobe of the gland, it is considered B_1 disease. B_2 cancer involves both lobes of the prostate. After the cancer has invaded into or beyond the prostate capsule, stage C disease is present. With metastases to distant sites, the patient has stage D cancer.[90] Survival is stage dependent. The ten-year survival rate for patients with stage A disease is 95%; for stage B is 80%; for stage C is 60%; for stage D (nodal metastases) is 40%; and for stage D (distant metastases) is 10%.[86]

Therapeutic Approaches and Nursing Care

Treatment options available for a particular patient are based on patient preference, PSA level, age, life expectancy, general medical condition, tumor grade (Gleason score), tumor volume (stage), potential treatment complications, and risk of relapse.[100,101] A patient may be offered watchful waiting (periodic observation), surgery, radiation therapy, combination therapy, hormonal manipulation, chemotherapy, or investigational drugs administered in a clinical trial setting.

Table 62-3 American Joint Committee on Cancer Staging for Prostate Cancer

Definition of TNM

Primary Tumor (T)

Clinical

TX	Primary tumor cannot be assessed
T0	No evidence of primary tumor
T1	Clinically inapparent tumor not palpable nor visible by imaging
T1a	Tumor incidental histologic finding in 5% or less of tissue resected
T1b	Tumor incidental histologic finding in more than 5% of tissue resected
T1c	Tumor identified by needle biopsy (e.g., because of elevated PSA)
T2	Tumor confined within prostate*
T2a	Tumor involves one-half of one lobe or less
T2b	Tumor involves more than one-half of one lobe but not both lobes
T2c	Tumor involves both lobes
T3	Tumor extends through the prostate capsule†
T3a	Extracapsular extension (unilateral or bilateral)
T3b	Tumor invades seminal vesicle(s)
T4	Tumor is fixed or invades adjacent structures other than seminal vesicles: bladder neck, external sphincter, rectum, levator muscles, and/or pelvic wall

*Tumor found in one or both lobes by needle biopsy, but not palpable or reliably visible by imaging, is classified as T1c.

†Invasion into the prostatic apex or into (but not beyond) the prostatic capsule is not classified as T3, but as T2.

Pathologic (pT)

pT2***	Organ confined
pT2a	Unilateral, involving one-half of one lobe or less
pT2b	Unilateral involving more than one-half of one lobe but not both lobes
pT2c	Bilateral disease
pT3	Extraprostatic extension
pT3a	Extraprostatic extension†
pT3b	Seminal vesicle invasion
pT4	Invasion of bladder, rectum

***There is no pathologic T1 classification.

†Positive surgical margin should be indicated by an R1 descriptor (residual microscopic disease).

Regional Lymph Nodes (N)

Clinical

NX	Regional lymph nodes cannot be assessed
N0	No regional lymph node metastasis
N1	Metastasis in regional lymph node or nodes

Pathologic

pNX	Regional nodes not sampled
pN0	No positive regional nodes
pN1	Metastases in regional node(s)

*Distant Metastasis (M)**

MX	Distant metastasis cannot be assessed (not evaluated by any modality)
M0	No distant metastasis
M1	Distant metastasis
M1a	Nonregional lymph node(s)
M1b	Bone(s)
M1c	Other site(s) with or without bone disease

*When more than one site of metastasis is present, the most advanced category is used. pM1c is most advanced.

Stage Grouping

Stage I	T1a	N0	M0	G1
Stage II	T1a	N0	M0	G2, 3–4
	T1b	N0	M0	Any G
	T1c	N0	M0	Any G
	T1	N0	M0	Any G
	T2	N0	M0	Any G
Stage III	T3	N0	M0	Any G
Stage IV	T4	N0	M0	Any G
	Any T	N1	M0	Any G
	Any T	Any N	M1	Any G

Used with permission of the American Joint Committee on Cancer (AJCC), Chicago, Illinois. The original source for this material is the *AJCC Cancer Staging Manual, Sixth Edition* (2002) published by Springer-Verlag New York, www.springer-ny.com.

Watchful Waiting or Periodic Observation for Early-Stage Prostate Cancer

Prostate cancer is a heterogenous disease and often slow growing. The challenge lies in differentiating those patients who will benefit from watchful waiting from those who should undergo therapy. Men with small-volume, well-differentiated cancers may die with, rather than from, prostate cancer. In the United States, there exists a group of 8 million men older than age 50 with potentially diagnosable prostate cancer. Of these 8 million men, 7.9 million will have an autopsy-discoverable cancer.[88] The remaining 100,000 men have a clinically diagnosable cancer.[88] Clinically diagnosable prostate cancer, if left untreated, will continue to grow and threaten the life of the patient. Latent or clinically unimportant cancers do not threaten the patient's life. Of men age 50 or older, approximately one-third will have malignant cells in their prostate.[102] As men age beyond 50 years, the incidence of cancer cells in the prostate increases. However, only 2%–3% of men who develop malignant cells in their prostate will die of the disease.[99] For men with early stage A and B_1 prostate cancer, this observation has led some physicians to offer periodic observation as a method of cancer management. Periodic observation involves monitoring PSA level and physical examination every three to six months to determine whether clinical disease progression has occured.

For patients with a limited life span, watchful waiting may be an appropriate treatment option.[98] Research has yet to demonstrate that for men who

Table 62-4 Comparison of the TNM and Whitmore-Jewett Staging Systems for Clinically Localized Prostate Cancer

TNM Staging System		Jewett Staging System (Modified)	
Tumor			
TX	Tumor cannot be assessed		
T0	No evidence of tumor		
T1s	Carcinoma in situ (PIN)		
T1a	Incidental, tumor ≤ 5%	Stage A1	Tumor ≤ 5%, Gleason score ≤ 4
T1b	Incidental, tumor > 5%	Stage A2	Tumor > 5%, Gleason score > 4
T1c	Identified by biopsy (PSA screening)		
T2a	Palpable or seen on TRUS; one lobe	Stage B1	Palpable, < one lob, ≤ 1.5 cm
T2b	Palpable or seen on Trus; both lobes	Stage B2	Palpable, both lobes, > 1.5 cm
T3a	Extracapsular extension	Stage C1	ECE, negative margins
		Stage C2	ECE, positive margins
T3b	Seminal vesicle involvement	Stage C3	Seminal vesicle involvement
T4	Bladder neck, external sphincter, rectal, levator muscles, or pelvic side wall involvement		
Node			
NX	Lymph nodes cannot be assessed	Stage D1	Microscopic pelvic lymph node involved
N0	No regional lymph node involved		
N1	Metastases, regional lymph node(s)		
Metastasis			
MX	Distant metastases cannot be assessed		
M0	No distant metastases		
M1a	Nonregional lymph node involvement	Stage D2	Disease outside pelvis
M1b	Bone involvement		
M1c	Other sites involved		

ECE, extracapsular extension; M, metastasis; N, node; PIN, prostatic intraepithelial neoplasia; PSA, prostate-specific antigen; T, tumor; TRUS, transrectal ultrasonography.

Reprinted with permission from Carroll PR, Lee KL, Fuks ZY, et al: Cancer of the prostate, in DeVita VT, Hellman S, Rosenberg SA (eds.): *Cancer: Principles and Practice of Oncology* (ed 6). Philadelphia, Lippincott, Williams and Wilkins, 2001, pp 1418–1479[90]

present with stage T1–2 cancer, radical prostatectomy is more beneficial than watchful waiting in terms of overall survival.[103] For men younger than age 70, a physician may often be reluctant to offer watchful waiting. There is also evidence that for younger men with moderately or poorly differentiated localized prostate cancer, treatment may offer a survival advantage.[104] For patients older than 70, treatment that produces side effects such as incontinence may be less beneficial.[104]

Treatment for localized prostate cancer may be presented as a means of preventing metastatic disease from developing.[102] However, there is no evidence that this is true. Currently for men in their forties and fifties, even with well-differentiated cancers, definitive treatment is almost always offered. Prostate cancer may behave in a more aggressive manner because of higher-grade tumors in younger men, so for this reason alone, definitive treatment is offered. Also, younger men have the potential to live longer and thus develop metastases that may be life-threatening.

The option of watchful waiting may not gain widespread support without evidence from large, prospective, randomized trials. Until such results are available, scientifically proven therapy with surgery or radiation therapy will be offered to patients with localized prostate cancer. Several studies have been conducted that address the concept of watchful waiting, both in Sweden and in the United States. However, some of these studies contain methodological flaws. Even though flawed, they are often cited as evidence that watchful waiting is an appropriate option in selected patients.

Albertsen and colleagues performed a retrospective cohort study of men age 65–75 diagnosed in Connecticut with localized prostate cancer during 1971–1976.[105] The cohort consisted of 451 men with an average age of 70.9 years. At the time of diagnosis, the patients were assessed with a status of TA1, TA2, TAx, or TBx based on chart content and pathologic information. Treatment, when offered, consisted of hormonal manipulation. Follow-up continued for 15.5 years, at which time 40 men (9%) were still alive. In only 34% of the cases in which men died could the cause of death be attributed to prostate cancer. The cause could not be determined in 8% of the deaths, and 49% had causes of death other than prostate cancer listed on the death certificate. The Gleason score was the most powerful predictor of death in this study. With a Gleason score of 8–10, 46% of men were dead in 10 years and 51% were dead in 15 years. The death rates at 10 and 15 years for Gleason scores of 5–7 were 24% and 28%, respectively; for Gleason scores of 2–4, the mortality rate was 9% at both intervals. Men with high Gleason scores lost 6–8 years of life and those with a Gleason score of 5–7 lost 4–5 years of life. Men with low-grade tumors did not experience loss of life-years.

Another study evaluated data from 828 patients who participated in six nonrandomized trials. The men received observation and delayed hormone therapy for localized stage A and B cancer.[106] The cancers were graded as 1 (well differentiated, Gleason score 2–4), 2 (moderately differentiated, Gleason score 5–7), or 3 (poorly differentiated, Gleason score 8–10). Grade 3 patients had a poorer survival ratio. At ten years, 34% of these men were alive and 26% were free of metastatic disease. The authors concluded that for grade 1–2 clinically localized cancer in men with a life expectancy of less than ten years, observation and delayed hormonal manipulation is an option for selected patients.

A recent study followed men aged 52–72 with small-volume prostate cancer defined as cT1c, no adverse findings, and a PSA density less than 0.15 ng/mL/cm^3. Adverse findings were a Gleason score of 7 or higher, three or more biopsy cores with prostate cancer, any core biopsy specimen containing 50% or more cancer cells, or any Gleason grade of 4 or 5.[107] The final study sample included 81 men. Follow-up consisted of twice-yearly PSA tests (total and free), and DRE, and annual TRUS-guided biopsy. Disease progression was defined as a Gleason score of 7 or higher, any Gleason grade of 4 or 5, more than two core biopsy specimens with cancer, or any core biopsy specimen containing 50% or more cancer on rebiopsy. At follow-up, 25 of 81 men (31%) had disease progression. Men with disease progression had shorter median follow-up times than those men without progression (14 months versus 25 months). Twelve of the 13 men who had a radical prostatectomy after disease progression had a curable cancer.

A prospective, randomized clinical trial compared radical prostatectomy and watchful waiting in men with early-stage prostate cancer.[100] Eligible patients were younger than age 75 with a newly diagnosed T0, T1, or T2 well- or moderately well-differentiated prostate cancer. Patients with poorly differentiated prostate cancer were not eligible, and those with any Gleason grade of 4 or 5 in the tumor needed to meet specific criteria. Other eligibility criteria included a negative preoperative bone scan, no obstructive upper urinary tract pathology, and a PSA level of less than 50 ng/mL. Patients then underwent radical prostatectomy or watchful waiting. Follow-up was done twice a year for two years, and then yearly. A physical exam was performed along with blood work and a PSA test. Annual bone scans and chest x-rays were also done. There were 348 men in the watchful waiting group and 347 men in the radical prostatectomy group. At 6.2 years, the medial follow-up, there was no difference in overall survival among the two groups, but the radical prostatectomy patients had significantly less disease-specific mortality. A second prospective randomized study confirmed the results of the first study[103] in terms of overall survival.[108] In terms of quality of life, the radical prostatectomy patients had more erectile dysfunction and urinary leakage, whereas the watchful waiting patients had more urinary obstruction.

Older patients may not be treated as aggressively as younger patients for a variety of reasons, including their shorter life expectancy. A recent analysis of the literature and data collected from 104 prostate cancer patients indicates that older patients can benefit from radiation therapy or surgery in terms of prolonged life expectancy.[109] More study is needed in the form of prospective randomized clinical trials. One study that may potentially shed light on this issue is the Prostate Cancer Intervention Versus Observation Trial (PIVOT). This trial will compare radical prostatectomy to observation in men with clinically localized prostate cancer.[110]

Patients on watchful waiting should have regular follow-up including a physical exam, DRE, and PSA test.[110,111] The exam should assess quality of life and urologic symptoms and be completed every three months for the first year and then twice each year. Bone scans should be done yearly. Patients need education and psychosocial support before making a decision to pursue watchful waiting and then afterward while on watchful waiting.[112]

Surgery

Transurethral resection of the prostate

Prostate cancer is not cured by transurethral resection of the prostate (TURP). Rather, the procedure is used to treat symptoms of bladder outlet obstruction. In some patients, it provides pathologic evidence that a cancer, previously unsuspected, is present. Using a transurethral resectoscope and electrocautery, the hypertrophic prostate is removed in pieces called *chips.* The procedure is performed under spinal anesthesia or general anesthesia with the patient in the dorsal lithotomy position. Potential immediate postoperative complications include clot retention, bleeding, and infection. The bladder is kept as free of blood and clots as possible using continuous saline irrigation through a three-way indwelling catheter. Bladder spasms can be problematic, and patients may require analgesics and antispasmodics. After the bleeding decreases, bladder irrigation is discontinued. As the urine becomes more normal in appearance, the catheter is removed. Rarely, patients may have difficulty initiating urination after catheter removal and may require recatheterization.

Nursing aspects of patient management include preoperative education about routine aspects of anesthesia, such as coughing, deep breathing, and early ambulation. The patient needs to know that he will have a catheter after surgery and that bladder irrigation will continue for approximately 24 hours or less. Pain management approaches using oral and rectal medications are discussed. The patient must drink large volumes of fluid, such as water, to promote urine formation. Accurate recording of intake and output is required until discharge. Large amounts of fluid may be absorbed through the cut prostatic capillaries during surgery, resulting in volumetric overload. This phenomenon, known as the *TUR syndrome,* may occur in the first 24 hours postoperatively. TUR syndrome is uncommon, affecting only in 0.2% of men who undergo TURP.[113] As a result of fluid shifts, electrolyte disturbances and hypoosmolality may precipitate neurologic and hypovolemic symptoms.[114] Supportive therapy is used to manage the patient. The nurse must monitor the patient for changes in mental status and cardiac and renal function.

The patient also needs to be aware that late complications, such as incontinence, impotence, and bladder neck contraction requiring urethral dilation, may occur.[77] Patients may have problems with recurrent bladder outlet obstruction; approximately 5% of men need to undergo repeat TURP. Table 62-5 presents an overview of the management of the TURP patient.

Radical prostatectomy

Radical prostatectomy involves removal of the prostate gland, ejaculatory ducts, seminal vesicles, and possibly the lymph nodes. This procedure is usually performed on patients staged with T1 or T2 disease.[77] With T3 disease, it may be more difficult to obtain tumor-free margins. The patient should be informed preoperatively by the physician about the potential for postoperative incontinence and impotence. Incontinence may occur after indwelling catheter removal and continues to be a problem for about 10% of men postoperatively.[117] Risk factors identified for the development of postoperative incontinence include age older than 65, development of anastomotic stricture, and stage T1a or T1b disease.[117] Urinary incontinence was assessed in 1291 men who underwent a radical prostatectomy during 1994–1995. Of these men, 8.4% were incontinent at 18 months after surgery. Younger men were more likely to be continent than men aged 75–79. Older men were also more likely to be incontinent more frequently than younger men.[117] Persistent incontinence requires urologic evaluation for bladder neck contracture, stricture, bladder dysfunction, or sphincter dysfunction.[117]

The autonomic nerves that control erectile function lie next to the prostate. Surgery may damage or sever these nerves. Currently, however, the right, left, or both neurovascular bundles may be preserved[118] (see Figure 62–1). Walsh developed and continues to refine the method of sparing the neurovascular bundles responsible for an erection.[119] With this nerve-sparing procedure, it is possible to retain potency; however, there will be no prostatic fluid and, therefore, no emission and ejaculation. This approach is recommended for patients with stage T1 or T2 disease who are eligible to undergo radical prostatectomy. In one study, the nerve-sparing procedure was performed in 503 men who were able to maintain an erection before surgery.[120] Sixty-eight percent of the patients were potent after surgery. Factors that promote sexual function after surgery include age younger than 50, stage of disease, and preservation of neurovascular bundles. In younger men (age 50 and younger), lower stage and surgical procedure were the factors associated with potency. When one bundle is intact in patients younger than 50, potency is preserved. In patients older than age 70, only 22% will regain potency postoperatively, even if both neurovascular bundles are spared. If disease is more advanced and there is involvement of the prostatic capsule or seminal vesicles at the time of surgery, resection may involve removal of or damage to the nerves. In the patients with stage B2 or C disease in the previously mentioned study, 51% had one bundle left intact. Age again becomes important, with men younger than 50 regaining potency and older patients having a reduced likelihood of potency.

A meta-analysis of the literature available on erectile dysfunction after surgery and radiation therapy indicates that the patients who were potent preoperatively were more likely to remain potent postoperatively. Also, patients were more likely to be potent after radiation therapy than surgery (probability 0.69 versus 0.42, $p < 0.0001$).[121]

Incontinence and impotence can place a heavy burden on male patients and their families. Increasingly, research is addressing concerns related to quality of life. Compared with normal age-matched men living in the same location, men who have undergone treatment for localized prostate cancer are more likely to have problems related to sexual, urinary, or bowel function.[122] Quality of life issues may be amenable to nursing interventions, such as patient education, and nurses need to accept responsibility for the assessment, management, and evaluation of these patient concerns.

Table 62-5 Nursing Management of the Patient Undergoing a TURP

Nursing Diagnosis	Etiology	Outcome	Nursing Management
Knowledge deficit, surgery	Lack of prior experience with surgery.	Patient will verbalize an understanding of preoperative and postoperative course.	1. Assess patient's understanding of cancer diagnosis, planned surgery to remove obstructing section of prostate gland around prostatic urethra compressing urethra and impeding release of urine from the bladder, expected outcome that patient will be able to void with reduced difficulty, potential complications of surgery including incontinence. 2. Educate patient regarding: • Care of indwelling catheter • Continuous bladder irrigation (CBI) • Drinking fluids • Ambulating first day postoperative • Coughing and deep breathing • Pain management with belladonna and opium suppositories for bladder spasms, oral narcotics for pain • Signs/symptoms of urinary tract infection (UTI) to report to physician after surgery — pain, burning, frequency, hematuria • Need to notify physician after discharge of inability to void, continued incontinence, bright red urine, numerous clots, chills, fever, decreased stream size and force
Incontinence	The urinary sphincter may be injured during surgery — may persist up to three months in elderly.	The patient will be able to manage incontinence.	• Methods for managing incontinence (see Table 62-6)
Indwelling catheter care	The patient is unable to void after indwelling catheter is removed postoperatively and requires recatheterization and discharge home with indwelling catheter.	The patient will demonstrate the skills necessary to maintain an indwelling catheter at home.	3. Educate patient to: • Wash around urinary meatus with soap and water, rinse and dry the area twice daily • Utilize leg bag during day, how to attach, disconnect, empty and cleanse bag to maintain a clean environment inside the equipment • Utilize straight drainage at night, how to cleanse bag to maintain a clean environment inside the equipment • Maintain a clean bag environment by rinsing the equipment, washing it with soapy water, rinsing well, and allowing it to air dry
Altered urinary elimination related to TURP and indwelling catheter	The patient has undergone TURP and requires a catheter to maintain prostate urethra patency and elimination of urine and blood. Clots have formed in the bladder, occluding the catheter/tubing lumen. As the bladder fills, clots slide down the outside of the catheter and out the meatus.	The catheter will remain patent. Urine output will be $\geq$ 30 mL/hr.	1. Maintain accurate I&O. 2. Empty urinary drainage bag when two-thirds full. 3. Maintain CBI at rate to keep urine clear using NSS 3 L irrigation bags. Do not allow bags to empty. Keep NSS running at all times to maintain pink-colored drainage. CBI is usually discontinued 24 hr postoperatively, but may by required for a longer period if some bleeding or clot formation persists beyond the first 24 hr. 4. Monitor for clots in the tubing, monitor for clot retention with subsequent bleeding around the catheter. Assess for bladder distention. Notify physician of clot retention. Irrigate Foley catheter manually with saline until free of clots. Do not forcefully irrigate catheter — notify surgeon. 5. Maintain IV fluids at prescribed rate of infusion. 6. Encourage fluid intake, usually 2000 mL/24 hr. 7. Maintain catheter tubing patency by unkinking tubing. 8. One to two days postoperatively, the catheter is removed. Accurately measure the first and each subsequent voiding until discharge. Notify physician if patient does not void in 8 hr.

(continued)

Table 62-5 Nursing Management of the Patient Undergoing a TURP (continued)

Nursing Diagnosis	Etiology	Outcome	Nursing Management
Bleeding related to TURP	The prostate is highly vascularized. Cauterization during the surgery does not seal all the bleeding capillaries, therefore bleeding occurs in the postoperative period.	The patient will have prompt recognition of and immediate intervention for increased bleeding. Bleeding will decrease daily.	1. Monitor hemoglobin and hematocrit values. Notify physician of ≥ 1 g reduction in hemoglobin. 2. Maintain traction with tape on catheter applied during surgery to assist in control of venous bleeding in prostatic bed. 3. Monitor color of urine. There should be a noted reduction in the amount of blood in the urine daily. If increased blood is present, notify physican. 4. Do not remove water from overfilled indwelling catheter balloon, as this helps to control bleeding. 5. Do not remove indwelling catheter until physician orders its removal. Premature removal may result in bleeding. 6. Monitor for bladder distention, which increases bleeding by pulling on capillaries
Potential for infection related to surgery and indwelling catheter	The presence of an indwelling catheter may promote bladder infection. The patient has undergone surgery under general anesthesia and may develop postoperative atelectasis, which may develop into pneumonia.	The patient will not develop a fever or other sign of infection	1. Encourage q1h coughing and deep breathing. 2. Use aseptic technique when emptying drainage bag and attaching new bladder irrigation bags. 3. Perform meatal care twice daily with soap and water. 4. Maintain catheter patency. Observe for clots, chips of tissue, mucus that can obstruct catheter lumen. Keep catheter and tubing straight and free of kinks. Keep drainage bag off floor. Hang with hook from bed. 5. Notify physician of temperature ≥ 38.5°C, tachycardia, tachypnea, decreased BP, other signs of infection. 6. Obtain urine, blood, or other cultures as prescribed.
Altered comfort related to pain, bladder spasms, or both	Pain or bladder spasms may be due to surgery, bladder distention, infection, clots, or the catheter balloon.	The patient will verbalize an acceptable level of analgesia.	1. Assess quantity, quality, and duration of pain. 2. Check for bladder distention, kinked tubing, freely flowing drainage. Palpate bladder after turning off CBI. Restart CBI if patient not distended. Otherwise, notify physician. 3. Administer prescribed narcotic for pain. 4. Administer belladonna and opium suppository, oxybutynin, or propantheline for bladder spasms. 5. Gently irrigate indwelling catheter if prescribed. Never force irrigation fluid — notify physician. 6. Remind patient not to tug or pull at the catheter. If the patient should pull out the catheter, notify physician immediately.
Potential for urethral stricture formation related to surgery	The urethra may heal with stricture formation if catheter is removed prematurely.	The patient will have a patent urethra.	1. The catheter is never to be removed without a physician's order. 2. Monitor for signs of stricture, such as small urine stream, straining to void, and difficulty voiding.
Potential for urinary retention after catheter removal	The patient is not able to void after catheter is removed.	The patient will not develop urinary retention.	1. The patient should void when he feels the urge and not wait, as this may produce urinary distention, which may cause retention.
Constipation related to antispasmodics used to manage bladder spasms	Anticholinergic drugs cause constipation. Straining can cause bleeding.	The patient will have an easy bowel movement.	1. Administer stool softeners/laxatives to reduce constipation and promote easy colon evacuation. 2. Educate patient not to strain on bowel movement.
Potential for altered fluid and electrolyte balance	Fluid balance and electrolyte alterations occur during surgery.	The patient will have prompt recognition of signs and symptoms of altered fluid and electrolyte balance.	1. Monitor electrolytes, BUN, creatinine. Notify physician of abnormal results. 2. Assess patient for changes in mental status, vital signs, tremor, vomiting, headache. 3. Monitor patient for change in renal or cardiac function..

Data from Mebust, Holtgrewe, Cockett, et al[113]; Chambers[114]; Meredith[115]; Volpe.[116]

Preoperative nursing care is similar to that provided to patients undergoing other surgical procedures of the abdomen and pelvis.[123] Many patients undergoing radical prostatectomy will be older than age 50, and special attention should be paid to the patient's co-morbid factors such as cardiopulmonary status. Additional routine preoperative care includes administering a bowel preparation to evacuate the colon, starting prescribed intravenous therapy, and ensuring that the patient eats or drinks nothing after midnight. Elderly patients should understand that they may have longer postoperative recovery times.

Intraoperatively, the prostate and its surrounding structures are removed via a perineal or retropubic incision.[77] One or more drains may be placed during surgery, and frequent dressing changes may be required to control drainage, reduce bacterial growth, and reduce the risk of skin maceration and resultant infection. The nurse must monitor incision and drainage sites for infection.

Depending on the surgical approach and degree of intraoperative findings, such as disease greater than expected, the patient may be immobilized on the operating room table for several hours. He is thus at risk for the usual postoperative complications. The nurse needs to encourage coughing, deep breathing, use of analgesics, and moving around in bed to promote lower extremity venous return to the heart. Compression stockings are typically used in the postoperative period to reduce the risk of thrombophlebitis and potentially fatal pulmonary embolus. In the presence of thrombophlebitis or suspected/proven pulmonary emboli, anticoagulant therapy is initiated with a heparin bolus and a heparin drip is started or low molecular weight heparin is used.

An indwelling urinary catheter is placed in the operating room and will remain in place postoperatively. Attention is needed to reduce the risk of infection with thorough hand washing, use of aseptic technique when emptying the drainage bag, and monitoring the catheter for patency. In addition to maintaining the indwelling catheter, the nurse must monitor the amount of hematuria.

In the initial postoperative period, a nasogastric tube may be placed to control gastric distention and remove gastric secretions. Management includes monitoring the type and amount of drainage, providing mouth care to promote oral comfort, and maintaining tube patency. Drains will collect serosanguineous drainage postoperatively. A sudden increase in the amount of drainage, the presence of increased bleeding, or the appearance of urine in the drains requires prompt physician notification.

Postoperatively, it is crucial that the patient maintain a urine output of greater than 30 mL/hr.[123] In addition to monitoring for hematuria and clots, maintaining a patent catheter, and ensuring an accurate intake and output, the nurse should assess the bladder for urinary retention and administer parenteral fluids. Also, the catheter taped to the patient's upper leg must be maintained securely to avoid catheter movement and tugging on the newly anastomosed urethra. The catheter provides support to the healing urethra and must not be removed without a physician's order.

Bladder spasms can be annoying and painful. They may be caused by kinking of the catheter, bladder distention, or the catheter itself.[118] Bladder spasms are commonly managed by administering antispasmodics such as oxybutynin and, if not contraindicated, belladonna and opium (B&O) suppositories.

Hematuria is common during the first 24 hours after surgery.[124] Frank bleeding and clots are abnormal and require physician notification. Frequent monitoring of vital signs is needed to assess the patient for signs of excess blood loss and temperature elevation, which may indicate a wound or urinary tract infection.

The patient is discharged with an indwelling catheter and needs to be educated in meatal care, attachment of a leg drainage bag, change to a straight drainage bag at bedtime, cleaning technique, and signs of urinary tract infection that would require physician notification. After the catheter is removed two to three weeks postoperatively, incontinence may be a problem for days, weeks, or months. A variety of management options are available. Simple devices, such as penile clamps or incontinence pads, may be suggested. Reducing the volume of fluid consumed after dinner may control problems with nighttime incontinence. Frequent emptying of the bladder (e.g., every hour) may provide a patient with enough control over his incontinence that he finds occasional incontinence tolerable. Instructing the patient to use Kegel exercises to strengthen the muscles also may prove beneficial.

Incontinence is a problem not only for patients undergoing prostate surgery but also for many other adults. The problem is so severe that the Agency for Health Care Policy and Research released urinary incontinence guidelines in 1992.[125] The guidelines provide an in-depth discussion of incontinence and its management (Table 62-6).

An additional burden placed on postprostatectomy men is the development of altered sexuality. See Chapter 35 for an in-depth discussion of sexual dysfunction and suggestions for nursing management. Table 62-7 presents helpful hints for starting sexual activity after prostate surgery.

Table 62-6 Assisting Patients to Manage Urinary Incontinence After Prostate Surgery

After prostate surgery, continence is maintained by the external urinary sphincter. This striated urethral sphincter prevents urinary leakage after prostate surgery.[126] Damage to the muscle controlling the sphincter or damage to its nerve supply can result in postoperative incontinence. The retropubic approach to prostatectomy may result in a lower rate of incontinence by avoiding injury to the cavernous nerves of the pelvic plexus.[127,128] After radical prostatectomy, 92% of patients achieve urinary control, 8% experience stress incontinence, and 6% wear one or fewer incontinence pads per day. Approximately 1% of men are incontinent after a TURP.[129]

Evaluation

Diagnostic studies are performed to evaluate incontinence after a history and physical exam are performed. Cystourethroscopy is used to evaluate the integrity of the external urinary sphincter under direct visualization. A voiding cystourethrogram looks for anatomical abnormalities, while urodynamic studies evaluate physiology.[130]

Management

Diapers, liners — these devices absorb urine. There are a variety available. Liners are useful for light to moderate incontinence. Adult diapers are needed for heavy urine loss. All devices should be changed frequently to avoid odor and skin maceration. Fungal infections can occur, and in summer, diapers can be hot and uncomfortable.[131] Cost can become a factor when absorbent products need to be changed frequently; for people with a limited income, this can be a financial burden. Bulky items may be noticed under clothing.

Drip collectors — The penis is placed inside the collector, which is worn underneath clothing in a garment holder designed to hold the disposable collecting device.[131]

Condom catheters — latex and nonlatex self-adhesive condom-shaped external urine collecting device. Problems include adhesive loss, skin breakdown, and urinary tract infections. The skin needs to be cleansed daily and monitored daily for irritation and infection.[125] Available in single-use and reusable models.

Indwelling catheters — closed sterile system that includes a catheter with a retaining water-filled balloon inserted into the urethra attached to a collection bag. Often left in place after surgery, these devices require daily cleansing and skin care to reduce the risk of infection and skin necrosis. They are not useful for long-term management of incontinence unless no other approach is successful.

Penile clamps — external urethral compressive device that occludes the urethra to reduce incontinence. The position of the clamp must be changed every 3 hr to prevent skin necrosis. Other complications include pain, edema, penile and urethral erosion, and urethral obstruction.[125]

Inflatable compression cuff[132] — band placed around penis and held in place with velcro. Inflated air bladder in band compresses urethra. Complications include tissue damage from compression. Bladder needs to be deflated every 3 hr.

Ostomy pouch — useful for a small or retracted penis. Clip the hair around where the adhesive is applied and attach pouch to a collection bag.

Fluid restriction — the patient who experiences incontinence mostly at night should restrict fluids after dinner to reduce the bladder urine volume and thus the risk of incontinence. Otherwise, 2 quarts of fluids per day are encouraged.

Timed voiding — at predetermined intervals, the patient empties the bladder. To develop a schedule, the patient needs to keep a diary for three or four days to identify times of incontinence. A schedule is then developed for the patient to void prior to the times identified as being at risk for incontinence.[125]

Kegel exercises — the pelvic floor muscles are crucial to maintaining continence. These muscles can be strengthened with exercise. The exercise consists of contracting the pelvic floor muscles by squeezing the pubococcygeus muscle.[125] Squeezing this muscle closes the urethra. The abdominal, pelvic, and thigh muscles must not be contracted during the exercises. Contracting the muscles involved in a bowel movement by pulling them in and holding for 10 seconds, followed by a 10-second rest, and repeated 30 to 80 times a day for a minimum of 6 weeks, can result in better bladder control.

Biofeedback — used in conjunction with Kegel exercises and timed voiding, biofeedback helps the patient become attuned to his physiology. Instruments help the person learn about bladder control.

Bladder dysfunction (detrusor instability) — symptoms include frequency, urgency, urge incontinence.[133] Treatment includes fluid restriction and medications:

Anticholinergics

Propantheline — blocks bladder contractions, dose 7.5 mg to 30 mg 3 to 5 times per day;[125] cost — inexpensive; effect — may reduce incontinence in as many as 53% of patients; side effects — urinary retention, dry mouth, blurred vision, nausea, constipation, confusion, drowsiness. Hyoscyamine is a newer drug.

Oxybutynin — also relaxes smooth muscle, dose 2.5 to 5 mg 3 to 4 times per day; effect — may reduce incontinence in as many as 56% of patients; side effects — dry skin, blurred vision, nausea, constipation.[125]

Muscarinic Receptor Antagonist — Tolterodine

Tolterodine — dose 2 mg 2 times per day PO — muscarinic receptor antagonist, new drug — expensive, lower incidence of dry mouth, better tolerated and as effective as oxybutynin.[134,135]

Antidepressants

Imipramine — anticholinergic properties, dose 10 to 25 mg 1 to 3 times per day; side effects — rare; effect — as many as 77% of patients may have reduced incontinence.[125]

Sphincter incompetence — symptoms include dribbling and stress incontinence.[133] Treatment includes alpha-adrenergic agonist drugs and surgery. The drugs increase sphincter resistance:

Phenylpropanolamine — dose 50 mg twice per day; effect — as many as 45% of patients are drier; side effects — nausea, dry mouth, rash, itching, restlessness, insomnia.[125]

Surgery — goal is urethral compression.[129] Artificial urinary sphincter — useful in patients with normal detrusor function and an incompetent sphincter[129] and after failure of previously discussed methods.[125] Approximately 80% of patients treated will be dry or almost dry requiring no incontinence pads.[129] Complications include infection, device malfunction, bleeding, erosion of cuff site, and urethral injury.[120] Injections of collagen or polytetrafluoroethylene may be useful in patients who are not surgical candidates.[134,135]

Table 62-7 Helpful Hints for Men Starting Sexual Activity After Prostate Surgery

With removal of the prostate, men may notice changes in their sexual functioning. Some men and their partners benefit from understanding these changes and learn how to adapt to them. Beginning with some definitions of the changes, methods of ways to adapt to these changes will be described.

Erection — stiff penis due to increased blood flow

Potency — ability to cause vaginal penetration

Orgasm — sexual climax or pleasure with ejaculation of semen

Semen — mixture of sperm, prostate secretions, and seminal vesicle fluid

Sperm — reproductive cells produced by testes

Radical prostatectomy — removal of prostate, seminal vesicles, and surrounding tissues to remove cancer. With removal of the prostate and seminal vesicles, the ejaculate will be reduced and may be retrograde into the bladder resulting in a dry ejaculation. The urine will become cloudy from the sperm. Orgasms may still occur without ejaculation but with the contractions that occur as part of ejaculation. Impotency can result from surgery or radiation therapy. This can be partial or complete inability to obtain an erection. Some men will regain potency postoperatively, especially those younger than age 50.

Nerve-sparing radical prostatectomy — depending on the size and location of the tumor, the surgeon spares one or both nerve bundles responsible for an erection. In the majority of men younger than 50 potency returns after wound healing occurs and all edema from the surgery subsides. This can take up to two years. Older men, over age 70, will probably not regain an erection.

Orgasms after prostate surgery may be weaker but are rarely completely absent. Alternative methods of obtaining pleasure need to be pursued if there is impotency.

To begin sexual activity after prostate surgery, wound healing must be complete; therefore, the urologist's permission is needed. This may occur six weeks to three months after surgery. Open, honest discussion of sexual issues with one's physician, nurse, and partner will help explore avenues of sexuality not previously considered. Open communication with the partner is the cornerstone of sexual recovery. Explore alternative methods of pleasure such as kissing, stroking, cuddling, massage, gentle rubbing, and fondling. Consider sexual counseling with a therapist if open discussion with the partner and other methods of pleasure are not successful. Couples need to understand that there is more to sexuality and pleasure than penis–vagina intercourse. The intimacy that develops between two partners who love each other will permit exploration. Beginning exploration produces trust and more intimacy that promotes the desire to find ways to pleasure the partner that may not have been previously considered. Failure to communicate desires and needs to one's partner is the greatest barrier to regaining sexual relations. It must also be understood that cancer of the prostate cannot be transmitted during sex or in the sperm. Cancer of the prostate is not a sexually transmitted disease.

Alternative methods of obtaining an erection include external and internal devices. Men in stable relationships with a previously good sex life are the best candidates. However, many of these couples have been able to substitute other sexual activity if erections are not able to penetrate the vagina.[136]

External Devices

Suction apparatus — vacuum erection device fits over the penis and air is removed by pumping it out with the device. Blood flows into the penis, making it rigid. A band is placed at the base of the penis to prevent blood from leaving the penis after the device is removed. After intercourse, the band is removed. (First-line therapy[137])

Injections of drugs into the spongy penile tissue increase blood flow to the area and produce an erection. Side effects include penile fibrosis and priapism. Drugs include prostaglandin E (alprostadil) and papaverine. (Second-line therapy[137,138])

Drug-impregnated pellets that are placed into the urethra also produce an erection.[202] Side effects include hypotension, urethral pain and burning, penile pain, and dizziness. (Second-line therapy[137])

Internal Devices (Implanted Penile Prostheses)

Semirigid — a variety of devices are available. The rod is placed in the spongy tissue of the penis but away from the urinary sphincter so that voiding is not affected. Heavy athletic undergarments will conceal the crotch bulge. Many of the devices available have a metal core that allows the device to be bent upward for sexual activity and downward for everyday activities. (Third-line therapy[137])

Self-containing prosthesis, semirigid — a self-contained device with a pump behind the head of the penis that is pumped to fill the rod with fluid from a reservoir. As the rod fills, an erection is produced. After sexual activity, a release valve drains the fluid back into the reservoir. Many of these devices can be placed under local anesthesia. Semirigid rods are the most commonly implanted penile prostheses. Success rates run about 95% for semirigid devices.[137] (Third-line therapy[137])

Inflatable penile prosthesis — consists of inflatable rods, reservoir, tubing, and pump. The reservoir for the fluid that fills the inflatable rods is placed in the abdomen with the pump in the scrotum. When the pump is activated manually, the fluid exits the reservoir and enters the rods, producing an erection. To release the fluid and deflate the rods at the end of intercourse, the release valve is activated. Mechanical problems occur in 10% to 20% of devices placed.[137] (Third-line therapy[138])

Medication — sildenafil 100 mg PO 1 hr prior to sexual activity. Effective in men with both neurovascular bundles intact.[139] Less effective in unilateral or non-nerve-sparing surgery.[139] Taken as needed 30–60 min prior to sexual activity.[137] Other agents include vardenafil and tadalafil. Side effects include flushing, indigestion, headache, color vision abnormalities. Contraindications — nitrates. Deaths have been reported in men taking both medications. May cause shock, myocardial infarction, or severe hypotension.[140] (First-line therapy.[137])

A rising PSA level after surgery indicates biochemical (PSA) failure of the disease to respond to treatment and evidence that prostate cancer recurrence may develop. The median time from the development of a rising PSA level to the emergence of metastatic disease is 8 years.[141] Immediate hormonal therapy has been compared with observation in 98 men who were treated with radical prostatectomy and pelvic lymphadenectomy.[142] The patients were prospectively randomized to hormonal treatment consisting of bilateral orchiectomy or goserelin or observation. Patients who received hormonal therapy immediately after radical prostatectomy had better survival than those patients on the observation arm.

Radiation therapy has also been used in the postoperative period for patients with high-Gleason-grade tumors, seminal vesicle involvement, lymph node metastasis, or extracapsular disease to reduce the risk of relapse.[143]

Cryosurgery

Cryosurgery to treat prostate cancer was revived and improved in the 1990s following the development of TRUS and improved surgical techniques that permit access to the prostate through a percutaneous approach.[144] Probes deliver a gaseous substance, which freezes the tissues, and are inserted percutaneously into the prostate. The urethra is kept warm with a urethral warmer that circulates warm water.[144] Ice balls form at the end of the probes, freezing the prostate tissue and killing the cancer cells. Freezing is done over two cycles to enhance cell kill. The procedure is monitored using TRUS. Candidates for cryoablation include patients with localized cancer (T1–4) and those with local recurrence after prior local therapy or hormonal therapy.[145] Large prostates (greater than 40 g) should be cytoreduced with hormonal therapy prior to cryosurgery.

Advantages associated with this approach include less pain, bleeding, and incontinence.[146] Possible complications include bleeding, infection, incontinence, fistula formation, urethral sloughing, urinary retention, urethral obstruction, urethral strictures, numbness of the penis, and impotence.[90,124] Also, not all the cancer cells may be killed.

In one study, 76 patients underwent cryosurgical ablation of the prostate.[147] After one or more treatments, 72 of 73 patients had negative biopsies. At five years, the overall survival rate was 89%. Complications included urethral sloughing, incontinence, and impotence. Long-term follow-up of these and other cryosurgery patients and additional trials are needed to determine the role of this procedure in the treatment of prostate cancer.

Nursing care includes preoperative teaching regarding the bowel preparation and home care of indwelling or suprapubic urinary drainage catheter.[102,123,146] Postoperative care includes monitoring vital signs, intake and output (I&O), administering IV fluids, assessing the urinary catheter drainage, and pain management.[148] Sequential compression stockings may be used to promote venous return. Ambulation is promoted on the first postoperative day. The patient must drink large amounts of fluid each day (2.5 L) and report signs of infection to the physician after discharge. Home care may be needed to assist with bladder retraining and care of the catheter, which may remain in place for three weeks to allow for urethral healing.[102]

Laparoscopic prostatectomy

Laparoscopic prostatectomy is a new surgical procedure developed in Europe that entails the removal of the prostate gland and associated structures, including the seminal vesicles and pelvic lymph nodes, which are removed first.[149] The procedure is performed under general anesthesia with the patient in a pronounced lithotomy position with the hips above the shoulders. An indwelling urinary drainage catheter is placed before the surgery begins. The abdomen is filled with carbon dioxide gas, and trochars are inserted into the gas-distended abdominal cavity through five stab wounds. The insertion of the instrumentation and removal of the organs occur through the wounds. A TV screen monitor is used to view the internal organs by means of one instrument. Robotics are used to hold the instruments. The urethral anastomosis is seen under magnification. A bag is passed through a trocar, the removed organs are placed inside the bag, and then the bag and contents are removed from the body. A drain is placed and the incisions are sutured.

Preoperative care includes patient education and routine care of the general anesthesia patient undergoing abdominal and pelvic surgery. Postoperative care includes monitoring for infection and bleeding, volume and type of wound drainage, care of the indwelling urinary catheter, monitoring of urine output, administration of antibiotics and parenteral fluids, and compression stockings. Because the patient has been immobilized in the lithotomy position, he is at risk for the hazards of immobility, including cardiopulmonary and venous thromboembolic complications. Ileus can be a postoperative complication, so the gastrointestinal system needs ongoing monitoring. The integrity of the indwelling urinary catheter must not be compromised, as it supports the ureteral anastomotic site. Lab work and vital signs are monitored. Pain is managed with parenteral narcotics and antispasmodics (e.g., oxybutynin) are used for bladder spasms.[150] The patient is not allowed any food or fluids and is kept on bed rest during the day of surgery. On the first postoperative day, the patient is gotten out of bed, switched to oral analgesics, and taught to care for and manage the indwelling urinary catheter at home.

Candidates for laparoscopic prostatectomy include patients with T1b–T2b disease.[151] Side effects and complications include the need to perform an open radical prostatectomy, bleeding, arterial injury, rectal injury, nerve damage, ileus, leaking anastomosis, uroma, myocardial infarction, infection, and urinary retention.[151–153] Advantages of the procedure include less pain, reduced risk of impotence and incontinence due to magnification of the operative site with increased visibility, less blood loss, fewer blood transfusions, and fewer indwelling catheter days.[152,154] A disadvantage is the surgeon learning curve — operative times become shorter as the individual surgeon performs the procedure more often. Cancer outcomes appear to be similar between laparoscopic prostatectomy and open radical prostatectomy.[154] However, because laparoscopic prostatectomy is a new surgical procedure, there is no long-term patient follow-up and no prospective randomized clinical trials comparing the outcomes of the two approaches.

Radiation Therapy

External beam radiation therapy may be administered in curative doses to treat men with early prostate cancer (T1, T2) confined to the gland itself. Radiation therapy is an option if a patient wishes to avoid surgery or is not a surgical candidate due to preexisting medical problems. There is no evidence that either radiation therapy or surgery is superior in treating early-stage disease (T1a–T2b).[155] As yet, no randomized trials have been completed to compare surgery and radiation therapy in patients with the same stage of disease.[155] Radiation therapy may also be used for locally advanced stage T3 or T4 disease.[116] The dose of radiation administered ranges from 73 to 77 Gy over seven to eight weeks and depends on tumor size, PSA level, Gleason score, and number of core biopsies positive for cancer.[156] Factors predicting postradiation treatment failure are the pre- and postradiation PSA levels and tumor characteristics.[157]

Conventional radiation therapy uses three-dimensional conformal radiation therapy to plan the treatment field and deliver the radiation using five to eight beams that are administered at different angles to spare normal tissues from radiation.[156] Intensity-modulated radiation therapy (IMRT) is the current state-of-the-art method for administering therapy. Using computer simulation, the area to be treated is identified; working in reverse, the number of beams and the intensity required to achieve the desired dose are determined.[158]

Radiation therapy also can be administered adjuvantly in the postoperative setting after radical prostatectomy. Indications often prompting use of such therapy include positive surgical margins, "close" surgical margins, and seminal vesicle involvement.[90,116] Patients who relapse after prostatectomy may also benefit from radiation therapy.[90] Of patients who are treated with radiation therapy after radical prostatectomy, 30%–65% will have undetectable PSA levels.[90] Patients with locally advanced disease benefit when goserelin is administered concurrently with radiation therapy.[159] Both local control and survival are improved. Radiation is also useful in managing complications of advanced prostate cancer, including hematuria, urinary obstruction, ureteral obstruction, and pelvic pain. Some patients who experience disease recurrence after radiation therapy may be eligible to receive additional treatment with brachytherapy.[90]

Side effects of radiation therapy may include fatigue, urinary frequency and dysuria, impotence, urinary incontinence, diarrhea, and rectal bleeding.[116] Diarrhea can be problematic, as part of the colon and rectum lie within the radiation field. The patient needs dietary counseling at the initiation of therapy. Teaching includes the need to consume a low-residue diet and management of diarrhea through regulation of the quantity of fiber consumed. Antidiarrheals, such as loperamide HCl, may be used to control diarrhea. Severe diarrhea may require opioid therapy.

The skin in the perineal area is thin and easily damaged by radiation therapy. Skin integrity is maintained through frequent perineal care, including gentle washing of the rectal area with soap and water after each bowel movement and applying a radiation-approved gel such as Natural Care Gel (Bard Patient Care Division) or a cream after treatment. All gels and creams should be washed off before treatment each day. The patient needs to avoid ointments and products that are difficult to remove until radiation therapy is completed. Silver sulfadiazine cream may be useful in promoting wound healing after radiation is completed.

Symptoms of radiation cystitis can be managed through the use of urinary antispasmodics such as oxybutynin, urinary analgesics such as phenazopyridine, $alpha_1$ blockers such as tamsulosin, frequent voiding, and management of urinary tract infections with antibiotic therapy. Fluids should be consumed in large volumes and caffeine should be avoided.

Altered sexual functioning probably is related to damage to the blood supplying the corpora cavernosa.[160] Potency is maintained in 20%–80% of patients receiving radiation[161] and may be related to age, with older men being at greater risk of impotency. Impotence begins months to years after completion of therapy. Cigarette smoking may have a negative effect on potency.[160] Diabetes, hypertension, and heart disease are also known to decrease potency.[162]

Proctitis and rectal bleeding require medical management, including sigmoidoscopy, fulguration of bleeding vessels, and hydrocortisone enemas. Blood transfusions may be required if bleeding causes the hemoglobin to drop to 8 g/dL.

Urethral strictures from inflammation are managed with periodic dilation or transurethral incision of the stenosis.[116] Repeated dilation may be needed. The incidence of urinary complications from radiation therapy is related to the dose of radiation delivered.[163]

Brachytherapy

Prostatic brachytherapy involves the placement of radioactive seeds directly into the prostate. Iodine-125 and palladium-103 seeds are frequently used as the sources of radiation.[164,165] In brachytherapy, a high dose of radiation is delivered to a smaller volume of tissue, with reduced doses being delivered to surrounding normal structures such as the bladder and rectum. Implants may be permanent or temporary. With the patient under general anesthesia and in the lithotomy position, a template is placed on the perineal area and needles are inserted into the target tissue. Radioactive seeds are left in place. Patients with early-stage disease may be offered brachytherapy as a single-modality therapy, or it can be used in locally advanced disease as a boost to the primary therapy.[166] In patients with local relapse, brachytherapy may be employed as salvage therapy.[167]

After insertion of the source, the principles of time, distance, and shielding should be utilized because iodine-125 emits gamma radiation. Side effects include discomfort from the needle and seed insertion, proctitis, dysuria, hematuria for 24 hours, and, in rare cases, infection.[164] Urine should be strained to locate any dislodged radioactive seeds if required by state or local ordinances or laws. Routine predischarge instructions for patients with permanent implants include teaching the patient to avoid close contact with children and pregnant women. A condom must be worn during sexual intercourse (when permitted by the physician) following implantation in case a radioactive seed is lost during intercourse.[164] In this way, the seed can be safely retrieved. Radiation safety precautions as determined by the radiation safety officer must be followed by the patient and his family members. Palladium-103 has a shorter half-life than iodine-125 and therefore produces fewer urinary and rectal side effects.[165]

Hormonal Therapy

Advanced prostate cancer is frequently managed by altering the patient's hormonal status. Tumors comprise a heterogenous population of cells. Three different cell populations constitute both normal and malignant prostate tissues: androgen dependent, androgen sensitive, and androgen independent.[168] When the androgen source is eliminated from androgen-dependent cells, they die, and the androgen-sensitive cells no longer divide.[169] In contrast, androgen-independent cells do not respond to the loss of hormones and continue to grow. The adrenal gland also produces hormones, which will continuously support hormone-independent cells and account for about 40% of the intraprostatic testosterone.[170]

The vast majority of androgen is produced by the testes. Androgen secretion is dependent on luteinizing hormone-releasing hormone (LHRH) released from the hypothalamus. LHRH stimulates the pituitary gland to produce luteinizing hormone (LH), which in turn stimulates the testes to produce testosterone (androgen).[171] The goal of hormone therapy for prostate cancer is to reduce the level of circulating androgens to castration levels, causing the death of androgen-dependent cells and inhibiting the growth of androgen-sensitive cells, thereby reducing tumor size. Although hormonal manipulation is not curative therapy, it can provide many patients with symptom control and palliation.

Both surgical and medical approaches are used to reduce serum testosterone levels. The oldest method is bilateral orchiectomy. With this procedure, testosterone levels are reduced quickly because 90%–95% of testosterone production is eliminated with removal of the testicles.[172]

Estrogen administration blocks LHRH and LH, resulting in reduced testosterone secretion. The estrogen diethylstilbestrol is rarely used as treatment for prostate cancer. The potential for cardiovascular side effects makes estrogen therapy less favored given the newer therapies available, which include LHRH agonists and antiandrogens. An estrogen compound is also found in estramustine, an oral antineoplastic.

LHRH agonists initially increase testosterone levels, but after several days of therapy testosterone levels fall to castration level. The surge of testosterone production after initiation of an LHRH agonist is called a *flare*. During a flare, patients need to be aware that symptoms can worsen and require prompt medical intervention. Pain may increase as well as symptoms of bladder outlet obstruction. Serious complications include spinal cord compression. Flutamide, an antiandrogen, may be administered prior to the initiation of an LHRH agonist to reduce the flare. Antiandrogens prevent the binding of testosterone to receptors on prostate cells.[171] Three antiandrogens are commercially available: flutamide, bicalutamide, and nilutamide. All have the side effect of hepatotoxicity. Liver function tests need to be monitored prior to the initiation of therapy, one month after therapy begins, and then every three months.

Combining antiandrogenic therapy with an LHRH agonist, such as leuprolide or goserelin, is called *combined androgen blockade (CAB)*. When a patient is a suitable candidate for hormonal manipulation, combination therapy is an often-used treatment option. However, a recent meta-analysis of CAB studies failed to demonstrate that CAB was superior to castration alone in terms of prolonging survival.[173] Hormonal manipulation may also be used with radiation therapy in patients with T2–3 disease.[171] Compared to radiation alone, patients receiving hormonal manipulation and radiation therapy have better local, distant, and PSA outcomes.

LHRH antagonists also cause castration levels of testosterone to develop. One agent, abarelix, is commercially available and is administered by intramuscular injection. It works by blocking LH and follicle-stimulating hormone (FSH) production and causes testosterone levels to fall without producing a flare.[174] Side effects include allergic reactions, increased values on liver function tests, reduced hemoglobin and hematocrit, and adverse effects on the gastrointestinal and central and peripheral nervous systems. This agent is useful in patients who should not experience a tumor flare with LHRH agonists.

All hormonal manipulations have the potential to produce side effects. The ones most commonly encountered include hot flashes, fatigue, impotence, and decreased libido.[175] Osteoporosis and bone metastasis are of significant concern in this patient population and may affect pain levels and the patient's quality of life. Metastatic lesions may develop due to concurrent osteoblastic and osteoclastic activity in sites of bone metastasis, so that the patient experiences an increase in both bone loss and bone formation. The new bone formed is not deposited at sites of bone loss, however. Osteoporosis in men on androgen ablative therapy results from increased loss of bone mineral density.[176,177] Risk factors for osteoporosis in men on a LHRH agonist taken either alone or in combination with an antiandrogen include white race and slender build.[178] Prior to starting hormonal therapy, a bone mineral density test should be performed and then repeated periodically.[178] The patient should receive dietary counseling regarding calcium and vitamin D supplements.[178] Physical activity should be initiated following a consultation with a physical therapist. Patient education includes instructing the patient to remove throw rugs and other objects that could precipitate falling, install safety devices in the bathroom, and avoid activities that could result in bone injury.

Bisphosphonates interfere with osteoclast function and increase bone strength. Zoledronic acid, a bisphosphonate, reduces skeletal-related events in patients with metastatic prostate cancer.[179] Clinical trials are needed to determine whether zoledronic acid can prevent bone metastasis, osteoporosis, or both in men with advanced prostate cancer.

Patients on hormonal therapy may have problems with altered self-esteem, loss of libido, and loss of sexual potency that may present a crisis for the patient and his sexual partner. Sensitive discussions allowing verbalization of feelings are encouraged before and during treatment.

Leuprolide and goserelin injections are administered parenterally every three to four months. Leuprolide acetate is given as an depot intramuscular injection available in a prefilled syringe. Special instructions are provided by the manufacturer for mixing the drug and diluent. This agent is also available as an injectable "gel" given subcutaneously and as a one-year implanted pump. Goserelin is a pellet given as a subcutaneous injection into abdominal fat.

Patients will respond well to hormonal therapy 70%–80% of the time, and responses can be several years in duration.[99] Progression of disease may be managed with palliative radiation therapy, with second-line hormonal manipulation, or with enrollment in a clinical trial. LHRH agonists need to be continued in non-orchiectomy patients to maintain testosterone castration levels.[180]

Hormone-refractory prostate cancer may respond to the withdrawal of flutamide.[181] Discontinuing flutamide in 36 patients who were receiving flutamide plus an LHRH agonist resulted in 10 patients having reduced PSA levels and improved clinical symptoms. Suppression of adrenal androgens can be achieved with ketoconazole. Ketoconazole and hydrocortisone combination therapy may be tried, or hydrocortisone may be used as a single agent given that it lowers testosterone levels.[180] Both high-dose (400 mg tid) and low-dose (200 mg tid) ketoconazole with hydrocortisone (10 mg bid) may be effective, with fewer side effects arising with the lower-dose ketoconazole regimen.[182] One study enrolled 28 patients with progressive prostate cancer after antiandrogen withdrawal and castration levels of testosterone. The participants received high-dose ketoconazole with hydrocortisone until disease progression occurred, at which time the dose of ketoconazole was increased to the high-dose level. Of the 28 patients, 13 demonstrated lower PSA levels (> 50%) with a median duration of response of at least 30 weeks (range 36–53 weeks). Toxicities noted included hepatotoxicity and depression. Side effects included nausea, dry skin, and fatigue.

Chemotherapy

For a patient with hormone-refractory prostate cancer (HRPC), antineoplastic therapy may be an option. Over the past several years, research has produced several drug regimens that can enhance the quality of life of patients with HRPC. Until recently, none of these drug combinations has improved survival.

When evaluating the response rates and research protocols used in HRPC, several factors must be taken into consideration. The trials need to disclose the hormone therapy the patient has received and control for ongoing hormonal therapy, as the withdrawal of antiandrogens during the research study may affect PSA levels rather than the agent being investigated.[181,183] PSA testing is often used as a method to measure research outcomes. PSA values need to be clearly described in the methodology section of the research report with respect to partial and complete responses and the length of time the response needs to be maintained in addition to how frequently blood levels are evaluated.[184] PSA results can be reduced by drug effect without evidence of a corresponding reduction in tumor size and therefore should be used with caution as means of evaluating tumor response in drug trials.[185,186] Likewise, soft tissue disease and bone metastases may not reflect response to treatment, as patients may not have adequate disease to measure on a CT scan and bone disease is slow to demonstrate response on a bone scan.[184,187]

Recently, palliative endpoints (specifically, pain) have been used to assess treatment outcome.[188,189] For example, different tools were used in the trials to evaluate the effect of mitoxantrone and prednisone on HRPC. In one trial, 27 men with HRPC received IV mitoxantrone 12 mg/m^2 every three weeks with prednisone 5 mg bid.[188] Hormonal therapy was continued throughout the trial. The patients completed a present pain intensity (PPI), a visual analog scale (VAS), and the European Organization for Research and Treatment of Cancer (EORTC) 32-item quality of life tool. A palliative complete response (CR) was defined as symptom absence for six weeks. A palliative partial response (PR) was defined as at least a 50% reduction in the analgesic score without a PPI increase or a PPI decrease without an analgesic score increase.[188] The CR rate was 36%, with one additional PR being observed. Side effects included neutropenia, nausea, anorexia, constipation, and alopecia. This trial demonstrated that mitoxantrone and low-dose prednisone can reduce pain and that pain assessments and quality of life indicators can be used to evaluate drug therapy outcomes.

Estramustine is a nornitrogen mustard conjugated with estradiol that demonstrates antimitotic and antimicrotubule activity.[190] Side effects include nausea, vomiting, breast tenderness, gynecomastia, and clotting problems.[191] Paclitaxel is a taxane that demonstrates antimitotic activity. Side effects include peripheral neuropathy, neutropenia, edema, fatigue, myalgia, and arthralgia.[192] Estramustine and paclitaxel have different but additive mechanisms of action.[193] Docetaxel is another taxane with antimitotic activity. Its side effects include increased liver function tests, neutropenia, stomatitis, fatigue, anemia, hyperglycemia, edema, and infection.[194] Both paclitaxel and docetaxel have been combined with estramustine in the treatment of HRPC.[195] Partial response rates for docetaxel and estramustine combination therapy range from 16% to 66% and for paclitaxel and estramustine combination therapy range from 27% to 46%.[195] Survival has not been affected by any of the regimens, even though these combinations show activity in the management of HRPC.[196] The efficacy of docetaxel and estramustine versus mitoxantrone and prednisone has been investigated in a cooperative group phase III trial. Patients were randomized by Petrylak and colleagues to receive 280 mg of estramustine (tid one hour before meals or 2 hours after) on days 1–5 and 60 mg/m^2 docetaxel on day 2.[197] Dexamethasone 20 mg tid (total dose 60 mg) was given the evening of day 1 prior to docetaxel. Of the eligible patients, 338 received estramustine and docetaxel (plus dexamethasone) and 336 received mitoxantrone (12 mg/m^2) plus prednisone (5 mg orally bid) on day 1. Cycles were repeated every 21 days. Doses of docetaxel or mitoxantrone were increased after cycle 1 if patients did not develop grade 3 or 4 toxicities. Two years into the study, the patients on the arm containing estramustine also started taking aspirin 325 mg plus warfarin 2 mg each day as prophylaxis against the vascular side effects due to estramustine.

Eligible patients showed evidence of progressive metastatic HRPC on bone scan, by PSA, or by bidimensional measurable disease.[197] Patients were stratified by the type of disease progression and severity of bone pain. Antiandrogens and bisphosphonates were stopped at least 4 weeks prior to starting therapy. Serious adverse events were more common in the docetaxel plus estramustine arm ($p < 0.001$).[197] They included cardiovascular side effects, nausea and vomiting, infection, metabolic problems, and neurotoxicites. Patients in the docetaxel plus estramustine arm had improved survival (17.5 months) compared to the mitoxantrone plus prednisone arm (15.6 months, $p = 0.02$).[178] In addition, the docetaxel arm had a 20% lower mortality rate.

In another study comparing docetaxel and mitoxantrone reported by Tannock and colleagues, all patients received 5 mg oral prednisone bid beginning on day 1.[198] Eligible patients had HRPC with evidence of disease progression. Antiandrogen therapy was stopped at least 4 weeks prior to therapy. Patients were stratified by pain severity and performance status. The standard therapy arm was mitoxantrone 12 mg/m^2 on day 1 IV every 21 days. There were two docetaxel arms. One arm was 75 mg/m^2 IV over 1 hour every 21 days; the other was 30 mg/m^2 IV weekly for 5 weeks followed by 1 week off therapy (6-week cycles). Side effects were more common in the docetaxel arm (neutropenia, peripheral edema, cutaneous changes) whereas there were more cardiac side effects in the mitoxantrone arm.[198] Patients in the docetaxel every 21 days arm had a median survival greater than the weekly docetaxel arm or the mitoxantrone arm (18.9 months versus 17.4 months versus 16.5 months). The docetaxel patients also had better pain control.

These two docetaxel-based studies are the first chemotherapy studies to demonstrate a survival advantage in patients with progressive HRPC. Hopefully, these results will translate into practice changes in community settings and that future studies will continue to build on this beginning success. Docetaxel-based therapy should now be considered the new standard against which other chemotherapy regimens will be compared.

Symptom Management and Supportive Care

Patients with advanced prostate cancer may experience a number of symptoms requiring nursing management. Problems include cachexia from weight loss, bone pain, spinal cord compression (SCC), fractures of long bones, leg or scrotal edema, coagulation disorders, and bladder or urethral obstruction.

Bone pain management includes a thorough assessment of the pain's location, onset, duration, and precipitating and alleviating factors. Analgesics useful in the management of bone pain include nonsteroidal anti-inflammatory drugs (NSAIDs) and narcotics, including opioids.[199] Routine long-acting narcotics supplemented by immediate-release, short-acting narcotics constitute a useful regimen. Doses are titrated to achieve maximal analgesia with minimal side effects. Expected narcotic side effects include constipation that requires management with routine laxatives and stool softeners. Additional side effects may include dry mouth, nausea, vomiting, and sedation. NSAID side effects include gastric distress, dizziness, and drowsiness. Higher doses produce more side effects but without enhancing analgesia. Other agents useful in the management of bone pain include the radionuclides strontium-89 and samarium-153.[199] Myelosuppression is the dose-limiting toxicity with these agents. Zoledronic acid is FDA approved for use in the management of patients with HRPC and at least one bone metastasis. This bisphosphonate reduces skeletal pain and skeletal-related events and plays a role in the management of patients with HRPC.[200,201] Radiation therapy is also effective in the management of bone pain.

All patients with bone metastasis are at risk for SCC. Prompt diagnosis and intervention are required to reduce the risk of permanent disability. Patients with SCC frequently experience back pain. This pain may have a radicular component, with the pain encircling the chest or abdomen. Leg weakness, sensory changes, and alterations in bowel or bladder function may be present. Diagnosis of SCC is made by MRI or myelogram. Treatment includes the use of pain management, dexamethasone, external bracing, radiation therapy, and, in selected cases, surgery.[202] Pretreatment performance status is a useful predictor of patient outcome. Of patients who are ambulatory at diagnosis, 75% will remain so, but only 28% of paraplegic patients will become ambulatory after treatment.[203] Nursing management focuses on preserving function, promoting restoration of lost function, and assisting the patient to adapt to changes in his ability to perform activities of daily living while monitoring for changes in neurologic functioning.

Leg and scrotal edema are distressing symptoms produced by advanced prostate cancer. A deep-vein thrombosis (DVT) must always be considered as a potential cause of unilateral or bilateral leg edema. Additional causes include lymphedema and medical conditions such as hypoalbuminemia or fluid overload. Elevation of the affected area may be useful but is often difficult to maintain. Compression therapy, exercise, skin care, and diuretics are all used in the management of lymphedema.[204]

In addition to DVT, patients with advanced prostate cancer may develop disseminated intravascular coagulation (DIC), which is characterized by the consumption of clotting factors and platelets resulting in concurrent hemorrhage and clotting. Patients experience bleeding from multiple body areas, abnormal laboratory results, and clotting throughout the body.[205] Nursing management includes frequent assessment of all body systems, administration of blood products, IV fluids, and medications, and monitoring of laboratory results.

Bladder outlet obstruction evidenced by the inability to void may be managed by intermittent or indwelling urinary bladder catheterization, TURP, or urethral stent. Ureteral stents or percutaneous nephrostomy tubes are used in the treatment of ureteral obstructions. Nursing management includes monitoring for infection and bleeding and educating the patient about catheter care.

Gradually, as the disease progresses and symptoms worsen, patients will find that they are less able to perform their usual activities of daily living. A palliative care team approach is useful in managing the progressive symptoms associated with advancing prostate cancer. A hospice referral provides optimal end-of-life care.

Conclusion

As the incidence and prevalence of prostate cancer continue to rise, it is imperative that nurses—particularly those in advanced nursing practice roles—become active in early detection programs that target high-risk individuals, especially black males. Participation in public education programs in the workplace will further demonstrate the nurse's role as educator and patient advocate. Helping families to understand the controversies involved in the management of prostate cancer continues to be a nursing priority.

References

1. Jemal, A, Tiwari RC, Murray T, et al: Cancer statistics, 2004. *CA Cancer J Clin* 54:8–29, 2004
2. Haas GP, Sakr WA: Epidemiology of prostate cancer. *CA Cancer J Clin* 47:273–287, 1997
3. Tiwari RC, Ghosh K, Jemal A, et al: A new method of predicting US and state-level cancer mortality counts for the current calendar year. *CA Cancer J Clin* 54:30–40, 2004
4. Weir HK, Thun MJ, Hankey BF, et al: Annual report to the nation on the status of cancer, 1975–2000, featuring the uses of surveillance data for cancer prevention and control. *J Natl Cancer Inst* 95:1276–1299, 2003
5. Potosky AL, Miller BA, Albertsen PC, et al: The role of increasing detection in the rising incidence of prostate cancer. *JAMA* 273:548–552, 1995
6. Wingo PA, Landis S, Ries LAG: An adjustment to the 1997 estimate for new prostate cancer cases. *CA Cancer J Clin* 47:239–242, 1997
7. Mettlin CJ, Murphy GP: Why is the prostate cancer death rate declining in the United States? *Cancer* 82:249–251, 1998
8. Surveillance, Epidemiology and End Results (SEER) Program: Age-adjusted U.S. cancer death rates. *J Natl Cancer Inst* 89:12, 1997
9. Parker SL, Davis KJ, Wingo PA, et al: Cancer statistics by race and ethnicity. *CA Cancer J Clin* 48:31–48, 1998
10. Shimizu H, Ross RK, Bernstein L, et al: Cancers of the prostate and breast among Japanese and white immigrants in Los Angeles County. *Br J Cancer* 63:963–966, 1991
11. American Cancer Society: *Cancer Facts and Figures 2003*. Atlanta, GA, American Cancer Society, 2003
12. Hsing AW, Tsao L, Devesa SS: International trends and patterns of prostate cancer incidence and mortality. *Int J Cancer (Pred Oncol)* 85:60–67, 2000
13. Kolonel LN, Nomura AMY, Cooney RV: Dietary fat and prostate cancer: current status. *J Natl Cancer Inst* 91:414–428, 1999
14. Rose DP: Dietary fatty acids and cancer. *Am J Clin Nutr* 66(suppl):998S–1003S, 1997
15. Boyle P, Severi G, Giles GG: The epidemiology of prostate cancer. *Urol Clin North Am* 30:209–217, 2003
16. De Stefani E, Deneo-Pellegrini H, Boffetta P, et al: α-Linolenic acid and risk of prostate cancer: a case-control study in Uruguay. *Cancer Epidemiol Biol Prev* 9:335–338, 2000
17. Lee MM, Wang RT, Hsing AW, et al: Case-control study of diet and prostate cancer in China. *Cancer Causes Control* 9:545–552, 1998
18. Amling CL, Riffenburgh RH, Sun L, et al: Pathologic variables and recurrence rates as related to obesity and race and men with prostate cancer undergoing radical prostatectomy. *J Clin Oncol* 22:1–7, 2004
19. Crawford ED: Epidemiology of prostate cancer. *Urology* 62(suppl 6A):3–12, 2003
20. Messina MJ: Emerging evidence on the role of soy in reducing prostate cancer risk. *Nutr Rev* 61:117–131, 2003
21. Giovannucci E, Clinton S: Tomatoes, lycopene, and prostate cancer. *Proc Soc Exp Biol Med* 218:129, 1998
22. Chan J, Giovannucci E: Vegetables, fruits, associated nutrients, and the risk of prostate cancer. *Epidemiol Rev* 23:82–85, 2001
23. Fleshner NE: Vitamin E and prostate cancer. *Urol Clin North Am* 29:107–113, 2002
24. Klein EA: Selenium: epidemiology and basic science. *J Urol* 171:S50–S53, 2004
25. Konety BR, Getzenberg RH: Vitamin D and prostate cancer. *Urol Clin North Am* 29:95–106, 2002
26. Peehl DM, Krishnan AV, Feldman D: Pathways mediating the growth-inhibitory actions of vitamin D in prostate cancer. *J Nutr* 133:2461S–2469S, 2003
27. Beer TM: Development of weekly high-dose calcitriol based therapy for prostate cancer. *Urol Oncol* 21:399–405, 2003
28. Goodman GE, Schaffer S, Omenn GS, et al: The association between lung and prostate cancer risk, and serum micronutrients: results and lessons learned from β-carotene and retinol efficacy trial. *Cancer Epidemiol Biomarkers Prev* 12:518–526, 2003
29. Alavanja MCR, Samanic C, Dosemeci M, et al: Use of agricultural pesticides and prostate cancer risk in the agricultural health study cohort. *Am J Epidemiol* 157:800–814, 2003
30. Stanford JL, Wicklund KG, McKnight B, et al: Vasectomy and risk of prostate cancer. *Cancer Epidemiol Biomarkers Prev* 8:881–886, 1999
31. Rosenblatt KA, Wicklund KG, Stanford JL: Sexual factors and the risk of prostate cancer. *Am J Epidemiol* 153:1152–1158, 2001
32. Carter HB, Piantadosi S, Isaacs JT: Clinical evidence for and implications of the multistep development of prostate cancer. *J Urol* 143:742–746, 1990
33. Carter BS, Beaty T, Steinberg G, et al: Mendelian inheritance of familial prostate cancer. *Proc Natl Acad Sci USA* 89:3367–3371, 1992
34. Verhage BAJ, Baffoe-Bonnie AB, Baglietto L, et al: Autosomal dominant inheritance of prostate cancer: a confirmatory study. *Urology* 57:97–101, 2001
35. Walsh PC, Partin AW: Family history facilitates the early diagnosis of prostate carcinoma. *Cancer* 80:1871–1874, 1997
36. Zeegers MPA, Jellema A, Ostrer H: Empiric risk of prostate carcinoma for relatives of patients with prostate cancer. *Cancer* 97:1894–1903, 2003
37. Carter BS, Bova GS, Beaty TH, et al: Hereditary prostate cancer: epidemiologic and clinical features. *J Urol* 150:797–802, 1993
38. Walsh PC, Partin AW: Family history facilitates the early diagnosis of prostate carcinoma. *Cancer* 80:1871–1874, 1997
39. Whittemore AS, Wu AH, Kolonel LN, et al: Family history and prostate cancer risk in black, white and Asian men in the United States and Canada. *Am J Epidemiol* 141:732–740, 1995
40. Hsieh K, Albertsen PC: Populations at high risk for prostate cancer. *Urol Clin North Am* 30:669–676, 2003
41. Jemal A, Thomas A, Murray T, et al: Cancer statistics, 2002. *CA Cancer J Clin* 52:23–47, 2002
42. Weinrich SP, Yoon S, Weinrich M: Predictors of participation in prostate cancer screening at worksites. *J Community Health* 15:113–129, 1998
43. Skar WA, Partin AW: Histological markers of risk and the role of high-grade prostatic intraepithelial neoplasia. *Urology* 57(suppl 4A):115–120, 2001
44. Powell IJ: Prostate cancer and African-American men. *Oncology* 11:599–605, 1997
45. Optenberg SA, Thompson IM, Friedrichs P, et al: Race, treatment, and long-term survival from prostate cancer in an equal-access medical care delivery system. *JAMA* 274:1599–1605, 1995

46. Robbins AS, Whittemore AS, VanDenEeden SK: Race, prostate cancer survival, and membership in a large health maintenance organization. *J Natl Cancer Inst* 90:986–990, 1998
47. Chu KC, Tarone RE, Freeman JP: Trends in prostate cancer mortality among black men and white men in the United States. *Cancer* 97:1507–1516, 2003
48. Stattin P, Lumme S, Tenkanen L, et al: High levels of circulating testosterone are not associated with increased prostate cancer risk: a pooled prospective study. *Int J Cancer* 108:418–424, 2004
49. Wu AH, Whittemore AS, Kolonel LN, et al: Serum androgen and sex hormone-binding globulins in relation to lifestyle factors in older African-American, white and Asian men in the United States and Canada. *Cancer Epidemiol Biomarkers Prev* 4:735–741, 1995
50. Linehan WM, Zbar B, Leach F, et al: Molecular biology of genitourinary cancers, in DeVita VT, Hellman S, Rosenberg SA (eds.): *Cancer: Principles and Practice of Oncology* (ed 6). Philadelphia, Lippincott, Williams and Wilkins, 2001, pp 1343–1361
51. Reichardt JKV, Makridakis N, Henderson BE, et al: Genetic variability of the human SRD5A2 gene: implications for prostate cancer risk. *Cancer Res* 55:3973–3975, 1995
52. Cooney KA, McCarthy JD, Lange E, et al: Prostate cancer susceptibility locus on chromosome 1q: a confirmatory study. *J Natl Cancer Inst* 89:955–959, 1997
53. Gronberg H, Xu J, Smith JR, et al: Early age at diagnosis in families providing evidence of linkage to the hereditary prostate cancer locus (HPC1) on chromosome 1. *Cancer Res* 57:4707–4709, 1997
54. Xu J, Meyers D, Freije D, et al: Evidence for a prostate cancer susceptibility locus on the X chromosome. *Nat Gen* 20:175–179, 1998
55. Schaid DJ: The complex genetic epidemiology of prostate cancer. *Hum Mol Genet* 13 (spec no 1): R103–R121, 2004
56. Silva APM, Salim ACM, Bulgarelli A, et al: Identification of 9 novel transcripts and two RGSL genes within the hereditary prostate cancer region (HPC1) at 1q25. *Gene* 310:49–57, 2003
57. Thompson IM, Goodman PJ, Tangen CM, et al: The influence of finasteride on the development of prostate cancer. *N Engl J Med* 349:215–224, 2003
58. Klein EA, Thompson IM, Lippman SM, et al: SELECT: the next prostate cancer prevention trial. *J Urol* 166:1311–1315, 2001
59. Thomas RD, Clejan S: Digital rectal examination–associated alteration in serum prostate-specific antigen. *Am J Clin Pathol* 97:528–534, 1992
60. Waldman AR, Osborne DM: Screening for prostate cancer. *Oncol Nurs Forum* 21:1512–1517, 1994
61. Littrup PJ, Lee F, Mettlin C: Prostate cancer screening: current trends and future implications. *CA Cancer J Clin* 42:198–211, 1992
62. McNeal JE, Price HM, Redwine EA, et al: Stage A versus stage B adenocarcinoma of the prostate: morphological comparison and biological significance. *J Urol* 139:61–65, 1988
63. Smith RA, Cokkinides V, Eyre HJ: American Cancer Society guidelines for the early detection of cancer, 2004. *CA Cancer J Clin* 54:41–52, 2004
64. Gretzer MB, Partin AW: PSA markers in prostate cancer detection. *Urol Clin North Am* 30:677–686, 2003
65. Ploch NR, Brawer MK: How to use prostate-specific antigen. *Urology* 43(suppl):27–35, 1994
66. Brawer M, Catalone W, McConnell J: Prostate cancer: is screening the answer? *Patient Care* 26:55–68, 1992
67. Balk SP, Ko Y-J, Bubley GJ: Biology of prostate-specific antigen. *J Clin Oncol* 21:383–391, 2003
68. Moul JW, Sesterhenn IA, Connelly RR, et al: Prostate specific antigen values at the time of prostate cancer diagnosis in African American men. *JAMA* 274:1277–1281, 1995
69. Morgan TO, Jacobsen SJ, McCarthy WF, et al: Age-specific reference ranges for serum prostate-specific antigen in black men. *N Engl J Med* 335:304–310, 1996
70. Gretzer MB, Partin AW: PSA markers in prostate cancer detection. *Urol Clin North Am* 30:677–686, 2003
71. Catalona WJ, Partin AW, Slawin KM, et al: Use of the percentage of free prostate specific antigen to enhance differentiation of prostate cancer from benign prostatic disease. *JAMA* 279:1542–1547, 1998
72. Catalona WJ, Smith DS, Ornstein DK: Prostate cancer detection in men with serum PSA concentrations of 2.6 to 4.0 ng/mL and benign prostate exam. *JAMA* 277:1452–1455, 1997
73. Carter HB, Pearson JD, Waclawiw Z, et al: Prostate-specific antigen variability in men without prostate cancer: effect of sampling interval on prostate-specific antigen velocity. *Urology* 45:591–596, 1995
74. Kadmon D, Weinberg AD, Williams RH, et al: Pitfalls in interpreting prostate specific antigen velocity. *J Urol* 155:1655–1657, 1996
75. Guess HA, Gormley GJ, Stoner E, et al: The effect of finasteride on prostate specific antigen: review of available data. *J Urol* 155:3–9, 1996
76. Punglia RS, D'Amico AV, Catalona WJ, et al: Effect of verification bias on screening for prostate cancer by measurement of prostate-specific antigen. *N Engl J Med* 349:335–342, 2003
77. Presti JC: Neoplasms of the prostate gland, in Tanagho EA, McAninch JW (eds.): *Smith's General Urology* (ed 15). New York, Lange Medical Books/McGraw-Hill, 2000, pp 399–421
78. Coley CM, Barry MJ, Mulley AG: Screening for prostate cancer. *Ann Intern Med* 126:480–484, 1997
79. Isola J, Auvinen A, Poutiainen M, et al: Predictors of biological aggressiveness of prostate specific antigen screening detected prostate cancer. *J Urol* 165:1569–1574, 2001
80. Labrie F: Screening and hormonal therapy of localized prostate cancer shows major benefits on survival. *Cancer J* 6(suppl 2):S182–S187, 2000
81. Brooks JD: Anatomy of the lower urinary tract and male genitalia, in Retik AB, Vaughan ED, Wein AJ, et al (eds.): *Campbells' Urology* (ed 8). Philadelphia, Saunders, 2002, pp 41–80
82. Bostwick DG, Junqu J, Schlesinger C: Contemporary pathology of prostate cancer. *Urol Clin North Am* 30:181–207, 2003
83. Skar WA, Haas GP, Cassin BF, et al: The frequency of carcinoma and intraepithelial neoplasia of the prostate in young male patients. *J Urol* 150:379–385, 1993
84. Sakr WA, Partin AW: Histological markers of risk and the role of high-grade prostatic intraepithelial neoplasia. *Urology* 57(suppl 4A):115–120, 2001
85. Gleason DF: Histologic grading of prostate cancer: a perspective. *Hum Pathol* 23:273–279, 1992
86. McNeal JE, Villers AA, Redwine EA, et al: Histologic differentiation, cancer volume, and pelvic lymph node metastasis in adenocarcinoma of the prostate. *Cancer* 66:1225–1233, 1990
87. Bluestein DL, Bostwick DG, Bergstralh EJ, et al: Eliminating the need for bilateral pelvic lymphadenectomy in selected patients with prostate cancer. *J Urol* 151:1315–1320, 1994
88. Scardino PT, Weaver R, Hudson MA: Early detection of prostate cancer. *Hum Pathol* 23:211–223, 1992
89. Kim ED, Grayhack JT: Clinical symptoms and signs of prostate cancer, in Vogelzang NJ, Scardino PT, Shipley WU, et al (eds.): *Comprehensive Textbook of Genitourinary Oncology* (ed 2). Philadelphia, Lippincott, Williams and Wilkins, 2000, pp 525–532
90. Carroll PR, Lee KL, Fuks ZY, et al: Cancer of the prostate, in DeVita VT, Hellman S, Rosenberg SA (eds.): *Cancer: Principles and Practice of Oncology* (ed 6). Philadelphia, Lippincott, Williams and Wilkins, 2001, pp 1418–1479
91. Degler MA: Assessment of renal and urinary tract function, in Smeltzer SC, Bare BG (eds.): *Brunner and Suddarth's Textbook of*

Medical-Surgical Nursing (ed 10). Philadelphia, Lippincott, Williams & Wilkins, 2004, pp 1250–1270

92. McAninch JW: Symptoms of disorders of the genitourinary tract, in Tanagho EA, McAninch JW (eds.): *Smith's General Urology* (ed 15). New York, Lange Medical Books/McGraw Hill, 2000, pp 31–40
93. Bates P: Nursing assessment urinary system, in Lewis SM, Heitkemper MM, Dirksen SR: *Medical-Surgical Nursing: Assessment and Management of Clinical Problems* (ed 5). St. Louis, Mosby, 2000, pp 1241–1260
94. Wilkes GM: Spinal cord compression, in Yarbro CH, Frogge MH, Goodman M (eds.): *Cancer Symptom Management* (ed 3). Sudbury, MA, Jones and Bartlett, 2004, pp 359–371
95. Partin AW, Mangold LA, Lamm DM, et al: Contemporary update of prostate cancer staging nomograms (Partin tables) for the new millennium. *Urology* 58:843–848, 2001
96. Roach M, Small E, Reese DM, et al: Urologic and male genital cancers, in Rubin P, Williams JP (eds.): *Clinical Oncology: A Multidisciplinary Approach for Physicians and Students* (ed 8). Philadelphia, W. B. Saunders, 2001, pp 523–564
97. Hanson KA: Diagnostic tests and tools in the evaluation of urologic disease: part II. *Urol Nurs* 23:405–414, 2003
98. Naya Y, Babaian RJ: The predictors of pelvic lymph node metastasis at radical retropubic prostatectomy. *J Urol* 170:2306–2310, 2003
99. Kirby RS, Christmas TJ, Brawer MK: *Prostate Cancer* (ed 2). London, Mosby, 2001
100. Tester W, Brouch MD: Treatment decision making, in Held-Warmkessel J (ed.): *Contemporary Issues in Prostate Cancer: A Nursing Perspective.* Sudbury, MA, Jones and Bartlett, 2000, pp 81–101
101. Scardino PT: Prostate cancer version 1.2002. National Comprehensive Cancer Network, Jenkintown, PA, 2002
102. Garnick MB: The dilemmas of prostate cancer. *Sci Am* 270:72–81, 1994
103. Holmberg L, Bill-Axelson A, Helgesen F, et al: A randomized trial comparing radical prostatectomy with watchful waiting in early prostate cancer. *N Engl J Med* 347:781–789, 2002
104. Fleming C, Wasson JH, Albertsen PC, et al: A decision analysis of alternative treatment strategies for clinically localized prostate cancer. *JAMA* 269:2650–2658, 1993
105. Albertsen PC, Fryback DG, Storer BE, et al: Long-term survival among men with conservatively treated localized cancer. *JAMA* 274:626–631, 1995
106. Chodak GW, Thisted RA, Gerber GS, et al: Results of conservative management of clinically localized prostate cancer. *N Engl J Med* 330:242–248, 1994
107. Carter HB, Walsh PC, Landis P, et al: Expectant management of nonpalpable prostate cancer with curative intent: preliminary results. *J Urol* 167:1231–1234, 2002
108. Steineck G, Helgesen F, Adolfsson J, et al: Quality of life after radical prostatectomy or watchful waiting. *N Engl J Med* 347:790–796, 2002
109. Alibhai SMH, Naglie G, Nam R, et al: Do older men benefit from curative therapy of localized prostate cancer? *J Clin Oncol* 21:3318–3327, 2003
110. Wilt TJ, Brawer MK: The Prostate Cancer Intervention Versus Observation Trial (PIVOT). *Oncology* 11:1133–1139, 1997
111. Schroder FH, de Vries SH, Bangma CH: Watchful waiting in prostate cancer: review and policy proposals. *BJU Int* 92:851–859, 2003
112. Wallace M: Uncertainty and quality of life of older men who undergo watchful waiting for prostate cancer. *Oncol Nurs Forum* 30:303–309, 2003
113. Mebust WK, Holtgrewe HL, Cockett ATK, et al: Transurethral prostatectomy: immediate and postoperative complications. A cooperative study of 13 participating institutions evaluating 3,885 patients. *J Urol* 141:243–247, 1989
114. Chambers A: Transurethral resection syndrome — it does not have to be a mystery. *AORN J* 75:156–170, 2002
115. Meredith C: Male genitourinary problems, in Lewis SM, Heitkemper MM, Dirksen SR (eds.): *Medical-Surgical Nursing: Assessment and Management of Clinical Problems* (ed 5). St. Louis, Mosby, 2000, pp 1553–1578
116. Volpe HM: Radiation therapy, in Held-Warmkessel J (ed.): *Contemporary Issues in Prostate Cancer: A Nursing Perspective.* Sudbury, MA, Jones and Bartlett, 2000, pp 137–169
117. Stanford JL, Feng Z, Hamilton AS, et al: Urinary and sexual function after radical prostatectomy for clinically localized prostate cancer: the Prostate Cancer Outcomes Study. *JAMA* 283:354–360, 2000
118. Waxman ES: Sexual dysfunction following treatment for prostate cancer: nursing assessment and intervention. *Oncol Nurs Forum* 20:1567–1571, 1993
119. Walsh PC: Anatomic radical prostatectomy: evolution of the surgical technique. *J Urol* 160:2418–2424, 1998
120. Quinlan DM, Epstein JI, Carter BS, et al: Sexual function following radical prostatectomy: influence of preservation of neurovascular bundles. *J Urol* 145:998–1002, 1991
121. Robinson JW, Dufour MS, Fung TS: Erectile functioning of men treated for prostate carcinoma. *Cancer* 79:538–544, 1997
122. Litwin MS, Hays RD, Fink A, et al: Quality of life in men treated for localized prostate cancer. *JAMA* 273:129–135, 1995
123. Maxwell M: Cancer of the prostate. *Semin Oncol Nurs* 9:237–251, 1993
124. Klimaszewski AD, Karlowicz KA: Cancer of the male genitalia, in Karlowicz KA (ed.): *Urologic Nursing: Principles and Practice.* Philadelphia, Saunders, 1995, pp 271–308
125. Urinary Incontinence Guideline Panel: *Urinary Incontinence in Adults: Clinical Practice Guidelines.* AHCPR Publication No. 92–0038. Rockville, MD, Agency for Health Care Policy and Research, 1992
126. Walsh PC: Anatomic radical retropubic prostatectomy, in Walsh PC, Retik AB, Vaughan ED, Wein AJ (eds.): *Campbell's Urology* (ed 8). Philadelphia, Saunders, 2002, pp 3107–3129
127. Steiner MS, Morton RA, Walsh PC: Impact of anatomic radical prostatectomy on urinary continence. *J Urol* 145:512–515, 1991.
128. Walsh PC, Quinlan DM, Morton RA, et al: Radical retropubic prostatectomy: improved anastomosis and urinary continence. *Urol Clin North Am* 17:679–684, 1990
129. Marks JL, Light JK: Management of urinary incontinence after prostatectomy with the artificial urinary sphincter. *J Urol* 142:302–304, 1989
130. Foote J, Yun S, Leach GE: Postprostatectomy incontinence: pathophysiology, evaluation and management. *Urol Clin North Am* 18:229–241, 1991
131. Thayer D: How to assess and control urinary incontinence. *Am J Nurs* 94:42–47, 1994
132. Fiers S, Thayer D: Management of intractable incontinence, in Doughty DB: *Urinary and Fecal Incontinence: Nursing Management* (ed 2). St Louis, Mosby, 2000, pp 183–207
133. Freedman A, Hahn G, Love N: Follow-up after therapy for prostate cancer. *Postgrad Med* 100:125–136, 1996
134. Appell RA: Clinical efficacy and safety of tolterodine in the treatment of overactive bladder: a pooled analysis. *Urology* 50(suppl):90–96, 1997
135. Abrams P, Freeman R, Anderstrom C, et al: Tolterodine, a new antimuscarinic agent: as effective but better tolerated than oxybutynin in patients with an overactive bladder. *Br J Urol* 81:801–810, 1998
136. Schrover LR: *Sexuality and Cancer: For the Man Who Has Cancer, and His Partner.* Atlanta, American Cancer Society, 2001

137. Lewis JH, Rosen R, Goldstein I, et al: Erectile dysfunction. *Am J Nurs* 103:48–57, 2003
138. Gontero P, Fontana F, Bagnasacco A, et al: Is there an optimal time for intracavernous prostaglandin E1 rehabilitation following nonnerve sparing radical prostatectomy? Results from a hemodynamic prospective study. *J Urol* 169:2166–2169, 2003
139. Raina R, Lankin MM, Agarwal A, et al: Long-term effect of sildenafil citrate on erectile dysfunction after radical prostatectomy. *Urology* 62:110–115, 2003
140. Albaugh J, Amargo I, Capelson R, et al: Healthcare clinicians in sexual health medicine: focus on erectile dysfunction. *Urol Nurs* 22:217–231, 2002
141. Pound CR, Partin AW, Eisenberg MA, et al: Natural history of progression after PSA elevation following radical prostatectomy. *JAMA* 281:1591–1597, 1999
142. Messing EM, Manola J, Sarosdy M, et al: Immediate hormonal therapy compared with observation after radical prostatectomy and pelvic lymphadenectomy in men with node-positive prostate cancer. *N Engl J Med* 341:1781–1788, 1999
143. Catalona WJ, Ramos CG, Carvalhal GF: Contemporary results on anatomic radical prostatectomy. *CA Cancer J Clin* 49:282–296, 1999
144. Han K-R, Belldegrun AS: Third-generation cryosurgery for primary and recurrent prostate cancer. *BJU Int* 93:14–18, 2004
145. Shinohara K, Carroll PR: Cryoablation of prostate cancer, in McConnell JD, Scardino P (eds.): *Atlas of Clinical Urology*. Philadelphia, Current Medicine, 1999, pp 14.1–14.13
146. Brenner ZR, Krenzer ME: Update on cryosurgical ablation for prostate cancer. *Am J Nurs* 95:44–48, 1995
147. Donnelly BJ, Saliken JC, Ernst DS, et al: Prospective trial of cryosurgical ablation of the prostate: five-year results. *Urology* 60:645–649, 2002
148. Leininger SM: Managing patients with cryosurgical ablation of the prostate and liver. *Medsurg Nurs* 6:359–386, 1997
149. Guillonneau B, Vallancien G: Laparoscopic radical prostatectomy: the Montsouris technique. *J Urol* 163:1643–1649, 2000
150. Bickert D, Frickel D: Laparoscopic radical prostatectomy. *AORN J* 75:762–782, 2002
151. Guillonneau B, Vallancien G: Laparoscopic radical prostatectomy: the Montsouris experience. *J Urol* 163:418–422, 2000
152. Abbou CC, Salomon L, Hoznek A, et al: Laparoscopic radical prostatectomy: preliminary results. *Urology* 55:630–634, 2000
153. Dahl DM, L'Esperance JO, Trainer AF, et al: Laparoscopic radical prostatectomy: initial 70 cases at a U. S. university medical center. *Urology* 60:859–863, 2002
154. Rassweiler J, Seemann O, Schulze M, et al: Laparoscopic versus open radical prostatectomy: a comparative study at a single institution. *J Urol* 169:1689–1693, 2003
155. Klein EA, Kupelina PA: Localized prostate cancer: radiation or surgery? *Urol Clin North Am* 30:315–330, 2003
156. Pollack A, Horwitz EM, Movsas B, et al: Mindless or mindful? Radiation oncologists' perspectives on the evolution of prostate cancer treatment. *Urol Clin North Am* 30:337–349, 2003
157. Crook JM, Bahadur YA, Bociek RG, et al: Radiotherapy for localized prostate cancer: the correlation of pretreatment prostate specific antigen and nadir prostate specific antigen with outcome as assessed by systematic biopsy and serum prostate specific antigen. *Cancer* 79:328–336, 1997
158. Horwitz EM, Hanks GE: External beam radiation therapy for prostate cancer. *CA Cancer J Clin* 50:349–375, 2000
159. Bolla M, Gonzalez D, Warde P, et al: Improved survival in patients with locally advanced prostate cancer treated with radiotherapy and goserelin. *N Engl J Med* 337:295–300, 1997
160. Goldstein I, Feldman MI, Deckers PJ, et al: Radation-associated impotence: a clinical study of its mechanism. *JAMA* 251:903–910, 1984
161. Siegel T, Moul JW, Spevak M, et al: The development of erectile dysfunction in men treated for prostate cancer. *J Urol* 165:430–435, 2002
162. Johannes CB, Araujo AB, Feldman HA, et al: Incidence of erectile dysfunction in men 40 to 69 years old: longitudinal results from the Massachusetts Male Aging Study. *J Urol* 163:460–463, 2000
163. Zelefsky MJ, Fuks Z, Hunt M, et al: High dose radiation delivered by intensity modulated conformal radiotherapy improves the outcome of localized prostate cancer. *J Urol* 166:876–881, 2001
164. Abel LJ, Blatt HJ, Stipetich RL, et al: Nursing management of patients receiving brachytherapy for early stage prostate cancer. *Clin J Oncol Nurs* 3:7–15, 1999
165. Cash JC, Dattoli MJ: Management of patients receiving transperineal palladium-103 prostate implants. *Oncol Nurs Forum* 24:1361–1367, 1997
166. Nag S, Beyer D, Friedland J, et al: American Brachytherapy Society (ABS) recommendations for transperineal permanent brachytherapy of prostate cancer. *Int J Radiation Biol Phys* 44:789–799, 1999
167. Beyer C: Salvage brachytherapy after external-beam irradiation for prostate cancer. *Oncology* 18:151–158, 2004
168. Isaacs JT, Lundmo PI, Berges R, et al: Androgen regulation of programmed cell death of normal and malignant prostatic cells. *J Androl* 13:457, 1992
169. Martikainen P, Kyprianou N, Tucker RW, et al: Programmed death of nonproliferating androgen-independent prostatic cancer cells. *Cancer Res* 51:4693–4700, 1991
170. Geller J, Albert JD, Nochstein DA, et al: Comparison of prostate cancer tissue dihydrotestosterone levels at the time of relapse following orchiectomy or estrogen therapy. *J Urol* 132:693–696, 1984
171. Hellestedt BA, Pienta KJ: The current state of hormonal therapy for prostate cancer. *CA Cancer J Clin* 52:154–179, 2002
172. Schroder FH: Endocrine treatment of prostate cancer, in Walsh PC, Retik AB, Vaughan ED, Wein AJ (eds.): *Campbell's Urology* (ed 7). Philadelphia, Saunders, 1998, pp 2627–2644
173. Prostate Cancer Trialists' Collaborative Group: Maximal androgen blockade in advanced prostate cancer: an overview of Randomised Trials. *Lancet* 355:1491–1498, 2000
174. Koch M, Steidle C, Brosman S, et al: An open-label study of abarelix in men with symptomatic prostate cancer at high risk of treatment with LHRH agonists. *Urology* 62:877–882, 2003
175. Stempkowski L: Hormonal therapy, in Held-Warmkessel J (ed.): *Contemporary Issues in Prostate Cancer: A Nursing Perspective*. Sudbury, MA, Jones and Bartlett, 2000, pp 170–194
176. Berruti A, Dogliotti L, Tucci M, et al: Metabolic bone disease induced by prostate cancer: rationale for use of bisphosphonates. *J Urol* 166:2023–2031, 2001
177. Townsend MF, Sanders WH, Northway RO, et al: Bone fractures associated with luteinizing hormone-releasing hormone agonists used in the treatment of prostate carcinoma. *Cancer* 79:545–550, 1997
178. Oefelein MG, Ricchuiti V, Conrad W, et al: Skeletal fracture associated with androgen suppression induced osteoporosis: the clinical incidence and risk factors for patients with prostate cancer. *J Urol* 166:1724–1728, 2001
179. Smith MR: Bisphosphonates to prevent skeletal complications in men with metastatic prostate cancer. *J Urol* 170:S55–S58, 2003
180. Smith DC: Secondary hormonal therapy. *Semin Urol Oncol* 15:3–12, 1997
181. Scher HI, Kelly WMK: Flutamide withdrawal syndrome: its impact on clinical trials in hormone-refractory prostate cancer. *J Clin Oncol* 11:1566–1572, 1993

182. Harris KA, Weinberg V, Bok RA, et al: Low dose ketoconazole with replacement doses of hydrocortisone in patients with progressive androgen independent prostate cancer. *J Urol* 168:542–545, 2002
183. Kelly WMK, Scher HI: Prostate specific antigen decline after antiandrogen withdrawal: the flutamide withdrawal syndrome. *J Urol* 149:607–609, 1993
184. Kelly WMK, Slovin S, Scher HI: Clinical use of posttherapy prostate-specific antigen changes in advanced prostate cancer. *Semin Oncol* 23(suppl):8–14, 1996
185. Thalmann GN, Sikes RA, Chang S–M, et al: Suramin-induced decrease in prostate specific antigen expression with no effect on tumor growth in the LNCaP model of human prostate cancer. *J Natl Cancer Inst* 88:794–801, 1996
186. Dreicer R: Metastatic prostate cancer: assessment of response to systemic therapy. *Semin Urol Oncol* 15:28–32, 1997
187. Newling D, Fossa SD, Andersson L, et al: Assessment of hormone refractory prostate cancer. *Urology* 49(suppl):46–53, 1997
188. Moore MJ, Osoba D, Murphy K, et al: Use of palliative end points to evaluate the effects of mitoxantrone and low-dose prednisone in patients with hormonally resistant prostate cancer. *J Clin Oncol* 12:689–694, 1994
189. Tannock IF, Osoba D, Stockler MR, et al: Chemotherapy with mitoxantrone plus prednisone or prednisone alone for symptomatic hormone-resistant prostate cancer: a Canadian randomized trial with palliative endpoints. *J Clin Oncol* 14:1756–1764, 1996
190. Tew KD, Stearns ME: Hormone-independent, non-alkylating mechanism of cytotoxicity for estramustine. *Urol Res* 15:155–160, 1987
191. Iversen P, Rasmussen F, Asmussen C, et al: Estramustine phosphate versus placebo as second line treatment after orchiectomy in patients with metastatic prostate cancer: DAPROCA study 9002. *J Urol* 157:929–934, 1997
192. Trivedi C, Redman B, Flaherty LE, et al: Weekly 1-hour infusion of paclitaxel. *Cancer* 89:431–436, 2000
193. Speicher LA, Barone L, Tew KD: Combined antimicrotubule activity of estramustine and taxol in human prostatic carcinoma cell lines. *Cancer Res* 52:4433–4440, 1992
194. Picus J, Schultz M: Docetaxel (Taxotere) as monotherapy in the treatment of hormone-refractory prostate cancer: preliminary results. *Semin Oncol* 26:14–18, 1999
195. Obasaju C, Hudes GR: Paclitaxel and docetaxel in prostate cancer. *Hematol/Oncol Clin North Am* 15:525–544, 2001
196. Hussain M, Petrylak D, Fisher E, et al: Docetaxel (Taxotere) and estramustine versus mitoxantrone and prednisone for hormone-refractory prostate cancer: scientific basis and design of Southwest Oncology Group Study 9916. *Semin Oncol* 17:55–60, 1999
197. Petrylak DP, Tangen CM, Hussain MHA, et al: Docetaxel and estramustine compared with mitoxantrone and prednisone for advanced refractory prostate cancer. *N Engl J Med* 351: 1513–1520, 2004
198. Tannock IF, de Wit R, Berry WR, et al: Docetaxel plus prednisone or mitoxantrone plus prednisone for advanced prostate cancer. *N Engl J Med* 351:1502–1512, 2004
199. Merterns WC, Filipczak LA, Ben-Josef E, et al: Systemic bone-seeking radionuclides for palliation of painful osseous metastases: current concepts. *CA Cancer J Clin* 48:361–374, 1998
200. Clarke NW: The management of hormone-relapsed prostate cancer. *BJU Int* 92:860–868, 2003
201. Saad F, Gleason DM, Murray R, et al: A randomized, placebo-controlled trial of zoledronic acid in patients with hormone-refractory metastatic prostate carcinoma. *J Natl Cancer Inst* 94:1458–1468, 2002
202. Chen TC: Prostate cancer and spinal cord compression. *Oncology* 15:841–854, 2001
203. Huddart RA, Rajan B, Law M, et al: Spinal cord compression in prostate cancer: treatment outcome and prognostic factors. *Radiother Oncol* 44:229–236, 1997
204. Cheville AL, McGarvey CL, Petrek JA, et al: Lymphedema management. *Semin Radiat Oncol* 13:290–301, 2003
205. Shuey K: Platelet-associated bleeding disorders. *Semin Oncol Nurs* 12:15–27, 1996

CHAPTER 63

Skin Cancer

Suzanne M. Mahon, RN, DNSc, AOCN®, APNG
Susan G. Yackzan, RN, MSN, AOCN®

Introduction

The skin is a large and very visible organ that serves both protective and aesthetic functions. Historically, these visible characteristics have served as indicators of social status and class. Until the second decade of the twentieth century, smooth, pale skin was valued as an indication of belonging to the more wealthy, leisure class. Those who worked as laborers and field hands had darker skin, tanned from exposure to the sun. During this century, outdoor leisure activities have become associated with a higher social status. This change in perception has led more people to seek tanned, bronze-colored skin. This change may also be one of the biggest factors contributing to the rise in the incidence of skin cancer.

The term *skin cancer* is used to describe several types of malignancies that occur in the skin. Basal cell carcinoma (BCC) and squamous cell carcinoma (SCC) are often combined and described as nonmelanoma skin cancer (NMSC). Malignant melanoma (MM) is usually addressed separately because of the differences in this malignancy when compared to NMSC in terms of treatment and prognosis. Most MMs are cutaneous; however, unusual presentations in the eye and viscera may occur. This chapter will focus on the cutaneous skin cancers.

Oncology nurses can have a significant impact on the morbidity and mortality associated with NMSC and MM. As educators, they can influence the public to practice primary and secondary prevention strategies. As clinicians, they can perform risk assessments and screening examinations to promote early detection of malignancies, ensure appropriate management of biopsies, administer therapies safely, manage symptoms, and provide appropriate psychosocial care. As researchers, they can improve strategies for education, management of symptoms, and knowledge acquisition through clinical trials.

Epidemiology

The incidence of skin cancer continues to grow both in the United States and throughout the world. Skin cancers account for approximately one-third of all diagnosed cancers. In the United States alone, the American Cancer Society (ACS) estimates that approximately 1 million cases of the highly curable BCCs and SCCs are detected annually.[1] Of the NMSCs, cases of BCC predominate over SCC by about five to one in males and ten to one in females.[2] Accurate figures on the incidence of these NMSCs are difficult to obtain, as many countries do not register these malignancies. In addition, these lesions are often removed in primary care practices and are treated without laboratory verification of the clinical diagnosis.[2,3] It is clear, however, that the incidence of these cancers has increased over the last few decades and that the increased incidence of NMSC is related to cumulative sun-exposure behaviors.

The annual incidence of the more serious form of skin cancer, MM, was estimated at 59,580 new cases in 2005 according to the ACS.[1] The annual incidence of MM has risen steadily from one in 1500 persons in 1930 to one in 75 persons in 2000, as shown in Figure 63-1.[4,5] For men, the lifetime risk of developing melanoma is one in 55; for women, the risk is one in 82.[1] From a public health perspective, it is vital to improve public awareness of MM. Better means are needed to identify high-risk persons and to detect MM early; more specific therapies are also needed. The incidence of MM continues to rise with age, as a consequence, lifetime prevention and early detection strategies are critical to decrease the morbidity and mortality associated with MM (Figure 63-2).[5]

Clearly, the dramatic rise in MM is real and not due to artifact. MM incidence is increasing worldwide at a faster rate than the incidence of any other cancer.[6] This trend is associated with increased morbidity, mortality, and rising healthcare costs. In Australia, direct healthcare costs for skin cancer are about $16 per person per year and exceed the expenditures for any other cancer.[6] In that country, the lifetime risk for developing MM is one in 25 for men and one in 34 for women. This increase is not due to better surveillance techniques. Rather, is hypothesized that the increase in MM incidence is related to the fact that people are going outdoors more often than in the past and are exposing themselves not only to sunlight but also increasingly to artificial ultraviolet radiation (UVR).[6,7] Incidence rates are approximately 20 times higher among whites as compared to blacks.

The mortality rate from the highly curable BCCs and SCCs is approximately 2000 persons per year according to ACS estimates.[1] These deaths are largely preventable, as most NMSCs are visible for long periods of time prior to metastasis. An estimated 7770 persons die annually from MM.[1] Although multiple factors influence survival, thickness of the tumor has been shown to be the most important factor across multiple studies.[3] The decreasing mean thickness of MMs at the time of diagnosis has resulted in an overall increased survival for localized MM, from about 50% in the 1950s to almost 90% in 2000. Note, however, that the absolute number of thicker MMs has also increased. The mortality rate from MM continues to increase, albeit not at the same rate as the emergence of new cases[1,5] (see Figures 63-1 and 63-2).

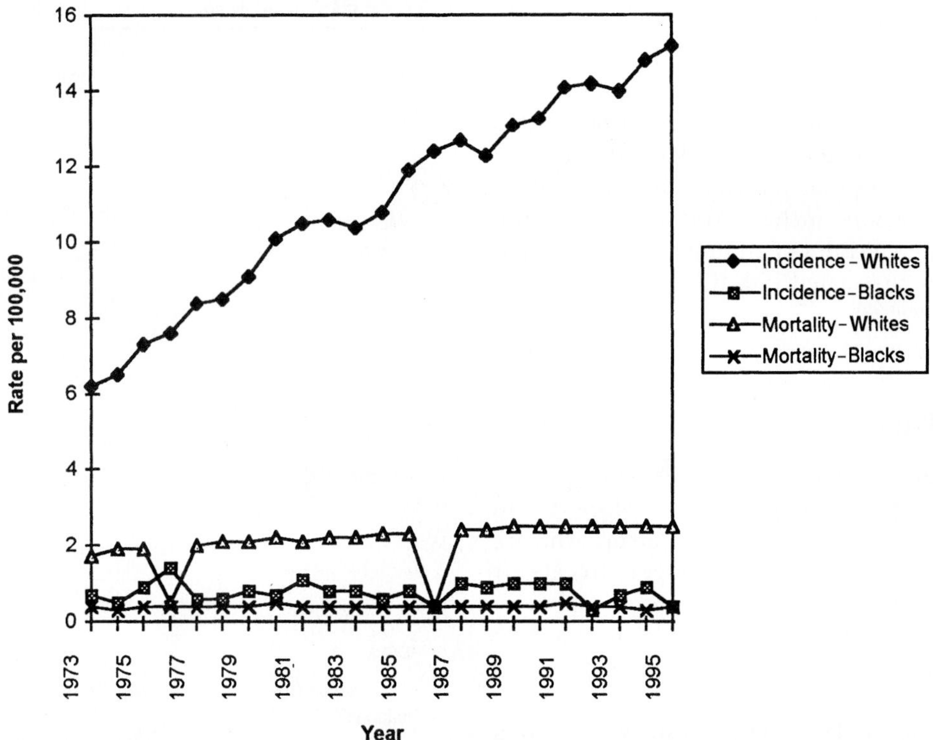

Figure 63-1 Incidence and mortality rates for malignant melanoma, United States, 1973–1995. (Ries LAG, Kosary CL, Hankey BF, et al: *SEER Cancer Statistics Review, 1973–1995*. Bethesda, MD, National Cancer Institute, 1998.[4])

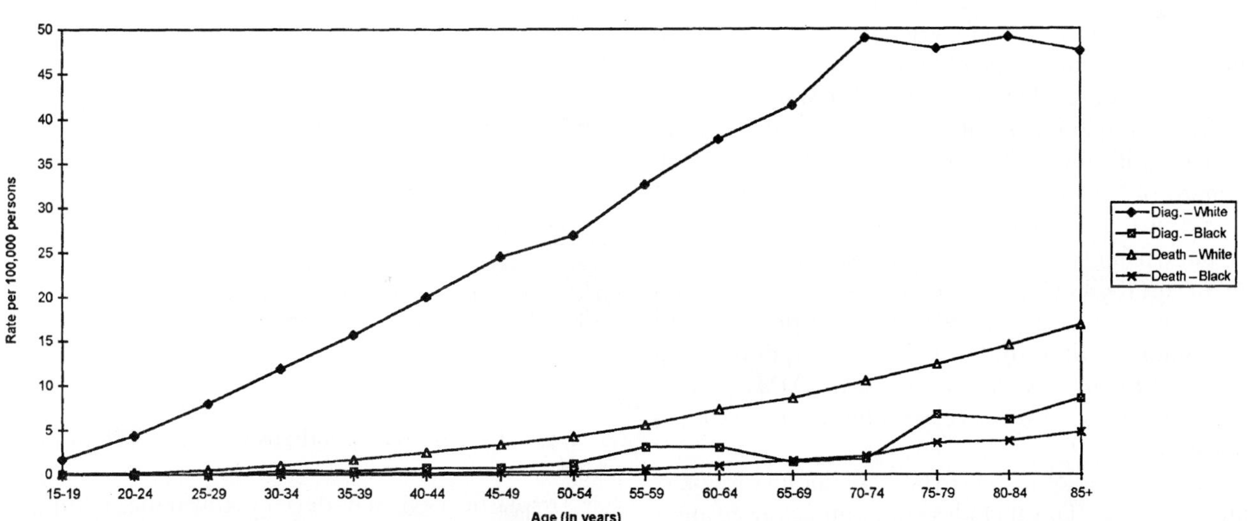

Figure 63-2 Age-specific rates – incidence and mortality for malignant melanoma, United States, 1973–1995. (Ries LAG, Kosary CL, Hankey BF, et al: *SEER Cancer Statistics Review, 1973–1995*. Bethesda, MD, National Cancer Institute, 1998.)[4]

Etiology

The etiology of skin cancer is multifactorial in nature. The likelihood that an individual might develop skin cancer during his or her lifetime depends on both constitutional factors and environmental exposures. Constitutional factors include the genotypic and phenotypic characteristics of an individual.[3] Different skin cancers are associated with different risk factors (Table 63-1).[3,5,8–10]

Genotypic Factors

Skin color is one of the most important genotypic features that places a person at risk for developing skin cancer. MM is very rare in blacks.[8,11,12] Persons who are light or fair complected, have a tendency to freckle, or burn easily are at higher risk. The development of melanocytic nevi in childhood is strongly related to characteristics of pigmentation associated with poor sun tolerance.[13]

The epidermis of blacks has been shown to have a natural sun protection factor (SPF) of 13.4, with the melanin in the epidermis filtering twice as much ultraviolet B (UVB) as the epidermis of a white person.[11] This protection, however, is not complete, and both NMSC and MM can develop in black persons. SCC is the most frequently seen skin cancer in blacks. BCCs in blacks are almost always pigmented. Furthermore, as many as 67% of MMs in the black population arise in non-sun-exposed skin such as on the palmer and plantar surfaces and even the mucous membranes. Blacks have proportionately greater percentages of the acral lentiginous type of MM and also tend to have poorer prognoses than do whites with MM.

Large congenital melanocytic nevi are also considered a significant risk factor associated with the development of MM and are estimated to occur in 1% of newborns.[14,15] This increase in risk has been reported to range from 0% to 42%. In most studies, the larger the nevus, the higher the lifetime risk.[15,16] Surgical removal of these large nevi is thought to decrease but not eliminate these individuals' risk for developing MM because approximately 50% of the MMs arise in extracutaneous sites. Therefore lifetime screening is important.

The number of melanocytic nevi (moles) is correlated with risk. This includes common acquired nevi, atypical nevi, and dysplastic nevi.[3,14,15] On the basis of nevus numbers and especially dysplastic nevi, clinicians can identify individuals at high risk for developing MM and implement aggressive screening and intervention programs. Higher nevus counts are associated with an increased risk of MM, with at least a tenfold greater risk for individuals who have 100 or more moles.

Table 63-1 Risk Factors for Skin Cancer

Risk Factor	Risk Factor for NMSC	Risk Factor for MM
Actinic keratoses*	+	+
Arsenic ingestion (well water, insecticides, medical)	+	
Chronic exposure to tar, soot, shale, or petroleum	+	
Cigarette or pipe smoking	+	
Congenital nevus		+
Family history of melanoma*		+
Geographic area where childhood was spent	+	+
History of NMSC in a first-degree relative	+	
History of three or more blistering sunburns before the age of 20 years*	+	+
Immunosuppression	+	+
Increasing age	+	+
Ionizing radiation (therapeutic or occupational)	+	
Large number of dysplastic nevi		+
Large number of melanocytic nevi		+
Male gender	+	+
Personal history of BCC	+	+
Personal history of MM	+	+
Personal history of SCC	+	+
Red or blond hair*	+	+
Scar related to heat burn, chemical burn	+	
Skin color	+	+
Tendency to freckle especially on the upper back area*	+	+
Three or more years of outdoor summer jobs during teenage years*	+	+
Xeroderma pigmentosum		+

*The presence of any one or two of these factors increases a person's risk for the development of MM threefold to fourfold and three or more of these factors increases the risk almost 20-fold.[5]

Data from Rigel[3,5]; Marks[8]; Hill, Ferrini.[9]

Dysplastic nevi may develop throughout life and show clinical features similar to normal moles and MMs (see Color Plates 9 and 10). These features include a size greater than 6–8 mm, irregular borders, variable pigmentation, and irregular surface characteristics. The identification of truly dysplastic nevi is more difficult to perform clinically than many epidemiologists realize, however, and in most cases requires a pathologic diagnosis.[14] Dysplastic nevi occur in approximately 10% of the general population, but the risk of progression to MM is not clear in this group.[13] The clinical importance of dysplastic nevi lies in their assocation with the risk of melanoma. The age-adjusted incidence of melanoma is approximately 15 times higher among persons with dysplastic nevi as compared to members of the general population.

Another important genotypic feature is family history. Approximately 10% of patients with MM describe a history of an affected family member.[17,18] People who have a family history of MM and/or dysplastic nevi, or who have a large number of nevi themselves, are at a very high risk (100-fold increase) of developing MM over their lifetime.[13] A hereditary predisposition to MM is sometimes associated with an earlier age of onset.[18] Sex distribution between males and females is usually about equal to those with a hereditary predisposition to MM.[19] In general, individuals with a hereditary predisposition to MM have malignancies that are clinically and histopathologically similar to those without such a family history.[20] Patients from these families are, however, often diagnosed with thinner lesions and generally have a better prognosis. This better outcome may be related to heightened awareness and increased surveillance. A second primary MM does develop in 17%–20% of patients from these families who survive their first MM.[21]

As the Human Genome Project continues, it is likely that a number of skin cancer susceptibility loci will be identified, for which genetic testing will ultimately become available. To date, a susceptibility gene has been clearly linked to chromosome 9p (a tumor suppressor gene), chromosome 1p, and CDKN2A.[17,22–25] Germ-line mutations in CDKN2A (on chromosome 9p21) have been found in 20%–40% of families in which at least three first-degree relatives are affected by melanoma. Research by family linkage studies identified an autosomal dominant melanoma gene located on chromosome 9p21.40. The tumor suppressor gene *p16* is involved in the regulation of cell growth. It regulates cell proliferation by inhibiting the CDK4 cell cycle protein kinase; thus, mutations in *p16* that disrupt function lead to unregulated cell growth.[19] An understanding of the genetics of MM is just beginning. It is speculated that a genetic predisposition to MM may be present on a number of genes. Because penetrance may be variable, the gene may not be expressed consistently.[20] It is also thought that the gene is transmitted in an autosomal dominant fashion, but the impact of environmental factors on the subsequent development of MM is not fully understood.[18] Therefore, even though the location of one or more susceptibility genes is now known, the usefulness of genetic testing is not completely clear. Genetic testing is commercially available for some CDKN2A mutations on both commercial and research bases. As genetic testing becomes available and the ramifications of testing are better understood, a number of education and counseling issues will emerge.

Several inherited syndromes are associated with BCC and SCC, including zeroderma pigmentosum, nevoid BCC syndrome, epidermodysplasia verruciformis, and albinism. Most of these syndromes are associated with other physical abnormalities.[26]

A personal history of BCC or SCC is associated with a much higher risk of MM.[2] The increase in relative risk has been reported to be anywhere from 2.8 to 17.0.[26] A personal history of a NMSC is associated with a much higher risk of developing a second NMSC, especially in persons with a history of significant sun exposure.

The importance of the immune system in controlling skin cancers, particularly MM, is not completely understood.[7] Persons with chronic immunosuppression are at higher risk for developing MM. Renal transplant recipients may have a fourfold increased risk for developing MM.[27] The risk may be as much as eight times higher in persons who have been successfully treated for cancers such as lymphoma.

Age itself is a risk factor for both NMSCs and MMs (see Figure 63–2).[2,6] It is difficult to separate the interaction of age from cumulative exposure to sunlight.

Environmental Factors

Frequent and prolonged exposure to UVR over a period of years will induce cellular changes in human skin. Ultraviolet radiation can act as an initiator, a promoter, a cocarcinogen, and an immunosuppressive agent.[7,28] Episodic high exposure resulting in sunburn, especially when it occurs in childhood, may be critical.[3,6,16,28]

Two adverse consequences are associated with UVR exposure. First, it leads to direct tissue and cellular damage. Second, exposure to UVR results in local and systemic immunosuppression.[3,7] The effects of UVR are both acute and chronic.[29] Acute changes include sunburn and discomfort. Chronic effects include photoaging, premalignant and malignant growths, and immunosuppression.[2,16,30] Immunosuppression is a significant risk factor for the development of both NMSC and melanoma.[2]

Solar keratoses, which are a direct result of chronic sun exposure, are major risk factors for both NMSC and MM. Data suggest that NMSCs are associated with cumulative sun exposure, whereas MM is associated with short, intense episodes of sun exposure, especially those involving sunburns.[9] Exposure to sunlight is the only environmental factor consistently linked to MM in most studies.[3] The exact link between sunlight exposure and risk of MM is not completely clear, but is probably a causal relationship that includes a complex relationship between dose-response, latent period, body site, genetics, and other unknown factors.[13,28]

Some occupations may be associated with a higher risk of developing MM. Persons who earn a higher salary and are employed in typical white-collar occupations may be at higher risk for developing MM than those who have more chronic occupational outdoor exposure to UVR.[2,3] These risks may be related to the fact that persons from this socioeconomic group have the financial means to travel to sunny climates on vacation, where they intermittently expose themselves to intense UVR resulting in sunburn, especially those associated with pain and blistering. This is probably related to the combination of reflected UVR from disturbed water and the cooling effect of water, which leads to a false sense of security. The same is true of cloudy days. Clouds give a false sense of security that is similar to the cooling effect of the water because clouds reduce the warming sensation of the sun. Another reason for the higher rate of MMs and NMSCs in this socioeconomic group is that people in these occupations may have better health insurance, a higher awareness of health issues, and ultimately better detection of lesions.[7,10] An association between high-paying jobs and MM may be due to confounding factors in recreational patterns rather than occupational choice.[10] Other environmental risk factors for the development of NSCC include exposure to ionizing radiation, phototherapy with psoralens, exposure to polycyclic hydrocarbons, and arsenic ingestion.[2]

High sun exposure at certain times of life confers higher risks for developing different types of skin cancer. Early sun exposure, particularly in childhood and adolescence, is associated with a much higher risk for developing BCC and is estimated to confer a tenfold elevated risk for developing SCC.[30–33] Sun exposure in the ten years prior to diagnosis may be important in accounting for many cases of SCC and is associated with a 2.5–fold increased risk when compared to those without this exposure.[2] Sun exposure during childhood and adolescence seems to have a substantial influence on the risk of developing MM.[28] Approximately 80% of lifetime sun exposure occurs before the age of 18 years. During this time, melanocytes may be more sensitve to the sun, resulting in alteration of their DNA and possibly leading to the formation of unstable moles that have a greater potential to become malignant. Sunlight exposure and blistering sunburns during youth may be more intense than those incurred later in life because of the recreation patterns of children.[28] Continued exposure in adulthood increases the risk for NMSC. For MM, the risk seems to increase with intermittent sun exposure on areas of skin only occasionally exposed.

The ocular structures can also be affected by UVR.[16] Repeated and prolonged exposure of the conjunctiva will lead to thickening and hypervascularity. There also appears to be a positive correlation between increased cataract formation, decreased latitude, increased UVB, and total sunlight exposure.[7,16,28]

UVR includes radiation wavelengths ranging from 200 nm to more than 18,000 nm.[28] Damage to the skin comes from UVR in the 200–400 nm range. Several types of UVR occur in this range. The two that have been studied the most in relation to the development of NMSC and MM are ultraviolet A (UVA) and ultraviolet B (UVB). UVA are longer waves (320–400 nm), resulting in deeper skin penetration. It is estimated that 50%–55% of UVA penetrates the dermis.[7] Although UVA carries significant risks, the risks of skin cancer are probably greatest in association with UVB.[7] UVB waves are the shortest (220–290 nm), make up about 5% of the sunlight striking the earth, and are probably the most biologically important component of UVR from the sun. Of UVB that reaches the skin, 85% is absorbed primarily in the epidermis, with only 10%–15% being transmitted to the deeper dermal layers.[7] UVB has a greater intensity in the summer than in the winter, at midday than in morning or late afternoon, in places closer to the equator, and at high altititudes. Sand, snow, concrete, and water can reflect as much as 85% of UVB, thus intensifying exposure.[7] Ultraviolet C (UVC) is largely blocked by the ozone layer. The physiologic effects of UVA and UVB on the skin are different and are summarized in Table 63-2.[3,5,7,10]

Erythema associated with a sunburn is due to excessive UVB. The minimal erythema dose (MED) is the amount of UVR necessary to cause the skin to change to shades of red or pink. MED is highly variable and depends on an individual's skin type, skin thickness, amount of melanin in the skin, and whether the UVR is short or long wave.[16] The erythema results from an increase in blood flow to the affected skin that begins about 4 hours after exposure, with peak erythema occurring 8–24 hours after exposure. The appearance of the erythema suggests that a threshold of UV damage has been reached sufficient to activate prostaglandin and other inflammatory pathways.

Wavelengths of UVR that produce the largest amount of erythema are also the most efficient at producing pyrimidine dimers. The inference is that the wavelengths that produce maximum erythema are most likely to be the wavelengths that produce the maximum number of carcinogenic mutations.

Table 63-2 Effects of Ultraviolet Light on the Skin

Effect	UVA (320–400 nm)	UVB (290–320 nm)
Immediate pigment darkening (usually fades within a few hours) due to photo-oxidation of melanin already in epidermis	Yes	Not as evident
Number of functioning melanocytes	No change	Increased number
Photosensitivity reactions	May occur quickly	May occur
Delayed tanning (occurs 36–72 hours after exposure)	Yes	Yes
Production of vitamin D from cholesterol precursors in the skin	None	Yes
Site of absorption	55% in dermis	Primarily the epidermis; 10%–15% in dermis
Radiant heat	Little to none	Moderate to large amount
Sunburn	Seldom evident except after large doses	May occur very quickly
Thickening of the stratum corneum	No	Yes
Carcinogen	Potentiates the effects of UVB	Yes
Distribution of melanosomes	Within dendrites of melanocytes only in basal cell layer	Within keratinocytes throughout the epidermis
Photoaging	Yes	Yes
Etiologic cause of NMSC	Role not completely clear	Yes
Immunosuppression	Yes	Yes
Etiologic cause of MM	Role not completely clear	Yes
Pathologic changes in the dermis	Yes	Yes

Data from Rigel[3,5]; Whiteman, Green[7]; U.S. Preventative Services Task Force.[10]

Two types of tanning occur in response to UVR exposure. Immediate tanning is a transient grayish, brown discoloration of the skin induced by UVA. It begins during exposure and is maximal at the end of exposure. Immediate tanning lasts a few hours to about 36 hours after exposure. Delayed tanning occurs 48–72 hours following UVR exposure, peaks in 7–10 days, and can persist for several days to months.

Photodamage (dermatoheliosis) is a spectrum of skin changes affecting the epidermis and the dermis. It includes the formation and growth of flat, brown spots on the skin (solar lentiges), fine and deep wrinkling, blackheads, telangiectasias, a yellow, sallow color to the skin, and loss of elasticity.[2,7,30] These changes can be prevented by the consistent and adequate application of sunscreen.

There appears to be an inverse relationship between increasing latitude and MM mortality. The closer a person lives to the equator, the higher the risk. For every decrease in latitude of two degrees, there is an associated 10% increase in the death rate from MM.[7,8]

Wavelengths of UVR that produce the largest amount of erythema are also the most efficient at producing pyrimidine dimers. A rough correlation exists between pyrimidine dimer yield and susceptibility to sun-induced erythema. Of the UVR that reaches the earth's surface, wavelengths of 290–310 nm are the most efficient for producing pyrimidine dimers. The maximum wavelength for erythema to be seen in humans is estimated to be 298.5 nm.[7,28] The inference is that wavelengths that produce the maximum erythema are most likely to produce the maximum number of carcinogenic mutations.

Stratospheric ozone depletion may also be a causative factor associated with both NMSC and MM. Ozone depletion may lead to increased terrestrial UVB levels for many populations. It has been estimated that for every 1% decrease in ozone, there is a 2% increase in UVB penetration to the earth. This increased UVB penetration is predicted to result in an additional 1%–3% increase per year in NMSC.[29] It has also been estimated that for each 1% decrease in the amount of ozone, MM incidence increases about 1%.[27]

Photosensitizing agents have also been associated with the development of skin cancer, as well as premature skin aging, reduced immunity, blood vessel damage, and allergic reactions.[34] Photosensitivity is defined as a chemically induced change in the skin that renders an individual unusually sensitive to light. Rashes, sunburn, or other adverse effects may occur from exposure to UVR of an intensity or duration that would not normally affect that individual. Many medications contain photosensitizing agents, including antihistamines, oral contraceptives and estrogen, nonsteroidal and anti-inflammatory drugs, phenothiazines, psoralens, sulfonamides, sulfonylureas, thiazide diuretics, tetracylines, tricyclic antidepressants, many chemotherapeutic agents, antiparasitic drugs, and oral hypoglycemics.[30,34–36] Persons who are taking a photosensitizing medication need to reduce UVR exposure whenever possible.

Prevention

Primary and secondary prevention are both important in regard to skin cancer. Primary prevention strategies are the steps taken to keep the malignancy from developing. In the case of skin cancer, these efforts include properly applying sunscreen, wearing protective clothing, and decreasing UVR exposure. Public education programs are an excellent means of addressing these primary prevention strategies. Secondary prevention efforts include attempts to detect skin cancer early in asymptomatic persons. Table 63-3 provides an overview of primary and secondary prevention strategies for both NMSCs and MMs and appropriate patient education points.

Primary Prevention

Public policy

The Healthy People 2010 Guidelines (*www.health.gov/healthypeople/Document/html*) aim to decrease the U.S. mortality rate from MM from 2.8 deaths per 100,000 persons to 2.5 deaths per 100,000 persons during the next ten years.[37] The Guidelines also seek to increase the proportion of people using skin cancer primary prevention strategies, which include at least one of the following protective measures: avoiding the sun between 10 A.M. and 4 P.M., wearing sun-protective clothing, using sunscreen with an SPF of 15 or higher, and decreasing or avoiding UVR exposure. Approximately 47% of the U.S. population age 18 and older currently use at least one of the measures; the goal is to increase this proportion to 75%. To make the Healthy People 2010 guidelines become a reality, increased efforts to implement primary, secondary, and tertiary skin cancer prevention are needed. As noted earlier, primary prevention strategies are the steps taken to keep the malignancy from developing through use of sun protection measures. Secondary prevention efforts include efforts to detect skin cancer early in asymptomatic persons and include total body skin examination by professionals and regular skin self-examination (SSE) by individuals. Tertiary prevention seeks to minimize the long-term consequences of cancer treatment and the detection of additional primary skin cancers early.

Public education programs

Public education programs need to include not only information about skin cancer and reducing UVR exposure, but also a behavioral component that ensures long-term adaptation of healthy behaviors.[38,39] All public education programs and health messages are most successful if they reflect regional and individual differences as well as the social context of culture and/or ethnicity.[10]

To reap the most benefits, public education programs need to be started early in a child's life, with the goal of having the individual adopt attitudes and practices that minimize UVR exposure. A number of such programs have demonstrated that even preschoolers can learn and practice behaviors that reduce UVR exposure.[37,40,41] The American Academy of Dermatologists (AAD) has recently launched a campaign that targets kindergarten through third grades called "Block the Sun, Not the Fun!"[34,35,42] More recently, the Centers for Disease Control and Prevention (CDC) has released Guidelines for School Programs to Prevent Skin Cancer.[36] These guidelines include the establishment of policies that reduce UVR exposure, establishment of safe environments, provision of health education for students and staff, involvement of the family, incorporation with other school services, and periodic evaluation.

Evidence suggests that to get children to change their practices and attitudes, their parents must first adopt more healthy behaviors.[34] Despite educational programs and knowledge about the dangers of exposure to UVR, many individuals fail to practice primary prevention strategies.[36] Some believe that fear of skin cancer is not a deterrent to sun-seeking behaviors and that until it becomes culturally acceptable to have untanned skin in the United States, there will not be a major decrease in MM and NMSC incidence and mortality rates. Some groups advocate that public messages should try to change this social norm and emphasize the photoaging effects of excessive UVR exposure.

Short-term goals for primary prevention programs should include an increase in knowledge about the importance of sun protection and a decreased desire for a suntan.[8] Until these goals are achieved, primary prevention strategies will not be implemented effectively.

Medium-term goals for primary prevention programs should include an increased use of hats, clothing, shade, and sunscreens that result in a decreased number of sunburns.[8] Truly effecting these changes in behavior so that they are practiced from childhood through adulthood can be very complicated and difficult to accomplish.

Ultimately, the long-term goals for primary prevention programs (which may not be evident for decades) include a decrease in the incidence of NMSC and MM as well as a decrease in mortality, especially from MM. Because most cases of BCC and SCC are induced by natural or artificial sources of UVR, primary prevention may be theoretically possible.[2,7] The exact role of UVR in the development of MM is not as clear, although it is speculated that primary prevention strategies remain important for this disease.

Sunscreens

There are two types of sunscreens: chemical sunscreens that provide protection by absorbing UVR and physical sunscreens that block UVR from reaching the skin.

Educating the public about sunscreens is more complicated than it appears. Controversies continue regarding the labeling, application, and effectiveness of these agents.

Chemical sunscreens. The primary goal of protecting the skin from UVR is not just to avoid a sunburn. Studies demonstrate that incremental damage occurs with each exposure to UVR regardless of whether there is clinical evidence of erythema.[27] It is impractical and impossible to think that humans can avoid sun exposure completely; therefore prevention with sunscreens and other protective clothing is necessary.

Epidemiologic studies suggest that recent UVR exposure may be more important than cumulative UVR exposure. Thus, even older individuals and those with high cumulative sun-exposure histories can benefit from sunscreen use by preventing the promoting influence of recent sun exposure and by avoiding new initiating mutations. Sunscreen clearly reduces further actinic damage in patients with such damage

Table 63-3 Primary and Secondary Prevention for Skin Cancer

Strategy	Patient Education	Strengths	Limitations
Risk assessment (secondary prevention)	Define and interpret individual risks for developing skin cancer	Patients who understand their personal risk for developing skin cancer may be more motivated to practice prevention strategies	Time-consuming Patient must be motivated to assist with and try to understand assessment Requires skilled healthcare providers
Reduce ultraviolet radiation exposure (primary prevention)	Decrease sun exposure between 10 A.M. and 3 P.M. Instruction that UVR is present on cloudy days Infants 6 mo of age and younger should not have direct UVR exposure	Decrease carcinogen exposure	Personal practices may be difficult to change
Avoid use of indoor tanning devices (primary prevention)	Large amounts of UVA are potentially carcinogenic Tanned skin is not healthy; rather it is a sign of injured skin Use of indoor tanning devices may lead to premature aging of skin and cataract formation	Large source of carcinogen exposure which can be avoided	Personal practices may be difficult to change — many persons believe they look healthier with a tan
Use chemical sunscreens correctly and consistently (primary prevention)	Use an SPF of at least 15–20 that is waterproof Apply a test dose to check for allergies Apply liberally (about an ounce for an adult in a swim suit) to all exposed skin surfaces 15–30 min prior to sun exposure Reapply sunscreen every 90 min and more frequently after toweling off	When used correctly, sunscreen will block most of the UVB exposure and a variable amount of UVA	Some consider sunscreens expensive and inconvenient to use Many persons do not apply products prior to exposure, apply them in inadequate amounts, and do not reapply when indicated, thereby limiting the effectiveness of the agents Personal practices may be difficult to change — many persons believe they look healthier with a tan May not apply on children younger than 6 mo of age

(continued)

Table 63-3 Primary and Secondary Prevention for Skin Cancer (continued)

Strategy	Patient Education	Strengths	Limitations
Apply zinc oxide (a physical block) to sun-exposed areas (primary prevention)	Apply a visible, liberal coat to sun-exposed areas Block is effective as long as a visible coat is seen on skin	Excellent for areas with a tendency to burn such as the nose, backs of ears Is more waterproof than chemical sunscreens	Unsuitable to be applied to all sun-exposed areas because of the amount of product necessary
Wear protective clothing (primary prevention)	Protective clothing with a tighter weave can provide an effective physical block against UVR Shirts with sleeves and hats with wide brims provide more protection	Provides a means to directly reduce direct UVR to skin surfaces Relatively inexpensive Easy to apply	Patients may forget to wear hats or not see the benefits of protective clothing as worth the effort
Take extra precaution to reduce UVR exposure when taking photosensitizing medications (primary prevention)	Teach patients about classes of photosensitizing medications and the need for extra protection	Reduces severe sunburns and UVR exposure	Patients may forget to take precautions or underestimate the dangers of photosensitizing medications
Practice monthly skin self-examination (secondary prevention)	Demonstrate technique on the patient Point out any potential problems that require extra monitoring Teach patients to perform in a well-lit area and to pay attention to hard-to-see areas as well as sun-exposed areas	Inexpensive Can be done in privacy of own home Patient may be able to note an early interval change	Patients often forget to do examination or do not see the value of self-examination Some areas of body may be difficult for patient to adequately examine Patients may lack confidence in ability to detect a change
Annual professional examination (secondary prevention)	Opportunity to review many primary prevention strategies Teach skin self-examination Detect lesions that may not be immediately obvious to the patient	May detect subtle, early changes in lesions	May result in removal of borderline lesions Dependent on the skill of the examiner Most cost-effective in higher-risk patients — cost-effectiveness in the general population is not known

when used consistently and adequately. These results can be evident in as little as two years.[2,39] Children and younger individuals benefit by avoiding the initiating mutations caused by UVR. It has been estimated that regular use of sunscreens (at least SPF 15) to the face, ears, neck, and upper extremities during the first 18 years of life could lead to a 78% reduction in the lifetime incidence of BCC and SCC.[2]

A study of 2458 Caucasian Americans revealed that only 47% routinely used sunscreen; of these individuals, half did not use sunscreen with an SPF of at least 15.[43] More recently, a national population-based telephone survey conducted by the ACS reported that among youth on sunny days, 32% report wearing sunglasses, 21% report wearing long pants, 22% report staying in the shade, and 31% report applying sunscreen.[44] In Australia, the use of sunscreens — a default option to be used only when other measures do not provide sufficient protection — is supported by clinical studies, which have recently reported that sunscreen use has been associated with a statistically significant reduced risk for MM.[45] The AAD recommends that patients be educated that the first defense against skin cancer is avoiding midday sun and using protective clothing when outdoors. Sunscreen should be used as an adjunct to other primary prevention measures.[46]

Chemical sunscreens. Currently, sunscreens are rated or classified by their sun protection factor (SPF). The SPF numbers that appear on a sunscreen's label refer to the product's ability to absorb, reflect, or scatter UVB. No uniformly acceptable standardized method currently exists to measure a sunscreen's ability to provide protection from UVA. UVA has a longer wavelength than UVB, which allows it to penetrate deeper into the skin.

Chemical sunscreens are designed to be applied generously to all exposed skin. Depending on the chemicals used, a laboratory SPF can range from 2 to 60. Sunscreens are rated for their UVR absorption under strict and ideal laboratory conditions. In a laboratory, a sunscreen with an SPF of 15 will absorb 92% of UVB, an SPF of 30 will absorb 96.7% of UVB, and an SPF of 40 will absorb 97.5% of UVB.[47] The effectiveness of a particular sunscreen agent is affected by an individual's body site of application, degree of normal skin color, thickness of the epidermis, time of day, time of year, cloud cover, ozone levels, reflection, and UVR scatter. Because most consumers typically apply less sunscreen than is used in laboratories to establish the SPF number, the actual SPF protection is often 20%–50% of the number on the label.[48]

Chemical sunscreens of sufficient SPF can substantially limit or prevent DNA damage and pyrimidine dimer formation. They contain one or more chemicals in a carrier base — either a gel, lotion, cream, or ointment. Some formulations are clear; others are available in milky or colored formulations. An estimated $3.4 billion is spent each year on sunscreen products worldwide.[45]

Chemical sunscreens usually contain a variety of products that protect primarily against UVB and, to a lesser extent, against UVA. Organic absorbers include PABA esters, camphor derivatives, salicylates, and cinnamates that absorb primarily UVB.[49] Parsol 1789 absorbs the longer UVA rays.[45] Other UVA absorbers include benzophenones, anthranilates, and dibenzoyl methanes. Each family has a different absorption spectrum, so these agents are used in combination to provide broader protection.

Effective December 31, 2002, the Food and Drug Administration (FDA) requires sunscreen manufacturers to comply with regulations to improve product labeling, including providing information on UVA protection.[50] In response to epidemiologic evidence suggesting that use of higher-SPF sunscreens can lead to consumer overconfidence and thus increased UVR exposure, the FDA has also recommended a cap on SPF claims greater than 30 so that such agents would be labeled as 30+. The AAD has further recommended that labels should include directions on how often to reapply sunscreen, how resistant it is to water, and how thickly to apply it. Sunscreens designated as "waterproof" may not, in fact, be completely waterproof. This designation requires merely that the sunscreen retain its waterproof effectiveness for 80 minutes of immersion. Consequently, the FDA is changing the label wording from "waterproof" to "very water resistant."

Most healthcare professionals recommend an SPF of at least 15 but preferably an SPF of 30, and consider the patient's formulation preference (e.g., gel, lotion). Ideally, a broad-spectrum sunscreen should be used to block some UVA as well as UVB. Waterproof/water-resistant sunscreens are usually preferred.

Many patient education points need to be emphasized regarding application of sunscreen.[26,29] To permit maximum absorption, sunscreens need to be applied 15–30 minutes before exposure, liberally (at least one ounce for an adult) and uniformly, and then should be allowed to dry. Products that are applied too thinly or rubbed vigorously into the skin will not provide the indicated protection. The technique of application greatly affects the effectiveness of the sunscreen product. In general, sunscreens should be reapplied every 90 minutes. Eyelids are commonly not covered to avoid skin irritation or stinging. Another facial area commonly missed is the ear. Sunscreen is now available in lipstick form to protect the lips. These products should also be applied liberally and reapplied frequently like chemical sunscreens.

When providing education about sunscreens, nurses need to instruct patients on how to read a label. One approach is to give samples to the patient, or examples of different agents with different labels for this education. It teaches the patient in a realistic setting how to be a better consumer and make good choices. Education must also include information about SPF, waterproof labeling, and ways to correctly apply and reapply the sunscreen. Most important, education should emphasize that sunscreen is an adjunct to other means to ultimately reduce UVR exposure.

When used properly, sunscreens with a high SPF are clearly effective in preventing sunburn.[39,49] Data are much more controversial as to whether sunscreen prevents BCC and MM, leading the International Agency for Research on Cancer (IARC) to state that sunscreens should not be the first choice for skin cancer prevention and should not be used as the sole means of sun protection.[46,49] In other words, sunscreen should not be used as a means to extend exposure to the sun. Current trends suggest, however, that may be the very thing that is happening.[45] The benefits of sunscreen should not be completely dismissed. Australians and Hawaiian Caucasians, who have some of the highest per capita uses of sunscreens, exhibit decreased incidence of MM, which is also related to other effective means of reducing UVR. The only real way to know with more certainty, the benefits of sunscreen would be to conduct a prospective randomized study, with some participants using sunscreen and others not using sunscreen. Because it is not feasible and is unethical to conduct such a trial, the controversy about sunscreen will continue.[42,50]

Physical sunscreens. Physical sunscreens physically block UVR from reaching the dermis and epidermis. These preparations contain molecules such as zinc oxide, talc, or titanium dioxide in an ointment base. They are considered inorganic chemical absorbers.[39,45] These sunscreens are available in white and neon colors and flesh tones. Physical sunscreens are effective and useful in protecting selected areas of the body such as the nose, cheeks, ears, and shoulders if applied thickly. The recent availability of physical sunscreens in bases that are cosmetically appealing (including titanium dioxide) has increased the use of these agents.[49] They are also sometimes combined with chemical sunscreens to create a more broad-spectrum product.

Protective clothing

The effectiveness of hats and shirts as a primary prevention measure should not be underestimated. A brim size of 10 cm can lead to a reduction of 70% of UVR exposure to the head and neck.[8] California was the first state to enact skin cancer legislation (SB310) that requires schools to allow students to wear sun-protective hats and other appropriate UVR-blocking clothing when outdoors.[51]

The weave of the material used in hats and clothing is very important. In general, synthetic materials provide better protection against UVA than cotton materials. Densely woven material provides a reflective barrier to UVR. Clothes designed to cover the most skin provide the most protection. Long-sleeved shirts with collars, long pants, and shoes and socks provide more coverage than tank tops, shorts, and sandals.[52] In general, synthetic materials provide better protection against UVA than cotton materials. Darker materials provide more protection.

Most clothes such as hats and summer wear offer an SPF of 2–6.5, although sun-protective clothing is available that offers an SPF of up to 30.[9,43] Clothing with an ultraviolet protection factor (UPF) is also available. This rating differs from an SPF rating, which is a measurement of sunburn or reddening time. The UPF provides information about the relative amount of UVR that penetrates the fabric and reaches the skin. The density of the fabric is the major determinant of UPF.[53] At this time, fabric UPF is not regulated by the FDA, but the Federal Trade Commission (FTC) carefully monitors advertising claims. The three classification categories for UPF are "good UVR protection" (UPF of 15–24), "very good UVR protection" (UPF of 25–39), and "excellent UVR protection" (UPF of 40–50+).[54] In some cases, fabrics may be treated with optical brighteners or chemical absorbers to increase UVR protectiveness before they are sold. Once purchased, clothes can be treated with detergents that contain optical brighteners to improve or retain UVR absorption. Spray-on treatments can also be used to increase UPF and last through repeated washings.

Nurses can educate patients about ways to assess the effectiveness of fabric as a sun protectant. A simple test of efficacy is to hold the material up to strong light and see whether it casts a dense shadow or whether it is easy to distinguish objects through the shadow.[16] Nurses should also educate patients that virtually all garments lose about one-third of their sun-protective ability when wet.[52]

Protection of the ocular structures is also important. Some sunglasses can offer protection against both UVA and UVB.[55] Consumers need to be instructed to read labels correctly and carefully before purchasing sunglasses to assure that they actually offer UVR protection. The label should state "blocks 99% of UVR." Some manufactures state "UVR up to 400 nm," which is equivalent to 100% UVR absorption. The color and degree of darkness do not provide any information about the ability of the lenses to block UVR.

Reducing UVR exposure

The best way to reduce the incidence of skin cancer is to reduce UVR exposure. Public policy may be one of the most important ways to ultimately achieve the goal of decreasing UVR exposure. UVR exposure comes from both outdoor exposure and artificial sources. There is a need to educate both individuals and the public as a whole about ways to reduce this exposure in places where children play. Key targets for policy development and public education include schools, camps, sporting events, other outdoor events, parks, pools, and workplaces.

Outdoor exposure. Approximately 60% of the total UVB exposure is received from 10 A.M. to 2 P.M. When possible, avoiding prolonged exposure during this time is recommended. Shade from trees and canopies can further reduce this exposure.[2]

In the United States, the National Weather Service (NWS) has developed an ultraviolet index (UVI) as one part of a national program of public education about the dangers of UVR.[56] This program was initiated in 1991. The public is informed by television and radio news and by newspapers of the day's solar ultraviolet intensity rating [a scale of 0 (minimal) to 10+ (very high)] and is given instructions on how to decrease UVR exposure. The long-term effectiveness of this program is not yet known.

In Australia, schools have a "no hat, no play" policies that restrict children who do not have hats from playing outdoors.[42,57] Sunscreen is provided at public places, and many towns have installed shade cloths over play structures and pools in parks and community centers. A shade cloth, which is relatively simple to install, can reduce sun exposure by 60%.[16] Shade produced by trees can substantially reduce UVR. Note that the higher the canopy is from the ground, the more opportunity there is for scattered UVR to reach people under the shelter. Efforts in countries such as the United States are much less extensive. In one survey, only 36% of child care centers had shade in more than half of the play area, and only 56% of the centers in another survey had implemented adequate sun protection policies.[16,58]

Artificial UVR exposure. Indoor tanning represents a relatively new area that public education programs need to target. Preliminary evidence suggests that there is an increase in MM risk for persons who regularly use artificial sources of UVA.[59] People who use artificial tanning expose their skin to 2.5-fold and 1.5-fold greater chances of developing SCC and BCC, respectively.[60,61]

Every day, more than 1 million Americans use tanning parlors that are largely unregulated. This $2.5 billion business features an estimated 24,000 salons in the United States. The FDA and the FTC share responsibilities in the regulation of sunlamps and tanning devices. The FDA enforces regulations concerning labels on the devices; the FTC investigates false, misleading, and deceptive advertising claims about the devices. When these agencies determine that device labels do not comply with the regulations or that advertisements are not truthful, they may take corrective action. The FDA has the authority to remove products from the market.

The most frequent users of artificial UVR exposure are adolescents and young adults, especially women. The UVA from these tanning parlors often amounts to five times more UVA per time unit than solar UVA.[29] Indoor tanning beds typically emit approximately 95% UVA and 5% UVB, which the parlors market as a "safe tan" because sunburning seldom occurs.[61] In reality, there is no known benefit from exposure to artificial UVA, and tanning actually represents the body's response to injury. Artificial tanning can substantially damage the skin, cause premature aging, cause loss of elasticity, and has been linked to ocular melanoma.[59,62]

Secondary Prevention

Early detection of BCC and SCC is important to prevent the disfiguring effects of these tumors and their treatment. Early detection of MM is an approach to control that, if used effectively and consistently, can have a relatively rapid impact on decreasing the mortality rate from this disease.[8] This approach is taken by most nations when implementing a public health control and awareness program for MM, even though the evolution of MM is not completely understood and it may not be completely preventable.[2,3] Table 63-4 provides an overview of approaches to screening. There are inherent strengths and weakness associated with each approach, so providers who design screening programs need to select one that is consistent with the goals of the program and the resources of the providers and their institution.

Skin cancer secondary prevention strategies are often defined as case finding, screening, and surveillance. Case finding is the incidental detection of cancer during a routine physical examination or visit to a healthcare professional for an unrelated medical problem. Skin cancer screening is the systematic cutaneous examination of a selected population, often from one geographic region, with individuals selected on the basis of age, sex, or other features. Screening may also be confined to those known to be at increased risk for skin cancer. Surveillance is the ongoing examination of individuals at regular intervals of three to six months for the development of new or changing lesions that might be early skin cancer. It may include photography of suspicious lesions. Presently there are no evidence-based guidelines for secondary skin cancer prevention.

Screening programs

A panel sponsored by the AAD and the CDC identified skin cancer control issues as a priority.[3] MM meets the criteria for a disease amenable to screening because it is a serious disease that is becoming increasingly common, it has an asymptomatic period, an available screening tool exists, and the disease can be detected and treated early. The panel concluded that primary care providers need to assume a major responsibility for skin cancer detection. These healthcare providers have an excellent opportunity either as part of a total physical examination or during focused examinations to assess for suspicious lesions and to refer for further evaluation when appropriate.

Data suggest, however, that total skin examinations are infrequently performed and documented in the primary care setting.[62] First, primary care physicians do not consistently examine the entire skin surface. Patients who are most likely to receive a skin examination from a primary care provider are those who request such an examination. Although managed care promotes health promotion and wellness services, in reality fewer patients may receive a total skin examination on a regular basis unless there is a clearly defined program directed toward screening, education, and prevention.[62,63]

The effectiveness of screening programs also reflects the skill of the provider performing the screening examination. In general, dermatologists and health professionals with special training in detecting skin lesions are better able to diagnose MM than

Table 63-4 Approaches to Screening for Skin

Approach	Characteristics	Strengths	Limitations
Skin self-examination	Regular (usually monthly) examination of all skin surfaces	Note interval changes Convenient Inexpensive	Patients often forget to do examination Some areas of body may be difficult for patient to adequately examine Patients may lack confidence in ability to detect a change
Opportunistic screening (case finding)	Sporadic examination of patients who present for other health reasons	Earlier detection of lesions that patient may be unaware of	Dependent on the skill of the health provider All skin surface areas may not be examined
Professional skin examination	Annual examination of all skin surfaces by a trained health professional with the goal of detecting skin cancers early	Trained professional may be able to detect a subtle sign or change Examination is focused on finding early changes or skin cancers Safe; noninvasive Usually includes an extensive educational component on ways to prevent skin cancer	Dependent on the skill of the health provider May result in increased removal of borderline lesions
Mass screening	Regular population-based screening of asymptomatic patients at a defined clinical site on a specific date	Large numbers of persons may be examined in a relatively short period of time Trained professionals may be able to detect a subtle sign or change Examination is focused on finding early changes or skin cancer	Dependent on the skill of the health provider May result in increased removal of borderline lesions May be difficult to ensure patients with suspicious lesions receive adequate follow-up
Surveillance	Regular examination (usually every 3–6 mo) of patients with a high risk of developing skin cancer May include medical photography of suspicious lesions	Earlier detection of tumors Usually includes an extensive educational component on ways to prevent skin cancer	May result in increased removal of borderline lesions More expensive
Genetic testing	DNA studies to determine whether a patient who has a hereditary predisposition to malignant melanoma carries susceptibility genes	More accurately select patients who will benefit from intense surveillance Usually includes extensive education on ways to reduce the risk of developing malignant melanoma	Expensive Patient may be psychologically disturbed by the results Results may be inconclusive A negative test does not mean the patient may not go on to develop malignant melanoma Results do not tell if, when, or where the patient will go on to develop malignant melanoma

primary care providers.[64] Over the last four decades, there has been a gradual improvement in the diagnostic accuracy of dermatologists in detecting MM. In programs with trained skin cancer screening specialists, reports suggest an overall sensitivity of 84%, a specificity of 99%, and a positive predictive value of 73% for the detection of MM.[62] Those who are not trained specifically in skin cancer detection and diagnosis have rates substantially lower than these figures (estimated to be about 59%).

A common criticism of skin self-examination is that people will be burdening the medical system with benign lesions, although research has not substantiated this criticism.[3] It is also important to note that a total skin examination and skin self-examination detect NMSCs. The high prevalence of these types of skin cancers suggests that a total skin examination will result in a higher yield of positive finds than screening of any other organ system. A properly conducted skin examination may be considered time-consuming by some, although it can be performed effectively in approximately seven minutes.[62] A risk assessment and total skin examination will identify persons at increased risk for developing NMSC and MM who may benefit from increased and more intensive surveillance. Often, these individuals can be referred to special clinics for pigmented lesions where intensive surveillance and education services are available.

While dependent on the population screened, rates of suspected melanoma in mass screening, case finding, and population-based screening range from 0 to 9 per 100 persons screened, with the most common findings between 1 and 3 cases per 100 population. Rates of confirmed melanoma and melanoma in situ are commonly in the range of 1–4 per 1000 persons screened. In total, 1%–5% of screened patients are confirmed to have NMSC.[63] The AAD has promoted free skin cancer education and screening programs in the United States since 1985. Screenings have averaged nearly 100,000 persons per year since 1990 and represent the largest dermatologic mass screening program in the country.

When skin cancer screening programs are designed, provisions for diagnostic and treatment services for those with positive screens need to be made available. Of great concern is the disposition of persons who have a positive screen.[62] Ultimately, the goal of such programs is that patients follow through with the recommended care. The utility and justifiability of any screening program depend on the extent to which those individuals with a positive screen can be followed and treated. If the financial resources necessary for such follow-up care and treatment are not included in the total budget for such screening programs, they will not achieve this goal.

Although dermatologists may have the most expertise in recognizing melanoma, their practice is often limited to persons at high risk for developing the disease.[63] Many melanomas do not occur in individuals with a family history or those with dysplastic nevi or fair skin. Thus, if early detection efforts are limited to this population, the overall impact to the population at large will be limited. To date, no randomized trials or case-controlled studies have examined whether screening by clinicians is associated with improved clinical outcomes such as reduced morbidity and mortality from skin cancer.[16,63] Some speculate that earlier treatment as a result of screening improves outcomes.[64]

Table 63-5 Components of Two Screening Checklists for the Early Detection of Skin Cancer

American System	Seven-Point Checklist
A Asymmetry	Major Features
B Border irregularity	• Change in size • Change in color
C Color irregularity	• Change in shape
D Diameter > 6 mm	Minor Features
E Elevation	• Diameter > 7 mm • Sensory change • Oozing/crusting/bleeding • Inflammation

Screening checklists

In clinical practice, decisions must be made regarding when to refer patients for further evaluation of suspicious skin lesions. Ideally, a screening checklist should detect abnormalities, without overreferring for benign lesions. A variety of checklist systems have been devised to make decisions for referral when screening for skin cancer. Two of the more common checklists are the American ABCDE system and the seven-point checklist (Table 63-5).

The seven-point checklist is reported to be a sensitive screening tool for MM.[65] This scale emphasizes changes in a lesion, particularly a change in size, shape, or color. Its usefulness in detecting BCC and SCC has not been reported. According to this checklist, the presence of one or more major features is an indication for referral. Suspicion for MM should be very high in the presence of two or more major features, but low when only minor features are identified. No studies have been located that compare the efficacy of the ABCDE system and the seven-point checklist.

Pathophysiology

Normal Skin Structures

The skin is the largest organ of the body and is responsible for vital functions such as protection from injury, maintenance of homeostasis, and regulation of temperature. This structure consists of two layers, the epidermis and the dermis (Figure 63-3). The epidermis is composed of stratified or layered epithelial cells, the majority of which are keratinocytes that are replaced every 15–30 days. The four layers of keratinocytic cells are named for either their morphology or their position: the stratum corneum (outermost layer), the stratum lucidum, the stratum granulosum, and the stratum spinosum.[66] Beneath these four layers is the stratum germinativum, or germinative layer consisting of basal cells that undergo mitosis in response to

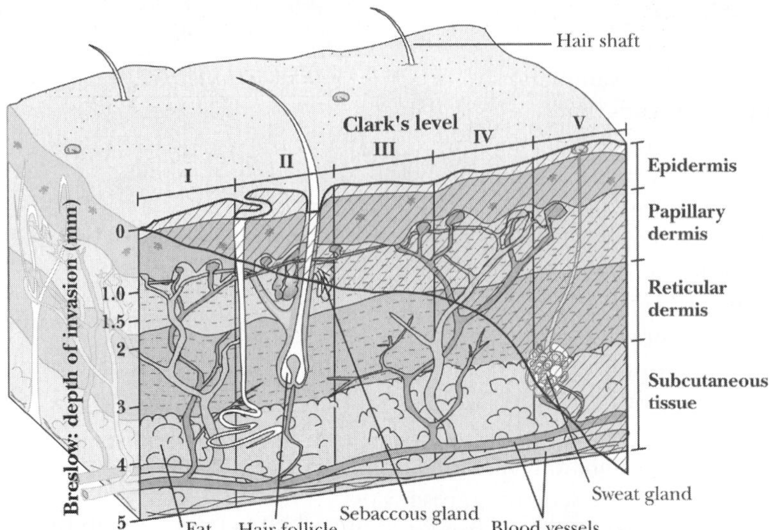

Figure 63-3 Anatomy of the skin demonstrating Clark's and Breslow's staging criteria.

growth-stimulating signals. Following mitosis, the newly produced cells are outwardly displaced from the germanitive layer and move toward the superficial layers. As they do so, they lose their nuclei and thus their proliferative ability and they begin to manufacture keratin. Upon reaching the stratum corneum, the epithelial cells are flat, dead cells filled with keratin.

In the stratum germinativum, basal cells grow in a single column attached to a basement membrane. Other cells that may be present in this layer of the epidermis include Merkel cells and melanocytes. *Melanocytes* are derived from the neural crest in embryology. Most migrate to the skin, but some populate the mucous membranes, uveal tract, meninges, and stria vascularis of the inner ear. Melanocytes of the retinal pigmented epithelium develop from the outer layer of the optic cup.[67,68] MMs arise from melanocytes.

Epidermal melanocytes possess dendrites that contact keratinocytes in more superficial layers of the epidermis. This relationship, termed the epidermal melanin unit, consists of several keratinocytes for each melanocyte. In response to UVR exposure, melanosomes are produced and transferred through melanocyte dendrites to the neighboring keratinocytes. Melanosomes synthesize melanin, a substance that helps protect the skin cells by absorbing UVR. Melanin is also the primary skin pigment. Persons with black skin have similar numbers of melanocytes as those with lighter skin, but their melanocytes have more and larger melanosomes that contain more melanin. In light-skinned persons, the melanosomes are smaller and contain less melanin.[67]

Immediately beneath the basement membrane lies the second layer of the skin, the dermis. This supportive, connective tissue network contains the vascular and lymphatic vessels, nerves, glands, hair follicles, and collagen-producing fibroblasts that give the skin much of its strength.[69] The dermis is also divided into two layers distinguished largely by the organization of the cells, nerves and vascular vessels, and connective tissue.[66] The upper layer is known as the *papillary dermis* because it forms projections (papilla) into the epidermis. It is usually no more than two times the thickness of the epidermis.[66] The lower layer, the *reticular dermis,* lies beneath the papillary dermis and is composed primarily of bundles of collagen. The reticular dermis lies above the subcutaneous fat and fascia that attaches the dermis to underlying structures.

Malignant Change

Nonmelanoma skin cancers

Basal cell carcinoma. BCC is a result of malignant transformation in cells of the basal layer of the epidermis. The cell of origin is not defined but is known to resemble basal cells. The hair follicle has been postulated as the cell of origin; BCCs rarely occur in non-hair-bearing areas of the skin.[70] BCCs may become locally invasive, rarely mestastasize, and usually contain both epidermal and dermal components within the tumor. BCCs transplanted beyond the skin without dermal tissue do not survive.[70] This may explain the usual slow-growing, nonmetastatic nature of BCCs.

Squamous cell carcinoma. SCC is a tumor of the epidermis that arises from malignant transformation of keratinocytes. It can occur anywhere on the skin or mucous membranes where there is squamous epithelium. Unlike BCC, SCC can rapidly progress to local tissue destruction by filling the epidermis, invading the dermis, and then infiltrating other tissues.[69] SCC has the potential to metastasize depending largely on the location, depth, and size of the tumor. Metastases from SCC are more likely with larger and deeper cutaneous lesions and with lesions of the hands, lips, or temple.[71]

Malignant melanoma

Most MM occurs in cutaneous sites after malignant transformation of melanocytes. The initial site of MM is known as the *primary tumor*. This disease may also occur in any melanocyte-containing tissue, including the meninges, the mucosa of the gastrointestinal (GI) and respiratory tracts, the uveal tract, and the vagina. MM may arise from preexisting lesions or occur in apparently healthy skin.[72]

Most MMs exhibit two growth phases: radial and vertical. In the radial phase, cells grow in a radial fashion from the primary site and do not metastasize.[73] This phase may continue for an extended period of time in superficial spreading and lentigo maligna MMs, or it may be of very short duration as in nodular MM. Eventually, the MM enters a vertical growth phase in which the cells invade down into and through the dermis and have the potential to metastasize. Although there are exceptions, MM tends to recur or metastasize in the stepwise manner of local recurrence, regional metastases, and distant metastases.[72,74]

Local recurrence is the reappearance of MM close to the surgical scar. The definition of local recurrence may be limited to recurrence within the scar or may include recurrence within 2 cm or even within 5 cm of the scar.[74] Local recurrence is presumed to represent failure to totally excise the primary tumor.[72,74]

Intransit or satellite metastases may occur anywhere between the primary tumor site and the regional lymph nodes. They may appear as multiple, small, bluish, or amelanotic nodules and represent tumor emboli that were in the lymph channels draining the primary lesion.[74]

Regional lymph node metastases may present as a clinically palpable lump or may be identified after either sentinel lymph node sampling or lymph node dissection. Regional lymph node metastases are one of the most important predictors of survival, with positive nodes being highly predictive of visceral metastasis.

Distant metastases more commonly involve nonvisceral sites, including the skin, subcutaneous tissue, and distant lymph nodes. The next most common sites (in descending order) are the lungs, liver, brain, bone, and small intestine. Brain metastases are the initial site of metastases in 20% of patients, and 50% of patients with other metastatic sites will eventually develop brain metastases.[75] With polymerase chain reaction (PCR) technique, it has been demonstrated that as many as 95% of patients with distant organ sites of metastases have circulating tumor cells and are theoretically likely to develop other metastases.

In less than 10% of all cases, MM may present as metastatic disease from an unknown primary site. In approximately two-thirds of these cases, the metastatic disease involves the lymph nodes; the other one-third of cases present in distant sites such as subcutaneous tissue, the lung, or the brain.[74] Patients who present with lymph node involvement with an unknown primary tumor have similar survival to those with a known primary tumor and lymph node involvement. A slight survival advantage may be seen in those patients with an unknown primary site beyond five years.[72] Median survival is also similar for those with unknown primary sites and visceral metastases as compared to those with known primary sites and visceral metastases.

Clinical Manifestations

Skin cancers have a wide variety of clinical presentations and signs and symptoms (Table 63-6). Tables 63-7 and 63-8 outline many of the common clinical characteristics of both NMSCs and MMs.[2,6,66,68,76–79] Many of these characteristics are shared among the malignancies and are difficult to distinguish with the naked eye. The signs and symptoms of different types of skin cancers can vary. SCC seems to be difficult to diagnose clinically.[62] BCCs have more distinctive features, facilitating their clinical diagnosis. Distinguishing between dysplastic nevi and true MM can prove very challenging. MM often presents on the lower extremities in women and on the trunk in men. The classic signs in a preexisting nevus include darkening or irregular color, increasing size, nodularity, ulceration, pruritus, and bleeding. A biopsy is necessary to determine the histopathologic characteristics of these different malignancies and to provide guidance for further treatment and follow-up recommendations.

Assessment

Patient and Family History

A risk assessment is the first step in any secondary prevention or cancer screening program. Assessment should include all of the factors identified in Table 63-1.[3,5,8–10] In particular, it is important to try to obtain an accurate history of sun exposure. This includes quantifying information about severe sunburns (especially in childhood), occupational history, use of indoor tanning devices, and overall cumulative exposure. In

Table 63-6 Signs and Symptoms of Skin Cancer

Nonmelanoma Skin Cancer	Malignant Melanoma
Nonhealing sore or ulcer	New pigmented nevus
Scaling red or pink patch that does not heal	New unpigmented nevus
Enlarging pink papule or nodule	A nevus that is asymmetrical
New nodule with or without scaling, erosion, ulceration, or crusting	A preexisting lesion that has developed notched or faded borders
Pearly papule with telangiectasia	A preexisting lesion that has developed irregular borders
	An unusual or prominent nevus that stands out from the rest of the nevi on the body
	A nevus that is persistently itching, tender, or bleeding
	A nevus that has grown in size or is greater than 6 mm
	A nevus that has changed in color or has multiple colors
	A preexisting nevus that has a change in surface (elevation, erosion, crusting, ulceration)

reality, it is very difficult to quantify lifetime exposure to UVR.[62] The history should also include a family history with particular emphasis on the number of cases of NMSCs, MMs (including specific pathology when available), dysplastic nevus syndrome, and other genetic diseases such as Gorlin syndrome or xeroderma pigmentosum. Finally, the assessment should include detailed information about any lesions that have been removed in the past. Particular attention should be given to determining whether the patient has had any of the following lesions: dysplastic nevi, congenital melanocytic nevi, actinic keratosis, Bowen's disease, solar keratoses, BCC, SCC, or MM. In some cases, pathology reports must be ordered to provide a more accurate assessment and to ultimately provide better screening recommendations.

Once the assessment is complete, screening recommendations can be discussed in light of the individual's specific risks. Patients with higher risk profiles will need screening more often than annually and may possibly need medical photography.[80] Prophylactic removal of suspicious lesions may be indicated. It is important to communicate to the patient that an accurate risk assessment provides more appropriate screening recommendations. It is also important for the patient to understand that the presence or absence of risk factors is not an absolute guarantee that he or she will or will not go on to develop malignancy. The risk assessment offers an opportunity to teach the patient about appropriate primary prevention strategies.[81] It also presents offers an opportunity to correct misconceptions about risk and offer reassurance about the benefits of early detection and primary prevention.

Before beginning the physical examination, it is important to determine whether the patient has noted any change in a lesion or if the patient has any concerns about a lesion. If such a history is elicited, further information should be obtained about any changes in size, shape, color, or other physical characteristics and when these changes were noted (see Table 63-6).

Physical Examination

Technical aspects

The mainstay for the early detection of both NMSC and MM is the physical examination. Clearly, the number of both NMSCs and MMs detected is greatly increased when the examiner focuses on that particular task and has a working knowledge of the different types of skin lesions (see Tables 63-7 and 63-8) as well as the signs and symptoms of skin cancer (see Table 63-6). Diagnostic methods that rely on inspection alone are 60%–80% effective in identifying MM.[6,62] Primary care providers need to be aware of high-risk persons and high-risk anatomical sites, as only 20% of MMs occur on sun-exposed body surfaces, in contrast to 85% of NMSCs.[63] Those who practice in the pediatric setting need to emphasize primary prevention strategies.

To be effective, the examination should be carried out in a well-lit room and include all skin surfaces. Dermatologic visual diagnosis is a skill that must be practiced to increase proficiency and appears to be based more on visual pattern recognition than on mastery of complex rules of logic.[63]

The physical examination of the skin should be performed systematically.[81] The areas to be assessed are the same as those covered in a skin self-examination. The patient should be taught the importance of and rationale for a total skin examination. All concealing cosmetics should be removed. To make the patient as comfortable as possible, only one area of the skin should be exposed at a time.

The lighting in the room should be carefully selected. Ideally, a total skin examination would be conducted in daylight, but this is impractical. A combination of incandescent and fluorescent light is probably best. Fluorescent light accentuates blue to yellow colors and incandescent light brings out red colors. Their combination can help bring out the wide range of colors sometimes seen in skin cancers. Tangential lighting will aid in the recognition of subtle elevations.[62,81]

Table 63-7 Characteristics of Premalignant and Nonmalignant Melanoma Skin Cancers

Type	Characteristics	Location	Other Features
Solar keratosis	Raised red papule or patch with roughened surface	Light-exposed surfaces such as face, dorsum of hand, bald scalp May occur on trunk	Premalignant lesions with variable degrees of dysplasia Increased risk for NMSC
Actinic chelilitis	Well-defined white patches (leukoplakia)	Lips, especially the lower lips Usually seen in men age 40–70	Range from epidermal dysplasia to invasive squamous cell carcinoma
Bowen's disease	Solitary lesion usually a well-defined, slightly raised red plaque with an adherent scale	Predominantly on the legs, backs of hands, finger, and face May occur on non-sun-exposed areas	Carcinoma in situ with full-thickness dysplasia When Bowen's disease occurs on non-sun-exposed areas it is associated with an increased frequency of internal malignancy
Paget's disease	Solitary red, slightly raised well-defined plaque	Nipple and areola	Epidermis is infiltrated by variable numbers of large cells
Squamous cell carcinoma	Nodule or ulcer May have a crusted surface	Sun-exposed areas including ears, lower lips, backs of hands, forearms	Grows more rapidly than BCC Well- to poorly differentiated variants
Basal cell — rodent ulcer	Small papule that subsequently ulcerates Ulcer margin is well defined and slightly raised with rolled, pearl-colored margin Most common skin cancer	Face	Locally invasive Rarely metastasizes Accounts for 70%–75% of BCC
Basal cell — cystic type	Central part of tumor does not break down until late in evolution	Face, especially the inner canthus of the eye	Often not detected early because it is mistaken for a benign cyst Accounts for about 5% of BCC
Basal cell — pigmented	Features similar to rodent ulcer except margins are heavily pigmented	Usually the face	Often misdiagnosed as malignant melanoma Accounts for 1%–3% of BCC
Basal cell — morphoeic type	Begins as a slightly elevated plaque	Usually the face	Often misdiagnosed because it spreads insidiously Accounts for 2%–4% of BCC
Basal cell — superficial	Red plaque with adherent scale Slightly raised, minute, well-defined margin that is rolled, pearly, and has telangiectasia	Usually the trunk	After a number of years it may become invasive Accounts for 13%–15% of BCC
Basal cell — nevus syndrome (Gorlin's syndrome)	Multiple lesions Multisystem disorder	Presence of palmar and planter pits	Dominantly inherited Begins in childhood

Data from Du Vivier[76]; Sober, Burstein[77]; Tong, Fitzpatrick[78]; McCormack, Kelly, Dorevitch.[79]

During the examination, all findings should be carefully documented on an anatomical chart. Characteristics to be documented include location, color(s), size (measured in millimeters), border characteristics, and presence or absence of elevation, telangiectasias, crusting, or ulceration. If the patient is being seen for follow-up screening, the anatomical chart from the most recent examination should be used for comparison to determine whether any characteristics of the lesions have changed.

Photography of lesions allows the clinician to accurately document the location and clinical characteristics for future reference. Total body photography is very important to assist in the identification of early MM in patients with dysplastic nevus syndrome. It usually requires about 24 different views.[80,81] In some cases, measuring tapes may be placed on the skin prior to photography to assess for changes in size.

Dermoscopy (epiluminescence microscopy, incident light microscopy, or surface microscopy) may be used as an adjunct to the physical examination in some clinical practices. The technique is not new but until recently was of limited use in the United States because of its timely and costly technical aspects and the lack of available formal training in its use.[82,83] Recently, improvements in the technique and equipment, consensus about terminology, and research validation have made the procedure more attractive. The diagnostic accuracy of the instrument directly

Table 63-8 Characteristics of Malignant Melanoma Skin Cancers

Type	Characteristics	Location	Other Features
Dysplastic nevus syndrome	Large number of atypical nevi with irregular margins and variable pigmentation	Sun-exposed and non-sun-exposed areas	Increased risk of developing MM May be sporadic or have a hereditary predisposition
Congenital nevus	May be giant or small Present at birth or shortly after birth	May occur anywhere on the body	Giant congenital nevus is rare, occurring in about 1 of 20,000 births, with a lifetime risk of malignant transformation of 2%–40% Small congenital nevus occurs in 1 of 100 births; lifetime risk of malignant transformation is not known
Lentigo maligna (Hutchinson freckle)	Flat, pigmented lesion that gradually enlarges Light tan to brown or black with irregular notched borders	Usually on the face, neck, or arms of the elderly	Begins as MM in situ and may take 5–50 yr to become invasive Usually occurs in the seventh decade of life Accounts for 5% of MM Three times more common in females
Superficial spreading malignant melanoma	Slightly raised lesion with an irregular border and variable, unevenly distributed pigmentation with shades of red, blue, brown, purple, and black	May be found anywhere on the body but usually on the upper back of men and women and the lower extremities of females	Most common of the MMs (about 70%–75%) With early diagnosis the five-year survival rate approaches 95% Long phase of horizontal growth prior to vertical growth and metastasis Usually occurs in the fifth decade of life Equally common in men and women
Acral lentinginous malignant melanoma	Initially the lesion is flat with irregular margins and pigmentation, but rapidly becomes raised and nodular	Soles, palms of hands, nailbeds, and oral mucosa	Early vertical growth and rapid metastasis May occur in Asians and blacks Accounts for 5%–10% of MM
Nodular malignant melanoma	Lesion is raised, nodular, and sometimes ulcerated Borders are irregular and color variegated Occasionally the tumor has no apparent visible pigmentation (amelanotic MM)	May occur on any part of the body, but most commonly on the legs and trunk	Does not seem to have a horizontal growth phase; grows vertically quickly with metastasis Twice as common in men Usually occurs in the fifth decade of life

Data from Weinstock[63]; Du Vivier[76]; Sober, Burstein.[77]

depends on the training and expertise of the clinician using the instrument.

Dermoscopy involves the application of oil to the surface of a lesion followed by examination. The oil eliminates some of the light reflection of skin and makes the surface of the skin more transparent.[82] Visual examination is aided by the use of various tools such as hand-held microscopes or computerized equipment that may include digital cameras.[83] This procedure may aid in the early detection of MM by assisting in distinguishing malignancy from benign pigmented skin lesions.[82]

Physical characteristics of lesions

Most BCCs begin as a small, firm, well-demarcated, dome-shaped papule (see Color Plate 11 and Table 63-7). A wide range of colors may be present, from pearly white to pink to red. Telangiectasias may or may not be present on the surface. Some lesions will have scaling plaques. As lesions progress, the center usually ulcerates and the borders develop a raised or rolled appearance.

The physical characteristics of SCC may not be as distinct (see Table 63-7). SCC often begins as a red, raised, firm papule. Crusting and ulceration is often seen (see Color Plate 12). It is not uncommon for the patient to report that the lesion is tender or painful.

A wide range of clinical characteristics may be noted in MM (see Table 63-8). It is often difficult to distinguish a dysplastic nevus from an MM. Within the different classifications of MM, a range of clinical characteristics may be observed (see Color Plates 13–16). Physical characteristics include asymmetrical, faded, or jagged borders; two or more colors in a lesion or a lesion that is a different color than the rest of the

Table 63-9 Biopsies for Suspicious Skin Lesions

Type	Indication	Purpose	Method	Healing	Advantage	Disadvantage
Punch	BCC Pigmented lesions	Incisional or excisional depending on size of lesion and instrument	Lesion is cut with a circular cutting instrument (punch); the cylinder of tissue is lifted and the base is transected with small scissors Specimen should not be removed with toothed forceps that may crush the tissue and interfere with pathologic examination of tissue Punch sizes range from 1.5–6 mm	By second intention or suture	Simple, easy to perform	Small specimen size may lead to difficult histopathologic examination Large (5–6 mm) punch biopsies may leave round, cosmetic defects
Shave	BCC	Removal of tissue that extends above the plane of surrounding skin	Injection of local anesthetic under the skin is used to elevate the lesion above the plane of surrounding tissue Scalpel or hand-held razor blade is used to shave off lesion Shave is made at depth between papillary and reticular dermis	By second intention	Simple Good cosmetic effect	Not enough tissue for histopathologic examination of suspected SCC or melanoma Nevi may return with central pigmentation
Saucerization	BCC Pigmented lesions SCC	Removal of tissue extending through dermis and down into subcutaneous fat	Scalpel or hand-held razor blade used to undercut the lesion at a 45° angle to the skin Incision carried down to fat	By second intention	Simple Provides complete dermal specimen	May result in hypopigmented, hyperpigmented, or hypertrophic scar Limited to areas of the skin that can close by second intention without cosmetic defect
Elliptical incision or excision	BCC Pigmented lesions SCC	Removal of large or deep lesions Removal of specimens with changes extending into the fascia	Scalpel is used to cut a fusiform or football-shaped incision with the lesion in the center Specimen is undercut with either scissors or scalpel and removed Blunt dissecting scissors are used to undermine the edges of the wound to maximize tissue healing and cosmesis	Sutures Some sites with concave surfaces such as facial areas heal better by second intention	Provides complete specimen for histopathologic examination Good cosmetic effect	More time-consuming and difficult Requires postsurgical wound care More discomfort and risk to the patient

Data from Robinson, Arndt, LeBoit, et al.[84]

pigmented lesions on a patient; diameter greater than 5 mm; nodular surface characteristics; and bleeding or ulceration.

Diagnostic Studies

Biopsy of the suspicious lesion is necessary for histologic examination. On occasion, the lesion may be so small that boundaries of excision are much the same as they would be for a biopsy. In this circumstance, the entire diagnostic and treatment phases may be carried out in one step. This is only prudent for small lesions when the lesion and disease-free margin can be obtained.

Biopsies can be accomplished using several techniques: punch (Figure 63-4), shave (Figure 63-5), saucerization (Figure 63-6), and incisional or excision (Figure 63-7) elliptical biopsies[84] (see Table 63-9). Although BCCs may be biopsied using any of those techniques, SCCs and lesions suspected of being MM — especially pigmented lesions — should be biopsied only using methods that remove the necessary tissue for complete dermatopathologic examination so that lesions may be correctly staged. Incisional or punch biopsies should be taken from the thickest portion of an elevated lesion and from the darkest area of a flat lesion.[74] Potential complications from biopsies include infection, bleeding, hyperpigmentation, hypopigmentation, adhesions, scarring, and problems with wound closure.

In some situations, immunohistochemistry (IHC) techniques must be used to assist with pathology study of the specimen. Biopsies that contain spindle cells, melanocytes without obvious characteristics of MM, or

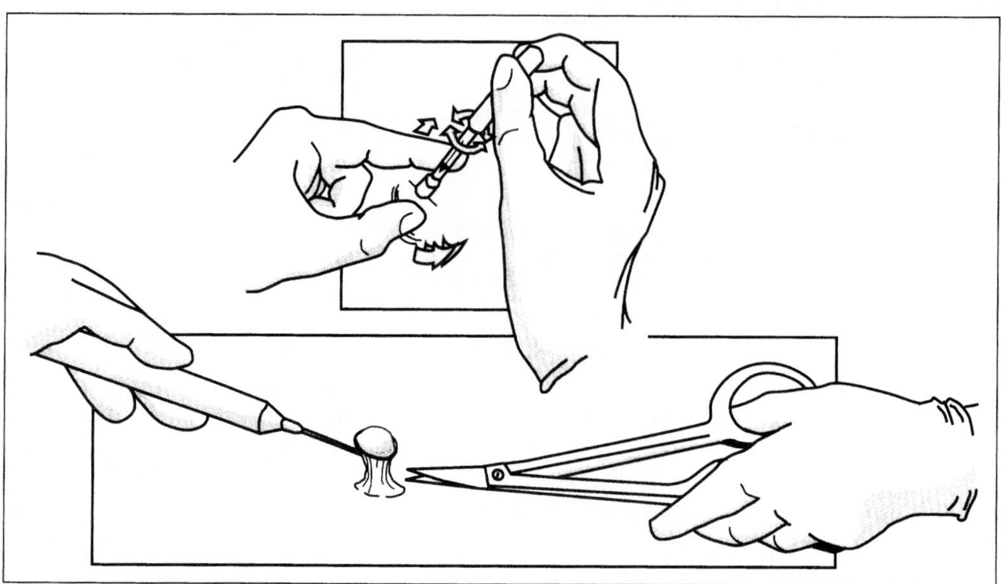

Figure 63-4 Punch biopsy of a lesion.

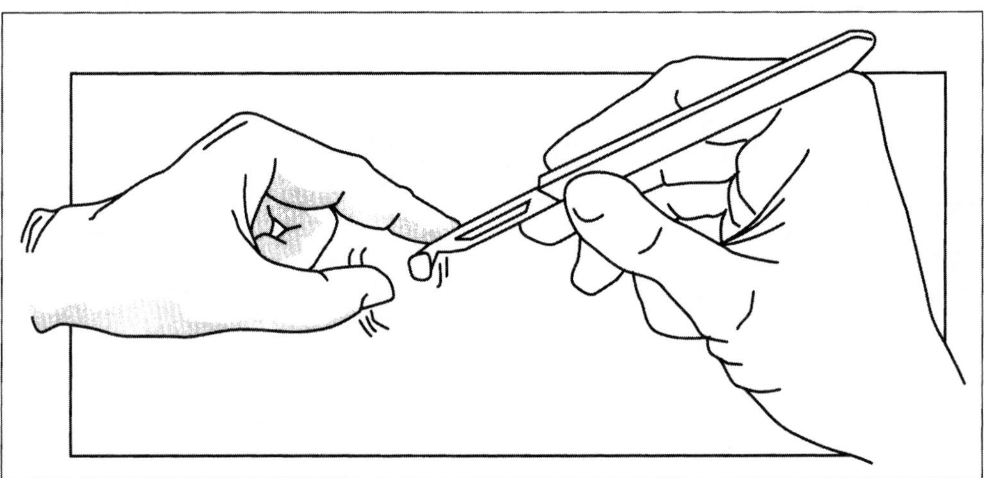

Figure 63-5 Shave biopsy of a lesion.

poorly differentiated specimens may require IHC techniques, for example. S-100, HMB-45, and MART-1 are molecules used in IHC review. S-100 is a calcium-channel-binding protein expressed in nearly all MMs. HMB-45 and MART-1 are markers for melanocytic-derived cells.[85,86]

A baseline chest x-ray may be part of the diagnostic work-up for primary cutaneous MM. Additional diagnostic studies may be necessary if regional or distant disease is suspected. Lymph node sampling is recommended for most MM patients with primary lesions greater than 1 mm in thickness, those who present with clinical lymphadenopathy, and those who present with other negative prognostic features. Blood tests such as complete blood count (CBC) and lactic dehydrogenase (LDH) may be performed. Liver scans or ultrasound may be indicated for persistent elevations in LDH to rule out liver metastases.[74] Additional studies may include computerized tomography (CT) scans, bone scans, magnetic resonance imaging (MRI), and positron emission tomography (PET) scans. More extensive work-up is necessary if patients complain of symptoms related to other body systems. For example, because MM may metastasize to the GI tract, patients with MM and GI symptoms should have further studies to rule out metastases.

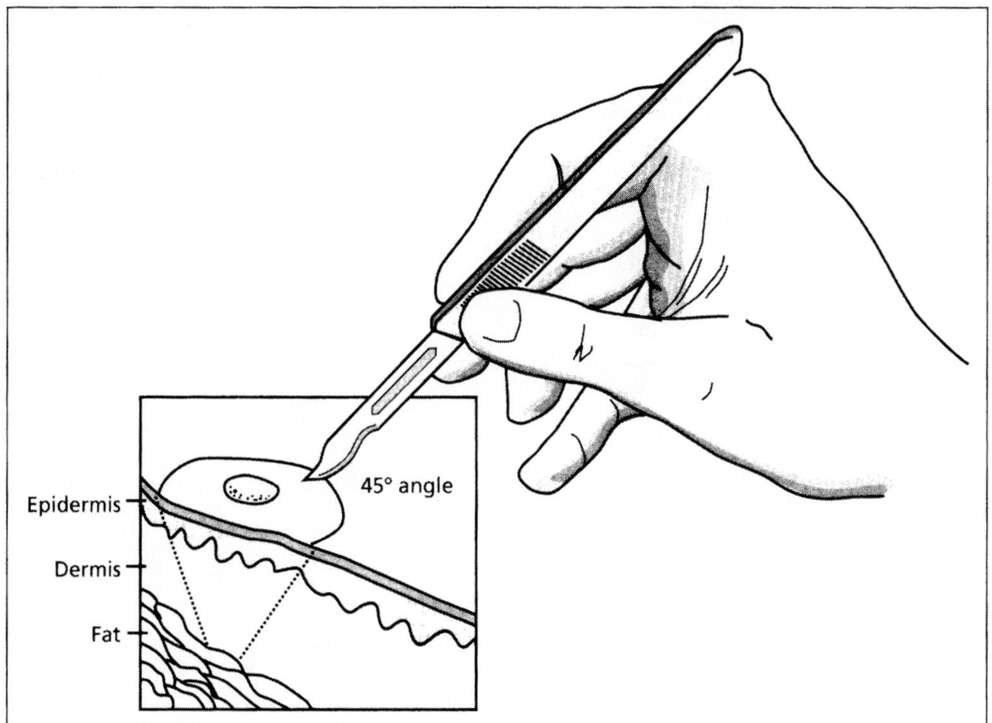

Figure 63-6 Saucerization biopsy of a lesion.

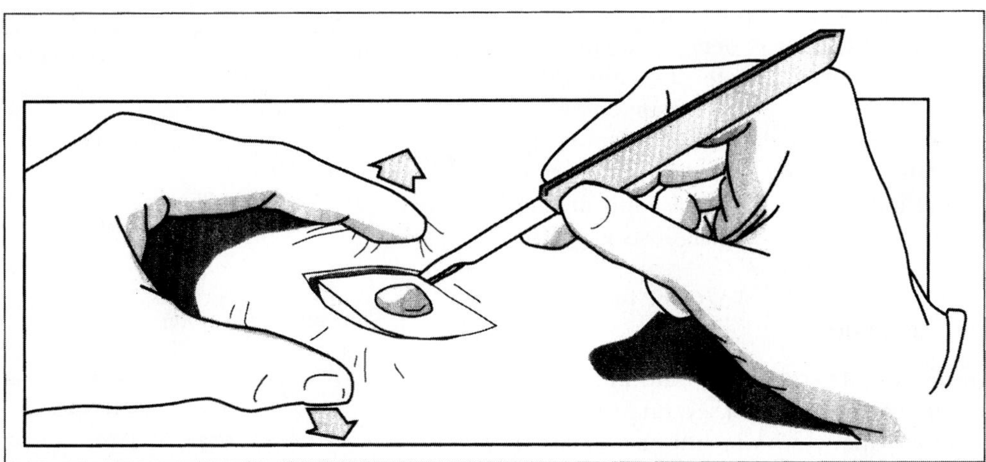

Figure 63-7 Incisional or excisional biopsy technique.

Prognostic Indicators

Nonmelanoma skin cancers

BCC is usually slow growing. Complete excision of a primary BCC suggests a 95% cure rate, and complete excision using Mohs surgery may further increase this percentage.[87] Primary lesions that are large and involve underlying structures, although rare, are more likely to have metastasized, in which case the prognosis is poorer. Extensive local invasion from BCC may cause significant cosmetic defects depending on the anatomical location of the lesion. For metastatic lesions, the one-year survival rate is less than 20%; the five-year survival rate is 10%.[87]

The course of SCC ranges along a continuum from slow-growing, locally invasive tumors to rapidly growing, widely invasive ones.[71] Overall, the five-year survival rate for SCC is 90% and its metastatic rate is 3%–6%. Dermal invasion and vertical tumor thickness are important prognostic indicators. Risk factors for recur-

Table 63-10 Survival Rates for Melanoma TNM and Staging Categories

Pathologic Stage	TNM	Thickness (mm)	Ulceration	Number of Positive Nodes	Nodal Size	Distant Metastasis	Number of Patients	Survival ± SE			
								1 Year	2 Years	5 Years	10 Years
IA	T1a	1	No	0	—	—	4510	99.7 ± 0.1	99.0 ± 0.2	95.3 ± 0.4	87.9 ± 1.0
IB	T1b	1	Yes or level IV, V	0	—	—	1380	99.8 ± 0.1	98.7 ± 0.3	90.9 ± 1.0	83.1 ± 1.5
	T2a	1.01–2.0	No	0	—	—	3285	99.5 ± 0.1	97.3 ± 0.3	89.0 ± 0.7	79.2 ± 1.1
IIA	T2b	1.01–2.0	Yes	0	—	—	958	98.2 ± 0.5	92.9 ± 0.9	77.4 ± 1.7	64.4 ± 2.2
	T3a	2.01–4.0	No	0	—	—	1717	98.7 ± 0.3	94.3 ± 0.6	78.7 ± 1.2	63.8 ± 1.7
IIB	T3b	2.01–4.0	Yes	0	—	—	1523	95.1 ± 0.6	84.8 ± 1.0	63.0 ± 1.5	50.8 ± 1.7
	T4a	> 4.0	No	0	—	—	563	94.8 ± 1.0	88.6 ± 1.5	67.4 ± 2.4	53.9 ± 3.3
IIC	T4b	> 4.0	Yes	0	—	—	978	89.9 ± 1.0	70.7 ± 1.6	45.1 ± 1.9	32.3 ± 2.1
IIIA	N1a	Any	No	1	Micro	—	252	95.9 ± 1.3	88.0 ± 2.3	69.5 ± 3.7	63.0 ± 4.4
	N2a	Any	No	2–3	Micro	—	130	93.0 ± 2.4	82.7 ± 3.8	63.3 ± 5.6	56.9 ± 6.8
IIIB	N1a	Any	Yes	1	Micro	—	217	93.3 ± 1.8	75.0 ± 3.2	52.8 ± 4.1	37.8 ± 4.8
	N2a	Any	Yes	2–3	Micro	—	111	92.0 ± 2.7	81.0 ± 4.1	49.6 ± 5.7	35.9 ± 7.2
	N1b	Any	No	1	Macro	—	122	88.5 ± 2.9	78.5 ± 3.7	59.0 ± 4.8	47.7 ± 5.8
	N2b	Any	No	2–3	Macro	—	93	76.8 ± 4.4	65.6 ± 5.0	46.3 ± 5.5	39.2 ± 5.8
IIIC	N1b	Any	Yes	1	Macro	—	98	77.9 ± 4.3	54.2 ± 5.2	29.0 ± 5.1	24.4 ± 5.3
	N2b	Any	Yes	2–3	Macro	—	109	74.3 ± 4.3	44.1 ± 4.9	24.0 ± 4.4	15.0 ± 3.9
	N3	Any	Any	4	Micro/macro	—	396	71.0 ± 2.4	49.8 ± 2.7	26.7 ± 2.5	18.4 ± 2.5
IV	M1a	Any	Any	Any	Any	Skin, SQ	179	59.3 ± 3.7	36.7 ± 3.6	18.8 ± 3.0	15.7 ± 2.9
	M1b	Any	Any	Any	Any	Lung	186	57.0 ± 3.7	23.1 ± 3.2	6.7 ± 2.0	2.5 ± 1.5
	M1a	Any	Any	Any	Any	Other visceral	793	40.6 ± 1.8	23.6 ± 1.5	9.5 ± 1.1	6.0 ± 0.9
Total							17,600				

Reprinted with permission from Balch CM, Buzaid AC, Soong SJ et al: final version of the American Joint Comittee on Cancer staging system for cutaneous melanoma. *J Clin Oncol* 19:3635–3648, 2001[88]

rence and metastasis are related to the cause, location, treatment, morphologic characteristics of the tumor, and immunocompetent status of the patient. SCC arising in areas of skin that have been irradiated or burned have a higher metastatic rate (20% and 18%, respectively). SCC arising in areas of sun-damaged skin rarely metastasize, although SCC of the lower lip has a metastatic rate of approximately 15%. SCC originating in the oral mucosa, on the penis, and on the vulva tend to be more invasive at diagnosis and also have a higher rate of metastases.[87]

Malignant melanoma

The prognosis of MM varies widely with the extent of disease and with consideration of several prognostic factors. In general, patients with in situ or very small (1.0 mm or smaller) lesions with favorable prognostic factors have almost a 90% ten-year survival rate, while patients with metastatic disease at presentation have a ten-year survival rate of less than 16%.[88] Survival rate by stage is listed in Table 63-10.[88] Prognostic factors are important in MM. Those that have been included in the revised staging system for MM are outlined in Table 63-11.[88] Additional prognostic factors have been suggested (Table 63-12[74,88,89]) and continue to be studied.

Table 63-11 Prognostic Factors for Malignant Cutaneous Melanoma by Stage

Stage	Factors	Prognostic Effect
I and II	Melanoma thickness	Worse prognosis with increasing thickness
	Ulceration	Increased risk of metastasis and decreased survival rates with ulceration
	Level of invasion (T1 lesions only)	Worse prognosis with increasing level of invasion
III	Regional lymph nodes (macroscopic or microscopically positive)	Worse prognosis with increasing number of positive lymph nodes
	Ulceration	Increased risk of metastasis and decreased survival rates with ulceration
	Intralymphatic metastasis	Worse prognosis when present
IV	Location of metastases	Worse prognosis with visceral versus extremity metastases; metastasis to the lung has an intermediate prognosis
	LDH	Worse prognosis with LDH elevation (measured by two or more values at least 24 hours apart)

Data from Balch, Buzaid, Soong, et al.[88]

Table 63-12 Additional Prognostic Factors for Cutaneous Malignant Melanoma

Factor	Prognostic Effect
Age	Better prognosis with younger age
Gender	Improved survival in females
Evidence of regression	Suggested better prognosis
Tumor site	Better prognosis with extremity lesions; worse prognosis with lesions on the hands and feet, acral lesions and intermediate-thickness lesions on the back, posterior arm, posterior neck, and scalp
Host immune response	Better prognosis with presence of tumor-infiltrating lymphocytes
Vascular invasion	Predictor of nodal metastasis
Mitotic rate	Worse prognosis with greater mitotic rate (number of mitoses/mm^2 in specimen)
Number of metastatic sites	Worse prognosis with increasing numbers of sites
Presence of resectable, solitary metastases	Better prognosis

Data from Langley, Barnhill, Mihm, et al.[74]; Balch, Buzaid, Soong, et al.[88]; Zettersten, Shaikh, Ramirez, et al.[89]

Table 63-13 American Joint Committee on Cancer Staging for Nonmelanoma Skin Cancers

Stage	Description
Stage 0 (Tis-N0-M0)	• Carcinoma in situ • No regional lymph node or distant metastasis
Stage I (T1-N0-M0)	• Tumor 2 cm or less in greatest dimension • No regional lymph node or distant metastasis
Stage II (T2-N0-M0 or T3-N0-M0)	• Tumor more than 2 cm but no more than 5 cm in greatest dimension (T2) or tumor more than 5 cm in greatest dimension (T3) • No regional lymph node or distant metastasis
Stage III (T4-N0-M0 or any T-N1-M0)	• Tumor invades deep extradermal structure (i.e., cartilage, skeletal muscle, or bone) or any tumor size with regional lymph node metastasis
Stage IV (any T-any N-M1)	• Any tumor size, any regional lymph node metastasis, and distant metastasis

Data from Fleming ID, Cooper JS, Henson DE, et al (eds.).[90]

Classification and Staging

Nonmelanoma Skin Cancers

Clinical staging is accomplished by inspection and palpation of lesions and involved lymph nodes plus imaging studies of any underlying bony structures.[90] Pathologic staging is accomplished by the examination of completely resected tumors and lymph nodes. The TNM categories for both clinical and pathologic classifications of NMSC are the same and are grouped as stages I–IV (Table 63-13). The histologic grade of specimens is described as grades 1–4. G1 is a well-differentiated tumor, G2 is a moderately well-differentiated tumor, G3 is a poorly differentiated tumor, and G4 is an undifferentiated tumor. GX denotes a grade that cannot be assessed.[91]

Malignant Melanoma

Clinical staging of MM is based on biopsy results, clinical examination, and radiological procedures.[86] Biopsied lesions may be described using either of two systems: Clark's level or Breslow's measurement (see Figure 63-3). Clark's level describes the lesion based on the depth of invasion into the dermis and subcutaneous fat. Level I (in situ) lesions do not penetrate the basement membrane. Level II lesions extend through the basement membrane and into the papillary dermis. Level III lesions reach into the reticular/papillary junction, and Level IV lesions invade the reticular dermis. The thickness of the dermis may vary depending on the anatomical site and individual differences and may affect the accuracy of Clark's level. The success of this method of microstaging depends on the examiner's ability to correctly recognize the microscopic anatomy of the skin.[72] The level of invasion is correlated to the metastatic potential of the lesion.[73]

Tumor thickness is described by the Breslow method. The lesion is measured and defined as the distance from the epidermis to the deepest identifiable layer of contiguous MM cells.[72] Measurements are reported in millimeters.

Surgical staging should follow in all cases for which surgery will offer a clinical benefit. Depending on the extent of disease, surgical staging may include wide local excision, sentinel lymph node biopsy, or lymph node dissection.

The American Joint Committee on Cancer (AJCC) has revised the MM staging system to encorporate research-proven prognostic factors and to organize subsets of patients by expected outcomes.[88] Several changes can be noted from the previous system: use of Clark's level for stage I MM only, inclusion of ulceration as a determinant of T and N staging, designation of satellite metastases as an N category, movement of lesions larger than 4.0 mm from stage IIIA to IIC, addition of the number of nodal metastases and metastatic tumor burden as N determinants, separation of lung metastasis into a distinct M category, and incorporation of sentinel lymph node sampling results (Table 63–14).[88] It is important not to confuse stage with Clark's level, both of which are reported in Roman numerals.

Table 63-14 AJCC Cancer Stage Grouping for Cutaneous Melanoma

	Pathologic Staging			
Stage	T	N	M	Criteria
0	Tis	N0	M0	In situ melanoma
IA	T1a	N0	M0	≤ 1.0 mm without ulceration and Clark's level II/III
IB	T1b	N0	M0	≤ 1.0 mm with ulceration or Clark's level IV/V
	T2a	N0	M0	1.01–1.0 mm without ulceration
IIA	T2b	N0	M0	1.01–1.0 mm with ulceration
	T3a	N0	M0	1.01–4.0 mm without ulceration
IIB	T3b	N0	M0	1.01–4.0 mm with ulceration
	T4a	N0	M0	> 4.0 mm without ulceration
IIC	T4b	N0	M0	> 4.0 mm with ulceration
IIIA	T1-4a	N1a	M0	Primary without ulceration, 1 microscopic* node
	T1-4a	N2a	M0	Primary without ulceration, 2–3 microscopic* nodes
IIIB	T1-4b	N1a	M0	Primary with ulceration, 1 microscopic* node
	T1-4b	N2a	M0	Primary with ulceration, 2–3 microscopic* nodes
	T1-4a	N1b	M0	Primary without ulceration, 1 macroscopic† node
	T1-4a	N2b	M0	Primary without ulceration, 2–3 macroscopic† nodes
	T1-4a/b	N2c	M0	Primary with or without ulceration, intransit metastasis without positive nodes
IIIC	T1-4b	N1b	M0	Primary with ulceration, 1 macroscopic† node
	T1-4b	N2b	M0	Primary with ulceration, 2–3 macroscopic† nodes
	Any T	N3	M0	Any size primary, 4 or more nodes, or matted nodes, or intransit metastasis/satellite(s) *with* positive nodes
IV	Any T	Any N	M1a	Distant skin, subcutaneous, or nodal metastasis with normal LDH
	Any T	Any N	M1b	Lung metastases with normal LDH
	Any T	Any N	M1c	All other visceral metastases with normal LDH *or* any distant metastasis with elevated LDH

*Micrometastases diagnosed after sentinel or elective lymphadenectomy.

†Macrometastases defined as clinically detectable nodal metastases confirmed by therapeutic lymphadenectomy or nodal metastases exhibiting gross extracapsular extension.

Data from Balch, Burzaid, Soong, et al.[88]

Therapeutic Approaches and Nursing Care

Initial treatment of both NMSC and MM relies on biopsy and histopathologic evaluation of the suspicious lesion. In the case of MM, removal of the entire lesion for histopathologic evaluation is the method of choice. This approach enables the pathologist to most accurately assess the primary lesion and prognostic indicators that will guide definitive treatment.

Nonmelanoma Skin Cancers

Complete removal of the lesion, including tumor-free margins, is the goal of treatment. Treatment choices depend on the tumor type, size, location, and extent of disease. Skin cancers usually begin as small, locally invasive lesions that can be easily removed via a variety of methods with minimal morbidity.[92] Extensive or recurrent skin cancer, however, may require complex surgical or radiation therapy, may be more expensive and difficult to treat, and has a less certain outcome. Treatments for NMSC include surgical excision, electrosurgery, Mohs micrographic surgery, cryosurgery, radiation therapy, and chemotherapy. Surgical excision and Mohs micrographic surgery yield a complete specimen that can be examined by a pathologist. Laser removal, cryosurgery, and electrosurgery should be used only when the diagnosis is certain and the lesion is small, as they will not produce a specimen for histopathologic diagnosis and evaluation for free margins.

Surgery

Surgical excision with tumor-free margins is the goal for most lesions. Primary closure or repair with skin graft or flaps usually produces good cosmetic results.[87] Margins of 4 mm around the visible tumor are recommended.[71] BCCs with tumor present in the lateral margins at the time of surgical excision may result in recurrence in approximately one-third of cases.[69] These recurrences usually present early and can often be surgically excised again. Positive deep BCC margins may result in deep, sometimes delayed recurrences at the tumor site and invasion of other structures.

Surgical excision may be recommended for SCC occurring within radiation fields. Further radiation therapy may be limited in those cases due to the exposure limits of normal tissue. Excision of the lesion and entire radiation scar removes any additional foci in the area.[71] SCCs should be removed with margins of 3–5 mm.[87] Margins of 6 mm are recommended for large tumors (> 3 cm), invasive tumors, and those on high-risk areas (scalp, ears, nose, eyelids, or lips). Surgical excision is often the treatment of choice for SCC overlying bone and cartilage and for SCC occurring in scars, ulcers, and sinuses.[87]

Electrosurgery. Electrosurgery involves the use of heat to cut tissue. It is fast, efficient, and relatively inexpensive but relies significantly on the expertise of the operator.[71,84] When combined with curettage, electrosurgery may be useful in the removal of distinct, superficial BCCs. SCCs that are small, located on flat surfaces, and do not invade past the dermis or upper subcutaneous tissue may also be removed in this manner.[71] Normal tissue around SCC that is transformed into radiation scars may be intolerable to additional radiation exposure. Electrosurgery may be useful in those cases. After the tumor is anesthetized, a sharp curette is used to scoop out the gelatinous carcinoma. Bleeding is stopped, and the perimeter of tissue is destroyed by using electrocautery or electrodessication. The wound is explored again with a curette to ensure complete removal of the lesion. Two or three cycles of curettage followed by electrodessication may be used.

Mohs micrographic surgery. This procedure is often used for tumors that are recurrent, are large, have indistinct margins, and are in a location where excision with wide margins of healthy skin removal would be surgically or cosmetically unacceptable.[71,93] With this procedure, the tumor is excised under local anesthesia using horizontal frozen sections that are microscopically examined during the surgery (Figure 63-8). Any margins of areas with residual tumor can continue to be selectively excised while normal tissues are preserved, until clear margins are obtained. For removal of primary skin cancer, Mohs offers a 95%–99% chance for complete removal without recurrence.[84]

Cryosurgery. Cryosurgery is the use of freezing temperatures to destroy tissue. It may follow shave excisions. A cryogen such as carbon dioxide, nitrous oxide, or liquid nitrogen must be used. The cryogen can be swabbed or sprayed on the lesion. Another method involves the use of a cryoprobe. It is cooled and then applied to the lesion for seconds or minutes. The deepest part of the tumor must reach at least –50°C during freezing. Cryosurgery for SCC may be used to treat superficial tumors and carcinoma in situ.[87]

Radiation therapy

Radiation therapy (RT) may be useful in treating both BCC and SCC lesions. Patients who are poor surgical candidates, elderly, or frail may still be able to undergo RT. This option may be the preferred treatment for small lesions in areas that would be difficult to excise, such as the eyelid, ear pinna, nasolabial fold, alar nasi, and lips.[71] RT for BCC lesions smaller than 5 cm in diameter may achieve good results, but lesions larger than 5 cm have higher recurrence rates when treated with RT alone.[87] Because SCCs have a tendency to follow embryonal planes of closure, tumors may invade deeply and not be amenable to cure by other treatments. Radiation therapy can penetrate through tissue and help destroy deeper tumors.[71] In both tumor types, doses between 4000 and 6000 cGy are often used and can be fractionated so as to decrease side effects. Treatment planning is based on the location and size of the lesion. Due to the risk of side effects to normal tissue, RT is rarely recommended for lesions overlying areas of bone or cartilage.[87] For recurrent skin cancers previously treated with RT, further radiation may not be an option owing to poor vascularization and exposure limits of normal tissue in the field.

Chemotherapy

Topical and intralesional fluorouracil (5-FU) has been used to treat BCCs. Topical applications are usually prescribed twice a day for several weeks for small, superficial tumors in patients who are unable to tolerate other treatments. Recurrence in patients treated with 5-FU is higher than that in patients treated with other therapies.[87] Intralesional 5-FU has been used in nodular lesions. Intralesional interferon has been used as an investigational treatment for both BCCs and SCCs.

Table 63-15 Surgical Margins and Sentinel Lymph Node Biopsy

Size of Primary Lesion	Surgical Margin (cm)	Sentinel Lymph Node Biopsy	Therapeutic Lymph Node Dissection
In situ	0.5–1	No*	No*
< 1 mm	1	No*	No*
1–4 mm	1–2	Yes/no	Yes *(if SLN + or presence of lymphadenopathy)*
> 4 mm	2–3	Yes *(may proceed to therapeutic lymph node dissection in some cases)*	Yes *(if SLN + or presence of lymphadenopathy)*

*In the absence of clinical data to suggest high-risk lesions or spread of disease.

Data from Morton, Essner, Kirkwood, Parker[72]; Morton, Essner[73]; Lamb, Halpern, Hwu[86]; Essner[94]; Karakousis[95]; Urist.[96]

1. Tumor is debulked by curettage

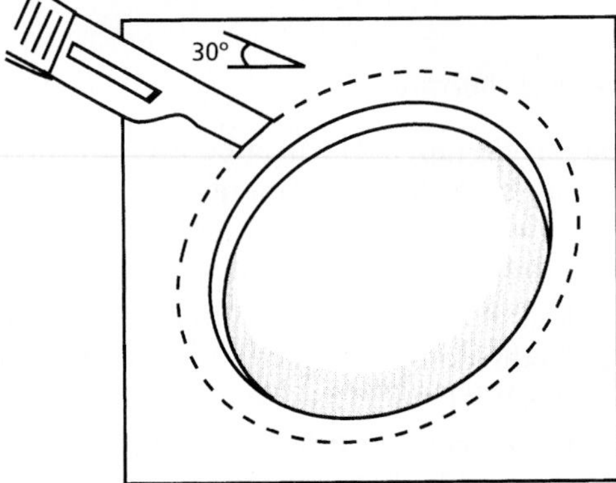

2. Wound base is excised

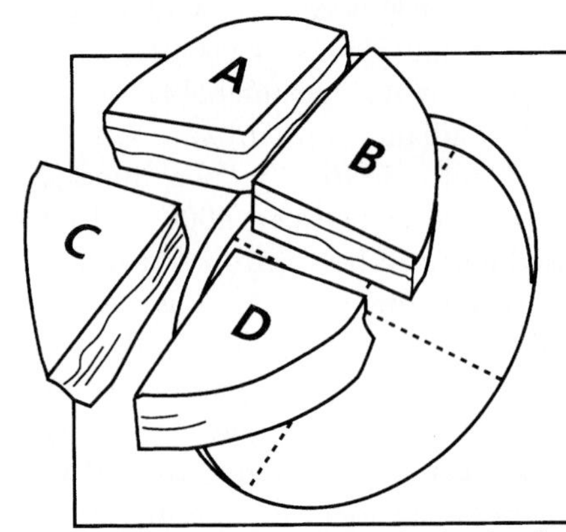

3. Excised wound base is divided and sectioned

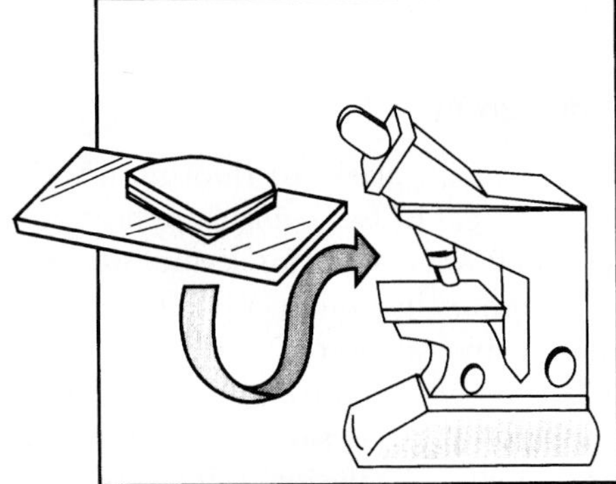

4. Each section is examined for residual tumor

Figure 63-8 Mohs' micrographic surgical technique.

Severe irritation may occur with topical 5-FU. Patients should apply the chemotherapy with a cotton-tipped applicator or latex glove to avoid contact with other skin surfaces. In general a dressing is not applied. If the physician requests a dressing, it should be gauze with tape instead of adherent-type dressings. Because topical 5-FU can lead to a significant photosensitizing reaction, patients must be instructed to avoid UVR exposure.

Retinoids

Oral isotretinoin has been studied as a treatment for SCC. Partial to complete regression of tumors has been noted. Isotretinoin has also been used as a chemoprevention agent to decrease the occurrence of second primary tumors in SCC.[87]

Malignant Melanoma

The treatment of MM is based on the location, appearance, and extent of disease and the condition of the patient. Initial treatment consists of complete excision of the primary lesion with disease-free margins. Decisions regarding lymph node sampling are based on the size of the primary lesion and clinical staging information. Lymph node sampling is rarely warranted for patients with nonulcerated, thin (≤1 mm) MM. For those with primary lesions larger than 1 mm or with ulcerated lesions, lymph node mapping and sentinel lymph node (SLN) biopsy are common recommendations (Table 63-15[72,73,86,94–96]).

There is no standard treatment for patients with locally recurrent or intransit metastases. Surgical excision, intralesional immunotherapy, regional chemotherapy, systemic chemotherapy and/or immunotherapy, and radiation therapy may all be of use in that setting.

Recommendations for treatment of metastatic MM are based on the number and location of metastases. Solitary lesions or those of a limited number may be amenable to surgical excision that can result in significant palliation and even long-term survival. For patients with multiple metastatic sites in multiple organs, chemotherapy, RT, and immunotherapy may be utilized.

Surgery

Surgical excision. Complete surgical excision should be wide and should include disease-free margins. Defects can usually be repaired by primary closure, although skin flaps may be necessary. The surgical margin size has been the subject of much controversy. In the past, margins of 3–5 cm were advocated for lesions of all sizes. Current recommendations are shown in Table 63-15. Excision of lesions larger than 4 mm should include skin and underlying adipose tissue. No improvements have been gained from the continuance of the excision through muscle fascia.[94] Amputation of the digit at the interphalangeal joint is necessary for subungual MM, and larger lesions may require more proximal amputation. Ear MMs may be successfully excised using a wedge excision and reconstruction without ear amputation.[72] Lesions on the face or vital structures may be excised with more limited margins depending on the situation. The use of Mohs micrographic surgery for MM is controversial but has been used for low-risk, thin MM on the face.[72,94]

Lymph node dissection. Lymph node dissection (LND) remains a controversial issue in the treatment of MM. The observation of the usual stepwise progression of melanoma from primary lesion to regional and then distant spread has been the basis for the use of LND. Elective lymph node dissection (ELND) is the removal of regional lymph nodes in the absence of clinical evidence of spread of disease. Theoretically, ELND should eliminate the most likely source of metastasis and translate into a survival advantage. Previous retrospective studies have shown that as many as 80% of patients with limited-stage MM who underwent ELND had uninvolved lymph nodes at the time of surgical excision of the primary tumor. Recommending ELND would, therefore, subject a large percentage of patients to an unnecessary procedure with potential complications and no benefit.[72,73] Although ELND may have benefits in patients with lesions of intermediate thickness (0.76–4.0 mm), it offers little or no benefit for those with thin MM lesions (< 0.76 mm); however, this has not been proven by randomized, propective studies.[72,94,96] ELND may not improve the survival of patients with tumors larger than 4 mm, as these individuals have a high incidence of distant as well as local metastases.[96] ELND has been largely abandoned in favor of sentinel lymph node biopsy.

Therapeutic lymph node dissection (TLND) should be performed when lymph nodes are found to be positive by physical examination or by biopsy.[96] TLND is often more extensive than ELND, involving the removal of both superficial and deep nodes. Modified dissections may be recommended in the neck to preserve cosmesis and function.[96] Infection, flap necrosis, seroma, and nerve dysfunction are all potential side effects of lymphadenectomy. Lymphedema may also occur. With axillary node dissection, lymphedema remains limited to the affected arm. Cervical lymphadenectomy has low morbidity. With inguinal node dissection, extremity edema is reported in as many as 39% of patients.[95] The majority of these patients exhibit mild lymphedema, but as many as 10% may develop debilitating edema.[72,73]

Lymphatic mapping and sentinel lymph node biopsy. Lymphatic mapping and SLN biopsy is a minimally invasive technique used to identify and sample regional lymph nodes. With this procedure, the first or "sentinel" lymph node(s) draining a primary MM lesion can be identified and sampled. If the SLN biopsy is negative, no further lymph node dissection is required. If the SLN is positive, a regional lymph node dissection is warranted.[97]

Lymphoscintigraphy may first be used to identify the draining basin and therefore improve the identification of the sentinel lymph node(s).[95] Extremity lesions usually drain into regional lymph basins in either the axilla or the groin.[73] Trunk, head, and neck lesions may flow to more than one lymph node basin. In lymphoscintigraphy, radiolabeled substances are injected preoperatively into the site of the primary MM. Hand-held gamma detectors are used to pick up the tracer and identify the draining nodes.[72,95] The skin is marked to identify the location of the SLN. This procedure can identify the regional lymph node basins at risk for metastases but cannot determine the presence or absence of metastases.

Intraoperative lymphatic mapping of the SLN can be accomplished by the injection of a tracer substance such as vital blue dye or a radiocolloid.[72] Injections of 0.5–1.0 mL are given into the primary MM site or on either side of the biopsy scar.[95] The dye may take 5–20 minutes to reach the SLN.[94] Injections may be repeated every 20 minutes due to the rapid venous drainage of the dye.[73] An incision is made over the identified lymph node basin (an area previously marked during lymphoscintography). As the injected blue dye first stains the lymphatic channel and then stains the draining lymph nodes, SLNs can be identified. These nodes can then be excised and examined by frozen or permanent section analysis.[72,94]

Using this method, 20% of patients with limited-stage MM are found to be positive for regional lymph node metastasis. They can be treated with lymphadenectomy, while the other 80% can be spared the complications of the procedure.[73] The incidence of wound infection, seroma, and necrosis following selective lymph node biopsy is less than 5%.

Surgery for site-specific metastasis. Surgical excision of intransit metastases can be an option. Patients with small numbers of lesions and slow-growing lesions may be candidates for such excision.[72,74]

In the majority of patients, distant metastases in MM present initially in one organ site. Most commonly, the initial metastasis is to the lung, followed by the skin, lymph nodes, brain, liver, and GI tract. Surgical resection in the setting of minimal morbidity and mortality risk may result in significant survival advantages in some patients. Those patients with small numbers of metastases in few sites are the optimal candidates for this procedure. Surgical resection of metastases is not usually considered a good option for those whose anticipated survival is imminently short.[94] Surgery may also be considered for palliation of symptoms. Resection of GI metastases may relieve bowel obstructions, for example.

Chemotherapy

Single-agent chemotherapy. Since the 1970s, dacarbazine (DTIC) has been the standard of comparison for all other antineoplastic agents used to treat MM. In patients with soft tissue metastases, overall response rates as high as 20% have been documented with single-agent DTIC.[75,98] Subcutaneous, lymph node, and pulmonary metastases are the most likely to respond to DTIC, but the therapy has been largely ineffective against visceral, bone, and brain metastases.[99] Complete remissions are rare, and the median duration of response has been 4–6 months.[99] Side effects of DTIC vary with the dose and may include mild hematologic toxicity, nausea and vomiting, photosensitivity, and liver toxicity.

Temozolomide is an analog of DTIC. At physiologic pH, it transforms to the active metabolite of DTIC. Because temozolomide can cross the blood–brain barrier, the potential exists for its use as a treatment of brain metastases. In clinical studies comparing DTIC with temozolomide in patients with metastatic melanoma, similar response rates and overall survival resulted for both agents. Regression of brain lesions in 25% of patients in a phase II study of temozolomide was noted.[99]

Nitrosoureas, vinca alkaloids, cisplatin, paclitaxel, and docetaxel have also been used in the treatment of MM.

Combination regimens. Regimens including several different chemotherapies have been the subject of clinical trials, sometimes showing modest improvement over single-agent DTIC. Of particular note is the Dartmouth regimen, which includes DTIC, BCNU, cisplatin, and tamoxifen. Initial response rates with this regimen were as high as 50%.[100] Other investigators have replicated this combination and obtained response rates of 27%–62%.[98,100] Although the improved response rate is encouraging, no improvement in overall survival was noted when compared to single-agent DTIC and the therapy causes significant toxicity.[99] Several additional combination regimens have been under investigation. In some cases, response rates showed some improvement. Few phase III randomized trials have been completed with these regimens; for those that have been completed, no survival advantage has been shown against single-agent DTIC.[99]

The combination of immunotherapy agents with chemotherapy regimens has also been the subject of investigation. Interferon alfa (IFN-α) and interleukin 2 (IL-2) were added to the Dartmouth regimen in a study of 42 patients, resulting in an overall response rate of 57%, with a 24% complete response and a 33% partial response rate.[74] The toxicity of this regimen was significant, however.

Dose intensification with and without stem cell support is another area of investigation in the treatment of MM. There is some indication that MM has a dose-responsive nature with a few chemotherapeutic agents, particularly cisplatin.

Regional chemotherapy. When a relatively confined area is the target of treatment, regional rather than systemic administration of chemotherapy may be a therapeutic avenue. With this approach, systemic side effects can be diminished or avoided and higher concentrations of drugs can be delivered to the tumor site. Liver metastases from MM, for example, may be treated by intrahepatic infusion of chemotherapy with or without chemoembolization. One regional approach to treatment for intransit metastases in the extremities, known as isolated limb perfusion (ILP), is usually combined with hyperthermia. Arterial inflow and venous outflow vessels in the targeted area are isolated and cannulated, and collateral circulation of the area is interrupted. Venous blood is collected from the cannulated veins, pumped through an oxygenated extracorporeal circuit, warmed, and then pumped back through the cannulated artery. Tissue temperatures are monitored during the procedure. After completion of the perfusion, an electrolyte solution is used as a rinse, cannulas are removed, and vessels are repaired.[101]

Chemotherapy can be injected into the blood at several points in the ILP procedure, increasing the exposure of the tumor to the chemotherapy. Single-agent melphalan is the most commonly used chemotherapy with regional perfusion, although other agents such as nitrogen mustard, cisplatin, tumor necrosis factor, and IL-2 have also been employed. Combinations of these agents have been studied as well. Overall response rates for these therapies have been as high as 65% with complete remission rates of 44%.[100] Acute local tissue reactions are possible and are graded based on their severity.[101] Despite the attempts to contain the chemotherapy to the targeted area, some systemic effects of the drugs may occur, as evidenced by severe hypotension in 10% of patients and a reaction similar to adult respiratory distress syndrome (ARDS) in 16% of patients receiving melphalan.[100,101]

Radiation therapy

Radiation therapy may be of use in the treatment of MM, although it is rarely the primary mode of therapy for this disease. Exceptions include cases involving patients who cannot undergo surgery because of physical limitations or patients whose lesions are not amenable to surgery. An example might be a case of extensive facial LMM requiring extensive reconstruction in an elderly person.[102] Radiation therapy may serve as an adjuvant treatment when combined with surgical resection for patients with lesions at particularly high risk of recurrence, including primary lesions larger than 4 mm, positive surgical margins, locally recurrent disease, multiple positive lymph nodes, and lymph nodes with extracapsular extension.[97,102] In those cases, RT would follow surgical excision. This therapy may also be useful for palliation of symptoms of metastases such as bone pain, obstruction, and spinal cord compression. Approximately 60%–70% of patients with brain metastases exhibit improved performance status after receiving RT.[97]

Immunotherapy

The potentially immunoresponsive nature of MM has been suggested by both clinical and histopathologic observations. Clinically, MM has a highly variable nature. The course of the disease may wax and wane over time.[75] Rarely, and usually in association with bacterial infections, spontaneous regressions have occurred in distant metastatic sites.[75,103] In addition, there is evidence of increased incidence of MM in immuncompromised individuals. These observations all point to a host immune response in case of MM. Lymphoid infiltrates are regularly found on histopathologic examination of MM specimens, suggesting an activated host response that occurs directly at the tumor site.[75]

Immunotherapy is an active area of research in the treatment of MM. Several agents, given either alone or in combination, have been examined. In many cases, these agents are used with chemotherapy in combined modality regimens. The two areas of greatest promise focus on the use of immunotherapy as adjuvant treatment for high-risk patients with surgical resection and for treatment of patients with metastatic disease. In either case, it is most effective as a treatment for patients with small tumor burden. As opposed to chemotherapy, the maximal effect from immunotherapy may not be seen until after 3–4 months of treatment, but the responses may be more durable.[103]

Immunotherapy of MM may be broadly classified as either specific or nonspecific. Specific immunotherapy agents target the tumor selectively; monoclonal antibody therapy is an example. Nonspecific immunotherapy agents (e.g., interferon) stimulate the immune system as a whole.

Interferon. Trials of alfa-inteferon (IFN-α) as a treatment for MM began in the late 1970s. This cytokine is thought to both directly affect malignant cells and indirectly affect them by augmenting and stimulating the host immune response.[104] IFN has been found to have synergistic activity with several chemotherapy agents and with other immunotherapy agents. It may be administered by subcutaneous, intravenous, and intralesional routes. The presence of visceral disease is a predictor of poor outcome because it signals the existence of a larger tumor burden. Central nervous system (CNS) disease is not well treated with IFN because of poor penetration of the drug into the CNS.[104]

In the adjuvant setting for high-risk patients with resected disease, systemic therapy has widely been unhelpful with the exception of IFN. A study by the Eastern Cooperative Oncology Group (EST1684) was the pivotal trial introducing this strategy. In this study, intensive intravenous IFN (20 MU/m^2/day) was administered to patients for 1 month followed by subcutaneous IFN (10 MU/m^2 three times per week) for 11 months. Considerable toxicity was experienced with this regimen. Fifty percent of subjects required dose adjustments in the first month, and more than 50% required such adjustments during the final 11 months.[105] However, a significant increase in relapse-free survival was demonstrated and a trend toward increased overall survival was observed.[105] After a median follow-up of

7 years, this regimen has been shown to significantly prolong overall survival (OS) and disease-free survival (DFS). The five-year relapse-free survival rate was 37% in patients who received high-dose IFN, compared to 26% in the observation group. The five-year OS rate was 47% in the treatment group versus 36% in the control group.[99] A subsequent trial (E1690) used a three-arm design to compare the EST1684 high-dose IFN regimen with low-dose IFN over 2 years against a control group. A DFS advantage was noted in the high-dose IFN group but no OS advantage was seen, bringing into question the use of high-dose IFN.[99,106] Several confounding variables were noted with this study, however.[99,106] In a later intergroup trial (E1694), high-dose IFN compared against a ganglioside vaccine showed increased relapse-free survival and OS in the IFN arm.[106] The toxicity of high-dose IFN regimens remains significant, however.[107] Clinical trials continue in an attempt to discern whether lower doses of IFN or alternate administration schedules can achieve similar or better results.[99,106]

Interleukin-2. Interleukin-2 (IL-2) stimulates several aspects of the immune system. It is another example of a nonspecific immunotherapy treatment for MM. In clinical trials, IL-2 has been given both alone and in combination with lymphokine-activated killer (LAK) cells and with tumor-infiltrating lymphocytes (TIL). It is thought to have some synergistic activity when given in combination with IFN and is part of many chemotherapy and hormonal therapy combination regimens for MM.

Clinical trials of IL-2 have employed different dosage ranges and administration routes. High-dose therapy (up to 720,000 IU/kg) given by intravenous bolus has resulted in response rates ranging from 5% to 22%.[108] In a pivotal study of high-dose IL-2, significant, life-threatening toxicities were observed, including sepsis, respiratory distress, and hypotension, which necessitated intensive monitoring during administration.[108,109] IL-2 given by continuous infusion is more toxic, so regimens employing this administration method must use lower doses. With this approach, life-threatening toxicities from the therapy have been decreased but response rates have also been lower in some trials.[108]

Bacille Calmette-Guérin. Bacille Calmette-Guérin (BCG) is a nonspecific immunotherapy agent used to treat MM. It may be administered intralesionally or as an epilesional scarification. When administered intralesionally, a 26-gauge needle is used and the BCG is directly injected into the site of disease. Complete saturation of the tumor is attempted.[105] Epilesional scarification is achieved by scratching the skin over the tumor nodules into a 5-cm square grid. BCG droplets are placed onto the grid, dried, and covered for 24 hours.[110]

The action of BCG in the lesion is hypothesized to follow two paths. First, its presence in the tissue causes a local inflammatory response at the site. The process of this local inflammation is thought to be the primary mechanism of destruction of tumor cells.[110] Second, its presence causes an immune response including cytokine production and lymphocyte activation that causes further destruction of the tumor.[110]

Injection of BCG into lesions is easily accomplished on the skin surface and can actually be done to any epithelial surface accessible by instrumentaton (e.g., bronchus, bladder). Injection into MM lesions has resulted in regression at other sites of disease, both regional and distant.[110] This effect may be the result of activation of the systemic immune response or, if the regression occurs in areas of lymphatic drainage of the BCG from the injected lesion, it may be a direct response to the BCG.

Prior to therapy, patients are skin tested with other microbial antigens such as mumps, *Candida*, and streptokinase.[110] Individuals who show a delayed hypersensitivity reaction to those antigens are more likely to respond to BCG. This skin testing serves as a measure of immune competence. Also prior to treatment, purified protein derivative (PPD) skin tests are administered to assess the patient's prior sensitization to mycobacterial antigens. Individuals who are PPD positive are at risk for acute and life-threatening hypersensitivity reactions following BCG administration. Doses of BCG are adjusted based on the patient's PPD status, his or her immunocompetence, and the strain of BCG used.

Side effects of BCG administration include local reactions, systemic reactions, and long-term effects on organs. Local reactions may include necrosis and ulceration, which may occur within 7–14 days. Healing may take 8–10 weeks. Acute systemic reactions may include fevers and flu-like symptoms. Hypersensitivity reactions are possible, and the risk increases with subsequent injections. BCG are living bacillus organisms and may, therefore, cause bacteremia. Long-term toxicities include the development of granulomas in the visceral organs, especially the lung.[110]

Monoclonal antibodies. Several antigens on the surface of MM cells have been identified, including melanotransferrin, GD3, GD2, and MM chondroitin sulfate (mCSP).[72,111] Monoclonal antibodies can be developed for those antigens and, when used to treat MM, cause a direct antigen–antibody cytotoxicity or complement-mediated cytotoxicity.

Monoclonal antibodies can be given systemically, intralesionally, and intravascularly during isolated limb perfusion, as well as intrathecally.[111] They are commonly conjugated with chemotherapy, toxins, or radionucleides to increase their cytotoxicity.

Vaccines. MM vaccines are a form of specific, active immunotherapy. They are manufactured using a variety of techniques and may contain autologous antigens (from the patient's own tumor). More commonly, allogeneic preparations of antigens derived from multiple MM cell lines are used. A more recent development has allowed for the development of cell-lysate vaccines. Vaccinia melanoma oncolysate is prepared by infecting melanoma cells with vaccinia virus, lysing the cells, and collecting the resulting cell lysate. Immunogenicity is enhanced by using the vaccinia virus in these vaccines.[103] Other types of vaccines are also available, including DNA and RNA vaccines and dendritic cell vaccines. Melanoma vaccines are given to to stimulate the immune system, causing it to actively seek out and destroy MM cells. Several phase III studies employing vaccine therapy for melanoma are currently under way.

MM vaccines may inhibit metastasis and are most effective for patients who have undergone complete resections of all sites of disease.[75] In patients with unresected MM sites, the best results arise when metastases are smaller than 2 cm in diameter.[75] In these patients, slowed tumor growth is a more common result.[75]

Time to response with vaccines is very different than the experience with chemotherapy. Because vaccines are weak antigens and have no direct cytotoxicity, patients must be repeatedly immunized for prolonged periods. Since they work by stimulating an immune response, they may require 6–8 months to induce a remission.[75] After initial immunization, the disease may actually progress for 4–8 weeks before tumor effects occur.[110] Patients who exhibit stimulation of humoral and cell-mediated responses are more likely to have a response to vaccine therapy.[110] Positive responses to vaccines are usually durable over months to years.[110]

Continuity of Care: Nursing Challenges

The management of patients with skin cancer provides many challenges for oncology nurses. A number of subspecialty disciplines are often involved, including prevention and detection specialists, dermatologists, and surgical, medical, and radiation oncologists. In addition, treatment of these cancers may involve the services of other specialists such as geneticists, dermatopathologists, vascular surgeons, and immunologists. Oncology nurses often assume the responsibility of communicating to the patient what the role of each of these specialists is in the patient's care and providing clarification about treatment. Communication and documentation between these disciplines is vital to ensure a positive outcome for the patient.

Follow-up After Screening Examinations

Follow-up after screening examinations is important, regardless of whether the screen was positive. It includes written communication to the patient and primary care provider(s) about the outcome of the screening and primary prevention recommendations. This includes information about the interval when screening should be repeated.

Those patients who have a hereditary predisposition to developing MM may benefit from in-depth education about the physiology of the skin, genetic transmission, and the benefits of employing more sophisticated screening techniques such as medical photography. Information about the benefits and limitations of genetic testing should be presented. Such information should also be communicated with primary care providers. In addition, information about primary prevention strategies and chemoprevention should be provided when available. Written reminders for follow-up screening examinations at more frequent intervals may motivate the patient to comply with the screening recommendations. Patients from these families often need reassurance. They need to understand that primary prevention efforts may prevent or delay the onset of the malignancy and that regular, thoughtful screening may result in the detection of lesions at an earlier stage, when treatment is most effective.

Follow-up After Treatment

The risk of developing a second BCC after resection is estimated to be 45%.[22,26] Clearly, patients with NMSC need to have lifelong screening for development of second primary malignancies. These individuals need to be reassured that with early detection a second primary malignancy is also curable, and that primary prevention efforts may be effective in preventing or delaying the development of a second NMSC.

The risk of recurrence of MM is a function of tumor thickness and other prognostic factors. A second primary MM is estimated to occur in 5% of persons who have already been diagnosed with MM.[3,5] These patients need to understand the importance of and rationale for lifelong follow-up for both recurrence and a second primary malignancy. If this follow-up is to be provided by a primary care physician, specific instructions need to be given to both the patient and the physician that outline the interval and specific tests to completed.

Psychosocial Care

Although NMSC is relatively common, little has been written about the psychological impact of its diagnosis and treatment.[8] Some patients delay seeking treatment because they have a misconception that all cancer is uniformly fatal, despite the excellent prognosis for nonmetastastic NMSC. NMSC often requires wide surgical excisions that are potentially disfiguring to obtain a good long-term prognosis. Careful psychological preparation may be necessary to help a patient accept such a treatment, and postoperative follow-up should consider assessment of adjustment, self-esteem, and socialization. If this assessment identifies difficulties with adjustment, referral to a mental health professional may be indicated.

Patients diagnosed with MM may face similar problems with disfiguring surgery. Often they also face issues related to undergoing extensive cytotoxic therapy, anxiety related to long-term follow-up and fears of recurrence, and ultimately concerns related to having a potentially fatal disease. Continuous assessment of these concerns is indicated and, in some cases, referral to a mental health professional may be helpful to improve quality of life for these patients.

Another area of psychological care for patients diagnosed with MM relates to fear of genetic susceptibility in relatives and particularly children. Education about primary and secondary prevention strategies and correction of misconceptions can be an effective intervention. Referral to a mental health professional with expertise in genetics and related counseling may help patients to better cope with these fears.

Conclusion

There is much still to be learned about skin cancer. Given that this disease's incidence is increasing at an alarming rate, much work remains to be done in the areas of public education and awareness of prevention. The biggest gains in decreasing the morbidity and mortality associated with skin cancer will come from the prevention of the disease. Because the skin is a highly visible organ, these malignancies lend themselves to early detection. Programs staffed by qualified practitioners could be an important means of reducing the morbidity and mortality associated with both NMSC and MM. Treatment of early lesions is relatively straightforward and usually effective, but further research is needed to improve the outcomes with recurrence and second primary tumors. Especially in the case of MM, treatment is often unsuccessful and new therapies are needed. Genetics represent a promising area of research, and much remains to be learned about both the genetic predisposition for these cancers and the use of gene therapy as a targeted treatment for them.

References

1. American Cancer Society: *Cancer Facts and Figures — 2005*. Atlanta, American Cancer Society, 2005
2. Albert RA, Weinstock MA: Keratinocyte carcinoma. *CA Cancer J Clin* 53:292–302, 2003
3. Rigel DS: Malignant melanoma: perspectives on incidence and its effects on awareness, diagnosis, and treatment. *CA Cancer J Clin* 46:195–198, 1996
4. Ries LAG, Kosary CL, Hankey BF, et al: *SEER Cancer Statistics Review, 1973–1995*. Bethesda, MD, National Cancer Institute, 1998
5. Rigel DS: Malignant melanoma: incidence issues and their effect on diagnosis and treatment in the 1990s. *Mayo Clin Proc* 72:367–371, 1997
6. Burton, RC: Malignant melanoma in the year 2000. *CA Cancer J Clin* 50:209–213, 2000
7. Whiteman D, Green A: The pathogenesis of melanoma induced by ultraviolet radiation. *N Engl J Med* 341:766–767, 1999
8. Marks R: Prevention and control of melanoma: the public health approach. *CA Cancer J Clin* 46:199–216, 1996
9. Hill L, Ferrini RL: Skin cancer prevention and screening: summary of the American College of Preventive Medicine's Practice Policy Statements. *CA Cancer J Clin* 48:232–235, 1998
10. U.S. Preventative Services Task Force: Screening for skin cancer: recommendations and rationale. *Am J Prev Med* 20:44–46, 2001
11. Halder RM, Bridgeman-Shah S: Skin cancer in African Americans. *Cancer* 75:667–673, 1995
12. Bellows CF, Belafsky P, Fortgang IS, Beech DJ: Melanoma in African Americans: trends in biological behavior and clinical characteristics over two decades. *J Surg Oncology*, 78:10–16, 2001
13. Luther H, Altmeyer P, Garbe C, et al: Increase of melanocytic nevus counts in children during 5 years of follow-up and analysis of associated factors. *Arch Dermatol* 132:1473–1478, 1996
14. Naeyaert JM, Brochez L: Dysplastic nevi. *N Engl J Med*, 349:2233–2240, 2003
15. Marghoob AA, Schoenbach SP, Kopf AW, et al: Large congenital melanocytic nevi and the risk for the development of malignant melanoma. *Arch Dermatol* 132:170–175, 1996
16. Emmons KM, Colditz GA: Preventing excess sun exposure: it is time for a national policy. *J Natl Cancer Inst* 91:1164–1165, 2001
17. Haluska FG, Hodi S: Molecular genetics of familial cutaneous melanoma. *J Clin Oncol* 16:670–682, 1998
18. Burden AD, Newell JA, Nicola KG, et al: Genetic and environmental influences in the development of multiple primary melanoma. *Arch Dermatol* 135:261–265, 1999
19. Kefford Rf, Newton Bishop JA, Bergman W, et al: Counseling and DNA testing for individuals perceived to be genetically

predisposed to melanoma: a consensus statement of the Melanoma Genetics Consortium. *J Clin Oncol* 17:3245–3251, 1999

20. Bishop DT, Demenais F, Goldstein AM, et al: Geographical variation in the penetrance of CDKN2A mutations for melanoma. *J Natl Cancer Inst* 94:894–903, 2002
21. Pollock PM, Trent JM: The genetics of cutaneous melanoma. *Clin Lab Med* 20:667–690, 2000
22. Greene MH: The genetics of hereditary melanoma and nevi. *Cancer* 86(suppl):2464–2477, 1999
23. Easton D: The role of atypical mole syndrome and cutaneous naevi in the development of melanoma. *Cancer Surv* 26:237–249, 1996
24. Greene MH: Genetics of cutaneous melanoma and nevi. *Mayo Clin Proc* 72:467–474, 1997
25. Meyer LJ, Zone JH: Genetics of cutaneous melanoma. *J Invest Dermatol* 103(suppl):112S–116S, 1994
26. Marghoob A, Slade J, Salopek TG, et al: Basal cell and squamous cell carcinomas are important risk factors for cutaneous malignant melanoma screening implications. *Cancer* 75:704–714, 1995
27. Liu T, Soong S: Epidemiology of malignant melanoma. *Surg Clin North Am* 76:1205–1222, 1996
28. American Academy of Pediatrics Committee on Environmental Health: Ultraviolet light: a hazard to children. *Pediatrics* 104:328–333, 1999
29. Oliveria SA, Christos PJ, Marghoob AA, et al: Skin cancer screening and prevention in the primary care setting: National Ambulatory Care Medical Survey 1997. *J Gen Intern Med* 16:297–301, 2001
30. Hill L, Ferrini RL: Skin cancer prevention and screening: summary of the American College of Preventive Medicine's practice policy statements. *CA Cancer J Clin* 48:232–235, 1998
31. Gallagher RP, Hill GB, Bajdik CD, et al: Sunlight exposure, pigmentation factors, and risk of nonmelanocytic skin cancer. I. Squamous cell carcinoma. *Arch Dermatol* 131:164–169, 1995
32. Gallagher RP, Hill GB, Bajdik CD, et al: Sunlight exposure, pigmentary factors, and risk of nonmelanocytic skin cancer. I. Basal cell carcinoma. *Arch Dermatol* 131:157–163, 1995
33. Katsambas A, Nicolaidou E: Cutaneous malignant melanoma and sun exposure. *Arch Dermatol* 132:444–450, 1996
34. Rodrigue JR: Promoting healthier behaviors, attitudes, and beliefs toward sun exposure in parents of young children. *J Consult Clin Psychol* 64:1431–1436, 1996
35. Martin SC, Jacobsen PB, Lucas DJ et al: Predicting children's sunscreen use: application of the theories of reasoned action and planned behavior. *Prev Med* 29:37–44, 1999
36. Glanz K, Saraiya M, Wechsler H: Guidelines for school programs to prevent cancer. *MMWR* 51:RR-4, 1–20, 2002
37. Centers for Disease Control and Prevention, National Institutes of Health: *Cancer. Healthy People 2010: Objectives for Improving Health.* Atlanta, GA, CDC, 2000
38. Stone VB, Parker V, Quarterman M, et al: The relationship between skin cancer knowledge and preventive behaviors used by parents. *Dermatol Nurs* 11:411–424, 1999
39. Dennis LK, Freeman LEB, VanBeek MJ: Sunscreen use and the risk of melanoma: a quantitative overview. *Ann Intern Med* 139:966–978, 2003
40. Boutwell WB: The Under Cover Skin Cancer Prevention Project. *Cancer* 75:657–660, 1995
41. Loescher LJ, Buller MK, Buller DB, et al: Public education projects in skin cancer. *Cancer* 75:651–656, 1995
42. Lamberg L: Dermatologists call for massive cover-up. *JAMA* 279:1426–1427, 1998
43. Koh HK: Sunbathing habits and sunscreen use among white adults: results of a national survey. *Am J Public Health* 87:1214–1217, 1997
44. Cokkinides VE, Johnston-Davis K, Weinstock M, et al: Sun exposure and sun-protection behaviors and attitudes among U.S. youth, 11–18 years of age. *Prev Med* 33:141–151, 2001
45. Autier P, Dore JF, Heike L: The case for sunscreens revisited. *Arch Dermatol* 134:509–511, 1998
46. Lamberg L: Sunscreen, in-office dispensing, surgery debated at annual dermatology meeting. *JAMA* 281:1363–1364, 1999
47. Farmer KC, Naylor MF: Sun exposure, sunscreens, and skin cancer prevention: a year-round concern. *Ann Pharmacother* 30:662–673, 1996
48. Mayer JA: Promoting skin cancer prevention counseling by pharmacists. *Am J Public Health* 88:1096–1099, 2000
49. Vainio H, Miller AB, Bianchini F: An international evaluation of the cancer-preventive potential of sunscreens. *Int J Cancer* 88:838–842, 2000
50. Gottlieb N: Sunscreen: bodies of research remain to be covered. *J Natl Cancer Inst* 92:637–638, 2000
51. State of California SB310. *http://leginfo.ca.gov/bilinfo.html.* Accessed January 24, 2004
52. ASPA Sun Safe Products: Sun safety information. *www. americansun.org/pages/clothing.htm.* Accessed January 26, 2004
53. Skin Cancer Foundation: UV protective clothing. *www. skincancer.org/prevention/dress.html.* Accessed January 26, 2004
54. Adam JE: Sun protective clothing. *J Cutan Med* 3:1–4, 1998
55. American Academy of Ophthalmology: Selecting the right sunglasses. *www.medem.com.* Accessed January 30, 2004
56. Centers for Disease Control and Prevention: Media dissemination of and public response to the Ultraviolet Index — United States, 1994–1995. *MMWR* 46:370–373, 1997
57. Milne E: Direct measurement of sun protection in primary schools. *Prev Med* 29:45–52, 1999
58. Martin CS, Jacobsen PB, Lucas DJ: Predicting children's sunscreen use: application of the theories of reasoned action and planned behavior. *Prev Med* 29:37–44, 1999
59. Glanz K, Saraiya M, Wechsler H: Guidelines for school programs to prevent cancer. *MMWR* 51:RR-4, 1–20, 2002
60. Karagas MR, Stannard LA, Mott MJ: Use of tanning devices and risk of basal cell and squamous cell skin cancer. *J Natl Cancer Inst* 94:224–226, 2002
61. American Academy of Dermatology: Dangers of artificial tanning. *www.aad.org/PressReleases/exposure.html.* Accessed January 30, 2004
62. MacKie RM, Koh HK, Geller P: Skin cancer and melanoma, in Reintgen DS, Clark RA (eds.): *Cancer Screening.* St. Louis, Mosby, 1996, pp 168–195
63. Weinstock MA: Early detection of melanoma. *JAMA* 284:886–889, 2000
64. Weinstock MA: Thorough skin examination for the early detection of melanoma. *Am J Prev Med* 17:169–175, 1999
65. Healsmith MF, Bourke JF, Osborne JE, et al: An evaluation of the revised seven-point checklist for the early diagnosis of cutaneous malignant melanoma. *Br J Dermatol* 130:48–50, 1994
66. Haake AR, Holbrook KA: The structure and development of skin, in Freedberg IM, Eisen AZ, Wolff K, et al (eds.): *Dermatology in General Medicine, vol 1* (ed 5). New York, McGraw-Hill, 1999, pp 70–114
67. Jimbow K, Quevedo WC Jr, Prota G, et al: Biology of melanocytes, in Freedberg IM, Eisen AZ, Wolff K, et al (eds.): *Dermatology in General Medicine, vol 1* (ed 5). New York, McGraw-Hill, 1999, pp 192–220
68. Mosher DB, Fitzpatrick TB, Ortonne JP, Hori Y: Normal skin color and general considerations of pigmentary disorders, in Freedberg IM, Eisen AZ, Wolff K, et al (eds.): *Dermatology in General Medicine, vol 1* (ed 5). New York, McGraw-Hill, 1999, pp 936–944

69. Vargo N: Basal cell and squamous cell carcinoma. *Semin Oncol Nurs* 19:12–21, 2003
70. Leffell DJ, Fitzgerald DA: Basal cell carcinoma, in Freedberg IM, Eisen AZ, Wolff K, et al (eds.): *Dermatology in General Medicine, vol 1* (ed 5). New York, McGraw-Hill, 1999, pp 857–864
71. Schwartz RA, Stoll HL Jr: Squamous cell carcinoma, in Freedberg IM, Eisen AZ, Wolff K, et al (eds.): *Dermatology in General Medicine, vol 1* (ed 5). New York, McGraw-Hill, 1999, pp 840–856
72. Morton DL, Essner R, Kirkwood JM, et al: Malignant melanoma, in Holland JF, Bast RC Jr, Morton DL, et al (eds.): *Cancer Medicine, vol 2* (ed 4). Baltimore, Williams and Wilkins, 1997, pp 2467–2499
73. Morton DL, Essner R: Skin cancers: melanoma, in Harvey JC, Beattie EJ (eds.): *Cancer Surgery*. Philadelphia, W. B. Saunders, 1996, pp 505–521
74. Langley R, Barnhill RL, Mihm MC, et al: Neoplasms: cutaneous melanoma, in Freedberg IM, Eisen AZ, Wolff K, et al (eds.): *Dermatology in General Medicine, vol 1* (ed 5). New York, McGraw-Hill, 1999, pp 1080–1116
75. Morton DL, Barth A: Vaccine therapy for malignant melanoma. *CA Cancer J Clin* 46:225–244, 1996
76. Du Vivier A: *Atlas of Skin Cancer*. New York, Gower Medical Publishing, 1991
77. Sober AJ, Burstein JM: Precursors to skin cancer. *Cancer* 75:645–650, 1995
78. Tong AKF, Fitzpatrick TB: Neoplasms of the skin, in Holland JF, Bast RC Jr, Morton DL, et al (eds.): *Cancer Medicine, vol 2* (ed 4). Baltimore, Williams and Wilkins, 1997, pp 2433–2464
79. McCormack CJ, Kelly JW, Dorevitch AP: Differences in age and body site distribution of the histological subtypes of basal cell carcinoma. A possible indicator of differing causes. *Arch Dermatol* 133:593–596, 1997
80. Jamora MJ, Wainwright BD, Meehan SA, Bystryn JC: Improved identification of potentially dangerous pigmented skin lesions by computerized image analysis. *Arch Dermatol* 139:195–198, 2003
81. Kopf AW, Salopek TG, Slade J, et al: Techniques of cutaneous examination for the detection of skin cancer. *Cancer* 75:684–690, 1995
82. Argenyi ZB: Dermoscopy (epiluminescence microscopy) of pigmented skin lesion. Current status and evolving trends. *Dermatol Clin* 15:79–95, 1997
83. Fleming MG: Digital dermoscopy. *Dermatol Clin* 19:359–367, 2001
84. Robinson JK, Arndt KA, LeBoit PE, et al: *Atlas of Cutaneous Surgery*. Philadelphia, W. B. Saunders, 1996
85. Liu V, Mihm MC: Pathology of malignant melanoma. *Surg Clin North Am* 83:31–60, 2003
86. Lamb LA, Halpern AC, Hwu WJ: Diagnosis and management of stage I/II melanoma. *Semin Oncol Nurs* 19:22–31, 2003
87. Neel VA, Sober AJ: Other skin cancers, in Kufe DW, Pollock RE, Weichselbaum RR, et al (eds.): *Cancer Medicine, vol 2* (ed 5). Baltimore, BC Decker, 2003, pp 1997–2013
88. Balch CM, Buzaid AC, Soong SJ, et al: Final version of the American Joint Committee on Cancer staging system for cutaneous melanoma. *J Clin Oncol* 19:3635–3648, 2001
89. Zettersten E, Shaikh L, Ramirez R, Kashani-Sabet M: Prognostic factors in primary cutaneous melanoma. *Surg Clin North Am* 83:61–76, 2003
90. Fleming ID, Cooper JS, Henson DE, et al (eds.): *AJCC Cancer Staging Handbook* (ed 5). Philadelphia, Lippincott-Raven, 1998
91. Otto SE: *Oncology Nursing* (ed 3). St. Louis, Mosby, 1997
92. Fleming ID, Amonette R, Monaghan T, Fleming MD: Principles of management of basal and squamous cell carcinoma of the skin. *Cancer* 75:699–704, 1995
93. Motley RJ: The technique of micrographic surgery for excising skin tumours. *J Wound Care* 4:380–382, 1995
94. Essner R: Surgical treatment of malignant melanoma. *Surg Clin North Am* 83:109–156, 2003
95. Karakousis CP: Surgical treatment of malignant melanoma. *Surg Clin North Am* 76:1299–1312, 1996
96. Urist MM: Surgical management of primary cutaneous melanoma. *CA Cancer J Clin* 46:217–224, 1996
97. Hollis G, Recio A, Schuchter L: Diagnosis and management of high-risk and metastatic melanoma. *Semin Oncol Nurs* 19:32–42, 2003
98. Ho RCS: Medical management of stage IV malignant melanoma. *Cancer* 75:735–741, 1995
99. Brown CK, Kirkwood JM: Medical management of melanoma. *Surg Clin North Am* 83:283–322, 2003
100. Nathan FE, Berd D, Mastrangelo MJ: Chemotherapy of melanoma, in Perry M (ed.): *The Chemotherapy Source Book* (ed 2). Baltimore, Williams and Wilkins, 1996, pp 1043–1069
101. Eggermont A, van Geel AN, deWilt J, tenHagen T: The role of isolated limb perfusion for melanoma confined to the extremities. *Surg Clin North Am* 83:371–384, 2003
102. Ballo MT, Ang KK: Radiation therapy for malignant melanoma. *Surg Clin North Am* 83:323–342, 2003
103. Kadison AS, Morton DL: Immunotherapy of malignant melanoma. *Surg Clin North Am* 83:343–370, 2003
104. Kirkwood JM: Melanoma, in DeVita VT, Hellman S, Rosenberg SA (eds.): *Biologic Therapy of Cancer* (ed 2). Philadelphia, Lippincott, 1995, pp 388–406
105. Kirkwood JM, Strawderman MH, Ernstoff MS, et al: Interferon alfa-2b adjuvant therapy of high-risk resected cutaneous melanoma: the Eastern Cooperative Oncology Group trial EST1684. *J Clin Oncol* 14:7–17, 1996
106. Agarwala SS, Kirkwood JM: Update on adjuvant interferon therapy for high-risk melanoma. *Oncology* 16:1177–1187, 2002
107. Kirkwood JM, Bender C, Agarwala S, et al: Mechanisms and management of toxicities associated with high-dose interferon alpha-2b therapy. *J Clin Oncol* 20:3703–3718, 2002
108. Marincola FM, Rosenberg SA: Melanoma, in DeVita VT, Hellman S, Rosenberg SA (eds.): *Biologic Therapy of Cancer* (ed 2). Philadelphia, Lippincott, 1995, pp 250–260
109. Morton DL, Barth A: Intralesional therapy, in DeVita VT, Hellman S, Rosenberg SA (eds.): *Biologic Therapy of Cancer* (ed 2). Philadelphia, Lippincott, 1995, pp 691–704
110. Houghton AN, Chapman PB: Melanoma, in DeVita VT, Hellman S, Rosenberg SA (eds.): *Biologic Therapy of Cancer* (ed 2). Philadelphia, Lippincott, 1995, pp 576–586
111. Akporiaye ET, Hersh EM: Immune adjuvants, in DeVita VT, Hellman S, Rosenberg SA (eds.): *Biologic Therapy of Cancer* (ed 2). Philadelphia, Lippincott, 1995, pp 635–646

CHAPTER 64

Stomach Cancer

Katherine G. O'Connor, RN, MS, ANP, OCN®

Introduction

Gastric cancer is a significant problem worldwide.[1] The high mortality associated with this malignancy is due to the late stage of disease at presentation and the lack of effective adjuvant therapies.[2] Although new diagnostic techniques and surgical treatments have improved the detection of gastric cancer, the mortality associated with it remains high. Early gastric cancer without lymph node metastasis is highly curable, whereas advanced-stage gastric cancer is associated with a poor prognosis.[3]

Epidemiology

There has been a continuing decline in the incidence and death rate from gastric cancer in the United States over the past 50 years.[4] An estimated 22,710 new cases of stomach cancer were expected to occur in 2004, with an estimated 11,780 deaths.[5] In the United States, gastric cancer is the twelfth most prevalent malignancy and ranks as the eleventh leading cause of cancer-related deaths.[6] While the incidence of distal gastric cancer has decreased in recent years, proximal gastric cancer incidence has increased and carries a poor prognosis despite surgical resection.[1] Gastric cancer ranks among the top five causes of cancer-related deaths among U.S. minority populations.[7]

Worldwide, the incidence of gastric cancer is highest in Japan, Chile, and Costa Rica.[6,8] Nordic countries, such as Scandinavia, have shown increased prevalence in recent decades, with an incidence rate two to three times that found in the United States. Recognizing that the highest rates of gastric cancer occur in Japan, officials there have implemented aggressive screening programs that have led to earlier diagnosis, improved surgical outcomes, and increased survival. Males have a higher incidence of gastric cancer than females; no country shows a greater incidence of women over men developing the disease.[6] Black Americans, Native Americans, and Hispanics are twice as likely to develop gastric cancer as whites in the United States.[5] The average age of onset is during the fifth to seventh decades of life.

Etiology

Several conditions are strongly linked to the development of gastric cancer, including dietary intake, infection with *Helicobacter pylori*, socioeconomic class, and prior gastric resection for benign peptic ulcer disease. Other factors associated with an increased risk of gastric cancer include blood type A, a history of pernicious anemia that is associated with achlorhydria, and atrophic gastritis. Cigarette smoking in combination with alcohol intake also has been proven to place an individual at a higher risk for developing adenocarcinoma of the gastric cardia.[1,6]

Dietary intake has been one of the most widely studied risk factors for the development of gastric cancer. The N-nitroso-compounds found in smoked, pickled, preserved, and cured foods have been implicated as contributing links to the development of this disease.[1,2] Salts contain caustic properties that may cause chronic atrophic gastritis, and hypertonic salts may cause delay in gastric emptying. Dietary salts facilitate the conversion of nitrates to carcinogenic nitrosamines in the stomach. With delayed emptying of gastric contents, the stomach is exposed to the nitrosamine compounds for longer periods of time, possibly contributing to the development of gastric cancer.[9] Conversely, diets high in vitamins A and C, fresh fruits, and vegetables are associated with a lower incidence of gastric cancer.[1] Ascorbic acid and beta-carotene function as antioxidants and nitrate neutralizers, thereby decreasing susceptibility to *H. pylori* gastritis.[6,10]

Low socioeconomic class has been reported to be a risk factor in the development of gastric cancer, but no specific link has been identified. Researchers suggest that this higher risk is related to dietary factors and environmental issues associated with poor housing conditions, including overcrowding and unsanitary settings, which may facilitate the transmission of *H. pylori* infection.[11] Advances in refrigeration and freezing techniques have replaced salting and smoking as primary methods of food preservation, and this approach has contributed to the decline in the incidence of gastric cancer.[1,12]

In recent years, a strong correlation has been noted between the development of distal stomach cancers and individuals who are infected with *H. pylori*, especially in China.[6] It is estimated that as much as one-third of the U.S. population is infected with the *H. pylori* organism, which is commonly transmitted during the childhood years.[11] *H. pylori* is a spiral-shaped, gram-negative bacillus that has been found to inhabit the gastric tissue between the mucous layer and the underlying epithelium. It is known to cause atrophic gastritis and intestinal metaplasia followed by chronic gastritis, which is an early inflammatory process that acts as a precursor to gastric cancer.[1,6,9–11,13]

Initially, when the *H. pylori* organism enters the stomach, acute inflammatory changes and mild to moderate dyspepsia occur over a period of days to weeks. This inflammatory reaction gradually converts to a chronic reaction characterized by the presence of neutrophils, eosinophils, monocytes, and lymphocytes, and ultimately the development of lymphoid follicles. After 10–15 years, atrophic gastritis develops. It initially involves the mucosa of the antrum, but gradually develops throughout the entire gastric mucosa.[11]

The eradication of *H. pylori* with an intensive antibiotic regimen is necessary in patients with gastric or duodenal ulcers because elimination of the bacteria prevents recurrent ulcer disease. In addition to having a strong association with the development of adenocarcinoma, infection with *H. pylori* has been implicated in the development of regional low-grade gastric mucosa–associated lymphoid tissue (MALT) lymphoma. The *H. pylori* infection has been observed in a large number of MALT lymphoma cases, and more than half of local nonbulky tumors will demonstrate complete histologic regression after eradication of the *H. pylori* organism.[10]

Chronic peptic ulcers not related to infection with the *H. pylori* bacteria have a small incidence of developing into gastric tumors. However, patients who have undergone past gastric resection for benign peptic ulcers have an increased incidence of gastric remnant carcinoma, which is specifically defined as a cancer that arises in the remaining gastric tissues five or more years after initial resection for benign peptic ulcer disease.[1,14] Gastric remnant carcinoma may result from the absence of normal gastric acid secretions, which permits the proliferation of bacteria, an inflammatory reaction, and the chronic atrophic gastritis reaction known to be the precursor for the development of adenocarcinoma. Other theories propose that gastric remnant carcinoma may result from duodenogastric reflux[14] or infection with the Epstein-Barr virus.[1,6,9,15,16] Careful screening of patients with known past gastric resection with endoscopy and biopsy may detect early carcinogenic changes, thereby allowing for curative surgical resection.[14,15]

Prevention, Screening, and Early Detection

In high-incidence areas such as Japan, mass screening programs for gastric cancer have improved survival rates. Screening tests usually include upper gastrointestinal series and endoscopy, which has 90% sensitivity and specificity. Regular screening with endoscopy has been recommended for patients who have undergone gastric resection for benign peptic ulcer disease to detect early carcinogenic changes.[14,15]

Because of the vagueness of early symptoms of gastric cancer, it is not unusual for misdiagnosis or a delay in treatment to occur. Although the incidence of gastric cancer is decreasing, aggressive preventive health care in high-risk populations is essential to maintain and even further decrease incidence and mortality.

Pathophysiology

Cellular Characteristics

Approximately 90% of all gastric cancers are adenocarcinomas.[12] The remaining 5% consist of leiomyosarcomas, lymphomas, carcinoid tumors, squamous cell carcinomas, or other rare histologic types.[7,8,17] It is essential to distinguish between gastric lymphoma and gastric adenocarcinoma because the staging, treatment plan, and prognosis will differ depending on the specific pathology. Those malignancies diagnosed as adenocarcinomas are further classified into one of four subcategories: papillary, tubular, mucinous, or signet-ring cell carcinomas.

Historically, the majority of gastric cancers were located in the antrum. However, over the past three decades, the incidence of tumors found in the cardia or upper third of the stomach has increased.[1,7] Approximately 10% of tumors involve the entire stomach, aggressively spreading through the submucosal layers and producing a nondistendible, rigid organ. This *linitis plastica* is usually a metastatic disease that carries a poor prognosis.[1,2,7]

The most widely used histologic classification system for gastric cancer is the Lauren system, which recognizes two distinct histologic types: intestinal and diffuse. The intestinal histologic type is more commonly found in underdeveloped countries, occurs in men more frequently than in women, presents in the older population, and is usually detected in the distal stomach (antrum and lesser curvature). *H. pylori* infection is associated with the intestinal histologic type.[10] The diffuse histologic type is characterized by poorly differentiated cells, shows a lack of organized gland formation, and is composed of signet-ring cells. Tumors of the diffuse histologic type usually have extensive submucosal spread and early metastasis with a more aggressive clinical course. Their incidence is equal among men and women, but the diffuse histologic type usually occurs at a younger age than does the intestinal histologic type.[9]

Medical reports from Japan, where mass screening programs have been established for detecting early gastric cancers, describe the pathology of gastric tumors that are confined to the mucosa. These tumors are small, discrete, single or multiple lesions that infrequently metastasize to local lymph nodes and are associated with a much improved five-year survival rate.[9]

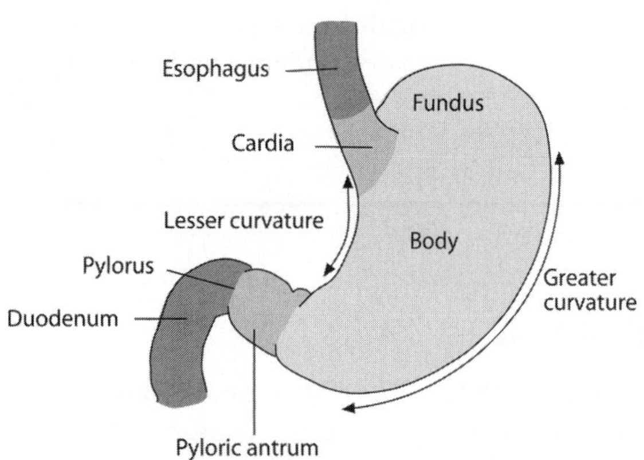

Figure 64-1 Divisions of the stomach.

Macroscopically, the early gastric carcinomas (all of which are T1 lesions) are classified as the following types:

Type I: polypoid—protrudes above the mucosal surface as a nodular or papillary growth
Type IIa: elevated—flat elevation, slightly thickens the mucosa by two or more times
Type IIb: flat—mass is at the same level as non-neoplastic gastric tissue
Type IIc: depressed—mass is slightly below the level of non-neoplastic gastric tissue
Type III: excavated—ulcer-like, often mistaken for a benign ulcer

These early gastric cancer lesions typically develop in the distal stomach, along the lesser curvature (Figure 64-1).[18] Early cancers may be as large as 10 cm in diameter, have any degree of differentiation, and be associated with regional lymph node involvement. Probably as a result of early detection, aggressive treatment, and extensive experience with the disease in Japan, nearly all patients with early gastric cancer who undergo gastrectomy are cured.

Progression of Disease

Progression and metastatic spread of gastric cancer occurs by direct extension and lymph node metastasis. The pattern of spread is closely correlated with the size and location of the primary tumor. Gastric cancer has the ability to metastasize through direct extension to adjacent organs such as the esophagus, pancreas, liver, transverse colon, and mesocolon.[9] Lesions of the distal stomach most commonly metastasize to subpyloric, inferior gastric, and celiac axis lymph nodes. Tumors of the proximal stomach will often metastasize to splenic, pancreatic, pericardial, and superficial diaphragmatic lymph nodes. Lymphatic spread of gastric cancer along the intrathoracic lymph channels may be manifested clinically by a metastatic lymph node in the left supraclavicular fossa (Virchow node) or in the left axilla (Irish node). Tumor spread to the lymphatics in the hepatoduodenal ligament can extend along the falciform ligament and result in subcutaneous periumbilical deposits in the lymph nodes known as Sister Mary Joseph's node. Krukenberg tumor, which is metastatic disease to the ovary, and Blumer shelf, a large peritoneal implant in the cul-de-sac palpable on digital rectal examination, are clinical findings representing evidence of diffuse peritoneal spread of gastric cancer.

Clinical Manifestations

Patients with early gastric cancers are essentially asymptomatic. Those with symptoms tend to report nonspecific complaints similar to those found with peptic ulcer disease or other gastrointestinal ailments, including reflux, indigestion, early satiety, nausea and vomiting, abdominal pain, weight loss, dysphagia, and anorexia. Gastric cancer often progresses to an advanced-stage before the patient develops obvious symptoms and seeks medical attention. The majority of patients with advanced-stage disease report experiencing symptoms for less than 12 months. Patients usually present with stage III tumors and complain of early satiety, postprandial fullness, rapid weight loss, anorexia, and fatigue, which is often secondary to anemia and obstruction. Vague abdominal pain is a common complaint with most gastric tumors, whereas dysphagia is a common complaint with proximal tumors. Presentation with major gastrointestinal bleeding is uncommon.[19] As the disease advances, weight loss is profound and problems with nutrition become significant. Ascites, hepatomegaly, and a palpable epigastric mass are significant findings for advanced disease, along with pulmonary, osseous, adrenal, and cutaneous metastases.[8,12]

Assessment

When the patient presents to the healthcare provider, a complete history and physical examination, complete blood count, and blood chemistries with liver function tests are performed. The history can provide valuable findings to direct the sequence of diagnostic studies. It may be necessary to perform radiographic, endoscopic, and surgical intervention to establish a diagnosis of gastric carcinoma.

No specific serum tumor markers for gastric cancer exists. The carcinoembryonic antigen (CEA) level is elevated in only 25%–30% of patients with gastric cancer; therefore, monitoring of patients with an elevated CEA level may be beneficial only for assessing response to treatment or as an indicator of recurrent disease. Assessing the CEA level is not helpful for screening purposes.[8]

Patient and Family History

To establish a clinical picture, a complete assessment of the individual's nutritional status, physical examination, and social and family history should be obtained. Particular attention should be directed to the following:

1. Oral intake (food and fluids), including amounts, frequency, calories, and supplements
2. Symptoms associated with eating, including pain, dysphagia, distention, nausea, vomiting, and fullness
3. Changes in appetite or dietary habits, including food intolerances, aversions, volumes, and consistency of foods ingested
4. Weight, including current weight, usual weight, weight six months and one year ago, and any intentional and unintentional weight loss
5. Bowel patterns and habits, including frequency, consistency, color, and flatulence
6. Medications, including over-the-counter, prescribed, vitamins, and homeopathic remedies
7. Past medical and surgical history, including childhood and adult illnesses

Physical Examination

The initial work-up of a presumed gastric cancer includes a complete physical examination to detect physical manifestations of primary and metastatic disease. Particular attention should be given to palpation of the abdomen for masses or hepatomegaly, and lymph node beds, particularly the supraclavicular and axillary lymph nodes. Palpate around the umbilicus for nodules is indicative of metastatic disease. A large ovarian mass palpable on pelvic exam or a large anterior shelf palpable on rectal examination would be indicative of peritoneal deposits. The presence of ascites or jaundice is also indicative of advanced or metastatic disease.

Diagnostic Studies

A computerized tomography (CT) scan is the diagnostic study most commonly used to evaluate abdominal malignancies. Scanning of the chest, abdomen, and pelvis is performed to stage the extent of disease, including extragastric extension, lymph node involvement, and peritoneal or hepatic metastasis. This scan, however, has little specificity in determining the depth of tumor penetration (T stage) of the gastric wall, and approximately 25% of patients will be found to be understaged by this method at the time of surgery.[20,21]

The barium swallow/upper gastrointestinal series is a noninvasive radiology procedure used to visualize the anatomical structures of the alimentary tract. Using double-contrast, hypotonic radio-opaque material, this test helps to identify polypoid masses, ulcerative lesions, and nondistendible lesions suggestive of cancer. It has limited capability for determining the depth of lesions and lymphadenopathy associated with malignancy.

The flexible upper gastrointestinal endoscopy is the procedure of choice for diagnostic purposes. This invasive procedure allows for the direct visualization of the gastric mucosa, biopsy of visible lesions, exfoliative cytology, and brush biopsies. With multiple biopsies and brushings, the endoscopy accurately detects more than 95% of gastric cancers.[18,22,23]

While executing the endoscopy, a simultaneous endoscopic ultrasound (EUS) of the gastric mucosa is performed by the gastroenterologist. The EUS, one of the newest technologic advances in imaging, allows the physician to evaluate tumor depth (T stage) through the layers of the stomach wall and the presence of lymph node involvement, allowing for more accurate disease staging[21,22] (Figure 64-2). The major disadvantage of this study is that the EUS cannot distinguish between benign and malignant tumors; this determination can be made only by pathologic study of the biopsy specimens.[21] The depth of tumor invasion has a great impact on prognosis, with the prognosis being directly correlated with the stage of disease.

The presence of *H. pylori* can be diagnosed by either invasive or noninvasive diagnostic tests. Endoscopic evaluation and biopsy of the gastric mucosa is an invasive procedure that allows for direct visualization and pathologic evaluation of tissue samples for the physical presence of the organism. Another study is the rapid urease test, which detects *H. pylori* by the presence of urease(not a normal gastric finding). The bacteria produce large amounts of urease, which neutralizes the normal acidity of the gastric environment, allowing the organism to proliferate and survive. When the biopsy tissue is applied to a combination urea substrate and pH-sensitive marker in the test kit, the urease is detected by its ability to convert urea to ammonia, which causes a change in color. Noninvasive methods of detecting *H. pylori* include carbon-labeled breath testing, which indirectly detects urease production, and elevated immunoglobulin G and immuno-

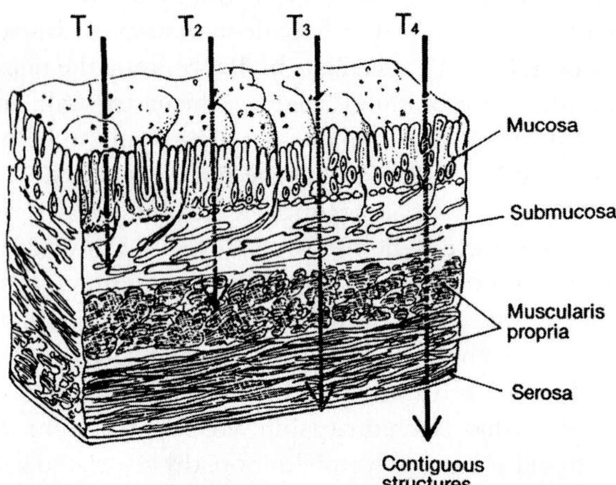

Figure 64-2 Depth of tumor through the gastric wall (T-stage). (Reprinted with permission from Alexander RH, Kelsen DG, Tepper JC: Cancer of the stomach, in DeVita VT, Hellman S, Rosenberg SA (eds.): *Principles and Practice of Oncology* (ed 5). Philadelphia, Lippincott-Raven, 1997, p 1031.[22])

globulin A antibodies from immunologic response in blood testing.[11,13]

Gastric acid studies should be part of the evaluation of any gastric ulcer, because benign ulcers do not occur in the presence of achlorhydria. Benign ulcers treated aggressively with proton pump inhibitors or H_2-blocking agents, when taken as prescribed, usually heal within six to eight weeks. If an ulcer persists despite aggressive therapy, a repeat biopsy should be performed to rule out gastric carcinoma because almost 15% of ulcers are malignant.[7]

Current radiographic imaging tools do not work well for detecting lymph node metastasis associated with metastatic gastric cancer. Research is ongoing into the value and efficacy of the positron emission tomography (PET) scan as a tool for evaluating primary gastric cancer as well as recurrent disease. Preliminary results suggest that gastric adenocarcinoma is a fluorodeoxy-glucose-avid tumor; however, studies have shown limited success in distinguishing perigastric lymphadenopathy from the primary gastric tumor and detecting peritoneal or pleural carcinomatosis and bone metastasis, necessitating further diagnostic workup.[23,24]

Table 64-1 TNM Staging of Stomach Cancer

Primary Tumor (T)	
TX	Primary tumor cannot be assessed
T0	No evidence of primary tumor
Tis	Carcinoma in situ: intraepithelial tumor without invasion of the lamina propria
T1	Tumor invades lamina propria or submucosa
T2	Tumor invades muscularis propria or subserosa
T2a	Tumor invades muscularis propria
T2b	Tumor invades subserosa
T3	Tumor penetrates serosa (visceral peritoneum) without invasion of adjacent structures
T4	Tumor invades adjacent structures

Regional Lymph Nodes (N)	
NX	Regional lymph nodes(s) cannot be assessed
N0	No regional lymph node metastasis
N1	Metastasis in 1–6 regional lymph nodes
N2	Metastasis in 7–15 regional lymph nodes
N3	Metastasis in > 15 regional lymph nodes

Distant Metastasis (M)	
MX	Distant metastasis cannot be assessed
M0	No distant metastasis
M1	Distant metastasis

Stage Grouping			
0	Tis	N0	M0
IA	T1	N0	M0
IB	T1	N1	M0
	T2a/b	N0	M0
II	T1	N2	M0
	T2a/b	N1	M0
	T3	N0	M0
IIIA	T2a/b	N2	M0
	T3	N1	M0
	T4	N0	M0
IIIB	T3	N2	M0
IV	T4	N1–3	M0
	T1–3	N3	M0
	Any T	Any N	M1

Histologic Grade (G)	
GX	Grade cannot be assessed
G1	Well differentiated
G2	Moderately differentiated
G3	Poorly differentiated
G4	Undifferentiated

Residual Tumor (R)	
RX	Presence of residual tumor cannot be assessed
R0	No residual tumor
R1	Microscopic residual tumor
R2	Macroscopic residual tumor

Classification and Staging

The current method of staging gastric cancer is based in the guidelines of the American Joint Committee on Cancer (AJCC) (see Table 64-1).[25] This system categorizes the stage of disease using a TNM designation, in which T refers to the depth of tumor invasion through the gastric wall regardless of tumor size (see Figure 64-2), N represents the extent of lymph node involvement, and M indicates the presence or absence of distant metastatic disease.

Therapeutic Approaches and Nursing Care

Once the diagnosis of gastric cancer is established, a thorough explanation of the disease, treatment options, and expected outcomes should be provided to the individual and family. The plan of therapy is dependent on the patient's health status, the stage of disease, and current options in surgery, radiation, chemotherapy, and biotherapy. The particular treatment must be individualized to the patient's nutritional status and cardiovascular, respiratory, renal, and hematologic state. The patient's potential for rehabilitation is another important consideration. The treatment plan selected depends on the location and extent of the lesion and presence of lymphatic spread.

In the absence of metastatic disease, localized gastric tumors are treated with aggressive surgical resection. However, because the majority of patients present initially with advanced disease, only 30%–40% are eligible for curative resection.[17,26] Advanced tumors that are unresectable are treated with combined modality therapy such as chemotherapy and surgical palliation. Combination chemotherapy has demonstrated transient improvement in control of the disease. Palliative surgical procedures include resection, gastric bypass, laser fulguration, and placement of gastrostomy drainage tubes or insertion of a jejunal feeding tube.

Surgery

Surgical resection is the only effective therapy for curing gastric cancer as well as an effective approach to provide palliation.[27–30] Consideration for surgical intervention is given to all patients with a good performance status and no major medical contraindications to surgery. Necessary considerations by both the healthcare team and the individual include morbidity, nutritional issues, and postoperative rehabilitation.

Prior to surgical intervention, it is necessary to correct abnormal hematologic conditions (such as anemia) and establish an adequate hydration and nutritional status. Patients should receive blood transfusions for significant anemia or oral iron supplementation for borderline anemia. Improving nutritional status requires extensive planning given that weight loss, emaciation, and malnutrition can adversely affect postoperative healing and recovery. Improvement of the nutritional status through enteral feeding is the preferred route, but more aggressive measures using hyperalimentation may be necessary in some cases.

The choice of the surgical resection procedure is based on the location and extent of disease.[2,31] Gastric neoplasms are not considered to be unresectable or incurable based on the size of the tumor, but may be deemed unresectable based on the involvement of other organs, involvement of vital blood vessels, and distant metastasis. Lymphatic spread is recognized as a major prognostic indicator of this disease,[8,32,33] although great controversy exists over the extent of lymph node dissection that should take place. In Japan, where the incidence of gastric cancer is high, extensive lymph node dissection is utilized during surgery and cure rates are higher than in the United States.[1,28,29] Nonetheless, it should be noted that due to the mass screening programs that have been employed throughout Japan for the past 25 years, gastric cancer is often detected at an early stage, allowing for improved survival rates. Researchers in the United States have studied this difference and concluded that a more extensive lymphadenectomy does not necessarily improve survival; in fact, it may increase the morbidity associated with surgery.[28,29] The use of sentinel node biopsy is under investigation in gastrointestinal cancers including gastric cancer; it might help establish definite need and benefits from an extended lymph node dissection. Total gastrectomy for tumors of the antrum or body of the stomach and prophylactic splenectomy are also being investigated.[30,33,34]

In many cases, the initial surgical approach will be a diagnostic/staging laparoscopic procedure to evaluate the primary tumor, obtain tissue for pathologic diagnosis, and detect metastatic tumor deposits. Laparoscopy also spares patients with unresectable or metastatic disease an unnecessary larger operation with extended recovery time, expediting their entry into adjuvant therapy.[35,36]

At the time of laparoscopy, those patients with stage I or II disease advance to an exploratory laparotomy and open surgical procedure to examine the stomach and regional lymph nodes, and to evaluate for evidence of extragastric extension of tumor or metastasis. With confined disease, the surgeon proceeds with en bloc resection of the tumor and appropriate locoregional lymphadenectomy. Patients with stage III or IV disease are referred for neoadjuvant chemotherapy before resection unless there is bleeding or a visible lesion that could potentially cause a gastric outlet obstruction that could be surgically relieved prior to the initiation of chemotherapy.

Total gastrectomy

A total gastrectomy may be performed for a resectable lesion in the midportion or body of the stomach. Linitis plastica is usually treated with a total gastrectomy because of the extensive tumor involvement of the stomach wall. The entire stomach is excised en bloc, along with the resected duodenum, a section of abdominal esophagus, supporting mesentery, and lymph nodes.[37] Reconstruction of the alimentary tract is achieved through the use of a jejunal segment anastomosed to the remaining esophagus. A jejunal loop is brought up, and an end-to-side Roux-en-Y jejunostomy is placed distally to provide flow for bile and pancreatic secretions. It is important for the surgical team to try to obtain adequate tissue margins around the tumor site that are free of malignant cells; this is a standard of surgical oncology. However, this margin free of cancer may not be possible in some cases due to the size of the tumor, surrounding vasculature, and location of the tumor.

Radical subtotal gastrectomy

Lesions located in the middle and distal portions of the stomach are treated with a radical subtotal gastrectomy. A Billroth I or Billroth II operation will be performed (see Figure 64-3).[38] The Billroth I procedure, or gastroduodenostomy, involves resection of the distal stomach, pylorus, first portion of the duodenum, and supporting lymph and vasculature. The remaining stomach is then anastomosed to the duodenum. The Billroth I procedure involves a limited amount of resection and as a result generally produces a lower cure rate than the Billroth II procedure. The Billroth I procedure is utilized primarily when the patient is debilitated and needs restricted intraoperative time.[22]

A Billroth II procedure is a wider resection that includes removing approximately 75% of the stomach, thereby decreasing the possibility of nodal or metastatic recurrence. It entails removal of the antrum, pylorus, first part of the duodenum, supporting vasculature, and all visible and palpable lymph nodes. The remaining stomach is anastomosed end-to-side to the jejunum. The duodenal stump is then oversewn with sutures. Gastric emptying is altered by both the Billroth I and II procedures, as well as with a total gastrectomy. There is also potential for a duodenal stump leak following the Billroth II procedure.[22]

Proximal subtotal gastrectomy

A proximal subtotal gastrectomy may be performed for a resectable tumor located in the proximal portion of the stomach or cardia. In many cases, a total gastrectomy or an esophagogastrectomy will be performed in place of this surgery to achieve a more extensive resection. Following resection of the stomach and distal esophagus, the esophagus is anastomosed to the duodenum of jejunum. Potential complications include pneumonia, anastomotic leak, infection, reflux aspiration, and esophagitis.[22]

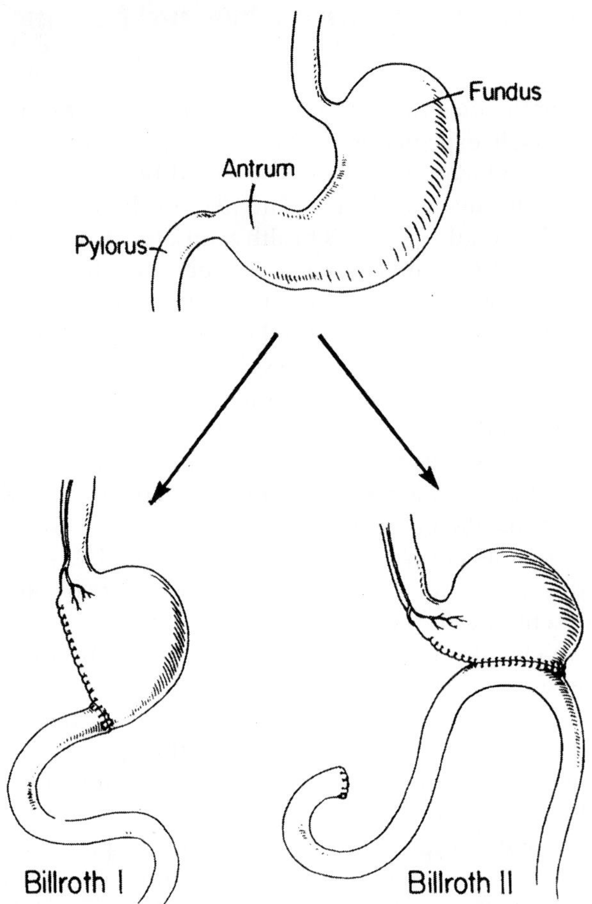

Figure 64-3 Reconstruction after gastrectomy. The Billroth I involves limited resection. The Billroth II is a wider resection of about 75% of the stomach. (Reprinted with permission from Seymour NE: Operations for peptic ulcer and their complications, in Feldman M, Scharschmidt BF, Sleisenger MH (eds.): *Sleisenger and Fordtran's Gastrointestinal and Liver Disease: Pathophysiology, Diagnosis, and Management, vol 1.* (ed 6). Philadelphia, Saunders, 1998, p 700.[38])

Palliative surgical procedures

Unfortunately, many patients with gastric cancer are not candidates for extensive curative resection. Often the symptoms of advanced gastric cancer are so severe that they significantly affect a person's quality of life and will require palliative surgical intervention. Gastric outlet obstruction, bleeding, and severe pain are common problems of advanced gastric cancer that can be well controlled with surgery. Gastric perforation is an emergency situation requiring surgery.

If the patient is deemed to be an acceptable surgical candidate, resection can be the most effective palliative treatment for advanced gastric cancer. The difficulty with performing a major operation, such as total gastrectomy, in the setting of metastatic disease is that this extensive procedure is associated with a high rate of mortality and complications, while ultimately providing no true survival benefit. Surgery also delays the patient from beginning systemic therapy. Although the survival time with palliative surgery is disappointing, it appears to be slightly longer than when no procedure is performed. The main benefit of a palliative resection is evident in the patient's quality of life. Relief of gastrointestinal symptoms, such as vomiting, can be achieved through palliative surgery. Placement of an enteral or esophageal stent may restore the patient's ability to swallow (particularly liquids) and aids in preventing aspiration of saliva. However, stents are associated with several risks, including stent migration, unobserved bleeding, tumor stenosis, and overgrowth.[39–41] With a skilled interventional radiologist performing the placement, general anesthesia is not required, and patients are usually able to return home on the same day.[39,40] Palliative procedures such as gastric or esophageal bypass, gastrostomy, or laparoscopic gastrojejunostomy[42] may temporarily alleviate symptoms but do not affect long-term survival. Laser surgery has been shown to benefit patients with tumors obstructing the esophagus and the gastroesophageal junction with satisfactory results.[30]

Postoperative care

Nursing care for individuals with gastric cancer who undergo surgical resection does not differ from care of individuals who undergo gastric surgery for benign disorders. The nurse must be acutely aware of the postoperative status of the patient and take necessary measures to maintain or improve the person's preoperative condition. Pneumonia, wound infection, deep-vein thrombosis, anastomotic leak, hemorrhage, sepsis, and reflux aspiration are the common postoperative complications following gastric surgery. Occasionally, a patient will develop a bezoar formation (i.e., ingested fibrous food clumping), causing a gastric outlet obstruction. A bezoar can be dissolved with enzymes, such as papain, or broken up through endoscopic intervention.

Weight loss is a major problem for patients with gastric cancer and for those who have undergone a gastric resection.[38] Preoperatively, inadequate food intake occurs from tumor bulk or compression; postoperatively, patients are unable to ingest high-carbohydrate or normal-size meals, leading to inadequate food intake. With decreased stomach size, foods may be inadequately absorbed due to the organ's inability to properly break down, churn, and mix foods. In response to this phenomenon, an enteral feeding tube may be placed during surgery for nutritional support. This measure is particularly advantageous for those individuals who have already experienced significant weight loss and are at greater risk for further weight loss with adjuvant therapy. The involvement of a registered dietitian is beneficial for determining enteral feeding solutions, for calculating and monitoring caloric requirements, and for patient and family teaching.

Surgical resection can lead to other nutritional problems. Anemia following gastrectomy can result from iron, vitamin B_{12}, or folate deficiency. Iron malabsorption may occur because of decreased gastric acid secretion, as gastric acid converts iron molecules into a substance that is more easily absorbed by the body. Iron absorption is further compromised in those patients who have undergone the Billroth II (gastrojejunostomy) reconstruction because the duodenum, where iron is normally absorbed, has been surgically resected.[43] Vitamin B_{12} deficiency is a complication that typically occurs several weeks after a gastrectomy due to the loss of parietal cells, which secrete an intrinsic factor needed to facilitate the absorption of vitamin B_{12}. Folate deficiency is directly related to poor nutritional intake or malnutrition. Management of these surgically induced problems includes oral iron and folate replacements and monthly vitamin B_{12} injections.

Many patients experience problems with their oral food intake after gastric resection. The most commonly reported problem is known as *postprandial dumping syndrome*. This syndrome begins with the rapid emptying of hypertonic/hyperosmolar chyme into the intestine approximately 10–20 minutes after eating. The influx causes a rapid shift of fluid from the vasculature into the small intestine, producing severe gastrointestinal and vasomotor symptoms. These symptoms include abdominal fullness and pain accompanied by vomiting, cramping, flushing, diarrhea, dizziness, and palpitations, all of which disappear once the bowels have emptied.

Most cases of dumping syndrome are remedied with dietary management, which involves eating small, frequent meals containing high-protein and low-carbohydrate foods. Patients should ingest minimal fluids with meals to reduce the volume ingested, reduce the possibility of triggering the syndrome, and thus allow for greater caloric intake from solid foods. Those who have undergone a proximal gastric resection or total gastrectomy should remain in the upright sitting position for at least one hour after meals because they no longer have a cardiac sphincter that prevents reflux of gastric contents into the upper esophagus and possibly into the lungs, causing an aspiration pneumonia. Patients with persistent dumping syndrome that does not respond to dietary modifications may require surgical modification to reconstruct the pylorus or revise the gastrojejunostomy to maintain their weight and adequate hydration.[43,44]

Radiation Therapy

Research into the benefits of radiation therapy in patients with gastric cancer is ongoing. The most significant change in practice is the use of radiation therapy in addition to chemotherapy as definitive therapy for patients who have undergone surgical resection of their primary disease, so long as no metastatic disease is present. The area of irradiation extends from the diaphragm to the umbilicus, including the gastric area in the left upper quadrant and the nodal beds in the right upper quadrant of the abdomen. The treatments are given by anterior and posterior fields, usually with a total dose of 4500 cGy. Advances in the field of radiation therapy have made it possible to deliver decreased doses to the extremely radiosensitive small intestine, while providing the necessary dose to the involved gastric area.

This change in therapy is based on the findings of the Gastric Cancer Intergroup trial (Intergroup 0116 trial), which focused on patients following curative gastric cancer resection for stage 1B–4 (M0) disease. The study randomized patients to a trial of surgery alone versus surgery followed by one cycle of 5-fluorouracil (5-FU) chemotherapy with leucovorin (LV), followed by five weeks of external beam radiotherapy with 5-FU/LV during the first and last week of therapy. Four weeks post-chemoradiation, another two cycles of 5-FU/LV were administered.[1,45–47] Results demonstrated an improvement in overall survival and prolonged median relapse-free survival.[47] Toxicities associated with this regimen included primarily gastrointestinal and hematological effects.[48]

In the setting of progressive disease, radiation therapy can be given for palliation to improve the patient's quality of life. It may benefit patients who have bulky proximal tumors causing obstruction, relieve chronic gastrointestinal bleeding secondary to tumor infiltration, and provide symptomatic relief.[8]

Special attention must be paid to the nutritional status of the patient with gastric cancer who is receiving radiation therapy. Excessive weight loss is the main dose-limiting toxicity that can lead to a delay or cessation of radiation therapy. Most patients receiving this treatment develop acute gastrointestinal symptoms including diarrhea, abdominal cramping, nausea, and gastritis. All of these reactions usually resolve within two weeks after completion of radiation treatments.[49] See Chapter 14 for additional information on the management of radiation toxicities.

Chemotherapy

A strong emphasis has been placed on the development of more effective systemic chemotherapy regimens because metastatic disease is a common problem with gastric cancer, either at presentation or later in the clinical course.[50] The risk of recurrence is directly related to the stage of disease after pathologic review, with patients who have advanced-stage disease (T3 or T4) and those who have lymph node metastasis being at a higher risk for recurrence.[51,52] Palliative chemotherapy is offered to individuals with surgically unresectable disease for control of symptoms and improved quality of life.

Adjuvant treatment with chemotherapy alone is not the standard approach for patients undergoing surgical resection;[1,50] it is reserved for patients diagnosed with advanced-stage disease. Unfortunately, few chemotherapeutic agents provide active benefits in gastric cancer. Single agents demonstrate response rates of less than 20%, and even that response is partial with a short duration of benefit.[50,53] Agents such as 5-FU, doxorubicin, cisplatin, etoposide, and mitomycin-c have been shown to have moderate activity in gastric cancer; over time, regimens have included different combinations of these drugs to yield improved response rates.[48]

Taxanes are cited as promising new chemotherapeutic agents in the treatment of advanced gastric cancer, both as single agents and in combination therapy.[54] Docetaxel in combination with platinol demonstrates partial response rates similar to nontaxane combination therapies, with studies revealing a nine-month time to progression interval.[54] Weekly doses of single-agent paclitaxel also demonstrate an acceptable toxicity profile. Ongoing studies are reviewing paclitaxel as first- and second-line therapy, as well as in conjunction with radiation therapy.[53]

For patients receiving chemotherapy, nursing assessment is an essential component of patient care. Stomatitis is an indication of toxicity in individuals receiving 5-FU. If stomatitis develops early in the course of treatment, it may be necessary to decrease the dose administered or withhold treatment until the sores resolve, depending on the degree of toxicity (grades 3 and 4 are most significant). Nursing staff should encourage meticulous oral hygiene, including rinsing with a sodium bicarbonate–saline solution four to six times daily. Instruct patients to notify their healthcare provider if mouth sores develop. These sores are quite painful for patients and may prevent them from eating and drinking, which in turn may compromise their nutritional status further. Symptoms may be improved with local analgesic preparations.

Patients with known cardiac dysfunction need ongoing monitoring while receiving chemotherapy consisting of doxorubicin or 5-FU. Doxorubicin is known to have dose-related cardiac toxicity at cumulative doses of 550 mg/m^2, so a baseline echocardiogram is essential, as well as echocardiograms at specified intervals to monitor the left ventricular ejection fraction (LVEF). If a significant change in LVEF occurs over time, the chemotherapy regimen may need to be changed to alternative agents. Those individuals receiving 5-FU as part of their chemotherapy regimen may require telemetry monitoring, as this drug may cause vasoconstriction and electrocardiogram (ECG) changes. Patients should be instructed to notify the nursing staff of chest pain or angina-like pain.

New therapies that may increase the potentially curative resection rates and decrease the risk of recurrence after surgery are currently under investigation. These approaches include preoperative (neoadjuvant) systemic chemotherapy and treatment with intraperitoneal adjuvant chemotherapy. Neoadjuvant regimens focus on reducing the tumor burden preoperatively to allow for a more complete resection of microscopic and macroscopic disease, thereby leading to lower rates of recurrence. Conversely, drug resistance may potentially develop from exposing tumors to the chemotherapy agents before surgery, thus blocking the effects of the subsequent chemotherapy given postoperatively. Some oncologists argue that neoadjuvant therapy delays local control of the primary tumor by surgery and therefore should not be considered.

Another approach for chemotherapy administration is regional therapy delivered through an intraperitoneal (IP) catheter.[55] The IP catheter is surgically placed, with the tip of the catheter lying in the peritoneum. Its port is accessed with a needle, which allows the chemotherapy to be delivered directly into the peritoneal cavity. The drug is dispersed through the peritoneum and then absorbed by the body over the course of a few days. Intraperitoneal therapy is directed at treating both peritoneal and hepatic metastases — common sites of recurrence for gastric cancer. Patients should be instructed that they may feel bloated after this therapy, as 2–3 L of fluid is instilled into the abdominal cavity. Intraperitoneal therapy is not associated with severe nausea and vomiting.

Symptom Management and Supportive Care

Advanced gastric cancer can result in rapid deterioration of an individual's health. Medical and nursing management aims to control symptoms and maintain optimal functioning. As gastric cancer progresses or recurs, nutritional problems usually become a serious issue. Without aggressive nutritional support, patients may be unable to receive further chemotherapy, cannot maintain strength, and cannot fully perform activities of daily living. Many of the advanced-stage problems are due to the dysfunction of the stomach, either from the lack of gastric secretions or the presence of tumor within or surrounding the stomach causing gastric outlet or intestinal obstruction. Nursing personnel and dietitians should make every effort to monitor the patient's nutritional intake and provide measures to supplement intake whenever possible.

Patients with progressive gastric cancer require supportive physical care depending on their symptoms. Common complications of advanced gastric cancer include pneumonia, deep-vein thrombosis from immobility, pulmonary emboli, ascites, sepsis, and anastomotic rupture. Any of these complications could potentially lead to death.

Many individuals and families feel a strong and long-lasting sense of regret, anger, and guilt as they may have ignored early symptoms or self-treated prior to seeking medical evaluation. Providing the individual and family with an opportunity to verbalize these feelings is an important nursing measure, as well as dispelling misconceptions and promoting a realistic sense of hope. Providing information and clarifying and explaining the multiple treatment modalities can help the individual and the family deal with physical problems and obtain assistance for emotional and economic issues. Strong nurse-to-nurse communication across the various disciplines can ensure a smooth transition in care, as many patients with this disease receive combined modality therapy. Nursing staff must be aware of the entire disease management treatment plan for individuals with gastric cancer. The nurse remains an advocate for the patient no matter which treatment options are chosen. To help prevent or treat complications that may hinder treatments, nurses must constantly evaluate and reevaluate patients with this disease for signs and symptoms of problems. Finally, compassionate care for individuals with gastric cancer can help to alleviate the physical and emotional pain of such a devastating illness.

Conclusion

The incidence of gastric cancer has been steadily decreasing in the United States, but the disease remains a significant challenge in many parts of the world, particularly Japan. Improvements in food preparation and mass screenings may contribute to a decline in incidence and mortality. The outcomes for treatment of early gastric cancer are positive when aggressive surgery and close follow-up surveillance are employed, yet the prognosis for stage III and IV disease remains poor because the unresectable disease is difficult to treat with chemotherapy and radiation. Less aggressive surgical procedures can be used to control or palliate advanced disease. Nutritional management is often one of the greatest challenges in the course of gastric cancer.

References

1. Alberts SR, Cervantes A: Gastric cancer: epidemiology, pathology and treatment. *Ann Oncol* 14(suppl 2):ii31–ii36, 2003
2. Yao JC, Ajani JA: Therapy of localized gastric cancer: preoperative and postoperative approaches. *Ann Oncol* 13 (suppl 4):7–12, 2002
3. Smith JW, Brennan MF: Surgical treatment of gastric cancer. *Surg Clin North Am* 72:333–345, 1992
4. Hanks JB, Jones RS, Minasi JS: Tumors of the stomach and duodenum, in Ritxhie WP Jr (ed.): *Shackelford's Surgery of the Alimentary Tract, vol 2* (ed 4). Philadelphia, Saunders, 1996, pp 88–95
5. Jemal A, Tiwari RC, Murray T, et al: Cancer statistics. *CA Cancer J Clin* 54:8–29, 2004
6. Neugut AI, Hayek M, Howe G: Epidemiology of gastric cancer. *Semin Oncol* 23:281–291, 1996
7. Luk GD: Tumors of the stomach, in Feldman M, Scharschmidt BF, Sleisenger MH (eds.): *Sleisenger and Fordtran's Gastrointestinal and Liver Disease: Pathophysiology, Diagnosis and Management, vol 1* (ed 6). Philadelphia, Saunders, 1998, pp 733–757
8. Haskell CM, Lavey RS, Ramming KP: Stomach, in Haskell CM (ed.): *Cancer Treatment* (ed 4). Boston, Little, Brown, 1995, pp 452–463
9. Fenoglio-Preiser CM, Nofsinger AE, Belli J, et al: Pathologic and phenotypic features of gastric cancer. *Semin Oncol* 23:292–306, 1996
10. Wisniewski RM, Peura DA: *Helicobacter pylori*: beyond peptic ulcer disease. *Gastroenterologist* 5:295–305, 1997
11. Schwesinger WH: Is *Helicobacter pylori* a myth or the missing link? *Am J Surg* 172:411–417, 1996
12. Tabbarah HJ: Gastrointestinal tract cancers, in Casciato DA, Lowitz BB (eds.): *Manual of Clinical Oncology* (ed 3). Boston, Little, Brown, 1995, pp 145–182
13. Cutler AF: Diagnostic tests for *Helicobacter pylori* infection. *Gastroenterologist* 5:202–212, 1997
14. Newman E, Brennan MF, Hochwald SN, et al: Gastric remnant carcinoma: just another gastric cancer or a unique entity? *Am J Surg* 223:292–297, 1997
15. Green FL: Management of gastric remnant carcinoma based on the results of a 15-year endoscopic screening program. *Ann Surg* 223:701–708, 1996
16. Yanamoto N, Tokunaga M, Uemura Y, et al: Epstein-Barr virus and gastric remnant carcinoma. *Cancer* 74:805–809, 1994
17. Staley CA: Gastric carcinoma, in Bears DH, Feig BW, Fuhrman GM (eds.): *The M. D. Anderson Surgical Oncology Handbook.* Boston, Little Brown. 1995, pp 120–141
18. Dempsey DT, Ritchie WP Jr: Anatomy and physiology of the stomach, in Ritchie WP Jr (ed.): *Shackelford's Surgery of the Alimentary Tract, vol 2* (ed 4). Philadelphia, Saunders, 1996, p 4
19. Lawrence M, Shiu MH: Early gastric cancer: twenty-eight year experience. *Ann Surg* 213:327–334, 1991
20. Conlon KC, Karpeh MS: Laparoscopy and laparoscopic ultrasound in the staging of gastric cancer. *Semin Oncol* 23:347–351, 1996
21. Catalano MF: Endoscopic ultrasonography for esophageal and gastric lesions. *Gastroenterologist* 5:3–9, 1997
22. Alexander R, Kelsen DG, Tepper JC: Cancer of the stomach, in DeVita VT, Hellman S, Rosenberg SA (eds.): *Principles and Practice of Clinical Oncology* (ed 5). Philadelphia, Lippincott-Raven, 1997, pp 1021–1050
23. Tschmelitsch J, Weiser MR, Karpeh MS: Modern staging of gastric cancer. *Surg Oncol* 9:23–30, 2000
24. Yoshioka T, Yamaguchi K, Kubota K, et al: Evaluation of 18F-FDG PET in patients with advanced, metastatic, or recurrent gastric cancer. *J Nucl Med* 44:690–699, 2003
25. American Joint Committee on Cancer: *The AJCC Cancer Staging Manual* (ed 6). New York, Springer-Verlag, 2002
26. Sun W, Haller, DG: Recent advances in the treatment of gastric cancer. *Drugs* 61:1545–1551, 2001
27. Ozmen MM, Zulfikogly B, Ozalp N, et al: Staging laparoscopy for gastric cancer. *Surg Laparosc Endosc Percutan Tech* 13:241–244, 2003
28. Roukos DH: Early-stage gastric cancer: a highly treatable disease. *Ann Surg Oncol* 11:127–129, 2004
29. Brennan MF, Karpeh MS: Surgery for gastric cancer: the American view. *Semin Oncol* 23:352–359, 1996
30. Lawrence W Jr, Zfass A: Gastric neoplasms, in Murphy GP, Lawrence W Jr, Lenhard RE Jr (eds.): *American Cancer Society Textbook of Clinical Oncology* (ed 2). Atlanta, American Cancer Society, 1995, pp 281–292
31. Boland CR: Gastrointestinal and pancreatic neoplasms, in Kelley WN (ed.): *Textbook of Internal Medicine* (ed 3). Philadelphia, Lippincott-Raven, 1997, pp 768–782
32. Roukos D, Kappas AM, Encke A: Extensive lymph node dissection in gastric cancer: is it of therapeutic value? *Cancer Treat Rev* 22:247–252, 1996
33. Kitagawa Y, Fujii H, Mukai M: Current status and future prospects of sentinel node navigational surgery for gastrointestinal cancer. *Ann Surg Oncol* 11 (suppl):242S–244S, 2004
34. Hiratsuka M, Miyashiro I, Ishikawa O, et al: Application of sentinel node biopsy to gastric cancer surgery. *Surgery* 129:335–340, 2001
35. Kelsen DG: Adjuvant and neoadjuvant therapy for gastric cancer. *Semin Oncol* 23:379–389, 1996
36. Burke EC, Karpeh MS, Conlon KC, et al: Laparoscopy in the management of gastric adenocarcinoma. *Ann Surg* 225:262–267, 1997
37. Harrison LE, Karpeh MS, Brennan MF: Proximal gastric cancers resected via transabdominal-only approach: results and comparison to distal adenocarcinoma of the stomach. *Ann Surg* 225:678–685, 1997
38. Seymour NE: Operations for peptic ulcers and their complications, in Feldman M, Scharschmidt BF, Sleisenger MH (eds.): *Sleisenger and Fordtran's Gastrointestinal and Liver Disease: Pathophysiology, Diagnosis, and Management,* vol I (ed 6). Philadelphia, Saunders, 1998, pp 696–710
39. Shand AG, Grieve DC, Brush T: Expandable metallic stents for palliation of malignant pyloric and duodenal obstruction. *Br J Surg* 89:349–352, 2002
40. Choi YB: Laparoscopic gastrojejunostomy for palliation of gastric outlet obstruction in unresectable gastric cancer. *Surg Endosc* 16:1620–1626, 2002
41. Ely CA, Arregui ME: The use of enteral stents in colonic and gastric outlet obstruction. *Surg Endosc* 17:89–94, 2003
42. Alam TA, Baines M, Parker MC: The management of gastric outlet obstruction secondary to inoperable cancer: an evaluation of laparoscopic gastrojejunostomy. *Surg Endosc* 17:320–323, 2003
43. Huether SE, McCance KL, Tarmina MS: Alterations in digestive function, in McCance KL, Huether SE (eds.): *Pathophysiology: The Biologic Response for Disease in Adults and Children* (ed 2). St. Louis, Mosby, 1994, pp 1320–1375
44. Eagon JC, Miedema BW, Kelly KE: Post gastrectomy syndromes. *Surg Clin North Am* 72:445–462, 1992

45. Park SH, Kim DY, Heo JS, et al: Postoperative chemoradiotherapy for gastric cancer. *Ann Oncol* 14:1373–1377, 2003
46. Wilke HJ, Van Cutsem E: Current treatments and future perspectives in gastric cancer. *Ann Oncol* 14(suppl 2):ii49–ii55, 2003
47. Hundahl SA, Macdonald JS, Benedetti J, et al: Surgical treatment variation in a prospective, randomized trial of chemoradiotherapy in gastric cancer: the effect of undertreatment. *Ann Surg* 9:278–286, 2002
48. Falcone A: Future strategies and adjuvant treatment of gastric cancer. *Ann Oncol* 14(suppl 2):ii45–ii47, 2003
49. Minsky BD: The role of radiation therapy in gastric cancer. *Semin Oncol* 23:390–396, 1996
50. Kelsen D, Atiq OT, Salz L, et al: FAMTX versus etoposide, doxorubicin and cisplatin: a random assignment trial in gastric cancer. *J Clin Oncol* 10:541–548, 1992
51. Kooby DA, Suriawinata A, Klimstra DS, et al: Biologic predictors of survival in node-negative gastric cancer. *Ann Surg* 237:828–835, 2003
52. Martin RC, Jaques DP, Brennan MF: Extended local resection for gastric cancer: increased survival versus increased mortality. *Ann Surg* 236:159–165, 2002
53. Schoffski P: New drugs for treatment of gastric cancer. *Ann Oncol* 13(suppl 4):13–21, 2002
54. Murad AM: Chemotherapy for advanced gastric cancer: focus on new agents and combinations. *Cancer Control* 6:361–368, 1999
55. Kelsen D, Karpeh MS, Schwartz, G, et al: Neoadjuvant therapy of high-risk gastric cancer: a phase II trial of preoperative FAMTX and postoperative intraperitoneal fluorouracil–cisplatin plus intravenous fluorouracil. *J Clin Oncol* 15:1818–1828, 1996

CHAPTER 65

Testicular Germ Cell Cancer

Eric Zack, RN, APRN, ACNP, AOCN®

Introduction

Testicular germ cell tumors (GCTs) account for 98% of all testicular malignancies and are the most common solid malignancy in men age 15–35.[1] Approximately 8980 new cases of testicular cancer will be diagnosed in the United States and 360 men will die of their disease in 2004.[2] Approximately 95% of patients with newly diagnosed GCT will be cured of their disease.[3] A direct correlation exists between early diagnosis, successful intervention, and lower cancer staging at the time of presentation. The optimal management of patients with GCT usually requires an interdisciplinary approach by medical, surgical, and (in the case of seminoma) radiation oncologists.

Table 65-1 Types and Descriptions of Testicular Cancer

Germ cell tumors (GCTs) (90%) occur in cells that make sperm
Seminoma (40% of GCTs)
Nonseminoma (60% of GCTs)
Teratoma Embryonal carcinoma Choriocarcinoma Yolk-sac tumors
Stromal cell tumors occur in cells in other parts of the testicle such as in cells that make hormones
Secondary testicular tumors occur from other types of cancer that have spread to the testicles from other parts of the body

Data from the American Cancer Society's website *www.cancer.org*.

Epidemiology

Testicular cancer accounts for approximately 1% of all male cancers. For unknown reasons, an increased worldwide incidence of testicular cancer has been observed in the last 30 years, primarily in industrialized regions such as North America, Europe, and Oceania.[4] Testicular cancer in blacks and Asians is rare. Although the disease can occur at any age, it most frequently affects men age 20–34. Testicular cancer occurs less frequently in adolescents, with an increased incidence being noted after age 40 and again after age 60.

Germ cell tumors are composed of seminomatous and nonseminomatous cell types. The different types of testicular tumors and their descriptions are noted in Table 65–1. Seminoma is the most common singular cell type, but mixed germ cell tumors are even more common. True seminomas do not differentiate, but rather they retain germ cell characteristics. Classic seminomas usually occur in men aged 40–50 years, whereas spermatocytic seminomas generally occur in men aged 60 or older. Nonseminomatous tumors are classified into four subtypes: teratomas, embyronal tumors, choriocarcinomas, and yolk-sac tumors.[5] Any seminoma associated with an increased alpha-fetoprotein (AFP) level is considered to be a nonseminomatous tumor.

In addition to GCTs, stromal cell tumors occur rarely, developing from the supportive structures of the testicle. Furthermore, secondary testicular tumors can result from metastases from different primary organ malignancies.

Fewer than 10% of all GCTs arise outside the gonads. These rare tumors occur (in descending order) most frequently in the retroperitoneum, mediastinum, and pineal gland and connote a poorer prognosis than a primary testicular cancer.[6]

Etiology

The exact cause of GCT is unknown, although several risk factors have been suggested for the development of this malignancy. These risk factors include prior history of testicular cancer, cryptorchidism, genetics, family history, environmental and dietary factors, and hormones.

Men who develop a GCT in one testis are 500 times more likely than the normal male population to develop testicular cancer in the contralateral testis.[7,8] This phenomenon occurs in approximately 1%–2% of males diagnosed with testicular cancer. Synchronous presentation of bilateral testicular cancer is uncommon and should suggest an infiltrative process resulting from secondary cancers such as leukemia or lymphoma.

Cryptorchidism (undescended testes) is associated with a 20- to 40-fold increased risk of developing testicular germ cell cancer compared to that of the normal male population. Controversies exist as to the best age at which to perform the surgery, if the surgery is necessary to fully prevent GCTs, and if cryptorchidism is directly implicated in the development of GCTs.[2] In some cases of cryptorchidism, a tumor is discovered in the scrotum while the testes are not.[9]

Twenty-five different hereditary disorders have been reported in patients who developed testicular cancer. Under these circumstances, other urogenital abnormalities were often present, possibly implicating hereditary etiologies to some degree in the development of testicular cancer.[10] Klinefelter's syndrome, a rare genetic disorder occurring in men and boys who possess one Y and two X chromosomes, is associated with an increased incidence of mediastinal GCTs.[11] Down's syndrome has also been associated in the development of GCTs.[12]

A familial tendency for the development of testicular germ cell cancer has been reported. One such report suggests a tenfold increase in risk for development of GCT in male siblings of testicular cancer patients, with a fourfold increase in risk for father–son transmission.[13] Caucasians have a 5–10 times greater risk of developing testicular GCTs than African American men.[2] Asian and African men have the lowest risk, while Hispanic men possess a risk level between that of Asian and non-Hispanic whites.

Environmental concerns, such as exposure to diethylstilbestrol (DES), have been widely studied. To date, no strong evidence links exposure in utero to the development of testicular cancer.

Strong evidence supports hormonal etiologies—primarily estrogen exposure during male development—as contributing to the development of testicular cancer. Another hormone-linked condition called gynecomastia, the most common benign breast condition in men, has been weakly associated with testicular GCTs.[14] However, it is not well understood whether gynecomastia contributes to the development of GCTs or results from the hormone imbalances caused by some GCTs. Syndrome X—a term describing a cluster of symptoms that include hypertension, elevated triglycerides, reduced high-density lipoprotein (HDL), and obesity—has shown a weak link in the development of testicular GCTs.[15]

Other possible etiologies have been postulated. Infection with human immunodeficiency virus (HIV) has been shown to be associated with an increased risk for the development of testicular cancer.[13] Researchers believe that GCTs develop due to impaired immune function and surveillance. To date, no substantial data have proved a direct viral etiology. Another risk factor may relate to low sperm count. A similar etiologic pathway with testicular cancer appears to correlate with lower sperm counts in certain men.[16] Dietary links have not been well established, although consumption of vitamin E has been associated with fewer seminoma cases.[17] Research investigating body type as a risk factor has yielded inconsistent findings. Environmental exposure to polyvinyl chloride has been weakly linked to testicular cancer development.[18] Conversely, research studies have failed to prove that men who have received vasectomies have an increased risk of developing testicular GCTs as compared to men in the general population.[19]

Prevention, Screening, and Early Detection

Testicular self-examination (TSE), not unlike breast self-examination (BSE), should be performed routinely. Given the nature of testicular GCTs, early diagnosis can lead to a more favorable outcome. Cure rates are highest for early-stage disease but decrease with more advanced disease. Unfortunately, there exist many barriers to TSE in men, particularly in diverse populations.[20] Given that testicular GCTs are the most common malignancies among men aged 15–35, testicular exams should be performed by the healthcare provider when accessible and taught to these men to perform monthly.[21] Moreover, healthcare providers need to educate themselves more fully to boost their confidence in promoting healthy screening behavior in younger men.[22] One tool that has been established in many physician and nurse training institutions includes a PowerPoint lecture, reading materials, video, and an artificial male model named "Zack" upon which to practice physical examinations and to teach male patients the proper technique.[23]

Educational programs beginning during the individual's teens should incorporate specific instructions on how to perform TSE. These exams should be performed after a warm shower/bath when the scrotum is relaxed and abnormalities can be more easily identified. While standing, each testicle should be examined for lumps, swelling, and any changes by rolling the testicle between the thumb and fingers. Any abnormality should be reported to a healthcare provider immediately. Both the American Cancer Society (ACS) and the National Cancer Institute (NCI) provide pamphlets explaining testicular cancer and TSE.

Certain physical characteristics in men should alert healthcare providers to the potential for development of testicular GCTs and the need to offer screening. These characteristics include the known risk factors for developing testicular GCT. For example, it is imperative that all males who present with gynecomastia be screened for testicular cancer.[24] Additionally, men who are overly physically active in their youth have been found to possess a higher incidence of testicular cancer.[25] Patients in their second or third decade of life who initially presented with seminoma are more likely to develop a second GCT later in their fourth or fifth decade of life and should be followed more closely.[26]

Massive screening campaigns for testicular cancer have not been deemed economically feasible because of the rarity of this disease. Nonetheless, public awareness through education is important.

Pathophysiology

As mentioned earlier, GCTs are classified into two histological categories: seminomas and nonseminomas. Upon diagnosis, these testicular GCTs can be moni-

Table 65-2 Common Serum Tumor Markers

Marker	Tumor
AFP (alpha-fetoprotein)	NSGCT (50%–60%)
B-hCG (beta-human chorionic gonadotropin)	Choriocarcinoma (100%) Embryonal tumor (80%) Pure seminoma (10-25%)
LDH (lactic acid dehydrogenase) isoenzyme	Advanced or large-volume disease Advanced pure seminoma
PLAP (placental alkaline phosphatase)	NSGCT
GCAP (germ cell-specific alkaline)	Seminoma
Inhibin-alpha	Leydig cell tumor

Data from Lee, Hamid, Arya, Patel.[27]

tored with specific tumor markers. Some tumor markers that are commonly used in assessing testicular cancer are outlined in Table 65–2.[27] Alpha-fetoprotein (AFP) and beta-human chorionic gonadotropin (B-hCG) are the two most useful tumor markers in cancer care.[28] Teratomas are benign tumors that do not secrete markers.

Germ cell tumors, similar to other cancers, start with the transformation of a single cell and evolve from its subsequent abnormal growth pattern. They are believed to be more responsive to chemotherapy (and, in the case of seminoma, to radiation therapy) because of their high tumor cell doubling time. More than 90% of GCTs will arise in the testicle. The spread of these cancers is generally predictable, with the initial spread occurring to the retroperitoneal lymph nodes. Once spread has occurred to the lymphatics, vascular spread follows. The lungs are the most common distant organ affected by this pattern of invasion.

Current research has identified a genetic mapping region that has been consistently linked to gains in the short arm of chromosome 12 (12p) given that all testicular GCTs, including seminomas, nonseminomas, and carcinoma in situ (CIS), are aneuploid.[29,30] Additionally, two distinct regions on the long arm of chromosome 17 (17q) have been identified that show elevated expression of genes attributed to extra copies in the pathogenesis of about half of all testicular GCTs.[31]

Clinical Manifestations

The most common presenting symptom of testis cancer is a painless, pea-sized swelling or enlargement of the testis. This symptom is often ignored because many patients may attribute this finding to recent trauma. Painful enlargement occurs in 30%–50% of patients and is often due to local hemorrhage within the tumor. Table 65–3 describes the local, metastatic, and hormonal presenting symptoms of testicular tumors. The most common metastatic site for testicular GCTs is the lungs, which correlates with the late presenting features. In the case of painful scrotal enlargement, diagnosis of testicular cancer may be delayed as a result of initially being treated for epididymitis or testicular torsion since these conditions occur more frequently than testicular GCTs.

Table 65-3 Presenting Symptoms Associated with Testicular Cancer

Local effects	Painless lump Testicular ache/discomfort Enlargement or firmness of testis Heaviness of scrotum Asymmetry Dull ache in lower abdomen or groin Sudden collection of fluid in scrotum
Metastatic effects	Back pain (paraaortic lymphadenopathy) Breathlessness or hemoptysis (pulmonary metastasis) Chest pain Coughing
Hormonal effects	Breast growth Tender or swollen breasts Reduced or loss of sex drive Growth of hair on face and/or body before puberty

Data from Lee F, Hamid R, Arya M, et al[27] and the American Cancer Society's website *www.cancer.org*.

Assessment

Patient and Family History

A thorough patient and family history are important components for establishing a plan of care. Patient histories of cryptorchidism, epididymitis, gynecomastia, back pain, and infertility should all be noted, as should a history of testicular cancer in the past given the 500–fold increase in risk. Additionally, individuals who have Down's syndrome, Klinefelter's syndrome, or HIV infection are at a greater risk for developing testicular GCTs. Other individuals who may have been exposed to testicular feminization, such as those with syndrome X, are also at greater risk for testicular cancers.[15] Family histories of male patients should be taken into account as well.

Physical Examination

A physical examination should incorporate a careful inspection of the scrotum. A mass that cannot be separated from the testis indicates a need for further evaluation, as do irregularities of tissue or nodularities.

Transillumination of the mass will reveal a hydrocele, an accumulation of fluid in any sac-like cavity or duct. Approximately 20% of patients with GCTs will have an associated hydrocele. A thorough assessment will pay close attention to symmetry of the testicles, their size, body hair growth, and lung sounds. Lymph nodes should be examined, especially the abdominal and supraclavicular lymph nodes. In general, adenopathy is not observed in the absence of prior surgical violation of the scrotum. Breasts should also be examined for gynecomastia.

Diagnostic Studies

Ultrasonography with a high-frequency transducer has become the imaging modality of choice for examination of the scrotum.[32] This technology can differentiate tissues in the scrotum with reliability and accuracy. However, ultrasonography is unable to determine whether a testicular mass is malignant. Seminomatous masses will appear hypoechoic when compared to adjacent tissue, whereas nonseminomatous masses may have an echo pattern that is hypoechoic, hyperechoic, or isoechoic.

Chest x-rays are valuable in determining whether a patient has gross metastases. If the chest x-ray is normal, a chest computerized tomography (CT) scan is warranted to rule out metastases within the lung or mediastinum.[33] Abdominal CT scans will provide information regarding retroperitoneal/pelvic disease.

Serum tumor markers such as AFP and B-hCG are elevated in approximately 85% of nonseminomatous GCTs. The lactate dehydrogenase (LDH) isoenzyme level is frequently elevated in patients with advanced disease. Other tests include bone scintigraphy, which has gained radiologists' confidence because it seems to be more sensitive in detecting the spread of GCT diseases.[34] Scintigraphy is a radiopharmaceutic procedure that utilizes a gamma camera to detect the amount of gamma-emitting substance that has gathered in a particular organ, tissue, or system. Magnetic resonance imaging (MRI) plays an important role in determining metastatic spread of testicular GCT into abdominal organ sites.[35] However, MRI is more typically utilized later during the follow-up period for evaluating treatment and monitoring for recurrence after surgery.[36] Positron emission tomography (PET) scans have not been shown to be more useful when compared to conventional imaging modalities and are more expensive.[37]

A fine-needle biopsy or transcrotal-approach orchiectomy of the testicular mass is contraindicated because of an increased risk of local recurrence or metastatic spread of disease to inguinal lymph nodes. Conversely, in the case of surveillance in a testicular cancer survivor in an attempt to diagnose early-stage GCTs such as testicular intraepithelium neoplasms (TINs), multiple biopsies are recommended from one particular surgical incision site as they may safely increase detection rates.[38]

Prognostic Indicators

The extent of disease and histology at the time of diagnosis determine the stage of disease and prognosis. Moreover, the percentage of embryonal carcinoma and vascular invasion appear to be the most significant prognosticators for GCTs based on the current data.[39] Virtually all patients with stage I (testis alone) or II (testis and retroperitoneal lymph nodes) seminomatous and nonseminomatous tumors should survive their disease. Approximately 70% of patients with testicular GCTs present with either stage I or II disease. The remaining patients present with stage III, disseminated disease characterized by hematologic spread to the lung, liver, bone, brain, or supradiaphragmatic region.

Patients with low serum markers or no evidence of pulmonary or mediastinal disease have an excellent prognosis. Those with low levels of tumor markers and/or limited disease will have a strong chance of cure if treated appropriately. Most patients with disseminated testicular cancer fall into the minimal or moderate disease category at the time of their diagnosis, which is associated with a greater than 90% cure rate with cisplatin-based combination chemotherapy. Prognosis is closely correlated with increased stage of disease and tumor burden.

Classification and Staging

Several systems exist for the classification and staging of testicular cancer and are often institution dependent. Table 65-4 details a staging system that the ACS has offered.[2] The International Germ Cell Collaborative Group developed a staging and prognostic system in 1997 that has remained the standard (Table 65–5).[40,41]

Therapeutic Approaches and Nursing Care

Nonseminoma Tumors

Nonseminomatous germ cell tumors (NSGCTs) account for about 60% of all GCTs and serve as an extraordinary example of how a multidisciplinary

Table 65-4 Testicular Cancer Staging

Stage 0	Carcinoma in situ (CIS) GCT found in only one place and has not spread to deeper tissues
Stage I	Cancer has not spread to lymph nodes or distant sites and blood tests are normal
Stage II	Cancer has spread to nearby lymph nodes, but not to lymph nodes in other parts of the body or to distant organs
Nonbulky stage II	Cancer has spread to lymph nodes in back of the abdomen, and lymph nodes are not larger than 2 inches (5 cm)
Bulky stage II	Cancer has spread to one or more lymph nodes behind the abdomen, and they are larger than 2 inches
Stage III	Cancer has spread to distant lymph nodes and/or distant organs such as the lungs or liver
Nonbulky stage III	Cancer cells are limited to lymph nodes and lungs; no tumor is larger than about 0.75 inches (2cm)
Bulky stage III	Organ metastases and lymph node metastases are larger than 0.75 inches and/or cancer has spread to other organs such as the liver or brain
Recurrent	Cancer has come back after treatment

Data from the American Cancer Society's website *www.cancer.org*.

Table 65-5 International Germ Cell Consensus Classification

Nonseminoma Tumors	Seminoma
Good Prognosis	
Testis/retroperitoneal primary	Any primary site
and	*and*
No nonpulmonary visceral metastases	No nonpulmonary visceral metastases
and	*and*
Good markers — all of AFP < 1000 ng/mL B-hCG < 5000 IU/L LDH < 1.5 × upper limit of normal	Normal AFP, any B-hCG, any LDH
Intermediate Prognosis	
Testis/retroperitoneal primary	Any primary site
and	*and*
No nonpulmonary visceral metastases	Nonpulmonary visceral metastases
and	*and*
Intermediate markers — any of AFP ≥ 1000 ng/mL and ≤ 10,000 ng/mL or B-hCG ≥ 5000 IU/L and ≤ 50,000 IU/L or LDH ≥ 1.5 and ≤ 10 × upper limit of normal	Normal AFP, any B-hCG, any LDH
Poor Prognosis	
Mediastinal primary	No patients classified as poor prognosis
or	
Nonpulmonary visceral metastases	
or	
Poor markers — any of: AFP > 10,000 ng/mL or B-hCG > 50,000 IU/L or LDH > 10 × upper limit of normal	

approach may ensure successful cancer management.[2] Early-stage disease primarily is approached surgically. Subsequent stages are treated with cisplatin-based chemotherapy with possible postsurgical resection of remaining tumor. The advent of cisplatin-based combination chemotherapy has dramatically affected the treatment of advanced disease. This success has, in turn, influenced the treatment of patients with earlier-stage disease. Stage I and early stage II disease can be managed well with primary surgery, but other options for selected patients are emerging. A discussion of the management of patients with NSGCTs follows.

Stage I

Stage I germ cell testis cancer is defined in Table 65-4 as disease that is confined to the testis. The choice for management for stage I NSGCT is one of the most controversial topics in urologic oncology. A retroperitoneal lymph node dissection (RPLND) following orchiectomy (a surgical procedure that removes the affected testicle and spermatic cord) has been the time-honored approach to the treatment of testicular cancer confined to the testis. Recently, another viable option, consisting of surveillance after orchiectomy without further treatment, has been offered to these men. Both options offer a cure rate approaching 100%, and the treatment selected is ultimately the patient's decision.[42]

The rationale for surgery is well grounded. RPLND in low-volume testis cancer is useful for staging because approximately 30% of patients with clinical stage I testis cancer, in fact, have pathological stage II disease. Surgery alone provides cure in approximately 90% of patients with pathological stage I and 70% of pathological stage II testis cancer with less than 1% chance of local recurrence.[41] Newer techniques have advanced RPLND in two major ways — nerve-sparing and laparoscopic procedures versus open RPLND. Nerve-sparing RPLND offers conventional surgery with strict emphasis on protecting all nerves, including those responsible for antegrade ejaculation, the major risk to fertility after surgery in these men. In addition, laparoscopic RPLND offers similar success rates with fewer scars and faster recovery time. However, controversy exists with this procedure because it has not been compared to conventional open RPLND in long-term studies despite being utilized by surgeons as a result of the demand voiced by male patients.

RPLND typically offers excellent postoperative results, but success largely depends on high volume and experience of the surgeon in dealing with early-stage NSGCTs.[43] Emphasis on improved management of NSGCTs has recently focused on identifying high-risk patient populations in an effort to base treatment decisions on a correlation between histological types of NSGCT and more aggressive disease requiring a more aggressive surgical approach. For example, patients with stage I embryonal carcinoma are at higher risk for developing metastatic disease (perhaps more than 80%) and therefore may be offered RPLND instead of surveillance.[44,45] Metastasis in stage I embryonal carcinoma rarely occurs to distant organs, but may be found in the retroperitoneum.[46] The likelihood of micrometastatic disease in the near lymph structures is greater in these patients, so the benefits of RPLND may begin to outweigh the risks in such cases.[47]

Teratomas, although benign, are the other type of stage I NSGCT that tends to recur more readily after chemotherapy. RPLND is used to remove the teratoma and often confers physical symptom relief for the patient.

Surveillance may be the preferred option for a man who has stage I NSGCT with a histological type other than carcinoma or teratoma. Because cisplatin-based chemotherapy will most likely cure this patient in the case of progressing disease or relapse, this option is gaining acceptance. Selection for surveillance must be considered carefully for individuals with stage I testicular cancer. Individuals must have normal serum AFP and B-hCG following orchiectomy, plus normal x-rays and scans. Meticulous follow-up consisting of monitoring currently identified serum tumor markers and CT scans can detect relapse while avoiding the morbidity that can occur in RPLND.[48] In one study, approximately 80% of relapses of NSGCT occurred in the first year, increasing to 95% within five years from the start of the surveillance period.[49] None of these patients died of their disease or the treatment.

Pathological stage IIA/B

As described in Table 65-4, metastasis to the retroperitoneal lymph nodes signifies pathological stage II disease with either microscopic (IIA or nonbulky disease) or gross (IIB or bulky disease) involvement. More than one-third of patients with stage II disease will not harbor metastatic disease.[50] However, the risk of relapse is not uncommon and adjuvant chemotherapy is generally offered. Virtually all of these patients will be cured with three or four cycles of chemotherapy depending on the stage at time of recurrence. Significant improvements in relapse rates have been observed with adjuvant cisplatin-based chemotherapy — usually consisting of bleomycin, etoposide, and cisplatin (BEP) — after complete resection of stage II disease. Indeed, this treatment has prevented relapse in nearly 100% of men diagnosed with testicular cancer. Without adjuvant chemotherapy, relapse rates are higher, but overall survival is unchanged.[51]

Surveillance after RPLND, rather than immediate postoperative chemotherapy, is another option for patients with pathological stage II disease. The obvious benefits of not having chemotherapy are that the 70% of patients who are cured by surgery are spared the experience as well as the long-term toxicities associated with such therapy.

Clinical stage IIB

Individuals who have a nonpalpable (smaller than 3 cm in transverse diameter) abdominal mass visualized on CT scan typically will have RPLND with complete resection followed by either observation or adjuvant chemotherapy. For patients with bulkier disease, primary chemotherapy is indicated. In patients who achieve a clinical complete remission, no further therapy is indicated. If a residual mass is present following three or four cycles of BEP, surgical resection via RPLND should be performed. Although the mortality is low, the morbidity associated with RPLND is acceptable in these cases.[52] The surgical finding in such cases may be necrosis (40%–45%), teratoma (40%–45%), or cancer (10%). In patients who are found to have cancer in the resected residual specimen, two additional cycles of etoposide and cisplatin (EP) should be administered.

Stage III/disseminated disease

A palpable mass with lymph nodes larger than 5 cm or involvement of more than five lymph nodes is designated as stage IIC disease. Abdominal disease of this magnitude will rule out initial surgical resection. Metastasis above the diaphragm or involvement of visceral organs, brain, or bone is classified as stage III disease. Chemotherapy is the preferred choice in this situation to reduce tumor burden before any other interventions are considered. Approximately 70% of men who initially present with stage III disease will be cured with conventional cisplatin-based chemotherapy. The remainder will require surgical interventions to rid the body of isolated metastatic disease that correlates with CT scan findings, as in the cases of pulmonary, mediastinal, and brain nodules.[53,54] In men who present with advanced or bulky disease, chemotherapy—most often BEP—is the mainstay of treatment.

Table 65-6 describes currently employed testicular cancer chemotherapy regimens. These chemotherapy regimens should always be given on schedule, generally every three weeks, regardless of myelosuppression, in view of the typically rapid tumor cell doubling time. Likewise, cytokines are used when indicated to avoid dose reductions. Because cisplatin is not myelosuppressive, it is rarely necessary to reduce the dose or delay treatment. Special circumstances, such as in the case of severe renal and/or pulmonary disease, may occasionally eliminate bleomycin as an option because of safety concerns. Nonetheless, these individuals should receive four cycles of etoposide and cisplatin (EP).

Table 65-6 Testicular Germ Cell Cancer Chemotherapy Regimens

Adjuvant Chemotherapy

Bleomycin 30 units IV weekly for 8 weeks
Cisplatin 20 mg/m^2 IV daily for 5 days
Etoposide 100 mg/m^2 IV daily for 5 days every 28 days for 2 cycles

Disseminated Disease Chemotherapy

Etoposide 100 mg/m^2 IV daily for 5 days (days 1–5)
+ Cisplatin 20 mg/m^2 IV daily for 5 days for 4 cycles administered at 21-day intervals

OR

Etoposide 100 mg/m^2 IV daily for 5 days,
Cisplatin 20 mg/m^2 IV daily for 5 days,
+ Bleomycin 30 units IV weekly on days 1, 8, 15 for 3 cycles administered at 21-day intervals

If a previously untreated patient is at intermediate or poor risk, then BEP for 4 cycles (not 3 as noted previously)

Salvage Chemotherapy

Ifosfamide 1.2 g/m^2 IV daily for 5 days
Mesna 400 mg/m^2 IV every 8 hours for 5 days
+ Cisplatin 20 mg/m^2 IV daily for 5 days
+ either vinblastine 0.11 mg/kg body weight IV on days 1 and 2, or etoposide 75 mg/m^2 IV daily for 5 days

OR

Paclitaxel 250 mg/m^2 IV day 1 followed by ifosfamide 1.5 g/m^2 IV and cisplatin 25 mg/m^2 IV daily on days 2–5
Mesna 500 mg/m^2 IV before and then 4 and 8 hours after each ifosfamide dose
Each is administered every 21 days for 4 cycles

Relapsed (Marker positivity, with or without radiographic evidence of disease)

ABMT
High-dose chemotherapy (carboplatin and etoposide) with ABMT or peripheral stem cell rescue
Some patients would receive 1–2 cycles of either BEP or VEP prior to ABMT

Seminomas

Seminomas account for approximately 40% of all testicular GCTs.[2] With the use of effective chemotherapy and radiation therapy, the overall cure rate for all stages exceeds 90%.[55] Unlike nonseminomatous testicular tumors, 80% of seminomas present as clinical stage I disease.[56] Seminomas are known to be exquisitely sensitive to radiotherapy. Both stage I and stage IIA/B disease are treated with external beam irradiation. Chemotherapy is the primary treatment of bulky stage IIC and disseminated disease. The management following chemotherapy remains controversial.

Stage I and stage IIA/B

Several management options consisting of adjuvant radiotherapy, surveillance, and adjuvant chemotherapy are available for stage I seminomas after orchiectomy.[57] Typically, radiotherapy is offered due to its overwhelming success in curing these patients. Oncology radiologists will determine the amount of radiation divided up into daily fractions that are delivered over a predetermined period of time. Higher doses of radiation are prescribed when more spread of disease is evident in the surrounding lymph nodes. Both anterior and posterior fields are treated. The area of treatment includes the paracaval and paraaortic nodes extending superiorly to the level of T10/11 and extending inferiorly to include the bilateral common iliac and the ipsilateral external iliac nodes. If the scrotum has been incised at the time of orchiectomy, if tumor spill has occurred, or if positive margins are present, the radiation field may be extended to include the ipsilateral hemiscrotum. If an inguinal approach to orchiectomy was utilized, the scrotum and contralateral testis are shielded to limit scatter irradiation to the remaining testicle. The bladder is also shielded.

Although surveillance may be an option following orchiectomy for stage I seminoma, excellent results with minimal side effects and morbidity make radiation the treatment of choice. Nonetheless, a very small risk of secondary malignancy is associated with radiotherapy; this risk should be taken into account but not overrated when compared to the long-term costs of surveillance.[58] Oligospermia or azoospermia may occur as a result of radiation even when appropriate radiation shields are employed. Spermatogenesis recovery is dose dependent, but generally resumes a few months later. Patients with stage I and IIA/B disease who are treated with radiation therapy have a 98% and greater than 93% chance of cure, respectively (survival past five years without evidence of disease).[59] Minor reductions in radiation doses and volumes (treatment fields) and their effects on long-term secondary malignancies have been investigated in randomized clinical trials.[55] Moreover, radiotherapy, when combined with reduced portals, yielded excellent control rates, minimal acute toxicity, and no late toxicity, making it the first-line treatment for patients with early-stage seminomas.[60]

Adjuvant chemotherapy with one or two cycles of single-agent carboplatin has been investigated as an alternative to adjuvant radiotherapy or surveillance for stage I seminomas.[61] This alternative treatment option proved highly effective and was well tolerated.[62]

Stage IIC

Treatment of bulky, localized retroperitoneal disease is controversial. Both chemotherapy and radiation therapy are effective after orchiectomy. Radiotherapy alone provides a cure for 30%–60% of patients with stage IIC disease.[56] However, a direct correlation exists between the volume of disease and the anticipated cure rate with radiotherapy. Individuals who present with large abdominal masses (larger than 10 cm) have a high relapse rate when treated with radiation alone. On the one hand, postorchiectomy radiation to areas where disease had been identified, such as in the mediastinum, significantly decreased the likelihood of relapse in stage IIA, IIB, and IIC seminomas.[63] On the other hand, men with bulky retroperitoneal disease (larger than 5 cm) who were treated with radiotherapy alone had recurrent disease outside the treatment field, altering the current recommendations to offer chemotherapy as first-line treatment.[64] Besides the risk of recurrence, men who have been treated with radiation therapy to the mediastinum have a higher incidence of death related to cardiac disease.[65] Salvage chemotherapy consisting of ifosfamide and cisplatin may be sufficient for control.[66]

Stage III/disseminated disease

Initial radiotherapy for metastasis to distant sites and bulky abdominal masses produces poorer survival rates when compared to cisplatin-based chemotherapy regimens. Given the nature of GCTs in advanced stages, when extranodal involvement and spread to distant organs such as the bone, lung, liver, or central nervous system are evident, combination chemotherapy using BEP (bleomycin, etoposide, cisplatin) is generally prescribed for three to four cycles. Management of residual disease following chemotherapy remains controversial.

Stromal Cell Tumors (Sertoli and Leydig Cell Tumors)

Stromal cell tumors originate from the supporting structures of the testicle such as adipose and spermatic cord tissues. These tumor types rarely occur and are often benign. Standard treatment consisting solely of orchiectomy typically cures the patient. Radiation and chemotherapy are usually not effective for these tumors.

Salvage Chemotherapy

The present emphasis in the treatment of disseminated, poor-risk disease is the exploration of cisplatin-intense regimens and the incorporation of innovative new agents. Common chemotherapy combinations include etoposide, ifosfamide, cisplatin, vinblastine, and bleomycin (VIP/VeB). Carboplatin has been studied as a replacement for cisplatin with solid evidence of support, especially in children.[67] Paclitaxel, gemcitabine, and cyclophosphamide have also been investigated with some success.[68–70] Carboplatin and cyclophosphamide have shown efficacy with mild toxicity in the treatment of metastatic seminomas.[71,72] Topoisomerase I (e.g., topotecan) and II inhibitor agents may be useful in chemorefractory GCTs, especially yolk-sac and some unresectable residual teratomas.[73] Similar to the situation in certain breast cancers, *HER2/NEU*, an oncogene that stimulates cell growth when overexpressed, can be present in some GCTs. Patients with this condition may derive benefit from the monoclonal antibody trastuzumab. However, the literature includes inconsistent reports on the clinical utility of screening and treating patients for which this agent might be of benefit.[74]

Surgical Salvage

Individuals with persistently elevated serum markers, indicative of viable disease following salvage chemotherapy, have not usually been considered surgical candidates because of the presumed systemic nature of their disease. However, after conventional treatment some men may show evidence of persistent localized tumors on CT scan and would benefit from surgical resection. Salvage surgeries should be performed at centers with significant experience with GCT management, as studies have shown that incomplete resection of residual masses may occur in more than 30% of cases.[75] Additionally, careful preoperative planning and intraoperative judgment are necessary to reduce the potential for serious vascular complications.[76]

High-Dose Chemotherapy with Rescue

Approximately 15% of individuals with persistent disease will not be cured with current treatment modalities.[77] These patients with cisplatin-refractory disease require a more aggressive approach consisting of combination high-dose chemotherapy with peripheral stem cell rescue, surgery, and sometimes radiation to cure or, at minimum, control their disease. High-dose chemotherapy followed by peripheral stem cell transplantation (PSCT) is a safe and effective treatment option for men with progressive disease or very late initial presentation.[78] Furthermore, patients with poor-prognosis diseases often will fail on conventional chemotherapy but may benefit from dose-intensive protocols using these newer agents with or without PSCT as first-line therapy.[79]

Nursing Care

The time of diagnosis and initiation of treatment are stressful. Education must begin early. Careful explanations of the nature of the disease, its treatment, goals of therapy, and side effects are essential.[80] Information must be provided and reinforced at various intervals along the treatment continuum. The patient's and family's anxiety levels may be elevated from perceived and real threats of mortality, alterations in life roles, and issues related to sexual identity, all of which require specialized attention. Consistent evaluations of the patient and family knowledge deficits are necessary to provide effective educational interventions.

Surgery

An inguinal orchiectomy is performed as an outpatient procedure for both diagnostic and therapeutic purposes — to establish a histological diagnosis and to remove the tumor. Nursing interventions should focus on postoperative teaching regarding pain management, activity level, and incisional wound care. Patients and family members need to learn how to change the dry, sterile dressing and how to recognize and report signs of infection and unusual bleeding. Men need to understand that neither sexual function nor fertility will be impaired or changed as a result of the orchiectomy. However, alterations in body image may result. Supportive interventions may be indicated to improve coping.

Care of the individual undergoing an RPLND, outside of the fertility issues, is similar to other abdominal surgeries. Paralytic ileus, a common side effect of abdominal surgery, may be prolonged for two to four days after RPLND depending on the extent of the abdominal resection performed and the length of time under anesthesia. Men are started on a clear liquid diet the day before surgery and undergo bowel preparation usually consisting of ingesting magnesium citrate or a full mechanical bowel preparation. A nasogastric tube is placed during surgery and remains in place until normal bowel sounds are present. After auscultation of normal bowel sounds, a clear liquid diet will be initiated, advancing to a regular diet as tolerated.

Fertility

The traditional bilateral RPLND results in the loss of antegrade ejaculation, thus producing infertility from subsequent retrograde ejaculation. New, more refined techniques for RPLND have focused on preserving the nerves responsible for antegrade ejaculation and hence maintaining fertility in this population. Current investigations are assessing the plausibility of sentinel lymph node biopsy in testicular GCTs.[81,82] Sentinel lymph node biopsy has shown diagnostic success in determining appropriate candidates for adjuvant treatments such as chemotherapy or radiation therapy in individuals with melanoma and breast cancer. Nevertheless, RPLND remains an important component of treatment for GCTs because it can eliminate any micrometastatic disease in the nearby surrounding lymph tissue, as predicted spread has been defined. The ability to experience a normal orgasm is not impaired because of RPLND.

Sperm banking prior to initiation of treatment may be an option depending on the stage of disease and sperm count at diagnosis. Because treatment of GCTs may include a combination of surgery, radiation, or chemotherapy, it is difficult to predict which men given different potential treatment options will develop fertility problems.[83] It is therefore necessary to offer sperm banking to all men in this situation. When successful, sperm banking allows men who will probably be cured of their disease to establish pregnancies with assisted reproductive techniques.[84] Nearly all semen samples collected from adolescents proved to be potentially useful in this regard.[85] On the downside, sperm banking can take weeks to obtain sufficient viable sperm. Men need to understand the risks of treatment delay, the cost of sperm collection and storage, and the potential costs of reproductive assistance such as in vitro fertilization if needed. Because of the aggressive nature of the disease, sperm banking may not be a viable option for some men due to their urgent need for therapy.

Testicular implants should be offered to all men who undergo orchiectomy procedures.[86,87] Men tend to experience more satisfaction with their prosthesis when they are given a choice when contemplating cosmetic issues such as size and elliptical shape.

Radiation

The resultant toxicities of abdominal radiotherapy for testicular cancer are less severe now than in the past due to lower effective doses, improved equipment, and computerized axial tomographic planning.[88] Problematic sequelae may include diarrhea, fatigue, nausea, fertility issues, myelosuppression, and occasionally bladder irritation, peptic ulcers, and lymphedema.

Gastrointestinal complications. Radiation to the abdominal and pelvic regions can cause diarrhea. Individuals should be instructed to manage radiation-associated diarrhea with a low-residue diet and over-the-counter antidiarrheals, but to seek medical attention if diarrhea continues despite these interventions. Prescriptive antidiarrheal medication is often required to manage this side effect. A low-residue diet is designed to reduce the amount of fiber in the intestinal tract by restricting indigestible carbohydrates such as milk products, high-fat-content foods, fruits and vegetables with seeds or skins, and high-fiber breads.

Unlike with radiation administered to other parts of the body, nausea and vomiting are not unusual with the first radiotherapy treatment for testicular cancer. Oral antiemetics administered one hour prior to the radiotherapy treatment and as needed usually control the associated mild nausea and vomiting.[89] Serotonin 5HT-3 antagonists used in combination with a steroid may prove useful. Other agents such as dopamine antagonists and anxiolytics may also help alleviate this problem. Light meals prior to treatment should be encouraged.

Myelosuppression. Radiation to the paraaortic lymph nodes and the pelvis often produces myelosuppression. Weekly complete blood counts with differential and platelets are monitored. Acute complications are uncommon. Information should be provided on the importance of seeking medical assistance for fever when neutropenia is present. Instruction should be provided to avoid medication that could potentially mask a fever. Patients should be told to call the physician's office if bruising or unusual bleeding occurs, as they could be a sign of thrombocytopenia, although transfusion is rarely performed. Also, individuals should be made aware that fatigue can occur and may interfere with normal activities. Pacing activities and allowing frequent rest periods will help patients cope with such fatigue.

Chemotherapy

Side effects resulting from chemotherapy are drug and dose dependent and must be managed accordingly. The extent of disease and history of prior therapy should also be taken into account. A thorough review of each medication's side-effect profile is necessary to successfully manage the patient's individual responses. Knowledge and experience in dealing with chemotherapy strengthen the nurse's ability to maximally assist each patient through his treatment continuum. Table 65-7 identifies the major side effects caused by common chemotherapeutic agents and their associated nursing interventions.[6,41] Potential side effects include nausea and vomiting, constipation, myelosuppression, nephrotoxicity, hemorrhagic cystitis, integumentary changes, reproductive changes, neurological changes, pulmonary complications, and body image changes. Other chemotherapeutic agents that have been investigated and show clinical efficacy against testicular GCTs include the following: vincristine, gleevec, methotrexate, paclitaxel, cyclophosphamide, carboplatin, gemcitabine, actinomycin D, and thiotepa.[90] Side effects of these agents should be reviewed before their administration.

Acute tumor lysis syndrome is a rare complication of chemotherapy directly caused by the rapid destruction of tumor cells (testicular cancer cells with a high tumor burden in this case) shortly after the initiation of treatment.[91] This oncologic emergency occurs when lysed cell particles consisting of certain electrolytes and uric acid flood the bloodstream and overwhelm the kidneys. Renal failure results when uric acid particles crystallize and create obstructions in the distal tubules and collecting ducts. Additionally, elevated serum levels of potassium and phosphorus can cause serious cardiac, neurologic, and gastrointestinal toxicities.

Acute pulmonary complications can occur primarily when bleomycin is used in the chemotherapeutic regimen. Bleomycin is an antibiotic that possesses antitumor activity and plays a major role in curing patients with testicular GCTs.[92] Pulmonary fibrosis is correlated with increasing doses of bleomycin to a maximum lifetime dose of 200 mg or 200 units. Furthermore, men who have poor renal function or who are 40 years and older have higher incidences of pulmonary toxicity.[93] Pulmonary fibrosis may lead to respiratory failure or death. Pulmonary function tests are often followed closely in men who have received bleomycin at some point in their treatment.

Acute electrolyte disturbances frequently occur and indirectly result from the side effects of chemotherapy such as nausea, vomiting, and diarrhea. In contrast, cisplatin may directly cause magnesium wasting and in effect increase the risk of seizures in

Table 65-7 Nursing Care and Educational Needs of Patients Receiving Chemotherapy for Testicular Cancer

Problem	Drug(s)	Nursing Interventions
Nausea/vomiting	Cisplatin Ifosfamide	• Administer prophylactic antiemetics with 5HT-3 antagonist and dexamethasone • Write down schedule for antiemetics regimen • Encourage and maintain adequate fluid intake • Consider supplemental IV hydration • Consider the use of music and relaxation therapy
Constipation	Vinblastine Etoposide	• Assess bowel function • Encourage fluids and high-fiber diet • Instruct patient to report significant bowel changes • Administer stool softeners and laxatives if patient is prone to constipation
Myelosuppression	Ifosfamide Vinblastine Etoposide	• Monitor complete blood count • Instruct patient to report signs of infection, fever, bleeding, shortness of breath, severe weakness, tachycardia • Instruct patient to avoid crowds and individuals with active infections. Encourage frequent hand-washing • Monitor incisions, wounds, catheter, sites for infection • Obtain blood and urine cultures, chest x-ray prior to administering antibiotics • Administer antibiotics as prescribed
Nephrotoxicity	Cisplatin Ifosfamide	• Monitor serum electrolytes, creatinine, and BUN daily intake and output • Provide aggressive pre- and posthydration and increase oral intake • Avoid aminoglycosides for the treatment of granulocytopenic fever when receiving cisplatin
Hemorrhagic cystitis	Ifosfamide	• Obtain urinalysis daily; if >10 RBCs per high-powered field, alert physician and hold drug • Provide aggressive pre- and posthydration and instruct patient to increase oral intake • Administer Mesna, a uroprotectant, as directed
Integumentary changes	Ifosfamide Bleomycin Etoposide	• Prepare patient for hair loss, reinforcing its temporary nature • Alert patient regarding skin hyperpigmentation and nail changes
Reproduction	Cisplatin Etoposide Bleomycin Ifosfamide Vinblastine	• Arrange for sperm banking if possible prior to chemotherapy • Reinforce that ejaculation/impotence will not change • Inform patients of azoospermia for at least 12 months with normal spermatogenesis returning in 50% of men within 2 years. Those treated with 3–4 cycles of BEP are at higher risk for persistent semen abnormalities.
Neurological changes	Cisplatin Vinblastine Bleomycin	• Instruct reporting of numbness and tingling of hands and feet (i.e., Raynaud phenomenon) • Inform patients to wear gloves and dress warmly in cold weather • Instruct patients to report hearing changes • Obtain baseline and serial audiometry for high-risk patients (i.e., > 50 years, total dose of > 400 mg cisplatin, abnormal renal function)
Pulmonary complications	Bleomycin	• Assess for bibasilar rates, inspirational lag, and cough • Evaluate men at high risk for fibrosis (i.e., smokers, decreased renal function, previous chest irradiation, and > 450 units of bleomycin)
Body image changes		• Encourage patient to verbalize feelings about hair loss and changes in appearance • Teach patient self-care activities related to body image disturbance • Reinforce any attempts to attend to the body part • Reinforce any verbalizations of feelings about actual or perceived loss • Provide consultation with hair stylist or barber

Data from Broch et al[6] and Poirier S, Rawl S.[41]

susceptible patients.[94] Frequent monitoring of magnesium and other critical electrolytes is necessary, and supplementation is required to avoid potential complications in organ systems that depend on specific electrolyte therapeutic ranges.

Sanctuary sites

In advanced testis cancer, the central nervous system (CNS) and the contralateral testicle are the most common sanctuary sites for malignancy.[56,95] Isolated cerebral metastases occurring after successful chemotherapy are curable.[96] Because of the blood–brain barrier, most chemotherapeutic agents cannot penetrate the structures of the brain. Therefore, other aggressive measures are taken, including stereotactic radiotherapy and resection, whole-brain radiation, and even surgical resection, in an attempt to cure the patient. Occult CNS metastases should be suspected if, in the presence of chest or abdominal radiological remission following therapy, new elevations or persistent tumor markers are present. In this situation, CT scan or MRI of the brain should be obtained even in the absence of clinical symptoms.

Current findings have suggested that it is unlikely that chemotherapy penetrates the testicle because of the blood–testis barrier.[97] This barrier functions to prevent germ cells from encountering harmful influences and contains three components: capillaries and Sertoli cells, an efflux pump with P glycoprotein, and an immunologic barrier consisting of FAS ligand on Sertoli cells. FAS ligand plays an important role in the maintenance of immune privilege by killing invading inflammatory cells.

Normally, the testis primary tumor is surgically resected prior to treatment. In the presence of advanced disseminated disease and positive tumor markers, however, chemotherapy may be initiated prior to a tissue diagnosis. At the completion of chemotherapy, the involved testis is removed. Whenever markers remain elevated following removal of the involved testicle (in the absence of radiographic evidence of disease), a second testis primary tumor should be investigated.

Symptom Management and Supportive Care

Disease Progression

Testicular GCTs arise from one cell, typically possess a fast cell doubling time, and can metastasize to distant sites in a matter of several months to years if left undiagnosed and untreated. Generally, the tumor inside the testicle will continue to grow with associated fluid accumulation and begin to cause local symptoms as discussed in the "Clinical Manifestations" section. As time passes, GCT cells move through the lymphatic and circulatory systems to reach distant sites that include, but are not limited to, the contralateral testicle, lungs, brain, liver, and bone. Here, GCTs acquire access to a blood supply for nutrition and waste removal purposes to support continued and unregulated growth and invasion. Testicular GCTs can become the cause of death in men because of their metastatic properties, but seldom do as a result of improved treatments.

Quality of Life and Psychosocial Issues

Quality of life and psychosocial issues have become important areas for nursing and medical research. As a consequence of the excellent cure rates for testicular GCTs, emphasis has now shifted in terms of optimizing the quality of life in these men post-treatment. The incidence of depression and anxiety in these patients is lower than that in patients diagnosed with different malignancies, but remains slightly higher than the incidence in the general population.[98,99]

Preserving fertility in this population greatly impacts quality of life. Awareness and sensitivity to the individual's and family's educational needs and initiating appropriate interventions to provide for psychosocial adjustment to the real or possible fertility changes will promote coping and acceptance. Additionally, men who underwent treatment and received information pertaining to their disease, treatment, and useful coping skills reported satisfactory quality of life scores by maintaining body image and controlling side effects.[100] Men who underwent unilateral RPLND reported minimal morbidity, excellent quality of life, and no long-standing effects.[101] However, in men who underwent a three-day chemotherapy regimen consisting of BEP, reports identified excess gastrointestinal toxicities and tinnitus as having a detrimental effect on quality of life.[102] Nursing interventions need to focus on controlling any and all disease- and chemotherapy-related symptoms that occur so as to maximize quality of life and help these men complete their treatment regimens without delay.

Follow-up Care and Survivorship

Because most men survive more than five years after the diagnosis of testicular GCT, follow-up care and survivorship issues need to be addressed. Follow-up care starts shortly after treatment and ultimately needs to become incorporated into lifelong strategies that promote healthy behaviors, maintenance, and well-being. This period is critical because therapy-related toxicities may occur at any time post-treatment, even several decades later in life. Some specific health problems that have been observed in this population include late effects of chemotherapy including but not limited to secondary malignancies, late relapse of original disease, long-term effects on fertility, and psychosocial consequences.[103–105]

Men who have been treated with cisplatin-based chemotherapy or radiation possess a higher risk for developing leukemia than the general population.[106] Surprisingly, trace levels of cisplatin can be detected in both plasma and urine of testicular cancer survivors almost 20 years after treatment.[107,108] Moreover, treatment with cisplatin confers a higher than normal risk for long-term nephrotoxicity.[109] Additionally, the risks for cardiovascular events and disease after successful treatment of testicular GCT are higher.[110] It remains unclear why this phenomenon occurs, but researchers have postulated that the lack of physical activity post-treatment may be partly responsible for these observed cardiovascular events.[110–112]

Vascular toxicities in the form of Raynaud's disease have been observed in cured patients and are suspected to be caused by chemotherapeutic agents, specifically bleomycin.[109] This phenomenon is characterized by transient episodes of vasoconstriction of the digital arteries that lead to fluctuations in color, warmth, and pain.[109] Occurrences range dramatically, but when present, Raynaud's disease may become long-lasting (e.g., more than ten years post-treatment).

Late relapse occurs in 2%–3% of men who have been diagnosed and successfully treated for GCTs in the past.[103] Patients who initially present with a high tumor burden and the presence of teratomatous components within the primary testicular cancer have a higher likelihood of developing a late disease relapse.[113] The vast majority of relapses occur within the first two years following therapy and become exceedingly rare once a patient is five years post-treatment. For this reason, close follow-up strategies generally cease after the five-year mark, except in the cases of patients presenting with metastatic NSGCT.[114] Conversely, most patients with advanced seminomas after relapse have a very poor prognosis despite further treatment.[115]

Several national organizations offer information and assistance programs for survivorship as well as other disease-related concerns. The following list includes major organizations, their associated Web sites, and their telephone numbers:

American Cancer Society: *www.cancer.org*, (800) 227-2345

Lance Armstrong Foundation: *www.laf.org*, (512) 236-8820

National Cancer Institute: *www.cancer.gov*, (800) 422–6237

National Coalition for Cancer Survivorship: *www.canceradvocacy.org*, (877) 622–7937

Conclusion

Current research in testicular GCTs has focused on several aspects of the disease. Identifying the testicular cancer genome is one area that may offer insight into improved treatment modalities through identification of chromosomal abnormalities and gene expression profiling.[31,116] Angiogenesis and tumorigenesis at the molecular level are other topics being actively funded and researched.[117] The information gained from these studies may explain why some tumors show resistance to current pharmaceutical therapies. Researchers may eventually suggest ways to manipulate specific signal pathways so as to overcome drug resistance.[118] One groundbreaking example resulting from genetic research highlights a defective mismatch repair pathway that leads to the microsatellite instability thought to be responsible for cisplatin drug resistance.[119] Microsatellite instability is a type of genetic error that results when the cell's DNA mismatch repair system fails to correct damaged DNA strands, thereby allowing stretches of DNA to hook up with the wrong partner.

Despite the many advancements brought by research, testicular cancer continues to be responsible for the deaths of many men. This disease, unlike many other malignancies, has the true potential to offer 100% cure if resources became more widely available.[120] As a result of ongoing education and greater public awareness, testicular self-examinations could significantly lessen its death toll.[121] These efforts would single out testicular GCTs as an excellent illustration of control that other malignancies could model as new research sheds light on them.

Although testicular cancer is a rare and devastating disease to the young population it affects, it is also one of the most highly curable malignancies. Testicular self-examination remains the best available tool for early diagnosis and treatment. Most males today can be successfully treated, with adverse side effects being vastly reduced compared to those produced by the therapy available 20 years ago. The high cure rate of testicular cancer can be attributed to dedicated clinical researchers who utilize combination modalities such as surgery, chemotherapy, radiation therapy, and bone marrow transplantation in the treatment of testicular cancer. Researchers continue to look for new ways to improve current treatment modalities and to reduce morbidity and mortality.

References

1. Weir HK, Thun MJ, Hankey BF, et al: Annual report to the nation on the status of cancer, 1975–2000, featuring the uses of surveillance data for cancer prevention and control. *J Natl Cancer Inst* 95:1276–1299, 2003
2. American Cancer Society: *Cancer Facts and Figures 2004.* Atlanta ACS, 2004
3. Miladi M, Peyromaure M, Remi J, et al: Testicular germ cell tumors: prognosis. *Prog Urol* 13:92–97, 2003
4. Huyghe E, Matsuda T, Thonneau P: Increasing incidence of testicular cancer worldwide: a review. *J Urol* 170:5–11, 2003
5. Mikuz G: [WHO classification of testicular tumors]. *Verh Dtsch Ges Pathol* 86:67–75, 2002
6. Brock DL, Fox SM: Testicular germ cell cancer, in Groenwald SM, Frogge MH, Goodman M, Yarbro CH (eds.): *Cancer Nursing: Principles and Practice* (ed 4). Sudbury, MA, Jones and Bartlett, 1997, pp 1374–1389
7. Montie J: Carcinoma in situ of the testis and bilateral carcinoma. *Urol Clin North Am* 20:127–132, 1993
8. Dieckmann K, Boeckman W, Brosig W, et al.: Bilateral testicular germ cell tumors. *Cancer* 51:1254–1258, 1986
9. Bani-Hani KE, Matani YS, Bani-Hani IH: Cryptorchidism and testicular neoplasia. *Saudi Med J* 24:166–169, 2003
10. Lutke Holzik MF, Sijmons RH, Sleijfer DT, et al: Syndromic aspects of testicular carcinoma. *Cancer* 97:984–992, 2003
11. Nichols C, Heerema NA, Palmer C: Klinefelter's syndrome associated with mediastinal germ cell neoplasms. *J Clin Oncol* 5:1290–1294, 1987
12. Hsiung Stripp DC, Vaughn D, Van Arsdalen K, et al: Three cases of advanced seminoma and Down's syndrome: a possible association. *Am J Clin Oncol* 26:197–199, 2003
13. Murty V, Chaganti RS: A genetic perspective of male germ cell tumors. *Semin Oncol* 25:133–144, 1998
14. Olsson H, Bladstrom A, Alm P: Male gynecomastia and risk for malignant tumours — a cohort study. *BMC Cancer* 2:26, 2002
15. Fukui M: Testicular cancer and syndrome X. *Lancet* 358:242, 2001
16. Jacobsen R, Bostofte E, Engholm G, et al: Risk of testicular cancer in men with abnormal semen characteristics: cohort study. *BMJ* 321:789–792, 2000
17. Bonner MR, McCann SE, Moysich KB: Dietary factors and the risk of testicular cancer. *Nutr Cancer* 44:35–43, 2002
18. Ohlson CG, Hardell L: Testicular cancer and occupational exposures with a focus on xenoestrogens in polyvinyl chloride plastics. *Chemosphere* 40:1277–1282, 2000
19. Moller H, Knudsen LB, Lynge E: Risk of testicular cancer after vasectomy: Cohort study of over 73,000 men. *Br Med J* 309:295–299, 1994
20. Wynd CA: Testicular self-examination in young adult men. *J Nurs Scholarsh* 34:251–255, 2002
21. Cook N: Testicular cancer: testicular self-examination and screening. *Br J Nurs* 9:338–343, 2000
22. Brenner JS, Hergenroeder AC, Kozinetz CA, et al: Teaching testicular self-examination: education and practices in pediatric residents. *Pediatrics* 111:e239–e244, 2003
23. Taylor JS, Dube CE, Pipas CF, et al: Teaching the testicular exam: a model curriculum from "A" to "Zack." *Fam Med* 36:209–213, 2004
24. Daniels IR, Layer GT: Testicular tumours presenting as gynaecomastia. *Eur J Surg Oncol* 29:437–439, 2003
25. Srivastava A, Kreiger N: Relation of physical activity to risk of testicular cancer. *Am J Epidemiol* 151:78–87, 2000
26. Che M, Tamboli P, Ro JY, et al: Bilateral testicular germ cell tumors: twenty-year experience at M. D. Anderson Cancer Center. *Cancer* 95:1228–1233, 2002
27. Lee F, Hamid R, Arya M, et al: Testicular cancer: current update and controversies. *Hospmed* 63:615–620, 2002
28. Duffy MJ: Clinical uses of tumor markers: a critical review. *Crit Rev Clin Lab Sci* 38:225–262, 2001
29. Looijenga LH, Zafarana G, Grygalewicz B, et al: Role of gain of 12p in germ cell tumour development. *Apmis* 111:161–171; discussion 172–173, 2003
30. Rosenberg C, Van Gurp RJ, Geelen E, et al: Overrepresentation of the short arm of chromosome 12 is related to invasive growth of human testicular seminomas and nonseminomas. *Oncogene* 19:5858–5862, 2000
31. Skotheim RI, Monni O, Mousses S, et al: New insights into testicular germ cell tumorigenesis from gene expression profiling. *Cancer Res* 62:2359–2364, 2002
32. Dogra VS, Gottlieb RH, Oka M, Rubens DJ: Sonography of the scrotum. *Radiology* 227:18–36, 2003
33. Bramley R: The role of chest X-ray and computed tomography thorax in the surveillance of testicular tumours. *Clin Oncol (R Coll Radiol)* 15:441–442, 2003
34. Braga FJ, Arbex MA, Haddad J, et al: Bone scintigraphy in testicular tumors. *Clin Nucl Med* 26:117–118, 2001
35. Sterpy MD, Tiutin LA: [Role of MRI tomography in testicular cancer]. *Vopr Onkol* 49:323–327, 2003
36. Corral DA, Varma DG, Jackson EF, et al: Magnetic resonance imaging and magnetic resonance angiography before postchemotherapy retroperitoneal lymph node dissection. *Urology* 55:262–266, 2000
37. Hofer C, Kubler H, Hartung R, et al: Diagnosis and monitoring of urological tumors using positron emission tomography. *Eur Urol* 40:481–487, 2001
38. Kliesch S, Thomaidis T, Schutte B, et al: Update on the diagnostic safety for detection of testicular intraepithelial neoplasia (TIN). *Apmis* 111:70–74; discussion 75, 2003
39. Heidenreich A, Srivastava S, Moul JW, et al: Molecular genetic parameters in pathogenesis and prognosis of testicular germ cell tumors. *Eur Urol* 37:121–135, 2000
40. International Germ Cell Cancer Collaborative Group: International Germ Cell Consensus Classification: a prognostic factor-based staging system for metastatic germ cell cancers. *J Clin Oncol* 15:594–603, 1997
41. Poirier S, Rawl S: Testicular germ cell cancer, in Yarbro CH, Frogge MH, Goodman M (eds.), *Cancer Nursing Practice and Principles* (ed 5). Sudbury, MA, Jones and Bartlett, 2000, pp 1494–1510
42. Heidenreich A: Clinical stage I nonseminomatous testicular germ-cell tumors: surgery or watchful waiting, still an issue? *Curr Opin Urol* 12:427–430, 2002
43. Leisinger HJ, Donohue JP: The role of retroperitoneal surgery in testis cancer. *Crit Rev Oncol Hematol* 44:71–80, 2002
44. Sweeney CJ, Hermans BP, Heilman DK, et al: Results and outcome of retroperitoneal lymph node dissection for clinical stage I embryonal carcinoma — predominant testis cancer. *J Clin Oncol* 18:358–362, 2000
45. Porcaro AB, Zecchini Antoniolli S, Novella G, et al: [Histopathologic risk factors in patients with non-seminomatous germ tumors of the testis in clinical stage 1. Retrospective study of 75 patients]. *Arch Ital Urol Androl* 73:177–180, 2001
46. Pohar KS, Rabbani F, Bosl GJ, et al: Results of retroperitoneal lymph node dissection for clinical stage I and II pure embryonal carcinoma of the testis. *J Urol* 170:1155–1158, 2003
47. Foster R, Bihrle R: Current status of retroperitoneal lymph node dissection and testicular cancer: when to operate. *Cancer Control* 9:277–283, 2002
48. Roeleveld TA, Horenblas S, Meinhardt W, et al: Surveillance can be the standard of care for stage I nonseminomatous testic-

ular tumors and even high risk patients. *J Urol* 166:2166–2170, 2001
49. Daugaard G, Petersen PM, Rorth M: Surveillance in stage I testicular cancer. *Apmis* 111:76–83, discussion 83–85, 2003
50. Albers P, Siener R, Kliesch S, et al: Risk factors for relapse in clinical stage I nonseminomatous testicular germ cell tumors: results of the German Testicular Cancer Study Group Trial. *J Clin Oncol* 21:1505–1512, 2003
51. Jones RH, Vasey PA: Part I: testicular cancer — management of early disease. *Lancet Oncol* 4:730–737, 2003
52. Thijssens K, Vaneerdeweg W, Schrijvers D, et al: Retroperitoneal lymph node dissection as adjuvant therapy in the treatment of non-seminomatous testicular cancer. *Acta Chir Belg* 103:599–602, 2003
53. Kesler KA: Surgical techniques for testicular nonseminomatous germ cell tumors metastatic to the mediastinum. *Chest Surg Clin North Am* 12:749–768, 2002
54. Horvath LG, McCaughan BC, Stockle M, et al: Resection of residual pulmonary masses after chemotherapy in patients with metastatic non-seminomatous germ cell tumours. *Intern Med J* 32:79–83, 2002
55. Bauduceau O, Souleau B, Le-Moulec S, et al: Radiotherapy in stage I testicular seminoma: retrospective study and review of literature. *Cancer Radiother* 7:386–394, 2003
56. Roth B, Nichols C, Einhorn L: Neoplasms of the testis, in Frei E, Holland J, Bast R, Kufe D, et al: *Cancer Medicine, vol 2* (ed 3). Philadelphia, Lea and Febiger, 1993, pp 1592–1619
57. Warde P, Specht L, Horwich A, et al: Prognostic factors for relapse in stage I seminoma managed by surveillance: a pooled analysis. *J Clin Oncol* 20:4448–4452, 2002
58. Warde P, Gospodarowicz MK, Panzarella T, et al: Long term outcome and cost in the management of stage I testicular seminoma. *Can J Urol* 7:967–972; discussion 973, 2000
59. Guden M, Ulutin C, Goktas S: Analyses of 98 seminoma cases: a review article. *Int Urol Nephrol* 33:529–531, 2001
60. Classen J, Schmidberger H, Meisner C, et al: Radiotherapy for stages IIA/B testicular seminoma: final report of a prospective multicenter clinical trial. *J Clin Oncol* 21:1101–1106, 2003
61. Porcaro AB, Antoniolli SZ, Schiavone D, et al: Management of clinical stage I testicular pure seminoma. Report on 42 patients and review of the literature. *Arch Ital Urol Androl* 74:77–80, 2002
62. Steiner H, Holtl L, Wirtenberger W, et al: Long-term experience with carboplatin monotherapy for clinical stage I seminoma: a retrospective single-center study. *Urology* 60:324–328, 2002
63. Zagars GK, Pollack A: Radiotherapy for stage II testicular seminoma. *Int J Radiat Oncol Biol Phys* 51:643–649, 2001
64. Fleshner N, Warde P: Controversies in the management of testicular seminoma. *Semin Urol Oncol* 20:227–233, 2002
65. Zagars GK, Ballo MT, Lee AK, et al: Mortality after cure of testicular seminoma. *J Clin Oncol* 22:640–647, 2004
66. Patel MI, Motzer RJ, Sheinfeld J: Management of recurrence and follow-up strategies for patients with seminoma and selected high-risk groups. *Urol Clin North Am* 30:803–817, 2003
67. Stern JW, Bunin N: Prospective study of carboplatin-based chemotherapy for pediatric germ cell tumors. *Med Pediatr Oncol* 39:163–167, 2002
68. Motzer RJ, Sheinfeld J, Mazumdar M, et al: Paclitaxel, ifosfamide, and cisplatin second-line therapy for patients with relapsed testicular germ cell cancer. *J Clin Oncol* 18:2413–2418, 2000
69. Hinton S, Catalano P, Einhorn LH, et al: Phase II study of paclitaxel plus gemcitabine in refractory germ cell tumors (E9897): a trial of the Eastern Cooperative Oncology Group. *J Clin Oncol* 20:1859–1863, 2002
70. Motzer RJ: Paclitaxel (Taxol) combination therapy for resistant germ cell tumors. *Semin Oncol* 27:33–35, 2000
71. Mardiak J, Salek T, Sycova-Mila Z, et al: Carboplatin and cyclophosphamide in the treatment of metastatic seminoma. *Neoplasma* 47:244–247, 2000
72. Amato RJ, Millikan R, Daliani D, et al: Cyclophosphamide and carboplatin and selective consolidation in advanced seminoma. *Clin Cancer Res* 6:72–77, 2000
73. Berney D, Shamash J, Gaffney J, et al: DNA topoisomerase I and II expression in drug resistant germ cell tumours. *Br J Cancer* 87:524–629, 2002
74. Soule S, Baldridge L, Kirkpatrick K, et al: HER-2/neu expression in germ cell tumours. *J Clin Pathol* 55:656–658, 2002
75. Flechon A, Bompas E, Biron P, Droz JP: Management of post-chemotherapy residual masses in advanced seminoma. *J Urol* 168:1975–1979, 2002
76. Sexton WJ, Wood CG, Kim R, et al: Repeat retroperitoneal lymph node dissection for metastatic testis cancer. *J Urol* 169:1353–1356, 2003
77. Salesi N, D. Cocco B, Alghisi F, et al: Testis cancer markers. Clinical use. *Minerva Med* 93:365–369, 2002
78. Miyazaki J, Miyanaga N, Kawai K, et al: High-dose chemotherapy with peripheral blood stem cell transplantation for advanced testicular cancer. *Int J Urol* 7:258–262, 2000
79. Jones RH, Vasey PA: Part II: testicular cancer — management of advanced disease. *Lancet Oncol* 4:738–747, 2003
80. Higgs D: The patient with testicular cancer: nursing management of chemotherapy. *Oncol Nurs Forum* 17:243–246, 1990
81. Horenblas S: Re: lymphatic mapping and gamma probe guided laparoscopic biopsy of sentinel lymph node in patients with clinical stage I testicular tumor. *J Urol* 169:2305–2306, author reply 2306, 2003
82. Tanis PJ, Horenblas S, Valdes Olmos RA, et al: Feasibility of sentinel node lymphoscintigraphy in stage I testicular cancer. *Eur J Nucl Med Mol Imaging* 29:670–673, 2002
83. Spermon JR, Kiemeney LA, Meuleman EJ, et al: Fertility in men with testicular germ cell tumors. *Fertil Steril* 79(suppl 3):1543–1549, 2003
84. Agarwa A: Semen banking in patients with cancer: 20-year experience. *Int J Androl* 23(suppl 2):16–19, 2000
85. Bahadur G, Ling KL, Hart R, et al: Semen quality and cryopreservation in adolescent cancer patients. *Hum Reprod* 17:3157–3161, 2002
86. Adshead J, Khoubehi B, Wood J, Rustin G: Testicular implants and patient satisfaction: a questionnaire-based study of men after orchiectomy for testicular cancer. *BJU Int* 88:559–562, 2001
87. Richie JP: Testicular implants and patient satisfaction: a questionnaire-based study of men after orchiectomy for testicular cancer. *J Urol* 168:1286, 2002
88. Boyer M, Raghavan D: Toxicity of germ cell tumors. *Semin Oncol* 19:128–142, 1992
89. Strohl R: Symptom management of acute and chronic reactions. *Oncol Nurs Forum* 15:429–434, 1988
90. Raghavan D: Testicular cancer: maintaining the high cure rate. *Oncology (Huntingt)* 17:218–228; discussion 228–229, 234–235, passim, 2003
91. Pentheroudakis G, O'Neill VJ, Vasey P, et al: Spontaneous acute tumour lysis syndrome in patients with metastatic germ cell tumours. Report of two cases. *Support Care Cancer* 9:554–557, 2001
92. Kawai K, Akaza H: Bleomycin-induced pulmonary toxicity in chemotherapy for testicular cancer. *Expert Opin Drug Saf* 2:587–596, 2003

93. O'Sullivan JM, Huddart RA, Norman AR, et al: DP, Horwich A: Predicting the risk of bleomycin lung toxicity in patients with germ-cell tumours. *Ann Oncol* 14:91–96, 2003
94. van de Loosdrecht AA, Gietema JA, van der Graaf WT: Seizures in a patient with disseminated testicular cancer due to cisplatin-induced hypomagnesaemia. *Acta Oncol* 39:239–240, 2000
95. Classen J, Dieckmann KP: Re: malignant germ cell tumor of the contralateral testis after radiotherapy for testicular intraepithelial neoplasia. *J Urol* 166:630–631, 2001
96. Crabb SJ, McKendrick JJ, Mead GM: Brain as sanctuary site of relapse in germ cell cancer patients previously treated with chemotherapy. *Clin Oncol* (*R Coll Radiol*) 14:287–293, 2002
97. Bart J, Groen HJ, van der Graaf WT, et al: An oncological view on the blood–testis barrier. *Lancet Oncol* 3:357–363, 2002
98. Fossa SD, Dahl AA, Loge JH: Fatigue, anxiety, and depression in long-term survivors of testicular cancer. *J Clin Oncol* 21:1249–1254, 2003
99. Trask PC, Paterson AG, Fardig J, et al: Course of distress and quality of life in testicular cancer patients before, during, and after chemotherapy: results of a pilot study. *Psychooncology* 12:814–820, 2003
100. Caffo O, Amichetti M, Tomio L, et al: Quality of life after radiotherapy for early-stage testicular seminoma. *Radiother Oncol* 59:13–20, 2001
101. Argirovic D, Hadzi-Djokic J, Micic S: [Quality of life after retroperitoneal lymphadenectomy in low clinical stages of nonseminomatous testicular tumors]. *Acta Chir Iugosl* 46:31–33, 1999
102. Fossa SD, de Wit R, Roberts JT, et al: Quality of life in good prognosis patients with metastatic germ cell cancer: a prospective study of the European Organization for Research and Treatment of Cancer Genitourinary Group/Medical Research Council Testicular Cancer Study Group (30941/TE20). *J Clin Oncol* 21:1107–1118, 2003
103. Vaughn DJ, Gignac GA, Meadows AT: Long-term medical care of testicular cancer survivors. *Ann Intern Med* 136:463–470, 2002
104. Tamboli CP: Long-term survivors of testicular cancer. *J Clin Oncol* 21:3888, author reply 3888–3889, 2003
105. Tong KT: Long-term medical care of testicular cancer survivors. *Ann Intern Med* 138:437, author reply 437, 2003
106. Travis LB, Andersson M, Gospodarowicz M, et al: Treatment-associated leukemia following testicular cancer. *J Natl Cancer Inst* 92:1165–1171, 2000
107. Gietema JA, Meinardi MT, Messerschmidt J, et al: Circulating plasma platinum more than 10 years after cisplatin treatment for testicular cancer. *Lancet* 355:1075–1076, 2000
108. Gerl A, Schierl R: Urinary excretion of platinum in chemotherapy-treated long-term survivors of testicular cancer. *Acta Oncol* 39:519–522, 2000
109. Chaudhary UB, Haldas JR: Long-term complications of chemotherapy for germ cell tumours. *Drugs* 63:1565–1577, 2003
110. Meinardi MT, Gietema JA, van der Graaf WT, et al: Cardiovascular morbidity in long-term survivors of metastatic testicular cancer. *J Clin Oncol* 18:1725–1732, 2000
111. Thorsen L, Nystad W, Dahl O, et al: The level of physical activity in long-term survivors of testicular cancer. *Eur J Cancer* 39:1216–1221, 2003
112. Sleijfer S, de Wit R: Physical activity in long-term survivors of germ-cell cancer. *Eur J Cancer* 39:1191–1193, 2003
113. Kuczyk MA, Bokemeyer C, Kollmannsberger C, et al: Late relapse after treatment for nonseminomatous testicular germ cell tumors according to a single center-based experience. *World J Urol* 22:55–59, 2004
114. Shahidi M, Norman AR, Dearnaley DP, et al: Late recurrence in 1263 men with testicular germ cell tumors. Multivariate analysis of risk factors and implications for management. *Cancer* 95:520–530, 2002
115. Bompas E, Flechon A, Biron P, et al: Management of advanced seminoma: retrospective study of 96 patients. *Bull Cancer* 89:877–885, 2002
116. Skotheim RI, Lothe RA: The testicular germ cell tumour genome. *Apmis* 111:136–150, discussion 50–51, 2003
117. Jones A, Fujiyama C, Turner K, et al: Angiogenesis and lymphangiogenesis in stage 1 germ cell tumours of the testis. *BJU Int* 86:80–86, 2000
118. Jones RH, Vasey PA: New directions in testicular cancer; molecular determinants of oncogenesis and treatment success. *Eur J Cancer* 39:147–156, 2003
119. Mayer F, Gillis AJ, Dinjens W, et al: Microsatellite instability of germ cell tumors is associated with resistance to systemic treatment. *Cancer Res* 62:2758–2760, 2002
120. Boyle P: Testicular cancer: the challenge for cancer control. *Lancet Oncol* 5:56–61, 2004
121. Whiteford A, Wordley J: Raising awareness and detection of testicular cancer in young men. *Nurs Times* 99:34–36, 2003

CHAPTER 66

Vulvar and Vaginal Cancer

Carol Guarnieri, RN, MSN

Introduction

Approximately 6,130 females in the United States were expected to be diagnosed with vaginal or vulvar cancer in 2004 and an estimated 1,640 deaths were expected to occur from these cancers in the same year.[1] Even though vulvar and vaginal cancers occur infrequently, nursing care for these women is very challenging. These cancers usually affect older, postmenopausal women. Treatment with surgery and radiation therapy will typically affect sexuality, and many women will face some degree of change in their body image. Nurses need to understand normal female genital anatomy because it is often affected or altered by treatment. Nurses play a vital role in the healthcare team by helping women to cope with changes in sexual functioning.

Vulvar and vaginal cancers are frequently preceded by a preinvasive intraepithelial neoplasia, and both can be curable if diagnosed in the early stages. Close follow-up care and education for women with preinvasive disease is crucial for early detection and to prevent progression to invasive disease.

VULVAR CANCER

Epidemiology

Vulvar carcinoma accounts for 3%–5% of all gynecologic cancers. It is largely a disease of elderly women, with peak incidence occurring in the seventh decade of life. Although the overall incidence of vulvar cancer has remained stable, a striking increase has been seen in women younger than 50 years of age.[2] Similar to cervical cancer, vulvar cancer can be preceded by a preinvasive intraepithelial neoplasia of the vulvar tissue. Vulvar intraepithelial neoplasia (VIN) is the term used to denote epithelial abnormalities of the vulva, which are classified into three categories (VIN I, II, or III) that differentiate the degree of epithelial involvement by neoplastic cells. The incidence of VIN has significantly increased during the past two decades. While VIN can develop at any age, the mean age at diagnosis has also fallen from women in their forties or fifties to women in their thirties.[3] The stable incidence of invasive carcinoma of the vulva, even as the overall number of cases of preinvasive disease increases, may suggest that the etiologic factors for VIN and invasive carcinoma are different, that diagnostic procedures have improved, or that treatment of VIN is effective in preventing invasive disease.[4]

Table 66-1 Two Subsets of Women with Squamous Cell Carcinoma of the Vulva

	Type I	Type II
Age	35–55 years	55–85 years
Associated with HPV infection	Yes	No
Preexisting disease	VIN	Lichen sclerosis, vulvar inflammation
Multifocal lesions	Yes	No
Histopathology of tumor	Poorly differentiated, nonkeratinizing	Well differentiated, keratinizing

Etiology

The etiology of VIN and invasive vulvar cancer is largely unknown. Even the relationship of VIN to invasive vulvar disease remains unclear and multifactorial. Recent evidence suggests that vulvar cancer consists of two separate diseases.

The first type is caused by the human papillomavirus (HPV), most commonly HPV type 16, and is associated with VIN. HPV infection has been found in 80%–90% of women with VIN, but concomitant occurrence of HPV infection decreases to 30% in women with invasive disease. HPV-positive tumors have a higher incidence among cigarette smokers than nonsmokers and are more commonly found in younger women, women who have their first sexual intercourse at a young age, and those who have multiple sexual partners. HPV lesions tend to be multifocal in nature.

The second type of vulvar cancer more often affects older women who generally have a history of vulvar inflammation or lichen sclerosis. Their tumors are usually unifocal, well differentiated, and keratinizing[3,5,6] (Table 66-1).

Research has shown that the *p53* tumor suppressor gene may play a role in the etiology of squamous cell carcinoma. This gene plays an important role in the regulation of the cell cycle. Studies have shown that *p53* mutations are more commonly seen in older women who are not infected by HPV. Younger patients rarely have *p53* mutations.[7,8]

Other risk factors for vulvar cancer include venereal warts and the presence of herpes simplex virus type 2. A history of chronic vulvar disease and previous malignancies of the lower genital tract are also seen in women with vulvar cancer. Preliminary reports suggest that immunosuppression may play an important role in development of this cancer. Individuals who have undergone organ transplants or individuals who are infected with the human immunodeficiency virus (HIV) may have an increased risk of vulvar cancer. Angiogenesis, the development of new blood vessels from

Table 66-2 Vulvar Cancer: Risk Factors and Preventive Measures

Risk Factors	Preventive Measures
Human papillomavirus	Pap smear per ACS guidelines
Herpes simplex virus type 2	Routine vulvar self-examination
History of smoking	Stop smoking
Multiple sexual partners	Limit number of sexual partners
Immunosuppression	Use barrier contraception
Chronic vulvar disease	
Previous malignancies of the lower genital tract	
Age > 60 years	

existing vasculature, is also being studied to determine how it may contribute to the development of vulvar cancer.[9–11] Table 66-2 summarizes the risk factors for this cancer.

Prevention and Screening

Screening for vulvar cancer should be performed when a woman has a Papanicolaou (Pap) smear done. Careful examination of the vulva is critical. Screening should focus on women who smoke, women with HPV infection, and women who have other preinvasive disease of the cervix, vagina, or perianal area. Nurses are often excellent resources to help educate women (especially older women) that a regular pelvic examination following American Cancer Society (ACS) guidelines is crucial. They can also teach women about performing vulvar self-examination, avoiding exposure to HPV, and the negative effects of smoking.

Women who are diagnosed with VIN or vulvar cancer at an early stage can benefit from early detection. If a woman has a lesion present, she should insist on a biopsy if the lesion persists despite treatment. With early detection, treatment morbidity is often decreased because physicians may be able to perform less radical surgery to eradicate the disease.[12] Stage I and II tumors have a low rate of recurrence. In addition, early detection remains crucial because the disease can have a significant impact on a woman's sexuality, particularly in its advanced stages.[7,13]

Pathophysiology

Cellular Characteristics

VIN commonly presents in a multifocal pattern. Discoloration of the vulva with white, gray, red, or brown lesions is usual. The lesions may be macular or papular and often present with a rough, warty-like surface.[4] On examination, the tumor may appear as an ulcerated mass and usually remains confined to the vulva for a long period of time. Histologically, squamous cell carcinoma accounts for more than 90% of all primary vulvar neoplasms. The remaining 10% of vulvar neoplasms include malignant melanoma, basal cell, adenocarcinoma, and sarcoma.[14]

Progression of Disease

VIN is divided into three categories: VIN I, VIN II, and VIN III. VIN I comprises mild dysplasia, while VIN II describes moderate dysplasia. VIN III or carcinoma in situ (CIS) includes severe dysplasia and suggests full-thickness changes of the epithelium. VIN III/CIS of the vulva does not appear to have the same malignant potential as preinvasive disease of the cervix. It is most likely to progress to invasive disease if the woman is elderly (older than 60 years of age), is immunosuppressed, or has multifocal disease.

The vulva includes the mons pubis, the labia majora and minora, the clitoris, the vestibule of the vagina, and the Bartholin glands. The mons pubis is the pad of fat anterior to the pubis symphysis and is covered by hair-bearing skin. The labia majora extends posterior from the mons into the vaginal opening. The labia minora consists of small folds of skin that lie between the labia majora and divides anteriorly to envelop the clitoris. The vestibule is the area into which the vagina opens. The bulbs of the vestibule are erectile tissue on each side of the vaginal opening. The vulva is surrounded by a network of lymphatics.

Although primary disease can develop anywhere on the vulva, approximately 70% of tumors arise on the labia majora. The labia minora, clitoris, and perineum are also common sites of disease development. Vulvar cancer usually remains a localized disease with well-defined margins.[14]

The most common routes of metastatic spread are through direct extension or dissemination to regional lymph nodes. Lymphatic spread of vulvar cancer usually follows a predictable pattern. From the superficial inguinal lymph nodes, the tumor usually spreads to the deep inguinal/femoral nodes and then to the pelvic lymph nodes[7,15,16] (Figure 66-1). Tumors involving the midline can metastasize to the groin nodes on both sides. Early-stage tumors rarely metastasize to the contralateral lymph nodes. At diagnosis, the overall incidence of positive lymph nodes is approximately 45%. Inguinal node metastases occur in 35%–40% of women, and the incidence of pelvic node metastases is 5%–10%.[4,15,17] In its advanced stages, vulvar cancer may spread to the urethra, vagina, anus, rectum, and

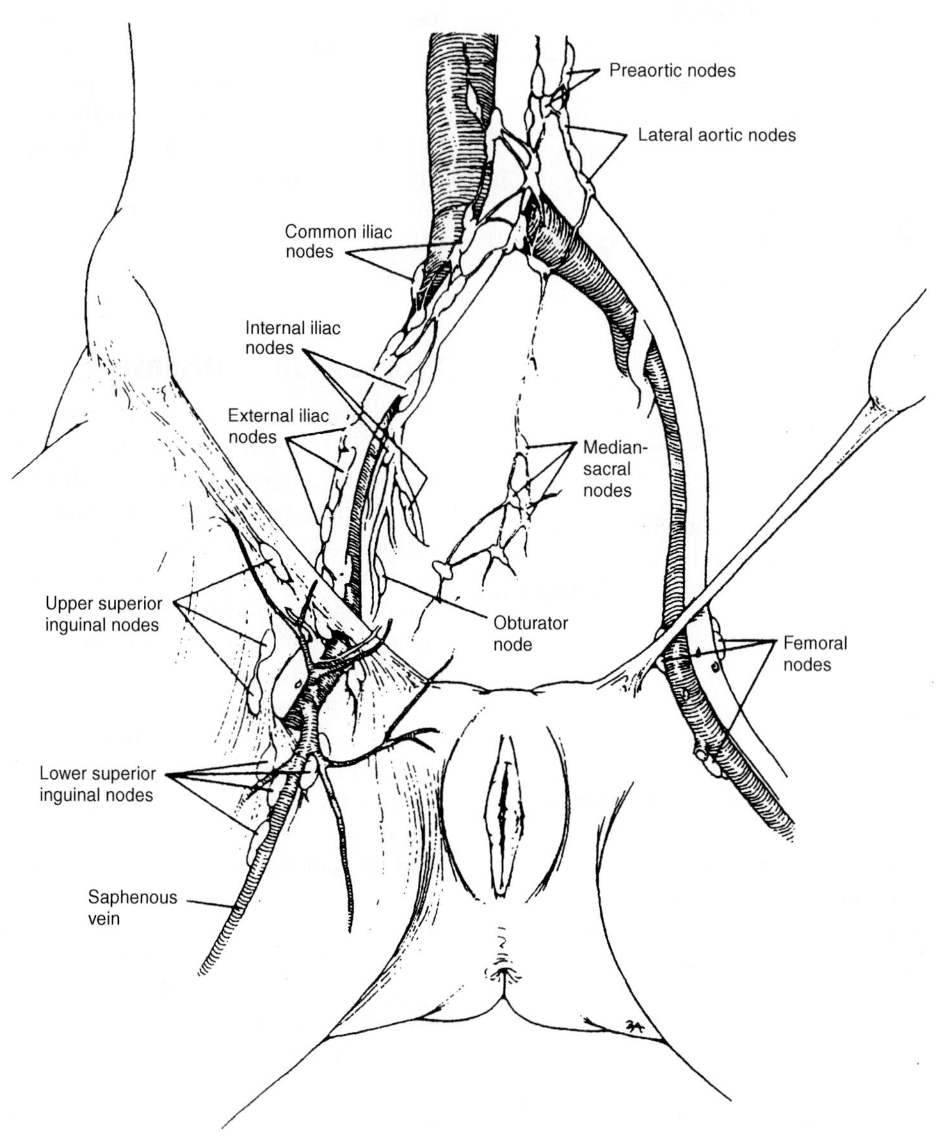

Figure 66-1 Inguinofemoral lymph nodes. [Reprinted with permission from Hacker NF: Surgery for malignant tumors of the vulva, in Gershenson DM, DeCherney AH, Curry SL (eds.): *Operative Gynecology*. Philadelphia, Saunders, 1996.[16]]

pubic bone. The most common site of distant metastasis is the lung.

Clinical Manifestations

The symptoms of VIN and invasive vulvar carcinoma are variable and insidious. Fifty percent of women with VIN are asymptomatic, whereas other women with VIN may complain of vulvar pruritus, irritation, or presence of a lesion. Less common presenting symptoms include vulvar bleeding, discharge, or dysuria. As many as 20% of women with vulvar cancer are asymptomatic, with lesions being detected only during routine pelvic examination.[18,19]

Delay in diagnosing a woman with vulvar cancer may occur because she is too embarrassed to seek medical assistance due to the intimate area of the body that is involved. As a result, the woman may have symptoms for 2–16 months before seeking medical attention.[19] A delay in definitive treatment may occur because symptomatic topical treatment for vulvar lesions can continue for 12 months or longer before the lesion is biopsied for definitive diagnosis, or because the healthcare provider fails to adequately assess a woman reporting symptoms of vulvar irritation.[15,19] Lesions are usually diagnosed and treated when they are small, which may suggest that women with vulvar cancer are being biopsied earlier.

Assessment

Patient and Family History

Women with VIN and invasive cancer should have a complete history that includes the duration and severity of signs and symptoms. They may have a history of a previous malignancy in the lower genital tract, so detailed questioning about gynecological history is warranted. Because cigarette smoking and multiple sexual partners are risk factors, a smoking and sexual history should be taken. A family history related to cancer is important; however, having a history of vulvar cancer in the family is not a potential risk factor.

Physical Examination

Careful inspection of the vulva during routine gynecologic examination is imperative because this practice remains the most productive diagnostic measure. Because the neoplasia is often multifocal, the entire vulva, perineum, and perianal area should be evaluated. Lymph nodes in the groin should be palpated. A Pap smear should be done to rule out cervical cancer. Colposcopic examination may help define the extent of the disease, and thorough examination under anesthesia with multiple biopsies is important to determine the extent of disease. Fine-needle aspiration biopsy of any suspicious lymph node can also be done at this time.[20,21]

Diagnostic Studies

All patients require a chest x-ray, complete blood count, and biochemical profile. Computerized tomography (CT) and magnetic resonance imaging (MRI) are used to evaluate patients for nodal metastasis and possible distant metastasis. In selected cases, cystoscopy and proctosigmoidoscopy may also be necessary. If the disease is thought to be advanced and the patient states that she has pelvic pain, skeletal radiographs should be done to rule out bone metastasis.[14]

Prognostic Indicators

The five-year survival rate for vulvar cancer is correlated with stage of disease and nodal involvement. Groin lymph node status is the best indicator of survival. In women with negative nodes, the five-year survival rate is as high as 90%. The survival rate decreases as the number of positive nodes increases. The five-year survival rate is approximately 40% when three to four nodes are positive but decreases to 20% with six or more positive nodes.[18,22] In addition to nodal status, tumors that show evidence of HPV infection have a better prognosis. HPV-negative tumors are correlated with a higher risk of recurrence and death rate from vulvar cancer than HPV-positive tumors.[23] Other major prognostic factors include the stage at time of diagnosis, tumor grade, and tumor size.

Classification and Staging

The International Federation of Gynecology and Obstetrics (FIGO) staging of vulvar cancer is shown in

Table 66-3 FIGO Staging of Vulvar Cancer

Stage	TNM	Clinical Findings
Stage 0		Carcinoma in situ (e.g., VIN III)
Stage I	TI, NO, MO TI, NI, MO	Tumor confined to the vulva or perineum, 2 cm or less in dimension, no nodal metastasis
Stage IA		Tumor confined to vulva or perineum, 2 cm or less, with stromal invasion no greater than 1.0 mm, no nodal metastasis
Stage IB		Tumor confined to the vulva or perineum, 2 cm or less, with stromal invasion greater than 1.0 mm, no nodal metastasis
Stage II	T2, N0, M0 T2, NI, M0	Tumor confined to vulva or perineum, more than 2 cm in greatest dimension, no nodal metastasis
Stage III	T3, N0, M0 T3, NI, M0 T3, N2, M0 TI, N2, M0 T2, N2, M0	Tumor of any size with adjacent spread to the urethra, vagina, or anus or with unilateral regional lymph node *metastasis*
Stage IVA	TX, N3, M0 T4, N0, M0 T4, NI, M0 T4, N2, M0 TX, NX, MIa TX, NX, MIb	Tumor invades upper urethra, bladder mucosa, rectal mucosa, pelvic bone, or bilateral regional node *metastases*
Stage IVB		Any distant metastasis, including pelvic lymph nodes

Reprinted with permission from Benedet JL, Bender H, Jones H 3rd: FIGO Staging classifications and clinical practice guidelines in the management of of gynecologic cancers. *Int J Gynecol Obstet* 70:209–262, 2000.[24]

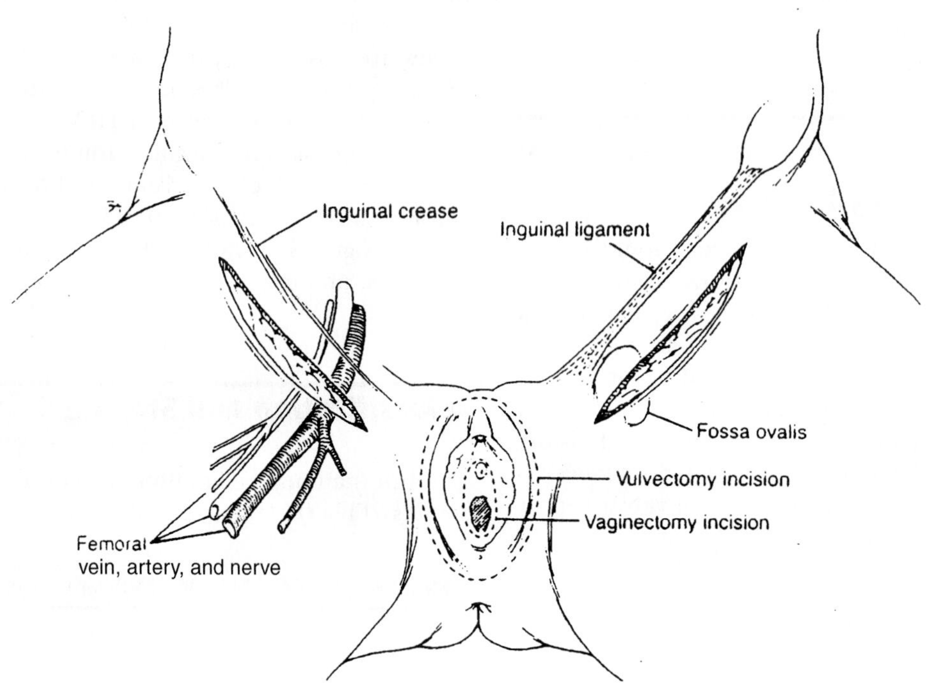

Figure 66-2 Vulvectomy and bilateral groin dissection through three separate incisions. [Reprinted with permission from Hacker NF: Surgery for malignant tumors of the vulva, in Gershenson DM, DeCherney AH, Curry SL (eds.): *Operative Gynecology*. Philadelphia, Saunders, 1996.[16]]

Table 66-3.[24] Surgical findings are incorporated into the staging evaluation. To make a diagnosis of invasive vulvar carcinoma, a wedge biopsy of the lesion is needed. The biopsy should be full thickness and include a margin of normal connective tissue. This biopsy will help in differentiating between stage I and stage II disease. Biopsy of the nodes should be done as well. In stage I and stage II disease, all lymph nodes are negative. In stage III disease, the tumor has spread to adjacent areas of the urethra and/or the vagina, perineum, and anus. Lymph nodes in the groin are clinically suspicious for tumor. Stage IV disease features a tumor that has infiltrated to the bladder and/or rectal mucosa and may be fixed to bone.[4]

Therapeutic Approaches and Nursing Care: VIN

Some controversy exists about the treatment of choice for patients with VIN. In the past, a total vulvectomy was done for the management of VIN. Today, a more conservative surgical approach is usually undertaken. A wide local excision of the lesion or lesions may be all that is necessary. This approach helps maintain the sexual and reproductive function of the vulva and may help women avoid the adverse physical and psychological effects of more extensive surgery. The effectiveness of wide local excision in eradicating VIN varies from 83% to 91%.[25]

For multicentric disease, a skinning vulvectomy (Figure 66-2)[16] is performed in which the vulvar skin is excised while conserving the fat, muscle, and glands below the skin.[25] A split-thickness skin graft reconstruction from the thigh or buttock is performed. The skinning vulvectomy has a success rate similar to that of other surgical treatment modalities.[26] The wide local excision and skinning vulvectomy provide excellent cosmetic and functional results.[25,26] A skinning vulvectomy may not be an option for elderly or debilitated women, however, because the healing of the skin graft requires prolonged bed rest.

An alternative to excision of the vulvar lesion is local treatment with cautery, CO_2 laser surgery, or cryosurgery. The advantages of these surgical techniques are outpatient management, sparing effect on surrounding tissue, and minimal scarring with good cosmetic and functional results. However, the procedures can result in painful ulcers and require several sequenced treatments. Healing time can be prolonged.[27,28] Comparative studies of excisional surgery and laser ablation demonstrate that both are equally effective in eradicating the disease, although some evidence suggests that relapse occurs more quickly after laser ablation.[26] Other promising treatments of VIN include cavitational ultrasonic surgical aspiration (CUSA), the topical application of imiquimod cream, and photodynamic therapy. While these treatments appear promising in helping to preserve the anatomy and function of the vulvar area, prospective, controlled studies need to be completed to confirm their efficacy.[20,29–31]

For women with VIN, education is an essential responsibility of nursing. Explaining the difference between VIN and invasive vulvar cancer is key. Given that several treatments are available, the nurse can help the woman understand the type of treatment recommended. Follow-up care by the nurse includes teaching the woman how to care for herself at home. When sexual intercourse is resumed in approximately four to six weeks following surgery, a water-soluble lubricant can be used for comfort. Sexual satisfaction is possible, and the nurse can discuss with the woman methods to maintain sexual activity. Due to the uncertain malignant potential of VIN and its potential for recurrence, close and long-term follow-up care should be stressed.

Therapeutic Approaches and Nursing Care: Invasive Disease

Surgery

The traditional treatment for women with cancer of the vulva has been surgical: en bloc dissection of the tumor along with contiguous skin, subcutaneous fat, regional inguinal and femoral nodes, and vulva (labia minora, labia majora, clitoris, and perineal body). Historically, physicians routinely recommended a pelvic node dissection. With such a dissection, wound closure was difficult to achieve. Today, many surgeons have abandoned the en bloc approach and perform the nodal dissections through separate groin incisions (Figure 66-2). Many studies have attested to the reduced morbidity associated with separate groin incisions without increasing recurrence rates.[32] In the absence of clinical suspicion of groin node involvement, unilateral lymphadenectomy may be sufficient.[25] The trend is to stay away from the radical surgery that has been associated with disturbances in sexual function and body image. Instead, more emphasis is placed on individualized treatment for each woman, taking into account her age, location of disease, extent of disease, and psychosocial consequences.[32,33]

Most stage I carcinomas of the vulva can be treated with wide local excision alone because the risk of nodal spread is small. For larger and more invasive tumors, ipsilateral inguinofemoral lymphadenectomy or postoperative radiation is recommended. For patients with midline lesions, bilateral node dissections using separate groin incisions are recommended. To further reduce the postoperative morbidity associated with groin dissections, intraoperative lymphatic mapping using the sentinel inguinal lymph node is being studied. In this procedure, isosulfan blue dye is injected into the dermis at the junction of the tumor and normal vulvar skin. This dye spreads to the nodes where the cancer has metastasized. By removing and examining only the blue-dyed nodes, the surgeon and pathologist can determine whether the cancer has spread. If the cancer has not metastasized, removal of additional lymph nodes is unnecessary. If this sentinel node method proves to be a reliable and accurate means of predicting nodal metastases, many women may be able to avoid extensive lymphadenectomies.[34,35]

Stage II vulvar cancer may require more extensive surgery, which usually involves a radical vulvectomy to obtain adequate tumor-free margins. If surgical margins of at least 1 cm are obtained, then the local recurrence rate for women with T2 tumors with radical local excision is identical to that of women with T1 tumors who received treatment.[14] For cancers that are more extensive, radical vulvectomy is performed. In this surgery, the labia minora, labia majora, and clitoris are removed. Bilateral node dissections are usually performed.[4,36]

In stage III disease, the tumor has spread to the urethra, vagina, anus, or lymph nodes in the inguinal area. Radical vulvectomy for such disease often involves removal of a portion of the distal urethra or vagina and may require excision of a portion of the anus. To prevent local recurrence, a course of radiation therapy alone or a combination of radiation therapy and chemotherapy is recommended.[18,37]

Women with stage IV disease may require pelvic exenteration in addition to a radical vulvectomy if the bladder or rectum is involved. A total pelvic exenteration removes the vagina, uterus, ovaries, fallopian tubes, bladder, and rectum. Patients will have a urinary conduit and colostomy. A neovagina is usually constructed. While the five-year survival rate for this surgery may be as high as 70%, many complications may follow, including a high psychological morbidity. Women should be carefully selected for this surgery. Usually, elderly women are not candidates. For women with locally advanced disease, many investigators combine surgery and radiation to spare critical structures.[19] If the tumor is fixed to the bone or distant metastases have occurred, treatment is usually palliative and mainly consists of radiotherapy.[38]

The major immediate complication after radical surgery is groin wound infection and breakdown. With the use of the separate incision approach for nodal resection, the incidence of wound breakdown decreased to about 44%; with an en bloc operation, it was reported to be as high as 85%. Major wound breakdown occurs in about 14% of patients. With proper debridement and wound care, the groin area can granulate and reepithelialize within a few weeks. Wet-to-dry dressings are usually recommended. Whirlpool therapy is also effective for areas of extensive breakdown.[14,20] Other early postoperative complications include urinary tract infection, deep-vein thrombosis, seromas in the femoral triangle, and pulmonary embolism.

The major late complication of radical surgery is chronic leg edema, which has been reported to occur in as many as 30% of women; the incidence of this problem decreases to 15% with the use of separate groin incisions.[39] The use of elastic stockings is recommended for 12 months after surgery to facilitate development of collateral pathways for lymph drainage. Recurrent cellulitis of the leg occurs in about 10% of women and usually responds to antibiotics. Urinary stress incontinence and genital prolapse occurs in about 10% of patients and may require corrective surgery. Numbness and paresthesia over the anterior thigh is common due to femoral nerve injury. This nerve injury usually resolves slowly.[20,40]

Radiation Therapy

The role of radiation therapy in the management of carcinoma of the vulva continues to evolve. To reduce the need for extensive radical surgery, this treatment is being used more often in combination with surgery. Radiation has become standard postoperative therapy for women who have undergone a resection of the primary lesion and are considered at high risk for recurrence due to inadequate resection of margins or positive nodes. Studies have demonstrated that women who have close or positive margins after surgery have significantly reduced local recurrence rates when they receive postoperative irradiation.[40] Women with two or more positive groin lymph nodes or positive pelvic lymph nodes are considered to be at high risk for recurrence and can also benefit from postoperative radiation.[20,38] While the use of radiation therapy has decreased recurrence rates, it cannot replace groin node dissection. Preoperative radiation in combination with chemotherapy for locally advanced cancer has been shown to be an effective approach to reduce the extent of radical surgery.[41,42]

Patients who receive external radiation to the vulva can develop severe erythema, moist desquamation, and swelling. Measures for managing these reactions include application of topical ointments, frequent sitz baths and exposure to air.[38] Maintaining skin integrity and management of pain and discomfort are the aims of nursing care.

Radiation cystitis may also occur with radiation treatment of the pelvis. In such cases, appropriate antibiotic therapy and antispasmodics are indicated to provide relief of symptoms. The woman should also be encouraged to increase her fluid intake.[43]

Severe late radiation effects, such as vulvar fibrosis, atrophy, or even necrosis, may occur. To prevent severe radiation effects, the total dose for postoperative radiation therapy is 4500–5000 cGy if there is no macroscopic residual disease. Higher doses of irradiation (6000–7000 cGy) can be given to known areas of gross residual tumor. When chemotherapy is used in combination with radiation therapy, the maximum dose is usually 6500 cGy.[38]

Chemotherapy

The concurrent use of radiation and chemotherapy for initial therapy of vulvar cancer shows promise in allowing a more conservative approach to surgery. The most common chemotherapy agents used are 5-fluorouracil (5-FU), cisplatin, and mitomycin C. The studies using concurrent radiation and chemotherapy have included only small samples, and further research needs to be completed. However, most studies have shown greater response rates when concurrent radiation and chemotherapy is given than when radiation is given alone.[44,45] Chemotherapy with radiation therapy is usually well tolerated by most women. However, patients with vulvar cancer, who typically are elderly and often have co-morbidities, should be closely monitored for evidence of side effects.[46] The use of chemotherapy alone in locally advanced or recurrent vulvar cancer yielded a response rate of 56% but the one-year survival rate was only 32%.[47]

Symptom Management and Supportive Care

Advanced/Recurrent Disease

About 80% of recurrences of vulvar cancer will develop within the first two years after initial treatment — a fact that demands initial close follow-up. Patients with fewer than three positive nodes generally have a low incidence of recurrence, whereas high recurrence rates are correlated with more than three positive nodes.[48] More than half of the recurrences are local and occur in close proximity to the original lesion. In many instances, local recurrences can be successfully treated using wide local excision with adequate tumor-free margins. For treatment of advanced recurrent disease, pelvic exenteration may be an option for selected women. For recurrent vulvar cancer, the five-year survival rate is 38%–50%.[15] Distant recurrence is difficult to treat, with an 8% survival rate at five years. A combination of radiation and chemotherapy may be used as a palliative treatment measure in metastatic disease.[4]

For the woman with advanced recurrent vulvar cancer, the physical symptoms can be distressing. The tumor can become very large, disfiguring, and painful. With a comprehensive assessment of the pain, an appropriate and effective pain management regimen can be developed. If the tumor becomes ulcerated, care should be taken to prevent infection. Meticulous skin care is important. Leg edema may become a problem for the woman with positive, enlarged lymph nodes. Elastic stockings are usually recommended. Massage and exercise of the legs may also help relieve discomfort. Skin care of the legs is essential to prevent infection and cellulitis. Moisturizing the skin can help.

Along with the physical symptoms, the patient and her family may be at risk for ineffective coping. The nurse and healthcare team can help the patient and family manage the many debilitating changes of advanced disease. Nurses in the hospital can make appropriate referrals to home care or hospice care. Continual education and reassurance can facilitate effective coping mechanisms to allow the patient to live as fully as possible.

Among women who are cured of their disease by vulvectomy, sexual satisfaction is low. Nurses can help by promoting open discussions about sexual concerns with the woman and her partner. Individualized sexual and reproductive counseling will be needed. Nurses, by providing expert knowledge, are in a vital position to address these sensitive issues.

Future Trends

For vulvar cancer prevention, HPV vaccines are being developed and tested. Some of these vaccines are intended to produce immunity to HPV so that women who are exposed to these viruses will not develop infections that persist for a long time. A woman's immune system could then destroy the virus before an infection occurs. Other vaccines are intended for women with established HPV infections and attempt to stimulate their immune systems to destroy the virus and cure the infection before a cancer develops.[49]

Because cancer of the vulva primarily affects elderly women and radical surgery may be involved, clinical trials are seeking to define the best way of combining radiation and chemotherapy with surgery to reduce the need for extensive surgery. One interesting clinical trial is examining the effectiveness of paclitaxel in locally advanced or recurrent carcinoma. Other trials are studying combinations of radiation with chemotherapy before surgery. The goal of these trials is to shrink the tumor initially so that a less radical surgery might be performed. The use of multimodality therapy will not only preserve organ function but also will likely extend the lives of women with vulvar cancer.[19] Photodynamic therapy involves injections of a chemical that cancer cells absorb, making them extremely sensitive to certain types of light. A special light is then focused on an area of the vulva where these cells exist, resulting in significant tumor cell death. In preliminary studies, this approach appears promising as a treatment for VIN and early vulvar cancers.[49]

VAGINAL CANCER

Epidemiology

Primary carcinoma of the vagina represents less than 2% of all gynecologic malignancies. Vaginal carcinomas should be classified as such only when the primary site of tumor growth is in the vagina. Any tumor that has extended to the cervical area and reached the external os should be classified as a cervical carcinoma. Secondary spread to the vagina from sites such as the cervix, vulva, endometrium, ovary, and rectum occurs more frequently than primary carcinoma of the vagina.[4]

The peak incidence of squamous carcinoma of the vagina, which is the most common cell type, occurs in women ages 50–70. It is rare that women younger than age 40 are diagnosed with vaginal cancer. In contrast, the peak incidence for clear cell adenocarcinoma of the vagina, which is associated with maternal use of diethylstilbestrol (DES), occurs in women ages 15–22.

Invasive squamous cell carcinoma of the vagina can be preceded by vaginal intraepithelial neoplasia (VAIN), just as cancer of the cervix and vulva are preceded by cervical and vulvar intraepithelial neoplasia, respectively. VAIN is much less common than cervical intraepithelial neoplasia (CIN) or VIN. However, its incidence is climbing and the mean age at diagnosis is decreasing.[50] VAIN is classified into three categories (I, II, III), with a higher number being indicative of increasing epithelial involvement. Although the natural history of VAIN is not well defined, VAIN III lesions are premalignant. The majority of women with VAIN III will have a history of CIN or invasive disease of the cervix. As many as 30% of women with primary vaginal carcinoma will have a history of in situ or invasive cervical cancer treated at least five years earlier.[4]

Table 66-4 Vaginal Cancer: Risk Factors and Preventive Measures

Risk Factors	Preventive Measures
Human papillomavirus	Pap smear per ACS guidelines
Long-term use of vaginal pessaries	Decrease use of vaginal pessaries
Prior radiation therapy to lower genital tract	Use of barrier contraception
Abdominal hysterectomy for benign disease	
Age > 60 years	
Maternal use of diethylstilbestrol	

Etiology

There is an association between HPV and vaginal cancer. HPV DNA has been found in more than 50% of women with vaginal cancer and in about 70% of cases of VAIN.[51] Other risk factors include a history of vaginal trauma due to pessarie use for coitus, which is believed to produce a chemical or physical irritation to the vaginal mucosa. Prior radiation therapy or abdominal hysterectomy may also be predisposing factors for primary vaginal carcinoma (Table 66-4).

Since 1971, the study of adenocarcinoma of the vagina has focused on young women who were exposed to DES in utero and who seemed to have an unusually high incidence of vaginal cancer. DES was used in the management of diabetic pregnancies, threatened abortion, and other high-risk obstetrical problems. From the late 1940s to 1970, an estimated 2 million pregnant women received DES. The risk of developing vaginal cancer in women who were exposed to DES in utero is about 1 in 1,000 up to age 35 and is the highest if the hormone was taken before 12 weeks' gestation.[52] There have been several cases of women with a history of in utero DES exposure who developed non-clear cell adenocarcinoma of the vagina. These vaginal cancers were found in older women and were more advanced than the clear cell adenocarcinoma associated with DES exposure.[53] Given that women appear to be developing cancer later in life, long-term surveillance of DES-exposed women is warranted.

Prevention and Screening

The incidence of vaginal cancer is 0.5 cases per 100,000 women.[14] Routine screening is probably not warranted given the low incidence. However, women should be encouraged to have a Pap smear following the ACS guidelines. At the time the Pap smear is done, inspection of the vagina should be performed. Because women who had cervical cancer, vulvar cancer, hysterectomy for benign disease, and exposure to DES before birth have a higher incidence of vaginal cancer, it is recommended that a Pap smear surveillance for vaginal cancer be performed yearly.[54] For women who have a history of VAIN, follow-up should include colposcopy as a part of every examination.[55] Avoiding HPV infection may reduce a woman's risk of vaginal cancer.

Pathophysiology

Cellular Characteristics

Squamous cell carcinoma accounts for 80%–90% of all vaginal cancers. Other histological types include verrucous, adenocarcinoma, melanoma, and sarcoma. A lesion may be red, white, or gray in color and have an ulcerated appearance.[4]

Progression of Disease

The vagina is lined throughout by stratified squamous epithelium. Embryologically, the upper two-thirds of the vagina develops separately from the lower one-third. The upper two-thirds grows downward and shares its blood supply and lymphatic drainage with the cervix. The lymphatics drain to the internal and external iliac and obturator nodes and to the common iliac and lower paraaortic nodes. The lower one-third of the vagina grows upward and shares its blood supply and lymphatic system with that of the vulva. The lymphatics drain to the inguinal and femoral nodes. All of the lymph nodes of the pelvis may at one time or another serve as potential sites of drainage from the vagina[56] (see Figure 66-1). Superiorly the cervix protrudes into the vaginal vault, and inferiorly the vagina meets the vulva. The bladder is positioned anterior to the vagina. The rectum and anus are posterior to the vagina[57] (Figure 66-3).

Similar to vulvar and cervical cancer, the preinvasive disease VAIN is divided into three categories. VAIN I describes mild dysplasia. VAIN II describes moderate dysplasia. VAIN III describes severe dysplasia and may be associated with microinvasive or invasive disease.[14]

Vaginal cancers occur most commonly in the upper third of the vagina. Early reports indicated that most tumors developed on the posterior wall of the vagina. However, more recent reviews noted that lesions were equally distributed on the posterior, anterior, and lateral walls. The tumor may spread along the vaginal wall to involve the cervix or vulva. As noted earlier, if the cervix is involved, the tumor is considered a primary cervical lesion. Anterior vaginal lesions can

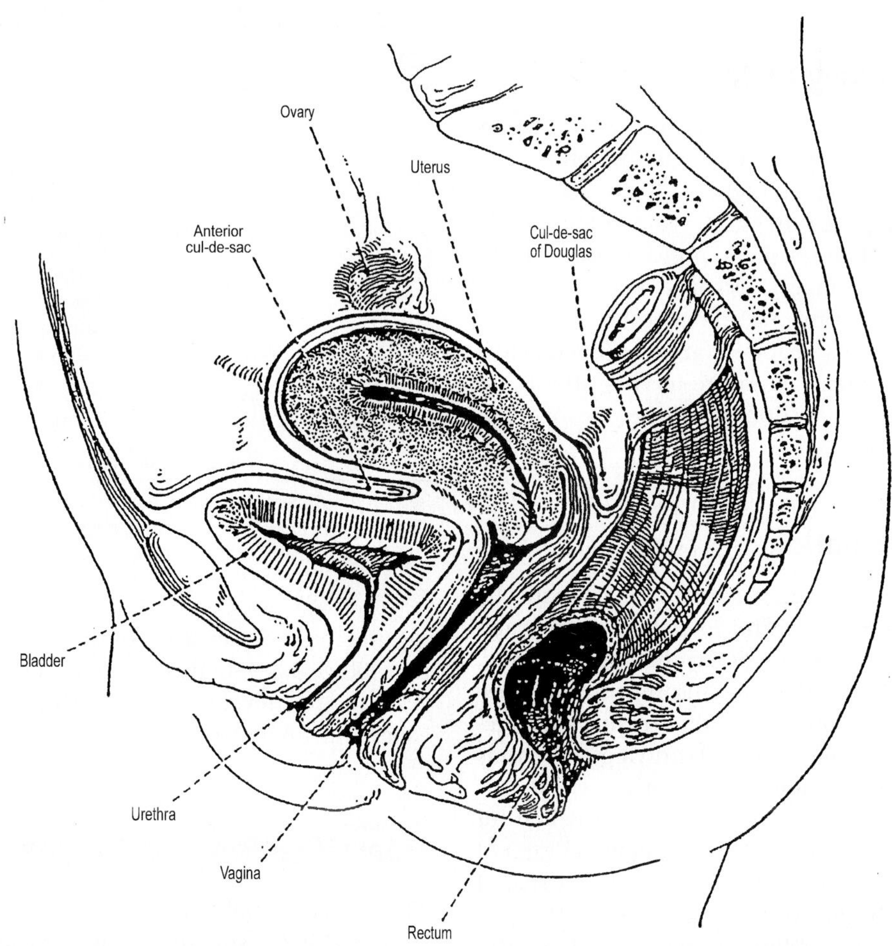

Figure 66-3 Sagittal section of the female pelvis. [Reprinted with permission from Bengton JM: The vagina, in Ryan KJ, Berkowitz RS, Barbieri RL (eds.): *Kistner's Gynecology Principles and Practice*. St. Louis, Mosby, 1996, p 82.[57]]

penetrate into the vesicovaginal septum during early stages of the disease. Posterior lesions can invade the rectum, although this spread usually occurs in the late stages.[20] Even though the urethra, bladder, and rectum are in close proximity to the vagina, fewer than 10% of vaginal tumors invade these structures, even in the later stages of disease.[20,58]

The lymphatic drainage of the vagina consists of a vast network that facilitates drainage into any of the local nodal groups regardless of the location of the vaginal lesion. The lymphatics in the upper portion of the vagina drain primarily via the lymphatics of the cervix; those in the lower portion either drain cephalad to the cervical lymphatics or follow the drainage pattern of the vulva into the inguinal and femoral nodes.[14]

Extension or metastasis of other malignancies to the vagina occurs more frequently than primary cancer of the vagina. Spread of cervical cancer to the vagina is the most common, but cancers of the endometrium, ovary, urethra, bladder, rectum, and malignant trophoblastic disease may also spread or metastasize to the vaginal area.[4]

Clinical Manifestations

The most frequently encountered initial symptom of invasive vaginal cancer is abnormal bleeding that may occur after coitus. Other symptoms may include foul-smelling discharge, pain in the perineum, or a palpable mass. With more advanced tumors, if the tumor presses on the bladder, urinary retention, bladder spasms, and hematuria may occur. Tumors developing on the posterior vaginal wall may produce rectal symptoms such as tenesmus, constipation, or blood in the stool.[59] Because many lesions are asymptomatic, an abnormal Pap smear may be the diagnostic event that initiates the search for a definitive diagnosis.

Assessment

Patient and Family History

All women should have a complete history regarding the duration and severity of their signs and symptoms. Because exposure to DES in utero is a major risk factor for developing vaginal cancer, all women should be questioned about their mothers' possible use of DES. For some women, a primary vaginal cancer may actually be a second pelvic cancer. A detailed history of the previous cancer and its treatment are necessary. Information about a woman's exposure to HPV should be obtained. Vaginal cancer does not have a known genetic predisposition.

Physical Examination

Clinical diagnosis of a vaginal neoplasm is made by careful visual examination and palpation of the vagina. This examination helps determine the location, number, and size of the lesions. This information is essential for planning appropriate therapeutic management. Pap smear is helpful for identifying squamous carcinoma, but not for adenocarcinoma because it is often subepithelial. Colposcopy is particularly helpful for performing directed biopsies of abnormal vaginal areas. The disease may then be evaluated and staged under anesthesia by the gynecologic oncologist and radiation therapist, and additional vaginal and cervical biopsies may be taken. Negative biopsies of the cervix are necessary to rule out cervical cancer and confirm the diagnosis of primary vaginal carcinoma.[4]

Diagnostic Studies

All patients require a chest x-ray, complete blood count, and biochemical profile. An intravenous pyelogram (IVP), barium enema, cystoscopy, and proctosigmoidoscopy may be helpful in determining extent of disease. An MRI or CT of the abdomen and pelvis is usually performed to assess local invasion and spread to the lymph nodes.

Prognostic Indicators

Clinical stage is the most important prognostic indicator in vaginal cancer. A better prognosis is associated with early diagnosis, small tumor burden, and negative nodal involvement. Conflicting reports have focused on the influence on outcome of histological grade, patient age, and location of tumor. Several studies indicate a poor prognosis with an increasing grade of squamous cell carcinoma and adenocarcinoma, tumors located in the lower third of the vagina, and age older than 60 years.[4,60] Eighty percent of women whose disease recurs develop pelvic recurrences within two years of primary treatment.[4]

Table 66-5 FIGO Staging of Vaginal Cancer

Stage	Clinical Findings
Stage 0	Carcinoma in situ, intraepithelial carcinoma.
Stage I	The carcinoma is limited to the vaginal wall.
Stage II	The carcinoma has involved the subvaginal tissues but has not extended onto the pelvic wall.
Stage III	The carcinoma has extended onto the pelvic wall.
Stage IV	The carcinoma has extended beyond the true pelvis or has clinically involved the mucosa of the bladder or rectum. Bullous edema as such does not permit a case to be designated as stage IV.
Stage IVA	Spread of the growth to adjacent organs, direct extension beyond the true pelvis, or both.
Stage IVB	Spread to distant organs.

Reprinted with permission from Benedet JL, Hacker NF, Ngen HYS: Staging classifications and clinical practice guidelines of gynecologic cancers. *Int J Gynecol Obstet* 70:207–312, 2000.[24]

Classification and Staging

The International Federation of Gynecology and Obstetrics (FIGO) staging of vaginal cancer is shown in Table 66-5.[24] Staging for vaginal cancer is achieved by clinical examination. Information from MRI or CT is not used to change the FIGO stage, but can prove helpful in planning treatment. The overall five-year survival rate for all stages of squamous cell vaginal carcinoma is 50%–65%. The survival rates are 80% for patients with stage I disease, 65% for those with stage II disease, 40% for those with stage III disease, and 15% for those with stage IV disease.[4,61–63] The ten-year survival rate in patients with adenocarcinoma is 79%. This relatively high rate may be related to the fact that females exposed to DES in utero have been followed closely due to their risk for developing adenocarcinoma, and are often diagnosed with early-stage disease. However, clear cell carcinoma has a greater tendency to recur late and develop metastases in distant sites more frequently than squamous cell carcinoma.[64]

Therapeutic Approaches and Nursing Care: VAIN

Location of the lesion, size of the lesion, and existence of a single focus or multiple foci are factors considered in determining treatment options. Women with VAIN I usually do not require any treatment, as these lesions often disappear without treatment. Women with VAIN II are usually treated with ablative treatment such as laser or 5-FU cream. With 5-FU cream, care must be taken to ensure direct contact with the entire lesion and to avoid contact with the vulva.[65] Laser therapy can cure between 69% and 80% of patients with vaginal intraepithelial lesions.[66,67] Both laser therapy and application of 5-FU cream are well tolerated by patients. Patients will often complain of a watery discharge for two to three weeks after laser therapy.

Because VAIN III lesions are considered to be premalignant, local excision is appropriate for single lesions or for several lesions clustered in a single portion of the vagina. For multifocal lesions or recurrent disease, or in poor surgical candidates, the treatment of choice is irradiation of the vagina with high-dose brachytherapy. Treatment is usually well tolerated and recurrence rates are low.[61,65]

Therapeutic Approaches and Nursing Care: Invasive Disease

Radiation Therapy

The anatomical position of the vagina, located between the urethra and bladder anteriorly and the rectum posteriorly, is the predominant factor in treatment planning. Radiation therapy is the most widely used treatment modality for all stages of vaginal cancer. Patients who have stage I small, superficial tumors may be treated with brachytherapy alone. A fractionated dose of 6000–7000 cGy to the whole vaginal mucosa is usually administered. For women with larger stage I or stage II tumors, a combination of external beam therapy and brachytherapy is recommended.[59]

In stage III and IV disease, tumors are large and may involve the bladder or rectum. A combination of external beam radiation and brachytherapy is recommended in such cases. Careful treatment planning is critical for shielding the bladder and rectum during high-dose radiation therapy. A total dose of 7000 cGy of external beam radiation and brachytherapy to the pelvis is usually given. The groin area is irradiated with 5000 cGy in women with positive nodes. In general, radiation treatment provides good control of tumor with limited morbidity.[38,61,63] Women with stage III and IV vaginal tumors have a high recurrence rate; to enhance the radiation therapy in such cases, radiosensitizers such as cisplatin, 5-FU, or hydroxyurea may be used.[38]

For women receiving radiation therapy to the vagina, vaginal fibrosis and scarring with a loss of blood supply and elasticity are the major adverse effects. The age of the woman diagnosed with vaginal cancer is usually advanced, and the typical low frequency of vaginal intercourse may increase the likelihood of significant stenosis. Frequent intercourse can minimize these effects. For patients who are not sexually active, the use of a vaginal dilator with water-soluble lubricants or prescribed estrogen cream starting two weeks after treatment is an effective prophylactic measure to minimize functional loss.[38]

Table 66-6 Skin Care of the Woman Receiving Radiation to the Lower Pelvis

- Wash the treated area with a mild soap. Use warm water, not hot.
- Do not rub skin dry; pat skin with a towel. Try to keep the skin free from moisture.
- Do not apply creams, lotions, or powder to the treated area.
- Do not shave skin.
- If skin becomes reddened, tell your nurse or physician. Application of a corticosteriod and/or antibiotic cream may be indicated. Apply medicated cream after the daily dose of radiation.

In the vulvar and groin area, desquamation of the skin from radiation therapy can be distressing to the patient. Educating the woman about meticulous skin care is imperative (Table 66-6). Application of corticosteroid and/or antibiotic cream can help prevent a skin infection. Once the radiation therapy is completed, the skin usually recovers quickly.

More serious complications include rectovaginal fistula, rectal ulceration, urethral stricture, and small bowel obstruction. The patient should be closely monitored for these complications. Fortunately, only a small percentage of women will develop these problems.[61]

Surgery

For a selected group of women, surgery may be an option. Because of the pelvic anatomy, curative surgery often means radical surgery. For superficial lesions in the upper part of the vagina, a radical vaginectomy or radical hysterectomy can be done.[4] With radical vaginectomy, vaginal reconstruction will be necessary for patients who wish to continue vaginal intercourse. For women who have had a reconstructed vagina, sexual intercourse or the use of vaginal dilators is also encouraged because the neovagina can be narrow. Open communication between the nurse and the patient about sexual concerns is essential. Sexual satisfaction can be achieved by women following treatment for cancer of the vagina.

For treatment of larger tumors without involvement of the pelvic sidewalls, a more extensive surgery may be warranted, such as pelvic exenteration.

However, many women with vaginal cancer are elderly and have other medical problems that may preclude this surgery. For women with recurrent disease or those who have received prior radiation therapy for cervical cancer, a pelvic exenteration may be the only option to achieve a cure.[68] For any patient who receives surgery, extensive preoperative counseling, postoperative care, and rehabilitation are necessary.

Chemotherapy

For patients who have metastatic or recurrent vaginal cancer, or if surgery or radiation therapy cannot be utilized, chemotherapy may be an option. Very few studies using chemotherapy to treat vaginal cancer have been reported. One promising study using methotrexate, vinblastine, doxorubicin, and cisplatin for advanced or recurrent vaginal cancer achieved high response rates with overall survival rates that appear promising.[69] More research is needed to better define the role of chemotherapy in vaginal cancer. 5-FU and cisplatin are the most common chemotherapeutic agents used concurrently with radiation therapy.

Symptom Management and Supportive Care

Advanced/Recurrent Disease

Women with stage III and IV vaginal cancer have a high recurrence rate. If the woman received radiation therapy as primary treatment, surgery might be an option if no evidence of distant metastases is found. The symptoms of advanced vaginal cancer depend on the location of the tumor. In tumors located anteriorly, the woman may experience urinary problems such as hematuria and urinary tract infections. Palliative radiotherapy can reduce hematuria from an ulcerating lesion. In addition to this radiation therapy, the patient may need continuous bladder irrigation to decrease the bleeding. Repeated urinary tract infections may be indicative of fistula formation and the patient may experience urinary incontinence, dysuria, and painful bladder spasms. For some women, surgery might be the best treatment choice to close the fistula.[70] For women who are too ill or when the tumor is too extensive, symptomatic treatment with appropriate antibiotics and antispasmodics is used. For larger draining fistulas, a urinary–vaginal prosthesis can be used to divert the drainage and to maintain the woman's skin integrity.

If the tumor grows posteriorly, blood in the stool and constipation may occur. For mild constipation, the use of stool softeners and laxatives may be all that is necessary. If complete obstruction occurs, surgery or radiation therapy is usually warranted. A rectovaginal fistula can cause distressing fecal incontinence. If the fistula is small, measures to keep the stool well formed may help the healing process. The use of vaginal tampons can help to control fistula discharge. For larger fistulas, a simple loop colostomy should be considered to provide relief of symptoms.[70]

Future Trends

Similar to vulvar cancer prevention, the use of HPV vaccines can help to reduce the incidence of vaginal cancer. Because the number of vaginal cancer patients is small, it is difficult to conduct clinical trials. Greater use of chemotherapy in vulvar and cervical cancer has shown promising results. This success might lead to clinical trials that could better define the role of chemotherapy for vaginal cancer. Combination radiation and chemotherapy is being studied in hope of being able to preserve anatomy and function. There are also studies under way to determine the most effective way to combine external beam radiation and brachytherapy to decrease damage to normal tissue.

The offspring (i.e., third generation) of DES daughters and sons are beginning to reach the age when relevant health problems can be studied. The potential risks associated with DES exposure in the third generation are being carefully monitored.

The majority of the women with vaginal cancer are treated with radiation therapy. Because radiation therapy to the lower pelvis can cause vaginal fibrosis, the radiation oncology nurse must address changes in body image, alteration in sexuality, and coping mechanisms with the woman. Most patients with vaginal cancer are elderly, so the probability of hospitalization or the need for home health care is high. The radiation therapy nurse can play a key role in helping facilitate communication between care settings.

Conclusion

While the emphasis is on individualized treatment for the woman who is diagnosed with vulvar or vaginal cancer, the treatment may be considered aggressive and can be disfiguring. Multimodal treatment has led to decreased recurrence rates. Effective communication across healthcare disciplines is necessary to achieve a successful and comprehensive approach for the patient. Nurses must consider the social, sexual, financial, and spiritual needs of all of these patients. To further improve the quality of care for women with vulvar or vaginal cancer, more nursing research on the management of treatment-related symptoms and care of the patient with advanced disease is essential. Nurses are also in the best position to address barriers to screening and to educate women to follow the ACS guidelines for obtaining regular Pap smears. If detected early, vulvar and vaginal cancers have high cure rates.

References

1. American Cancer Society: *www.cancer.org*. Accessed January 25, 2004
2. Joura EA, Losch A, Haider-Angeler MG, et al: Trends in vulvar neoplasia. Increasing incidence of vulvar intraepithelial neoplasia and squamous cell carcinoma of the vulva in young women. *J Reprod Med* 45:613–615, 2000
3. Jones RW: Vulvar intraepithelial neoplasia: current perspectives. *Eur J Gynaecol Oncol* 22:393–402, 2001
4. Eifel PJ, Berek JS, Thigpen JT: Cancer of the cervix, vagina, and vulvar, in Devita VT, Hellman S, Rosenberg SA (eds.): *Cancer: Principles and Practice of Oncology* (ed 6). Philadelphia, Lippincott-Raven, 2001, pp 1526–1572
5. Hildesheim A, Han CL, Brinton LA, et al: Human papillomavirus type 16 and risk of preinvasive and invasive vulvar cancer: results from a seroepidemiological case-control study. *Obstet Gynecol* 90:748–754, 1997
6. Canavan TP, Cohen D: Vulvar cancer. *Am Fam Physician* 66:1269–1274, 2002
7. Chambers SK: Molecular biology of gynecologic cancers, in Devita VT, Hellman S, Rosenberg SA (eds.): *Cancer: Principles and Practice of Oncology* (ed 6). Philadelphia, Lippincott-Raven, 2001, pp 1519–1525
8. Rosenthal AN, Hopster D, Ryan A, et al: Immunohistochemical analysis of p53 in vulvar intraepithelial neoplasia and vulvar squamous cell carcinoma. *Br J Cancer* 88:251–256, 2003
9. Joura EA: Epidemiology, diagnosis and treatment of vulvar intraepithelial neoplasia. *Curr Opin Obstet Gynecol* 14:39–43, 2002
10. Baker VV: Vulvar: pathogenesis and epidemiology of vulvar cancer, in Shingleton HM, Fowler WC Jr, Jordan JA, et al (eds.): *Gynecologic Oncology — Current Diagnosis and Treatment.* Philadelphia, Saunders, 1996, pp 239–245
11. Bamberger ES, Perrett CW: Angiogenesis in benign, pre-malignant and malignant vulvar lesions. *Anticancer Res* 22:3853–3865, 2002
12. Tyring SK: Vulvar squamous cell carcinoma: guidelines for early diagnosis. *Am J Obstet Gynecol* 189:S17–S23, 2003
13. Cardosi RJ, Bomalaski JJ, Hoffman MS: Diagnosis and management of vulvar and vaginal intraepithelial neoplasia. *Obstet Gynecol Clin North Am* 28:685–702, 2001
14. Chi DS, Mychalczak B, Hoskins WJ: Cancer of the vulvar and vagina, in Bland KI, Daly JM, Karakouis CP (eds.): *Surgical Oncology — Contemporary Principles and Practices.* New York, McGraw Hill, 2001, pp 852–882
15. Chan KK, Helm CW: Invasive vulvar cancer, in Shingleton HM, Fowler WC, Jordan JA, et al (eds.): *Gynecologic Oncology — Current Diagnosis and Treatment.* Philadelphia, Saunders, 1996, pp 264–271
16. Hacker NF: Surgery for malignant tumors of the vulva, in Gersherson DM, DeCherney AH, Curry SL (eds.): *Operative Gynecology.* Philadelphia, Saunders, 1996, pp 175–181
17. Dhar KK, Woolas RP: Changes in the management of vulval cancer. *Best Pract Res Clin Obstet Gynaecol* 17:529–542, 2003
18. Rosen C, Malmstrom H: Invasive cancer of the vulva. *Gynecol Oncol* 65:213–217, 1997
19. Coleman RL, Santoso JT: Vulvar carcinoma. *Curr Treat Options Oncol* 1:177–190, 2000
20. Hacker NF: Vulvar cancer, in Berek JS, Adashi EY, Hillard PA (eds.): *Gynecology* (ed 12). Philadelphia, Williams and Wilkins, 1996, pp 1231–1260
21. August CZ, Ganji M, Froula E: Misdiagnosis of high-grade vulvar intraepithelial neoplasia (VIN III) as mild cervical intraepithelial neoplasia (CIN I) on Papanicolaou tests. *Arch Pathol Lab Med* 127:68–70, 2003
22. Homesley HD, Bundy BN, Sedles A, et al: Assessment of current International Federation of Gynecology and Obstetrics staging of vulvar carcinoma relative to prognostic factors for survival (a Gynecologic Oncology Group study). *Am J Obstet Gynecol* 174:997–1004, 1991
23. Rouzier R, Morice P, Haie-Meder C, et al: Prognostic significance of epithelial disorders adjacent to invasive vulvar carcinoma. *Gynecol Oncol* 81:414–419, 2001
24. Benedet JL, Bender H, Jones H 3rd, et al: FIGO Staging classifications and clinical practice guidelines in the management of of gynecologic cancers. *Int J Gynecol Obstet* 70:209–262, 2000
25. Morrow CP, Curtin JP: Surgery for vulvar neoplasia, in Morrow CP, Curtin JP (eds.): *Gynecologic Cancer Surgery.* New York, Churchill Livingstone, 1996, pp 381–450
26. Warwick A, Luesley DM: Vulvar intraepithelial lesions, in Shingleton HM, Fowler WC, Jordan JA, Lawrence WD (eds.): *Gynecological Oncology — Current Diagnosis and Treatment.* Philadelphia, Saunders, 1996, pp 259–263
27. Sideri M, Spinaci L, Spolti N, et al: Evaluation of CO_2 laser excision or vaporization for the treatment of vulvar intraepithelial neoplasia. *Gynecol Oncol* 75:277–281, 1999
28. Penna C, Fallani MG, Fambrini M, et al: CO_2 laser surgery for vulvar intraepithelial neoplasia. Excisional, destructive and combined techniques. *J Reprod Med* 47:913–918, 2002
29. Todd RW, Etherington IJ, Luesley DM: The effects of 5% imiquimod cream on high-grade vulval intraepithelial neoplasia. *Gynecol Oncol* 85:67–70, 2002
30. Miller BE: Vulvar intraepithelial neoplasia treated with cavitational ultrasonic surgical aspiration. *Gynecol Oncol* 85:114–118, 2002
31. Fehr MK, Hornung R, Degen A, et al: Photodynamic therapy of the vulvar and vaginal condyloma and intraepithelial neoplasia using topically applied 5-aminolevuline acid. *Lasers Surg Med* 30:273–279, 2002
32. Nash JD, Curry S: Vulvar cancer. *Surg Oncol Clin North Am* 7:335–346, 1998
33. Edwards CL, Tortolero-Luna G, Linares AC, et al: Vulvar intraepithelial neoplasia and vulvar cancer. *Obstet Gynecol Clin North Am* 23:295–324, 1996
34. Gotlieb WH: The assessment and surgical management of early-stage vulvar cancer. *Best Pract Res Clin Obstet Gynaecol* 17:557–569, 2003
35. Sliutz G, Reinthaller A, Lantzsch T, et al: Lymphatic mapping of sentinel nodes in early vulvar cancer. *Gynecol Oncol* 84:449–452, 2002
36. Siller BS, Alvarez RD, Conner WD, et al: T2–3 vulvar cancer: a case control study of triple incision versus en bloc radical vulvectomy and inguinal lymphadenectomy. *Gynecol Oncol* 57:335–339, 1995
37. Leiserowitz GS, Russell AH, Kinney WK: Prophylactic chemoradiation of inguino-femoral lymph nodes in patients with locally extensive vulvar cancer. *Gynecol Oncol* 66:509–514, 1997

38. Thomas GM, Murphy KJ: Vulvar and vaginal carcinoma, in Gunderson LL, Teppe JE (eds.): *Clinical Radiation Oncology.* New York, Churchill Livingstone, 2000, pp 920–938
39. Magrina JF, Gonzalez-Bosquet J, Weaver AL, et al: Primary squamous cell cancer of the vulva: radical versus modified radical vulvar surgery. *Gynecol Oncol* 71:116–121, 1998
40. Faul CM, Mirmow D, Huang Q, et al: Adjuvant radiation for vulvar carcinoma: improved local control. *Int J Radiat Oncol Biol Phys* 38:381–389, 1997
41. Hoffman MS: Squamous-cell carcinoma of the vulva: locally advanced disease. *Best Pract Res Clin Obstet Gynaecol* 17:635–647, 2003
42. Blake P: Radiotherapy and chemotherapy for carcinoma of the vulva. *Best Pract Res Clin Obstet Gynaecol* 17:649–661, 2003
43. Door A: Less common gynecologic malignancies. *Semin Oncol Nurs* 18:207–222, 2002
44. Moore DH, Thomas GM, Montana GS, et al: Preoperative chemoradiation for advanced vulvar cancer: a phase II study of the Gynecologic Oncology Group. *Int J Radiat Oncol Biol Phys* 42:79–85, 1998
45. Cunningham MJ, Goyer RP, Gibbons SK, et al: Primary radiation, cisplatin, and 5-fluorouracil for advanced squamous carcinoma of the vulva. *Gynecol Oncol* 66:258–261, 1997
46. Kim RY, Alvarez RD, Omura GA: Advances in the treatment of gynecologic malignancies. Part 1: cancers of the cervix and vulva. *Oncology* 11:1510–1517, 2002
47. Wagenaar HC, Colombo N, Vergote I, et al: Bleomycin, methotrexate, and CCNU in locally advanced or recurrent inoperable, squamous-cell carcinoma of the vulva: an EORTC Gynaecological Cancer Cooperative Group Study. *Gynecol Oncol* 81:348–354, 2001
48. Rouzier R, Haddad B, Plantier F, et al: Local relapse in patients treated for squamous cell carcinoma: incidence and prognostic value. *Obstet Gynecol* 100:1159–1167, 2002
49. American Cancer Society: What's new in vulvar cancer research and treatment? *www.nlm.nih.gov/medlineplus/vulvarcancer.html.* Accessed January 31, 2004
50. Dodge JA, Eltabbakh GH, Mount SL, et al: Clinical features and risks of recurrences among patients with vaginal intraepithelial neoplasia. *Gynecol Oncol* 83:363–369, 2001
51. Sugase M, Matsukurat T: Distant manifestations of human papillomaviruses in the vagina. *Int J Cancer* 72:412–415, 1997
52. Herbst AL, Anderson S, Hubby MM, et al: Risk factors for the development of diethylstilbestrol-associated clear cell adenocarcinoma: a case-control study. *Am J Obstet Gynecol* 154:814–822, 1986
53. DeMars LR, Van Le L, Huang I, et al: Primary non-clear-cell adenocarcinoma of the vagina in older DES-exposed women. *Gynecol Oncol* 58:389–392, 1995
54. American Cancer Society: Can vaginal cancer be prevented? *www.nlm.nih.gov/medlineplus/vaginalcancer.html.* Accessed January 31, 2004
55. Kalogiroud D, Antoniou G, Karakitsos P, et al: Vaginal intraepithelial neoplasia (VAIN) following hysterectomy in patients treated for carcinoma in situ of the cervix. *Eur Gynaecol Oncol* 18:188–191, 1997
56. Hammond CB: Gynecology: the female reproductive organs, in Sabiston DC, Lyerly HK (eds.): *Textbook Surgery: The Biological Basis of Modern Surgical Practice* (ed 15). Philadelphia, Saunders, 1996, pp 1490–1505
57. Bengton JM: The vagina, in Ryan KJ, Berkowitz RS, Barbieri RL (eds.): *Kistner's Gynecology Principles and Practice.* St. Louis, Mosby, 1996, pp 80–93
58. Perez CA, Grigsby PW, Garipagaoglu M, et al: Factors affecting long-term outcome of irradiation in carcinoma of the vagina. *Int J Radiat Oncol Biol Phys* 44:37–45, 1999
59. Hatch KD, Fu YS: Cervical and vaginal cancer, in Berek JS, Adashi EY, Hillard PA (eds.): *Gynecology* (ed 12). Philadelphia, Williams and Wilkins, 1996, pp 1111–1154
60. Perez CA, Garipagasglu M, Grigsly PW, et al: Vagina, in Hoskins WJ, Perez CA, Young RC, et al (ed.): *Gynecologic Cancer Surgery* (ed 2). Philadelphia, Lippincott-Raven, 1997, pp 753–783
61. Chyle V, Zagars GK, Wheeler JA, et al: Definitive radiotherapy for carcinoma of the vagina: outcome and prognostic factors. *Int J Radiat Oncol Biol Phys* 35:891–905, 1996
62. Kirkbridge P, Fyles A, Rawlings GA, et al: Carcinoma of the vagina: experience at the Princess Margaret Hospital (1974–1989). *Gynecol Oncol* 56:435–443, 1995
63. Fine BA, Piver MS, McAuley M, et al: The curative potential of radiation therapy in the treatment of primary vaginal carcinoma. *Am J Clin Oncol* 19:39–44, 1996
64. Helm CW, Chan KK: Vaginal cancer, in Shingleton HM, Fowler WC, Jordan JA, et al (eds.): *Gynecologic Oncology — Current Diagnosis and Treatment.* Philadelphia, Saunders, 1996, pp 109–116
65. Rome RM, England PG: Management of vaginal intraepithelial neoplasia: a series of 132 cases with long-term follow-up. *Int J Gynecol Cancer* 10:382–390, 2000
66. Campagnutta E, Parin A, DePiero G, et al: Treatment of vaginal intraepithelial neoplasia (VAIN) with the carbon dioxide laser. *Clin Exp Obstet Gynecol* 26:127–130, 1999
67. Yalcin OT, Rutherford TJ, Chambers SK, et al: Vaginal intraepithelial neoplasia: treatment by carbon dioxide laser and risk factors for failure. *Eur J Obstet Gynecol Reprod Biol* 106:64–68, 2003
68. Tjalma WA, Monaghan JM, Lopes AB, et al: The role of surgery in invasive squamous carcinoma of the vagina. *Gynecol Oncol* 81:360–365, 2001
69. Long HJ 3rd, Rayson S, Podratz KC, et al: Long-term survival of patients with advanced/recurrent carcinoma of the cervix and vagina after neoadjuvant treatment with methotrexate, vinblastine, doxorubicin, and cisplatin with or without the addition of molgramostim, and review of the literature. *Am J Clin Oncol* 25:547–551, 2002
70. Regnard CFB, Comiskey MC: Advanced cancer: the hospice approach, in Shingleton HM, Fowler WC, Jordan JA, Lawrence WD (eds.): *Gynecologic Oncology — Current Diagnosis and Treatment.* Philadelphia, Saunders, 1996, pp 397–415

PART VII

Dimensions of Cancer Survivorship

CHAPTER 67

Cancer Survivorship: A Critical Aspect of Care

Karen Hassey Dow, PhD, RN, FAAN
Victoria Wochna Loerzel, RN, MSN, OCN®

Introduction

Survival rates from cancer have steadily increased over the past 30 years. Increased survival is the result of multiple factors, including changes in our basic understanding about the disease, growth of translational research to practice, changes in dose-limiting treatment toxicities, development of new targeted therapies, increased screening and early detection activities, enhanced rehabilitation and support interventions, and changes in sociocultural factors.[1,2] We have likewise witnessed a change in the long-term and late effects of cancer requiring a larger perspective on cancer survivorship. Oncology nursing has as its ultimate goal enhancing the length and quality of survival of all cancer survivors. The purpose of this chapter is to (1) provide an overview of cancer survivorship, (2) describe the historical perspective of cancer survivorship, (3) explore current views, and (4) describes challenges in cancer survivorship for the future.

Overview of Cancer Survivorship

The most recent cancer survivorship figures, compiled by the National Cancer Institute (NCI) in April 2003, show that there are now 9.6 million persons living with a history of cancer in the United States (*http://plan.cancer.gov/public/survivor.htm*). The definition of a cancer survivor, put forward by the National Coalition for Cancer Survivorship in 1986, says "anyone who has been diagnosed with cancer is a survivor, from the time of diagnosis and for the balance of that individual's life."[3] The Office of Cancer Survivorship at the NCI also considers caregivers and family members as secondary survivors because they are also touched by the experience of cancer in a family member or loved one.

The population of cancer survivors is increasing, with 60% of adults and 77% of children surviving now beyond five years after their diagnosis. Fourteen percent of all survivors alive today were diagnosed more than 20 years ago. Of the 24,040 households in the 1992 National Health Interview Survey, 63% of respondents had a cancer diagnosis more than 5 years and 10% had a cancer diagnosis more than 25 years.[4]

Demographic trends show that cancer survivors in the future will be older and more ethnically diverse. First, both males and females are now older at the time of diagnosis — ages 68 and 67 years, respectively.[2] This trend, coupled with the growing elderly population in the United States, which is expected to double from 1.3 million to 2.6 million by 2050, suggests that cancer rates in the elderly will also double.[5] Second, we can expect a racially and ethnically diverse population. Hispanics will account for 25% of the U.S. population by 2050, while African Americans, Asian Americans, and Native Americans combined are projected to constitute an additional 25% of the population in that year.[6]

In the past, "unwarranted pessimism" has been prevalent in the treatment of older patients with cancer. While uncertainty exists about the value of cancer treatment in older patients, Saltzstein and Belling[7] surprisingly found that survival among older patients is not affected for up to ten years after treatment. The authors used data from the NCI's Surveillance, Epidemiology, and End Results (SEER) Program.[8] For the period 1973–1998, they located 37,318 records of individuals age 90 and older and then compared their records with those of two other age groups, 0–69 and 70–89. The results showed that relative survival data for all three age groups were similar after the first year of diagnosis. The largest number of deaths occurred during the first year after diagnosis, particularly within the first four months after diagnosis. Once past the first year post-diagnosis, patients 90 years of age and older did well compared to their younger counterparts. The oldest patients will benefit from treatment as much as younger ones within the first year. Thus, older age alone may not be a contraindication for treatment.

Late Effects in Cancer Survivors

While children and adults with a history of cancer are living longer, there is a growing body of evidence demonstrating long-term and late physiologic effects such as secondary cancers; cognitive changes; cardiac dysfunction; respiratory late effects; infertility and sexual dysfunction; psychosocial late effects such as depression, anxiety, uncertainty, isolation, and altered body image; social late effects such as changes in interpersonal relationships, health and life insurance issues, and financial burden; and existential issues such as changes in life purpose and meaning, and spiritual effects.[9,10] These effects may be **acute**, meaning that they are short-lived and time-limited; **long-term,** meaning that they persist for various periods of time even after treatment ends; or **late**, meaning that they occur months or years after treatment. The long-term and late effects are of greatest consequence to long-term cancer survivors. Chapter 68 discusses the physical late effects of cancer. This chapter focuses on quality of life in relationship to psychosocial late effects in adult cancer survivors.

Quality of Life and Cancer Survivors

Quality of life issues for long-term cancer survivors differ from the problems faced at the time of diagnosis and treatment.[11–15] Zebrack[16] provided an excellent and comprehensive overview of the literature on quality of life and cancer survivors. He discussed the differences in the meaning of quality of life, as this definition has changed over the past 30 years. In the 1970s, quality of life research showed that how people survive is just as critical as how long they survive. Quality of life research in the 1980s examined the relationship between psychosocial effects of cancer (e.g., psychological, behavioral, and environmental factors) in relationship to causes of cancer. The predominant conceptual framework was the stress-coping paradigm. Studies identified individuals at high risk for poor psychosocial adjustment, with clinical interventions being designed to help buffer or prevent these effects. In the 1990s, studies continued to focus on problems of adjustment and psychological distress, with less attention being paid to personal growth and well-being.[16] By the late 1990s, however, the focus on the positive psychosocial outcomes of resilience, hardiness, enhanced appreciation for life, and spiritual growth helped counterbalance the negative psychosocial effects of cancer and survivorship.[16,17] The next section profiles the psychosocial late effects commonly seen in cancer survivors.

Psychosocial Late Effects in Cancer Survivors

Fear of Recurrence

Regardless of the type of cancer and its stage at diagnosis, fears — and more often fears of recurrence — can play a profound role in cancer survivorship and quality of life. This topic has been reported extensively in the literature,[18–22] most often with survivors of breast cancer.[23–27] Other cancer survivors also experience fears of recurrence, though survivors other than those with breast cancer are often underrepresented in quality of life studies. Thus, further research regarding fears of recurrence and quality of life in relation to other cancer survivors is needed.

There are different levels of fear of recurrence. Vickberg[23] reported that the majority of women in her study had moderate levels of fear related to breast cancer recurrence. These include fears of death, further treatment such as chemotherapy, pain, difficult emotions, potential for progression of disease, loss of a breast with mastectomy, and suffering of family members. At the same time, several women identified certain life circumstances that had more impact than the potential for recurrence. For example, family issues, such as the health of a spouse or child, and other personal chronic conditions could take precedence over their own fear of recurrence. Interestingly, cancer stage, time since diagnosis, and type of surgery were not related to fears of recurrence.[26]

Breast cancer survivors also identified "triggers" of their fear of recurrence: being around other people newly diagnosed with cancer or hearing about cancer, attending support groups where women discussed more aggressive treatment, and second-guessing their own conservative treatment choices. In addition, survivors became more fearful in situations where cancer or recurrence could be detected, such as follow-up mammography and testing, or when they felt something new or different in their breasts.[21,23]

Fear of recurrence influences family quality of life as well. Caregivers report fear of recurrence for their family members. Other shared concerns include: treatment distress, concerns over future diagnostic tests, and uncertainties about the future.[28] Mellon and Northouse[20] found a direct relationship between family members' fear of recurrence and the family's quality of life.

While many survivors continue to have thoughts concerning the possibility of recurrence, others recognize positive changes that their illness has made on their lives. In a study that examined quality of life in long-term survivors of non-small cell lung cancer, Sarna and colleagues[29] noted that 50% of their participants believed that their illness had made positive changes in their lives. Additionally, the majority of their participants (71%) described themselves as being very hopeful about the future.

Wenzel and colleagues[21] note high quality of life in their population of early-stage ovarian cancer survivors. Although the participants reported fears of recurrence, a second cancer diagnosis, and future diagnostic tests, 43% of their sample members stated that they had no current survivorship concerns. A notable aspect of this study, according to the authors, was that many participants reported having a positive attitude concerning their diagnosis and showed signs of growth and resilience as a result of their cancer experience.

Depression

Cancer-related intrusive thoughts have been linked with poor psychological adjustment and quality of life. Lewis et al[30] examined the link among cancer-related intrusive thoughts, quality of life, and perceived social support. For women who reported high levels of social support, intrusive thoughts did not affect their quality of life. However, a significant relationship was identified between cancer-related thoughts and poor quality of life among women having low levels of social support. Matsuoka et al[31] further noted that intrusive thoughts and psychological adjustment persisted several years after diagnosis in cancer survivors.

Deimling and colleagues[32] explored physiologic effects, psychological distress, and post-traumatic stress in cancer survivors. While acute symptoms from treatment may decline, the persistence of late and long-term physiologic sequelae contribute to psychological distress. These long-term physiologic effects may include lymphedema among breast cancer survivors, urinary changes in prostate cancer survivors, elimination problems in colorectal cancer survivors, and persistent dry mouth among head and neck cancer survivors.

Depression is not uncommon in the presence of late physiologic effects. Deimling et al[32] noted that 25% of older adult survivors were depressed. Distress was found to be directly related to current illness symptoms, regardless of whether it was related to cancer. Individuals who continued to experience cancer-related long-term effects as well as new conditions had higher levels of depression and post-traumatic stress characteristics. Sarna et al[29] also noted a relationship between the number of co-morbid conditions that lung cancer survivors experienced and their perception of quality of life. The more co-morbid conditions reported by participants, the poorer they rated their quality of life. These results show the need for nurses and other oncology providers to acknowledge that those patients who continue to have cancer-related symptoms, even many years after treatment, are at risk for depression and psychological distress related to their current condition and may benefit from counseling.

Uncertainty in Illness

Uncertainty in illness is very common in long-term cancer survivorship. Mast[33] found that uncertainty in illness was rated moderately high even several years after breast cancer treatment. Uncertainty is highly related to fear of recurrence. Mast also noted that older women who have faced other difficulties and losses throughout their lives were less likely than younger women to fear the uncertainty of cancer. Persistent symptoms contribute to fear of recurrence and feelings of uncertainty that may lead to emotional distress in women.

Lee-Jones and colleagues[19] proposed a cognitive formulation to explain exacerbation of fear of recurrence. The authors viewed fear of recurrence as consisting of cognitions, beliefs, and emotions and suggested that outcomes are not unidirectional but rather continually evolving. Their model demonstrates how internal and external cues act as antecedents to fear of recurrence. These antecedents lead to a perception of risk for a recurrence. Ultimately, fear of recurrence leads to consequences that can have a profound effect on survivors. Behavioral responses, which may be either positive or negative, include the positive aspect of seeking advice from professionals, family, and friends, and the negative aspect of limited planning for the future. Fear of recurrence may also increase survivors' anxiety if they have a tendency to misinterpret symptoms, giving them a preoccupation with thoughts of recurrence.

Coping with these psychosocial late effects can also pose a challenge for survivors. Cognitive strategies such as thinking positive thoughts or avoiding thinking about recurrence may be used. Distraction techniques, exercise, religious and spiritual activities, and having regular follow-up mammograms are behavioral coping strategies used by women.[23]

Several authors suggest interventions for patients and families concerning fears of recurrence.[19,20,34] These interventions include offering reassurance to the patient concerning the effectiveness of available treatments, providing information on recurrence rates and helping the patient interpret this information, and assisting the patient in identifying precipitating factors that influence or trigger fears of recurrence.[19] The need for healthcare professionals to recognize the common distressors experienced by patients is important so that nurses and other providers can support and assist them with coping strategies to improve their quality of life.[35]

Meaning and Appraisal

A positive aspect of long-term survivorship is the appraisal of the cancer experience. Long-term survivors have had an opportunity to reflect about their cancer experience, and their appraisal can be either positive or negative. For some survivors, appraisal and meaning of illness may result in a new identity and social role.[36] Having cancer involves incorporating the experience into a sense of self and may change the way survivors view themselves. This view continues for the rest of the survivor's life. Zebrack[36] described the cancer survivor as being on a trajectory that starts with diagnosis, continues through a treatment trajectory, and then moves into a survivor trajectory. Each of these trajectories has its own experiences and challenges, and each can influence the sense of self, appraisal of the cancer experience, and perceived quality of life.

Bowman and colleagues[37] examined how survivors viewed the cancer experience over time and noted that appraisal of the experience changed with the passage of time. Many survivors believed that having cancer was both a stressful life event and "just part of living." Older survivors demonstrated a less stressful appraisal of the cancer experience. As the appraisal of the illness changes over time, coping may be affected in relation to perceived threats that may appear. This may, in turn, affect quality of life. Threats that may be related to the cancer experience include concerns regarding employment or insurability, reproductive limitations, and reminders of the cancer experience such as follow-up tests.[36]

In studying breast cancer survivors one year after their diagnosis, Stanton and colleagues[38] found that women who coped by actively accepting their diagnosis had a more positive adjustment over time, whereas women who used the coping style of avoidance had greater fears of recurrence. Acceptance of the diagnosis may enable women to take an active approach toward their treatment and recovery, assisting in their adaptation to the disease.

Utley[39] also evaluated the meaning of cancer in long-term survivors of breast cancer. In this phenomenological study, the meaning of cancer evolved over time for the women. Initially, the women viewed cancer as sickness and death based on their previous experiences and memories of those they had known who had experienced cancer. When they were diagnosed themselves, many saw cancer as an obstacle that they had to deal with before living the rest of their lives. Finally, as the women continued to survive and make it through the obstacle of cancer, the experience was viewed as transforming. Several viewed the cancer as benefiting them and bringing about positive experiences. Many reported gaining a greater appreciation for life after the cancer.

Understanding the meaning of the cancer experience for survivors is very important for assisting healthcare professionals and nurses in relating to survivors. This knowledge can help facilitate an understanding of a patient's goals and informational needs, thereby fostering communication.[39]

Vachon[40] outlines several approaches to survivorship representing both positive and negative coping strategies. For some people, cancer is considered a non-issue; these people plan to return to their normal lives after treatment. Others minimize and deny the problem of cancer. Denial may result in not attending appropriate follow-up visits with healthcare providers as people try to get on with their normal lives. Still other individuals see surviving cancer as a strong part of their self-concept. Some view the experience as positive, using their experiences constructively by working as an individual advocate or as a member of a cancer group such as a support group or by becoming involved with the American Cancer Society (ACS). Other people allow their lives to revolve around the fact they had cancer and focus on the suffering they have experienced. These patients may even be hesitant to give up their illness role. Many others see cancer as a turning point in their lives and seize the opportunity to reflect on their lives and mull over future directions.

Whatever the evaluation, cancer has a profound impact on the lives of cancer survivors and their families. Having an understanding of patients' differing perspectives and experiences of the illness can give oncology nurses and healthcare providers the appropriate knowledge necessary to assist survivors through the experience while also assisting them to find meaning in the illness. Familiarizing nurses and healthcare professionals with the emotional and psychological aspects of illness and survivorship can facilitate interventions to assist patients in lessening distress and achieving good quality of life.

In January 2004, the Institute of Medicine[41] issued a report examining the psychosocial needs of women with breast cancer (*http://www.iom.edu/report.asp?id=18136*). Breast cancer survivors were chosen because they represent the largest group of cancer survivors and have been studied extensively. According to this report, strong data from clinical trials show that psychosocial interventions assist women with breast cancer in experiencing a better quality of life; however, these measures have not been widely integrated into routine cancer care. The report recommends incorporating psychosocial services into treatment plans as an integral part of high-quality cancer care. The information contained in the report is also seen as having value in other patient populations, not just with breast cancer survivors.[42] Additionally, the report urges professional organizations such as the Oncology Nursing Society, the National Cancer Institute, the American Cancer Society and the American Society of Clinical Oncology to focus on the psychosocial needs of patients and to provide resources to meet the needs of patients on both national and local levels. Further research is needed to determine the benefits of specific interventions and the most effective way to deliver the intervention to the patient.

In summary, the vast majority of research concerning quality of life, psychosocial clinical issues, and research-based interventions has been primarily conducted in breast cancer survivors. While a few reports focus on cancer survivors in general, there is little diversity in the quality of life literature. Thus, there is a great need to study cancer survivors who are dealing with other diagnoses and who might have different quality of life issues related specifically to their disease and treatment. Further research concerning disease-specific quality of life issues might enable interventions to be designed to improve quality of life for all cancer survivors.

Rural Cancer Survivors

While a growing body of evidence demonstrates the positive and negative aspects of survivorship, these data have been obtained primarily from urban dwellers. We have few data on rural cancer survivorship, as the majority of rural research has focused on screening and prevention activities. What we do know is that rural cancer survivors report feeling poorly treated by the healthcare system and voice a strong desire for increased support and educational services.[43] Rural cancer survivors identify several obstacles to survival, including a lack of insurance, out-of-pocket costs, delayed diagnosis, and transportation issues.[44] A few investigators have identified positive aspects of rural cancer survivorship.[45,46]

A review of the literature on rural cancer shows that the few available studies have focused on psychosocial unmet needs after treatment. Wilson and colleagues[43] conducted focus groups with 128 cancer survivors in rural Washington state communities and explored ways to improve services to breast cancer survivors. Survivors, particularly those with advanced-stage disease, reported both positive and negative outcomes. They reported feeling poorly treated by the healthcare system and voiced a strong desire for increased support and educational services. According to the investigators, rural breast cancer survivors also needed more emotional support after the end of treatment. Braun et al[44] conducted focus groups to examine rural and urban perspectives of Native Hawaiian survivors' concerns in survivorship. Obstacles to survival included a lack of insurance, out-of-pocket costs, delayed diagnosis, and transportation issues. Survival-supportive factors included personal advocacy.

Burman and Weinert[47] examined interpersonal relationships, self-image, healthcare interactions, and occupational concerns of rural men and women with cancer or with family members. In their study, they used a mail survey that was sent to rural areas in the northern Rocky Mountain region. The sample included 294 people with cancer and 294 family caregivers in Montana. Fifty-two percent were women, and almost all were white. Results showed that women were more likely than men to report relationship problems and lack of support. People with cancer, as compared with caregivers, were more likely to report feeling alone and to say that other people avoided them and were afraid to talk to them. Men with cancer were more likely than women with cancer and caregivers to feel that their job security was threatened. However, only a small percentage of all participants felt discriminated against at work.

Burman and Weinert[48] further explored differences in cancer fears and perceptions of cancer treatment among four rural groups: men with cancer, men caregivers, women with cancer, and women caregivers ($N = 590$). The four groups differed in their cancer fears. Approximately half feared pain, nausea, body disfigurement, and sexual problems from cancer. More than two-thirds were worried about finances and decreases in quality of life. They expressed more worries about separation from loved ones than worries about death.

While the few studies of rural cancer survivors emphasized the negative aspects of the illness experience, Rogers-Clark[45] found that resilience was a unique strength among rural women with breast cancer. Her findings suggest that "rurality" in the context of health and illness must be considered as a multifaceted dimension, with resources to support cancer survivors building on the existing strengths in rural communities. Similarly, Winstead-Fry and Schultz[49] found that rural residents in two northeastern rural states had higher quality-of-life scores on the FACT-G compared with urban dwellers. Curran and Church[46] found that a pilot project to facilitate a self-help peer support group network using audio teleconferencing was very useful with rural breast cancer survivors.

Surveillance of Cancer Survivors

There are many challenges when undertaking surveillance of cancer survivors. Hobbie and Ogle[50] identified four transitional care models: disease-specific, generic, primary care, and single-site models. In the disease-specific model, patients move from a pediatric specialist to a transition team of pediatric and adult specialists. Generic models are adolescent focused, and survivors migrate from pediatric to adolescent to adult health services. Primary care models use a family physician or general practitioner as the care coordinator. Single-site models use the same clinical environment, and the young person moves from pediatric to adolescent to adult within the same system. For childhood cancer survivors, the two most frequently used models are the disease-specific and single-site models. For the adult, the most commonly used model is the primary care model.

They also found that some programs have not demonstrated great success because of their inability to locate adult survivors of childhood cancer, patient unwillingness to seek follow-up care, lack of insurance, long distance to the follow-up clinic, lack of funding,

Table 67-1 Suggestions for Cancer Surveillance

- Stay in regular contact with your oncology team and keep a personal copy of your cancer treatment history.
- Stay informed. Learn about the different types of cancer surveillance procedures, such as blood studies, tumor markers, x-ray studies, scans, and other tests.
- Cancer surveillance time varies. Generally a visit twice a year for the first two years may be suggested. Follow-up visits may be suggested annually thereafter.
- Keep track of your out-of-pocket expenses.
- Use advocacy resources available on the Internet and through your local organizations.

lack of dedicated provider time, financial problems, and lack of institutional support.

Tesauro and colleagues[51] examined the scope of services and resources available to cancer survivors who had completed active treatment at an NCI-designated comprehensive cancer center. Patient education program contacts from 37 NCI-designated comprehensive cancer centers participated in a telephone interview. The following services were provided: lymphedema management (70%), professionally led support groups (49%), long-term medical care (49%), school reentry programs (19%), nutritional counseling (14%), and fertility and sexual counseling (14%). One program offered fatigue management. Of the long-term follow-up clinics, the majority focused on pediatric cancer ($n = 12$), with three focusing on adult cancer survivors.

While follow-up surveillance of cancer survivors is certainly needed, no uniform guidelines for specific follow-up exist. Suggestions are for regular surveillance with the oncology team at more frequent intervals within the first two years after treatment has ended. Thereafter, a minimum of annual surveillance may be recommended. In addition, as Tesauro indicated, there is a need for programs specific to symptoms and needs of cancer survivors. Table 67-1 provides suggestions for cancer surveillance.

Health Promotion in Cancer Survivors

Cancer survivors may benefit from additional health-promoting behaviors.[52] Long-term disease-free cancer survivors are interested in weight management through physical activity and healthy nutritional choices, as well as smoking cessation programs. The ACS recently released nutrition and physical activity recommendations for cancer survivors. Although the nutrition and physical activity guidelines established by ACS for the prevention of cancer are likely to be beneficial to survivors, the new report has recommendations specifically geared toward cancer survivors.[53] Table 67-2 summarizes these recommendations.

Table 67-2 Recommendations for a Health-Promoting Lifestyle

- Physical activity may be beneficial for people with advanced cancer by increasing appetite and reducing constipation and fatigue.
- A standard multivitamin and mineral supplement in amounts equivalent to 100% of the daily value can help survivors meet their nutrient needs. Supplements that contain high levels of folic acid or antioxidants may be harmful during cancer treatment.
- A vegetarian diet may have health-promoting features, but no direct evidence indicates that it can prevent cancer recurrence. Survivors who eat a vegetarian diet need to ensure adequate nutrient intake.
- Alcohol can have positive and negative effects, increasing the risk of new cancers in survivors while reducing the risk of heart disease.

Data from ACS nutrition and physical activity during and after cancer treatment. Available online at *CAonline.AmCancerSoc.org*.[53]

In general, data support the combined use of good nutrition and exercise and resistance training for cancer survivors. A diet rich in vegetables, fruit, whole grains, and low-fat dairy products combined with exercise to preserve or increase lean muscle mass is recommended.

Smoking Cessation

When patients with cancer smoke, they may be at increased risk for reduced survival, recurrence, and development of secondary cancers. Higher rates and longer duration of symptoms occurring during treatment (e.g., loss of taste, dry mouth, impaired pulmonary function, and mucositis) are noted in patients with lung and head and neck cancers who continue to smoke after treatment. Thus, smoking cessation during and after treatment is a high priority.[54]

Lifestyle choices of cancer survivors may influence their risk of late cardiac and pulmonary damage. Emmons and colleagues[55] examined smoking behavior among five-year survivors in the Childhood Cancer Survival Study (CCSS) cohort. They found that 28% of patients reported ever smoking and 17% reported current smoking. While these figures are lower than the corresponding rates in the general population, they need to be reduced because of the greater risk of secondary cancers in this population. Factors that were related to the relative risk of smoking initiation included older age at cancer diagnosis, lower household income, less education, not having a pulmonary-related cancer treatment, and not having had brain radiation.

In a follow-up study, the same investigators describe baseline data collection for the Partnership for Health, a smoking cessation intervention for smokers in the CCSS.[56] Initial results showed that smokers had an average of 14 cigarettes per day, 53.2% were nicotine dependent, and 58% had made at least one attempt to quit smoking. Smoking behaviors were related to age at cancer diagnosis and perceived vulnerability to smoking-related illnesses.

Hecht and colleagues[57] identified strategies for oncology nurses to assist patients with cancer in modifying their smoking behaviors by assessing smoking status and patients' readiness to quit; providing brief, supportive messages consistently over time; offering or referring patients to appropriate resources; and providing continued follow-up.

One study[58] evaluated the effectiveness of a nurse-managed minimal smoking cessation intervention among 28 hospitalized patients with cancer. At admission, 64% of the intervention group and 71% of the usual-care group reported an intention to quit smoking. At six weeks post-intervention, 21% and 14% of the intervention and usual-care groups, respectively, abstained from smoking. More than 90% of the intervention group members who resumed smoking did so within the first week after their discharge. It may be that a more intensive intervention is necessary to help patients in quit smoking.

Another study[59] evaluated the effectiveness of a nurse-managed smoking cessation intervention based on the Agency for Health Care Policy and Research's (AHCPR) Smoking Cessation Guidelines. Subjects in the intervention group received a nurse-delivered, AHCPR-based smoking cessation intervention that included face-to-face and phone follow-up contact beginning with the first preoperative clinic consultation. Browning found that smokers diagnosed with lung cancer wanted to quit smoking and may benefit from an intensive smoking cessation intervention implemented at the time of diagnosis.

Smoking prevention or cessation to reduce tobacco-related cardiac and pulmonary disease is another important area of health promotion for cancer survivors. Unfortunately, many young cancer survivors are not taught about the adverse health effects of smoking and the increased risks to themselves posed by smoking after cancer treatment. Smoking behaviors are related to age at cancer diagnosis and the perception that survivors are vulnerable to smoking-related illnesses. Strategies to help patients with cancer quit smoking include assessing smoking status and the survivors' readiness to quit; providing brief, supportive messages consistently over time; offering or referring patients to appropriate resources; and providing continued follow-up. In addition, the AHCPR and ACS smoking cessation guidelines can be used effectively with cancer survivors.

Return-to-Work Issues

Cancer survivors either continue to work or return to work and lead full, productive lives after treatment.[13] Generally, cancer survivors want to return to work because it is an important part of their lives. In other circumstances, cancer survivors may have long-term disability or dysfunction that requires changes in their type or place of employment. Most often, survivors return to work with very little job adjustment needed. Flexibility in hours, particularly for follow-up care, may be needed. Unfortunately, some employers may mistake a survivor's need to follow up care as interfering with job responsibilities or may consider a survivor a poor risk for promotion.

The Americans with Disabilities Act (ADA), enacted by Congress in 1990, protects individuals with disabilities, including cancer survivors, from workplace discrimination. Organizations with at least 15 employees must comply with the ADA guidelines. Cancer survivors must disclose their diagnosis to their employer to be protected by the ADA. The act also provides protection for cancer survivors when they apply for a job. In particular, it prohibits a potential employer from asking questions about an individual's health history or current health status during an interview. Cancer survivors are not required to disclose a cancer history. However, when a cancer survivor is hired and must undergo a physical examination, it is prudent to disclose one's cancer history.

Advocacy

Survivorship is not a static process.[60] Reflecting on their own cancer experience and experiences of others may encourage some survivors to become advocates for others. The National Coalition for Cancer Survivorship (NCCS; *http://www.canceradvocacy.org/advocacy/*) defines advocacy as a continuum. It can begin with self-advocacy, as the cancer patient or a family member becomes an active participant in care. Many survivors find they become an advocate for others as the unofficial designated community ''authority'' on cancer and help others through the experience when they or a family member has been diagnosed with cancer. Support groups also create a forum for cancer survivors to advocate for one another. Many survivors benefit from hearing the experiences of others in similar situations.[61]

Advocacy can also be seen at the community level in support groups or as survivors share their experiences with friends. Also at the community level, many survivors volunteer in hospitals or cancer support organizations. Others participate in research studies or

Table 67-3 Internet Resources for Cancer Survivors

- American Cancer Society: 800-ACS-2345 or *www.cancer.org*. The ACS's Cancer Survivors Network (*www.cancer.org* or *www.acscsn.org/*) provides online discussions for survivors.
- Childhood Cancer Survivors: *www.patientcenters.com/survivors/*.
- Lance Armstrong Foundation: *http://www.laf.org/*.
- National Cancer Institute Office of Cancer Survivorship: *dccps.nci.nih.gov/ocs/follow.html*. NCI has a publication called "Facing Forward: Life after Cancer Treatment" that is available at *www.cancer.gov/cancerinfo/life-after-treatment*.
- National Coalition for Cancer Survivorship: 800-828-7866 or *www.canceradvocacy.org*. The *Cancer Survival Toolbox* consists of audiocassettes with basic guidelines to help navigate through survivorship and an *Essential Care Resource Guide*. The toolkit and the guide are available at the NCCS Web site.
- OncoChat is an online peer support for patients, families, and friends at *http://www.oncochat.org/*.
- Susan G. Komen Breast Cancer Foundation: 972-885-9600 or *www.komen.org*. It provides information specific to breast cancer survivors.

cancer awareness events such as "fun runs" and other sporting events.[61] In addition, advocacy can be found at the state and federal levels. Organizations such as the NCCS serve as the voice of cancer survivors and caregivers, assisting in the legislative process and promoting public policy decisions that affect people with cancer. Approximately 300 organizations participate in organized efforts to effect changes and to make sure that the needs and concerns of cancer survivors are met.[61] Table 67-3 lists some Internet resources of interest to cancer survivors.

Nurses and other healthcare professionals are also in a position to be advocate partners by promoting educational programs for cancer survivors and their families and by helping to empower survivors to be advocates for themselves and make the best possible care decisions.[60] Through the involvement of special-interest groups such as the Oncology Nursing Society's Survivorship SIG and through the literature, nurses can learn about and support survivorship issues.

Cancer Survivorship Research

Cancer survivorship research encompasses the "physical, psychosocial, and economic sequelae of cancer diagnosis and its treatment among both pediatric and adult survivors of cancer" (*http://dccs.nci.nih.gov/ocs.definitions.html*). Cancer survivorship research focuses on (1) health beyond acute diagnosis and treatment; (2) prevention and control of adverse outcomes, late effects, second cancers, and poor quality of life; and (3) optimizing follow-up, surveillance, and health after treatment. The ultimate goal of cancer survivorship research is to identify adverse effects and to develop effective prevention or intervention strategies so that cancer survivors will have the best chance for attaining a long and healthy life.[62]

Table 67-4 Quality of Life Directions in Cancer Survivorship Research

- Need to address methodological issues in long-term cancer survivorship research
- Need to understand long-term impact of different treatments on quality of life
- Need to assess quality of life in survivors experiencing second cancers
- Need to assess more diverse populations
- Need to examine the impact of long-term survival on the family
- Need to ask survivors what they need and want

Data from Gotay & Muraoka.[14]

Researchers who evaluate the psychosocial needs of survivors advocate an improved understanding of the phased nature of the cancer experience and the coping issues that are pertinent to each phase. Integrating the cancer experience into one's self-concept is vital to improve quality of life for long-term survivorship.[16] The pediatric cancer survivorship literature, for example, shows that resilience is a concept most often associated with positive appraisal, flexibility, and adaptation.[63–66] These positive coping styles are just beginning to be seen in the adult cancer survivorship literature.

The NCI's cancer survivorship research portfolio focuses on studies about the health and life of a person with a history of cancer *beyond* the acute diagnosis and treatment phase. Studies that examine newly diagnosed survivors or those in active treatment are included in the survivorship portfolio if follow-up extended at least two months or longer post-treatment. Studies addressing recurrence or end-of-life research are not included in the current portfolio. In fiscal year (FY) 2001, which includes the most recent data, 124 of the 142 research grants focusing on cancer survivorship were funded through or jointly with NCI. The remaining 17 were funded or cofunded through other NIH mechanisms. The Office of Cancer Survivorship Web site provides detailed identification of the research topics covered by these studies (*http://dccps.nci.nih.gov/ ocs/*).

Gotay and Muraoka[14] provided an excellent review of research on the quality of life in long-term cancer survivors who have survived beyond five or more years and suggested additional avenues for quality of life research. Table 67-4 outlines the pertinent research areas.

In summary, cancer survivorship research represents a major area of research opportunity. The majority of survivorship grants to date have focused on breast cancer, with a limited number targeting other high-incidence cancers such as prostate, colorectal, lung, and gynecologic cancers. A small but very important part of the NCI survivorship portfolio targets family research. National Institute of Nursing Research does not have a specific thrust in cancer survivorship, though its broad areas of research priority fit with cancer survivorship research.

Conclusion

Survival rates from cancer have steadily increased over the past 30 years. The growing number of cancer survivors presents a tremendous opportunity for clinical practice, education, and research. Cancer survivors are living longer, but their long-term survival is tempered by the prospect of late effects. At the same time, these individuals are eager to learn ways to improve their health through physical activity and nutrition and to monitor their progress through cancer surveillance. This chapter provided an overview of cancer survivorship, described the historical perspectives on cancer survivorship, explored late psychosocial effects, and described challenges in cancer survivorship research for the future.

Acknowledgment

The authors would like to thank Sharon Austin for her assistance in manuscript preparation.

References

1. Dow KH: Challenges and opportunities in cancer survivorship research. *Oncol Nurs Forum* 30:455–469
2. Rowland JH, Aziz N, Tesauro G, et al: The changing face of cancer survivorship. *Semin Oncol Nurs* 17:236–240, 2001
3. National Cancer Institute: News brief on office of cancer survivorship. *J Natl Cancer Inst* 88:713, 1996
4. Hewitt M, Breen N, Devesa S: Cancer prevalence and survivorship issues: Analyses of the 1992 National Health Interview Survey. *J Natl Cancer Inst* 91:1480–1486, 1999
5. Simmonds MA: Cancer statistics, 2003: Further decrease in mortality rate, increase in persons living with cancer. *CA: Cancer J Clin* 53:5–26, 2003
6. Aziz N, Rowland J: Cancer survivorship research among ethnic minority and medically underserved groups. *Oncol Nurs Forum* 29:788–801, 2001
7. Saltzstein SL, Behling CA: 5- and 10-year survival in cancer patients aged 90 and older: A study of 37,318 patients from SEER. *J Surg Oncol* 81:113–117, 2002
8. *SEER Cancer Incidence Public-Use Database, 1973–1998* (CD-ROM) [computer program]. Bethesda, MD; National Cancer Institute, DCCPS, Cancer Surveillance Research Program, Cancer Statistics Branch, April 2001
9. Ganz PA: Late effects of cancer and its treatment. *Semin Oncol Nurs* 17:241–248, 2001
10. Donaldson SS, Hancock SL, Hoppe RT: The Janeway lecture. Hodgkin's disease — finding the balance between cure and late effects. *Cancer J Sci Am* 5:325–333, 1999
11. Dow KH, Ferrell BR, et al: The meaning of quality of life in cancer survivorship. *Oncol Nurs Forum.* 26:519–528, 1999
12. Ferrell BR, Dow KH: Quality of life among long-term cancer survivors. *Oncology* 11:565–576, 1997
13. Dow KH, Ferrell BR, Leigh S, et al: An evaluation of the quality of life in long-term breast cancer survivors. *Breast Cancer Res Treat* 39:261–273, 1996
14. Gotay CC, Muraoka MY: Quality of life in long-term survivors of adult-onset cancers. *J Natl Cancer Inst* 90:656–667, 1998
15. Harpham W: Long-term survivorship: Late effects. In Berger A, Portenoy R, Weissman D (eds.): *Principles and Practice of Supportive Oncology.* Philadelphia, Lippincott Williams & Wilkins, 1998, pp 889–897
16. Zebrack B: Cancer survivors and quality of life: A critical review of the literature. *Oncol Nurs Forum* 27:1395-1401, 2000
17. Aaronson NK, Meyerowitz BE, Bard M, et al: Quality of life research in oncology. Past achievements and future priorities. *Cancer* 67:839–843, 1991
18. Ferrell BR, Dow KH, Leigh S, et al: Quality of life in long-term cancer survivors. *Oncol Nurs Forum* 22:915–922, 1995
19. Lee-Jones C, Humphris G, Dixon R, et al: Fear of cancer recurrence — a literature review and proposed cognitive formulation to explain exacerbation of recurrence fears. *Psychooncology* 6:95–105, 1997
20. Mellon S, Northouse LL: Family survivorship and quality of life following a cancer diagnosis. *Res Nurs Health* 24:446–459, 2001
21. Wenzel LB, Donnelly JP, Fowler JM, et al: Resilience, reflection, and residual stress in ovarian cancer survivorship: A gynecologic oncology group study. *Psychooncology* 11:142–153, 2002
22. Northouse LL, Schafer JA, Tipton J, et al: The concerns of patients and spouses after the diagnosis of colon cancer: a qualitative analysis. *J Wound Ostomy Continence Nurs* 26:8–17, 1999
23. Vickberg SM: Fears about breast cancer recurrence: Interviews with a diverse sample. *Cancer Pract* 9:237–243, 2001
24. Fredette SL: Breast cancer survivors: Concerns and coping. *Cancer Nurs* 18:35–46, 1995
25. Steginga S, Occhipinti S, Wilson K, et al: Domains of distress: The experience of breast cancer in Australia. *Oncol Nurs Forum* 25:1063–1070, 1998
26. Vickberg SM: The Concerns About Recurrence Scale (CARS): A systematic measure of women's fears about the possibility of breast cancer recurrence. *Ann Behav Med* 25(1):16–24, 2003
27. Lyons MA, Jacobson SS, Prescott B, et al: Women's experiences during the first year following diagnosis of breast cancer. *Southern Online J Nurs Res* 3:26, 2002
28. Matthews BA: Role and gender differences in cancer-related distress: A comparison of survivor and caregiver self-reports. *Oncol Nurs Forum* 30:493–499, 2003
29. Sarna L, Padilla G, Holmes C, et al: Quality of life of long-term survivors of non-small cell lung cancer. *J Clin Oncol* 20: 2920–2929, 2002
30. Lewis JA, Manne SL, DuHamel KN, et al: Social support, intrusive thoughts, and quality of life in breast cancer survivors. *J Behav Med* 24:231–245, 2001
31. Matsuoka Y, Nakano T, Inagaki M, et al: Cancer-related intrusive thoughts as an indicator of poor psychological adjustment at 3 or more years after breast surgery: A preliminary study. *Breast Cancer Res Treat* 76:117–124, 2002
32. Deimling GT, Kahana B, Bowman KF, et al: Cancer survivorship and psychological distress in later life. *Psychooncology* 11: 479–494, 2002

33. Mast ME: Survivors of breast cancer: Illness uncertainty, positive reappraisal, and emotional distress. *Oncol Nurs Forum* 25:555–562, 1998
34. Dow KH: The growing phenomenon of cancer survivorship. *J Prof Nurs* 7:54–60, discussion 60–51, 1991
35. Ferrell B, Smith SL, Cullinane CA, et al: Psychological well being and quality of life in ovarian cancer survivors. *Cancer* 98:1061–1070, 2003
36. Zebrack B: Cancer survivor identity and quality of life. *Cancer Pract* 8:238–242, 2000
37. Bowman KF, Deimling GT, Smerglia V, et al: Appraisal of the cancer experience by older long-term survivors. *Psychooncology* 12:226–238, 2002
38. Stanton AL, Danoff-Burg S, Huggins ME: The first year after breast cancer diagnosis: Hope and coping strategies as predictors of adjustment. *Psychooncology* 11:93–102, 2002
39. Utley R: The evolving meaning of cancer for long-term survivors of breast cancer. *Oncol Nurs Forum* 26:1519–1523, 1999
40. Vachon ML: The meaning of illness to a long-term survivor. *Semin Oncol Nurs* 17:279–283, 2001
41. Institute of Medicine: Meeting psychosocial needs of women with breast cancer *www.iom.edu/report.asp?id=18136.* Accessed April 5, 2004
42. Tuma RS: 10M: Psychosocial care in breast cancer improves quality of life, but more attention required. *Oncol Times* 26:7–8, 2004
43. Wilson SE, Andersen MR, Meischke H: Meeting the needs of rural breast cancer survivors: What still needs to be done? *J Womens Health Gend Based Med* 9:667–677, 2000
44. Braun K, Mokuau N, Hunt G, et al: Supports and obstacles to cancer survival for Hawaii's native people. *Cancer Pract* 10:192-200, 2002
45. Rogers-Clark C: Living with breast cancer: The influence of rurality on women's suffering and resilience. A postmodern feminist inquiry. *Australian J Adv Nurs* 20:34–39, 2003
46. Curran VR, Church JG: A study of rural women's satisfaction with a breast cancer self-help network. *J Telemed Telecare* 5:47–54, 1999
47. Burman ME, Weinert C: Concerns of rural men and women experiencing cancer. *Oncol Nurs Forum* 24:1593–1600, 1997
48. Burman ME, Weinert C: Rural dwellers' cancer fears and perceptions of cancer treatment. *Pub Health Nurs* 14:272–279, 1997
49. Winstead-Fry P, Schultz A: Psychometric analysis of the Functional Assessment of Cancer Therapy–General (FACT-G) scale in a rural sample. *Cancer* 79:2446–2452, 1997
50. Hobbie W, Ogle S: Transitional care for young adult survivors of childhood cancer. *Semin Oncol Nurs* 17:268–273, 2001
51. Tesauro GM, Rowland JH, Lustig C: Survivorship resources for post-treatment cancer survivor. *Cancer Pract* 10:277–283, 2002
52. Demark-Wahnefried W, Peterson B, McBride C, et al: Current health behaviors and readiness to pursue life-style changes among men and women diagnosed with early stage prostate and breast carcinomas. *Cancer* 88:674–684, 2000
53. American Cancer Society: ACS nutrition and physical activity during and after cancer treatment. www.CAonline.AmCancerSoc.org. Accessed April 9, 2004
54. Gritz ER, Carmack CL, de Moor C, et al: First year after head and neck cancer: Quality of life. *J Clin Oncol* 17:352–360, 1999
55. Emmons K, Li FP, Whitton J, et al: Predictors of smoking initiation and cessation among childhood cancer survivors: A report from the childhood cancer survivor study. *J Clin Oncol* 20:1608–1616, 2002
56. Emmons KM, Butterfield RM, Puleo E, et al: Smoking among participants in the childhood cancer survivors cohort: The partnership for health study. *J Clin Oncol* 21:189–196, 2003
57. Hecht JP, Emmons KM, Brown RA, et al. Smoking interventions for patients with cancer: Guidelines for nursing practice. *Oncol Nurs Forum* 21:1657–1666, 1994
58. Griebel B, Wewers ME, Baker CA: The effectiveness of a nurse-managed minimal smoking-cessation intervention among hospitalized patients with cancer. *Oncol Nurs Forum* 25:897–902, 1998
59. Browning KK, Ahijevych KL, Ross P, et al: Implementing the Agency for Health Care Policy and Research's smoking cessation guideline in a lung cancer surgery clinic. *Oncol Nurs Forum* 27:1248–1254, 2000
60. Clark EJ, Stovall EL: Advocacy: The cornerstone of cancer survivorship. *Cancer Pract* 4:239–244, 1996
61. Zebrack B. An advocate's perspective on cancer survivorship. *Semin Oncol Nurs* 17:284–287, 2001
62. Vaughn DJ, Meadows AT: Cancer survivorship research: The best is yet to come. *J Clin Oncol* 20:888–890, 2002
63. Dyer J, McGuinness T: Resilience: Analysis of a concept. *Arch Psych Nurs* 10:276–282, 1996
64. Hunter AJ, Chandler GE: Adolescent resilience. *Image: J Nurs Schol* 31:243–247, 1999
65. Haase JE: Hopeful teenagers with cancer; living courage. *Reflections* 32:20, 1997
66. Haase JE, Heiney SP, Ruccione KS, et al: Research triangulation to derive meaning-based quality-of-life theory: Adolescent resilience model and instrument development. *Int J Cancer Suppl* 12:125–131, 1999

CHAPTER 68

Late Effects of Cancer Treatment

Linda A. Jacobs, PhD, RN
Wendy Hobbie, MSN, RN
Ida Marie (Ki) Moore, DNS, RN, FAAN

Introduction

One of oncology's greatest success stories is the treatment and cure rate for childhood cancer. Consequently, the identification of late effects of treatment and subsequent need for specialized care for cancer survivors began more than 20 years ago among children who survived cancer.[1] There are few data focusing on the late effects of cancer treatment or surveillance guidelines for adult cancer survivors. Indeed, most of what we know about these issues today has come from studies that focused on survivors of pediatric cancer. Improvements in prevention, early detection, and treatment strategies, including surgery, chemotherapy, and radiotherapy, have led to enhanced survival and cure rates for many adult as well as pediatric cancers. Today it is estimated that there are more than 9.6 million cancer survivors, representing approximately 3% of the U.S. population. Of these survivors, 61% are 65 years of age or older. As long-term disease-free survival improves, it is interesting to note that approximately 14% of the 9.6 million estimated cancer survivors were diagnosed more than 20 years ago, creating a large number of cancer survivors with significant issues that must be addressed.[2]

In 1996, the National Cancer Institute (NCI) established the Office of Cancer Survivorship (OCS) to provide a focus within the National Institutes of Health (NIH) for the support of research and education aimed at professionals who deal with cancer patients and survivors. In doing so the NCI recognized the large number of individuals surviving cancer and their unique concerns.

The OCS objectives were as follows:

1. To develop an agenda for the continuous acquisition of knowledge concerning the problems facing cancer survivors, including the medical, psychological, and economic late effects of treatment;
2. To support studies that aim to increase the length of survival for cancer patients, including those that involve prevention of subsequent disease and disability;
3. To enable the dissemination of information to treating professionals concerning the problems and needs of cancer survivors;
4. To assist in providing information to the public concerning the issues of concern to survivors;
5. To improve the quality of survival of all individuals diagnosed with cancer.[3]

In June 2003, the Centers for Disease Control and Prevention (CDC) and the Lance Armstrong Foundation (LAF) conducted a workshop, "Building Partnerships to Advance Cancer Survivorship and Public Health," which focused on developing an action plan that outlined how public health can address critical cancer survivorship issues, including the underrecognized late effects of treatment. Survivorship has also been identified as a new priority for the NCI, and an action plan on this issue was outlined by the NCI for fiscal year 2004.

The pediatric oncology literature provides the foundation for the identification of late effects of treatment that are currently being explored in adult oncology. In addition, the population of adult survivors of childhood cancers has grown dramatically. This group, estimated to include 1 in 640 adults ages 20–39, will continue to increase, adding to the expanding population of adults with late effects related to their cancer treatment.[2]

Scope of the Problem

Biological cure refers to a patient who has no evidence of disease, has the same life expectancy as a person who never had cancer, and ultimately dies of unrelated causes.[4] Because of the aggressive nature of cancer treatment, cure is not without consequences. The consequences (or late effects) of cancer result from the physiological effects of particular treatments or from the interactions among treatment, the individual, and the disease. In contrast to the acute side effects of chemotherapy and radiation, which are due to the death of proliferative cells in tissues with relatively rapid renewal, late biological toxicity is believed to progress over time and by different mechanisms.

Most patients appear clinically healthy shortly after the completion of cancer therapy, but they may have subclinical tissue damage that may be detected by sensitive screening tests. Individuals with subclinical tissue damage can function well and be asymptomatic if compensatory mechanisms are adequate. Late effects—that is, the late expression of tissue damage—occur when physiological stress or developmental changes overwhelm compensatory mechanisms.[5] Late effects can appear months to years after treatment and can range from mild to severe to life-threatening. Their impact depends on the age and developmental state of the patient. Younger individuals may be more resilient than older adults to the acute side effects of treatment, but children are often at greater risk than adults for developing late effects. Little is known regarding the late effects of cancer treatment experienced by individuals who are surviving for decades as a result of better treatments and supportive cancer care. Although we may not be able to detect any obvious side effects soon after the completion of treatment, the influence of even subtle tissue damage on the process of aging is unknown. For adults, the cumulative effects of treatment toxicity combined with hereditary predisposition to particular health problems and exposure to damaging agents such as alcohol, cigarette smoke, or pollutants on organ systems are also unknown. This chapter provides an overview of what is currently known about these late effects by providing reference to both the pediatric and the adult oncology literature.

Central Nervous System

Neuropsychological, neuroanatomical, and neurophysiological changes can all occur as a result of central nervous system (CNS) treatment. These late effects have been observed in survivors of acute lymphoblastic leukemia (ALL) and brain tumors, and following bone marrow transplant.

Neuropsychological Late Effects

Declines in general intellectual abilities (intelligence quotient, IQ) and academic achievement, as well as deficits in visual-motor integration, attention, memory, visual-motor skills, and verbal fluency are the most frequently reported neuropsychological late effects of CNS treatment.[6–16] Nonverbal skills are especially vulnerable to the deleterious effects of CNS treatment, and deficits in these areas may be among the first to appear.

Neuropsychological late effects progress over time and become observable as cognitive abilities begin to lag behind age and developmental expectations. Age at time of CNS treatment is an important consideration because of the vulnerability of the developing brain to the damaging effects of radiation and chemotherapy. Children with ALL who receive cranial radiation at a young age (e.g., five years or younger) are at greatest risk for cognitive deficits. The majority of children with brain tumors who receive radiation therapy before age three, for example, experience significant cognitive impairments, such as a decline in full-scale IQ of 15–25 or more standard score points.[17,18]

The type of CNS treatment that has been most closely associated with neuropsychological deficits is cranial radiation administered alone or in combination with intrathecal (IT) chemotherapy. Children and adults treated for brain tumors with relatively high doses of cranial radiation consistently demonstrate deficits in intellectual abilities, memory, reasoning, visual-spatial abilities, and mathematical skills. A relationship also exists between the radiation dose and the severity of late effects. Survivors of brain tumors often have the most serious cognitive deficits, while children who receive lower cranial radiation doses as part of bone marrow conditioning regimens experience mild to no observable impairments.[7,19] In addition to age at time of CNS treatment and radiation dose, gender may be an important risk factor. For some late effects, such as verbal skills, females treated at an early age may be more vulnerable than males.[16]

There is a growing body of evidence about the effects of IT chemotherapy given alone or in combination with moderate- to high-dose systemic chemotherapy on long-term cognitive and academic abilities. Findings from several studies document that IT chemotherapy combined with systemic methotrexate (1 g/m^2) for treatment of ALL is also associated with long-term cognitive and academic problems, especially in math.[8–11,14,15,20]

Neuroanatomical Changes

Computerized tomography (CT) and magnetic resonance imaging (MRI) have been used to evaluate structural changes after CNS treatment. Atrophy, leukoencephalopathy, and white matter changes or calcifications have been found in children with ALL who received either systemic medium- to high-dose methotrexate (2 g/m^2) or systemic and IT methotrexate plus cranial radiation. Structural abnormalities have also been observed in children treated for brain tumors. A greater percentage of abnormal scans occurred in children who received radiation.[21–26]

Diffuse brain atrophy, as measured by the size of the CNS compartments, has also been documented in children who had either completed or were receiving ALL treatment. The highest incidence of brain atrophy (71% overall) occurred during the administration of IT chemotherapy, suggesting that CNS damage begins during treatment.[22] In addition to atrophy, perfusion defects have been identified in children with ALL whose treatment regimens included either IT and intravenous methotrexate or cranial radiation.[23] Reduced cerebellar and prefrontal cortex volumes also support the hypothesis that brain atrophy is an important neuroanatomical change following CNS treatment.[27] White matter deficits have been observed by quantitative MRI, and linked to deficits in attentional abilities in children with brain tumors.[18]

Mechanisms of Injury

Several mechanisms have been proposed by which radiation and chemotherapy might damage nonmalignant CNS tissue. Radiation injury to endothelial cells in small and medium-sized cerebral vessels causes deposition of calcium and mineralized debris. The result is some degree of occlusion, depending on the lumen size of the vessel. Dystrophic calcification of surrounding neural tissue also occurs.[21] Vascular endothelial damage can also perturb the normally tight junctions of the blood–brain barrier, allowing greater concentrations of systemic chemotherapy to penetrate the CNS.

Radiation and methotrexate may damage oligodendroglia, the myelin-producing cells in the CNS. Occlusive changes in vessels and decreased perfusion cause necrosis of glial cells and neurons.[26] Methotrexate also causes myelin damage. This drug blocks the synthesis of tetrahydrofolate by inhibition of the enzyme dihydrofolate reductase. Tetrahydrofolate is required as an intermediate carrier of one-carbon groups necessary for the synthesis of many biological macromolecules, such as myelin proteins and lipids.[28,29] Injury to gray matter structures can also occur but is thought to be less common than vascular or white matter damage. Vascular endothelial damage and decreased perfusion may contribute to gray matter damage.[26]

Vision and Hearing

Visual defects and hearing loss can occur following CNS treatment. Enucleation, which may be necessary in the treatment of ocular tumors such as retinoblastoma, is the most disabling visual deficit. Cataracts have been associated with cranial irradiation (2–16 Gray [Gy]) and long-term corticosteroid therapy. They result from radiation damage to the germinative zone of lens epithelial cell DNA as well as direct cytoplasmic effects such as disruption of membrane channels.[30]

Retinopathy can occur following radiation to the eye, orbit, nasal cavity, paranasal sinus, or nasopharyngeal area.[31,32] The mean time to onset of symptoms in one study was 2.8 years after treatment, and the earliest symptom was usually diminished vision.[31] The risk of radiation retinopathy increased with doses in the 45–55 Gy range. However, chemotherapy and concurrent chronic illness, such as diabetes mellitus, may increase the risk.[31] Radiation retinopathy is primarily due to vascular changes such as thickened arteriolar walls, lumenal narrowing and occlusion, and ischemia.[30]

The pathogenesis of radiation retinopathy involves obstruction of small vessels, resulting in ischemia, edema, and neovascularization of the optic disk.[32] Conjunctivitis, telangiectasis, corneal ulceration, optic neuropathy, and atrophy or stenosis of the lacrimal system can also occur, but at radiation doses between 30 and 75 Gy.[30]

Chemotherapy can cause ocular effects that may or may not be reversible. Conjunctivitis, keratitis, retinal hemorrhage, retinopathy, optic neuritis, and blurred vision are the more commonly reported ocular toxicities of systemic chemotherapy.[30,33] Less has been written about the mechanisms of ocular toxicity following chemotherapy, although one study suggests direct vascular injury may be at fault.[34]

Visual defects can be assessed by visual examination, slit-lamp examination, ultrasound, fluorescein angiogram, or MRI.[30] Visual evoked potentials may prove helpful in monitoring changes in sensory visual pathway or visual pathway damage in young children who cannot communicate visual symptoms or cooperate with more standard vision assessment methods.[35]

Hearing loss, especially in the high-tone range, is most closely associated with the administration of cisplatin.[36–38] One study of children with brain tumors who were treated with dose-intensive induction chemotherapy suggested that carboplatin-based high-dose therapy likewise results in significant ototoxicity.[39] Treatment regimens that combine cranial radiation and cisplatin-based chemotherapy increase the risk for sensorineural hearing loss.[40,41] Concurrent ifosfamide therapy also can exacerbate cisplatin-induced hearing loss. Patients who receive ifosfamide in combination with cisplatin are more likely to require amplification than those who receive cisplatin in combination with other drugs such as methotrexate and doxorubicin.[42]

One of the most consistently reported risk factors for cisplatin-based ototoxicity is drug dose. A cumulative dose of more than 600 mg/m^2 greatly increases the risk for persistent hearing loss in both adults and children.[36,38] High cumulative doses of cisplatin can impair renal function as well. In one study, children with malignant brain tumors who were treated with eight drugs (including cisplatin) in one day and who developed severe renal insufficiency were at greatest risk for significant hearing loss.[43] Iris and skin pigmentation may also affect cisplatin-induced ototoxicity. In a study of 19 children who had audiological assessments before and after cisplatin therapy for various solid tumors, researchers found a weak association between iris pigmentation and decreased auditory threshold. Children with brown or black eyes developed a greater hearing loss than did those with blue or hazel eyes, suggesting that pigmentation influences host susceptibility to cisplatin ototoxicity.[44] History of noise exposure has also been found to be a risk factor for adults.[37]

Periodic audiometric evaluations can be used to monitor for ototoxicity that is manifested as a deterioration of pure-tone thresholds. Acoustic reflex threshold measures may prove useful for detecting early sensorineural hearing loss.[45]

Damage to the hair cells of the cochlea is the most common mechanism of ototoxicity following cisplatin therapy.[46] Post-irradiation hyperemia may increase the sensitivity of the cochlea to cisplatin damage.[42] Recurrent otitis media, as well as the use of antibiotics that are ototoxic, also can contribute to hearing loss.

Little is known about effective methods for protecting the auditory system from the damaging effects of chemotherapy and radiation. However, two studies reported an otoprotective effect with sodium thiosulfate (SDS). In these studies, high doses of SDS were administered to patients with malignant brain tumors after recovery of blood–brain barrier disruption. This drug is thought to bind and inactivate DNA alkylating agents such as cisplatin and carboplatin. In both studies, hearing loss was decreased in patients who were treated with SDS.[46,47]

Immune System

Immunosuppression is one of the most serious acute toxic effects of chemotherapy and radiation. Some aspects of immune function can remain impaired for years after treatment. For example, high-dose chemotherapy followed by bone marrow transplantation has been found to induce a profound and prolonged impairment of hematopoiesis.[48] Radiation in conjunction with multiagent chemotherapy can result in more frequent and more severe immune system impairment.[49,50]

The clinical significance of these long-term alterations in immune function is not well understood. There is no evidence that patients with persistent immunologic abnormalities are at greater risk for infection. One group of patients who are known to be at increased risk of infection are those who have undergone splenectomy. Overwhelming bacterial infections, primarily pneumococcal, are a major concern to these individuals because of the protective role that the spleen plays against encapsulated organisms. Persistent immune defects have not been linked to the occurrence of second malignancies. This may change, however, as survival time increases for larger numbers of patients.

Cardiovascular System

Anthracyclines, such as daunorubicin and doxorubicin, have improved survival in patients with acute leukemias, lymphomas, solid tumors, and other cancers. One of the most serious late effects of these drugs (as well as cisplatin, which has been recently implicated), is cardiac toxicity, which typically presents as cardiomyopathy, with clinical signs of congestive heart failure.[51,52] Pathophysiological changes associated with cardiomyopathy include decreased contractility and stroke volume, increased left ventricular afterload, and increased end systolic wall stress. Recent evidence indicates that structural damage to the heart can precede the onset of symptoms.[53,54]

The risk and severity of cardiotoxicity is related to cumulative dose,[54–56] schedule of administration (continuous versus intermittent), and presence of other factors such as mediastinal irradiation. Cumulative doses of 550 mg/m^2 have been associated with cardiac toxicity in adults; similar abnormalities can occur after lower doses in children. The cumulative dose of doxorubicin, male gender, and concurrent mediastinal radiation are the most significant predictors of abnormal cardiac function.

Individuals who received radiation therapy to a field that includes the heart, such as mediastinal radiation for Hodgkin's disease or other lymphomas, also are at risk for cardiotoxicity. Delayed radiation injury to the heart can be manifested as pericardial disease, myocardial disease, or coronary heart disease.[57,58] An acceleration of coronary artery disease that results in angina and myocardial infarction may occur in some patients. Patients with pericardial damage secondary to mediastinal irradiation may have overt symptoms and abnormalities that are visible on x-ray examination. Although pericardial damage may be self-limiting, life-threatening pericardial effusions with tamponade can occur long after treatment has ended.[50,59] Current radiation-blocking techniques may protect some portions of the ventricles from irradiation, thereby resulting in more modest and less frequent cardiac toxicity.[57]

In general, cardiovascular late effects have not been examined thoroughly in long-term cancer survivors. Nevertheless, an unfavorable cardiovascular risk profile has been identified in patients with germ cell tumors of the testes treated with cisplatin and bleomycin. This profile includes hypertension, increased weight, and an elevated lipid profile. These survivors also report Raynaud's phenomenon-like symptoms.[53,54]

The mechanisms of cardiac damage following anthracycline therapy include inhibited expression of genes encoding for cardiac muscle protein, binding to membranes rich in cardiolipin, and the formation of free radicals.[55] The heart is particularly sensitive to free radical-induced damage because of the low levels of free radical scavengers there. Drugs that prevent the formation of superhydroxide radicals continue to be investigated for efficacy, and a number of drugs are currently being used to prevent doxorubicin-induced cardiotoxicity.[55,60,61]

Pulmonary System

Pneumonitis and pulmonary fibrosis are the major biological late effects of cancer treatment that affect the pulmonary system. Lung injury can be caused by chemotherapy, radiation therapy, and recurrent respiratory infections in immunosuppressed patients.[62,63] Alkylating agents (primarily busulfan), nitrosourea agents (e.g., lomustine and carmustine), and bleomycin have all been associated with the development of pulmonary fibrosis. The mechanisms of bleomycin injury include formation of free radicals and lipid peroxidation of phospholipid membranes. Subsequently, interstitial edema and damage to type 1 pneumocytes occur. Late lung injury is characterized by progressive fibrosis and collapse of alveoli.[62]

Pulmonary fibrosis is the most common type of chronic lung damage following radiation therapy. Obstructive lung disease can occur as well. Lung injury is more likely when higher radiation doses are used and when larger lung volumes are irradiated.[64] Radiation therapy also can potentiate the long-term toxicity induced by other agents such as bleomycin and nitrosoureas.[50]

Benign pleural effusions have been reported years after treatment with mantle radiation therapy due to enlarged lymphatic channels in the visceral pleura. These effusions can usually be treated with pleural aspiration, although they can become a chronic problem and require more aggressive treatment.[64,65] Chemotherapy dose reduction, medications currently under investigation, and sophisticated radiation therapy planning and delivery methods all hold promise to reduce the incidence of long-term treatment-related lung injury.[66–68]

Gastrointestinal System

Radiation and radiation-enhancing chemotherapeutic agents can have long-term effects on the gastrointestinal tract and the liver. Late effects of radiation on the esophagus result primarily from damage to the esophageal wall, although mucosal ulcerations may persist.[69,70] The major late effect of gastric irradiation is ulceration due to destruction of mucosal cells of the gastric mucosa. Although rare, vascular abnormalities and altered digestive system activity can result in malabsorption.

Moderate to severe intestinal injury following pelvic radiation usually appears within two to five years after irradiation. Late radiation injury to the small and large intestines can result in increased frequency of bowel actions and greater stool weight; decreased bile acid, vitamin B_{12}, and fat absorption; more rapid gastric emptying and small bowel transit; and bleeding, pain, fistula formation, and obstruction.[70,71] Histologic changes due to radiation injury include atypical epithelial cells, intestinal wall fibrosis, serosal thickening, and vascular sclerosis.[71] The technique and field of radiation both affect the probability of late gastrointestinal injury. For example, conformal radiation therapy allows for a higher tumor dose while irradiating a smaller volume of normal tissue. Therefore, the incidence and severity of injury to normal gastrointestinal tissues should be less with this type of treatment.[70,72] Although chemotherapy can augment acute gastrointestinal radiation toxicity, the effect of chemotherapy on late toxicity remains poorly established. The role of proton pump inhibitors for prophylaxis as well as treatment for mucosal damage caused by cancer treatment is being investigated and shows promise.[70]

Late effects in the liver are more common and include hepatic fibrosis, cirrhosis, portal hypertension, and venoocclusive liver disease. Radiation therapy in combination with radiation-enhancing agents, such as actinomycin D and possibly vincristine, can result in hepatic fibrosis. If the fibrosis is severe, portal hypertension can occur. Hepatic arterial infusion chemotherapy for management of liver metastases can result in significant hepatotoxicity. Chemotherapy-induced hepatic injury is usually due to the breakdown of drugs into free radicals that impair cell function and result in cell death.[73,74]

The administration of blood products as part of the supportive care of myelosuppressed patients can cause chronic hepatitis. Hepatitis C, transmitted by blood transfusions or by lifestyle practices, is now the most common chronic blood-borne infection in the United States and has emerged as an important cause of late gastrointestinal toxicities.[75,76]

Renal System

Nephritis, cystitis, reduced bladder capacity, and contractility and fibrosis of the ureter, bladder, and urethra are all long-term renal toxicities that result from cancer treatment. Damage to the nephrons and bladder has been documented in patients treated with cyclophosphamide, ifosfamide, and cisplatin.[77] Hemorrhagic cystitis following cyclophosphamide therapy may persist after treatment is completed, and the risk of this condition is increased by concurrent pelvic radiation. Acrolein, a metabolite of cyclophosphamide, is thought to be responsible for hemorrhagic cystitis. Mesna, a sulfhydryl compound, binds to acrolein within the urinary tract, thereby decreasing the incidence of renal toxicity associated with cyclophosphamide and ifosfamide therapy.[77] Pharmacological strategies that may prove effective in protecting the kidney from chemotherapy-related injury include administration of calcium chloride, N-acetylcysteine, and amifostine.[77–80]

Radiation doses of 20 Gy or less may minimize the risk of renal toxicity, whereas concurrent administration of radiation-enhancing drugs may increase this risk.[80] Clinical manifestations of nephritis include proteinuria, hypertension, anemia, and progressive renal failure, although early detection and intervention may prevent irreversible damage.[81]

The bladder, ureters, and urethra can be damaged by radiation and chemotherapy. Fibrosis of the bladder, reduction in capacity, and contractility are noted following the treatment of prostate cancer, cervical cancer, and other diseases utilizing pelvic irradiation.[82-84] The combination of chemotherapy agents such as cyclophosphamide and ifosfamide may have a synergistic effect, thereby placing long-term cancer survivors at greater risk. Radioenhancers such as actinomycin-D also potentiate the radiation effects on these organs.[80] The dose of radiation and the area treated influence the degree of fibrosis and ultimately the degree of scarring, and dysfunction.[84–86] Symptoms of bladder, ureter, and urethra damage include frequent urination, urgency, stress incontinence, and incontinence.

Endocrine System

Cancer treatment can adversely affect a number of endocrine functions, including metabolism, growth, secondary sexual development, and reproduction. These late effects result from damage to the target organ (i.e., thyroid, ovary, and testis) and the hypothalamic pituitary axis. Table 68-1 summarizes endocrine late effects, risk factors, and evaluation methods.

Thyroid

Direct damage to the thyroid gland causes primary hypothyroidism, thyroiditis, and, less frequently, hyperthyroidism. With primary hypothyroidism, there is a decreased production of thyroxine (T_4) and triiodothyronine (T_3). These hormones have biological effects on oxygen consumption, the central and peripheral nervous systems, skeletal and cardiac muscle, carbohydrate and cholesterol metabolism, and growth and development.[87] Primary hypothyroidism can be compensated when only partial organ damage occurs and some function is preserved. The compensated state is maintained by an increased production of thyrotropin-releasing factor (TRF) and thyroid-stimulating hormone (TSH) from the hypothalamus and pituitary. This chronic overstimulation is believed to increase the risk of malignant transformation in previously damaged cells.[88,89] Overt or compensated primary hypothyroidism has been documented in 4% to 80% of patients who received radiation to the neck for Hodgkin's disease, other lymphomas, and carcinomas or total body irradiation for transplant.[90–94]

Damage to the thyroid gland usually occurs after radiation doses of more than 20 Gy administered in multiple fractions.[95] In general, the incidence and severity of thyroid dysfunction appear to increase with higher radiation doses and may be due to damage to thyroid follicular cells, thyroid vasculature, or connective tissue. To date, no chemotherapeutic agents have been conclusively associated with long-term thyroid damage.[95] Although hypothyroidism usually develops three to four years after treatment, it can occur as late as 7 to 14 years later.[95] However, some data now suggest an increased lifetime risk of thyroid gland dysfunction following radiation.[96]

When the hypothalamic pituitary axis is in the field of radiation to the nasopharynx of the CNS, secondary hypothyroidism can occur. Decreased levels of TRF, TSH, T_3, and T_4 have been reported in patients who received at least 55 Gy of external beam radiation for nasopharyngeal, paranasal sinus, or brain tumors that did not involve the hypothalamus or pituitary.[95,97] These studies found no difference in the development of secondary hypothyroidism between children and adults, although most subjects were adults. As with primary thyroid dysfunction, secondary hypothyroidism may not develop until years after the completion of therapy.

Hyperthyroidism has also been reported after radiation to the mantle region. The incidence is low, however, and the mechanism of action remains unclear.[95]

Growth

Pituitary dysfunction requires radiation doses of at least 40 Gy, but damage to the hypothalamus may occur even with lower doses.[95] The belief has been that growth disturbances as a result of hypothalamic damage require doses of at least 24 Gy.[98,99]

Growth hormone deficiency in adults is a growing area of research. As linear growth is complete in adults, other properties of growth hormone take on greater significance in the adult cancer survivor population. The activities of growth hormone that are important in adulthood include definition of body composition, bone mineral density, muscle strength,

Table 68-1 Endocrine Late Effects, Risk Factors, and Evaluation Methods

Organ	Chemotherapy	Radiation	Risk Population	Evaluation
Thyroid	None known	>2000 cGy or >750 cGy TBI = overt or compensated hypothyroidism Graves' disease	Young children Tumors of head and neck Brain tumors Leukemia with cranial radiation BMT Lymphomas (HL, NHL)	T_4, free T_4, TSH, T_3
Ovaries	MOPP/COPP Cyclophosphamide Ifosfamide Busulfan BCNU/CCNU (age and dose dependent)	400–1000 cGy (age dependent)	>40 yr Abdominal and pelvic tumors HL Spinal radiation	LH, FSH, estradiol drawn on days 5–8 of menstrual cycle
Testes	MOPP/COPP Cyclophosphamide Ifosfamide Busulfan BCNU/CCNU	<400 cGy = azoospermia, possible recovery >600 cGy = permanent azoospermia >2400 cGy = Leydig cell damage, decreased testosterone	HD and NHL Pelvic tumors Testicular tumors Leukemia with testicular infiltrates	LH, FSH, testosterone, semen analysis
Hypothalamic pituitary axis	None currently identified	>2400 cGy = hypothalamic dysfunction >4000 cGy = pituitary dysfunction	Leukemia with CNS radiation CNS tumors Head and neck tumors	Growth charts (sitting and standing height) Somatomedin-C LH, FSH, estradiol, testosterone, prolactin T_4, TSH, free T_4, T_3 Bone age Cortisol levels Growth hormone (even in adults at risk)

Abbreviations:
TBI: total body irradiation
BMT: bone marrow transplant
HD: Hodgkin's disease
NHL: non-Hodgkin's lymphoma
TSH: thyroid-stimulating hormone
LH: luteinizing hormone
FSH: follicle-stimulating hormone
CNS: central nervous system
MOPP: nitrogen mustard, vincristine, procarbazine, prednisone
COPP: cyclophosphamide, vincristine, procarbazine, prednisone

exercise performance, cardiovascular system function, metabolism, and immune function.[100,101] Studies have documented that growth hormone-deficient adults are at increased risk for osteoporotic fractures, heart disease, decreased lean body mass, and muscle strength. Studies in adults with growth hormone deficiency document improvement in lean body mass, fasting cholesterol, physical performance, basal metabolic rate, and psychological well-being when treated with growth hormone replacement therapy.[102–104] Therefore, it is important that at-risk adults be evaluated for growth hormone deficiency and be referred to an endocrinologist for evaluation and consideration for hormone replacement therapy.[100,101]

In recent years, controversy has surounded the use of growth hormone in children treated for malignancies. The concerns stem from the potential side effects of growth hormone administration, including the development of leukemia. A related concern is the fear that growth hormone therapy may stimulate cancer cell growth and result in a relapse or recurrence of the primary disease. However, recent studies indicate that the incidence of relapse or recurrence is not higher in children who receive growth hormone when compared to untreated controls.[105,106] Whether these concerns regarding tumor recurrence, leukemia, and the long-term implications of growth hormone use in adults are justified has yet to be determined.

Secondary Sexual Development and Reproduction

Chemotherapy, specifically alkylating agents (e.g., cyclophosphamide, mechlorethamine, busulfan, and procarbazine), and radiation can cause permanent damage to the gonads. Age at the time of treatment, gender, total drug dose, use of combinations of alkylating agents, and dose and site of radiation are important risk factors for gonadal dysfunction. The quiescence of the pre-pubertal gonad provides some protection, whereas the incidence of gonadal damage increases with age and stage of pubertal development.[107]

Ovary

Primary ovarian failure, along with amenorrhea, decreased estradiol, and elevated gonadotropins (luteinizing hormone [LH] and follicle-stimulating hormone [FSH]), has been reported in women who received these agents for treatment of Hodgkin's disease, breast cancer, and ovarian germ cell tumors.[108–110] In addition, those women who retain ovarian function following treatment with gonadotoxic agents are expected to be at risk for premature ovarian failure, a condition also seen in the adolescent population.[111] Tamoxifen used in treatment of breast cancer can result in hot flashes, night sweats, and vaginal discharge, itching, and dryness.[112]

Pathological changes in women who receive radiation to the ovaries include reduced numbers of oocytes, inhibited follicle development, atrophic ovaries, and strong fibrohyalinization.[113,114] Older women are at greater risk for ovarian failure following radiation. Ovarian function may be preserved in girls who receive 8 Gy of radiation; however, ovarian failure has been reported in 100% of women older than 40 years of age who were treated with 400 cGy.[115] Scatter to the ovaries as a result of abdominal or cranio-spinal irradiation can result in long-term damage as well.[116]

Testis

Damage to the germinal epithelium of the testis with decreased or absent spermatogonia can occur in males who are treated with alkylating agents and radiation. Leydig cell damage is unusual; thus, testosterone production and pubertal development are usually not affected.[117,118] Testicular damage with azoospermia is most frequently observed in males with Hodgkin's disease who received MOPP (mechlorethamine, vincristine, procarbazine, and prednisone) or COPP (cyclophosphamide, vincristine, procarbazine, and prednisone) therapy, but has also been observed in males with ALL or rhabdomyosarcoma who were treated with cyclophosphamide and cytosine arabinoside.[107,119] Impaired testicular function has also been documented in men who received higher-dose cisplatin and etoposide therapy for germ cell cancer.[120]

The testis appears to be more sensitive than the ovary to the damaging effects of therapy. Byrne et al found that the fertility of men who were treated with alkylating agents was half the fertility of control subjects, whereas the fertility of women was unimpaired.[121] The risk of gonadal failure also increases with greater total doses of alkylating agents and the use of more than one drug, such as in MOPP therapy. The cumulative cyclophosphamide dose is an important risk factor for recovery of spermatogenesis.[107,108,122] Cumulative doses exceeding 7.5 g and 9 g are associated with the highest risk of infertility.[123,124]

The testis is extremely sensitive to the damaging effects of radiation. The threshold dose required to damage the germinal epithelium is as low as 3–4 Gy, while the Leydig cells are more resistant, with permanent damage occurring only following doses at 20 Gy.[125,126]

In addition to the damaging effects of chemotherapy and radiation therapy on stem cells, retroperitoneal lymph node dissection can contribute to ejaculatory dysfunction.[127] Following radiation for prostate cancer, ejaculatory function may be dramatically affected as well as sexual functioning.

Central Gonadal Dysfunction

Radiation to the cranium or nasopharynx can damage the hypothalamic pituitary axis, causing secondary gonadal failure. Subnormal levels of LH, FSH, and prolactin-inhibiting factor (PIF) have been found in both males and females treated for head and neck tumors with 4–78 Gy of radiation.[128] In addition to the effects of low LH and FSH levels on ovarian and testicular function, the decrease in PIF and resultant increase in prolactin causes irregular menses, anovulatory periods, low testosterone, reduced libido, and impotence.[129]

Sexual Dysfunction

In addition to gonadal failure, a number of treatment-related factors may impair sexual functioning. Sexual issues are complex and include both physiological and psychological components. Although sexual functioning effects are more often noted in adult survivors of cancer, they may also become apparent in childhood survivors as they enter adulthood. The most common problems include decreased libido, erectile dysfunction, and dyspareunia. Cancer-related therapies that often lead to the development of sexual dysfunction include radiation to the pelvis, surgical changes, and removal of gonads, which can result in decreased hormonal production, fibrosis of tissue, decreased blood flow, and nerve damage.[130–132] Researchers have reported sexual dysfunction in approximately 50% of women who survive breast cancer.[133] These findings are similar to those noted in survivors of gynecological cancer.[134,135] Seventy percent of men who have undergone radical prostatectomies report erectile dysfunction.[136,137]

Lack of physical energy or syndromes resulting in chronic pain and psychological concerns may compound the complex issues of sexual dysfunction.[133] Questions regarding sexual functioning and satisfaction should be incorporated into routine follow-up visits so that a treatment plan can be developed if problems arise.

Treatment programs are influenced by many factors, including the initial diagnosis, type of treatment, available intervention, and willingness of the survivor. For example, some women who are diagnosed with breast cancer cannot receive estrogen replacement therapy. However, less risky alternatives (estrin vaginal ring and water-based lubricants) to combat certain menopausal symptoms are available.[138] In contrast, interventions for erectile dysfunction have poor acceptance in general. Penile injections, vacuum devices, and intraurethral medications have low satisfaction and high dropout rates.[139,140] Although sildenafil has a high acceptance rate among patients, many cancer survivors will not achieve an adequate erection with this medication alone.[139–141] Although treatment programs may be difficult to develop due to the multifaceted aspects of sexual dysfunction, the healthcare provider's approach to this subject matter may greatly increase patient awareness and compliance with intervention programs.

Offspring

There has long been concern regarding the effects of cancer therapy on the offspring of survivors. The effects of antineoplastic therapy on a fetus in the first and second trimesters can be devastating.[142,143] However, the potential mutagenic effects of cancer therapy on offspring years after the completion of treatment have been less well elucidated due to the relatively small numbers of offspring of long-term survivors. The largest study to date involved 5847 offspring of 14,652 survivors of childhood cancer. These researchers found no increased risk of nonhereditary cancers among offspring. Likewise, no increased risk of birth defects was observed.[144] The majority of studies involving offspring of survivors have utilized pediatric data. These studies examined a variety of diagnosis and treatment regimes, but generally failed to find any increased risk of malignancies or anomalies in the offspring.[144–147] To date no large cohort studies have examined the effects of chemotherapy and radiation on offspring following the treatment of cancer during adulthood. Nevertheless, the data from the pediatric survivor community are encouraging.

Another concern for survivors of breast cancer is the risk of recurrence with pregnancies following treatment. To date, studies have not found an association with pregnancy and the risk of recurrence of disease.[148]

Musculoskeletal System

Late effects in the musculoskeletal system and related tissues are most frequently associated with radiation. Cosmetic and functional alterations of the bone, soft tissue, and teeth are frequently reported in children who have been treated with radiation. Factors that can dramatically affect the degree of disfigurement include age at diagnosis, total dose and volume of tissue irradiated, and fraction size.[149]

Surgical procedures such as amputation or limb disarticulation have obvious immediate and lasting cosmetic as well as physical and psychological consequences. Physical problems that may arise following these procedures include, but are not limited to, recurrent infections, the need for surgical revisions of an internal prosthesis, and poorly fitting external prosthetics.[150] The decision regarding amputation versus limb salvage has been controversial for years. Advocates of limb salvage focus on the survivor's desire to maintain his or her limb whereas advocates of amputation focus on the quality of life issues and high functioning of amputees. This issue is not likely to be resolved easily, because prognosis is not affected by the procedure used at time of diagnosis.[151,152]

Treatment-induced osteopenia and osteoporosis can be caused by many factors including treatment-specific effects like those produced by glucocorticoids, premature gonadal failure, growth hormone deficiency, and thyroid dysfunction resulting in hormone-related losses.[153] Chemotherapeutic agents linked to loss of bone mineral density through a variety of mechanisms include glucocorticoids, cyclophosphamide, ifosfamide, doxorubicin, methotrexate, and interferon-alfa.[154–158] At-risk individuals should be encouraged to utilize strategies that have proven useful in postmenopausal osteoporosis, such as smoking cessation, weight-bearing exercise, and calcium and vitamin D supplementation.[159] Bisphosphonates are being used to improve bone density in both men and women who have premature gonadal dysfunction accompanying with hormone-sensitive tumors such as breast and prostate cancer.[160,161]

Late radiation damage to muscle can occur, especially following treatment of soft tissue sarcomas of the extremities. Mechanisms of injury that have been identified (primarily from animal studies) include a direct effect on myocytes resulting in cell death; vascular damage with ischemia; atrophy and fibrosis; and inflammation with a preferential increase in type III collagen.[162] Muscle damage can progress over time; the risk of this complication increases with larger radiation doses and decreases with dose fractionation.

Skin, hair, and breast tissue may be affected by radiation as well. Permanent alopecia can occur following higher doses of radiation (more than 40 Gy), such as are used in treatment of brain tumors. Following breast-conserving surgery and radiation, women have achieved lactation in the treated breast although the milk production seems inadequate.[163,164] Other skin and related changes include contractures noted following infiltrations and edema secondary to disrupted lymphatic flow.[165] Lymphedema is a significant effect noted in 10% to 25% of women post-mastectomy.[166] Its incidence is greater with high-dose radiation therapy, a history of one or more infections, and radical lymph-node dissection.[167,168] Other factors that appear to play a role in the degree of lymphedema experienced include obesity and weight gain after treatment.[169] A variety of interventions for lymphedema, such as sequential pneumatic compression sleeve and manual massage, are available, but results with these treatments have been variable.[170] The role potential for alternative treatments is currently being examined, but to date nothing has proven more successful than conservative intervention.[171]

Fatigue

Fatigue continues to be the most prevalent and disruptive symptom identified by patients in active cancer treatment. This symptom may persist long after treatment has ended. Many causes of cancer-related fatigue exist, including physiological and psychological preexisting conditions as well as conditions caused by cancer and cancer treatments such as chemotherapy and radiation therapy.[172–174] Although fatigue is one of the most common complaints of patients with cancer, it remains poorly understood and interventions have not been adequately studied.[175] Anemia has been identified as a common cause of cancer-related fatigue, and pharmacologic and nonpharmacologic treatments for anemia and fatigue as well as valid tools for measuring fatigue continue to be explored.[176–178] Several studies have documented fatigue in survivors years following the completion of treatment. For example, Whedon et al documented fatigue in survivors of bone marrow transplantation 1 to 18 years after treatment.[179] Fatigue also plays a significant role in a survivor's perception of quality of life post-treatment.[179] Ferrell et al noted that among 687 survivors, fatigue was perceived as one of the most negative items affecting quality of life.[180]

Although the etiology of fatigue in the cancer survivor population is poorly understood, it is imperative that the prevalence of this problem be explored. Questions regarding this symptom should be incorporated into the annual follow-up evaluation. Physiological causes for fatigue should be ruled out when possible, and strategies for decreasing fatigue — such as adequate nutrition and hydration, modified activity and rest patterns, stress management, and cognitive therapies — should be used.[172]

Second Malignant Neoplasms

It has been clearly established that adults and children who have received chemotherapy or radiation for a primary malignancy are at increased risk for the development of a second malignant neoplasm.[181] Malignant transformation of normal cells results from nonlethal damage to the DNA that is not repaired.[182] Alkylating agents and ionizing radiation are the treatments most closely linked to a second malignant neoplasm. In addition to the type and dose of treatment received, the risk of the development of a second cancer depends on several predisposing factors. Environmental exposures such as tobacco and diet, as well as hormonal exposures and genetic predisposition, contribute to the risk profile of any patient.[181] For example, the *BRAC1* and *BRAC2* genes have been linked to breast and ovarian cancer. Women who carry these genes are also at risk for developing colon cancer.[183]

Following Chemotherapy

Acute nonlymphocytic leukemia (ANL) following treatment with alkylating agents in the most common chemotherapy-related second malignant neoplasm. However, acute lymphoblastic leukemia, chronic myelogenous leukemia, and myelodysplastic syndrome have also been reported.[184] Acute nonlymphocytic leukemia following Hodgkin's lymphoma has been studied intensively in large cohorts of patients. The overall cumulative risk has been reported to be 3.3% at 15 years post-diagnosis, but varies from 0.6% in patients who received only radiation therapy to 17% in those treated with combination chemotherapy.[185–189] The treatment regimen with the greatest leukemogenic potential is MOPP, presumably due to the mechlorethamine and procarbazine.[185,186,189]

Although the incidence is not as great as with Hodgkin's lymphoma or multiple myeloma, treatment-related acute leukemia has occurred in patients with non-Hodgkin's lymphoma,[190] breast cancer,[191] lung cancer,[192] and ovarian cancer.[193] There is also concern among some cancer researchers that etoposide may increase the risk for ANL.[192] Intercalating topoisomerase II inhibitors (doxorubicin, dactinomycin), when combined with alkylating agents and radiation, may cause secondary AML.[194,195]

Following Radiation

Sarcomas of the bone and soft tissue are the most common second malignant neoplasms after radiation therapy. Although the latency period can be as short as 5 months, it ranges from 10 to 20 years following radiation.[196] The incidence of these neoplasms has been found to peak at 15 to 20 years after the initial diagnosis.[196] Malignant transformation can occur in doses ranging from 10 to 80 Gy. The relative risk increases from 8% following doses of 10 to 20 Gy to 40% following doses of 60 Gy.[196] It has been postulated that the decreased risk following doses of 80 Gy is due to the phenomenon of cell killing rather than nonlethal cell damage.[189]

Acute nonlymphocytic leukemia following radiation therapy is uncommon. Nevertheless, women with breast cancer treated with postoperative radiation have a slightly increased risk of ANL.[191]

In addition to sarcomas and leukemia, a variety of other solid tumors have been linked to treatment with radiation. Slightly excessive numbers of tumors of the bladder, rectum, uterus, bone, and connective tissue have been reported in women who received radiation for gynecologic cancer, for example.[192] In a study of survivors of Hodgkin's lymphoma, a 17% cumulative risk of second cancers was noted 20 years post-treatment. The most common tumors were thyroid, lung, and breast cancer, with 77% occurring in or adjoining the field of radiation.[197] In a recent study of women younger than 30 years of age who had received chest irradiation, breast cancer was the most frequent solid tumor in this population.[198] In another study of childhood survivors of Hodgkin's lymphoma, breast cancer was the most common solid tumor. Individuals at highest risk were girls who received mantle radiation between the ages of 10 and 16 years and patients who received higher doses (more than 30 Gy).[199,200]

With the recently observed increased risk for breast cancer following radiation, routine evaluation has become controversial in young women (younger than 30 years of age). Currently, mammography is thought to be the best available technique for breast cancer screening. However, with younger women concern has arisen about the accuracy of mammography in dense breast tissue. Some clinicians now recommend baseline mammography 10 years after radiation or the age of 25. Others recommend chemoprevention with tamoxifen and retinoids for individuals in the highest risk categories.[199,200] In any event, there is consensus that women who receive radiation to the breast (especially those treated between the ages of 10 and 16 years and who receive higher radiation doses) need close monitoring. Aggressive evaluation of any breast mass and examination of the contralateral breast (due to the increased risk of synchronous bilateral disease) is imperative.[198–200]

Early Detection and Prevention, Health Maintenance, and Health Promotion

"Comprehensive care of cancer survivors demands maximum efforts to prevent, minimize, and effectively treat long-term medical sequelae through the survivorship trajectory."[201]

Early detection and prevention of late toxicities is a relatively new area of investigation. If early indicators of late tissue damage are identified, interventions designed to diminish the severity and overall impact of the toxicity can be developed and tested. Knowledge of the mechanisms responsible for delayed tissue damage following radiation and chemotherapy is increasing and provides the basis for interventions designed to inhibit specific pathways or scavenge toxic by-products. In addition, understanding the etiology of post-treatment effects will assist in the development of treatment modifications that will decrease late effects for future generations without compromising disease control and overall survival rates.

Researchers in pediatric oncology have led the way in developing comprehensive care clinics that meet the unique needs of childhood cancer survivors. Since the early 1980s, Meadows and Hobbie have focused on the role of the healthcare team in post-treatment management of survivors.[202] Since that time, numerous pediatric, young adult, and, more recently, adult survivorship programs have beem established across the United States.[203] These follow-up programs focus on health education, promotion, and maintenance, as well as modifiable risk factors among the population of cancer survivors.[204]

In an effort to provide organization for follow-up care and universal guidelines, cooperative organizations that initiate and coordinate multicenter clinical trials have formed specific subcommittees to develop standard criteria for monitoring the late effects of cancer treatment.[205] Survivors of cancer require lifelong follow-up care to maximize the opportunities to provide education about previous treatment, potential and actual late effects, and lifestyle choices that may modify the expression of late effects. In particular, the healthcare team should focus on modifiable risk factors such as smoking, drinking, dietary habits, and exercise.[204,206]

Follow-up programs for adult cancer survivors are rare. At completion of treatment, the individual with cancer returns to a primary care provider and makes episodic visits to the oncologist to rule out disease recurrence. Insurance issues, institutional resistance, and financial constraints are often cited as common causes for the lack of follow-up programs.

Conclusion

This chapter provides a comprehensive review of the biological late effects that can be caused by curative cancer therapy. Long-term surveillance for these toxic effects is a relatively new and challenging area for oncology nurses and physicians. A long-range perspective is essential because the latency period for some late effects can last many years after completion of treatment, and the consequences of permanent tissue damage across the lifespan remain largely unknown.

General recommendations for long-term follow-up include an annual physical examination with a complete blood cell count and urinalysis. Evaluation of specific toxicity to organ systems and second malignancies depends on the initial diagnosis, type and amount of treatment received, and a host of risk factors. Currently, specific surveillance guidelines for adult cancer survivors are just beginning to be explored. A careful balance between monitoring and the creation of needless anxiety that could hinder the patient's overall rehabilitation and emotional adjustment is essential. Tempering information regarding late effects with modifiable risk factors, wellness, and health promotion offers the best opportunity for early identification of late effects and maximizes survivor compliance and sense of well-being.

References

1. Schwartz CL, Constine LS, Hobbie WL: Overview, in Schwartz CL, Constine LS, Hobbie WL, Ruccione KS (eds): *Survivors of Childhood Cancer: Assessment and Management,* Philadelphia, W. B. Mosby, 1994, pp 5–6
2. Ries LAG, Eisner MP, Kosary CL, et al (eds): *SEER Cancer Statistics Review, 1975–2000,* Bethesda, MD, National Cancer Institute, *http://seer.cancer.gov/csr/,* 1975, 2000, 2003
3. Meadows AT, Varricchio C, Crossen K, et al: Meeting report-research issues in cancer survivorship: report of a workshop sponsored by the office of cancer survivorship, National Cancer Institute. *Cancer Epidemiol, Biomarkers Prevent,* 7:1145–1151, 1998
4. Van Eys J: Living beyond cure: transcending survival. *Am J Pediatr Hematol Oncol* 9:114–118, 1987
5. Schwartz CL: Late effects of treatment in long-term survivors of cancer. *Cancer Treat Rev* 21:355–366, 1995
6. Anderson V, Smibert E, Ekert H, et al: Intellectual, educational, and behavioural sequelae after cranial irradiation and chemotherapy. *Arch Dis Child* 70:476–485, 1994
7. Kupst MJ, Penati B, Debban B, et al: Cognitive and psychosocial functioning of pediatric hematopoietic stem cell transplant patients: a prospective longitudinal study. *Bone Marrow Transplant* 30:609–617, 2002
8. Hill DE, Ciesielski KT, Sethre-Hofstad L, et al: Visual and verbal short-term memory deficits in childhood leukemia survivors after intrathecal chemotherapy. *J Pediatr Psychol* 22:861–870, 1997
9. Langer T, Martus P, Ottensmeier H, et al: CNS late-effects after ALL therapy in childhood. Part III: Neuropsychological performance in long-term survivors of childhood ALL: impairments of concentration, attention, and memory. *Med Pediat Oncol* 38:320–328, 2002
10. Rodgers J, Marckus R, Kearns P, et al: Attentional ability among survivors of leukaemia treated without cranial radiation. *Arch Dis Child* 88:147–150, 2003
11. Von der Weid N, Mosimann I, Hirt A, et al: Intellectual outcome in children and adolescents with acute lymphoblastic leukemia treated with chemotherapy alone: age- and sex-related differences. *Eur J Cancer* 39:359–365, 2003
12. MacLean WE, Noll RB, Stehbens JA, et al: Neuropsychological effects of cranial irradiation in young children with acute lymphoblastic leukemia 9 months after diagnosis. *Arch Neurol* 52:156–160, 1995
13. Smibert E, Anderson V, Godber T, et al: Risk factors for intellectual and educational sequelae of cranial irradiation in childhood acute lymphoblastic leukemia. *Br J Cancer* 73:825–830, 1996
14. Brown RR, Sawyer MB, Antoniou G, et al: A 3 year follow-up of the intellectual and academic functioning of children receiving central nervous system prophylactic chemotherapy for leukemia. *J Dev Behav Pediatr* 17:392–398, 1996
15. Copeland DR, Moore BD, Francis DJ, et al: Neuropsychologic effects of chemotherapy on children with cancer — a longitudinal study. *J Clin Oncol* 14:2826–2835, 1996
16. Christie D, Leiper AD, Chessells JM, et al: Intellectual performance after presymptomatic cranial radiotherapy for leukaemia: Effects of age and sex. *Arch Dis Child* 73:136–140, 1995
17. Kramer JH, Crowe AB, Larson DA, et al: Neuropsychological sequelae of medulloblastoma in adults. *Int J Radiat Oncol Biol Phys* 38:21–26, 1997
18. Reddick WE, White HA, Glass JO, et al: Developmental models relating white matter volume to neurocognitive deficits in pediatric brain tumor survivors. *Cancer* 97:2512–2519, 2003

19. Cool VA: Long-term neuropsychological risks in pediatric bone marrow transplant: what do we know? *Bone Marrow Transplant* 18:S45–49, 1996
20. Andrews-Espy K, Moore IM, Kaufmann PM, et al: Neuropsychological declines in survivors of childhood ALL. *J Pediatr Psychol* 26:1–9, 2001
21. Hertzberg H, Huk WJ, Ueberall MA, et al: CNS late effects after ALL therapy in childhood. Part I: neuroradiological findings in long-term survivors of childhood ALL: an evaluation of the interferences between morphology and neuropsychological performance. *Med Pediatr Oncol* 28:387–400, 1997
22. Prassopoulos P, Cavouras D, Golfinopoulos S, et al: Quantitative assessment of cerebral atrophy during and after treatment in children with acute lymphoblastic leukemia. *Invest Radiol* 31:749–754, 1996
23. Harila-Saari AH, Ahonen KA, Vainionpää LK, et al: Brain perfusion after treatment of childhood acute lymphoblastic leukemia. *J Nucl Med* 38:82–88, 1997
24. Chen CY, Zimmerman RA, Faro S, et al: Childhood leukemia: Central nervous abnormalities during and after treatment. *Am J Neuroradiol* 17:295–310, 1996
25. Davidson A, Payne G, Leach MO, et al: Proton magnetic resonance spectroscopy (^{1}H-MRS) of the brain following high-dose methotrexate treatment for childhood cancer. *Med and Pediatr Oncol* 35:28–34, 2000
26. Ueberall MA, Wenzel D, Hertzberg H, et al: CNS late effects after ALL therapy in childhood. Part II: conventional EEG recordings in asymptomatic long-term survivors of childhood ALL — an evaluation of the interferences between neurophysiology, neurology, psychology, and CNS morphology. *Med Pediatr Oncol* 29:121–131, 1997
27. Lesnik PG, Ciesielski KT, Hart BL, et al: Evidence of cerebellar-frontal system changes in children treated with intrathecal chemotherapy for leukemia. *Arch Neurol* 55:1561–1568, 1998
28. Surtees R, Clelland J, Hann I, et al: Demyelination and single-carbon transfer pathway metabolites during the treatment of acute lymphoblastic leukemia: CSF studies. *J Clin Oncol* 16:1505–1511, 1998
29. Quinn CT, Griener JC, Bottiglieri T, et al: Elevation of homocysteine and excitatory amino acid neurotransmitters in the CSF of children who receive methotrexate for the treatment of cancer. *J Clin Oncol* 15:2800–2806, 1997
30. Gordon KB, Char DH, Sagerman RH, et al: Late effects of radiation on the eye and ocular adnexa. *Int J Radiat Oncol Biol Phys* 31:1123–1139, 1995
31. Parsons JT, Bova FJ, Fitzgerald CR, et al: Radiation retinopathy after external-beam irradiation: analysis of time-dose factors. *Int J Radiat Oncol Biol Phys* 30:765–773, 1994
32. Coucke PA, Schmid C, Balmer A, et al: Hypofractionation in retinoblastoma: an increased risk of retinopathy. *Radiother Oncol* 28:157–161, 1993
33. Al-Tweigeri T, Nabholtz JM, Mackey JR, et al: Ocular toxicity and cancer chemotherapy. *Cancer* 78:1359–1373, 1996
34. Defer G, Fauchon F, Schaison M, et al: Visual toxicity following intra-arterial chemotherapy with hydroxyethyl-CNU in patients with malignant gliomas. *Neuroradiology* 33:432–437, 1991
35. Taylor MJ, McCulloch DL: Visual evoked potentials in infants and children. *J Clin Neurophysiol* 3:357–372, 1992
36. Bokemeyer C, Berger CC, Kuczyk MA, et al: Evaluation of long-term toxicity after chemotherapy for testicular cancer. *J Clin Oncol* 14:2923–2932, 1996
37. Bokemeyer C, Berger CC, Hartmann JT, et al: Analysis of risk factors for cisplatin-induced ototoxicity in patients with testicular cancer. *Br J Cancer* 77:1355–1362, 1998
38. Skinner R, Pearson ADJ, Amineddine HA, et al: Ototoxicity of cisplatinum in children and adolescents. *Br J Cancer* 61:927–931, 1990
39. Freilich RJ, Kraus DH, Budnick AS, et al: Hearing loss in children with brain tumors treated with cisplatin and carboplatin-based high-dose chemotherapy with autologous bone marrow rescue. *Med Pediatr Oncol* 26:95–100, 1996
40. Walkwe DA, Pillov J, Waters KD, et al: Enhanced cisplatin ototoxicity in children with brain tumors who have received simultaneous or prior cranial irradiation. *Med Pediatr Oncol* 17:48–52, 1989
41. Miettinen S, Laurikainen E, Johansson R, et al: Radiotherapy enhanced ototoxicity of cisplatin in children. *Acta Otolaryngol (Stockh)* 529:90–94, 1997
42. Meyer WH, Ayers D, McHaney VA, et al: Ifosfamide and exacerbation of cisplatin-induced hearing loss. *Lancet* 341:754–755, 1993
43. Ilveskoski I, Saarinen UM, Wiklund T, et al: Ototoxicity in children with malignant brain tumors treated with the "8 in 1" chemotherapy protocol. *Med Pediatr Oncol* 27:26–31, 1996
44. Todd NW, Alvarado CS, Brewer DB, et al: Cisplatin in children: Hearing loss correlates with iris and skin pigmentation. *J Laryngol Otol* 109:926–929, 1995
45. Park KR: The utility of acoustic reflex thresholds and other conventional audiologic tests for monitoring cisplatin ototoxicity in the pediatric population. *Ear Hear* 17:107–115, 1996
46. Neuwelt EA, Brummett RE, Doolittle ND, et al: First evidence of otoprotection against carboplatin-induced hearing loss with a two-compartment system in patients with central nervous system malignancy using sodium thiosulfate. *J Pharmacol Exp Ther* 286:77–84, 1998
47. Madasu R, Ruckenstein MJ, Leake F, et al: Ototoxic effects of supradose cisplatin with sodium thiosulfate neutralization in patients with head and neck cancer. *Arch Otolaryngol Head Neck Surg* 123:978–981, 1997
48. Domenech J, Linassier C, Gihana E, et al: Prolonged impairment of hematopoiesis after high-dose therapy followed by autologous bone marrow transplantation. *Blood* 85:3320–3327, 1995
49. Van Rijswijk RF, Sybesma JPH, Kater L: A prospective study of the changes in the immune status before, during and after multiple agent chemotherapy for Hodgkin's disease. *Cancer* 51:637–644, 1983
50. Brusamolino E, Lunghi F, Orlandi E, et al: Treatment of early-stage Hodgkin's disease with four cycles of ABVD followed by adjuvant radiotherapy: analysis of efficacy and long-term toxicity. *Haematologica* 85:1032–1039, 2000
51. Heidenreich PA, Hancock SL, Lee BK, et al: Asymptomatic cardiac disease following mediastinal irradiation. *J Am Coll Cardiol* 42:743–749, 2003
52. Clements IP, Davis BJ, Wiseman GA: Systolic and diastolic cardiac dysfunction early after the initiation of doxorubicin therapy: significance of gender and concurrent mediastinal radiation. *Nucl Med Commun* 23:521–527, 2002
53. Meinardi JA, Gietema WTA, van der Graaf DJ, et al: Cardiovascular morbidity in long-term survivors of metastatic testicular cancer. *J Clin Oncol* 18:1725–1732, 2000
54. Strumberg D, Brugge S, Korn MW, et al: Evaluation of long-term toxicity in patients after cisplatin-based chemotherapy for non-seminomatous testicular cancer. *Ann Oncol* 13:229–236, 2002
55. Noori A, Lindenfeld J, Wolfel E, et al: Beta-blockade in adriamycin-induced cardiomyopathy. *J Card Fail* 6:115–119, 2000
56. Steinherz LJ, Steinherz P, Tan G, et al: Cardiac toxicity 4–20 years after completing anthracycline therapy. *Proc Am Soc Clin Oncol* 8:296, 1989 (abstr)

57. Miltenyi Z, Gergely L, Illes A: Chronic pericarditis in Hodgkin disease. *Orv Hetil* 143:2687–2689, 2002
58. Deist TJ, Freytag A: Therapy of abdominal and thoracic chylous effusions 18 years after radiation therapy. *Z Gastroenterol* 39:523–527, 2001
59. Constine LS, Schwartz RG, Savage DE, et al: Cardiac function, perfusion, and morbidity in irradiated long-term survivors of Hodgkin's disease. *Int J Radiat Oncol Biol Phys* 39:897–906, 1997
60. Abou-El-Hassan AM, Rabelink, MJ, van der Vijgh WJ, et al: A comparative study between catalase gene therapy and the cardioprotector monohydroxyethylrutoside (MonoHER) in protecting against doxorubicin-induced cardiotoxicity in vitro. *Br J Cancer* 89:2140–2146, 2003
61. Laws PE, Spark JI, Cowled PA, et al: The role of statins in vascular disease. *Eur J Vasc Endovasc Surg* 27:6–16, 2004
62. McDonald S, Rubin P, Phillips TL, et al: Injury to the lung from cancer therapy: Clinical syndromes, measurable endpoints, and potential scoring systems. *Int J Radiat Oncol Biol Phys* 31:1187–1203, 1995
63. Morgan GW, Breit SN: Radiation and the lung: A reevaluation of the mechanisms mediating pulmonary injury. *Int J Radiat Oncol Biol Phys* 31:361–369, 1995
64. Morrone N, Gama e Silva Volpe VL, Dourado AM, et al: Bilateral pleural effusion due to mediastinal fibrosis induced by radiotherapy. *Chest* 104:1276–1278, 1993
65. Cwikiel M, Albertsson M, Hambraeus G: Acute and delayed effects of radiotherapy in patients with oesophageal squamous cell carcinoma treated with chemotherapy, surgery and pre- and postoperative chemotherapy. *Acta Oncol* 33:49–53, 1994
66. Marks LB, Yu X, Vujaskovic Z, et al: Radiation-induced lung injury. *Semin Radiat Oncol* 13:333–345, 2003
67. Dik WA, McAnulty RJ, Versnel MA, et al: Short course dexamethasone treatment following injury inhibits bleomycin induced fibrosis in rats. *Thorax* 58:765–771, 2003
68. Gunther A, Lubke N, Ermert M, et al: Prevention of bleomycin-induced lung fibrosis by aerosolization of heparin or urokinase in rabbits. *Am J Respir Crit Care Med* 168:1268–1269, 2003
69. Coia LR, Myerson RJ, Tepper JE: Late effects of radiation therapy on the gastrointestinal tract. *Int J Radiat Oncol Biol Phys* 31:1213–1236, 1995
70. Steer CB, Harper PG: Gastro-oesophageal complications in patients receiving cancer therapy: the role of proton pump inhibitors. *Eur J Gastroenterol Hepatol* 14 S:S17-S21, 2002 (suppl)
71. Saclarides TJ: Radiation injuries of the gastrointestinal tract. *Surg Clin North Am* 77:261–267, 1997
72. Song DY, Lawrie WT, Abrams RA, et al: Acute and late radiotherapy toxicity in patients with inflammatory bowel disease. *Int J Radiat Oncol Biol Phys* 51:455–459, 2001
73. Czauderna P, Katski K, Kowalczyk J, et al: Venoocclusive liver disease (VOD) as a complication of Wilms' tumour management in the series of consecutive 206 patients. *Eur J Pediatr Surg* 10:300–303, 2000
74. Kristal O, Rassnick KM, Gliatto JM, et al: Hepatotoxicity associated with CCNU (lomustine) chemotherapy in dogs. *J Vet Intern Med* 18:75–80, 2004
75. Alter MJ, Mast EE, Moyer LA, et al: Hepatitis C. *Infect Dis Clin North Am* 12:13–25, 1998
76. Hubbard P: Hepatitis C. *Hepatology* 2:17–18, 23–26, 29–31, 1998
77. Sheikh-Hamad D, Timmins K, Jalali Z: Cisplatin-induced renal toxicity: possible reversal by N-acetylcysteine treatment. *J Am Soc Nephrol* 8:1640–1645, 1997
78. Foster-Nora JA, Siden R: Amifostine for protection from antineoplastic drug toxicity. *Am J Health Syst Pharm* 54:787–800, 1997
79. Capizzi RL, Oster W: Protection of normal tissue from the cytotoxic effects of chemotherapy and radiation by amifostine: Clinical experiences. *Eur J Cancer* 31A:S8-S13, 1995
80. Tefft M, Laffin PB, Jereb B, et al: Acute and later effects on normal tissues following combined chemo- and radiotherapy for childhood rhabdomyosarcoma and Ewing's sarcoma. *Cancer* 37(2 Suppl):1201–1217, 1976
81. Cassady JR: Clinical radiation nephropathy. *Int J Radiat Oncol Biol Phys* 31:1249–1256, 1995
82. Marks LB, Carroll PR, Dugan TC, et al: The response of the urinary bladder, urethra, and ureter to radiation and chemotherapy. *Int J Radiat Oncol Biol Phys* 30:1257–1280, 1995
83. Stewart DJ, Mikhael NZ, Nanji AA, et al: Renal and hepatic concentrations of platinum: Relationship to cisplatin time, dose and nephrotoxicity. *J Clin Oncol* 3:1251–1256, 1985
84. Suresh UR, Smith VJ, Lupton EW, et al: Radiation disease of the urinary tract: histological features of 18 cases. *J Clin Pathol* 43:228–231, 1993
85. Buglione M, Toninelli M, Pietta N, et al: Post-radiation pelvic disease and ureteral stenosi: pathophysiology and evolution in the patient treated for cervical carcinoma. Review of the literature and experience of the Radium Institute. *Arch Ital Urol Androl* 74:6–11, 2002
86. Stewart FA: Mechanism of bladder damage and repair after treatment with radiation and cytostatic drugs. *Br J Cancer* 53: 280–291, 1986
87. Ganong WF: The thyroid gland, in Ganong WF (ed): *Review of Medical Physiology*. Palo Alto, CA, Appleton & Lange, 1987, pp 262–275
88. Morgan GW, Freeman AP, McLean RG, et al: Late cardiac, thyroid and pulmonary sequelae of mantle radiotherapy for Hodgkin's disease. *Radiat Oncol Biol Phys* 11:1925–1931, 1985
89. Moroff SV, Fluks JZ: Thyroid cancer following radiotherapy for Hodgkin's disease: a case report and review of the literature. *Med Pediatr Oncol* 14:216–220, 1986
90. Joensuu H, Viikari J: Thyroid function after postoperative radiation therapy in patients with breast cancer. *Acta Radiol Oncol* 25:167–170, 1986
91. Knobel H, Loge JH, Lund MB, et al: Late medical complication and fatigue in Hodgkin's disease survivors. *J Clin Oncol* 19:3226–3233, 2001
92. Daniell HW: Hypothyroidism: a frequent event after radiotherapy for patients with head and neck carcinoma. *Cancer* 95:673–674, 2002
93. Illes A, Keresztes K, Varoczy L, et al: Hypothyroidism and thyroiditis after therapy for Hodgkin's disease. *Acta Haematol* 109: 11–17, 2003
94. Kantsanis E, Shapiro RS, Robison LL, et al. Thyroid dysfunction following bone marrow transplantation: long-term follow-up of 80 pediatric patients. *Bone Marrow Transplant* 5:335–340, 1990
95. Sklar CA, Constine LS: Chronic neuroendocrinological sequelae of radiation therapy. *Int J Rad Oncol Biol Phys* 31:1113–1121, 1995
96. Sklar CA, Whitton J, Mertens A, et al: Abnormalities of the thyroid in survivors of Hodgkin's disease: data from the Childhood Cancer Survivor Study. *J Clin Endocrinol Metab* 85:3227–3232, 2000
97. Constine LS, Rubin P, Woolf PD: Hyperprolactinemia and hypothyroidism following cytotoxic therapy for central nervous system malignancies. *J Clin Oncol* 5:1841–1851, 1987
98. Robison LL, Nesbit ME, Sather HN, et al: Height of children successfully treated for acute lymphoblastic leukemia: a report from the Late Effects Study Committee of Children's Cancer Study Group. *Med Pediatr Oncol* 13:13–21, 1985

99. Cicognani A, Cacciari E, Veechi V, et al: Differential effects of 18- and 24-Gy cranial irradiation on growth rate and growth hormone release in children with prolonged survival after acute lymphoblastic leukemia. *Am J Dis Child* 141:550–552, 1986
100. Carroll PV, Emanuel CR, Thorner M, et al: Growth hormone deficiency in adulthood and the effects of growth hormone replacement: a review. *J Clin Endocrinol Metab* 83:382–395, 1998
101. Chipman JJ, Attanasio AF, Birkett MA, et al: The safety profile of growth hormone replacement therapy in adults. *Clin Endocrinol (Oxf)* 46:473–481, 1997
102. Salomon R, Cuneo RC, Hesp R, et al: The effects of treatment with recombinent human growth hormone on body composition and metabolism in adults with growth hormone deficiency. *N Engl J Med* 321:1797–1803,1989
103. Stouthart PJ, Deijen JB, Roffel M, Delemarre-van de Waal HA: Quality of life in growth hormone deficient young adults during discontinuation and restart of GH therapy. *Psychoneuroendocrinology* 28:612–626, 2003
104. Shimon I: Growth hormone replacement for adult growth hormone deficiency. *Exp Opin Pharmacother* 4:1977–1983, 2003
105. Moshang T, Rundle AM, Graves DA, et al: Brain tumor recurrence in children treated with growth hormone: The National Cooperative Growth Study experience. *J Pediatr* 128:S4–7, 1996 (suppl)
106. Shalet SM, Brennan BD: Growth and growth hormone treatment for childhood leukemia. *Hormone Res* 50:1–10, 1998
107. Rivkees SA, Crawford JD: The relationship of gonadal activity and chemotherapy-induced gonadal damage. *JAMA* 259:2123–2125, 1988
108. Morgenfeld MC, Pavlovsky A, Suarez A, et al: Combined cyclophosphamide vincristine, procarbazine, and prednisone (COPP) therapy of malignant lymphoma. Evaluation of 190 patients. *Cancer* 36:1241–1249, 1975
109. Goodwin PJ, Ennis M, Pritchard KI, et al: Risk of menopause during the first year after breast cancer diagnosis. *J Clin Oncol* 17:2365–2370, 1999
110. Weber B, Luporsi E: Ovarian toxicity of breast cancer chemotherapy. *Eur J Cancer* 34: S42, 1998 (abstr) (suppl)
111. Byrne J, Fears FR, Gail MH, et al: Early menopause in long term survivors of cancer during adolescence. *Am J Obstet Gynecol* 166:788–793, 1992
112. Day R, Ganz PA, Constantino JP, et al: Health related quality of life and tamoxifen in breast cancer prevention: a report from the National Surgical Adjuvant & Bowel Project P-1 Study. *J Clin Oncol* 17:2659–2669, 1999
113. Nicosia S, Matus-Ridley M, Meadows AT: Gonadal effects of cancer therapy in girls. *Cancer* 55:2364–2372, 1985
114. Fischer B, Bheung A: Delayed effect of radiation therapy with or without chemotherapy on ovarian function in women with Hodgkin's disease. *Acta Radiol Oncol* 23:43–48, 1984
115. Kreuser E, Hetzel W, Heit W, et al: Reproductive and endocrine gonadal functions in adults following multidrug chemotherapy for acute lymphoblastic or undifferentiated leukemia. *J Clin Onco* 6:588–595, 1988
116. Hamre MR, Robison LL, Nesbit ME, et al: Effects of radiation on ovarian function in long term survivors of childhood acute lymphoblastic leukemia: a report from the Children's Cancer Study Group. *J Clin Oncol* 5:1759–1765, 1987
117. Sklar C: Reproductive physiology and treatment-related loss of sex hormone production. *Med Pediatr Oncol* 1:2–8, 1999
118. Shalet SM, Tsatsoulis A, Whitehead E, et al: Vulnerability of the human Leydig cell to radiation damage is dependent upon age. *J Endocrinol* 1:161–165, 1989
119. Heyn R, Raney RB, Hays DM, et al: Late effects of therapy in patients with paratesticular rhabdomyosarcoma. *J Clin Oncol* 10:614–623, 1992
120. Petersen PM, Hansen SW, Giwercman A, et al: Dose-dependent impairment of testicular function in patients treated with cisplatin-based chemotherapy for germ cell cancer. *Ann Oncol* 5:355–358, 1994
121. Byrne J, Mulvihill JJ, Myers MH, et al: Effects of treatment on fertility in long-term survivors of childhood or adolescent cancer. *N Engl J Med* 317:1315–1321, 1987
122. Charak BS, Gupta R, Mandrekar P, et al: Testicular dysfunction after cyclophosphamide-vincristine-procarbazine-prednisolone chemotherapy for advanced Hodgkin's disease. A long-term follow-up study. *Cancer* 65:1903–1906, 1990
123. Aubier F, Flamamant F, Brauner R, et al: Male gonadal function after chemotherapy for solid tumors in childhood. *J Clin Oncol* 7:304–309, 1989
124. Kenney LB, Laufer MR, Grant FD, et al: High risk of infertility and long term gonadal damage in males treated with high dose cyclophosphamide for sarcoma during childhood. *Cancer* 91:613–621, 2001
125. Ash P: The influence of radiation on fertility in man. *Br J Radiol* 53:271–278, 1980
126. Rowley MM, Leach DR, Warner GA, et al: Effects of graded doses of ionizing radiation on the human testes. *Radiat Res* 59:665–678, 1974
127. Green DM, Hall B, Zevon M: Pregnancy outcome after treatment for acute lymphoblastic leukemia during childhood or adolescence. *Cancer* 64:2335–2339, 1989
128. Samaan N, Vieto R, Schultz B, et al: Hypothalamic, pituitary and thyroid dysfunction after radiotherapy to the head and neck. *Int J Radiat Oncol Biol Phys* 11:1857–1867, 1982
129. Buvat J, LeMarie A, Burat-Herbaut M, et al: Hyperprolactinemia and sexual function in men. *Hormone Res* 22:196–203, 1984
130. Davis JW, Kuban DA, Lynch DF, et al: Quality of life after treatment for localized prostate cancer: differences based on treatment modality. *J Urol* 166:947–952, 2001
131. Bastasch MD, Teh BS, Mai WY, et al: Post-nerve sparing prostatectomy, dose-escalated intensity-modulated radiotherapy: effect on erectile function. *Int J Radiat Biol Phys* 54:101–106, 2002
132. Schover LR, Fouladi RT, Warneke CL, et al: Defining sexual outcomes after treatment for localized prostate carcinoma. *Cancer* 95:1773–1785, 2002
133. Schover LR, Montague DK, Lakin MM: Sexual problems, in DeVita VT, Hellman S, Rosenberg SA (eds): *Cancer: Principles and Practice of Oncology* (ed 5). Philadephia, Lippincott-Raven, 1997, pp 2857–2872
134. Ganz PA, Rowland JH, Desmond K, et al: Life after breast cancer: understanding women's health related quality of life and sexual functioning. *J Clin Oncol* 16:501–514, 1998
135. Andersen BL: Quality of life for women with gynecologic cancer. *Curr Opin Obstet Gynecol* 7:69–76, 1995
136. Fossa SD, Woehre H, Kurth KH, et al: Influence of urologic morbidity on quality of life in patients with prostate cancer. *Eur Urol* 31:3–8, 1997
137. Robinson JW, Dufour MS, Fung TS: Erectile functioning of men treated for prostate carcinoma. *Cancer* 79:538–544, 1997
138. Rogers M, Kristjanson L: The impact on sexual functioning of chemotherapy-induced menopause in women with breast cancer. *Cancer Nurs* 25:57–65, 2001
139. Hanash KA: Comparative results of goal oriented therapy for erectile dysfunction. *Br J Urol* 157:2135–2138, 1997
140. Dewire DM, Todd E, Meyers P: Patient satisfaction with current impotence therapy. *Wis Med J* 94:542–544, 1995

141. Jarow JP, Nana-Sinkam P, Sabbagh M, et al: Outcome analysis of goal directed therapy for impotence. *J Urol* 155:1609–1612, 1996
142. Nicholson HO: Cytotoxic drugs in pregnancy. *J Obstet Gynaecol Brief Comm* 75:307–312, 1968
143. Sokal JE, Lessmann EM: Effects of cancer chemotherapeutic agents on the human fetus. *JAMA* 172:1765–1771, 1960
144. Sankila R, Olsen J, Anderson H, et al: Risk of cancer among offspring of childhood cancer surivivors. *N Engl J Med* 338:1339–1344, 1998
145. Green DM, Whitton JA, Stovall M, et al: Pregnancy outcome of female survivors of childhood cancer. A report from the Childhood Cancer Survivors Study. *Am J Obstet Gynecol* 187:1070–1080, 2002
146. Green DM, Whitton JA, Stovall M, et al: Pregnancy outcome of partners of male survivors of childhood cancer. A report from the Childhood Cancer Survivor Study. *J Clin Oncol* 21:716–721, 2003
147. Holmes GE, Holmes FF: Pregnancy outcome of patients treated for Hodgkin's disease. *Cancer* 41:1317–1322, 1978
148. Blakely LJ, Buzdar AU, Lozasa JA, et al: Effects of pregnancy after treatment for breast carcinoma on survival and risk of recurrence. *Cancer* 100:465–469, 2004
149. Silber JH, Littman PS, Meadows AT: Stature loss following skeletal irradiation for childhood cancer. *J Clin Oncol* 8:304–312, 1990
150. Mosher RB, McCarthy BJ: Late effects in survivors of bone tumors. *J Pediatr Oncol Nurs* 15:72–84, 1998
151. Marcove RC, Sheth DS, Healey J, et al: Limb sparing surgery for extremity sarcoma. *Cancer Invest* 12:497–504, 1994
152. Greenberg DB, Goorin A, Gebhardt MC, et al: Quality of life in osteogenic survivors. *Oncology* 8:19–25, 1994
153. Pfeilschifter J, Diel IJ: Osteroporosis due to cancer treatment: pathogenesis and management. *J Clin Oncol* 18:1570–1593, 2000
154. Burk CD, Restaino I, Kaplan BS, et al: Ifosfamide-induced renal tubular dysfunction and rickets in children with Wilms' tumor. *J Pediatr* 117:331–335, 1990
155. Wang TM, Shih C: Study of histomorphometric changes of the mandibulare condyles in neonatal and juvenile rates after administration of cyclophosphamide. *Acta Anat* 127:93–99, 1986
156. Friedlander GE, Tross RB, Doganis AC, et al: Effects of chemotherapeutic agents on bone: short-term methotrexate and doxorubicin treatment in the rat model. *J Bone Joint Surg* 66:602–607, 1984
157. Tsuda-Futami E, Shioi A, Jono S, et al: Lymphoblastoid interferon-alpha downregulates parathyroid hormone (PTH)/PTH-related peptide (PTHrP) receptor expression in human osteoblastic cells. *Bone* 23A:205–211, 1998
158. Canalis E: Mechanisms of glucocorticoid action in bone: implications to glucocorticoid-induced osteoporosis. *J Clin Endocrinol Metab* 81:3441–3447, 1996
159. Eastell R: Treatment of postmenopausal osteoporosis. *N Engl J Med* 338:736–746, 1998
160. Powles TJ, McCloskey E, Paterson AHG, et al: Oral clodronate and reduction in loss of bone mineral density in women with operable primary breast cancer. *J Natl Cancer Inst* 90:704–708, 1998
161. Holmes SJ, Whitehouse RW, Clark ST, et al: Reduced bone mineral density in men following chemotherapy for Hodgkin's disease. *Br J Cancer* 70:371–375, 1994
162. Gillette EL, Mahler PA, Powers BE, et al: Late radiation injury to muscle and peripheral nerves. *Int J Radiat Oncol Biol Phys* 31:1309–1318, 1995
163. Higgins S, Haffly BG: Pregnancy and lactation after breast conserving therapy for early stage breast cancer. *Cancer* 73:2175–2180, 1994
164. Tralins AH: Lactation after conservative breast surgery combined with radiation. *Am J Clin Oncol* 18:40–43, 1995
165. Marcus RB, McGrath B, O'Conner K, et al: Long term effects on the musculoskeletal and integumentary systems and the breast, in Schwartz CL, Hobbie WL, Constine LS, Ruccione KS (eds): *Survivors of Childhood Cancer: Assessment and Management.* Philadelphia, Mosby-Yearbook, 1994, pp 263–292
166. Petrick JA, Lerner R: Lymphedema, in Harris JR, Lippman ME, Morrow M, Osborne K (eds): *Disease of the Breast.* (ed 2). Philadelphia, Lippincott Williams & Wilkins. 2000, pp 1033–1040
167. Schuster RH, Kuske RR, Young VL, et al: Breast reconstruction in women treated with radiation for breast cancer: cosmesis, complications and tumor control. *Plast Reconstr Surg* 90:445–452, 1992
168. Evans GRK, Schusterman MA, Kroll SS, et al: Reconstruction and the irradiated breast: is there a role for implants? *Plast Reconstr Surg* 96:1111–1115, 1995
169. Burnstein H, Winer E: Primary care for survivors of breast cancer. *N Engl J Med* 343:1086–1093, 2004
170. Bertelli G, Venturini M, Forno G, et al: Conservative treatment of post mastectomy lymphedema: A controlled randomized trial. *Ann Oncol* 2:575–578, 1991
171. Rockson SG: Precipitating factors in lymphedema: myths and realities. *Cancer* 83:2814–2816, 1998
172. Miakowski C, Portenoy RK: Update on the assessment and management of cancer-related fatigue. *Prin Pract Supp Oncol Updates* 1:1–10, 1998
173. Visovsky C, Schneider SM: Cancer-related fatigue. *Online J Issues Nurs* September 23, 2003
174. Jereczek-Fossa BA, Marsiglia HR, Orecchia R: Radiotherapy-related fatigue. *Crit Rev Oncol Hematol* 41:317–325, 2002
175. Stasi R, Abriani L, Beccaglia P, et al: Cancer-related fatigue: evolving concepts in evaluation and treatment. *Cancer* 98:1786–1801, 2003
176. Stein KD, Jacobsen PB, Blanchard CM, et al: Further validation of the multidimensional fatigue symptom inventory–short form. *J Pain Symptom Manage* 27:14–23, 2004
177. Abdel-Razeq HN: Cancer-related anemia. *Saudi Med* 25:15–20, 2004
178. Mock V, Olsen M: Current management of fatigue and anemia in patients with cancer. *Semin Oncol Nurs* 19:36S-41S, 2003 (suppl)
179. Whedon M, Stearns D, Mills LE: Quality of life of long-term adult survivors of autologous bone marrow transplantation. *Oncol Nurs Forum* 22:1527–1535, 1995
180. Ferrell BR, Grant M, Dean GE, et al: Bone tired: the experience of fatigue and its impact on quality of life. *Oncol Nurs Forum* 23:1539–1547, 1996
181. Rheingold S, Neugut A, Meadows AT: Second cancers: incidence, risk factors and management, in Kufe D, Pollack R, et al (eds): *Cancer Medicine,* vol 2. Hamilton, Ontario, BC Decker, 2003, pp 2623–2631
182. Moolgavkar SH , Knudson AG Jr: Mutation and cancer: a model for human carcinogenesis. *J Natl Cancer Inst* 66:1037–1052, 1981
183. Shih HA, Couch FJ, Nathanson KL, et al: BRCA1 and BRCA2 mutations' frequency in women evaluated in breast cancer risk evalutation clinic. *J Clin Oncol* 20:994–999, 2002
184. Bhatia S, Davies SM, Robison LL: Leukemia, in Neugut AI, Meadows AT, Robinson E (eds): *Multiple Primary Cancers.* Philadelphia, Lippincott Williams & Wilkins, 1999 pp 257–276
185. Kaldor JM, Day NE, Clarke EA, et al: Leukemia following Hodgkin's disease. *N Engl J Med* 322:7–13, 1990

186. Tucker MH, Coleman CN, Cox RS, et al: Risk of second cancers after treatment for Hodgkin's disease. *N Engl J Med* 318:76–81, 1988
187. Valagussa P, Santoro A, Fossati-Bellani F, et al: Second acute leukemia and other malignancies following treatment for Hodgkin's disease. *J Clin Oncol* 4:830–837, 1986
188. Coleman M, Easton DF, Horwich A, et al: Second malignancies and Hodgkin's disease: The Royal Marsden Hospital experience. *Radiother Oncol* 11:229–238, 1988
189. Meadows AT: Second malignant neoplasms. *Clin Oncol* 4:217–261, 1985
190. Pedersen-Bjergaard J, Ersboll J, Sorensen HM, et al: Risk of acute nonlymphocytic leukemia and preleukemia in patients treated with cyclophosphamide for non-Hodgkin's lymphomas. *Ann Intern Med* 103:195–200, 1985
191. Curtis RE, Boice JE Jr, Stovall M, et al: Risk of leukemia after chemotherapy and radiation treatment for breast cancer. *N Engl J Med* 326:1745–1751, 1992
192. Ratain MJ, Kaminer LS, Bitran JD, et al: Acute nonlymphocytic leukemia following etoposide and cisplatin combination chemotherapy for advanced non-small cell carcinoma of the lung. *Blood* 70:1412–1417, 1987
193. Kaldor JM, Day NE, Pettersson F, et al: Leukemia following chemotherapy for ovarian cancer. *N Engl J Med* 322:1–6, 1990
194. Felix CA: Chemotherapy related second cancers, in Neugut AI, Meadows AT, Robinson E, (eds): *Multiple Primary Cancers.* Philadelphia. Lippincott Williams & Wilkins, 1999, pp 137–164
195. Smith MA, Rubinstein L, Anderson JR, et al: Secondary leukemia or myelodysplastic syndrome after treatment with epipodophyllotoxins. *J Clin Oncol* 17:569–577, 1999
196. Tucker MA, D'Angio GJ, Boice JD, et al: Bone sarcomas linked to radiotherapy and chemotherapy in children. *N Engl J Med* 317:588–593, 1988
197. Nyandoto P, Muhonen T, Joensuu H: Second cancers among long term survivors from Hodgkin's disease. *Int J Radiat Biol Phys* 42:373–378, 1998
198. Travis L, Hill DA, Dores GM: Breast cancer following radiotherapy and chemotherapy among young women with Hodgkin disease. *JAMA* 290:654–475, 2003
199. Bhatia S, Robison LL, Oberlin O, et al: Breast cancer and other second neoplasms after childhood Hodgkin's disease. *N Engl J Med* 334:745–751, 1996
200. Dershaw DD, Yahalom J, Petick JA: Breast carcinoma in women previously treated for Hodgkin's disease: mammographic evaluation. *Radiology* 184:421–423, 1992
201. Harpham WS: Long term survivors, in Berger A, Portenoy RK, Weismann DS (eds): *Principles and Practice of Supportive Oncology.* Philadelphia, Lippincott-Raven, 1998, pp 889–908
202. Meadows AT, Hobbie WL: Medical consequences of cure. *Cancer* 58:524–528, 1986
203. Oeffinger KC, Eshelman DA, Tomlinson GE, Buchanan GR: Programs for adult survivors of childhood cancer. *J Clin Oncol* 16:2864–2867, 1998
204. Jacobs LA, Hobbie W: The Living Well After Cancer Program: An advanced practice model of care. *Oncol Nurs Forum* 29:637–638, 2002
205. Pavy JJ, Denekamp J, Letschert J, et al: Late effects of toxicity scoring: the SOMA scale. *Int J Radiat Oncol Biol Phys* 31:1043–1047, 1995
206. Vaughn DJ, Gignac G, Meadows AT: Long-term medical care of testicular cancer survivors. *Ann Internal Med* 136:463–470, 2002

CHAPTER 69

Physical, Economic, and Social Issues Confronting Patients and Families

Cathy J. Bradley, PhD
Barbara A. Given, PhD, RN, FAAN
Charles W. Given, PhD
Sharon Kozachik, RN, MSN

Introduction

Increased awareness of certain types of cancer (e.g., prostate, breast) and improved detection methods and treatment regimens have led to more — and younger — people being diagnosed, treated, and surviving cancer. Increasing numbers of patients with cancer are either cured or have longer disease-free survival. The five-year survival rate for all cancers is 64%.[1] Nearly 10 million people have survived their initial diagnosis and episode of cancer treatment. Approximately 13% of these survivors were diagnosed more than 20 years ago.

Survival rates are commonly used to monitor progress in the treatment of cancer. These rates include all persons who are in remission, disease free, dying, or currently under treatment. While these rates indicate some improvement in cancer survival, they are an inadequate measure of overall progress toward minimizing the disease burden. The rates tell us nothing about the quality of survival or cancer's effects on the lives of patients and their families. For patients and their families, treatment decisions are merely the beginning of long-term dilemmas that may lead to changes in employment, diminished social and psychological functioning, reorganization of family relationships, and diminished economic viability.

Who is considered a cancer survivor? The traditional medical definition of a *cancer survivor* is one who has remained free from disease five years or more after diagnosis. However, many reject this definition and argue that survival begins at diagnosis and continues for the rest of the person's life.[2] The National Coalition for Cancer Survivorship (NCCS) defines survivorship this way: "From the time of [the cancer's] discovery and for the balance of life, an individual diagnosed with cancer is a survivor." The National Cancer Institute's Office of Cancer Survivorship adds that survivorship encompasses physical, psychological, social, and economic sequelae of cancer diagnosis and treatment beyond the acute diagnosis and treatment phase.[3] In the spirit of these definitions, this chapter refers to *survivorship* as the period beginning once initial treatment of the cancer ends and continuing throughout the remainder of the person's life. Nurses involved in cancer care should seek to prevent and control adverse outcomes that include late effects of the cancer, subsequent cancers, and poor quality of life for those who experience cancer.

In the past, little emphasis has been placed on how the postdiagnosis and treatment period affects patients and their families. Few long-term guidelines exist for the survivorship period, and survivors are not followed into perpetuity by oncologists and other cancer specialists. In fact, once the initial treatment period ends, healthcare delivery shifts from inpatient and specialty care to ambulatory treatment centers and the home setting. Patient care is returned to the purview of the primary care system. Yet the work of Hewitt and others suggests that compared with noncancer survivors, cancer survivors are more likely to be in poor or fair health and to have a psychological disability, limitations in daily living, or instrumental activities of daily living and functional disabilities.[4] Insufficient evidence exists about how these patients and their families adapt to the longer-term survival period.[5]

Nurses play a critical role in coordinating care in the survivorship phase of cancer. These nurses may be part of the primary care system and must recognize patients' and family members' needs, make appropriate referrals for care, and prepare patients and their families for situations they are likely to face as cancer survivorship begins. They should also provide education and counseling to patients and families for symptom management and monitoring, coordination of services, and guidance about how to function at home and in their jobs after having been treated for cancer. Recovery and return to normal function should be the focus of concern when working with patients as they make the transition to survivorship status.

The goal of this chapter is to increase the reader's awareness of several important issues faced by patients with cancer and their families, as patients increasingly live beyond initial diagnosis and treatment and return to their usual lives. Nurses should consider these issues as they assist patients in their transition from the active treatment and follow-up phase to a phase where direct contact with oncology specialists is sporadic, patients may experience unmet needs, and new health-related problems might arise. Focus is placed on how cancer care professionals can guide patients and families into problem solving and decision making about how they will integrate the effects of cancer into their lives. Patients and families face several daunting situations, including adjustment to physical disability, psychosocial needs, employment changes, insurance challenges, and ongoing medical care needs and associated costs.[6] Special attention is given to these issues, and suggestions and strategies are provided for nurses who are assisting patients and their families during the transition from acute cancer care to longer-term survivorship.

Physical Disability and Impaired Physical Function: Implications for the Family

Although cancer treatment extends life expectancy, the treatment itself often leaves patients with functional deficits that can have long-term medical,

Table 69-1 Functional Impairments

Common Functional Deficits Among Persons Treated for Cancer	Often Associated with
Impaired cognition and memory loss	Radiation, chemotherapy
Loss of motor control	Surgery, radiation, chemotherapy
Cranial nerve deficits, peripheral neuropathy, neuropathy motor and sensory	Surgery, radiation/head and neck cancer, chemotherapy
Speech difficulties	Surgery/head and neck cancer
Problems with swallowing and feeding	Surgery, pulmonary radiation/head and neck and esophageal cancers
Fatigue	All treatments
Severe weakness	Chemotherapy, surgery
Scarring and fibrosis	Surgery/breast cancer
Sensory loss, reduction in fine motor skills (hyperesthetic parathesis)	All treatments
Loss of bowel and bladder control	Surgery/bladder cancer, prostate cancer, chemotherapy

psychosocial, vocational, and economic implications. Symptoms of fatigue, pain, anemia, neutropenia, and changes in weight or appetite may continue indefinitely.[5] As levels of impairment increase during the survivorship phase, psychological distress will likewise increase.[4,6,7]

Most patients will experience some disability as a result of cancer and its treatment. Patients' prior disposition will influence their response to treatment and the time until they recover from treatment. Those with compromised health or co-morbid conditions (particularly as found in older adults) prior to diagnosis may have few reserves or little resilience to the effects of cancer and its treatment. The severity of their disability will ultimately influence a sequence of psychosocial events for patients and their families.

Patients' disabilities vary by individual characteristics, cancer site and stage, and treatment modality. Common disabilities and their causes are listed in Table 69-1. Fatigue, nausea, and severe deconditioning are perhaps the most common functional problems for all patients recovering from treatment.[8] These symptoms persist long after chemotherapy and radiation are administered. Some patients may require medications for many months or even years after the initial acute treatment phase; the effects of these medications may hinder their abilities to fully recover.

Once patients have moved from the acute treatment phase to the maintenance or remission phase, nurses caring for these individuals must be aware of functional problems and make appropriate referrals for rehabilitation, palliative care, and long-term follow-up. Patient and family education can also play an important role in maintaining or restoring physical function. For example, maintenance of strength and range of motion in the upper extremity of the affected side following breast cancer surgery might be affected by lymphedema or numbness (i.e., peripheral neuropathy) from the chemotherapy drugs. Aerobic exercise following bone marrow transplantation is vital to prevent further disability.[9] Encouraging physical exercise for patients experiencing fatigue is also important for return to normal functioning.[9,10] Compliance with these rehabilitative plans will largely be the responsibility of patients and their families because the healthcare system is not designed to oversee patients long term. Nurses must emphasize the importance of maintaining a routine of follow-up care and develop a means for communicating expectations for physical functioning that patients and families can understand, assess within the home, and communicate about to nurses and other healthcare providers.

One method to communicate objectively and assess functional status is through the use of validated questionnaires. Measures of functioning include the Karnofsky Performance Scale, Functional Independence Measures, the Cancer Inventory and Problem Situations,[8] Functional Assessment of Cancer Treatment,[11] the Brief Pain Inventory,[12] and the Medical Outcomes Short Form-36.[13] Based on the patient's functional status, a plan may be devised to promote recovery of physical functioning and to prevent further deterioration. Responses to these scales provide an indication of physical and, to a lesser extent, role and emotional functioning.

Nurses need to assess family members as well as patients to fully ascertain the effects of disability on the family. The assessment measures noted above are not universally applicable to caregivers and family members. While the healthcare system focuses its health and wellness efforts on the cancer survivor, family caregivers who provide both direct care assistance and standby monitoring of cancer treatment effectiveness and side effects frequently have unmet health needs. Caregivers are not immune to chronic health conditions (e.g., diabetes, hypertension); they may need to provide physically and emotionally demanding tasks, such as lifting and turning; and they have interrupted nocturnal sleep and experience fatigue.[14,15]

The family caregiver's attention is focused on providing comfort, symptom management, and emotional support to the patient with cancer; in the process, the family caregiver's own physical and mental well-being may suffer.[16,17] Braithwaite showed a correlation between caregiver burden and minor psychiatric symptoms.[18] Krach and Brooks found that caregiving responsibilities interfered with rest and that caregivers reported experiencing headaches, nervousness, insomnia, weight changes, and unusual drowsiness.[19] In addition, Hoyert and Seltzer found that caregiving women reported poorer health and were more depressed than other women, and that female spousal caregivers reported the poorest health and greatest levels of depression — more so than those caring for a parent or child, or a noncaregiver.[20]

Successful rehabilitation and future survival often depend on patients' abilities to get the care they need. In this era of constrained costs and limited use of services, the spouse and family play essential roles in encouraging patients to return to their usual daily functioning, to engage in limited exercise, and to implement prescribed regimens of care. The healthcare environment places considerable responsibility on the family to become active participants in the care of the person with cancer. The effectiveness of this approach depends partially on patients' and families' understanding and awareness of the disease, their financial resources to obtain the care they need, and access to the healthcare system. Nurses can greatly enhance the ability of patients and family members to understand how to access resources and get the most possible support from the healthcare system. Family members may not be aware of existing community resources or may assume that they and the patient are not eligible for such resources.

Cancer Survival and Employment

The prevalence of early-stage disease is rising in working-age people, as screening is routinely recommended for younger individuals, and suspicious cells that would have gone unnoticed in the past are now detected and treated. For example, nearly 140,000 women younger than age 65 were diagnosed with breast cancer in 2001.[1] In addition, treatment for cancer has become considerably more aggressive, even for early-stage tumors.[21] Due to these changes in detection and treatment, patients have become more likely to bear the consequences of cancer during their working years when they may have otherwise lived and functioned for some time without knowledge or effects of their disease. Cancer-specific empirical studies have pointed to some key questions in understanding the direction of influence that cancer is likely to have on employment, but they are far from decisive.

Cancer survivors often want and need to work and to perform in their customary roles, regardless of their physical and emotional limitations. Studies have shown that patients employed at the time of diagnosis are strongly motivated to return to work.[22–24] Return to work may be one of the main objectives of rehabilitation and recovery and can be an important indication of how well patients are coping. However, the ability to return to work can vary by cancer site, treatment modality, and characteristics inherent to patients and their jobs.

Kornblith reports the following unemployment percentages by site among cancer survivors: 19%, Hodgkin's disease; 25%, leukemia; 19%, breast cancer; 11%, prostate cancer; 22%, colon cancer; and 40%, lung cancer.[24] Razavi and associates found that patients treated for lymphoma often have difficulty returning to their jobs.[25] Of lymphoma patients in remission and able to work, only 54% actually returned to work. Anxiety, depression, and issues related to treatment were cited as reasons that patients refused to reenter the work force.[25] Because the incidence of Hodgkin's lymphoma peaks between ages 15 and 34 and after age 50, professional rehabilitation and return to function are extremely important for these individuals. Only 41% of patients with head and neck cancer return to work, most likely due to the nature of the surgery required and resulting disfigurement.[26]

Overwhelmingly, studies have focused on survivors' subjective impressions of the impact of cancer on their lives. These studies suggest negative factors that can reduce employment, including physical disability (e.g., limitations in upper body strength),[8] memory loss,[27] lack of control over schedules, need for transportation, and type of work performed,[28,29] and in some cases discrimination on the part of employers.[30,31] Nurses must first consider the short-term employment-related disabilities that are due to the effects of cancer treatment. These disabilities are likely to be most pronounced during the first year following diagnosis. Once these disabilities are partially or totally resolved, nurses must then consider the long-term needs and decisions patients face with regard to employment. For example, in a study of breast and prostate cancer survivors, Bradley and associates[32] found that employment and weekly hours worked were lowest for cancer patients 6 months following diagnosis, whereas at 12 and 18 months more cancer patients returned to work and their average weekly hours increased, albeit not to the levels observed prior to diagnosis.

The employment effects of cancer, both short- and long-term, are well described for women with breast cancer. The National Comprehensive Cancer Network (NCCN) treatment guidelines for breast cancer recommend a combination of surgery, radiotherapy, and chemotherapy depending on cancer stage, histology, and other clinical factors. These aggressive treatment regimens are believed to reduce the chances of recurrence and prolong survival,[21] but can also cause impairments such as loss of range of motion in the arm on the affected side, lymphedema, reduced concentration and cognition, pain, and fatigue.[33–35] As many as

80% of women who undergo breast-conserving surgery, axillary dissection, and breast radiation experience arm and psychological distress.[36,37]

In a longitudinal study, Bradley and associates[38] examined the consequences of breast cancer on women's employment for the six-month period following diagnosis. Women with breast cancer, with the exception of those having in situ cancer, were 17 percentage points less likely to work six months following diagnosis relative to a control sample of women. For those women who continued working, women with local and regional/distant cancers reduced their hours relative to women in the control group. The negative employment and reduction in hours worked were not observed for women with in situ cancers—lending economic support to arguments for early detection and treatment.

The long-term effects (e.g., three or more years) of breast cancer on employment are less certain. In a study of patients two and three years after their primary treatment, Ganz and associates[39] found that 65% of breast cancer survivors were either working for pay or volunteering their services. The mean numbers of hours worked were 34.4 and 33.2 hours per week among women who were two and three years post-treatment, respectively. This study concluded that women continue to work and perform their usual roles after treatment for breast cancer. In a separate study, Ganz and associates[40] reported that 80% of five- to seven-year breast cancer survivors had no change in employment. The authors found that the 20% of women who had a change in work status went from full-time to part-time employment or retired. They also found that survivors' long-term physical functioning had not diminished over time.[40]

Relying on data from the Health and Retirement Study (HRS) linked to longitudinal Social Security earnings data, Bradley and associates[41] examined differences between breast cancer survivors and a non-cancer control group in terms of employment, hours worked, wages, and earnings. This study found that breast cancer survivors were statistically significantly less likely to work (by approximately 9 percentage points) relative to women who never had cancer. This may have been due to morbidity imposed by the disease or perhaps changes in desire to work. Surprisingly, the researchers also found that women with breast cancer who were employed after their diagnosis worked more hours (between three and four additional hours per week) and had higher wages and earnings relative to the noncancer control group. The authors speculated that breast cancer's influence on employment is multifaceted, involving physical impairments (i.e., morbidity imposed by the disease and treatment) that produce a negative employment effect, as well as attitudinal and financial components that could lead survivors that remain in the work force to work additional hours.[41] Approximately one-fourth of the participants in a study of long-term breast cancer survivors reported that cancer made them more goal focused.[42]

In contrast, Chirikos and associates found that 41% of breast cancer survivors required special accommodations to perform their jobs.[43] These survivors were nearly three times more likely to be impaired relative to their non-cancer-affected peers. Similarly, Stewart and associates[42] found that 41% of a sample of long-term breast cancer survivors who were employed prior to their diagnosis no longer worked. One study conducted in the Netherlands examined changes in employment and earnings among adult five-year cancer survivors ($n = 649$)[26] and found that one-third of these individuals had a change in their employment status from employed to either homemakers, retired, or unemployed. The percentage of patients who were employed part-time at the end of five years doubled from the time of diagnosis.

Nurses need to consider the long-term implications of unemployment as they assist patients and families in planning for these likely events. To avoid unnecessary patient disability and unemployment, they can help develop a plan to ensure that patients get the maximum recovery and rehabilitation services available so that permanent unemployment is not necessary.

Patients, nurses and other healthcare providers, and employers need to be informed about possible periods of nonemployment that may have long-term consequences, such as limiting one's ability to return to the labor force, affecting the ability to obtain or retain health insurance, and reducing earnings. Patients and families require guidance and counseling to address how altered function or disability will affect their lives, finances, and roles. Identifying problems with employment and intervening appropriately pose a significant challenge for nurses, but should be considered and discussed with all patients at risk for long-term survivorship problems.

The following sections discuss specific problems (i.e., physically demanding jobs, barriers to job reentry, inability to change jobs, early retirement, and problems specific to self-employment) that can occur at the work site, regardless of patient characteristics, job type, or disability.

Physically Demanding Jobs

Because job requirements are often related to workers' gender, education, and local economic conditions, certain groups of patients may be disproportionately and adversely affected by cancer- and treatment-related disability. To illustrate this point, one study found that functional limitations and health impairments have significant negative effects on employment for men.[44] Among employed men who reported having a neoplasm, 62% reported a functional disability, and 50% reported a work disability. Among employed women with a neoplasm, 67% had a functional disability, but only 38% had a work disability. Even though both genders reported approximately the same percentage of functional disability, disability prevented more men from working than women, perhaps because more men are employed in physically demanding jobs than women.

In general, persons employed in physically demanding jobs are more likely to become unemployed due to the functional limitations resulting from cancer and its treatment than are people employed in sedentary jobs. These individuals may not be able to perform at their former pace or may have to exert greater effort in carrying out activities. Because of physical disability, fewer blue-collar workers return to their previous jobs than do white-collar workers.[24]

For those who perform physical work or whose work requires use of machinery, safety may be a concern. Some chemotherapeutic agents and radiation therapy cause paresthesia and neurological and cognitive deficits that may endanger the worker. For other patients, nerve damage or the peripheral neuropathy to an extremity such as an arm or leg may result from surgical procedures or from radiation and interfere with job responsibilities. Unfortunately, these laborers are more likely to have low wages and are less likely to have adequate insurance coverage; thus, their inability to work can have dramatic consequences for their families if all members become uninsured due to job loss by the primary wage earner. Men, particularly men of minority races or ethnic groups, are more likely to be employed in physically demanding jobs and are more likely to report limitations in their ability to work after a cancer diagnosis than are white men.[45]

Work Site Barriers to Job Reentry

Of survivors who report problems returning to work, many report instances of gross discrimination in which they were fired or laid off because of their cancer diagnosis. Others report that they were encouraged to leave, transferred to less desirable jobs, demoted, had difficulty finding a new job, or found that their work responsibilities were unwillingly curtailed.[5,24] Nurses and other healthcare professionals must work with patients and their families to prepare them for possible discrimination and to help them develop strategies to thwart its effects. These strategies must be consistent with survivors' goals, expectations, and capabilities.

Breast cancer survivors identified four situations that hindered successful job reentry: (1) breach of confidentiality of medical information; (2) absence of support from coworkers and managers to assist in reentry, and management of the stigma associated with cancer; (3) difficulty talking to colleagues about health; and (4) difficulty asking for and receiving assistance.[30] It is important to note that one cannot assume that employers or employees are aware of or will adhere to federal regulations such as the Americans with Disabilities Act (1990). Common violations include disclosure of health history information and failure to provide reasonable accommodation for patients returning to work. However, the return to work does not have to be a negative experience. Some survivors report positive experiences of being relieved of difficult physical tasks, job sharing, and opportunities for holding other types of jobs within the same organization.

Inability to Change Jobs

Simply considering whether a patient can return to work is insufficient. The inability to change jobs, or *job lock*, is another important outcome that may result from having been treated for cancer. Job lock entails a reluctance to change jobs for fear of not finding comparable insurance coverage or an employer willing to hire someone with cancer. Lack of career mobility is part of many cancer survivors' experience.[5]

Job lock can lead to reduced worker productivity, less job satisfaction, and limited income. Also, some patients may stay in jobs they are no longer able to perform in an effort to preserve their insurance coverage. One study reported that 44% of breast cancer survivors felt "locked in" to their current job because they needed to retain their insurance coverage.[46] Particularly troubling is a situation in which patients survive cancer but they (or another wage earner in the household) cannot seek better employment for fear of losing insurance coverage.

Insurance-related reasons for not changing jobs include waiting periods, preexisting conditions, incomparable coverage, and higher premiums. Employers, particularly small firms, may not find potential employees (or their family members) with medical risks desirable because the employer's risk rating and premiums will dramatically increase. The risk of losing insurance coverage is greatest for workers with less experience and limited skills.[47]

Job lock can be a frustrating experience for cancer survivors. These individuals may not be able to attain the career goals they have set for themselves. Until public policies such as health insurance portability are adopted, little can be done to remedy job lock. Coping strategies that refocus priorities away from career achievement to another meaningful goal are perhaps the only means to alleviate frustration. Job counseling and training for new skills may also be appropriate, in some cases.

Early Retirement

For many patients who are nearing retirement and who have the financial means to do so, early retirement may be an option for coping with the cognitive and functional disabilities resulting from cancer and its treatment. However, this decision may not be without consequences. Palmore and associates found that when someone retires for health reasons, his or her income and standards of living dramatically decrease compared to other retirees, even after controlling for preretirement characteristics.[48] Such individuals also suffer more dissatisfaction with their living situations and experience decreased happiness.

Conversly, Bednarek and Bradley[49] found that the retirement experience for some cancer survivors was quite positive. These researchers compared patients who retired before versus after their cancer diagnosis. Those who retired following such a diagnosis were close to the traditional retirement age of 65 rather than a much younger age. These retirees' subjective impressions of retirement were not very different from the impressions of patients who retired prior to diagnosis. One might have anticipated that those who retired after their cancer diagnosis would have a more positive impression of retirement than those who had enjoyed some time of cancer-free retirement, but this was not the case.

Often nurses are asked to anticipate changes that patients and families may need to make in their lives in response to cancer. A patient's ability to adapt to both the immediate distress of diagnosis and treatment and then adjust to longer-term life changes is an important aspect of cancer survivorship.[50] Some encouraging evidence suggests that cancer may neither deter patients from continuing to work nor affect the quality of the retirement experience for those who decide to leave the labor force. Nevertheless, nurses may need to advise patients not to make decisions too hastily. Patients may be tempted to make lasting decisions when they are in the midst of aggressive treatment and before they know whether they can return to previous functioning levels. All patients should be encouraged to seek career and financial counseling before making retirement decisions. The knowledge that an enjoyable retirement experience is possible may relieve patients' distress with regard to psychosocial aspects of cancer and help them to adapt to survivorship.

Self-Employment

Individuals who are self-employed, especially those in sole proprietorships, are not likely to have many options for job sharing, retirement, or working fewer hours. These individuals require special attention and counseling from the healthcare system and nurses. Some may need to sell their business, hire someone to resume their previous responsibilities, or rely on other members of their families to take over the business either permanently or temporarily. This transition can cause worry, a sense of loss, and financial and emotional hardships. Because of the personal nature of owning and growing a business, letting go of some or all responsibilities and control may be extremely difficult. In addition, a number of legal concerns regarding ownership and decision making may need to be resolved. Anticipating the problems and emphasizing reasoned decisions rather than hasty decisions should be a part of the nurse's discussion with patients prior to treatment.

Recommendations

Nurses need to urge patients and their family members to consider the possible effects that cancer and its treatment may have on their ability to work *prior* to receiving treatment. They need to assist the patient and family to consider what adaptations or adjustments may be needed and to request community service programs that might assist the patient in rehabilitation and recovery.

Many patients require treatments that can affect concentration and mental alertness. These individuals may need attention-building exercises so that they can return to their usual cognitive functioning level. At times, patients may need change job positions until their cognitive abilities return. Some long-term treatments such as steroids can cause mood swings and depression. Patients may require pain, sleeping, and antiemetic medications that may interfere with cognitive functioning. These treatments may last for months or years, and their effects may linger for as long as six months after treatment stops. This persistence may decrease survivors' accuracy and efficiency or general ability to do cognitive work. Patients need to work proactively with their employers so that a constructive plan for temporary absences or job restructing is in place.

Fatigue and lack of endurance can also prevent patients from attaining their former productivity levels. Nurses can play a pivotal role in helping patients and families prepare for treatment and anticipate what work-related adaptations might be needed. They can assist patients in learning strategies that increase the attention and cognitive capacity so they can return to work.[51] Such preparation minimizes lost work time and helps families plan to provide care and to assist with recovery.

While employment issues can be quite formidable, nurses can aid patients first by making them aware of potential difficulties, and then by helping them think about solutions and plan ahead. For example, some coworkers may be willing to job share with the patient during the acute treatment phase; such options should be considered at the beginning of treatment. Some employers may be willing to assist the patient with internal placement in less physically and emotionally demanding jobs. If these changes are initiated by the survivor, chances are greater that he or she will feel more in control of the situation than if the change were imposed on the patient. Long-term strategies might include taking early retirement, finding a new job, or reducing the number of hours worked. Family members who were not previously working may need to work, or if they were working they may need to plan for time away from work to care for the patient. Nurses can prompt families to discuss and consider options that maintain the family status and prevent financial vulnerabilities. These strategies help patients and their families to become proactive and more prepared for inevitable changes. Patients and family members should be encouraged to consider who has health insurance benefits and how the treatment, both short- and long-term, might affect employment.

The following section discusses the Americans with Disabilities Act and the Family Medical Leave Act, both of which may prove useful to cancer survivors and their family members. Other legislation may also be pertinent, but these two acts apply to the immediate concerns of taking time away from a job to seek care and possible job discrimination.

Legislative Protection

Fortunately, legislative protection exists for some of the challenges that may confront the cancer survivor in the workplace. It is essential that nurses and other healthcare professionals be aware of these protections and provide patients and families with information about their rights. Survivors and their family members are protected at the workplace by the Americans with Disabilities Act (ADA) and the Family Medical Leave Act (FMLA).

Cancer is considered a disability under the ADA. This act requires employers to make "reasonable accommodation" for employees with a disability. Scheduling changes would be considered reasonable, for example, but turning a full-time job into a part-time job is not required.[52] The ADA specifies that employers may ask only job-related medical questions, prohibits employers from firing an employee with a disability without first making a reasonable accommodation on the job, and requires that employers treat all employees the same. Thus, an employer that provides insurance benefits to all employees, with the exception of a employee with a disability, violates the ADA requirement for equitable treatment of all employees. In addition, the ADA prohibits exclusion of an applicant for a job or from a training program because of disability.

The ADA has some noteworthy restrictions. It applies to employers with 15 or more employees, so persons with disabilities who are employed by small businesses are not protected. This may impose a greater hardship on those living in rural communities where small businesses are the principal employers. In addition, a 180-day statute of limitations on filing complaints from the date of discrimination exists. Patients with cancer must be proactive in making their needs known to their employer — becoming their own advocates to ensure their needs are met. If a court finds in favor of an employee, the remedy may include back pay, an injunction, and attorney's fees.

The FMLA gives employees the right to take time off due to their own illness or if they are caring for an ill dependent, without the threat of losing their jobs. Currently, this law provides for 12 weeks of unpaid leave per year for serious illness. A *serious health condition* is defined as one that incapacitates the patient for more than three consecutive days, requires a doctor's or other healthcare professional's care, or requires a regimen of continuous treatment. Cancer is a condition generally considered serious enough for FMLA to apply to both patients and family members needing to care for them.

The 12-week leave does not have to be taken all at once, but can instead be taken in blocks of time. For example, taking several hours of leave per day over a period of weeks for treatments or follow-up tests receives the same protection as a more extensive leave of 12 consecutive weeks. During this time, the employer is required to continue providing health benefits. Taking blocks of time off may be particularly beneficial for patients requiring treatment over long periods of time. Nurses can help patients plan the time they will need to be away from their jobs to maximize FMLA's benefits.

An important limitation of FMLA is that it applies only to employers with 50 or more employees. Therefore, cancer patients and family members employed by most small businesses will not be covered. These individuals are likely to suffer greater hardships due to discrimination and may even lose their jobs because of their need for medical care and time away from work.

Table 69-2 Provisions of the Americans with Disabilities Act and the Family Medical Leave Act

	Americans with Disabilities Act
Applies to:	Patients
Protection:	1. Requires reasonable accommodation for disability 2. Restricts employer inquiries to job-related medical questions 3. Provides for equitable insurance benefits 4. Prohibits exclusions from hiring decisions or training programs due to disability
Restrictions:	Applies to employers with 15 or more employees 180-day statute of limitations
	Family Medical Leave Act
Applies to:	Patients and family members
Protection:	12 weeks of unpaid leave without losing job or benefits Leave can be taken all at once or in blocks of time
Restrictions:	Applies to employers with 50 or more employees

Nurses need to assist patients and their families to understand their rights and legal protections. This assistance may simply involve providing information to the patient or it may require documenting a patient's illness and treatment for his or her employer. Table 69-2 summarizes the benefits and restrictions of the ADA and FMLA.

Cancer and its treatment may create numerous workplace challenges for the survivor. These challenges can apply to family members as well and may lead to considerable hardship. In most situations, cancer survivors and their family members face difficult decisions that can have serious emotional and financial implications. Fortunately, some patients report positive experiences at the work site. The realities of disability and physical, emotional, and cognitive limitations need to be discussed with patients. Oncology nurses can play an important role in helping families plan for the inevitable work challenges and the possibility of financial hardships before patients receive treatment. In addition, primary care nurses need to be aware of and plan for the long-term employment implications of the patient's cancer and its treatment.

Health Insurance Challenges

In the United States, insurance status is closely tied to employment for individuals younger than age 65. Therefore, all of the problems associated with having been treated for cancer and employment—specifically, presence of physical disability, physically demanding job, minority race, low-income or low-skilled job—affect one's ability to obtain and keep insurance coverage. For example, in a study by Guidry and associates, 26% of white patients and 46% of black patients lost their insurance coverage after they were diagnosed with cancer.[53] The difference arose because African Americans were employed in lower-paying and physically demanding jobs. Twenty-one percent of white patients were denied insurance coverage after changing jobs, whereas 55% of black patients were denied insurance coverage after changing jobs. Inability to work often translates into lack of insurance coverage for medical care and lost wages.

Survivors and their families have constant concerns about future health and the possibility of cancer recurrence and progression. Because medical costs are increasing, the need for adequate health insurance is critical. Given that lack of insurance is associated with physical, emotional, and financial burdens,[54,55] health insurance coverage is extremely important to these individuals.

Transitions from private to public insurance may occur for people with cancer. A change in patient insurance status will likely lead to a change in healthcare provider and subsequently to an interruption in continuity of care. A change in insurance status may also affect access to pharmaceuticals, particularly if the new insurer does not include certain drugs on its formulary.

Specific challenges to insurability include refusal, policy cancellation, higher premiums, and extended waiting periods.[56] For some patients, the price to obtain insurance may become prohibitive once their health history is known. According to 2000 National Health Interview Survey data, approximately 17% of Americans younger than age 65 have no health insurance.[1] For adults younger than age 65 who are not pregnant or caring for young children and who seek Medicaid enrollment because they do not have health insurance through an employer, they must have a disabling condition expected to last at least one year and they must meet asset and income requirements to qualify for Medicaid. If cancer is a Medicaid enrollee's qualifying condition, then the cancer, by definition, has to be advanced. Treatments for late-stage cancers, even if they are "state-of-the-art," are less likely to offer a survival benefit. The Medicaid enrollment process in itself can have serious psychosocial consequenes for patients and their family members. In addition, some healthcare providers may not accept patients who are covered under Medicaid or who have no insurance. This may subsequently lead to fragmented care and perhaps worsening of disease.

Insurance coverage for cancer care often is not comprehensive. Coverage for anticancer drugs, investigational medications, and mental health and rehabilitation services and therapies are frequently lacking.[57] For patients older than age 65, Medicare pays for a substantial portion of the care. However, only drugs administered in the physician's office and drugs administered by infusion pump are covered by Medicare; oral drugs and injectable drugs that are self-administered by the patient are not reimbursed. Medicare does not pay for prescription medications and other out-of-pocket expenditures, although some prescription drug benefits are expected in 2006 for Medicare beneficiaries who qualify for these benefits and enroll in the prescription drug benefit program. Therefore, by the time patients enter into the survivorship phase, they have already incurred many expenses. Insufficient funds may hinder patients' ability to obtain the rehabilitation care they require to recover to the fullest extent possible.

Even though currently Medicare pays 80% of the average wholesale price of drugs administered in a physician's office or by infusion pump, this benefit is restrictive. For example, the use of a well-known chemotherapeutic agent for an indication not specified by the Food and Drug Administration (FDA) is prohibited by Medicare. This restriction is particularly problematic: a General Accounting Office study found that one-third of chemotherapy use was for an indication other than the one approved by the FDA. At least 56% of patients in this study received one "off-label" drug (a drug used for an indication not specifically approved by the FDA) as part of their treatment.[58,59]

For patients who cannot receive state-of-the-art care due to health insurance and financial restrictions, survivorship may become difficult. These individuals may lack access to medications including drugs that can ease the effects of cancer treatments or that can slow disease progression. Therefore, patients with insufficient insurance are more likely to experience adverse events, cancer recurrences, and disease progression due to the use of less effective therapies.

Under many managed care arrangements, specialists such as oncologists are paid on a discounted fee-for-service basis.[60] The primary care physician's income may be capitated, and he or she may receive financial incentives to curtail referrals to specialists such as oncologists. Under this arrangement, patients are likely to experience discontinuity in their care and must assume much of the responsibility for managing their symptoms and seeking treatment.

Medicaid is one option for financially indigent people meeting fairly stringent criteria that are set on a state-by-state and sometimes case-by-case basis. However, less than 45% of the population below the federal poverty level is eligible for Medicaid. This program is designed for acute care needs and is not meant to provide for patients' long-term chronic needs. For example, once patients are able to work (according to standards set by the state in which they reside) or are disease free for a specified period of time, Medicaid may cancel their coverage. Social Security Disability Insurance, a program offered under Medicare, is available to patients who are disabled depending on the site, stage, and type of cancer. This insurance is canceled if the patient remains disease free for three years. Thus, survivors with this type of insurance soon find that their ongoing medical care needs are not covered by Medicare and that they are responsible for paying for their care out-of-pocket.

Understanding patients' insurance coverage can offer clues about access to care, utilization of services, and quality of care. Nurses face considerable challenges in trying to understand the many different plans and their specific limitations. Coordinating care while navigating through insurance provisions can be quite difficult, but it is critical to ensure that patients have access to the most appropriate care available. Primary care nurses have a unique opportunity to devise a plan of care for survivors and to follow them over time. These nurses need to incorporate survivorship and rehabilitation issues into their conceptual framework of primary care, which traditionally focuses on wellness. For example, nurses could educate patients to monitor their symptoms for possible cancer recurrences. They could also help patients prevent long-term disability by developing regimens for rehabilitation and health maintenance. By doing so, nurses help patients and their families avoid long-term healthcare costs.

Cost-of-Care Considerations: Influences on Treatment Decisions and Long-Term Impact

The National Institutes of Health estimated that the overall costs for cancer in 2002 amounted to $171.6 billion: $60.9 billion for direct medical costs; $15.5 billion for lost productivity due to illness; and $95.2 billion for productivity losses due to premature death.[1] Many of the recently adopted cancer treatment regimens are particularly expensive. Examples of these therapies include stem cell transplantation for hematological disorders, transplant procedures, paclitaxel for palliative chemotherapy, serotonin-antagonist antiemetics, and growth factors for supportive care during treatment. Often new therapeutic agents (e.g., antinausea drugs) are not on formularies. Given the existence of gaps in insurance plan coverage and managed care organizations that have capitated payment systems, both patients and healthcare providers must understand the relative value of different treatment options. This is no easy task. Many new treatments may offer outcomes comparable to those achieved with standard therapies or may provide only marginal gains in life expectancy and symptom relief. If the economic impact of cancer treatment on patients is not considered, many may receive expensive therapies that offer little benefit or that leave them with limited resources to pay for future healthcare services. Many of the drugs have to be given in a cancer setting for reimbursement purposes.

In recent years, out-of-pocket expenses for healthcare have been rising as health insurance deductibles and co-payments increase and coverage for some types of care (e.g., rehabilitation) becomes more limited. This financial responsibility may prove particularly burdensome for cancer survivors and their families. One study found that insured cancer patients younger than age 65 paid $549 out-of-pocket for cancer care and that uninsured cancer patients paid $1343 out-of-pocket for cancer care in a *six-month period.*[61] Over the expected lifetime of cancer survivors, it is easy to imagine how these expenses can become unmanageable — especially for patients who are uninsured.

Another out-of-pocket expense that cancer patients younger than age 65 may need to consider is the cost of participation in a clinical trial. Many health insurance plans (Medicare being the major exception), may not include some or all of the patient care costs associated with a clinical trial.[3] Some states have passed legislation or instituted special agreements requiring health plans to pay the cost of routine medical care provided to a clinical trial participant. Nurses need to guide patients who are interested in participating in a clinical trial about the health risks and benefits as well as the financial costs associated with the trial, because costs can present a significant barrier to participation in such studies. One estimate for the cost of care for participation in a clinical trial over 2.5 years was $35,418.[62] Patients need to know about the experience of other patients in the trial and if their plans paid for their care, the presence of any persistent problems with coverage, and the trial's administrators' success (if any) in getting plans to cover patient care costs. Nurses can help patients understand what their policy covers and request and carefully review the actual contract language. Claims for service may need to be filed in a particular way for reimbursement purposes, and nurses may need to send an information package to the patient's healthcare plan that includes study results supporting the clinical trial's safety, benefits, and medical appropriateness. This package might include publications from peer-reviewed literature about the proposed therapy that demonstrate patient benefits; a letter that uses the insurance contract's own language to explain why the treatment should be covered; and letters from researchers that explain the clinical trial.[3]

Economic evaluation of cancer treatments has become more relevant in recent years. In 1996, the FDA announced an initiative to accelerate the approval process for cancer treatments.[63] This initiative allows the agency to approve new products based on evidence of increased survival or improved quality of life. Thus, a survivor may undergo treatment simply because it provides quality-of-life improvements, realizing there is no chance for improved survival. As might be expected, many new and often expensive therapies are becoming available, and the challenge to healthcare providers and patients is to determine the *value* of the new therapies compared to standard treatment regimens.

Economic concerns are likely to play an important role in the treatment decisions of healthcare providers and patients. Cost-effectiveness analysis is an increasingly popular technique that compares the costs and effects among treatment strategies. *Effects* are health outcomes such as cases of disease prevented, years of life gained, or quality-adjusted life-years.[64] The quality-adjusted life-year incorporates patients' symptoms and disability over time, but does not consider family burden. Furthermore, the costs to keep the survivor alive in a compromised health state are typically estimated from the perspective of the payer (i.e., insurance provider), not from the perspective of the patient. The results of a cost-effectiveness analysis provide the incremental or additional cost of obtaining a unit of effect, such as a life-year, from one medical intervention compared to another.

Cost-effectiveness analysis is likely to affect survivors in two ways: (1) by making treatments more (or less) available, and (2) by defining an economic dimension for treatment choices. Managed care organizations may use economic evaluations to develop treatment practice guidelines and to make formulary decisions for the inclusion of medications. These practice guidelines and formulary decisions may dictate the type of treatment patients receive and the availability of certain medications. Patients need to know their options for obtaining "off-formulary" medications and alternative medical procedures. Cost-effectiveness analysis available in the literature can be evaluated using the criteria shown in Table 69-3. Perhaps the most important of these criteria are the clarity of the research question, the inclusion of all pertinent costs and consequences (including those incurred by family members), and the relevance to clinical practice. Regardless of the methodological rigor, if the study is not relevant to clinical practice and the alternatives are not reasonable comparisons (i.e., placebo may not be a reasonable comparison), the study has limited application. In a practical sense, studies of cost-effectiveness can help patients understand why certain therapies are available and others are not and may prove useful for helping patients make treatment decisions. Nurses can use these studies to help patients understand their treatment alternatives and the costs and consequences of each alternative. For example, a cost-effectiveness analysis may be the only source of information that incorporates time away from work and lost wages, long-term medical care required and its costs, and quality-adjusted survival into a single study.

Table 69-3 Criteria for Evaluating Cost-Effectiveness Analysis to Assist Patients with Treatment Decisions

Checklist	Comments
1. Research question is well-defined	Is it clear what the researchers were trying to accomplish?
2. Alternative therapies are well-defined and explained	Each alternative therapy and its sequelae are fully explained.
3. Alternative therapies are reasonable comparisons	Is this something that would normally be used in routine practice? Or is the comparison to a therapy rarely used?
4. Target population is well-defined	Is the target population a high-risk group? Is the target population the "typical" patients treated for the illness under question? Who was *excluded* from the analysis?
5. Perspective of the analysis is stated	Was the analysis conducted from the perspective of the payer? Society? Patient?
6. All important costs and consequences are identified for each strategy	Were all direct medical care costs (including additional diagnostic tests) and productivity costs (i.e., time away from work) fully estimated? Were all consequences, including side effects, long-term disabilities, and benefits, included?
7. Sources for obtaining costs and outcomes are stated	Are the sources credible? Are they applicable to other treatment settings?
8. Sensitivity analysis is performed	Were other reasonable costs and survivorship outcomes considered in the analysis?
9. Results are expressed as incremental costs and outcomes	Were the results expressed in terms of cost per life-year gained for each alternative studied?
10. Study limitations are stated	Were any of the limitations stated a "fatal flaw" of the analysis?
11. Study conclusions have relevance to clinical practice and are clinically meaningful: Was there a quality of life improvement in addition to (or instead of) tumor reduction and small survival benefits (less than one month)?	Were the results relevant to clinical practice? For example, if the study was conducted in a clinical trial setting, are the results applicable to routine practice and to survivorship?
12. Published in a peer-reviewed journal	Is the publication source credible?

Ongoing Medical Care Needs of Survivors and Their Impact on Family Members

An understanding of the economic implications of medical treatment is important because the medical care needs of patients and families extend far beyond the initial treatment episodes and, as previously discussed, insurance benefits are often limited. Long-term treatment of individuals with cancer involves periodic medical visits to monitor patients' conditions and may require prolonged use of medications, medical supplies, durable medical equipment, and lifestyle alterations to manage the symptoms and side effects (e.g., pain) of cancer and treatment. In addition, inpatient care to combat other concomitant conditions (e.g., bowel obstructions, fistulas) or cancer recurrences may be necessary. Hewitt and associates compared 4878 cancer survivors to subjects without a history of cancer.[4] Those individuals with a cancer history had more other chronic diseases, and were more likely to report being in poor or frail health, having a psychological disability, or having limitations in activities of daily living or limitations in instrumental activities of daily living. For those subjects younger than age 65, more cancer patients than other patients were unable to work due to health. Younger individuals diagnosed before age 45 were more likely to have psychological problems as compared to those who were older than 65 at time of diagnosis.

Kornblith[24] examined the long-term (median 20 years) impact of breast cancer on patients. Only 5% of survivors had scores indicating clinical depression, but 15% had two or more symptoms of post-traumatic stress disorder (PTSD). Twenty-nine percent had sexual problems. Survivors with lower educational attainment and less adequate social support, more negative life events, and greater dissatisfaction with their medical care had worse PTSD symptoms compared to other survivors. Thirteen percent of this group said they had employment problems attributed to cancer, 26% had insurance problems attributed to cancer, 22% had interference due to lymphedema, and 9% felt they could not change their jobs for fear of losing their health insurance. Ganz and associates[65] reported a substantial degree of psychological distress in younger women after breast cancer that persists for years. African American, partnered women, and those with better emotional and physical functioning were associated with better emotional and physical outcomes.

Finding a balance between the long-term negative effects and costs of aggressive treatment and the anticipated benefits must be uppermost in the minds of those making treatment decisions. For example, increased use of palliative care may lower total costs by preventing or delaying hospitalization. Patients with cancer, in particular, can benefit from the assistance of a nurse case manager, who provides assessment, education, and support as well as referral to medical treatment, supportive services, and community resources. In recent years, the burden of locating and paying for supportive services has been largely shifted to patients and their families. Therefore, the role of the nurse is to identify where gaps exist in patients' care and to help them evaluate their alternatives.

Examples of ongoing care include medications, treatment for second malignant neoplasms, and rehabilitation. Rehabilitation can occur in many settings, including inpatient, acute care, subacute rehabilitation, outpatient, nursing homes, and home. In addition, psychological counseling and participation in support groups for patients and family members are often important parts of the recovery process. Many communities have resources and advocacy groups that can help survivors and their families locate the care they need.

Because patients and their family members are responsible for their care, they need to have an awareness of potential side effects and long-term problems associated with treatment so that difficulties can be quickly recognized and acted on before they become difficult to manage. For example, pain, compromised immunity, significant fatigue and endurance problems, and psychosocial problems are best addressed proactively. Nurses can take a leadership role in assessing patients' needs and offering guidance for meeting long-term medical requirements.

For cancer survivors who require ongoing care and monitoring in the home setting, family members are frequently asked to provide both direct care, such as bathing, feeding, dressing changes, and medication administration, and indirect care, such as emotional support, transportation, and monitoring and standby care. The caregiving role may be disruptive to family members' developmental needs, however. Many patients with breast cancer have reported that their family members were tired of talking about cancer and its symptoms because these family members were ready to move past the cancer experience.[51]

Employed young and middle-aged adult caregivers must balance work roles with caregiving tasks. Stommel and associates documented that the care provided by family members during and immediately after the treatment phase can be equivalent to a part-time job.[66] They found that family caregivers devoted as many as 6 hours per day in the provision of care to their family member with cancer. Seventy-two percent of unpaid caregivers are women, and most continued to be employed on a part-time or full-time basis outside of the home.[67] Hayman and associates[68] reported that subjects who had a cancer diagnosis but who had not received treatment in the last year required an average of 6.8 hours per week of informal care. Krach and Brooks found that the average amount of time spent in caregiving activities was 5 hours per week (range, 1–30 hours per week).[19] Forty percent of their sample of employed caregivers reported that they received no assistance in the caregiving tasks from either formal or informal supports, and 48% of these employed caregivers reported missing an average of 4 days of work over a 6-month period due to their caregiving activities.

Caregivers who are employed in minimum-wage positions or who work part-time may not have paid time off as part of their benefits and may not be employed in settings where the FMLA applies. Therefore, these individuals may need to (1) arrange for secondary caregivers to stay with the patient when the primary caregiver is working, (2) take days off from work without pay, or (3) negotiate with their supervisors to rearrange work schedules so that they are able to be at home during times when the patient with cancer requires the greatest amount of care. Employed caregivers may not have enough time available for caregiving, and their job performance may be negatively affected through decreased productivity and quality of work. Caregivers' health and social roles may also change. Nurses need to be cognizant of the needs of these family members and must help them prepare for the immediate and ongoing requirements of caregiving. They can also assist family members by ensuring that patient appointments are not delayed and by being available for questions or care after normal working hours.

For many patients and their families, cancer survivorship may bring financial problems. In addition to direct medical treatment costs, patients spend a significant amount of their earnings and savings for "ancillary" expenditures. Some patients may even be required to modify their homes to accommodate special beds, wheelchairs, or other durable equipment. Lost earnings due to the inability to work is included in patients' expenses as well. Other family members may also be required to miss work. Therefore, even those who are insured can be financially crippled by substantial gaps in coverage.

Persons with few financial resources are more likely to be diagnosed with cancer when the disease is advanced and treatment options are limited. Because they have limited access to treatment, they may also have limited access to community services and ongoing care because referrals for these services are often made from within the medical care system. Financial problems may inhibit treatment, making cancer more costly in the long run. These patients are likely to experience greater morbidity and shorter survival.

Regardless of their socioeconomic status, all families are likely to experience financial burdens due to gaps in insurance coverage, lost wages, and out-of-pocket expenditures for rehabilitation, special equipment, and/or special clothing. In a study of survivors of breast cancer, Polinsky reported that 19% reported their income was inadequate to cover their medical care, 63% reported that they had inadequate insurance, and 44% worried about future health expenditures because they were concerned that they would not be able to afford the escalating cost.[46] Nurses, patients, and family members together must consider future care needs. Nurses can help patients and families devise a plan to prepare for future expenditures.

Summary of Recommendations for Care

Throughout the care trajectory, family members will have to assume new roles and reorganize established and familiar roles due to the nature of the needs of the patient with cancer. Recommendations for nurses caring for cancer survivors can be summarized as follows:

- Educate patients and their families on the disease and its anticipated trajectory.
- Educate patients and their families on treatment modalities and long-term consequences of those treatments and on the necessity for long-term follow-up.
- Equip patients with skill-building activities aimed at enhancing self-efficacy and improving self-management behaviors.
- Educate patients and their families on common symptoms and adverse effects of treatment and provide strategies for their management.
- Foster a spirit of teamwork among patients, families, and healthcare providers, especially with relation to the long-term effects of cancer and its treatment.
- Help patients learn the communication styles that are necessary to express economic, social, and psychological needs so that healthcare providers can respond.
- Help patients and their families anticipate and plan for time away from work, and advise them to be prepared for long-term accommodations.
- Make patients and family members aware of their rights at work. Help them understand and anticipate problems so they can proactively problem solve before discrimination or other problems occur.
- Become knowledgeable in studies of cost-effectiveness of alternative therapies so that treatment decisions incorporate economic concerns.
- Understand patients' insurance limitations in coverage and advocate for patients with their insurance providers, where possible.
- Help patients project their out-of-pocket expenses and develop strategies to minimize these costs (e.g., physician prescriptions for equipment and supplies that are needed for long-term effects).
- Develop a transition plan for each patient as he or she leaves the active treatment phase and moves to survivorship.
- Assist patients and families in taking responsibility for their healthcare through self-advocacy, and make patients and their families aware of resources available to them. Patients need to be assisted to develop a personal wellness plan to improve their overall functioning and quality of life. This will include paying attention to exercise and nutrition for improved energy, restoration of mental energy, and stress reduction strategies.
- Assist patients to develop strategies for obtaining needed support following completion of treatment, including the return to social relationships foregone during the treatment. It is important to plan such a return to social function. Communication skills that ease interpersonal and social adjustments should also be encouraged.
- Develop a discharge plan for follow-up care.
- Become familiar with survivor groups (both general and disease-specific) that may further assist patients and their families and help them to become advocates for their own healthcare.
- Encourage patients to talk to job counselors so that employment options or creative work changes can be considered.
- All patients should be given documents on employment rights of cancer survivor and financial help for cancer survivors.

Table 69-4 Survivorship Worksheet

Employment

1. How much time should the patient plan to be away from work during the acute treatment phase?
2. What are the expected side effects from treatment?
3. Will the side effects of treatment affect the patient's ability to perform his or her job in the short term? The long term?
4. Will the side effects of treatment interfere with the patient's ability to perform his or her job? How long will treatment continue?
5. What can be done to reduce the impact on the patient's job? Is job sharing an option?
6. Should the patient consider a job change? Different job? Fewer hours?
7. How much time should the caregiver plan to be away from work while the patient is undergoing treatment?
8. If the patient decides to quit his or her job, has he or she considered how such a decision will affect health insurance and retirement benefits?
9. Is the patient aware of legislative protections under the Americans with Disabilities Act and the Family Medical Leave Act?

Insurance

1. Will patient's health insurance coverage be affected by a change in his or her employment?
2. If yes, is the patient a candidate for Medicaid or Social Security Disability Insurance?
3. If yes, will the patient have to change healthcare providers?
4. If no, what are the patient's alternative plans for health insurance?

Estimate of Out-of-Pocket Expenses

Co-payments
Visits per month @ $xx.xx/per visit
Deductible
Prescription medication
Over-the-counter medication
Equipment, supplies, wigs
Transportation costs
Child care costs
Lost wages
Clinical trial participation
Monthly total

Rehabilitation Needs/Referrals

1. Physical therapy
2.
3.

Supportive Services/Referrals

1. Self-advocacy training
2. Support groups

Psychosocial Assessment

Date:
Findings:

Community Services/Referrals

1. Home care and chore services
2. Transportation
3. Meals

Other Resources (Books, Web Sites)

1.
2.

When the patient is unable to participate in self-care activities, such as during chemotherapy, family caregivers will need to reassign or relinquish long-held roles to assist the patient and to ensure that care needs are being met. As the patient regains the ability to perform self-care tasks, the caregiver may be able, to some extent, reclaim previously reassigned and relinquished roles. Nevertheless, throughout the care trajectory, family members will have to assume some new roles and reorganize established and familiar roles due to the nature of the needs of the patient with cancer. The unpredictability and fluid nature of the caregiving role make it difficult for family caregivers to plan for their own needs for social and leisure time. Nurses need to be aware of the needs of family members and provide information on support groups and resources that are available in their community. Helping them to adjust and reduce care when the patient has recovered is also important. Nurses need to assist family members in understanding the long-term effects, as often the family members are ready for care to cease and return to normalcy once the treatment is complete. Family members may not understand the long-term effects of fatigue, depression, cognitive alterations, or disability of an arm or numbness that result from use of certain types of drugs.

Because of improved treatment regimens and greater longevity following a cancer diagnosis, an understanding of survivorship issues will become increasingly more important for patients, families, and healthcare professionals alike. Nurses in cancer care need to continue examining survivorship issues as they develop plans of care because this phase, whether short or long, is vitally important to those who have endured the diagnosis and treatment.

Oncology nurses must be sensitive to survivorship issues in their discharge plans and as they refer patients back to their primary care provider at the close of active treatment. Psychosocial assessment is as important as biomedical examinations. Programs geared toward the survivor must address not only patients' physical activities, but also the daily demands (e.g., employment, insurance) they are likely to face once they leave the acute treatment phase. The worksheet in Table 69-4 can serve as a template for the survivorship plan.

Most cancer survivors will seek long-term care from primary care providers (physicians and nurse practioners).[68] Correct identification of patients with a cancer history is the first step toward making an accurate assessment of their needs. Nurses can take a lead role in trying to determine the history of cancer patients and in considering cancer and its effects in their usual plan of primary care and health promotion and health maintenance activities. Information about the treatment regimen and potential long-term sequelae, including second malignancies or recurrences, helps to prepare survivors to recognize the importance of monitoring symptoms[67] and being vigilant in their follow-up care. Nurses can assume a leadership role in the continuity of care geared toward the social, economic, and psychological needs of survivors. Given the high percentage of patients who have unmet psychological and socioeconomic needs, more attention is needed to guide patients to report a history of cancer. Nurse practioners in primary care and primary care providers are well suited to perform this assessment and to provide follow-up care.

Part of the nurse's challenge is to educate survivors and their families to access information and resources appropriate to their needs, values, and beliefs.[56] Because such a diversity of resources exists, patients must be prompted to become active participants in their health care. Nurses should prepare patients and their family members to advocate for themselves in matters concerning their health and to include the previous diagnosis of cancer and cancer treatment in discussions with healthcare providers. These individuals need to feel empowered so that they can communicate effectively and access the care they need. It is critical that survivors enjoy a sense of control in their lives and continue to face the challenges inherent in managing cancer and navigating the healthcare system.

The NCCS stresses the need for rehabilitative services, psychosocial services, and a choice of interventions and training in cancer-related self-advocacy, information-seeking, negotiation, communication, and problem-solving skills. For many patients, self-advoca-

Table 69-5 Internet Sites and Telephone Numbers for Cancer Information

National Cancer Institute (NCI)	*www.cancer.gov*	800-4-CANCER
NCI publications list	*http://cissecure.nci.nih.gov/ncipubs*	800-4-CANCER
NCI clinical trials information	*http://nci.nih.gov/clinicaltrials*	800-4-CANCER
NCI cancer information	*http://nci.nih.gov/cancerinfo*	800-4-CANCER
OncoLink	*http://oncolink.upenn.edu*	
American Cancer Society	*www.cancer.org*	800-ACS-2345
National Coalition for Cancer Survivorship	*www.canceradvocacy.org*	888-937-6227 (888-YES-NCCS)
Association of Community Cancer Centers	*www.accc-cancer.org*	301-984-9496
Oncology Nursing Society	*www.ons.org/*	
Wisconsin Cancer Pain Resource Center	*www.wisc.edu/molpharm/wcpi*	
National Comprehensive Cancer Network	*www.nccn.org*	888-909-NCCN
Family Care Research Program	*www.healthteam.msu.edu/fcrp/*	888-353-0306
Candlelighters Childhood Cancer Foundation	*www.candlelighters.org*	800-366-2223
Health Insurance Association of America	*www.hiaa.org/consumer/insurance_counsel.cfm*	202-824-1600
Cancer Care, Inc.	*www.cancercare.org*	800-813-HOPE
Patient Advocate Foundation	*www.patientadvocate.org/*	757-873-6668
Medicare Helpline	*www.cms.hhs.gov/*	800-444-4606
American Association of Health Plans	*www.aahp.org/template.cfm*	202-778-3200

cy and problem solving are skills that must be acquired. Fortunately, many survivorship groups offer classes in communication, negotiation, information seeking, and problem solving. Referral to these groups may be appropriate for many patients. Table 69-5 lists Internet sites and telephone numbers that may be useful in locating resources that may be of benefit over the longterm.

Conclusion

Despite the many challenges, cancer survivorship is cause for celebration for patients and their families. Nurses can play an important role in guiding patients and their families through the survivorship phase. The most visionary institutions are those that successfully combine state-of-the-art treatment programs with strong, active survivor programs.[56] The physical, economic, and social issues confronting patients and their families during the survival period are an integral part of cancer care. The care of the cancer patient does not end after the initial treatment phase.

References

1. American Cancer Society: *Cancer Facts and Figures.* Atlanta, American Cancer Society, 2003
2. Tamlyn-Leaman K: Adult cancer survivorship issues and challenges. *Can Oncol Nurs J* 5:45–47, 1995
3. National Cancer Institute: Office of Cancer Survivorship, Fact Sheet, *:http://survivorship.cancer.gov.* Accessed February 18, 2004
4. Hewitt M, Rowland J, Yancik R: Cancer survivors in the US: age, health and disability. *J Gerontol Med Sci* 58:82–91, 2003
5. Quigley KM: The adult cancer survivor: psychosocial consequences of cure. *Semin Oncol Nurs* 5:63–39, 1989
6. Leigh S: Survivorship, in Sigler B, George LM (eds.): *Psychosocial Dimensions of Oncology Nursing Care.* Pittsburgh, Oncology Nursing Press, 1998, pp 130–148
7. Stafford RS, Cyr PL: The impact of cancer on the physical function of the elderly and their utilization of health care. *Cancer* 80:1973–1980, 1997
8. Fow NR: Cancer rehabilitation: an investment in survivorship. As more people survive the disease, focus shifts on improving quality of life. *Rehabil Manage* 9:48–53, 1996
9. Mock V: Fatigue management: evidence and guidelines for practice. *Cancer* 92(suppl):1699–1707, 2001
10. Schwartz AL, Mori M, Gao R, et al: Exercise reduces daily fatigue in women with breast cancer receiving chemotherapy. *Med Sci Sports Exerc* 33:718–723, 2001
11. Cella D, Tulsky D, Gray G, et al: The functional assessment of cancer therapy scale: development and validation of the general measure. *J Clin Oncol* 11:570–579, 1993
12. Twycross R, Harcourt J, Bergl S: A survey of pain in patients with advanced cancer. *J Pain Symptom Manage* 12:273–282, 1996
13. Ware J, Sherbourne C: The SF-36 short-form health status survey. I. Conceptual framework and item selection. *Med Care* 30:473–483, 1992
14. Jensen S, Given B: Fatigue affecting family caregivers of cancer patients. *Support Care Cancer* 1:321–325, 1993
15. Shulz R: Caregiving as a risk factor for mortality: the Caregiver Health Effects Study *JAMA* 282:2215–2219, 1999
16. Kurtz M, Kurtz J, Given C, et al: Relationship of caregiver reaction and depression to cancer patients, symptoms, functional status and depression — a longitudinal view. *Soc Sci Med* 40:837–846, 1995
17. Given C, Given B, Stommel M, et al: The impact of new demands for assistance on caregiver depression: tests using an inception cohort. *Gerontologist* 39:76–85, 1999
18. Braithwaite V: Between stressors and outcomes: can we simplify the care-giving process variables? *Gerontologist* 36:42–53, 1996
19. Krach P, Brooks JA: Identifying the responsibilities and needs of working adults who are primary caregivers. *J Gerontol Nurs* 21:41–50, 1995
20. Hoyert DL, Seltzer MM: Factors relating to the well-being and life activities of family caregivers. *Fam Relations* 41:74–81, 1992
21. Fisher B, Dignam J, Tan-Chiu E, et al: Prognosis and treatment of patients with breast tumors of one centimeter or less and negative axillary lymph nodes. *J Natl Cancer Inst* 93:112–120, 2001
22. Craig TJ, Comstock GW, Geiser PB: The quality of survival in breast cancer: a case-control comparison. *Cancer* 33:1451–1457, 1974
23. Van Tulder MW, Aaronson NK, Bruning PF: The quality of life of long-term cancer survivors of Hodgkin's disease. *Ann Oncol* 5:153–158, 1994
24. Kornblith AB: Psychosocial adaptation of cancer survivors, in Holland JC, Rowland J (eds.): *Psycho-oncology.* New York, Oxford University Press, 1998, pp 223–241
25. Razavi D, Delvaux N, Bredart A, et al: Professional rehabilitation of lymphoma patients: a study of psychosocial factors associated with return to work. *Support Care Cancer* 1:276–278, 1993
26. van der Wouden MC, Greaves-Otte JGW, Greaves J, et al: Occupational reintegration of long-term cancer survivors. *J Occup Med* 34:1084–1089, 1992
27. Schagen SB, Frits SAM, van Dam M, et al: Cognitive deficits after postoperative adjuvant chemotherapy for breast carcinoma. *Cancer* 85:640–650, 1999
28. Satariano WA, DeLorenze GN: The likelihood of returning to work after breast cancer. *Public Health Rep* 111:236–241, 1996
29. Greenwald HP, Dirks SJ, Borgatta EF, et al: Work disability among cancer patients. *Soc Sci Med* 29:1253–1259, 1989
30. Carter B: Surviving cancer: a problematic work re-entry. *Cancer Pract* 2:135–140, 1994
31. Berry DL: Return-to-work experiences of people with cancer. *Oncol Nurs Forum* 20:905–911, 1993
32. Bradley, C., Neumark, D., Bednarek, H., et al: Combining registry, primary, and secondary data sources to identify the impact of cancer on labor market outcomes. *Med Decis Making* (in press)
33. Ashles TA, Saykin AJ, Furstenberg CT, et al: Neuropsychologic impact of standard dose systemic chemotherapy in long-term survivors of breast cancer and lymphoma. *J Clin Oncol* 20:485–493, 2002
34. Lippman ME, Hayes DF: Adjuvant therapy for all patients with breast cancer? *J Natl Cancer Inst* 93:80–82, 2001
35. Olin JJ: Cognitive function after systemic therapy for breast cancer. *Oncology* 15:613–618, 2001
36. Maunsell E, Brisson J, Deschenes L: Arm problems and psychological distress after surgery for breast cancer. *Can J Surg* 36:315–320, 1993
37. Yap KP, McCready DR, Narod S, et al: Factors influencing arm and axillary symptoms after treatment for node negative breast carcinoma. *Cancer* 97:1369–1375, 2003

38. Bradley CJ, Bednarek HL, Neumark D, et al: Short-term effects of breast cancer on labor market attachment: results from a longitudinal study. *J Health Econ* 24:137–160, 2005
39. Ganz PA, Coscarelli A, Fred C, et al: Breast cancer survivors: psychosocial concerns and quality of life. *Breast Cancer Res Treat* 38:183–199, 1996
40. Ganz P, Desmond K, Leedham B, et al: Quality of life in long-term, disease-free survivors of breast cancer: a follow-up study. *J Natl Cancer Inst* 94:39–49, 2002
41. Bradley C, Bedarek H, Neumark D, et al: Breast cancer survival, work, and earnings. *J Health Econ* 21:757–779, 2002
42. Stewart DE, Cheung AM, Duff S, et al: Long-term breast cancer survivors: confidentiality, disclosure, effects on work and insurance. *Psychooncology* 10:259–263, 2001
43. Chirikos TN, Russell-Jacobs A, Cantor AB: Indirect economic effects of long-term breast cancer survival. *Cancer Pract* 10:248–255, 2002
44. Loprest P, Rupp K, Sandell SH: Gender, disabilities, and employment in the health and retirement study. *J Hum Resources* 30(suppl):S293–S318, 1995
45. Bound J, Schoenbaum M, Waidmann R: Race and education differences in disability status and labor force attachment in the health and retirement study. *J Hum Resources* 30(suppl): S227–S267, 1995
46. Polinsky ML: Functional status of long-term breast cancer survivors: demonstrating chronicity. *Health Soc Work* 19:165–173, 1944
47. Cooper PF, Monheit AC: Does employment-related health insurance inhibit job mobility? *Inquiry* 30:400–416, 1993
48. Palmore E, Burchett B, Fillenbaum G, et al (eds.): *Retirement: Causes and Consequences.* New York, Springer, 1985
49. Bednarek H, Bradley, C: Work and retirement beyond cancer diagnosis. *Res Nurs Health* (in press)
50. Sivesind D, Rohaly-Davis J: Coping with cancer: patient issues, in Burke C (ed.): *Psychosocial Dimensions of Oncology Nursing Care.* Pittsburgh, Oncology Nursing Press, 1998, pp 3-26
51. Cimprich B, Ronis D: Attention and symptom distress in women with and without breast cancer. *Nurs Res* 50:86–94, 2001
52. Abeloff MD (ed.): Lawyer tells cancer patients how to fight job discrimination. *Oncol News Int* 7:34–35, 1998
53. Guidry JJ, Aday L, Zhang D, et al: Cost considerations as potential barriers to cancer treatment. *Cancer Pract* 6:182–187, 1998
54. Glajchen M: Psychosocial consequences of inadequate health insurance for patients with cancer. *Cancer Pract* 2:115–120, 1994
55. Franks P, Nutting PA, Clancy CM: Health care reform, primary care, and the need for research. *JAMA* 270:1449–1453, 1993
56. Leigh S: Cancer survivorship: a consumer movement. *Semin Oncol* 21:783–786, 1994
57. Card IC: National coalition for cancer survivorship perspective. *Proc Am Cancer Soc Workshop on Children.* Atlanta, American Cancer Society, 1991
58. Boring CG, Squires TS, Tong T: Cancer statistics. *CA Cancer J Clin* 42:19–38, 1992
59. Leake AR: The economic impact of cancer. *Nurse Pract Forum* 6:207–214, 1995
60. Berkman BJ, Sampson SE: Psychosocial effects of cancer economics on patients and their families. *Cancer* 72(suppl): 2846–2849, 1993
61. Thorpe KE, Howard D: Health insurance and spending among cancer patients. *Health Aff* W3-189–98(suppl), 2003
62. Goldman DP, Berry SH, McCabe MS, et al: Incremental treatment costs in National Cancer Institute–Sponsored clinical trials. *JAMA* 289:2970–2977, 2003
63. Beltz SE, Yee GC: Pharmacoeconomics of cancer therapy. *Cancer Control* 5:415–424, 1998
64. Gold MR, Siegel JE, Rusell LB, Weinstein MC (eds.): *Cost-Effectiveness in Health and Medicine.* New York, Oxford University Press, 1996
65. Ganz PA, Greendale GA, Petersen L, et al: Breast cancer in younger women: reproductive and late health effects of treatment. *J Clin Oncol* 21:4184–4193, 2003
66. Stommel M, Given CW, Given BA: The cost of cancer home care to families. *Cancer* 71:1867–1874, 1993
67. Robinson KM: Family caregiving: who provides the care, and at what cost? *Nurs Econ* 15:243–247, 1997
68. Hayman JA, Langa KM, Kabeto MU, et al: Estimating the cost of informal caregiving for elderly patients with cancer. *J Clin Oncol* 19:3219–3225, 2001

CHAPTER 70

Spiritual Responses to Cancer

Elizabeth Johnston Taylor, PhD, RN

Introduction

> I had to do a crash course in spirituality. I mean, you may be facing the end of your life. . . . I started going back to church and trying to investigate my feelings about God, and about what would happen after I die. . . . At one point you're facing death, and then the next point you're like facing, "What am I going to eat for breakfast tomorrow morning?" . . . That's what I think I came to terms with after crying for 6 months, that, you know, either this is it and you might as well die right now, or you can have a life. It's your choice. So I said, "OK, I'm going to have a life."

This statement about living with breast cancer by a 40-year-old woman poignantly describes a pervasive experience among cancer survivors. When diagnosed with cancer, individuals inevitably become more aware of their personal vulnerability and mortality. Heightened spiritual awareness is a typical response to this threat to self. The cancer experience not only prompts spiritual questions, struggles, and triumphs, but may also inspire continued or renewed use of spiritual resources for coping. Because the spirit is an innate and influential aspect of being human, it is valuable for nurses to consider how spiritual responses to cancer might affect the illness experience.

This chapter reviews recent research that describes spiritual responses across the cancer continuum. The spiritual perspectives of cancer patients, family caregivers, and oncology nurses are discussed. The chapter concludes with a brief discussion of fundamental skills that nurses must practice to provide care that nurtures the spiritual health of patients and their family members. First, however, it is necessary to define what spirituality is and examine why it is important to address in oncology nursing care.

Definitions

Before a discussion using the easily misunderstood terms of *spirituality* and *religiosity* proceeds, the terms must be defined. *Spirituality* refers to that dimension of being human that motivates meaning-making and self-transcendence — or intra-, inter-, and transpersonal connectedness.[1,2] In nursing literature that defines related terms such as spiritual distress, need, or well-being; one will find spirituality described as an integrating energy, a life principle, an innate human quality.[3] Spirituality prompts individuals to make sense of their universe and to relate harmoniously with self, nature, and others — including any god(s), as conceptualized by each person.

In contrast to spirituality, *religiosity* often is viewed as a narrower concept.[3,4] Religion is a representation and expression of spirituality. A religion offers an individual a specific worldview and an explanation that seeks to provide answers to the questions of ultimate meaning; it also may recommend how one is to live harmoniously with self, others, nature, and god(s). Such explanations and recommendations are presented in a religion's belief system (e.g., myths/stories, doctrines, dogmas) and are remembered and appreciated with rituals and other religious practices or observances. One's religion may or may not be of an institutional nature.

Why Address Spirituality?

Numerous reasons could be given for why oncology nurses must include spiritual care in nursing practice. Taylor[5] identified four reasons:

1. Spirituality is part of the whole person. Given that nursing appreciates the necessity of providing holistic care, spiritual care is fundamental to nursing care. It will nurture health in general, too.
2. Spiritual awareness increases when life is threatened — that is, when the sense of self is threatened. Nurses must be sensitive to such responses to illness and understand how they affect patients.
3. Empirical studies have demonstrated significant relationships between spirituality and other health-related variables (e.g., quality of life) among people with cancer. If nurses are interested in addressing factors that relate directly to health and quality of life, then they must address patients' spirituality.
4. Pragmatic reasons for addressing spirituality in oncology nursing include mandates (such as the Joint Commission's demand that all institutions assess spiritual beliefs and practices and make spiritual support available), and potential marketing and economic benefits.

These reasons are complemented by the fact that the role of nursing lends itself well to at least an initial level of spiritual caregiving. For example, nurses are in a position to have established rapport with patients, and nurses' constant presence allows them to observe and address spiritual needs.

Spirituality Throughout the Cancer Experience

A review of research between 1990 and 1999 published in three oncology nursing journals revealed that 17% of all studies investigated some aspect of spirituality or religion.[6] Empirical research studying spirituality in the context of health has, indeed, flourished during the past decade; much of it investigates the spirituality of persons living or dying with cancer.[3] Although much of this research has focused on women (especially those with breast cancer) and whites, some studies have examined persons newly diagnosed, actively living with cancer or in treatment, surviving, and dying from cancer. A few studies have explored how spirituality may influence cancer screening and prediagnostic experiences of cancer. Following is a summary of research from the past decade that provides evidence about spirituality during different phases of the cancer experience.

Cancer Screening and Prediagnosis

A handful of studies suggest that religion may play a significant role in cancer screening practices among women. Strickland and colleagues[7] conducted three years of participant observation in a Yakima Indian community to understand how these Native Americans' religion could assist in designing a cervical cancer prevention project. These nurses learned that a health promotion project in this community would be culturally sensitive if three criteria were met: (1) goals were holistic and wellness oriented, (2) the community's elders were involved, and (3) role models, storytelling, talking circles, and other circular symbols were used when teaching. Yi[8] observed that Vietnamese women living in Massachusetts were less likely to have had a Pap smear if they were Buddhist compared to the Christian subjects ($p = 0.028$). It is possible that the women who ascribed to the Western religion of Christianity also ascribed to Western medical recommendations. Pakistani researchers[9] found that 53% of women recently diagnosed with breast cancer delayed seeking medical help; 15% reported using various spiritual therapies in attempts to rid themselves of the breast lump. Although not systematically researched, clinical observation taught Underwood and colleagues[10] that the religio-cultural beliefs of Muslims about modesty deterred women from performing and receiving breast examinations.

A few researchers have recognized that a fatalistic attitude toward cancer does occur in some cultural groups and presumably affects what one believes about cancer screening and how one treats cancer. Fatalism essentially reflects one's worldview, or personal philosophical framework that is shaped largely by spirituality. A fatalistic attitude is illustrated by comments such as "My cancer is God's will, so there is nothing I can do about it." The belief that God determines whether one will die or be cured of cancer was found to be stronger among African Americans than whites in the southern United States.[11] Phillips[12] described how low- and middle-income African American women are fearful, fatalistic, and silent about breast cancer. Holt and colleagues[13] observed a strong active and passive spiritual locus of control [i.e., believing God empowers individuals to take care of themselves (active) versus believing that control rests with God (passive)] among 1227 African American women surveyed about mammography. Although the study used weak instrumentation, the findings indicated that God orientation among black women may be associated with perceiving more barriers and fewer benefits to mammography, which in turn influences mammography utilization. These attitudes presumably contribute to African American women's tendency to delay their visits to healthcare centers for cancer screening and treatment and, therefore, they have higher mortality rates for breast cancer compared to American women of European descent. A fatalistic attitude toward breast cancer was also observed, however, in one small study of Jewish Israeli women among those from Muslim countries but not their cohorts from U.S. or European backgrounds.[14] VandeCreek and colleagues[15] found that fatalism was positively correlated with use of prayer in a large sample of mostly Euro-American women with breast cancer. Although fatalism may be pronounced among certain ethnic groups, these studies suggest it may be present in many and diverse cultures.

Diagnosis

Nearly 30 years ago, Weisman and Worden[16] described the first 100 days after a diagnosis of cancer as an "existential plight." Subsequently, very little research has focused on the spiritual responses to the diagnostic phase. Because receiving the diagnosis of cancer is typically devastating, or unsettling at best, it is likely that it can be a time of petitionary prayer or invocations of magic, questions about the nature of God, or calls for support from a spiritual community. A study of 73 women diagnosed within the past three months indicated that religious beliefs were considered very helpful in coping with treatment (mean of 7.8 on scale of 1–9).[17] Conversely, two studies with inadequately small samples provided tentative evidence that newly diagnosed persons with cancer may rely on their "faith" less than counterparts with advanced cancer.[18,19]

A qualitative study of 33 elderly women who had been diagnosed with breast cancer during the past six months found that spirituality and religion gave these women emotional and social support, as well as meaning during a frightening and despairing time.[20] For example, attending religious services, doing religious volunteer work, and having a warm relationship with a religious leader functioned to provide social support. Relating to God brought comfort, companionship, inner strength, guidance, and well-being to these women, who often feared sharing their inner thoughts and worries with their families. Feher and Maly,[20] who initially asked these informants about their emotional responses to diagnosis, noted that it was not until they asked about spiritual responses that a stoic façade was dropped and informants divulged the degree of distress they had experienced.

The diagnostic phase usually includes the process of determining how to treat the cancer. A case study of one woman's decision-making after a diagnosis of leukemia identified spirituality as a factor contributing to this challenging process.[21] Shannon-Dorcy and Wolfe[21] noted that spiritual questions arise, such as "Where is God in the midst of this?"; "Does my faith answer questions or create them?"; and "Do I use my spirituality to help me make decisions?". A qualitative study revealed that cancer patients may pray about these decisions; they bring to God the questions of which physician and which treatment plan, and ask for providential guidance.[22] In a study of 218 patients designed to determine why African Americans infrequently join clinical trials, Advani and colleagues[11] found that a belief in God, along with low income and education, predicted unwillingness to participate in a cancer clinical trial. These findings suggest how spiritual beliefs can determine not only whether persons seek screening, but also which decisions about cancer treatment are made.

Living with Cancer

Research and clinical observations suggest that individuals living with cancer have a heightened spiritual awareness.[20,23,24] This heightened awareness of personal spirituality may manifest itself as spiritual or existential distress or increased spiritual well-being.

Spiritual needs

Regardless of whether patients experience spiritual distress or eustress, spiritual needs are an inherent part of living.[3] A qualitative study of 28 cancer patients and family caregivers identified seven categories of spiritual needs.[25] These categories, along with their respective themes, are presented in Table 70-1. Although no other investigations have scientifically inducted the spiritual needs of nonterminal patients with cancer, a survey of 248 cancer patients showed that more than 40% wanted help with overcoming fears, finding hope, and finding meaning in life and peace of mind.[26] Those with the highest self-reported spiritual needs were those who were unmarried, recently diagnosed, or Hispanic American or African American. Ethnicity, in fact, was found to be the best predictor of many spiritual needs.

Search for meaning

The spiritual needs of persons living with cancer are not only varied, but often deeply painful and distressing. The search for meaning, or the yearning to make sense of a senseless disease and suffering, can plague many patients.[27] Inner questions that may be discomforting to voice (or thought to be forbidden by religion) may include "Why do bad things happen, especially since I was good?" and "Why me? Why now?" The search for meaning can include an attempt to attribute causality (what caused the cancer), selective incidence (why a certain person got it), blame (what is responsible), or significance (positive meanings of an ultimate nature).

Although most of the research describing the search for meaning has focused on cancer survivors, a few studies have described it among persons living with active disease. For example, a qualitative study of 9 women with ovarian cancer identified "finding meaning in life" as the care category in the data.[28] Finding meaning involved self-reflection, reappraisal of life, and development of new short-term life goals. Although patients can get "stuck" attempting to find meaningfulness in having cancer (28% in a study of 60 women surviving breast cancer), many are able to ascribe positive meanings in a way that is spiritually transformative.[29] A qualitative study of 24 women with breast cancer described the process and outcomes of transforming the tragedy of cancer.[30] Stages of this transformative process included the following:

- "Encountering the darkness": entertaining the painful doubts and "why?" questions; often experiencing depression
- "Converting the darkness": beginning to live beyond the questions, recognizing they may be unanswerable; considering "wherefore?" rather than "why?"
- "Encountering the light": finding positive meanings or outcomes; ascribing significance
- "Reflecting the light": behaving in ways that reflect the inner experience of spiritual transformation, such as helping others with cancer more or being more empathic toward others' suffering

Taylor[30] identified several categories of significance or positive meanings that these women ascribed to their cancer: reevaluating and reprioritizing personal values; reconsidering the direction and mission of life; having a sense of urgency, intentionality, and immediacy about life; appreciating profoundly with

Table 70-1 Themes and Categories of Spiritual Needs

Categories	Themes/Spiritual Needs
Needs associated with relating to an Ultimate Other	Need to . . . • Know God's will • Resign yourself to God being in control of your/your loved one's illness • Get right with God • Believe that God has or will heal • Remember how God has guided or helped you/your loved one • Feel that there is Something out there looking after you/your loved one • Know that your/your loved one's situation is in God's hands
Need for positivity, gratitude, and hope	Need to . . . • Have hope that you/your loved one will be well • Keep a positive outlook • Count your blessings • Tell others about the good things in your life • Just enjoy life • Have confidence/faith within yourself • Not take life for granted
Need to give and receive love from other persons	Need to. . . • Make the world a better place • Return others' kindnesses • Protect your family from seeing you suffer • Try to help others • Get right with others (e.g., forgiving or being forgiven) • Become more gracious about receiving care from other people • Know that others are praying (or thinking positive thoughts) for you • Be appreciated by others • Be with others you consider to be family • Not be a burden to others
Need to review beliefs	Need to . . . • Review what you believe • Wonder if your beliefs about God are correct • Think about what it means to live spiritually (e.g., to have faith, to forgive) • Ask "Why?" questions (e.g., Why me/us? Or why not me? Or what did I/we do to deserve this?) • Think about the unfairness of what has been happening to you
Creating meaning, finding purpose	Need to . . . • Get over or past asking "Why me?" • Find helpful explanations for why this illness happened • Become aware of positive things that have come with this illness • Realize that other people are worse off • Sense that there is a reason for being alive now • Try to make life count • Lessen the frustration of not being able to do meaningful things • Reevaluate your life
Religious needs	Need to . . . • Participate in a religious or spiritual meeting (e.g., worship at a church) • Listen to religious programs or music on TV or radio • Pray privately • Read scripture or spirit-nurturing material • Have quiet time or space to reflect or meditate
Preparing for Death	Need to . . . • Make sure personal business is in order, just in case of death • Balance thoughts about dying with hoping for health • Know that there will be a purpose for your/your loved one's death, whenever it happens

Reprinted with permission from Taylor, EJ: Spiritual needs of cancer patients and family caregivers. *Cancer Nurs* 26:260–266, 2003[25] joy the gifts of life and nature; having a more intense spiritual awareness; and becoming more self-respectful or self-aware.

Forgiveness

One of the spiritual needs of persons living with cancer identified in the Taylor study was the need to give and receive love by "getting right" in wronged relationships.[25] Only one study explored this spiritual response among persons with cancer. Mickley and Cowles's[31] qualitative study of 25 living and dying patients described how forgiveness was used to heal the tension between living with negative emotions and personal values that condemn the angry and bitter response toward another. These investigators observed that patients processed through phases of "I won't forgive" to "I can't forgive" to "Should I forgive?" before they reached a resolution involving forgiveness.

Hope

A few studies of persons living with cancer link hope with various aspects of spirituality.[17,23] Post-White and colleagues[32] interviewed 32 individuals who were actively or palliatively being treated for cancer. These data, like previous research, demonstrated that spiritual beliefs and practices and finding meaning were integral to maintaining hope. Fehring and colleagues[33] also observed among 100 elders with cancer that intrinsic religiosity (i.e., an integrated, lived religion rather than an extrinsic religion used for social or other gain) and spiritual well-being were highly correlated with hope ($r = 0.58$ and $r = 0.75$, respectively).

Use of prayer and other spiritual resources

A number of studies have documented the pervasive use of religious or spiritual beliefs and practices among persons living with cancer.[23,34–36] For example, in a survey of 108 women with various stages of gynecologic cancer, 76% reported religion to be important, and 49% indicated they had become more religious since their diagnosis.[23] Religious beliefs and practices are often considered coping strategies by researchers.[34,35] A qualitative study of 143 Hawaiian cancer patients, however, enumerated other reasons for why patients use these spiritual resources.[36] Tatsumura and colleagues[36] noted that spiritual resources not only supported treatment or cure, but also provided the possibility of treatment or cure, and were used simply because they were part of the patients' lives.

Several studies of complementary and alternative medicine (CAM) used by persons with cancer have documented the frequency and perceived helpfulness of prayer and other spiritual resources or "therapies."[15,36–41] The CAM options that appear to most reflect spirituality and religiosity include prayer (personal and from others), "spiritual healing," church-related activities, personal faith, counseling with religious leader, scripture reading, attending religious services, meditation, spending time where spiritual energy is felt, and help from ancestors. Prayer is a common CAM, with 59%–76% reporting use of it—a significantly higher percentage than reported by samples of the general population surveyed regarding CAM use.[15,42]

A study of 30 cancer patients found that for some persons with cancer, the intensity and frequency with which they pray increased as they lived with cancer.[22] These informants prayed for many things, including both physical concerns (especially pain and distressing symptoms) and spiritual concerns ("Why?"). While some denied petitioning God for a cure, others prayed for healing in a vague way or for "God's will." A secondary analysis of these data revealed that beliefs about prayer can also contribute to spiritual distress, such as questions about why God doesn't "answer" or whether God exists.[43]

Spiritual well-being and quality of life

While much of the research about spirituality in the context of cancer describes spiritual responses and needs or the use of spiritual resources to cope, a number of studies have investigated the relationship between spirituality and quality of life among persons with cancer. Five quality of life instruments designed for use among persons with cancer include spirituality subscales.[44] This research indicates that persons living with cancer typically rank spiritual quality of life second highest in importance, after physical quality of life.[45–47]

Several studies have also documented that spiritual well-being or spiritual quality of life is strongly and positively correlated with overall quality of life.[44] For example, Fisch and colleagues[48] found that more than half of 163 patients with noncurable cancer receiving therapies in an ambulatory care clinic had high spiritual well-being and that spiritual quality of life correlated with overall quality of life ($r = 0.56$, $p < 0.0001$). Other studies have suggested that spiritual well-being is directly correlated with a fighting spirit, hope, life satisfaction, happiness, and other positive moods. Conversely, spiritual well-being is negatively correlated with depression, anxiety, pain level, demands of illness, and negative moods.[44] Certain demographic factors have also been found to correlate with spiritual quality of life—namely, being female, older, married, or living with children may be related to higher spiritual quality of life.[49–52] Although spiritual well-being consistently correlates with overall quality of life and adjustment, a study of 142 women with breast cancer suggests that spiritual well-being may not predict quality of life much, once adjustment style and demographic factors are controlled.[53]

Surviving Cancer

Many studies examining spirituality among persons with cancer actually sample cancer survivors — that is, persons who have completed treatment and are disease free. This body of research includes mostly descriptive studies about the positive meanings of having cancer and spiritual quality of life among survivors. Many of the findings about how cancer survivors ascribe meaning and are spiritually transformed parallel the findings from studies about persons with active disease. This relationship is likely explained by the inclusion of some survivors in the samples of persons with cancer, by sampling of survivors who have recently lived with active disease, or by spiritual responses remaining somewhat static even after the disease no longer actively threatens study participants.

The ability to make meaning and positively reframe the illness experience contributes to long-term adjustment and quality of life among cancer survivors.[54–59] One study surveying 200 ovarian cancer survivors found that two-thirds reported appreciating others more and wanting to be more involved in helping others, believing that their lives had been enriched and that they were strengthened by the cancer, and appreciating things in life more than ever.[60] Two studies compared the spiritual quality of life between breast cancer survivors and women without cancer.[57,58] Andrykowski and colleagues[57] found that although the survivors had poorer physical health, their psychological distress levels were not different and they reported greater psychosocial adaptation. These survivors had an improved life outlook, better interpersonal relationships, and more spiritual and religious satisfaction. Tomich and Helgeson,[58] however, found weak evidence for survivors construing more personal growth or meaning than matched controls who were asked to consider their most stressful events. Although the experience of cancer may not be unique in its ability to prompt spiritual growth, it nevertheless often does.

In contrast to the quality of life studies of persons with active disease, two studies measuring spiritual well-being among survivors suggested it could be less important once the immediate threat of illness passes.[51,61] Another study, however, ranked spiritual well-being second in importance, after physical concerns.[52] Regardless of rank, spirituality definitely has an impact on survivors' adjustment and quality of life.

A team of researchers has explored how survivors' perceptions of God affect their adjustment.[55,62] Content analysis of 39 breast cancer survivors' written responses to a query about how spirituality affected adjustment revealed that a relationship with God offered meaning, guidance, emotional support, positive attitude, inner strength, and diminished emotional distress.[55] Although the sample was inadequately small, Gall and colleagues[62] found that the specific nature of these survivors' relationship with God correlated with adjustment ($r = 0.50$). That is, the survivors with a benevolent attitude toward God had less psychological distress, and those who experienced God as present and in control were more optimistic.

Dying with Cancer

Dying entails facing an unknown, the loss of self, the desire to leave a legacy, the yearning to know that life — and death — possess purpose, and many other experiences that are inherently spiritual. Although numerous articles have been published about the import of spiritual care for terminally ill patients, few have reported research about the spiritual responses to dying with cancer. One study, however, documented how terminally ill cancer patients find spiritual and existential concerns to be extremely important. Greisinger and colleagues[63] found 92%–99% of 120 patients rated these concerns as extremely or very important.

Although terminal illness may be a time of extreme spiritual pain,[64] it can also be a time for spiritual growth. Thomas and Retsas[65] concluded from interviews with 19 Australian patients with terminal cancer that the experience fostered increased self-understanding and, in turn, increased spiritual awareness. Another study illustrated how spiritual responses to dying do not necessarily involve religiosity. Hermann[66] interviewed 19 hospice patients (14 of whom had cancer) to determine what were their specific spiritual needs. The 29 resulting spiritual needs were categorized under the following themes: need for involvement and control, need for companionship, need to finish business, need to experience nature, need for a positive outlook, and need for religion.

Several studies have explored spirituality in relation to quality of life in the context of terminal cancer.[44] Two studies measuring various domains of quality of life found spiritual well-being to rank highest among samples of hospice patients.[67,68] McClain and colleagues[69] observed that spiritual well-being functioned to protect terminal cancer patients against end-of-life despair. They found spiritual well-being to have moderately strong inverse relationships with the desire for a hastened death, hopelessness, and suicidal ideation. A study of 44 terminally ill cancer patients found that 28% of the variance in quality of life was explained by level of faith maturity.[70]

Caregiver Perspectives

Although the experience of living with cancer in one's body is challenging, if not traumatizing, the experience of caring for someone with cancer is difficult as well. Family and nurse caregivers alike witness the challenges and inevitably have their own spiritual responses to watching life with cancer.

Family Caregiver Perspectives

Being the family caregiver can be an emotionally and physically exhausting role. Family caregivers' spiritual questions may include "Why does my loved one have to suffer?"; "Where can I get my need for love filled when all I do is give care?"; and "What did I do to deserve this?" Harrington and colleagues[71] documented that spiritual needs, alongside informational needs, were ranked as most important by 55 family caregivers. Findings from two studies suggest there may be little difference between the spiritual needs of cancer patients and those of their family caregivers.[25,72] It is likely, however, that family caregivers may receive spiritual nurture from their nurses less often than do their loved ones, according to two descriptive Scandinavian studies.[73,74]

Spirituality is a resource for this stressful caregiving role.[75] This likely explains why family caregivers' sense of meaningfulness and spiritual well-being are associated with emotional health.[76,77] "Prayer or putting trust in God"—examples of spiritual resources—were identified by Steele and Fitch[78] as a coping strategy used and found effective by hospice family caregivers (N = 18). The import and nature of the relationship a caregiver has with God, however, may influence this coping and quality of life.[79–81] For example, among 125 family caregivers of hospice patients, Mickley and colleagues[80] found that those who viewed God as apathetic or unfair were more anxious, were more depressed, and perceived less purpose in life. Abernethy and colleagues[81] found that the relationship between religious coping and depression among 156 spouses of lung cancer patients was significant but not linear; that is, those who used moderate amounts of religious coping were less depressed than those who used either high or low amounts of such coping.

Oncology Nurse Perspectives

Inherent in oncology nursing is sharing with care recipients the profound and humbling experiences of life, both the sacred and the profane. This role can be burdensome and draining; at the same time, it can be a privilege. A survey of 813 hospice and oncology nurses revealed that most acknowledged that working with cancer-care recipients had influenced their own spirituality either a great deal (65%) or somewhat (24%).[82] While working with patients influences nurses, it is also true that hospice and oncology nurses' personal spirituality and religiousness influence if and how spiritual care is delivered to care recipients. Taylor and colleagues[83] found that self-reported spirituality and attitudes about spiritual care were predictors of how frequently and how comfortably cancer nurses provided spiritual care.

Three studies provide insight about what oncology nurses think constitutes spiritual care.[84–86] A survey of 181 clinicians reported the following categories of spiritual caregiving: verbally communicating about spiritual or religious concerns, involving spiritually supportive others in patient care, facilitating or initiating prayer, attending to family, providing or suggesting religious materials, being therapeutically present, touching, and conveying a benevolent attitude.[84] When Kristeller and colleagues[85] surveyed 267 oncology nurses, they found that 47% viewed themselves as the primary professional responsible for addressing spiritual distress. These respondents identified the following interventions for spiritual needs: suggesting patients seek help (11%), giving an educational brochure (7%), informing clients of local resources (27%), discussing an issue in depth (39%), and making a referral (37%).

The findings of Sellers and Haag[86] provide reinforcement of this role. These nurse researchers surveyed 208 Midwestern nurses, 27% of whom were oncology or hospice nurses, about what spiritual care nursing interventions they utilized in practice. The 10 most frequently used interventions (of 95 identified) included referral to spiritual care experts, different types and methods of prayer, active listening, facilitating and validating client feelings and thoughts, acceptance and nonjudgmental attitude, instilling hope, clarification of values and experiences by doing a spiritual history or assessment, touch, and referral to community resources. Although numerous other creative interventions were identified, 14% of the respondents did not identify any interventions.

Providing Spiritual Care

This review of recent research validates the contentions that persons with cancer and their family members often use spiritual coping strategies and that spiritual well-being contributes to adjustment and quality of life. It follows that nurses should support these coping strategies and nurture spiritual well-being. That is, oncology nurses should provide spiritual care.

Although this idea is accepted and promoted in nursing practice and education, little evidence exists regarding what clients desire in terms of nurses providing spiritual care. When Taylor[87] interviewed 28 patients and family members living with cancer about what spiritual care they might want from a nurse, some responded that they would not want or expect it, while others stated "it depends" or were enthusiastic about receiving spiritual care. Two dated small studies found that oncology patients ranked nurses fourth for preference as spiritual care providers, after friends and family, chaplains, and clergy.[88,89] When Reed[90] asked 100 cancer patients, "In what ways could hospital nurses help you in your spiritual needs?" only a minority agreed they would want something. Whereas 14% agreed that they would want a nurse to talk with them about their beliefs, only 7% wanted the nurse to read to or with them. The most frequent (yet not that frequent) responses were interventions not requiring direct nurse involvement: arranging for clergy (27%), allowing time for prayer (17%), providing time for family (15%), and helping them to attend chapel (12%).

These findings suggest that although many clients want and seek spiritual support, they may not always expect it from a nurse. An oncology nurse, therefore, must conduct a spiritual assessment that includes questions such as "How can we nurses best support your spiritual health?" Taylor's findings also indicate that a client may not be receptive to spiritual care from a nurse unless some degree of rapport and respectful relationship are established first.[87]

Organizational Approaches

Although most discussions of spiritual care describe how a nurse can provide care on a one-to-one basis, other approaches to spiritual care have been provided by cancer care institutions. For example, a cancer center in Ohio has instituted measures designed to nurture the spirit, including a healing garden on the premises (which includes a waterfall, labyrinth, and lush landscaping).[91] Wellness Centers across the United States offer a myriad of experiences that support the spirit of cancer patients and their family members. These often include classes such as yoga, journal writing, meditation, and dream analysis. Others have created weekends of renewal (e.g., Healing Odyssey Retreats[92]) or support groups[93] that include spiritual nurturing for patients or family members. While most hospitals maintain a chapel, some hospital chaplaincy departments have also instituted unique approaches that provide spiritual care to oncology patients as well as others, such as mobile carts with spiritually edifying tapes, books, and other resources.

Individual Approaches

Although not a spiritual care specialist, the nurse can be a spiritual care generalist. A nurse must possess basic spiritual assessment skills, be able to provide fundamental spiritual care such as presencing and empathic listening, and be able to make referrals to diverse spiritual care experts when unable to address spiritual needs adequately. Experts who nurses may consult, or to whom they can make referrals, include chaplains, clergy, folk healers, lay ministers, spiritual directors, parish nurses, mental health professionals with sensitivity toward spirituality, or others with knowledge about various spiritual practices such as meditation. Sometimes, however, family and friends may be the persons best suited to meet the patient's spiritual needs.[3]

Some evidence indicates that many persons with cancer do want their physicians to inquire about their spirituality and possibly address spiritual concerns.[35,94,95] There is, however, little information about patients' receptivity toward nurses addressing spiritual matters. Unpublished data collected by this chapter's author indicated that roughly half of 156 cancer patients and 68 family caregivers surveyed wanted spiritual care from a nurse, while the other half did not. The spiritual care nursing interventions that generated the greatest enthusiasm among these respondents were those that allowed for personal spiritual development in an independent way (e.g., help to have quiet times, tell me about spiritual resources) and humor (i.e., help me laugh, bring me humorous things). In contrast, the lowest-ranked items were interventions that involved approaching a client in a very personal way, with nontraditional methods for spiritual nurturing, and even inferring a hierarchal position in the nurse–client relationship (i.e., help me to think about my dreams, teach me about ways to draw or write about my spirituality, talk about difficulties of praying when sick). Generally, interventions that were less intimate, commonly used, and not overtly religious found the most approval.[96]

Assessment

Before any spiritual care generalist or specialist can provide appropriate care, a spiritual assessment is necessary. A two-tiered approach to spiritual assessment is recommended for nurses.[3] Because it is impossible, if not inappropriate, to conduct a thorough spiritual assessment on every patient, an initial assessment of patient spirituality should glean basic information about spiritual care requirements and function as a screening tool for spiritual distress. Taylor suggested the following components for this initial spiritual assessment: general spiritual status (e.g., "How are your spirits now?''); spiritual needs (e.g., ''What kinds of spiritual concerns bother you most?''); and spiritual resources (e.g., ''What do you think might help you with these concerns? In what ways can members of your health-care team boost your spirits?''). An alternative to interviewing patients is a paper-and-pencil questionnaire about spirituality that may be appropriate for patients who are capable of reading and writing (see Table 70-2).[3]

Table 70-2 Patient Spiritual Self-Assessment Form

Often when people confront health challenges, they become more aware of their spirituality. For some, spiritual ways of thinking or living are especially helpful when health concerns emerge. For others, spiritual questions or doubts arise.

This form will guide you to think about spiritual issues. After completing it, you may choose to keep it or give it to your nurse, who may want to share it with other health care professionals who will be caring for you.

NAME: ______________________________

ROOM NUMBER: ________________

Place an "X" on the lines to show the answer that comes closest to describing your feelings.

Recently, my spirits have been . . .

____

Awful. . . .	Low. . . .	Okay. . . .	Good. . . .	Great

In general, I see myself as . . .

____

Not at all. . . . Spiritual	A little. . . . . Spiritual	Somewhat. . . . . Spiritual	Fairly. . . . . Spiritual	Very Spiritual

In general, I see myself as . . .

____

Not at all. . . . Religious	A little. . . . . Religious	Somewhat. . . . . Religious	Fairly. . . . . Religious	Very Religious

What can a nurse do that would help to nurture or boost your spirits? (Check all that apply.)

____ Spend quiet time with you
____ Have prayer with you
____ Help you meditate
____ Allow time and space for your private prayer or meditation
____ Let you know nurse(s) are praying privately for you

____ Read spiritually helpful literature to you
____ Bring art or music to you that nurtures your spirit
____ Bring you literature that you feel is spiritually helpful

____ Help you to stay connected to your spiritual community
____ Help you to observe religious practices

____ Listen to your thoughts about certain spiritual matters
____ Help you to remember how you have grown from previous difficult life experiences
____ Help you to tell your life story
____ Help you to face painful questions, doubts, or suffering

____ Just be with you, not necessarily talking with you
____ Just show a genuine and personal interest in you

I would also like help in boosting my spirits from:
____ My friends and family
____ Other healthcare professionals
____ My own clergy or spiritual mentor
____ Other clergy or spiritual leader
____ A chaplain at this institution

What would you like your nurse to know about your prayer or meditation beliefs and practices?

____

____

____

What literature, art, or music nurtures your spirit?

____

____

How can the nurse assist you with religious practices or fellowship?

____

____

What spiritual matters would you like to talk about most?

____

____

In what other ways can the nurse help to boost your spirits?

____

____

If there is anyone in particular you would like to meet with for spiritual fellowship, please so state. If there is someone you would like us to contact for you, please share what contact information you know:

____

____

Reprinted with permission from Taylor, EJ: Spiritual care: nursing theory, research, and practice, 1st edition,© 2002, Pearson Education, Inc. Upper Saddle River, NJ.[3]

The second tier of assessment can occur when the nurse observes a need for detailed assessment. For example, if a patient remarks, "Sometimes I wonder if God hears me, because He's not answering me," the nurse will support spiritual health if further assessment is conducted. In this case, the nurse would query the patient about prayer experience and beliefs about relating to God. Assessment questions could include the following: "Tell me more about how you believe God hears and answers people." (Note the use of language that mirrors the patient's wording.) "How are you finding that illness affects your praying?" (Note the nonthreatening and nonbiasing tone.) "At times like these, exploring doubts can help to build faith. Could we do anything to assist you in this process?" (Assess not only what the problem is, but also what intervention would be acceptable.) The spiritual assessment not only provides data with which to determine appropriate interventions, but also functions to provide care. Prompting clients to consider their spirituality in this way often allows them to begin an internal journey toward spiritual healing.

Empathic listening and presencing

The two skills that are probably the most fundamental to providing spirit-nurturing care are empathic listening and presencing. Because more detailed information about these "interventions" can be found elsewhere,[97] a brief review will suffice here. Four levels of empathic listening have been identified: (1) listening intellectually; (2) listening intellectually and emotionally; (3) listening intellectually, emotionally, and physically; and (4) listening intellectually, emotionally, physically, and spiritually. A holistic listener, one who listens at this fourth level, is a "holy" listener.[3] Key components of empathic listening to promote spiritual health are striving to hear all aspects of patients' message, recognizing your inner response, and helping patients to listen to the self who is speaking and make sense of what they have heard.

In a classic discussion about presencing, Pettigrew[98] delineated the components of presence as vulnerability and silence, invitation and privilege. Willingness to "just" be with a patient in pain is extremely difficult. Nurses can easily escape this discomfort by literally avoiding patients in pain or by "hid[ing] behind the facade of professionalism or the technology or traditions of [their] role."[98, p. 505] Indeed, *being* with patients in pain can be avoided by engaging in *doing*. Being present to a patient therefore requires vulnerability, presence in a helpless situation. Being present to someone in pain also challenges the developed and practiced instinct to say "the right thing." Because words are often inadequate to comfort, nurses must learn to share silence. Likewise, because suffering is so private, nurses must never force their presence upon an individual. Indeed, Pettigrew posits that it is a privilege to be present for and with persons who suffer.

Fostering positive meaning

Perhaps the most pressing spiritual need for those with cancer, according to several studies cited earlier, is the need to create positive meanings — to transform the tragedy and experience spiritual growth. Although the research suggests that it may happen without professional intervention for many patients, it also indicates that some individuals may get "stuck" searching and experience spiritual distress ruminating about "why" questions. Taylor[3] identified some specific strategies nurses can employ to assist persons searching for meaning:

- Encourage resiliency (e.g., assist clients to remember how previous traumatic life events were surmounted, help clients to find an inspirational role model who similarly made good from bad circumstances).
- Encourage disclosure, remembering that one must encounter the darkness of this process before passing through it (e.g., "What kinds of questions are you finding yourself wondering about?" or "Who suffers with you?").
- If the client is ready, prompt a movement toward asking "Wherefore?" instead of "Why?" (e.g., ask the client questions like "What are some of the good things that have come out of your illness experience?" or "What sorts of lessons has this taught you?" or "What have you learned about yourself?").
- Avoid inappropriate responses such as imposing your beliefs about why cancer happens or avoidance and minimizing strategies like "It's God's will."
- Facilitate meaning-making activities (e.g., have clients get in involved with altruistic work such as volunteering or dedicating themselves to a social, religious, scientific, or other cause).

With any attempts to promote positive meaning, the nurse must remember that only the client can ascribe the meaning. This positive meaning cannot be forced; it cannot be fed.

Supporting religiosity

After assessment, the nurse may determine that religious beliefs or practices need to be supported. Prayer is likely the most frequent religious practice benefiting from support. Other religious beliefs and practices may need to be respected or incorporated in the plan of care.

Prayer. Because many persons with cancer use prayer, oncology nurses may need to support patients' prayer practices. Many patients may even appreciate a nurse praying with or for them.[99] Although two-thirds of one oncology nurse sample (N = 181) reported praying privately for their patients,[84] many nurses may feel discomfort with the idea of praying with patients. Tips for praying with clients follow:

- Determine whether it would be ethical to pray with a client.[99] Ask whether the patient wants it. Reflect on whether you have an improper, hidden agenda in your offer to pray.
- Assess the patient's desire for this intervention with a question such as "Many people at times like this want someone to pray with them. Would you feel comfortable with me praying with you?" Make sure the patient will be comfortable declining any offer.
- Assess the type of prayer experience from which the client would benefit. Introverts may prefer a shared time of silence. Others may prefer a conversational or ritual style of prayer. If petitionary prayer is preferred, inquire for what the patient desires prayer so that it can be included. (Styles of prayer are further described in Taylor's text on spiritual caregiving.)
- Pray by acknowledging the realities of the patient's current situation and feelings.
- Remember that the patient may also want to pray for the nurse. This can be a very spiritually intimate experience and the nurse should be prepared to receive this gift graciously.
- Know that prayer with a patient can be a springboard for further spiritual caregiving. Do not use prayer as an avoidance strategy to bring premature closure to an uncomfortable conversation.[3,99]

Although a nurse may not share the religious beliefs of the patient, these tips assume that the nurse's spiritual beliefs overlap in some fundamental way with those of the patient. For example, they both accept that there is an Ultimate Other with whom they can interact through prayer.

Religious beliefs and practices. Although a nurse is unlikely to have extensive knowledge about diverse religions, a broad appreciation for the general tenets of the basic world religions will be helpful. Some of the religious peculiarities that can affect cancer care are summarized in Table 70-3. For more information, the reader is referred to texts on spiritual care[3,100] or a handbook of religion.

On occasion, a patient's spiritual beliefs may create conflict with the healthcare team, which is trying to benevolently impose the best of healthcare. For example, a Jehovah's Witness with leukemia may refuse a blood transfusion. The oncology nurse can play a pivotal role in creating a resolution between the conflicting parties. Taylor[101] adapted anthropologist Kleinman's steps to managing conflicting cultural values, as follows:

1. Assess the patient's "model" that determines the approach to explaining illness and choosing a response to it (e.g., What do you think has caused your illness [or distressed your spirit]? What do you think your sickness does to you [spiritually]? How does it work? What do you think are the best things to do for your illness [or spiritual health]? What [spiritual] concerns has your illness caused you? What do you do about them?)
2. Explain simply to the client your model and beliefs about etiology (or meaning) and how best to respond to (or cope with) this illness.
3. Openly discuss with patients how your model differs from theirs. Objectively discuss how your different cultural backgrounds and spiritual beliefs contribute to the contrast in models.
4. Encourage the patient to ask questions about your model.
5. Support client beliefs and practices that are healthful (from your perspective).
6. Accommodate client beliefs and practices that are neither helpful nor harmful.
7. Change and provide alternatives for client beliefs and practices that are harmful without trying to change the underlying belief system, if possible. Engage family member(s) and religious clergy as therapeutic allies.

Conclusion

Recent research about the experience of living with cancer documents that spiritual responses to the illness affect both adjustment and overall quality of life. Personal spiritual factors, such as degree of faith development and perceptions about God, likely contribute to how healthy the adjustment is. It is expedient—even vital—that oncology nurses provide care that recognizes these personal spiritual variables and promotes spiritual well-being. Although many approaches to spiritual caregiving are possible, the most effective care may be dependent on a spiritually sensitive and aware nurse who creates a spiritually healing

Table 70-3 Selected Religious Beliefs and Practices Pertinent to Cancer Care

Religion	Selected Beliefs and Practices
Amish	Unless employed by non-Amish employer, will not have health insurance. Will rely on personal/family savings and Amish community resources. Extended family very involved during illness.
Baha'i	Cremation and embalming prohibited (unless civic law or exemption directs otherwise).
Buddhist	Health-related decisions (e.g., medical treatment, euthanasia, organ donation) are based on ultimate goal of Enlightenment (e.g., attainment of wisdom, truth, peace): If outcome allows continued pursuit of Enlightenment, it is encouraged. After death, reincarnated unless Enlightenment is attained.
Catholic Roman	"Sacrament of the Sick" is a ritual for all those who seek healing (not just for time of death). Lay ministers may bring Holy Communion to the sick. Ordinary (but not extraordinary) means for preserving life are an obligation.
Christian Science	Illness results from imperfect understanding of God's spiritual creation. Cure comes with prayer and spiritual regeneration. Seek assistance with healing from church-approved practitioners and nurses. Generally avoid medical procedures and therapies.
Latter-Day Saints (Mormons)	May wear temple garments under clothing. Church offers strong social support network (including a Relief Society). Ordinance for the sick involves anointing and prayer. Use only King James Version of Bible.
Hinduism	Reincarnation occurs after death. Eating meat is forbidden, especially beef. Cremation is common.
Islam	Ablutions and ritual prayer five times every day (facing Mecca) part of "pillars of faith." Eat no pork. Burial is compulsory and procedure is specified; should occur as soon as possible after death. Modesty (remaining covered) is critically important for women, especially in the presence of men.
Jehovah's Witness	Blood and blood products are forbidden. Giving blood would be "medical rape." Blood volume expanders, hematopoietic agents, and blood-conserving equipment are used. Reading Jehovah's Witness version of Bible can comfort and bring spiritual healing.
Judaism	Practices vary widely among Orthodox, Conservative, and Reform branches. Observant Jews keep Shabbat (observe Friday sunset to Saturday sunset as a holy day) and refrain from specified activities of work. Refrain from medical/surgical procedures on Shabbat unless life is threatened. Dietary law proscribes never eating pork, certain fowl, and seafoods; never mixing meat and dairy foods at same meal; and eating only ritually slaughtered meats. After death: ritual washing, no embalming, undelayed burial, family "sitting shiva" for seven days to mourn and receive social support.
Native American	Illness may result from natural or supernatural causes. Often use native healing practices and consult a medicine man. May disbelieve in efficacy of Western medicines and refuse blood.
Orthodox, Eastern	May request Holy Communion, confession, or anointing. Shave males only if necessary. May oppose autopsy, embalming, or cremation.
Seventh-Day Adventist	Observe Sabbath. Often vegetarian and refrain from caffeine and tobacco. Hypnotism viewed negatively. May request ritual anointing.

Many religious traditions observe fasts; ill persons, however, are exempted from observing these fasts. Many religions discourage or forbid use of alcohol and narcotics, but support their use for the medically ill. Religions that have restrictions on autopsies and biopsies permit them for medical or legal reasons. Most religions oppose euthanasia.

Reprinted from Taylor EJ: Spirituality, culture and cancer care. *Seminars in Oncology Nursing* 17:202–203, 2001.[101]

environment through a therapeutic use of self in a respectful nurse–client relationship.

References

1. Golberg B: Connection: an exploration of spirituality in nursing care. *J Adv Nurs* 27:836–842, 1998
2. Reed PG: An emerging paradigm for the investigation of spirituality in nursing. *Res Nurs Health* 15:349–357, 1992
3. Taylor EJ: *Spiritual Care: Nursing Theory, Research, and Practice.* Upper Saddle River, NJ, Prentice Hall, 2002
4. Indinopulus TA, Wilson BC (eds.): *What Is Religion? Origins, Definitions, and Explanations.* Boston, Brill, 1998
5. Taylor EJ: Spirituality and the cancer experience, in Carroll-Johnson RM, Gorman LM, Bush NJ (eds.): *Psychosocial Nursing Care Along the Cancer Continuum.* Pittsburgh, Oncology Nursing Society (in press)
6. Flannelly LT, Flannelly KJ, Weaver AJ: Religious and spiritual variables in three major oncology nursing journals: 1990–1999. *Oncol Nurs Forum* 29:679–685, 2002
7. Strickland CJ, Squeoch MD, Chrisman NJ: Health promotion in cervical cancer prevention among the Yakima Indian women of the Wa'Shat longhouse. *J Transcult Nurs* 10:190–196, 1999
8. Yi JK: Factors associated with cervical cancer screening behavior among Vietnamese women. *J Community Health* 19:189–199, 1994
9. Malik IA, Gopalan S: Use of CAM results in delay in seeking medical advice for breast cancer. *Eur J Epidemiol* 18:817–822, 2003
10. Underwood SM, Shaikha L, Bakr D: Veiled yet vulnerable: breast cancer screening and the Muslim way of life. *Cancer Pract* 7:285–290, 1999
11. Advani AS, Atkeson B, Brown CL, et al: Barriers to the participation of African-American patients with cancer in clinical trials: a pilot study. *Cancer* 97:1499–1506, 2003

12. Phillips JM: Breast cancer and African American women: moving beyond fear, fatalism, and silence. *Oncol Nurs Forum* 26:1001–1007, 1999
13. Holt CL, Clark EM, Kreuter MW, et al: Spiritual health locus of control and breast cancer beliefs among urban African American women. *Health Psychol* 22:294–299, 2003
14. Baider L, Sarell M: Perceptions and causal attributions of Israeli women with breast cancer concerning their illness: the effects of ethnicity and religiosity. *Psychother Psychosom* 39:136–143, 1983
15. VandeCreek L, Rogers E, Lester J: Use of alternative therapies among breast cancer outpatients compared with the general population. *Altern Ther Health Med* 5:71–76, 1999
16. Weisman AD, Worden JW: The existential plight in cancer: significance of the first 100 days. *Int J Psychiatr Med* 7:1–15, 1976
17. Ebright PR, Lyon B: Understanding hope and factors that enhance hope in women with breast cancer. *Oncol Nurs Forum* 29:561–568, 2002
18. Ballard A, Green T, McCaa A, et al: A comparison of the level of hope in patients with newly diagnosed and recurrent cancer. *Oncol Nurs Forum* 24:899–904, 1997
19. Gotay CC: The experience of cancer during early and advanced stages: the views of patients and their mates. *Soc Sci Med* 18:605–613, 1984
20. Feher S, Maly RC: Coping with breast cancer in later life: the role of religious faith. *Psychooncology* 8:408–416, 1999
21. Shannon-Dorcy K, Wolfe V: Decision-making in the diagnosis and treatment of leukemia. *Semin Oncol Nurs* 19:142–149, 2003
22. Taylor EJ, Outlaw FH: Use of prayer among persons with cancer. *Holist Nurs Pract* 16:46–60, 2002
23. Roberts JA, Brown D, Elkins T, Larson DB: Factors influencing views of patients with gynecologic cancer about end-of-life decisions. *Am J Obstet Gynecol* 176(pt 1):166–172, 1997
24. Taylor EJ: Spiritual and ethical end-of-life concerns, in Groenwald SL, Frogge MH, M. Goodman M, Yarbro CH (eds.): *Cancer Nursing: Principles and Practice* (ed 4). Sudbury, MA, Jones and Bartlett, 1997, pp 1421–1434
25. Taylor EJ: Spiritual needs of cancer patients and family caregivers. *Cancer Nurs* 26:260–266, 2003
26. Moadel, A, Morgan C, Fatone A, et al: Seeking meaning and hope: self-reported spiritual and existential needs among an ethnically-diverse cancer patient population. *Psychooncology* 8:378–385, 1999
27. Taylor EJ: Whys and wherefores: adult patient perspectives of the meaning of cancer. *Semin Oncol Nurs* 11:32–40, 1995
28. Bowes DE, Tamlyn D, Butler LJ: Women living with ovarian cancer: dealing with an early death. *Health Care Women Int* 23:135–148,2002
29. Carpenter JS, Brockop DY, Andrykowski MA: Self-transformation as a factor in the self-esteem and well-being of breast cancer survivors. *J Adv Nurs* 29:1402–1411, 1999
30. Taylor EJ: Transformation of tragedy among women surviving breast cancer. *Oncol Nurs Forum* 27:781–788, 2000
31. Mickley JR, Cowles K: Ameliorating the tension: use of forgiveness for healing. *Oncol Nurs Forum* 28:31–37, 2001
32. Post-White J, Ceronsky C, Kreitzer MJ, et al: Hope, spirituality, sense of coherence, and quality of life in patients with cancer. *Oncol Nurs Forum* 23:1571–1579, 1996
33. Fehring RJ, Miller JF, Shaw C: Spiritual well-being, religiosity, hope, depression, and other mood states in elderly people coping with cancer. *Oncol Nurs Forum* 24:663–671, 1997
34. Pargament KI: *The Psychology of Religion and Coping*. New York, Guilford, 1997
35. Bowie J, Sydnor KD, Granot M: Spirituality and care of prostate cancer patients: a pilot study. *J Natl Med Assoc* 95:951–954, 2003
36. Tatsumura Y, Maskarinec G, Shumay DM, et al: Religious and spiritual resources, CAM, and conventional treatment in the lives of cancer patients. *Altern Ther Health Med* 9:64–71, 2003
37. Lengacher CA, Bennett M, Kip KE, et al: Frequency of use of complementary and alternative medicine in women with breast cancer. *Oncol Nurs Forum* 29:1445–1452, 2002
38. Lengacher CA, Bennett MP, Kip KE, et al: Design and testing of the use of a complementary and alternative therapies survey in women with breast cancer. *Oncol Nurs Forum* 30:811–821, 2003
39. Alferi S, Antoni M Ironson G, et al: Factors predicting the use of complementary therapies in a multi-ethnic sample of early-stage breast cancer patients. *J Am Med Women's Assoc* 56:120–123, 2001
40. Balneaves LG, Krisjanson LJ, Tataryn D: Beyond convention: describing complementary therapy use by women living with breast cancer. *Patient Educ Counsel* 38:143–153, 1999
41. Lee MM, Lin SS, Wrensch MR, et al: Alternative therapies used by women with breast cancer in four ethnic populations. *J Natl Cancer Inst* 92:42–47, 2000
42. Eisenberg DM, Kessler RC, Foster C, et al: Unconventional medicine in the United States: prevalence, costs, and patterns of use. *New Engl J Med* 328:246–252, 1993
43. Taylor EJ, Outlaw FH, Bernardo T, et al: Spiritual conflicts of cancer cancer patients who pray. *Psychooncology* 8:386–394, 1999
44. Taylor EJ: Spiritual quality of life, in King CR, Hinds PS (eds.): *Quality of Life: From Nursing and Patient Perspectives* (ed 2). Sudbury, MA, Jones and Bartlett, 2003, pp 93–116
45. Ersek M, Ferrell BR, Dow KH, et al: Quality of life in women with ovarian cancer. *West J Nurs Res* 19:334–350, 1997
46. Cohen SR, Mount BM, Tomas JJN, et al: Existential well-being is an important determinant of quality of life. *Cancer* 77:576–586, 1996
47. Saleh US, Brockopp DY: Quality of life one year following bone marrow transplantation: psychometric evaluation of the Quality of Life Bone Marrow Transplant Survivors Tool. *Oncol Nurs Forum* 28:1457–1464, 2001
48. Fisch MJ, Titzer ML, Kristeller JL, et al: Assessment of quality of life in outpatients with advanced cancer: the accuracy of clinician estimations and the relevance of spiritual well-being — a Hoosier Oncology Group Study. *J Clin Oncol* 21:2754–2759, 2003
49. Schnoll RA, Harlow LL, Brower L: Spirituality, demographic and disease factors, and adjustment to cancer. *Cancer Pract* 8:298–304, 2000
50. Ferrell BR, Dow KH, Leigh S, et al: Quality of life in long-term cancer survivors. *Oncol Nurs Forum* 22:915–922, 1995
51. Gioiella ME, Berkman B, Robinson M: Spirituality and quality of life in gynecologic oncology patients. *Cancer Pract* 6:333–338, 1998
52. Wyatt G, Friedman LL: Long-term female cancer survivors: quality of life issues and clinical implications. *Cancer Nurs* 19:1–7, 1996
53. Cotton SP, Levine EG, Fitzpatrick CM, et al: Exploring the relationships among spiritual well-being, quality of life, and psychological adjustment in women with breast cancer. *Psychooncology* 8:429–438, 1999
54. Mast ME: Survivors of breast cancer: illness uncertainty, positive reappraisal, and emotional distress. *Oncol Nurs Forum* 25:555–562, 1998
55. Gall TL, Cornblat MW: Breast cancer survivors give voice: a qualitative analysis of spiritual factors in long-term adjustment. *Psychooncology* 11:524–535, 2002
56. Halstead MT, Hull M: Struggling with paradoxes: the process of spiritual development in women with cancer. *Oncol Nurs Forum* 28:1534–1544, 2001

57. Andrykowski MA, Curran SL, Studts JL, et al: Psychosocial adjustment and quality of life in women with breast cancer and benign breast problems: a controlled comparison. *J Clin Epidemiol* 49:827–834, 1996
58. Tomich PL, Helgeson VS: Five years later: a cross-sectional comparison of breast cancer survivors with healthy women. *Psychooncology* 11:154–169, 2002
59. Carpenter JS: Self-transformation as a factor in the self-esteem and well-being of breast cancer survivors. *J Adv Nurs* 29:1402–1411, 1998
60. Stewart MD, Wong F, Duff S, et al: "What doesn't kill you makes you stronger," an ovarian cancer survivor survey. *Gynecol Oncol* 83:537–542, 2001
61. Wenzel LB, Donnelly JP, Fowler JM, et al: Resilience, reflection, and residual stress in ovarian cancer survivorship: a Gynecologic Oncology Group study. *Psychooncology* 11:142–153, 2002
62. Gall TL, deRenart RMM, Boonstra B: Religious resources in long-term adjustment to breast cancer. *J Psychosoc Oncol* 18:21–37, 2000
63. Greisinger AJ, Lorimor RJ, Aday L, et al: Terminally ill cancer patients: their most important concerns. *Cancer Pract* 5:147–154, 1997
64. McGrath P: Spiritual pain: a comparison of findings from survivors and hospice patients. *Am J Hosp Palliat Care* 20:23–33, 2003
65. Thomas J, Retsas A: Transacting self-preservation: a grounded theory of the spiritual dimensions of people with terminal cancer. *Int J Nurs Stud* 36:19–201, 1999
66. Hermann CP: Spiritual needs of dying patients: a qualitative study. *Oncol Nurs Forum* 28:67–72, 2001
67. Thomson JE: The place of spiritual well-being in hospice patients' overall quality of life. *Hospice J* 15:13–27, 2000
68. McMillan SC, Weitzner M: How problematic are various aspects of quality of life in patients with cancer at the end of life? *Oncol Nurs Forum* 27:817–823, 2000
69. McClain CS, Rosenfeld B, Brietbart W: Effect of spiritual well-being on end-of-life despair in terminally ill cancer patients. *Lancet* 361:1603–1607, 2003
70. Swenson CH, Fuller S, Clements R: Stage of religious faith and reactions to terminal cancer. *J Psychol Theol* 21:238–245, 1993
71. Harrington V, Lackey NR, Gates MF: Needs of caregivers of clinic and hospice cancer patients. *Cancer Nurs* 19:118–125, 1996
72. Mellon S: Comparisons between cancer survivors and family members on meaning of the illness and family quality of life. *Oncol Nurs Forum* 29:1117–1125, 2002
73. Kuuppelomaki M: Spiritual support for families of patients with cancer: a pilot study of nursing staff assessments. *Cancer Nurs* 25:209–218, 2002
74. Strang S, Strang P, Ternestedt BM: Existential support in brain tumour patients and their spouses. *Support Care Cancer* 9:625–633, 2001
75. Petrie W, Logan J, DeGrasse C: Research review of the supportive care needs of spouses of women with breast cancer. *Oncol Nurs Forum* 28:1601–1607, 2001
76. Ferrell BR, Ervin K, Smith S, et al: Family perspectives of ovarian cancer. *Cancer Pract* 10:269–276, 2002
77. Strang S, Strang P: Spiritual thoughts, coping and "sense of coherence" in brain tumour patients and their spouses. *Palliat Med* 15:127–134, 2001
78. Steele RG, Fitch MI: Coping strategies of family caregivers of home hospice patients with cancer. *Oncol Nurs Forum* 23:955–960, 1996
79. Germino BB, Mishel MH, Belyea M, et al: Uncertainty in prostate cancer: ethnic and family patterns. *Cancer Pract* 6:107–113, 1998
80. Mickley JR, Pargament KI, Brant CR, et al: God and the search for meaning among hospice caregivers. *Hospice J* 13:1–17, 1998
81. Abernethy AD, Chang HT, Seidlitz L, et al: Religious coping and depression among spouses of people with lung cancer. *Psychosomat* 43:456–463, 2002
82. Highfield MEF, Taylor EJ, Amenta MO: Preparation to care: the spiritual care education of oncology and hospice nurses. *J Hospice Palliat Nurs* 2:53–63, 2000
83. Taylor EJ, Highfield MF, Amenta MO: Predictors of oncology and hospice nurses spiritual care perspectives and practices. *App Nurs Res* 12:30–37, 1999
84. Taylor EJ, Amenta MO, Highfield MF: Spiritual care practices of oncology nurses. *Oncol Nurs Forum* 22:31–39, 1995
85. Kristeller JL, Zumbrun CS, Schilling RF: "I would if I could"; how oncology nurses address spiritual distress in cancer patients. *Psychooncol* 8:451–458, 1999
86. Sellers SC, Haag BA: Spiritual nursing interventions. *J Holist Nurs* 16:338–354, 1998
87. Taylor EJ: Nurses caring for the spirit: patients with cancer and family caregiver expectations. *Oncol Nurs Forum* 30:585–590, 2003
88. Highfield MF: Spiritual health of oncology patients: nurse and patient perspectives. *Cancer Nurs* 15:1–8, 1992
89. Sodestrom KE, Martinson IM: Patients' spiritual coping strategies: a study of nurse and patient perspectives. *Oncol Nurs Forum* 14:41–46, 1987
90. Reed PG: Preferences for spiritually related nursing interventions among terminally ill and nonterminally ill hospitalized adults and well adults. *Appl Nurs Res* 4:122–128, 1991
91. Abdallah-Baran R: Nurturing spirit through complementary cancer care. *Clin J Oncol Nurs* 7:468–470, 2003
92. Rutledge DN, Raymon NJ: Changes in well-being of women cancer survivors following a survivor weekend experience. *Oncol Nurs Forum* 28:85–91, 2001
93. Coward DD: Facilitation of self-transcendence in a breast cancer support group: II. *Oncol Nurs Forum* 30:291–300, 2003
94. Hart A, Kohlwes RJ, Deyo R, et al: Hospice patients' attitudes regarding spiritual discussions with their doctors. *Am J Hosp Palliat Care* 20:135–139, 2003
95. Miller BE, Pittman B, Strong C: Gynecologic cancer patients' psychosocial needs and their views of the physician's role in meeting those needs. *Int J Gynecol Cancer* 13:111–119, 2003
96. Taylor EJ, Mamier I: Spiritual care nursing: What cancer patients and family caregivers want. *J Adv Nurs* (in press)
97. Burkhardt MA, Nagai-Jacobson MG: *Spirituality: Living Our Connectedness.* Albany, NY, Delmar, 2002
98. Pettigrew J: Intensive nursing care: the ministry of presence. *Crit Care Nurs Clin North Am* 2:503–508, 1990
99. Taylor EJ: Prayer's clinical issues and implications. *Holist Nurs Pract* 17:179–188 2003
100. Mauk KL, Schmidt NK: *Spiritual Care in Nursing Practice.* Philadelphia, Lippincott, Williams and Wilkins, 2004
101. Taylor EJ: Spirituality, culture, and cancer care. *Semin Oncol Nurs* 17:197–205, 2001

PART VIII

End-of-Life and Palliative Care

CHAPTER 71

Principles and Issues in Palliative Care

Peg Esper, MSN, RN, CS, AOCN®

> A person's dying may not be easy, but what of value in life is? Similarly, caring for our loved ones as they die is simply part of full and healthy living. It is rarely "fun," indeed is often hard — but it is as important as any experience in life.
>
> Ira Byock

Introduction

Many exciting changes are taking place in the treatment of individuals with a cancer diagnosis. Even so, cancer continues to claim the lives of more than 550,000 people in the United States each year.[1] While interest soars in new strategies at the molecular level designed to treat this disease, the larger population of affected individuals need and deserve a greater focus on quality palliative care.

Palliative care is a concept that has been defined with some degree of ambiguity. As more efforts have been concentrated in this area, various groups have struggled over the continuum of care to be encompassed by this term. How would palliative care differ from hospice care or end-of-life care or supportive care — or would it?

The differences in how these concepts are applied vary based on the geographical and cultural frameworks from which they are applied. The term *supportive care* has often had a *treatment-focused* correlative encompassing those measures taken to support the patient during active therapy. These measures may include interventions such as growth factor administration, blood transfusions, and antiemetics. More recently, supportive care has taken on some of the psychosocial and spiritual components of care. It typically is identified as having its endpoint at the time of patient death.[2]

Hospice care, particularly in the United States, has been identified primarily in legalistic fashion and, because of governmental definition, as being a "time-specific" point in the care of terminally ill individuals. This term is derived from the Latin word *hospitium,* which in its medieval roots referred to a place of shelter or rest and implied what we now refer to as "hospitality." Those who were acutely ill were cared for in *hospitals,* and those with illnesses for which no cure existed were cared for in *hospices.*[3] More traditionally, hospice care places the patient and family at the center of an interdisciplinary model of caring for individuals in the final stages of an illness.[4]

The World Health Organization has defined *palliative care* as "an approach that improves the quality of life of patients and their families facing the problems associated with life-threatening illness, through the prevention and relief of suffering by means of early identification and impeccable assessment and treatment of pain and other problems, physical, psychosocial and spiritual."[5] Palliative care begins with the initial identification of an incurable illness and concludes as the illness ends in death and bereavement. Its fundamental precept is that the goals of care are patient directed and quality oriented. Palliative care follows a design that neither hastens nor prolongs death, but allows individuals to "live with their illness" as long as possible prior to "dying from it" (Figure 71-1). The relationship between these three models of care is overlapping and occasionally the subject of debate (Figure 71-2).

Historical Perspectives

The word "palliative" has its origin in the Latin word *pallium,* meaning "a cloak." When discussing palliative care, one refers to the *covering* of the effects of illness rather than addressing the actual cause of the illness. Palliation provides protection from the internal and external threats to the individual precipitated by the disease and its treatment.[6]

The provision of care with the same intent as what we now refer to as palliative care is not unique to the last few decades. Reference to this type of treatment for the sick can be found dating back to the fourth century A.D. and before. Hostels for those with incurable illnesses such as leprosy were among those early efforts in palliative care.[3]

Modern-day palliative care acknowledges the tremendous efforts of a number of individuals, but specifically the contributions of Jeanne Garnier, Dame Cicely Saunders, Elisabeth Kubler-Ross, and, more recently, proponents of palliative care such as Russell Portenoy,

Places the patient at the center of care

Acknowledges dying as a normal part of life

Seeks to provide relief from symptoms that cause distress

Provides care that doesn't hasten or postpone death

Offers support to family following the patients death

Figure 71-1 Goals of Palliative care.

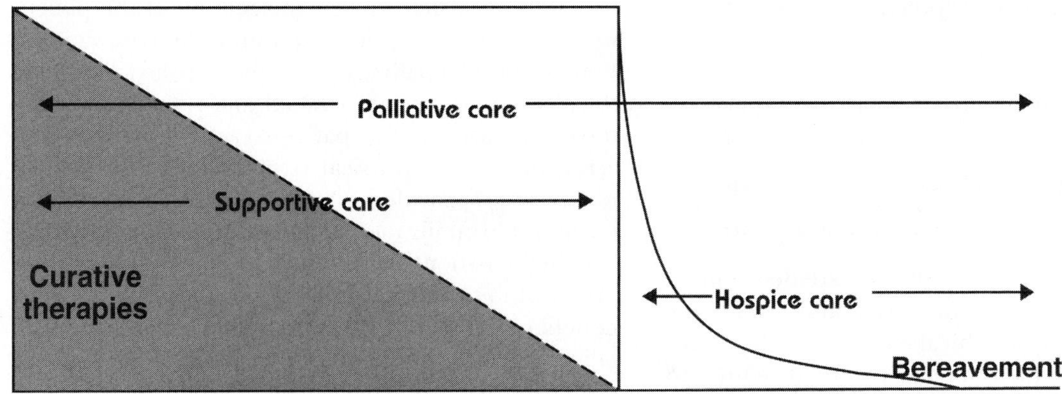

Figure 71-2 Overlap of concepts related to care of individuals with a terminal diagnosis.

Eduardo Bruera, Robert Twycross, and Ira Byock. Saunders describes her passion for the care of the dying as stemming from her interactions with a patient who died of cancer in the late 1940s when she was a nurse. A surgeon recognized her interest in learning more about pain management and symptom control and persuaded her to go to medical school, which she did at age 33. Her continued practice in this area led to the founding of the first modern hospice — St. Christopher's Hospice, in a London suburb in 1967.[7]

It was just two years later that Kubler-Ross published *On Death and Dying*. This book represented the culmination of more than 500 interviews with dying patients in which she theorized that there were five stages to the process of death and dying. Kubler-Ross was one of the first people to promote the concept of dying at home and letting patients have a choice in decisions related to their own care at the end of life.[8] Balfour Mount opened the first hospital-based palliative care service at the Royal Victoria Hospital at McGill University in Montreal in 1975. It was the first to include research and education in the area of symptom management.[9]

Interest in hospice care was growing in the United States as well. An early leader in the U.S. movement was Florence Wald, the dean of the Yale University graduate nursing program. Wald and Saunders met in 1963 when Saunders was a guest lecturer at the Yale School of Medicine. This meeting ultimately led to Wald opening the New Haven Hospice, which provided home care, in 1974.[3] Over the next 30 years, governmental efforts specific to hospice and end-of-life care received various levels of support (Table 71-1).

Models of Palliative Care

The goals of palliative care remain constant despite the model being used. Five precepts of palliative care have been identified as part of a multimillion-dollar, multiple-year campaign named *Last Acts*. The mission of Last Acts, which is funded by the Robert Wood Johnson Foundation, is to promote improvements in care and caring near the end of life. These five precepts were identified by the Palliative Care Committee of Last Acts as key areas for humane and technically competent end-of-life care:[10]

Table 71-1 Hospice-Related Legislative Activity, 1972–2000

	Legislative Activity
1972	Elisabeth Kubler-Ross testifies before the U.S. Senate Special Committee on Aging. She supports helping patients and families remain in their homes for terminal care.
1979	The Health Care Financing Administration (HCFA) evaluates the cost-effectiveness of hospice care using 26 hospice programs across the country.
1982	Medicare hospice benefit is introduced in the Tax Equity and Fiscal Responsibility Act of 1982.
1984	Hospice accreditation by JCAHO begins.
1986	Medicare hospice benefit made permanent by Congress.
1989	Omnibus Budget Reconciliation Act of 1989 ties reimbursement increases to the annual increase in the hospital market basket.
1993	Hospice becomes a nationally guaranteed benefit under the healthcare reform proposal during the Clinton administration.
1996	Bills introduced in the Senate and House of Representatives seek to improve the Medicare hospice benefit.
1997	Legislation passed by Congress prohibits taxpayer dollars from funding physician-assisted suicide. This same year, Oregon voters pass the "Death with Dignity Act" for the second time, sanctioning physician-assisted suicide in that state.
1999	HCFA releases the Hospice Cost Report.
2000	Hospice rate increase approved by Congress.

- Respecting patient goals, preferences, and choices
- Comprehensive caring
- Utilizing the strengths of interdisciplinary resources
- Acknowledging and addressing caregiver concerns
- Building systems and mechanisms of support

The particular models of care utilized are determined largely by the population being served and by the associated facility and geographical constraints identified. In the broad sense, these models can be divided into inpatient and outpatient services. They include the following elements[11–13]:

- Dedicated inpatient palliative care unit
- Consultation service within the acute care setting
- Combined consultative service with designated inpatient beds
- Combined hospital palliative care unit (with or without a community-based hospice program)
- Outpatient palliative care clinic
- Community-based hospice program
- Nursing home palliative care

Inpatient Services

Palliative care can be provided within the confines of the acute care setting. In this model, there may be a designated unit managed by a team of specialists in palliative care including physicians, nurses, therapists, social workers, and other caregivers. The design of the unit allows for great flexibility in visitation and participation in care by family and friends of the individual. Admission to the inpatient palliative care unit generally results from an exacerbation of symptoms that require more intensive management to control or offers a means of providing respite care to overburdened caregivers.[14,15] Funding of such units is often a limiting factor for institutions, as is their ability to designate an entire unit for this type of service.

Inpatient palliative care can also be provided across all units of an inpatient facility with the support of a consultative team. The team in this model will often include anesthesiologists, radiologists, and possibly a consultant from an outpatient palliative care program, as well as physicians, nurses, and social workers who have specialized expertise in palliative care. In this model, patients admitted to any inpatient unit can benefit from a consultation from the palliative care team.[16,17] Upon evaluation, recommendations from the team may be either recommended or the team may jointly participate in management of the patient with the medical service requesting the consultation. Limitations of a palliative consultation service include the absence of specially trained staff providing round-the-clock care for the patient. Limitations may also arise due to the physical structure of the units on which care is provided. There may be little or no room for multiple family members to be present and participate in the patient's care. The condition of roommates may prohibit flexibility in established visiting hours. A benefit of this model, however, is that specialist consultation can be made available to patients throughout the facility and, in effect, may broaden the reach of palliative care services across multiple specialty units.[9,16,18]

A combination of the two aforementioned models may also exist. A small number of designated palliative care beds may be provided on a particular unit for those patients needing various levels of crisis intervention. A consultative team remains available for those patients throughout the institution who have palliative care needs to be addressed by the team. This is frequently a very workable model for facilities that do not have the ability to devote an entire unit to palliative care patients, but would benefit from having "swing beds" that can be assigned to a unit where staff have an identified interest and additional education in the clinical management of these patients. This model of care may or may not be associated with a community-based hospice program.[9,16,17]

Outpatient Services

Ambulatory palliative care clinics may exist within the scope of services provided by an established ambulatory care clinic. These clinics primarily serve as symptom management clinics. Visits may be based on preset appointments for the ongoing management of problems such as cachexia or lymphedema, or they may be scheduled for urgent care needs outside of regularly scheduled physician appointments. These clinics may be staffed by physicians or advanced practice nurses who have additional expertise in palliative care. Once again, revenue to justify providing this service within an ambulatory care clinic may be a limitation in utilizing this model.

Palliative day care centers are not as popular in the United States, but have found more widespread use in the United Kingdom. These centers allow a small number of patients (generally 10–15) to attend during the day to provide both respite for caregivers and a social break for patients. Patients have access to medical support in the day care center as well as services such as manicures, massages, and hairstyling.[14,18] *Rapid response teams* and *respite care teams* are also unique to the

United Kingdom. Rapid response teams go into the home to provide urgently needed care and stay until the crisis is resolved. Such a team is typically contacted by a terminally ill patient's family physician to respond to an acute need. Respite care teams take over the care of patients for a couple of hours daily to provide relief for caregivers.[13,19]

Probably the best-known and most widely employed model of palliative care in the United States is the home hospice model of care. In its purest form, this model can be defined as an interdisciplinary "model for quality, compassionate care at the end of life. Hospice care places an emphasis on managing a patient's pain and symptoms, and provides psychosocial/spiritual support"[20] using the expertise of a team of professionals and volunteers. Care is provided on a 24-hour, 7-day-a-week availability basis.

Much to the consternation of most palliative care providers, hospice care in the United States has taken on its persona as a result of government regulations rather than because of the scope of services provided. The interdisciplinary team is made up of physicians, nurses, social workers, and counselors. The patient's own primary physician may also be a member of the team. Four levels of hospice care exist based on Medicare hospice regulations; they are outlined in Table 71-2.[21] The establishment of a Medicare hospice benefit has placed a number of regulations on hospice care: an expected prognosis of 6 months or less; patient's decision to choose hospice care rather than curative therapy for their illness; and enrollment in an accredited Medicare hospice program. Additional requirements that the individual hospice program may apply can specify that a primary caregiver be present in the home, and that patients agree to a "do not resuscitate" status. Those patients without Medicare coverage may have hospice home care coverage through their third-party insurance provider or may agree to pay out-of-pocket for services.[22,23]

Hospice home care has typically been viewed as the final trajectory of an incurable illness, and there are those in the field who have difficulty with the current overlapping of the terms "palliative" and "hospice." Those who embody the ideals of the modern hospice movement, however, expand the initially limited scope of hospice care from management of terminal symptoms to an approach that seeks to address the multidimensional plethora of issues concerning patients and their caregivers.[24]

Hospices are also forming partnerships with hospitals in an effort to promote a more seamless continuum of care for patients. This collaboration allows hospitals to benefit from the expertise of hospices in providing end-of-life care and maintaining high levels of satisfaction among patients and families. It allows hospices to gain greater exposure to the hospital setting, thereby engendering a greater appreciation for the intricacies of caring for the acutely terminally ill. Ultimately, patients probably stand to gain the most from such partnerships, as they receive more specialized care within the inpatient setting that can transfer into the home setting in a more streamlined fashion. Much work remains, however, if we are to address the multitude of regulatory and revenue-related issues pertaining to this model of care.[25]

Another combined effort being seen on a much more frequent basis is the "bridge"-type program for home care and hospice. Patients who do not fully meet the requirements for hospice eligibility or who are reluctant to sign on to a hospice benefit with their insurance provider can receive traditional home care from an agency that has the joint accreditation for both

Table 71-2 Levels of Hospice Care (Medicare Hospice Regulations)

Level of care	Description
Mandated Services	
Routine home care	Care typically provided in the patient's home with hospice staff providing the full scope of services.
Continuous home care	More intensive care in the home requiring skilled nursing for at least 8 of 24 hours per day. Typically used for acute symptom management to prevent the need for hospitalization.
Respite care	Patients are transferred to an inpatient facility to give caregivers a break from the physical and emotional stresses of caring for a terminally ill individual.
Inpatient care	Admission to an inpatient facility when acute problems require medical and nursing management (limitations on days exists).
Optional Services (Funding Not Provided by Medicare)	
Residential care	Care provided in an inpatient setting for patients who are unable to meet their own self-care needs and for whom caregivers are either not able or available to do so for them. Skilled care should not be required to qualify for this level of care.
Day care	Patients are taken to a day care site where planned activities, meals, socialization, and supervision are available.
Extended caregiver services	In-home respite care offers shifts of nursing home assistance to patients to substitute for or supplement caregivers.

Data from Kitzes, Sehmoll, Dixon.[21]

standard and hospice home care. Patients can transition within the same organization to hospice home care as their condition warrants. Many times the staff of these agencies will maintain the care of patients on both sides of the "bridge." This allows patients to have the benefit of receiving home care from nurses who have palliative care skills earlier in their care and then to enjoy the continuity of caregivers as they enter into a more terminal stage of their illness.[22]

Extended Care Services

Somewhere along the continuum of models is the care of patients in extended care facilities. A Robert Wood Johnson Foundation report, *Means to a Better End,* determined that at least 25% of nursing home residents experienced pain for a minimum of two months without appropriate pain management.[26] These patients with chronic illnesses often have similar needs but may or may not receive specialized palliative care. There is a growing trend at this time for hospices to contract with long-term care facilities to allow for cooperative efforts. Such liaisons should prove beneficial for patients as well as the long-term care facility and hospice organizations.[21,27]

Barriers to Providing Quality Palliative Care

The incentive for taking a harder look at how end-of-life and palliative care are provided in this country had one of its most poignant moments, when the report of the Study to Understand Prognoses and Preferences for Outcomes and Risks of Treatments (SUPPORT) was released in 1995.[28,29] This report, funded by the Robert Wood Johnson Foundation, heralded the shortcomings in the care of hospitalized patients related to end-of-life care and set the stage for a nationwide evaluation of how palliative care is provided. The results of this study provided a number of disturbing findings:[28]

- Only 47% of physicians knew that their patients did not want cardiopulmonary resuscitation (CPR).
- Approximately 46% of do-not-resuscitate orders were written within two days of death.
- Intensive care unit (ICU) stays of 10 days or more were noted for 38% of patients who died.
- Family members of conscious patients who died in the hospital reported that 50% of patients experienced moderate to severe pain at least half the time.

While this study was never intended to unmask such a deficit in the provision of end-of-life care, it became the cornerstone for further research and initiatives to determine what went wrong and how to correct the problem.

A number of barriers to providing quality palliative care persist. These barriers overlap to some degree, but have been divided into four categories (Figure 71-3). While each will be discussed for its own merit, the barriers are typically not found in isolation from one another.

Access to Care

Issues surrounding access to care are not unique to the palliative care environment, but are oftentimes an overlooked barrier to quality care in this setting. The lack of access to palliative care can be related to social as well as geographical factors. Minority groups such as African Americans are already known to experience inadequate access to health care in general. African Americans have higher cancer incidence and mortality rates than their Caucasian counterparts. While they make up approximately 14% of the total population, they make up only 5%–7% of hospice patients.[29,30] This disparity holds true for other vulnerable populations.[31,32] The reasons underlying this issue are multifactorial, but need further exploration. Specific cultural barriers for these populations are discussed later in this chapter.

The lack of palliative care resources in the inner city and rural areas is another factor that limits access to palliative care. Resources, both in personnel and arising from economic constraints, restrict the availability of palliative care services in these areas.[29,33]

Economics

A diagnosis of cancer is no longer necessarily synonymous with a "death sentence." The advent of new therapies and new technologies has enabled individuals to receive multiple therapies and often experience longer remissions prior to a determination being made that further attempts at cure are futile. While most would agree that philosophically this is a positive advancement, from an economic perspective it has placed a considerable drain on an already-overstressed healthcare system. Few data are available regarding how to accurately calculate cost-effectiveness ratios in palliative care.[34]

Questions are also posed about whether multiple successive treatments have any impact on quality or quantity of life for individuals with an advanced cancer diagnosis and how this potential abuse of resources

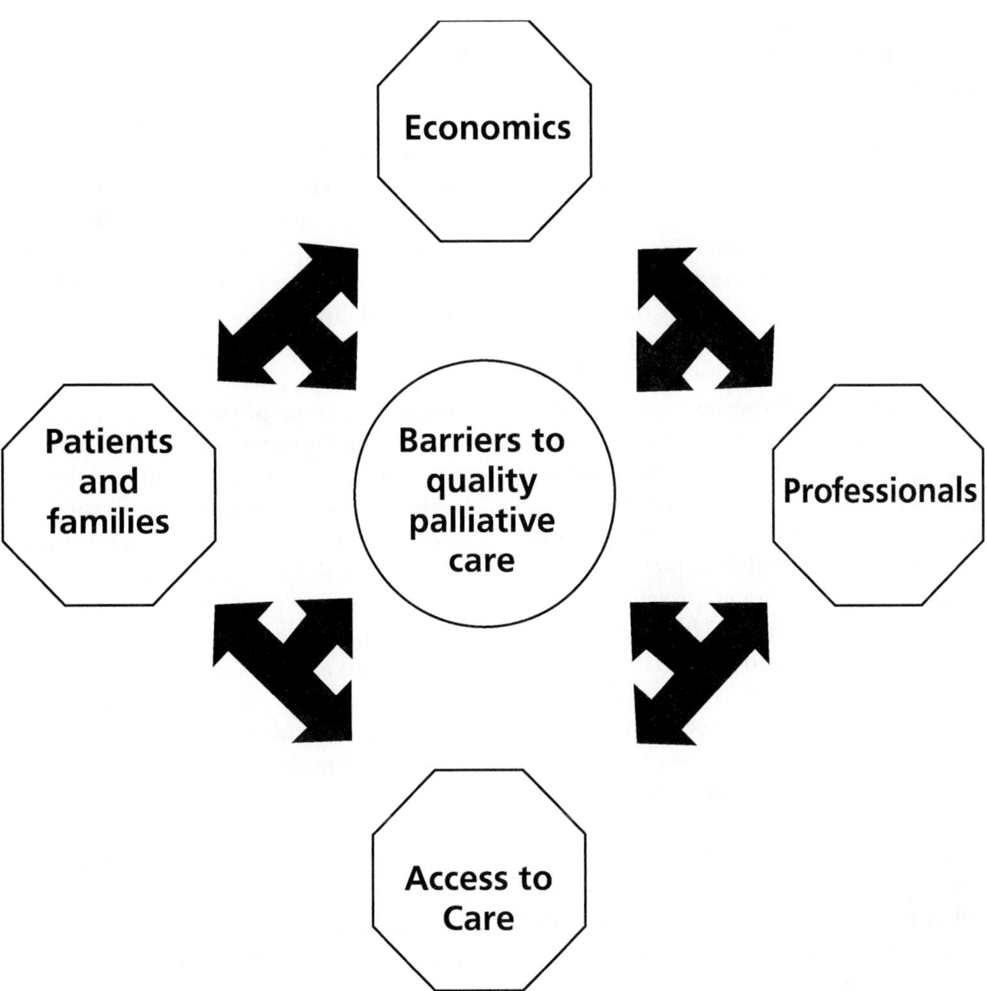

Figure 71-3 Barriers to quality palliative care.

should be handled.[35,36] Throughout the treatment period, patients are in need of various degrees of palliative support. While physicians may hesitate to make treatment decisions based on the costs of two equally effective therapies, it may be wise for them to do so before the decision is made for them.[36] Unfortunately, in the United States the incentive to use more expensive technologies that have little hope of improving the patient's survival is driven both by physician eagerness to gain experience with these modalities and even more by fears of litigious retribution when all possible modalities have not been exhausted.[37,38]

Most patients in the United States fall into one of three categories: the insured, the underinsured, and the uninsured. A single patient may move between these categories during the course of illness based on his or her disease trajectory. Many patients are employed when they receive a cancer diagnosis. As they begin to explore treatment options, concerns are often expressed about maintaining healthcare coverage by their employers. This issue can have a significant impact not only on the patient, but also for entire families when the patient is the insurance carrier for the family. Patients making the transition between treatments being provided with curative intent and treatments provided with palliative intent face unique economic issues. The changeover for these patients to a Medicare benefit (specifically Medicare disability insurance) may mean a loss of coverage for office visits and for prescription coverage prior to initiation of the Medicare hospice benefit. The subsequent financial strain on patients can be overwhelming when coupled with the stresses already induced by their diagnosis and treatment. In contrast, patients who elect to transfer into a home hospice program may be required to forgo some costly palliative strategies due to the hospice program's inability to financially offset the costs of such therapies as part of the per diem received from Medicare and other third-party payers.[39] For instance, patients who have achieved optimal control of pain by using a specific long-acting analgesic such as a fentanyl patch may be told that enrollment into a particular home hospice program requires that they switch to another agent that is part of that hospice's contracted pharmaceutical formulary. Only if they have documented evidence that the new agent is ineffective can they go back to the original treatment. Those unwilling to change may be asked to pay for the prescription out-of-pocket.[40]

Palliative care is no longer limited to administration of morphine. As research in the area of symptom management continues, the use of newer therapies to improve symptoms and quality of life such as antiemetics and analgesics has increased almost logarithmically. The cost of these therapies, however, has increased substantially, turning optimal pain and symptom management into a significant challenge for patients and healthcare providers alike. The cost of palliative care services is also affected by the location where that care is delivered. The SUPPORT study[28] depicted the inadequacies of end-of-life care being provided in the ICU. Resource allocation in the ICU involves modalities such as renal dialysis, antiendotoxin therapy, and thromboplastin administration. Ethical issues may clash with economic issues as decisions regarding patient condition and appropriateness of resource utilization are made, as well as who should be making those decisions.[34]

Limited research currently exists on the cost-effectiveness of moving some of the higher-technology services provided in the hospital setting to the home setting.[38] Palliative measures such as intravenous hydration and analgesia may be reasonable to provide in the home setting with home care nursing support. Other studies have attempted to demonstrate the cost-effectiveness of providing palliative or supportive care services earlier in the course of treatment for terminal illnesses. For example, the staff may initiate home care services as patients begin what is felt to be palliative therapies for advanced cancer. These staff are educated in the intricacies of therapeutic cancer treatment but also have expertise in palliative symptom management. Their efforts help to bridge the movement of patients from acute to palliative care and diminish feelings of abandonment perceived by patients and families.[41]

Patient and Family Barriers

The patient and family barriers to quality palliative care can be grouped under the general headings of "lack of knowledge" and "fear." With attention to these barriers, great strides can be made in the quality of the dying experience.

Patients and their families may start with a lack of basic knowledge about palliative care. Even more fundamental is the recognition that the patient is the central controlling force in care. Misconceptions related to what palliative care involves can lead to patients not seeking this support or, in worse scenarios, refusing support made available to them.[42]

Misunderstandings may also emerge regarding how insurance benefits are handled. Patients and families who are not familiar with the Medicare hospice benefit may have concerns that they will have no insurance coverage if they participate in hospice care.[43] Patients and families should be referred to social workers or other personnel who can assist them with insurance issues. Those patients who have established strong bonds with their physician and healthcare team may also be reluctant to enter a hospice program if they fear that their care will managed by a new group of healthcare workers with whom they have not developed a trust relationship. In fact, hospice care encourages the participation of and continued management by the referring physician. Those physicians and nurses who maintain responsibility for their patients even as they enter hospice care should make this continuity of care very clear to patients and families when beginning discussions concerning referral.

Another major way in which patients become barriers to quality palliative care is the absence of advance directives. Advance directives are intended to provide very specific instructions regarding the medical care that an individual would want to receive if unable to express his or her wishes at a future date.[44] Advance directives may be written or verbal and include documents such as a living will and durable power of attorney. A living will is a type of advance directive which describes specific types of care that should and should not be used in particular situations. The durable power of attorney for health care identifies a specific person who the individual trusts to make these types of decisions in the event that the appointing person becomes incapable of doing so.[39] Advance directives do more than merely state whether the patient wants to be resuscitated. They should encompass a range of scenarios that are possible in the event of an illness that incapacitates the patient and leaves the individual unable to express his or her desires.[45] At the time of this writing, 35 states did not mandate specific forms or particular language be used for advance directives, allowing individuals to express their wishes as they desire.

In 1991, the Patient Self-Determination Act (PSDA) was passed. This act requires that patients be informed on admission that they have the right to refuse or accept medical treatment and to specify in advance what their wishes are.[46] Thus advance directives can encompass patient preferences pertaining to issues such as CPR, use of invasive procedures, intubation, nutritional support provided by nonoral means, and transfusions. The expression of these desires in advance can decrease patients' concerns over what may happen to them if they are in a state that prevents their direct decision making. It also decreases potential guilt feelings of family members who are left to make these decisions in the absence of knowing specifically what type of care is desired by the individual.[47]

Documentation in some form, however, is critical in trying to assure that the patient's desires are followed. The absence of this documentation can lead to conflicts between the healthcare team and the patient's family as well as among family members. State-specific advance directives are available online through the Partnership for Caring Web site, *(www.partnershipforcaring.org/Advance/documents_set.html).*

Patients bring many fears with them into the healthcare arena. In the case of minority patients such as those of African American descent, there are historical events. A general mistrust of the healthcare system has been shared by many African Americans as a result of the atrocities that took place as part of the National Public Health Service Syphilis Study at Tuskeegee Institute. Discussions surrounding palliative or hospice care may be interpreted as withholding of the best medical treatment.[30,48–50] This same mistrust exists in many minority groups, who question whether their best interests are being taken into consideration as part of care planning.

Patient fears are also well documented pertaining to their reporting of pain and other symptoms. Concerns that lead to underreporting specifically of pain can involve a number of factors. Patients often fear addiction to pain medication and, as a result, will give inaccurate representations of pain scores.[51] For some patients, admitting that they have pain or other symptoms related to their illness forces them to abandon their denial of the extent of their disease.[52] At the most basic level, the patient's fear of death may block communication in discussing it. Some patients fear that just the act of discussing their death may hasten it.[53]

All members of the healthcare team have a responsibility to assess for patient-related barriers to care and implement approaches to address them. The importance of open communication cannot be overstressed. Only when open exchange of information and an atmosphere of trust exist can these barriers be broken.

Professionals as Barriers

Recent research has uncovered a number of roadblocks to successful palliative care that pertain to healthcare professionals. These barriers include inadequate knowledge related to palliative care, lack of cultural awareness and sensitivity, difficulty with issues related to death and dying, and delays in referral for hospice services.

A survey was conducted in 1998 by the American Society of Clinical Oncology to evaluate experiences of U.S. oncologists in end-of-life care. A key finding of this survey was the identification of a lack of formal training in palliative care.[54] This theme carried over to nurses, who identified an overall lack of formal preparation in dealing with a number of end-of-life topics.[55] The issue led to sentinel research on end-of-life content found in medical and nursing textbooks conducted by Ferrell and colleagues[56] and Rabow and colleagues,[57] which has prompted a major education initiative. Their studies demonstrated that the end-of-life content in both medical and nursing textbooks was extremely limited. Physicians and nurses have typically lacked the basic preparation needed to manage patients at the end of life. Much of what has been learned has been gleaned via "on-the-job training."

Based on these studies, programs have now been developed in medicine and nursing to provide education for healthcare professionals in palliative care. The End-of-Life Nursing Education Consortium (ELNEC) was a three-year project that began in February 2000 and was funded with grants from the Robert Wood Johnson Foundation. Through this "train the trainer" program, nurse educators in all 50 states have received training through ELNEC that they are now sharing in a variety of settings.[58] The core content is divided into nine modules (Figure 71-4). The physician counterpart to this educational effort is the Education for Physicians on End-of-Life Committee (EPEC). Also funded by the Robert Wood Johnson Foundation, EPEC has as its goal the education of physicians in the critical clinical competencies needed for quality end-of-life care.[59] Palliative care fellowships provide a focused experience in which the individual is involved in care and research activities. One such program supported by the Project on Death in America, called the Faculty Scholars Program, funds five to eight 2-year fellowships for this purpose.[60] Programs focusing on end-of-life care for social workers are also being developed.

The need for culturally competent care is not unique to palliative care, but inattention as to how it impacts those with a terminal diagnosis will severely limit the effectiveness of healthcare providers. Even practitioners with the purest motives may become insular as they care for individuals outside of their own culture. It is predicted that by 2050, half of Americans will identify with a specific ethnic minority group.[61] The concept of culture, however, is much broader than an individual's race or ethnicity; it encompasses a multitude of personal variables such as age, gender, religious preferences, socioeconomic status, and educational background.[62] There is a tendency to become

ELNEC Modules
Nursing Care at the End of Life
Pain Management
Symptom Management
Ethical/Legal Issues
Cultural Considerations in End-of-Life Care
Communication
Grief, Loss, Bereavement
Achieving Quality Care at the End of Life
Preparation and Care for the Time of Death

Figure 71-4 End-of-life Nursing Education Consortium (ELNEC) modules.

ethnocentric as we provide care to individuals. Unfortunately, this can create barriers in the way in which patients and families communicate with the healthcare team. Differences may arise between what is considered to be traditional medical practice and what the patient wants to have done. Individuals who are made to feel that their beliefs and practices are not valued will be less likely to share essential information that can influence the quality of their care.[62–64]

In our society's efforts to wage a "war on drugs," there has been an increase in "opiophobia" on the part of patients, but more importantly on the part of healthcare providers, including both doctors and nurses. Despite the efforts of state Cancer Pain Initiatives to recognize pain as a fifth vital sign, pain medications are being withheld from individuals due to fear of patients becoming addicted or "selling" their narcotics on the street.[18] Education of healthcare professionals on pain and symptom management principles is essential. While mandates such as the Joint Commission on Accreditation of Healthcare Organizations (JCAHO) standards for pain management[65] are wonderful from a broad institutional perspective, the fears that exist in individuals who are responsible for care must be addressed. Nurses have admitted withholding doses of morphine out of concern that they would cause too much respiratory depression and actually provoke a patient's death.[55] It is critical that nurses take the lead in removing this barrier. There are no symptoms that should be endured solely because the patient is "terminal."

Another significant barrier to quality care stems from difficulties in discussing issues related to death. Patients admitted to an acute care facility in a crisis situation who are then found to have a terminal prognosis may be at the mercy of hospital staff who are unable to communicate this information to the patient and their family due to their own lack of comfort with the prognosis. Patients may have to endure unnecessary procedures and lose valuable time with family members as a result.[66] The dichotomy of inciting death versus allowing death may lead to paralysis in making decisions that can have an enormous impact on the quality of death. As caregivers, each of us must reflect on the issues we may have with our own mortality. It is nearly impossible to discuss concerns related to the patient's death and the dying process if that is ground where we ourselves, fear to tread. The pinnacle of quality palliative care is reached through open and honest communication with patients.[18]

Difficulties in discussing end-of-life issues with patients and families can result in delays in referral to hospice care. While 70% of Americans state that they want to die at home, only 25% actually do so. Most states in the United States have less than optimal use of hospice services, with only 12%–25% of deaths including a hospice stay.[67] The causes underlying this trend are likely to be multifactorial. Physicians may be unaware that they can continue to follow their patients after enrollment into a hospice program and, as a result, may have a sense of abandoning them, which prevents earlier referral. Members of the acute healthcare team may not have an appreciation for the depth of services provided by hospice, leading to impediments in discussing these services with patients and families.[68–70] A recent report funded by the Robert Wood Johnson Foundation, *Means to a Better End*, rates states in eight areas related to the availability and quality of palliative care they provide (*www.rwjf.org*).

Ethical and Legal Issues in Palliative Care

The four ethical principles guiding clinical practice — autonomy, nonmaleficence, beneficence, and justice — must also be utilized in the practice of palliative care.[18,71] *Autonomy* refers to the process of helping patients make the decisions that are right for them.[72] Nurses are in the position to advocate for patients. It is our responsibility to ensure that patients have the knowledge they need to weigh the pros and cons of proposed treatment decisions. It also means making a concerted effort to allow patients to control as many aspects of their care as possible.

Nonmaleficence in palliative care involves avoiding practices that will do harm to the individual. An example of harm would be ordering inappropriate diagnostic tests that cause discomfort but have no real clinical merit.[73] Inappropriate care could also entail withholding pain medication for a patient in pain. The opposite of this would be *beneficence,* which seeks to help the patient while balancing the benefits against the risk of harm. Turning a patient to prevent skin breakdown seems like a reasonable activity unless the patient is imminently dying and has widespread bony metastasis causing severe pain with any movement.

Justice refers to the distribution of resources in a fair and reasonable way. How should healthcare dollars be spent? Should more funding be devoted to research in palliative care? Should a patient with a terminal diagnosis receive care that is comprehensive but devoid of the more expensive tests? How are staffing assignments made in relation to high-acuity patients receiving end-of-life care?[74]

How these principles are applied in physician-assisted suicide and euthanasia is the subject of continued debate. Active euthanasia has been defined as "the direct administration of a lethal agent to the patient by another party with a merciful intent."[75] In 1994, the state of Oregon passed the Death with Dignity Act, a legislative effort that allows physician-assisted suicide.[76] These measures should not be confused with terminal sedation and the withholding or discontinuation of life-sustaining therapy. The latter is typically employed in palliative care as a means of providing dignity to a patient when there is believed to be no chance for recovery.[77] This practice gained extensive media coverage as the family of Karen Ann Quinlan fought to gain the right to remove her from a respirator following a respiratory arrest in 1975 that left Quinlan in a permanent vegetative state.[78] Terminal sedation is a means of palliating symptoms that have become refractory to all other measures which may ultimately have the unforeseen side effect of death.[79] Unfortunately, there are times when conflict occurs between good clinical judgment, ethics, and the law. It is important that healthcare professionals have an understanding of what is fact and what is myth so as to provide optimal care.[80] Proponents of palliative care are hopeful that increased efforts and success in providing quality end-of-life care will eliminate the need for physician-assisted suicide as an alternative.

Challenges for the Future of Palliative Care

Whenever a major need is identified in a society, multiple groups inevitably begin to independently try to meet that need. The same has been true of palliative care. Since the SUPPORT data[28] were released and the inadequacies of care in this area were identified, a number of local and national efforts have sought to address these issues. While this movement has in general been very positive, it has also resulted in disagreements about what the issues are and what the best approaches to deal with them are by those who deem themselves to be experts in the field. This section of the chapter addresses a number of issues that will help shape the future of palliative care, including consistency in practice, research efforts, and outcome measures.

Consistency in Practice

Determining how to provide consistency in the delivery of care is a daunting task. It is frequently attempted via the use of policy, nationally accepted standards of practice, and the formation of consensus panels. Standards for specialization in a given field are often addressed by means of specialty certification.

Scope and Standards of Hospice and Palliative Nursing Practice provides guidelines on nursing care delivered in the palliative care setting. This text is useful in formulating programmatic planning and evaluation and in the development of individual state guidelines.[81] The Hospice and Palliative Nurses Association (HPNA) was originally formed in 1987 (at that time it was called the Hospice Nurses Association) as an organization to promote excellence in hospice nursing practice. Out of that organization came what is now known as the National Board for the Certification of Hospice and Palliative Nurses (NBCHPN). Certification in the palliative care specialty for nurses is currently provided through this board for registered nurses and nursing assistants.[82] In 2003, the first certification for advanced practice nurses in palliative care was offered through the joint efforts of HPNA and the American Nurses Credentialing Center (ANCC).[83] A specialty for physicians practicing in palliative care exists through the American Board of Hospice and Palliative Medicine, which was formed in 1995.[84]

On a more global level, the goal of the National Consensus Project for Quality Palliative Care (NCP; *www.nationalconsensusproject.org*) is to improve the delivery of palliative care in the United States by developing clinical practice guidelines by voluntary consensus. The steering committee for this project was formed following a 2001 national leadership conference in New York City. This committee is charged with document development, fund raising, administrative oversight, and comprehensive communication. Five organizations have formed a consortium that will oversee and ensure the success of NCP:

- American Academy of Hospice and Palliative Medicine
- Center to Advance Palliative Care

- Hospice and Palliative Nurses Association
- National Hospice and Palliative Care Organization
- Partnership for Caring: America's Voices for the Dying

Research Issues in Palliative Care

The paucity of data available in the area of palliative care has a multifactorial etiology. Frequently cited as a barrier to research in palliative care is the concern that patients at the end of life are too vulnerable and that it is not ethical to place them in a position where they can be exploited.[85] The concern with vulnerability is associated with decreased decision-making capability and volunteerism. Patients in the palliative setting, however, are not inimitable to this threat and researchers must use strategies to determine if the patient is capable of making an informed decision to participate. A fear that patients will volunteer to participate in research because of a closeness established with the researcher or solely out of desperation is also not unique to this population. Phase I clinical studies can be said to offer the same risk for patients.[86] Other ethical issues arise from conflicts for investigators as they attempt to wear the hats of both researcher and clinician. For instance, if the nurse researcher identifies that an intervention in one group of patients has an enormous benefit for symptom management and the other group of patients continues to experience suffering while receiving another intervention, what should be done? These are difficult, but not unanswerable, questions. Research design must take the potential for such issues into consideration prior to study implementation.[87]

Another identified concern is that the risks and benefits of research in the palliative care setting are more difficult to determine. The risk of a terminally ill patient responding to interview questions for 15 minutes may appear minimal on a superficial level, but may be intolerable for a patient who feels that it takes away precious time with his or her loved ones.[86,88] Additional study is clearly needed that focuses on the identification of what patients and families view to be the risks and benefits associated with research.

Outcome Measurement

One must rethink the traditional concept of outcome measurement when application is made to palliative care. This creates another exigency in advancing this science. While the anticipated outcome is not resolution of the illness, the assorted maladies seen concomitantly are appropriate targets on which to focus.[88] Reports of economic outcomes of palliative care are not easily found. Studies have suggested, however, that clinical outcomes of palliative care were maintained by nurses coordinating care with a 40% cost savings.[89] Outcomes pertaining to the provision of palliative care that have been discussed in the literature include patient and family satisfaction, quality of life, relief of symptoms, provider continuity, comfortable dying, self-determined life closure, and effective grieving, among others.[90–92]

Critical in outcome measurement is making sure that the focus is on areas which the patient and family believe to be important. Measures of patient satisfaction have been criticized because this area remains difficult to both quantify and define. There are also a number of inconsistencies across such studies.[93] Additional work is required to substantiate the results in a meaningful way.

Quality of life questionnaires have been used more frequently over the last decade as an a multidimensional approach in the evaluation of care. Quality of life essentially becomes the primary goal in end-of-life care. A number of instruments have been developed that are specific for the palliative care population (Table 71-3).[94–99] Another resource is available through the Center for Gerontology and Health Care Research at Brown University. The *Toolkit of Instruments to Measure End of Life Care (TIME)* provides an annotated bibliography of instruments currently available to measure quality of care at the end of life and is available online (*www.chcr.brown.edu/pcoc/toolkit.htm*). In determining how to measure quality of care, consideration must be given to the purpose of measurement, the patient population involved, the timing of the measurement, the source of the information, and the setting in which care is to be measured.[100] Some criticism has targeted the use of measurement instruments that attempt to evaluate excessive numbers of outcomes, as their psychometric utility may be compromised.[101]

An Institute of Medicine report entitled *Describing Death in America* reviewed the data related to quality assessment in the months just prior to death. This report indicated that there are wide gaps between what we should know and what we actually know. It recommended several initiatives to address the problem. One of these involves interviewing the next-of-kin identified on death certificates one month after the patient's death to focus on the period of dying. This would be part of an ongoing National Mortality Followback Survey program. These surveys provide a great deal of information regarding the dying process. Oversampling of children and minorities, two understudied populations, was recommended.[102]

Table 71-3 Quality of Life Instruments for Palliative Care

Instrument	Brief Description
Missoula-Vitas Quality of Life Index[94]	25-item survey validated in a hospice setting; covers five domains, including spirituality
McGill Quality of Life Questionnaire[95]	17-item questionnaire including five subscales that measure physical well-being, physical symptoms, psychological symptoms, existential well-being, and support
FAMCARE[96]	20-item scale that measures family satisfaction with health care provided to the patient and to them
Life Evaluation Questionnaire[97]	45-item questionnaire evaluating aspects not measured by existing surveys; five domains covered include appreciation of life, contentment, resentment, social interaction, and freedom versus restrictions
McMaster Quality of Life Scale[98]	32-item questionnaire measuring four domains from patient's perspective
After-Death Bereaved Family Member Interview[99]	Retrospective telephone-administered survey with bereaved family members; seven domains included; full instrument contains 133 questions; shortened and adapted for specific sites of care (hospice, hospital, nursing home)

Conclusion

Great progress has been made in collective efforts to advance the practice of palliative care in the United States and around the world. Major sources of funding have been allocated by the government and charitable organizations such as the Robert Wood Johnson Foundation, which have supported efforts to identify and address the inadequacies associated with end-of-life care reported in the literature. Much work still remains, but the accomplishments of recent years provide hope for the future of palliative care for this and coming generations.

References

1. National Cancer Institute: Cancer progress report — 2003 update. *http://progressreport.cancer.gov/doc.asp?pid=1&did=21&chid=14&coid=35&mid=vpco#most.* Accessed February 20, 2004
2. Senn HJ, Glaus A: Supportive care in cancer — 15 years thereafter. *Support Care Cancer* 10:8–12, 2002
3. Bennahum DA: The historical development of hospice and palliative care, in Forman WB, Kitzes JA, Anderson RP, et al (eds.): *Hospice and Palliative Care.* Sudbury, MA, Jones and Bartlett, 2003, pp 1–12
4. Homant SF: Hospice care, in Kuebler KK, Esper P (eds.): *Palliative Practices from A–Z for the Bedside Clinician.* Pittsburgh, Oncology Nursing Society, 2002, pp 147–150
5. World Health Organization: What is palliative care? *www.who.int/cancer/palliative/definition/en/.* Accessed December 18, 2003
6. Faull C: The history and principles of palliative care, in Faull C, Carter Y, Woof R (eds.): *Handbook of Palliative Care.* Malden, MA, Blackwell, 1998, pp 1–12
7. Saunders C: The evolution of palliative care. *Patient Educ Couns* 41:7–13, 2000
8. National Hospice and Palliative Care Organization: Hospice and palliative care — history of hospice care. *www.nhpco.org/i4a/pages/index.cfm?pageid=3285.* Accessed January 30, 2004
9. Mount BM: The Royal Victoria Hospital palliative care service: a Canadian experience, in Saunders C, Kastenbaum R (eds.): *Hospice Care in the International Scene.* New York, Springer, 1997, pp 73–85
10. Fins JJ, Renes LC, Schumacher JD, et al: On the road from theory to practice — progressing toward seamless palliative care near the end-of-life. *www.lastacts.org,* Washington, Last Acts, 2003. Accessed December 18, 2003
11. Center to Advance Palliative Care: *http://old.capc.org/topic/5/.* Accessed Febuary 10, 2004
12. von Gunten CF, Martinez J: Hospice and palliative care. *www.galter.nwu.edu/Geriatrics/chapters/hospice_palliative_care.cfm.* Accessed February 10, 2004
13. Abu-Saad HH: Palliative care: an international view. *Patient Educ Couns* 41:15–22, 2000
14. Twycross R: *Introducing Palliative Care* (ed 4). Oxford, Radcliffe Medical Press, 2003
15. Santa-Emma PH, Roach R, Gill MA, et al: Development and implementation of an inpatient acute palliative care service. *J Palliat Med.* 5:93–100, 2002
16. Bascom PB: A hospital-based comfort care team: consultation for seriously ill and dying patients. *Am J Hospice Pall Care* 14: 57–60, 1997
17. Woof R, Carter Y, Faull C: Palliative care: the team, the services, and the need for care, in Faull C, Carter Y, Woof R (eds.): *Handbook of Palliative Care.* Malden, MA, Blackwell, 1998, pp 13–32
18. Twycross RG: Palliative care: an international necessity. *J Pain Palliat Care Pharmacother* 16:61–80, 2002
19. Faull C, Woof R: *Palliative Care: An Oxford Core Text.* Oxford, Oxford University Press, 2002
20. National Hospice and Palliative Care Organization: NHPCO facts and figures. *www.nhpco.org/files/public/facts_and_figures_0703.pdf.* Accessed January 25, 2004
21. Kitzes JA, Sehmoll BL, Dixon CE: Hospice/palliative care settings, in Forman WB, Kitzes JA, Anderson RP, et al (eds.): *Hospice and Palliative Care.* Sudbury, MA, Jones and Bartlett, 2003, pp 47–55
22. Billings JA: Definitions and models of palliative care, in Berger AM, Portenoy RK, Weissman DE (eds.): *Principles and Practice of Palliative Care and Supportive Oncology.* Philadelphia, Lippincott, Williams and Wilkins, 2002, pp 635–646
23. Eustler NE, Martinez JM: The interdisciplinary team, in Forman WB, Kitzes JA, Anderson RP, et al (eds.): *Hospice and Palliative Care.* Sudbury, MA, Jones and Bartlett, 2003, pp 13–33
24. Miller SC, Teno JM, Mor V: Hospice and palliative care in nursing homes. [review] [80 refs]. *Clin Geriatr Med* 20:717–734; 2004
25. National Hospice and Palliative Care Organization and the Center to Advance Palliative Care: Hospital–hospice partner-

ships in palliative care: creating a continuum of service. *www.capc.org/Files/tmp_134090747.pdf.* Accessed December 2001

26. Robert Wood Johnson Foundation: Means to a better end. *www.lastacts.org.* Accessed January 20, 2004
27. Zerzan J, Stearns S, Hanson L: Access to palliative care and hospice in nursing homes. *JAMA* 284:2489–2494, 2000
28. SUPPORT Study Investigators: A controlled trial to improve care for seriously ill hospitalized patients: SUPPORT. *JAMA* 274:1591–1598, 1995
29. Foley KM, Gelband H (eds.): *Improving Palliative Care for Cancer.* Washington, National Academy Press, 2001
30. Payne R: Palliative care for African Americans and other vulnerable populations: access and quality issues, in Foley KM, Gelband H (eds.): *Improving Palliative Care for Cancer.* Washington, National Academy Press, 2001, pp 153–160
31. Krakauer EL, Crenner C, Fox K: Barriers to optimum end-of-life care for minority patients. *J Am Geriatr Soc* 50:182–190, 2002
32. McCarthy EP, Burns RB, David RB, et al: Barriers to hospice care among older patients dying with lung and colorectal cancer. *J Clin Oncol* 21:728–735, 2003
33. Lipman AG: Calls for improved cancer symptom control . . . and some responses. *J Pain Palliat Care Pharmacother* 17:71–76, 2003
34. Pronovost P, Angus DC: Economics of end-of-life care in the intensive care unit. *Crit Care Med* 29(2 suppl): N46–N51, 2001
35. Smith TJ, Hillner BE, Desch CE: Efficacy and cost-effectiveness of cancer treatment: rational allocation of resources based on decision analysis. *J Natl Cancer Inst* 85:1460–1474, 1993
36. Lynn J, O'Mara A: Reliable, high quality, efficient end-of-life care for cancer patients: economic issues and barriers, in Foley KM, Gelband H (eds.): *Improving Palliative Care for Cancer.* Washington, National Academy Press, 2001, pp 65–95
37. Whynes D: Costs of palliative care, in Clark D, Hockley J, Ahmedzai S (eds.): *New Themes in Palliative Care.* Buckingham, Open University Press, 1997, pp 34–48
38. Witteveen PO, van Groenestijn MA, Blijham GH, et al: Use of resources and costs of palliative care with parenteral fluids and analgesics in the home setting for patients with end-stage cancer. *Ann Oncol* 10:161–165, 1999
39. Taylor C: Advance directives, in Kuebler KK, Esper P (eds.): *Palliative Practices from A–Z for the Bedside Clinician.* Pittsburgh, Oncology Nursing Society, 2002, pp 1–4
40. Field MJ, Cassel CK (eds.): Financial and economic issues in end-of-life care, in *Approaching Death: Improving Care at the End of Life.* Washington, DC, Institute of Medicine, National Academy Press, 1997
41. Esper P, Hampton JN, Finn J, et al: A new concept in cancer care: the supportive care program. *Am J Hospice Palliat Care* 16:713–722, 1999
42. Wilke P: The person, the patient and their caregivers, in Faull C, Carter Y, Woof R (eds.): *Handbook of Palliative Care.* Malden, MA, Blackwell, 1998, pp 55–63
43. Longaway D: Death education and family support, in Forman WB, Kitzes JA, Anderson RP, et al (eds.): *Hospice and Palliative Care.* Sudbury, MA, Jones and Bartlett, 2003, pp 13–33
44. Leland JV, Schonwetter RS: Hospice, in Berger AM, Portenoy RK, Weissman DE (eds.): *Principles and Practice of Palliative Care and Supportive Oncology.* Philadelphia, Lippincott, Williams and Wilkins, 2002, pp 647–652
45. Emanuel LL: Advance directives, in Berger AM, Portenoy RK, Weissman DE (eds.): *Principles and Practice of Palliative Care and Supportive Oncology.* Philadelphia, Lippincott, Williams and Wilkins, 2002, pp 861–879
46. Balus ME: Palliative care: ethics and the law, in Berger AM, Portenoy RK, Weissman DE (eds.): *Principles and Practice of Palliative Care and Supportive Oncology.* Philadelphia, Lippincott, Williams and Wilkins, 2002, pp 902–914
47. Gomez D: Advance directives and CPR, in Kinzbrunner BM, Weinreb NJ, Policzer JS, et al (eds.): *20 Common Problems in End-of-Life Care.* New York, McGraw-Hill Medical Publishing, 2002, pp 297–311
48. Freimuth VS, Quinn SC, Thomas SB, et al: African Americans' views on research and the Tuskegee Syphilis Study. *Soc Sci Med* 52:797–808, 2001
49. Shavers VL, Lunch CF, Burmeister LF: Knowledge of the Tuskegee study and its impact on willingness to participate in medical research studies. *J Natl Med Assoc* 92:563–572, 2000
50. Farnon C, Hofmann M: Factors contributing to late hospice admission and proposals for change. *Am J Hospice Palliat Care* 14: 212–218, 1997
51. Esper P: Pain management in patients with advanced malignancies. *Home Health Consultant* 7:11–18, 2000
52. Murphy-Ende K: Barriers to palliative and supportive care. *Nurs Clin North Am* 36:843–853, 2001
53. Jeffrey D: Communication skills in palliative care, in Faull C, Carter Y, Woof R (eds.): *Handbook of Palliative Care.* Malden, MA, Blackwell, 1998, pp 88–98
54. Gelband H: Professional education in palliative and end-of-life care for physicians, nurses, and social workers, in Foley KM, Gelband H (eds.): *Improving Palliative Care for Cancer.* Washington, National Academy Press, 2001, pp 277–310
55. Ferrell BR, Virani R, Grant M, et al: Beyond the Supreme Court decision: nursing perspective on end-of-life care. *Oncol Nurs Forum* 27:445–455, 2000
56. Ferrell BR, Grant M, Virani R: Strengthening nursing education to improve end-of-life care. *Nurs Outlook* 47:252–256, 1999
57. Rabow MW, Hadie GE, Fair JM, McPhee SJ: End-of-life care content in 50 textbooks from multiple specialties. *JAMA* 283:771–778, 2000
58. American Association of Colleges of Nursing: ELNEC project, 2003. *www.aacn.nche.edu/ELNEC/.* Accessed February 4, 2004
59. Feinberg School of Medicine, Northwestern University: The EPEC project, 2003. *http://epeconline.net/EPEC/webpages/index.cfm.* Accessed February 4, 2004
60. Soros Foundation: Project on death in America. New York, Open Society Institute, 2004. *www.soros.org/initiatives/pdia.* Accessed February 22, 2004
61. Ersek M, Kegawa-Singer M, Barnes D, et al: Multicultural considerations in the use of advance directives. *Oncol Nurs Forum* 25:1683–1701, 1998
62. Mazanec P, Tyler MK: Cultural considerations in end-of-life care: how ethnicity, age, and spirituality affect decisions when death is imminent. *Am J Nurs* 103:50–58, 2003
63. Crawley LM, Marshall PA, Lo B, et al: Strategies for culturally effective end-of-life care. *Ann Intern Med* 136:673–679, 2002
64. Rhymes JA: Barriers to effective palliative care of terminal patients. An international perspective. *Clin Geriatr Med* 12:407–416, 1996
65. Phllips D: JCAHO pain management standards are unveiled. *JAMA* 284:726–733, 2000
66. Seymour JE: Negotiating natural death in intensive care. *Soc Sci Med* 51:1241–1252, 2000
67. Anonymous: U.S. end-of-life care gets a (barely) passing grade. *Healthcare Benchmarks and Quality Improvement* 10:9–10, 2003
68. Ogle K, Mavis B, Want T: Hospice and primary care physicians: attitudes, knowledge, and barriers. *Am J Hosp Palliat Care* 20:41–51, 2003
69. Ogle KS, Mavis B, Wyatt GK: Physicians and hospice care: attitudes, knowledge, and referrals. *J Palliat Med* 5:85–92, 2002
70. Miller KE, Miller MM, Single N: Barriers to hospice care: family physicians' perceptions. *Hospice J* 12:29–41, 1997

71. Beauchamp TL, Childress JF: *Principles of Biomedical Ethics* (ed 5). New York, Oxford University Press, 2001
72. Hermsen MA, ten Have AMJ: Moral problems in palliative care practice: a qualitative study. *Med Health Care Philos* 6:263–273, 2003
73. Weinreb NJ: Diagnostic tests and invasive procedures, in Kinzbrunner BM, Weinreb NJ, Policzer JS, et al (eds.): *20 Common Problems in End-of-Life Care.* New York, McGraw-Hill Medical Publishing, 2002, pp 329–364
74. Farsides C, Garrard E: Resource allocation and palliative care, in Clark D, Hockley J, Ahmedzai S: *New Themes in Palliative Care.* Buckingham, Open University Press, 1997, pp 49–59
75. Supanich BA: Palliative care and physician-assisted death, in Berger AM, Portenoy RK, Weissman DE (eds.): *Principles and Practice of Palliative Care and Supportive Oncology.* Philadelphia, Lippincott, Williams and Wilkins, 2002, pp 891–901
76. Barnard D: Ethical issues in hospice care, in Forman WB, Kitzes JA, Anderson RP, et al (eds.): *Hospice and Palliative Care.* Sudbury, MA, Jones and Bartlett, 2003, pp 87–101
77. Neumann JL: Ethical issues confronting oncology nurses. *Nurs Clin North Am* 36:827–841, 2001
78. McKeever L: Legal issues in hospice and palliative care, in Forman WB, Kitzes JA, Anderson RP, et al (eds.): *Hospice and Palliative Care.* Sudbury, MA, Jones and Bartlett, 2003, pp 103–117
79. McHale HK: Terminal sedation, in Kuebler KK, Esper P (eds.): *Palliative Practices from A–Z for the Bedside Clinician.* Pittsburgh, Oncology Nursing Society, 2002, pp 231–234
80. Meisel A, Snyder L, Quill T: Seven legal barriers to end-of-life care: myths, realities, and grains of truth. *JAMA* 284:2495–2501, 2000
81. Hospice and Palliative Nurses Association: *Scope and Standards of Hospice and Palliative Nursing Practice.* Washington, DC, American Nurses Association, 2002
82. National Board for Certification of Hospice and Palliative Nurses: *www.nbchpn.org.* Accessed February 10, 2004
83. American Nurses Credentialing Center: *http://nursingworld.org/ancc/.* Accessed February 10, 2004
84. American Board of Hospice and Palliative Medicine: *www.abhpm.org/.* Accessed February 10, 2004
85. Lee S, Kristjanson L: Human research ethics committees: issues in palliative care research. *Int J Palliat Nurs* 9:13–18, 2003
86. Casarett DJ, Karlawish HT: Are special ethical guidelines needed for palliative care research? *J Pain Symptom Manage* 20:130–139, 2000
87. Fine PG: Maximizing benefits and minimizing risks in palliative care research that involves patients near the end-of-life. *J Pain Symptom Manage* 25:S53–S62, 2003
88. Sanoshy J: Outcomes benefit patients by helping nurses to incorporate proven therapies. *ONS News* 14:1–5, 1999
89. Payne SK, Coyne P, Smith TJ: The health economics of palliative care. *Oncology* 16:801–808, 2002
90. Merriman MP: Measuring outcomes and quality of life, in Kinzbrunner BM, Weinreb NJ, Policzer JS, et al (eds.): *20 Common Problems in End-of-Life Care.* New York, McGraw-Hill Medical Publishing, 2002, pp 73–88
91. Lynn J: Measuring quality of care at the end-of-life: a statement of principles. *J Am Geriatr Soc* 45:526, 1997
92. National Hospice Workgroup: *www.nhwg.org/.* Accessed January 20, 2004
93. Aspinal F, Addington-Hall J, Hughes R, Higginson IJ: Using satisfaction to measure the quality of palliative care: a review of the literature. *J Adv Nurs* 43:533–534, 2003
94. Byock IR, Merriman MP: Measuring quality of life for patients with terminal illness: the Missoula-VITAS quality of life index. *Palliat Med* 12:231–244, 1998
95. Cohen SR, Mount BM, Strobel MG, et al: The McGill Quality of Life Questionnaire: a measure of quality of life appropriate for people with advanced disease. A preliminary study of validity and acceptability. *Palliat Med* 9:207–219, 1995
96. Ringdal GI, Jordhoy MS, Kaasa S: Measuring quality of palliative care: psychometric properties of the FAMCARE scale. *Qual Life Res* 12:167–176, 2003
97. Salmon P, Manzi F, Valori RM: Measuring the meaning of life for patients with incurable cancer: the life evaluation questionnaire (LEQ). *Eur J Cancer* 32A:755–760, 1996
98. Sterkenburg C: A reliability and validity study of the McMaster Quality of Life Scale (MQOLS) for a palliative population *J Palliat Care* 12:18–25, 1996
99. Teno JM, Clarridge B, Casey V, et al: Validation of Toolkit After-Death Bereaved Family Member Interview. *J Pain Symptom Manage* 22:752–758, 2001
100. Donaldson MS, Field MJ: Measuring quality of care at the end of life. *Arch Intern Med* 158:121–128, 1998
101. Kaasa S, Loge JH: Quality of life in palliative care: principles and practice. *Palliat Med* 17:11–20, 2003
102. Institute of Medicine: Describing Death in America, 2003. *www.nap.edu/books/0309087252/html/.* Accessed February 22, 2004

CHAPTER 72

Delivery of Comfort Care

Judith A. Paice, PhD, RN, FAAN

Introduction

Many people living with a cancer diagnosis will ultimately die of their disease. Because of their strong training in symptom control, oncology nurses are uniquely prepared to care for those patients who are in their final days of life. Furthermore, oncology nurses understand the psychological and spiritual distress expressed by these patients and their families and are able to address these concerns. Oncology nurses often have long-term relationships with these patients and their loved ones, thus providing continuity of care during what can be a very stressful time.

To be equipped to provide this care, oncology nurses must be aware of the common symptoms experienced during the final days of life, as well as the appropriate assessment and management of these symptoms. Although many dying patients have few symptoms that can be easily managed, difficult situations can arise that can complicate the dying process. Well-trained oncology nurses can ensure a peaceful death for these patients, ultimately improving the experience for the patient as well as for all the loved ones in attendance during this process. Finally, as societal changes have moved death out of the home and into institutions, many people have little understanding of the dying process. Oncology nurses must provide education for patients and their family members to alleviate fear and foster the relationship work that may take place during this time.

Symptoms During the Final Days of Life

Prevalence of Symptoms

Certain symptoms are common during the final days of life, although their prevalence and other characteristics have not been extensively investigated. In a study of patients with colon and lung cancer during the last three days of life, pain was prevalent in more than 40%, while delirium occurred in more than 25% of these patients.[1] Noisy breathing (''rattle''), pain, and urinary dysfunction were the most common symptoms of 200 patients, most with cancer, during the last 48 hours of life.[2] In a study of patients dying in long-term care facilities (some with cancer), pain, noisy breathing, dyspnea, and delirium were common during the final days of life.[3] Studies of patients in various stages of the dying process who had been referred to palliative care services, many of whom had cancer, affirm the prevalence of these symptoms. These studies and others assert that the most common symptoms are pain, anorexia, constipation, weakness, rattle, dyspnea, cough, and delirium.[4–6]

Children also experience an increased symptom burden during the final days of life. In a study of 30 children, more than half with cancer, the mean number of symptoms was 11.1 during the last week of life.[7] In another study of children who died from cancer, pain, fatigue, and dyspnea were the most common symptoms during the final days of life, and 89% suffered ''a lot'' or ''a great deal'' from at least one symptom.[8]

Two ''roads'' to death have been described.[9] The ''usual death'' includes a continuum where patients become sleepy and withdrawn, lethargic, and obtunded, gradually progressing to coma and death. The ''difficult death'' is one where the patient develops confusion and restlessness, followed by hallucinations, delirium, myoclonus, seizures, and eventually, coma and death.[9,10] The degree to which patients travel each of these roads is not known, yet even if less common, clinicians need to be prepared to manage the very disturbing ''difficult death.''

Thus, a wide range of symptoms are common during the final stages of life. Oncology nurses with knowledge and skills regarding palliative care can effectively manage these symptoms, reducing the prevalence of the ''difficult death'' and ultimately relieving distress experienced by patients and their families. This chapter addresses those symptoms commonly seen in the final days of life. For a complete review of symptoms common in those with cancer at other times during the disease trajectory, see Part IV, Cancer Symptom Management, Chapters 25–35.

Management of Specific Symptoms

Pain

Pain is common throughout the cancer continuum yet is particularly prevalent toward the end of life. The assessment and management of pain are thoroughly discussed in Chapters 26 and 27, and the strategies offered are pertinent to individuals during the final days of life. Unique aspects of pain control at the end of life include assessment in the cognitively impaired, delivery of drugs when the oral route is no longer feasible, and concerns by family and professionals that opioids hasten death.

Assessment of pain. Assessment of pain in the final days of life may be complicated when the patient is no longer able to report the intensity or presence of pain. In nonverbal patients, examine the brow for tightening or furrowing.[9] Treat the pain empirically and reassess. If the furrowed brow becomes smooth,

Table 72-1 Routes of Administration During the Final Days of Life

Route	Considerations
Enteral administration via tubes	• Caution when using long-acting opioid "sprinkles" to avoid plugging small lumen tubes
Oral	• Possible even in last days of life • Liquid placed sublingually is absorbed via the gastrointestinal tract
Parenteral • Intravenous	• IM route not indicated • Vascular access may be complicated in home environment due to need for complex technology (yet delivery is ensured)
• Subcutaneous	• Subcutaneous infusion is a useful alternative
Rectal/stomal/vaginal	• Not recommended in patients with thrombocytopenia or rectal lesions • May be physically difficult for family members to place
Spinal • Epidural • Intrathecal	• Allows administration of other agents such as local anesthetics • May increase level of care due to high-tech nature of equipment
Transdermal	• Ease of administration, yet may be difficult to titrate for patient with rapidly changing pain

Data from McCaffery M, Martin L, Ferrell BR[12]; American Pain Society[13]; Nelson KA, Glare PA, Walsh D, et al[14]; Watanabe S, Pereira J, Hanson J, et al[15]; Smith TJ, Staats PS, Deer T, et al.[16]

assume that the patient was in pain and continue treatment. If the brow remains furrowed, consider other causes of discomfort, such as impaction, a distended bladder, or spiritual concerns.

Routes of administration. Many routes of administration are available when patients can no longer swallow, including transdermal, transmucosal, rectal, vaginal, topical, epidural, and intrathecal delivery (see Table 72-1). In a study of cancer patients at 4 weeks, 1 week, and 24 hours before death, the oral route of opioid administration was continued in 62%, 43%, and 20% of patients, respectively.[11] Intermittent subcutaneous injections and intravenous or subcutaneous infusions were most commonly used when patients were no longer able to swallow.[11]

Preexisting enteral feeding tubes can be used to access the gut when patients can no longer swallow. The rectum, stoma, or vagina also can be used to deliver medication, although thrombocytopenia or painful lesions preclude the use of these routes. Nurses must assess for the possibility that family members may have physical or cultural barriers to delivering medications by these routes.[12] Transdermal delivery is another useful alternative.

Parenteral administration includes subcutaneous and intravenous delivery (intramuscular opioid delivery is inappropriate and not indicated at any time, but particularly during end of life). The intravenous route provides rapid drug delivery but requires vascular access, occasionally a problem for patients in the final days of life. Subcutaneous boluses have a slower onset and lower peak effect when compared with intravenous boluses.[13] Subcutaneous infusions may include up to 10 mL/hour (although most patients absorb 2 to 3 mL/hour with the least difficulty).[14,15]

Epidural or intrathecal routes of delivery allow the administration of several analgesic agents, including opioids, local anesthetics, and/or α_2-adrenergic agonists (such as clonidine). A recent randomized controlled trial demonstrated benefit for cancer patients experiencing pain.[16] Although an external epidural catheter may be placed to assist in intractable pain control during the final days of life, implanted devices should not be initiated at this time.

Opioids and time of death. Family members and clinicians express great fear that they will hasten the patient's death through the use of opioids. In fact, many family members and less experienced nurses have commented that they do not want to be the one to give the "last dose" of opioid. These fears may lead to undertreatment of pain during the dying process. There will always be a last dose of opioid. Furthermore, the literature does not support the concern that opioids hasten death. In an analysis of 17 studies employing opioids at the end of life, patterns of delivery, dose, type of opioid, and survival were examined.[17] None of the five studies that explored the effect of opioids on survival found any association.[18] This finding also is consistent with sedative use and survival.[19] The implication for oncology nurses is that patients can obtain good control of pain and other symptoms through appropriate titration of opioids. Because of this lack of association, the often cited (and frequently misunderstood) "doctrine of double effect" is not relevant to opioids and care delivered at the end of life.[17]

Myoclonus

Myoclonus, characterized by sudden, uncontrollable, and nonrhythmic jerking, usually of the extremities, is common at the end of life and is generally associated with opioid use.[20] Given in high doses, opioids, including morphine, hydromorphone, methadone,[21] meperidine,[22] and transdermal fentanyl[23,24] may result in myoclonus.[25] Patients may first present with nocturnal myoclonus, and thus nurses should be attuned to early identification of this syndrome, particularly in patients receiving high doses of opioids.[26]

Specifically, neuroexcitatory metabolites of the opioids have been implicated in the development of opioid-induced myoclonus.[25,27] The best studied of these metabolites are morphine-3-glucuronide and hydromorphone-3-glucuronide.[28,29] Serum and cerebrospinal fluid levels of these metabolites are elevated in patients receiving morphine for cancer and nonmalignant pain, particularly individuals with renal dysfunction.[30,31] However, metabolites alone do not explain the etiology of myoclonus, as other opioids with no known metabolites have also been shown to produce myoclonus.[32]

Hyperalgesia may also occur as a result of metabolite accumulation. In this case, patients will report increased pain with additional doses of the opioid. The first response by well-meaning clinicians is often to increase the opioid dose. This generally results in greater pain, with potential progression to delirium and possibly seizures.

Other reported causes of myoclonus include surgery to the brain,[33] placement of an intrathecal catheter,[34] AIDS dementia,[35] hypoxia,[36] chlorambucil,[37] and a rare paraneoplastic syndrome called opsoclonus-myoclonus that occurs in fewer than 1% of people with cancer.[38]

Assessment includes asking the patient and his or her family about a jerking sensation, particularly in the extremities. A physical exam will reveal jerking of the extremities that is uncontrolled by movement or other activities. Jerking can also be elicited by single or repeated tapping of an isolated muscle group.

Unfortunately, strategies to relieve myoclonus have not been well studied, particularly at the end of life. If the patient is receiving opioids, the primary treatment includes changing the opioid, reducing the dose when possible, and adding a benzodiazepine (see Table 72-2). Rotation to another opioid is the primary treatment of myoclonus, particularly if the patient is receiving higher doses and has renal dysfunction.[20] Calculate the equianalgesic dose, using standardized tables, and reduce by 25%–50% to account for cross-tolerance between agents.[41] Pain reassessment is critical as opioids are rotated, since equianalgesic conversions are approximations and wide variability exists. Methadone has been used as an alternative agent with success,[30] although titration must be done slowly to avoid adverse effects. Furthermore, myoclonus has been reported with methadone use.[21] Other strategies include adding adjuvant analgesics, with the goal of reducing the overall opioid dose. Of the benzodiazepines, clonazepam is most frequently recommended, although its use is limited during the final days of life

Table 72-2 Management of Myoclonus

1. ***Rule out potential causes***
   - Opioids, metoclopramide, and chlorambucil are the most common pharmacologic causes
   - Nonpharmacologic causes include hypoxia, AIDS dementia, surgery to the brain, and paraneoplastic syndrome
2. ***Rotate the opioid***
   - Calculate the equianalgesic dose of the existing opioid, using a standard table
   - Convert to another opioid, based upon the patient's past experiences with these medications
   - Reduce the dose by 25%–50% to account for cross-tolerance
   - Reassess frequently, as these equivalents are only a guide; there is significant variation in response among individuals
3. ***Reduce the dose of the opioid by:***
   - Adding adjuvant analgesics
   - Considering interventional therapies
4. ***Add a benzodiazepine***
   - Clonazepam 0.5 mg orally twice daily, and increase upward
   - Midazolam 0.5 mg intravenous or subcutaneous if unable to swallow, and titrate upward

Data from Mercadante S[20]; End of Life/Palliative Education Resource Center[39]; Golf M, Paice JA, Feulner E, et al.[40]

by the absence of a parenteral formulation. Other benzodiazepines, including diazepam and midazolam, are also recommended and available in parenteral forms.[20,42] The antispasmodic baclofen has been used to treat myoclonus due to intraspinal opioid administration.[44]

As was mentioned earlier, opioid-induced myoclonus can progress to seizures. When more severe neurotoxicities occur, the opioid dose should be reduced by at least 50% or more.[39] Naloxone is not effective in reversing this toxicity. If seizures occur, first- and second-line therapies include phenytoin and benzodiazepines, such as diazepam or lorazepam.[43] If seizures are refractory to treatment, or if they advance to status epilepticus, then midazolam, barbiturates, or propofol may be indicated (see Table 72-3).[40,45] Midazolam has a fairly rapid onset and short duration and can be given subcutaneously, intravenously, orally, bucally, sublingually, or rectally. Furthermore, particularly important in the end-of-life period, when numerous medications are given, the only known drug incompatibility for midazolam is with corticosteroids, particularly betamethasone, dexamethasone, and methylprednisolone.[40] The standard dose of phenobarbital in the management of seizures is 20 mg/kg intravenous infusion, with a maximum rate of 50–100 mg/minute. The recommended dose of propofol to treat refractory status epilepticus is 1–2 mg/kg via intravenous injection over five minutes, then starting a continuous intravenous infusion of 2–10 mg/kg per hour.[40]

Table 72-3 Management of Seizures

Assessment
Consider reversible causes, including:
- Hypoglycemia
- Metabolic conditions (e.g., hyponatremia, hypercalcemia, hypoxia, withdrawal from opioids, benzodiazepines, or alcohol)

Management
Pharmacologic
- Lorazepam 1–2 mg intravenous or 4 mg rectally (alternatives include rectal diazepam available in suppository or rectal gel)
- Phenytoin 18 mg/kg intravenous over 30 minutes (monitor for bradycardia and hypotension); if able to swallow, 300 mg orally every 2–3 hours for 3 doses, followed by 300 mg/day (alternatives, include fosphenytoin)

If ineffective:
- Phenobarbital 20 mg/kg intravenous infusion; maximum rate 50–100 mg/minute
- Midazolam 0.5 mg/kg/hour with upward titration (can be given subcutaneously, intravenously, orally, bucally, sublingually, or rectally)
- Propofol 1–2 mg/kg intravenous loading dose, followed by infusion of 2–10 mg/kg/hour (incompatible with most other drugs; contraindicated in patients with egg allergies or soya lecithin hypersensitivity)
- Lidocaine infusions 1–2 mg/kg/hour intravenous

Nonpharmacologic
- Pad side rails with pillows
- Provide calm, soothing, and safe environment
- Instruct family and caregivers not to place items in mouth

Data from Golf M, Paice JA, Feulner E, et al[40]; Eisele JH, Jr., Grigsby EJ, Dea G[42]; Stayer C, TronnierV, Dressnandt J, et al[43]; Lowenstein DH, Alldredge BK.[45]

Table 72-4 Causes of Dyspnea

Cancer-Related Causes (Direct or Indirect)
Anemia
Ascites
Cachexia
Electrolyte abnormalities
Hepatomegaly
Pericardial effusion
Pleural effusion
Pneumonia
Superior vena cava syndrome
Tracheal esophageal fistula
Tumor, either primary or metastatic

Treatment-Related Causes
Surgery
Radiation
Chemotherapy

Causes Unrelated to Cancer or Its Treatment
Anxiety
Arrhythmias
Asthma
Cardiac ischemia
Chronic obstructive pulmonary disease
Congestive heart failure
Neuromuscular disorders (e.g., ALS, multiple sclerosis)
Pneumothorax
Obesity

Nursing interventions include safety measures such as padding around the bed rails and assistive devices if the patient is ambulatory. Interventions designed to reduce fatigue are critical, including the provision of a relaxing and calm environment.

Dyspnea

Dyspnea is a common symptom in people diagnosed with cancer. Often described as shortness of breath or air hunger, this symptom shares many attributes with pain in that self-report is the only reliable strategy for assessment. Laboratory values (e.g., oxygen saturation) do not necessarily correlate with the intensity of the symptom, and opioids are the primary treatment for both dyspnea and pain. As with pain, patients may be reluctant to report the presence of dyspnea. As a result, oncology nurses must routinely ask patients about this symptom.

Although dyspnea can occur in a variety of cancer diagnoses and throughout the disease trajectory, this symptom is more common in those with advanced lung or breast cancer.[4,46] Other risk factors for dyspnea include ascites, congestive obstructive pulmonary disease (COPD), and pneumonia (see Table 72-4). However, it is important to note that the National Hospice Study determined that approximately one-quarter of patients reporting dyspnea had no underlying cardiopulmonary pathology.[47] Dyspnea also is extremely common in children who die from cancer, occurring in more than 80% of the patients.[8] In general, dyspnea occurs when there is either an increase in respiratory effort necessary to overcome obstruction or restrictive disease (e.g., tumor or pleural effusions), an increase in the amount of respiratory muscles required to maintain adequate breathing (e.g., neuromuscular weakness or cachexia), or an increase in ventilatory need (e.g., hypercapnia, metabolic acidosis).[48]

Because of its prevalence during the final days of life, and because of the distress it causes patients, screening for and assessment of dyspnea is critical. Patients can be asked to rate their level of dyspnea at rest and during activity using a 0 to 10 scale, where 0 equals "no breathlessness" and 10 indicates the "worst possible breathlessness." Patients often use phrases such as "I cannot get enough air," "I feel tightness in my lungs," or "I feel as if I am drowning."[49] A thorough assessment of dyspnea should include past medical history, smoking history, exposure to occupational hazards that may affect pulmonary function, and past medication use, as well as cancer treatments. Questions that incorporate the psychosocial and spiritual domains of the individual's life might include "What does this symptom mean to you?" and "What effect does this have on your daily life?"[50]

Physical examination, with attention to auscultation and percussion of the lung fields, can assist in identifying the underlying cause of dyspnea. Diagnostic evaluation may also be helpful; however, in the final days of life, the goals of care should always be considered when ordering these tests. For example, pneumonia may potentially be treatable with antibiotics, leading to relief of shortness of breath.[51] Yet this treatment may not be consistent with the patient's goals of care. Furthermore, CT scans, arterial blood gases, and pulmonary function tests do not provide useful information about the patient's dyspnea and are unlikely to reveal treatable causes of this symptom at this time in the patient's life.[52] Additionally, conducting these tests will likely result only in pain and discomfort for the patient, as well as reducing time spent with loved ones. An important nursing consideration is that although continuous pulse oximetry is widely available on most oncology units, patients and family members often focus on the monitor. This serves only to exacerbate existing fear and anxiety and yields little meaningful information during the final days of life. Therefore, reliance upon pulse oximetry should be minimal.[50]

During the final days of life, the goal of dyspnea management is to lessen the sensation of breathlessness. Opioids are the first-line therapy in relieving dyspnea.[48,53] Opioids decrease the intensity of dyspnea, regardless of the underlying pathophysiology, without causing respiratory depression.[48,53,54] Very low doses of an opioid administered on an as-needed basis are generally very effective in patients with mild to moderate dyspnea who have previously not been taking opioids. Individuals with more persistent or severe dyspnea, or those patients currently using opioids for pain relief, may require higher doses.[50] As with pain control, titrate the dose as needed to provide relief, and develop a plan to prevent opioid-induced side effects, particularly constipation. A stimulant laxative and stool softener, administered nightly and increased as needed, will reduce straining necessary to produce a bowel movement, which can exacerbate dyspnea.

The route of opioid administration does not seem to correlate with relief of dyspnea, and thus oral, parenteral, and transdermal routes can all be effective. A controversial delivery method is nebulized opioids for control of dyspnea. The rationale for administering opioids via nebulizer is based upon the presence of opiate receptors within the lung. Delivering the drug directly to the lung might provide relief while preventing systemic side effects of the opioids.[55] However, although uncontrolled clinical trials and case reports described benefits of using this technique,[56] controlled trials have not confirmed these positive results.[48,57]

Other treatment options in relieving dyspnea include benzodiazepines to treat the anxiety that often is associated with dyspnea, but only after using opioids to manage the primary symptom. Initial doses should be low and titrated upward as indicated. Glucocorticoids or bronchodilators can relieve bronchospasm, although bronchodilators should be used cautiously due to their potential to cause anxiety and worsen dyspnea. In patients with pleural effusions, thoracentesis may provide relief.[58]

Supplemental oxygen may be useful, but only in the face of hypoxemia. In those patients with relatively normal oxygenation, oxygen is not effective in reducing the sensation of dyspnea.[46,59] Nursing interventions include providing a cool fan blowing on the patient's face and repositioning the patient so he or she is sitting upright. Nurses may also recommend and guide patients in the use of cognitive behavioral therapies that have been shown to be effective in relieving dyspnea, including relaxation, breathing control exercises, and psychosocial support.[60] The use of behavioral therapies requires patient involvement, which in many cases may be difficult during the final days of life due to cognitive changes or extreme weakness. Complementary therapies, such as acupuncture and acupressure, may also be of benefit in relieving dyspnea, although controlled studies are needed.[61]

Anxiety

Anxiety is common during the final days of life and is highly correlated with other symptoms, such as unrelieved pain and dyspnea.[62] Thus, a thorough assessment of anxiety includes screening for these and other symptoms, as well as a complete review of current pharmacologic therapies. Medications commonly used in palliative care can contribute to the sense of anxiety, including corticosteroids, neuroleptics (e.g., metoclopramide), bronchodilators, antihistamines, digitalis, and occasionally benzodiazepines (which can cause a paradoxical reaction in elderly patients). The nurse should also consider the patient's risk for withdrawal from alcohol, opioids, benzodiazepines, and nicotine, which can also produce agitation.[63] Other factors to be considered include hypoxia, pulmonary embolus, sepsis, hypoglycemia, thyroid abnormalities, and heart failure, as well as certain tumors, including pheochromocytomas and some pancreatic cancers. During the final days of life, spiritual or existential distress, as well as fear of the unknown, can manifest as anxiety.

The pharmacologic management of anxiety often includes benzodiazepines, particularly lorazepam, as it has a short duration of action and generally produces fewer adverse effects. A common initial dosage is 0.5 to 2 mg orally three or four times daily, with upward titration as needed. Lorazepam can be placed sublingually, which is useful when patients have difficulty swallowing, or given parenterally as a bolus or infusion. Haloperidol is frequently used for short-term management of severe anxiety and as an antipsychotic (as discussed in the section on delirium), with the initial dosage starting at 0.5 to 1 mg orally twice daily.[62]

Nurses should foster frank discussion of the patients' fears in a supportive environment. Relaxation strategies, such as massage, audiotapes, breathing exercises, and guided imagery, may also alleviate anxiety if the patient is able to participate at this time.[64,65]

Delirium

Delirium is common during the final days of life and includes altered perception, impaired memory, emotional lability, hallucinations, incoherent speech, and disorientation to time, place, and person.[3,66,67] These symptoms may be misdiagnosed as anxiety or depression, particularly when mild or in the early stages. Common causes of delirium at the end of life include medications, such as opioids, corticosteroids, benzodiazepines, and adjuvant analgesics, as well as metabolic changes resulting from hypercalcemia and hyperglycemia, sepsis, central nervous system involvement by tumor, encephalopathy, and other organ system failure.[68]

Careful assessment includes a review of the onset and character of symptoms with family members and caregivers. Standardized tests of cognition frequently used in clinical practice, such as the Mini-Mental Status Exam, can help to determine the degree of impairment. Delirium has been characterized as two subtypes, including hyperactive and hypoactive. Signs and symptoms of hyperactive delirium include agitation, hyperarousal, hallucinations, and delusions. Withdrawal from benzodiazepines or alcohol can result in this type of delirium. Hypoactive delirium leads to lethargy and withdrawal and is more commonly related to encephalopathies and organ system failure.[69]

Treatment includes reversing the underlying cause whenever possible. Pharmacologic therapy includes haloperidol, an agent that blocks dopamine. Low doses (0.5 to 1 mg) can be given orally, intravenously, rectally, or subcutaneously. Risperidone and olanzapine are also used, but are not yet available parenterally.[70] Benzodiazepines such as lorazepam have been found to worsen delirium and cognitive impairment and, therefore, are not recommended.

Nursing management includes fostering a safe, quiet environment. Keep the patient's room well lit during the day, with visible clocks. At night, dim the lights and minimize interruptions to sleep, as a normal pattern of waking and sleeping is believed to help prevent disorientation. Reality orientation is no longer considered beneficial in actively hallucinating patients. In fact, correcting the patient's perceptions may only increase anxiety and agitation. Rather, speak in a calm, relaxed tone, ask questions gently, and offer support. Also, be open to comments by dying patients about "going home" or seeing loved ones who have previously died. These are common behaviors seen during the dying process and are very beautifully described by Callanan and Kelley in the book *Final Gifts.*[71]

Rattle

Excessive respiratory tract secretions, often called "death rattle" or "rattle," are common during the last hours of life. Although not likely painful to the patient, rattle is extremely disturbing to family members and other loved ones in attendance during this time. This may be due in part to the meaning of this symptom, as rattle is a strong indicator that the patient is actively dying. Studies indicate that rattle typically occurs within 16–57 hours before death, often preceding other symptoms such as cyanosis.[72–74] The prevalence of rattle varies greatly (ranging from 23% to 50%), likely as a result of practice variations, particularly in relation to hydration.[73,75] In people with cancer, risk factors for the development of death rattle include neoplasms of the brain and lung, as well as pulmonary infection, or edema.[72,76]

Two categories of rattle have been identified. Type I rattle originates from salivary secretions and appears to respond well to anticholinergic and other drying agents, with more than 90% of patients obtaining relief.[73] Type II secretions originate in the bronchi and are likely due to pulmonary pathology, such as infection, tumor, fluid retention, or aspiration. These secretions do not seem to respond well to treatment.[73,75]

Few studies have explored the most effective pharmacologic treatment of rattle, and therefore, treatment is often empiric (see Table 72-5).[77,78] Hyoscine (scopolamine) is available in transdermal and parenteral formulations. Originally released to reduce motion sickness, the scopolamine patch (Transderm Scop) is available in the United States in a 1.5-mg dose that is changed every three days. If two patches are ineffective, a continuous intravenous or subcutaneous scopolamine infusion is started.[73] The infusion is often started at 50 micrograms/hour, with doubling of the dose every hour until the secretions are reduced, to a maximum dose of 200 to 300 micrograms/hour. One study suggested that higher doses may be needed in patients with cerebral metastases.[75] Glycopyrrolate 0.2 mg (Robinul) with upward titration to relieve the noisy breathing is another option.[79] Other agents reported to reduce these secretions include atropine 0.4 mg subcutaneously every 15 minutes as needed or

Table 72-5 Management of Rattle

- Atropine 0.4 mg subcutaneous every 15 minutes until relief
- Scopolamine transdermal patch 1.5 mg
  - Increase to 2 patches after 24 hours
  - If inadequate relief, begin scopolamine infusion 50 micrograms/hour intravenous or subcutaneous and double every hour to a maximum dose of 200–300 micrograms/hour
- Glycopyrrolate 1–2 mg orally or 0.1 mg–0.2 mg intravenous or subcutaneous every 4 hours as needed or 0.4–1.2 mg continuous infusion
- Hyoscyamine 0.125–0.25 mg orally every 4 hours
- Stop or reduce parenteral or enteral fluids
- Diuretics may reduce overhydration
- Reposition to avoid accumulation of fluid

Data from Callanan M, Kelley P[72]; Wildiers H, Menten J[73]; Kass RM, Ellershaw J[74]; Bennett MI[75]; Morita T, Tsunoda J, Inoue S, et al[76]; Bennett M, Lucas V, Brennan M, et al[77]; Spiess JL, Scott SD[78]; Back IN, Jenkins K, Blower A, et al.[79]

hyoscyamine (Levsin) 0.125–0.25 mg orally every four hours. Because most patients cannot swallow at this time, the oral liquid can be placed sublingually.

Parenteral and enteral fluids contribute to respiratory secretions and should be discontinued whenever possible. If this is not feasible, the volume should be minimized to less than 500 mL in 24 hours. When patients have received large amounts of fluid, often during resuscitation efforts, diuretics may be useful in reducing the excess volume. Nursing measures such as altering the patient's position in bed may reduce pooling of secretions and the resultant rattle. Although suctioning may seem an appropriate intervention, this technique often elicits gagging and can be painful for patients. In those rare cases when suctioning is necessary, soft catheters should be used to suction only the oral cavity. Family members may require education, particularly if they request that suctioning be performed.

General Changes as Death Nears

In addition to the symptoms just described, patients will develop weakness, fatigue, and anorexia. Nausea and vomiting may also occur. Patients may become incontinent of urine or feces. Greater assistance with the activities of daily living and hygiene will be required, until total care must be provided. Family members require additional support as they witness their loved ones dying.

Patients' lack of interest in food or fluids is particularly distressing to loved ones, as nutrition holds such meaning of nurturance in our culture.[10] Family members may inadvertently try to force patients to eat or drink, leading to aspiration or simply to discomfort for the patient. Some loved ones may demand the placement of intravenous lines, total parenteral nutrition, or tube feedings, expressing fears that we are "starving" their loved one to death. Studies demonstrate that tube feeding does not prolong survival (with the possible exception of those with amyotrophic lateral sclerosis or ALS) and actually may increase the risk of aspiration. In fact, in several studies of patients with advanced cancer, tube feedings may actually have decreased survival.[80] Other data support the lack of suffering or discomfort associated with dehydration, thus negating the need for hydration.[81] Oncology nurses must be aware of these findings to support patients and family as they are faced with difficult decisions regarding artificial nutrition and hydration. The Hospice and Palliative Nurses Association has developed a position paper, "Artificial Nutrition and Hydration in End-of-Life Care," that can be accessed at *www.hpna.org*.

Spiritual suffering is not uncommon as patients review their lives and reflect on their meaning. This appraisal can raise feelings of guilt, regret, or sadness. Oncology nurses can provide comfort simply through their presence, allowing the patient to express these thoughts in a nonjudgmental environment. Rituals are useful for some, and consults with chaplains, social workers, or other team members can be beneficial.

As the dying process progresses, patients will become more withdrawn and less interactive with loved ones and caregivers. They may develop decreased perfusion in their extremities, leading to coolness, mottling, and a bluish cast to the skin. Changes in breathing, with periods of apnea, may also occur. Family members and loved ones often question whether they should leave the bedside, hoping to be present at the time of death. Because prognostication is so difficult, it is important to avoid giving a specific time frame. One helpful communication strategy that can be used throughout the disease process is to give a range of time, such as "hours to days," "days to weeks," or "weeks to months." Family members also need to be cautioned that some patients wait for loved ones to leave the room to die, sparing them the pain of witnessing their death, so that the timing of death can be very unpredictable.

After-Death Care

After-death care includes preparing the body so that loved ones can see the patient in as natural a state as possible. Cleaning and redressing the patient, as well as removing tubes and equipment, assists family members in developing a less painful memory of their loved one, fostering a healthy bereavement process. Cultural practices need to be considered. For example, Jewish and Muslim families may refuse autopsies, on the belief that the body belongs to God or Allah and must remain whole, even in death.[82,83] In Islam, a male patient can be cared for only by another male, and in Buddhism the body should not be moved for several hours to allow the spirit to leave without becoming confused.[84] Family members can provide guidance, and chaplains may be consulted.

Oncology nurses may offer to assist family members and friends with phone calls and notification. Some may need time to adjust to the death before making these calls, yet others may find healing and comfort in telling the story to those who were important to the patient.

Oncology nurses who are knowledgeable regarding the physical changes that occur in those who are actively dying, as well as the emotional and cultural needs of the patient and family, can greatly affect the final hours of life for those in their care. They can also significantly improve the memories of loved ones witnessing this death, fostering the bereavement process.

Difficult Cases

Although excellent symptom control and attention to psychosocial and spiritual concerns generally provide relief, for some the dying process can be quite difficult. These difficult situations can include sudden death from events such as hemorrhage, or intractable symptoms including pain, dyspnea, nausea, and vomiting.

A particularly difficult death may be due to sudden, fatal hemorrhage.[85] For patients with hematologic malignancies, bleeding from any orifice, such as the mouth, nose, eyes, rectum, urethra, or vagina can be due to thrombocytopenia or other coagulopathies.[86] Sudden death also may involve massive hemoptysis due to pulmonary or aerodigestive tumors or external hemorrhage from carotid involvement by tumor.[87] These scenarios are frightening to patients and family members. Rapid sedation using parenteral benzodiazepines is warranted. Offer a comforting environment through calm communication, reassuring the patient that he or she will not be left alone, covering wounds or secretions with dark towels, cleansing the area frequently, and rapidly disposing of soiled linens to reduce offensive odors.[88] A standing order for these types of unexpected events, particularly in patients at risk, may be helpful to ensure rapid management.

Palliative, or controlled, sedation at the end of life is an important option for patients with intractable pain and suffering. In one study, 16% of patients in an inpatient palliative care unit required treatment to relieve symptoms that resulted in sedation to a level of unresponsiveness.[89] In other studies, as many as 15%–30% of dying patients may require this therapy.[90,91] However, this approach is not without controversy. Some fear hastened death or believe this practice is the same as assisted suicide.[92] To mediate these concerns and provide a guide to clinicians, the Hospice and Palliative Nurses Association has developed a position paper that addresses these concerns. "Palliative Sedation at the End of Life" can be found at *www.hpna.org*.[93]

Education and informed consent of the patient (if possible) and family is essential. They should understand the benefits and risks of initiating therapy and should never feel coerced into making a decision. A Do Not Resuscitate order should be discussed and, if desired, should be in place, and discussions regarding other life-prolonging therapies (such as dialysis or implanted defibrillators) should occur.[92] A team approach is critical, along with consultation from pain and palliative care specialists and, in some circumstances, the ethics team.

The literature describing specific agents used to provide sedation at the end of life is largely anecdotal and refers to a wide variety of drugs, including opioids, neuroleptics, benzodiazepines, ketamine (a dissociative anesthetic), barbiturates, and propofol.[45,68,94,95] Because there are no randomized, controlled clinical trials, guidelines for drug selection do not exist, and therefore, the choice of agent is often empirical.

Regardless of the drug selected, titration is necessary to provide relief from intractable symptoms, followed by ongoing therapy to maintain the desired effect. The depth of sedation necessary to control symptoms varies greatly, so that a few patients may retain consciousness. Once adequate relief is obtained, ongoing monitoring is determined by the goal of care. If the goal of care is to ensure comfort until death, vital signs or other indicators may be taken infrequently. However, comfort care of the patient and family remains critical. Turning, cleansing, massaging, or other measures that provided relief prior to sedation should continue. Family members require support during this time as they observe their loved one alive but unable to respond. Chaplains and social workers should be consulted prior to beginning this therapy to assist in decision making and support.

Each agent used to provide palliative sedation has different side effects. Haloperidol is particularly useful for the patient with delirium at the end of life and can be given by the oral, subcutaneous, or intravenous routes. The oral or parenteral starting dose is generally 0.5 mg and can be increased to as much as 5 mg/hour continuous infusion.

Benzodiazepines, such as lorazepam or midazolam, produce sedation and can treat neurotoxicity related to opioids. Both have short half-lives. Lorazepam can be given orally, sublingually, or intravenously (starting at 0.5–5 mg every hour), while midazolam can be given parenterally (starting with a loading dose of 0.5 mg or higher). Benzodiazepines can produce paradoxical reactions, including increased agitation, particularly in the elderly.[92]

Barbiturates have been used for decades, yet their long half-lives complicate their administration. Additionally, their lack of analgesic efficacy and their numerous incompatibilities make their use more complicated. Pentobarbital can be given rectally (usual starting dose 60–200 mg) or via the intravenous route (with a usual loading dose of 2–3 mg/kg and 1–2 mg/kg per hour continuous infusion). Phenobarbital can be given by subcutaneous or intravenous routes, with a loading dose of 200 mg followed by 0.5 mg/kg/hour.[92]

Propofol is an anxiolytic, antiemetic, anticonvulsant, and anesthetic. Although generally used in the operating room, propofol can provide relief of intractable symptoms, such as pain, myoclonus, and seizures.[45] Usual starting doses begin at 2.5 micrograms/kg/minute, titrating every 10 minutes.[92] Patients allergic to lipids should not be given propofol, and the solution is not compatible with other compounds. There is no literature at this time regarding the safety of subcutaneous infusion.[45]

Parenteral administration of ketamine may be useful for some patients with refractory pain at the end of life. Ketamine is a potent analgesic at low doses and a dissociative anesthetic at higher doses.[96] It has been reported to relieve intractable pain and, in some cases, results in a significant decrease in the dose of opioids and sedatives, allowing the patients to interact with loved ones. However, ketamine can produce rapidly developing tolerance and hallucinations, dysphoria, or nightmares that may occur with higher doses and with drug accumulation.[97,98] Haloperidol can be used to treat the hallucinations, and scopolamine may be needed to reduce the excess salivation seen with this drug.

The oncology nurse should investigate whether institutional policies exist regarding palliative sedation. If not, an interdisciplinary team may develop such policies and educate colleagues throughout the institution regarding this type of care.[94] For more information regarding palliative sedation, access the Web site *www.eperc.mcw.edu.*

Patient and Family Education

The patient and family are the center of care, particularly during the final days of life. Patients may be aware that they are dying, and honest communication is needed between patient, family, and clinicians. Education and open communication help build trust and empower the patient and family regarding end-of-life decision making. Patients and family may fear the dying process. Many people in our society have never witnessed death and, therefore, need explicit guidance regarding the physical and emotional changes that occur during this time. Assess the family's level of understanding regarding their loved one's condition, as well as their readiness to discuss these issues. Caregiver fatigue and stress may preclude the ability to fully comprehend complex medical information, and repetition may be indicated. Written materials and role modeling, provided in an unhurried manner, are essential. Assist families to be involved in the care of their loved one, if appropriate, as this facilitates coping after death. Family meetings help ensure that consistent information is provided and heard by all present. These meetings may need to be repeated as the patient's condition changes or as the family is gradually able to assimilate the information. All of these interventions ease the dying process for the patient and support bereavement in loved ones.

Conclusion

Oncology nurses are well prepared to provide care to cancer patients facing the end of life. Because of their long-term relationships with these patients and their loved ones, oncology nurses can provide continuity of care during what can be a very stressful time. To be equipped to provide end-of-life care, oncology nurses must be aware of the common physical, psychological, and spiritual symptoms experienced during the final days of life, as well as the appropriate assessment and management of these symptoms. Oncology nurses can ensure a peaceful death for these patients, ultimately improving the experience for the patient as well as all the loved ones in attendance during this process. By being present and educating patients and families, nurses can help alleviate fear and can foster the relationship work that may take place during this time period. This care relieves the patient's distress and facilitates the bereavement process of family and loved ones.

References

1. McCarthy EP, Phillips RS, Zhong Z, et al: Dying with cancer: patients' function, symptoms, and care preferences as death approaches. *J Am Geriatr Soc* 48:S110–S121, 2000
2. Lichter I, Hunt E: The last 48 hours of life. *J Palliat Care* 6:7–15, 1990

3. Hall P, Schroder C, Weaver L: The last 48 hours of life in long-term care: a focused chart audit. *J Am Geriatr Soc* 50:501–506, 2002
4. Potter J, Hami F, Bryan T, et al: Symptoms in 400 patients referred to palliative care services: prevalence and patterns. *Palliat Med* 17:310–314, 2003
5. Ng K, von Gunten CF: Symptoms and attitudes of 100 consecutive patients admitted to an acute hospice/palliative care unit. *J Pain Symptom Manage* 16:307–316, 1998
6. Morita T, Ichiki T, Tsunoda J, et al: A prospective study on the dying process in terminally ill cancer patients. *Am J Hospice Palliat Care* 15:217–222, 1998
7. Drake R, Frost J, Collins JJ: The symptoms of dying children. *J Pain Symptom Manage* 26:594–603, 2003
8. Wolfe J, Grier HE, Klar N, et al: Symptoms and suffering at the end of life in children with cancer. *N Eng J Med* 342:326–333, 2000
9. Education for Physicians on End-of-life Care Project (EPEC). *www.epec.net*. Accessed December 17, 2004
10. Furst CJ, Doyle D: The terminal phase, in Doyle D, Hanks G, Cherny N, et al (eds.): *Oxford Textbook of Palliative Medicine* (ed 3). Oxford, Oxford University Press, 2004, pp 1119–1133
11. Coyle N, Adelhardt J, Foley KM, et al: Character of terminal illness in the advanced cancer patient: pain and other symptoms during the last four weeks of life. *J Pain Symptom Manage* 5:83–93, 1990
12. McCaffery M, Martin L, Ferrell BR: Analgesic administration via rectum or stoma. *J Enterostom Nurs* 19:114–121, 1992
13. American Pain Society: *Principles of Analgesic Use in the Treatment of Acute Pain and Cancer Pain (ed 5)*. Glenview, IL, American Pain Society, 2003
14. Nelson KA, Glare PA, Walsh D, et al: A prospective, within-patient, crossover study of continuous intravenous and subcutaneous morphine for chronic cancer pain. *J Pain Symptom Manage* 13:262–267, 1997
15. Watanabe S, Pereira J, Hanson J, et al: Fentanyl by continuous subcutaneous infusion for the management of cancer pain: a retrospective study. *J Pain Symptom Manage* 16:323–326, 1998
16. Smith TJ, Staats PS, Deer T, et al: Randomized clinical trial of an implantable drug delivery system compared with comprehensive medical management for refractory cancer pain: impact on pain, drug-related toxicity, and survival. *J Clin Oncol* 20:4040–4049, 2002
17. Sykes N, Thorns A: The use of opioids and sedatives at the end of life. *Lancet Oncol* 4:312–318, 2003
18. Thorns A, Sykes N: Opioid use in last week of life and implications for end-of-life decision-making. *Lancet* 356:398–399, 2000
19. Sykes N, Thorns A: Sedative use in the last week of life and the implications for end-of-life decision making. *Arch Intern Med* 163:341–344, 2003
20. Mercadante S: Pathophysiology and treatment of opioid-related myoclonus in cancer patients. *Pain* 74:5–9, 1998
21. Sarhill N, Davis MP, Walsh D, et al: Methadone-induced myoclonus in advanced cancer. *Am J Hosp Palliat Care* 18:51–53, 2001
22. Kaiko RF, Foley KM, Grabinski PY, et al: Central nervous system excitatory effects of meperidine in cancer patients. *Ann Neurol* 13:180–185, 1983
23. Han PK, Arnold R, Bond G, et al: Myoclonus secondary to withdrawal from transdermal fentanyl: case report and literature review. *J Pain Symptom Manage* 23:66–72, 2002
24. Bruera E, Pereira J: Acute neuropsychiatric findings in a patient receiving fentanyl for cancer pain. *Pain* 69:199–201, 1997
25. Hagen N, Swanson R: Strychnine-like multifocal myoclonus and seizures in extremely high-dose opioid administration: treatment strategies. *J Pain Symptom Manage* 14:51–58, 1997
26. Nunez-Olarte J: Opioid-induced myoclonus. *Eur J Palliat Care* 2:146–150, 1995
27. Hemstapat K, Monteith GR, Smith D, et al: Morphine-3-glucuronide's neuro-excitatory effects are mediated via indirect activation of N-methyl-D-aspartic acid receptors: mechanistic studies in embryonic cultured hippocampal neurones. *Anesth Analg* 97:494–505, 2003
28. Smith MT: Neuroexcitatory effects of morphine and hydromorphone: evidence implicating the 3-glucuronide metabolites. *Clin Exper Pharmacol Physiol* 27:524–528, 2000
29. Wright AW, Mather LE, Smith MT: Hydromorphone-3-glucuronide: a more potent neuro-excitant than its structural analogue, morphine-3-glucuronide. *Life Sci* 69:409–420, 2001
30. Sjögren P, Thunedborg LP, Christrup L, et al: Is development of hyperalgesia, allodynia and myoclonus related to morphine metabolism during long-term administration? Six case histories. *Acta Anaesthesiol Scand* 42:1070–1075, 1998
31. Lee MA, Leng ME, Tiernan EJ: Retrospective study of the use of hydromorphone in palliative care patients with normal and abnormal urea and creatinine. *Palliat Med* 15:26–34, 2001
32. Gong QL, Hedner J, Bjorkman R, et al: Morphine-3-glucuronide may functionally antagonize morphine-6-glucuronide induced antinociception and ventilatory depression in the rat. *Pain* 48:249–255, 1992
33. Nishigaya K, Kaneko M, Nagaseki Y, et al: Palatal myoclonus induced by extirpation of a cerebellar astrocytoma: case report. *J Neurosur* 88:1107–1110, 1998
34. Ford B, Pullman SL, Khandji A, et al: Spinal myoclonus induced by an intrathecal catheter. *Mov Disord* 12:1042–1045, 1997
35. Maher J, Choudhri S, Halliday W, et al: AIDS dementia complex with generalized myoclonus. *Mov Disord* 12:593–597, 1997
36. Werhahn KJ, Brown P, Thompson PD, et al: The clinical features and prognosis of chronic posthypoxic myoclonus. *Mov Disord* 12:216–220, 1997
37. Wyllie AR, Bayliff CD, Kovacs MJ: Myoclonus due to chlorambucil in two adults with lymphoma. *Ann Pharmacother* 31:171–174, 1997
38. Pranzatelli MR, Tate ED, Kinsbourne M, et al: Forty-one year follow-up of childhood-onset opsoclonus-myoclonus-ataxia: cerebellar atrophy, multiphasic relapses, and response to IVIG. *Mov Disord* 17:1387–1390, 2002
39. End of Life/Palliative Education Resource Center: Fast Fact and Concept #58: Neuroexcitatory effects of opioids: treatment. *www.eperc.mcw.edu*. Accessed December 17, 2004
40. Golf M, Paice JA, Feulner E, et al: Refractory status epilepticus. *J Palliat Med* 7:85–88, 2004
41. Indelicato RA, Portenoy RK: Opioid rotation in the management of refractory cancer pain. *J Clin Oncol* 20:348–352, 2002
42. Eisele JH, Jr., Grigsby EJ, Dea G: Clonazepam treatment of myoclonic contractions associated with high-dose opioids: case report. *Pain* 49:231–232, 1992
43. Stayer C, Tronnier V, Dressnandt J, et al: Intrathecal baclofen therapy for stiff-man syndrome and progressive encephalomyelopathy with rigidity and myoclonus. *Neurology* 49:1591–1597, 1997
44. Chang BS, Lowenstein DH: Epilepsy. *N Engl J Med* 349:1257–1266, 2003
45. Lowenstein DH, Alldredge BK: Status epilepticus. *N Engl J Med* 338:970–976, 1998
46. Bruera E, Schmitz B, Pither J, et al: The frequency and correlates of dyspnea in patients with advanced cancer. *J Pain Symptom Manage* 19:357–362, 2000
47. Reuben DB, Mor V: Dyspnea in terminally ill cancer patients. *Chest* 89:234–236, 1986

48. Ripamonti C: Management of dyspnea in advanced cancer patients. *Support Care Cancer* 7:233–243, 1999
49. O'Driscoll M, Corner J, Bailey C: The experience of breathlessness in lung cancer. *Eur J Cancer Care* 8:37–43, 1999
50. Thomas JR, von Gunten CF: Management of dyspnea. *J Support Oncol* 1:23–34, 2003
51. Dudgeon DJ, Kristjanson L, Sloan JA, et al: Dyspnea in cancer patients: prevalence and associated factors. *J Pain Symptom Manage* 21:95–102, 2001
52. Mosenthal AC, Lee KF: Management of dyspnea at the end of life: relief for patients and surgeons. *J Am Coll Surg* 194:377–386, 2002
53. LeGrand SB, Khawam EA, Walsh D, et al: Opioids, respiratory function, and dyspnea. *Am J Hospice Palliat Care* 20:57–61, 2003
54. Bruera E, MacEachern T, Ripamonti C, et al: Subcutaneous morphine for dyspnea in cancer patients. *Ann Intern Med* 119:906–907, 1993
55. Zebraski SE, Kochenash SM, Raffa RB: Lung opioid receptors: pharmacology and possible target for nebulized morphine in dyspnea. *Life Sci* 66:2221–2231, 2000
56. Farncombe M, Chater S, Gillin A: The use of nebulized opioids for breathlessness: a chart review. *Palliat Med* 8:306–312, 1994
57. Foral PA, Malesker MA, Huerta G, et al: Nebulized opioids use in COPD. *Chest* 125:691–694, 2004
58. Brubacher S, Gobel BH: Use of the pleurx pleural catheter for the management of malignant pleural effusions. *Clin J Oncol Nurs* 7:35–38, 2003
59. Booth S, Wade R: Oxygen or air for palliation of breathlessness in advanced cancer. *J R Soc Med* 96:215–218, 2003
60. Bredin M, Corner J, Krishnasamy M, et al: Multicentre randomised controlled trial of nursing intervention for breathlessness in patients with lung cancer. *BMJ* 318:901–904, 1999
61. Pan CX, Morrison RS, Ness J, et al: Complementary and alternative medicine in the management of pain, dyspnea, and nausea and vomiting near the end of life: a systematic review. *J Pain Symptom Manage* 20:374–387, 2000
62. Payne DK, Massie MJ: Anxiety in palliative care, in Chochinov HM, Breitbart W (eds.): *Handbook of Psychiatry in Palliative Medicine.* New York, Oxford University Press, 2000, pp 63–74
63. Bruera E, Moyano J, Seifert L, et al: The frequency of alcoholism among patients with pain due to terminal cancer. *J Pain Symptom Manage* 10:599–603, 1995
64. Buckman R: Communication in palliative care: a practical guide, in Doyle D, Hanks G, MacDonald N (eds.): *Oxford Textbook of Palliative Medicine* (ed 2). New York, Oxford University Press, 1998, pp 141–156
65. Stephenson NL, Weinrich SP, Tavakoli AS: The effects of foot reflexology on anxiety and pain in patients with breast and lung cancer. *Oncol Nurs Forum* 27:67–72, 2000
66. Lawlor PG, Gagnon B, Mancini IL, et al: Occurrence, causes, and outcome of delirium in patients with advanced cancer: a prospective study. *Arch Intern Med* 160:786–794, 2000
67. Lawlor PG, Bruera ED: Delirium in patients with advanced cancer. *Hematol Oncol Clin North Am* 16:701–714, 2002
68. Fainsinger RL, Waller A, Bercovici M, et al: A multicentre international study of sedation for uncontrolled symptoms in terminally ill patients. *Palliat Med* 14:257–265, 2000
69. Breitbart W, Gibson C, Tremblay A: The delirium experience: delirium recall and delirium-related distress in hospitalized patients with cancer, their spouses/caregivers, and their nurses. *Psychosomatics* 43:183–194, 2002
70. Breitbart W, Tremblay A, Gibson C: An open trial of olanzapine for the treatment of delirium in hospitalized cancer patients. *Psychosomatics* 43:175–182, 2002
71. Callanan M, Kelley P: *Final Gifts: Understanding the Special Awareness, Needs, and Communications of the Dying.* New York, Bantam Books, 1992
72. Morita T, Tsunoda J, Inoue S, et al: Risk factors for death rattle in terminally ill cancer patients: a prospective exploratory study. *Palliat Med* 14:19–23, 2000
73. Wildiers H, Menten J: Death rattle: prevalence, prevention and treatment. *J Pain Symptom Manage* 23:310–317, 2002
74. Kass RM, Ellershaw J: Respiratory tract secretions in the dying patient: a retrospective study. *J Pain Symptom Manage* 26:897–902, 2003
75. Bennett MI: Death rattle: an audit of hyoscine (scopolamine) use and review of management. *J Pain Symptom Manage* 12:229–233, 1996
76. Morita T, Tsunoda J, Inoue S, et al: Contributing factors to physical symptoms in terminally-ill cancer patients. *J Pain Symptom Manage* 18:338–346, 1999
77. Bennett M, Lucas V, Brennan M, et al: Using anti-muscarinic drugs in the management of death rattle: evidence-based guidelines for palliative care. *Palliat Med* 16:369–374, 2002
78. Spiess JL, Scott SD: Anticholinergic agents for the treatment of "death rattle" in patients with myasthenia gravis. *J Pain Symptom Manage* 26:684–686, 2003
79. Back IN, Jenkins K, Blower A, et al: A study comparing hyoscine hydrobromide and glycopyrrolate in the treatment of death rattle. *Palliat Med* 15:329–336, 2001
80. Ersek M: Artificial nutrition and hydration: clinical issues. *J Hospice Palliat Nurs* 5:221–230, 2003
81. Huang ZB, Ahronheim JC: Nutrition and hydration in terminally ill patients: an update. *Clin Geriatr Med* 16:313–325, 2000
82. Salahi H, Ghahramani N, Malek-Hosseini SA, et al: Religious sanctions regarding cadaveric organ transplantation in Iran. *Transplantation Proc* 30:769–770, 1998
83. Rappaport ZH, Rappaport IT: Brain death and organ transplantation: concepts and principles in Judaism. *Adv Exp Med Biol* 550:133–137, 2004
84. Hardacre H: Response of Buddhism and Shinto to the issue of brain death and organ transplant. *Camb Q Healthc Ethics* 3:585–601, 1994
85. Black M, Graham DI: Sudden unexplained death in adults. *Curr Top Pathol* 95:125–148, 2001
86. Enck RE: Dying from hematological cancers. *Am J Hospice Palliat Care* 19:79–80, 2002
87. Whedon MB: Revisiting the road not taken: integrating palliative care into oncology nursing. *Clin J Oncol Nurs* 6:27–33, 2002
88. Ferrell BA: *ELNEC: Promoting Palliative Care in Oncology Nursing.* Duarte, CA, City of Hope, 2004, *www.aach.nche.edu/elnec.* Accessed January 21, 2005
89. Fainsinger R, Miller MJ, Bruera E, et al: Symptom control during the last week of life on a palliative care unit. *J Palliat Care* 7:5–11, 1991
90. Cowan JD, Palmer TW: Practical guide to palliative sedation. *Curr Oncol Rep* 4:242–249, 2002
91. Cowan JD, Walsh D: Terminal sedation in palliative medicine: definition and review of the literature. *Support Care Cancer* 9:403–407, 2001
92. Lynch M: Palliative sedation. *Clin J Oncol Nurs* 7:653–657, 667, 2003
93. Palliative sedation at the end of life. *J Hosp Palliat Nurs* 5:235–237, 2003
94. Braun TC, Hagen NA, Clark T: Development of a clinical practice guideline for palliative sedation. *J Palliat Med* 6:345–350, 2003
95. Hanks-Bell M, Paice J, Krammer L: The use of midazolam hydrochloride continuous infusions in palliative care. *Clin J Oncol Nurs* 6:367–369, 2002

96. Hocking G, Cousins MJ: Ketamine in chronic pain management: an evidence-based review. *Anesth Analg* 97:1730–1739, 2003
97. Bell RF, Eccleston C, Kalso E: Ketamine as adjuvant to opioids for cancer pain: a qualitative systematic review. *J Pain Symptom Manage* 26:867–875, 2003
98. Fine PG: Low-dose ketamine in the management of opioid nonresponsive terminal cancer pain. *J Pain Symptom Manage* 17:296–300, 1999

PART IX

Professional Issues for the Cancer Nurse

CHAPTER 73

The Oncology Advanced Practice Nurse

Susan Moore, RN, MSN, ANP, AOCN®

Introduction

Oncology nursing is rapidly becoming a field of unlimited opportunity for advanced practice nurses. Recent developments in cancer prevention and treatment have opened new areas of specialization for advanced practice nurses in private practice, ambulatory clinics, and tertiary care centers. Increased practice autonomy encourages advanced practice nurses to become entrepreneurs, establishing nurse-managed clinics and consulting services. This chapter describes the educational preparation required for oncology advanced practice and reviews issues critical to advanced nursing practice, including regulation of advanced practice and third-party reimbursement. Finally, trends and emerging roles for oncology advanced practice nurses are explored.

Advanced Practice Nursing Defined

Advanced practice nurse

The title advanced practice nurse (APN) is given to any registered nurse (RN) who has met specific graduate degree educational requirements, has expert clinical knowledge, and provides direct care to patients.[1] Regulatory bodies in the United States recognize four distinct types of APNs: certified nurse anesthetists (CRNA), certified nurse midwives (CNM), clinical nurse specialists (CNS), and nurse practitioners (NP). The American Association of Colleges of Nursing (AACN) has defined advanced practice nurse as an umbrella term appropriate for a licensed registered nurse prepared at the graduate degree level as either a CNS, CRNA, CNM, or NP.[2] This chapter addresses issues related to the CNS and NP role in oncology nursing.

Nurse practitioner. A nurse practitioner is a registered nurse who has advanced education and clinical training in a specialty area such as acute care, adult or family health, or women's health. The NP practice specialty can be identified by the initials included in the credential: adult (ANP), family (FNP), pediatric (PNP), or acute care (ACNP). Except for FNP, a master's degree is now considered the minimum education required for entry; FNP requires a clinical doctorate in nursing (ND) due to the extended content in order to care for all age groups. Within ANP programs, further subspecialties are available: geriatric (GNP) and women's health (WHNP) are just two examples of educational tracks available in NP programs. NP education has gradually shifted away from certificate programs, although most states allow practicing NPs who attained credentialing through certificate programs to become licensed APNs if they apply during a limited grandfathering phase of new legislation. Today, most nurse practitioner programs are graduate-level programs in schools of nursing. By the year 2007, all NP certifying bodies will require a master's degree for certification eligibility.[3] Nurse practitioners are strongly focused on a medical model. NPs obtain medical histories, perform physical examinations, make medical and nursing diagnoses, and treat persons with common health problems and chronic diseases. Nursing practice is regulated by the nurse practice statutes of the state in which the NP is employed; therefore, the amount of autonomy the NP has in performing these functions varies from state to state.

Clinical nurse specialist. The clinical nurse specialist (CNS) role is based on nursing models. A CNS is a master's-prepared registered nurse who has expert knowledge and skill in caring for a population of patients within a given specialty. The four functional components of the CNS role are clinical practice, education, consultation, and research. The majority of CNSs work within tertiary care centers, primarily in inpatient settings, as staff and patient/family educators and consultants. As economic changes forced efficient use of resources, many CNS roles in tertiary care sites were eliminated. Some CNSs chose case management for managed care organizations as a way to advocate for patients and for quality, cost-effective care.[1]

Oncology advanced practice nurse. The oncology advanced practice nurse (OAPN) is not a regulatory title, but is one that reflects the merged or blended role of an APN who has graduate-level education as an oncology CNS and as an adult or acute-care NP. This role may also carry the title of oncology nurse practitioner (ONP). Although early NP education prepared NPs for primary care practice, the oncology specialty reflects components of both traditional primary NP care and acute care. The current ONP role reflects the shifting healthcare changes and expands ONP services to cover the continuum of care for cancer patients and families.[4]

Blended Clinical Nurse Specialist–Nurse Practitioner Role

In 1994, the American Cancer Society published a curriculum guideline for CNS and NP education, thus acknowledging the merged or blended role of a specialist in oncology nursing who is jointly educated in the roles of CNS and NP.[1] The oncology advanced practice nurse (OAPN) would have specialized knowledge in oncology nursing as well as the medical, physical assessment, and diagnostic knowledge of a nurse practitioner.

Many medical centers have grouped both CNSs and NPs under a single title, advanced practice nurse. Tertiary care centers in particular have blended the roles in order to maximize the use of master's-prepared nurses.[5] Within both groups, CNS and NP, are many APNs who feel the roles are quite distinct and should be maintained as such.[6] The Oncology Nursing Society (ONS) endorses the title "advanced practice nurse" to designate both CNS and NP roles. According to ONS's position statement, APNs are prepared, at a minimum, with a master's degree in nursing, with specialty education and precepted clinical experience in oncology. The oncology APN coordinates and provides direct and indirect care to people affected by cancer and collaborates with nurse colleagues and other members of the healthcare team.[7]

The ONS has defined the various titles in oncology nursing by adding position attributes and clarifying educational preparation required for each title, as follows:

> ONS recognizes nurses who have become experts in coordinating and providing direct and indirect care to people affected by cancer through study and precepted clinical practice in oncology at the graduate level as oncology CNSs. The term NP describes the nurse whose educational preparation includes completion of a NP program at the master's or doctorate level. The role of the NP is to provide comprehensive clinical care to individuals, with an emphasis on health promotion, disease prevention, diagnosis, and management of acute and chronic diseases. ONS recognizes NPs who have expertise in the specialty of oncology as oncology NPs.[8]

Legislative and Regulatory Issues in Advanced Practice Nursing

The legal regulation of nursing, including advanced practice, is the responsibility of state boards of nursing. Each state's board is vested with this authority by the state legislature that enacts the state's nurse practice act. This approach has resulted in tremendous variability among states. Although there is a trend in RN licensure toward a compact agreement between states allowing nurses licensed in any state participating in the compact agreement to practice in any other compact state,[9] the regulation surrounding advanced practice nursing is far less confluent. There is a great deal of inconsistency from state to state in the educational/certification requirements, scope of practice, physician oversight, prescriptive authority, and level of regulatory oversight. Despite position statements from the American Nurses Association (ANA), American Nurses Credentialing Center (ANCC), American Academy of Nurse Practitioners (AANP), and American College of Nurse Practitioners (ACNP), inconsistency regarding the definition of an advanced practice registered nurse persists. These inconsistencies create barriers to practice for APNs moving to other states or working in practices that span state lines.

Levels of Regulation

There are four levels of regulation: designation/recognition, registration, certification, and licensure. *Designation/recognition* is the least restrictive method of regulation and consists of recognition of credentials by a state's board of nursing. It does not involve an inquiry into the competence of the APN by the board. *Registration* is the placement of names of APNs on an official board roster. *Certification* involves title regulation. The APN must meet specified, predetermined requirements, and only those who meet the requirements may use the title. However, a title carries legal status only if it is recognized or authorized in statute or regulation. Certification attempts to measure competence. Certification examinations are required for licensure in most situations. Certification examinations are administered by outside organizations recognized by the licensing body as a provider of competency examinations. *Licensure* specifies scope of practice, and applications for licensure are evaluated to ensure that predetermined requirements are met. Licensure also allows the grantor, such as the board of nursing, to take disciplinary action for violation of laws or rules.

Certification as an Advanced Practice Nurse

Certification has been used by the ANA and various specialty organizations, including ONS, for a range of purposes, from recognizing excellence or professional achievement to denoting minimum competency to practice a specialty. There are more than 30 specialty nursing organizations that grant certification to nurses with training beyond the entry level. The Oncology Nursing Certification Corporation (ONCC) is one such organization and offers both basic and advanced oncology nursing certification examinations.

The term *certification* is confusing, since it is used to refer to both specialty and advanced practice certification. For example, ONCC offers two levels of certification in oncology nursing. Oncology Certified Nurse (OCN®) certification is open to any nurse who regularly cares for oncology patients in any setting and meets other practice requirements. RN licensure is the only education requirement; a graduate-level or BSN degree is not required.[10] Advanced practice certification from any certifying body requires education beyond the entry level, usually at the graduate level. In the past, ONCC has had only a single advanced oncology nursing certification examination that was used for all oncology APNs regardless of nursing role. AOCN® role delineation studies and focus groups meeting to discuss the AOCN® examination led to agreement that test items on the AOCN® examination did not accurately reflect the competencies and expectations of the separate roles. Beginning in 2005, ONCC will offer two separate advanced oncology nursing certification examinations, one for oncology CNSs and another for oncology NPs. OAPNs who have already attained AOCN® certification may elect to renew as an AOCN® or may take the appropriate new test at the next renewal. Nurses who are currently AOCN® certified will not be granted the new credential without successful testing, nor will the general AOCN® test be offered in the future.[10]

The eligibility criteria for the new advanced oncology nursing certification examinations are as follows:

Advanced Oncology Clinical Nurse Specialist (AOCNS®)

- Current, active, unrestricted RN license at time of application and examination
- Master's or higher degree in nursing from an accredited institution
- Minimum of 500 hours of supervised practice in an advanced practice role in oncology nursing. These hours may be obtained within the NP program or following graduation from the program.

Advanced Oncology Nurse Practitioner (AOCNP®)

- Current, active, unrestricted RN license at time of application and examination
- Master's or higher degree in nursing from an accredited institution
- Successful completion of an accredited nurse practitioner program
- Minimum of 500 hours of supervised clinical practice as an oncology nurse practitioner. These hours may be obtained within the NP program or following graduation from the program

Many professional nursing organizations, including the ANA, have supported the regulation of advanced practice, through the mechanism of voluntary certification as opposed to securing a second nursing license as an APN. The RN license would be the only nursing license required. Advanced practice would be recognized through certification. This mechanism was established and is operated by professional nursing specialty organizations and mirrors the credentialing process for physicians who seek specialty board certification. Through certification, the profession maintains autonomy and responsibility for the regulation of advanced practice, whereas through second licensure that control is assumed by state boards of nursing. The National Council of State Boards of Nursing (NCSBN) advocates licensure of APNs on the basis that the degree of autonomy and level of care provided by the APN warrants that level of regulation.[3]

A standardized national certification process for advanced practice nursing would eliminate much of the criticism of the current certification process and would potentially abolish the need for a second license to regulate nursing practice. Movement toward such a standardized certification process has begun. In 1991, the ANCC and other certification boards formed the American Board of Nursing Specialties (ABNS). Membership in the ABNS is limited to advanced practice nursing certification bodies that meet ABNS standards. This board is analogous to the American Board of Medical Specialties and other professional boards that certify individuals to specialize in a particular practice area. In 2000, NCSBN launched an advanced practice task force to examine the issue of regulatory sufficiency of advanced practice certification examinations. The resulting NSCBN recommendations were published in a position paper in 2002 that supported certification through recognized agencies.[3] At this time, the AOCN®, AOCNS®, and AOCNP® certification examinations through ONCC or a nurse practitioner certification examination through ACNP or AANP are the only examinations that would qualify an APN to be licensed as an oncology CNS or oncology NP.

Licensure

Current legal requirements for practice as an APN require current, unrestricted RN licensure, graduate-level nursing education, and completion of a minimum number of clinical hours as a graduate student before applying for the APN license. The requirement of clinical hours prevents recipients of nonclinical master's degrees, such as health administration or health information systems, from obtaining APN licenses. The APN must also submit proof of successful completion of an approved certification examination in the specialty area (for the CNS) or as a nurse practitioner (for the NP). Some states may grant separate licenses to CNS and NP candidates. In this situation, APNs with blended roles, having completed both a master's in a specialty such as oncology nursing and a post-master's NP certification, can either choose one

Table 73-1 Nurse Licensure Compact Implementation

State	Implementation	APN Approved
Arizona	7/1/2002	
Arkansas	7/1/2000	
Delaware	7/1/2000	
Idaho	7/1/2001	
Iowa	7/1/2000	
Maine	7/1/2001	
Maryland	7/1/1999	
Mississippi	7/1/2001	
Nebraska	1/1/2001	
New Mexico	1/1/2004	
North Carolina	7/1/2000	
North Dakota	1/1/2004	
South Dakota	1/1/2001	
Tennessee	7/1/2003	
Texas	1/1/2000	
Utah	1/1/2000	3/15/04
Wisconsin	1/1/2000	

Data from NCSBN.[3] Updated information can be found on the NSCBN Web site: *www.nscbn.org/nlc/rnlpbvncompact_mutual_recognition_state.asp.*

Table 73-2 Level of Prescriptive Authority by State

Independent Prescriptive Authority Including Controlled Substances
Alaska, Arizona, Delaware, DC, Idaho, Iowa, Maine, Montana, Nebraska, New Hampshire, New Mexico, New York, Oregon, Vermont, Wisconsin, Wyoming

Dependent Prescriptive Authority Including Controlled Substances
Arkansas, California,* Connecticut, Colorado, Hawaii, Illinois, Indiana, Louisiana, Maryland, Massachusetts, Minnesota, Mississippi,* Nevada, New Jersey,* New York, North Carolina, North Dakota, New York, Ohio,* Pennsylvania, Rhode Island, South Carolina,* South Dakota, Tennessee, Texas, Utah, Washington, West Virginia

Dependent Prescriptive Authority Excluding Controlled Substances
Alabama, Florida, Georgia, Kansas, Kentucky, Missouri, Oklahoma, Virginia

No Prescriptive Authority
All states have some degree of prescriptive authority for APNs as of 2003.

*In specific situations — see state regulations for complete information. Note: Some states differentiate between prescriptive authority for NPs and for other APNs. Check individual state regulations for details.

Data from Pearson.[11]

license over the other or submit paperwork and fees to obtain both licenses. Illinois is one such state.

Depending on the individual state licensing agency, a second APN license may be required in order to obtain prescriptive authority. If so, the license may be applied for at the same time as the APN license. Other states have a single application for APN-prescriber, and no second license is required. Wisconsin is one example of the combined license. APNs completing their educational and clinical requirements should obtain current certification and licensing requirements from the state in which they intend to practice in order to determine license requirements. An excellent source for current legislative and regulatory practice requirements for APNs, listed by state, is published annually in the January issue of *The Nurse Practitioner* journal.[11]

The Nurse Licensure Compact has not met with nationwide approval for basic RN or APN licensure. The Advanced Practice Registered Nurse (APRN) Compact addresses the need to promote consistent access to quality advanced practice nursing care within states or across state lines. NSCBN published a position paper in 2002 supporting (1) APN practice under the RN license after successful completion of a recognized certification exam, rather than second licensure, and (2) support of the Uniform Advanced Practice Registered Nurse Licensure/Authority to Practice (APRN Compact Agreement) adopted in August 2002.[3] As of March 2004, the states shown in Table 73-1 have agreed to the RN or APRN compact, and nurses licensed in those states may practice in any other compact state without relicensure in the second state.[3]

Prescriptive Authority

The authority for the APN to prescribe is regulated at the state level but also involves the Drug Enforcement Administration (DEA) if prescriptive authority for controlled substances is desired. The level of authority varies from independent prescriptive authority including controlled substances to dependent prescriptive authority excluding controlled substances (see Table 73-2). The dependent authority requires that the APN be under supervision of a physician when performing this task. As of 1999, all 50 states and the District of Columbia provide for some level of prescriptive authority for APNs. Some states may require documentation of a certain amount of pharmacology coursework, either as part of the graduate program or independently, for a prescriber's license. Many states and nearly all certifying agencies require documentation of pharmacology primary or continuing education for license or certification renewal.

Controlled substances

In states where APNs are allowed to prescribe controlled substances, DEA registration numbers are required. The DEA has established a midlevel practitioner registration category under which APNs, physician assistants (PAs), and others are given individual DEA registration numbers. These numbers begin with the letter ''M'' to allow responsible parties in the controlled substance distribution chain (e.g., pharmacists) to contact appropriate state officials to verify the authority the practitioner has been granted. DEA registration allows a wide variety of acts, including purchasing, storing, administering, dispensing, and prescribing controlled substances; however, the APN may engage in only those activities authorized by the state in which he or she practices.[5] Figure 73-1 outlines the procedure for obtaining a DEA registration number.

> An application for registration with the Drug Enforcement Administration (DEA) may be obtained, along with the *Mid-Level Practitioner's Manual*, by mailing or telephoning a request to:
>
> United States Department of Justice
> Drug Enforcement Administration
> Central Station
> PO Box 28083
> Washington DC 20038-8083
> 202-307-7255
>
> The application for registration with the DEA also can be accessed online at *www.deadiverson.usdoj.gov/online_forms.htm*. The forms can be viewed and printed or completed online with payment by credit card.
>
> Some states require a state controlled-substance registration number prior to applying for the DEA registration number. In that situation, the address shown on the state controlled-substance license must match the address on the DEA registration, which is generally the place of business, not the residential address. Contact the DEA for further information.

Figure 73-1 Obtaining a DEA registration number

Many states restrict controlled-substance prescriptive authority to schedules III–V for APNs. For oncology APNs, especially those who care for patients throughout the trajectory of disease, or for palliative care specialists, the restriction on prescribing schedule II narcotics for pain relief is viewed as a significant barrier to effective practice. Numerous task forces have addressed these issues before state legislatures in an effort to allow all APNs full prescriptive authority in all states.

Reimbursement of Advanced Practice Nursing Services

APNs provide direct patient care in a variety of settings. Inpatient or hospice APNs are generally paid directly by the medical center or hospice organization and do not bill directly for their services. The cost of their salary is considered part of the operational expense of the institution. Health systems subsidize the nonreimbursable activities of their employees through reimbursement for services by providers able to bill directly.[12] APNs who work in private practice, in ambulatory clinics, as hospitalists, or in independent practice must be able to bill and collect for the services rendered in order to maintain a financially viable practice. In private practice, the contract between the APN and the collaborating physician may require the APN to bring in a certain percentage of the annual salary for continued employment.

The effective utilization of an APN is, in part, tied to reimbursement of services provided. Reimbursement for direct patient care is provided through federal and state programs such as Medicare or Medicaid or through private insurers, including health maintenance organizations (HMOs) and preferred provider organizations (PPOs). Title XVIII of the Social Security Act[13] determines reimbursement eligibility under Medicare and is referred to as provider status. Public and private insurers refer to the Social Security Act to define covered medical and health services.[12]

Reimbursement for APN services decreases the financial burden assumed by the private practice or organization that hires the APN. In addition to the salary paid to the APN, most employers provide paid vacation, medical and disability insurance, education and conference reimbursement, and retirement benefits such as a contributory pension fund or access to 403(b) or, in the case of for-profit companies, 401(k) accounts. The average salary for an APN ranges from $50,000 to $85,000 per year.[14,15] This figure varies considerably based on geographic location, experience, and practice setting. If the practice routinely provides productivity bonuses for physicians, the APN may also share in the bonus system. APNs may also share in the equity of a private practice. If a collaborative practice is required by the state or is desired by the physician or APN, a legal contract may be a condition of practice. The contract will spell out salary, expectations in terms of APN contributions to the practice, benefits, hours, on-call requirements, and other details specific to the practice. APNs who enter into practice contracts are advised to seek legal counsel before finalizing any employment contract.[16]

Medicare payment

Medicare is a federal health insurance program for individuals who are disabled or older than age 65. It is funded through payroll deductions from Social Security. Part A of the program pays for costs incurred during hospitalizations; Part B pays for outpatient services of physicians and some other healthcare providers, including APNs.

Prior to January 1, 1998, APNs were eligible to receive direct reimbursement for services only in rural settings; they received indirect reimbursement for services provided in a nursing home or under the direct supervision of a physician, services termed incident to a physician's services (referred to as "incident-to services"). With passage of the Balanced Budget Act of 1997,[17] APNs became eligible for direct reimbursement of Medicare Part B services in all practice sites and geographic locations, except for rural health centers and federally qualified health centers. Payment is excluded in these two settings because payment to these types of facilities is made under an all-inclusive rate.

In November 1998, the Health Care Financing Administration (HCFA), now the Center for Medicare and Medicaid Services, published the changes and revisions to the Medicare Physician's Fee Schedule, including the regulations covering reimbursement for services provided by APNs.[18] This final rule clarified the definition of collaboration, educational requirements, and practice settings for APNs. In order to apply for a Medicare provider number and bill for services, the APN must:

- Possess a master's or doctorate degree in nursing
- Be a registered professional nurse who is authorized by the state in which the services are furnished to practice as an APN in accordance with state law
- Be nationally certified as an APN by a recognized national certifying body that has established standards for APNs[19]

Under the Balanced Budget Act of 1997, direct payment to APNs is equal to 80% of the lesser of either the actual charge or 85% of the fee schedule amount for the same service if provided by a physician. For services provided by an APN in a hospital outpatient department, payment is made to that department both for the professional services of the APN and for the facility component of the hospital outpatient department service.

The degree of APN-physician collaboration that is necessary for reimbursement is defined by the requirements in each state's nurse practice act. In states without laws or guidelines requiring collaboration, APNs must document their scope of practice and indicate the collaborative relationships they have with physicians to deal with issues outside their scope. It is permissible in these states for the APN to bill directly for his or her services as well as for all of the ancillary services provided to a patient by staff working under the APN's direct supervision. In instances where the APN is employed by a physician, the physician is able to bill 100% of the Medicare fee schedule for the services provided by the APN as long as certain requirements for incident-to services are met:

- The collaborating physician must be present in the same office suite in which the services are provided.
- The patient must have been seen by the physician at least once, and a plan of care must have been documented by the physician.
- The patient must not have a new problem.
- Services must be of the type commonly provided in a physician's office, which means incident-to billing cannot be used for inpatient or home visits. Administration of chemotherapy and insertion of central lines are considered hospital-type services.
- The physician need not countersign the patient's chart, but the office schedule must document the physician's presence in the office at the time of the patient's visit.

Conditions for incident-to billing are restrictive; all conditions must be met, or billing in this manner would be considered Medicare fraud. The additional expense, availability of the collaborating physician, and compliance issues incurred by the practice in order to meet the incident-to billing rate of 100% of the physician fee versus the lower 80% or 85% directly billed by the APN usually encourages practices to bill directly under the APN's Medicare number. In addition, billing on an incident-to basis exposes a practice to more frequent and intensive audits of Medicare compliance, since Medicare wants to ensure that practices abide by the incident-to rules.[20]

APNs wishing to bill Medicare directly for their services and avoid the issues of incident-to billing must have their own provider identification number (PIN), even in cases when the APN is an employee and the employer has always billed for the APN's services using the employer's PIN with a modifier. Figure 73-2 provides information on obtaining a Medicare provider number. The process of applying for a Medicare PIN is quite complicated, and new APNs may wish to use the employing facility's medical credentialing office to assist with completion of the necessary forms. Once obtained, the PIN remains unique to the APN and can be used in any practice in the future, so long as Medicare is notified of the practice change.

Medicaid payment

Medicaid is a joint state and federally funded healthcare program for lower-income Americans. Direct reimbursement to pediatric (PNP) and family nurse practitioners (FNP) for services provided to children is federally mandated. Other healthcare services provided by other APNs may be reimbursed at the discretion of the state, although many states have refused

To receive direct reimbursement for services covered by Medicare or Medicaid, an advanced practice nurse must have a billing or provider number.

Medicare Provider Number
Contact the local Medicare carrier to obtain the registration form to apply for a Medicare billing number, or contact the Social Security Office at 800-772-1213.

Medicaid Provider Number
To obtain a registration form to apply for a Medicaid provider number, contact the local Medicaid office within the state health department.

CHAMPUS Provider Information
To obtain a CHAMPUS provider application, write to the following address:
CHAMPUS
Provider File Operations
PO Box 100558
Florence, SC 29501-0558
Telephone numbers for CHAMPUS area offices:
Mid-Atlantic Region 800-467-8500
Western Region 800-225-4816
MN, WI, IA, WV, KY, OH 800-471-0704

Figure 73-2 Obtaining a provider number.

to credential CNSs and ANPs. The reimbursement rate for covered services is determined by each state. Many states have requested and have been given waivers that preempt federal Medicaid regulation and allow the state to develop managed care organizations (MCO) for the provision of their Medicaid services. Since the majority of MCOs exclude APNs from their provider panels, APNs are unable to bill Medicaid for services.

Payment by other providers

Private insurers include indemnity plans and HMOs. No standard rules exist for private insurers in regard to billing by APNs. Each company can establish its own policies. Most have chosen not to issue rules regarding care and billing by APNs or to credential APNs, although some companies have begun to include FNPs in their provider panels. Many private insurers allow APNs to bill under the physician's number without restriction. The only way to know if the APN can become a provider is to contact each individual insurance company to determine its policy regarding nonphysician providers. Insurers who agree to credential APNs will have specific forms to complete, which must be submitted with a copy of the RN and APN licenses as well as a copy of the NP-physician collaborative agreement, if required by the state.

HMOs provide care to enrollees at a capitated annual rate regardless of the type of provider or the level of services provided. APNs who work in collaboration with a physician are eligible for reimbursement. The HMO receives a fixed, monthly payment per enrollee. The APN may contract directly with the HMO to provide services and be paid by the HMO or may bill under the physician's number.

The Civilian and Medical Program of the Uniformed Services (CHAMPUS) is a federal program that provides services to members of the uniformed services and their families when these services cannot be provided by a military hospital. NPs as well as psychiatric and mental health CNSs are eligible for direct reimbursement under CHAMPUS.

The Federal Employee Health Benefit Plan (FEHBP) offers health insurance plans to federal employees and retirees. Coverage of APN services is mandated, and direct reimbursement of services is provided. Prepaid health insurance plans that are part of the FEHBP network are not required to include APNs in their provider network. If APNs are part of the provider network, the specific health insurance plan determines the level of payment for APN services.

Collaboration and Consultation

Except in states allowing independent practice for APNs, a collaborative agreement is required between a physician and the APN. A collaborative agreement is not a contract of employment; rather, it states the conditions of the APN practice, including:

- Scope of practice
- Name(s) of collaborating physician(s) and contact information
- License information for the APN
- Certification information for the APN
- Resources for other consultations
- Practice protocols, if required or desired
- Invasive procedures for which the APN is certified or has been credentialed by the institution (for example, lumbar puncture, bone marrow aspiration and biopsy)
- Malpractice insurance, if required or desired

Some states restrict the number of APNs in collaborative practice with an individual physician or the number of physicians with whom an individual APN may have a collaborative practice. The Board of Nursing in each state will have information regarding any restrictions to collaborative practice. When a collaborative agreement is required by the state or desired by the physician or APN, it must be written and signed by both parties. Some medical institutions require annual renewal of the collaborative agreement by both parties. The collaborative agreement should be as general as allowed by regulatory statute in order to avoid practicing outside the confines of the agreement. Some states require APNs to practice only within defined protocols; if so, these protocols should be clearly stated within the collaborative agreement. If procedures are allowed under the agreement, they should also be clearly stated. A sample collaborative agreement is given in Appendix A at the end of this chapter.

The OAPN possesses outstanding clinical skills that serve as the foundation for practice. He or she is expert in the process of patient and family education, skilled in the use of evidence-based practice, is able to negotiate complex organizations, and possesses specialized, in-depth knowledge that is utilized to care for cancer patients and families. In the process of consultation, the OAPN seeks the help of an expert to either manage a patient problem or solve an organizational problem. An external or internal approach to consultation can be utilized. In the former, consultation is the focus of the APN's job, whereas in the latter, it is one of the subroles of the APN's position. In either approach, the APN acts as a catalyst for change.

Oncology Advanced Practice Nursing Roles

The CNS role has traditionally been conceptualized as integrating the subroles of expert practitioner, educator, consultant, researcher, and manager/leader and has predominantly been actualized in inpatient, tertiary settings. In contrast, the nurse practitioner (NP) role has emphasized the role of direct care provider. Historically, the CNS's primary responsibility has been to the employing organization, whereas the NP's primary responsibility has been to the patient. Acknowledging the recent paradigm shift toward a blended role, ONS has revised its position paper on the role of APNs in oncology care to recommend full inclusion of OAPNs in all aspects of cancer care and health policy reform.[7]

The dramatic shift toward a merged or blended role for APNs has led to a decision in many states to grant APN licensure to both CNSs and NPs without restriction as to the location of practice or manner of patient care. In the ambulatory cancer center in one large midwestern academic medical center, CNSs and NPs see patients for physical examinations and patient management in seemingly equivalent roles. Therefore, it seems appropriate to consider practice focus as the primary component when describing the basic role of the OAPN. The OAPN specializes in the care of individuals and families with or at high risk for cancer. Within that general practice, the OAPN often develops a practice focus. For example, the focus can be in a particular area of oncology advanced practice, such as prevention and early detection, genetic predisposition to cancer, or symptom management, or it can be in the care of individuals with a specific malignancy, such as breast or lung cancer.

Many of today's OAPN roles involve responsibilities that traditionally have fallen within the realm of medicine, such as physical examination, interpretation of diagnostic tests, and prescription of medication, but still include concepts of health promotion, disease prevention, and patient/family advocacy. Successful advanced practice involves expanding nursing's traditional boundaries while preserving the essence of nursing. It is not only the ability to perform a physical examination and prescribe medication, it is also the ability to translate to the patient and family the impact the treatment will have on their lives. It is the ability to identify trends, predict outcomes, and anticipate needs. Appendix B at the end of this chapter provides a sample position description for an oncology nurse practitioner.

Primary Care

Prevention, screening, and risk assessment

Intervention for primary prevention of cancer is one of the most effective means of reducing the incidence, morbidity, and mortality of cancer.[21] Cancer screening activities are routinely taught in APN education programs, and most practitioners see these activities as consistent with their role, regardless of practice setting. The physical examination for cancer screening and defining an individual's risk profile requires specialized and continuing education. Routine screening for skin, breast, testicular, and colorectal cancers may be performed in primary care offices, or patients may be referred to cancer centers for surveillance. The OAPN is in a unique position to educate healthcare consumers and healthcare providers alike about barriers to cancer screening and to advocate for patients to obtain timely screening procedures such as mammograms and colonoscopies. The OAPN is involved in many aspects of cancer screening, from identifying individuals at risk to performing physical examinations focusing on cancer screening. The OAPN also develops and implements educational programs in school, community, and employment settings on cancer risk factors, prevention, and early detection practices. OAPNs teach self-examination, offer counseling on lifestyle and risk-factor modification, and sponsor programs aimed at risk reduction, such as nutritional and smoking cessation programs. They develop educational materials and conduct research in the area of prevention and early detection. OAPNs have been responsible for establishing breast cancer screening clinics,[22] providing access to clinical breast examinations, and screening mammograms for low-income women. Women at high risk for breast cancer may benefit from care by OAPNs in a high-risk breast cancer screening clinic where they have access not only to skilled OAPNs but to nurse geneticists as well.[21]

Cancer genetic predisposition testing

The rapid expansion of knowledge regarding the role of genetics in the development of cancer and the identification of cancer susceptibility genes has led to a role for the OAPN in cancer genetics.[23] Testing and counseling for a genetic predisposition to cancer initially was limited to individuals and families with a hereditary tendency to develop cancer. However, as genetic testing for certain cancers has become commercially available, the demand for testing has increased. Genetic testing requires a precise sequence of patient screening, education, and informed consent prior to testing. Regardless of the outcome of the test, whether or not a deleterious mutation has been identified, disclosure of the results involves counseling and further follow-up with the patient and family regarding the test results. OAPNs with specific knowledge of genetics frequently provide the bulk of patient education and counseling and also obtain informed consent for genetic testing.[23]

Secondary Care

Active treatment

OAPNs are involved in the care of patients receiving treatment for cancer as either direct care providers or consultants. If independent practice is allowed, the OAPN can see newly diagnosed patients and outline a plan of care. If collaborative practice is required, the OAPN may work with the physician during the initial visit to obtain the patient's health history and perform the physical examination. The OAPN reviews the results of radiological and laboratory studies, including pathology, and devises a treatment plan in collaboration with the oncologist. He or she then discusses the treatment plan and expected outcomes with the patient and family. Side effects and self-care management strategies are reviewed in detail. In many settings, the OAPN orders laboratory and radiological studies and prescribes medications.

During the phase when the patient is receiving active treatment, the OAPN meets the patient's medical and nursing needs. The OAPN usually sees patients who are actively undergoing chemotherapy or radiation therapy at regular intervals, managing any treatment-related side effects. The OAPN also manages concomitant medical problems such as diabetes mellitus and hypertension and provides ongoing education and psychosocial support. Because chemotherapy is not considered a physician-provided service, most OAPNs do not administer chemotherapy in conjunction with an examination but serve as a consultant to the infusion room staff should problems arise.

As a consultant, the OAPN in secondary care is involved in planning and implementing initiatives aimed at supporting and educating patients and their families. Educational initiatives usually focus on helping patients and families understand the disease process, its treatment, and the potential side effects. The OAPN's expertise is also used in symptom management as an important part of a multidisciplinary pain and symptom management team. He or she also may act as a consultant to the institution in establishing standards for oncology practice and developing critical pathways. Patients receive care from OAPNs in a variety of settings, ranging from office, hospital, ambulatory clinic, radiation facility, and home or hospice.

Follow-up care

At the conclusion of initial treatment, the patient enters the follow-up phase of care. The healthcare focus shifts to returning the patient to his or her premorbid condition, moving into the survivor phase of the disease, identifying and managing the long-term effects of therapy, and monitoring for disease recurrence. Many oncologists have limited time to spend caring for patients during this phase of their disease, as their focus is on patients receiving active treatment. OAPNs have assumed care for this patient population in many settings. In states where independent practice is allowed, the physician may refer the patient to a nurse-managed clinic for follow-up. In others, the patient is collaboratively cared for by the oncologist and OAPN, with the OAPN assuming the role of primary provider when the patient moves into the follow-up phase. The OAPN is responsible for performing physical examinations, ordering and interpreting laboratory and radiological studies, and referring patients for diagnostic studies as needed. Additionally, the OAPN maintains communication with the patient's primary care provider and referring physician.

Tertiary Care

Acute care

Oncology CNSs have traditionally fulfilled the role of acute care practitioners; however, in recent years organizational needs have changed and the role of the acute care NP has developed.[24] Several recent trends have led to the development of this role. Changes in medical residency training programs, the shift from fee-for-service to capitated payment plans for health care, and economic downturns in health care have created new acute care roles for APNs.

Medical education has placed a renewed emphasis on primary care, shifting the focus of training away from the inpatient setting toward the ambulatory setting. In recent years, some states have placed legal limits on the number of hours that can be worked by medical residents. Cutbacks in the federal funding of residency training programs have led to a downsizing of such programs. The shift away from fee-for-service-based care and the reduced levels of reimbursement for physician services have resulted in physicians' caring for more patients for less revenue. The net result is that the physician has become less available to the patient and his or her family. These forces have combined to create the need for qualified providers in the acute care setting, and APNs have stepped in to fill that need. Some APNs have secured positions in acute care settings as NP hospitalists. In this role, the APN performs the admission history and physical examination and oversees patient care in collaboration with the attending physician. Acute care facilities that do not participate in residency programs have found this APN role to be efficacious.

The needs of the organization determine whether the OAPN role is more similar to that of a CNS or an NP. Complex organizations such as academic medical centers and comprehensive cancer centers that traditionally have relied on medical residents to provide acute care services have been most affected by changes in medical residency programs. These organizations use both types of OAPNs in the acute care setting.[4]

The OAPN with a direct care emphasis is responsible for managing a caseload of patients from admission through discharge. He or she has medical staff privileges and obtains the patient's health history, performs a physical examination, interprets laboratory and radiological studies, prescribes medications, and coordinates discharge and follow-up care. Invasive procedures such as bone marrow aspiration and biopsy, lumbar puncture, thoracentesis, and paracentesis may also be the responsibility of the OAPN, as permitted by the state's nurse practice act.[25] Routine management of acute care patients requiring anticoagulation monitoring are excellent areas for APN responsibility.[26] In essence, the OAPN is responsible for the minute-to-minute care of the patient, in collaboration with the attending physician.

The OAPN with an organizational focus performs functions such as acting as a mentor to nursing staff, consulting with nursing staff on the care of patients with complex needs, developing staff and patient educational programs, facilitating support groups, and implementing research-based changes in practice. This type of OAPN often has nursing department and hospital responsibilities such as committee representation.

Nurse case manager

Another OAPN role that has emerged, due primarily to changes in healthcare reimbursement, is that of the case manager. The economic and clinical demands of case management in tertiary care are best served by a nurse who possesses a master's degree. Case managers do not provide direct care but coordinate care provided by others. The case manager may be employed or retained by a patient's insurance carrier in order to provide quality, cost-effective care or can be an independent case manager–consultant working directly for the patient or family. When contracted to work directly with the patient, the case manager–consultant serves in an advisory capacity to guide the family through an often-confusing healthcare system. The case manager–consultant may provide information on access to clinical trials, offer referral information to medical centers providing specialized care outside the patient's residential area, or help secure ancillary services. Regardless of the case manager's focus, the goal of case management is to ensure the effective use of resources and to meet outcomes within an appropriate length of stay. Thus, a case manager also identifies trends in patient outcomes and implements measures to correct variances.

Palliative, Hospice, and Bereavement Care

End-of-life (EOL) care in our society is often engaged late in the dying process, resulting in fragmented care. Unfortunately, many cancer patients will experience the shift of treatment from cure to care, and the services of an OAPN with an expertise in palliative and hospice care can improve quality of life.[27] The OAPN in palliative and hospice care is an expert in aggressive pain and symptom management, psychosocial and spiritual care, and end-of-life ethical and legal issues. Palliative care should be initiated throughout the course of advanced disease. The experience of palliative care can be enhanced by the services of an expert

OAPN.[27,28] By the year 2030, for the first time in history, the old will outnumber the young; the aging population is living longer but with more chronic illness.[29] Recent developments in cancer treatment mean that many cancer patients are living longer with chronic advanced disease rather than dying quickly with acute disease, necessitating a paradigm shift that should include palliative care over a longer time span than is currently employed. The World Health Organization has suggested that active palliative care be incorporated into care from the time of diagnosis.[30]

The APN who integrates palliative practices into the patient's care has advanced knowledge in pathophysiology, pharmacology, pharmacokinetics, pharmacodynamics, and the application of evidence-based interventions. The palliative APN is skilled at managing the complex symptoms of advanced illness, in promoting quality of life,[27,28] and in providing cost-effective and appropriate palliative care.[27,31]

Several different models are used for the delivery of palliative and hospice care. In the inpatient direct care model, the OAPN is a staff member of a palliative care or hospice unit. Patients are examined daily by the OAPN, and orders for medications and treatments are written as needed. Palliative care may also be used as a consulting interdisciplinary service. In this model, the OAPN is a member of a palliative care team that sees patients as requested by physicians and nurses in various locations in the hospital or outpatient department. The OAPN acts as a consultant to the patient's primary care team. Recommendations are made for interventions, but orders are usually written by the referring physician. The patient is revisited daily or as often as necessary to reevaluate the efficacy of the intervention. In the community-based model, the OAPN may be employed by a hospice or home care agency and utilized as a consultant for complex patients and families with difficult management issues. In some instances, the OAPN may make home visits. Because hospice reimbursement is made on a per diem basis, APNs in hospice settings do not bill directly for services rendered; rather, they are paid on a salary basis directly by the hospice organization. Regardless of the setting in which patient care occurs, the OAPN acts as a role model and provides informal teaching to less experienced nurses as well as to patients and their care providers.

Industry and Research

Industry

Employment opportunities for OAPNs outside of traditional hospital- or office-based clinical practice include a variety of diverse roles in the healthcare industry. They are employed by insurers as case managers, by consulting firms as healthcare consultants, and by pharmaceutical and biotechnology firms in roles ranging from company sales representatives to educational consultants. OAPNs are also combining their clinical expertise with a knowledge of information systems in roles as nursing informatics specialists in developing cancer practice software, coding and billing support systems, and online educational programs.

Research

The OAPN is involved in research by using research results, implementing independent research projects, and collaborating on medical research. The OAPN can function as director or manager of the organization's clinical research program assuming responsibility for preparing grant proposals, implementing protocols, accruing patients, and complying with regulations. OAPNs are also employed by clinical research management companies or by pharmaceutical firms as clinical research associates. In this role, the OAPN supervises and monitors clinical trials, often at different sites, to ensure the integrity of the research data.

Outcomes Measurement

Given the current tight economic budget for health care in the United States, OAPNs seeking positions in private practice or medical centers are often asked to prove that their services will be cost-effective and provide a financial incentive for the creation or retention of the positions. On many occasions in the past five to ten years, administrators have globally eliminated CNS positions from tertiary care centers, citing increased cost without apparent financial benefit to the medical center. Outcomes measurement is one method for proving clinical and financial benefit for APN services.[32] Mundinger and colleagues[33] published a landmark randomized trial evaluating care by NPs or physicians in a primary, ambulatory care setting in which patient outcomes were found to be comparable. Although one cannot generalize a study conducted in a primary care setting to the care provided in specialty practices, the foundation for the argument that NPs can provide care comparable to that provided by physicians is certainly there. Cunningham[34] reviewed selected empirical literature examining outcomes of advanced practice nursing with a specific focus on OAPNs to provide evidence supporting the effectiveness of OAPNs. A conceptual framework for evaluating the ACNP role may be needed, both for annual performance evaluation and as a basis for future

Table 73-3 Nurse-Sensitive Outcomes of Advanced Practice

1. Satisfaction with care delivery
2. Symptom resolution/reduction
3. Perception of being well cared for
4. Compliance/adherence with treatment plan
5. Knowledge of patients and families
6. Trust of care provider
7. Collaboration among care providers
8. Care provider recommendation according to need
9. Frequency and type of procedures ordered
10. Quality of life

Data from Ingersoll et al.[37]

outcomes studies.[35] The lack of randomized outcomes research in APN specialty practices should provide an incentive for OAPNs to initiate such studies.

Linking outcomes data with cost analysis, a business tool that can be used by any practitioner in any healthcare system, can be used to examine business practices to determine the cost-effectiveness of services provided. Understanding and managing operational costs are crucial in attaining financial stability. Cost analysis is particularly important in independent nurse-managed clinic settings where NPs are in direct competition with physician practices.[36]

The AANP has a fact sheet available that provides numerous references concerning the cost-effectiveness of quality care provided by NPs. This and other outcomes information is available through the AANP Web site at *www.aanp.org*. Finally, it is important to identify outcome indicators for APN practice. Ingersoll and colleagues[37] conducted a modified Delphi survey from 1997 to 1998 to determine the outcome indicators that APNs recommend for use in measuring their effect on care delivery outcomes. Table 73-3 lists the ten highest-ranked outcome indicators in a sample of APNs in the Ingersoll study.

Looking to the Future

Advanced practice nurses have made great strides since the first nurse practitioner training program was started at the University of Colorado in 1965. NPs and CNSs play an increasingly important role in promoting and maintaining health in both rural and urban areas in the United States. Once welcomed only in areas unable to secure physician services, APNs have now begun to appear in practices throughout the spectrum of health care. In order to continue to promote advanced practice nursing in this country, APNs must focus on three areas of change: education, regulation, and independent practice with full reimbursement.

Education

One concern is the lack of consistency in content from one APN educational program to another.[38] Unlike medical schools, where content is mandated by preparation for the United States Medical Licensing Examinations (USMLE), graduate-level APN program content tends to vary from one institution to another, although the total number of preparation hours is consistent. In some cases, content has been dictated by tailoring a program to secure federal or private grant funds in order to continue to operate. By promoting consistent course content across the board, APNs will be properly prepared for board certification at the completion of the program and will be on a par with other APNs from different institutions following certification. The development of a model core curriculum for OAPNs and support for increased federal funding for OAPN programs have been recommendations of ONS since 1994.[1] Alpert and colleagues[38] recommend three levels of education for the NP role, beginning at the baccalaureate level and extending into doctorate education.

Regulation

Without exception, the major nursing groups including ONS, have supported the use of the term "advanced practice nurse" as the single official designation for the CNS and NP, but they do not infer the merger of the two roles. Once titles are agreed upon, the next task of APNs and their supporting groups should be to attain a single, national licensure for all APNs through the adoption of the compact agreement by all states for all levels of nursing. Although the compact agreement is being approved for RN licensure, approval for APNs lags far behind. In addition, only nineteen states accept the AOCN® certification for licensure as an APN. The compact agreement should also have a common list of approved certifications so that APNs who move from one state to another can practice without relicensure or without seeking another certification in order to meet individual state APN licensure requirements. State laws are not uniform in scope of practice; some states allow fully independent practice with full prescriptive authority for APNs, while others restrict both severely. National licensing with the right to independent practice can amend this situation.

Reimbursement

As APNs achieve independent practice, full reimbursement for services rendered must follow. APNs provide quality, cost-effective care, and insurance providers will have to acknowledge this level of care by reimbursing nurse-provided services at the same level at which they currently reimburse physician services. In the interim, OAPNs can continue to meet the needs of patients by marketing services to insurers, oncologists, and patients. The addition of an OAPN to an oncology practice can result in a larger volume of patients being seen and more comprehensive care being provided. The OAPN can assume the follow-up care of patients, enabling the practice to increase volume without significant cost. Alternatively, the OAPN can help the oncology practice compete in an increasing competitive market by offering a variety of types of education and support. Nurse-managed centers will play an important role in health services delivery by offering a unique approach to primary and specialty care, but this can be done only if services are appropriately reimbursed by all insurers.[39]

Conclusion

Private consumer expenditures for both ambulatory and inpatient care have increased to 14% of the gross national product and will continue this upward trend, driven by scientific and technological advances as well as general inflation. As the population also increased by approximately 75 million people from 1990 to 2000, projected demands on the healthcare system will also increase.[40] Although physicians and APNs have many overlapping roles, each has something unique to offer the consumer that broadens the spectrum of healthcare delivery. Independent practice, unencumbered by artificial regulatory barriers, will afford OAPNs new and challenging opportunities, increasing responsibilities and the skills to be mastered and leading to new relationships with patients, administrators, the economic environment, and nursing and medical colleagues. OAPNs are in a unique position to bring together two distinct but overlapping disciplines — nursing and medicine — that share the common goal of patient well-being.

APPENDIX A: ADVANCED PRACTICE NURSING COLLABORATIVE AGREEMENT

RUSH UNIVERSITY MEDICAL CENTER CHICAGO, ILLINOIS 60612

ADVANCED PRACTICE NURSING WRITTEN COLLABORATIVE AGREEMENT

A. ADVANCED PRACTICE NURSE INFORMATION

NAME:

ILLINOIS RN LICENSE NUMBER:

ILLINOIS APN LICENSE NUMBER:

ILLINOIS MIDLEVEL PRACTITIONER LICENSE NUMBER:

FEDERAL MIDLEVEL PRACTITIONER DEA NUMBER:

AREAS OF CERTIFICATION:

CERTIFYING ORGANIZATION:

CERTIFICATION EXPIRATION DATE:

CERTIFICATION NUMBER:

PRACTICE SITES: ***See Attachment A.***

CONTACT NUMBER:

FAX NUMBER:

E-MAIL ADDRESS:

EMERGENCY CONTACT NUMBERS:
(e.g., pager, answering service)

Attachments:
Copy of Certification/Recertification
Copies of RN & APN License
Copy of Certificate of Insurance
Copy of Midlevel Practitioner License

B. COLLABORATING PHYSICIAN INFORMATION

NAME:

ILLINOIS LICENSE NUMBER:

PRACTICE AREA OR CONCENTRATION:

BOARD CERTIFICATION (IF ANY):

CERTIFYING ORGANIZATION:

PRACTICE SITES: ***See Attachment A.***

CONTACT NUMBER:

FAX NUMBER:

EMERGENCY CONTACT NUMBERS:
(e.g. pager, answering service)

C. ADVANCED PRACTICE NURSE–COLLABORATING PHYSICIAN WORKING RELATIONSHIP

1. SCOPE OF PRACTICE

Under this agreement, the advanced practice nurse will work with the collaborating physician in an active practice to deliver healthcare services to ____________________ . This includes, but is not limited to, the diagnosis, treatment and management of acute and chronic health problems; ordering, interpreting and performing laboratory and radiology tests; prescribing medications, including controlled substances, to the extent delegated; receiving and dispensing stock and sample medications; and performing other therapeutic or corrective measures as indicated.

If applicable, the advanced practice nurse shall maintain allied health personnel privileges at the following hospital(s) for the designated services:
Hospitals:

____

This written collaborative agreement shall be reviewed and updated annually. A copy of this written collaborative agreement shall remain on file at all sites where the advanced practice nurse renders service and shall be provided to the Illinois Department of Professional Regulation upon request.

Any joint orders or guidelines are set forth or referenced in Attachment B.

2. MEDICAL DIRECTION

Physician medical direction shall be adequate with respect to collaboration with certified nurse practitioners, certified nurse midwives, and certified clinical nurse specialists if a collaborating physician:

(A) participates in the joint formulation and joint approval of orders or guidelines with the advanced practice nurse and periodically reviews such orders and the services provided patients under such orders in accordance with accepted standards of medical practice and advanced practice nursing practice;

(B) is on site at least once a month to provide medical direction and consultation; and

(C) is available through telecommunications for consultation on medical problems, complications, or emergencies or patient referral. (225 ILCS 60/54.5(6))

The written collaborative agreement shall be for services the collaborating physician generally provided to his or her patients in the normal course of clinical practice.

3. COMMUNICATION, CONSULTATION, AND REFERRAL

   The advanced practice nurse shall consult with the collaborating physician by telecommunication or in person as needed. In the absence of the designated collaborating physician, another physician shall be available for consultation.

   The advanced practice nurse shall inform each collaborating physician of all written collaborative agreements he or she has signed with other physicians, and provide a copy of these to any collaborating physician upon request.

4. DELEGATION OF PRESCRIPTIVE AUTHORITY

   As the Collaborating Physician, any prescriptive authority delegated to the Advanced Practice Nurse is set forth in Attachment C.
   NOTE: ADVANCED PRACTICE NURSE MAY ONLY PRESCRIBE CONTROLLED SUBSTANCES UPON RECEIPT OF AN ILLINOIS MIDLEVEL PRACTITIONER CONTROLLED SUBSTANCE LICENSE.

WE, THE UNDERSIGNED, AGREE TO THE TERMS AND CONDITIONS OF THIS WRITTEN COLLABORATIVE AGREEMENT.

____

Collaborating Physician's Typed Name

____

Collaborating Physician Signature/Date

____

Advanced Practice Nurse's Typed Name

____

Advanced Practice Nurse Signature/Date

ATTACHMENT A
PRACTICE SITES

[Practice sites should be listed in this section with full name and address of each facility]

ATTACHMENT B
JOINT ORDERS OR GUIDELINES

1. The Advanced Practice Nurse is authorized to perform all of those procedures that are performed by registered nurses in accordance with generally accepted standards of nursing practice. In addition to which, the Advanced Practice Nurse is authorized to perform the following procedures (Please specify which, if any, of the procedures listed below require a physician's presence):

NOTE: Although not delineated above, the Advanced Practice Nurse is also authorized to perform such additional procedures which are within the scope of practice of the Collaborating Physician and which may be performed in accordance with accepted standards of advanced nursing practice, and commensurate with the skills and training of the Advanced Practice Nurse.

2. [The completion of Paragraph 2 is optional]
   The Advanced Practice Nurse may rely upon the following references in providing healthcare services:
3. [The completion of Paragraph 3 is optional]
   The following restrictions, if any, are imposed upon the Advanced Practice Nurse:

ATTACHMENT C
DELEGATION OF PRESCRIPTIVE AUTHORITY

The Advanced Practice Nurse may prescribe medications in association with the scope of services described in the written collaborative agreement, page 2, section C.1.

1. The Advanced Practice Nurse may not prescribe the following medications (if none, state none):
2. The Advanced Practice Nurse may prescribe controlled substances, Schedule III, IV, or V, in association with the scope of services described in attachment B (if none, state none):

Provided courtesy of Rush University Medical Center, Chicago, Illinois.

APPENDIX B: ONCOLOGY NURSE PRACTITIONER POSITION DESCRIPTION

General Description

A nurse practitioner (NP) is a registered nurse who has completed an accredited graduate-level NP program. NP practice includes health supervision of well individuals, episodic care of individuals with acute, commonly occurring illnesses, and the long-term management of individuals with chronic conditions. NPs work collaboratively with physicians and other members of the healthcare team.

The oncology NP cares for individuals with cancer who are either receiving treatment or being monitored for disease progression, for relapse, or for long-term side effects of therapy. Only those individuals whose disease, treatment, and side effects can be managed primarily in an ambulatory care setting are cared for by the oncology NP.

Major Duties

The oncology NP functions independently as the care provider for a select group of individuals with cancer under the general supervision of an attending physician. Major duties fall into three broad categories: clinical practice, research, and education.

Clinical Practice

1. Obtains a health history and assesses the patient's physical status through the performance of a physical examination.
2. Assesses the psychosocial situation, coping strategies, and learning needs of patients and their significant others.
3. Develops and implements a plan of care based on clinical findings and disease process. This includes a plan for treatment, counseling, and education.
4. Communicates the plan of care to other members of the healthcare team.
5. Evaluates patient response to treatment and revises the plan of care as necessary and in collaboration with the attending physician.
6. Prescribes medications, laboratory, and diagnostic tests.
7. After successful performance of three supervised diagnostic procedures (i.e., bone marrow biopsies, thoracentesis, or paracentesis), the NP will independently perform these procedures on his or her patient population according to written guidelines.
8. Coordinates patient care with other departments and disciplines.
9. Requests consultation and/or initiates referrals for complex problems or specialized care as necessary.
10. Maintains complete and current medical records and flow sheets.
11. Provides follow-up letters to primary care and referring physicians.

Research

12. Assists with the design and implementation of clinical trials.
13. Acts as co-investigator on medical clinical trials and as primary investigator on nursing research studies.
14. Acts as a patient advocate.
15. Evaluates and reports adverse effects and complications of treatment.

Education

16. Serves as an expert resource in cancer to nursing staff, medical staff, patients, and families.
17. Conducts professional and patient educational programs.
18. Participates in patient care rounds and care conferences.
19. Acts as a preceptor for graduate students in NP and oncology nursing programs.
20. Acts as a role model and consultant to other members of the nursing staff.

Qualifications

1. Graduate of an accredited NP program.
2. Current licensure as a registered nurse and NP.
3. Minimum of five years of oncology nursing experience.
4. Advanced oncology nursing certification.
5. Clinical expertise in caring for individuals with cancer.
6. Knowledge of current nursing and medical practice and research related to medical oncology.
7. Demonstrated commitment to continued professional growth as evidenced by membership in professional organizations and attendance at continuing education offerings.
8. Demonstrated strong written and verbal communication skills. Public speaking and publishing experience strongly preferred.

Used with permission from Galassi.[41]

References

1. Murphy-Ende K: Advanced practice nursing: reflections on the past, issues for the future. *Oncol Nurs Forum* 29:106–112, 2002

2. American Nurses Association: *Scope and Standards of Advanced Practice Nursing*. Washington DC, American Nurses Association, 1995
3. Nursing Council of State Boards of Nursing. *Nursing Regulation: Nursing Licensure and Certification*. Chicago, National Council of State Boards of Nursing, 2004
4. Bush NJ, Watters T: The emerging role of the oncology nurse practitioner: a collaborative model within the private practice setting. *Oncol Nurs Forum* 28:1425–1431, 2001
5. Quall SJ: Clinical nurse specialist: role restructuring to advanced practice registered nurse. *Crit Care Nurs Q* 21:37–49, 1999
6. Loftus LA, McDowell J: The lived experience of the oncology clinical nurse specialist. *Int J Nurs Stud* 37:513–521, 2000
7. Oncology Nursing Society: The role of the advanced practice nurse in oncology care. *Oncol Nurs Forum* 30:549–550, 2003
8. Oncology Nursing Society: *The Use of Titles in Oncology Nursing Practice*. Pittsburgh, Oncology Nursing Society, 1997
9. National Council of State Boards of Nursing. Chicago, 2003. Nursing regulation. *www.nscbn.org/regulation/nlc_licensure_aprn. asp*. Accessed June 22, 2004
10. Oncology Nursing Certification Corporation. *2005 Oncology Nursing Certification Bulletin*. Pittsburgh, Oncology Nursing Certification Corporation, 2004
11. Pearson L: Sixteenth annual legislative update. *Nurse Pract* 29:26–51, 2004
12. O'Brien JM: How nurse practitioners obtained provider status: lessons for pharmacists. *Am J Health Syst Pharm* 60:2301–2307, 2003
13. Sec 1861(s)(2)(k)(42 U.S.C. 1395x)(s)(2)(k) Social Security Act of 1935, 18 USC, 1999
14. Tumolo J, Rollet J: Gliding higher. NP salaries ascend at a steady pace. *Adv Nurse Pract* 12:32–38, 2004
15. Pilla L: Money matters: results of the 2002 NP salary survey. *Nurse Pract* 28:32–36, 2003
16. Buppert C: Billing for nurse practitioner services: guidelines for NPs, physicians, employers and insurers. Medscape Nurses, 2002. *www.medscape.com/viewarticle/422935*. Accessed June 22, 2004
17. Balanced Budget Act of 1997, Pub L No. 105–33, 1997
18. Health Care Finance Authority: Medicare program: revisions to payment policies and adjustments to the relative value units under the physician fee schedule for calendar year 1999. *Federal Register* 63:58813–59187, 1998
19. Towers J: Medicare reimbursement for NPs. *J Am Acad Nurse Pract* 11:289–292, 1999
20. Illinois Society for Advance Practice Nursing: FAQ: Illinois issues. Chicago: ISAPN, 2002. *www.isapn.org/reimburse.php*. Accessed December 17, 2004
21. Vogel WH: The advanced practice nurse role in a high-risk breast cancer clinic. *Oncol Nurs Forum* 30:115–122, 2003
22. Edge RM, Peterson C, James Ward S: The development of a community breast center. *Radiol Manage* 21:38–43, 1999
23. Burrer CV, Bauer SM: Insights into genetic testing for colon cancer: the nurse practitioner role. *Clin Excellence Nurse Pract* 4:349–355, 2000
24. Counsell C, Gilbert M: Implementation of a nurse practitioner role in an acute care setting. *Crit Care Nurs Clin North Am* 11:277–282, 1999
25. Trewhitt KG: Bone marrow aspiration and biopsy: collection and interpretation. *Oncol Nurs Forum* 28:1409–1415, 2001
26. Porter B: The role of the advanced practice nurse in anticoagulation. *AACN Clin Issues* 13:221–233, 2002
27. Williams D, Sidani S: An analysis of the nurse practitioner role in palliative care. *Can J Nurs Leadership* 14:13–19, 2001
28. Kuebler KK: The palliative care advanced practice nurse. *J Palliat Med* 6:707–714, 2003
29. Overberg P: Other studies of density and growth. *USA Today* 07A, February 22, 2001
30. Sepulveda C, Marlin A, Yoshida T, et al: Palliative care: the World Health Organization's global perspective. *J Pain Symptom Manage* 24:91–96, 2002
31. Payne P, Coyne P, Smith T: The health economics of palliative care. *Oncology* 16:801–808, 2002
32. Oermann MH, Floyd JA: Outcomes research: an essential component of the advanced practice nurse role. *Clin Nurse Spec* 16:140–144, 2002
33. Mundinger MO, Kane R, Lenz ER, et al.: Primary care outcomes in patients treated by nurse practitioners or physicians: a randomized trial. *JAMA* 283:59–68, 2000
34. Cunningham RS: Advanced practice nursing outcomes: a review of selected empirical literature. *Oncol Nurs Forum* 31:219–230, 2004
35. Sidani S, Irvine D: A conceptual framework for evaluating the nurse practitioner role in acute care settings. *J Adv Nurs* 30:58–66, 1999
36. Vincent D: Using cost-analysis techniques to measure the value of nurse practitioner care. *Int Nurs Rev* 49:243–249, 2002
37. Ingersoll GL, McIntosh E, Williams M: Nurse-sensitive outcomes of advanced practice. *J Adv Nurs* 32:1272–1281, 2000
38. Alpert PT, Fjone A, Candela L: Nurse practitioner: Reflecting on the future. *Nurs Adm Q* 26:79–89, 2002
39. McIntosh E, Nagelkerk J, Vonderheid SC, et al.: Financially viable nurse-managed centers. *Nurs Pract* 28:40–51, 2003
40. United States Bureau of the Census. *U.S. Census 2000*: Resident Population, 2001. Available online at *www.census.gov/main/www/census2000*. Accessed June 21, 2004
41. Galassi A: Role of the oncology advanced practice nurse, in Yarbro CH, Frogge MH, Goodman M, et al. (eds.) *Cancer Nursing: Principles and Practice* (ed 5). Sudbury, MA, Jones and Bartlett, 2000, pp 1712–1727

CHAPTER 74

Evidence-Based Oncology Nursing

Dana N. Rutledge, RN, PhD

Introduction

Information use in clinical decisions has to be viewed in the context of a service environment in which nurses are prevented from developing their decisions by the competing demands made on their time and skills by the sheer volume of workload. It is little wonder that nurses see clinical information use in routine decision making as a fairly low priority.[1]

On any given day, an oncology nurse working in an ambulatory infusion clinic may face several decisions, such as:

- How to determine whether a woman with stage III breast cancer would be a candidate for exercise treatment aimed at preventing or ameliorating cancer-related fatigue.
- Whether to recommend around-the-clock dosing of a patient's pain medication.
- How best to discuss advance directives with a person newly diagnosed with metastatic lung cancer.
- A dilemma in understanding, and knowing how to respond to, a patient who has missed four clinic appointments.

Every day, this oncology nurse, along with most nurses, needs evidence to help give good patient care. A recent British study of nurses in three diverse medical surgical settings[1] found that nurses make clinical decisions in several key areas. These include decisions related to (1) type of intervention or effectiveness of an intervention, (2) choice and implementation of interventions (including their timing) to enhance benefits to patients, (3) selection of communication strategies to and from patients, families, and colleagues, (4) configuration of service organization, delivery, and management, and (5) interpretation of cues in the process of delivering patient care.

Unfortunately, oncology nurses, like the acute care nurses in the British study,[1] may not seek out the optimal evidence in making decisions regarding patient care. They may instead rely upon easily accessible evidence, which is that provided by their nursing colleagues and peers (see Table 74-1). Using peers as a sole source of evidence excludes the potential effectiveness of using research-based evidence that may help nurses make decisions and use tools that optimize patient outcomes, decrease variations in care delivery, and promote patient satisfaction. In fact, evidence-based practice (EBP) has not become a reality for nurses in many areas of practice.[2] It is imperative that nurses go beyond easy access to find potentially important information that can enhance patient care. Practice based upon good evidence serves to improve patient care.

Table 74-1 Advantages and Disadvantages of Information Obtained from Nursing Peers

Advantages
• Easy to access
• Fast retrieval
• Cheap
• Tailored to the needs of the person asking
• Usually easy to understand
• Does not usually require appraisal by the person asking
Disadvantages
• May be vague
• May be out of date
• May be wrong
• May be based upon inappropriate sources
• Nursing peer may have biases

Evidence-Based Nursing

What is evidence-based nursing? It is the integration of the best evidence available, combined with nursing expertise and the values and preferences of the individuals, families, and communities that are served.[3] Evidence-based nursing requires three things: (1) that nurses have access to the evidence; (2) that a consensus of opinion exists on the implications of the evidence; and (3) that nurses in a work setting have the authority to exercise their judgment in planning and providing care. Thus, making evidence-based decisions requires access to research and other sources of evidence, the use of clinical expertise, and an understanding and acknowledgment of patient preferences.[1]

In "Nursing's Agenda for the Future,"[4] the American Nurses Association notes that decision making and positive change in nursing need to be driven by reliable data, and that selected nursing practices should lead to quality patient care. This should encourage nurses who want to deliver excellent nursing care to find out how to access all sources of evidence appropriate for their situation, and then to find out how to best implement and evaluate EBP changes or innovations.

A Framework: Implementation of Evidence-Based Practice

Out of Great Britain has come a model that seeks to explain what is necessary for EBP to occur. Basically, an EBP change is most likely to be successfully implemented when three things occur:[5,6]

1. The evidence is strong and matches the professional consensus and patient need.
2. The work setting or context is receptive to change, with strong leadership, decentralized decision making, and appropriate quality monitoring systems.
3. The proposed change is appropriately facilitated through the system by skilled internal or external facilitators or change agents.

Evidence is defined as a combination of research, professional expertise, and patient preference.[7] Context is the environment or setting where a proposed change may be implemented. Each setting has its own organizational culture, unique leadership team and system, and degree of measurement for quality outcomes. Ideal facilitators or persons in charge of facilitating a change are clearly authorized by a system to initiate change, are credible or respected in the eyes of the users of a change, and have a flexible style of relating to others. Facilitators enable people to understand what must be changed and how to achieve the desired outcomes, to make sense of the "evidence" to be implemented;[6] to do this, they consciously use a set of interpersonal and group skills to cross professional and organizational boundaries and, eventually, to achieve change.[5] A basic assumption of the model is that level of evidence, factors related to context, and facilitation are all important for an EBP change to occur.

Becoming a Nurse Who Bases Care upon Evidence

Oncology nurses who question the way things are done, who ask themselves, "What is the best way to accomplish this goal?" and who seek to understand why patients behave the way they do are already seeking EBP. Nurses in many roles are important to promoting and assuring that EBP occurs. Roles integral to the EBP process are listed in Table 74-2.[1,8–10] Many sources of information are available to help nurses obtain the most truthful or valid information, that is, to get the "evidence" to answer particular questions. Several steps are involved between obtaining the evidence and implementing a practice change. Barriers to fully implementing EBP are shown in Table 74-3.[12-18] Nurses must be aware that these barriers may exist and must be addressed. Note that advanced practice nurses who are seeking evidence related to treatment decisions for individual patients may have different needs in implementing EBP. Besides those mentioned in this chapter, multiple resources related to evidence-based medicine will assist advanced practice nurses in coming up with good decisions. Some of these resources are listed in Figure 74-1.

Asking Good Questions

Oncology nurses deliver care in a multitude of environments, so their clinical questions will vary depending upon setting and other factors. Focusing an inquiry on a specific area or topic assists in finding appropriate evidence. If a search is too broad, the amount of evidence found can be overwhelming, while a too-narrow focus can lead to insufficient evidence. Different types of inquiries lead to seeking different types of evidence. For example, questions such as What works? or What works best? will send nurses to sources such as experimental or clinical trial studies. On the other hand, trying to determine communication techniques to enhance adherence to oral chemotherapeutic agents may require reading findings from correlational studies (predictors of patients likely to be adherent or nonadherent) or qualitative studies (patient experiences with taking oral chemotherapy). For some clinical questions, especially those involving comparisons among strategies, oncology nurses may find it helpful to use the PICO method of question framing: *P*opulation, *I*ntervention, *C*omparison intervention, *O*utcome.[19] For example, if a nurse is interested in evaluating the accuracy of one tool versus another in assessing cognitive impairment in persons who have terminal cancer, PICO could be applied as follows:

- Population: terminally ill persons with cancer; the group that the question is about, the patients similar to the nurse's patients
- Intervention or tool: cognitive impairment assessment tool A, the tool the nurse is interested in or is considering
- Comparison intervention or tool: tool B, the alternate tool that can be compared with tool A
- Outcome: accuracy in measuring cognitive impairment

The oncology nurse seeks evidence that contains all elements of PICO, when possible; for example, studies that compare the accuracy of tool A to that of tool B in terminally ill cancer patients.

Obtaining Evidence

Ideally, once a nurse or group of nurses determines a clinical focus, they would determine what type of evidence is necessary to help them find an answer. Besides clinical expertise and patient preferences, other

Table 74-2 Potential Roles of Nurses in Evidence-Based Practice Process

Role	Description
Information brokers	Nurses who maintain up-to-date knowledge in a clinical area; they influence others' attitudes or behaviors in a desired manner and may be called opinion leaders.* Clinical nurse specialists are often information brokers.
Interested nurses	Nurses who want to practice from a solid evidence base will read nursing literature, particularly systematic reviews and research reports in areas of interest to them. Nurses will attend presentations where research findings are offered. Becoming a research consumer is a skill that can be taught.
Systems savvy nurses	Nurses who truly understand the workings of a work setting and how changes happen there. They know who the powerful people are and the mechanisms necessary to adopt and maintain change.
Change agents or facilitators	Nurses who facilitate appropriate use of promising new knowledge. Going beyond dissemination of new knowledge, they assist with diffusion and implementation of practices. They may serve as project leaders or may be external consultants. They flex between being nurses or patient advocates and project advocates. When successful, change agents may be considered opinion leaders.
Retrievers	Nurses who are experienced in using libraries and retrieving manuscripts can be vital to getting started in accessing evidence. Librarians may also be useful in this role. Manuscript retrieval can be a stumbling block early in an EBP project unless retrievers are identified.
Critiquers	Nurses who are excellent evaluators of nursing research have often had graduate research courses or gained much experience reading research studies. Critiquers enjoy reading and have good analytic and synthesis skills.
Early new practice users	Early adopters of EBP changes may tend to be leaders, although not by job description. They like learning about and trying out new ideas. Subsequently, they serve as role models for other nurses who see them using new practices.
Later new practice users	Nurses who follow others in using new practices may be considered early majority or later adopters. These nurses need to understand the rationale behind practice changes. As early majority users adopt a practice after seeing early new practice users, diffusion of the practice amplifies, and the overall rate of adoption increases. The late majority eventually use a practice change but may need authoritative pressure to maintain it.
Nurse educators	EBPs can be taught by educators who emphasize the research or evidence base behind an innovation. Teaching needs to emphasize that a practice or tool has been tested and found useful — that is, its research or evidence base. It should include rationales for patient care practices.

*Opinion leadership is the degree to which an individual is formally able to influence the attitudes and behavior of others in a specific direction and with relative frequency.[10]

Data from Thompson, McCaughan, Cullum, et al[1]; Rutledge, DePalma, Cunningham[8]; Rutledge[9]; Rogers[10]; Funk, Tornquist, Champagne.[11]

types of evidence have been deemed helpful to supplement the research core of evidence.[20] These sources include national benchmarking data, cost-effectiveness analyses, pathophysiology, chart review data, quality improvement and risk management trends, standards of care, and infection control data. For a question related to central venous catheter (CVC) site care, oncology nurses would benefit by seeking out local CVC infection rates and policies or standards of care. With any search, sources of evidence must be identified and a plan for retrieval developed, including how time will be found to obtain, read, and evaluate evidence sources (see Table 74-3 for barriers related to obtaining and appraising evidence).

For any topic, finding a recent systematic review or clinical practice guideline based upon a systematic review related to the topic can help in understanding the evidence. A *systematic review* is an information analysis and synthesis that summarizes a body of literature, focuses on findings, and draws conclusions about the clinical implications of the findings. Systematic reviews follow particular steps, from identifying the focus area to determining what outcome data are extracted from

Table 74-3 Barriers to Carrying Out Research Utilization or Evidence-Based Practice

Seeking/Appraising Evidence Phase
Lack of time to read research
Difficulty reading and interpreting research studies
Unclear implications for practice from research studies
Inability to find all of the relevant research studies
Lack of awareness of research findings
Staff does not see the value of research for practice
Isolation of nurses from knowledgeable colleagues with whom to discuss the research
Implementation/Evaluation Phase
Lack of authority to change patient care
Lack of time to implement new ideas
Lack of support of administration, staff, or physicians
Research findings not generalizable to work setting
Staff unwilling to change or try new ideas
Inadequate resources for implementation of practice changes

Data from Rutledge, Ropka, Greene, et al[12]; Funk, Tornquist, Champagne[13]; Carroll, Greenwood, Lynch, et al[14]; McCleary, Brown[15]; Nilsson Kajermo, Nordstrom, Krusebrant, et al[16]; Parahoo, McCaughan[17]; McCaughan, Thompson, Cullum, et al.[18]

Conn VS, Isaramalai SA, Rath S, et al: Beyond Medline for literature searches. *J Nurs Scholarship* 35:177–182, 2003

DePalma JA, McGuire DB: Research, in Hamric AB, Spross JA, Hanson CM (eds.): *Advanced Nursing Practice: An Integrative Approach* (ed 3). Philadelphia, Saunders, 2004, pp 257–300

Glanville I, Schirm V, Wineman NM: Using evidence-based practice for managing clinical outcomes in advanced practice nursing. *J Nurs Care Qual* 15:1–11, 2000

Guyatt G, Rennie D (eds.): *The Evidence-Based Medicine Working Group: Users' Guides to the Medical Literature. Essentials of Evidence-Based Clinical Practice*. Chicago, AMA Press, 2002

Jacobs SK, Rosenfeld P, Haber J: Information literacy as the foundation for evidence-based practice in graduate nursing education: a curriculum-integrated approach. *J Prof Nurs* 19:320–328, 2003

Jadad AR: The Cochrane Collaboration: advances and challenges in improving evidence-based decision making. *Med Dec Making* 18:2–9, 1998

Morrisey LJ, DeBourgh GA: Finding evidence: refining literature searching skills for the advanced practice nurse. *AACN Clin Issues* 12:5760–577, 2001

Savoie I, Helmer D, Green CJ, et al: Beyond Medline: reducing bias through extended systematic review search. *Int J Technol Assess Health Care* 19:168–178, 2003

Soukop SM: The Center for Advanced Nursing Practice evidence-based practice model: promoting the scholarship of practice. *Nurs Clin North Am* 35:301–309, 2000

Figure 74-1 Resources for Advanced Practice Nurses

selected studies. Using a systematic review as a starting point is efficient because reviewing primary studies takes longer and may require skills that many clinicians do not have.[21] Also, the authors of a systematic review have "already done the work of accumulating and summarizing the best of the published (and ideally unpublished) evidence," according to McKibbon and colleagues.[22] Systematic reviews may be quantitative (meta-analysis) or qualitative (narrative). In quantitative reviews, a collection of study results from individual studies is statistically analyzed in order to integrate findings. In qualitative reviews, primary study results are summarized with no statistical combination of results, but with an attempt to reduce the likelihood of bias.[23] All reviews are subject to bias and thus should be read critically. When a review is prepared carefully using specific steps, it is less likely that author bias has occurred. When reviews are older than a couple of years, nurses should supplement their search with studies done since the oldest study cited in the review to assure the timeliness of recommendations based upon the review.

Where can systematic reviews be found? Figure 74-2 shows sources for reviews, with examples that might be of interest to oncology nurses. Reviews can also be sought by using computerized databases such as Medline and CINAHL, and limiting searches to review articles. Examples of searches using PubMed and CINAHL are given in Figure 74-3.

Cochrane Library Database of Systematic Reviews
(*www.thecochranelibrary.com*) This subscription-only database contains full-text reviews that are highly structured, systematically prepared, and done using meta-analyses, when possible. Done by international groups made up predominantly of physicians, the reviews may be biased toward randomized clinical trials. These reviews are also indexed in Medline and CINAHL.

Examples

Fellowes D, Wilkinson S, Moore P, et al: Communication skills training for health care professionals working with cancer patients, their families and/or carers. *Cochrane Database Syst Rev.* 2:CD003751, 2003

Murray SM, Pindoria S: Nutrition support for bone marrow transplant patients. *Cochrane Database Syst Rev.* 2:CD002920, 2002;

Quigley C: Hydromorphone for acute and chronic pain. *Cochrane Database Syst Rev.* 1:CD003447, 2002

Database of Abstracts of Reviews of Effectiveness (DARE)
(*http://nhscrd.york.ac.uk/darehp.htm*) This is a database of quality assessed reviews, developed and updated by the National Health Service Centre for Reviews and Dissemination (CRD) at the University of York. In a search on 1/6/04 using the search terms, "sexual" and "cancer," 22 hits were obtained. The first three are listed as examples; structured abstracts written by CRD reviewers are linked to the titles on the DARE database.

Examples

Robinson JW, Dufour MS, Fung TS: Erectile functioning of men treated for prostate carcinoma. *Cancer 79:538–544, 1997 (Record 1)*

Wessex Institute for Health Research and Development: Psychosocial interventions in oncology: counselling services for women with breast cancer. Southampton, Wessex Institute for Health Research and Development, 1998 (Record 2)

Irwig L, Bennetts A: Quality of life after breast conservation or mastectomy: a systematic review. *Austral N Z J Surg* 67: 750–754, 1997 (Record 3)

Online Journal of Clinical Innovations
(*www.cinahl.org*) CINAHL's online journal contains reviews of clinically relevant nursing topics that include research studies along with quality improvement and research utilization efforts. Reviews highlight analyses of innovation adoption tactics; evidence of cost, quality, or outcome improvements following implementation; and evaluation of new protocols or staff education programs. Some examples of topics are Readability of Print Materials, Fall Prevention, and Restraints in Acute Care Settings.

Online Journal of Knowledge Synthesis in Nursing
(*www.stti.iupui.edu/VirginiaHendersonLibrary/OJKSNMENU*) This online journal from the Sigma Theta Tau Institute presents current scientific evidence to inform clinical decisions and ongoing discussions of issues, methods, clinical practice, and teaching strategies for evidence-based practice. Some examples of topics are Exposure Risk in the Handling and Administration of Chemotherapy Agents, Efficacy of Cold for Pain, and Adult Patient Decision Making about Withholding or Withdrawing Nutrition and/or Hydration.

Figure 74-2 Sources and Examples of Systematic Reviews

Database	Search Terms	Limits	Number of Hits
1. PubMed	Breast Self Examination AND Breast Cancer	Meta-analysis	1
2. PubMed	Breast Self Examination AND Breast Cancer	Review	20 (did not include Ku article found in search 1)
3. CINAHIDirect	Breast Self Examination AND Breast Neoplasm	Systematic review	2

Search 1

Ku YL: The value of breast self-examination: meta-analysis of the research literature. *Oncol Nurs Forum* 28:815–822, 2001

Search 2 — First 5 Hits

Smalley SM: Breast implants and breast cancer screening. *J Midwifery Womens Health* 48:329–337, 2003

Champion VL: Breast self-examination: what now? *Oncol Nurs Forum* 30:723–724, 2003

Feldhusen AE: Breast health. *Midwifery Today Int Midwife* 59:44–49, 69, 2001

Bailey K: The nurse's role in promoting breast awareness. *Nurs Stand* 14:34–36, 2000

George SA: Barriers to breast cancer screening: an integrative review. *Health Care Women Int* 21:53–65, 2000

Search 3 — 2 Hits

1. Kösters JP, Gøtzsche PC: Regular self-examination or clinical examination for early detection of breast cancer. *The Cochrane Library* (Oxford), 2003, issue 2 (CD003373)
2. Yarbrough SS, Braden CJ: Utility of health belief model as a guide for explaining or predicting breast cancer screening behaviours *J Adv Nurs* 33:677–688, 2001

Figure 74-3 Searches (1/6/04) for Reviews on the Effectiveness of Breast Self-Examination in Detecting Breast Cancer

Some topics are of such importance to organizations that *clinical practice guidelines* (CPG) have been developed following a systematic review. CPGs contain recommendations based upon systematic reviews and expert consensus that aim to help healthcare providers and patients make decisions in specific clinical situations, such as with cancer pain.[24] When done well, CPGs can be a great resource for nurses seeking answers to clinical questions. An excellent resource for those seeking CPGs is the National Guideline Clearinghouse™ (NGC™), a public resource for evidence-based CPGs (*www.guideline.gov*). It includes guideline summaries with information about development along with available links to full-text guidelines and ordering information for print copies. CPGs are developed by many different organizations and individuals, so nurses are urged to closely evaluate them for quality and appropriateness.

Evaluating the Evidence and Determining Clinical Recommendations

Once the review(s) or primary studies have been gathered, they must be read and interpreted using some method of critical appraisal. Critical appraisal is a means of assessing the strengths and weaknesses of information in order to determine which information most reliably or "best" answers the question being posed. It is this "best" information that constitutes "evidence"; the type of information providing such evidence will depend on the question and the circumstances.[25] At this point, collaboration with others who are interested in the area can be important in assuring that the evidence is interpreted appropriately.[8] Nurses who lack expertise in evaluating research and research-based evidence can partner with others who have this knowledge or can gain expertise from courses or working with others.[21,26,27]

Desirable attributes of reviews have been determined.[28] These include development by a group rather than a single reviewer, indication of inclusion/exclusion criteria for the quality of the studies included, inclusion of tables with critical information for applicability, meaningful display of different aspects of the studies' findings, and communication with experts in the field by the review group.

The desirable attributes of primary studies vary with clinical questions and types of evidence. Hierarchies of quality of evidence have been developed, primarily for use in medical EBP or for questions regarding the effectiveness of treatments. A hierarchy developed by nurses is that used in the Priority Symptom Management efforts.[23] These hierarchies typically put meta-analyses, systematic reviews, and randomized clinical trials (RCTs) as the top levels of evidence, because the degree of bias in these types of investigations is less than in other types. However, many clinical questions of interest to oncology nurses cannot be answered with clinical trials. For instance, a question related to understanding how a particular treatment (e.g., cryotherapy) leads to decreased mucositis outcomes could not be addressed based upon RCT findings. The importance of context, patient characteristics, and clinical expertise are not addressed in most RCT data. Other types of studies, including qualitative ones, may be necessary to address issues of concern to nurses. For example, an ongoing problem in oncology care is the disconnect between hospital and nonhospital caregivers in patient transfers. Qualitative studies involving interviews with nurses involved in the discharge process[29] may give insights into expectations and satisfaction with the referral process that no clinical trial can give. In any case, nurses seeking good evidence must evaluate the quality of all studies in order to determine their usefulness in leading to practice recommendations.

A variety of tools are available to assist in appraisal. Davies and Logan[30] authored a user-friendly guide for health professionals on reading research. The guide includes helpful tips for reading both quantitative and qualitative research articles. Worksheets for critical appraisal from the guide were found useful by nurses participating in the Oncology Nursing Society Research Utilization Short Course.[21] These worksheets are also available at *www.elsevier.ca/ReadingResearch/instructor_worksheets.htm.*

Brown's *Knowledge for Health Care Practice: A Guide to Using Research Evidence* contains tools for appraising the findings of several types of studies and for summaries such as meta-analyses, integrative reviews, and clinical practice guidelines. The tools are clearly written, practical, and geared to clinicians. Brown suggests that the bottom line is whether the nurses contemplating a research-based practice change believe they should change their practice based upon the evidence reviewed and whether they can determine how patients will benefit once the practice change is made.[31]

Translating the findings from the evidence search and appraisal into practice often requires the development of written guidelines for nurses to use when learning about or implementing a new or modified procedure.[9] These guidelines or protocols usually give step-by-step instructions for the procedure. Each work setting has norms about guideline or procedure format. As much as possible, guideline development should be driven by research findings, with citations of key articles or sources that support the nursing practice.

Evaluating the Context Where a Change Is Being Contemplated

Implementing and evaluating an EBP change is not a simple process. Most nurses work in organized nursing service settings, which may limit their individual adoption of many practice changes. Organizational adoption of an evidence-based change or innovation requires educating staff, disseminating policy/procedure or protocol documentation, and creating a climate that facilitates or rewards change that improves performance and outcomes.[27] The documented barriers identified in Table 74-3 were reiterated by alumni of Oncology Nursing Society–sponsored short courses aimed at assisting nurses to complete research utilization projects.[21] The alumni identified multiple barriers to project completion in nonsupportive clinical environments — specifically staffing changes, lack of administration support, high patient loads or acuity, competing time commitments, and the difficulties of staff "unlearning." Factors facilitating the successful implementation of practice changes identified by alumni were institutional and peer support, multidisciplinary support, a nursing research department in the work setting, autonomy in one's role, and access to knowledge and resources about implementing EBP change.[21] Nurses embarking upon an EBP project need to determine what barriers exist in their own work setting and to develop or gain access to resources or strategies to overcome these.

Early in the planning phase of a specific practice implementation, stakeholders for whom the practice change is important must be identified. Stakeholders are persons beyond the primary group who are in one of the following categories: (1) care whether the problem is solved; (2) may be affected by the problem or issue; (3) can help solve or address the issue; (4) bring knowledge of or skills related to the issue; (5) may benefit if the problem is solved or the issue is addressed; and (6) would bring a diverse viewpoint to the group.[32] For example, a decision to use a new dressing change procedure post-colectomy would require input from physicians, nurses, and pharmacy, with acknowledgment by the hospital supply service. A change involving the way in which the assessment of a common set of symptoms is documented in an ambulatory clinic would involve nurses, physicians, and ancillary staff, with acknowledgment from a documentation (forms) approval group. Achieving stakeholder buy-in early during implementation maximizes the chance that all aspects of the practice change will be considered.

Implementing and Evaluating an Evidence-Based Practice Change

Implementation of a practice change may begin with the use of a pilot unit. Conducting a trial with a small group of patients or nurses prior to adoption by a whole system allows assessment of whether the protocol will actually work in the target setting.[9] Some types of changes lend themselves to trials better than others. For example, adopting a new skin integrity assessment tool or initiating of hypnosis for management of anticipatory nausea can be tried on a unit or two or on a group of patients prior to general adoption.

The pilot evaluation may determine that a practice innovation is ready for implementation or that alterations are needed in the protocol, in requested resources, or in training. Once alterations occur, implementation can proceed according to the developed strategic plan. The length of time for project completion will vary with the complexity of the change involved. Implementation of strategies aimed at optimal pain management in oncology areas can take up to two years,[33] while changing a print pamphlet for use related to advanced directives may take little time beyond that needed for development and printing.

Evaluating evidence-based changes in work settings in which nurses are integrally involved in ongoing quality improvement processes may be easier than in settings where quality monitoring is not entrenched practice.[6] Monitoring processes of care that have been changed, along with outcomes predicted by an EBP, is necessary to determine whether a change was enacted and what its effects were. That is, if a project requires that nurses change their handwashing techniques, their compliance with the new method should be checked. Also, the potential outcomes of the change, altered nosocomial infection rates, should be monitored to make sure changes occur as predicted. Thus, it is necessary to evaluate whether the practice change has been implemented as planned and whether the expected outcomes have been achieved.

Conclusion

Oncology nurses who seek to accomplish truly evidence-based practice must be able to identify, obtain, and evaluate information that comes in a variety of forms and formats.[34] They then must be able to inform clinical decision making and develop practical protocols following critical appraisal of the evidence gathered and read. Challenging these nurses is an educational system that may not have prepared them for seeking evidence, the pressure of time, the demands of informed patients, and the lack of role models who are "trained" in EBP.[2,35] Furthermore, these nurses must be excellent team builders who know how to rally their stakeholders in cancer care, plan strategically to implement evidence-based changes, and evaluate the processes necessary for changing practice and the desired outcomes. In order to move forward the reality of EBP, oncology nurses must demand the resources necessary to help them improve the care they deliver via incorporating evidence-based protocols into healthcare systems. Managers and administrators must ensure that giving evidence-based care is a work setting priority, and they must then support nurses and others in their efforts.

References

1. Thompson C, McCaughan D, Cullum N, et al: Nurses' use of research information in clinical decision making: a descriptive and analytical study. Centre for Evidence Based Nursing, Department of Health Studies, University of York, 2002. *www.york.ac.uk/healthsciences/centres/evidence/decrpt.pdf.* Accessed January 5, 2004
2. Young KM: Where's the evidence? [Viewpoint]. *Am J Nurs* 103:11, 2003
3. Sigma Theta Tau International: STT's position statement on evidence-based nursing. *www.nursingsociety.org/research/main.html#ebp.* Accessed January 14, 2004
4. American Nurses Association: Nursing's agenda for the future. A call to the nation *www.nursingworld.org/naf/nafa.pdf.* Accessed January 5, 2004
5. Kitson A, Harvey G, McCormack B: Enabling the implementation of evidence-based practice: a conceptual framework. *Qual Health Care* 7:149–158, 1998
6. Rycroft-Malone J, Kitson A, Harvey G, et al: Ingredients for change: revisiting a conceptual framework. *Qual Safety Health Care* 11:174–180, 2002
7. Sackett DL, Rosenberg WMC, Gray JAM, et al: Evidence based medicine: what it is and what it isn't. *BMJ* 312:71–72, 1996
8. Rutledge DN, DePalma JA, Cunningham M: A process model for evidence-based literature syntheses. *Oncol Nurs Forum* 31:543–550, 2004
9. Rutledge DN: Research utilization in oncology nursing. *Oncol Nurs: Pt Treatment Support* 4:1–14, 1995
10. Rogers EM: *Diffusion of Innovations.* New York, Free Press, 1995
11. Funk SG, Tornquist EM, Champagne MT: The listener's guide to research presentations. *J Pediatr Nurs* 7:141–144, 1992
12. Rutledge DN, Ropka M, Greene PE, et al: Barriers to research utilization for oncology staff nurses and nurse managers/clinical nurse specialists. *Oncol Nurs Forum* 25:497–506, 1998
13. Funk S, Tornquist EM, Champagne MT: Barriers and facilitators of research utilization: an integrative review. *Nurs Clin North Am* 30:395–407, 1995
14. Carroll DL, Greenwood R, Lynch KE, et al: Barriers and facilitators to the utilization of nursing research. *Clin Nurs Specialist* 11:207–212, 1997
15. McCleary L, Brown GT: Barriers to paediatric nurses' research utilization. *J Adv Nurs* 42:364–372, 2003
16. Nilsson Kajermo K, Nordstrom G, Krusebrant A, et al: Barriers to and facilitators of research utilization, as perceived by a group of registered nurses in Sweden. *J Adv Nurs* 27:798–807, 1998
17. Parahoo K, McCaughan EM: Research utilization among medical and surgical nurses: a comparison of their self reports and perceptions of barriers and facilitators. *J Nurs Manage* 9:21–30, 2001
18. McCaughan D, Thompson C, Cullum N, et al: Acute care nurses' perceptions of barriers to using research information in clinical decision-making. *J Adv Nurs* 39:46–60, 2002
19. Craig JV, Smyth RL (eds.): *The Evidence-Based Practice Manual for Nurses.* Philadelphia, Churchill Livingstone, 2002
20. Goode CJ: What constitutes the "evidence" in evidence-based practice? *Appl Nurs Res* 13:222–225, 2000
21. Rutledge DN, Mooney KH, Grant M, et al: Implementation and refinement of a research utilization course for oncology nurses. *Oncol Nurs Forum* 31:121–126, 2004
22. McKibbon A, Hunt D, Richardson S, et al: Finding the evidence, in Guyatt GH, Rennie D (eds.): *Users' Guides to the Medical Literature: Essentials of Evidence-Based Clinical Practice.* Chicago, American Medical Association, 2002, pp 21–71

23. Ropka ME, Spencer-Cisek P: PRISM: Priority Symptom Management Project, phase I: assessment. *Oncol Nurs Forum* 28:1585–1594, 2001
24. Jacox A, Carr DB, Payne R, et al: *Management of Cancer Pain: Clinical Practice Guideline No. 9.* Rockville, MD, Agency for Health Care Policy and Research, U.S. Department of Health and Human Services, 1994
25. The CASP Team: Critical skills appraisal workshop [Powerpoint slides], Aggressive Research Intelligence Facility, University of Birmingham, Great Britain. *www.bham.ac.uk/arif/casp/caspslides_files/frame.htm.* Accessed January 5, 2004
26. Barnsteiner JH: Research-based practice. *Nurs Admin Q* 20:52–58, 1996
27. Rutledge DN, Donaldson NE: Building organizational mechanisms for research utilization. *J Nurs Admin* 25:12–16, 1995
28. Stetler CB, Morsi D, Rucki S, et al: Utilization-focused integrative reviews in a nursing service. *Appl Nurs Res* 11:195–206, 1998
29. Pateman B, Wilson K, McHugh G, et al: Continuing care after cancer treatment. *J Adv Nurs* 44:192–199, 2003
30. Davies B, Logan J: Reading research: *A user-friendly guide for nurses and other health professionals* (ed 3). Toronto, Canada, Elsevier, 2003
31. Brown SJ: *Knowledge for Health Care Practice: A Guide to Using Research Evidence.* Philadelphia, W.B. Saunders, 1999
32. Rinehart TA, Laszlo AT, Briscoe GO: *Collaboration Toolkit: How to Build, Fix, and Sustain Productive Partnerships.* Washington DC, Department of Justice, Office of Community Oriented Policing Services, 2001
33. Bookbinder M, Kiss M, Coyle N, et al: Improving pain management practices, in McGuire DB, Yarbro CH, Ferrell BR (eds.): *Cancer Pain Management.* Boston, Jones and Bartlett, 1995, pp 321–361
34. Jacobs SK, Rosenfeld P, Haber J: Information literacy as the foundation for evidence-based practice in graduate nursing education: a curriculum-integrated approach. *J Prof Nurs* 19: 320–328, 2003
35. Rosenfeld P, Salazar-Riera N, Vieira D: Piloting an information literacy program for staff nurses: lessons learned. *Computers Inform Nurs* 20:236–241, 2002

CHAPTER 75

Legal Issues

Lisa Schulmeister, RN, MN, CS, OCN®

Introduction

A major goal of oncology nursing practice is the safe delivery of patient care. Many mechanisms exist to help ensure that this goal will be met, such as federal laws, state licensing requirements for professional nursing practice, technological advancements (e.g., safer medical equipment), institutional procedures (e.g., computerized medication ordering), and personal practices (e.g., double-checking medications). However, because health care is a complex system of people and processes, risk is inherent in its delivery.

Oncology nurses practice in high-risk environments. Patients with cancer are often weak, fatigued, and mobility-impaired, thus increasing their risk of injury from falls. Most cancer treatments, such as chemotherapy, biotherapy, and radiation therapy, are based on individual rather than standardized dosing, and the potential for dosing or delivery errors is high. Some patients receive chemotherapy or monoclonal antibody treatments that can cause anaphylaxis or infusion-related reactions, so these patients are at risk for life-threatening adverse events. In addition, vesicant chemotherapy agents have the potential to cause severe tissue necrosis if they extravasate. Patient harm, and even death, can potentially result from medical errors and events. Legal action can also ensue.

Litigation involving oncology nurses may be prompted by patient falls, medication errors, hypersensitivity and infusion-related reactions, and vesicant chemotherapy extravasations, as well as other situations, such as failure to monitor a patient, privacy and confidentiality violations, inappropriate triage or management of patient-reported complaints, and undertreatment of pain. Oncology nurses play a key role in preventing these errors and adverse events.

Patient Safety

Patient safety received increased attention following the publication of the Institute of Medicine's (IOM) report *To Err Is Human: Building a Safer Health System* in 2000, which closely examined the problem of medical errors and estimated that they cause 44,000–98,000 deaths per year in the United States.[1] Medical errors can occur when the wrong plan is used to achieve an aim (error in planning), a planned action is not completed (error of omission), or an action is performed incorrectly (error of execution or commission). Medical errors are costly, preventable adverse events and include errors associated with medication or treatment administration, healthcare-acquired infections, restraint-related injuries, falls, burns, and pressure sores.[2–4] A subset of adverse events, termed sentinel events, are defined as unexpected occurrences that result in death or serious physical or psychological risk or injury not present on admission or related to the natural course of illness or underlying condition.[5] Events categorized as sentinel events by the Joint Commission on Accreditation of Healthcare Organizations (JCAHO) include medication errors, rape or patient suicide in a healthcare facility, hemolytic transfusion reactions, wrong-site or wrong-patient surgery, and infant abduction or discharge to the wrong family.[6]

In 2001, the IOM identified potential solutions to the problem of medical errors and recommended a redesign of the U.S. healthcare system in *Crossing the Quality Chasm: A New Health System for the 21st Century*. In order to provide continuous, customized care, with patients in control of their care, the IOM advocates organizational support for change, evidence-based healthcare delivery, the use of information technology, and the alignment of legislative and payment policies with quality improvement in healthcare.[7]

In 2003, JCAHO issued six national safety goals and recommendations (see Table 75-1).[8] A seventh goal, to reduce the risk of healthcare-acquired infection, was added in 2004. Examples of healthcare-acquired (also termed nosocomial) infections include ventilator-associated pneumonia and device-associated infections in patients with urinary or intravenous catheters. A major factor in the development of healthcare-acquired infections is increasing antimicrobial resistance, and the greatest number of healthcare-acquired infections occur in the intensive care unit (ICU), followed by non-ICU inpatient areas and outpatient areas. According to the Centers for Disease Control, nosocomial infections affect two million patients annually in acute care facilities in the United States. It is estimated that at least one third of these infections can be prevented by simple infection-control strategies, such as handwashing.[1,9]

Despite nurses' awareness of the importance of handwashing in infection control, rates of compliance remain low.[1,9,10] Several factors are responsible for this, such as empty soap dispensers, broken or inconveniently located sinks, and nurses being hurried or forgetful. Increased education on the importance of handwashing or sanitizing, combined with more stringent surveillance programs, are strategies that may decrease healthcare-acquired infection rates and reduce the risk of institutional liability.[10]

Numerous texts and articles have recently been published on preventing medical error and healthcare-acquired infection, and patient safety is now considered a priority in healthcare delivery. However, despite the growing body of knowledge of risk reduction strategies, adverse events still occur and may result in patient harm and legal action. While many of these events, such as patient falls and medication errors, are

Table 75-1 Joint Commission on Accreditation of Healthcare Organizations National Patient Safety Goals and Recommendations for 2004

Goal	Recommendations
Improve patient identification procedures	Use at least two patient identifiers other than room number to ensure correct patient identification
Improve communication	Develop institutional procedures to standardize communication processes, such as verbal orders and use of abbreviations
Improve safety when stocking, ordering, and dispensing medications associated with a high risk of medication errors	Limit the number of different drug concentrations in stock, clearly label all storage areas and drugs, use generic drug names, be familiar with "look-alike" or "sound-alike" medications, develop additional procedures to reduce the potential for medication errors
Perform the correct surgical procedure on the correct patient and correct site	Verify patient identity, procedure scheduled, and body site. Consider identifying correct site on body with a marker or pen
Improve safety when using infusion pumps	Use pumps with free-flow protection for general use and patient-controlled analgesia
Improve the effectiveness of alarm systems in patient care areas	Frequently test alarm and alerting systems, such as call bells and patient monitoring equipment
Reduce the risk of healthcare-acquired infection	Comply with current Centers for Disease Control hand hygiene guidelines. Manage unanticipated death or permanent disability associated with healthcare-acquired infection as a sentinel event

Data from Joint Commission on Accreditation of Healthcare Organizations.[8]

not unique to the practice of oncology nursing, some errors and events are specific to oncology nursing practice, such as chemotherapy medication errors, chemotherapy-induced hypersensitivity reactions, monoclonal antibody infusion–related reactions, and vesicant extravasations.

Chemotherapy Medication Errors

The incidence and severity of chemotherapy medication errors are unknown. Sometimes these errors, especially those involving lethal overdoses of chemotherapy, prompt litigation and are publicized in the media. For example, in 1999, newspapers reported that a patient with testicular cancer died after receiving a fourfold overdose of cyclophosphamide, and the family agreed to a $7.9 million settlement with the hospital.[11]

Chemotherapy medication errors often are reported only internally and are not reported to national medication error reporting programs or published in the literature. The low external error reporting rate, reported to be 3% in one study,[12] is attributable to several factors, such as fear of employer punishment, coworker disapproval, concern that a lawsuit may be filed, feelings of guilt and inadequacy, and lack of awareness of the process for externally reporting errors. In addition, there is a prevailing perception that medication errors causing minimal or no harm do not need to be reported externally.[13,14]

Chemotherapy medication errors include incorrect preparation, wrong drug, dose errors (including under- and overdosing), incorrect administration time or route, and chemotherapy administered to the wrong patient.[12] Examples of these errors include mixups caused by similar drug names (e.g., cisplatin administered instead of carboplatin, which caused three patient deaths reported in a review of 469 fatal medication errors[15]) or "look-alike" vial labels, dose miscalculations (e.g., underdosing that occurred when one day's dose of cladribine was administered over one week, which resulted in two patients with hairy-cell leukemia not responding to treatment,[16] and overdosing that occurred when a nurse thought she had used five 10-mg vials of vinorelbine to prepare a 50-mg dose but inadvertently used two 50-mg and three 10-mg vials[17]), mistakes in interpreting orders (e.g., infusion of doxorubicin and vincristine over one day instead of four days[18]), and lack of patient understanding (e.g., oral chemotherapy dose for one week taken all at one time).

Many of these errors are preventable. Education is paramount so that individuals who prescribe, prepare, handle, and administer chemotherapy are well informed about the drugs' properties, toxicities, cumulative doses, and effects. The environment in which chemotherapy is prepared and administered needs to be uncluttered and nondistracting. The individuals involved in these processes need to be focused, consult available resources, and strictly adhere to principles of practice (e.g., the "five rights" of medication administration) and institutional procedures. Applicable risk reduction strategies include not storing chemotherapy drugs with similar names or labels side by side, being familiar with the generic and trade names of chemotherapy agents, triple-checking dose calculations and checking doses against reference sources such as the treatment protocol, clearly labeling the route of administration, verifying patient identity, clarifying unclear orders, and dispensing one course of oral chemotherapy at a time. Several publications describe additional strategies that can be used to prevent chemotherapy medication errors.[19–21]

Chemotherapy medication errors can result in various actions. Employers may initiate remedial actions (e.g., staff education) or disciplinary actions (e.g., termination of employment). State licensing boards may take action and mandate staff education and institutional procedural improvements, or may revoke or restrict professional licensure. Patients and their families may initiate legal action following chemotherapy medication errors, especially those associated with patient injury, and sometimes file criminal charges against healthcare providers as well. For instance, a review of 17 lethal medication errors that occurred in the United Kingdom from 1970 to 1999 describes two incidents involving cases in which vincristine for intravenous use was erroneously administered intrathecally, and the physicians involved were charged with manslaughter.[22]

Being well informed about the chemotherapy administration process, adhering to institutional procedures, employing risk reduction strategies, and openly communicating with patients and other staff members are key strategies for reducing the likelihood that a chemotherapy medication error will be made and legal action will ensue.

Hypersensitivity and Infusion-Related Reactions

Hypersensitivity, defined as an unexpected reaction with signs and symptoms not consistent with known toxicity of the drug,[23] may be experienced by patients when they receive asparaginase, bleomycin, taxanes, platinum compounds, and monoclonal antibodies. The severity of these reactions can range from mild symptoms, such as urticaria and rash, to life-threatening dyspnea and bronchospasm.

Asparaginase is an enzyme derived from *Escherichia coli (E. coli)* or *Erwinia* that is primarily used to treat acute lymphoblastic leukemia. Its risk of hypersensitivity when administered intravenously is well known and is estimated to occur in 20%–30% of patients. Test dosing (0.1 mL of a 20 units/mL dilution of drug given intradermally) is advocated, and educating the patient about the risk of hypersensitivity and the importance of reporting early symptoms of this reaction is essential.[23,24] However, skin testing is not standardized in clinical practice, and reactions have occurred in patients with negative skin tests, so the drug needs to be administered in a facility that is capable of treating anaphylaxis. The drug is often given intramuscularly or subcutaneously; these routes of administration are associated with a lower reaction rate. Patients sensitive to asparaginase may need to undergo desensitization, switch from the *E. coli* form to the *Erwinia* product, or change to the polyethylene glycolated (PEG) form of the drug, pegaspargase, which is better tolerated, especially when given intramuscularly.[25]

Bleomycin is another agent with hypersensitivity potential. Reactions can occur in any patient receiving the drug, but they occur more often in patients with lymphoma during or after the first or second dose of the drug. Symptoms of a bleomycin-induced hypersensitivity reaction include hypotension, tachycardia, wheezing, confusion, and facial edema. In some settings, test dosing (0.5–1 unit administered intravenously or intradermally) is performed on all patients scheduled to receive bleomycin, and in other settings, only patients with lymphoma are test-dosed.[24] Both asparaginase and bleomycin increase leukotriene production, which is thought to explain the etiology of hypersensitivity to these agents, since leukotriene activation of the mast cells causes febrile and inflammatory responses, including anaphylactic reactions.[26]

Paclitaxel is a newer agent that induces a hypersensitivity reaction in 1%–10% of patients.[24,27,28] Docetaxel, another taxane, induces hypersensitivity in about 2% of patients.[23] It is unclear if reactions occur because of sensitivity to these agents or to excipients added to solubilize these agents (e.g., Cremophor EL in paclitaxel and polysorbate-80 in docetaxel).[23] All patients require pretreatment with steroids and antihistamines before *each dose* of either drug.[23] Reactions may be mild (dyspnea, hypotension) to severe (angioedema, tachycardia, chest pain). Some patients experiencing mild reactions to paclitaxel are rechallenged with paclitaxel infusing at a lower rate,[24] some are switched to docetaxel, which is tolerated by most patients who have had reactions to paclitaxel,[23] and some have required treatment using a desensitization protocol in order to receive subsequent infusions of paclitaxel.[27]

Another newer agent, carboplatin, can cause hypersensitivity after multiple cycles of the drug have been administered in 16%–27% of patients.[29–31] Clinical features of carboplatin-induced hypersensitivity include diffuse rash, tachycardia, dyspnea, wheezing, facial swelling, and chest tightness.[30,31] Some patients become hypotensive while others become hypertensive. In half of the patients, the reaction develops after 50% or more of the carboplatin has been infused.[30] Reactions are treated by stopping the infusion and administering steroids, antihistamines, benzodiazepines, nebulized beta-agonists, and/or vasopressors.[32]

Patients who have had a hypersensitivity reaction to a platinum agent will often have a repeat reaction with rechallenge, and pretreatment with steroids or antihistamines has not prevented these reactions.[23] Skin-testing protocols, such as the use of a 0.02 mL intradermal injection of an undiluted aliquot of the planned carboplatin dose one hour before each course of the drug, have been developed to help predict which patients are hypersensitive to carboplatin.[33] Desensitizing carboplatin infusion regimens may be required for patients with moderate to severe carboplatin hypersensitivity.[34,35] Subsequent treatment with cisplatin, using a cisplatin desensitization protocol, has also been successful for patients who cannot continue carboplatin because of an allergic reaction to the drug.[36,37]

The monoclonal antibodies alemtuzumab, cetuximab, rituximab, and tositumomab have the potential to cause rare but life-threatening anaphylaxis. Mouse antibodies that are used in the production of monoclonal antibodies are foreign substances and may stimulate anaphylaxis. The fusion protein denileukin difitox also has the potential to cause acute hypersensivity reactions.[24]

Infusion reactions are common when alemtuzumab is administered, and premedication is required to prevent them. Common symptoms include fever and chills (80%), nausea (60%), rash (50%), and hypotension (16%). Infusion reactions usually resolve after a week of treatment. Premedications, including acetaminophen and diphenhydramine, are often prescribed, and the dose of alemtuzumab is escalated during treatment (started at 3 mg and gradually increased as tolerated to 10 mg and then 30 mg).[24,38]

Mild infusion-related reactions, including chills, fever, and dyspnea, occur in 23% of patients who receive single-agent cetuximab and in 16% who receive this agent in conjunction with irinotecan. About 3% of patients experience severe cetuximab infusion-related reactions characterized by the rapid onset of airway obstruction, rash, and hypotension. Most of these infusion-related reactions occur on the first day of initial dosing. Premedication with 50 mg diphenhydramine IV is recommended. Patients who experience mild to moderate infusion-related reactions should have the rate of infusion reduced by 50%, and those who experience severe infusion reactions should not receive further therapy with this agent.[24,39,40]

Gemtuzumab ozogamicin is a monoclonal antibody conjugated to the cytotoxic antibiotic calicheamicin. Patients receiving this agent for the first time often experience a post-infusion syndrome that occurs within 24 hours and is characterized by chills and fever (60%), nausea and vomiting (35%), and headache (12%). It resolves with supportive therapy of acetaminophen, diphenhydramine, and fluids. Patients are less likely to experience this post-infusion syndrome with subsequent treatments and are typically premedicated with acetaminophen and diphenhydramine prior to treatment.[24,41]

Infusion-related reactions occur in about 80% of patients receiving the first dose of rituximab and 40% of patients receiving subsequent infusions. Fever and chills commonly occur, and other symptoms include nausea, headache, and throat irritation. Reactions generally occur within 30 minutes to 2 hours of the start of the first infusion and resolve when the infusion is slowed or interrupted and supportive care (e.g., diphenhydramine, acetaminophen, fluids) is provided. Initial infusions of rituximab are started at 50 mg/hour. If tolerated, the rate is escalated in 50 mg/hour increments every 30 minutes to a maximum of 400 mg/hour. Subsequent infusions, if the patient tolerated the first infusion well, are initiated at 100 mg/hour and increased by 100 mg/hour increments at 30-minute intervals to a maximum of 400 mg/hour as tolerated.[24,42]

Treatment with tositumomab and iodine-131 tositumomab is dual action (immunotherapy with a monoclonal antibody and radiotherapy with iodine-131). Rare but potentially life-threatening reactions during the two-step treatment may occur. The first step, the dosimetric step, is followed 7–14 days later by the therapeutic step. Approximately 8% of patients experience fever and/or chills during the infusion and require a 50% reduction in the infusion rate. Infusions are interrupted if severe infusion-related reactions occur.[24]

Denileukin difitox, a recombinant protein containing diphtheria toxin fragments and interleukin-2, can cause acute hypersensitivity reactions. In clinical trials, 69% of patients experienced a hypersensitivity reaction during or within 24 hours of the infusion. Most reactions occur during the first day of dosing of each treatment cycle and are characterized by hypotension (50%), back pain (30%), dyspnea (28%), and rash (25%).[24,43]

Patient injury has occurred, and litigation has been initiated, when patients who were treated with agents with known hypersensitivity potential, but who were not premedicated when premedication was indicated or not test-dosed when test dosing was indicated, experienced a hypersensitivity or infusion-related reaction. Legal actions also have been filed when reactions occurred but were not promptly recognized or properly treated.

Risk reduction measures include educating staff about chemotherapy agents and side effects, using appropriate test-dose or premedication procedures, immediately stopping an infusion if a hypersensitivity reaction is suspected, being prepared for emergencies (e.g., having oxygen, medications, etc., available), issuing standing orders to administer emergency medications, having written policies on emergency management procedures, educating patients regarding the risk of hypersensitivity and its symptoms, and closely monitoring patients during chemotherapy and administration of monoclonal antibodies (including monitoring and recording vital signs when indicated). With both paclitaxel and carboplatin, patients with a prior history of systemic hypersensitivity to medications or environmental causes (e.g., bee stings) were noted to be at increased risk for experiencing allergic reactions to these agents.[44] Therefore, nurses also need to obtain an allergy history when assessing patients scheduled to receive chemotherapy agents that have the potential for hypersensivity.

Vesicant Extravasation

A number of vesicant chemotherapy agents cause extensive damage if they extravasate out of the vein into the tissue. Extravasation may occur with peripherally administered vesicants, as well as vesicants administered via indwelling central venous access devices, such as percutaneously placed central venous catheters and implanted ports. Peripheral extravasations may occur following inaccurate device placement, vein damage, patient movement, and other factors. Catheter rupture or fracture, or backtracking of the vesicant along the catheter because of thrombus formation at the catheter tip can cause extravasations from central venous catheters. Port-related extravasations can occur from perforation of the superior vena cava, incomplete needle placement, needle dislodgment, thrombus formation, catheter fracture, and catheter/portal septum separation.[45]

Extravasation-related injuries may resolve with time and symptomatic management or may be extensive, in some cases requiring surgery and skin grafting. Extensive injury often delays or prevents cancer treatment, may cause functional impairment of the affected body part, renders the patient vulnerable to infection, and may cause related problems, such as the patient's inability to perform daily activities. Consequently, the physical and emotional impact of an extensive extravasation injury may prompt legal action. Although extravasation is a known risk of vesicant administration, attorneys may allege that the nurse administering the vesicant was negligent. The circumstances surrounding the administration of the vesicant are closely examined to ascertain whether the nurse deviated from the institution's procedures or the level of care that nurses in similar situations would provide. For instance, administering a vesicant through a device that lacks a blood return without taking further action to verify placement and patency deviates from safe practice. A case example is an account of an implanted port lacking a blood return that was used to administer vesicant chemotherapy. The nurse's rationale for using the port despite a lack of blood return or other evidence of placement and patency was that the port was newly inserted. Although an anterior-posterior chest x-ray was interpreted as showing the port's catheter tip in good position, the catheter had perforated the superior vena cava, and an intrathoracic extravasation subsequently occurred. The patient became septic and died. The family filed a malpractice claim, which was settled for nearly $500,000.[46]

The best defense against claims of negligence related to extravasation injuries is to prevent them from occurring to the extent possible, to detect them quickly should they occur, and to intervene promptly. Guidelines and recommendations for vesicant administration, such as those published by the Oncology Nursing Society,[47] and institutional policies should guide vesicant administration. Vesicants should never be administered without evidence of proper device placement and patency. Clinical resources, such as experienced staff members, along with institutionally defined procedures for using declotting agents and radiologic studies, should be used to evaluate devices with questionable placement or patency. Patients receiving vesicants need close monitoring during vesicant administration and should be instructed regarding actions to take, such as not moving the arm during peripheral vesicant administration, and signs and symptoms to report. Patients need to be informed that extravasation is a risk of vesicant administration, and they should be reminded of this risk with each course of treatment. Nurses should document ease of device insertion (when applicable), number of attempts to insert the device, detailed location of the device, assessment of the device and patient during the infusion, and the patient's response. If an extravasation occurs or is suspected, the vesicant should be stopped immediately and institutional policies for managing extravasations initiated. The area involved should be measured and, ideally, photographed. Close follow-up of the patient for the next several days, and possibly weeks, along with referral to a plastic or hand surgeon, may be needed.[45,47]

Responding to Errors and Adverse Events

When an error contributes to or causes an injury, patients and their families are entitled to a prompt explanation of how the event occurred and its short

Food and Drug Administration (FDA) MedWatch program provides an online voluntary reporting form to report serious adverse events, potential and actual medical product errors, and product quality problems associated with the use of FDA-regulated drugs, biologics, devices, and dietary supplements. Phone 800-FDA-1088, *www.accessdata.fda.gov/scripts/medwatch/medwatch_online.cfm.*

Institute for Safe Medication Practices (ISMP) Medication Errors Reporting Program (MERP), operated by the United States Pharmacopeia (USP) in cooperation with ISMP, is a confidential national voluntary reporting program that collects information about medication errors, provides analysis of the system causes of these errors, and disseminates recommendations to healthcare providers. Phone 800-FAIL-SAF(E) (800-324-5723), *www.ismp.org/pages/mederr_usa.html.*

United States Pharmacopeia (USP) Medication Errors Reporting Program, operated in cooperation with ISMP, is an FDA MedWatch partner. Phone 800-23 ERROR (800-233-7767), *secure.usp.org/patientsafety/reporting/merform.html.*

Joint Commission on Accreditation of Healthcare Organizations provides tools for conducting a root cause analysis and a self-report form to describe and report sentinel events occurring in healthcare facilities: *www.jcaho.org/accredited+organizations/hospitals/sentinel+events/forms+and+tools/index.htm.*

Figure 75-1 Sources for reporting medical errors and adverse events.

and long-term effects. Patients and family members should receive an honest, compassionate explanation of the error and the treatment or remedies that are available. They should be informed that the event and the factors contributing to the event will be investigated so that action can be taken to reduce the likelihood of similar events occurring in the future.[48] Truthful and complete disclosure is the healthcare provider's only appropriate ethical response to a medical error or adverse event.[49]

It is unknown whether full disclosure influences malpractice liability (e.g., whether a lawsuit is filed or not)[50]; however, legal action is sometimes initiated by patients or their families in an effort to obtain information about what happened when they perceive that healthcare providers are withholding or concealing information. The patient's perception of lack of communication or poor communication is frequently the impetus for filing a lawsuit.[51]

A systems approach is advocated for investigating and responding to errors and adverse events. The basic premise of a systems approach is that humans are fallible and errors are to be expected. Errors are viewed as consequences of an ineffective system.[52] A systems approach represents the philosophical belief that it was not the nurse who failed, but rather the system.

A root cause analysis (RCA) is the process of defining the underlying cause of an event and involves repeatedly asking why an event occurred. An RCA is a retrospective evaluation of an incident that considers several perspectives, including, in most instances, that of the patient and family. The goal of this analysis is to identify the many factors that contribute to an error. After an incident occurs, a particular action or omission of action may at first appear to be the cause of the incident; however, closer analysis often reveals a cascade of events and a multitude of contributing factors.[53,54] JCAHO requires hospitals to conduct RCAs of adverse events as part of its accreditation program, and encourages reporting these events to JCAHO. In addition, many states mandate adverse event reporting.[55] Medical errors and adverse events should be reported internally and externally to appropriate agencies as soon as possible following the incident (see Figure 75-1).

A procedure that often is used in conjunction with RCAs is failure mode and effects analysis (FMEA), which proactively identifies potential problems within systems or processes. An FMEA can be conducted after an RCA to identify other potential problems related to the system under scrutiny, or can be performed independently to prevent errors.[40,41] For instance, FMEA can be used proactively to examine high-risk areas, such as chemotherapy prescribing, dispensing, and administering.

When a medical error or adverse event occurs, even in organizations that purport to embrace a systems approach to examining those events, a subtle undercurrent to assign some degree of blame to the individual involved may occur. A survey of 1400 hospitals conducted by the American Hospital Association, Health Research and Education Trust, and Institute for Safe Medication Practices found that only 46% of respondents reported full confidence that error reduction strategies at their institutions targeted the system and not the individual. Only 23% indicated that they felt they could openly report and discuss errors without undue embarrassment or fear of reprisal.[56] The implication of this study's findings is that despite the widespread promotion of a systems-based approach to reducing medication error, truly nonpunitive environments are not yet the norm. It also has been recognized that the individual involved in a medical error is the "second victim" of the error. Unconditional sympathy and support for this individual is needed but often not provided by coworkers and supervisory staff after a medical error occurs.[57]

Risk Management

The healthcare delivery system has been compared to the aviation industry because of their similar complex environments, extensive use of technology, and the potential for human error. Consequently, many risk management procedures used in health care are modeled after those used in aviation, including proactively examining environmental, organizational, individual, team, and patient factors that can cause or contribute to the occurrence of medical errors and close calls (often termed "near misses"). Error prevention is based on understanding the nature and extent of potential errors, changing the conditions that can induce errors, determining behaviors that prevent or mitigate errors, and training personnel.[58–60]

Institutions can conduct periodic self-assessments of their error prevention programs. These programs should demonstrate evidence of organizational commitment, utilize clearly delineated policies and procedures, include staff education (both initial and ongoing), and contain detailed assessment parameters specific to the area being assessed. For instance, medication error prevention may include assessing environmental factors such as storage, dispensing, and administration areas; organizational factors such as the prescription, preparation, and administration processes; individual and team factors such as education and information resources; and patient factors such as patient education and partnership.

In 2003, the National Academy of Sciences published *Patient Safety: Achieving a New Standard for Care*, a report describing a detailed plan developed by representatives from the public and private sectors. The report recommends that all healthcare settings establish comprehensive patient safety programs that include detecting and analyzing adverse events and near misses. In addition, it recommends that the federal government support a research agenda for patient safety focused on increasing knowledge, creating data collection tools, and disseminating results. Lastly, the report recommends that a standardized vocabulary and reporting format be developed to better capture data related to medical errors.[55]

Although a variety of specific strategies have been advocated by safety experts (see Table 75-2), concepts integral to risk reduction in health care include the need to simplify and standardize, proactively examine systems, educate for safety, train for teamwork, and create and support a culture of safety.[95] Some "fixes" are simple and require only a practice change, such as requiring that generic drug names be written on prescriptions in block letters. More sophisticated solutions, such as an automated medication dispensing system, involve large financial investments and may require workplace renovations, additional manpower, equipment training and maintenance, and so forth.

Sophisticated automated systems do not eliminate the potential for error; they merely reduce the potential for error, because these systems are operated by people and, therefore, are vulnerable to human error. Many systems can also be manually overridden, increasing the potential for error. In a study of 3481 computerized order entry alerts, physicians overrode 91.2% of drug allergy and 89.4% of high-severity drug interaction alerts. No adverse drug events occurred when physicians observed the alerts, and three occurred in patients who received medications with alerts that were overridden.[96] This study's findings suggest that the threshold level for alerting may have been low, prompting the high frequency of manual overrides. When purchasing and using automated systems, it is important to be aware of the ability to manually override the systems and to recognize that this is a limitation of their use.

In 2003, the National Patient Safety Foundation published the results of a national educational needs assessment for improving patient safety. Physicians and nurses indicated the need for information on the role of technology in reducing errors, communication (especially on disclosure of errors to patients and families), reporting errors and following up on them, the relationship between staffing levels and error occurrence, and strategies to minimize the influence of human factors, such as complacency, fatigue, and stress, on medical errors.[97] These and other related safety topics are appropriate subjects that staff educators should consider addressing in safety programs.

It is also important to note that safety changes are often as much cultural as they are technical. Creating a culture of safety requires attention to the conditions in which employees work and support for processes and programs designed to promote safety. In order to foster a culture of safety, effective leadership must be present, team building needs to be emphasized, and quality improvement objectives must align with the institution's core values.[98] An additional error prevention strategy is to design jobs for safety by considering length of work hours, workload, staffing ratios, and so forth. Staffing issues also encompass insufficient staffing and the use of inexperienced staff, floating and temporary staff, and unlicensed assistive personnel.

Some safety experts recommend developing a strategic plan for safety. To formulate short and long-term goals, the plan should assess the institution's internal processes and capabilities. The goals should be measurable to allow tracking of progress and allow for modification as needed, be compatible with the organization's culture, and be able to remain applicable over the long term despite anticipated changes in the

Table 75-2 Risk Management Strategies Applicable to Oncology

Action	Examples
Use automated systems and information technology[61–69]	Automated dispensing machines, electronic communication and medical records, computerized physician order entry, computerized medication administration records, computerized clinical decision support systems, personal data assistants, bar coding, use of robots
Reduce complexity[70–74]	Minimize and standardize stock inventory, use one type or brand of equipment (e.g., infusion pumps), streamline procedures, simplify systems, unify the prescribing vocabulary, and use generic rather than trade names for medications
Include constraints in systems[73,75,76]	Restrict actions that can result in error (e.g., avoid use of abbreviations, delineate who can order and administer chemotherapy, etc.), remove concentrated electrolytes from patient care areas, use automated medication ordering systems with alerts for higher-than-standard doses
Utilize human resources[75,77–82]	Require pharmacist verification of order entry, have pharmacists and nurses on rounding teams, place advanced practice nurses in clinical decision support roles, involve patients in the treatment verification process, create a patient safety committee, utilize medical librarians to obtain information
Educate healthcare providers[83,84]	Provide formal instruction on safety in schools of nursing, hospital teaching rounds, and conferences; perform comprehensive orientation of new employees, offer ongoing staff education programs, encourage and reward specialty certification
Monitor patients closely and promote continuity of care[85–89]	Ensure adequate patient/staff ratios, employ qualified staff, have an appropriate skill mix of personnel, conduct change-of-shift rounds and reports in patients' rooms, use reliable, well-maintained equipment, provide alarm and alerting mechanisms when indicated (e.g., call bells, bed alarms, etc.)
Optimize infection control practices[89,90]	Comply with CDC hand hygiene and infection control recommendations, monitor personnel and the environment, use proper medical device sterilization and environmental disinfection
Periodically assess procedures, risks, and emergency preparedness[78,91,92]	Self-assess or have policies and procedures externally reviewed; update as needed. Identify high-alert medications and high-risk procedures, conduct mock emergency drills
Improve communication[93]	Delineate who is "in charge" during medical emergencies, identify channels of communication, communicate openly and honestly with patients and their families, fully disclose medical errors and adverse events
Implement voluntary, nonpunitive error reporting[94]	Identify what to report, such as actual events and near misses, delineate staff involvement, educate staff, provide positive reinforcement, promote accountability, support culture of learning from mistakes instead of hiding or minimizing them

organization and healthcare delivery. External influences should be examined, including the current and projected economy, reimbursement patterns, trends in technology, applicable laws, regulatory and accreditation requirements, the legal climate, and healthcare trends such as staffing shortages.[99]

Complaints and Litigation

Although the prevailing philosophy of examining medical errors has changed from one of "naming, blaming, and shaming"[52] to a nonpunitive systems approach, the desire to find fault continues in the legal arena. Legal action following a medical error or adverse event is intended to identify and punish those perceived to be at fault.

Formal complaints are sometimes filed with state licensing boards. Licensing boards are charged with protecting the public by licensing and regulating healthcare providers under their jurisdiction. They also investigate complaints filed against healthcare providers by patients, their family members, or the general public to determine whether the healthcare providers violated state practice acts. Professional practice acts enumerate the infractions that could result in disciplinary actions such as formal reprimands or consent orders to restrict or revoke licensure. In many states, licensing boards have the right to (and usually do) publish the circumstances of a consent order in local newspapers. Licensing boards are also required to disclose adverse actions to the National Practitioner Data Bank.

Patients and/or their families sometimes retain legal counsel to explore filing a lawsuit against healthcare providers when they perceive that an injury has occurred as a result of negligence or malpractice. Lawsuits alleging patient injury following medication errors, vesicant chemotherapy extravasations, chemotherapy-induced hypersensitivity reactions, and other events often specifically name the nurses involved and may include others, such as supervisory personnel. Plaintiffs (the parties initiating the lawsuit) typically allege incorrect or improper actions (acts of commission) but also may sue for injuries related to acts of omission, such as failure to monitor a patient. Litigation can be physically and emotionally draining for the nurses involved, and costly. Jury awards in medical malpractice cases often exceed $1 million.[100]

The documentation of an error or event is scrutinized when a lawsuit is filed. It has been said that "if it wasn't charted, it wasn't done" and that "the palest ink is better than the best memory." Although the primary purpose of documentation is to provide communication among the healthcare team, it also provides a legal record of the care rendered to a patient. It is essential that documentation in medical records be accurate. Inaccurate, incomplete, or contradictory documentation creates confusion for healthcare providers, increases legal liability, and decreases the credibility of healthcare providers, especially when medical record entries are scrutinized in the courtroom.

Nurses named as defendants may find the fault-finding nature of the courtroom to be distressing and in stark contrast to their supportive, understanding work environments. This dichotomy between the U.S. legal system and patient safety initiatives has prompted concern about the role of adversarial dispute resolution in healthcare.[101] It is a factor in the current malpractice crisis, in which healthcare providers are unable to afford liability insurance premiums or choose not to practice in a litigious environment.[102] It has also been the impetus for recommendations to abolish the National Practitioner Data Bank, establish a national patient safety authority, cap noneconomic damages (limit monetary awards for metal anguish, pain, and suffering), and utilize medical review panels and mediation committees to evaluate allegations of healthcare-related injuries.[103,104] Compensation for these injuries needs to be appropriately structured, fair, timely, and, ideally, funded as an intrinsic component of healthcare.[105] An example of this type of system exists in Finland, where injured patients do not sue in court but rather submit claims to the Patient Insurance Association. Median compensation under this system is $1970 per claim.[106]

Lawsuits filed against healthcare organizations are increasingly including short staffing as a contributing factor or cause of patient injury.[107] State legislation is pending or has been enacted in some states, such as California, to mandate nurse/patient staffing ratios, and a federal safe staffing bill was introduced in 2003.[108,109] Defensive administrative strategies to reduce the risk of litigation include appropriate and adequate staffing, use of qualified healthcare providers, extensive staff education and close supervision, clear role delineation, open communication, and truthful documentation.

Privacy Protection

When the U.S. Congress enacted the Health Insurance Portability and Accountability Act (HIPAA) of 1996, it mandated regulations to protect the privacy, security, and confidentiality of health information. Title II of HIPAA, the Privacy Rule, became effective April 14, 2001, and provides comprehensive protections against inappropriate or unintended disclosure of personal health information. Provisions of the Privacy Rule include patient control of the use of health information, patients' rights to review and amend their health information, standards limiting the disclosure of health information, requirements for patients to be informed of providers' health information disclosure policies, and penalties for noncompliance with the law. The Privacy Rule applies to personally identifiable health information in any form, communicated electronically, on paper, or verbally by healthcare providers, health plans, and healthcare clearinghouses. However, the rule does not preempt state laws that provide more stringent privacy protection. Therefore, in some areas, healthcare providers need to comply with multiple layers of federal and state law.[110–113]

The specific procedures used to protect patients' privacy vary by institution but generally involve not posting patients' names or health information in public or prominent places, such as large wipe-off boards in nurses' stations or hallways, using "sign-in" procedures that promote privacy, such as covering names of patients who have already signed in, maintaining medical records in secure locations, and using password-protected computer access. In addition, healthcare providers cannot sell or provide patients' names and addresses to product or pharmaceutical manufacturers. Under the Privacy Rule, patients are given information about the law and the healthcare providers' privacy practices and are able to specifically stipulate how their health information will be used.

Telephone and Electronic Communication

Oncology nurses who provide home care or care for patients in outpatient settings frequently receive telephone calls from patients or family members to ask questions, express concerns, notify nurses of problems, or request renewal of medications. Nurses working in acute care settings often place telephone calls to patients post-discharge.[114,115] Patients' questions and problems are also sometimes addressed via electronic mail or other electronic communication devices, such as video-phones.[116,117] Because nurses cannot physically assess patients under these circumstances, they must rely on their interviewing skills in order to obtain information and intervene appropriately and effectively.

Telephone triage raises many issues, such as how best to protect patient privacy and ensure that information obtained via the telephone is accurate and complete. There is also the need to ensure that nurses providing advice to patients are qualified to do so, and that they dispense instructions that are within their scope of practice. Differentiation between medical, nursing, and secretarial responsibilities needs to be delineated. Telephone triage guidelines and clinical decision trees or protocols can be used to promote the comprehensiveness and consistency of information provided to patients. These guidelines should be evidence-based, reviewed at least annually, and updated when indicated. Telephone calls and electronic communication to and from patients need to be documented in the patients' medical records. In addition, nurses should follow up on instructions relayed via the telephone in order to determine the patient's response, and should communicate their interactions to the appropriate healthcare providers when applicable, such as informing the physician on call about patients with problems or conditions that may worsen after hours.[118–121]

Pain Management

In recent years, the undertreatment of pain has received media attention and in some cases has prompted litigation and state licensing board action. Chronic pain is a common problem experienced by 30%–50% of patients with cancer undergoing active treatment and 70%–90% of patients with advanced disease.[122] Patients with cancer and, in particular, older patients with cancer, are at high risk for undertreatment of pain.[123,124] Inadequate pain management occurs frequently and has been attributed to healthcare providers' lack of knowledge, inappropriate concerns about opioid side effects and addiction, focus on disease treatment rather than symptom management, and other factors.[122,125]

Physicians have been cited for negligent pain management. For instance, a physician was disciplined by a state board of medical examiners in 1999 after he used acetaminophen to treat an elderly man's cancer-related pain. In another case, a jury found a nurse liable for failure to medicate and control pain in a patient dying of cancer. The nurse withheld the prescribed opioid analgesics and substituted a placebo instead. In a case involving inadequate pain management experienced by an elderly patient with cancer, the patient's family alleged elder abuse as well as medical malpractice, and the case went to trial as an elder abuse charge. A jury awarded the family $1.5 million.[126]

Nurses are liable for the undertreatment of pain. They need to be proactive in managing pain effectively and protecting themselves from lawsuits claiming inappropriate or inadequate pain management. Nurses should treat a patient's level of pain as the "fifth vital sign"; use the World Health Organization's analgesic ladder, which serves as a basis for the Agency for Healthcare Policy and Research's pain management guidelines, to assess and treat pain; individualize the pain treatment to the patient; and advocate for treatment modification as needed in order to effectively control pain.[127] Nurses also play an important role in implementing state pain initiatives that enhance the knowledge and skills of healthcare providers, support institutional change, and stress the importance of patient and family involvement in effective pain control.[128]

Conclusion

Oncology nurses are instrumental in promoting patient safety. Strategies for ensuring safety include implementing national safety recommendations and adhering to principles of practice and institutional policies. A high-risk area of practice is chemotherapy administration, since the potential exists for chemotherapy medication errors, hypersensitivity reactions, and vesicant extravasations. Other areas of liability include documentation, privacy, communication via telephone, and pain management. By employing risk management strategies, nurses can reduce the risk of legal action and, more importantly, deliver safe patient care.

References

1. Kohn LT, Corrigan JM, Donaldson MS (eds.): *To Err Is Human: Building a Safer Health System.* Washington, DC, National Academies Press, 2000
2. Kanjanarat P, Winterstein AG, Johns TE, et al: Nature of preventable adverse drug events in hospitals: a literature review. *Am J Health Syst Pharm* 60:1750–1759, 2003
3. Kellogg VA, Havens DS: Adverse events in acute care: an integrative literature review. *Res Nurs Health* 31:398–408, 2003

4. Lassetter JH, Warnick ML: Medical errors, drug-related problems, and medication errors: A literature review on quality of care and cost issues. *J Nurs Care Qual* 18:175–181, 2003
5. Radtke K: Take the fear out of sentinel events. *Nurs Manag* 34:24–25, 2003
6. Joint Commission on Accreditation of Healthcare Organizations: sentinel event statistics. *www.jcaho.org/accredited+organizations/office+based¢rgery/sentinel+events/se_stats.pdf.* Accessed December 3, 2003
7. Committee on Quality of Healthcare in the United States, Institute of Medicine: *Crossing the Chasm: A New Health System for the 21st Century*. Washington, DC, National Academies Press, 2001
8. Joint Commission on Accreditation of Healthcare Organizations: *Facts about the 2004 National Patient Safety Goals. www.jcaho.org/accredited+organizations/patient{fety/04+npsg/facts+about+the+04+npsg.htm.* Accessed December 23, 2003
9. National Nosocomial Infections Surveillance (NNIS) system report, data summary from January 1992 through June 2003, issued August 2003. *www.cdc.gov/ncidod/hip/nnis/2003nnisreport_ajic.pdf.* Accessed 12/23/03
10. Schulmeister L: I know handwashing is important, but... *Clin J Oncol Nurs* 3:4–5, 1999
11. Associated Press: Fatal dosage costs hospital millions. *Times Picayune* 10/9/99:A6
12. Schulmeister L: Chemotherapy medication errors: Descriptions, severity, and contributing factors. *Oncol Nurs Forum* 26:1033–1042, 1999
13. Crawford SY, Cohen MR, Tafesse E: Systems factors in the reporting of serious medication errors in hospitals. *J Med Syst* 27:543–551, 2003
14. Wakefield DS, Wakefield BJ, Uden-Holman T, et al: Understanding why medication administration errors may not be reported. *Am J Med Qual* 14:81–88, 1999
15. Phillips J, Beam S, Brinker A, et al: Retrospective analysis of mortalities associated with medication errors. *Am J Health Syst Pharm* 58:1835–1841, 2001
16. Golde DW, Jakubowiak A, Caggiano J, et al: Cladribine underdosing in hairy-cell leukemia: a cause for apparent response failure. *Leuk Lymphoma* 43:365–367, 2002
17. Institute for Safe Medication Practices: Cancer patients deserve the safest practices, regardless of where they are treated. *ISMP Medication Safety Alert* 8(17):3, 2003
18. Waddell JA, Coleman TA: Clinical response to unintended infusion of doxorubicin and vincristine over one instead of four days. *Am J Health Syst Pharm* 57:1242–1244, 2000
19. Boyle DA, Schulmeister L, Lajeunesse JD, et al: Medication misadventure in cancer care. *Semin Oncol Nurs* 18:109–120, 2002
20. Kohler DR, Ontello MJ, Green L, et al: Standardizing the expression and nomenclature of cancer treatment regimens. *Am J Health Syst Pharm* 55:137–144, 1998
21. Ross TW, Wojdylo JR: Identifying sources and reducing the potential for chemotherapy-related errors: mission impossible? *Cancer Control J* 4:528–536, 1997
22. Ferner RE: Medication errors that have led to manslaughter charges. *BMJ* 321:1212–1216, 2000
23. Shepherd GM: Hypersensitivity reactions to chemotherapeutic drugs. *Clin Rev Allergy Immunol* 24:253–262, 2003
24. Wilkes GM, Ingwersen K, Barton-Burke M (eds.): *Oncology Nursing Drug Handbook*. Subdury, MA, Jones and Bartlett, 2002
25. Graham ML: Pegaspargase: a review of clinical studies. *Adv Drug Deliv Rev* 55:1293–1302, 2003
26. Geuenich S, Haberl C, Egger D, et al: Induction of leukotriene production by bleomycin and asparaginase in mast cells in vitro and in vivo. *Biochem Pharmacol* 55:447–453, 1998
27. Markman M, Kennedy A, Webster K, et al: Paclitaxel-associated hypersensitivity reactions: experience with the gynecologic oncology programs of the Cleveland Clinic Cancer Center. *J Clin Oncol* 18:102–105, 2000
28. Myers J: Hypersensitivity reaction to paclitaxel: nursing interventions. *Clin J Oncol Nurs* 4:161–163, 2000
29. Markman M, Zanotti K, Peterson G, et al: Expanded experience with an intradermal skin test to predict for the presence or absence of carboplatin hypersensitivity. *J Clin Oncol* 21:4611–4614, 2003
30. Markman M, Kennedy A, Webster K, et al: Clinical features of hypersensitivity reactions to carboplatin. *J Clin Oncol* 17:1141, 1999
31. Polyzos A, Tsavaris N, Kosmas C, et al: Hypersensitivity reactions to carboplatin administration are common but not always severe: a 10-year experience. *Oncology* 61:129–133, 2001
32. Robinson JB, Singh D, Bodurka-Bevers DC, et al: Hypersensitivity reactions and the utility of oral and intravenous densensitization in patients with gynecologic malignancies. *Gynecol Oncol* 82:550–558, 2003
33. Zanotti KM, Rybicki LA, Kennedy AW, et al: Carboplatin skin testing: a skin-testing protocol for predicting hypersensitivity to carboplatin chemotherapy. *J Clin Oncol* 19:3126–3129, 2001
34. Markman M, Hsieh, F, Zanotti K, et al: Initial experience with a novel desensitization strategy for carboplatin-associated hypersensitivity reactions. *J Cancer Res Clin Oncol* 130:25–28, 2004
35. Rose PG, Fusco N, Smrekar M, et al: Successful administration of carboplatin in patients with clinically documented carboplatin hypersensitivity. *Gynecol Oncol* 89:429–433, 2003
36. Jones R, Ryan M, Friedlander M: Carboplatin hypersensitivity reactions: re-treatment with cisplatin desensitization. *Gynecol Oncol* 89:112–115, 2003
37. Ottaiano A, Tambaro R, Greggi S, et al: Safety of cisplatin after severe hypersensitivity reactions to carboplatin in patients with recurrent ovarian carcinoma. *Anticancer Res* 23:3465–3468, 2003
38. Berlex Laboratories: Campath® (alemtuzumab) prescribing information. *www.campath.com.* Accessed March 14, 2004
39. ImClone Systems, Inc. and Bristol-Myers Squibb Co.: Erbitux™ (cetuximab) prescribing information. *www.ERBITUX.com.* Accessed March 14, 2004
40. Needle, MN: Safety experience with IMC-C225, an anti-epidermal growth factor receptor antibody. *Semin Oncol* 29(5 suppl 14):55–60, 2002
41. Wyeth Laboratories: Mylotarg® (gemtuzumab ozogamicin) prescribing information. *www.wyeth.com/content/ShowLabeling.asp?id=119.* Accessed April 14, 2004
42. Genentech, Inc. and IDEC Pharmaceuticals Corp.: Rituxan® (rituximab) prescribing information. *www.rituxan.com.* Accessed March 14, 2004
43. Ligand Pharamceuticals: ONTAK® (denileukin difitox) prescribing information. *www.ligand.com/pdf/Ontak_PI_Rev_1099.pdf.* Accessed March 14, 2004
44. Markman M, Zanotti K, Kulp B: Relationship between a history of systematic allergic reactions and risk of subsequent carboplatin hypersensitivity. *Gynecol Oncol* 89:514–516, 2003
45. Schulmeister L, Camp-Sorrell D: Chemotherapy extravasation from implanted ports. *Oncol Nurs Forum* 27:531–538, 2000
46. Schulmeister L: A complication of vascular access device insertion: a case study and review of subsequent legal action. *J Intraven Nurs* 21:197–202, 1998
47. Brown KA, Esper P, Kelleher L, et al (eds.): *Chemotherapy and Biotherapy Guidelines and Recommendations for Practice*. Pittsburgh, Oncology Nursing Society, 2001
48. National Patient Safety Foundation: Talking to patients about health care injury. *Focus Patient Safety* 4(1):3, 2001
49. Banja JD: Disclosing medical error: how much to tell. *J Healthc Risk Manag* 23(1):11–14, 2003

50. Kachalia A, Shojania KG, Hofer TP, et al: Does full disclosure of medical errors affect malpractice liability? *Jt Comm J Qual Safety* 29:503–511, 2003
51. Wissow LS: Communication and malpractice claims-where are we now? *Patient Educ Couns* 52:3–5, 2004
52. Reason J: Human error: models and management. *BMJ* 320:768–770, 2000
53. Gluck PA: Root cause analysis studies incidents to reveal system failures. *Focus Patient Safety* 6:1–5, 2003
54. Vincent C, Taylor-Adams S, Chapman EJ, et al: How to investigate and analyse clinical incidents: Clinical Risk Unit and Association of Litigation and Risk Management protocol. *BMJ* 320:777–781, 2000
55. National Academy of Sciences: *Patient Safety: Achieving a New Standard for Care.* Washington, DC, National Academies Press, 2003
56. Smetzer J: Pathways for medication safety project background: ISMP survey pinpoints weaknesses in medication practices. *Pathways for Medication Safety™. www.medpathways.info.* Accessed January 2, 2004
57. Wu AW: Medical error: the second victim. *BMJ* 320:726–727, 2000
58. Barach P, Small SD: Reporting and preventing medical mishaps: lessons from non-medical near miss reporting systems. *BMJ* 320:759–763, 2000
59. Cohoon BD: Learning from near misses through reflection: a new risk management strategy. *J Healthc Risk Manag* 23(2):19–25, 2003
60. Helmreich RL: On error management: lessons from aviation. *BMJ* 320:781–785, 2000
61. Bates DW: Using information technology to reduce rates of medication errors in hospitals. *BMJ* 320:788–791, 2000
62. Bates DW, Gawande AA: Improving safety with information technology. *N Engl J Med* 348:2526–2534, 2003
63. Chung K, Choi YB, Moon S: Toward efficient medication error reduction: error-reducing information management systems. *J Med Syst* 27:553–560, 2003
64. Gray MD, Felkey BG: Computerized prescriber order-entry systems: evaluation, selection, and implementation. *Am J Health Syst Pharm* 61:190–197, 2004
65. Healthcare Information and Management Society: Bar coding fact sheet. *www.himss.org/content/files/whitepapers/wp_barcoding .pdf.* Accessed January 28, 2004
66. Kaushal R, Shojania KG, Bates DW: Effects of computerized physician order entry and clinical decision support systems on medication safety: a systematic review. *Arch Intern Med* 163:1409–1416, 2003
67. Larrabee S, Brown MM: Recognizing the institutional benefits of bar-code point-of-care technology. *Jt Comm J Qual Safety* 29:345–353, 2003
68. Oren E, Shaffer ER, Guglielmo BJ: Impact of emerging technologies on medication errors and adverse drug events. *Am J Health Syst Pharm* 60:1447–1458, 2003
69. Schumock GT, Nair VP, Finley JM, et al: Penetration of medication safety technology in community hospitals. *J Med Syst* 27:531–541, 2003
70. Adamson AJ: Infusion devices: characteristics, limitations and risk management. *Nurs Stand* 17:45–52, 2003
71. Hoffman J, Prouix S: Medication errors cause by confusion of drug names. *Drug Safety* 26:445–452, 2003
72. Keselman A, Patel VL, Johnson TR, et al: Institutional decision-making to select patient care devices: identifying venues to promote patient safety. *J Biomed Informat* 36:31–44, 2003
73. Nolan TW: System changes to improve patient safety. *BMJ* 320:771–773, 2000
74. Schwab M, Oetzel C, Morike K, et al: Using trade names: a risk factor for accidental drug overdose. *Arch Intern Med* 162:1065–1066, 2002
75. George D, Austin-Bishop N: Error rates for computerized order entry by physicians versus nonphysicians. *Am J Health Syst Pharm* 60:2250–2252, 2003
76. Karch AM: Looks can be deceiving: use caution when using abbreviations. *Am J Nurs* 103:73, 2003
77. Awe C, Lin SJ: Patient empowerment model to prevent medication errors. *J Med Syst* 27:503–517, 2003
78. Cohen HS: Developing a patient safety committee: one hospital's experience. *Focus Patient Safety* 6:6–7, 2003
79. Gandhi TK, Graydon-Baker E, Barnes JN, et al: Creating an integrated patient safety team. *Jt Comm J Qual Safety* 29:383–390, 2003
80. Kucukarsian SH, Peters M, Mlynarek, et al: Pharmacists on rounding teams reduce preventable adverse drug events in hospital general medicine units. *Arch Intern Med* 138: 2014–2018, 2003
81. Rucker NL: ''Risk, respect, responsibility'': educational strategies to promote safe medication use. *J Med Syst* 27:519–530, 2003
82. Williams L, Zipperer L: Improving access to information: librarians and nurses team up for patient safety. *Nurs Econ* 21:199–201, 2003
83. Papastrat K, Wallace, S: Teaching baccalaureate nursing students to prevent medication errors using a problem-based learning approach. *J Nurs Educ* 42:459–464, 2003
84. Pierluissi E, Fischer MA, Campbell AR, et al: Discussion of medical errors in morbidity and mortality conferences. *JAMA* 290:2838–2842, 2003
85. Clarke SP: Balancing staffing and safety. *Nurs Manage* 34:44–48, 2003
86. Moore C, Wisnivesky J, Williams S, et al: Medical errors related to discontinuity of care from an inpatient to outpatient setting. *J Gen Intern Med* 18:646–651, 2003
87. Sasichay-Akkadechanunt, T, Scalzi CC, Jawad AF: Relationship between nurse staffing and patient outcomes. *J Nurs Admin* 33:478–485, 2003
88. Stone PW, Tourangeau AE: Measuring nursing services in patient safety research. *Appl Nurs Res* 16:131–132, 2003
89. Cozad A, Jones, RD: Disinfection and the prevention of infectious disease. *Am J Infect Control* 31:243–254, 2003
90. Pittet D: Hand hygiene: improved standards and practice for hospital care. *Curr Opin Infect Dis* 16:327–335, 2003
91. ECRI: medication safety: self assessment questionnaire. *Healthc Risk Contr* 1(SAQ 31):1–24, 2003
92. Smetzer JL, Vaida AJ, Cohen, MR, et al: Findings from the ISMP Medication Safety Self Assessment for hospitals. *Jt Comm J Qual Safety* 29:586–597, 2003
93. Poor communication cited in patient deaths at Boston hospital. *Patient Safety* 4:103, 2003
94. ECRI: nonpunitive error-reporting programs: overcoming the problem of fear. *Risk Manage Reporter* 22:3–9, 2003
95. Schulmeister L: Risk-reduction strategies. *Sentinel Events Toolkit.* Pittsburgh, Oncology Nursing Society, 2002
96. Weingart SN, Toth M, Sands DZ, et al: Physicians' decisions to override computerized drug alerts in primary care. *Arch Intern Med* 163:2625–1631, 2003
97. VanGeest JB, Cumins DS: *An Educational Needs Assessment for Improving Patient Safety: Results of a National Study of Physicians and Nurses* [white paper report issued 3/20/03 by the National Safety Foundation®]. *www.npsf.org/download/EdNeedsAssess .pdf.* Accessed January 15, 2004

98. Cohen MM, Eustis, MA, Gribbins RE: Changing the culture of patient safety: leadership's role in health care quality improvement. *Jt Comm J Qual Safety* 29:329–335, 2003
99. American Hospital Association, Health Research & Education Trust, and the Institute for Safe Medication Practices: *Creating an Organization-Specific Strategic Plan for Medication Safety. www.medpathways.info.* Accessed January 6, 2004
100. Santana S: Malpractice update: states say federal help needed to deal with spiraling costs. *AAMC Reporter. www.aamc.org/newsroom/reporter/oct02/malpractice.htm* Accessed January 4, 2004
101. Brennan TA, Mello, MM: Patient safety and medical malpractice: a case study. *Ann Intern Med* 139:267–273, 2003
102. Liang BA: Layperson and physician perceptions of the malpractice system: implications for patient safety. *Soc Sci Med* 57:147–153, 2003
103. Hatlie MJ, Sheridan SE: Medical liability crisis of 2003: must we squander the change to put patients first? *Health Aff* 22:37–43, 2003
104. Runciman WB: Error, blame, and the law in health care: an antipodean perspective. *Ann Intern Med* 138:997–998, 2003
105. Sage WM: Medical liability and patient safety. *Health Aff* 22(4):26–36, 2003
106. Nyandoto P, Muhonen T, Hakala T, et al: Financial compensation for radiotherapy-related adverse events in a judicial system where proof of medical negligence is not required. *Int J Radiat Oncol Biol Phys* 51:209–121, 2001
107. Borg E: Professional liability during the shortage. *Can Nurse* 97:34–35, 2001
108. Federal safe staffing bill introduced. *Am Nurs* 35:1, 5, 2003
109. Reilly P: California moves ahead on ratios: Davis issues controversial nurse-staffing regulations. *Mod Healthc* 32:17, 2002
110. Blechner B, Butera A: Health Insurance Portability and Accountability Act of 1996 (HIPAA): a provider's overview of new privacy regulations. *Conn Med* 66:91–95, 2002
111. Gostin LO: National health insurance information privacy: regulations under the Health Insurance Portability and Accountability Act. *JAMA* 285:3015–3021, 2001
112. Maddox PJ: HIPAA: Update on rule revisions and compliance requirements. *Nurs Econ* 20:88–92, 2002
113. Office for Civil Rights, Department of Health and Human Resources: Standards for privacy of individually identifiable health information: final rule. *Federal Register* 67: 53181–53273, 2002
114. Dudas V, Bookwalter T, Kerr KM, et al: The impact of follow-up telephone calls after hospitalization. *Am J Med* 111(9B): 26S–30S, 2001
115. Ferrer-Roca O, Subirana R: A four-year study of telephone support for oncology patients using a non-supervised call centre. *J Telemed Telecare* 8:331–336, 2002
116. Liedermann EM, Morefield CS: Web messaging: a new tool for patient-physician communication. *J Am Med Inform Assoc* 10:260–270, 2003
117. Miyazaki M, Stuart M, Liu L, et al: Use of ISDN video-phones for clients receiving palliative and antenatal home care. *J Telemed Telecare* 9:72–77, 2003
118. Anastasia PJ, Blevins MC: Outpatient chemotherapy: telephone triage for symptom management. *Oncol Nurs Forum* 24(suppl 1):13–22, 1997
119. Coleman A: Where do I stand? Legal implications of telephone triage. *J Clin Nurs* 6:227–231, 1997
120. Cox K, Wilson E: Follow-up for people with cancer: nurse-led services and telephone interventions. *J Adv Nurs* 43:51–61, 2003
121. Preston FA: Telephone triage. *Clin J Oncol Nurs* 4:294–296, 2000
122. Portenoy RK, Lesage P: Management of cancer pain. *Lancet* 353:1695–1700, 1999
123. Miller LL, Talerico KA: Pain in older adults. *Annu Rev Nurs Res* 20:63–68, 2002
124. Schilling ML: Pain management in older adults. *Curr Psychiatry Rep* 5:55–61, 2003
125. Resnik DB, Rehm M, Minard RB: The undertreatment of pain: scientific, clinical, cultural, and philosophical factors. *Med Health Care Philos* 4:277–288, 2001
126. Frank-Stromborg M, Christensen A: A serious look at the undertreatment of pain: part I. *Clin J Oncol Nurs* 5:235–236, 2001
127. Frank-Stromborg M, Christensen A: The undertreatment of pain: a liability risk for nurses. *Clin J Oncol Nurs* 4:41–44, 2000
128. Dahl JL, Bennett ME, Bromley MD, et al: Success of the state pain initiatives: moving pain management forward. *Cancer Pract* 10(suppl 1):S9–S13, 2002

CHAPTER 76

Informatics

Heidi E. Ehrenberger, PhD, RN, AOCN®
Elizabeth G. Gomez, MSN, RN, AOCN®

Introduction

The substance of informatics is information, a capital good of immense value to cancer care. A solid foundation of information used during cancer care and as a source of scientific data on which to base rational healthcare policies is essential to improving quality, reducing cost, and ensuring access to care. The rapid advancement and proliferation of computer technology, as a vehicle to manage and process information, is enabling us to advance cancer care. This chapter describes the contributions of informatics to the delivery of cancer care. It first gives an academic overview of informatics, highlighting select topics of relevance within the science. The chapter then focuses specifically on the use of the Internet in advancing cancer care.

The Significance of Informatics

The word "informatics" is derived in part from the French *informatique*, which refers to the computer milieu.[1,2] Informatics integrates information science and computer science. It denotes activities involved in managing and processing information. Nearly all informatics activities are dependent on information technology (IT) such as computers and telecommunications. Yet, the essence of informatics is the information — not the technology. When the name of a discipline is used in combination with the term "*informatics*," it implies an application of computer science and information science to the management and processing of information in the named discipline (e.g., nursing informatics).[3] Health informatics, as a broad science, encompasses medical, nursing, dental, and pharmacy informatics, among others. Informatics nurses, using clinical experience and knowledge, add the dimension of nursing to the health informatics viewpoint.[4,5] The significance of informatics lies in part in its ability to transform data to make it meaningful and useful to multiple constituencies within the healthcare system. With IT, the transformation is expedited.

During the 1990s, major federal initiatives were implemented in the United States to greatly expand the accessibility and use of information technologies in all sectors of the economy, including health care.[6] These initiatives, to build the nation's technology infrastructure and to enable nurses to use technology routinely in delivering care, highlighted the need for a strategic agenda targeting the informatics needs of nursing nationally. A report, titled *A National Informatics Agenda for Nursing Education and Practice,*[7] established five informatics goals for nursing (see Table 76-1).

Table 76-1 Strategic Goals for Nursing to Manage Information

- Educate nursing students and practicing nurses to achieve core informatics competencies
- Prepare nurses with specialized skills in informatics
- Enhance nursing practice and education through informatics projects
- Prepare nursing faculty in informatics
- Increase collaborative efforts in nursing informatics

Data from National Advisory Council on Nurse Education and Practice.[7]

Nursing Informatics as a Specialty

The American Nurses Association (ANA) recognized nursing informatics as a specialty in 1992. Work has been done to identify the scope and standards of nursing informatics practice.[8] Nursing informatics supports the practice of all nursing specialties (e.g., oncology nursing) at the basic or advanced practice level, in all sites and settings of health care. Informatics activities include developing and evaluating applications for managing and processing nursing data, information, and knowledge in cancer care. Nursing informatics is different from other specialties because of its special focus on the structure, acquisition, and use of information.[9] In specialties such as oncology nursing, the focus is on the substance of the information in the care of cancer patients. An oncology nurse who is also an informatician is likely to be better able than other informaticians to represent the concepts of oncology nursing and their relationships in the structure of informatics applications to support oncology nursing.

Research Priorities

As early as 1986, a research framework for nursing informatics was proposed.[10] Research priorities for nursing informatics have since been formalized by the National Institute of Nursing Research (NINR). Since 1993, NINR has supported a program initiative called *Enhancing Clinical Care Through Nursing Informatics.* The intent of this program is to generate research that will examine systems to manage and process data, information, and knowledge with the goal of facilitating appropriate and effective clinical care. This initiative built directly on the work of a panel of experts on nursing informatics. The panel proposed six program goals for informatics research that are detailed in a 1993 report, "*Nursing Informatics: Enhancing Patient Care.*"[11] Since then, research in clinical nursing informatics has proceeded along three important dimensions: (1) identifying and defining nursing's language; (2) understanding how clinical judgment and decision making can be facilitated by computer-based systems; and (3) determining how well-designed systems can transform nursing practice.[12] In 1997, given the rapid changes in health care and technology, a survey was conducted to reevaluate the established NINR program goals and to determine whether new priorities exist.[13] The findings reaffirmed the six NINR program goals. Newly identified priorities included patient use of IT, telecommunications for nursing practice, issues of privacy and confidentiality, and innovative nursing interventions such as the electronic delivery of nursing interventions.[14,15] In 2000, NINR supported a program initiative known as *Telehealth Interventions to Improve Clinical Nursing Care.*[16] The goal of this program is to move beyond nursing language and hospital-based clinical information systems by stimulating research on innovative nursing telehealth interventions.[17]

Standardized Vocabularies

The importance of standardized vocabularies designed to represent nursing data cannot be overstated.[18] Historically, nurses have used different terms when documenting patient experiences and nursing actions. But when different terms are used, the data are essentially not comparable. For example, at the Vanderbilt Medical Center, analysis of standardized documents used to plan and document nursing care showed 17 different ways to convey the information "nausea and vomiting controlled."[19] When this occurs, we cannot compare data to identify effective nursing interventions, and our contribution to patient outcomes is compromised. It is clear that structured, coded data are needed to ensure comparability of nursing observations and records across time and location.

As early as 1985, a group of national experts designed the Nursing Minimum Data Set (NMDS), a system for collecting uniform, standard, comparable minimum nursing data in any setting where nursing care is provided.[20] In 1989, the ANA Steering Committee on Databases to Support Clinical Nursing Practice was established to monitor and ensure the development and use of multiple nursing vocabularies and classification schemes within the framework of the NMDS.[21] Nursing vocabularies have since evolved as appropriate to support clinical practice.[22,23] As of 2004, there were 13 ANA-recognized languages for nursing. A current listing is available on the ANA Web site.[24] For example, SNOMED Clinical Terms® (SNOMED CT®)[25] is a clinical language standard that supports nursing and is available for free through the National Library of Medicine. Ultimately, the optimal use of standardized languages within computerized patient records allows us to document care and to aggregate data to determine costs, quality of care, and health policy.[26]

Computer-Based Patient Records

Overview

In 1989, the National Academy of Science's Institute of Medicine (IOM) launched a study to examine how IT could improve the paper-based patient record. The two-year study resulted in a seminal report, "*Computer-Based Patient Records: An Essential Technology for Health Care.*"[27] Computer-based patient records (CPRs), also referred to as electronic health records (EHRs) or electronic medical records (EMRs),[28] are essential to improving the quality and reducing the cost of delivering health care in the 21st century. The IOM report on CPRs, revised in 1997, continued to provide a compelling case for recognizing the CPR as the standard patient record.[29] Additional reports focus, in part, on the key steps needed to strengthen clinical information systems.[30]

In 2003, a committee of the IOM issued a report titled "*Key Capabilities of an Electronic Health Record System.*"[31] This report identified a set of eight core functions that EHRs should be capable of performing in order to promote greater safety, quality, and efficiency in healthcare delivery (see Table 76-2). It also detailed key capabilities to be used by Health Level Seven (HL7), one of the world's leading developers of healthcare standards.[32] A common industry standard for EHRs would guide the efforts of software developers and the widespread adoption of EHRs. In 2004, the passage of an EHR draft standard represented a significant development in healthcare IT. By 2010, it is anticipated that comprehensive EHR systems will be available and implemented in many health systems and regions.

Application to Cancer Care

As early as 1991, Hendrickson and colleagues described how computerized clinical information systems could assist oncology nurses in providing integrated care by aiding in the collection, organization, and storage of patient data.[33] Because persons with cancer frequently require complex care and numerous encounters in various settings, the available data surrounding their care becomes complex as well. The presence of a comprehensive CPR system with an integrated view of patient data can assist oncology nurses through automated care planning, patient monitoring, and tracking of patients' comfort, therapeutic, and educational needs.[34] As one example, IMPAC

Table 76-2 Core Functions of an Electronic Health Record

Health information and data: provides immediate access to key patient information.
Results management: allows all providers participating in the care of a patient in multiple settings to quickly access new and past test results.
Order entry/management: allows providers to enter and store orders for prescriptions, tests, and other services in a computer-based system.
Decision support: permits the use of reminders, prompts, alerts, and computerized decision support systems.
Electronic communication and connectivity: allows efficient, secure, and readily accessible communication among providers and patients.
Patient support: offers tools that give patients access to their health records, provide interactive patient education, and help them carry out home monitoring and self-testing.
Administrative processes: provides computerized administrative tools, such as scheduling systems, to improve hospitals' and clinics' efficiency and provide more timely service to patients.
Reporting: enables electronic data storage that employs uniform data standards.

Data from Institute of Medicine.[31]

Medical Systems, a commercial vendor, produces a product called eCHART™, a CPR that is the clinical foundation for its integrated oncology management system.[35] The eCHART™ is tailored for radiation and medical and surgical oncology, and can be customized to the practice setting or enhanced with other product offerings.

A comprehensive CPR system can also provide cancer care providers with alerts and reminders about policies and procedures while efficiently integrating clinical practice guidelines and tools to measure oncology outcomes.[36] In outpatient care, randomized controlled clinical trials have been conducted that have demonstrated the efficacy of CPR systems for both healthcare providers and patients alike.[37] Today, many cancer care facilities have some aspect of a CPR system in place. Widespread integration of comprehensive CPR systems into cancer care provides high-quality data for computer-based population databases essential to the healthcare management of individuals, data for cancer research, data to support public health initiatives, and data that can be used to track the performance of individual cancer care providers and institutions. As consumers and persons with cancer become more actively involved in managing their own health care, and as IT becomes available in more homes, individuals will increasingly use elements of the CPR and CPR-related technology to search through the scientific literature, communicate with their healthcare providers via e-mail, access data on their medical history, monitor the financial costs and the value of services they receive, and diagnose acute health problems while managing chronic health problems.

Decision-Support Systems

Overview

Decision-support systems (DSSs) function as tools for the user during the decision-making task.[38] These tools vary in size and function. They may be part of a CPR system or serve as a stand-alone system, and can range from general to patient-specific. For example, DSSs can function as tools for information management, tools for focusing attention, and tools for providing patient-specific recommendations.[39] Information-management tools provide the user with necessary data and knowledge for making a decision; however, the tools do not help the user apply the information to the decision at hand. Such tools can provide, for example, access to electronic textbooks. Tools that focus the user's attention are computer programs designed to remind the user of problems as well as diagnoses that might have been inadvertently omitted or overlooked. These tools can be viewed as monitoring tools. Finally, tools that provide patient-specific recommendations are based on a database of patient-specific data.

Those who design and implement DSSs use various underlying methodologies. These include protocols and algorithms such as clinical guidelines, clinical databanks, mathematical models, statistical pattern recognition and neural networks, Bayesian statistics and Bayesian networks, decision analysis, and artificial intelligence. In medicine, several types of patient-specific consultation systems have been designed and are commercially available. In nursing, DSSs to provide patient-specific recommendations have also been specifically designed for clinical nursing practice.[40,41] Many have used knowledge-based systems, an area of artificial intelligence, as the underlying methodology. Knowledge-based systems incorporate the judgment and advice of expert nurses; these systems have also been described as "expert systems." Such systems developed by nurses and their colleagues include the *Creighton Online Multiple Modular Expert System*, an effort that evolved into what is now the *Patient Care Expert*, designed to support nursing clinical decision making about individual patient conditions.[42] Ultimately, the development of DSSs results in the creation of tools to support our practice by making nursing knowledge more explicit and more accessible.[43]

At the consumer level, the development of DSSs by the government and private sector has resulted in widespread dissemination of health informatics tools for patient treatment decisions.[44] These tools transform the traditional delivery of healthcare information by providing, for example, cancer treatment information or other disease-specific health information to patients when they are making decisions about how best to manage their illness, and may result in improved treatment outcomes and quality of life. With the advent of the Internet, DSSs designed specifically for patient use can be accessed directly from home, 24 hours a day, for the promotion of self-care and prevention. Consumers typically have not had the tools necessary to become active and informed participants in their own health care. Clearly, this area is key for nursing involvement, given our focus on patient education, the advent of consumer health informatics, and the evolving significance of self-care.

Application to Cancer Care

Various types of DSSs have been designed for cancer care, and their use continues to be refined. For example, the Oncology Clinical Information System (OCIS), a computer-based DSS for the clinical management of cancer patients, was developed and implemented at the Johns Hopkins Oncology Center during the 1970s.[45] In developing the OCIS, the goal was to provide reliable, complete, and timely information that presented itself in a manner that led the clinician most directly to the correct decision; it was to be considered first and foremost as a tool to support clinical decision making in a large healthcare setting. Over the past 30 years, the OCIS has evolved to be viewed more as the core of a CPR, linked with the operational, clinical, and administrative functions of cancer care.

Another example of an oncology DSS is ONCOCIN, developed at Stanford University in the 1980s for the purpose of facilitating adherence to complex protocol regimens.[46] ONCOCIN integrated a clinical data management environment with a DSS in order to provide customized treatment advice for cancer patients and clinical trials management. Although ONCOCIN is no longer in clinical use, its development represented a scientific research endeavor, and its use by clinicians led to improvements in data collection for complex protocol regimens while enhancing quality care for patients through decision support.[47] Newer DSSs continue to be developed.[48]

While DSSs in cancer care were initially intended for clinician use, they have also become increasingly viable for patient use. For example, Williams and colleagues tested the effectiveness of a patient-oriented DSS for improving cancer screening rates in a randomized, controlled trial.[49] The researchers concluded that the system enhanced the provision of patient-specific preventive service recommendations and facilitated clinic work flow to increase the completion of the screenings. At the University of Wisconsin-Madison, researchers developed the *Comprehensive Health Enhancement Support System*, a noncommercial computer system that provides patients with disease-specific information, emotional support, and skill-building tools.[50] This computer-based system is designed to help individuals cope with various health problems, including breast cancer. DSSs of any scope can facilitate the complexity of cancer care. Nurses, in particular, can seek to gain by being involved in developing and testing consumer- and patient-oriented DSSs, as well as knowledge-based delivery systems that are appropriate for nurses' needs.

Telemedicine and Telehealth

Overview

Telemedicine is an aspect of telehealth that focuses specifically on the provider aspects of healthcare telecommunications. The focus appropriately is on the remote communication of information to facilitate clinical care.[51,52] Numerous terms have been coined to specify the specialty to which telemedicine is then applied: teledermatology, teleophthalmology, teleoncology, tele-home health. In addition, some have used the term "*telenursing*" to specify the use of telemedicine technology in the delivery of nursing care. While the term "*telemedicine*" remains in common usage, many in the healthcare field recognize and embrace the broader perspective of the term "*telehealth*," as it more clearly delineates the systematic application of telecommunication technology to all healthcare.[53,54]

The benefits and applications of telemedicine are numerous. Telemedicine is viewed as a partial solution for reducing escalating healthcare costs while simultaneously providing innovative healthcare to rural areas, correctional facilities, military settings, home care, and international agencies. Indeed, one of the largest reported applications of telemedicine is the delivery of healthcare to rural areas. By using telemedicine, healthcare providers can consult with specialists thousands of miles away, upgrade their education and skills, and share medical records. This results in an increased access to specialists and savings in treatment time and travel costs.[55] For example, cost savings were examined in a telehealth project at the University of Arkansas during 1998–2002. Results suggested that without telemedicine, 94% of the patients would have traveled more than 70 miles for medical care, 84% would have missed one day of work, and 74% would have spent $75–$150 for additional family expenses.[56] Another significant area of growth where nursing can play a vital role is in the home care segment of telemedicine.[57] One study suggested that in the United States approximately 45% of home nursing visits could be done via telemedicine.[58]

Barriers related to implementing telehealth include reimbursement, licensing of healthcare providers, malpractice, and privacy and confidentiality of patient data, as well as technology costs.[59] Despite these issues, the evolution of telemedicine is reengineering the traditional delivery of health care.

Application to Cancer Care

The application of telemedicine to cancer care is increasingly visible.[60,61] For example, Allen and colleagues[62] described how medical oncologists from an urban, university-based hospital provided oncology care to rural patients using interactive video clinics, which they described as "tele-oncology." Surveys were performed after the video encounters as well as after a limited number of subsequent clinical encounters on site in order to assess physician satisfaction with this form of outreach. The results suggested that there was a reasonable level of physician satisfaction with, and confidence in, the use of video to replace some on-site oncology consultations. Doolittle and colleagues[63] report monitoring and evaluating costs of different types of oncology practice, including a telemedicine clinic and a fly-in outreach clinic, both held in rural areas. Findings showed that it was less expensive to use telemedicine than to fly in oncology support for the practice. The University of Wisconsin Hospital and Clinics and regional oncology affiliates are using telemedicine to promote and enhance cancer treatment and clinical research.[64] Their system encompasses several forms of technology in order to provide professional education and training, patient evaluation and protocol eligibility, data transfer for radiation therapy treatment planning, quality assurance, and peer review programs for medical oncology and radiation oncology. In other parts of the United States, home telemedicine is being used with pediatric bone marrow transplant patients, as well as in the care of hospice patients located in geographically rural areas.[65] Ultimately, innovative applications of telehealth to the delivery of high-quality cancer care will continue to grow.[66] A list of telehealth resources is provided in Table 76-3.

Table 76-3 Select Resources in Telehealth

Association of Telehealth Service Providers (*www.atsp.org*)
International membership-based organization dedicated to improving health care through the growth of the telehealth industry.

American Telemedicine Association (*www.atmeda.org*)
A leading resource and advocate promoting access to medical care for consumers and health professionals via telecommunications technology.

Telemedicine Information Exchange (*www.telemed.org*)
A comprehensive, international resource without bias for information about telehealth and telehealth-related activities.

The Center for Telemedicine Law (*www.ctl.org*)
A nonprofit entity founded by organizations committed to providing high-quality patient services through the use of telemedicine systems throughout the United States and the world.

VHA Telehealth (*www.va.gov/telehealth*)
This portal provides access to telehealth resources and educational resources that exist within the Veterans Health Administration.

VHA Telehealth Toolkits (*www.va.gov/telehealth/toolkits_home.htm*)
Provides free informational and developmental resources when establishing a telehealth project or program.

Privacy and Security

Overview

As the application of IT to the healthcare industry becomes increasingly important, the actual storage and dissemination of health information in electronic form raises concerns about patient privacy and data security. These concerns have increased as more sensitive material is stored in medical records, such as HIV status, psychiatric records, and genetic information.[67] The fear is that electronically storing and transmitting such information over the National Information Infrastructure (NII) will further compromise individual privacy. The problem is complex; however, the complexity of the issue resides not so much with the technology itself but with the absence of a global, cohesive informational security policy.[68]

Implementing policy has been difficult for numerous reasons: the legal meaning of privacy is apt to shift periodically to reflect society's public versus private interests, ownership and control of health information is not always readily identifiable, and the patient's informed consent to disclosure of information is arguably a misnomer. While individual institutions and organizations employ a wide variety of technical and nontechnical practices for protecting electronic health information, a relatively unregulated dissemination of information has occurred among institutions in the healthcare industry, including healthcare providers, payers, managers of pharmaceutical benefits programs, equipment suppliers, researchers, and oversight agencies. Although information is primarily collected for legitimate reasons, the potential threat of misuse of accessed information from both authorized and unauthorized outsiders exists.

In order to protect health information, the Health Insurance Portability and Accountability Act (HIPAA) of 1996 (H.R. 3103) was signed into law. HIPAA provides guidelines for electronic healthcare transactions, unique health identifiers, code sets, security, confidentiality, and privacy. In 1998, the U.S. Department of Health and Human Services issued new electronic data security standards, as mandated under HIPAA.[69] These standards included, for example, a call for universal encryption of medical data when electronically distributed, the use of digital signatures, and strict control over online access to records. By issuing such standards and regulations for security and privacy, HIPAA began to fill the gap in existing legislation for protecting health information. On April 14, 2003, the first federal privacy standards to protect patients' health information took effect. The security standards go into effect on April 21, 2005.

The need for dedicated individuals (e.g., chief privacy officers) and sophisticated security technologies to protect privacy will increase as more healthcare organizations take greater advantage of IT.[70,71] While the technological implementation of such measures can protect privacy, technology remains limited in that it cannot control what the individual eventually does with the information.

Application to Cancer Care

Clearly, the issues of privacy and security as they relate to electronic health information are relevant in the delivery of cancer care. This is particularly true for those individuals who have undergone genetic testing and are identified as being at risk for developing cancer.[72] Mounting concerns by consumers reveal justified apprehension about potential genetic discrimination resulting from the release of predictive and presymptomatic genetic test results to employers, insurers, and others.[73] As the use of CPR systems expands, it is paramount to keep such sensitive information secure. Unfortunately, individual fear of employment discrimination through employer access to such health information may discourage at-risk individuals from undergoing testing. The individual may also fear discriminatory actions by insurance companies if he or she is identified as being at risk.

While HIPAA mandates security and privacy regulations for electronic health information, it also permits the use of a common identifier for indexing patient records. A common identifier has the potential to improve the quality and reduce the costs of health care by making a more complete patient record available to providers, to facilitate the creation of a longitudinal patient record for healthcare researchers, and to simplify the administration of healthcare benefits. However, particularly for those individuals with sensitive genetic information, it could also facilitate the assembly of information about patients without their consent.[74] Because the issue of genetic discrimination is a major challenge, healthcare professionals will need knowledge of federal and state laws that provide some measure of protection against discrimination. The potential risk of improper disclosure of sensitive information remains a reality. Only through the enforcement of strong legal penalties, as well as other measures, will such actions be deterred.

The Internet and the World Wide Web

Overview

The first goal identified in *A National Nursing Informatics Agenda* is that nursing students and practicing nurses achieve core informatics competencies. Nurses need to have these competencies to practice effectively in the 21st century.[75] The skills involved include the ability to use word processing, e-mail, spreadsheets, presentation graphics software, databases, bibliographic retrieval, the Internet, and the Web.

Understanding the Internet

The word *Internet* means different things to different people. It can most simply be described as a network of computers. It is also known as the Information superhighway and to some, the Web. The Web is the graphical portion of the Internet that one accesses with a software program called a browser. Some consider simply using electronic mail (e-mail) the Internet. Still others will tell you that they ''surf the net'' by ''logging on'' to America Online®. In part, all of these definitions are true.

At the core of the Internet are ''backbones.'' Backbone networks provide the speed of communications, the ability to transfer large amounts of data (high bandwidth), and the reliability necessary to connect computers on the Internet. The high-speed transfer of data around the globe is accomplished by fiber-optic cabling and, increasingly, by the use of satellites. Computers on the Internet are connected via a leased-line fee structure, effectively eliminating long-distance charges. Data on the Internet may be routed through several computers to reach its final destination. The evolution of the Internet continues. In the early days, when the Advanced Research Projects Agency Network (ARPANET) was the backbone network for the Internet, only academics could connect and use it. Today, the Internet is a very successful commercial venture that is changing the way we work, learn, shop, and define community.

Communication Tools

Electronic mail

E-mail can be thought of as a hybrid between letter writing and the spoken word. It is more spontaneous than letter writing, less likely to get lost, and self-documenting. The use of e-mail, the very first Internet application, has increased significantly in recent years. With millions of e-mail messages being sent around the world each day, it is becoming the preferred method for healthcare professionals to communicate with one another. Nurses are increasingly seeking more rapid, efficient communications with each other, and as a result, electronic mail and online interactive messaging are becoming more important. Patients are also increasingly using e-mail to communicate with their healthcare providers. Because this presents a new method of communication, guidelines for the clinical use of patient-provider e-mail were published by the American Medical Informatics Association in 1998.[76] These guidelines address two interrelated aspects of electronic communication: effective communication between the clinician and patient and judicious regard of medicolegal issues.

Newer issues surround Web messaging, a tool for patient–physician communication that is gaining acceptance.[77] Secure messaging portals solve some of the problems with traditional e-mail, which lacks the design and security necessary for effective and protected electronic communication. Some of these portals can merge with electronic health records and allow patients to review medications and correct errors, make appointments and request refills, access lab results, and review educational materials forwarded to them by clinicians.

Mailing lists

Mailing lists, commonly known as listservs, are the most accessible of the Internet resources discussed here. Users need only to have e-mail access. Each listserv, no matter what the topic, functions in virtually the same way. Listservs are based on the concept of a shared distribution list. Every e-mail sent to the list is distributed to everyone else who is "subscribed" to the list. One person, usually the list owner or postmaster, is responsible for maintaining the listserv software and answering questions about the list. The software program keeps track of subscribers and sends copies of messages. The original software program was called Listserv™, and this is the reason that mailing lists are often referred to as listservs. Cancer-related mailing lists are a very effective way of distributing and obtaining cancer information. For example, the Association of Cancer Online Resources® (ACOR) hosts a Web site with more than 130 public cancer-related mailing lists.[78]

Newsgroups

Newsgroups are electronic discussion forums in which anyone can participate in a public dialogue on a topic of interest. Usenet, a network of computers, was developed to carry messages and replies that are posted to newsgroups. Usenet is supported in nearly all countries and reaches millions of users. No single person or group controls Usenet, and no authority manages it. A newsreader, as its name implies, is a piece of software designed to let you read the messages posted to the newsgroup. The latest versions of most web browsers have newsreaders built into them. Newsreaders obtain the news for you and sort it into threads. A single message posted to a newsgroup usually generates responses along the same line. The sequence of messages following the initial message is called a thread. Additionally, Usenet newsgroups have a hierarchical naming system. The *alt.support* groups and the *sci.med* groups generally covers nursing and health-related discussions.

Internet relay chat

Most Internet applications work asynchronously. You rarely read your e-mail while parts of it are being sent. As the nearly 100% penetration rate of telephony around the globe proves, real-time synchronous communications between two geographically distant people is very valuable. Internet relay chat (IRC) is one example of the Internet's answer to the phone call. IRC is simply a network of IRC servers ("nets") that allow users to connect to ongoing chats. The largest nets are EfNet (the original IRC net, often having more than 32,000 people use it at once), Undernet, IrcNet, DalNet, and NewNet. Once connected to an IRC net, you will usually join one or more "channels" and converse with the others gathered there. Conversations may be public (where everyone in a channel can see what you type) or private (messages travel between only two people, who may or may not be on the same channel). Client software to access IRC is readily available and free. IRC has a reputation for being a "time waster" because of the amount of frivolous discussions that take place and the interactive games found on these servers, but in actuality it is a valuable news distribution source and a place where meetings are being held.

Searching the Internet

While the Internet has a great many qualities, organization is not one of them. Locating information on the

Internet can be an extremely frustrating experience. Because no one body controls the Internet, it lacks certain bibliographic control standards such as international standard book numbers (ISBNs), commonly used to identify and catalog print documents. The majority of Internet materials lack the name of the author and the date of "publication." Moreover, a Web site can be here today and gone tomorrow, and the issues surrounding archiving Internet data have yet to be resolved.

Universal resource locators

Every Web-based document has its own unique address—a universal resource locator (URL). A URL specifies the location of the computer hosting a Web document. Web documents can be found by typing their URLs into a browser program. URLs always have two or more parts, separated by dots. The part on the left reveals the most specific information, for example, "ons" in the URL *http://www.ons.org.* This may reveal the geographic location of the computer, company, or department, or an individual name may be found here. The part on the right is the most general and describes the type of information or domain, such as "org" for an organization, "edu" for an educational institution, "gov" for a government agency, and "com" for a commercial organization. Usually, all of the computers on a given network will have the same characters as the right-hand portion of their URL. Knowledge of the URL, or at least of part of it, can make searching easier.

If the URL is entered correctly into a browser program and you get an error message, you might want to "deconstruct" the URL. This process can help you find Web pages that are still on the same site, but have moved. Start deconstructing a URL by removing portions of the address from the right, one item at a time. As you remove each item, click on the address to see what happens. Addresses or locations of pages on Web sites may change. Working your way backward through a site often will uncover those new links.

Search tools

The Internet itself provides different tools to search the Web: search engines, directories, and metasearch engines. Search engines allow the user to enter keywords that are then matched against a large database of Web pages. Search engines have software packages called "spiders," "crawlers," or "robots" that create these databases automatically by searching the Internet for new documents. Because spiders run constantly and index so many Web pages, the search engine databases frequently have information that is not listed in directories. While all search engines perform the same task, each does it in a slightly different way, leading to very different results. Factors that influence results include the size of the database, the frequency of updating, and the "weight" given to the placement key words. Search engines also differ in how fast they search, the user interface for input and output features, and the amount of help they offer.

Directories are hierarchically organized indexes of subject categories that allow the searcher to browse through lists of Web sites by subject. Unlike search engines, these subject directories are created by humans and can often provide better results than search engines because of the human intervention. Directory databases tend to be smaller than the results from search engines because they rely mostly on user submissions and recommendations. A directory is also more likely to provide a link only to the site's home page. They lend themselves best to searching for general information.

Metasearch tools combine the searching of several search engines. Instead of using spiders to build listings, metasearchers send the query to several search engines. Depending on the metasearch engine, the database searches are then performed either simultaneously or sequentially, and the results are combined onto one page. Some metasearch engines also provide the convenience of using only one input form for searching numerous databases. Metasearch engines are powerful tools for finding very specific information.

Identifying the correct search tool to use depends on the information you need; however, the difference is less distinct now than it once was because more search engines are incorporating directories into their sites. Learning simple search strategies is also important and will help you retrieve better results. Many search tools now allow the user to simply type in a question. Finally, because search tools and techniques change regularly, the Web site Search Engine Watch exists to keep Internet users aware of ongoing changes.[79]

Information-Retrieval Systems

The ability to search the literature is an important skill for improving the quality of cancer nursing care.[80] Traditionally, print formats such as card catalogs have been used to search the literature. This time-consuming format gave way to computerized database systems that could be searched electronically. Today, different types of information-retrieval systems are readily accessible via the Web. Bibliographic-retrieval systems contain citations to the relevant literature, while full-text retrieval systems contain the complete textual content of the source. Information from Web-based database systems can rapidly answer queries posed by healthcare providers, researchers, and, increasingly, consumers and patients.[81,82]

The National Library of Medicine (NLM) provides a wide variety of resources related to the biomedical and health sciences, both past and present. The format of these resources varies: searchable databases and databanks, bibliographic citations, full text (when available), archival collections, and images. The NLM's MEDLINE® is its premier bibliographic database, containing more than 11 million references, citations, and abstracts to articles in biomedical and life sciences journals, published mostly since 1966 in 4600 biomedical journals.

On June 26, 1997, the NLM announced that the MEDLINE database would be accessible on the Web free of charge. PubMed provides access to bibliographic information drawn from MEDLINE and links to the full text of selected journal articles from collaborating publishers with Web sites. A powerful feature of PubMed is that most of its records are linked to other records, and users can retrieve related articles for each citation displayed. In addition, "Cancer Topic Searches" are prepared literature searches from the PubMed database. Literature citations on more than 100 different cancer topics can be obtained via these searches.

Since MEDLINE became freely available on the Web, the NLM reports that many members of the public are willing to make the effort to read scientific articles for guidance on treatment or management of health conditions, whether for themselves, family members, or friends.[83] Although little evidence exists to support the notion that public access to the scientific literature improves health outcomes, numerous anecdotal reports document ways that the scientific literature has helped lay persons find a physician with special experience relevant to their concerns. Thus, the NLM continues to enhance consumer access to health information while devising new evaluation strategies. On October 22, 1998, the NLM introduced MEDLINEplus, which provides consumers with specific subject access to selected sources of health information from government and select nongovernmental agencies. Increasingly, there are links between article references and the full text. Another service called PubMed Central allows free access to a central repository of journal articles. PubMed Central aims to fill the role of a world class library in the digital age.

The National Cancer Institute (NCI) also provides a database, PDQ (Physician Data Query), accessible via the NCI's Web site.[84] PDQ is a comprehensive full-text retrieval system of current, peer-reviewed syntheses of state-of-the-art information on cancer care. It contains peer-reviewed summaries on cancer treatment, screening, prevention, genetics, and supportive care, and complementary and alternative medicine; a registry of approximately 2000 open and 13,000 closed cancer clinical trials from around the world; and directories of physicians, professionals who provide genetics services, and organizations that provide cancer care.

Table 76-4 Organizations Involved in Ensuring the Quality of Online Health Information

eHealth Code of Ethics (*www.ihealthcoalition.org*)
Health Internet Ethics (*www.hiethics.com*)
Health on the Net Foundation (*www.hon.ch*)
Health Summit Working Group (*www.mitretek.org*)
URAC Health Web Site Accreditation Program (*www.urac.org*)

Several other valuable information-retrieval systems exist for nurses, such as the Cumulative Index to Nursing and Allied Health (CINAHL). Although a bibliographic database, CINAHL also includes selected original and full-text material. Full text is included for selected state nursing journals and some newsletters, standards of practice, practice acts, government publications, research instruments, and patient education material.

Quality of Online Cancer Information

The major concern with the public's access to cancer Web sites is that someone might be harmed should they act on information obtained from a site. The rapid growth of healthcare Web sites in the 1990s was accompanied by numerous initiatives to rate their quality, including awardlike symbols on Web sites. A systematic review of the reliability and validity of such rating instruments, published in 1998, showed that they were incompletely developed.[85] Although there is no universally accepted method for evaluating the credibility of any Internet resource, various standards have emerged.[86] Many sources of cancer information are authoritative and reliable. Others are not. The most vulnerable populations are patients and their families, who in a time of great distress may be downloading an enormous amount of information from cancer-related Web sites.[87] Examples of organizations that provide guidelines, rating criteria, or accreditation for evaluating health-related Web sites are listed in Table 76-4. These criteria can be applied when evaluating the quality of online cancer information.

Conclusion

The delivery of cancer care will continue to be affected by developments in the field of healthcare informatics and rapid changes in IT.[88,89] Computer-processing

LIBRARY, UNIVERSITY OF CHESTER

power doubles in performance and halves in cost about every two years. We can expect to see communication network speeds increase tenfold within the next five to ten years, while robust compact portable systems replace the simple hand-held computers and wireless communications.[90] Automated clinical systems will achieve their greatest value when CPRs, decision support tools, and other clinical applications are integrated seamlessly across systems and sites.[91] Standardization of vocabulary will greatly facilitate the effort to measure outcomes and treatment efficacy. Nursing innovations testing the effects of the electronic delivery of nursing interventions will flourish and improve the delivery and cost of health care.

Finally, healthcare consumerism will continue to shift competition in the industry. Sophisticated informatics tools are already being used by motivated persons with cancer to maintain their own records and observations.[92] We do not know when the next innovation will transform our world as rapidly as the Internet has. For the present, we can develop our own informatics competencies, ensure that consumers and persons with cancer get connected to the right set of electronic information, and be involved in developing and testing nursing innovations.

Glossary

Browser A software program that accesses the Web and reads hypertext.

Classification A systematic arrangement of classes; a structural framework arranged according to similar groups.

Computer-based Patient Record (CPR) A repository of electronically maintained information about an individual's lifetime health status and health care, stored such that it can serve the multiple legitimate users of the record.

CPR Systems The hardware and software used to create, maintain, edit, display, and manipulate all the data stored in an individual's CPR. These systems provide availability to complete and accurate patient data, clinical reminders and alerts, decision support, and links to bodies of related data and knowledge bases.

Data Element The smallest unit of data that has meaning without interpretation; a raw fact, material, or observation.

Data Repository A database acting as an information storage facility.

Data Set A collection of related data items, a directory.

Database A collection of interrelated files with records organized and stored together in a computer system.

Decision Support System Any computer program designed to help health care professionals and/or patients, as users of the system, make clinical decisions.

E-mail A form of communication, usually a text message sent from one person to another over a computer network. E-mail also may contain enclosed files and graphics.

Electronic Health Record (EHR) (see Computer-based Patient Record)

Encryption Coding attached to data with the intent to keep the information secure from anyone but the addressee.

Firewall A security device situated between a private network and outside networks.

Hypertext A document containing words or phrases, usually highlighted in a different color, that are electronically linked to text elsewhere.

Hypertext Markup Language (HTML) The basic programming language for sites on the Web.

Informatics The science that studies the use and processing of data, information, and knowledge.

Information Technology (IT) Refers to systems (e.g., computers, software packages, decision support systems) used to manage and process information.

Internet A worldwide distributed network of computers.

Internet Relay Channel (IRC) A program that allows you to carry on "live" conversations with people all over the world by typing messages back and forth across the Internet.

Internet Service Provider (ISP) A service or company that allows access to a larger computer that is connected continuously to the Internet.

Language In computing and communications, a set of characters (symbols, alphabets, codes and syntax), conventions, and rules used to convey ideas and information.

Mailing List Commonly known as a "listserv," a communication medium based on e-mail. It allows for a sender's single message to be distributed automatically to all subscribers to a list.

Newsgroup Electronic discussion groups, similar to traditional bulletin boards.

Nursing Informatics The specialty that integrates nursing science, computer science, and information science in identifying, collecting, processing, and managing data and information to support nursing practice, administration, education, research, and the expansion of nursing knowledge.

Search Engine A database of Web sites, available to all users on the Web, that can be searched using keywords.

Taxonomy A method of classifying a vocabulary of terms for a specific topic.

Telecommunications The electronic transmission of voice signals and other data over telephone-based carrier lines.

Telehealth A broad term describing the combined efforts of information technology, health communication, and health education to improve the efficiency and quality of health care.

Telemedicine As a segment of telehealth, telemedicine uses telecommunications technology to send data, graphics, audio, and video images between participants who are physically separated (i.e., at a distance from one another) for the purpose of clinical care.

Universal Resource Locator (URL) An address that specifies the location of a file on the Internet.

Usability The measure of the quality of a user's experience when interacting with a product or system—whether a Web site, a software application, mobile technology, or any user-operated device.

Vocabulary (Nomenclature) A consistent method for assigning names to elements of a system.

Web Page A computer file written in HTML.

Web Site A group of related Web pages. Accessed by typing its unique address, a site usually includes layers of supporting pages as well as a home page.

World Wide Web (WWW or Web) The component of the Internet that integrates text, graphics, audio, and video.

References

1. Collen MF: The origins of informatics. *MD Comput* 16:104, 1999
2. Saba VK, McCormick KA: *Essentials of Computers for Nurses: Informatics for the New Millenium* (ed 3). New York, McGraw-Hill, 2000
3. Graves JR, Corcoran S: The study of nursing informatics. *Image J Nurs Sch* 21:227–231, 1989
4. Hannah KJ, Ball MJ, Edwards M: *Introduction to Nursing Informatics* (ed 2). New York, Springer-Verlag, 1999
5. Delaney C: Health informatics and oncology nursing. *Semin Oncol Nurs* 17:2–6, 2001
6. Gassert CA: The challenge of meeting patients' needs with a national nursing informatics agenda. *J Am Med Inform Assoc* 5:263–268, 1998
7. National Advisory Council on Nurse Education and Practice: Report to the Secretary of the Department of Health and Human Services: a national informatics agenda for nursing education and practice, December 1997. *bhpr.hrsa.gov/nursing/nacnep/informatics.htm.* Accessed December 22, 2004
8. American Nurses Association: *Scope and Standards of Nursing Informatics Practice.* Washington, DC, American Nurses Publishing, 2001
9. Staggers N, Thompson CB: The evolution of definitions for nursing informatics: a critical analysis and revised definition. *J Am Med Inform Assoc* 9:255–261, 2002
10. Schwirian PM: The NI pyramid: a model for research in nursing informatics. *Comput Nurs* 4:134–136, 1986
11. National Institute of Nursing Research: Nursing informatics: enhancing patient care. *www.nih.gov/ninr/vol4/Execsum.html.* Accessed December 22, 2004
12. Ozbolt J, Graves J: Clinical nursing informatics: developing tools for knowledge workers. *Nurs Clin North Am* 28:407–425, 1993
13. Brennan PF, Zielstroff R, Ozbolt JG, et al: Setting a national research agenda in nursing informatics, in Cesnik B, McCray A, Scherrer J (eds.): *MedInfo'98, Seoul, Korea.* Burke, VA, IOS Press, 1998, pp 1188–1191
14. Ehrenberger H, Murray P: An overview of the issues in the use of communication technologies in nursing research. *Oncol Nurs Forum* 25(suppl 2):11–15, 1998
15. Ehrenberger HE, Brennan, PF: Nursing informatics as a support function for oncology nursing research. *Oncol Nurs Forum* 25(suppl 2):21–26, 1998
16. National Institute of Nursing Research: Telehealth interventions to improve clinical nursing care. *grants.nih.gov/grants/guide/pa-files/PA-00-138.html.* Accessed December 22, 2004
17. Jones JF, Brennan PF: Telehealth interventions to improve clinical nursing of elders. *Annu Rev Nurs Res* 20:293–322, 2002
18. Elfrink V, Bakken S, Coenen A, et al: Standardized nursing vocabularies: a foundation for quality care. *Semin Oncol Nurs* 17:18–23, 2001
19. Ozbolt J: Testimony to the NCVHS Hearings on Medical Terminology and Code Development, 1999. *www.mc.vanderbilt.edu/nursing/informatics/pdf/NCVHS10_99.pdf.* Accessed December 22, 2004
20. Werley HH, Lang NM (eds.): *Identification of the Nursing Minimum Data Set.* New York, Springer, 1988
21. American Nurses Association: *An Emerging Framework: Data System Advances for Clinical Nursing Practice.* Washington, DC, American Nurses Publishing, 1995
22. Henry SB, Warren JJ, Lange L, et al: A review of major nursing vocabularies and the extent to which they have the characteristics required for implementation in computer-based systems. *J Am Med Inform Assoc* 5:321–328, 1998
23. Payne J: The nursing interventions classification: a language to define nursing. *Oncol Nurs Forum* 27:99–103, 2000
24. American Nurses Association: NIDSEC Web site. *www.nursingworld.org/nidsec.* Accessed December 22, 2004
25. SNOMED International: SNOMED Web site. *www.snowmed.org.* Accessed December 22, 2004

26. Button P, Androwich I, Hibben L, et al: Challenges and issues related to implementation of nursing vocabularies in computer-based systems. *J Am Med Inform Assoc* 5:332–334, 1998
27. Dick RS, Steen EB (eds.): *The Computer-Based Patient Record: An Essential Technology for Health Care* (ed 1). Washington, DC, National Academy Press, 1991
28. Marietti C: Will the real CPR/EMR/EHR please stand up? *Healthcare Inform* 15:77–81, 1998
29. Dick RS, Steen EB, Detmer DE (eds.): *The Computer-Based Patient Record: An Essential Technology for Health Care* (ed 2). Washington, DC, National Academy Press, 1997
30. Institute of Medicine: *Crossing the Quality Chasm: A New Health System for the 21st Century.* Washington, DC, National Academies Press, 2001
31. Institute of Medicine: *Key Capabilities of an Electronic Health Record System: Letter Report.* Washington, DC, National Academies Press, 2003
32. Health Level Seven: Web site. *www.hl7.org.* Accessed December 22, 2004
33. Hendrickson G, Kelly JB, Citrin L: Computers in oncology nursing: present use and future potential. *Oncol Nurs Forum* 18:715–723, 1991
34. Chamorro T: Computer-based patient record systems. *Semin Oncol Nurs* 17:24–33, 2001
35. IMPAC Medical Systems: Web site. *www.impac.com.* Accessed December 22, 2004
36. McCormick KA: Including oncology outcomes of care in the computer-based patient record. *Oncology* 9(suppl):161–167, 1995
37. Balas EA, Austin SM, Mitchell JA, et al: The clinical value of computerized information services. *Arch Fam Med* 5:271–278, 1996
38. Hunt DL, Haynes RB, Hanna SE, et al: Effects of computer-based clinical decision support systems on physician performance and patient outcomes: a systematic review. *JAMA* 280:1339–1346, 1998
39. Musen M, Shahar Y, Shortliffe E: Clinical decision-support systems, in Shortliffe E, Perreault L (eds.): *Medical Informatics: Computer Applications in Health Care.* New York, Springer-Verlag, 2000, pp 573–609
40. Chang BL, Roth K, Gonzales E, et al: CANDI: a knowledge-based system for nursing diagnosis. *Comput Nurs* 6:13–21, 1988
41. Larson DE: Development of a microcomputer-based expert system to provide support for nurses caring for AIDS patients, in Daly N, Hannah KJ (eds.): *Proceedings of Nursing and Computers: The Third International Symposium on Nursing Use of Computers and Information Science.* St. Louis, Mosby, 1988, pp 682–690.
42. Evans S: *The PACE System: An Expert Consulting System for Nursing.* New York, Springer-Verlag, 1997
43. Ozbolt J, Vandewal D, Hannah K (eds.): *Decision Support Systems in Nursing.* St. Louis, Mosby, 1990
44. Hersey JC, Matheson J, Lohr KN: *Consumer Health Informatics and Patient Decision-Making* (AHCPR Publication No. 98-N001). Springfield, VA, National Technical Information Service, 1997
45. Enterline JP, Lenhard RE, Blum BI: *A Clinical Information System for Oncology.* New York, Springer-Verlag, 1989
46. Hickham DH, Shortliffe EH, Bishoff MB, et al: The treatment advice of a computer-based chemotherapy protocol advisor. *Ann Intern Med* 103:928–936, 1985
47. Kent DL, Shortliffe EH, Carlson RW, et al: Improvements in data collection through physician use of a computer-based chemotherapy treatment consultant. *J Clin Oncol* 3:409–417, 1985
48. Breitfeld PP, Weisburd M, Overhage JM, et al: Pilot study of a point-of-use decision support tool for cancer clinical trials eligibility. *J Am Med Inform Assoc* 6:466–477, 1999
49. Williams RB, Boles M, Johnson RE: A patient-initiated system for preventive health care: A randomized trial in community-based primary care practices. *Arch Fam Med* 7:338–345, 1998
50. Comprehensive Health Enhancement Support System: Web site. *http://chess.chsra.wisc.edu/Chess.* Accessed December 22, 2004
51. Coiera E: *Guide to Medical Informatics, the Internet and Telemedicine.* London, Chapman & Hall Medical, 1997
52. Brecht RM, Barrett JE: Telemedicine in the United States, in Viegas S, Dunn K (eds.): *Telemedicine: Practicing in the Information Age.* Philadelphia, Lippincott-Raven, 1998, pp 25–30
53. American Nurses Association: *Core Principles on Telehealth.* Washington, DC, American Nurses Publishing, 1999
54. American Nurses Association: *Competencies for Telehealth Technologies in Nursing.* Washington, DC, American Nurses Publishing, 1999
55. Johnston BL, Wheeler L, Deuser J, et al: Outcomes of the Kaiser Permanente tele-home health research project. *Arch Fam Med* 9:40–45, 2000
56. Bynum AB, Irwin CA, Cranford CO, et al: The impact of telemedicine on patients' cost savings: some preliminary findings. *Telemed J E-Health* 9:361–367, 2003
57. Warner I: Introduction to telehealth home care. *Home Healthc Nurse* 14:791–796, 1996
58. Wootton R, Loane M, Mair F, et al: A joint US–UK study of home telenursing. *J Telemed Telecare* 4(suppl 1):83–85, 1998
59. Guttman-McCabe C: Telemedicine's imperilled future? Funding, reimbursement, licensing and privacy hurdles face a developing technology. *J Contemp Health Law Policy* 14:161–186, 1997
60. London JW, Morton DE, Marinucci D, et al: The implementation of telemedicine within a community cancer network. *J Am Med Inform Assoc* 4:18–24, 1997
61. Allen A, March A: Telemedicine at the community cancer center. *Oncol Issues* 17:18–24, 2002
62. Allen A, Hayes J, Sadasivan R, et al: A pilot study of the physician acceptance of tele-oncology. *J Telemed Telecare* 1:34–37, 1995
63. Doolittle GC, Harmon A, Williams A, et al: A cost analysis of a tele-oncology practice. *J Telemed Telecare* 3(suppl 1):20–22, 1997
64. Stitt JA: A system of tele-oncology at the University of Wisconsin Hospital and clinics and regional oncology affiliate institutions. *WMJ* 97:38–42, 1998
65. Doolittle GC, Yaezel A, Otto F, et al: Hospice care using home-based telemedicine systems. *J Telemed Telecare* 4(suppl 1):58–59, 1998
66. Schlachta-Fairchild L: Telehealth: a new venue for health care delivery. *Semin Oncol Nurs* 17:34–40, 2001
67. National Research Council: *For the Record: Protecting Electronic Health Information.* Washington, DC, National Academy Press, 1997
68. Barrows RC, Clayton PD: Privacy, confidentiality, and electronic medical records. *J Am Med Inform Assoc* 3:139–148, 1996
69. U.S. Department of Health and Human Services, Office for Civil Rights: HIPAA Web site. *www.hhs.gov/ocr/hipaa.* Accessed December 22, 2004
70. Epstein MA, Pasieka MS, Lord WP, et al: Security for the digital information age of medicine: issues, applications, and implementation. *J Digit Imaging* 11:33–44, 1998
71. Health Privacy Project: Web site. *www.healthprivacy.org.* Accessed December 22, 2004
72. Jacobs L: At-risk for cancer: genetic discrimination in the workplace. *Oncol Nurs Forum* 25:475–480, 1998
73. Lapham EV, Kozma C, Weiss JO: Genetic discrimination: perspectives of consumers. *Science* 274:621–624, 1996
74. Hodge JG Jr: Ethical issues concerning genetic testing and screening in public health. *Am J Med Genet* 15:66–70, 2004

75. Travis L, Brennan PF: Information science for the future: an innovative nursing informatics curriculum. *J Nurs Educ* 37: 162-168, 1998
76. Kane B, Sands D: White paper: guidelines for the clinical use of electronic mail with patients. *J Am Med Inform Assoc* 5:104–111, 1998
77. Liederman EM, Morefield CS: Web messaging: a new tool for patient-physician communication. *J Am Med Inform Assoc* 10:260–270, 2003
78. Association of Cancer Online Resources: Web site. *www.acor.org*. Accessed December 22, 2004
79. Search Engine Watch: Web site. *www.searchenginewatch.com*. Accessed December 22, 2004
80. Graves JR: Electronic access to scientific nursing knowledge: The Virginia Henderson international nursing library. *Semin Oncol Nurs* 17:62–68, 2001
81. National Center for Biotechnology Information: Entrez life sciences search engine. *www.ncbi.nlm.nih.gov/gquery*. Accessed December 22, 2004
82. National Center for Biotechnology Information: literature databases. *www.ncbi.nlm.nih.gov/literature*. Accessed December 22, 2004
83. Lindberg DA, Humphreys BL: A time of change for medical informatics in the USA, in van Bemmel JH, McCray AT (eds.): *Yearbook of Medical Informatics*. Stuttgart, Germany, Schattauer, 1999, pp 53–57
84. National Cancer Institute: Physician Data Query database. *www.cancer.gov*. Accessed December 22, 2004
85. Gagliardi A, Jadad AR: Examination of instruments used to rate quality of health information on the Internet: chronicle of a voyage with an unclear destination. *BMJ* 324:569–573, 2002
86. Schloman B: Quality of health information on the Web: where are we now? *Online J Issues Nurs*, 2002. *nursingworld.org/ojin/infocol/info_10.htm*. Accessed December 22, 2004
87. Gomez EG: How to find and evaluate Internet information. *Clin J Oncol Nurs* 7(suppl 1):14–23, 2003
88. Eysenbach G: The impact of the Internet on cancer outcomes. *CA Cancer J Clin* 53: 356–371, 2003
89. Covitz PA, Hartel F, Schaefer C, et al: caCORE: a common infrastructure for cancer informatics. *Bioinformatics* 19:2404–2412, 2003
90. Rindfleisch TC: (Bio)Medical informatics in the next decade. *J Am Med Inform Assoc* 5:416–420, 1998
91. Westberg EE, Miller RA: The basis for using the Internet to support the information needs of primary care. *J Am Med Inform Assoc* 6:6–25, 1999
92. Houston TK, Ehrenberger HE: The potential of consumer health informatics. *Semin Oncol Nurs* 17:41–47, 2001

CHAPTER 77

Oncology Nursing and Professional Advocacy

Pamela J. Haylock, RN, MA

Introduction

The 1999 report issued by the Institute of Medicine (IOM), *Ensuring Quality Cancer Care,* acknowledged that most of cancer care entails the management of physical and emotional sequelae of the disease.[1] Thus, it is important to note that most of cancer care, as defined by the IOM, is *not* the diagnosing and prescription of treatment, which lie in the domain of medicine, but instead falls squarely within the scope of oncology nursing practice.[2] Oncology nurses hold the key to enhancing the effectiveness and efficiency of cancer care.

In the United States, cancer-related research and care delivery exist within the political and environmental context of the nation and are therefore susceptible to the twists and turns of American and global economies and politics and the unique American healthcare system. Health care in America is a business based on market-driven forces. The values of for-profit healthcare are rooted in self-interest, not on a sense of corporate social responsibility.[3] Free-market vendors are under no obligation to determine and provide what is truly needed.[3] Nevertheless, influential forces within free-market enterprises often can and do advocate for what is truly needed, and this, ultimately, is what professional nursing can bring to the table.

American-style health care is increasingly recognized as a "broken health care nonsystem in which nursing is seldom practiced as the nurses who are there would prefer to practice."[4] For many if not most nurses, the status quo is unacceptable, and thousands of nurses contribute efforts to enhancing the effectiveness and efficiency of healthcare services, focusing on the needs of individual patients, groups, and communities.[3–5] There is also growing evidence that consumers of healthcare services want healthcare delivery that is holistic and directed toward wellness.[6–8] An exploration of what American citizens need, fear, want, and will accept with regard to health and health care affords the profession opportunities to envision and create its new future[9] that is also in the best interest of those served by nursing.

Professional Advocacy and Oncology Nursing

Nursing has been dominated by medicine since Nightingale's time and has historically conceded to the medical model that does not (yet) embrace a holistic approach to health care or support the maximum application of nursing knowledge, wisdom, and skills. The majority of today's practicing nurses have been socialized in nursing education programs modeled on the principle of health as a basic human right promoted by Hildegard Peplau.[10] The philosophical foundation of American nursing, *The Code of Ethics for Nurses,* is based on nursing's tradition of concern for the welfare of the sick, injured, and vulnerable, and for social justice.[11] This tradition is philosophically and practically at odds with the for-profit model of healthcare delivery used in the United States. This incongruity characterizes the situation in which most American nurses find themselves today.

The role of "patient advocate" is generally seen as a foundational construct of contemporary professional nursing. *The Code of Ethics for Nurses* alludes to nurses' responsibilities as patient advocate[11] but fails to clearly define the term, delineate roles and preparation, or clarify expectations of nurses as patient advocates. One of the first nursing leaders to use the term "patient advocate" was nurse-historian Theresa Christy, writing in 1973:

> Nurses should and can become patients' advocates in the truest sense, the intermediaries for the befuddled civilian who is thrust into the maze of an alien world . . . the American health care system.[12]

If civilians were befuddled in 1973's American healthcare system, what must they be experiencing today? Is it not ironic that U.S. society, based on constitutionally defined notions of justice and equal opportunity, should support a healthcare system in which so many citizens are left vulnerable?

It has been suggested that every nurse, by virtue of his or her decision to enter the nursing profession, is obligated to assume an advocacy role.[13] Grace asserts that healthcare professions such as nursing exist to serve society and are morally obligated to address health-related shortcomings.[13] Grace clarifies that these shortcomings are related to individual patients and future patients, groups of people, communities, and society as a whole. Changes in social and health policy are often required to fully address the needs of future patients, and thus Grace offers the term "professional advocacy" to more fully encompass the professions' obligations to society, suggesting that the term "patient advocate" is more relevant to a scenario in which one nurse addresses the needs of one patient.[13]

The Oncology Nursing Society (ONS), in its *Statement on the Scope of Oncology Nursing Practice,* also directs nurses to be advocates, confirming that "acting as patient advocate through assisting with information seeking, assurance of informed consent, and promotion of maximal patient independence" is central to the defined scope of oncology nursing practice.[2] The *ONS Position on Quality Cancer Care* directs nurses to address social and policy-related barriers to the provision of quality cancer care, defined as "services that are effective, comprehensive and safe."[14]

Every nurse has ideas or opinions about politics and policy that affect health in his or her community or work setting — whether it is a local city council decision to ban smoking in public spaces, a facility's obligation to support a cancer screening program for low-income citizens, a school board's decision to create (or eliminate) a school nurse position, or a decision by a healthcare facility's board of directors to address nurse–patient ratios. There are literally thousands of issues that arouse citizens' political passions. Yet we would render ourselves totally ineffective if we tried to address every shortcoming that affects how we, as nurses, perform our work. Wise mentors often tell us to "pick our battles," but how does one decide which battle to pick?

Professional nursing organizations, including international associations such as the International Council of Nurses and the International Society of Nurses in Cancer Care, provide guidance regarding health-related situations that the world's nurses could address, including tobacco control,[15] pain management,[16] and prevention and early detection of cervical cancer.[17] Nurses in the United States have at their disposal the guidance and resources of the ONS, the world's largest oncology membership association. Composed of more than 30,000 nurses and other healthcare professionals,[18] the ONS has a long history of direct involvement in government relations. Annually, the ONS board of directors establishes its Health Policy Agenda — a document identifying policy and programmatic issues that are of special importance to oncology care in general and to oncology nursing in particular. Other supporting documents, such as organizations' position statements, offer nurses background and direction with regard to policy-directed efforts.

Although there are many issues that affect cancer care, in crafting its Health Policy Agenda, the ONS board gives priority to issues that are likely to be considered in national political discourse.[19] Identifying priorities is important in minimizing "wheel spinning" and provides nurses the greatest potential to influence political debate to produce outcomes that are consistent with oncology nursing values and experience.

In recent years, the ONS Health Policy Agenda has highlighted three major areas of focus for its health policy efforts,[19] which generally guide the content for this chapter:

- Bolster and expand the nursing workforce to safeguard public health
- Advance cancer prevention and early detection
- Ensure access to quality care and reduce suffering for people with cancer

Oncology Nursing Workforce and Safeguarding Public Health

It has been known for some time that nurses' work satisfaction is linked to patient satisfaction and patient outcomes.[20] The nursing shortage experienced in America in the 1980s prompted a formal study led by nurse fellows of the American Academy of Nursing of hospitals that maintain an ability to attract and retain highly qualified nurses — designated "magnet" hospitals. The American Nurses Credentialing Center (ANCC) established the Magnet Nursing Services Recognition Program to acknowledge excellence in nursing services. In 2000, Aiken and colleagues compared the outcomes of the originally recognized magnet hospitals with those that are currently designated as ANCC-recognized magnet hospitals.[21] In both investigations, the magnet characteristics were consistent: Overall, magnet hospitals have better outcomes (i.e., lower mortality rates, higher levels of patient satisfaction, lower rates of nurse burnout, and lower rates of needle-stick injuries among nurses) than nonmagnet hospitals.

Work Satisfaction and Oncology Care Outcomes

Advances in technology and changes in financial incentives have been the catalysts for a dramatic shift in the paradigm of practice within the cancer care arena. Data indicate that 80% of encounters with cancer patients for the four most common cancers are concentrated in the community-based office setting,[22] but studies of factors relating to nurse satisfaction have primarily been carried out in acute, hospital-based environments. In addition, there is no empiric approach to the delivery of cancer care in these settings.[22] Work to determine whether hospital-based "magnet" traits are valid in ambulatory and physician office–based practice settings has yet to be reported. Recognition of the importance of work satisfaction to maintaining an adequate nursing workforce necessitates attention to the creation and sustenance of healthy, healing work cultures as an imperative for all nurses[9,23,24] and particularly for those working in emerging, nonhospital settings.

The Nursing Shortage and Oncology Care

The oncology sector is vulnerable to the nursing shortage affecting most of America.[25–27] An ONS-sponsored workforce survey demonstrated increased patient acuity, decreased lengths of hospital stay for all patients, increased paperwork, and a perception that too few RNs are practicing in the United States.[26,27] The ONS endorsed the Nurse Reinvestment Act, designed to address the nursing shortage, which was signed into law by President Bush in 2002.[28] This legislation creates scholarship programs for nursing students, public service announcements to highlight the advantages and rewards of nursing, nurse education, retention and practice grants, geriatric nurse training grants, and faculty loan repayment grants.[28] However, the legislation, which met with much rejoicing in the nursing community when it was signed by the president, remains underfunded. Organized nursing, in an initiative titled Americans for Nursing Shortage Relief (ANSR) composed of more than 30 professional associations, has mounted a collective response calling for $205 million to fund the Nursing Workforce Development Programs in the fiscal year 2005 federal budget.[29] Under the auspices of ANSR, nurses have testified in hearings and created a letter-writing campaign to encourage members of Congress to invest in the future health and well-being of our nation.[29] Funding beyond one fiscal year is obviously necessary if we are to strengthen the nation's nursing workforce.

The Nursing Workforce and Patient Safety

Patient well-being and safety are of concern to oncology nurses, and the IOM report *To Err Is Human: Building a Safer Health System*[30] focuses attention on systematic errors that can harm patients. The Agency for Healthcare Research and Quality (AHRQ) identifies four types of errors that occur in healthcare settings: (1) blood transfusion errors, (2) diagnostic errors including misdiagnosis or misinterpretation, (3) equipment failures, and (4) infections.[31] In oncology care, patient safety can be compromised by any and all of these types of errors. Most data on adverse events has been collected in acute care settings; few data exist on adverse events among outpatients in any setting,[32] and a review of the literature reveals little adverse-event data specific to cancer care. Yet the complex, multidrug chemotherapy protocols; the combination therapies and their wide variability of interactions and therapeutic outcomes; and the number of invasive procedures performed on oncology patients are just a few of the risks for adverse events that occur in oncology care settings. The risk of adverse drug events in the busy and high-volume setting that characterizes today's outpatient clinics and physician offices would seem particularly high, though a search of the literature fails to identify published data. McGee and Gould found, for example, that up to 26% of adult patients with central venous catheters experience mechanical, infectious, and/or thrombotic complications.[33] The "ONS Position on Prevention and Reporting of Medication Errors" advises oncology nurses to take an active role in preventing medication errors.[34]

"Failure to rescue" has been used to assess medical care and is more recently being used to describe "clinicians' inability to save a hospitalized patient's life when he experiences a complication not present on admission."[35] Failure to rescue is applicable to oncology care — not just in acute care but in the vast variety of oncology care settings, including outpatient clinics, physician offices, and even the home-care environment. Untoward drug reactions, the rapid progression from fever to sepsis, and hemodynamic shifts are examples of the critical importance of astute surveillance and quick action[35] on the part of oncology nurses.

Nurses who provide cancer care are obligated to advocate for policies — both public health policies and institutional policies — that enhance patient safety. Nurses must understand the nature of errors in delivery systems in general and in nursing systems in particular, and must be able to analyze critical incident reports.[36] Fostering a culture of safety is also an important element of professional advocacy, requiring the ability to assess organizational factors and to apply critical thinking to problem solving and risk management programs.[37] Mrayyan and Huber note that three aspects of patient safety are relevant to public policy: public fear, system problems, and the association of errors with staffing cutbacks.[37] According to the model for political influence proposed by Maynard, nurses need to be informed about current healthcare policies; must have the commitment, responsibility, and initiative to act; and must be involved in setting and accomplishing a healthcare agenda based on nurses' primary concerns for patients and their safety.[38]

Cancer Prevention and Early Detection

Nurses have the potential to promote health and reduce risks of cancer and other acute and chronic illnesses. Despite their importance, and the ONS's designation as a major component of quality cancer care,[14] prevention and early detection activities seem to be of only minor interest to the vast majority of members. Sessions presented during ONS's annual meetings that deal with prevention and early detection activities continue to have limited attendance when compared to sessions that deal with emerging treatment modalities and interventions employing high technology.[39] A perusal of the annual index issues of leading oncology nursing journals (*Oncology Nursing Forum, Clinical Journal of Oncology Nursing, Cancer Nursing,* and *Seminars in Oncology Nursing*) reveals a telling paucity of attention paid to prevention and early detection by oncology nurse authors and, presumably, oncology nurse readers.

Oncology nurses, however, are not unique in their inattention to prevention and early detection issues, and in fact, their focus on therapeutic interventions is clearly in line with the nation's overall cancer research priorities. A report in *Fortune* magazine found that Americans have spent nearly $200 billion (in inflation-adjusted dollars) in taxes, charitable donations, and private research and development on the so-called war on cancer since it was declared by President Nixon in 1971.[40] The vast majority of these research efforts are directed to discovering new compounds that add only months to the lives of people with cancer. Yet relatively simple and far less costly gains in cure rates and longevity come from behavioral changes (such as smoking prevention and cessation efforts) and early detection measures such as screening for prostate, colon, and cervical cancer and mammography. The conclusion of many researchers, physicians, epidemiologists, biostaticians, and government officials is that the nation's research incentives promoting a research agenda focused on "tiny improvements" in treatment rather than genuine breakthrough, are "out of whack."[40] Michael Sporn, professor of pharmacology and medicine at Dartmouth Medical School, points out the need to intervene early in the carcinogenic process, asserting that "we have to break away from the notion that people in early stages of carcinogenesis are healthy and shouldn't be treated."[40] On the contrary, Sporn says, "People are not healthy if they are on a path toward cancer."[40] Finally, Sporn advises, "All these people who are obsessed with cures, cures, cures, and the miraculous cure which is still eluding us, they're being . . . selfish by ignoring what could be done in terms of prevention."[40] To win the war on cancer, many researchers advocate a coordinated assault in which we "work as an army, not as individuals fighting on their own."[40]

Nurse-Led Cancer Control Programs

Nurses, using a model that is more holistic than the traditional medical model, recognize the complex mix of environmental, social, familial, genetic, economic, and behavioral factors that foster or undermine health behaviors to create human responses to illness. Nurses are increasingly likely to know and employ community assessment skills as they plan and coordinate programs for a variety of populations.[41] Consequently, examples abound in which nurses create, lead, or participate in innovative, imaginative programs to assist individual patients and communities in addressing barriers to quality cancer care.

Tobacco control

Global and local efforts to control the use of tobacco have benefited from nurses' individual and collective efforts.[42] Tobacco is responsible for at least 4 million unnecessary deaths each year, and its impact is a recognized global public health crisis.[43] The International Society of Nurses in Cancer Care (ISNCC) position on tobacco[15] addresses prevention, cessation, and exposure to secondhand smoke, and endorses nurses' efforts in crafting and supporting tobacco control legislation. Further, the ISNCC position supports the concept of nurses as nonsmoking role models.[15] A handful of nurses plan, develop, and deliver tobacco control programs, but given the magnitude of the tobacco epidemic, there is much more that can and must be done.

Lung cancer, an almost entirely preventable cancer, is the leading cause of cancer mortality among American men and women. The "ONS Position on Global and Domestic Tobacco Use and Proposals for Tobacco Control Policies"[44] endorses the World Health Organization's Framework Convention on Tobacco Control (FCTC), a measure committing world governments to action on tobacco. This ONS position challenges nurses to address other elements of tobacco control, including marketing restrictions, regulation and taxation of tobacco products, prevention of exposure to secondhand smoke, and insurance coverage for cessation services.[44]

Ruth Malone, PhD, RN, and associate professor at the University of California, San Francisco School of Nursing, is the organizer of a nurses' advocacy group called the Nightingales (Nurses in Groups Highlighting Tobacco Industry Nastiness, Greed and Lies [to] End Suffering), dedicated to using "the voice of nursing to contribute to the delegitimazation of the tobacco industry" and challenging the idea that the tobacco industry's "business as usual can go on indefinitely." (Malone, personal communication, May 12, 2004). The Nightingales are not aligned with any nursing organization but nevertheless "do what they can." In 2004, a dozen nurses donned white lab coats with black armbands to attend the annual shareholders' meeting of Philip Morris–Altria Group, Inc., in East Hanover, New Jersey, calling on the company to "show genuine corporate social responsibility by voluntarily ending active promotion of cigarettes."[45] The

Nightingales intend to pursue a variety of tobacco control advocacy efforts, including ongoing annual attendance at tobacco companies' corporate board meetings, and they welcome American nurses' involvement.

Rural dwellers and cancer

Rural dwellers face unique challenges when dealing with potential and actual cancer diagnoses. There are several models of rural cancer care delivery,[46] but the variations in defining ''rurality'' contribute to the difficulties in adapting models developed in one setting for use in another.[47] Nevertheless, nurses living and working in rural communities have the potential to make significant contributions to cancer control efforts in otherwise underserved settings. For example, rural women are at higher risk of dying from breast cancer. A group of nurses in rural southeastern Indiana created a community-based project focusing on breast health, based on the Logic Model, that addresses issues of access in an acknowledged underserved population.[48] Outcomes appeared to influence women in the community, nurses in community-health roles, and the organization in which nurses are employed.[48]

Nurses living in vastly different settings have collaborated to explore the nursing implications of Native American traditional medicine in 21st century rural nursing.[49] Their work, highlighting the insight into the complexities of providing health care in a volatile, changing environment yet honoring tradition and culture, could apply in nearly all cancer settings, but offers particular inspiration to those working in rural settings.[49]

Cancer prevention and the elderly

Older men and women are often among the underserved populations, a phenomenon that is complex but seems to be linked to the elders' perception of declining health status and erroneous explanations for symptoms.[50] Nurses are involved in programmatic approaches to prevention and early detection among the elderly, addressing physical activity, diet, tobacco and alcohol use, and promotion of cancer-related screening.[50–52]

Access to Quality Cancer Care

People with cancer, their family members, and caregivers (professional and lay) face emotional, financial, spiritual, psychosocial, racial, ethnic, and gender-related needs that quite often go unmet or unaddressed.[1,7] The President's Cancer Panel reported in 2002 that there is a ''critical disconnect between our cancer research discoveries and the type, timeliness and continuity of cancer care that people actually receive.''[53]

Socioeconomic Status and Cancer

Despite enormous investments and expenditures for research, services, and products relating to preventing and managing cancer, socioeconomic forces create barriers that limit or deny services to many American citizens.[53,54] Socioeconomic status is specifically related to the incidence of cancer and the outcomes of cancer management.[53] Low socioeconomic status is associated with a higher incidence of cancer, later stage (and therefore less curable) at diagnosis, higher morbidity from cancer and its treatment, and higher mortality rates.[55,56] Women of racial and ethnic minorities and low-income groups have higher mortality rates from breast and cervical cancer, and the same can be said of men who are affected by prostate cancer.[57] Access issues highlight racial, ethnic, and socioeconomic issues: Black and Hispanic patients in nonwhite neighborhoods are often unable to get prescribed opioids from neighborhood pharmacies.[58] Racial differences exist regarding treatment recommendations, patient comprehension of recommendations, trust in providers, and outcomes.[59,60] Disparities in access to services, health, and outcomes also exist for older people diagnosed with cancer[61] and individuals living in rural settings.[62] In fact, there is growing evidence of inferior health care for African-Americans when compared to their white counterparts, even when the two groups are socioeconomically similar — differences in access to treatment and quality of care offered — that many experts believe to be at least partially responsible for variations in morbidity and mortality outcomes.[63]

Insurance Status and Cancer

Health insurance status, access to services, and cancer outcomes are clearly linked. Cancer patients without insurance are at risk for receiving inadequate cancer care. An analysis derived from the Medical Expenditure Panel Survey for 1996–1999 revealed that spending for cancer patients without insurance was 57% of the amount spent for privately insured patients.[64] Ten percent of cancer patients under 65 and 20% of Hispanic cancer patients under 65 are uninsured.[64]

The Medicare Program and Cancer Care

Nearly 60% of new cancer diagnoses and 50% of all cancer-related deaths occur in the 65 and older population,[65] making Medicare the single largest payer for cancer care in the United States. In 2003, Medicare paid for about 450 drugs that are administered on an outpatient basis, but just 35 of those drugs, mostly cancer cytotoxic agents, accounted for the bulk of Medicare's expenditures.[66] Physicians, including hematologists and oncologists, purchase most of these drugs, deliver them to patients in clinics and offices, and are reimbursed by Medicare. The oncology community—including cancer care professionals and national and grassroots advocacy groups—is concerned about the increase in pharmaceutical costs and the uncertainties of Medicare drug benefits enacted in 2003 and 2004.

The Medicare Prescription Drug Discount Card and Transitional Assistance Program is part of the Medicare Prescription Drug, Improvement, and Modernization Act of 2003. This voluntary drug discount program was devised to give immediate relief to Medicare beneficiaries, reducing prescription drug costs, before a new Medicare drug benefit is implemented on January 1, 2006. Prior to this legislation, Medicare beneficiaries without outpatient drug coverage paid as much as 20% more than people with prescription drug coverage for prescribed medications. Proponents contend that the program, which began in May 2004, offers Medicare beneficiaries (except for those who also have Medicaid drug coverage) the opportunity to enroll in Medicare-approved prescription drug discount card programs, thereby lowering prescription drug costs. Opponents are disappointed in the narrow scope of the changes and also contend that the Bush administration's $400 billion price tag is deceptively low.[67] Still, aspects of the bill important to consumers, patients, and caregivers include reimbursement for mammography and screening activities, funding for comparative drug effectiveness studies, improved payment schemes for rural health facilities, extended needle-stick protections, and increased payments to nurse practitioners and clinical nurse specialists.[68]

Although Medicare beneficiaries have sought prescription drug benefits for some time, the "devil in the details" of the new Medicare plan is a source of contention and confusion among healthcare providers and consumers and a source of heated debate among policy makers and advocacy groups.[69] Some 70 prescription drug discount cards have been approved by Medicare, offering a number of plans from a variety of companies and organizations, including drugstore chains and grocery stores.[69]

Payment for oral agents

Medicare covers more than 90% of cancer drugs, most of which are administered intravenously. It also has paid for oral agents that have an intravenous (IV) equivalent. However, many emerging therapies, believed to be less toxic and more effective, are available only for oral administration. By 2010, it is projected that oral agents will represent 25% of the market.[70] Yet Medicare has resisted paying for the newer targeted therapies. Advocates, including the ONS and National Coalition for Cancer Survivorship, encourage Medicare to update its payment schedule to include oral cytotoxic agents.[70,71]

Medicare, practice expense provisions, and oncology nursing

Whether the final expense of Medicare's prescription drug benefits is $400 billion or much more, as many believe will be the case, the costs will reduce spending in other areas. Cancer advocates believe that as much as $11 billion will be cut from cancer care over the first ten years of the prescription drug benefit, and they stress that cuts in Medicare spending should not come at the expense of quality care for cancer patients.[70]

Medicare is changing the calculation and payment on drugs and biologicals, which will directly affect practice expense reimbursements to oncologists. Debate over practice expenses, what they are, and how they are paid for has been a matter of great concern for at least the past decade. Medicare's oversight agency, the Center for Medicare/Medicaid Services (CMS), acknowledges overpayment for oncology drugs based on a payment system using the average wholesale price (AWP) of drugs. Community-based oncology practices generally purchase drug inventory at reduced prices through group purchasing agreements and are reimbursed by Medicare at a rate based on the AWP minus 5%, or 95% of the AWP. The difference between the amounts reimbursed and the actual cost of the drugs has been used to support practice expenses, including the costs associated with recruiting, hiring, educating, and maintaining skilled nurses and other practice staff such as dieticians, social workers, and psychologists. Practice expenses also include rent, utilities, equipment, supplies, and the salaries of technicians, administrative, and clerical staff. Funds not used for practice expense become practice revenue.[72]

Under the current Medicare system, outpatient oncology nursing services are classified and paid for as a practice expense. One factor contributing to Medicare's failure to recognize and reimburse for oncology nursing services in the outpatient setting is that the actual costs associated with skilled oncology nursing care remain obscure, and nursing care costs traditionally have been assumed by the setting's reimbursement for drugs and supplies. Activities performed by nurses in office-based settings and how they are classified for potential payment are important considerations that have yet to be explored and reported. The Physician's

Current Procedural Terminology (CPT) comprises more than 7000 codes designed to classify the reimbursement of services provided by physicians. The Nursing Interventions Classification (NIC) is a categorization of direct and indirect care activities performed by nurses.[73] However, when they compared NIC and CPT codes, Henry and colleagues found that CPT offered incomplete documentation of routine nursing activities,[74] another indicator that physician-specific language is not a particularly useful indicator of nursing activities.

The ONS advocates that Medicare reimbursement for oncology nursing practice expenses be based on current practice data, using bottom-up methodology detailing local, practice-level expenses.[75] Further, ONS suggests that CMS support work sampling studies and the incorporation of results into practice expense calculations, thereby ensuring that reimbursement is based on real costs and practice patterns.[75] The ONS recommendation is mindful of Medicare solvency issues as well as threats to patients' access to expert oncology specialty nurses. A number of organizations representing professional provider organizations, cancer-related nongovernmental organizations, and several grassroots survivor advocacy groups have indicated support for this perspective.[70,71,75,76]

Congress issued its interim final rule for "Manufacturer Submission of Manufacturer's Average Sales Price Data for Medicare Part B Drugs and Biologicals" in early 2004 with a comment period.[77] The cancer community, including professional associations and grassroots consumer advocacy groups such as the ONS, the American Society of Clinical Oncologists, and the National Coalition for Cancer Survivorship, has mounted a response, including a flurry of stories in the media highlighting fears of diminished access to services such as expert oncology nursing, social work, and other supportive care services.[78] Oncology nurses, through ONS-directed efforts, have contributed letters describing potential consequences and have been involved in providing testimony to policy makers. The actual outcome remains to be seen but will undoubtedly affect other payers that traditionally follow the lead set by the Medicare program. The complexities of the new Medicare provisions, Medicare's financial limitations, and the target offered by high-visibility oncology expenditures ensure that Medicare will continue to be in the political spotlight for some time.

Health Savings Accounts

Alternative means of assuring access to insurance and subsequent care include health savings accounts (HSAs). Changes signed into law in 2004 by President Bush offer a new version of the medical savings account (MSA) mechanism and include three major changes:[79,80]

- Lower deductibles
- 100% of the deductible amount can be contributed to the savings account
- Almost everyone will be eligible for an HSA

The HSA is a tax-sheltered savings account similar to the IRA but earmarked for medical expenses. Deposits are 100% tax-deductible for the self-employed (and now for almost everyone with an HSA) and can easily be withdrawn by check or debit card to pay routine medical bills with tax-free dollars. Larger medical expenses are covered by a low-cost, high-deductible health insurance policy. What is not used from the account each year stays in the account and continues to earn interest on a tax-favored basis to supplement retirement, just like an IRA.

When combined with the required low-cost, high-deductible health insurance policy, the health savings account is meant to replace a traditional high-cost health insurance policy, with low co-payments and restrictions on medical choices. Theoretically, the HSA plan restores a high degree of freedom of choice by allowing consumers to choose their physicians (typically from an extensive preferred provider directory) without the extensive restrictions imposed by HMO-type plans.[79,80]

Cancer Survivorship and Quality Cancer Care

Notable in its absence from the ONS Health Policy Agenda is a recognition of the unmet needs of long-term survivors of cancer. The term "cancer survivor" was coined and defined in the 1970s in this way: "From the time of discovery and for the balance of life, an individual diagnosed with cancer is a survivor."[81] More than 9 million Americans alive today are, using this definition, considered cancer survivors.[82] Although oncology nurses are among the first of the healthcare disciplines to recognize rehabilitation needs,[83] have recognized the need for long-term follow-up among survivors,[14] and claim the most intimate relationships with patients and survivors, organized oncology nursing has yet to exhibit a prominent focus on the needs of long-term survivors.

The millions of American survivors are, for the most part, alive today as the result of improvements in early detection, therapeutic advances, and, many nurses contend, the care offered by expert nurses.[84] People with cancer in active treatment generally have access to resources in acute care settings. Once treatment concludes, however, supportive services phase out or are nonexistent, yet it is increasingly clear that survivors have a unique set of needs.[85–88] Cancer care delivery systems, particularly for survivors of adult cancers, have not focused on long-term issues. As a result, little is known about the healthcare needs of survivors, and their needs often go unmet.[89] The cancer survivorship movement, initiated by survivors in the 1970s and given life by the NCCS, has become a political force to be reckoned with. The NCCS Cancer Survivors' Bill of Rights calls public attention to the needs of survivors,[86] and the NCCS Imperatives for Quality Cancer Care outline access, advocacy, action, and accountability in three specific domains: quality cancer care, physiologic long-term and late effects of cancer treatment, and psychosocial issues associated with cancer survivorship.[90]

A growing number of nurse-led programs are available to enhance coping among various survivor populations. I Can Cope™, one of the first programs to combine psychosocial support with information, was devised by Judith Bond Johnson and is now used throughout the world.[91] Nurses are involved in creating immersion retreats for survivor populations, including low-income groups, that address the emotional and psychosocial effects of cancer diagnoses.[92,93] Nurses and social work colleagues have been the dominant force in the development and success of support groups and other supportive care offerings.[94] It is becoming clear, however, that existing support mechanisms fall short of the mark for many survivors, and oncology nurses have the knowledge and skills to partner with individuals and groups of survivors to address these shortcomings in cancer care.

Conclusion

Oncology nursing workforce initiatives that promote a work environment that supports nurses' best work, including an emphasis on patient well-being and positive outcomes, are imperative to the future of oncology nursing practice. Efforts by oncology nurses to promote prevention and early detection, revolving around the realization of the significance of health behaviors and interruption of early carcinogenic processes, have been slow to evolve but are essential to nurses' commitment to health promotion. Access issues, starting with America's "nonuniversal" and market-driven healthcare system and mechanisms that pay for care, cannot be affected by unilateral nursing action. However, nurses, in collaboration with other healthcare disciplines, can continue to advocate for delivery systems that assure access to quality care services. In the absence of broad-based change in the American healthcare system, nurses' application of critical thinking and imaginative, innovative strategies to enhance community-based access will continue to be of utmost importance. Finally, oncology nurses must partner with cancer survivors, other healthcare disciplines, and policy makers to explore, understand, and create systematic approaches to the needs of cancer survivors throughout the phases of cancer survivorship.

Organized oncology nursing, including the Oncology Nursing Society and the International Society of Nurses in Cancer Care, is to be commended for advancing oncology nursing education, administration, practice, and research. Political and economic realities pose significant challenges to oncology nursing, and nurses must continue to be cognizant of issues affecting their ability to provide quality cancer care services. Oncology nurses continue to report "making a difference," "opportunities to accompany patients on the cancer journey," and "the ability to find purpose in nursing" as reasons to be an oncology nurse.[95] By advocating for environments that support the true scope of nursing practice, oncology nurses will continue to advance our professional specialty in ways that also fulfill the needs of people affected by cancer.[96] Nurse leader Virginia Henderson noted that Florence Nightingale and "subsequent nursing leaders conceived of professional nursing as a social service with revolutionary capabilities."[97] Efforts to convert oncology nursing's capabilities to realities will surely serve humanity well.

References

1. Hewitt M, Simone JV (eds.): *Ensuring Quality Cancer Care.* National Cancer Policy Board, Institute of Medicine. Washington, DC, National Academy Press, 1999
2. American Nurses Association and Oncology Nursing Society. *Statement on the Scope and Standards of Oncology Nursing Practice.* Washington, DC, American Nurses Publishing, 1996
3. Mohr WK, Mahon MM: Dirty hands: the underside of marketplace health care. *Adv Nurs Sci* 19:28–37, 1996
4. Chinn PL: From the editor. *Adv Nur Sci* 26:161, 2003
5. Schroeder C: The tyranny of profit: concentration of wealth, corporate globalization, and the failed US health care system. *Adv Nurs Sci* 26:173–184, 2003
6. Hall BA: An essay on an authentic meaning of medicalization: the patient's perspective. *Adv Nurs Sci* 26:53–62, 2003
7. Hoffman B (ed.): *A Cancer Survivor's Almanac: Charting Your Journey.* Hoboken, NJ, John Wiley, 2004
8. Spingarn ND: *The New Cancer Survivors.* Baltimore, Johns Hopkins Press, 1999
9. Porter-O'Grady T: Profound change: 21st century nursing. *Nurs Outlook* 49:182–186, 2001.
10. Peplau H: Is healthcare a right? [original 1974 article condensed for republication]. *Image: J Nurs Schol* 29:220–224, 1997

11. American Nurses Association: *Code of Ethics for Nurses with Interpretive Statements.* Washington, DC, American Nurses Association, 2001
12. Christy TE: New privileges . . . new challenges . . . new responsibilities. *Nursing* 3:8, 11, 1973
13. Grace PJ: Professional advocacy: widening the scope of accountability. *Nurs Philosophy* 2:151–162, 2001
14. Oncology Nursing Society: ONS position on quality cancer care. *www.ons.org.* Accessed April 24, 2004
15. International Council of Nurses: Tobacco use and health. *www.icn.ch/pssmoking99.htm.* Accessed February 19, 2004
16. International Society of Nurses in Cancer Care: Cancer pain position statement. *www.isncc.ch.* Accessed February 19, 2004
17. International Society of Nurses in Cancer Care: Position statement on cervical cancer screening. *www.isncc.ch.* Accessed February 19, 2004
18. Oncology Nursing Society: Memorandum to leadership: Membership demographics report, 1st quarter 2004. Pittsburgh, April 26, 2004
19. Oncology Nursing Society: Health Policy Agenda, 108th Congress, 2nd Session. *www.ons.org.* Accessed February 19, 2004
20. Weisman CS, Nathanson CA: Professional satisfaction and client outcomes. *Med Care* 23:1179–1192, 1985
21. Aiken LH, Havens DS, Sloane DM: The Magnet Nursing Services Recognition Program: a comparison of two groups of magnet hospitals. *Am J Nurs* 100:26–35, 2000
22. Herzlinger RE: Cancer care in America: description and implications of outpatient community-based care. 2000. *www.usoncology .com.* Accessed February 19, 2004
23. Scott JG, Sochalski, J, Aiken LH: Review of magnet hospital research: findings and implications for professional nursing practice. *J Nurs Admin* 29:9–19, 1999
24. Snyder-Halpern R, Corcoran-Perry S, Narayan S: Developing clinical practice environments supporting the knowledge work of nurses. *Computers Nurs* 19:17–23, 2001
25. Corbett S: The last shift. *New York Times Magazine.* March 16, 2003:58–61
26. Lamkin L, Rosiak J, Buerhaus P, et al: Oncology Nursing Society workforce survey (part II): perceptions of the nursing workforce environment and adequacy of nurse staffing in outpatient and inpatient oncology settings. *Oncol Nurs Forum* 29:93–100, 2001
27. Buerhaus P, Donelan, K, DesRoches C, et al: State of the oncology nursing workforce: problems and implications for strengthening the future. *Nurs Econ* 19:198–208, 2001
28. Oncology Nursing Society: Summary of the Nurse Reinvestment Act (Public Law 107-205). *www.ons.org.* Accessed May 30, 2004
29. Oncology Nursing Society: Americans for Nursing Shortage Relief letter, April 27, 2004. *www.ons.org.* Accessed May 30, 2004
30. Institute of Medicine: *To Err Is Human: Building a Safer Health System.* Washington, DC, Academy Press, 2000
31. U.S. Department of Health and Human Services: *Medical Errors: The Scope of the Problem.* AHRQ publication 00-P037. Rockville, MD, AHRQ Clearinghouse, August 2000.
32. Gandhi T, Weingart SN, Borus J, et al: Adverse drug events in ambulatory care. *N Engl J Med* 348:1556–1564, 2003
33. McGee DC, Gould MK: Preventing complications of central venous catheterization. *N Engl J Med* 348:1123–1133, 2003
34. Oncology Nursing Society. ONS position on prevention and reporting of medication errors. *www.ons.org.* Accessed April 14, 2004
35. Clarke SP, Aiken LH: Failure to rescue: needless deaths are prime examples of the need for more nurses at the bedside. *Am J Nurs* 103:42–47, 2003
36. Meurier CE: Understanding the nature of errors in nursing: using a model to analyze critical incident reports of errors which had resulted in an adverse or potentially adverse event. *J Adv Nur* 32:202–207, 2000
37. Mrayyan M, Huber DL: The nurse's role in changing health policy related to patient safety. *JONA's Healthcare Law, Ethics, Regul* 5:13–18, 2003
38. Maynard CA: Political influence: A model for advanced nursing education. *Clin Nurse Specialist* 13:191–195, 1999
39. Haylock PJ: Nurses against tobacco [viewpoint]. *Am J Nurs* 104:13, 2004
40. Leaf C: Why we're losing the war on cancer [and how to win it]. *Fortune* 149(6):76–97, 2004
41. Bosworth TW: *Community Health Needs Assessment.* Chicago, Irwin Professional Publishing, 1996
42. World Health Organization: Tobacco Free Initiative. *www.who.int/tobacco/en.* Accessed March 15, 2004
43. Sarna L, Bialous SA: Tobacco control policies of oncology nursing organizations. *Semin Oncol Nurs* 20:101–110, 2004
44. Oncology Nursing Society: ONS position on global and domestic tobacco use and proposals for tobacco control policies. *www.ons.org/Positions/Tobacco.pdf.* Accessed July 19, 2003
45. Nightingales, voices from across the country. *www.nightengalesnurses.org/voices.html.* Accessed January 15, 2005
46. Curtiss CP: Trends and issues for cancer care in rural communities. *Nurs Clin North Am* 28:241–251, 1993
47. Couto RA, Simpson NK, Harris G, et al: *Sowing Seeds in the Mountains: Community-Based Coalitions for Cancer Prevention and Control.* Bethesda, MD, NIH publication 94-3779, September 1994
48. Lane A, Martin M, Uhler J, et al: Enhancing breast health in rural populations: clinical nurse specialist as the key. *Clin Nurs Spec* 17:292–297, 2003
49. O'Brien BL, Anslow RM, Begay W: Century rural nursing: Navajo traditional and Western medicine. *Nurs Admin Q* 26:47–57, 2002
50. Yarbrough SS: Older women and breast cancer screening: research synthesis. *Oncol Nurs Forum, Online Exclusive. www. ons.org/xp6/ONS/Library.xml/ONS_Publications.xml/ONF.xml. 2004.* Accessed March 15, 2004
51. Dessner SH: Prevention and detection, in Luggen AS, Meiner SE (eds.): *Handbook for the Care of the Older Adult with Cancer.* Pittsburgh, Oncology Nursing Press, 2000
52. Fitch M, Greenberg M, Levstein L, et al: Health promotion and early detection of cancer in older adults: assessing knowledge about cancer. *Oncol Nurs Forum* 24:1743–1748, 1997
53. President's Cancer Panel: *Voices of a Broken System: Real People, Real Problems.* Bethesda, MD, National Cancer Institute, 2002
54. Freeman HP: Cancer in the socioeconomically disadvantaged. *CA Cancer J Clin* 39:266–288, 1989
55. Ward E, Jemal A, Cokkinides V, et al: Cancer disparities by race/ethnicity and socioeconomic status. *CA Cancer J Clin* 54:78–93, 2004
56. Freeman HP: Poverty, culture and social injustice: determinants of cancer disparities. *CA Cancer J Clin* 54:72–77, 2004
57. Jones LA: Speaking with one voice: solutions to the problem. *Cancer* 83 (suppl):1696–1700, 1998
58. Morrison RS, Wallenstein S, Natale DK, et al: "We don't carry that": failure of pharmacies in predominantly nonwhite neighborhoods to stock opioids analgesics. *N Engl J Med* 342:1023–1026, 2000

59. Bach PB, Cramer LD, Warren JL: Racial differences in the treatment of early-stage lung cancer. *New Engl J Med* 341:1198–1233, 1999
60. Phillips DA, Drevdahl D: "Race" and the difficulties of language. *Adv Nurs Sci* 26:17–29, 2003
61. Lee-Feldstein A, Feldstein PJ, Buchmueller T: Breast cancer outcomes among older women: HMO, fee-for-service, and delivery system comparisons. *J Gen Intern Med* 16:189–199, 2001
62. Friedell GH, Rubio A, Maretzki A, et al: Community cancer control in a rural, underserved population: The Appalachian Leadership Initiative on Cancer Project. *J Health Care Poor Underserved* 12:5–19, 2001
63. Freeman HP, Payne R: Racial injustice in health care. *N Engl J Med* 342:1045–1046, 2000
64. Thorpe KE, Howard D: Health insurance and spending among cancer patients. *Health Affairs* (Web exclusive). W3-189-197, April 9, 2003 *www.healthaffairs.org/webexclusives/thorpesweb-excl-04093.htm.* Accessed January 27, 2004
65. American Cancer Society: *Cancer Facts and Figures.* Atlanta, GA, American Cancer Society, 2004
66. Iglehart JK: Medicare and drug pricing. *N Engl J Med* 348:1590–1597, 2003
67. Connolly C: New drug law's cost impact debated. *Washington Post.* A03. *www.washingtonpost.com.* Accessed April 9, 2004
68. Disch J: Why *did* AARP back the Medicare drug plan? *J Prof Nurs* 20:79, 2004
69. Budge RM: Medicare drug plan causing headaches. *San Antonio Express-News.* May 29, 2004: 1A, 11A
70. National Coalition for Cancer Survivorship: Web site. *www.canceradvocacy.org.* Accessed 5/31/04
71. Oncology Nursing Society: Position on ensuring high-quality cancer care in the Medicare program. *www.ons.org.* Accessed May 31, 2004
72. Dummit LA: Medicare Chemotherapy payments: new drug and administration fees are closer to providers' costs. GAO-05-142R Medicare payments to oncologists. Dec. 1, 2004 *www.gao.gov/new.hemsld05142r.pdf.* Accessed January 5, 2005
73. McClosky JC, Bulechek GM (eds.): *Nursing Interventions Classification (NIC)* (ed 3). St. Louis, Mosby, 2000
74. Henry SB, Holzemer WL, Randell C, et al: Comparison of nursing interventions classification and current procedural terminology codes for categorizing nursing activities. *Image: J Nurs Schol* 29:133–138, 1997
75. Oncology Nursing Society: General principles and policies regarding Medicare reimbursement for oncology nursing practice expenses. *www.ons.org.* Accessed April 15, 2003
76. LegisLink: Advocacy Watch. *www.usoncology.com.* Accessed May 30, 2004
77. Medicare program: manufacturer submission of manufacturer's average sales price (ASP) data for Medicare part B drugs and biologicals. *Federal Register,* April 6, 2004: 42 CFR, Part 414 Vol. 69, pp 17935-17941
78. Hall S: Reforms may weaken cancer patient care: doctors fear cuts in Medicare drug payments will lead to less personalized treatment. *Detroit News,* April 20, 2004
79. Beck E: Critics: health savings accounts flaw. *UPI Science News. www.upo.com/view.cfm.* Accessed January 27, 2004
80. Richard D: Medical and health savings accounts. *www.msainfo.net.* Accessed January 27, 2004
81. National Coalition for Cancer Survivorship: Web site. *www.canceradvocacy.org.* Accessed January 15, 2004
82. National Cancer Institute: *SEER Cancer Statistics Review, 1973–1997.* Bethesda, MD, National Cancer Institute NIH publication 00-2789, 2000
83. Association of Rehabilitation Nurses, Oncology Nursing Society: Position on rehabilitation of people with cancer, 2003. *www.ons.org.* Accessed May 31, 2004
84. Clark J: Expert nursing: a necessary extravagance. *Euro J Cancer Care* 4:109–117, 1995
85. McKinley ED: Under toad days: surviving the uncertainty of cancer recurrence. *Ann Intern Med* 133:479–480, 2000
86. Spingarn ND: Living with spirit: the rights of cancer survivors. *Illness, Crisis Loss* 10:6–9, 2002
87. Rowland JH, Aziz N, Tesauro G, et al: The changing face of cancer survivorship. *Semin Oncol Nurs* 17:236–240, 2001
88. Ganz PA: Late effects of cancer and its treatment. *Semin Oncol Nurs* 17:241–248, 2001
89. Aziz, NM: Cancer survivorship research: challenge and opportunity. *J Nutri* 132:3494S–3503S, 2002
90. Clark EJ, Stovall EL, Leigh S, et al: *Imperatives for Quality Cancer Care: Access, Advocacy, Action and Accountability.* Silver Spring, MD, National Coalition for Cancer Survivorship, 1996. *www.canceradvocacy.org/policy/imperatives.html.* Accessed February 10, 2003
91. Zuckerman B, Preskill H, Levenson C: An evaluation of I Can Cope: insights into program design and implementation. *Cancer Pract* 9(suppl 1):S31–6, 2001
92. Rutledge DN, Raymon NJ: Changes in well-being of women cancer survivors following a survivor weekend experience. *Oncol Nurs Forum* 28:85–91, 2001
93. Levine EG, Levenberg S, Wardlaw L, et al: The efficacy of a retreat for low-income women with breast cancer. *Health Promotion Pract* 2:143–154, 2001
94. Walsh-Burke K, Marcusen C: Self-advocacy training for cancer survivors: the cancer survival toolbox. *Cancer Pract* 7:297–301, 1999
95. Medland J, Howard-Ruben J, Whitaker E: Fostering psychosocial wellness in oncology nurses: addressing burnout and social support in the workplace. *Oncol Nurs Forum* 31:47–54, 2004
96. Smith AP: Patient advocacy: roles for nurses and leaders. *Nurs Econ* 22:88–90, 2004
97. Henderson V: Nursing as an aspect of health care, in Halloran EJ (ed.): *A Virginia Henderson Reader: Excellence in Nursing.* New York, Springer, 1995, pp 307–378

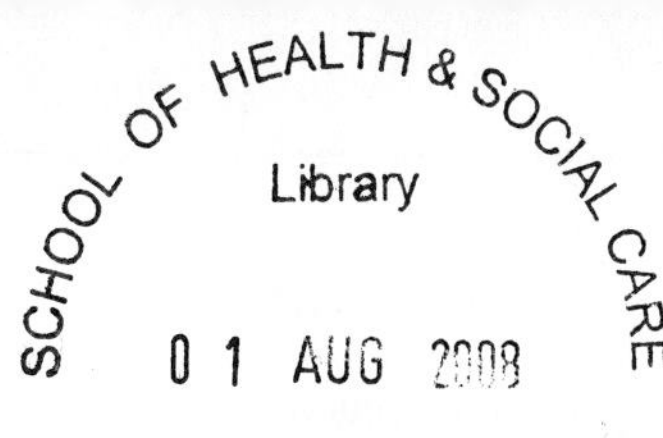

Index

Note: page numbers followed by t indicate tables; those followed by f indicate figures

A

B

C

D

F

H

I

J

K

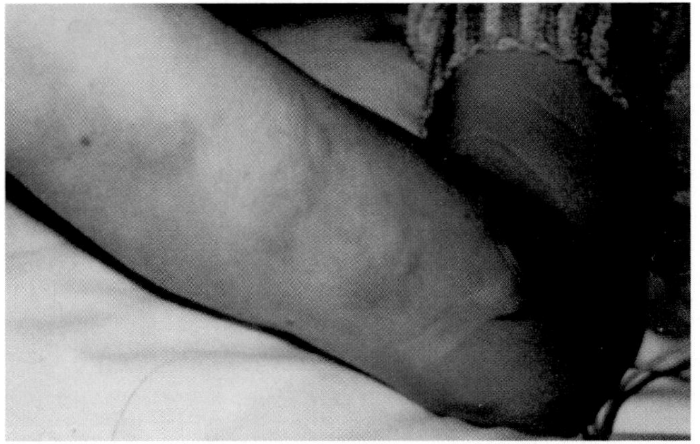

PLATE 1 Venous flare (doxorubicin).

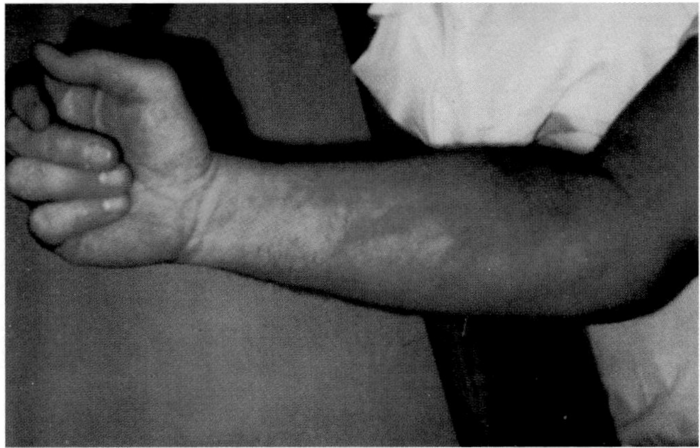

PLATE 2 Venous extravasation 2½ weeks after doxorubicin extravasation.

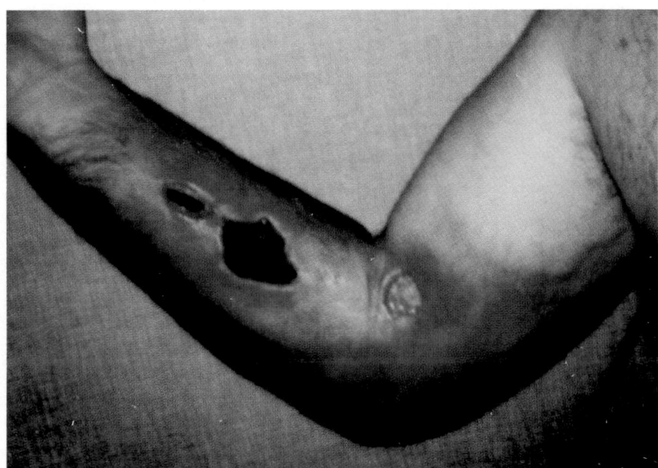

PLATE 3 ◀ Same patient 4½ months after doxorubicin extravasation.

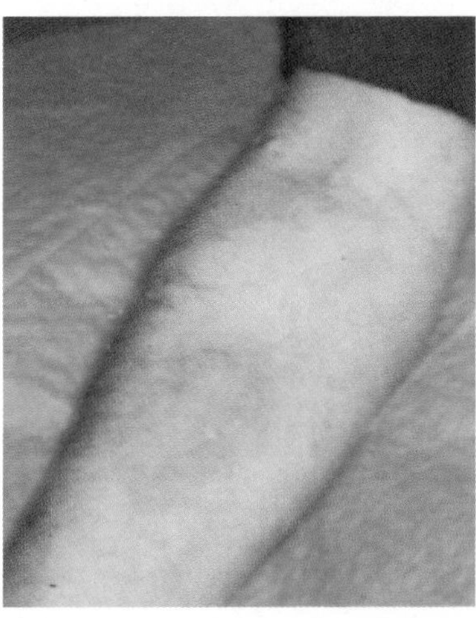

PLATE 4 ▶ Doxorubicin extravasation after 12 days. No pain with movement. Healed spontaneously.

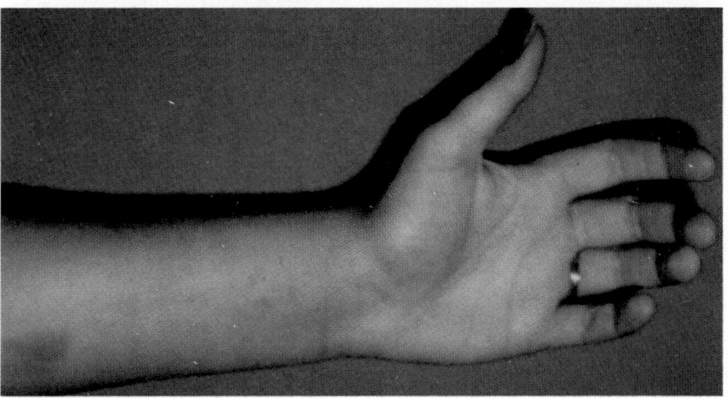

PLATE 5 Erythema and edema at injection site one week after doxorubicin administration.

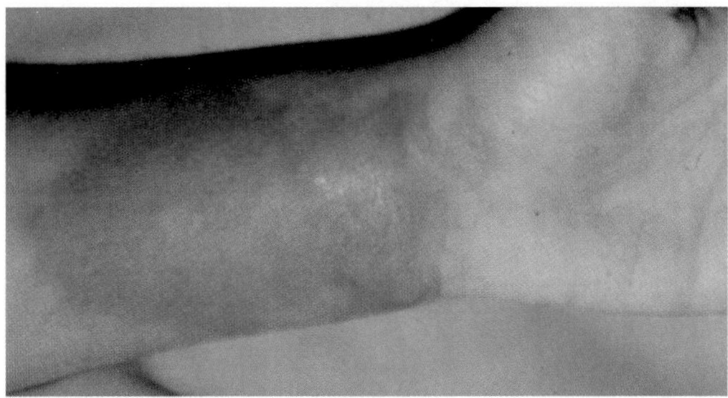

PLATE 6 At three weeks, blister formation and demarcation are present.

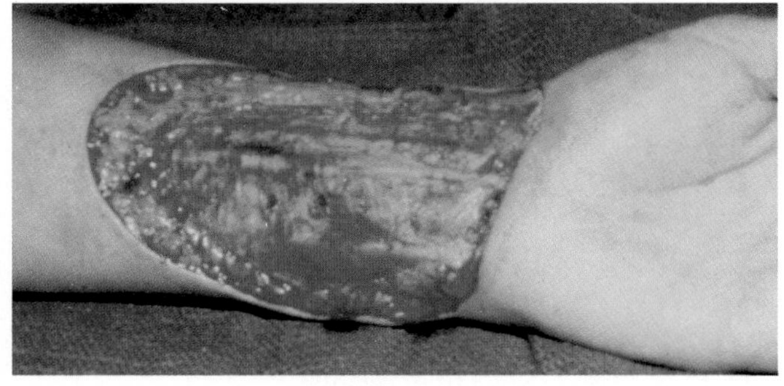

PLATE 7 Tissue surgically excised after doxorubicin extravasation.

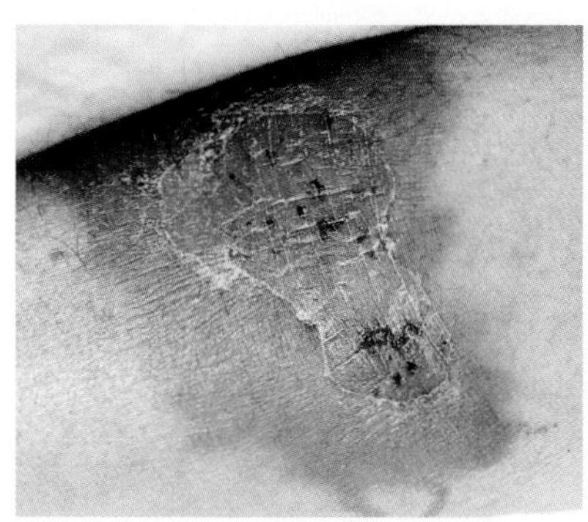

PLATE 8 ◀ Docetaxel infiltration.

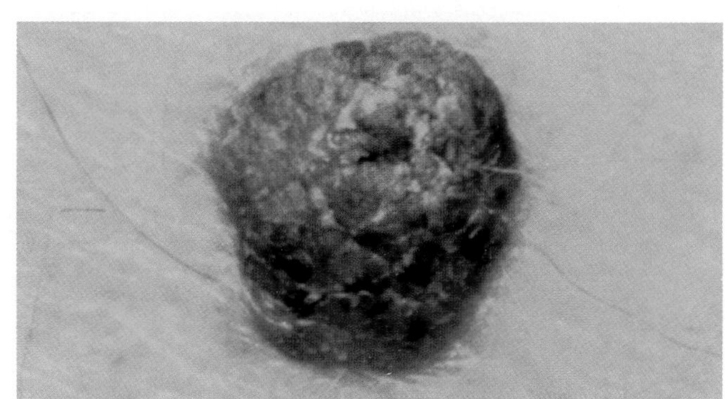

PLATE 9 ▶ Normal mole.

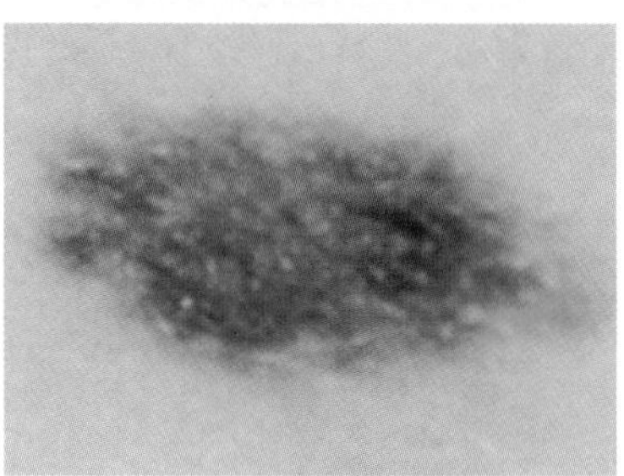

PLATE 10 ◀ Dysplastic nevus.

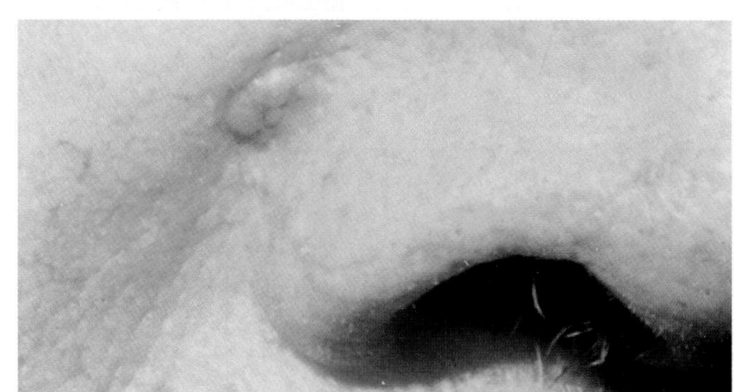

PLATE 11 ▶ Basal cell carcinoma.

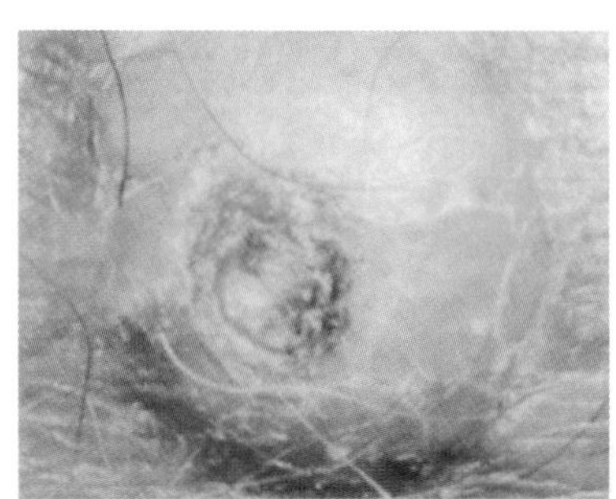

PLATE 12 ◀ Squamous cell carcinoma of the skin.

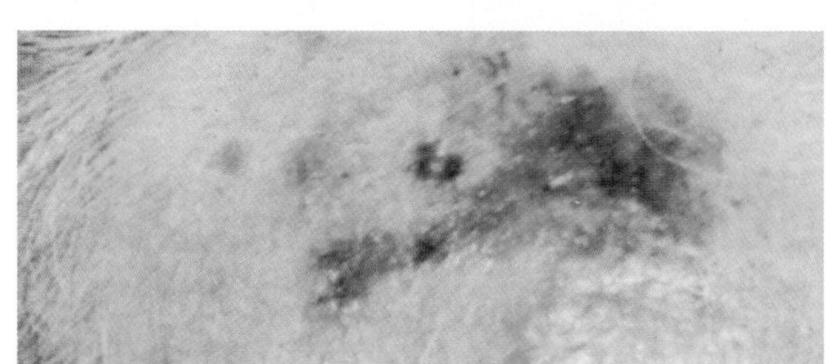

PLATE 13 Lentigo malignant melanoma.

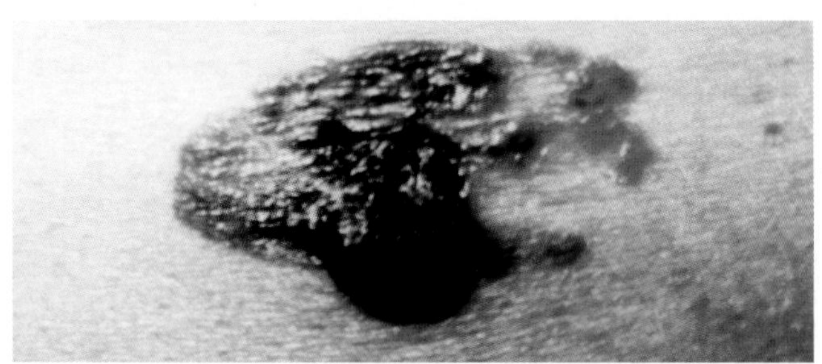

PLATE 14 Superficial spreading melanoma.

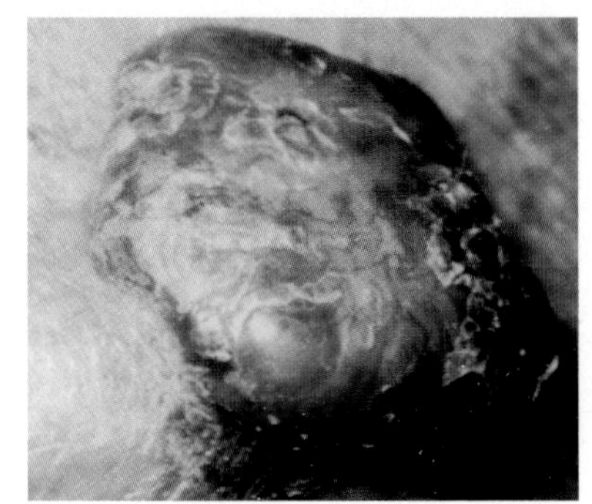

PLATE 15 ▶ Nodular melanoma.

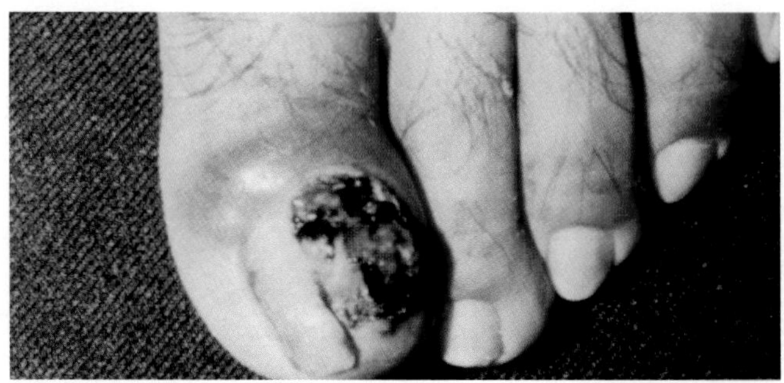

PLATE 16 ◀ Acral lentiginous melanoma.

L

N

O

P

Q

R

S

T

U

W

X

Y

Z